AF615320

Principles and Practice of Pain Medicine

NOTICE

Medicine is an ever-changing science. As new research and clinical experience broaden our knowledge, changes in treatment and drug therapy are required. The authors and the publisher of this work have checked with sources believed to be reliable in their efforts to provide information that is complete and generally in accord with the standards accepted at the time of publication. However, in view of the possibility of human error or changes in medical sciences, neither the authors nor the publisher nor any other party who has been involved in the preparation or publication of this work warrants that the information contained herein is in every respect accurate or complete, and they disclaim all responsibility for any errors or omissions or for the results obtained from use of the information contained in this work. Readers are encouraged to confirm the information contained herein with other sources. For example and in particular, readers are advised to check the product information sheet included in the package of each drug they plan to administer to be certain that the information contained in this work is accurate and that changes have not been made in the recommended dose or in the contraindications for administration. This recommendation is of particular importance in connection with new or infrequently used drugs.

Principles and Practice of Pain Medicine

Third Edition

Editors

Zahid H. Bajwa, MD
Director, Boston Headache Institute
Director, Clinical Research at Boston PainCare
Tufts University School of Medicine
Boston, Massachusetts

R. Joshua Wootton, MDiv, PhD
Director of Pain Psychology
Arnold-Warfield Pain Center
Beth Israel Deaconess Medical Center
Brookline, Massachusetts
Assistant Professor
Department of Anesthesia
Harvard Medical School
Boston, Massachusetts

Carol A. Warfield, MD
Lowenstein Distinguished Professor of Anesthesia
Harvard Medical School
Department of Anesthesia, Critical Care and Pain Medicine
Beth Israel Deaconess Medical Center
Boston, Massachusetts

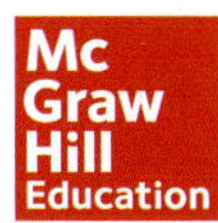

New York Chicago San Francisco Athens London Madrid Mexico City
Milan New Delhi Singapore Sydney Toronto

Principles and Practice of Pain Medicine, Third Edition

Copyright © 2017 by McGraw-Hill Education. All rights reserved. Printed in China. Except as permitted under the United States Copyright Act of 1976, no part of this publication may be reproduced or distributed in any form or by any means, or stored in a data base or retrieval system, without the prior written permission of the publisher.

Previous edition copyright © 2004 by The McGraw-Hill Companies, Inc.

1 2 3 4 5 6 7 8 9 DSS 21 20 19 18 17 16

ISBN 978-0-07-176683-8
MHID 0-07-176683-9

This book was set in Minion Pro 9/10.5 by MPS Limited.
The editors were Brian Belval, Karen G. Edmonson, and Robert Pancotti.
The production supervisor was Catherine H. Saggese.
Project management was provided by Shubham Dixit, MPS Limited.
The text designer was Alan Barnett; the cover designer was Thomas DePierro.
RR Donnelley was the printer and binder.

Library of Congress Cataloging-in-Publication Data

Principles and practice of pain medicine / editors, Zahid H. Bajwa, R. Joshua Wootton, Carol A. Warfield. — Third edition.
p. ; cm.
Includes bibliographical references.
ISBN 978-0-07-176683-8 (hardcover) — ISBN 0-07-176683-9 (hardcover)
I. Bajwa, Zahid H., editor. II. Wootton, R. Joshua (Raymond Joshua), editor. III. Warfield, Carol A., editor.
[DNLM: 1. Pain Management. 2. Analgesia—methods. 3. Pain. WL 704.6]
RB127
616'.0472—dc23

2015008912

McGraw-Hill Education books are available at special quantity discounts to use as premiums and sales promotions or for use in corporate training programs. To contact a representative, please visit the Contact Us pages at www.mhprofessional.com.

This book is dedicated to my wife Fatima and children Ahmad, Tania, Sarah, and Zaydan, "for I have learned that every heart will get what it prays for most." (Hafez).

Zahid H. Bajwa, MD

This book is dedicated to my wife Lois for her "faith, hope, and love; and the greatest of these is love." (I Cor 13:13).

R. Joshua Wootton, MDiv, PhD

To my husband Gordon and my children Richard, Chris, and Alexandra for their love and support.

Carol A. Warfield, MD

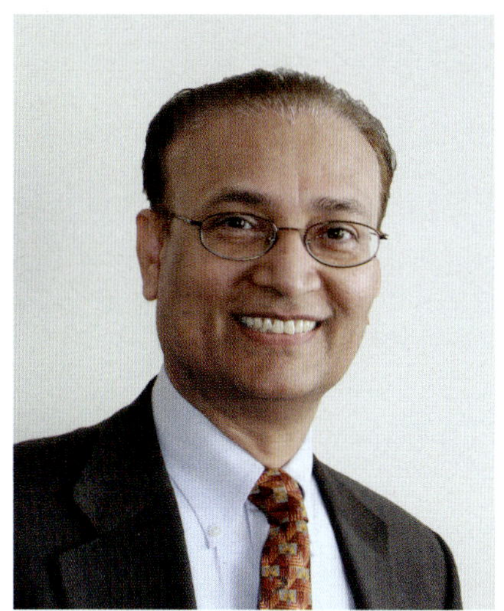

Zahid H. Bajwa

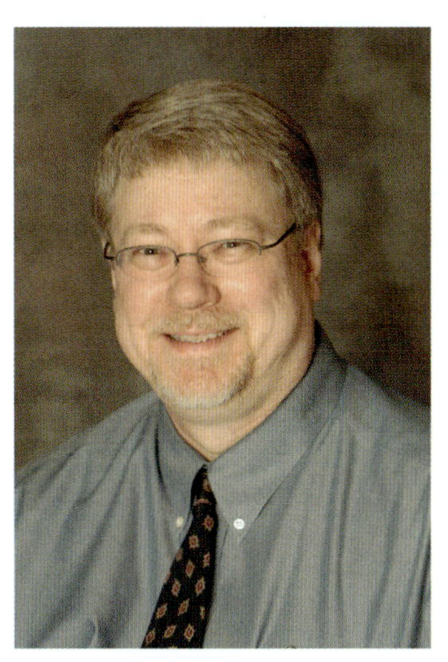

R. Joshua Wootton

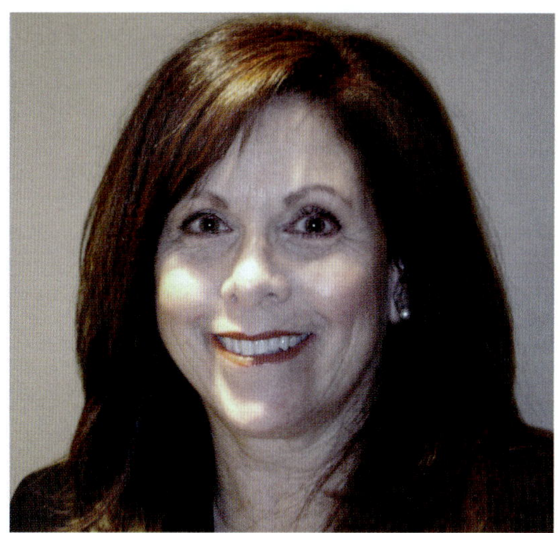

Carol A. Warfield

Contents

Contributors

Ayesha Abdeen, MD, FRCSC
Department of Orthopaedics
Beth Israel Deaconess Medical Center
Harvard Medical School
Boston, Massachusetts

Salahadin Abdi, MD, PhD
Professor, Chair, and Clinical Medical Director
Department of Pain Medicine
The University of Texas MD Anderson Cancer Center
Houston, Texas

Vimal K. Akhouri, MBBS, MD
Instructor, Department of Anesthesiology
Harvard Medical School
Beth Israel Deaconess Medical Center
Boston, Massachusetts

Nina K. Anderson, PhD
Director, Pre-doctoral Research
Harvard School of Dental Medicine
Boston, Massachusetts

Moris Aner, MD
Anesthesiologist and Pain Management Specialist
Arnold-Warfield Pain Center
Beth Israel Deaconess Medical Center
Assistant Professor
Department of Anesthesia
Harvard Medical School
Boston, Massachusetts

Amit Asopa, MD
Staff Physician, Pain Management
Anesthesiology Institute
Cleveland Clinic Abu Dhabi
Abu Dhabi, United Arab Emirates

Joseph F. Audette, MD
Chief, Department of Pain Medicine
Harvard Vanguard Medical Associates
Assistant Professor
Harvard Medical School
Boston, Massachusetts

Fadi Badlissi, MD, MSc, RhMSUS
Assistant Professor of Medicine, Harvard Medical School
Director of The Musculoskeletal Medicine Unit
Department of Orthopedics and Division of Rheumatology
Beth Israel Deaconess Medical Center
Boston, Massachusetts

Zahid H. Bajwa, MD
Director, Boston Headache Institute
Director, Clinical Research, Boston PainCare
Tufts University School of Medicine
Boston, Massachusetts

Andrew P. Baranowski, MD, FFPMRCA, FRCA, MBBS, BScHons
Consultant UCLH and Honorary Senior Lecturer UCL
The Pain Management Centre
National Hospital for Neurology and Neurosurgery
University College London Hospitals
London, England

Rodrigo Benavides, MD
Department of Anesthesiology, Perioperative and Pain Medicine
Brigham and Women's Hospital, Harvard Medical School
Boston, Massachusetts

Charles B. Berde, MD, PhD
Sara Page Mayo Chair and Chief
Division of Pediatric Pain Medicine
Department of Anesthesiology, Perioperative and Pain Medicine
Boston Children's Hospital
Professor of Anesthesia, Harvard Medical School
Boston, Massachusetts

Chantal Berna Renella, MD, PhD
Centre d'Antalgie, Service d'Anesthésiologie
Centre Hospitalier Universitaire Vaudois (CHUV)
Université de Lausanne
Lausanne, Switzerland

David M. Biondi, DO
Adjunct Associate Professor, Department of Biomedical Sciences and Center of Excellence in Neuroscience
University of New England, College of Osteopathic Medicine
Biddeford, Maine
Senior Director, Medical Affairs and Clinical Research for North America OTC
Johnson & Johnson Consumer, Inc.
Fort Washington, Pennsylvania

Donna Bloodworth, MD
Specialist in Pain Medicine
Quentin Mease Hospital
Houston, Texas

Joanne Borg-Stein, MD
Associate Professor of Physical Medicine and Rehabilitation
Harvard Medical School
Boston, Massachusetts

Jonathan M. Borkum, PhD
Department of Psychology
University of Maine
Orono, Maine
Health Psych Maine
Waterville, Maine

David Borsook, MD, PhD
Professor, Harvard Medical School
The Mayday Fund/Louis Herlands Chair in Pain Systems Neuroscience
Director, The Center for Pain and the Brain, Harvard Medical School
Director, P.A.I.N. Group, Boston Children's Hospital
Boston, Massachusetts

Daniel B. Carr, MD
Director, Tufts Program on Pain Research, Education and Policy
Professor, Public Health and Community Medicine (primary appointment)
Professor of Anesthesiology, Medicine and Molecular Physiology and Pharmacology (secondary appointments)
President, American Academy of Pain Medicine
Boston, Massachusetts

Margaret A. Caudill-Slosberg, MD, PhD, MPH
Clinical Associate Professor of Community and Family Medicine
Dartmouth Geisel School of Medicine
Instructor in Anesthesiology
Department of Anesthesiology
Dartmouth Hitchcock Medical Center
Lebanon, New Hampshire

James Celestin, MD
Orthopedic Surgery, Physiatry
Reliant Medical Group
Southborough, Massachusetts

Thomas Chai, MD
Assistant Professor
Department of Pain Medicine
Division of Anesthesiology and Critical Care
The University of Texas MD Anderson Cancer Center
Houston, Texas

Ronil V. Chandra, MBBS, MMed, FRANZCR
Interventional Neuroradiology
Monash Imaging, Monash Health
Monash University
Melbourne, Victoria, Australia

Lucy Chen, MD
Associate Professor, Harvard Medical School
Department of Anesthesia, Critical Care, and Pain Medicine
Massachusetts General Hospital
Boston, Massachusetts

Michael R. Clark, MD, MPH, MBA
Vice Chair, Clinical Affairs and Director, Chronic Pain Treatment Program
Department of Psychiatry and Behavioral Sciences
Johns Hopkins Medicine
Baltimore, Maryland

Robert I. Cohen, MD, MS
Assistant Professor of Anesthesia
Harvard Medical School
Department of Anesthesia, Critical Care, and Pain Medicine
Beth Israel Deaconess Medical Center
Boston, Massachusetts

Stephen A. Cohen, MD, MBA
Instructor in Anesthesia
Harvard Medical School
Director of Ambulatory Anesthesia
Beth Israel Deaconess Medical Center
Boston, Massachusetts

Steven P. Cohen, MD
Director of Medical Education, Pain Medicine Division
Professor of Anesthesiology and Critical Care Medicine
The Johns Hopkins Hospital
Baltimore, Maryland

David J. Copenhaver, MD, MPH
Faculty, Division of Pain Medicine
Anesthesiology and Pain Medicine
University of California, Davis Medical Center
Sacramento, California
Director of Cancer Pain Management and Supportive Care
Director of Pain Medicine Telehealth
Sacramento, California

F. Michael Cutrer, MD
Associate Professor of Neurology
Mayo Foundation for Medical Education and Research
Rochester, Minnesota

Peter P. Czakanski, MD
Department of Gynecology and Obstetrics
University of Alabama at Birmingham
Birmingham, Alabama

Alexander F. Debonet, MD
Specialist in Anesthesia and Pain Medicine
Martin Medical Group
Stuart, Florida

Timothy R. Deer, MD
President and CEO, Center for Pain Relief, Inc.
Clinical Professor, Anesthesiology Department
West Virginia University School of Medicine
Charleston, West Virginia

Thanh Dinh, DPM
Assistant Professor of Surgery
Harvard Medical School
Program Director
Podiatric Surgical Residency Program
Beth Israel Deaconess Medical Center
Boston, Massachusetts

Larry C. Driver, MD
Professor, Department of Pain Medicine
The University of Texas MD Anderson Cancer Center
Houston, Texas

Jennifer Earle, MD
Physical Medicine and Rehabilitation
Harvard Medical School
Boston, Massachusetts

Robert R. Edwards, PhD, MSPH
Associate Professor
Department of Anesthesiology
Brigham and Women's Hospital
Boston, Massachusetts

Mohamed Elkersh, MD
Department of Anesthesia
Harvard Medical School
Beth Israel Deaconess Medical Center
Boston, Massachusetts

Jennifer A. Elliott, MD
Associate Professor
Department of Anesthesiology
University of Missouri-Kansas City School of Medicine
Kansas City, Missouri

Gilbert J. Fanciullo, MD, MS
Director, Pain Management Center
Dartmouth-Hitchcock Medical Center
Lebanon, New Hampshire

Ephrem Fernandez, PhD
Professor, Department of Psychology
University of Texas at San Antonio
San Antonio, Texas

Lauren J. Fisher, MD
Department of Anesthesia, Critical Care, and Pain Medicine
Beth Israel Deaconess Medical Center
Boston, Massachusetts

Scott M. Fishman, MD
Professor of Anesthesiology and Pain Medicine
Chief, Division of Pain Medicine
Vice Chair, Department of Anesthesiology and Pain Medicine
Director, Center for Advancing Pain Relief
University of California, Davis School of Medicine
Sacramento, California

Jillian B. Frank, PhD
Clinical Psychologist
Brookline, Massachusetts

Preeti Gandhi, MBBS
Attending Physician
Pain Management, Department of Anesthesiology
Metrohealth Medical Center
Cleveland, Ohio

Janice E. Gellis, MD
Pain Management Center
Dartmouth-Hitchcock Medical Center
Lebanon, New Hampshire

Donald B. Giddon, MA, DMD, PhD
Professor of Developmental Biology (Behavioral Medicine)
Emeritus Faculty of Medicine, Harvard University
Consultant in Psychology, Brigham and Women's Hospital, Pain Management Center Department of Anesthesiology, Perioperative and Pain Medicine
Boston, Massachusetts

Jatinder S. Gill, MD
Anesthesiologist and Pain Management Specialist
Arnold-Warfield Pain Center
Beth Israel deaconess Medical Center
Assistant Professor
Department of Anesthesia
Harvard Medical School
Boston, Massachusetts

Chris Gilligan, MD, MBA
Chief, Division of Pain Medicine
Department of Anesthesia, Critical Care, and Pain Medicine
Beth Israel Deaconess Medical Center
Assistant Professor of Anesthesia
Harvard Medical School
Boston, Massachusetts

Jeremy Goodwin, MS, MD
Chief, Division of Pain Medicine
Oregon Health & Science University (OHSU)
Chief of the Division of Pain Medicine and A Senior Attending Physician
Oregon Health and Science University
Portland, Oregon

Leonidas C. Goudas, MD, PhD
Assistant Professor of Anesthesiology
Tufts University School of Medicine
Special and Scientific Staff
New England Medical Center
Boston, Massachusetts

Abhishek Gowda, MD
Pain Management Fellow
Stanford Health Care
Redwood City, California

Martin Grabois, MD
Specialist in Physical Medicine and Rehabilitation
Baylor College of Medicine
Houston, Texas

Daniel P. Gray, MD
Academic Anesthesiology and Pain Medicine
Edmonton, Canada

Christine D. Greco, MD
Senior Associate in Pain Medicine, Department of Anesthesiology, Perioperative and Pain Medicine
Boston Children's Hospital
Assistant Professor of Anesthesia
Harvard Medical School
Boston, Massachusetts

Brian M. Grosberg, MD
Director, Montefiore Headache Center
Associate Professor of Neurology
Albert Einstein College of Medicine
Montefiore Headache Center
Bronx, New York

David B. Hackney, MD
Professor of Radiology, Harvard Medical School
Chief, Neuroradiology
Beth Israel Deaconess Medical Center
Boston, Massachusetts

Joshua A. Hirsch, MD, PhD
Specialist in Diagnostic Radiology
Massachusetts General Hospital
Boston, Massachusetts

Charles C. Ho, MD
Beverly Anesthesia Associates
Beverly, Massachusetts

Stuart W. Hough, MD
Anesthesiologist (pain control)
Pain Management Specialists
Rockville, Maryland

Jessica B. Jameson, MD
Medical Director
Northwest Pain Management
Post Falls, Idaho

Robert N. Jamison, PhD
Professor, Departments of Anesthesiology and Psychiatry, Brigham and Women's Hospital, Harvard Medical School
Boston, Massachusetts

Gaurav Jindal, MD
Clinical Fellow (2011–2012), Neuroradiology
Department of Radiology
Beth Israel Deaconess Medical Center
Boston, Massachusetts

Ronald M. Kanner, MD, FAAN, FACP
Associate Dean for Career Advisement
Professor and Chairman Emeritus, Department of Neurology
Hofstra Northwell School of Medicine
Hempstead, New York

John C. Keel, MD
Department of Orthopaedics
Beth Israel Deaconess Medical Center
Harvard Medical School
Boston, Massachusetts

Douglas Keene, MD
Pain Medicine Specialist, Attending Anesthesiologist and Clinical Informaticist
Boston Pain Care Center, Greater Boston Anesthesia Associates
Waltham, Massachusetts

John M. Kelley, PhD
Associate Professor, Psychology Department
Endicott College
Beverly, Massachusetts
Deputy Director, Program in Placebo Studies
Harvard Medical School
Boston, Massachusetts
Staff Psychologist, Psychiatry Department
Massachusetts General Hospital,
Boston, Massachusetts

Robert D. Kerns, PhD
Departments of Psychiatry, Neurology and Psychology, Yale University
Pain Research, Informatics, Multimorbidities and Education (PRIME) Center, VA Connecticut Healthcare System
New Haven, Connecticut

Matthew G. Kestenbaum, MD
Medical Director, Health Information and Training, Capital Caring
Falls Church, Virginia

Soorena Khojasteh, MD
Specialist in Pain Medicine
Boston Children's Hospital
Boston, Massachusetts

Harrison Kibe, MD, MPH
Clinical Fellow
Division of Pain Management
Beth Israel Deaconess Medical Center
Harvard Medical School
Boston, Massachusetts

Dhanalakshmi Koyyalagunta, MD
Professor, Department of Pain Medicine
Division of Anesthesiology and Critical Care
The University of Texas MD Anderson Cancer Center
Houston, Texas

Ronald J. Kulich, PhD
Professor, Tufts School of Dental Medicine
Tufts Craniofacial Pain Center
Lecturer, Harvard Medical School
Boston, Massachusetts

Amaro J. Laria, PhD
Clinical Instructor, Department of Psychiatry
Cambridge Health Alliance, Harvard Medical School
Boston, Massachusetts
Co-Founder and Director of Training, Boston Behavioral Medicine
Brookline, Massachusetts

Katharine M. Larsson, RN, CS, PhD
Co-Founder and Clinical Director
Boston Behavioral Medicine
Brookline, Massachusetts

John M. Lavelle, DO
Spine Physiatrist
Tennessee Orthopaedic Clinics
Knoxville, Tennessee

Alyssa A. LeBel, MD
Senior Associate, Anesthesiology and Neurology
Boston Children's Hospital
Assistant Professor, Anesthesiology
Harvard Medical School
Boston, Massachusetts

Anthony C. Lee, MD
Physiatrist and Pain Management Specialist
Arnold-Warfield Pain Center
Beth Israel Deaconess Medical Center
Instructor in Anesthesia
Harvard Medical School
Boston, Massachusetts

Steve C. Lee, MD
Specialist in Anesthesiology
Comprehensive Neurological Solutions
Hammond, Louisiana

Lance J. Lehmann, MD
Medical Director, Pain Consultants of Florida
Medical Director, Hallandale Outpatient Surgical Center
Hollywood, Florida

Thabele M. Leslie-Mazwi, MD
Specialist in Neurology
Massachusetts General Hospital
Boston, Massachusetts

Danijela Levačić, MD
Attending Neurologist, Division of Neuro-Oncology, Northwell Health
Manhasset, New York
Assistant Professor of Neurology, Hofstra Northwell School of Medicine
Manhasset, New York

Morris Levin, MD
Professor, Department of Neurology
University of California, San Francisco School of Medicine
San Francisco, California

Yuan-Chi Lin, MD, MPH
Senior Associate in Anesthesia and Pain Medicine
Department of Anesthesiology, Perioperative and Pain Medicine
Boston Children's Hospital
Associate Professor of Anesthesia (Pediatrics)
Harvard Medical School
Boston, Massachusetts

Arthur G. Lipman, Pharmd
Professor, College of Pharmacy
Director of Clinical Pharmacology, Pain Management and Research Centers
University of Utah Health Sciences Center
Salt Lake City, Utah

Jennifer Luz, MD
Department of Physical Medicine and Rehabilitation
Spaulding Rehabilitation Hospital
Harvard Medical School
Boston, Massachusetts

Sania Mahmood, MS, MD
Drexel University College of Medicine
Philadelphia, Pennsylvania

Atif B. Malik, MD
Board of Directors
American Spine
Frederick, Maryland

Jianren Mao, MD, PhD
Richard J. Kitz Professor of Anesthesia Research, Harvard Medical School, Harvard University
Department of Anesthesia, Critical Care, and Pain Medicine
Massachusetts General Hospital
Boston, Massachusetts

Norman J. Marcus, MD
Associate Professor of Anesthesiology and Psychiatry
Director, Division of Muscle Pain Research
New York University School of Medicine
Director, Norman Marcus Pain Institute
New York, New York

Paul G. Mathew
Director of Continuing Medical Education
Brigham and Women's Hospital
Harvard Medical School
Department of Neurology
John R. Graham Headache Center
Boston, Massachusetts
Director of Headache Medicine
Cambridge Health Alliance
Harvard Medical School
Division of Neurology
Cambridge, Massachusetts

William McCarberg, MD
Chronic Pain Management Program
Kaiser Permanente
San Diego, California

Robert M. McCarron, DO
Associate Professor
Director, Pain Psychiatry and Behavioral Sciences
Director, Internal Medicine/Psychiatry Residency Program
Department of Anesthesiology, Division of Pain Medicine
Department of Psychiatry and Behavioral Sciences
Department of Internal Medicine
University of California, Davis School of Medicine
Davis, California

Brant McCartan, DPM, MBA, MS
Milwaukee Foot and Ankle Specialists
Milwaukee, Wisconsin

Cristin A. McMurray, MD
Blue Hill Pain Care, PLLC
Braintree, Massachusetts

Noshir R. Mehta, DMD, MDS, MS
Professor and Associate Dean
International Relations Chairman
General Dentistry Director
Tufts University School of Dental Medicine
Boston, Massachusetts

Siegfried Mense, Prof. Dr. med.
Department of Neurophysiology, CBTM
Medical Faculty Mannheim
University of Heidelberg
Mannheim, Germany

Natalie Moryl, MD
Specialist in Pain Medicine
Memorial Neurology Group
New York, New York

J. Cameron Muir, MD, FAAHPM
EVP and CMO, Capital Caring
Washington, DC
Clinical Associate Professor of Oncology, Johns Hopkins Medicine
Baltimore, Maryland

Nicholas K. Muraoka, DO
Physical Medicine and Rehabilitation Specialist
The Queen's Medical Center, Straub Clinic & Hospital, Pali Momi Medical Center
Honolulu, Hawaii

Jyotsna V. Nagda, MD
Assistant Professor
Department of Anesthesiology, Critical Care, and Pain Medicine
Beth Israel Deaconess Medical Center
Boston, Massachusetts

Umer Najib, MD
Department of Neurology
West Virginia University
Morgantown, West Virginia

Christopher Noto, MD
Department of Anesthesiology
Division of Pain Medicine
University of California, San Diego School of Medicine
La Jolla, California

Akiko Okifuji, PhD
Professor, Department of Anesthesiology
Pain Research and Management Center
University of Utah
Salt Lake City, Utah

Said Osman, MD
Director of Orthopedics
American Spine
Frederick, Maryland

Einar Ottestad, MD
Clinical Assistant Professor
Department of Anesthesiology, Perioperative and Pain Medicine
Stanford University School of Medicine
Redwood City, California

Amar Parikh, MD
Anesthesiologist and Interventional Pain Management Physician
OrthoNY
Albany, New York

Josemaria Paterno, MD
Specialist in Pain Medicine
Washington Center for Pain Management
Puyallup, Washington

Nagamani Peri, MD
Instructor, Harvard Medical School
Staff Radiologist, Neuroradiology
Department of Radiology
Beth Israel Deaconess Medical Center
Boston, Massachusetts

Jason E. Pope, MD
President and CEO, Summit Pain Alliance
Santa Rosa, California

Russell K. Portenoy, MD
Department of Pain Medicine and Palliative Care
Beth Israel Medical Center
New York, New York

James D. Rabinov, MD
Departments of Radiology and Neurosurgery
Massachusetts General Hospital
Boston, Massachusetts

Alan M. Rapoport, MD
Clinical Professor of Neurology
David Geffen School of Medicine
University of California, Los Angeles
Los Angeles, California

James P. Rathmell, MD
Professor of Anesthesia, Harvard Medical School
Chair, Department of Anesthesiology, Perioperative and Pain Medicine
Brigham and Women's Hospital
Boston, Massachusetts

Melissa L. Rayhill, MD
Brigham and Women's Hospital
Harvard Medical School
Department of Neurology
John R. Graham Headache Center
Boston, Massachusetts

Steven H. Richeimer, MD
Chief, Division of Pain Medicine
Associate Professor, Departments of Anesthesiology and Psychiatry
Keck School of Medicine, University of Southern California
Los Angeles, California

Joseph Rigby, PT, DPT
Spine & Sports Injury Center
Boston, Massachusetts

Daniel Rockers, PhD
President, Sacramento Valley Psychological Association
Psychologist/Psychotherapist
Sacramento, California

Joshua M. Rosenow, MD, FAANS, FACS
Director, Functional Neurosurgery
Associate Professor of Neurosurgery, Neurology and Physical Medicine and Rehabilitation
Northwestern University Feinberg School of Medicine
Chicago, Illinois

Edgar L. Ross, MD
Director of Pain Center
Brigham and Women's Hospital
Associate Professor of Anesthesia
Harvard Medical School
Boston, Massachusetts

Seward B. Rutkove, MD
Department of Neurology
Beth Israel Deaconess Medical Center
Boston, Massachusetts

Christine N. Sang, MD, MPH
Associate Professor of Anesthesia, Harvard Medical School
Director, Translational Pain Research, Department of Anesthesiology, Perioperative and Pain Medicine
Brigham and Women's Hospital
Boston, Massachusetts

Jerome Schofferman, MD
SpineCare Medical Group
Daly City and San Francisco, California

Daniel P. Schwartz, MD
Department of Neurology
National Institutes of Health
Bethesda, Maryland

Richard Scott Stayner, MD, PhD
St. Vincent Healthcare Pain Center
Billings, Montana

Steven J. Scrivani, DDS, DMSC
Director, Division of Oral and Maxillofacial Pain
Director, Orofacial Pain Residency Program
Massachusetts General Hospital
Boston, Massachusetts

Anna Serels, MD
Department of Physical Medicine and Rehabilitation
Spaulding Rehabilitation Hospital
Harvard Medical School
Boston, Massachusetts

Vinil Shah, MD
Specialist in Neuroradiology
Massachusetts General Hospital Diagnostic Radiology
Boston, Massachusetts

Huma Sheikh, MD
Neurology Department, BWH
Harvard Medical School, Boston

Sandeep Sherlekar, MD
Clinical Associate Department of Anesthesiology and Pain Medicine at Johns Hopkins University
Medical Director, Advanced Pain Surgery Center
Founder and Board of Directors, American Spine
Frederick, Maryland

Samir J. Sheth, MD
Assistant Professor
Director of Neuromodulation and Director of Student and Resident Training
University of California, Davis
Sacramento, California

Imran J. Siddiqui, MD
Department of Physical Medicine and Rehabilitation
Spaulding Rehabilitation Hospital
Harvard Medical School
Boston, Massachusetts

Lee S. Simon, MD
Co Managing Director
SDG LLC
Cambridge, Massachusetts

Thomas T. Simopoulos, MD, MA
Director, Implantable Devices Program
Arnold-Warfield Pain Center
Beth Israel Deaconess Medical Center
Assistant Professor
Department of Anesthesia
Harvard Medical School
Boston, Massachusetts

Konstantin V. Slavin, MD
Professor, Department of Neurosurgery
University of Illinois at Chicago
Chicago, Illinois

Gerald W. Smetana, MD
Division of General Medicine and Primary Care
Beth Israel Deaconess Medical Center, and Harvard Medical School
Boston, Massachusetts

Howard S. Smith, MD (deceased)
Professor, Department of Anesthesiology
Albany Medical College
Albany, New York

Maaz Sohail, MD
Diagnostic Radiologist
Columbia, Missouri

Abhilasha Solanki, MBBS, MD
Interventional Pain Management Specialist
WRMC Pain Management Clinic
Batesville, Arkansas

Mark Sollars, MS
Research Coordinator
Montefiore Headache Center
Bronx, New York

Jean C. Solodiuk, RN, PhD
Boston, Massachusetts

Egilius L.H. Spierings, MD, PhD
Department of Neurology
Brigham and Women's Hospital
Harvard Medical School
Boston, Massachusetts

Steven Stanos, DO
Specialist in Pain Medicine
RIC Center for Pain Management
Chicago, Illinois

Michael Stanton-Hicks, MD
Pain Management Department, Center for Neurological Restoration
Consulting Staff, Children's Hospital CCF Shaker Campus
Pediatric Pain Rehabilitation Program
Cleveland, Ohio

Melissa T. Stone, PsyD
Psychologist
Child and Family Psychological Services
Norwood, Massachusetts

Scott Strassels, PharmD, BCPS
Pharmaceutical Outcomes Research and Policy Program
Department of Pharmacy
University of Washington
Seattle, Washington

Lisa R. Strauss, PhD
Private Practice
Brookline, Massachusetts

Shannon Suo, MD
Associate Clinical Professor
Department of Psychiatry and Behavioral Sciences
University of California, Davis
Davis, California

Dennis C. Turk, PhD
John and Emma Bonica Endowed Chair for Anesthesiology and Pain Research
Director, Center for Pain Research on Impact Measurement, and Effectiveness (C-PRIME)
Editor-in-Chief, Clinical Journal of Pain
Department of Anesthesiology and Pain Medicine
University of Washington
Seattle, Washington

Lisa Victor, PhD (deceased)
Assistant Professor of Anesthesiology and Psychiatry
Keck School of Medicine, University of Southern California
Los Angeles, California

Jaya Vijayan, MD
Medical Director, Palliative Care
Holy Cross Health
Silver Spring, Maryland

Sarah E. Vollbracht, MD
Assistant Professor of Neurology
Albert Einstein College of Medicine
Montefiore Medical Center
Bronx, New York

Steven D. Waldman, MD, JD, MBA
Associate Dean International Programs
Chair and Professor, Department of Medical Humanities and Bioethics
Clinical Professor of Anesthesiology
University of Missouri-Kansas City School of Medicine
Kansas City, Missouri

Mark S. Wallace, MD
Professor of Clinical Anesthesiology
Chair, Division of Pain Medicine
Department of Anesthesiology
University of California, San Diego
San Diego, California

Thomas N. Ward, MD
Dartmouth Hitchcock Medical Center
Professor of Medicine and Neurology
Dartmouth Medical School
Hanover, New Hampshire

Alan A. Wartenberg, MD, FACP, FASAM
Affiliated Faculty, Brown University Center for Alcohol and Addiction Studies
Consulting Physician, Substance Abuse Treatment Program/Opioid Treatment Program
Department of Veterans Affairs Medical Center
Providence, Rhode Island

Ajay Wasan, MD
Department of Anesthesiology
Perioperative and Pain Medicine
Brigham and Women's Hospital
Harvard Medical School
Boston, Massachusetts

Nicholas R. Wasson, MD
Instructor in Anesthesiology
Northwestern University Feinberg School of Medicine
Chicago, Illinois

Lynn R. Webster, MD
Vice President of Scientific Affairs, PRA Health Sciences
Past President, American Academy of Pain Medicine
Salt Lake City, Utah

Faye M. Weinstein, PhD
Assistant Professor, Department of Anesthesiology and Psychiatry
Keck School of Medicine, University of Southern California
Los Angeles, California

Ursula Wesselmann, MD, PhD
Professor of Anesthesiology and Neurology
Department of Anesthesiology/Division of Pain Medicine
University of Alabama at Birmingham
Birmingham, Alabama

Harriët Wittink, PhD, MSc, PT
Chair, Research Group Lifestyle and Health
Faculty of Health Care
Utrecht University of Applied Sciences
Utrecht, the Netherlands

Edison H. Wong, MD
Physiatrist, Pain Medicine
Waltham, Massachusetts

R. Joshua Wootton, MDiv, PhD
Director of Pain Psychology
Arnold-Warfield Pain Center
Beth Israel Deaconess Medical Center
Brookline, Massachusetts
Assistant Professor
Department of Anesthesia
Harvard Medical School
Boston, Massachusetts

Jason C. Wu, MD
Clinical Fellow, Harvard Medical School
Department of Physical Medicine and Rehabilitation
Boston, Massachusetts

Tony L. Yaksh, PhD
Professor of Anesthesiology and Pharmacology
University of California, San Diego
La Jolla, California

Aaron J. Yang, MD
Assistant Professor, Department of Physical Medicine and Rehabilitation
Vanderbilt University Medical Center
Nashville, Tennessee

Albert J. Yoo, MD
Specialist in Diagnostic Radiology
Massachusetts General Hospital
Boston, Massachusetts

Sean R. Zion, MA
Department of Anesthesiology, Perioperative and Pain Medicine
Brigham and Women's Hospital
Harvard Medical School
Boston, Massachusetts

Foreword

The alleviation of pain has been central to the humane practice of medicine since its ancient beginnings. How this essential mission has been carried out, however, has evolved exponentially with time, driven by the expansion of medical knowledge, the invention of new treatments, and ongoing changes in the practice of medicine itself. Today, this evolution is unfolding in the United States against the backdrop of radical changes in the way in which healthcare is practiced and financed.

The rapid pace of change in the knowledge and care of pain has motivated this revised and expanded third edition of *Principles and Practice of Pain Medicine*. Since the previous edition was published in 2004, new treatments and treatment modalities have been created; a major paradigm shift has occurred in the use of opioid analgesics; and substantial progress has been made in how pain is studied, taught, and treated.

What has not changed is the demand for pain relief. If anything, the tide of patients in pain has swelled: the Institute of Medicine (IOM) reported in 2011 that about 100 million American adults suffer from chronic pain, more than those suffering from diabetes, heart disease, and cancer combined.[1] The annual direct and indirect cost is estimated to exceed $600 billion annually;[1] and these estimates do not include the burdens of acute pain, pain in pediatric populations, cancer-related pain, or pain at the end of life. Opioid analgesics, which have been widely deployed in the past decade against this onslaught of chronic pain, continue to be associated with efficacy data that is weak to inadequate. In addition, these agents have proven to pose substantial risks and to require greater caution than was widely recognized prior to publication of the second edition. Since then, data have convincingly shown a trend toward the excessive prescribing of opioids, as well as the dramatic scope of the U.S. epidemic of prescription drug abuse, which only recently has shown signs of easing.[2]

Viewing the IOM findings of high prevalence and costs of pain, in the light of both the epidemic of prescription opioid abuse and the fact that the U.S. presently consumes the vast majority of the world supply of prescription opioids, strongly suggests that many patients are being inadequately treated for their pain. It has become clear that inadequate treatment may result from too *much* as well as too *little* treatment. We are reminded that the enthusiasm for the benefits of analgesic therapies must be tempered by a clear-eyed appreciation for their risks. This is just one of the important attitudinal shifts that have been reflected in the revisions of this third edition—shifts that may also apply to procedural and psychosocial options for pain management.

Currently, medicine possesses greater knowledge and more tools to manage pain than ever before. Yet the foundational scientific knowledge base for pain is still insufficient to fully support treatment decisions and major health policies. The National Institutes of Health continues to spend a disproportionately small fraction of its budget on pain relative to the substantial burden of pain on patients and society at large. In addition to inadequate funding of research in pain medicine, education about pain and its safe and effective management is astonishingly under-represented in the curricula for most pre-licensure healthcare professional schools, as well as post-graduate and continuing education programs. According to the 2011 IOM report on Pain in America: *"Despite the large role that care of patients with pain will play in their daily practice, many health professionals, especially physicians, appear underprepared for and uncomfortable with carrying out this aspect of their work. These professionals need and deserve greater knowledge and skills so they can contribute to the necessary cultural transformation in the perception and treatment of people with pain."* The transformation for pain care envisioned by the IOM will require recognizing pain and its management as a core component of the education for every health professional.

Many of the obstacles that impede progress in addressing pain may be attributed to its omnipresence throughout healthcare, which confounds division into neat partitions and units. The traditional organizations that are intended to support patient care, education, and research are often unable to fully integrate the vast dimensions of pain, too often leading to fragmented organizations and programs. It is no surprise that pain remains poorly integrated within the siloed departmental structure of traditional medicine or the vital institutions that support research and education. These systemic failings mean that clinicians (generalists *and* specialists), as well as educators, researchers, and students, are too often ill-equipped to effectively deal with the challenge of helping the millions of Americans who have complex, multi-dimensional pain conditions.

In the midst of massive economic uncertainty in U.S. healthcare, it might appear that we simply cannot afford to make such foundational changes. However, evidence of the costs associated with the current epidemic of prescription drug abuse, as well as the substantial costs associated with inadequately treated pain, suggests that we cannot afford *not* to make these changes. Doing so will require intensified partnerships and integration within our health systems and with the organizations that fund our research, accredit our schools for health professionals, and license and certify our clinicians and healthcare facilities.

It could be easy to despair in the face of these challenges. Yet the years since the previous edition of *Principles and Practice* have also witnessed many hopeful changes. Science continues its steep growth in knowledge of pain, and pain management is increasingly recognized as integral to healthcare. Both of these perspectives drive the advancement of treatment forward. Recent thoughtful policy and regulatory changes raise hope that we are in the process of reversing our excessive reliance on opioids for chronic pain, which may stem the current epidemic of prescription opioid abuse and overdose. Substantial efforts at the federal level are currently underway, holding the promise of an integrated national strategy for pain care, research, and education.

The third edition of this textbook represents over two decades of sustained commitment to interdisciplinary pain education by many thought leaders including Dr Bajwa, Dr Wootton, and Dr Warfield. With its many revisions and updates, this volume presents a review of current perspectives that will be invaluable to specialists and generalists across many health professions. The principles and practice of pain medicine will continue to evolve, of course, but the authors of future editions may look back on this edition as reflecting an important time in medical history. Perhaps they will see that we were at a tipping point beyond which pain care would be solidly founded on quality evidence, comprehensive education, and integration throughout healthcare.

Scott M. Fishman, MD
Chief, Division of Pain Medicine
Professor and Vice Chair for Pain Medicine & Faculty Development
Department of Anesthesiology
University of California, Davis Health System
Sacramento, California

[1]Institute of Medicine. *Relieving pain in American: a blueprint for transforming prevention, care, education, and research.* June 2011.

[2]Centers for Disease Control and Prevention. National Vital Statistics Report: Deaths: Final Data for 2013.

Preface

Dr Carol A. Warfield published the first edition of this book in 1992 as *Principles and Practice of Pain Management* with 39 chapters. At around the same time, the Accreditation Council for Graduate Medical Education (ACGME) began the process of formally accrediting pain medicine fellowship training programs. The majority of ACGME-accredited pain programs were based in anesthesia departments, but within a few years, physicians from other specialties were welcomed into inter-disciplinary pain fellowship programs. The International Association for the Study of Pain (IASP) was soon joined by many other professional pain societies with the mission of bringing clinicians and researchers to think and work together to understand pain and help find better treatments for patients in pain.

From the "decade of the brain" to the "decade of pain control and research," our improved understanding of pain mechanisms led to more and generally better treatments for our patients. The second edition of this book, published in 2004, was a larger and more comprehensive text reflecting those advances and was entitled *Principles and Practice of Pain Medicine.* Not only had it expanded to 87 chapters, including emphasis on headache disorders, cancer pain, and palliative medicine, but it had also enhanced the multidisciplinary collaborative spirit among editors and authors. Since the publication of the second edition of *Principles and Practice of Pain Medicine,* the field of pain medicine has matured even further as a multidisciplinary specialty with a broad scientific and clinical knowledge base. This third edition seeks to capture the essentials of this knowledge and understanding in a comprehensive review of pain medicine. Since the topic of analgesia is the domain of no single discipline, the content of this book is authored by leaders who represent the many disciplines that constitute this evolving field. One could easily write entire volumes about the topics of each of the chapters in this text, but the task of the authors and editors here was to assimilate this large body of information on pain medicine and condense it into a useful textbook of manageable size. Each chapter represents a careful distillation of current science, key concepts, and clinical treatments of the subject at hand into an accessible format. For those readers seeking to expand their horizons further, the authors have prepared extensive lists of references at the end of each chapter to provide the reader with further details.

This third edition discusses the fundamental dimensions of pain, the various disorders in which pain poses a major problem, and the methods employed in its management, with special emphasis on the use of injections and nerve blocks as an aid to diagnosis, prognosis, and therapy. It covers the biology of pain and the principles of physical and psychological evaluation of chronic pain. It goes on to discuss pain categorized by anatomic location, as well as by syndrome, such as acute and peri-operative pain, neuropathic pain, pain in the terminally ill, and pediatric and geriatric pain. The authors have been careful to incorporate vivid illustrations depicting the physical symptoms and anatomy of each site, as well as key findings from MRI, CT, X-rays, and other imaging and diagnostic technology. The next group of chapters discusses pain therapies and includes detailed attention to pharmacologic treatments, interventional therapies, and complementary and physical treatments of pain. Lastly, because pain medicine has now grown beyond its clinical bounds, we have introduced chapters covering the new areas of pain and law, ethics, and business administration.

The breadth and rapidity of change in this specialty has prompted the publication of this edition, reflecting the expansion of pain medicine with former chapters updated and new chapters added. We have also attempted to be comprehensive in our consideration of pain medicine from a multidisciplinary perspective, with the idea that, regardless of the reader's background and training—whether anesthesiology, medicine, neurology, physical medicine and rehabilitation, neurosurgery, psychology, or other specialties—a picture of pain medicine as a multifaceted and continually evolving field emerges.

We extend our thanks to all of the chapter authors for their tireless work on this project and extend a special thanks to Dr Scott M. Fishman for writing the foreword to the third edition of this textbook and to Drs Thomas T. Simopoulos and John Keel for their help in developing content and multiple contributions. We welcome comments, suggestions, and constructive criticism from all our readers.

Zahid H. Bajwa, MD
R. Joshua Wootton, MDiv, PhD
Carol A. Warfield, MD

PART 1

Pain: Biology, Anatomy, and Physiology

Molecular Biology of Pain

Tony L. Yaksh

"Stimuli become adequate as excitants of pain when they are of such intensity as threatens damage to the skin."

—Sherrington (1906)[1]

OVERVIEW

The acute activation of small sensory afferent axons by high-intensity thermal and mechanical stimuli evokes locally organized spinal motor reflexes (nociceptive reflexes), autonomic responses, and pain behavior in animals and humans. This effect is mediated by the local encoding of afferent input at the level of the dorsal horn and the activation of spinofugal projection neurons. These projection systems travel both ipsilaterally and contralaterally in the ventrolateral aspect of the spinal cord, projecting supraspinally into the medulla, mesencephalon, and diencephalon. Medullary projections serve to activate spinobulbospinal reflexes that influence autonomic tone. Other projections into the mesencephalon and thalamus are assumed to contribute to the perceptual and complex emotive and discriminative components of the pain state. It is important to appreciate that encoding by the sensory afferent and the spinal dorsal horn of the nociceptive stimulus is the first step in nociceptive processing, and this encoding process contributes properties that are important to the understanding of the behavioral correlates of nociception. The following sections consider aspects of the mechanisms whereby injury leads to an ongoing pain state from the perspective of the organization of the sensory afferents and the spinal dorsal horn. Of particular importance is the appreciation that these linkages have distinct pharmacologies and that these systems can be regulated to display prominent increases (hyperalgesia) and decreases (analgesia) in the input–output function.

PRIMARY AFFERENTS

MORPHOLOGY

Sensory afferents represent the first link between the nervous system and the peripheral milieu. Whether they are enteroceptive organs such as viscera or blood vessels, the meninges, deep structures such as muscle or joint, or the skin, all surfaces are innervated by axons that transduce the local milieu to generate action potentials that provide input to the neuraxis. These primary afferent axons are made up of the central (root) and peripheral (nerve) projections and the dorsal root ganglion cell body that is connected to the root by a sinuous glomerulus. With the exception of several cranial nerves, all axons have their primary cell body in the dorsal root ganglia that lie outside of the neuraxis proper.[2]

NORMAL SENSORY AFFERENT ACTIVITY

Classification of Sensory Afferents These axons may be classified according to the nature of the peripheral terminals, their size (large or small), and state of myelination (myelinated or unmyelinated), as well as, functionally, their conduction velocity (large axons are rapid; small axons are slower) and the modality of stimulation that most effectively results in activity in the associated axon.

Sensory Nerve Endings It is important to emphasize that the peripheral afferent terminal is an exceedingly specialized region. The terminal provides the transduction properties that convert stimulus of a given modality into a local sodium channel–mediated depolarization that leads to activity in the afferent axon.[3] This degree of depolarization leads to activation of the axon, the frequency of which is proportional to the stimulus intensity. Large axons typically display complex, specialized structures, such as pacinian corpuscles or stretch sensitive organs, that transduce mechanical stimuli and define the nature of the afferent response—for example, a rapidly adapting response in which a continued stimulus may evoke an output when the stimulus is applied and then again when it is removed (i.e., rapidly adapting, as compared with slowly adapting). Small afferents may not display evident specialization and, hence, are commonly referred to as being "free" nerve endings. These free nerve endings are, however, extremely complex, providing a transduction of different modalities and various chemical stimuli.[4]

TABLE 1-1 Primary Afferents Classed by Conduction Velocity and Physical Nature of the Effectivew Stimulus

Fiber Class[a]	Velocity	Effective Stimuli
Aβ (myelinated) (12–20 μ dia)	Group II (>40–50 m/sec)	Low-threshold mechanoreceptors
		Specialized nerve endings (pacinian corpuscles)
Aδ (myelinated) (1–4 μ dia)	Group III (10< × <40 m/sec)	Low-threshold mechanical or thermal
		High-threshold mechanical or thermal
		Specialized nerve endings
C (unmyelinated) (0.5–1.5 μ dia)	Group IV (<2 msec)	High threshold thermal, mechanical, and chemical
		Free nerve endings

[a]Aβ/Aδ/C is the Erlanger-Gasser classification and refers to axon size; II/III/IV is the Lloyd-Hunt classification and is defined on conduction velocity in muscle afferents. Because of the relationship between size and state of myelination with conduction velocity, these designations are often used interchangeably.

Effective Stimuli Under normal conditions, the cardinal observation is that sensory afferents show minimal, if any, spontaneous activity. However, the brief application of a peripheral mechanical or thermal stimulus will often evoke intensity-dependent increases in firing rates. As outlined in **Table 1-1**, recording from fibers identified according to their conduction velocity reveals that large Aβ (group II) fibers are typically activated by low thresholds (i.e., mechanoreceptors). Small, lightly myelinated axons A∂ (group III) fibers that conduct at a lower velocity may belong to populations that are heterogeneous, responding to low or high thresholds, mechanical or thermal. Thus, low-threshold afferents may begin firing at temperatures that are not noxious (30°C) and increase their firing rate monotonically as the temperature rises. Other populations of A∂ fibers may begin to fire at temperatures that are mildly noxious and increase their firing rates up to very high temperatures (52–55°C). These would be referred to as thermal nociceptors. Small, unmyelinated, slowly conducting afferents (C fiber or group IV) constitute the largest population of sensory axons. The large majority of these small afferents are activated by high-threshold thermal, mechanical, and chemical stimuli and are, therefore, called C-polymodal nociceptors.[5] Accordingly, the afferent input from a given stimulus will reflect on (1) the modality of the stimulus (e.g., thermal, mechanical, or chemical) and (2) the coactivation of several populations of afferents, which transduce that stimulus energy and a discharge frequency that covaries with stimulus intensity over a range reflecting a low versus high stimulus-intensity threshold (**Fig. 1-1**).

Psychophysical Correlates of Afferent Activity In normal, uninjured tissue, stimuli that give rise to activity in small sensory afferents evoke a psychophysical report of pain sensation in humans and a somatotopically organized escape response in animals (e.g., withdrawal of the stimulated limb). The intensity of the report and the vigor of the escape are typically monotonically correlated with stimulus intensity and, hence, with the frequency of discharge in a given sensory axon. Conversely, electrical activation of Aδ nociceptors produces a short-lasting pricking sensation (first pain), whereas activation of C fibers results in a poorly localized burning sensation (second pain). In the absence of tissue injury, the removal of the stimulus leads to rapid abatement of the afferent input and disappearance of the pain sensation.

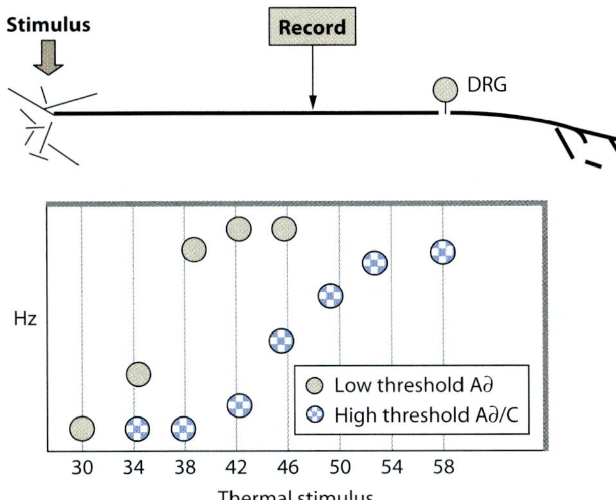

FIGURE 1-1. (**Top**) Schematic of sensory axon fiber with peripheral nerve ending. (**Bottom**) Two types of fibers—low-threshold A∂ and high-threshold A∂ and C fibers—typically show little, if any, spontaneous activity but show a monotonic increase in response to increasing stimulus intensities. For the high-threshold afferents, the triggering threshold usually reflects temperatures that would correspond to a temperature at which a pain report would be elicited.

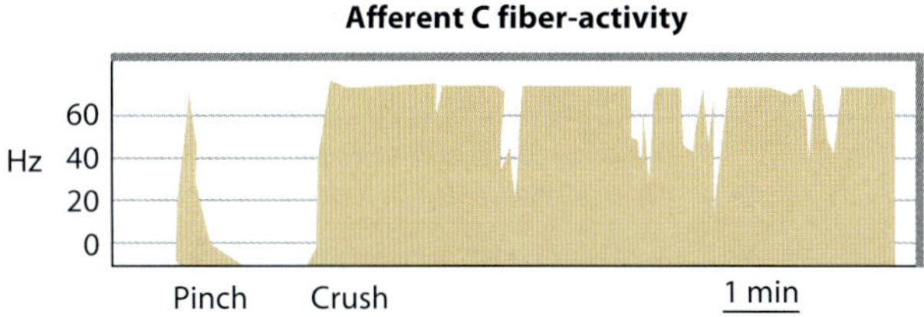

FIGURE 1-2. Schematic presenting the firing rate to pinch and to tissue crush of a single, small, cutaneous afferent axon. Note that in the absence of stimulation, there is no spontaneous activity in this small afferent axon. After a brief pinch, there is a brief stimulus-linked discharge. Creation of tissue injury by a mechanical crush leads to a prolonged, ongoing discharge.

AFFERENT ACTIVITY AFTER TISSUE INJURY

Afferent Response After Tissue Injury If a stimulus produces a local injury, as in a tissue crush or incision, two events are observed to occur.

1. The normally silent sensory afferent begins to display a persistent bursting discharge that continues for an extended interval (minutes to hours) after the injuring stimulus is removed (**Fig. 1-2**).
2. The stimulus intensity required for activating the otherwise high-threshold afferent may fall significantly, such that otherwise moderately intense stimuli will be highly effective. In effect, this serves to shift the relationship between response (frequency of discharge) and stimulus intensity up, to the left, and increases its slope. The extreme example of this peripheral sensitization is the population of afferent C fibers referred to as silent nociceptors. These afferents are normally only poorly activated by even extreme mechanical stimuli. In the presence of tissue injury or inflammation, these previously silent afferents may develop spontaneous activity and a low mechanical threshold.

Origin of Persistent Afferent Activity The ongoing activity observed after injury originates from the terminal region of the sensory afferent and appears to have two sources:

1. Afferent terminals that are in the vicinity of the injury may develop spontaneous activity, in part because of local damage to the terminal that may result in an increase in local sodium channel activation.
2. A tissue-injuring stimulus will lead to the release of local factors that (a) directly activate the local terminals of afferents (that are otherwise silent), and (b) facilitate the discharge of the afferent in response to otherwise submaximal stimuli (**Fig. 1-3**). Some of these local factors are enumerated in **Table 1-2**. Importantly, exogenous administration of these products has been shown to directly excite

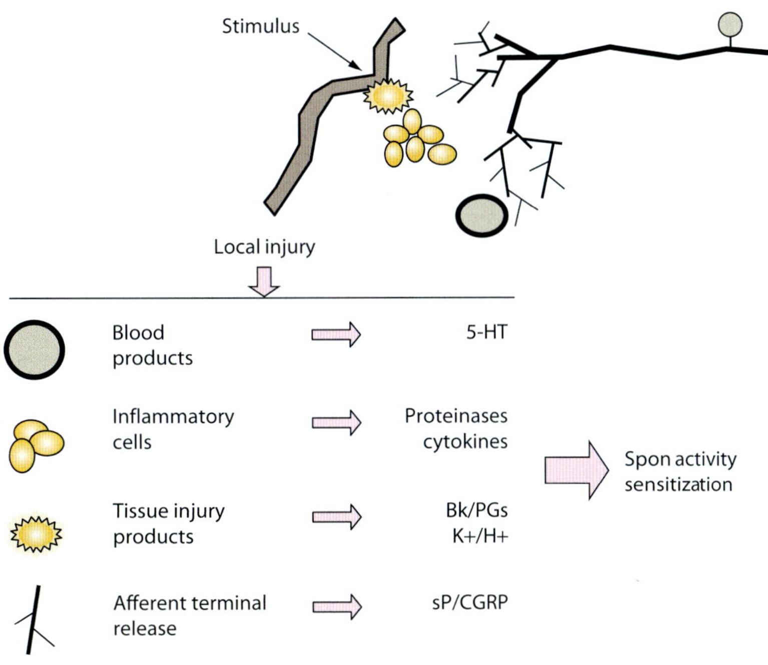

FIGURE 1-3. Schematic of local organization causing changes in the chemical milieu in the region of a local injury that lead to afferent activation and sensitization. Primary afferent terminal A: Local damaging stimulus leads to activation of the fine sensory afferent (C fiber). Activity proceeds orthodromically to the spinal cord and antidromically to invade local peripheral collaterals. This antidromic activity can depolarize the peripheral terminals and locally release their peptide content. The orthodromic traffic reaches the spinal cord and may serve to produce sufficient local depolarization in the dorsal horn that an antidromic action potential is generated in the terminals of an adjacent sensory axon. The antidromic activity generated by a local axon reflex and by the spinal component invades the distal terminal region locally to release neuropeptides (substance P [sP], calcitonin gene–related peptide [CGRP]). Local injury and the released hormones serve to activate local inflammatory cells. Hormones, such as bradykinin, prostaglandins, and cytokines, or K^+/H^+ released from inflammatory cells and plasma extravasation products result in stimulation and sensitization of free nerve endings.

TABLE 1-2 Classes of Agents Released After Tissue Injury That Influence Activity in Small Primary Afferent Fibers[a]

Agents	Action
Amines	Histamine (granules of mast cells, basophils, and platelets) and serotonin (mast cells and platelets) are released by a variety of stimuli, including mechanical trauma, heat, radiation, certain byproducts of tissue damage, thrombin, collagen, epinephrine, and members of the arachidonic acid cascade, leukotrienes, and prostanoids.
Kinin	A variety of kinins, notably bradykinin, are released by physical trauma. Peptide is synthesized by a cascade that is triggered by the activation of factor XII by agents such as kallikrein and trypsin. Bradykinin acts by specific bradykinin receptors (B1/B2) to activate free nerve endings.
Lipid acids	Agents are synthesized by lipoxygenase or cyclooxygenase (prostanoids) upon the release of cell membrane–derived arachidonic acid secondary to the activation of phospholipase A_2. A number of prostanoids, including PGE_2, can directly activate C fibers. Others such as PGI_2 and TXA_2, and several leukotrienes, can markedly facilitate the excitability of C fibers. These effects are also mediated by specific membrane receptors.
Cytokines	Cytokines such as the interleukins are formed as part of the inflammatory reaction involving macrophages and have been shown to exert powerful sensitizing effects on C fibers. Interleukins such as Il-1 may sensitive C fibers via a prostaglandin intermediary.
Primary afferent peptides	CGRP and sP are found in and released from the peripheral terminals of C fibers and will produce local cutaneous vasodilation, plasma extravasation, and sensitization in the region of skin innervated by the stimulated sensory nerve.
[H]/[K]	Elevated H^+ (low pH) and high K^+ are found in injured tissue. These ions can directly stimulate C fibers and facilitate the discharge produced by a given stimulus (e.g., hyperalgesia activates the local axon reflex and results in the local release of CGRP, a potent vasodilator and modulator of plasma extravasation). A population of C nociceptors sensitive to noxious intensities of mechanical and thermal stimuli also responds in a stimulus-released fashion to solutions of increasing proton concentration injected into their receptive fields. These receptors develop a lower threshold and enhanced response to mechanical stimuli. Similar injections in humans induce a sustained graded pain and hyperalgesia. Increasing evidence suggests that agents such as capsaicin may interact directly with peripheral terminal membranes to increase proton conductance.
Proteinases	Thrombin or trypsin, among others, are released from inflammatory cells and can cleave tethered peptide ligands that exist on the surface of small primary afferents. These tethered peptide act upon adjacent receptors (PARs) that can serve to depolarize the terminal, causing an orthodromic input and the local release of sP and CGRP into the injured tissues.

[a]CGRP, calcitonin gene–related peptide; PAR, proteinase-activated receptor; PGE_2, prostaglandin E_2; PGI_2, prostaglandin I_2; sP, substance P; TXA_2, thromboxane A_2.[6-8]

C fibers and facilitate C-fiber firing, resulting in a shift to the left and increased slope of its frequency response curve.[6] For the substances in which it has been examined, these agents, when applied to the skin of humans and animals, usually evoke pain behavior and increase the magnitude of the reported pain response evoked by a given stimulus (hyperalgesia) (**Fig. 1-4**).[7,8]

In short, peripheral mechanical and thermal stimuli will evoke intensity-dependent increases in firing rates of small afferents, and this response corresponds to the psychophysical report of pain sensation in humans and the vigor of the escape response in animals. Such stimuli may result in local injury and the subsequent elaboration of active products that directly activate the local terminals of afferents (which are otherwise essentially silent) innervating the injury region and facilitate their discharge in response to otherwise submaximal stimuli.

SPINAL SYSTEMS ENCODING SENSORY INPUT EVOKED BY INJURY

Sensory afferents project into the spinal dorsal horn and make synaptic contact with dorsal horn neurons. Two issues pertinent to our understanding of spinal organization should be considered: (1) the organization of the afferent termination in the dorsal horn and (2) the classes of neurons that receive these projections.

GENERAL ORGANIZATION OF THE SPINAL DORSAL HORN

The spinal cord is divided into several broad anatomic regions (dorsal root entry zone, dorsal horn, and ventral horn; gray and white matter). These regions are further divided on the basis of descriptive anatomy into spinal lamina (Rexed)[9,10] (**Fig. 1-5**).

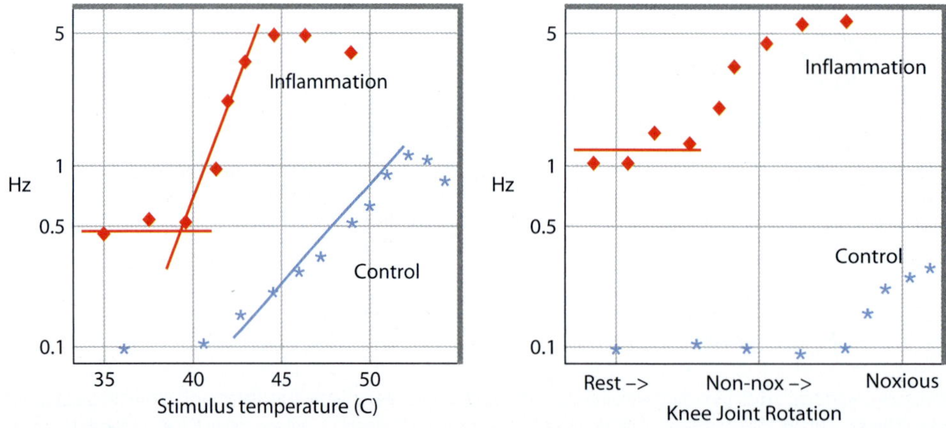

FIGURE 1-4. Representation of the response of small axons innervating the skin to thermal stimuli before and after the injection of a local inflammatory substance (**left**) and the activity in an afferent to a range of knee joint motion before and after inflammation of the knee joint (**right**). Following the initiation of cutaneous inflammation, the afferent shows increasing spontaneous activity, a left shift, and an increase in the slope in the stimulus-response curve, indicating a facilitated response to the thermal stimulus. In the knee, the articular afferent shows little response to normal rotation and only fires in response to extreme rotation. After the initiation of joint inflammation, even mild rotation results in a significant discharge.

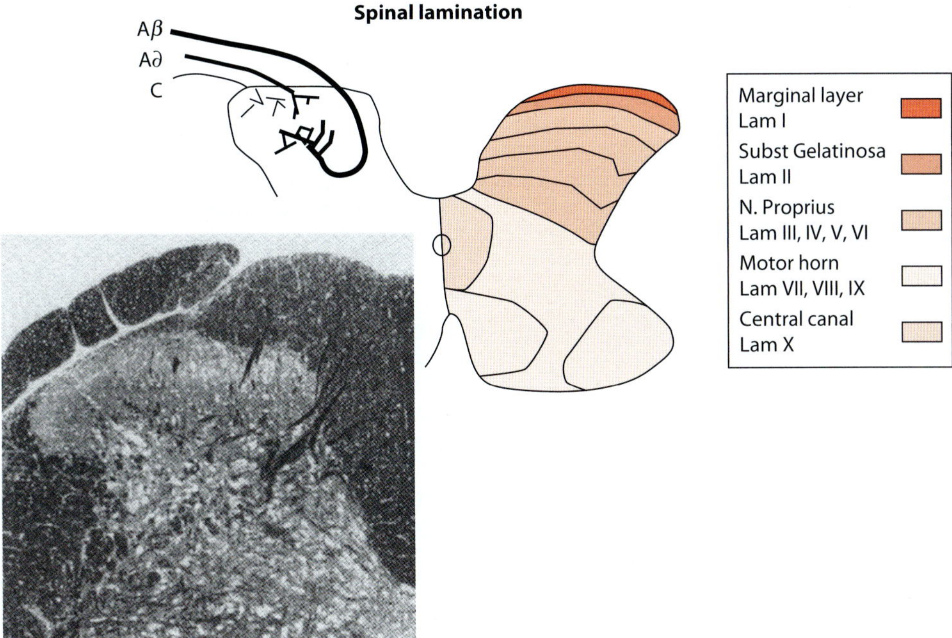

FIGURE 1-5. Schematic showing the Rexed lamination (**right**) and the approximate organization of the approach of the afferent to the spinal cord (**left**) as they enter at the dorsal root entry zone and then penetrate into the dorsal horn to terminate in laminae I and II (A/C) or penetrate more deeply to loop upward to terminate as high as the dorsum of lamina III (Aβ). Inset in lower left shows histologic appearance of the left dorsal quadrant. Note root entry zone, substantia gelatinosa, and large, myelinated axons.

SPINAL TERMINALS OF PRIMARY AFFERENTS

Spinal Trajectory of Afferent Axons In the peripheral nerve, afferents are anatomically intermixed. As the sensory root approaches the spinal dorsal root entry zone, large afferents tend to move medially, and these displace smaller, unmyelinated afferents laterally. Upon entering the spinal cord at the dorsal root entry zone, the central processes of the afferents collateralize, sending fibers rostrally and caudally up to several segments in Lissauer's tract (small, C-fiber afferents) or in the dorsal columns (large afferents) and into the segment of entry. Upon penetrating into the parenchyma, the terminal fields ramify rostrally and caudally for several millimeters[10] (**Fig. 1-6**).

Spinal Terminals of Afferent Axons In the spinal cord, terminals from the large, myelinated afferents are found in the deeper laminae (Rexed III–VI). Smaller myelinated fibers terminate in the marginal zone (Rexed lamina I), the ventral portion of lamina II, and throughout lamina III. Small-diameter, unmyelinated fibers (C fibers) largely terminate throughout lamina II and in lamina X around the central canal.

From a functional standpoint, this ramification emphasizes that neurons that lie distal to the segment of entry of the afferent will receive excitatory input. Electrophysiologic studies have shown that whereas the strongest excitation is observed in neurons in the segment of entry, excitation from the L5 root may be observed in cells as far as five to seven segments rostrally. As discussed later in this chapter, factors that alter

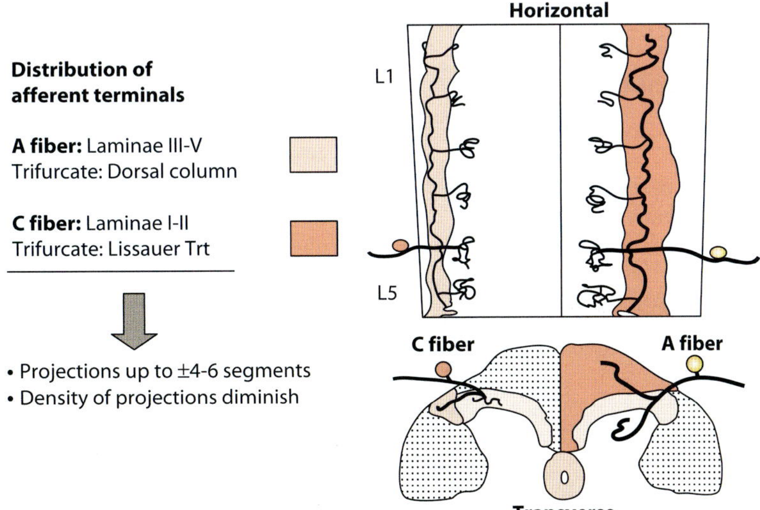

FIGURE 1-6. Schematic displaying the ramification of C fibers (**left**) into the dorsal horn and collateralization into Lissauer's tract and of Aβ fibers (**right**) into the dorsal columns and into the dorsal horn. Note that the densest terminations are within the segment of entry and that there are less-dense collateralizations into the dorsal horns at the more distal spinal segments. This density of collateralization corresponds to the potency of the excitatory drive into these distal segments.

TABLE 1-3 Summary of Several Products Contained and Released from Small Primary Afferents

Peptides	Excitatory Amino Acids	Other
Substance P	Glutamate	Purines (ATP)
Calcitonin gene–related peptide	Aspartate	
Galanin		
Vasoactive intestinal polypeptide		
Somatostatin		

ATP, adenosine triphosphate.

the excitability of these distant neurons may thus increase the apparent size of the receptive field for a given neuron.[11,12]

PRIMARY AFFERENT TRANSMITTERS

Activation of primary afferents typically induces a postsynaptic excitation. Excitation is mediated by the release of neurotransmitters from the afferent terminal. Considerable effort has been directed at establishing the identity of the excitatory neurotransmitters in the primary afferent. Some of these are listed in **Table 1-3**.[13]

Characteristics of Primary Afferent Transmitters A number of properties characterize the transmitters that are contained in and released from the primary afferent. Peptides and glutamate have been shown to exist within subpopulations of small, type B dorsal root ganglion cells (giving rise to C fibers) and are in laminae I and II of the dorsal horn of the spinal cord, where the majority of primary afferent terminals are found (**Fig. 1-7**). These levels in the dorsal horn are reduced by rhizotomy or ganglionectomy, or both, or by treatment with the small afferent neurotoxin, capsaicin.

Many peptides present in large, dense core vesicles (e.g., substance P and calcitonin gene–related peptide) as well as excitatory amino acids in small, clear core synaptic vesicles (glutamate) are present in and released from the same terminal. Iontophoretic application onto the dorsal horn of the several amino acids and peptides found in primary afferents has been shown to produce excitatory effects. Amino acids produce a very rapid, short-lasting depolarization. Peptides produce a delayed and long-lasting depolarization. Local spinal administration of several agents, such as substance P and glutamate, does yield pain behavior, suggesting their possible role as transmitters in the pain process.[14]

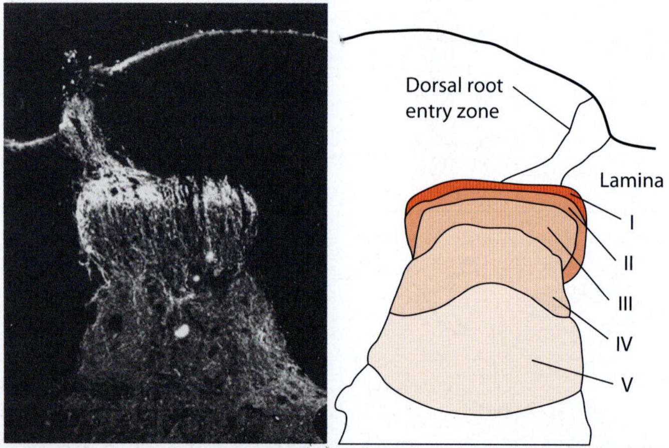

FIGURE 1-7. Histochemistry showing distribution of substance P immunoreactivity in laminae I and II (substantia gelatinosa) of the dorsal horn.

A large proportion of nociceptive dorsal horn neurons are contacted by substance P–containing terminals. Administration of noxious, but not innocuous, stimulation to the tissue results in release of several of these peptides into the spinal dorsal horn. With regard to the excitatory amino acids, their release has been evoked by acute and chronic nociceptive stimuli, including joint inflammation. Unlike the peptides, amino acids are also present in large primary afferents, and their spinal release can also be induced by activation of Aβ fibers.

CLASSES OF DORSAL HORN NEURONS

Anatomically, dorsal horn neurons may be broadly described in terms of their location (marginal layer, substantia gelatinosa, and the nucleus proprius), size (small, magnocellular), and functional response properties and neurochemistry. The complexity of this region accordingly cannot be overstated. For practical purposes related to nociceptive processing, it is reasonable to consider the functional properties of two principal classes of neurons. Electrophysiologic recording from single neurons in the spinal dorsal horn reveals several populations that are activated by high-intensity stimuli: nociceptive specific (marginal cells) and wide dynamic range (lamina V neurons) (**Fig. 1-8**).

Nociceptive-specific Neurons Marginal neurons, located in lamina I of the dorsal horn, are large neurons that are oriented transversely across the cap of the dorsal gray matter and receive input from small unmyelinated and lightly myelinated afferents (see Fig. 1-5). Some project to the thalamus via ipsilateral and contralateral ascending pathways, and others project intra- and intersegmentally along the dorsal and dorsolateral white matter. Populations of these neurons respond selectively to intense cutaneous and muscle stimulation. Whereas some are modality specific (e.g., firing in response only to thermal or mechanical stimuli), others respond to both types of stimuli. Activity in these subpopulations of neurons provides an unambiguous message that nociceptors have activated. Other prominent cell types in lamina I include (1) thermoreceptive "cool" cells that are activated and inhibited by innocuous cooling and warming, respectively, and (2) heat, pinch, and cold cells that are similar to traditional marginal cells but also are excited by noxious cold.[15]

Wide-dynamic-range (WDR) Neurons The cell bodies of lamina V cells are located in the nucleus proprius of the dorsal horn and send their apical dendrites up into laminae II and III (see Fig. 1-8). An important property of these cells is that they receive convergent input from a variety of functionally distinct primary afferents.[16] Practically, these cells demonstrate three kinds of convergence.

1. *Fiber response properties.* As indicated schematically in Figure 1-8, WDR-type cells receive input both from large, typically low-threshold afferents that project deep into the dorsal horn and from small, typically high-threshold afferents that project only into laminae I and II. As suggested schematically, some of this input, particularly that which is superficial, is mediated by excitatory interneurons. These WDR cells accordingly display a graded increase in the frequency of response to stimuli that are progressively more intense and recruit increasingly higher threshold populations of afferents Aβ to A∂ and C. This convergence thus permits these single cells to integrate input activated by a wide range of stimuli that vary in intensity, with higher frequency firing being noted as stimulus intensity rises.
2. *Spatial convergence.* As outlined earlier in Figure 1-6, primary afferents entering a specific segment have their primary excitatory input on dorsal horn neurons in that segment of entry. Still, it is clear that such axons can collateralize and mediate an excitatory effect on cells that lie in distal dermatomes. Accordingly, the size of the dermatome of that segment is actually larger than the peripheral distribution of the afferents in the root of that respective segment. As noted later in this discussion, it is likely that the size of the receptive field of a given neuron may be increased by conditions that lead to an enhancement of its excitability as inputs that are relatively weak become able to drive activity in that now-"sensitized" spinal neuron.

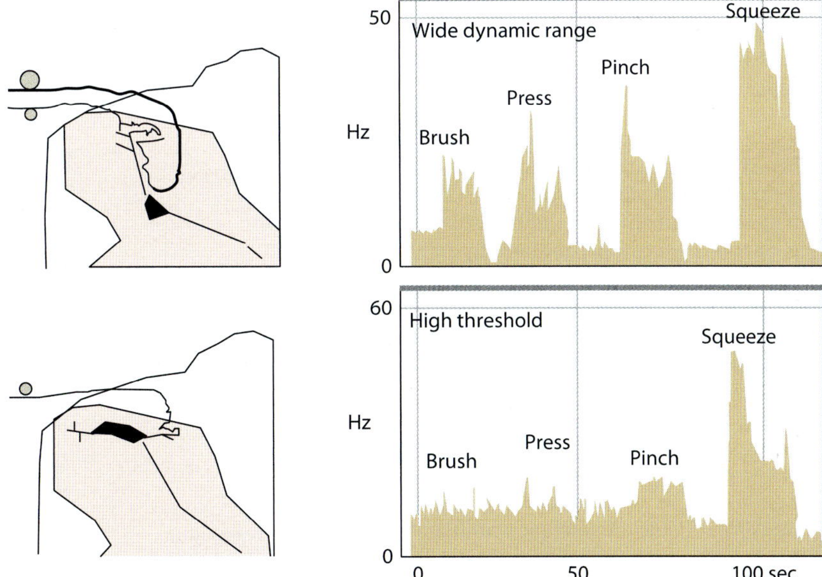

FIGURE 1-8. Schematic representing the morphology and dendritic pattern (**left**) of a lamina V, wide-dynamic-range neuron (**top**) and a lamina I, marginal neuron (**bottom**). The firing patterns of the respective classes of neurons are indicated in the representation on the right, in which a poststimulus time histogram shows the frequency of firing in response to four graded, mechanical stimuli ranging from innocuous (brush/press) to noxious (pinch/squeeze).

3. *Organ convergence.* Depending on the spinal level, a WDR neuron can be activated by input traveling with the sympathetics (e.g., as activated by distention of hollow viscera [bladder, small intestine, and gallbladder]), injection of bradykinin into the mesenteric artery, close intraarterial administration of bradykinin or the injection of hypertonic saline into muscle/tendon, or group III afferent stimulation from the gastrocnemius. The same WDR neuron can thus be excited by cutaneous or deep (muscle and joint) input applied within the dermatome that coincides with the segmental location of these spinal cells. Thus, stimulation of the skin and muscles of the left shoulder and upper arm (T_1–T_5 dermatome) activates WDR neurons that are also excited by coronary artery occlusion. These results indicate that the phenomenon of *referred* visceral pain, for example, has its substrate in the anatomic convergence of input from viscera, muscle, and skin onto the same populations of dorsal horn neurons.[17] Migraine is another example of such organ convergence. The migraine pain referred to the head arises from activation of dural afferents that project to neurons in the nucleus caudalis which receive input from afferents arising from homologous extracranial tissues. Accordingly, the migraine pain is referred to those extracranial regions.

ASCENDING SPINAL TRACTS

Clinical experience based on local spinal lesions of the ventrolateral quadrant suggests that pain is a "crossed" pathway with relevant projections traveling in the contralateral ventrolateral white matter. Midline myelotomies that destroy fibers crossing the midline at the levels of the cut produce bilateral pain deficits. These observations suggest that the relevant pathways for nociception are predominantly crossed. Similarly, stimulation of the ventrolateral tracts in awake subjects undergoing percutaneous cordotomies results in reports of contralateral warmth and pain. In accord with these observations, tract-tracing studies and electrophysiologic investigations emphasize that activity evoked in the spinal cord by high-threshold stimuli reaches supraspinal sites by several long and tract systems that travel within the ventrolateral quadrant[18] (**Fig. 1-9**).

Spinoreticular Fibers Spinoreticular axons originating in laminae V through VIII terminate ipsilaterally and contralaterally to their spinal site or origin. In the medulla, the fibers aggregate laterally, and collaterals of these fibers terminate in the more medially situated brainstem reticular nuclei. Reticulothalamic afferents excited by this input then project to the thalamus.

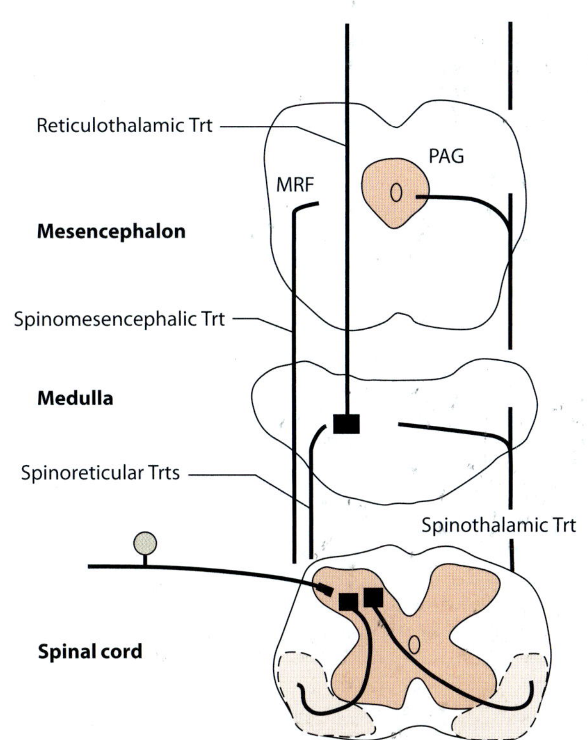

FIGURE 1-9. Schematic demonstrating the ascending crossed projections from dorsal horn neurons into the brainstem (spinoreticular) and into the thalamus (spinothalamic). The ventrobasal thalamus receives somatically mapped input from the spinal cord and projects this input into the somatosensory cortex, where the somatotopy is preserved. Other projections go to the medial thalamus and, from there, to a variety of limbic forebrain sites.

Spinomesencephalic Fibers Spinomesencephalic tracts originate primarily in lamina I, with a smaller component from laminae VI through VIII and X. They project into the mesencephalic reticular formation and the lateral periaqueductal gray matter.

Spinothalamic Fibers The cells of origin of this tract, the most extensively studied of the ventrolateral tract systems, are not limited to the dorsal gray matter, but are found throughout laminae I through VII and X of the spinal gray matter. Axons originating in the marginal layer and the neck of the nucleus proprius ascend predominantly in the contralateral ventral quadrant. Spinothalamic axons differentiate into a lateral and medial component in the posterior portion of the thalamus: The medial component passes through the internal medullary lamina to terminate in the nucleus parafascicularis and in the intralaminar and paralaminar nuclei. The majority of fibers pass laterally to terminate throughout the nucleus ventralis posterolateralis, the medial aspect of the posterior nucleus complex, and the intralaminar nuclei. A significant proportion of the neurons projecting laterally in the thalamus (ventral posterior lateral complex) also project to the medial thalamic regions such as the VMpo (ventromedial pars oralis) and Mediodorsalis portion (**Fig. 1-10**).

Suprathalamic Projection Projections to higher centers include specific mapping of input from the ventrobasal complex into the somatosensory cortex and multiple outputs particularly from the medial (VMpo/Mediodorsalis) and intralaminar nuclei projects diffusely to wide areas of the cerebral cortex, including the frontal, parietal, and limbic regions. Positron emission tomographic (PET) scanning studies in humans have confirmed that noxious stimuli will activate the appropriate cortical regions in the somatosensory cortex and limbic forebrain regions such as the insula and anterior cingulate gyrus[19] (see Fig. 1-10).

SIGNIFICANCE OF ASCENDING PATHWAYS: SENSORY-DISCRIMINATIVE AND AFFECTIVE-MOTIVATIONAL

Early thinking made the useful conjecture that pain could be considered in terms of two principal components: the sensory-discriminative and the affective-motivational components.[20] An important question is whether this functional distinction finds parallels in the underlying physiology and connectivity of the substrates thus far examined as being relevant to nociceptive processing.

At present, it is appreciated that the WDR neurons typically project into the ventrobasal thalamus, where their input is mapped precisely onto a sensory homunculus. These cells then project rostrally to the somatosensory cortex, where that input is similarly mapped onto a sensory homunculus.

In this system, each site on the body surface is faithfully mapped, and this map is maintained to the cortex. This system is uniquely able to preserve anatomic information and information regarding the intensity of the stimulus (as initially provided by the frequency response characteristics of the WDR neuron). This system is able to provide the information necessary for mapping the *sensory-discriminative* dimension of pain.

On the other hand, it has become evident that marginal, nociceptive-specific neurons also project contralaterally into the thalamus. This input thus provides one aspect of a circuit that appears to be activated by only particularly intense stimuli. This input function is defined by the response properties of the spinal marginal cell. It might be speculated that this circuit may underlie the *affective-motivational* component of the pain pathway.

The preceding recitation of the pathways through which afferent information evoked by high-threshold information travels reflects what traditionally is known as the pain pathway. In fact, this schematic, although correct, vastly oversimplifies the true organization. At every synapse, the transmission through the dorsal horn and brainstem is subject to significant modulation.

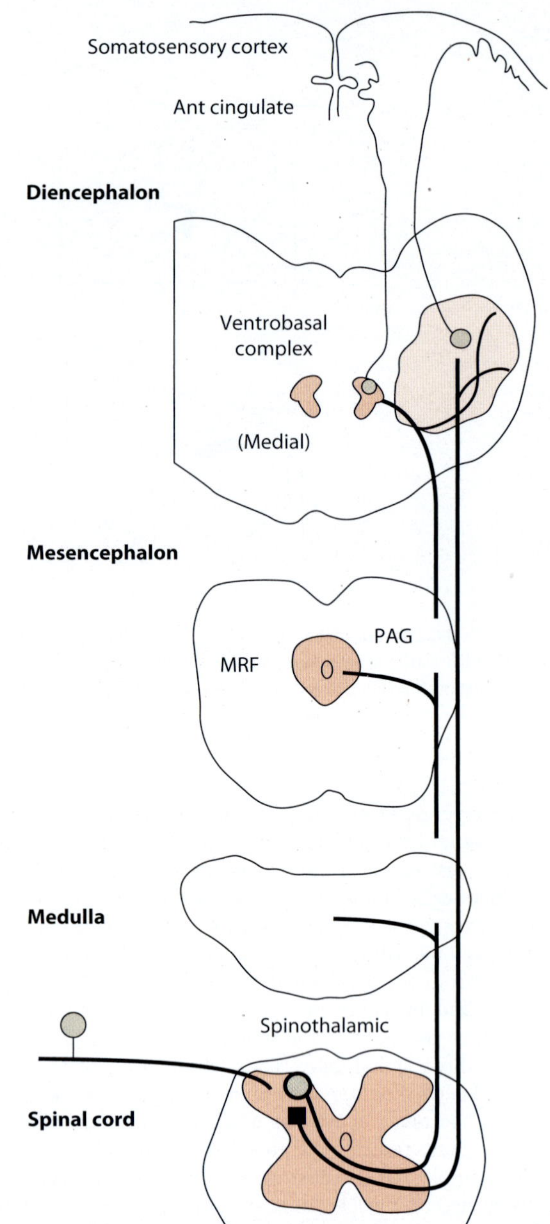

FIGURE 1-10. Sensory input into the spinal cord leads to the local activation of complex linkages that eventually project rostrally in the contralateral-ventrolateral pathways to medullary and diencephalic structures. In this schematic organization, it is emphasized that these ascending projections provide input in the lateral thalamus, which is somatotopically organized and projects from there into the somatosensory cortex. Importantly, a significant portion of the ascending traffic travels medially and makes synaptic contact in these medial regions with ascending projections that travel to the limbic cortex, such as the anterior cingulate cortex. Organizationally, it has been suggested that these different projection targets reflect upon substrates that underlie the "sensory-discriminative" and "affective-motivational" aspects of the pain experience.

In some instances, it is believed that the modulation may serve to diminish the pain message (i.e., endogenous analgesic systems). However, as subsequently discussed, there are several circumstances in which a repetitive afferent drive results in the involvement of an active facilitation of the message. In other cases, the nonaversive nature of large afferent stimulation (Aβ) reflects the continued presence of small inhibitory interneurons that alter large afferent input, but have no effect on activity in C fibers.

DYNAMIC ASPECTS OF ENCODING OF INJURY-GENERATED INPUT

The preceding section emphasized that tissue injury yielded activity in small primary afferents and that small afferent input resulted in monosynaptic and polysynaptic excitation of dorsal horn neurons that projected to the brainstem and higher centers. Importantly, the pathway appears to preserve several properties of the stimulus, the anatomic sign (localization), and intensity. Thus, input from an area of skin might be expected to activate a given population of spinal neurons that received afferent input from that part of the body surface, and the intensity of the stimulus was mirrored either by the specific neuronal population activated (e.g., nociceptive specific cells) or by the frequency of the discharge (as with the WDR neurons), or both. This linkage, even in its simplest form, would be described as the "pain pathway" as it reflects the connectivity by which afferent traffic generated by tissue injury reaches higher centers and the conscious state. This afferent substrate, in fact, represents only one component of the system that is essential to the processing of nociceptive input. The excitation of dorsal horn neurons evoked by small afferent input is subject to modulation by a number of receptor systems within the spinal cord. Technically, this modulation may be thought of in terms of those systems that increase or decrease the efficacy of synaptic connections of the afferent pathway.

PLASTICITY OF THE ENCODING OF PERSISTENT AFFERENT INPUT

Acute activation of small afferents by high-intensity mechanical or thermal stimuli will result in a clearly defined pain behavior in humans and animals. This event is believed to be mediated by the release of the excitatory afferent transmitters outlined earlier and, consequently, the depolarization of projection neurons. The magnitude of the response of a dorsal horn neuron, either WDR or nociceptive specific, is related to the frequency (and identity) of the afferent input.

The frequency of the afferent input is proportional to the magnitude of the acutely applied stimulus. The organization of this system's response to an acute stimulus is thus typically modeled in terms of a monotonic (linear) relationship between activity in the peripheral afferent and the activity of neurons that project out of the spinal cord to the brain.

As previously noted, in the face of tissue injury, the afferent input is characterized by a persistent afferent barrage. As discussed subsequently, such input reveals the initiation of a variety of inhibitor and facilitatory processes that lead to a nonlinear increase in spinal output.

INTRINSIC MODULATORY PROCESSES

The activation of dorsal horn neurons by afferent input can be modulated in such a fashion as to be decreased by several discrete systems.

Large Afferent Axon Interactions Dorsal horn WDR neurons can be inhibited by transient activation of large primary afferents. Such inhibition is mediated by a local spinal circuit that produces primary afferent depolarization (PAD), which exerts an inhibitory effect on the terminals of adjacent afferents. This serves to reduce the amount of neurotransmitter released from the afferent fibers in response to a fixed input. PAD is mediated by release from local interneurons in the substantia gelatinosa of the inhibitory amino acids, γ-aminobutyric acid (GABA) and glycine.[21] In human psychophysical studies, vibratory stimuli applied to a painful area served to activate large myelinated fibers and reduced perception of chronic musculoskeletal pain. Dorsal column stimulation by antidromically activating collaterals of large primary afferent fibers would also induce PAD, and this mechanism may account for some of the antinociceptive actions of dorsal column stimulation.

It is important to appreciate that the presence of these small inhibitory interneurons is crucial for the ongoing encoding of large afferent input. Thus, the spinal action of $GABA_A$ and glycine receptor inhibitors will induce a potent tactile allodynia. These results suggest that the non-aversive characteristics of large afferent stimulation depend upon this ongoing modulation. Studies in nerve injury–induced pain states have suggested that there is a loss of glycine or GABAergic inhibition secondary to the loss of dorsal horn neurons. The reduction in such inhibition may provide a partial explanation of the potent allodynia that accompanies such nerve injury states. An alternative event is that in the face of chronic inflammation and nerve injury, that there is a change in the expression of a neuronal chloride transporter that leads to an increase in intracellular Cl. In this case, opening a chloride ionophore will lead to an *exit* of anions that results in membrane *depolarization*. This anomolous event results in the GABA A and Glycine channels transitioning from an inhibitory to an excitatory phenotype.[22] Thus, the very circuit that would otherwise reduce large afferent excitation would itself become facilitatory.

Bulbospinal and Spinal Modulation Considerable evidence indicates that a variety of spinal terminal systems may serve to modulate nociceptive processing at the level of the spinal dorsal horn. Early work demonstrated that activation of bulbospinal pathways would suppress spinal nociceptive processing and produce a behaviorally defined analgesia by the release of noradrenaline and the activation of dorsal horn α_2 receptors. Evidence that small afferent activation could indirectly activate systems that mediated the spinal release of hormones, such as enkephalin or noradrenaline, which could act at such modulatory receptors, supported the perspective that nociceptive processing was under a tonic endogenous inhibition. In spite of the observation that activating these receptors (e.g., spinal injection of opiate and α_2 agonists) could yield a powerful analgesia by an action pre- and postsynaptic to the small afferent terminal, the delivery of antagonists for these receptors has surprisingly modest effects on spontaneous pain thresholds. This suggests that however potent a modulatory system these several receptors represent, these endogenous systems are not in a tonically active mode, and downregulation of small afferent input is not a pervasive component of the ongoing processing of input generated by tissue injury.

INTRINSIC FACILITATORY PROCESSES: REPETITIVE SMALL AFFERENT INPUT

WDR neurons in the spinal and medullary dorsal horn display a stable response to the discrete, periodic activation of afferent C fibers. However, repetitive stimulation of C (but not A) fibers at a moderately faster rate results in a progressively facilitated discharge. This facilitated response is called "wind-up" (see Fig. 1-9). This condition has three properties:

1. The conditioning serves to enhance the response of the dorsal horn neuron to subsequent input, such that a given stimulus yields a greater response that would otherwise be anticipated from that stimulus.
2. The conditioning of the spinal cord with repetitive small afferent stimulation has the additional effect of increasing the receptive field size of the neuron. Thus, afferent input from dermatomal areas that previously did not activate the WDR neuron being studied now evokes a prominent response. The anatomic substrate for this increased receptive field size is believed to reflect the otherwise weak excitatory input that comes from collaterals of afferents innervating the skin areas adjacent to the injury. In the face of the induction of a facilitated state in the specific neuron under study, this otherwise ineffective excitatory drive becomes adequate to drive depolarization. Intracellular recording reveals that the facilitated state reflects a progressive and sustained partial depolarization of the cell, rendering the membrane increasingly susceptible to afferent input.
3. Low-threshold tactile stimulation also becomes increasingly effective in driving these neurons. This facilitation by repetitive C-fiber input, therefore, increases the subsequent neuronal response to low-threshold afferent input and enhances the response generated by a given noxious afferent input. These mechanisms are discussed further in the next sections.

WIND-UP AND CENTRAL FACILITATION

In animal studies, WDR neurons in the dorsal horn display a stimulus-dependent response to discrete activation of afferent C fibers. Repetitive stimulation of C (but not A) fibers at a moderately faster rate results in a progressively facilitated discharge.

The exaggerated discharge was dubbed *wind-up* by Mendell[23] (**Fig. 1-11**). Intracellular recording has indicated that the facilitated state is represented by a progressive and long-sustained partial depolarization of the cell, rendering the membrane increasingly susceptible to afferent input.[24]

Given the likelihood that WDR discharge frequency contributes to the encoding of a high-threshold stimulus as aversive, and that many of these WDR neurons project through the ventrolateral quadrant of the spinal cord (i.e., spinobulbar or spinothalamic projections), this augmented response is believed to be an important component of the pain message. In addition, the conditioning of the afferent input as described has the added effect of increasing the receptive field size of the neurons, such that afferent input from dermatomal areas that previously did not activate the WDR neuron now evokes a prominent response. Moreover, low-threshold tactile stimulation also becomes increasingly effective in driving these neurons.

This facilitation by repetitive C-fiber input, therefore, increases the subsequent neuronal response to low-threshold afferent input, enhances the response generated by a given noxious afferent input, and increases the size of the receptive field at which a stimulus can evoke activity in that neuron. Given the likelihood that WDR discharge frequency is part of the encoding of the intensity of a high-threshold stimulus, and that many of these WDR neurons project in the ventrolateral quadrant of the spinal cord (i.e., spinobulbar projections), this augmented response is believed to be an important component of the pain message.

The enhanced responsiveness reflects an augmented sensitization of the neuronal membrane leading to an enhanced response for a given depolarization. The pharmacology leading to this sensitization is examined in the discussion that follows. The enlarged receptive field is believed to reflect, in part, on the collateral input from distal segments (see Fig. 1-6). In the presence of sensitization, these distal inputs that exert a degree of excitation that is otherwise inadequate to activate the neuron will become sufficient. This combination of spinal events results in an apparent increase in the size of the neuronal receptive field.

FUNCTIONAL CORRELATES OF INJURY-EVOKED CENTRAL FACILITATION

Protracted pain states, such as those that may occur with inflamed or injured tissue (leading to the peripheral release of active factors), would routinely result in such an augmented afferent drive of the WDR neuron and, thence, to the ongoing facilitation. Such observations are consistent with the speculation that the afferent C-fiber burst may initiate long-lasting events, resulting in changes in spinal processing that will alter the response to subsequent input. The preceding observations regarding this dorsal horn system have been shown to have behavioral consequences. This phenomenon has clear functional correlates.

Studies in animals have shown that the acute injection of an irritant such as formalin will induce an acute afferent barrage followed by a prolonged low level of afferent activity. During this later period after formalin injection, WDR dorsal horn neurons show an unexpected level of activity, given the modest afferent input (e.g., a central facilitation). Finally, examination of behavior has shown that the animal displays an exaggerated response (flinching) during the second phase, consistent with the activity in dorsal horn neurons but, again, greater than might be anticipated based on the afferent traffic[25] (**Fig. 1-12**).

The role of this afferent-evoked facilitation in the postinjury pain state cannot be minimized. After tissue injury, in animals and in humans, inflammation and cellular/vascular injury lead to the local peripheral release of active factors. Such active factors will produce a prolonged activation of C fibers that evoke a facilitated state of processing in WDR neurons, and, thence, an ongoing facilitation of nociceptive perception. Such observations are consistent with the speculation that the afferent C-fiber burst may initiate long-lasting events, resulting in changes in spinal processing, which will alter the response to subsequent input.

The relevance of this C-fiber–evoked facilitation to humans has been emphasized by psychophysical studies. To observers, the activation of C fibers by the intradermal injection of capsaicin will lead to an initial pain state followed for an extended period of time by a large region of profoundly enhanced mechanical and thermal sensitivity.[26] This phenomenon is referred to as secondary hyperesthesia (**Fig. 1-13**). Thus, in humans, following local injury where C fibers are similarly activated, there is every reason to believe that similar processes apply and that important components of the postinjury pain state are the events consequent to the afferent barrage and not, strictly speaking, the input present in the postinjury phase.

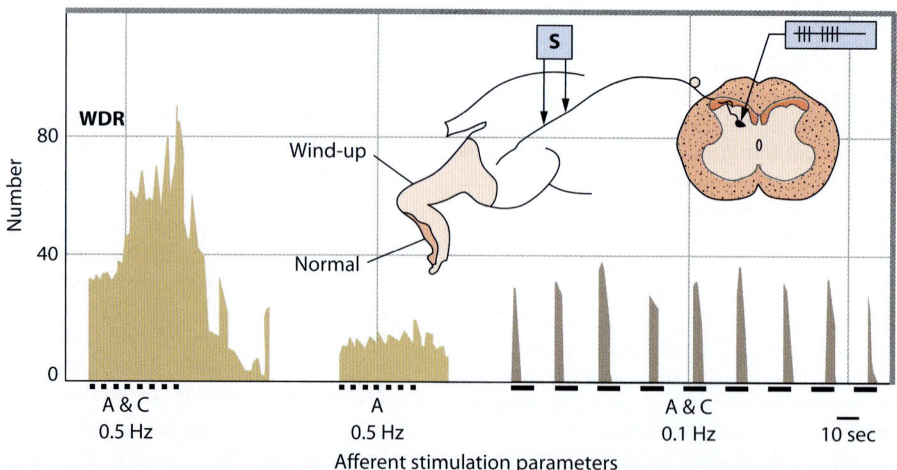

FIGURE 1-11. Schematic showing a single unit recording from wide-dynamic-range neurons in response to an electrical stimulus delivered at 0.1 Hz (**right**). A very reliable, stimulus-linked response is evoked at this frequency. In contrast, when the stimulation rate is increased to 0.5 Hz, there is a progressive increase in the magnitude of the response generated by the stimulation (**left**). This facilitation results from the C-fiber input and not an A-fiber input (**middle**) and is called "wind-up."

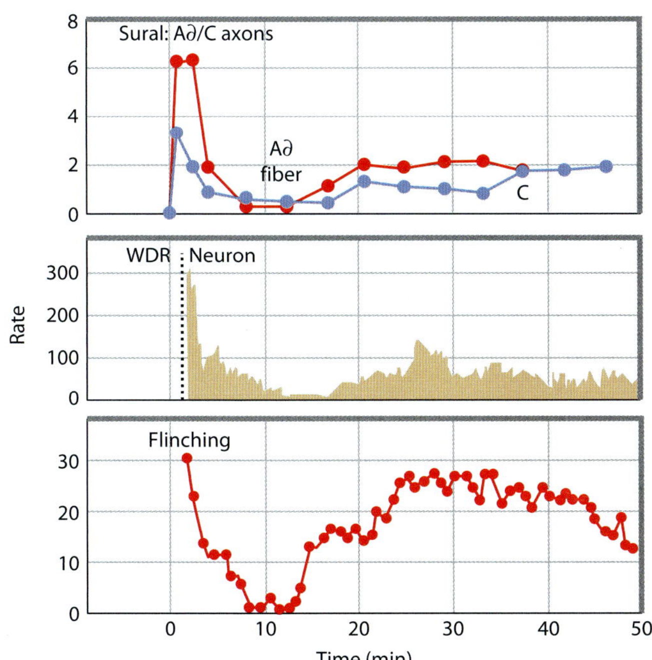

FIGURE 1-12. C-fiber activity (firing rate/sec; **top**) measured in the sural nerve of the anesthetized rat; firing of a wide-dynamic-range neuron (anesthetized rat; **middle**) and number of flinches in the unanesthetized rat (**bottom**) measured before and after the ipsilateral subcutaneous injection of formalin into the hind paw at the time indicated by the vertical dashed line. Note the low level of input during the second phase, in which behavior suggestive of pain is particularly high. Importantly, the second phase of the formalin test persists in spite of the animal being deeply anesthetized during the first phase.

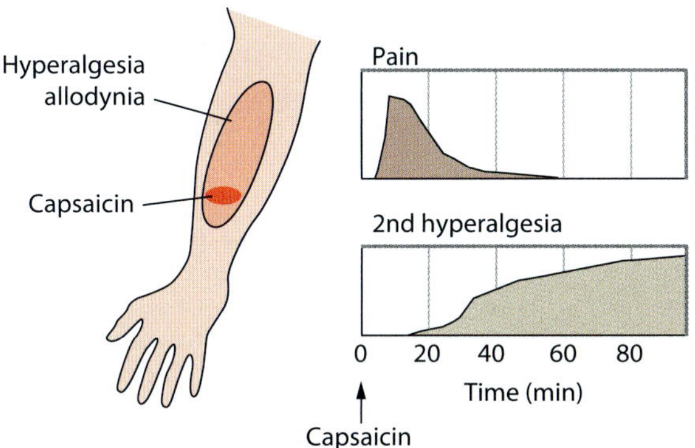

FIGURE 1-13. Schematic illustrating the effects of injecting the C-fiber stimulant, capsaicin, under the skin. This generates an intense local pain sensation that persists for about 20 to 30 minutes. This sensation diminishes, and it is possible to demonstrate that the patient/observer reports a large area of secondary hyperalgesia that persists for hours. Importantly, if the area of the injection is anesthetized with local anesthetic prior to capsaicin delivery, then when the initial capsaicin effect is gone and the local anesthesia reverses, the observer reports no secondary allodynia.

PHARMACOLOGY OF CENTRAL FACILITATION

The pharmacology of this central facilitation suggests that the wind-up state reflects more than simply the repetitive activation of a simple excitatory system. The first real demonstration of this unique pharmacology was presented by showing that the phenomenon of spinal wind-up was prevented by the spinal delivery of antagonists for the *N*-methyl-D-aspartate (NMDA) receptor[27] (**Fig. 1-14**). Importantly, this agent had no effect on acute evoked activity, but reduced the wind-up.

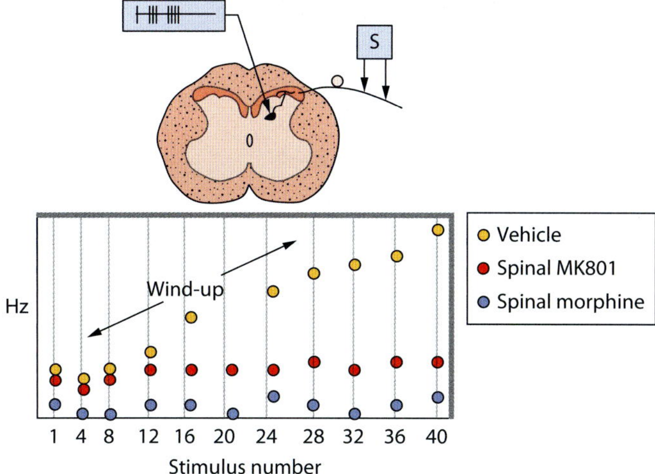

FIGURE 1-14. Repetitive C-fiber stimulation was repeated 40 times at 2 Hz, and the response of a spinal wide-dynamic-range (WDR) neuron was counted. As indicated under control conditions, there was a progressive increase in the number of discharges counted with each subsequent stimulus. Addition of morphine resulted in a block of the initial C-fiber–evoked discharge, and there was no subsequent increase. In contrast, the delivery of *N*-methyl-D-aspartate (NMDA) antagonists resulted in no change in the initial discharge but prevented the subsequent wind-up.

Subsequent behavioral work demonstrated that such drugs had no effect on acute pain behavior, but reduced the facilitated states induced after tissue injury.

Protracted pain states, such as those that may occur with inflamed or injured tissue (leading to the peripheral release of active factors), will routinely result in such an augmented afferent drive of the WDR neuron and, thence, to an ongoing facilitation (e.g. the wind-up described in Fig. 1-14). Such observations are consistent with the speculation that the afferent C-fiber burst may initiate longer-lasting events, resulting in changes in spinal processing that will alter the response to subsequent input. The pharmacology of the central facilitation suggests that the state of central facilitation reflects more than the repetitive activation of a simple excitatory system. Based on studies examining the spinal pharmacology of the electrophysiologic and behavioral response to the postinjury stimulus state, it has become apparent that the arrival of the first small afferent barrage appears to trigger a cascade of events that serve to facilitate the response to subsequent peripheral stimuli.[28]

Aspects of the complex pharmacology of central facilitation in the dorsal horn are presented in **Figure 1-15**. The following points may be made that define components of spinal systems involved in the postinjury pain state. For review purposes, the cascade may be thought of in terms of i) primary afferent; ii) second order neuronal systems and, iii) non neuronal systems.

Primary Afferent Systems The initial activation generated by small afferent input is mediated by specific primary afferent transmitters. Primary afferent C fibers release peptide (e.g., substance P, calcitonin gene–related peptide, and others) and excitatory amino acid (glutamate) products. These substances evoke excitation in second-order neurons.

Substance P Receptors The spinal delivery of substance P results in a mild acute "pain behavior" and a subsequent reduced response latency to thermal stimuli (thermal hyperalgesia). These effects are believed to be mediated by neurokinin 1 (NK-1) receptors that are located in the superficial dorsal horn on second-order neurons. Blockade of the NK-1 receptor by intrathecal antagonists or downregulation of NK-1 receptor expression by intrathecal treatment with NK-1 receptor mRNA antisense has little effect on acute nociceptive thresholds, but it reduces

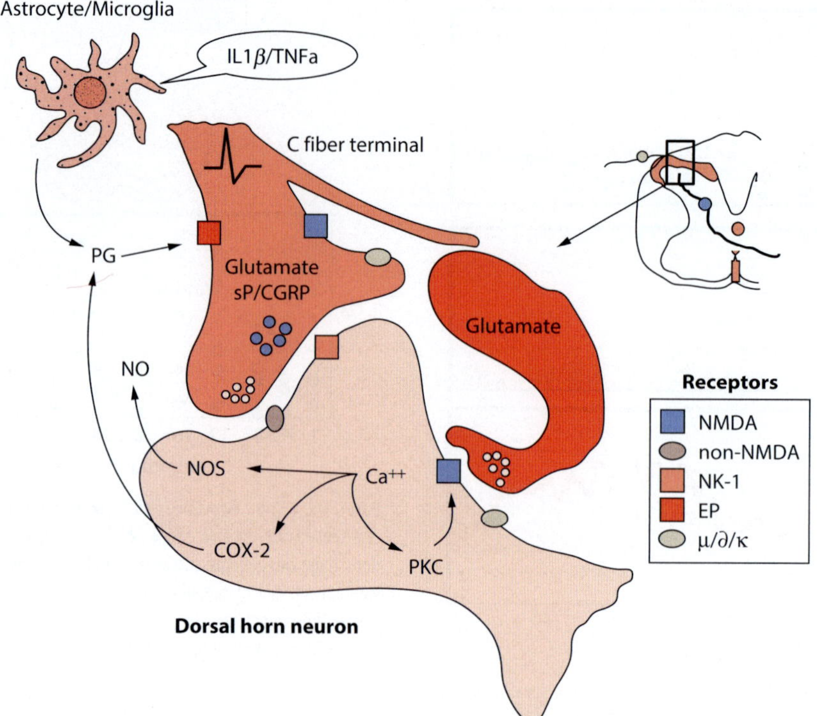

FIGURE 1-15. Schematic summarizing the organization of dorsal horn systems that contribute to the processing of nociceptive information. (1) Primary afferent C fibers release peptide (e.g., substance P [sP], calcitonin gene–related peptide [CGRP], and so on) and excitatory amino acid (glutamate) products. Small dorsal root ganglion (DRG) cells, as well as some postsynaptic elements contain nitric oxide synthase (NOS) and are able, upon depolarization, to release NO (nitric oxide). (2) Peptides and excitatory amino acids evoke excitation in second-order neurons. For glutamate, direct monosynaptic excitation is mediated by non–*N*-methyl-D-aspartate (NMDA) receptors (i.e., acute primary afferent excitation of WDR neurons is not mediated by the NMDA or neurokinin 1 [NK-1] receptor). (3) Interneurons excited by afferent barrage induce excitation in second-order neurons via an NMDA receptor. This leads to a marked increase in intracellular Ca^{2+} and the activation of kinases and phosphorylating enzymes. Prostaglandins (PG) generated by cyclooxygenase-2 (COX-2) and NO by NOS are formed and released. These agents diffuse extracellularly and facilitate transmitter release (retrograde transmission) from primary and nonprimary afferent terminals, either by a direct cellular action (e.g., NO) or by an interaction with a specific class of receptors (e.g., EP receptors for prostanoids). (4) Non-neuronal sources of prostaglandins may include activated astrocytes and microglia that are stimulated by circulating cytokines, which are released secondary to peripheral injury and inflammation. Terminal excitability can be altered by activation of a variety of receptors located on the sensory terminal, including those for μ, ∂ and κ opioids. See text for other details.[28]

the facilitated state and the behaviorally defined hyperalgesia (as in the second phase of the formalin test) induced by peripheral injury.[29]

Glutamate Receptors For glutamate, direct monosynaptic excitation of the second-order neuron is believed to be mediated by the ionotropic non-NMDA (AMPA) receptors (i.e., acute primary afferent excitation of dorsal horn neurons is not mediated by the NMDA receptor). The spinal delivery of agonists for the alpha-amino-3-hydroxy-5-methyl-4-isoxazole propionic acid and NMDA receptors will evoke a potent spontaneous pain behavior and a subsequent hyperalgesia and tactile allodynia.[30]

Opiates targeted at the spinal cord serve to block the release of transmitter from C fibers by acting presynaptically on the terminals of C fibers to prevent the opening of voltage-sensitive calcium channels responsible for the depolarization-evoked release of terminal transmitters. Opioid receptors have been demonstrated to be present on small afferent terminals, with the highest density of opioid binding present in the substantia gelatinosa.

Second Order Systems Following the initial excitation, it is appreciated that the spinal dorsal horn displays a prominent facilitation of its input–output function. This central facilitation represents a cascade that is initiated by the ongoing afferent drive.

Glutamate As indicated earlier, wind-up as evoked by repetitive small afferent input is diminished by NMDA receptor antagonists. Repetitive small afferent input (as occurs after tissue injury) will evoke spinal glutamate release (see Fig. 1-14). Blockade of spinal AMPA receptors by intrathecal antagonists will elevate acute nociceptive thresholds, as well as the first and second phase of the formalin test. In contrast, intrathecal NMDA antagonists have little effect on acute nociception but diminish facilitated states of processing. It is appreciated that the channel associated with the NMDA receptor is blocked by normal, resting physiologic levels of magnesium, so no change in excitability of the neurons possessing NMDA receptors can occur until this is removed (**Fig. 1-16**).

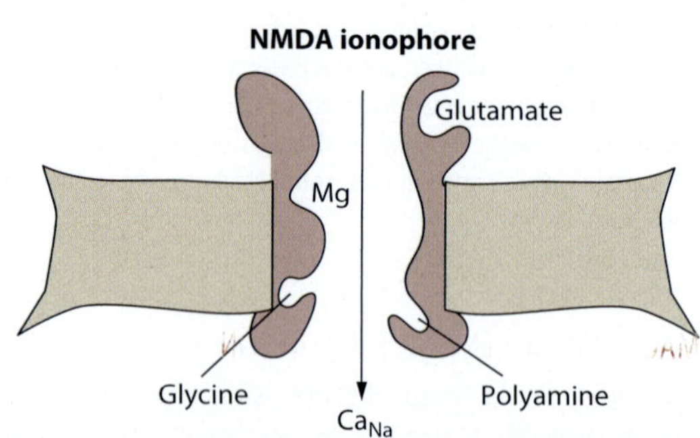

FIGURE 1-16. As indicated in the text, the *N*-methyl-D-aspartate (NMDA) receptor is a Ca^{2+} ionophore that, when activated, results in an influx of Ca^{2+}. To be activated, the receptor requires the occupancy by glutamate, the removal of the magnesium block by a mild membrane depolarization, and the occupancy of the "glycine site," along with several allosterically coupled elements, including the "polyamine site." Together, these events permit the ionophore to be activated.

The magnesium block is only removed by a shift in the membrane voltage toward depolarization. Thus, the binding of glutamate to the receptor alone is insufficient to activate the channel. The receptor channel complex is unique because of this dual requirement: The channel is gated by both ligand binding to the receptor and by the membrane voltage. An added degree of complexity is that glycine is a required coagonist with glutamate for activation of the receptor, acting at a strychnine-insensitive site closely associated with the NMDA receptor. Thus, for the NMDA receptor channel to operate, certain conditions need to be met: The release and binding of glutamate and the binding of glycine at the strychnine-insensitive site on the NMDA ionophore are needed, together with a non-NMDA–induced depolarization to remove the tonic magnesium block. C-fiber stimulation will induce the release of glutamate but also with excitatory peptides, and the latter may provide the required depolarization. Hence, as noted in the discussion that follows, the events mediated by NMDA-receptor activation occur secondary to an initial conditioning input. Mechanistically, the NMDA receptor is a Ca^{2+} ionophore that, when activated, will lead to a significant increase in intracellular Ca^{2+}. As emphasized later, it is in part due to this increase in intracellular Ca^{2+} that the cascade initiated by repetitive afferent input is initiated.[31] Aside from the NMDA receptor, it has become evident that in the face of ongoing small afferent input, there is a change in the properties of the membrane ionophores. Thus, with repetitive input the AMPA ionophore changes from sodium channel to one that allows the passage of Calcium (as does the NMDA ionophore). This conversion contributes to an enhanced response of the second order neuron.

Prostaglandins Cyclooxygenase is found in the spinal dorsal horn and inhibitors, and prostaglandin-receptor antagonists given intrathecally will diminish hyperalgesia induced in the postinjury pain state. This reaction reflects on the important role of prostaglandins released from the spinal cord. Dialysis of the spinal cord has emphasized that, in the postinjury pain state, there is an increase in prostaglandin E_2 release. Prostanoids will facilitate release of C-fiber transmitters such as substance P. Consistent with the observation that NMDA antagonists can block a hyperalgesic state, spinal NMDA agonists evoke a hyperalgesic state, and this hyperalgesia is blocked by spinal cyclooxygenase inhibitors. Further, it has been shown that prostaglandins can serve to inhibit glycine receptor function, thereby reducing the inhibition that otherwise regulates large afferent evoked excitation. Such observations suggest that spinal activation can evoke the release of prostanoids that, in turn, augments spinal nociceptive processing.[32]

It is currently appreciated that there are two cyclooxygenase enzymes. The present data emphasize that the cyclooxygenase-2 (COX-2) isozyme is constitutively in the spinal cord, and it is COX-2 that is primarily responsible for the prostaglandin E_2 release generated by small afferent input.

An additional interesting variant, suggested in Figure 1-15, is that COX-2 (and likely other proteins) expression may be elevated by circulating factors, released by inflammation and septic process—such as interleukin-1β, tumor necrosis factor-α, and lipopolysaccharide—that activate spinal astrocytes and microglia. Such activation may lead to an enhanced expression of a variety of enzymes (such as COX-2), channels, and receptors. The relevance of this non-neuronal expression in the central nervous system is not certain, but these cells may serve as a source of neuraxial prostaglandins. Such material would likely result in an enhanced release from neuronal terminals. It suggests an additional and intriguing role played by the central COX-2 isozyme and its selective inhibitors. Interestingly, these factors are believed to work on terminals that may lie distant from the site of synthesis and release. As such, they are referred to as volume transmitters.[33]

Nitric Oxide (NO) Small dorsal root ganglion cells as well as some postsynaptic elements contain NO synthase (NOS). NOS inhibitors given intrathecally will diminish hyperalgesia induced by intrathecal NMDA and by the postinjury pain state. Increased citrulline (a product of NO formation) is released from the spinal cord in the postinjury pain state. NO has been shown to facilitate terminal release of glutamate.[34]

Kinases and Phosphorylation Increasing intracellular Ca_i^{2+}—through the inositol 1,4,5-triphosphate (IP_3) pathway by neurokinin receptor or by the influx of Ca^{2+} through voltage-gated Ca^{2+} channels or ionophores (NMDA receptor)—activates kinases that phosphorylate and phosphatases that dephosphorylate local proteins. Phosphorylating enzyme systems consist of several classes of kinases that are distinguished by the structure and pharmacology of their inhibitors. In the spinal dorsal horn, mitogen-activated kinases (e.g., MAP kinases), cAMP-dependent kinase, and camkinase II have been observed in the spinal dorsal horn and dorsal root ganglia. Protein kinase C (PKC) consists of a large family of isozymes. Although some or all of the previously noted phosphorylating enzymes may play a role, the use of inhibitors for protein kinase A (PKA) and PKC have shown the particular importance of this family of kinases in regulating spinal facilitation. Many hyperalgesic states are mediated by a spinal NMDA receptor. The NMDA receptor is multiply phosphorylated by PKA and PKC. Intrathecal delivery of PKC inhibitors has been shown stereospecifically to diminish injury-induced hyperalgesia.[35,36]

Non-neuronal cells While it is evident that the neurotransmission involves the pre and post-synaptic neuron. There is ample evidence now that non-neuronal cells may play an important regulatory role in the excitability of the neuronal linkage. These non-neuronal cells may be though of in terms of those that are resident and those that migrate into the neuraxis.

Resident cells In recent years, it has been appreciated that glial cells (astrocytes/microglia) can also influence neuronal responses apart from being just support cells. The involvement of spinal glial cells in initiating and maintaining hyperalgesic states has been implicated. Following persistent inflammation and nerve injury, the spinal primary afferents apart from releasing pro-inflammatory neuropeptides (CGRP, sP) and neurotransmitters (glutamate, ATP) also releases molecules such as HMGB1and HSP60 that activates the neighboring glial cells. Astrocytes and microglia both expresses wide range of pattern recognition-sites such as toll like receptors (TLRs). HMGB1 and HSP60 act on toll like receptor-4 (TLR-4) that initiate immune like responses and releases a plethora of pro-inflammatory cytokines (IL-1b, IL-6, TNF) and growth factors (BDNF) each promoting nociceptive hypersensitivity. For e.g. IL-1b enhances phosphorylation of NR1 subunit of NMDAR and facilitate its activation in neurons. Similarly, TNF can maintain the augmented responsive state of glial cells by increasing phosphorylation of JNK and release of chemokine CCL2 also known to contribute enhanced pain signaling. Further, BDNF that acts on TRKB receptor, down regulates K+-Cl− co-transporter (KCC2) in inhibitory neurons (GABA/Glycine) required for maintaining the Cl homeostasis. As noted above, down regulation of KCC2 impairs the intracellular Cl gradient in neurons, causing a depolarizing shift and thus enhancing the excitation of otherwise inhibitory neurons. Thus, activation of glial cells can alter glial–neuronal/glial-glial interaction, developing an excitatory positive-feedback in pain pathway.[37,38,39]

Non-resident cells The presence of lymphocytes (T cells) and macrophages have been observed in the DRG and spinal cord following remote damage in the periphery (inflammation or nerve injury). Convincing evidences suggest that these non-resident cells contribute to central sensitization. Exposure of inflammatory cytokines to neurons and endothelial cells induces the release of chemokines, fractalkine (FKN) and CCL2 that binds to its receptor CX3CL1 and CCR2, respectively that are present on both, microglial and endothelial cells. As a consequence, these chemokine: receptor interaction acts as adhesion molecule for lymphocytes/macrophages and mediating trans-endothelial migration of these non-resident cells. Following infiltration, these cells initially provide short-term support to the damaged neuron in DRG and spinal cord and their long-term presence plays a role in glial activation and pain facilitation by potentially releasing excitatory cytokines. These cells have shown to play a major role in chronic neuropathic pain conditions.[40,41]

SYSTEM INTERACTION

After local tissue injury, the components of post-tissue injury pain reflect an increased receptive field and a left shift in the stimulus response curve for spinal dorsal horn neurons that is evoked initially and then sustained in part by persistent small afferent input. The contribution of these changes in spinal function to the behaviorally relevant nociceptive state is substantiated by comparing the pharmacology associated with the effects on the behavior of the unanesthetized animal with the effects of the drugs on the underlying electrophysiology. Based on such observations, it is possible to formulate a heuristic picture of the organization of several pharmacologically defined spinal systems that mediate the response of the animal to a strong and tissue-injurious stimulus. Thus, repetitive afferent input increases excitatory amino acid and peptide release from primary afferents that serve initially to depolarize dorsal horn neurons. Persistent depolarization serves to increase intracellular calcium, activating a variety of intracellular enzymes (COX-2, NOS) and various kinases (PKC). Prostaglandins and nitric oxide are released spinally and serve acutely to enhance the subsequent release of afferent peptides and glutamate. Activation of local kinases serves to phosphorylate membrane receptors and channels. As an example, the NMDA receptor when phosphorylated displays an enhanced calcium flux (see Fig. 1-5). The role of these system-level changes in spinal nociceptive processing in "pain behavior" is supported by the analgesic effects of spinally delivered agents known to reduce small afferent transmitter release (μ, ∂ opioid, and α_2-adrenergic agonists) and the antihyperalgesic actions of spinally delivered neurokinin-1 and NMDA-receptor antagonists, as well as inhibitors of spinal COX-2, NOS, and PKC.

It is important to note that the WDR-wind-up studies discussed earlier are carried out in animals that are under 1 minimum alveolar concentration anesthesia. The relevance of the observations to the performance of surgery on volatile "anesthetized" patients is clear. The implication of the afferent-evoked facilitation is that it is better to prevent small afferent input than to deal with its sequelae. This is believed to represent the basis of the consideration of the use of preemptive analgesics.[42]

ACUTE TO CHRONIC PAIN TRANSITION

The above commentary has focused on the role of acute nociception and tissue injury. Acute pain is adaptive in that it indicates the presence of a potentially tissue inuring stimulus. In the face of tissue injury, infection, or inflammation, the ongoing pain and the facilitated state is typically considered to resolve with time, e.g., healing. In each case, however, the inflammatory pain can sometimes transition to a chronic, pain condition, persisting beyond the resolution of the initiating stimulus.[43] This transition to a persistent, maladaptive pain state is the focus of much research. For instance, it is now evident that, in the face of persistent inflammation, peripheral afferent terminals may display sprouting and markers similar to those observed in neuromas.[44] This indicates that, with persistent inflammation, a neuropathic pain phenotype may develop.[45] Additionally, in recent years, research has increasingly focused on the involvement of immunocompetent cells (e.g. T-cells, microglia/macrophages, and astrocytes) in producing a facilitated pain state, as described above. The involvement of these cell types has led to implication of a role of both the innate and adaptive immune systems in the development of chronic pain.[46]

Innate Immune Signaling The innate immune system is responsible for detecting both damage and pathogens and does so in part through Toll-like receptors (TLRs). Of the TLRs, much pain-related research has focused specifically on TLR4.[47] Upon ligand binding, TLR4 activation results in the induction of pro-inflammatory cytokines (TNF and IL-1β) and Type 1 interferon (IFNβ). These pro-inflammatory cytokines can increase glutamate levels, increase AMPA-R signaling, and increase calcium permeability of the NMDA-R, leading to increased synaptic transmission, and nociceptive hypersensitivity. Of particular interest, TLR4 has been shown to mediate the transition from an acute to a chronic pain state in preclinical models; animals deficient in TLR4 do not develop a chronic pain phenotype despite the presence of an initial inflammatory pain. Additionally, TLR4 signaling has been implicated in the development and maintenance of a variety of pathological pain conditions including inflammatory pain, mononeuropathy (e.g., nerve injury), and polyneuropathy (e.g., chemotherapy-induced peripheral neuropathy, arthritis), indicating this may be a target of new drug development.

Adaptive Immune Signaling As with the innate immune system, the adaptive immune system is responsible for detection of invading pathogens and damage within the system. Here, the main cell types responsible for responding are B- and T-cells. There are a variety of T-cell subtypes, each with a distinct function, yet their role in pain has not been well defined. In general, however, T-cells have a number of chemokine receptors (CCR7, CX3CR1, CCR2) involved in pain transmission and neuron-glial interactions and secrete pro-inflammatory cytokines.[48] Recent work has demonstrated a role for T-cells in the development of chronic pain. Specifically, animals deficient in T-cells show less neuropathic pain after SNI. This effect seems to depend on the presence of IFNγ, secreted by Th1 T-cells and NK cells.[49] Further investigation into the interactions of the innate and adaptive immune systems in contributing to persistent pain are promising.

CONCLUSION

The preceding comments have provided a general overview of components of the neuraxis that contribute to the encoding of the pain state. It is clear that there are a number of discrete substrates through which such information generated by a high-intensity stimulus may travel. It is equally clear that the process of encoding is plastic and the throughput function at every level is subject to alteration, which can significantly modify the message generated by a given stimulus. The developing appreciation of this complex biology has been briefly touched on here, but it can be appreciated that this complex pharmacology provides an increasing number of venues whereby afferent input can be regulated. The current work showing the role of non-neuronal cells as well as inflammatory components typically associated with innate and adaptive immunity emphasizes the complexity of the processing system. We would note that such complexity is consistent with the deep integration that pain processing has with system biology. Such deep integration emphasizes why the effective control of pain poses such a difficult challenge.

REFERENCES

1. Sherrington CS. *The Integrative Action of the Nervous System*. New Haven, Conn: Yale University Press; 1906.
2. Myers RR, Olmarker K. Anatomy of DRG, intrathecal nerve roots, and epidural nerves with emphasis on mechanisms of neurotoxic injury. In: Yaksh TL, ed. *Spinal Drug Delivery*. Amsterdam, Netherlands: Elsevier Science BV; 1999.
3. Waxman SG, Cummins TR, Dib-Hajj S, et al. Sodium channels, excitability of primary sensory neurons, and the molecular basis of pain. *Muscle Nerve*. 1999;22:1177-1187.
4. Myers RR. Morphology of the peripheral nervous system and its relationship to neuropathic pain. In: Yaksh TL, Lynch C III, Zapol WM, et al., eds. *Anesthesia: Biologic Foundations*. Philadelphia, Pa: Lippincott-Raven; 1997.
5. Raja SN, Meyer RA, Campbell JN. Transduction properties of the sensory afferent fibers. In: Yaksh TL, Lynch C III, Zapol WM, et al., eds. *Anesthesia: Biologic Foundations*. Philadelphia, Pa: Lippincott-Raven; 1997.

6. Dray A. Pharmacology of peripheral afferent terminals. In: Yaksh TL, Lynch C III, Zapol WM, et al., eds. *Anesthesia: Biologic Foundations.* Philadelphia, Pa: Lippincott-Raven; 1997.
7. Schaible HG, Grubb BD. Afferent and spinal mechanisms of joint pain. *Pain.* 1993;55:5-54.
8. Watkins LR, Wiertelak EP, Goehler LE, et al. Characterization of cytokine-induced hyperalgesia. *Brain Res.* 1994;654:15-26.
9. Rexed B. The cytoarchitectonic organization of the spinal cord in the cat. *J Comp Neurol.* 1952;96:415-495.
10. Kerr FW. Neuroanatomical substrates of nociception in the spinal cord. *Pain.* 1975;1:325-356.
11. Shortland P, Wall PD. Long-range afferents in the rat spinal cord, II: arborizations that penetrate grey matter. *Philos Trans R Soc Lond B Biol Sci.* 1992;337:445-455.
12. Wall PD, Shortland P. Long-range afferents in the rat spinal cord, 1: numbers, distances and conduction velocities. *Philos Trans R Soc Land B Biol Sci.* 1991;334:85-93.
13. Sorkin LS, Carlton SM. Spinal anatomy and pharmacology of afferent processing. In: Yaksh TL, Lynch C III, Zapol WM, et al., eds. *Anesthesia: Biologic Foundations.* Philadelphia, Pa: Lippincott-Raven; 1997.
14. Yaksh TL, Malmberg AB. Central pharmacology of nociceptive transmission. In: Wall P, Melzack R, eds. *Textbook of Pain.* 4th ed. Edinburgh, Scotland: Churchill Livingstone; 1999.
15. Craig AD, Krout K, Andrew D. Quantitative response characteristics of thermoreceptive and nociceptive lamina I spinothalamic neurons in the cat. *J Neurophysiol.* 2001;86:1459-1480.
16. Willis WD, Westlund K. Neuroanatomy of the pain system and of the pathways that modulate pain. *J Clin Neurophysiol.* 1997;14: 2-31.
17. Cervero F. Mechanisms of acute visceral pain. *Br Med Bull.* 1991;47:549-560.
18. Hodge CJ Jr, Apkarian AV. The spinothalamic tract. *Crit Rev Neurobiol.* 1990;5:363-397.
19. Schnitzler A, Ploner M. Neurophysiology and functional neuroanatomy of pain perception. *J Clin Neurophysiol.* 2000;17: 592-603.
20. Melzack R, Casey KL. Sensory, motivational, and central control determinants of pain: a new conceptual model. In: Kenshalo D, ed. *The Skin Senses.* Springfield, Ill: Charles C Thomas; 1968:423-443.
21. Rudomin P, Schmidt RF. Presynaptic inhibition in the vertebrate spinal cord revisited. *Exp Brain Res.* 1999;129:1-37.
22. Fields HL. Pain modulation: Expectation, opioid analgesia and virtual pain: review. *Prog Brain Res.* 2000;122:245-253.
23. Mendell LM, Wall PD. Responses of single dorsal cord cells to peripheral cutaneous unmyelinated fibers. *Nature.* 1965;206: 97-99.
24. Woolf CJ, Thompson SW. The induction and maintenance of central sensitization is dependent on *N*-methyl-d-aspartic acid receptive activation; implications for the treatment of post-injury pain hypersensitivity states. *Pain.* 1991;44:293-299.
25. Yaksh TL, Ozaki G, McCumber D, et al. An automated flinch detecting system for use in the formalin nociceptive bioassay. *J Appl Physiol.* 2001;90:2386-2402.
26. LaMotte RH, Torebjork HE, Robinson CJ, et al. Time-intensity profiles of cutaneous pain in normal and hyperalgesic skin: a comparison with C-fiber nociceptor activities in monkey and human. *J Neurophysiol.* 1984;51:1434-1450.
27. Dickenson AH, Sullivan AF. Evidence for a role of the NMDA receptor in the frequency dependent potentiation of deep rat dorsal horn nociceptive neurones following C fibre stimulation. *Neuropharmacology.* 1987;26:1235-1238.
28. Yaksh TL, Hua X-Y, Kalcheva I, et al. The spinal biology in humans and animals of pain states generated by persistent small afferent input. *Proc Natl Acad Sci U S A.* 1999;96:7680-7686.
29. Saria A. The tachykinin NK1 receptor in the brain: pharmacology and putative functions. *Eur J Pharmacol.* 1999;375:51-60.
30. Madsen U, Stensbol TB, Krogsgaard-Larsen P. Inhibitors of AMPA and kainate receptors. *Curr Med Chem.* 2001;8:1291-1301.
31. Klein RC, Castellino FJ. Activators and inhibitors of the ion channel of the NMDA receptor. *Curr Drug Targets.* 2001;2:323-329.
32. Svensson CI, Yaksh TL. The spinal phospholipase-cyclooxygenase-prostanoid cascade in nociceptive processing. *Annu Rev Pharmacol Toxicol.* 2002;42:553-583.
33. Watkins LR, Milligan ED, Maier SF. Glial activation: a driving force for pathological pain. *Trends Neurosci.* 2001;24:450-455.
34. Sorkin LS. NMDA evokes an L-NAME sensitive spinal release of glutamate and citrulline. *Neuroreport.* 1993;4:479-482.
35. Akinori M. Subspecies of protein kinase C in the rat spinal cord. *Prog Neurobiol.* 1998;54:499-530.
36. Zhuo M. Silent glutamatergic synapses and long-term facilitation in spinal dorsal horn neurons. *Prog Brain Res.* 2000;129:101-113.
37. Agalave NM, Svensson CI. Extracellular HMGB1 as a mediator of persistent pain. *Mol Med* 2015;20(1):569-578.
38. Milligan ED, Watkins LR. Pathological and protective roles of glia in chronic pain. *Nat Rev Neurosci* 2009;10:23-36.
39. Coull JA, Beggs S, Boudreau D, Boivin D, Tsuda M, Inoue K, et al.: BDNF from microglia causes the shift in neuronal anion gradient underlying neuropathic pain. *Nature* 2005;438:1017-1021.
40. Clark AK, Malcangio M. Fractalkine/CX3CR1 signaling during neuropathic pain. *Front Cell Neurosci* 2014;8:121.
41. Kiguchi N, Kobayashi Y, Kishioka S. Chemokines and cytokines in neuroinflammation leading to neuropathic pain. *Curr Opin Pharmacol* 2012;12:55-61.
42. Wilder-Smith OH. Pre-emptive analgesia and surgical pain. *Prog Brain Res.* 2000;129:505-524.
43. Kehlet H, Rathmell JP. Persistent Postsurgical pain. The path forward through better design of clinical studies. *Anesthesiology* 2010;112(3):514-515.
44. Jimenez-Andrade JM, Mantyh PW. Sensory and sympathetic nerve fibers undergo sprouting and neuroma formation in the painful arthritic joint of geriatric mice. *Arthritis Res Ther.* 2012;14(3):R101.
45. Xu Q, Yaksh TL. A brief comparison of the pathophysiology of inflammatory versus neuropathic pain. *Curr Opin Anaesthesiol.* 2011;24(4):400-407. PMCID: PMC3290396.
46. Grace PM, Hutchinson MR, Maier SF, Watkins LR. *Exp Neurol.* 2012;234(2):316-329.
47. Nicotra L, Loram LC, Watkins LR, Hutchinson MR. Toll-like receptors in chronic pain. *Exp Neurol.* 2012;234(2):316-329.
48. Duffy SS, Lees JG, Moalem-Taylor G. The contribution of immune and glial cell types in experimental autoimmune encephalomyelitis and multiple sclerosis. *Mult Scler Int.* 2014;2014:285245.
49. Costigan M, Moss A, Latremoliere A, Johnston C, Vera-Gandhu M, Herbert TA, Barrett L, Brenner GJ, Vardeh D, Woolf CJ, Fitzgerald M. T-cell infiltration and signaling in the adult dorsal spinal cord is a major contributor to neuropathic pain-like hypersensitivity. *J Neurosci.* 2009; 29(46):14415-14422.

Anatomy and Physiology of Pain

Robert I. Cohen

Understanding the anatomy and physiology of pain transmission systems is important for the pain management specialist because it informs diagnostic and treatment decisions for the common pain syndromes for which patients seek help (e.g., diabetic neuropathy and migraine headache). Interventions to provide the relief the patient seeks (nerve blocks, implantable devices) are available at distinct anatomic sites. As ongoing research reveals new modalities and pharmaceutical agents to provide relief, the provider with this knowledge base will better understand their mechanism and application. Designed as an overview to be read in one sitting, the clinician will find it an efficient way to review the large body of knowledge acquired in medical school and residency.

This chapter reviews the transmission of a nociceptive or pain impulse from the site of stimulus in the periphery to the central nervous system. The basic anatomic pathways of nociceptive transmission and of descending nociceptive modulations are described. While some basic physiology is discussed, the fundamentals of neuronal transduction, such as action potential propagation and the relationship of the cell body to the dendrites and axon, are not. While mention is made here of pathophysiology and disease states, the details follow in the subsequent chapters.

This chapter focuses on the neuronal components of the nervous system that transmit and modulate nociceptive stimuli. Although attention is focused on primary afferents and descending pathways, interneurons in the dorsal horn of the spinal cord and at higher levels in the central nervous system play important roles in signal processing, transmission, plasticity, and, ultimately, in the way pain is experienced, including its emotional components. The complexities of chronic pain syndromes, including such theories as chronic pain as a variant of depressive disorders,[1,2] are discussed elsewhere.

Knowledge of nociceptive transmission has advanced considerably since Descartes outlined his concept of the nerve as tubes with delicate threads to convey a painful impulse.[3] It is now widely believed that stimulation of a primary afferent neuron in the peripheral nervous system results in patterns of activation of neurons in the dorsal horn of the spinal cord and then in transmission(s) rostrally to the brain.

PRIMARY AFFERENTS

Sensory neurons, called primary afferents, have a cell body in the dorsal root ganglia (DRG) of the spinal cord or in the ganglia of the cranial nerves. Cranial nerves V, VII, IX, and X receive inputs from primary afferents and, thus, sensory information from the head, face, and throat. Nerve cells in the DRG are a heterogeneous population of size and function—a reflection of the heterogeneity of the sensory inputs processed by the central nervous system.[4] Central nervous system pain processing is also influenced by immune and surrounding glial cells.[5]

The classic nomenclature of peripheral neurons relies on the size of the axon and presence or absence of myelin as distinguishing characteristics. This taxonomy is referred to as the Erlanger-Gasser classification.[6] There are three major groups, A, B, and C, in order of diminishing axonal diameter. Group A is further divided into four subgroups: Aα, or primary muscle spindle and motor to skeletal muscles; Aβ, which are cutaneous touch and pressure afferents; Aγ, which are motor to muscle spindles; and Aδ, which are mechanoreceptors, nociceptors, thermoreceptors, and sympathetic postganglionic fibers. Group B is sympathetic preganglionic fibers. Group C refers to mechanoreceptors, nociceptors, and thermoreceptors, as well as sympathetic postganglionic fibers.

Classification of primary afferents on the basis of size and morphology has been refined.[4] Most pain management practitioners are familiar with the traditional classification and are acquainted with the terms *Aδ* and *C fibers* as pain transmission fibers. An alternative classification based on size of axon cross-section—type Ia/b, II, III, and IV, from large myelinated to smaller and more slowly conducting fibers—is not used in this.

Thus, the sensory neurons of greatest interest to the pain clinician are the Aδ and C fibers have cell bodies in the DRG and project to the dorsal horn of the spinal cord (or the equivalent nuclei for the cranial nerves).[7] The morphology of the peripheral termination of the axon is a reflection of the neuron's function: Mechanoreceptors end in specialized structures, whereas nociceptors have free endings. Although the majority of Aδ fibers respond to low-intensity mechanical, chemical, or thermal stimuli, the free nerve endings of the Aδ and C-type neurons likely allow a less specialized response to hazardous, potentially dangerous, and damaging stimuli.[8] As a nociceptive stimulus persists, cells along the transmission pathway undergo change, which can lead to the formation of a chronic pain state.[9] This chapter focuses primarily on the anatomy and physiology of early acute pain before nervous system structure is altered by a persisting pain state.

The nociceptive primary afferents supply all the areas of the body: skin and subcutaneous tissue, muscle, joints, the periosteum, and the viscera. The skin, subcutaneous tissue, and fascia are supplied by mechanical nociceptors (Aδ high-threshold mechanoreceptors), polymodal nociceptors (C-fiber nociceptors), and myelinated mechanothermal nociceptors (Aδ heat nociceptors).[8] The latter respond to both noxious heat and intense mechanical stimuli, and these Aδ fibers are likely responsible for the first pain perceived after heat stimulation. This is in contrast to the high-threshold Aδ mechanoreceptors, which respond to repeated stimuli and not to the initial noxious stimulus of heat or cold and may be the first nociceptors involved in peripheral sensitization.[10] The C-polymodal nociceptors, which also respond to high-intensity stimuli, whether mechanical or heat, respond by sensitizing to heat but, interestingly, fatigue in response to repeated mechanical stimuli.[11,12]

A brief, noxious stimulus that results in an immediate but transient epicritic sensation that is mediated by Aδ fibers also evokes the slow onset of a protopathic burning pain sensation that is C-fiber dependent.[13]

Muscle, fascia, and tendons are innervated by Aδ and C fibers. Activation of these neurons by noxious stimulation produces diffuse, aching pain that is poorly localized. Ischemic contraction of muscle may result in C-fiber activation. The muscle nociceptors are also activated by chemical stimulation.[14,15] Joints are innervated by Aδ and C fibers, which, when activated in a normal joint, result in deep aching pain. In an arthritic joint or during acute inflammation, however, even normal and minimal activities result in pain.[16] There has long been interest in the pathogenesis of arthritis and the interaction between inflammatory changes and the development of chronic pain.[17]

The periosteum of bone is acutely sensitive to noxious stimuli and nociceptors capable of releasing substance P are present in both cortex and marrow.[18] Teeth are innervated by nociceptive and mechanical afferents. Both the inner and outer aspects of the tooth are innervated.[19] Immunohistochemical labeling demonstrates that most dental primary afferents are C nociceptors, that Aδ fibers are present, and that a quarter of the fibers appear to be low-threshold Aβ mechanoreceptors capable of the mechanical allodynia responsible for tooth pulp hypersensitivity.[20] The Aδ neurons projecting to the trigeminal nucleus are stimulated by noxious thermal stimulation of tooth pulp and may contribute to peripheral sensitization in pulpitis.[21]

The viscera are innervated by nociceptors as well as parasympathetic and sympathetic fibers, some of which may also be nociceptors. In contrast to cutaneous innervation, visceral structures are sparsely innervated so that few fibers respond to stimuli over a large area.[22] Clinically, patients with visceral conditions are likely to complain of diffuse discomfort or poorly localized pain except under conditions of extremes (e.g., appendicitis, pleurisy). Very often, even extreme perturbations are interpreted with the less common pain descriptors such as discomfort, pressure, crushing, and squeezing. These patients may even reject "pain" as a descriptor (e.g., acute myocardial infarction). Convergence of deep somatic (muscle, joints) and visceral nociceptive information at higher midbrain structures[23] and convergence of cutaneous and visceral projections contribute to the poor localization of noxious stimuli in the viscera.

The heart has Aβ, Aδ fibers, and C fibers[24] involved in cardiovascular reflex responsiveness and nociception. The classic pain of myocardial ischemia—angina—was postulated to be mediated via chemical sensitization of afferents by substances released by the damaged cells (potassium, hydrogen ions) as well as humoral factors (bradykinin and prostaglandins).[9,12] Cardiac nociceptors project as vagal afferents into the nodose ganglia[25] and as sympathetic afferents into the superior cervical ganglion and dorsal horn of the spinal cord.[26]

The lungs and bronchi are also innervated by Aδ and C fibers. These fibers play a diverse role, serving to warn of irritants in the airway that are either mechanical or chemical. Furthermore, such distinct stimuli as pulmonary edema, embolism, and changes in oxygen tension may give rise to the sensation of dyspnea.

The abdominal viscera include such diverse structures as the stomach and intestines, gallbladder, and urinary bladder. Direct activation of nociceptors may occur; for example, hypersensitivity is noted in acid-sensing nociceptors present in lamina propria in nonerosive esophagitis.[27] Transmission of acid-injury–related visceral nociceptor signals into the CNS can be enhanced by descending pathways from midbrain structures.[28] Two common clinical manifestations of visceral pain states are chronic pelvic pain and interstitial cystitis. Both syndromes may be disabling to patients and are frustratingly difficult to treat. Both myelinated and unmyelinated sensory fibers project from the bladder to the lumbar and sacral dorsal horn of the spinal cord, and immunohistologic studies have identified their possible role in pain transmission.[29] Mechanoreceptors transmitting stretch/distention may also become sensitized by local bladder irritants, especially in the setting of erosive tissue damage.[29]

Nociceptors, sensitive to diverse extracellular signals and able to project with release of an array of molecular signals,[30] are but the first in the highly integrated systems of neuronal, glial hormonal, and inflammatory cells that process their signals.

SPINAL DORSAL HORN LAMINAE

The primary afferents, which have their cell bodies in the DRG, extend from the periphery to terminate centrally in the dorsal horn. The fibers that enter the dorsal horn are segregated by size as they form small bands or rootlets and approach the dorsal horn. Lissauer observed that the smaller fibers are segregated laterally and then terminate in the first layers of the dorsal horn. This area has come to be known as Lissauer's tract. There are clinical applications of knowledge of the anatomy of the dorsal horn and dorsal root entry zone. Neurosurgeons may perform a selective posterior rhizotomy in the hopes of ablating otherwise intractable, unrelenting chronic pain. These techniques are discussed further in the chapters on clinical pain management.

It is important to note that many cells in the DRG have more than one process.[31] Thus, a fiber may receive input from two distinct areas, such as the dura mater and part of the face. The connections that appear to subserve sensory processing during migraine, for example, are complex.[32] The terminal connections may also branch and innervate multiple spinal levels.[33] There is also evidence that sensory fibers may travel in the ventral roots, as well. There are certainly small unmyelinated fibers in ventral tracts. Thus, the anatomy is more complex than a simple schema can represent. These complexities may explain why selective posterior rhizotomy is, clinically, rarely successful in providing complete relief of unrelenting pain. But, as understanding of the peripheral nervous system grows, so does an appreciation of its complexity. Injury to peripheral nerves may result in chronic changes. Initial injury and acute changes may develop into chronic ectopic inputs, which may induce a state of central sensitization and structural reorganization of dorsal horn synapse.[10] Thus, there are profound physiologic reasons why a surgical anatomic approach to pain management may not be sufficient.

The majority of primary afferents terminate in the ipsilateral dorsal horn. The process of the spinal neurons bifurcates into an ascending and a descending branch, thus innervating the spinal cord over several spinal segments. Some processes travel dorsal to the central canal to end in the contralateral dorsal horn. The terminus of each primary afferent is the reflection of its function because the dorsal horn neurons are segregated by physiology. Rexed divided the gray matter of the spinal cord into ten laminae.[34] This classic cytoarchitectural segregation yields six subdivisions of the dorsal horn (laminae I through VI) and three subdivisions of the ventral horn (laminae VII through IX.) Lamina X describes the column of cells around the central canal.

The dorsal laminae of the spinal cord run its entire length and, in the medulla, become the medullary dorsal horn. The marginal layer of the dorsal horn refers to lamina I. Lamina II, or the substantia gelatinosa, is subdivided into outer and inner areas (IIo and IIi). The substantia gelatinosa is of interest to clinicians and researchers.[35] Laminae III through V are referred to as the nucleus proprius or the magnocellular layer.

Dorsal horn neurons, which process nociceptive information, are a heterogenous population. Laminae I and V have nociceptive specific neurons. There are two populations of nociceptive-specific neurons. One type receives inputs from Aδ fibers, both high-threshold mechanoreceptors and temperature-sensitive receptors and from polymodal C fibers. The second type of nociceptive-specific neuron appears to receive inputs only from high-threshold Aδ mechanoreceptors. The other neuron type that processes nociceptive input is the wide-dynamic-range (WDR) neuron. Found predominantly in lamina V (and to a lesser degree in lamina I), the WDR neuron receives input from Aδ fibers of both high-threshold mechanoreceptors and temperature-sensitive neurons and also from polymodal C fibers, as well as from Aβ low-threshold mechanoreceptors.[32]

The physiology of the dorsal horn explains the heterogeneity of function. Lamina I cell projection pathways have been shown to be concerned with long-latency, long-duration reactions to prolonged events, rather than to brief stimuli.[33] Lamina I neurons, which project via the spinothalamic tract, are an integral component of the central representation of pain and temperature. These nociceptive-specific neurons, both the high-threshold mechanoreceptors and the temperature-sensitive polymodal C fibers, are inhibited by morphine in a dose-dependent manner.[36,37] This suggests that opiate-modulation of nociceptive transmission is functionally organized. Both substance P and neurokinin A are released by neurons in the substantia gelatinosa when a noxious impulse is transmitted.[38] Somatostatin is released following noxious thermal but not noxious mechanical stimuli, which implies some encoding of information by the dorsal horn.[10]

The fibers of greatest interest to pain clinicians are Aδ and C fibers. The Aδ nociceptors terminate in laminae I and IIo and have collateral branches that terminate in laminae V and X. Similarly, the C fibers, which enter the spinal cord via the lateral aspect of Lissauer's tract, also terminate in laminae I and IIo, as well as lamina V. The termination of the large, myelinated Aβ fibers is in laminae III and IV, as well as lamina V.[34]

Following an injury, however, there may be marked alterations in the cytoarchitecture of the dorsal horn. Woolf reported that following nerve injury, large-diameter fibers may invade laminae I and IIo.[10] This may provide a mechanism to explain the clinical finding of allodynia and the physiologic alterations in neuropathic pain syndromes.[10,39,40] This subject is discussed in detail in subsequent chapters.

The information conveyed by the primary afferents travels first to the dorsal horn and then from the dorsal horn rostral via the ascending tracts.[41] A variety of neurotransmitters are used to convey noxious information.[37,42] There are distinct areas of dopamine-containing neurons.[43] The peptide substance P is found in the dorsal horn.[44,45] There is evidence that glutaminergic neurons are also involved, as well as neurons that respond to γ-aminobutyric acid (GABA), although these neurons are not as prevalent.[46] A segmental chronic pain syndrome can be induced in rats by an intrathecal infusion of *N*-methyl-D-aspartate (NMDA)[47] or by amputating large mylenated neurons at the dorsal root ganglia.[48]

New possibilities for targeting specific receptors to provide relief from pain continue to generate a great deal of excitement from clinicians. In 2013, Gohlke and colleagues performed data mining of the entire Medline/PubMed NBCI FTP database, using computational linguistics on titles and abstracts, sometimes on full texts, to identify possible receptors and ligands associated with pain transmission; built a web engine to link the human-reviewed results with molecular databases (BindingDB and PubChem); and designed a user-friendly graphical and text interface to search among 8700 molecules likely to increase or decrease pain or 100,000 that may possibly have an effect.[49] The website and database, known as "SuperPain,"[50] allows sharing and adapting content for noncommercial purposes.

SPINAL TRACTS

The spinothalamic tract (STT) and the trigeminothalamic tract transmit primarily pain and temperature information.[51,52] Neither tract, however, transmits exclusively noxious stimuli: The tracts are heterogenous and transmit some innocuous stimuli such as light touch, as well.[53] Furthermore, it is now accepted that other ascending tracts also convey noxious information, as well.[54-56]

The lateral and ventral STTs travel in the anterior lateral quadrant of the spinal cord. The spinomesencephalic tract (SMT) is located in the anterior lateral quadrant and in the dorsolateral funiculus.[52] The dorsal column postsynaptic spinomedullary system is a second-order dorsal column pathway that is located appropriately in the dorsal column.[57,58] This propriospinal multisynaptic ascending system is a more complicated network of short chains of neurons, which may play a role in nociceptive transmission.[57,59]

A lesion of the anterior lateral quadrant (which disrupts the STT and SMT) results in the abolition of pain sensation on the side contralateral to the lesion, below the spinal segment.[60] There is also some mild decrease in responsiveness to noxious stimuli on the ipsilateral side. The neurons of the STT are located throughout the dorsal horn, but with the greatest concentration in lamina I.[61] As it ascends, the STT widens as fibers are added along the anteromedial border. Thus, the STT has somatotropic organization, with axons originating in the sacral region lateral to those of the lumbar region and so forth, and with the cervical region representing the most medial aspect in the spinal cord, but with the facial area being the most medial in the medulla. As the STT travels rostrally, it divides, at the mesencephalon, into a medial component that innervates the medial thalamic region and a lateral component that projects to the ventrobasal and posterior thalamus. The ventroposterolateral (VPL) nucleus of the thalamus is somatotropically organized, in contrast to the other thalamic nuclei, and receives the majority of the lamina I projections.[61]

The spinoreticular tract (SRT) conveys impulses from the spinal cord to the reticular formation.[62] The reticular formation triggers arousal, so the SRT may convey information that contributes to the affective aspect of pain. The SRT may be important for the motivational and emotional aspect of pain, as well as for autonomic and somatic motor reflexes. The SMT projects to the midbrain reticular formation. Thus, its function may be similar to that of the SRT. These tracts, the SRT and the SMT, may be involved in the perpetuation of chronic pain. In their classic neurosurgery text, White and Sweet report that lesioning medial to the STT in the midbrain results in relief of chronic pain.[60]

Evidence exists of alternative ascending pathways that convey nociceptive impulses. A small percentage of neurons in the dorsal column postsynaptic system respond to noxious stimuli.[54] The spinocervical tract (SCT) has neurons that respond to tactile stimuli as well as noxious stimuli. Although the SCT appears to play a role in the transmission of nociceptive impulses in the cat, its role in the transduction of pain in humans is unclear.[53] In cats, there is a convergence of visceral and somatic inputs in the medulla.[56] The propriospinal multisynaptic ascending system is composed of neurons with short axons that make multiple synaptic contacts with other short-axon neurons. Basbaum proposed a role for this multisynaptic ascending system in the maintenance of chronic pain.[57]

The anatomy and physiology of the neurons that serve the head and face are similar to the systems that transmit impulses from the body.[63] The cranial nerves that transmit noxious stimuli include the trigeminal (CN V), facial (CN VII), glossopharyngeal (CN IX), and vagus (CN X) nerves. The area of the medulla that receives these inputs is often referred to as the medullary dorsal horn. Because the trigeminal system is the one most important to pain clinicians, it is the system reviewed here.

The trigeminal nerve system is of particular interest to pain clinicians because of a number of chronic pain states, such as tic douloureux and migraine.[64] The trigeminal ganglion divides into three branches: the ophthalmic, maxillary, and mandibular nerves. Each division carries information about proprioception, touch and pressure, and pain and temperature. Also known as the gasserian ganglion, it has somatotropic organization, and this is preserved as the fibers course to their unique terminations. The somatotropic laminar organization is true for both myelinated and unmyelinated fibers. The large-diameter fibers terminate in the main sensory nucleus, whereas the Aδ and C fibers terminate in the subnucleus caudalis.[65]

The trigeminal subnucleus caudalis can be subdivided by its cytoarchitecture into three layers. These three layers have been termed the *marginal layer*, the *substantia gelatinosa*, and the *magnocellular layer* and correlate with their dorsal horn counterparts in both form and function. Thus appropriately called the *medullary dorsal horn*, it receives convergent sensory information, including Aδ and C nociceptors from the face and dura implicated in migraine pathophysiology.[66] Although analogous, the medullary dorsal horn may be less responsive to descending inhibition pathways than the spinal dorsal horn cells.[67] Trigeminal nociceptors project via the ventral (anterior or neo) trigeminothalamic tract to the ventral posterolateral thalamus and the cortex.[68] Like the ventral (anterior or neo) spinothalamic tract, to which it is analogous, it also conveys somatotrophic organized information about pain and temperature.

There is also a paleotrigeminothalamic system (pTTS). Some fibers from the subnucleus caudalis project to a variety of terminations, thus, having both ipsilateral and contralateral connections to the brainstem reticular formation, as well as to the periaqueductal gray matter, hypothalamus, and medial and intrathalamic nuclei. As these structures project diffusely, including to the limbic system, the pTTS likely plays a role in the affective qualities of pain.[69]

Trigeminal and visceral afferents project to the parabrachial region which may be an important relay station for further processing of nociceptive information.[70] In certain species, pain and tonic immobility may be modulated here and analgesia (or pain) may reinforce immobility as a defense mechanism during predator–prey confrontation.[71] It is uncertain if an analogous function exists in humans.

SUPRASPINAL SYSTEMS: THALAMUS

The thalamus is both an end point and the transition area for the sensory input traveling to the sensory cortex.[72,73] The medial and intralaminar nuclei of the thalamus receive input from the spinal cord and the reticular formation but are not somatotropically organized. The nuclei receive input from the ascending spinal (and trigeminal) systems and the reticular formation and innervate a wide area of the brain.[74] In contrast, the ventrobasal complex of the thalamus is somatotropically organized. The ventrobasal thalamus receives input from the neospinothalamic tract and the neotrigeminothalmic tract and projects to the primary somatosensory (SI) and secondary somatosensory (SII) region of the somatosensory cortex, allowing localization and sensory discrimination.[72,75]

The ventrobasal complex of the thalamus refers to the region composed of the ventral and the posterior thalamic nuclei. It is subdivided into a lateral division (the ventroposterolateral nucleus) and a medial division (the ventroposteromedial nucleus). These neurons respond primarily to stimuli on the contralateral surfaces of the body or face.[76] The thalamus may have a modulatory role on nociceptive transmission during varied states of arousal.[77] White and Sweet reported that the lesions in this area of the thalamus produced transient analgesia but a marked interference of a patient's ability to perceive spatial discrimination.[60] In patients with spinal cord transection, somatotropic organization and spontaneous neuronal activity in thalamic nuclei has been described.[78]

SUPRASPINAL SYSTEMS: RETICULAR FORMATION

The reticular formation is involved with the affective component of pain. The aversive response and the motivational aspect of pain are modulated via reticular activation. Similarly, the motor, autonomic, and sensory functions that are a response to noxious stimuli are mediated by the pathways through the reticular formation. Casey proposes that one way in which opiates may relieve suffering without altering an individual's ability to recognize a stimulus as noxious is via the reticular formation.[79,80]

SUPRASPINAL SYSTEMS: HYPOTHALAMUS

The hypothalamus has a role in both the autonomic nervous system and the neuroendocrine response. The hypothalamus probably plays a role in the response both to somatic and visceral tissue damage and to pain.[81] Thus, the emotional response and autonomic arousal elicited by pain is likely mediated, at least in part, by the hypothalamus. There are STT neurons that provide nociceptive input to the many areas that are involved in producing the multifaceted response to pain, which is familiar to clinicians.[82]

SUPRASPINAL SYSTEMS: LIMBIC SYSTEM

The limbic system refers to a wide array of structures that are part of the telencephalon, diencephalon, and mesencephalon. The parts of the telencephalon that contribute to the limbic system are the amygdala, hippocampus, nucleus accumbens, and preoptic regions. In the diencephalon, the hypothalamus and parts of the thalamus contribute to the limbic system. The limbic area also encompasses the ventral tegmental area, the dorsal tegmental nucleus, and parts of the midbrain raphe nuclei and periaqueductal gray matter. The interconnections between these areas and wider areas of the cortex are complex and diverse.[83] This organization explains the allowable diversity of response to painful stimuli.

SUPRASPINAL SYSTEMS: CEREBRAL CORTEX

The human cortex has two main areas that receive sensory inputs: SI and SII. SI, on the postcentral gyrus, receives direct somatotropically organized input from the ipsilateral ventrobasal complex of the thalamus (the ventroposterolateral and the ventroposteromedial nuclei). The SII area is smaller than the SI area and is located on the parietal lobe of the cortex. The somatosensory cortex allows the discrimination of sensation. The somatotropic organization of the somatosensory cortex was mapped in the first half of the last century by Penfield and Rasmussen.[83] The illustrated representation of this mapping, the homunculus, is familiar to any medical student.

The role of the sensory cortex in nociceptive processing is the subject of renewed research and debate. Although early studies revealed that many SI neurons respond to noxious stimuli, these responses were putatively only localizing in nature. Further investigation suggested that the SI neurons actually have an integrative function whereby the intensity of a stimulus is encoded and processed.[82,84-86]

DESCENDING PATHWAYS

The descending nociceptive modulatory system is of interest to researchers and clinicians. Melzack and Wall proposed the existence of a nociceptive modulating system in their seminal article in *Science* in 1965.[87] The gate-control hypothesis of pain proposed that dorsal horn processing could be modified not only by stimulation that arrived from the periphery, but also from putative descending pathways. A few years later, Reynolds demonstrated the effect of electrical stimulation in the periaqueductal gray matter (PAG) on the nocifensive responses of the rat.[88] A nocifensive response is a behavior to avoid pain.[89] It is now widely believed that descending antinociceptive mechanisms are an important part of an animal's defense system.[90]

The remarkable effect of PAG electrical stimulation is to diminish or ablate the animal's response to a noxious stimulus while preserving the sensation of light touch.[91] During PAG electrical stimulation, the animal maintains normal motor control and the ability to eat. Electrical stimulation of the PAG completely inhibits the nocifensive response of an animal to a variety of noxious stimuli, not limited to somatic stimuli, but including visceral and tooth pulp stimulation. The analgesic response endures for a brief time following termination of the stimulation. Electrical stimulation of the PAG results in analgesia that is naloxone reversible, implying an opiate-mediated response.[92] Stimulation of the PAG has been shown to provide pain relief to humans with a variety of intractable pain diagnoses.[93,94]

The electrical stimulation and, thus, the activation of neurons in the PAG results in suppression of activity of dorsal horn neurons.[95] Basbaum and Fields published extensively both together and independently on descending nociceptive modulatory systems and elucidated the anatomic and physiologic pathways of descending inhibition of nociception.[96,97] The PAG has connections to the nucleus raphe magnus in the medulla, as well as to the parabrachial nucleus (PBN), a proposed site of behavior modification.[98] The PBN also processes aversion to bad taste,[99] loss of apetite,[100,101] respiratory coupling to vocalization,[102] and sleep apnea arousal.[103] The nucleus raphe magnus is served by a group of nearby structures within the rostral ventromedial medulla (RVM). The information from these rostral areas is conveyed to the dorsal horn by way of the dorsal lateral funiculus. If any of these structures or their connections are ablated, so is the inhibition of nocifensive reflexes.[104]

The PAG and the RVM are also involved in opiate analgesia.[105] Microinjection of morphine or of selective μ-opioid agonists into the PAG or RVM results in potent naloxone-reversible antinociception. Lesioning the dorsal lateral funiculus unilaterally diminishes the opiate analgesia produced by PAG microinjection, and bilateral lesions of the dorsal lateral funiculus ablate the opiate effect on nocifensive reflexes. Thus, a system of descending endogenous opioid analgesia can be elucidated, and a pathway from the PAG to the dorsal horn, by way of the RVM and the dorsal lateral funiculus, has been demonstrated.[106,107] The PAG and RVM are also endocanabanoid targets, for example, responding to metamizol, a nonopioid COX inhibiting analgesic used in Europe, which increases descending inhibition and projects an antinociceptive effect to the spinal cord.[108]

The connections of the neurons in the medulla are complex, but it appears as if serotonergic cell projections to brainstem sites may contribute to the integration of sensory, autonomic, and motor modulation at the brainstem level.[109] There are other loci, such as the nucleus cuneiformis, which may also play a role in sensory and motor integration of responses to noxious stimuli.[110]

Fields and Heinricher noted that the electrophysiologic responses of neurons in the RVM to microinjection or iontophoresis of opiates was mixed: some neurons became less active and others became more active.[111] Certain neurons in the RVM are activated by noxious stimuli. Called "on-cells," these neurons fire more rapidly during noxious stimuli, and if these cells are spontaneously firing and a noxious stimulus is applied, the nocifensive reflex time is shortened. In addition, μ-opioid agonists diminish or ablate the firing of on-cells. Other neurons stop firing before a nocifensive reflex response occurs. These "off-cells" are activated by opiates, and if a noxious stimulus is applied during the spontaneous firing of an off-cell, the nocifensive reflex time is lengthened.[111] In the early stages of acute pain due to inflammation, "on-cell" baseline activity increases promoting hyperalgesia, while "off-cell" activity predominates as inflammation persists (becomes chronic.)[112]

The circuitry of the RVM involves excitatory amino acids, GABA and opioids, as well as serotonergic and noradrenergic neurons.[113] Neurotensin microinjected into the RVM has either a facilitatory or an inhibitory effect on the response of spinal neurons to noxious thermal stimulation, depending on the dose of the neurotensin.[114] During conditions of analgesia, the removal of the RVM predictably lessens the analgesic response of the animal. During conditions of hyperalgesia, the temporary blocking of the RVM with local anesthetic actually attenuates the hyperalgesic response.[115] Thus, the RVM contains a heterogenous population of neurons that has the potential to either ameliorate or facilitate nociceptive transmission.

SUMMARY

The anatomy and physiology of the cellular systems of the primary afferents, dorsal horn laminae, spinal tracts, supraspinal systems, and descending pathways reviewed in this chapter at once suggest the wealth of potential targets for pain treatment and the limitation of our current knowledge.

The author wishes to thank Hilary J. Fausett, who prepared a prior version of this manuscript.

REFERENCES

1. Blumer D, Heilbronn M. Chronic pain as a variant of depressive disease: the pain-prone disorder. *J Nerv Ment Dis.* 1982;170(7):381-406.
2. Blumer D, Heilbronn M. Chronic pain as a variant of depressive disease: a rejoinder. *J Nerv Ment Dis.* 1984;172(7):405-407.
3. Decartes R. *L'homme et un traitté de la formation du foetus.* France: 1664.
4. Yaksh TL, Hammond DL. Peripheral and central substrates involved in the rostrad transmission of nociceptive information. *Pain.* 1982;13(1):1-85.
5. Watkins LR, Maier SF. Beyond neurons: evidence that immune and glial cells contribute to pathological pain states. *Physiol Rev.* 2002;82(4):981-1011.
6. Gasser H. The classification of nerve fibers. *Ohio J Sci.* 1941;41(3):145-159.
7. Wilkinson SV, et al. The neuroanatomy of pain. *Clin Podiatr Med Surg.* 1994;11(1):1-13.
8. Adriaensen H, et al. Response properties of thin myelinated (A-delta) fibers in human skin nerves. *J Neurophysiol.* 1983;49(1):111-122.
9. Diamond J, Holmes M, Coughlin M. Endogenous NGF and nerve impulses regulate the collateral sprouting of sensory axons in the skin of the adult rat. *J Neurosci.* 1992;12(4):1454-1466.
10. Woolf CJ. The pathophysiology of peripheral neuropathic pain–abnormal peripheral input and abnormal central processing. *Acta Neurochir Suppl (Wien).* 1993;58:125-130.
11. Hallin RG, Torebjork HE, Wiesenfeld Z. Nociceptors and warm receptors innervated by C fibres in human skin. *J Neurol Neurosurg Psychiatry.* 1982;45(4):313-319.
12. Van Hees J, Gybels J. C nociceptor activity in human nerve during painful and non painful skin stimulation. *J Neurol Neurosurg Psychiatry.* 1981;44(7):600-607.
13. Price DD, et al. Peripheral suppression of first pain and central summation of second pain evoked by noxious heat pulses. *Pain.* 1977;3(1):57-68.
14. Chen CC, Wong CW. Neurosensory mechanotransduction through acid-sensing ion channels. *J Cell Mol Med.* 2013;17(3):337-349.
15. Kniffki KD, Mense S, Schmidt RF. Responses of group IV afferent units from skeletal muscle to stretch, contraction and chemical stimulation. *Exp Brain Res.* 1978;31(4):511-522.
16. Schaible HG, Ebersberger A, Natura G. Update on peripheral mechanisms of pain: beyond prostaglandins and cytokines. *Arthritis Res Ther.* 2011;13(2):210.
17. Coggeshall RE, et al. Discharge characteristics of fine medial articular afferents at rest and during passive movements of inflamed knee joints. *Brain Res.* 1983;272(1):185-188.
18. Amadesi S, et al. Role for substance p-based nociceptive signaling in progenitor cell activation and angiogenesis during ischemia in mice and in human subjects. *Circulation.* 2012;125(14):1774-1786, S1-S19.
19. Kovacic U, et al. Dental pulp and gingivomucosa in rats are innervated by two morphologically and neurochemically different populations of nociceptors. *Arch Oral Biol.* 2013;58(7):788-795.
20. Vang H, et al. Neurochemical properties of dental primary afferent neurons. *Exp Neurobiol.* 2012;21(2):68-74.
21. Ahn DK, et al. Functional properties of tooth pulp neurons responding to thermal stimulation. *J Dent Res.* 2012;91(4):401-406.
22. Melzack R, Wall PD. *The Challenge of Pain.* Completely rev. ed. New York: Basic Books; 1983:447.
23. Keay KA, et al. Convergence of deep somatic and visceral nociceptive information onto a discrete ventrolateral midbrain periaqueductal gray region. *Neuroscience.* 1994;61(4):727-732.
24. Tan Y, et al. Characteristics of ATP-activated current in nodose ganglion neurons of rats. *Neurosci Lett.* 2009;459(1):25-29.
25. Wang Y, et al. Expressions of P2X2 and P2X3 receptors in rat nodose neurons after myocardial ischemia injury. *Auton Neurosci.* 2009;145(1-2):71-75.
26. Li G, et al. Increased sympathoexcitatory reflex induced by myocardial ischemic nociceptive signaling via P2X2/3 receptor in rat superior cervical ganglia. *Neurochem Int.* 2010;56(8):984-990.
27. Yoshida N, et al. Role of nociceptors/neuropeptides in the pathogenesis of visceral hypersensitivity of nonerosive reflux disease. *Dig Dis Sci.* 2013;58(8):2237-2243.
28. Kang Y, et al. Activation of ERK signaling in rostral ventromedial medulla is dependent on afferent input from dorsal column pathway and contributes to acetic acid-induced visceral nociception. *Neurochem Int.* 2013;63(5):389-396.
29. Forrest SL, Osborne PB, Keast JR. Characterization of bladder sensory neurons in the context of myelination, receptors for pain modulators, and acute responses to bladder inflammation. *Front Neurosci.* 2013;7:206. doi:10.3389/fnins.2013.00206.
30. Reichling DB, Green PG, Levine JD. The fundamental unit of pain is the cell. *Pain.* 2013;154(Suppl 1):S2-9. doi: 10.1016/j.pain.2013.05.037. Epub 2013 May.
31. Langford LA, Coggeshall RE. Branching of sensory axons in the peripheral nerve of the rat. *J Comp Neurol.* 1981;203(4):745-750.
32. Goadsby PJ, Zagami AS, Lambert GA. Neural processing of craniovascular pain: a synthesis of the central structures involved in migraine. *Headache.* 1991;31(6):365-371.
33. Strassman AM, Raymond SA, Burstein R. Sensitization of meningeal sensory neurons and the origin of headaches. *Nature.* 1996;384(6609):560-564.
34. Rexed B. A cytoarchitectonic atlas of the spinal cord in the cat. *J Comp Neurol.* 1954;100(2):297-379.
35. Strassman AM, Potrebic S, Maciewicz RJ. Anatomical properties of brainstem trigeminal neurons that respond to electrical stimulation of dural blood vessels. *J Comp Neurol.* 1994;346(3):349-365.
36. Craig AD, Serrano LP. Effects of systemic morphine on lamina I spinothalamic tract neurons in the cat. *Brain Res.* 1994;636(2):233-244.
37. Iggo A, Steedman WM, Fleetwood-Walker S. Spinal processing: anatomy and physiology of spinal nociceptive mechanisms. *Philos Trans R Soc Lond B Biol Sci.* 1985;308(1136):235-252.
38. Cervero F, Iggo A. The substantia gelatinosa of the spinal cord: a critical review. *Brain.* 1980;103(4):717-772.

39. Aminoff MJ. Sensory modulation and the spinal cord. *Ann Neurol.* 1993;34(4):511-512.

40. Wall PD, Bery J, Saade N. Effects of lesions to rat spinal cord lamina I cell projection pathways on reactions to acute and chronic noxious stimuli. *Pain.* 1988;35(3):327-339.

41. Coggeshall RE, et al. Primary afferent axons in the tract of Lissauer in the monkey. *J Comp Neurol.* 1981;196(3):431-442.

42. Bennett GJ, et al. Physiology and morphology of substantia gelatinosa neurons intracellularly stained with horseradish peroxidase. *J Comp Neurol.* 1980;194(4):809-827.

43. Lindvall O, Bjorklund A, Skagerberg G. Dopamine-containing neurons in the spinal cord: anatomy and some functional aspects. *Ann Neurol.* 1983;14(3):255-260.

44. Ding YQ, et al. Spinoparabrachial tract neurons showing substance P receptor-like immunoreactivity in the lumbar spinal cord of the rat. *Brain Res.* 1995;674(2):336-340.

45. Duggan AW, Furmidge LJ. Probing the brain and spinal cord with neuropeptides in pathways related to pain and other functions. *Front Neuroendocrinol.* 1994;15(3):275-300.

46. Lekan HA, Carlton SM. Glutamatergic and GABAergic input to rat spinothalamic tract cells in the superficial dorsal horn. *J Comp Neurol.* 1995;361(3):417-428.

47. Zochodne DW, et al. A segmental chronic pain syndrome in rats associated with intrathecal infusion of NMDA: evidence for selective action in the dorsal horn. *Can J Neurol Sci.* 1994;21(1):24-28.

48. Devor M. Ectopic discharge in Abeta afferents as a source of neuropathic pain. *Exp Brain Res.* 2009;196(1):115-128.

49. Gohlke BO, Preissner R, Preissner S. SuperPain–a resource on pain-relieving compounds targeting ion channels. *Nucleic Acids Res.* 2013; 42:Database issue D1107–D1112 doi:10.1093/nar/gkt1176.

50. Gohlke BO, Preissner R, Preissner S. SuperPain–a resource on pain-relieving compounds targeting ion channels. 2013; Available from: http://bioinformatics.charite.de/superpain/index.php.

51. Brodal A. *Neurological Anatomy in Relation to Clinical Medicine.* 3rd ed. New York: Oxford University Press; 1981:xvii, 1053.

52. Young PA. The anatomy of the spinal cord pain paths: a review. *J Am Paraplegia Soc.* 1986;9(3-4):28-38.

53. Willis WD. Nociceptive pathways: anatomy and physiology of nociceptive ascending pathways. *Philos Trans R Soc Lond B Biol Sci.* 1985;308(1136):253-270.

54. Ekerot CF, Garwicz M, Schouenborg J. The postsynaptic dorsal column pathway mediates cutaneous nociceptive information to cerebellar climbing fibres in the cat. *J Physiol.* 1991;441:275-284.

55. Ness TJ. Evidence for ascending visceral nociceptive information in the dorsal midline and lateral spinal cord. *Pain.* 2000;87(1):83-88.

56. Roy JC, et al. Convergence of visceral and somatic inputs onto subnucleus reticularis dorsalis neurones in the rat medulla. *J Physiol.* 1992;458:235-246.

57. Basbaum AI. Conduction of the effects of noxious stimulation by short-fiber multisynaptic systems of the spinal cord in the rat. *Exp Neurol.* 1973;40(3):699-716.

58. Bennett GJ, et al. The morphology of dorsal column postsynaptic spinomedullary neurons in the cat. *J Comp Neurol.* 1984;224(4):568-578.

59. Basbaum A. Anatomical substrates of pain and pain modulation and their relationship to analgesic drug action. In: *Analgesics: Neurochemical, behavioral, and clinical perspectives.* Central Nervous System Pharmacology. In: Kuhar MJ, Pasternak GW, eds. New York: Raven Press; 1984:x, 341.

60. White JC, Sweet WH. *Pain and the Neurosurgeon; A Forty-Year Experience.* Springfield, Ill: C. C. Thomas; 1969:xxxi, 1000.

61. Ralston H. Synaptic organization of the spinothalamic tract projection to the thalamus with special reference to pain. In: Kruger L, Liebeskind JC, Intra-Science Research Foundation. Symposium, eds. *Neural Mechanisms of Pain: Advances in Pain Research and Therapy.* New York: Raven Press; 1984:xx, 364.

62. Jr, WDW, Coggeshall RE. *Sensory Pathways in the Ventral Quadrant, in Sensory Mechanisms of the Spinal Cord.* Vol. 2. *Ascending Sensory Tracts and Their Descending Control.* New York: Kluwer Academic/Plenum Publishers; 2004:705-788.

63. Sessle BJ. Neural mechanisms of oral and facial pain. *Otolaryngol Clin North Am.* 1989;22(6):1059-1072.

64. Noseda R, Burstein R. Migraine pathophysiology: anatomy of the trigeminovascular pathway and associated neurological symptoms, CSD, sensitization and modulation of pain. *Pain.* 2013;154(Suppl 1): S44-S53. doi: 10.1016/j.pain.2013.07.021. Epub 2013 Jul 25.

65. Price DD, Dubner R, Hu JW. Trigeminothalamic neurons in nucleus caudalis responsive to tactile, thermal, and nociceptive stimulation of monkey's face. *J Neurophysiol.* 1976;39(5):936-953.

66. Bernstein C, Burstein R. Sensitization of the trigeminovascular pathway: perspective and implications to migraine pathophysiology. *J Clin Neurol.* 2012;8(2):89-99.

67. Aicher SA, et al. Descending projections from the rostral ventromedial medulla (RVM) to trigeminal and spinal dorsal horns are morphologically and neurochemically distinct. *J Chem Neuroanat.* 2012;43(2):103-111.

68. Young RF. Effect of trigeminal tractotomy on dental sensation in humans. *J Neurosurg.* 1982;56(6):812-818.

69. Hayashi H. Morphology of terminations of small and large myelinated trigeminal primary afferent fibers in the cat. *J Comp Neurol.* 1985;240(1):71-89.

70. Wang LG, Li HM, Li JS. Formalin induced FOS-like immunoreactive neurons in the trigeminal spinal caudal subnucleus project to contralateral parabrachial nucleus in the rat. *Brain Res.* 1994;649(1-2):62-70.

71. Menescal-de-Oliveira L, Hoffmann A. The parabrachial region as a possible region modulating simultaneously pain and tonic immobility. *Behav Brain Res.* 1993;56(2):127-132.

72. Martin RJ, Apkarian AV, Hodge CJ Jr., Ventrolateral and dorsolateral ascending spinal cord pathway influence on thalamic nociception in cat. *J Neurophysiol.* 1990;64(5):1400-1412.

73. Penny GR, Itoh K, Diamond IT. Cells of different sizes in the ventral nuclei project to different layers of the somatic cortex in the cat. *Brain Res.* 1982;242(1):55-65.

74. Rub U, et al. The intralaminar nuclei assigned to the medial pain system and other components of this system are early and progressively affected by the Alzheimer's disease-related cytoskeletal pathology. *J Chem Neuroanat.* 2002;23(4):279-290.

75. Morrow TJ, Casey KL. Suppression of bulboreticular unit responses to noxious stimuli by analgesic mesencephalic stimulation. *Somatosens Res.* 1983;1(2):151-168.

76. Desbois C, Villanueva L. The organization of lateral ventromedial thalamic connections in the rat: a link for the distribution of nociceptive signals to widespread cortical regions. *Neuroscience.* 2001;102(4):885-898.

77. Morrow TJ, Casey KL. Modulation of the spontaneous and evoked discharges of ventral posterior thalamic neurons during shifts in arousal. *Brain Res Bull.* 1988;21(3):433-438.

78. Lenz FA, et al. Characteristics of somatotopic organization and spontaneous neuronal activity in the region of the thalamic principal sensory nucleus in patients with spinal cord transection. *J Neurophysiol.* 1994;72(4):1570-1587.

79. Casey KL, Morrow TJ. Effect of medial bulboreticular and raphe nuclear lesions on the excitation and modulation of supraspinal nocifensive behaviors in the cat. *Brain Res.* 1989;501(1):150-161.
80. Casey KL, et al. Selective opiate modulation of nociceptive processing in the human brain. *J Neurophysiol.* 2000;84(1):525-533.
81. Bester H, et al. Spino (trigemino) parabrachiohypothalamic pathway: electrophysiological evidence for an involvement in pain processes. *J Neurophysiol.* 1995;73(2):568-585.
82. Kenshalo DR, et al. Response properties and organization of nociceptive neurons in area 1 of monkey primary somatosensory cortex. *J Neurophysiol.* 2000;84(2):719-729.
83. Penfield W, Rasmussen T. *The Cerebral Cortex of Man: A Clinical Study of Localization of Function.* New York: Macmillan; 1950:xv, 248.
84. Jeffrey-Gauthier R, Guillemot JP, Piche M. Neurovascular coupling during nociceptive processing in the primary somatosensory cortex of the rat. *Pain.* 2013;154(8):1434-1441.
85. Lanz S, Seifert F, Maihofner C. Brain activity associated with pain, hyperalgesia and allodynia: an ALE meta-analysis. *J Neural Transm.* 2011;118(8):1139-1154.
86. Ploner M, et al. Differential organization of touch and pain in human primary somatosensory cortex. *J Neurophysiol.* 2000;83(3):1770-1776.
87. Melzack R, Wall PD. Pain mechanisms: a new theory. *Science.* 1965;150(3699):971-979.
88. Reynolds DV. Surgery in the rat during electrical analgesia induced by focal brain stimulation. *Science.* 1969;164(3878):444-445.
89. Sulkowski MJ, Kurosawa MS, Cox DN. Growing pains: development of the larval nocifensive response in Drosophila. *Biol Bull.* 2011;221(3):300-306.
90. Harris JA. Descending antinociceptive mechanisms in the brainstem: their role in the animal's defensive system. *J Physiol Paris.* 1996;90(1):15-25.
91. Reichling DB, Kwiat GC, Basbaum AI. Anatomy, physiology and pharmacology of the periaqueductal gray contribution to antinociceptive controls. *Prog Brain Res.* 1988;77:31-46.
92. Thorn BE, Applegate L, Johnson SW. Ability of periaqueductal gray subdivisions and adjacent loci to elicit analgesia and ability of naloxone to reverse analgesia. *Behav Neurosci.* 1989;103(6):1335-1339.
93. Hosobuchi Y. Subcortical electrical stimulation for control of intractable pain in humans. Report of 122 cases (1970–1984). *J Neurosurg.* 1986;64(4):543-553.
94. Meyerson BA, Boethius J, Carlsson AM. Percutaneous central gray stimulation for cancer pain. *Appl Neurophysiol.* 1978;41(1-4):57-65.
95. Willis WD Jr. Anatomy and physiology of descending control of nociceptive responses of dorsal horn neurons: comprehensive review. *Prog Brain Res.* 1988;77:1-29.
96. Basbaum AI, Fields HL. The origin of descending pathways in the dorsolateral funiculus of the spinal cord of the cat and rat: further studies on the anatomy of pain modulation. *J Comp Neurol.* 1979;187(3):513-531.
97. Fields HL, Basbaum AI. Brainstem control of spinal pain-transmission neurons. *Annu Rev Physiol.* 1978;40:217-248.
98. Krout KE, Jansen AS, Loewy AD. Periaqueductal gray matter projection to the parabrachial nucleus in rat. *J Comp Neurol.* 1998;401(4):437-454.
99. Dayawansa S, Ruch S, Norgren R. Parabrachial-hypothalamic interactions are required for normal conditioned taste aversion. *Am J Physiol Regul Integr Comp Physiol.* 2014;306(3):R190-R200.
100. Wu Q, Clark MS, Palmiter RD. Deciphering a neuronal circuit that mediates appetite. *Nature.* 2012;483(7391):594-597.
101. Wu Q, et al. NR2B subunit of the NMDA glutamate receptor regulates appetite in the parabrachial nucleus. *Proc Natl Acad Sci U S A.* 2013;110(36):14765-14770.
102. Smotherman M, et al. A mechanism for vocal-respiratory coupling in the mammalian parabrachial nucleus. *J Neurosci.* 2006;26(18):4860-4869.
103. Kaur S. et al. Glutamatergic signaling from the parabrachial nucleus plays a critical role in hypercapnic arousal. *J Neurosci.* 2013;33(18):7627-7640.
104. Basbaum AI, Clanton CH, Fields HL. Opiate and stimulus-produced analgesia: functional anatomy of a medullospinal pathway. *Proc Natl Acad Sci U S A.* 1976;73(12):4685-4688.
105. Fields HL, et al. Nucleus raphe magnus: a common mediator of opiate- and stimulus-produced analgesia. *Trans Am Neurol Assoc.* 1976;101:208-210.
106. Basbaum AI, Fields HL. Endogenous pain control systems: brainstem spinal pathways and endorphin circuitry. *Annu Rev Neurosci.* 1984;7:309-338.
107. Watkins LR, Mayer DJ. Organization of endogenous opiate and nonopiate pain control systems. *Science.* 1982;216(4551):1185-1192.
108. Escobar W, et al. Metamizol, a non-opioid analgesic, acts via endocannabinoids in the PAG-RVM axis during inflammation in rats. *Eur J Pain.* 2012;16(5):676-689.
109. Gao K, Mason P. Somatodendritic and axonal anatomy of intracellularly labeled serotonergic neurons in the rat medulla. *J Comp Neurol.* 1997;389(2):309-328.
110. Zemlan FP, Behbehani MM. Nucleus cuneiformis and pain modulation: anatomy and behavioral pharmacology. *Brain Res.* 1988;453(1-2):89-102.
111. Fields HL, Heinricher MM. Anatomy and physiology of a nociceptive modulatory system. *Philos Trans R Soc Lond B Biol Sci.* 1985;308(1136):361-374.
112. Cleary DR, Heinricher MM. Adaptations in responsiveness of brainstem pain-modulating neurons in acute compared with chronic inflammation. *Pain.* 2013;154(6):845-855.
113. Heinricher MM, McGaraughty S. Analysis of excitatory amino acid transmission within the rostral ventromedial medulla: implications for circuitry. *Pain.* 1998;75(2-3):247-255.
114. Urban MO, Gebhart GF. Characterization of biphasic modulation of spinal nociceptive transmission by neurotensin in the rat rostral ventromedial medulla. *J Neurophysiol.* 1997;78(3):1550-1562.
115. Kaplan H, Fields HL. Hyperalgesia during acute opioid abstinence: evidence for a nociceptive facilitating function of the rostral ventromedial medulla. *J Neurosci.* 1991;11(5):1433-1439.

CHAPTER 3

Pathophysiology of Pain

Stephen A. Cohen

The Decade of Pain Control and Research (DPCR) legislation passed by the 106th Congress helped promulgate an extraordinary number of scientific inquiries into the mechanisms and treatment of pain. In the decade before Senator Hatch introduced the Bill, a PubMed search of the term "pathophysiology of pain" retrieved 53 articles. In the DPCR, the same search yielded 32,283 articles. In the ten years since the publication of the second edition of this textbook in 2004, nearly 48,000 articles have been published. The accelerated rate of publications has begun to slow; but it was hoped that such research growth would continue for three reasons: (1) For humane considerations, we simply need more effective and safer medications for better pain management. (2) The cost of pain to society is colossal–nearly $55 billion per year by one estimate. (3) Improved scientific and technological knowledge about pain pathways drives pain drug discovery research and development to meet demand.[1] However, by the end of the DPCR, many impediments to using evidence-based pain management methods still remained, and federal economic support was waning.[2,3]

Acute pain results from the complex convergence of many signals traveling up and down the neuraxis and serves to warn us of potential impending harm. For example, noxious stimuli activate nociceptors in the periphery. The signal travels centrally, carried by the axons of the primary sensory neurons, the dorsal root ganglia (DRG), which are relatively quiescent unless specifically stimulated by sensory input. The pain response can also harm rather than help the individual. Injured DRG may become hyperexcitable and display considerable spontaneous electrical activity. Such increased activity results from the expression of a dramatically different constellation of cell-specific molecules in injured cells compared with normal ones. Ultimately, the operation of complex neuronal circuits may be markedly altered. Chronic pain sensation can result from such injury.

Woolf describes a classification system that separates pain into two major divisions: adaptive and maladaptive. The former serves to protect the organism, but the latter can lead to pathological pain maintained as a disease state. Woolf's framework then distinguishes four different types of pain: nociceptive, inflammatory, neuropathic, and functional (abnormal central processing). Investigators have delineated some, but far from all, of the many mechanisms operative in the generation of these types of pain and the etiologies that cause them.[4]

Considerable knowledge has accrued, which has given some insight into the mechanisms responsible for the development of acute and chronic pain. Understanding the changes that follow injury at a cellular and molecular level may help lead to new therapeutic interventions. This chapter highlights, rather than exhaustively chronicles, some of these findings. The peripheral sensitization changes seen in inflammatory pain are described first, then the central mechanisms of sensitization, followed by the role of neurotrophic factors, the effects on neuronal ionic channels, higher neural mechanisms, central pain, and genetics. The chapter concludes with some remarks.

PERIPHERAL SENSITIZATION

Unmyelinated C or thinly myelinated Aδ afferent fibers convey nociceptive pain sensation. Minor irritation of tissue in a neuron's receptive field also results in the release of inflammatory mediators, which is often accompanied by a reduction in the nociceptor threshold. Such a change, called *peripheral sensitization*, renders the nerve ending responsive to weak, normally nonpainful stimuli (allodynia). Stronger stimuli typically provoke exaggerated pain (hyperalgesia). Sensitization involves not only normal nociceptive fibers, but also the recruitment of so-called silent nociceptors, which are not usually sensitive to painful stimuli or inflammatory substrates such as prostaglandins or bradykinin.

Bradykinin can sensitize C and Aδ fibers to prostaglandins, protons, serotonin, heat, and mechanical stimuli.[5-8] Because its algesic effect displays considerable tachyphylaxis, however, bradykinin alone cannot account for the hyperalgesia seen in inflammation.[7] Bradykinin also appears to facilitate the production of prostaglandins.[9] Similarly, prostaglandins sensitize nerve afferents to bradykinin action.[10] Blockade of such sensitization accounts for the clinical efficacy of antiinflammatory drugs such as aspirin and cyclooxygenase-1 and -2 inhibitors.

Some light has been shed on cellular transduction mechanisms that may be involved in the development of this type of sensitization. For example, the afterhyperpolarization of primary afferent fibers decreases, which renders the cell more likely to fire repetitive action potentials in response to subsequent stimuli. The process appears to involve adenyl cyclase and the second messenger cyclic adenosine monophosphate (cAMP). The latter provokes the phosphorylation of potassium (K) channels, which is catalyzed by protein kinase A (PKA). Excitability increases as K conductance decreases. Some investigators have proposed a universal role for cAMP in producing sensitization in response to multiple physical and chemical noxious stimuli.[11-13] Some evidence suggests the role of cAMP-PKA in decreasing the activation threshold and increasing the size and rate of activation of a tetrodotoxin-resistant sodium (Na) channel in nociceptive neurons, too.[14] The decrease in inflammatory pain seen in mice that have a point mutation in a PKA subunit supports the importance of this cAMP-PKA mechanism.[12]

Phospholipase C induction by the activation of bradykinin or neurokinin (NK) receptors can ultimately lead to increased electrical activity of primary afferent nerve terminals. Intracellular calcium (Ca) increases, which may increase adenyl cyclase activity and cAMP levels. Phosphorylation of specific cation channels and their subsequent increased activity results.[15]

Primary afferent nerve fibers have many 5-HT_{2A} receptors,[16] the activation of which produces a G protein–mediated decrease in K currents.[17,18] Hence, 5-HT_{2A} receptor blockade can antagonize this component of inflammatory pain.[17] Prostaglandins may also provoke a separate type of decrease in outward K current, mediated by cAMP-PKA.[12]

Inflammation leads to an upregulation of nitric oxide (NO) synthetase in DRG and other cells. Ultimately, neuropeptides may be released from nociceptive nerve terminals, which can produce inflammatory hyperalgesia.[8] Whereas subcutaneous injection of NO produces pain,[19] interruption of NO synthetase blocks the hyperalgesia.[20] These findings oversimplify the role of NO in peripheral sensitization, however, because some data suggest an antinociceptive role for NO.[8,21,22] Although NO generates cyclic guanosine monophosphate (cGMP) as an intracellular second messenger, the cyclic nucleotide does not seem to contribute to the sensitization of the nerve terminals.[11,23] Recent data suggest that NO may exert its action on peripheral nerve terminals indirectly. Moreover, NO synthetase may be involved early in the inflammatory response, but NO itself does not participate in chronic inflammation.[24] This indirect action, which may be mediated by its effect on blood vessels, coupled with its direct action on nerve terminals, has led some investigators to postulate a role for NO in triggering migraine headaches.[25]

Considerable evidence exists for the role of neurotrophic factors in the long-term development of neuropathic pain (see later discussion). Recent data have suggested that neurotrophins can also affect neuronal function in the short term. Although not studied directly in C-fiber terminals, changes in ionic current flow, intracellular Ca level, and protein phosphorylation have been shown to lead to altered neuronal excitability, neurotransmitter release, receptor distribution, and synaptic efficacy in other systems.[8,26-30]

The recruitment of previously mechanically silent nerve fibers that become sensitive to mechanical or thermal stimuli after exposure to inflammatory mediators such as bradykinin suggests another mechanism of peripheral sensitization.[31,32] Investigators have proposed that primary afferent substance P–containing neurons are involved in developing hyperalgesia. The demonstration that prostaglandins can increase the number of bradykinin-responsive, substance P–containing fibers is consistent with this finding.[33]

Transient receptor potential (TRP) channels constitute a group of ligand-activated, nonselective cation channels. It has been known for some time that the transient receptor potential vanilloid 1 (TRPV1) receptor, a member of this family, plays a role in the transduction of noxious thermal and chemical stimuli such as acids and vanilloids (e.g., capsaicin) and inflammation-induced hyperalgesia.[34-36] More recently, using a genetic knock-out mouse model, Vardanyan and colleagues demonstrated that TRPV1 receptors also play a role in opioid-induced hyperalgesia.[37]

In summary, multiple mechanisms modulate the functioning of primary afferent nerve terminals. The final common pathway appears to involve the increase in intracellular Ca and protein kinase levels. Both Ca and protein kinases exert a profound influence on the control of gene transcription (see later discussion).

CENTRAL SENSITIZATION

Central sensitization refers to the plasticity displayed by central neural structures involved in pain perception. Some of these physiologic neuronal changes can occur within a few minutes. These may not be maintained once the stimulus is removed. Still other changes remain long after the noxious stimuli cease and may reflect irreversible processes. Two prominent features of peripheral tissue injury include pain and an exaggerated response to noxious stimuli, such as heat. However, the hallmark of clinical pain, mechanical allodynia, cannot easily be explained without invoking central neuronal plasticity. Central mechanisms must also be considered in describing referred pain.[8]

One clinical example of central sensitization is seen in amputees who exhibit phantom limb pain, which is similar to that experienced prior to the amputation. The pain can remain long after the inciting peripheral stimulus is removed. Surgical patients who have derived benefit from preemptive analgesia constitute another example. In these patients, the short- and long-term central neural structure changes that might lead to sensitization are blocked.

Considerable experimental data support the concept that mechanical allodynia results from the activation of Aβ nerve fibers, which normally subserve light touch or vibration, not pain. Some of the evidence is indirect but includes the following.[8] Primary afferent nerve fiber injury leads to abnormal electrical excitability of both small and large fibers, including Aβ fibers. The latter exhibit exquisite sympathetic sensitivity after injury, and pharmacologic or surgical sympathectomy can ameliorate mechanical allodynia.[38,39] High-threshold C or Aδ fibers do not seem responsible for the allodynia because the transduction sensitivity of these single fibers remains stable before and after injury.[38,40] The time course of onset of allodynia correlates with the more rapid conduction velocity of the larger fibers.[38] Blockade of only Aβ fibers extinguishes allodynia.[41] Aβ fibers activate AMPA (DL-α-amino-2,3-dihydro-5-methyl-3-oxo-4-isoxazolepropanoic acid)/kainic acid receptors in the dorsal horn (DH) of the spinal cord. Such receptors have not been found on C fibers, and their specific antagonism reduces allodynia.[42] The time course of the appearance of allodynia following nerve injury corresponds to that of the upregulation of AMPA receptors.[8] Finally, without inflammation, normal touch does not lead to changes in gene expression.[43] In summary, although some of the evidence is indirect, Aβ fibers appear to play a powerful role in the mediation of mechanical allodynia.

Reports have demonstrated secondary hyperalgesia to only mechanical stimuli. The investigators suggested that independent peripheral mechanisms accounted for the evoked pain and central sensitization.[44] The involvement of Aβ fibers in mechanical allodynia, as noted earlier, also suggests that central, rather than peripheral, mechanisms must be operative.[8]

Data suggest that maintained pain can result from several specific processes that converge on the DH of the spinal cord. They include neuronal sensitization, reduction in inhibitory interneuron activity, and a modulation of descending pathway activity.[8] Brief descriptions of each follow.

NEURONAL SENSITIZATION

DH neuron changes resembling long-term potentiation and long-term depression can result from high-frequency stimulation of C fibers or low-frequency stimulation of Aδ fibers, respectively.[45-47] Intense electrical or noxious stimulation of C fibers can promote wide-dynamic-range (WDR) neuron hyperexcitability in the DH. *N*-methyl-D-aspartate (NMDA) receptors and levels of intracellular Ca and protein kinases play a crucial role in this sensitization.[45,48] Sensitization may involve two qualitatively different actions at synapses. At one type of synapse, transmission efficacy increases in a graded fashion. At the other, so-called silent synapses switch to become active.[49,50]

Sensitization can be demonstrated in DH neurons even after short periods of electrical or noxious stimulation. For example, repetitive electrical stimulation provokes increased excitability, lasting about an hour. Such action potential "wind-up" has been used to model "pain" at the cellular level. Wind-up refers to the slow, prolonged depolarization and ultimate burst of action potentials seen with stimulation.[51] It can be demonstrated in only a few cells, which suggests a cell-specific mechanism of generation.[48] During such hyperexcitability, several neuronal changes occur, with presumptive clinical correlates. First, subsequent stimuli evoke a longer and more intense period of action potential firing, which qualitatively resembles hyperalgesia. Second, receptive fields increase in size, which is consistent with secondary hyperalgesia. Finally, the threshold for firing action potentials is decreased and responses to Aβ fibers appear, which resembles allodynia.[8]

Temporal and spatial summation of fast and slow synaptic potentials and action potential wind-up can explain the period of DH neuronal hyperexcitability. Heterosynaptic facilitation also develops whereby the increased excitability derived from one synaptic input increases the response amplitude from a second, separate input.[45]

Most of the recent work on unraveling the molecular mechanisms of WDR neuron sensitization has focused on three classes of agents: excitatory amino acids, tachykinins, and calcitonin gene–related peptide (CGRP). Other compounds have been less well studied. These transmitters and neuromodulators affect DH neuron activity by directly increasing cation fluxes, impinging on intracellular transduction mechanisms, and modulating receptor and transmitter gene transcription. Synaptic transmission augmentation at NMDA receptors is the final common pathway.[8,52-54]

Because the central role of NMDA receptors in sensitization cannot be overemphasized, its following properties may lend some insight.[8] Magnesium (Mg) blocks the ionic channel at rest but can be displaced by adequate depolarization.[55,56] Ca readily permeates its ionic channel; hence its activation increases intracellular Ca levels.[57] Increased intracellular Ca levels augment protein kinase activity.[58] Phosphorylation antagonizes the Mg-channel blockade, which then can function at hyperpolarized levels.[59] Bursts of action potentials can result from NMDA receptor activation, which greatly increases transmitter release at higher levels in the nervous system. Activation of presynaptic NMDA receptors causes increased release of excitatory amino acids and substance P.[60] Hence, several mechanisms serve to amplify signals transmitted through NMDA receptors.

NMDA receptors consist of the subunit NR1 and at least one of the subunits NR2A-D. Recently, Qu and colleagues reported that intrathecal application of a selective NR2B-containing NMDA (NMDA-2B) receptor antagonist both alleviated neuropathic pain selectively, without affecting motor function, and inhibited the induction of long-term potentiation (LTP) in dorsal horn WDR neurons.[61]

AMPA, NK, metabotropic glutamate (mGlu), and CGRP receptors also play roles in the sensitization of DH neurons.[8] Activation of AMPA receptors leads to increased intracellular Ca and depolarization. In other areas of the nervous system, AMPA and NMDA receptors reciprocally activate one another. AMPA receptors are ultimately phosphorylated over a time course of 10 to 15 minutes, which increases their responsiveness. Some investigators have proposed a role for them in maintaining long-term potentiation.[62,63]

Substance P and neurokinin A (NKA), which are released by stimulation of C fibers, exert their actions at neurokinin-1 (NK-1) and neurokinin-2 (NK-2) receptors, respectively.[64] Activation of these receptors supplements DH neuron sensitization. Moreover, NK-1 receptors appear to strengthen the sensitizing actions mediated by NMDA receptors. Consequently, administering specific antagonists of both receptors can ameliorate certain painful states.[65,66]

Subtypes of mGlu receptors are coupled to phospholipase C, which suggests that their activation increases intracellular Ca levels. In the cerebral cortex, evidence exists that mGlu receptors augment the sensitizing actions of NMDA receptors.[67,68] They also increase AMPA receptor excitability.[69] Their appearance at high density in lamina II of the DH indirectly suggests a role for them in pain transmission. The action of CGRP in the spinal cord remains poorly understood, but investigators have suggested that it potentiates NMDA and NK-1 receptor opening.[70]

The preceding cell-surface receptor actions suggest that intracellular Ca levels, Ca influx, and protein kinase activation play an important intracellular role in DH neuron sensitization.[8] Different intracellular stores of Ca may promote different events in the neurons. On balance, the increased levels of intracellular Ca generate sensitization, but suitable negative feedback mechanisms are activated to minimize the likelihood of cell death resulting from toxic intracellular levels of free Ca. Calcium levels induce protein kinase activity in the neuronal soma, which leads to phenotypic and ultimately genotypic changes. For example, under the influence of high intracellular Ca, protein kinase C phosphorylates NMDA receptors, which promotes long-term potentiation.[58,71] Activation of nuclear transcription factors and gene transcription also occurs.[72,73]

REDUCTION IN INHIBITORY INTERNEURON ACTIVITY

Diminution of the inhibitory influences supplied by inhibitory interneurons results in increased WDR neuron excitability consistent with clinical hyperalgesia and mechanical allodynia.[74] The loss of γ-aminobutyric acidergic (GABAergic) and glycinergic activity in the DH produces a state of neuronal hyperexcitability. Such inhibitory loss amplifies the excitability of WDR projections.[75,76] As would be expected, pharmacologic antagonism of GABAergic and glycinergic receptors with bicuculline and strychnine produces a functional state resembling clinical allodynia. Conversely, the allodynia produced by injury is ameliorated by GABA agonist administration.[77]

Considerable research has addressed the possible mechanisms responsible for the reduction in inhibitory interneuron activity.[8] If a decrease in GABAergic and glycinergic activity can mimic allodynia, does such a diminution actually cause chronic pain? Although the final verdict is not yet in, it appears that primary afferent fiber injury leads not only to NMDA receptor activation, with consequent sensitization of WDR neurons, but also to a huge outpouring of excitatory amino acid neurotransmitters at inhibitory interneuron NMDA synapses. Such release has been postulated to cause massive accumulation of intracellular Ca and NO, which ultimately leads to cell death.[78,79] Other speculation attributes the decrease in inhibitory interneuron activity to loss of neurotrophic factors from injured primary afferent fibers.[80] In this regard, the role of GABA attracts attention because primary afferent terminal degeneration provokes a biphasic response of GABAergic neurons, which suggests a trophic role for GABA itself in the reorganization of spinal networks.[81]

MODULATION BY DESCENDING PATHWAYS

For some time, neuroscientists have envisaged a role for descending input from supraspinal pathways in controlling nociceptive signaling in the DH of the spinal cord.[82] Signals transmitted to higher centers depend on tremendous afferent and efferent integration of information processing at lower centers.[83] Investigators have examined the role of supraspinal structures in the development of secondary allodynia.[84] Blocking allodynia with precisely localized microinjections of lidocaine, they concluded that brainstem pathways immediately adjacent to the raphe magnus contribute to the development of secondary allodynia.

Several neurotransmitter systems appear to be involved in the increases or decreases in descending facilitation or inhibition, respectively.[8,85] Recent data suggest that augmentation of serotonergic systems contributes to DH neuron sensitization. Primary afferent nerve terminals, excitatory interneurons, and projection neurons exhibit multiple types of 5-HT receptors over their plasmalemmae. Evidence suggests that the 5-HT_3 receptor subtype accounts for the facilitatory action of 5-HT on the evoked release of substance P–like immunoreactive materials. NO mediates the intracellular signal transduction by promoting an increase in cGMP production.[86] Stimulation of the 5-HT_{1A} subtype enhances K currents and suppresses Ca currents.[87] These data have led to the suggestion that inhibition of inhibitory interneuron 5-HT_{1A} receptors reinforces DH neuron sensitization and, therefore, allodynia.[85]

Recently, using a spinal nerve ligation (SNL) rat model of neuropathic pain, Wang and colleagues reported that the $5HT_3$ receptor antagonist ondansetron blocked SNL-induced pain.[88]

Descending dopaminergic systems also play a role in regulating spinal neuron excitability. Two families of dopamine receptors have been defined based on their properties. One includes dopaminergic receptors that are D_1-like, which consists of D_1 and D_5, and another that are D_2-like, which consists of D_2, D_3, and D_4. Stimulation of members of the first group increases adenyl cyclase and potentiates neuronal excitability.[89] Stimulation of members of the second group inhibits neuronal excitability by inhibiting adenyl cyclase and Ca currents and augmenting K currents. Such changes may play a role in the sensitization of WDR neurons. D_1 agonists provoke release of CGRP and substance P from the spinal cord, which correlates with their ability to increase nociception at the level of the projection neurons.[90]

Inhibition of nociception involves mesolimbic, mesocortical, and nigrostriatal dopaminergic circuits.[91-93] An understanding of how these functionally impinge on lower centers remains incomplete.[94,95]

Descending adrenergic pathways innervating the spinal cord derive primarily from the locus ceruleus, subceruleus, and medullary raphe nuclei.[96-99] They exert descending inhibitory and facilitatory influence on spinal neurons by action on specific adrenoreceptors. The three major classes of such receptors, α_1, α_2, and β, can be further divided into ten subtypes, which are designated α_{1A}, α_{1B}, α_{1D}, α_{2A}, α_{2B}, α_{2C}, β_1, β_2, β_3, and β_4. The first three promote mobilization of intracellular Ca by coupling to phospholipase C and voltage-dependent Ca channels. The α_2 class inhibits adenyl cyclase, facilitates K currents, and inhibits Ca currents, and the β class stimulates adenyl cyclase and, hence, neuronal excitability.

Under normal conditions, descending noradrenergic pathways display little spontaneous activity. Various events can provoke considerable change in their activity, which plays a significant role in the modulation of descending inhibition.[85,100] For example, noxious stimuli activate release of noradrenaline in the DH of the spinal cord, which excites α_2 receptors to effect "pain-induced analgesia." Some investigators have developed a model of allodynia in which locus ceruleus neurons become activated.[101] Such activation also potentiates descending noradrenergic inhibitory circuits.

Evidence exists for the facilitation of efferent antinociceptive adrenergic systems provoked by acute and chronic noxious stimuli. Much of this research has focused on the inhibition of nociception mediated by α_{2A} receptors, which are negatively coupled to adenyl cyclase.[97] On the contrary, data also suggest that higher nervous centers cause hyperexcitation of spinal neurons by increasing intracellular Ca, an effect that is mediated by the activation of α_1 adrenoreceptors.[97,102] Recent data corroborate these findings. Destruction of p75 nerve growth factor (NGF) receptor afferents (see later discussion) does not interfere with the hypersensitivity to mechanical stimuli that results from nerve injury. Such injury does disrupt the inhibitory action of descending α_2 circuits, however, which exerts net reinforcement of hypersensitivity and neuropathic pain states.[103]

Descending facilitation also plays an important role in the pathophysiology of pain. For example, diminished cerebral GABAergic tone, such as may occur with direct brain injury, can lead to the disinhibition of descending facilitation.[104] The rostromedial area of the ventral medulla seems to be involved because blocking electrical transmission there with lidocaine ameliorates experimental allodynia.[8]

Neurotensin (NT) is a 13–amino acid neuropeptide that is widely distributed throughout the central nervous system. It exerts its actions via NT receptors (NTRs), which consist of three subtypes: high affinity NTS1, low affinity NTS2, and NTS3. NT and NTRs regulate nociception at several levels in the descending CNS pathways. From a molar perspective, NT is a more potent analgesic than morphine. Investigators have reported that spinal injection of NT or one of its analogs modulates pain perception in rodent models of both persistent and neuropathic pain.[105,106] Other studies have shown NT analog effectiveness in treating thermal, visceral, and persistent inflammatory pain, but there appears to be variability of efficacy depending on NTS1 or NTS2 selectivity, the animal pain model, and animal species.[107-110]

NEUROTROPHIC INTERACTIONS

In addition to the rapid (msec time course) electrical signaling that occurs in the nervous system, neuron-neuron, neuron-glia, and neuron-muscle communication also occurs over a much longer time course. This has been perhaps most apparent at the skeletal neuromuscular junction, where disruption of the nerve innervating the muscle not only causes absence of voluntary movement, but also leads to profound changes in the muscle cell. We say that the nerve exerts a "trophic," or nourishing effect, on the muscle. Without activity and the so-called neurotrophic influences of the nerve, the muscle loses many specialized features and becomes "atrophic." Profound molecular changes occur, for example, in the muscle membrane's electrical properties; the number, type, and distribution of acetylcholine receptors over the surface of the muscle fiber; and the proteins of the contractile mechanism in the sarcomeres.

A number of so-called trophic factors have been studied. Considerable information exists about the mechanisms and actions of NGF. More than 50 years ago, the requirement of NGF for the development of sensory and sympathetic neurons was described by Rita Levi-Montalcini.[111-113] According to the theory, the neurotrophic factors made by target postsynaptic cells are transported retrogradely to the presynaptic neuronal soma, where they are required for the survival, development, and differentiation of the presynaptic neurons. Over the last half-century, many lines of research have tended to support Levi-Montalcini's seminal theory.

Many neurotrophic factors besides NGF have been identified as playing a role in the integrity of nerve and muscle cells. More recently, investigators have realized the importance of such factors not only in the growth and development of immature cells, but also in the maintenance of differentiated properties of mature cells. Hence, the definition of neurotrophic factors in the sensory nervous system has been broadened to include those factors that permit the long-term growth, survival, or differentiation of neurons. The current knowledge of factors important in sensory nerve integrity focuses on the neurotrophin family and the glial cell line–derived neurotrophic factor (GDNF) family of factors.

The neurotrophin family consists of NGF, brain-derived neurotrophic factor (BDNF), neurotrophin-3 (NT3), neurotrophin-4/5 (NT4/5), and, in teleost fish *Xiphophorus*, neurotrophin-6 (NT6). The factors are basic proteins of about 120 amino acids and weigh about 13 kDa. Family members display considerable (~50%) homology of amino acids and exist as homodimers. The GDNF family of trophic factors belongs to the transforming growth factor-β (TGF-β) superfamily and includes GDNF, neurturin, persephin, and artemin. They signal by way of a complex composed of a tyrosine kinase transduction domain (RET) and a ligand-binding domain, the GDNF family receptor-α (GFR-α).[114]

All neurotrophins bind specifically, selectively, and with high affinity to one or more of the three known tyrosine kinase (Trk) receptors: TrkA, TrkB, and TrkC. NGF binds preferentially to TrkA, NT3 binds to all three Trks but exerts its effects mainly through TrkC, and both BDNF and NT4/5 bind preferentially to TrkB. In general, high-affinity binding (K_d ~ 10^{-11} M) constitutes only 10% to 30% of the total binding to Trk receptors, with the remainder being low affinity. Moreover, all members of the family bind with low affinity (K_d ~ 10^{-8}–10^{-9} M) and somewhat different characteristics to a so-called low-affinity nerve growth factor receptor (LNGFR) or p75, which is also a member of the tumor necrosis factor receptor family.[114,115]

Structurally, Trk receptors consist of four main regions: The first is extracellular for ligand binding; the second is immunoglobulin G–like; the third spans the membrane (transmembrane domain); and the fourth is the kinase domain.[115-117] Different isoforms can be distinguished on the basis of different amino acid residues of the extracellular domain.[115,117] Still other isoforms have been identified that lack the kinase domain.[115] The significance of these differences remains to be determined.

NERVE GROWTH FACTOR

Based largely on studies of the action of NGF on PC-12 cells (a pheochromocytoma cell line), some of the steps of signal transduction following Trk activation have been described. Neurotrophin-receptor interaction activates multiple pathways. After ligand binding, receptor autophosphorylation of tyrosine residues occurs, which is likely mediated by dimerization as an obligatory step in the activation process.[118,119] Other substrates such as phospholipase C (PLC-γ) are also phosphorylated.[114] Interaction between phosphatidylinositol-3 kinase and the Trk domain occurs, but its significance is not clear.

The p75 receptor spans the cell membrane and contains both an intracellular region and an extracellular glycoprotein moiety. It appears to act, at least in part, to facilitate high-affinity neurotrophin-Trk binding. Although some investigators refute the role of p75 alone in neurotrophin signaling, others suggest that it may mediate NGF signal transduction through TrkA receptors.[115,116] In cultured Schwann cells, the induction of NF-κB nuclear staining by NGF depends on the presence of the p75 receptor.[120] NF-κB is a transcription factor, which translocates to the nucleus and regulates gene transcription after suitable activation.[121] Such activation also enables NF-κB to bind particular DNA chains.[120] It has also been hypothesized that NGF-p75-NF-κB activation is involved in the generation of hyperalgesia.[120,122]

Neurotrophin receptors are distributed widely and specifically throughout the nervous system. For example, so-called small, dark DRG, which display the neuropeptide marker CGRP, express predominantly TrkA receptors. So-called large, light DRG, which stain with the neurofilament antibody RT97, express TrkC. TrkB receptors appear only on certain types of DRG, which are not distinguishable by any histochemical staining property. For the most part, DRG expressing a Trk also express a p75. About one-third of DRG do not express either a Trk or a p75.

More recent investigation has promoted the concept that NGF also plays an important role in persistent pain states. Some studies suggest that NGF can not only modulate the sensitivity of sensory neurons, but can also mediate inflammatory pain. The precise mechanisms remain unclear, but some of the data are presented in the discussion that follows.

Different neurotrophins affect functionally different groups of DRG. Small-diameter DRG require NGF for survival. Two methods have been used to eliminate NGF during development: gene deletion and in utero antibody application.[123,124] The resultant absence of NGF during development renders animals virtually devoid of small-diameter DRG, which express the nociceptive mediators CGRP and substance P. Such animals display significant hypoalgesia.[114]

Adult DRG do not possess the developmental requirement of NGF for survival. However, they are still exquisitely sensitive to NGF. For example, exogenous NGF added to cultured DRG elicits prolific neurite outgrowth[125] and regulates the expression of both CGRP and substance P as well as the chemosensitivity of the ganglion cells.[28] Interestingly, in the absence of NGF, capsaicin sensitivity, a specific proton-evoked current, and GABA sensitivity were diminished, but adenosine triphosphate (ATP) sensitivity was unaffected. NGF has recently been shown to increase selectively the expression of bradykinin-binding sites on cultured DRG mediated by a mechanism, which requires the p75 receptor.[126] Such an increase has been associated with the increased excitability of nociceptors seen in chronic pain.[15]

Injection of minute amounts of NGF can produce pain and hyperalgesia at the site of injection.[122,127] Because of the localization of these effects, some investigators have suggested that the NGF may also exert its actions on the peripheral terminals of nociceptors.[127]

Nerve activity regulates both neurotrophin synthesis and release from dendrites. Neurotrophins also promote transmitter release, which is mediated by the specific Trk receptor, from corresponding neurons. Hence, the suggestion has been made that neurotrophins act as retrograde messengers and regulate synaptic efficacy and neuronal plasticity.[128]

An interaction between NGF and sympathetic neurons during inflammation has been proposed. Sympathectomy leads to reduction of the short latency hyperalgesia produced by NGF.[129,130] NGF may also cause peripheral sensitization by activating 5-lipoxygenase to generate leukotrienes. Martin and colleagues[131] showed that leukotriene B_4 sensitizes pain afferents to thermal and mechanical stimuli. Conversely, inhibition of 5-lipoxygenase prevents NGF-injection–produced hyperalgesia.[132] Curiously, indomethacin does not prevent such hyperalgesia.[133]

Although systemically administered NGF does not penetrate the spinal cord, it does appear to affect central pain pathways.[114] NGF may also produce increased neurotransmitter release from nociceptive afferents.[134] Finally, NGF appears able to upregulate BDNF synthesis in some pain sensory cells. Hence, NGF seems to induce central sensitization in resetting the sensitivity of spinal processing of noxious stimuli.

Nerve injury as modeled by axotomy provokes a multitude of biochemical responses. Although traumatic plexus and root lesions do constitute serious clinical problems, frank nerve section does not account for many of the clinical syndromes seen. Some, but not all, of the neuronal changes provoked by axotomy are also seen in other neuropathies. For example, normal retrograde flow of neurotrophic substances ceases. About 30% of sensory neurons degenerate and die.[135] *C-jun* gene expression increases[136] but can be blocked by NGF treatment.[137] Substance P and CGRP levels are reduced, and vasoactive intestinal peptide and galanin levels are increased.[138] Neurofilament production is reduced. Axon diameter and conduction velocity decrease. DRG produce more of the phosphoprotein, GAP-43, which is important in neuronal development and plasticity.[139] Some of these changes can be partly ameliorated by the exogenous administration of NGF. Other axotomy induced effects such as downregulation of isolectin B4 binding, thiamine monophosphatase activity, and somatostatin expression can be reversed by GDNF, but not NGF, administration.[114,140]

Because the most commonly seen clinical neuropathies do not involve overt transection of the peripheral nerve, axotomy may not provide a suitable model for studying the mechanisms of chronic pain development. Rather, diabetic neuropathy is the most common neuropathy seen clinically and is usually seen as a distal symmetric sensorimotor neuropathy. It progresses by a nerve terminal dying-back phenomenon. Recently, investigators have studied the actions of trophic factors in both animal models and human clinical trials of diabetic neuropathy. Streptozotocin treatment of rats to produce a model of diabetic neuropathy provokes a number of neuronal changes, such as elevation of tail-flick threshold (thermal hypoalgesia); increase in compound action potential latency; decrement in C-fiber conduction velocity; and fall in substance P, CGRP, and CGRP mRNA levels.[141] NGF can at least partially reverse some of these changes.[114]

Some researchers have begun administering neurotrophic factors in clinical trials for the treatment of diabetic neuropathy. One such phase II trial using recombinant human NGF (rhNGF) showed improvement in the sensory component of the neurologic examination, two quantitative sensory tests, and the subjective impression of the patients who received rhNGF compared to those subjects who received placebo.[142] Efficacy of rhNGF failed statistical significance, however, in a large phase III trial.[143] In this trial, subjects received 0.1 μg/kg of rhNGF subcutaneously three times a week. Doses reported to be effective in animal studies ranged from 3 to 5 mg/kg. Moreover, the serum half-life of NGF has been calculated to be only 7.2 minutes. Hence, it has been suggested that the lack of effect shown in the phase III trial might be the result of inadequate dose. In this context, the recent publication using genomic virus-mediated gene transfer of neurotrophin to protect against pyridoxine neuropathy in the rat elicits optimism.[144] Such gene transfer of the coding sequences for specific trophic substances may circumvent the dose and delivery problem and enable the factors' therapeutic abilities.

Two strategies have been used to elucidate the role of endogenous NGF in the pathophysiology of pain. One involves genetic manipulation to eliminate either NGF or its receptor ("knock-out"), and the other involves inhibiting the actions of NGF by adding selective blockers. For example, blocking NGF for 10 to 12 days leads to fewer nociceptors responding to heat and to a right-shifted, flatter stimulus-response curve generated by measuring the neural firing to intracutaneous heat application. The mechanical stimulus threshold remained unchanged.[145] Taken together, the two kinds of experiments support the notion that native NGF modulates pain sensitivity.[114]

Considerable experimental evidence supports the hypothesis that NGF plays an important role acting as a mediator in inflammatory pain. In both human and animal studies, data suggest that inflammation generally causes increased NGF levels and consequent hyperalgesia.[146,147] Such increase appears to depend on the synthesis and release of NGF *de novo* in the affected cells.[148]

How NGF may play a role in the development of neuropathic pain, however, remains speculative. In many neuropathic conditions, abnormal sympathetic nerve sprouting creates basketlike arborizations around large-diameter DRG, which resemble the connections that develop in animals exposed to excessive NGF.[149-151] Hence, one hypothesis suggests that such NGF abundance, per se, can produce maintained pain.[150,152-154] In axotomy, however, NGF levels are reduced, which has led to the hypothesis that merely an imbalance of NGF can produce chronic pain.[114] Wallerian degeneration of injured nerves appears to be linked to both pain development and sympathetic sprouting. Ramer and colleagues have speculated that NGF serves as a mediator for both processes.[155]

Decreased NGF levels seen after nerve injury have been reputed to be responsible for changes in spinal cord connectivity, too.[114] Normally, only unmyelinated C fibers, many of which are nociceptors, terminate on lamina II of the DH and myelinated A fibers terminate exclusively on laminae I, III, IV, and V. However, after nerve injury, myelinated nerve fibers sprout into lamina I and II.[156,157] Investigators have suggested that this anatomic reorganization may play a role in pain mediated by A fibers.[157] NGF administration prevents such sprouting.[158,159]

BRAIN-DERIVED NEUROTROPHIC FACTOR

BDNF levels also increase in small DRG during inflammation.[114] Unlike NGF, its transport away from the neuronal soma occurs in the anterograde direction.[160-162] In this regard, BDNF resembles prototypal neurotrophic factors collectively called neuregulins, which are seen in the motor, rather than sensory, system.[163] It has been suggested that the binding of BDNF to TrkB, which activates NMDA receptor phosphorylation, may ultimately lead to central neuronal hyperexcitability.[164,165] Such heightened excitability might play a role in the maintenance of pain. To test this idea, a molecular tool has been synthesized, a TrkB-IgG complex, that specifically binds BDNF and effectively renders it inactive. The probe was shown to have binding characteristics similar to intact Trks. When the complex is applied to the spinal cord after inflammation, the hyperexcitability subsides,[114,166] thus implicating BDNF as a mediator of central sensitization.

NEUROTROPHIN-3 AND NEUROTROPHIN-4/5

Less information exists regarding the roles of NT3 and NT4/5 in the development of chronic pain. In inhibiting the electrically evoked release of substance P–like immunoreactivity from isolated rat spinal cords, investigators have recently suggested that NT3 displays antinociceptive properties.[134] They further argued that enkephalins in DH neurons mediate such NT3-induced hypoalgesia because the effect can be blocked by naloxone. Indeed, injected NT3 can transiently reverse experimentally induced inflammatory hyperalgesia.[167] NT3 also increased substance P release from high-threshold (C) fibers in rat spinal cords by electrical stimulation and capsaicin superfusion. Such release was not associated with the development of thermal hyperalgesia.[134,168] Electrophysiologic and behavioral studies in intact rats confirmed that only the TrkB agonists NGF, BDNF, and NT4/5 induced thermal hyperalgesia, whereas the TrkC agonist NT3 had no effect.[169] Hence, investigators have tested and found that NT3 can reverse some injury-induced neuronal changes.[170] Systemic administration of NT3 did produce mechanical hyperalgesia acutely, however, which the authors attributed to autonomic nervous system activation mediated by a relatively nonspecific action on TrkA receptors caused by a transient high concentration.[134,168] They speculated that neurotrophic factor application may have some efficacy in treating nerve root avulsion injuries.[168]

Another report claimed that DRG satellite cells synthesize NT3, which contributes to the sprouting of the sympathetic baskets mentioned earlier around injured neurons.[171] Blocking NT3 with a specific antibody reduces the sprouting by more than 50%.

GLIAL CELL LINE–DERIVED NEUROTROPHIC FACTOR

GDNF has been recently shown to exert an effect on adult sensory neurons, at least some of which is mediated by purinergic receptors. These receptors are important in the activation of peripheral nociceptors[163,172] by nucleotides and nucleotide phosphates. The two different subtypes of purinoreceptors, P1 and P2, display differential sensitivity to adenosine and adenosine triphosphate/adenosine diphosphate (ATP/ADP), respectively. The P2 receptors can be further divided into P2X, which are agonist-induced ionic channels, and P2Y families. P2X receptors are usually distributed widely in the central nervous system. One subtype, however, called $P2X_3$, can be found only on small, nociceptive, peripheral sensory neurons that bind isolectin B4.[173,174] At low doses, adenosine selectively modulates prejunctional nociceptive transmission. At high doses, it appears to act synergistically with the $P2X_3$ ATP receptor to stimulate pain.[163]

GDNF plays an important role in the regulation of $P2X_3$ receptors and, hence, in the development of pain. After axotomy, $P2X_3$ expression decreases by at least 50%. Intrathecal GDNF administration reverses this downregulation of $P2X_3$ receptors[175] and prevents, as well, the decrease of isolectin B4 binding, the number of cells showing thiamine monophosphatase activity, and somatostatin expression. It also prevents the sprouting of A fibers into lamina II of the spinal cord and the slowing of conduction velocity.[158]

IONIC CHANNELS

The dramatic changes in electrical properties of primary sensory neurons seen after injury have led researchers to investigate the role that various neuron-specific ionic channels might play in the development of chronic pain.

SODIUM CHANNELS

In one line of inquiry, the importance of Na channels in the development of the hyperexcitability seen after nerve injury has been evaluated. Recent data suggest that at least ten distinct subtypes of Na channels exist.[176-179] These channels have been classified on the basis of their differential sensitivity to the Na channel–blocking drug tetrodotoxin (TTX), their voltage dependence, and their kinetics. Primary sensory neurons express at least six of these channel types, and DRG and trigeminal ganglion cells express three. A single DRG can express more than one type of Na channel. Discrete genes encode for each type. Using reverse transcription–polymerase chain reaction (RT-PCR) or hybridization technologies, α-subunit mRNAs for ten different Na channels have been demonstrated.[178] Large and medium-size DRG produce two TTX-sensitive (TTX-S) channels, which are denoted $Na_V1.6$ and Na_x. Another TTX-S channel called $Na_V1.7$ is found near DRG terminals.[180] DRG also show TTX-resistant (TTX-R) channels, which have been designated $Na_V1.9$ and $Na_V3.1$. Small, nociceptive DRG also express $Na_V1.8$ and $Na_V3.1$channels.

The various Na channels are distributed differently over different populations of DRG. Because they also have different voltage dependencies and kinetics, they confer markedly different electrophysiologic properties on the various populations of neurons that express them. Axotomy has been shown to modulate DRG electrogenesis considerably.[181] The demonstration of abnormal collections of Na channels on injured axons and the partial efficacy of Na channel blockers in ameliorating experimental models of neuropathic pain have led to the suggestion that Na channel activation plays a role in the hyperexcitability seen in chronic pain.[176]

Recent studies have shown that $Na_V1.8$ (formerly denoted SNS/PN3)[182] and $Na_V1.9$ (formerly denoted NaN)[183] channel genes are downregulated after axotomy, and a normally silent $Na_V1.3$ (formerly denoted α-III)[184] gene is upregulated. Hence, there is a decrease in TTX-R Na channels but an increase in TTX-S currents that recover much more rapidly from inactivation (the $Na_V1.3$ channel).[185] The net effect has been postulated to produce abnormal action potential activity with a lower threshold for firing.[176]

Neurotrophins mediate at least some of the changes in Na channel expression. For example, *in vitro* application of NGF promotes downregulation and upregulation of $Na_V1.3$ and $Na_V1.8$ mRNA expression, respectively.[186] The meaning of the apparent opposing effects of NGF on the membrane excitability of small DRG remains yet unexplained. *In vivo,* NGF effects an incomplete rescue of the $Na_V1.8$ mRNA downregulation seen after axotomy.[187] GDNF appears to at least partly reverse the fall in $Na_V1.9$ mRNA levels seen after axotomy.[188] BDNF appears to have little effect on Na channel expression in DRGs but does play a role in GABA receptor expression.[189]

Inflammatory pain states also demonstrate abnormal Na channel expression. For example, in such models, $Na_V1.8$ mRNA levels increase dramatically in the DRG projecting to the affected extremity.[190] Correlative electrophysiologic studies revealed an increase in both the amplitude and current density of TTX-R Na currents. $Na_V1.9$ mRNA levels also increase.[191]

Some of these changes seem likely mediated by neurotrophins, but the precise sequence of events has not yet been determined. Recently, GDNF and NGF have been shown to reverse the changes seen in repriming of TTX-S Na currents after axotomy.[192] As previously suggested, intact, noninjured DRG normally display two TTX-R Na channel genes ($Na_V1.8$ and $Na_V1.9$) and a silent TTX-S one ($Na_V1.3$). The TTX-R currents inactivate slowly and the TTX-S ones inactivate rapidly. The TTX-R and TTX-S channels also have different kinetics, which allows analysis of recovery from inactivation of Na currents, so-called repriming. The different repriming kinetics permit separation of the TTX-R and TTX-S Na channel currents. The rapidly repriming TTX-S Na currents predominate after axotomy. Both NGF and GDNF can partially ameliorate this shift in repriming current kinetics. Coadministration of NGF and GDNF resulted in complete restoration of the Na channel repriming kinetics.

POTASSIUM CHANNELS

Using human DRG cells obtained from trauma patients and dissociated cultured rat DRG, reports have shown changes in specific types of K channels after injury, too.[193] Calcium-activated K channels can be divided into three main classes, which display a "small" (SK), "intermediate" (IK), or "big" (BK) conductance. The classes can be further divided into different subtypes.[194] Intracellular Ca gates all of them. SK channel activation partly causes the prolonged membrane hyperpolarization, called the *slow afterhyperpolarization*, which inhibits or limits action potential generation.

Employing immunohistochemical techniques, investigators have demonstrated the presence of a human SK type 1 (hSK1) and a human IK type 1 (hIK1) on the soma of small to medium-sized DRG. The hSK1 immunoreactivity decreased in traumatically avulsed DRG. The hIK1 reactivity decreased mostly in large DRG acutely and all-sized DRG chronically. NGF increased the number of hSK1-positive cells in the cultured neurons, whereas NT3 and GDNF did not. NGF also stimulated the expression of the voltage-gated Na channel ($Na_V1.8$). NT3 stimulated the expression of hIK1, but NGF and GDNF did not. The authors suggest that the decreased retrograde transport of the neurotrophic factors that may be seen with injury significantly contribute to the reduced expression of these specific ionic channels and, hence, increased neuronal excitability. They further speculate that novel K channel opener molecules may prove to have therapeutic benefit. Along these lines, the facilitation of K currents by drugs such as mexiletine has been postulated to account for its role in diminishing neuropathic pain.[195,196]

Nerve injury does not invariably lead to neuropathic pain. The risk differs depending on at least the extent of the nerve damage, a person's age, and the expression of the potassium channel alpha subunit KCNS1, which is involved in neuronal excitability and is downregulated after nerve injury. Calling KCNS1 a "putative pain gene," Costigan and colleagues recently demonstrated that the "valine risk allele," an amino acid–changing allele, was significantly associated with higher pain scores.[197]

Investigators have also just identified a mechanosensitive (MS) potassium current (I_{Kmech}) that regulates mechanical threshold and adaptation of a number of mechanoreceptors. I_{Kmech} is carried by the potassium channels Kv1.1–Kv1.2. Being expressed in high-threshold C-mechanonociceptors (C-HTMRs) Aβ-mechanoreceptors, I_{Kmech} shifts mechanical threshold to higher values, thereby acting as a mechanical brake in pain sensation.[198]

CALCIUM CHANNELS

Calcium channels have been variously classified as L-, P/Q-, N-, R-, and T-type depending on their different α subunit composition.[199] N-type Ca channels mediate excitation-secretion coupling at sensory, sympathetic, and central neurons.[200,201] Specific Ca channel blockers can partially relieve neuropathic pain and decrease ectopic electrical activity in DRG, hence implicating a role for the channel's overactivity in chronic pain states.[202] However, blocking L-type Ca channels appears not to ameliorate nociceptive pain. The clinical efficacy of anticonvulsants such as carbamazepine and gabapentin in the treatment of neuropathic pain has been related to their interactions with Ca channels.[203-205]

HIGHER NEURAL MECHANISMS

In addition to the changes seen in peripheral neural structures, nociceptive, inflammatory, and neuropathic pain can modulate neuronal function in supraspinal centers such as the thalamus and somatosensory cortex.[8] For example, Faggin and colleagues[206] demonstrated extensive reorganization of the nervous system in response to reversible peripheral sensory deactivation by making concurrent recordings of ventroposteromedial thalamic nuclei and somatosensory cortical neurons. They could not attribute their results to plasticity of cortical circuits alone, but rather needed to invoke the changes in the thalamus as necessary to the cortical reorganization. Other investigators have emphasized the importance of both thalamocortical and corticothalamic signaling in the modulation of supraspinal centers important in the sensation of pain.[207–209] The picture that emerges suggests considerable bidirectional processing of information rather than simply a relay mechanism as nociceptive impulses ascend the neuraxis.[210]

In a strychnine-induced rat model of allodynia, Sherman and colleagues[211] demonstrated alterations in receptive fields and sensory modalities of ventroposterolateral thalamic neurons. After intrathecal strychnine administration, innocuous tactile stimuli elicited painful responses, the spinal afferent neuron cutaneous receptive fields expanded, and the nociceptive-specific ventroposterolateral neurons displayed lower threshold responsiveness. Because strychnine antagonizes glycine action, their data implicate glycinergic inhibitory interneurons as important mediators of allodynia.

Recently, the activity state of rats has been shown to affect tactile stimuli signal processing in the thalamus.[212] Thalamic neurons in rats display low-pass filter characteristics in quiescent animals so that stimulation above frequencies of 2 Hz are cut off and not transmitted to the somatosensory cortex. The same neurons in active animals pass frequencies at up to 40 Hz.

Clinical experience has led to insight about the pathophysiology of thalamic pain signal processing. For example, using single-unit microelectrode recordings of human sensory thalamic neurons in a variety of patients, Hua and colleagues[213] have shown the alteration of receptive fields in limb amputation victims. Their studies document the plasticity of the human thalamus in processing both painful and nonpainful stimuli.

Basal ganglia also appear to play a role in nociception. Clinicians have noticed that patients with basal ganglionic disorders such as Parkinson's or Huntington's disease display abnormal pain sensation. Ganglionic neurons appear to encode stimulus intensity well but not stimulus location. Hence, investigators have proposed that the basal ganglia function in the sensory-discriminative, affective, and cognitive dimensions of pain.[214]

Some somatosensory cortical neurons display variable integration of pain signaling. It has been known for some time that firing patterns characteristic of sensitization, such as paroxysmal bursts seen in the thalamus, are not seen in somatosensory neurons.[215] More recently, some somatosensory cells have been shown to display much less sensitization to sustained application of heat stimuli than heat-responsive neurons in the thalamus. Some somatosensory thermal nociceptive cortical neurons encode the magnitude of heat intensity by continuously varying their mean discharge frequency. Significant numbers of high-threshold and wide-range thermoreceptive neurons, however, do not display such encoding.[216] Still other reports have documented sensitization that is more marked in the cortex than in the thalamus.[217] Finally, in a rat model of chronic arthritis, both sensitized thalamic and somatosensory cortical neurons displayed activation to non-nociceptive stimulation.

GABAergic, NMDA, excitatory amino acid, and glutamatergic neurotransmitter systems have been implicated in supraspinal pain sensation neuronal modulation.[8] For example, recent data have demonstrated the prevention of an extreme type of neuronal hyperexcitability, kainic acid–induced seizures, by the $GABA_A$ agonist, muscimol.[218] Kao and Coulter[219] showed corticothalamic excitatory postsynaptic currents, which displayed electrophysiologic and pharmacologic properties of NMDA-receptor mediated currents; moreover, an NMDA antagonist blocked them. They also found inhibitory postsynaptic currents, components of which showed sensitivity to bicuculline and a $GABA_B$ antagonist. Because at least some thalamocortical sensory transmission seems to be mediated by NMDA receptors, investigators have proposed that NMDA plays a significant role in the sensitization of the thalamus and somatosensory cortex seen in pain states.[49] Data suggest that the NMDA system maintains the hyperalgesia seen from inflammation, which is perhaps mediated by NO.[220] Researchers have proposed other potential candidates—such as neuropeptides, neurotrophins, or cytokines—that might exert a neuromodulatory action on higher pain sensation centers, but further study remains.

Clearly, we have only just begun to unravel the complexity of supraspinal pain signal processing and modulation.

CENTRAL PAIN

Damage to, or altered function of, the central nervous system itself can lead to so-called central pain. In such cases, rather than diminishing pain, injury to central pain processing centers often exacerbates the pain sensation, which can be exceedingly difficult to treat. Disease processes such as cerebrovascular ischemia, malignancies, and neurodegenerative disorders can all lead to the development of a central pain syndrome.[8]

For a long time, neuronal events such as proliferation, maturation, neurite outgrowth, and apoptosis have been known to be critical during the formation and development of the brain. These processes were not thought to be significant in the adult. Recent studies have emphasized, however, that central nervous system plasticity continues in the adult and plays a role in the development of central pain. After brain injury, neuronal connections change and form new synapses to occupy the empty places left by degenerating synaptic boutons. Moreover, axonal sprouting may lead to entirely new sites of synaptic contact being made.[221] Indeed, a balance is struck between certain kinds of axonal sprouting being promoted and other types being repelled. The authors speculate that reactive astrocytes may elaborate extracellular matrix molecules such as tenascin-C, proteoglycans, neurocan, or brevican to guide the process.[221] Mechanistically, such injury elicits a response of neurotrophins, adhesion molecules, glia, and many other cellular mediators, which is qualitatively similar to that seen in the periphery.

Brain injury stimulates cytokine production in intrinsic neuroglial cells as well as extrinsic migrating inflammatory macrophages and mast cells.[221] The roles of NGF, BDNF, and tumor necrosis factor (TNF-α) in the development of central pain have drawn attention, but precise mechanisms have not yet been worked out.

Investigators have also focused on the role of the neuronal growth associated phosphoprotein, GAP-43 (neuromodulin), in regulating nerve terminal growth. Experimentally induced excess of GAP-43 provokes *de novo* synaptogenesis and more profuse axonal sprouting after injury.[222] It seems to exert a powerful influence in particular on the neuron's cytoskeleton. Protein kinase C phosphorylation appears to mediate the transduction of intra- and extracellular signals regulating nerve terminal sprouting and long-term potentiation in response to injury. Moreover, it has been shown that radiolabeled phosphate incorporation into GAP-43 correlates with the extent of synaptic enhancement.[223] An NMDA receptor antagonist that blocks long-term potentiation has been shown to inhibit the increase in phosphorylation.[224] Thus, it appears that some postsynaptic event requiring NMDA-receptor activation leads to GAP-43 phosphorylation and then to a retrograde signal, which modulates presynaptic GAP-43.[225]

GENETICS

For a long time, researchers have recognized a heritable component of pain perception. It has been recently estimated, for example, that up to 50% of the differences in degenerative disc disease pain perception among individuals can be attributed to genetic influences. Of that 50%, genetic influences account for about 75% of the variability, and the remaining 25% is due to actual structural abnormalities.[226]

Currently, investigators regard genes for the enzymes catechol-O-methyltransferase (COMT) and GTP cyclohydrolase 1 (GCH1) as determining the "set point" of pain sensitivity. The enzyme gene product, COMT, terminates the action of catecholamines such as noradrenaline and dopamine. Hence, inhibition of COMT produces a significant increase in pain threshold (i.e., becoming less sensitive to noxious stimuli).[227] For example, in an arthritis database, persons with the 158-MetCOMT variant displayed a threefold higher risk for pain compared to other genotypes, and women with the 158-MetVal allele had 4.9 times the risk.[228] Conversely, GCH1 limits tetrahydrobiopterin synthesis, which is required to synthesize catecholamines, serotonin, and nitric oxide. Increase in its activity should produce a decrease in pain threshold. Single nucleotide polymorphism (SNP) studies have identified a GCH1 haplotype in individuals who were less sensitive to noxious stimuli.[229]

It is hoped by some investigators that other genes will be discovered that may play a role in pain sensitivity and perception. Epigenetic factors must also be taken into account in the attempt to individualize analgesia regimens.

CONCLUSION

In conclusion, during the Decade of Pain Control and Research, and beyond, investigators have shed light on the neurobiologic mechanisms underlying certain aspects of pain. Ionic channels and neurotransmitter receptor system mechanisms have been discovered and further elucidated. Numerous studies have shown that many aspects of pain are genetically determined. As a result, future clinicians may be able to provide individualized analgesic regimens for their patients. The basic research has created incremental improvements in our understanding of the pathophysiology of pain but has failed to produce any disjunctive insights. Even rethinking the validity and sensitivity of existing pain assessment techniques needs attention. Moreover, scientific discoveries have diffused only slowly into clinical practice so that pain management today has not dramatically improved over the last decade. What we have indeed learned, however, is that we need to do far better in treating both acute and chronic pain.

REFERENCES

1. Luo AD. *Advancements in Pain Research. Pain Research: Methods and Protocols, Methods in Molecular Biology*. Vol. 851. Springer Science + Business Media, LLC 2012.
2. Bradshaw DH, Empy C, Davis P, et al. Trends in funding for research on pain: a report on the National Institutes of Health grant awards over the years 2003 to 2007. *J Pain*. 2008;9:1077-1087.
3. Green CR. The healthcare bubble through the lens of pain research, practice, and policy: advice for the new President and Congress. *J Pain*. 2008;9:1071-1073.
4. Woolf CJ. Pain: moving from symptom control toward mechanism-specific pharmacologic management. *Annals of Internal Medicine*. 2004;140:441-451.
5. Khan AA, Raja SN, Manning DC, Campbell JN, Meyer RA. The effects of bradykinin and sequence-related analogs on the response properties of cutaneous nociceptors in monkeys. *Somatosens Mot Res*. 1992;9:97-106.
6. Lang E, Novak A, Reeh PW, Handwerker HO. Chemosensitivity of fine afferents from rat skin in vitro. *J Neurophysiol*. 1990;63:887-901.
7. Manning DC, Raja SN, Meyer RA, Campbell JN. Pain and hyperalgesia after intradermal injection of bradykinin in humans. *Clin Pharmacol Ther*. 1991;50:721-729.
8. Millan MJ. The induction of pain: an integrative review. *Prog Neurobiol*. 1999;57:1-164.
9. Prado GN, Taylor L, Polgar P. Effects of intracellular tyrosine residue mutation and carboxyl terminus truncation on signal transduction and internalization of the rat bradykinin B2 receptor. *J Biol Chem*. 1997;272:14638-14642.
10. Coleman RA, Smith WL, Narumiya S. International Union of Pharmacology classification of prostanoid receptors: properties, distribution, and structure of the receptors and their subtypes. *Pharmacol Rev*. 1994;46:205-229.
11. Kress M, Rodl J, Reeh PW. Stable analogues of cyclic AMP but not cyclic GMP sensitize unmyelinated primary afferents in rat skin to heat stimulation but not to inflammatory mediators, in vitro. *Neuroscience*. 1996;74:609-617.
12. Malmberg AB, Brandon EP, Idzerda RL, Liu H, McKnight GS, Basbaum AI. Diminished inflammation and nociceptive pain with preservation of neuropathic pain in mice with a targeted mutation of the type I regulatory subunit of cAMP-dependent protein kinase. *J Neurosci*. 1997;17:7462-7470.
13. Levine JD, Reichling DB. Peripheral mechanisms of inflammatory pain. In: Wall PD, Melzack R, eds. *Textbook of Pain*. 4th ed. New York, NY: Churchill Livingstone; 1999:59-84.
14. Gold MS, Reichling DB, Shuster MJ, Levine JD. Hyperalgesic agents increase a tetrodotoxin-resistant Na+ current in nociceptors. *Proc Natl Acad Sci U S A*. 1996;93:1108-1112.
15. Dray A, Perkins M. Bradykinin and inflammatory pain. *Trends Neurosci*. 1993;16:99-104.
16. Carlton SM, Coggeshall RE. Immunohistochemical localization of 5-HT2A receptors in peripheral sensory axons in rat glabrous skin. *Brain Res*. 1997;763:271-275.
17. Abbott FV, Hong Y, Blier P. Persisting sensitization of the behavioural response to formalin-induced injury in the rat through activation of serotonin2A receptors. *Neuroscience*. 1997;77:575-584.
18. Todorovic SM, Scroggs RS, Anderson EG. Cationic modulation of 5-HT2 and 5-HT3 receptors in rat sensory neurons: the role of K+, Ca2+, and Mg2+. *Brain Res*. 1997;765:291-300.
19. Holthusen H, Arndt JO. Nitric oxide evokes pain in humans on intracutaneous injection. *Neurosci Lett*. 1994;165:71-74.

20. Lawand NB, Willis WD, Westlund KN. Blockade of joint inflammation and secondary hyperalgesia by L-NAME, a nitric oxide synthase inhibitor. *Neuroreport*. 1997;8:895-899.
21. Duarte ID, dos Santos IR, Lorenzetti BB, Ferreira SH. Analgesia by direct antagonism of nociceptor sensitization involves the arginine-nitric oxide-cGMP pathway. *Eur J Pharmacol*. 1992;217:225-227.
22. Kawabata A, Manabe S, Manabe Y, Takagi H. Effect of topical administration of L-arginine on formalin-induced nociception in the mouse: a dual role of peripherally formed NO in pain modulation. *Br J Pharmacol*. 1994;112:547-550.
23. Holthusen H, Kindgen-Milles D, Ding ZP. Substance P is not involved in vascular nociception in humans. *Neuropeptides*. 1997;31:445-448.
24. Fletcher DS, Widmer WR, Luell S, et al. Therapeutic administration of a selective inhibitor of nitric oxide synthase does not ameliorate the chronic inflammation and tissue damage associated with adjuvant-induced arthritis in rats. *J Pharmacol Exp Ther*. 1998;284:714-721.
25. Fozard JR. The 5-hydroxytryptamine-nitric oxide connection: the key link in the initiation of migraine? *Arch Int Pharmacodyn Ther*. 1995;329:111-119.
26. Berninger B, Garcia DE, Inagaki N, Hahnel C, Lindholm D. DNF and NT-3 induce intracellular Ca2+ elevation in hippocampal neurones. *Neuroreport*. 1993;4:1303-1306.
27. Berninger B, Poo M. Fast actions of neurotrophic factors. *Curr Opin Neurobiol*. 1996;6:324-330.
28. Bevan S, Winter J. Nerve growth factor (NGF) differentially regulates the chemosensitivity of adult rat cultured sensory neurons. *J Neurosci*. 1995;15(pt 1):4918-4926.
29. Winter J. Brain derived neurotrophic factor, but not nerve growth factor, regulates capsaicin sensitivity of rat vagal ganglion neurones. *Neurosci Lett*. 1998;241:21-24.
30. Sherwood NT, Lesser SS, Lo DC. Neurotrophin regulation of ionic currents and cell size depends on cell context. *Proc Natl Acad Sci U S A*. 1997;94:5917-5922.
31. Handwerker HO, Kilo S, Reeh PW. Unresponsive afferent nerve fibres in the sural nerve of the rat. *J Physiol*. 1991;435:229-242.
32. Meyer RA, Davis KD, Cohen RH, Treede RD, Campbell JN. Mechanically insensitive afferents (MIAs) in cutaneous nerves of monkey. *Brain Res*. 1991;561:252-261.
33. Stucky CL, Thayer SA, Seybold VS. Prostaglandin E2 increases the proportion of neonatal rat dorsal root ganglion neurons that respond to bradykinin. *Neuroscience*. 1996;74:1111-1123.
34. Catarina MJ, Julius D. The vanilloid receptor: a molecular gateway to the pain pathway. *Annu Rev Neurosci*. 2001 24:487-517.
35. Catarina MJ, Schumacher MA, Rominaga M, et al. The capsaicin receptor: a heat-activated ion channel in the pain pathway. *Nature*. 1997;389:816-824.
36. Davis JB, Gray J, Gunthorpe MJ, et al. Vanilloid receptor-1 is essential for inflammatory thermal hyperalgesia. *Nature*. 2000;405:183-187.
37. Vardanyan A, Wang R, Vanderah TW, et al. TRPV1 receptor in expression of opioid-induced hyperalgesia. *J Pain*. 2009;10(3):243-252.
38. Handwerker HO, Kobal G. Psychophysiology of experimentally induced pain. *Physiol Rev*. 1993;73:639-671.
39. Treede RD, Davis KD, Campbell JN, Raja SN. The plasticity of cutaneous hyperalgesia during sympathetic ganglion blockade in patients with neuropathic pain. *Brain*. 1992;115(pt 2):607-621.
40. Gracely RH, Lynch SA, Bennett GJ. Painful neuropathy: altered central processing maintained dynamically by peripheral input. *Pain*. 1992;51:175-194.
41. Koltzenburg M. Stability and plasticity of nociceptor function and their relationship to provoked ongoing pain. *Semin Neurosci*. 1995;7:199-210.
42. Sang CN. NMDA-receptor antagonists in neuropathic pain: experimental methods to clinical trials. *J Pain Symptom Manage*. 2000;19(1)(Suppl S21-25).
43. Ma Z-P, Woolf CJ. Basal and touch-evoked fos-like immunoreactivity during experimental inflammation in the rat. *Pain*. 1996;67:307-316.
44. Ali Z, Meyer RA, Campbell JN. Secondary hyperalgesia to mechanical but not heat stimuli following a capsaicin injection in hairy skin. *Pain*. 1996;68:401-411.
45. Woolf CJ. A new strategy for the treatment of inflammatory pain: prevention or elimination of central sensitization. *Drugs*. 1994;47(Suppl 5):1-9; 46-47.
46. Gozariu M, Bouhassira D, Willer JC, Le Bars D. The influence of temporal summation on a C-fibre reflex in the rat: Effects of lesions in the rostral ventromedial medulla (RVM). *Brain Res*. 1998;792:168-172.
47. Guirimand F, Dupont X, Brasseur L, Chauvin M, Bouhassira D. The effects of ketamine on the temporal summation (wind-up) of the R(III) nociceptive flexion reflex and pain in humans. *Anesth Analg*. 2000;90:408-414.
48. Baranauskas G, Nistri A. Sensitization of pain pathways in the spinal cord: cellular mechanisms. *Prog Neurobiol*. 1998;54:349-365.
49. Isaac JT, Crair MC, Nicoll RA, Malenka RC. Silent synapses during development of thalamocortical inputs. *Neuron*. 1997;18:269-280.
50. Malenka RC, Nicoll RA. Silent synapses speak up. *Neuron*. 1997;19:473-476.
51. King AE, Thompson SWN. Brief and prolonged changes in spinal excitability following peripheral injury. *Semin Neurosci*. 1995;7:233-243.
52. Lin Q, Peng YB, Wu J, Willis WD. Involvement of cGMP in nociceptive processing by and sensitization of spinothalamic neurons in primates. *J Neurosci*. 1997;17:3293-3302.
53. Sluka KA, Milton MA, Willis WD, Westlund KN. Differential roles of neurokinin 1 and neurokinin 2 receptors in the development and maintenance of heat hyperalgesia induced by acute inflammation. *Br J Pharmacol*. 1997;120:1263-1273.
54. Sluka KA, Rees H, Chen PS, Tsuruoka M, Willis WD. Capsaicin-induced sensitization of primate spinothalamic tract cells is prevented by a protein kinase C inhibitor. *Brain Res*. 1997;772:82-86.
55. Chizh BA, Cumberbatch MJ, Herrero JF, Stirk GC, Headley PM. Stimulus intensity, cell excitation and the N-methyl-D-aspartate receptor component of sensory responses in the rat spinal cord in vivo. *Neuroscience*. 1997;80:251-265.
56. Sharma G, Stevens CF. A mutation that alters magnesium block of N-methyl-D-aspartate receptor channels. *Proc Natl Acad Sci U S A*. 1996;93:9259-9263.
57. Reichling DB, MacDermott AB. NMDA receptor-mediated calcium entry in the absence of AMPA receptor activation in rat dorsal horn neurons. *Neurosci Lett*. 1996;204:17-20.
58. Zheng X, Zhang L, Wang AP, Bennett MV, Zukin RS. Ca2+ influx amplifies protein kinase C potentiation of recombinant NMDA receptors. *J Neurosci*. 1997;17:8676-8686.
59. Lerea LS. Glutamate receptors and gene induction: signalling from receptor to nucleus. *Cell Signal*. 1997;9:219-226.
60. Coggeshall RE, Carlton SM. Receptor localization in the mammalian dorsal horn and primary afferent neurons. *Brain Res Brain Res Rev*. 1997;24:28-66.

61. Qu X-X, Cai J, Li M-J, et al. Role of the spinal cord NR2b-containing NMDA receptors in the development of neuropathic pain. *Exp Neurol.* 2009;215:298-307.

62. Barria A, Muller D, Derkach V, Griffith LC, Soderling TR. Regulatory phosphorylation of AMPA-type glutamate receptors by CaM-KII during long-term potentiation. *Science.* 1997;276:2042-2045.

63. Lisman J, Malenka RC, Nicoll RA, Malinow R. Learning mechanisms: the case for CaM-KII. *Science.* 1997;276:2001-2002.

64. Abbadie C, Trafton J, Liu H, Mantyh PW, Basbaum AI. Inflammation increases the distribution of dorsal horn neurons that internalize the neurokinin-1 receptor in response to noxious and non-noxious stimulation. *J Neurosci.* 1997;17:8049-8060.

65. Chapman V, Buritova J, Honore P, Besson JM. Physiological contributions of neurokinin 1 receptor activation, and interactions with NMDA receptors, to inflammatory-evoked spinal c-Fos expression. *J Neurophysiol.* 1996;76:1817-1827.

66. Clayton JS, Gaskin PJ, Beattie DT. Attenuation of Fos-like immunoreactivity in the trigeminal nucleus caudalis following trigeminovascular activation in the anaesthetised guinea-pig. *Brain Res.* 1997;775:74-80.

67. Huber KM, Sawtell NB, Bear MF. Effects of the metabotropic glutamate receptor antagonist MCPG on phosphoinositide turnover and synaptic plasticity in visual cortex. *J Neurosci.* 1998;18:1-9.

68. Vickery RM, Morris SH, Bindman LJ. Metabotropic glutamate receptors are involved in long-term potentiation in isolated slices of rat medial frontal cortex. *J Neurophysiol.* 1997;78:3039-3046.

69. Budai D, Larson AA. The involvement of metabotropic glutamate receptors in sensory transmission in dorsal horn of the rat spinal cord. *Neuroscience.* 1998;83:571-580.

70. Miletic V, Tan H. Iontophoretic application of calcitonin gene-related peptide produces a slow and prolonged excitation of neurons in the cat lumbar dorsal horn. *Brain Res.* 1988;446:169-172.

71. Rostas JA, Brent VA, Voss K, Errington ML, Bliss TV, Gurd JW. Enhanced tyrosine phosphorylation of the 2B subunit of the N-methyl-D-aspartate receptor in long-term potentiation. *Proc Natl Acad Sci U S A.* 1996;93:10452-10456.

72. Bito H, Deisseroth K, Tsien RW. Ca2+-dependent regulation in neuronal gene expression. *Curr Opin Neurobiol.* 1997;7:419-429.

73. Deisseroth K, Heist EK, Tsien RW. Translocation of calmodulin to the nucleus supports CREB phosphorylation in hippocampal neurons. *Nature.* 1998;392:198-202.

74. Lin Q, Peng YB, Willis WD. Inhibition of primate spinothalamic tract neurons by spinal glycine and GABA is reduced during central sensitization. *J Neurophysiol.* 1996;76:1005-1014.

75. Malcangio M, Bowery NG. GABA and its receptors in the spinal cord. *Trends Pharmacol Sci.* 1996;17:457-462.

76. Todd AJ, Watt C, Spike RC, Sieghart W. Colocalization of GABA, glycine, and their receptors at synapses in the rat spinal cord. *J Neurosci.* 1996;16:974-982.

77. Hwang JH, Yaksh TL. The effect of spinal GABA receptor agonists on tactile allodynia in a surgically-induced neuropathic pain model in the rat. *Pain.* 1997;70:15-22.

78. Gu ZZ, Pan YC, Cui JK, Klebuc MJ, Shenaq S, Liu PK. Gene expression and apoptosis in the spinal cord neurons after sciatic nerve injury. *Neurochem Int.* 1997;30:417-426.

79. Nishio E, Watanabe Y. NO induced apoptosis accompanying the change of oncoprotein expression and the activation of CPP32 protease. *Life Sci.* 1998;62:239-245.

80. Oliveira AL, Risling M, Deckner M, Lindholm T, Langone F, Cullheim S. Neonatal sciatic nerve transection induces TUNEL labeling of neurons in the rat spinal cord and DRG. *Neuroreport.* 1997;8:2837-2840.

81. Dumoulin A, Alonso G, Privat A, Feldblum S. Biphasic response of spinal GABAergic neurons after a lumbar rhizotomy in the adult rat. *Eur J Neurosci.* 1996;8:2553-2563.

82. Basbaum AI, Fields HL. Endogenous pain control systems: brainstem spinal pathways and endorphin circuitry. *Annu Rev Neurosci.* 1984;7:309-338.

83. Melzack R, Wall PD. Pain mechanisms: A new theory. *Science.* 1965;150:971-979.

84. Mansikka H, Pertovaara A. Supraspinal influence on hindlimb withdrawal thresholds and mustard oil-induced secondary allodynia in rats. *Brain Res Bull.* 1997;42:359-365.

85. Millan MJ. Descending control of pain. *Prog Neurobiol.* 2002;66:355-474.

86. Inoue A, Hashimoto T, Hide I, Nishio H, Nakata Y. 5-Hydroxytryptamine-facilitated release of substance P from rat spinal cord slices is mediated by nitric oxide and cyclic GMP. *J Neurochem.* 1997;68:128-133.

87. Yang SW, Guo YQ, Kang YM, Qiao JT, Laufman LE, Dafny N. Different gaba-receptor types are involved in the 5-ht induced antinociception at the spinal level: a behavioral study. *Life Sci.* 1998;62:PL143-PL148.

88. Wang R, King T, De Felice M, et al. Descending facilitation maintains long-term spontaneous neuropathic pain. *J Pain.* 2013;14(8); 845—53.

89. Vallone D, Picetti R, Borrelli E. Structure and function of dopamine receptors. *Neurosci Biobehav Rev.* 2000;24:125-132.

90. Bourgoin S, Pohl M, Mauborgne A, et al. Monoaminergic control of the release of calcitonin gene-related peptide- and substance P-like materials from rat spinal cord slices. *Neuropharmacology.* 1993;32:633-640.

91. Gao K, Mason P. Serotonergic raphe magnus cells that respond to noxious tail heat are not ON or OFF cells. *J Neurophysiol.* 2000;84:1719-1725.

92. Gear RW, Aley KO, Levine JD. Pain-induced analgesia mediated by mesolimbic reward circuits. *J Neurosci.* 1999;19:7175-7181.

93. Gilbert AK, Franklin KB. Characterization of the analgesic properties of nomifensine in rats. *Pharmacol Biochem Behav.* 2001;68:783-787.

94. Ciliax BJ, Nash N, Heilman C, et al. Dopamine D(5) receptor immunolocalization in rat and monkey brain. *Synapse.* 2000;37: 125-145.

95. Kitahama K, Nagatsu I, Geffard M, Maeda T. Distribution of dopamine-immunoreactive fibers in the rat brainstem. *J Chem Neuroanat.* 2000;18:1-9.

96. Hokfelt T, Arvidsson U, Cullheim S, et al. Multiple messengers in descending serotonin neurons: localization and functional implications. *J Chem Neuroanat.* 2000;18:75-86.

97. Millan MJ. The role of descending noradrenergic and serotoninergic pathways in the modulation of nociception: focus on receptor multiplicity. In: Dickenson A, Besson JM, eds. *The Pharmacology of Pain: Handbook of Experimental Pharmacology.* Vol. 130. Berlin, Germany: Springer-Verlag; 1997:385-446.

98. Schreihofer AM, Guyenet PG. Identification of C1 presympathetic neurons in rat rostral ventrolateral medulla by juxtacellular labeling in vivo. *J Comp Neurol.* 1997;387:524-536.

99. Simpson KL, Altman DW, Wang L, Kirifides ML, Lin RC, Waterhouse BD. Lateralization and functional organization of the locus coeruleus projection to the trigeminal somatosensory pathway in rat. *J Comp Neurol.* 1997;385:135-147.

100. Martin WJ, Gupta NK, Loo CM, Rohde DS, Basbaum AI. Differential effects of neurotoxic destruction of descending noradrenergic pathways on acute and persistent nociceptive processing. *Pain*. 1999;80:57-65.
101. Milne B, Hall SR, Sullivan ME, Loomis C. The release of spinal prostaglandin E2 and the effect of nitric oxide synthetase inhibition during strychnine-induced allodynia. *Anesth Analg*. 2001;93:728-733.
102. Jones SL. Noradrenergic modulation of noxious heat-evoked fos-like immunoreactivity in the dorsal horn of the rat sacral spinal cord. *J Comp Neurol*. 1992;325:435-445.
103. Paqueron X, Li X, Eisenach JC. P75-expressing elements are necessary for anti-allodynic effects of spinal clonidine and neostigmine. *Neuroscience*. 2001;102:681-686.
104. Hammond DL. Inhibitory neurotransmitters and nociception: Role of GABA and glycine. In: Dickenson A, Besson J-M, eds. *The Pharmacology of Pain: Handbook of Experimental Pharmacology*. Vol. 130. Berlin, Germany: Springer-Verlag; 1997:361-384.
105. Roussy G, Dansereau MA, Belleville K, et al. NTS1-preferring agonists produce spinal antinociception in a formalin tonic pain model. 2006; Society for Neuroscience Annual Meeting, Atlanta, GA.
106. Dansereau MA, Roussy G, Belleville K, et al. Potent antinociceptive effects of NTS1 agonists in a model of neuropathic pain. 2006; Society for Neuroscience Annual Meeting, Atlanta, GA.
107. Boules M, Shaw A, Liang Y, et al. NT69L, a novel analgesic, shows synergy with morphine. *Brain Res*. 2009;1294:22-28.
108. Boules M, Liang Y, Briody S, et al. NT79: a novel neurotensin analog with selective behavioral effects. *Brain Res*. 2010;1308:35-46.
109. Bredeloux P, et al. Synthesis and biological effects of c(lys-lys-pro-tyr-ile-leu-lys-lys-pro-tyr-ile-leu) (JMV2012), a new analogue of neurotensin that crosses the blood-brain barrier. *J Med Chem*. 2008;51:1610-1616.
110. Mechanic JA, Sutton JE, Berson AE, et al. Involvement of the neurotensin receptor 1 in the behavioral effects of two neurotensin agonists, NT-2 and NT69L: lack of hypothermic, antinociceptive and antipsychotic actions in receptor knock-out mice. *Eur Neuropsychopharmacol*. 2009;19:466-475.
111. Levi-Montalcini R. The nerve growth factor: its mode of action on sensory and sympathetic nerve cells. *Harvey Lect*. 1966;60:217-259.
112. Levi-Montalcini R. The saga of the nerve growth factor. *Neuroreport*. 1998;9:R71-R83.
113. Levi-Montalcini R, Dal Toso R, della Valle F, Skaper SD, Leon A. Update of the NGF saga. *J Neurol Sci*. 1995;130:119-127.
114. McMahon SB, Bennett DLH. Trophic factors and pain. In: Wall PD, Melzack R, eds. *Textbook of Pain*. 4th ed. New York, NY: Churchill Livingstone; 1999:105-128.
115. Chao MV. The p75 neurotrophin receptor. *J Neurobiol*. 1994;25:1373-1385.
116. Barbacid M. The Trk family of neurotrophin receptors. *J Neurobiol*. 1994;25:1386-1403.
117. Barbacid M. The Trk family of neurotrophin receptors: molecular characterization and oncogenic activation in human tumors. In: Levine AJ, Schmidek HH, eds. *Molecular Genetics of Nervous System Tumors*. New York, NY: Wiley and Sons;1993:123-135.
118. Clary DO, Weskamp G, Austin LR, Reichardt LF. TrkA cross-linking mimics neuronal responses to nerve growth factor. *Mol Biol Cell*. 1994;5:549-563.
119. Ibanez CF, Ilag LL, Murray-Rust J, Persson H. An extended surface of binding to Trk tyrosine kinase receptors in NGF and BDNF allows the engineering of a multifunctional pan-neurotrophin. *EMBO J*. 1993;12:2281-2293.
120. Carter BD, Kaltschmidt C, Kaltschmidt B, et al. Selective activation of NF-kappa B by nerve growth factor through the neurotrophin receptor p75. *Science*. 1996;272:542-545.
121. Baeuerle PA, Henkel T. Function and activation of NF-kappa B in the immune system. *Annu Rev Immunol*. 1994;12:141-179.
122. Lewin GR, Ritter AM, Mendell LM. Nerve growth factor-induced hyperalgesia in the neonatal and adult rat. *J Neurosci*. 1993;13:2136-2148.
123. Crowley C, Spencer SD, Nishimura MC, et al. Mice lacking nerve growth factor display perinatal loss of sensory and sympathetic neurons yet develop basal forebrain cholinergic neurons. *Cell*. 1994;76:1001-1011.
124. Ruit KG, Elliott JL, Osborne PA, Yan Q, Snider WD. Selective dependence of mammalian dorsal root ganglion neurons on nerve growth factor during embryonic development. *Neuron*. 1992;8:573-587.
125. Lindsay RM, Harmar AJ. Nerve growth factor regulates expression of neuropeptide genes in adult sensory neurons. *Nature*. 1989;337:362-364.
126. Petersen M, von Banchet S, Heppelmann B, Koltzenburg M. Nerve growth factor regulates the expression of bradykinin binding sites on adult sensory neurons via the neurotrophin receptor p75. *Neuroscience*. 1998;83:161-168.
127. Petty BG, Cornblath DR, Adornato BT, et al. The effect of systemically administered recombinant human nerve growth factor in healthy human subjects. *Ann Neurol*. 1994;36:244-246.
128. Thoenen H. Neurotrophins and neuronal plasticity. *Science*. 1995;270:593.
129. Andreev NY, Dimitrieva N, Koltzenburg M, McMahon SB. Peripheral administration of nerve growth factor in the adult rat produces a thermal hyperalgesia that requires the presence of sympathetic post-ganglionic neurones. *Pain*. 1995;63:109-115.
130. Woolf CJ, Ma QP, Allchorne A, Poole S. Peripheral cell types contributing to the hyperalgesic action of nerve growth factor in inflammation. *J Neurosci*. 1996;16:2716-2723.
131. Martin HA, Basbaum AI, Goetzl EJ, Levine JD. Leukotriene B4 decreases the mechanical and thermal thresholds of C-fiber nociceptors in the hairy skin of the rat. *J Neurophysiol*. 1988;60:438-445.
132. Amann R, Schuligoi R, Lanz I, Peskar BA. Effect of a 5-lipoxygenase inhibitor on nerve growth factor-induced thermal hyperalgesia in the rat. *Eur J Pharmacol*. 1996;306:89-91.
133. Bennett G, al-Rashed S, Hoult JRS, Brain SD. Nerve growth factor induced hyperalgesia in the rat hind paw is dependent on circulating neutrophils. *Pain*. 1998;77:315-322.
134. Malcangio M, Garrett NE, Cruwys S, Tomlison DR. Nerve growth factor- and neurotrophin-3-induced changes in nociceptive threshold and the release of substance P from the rat isolated spinal cord. *J Neurol Sci*. 1997;17:8459-8467.
135. Rich KM, Luszczynski JR, Osborne PA, Johnson EM Jr. Nerve growth factor protects adult sensory neurons from cell death and atrophy caused by nerve injury. *J Neurocytol*. 1987;16:261-268.
136. Mulderry PK, Dobson SP. Regulation of VIP and other neuropeptides by c-Jun in sensory neurons: implications for the neuropeptide response to axotomy. *Eur J Neurosci*. 1996;8:2479-2491.
137. Gold BG, Storm-Dickerson T, Austin DR. Regulation of aberrant neurofilament phosphorylation in neuronal perikarya. IV. Evidence for the involvement of two signals. *Brain Research*. 1993;626:23-30.
138. Hokfelt T, Zhang X, Wiesenfeld-Hallin Z. Messenger plasticity in primary sensory neurons following axotomy and its functional implications. *Trends Neurosci*. 1994;17:22-30.

139. Woolf CJ, Reynolds ML, Molander C, O'Brien C, Lindsay RM, Benowitz LI. The growth-associated protein GAP-43 appears in dorsal root ganglion cells and in the dorsal horn of the rat spinal cord following peripheral nerve injury. *Neuroscience.* 1990;34:465-478.

140. Bennett DLH, Michael GJ, Ramachandran N, et al. A distinct subgroup of small DRG cells express GDNF receptor components and GDNF is protective for these neurons after nerve injury. *J Neurol Sci.* 1998;18:3059-3072.

141. McMahon SB, Priestley JV. Peripheral neuropathies and neurotrophic factors: animal models and clinical perspectives. *Curr Opin Neurobiol.* 1995;5:616-624.

142. Apfel SC, Kessler JA, Adornato BT, Litchy WJ, Sanders C, Rask CA. Recombinant human nerve growth factor in the treatment of diabetic polyneuropathy. NGF Study Group. *Neurology.* 1998;51:695-702.

143. Apfel SC, Schwartz S, Adornato BT, et al. Efficacy and safety of recombinant human nerve growth factor in patients with diabetic polyneuropathy: a randomized controlled trial. rhNGF Clinical Investigator Group. *JAMA.* 2000;284:2215-2221.

144. Chattopadhyay M, Wolfe D, Huang S, et al. In vivo gene therapy for pyridoxine-induced neuropathy by herpes simplex virus-medicated gene transfer of neurotrophin-3. *Ann Neurol.* 2002;51: 19-27.

145. Bennett DL, Koltzenburg M, Priestley JV, Shelton DL, McMahon SB. Endogenous nerve growth factor regulates the sensitivity of nociceptors in the adult rat. *Eur J Neurosci.* 1998;10:1282-1291.

146. Aloe L, Tuveri MA, Carcassi U, Levi-Montalcini R. Nerve growth factor in the synovial fluid of patients with chronic arthritis. *Arthritis Rheum.* 1992;35:351-355.

147. Lowe EM, Anand P, Terenghi G, Williams-Chestnut RE, Sinicropi DV, Osborne JL. Increased nerve growth factor levels in the urinary bladder of women with idiopathic sensory urgency and interstitial cystitis. *Br J Urol.* 1997;79:572-577.

148. Bennett DLH, McMahon SB, Rattray M, Shelton D. Nerve growth factor and sensory nerve function. In: Brain SD, Moore PK, eds. *Pain and Neurogenic Inflammation Berlin,* Germany: Springer-Verlag; 1999.

149. Deng YS, Zhong JH, Zhou XF. Effects of endogenous neurotrophins on sympathetic sprouting in the dorsal root ganglia and allodynia following spinal nerve injury. *Exper Neurol.* 2000;164:344-350.

150. Ramer MS, Kawaja MD, Henderson JT, Roder JC, Bisby MA. Glial overexpression of NGF enhances neuropathic pain and adrenergic sprouting into DRG following chronic sciatic constriction in mice. *Neurosci Lett.* 1998;251:53-56.

151. Ramer MS, Thompson SWN, McMahon SB. Causes and consequences of sympathetic basket formation in dorsal root ganglia. *Pain Supp.* 1999;6:S111-S120.

152. Davis BM, Albers KM, Seroogy KB, Katz DM. Overexpression of nerve growth factor in transgenic mice induces novel sympathetic projections to primary sensory neurons. *J Comp Neurol.* 1994;349:464-474.

153. Davis BM, Goodness TP, Soria A, Albers KM. Over-expression of NGF in skin causes formation of novel sympathetic projections to trkA-positive sensory neurons. *Neuroreport.* 1998;9:1103-1107.

154. Jones MG, Munson JB, Thompson SW. A role for nerve growth factor in sympathetic sprouting in rat dorsal root ganglia. *Pain.* 1999 Jan;79(1):21-29.

155. Ramer MS, French GD, Bisby MA. Wallerian degeneration is required for both neuropathic pain and sympathetic sprouting into the DRG. *Pain.* 1997;72:71-78.

156. Shortland P, Woolf CJ. Chronic peripheral nerve section results in a rearrangement of the central axonal arborizations of axotomized A beta primary afferent neurons in the rat spinal cord. *J Comp Neurol.* 1993;330:65-82.

157. Woolf CJ, Shortland P, Coggeshall RE. Peripheral nerve injury triggers central sprouting of myelinated afferents. *Nature.* 1992;355:75-78.

158. Bennett DL, French J, Priestley JV, McMahon SB. NGF but not NT-3 or BDNF prevents the A fiber sprouting into lamina II of the spinal cord that occurs following axotomy. *Mol Cell Neurosci.* 1996;8:211-220.

159. Eriksson NP, Aldskogius H, Grant G, Lindsay RM, Rivero-Melian C. Effects of nerve growth factor, brain-derived neurotrophic factor and neurotrophin-3 on the laminar distribution of transganglionically transported choleragenoid in the spinal cord dorsal horn following transection of the sciatic nerve in the adult rat. *Neuroscience.* 1997;78:863-872.

160. Cho HJ, Kim JK, Zhou XF, Rush RA. Increased brain-derived neurotrophic factor immunoreactivity in rat dorsal root ganglia and spinal cord following peripheral inflammation. *Brain Res.* 1997;764:269-272.

161. Cho HJ, Kim SY, Park MJ, Kim DS, Kim JK, Chu, MY. Expression of mRNA for brain-derived neurotrophic factor in the dorsal root ganglion following peripheral inflammation. *Brain Res.* 1997;749:358-362.

162. Michael GJ, Averill S, Nitkunan A, et al. Nerve growth factor treatment increases brain-derived neurotrophic factor selectively in TrkA-expressing dorsal root ganglion cells and in their central terminations within the spinal cord. *J Neurosci.* 1997;17:8476-8490.

163. Burnstock G, Wood JN. Purinergic receptors: their role in nociception and primary afferent neurotransmission. *Curr Opin Neurobiol.* 1996;6:526-532.

164. Levine ES, Crozier RA, Black IB, Plummer MR. Brain-derived neurotrophic factor modulates hippocampal synaptic transmission by increasing N-methyl-D-aspartic acid receptor activity. *Proc Natl Acad Sci U S A.* 1998;95:10235-10239.

165. McMahon SB, Lewin GR, Wall PD. Central hyperexcitability triggered by noxious inputs. *Curr Opin Neurobiol.* 1993;3:602-610.

166. Shelton DL, Sutherland J, Gripp J, et al. Human trks: molecular cloning, tissue distribution, and expression of extracellular domain immunoadhesins. *J Neurosci.* 1995;15(pt 2):477-491.

167. Watanabe M, Endo Y, Kimoto K, Katoh-Semba R, Arakawa Y. Inhibition of adjuvant-induced inflammatory hyperalgesia in rats by local injection of neurotrophin-3. *Neurosci Lett.* 2000;282:61-64.

168. Ramer MS, Priestley JV, McMahon SB. Functional regeneration of sensory axons into the adult spinal cord. *Nature.* 2000;403:312-316.

169. Shu XQ, Llinas A, Mendell LM. Effects of trkB and trkC neurotrophin receptor agonists on thermal nociception: a behavioral and electrophysiological study. *Pain.* 1999;80:463-470.

170. Ohara S, Tantuwaya V, DiStefano PS, Schmidt RE. Exogenous NT-3 mitigates the transganglionic neuropeptide Y response to sciatic nerve injury. *Brain Res.* 1995;699:143-148.

171. Zhou XF, Deng YS, Chie EC, et al. Satellite-cell-derived nerve growth factor and neurotrophin-3 are involved in noradrenergic sprouting in the dorsal root ganglia following peripheral nerve injury in the rat. *Eur J Neurosci.* 1999;11:1711-1722.

172. Bland-Ward PA, Humphrey PP. Acute nociception mediated by hindpaw P2X receptor activation in the rat. *Br J Pharmacol.* 1997;122:365-371.

173. Chen CC, Akopian AN, Sivilotti L, Colquhoun D, Burnstock G, Wood JN. A P2X purinoceptor expressed by a subset of sensory neurons. *Nature.* 1995;377:428-431.

174. Lewis C, Neidhart S, Holy C, North RA, Buell G, Surprenant A. Coexpression of P2X2 and P2X3 receptor subunits can account for ATP-gated currents in sensory neurons. *Nature*. 1995;377:432-435.
175. Bradbury EJ, Burnstock G, McMahon SB. The expression of P2X3 purinoreceptors in sensory neurons: effects of axotomy and glial-derived neurotrophic factor. *Mol Cell Neurosci*. 1998;12:256-268.
176. Waxman SG, Cummins RR, Dib-Hajj S, Fjell J, Black JA. Sodium channels, excitability of primary sensory neurons, and the molecular basis of pain. *Muscle Nerve*. 1999;22:1177-1187.
177. Goldin AL. Diversity of mammalian voltage-gated sodium channels. *Ann N Y Acad Sci*. 1999;868:38-50.
178. Goldin AL. Resurgence of sodium channel research. *Annu Rev Physiol*. 2001;63:871-894.
179. Goldin AL, Barchi RL, Caldwell JH, et al. Nomenclature of voltage-gated sodium channels. *Neuron*. 2000;28:365-368.
180. Toledo-Aral JJ, Moss BL, He ZJ, et al. Identification of PN1, a predominant voltage-dependent sodium channel expressed principally in peripheral neurons. *Proc Natl Acad Sci U S A*. 1997;94:1527-1532.
181. Gurtu S, Smith PA. Electrophysiological characteristics of hamster dorsal root ganglion cells and their response to axotomy. *J Neurophysiol*. 1988;59:408-423.
182. Dib-Hajj S, Black JA, Felts P, Waxman SG. Down-regulation of transcripts for Na channel alpha-SNS in spinal sensory neurons following axotomy. *Proc Natl Acad Sci U S A*. 1996;93:14950-14954.
183. Dib-Hajj SD, Black JA, Cummins TR, Kenney AM, Kocsis JD, Waxman SG. Rescue of alpha-SNS sodium channel expression in small dorsal root ganglion neurons after axotomy by nerve growth factor in vivo. *J Neurophysiol*. 1998;79:2668-2676.
184. Waxman SG, Kocsis JD, Black JA. Type III sodium channel mRNA is expressed in embryonic but not adult spinal sensory neurons, and is reexpressed following axotomy. *J Neurophysiol*. 1994;72:466-470.
185. Cummins TR, Waxman SG. Downregulation of tetrodotoxin-resistant sodium currents and upregulation of a rapidly repriming tetrodotoxin-sensitive sodium current in small spinal sensory neurons after nerve injury. *J Neurosci*. 1997;17:3503-3514.
186. Black JA, Langworthy K, Hinson AW, Dib-Hajj SD, Waxman SG. NGF has opposing effects on Na+ channel III and SNS gene expression in spinal sensory neurons. *Neuroreport*. 1997;8:2331-2335.
187. Dib-Hajj SD, Tyrrell L, Black JA, Waxman SG. NaN, a novel voltage-gated Na channel, is expressed preferentially in peripheral sensory neurons and down-regulated after axotomy. *Proc Natl Acad Sci U S A*. 1998;95:8963-8968.
188. Fjell J, Cummins TR, Dib-Hajj SD, Fried K, Black JA, Waxman SG. Differential role of GDNF and NGF in the maintenance of two TTX-resistant sodium channels in adult DRG neurons. *Brain Res Mol Brain Res*. 1999;67:267-282.
189. Oyelese AA, Rizzo MA, Waxman SG, Kocsis JD. Differential effects of NGF and BDNF on axotomy-induced changes in GABA(A)-receptor-mediated conductance and sodium currents in cutaneous afferent neurons. *J Neurophysiol*. 1997;78:31-42.
190. Tanaka M, Cummins TR, Ishikawa K, Dib-Hajj SD, Black JA, Waxman SG. SNS Na+ channel expression increases in dorsal root ganglion neurons in the carrageenan inflammatory pain model. *Neuroreport*. 1998;9:967-972.
191. Tate S, Benn S, Hick C, et al. Two sodium channels contribute to the TTX-R sodium current in primary sensory neurons. *Nat Neurosci*. 1998;1:653-655.
192. Leffler A, Cummins TR, Dib-Hajj SD, Hormuzdiar WN, Black JA, Waxman SG. GDNF and NGF reverse changes in repriming of TTX-sensitive Na+ currents following axotomy of dorsal root ganglion neurons. *J Neurophysiol*. 2002;88:650-658.
193. Boettger MK, Till S, Chen MX, et al. Calcium-activated potassium channel SK1- and IK1-like immunoreactivity in injured human sensory neurones and its regulation by neurotrophic factors. *Brain*. 2002;125(pt 2):252-263.
194. Vergara C, Latorre R, Marrion NV, Adelman JP. Calcium-activated potassium channels. *Curr Opin Neurobiol*. 1998;8:321-329.
195. Khandwala H, Hodge E, Loomis CW. Comparable dose-dependent inhibition of AP-7 sensitive strychnine-induced allodynia and paw pinch-induced nociception by mexiletine in the rat. *Pain*. 1997;72:299-308.
196. Sato T, Shigematsu S, Arita M. Mexiletine-induced shortening of the action potential duration of ventricular muscles by activation of ATP-sensitive K+ channels. *Br J Pharmacol*. 1995;115:381-382.
197. Costigan M, Belfer I, Griffin RS, et al. Multiple chronic pain states are associated with a common amino acid-changing allele in KCNS1. *Brain*. 2010;133:2519-2527.
198. Hao J, Padilla F, Dandonneau M, et al. Kv1.1 channels act as mechanical brake in the senses of touch and pain. *Neuron*. 2013;77:899-914.
199. Fisher TE, Bourque CW. The function of Ca(2+) channel subtypes in exocytotic secretion: new perspectives from synaptic and non-synaptic release. *Prog Biophys Mol Biol*. 2001;77:269-303.
200. Diaz A, Dickenson AH. Blockade of spinal N- and P-type, but not L-type, calcium channels inhibits the excitability of rat dorsal horn neurones produced by subcutaneous formalin inflammation. *Pain*. 1997;69:93-100.
201. Wright CE, Angus JA. Effects of N-, P- and Q-type neuronal calcium channel antagonists on mammalian peripheral neurotransmission. *Br J Pharmacol*. 1996;119:49-56.
202. Bowersox SS, Gadbois T, Singh T, Pettus M, Wang YX, Luther RR. Selective N-type neuronal voltage-sensitive calcium channel blocker, SNX-111, produces spinal antinociception in rat models of acute, persistent and neuropathic pain. *J Pharmacol Exp Ther*. 1996;279:1243-1249.
203. Field MJ, Oles RJ, Lewis AS, McCleary S, Hughes J, Singh L. Gabapentin (neurontin) and S-(+)-3-isobutylgaba represent a novel class of selective antihyperalgesic agents. *Br J Pharmacol*. 1997;121:1513-1522.
204. Todorovic SM, Lingle CJ. Pharmacological properties of T-type Ca2+ current in adult rat sensory neurons: effects of anticonvulsant and anesthetic agents. *J Neurophysiol*. 1998;79:240-252.
205. Todorovic SM, Perez-Reyes E, Lingle CJ. Anticonvulsants but not general anesthetics have differential blocking effects on different T-type current variants. *Mol Pharmacol*. 2000;58:98-108.
206. Faggin BM, Nguyen KT, Nicolelis MA. Immediate and simultaneous sensory reorganization at cortical and subcortical levels of the somatosensory system. *Proc Natl Acad Sci U S A*. 1997;94:9428-9433.
207. Castro-Alamancos MA, Calcagnotto ME. Presynaptic long-term potentiation in corticothalamic synapses. *J Neurosci* 1999;19:9090-9097.
208. Gil Z, Amitai Y. Adult thalamocortical transmission involves both NMDA and non-NMDA receptors. *J Neurophysiol*. 1996;76:2547-2554.
209. Gil Z, Amitai Y. Properties of convergent thalamocortical and intracortical synaptic potentials in single neurons of neocortex. *J Neurosci*. 1996;16:6567-6578.
210. Sherman SM, Guillery RW. Functional organization of thalamocortical relays. *J Neurophysiol*. 1996;76:1367-1395.

211. Sherman SE, Luo L, Dostrovsky JO. Altered receptive fields and sensory modalities of rat VPL thalamic neurons during spinal strychnine-induced allodynia. *J Neurophysiol.* 1997;78:2296-2308.

212. Castro-Alamancos MA. Different temporal processing of sensory inputs in the rat thalamus during quiescent and information processing states in vivo. *J Physiol Soc.* 2002;539:567-578.

213. Hua SE, Garonzik IM, Lee JI, Lenz FA. Microelectrode studies of normal organization and plasticity of human somatosensory thalamus. *J Clin Neurophysiol.* 2000;17:559-574.

214. Chudler EH, Dong WK. The role of the basal ganglia in nociception and pain. *Pain.* 1995;60:3-38.

215. Lamour Y, Guilbaud G, Willer JC. Altered properties and laminar distribution of neuronal responses to peripheral stimulation in the SmI cortex of the arthritic rat. *Brain Res.* 1983;273:183-187.

216. Dong WK, Chudler EH, Sugiyama K, Roberts VJ, Hayashi T. Somatosensory, multisensory, and task-related neurons in cortical area 7b (PF) of unanesthetized monkeys. *J Neurophysiol.* 1994;72:542-564.

217. Guilbaud G, Benoist JM. Thalamic and cortical processing in rat models of clinical pain. In: Besson J-M, Guilbaud G, Ollat H, eds. *Forebrain Areas Involved in Pain Processing Paris.* France: John Libbey Eurotext; 1995:79-92.

218. Zhang X, La Salle G, Ridoux V, Yu PH, Ju G. Prevention of kainic acid-induced limbic seizures and Fos expression by the GABA-A receptor agonist muscimol. *Eur J Neurosci.* 1997;9:29-40.

219. Kao CQ, Coulter DA. Physiology and pharmacology of corticothalamic stimulation-evoked responses in rat somatosensory thalamic neurons in vitro. *J Neurophysiol.* 1997;77:2661-2676.

220. Shaw PJ, Salt TE. Modulation of sensory and excitatory amino acid responses by nitric oxide donors and glutathione in the ventrobasal thalamus of the rat. *Eur J Neurosci.* 1997;9:1507-1513.

221. Deller T, Frotscher M. Lesion-induced plasticity of central neurons: sprouting of single fibres in the rat hippocampus after unilateral entorhinal cortex lesion. *Prog Neurobiol.* 1997;53:687-727.

222. Benowitz LI, Routtenberg A. GAP-43: An intrinsic determinant of neuronal development and plasticity. *Trends Neurosci.* 1997;20:84-91.

223. Ramakers GM, De Graan PN, Urban IJ, et al. Temporal differences in the phosphorylation state of pre- and postsynaptic protein kinase C substrates B-50/GAP-43 and neurogranin during long-term potentiation. *J Biol Chem.* 1995;270:13892-13898.

224. Linden DJ, Wong KL, Sheu FS, Routtenberg A. NMDA receptor blockade prevents the increase in protein kinase C substrate (protein F1) phosphorylation produced by long-term potentiation. *Brain Res.* 1988;458:142-146.

225. Linden DJ, Routtenberg A. The role of protein kinase C in long-term potentiation: a testable model. *Brain Res Brain Res Rev.* 1989;14:279-296.

226. Battie MC, Videman T, Levalahti E, et al. Heritability of low back pain and the role of disc degeneration. *Pain.* 2007;131:272-280.

227. Nackley AG, Shabalina SA, Tchivileva IE, et al. Human catechol-O-methyltransferase haplotypes modulate protein expression by altering mRNA secondary structure. *Science.* 2006;314:1930-1933.

228. Van Meurs JB, Uitterlinden AG, Stolk L, et al. A functional polymorphism in the catechol-O-methyltransferase gene is associated with osteoarthritis-related pain. *Arthritis Rheum.* 2009;60:628-629.

229. Tegeder I, Costigan M, Griffin RS, et al. GTP cyclohydrolase and tetrahydrobiopterin regulate pain sensitivity and persistence. *Nat Med.* 2006;12:126-177.

Inflammation in Pain Disorders

John C. Keel
John M. Lavelle

INTRODUCTION

Pain is indeed an unpleasant experience; the perception of pain feels like damage or injury. Whether such damage is actual or potential, pain is usually described with the idioms of injury, including *inflammation*. The word itself conjures flames, fire, burning, redness, swelling...ouch! As students of the body, we know that *inflammation* refers to a complex biochemical process and is not a colloquialism to be used loosely. How often do patients describe their pain as swelling or fire, or ask "is it inflammation?" or "will this injection make the disc swelling go down?" How often are treatments variations of anti-inflammatories? Is inflammation truly there? This chapter serves as a review of evidence that there is a process of inflammation involved in some of the major conditions seen in the pain clinic: musculoskeletal pain and neuropathic pain. The general principles applicable are illustrated in detail by the specific examples of intervertebral disc disorders and complex regional pain syndrome.

Celsus' ancient description of the cardinal signs of inflammation includes rubor, calor, tumor, and dolor. These are, respectively, redness, heat, swelling, and pain. Others, including Virchow, later added loss of function as part of the cardinal descriptors of inflammation. Two thousand years after Celsus, we are beginning to understand the biochemical substrates underlying the cardinal properties of inflammation. Increasingly, inflammatory biochemical profiles are being discovered in association with all afflictions, from Alzheimer's to zoster. While disorders such as rheumatoid arthritis or gout have long been managed as inflammatory conditions, new knowledge of the inflammatory mechanisms underlying "noninflammatory" disorders gives hope that new treatments may be on the horizon.

REVIEW OF INFLAMMATION

Inflammation types include acute and chronic. The inflammation response may result from a variety of types of damage to body tissue; inflammation itself may perpetuate damage. Vascular response is a critical component of inflammation and includes vasodilation, increased small blood vessel flow adjacent to tissue damage, and increased permeability of blood vessels. These vascular changes are caused by chemical mediators histamine and prostaglandin, and the kinin and complement enzyme systems. Polymorphonuclear lymphocytes migrate first, then macrophages, through permeable blood vessels, and into the damaged tissue. Plasma proteins flow through permeable vessels into tissue, resulting in increased osmotic pressure there, and tissue edema by a process of exudation. Fibrinogen is converted into fibrin, which forms acute inflammatory exudate (and aids in clotting).

Chemical mediators are numerous in inflammation. Histamine causes the immediate dilation of vessels. Histamine is stored in mast cells, basophils, eosinophils, and platelets. Histamine release is activated by complement C3a and C5a and lysosomal protein from neutrophils. Complement proteins are glycoproteins that may form a membrane attack complex, and may amplify immune response. Serotonin is also a vasoactive mediator released by mast cells and basophils. Phospholipase, contained in cell membranes, produces arachadonic acid during inflammation. Arachadonic acid is rapidly formed into (1) prostaglandins, prostacyclins, thromboxanes, via the cyclooxygenase pathway, and (2) and leukotrienes and lipoxins, via the lipoxygenase pathway. Cytokines are a diverse group of locally acting glycoproteins with short half-lives that act on specific receptors to regulate cell function in inflammation. Cytokine categories include interleukins, interferons, tumor necrosis factors, growth factors, and chemokines.[1]

Enzyme systems involved in inflammation are alluded to earlier. The four major enzyme systems are complement proteins, kinins, coagulation factors, and the fibrinolytic system. The complement system may be involved in tissue necrosis, may be activated by antigen–antibody complexes in the classic pathway (or endotoxin is in alternate pathway), and are involved in the opsonization of bacteria. The kinins, such as bradykinin, are activated by coagulation factor XII and are mediators of vascular permeability and pain.

Many cell types are involved in inflammation. B lymphocytes secrete the antibodies that bind antigens to form a complex that activates complement. T lymphocytes secrete the cytokines and chemokines. Neutrophils, basophils, and eosinophils are known as granulocytes. Neutrophils are polymorphonuclear leukocytes (PML) and are the main cell of inflammation response, being the first cells drawn to the site of inflammation. They have granules containing cytotoxic substances as well as tissue remodeling substances. Neutrophils are next to respond, and both synthesize and are regulated by cytokines. Arachadonic acid and derivatives such as leukotrienes and prostaglandins are abundant in neutrophils. Macrophages derive from mononuclear phagocytes, known as monocytes. Macrophages may be primed, with enhanced major histocompatibility complex (MHC) class II expression. Such activated macrophages are important producers of inflammatory mediators such as arachadonic acid and derivatives. Macrophages play a role in neovascularization when activated by low oxygen conditions, such as in wounds, or cytokines. Mast cells occur in connective tissue typically (versus circulating in the bloodstream). The process of degranulation is the release of inflammatory mediators, contained in cytoplasmic granules, from mast cells and basophils. Mast cells and basophils are known for roles in allergic reactions. Eosinophils are leukocytes recruited to tissue sites of immune reaction; these are also known for allergic states. Chronic inflammation may differ from acute inflammation, although both may be present simultaneously; chronic inflammation may involve a predominance of monocytes and lymphocytes, rather than granulocytes.[2]

INFLAMMATION IN DISC DISORDERS

One of the most common examples of musculoskeletal pain is the painful intervertebral disc. Disc degeneration is actually a normal, expected part of the human experience. Disc degeneration is not always painful, but there may be increased likelihood of pain in those with magnetic resonance imaging (MRI) evidence of disc degeneration.[3] Clinical, animal, and tissue studies have implicated a number of inflammatory substances in painful disc disorders. In association with inflammatory processes, herniated nucleus pulposus alters nerve conduction and discharge, causes nerve fiber degeneration, alters intraneural capillary permeability and blood flow, and induces an inflammatory cascade.[4]

The normal structure of the intervertebral disc follows from its components, resulting in an orderly functional arrangement. The normal disc morphology allows the performance of its physiological functions, including movement and load bearing. In early life, the disc is arranged as a very ordered structure: It is comprised of a central gelatinous nucleus pulposus contained within a series concentric bundles of collagen fibers, which make up the annulus fibrosus.[5] With age and variations of stress through load bearing, the collagen bands (lamellae) develop increased complexity, including variations in the number and size. Thus, throughout life, as more stress is placed on the disc, there is a perpetuating cycle of disruption to disc morphology and cell organization resulting in degeneration.[5]

The lumbar intervertebral disc has a molecular and cellular makeup similar to articular cartilage. The nucleus pulposus' matrix is a combination of type II collagen, proteoglycans, and noncollagenous proteins synthesized from chondrocyte-like cells. The annulus fibrosus is primarily type I (and includes type II) collagen produced by fibroblast-like cells.[6] The proteoglycans consist of a central protein from which there are branching chains of glycosaminoglycans. Multiple proteoglycans are joined to a hyaluronic acid chain to form aggregates, held together by type II and IX collagen.[7] The proteoglycan matrix has hygroscopic properties which allow it to hold water molecules giving the nucleus hydrostatic properties, and thus, the nucleus can bear compressive forces. The matrix components fluctuate and are continually degraded by enzymes called the matrix metalloproteinases (MMPs).[8-10] Intervertebral disc herniation is likely preceded by physiologic degeneration of the disc caused by MMPs.[11]

Disc degeneration is a biochemical process involving altered rate of matrix breakdown and synthesis, change from type II to type I collagen, decreased aggrecan, and chondrocyte death.[12] Matrix metalloproteinases (MMPs), aggrecanase, and interleukin 1 (IL-1) have been strongly implicated in the degeneration, inflammation, and tissue destruction of the intervertebral disc.[13] IL-1 is the stimulator of chondrocytes to produce the matrix-degrading MMPs.[8,14,15] MMPs degrade matrix and produce matrix fragments, which in turn propagate further tissue destruction by activating cell-signaling pathways.[16] Cytokines, such as IL-1, interferon (IFN), and tumor necrosis factor-α (TNF-α) are produced by macrophages that invade the disc in response to injury.[17] The ability to invade the disc is due to the increased vascularity that develops as the normally avascular disc in the healthy adult becomes increasingly vascularized with degeneration. This leads to an increased supply of molecules such as cytokines.[5,18] Cytokines cause secretion of growth factors by disc cells, leading not only to this neovascularization, but also to an ingrowth of nerve fibers, altered sensitivity of nerve fibers, and granulation tissue formation. Macrophages secrete superoxide (O_2^-), which causes degradation of the proteoglycans, forcing them to deaggregate. That is, glycosaminoglycans of the extracellular matrix, especially aggrecan, are broken down by enzymes such as aggrecanase. Furthermore, superoxide will inhibit chondrocyte proliferation and synthesis. TNF-α and IL-1 stimulate the production of produce nitric oxide, which affects the matrix components directly via promotion of matrix degradation and inhibition of matrix synthesis.[19] Degeneration includes the production of abnormal components of the matrix and an increase in the mediators of matrix degradation (IL-1, TNF-α, superoxide, nitric oxide, MMPs).[20,21]

Herniated intervertebral disc tissue has been shown to produce a number of proinflammatory mediators and cytokines, although studies are not without controversy. Specifically, herniated intervertebral disc specimens have been shown to produce increased amounts of nitric oxide, interleukins-6 and 8 (IL-6 and IL-8), prostaglandin E2 (PGE2), and matrix metalloproteinases.[19,22] Burke and colleagues demonstrated a statistically significant difference between levels of production of IL-6 and IL-8 in the herniated discs of sciatica and low back pain groups ($p < 0.006$ and $p < 0.003$, respectively) compared to nonherniated discs.[22] These inflammatory markers found in disc tissue suggest that production of proinflammatory mediators within the nucleus pulposus may be a cause of the painful intervertebral disc. However, a study of cerebrospinal fluid in patients with lumbosacral radicular pain demonstrated no difference in IL-6 or TNF-α, and only 12 of 39 patients had an increase in IL-8, and, of those, no correlation was found with pain intensity.[23] Another study of cerebrospinal fluid concentrations of IL-1β, IL-6, and TNF-α found only increased concentration of IL-6 in patients with cervical myelopathy and lumbar radiculopathy but no clinical correlation involving the concentration of IL-6.[24]

Some studies do suggest a quantifiable relation of proinflammatory mediators with degree of disc abnormality. Using magnetic resonance imaging, Kanemoto and colleagues determined that MMPs were significantly correlated with the grade of intervertebral disc degeneration, and levels of MMPs observed in prolapsed lumbar intervertebral discs were significantly higher than that in nonprolapsed discs. Such a relation has also been demonstrated in cervical intervertebral discs, in that MMPs have been correlated with the size of osteophyte formation.[21,25]

Herniated disc tissues demonstrate high activity—for example, a 20- to 100,000-fold increase—of inflammatory phospholipase A2, revealing the occurrence of inflammation and an immune reaction in disc herniations.[26] Prostaglandins and leukotrienes are strong mediators of inflammation and are produced when phospholipase A2 releases arachidonic acid from cell membranes, causing inflammation, in this case at the site of disc herniations.[27] Cytokines induce phospholipase A2 activation: Nygaard showed there is a significantly higher concentration of leukotriene B4 and thromboxane B2 in noncontained versus contained disc herniation.[28] Therefore, varying inflammatory mechanisms are involved in different types of disc herniations. There are data suggesting that cumulative damage and elevated cytokine levels may be connected to incidence of low back pain: Ulrich demonstrated that recurrent disc injury results in persistent inflammation and enhanced disc degeneration.[29]

Inflammation of disc tissue may be a major factor in radicular pain. When the disc extrudes into the epidural space, it becomes like a foreign material and an immune response occurs, leading to an inflammatory cascade. The extruded discs express anti-interleukin-1, intracellular adhesion molecule-1, lymphocyte function-associated antigen, and basic fibroblast growth factor. These extruded discs express inflammatory mediators that could induce neovascularization and persistence of inflammation.[30] Woertgen analyzed the discs of patients who had undergone discectomy and found that those who did better after having the herniated disc material removed had a statistically significant correlation between the histologically proven inflammation and the outcome, as shown by the pain grading scale.[31] That is, when an inflamed disc was removed, the patient had a better outcome because it was likely the etiology of pain. Sequestered discs have been shown to be associated with a higher level of prostaglandin E2 content than extruded discs, while, in turn, extruded discs have been associated with higher prostaglandin E2 content than disc protrusions. Clinically, a positive straight leg raising test has been associated with a higher prostaglandin E2.[32]

Inflammatory markers have also been demonstrated in lumbosacral spinal stenosis. Cerebrospinal fluid concentration of IL-6 is increased in lumbosacral spinal stenosis, but studies are not consistent in correlating this with pain severity for this function.[33]

Animal model evidence supports the notion of inflammation in disc herniation and radiculopathy. In animal models, TNF-α causes neuropathologic injury in nerve roots and neuropathic pain, as when exogenous TNF-α is applied *in vivo* to rat nerve roots, resulting in behavior deficits that mimic experimental studies with herniated nucleus pulposus applied to nerve roots.[34] Also, TNF-α inhibitors prevent the injury-associated reduction of nerve conduction velocity and intraneural edema formation.[35] In a pig study of radiculopathy, wherein study animals had spinal nerve roots exposed to exogenous nucleus pulposus, application of aminoguanidine, a nitric oxide synthase inhibitor, significantly reduced the injurious effect of nucleus pulposus on nerve-conduction velocity in spinal nerve roots. Nucleus pulposus exposure (disc herniation) increases nitric oxide synthase activity in spinal nerve roots, and by inhibiting nitric oxide synthase, nucleus pulposus–induced edema and abnormalities in nerve-conduction velocity are countered. Such activity strongly suggests that nitric oxide, an inflammatory marker, is involved in the pathophysiology of the nucleus pulposus in disc herniation.[36] Other inflammatory markers are also implicated. For example, Kawakami demonstrated that thromboxane A2 and leukotriene B4 result in the hyperalgesia induced by application of nucleus pulposus to the lumbar nerve root in the rat. He applied thromboxane A2 synthetase inhibitor and leukotriene B4 receptor antagonist by injection into the epidural space and demonstrated decreased mechanical hyperalgesia after such epidural injection.[37]

Regulation of gene expression via signaling pathways may be involved in a variety of inflammatory conditions, including intervertebral disc disorders. For example, NF-κB and MAP kinases are known to be involved in disc degeneration. Expression of the proinflammatory cytokines such as TNF and interleukins are all upregulated by NF-κB. MAP kinases may be involved in maintenance of the extracellular matrix of the disc by regulation of anabolic and catabolic gene products. Targeting NF-κB and MAP kinases may be promising for future therapies for disc disorders.[38]

The preceding is a selection of human and animal evidence demonstrating that inflammation is involved in disc-related pain and degeneration. There is evidence of inflammation in disc disorders, in spite of the fact that the disc is a relatively avascular structure. In fact, it may be the inflammatory component of disc herniation or disruption, and not the physical or compressive component, that is most important in pathology of disc disorders. However, the existing evidence is not entirely consistent. It is rational to target the inflammation involved when treating pain related to discs not only with current modalities, but with future research. For example, studies have evaluated biomarkers as predictors in response to epidural steroid injection, and therapies involving gene, stem cell, and antibodies have been proposed.[39,40] TNF-α inhibition has been studied as a therapy for disc disorders, *in vitro* and *in vivo*, with mixed results.[39,41] There is also promising work under way on new MRI techniques that highlight inflammatory signals, which may distinguish painful discs versus nonpainful degenerated discs.[42] In fact, many of the MRI features of degeneration can already be understood as markers of inflammation. The breakdown of the hydrophilic extracellular matrix leads to loss of water content, resulting in the "dark disc" and decreased disc height seen on MRI. Cytokines migrate through the end plates into adjacent vertebral bone, leading to inflammatory response there, including marrow edema, seen as Modic changes on MRI.

INFLAMMATION IN NEUROPATHIC PAIN

Neuropathic pain is a major cause of suffering treated by pain physicians, but it has often been considered as a special class of pain, in contrast with the more commonly understood "normal" or nociceptive pain. Per the revised definition of the Neuropathic Pain Special Interest Group of the International Association for the Study of Pain, *neuropathic pain* is "pain arising as direct consequence of a lesion or disease affecting the somatosensory system," and may be graded as "definite," "probable," or "possible."[43] Common examples of neuropathic pain include postherpetic neuralgia, peripheral neuropathy, tic douloureux, and complex regional pain. What is often forgotten is that the lesion or disease affecting the somatic sensory system, resulting in neuropathic pain, may involve inflammation.

Immunologic pathways have a role in normal neurophysiology as well as pathologic states. Cells of both the central and peripheral nervous systems release cytokines and chemokines and have receptors for these molecules. For example, in response to injury, neurons produce molecules that activate microglia, which, in turn, produce cytokines and chemokines. The cytokines trigger the inflammatory cascade, while the chemokines induce chemotaxis of inflammatory cells such as monocytes, T cells, neutrophils, and granulocytes. Such immune activation is known to be associated with a wide spectrum of diseases of the nervous system, and a common feature is the previously discussed cytokine and chemokine activation.[44]

Tissue trauma may lead to both classic and neurogenic inflammation. Classic inflammation involves leukocyte release of cytokines such as IL-β, IL-2, and IL-6. In neurogenic inflammation, cytokines are released from neurons themselves. TNF-α may be elevated in neuropathic pain specifically presenting with allodynia; TNF-α further stimulates production of IL-1β and IL-6.[45,46] Neurons also may release neuropeptides such as substance P, calcitonin gene–related peptide (CGRP), bradykinin. These substances also produce the cardinal signs of inflammation.[47] Cytokines increase the amount of neuropeptide in primary afferents.[48] Neurogenic inflammation follows excitation of these primary afferents, consists of plasma extravasation and vasodilatation, and is mediated by CGRP and substance P. CGRP facilitates vasodilation. Substance P induces protein extravasation.[48] Nerve injury also leads to release of NGF, which is proinflammatory.[48]

When peripheral tissue is inflamed, sustained nociception induces cortex neuroplastic changes, or *central sensitization*. When peripheral nerves are injured, activated microglia produce cytokines and chemokines, which recruit neutrophils and macrophages and which themselves alter the blood–nerve barrier and directly damage nerves. For example, peripheral nerve excitability becomes increased directly by cytokines. In peripheral nerve injury states, Schwann cells can induce a T-cell and monocyte inflammatory response via production of chemokine CCL2. There are chemokine receptors in neurons such as primary afferents, dorsal root ganglia, and dorsal horn neurons. For example, in animal models, both peripheral tissue inflammation as well as peripheral nerve injury are associated with macrophage migration into dorsal root ganglia.[49-51] In peripheral nerve injury, migration of inflammatory cells may continue into the central nervous system itself, as the blood–brain barrier is transiently compromised (also demonstrated in animal models).[52,53] Chemokines such as CCL2 interact directly with receptors on these neurons, while also continuing to recruit inflammatory cells. Chemokine receptors may interact directly with μ-opioid receptors to increase pain. Interleukins accelerate neuropathic pain. For example, IL-1β sensitizes nociceptors in primary afferents, IL-1 induces substance P release in dorsal root ganglia, and IL-6 activates dorsal horn pathways after peripheral nerve injury.[44] Thus, *peripheral sensitization* also results after tissue trauma. Peripheral primary afferents release mediators such as substance P and bradykinin, increasing the irritability of these nerves. Clinically, this results in hyperalgesia or allodynia.[47]

Complex regional pain syndrome (CRPS) is a specific example of neuropathic pain illustrating the involvement of inflammation. CRPS type I (reflex sympathetic dystrophy) may follow trauma such as fracture, and CRPS type II (causalgia) may develop after definite peripheral nerve injury, but both types likely involve nerve injury. CRPS is characterized by sensory features including allodynia, hyperalgesia, distal sensory abnormalities, and disproportionate pain. Autonomic features of CRPS may include edema, perfusion abnormalities, and sweat gland and temperature changes of skin. CRPS may be associated with motor dysfunction as well. Sympathetically mediated pain may be a feature of CRPS. Trophic abnormalities may be present in bone or skin. Being truly complex and heterogeneous in presentation, many mechanisms are likely involved in CPRS, such as abnormalities of the central nervous system and sympathetic nervous system. Inflammatory factors are also involved in the development of CRPS at the local, systemic, and central nervous system levels.[47] Genetic variations in the inflammatory system, such as human leukocyte antigens and chemokine expression genes, are associated with CRPS.[47] Treatments targeting inflammation demonstrate benefit in CRPS (e.g., clinical trials of corticosteroids).[47]

CRPS-I animal modeling may involve controlled fracture of a large bone, whereas CRPS-II is modeled with sciatic nerve lesion.[48] An animal model involving reperfusion injury to a rat hindlimb is also used to model CRPS-I. Reperfusion injury is known to create inflammatory conditions, in general. Cytokines such as TNF-α, IL-1, IL-6, and transcription factor NF-κB, are elevated in the reperfusion limb model in the rat. In animal models of neuropathic pain, countering TNF-α reduces pain behavior.[54] Skin warmth, edema, and pain are reduced with glucocorticoid, and with NK1 (substance P receptor) antagonism, in animal models.[48] Pain behaviors are reduced with N-acetyl-L-cysteine, and 4-hydroxy-2,2,6,6-tetramethylpiperydine1-oxyl, and with IL-1 receptor antagonist and an NF-κB inhibitor, pyrrolidine dithiocarbamate.[55] In the animal model of CRPS-I in involving ischemia/reperfusion injury, evidence of increased nociception suggests that NF-κB and enhanced inflammatory response is involved in the development of CRPS. The postfracture rat model of CRPS-I also demonstrates inflammatory response including cytokines and clinical cardinal changes of inflammation.[47]

Clinical studies demonstrate increased proinflammatory cytokines such as TNF-α, IL-1β, IL-2, and IL-6, locally, in circulation, and in CSF, in patients with CRPS.[56-59] Patients with CRPS have reduced systemic mRNA for anti-inflammatory cytokines IL-4 and IL-10.[58] Levels of TNF-α and its receptor may be related to hyperalgesia and allodynia seen in neuropathic pain, including CRPS. Clinical studies demonstrate elevated TNF-α receptor type I in patients with CRPS who specifically suffer with hyperalgesia.[57] A single case report of TNF-α antibody (infliximab) demonstrates dramatic, prolonged improvement in pain intensity, temperature difference, and range of motion of the wrist in a patient with CPRS.[60] Elevated systemic CGRP has been found in patients with CRPS in several clinical studies.[61,62] Elevated bradykinin and substance P have been found in patients with CRPS.[62] Elevated substance P receptor NK1 expression in keratinocytes has been documented in skin biopsies of a patient with CPRS (and this has also been found in a rat tibia fracture model of CRPS).[63] A study of intradermal application of substance P in comparing controls to patients with CRPS found plasma protein extravasation increase in patients on both the affected and unaffected limbs, suggesting that inactivation of substance P may be impaired in patients with CRPS.[64] In summary, these cytokines and neuropeptides produce the cardinal signs of inflammation such as edema, warmth, and pain.[47,55] Neurogenic inflammation in CRPS is likely increased due to less deactivation of inflammatory neuropeptides, as well as increased receptors for inflammatory cytokines.[65]

Vasomotor, sudomotor, and trophic features of CRPS may also be explained by neuroinflammation and associated cytokines and neuropeptides. Endothelin-1 is a neuropeptide secreted from inflammatory cells that regulates vasoconstriction and also sensitizes primary and secondary afferents, in general.[66] Endothelin-1 is increased in patients with "cold" CRPS.[48] Chemokines and neuropeptides may be responsible for trophic changes seen in CRPS. These include hair and skin changes as well as patchy local osteoporosis. CGRP activates sweat glands and may be related to the hyperhydrosis seen in about 50% of CRPS cases.[48,67] Osteoclasts are activated by cytokines and substance P, explaining the local patchy osteoporosis seen in CRPS. CGRP causes hair growth.[48,47]

There is clinical evidence consistent with the reperfusion injury hypothesis of CRPS and the inflammatory process. Amputated limbs of patients with CRPS demonstrate findings consistent with reperfusion injury, including lipofuscin deposits, atrophic fibers, and thickened capillary basal membranes.[55]

In contrast to evidence regarding neuroinflammation, there is little evidence of a cell-mediated immune response in CRPS.[65] WBC and CRP are normal in CRPS.[68] Flow cytometry of lymphocytes, including activated T cells, showed no difference in patients with CRPS.[69] Patients with chronic CRPS may have higher percentages of proinflammatory CD14(+)CD16(+) monocytes.[70] There may be autoimmune mechanisms involved in CRPS, but the evidence is unclear at present.[65]

A systematic review and meta-analysis found several consistent specific systemic inflammatory features associated with CRPS. In acute CRPS, there are elevated blood concentrations of IL-8 and TNF-α receptors. In chronic CRPS, there are elevations of numerous cytokines—but, especially, TNF-α and bradykinin—in blood, blister fluid, and CSF. The meta-analysis found that not only is CRPS a systemic inflammatory condition, but that the inflammatory states differ in chronic and acute CRPS. This meta-analysis did not find consistent strong markers of neurogenic inflammation.[71]

Systematic reviews of treatments directed at inflammation for CRPS are inconclusive but do contain some promising results. For examples, in CRPS-I, randomized controlled trials demonstrate that free radical scavengers including N-acetylcysteine and dimethyl sulfoxide (DMSO) may be comparable in efficacy for pain, range of motion, and global improvement, while mannitol has no benefit. Randomized controlled trials and case series demonstrate pain reduction and global improvement with oral prednisolone, but no change in range of motion.[72]

Interest remains in exploiting inflammation with imaging modalities in the diagnosis of pain. Examples include functional MRI and PET imaging to highlight receptor activity and glial cell systems.[73]

INFLAMMATION IN OTHER PAIN CONDITIONS

While some pain conditions are readily associated with inflammation, such as rheumatoid arthritis, seronegative spondyloarthropathies, polymyalgia rheumatica, or inflammatory neuropathies, inflammation plays a wider role in pain disorders. The preceding sections present general principles of inflammation that are applicable in common musculoskeletal and neuropathic pain disorders by outlining specific evidence of inflammation in disc disorders and CRPS. However, elevation of inflammatory cytokines and reduction of anti-inflammatory cytokines may be characteristic of chronic pain in general.[74,75]

Osteoarthritis may be the classic "noninflammatory" pain. However, features of inflammation are found in osteoarthritis. Cardinal signs of inflammation are typical of acute pain flares in osteoarthritis, and these exacerbations respond to treatments directed at inflammation, such as systemic anti-inflammatory medications or joint injections. Synovitis may be detected at all stages of osteoarthritis: Inflammatory cell infiltration, including macrophages and T cells, as well as angiogenesis, are evident on histology of synovium. IL-6 is increased in synovial fluid in osteoarthritis and may activate systemic CRP elevation. C-reactive protein may be elevated osteoarthritis. Calcium pyrophosphate crystals may occur in osteoarthritis, and may induce chondrocyte expression of cytokines TNF-α, IL-6, and IL-8. Substance P, CGRP, bradykinin, histamine, 5-HT, PGE2, and others may be present in joints and periarticular tissues, where they mediate inflammation and pain itself. Inflammatory cytokines and nerve growth factor promote more inflammation, as well as facilitate peripheral and central sensitization. Cytokines stimulate chondrocytes to produce MMPs, and resulting breakdown products stimulate further tissue destruction. Acute osteoarthritis likely has a different inflammatory profile compared to chronic osteoarthritis.[76] Sound familiar?

Inflammatory cytokines are implicated in other common musculoskeletal conditions such as bursitis and tendonitis. IL-1β is expressed in inflamed tissue, is believed to correlate with the magnitude of inflammation, and also affects articular cartilage in the nearby joint. Production of IL-1β is increased in the synovium of the glenohumeral joint in patients with anterior instability, suggesting the presence of chronic inflammation at the site.[77] Inflammation in the subacromial bursa causes pain in patients suffering from rotator cuff tear, with chronic inflammation leading to fibrosis and thickening of the subacromial bursa. Both inflammatory cytokines and mechanical stress, and impingement in the subacromial space, might induce and worsen this inflammation. Immunohistological staining demonstrates expression of the proinflammatory markers IL-1β, TNF-α, TGF-β, and basic fibroblast growth factor (bFGF) in the subacromial bursa of patients suffering from a rotator cuff tear. In comparison, the expression of these inflammatory cytokines and growth factors was detected to only a small degree in subjects without anterior instability, severe shoulder pain, or impingement in the subacromial space. This suggests that those inflammatory markers may play an important role in inflammation of the subacromial bursa.[78]

Inflammation has been demonstrated with peripheral sensitization effect on meningeal nociceptors in migraine headache.[79] Inflammatory mediators such as bradykinin, histamine, serotonin (5-HT), and prostaglandin E2 (PGE2) have action on meningeal nociceptors, as seen in animal models.[80] Cytokines are believed to play a role in peripheral sensitization in migraine, especially IL-1, IL-6, IL-8, and TNF-α.[79] Inflammatory mechanisms may also play a role in central sensitization seen in migraine.

Diabetic peripheral neuropathy may result in part due to inflammation. Animal models indicate that microglia activation, in part via kinin B1 receptor, leads to release of pro-inflammatory substances that also alter neuronal excitability (and blocking the microglial kinin B1 receptor may be a treatment strategy.)[81] In a mouse model, anti-inflammatory stem cells had partial clinical improvement and along with decreased serum levels of inflammatory cytokines.[82] In a rat model, inhibition of the NF-κB inflammatory pathway using BAY 11-7082 resulted in clinical improvement and normalization of biochemical markers of neuroinflammation.[83] Clinical evidence comparing patients with diabetic peripheral neuropathy to control subjects correlates diabetic neuropathy with increased presence of CD14(+)CD16(+) monocytes, increased serum IL-6 and elevated CRP, and NF-κB activation.[84] Inflammation may be linked with the microvascular mechanisms associated with complications of diabetes, including retinopathy, nephropathy, and neuropathy.[85]

Sequelae of inflammation are found in herpes zoster and postherpetic neuralgia. The viral reactivation that defines zoster consists of inflammation and cell death of glial cells and neurons. The virus also travels to skin and causes local neural and skin inflammation. Immunostaining of sensory ganglia donated by patients with zoster demonstrate persistent inflammatory infiltrate.[86] Local spread of the inflammatory process under way in somatosensory cells to nearby motor cells can lead to the weakness and organ dysfunction sometimes seen in zoster.[87]

Alterations of inflammatory cytokines appear in fibromyalgia. A clinical study of serum markers found elevated CRP (high-sensitivity type), and these levels correlated with IL-6, IL-8, and ESR, as well as body mass index, in patients.[88] Substance P and CGRP levels in CSF are both elevated threefold in patients with fibromyalgia.[89,90] In a controlled study of women with fibromyalgia, IL-8 and CRP were elevated. This study also found increased monocyte release of cytokines IL-1β, TNF-α, IL-6, IL-10, IL-18, and MCP-1.[91] In particular, elevated serum IL-8 seems to be a consistent finding in such studies.[92-95]

Inflammation and its mediators are present in numerous other pain conditions. Sickle cell crises are partly mediated by endothelin receptors.[96] Endothelins also regulate cancer pain. NFKB activation contributes to pain in cancer patients, as does TNF-α (hence, the name, *tumor* necrosis factor).[97,98] Central pain results from mechanisms of inflammation. For example, in spinal cord injury, increased extracellular glutamate initiates an inflammatory cascade and formation of reactive oxygen species and neutrophil-mediated inflammation. The injury process produces activated glial cells, which express inflammatory cytokines and neuropeptides.[99] Peripheral vascular disease is considered an inflammatory disorder, much as is atherosclerosis.[100] Delayed-onset muscle soreness (DOMS) is a type of hyperalgesia in muscle that occurs about one day after eccentric exercise. Bradykinin, nerve growth factor, IL-6 receptor, and neutrophil migratory activity—all are inflammatory features that have been implicated in DOMS.[101,102,104]

Is there any "noninflammatory" pain left to consider? *Tendinopathy* may provide a distinct example. Tendinopathy is a common, painful degeneration process, often seen in rotator cuff, Achilles tendon, or other locations, and may be associated with pain, dysfunction, calcification, and rupture. Tendinopathy appears to be a chondrocyte and fibroblast cell-mediated abnormal or failed healing process, wherein neovascularization and inflammatory cells are sparse.[103] Tendinopathy is characterized by a disorganized proliferation of cells, including tenocytes, with a disorganized collagen structure and extracellular matrix.

We conclude by pointing out that this chapter is only an introduction to understanding inflammation. Inflammation is increasingly appreciated as a mechanism underlying much of human suffering, including pain disorders. The table outlines evidence for involvement of inflammation in a variety of pain conditions (**Table 4-1**).

TABLE 4-1 Evidence of Inflammation in Pain Disorders

Pain Condition	Selected Evidence of Inflammation
Intervertebral disc	• Cytokines stimulate chondrocyte production of MMPs, resulting breakdown products further promote inflammation • Neovascularization • Nerve ingrowth
Complex regional pain syndrome	• Cytokines and neuroinflammatory peptides • Neuroinflammation
Diabetic peripheral neuropathy	• Microglia activation via kinin B1R • Neuroinflammation
Zoster and postherpetic neuralgia	• Inflammation in glia, ganglia, peripheral neurons, skin • Spread of inflammation
Headaches	• Peripheral sensitization via inflammatory mediators and cytokines act on meningeal nociceptors.

(Continued)

TABLE 4-1 Evidence of Inflammation in Pain Disorders (*Continued*)

Pain Condition	Selected Evidence of Inflammation
Fibromyalgia	• Elevated CRP, ESR • Cytokine elevation, especially IL-8 • Neuropeptide elevation, substance P and CGRP (threefold)
Osteoarthritis	• Cardinal signs, synovitis • Cytokines stimulate chondrocyte production of MMPs, resulting breakdown products further promote inflammation • Neovascularization • Nerve ingrowth
Bursitis, tendinitis	• Cytokines, growth factors
Tendinopathy, enthesopathy	• Failed healing reponse
Delayed-onset muscle soreness	• IL-6 receptor decreased
Peripheral vascular disease	• Cigarette smoking, diabetes mellitus, promote oxidative stress • Multifactorial
Cancer pain	• NF-κB activation • TNF-α
Sickle cell	• Partly mediated by endothelin receptors
Central pain, spinal cord injury (SCI)	• Reactive oxygen species

REFERENCES

1. Leung L, Cahill C. TNF-α and neuropathic pain: a review. *Journal of Neuroinflammation*. 2010;7:27.
2. Kang JD, Hanks S. Chapter 3: Inflammatory basis of spinal pain. In: Slipman CW, et al., eds. *Interventional Spine: An Algorithmic Approach*. Saunders Elsevier;2008.
3. Chou D, Samartzis D, Bellabarba C, et al. Degenerative magnetic resonance imaging changes in patients with chronic low back pain: a systematic review. *Spine (Phila Pa 1976)*. 2011 Oct 1;36 (21 Suppl):S43-S53.
4. Brisby H. Pathology and possible mechanisms of nervous system response to disc degeneration. *J Bone Joint Surg Am*. 2006 Apr 01;88(Suppl 2):68-71.
5. Roberts S. Disc morphology in health and disease. 677th Meeting Held at Cardiff University, Wales, 16–18 July 2002 Speaker Manuscript. *Biochemical Society Transactions*. 2002;30:864-869.
6. Hadjipavlou AG. The pathophysiology of disc degeneration: a critical review. *J Bone Joint Surg Br*. October 2008;90-B(10): 1261-1270.
7. Eyre DR, Matsui Y, Wu JJ. Collagen polymorphisms of the intervertebral disc. *Biochem Soc Trans*. 2002;30:844-848.
8. Ito A, Mukaiyama A, Itoh Y, et al. Degradation of interleukin 1 beta by matrix metalloproteinases. *J Biol Chem*. 1996;271:14657-14660.
9. Matrisian LM. Metalloproteinases and their inhibitors in matrix remodeling. *Trends Genet*. 1990;6:121-125.
10. Urban JP, Maroudas A. Swelling of the intervertebral disc in vitro. *Connect Tissue Res*. 1981;9:1-10.
11. Goupille P, Jayson MI, Valat JP, Freemont AJ. Matrix metalloproteinases: the clue to intervertebral disc degeneration? *Spine*. 1998;23:1612-1626.
12. Freemont AJ. The cellular pathobiology of the degenerate intervertebral disc and discogenic back pain. *Rheumatology (Oxford)*. 2009;48(1):5-10.
13. Anderson DG, Tannoury C. Molecular pathogenic factors in symptomatic disc degeneration. *Spine J*. 2005;5(6 Suppl): 260S-266S.
14. Matsui Y. The involvement of matrix metalloproteinases and inflammation in lumbar disc herniation. *Spine*. 15 April 1998;23(8): 863-868.
15. Ohshima H, Urban JPG. The effect of lactate and pH on proteoglycan and protein synthesis rates in the intervertebral disc. *Spine*. 1992;17:1079-1082.
16. Feng H, Danfelter M, Strömqvist B, et al. Extracellular matrix in disc degeneration. *J Bone Joint Surg Am*. 2006;88(Suppl 2):25-29.
17. Shinmei M, Masuda K, Kikuchi T, Shimomura Y. Interleukin-1, tumour necrosis factor, and interleukin-6 as mediators of cartilage destruction. *Semin Arthritis Rheum*. 1989;18:27-32.
18. Kobayashi M, Squires GR, Mousa A, et al. Role of interleukin-1 and tumor necrosis factor alpha in matrix degradation of human osteoarthritis cartilage. *Arthritis Rheum*. 2005;52:128-135.
19. Kang JD, Stefanovic-Racic M, McIntyre LA, Georgescu HI, Evans CH. Toward a biochemical understanding of human intervertebral disc degeneration and herniation: contributions of nitric oxide, interleukins, prostaglandin E2, and matrix metalloproteinases. *Spine*. 1997;22:1065-1073.
20. Burke JG, Watson GRW, Conhyea D, McCormack D, Dowling FE, Walsh MG, Fitzpatrick JM. Human nucleus pulposis can respond to a pro-inflammatory stimulus. *Spine*. 2003 Dec 15;28(24):2685-2693.
21. Kanemoto M, Hukuda S, Komiya Y, Katsuura A, Nishioka J. Immunohistochemical study of matrix metalloproteinases-3 and tissue inhibitor of metalloproteinase-1 human intervertebral discs. *Spine*. 1996;21:1-8.
22. Burke JG, Watson RW, McCormack D, et al. Intervertebral discs which cause low back pain secrete high levels of proinflammatory mediators. *J Bone Joint Surg [Br]*. 2002;84-B:196-201.
23. Brisby H, Olmarker K, Larsson K, et al. Proinflammatory cytokines in cerebrospinal fluid and serum in patients with disc herniation and sciatica. *Eur Spine J*. 2002;11:62-66.
24. Nagashima H, Morio Y, Yamane K, et al. Tumor necrosis factor-α, interleukin-1β, and interleukin-6 in the cerebrospinal fluid of patients with cervical myelopathy and lumbar radiculopathy. *Eur Spine J*. 2009;18:1946-1950.
25. Peng B, Hao J, Hou S, et al. Possible pathogenesis of painful intervertebral disc degeneration. *Spine*. 2006;31:560-566.
26. Habtemariam, A. Immunocytochemical localization of immunoglobulins in disc herniations. *Spine*. 15 August 1996;21(16): 1864-1869.
27. Saal JS. High levels of inflammatory phospholipase A2 activity in lumbar disc herniations. *Spine*. 1990;15(7):674-678.
28. Nygaard, Ø. The inflammatory properties of contained and noncontained lumbar disc herniation. *Spine*. 1 November 1997;22(21):2484-2488.
29. Ulrich, J. ISSLS prize winner: repeated disc injury causes persistent inflammation. *Spine*. 1 December 2007;32(25):2812–2819.
30. Doita M, Kanatani H, Harada T, Mizuno K. Immunohistologic study of the ruptured intervertebral disc of the lumbar spine. *Spine*. 1996;21:235-241.
31. Woertgen, C. Influence of macrophage infiltration of herniated lumbar disc tissue on outcome after lumbar disc surgery. *Spine*. 1 April 2000;25(7):871-875.
32. O'Donnell JL. Prostaglandin E2 content in herniated lumbar disc disease. *Spine*. 15 July 1996;21(14):1653-1655.

33. Ohtori S, Suzuki M, Koshi T, et al. Proinflammatory cytokines in the cerebrospinal fluid of patients with lumbar radiculopathy. *Eur Spine J.* 2011 June;20(6): 942-946.
34. Igarashi T, Kikuchi S, Shubayev V, Myers RR. 2000 Volvo Award winner in basic science studies: exogenous tumor necrosis factor-alpha mimics nucleus pulposus-induced neuropathology. Molecular, histologic, and behavioral comparisons in rats. *Spine.* 2000 Dec 1; 25Room(23):2975-2980.
35. Olmarker K, Rydevik B. Selective inhibition of tumor necrosis factor-alpha prevents nucleus pulposus-induced thrombus formation, intraneural edema, and reduction of nerve conduction velocity: possible implications for future pharmacologic treatment strategies of sciatica. *Spine.* 2001 Apr 15;26(8):863-869.
36. Brisby H, Byrod G, Olmarker K, Miller VM, Aoki Y, Rydevik B. Nitric oxide as a mediator of nucleus pulposus-induced effects on spinal nerve roots. *J Orthop Res.* 2000 Sep;18(5):815-820.
37. Kawakami M. Roles of thromboxane A2 and leukotriene B4 in radicular pain induced by herniated nucleus pulposus. *Journal of Orthopaedic Research.* 2001;19:472-477.
38. Wuertz K, Vo N, Kletsas D, et al. Inflammatory and catabolic signalling in intervertebral discs: The roles of NF-κB and MAP kinases. *European Cells and Materials.* 2012;23:103-120.
39. Cohen SP, White RL, Kurihara C, et al. Epidural steroids, etanercept, or saline in subacute sciatica: a multicenter, randomized trial. *Ann Intern Med.* 2012 Apr 17;156(8):551-559.
40. Golish SR, Hanna LS, Bowser R, et al. Outcome of lumbar epidural steroid injection is predicted by assay of a complex of fibronectin and aggrecan from epidural lavage. *Spine.* 15 August 2011;36(18):1464-1469.
41. Sinclair SM, Shamji MF, Chen J, et al. Attenuation of inflammatory events in human intervertebral disc cells with a tumor necrosis factor antagonist. *Spine (Phila Pa 1976).* 2011 July 1;36(15): 1190-1196.
42. Lotz JC, Haughton V, Boden SD, et al. New treatments and imaging strategies in degenerative disease of the intervertebral disks. *Radiology.* July 2012;264(1):6-19.
43. Geber C, Baumgärtner U, Schwab R, et al. Revised definition of neuropathic pain and its grading system: an open case series illustrating its use in clinical practice. *Am J Med.* 2009 Oct;122(10 Suppl):S3-S12.
44. Ramesh G, Maclean AG, Philipp MT. Cytokines and chemokines at the crossroads of neuroinflammation, neurodegeneration, and neuropathic pain. *Mediators Inflamm.* 2013;2013, Article 480739, 20 pages.
45. Ludwig J, Binder A, Steinmann J, et al. Cytokine expression in serum and cerebrospinal fluid in non-inflammatory polyneuropathies. *J Neurol Neurosurg Psychiatry.* 2008;79:1268-1273.
46. Sommer C, Kress M. Recent findings on how proinflammatory cytokines cause pain: Peripheral mechanisms in inflammatory and neuropathic hyperalgesia. *Neurosci Lett.* 2004;361:184-187.
47. Bruehl S. An update on the pathophysiology of complex regional pain syndrome. *Anesthesiology.* 2010;113:713-725.
48. Birklein F, Schmelz M. Neuropeptides, neurogenic inflammation and complex regional pain syndrome (CRPS). *Neuroscience Letters.* 2008;437:199-202.
49. von Banchet GS, Boettger MK, Fischer N, et al. Experimental arthritis causes tumor necrosis factor-alpha-dependent infiltration of macrophages into rat dorsal root ganglia which correlates with pain-related behavior. *Pain.* 2009;145(1-2):151-159.
50. Hu P, McLachlan EM. Macrophage and lymphocyte invasion of dorsal root ganglia after peripheral nerve lesions in the rat. *Neuroscience.* 2002;112(1):23-38.
51. Morin N, Owolabi SA, Harty MW, et al. Neutrophils invade lumbar dorsal root ganglia after chronic constriction injury of the sciatic nerve. *J Neuroimmunol.* 2007;184(1-2):164-171.
52. Beggs S, Liu XJ, Kwan C, Salter MW. Peripheral nerve injury and TRPV1-expressing primary afferent C-fibers cause opening of the blood-brain barrier. *Mol Pain.* 2010 Nov 2;6:74.
53. Sweitzer SM, Hickey WF, Rutkowski MD, et al. Focal peripheral nerve injury induces leukocyte trafficking into the central nervous system: potential relationship to neuropathic pain. *Pain.* 2002;100(1-2):163-170.
54. Sommer C, Lindenlaub T, Teuteberg P, et al. Anti-TNF-neutralizing antibodies reduce pain-related behavior in two different mouse models of painful mononeuropathy. *Brain Res.* 2001;913:86-89.
55. Coderre TJ, Bennett GJ. A hypothesis for the cause of complex regional pain syndrome-type i (reflex sympathetic dystrophy): pain due to deep-tissue microvascular pathology. *Pain Medicine.* 2010;11:1224-1238.
56. Alexander GM, van Rijn MA, van Hilten JJ, et al. Changes in cerebrospinal fluid levels of pro-inflammatory cytokines in CRPS. *Pain.* 2005;116:213-219.
57. Maihofner C, Handwerker HO, Neundorfer B, et al. Mechanical hyperalgesia in complex regional pain syndrome: a role for TNF-alpha? *Neurology.* 2005;65:311-313.
58. Uçeyler N, Eberle T, Rolke R, et al. Differential expression patterns of cytokines in complex regional pain syndrome. *Pain.* 2007 Nov;132(1-2):195-205. Epub 2007 Sep 24.
59. Wesseldijk F, Huygen FJ, Heijmans-Antonissen C, et al. Tumor necrosis factor-alpha and interleukin-6 are not correlated with the characteristics of Complex Regional Pain Syndrome type 1 in 66 patients. *Eur J Pain.* 2008;12:716-721.
60. Bernateck M, Rolke R, Birklein F, et al. Successful intravenous regional block with low dose tumor necrosis factor-alpha antibody infliximab for treatment of complex regional pain syndrome 1. *Anesth Analg.* 2007;105:1148-1151.
61. Birklein F, Schmelz M, Schifter S, et al. The important role of neuropeptides in complex regional pain syndrome. *Neurology.* 2001;57:2179-2184.
62. Blair SJ, Chinthagada M, Hoppenstehdt D, et al. Role of neuropeptides in pathogenesis of reflex sympathetic dystrophy. *Acta Orthop Belg.* 1998;64:448-451.
63. Kingery WS. Role of neuropeptide, cytokine, and growth factor signaling in complex regional pain syndrome. *Pain Med.* 2010;11:1239-1250.
64. Leis S, Weber M, Isselmann A, et al. Substance-P-induced protein extravasation is bilaterally increased in complex regional pain syndrome. *Exp Neurol.* 2003;183:197-204.
65. Marinus J, Moseley GL, Birklein F, et al. Clinical features and pathophysiology of complex regional pain syndrome. *Lancet Neurol.* 2011;10: 637-648.
66. Mujenda FH, Duarte AM, Reilly EK, et al. Cutaneous endothelin-A receptors elevate post-incisional pain. *Pain.* 2007;133:161-173.
67. Schlereth T, Dittmar JO, Seewald B, Birklein F. Peripheral amplification of sweating—a role for calcitonin generelated peptide. *J Physiol.* 2006;576:823-832.
68. Schinkel C, Gaertner A, Zaspel J, et al. Inflammatory mediators are altered in the acute phase of posttraumatic complex regional pain syndrome. *Clin J Pain.* 2006;22:235-239.
69. Ribbers GM, Oosterhuis WP, van Limbeek J, et al. Reflex sympathetic dystrophy: is the immune system involved? *Arch Phys Med Rehabil.* 1998 Dec;79(12):1549-1552.

70. Ritz BW, Alexander GM, Nogusa S, et al. Elevated blood levels of inflammatory monocytes (CD14(+) CD16(+)) in patients with complex regional pain syndrome. *Clin Exp Immunol.* 2011;164:108-117.
71. Parkitny L, McAuly JH, Di Pietro F, et al. Inflammation in complex regional pain syndrome: A systematic review and meta-analysis. *Neurology.* 2013 Jan 1;80(1):106-117.
72. Fischer S, Zuurmond WWA, Birlein F, et al. Anti-inflammatory treatment of Complex Regional Pain Syndrome. *Pain.* 2010;151:251-256.
73. Linnman C, Becerra L, Borsook D. Inflaming the brain: CRPS a model disease to understand neuroimmune interactions in chronic pain. *J Neuroimmune Pharmacol.* 2013 Jun;8(3)547-563.
74. Koch A, Zacharowski K, Boehm O, et al. Nitric oxide and proinflammatory cytokines correlate with pain intensity in chronic pain patients. *Inflamm Res.* 2007;56:32-37.
75. Uçeyler N, Valenza R, Stock M, et al. Reduced levels of antiinflammatory cytokines in patients with chronic widespread pain. *Arthritis Rheum.* 2006;54:2656-2664.
76. Bonnet CS, Walsh DA. Osteoarthritis, angiogenesis and inflammation. *Rheumatology* (Oxford). 2005 Jan;44(1):7-16. Epub 2004 Aug 3.
77. Gotoh M, Hamada K, Yamakawa H, Nakamura M, Yamazaki H, Inoue A, Fukuda H. Increased interleukin-1beta production in the synovium of glenohumeral joints with anterior instability. *J Orthop Res.* 1999 May;17(3):392-397.
78. Sakai H, Fujita K, Sakai Y, Mizuno K. Immunolocalization of cytokines and growth factors in subacromial bursa of rotator cuff tear patients. *Kobe J Med Sci.* 2001 Feb;47(1):25-34.
79. Burstein R, Jakubowski M, Rauch SD. The science of migraine. *J Vestib Res.* 2011;21(6): 305-314.
80. Levy D, Strassman AM. Distinct sensitizing effects of the cAMP-PKA second messenger cascade on rat dural mechanonociceptors. *J Physiol.* 2002;538:483-493.
81. Talbot S, Couture R. Emerging role of microglial kinin B1 receptor in diabetic pain neuropathy. *Exp Neurol.* 2012 Apr;234(2):373-381.
82. Waterman RS, Morgenweck J, Nossaman BD, et al. Anti-inflammatory mesenchymal stem cells (MSC2) attenuate symptoms of painful diabetic peripheral neuropathy. *Stem Cells Transl Med.* 2012 Jul;1(7):557-565.
83. Kumar A, Negi G, Sharma SS. Suppression of NF-κB and NF-κB regulated oxidative stress and neuroinflammation by BAY 11-7082 (IκB phosphorylation inhibitor) in experimental diabetic neuropathy. *Biochimie.* 2012 May;94(5):1158-1165.
84. Yang M, Gan H, Shen Q, et al. Proinflammatory CD14+CD16+ monocytes are associated with microinflammation in patients with type 2 diabetes mellitus and diabetic nephropathy uremia. *Inflammation.* 2012 Feb;35(1):388-396.
85. Kaul K, Hodgkinson A, Tarr JM, et al. Is inflammation a common retinal-renal-nerve pathogenic link in diabetes? *Curr Diabetes Rev.* 2010 Sep;6(5):294-303.
86. Gowrishankar K, Steain M, Cunningham AL, et al. Characterization of the host immune response in human ganglia after herpes zoster. *J Virol.* 2010 Sep;84(17):8861-8870.
87. Oaklander AL. Mechanisms of pain and itch caused by herpes zoster (shingles). *The Journal of Pain.* 2008 January;9(1 Suppl. 1):S10-S18.
88. Xiao Y, Haynes WL, Michalek JE, Russell IJ. Elevated serum high-sensitivity C-reactive protein levels in fibromyalgia syndrome patients correlate with body mass index, interleukin-6, interleukin-8, erythrocyte sedimentation rate. *Rheumatol Int.* 2013;33:1259-1264.
89. Russell IJ, Orr MD, Littman B, et al. Elevated cerebrospinal levels of substance P in patients with the fibromyalgia syndrome. *Arthritis Rheum.* 1994;37:159-1601.
90. Fischer HP, Eich W, Russell IJ. A possible role for saliva as a diagnostic fluid in patients with chronic pain. *Semin Arthritis Rheum.* 1998;27:348-359.
91. Bote ME, Garcia JJ, Hinchado MD, et al. Inflammatory/stress feedback dysregulation in women with fibromyalgia. *Neuroimmunomodulation.* 2012;19:343-351.
92. Wallace DJ, Linker-Israeli M, Hallegua D, et al. Cytokines play an aetiopathogenetic role in fibromyalgia: a hypothesis and pilot study. *Rheumathology.* 2001;40:743-749.
93. Gür A, Karakoç M, Nas K, Cevik R, et al. Cytokines and depression in cases with fibromylagia. *J Rheumatol.* 2002; 29:358-361.
94. Ortega E, García JJ, Bote ME, et al. Exercise in fibromialgia and related inflammatory disorders: known effects and unknown chances. *Exerc Immunol Rev.* 2009;15:42-65.
95. Bazzichi L, Rossi A, Massimetti G, et al. Cytokine patterns in fibromyalgia and their correlation with clinical manifestations. *Clin Exp Rheumatol.* 2007;25:225-230.
96. Khodorova A, Montmayeur JP, Strichartz G. Endothelin receptors and pain. *J Pain.* 2009 January;10(1):4-28.
97. Gupta SC, Kim JH, Kannappan R, et al. Role of nuclear factor-κB-mediated inflammatory pathways in cancer-related symptoms and their regulation by nutritional agents. *Exp Biol Med (Maywood).* 2011 June 1;236(6):658-671.
98. Bennett GJ. Pathophysiology of cancer-related painful neuropathy. *The Oncologist.* 2010;15(suppl 2):9-12.
99. Hulsebosch CE, Hains BC, Crown ED, et al. Mechanisms of chronic central neuropathic pain after spinal cord injury. *Brain Res Rev.* 2009 April;60(1):202-213.
100. Brevetti G, Giugliano G, Brevetti L, et al. Inflammation in peripheral artery disease. *Circulation.* 2010;122:1862–1875.
101. Murase S, Terazawa E, Queme F, et al. Bradykinin and nerve growth factor play pivotal roles in muscular mechanical hyperalgesia after exercise (delayed-onset muscle soreness). *J Neurosci.* 2010 Mar 10;30(10):3752-3761.
102. Robson-Ansley P, Cockburn E, Walshe I, et al. The effect of exercise on plasma soluble IL-6 receptor concentration: a dichotomous response. *Exerc Immunol Rev.* 2010;16:56-76.
103. Oliva F, Giai Via A, Nicola M. Physiopathology of intratendinous calcific deposition. *BMC Medicine.* 2012;10:95.
104. Kanda K, Sugama K, Hayashida H, et al. Eccentric exercise-induced delayed-onset muscle soreness and changes in markers of muscle damage and inflammation. *Exerc Immunol Rev.* 2013; 19:72-85.

CHAPTER 5

Physiologic and Pathologic Gait

Anthony C. Lee

GAIT ANALYSIS

Analysis of a patient's gait (the way a person walks) can reveal biomechanical deficits that could be addressed by physical therapy, prescribed medical equipment, interventional procedures, or even surgery. While a gait defect alone does not warrant treatment, the combination of pain and neurological deficits from nerve involvement, including muscle weakness that results in a gait deficit, can all improve with proper management.

We must distinguish between a *gait abnormality*, which is caused by a particular myotomal deficit that is either compensated by other myotomal activity or not compensated, versus an *antalgic gait*, which is an inconsistent alteration in gait in a nonmyotomal pattern that serves as an expression of the degree of pain.

Before a practitioner can analyze gait, understanding the basic features of gait is paramount so that a deficit can readily be identified.

DEFINITIONS

Stride length: The linear distance between any point along the contact surface of the foot with the ground with the same point of contact of the same foot with the ground after taking two steps. For example, the distance from right heel strike to the next right heel strike is the stride length. Normal stride length is approximately 56 inches. (See **Fig. 5-1**.)

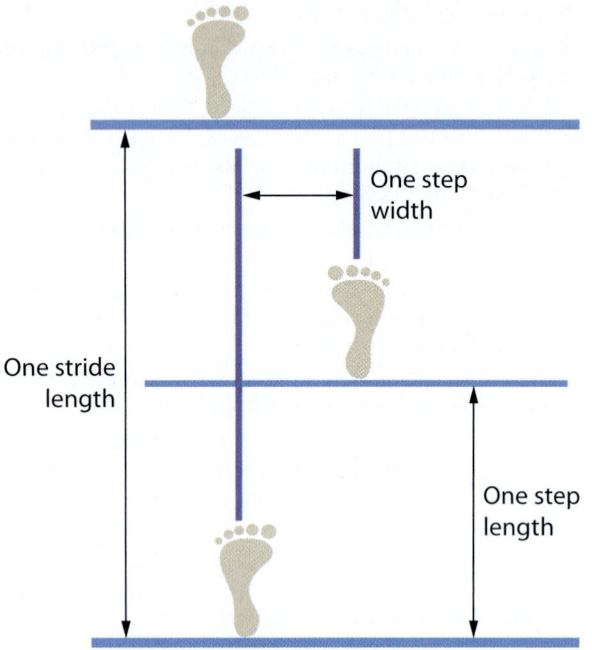

FIGURE 5-1. Stride length, step length, and step width.

Step length: The longitudinal (the net direction of ambulation) projection of the linear distance between any point along the contact surface of the foot with the ground with the same point of contact of the contralateral foot with the ground after taking one step. For example, the longitudinal distance from right heel strike to the next left heel strike is the step length. Not taking hypotenuse distances in consideration, roughly two step lengths equal one stride length. Normal step length is approximately 28 inches. (See Fig. 5-1.)

Step width: The lateral (orthogonal to the longitudinal direction) projection of the linear distance between any point along the contact surface of the foot with the ground with the same point of contact of the contralateral foot with the ground after taking one step. Normal step width is approximately 3 inches. This measurement is also known as the walking base. (See Fig. 5-1.)

Gait cycle: All the musculoskeletal activities that occur during the time it takes to traverse one stride length. The gait cycle consists of the stance phase and the swing phase.

Cadence: The number of steps per minute. Normal cadence is approximately 115 steps per minute.

Normal walking speed: Approximately 80 meters per minute or 3 mph.

Center of gravity: The center of gravity for a normal human standing upright is located approximately 5 cm anterior to the S2 vertebral body. During the gait cycle, this center of gravity moves 5 cm horizontally and 5 cm vertically. Maximum gait efficiency results in optimization of this movement to allow for the lowest possible energy expenditure during ambulation. Deviation from this optimization results in increased energy expenditure and decreased walking distances due to fatigue.

THE GAIT CYCLE (FIG. 5-2)

Stance phase: The period of time that the foot is in contact with the ground. It is subdivided into five phases: initial contact, loading response, midstance, terminal stance, and preswing. The stance phase makes up approximately 60% of the gait cycle.

Swing phase: The period of time that the foot is not contacting the ground. It is subdivided into three phases: initial swing, midswing, and terminal swing. The swing phase makes up approximately 40% of the gait cycle.

Double support: The period of time that both feet are in contact with the ground (i.e., the heel of the anterior foot and the ball/toes of the posterior foot). Approximately 20% of the gait cycle is spent in double support. The quicker the ambulation, the lower the percentage of time that is spent in double support. There is no double support in running.

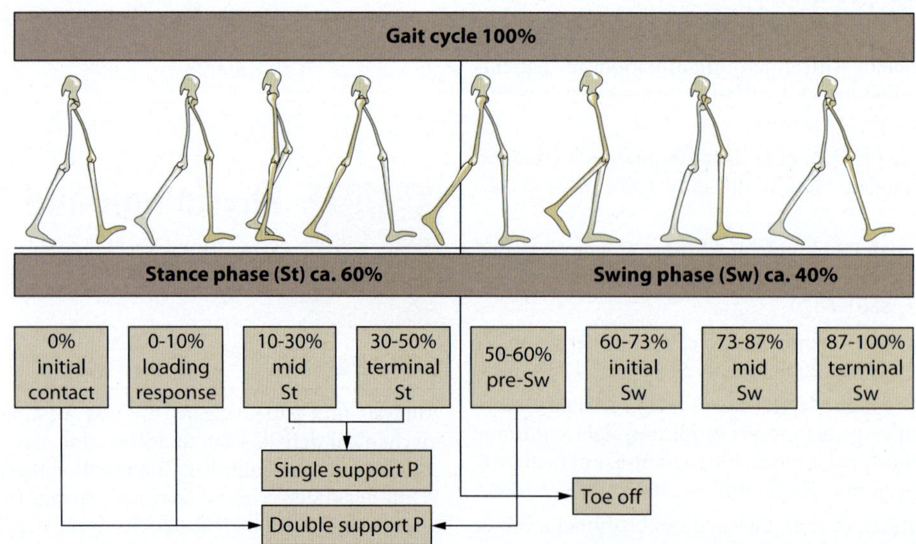

FIGURE 5-2. The gait cycle. (M. Hartmann, F. Kreuzpointner, R. Haefner, H. Michels, A. Schwirtz, and J. P. Haas: Effects of Juvenile Idiopathic Arthritis on Kinematics and Kinetics of the Lower Extremities Call for Consequences in Physical Activities Recommendations. International Journal of PediatricsVolume 2010 (2010). Hindawi Publishing Corporation.)

Stance-Phase Components **Initial contact:** Appearing when the heel strikes the ground, this phase consists of the first 0% to 2% of the gait cycle and is facilitated by eccentric contraction of the gluteus maximus (L5-S2, inferior gluteal nerve), gluteus medius (L4-S1, superior gluteal nerve), hamstrings (L5-S2, tibial division of the sciatic nerve), quadriceps (L2-4, femoral nerve), and dorsiflexors (L4-5, deep peroneal nerve).

Loading response: Appearing as the period between heel strike and flat foot, this phase consists of the next 2% to 10% of the gait cycle and is facilitated by the eccentric contraction of the gluteus medius (L4-S1, superior gluteal nerve), hamstrings (L5-S2, tibial division of the sciatic nerve), quadriceps (L2-4, femoral nerve), and dorsiflexors (L4-5, deep peroneal nerve).

Midstance: Appearing as flat foot, this phase consists of the next 10% to 30% of the gait cycle and is facilitated by the eccentric contraction of the gluteus medius (L4-S1, superior gluteal nerve) and plantarflexors (S1-2, tibial nerve).

Terminal stance: Appearing when the heel moves off the ground, this phase consists of the next 30% to 50% of the gait cycle and is facilitated by the eccentric contraction of the gluteus medius (L4-S1, superior gluteal nerve) and concentric contraction of the iliopsoas (L1-L3, iliopsoas nerve and femoral nerve) and plantarflexors (S1-2, tibial nerve).

Preswing: Appearing when the toe pushes off, this phase consists of the next 50% to 60% of the gait cycle and is facilitated by the concentric contraction of the planarflexors (S1-2, tibial nerve) and iliopsoas (L1-L3, iliopsoas nerve and femoral nerve) and the eccentric contraction of the gluteus medius (L4-S1, superior gluteal nerve).

Swing-Phase Components **Initial swing:** Appearing when the swinging limb accelerates through the swing phase, this phase consists of the next 60% to 73% of the gait cycle and is facilitated by the concentric contraction of the iliopsoas (L1-L3, iliopsoas nerve and femoral nerve) and dorsiflexors (L4-5, deep peroneal nerve, to clear the ground) and the eccentric contraction of the hamstrings (L5-S2, tibial division of the sciatic nerve) and quadriceps (L2-4, femoral nerve).

Midswing: Appearing when the swinging limb is at its maximum velocity, this phase consists of the next 73% to 87% of the gait cycle and is facilitated by the concentric contraction of the iliopsoas (L1-L3, iliopsoas nerve and femoral nerve) and dorsiflexors (L4-5, deep peroneal nerve) and eccentric contraction of the hamstrings (L5-S2, tibial division of the sciatic nerve).

Terminal swing: Appearing when the swinging limb begins to slow down, this phase consists of the final 87% to 100% of the gait cycle and is facilitated by the eccentric contraction of the hamstrings (L5-S2, tibial division of the sciatic nerve) and concentric contraction of the dorsiflexors (L4-5, deep peroneal nerve).

DETERMINANTS OF GAIT

The optimal movement of the center of gravity is determined by six factors, otherwise known as the six determinants of gait. They are pelvic rotation, pelvic tilt, pelvic lateral displacement, knee flexion in stance, knee mechanisms, and foot ankle mechanisms.

1. **Pelvic rotation:** When the swinging leg moves anteriorly, the pelvis rotates up to 4 degrees such that the ipsilateral side of the pelvis also moves anteriorly, effectively lengthening the leg and allowing the foot to touch the ground, minimizing the simultaneous pelvic tilt and drop in the center of gravity. (See **Fig. 5-3**.)
2. **Pelvic tilt:** While the pelvis rotates in the direction of the swinging leg, it also tilts 4 to 5 degrees to effectively lengthen the leg. The center of gravity is the lowest when the contralateral leg is at midstance. (See **Fig. 5-4**.)
3. **Pelvic lateral displacement:** While the pelvis rotates anteriorly and tilts inferiorly toward the direction of the swinging foot, it also moves laterally toward the standing foot, placing the center of gravity directly over the leg of support. With large knee varus, the step width increases, and lateral displacement is larger (left image of **Fig. 5-5**). Increasing knee valgus decreases step width, and lateral displacement is smaller (right image of Fig. 5-5).
4. **Knee flexion in stance:** When the heel strikes the ground, the knee is flexed at 15 degrees. This minimizes upward movement of the center of gravity and also absorbs impact force transmission from the ground through the heel and hip. (See **Fig. 5-6**.)
5. **Knee mechanisms:** During pushoff, extension of the knee together with plantarflexion provide the force to propel the ambulating person forward and also raises the center of gravity from its lowest position at

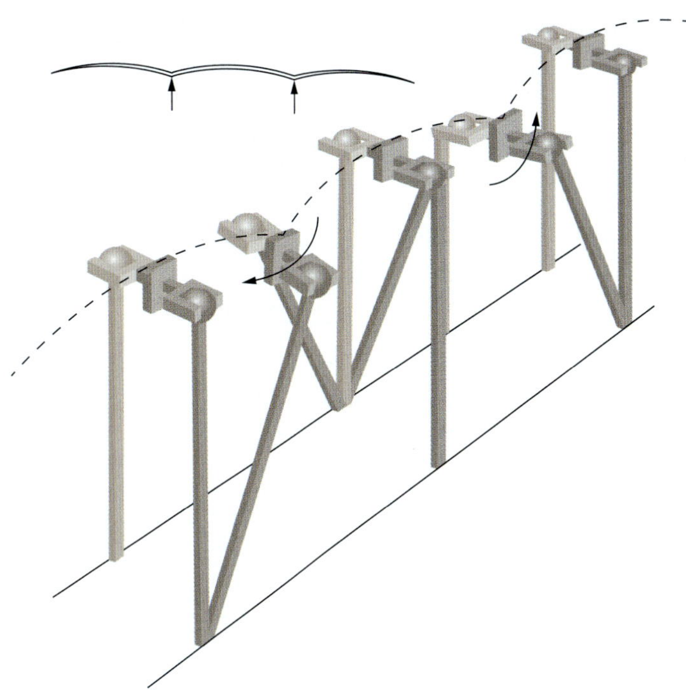

FIGURE 5-3. The effect of pelvic rotation on center of gravity. (From Inman, VT, Ralston, HJ, Todd, F. (1981), Human Walking, Baltimore: Williams and Wilkins.)

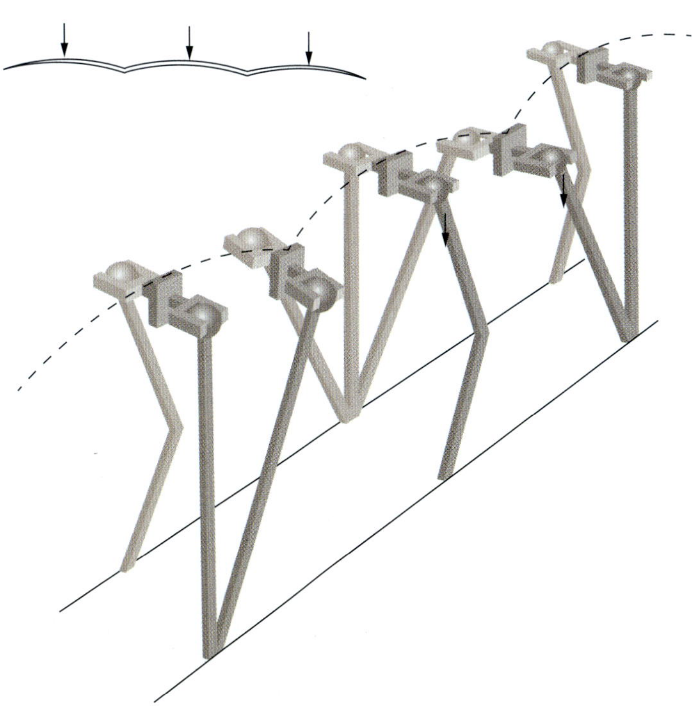

FIGURE 5-4. The effect of pelvic tilt on center of gravity. (From Inman, VT, Ralston, HJ, Todd, F. (1981), Human Walking, Baltimore: Williams and Wilkins.)

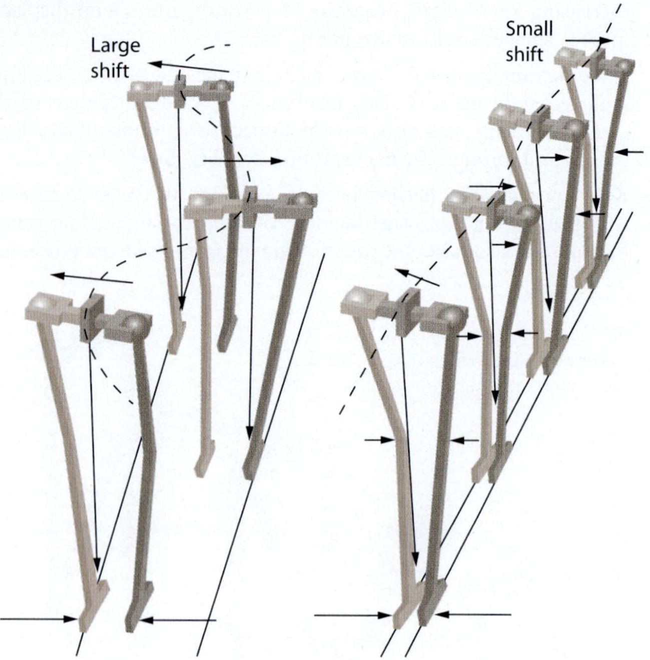

FIGURE 5-5. Effect of pelvic lateral displacement. (From Inman, VT, Ralston, HJ, Todd, F. (1981), Human Walking, Baltimore: Williams and Wilkins.)

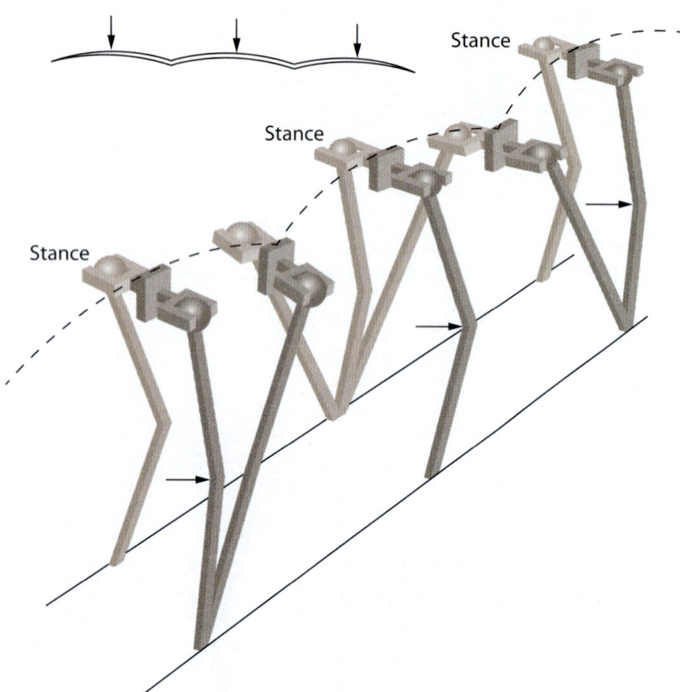

FIGURE 5-6. The effect of knee flexion in stance phase on center of gravity. (From Inman, VT, Ralston, HJ, Todd, F. (1981), Human Walking, Baltimore: Williams and Wilkins.)

midstance. Knee flexion in early stance is approximately 15 degrees, and at preswing it is approximately 30 to 40 degrees. (See **Fig. 5-7**.)

6. **Ankle mechanisms:** Initial contact forces the ankle to plantarflex with eccentric contraction of the dorsiflexors. This facilitates a controlled weight transfer from the heel of the foot to the entire foot during the progression to midstance. During pushoff, concentric plantarflexion together with knee extension provide the force to propel the ambulating person forward and also raise the center of gravity from its lowest position at midstance. (See Fig. 5-7.)

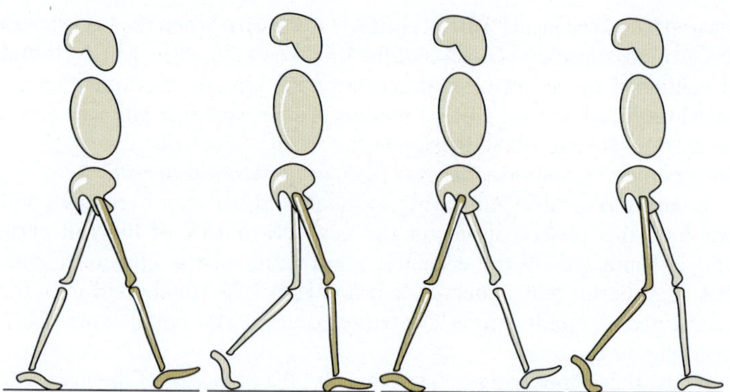

FIGURE 5-7. Knee and ankle mechanisms. (Modified from Perry J and Burnfield J. 2010. Gait Analysis: Normal and Pathological Function. Series, SLACK Incorporated.)

GAIT ABNORMALITIES

Gait abnormalities can give clues that allow isolation of the involved nerve root. Gait abnormalities result in increased energy expenditure per unit distance and overall slower walking speed. Keep in mind that a limited walking distance of a patient may be due to shortness of breath or fatigue because of a large energy expenditure with an inefficient gait in addition to pain.

Trendelenburg gait: With L4, L5, or S1 nerve root impingement, gluteus medius function is compromised. This produces a gluteus medius gait, known more commonly as a Trendelenburg gait. A weak gluteus medius muscle cannot eccentrically contract to resist adduction forces during the loading response phase. This forces the center of gravity downward and medial, away from the required position of being over the supporting limb. This causes lateral trunk bending to avoid a fall. When standing still, this "pelvic drop" can be found on a physical exam. To compensate for this, the person leans to the side of weakness, moving the center of gravity upward and laterally, placing the center of gravity back to where it should be, over the supporting limb. What is seen during ambulation is truncal sway toward the side of weakness, producing the Trendelenburg gait. For bilateral gluteus medius weakness, the patient appears to have a waddling gait. Ipsilateral hip pain may also be present. Other causes for truncal sway include hip pain, dislocated hip, poor balance, or significant leg length discrepancy. A cane on the opposite side of a weak gluteus medius can correct the gait deficiency and increase gait efficiency. The height of the cane should be such that the elbow is at a 20- to 30-degree angle. (See **Fig. 5-8**.)

Hip hiking: While weak hip abductors result in ipsilateral pelvic drop and produce a Trendelenburg gait, the opposite phenomenon, hip hiking (ipsilateral pelvic raising), results from weak hamstrings (L5-S2, tibial division of the sciatic nerve). Hamstrings are inactive in initiating swing; nevertheless, the knee flexes in response to active hip flexion. Hip hiking can also result from a longer ipsilateral limb (circumduction is also a compensatory motion for a long limb), a stiff knee (swollen or pain with knee flexion), quadratus lumborum shortening or spasms (T12-L4 nerve roots), or, most commonly, dorsiflexor weakness. (see **Fig. 5-9**.)

Foot slap: With L4 or L5 nerve root impingement or deep peroneal nerve impingement, dorsiflexor function can be compromised. Instead of eccentric contraction of the dorsiflexors to counteract plantarflexion during the initial contact phase, the ankle rapidly plantarflexes, causing the plantar surface to slap the ground. This is known as foot slap. Patients may describe difficulty ambulating because their foot catches on elevated surfaces or uneven ground. Treatment may include an ankle-foot orthosis to prevent foot slap.

Steppage gait: If dorsiflexors are severely weakened, foot drop occurs and the patient must lift the foot high to clear the ground during the swing phase by excessive hip flexion (which causes knee flexion) and then placing the foot forward. This is commonly known as a steppage

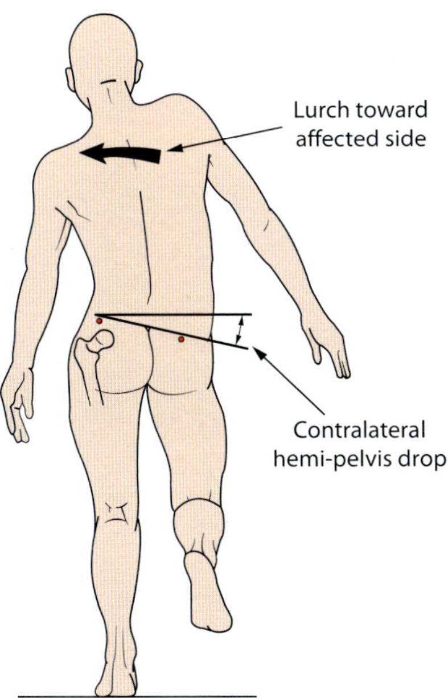

FIGURE 5-8. Trendelenburg gait. (Modified from Hoppenfeld S. Physical Examination of the Spine and Extremities. Upper Saddle, NJ: Pearson Education, 1976, p. 164.)

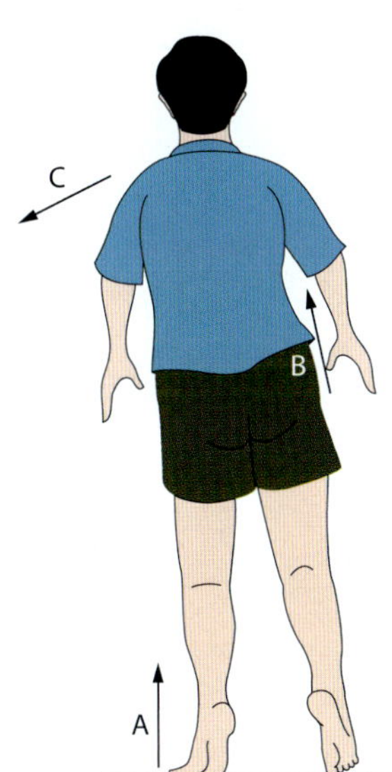

FIGURE 5-9. Hip hiking.

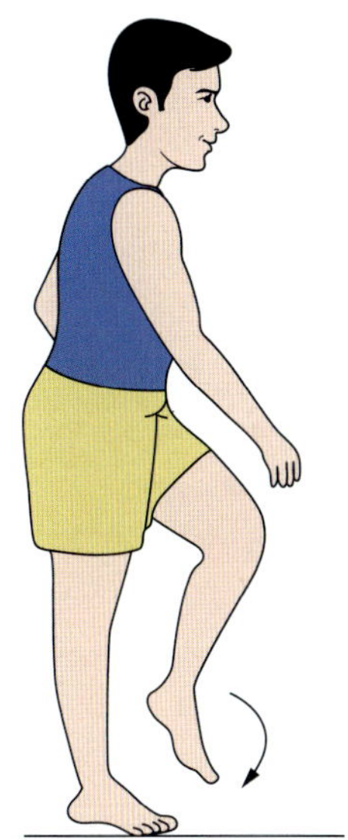

FIGURE 5-10. Steppage gait.

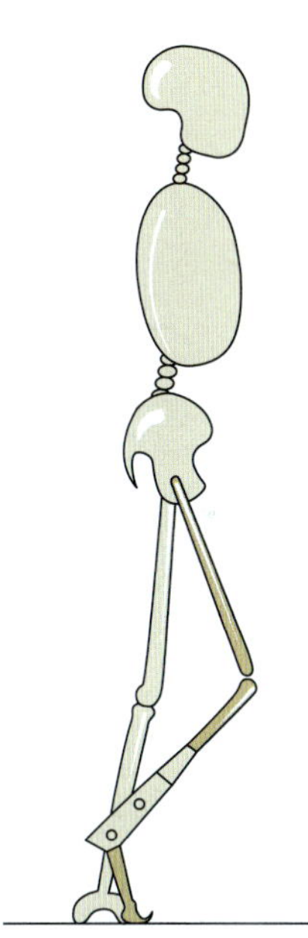

FIGURE 5-11. Plantarflexor (toe walking) gait. (Modified from Perry J and Burnfield J. 2010. Gait Analysis: Normal and Pathological Function. Series, SLACK Incorporated.)

gait. Steppage gait can also be found in plantarflexor spasticity caused by upper motor neuron disease or Achilles tendon contracture. With plantarflexor spasticity or Achilles tendon contracture, genu recurvatum (discussed later) can also be present. (See **Fig 5-10**.)

Toe walking: Weak dorsiflexors can also result in compensatory toe walking. It can also result from hip or knee flexion contracture or a shortened limb as a way to lengthen the total leg length and minimize vertical movement of the center of gravity. Plantar spasticity can result in either tiptoe walking or steppage gait. Finally, heel pain can cause a patient to toe walk in order to avoid weight bearing on the painful heel. (See **Fig. 5-11**.)

Genu recurvatum: The literary meaning is "knee backward," or hyperextended knee. This occurs with weak quadriceps due to L2-L4 nerve root or femoral nerve impingement or quadriceps myopathy. A person who has weak quadriceps compensates by locking the knee in hyperextension (via contraction of the gluteus maximus and soleus). This prevents inadvertent knee flexion ("buckling") during initial contract through midstance. This also keeps the center of gravity over the ipsilateral foot. Other reasons for genu recurvatum include laxed knee ligaments, contracted quad tendon, or spastic quadriceps (isolated or in synergy with hip or ankle extension), possibly due to upper motor neuron disorder. (See **Fig. 5-12**.)

Excessive trunk (not only lumbosacral) flexion: During initial contact through midstance, excessive trunk flexion occurs as a compensation for weak quadriceps. Leaning forward places the center of gravity anterior to the knees, forcing them into extension and minimizing the chance of buckling. This can also be caused by weak hip flexors (L1-L3 nerve root impingement) that force the ambulator to lean forward to compensate for poor control of the overpowering hip extensors. The

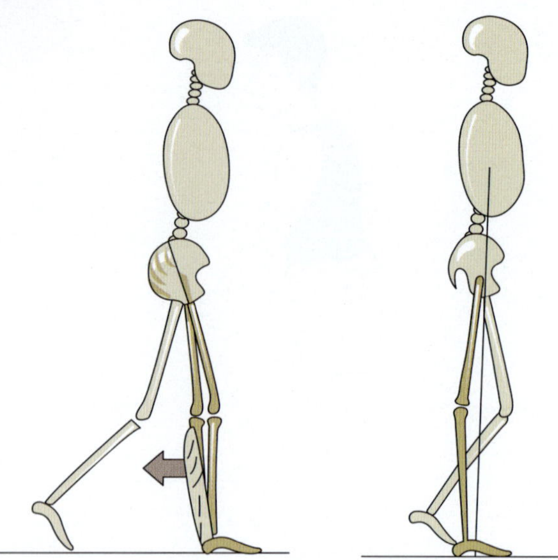

FIGURE 5-12. Genu recurvatum. (Modified from Perry J and Burnfield J. 2010. Gait Analysis: Normal and Pathological Function. Series, SLACK Incorporated.)

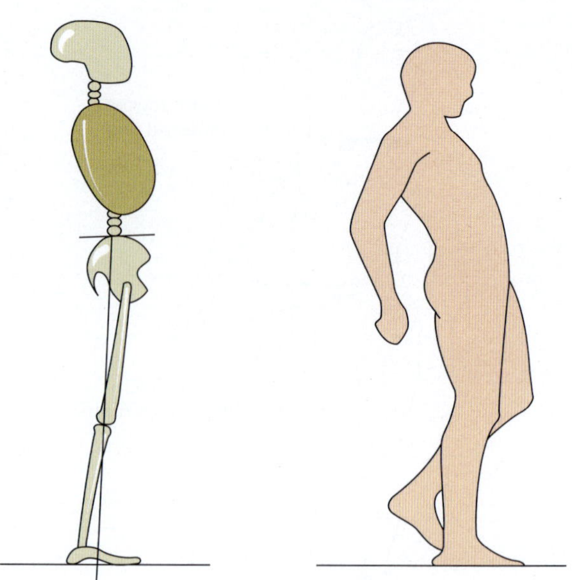

FIGURE 5-14. Excessive lumbosacral extension. (Modified from Perry J and Burnfield J. 2010. Gait Analysis: Normal and Pathological Function. Series, SLACK Incorporated.)

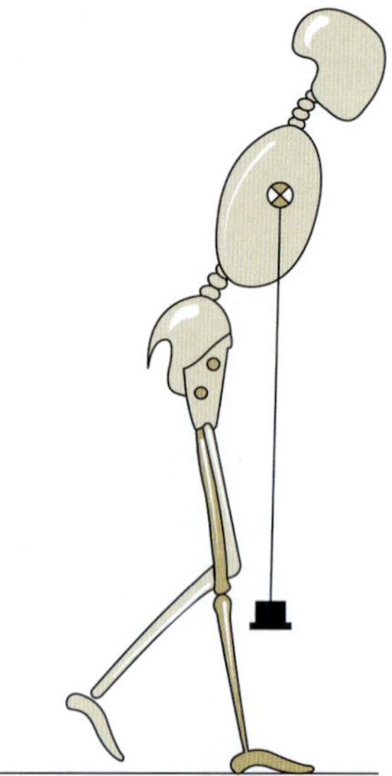

FIGURE 5-13. Excessive lumbosacral flexion. (Modified from Perry J and Burnfield J. 2010. Gait Analysis: Normal and Pathological Function. Series, SLACK Incorporated.)

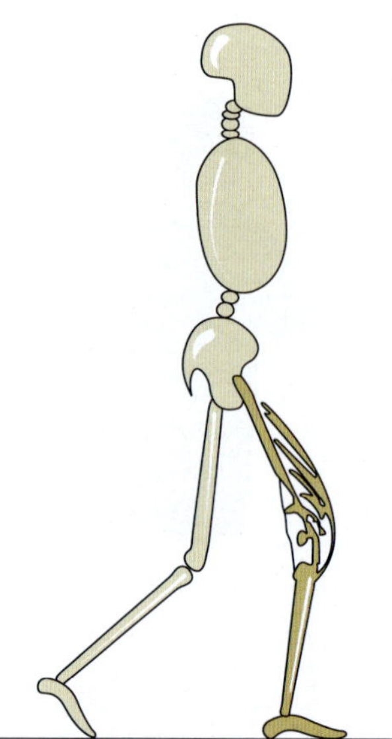

FIGURE 5-15. Flexed knee gait. (Modified from Perry J and Burnfield J. 2010. Gait Analysis: Normal and Pathological Function. Series, SLACK Incorporated.)

angle of forward flexion is the result of balancing the forces over the hip joint produced by the forward center of gravity and extension forces produced by the hip extensors. Hip flexor contractures can also create excessive lumbosacral flexion. (See **Fig. 5-13**.)

Excessive lumbosacral extension (lumbar lordosis): Also during initial contact through midstance, excessive lumbosacral extension occurs with weak gluteus maximus muscles (L5-S1 nerve roots or inferior gluteal nerve impingement) and results in difficulty generating eccentric hip extension force required to resist forward movement of the torso. To compensate, the ambulator leans backward to prevent falling forward. Excessive lumbosacral extension can also occur with hip pain and is a pain compensation strategy rather than true muscle weakness. Testing of the hip extensor strength in isolation can make the distinction. Knee flexion contracture (discussed next) can also result in excessive lumbosacral extension as can knee ankylosis. (See **Fig. 5-14**.)

Excessive knee flexion: While hamstring contracture is an obvious cause of excessive knee flexion, quad weakness (L2-L4 or femoral nerve impingement) is a major cause of excessive knee flexion. Weak plantarflexors (S1-S2 or tibial nerve impingement) resulting in excessive ankle dorsiflexion forces the knee to bend in order to maintain the center of gravity over the weight-bearing portion of the foot (behind the knee in this case). Bending the knee is also useful when trying to achieve flat foot during progression toward midstance. This enhances compensatory pushoff by the quads during terminal stance and preswing when the plantarflexors are unable to provide this force. Hip flexion contracture can likewise force the knee to bend in order to achieve flat foot during progression toward midstance and to facilitate pushoff if plantarflexors are functional. A synergistic hip-knee flexion may also be present, as seen in patients with cerebral palsy. An ipsilateral long limb or contralateral short limb can also force the ipsilateral knee to bend to minimize sudden upward movement of the center of gravity and smooth the curve of the center of gravity as the patient ambulates forward. Finally, knee pain can prevent full extension of the knee. (See **Fig. 5-15**.)

Insufficient pushoff/failure of weight-bearing transfer from heel to forefoot: During midstance through preswing, insufficient pushoff is often attributed to weak plantarflexors (S1-S2 or tibial nerve impingement); a weak flexor hallucis longus (S2-S3) may also be a contributing factor. Achilles tendon rupture can also significantly impair or prevent pushoff as well. In addition, metatarsalgia and hallux rigidus can also significantly impair a strong pushoff.

Bouncing, circumduction, or exaggerated pushoff (vaulting): This is caused by any disorder that makes the ipsilateral leg functionally or actually longer than the contralateral limb. Common sources are plantarflexor spasticity (in isolation or in synergy with hip or knee extensors), which in turn can be caused by upper motor neuron disease. It can also be caused by contracture of the Achilles tendon, weak hip flexors, weak dorsiflexors, shorter contralateral leg, or contralateral hip or knee flexion contractures.

STANDING

A word on standing. While standing appears to be a static activity, microscopic activation of alternating plantarflexors and dorsiflexors, as well as trunk muscles, occurs, and, therefore, standing is actually a dynamic process. Consider that the center of gravity of a normal adult passes anterior to the knee (forcing activation of the quads) and anterior to the ankle (forcing activation of the plantarflexors to prevent falling forward). (See Fig. 5-8.) Weakness of muscle groups that reinforce this posture (hip musculature, quads, plantarflexors) can predispose patients to falling and patients often adopt compensatory postures or rely on a cane or walker. Observation of these postures in addition to observing the patient's gait can help isolate muscle group weakness, which may go unnoticed by a gross motor exam. (See **Fig. 5-16.**)

CASE STUDY

A 46-year-old man presents with subacute (duration less than 6 weeks) low back pain without a known precipitating event. You decide to observe his gait as part of your physical exam and find that he is locking his right knee (genu recurvatum) during the stance phase. His wife confirms that he has been "walking funny" over the last week.

1. How would you evaluate this particular finding?

   A thorough evaluation, as described in chapter 38 should be performed. Consider that given the patient's age and probable etiology (herniated nucleus pulposus), he likely has an L3 nerve root impingement from said herniated disc. Subsequent to the initial onset of pain, the patient developed right quadracep weakness. For most practitioners, observing a patient's gait is unfortunately not usually a part of a routine physical exam for low back pain, and, therefore, this finding would be missed.

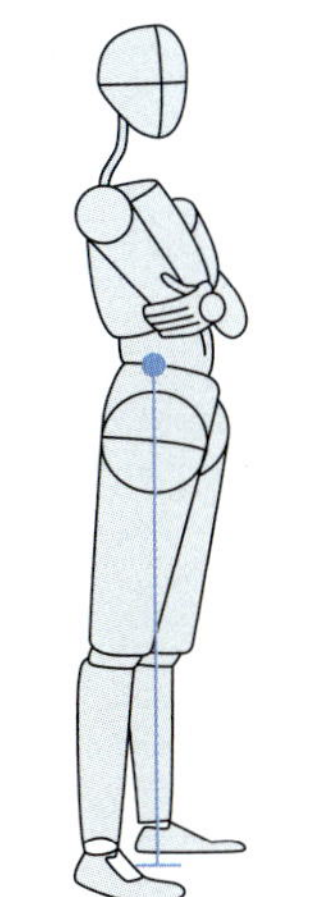
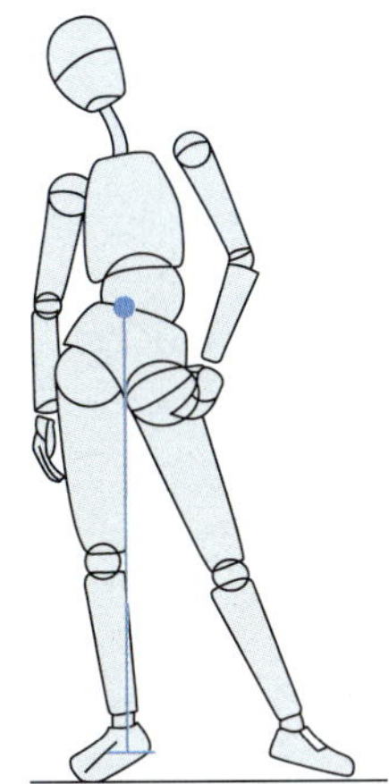

FIGURE 5-16. Normal standing.

   Furthermore, strength testing of the quadriceps is usually done by having the patient extend his or her knee against resistance provided by the examiner's triceps, a significantly weaker muscle group. This usually results in a "5/5" finding because the triceps are easily overcome by the quadriceps, even if the quadriceps are relatively weakened. Keep in mind that a single quadriceps muscle group can lift the center of gravity of a 100- to 250-pound person above the knee, despite the long moment arm of the femur. In contrast, it would be very difficult to lift the same mass with the same moment arm with a single triceps muscle group. Imagine (but do not perform) doing a one-handed push up while positioned upside down such that your legs are not supporting your weight. This would prove to be difficult for most people.

   The proper way to test the quadriceps is to utilize the sit-to-stand test, outlined in the Low Back Pain chapter. It is 50% sensitive and 77% specific for an L3 nerve root impingement. Measuring thigh circumference is also crucial to detect atrophy.

2. After a thorough assessment of the patient, you conclude that he likely has a right L3 nerve root impingement from a herniated disc. How would you manage this patient?

   During your evaluation, consider the possibility of diabetic amyotrophy if the patient is diabetic or has a family history of diabetes. Referral to the primary care physician for a diabetic workup is warranted if it hasn't already been done. Also, consider the fact that because the herniated disc is subacute, the benefits of physical therapy are debatable. The symptoms of disc herniation usually resolve with observation only.

   However, progressive weakness, a surgical indication, should not be missed. Therefore, a reasonable approach could be to provide medication management, offer reassurance that nothing catastrophic is immediately happening, and have the patient follow-up in 2 to 3 weeks. This follow-up is crucial. A repeat sit-to-stand test should be performed as well as remeasuring the thigh circumference at a location identical to the one used on the initial visit. If there is progressive weakness or atrophy, a surgical referral is warranted. If weakness and thigh circumferences are stable compared to the first visit, then only further observation is warranted. Note that the weakness has already occurred prior to the initial visit and only spontaneous recovery can be expected. The patient may ask if working out the quadriceps will strengthen it; however, this approach results only in limited gains for true neurological compromise. Spontaneous recovery can take as long as 2 years.

   Consider, though, that at the time of the follow-up visit, if the low back pain persists, it has now crossed over from being subacute to chronic because the duration is now longer than 6 weeks. When low back pain becomes chronic, physical therapy begins to have a greater benefit and should be prescribed. This is by no means a rule of thumb as clinical judgment takes precedence.

3. An 86-year-old woman presents to your clinic because her daughter is concerned that the patient is now walking backward down stairways. This has been going on for at least 6 months. The patient states that she does this because "this makes it easier to go down stairs." She has no particular pain complaints. How would you manage this patient?

   Consider the nonmyotomal reasons for an altered gait. The most common reason is to minimize pain, particularly in the joints, but pain can occur anywhere. This patient has no particular pain complaints but her compensatory strategy can minimize arthritic knee pain by minimizing hyperextension of the knee or minimize painful stenosis or facet pain by keeping the lumbosacral spine in a relatively flexed position without falling forward down the stairs due to an altered center of gravity.

   Another common reason for the altered gait is to minimize energy, an adaptation or strategy found throughout the animal kingdom. An example is when a horse goes from a walk to a trot and then to a gallop with increasing speed. Compensating for multiple sources of myotomal and/or nonmyotomal weakness and fatigue often results in an altered gait because using the weak muscles as one normally would costs more energy overall than utilizing an altered gait.

On the other hand, in a patient with multiple levels of stenosis, there is a possibility of multiple levels of myotomal weakness that can alter gait. It is important to test for these weaknesses with a very detailed physical exam, as described in the Low Back Pain chapter. Electromyography can also be utilized, but this is usually not necessary. Surgical referral may be indicated for spinal stenosis, as also described in the Low Back Pain chapter. If surgery is not indicated, observation would be the best course of action. There is no requirement that the patient descends stairs "normally," and her adaptation is a perfectly valid way to compensate for her impairments. An attempt to "correct" her way of descending stairs could lead to increased pain and falls; thus, leaving well enough alone is often the best course of action. With the patient's permission, the daughter must be educated on this fact and reassured that nothing catastrophic is happening.

SELECTED REFERENCES

1. Cuccurullo SJ. *Physical Medicine and Rehabilitation Board Review*. 2nd ed. New York: DemosMedical Publishing; 2010.
2. Braddom RL. *Physical Medicine and Rehabilitation*. 3rd ed. Philadelphia: Saunders Elsevier; 2007.
3. The Rusk Institute of Rehabilitation Medicine. Department of Rehabilitation Medicine Post-Graduate Medical School, 2011.
4. Gage WH, Winter DA, Frank JS, Adkin AL. Kinematic and kinetic validity of the inverted pendulum model in quiet standing. *Gait Posture*. April 2004;19(2):124-132.
5. Inman VT, Ralston HJ, Todd F. *Human Walking*. Baltimore: Williams and Wilkins; 1981.
6. Hartmann M, Kreuzpointner F, Haefner R, Michels H, Schwirtz A, Haas JP. Effects of Juvenile Idiopathic Arthritis on Kinematics and Kinetics of the Lower Extremities Call for Consequences in Physical Activities Recommendations.
7. Hoppenfeld S. *Physical Examination of the Spine and Extremities*. Upper Saddle, NJ: Pearson Education; 1976:164.
8. From http://hippie.nu/~unicorn/tut/xhtml-chunked/ch02s08.html
9. Bensoussan L, Viton JM, Barotsis N, Delarque A. Evaluation of patients with gait abnormalities in physical medicine and rehabilitation medicine settings. *J Rehabil Med*. 2008;40:497-507.
10. Siegel KL, Kepple TM, Stanhope SJ. A case study of gait compensations for hip muscle weakness in idiopathic inflammatory myopathy. *Clin Biomech (Bristol, Avon)*. 2007 March;22(3):319-326.
11. Perry J, Burnfield J. *Gait Analysis: Normal and Pathological Function*. Series, SLACK Incorporated. 2010.

PART 2

Pain: General Principles and Evaluation

CHAPTER 6

Definitions and Classification of Pain

Jyotsna V. Nagda
Zahid H. Bajwa

"For all the happiness Mankind can gain; Is not in pleasure, But in rest from pain."
—John Dryden (1631–1701)

Relief of pain is one of the great objectives of medicine. Pain is the most common symptom reported to physicians; more than 80% of all patients who see physicians do so because of pain. It has been a predominant concern of humankind since the beginning of recorded history. Chronic pain affects hundreds of millions of people worldwide, altering their physical and emotional functioning, decreasing their quality of life, and impairing the ability to work. According to an Institute of Medicine report released in 2011, one in three Americans experiences chronic pain—more than the total affected by heart disease, cancer, and diabetes combined. In Europe, the prevalence of chronic pain is 25% to 30%. It affects general health, psychological health, and social and economic well-being. Pain as a symptom—now considered the fifth vital sign—accounts for approximately 80% of physician visits and is estimated to cause $650 billion (in U.S. dollars) annually between health care expenditures and lost productivity percentage. More than 550 million workdays are lost every year because of chronic pain.

In October 2000, the 106th U.S. Congress passed HR 3244, which was then signed into law. Title VI, Section 1603, provides for the "Decade of Pain Control and Research," to begin in January 2001. It follows the "Decade of the Brain" and is only the second congressionally declared, medically related decade. Pain is now designated as a public health problem of national significance. Beginning in 2001, the Joint Commission on Accreditation of Healthcare Organizations (JCAHO) implemented new standards to assess and treat pain. To qualify for accreditation, all facilities—including rehabilitation centers, outpatient surgical centers, hospitals, and nursing homes—must recognize the right of patients to appropriate assessment and management of pain. All health care facilities must identify pain in patients during initial assessment and, where required, during ongoing periodic assessments and must educate patients and their families about pain management.

The word *pain* is derived from the Latin *poena,* meaning punishment. The International Association for the Study of Pain (IASP) defines pain as "an unpleasant sensory and emotional experience associated with actual or potential tissue damage, or described in terms of such damage." This definition may appear somewhat convoluted, but it clearly states that pain is subjective. It is both a physiologic sensation and an emotional reaction to that sensation. Viewed from an evolutionary prospective, pain is perceived as a threat or damage to one's biological integrity and has three components: sensory-discriminative, motivational-affective, and cognitive-evaluative.

The concepts of pain and suffering are frequently mixed and sometimes confused in the dialogue between patient and physician, especially because pain is commonly used as if it were synonymous with suffering. However, pain and suffering are distinct phenomena. *Suffering* is loosely defined as a "state of severe distress associated with events that threaten the intactness of person." Not all pain causes suffering, and not all suffering expressed as pain or coexisting with pain, stems from pain.

Pain has a protective role. It warns us of imminent or actual tissue damage. If tissue damage is unavoidable, a set of excitability changes in the peripheral and central nervous systems establish profound but reversible pain hypersensitivity in inflamed and surrounding tissue. This process avoids further damage until wound healing has occurred. In contrast, chronic pain syndromes offer no biologic advantage and cause suffering and distress.

DEFINITIONS

Acute pain: Signifies the presence of a noxious stimulus that produces actual tissue damage or possesses the potential to do so. The presence of acute pain implies the presence of an intact nervous system and is associated with autonomic hyperactivity: hypertension, tachycardia, sweating, and vasoconstriction. A common definition of acute pain is "the normal, predicted physiologic response to an adverse chemical, thermal, or mechanical stimulus...associated with surgery, trauma, and acute illness." Acute pain is short lived.

Allodynia: Pain in response to a non-nociceptive stimulus. *Allo* means "other" in Greek and is a common prefix for medical conditions that diverge from the expected. *Odynia* is derived from the Greek word "odune" or "odyne," which is used in "pleurodynia" and "coccydynia" and is similar in meaning to the root from which we derive words with *-algia* or *-algesia* in them. Allodynia is common in many neuropathic conditions, such as postherpetic neuralgia, chronic regional pain syndromes, and certain peripheral neuropathies. Allodynia can be produced in two ways: by the action of low-threshold myelinated Aβ fibers on an altered central nervous system and by a reduction in the threshold of nociceptor terminals in the periphery. As allodynia is used in the terms of clinical diagnosis, it can be also used to subclassify the broader symptoms of hyperalgesia, which may help identify the mechanisms causing it.

Analgesia: Implies absence of pain in response to stimulation, which would normally be painful. Analgesia can be produced peripherally (at the site of tissue damage, receptor, or nerve) or centrally (in the spinal cord or brain).

Anesthesia dolorosa: Implies pain in an area or region, which is anesthetic. Anesthesia dolorosa is more common after lesions that totally denervate a region. It is most commonly noted after surgery for atypical facial pain but can occur after surgery for tic douloureux or after traumatic nerve injury.

Catastrophizing: A distinct phenomenon characterized by feelings of helplessness, active rumination, and excessive magnification of cognitions and feelings toward the painful situation. Pain catastrophizing has been shown to be an important predictor of response to both acute and chronic pain.

Central pain: Pain initiated or caused by a primary lesion or dysfunction in the central nervous system. Any type of vascular, demyelinating, infectious, inflammatory, or traumatic lesion in the brain or spinal cord can produce central pain syndrome.

Chronic pain: Defining when a pain becomes chronic is always difficult. Pain that is unlikely to resolve or pain that lasts longer than the usual healing time is defined as chronic pain. From a temporal perspective, pain is deemed to be chronic when it persists beyond 3 months. Function of the nervous system becomes reorganized (neuroplasticity) with the potential for spontaneous and atopic nerve excitation.

Complex regional pain syndrome (CRPS): CRPS is a syndrome characterized by a continuing (spontaneous and/or evoked) regional pain that is seemingly disproportionate in time or degree to the usual course of any known trauma or other lesion. The pain is regional (not in a specific nerve territory or dermatome) and usually has a distal predominance of abnormal sensory, motor, sudomotor, vasomotor, and/or trophic findings. The syndrome shows variable progression over time. Used to describe the painful syndromes that formerly were described under the title of reflex sympathetic dystrophy and causalgia. The term *reflex sympathetic dystrophy* was a misnomer because not all cases have sympathetically maintained pain and not all were dystrophic. Thus, in 1993, a consensus group of pain medicine experts (a special consensus workshop of the IASP) gathered with the task of redefining causalgia and reflex sympathetic dystrophy. The diagnostic criteria proposed are purely clinical, with no laboratory test or diagnostic blocks. The consensus group divided the disorders based on the type of injury that initiated the disorder: type I, following a soft tissue injury, similar to reflex sympathetic dystrophy (RSD), and type II, following well-defined nerve injury.

IASP criteria are as follows:

CRPS I

1. The presence of an initiating noxious event or a cause for immobilization.*
2. Continuing pain, allodynia, or hyperalgesia in which the pain is disproportionate to any known or inciting event.
3. Evidence at some time of edema, changes in the skin blood flow, or abnormal sudomotor activity in the region of pain.
4. The diagnosis is excluded by the existence of other conditions that would otherwise account for the degree of dysfunction.

CRPS II

1. Type II is a syndrome that develops after nerve injury. Spontaneous pain or allodynia/hyperalgesia occurs and is not necessarily limited to the territory of the injured nerve.
2. There is or has been evidence of edema, skin blood flow abnormality, or abnormal sudomotor activity in the region of the pain since the inciting event.
3. This diagnosis is excluded by the existence of the conditions that would otherwise account for the degree of pain and dysfunction.

Ten years after the IASP conference, new diagnostic criteria were defined by the Budapest task force in a consensus conference. Also, there is more recent evidence that both CRPS type I and CRPS type II may be associated with nerve injury, and CRPS I may represent a small fiber predominant mono- or oligoneuropathy that is initiated by limb trauma.

The IASP criteria as written (i.e., criteria can be met by either self-reported symptoms or objective signs) were highly sensitive but had poor specificity.

Budapest clinical diagnostic criteria:

1. Continuing pain, which is disproportionate to any inciting event
2. Must report at least one symptom in three of the four following categories:
   - Sensory: reports of hyperesthesia and/or allodynia
   - Vasomotor: reports of temperature asymmetry and/or skin color changes and/or skin color asymmetry
   - Sudomotor/edema: reports of edema and/or sweating changes and/or sweating asymmetry
   - Motor/trophic: reports of decreased range of motion and/or motor dysfunction (weakness, tremor, dystonia) and/or trophic changes (hair, nail, skin)
3. Must display at least one sign at time of evaluation in two or more of the following categories:
   - Sensory: evidence of hyperalgesia (to pinprick) and/or allodynia (to light touch and/or deep somatic pressure and/or joint movement)
   - Vasomotor: evidence of temperature asymmetry and/or skin color changes and/or asymmetry
   - Sudomotor/edema: evidence of edema and/or sweating changes and/or sweating asymmetry
   - Motor/trophic: evidence of decreased range of motion and/or motor dysfunction (weakness, tremor, dystonia) and/or trophic changes (hair, nail, skin)
4. There is no other diagnosis that better explains the signs and symptoms

*Not required for diagnosis.

Deafferentation pain: Pathological pain condition associated with a partial or complete loss of sensory input from a part of the body after lesions in somatosensory pathways, often as a result of reorganization in the central nervous system.

Dysesthesia: An unpleasant abnormal sensation, whether spontaneous or evoked. Examples include the burning feet that may be felt in alcoholic neuropathy.

Hyperalgesia: Increased pain sensitivity. It may include both a decrease in threshold and an increase in suprathreshold response. Stimulus-evoked hyperalgesias are commonly classified into subgroups on the basis of modality (i.e., mechanical, thermal, or chemical). Mechanical hyperalgesias are further classified as brush-evoked (dynamic), pressure-evoked (static), and punctuate hyperalgesia. Brush-evoked (dynamic) hyperalgesia is a consequence of increased central response to Aβ fiber input.

Hyperesthesia: Increased sensitivity to stimulation, excluding special senses.

Hyperpathia: A painful syndrome characterized by an abnormally explosive painful reaction to a stimulus, especially a repetitive stimulus, as well as an increased threshold. Faulty identification and localization of the stimulus, delay, radiating sensation, and after sensation may occur.

Hypoalgesia: Diminished response to a normally painful stimulus.

Hypoesthesia: Decreased sensitivity to stimulation, excluding the special senses.

Neuralgia: Pain in the distribution of a peripheral nerve, typically described as lancinating or electric shock–like sensation.

Neuritis: A special type of neuropathy; the term is reserved primarily for describing inflammatory process affecting nerves.

Neurogenic pain: Pain initiated or caused by a primary lesion or dysfunction or by transitory perturbation in the peripheral or central nervous system.

Neuropathic pain: Pain caused by a lesion or disease of the somatosensory system. Neuropathic pain syndromes can originate at any point or points along the somatosensory pathways, from the most distal nerve endings in the skin to the somatosensory cortex in the parietal lobe. Examples of neuropathic pain include painful polyneuropathy, postherpetic neuralgia, trigeminal neuralgia, and poststroke pain.

> **Peripheral neuropathic pain:** Pain arising as a direct consequence of a lesion or disease of the peripheral somatosensory system.
>
> **Central neuropathic pain:** Pain caused by lesion or disease of the central somatosensory system.

Neuropathy: A disturbance of function or pathologic change in nerves. It may be in a single nerve (mononeuropathy), in several nerves (mononeuropathy multiplex), or symmetric and bilateral (polyneuropathy).

Neuroplasticity: Nociceptive input leading to structural and functional changes that may cause altered perceptual processing and contribute to pain chronicity.

Nociception: The neural process of encoding and processing noxious stimuli. Nociception and pain should be distinguished as each can occur without the other. Pain is a subjective phenomenon, whereas nociception is the object of the sensory physiology.

Nociceptive neuron: A central or peripheral neuron that is capable of encoding noxious stimuli. Non-nociceptive neurons may respond to noxious stimuli, when these stimuli are above their respective threshold; however only nociceptive neurons are capable of encoding the relevant properties of those stimuli.

Nociceptive pain: Pain arising from activation of nociceptors.

Nociceptor: A sensory receptor that is capable of transducing and encoding noxious stimuli.

Noxious stimulus: An actually or potentially tissue-damaging event.

Pain threshold: The minimal intensity of a stimulus that is perceived as painful.

Pain tolerance level: The maximum intensity of a stimulus that evokes pain and that a subject is prepared to tolerate.

Paresthesia: An abnormal sensation, whether spontaneous or evoked. The most common paresthesia is the sense of "pins and needles."

Peripheral neurogenic pain: Pain initiated or caused by a primary lesion or dysfunction, or by transitory perturbation in the peripheral nervous system.

Phantom pain: Pain in a part of the body that has been surgically removed or is congenitally absent. Although best described after limb amputations, phantom pain can occur after a wide variety of amputation.

Referred pain: Pain localized not to the site of its cause but to an area that may be adjacent to or at a distance from such a site. An example is shoulder pain caused by diaphragmatic irritation.

Sensitization: Increased responsiveness of neurons to their neurons to their normal input or recruitment of a response to normally subthreshold inputs. Spontaneous discharges and increases in receptive field size may also occur.

> **Peripheral sensitization:** Increased responsiveness and reduced threshold of of nociceptors to stimulation of their receptive fields.
>
> **Central sensitization:** Increased responsiveness of nociceptive neurons in central nervous system to their normal or subthreshold afferent input.

Windup: Progressive increase in the frequency and magnitude of firing of dorsal horn neurons produced by repetitive activation of C fibers above a critical threshold, leading to a perceived increase in intensity.

CLASSIFICATION OF PAIN

The most recognized categories of classification are based on neurophysiologic mechanism, temporal aspects, etiology, or region affected.

NEUROPHYSIOLOGIC

The neurophysiologic classification is based on inferred mechanism of pain. There are essentially three broad categories-: nociceptive pain, inflammatory pain, and pathological pain.

The term *nociceptive* is applied to pain that is presumed to be maintained by continual tissue injury. Nociceptive pain results from the activation or sensitization of high-threshold, unmyelinated C or thinly myelinated Aδ primary sensory neurons that feed into nociceptive pathways of the central nervous system. Four physiologic processes are involved in the somatic nociception: (1) transduction, (2) transmission, (3) modulation, and (4) perception. Nociceptive pain occurs in response to the noxious stimuli and continues only in the maintained presence of noxious stimuli. In the absence of ongoing tissue injury, the heightened sensitivity returns over to normal baseline, where high-intensity stimuli are again required to initiate nociceptive pain. It has a warning function and signalizes imminent or actual tissue damage. It is, therefore, essential for maintaining bodily integrity. Examples include angina, ischemic claudication, and the like. Loss of nociception, as in hereditary disorders associated with congenital insensitivity to pain, leads to repeated injury and inadvertent self mutilation.

Certain diseases like osteoarthritis may generate recurrent or ongoing noxious stimuli to produce chronic nociceptive pain.

The second kind of pain is the *inflammatory* pain, which is also adaptive and protective. This pain is caused by activation of the immune system by tissue injury or infection. Inflammatory pain occurs in response to tissue injury and the subsequent inflammatory response. It assists in healing of the injured part by creating a situation that discourages physical contact. The sensory nervous system undergoes a profound change in its responsiveness: Normally innocuous stimuli produce pain and responses to noxious stimuli are both exaggerated and prolonged. Due to the plasticity in peripheral and central nociceptive pathways, pain can be activated by low-threshold innocuous inputs. Typically, inflammatory pain disappears after resolution of tissue injury; however, in some diseases like rheumatoid arthritis, pain may persist as long as the inflammation is active.

The third type of pain is *pathological* pain, which is maladaptive resulting from abnormal functioning of the nervous system. It can occur after damage to the nervous system *(neuropathic pain)* but also in conditions where there is no such damage or inflammation *(dysfunctional pain)*.

In neuropathic pain, there is no transduction (conversion of a nociceptive impulse into an electrical impulse). It is an expression of maladaptive plasticity within the nociceptive system with multiple alterations across the nervous system. These alterations include ectopic generation of action potentials, facilitation and disinhibition of synaptic transmission, loss of synaptic connectivity, and formation of new synaptic circuits and neuroimmune interactions. Neuropathic pain typically manifests with continuous pain (burning, squeezing, pressure) or paroxysmal pain (electric shock–like sensations, stabbing pain) and provoked (brush evoked, pressure evoked, cold evoked) or paresthetic and dysesthetic (tingling, pins and needle) sensations. There are two subsets of neuropathic pain: peripheral and central. Examples of peripheral neuropathic pain includes various polyneuropathies, trigeminal neuralgia, postherpetic neuralgia, diabetic neuropathy, focal neuropathies related to trauma (such as traumatic brachial plexus injuries), and pain following surgical interventions (thoracotomy, breast surgery, etc). Central nervous system diseases that commonly cause neuropathic pain include stroke, multiple sclerosis, spinal cord injury, Parkinson's disease, and so forth.

Examples of dysfunctional pain include fibromyalgia, irritable bowel syndrome, tension type headache, temporomandibular disorders, interstitial cystitis, and other syndromes where there are no noxious stimuli or minimal peripheral inflammatory pathology but there is significant pain.

The major characteristics of inflammatory and pathological pain are that noxious stimuli are no longer required to generate pain. Inflammatory pain represents hypersensitivity reaction to a defined peripheral pathology, whereas pathological pain results from altered neural processing.

Pain can also be divided into somatic and visceral pain. Somatic pain is characterized as being well localized topographically, intermittent, or constant and is described as "aching, stabbing, gnawing, or throbbing."

Visceral pain has five important clinical characteristics:

1. It is not evoked from all visceral organs, such as liver; kidney, most solid viscera, and lung parenchyma are not sensitive to pain.
2. It is not always linked to visceral injury (cutting the intestine causes no pain, whereas stretching of the bladder causes pain).
3. It is diffuse and poorly localized, owing to organization of visceral nociceptive pathways in the central nervous system, particularly the absence of a separate visceral sensory pathway and the low proportion of the visceral afferent nerve fibers.
4. It is referred to other locations.
5. It is accompanied by motor and autonomic reflexes, such as the nausea, vomiting, and lower back muscle tension that occur in renal colic. Discrete nociceptors in the cardiovascular, respiratory, gastrointestinal, and genitourinary systems mediate visceral pain. Although its neural pathways are less well defined than those of somatic pain, the visceral pathways share some of the features with somatic pathways. Visceral pain is less topographically distinct and is described as diffuse. It may be intermittent or constant and is often described as "dull, colicky, or squeezing."

TEMPORAL

The temporal classification is based on the duration of symptoms and is usually divided into acute and chronic categories. The major shortcoming is that distinction between *acute* and *chronic* is arbitrary, and the two most common chronological markers used to denote chronic pain have been 3 months and 6 months. Cancer pain includes pain associated with the disease progression, treatment, and concurrent conditions. Hence, the pain associated with cancer may be acute or chronic. Some clinicians advocate cancer pain as a third category, distinct from acute and chronic pain.

MECHANISM-BASED

In 1998, Woolf and his colleagues suggested implementation of a mechanism-based classification of pain. They believed it could have profound implications: Drugs could be developed that target distinct mechanisms, basic scientists could have new guidelines for experimental design, and clinicians could be armed with more reliable and valid diagnostic tools for treatment and clinical investigation. Although there are still important hurdles, several research groups across the world are systematically analyzing sensory profiles and clinical presentation to correlate with the underlying mechanism.

ETIOLOGIC

The etiologic classification pays more attention to the primary disease process in which the pain occurs, rather than to the neurophysiologic basis. Examples include cancer pain, arthritis pain, and pain in sickle cell disease. Therapeutically, it is less useful than the neurophysiologic classification.

REGIONAL

The regional classification is strictly topographic and does not infer pathophysiology or etiology. It is defined by the part of the body affected.

MULTIAXIAL

An alternative to the one-dimensional approach is the multidimensional approach. The IASP has published an expert-based multiaxial classification of chronic pain with the goals of standardization and provision of a point of reference. The published taxonomy classifies chronic pain patients according to five axes based on the best-published information and consensus:

1. Region of the body affected (axis I)
2. System whose abnormal functioning could conceivably produce pain (axis II)
3. Temporal characteristics of pain and pattern of occurrence (axis III)
4. Patient's statement of intensity and time since the onset of pain (axis IV)
5. Presumed etiology (axis V)

CONCLUSION

Chronic pain affects billions of lives and is a major public health problem. However, pain management is still a challenging task due to a lack of understanding of the fundamental mechanisms of pain. Pain management has been a rapidly advancing field. Many concepts and terminologies that were a source of confusion in the past have now been more clearly defined. However, more work clearly needs to be done in classification and taxonomy to simplify the communication and meet the objectives of basic scientists, researchers, and clinicians providing patient care.

BIBLIOGRAPHY

Albrecht PJ, Hines S, Eisenberg E, Pud D, Finlay DR, Connolly MK, Pare M, Davar G, Rice FL. Pathologic alterations of cutaneous innervation and vasculature in affected limbs from patients with complex regional pain syndrome. *Pain*. 2006;120:244-266.

Backonja MM. Defining neuropathic pain. *Anesth Analg*. 2003;97:785-790.

Bonica JJ. *Pain Terms and Taxonomies of Pain. The Management of Pain*. 3rd ed. Philadelphia, PA: John D Loeser; 2001.

Cervero F, Merskey H. What is a noxious stimulus? *Pain Forum*. 1996;5:157-161.

Cervero F, Laid J. Visceral pain. *Lancet*. 1999;353:2145-2148.

Gatchel RJ, Peng YB, Peters ML, Fuchs PN, Turk DC. The biopsychosocial approach to chronic pain: scientific advances and future directions. *Psychol Bull*. 2007;133(4):581-624.

Institute of Medicine Report from the Committee on Advancing Pain Research, Care, and Education. *Relieving Pain in America. A Blueprint for Transforming Prevention, Care, Education and Research*. National Academies Press; 2011.

Leadley RM, Armstrong N, Lee YC, Allen A, Kleijnen J. Chronic diseases in the European Union: the prevalence and health cost implications of chronic pain. *J Pain Palliat Care Pharmacother*. 2012;26:310-325.

Jensen TS, Sindrup SR, Bach FW. Test the classification of pain: reply to Mitchell Max. *Pain*. 2002;96:407-408.

Julius D, Basbaum AI. Molecular mechanisms of nociception. *Nature*. 2001;413:203-210.

Max MB. Clarifying the definition of neuropathic pain. *Pain*. 2002;96:406-407.

Melzack R. The short McGill Pain Questionnaire. *Pain*. 1987;30:191-197.

Merskey H, Bogduk N. *International Association for the Study of Pain (IASP): Classification of Chronic Pain*. 2nd ed. Seattle. IASP Press.

Merskey H. Terms and taxonomy: paper tools at the cutting edge of study. In: Merskey H, Loeser JD, Dubner R, eds. *The paths of pain 1975–2005*. Seattle: IASP Press; 2005:329-337.

Merskey H, Albe-Fessard D, Bonica JJ, Carmon A, Dubner R, Kerr FWL, et al. Pain terms: a list with definitions and notes on usage. Recommended by the IASP subcommittee on taxonomy. *Pain*. 1979;6:249-252.

Meyer RA, Campbell JN, Raja SN. Peripheral neural mechanisms of nociception. In: Wall PD, Melzack R, eds. *Textbook of pain*. Edinburgh: Churchill Livingstone; 1994:13-44.

Oaklander AL, Rissmiller JG, Gelman LB, Zheng L, Chang Y, Gott R. Evidence of focal small-fiber axonal degeneration in complex regional pain syndrome-I (reflex sympathetic dystrophy). *Pain*. 2006;120:235-243.

Raja SN, Grabow TS. Complex regional pain syndrome I (reflex sympathetic dystrophy). *Anesthesiology*. 2002;96:1254-1260.

Todd M, Raja SN, Eisenach J. International Association for the Study of Pain, 9th World Congress on Pain. *Anesthesiology*. 2000;92:292-294.

Treede RD, Handwerker HO, Baumgärtner U, Meyer RA, Magerl W. Hyperalgesia and allodynia: taxonomy, assessment, and mechanisms. In: Brune K, Handwerker HO, eds. Hyperalgesia: molecular mechanisms and clinical implications. Seattle: IASP Press; 2004:1-15.

Treede RD, Jensen TS, Campbell JN, Cruccu G, Dostrovsky JO, Griffin JW, et al. Neuropathic pain: redefinition and a grading system for clinical and research diagnostic purposes. *Neurology*. 2008;70:1630-1635.

Willis WD. *The Pain System*. Basel: Karger; 1985.

Woolf CJ. Pain: moving from symptom control toward mechanism-specific pharmacologic management. *Ann Intern Med*. 2004;140:441-451.

Woolf CJ. What is this thing called pain? *Journal of Clinical Investigation*. 2010 Nov;120(11):3742-3744.

Woolf C, Max ML. Mechanism-based pain diagnosis: Issues for analgesic drug development. *Anesthesiology*. 2001;95:241-249.

Woolf CJ, Bennett GJ, Doherty M, et al. Towards a mechanism based classification of pain? *Pain*. 1998;77:227-229.

Woolf CJ, Mannion RJ. Neuropathic pain: etiology, symptoms, mechanisms, and management. *Lancet*. 1999;353:1959-1964.

Woolf CJ, Walters ET. Common patterns of plasticity contributing to nociceptive sensitization in mammals and aplysia. *Trends and Neuroscience*. 1991;14:74-78.

CHAPTER 7 Understanding the Patient with Chronic Pain

Jeremy Goodwin
Zahid H. Bajwa

"It is not suffering that diminishes man, but suffering without meaning."

—Victor Frankl

Asked to describe their pain, especially chronic, noncancer pain, patients often appear perplexed, stating, "I don't know. It just hurts." Clearly, more information is needed, and obtaining the necessary details is an art. While subjective and objective methods of psychological evaluation provide one of the cornerstones of diagnosing factors important in the perpetuation of pain beyond the otherwise apparent state of healing—not to mention executing and monitoring the results of multimodal and interdisciplinary approaches to pain control and functional rehabilitation—it is vital that the treating medical professional develops a sound rapport with the patient independently of the mental health specialist. This comes about via empathy and an understanding of the patient that is best summed up by stating that the person suffering from chronic, noncancer pain needs to be *heard* and his or her pain *validated* as real. Only then can an accurate diagnosis be made to form the foundation upon which a rational treatment program can be built.

By the time most patients are referred to a pain specialist, they are often frustrated, sleep deprived, anxious, and depressed and feel angry toward those they feel have not really listened to how they have been compromised by persistent pain. To many sufferers, the message has come across as "it is in your head," even when not intended as such. Much of that anger dissipates when patients truly feel as if they have been heard. They are then far easier to work with, and the likelihood of progress significantly increases. When such a rapport is achieved, patients generally become more open to understanding that the locus of control lies within themselves to a considerable degree and cannot be expected to appear magically from an outside source even if that source is able to guide and to provide tools useful in the healing process.

A few basic pointers are worth emphasizing here. These are not insignificant and are often noted by patients as some of the reasons that they did not feel heard. It is important to maintain eye contact and body language that emphasizes that, at least for the time spent together, the patient is the clinician's sole concern. Typing or dictating into an electronic medical record should be avoided while the patient is talking or before the interview and examination are complete. Furthermore, providing verbal feedback shows that the clinician has really grasped the essence of the patient's experience of suffering as well as the details of the pain syndrome in terms of its time of onset and the events leading up to it. Such feedback supports the notion that the patient is being taken seriously with respect to what *he or she* feels is important, regardless of whether or not the clinician wishes to steer the focus over time in a different direction. This cannot be emphasized enough, and the extra time taken will pay off in making future interviews shorter, mainly because trust and hope will have been established.

It is worth noting here that teenage and adult patients with cancer often fear insufficiently treated pain more than they fear death. Younger children, on the other hand, generally fear potentially painful procedures more than the disease or condition for which the intervention is indicated. Procedures should, therefore, not be performed on pediatric patients outside of a procedure room, making their hospital bed a relatively safe place. Parents often fear the presence of a cerebral tumor that might explain a child's headache but may be too afraid to ask about this. They might also assume that opioids given in a pediatric setting may predispose their children to illicit drug use in adolescence. As a final point, geriatric patients may associate opioids with the imminent end of life, just as they may fear addiction even when a terminal illness has been diagnosed. These points should always be brought up and clarified, even if the questions or fears have not been vocalized.

CLASSIFICATION OF PAIN

Before we focus in more detail on the patient with chronic pain and a general approach to pain management, basic nosology and terminology require clarification. There is much confusion over this, both within the lay public and within the medical and associated professions.

There are a number of ways to classify pain. Some pain specialists broadly separate it into *cancer pain* and *noncancer pain* (the term "nonmalignant pain" can be misinterpreted as benign when clearly the risk of medication overuse and even suicide strongly suggests otherwise). Others divide it into acute, recurrent acute, and chronic pain. *Acute pain* is short-lived and follows disease, injury, or near injury to tissue. It resolves with healing. *Recurrent-acute pain* is similar in duration but tends to recur. It need not involve injury. Examples are migraine headache and sickle cell vasoocclusive episodes, previously known as "sickle cell crises." Depending on the injury, *chronic pain* is variably defined as that persisting 1 to 6 months after the tissue has healed. One example of chronic, noncancer pain is postherpetic neuralgia following a breakout of shingles.

Pain can also be classified in terms of mechanism. *Nociceptive pain* denotes pain arising from tissue injury, and the degree of pain is usually somewhat proportional to the degree of injury. Nociceptive pain itself may be subcategorized into *visceral pain*, a dull, crampy, and poorly localizable discomfort—as might be experienced in gastroenteritis—or *somatic pain*, a sharper and more localizable sensation of the body wall—as might be felt after a laceration. Each type of pain may be mild or intense.

Neuropathic pain is not nociceptive, and the degree of pain is not proportional to the degree of injury; it is caused by disordered sensory processing of the nervous system and is a pathologic persistence of normal sensitizing mechanisms that can, under normal circumstances, be useful in the setting of acute pain. Neuropathic pain can be subcategorized into *central neuropathic pain*, which can originate at any level of the central nervous system, and *peripheral neuropathic pain*, which is generated at the level of a nerve, plexus, or nerve root. The most famous example of central pain is poststroke thalamic pain; common examples of peripheral neuropathic pain are neuromas, diabetic neuropathy, and complex regional pain syndrome, types 1 and 2 (previously known as reflex sympathetic dystrophy and causalgia). As with central pain, a number of different mechanisms may be involved. Even when the damage occurs in the periphery, such as injury to a nerve, the constant bombardment of sensory neurons in the spinal cord with pain signals from the periphery renders the wide-dynamic-range (WDR) sensory neurons in the spinal cord hypersensitive to all input, even to non-noxious stimuli from distal regions to which little attention is usually paid. Neurons then almost continuously "fire up" the pain pathway, no matter the type of sensory input, resulting in allodynia (discussed later). Although this is a normal sequence of events in acute injury (i.e., temporarily sensitizing injured areas so that they may be protected from further harm), when it fails to abate with healing, it becomes pathologic. This process is called central sensitization of pain and is related to the concept of wind-up, both of which are discussed elsewhere in this textbook.

Other relevant terminology includes:

- *Hyperpathia:* an elevated sensory threshold above which is generated an abnormally intense and prolonged response to pain.
- *Hyperalgesia:* which is secondary to a lowered threshold to pain.
- *Allodynia:* a painful response to a nonpainful stimulus.
- *Hyperesthesia:* caused by a lowered threshold to any stimuli.
- *Hypoesthesia:* the opposite of hyperesthesia.
- *Analgesia:* without pain.
- *Anesthesia:* without sensation.

Incident pain is generated by mechanical factors characteristic of movement and position. Incident pain commonly occurs in cancer patients in whom, for example, metastatic spread of the cancer involves the skeleton. Such pain may be neuropathic or nociceptive, depending on the structures involved. For example, a pathologic or metastatic rib fracture results in nociceptive bone pain and neuropathic pain in the distribution of the rib's intercostal nerve.

SPECIAL POPULATIONS AFFECTED BY MISCONCEPTIONS ABOUT PAIN

INFANTS AND CHILDREN

Patients within certain age groups are often subjected to unnecessary pain and suffering that may have long-term consequences. Children are still relatively undermedicated compared with adults, and although the situation is improving, there continues to be room for improvement. Surgeons were operating on infants who were only partially anesthetized as late as the early to mid-1980s.

Misconceptions about pain and the consequences of its treatment continue to impede patient care. For example, nurses concerned about the risk of addiction may read a physician's "prn" order to mean "as little as possible" rather than "as needed." Or they may rely too much on changes in vital signs, such as quickened heart rate or increased blood pressure, to decide if a child's complaint of pain is "real" or not and may thus withhold "prn" medications inappropriately. We are aware of no evidence that appropriate opioid use in pediatric pain management leads to addiction in childhood or adulthood. And we now know that there is great variability in individual pain thresholds and ability to cope with pain, so that *vital signs may not correlate as well with the level of pain as previously thought*. This is especially so in newborn babies. Even in infants and children, fluctuating levels in vital signs may be a better indicator of pain than absolute levels. It is, therefore, wise to combine several methods of pain evaluation, no matter the patient's age. Verbal or visual analog pain scores (from 0 to 10), a developmentally sensitive analysis of general behavior and body language, and recording of facial expression can provide valuable information for the assessment of pain.

Some practitioners believe that infants feel little pain because their nervous systems are immature. This is a false assumption. The anatomic, biochemical, and physiologic apparatus necessary for the perception of pain is present 2 to 3 months before term, but because the descending inhibitory modulating system is immature, and because of a higher-than-adult level of cutaneous pain receptor density, babies and infants may, in fact, be hyperalgesic. They may have a lower average threshold to pain than adults. The main consequence of immature central and peripheral myelination is *not* poor transmission of pain signals, given that such pathways are unmyelinated or only thinly so, but poorly coordinated nocifensive (defensive) motor behavior, which is reflexive and modified by experience. Newborns quickly learn to squirm and kick during a heel stick blood draw. Facial grimacing and fluctuating vital signs belie their experience of pain. There is even growing evidence that infants subjected to long and painful treatments without pain management in intensive care units are more likely to develop problems of somatization in school compared with those given intermittent or constant infusions of carefully adjusted opioid medications.[1]

ELDERLY PATIENTS

Geriatric patients also suffer from caregivers who have been misinformed about pain management. Although those aged 70 or older may, in general, be more susceptible to medication side effects, it does not mean that they should be left untreated for pain. It is wise to note that older generations might associate pain medication, especially those related to morphine, as a sign that they have little time left to live. Historically, in many settings, it was offered only at the time of death. Clarification here is the responsibility of the prescribing clinician.

Careful dose adjustment is key to good pain management, as is awareness of the various delivery systems that might minimize systemic side effects. "Start low and go slow" is a principle worth attending to. Realize, as well, that elderly patients long treated with controlled substances may have developed a high level of physical tolerance to medication effects such that aggressive treatment can be used with some in this age group, at least within reason. Each person must be assessed individually.

Selected patients who experience intolerable side effects from high-dose oral opioids prescribed for persistent cancer or noncancer pain—spinal pain being a common example—may benefit from the implantation of an intrathecal opioid pump through which relatively tiny amounts of medication are placed directly into the cerebrospinal fluid. It then enters the spinal cord and brain quickly and efficiently, minimizing spread to other systems and thereby minimizing side effects. Falls with potentially fatal hip fractures may be averted. Similarly, a well-placed epidural catheter may provide better, short-term, postoperative analgesia with fewer side effects than intermittent, nurse-given intravenous or oral opioids or even boluses delivered by a patient-controlled analgesia (PCA) device. When dementia is of concern, the dose must be titrated even more carefully and adjuvant medications or techniques employed that might prove opioid sparing. It must be remembered that in this group of patients, even normally well-tolerated medications may have adverse effects on mentation, as well as on the gastrointestinal and cardiovascular systems.

EFFECTIVE APPROACHES TO CHRONIC PAIN

It is a little appreciated but important concept that chronic pain is *not* merely a protracted form of acute pain and is often preventable. Chronic pain is not a symptom, from this perspective, but rather a disease and should be treated as such. There is a general consensus that a multimodal, interdisciplinary, or multidisciplinary approach to pain management is most effective. Nonetheless, prevention is still the key to minimize the likelihood of avoiding the development and consequences of chronic pain.

In addition to the effect that persistent pain has on the sufferer and his or her immediate family, it affects the greater community. The financial burden to society from lost productivity resulting from recurrent acute and chronic pain is staggering. Estimates range from $50 billion to $100 billion yearly for headache and low back pain alone. But the problem is wider and more serious than that. Failure to alleviate unnecessary suffering creates distrust between clinicians and patients, and this, in turn, diminishes the efficacy of our medical system. If patients feel forced to seek alternative and what they often interpret as more personal and caring forms of treatment, they may fail to seek appropriate care for other serious conditions when an allopathic approach is needed. The systems can work in harmony. More people than ever before are seeking alternatives to allopathic medicine because prevention, healing, and caring are emphasized over the concept of cure, but it is not always to their advantage. Missing the opportunity for early cancer detection, for example, may have tragic consequences. The modern concept of *integrative care* is important because it affords communication between all concerned, both patients and caregivers, and because the *combination* of allopathic and alternative approaches to care employed in concert may maximize positive results while minimizing the side effects of what might otherwise be a need for higher doses of allopathic medication with unwanted side effects. It is a more thorough form of interdisciplinary care where acupuncture, osteopathic, or chiropractic manipulation and herbal medicine, among other modalities, may assist with pain management and even the curative process. Employing a rational mixture of different treatments can decrease the daily amount of medication, as well as the duration of time spent taking controlled substances, thus minimizing the likelihood of accidental overdose or illicit drug use.

The public's trust must be regained. It has been lost with respect to allopathic medicine in many quarters for complex reasons, many of which can be traced to feelings of lack of control. This can lead to aberrant behavior sometimes unconsciously induced by the clinician, resulting in a loss of connection and, therefore, communication. Ultimately, the patient may be blamed when the problem was really the result of a dynamic between the treating staff and the patient. Medical providers must be willing to examine their own roles in the breakdown of communication and trust, eschewing the routine blame of patients.

Patients become anxious and distraught as their pain persists, and they become frustrated with the inability of medical professionals to alleviate it. Therefore, realistic expectations should be offered and periodically clarified or reinforced. Clinicians, in turn, become frustrated with their own lack of understanding of pain and their inability to control it. Sometimes, these feelings of frustration and inadequacy are turned against the patient in the form of "there is nothing more that can be done" or "obviously something else is going on, so I'm sending you to a psychiatrist." At such times, it may be more appropriate (and less worrying to the patient) to state that "there is little more that *I* am able to do" or, preferably, "your situation is quite complex and involves suffering beyond that of the physical pain alone, so we need to have it assessed more fully to formulate a better plan for pain management." This last comment, of course, needs expansion and explanation because a common interpretation of it is that "the doctor thinks that it is all in my head." Trust takes considerable effort and risk on both sides. It requires empathy. The adage "to hear about pain is to have doubt, but to experience it is to have certainty" is poignant and true.

WHAT IS CHRONIC PAIN IF NOT PROTRACTED ACUTE PAIN?

There are certain concepts that need emphasis to answer this question. The first of these is that *pain and suffering are not synonymous*. Although pain has been described as an unpleasant sensory and emotional experience arising from actual or potential damage to tissue, only when the consequences of pain—usually prolonged—begin to interfere negatively with the physical and emotional experience of life is suffering said to occur. In this way, pain may be likened to stress. A little pain is not necessarily a terrible thing. It may serve to focus attention on a stimulus and foster an appropriate response to it, but too much pain may prove overwhelming, exhausting, and demoralizing. It may lead to depression, which may further intensify the experience. And depression is not benign. With little warning, it may lead to suicide. Saying that "there is nothing more that can be done" may take away the only hope the patient has that he or she can keep going.

Continuing the analogy to stress, pain is difficult to study. It is not easily monitored or reliably objectively assessed, nor are its effects predictable from one individual to another. Indeed, pain thresholds may vary, not only among people, but also within the individual person over time according to mood, previous experience, and expectations. This complexity, fortunately, provides multiple levels or points at which pain management may prove successful. Appropriate interventions may be pharmacologic, invasive (i.e., surgery or nerve block), behavioral, or a combination of all three.

What, then, is the difference between pain and suffering? To answer this question, it must be understood that pain may affect a person's life in different ways according to his or her general state of well-being. Someone who is tired, hungry, anxious, or depressed reacts to an unpleasant sensation differently from someone who is well rested, in excellent shape, and in high spirits. When pain persists and overwhelms a person's coping mechanisms, it is likely to be seen as insurmountable and may take on a life of its own. Eventually, the tail wags the dog, as the saying goes. With this loss of control and autonomy and a growing feeling of helplessness, the person begins to experience a downward spiraling of emotional and physical well-being, in which severe deconditioning threatens normal functioning at home, work, and play. The consequence is a state of suffering of which only a portion is physical pain. This is why pain management clinicians do not advocate simply prescribing the strongest medication possible when the patient states, "If you just give me something to kill the pain, I will go back to work and everything will be OK." If only it were so simple! The wise practitioner tries to convince the patient that going back to work first—in graded increments—may offer a useful distraction from the pain and explains why a concurrent and multifaceted approach to pain management is needed. Although no single physician is capable of all aspects of care, in a multidisciplinary setting, there needs to be one clinician in overall charge of each patient's regimen to avoid processing patients "by committee." It is well to remember that pain management needs may change rapidly or slowly over time where progressive conditions such as cancer require frequent reevaluation. This is less the case in more static or far-more-slowly progressive syndromes such as those following spinal fusion.

CLINICAL EXAMPLE: THE DOWNWARD SPIRAL THAT TURNS PAIN INTO SUFFERING

To illustrate how a fairly minor event may lead to catastrophic results if early warning signs of chronic pain are not recognized and responded to appropriately, we will use the common scenario of a 50-year-old citizen sitting in a stationary car, hit from behind. There is no apparent injury at the time. Over the next few days, the patient experiences tightening up of muscles and low back pain, described as "spasms." These get worse over time. The family practitioner reassures the patient that it is only a muscular problem. Although the patient is willing to accept this for a while, a friend suggests initiating a lawsuit just in case something is more seriously wrong. An attorney, who states that he or she has seen many patients settle a case too early only to find out later that they have a lifelong disability for which they have no financial coverage, reinforces that philosophy.

The driver now sues and becomes hypervigilant about symptoms, becoming anxious every time pain is felt. The family physician reasserts that there is no neurologic dysfunction and that x-ray studies fail to show any skeletal injury. The patient disagrees. The pain is prolonged and is seemingly becoming intensified. He or she seeks a second opinion and, not satisfied with it, seeks a third, fourth, and so on, until a practitioner is found who echoes his or her concerns and who is willing to order a magnetic resonance imaging (MRI) scan. MRI then reveals degenerative changes not apparent on x-ray films, but probably consistent with age, such as "bulging discs," that do not clearly impinge a nerve root or the spinal cord but nonetheless are read correctly as just "touching" a nerve root. For the sake of argument, we shall assume that provocative discography, which measures pain within the disk itself, if performed, was negative in terms of reliably reproducing the pain. The consulting surgeon, wanting to help the patient, offers to operate to see if he or she can remove the tissue that "might" be touching a nerve, thus setting off the pain. The patient agrees, giving consent, *but doesn't hear or truly appreciate the qualification "might."* It may take several times before the patient understands that point—physicians likewise find it hard to recall all that has been explained to them. A physician must take the possibility of emotional shock into account and be patient when explaining his or her impression and plan.

As often happens, the surgery does not ameliorate the pain, and within a few months, a new pain begins. Subsequent MRI reveals evidence of scarring around the nerve root, one of the possible complications of invasive surgery. As the scar contracts, it pulls and irritates the nerve root, causing radicular pain along the upper or lower extremity in the dermatomal and sclerotomal (skeletal) distribution of the corresponding peripheral nerve and nerve root. The patient becomes frustrated, despondent, and depressed. The family physician then prescribes antidepressants for pain, but they seem to negatively affect the patient's ability to think clearly at work. The patient now no longer trusts the family physician's judgment (or prescriptions) and begins to take multiple over-the-counter drugs or uses "alternative" therapy that may, for the sake of argument, be expensive and of dubious value in this particular scenario. The pain persists.

Eventually, the family physician is forced to prescribe a mild narcotic for ongoing and worsening pain. This is taken over the next few months, with escalating dose requirements because the patient develops tolerance to the drug, leading to stronger medications, a pattern to which the clinician responds with concern, stating that he or she is not going to prescribe these medicines any more "because you are becoming addicted to them." They argue, and the patient is forced to seek care elsewhere. By now, having missed work so often and failing as well in personal relationships, the patient is fired at work and unhappy at home. Marriages and partnerships may fall apart. The patient becomes more depressed and cannot sleep well, escalating the pain.

Having been physically inactive now for several months, the patient is physically deconditioned and the ensuing poor posture and ill-functioning core musculature (some muscles being chronically contracted to minimize painful movements while others are weak and flaccid from disuse) induces myofascial or soft-tissue pain, worsening the situation. Now, an extra source of pain has developed—one that often goes unrecognized, which further invalidates the patient's complaints in the eyes of the clinician. The patient is no longer able to go out with friends or to visit family because of neck and back pain that prohibits driving. Sitting or standing in any one place for too long brings on the pain. The family withdraws, unable to console the patient, and feels inadequate. The patient ends up at a multidisciplinary pain management clinic, diagnosed with failed back surgery syndrome complicated by depression and severe deconditioning. A fairly long and expensive treatment program is now required to help the patient pick up the pieces. *The pain has become a state of suffering.*

Without overanalyzing this scenario, it is clear that a fairly innocuous event initiated a domino effect, resulting in biological, psychological, and social disruption of the patient's life. *This is why a biopsychosocial approach to pain management is necessary.* Early recognition of this downward spiral might have helped the patient if a brief period of pain management–oriented counseling or relaxation-based and or cognitive behavioral therapy was initiated earlier to help the patient look at the pain from a different perspective as well as to help alter his or her behavior. Self-reflection by the clinician might have helped as well. Furthermore, a more successful pain management program might have incorporated carefully focused physical therapy and/or warm pool exercises early on to minimize the deconditioning process. Short-term use of nonsteroidal anti-inflammatory drugs (NSAIDs), TCAs (tricyclic antidepressants) or SNRIs (serotonin norepinephrin reuptake inhibitor), and/or muscle relaxants might have decreased pain and improved sleep, minimizing the potential for depression. Potential sleep disorders should also have been assessed. This is especially important when pain has become chronic, given that restorative sleep is vital to a person's sense of well-being. Restful sleep can also raise the threshold of pain or fortify a person's tolerance of it. However, some of the commonly applied treatments for sleep disorders may actually prove counterproductive in this regard (as discussed later).

Close communication between the clinician and patient is therefore needed to develop mutual trust. Limits need to be specified with regard to medication refill requests and self-adjustments of dose to avoid misunderstandings that might lead to suspicion of addictive behavior and the firing of a patient. *Prescribing medications without adequate thought and discussion followed by abruptly stopping them simply generates patient frustration, bewilderment, and resentment.* Setting limits early and paying firm attention to them fosters the patient's respect and trust. With the rules established at the outset, perhaps in the form of a signed agreement or "contract," and agreed-upon random urine toxicology screening, the chance for misunderstanding is minimized. Such agreements, coupled with appropriate education about the pros and cons of using controlled substances, satisfy the *requirement of informed consent.*

PSYCHIATRIC COMORBIDITY AND CHRONIC PAIN

A common misconception is that chronic pain is the result of psychiatric disease. No doubt, the two often coexist, but psychiatric illness is more often a reaction to poorly controlled, life-affecting chronic pain. The prevalence and incidence of psychiatric comorbidity in patients with chronic pain is probably no greater than that seen in other patients with chronic medical disorders (e.g., epilepsy). A history of sexual, physical, or emotional abuse, with the resultant psychological ramifications, is astonishingly prevalent in a wide range of clinical settings, though, if the pratictioner takes the time to look. These issues may have special relevance to patients for whom invasive treatments are being contemplated, and this is one of the reasons such histories are pursued (and found to exist) in the pain clinic.

Poor coping skills and mood disorders may affect the experience of pain, but *the decision that depression, for example, is causing a person's pain should be made with the help of a trained mental health professional.* Even somatoform pain is real pain; it is simply treated from a more behavioral perspective. Assuming somatization without the assistance of a mental health professional may prove incorrect and result in invalidation of the patient's complaint. Worse, somatization may be confused with malingering and may unjustly and significantly influence legal and disability compensation issues. Thus, care must be taken when using terms such as "psychogenic" or "somatoform pain."[2] According to the *Diagnostic and Statistical Manual of Mental Disorders* (DSM-IV), the former term is no longer acceptable and the latter is relatively uncommon. The current terminology is "pain disorder associated with psychological factors." When a medical condition also affects the patient's experience of pain, it is termed "pain disorder associated with both psychological factors and a general medical condition."

Evaluating pain as physical ("real") or psychological ("unreal") is a simplistic and limited approach that serves no useful purpose: "Absence of evidence is not evidence of absence." For example, when MRI and a nerve conduction test fail to reveal a cause of a person's chronic low back pain, it is often assumed that there is no observable lesion. The problem is then usually treated with physical therapy and often with psychotherapy. Recent work has demonstrated that focal pathology may, in fact, exist but be out of the reach of the technology used to find it. For example, although MRI of a disk may appear normal, this technology cannot evaluate the inside of the disk: It will not reveal internal disk disruption, a painful tear. Thus, some specialists inject disks with a contrast agent (provocative discography), pressurizing it to determine if the pain induced is concordant with the clinical complaint. A normal disk—and some "wear and tear" is normal—is not painful during this procedure; however, although this is true of the lumbar region, it is controversial in the cervical spine. Specially guided computer-assisted tomography (CT scans) of these contrast-injected disks may then reveal fissures within the disk, some grades of which correlate well with the pain and may prove predictive of success with further intervention.

Elimination of the discogenic pain might be achieved (rarely) by corticosteroid injection into the disk; ablation of the sensory nerves subserving the disk; stiffening the disk by intradiskal electrothermal therapy (IDET), sometimes referred to as intradiskal electrothermal annuloplasty (IDEA); or disk removal with fusion of the vertebrae. There can be long-term negative consequences to such fusions of vertebrae, and rarely will a surgeon fuse more than two when neurologic compromise is not a risk. IDET was approved by the U.S. Food and Drug Administration (FDA) in 1998 and was found useful in workers' compensation and non–workers' compensation patients in a well-controlled study.[3] In recent years, artificial disk replacement (ADR) has become an option, using motion preserving surgery at one or more levels. In Germany, up to five levels of ADR have been performed with a high degree of success for many years, even in the face of osteoporosis (Bertagnoli, R. personal communication). It is good to know that the criteria for single- or multiple-level ADR differs from country to country as does the experience, rate of success, and level of skill (see Yue & Bertagnoli in this chapter's Bibliography).

Similarly, facet joint–mediated spinal pain may be missed without precision spine injections because there is a relatively poor correlation among the reported symptoms, physical examination, and electrodiagnostic and/or imaging test results. Currently, there is renewed interest in this controversial approach to the diagnosis and treatment of spine pain because improvements in patient selection and procedure technique have begun to help a significant number of those with "whiplash" and other so-called minor strain injuries.[4,5] These techniques will be described in detail in subsequent chapters.

To summarize, *a patient's pain need not be attributed to organic pathology in order to validate it as real.* Pain is what the patient says it is. Moreover, if psychological factors are found to be important in a patient's experience of pain, their importance should not be underestimated. Depression kills. Conversely, unless the diagnostic workup is well thought out, important physical pain generators may be missed; centralization of pain, however, may still prove problematic. Therefore, the question should not be "is this person's pain real (physical), or unreal (psychological)?" but "will this person's pain most likely respond to medical, invasive, or psychological intervention?"

ARE PLACEBOS USEFUL IN THE DIAGNOSIS OF PAIN?

The systematic use of placebo control is important in clinical research, but it is controversial in diagnostic medicine. This is another deceptively complex topic, fraught with misunderstanding. The placebo response has no bearing on whether pain is real or not; it merely defines the sufferer as a placebo responder or nonresponder. It neither confirms a psychogenic cause nor rules out physical pathology. In addition, there is no clear correlation of personality type with the likelihood of placebo response. A person may respond to placebo on one occasion but not on another. There may even be a spectrum of responses. Contrary to popular belief, the placebo response does not predictably occur one-third of the time or in one-third of the subjects. This notion stems from a paper in the *Journal of the American Medical Association* in which the author averaged the results of 11 studies to come up with 35.2%.[6] More recent studies estimate the rate to vary between 0% and 100%.[7] Placebo response varies widely between and within groups according to the expectations of both examiners and examinees. Its mechanism is controversial and incompletely understood, although it may, in part, result from the release of endorphins. The use of placebo under certain circumstances may prove damaging. When used without consent, it may be viewed by the patient as trickery. It can undermine the patient–clinician relationship, resulting in loss of trust. We have already established that trust is necessary for a good therapeutic outcome. Using a placebo may even violate the spirit of informed consent, if the placebo-controlled part of a procedure is not disclosed. Disclosure will not necessarily interfere with the placebo's usefulness. The clinician simply explains to the patient that response to treatment is complicated and may be influenced by patient expectation. The patient should be reassured that the medicine will be given, but in a manner and timing of which the patient will be unaware. The reassurance that he or she *will* receive the medication (not just placebo) is important. As Patrick Wall noted, the power of suggestion is a tool that may be employed benevolently and appropriately: "Mummy will kiss it better" is a wonderfully effective remedy.[8]

WHAT ABOUT OPIOIDS AND SUBSTANCE ABUSE?

The use of opioid medication in the management of noncancer pain remains controversial, despite more than a decade or two of active debate. There is still much prejudice and misunderstanding that governs clinical decision making in this area. Opioid medications actually have a lower risk for *addiction* than previously thought, at least if used appropriately in the management of pain. That last point is key. This is especially true in patients without a history of substance abuse by age 30, although it applies to infants and children, as well as adults. Unfortunately, many clinicians have not employed the use of such medication within a well-enough-constructed plan or with frequent-enough reviews. This problem, coupled with the increasing availability of prescription-controlled substances on the street, often taken with other psychoactive agents such as benzodiazepines and alcohol, has resulted in an exponential increase in accidental overdoses. This, too, will be discussed later in this text.

Some of the confusion regarding addiction concerns terminology. *Tolerance* is defined as an increasing dose requirement to maintain the same therapeutic effect. This may or may not occur in an individual on opioid therapy, but when it does, it does not necessarily equate with addiction. *Physical dependence* is another confusing term that is often misapplied as a synonym for addiction. It merely describes the potential for developing a physical state of withdrawal if the medication is weaned or withdrawn too quickly. Patients can usually be weaned successfully from drug therapy without inducing symptoms of withdrawal. Furthermore, tolerance and physical dependence together do not make for addiction per se. *Psychological dependence*, however, is equivalent to addiction, but there are strong underpinning neurobiological mechanisms responsible for it such that "free will" has less to do with relapse after detoxification than is commonly thought. Some of the mechanisms involve genetic predisposition, but arguably less so than recently thought.

Psychosocial and developmental events in life, such as neglect, physical, emotional, or sexual abuse, affect the development of neurochemical and neuroanatomical systems within the brain at very early ages, turning certain genes on or off in the process and increasing the likelihood of a medication-induced "high" and subsequent compulsive behavior with poor impulse control that leads to another downward spiral, addiction. Therefore, genes may have less to do with predisposition to addiction than the events in a person's life starting in early childhood. For this reason, it is vital that an accurate psychosocial history is obtained (see Gabor Mate in the Bibliography for a highly readable and current review of this concept). Psychological dependence or addiction may remain long after the weaning process has been completed and long after tolerance and physical dependence abate. It is somewhat controversial as to whether addiction can be reversed in whole or in part, or to what degree.

Psychological dependence is defined as a psychological fixation on a drug; the behavioral manifestation being compulsive and continued use of it, *despite known potential harm.* This problem is estimated to occur less than one-tenth of 1% of the time with short-term treatment following surgery using strong narcotics when there is no history of substance abuse. Even with long-term treatment, the addiction rate is probably between 3% and 16%; with the vast majority of those addicted having a history of substance abuse.[9,10] This means that there is unlikely to be a problem with addiction 84% to 97% of the time *in carefully selected and monitored patients.*

The role of cigarette smoking is yet unknown, but it is not generally considered to be an indicator of potential medication abuse problems, although some would disagree. Importantly, a history of addiction does not mean that patients in pain should go untreated or be denied opioids or other controlled substances, but a high state of vigilance by the prescribing clinician is recommended, as would be the inclusion on the team of a pain-specializing psychologist and/or an addictionologist whenever possible. In such cases, the clinician must monitor the patient more closely than usual for signs of addictive behavior. In general, it is good advice to have the patient sign a contract or an agreement that clearly outlines the parameters within which the relationship of prescriber to prescribee may operate smoothly. A copy should be given to the patient and highlighted where appropriate. Breaking this agreement is grounds for dissolution of the relationship. In selected cases, a zero tolerance approach is recommended with the relationship being discontinued with a carefully monitored wean of the prescribed substance. If this happens, there is an ethical obligation on the part of the physician to reasonably help the patient find care elsewhere.

Of note is that drug-seeking behavior is *not* synonymous with pain avoidance behavior (otherwise known as pseudo-addiction). The main difference between the two is that a person who is initially undermedicated and protests such treatment as though he or she is drug-seeking will likely stop such demands once the pain is controlled. His or her protests and pain behaviors are rational. The psychologically dependent (addicted) person may never seem to be appeased. When there is concern over patient behavior, it is appropriate to ask for help from a pain specialist or an addictionologist to evaluate and interpret the situation.

MEDICATIONS, ALTERNATIVE DELIVERY SYSTEMS, AND SURGERY

Pharmacotherapy is one of the mainstays of treatment of pain. Only brief mention of it is made here. The reader is directed to Fields and Liebeskind and Smith[11,12] for detailed overviews. In addition to the anti-inflammatory agents and opioids, certain antidepressant and antiepilepsy medications may prove useful for a variety of painful conditions. Those agents that elevate serotonin *and* norepinephrine in the brain, primarily the tricyclic (TCAs) and several atypical antidepressants such as SNRIs, may activate a descending pain modulatory system, thereby diminishing some forms of pain. SNRIs such as duloxetine (Cymbalta) and venlafaxine (Effexor) have proven effective with some pain disorders and tend to have fewer sexual, gastrointestinal, or motor side effects. Antidepressants may also diminish anxiety and improve sleep, reducing irritability and the negative affective ramifications of chronic pain. Note that bupropion hydrochloride (Wellbutrin) may occasionally help with pain, facilitate weight loss and cessation of cigarette smoking, and even improve sexual responsiveness; however, at higher doses, it can increase anxiety and interfere with sleep. Pain relief with antidepressants usually occurs independently of the drug's effect on mood. Antidepressants attenuate pain more quickly and at lower doses than is commonly needed for depression. Of the selective serotonin reuptake inhibitors (SSRIs), only paroxetine hydrochloride (Paxil) has a clinically demonstrable effect on neuropathic pain, but the evidence is weak. Some antidepressants increase the manifestation of restless legs syndrome (RLS) and the often concomitant periodic limb movements of sleep (PLMS) disorder. This is true mostly for the SSRIs and TCAs. Even those that make the patient sleepy might thereby negatively affect the quality of restorative sleep. A thorough sleep history is always indicated.

Some antiepilepsy medications and tricyclic antidepressants act as membrane-stabilizing agents, elevating the threshold for neuronal firing. They, too, may help diminish neuropathic pain. It is unlikely that membrane stabilization is the only mechanism for their analgesic effect because each drug may have multiple mechanisms of action. And, although it is often taught that tricyclic depressants are best for treatment of burning neuropathic pain with anticonvulsants being best for paroxysmal or shooting pain, either class can be used with some and perhaps comparable efficacy and should be selected on the basis of cost, side-effect profile, and likelihood of compliance. Antidepressants are commonly tried first because of their potential effect on problems other than pain, especially those that may exacerbate pain. The only clear indication for a specific medication to treat neuropathic pain is carbamazepine (Tegretol) or oxcarbazepine (Trileptal) for trigeminal neuralgia. In this case, there is well-documented evidence for their superiority over other agents. Likewise, the majority of the literature supports the use of tricyclic antidepressants over other agents for treatment of postherpetic neuralgia, although a number of viable options exist. These include opioids, gabapentin (Neurontin), pregabalin (Lyrica), and topical lidocaine (Lidoderm 5% patches), among others.

There are many other medications for which empirical and anecdotal evidence for efficacy in pain control exists, and the approach differs with chronic, recurrent acute, and acute pain. The skillful practitioner should be able to use combinations of these agents to minimize pain and suffering in patients for whom single agents have proven ineffective. It also pays to be aware of the different delivery systems available for some of these agents. Epidural and subarachnoid catheters; PCA devices; and the use of oral, rectal, sublingual, buccal, subcutaneous, intravenous, and intramuscular routes of administration all have their place in pain management.

Added to these modes of delivery is the neurosurgical approach to pain management. Under appropriate circumstances, pain pathways may be cut or neurostimulatory devices used with considerable efficacy at the level of the peripheral nerve, spinal cord, and subcortical and neocortical brain regions. Even ablation of the pituitary gland may significantly diminish the whole-body pain of metastatic cancer, but it is rarely performed today. Implanted intrathecal medication pumps and intraventricular catheters are useful modes of treatment in selected cases. Pain-oriented neurosurgery may prove valuable to multidisciplinary pain management teams. And, because some of the procedures are reversible (e.g., spinal cord stimulation and intrathecal pumps), neurosurgical intervention is *not* necessarily a "last resort." Use of it early in the course may preclude medication side effects and toxicity and may buy time for improvement of more definitive invasive approaches that are still in the experimental stage. Surgical treatment of pain is thoroughly addressed elsewhere.[13]

BRINGING IT ALL TOGETHER

What we have discussed here is a multimodal and interdisciplinary approach to the patient with chronic pain. The most important point is that the patient needs to feel *heard.* A biopsychosocial approach (however fuzzy that sounds) is useful to analyze and effectively manage the physical, emotional, and social aspects of patients' pain and suffering. Reasonable goals should be set with respect to diminution of pain and improvement in function. A good interdisciplinary team should include one or two physicians well-versed in pharmacologic and interventional procedures; a counselor, psychologist, social worker, psychiatric nurse practitioner, or psychiatrist to diagnose and treat or to help manage social and psychiatric conditions that may result from, cause, or exacerbate the pain; a physical therapist or rehabilitation specialist to assess physical conditioning requirements; complementary and alternative medical programs integrated with allopathic ones; and nurses knowledgeable about how these approaches may be applied to specific patients' multifaceted pain disorders.

Expertise in nursing requires emphasis here. Nurses help move clinics along efficiently and allay patient anxiety by being able to return calls promptly and expertly. Their skill in patient triage and procedure and postprocedural evaluation may prove invaluable to successful pain management. Patients often tell nurses information not disclosed to physicians. From the patient's perspective, the quality and responsiveness of the nursing staff may make the difference between an overall positive or negative clinical experience.[14]

Pain management teams that have frequent multidisciplinary meetings to discuss individual patients and their diagnoses and progress are more likely to be effective in carrying out a reasonable plan. However, there are too many patients with chronic pain to expect pain specialists alone to care for them. Primary care physicians are also well suited to the task and can be highly successful if some of the principles discussed in this chapter are followed. Note, however, that *success does not always mean cure*. If an approach to pain management diminishes a person's pain score by 1 point out of 10, then applying three or four approaches in concert may drop a person's pain score from 8 to 4, marking the difference between a state of suffering and one of simple pain. If this allows that person to return to school or to work with an improved level of function, then the pain management program may be called a success.

ACKNOWLEDGMENT

The authors wish to express their gratitude to Julie A. Brady (aka Wesley), RN, whose experience and comments proved invaluable to the production of this chapter.

REFERENCES

1. McGrath PA, et al. Controlling Children's Pain: A Practical Approach to Assessment and Management. 8th World Congress of Pain. Refresher course syllabus, 157-170. International Association for the Study of Pain (IASP), Vancouver, Canada; 1996.
2. Covington EC. Psychogenic pain—what it means, why it does not exist, and how to diagnose it. *Pain Med.* 2000;1:287-294.
3. Karasek M, Bogduk N. Twelve-month follow-up of a controlled trial of intradiscal electro thermal annuloplasty for the treatment of low back pain due to internally disrupted discs. *Spine.* 2000;25:2601-2607.
4. Bogduk N, et al. Precision Diagnosis of Spinal Pain. 8th World Congress of Pain. Refresher course syllabus, 313-323. International Association for the Study of Pain (IASP), Vancouver, Canada; 1996.
5. Goodwin J. Current concepts in the neurologic assessment of spinal pain: cancer and non cancer pain. In: Burchiel KJ, ed. *Surgical Management of Pain*. New York, NY: Thieme Medical Publishers; 2002:98-127.
6. Beecher HK. The powerful placebo. *JAMA*. 1955;159:1602-1606.
7. Wall PD. The placebo and the placebo response. In: Wall PD, Melzack R, eds. *Textbook of Pain*. 4th ed. Philadelphia, Pa: Churchill Livingstone; 1999:1419-1430.
8. Wall PD. The placebo and the placebo response. In: Wall PD, Melzack R, eds. *Textbook of Pain*. 3rd ed. Philadelphia, Pa: Churchill Livingstone; 1994:1297-1308.
9. Portenoy RK. Chronic opioid therapy in nonmalignant pain. In: Fields, HL, Liebeskind JC, eds. *Pharmacological Approaches to the Treatment of Chronic Pain: New Concepts and Critical Issues*. Seattle, Wash: International Association for the Study of Pain (IASP) Press; 1994.
10. Fishbain DA, et al. Drug abuse, dependence, and addiction in chronic pain patients. *Clin J Pain*. 1992;8:77-85.
11. Fields HL, Liebeskind JC, eds. *Pharmacological Approaches to the Treatment of Chronic Pain: New Concepts and Critical Issues*. Seattle, Wash: International Association for the Study of Pain (IASP) Press; 1994.
12. Smith HS, ed. *Drugs for Pain*. Philadelphia, PA: Hanley & Rufus, Inc. (pubs); 2003.
13. Burchiel KJ, ed. *Surgical Management of Pain*. New York, NY: Thieme Medical Publishers; 2002.
14. Brady JA, Jeffreys LK. Role of the nurse clinician. In: Burchiel KJ, ed. *Surgical Management of Pain*. New York, NY: Thieme Medical Publishers; 2002:246-256.

BIBLIOGRAPHY

Ballantyne JC, ed. *The Massachusetts General Hospital Handbook of Pain Management*. 3rd ed. Philadelphia, Pa: Lippincott, Williams and Wilkins Handbook Series; 2006.

A useful manual giving special attention to selected procedures; headache, adult and pediatric, as well as AIDS-related pain.

Burchiel KJ, ed. *Surgical Management of Pain*. New York, NY: Thieme Medical Publishers; 2002.

The most current and authoritative textbook on surgical approaches to pain management. A number of chapters pertain to issues discussed in this chapter.

Diagnostic and Statistical Manual of Mental Disorders (DSM-IV revised). Washington, DC: American Psychiatric Association; 1994.

Ferrell BR, Terrell BA. Pain in the elderly. In: *Task Force on Pain in the Elderly*. Seattle, Wash: International Association for the Study of Pain (IASP) Press; 1996:1-130.

Fishman SM, Ballantyne JC, Rathmell JP eds. *Bonica's Management of Pain*. 4th ed. Philadelphia, Pa: Lippincott Williams & Wilkins; 2009.

A highly comprehensive and resourceful reference textbook on pain management.

Goodwin J. Current concepts in the neurologic assessment of spinal pain: cancer and non cancer pain. In: Burchiel KJ, ed. *Surgical Management of Pain*. New York, NY: Thieme Medical Publishers; 2002:98-127.

An extensive review of diagnostic and therapeutic techniques pertaining to persistent spinal pain.

Goodwin J, Kraemer J, Bajwa Z. The Use of Opioids in the Treatment of Osteoarthritis: Why, When and How. *Curr Pain Headache Rep*. 2005 Dec;9(6):390-398.

Overview of a rational and integrative approach to caring for refractory osteoarthritis.

Kandel ER. *The Age of Insight: The Quest to Understand the Unconscious in Art, Mind, and Brain*. New York, NY: Random House; 2012.

An exceptionally brilliant and readable synthesis of the ways in which medicine, psychology, history, literature, and art have influenced one another over the last 110 years. By analogy, this Nobel Laureate and world renowned neuroscientist uses the thinking processes that all pain specialists should strive to reach in connecting the dots seen by most others as disparate rather than lying along an interwoven and multidimentional continuum.

Mate G. *In The Realm of the Hungry Ghosts*. Berkeley, Calif: North Atlantic Books; 2010.

A very readable and useful overview of the psychosocial, genetic and biological underpinnings of addiction by one of Canada's foremost experts.

McMahon SB, Koltzenburg M, eds. *Wall and Melzack's Textbook of Pain*. 5th ed. New York, NY: Churchill Livingstone; 2006.

A highly comprehensive and resourceful reference textbook on pain management.

Schecter NL, Berde CB, Yaster M, eds. *Pain in Infants, Children, and Adolescents*. 2nd ed. Philadelphia, Pa: Lippincott Williams & Wilkins; 2003.

The definitive textbook of pain management pertaining to the pediatric and adolescent years.

Yue JJ, Bertagnoli R, et al. eds. *Motion Preservation Surgery of the Spine*. Philidelphia, Pa: Saunders Elsevier; 2008.

The definitive textbook on the history and current developments in artificial disk replacement and other motion-preserving techniques in spinal surgery with a worldwide view.

Evaluating the Patient with Chronic Pain

Jeremy Goodwin
Umer Najib
Zahid H. Bajwa

Pain is a complex multidimensional symptom. It is determined not only by actual or potential tissue injury and normal and abnormal activity of the nervous system, but also by the patient's personal beliefs, mood, previous painful experiences, psychosocial stressors, coping mechanisms, and motivational factors. Evaluation of a patient with chronic pain should take into consideration all of these factors. Unfortunately, there is no single test or scale that can measure pain comprehensively, reliably, or objectively. A thorough history and physical examination, in combination with other diagnostic tools, are critical in the evaluation of pain patients to identify anatomic and physiologic pain generators. Several visits may be required to elucidate relevant medical and pyschosocial factors. The patient's motivation for the evaluation must be clarified early (i.e., whether there are issues of litigation or disability affecting the patient's pain and whether the patient perceives the potential to control pain as coming from within or without). To do this, it is important to listen well, develop the patient's trust, and not overly structure the interview. Chronic pain patients need validation. Without it, they cannot offer their trust, and trust is vital for treatment compliance and a successful outcome.

Pain assessment is a dynamic process that evolves with the pain management plan. The pain evaluation should be used to localize the source of pain; to determine its quality, pattern, and intensity; to define exacerbating and attenuating factors; and to assess how environmental and behavioral influences affect the pain. Clinicians should always try to make a diagnosis before implementing a treatment plan, recognizing that jumping to a premature conclusion might result in inappropriate treatment or harm to the patient. It is also necessary, at times, to rethink the diagnosis, despite previous and thorough workups. In this chapter, we focus on the history taking and targeted physical examination of a pain patient, pertinent diagnostic testing, pain measurement tools, and models of pain assessment and management.

HISTORY AND PHYSICAL EXAM

DEFINING THE TYPE OF PAIN

Pain should be broadly defined as nociceptive (somatic or visceral), neuropathic, or idiopathic. Toward this end, pain *location* is of utmost importance to accurate diagnosis. It may be well localized, as in entrapment neuropathy (e.g., carpal tunnel syndrome), widespread and diffuse (e.g., fibromyalgia), or regional (e.g., musculoskeletal pain). Patterns of *radiation* may help determine the site of pathology, such as in cervical or lumbar radiculopathy. Radicular pain (along a dermatome) implies involvement of a nerve root. Pain may also be *referred*, as in visceral pain, when it is felt over a particular area of skin that is embryologically associated with but anatomically distant from the source of irritation. Accurate characterization of the pain's location and pathophysiology provides the rationale for treatment. **Tables 8-1, 8-2,** and **8-3** provide examples of referred pain contrasted with clinical findings associated with nerve root versus peripheral nerve pathology.

TABLE 8-1 Patterns of Referred Pain

Origins of Pain	Region of Pain Referral
Heart	Chest, left arm, jaw, epigastrium (C8–T8)
Esophagus	Substernal region
Diaphragm/liver capsule	Shoulder (C4)
Kidney	Lower thorax and back (T11–L1)
Ureter (upper)	Groin, testes, or ovary
Ureter (terminal)	Scrotum, labia
Prostate	Lower back (T10–T12)
Uterus	Lower back (T10–T12)
Ovary	Anterior thigh
Upper cervical facets	Occiput, vertex, and toward frontal region of head
Lower cervical facets	Shoulder, neck, and scapulae
Lumbar facets	Groin, buttocks, anterior and posterior thighs, calves; can be felt above L5, midline
Sacroiliac joints	Groin, buttocks, anterior and posterior thighs, calves; should not refer above L5, midline

TAKING THE HISTORY

Detailed history taking at the first visit and a focused history (with emphasis on response to recent intervention) on subsequent visits is extremely beneficial. In many pain centers, the physician obtains a history after reviewing forms (see Appendix B) completed by the patient before the first interview. Some of the important points to be covered in this part of the evaluation are:

1. Location of pain.
2. Character of pain.
3. How and when the pain started.
4. If the pain is continuous or intermittent.
5. Exacerbating and relieving factors.
6. Effect of certain positions and activities on pain.
7. Effect of stress on the pain.
8. Effect of alcohol and other substances on pain.
9. If there is an associated sleep disturbance.
10. If there is an associated mood disturbance.
11. Effect of pain on functioning at work or school.
12. Effect of pain on quality of life, including social, sexual, and family interactions.
13. Effect of pain *treatment* on cognitive, social, and sexual function.
14. Motivation: issues of secondary gain (i.e., disability or psychological attention from partner, parents, or spouse).
15. If a lawsuit is involved.
16. If there is anyone the patient blames for the pain.

Beware of attributing new pain to an already defined process. For example, someone with ankylosing spondylitis can still develop a herniated disk, and cancer pain may change or worsen because of disease spread, tolerance to medications, side effects of treatment, or a new psychosocial stressor.

GENERAL PHYSICAL EXAMINATION

The physical examination starts with the first clinical interaction between the patient and clinician. It begins with how the patient responds to the initial greeting: getting up, walking, sitting down, and posture during these activities. Appearance (general health, weight, muscle bulk, and grooming), attitude and behavior (degree of distress and reactions to specific examination maneuvers), and gait (ataxia, walking with a limp, or requiring a cane or walker) can provide

TABLE 8-2 Clinical Manifestations of Root Versus Nerve Lesions in the Arm

Roots	C5	C6	C7	C8	T1
Sensory supply	Lateral border of upper arm	Lateral forearm, including finger 1	Over triceps, midforearm, and finger 3	Medial forearm to finger 5	Axilla down to elbow
Reflex affected	Biceps reflex	None	Triceps reflex	None	None
Motor loss	Deltoid	Biceps	Latissimus dorsi	Finger extensors	Intrinsic hand muscles (in some thenar muscles through C8)
	Infraspinatus Rhomboids Supraspinatus	Brachialis Brachioradialis	Pectoralis major Triceps Wrist extensors	Finger flexors Flexor carpi ulnaris Wrist flexors	
Nerves	**Axillary (C5, C6)**	**Musculocutaneous (C5, C6)**	**Radial (C5–C8)**	**Median (C6–C8, T1)**	**Ulnar (C8, T1)**
Sensory supply	Over deltoid	Lateral forearm to wrist	Lateral dorsal and back of thumb and finger 2	Lateral palm and lateral fingers 1, 2, 3, and half of 4	Medial palm and fingers and medial half of finger 4
Reflex affected	None	Biceps reflex	Triceps reflex	None	None
Motor loss	Deltoid	Biceps brachialis	Brachioradialis Finger extensors Forearm supinator	Abductor pollicis brevis Long flexors of fingers 1, 2, 3	Intrinsic hand muscles Flexor carpi ulnaris
			Triceps Wrist extensors	Pronators of forearms Wrist flexors	Flexors of fingers 4 and 5

From Patten J. *Neurological Differential Diagnosis*. New York, NY: Springer-Verlag; 1977.

important information. The presence or absence of masses or lesions, signs of injury or trauma, and limb asymmetry regarding skin, hair, nails, or temperature changes should be noted. Alignment of the spine (scoliosis, kyphosis, loss of curvature) and range of motion (ROM) should be noted. Joint shape, swelling, redness, and tenderness should also be noted. Measurement of vital signs may prove useful in evaluating stress, pain (which alters vital signs in young children), and side effects of medication.

PERTINENT NEUROLOGICAL AND PSYCHIATRIC EXAMINATIONS

Focused neurologic and psychiatric examinations also start with the first clinic visit. If the patient is able to give a clear and adequate history, a formal mental status examination is usually unnecessary, but range of affect (facial expression) and its congruency with language content and mood can provide important clues to the presence or absence of depression or anxiety. The effect of analgesics on higher intellectual function should be documented to help with future medication trials and to interpret problems of mental status. And unless the patient suffers from a headache or cranial nerve pain or dysfunction (i.e., trigeminal neuralgia or trigeminal neuropathy), the cranial nerve examination can generally be simplified by checking facial symmetry and eye movements (for a detailed outline, see **Table 8-4**). Experience best guides the clinician in the directed examination; however, subtle and sometimes significant findings may be missed by using a screening technique.

Results of the motor, sensory, and deep tendon reflex examination should be viewed together. Patients with lumbar or cervical radiculopathy may have more than one measurable objective sign or abnormality, although pain in a nerve root distribution may be the only symptom. If a

TABLE 8-3 Clinical Manifestations of Root Versus Nerve Lesions in the Leg

Roots	L2	L3	L4	L5	S1
Sensory supply	Across upper thigh	Across lower thigh	Across knee to medial malleolus	Side of leg to dorsum and sole of foot	Behind lateral malleolus to lateral foot
Reflex affected	None	None	Patellar reflex	None	Achilles tendon reflex
Motor loss	Hip flexion	Knee extension	Inversion of foot	Dorsiflexion of toes and foot	Plantar flexion and eversion of foot
Nerves	**Obturator (L2–L4)**	**Femoral (L2–L4)**	**Peroneal division of sciatic nerve (L4, L5, S1–S3)**	**Tibial division of sciatic nerve (L4, L5, S1–S3)**	
Sensory supply	Medial thigh	Anterior thigh to medial malleolus	Anterior leg to dorsum of foot	Posterior leg to sole and lateral aspect of foot	
Reflex affected	None	Patellar reflex	None	Achilles tendon reflex	
Motor loss	Adduction of thigh	Extension of knee	Dorsiflexion, inversion, and eversion of foot	Plantar flexion and inversion of foot	

From Patten J. *Neurological Differential Diagnosis*. New York, NY: Springer-Verlag; 1977.

TABLE 8-4 Clinical Evaluations of Cranial Nerve Function

Cranial Nerve	Name	Evaluation Procedures
I	Olfactory	Test ability to identify familiar aromatic odors (e.g., coffee grounds, vanilla extract), one naris at a time and with eyes closed. Not routinely tested.
II	Optic	Test vision with Snellen chart or Rosenbaum near-vision chart. Perform ophthalmoscopic examination of fundi. Recognize papilledema and retinal hemorrhages. Test fields of vision using confrontation and double simultaneous stimulation. Is color vision equal for both eyes?
III, IV	Oculomotor, trochelar	Inspect eyelids for drooping (ptosis). Inspect pupil reactivity and size for equality (direct and consensual response) and rule out paradoxical dilation or afferent pupillary defect with swinging flashlight test (optic neuritis). Check for nystagmus of immediate, delayed, and attenuating type. Assess basic fields of gaze. Note asymmetric extraocular movements. Test ability to bury sclera when right or left eye looks toward nose.
V	Trigeminal	Test corneal reflex. Test superficial pain and touch sensation in each branch: V_1, V_2, V_3.
VI	Abducent	Test ability to bury sclera when right or left eye looks to side.
VII	Facial	Palpate jaw muscles for tone and strength while patient clenches teeth. Inspect symmetry of facial features. Test adequacy of closed-eye strength. Have patient smile, frown, puff cheeks, wrinkle forehead to test symmetry. Watch for spasmodic, jerking movements of face.
VIII	Vestibulocochlear	Test sense of hearing with watch or rubbing fingers 6 in. from ear. Compare bone and air conduction of sound (Weber's and Rinne tests).
IX	Glossopharyngeal	Test gag reflex and ability to swallow.
X	Vagus	Inspect palate for symmetry of evaluation when patient says "ahhhh." Observe for swallowing difficulty. Have patient take small sip of water. Watch for nasal or hoarse quality of speech. Can patient make a quick, clear "cough"?
XI	Spinal accessory	Test trapezius strength (have patient shrug shoulders against resistance). Test sternocleidomastoid muscle strength (have patient turn head against resistance).
XII	Hypoglossal	Inspect tongue in mouth and while protruded for symmetry, fasciculations, and atrophy. Test tongue strength with index fingers when tongue is pressed against cheek.

Note: Taste, like smell, is not routinely assessed. When necessary, it should probably be assessed by a neurologist.

Modified from Donohoe CD. Targeted history and physical examination. In: Waldman SD, ed. *Interventional Pain Management.* 2nd ed. Philadelphia, Pa: WB Saunders; 2001:90.

TABLE 8-5 Deep Tendon Reflex Scale

0	No response
1+	Sluggish
2+	Active or normal
3+	More brisk than expected, slightly hyperactive
4+	Abnormally hyperactive, with intermittent clonus

From Seidel HM, et al. *Mosby's Guide to Physical Examination.* 3rd ed. St. Louis, Mo: Mosby-Yearbook; 1995.

single nerve or nerve root is involved, motor, sensory, and reflex abnormalities should coincide with and not contradict one another (see Tables 8-2, 8-3, **8-5,** and **8-6**). If a nerve plexus is involved, the situation is more complex and may require more extensive neurologic or electrodiagnostic evaluation. It is helpful to know that the boundaries of sensory-motor deficits are less clear in plexopathies than they are in peripheral nerve injury and that pain can occur without such deficits. Progression of sensory dysfunction, even outside of the originally involved area (i.e., allodynia) may indicate centralization of pain or disordered sensory processing in the spinal cord and not necessarily psychiatric overlay, as is often supposed.

We recommend *functional* motor assessment as an initial evaluative tool for the motor system, followed by a more focused examination of any abnormal findings (Tables 8-2 through **8-7**). For example, if patients with back pain can rise from a chair without using their arms and can easily walk on tip-toes and heels, they are unlikely to have lower extremity weakness on manual-motor testing.

Some tests are more nerve root–specific than others. Great toe extension is mostly controlled by the L5 nerve root, whereas dorsiflexion of the foot involves nerve roots L4 through S1. It is vital to distinguish true muscle weakness from pain-limited strength and lack of effort. "Giveway" weakness may be indicative of either. Feigned unilateral weakness, an uncommon problem, is harder to maintain when both limbs are assessed at the same time. Table 8-7 summarizes some likely "nonorganic" signs and symptoms that are referred to as "illness or pain behavior."

The sensory examination should include response to light touch, light pressure, pinprick or cold (i.e., metal object or alcohol swab because pain and temperature are carried in the same pathway), and vibration and assessment of proprioception or joint position sense. If the patient's Romberg stance is stable, significant loss of vibratory and position sense is unlikely but still possible. The affected skin area, which

TABLE 8-6 Grading of Muscle Strength

Clinical Finding	Grade	% of Normal Response
No evidence of contractility	0	0
Slight contractility, no movement	1	10
Full range of motion with gravity eliminated	2	25
Full range of motion with gravity	3	50
Full range of motion against gravity, some resistance	4	75
Full range of motion against gravity, full resistance	5	100

From Chipps EM, et al. *Neurologic Disorders.* St. Louis, Mo: Mosby-Yearbook; 1992.

TABLE 8-7 Chronic Low Back Pain: Symptoms and Signs of Physical Disease Versus Abnormal Illness Behavior

	Physical Disease	Abnormal Illness Behavior
Symptoms		
Pain	Anatomic distribution	Whole leg pain
Numbness	Dermatomal	Whole leg numbness
Weakness	Myotomal	Whole leg giving way
Time pattern	Varies with time	Never free of pain
Response to treatment	Variable benefit	Intolerance of treatments
Signs		
Tenderness	Anatomic distribution	Superficial Widespread, nonanatomic
Axial loading	No lumbar pain	Lumbar pain
Simulated rotation	No lumbar pain	Lumbar pain
Straight-leg raising	Limited on distraction	Improves with distraction
Sensory	Dermatomal	Regional, but patchy numbness may indicate spinal cord lesion
Motor	Myotomal	Regional, jerky, giving way

Modified from Waddell G, et al. Clinical evaluation of disability in low back pain. In: Frymoyer JW, et al., eds. *The Adult Spine: Principles and Practice.* 2nd ed. Philadelphia, Pa: Lippincott-Raven; 1997:171-184.

almost always manifests hyperesthesia, should be tested at the end of the examination. Allodynia should be sought in terms of light touch, light tapping, mechanical movement, and cold stimuli. Hyperpathia is elicited by fairly rapidly applying pinpricks to the focal area. What at first appears to be a diminution in pain sensation suddenly becomes an abnormally intense and prolonged discomfort lasting beyond the time of stimulation. When pain has become chronic and local tissue injury has healed, the persistence of allodynia, with or without hyperpathia, points to a neuropathic rather than nociceptive pain process. This may have important implications for further workup and treatment. Nociceptive pain, on the other hand, is generally associated with hyperesthesia that resolves with healing.

Examination of gait is not only helpful in screening for motor, sensory, or balance dysfunction, but it can also help evaluate the toxicity of some analgesic medications (high levels of some antiseizure medications used for pain may cause a broad-based gait and loss of balance, otherwise known as truncal ataxia). Conversely, the *absence* of a widely based gait in a patient complaining of difficulty balancing raises the question of astasia-abasia or functional sway. If present, the latter does not negate a physical basis for pain, but raises the question as to whether psychologic factors influence the degree of patient suffering.

PROVOCATIVE TESTS

Pain-exacerbating maneuvers—such as the cervical distraction and compression tests, Spurling's maneuver of the neck, drop-arm test for evaluation of rotator cuff, Yergason test for the integrity of the biceps tendon, tennis elbow test, Tinel's and Phalen's sign tests for median nerve dysfunction, straight-leg raising test, facet loading maneuvers, Patrick Faber test for sacroiliac joint dysfunction, tests for piriformis syndrome (Pace, Laseque, and Freiberg test), and spinal ROM tests—may yield important diagnostic information. The examiner should keep in mind that the validity of provocative tests is compromised by lack of patient participation and presence of secondary gains. Maneuvers such as Hoover's sign and Waddell's signs can help differentiate organic from nonorganic components of pain (see Table 8-7 for other nonorganic signs and symptoms).

DIAGNOSTIC TESTING

ELECTRODIAGNOSTIC TESTING, SPINAL INJECTIONS, AND NEURAL BLOCKAGE

Methods of evaluation may not be as equivalent as they first appear. Electromyography and neural blockade is a case in point. Electromyography, including the electromylogram (EMG) and nerve conduction tests (NCT), can help rule in or out a myopathy, neuropathy, radiculopathy, or plexopathy accompanying a painful condition. It can also help determine chronicity. Several spinal and nerve root levels may be tested in a single session. Reflex arcs of the spinal cord can be evaluated and peripheral neurologic findings on the physical examination confirmed, but EMG cannot measure pain. EMG cannot measure small-fiber dysfunction (i.e., as caused by diabetes) and should not be attempted until 2 to 3 weeks after the onset of symptoms. This minimizes the chance of false-negative results. EMG and NCT are extremely operator dependent, in terms of both technique and interpretation.

Selective nerve root blockade and spinal injection into vertebral disks (diskograms) and zygahypophyseal (facet) joints or the epidural space may prove diagnostic or therapeutic but offer no clues to chronicity. Except for diskography, multiple levels of testing are not easily or wisely done during a single visit because specificity is lost. Although the usefulness of EMG, NCT, and selective nerve root blockade may overlap, information obtained through one does not necessarily negate the need for the other. If in doubt about which diagnostic test is most appropriate, ask a colleague with advanced understanding of that particular field.

IMAGING STUDIES

Choosing the appropriate mode of imaging can be difficult, the consequence of which may hasten or slow the time to accurate diagnosis. A general guide to the commonly used techniques is presented in **Table 8-8**. Advice should be sought from knowledgeable colleagues for specific case applications.

TABLE 8-8 Imaging Procedures with Best Diagnostic Value by Body Region

Body Region	Recommended Procedure(s)*
Head and brain	**MRI** CT scan Angiography Plain films
Neck and spine	**MRI** Plain films Myelography CT scan
Extremities, soft tissues (including muscle, excluding bone)	**MRI** Plain films Ultrasonography CT scan Venography
Bone	**Plain films** **Bone scintigraphy** **CT scan** **MRI**
Joint	**MRI** Plain films Arthrography

(*Continued*)

TABLE 8-8 Imaging Procedures with Best Diagnostic Value by Body Region (*Continued*)

Body Region	Recommended Procedure(s)*
Chest	**Plain films** **CT scans** MRI Radionuclide studies Coronary arteriography Aortography
Abdomen	**Ultrasonography** **CT scan** **Contrast studies (barium meal or enema, IV pyelography)** Plain films MRI Radionuclide studies
Pelvis	**Ultrasonography** **MRI** CT scan

*Boldface indicates procedure of choice. CT, computed tomography; MRI, magnetic resonance imaging.

Modified from Banitzky S, et al. Radiologic testing in patient evaluation. In: Waldman SD, ed. *Interventional Pain Management,* 2nd ed. Philadelphia, Pa: WB Saunders; 2001:129.

PAIN MEASUREMENT TOOLS

No single tool or instrument can measure pain fully and objectively in a clinical setting. But several measurement instruments have been developed to assess the most clinically relevant aspects of pain and ways in which it affects the patient's life. These tools are either easily used but limited in what they measure (unidimensional scales) or require time to apply and psychological expertise to interpret (multidimensional scales).

UNIDIMENSIONAL INSTRUMENTS, SCALES, AND INDICES

In clinical practice, unidimensional and self-report scales offer a simple, useful, and valid method for assessment and monitoring of a patient's pain. Unidimensional scales measure only the intensity of pain.

Numeric Rating Scale (NRS) or Verbal Rating Scale (VRS) This is the simplest and most commonly used scale to evaluate pain. On a scale of 0 to 10, where 0 represents "no pain" and 10 the "worst imaginable pain," the patient chooses a number to describe the pain intensity. Advantages of this scale are that it is simple and reproducible, it is easily understood by most patients, and small changes in pain can be measured. Its major disadvantage is its inability to reflect anything more than the intensity of pain. Ramifications of pain on mood (or vice versa) are not so easily measured.

Visual Analog Scale (VAS) The VAS is very similar to the NRS or VRS except that the patient puts a mark on a *nongradated* 10-cm line, with one end labeled as "no pain" and the other as "worst pain imaginable." Using the VAS, pain can be evaluated on a 0 to 10 scale and can be described as such. The advantages and disadvantages are very similar to the NRS, but the VAS is used more commonly in clinical pain research. VAS results do not always match, but the discrepancy itself can prove useful because it stimulates a more in-depth evaluation.

Verbal Descriptor Scales With verbal descriptor scales, patients are asked to describe their pain by choosing descriptors from a list of adjectives reflecting pain intensity. One example is a five-word scale denoting pain as *mild, uncomfortable, distressing, horrible,* or *excruciating.* A major limitation of this scale is that patients often select moderate descriptors rather than extremes to appear more "reasonable" or may select extremes rather than more moderate descriptors when their level of distress is very high. This should prompt a search for confounding factors, such as anxiety or fear, which can greatly affect the level of pain or suffering.

Faces Pain Rating Scale Evaluating pain in children younger than 8 years old is extremely challenging because of their inability to fully describe pain or understand pain assessment forms. The faces pain rating scale depicts sketches of facial expression, ranging from a happy, smiley face to a very distressed and teary face. Several versions are in common use. In evaluating children in pain, their cognitive-developmental level, pain self-support, pain behavior, and physiologic parameters, such as variation in blood pressure and heart rate, must also be taken into account. The faces pain rating scale may also be useful in developmentally disabled patients, cognitively impaired geriatric patients, and sometimes in patients who do not speak English (when no interpreter is available).

MULTIDIMENSIONAL INSTRUMENTS, SCALES, AND INDICES

These instruments provide more detailed information about the patient's pain than do unidimensional scales. They are especially useful in the evaluation of complex pain in patients whose suffering is likely multifactorial in origin. However, these tools are relatively cumbersome and time-consuming, requiring expert interpretation. They are usually reserved for use in clinical research or in-depth multidisciplinary evaluations at comprehensive pain management centers. Pain psychologists often employ a battery of such tests in conjunction with the psychiatric interview. Only a few are mentioned here for the purpose of illustration.

It is important to reemphasize that no single assessment tool can fully evaluate a person's pain. Just as magnetic resonance imaging cannot replace the acumen of the clinician, so these measurement tools are limited to an adjunctive role in evaluation of the neuropsychologic pain. The value of these tests lies in their appropriate use by trained individuals.

Minnesota Multiphasic Personality Inventory (MMPI) This instrument is a long and complex questionnaire that requires caution in interpretation (its scales are based on the general population, not a chronic pain patient population). A number of scales are generated, which may lead to a false sense of confidence in the ability of the test to assess pain. The ability to predict outcome of treatment is variable. The test is better at predicting who is not likely to return to work than who is. Thus, the degree to which this tool is helpful depends greatly on the application, knowledge, and skill of the clinician using it. Many pain centers use an abbreviated and modified version called the MMPI-2.

McGill Pain Questionnaire (MPQ) Historically, this is one of the most commonly used multidimensional instruments. Patients select descriptive terms from groups of words ranked in order of severity. Pain location is also sketched on a human figure drawing. Present and previous pain experiences are noted, and all of this is integrated into a general analysis of the patient's pain experience. The MPQ requires some patient sophistication in the use of language, reducing the value of the test considerably if applied indiscriminately.

Brief Pain Inventory (BPI) The BPI asks patients to rate the pain at its worst, least, and average intensity, as experienced at the time of evaluation. It also asks patients to present the location of their pain on a schematic diagram of the body. The BPI is a cross-cultural instrument and is particularly useful in clinical pain research.

TWO MODELS OF PAIN ASSESSMENT AND MANAGEMENT

As we have discussed, no single scale or test is able to fully evaluate a patient with chronic pain, but a combination of the patient's history and physical examination, diagnostic tests, and some of the assessment tools can be very helpful. Each pain center or clinician can develop a pain assessment form dictated by the type of pain problems most often encountered in their referral group. Appendix A is the pain assessment form used by the pain management center at the Beth Israel-Deaconess Medical Center (BIDMC) in Boston. Patients complete the center's assessment form before their first appointment. This approach is a classic consultative model. Referral is made by primary care or treating clinician, via a referral letter or form provided by the BIDMC pain center. Once the referral is received, a pain management specialist reviews the information and decides on the best line of action, based on the nature of the pain and urgency of the situation. Urgent appointments are scheduled with patients for whom immediate interventions may prevent chronic pain and disability, such as patients in the early stages of reflex sympathetic dystrophy (complex regional pain syndrome, type 1) or postherpetic neuralgia.

All patients are required to complete the assessment form before their first visit. Some patients are selected for a "comprehensive pain evaluation" based on the chronicity and complexity of their pain, response to previous interventions, and complicating factors, such as substance abuse, psychiatric illness, or factors associated with possible secondary gain. The comprehensive pain evaluation requires completion of modified versions of the Beck Depression Inventory (BDI), the MMPI, and other behavior assessment tools before the first visit. These patients are then scheduled to see a team composed of one or two physicians, a nurse, a psychologist, and a physical or occupational therapist, all on the same day. Then, the full multidisciplinary team (i.e., clinicians who have personally seen the patient plus those who have not) discusses the evaluation team's findings and impressions and arrives at a realistic, practical, and long-term plan.

The cornerstone of this model is that pain specialists act as *consultants* in coordinating short-term and long-term care of a variety of patients with chronic pain. Once the patient is stabilized on a certain regimen or has reached a medical end point, patient management is taken over by the referring clinician. The patient must have a primary care clinician to be seen. The pain specialist does not "take over" responsibility of the patient's care but may be heavily involved in it, at least initially. Where possible, the primary care clinician should prescribe the pain medications, once the dose has been stabilized. This allows closer monitoring of a patient's health over time and minimizes the chance of accidental drug-to-drug interactions. The fewer providers prescribing for a patient, the better it is for long-term care.

A modification of this approach (used where state health plans or insurance coverage is more restrictive) begins with the pain physician's initial evaluation on referral by another clinician. The pain physician then refers to other clinicians (not necessarily in his or her clinic) as necessary and as authorized by the third-party payer. As the third-party payer milieu continues to evolve, more pain centers may have to adopt this potentially less expensive and slower approach. One of the authors (Goodwin) and Kim J. Burchiel, MD, Chairman of the Department of Neurological Surgery at the Oregon Health and Science University, believe that a potentially successful means of doing this is via a coordinated network of persons, clinicians, and services who are financially independent of each other yet complementary in terms of skills, philosophy, and training. Such interdisciplinary or interdepartmental cooperation could provide a depth and breadth of resources unlikely to be available in a smaller, single department–funded multidisciplinary pain center. If alternative medicine is specifically and *openly* included in interdisciplinary patient care and not just used as an adjunctive complementary or alternative approach, the care can then rightly be referred to as *integrative* pain medicine.

Finally, in some states, such as Oregon, patient evaluation by a pain specialist, or an expert on the physiologic or anatomic system that is painful (e.g., urologist, orthopedist, gastroenterologist), is required by law so that a primary care provider can prescribe long-term opioids for the management of nonmalignant pain without concern of criticism by the medical board of examiners. This particular type of evaluation may or may not require a team approach, depending on the complexity of the situation.

PUTTING IT ALL TOGETHER

Evaluating a patient with chronic pain can be time-consuming and frustrating, because clinicians must rely greatly on the patient's subjective report and the somewhat limited results of objective tests. An understanding of central and peripheral neuroanatomy and pathophysiology, visceral innervation, and musculoskeletal function is essential for interpretation of findings by review of the history, physical examination, and other diagnostic tools. If done correctly, the evaluation alone can prove therapeutic; just having a diagnosis can alleviate stress. It is the first step in building the physician–patient relationship and therapeutic alliance. It is important always to listen to and believe in your patients and involve them in the decision-making process. The clinician should be empathic, supportive, and honest, neither promising too much nor removing all hope. There is a big difference between stating, "There is nothing I can do," and, "There is nothing more that can be done." The suffering patient is a human being in distress, not a disease. Tests and measurement tools aid in diagnosis and treatment but cannot replace a thorough history and physical examination. Several visits may be necessary before the picture becomes clear. If the preceding approach is followed, especially within a multidisciplinary or interdisciplinary setting, then there is a reasonable chance that correct diagnoses will be made, followed by appropriate management.

BIBLIOGRAPHY

Aprill C. Diagnostic disc injections I (cervical) and II (lumbar). In: Frymoyer JW, ed. *The Adult Spine*. Philadelphia, Pa: Lippincott-Raven; 1997:523-562.

Cipriano JJ. *Photographic Manual of Regional Orthopaedic and Neurological Tests*. 3rd ed. Baltimore, Md: Williams & Wilkins; 1997.

Donohoe CD. Targeted history and physical examination. In: Waldman SD, ed. *Interventional Pain Management*. 2nd ed. Philadelphia, Pa: WB Saunders; 2001:83-94.

Finley GA, McGrath PJ, eds. *Measurement of Pain in Infants and Children. Progress in Pain Research and Management*. Vol IV. Seattle, Wash: International Association for the Study of Pain (IASP) Press; 1998.

Gagliese L, Melzack R. The assessment of pain in the elderly. In: Mostofsky DI, Lomranz J, eds. *Handbook of Pain and Aging*. New York, NY: Plenum Press; 1997:69-96.

Goodwin JLR. Current concepts in the neurologic assessment of spinal pain: cancer and noncancer pain. In: Burchiel KJ, ed. *Surgical Management of Pain*. New York, NY: Thieme Medical Publishers; 2002:98-127.

Karasek M, Bogduk N. Twelve-month follow-up of a controlled trial of intradiscal electro thermal annuloplasty for the treatment of low back pain due to internally disrupted discs. *Spine*. 2000;25:2601-2607.

Klein JD, Garfin SR. Clinical evaluation of patients with suspected spine problems. In: Frymoyer JW, ed. *The Adult Spine: Principles and Practice*. 2nd ed. Philadelphia, Pa: Lippincott-Raven; 1997: 319-340.

Menses S, Simons DG, eds. *Muscle Pain: Understanding Its Nature, Diagnosis, and Treatment*. Philadelphia, Pa: Lippincott Williams & Wilkins; 2001.

Waldman SD, ed. *Interventional Pain Management*. 2nd ed. Philadelphia, Pa: WB Saunders; 2001.

Spine, Neuromuscular, and Musculoskeletal Exam of the Chronic Pain Patient

John C. Keel
Imran J. Siddiqui
John M. Lavelle

INTRODUCTION

Most patient assessment is the taking of the history itself: *Listen to the patients; they will tell you what is wrong with them.* Physical examination then serves as a confirmation of your suspicions. Spine, neuromuscular, and musculoskeletal disorders comprise the bulk of conditions seen in the pain clinic, so basic physical exam is reviewed here. The reader is urged to refer to classic texts for more detail regarding this expansive topic: The single *vade mecum* is Hoppenfeld's *Physical Examination of the Spine and Extremities.*[1] Comprehensive instruction in all musculoskeletal examination maneuvers is found in Magee's *Orthopedic Physical Assessment.*[2] Musculoskeletal examination as well as anatomy, imaging, and management are covered in detail in the "Essentials."[3] A complete text for neurological exam is *DeJong's The Neurologic Examination.*[4] Beyond reading, practice over years is encouraged to attain mastery. We cite utility of common tests in terms of sensitivity and specificity when available. Beyond the science, the art and the truth are that the physical examination is a bonding ritual with patients.

The physical exam begins as soon as you see the patient walking into the room, with the assessment of gait. For the most careful assessment, it is best to have the patient disrobe. Common themes of physical examination include *inspection, palpation, motion testing,* and *provocation* or special tests, which are often eponymous. Spine and musculoskeletal range of motion values are not universally agreed upon, and values here are for reference. Many special physical exam protocols exist, and a few with practical application in pain are included at the close of this chapter.

SPINE, ALL LEVELS

Inspection: Visually inspect spine alignment, including normal curvatures, sagittal and coronal balance, or any scoliosis or excess kyphosis. The four normal curves exist only in the sagittal plane and include cervical lordosis, thoracic kyphosis, lumbar lordosis, and sacral kyphosis. Normal sagittal balance is the arrangement of these curves so that an imagined plumb line from C7 would pass through S1.

Scoliosis is a three-dimensional curvature of the spine as the spine deviates from midline in the coronal plane with maximal rotation occurring at the apex of the curve—the majority of which are idiopathic and seen in the thoracic and lumbar spine. The curve is named for the side of the apex. To evaluate for spinal curves, the patient slowly bends forward at the waist with knees straight. Paraspinal or rib humping correlates with the apex of the curve (hump on the left is levoscoliosis, on the right is dextroscoliosis).

Palpation: Palpate bony landmarks and paraspinal regions. Cervical and thoracic bony landmarks include spinous process, mastoid process, inion, and paraspinal regions corresponding to facet joints. Lumbosacral bony landmarks include spinous process, coccyx, iliac bone including posterior superior iliac spine, and paraspinal regions corresponding to sacroiliac and facet joints.

Provocation: Provocation includes range of motion testing as well as special tests (**Table 9-1**). Range of motion in the cervical and lumbar spine includes flexion, extension, rotation, and lateral bending. In the cervical spine, 50% of flexion and extension occurs between the occiput and C1, and the other 50% is distributed throughout the cervical spine; 50% rotation is at C1–C2, with the other 50% evenly distributed again. Normal range of motion in the cervical spine is 65° of flexion (chin to chest), 45° extension (look at ceiling), 35–45° lateral flexion, and 50° or more rotation (chin to shoulder). Normal ranges for the lumbar spine include 85° of true lumbar flexion (not including hip motion), 60° extension, 40° lateral flexion, and 50° rotation.[1,5] Lumbopelvic rhythm refers to the ratio of motion when a patient bends at the waist to touch the toes. Most of the initial arc is motion in the lumbar spine, while the latter portion involves hip joint flexion.[5] In contrast, there is very little motion appreciated in the thoracic and sacral regions.

TABLE 9-1 Spine Range of Motion

	Cervical	True Lumbar
Flexion	65	85
Extension	40	60
Lateral flexion	35	40
Rotation	80	50

Schuenke M, Schult E, Schumacher U. *Thieme Atlas of Anatomy: General Anatomy and Musculoskeletal System*. New York, NY: Thieme; 2010.

We routinely use inclinometry to document lumbar and cervical spine range of motion. Total lumbosacral flexion is easily measured by holding an inclinometer at T12–L1 and having the patient bend forward at the waist while keeping the legs (knees) straight. This measures true lumbar flexion plus flexion due to hip motion. This simple measure correlates well with true lumbar flexion, is easier to obtain, and may be more correlated with disability measures in patients with back pain.[6] Many techniques have been described for cervical spine inclinometry, including simple methods.[7]

Surface landmarks of the spine for inspection, palpation, and provocation are noted in **Table 9-2**.

There are numerous special tests of the spine. The modified Schober's test evaluates true lumbar flexion. A line is drawn between right and left posterior superior iliac spines (L5), and mark number one is made 5 cm below and mark number two 10 cm above this line. The patient bends forward, and the distance between mark numbers one and two should increase at least an additional 5 cm. An abnormal test indicates decreased lumbar mobility.[1,5] The modified Schober's test is thought to be abnormal in conditions such as ankylosing spondylitis.

There are perhaps dozens of eponymous tests for the sacroiliac joint. Patrick's test, also known as FABER (flexion, abduction, external rotation), can test for sacroiliac or femoroacetabular (hip) joint problems. With the symptomatic side hip joint flexed, abducted, and externally rotated, inguinal pain suggests hip arthritis, or pain from surrounding muscles. The ipsilateral sacroiliac joint can be stressed by simultaneously pressing the ipsilateral knee and contralateral anterior superior

TABLE 9-2 Surface Anatomy

Landmark	Structure
C3	Hyoid bone
C4/5	Thyroid cartilage
C6	Cricoid cartilage, carotid tubercle
T3	Spine of scapula
T7	Inferior angle of scapula
L4/5	Iliac crest
S2	PSIS
Coccyx	Coccyx
Inion	Inion
Mastoid process	Mastoid process
Paraspinal region	Facets

iliac spine. The sensitivity and specificity of the Patrick test alone for sacroiliac joint origin are poor. Sensitivity ranges from 48% to 77% and specificity has been reported to be as low as 16%.[8,9] However, if Patrick's test is combined with other tests for sacroiliac pain source, such as Gaenslen's test, thigh thrust, distraction test, compression test, or sacral thrust, and if three or more tests are positive, the sensitivity and specificity of the combination of tests increase to 91% and 87%, respectively.[10]

Facet joint tests include facet loading maneuvers and paraspinal tenderness. The latter may be more valid, and anesthetic blocks under fluoroscopic guidance may be more valid still. Facet loading maneuvers, like sacroiliac provocation, are very nonspecific.[11,12]

Tenderness upon percussion of the midline is 87.5% sensitive and 90% specific for acute vertebral compression fractures.[13]

UPPER LIMB

SHOULDER

Four "joints" make up the shoulder girdle: sternoclavicular, acromioclavicular, glenohumeral, and the scapulothoracic articulation. Inspect and compare side to side, for bony prominences, muscle bulk, and limb position, as well as motion of the shoulders. Normal range of motion is 170–180° flexion, 40–45° extension, 180° abduction, 40–45° adduction, 45–90° external rotation, and 55–70° internal rotation. Internal and external rotation varies, depending on the degree of abduction. Inspect for symmetry of scapula position or any winging of the scapula. Medial winging indicates serratus anterior dysfunction, while lateral winging is suggestive of the trapezius.

Palpable structures include clavicle, acromion, coracoid, spine of scapula, and greater and lesser tuberosities of the humerus. Palpable joints include sternoclavicular and acromioclavicular.

Special tests: Motion of the shoulder girdle includes abduction, adduction, extension, flexion, internal rotation, and external rotation. The Apley scratch test assesses active shoulder range of motion, wherein the patient reaches first behind the head for the superior contralateral scapula, then in front across to the contralateral acromion, and then inferiorly behind to the inferior aspect of contralateral scapula; sides are compared. Scapulohumeral rhythm is the normal 2:1 ratio of motion of the glenohumeral and scapulothoracic articulations during abduction and adduction of the shoulder. For example, abnormal scapulohumeral rhythm, such as a 1:1 ratio, would suggest a possible "frozen shoulder" or adhesive capsulitis.

The apprehension test involves abduction and external rotation of the arm. The patient may exhibit apprehension, expecting dislocation of the shoulder, especially if the patient experiences chronic shoulder dislocations.

The Yergason test assesses the biceps tendon in his position in the bicipital groove, between the greater and lesser trochanters. The patient flexes the elbow. The patient's arm is externally rotated while pulling down the elbow, all while the patient resists. If the biceps tendon subluxes, it will reproduce symptoms. The Yergason test will also be positive, eliciting shoulder pain, when superior labral tears are present (as this is the origin of the long head of biceps). In general, Yergason's test has low sensitivity (9–43%), but high specificity (79–96%).[14-16]

The drop arm and empty can tests assess the rotator cuff, particularly the supraspinatus. In the drop arm, the patient starts with arm abducted and slowly lowers the arm to the side. With a supraspinatus tear, the patient will not be able to do this in a smooth motion because the rotator cuff ordinarily provides much of the action in the lowest part of the abduction arc. The position for the empty can test, also known as the Jobe test, involves bilateral shoulders abducted to 90°, forward flexed 30°, and internally rotated so the thumbs are down. Resistance is applied and is positive for a rotator cuff tear if it produces pain or demonstrates weakness. Sensitivity is high (89–99%), but it is not very specific (43–50%).[17,18]

Neer and Hawkins-Kennedy tests are used to aid in the diagnosis of subacromial impingement. The Neer test is passive full flexion of the shoulder, while the arm is pronated and while the examiner stabilizes the scapula with one hand. A positive test is shoulder pain at the end range.[19] For impingement, the test is relatively sensitive (68–86%) but not very specific (30–68%).[20-22] Hawkins-Kennedy test (often called "Hawkins") is shoulder flexion to 90° combined with passive internal rotation, which reproduces pain when supraspinatus tendon impingement is present. The sensitivity (63–74%) and specificity (50–66%) for impingement with Hawkins are slightly lower than Neer.[20,22,23] While both Neer and Hawkins tests are most sensitive and specific for subacromial impingement, they can also be positive in labral and biceps tears.[19]

The cross-arm test is forward flexion of the shoulder to 90° and active adduction, also known as cross-body adduction, which elicits pain from acromioclavicular joint. Cross-arm has a sensitivity and specificity of 77% and 79%, respectively.[24]

ELBOW

Inspect the elbow for the carrying angle—that is, the angle between the forearm and the humerus. This is typically a valgus angle, more pronounced in women than men. Palpable structures include medial and lateral epicondyles, olecranon, and radial head. Flexion of the elbow should be such that the hand can touch the ipsilateral shoulder, or 130–150°, and extension is 0–10° of hyperextension. Supination and pronation together total 180°.[1,5]

A common special test is the tennis elbow test, or Cozen's test. With elbow extended, the patient makes a fist and extends the wrists against resistance while the examiner palpates the lateral epicondyle. This will reproduce the pain of tennis elbow at the common origin of the wrists extensors at the lateral epicondyle—that is, at the origin of extensor carpi radialis longus and brevis. There are few data in the literature on the sensitivity or specificity of this maneuver.[19]

HAND

Inspect the hand for bony integrity, symmetry, and condition of nails and skin. Inspect for Heberden and Bouchard nodes. A Heberden node is hypertrophy of the distal interphalangeal (DIP) joint and is associated with osteoarthritis; a Bouchard node is hypertrophy of the proximal interphalangeal (PIP) joint and is associated with rheumatoid arthritis (RA).

Inspect for mallet finger, swan neck, or boutonniere deformities. In mallet finger, the distal phalanx remains in flexion when the finger is extended, due to rupture or avulsion of the DIP extensor tendon. Swan neck is flexion of the metacarpophalangeal (MCP) and DIP joints and extension of the PIP joint caused by contracture of the intrinsic muscles. A boutonniere deformity is extension of the MCP and DIP joints and flexion of the PIP joint from rupture of the extensor hood. Both swan neck and boutonniere deformities can be secondary to trauma or RA.

Palpate the radial and ulnar styloid processes, and the anatomic snuffbox, the floor of which is the navicular (scaphoid) bone. Tenderness can indicate scaphoid fracture, which is often missed on x-ray. In Cascade sign, the flexed fingertips should converge toward the scaphoid tubercle on the radial side of the wrist. A deviation indicates that the finger may have been fractured.

Palpate for ganglion cysts on the dorsal or volar surface of the wrists. These are swellings around tendons and joints, of uncertain clinical significance. Palpate for trigger finger, a nodule of the finger flexor tendon. Finkelstein's test for de Quervian's tenosynovitis is performed by the patient closing a fist around his or her thumb while deviating the wrist to the ulnar side. A positive test elicits pain in abductor pollicis longus or extensor pollicis brevis tendons along the anatomic snuff box.

LOWER LIMB

HIP

Assess gait and test for the Trendelenburg sign, caused by weakness of the hip abductors of the leg in stance, especially the gluteus medius. For example, a positive Trendelenburg on the left is a drop of the right hip while standing on the right leg; this can also be accompanied by a lean to the left in order to maintain balance. Observe stance for symmetry, and note any apparent pelvic obliquity. Assess for leg length discrepancy (discussed later).

Palpate the anterior superior iliac spine, iliac crest and tubercle, greater trochanter, posterior superior iliac spine, and ischial tuberosity.

Passive internal rotation of the hip is the most common method of assessing for hip arthritis. Normal range of motion for hip internal rotation is 30–40° with the knee flexed at 90°.[1,5] Limited range of motion and reproduction of pain, typically inguinal pain, is associated with hip arthritis. Limited range of motion with internal rotation alone has only a sensitivity and specificity of 66% and 72%, respectively. However, if the patient has also either decreased hip flexion (<115°) or the triad of pain with internal rotation, prolonged morning stiffness, and and is over 50 years old, then the sensitivity and specificity increase to 86% and 75%, respectively.[25] "Hip scour" is a variant of passive hip range of motion (ROM) in which in which the examiner flexes the hip to 90° and flexes the knee to end range. The examiner then applies a downward force through the femur while internally and externally rotating the hip. A positive test is pain, apprehension, or catching and can indicate almost any intra-articular hip pathology. These hip provocation tests should be done with care because they can cause great pain in a patient with hip arthritis.

The Thomas test assesses for hip flexion contractures as well as hip range of motion. In this test, the patient in a supine position flexes one hip as far as possible up toward the trunk, and the presence of contralateral flexion contractures is confirmed if the other leg is unable to remain extended on the table. The Ober test has the patient lie in a lateral decubitus position with the symptomatic side up. This symptomatic leg is abducted toward the table with the knee flexed in an attempt to drop the knee down to the table. If the knee does not reach the table, it suggests decreased range of motion of the iliotibial band. Sensitivity or specificity are not established for the Thomas or Ober tests, although studies have demonstrated their reliability.[19]

KNEE

Inspect the knee during gait. Note the alignment of the knee in stance, including varus or valgus angulation in the coronal plane as well as either recurvatum or incomplete extension in the sagittal plane. Note the Q angle, the physiologic knee valgus angle between the tibia and a straight line through the femur to the ground. The normal Q angles are 11–17° for men and 14–20° for women.[5] Inspect for any swelling. Note the muscle bulk, particularly the vastus medialis. Palpate the joint line of the knee medially and laterally. Test the patella for mobility. Palpate to assess for temperature symmetry and for effusion or bursa swelling.

Provocative tests of the knee include varus and valgus stress to test the lateral and medial collateral ligaments, respectively. Drawer signs test the cruciate ligaments. The anterior drawer sign tests the anterior cruciate ligament. The patient lies supine with knee flexed 90° as the examiner stabilizes the foot and pulls the tibia anteriorly. Sides are compared, and a positive test is increased laxity in the affected knee. The Lachman test is performed in a similar manner, but at only 15° of knee flexion; it has superior sensitivity and specificity.[19] Anterior drawer and Lachman's tests have specificity of 86–100% and 100%, respectively, but the anterior drawer's sensitivity is only 52–78% while the Lachman's is 91–96%.[26,27] Posterior drawer sign uses the same positioning as anterior drawer, but with posterior pressure on the tibia. Asymmetry or laxity with these tests suggests cruciate ligament damage. Range of motion should include flexion to 130–135° and extension neutral to −10° of hyperextension.[1,5] Extension lag is decreased extension at the end range, which frequently suggests pathology.

FOOT AND ANKLE

Inspect the alignment of the foot and ankle in stance. Inspect the shape of the foot, including the arch; identify pes planus or pes cavus. Inspect and palpate for edema. Palpate the dorsalis pedis and posterior tibial pulses. Like the hand, the dorsum of the foot can also have ganglion cysts. Inspection of the feet may also include inspection of the wear pattern of the shoes, which can help determine if there is subtle gait dysfunction. Compare right and left passive range of motion and stability. Palpate the major ligaments, including anterior and posterior talofibular, calcaneofibular, and deltoid. Tenderness may indicate sprain.

Anterior drawer of the ankle tests for sprain of the anterior talofibular ligament. The examiner provides an anterior force to the talus and calcaneus at the heel while stabilizing the tibia. Sides are compared, and increased laxity is a positive test. The sensitivity and specificity are 78% and 75%, respectively. The talar tilt test also tests for laxity in the lateral ligaments and is performed by the examiner applying medial pressure to the calcaneus while stabilizing the ankle at the malleoli. Again, sides are compared, and a positive test is increased laxity. The sensitivity is lower than the anterior drawer (67%), but the specificity is comparable (75%).[28]

NEUROLOGIC EXAMINATION

The traditional neurological exam consists of six basic elements: mental, cranial nerve, cerebellar, motor, sensory, and reflex. Tables are used here to summarize this vast topic in a practical format.

- Mental (**Table 9-3**).
- Cranial nerve (**Table 9-4**).
- Cerebellar (**Table 9-5**).
- Motor (**Table 9-6**).

In a prospective study, forearm pronation weakness was found to be the most common and most sensitive motor deficit in C6 radiculopathies but was also found in some C7 radiculopathies, so it is not specific for C6.[29]

TABLE 9-3 Mental Status

Appearance and Behavior	
Grooming	Observe hygiene, appearance, appropriate attire
Emotional state	Appropriate behavior for the situation
Body language	Eye contact; appropriate facial expressions and posture
Cognitive Abilities (consider MMSE)	
Level of consciousness	Oriented to person, place, and time
Analogies	Ability to describe simple analogies (apples and oranges)
Abstract thinking	Ability to describe a metaphor (raining cats and dogs)
Calculations	Serial 7's
Writing	Write name or phrase
Motor skills	Ask patients how they would brush their teeth
Memory	Ability to repeat three words immediately and at 5 minutes; ability to recall family events/history
Attention	Follow 3-step commands; spell "world" backwards
Judgment	Ability to respond appropriately to hypothetical situations (burning building)
Emotions	
Mood	Observe mood and expressions
Thought process	Observe thinking and coherence
Perception	Hallucinations or delusions
Language	
Voice quality	Sounds
Articulation	Fluency, pronunciation, and rhythm
Comprehension	Ability to follow commands

Seidel, Henry M. *Mosby's Guide to Physical Examination,* 5th ed. Philadelphia, Pa: Elsevier; 2003.

TABLE 9-4 Cranial Nerves

Cranial Nerve	Name	Testing	Function
CN1	Olfactory	Check each nostril at a time with smell familiar odors (coffee, orange)	Sensory: smell
CN2	Optic	(1) Visual acuity with the Snellen chart (2) Visual fields with confrontation and extinction of vision (3) Fundoscopic exam	Sensory: visual acuity and visual fields
CN3	Oculomotor	(1) Check eye movements by having patient follow examiner's finger (2) Direct and consensual pupillary constriction to light and accommodation	Motor: raise eyelids, most extraocular Movements Parasympathetic: pupillary constriction
CN4	Trochlear	Check eye downward/inward gaze by having patient follow examiner's finger	Motor: downward/inward eye movement
CN5	Trigeminal	(1) Check sensation along ophthalmic, maxillary and mandibular divisions (2) Check muscles of mastication (3) Check corneal blink reflex	Sensory: cornea, face Motor: jaw opening, mastication
CN6	Abducens	Check eye abduction by having patient follow examiner's finger	Motor: lateral eye movement
CN7	Facial	(1) Check forehead wrinkling, eye closure, puffed cheeks, and smile (2) Taste to anterior 2/3 of tongue	Sensory: taste to anterior 2/3 of tongue and pharynx Motor: movement of facial expression Muscles Parasympathetic: secretion of tears and saliva
CN8	Vestibulocochlear	Check hearing with tuning fork: Rinne and Weber tests	Sensory: hearing and equilibrium
CN9	Glossopharyngeal	(1) Taste to posterior 1/3 of tongue (2) Gag reflex and ability to swallow	Sensory: taste to posterior 1/3 of tongue and nasopharynx, gag reflex Motor: muscles of swallowing Phonation Parasympathetic: secretion of salivary glands, carotid reflex
CN10	Vagus	(1) Palate and uvula symmetry (2) Observe swallow	Motor: muscles of phonation and Swallowing Sensory: behind ear Parasympathetic: peristalsis, carotid reflex, involuntary action of heart, lungs, and GI tract
CN11	Accessory	Check shoulder shrug and head turn	Motor: turn head, shrug shoulders
CN12	Hypoglossal	Check tongue protrusion	Motor: tongue movement for speech

Seidel, Henry M. *Mosby's Guide to Physical Examination*, 5th ed. Philadelphia, Pa: Elsevier; 2003.

TABLE 9-5 Cerebellar

Rapid movements—diadochokinesia		
	Rapid finger movement	Touch thumb to each finger in sequence repeatedly
	Rapid hand movement	Rapidly, pat the knees with both hands alternating from palm to the dorsum of hand
Accuracy of movement—dysmetria	Finger to nose testing	Patient touches examiner's finger then his or her own nose and the finger again
	Heel to shin testing	Patient drags his or her heel down the shin proximally at knee to the ankle
Balance		
	Romberg test	Patient stands feet together, eyes closed and arms outstretched
	Single leg stance	Patient balances/hops on one leg
Gait	Standard gait	Patient walks down the hall
	Tandem gait	Patient walks heel to toe

TABLE 9-6 Motor

Manual Muscle Testing			
Grade 0	No movement		
Grade 1	Palpable muscle contraction but no movement		
Grade 2	Movement with gravity eliminated		
Grade 3	Full range of motion against gravity but not against resistance		
Grade 4	Full range of motion against gravity but decreased strength against resistance		
Grade 5	Full strength against resistance		
Upper Extremity			
Muscle	Nerve root	Nerve	Action
Deltoid	C4–C5	Axillary	Shoulder abduction
Biceps	C5	Musculocutaneous	Elbow flexion
Extensor carpi radialis Longus	C6	Radial	Wrist extension
Pronators	C6	Median	Forearm pronation
Triceps	C7	Radial	Elbow extension
Flexor digitorum Profundus	C8	Anterior Interosseus Nerve	DIP flexion
Abductor digiti minimi	T1	Ulnar nerve	5th digit abduction
Lower Extremity			
Iliopsoas	L2	Femoral	Hip flexor
Quadriceps muscles	L3	Femoral	Knee extension
Tibialis anterior	L4	Deep peroneal	Ankle dorsiflexion
Extensor hallucis longus	L5	Deep peroneal	Great Toe extension
Tensor fasciae latae	L5	Superior gluteal	Hip abduction
Gastrocnemius-soleus complex	S1	Tibial	Ankle plantarflexion

In a prospective study of patients with L3 and L4 radiculopathies, unilateral quadriceps weakness was best detected by a single leg sit-to-stand test, whereas patients with L5 or S1 radiculopathies could perform this test.[30]

- Sensory (**Table 9-7**).
- Reflex (**Table 9-8**).

Table 9-7 Sensory

Nerve Root	Location
C2	Occipital protuberance
C3	Supraclavicular fossa
C4	Top of AC joint
C5	Lateral antecubital fossa
C6	Dorsal proximal thumb
C7	Dorsal proximal middle finger
C8	Dorsal proximal 5th finger
T1	Medial antecubital fossa
T2	Apex of axilla
T4	Medial to nipple
T5	
T6	Level of xiphoid process along nipple line
T10	Level of umbilicus process along nipple line
T12	Inguinal ligament
L1	Between T12 and L2
L2	Medial anterior thigh
L3	Medial anterior knee
L4	Medial malleolus
L5	Medial dorsal foot
S1	Inferior lateral malleolus
S2	Popliteal fossa
S3	Ischial tuberosity
S4-5	Anal mucocutaneous junctions

- Upper motor neuron signs (**Table 9-9**).
- Special tests: Spurling, Lhermitte, Phalen, Tinel, SLR, femoral stretch, Rainville Pronation test, Rainville Single Leg Stance test (**Table 9-10**).
- Neuropathic pain examination findings.

TABLE 9-8 Muscle Stretch Reflexes

0	Mute
1+	Hypoactive/trace
2+	Normal
3+	Hyperactive/brisk
4+	Sustained clonus
Reflex nerve root levels:	
Biceps	C5
Brachioradialis	C6
Pronator	C6
Triceps	C7
Finger flexors	C8–T1
Quadriceps femoris/patellar tendon	L4
Medial hamstring	L5
Gastrocnemius/Achilles tendon	S1

TABLE 9-9 Upper Motor Neuron Tests

Sign		
Hoffman	Flicking the nail on the third. Positive if involuntary thumb flexion. Normally, no reflex response.	Indicates myelopathy
Babinski	Lateral sole of the foot is stroked from heel to toe, curving medial to big toe. Positive if big toe extends upward. Normally toes flex/curl downward.	CNS/UMN dysfunction
Clonus	Rapidly flexing the foot into dorsiflexion.	UMN dysfunction, spasticity

TABLE 9-10 Special Tests

Test		Significance
Spurling	Extend and rotate patient's head to the affected side and apply axial compression. Positive test elicits radicular pain.	Nerve root compression
Lhermitte	Patient sits, flexes head, and slouches forward. Positive if electrical sensation shoots down the back and into the limbs.	Lesion of the dorsal column of the cervical cord/myelopathy
Slump	Patient sits and performs thoracolumbar and cervical flexion then extends knees and dorsiflexes their ankles. Positive if shooting sensation down the legs.	Nerve root tension/ radiculopathy
SLR	Patient supine and the examiner lifts the patient's leg with knee extended. Positive if shooting sensation down the legs between 30–70°.	Nerve root tension/ radiculopathy (L4–S1)
Femoral stretch	Patient prone and the examiner extends the hip. Positive if shooting pain down anterior thigh.	Nerve root tension/ radiculopathy (L2–L3)
Valsalva	Patient sitting and forcefully exhales air into closed fist. Positive if reproduction of back pain.	Discogenic pain/ radiculopathy
Phalen	Patient forcefully pushes the dorsum of the hands together, flexing the wrist, for 60 seconds. Positive if shooting sensation into thumb, 2nd or 3rd finger.	Median nerve compression at carpal tunnel
Tinel	Median nerve: Tap with a reflex hammer over median nerve at level of transverse carpal ligament at the wrist. Positive if shooting sensation into thumb, 2nd, or 3rd finger. Ulnar Nerve: Tap with reflex hammer over ulnar nerve at level of the cubital tunnel at the flexed elbow. Positive is shooting sensation into 4th or 5th finger.	Median nerve compression at carpal tunnel Ulnar nerve compression at cubital tunnel
Rainville pronation test	Patient in sitting position with elbow flexed to 90° and against trunk; examiner forcefully supinates the pronated forearm. Assess for forearm pronation weakness per manual muscle testing grading scale.	C6 and C7 radiculopathy
Rainville single leg stance test	Patient performs a sit-to-stand on one leg without using arms. Positive if quadriceps weakness compared to opposite leg.	L3 and L4 radiculopathy

Rainville J, Noto DJ, Jouve C, et al. Assessment of forearm pronation strength in C6 and C7 radiculopathies. *Spine.* 2007;32(1):71-75.

Rainville J, Jouve C, Finno M, et al. Comparison of four tests of quadriceps strength in L3 or L4 radiculopathies. *Spine.* 2003;28(21):2466-2471.

SPECIAL EXAMINATIONS

18-POINT FIBROMYALGIA EXAM

We must mention the famous 18 tender points. The reader is referred to the chapter on fibromyalgia for more details. Palpation with the thumb of the dominant hand with 4-kg pressure, enough to blanch the nail, should produce pain (not just tenderness) in 11 of 18 points, according to the strict ACR criteria.[31] However, the validity of the tender points is questionable, and in reality, they are not often used to make the diagnosis of fibromyalgia.[32] The ACR criteria continue to evolve.[33]

14-POINT SPORTS ASSESSMENT SCREEN

Range of motion of major joints and strength of major muscle groups are quickly assessed with a 14-point musculoskeletal screening (**Table 9-11**). Although intended for preparticipation screening for sports and not validated in the chronic pain population, this may be a useful and expeditious battery of maneuvers that can exclude major pathology.[34,35]

NINE-JOINT HYPERMOBILITY ASSESSMENT WITH THE BEIGHTON SCORE

Most chronic pain patients are afflicted with decreased range of motion; however, abnormally increased range of motion can also be a problem. For example, benign joint hypermobility and Marfan and Ehlers-Danlos syndromes are associated with joint hypermobility. Beighton described a score for hypermobility in nine major joints. If four or more are positive, and the patient has had arthralgias for longer than 3 months, then the patient fulfills the criteria for a diagnosis of benign joint hypermobility syndrome.[36] It is helpful for pain physicians to be aware of the phenomenon of joint hypermobility, so these items are included here in **Table 9-12**.

LEG LENGTH DISCREPANCY MEASUREMENT

Leg length discrepancy (LLD) may be (1) structural, due to different lengths of femur or tibia, or (2) functional, due to alignment or mechanics in limb or spine joints. The significance of LLD is controversial, especially in low back pain, but it remains an obsession nonetheless. Clinical measurement is considered reliable and valid as a screening method, performed with the patient supine, measuring on each side the distance from anterior superior iliac spine to medial malleolus.[37] Radiography is the gold standard, and in our clinic is reserved for instances where clinical measurement reveals LLD at least 2 cm and where the outcome of the x-ray would make a difference in management of the patient.

TABLE 9-11 14-Point Sport Examination

Patient Action	Assessment
1. Face physician	General habitus, acromioclavicular joints
2. Look at ceiling, floor, to both shoulders, ears to shoulders	Cervical spine ROM
3. Shrug shoulder vs. resistance	Trapezius strength
4. Abduct shoulder to 90° vs. resistance	Deltoid strength
5. Internal and external rotation of shoulders with elbows flexed	Shoulder ROM
6. Flex and extend elbows	Elbow ROM
7. Supinate and pronate forearms	Elbow and wrist ROM
8. Abduct fingers, then make a fist	Hand and finger ROM, defects
9. Face away from physician	Trunk and limb alignment
10. Extend back with straight legs	Test for pain (spondylolysis, etc.)
11. Flex back with straight legs	Spine/hip/hamstring ROM, scoliosis
12. Contract and relax quadriceps	Lower limb alignment
13. Duck walk	ROM, strength, balance
14. Heel and toe walk	Dorsiflexion/plantar flexor strength; balance

TABLE 9-12 Beighton Hypermobility Score

Joint	Positive Finding	Possible Points
Little (5th) fingers	Passive dorsiflexion beyond 90°	2 (1 each side)
Thumbs	Passive dorsiflexion to the flexor aspect of the forearm	2 (1 each side)
Elbows	Hyperextends beyond 10°	2 (1 each side)
Knees	Hyperextends beyond 10°	2 (1 each side)
Forward flexion of trunk with knees fully extended	Palms and hands can rest flat on the floor	1

Bouwien Smits-Engelsman, PhD, Mariëtte Klerks, MS, and Amanda Kirby, MRCGP, PhD. Beighton Score: A Valid Measure for Generalized Hypermobility in Children. *J Pediatr* 2011;158(1):119-123.

ASIA EXAM

The American Spinal Injury Association (ASIA) produces the International Standards for Neurological Classification of Spinal Cord Injury, commonly called the "ASIA exam," which was last revised in 2011. All physiatrists hone their examination skills through fastidious performance of this exam to determine and document the neurological level and degree of severity of spinal cord injury in patients. This document summarizes dermatomes, myotomes, and sensory and motor examination in a manner that is generally practical for neurological examination, especially for pain physicians, because it is organized by spinal neurological level.[38]

WADDELL'S SIGNS

The original meanings of Waddell's signs are worth revisiting. Waddell described and standardized a group of nonorganic physical signs that could be unobtrusively added to the usual physical exam, and that were reproducible and stable over time. Waddell found that these signs correlate well with other nonorganic assessment, such as psychological unsuitability for surgery.[39] See **Table 9-13**. Over time, Waddell's signs have come to encompass a variety of meanings, including malingering, symptom magnification, and secondary gain. Evidence-based reviews have since found that Waddell's signs may more closely correlate with

TABLE 9-13 Waddell's Signs

Categories	Subtests	Description
Tenderness	Superficial	Pain with light pinch over large lumbar area
	Nonanatomic	Deep tenderness not localized to an anatomic structure
Simulation tests	Axial loading	Pain with loading the spine by pressure on the head of an erect patient
	Rotation	Pain with rotating the spine and pelvis together in the same plane of an erect patient
Distraction tests	Straight leg raise	Perform a straight leg raise while distracting the patient by checking plantar reflexes
Regional disturbances	Pain	Pain in a wide region, such as entire leg
	Weakness	Weakness in a nonanatomic distribution or low effort on testing
	Sensation	Deficits in nonanatomic distribution
Overreaction		Pain disproportionate to examination or overexaggerated vocalization or facial expressions

Waddell G, McCulloch JA, Kummel E, Venner RM. Nonorganic physical signs in low-back pain. *Spine.* 1980;5(2):117-125.

poor nonsurgical outcome than with poor surgical outcome.[40] Although methodological weaknesses abound in the evidence regarding his signs, Waddell's caveat to carefully assess and examine patients still rings true, and is a perfect conclusion here:

The minutes thus spent, to "operate on a patient, not a spine" may save years of coping with the human wreckage caused by ill-considered surgery on the lumbar discs.

REFERENCES

1. Hoppenfeld S. *Physical Examination of the Spine and Extremities.* Upper Saddle River, NJ: Prentice Hall; 1976.
2. Magee DJ. *Orthopedic Physical Assessment.* 5th ed. St. Louis, Mo: Saunders Elsevier; 2008.
3. Sarwark JF, ed. *Essentials of Musculoskeletal Care.* 4th ed. Rosemont, Ill: American Academy of Orthopaedic Surgeons; 2010.
4. Campbell WW. *DeJong's The Neurologic Examination.* 7th ed. Philadelphia, Pa: Lippincott Williams & Wilkins; 2013.
5. Schuenke M, Schult E, Schumacher U. *Thieme Atlas of Anatomy: General Anatomy and Musculoskeletal System.* New York, NY: Thieme; 2010.
6. Rainville J, Sobel JB, Hartigan H. Comparison of total lumbosacral flexion and true lumbar flexion measured by a dual inclinometer technique. *Spine.* 1994;19(23):2698-2701.
7. Moffett JAK, Hughes I, Griffiths P. Measurement of cervical spine movements using a simple inclinometer. *Physiotherapy.* 1989;75(6):309-312.
8. Dreyfuss P, Dreyer S, Griffin J, et al. Positive sacroiliac screening tests in asymptomatic adults. *Spine.* 1994;19(10):1138-1143.
9. Ozgocmen S, Bozgeyik Z, Kalcik M, Yildirim A. The value of sacroiliac pain provocation tests in early sacroilitis. *Clin Rheumatol.* 2008;27:1275-1282.
10. Laslett M, Young SB, Aprill CN, McDonad B. Diagnosing painful sacroiliac joints: a validity study of a McKenzie evaluation and sacroiliac provocation tests. *Aust J Physiotherapy.* 2003;49:89-97.
11. Schwarzer AC, Derby R, Aprill CN, et al. Pain from the lumbar zygopophyseal joints: a test of two models. *J Spine Disord.* 1994;7:331-336.
12. Laslett M, Oberg B, Aprill CN, McDonald B. A study of clinical predictors of lumbar provocation discography: a study of clinical predictors of lumbar provocation discography. *Eur Spine J.* 2006;15(10):1473-1484.
13. Langdon J, Way A, Heaton S, Bernard J, Molloy S. Vertebral compression fractures: new clinical signs to aid diagnosis. *Ann R Coll Surg Engl.* 2010;92(2):163-166.
14. Holtby R, Razmjou H. Accuracy of the Speed's and Yergason's tests in detecting biceps pathology and SLAP lesions: comparison with arthroscopic findings. *Arthroscopy.* 2004;20(3):231-236.
15. Guanche CA, Jones DC. Clinical testing for tears of the glenoid labrum. *Arthroscopy.* 2003;19(5):517-523.
16. Oh JH, Kim JY, Kim WS, Gong HS, Lee JH. The evaluation of various physical examinations for the diagnosis of type II superior labrum anterior and posterior lesion. *Am J Sports Med.* 2008;36(2):353-359.
17. Itoi E, Kido T, Sano A, Urayama M, Sato K. Which is more useful, the "full can test" or the "empty can test," in detecting the torn supraspinatus tendon? *Am J Sports Med.* 1999;27(1):65-68.
18. Kim E, Jeong HJ, Lee KW, Song JS. Interpreting positive signs of the supraspinatus test in screening for torn rotator cuff. *Acta Med Okayama.* 2006;60(4):223-228.
19. Cook CE, Haggedus JE. *Orthopedic Physical Examination Tests: An Evidence Based Approach.* 2nd ed. Upper Saddle River, NJ: Pearson Education, Inc; 2013.
20. Michener LA, Walsworth MK, Doukas WC, Murphy KP. Reliability and diagnostic accuracy of 5 physical examination tests and combination of tests for subacromial impingement. *Arch Phys Med Rehabil.* 2009 Nov;90(11):1898-1903.
21. Silva L, Andréu JL, Muñoz P, Pastrana M, Millán I, Sanz J, Barbadillo C, Fernández-Castro M. Accuracy of physical examination in subacromial impingement syndrome. *Rheumatology* (Oxford). 2008 May;47(5):679-683.
22. Park HB, Yokota A, Gill HS, El Rassi G, McFarland EG. Diagnostic accuracy of clinical tests for the different degrees of subacromial impingement syndrome. *J Bone Joint Surg Am.* 2005 Jul;87(7): 1446-1455.
23. Kelly SM, Brittle N, Allen GM. The value of physical tests for subacromial impingement syndrome: a study of diagnostic accuracy. *Clin Rehabil.* 2010 Feb;24(2):149-158.
24. Chronopoulos E, Kim TK, Park HB, Ashenbrenner D, McFarland EG. Diagnostic value of physical tests for isolated chronic acromioclavicular lesions. *Am J Sports Med.* 2004 Apr-May;32(3): 655-661.
25. Altman R, Alarcón G, Appelrouth D, Bloch D, Borenstein D, et al. The American College of Rheumatology criteria for the classification and reporting of osteoarthritis of the hip. *Arthritis Rheum.* 1991 May;34(5):505-514.
26. Torg JS, Conrad W, Kalen V. Clinical diagnosis of anterior cruciate ligament instability in the athlete. *Am J Sports Med.* 1976 Mar-Apr;4(2):84-93.
27. Lee JK, Yao L, Phelps CT, Wirth CR, Czajka J, Lozman J. Anterior cruciate ligament tears: MR imaging compared with arthroscopy and clinical tests. *Radiology.* 1988 Mar;166(3):861-864.
28. Hertel J, Denegar CR, Monroe MM, Stokes WL. Talocrural and subtalar joint instability after lateral ankle sprain. *Med Sci Sports Exerc.* 1999 Nov;31(11):1501-1508.
29. Waddell G, McCulloch JA, Kummel E, Venner RM. Nonorganic physical signs in low-back pain. *Spine.* 1980;5(2):117-125.
30. Fishbain DA, Cole B, Cutler RB. A structured evidence-based review on the meaning of nonorganic physical signs: Waddell signs. *Pain Medicine.* 2003;4(2):141-181.
31. The Physician and Sportsmedicine Staff. *Preparticipation Physical Evaluation.* 3rd ed. New York, NY: McGraw-Hill; 2004.
32. McKeag D, Moeller JL. *ACSM's Primary Care Sports Medicine.* 2nd ed. Lippincott Williams & Wilkins: Philadelphia, Pa; 2007.
33. Beighton PH, Horan F. Orthopedic aspects of the Ehlers-Danlos syndrome. *J Bone Joint Surg* [Br]. 1969;51:444-453.
34. Burke G. Leg length discrepancy. *Gait Post.* 2002;15: 195-206.
35. Rainville J, Jouve C, Finno M, et al. Comparison of four tests of quadriceps strength in L3 or L4 radiculopathies. *Spine.* 2003;28(21): 2466-2471.
36. Rainville J, Noto DJ, Jouve C, et al. Assessment of forearm pronation strength in C6 and C7 radiculopathies. *Spine.* 2007;32(1):71-75.
37. http://www.asia-spinalinjury.org
38. Wolfe F, Smythe HA, Yunus MB, et al. The American College of Rheumatology 1990 criteria for the classification of fibromyalgia. Report of the Multicenter Criteria Committee. *Arthritis Rheum.* 1990;33:160-172.
39. Wolfe F. Stop using the American College of Rheumatology criteria in the clinic. *J Rheumat.* 2003;30:1671-1672.
40. Wolfe F. Clauw DJ, Fitzcharles MA, et al. The American College of Rheumatology Preliminary Diagnostic Criteria for Fibromyalgia and Measurement of Symptom Severity. *Arthritis Care.* 2010;62(5): 600-610.

CHAPTER 10 Radiologic Evaluation of Spinal Disease

Nagamani Peri
Gaurav Jindal
David B. Hackney

INTRODUCTION

Spinal disease is a very common cause of neck and back pain. Patients presenting with spinal pain form a very important group at the Pain Clinic. Hence, appropriate evaluation of spinal disease is essential to provide excellent care to the patients.

This chapter describes the different imaging modalities available for the evaluation of spinal disease and imaging appearance of different spinal abnormalities. Emphasis will be laid on degenerative disease and postoperative changes with a brief note on nondegenerative diseases of the spine and diseases of the spinal cord.

IMAGING MODALITIES FOR THE EVALUATION OF SPINAL DISEASE

PLAIN RADIOGRAPH

Plain radiography (PXR) is easily available and less expensive. It can be used as a screening study in patients presenting with pain to identify gross osseous and soft-tissue abnormalities related to degenerative changes, and for evaluation of hardware. Flexion and extension views are helpful in assessing instability and intersegmental mobility. Composite views are helpful in the evaluation of scoliosis. However, plain radiographs are not ideal for detailed evaluation of the spine and spinal contents.

COMPUTED TOMOGRAPHY

Computed tomography (CT) provides very good anatomic and structural details of the spine, in particular, the osseous details related to degenerative changes, trauma, and tumors. The spatial resolution is very good; however, the contrast resolution is low. Hence, it is not ideal for the evaluation of cord, nerve, and soft-tissue abnormalities, although gross abnormalities can be identified based on the alteration of the normal outlines of the structures and natural contrast among fat, bone, and disk. Usually, noncontrast studies are performed for evaluation of osseous details. Intravenous iodinated contrast medium is used for obtaining postcontrast CT images for evaluation of infection and tumors if Magnetic Resonance Imaging (MRI) cannot be performed. MRI is a better modality for these indications.

With the advent of newer generation scanners with multiple detectors, studies can be performed very rapidly and can include larger segments of the spine. Postprocessing methods help obtain very good reformations in multiple planes and form part of the standard algorithm of spinal imaging.

CT does have certain disadvantages that include risk of ionizing radiation, allergic reaction to intravenous contrast (IV) agent, and low-contrast resolution for assessment of intrathecal and soft-tissue abnormalities.

MAGNETIC RESONANCE IMAGING

Magnetic resonance imaging studies are performed using radiofrequency waves and, hence, have no risk of ionizing radiation. MRI is mostly used for detailed assessment and characterization of spinal disease, including cord and neural structures. It provides excellent anatomical details with high-contrast resolution. Acquisition of images using different sequences and in different planes helps in better characterization and localization of abnormalities compared to CT studies. Intravenous contrast agents such as gadolinium-based agents are helpful in the characterization of infective, inflammatory, vascular, and neoplastic lesions. For the evaluation of traumatic, degenerative, and congenital abnormalities, there is no need for IV contrast agents. The usual sequences that are performed are sagittal and axial T1-weighted (T1W) and T2-weighted (T2W) sequences, gradient echo, and short-time inversion recovery (STIR) sequences, which help in better characterization of the abnormalities. Wider and open-bore scanners are very helpful with claustrophobic patients and are increasing in availability and popularity. Dynamic MRI scanners and techniques help in assessing the spine and cord in different physiologic positions of the spine. These techniques can help identify latent abnormalities and subtle signs of instability.

The presence of certain implants or foreign bodies such as certain pacemakers, brain/cord stimulators, metallic foreign bodies in orbits, certain prostheses, and the like is not considered safe for MRI and precludes patients from undergoing MRI scan. It is essential to assess the safety of these by obtaining details of the implants from the manufacturer and obtaining screening radiographs, if necessary, in order to identify types of implants and any foreign bodies near vital organs. There are online resources to determine the MRI safety of various implants, such as www.mrisafety.com, that can be used as quick references when needed, in addition to the product manuals.

CONTRAST AGENTS FOR CT AND MRI

Intravenous contrast agents used for CT are iodinated contrast agents. Due to the risk of allergic reactions and renal failure, these are either contraindicated or to be used with certain precautions in patients with history of allergy to these agents and those with renal failure.

The intravenous contrast agents used for MRI are gadolinium based. There have been reports of association between gadolinium administration in patients with renal failure and a systemic syndrome called nephrogenic systemic fibrosis (NSF) that can be fatal. Hence, gadolinium agents must be used with caution in patients with acute or significant chronic kidney disease (estimated glomerular filtration rate (eGFR) $<30\,\text{mL/min/1.73}\,\text{m}^2$), recent significant decrease in eGFR, recent liver or renal biopsy, hepatorenal syndrome, and so on. If the benefits outweigh the risk in these patients, it is usually recommended that appropriate precautions be taken for immediate dialysis after injection of gadolinium agent.[1] Note, however, that the protective effects of dialysis for prevention of NSF are unknown. Gadolinium is also to be used with caution in pregnant patients to avoid any potential harm to the fetus.[2]

FLUOROSCOPY

Fluoroscopic guidance is commonly used for performing image-guided procedures such as epidural and facet joint injections, for performing lumbar puncture in difficult situations, for myelography, and in the operating room for guidance and confirmation of position of hardware.

MYELOGRAPHY, CT MYELOGRAPHY

In patients who cannot undergo MRI and MR myelography, assessment of the extent of spinal canal stenosis, deformity on the cord, and extent of obstruction to flow of cerebrospinal fluid (CSF) can be performed by myelography and CT myelography. Iodinated contrast medium is injected into the CSF space of the thecal sac under fluoroscopic guidance. After allowing the contrast medium and CSF to flow in the thecal sac by appropriate positioning if necessary, fluoroscopic spot images are taken. At the completion of myelography, CT scan images of spine are obtained in the area of interest. Early and delayed CT images can be obtained until adequate information about the level and extent of obstruction to CSF flow is obtained.

Myelographic images can be obtained with MRI without the use of intrathecal contrast. To date, there are limited data comparing noncontrast to contrast-enhanced MR myelography.

DISKOGRAPHY

In this procedure, iodinated contrast agent is injected directly into the nucleus of the disc under fluoroscopic guidance and plain radiographs or CT images are obtained soon after injection. Extension of the contrast

TABLE 10-1 Advantages and Disadvantages of Different Spine-Imaging Modalities

No.	Modality	Advantages	Disadvantages
1	Plain radiography	Less expensive Easily available Screening for pain, hardware, and scoliosis	Cannot provide detailed evaluation of osseous structures
2	Fluoroscopy	Real-time guidance for procedures such as lumbar puncture, CT myelography, epidural and facet injections, etc.	Low resolution for diagnostic information
3	CT	Very good spatial resolution Rapid Multiplanar reformations Different algorithms for bone, soft-tissue, and lung display Very good for osseous details	Radiation risk Lower-contrast resolution Not good for evaluation of cord, nerves, and soft-tissue details
4	MRI	High-contrast resolution Excellent anatomic details Detailed evaluation of cord, nerves Better tissue characterization of lesions	Contraindicated with some implants Risk of NSF

agent into the annulus fibrosus or epidural space indicates annular tear. Diskography is not routinely performed and is of controversial significance. It may be useful in patients with pain and no definitive imaging findings or in patients with degenerated discs at multiple levels to identify the most symptomatic level.[3,4]

In patients allergic to iodinated contrast material, dilute gadolinium (off-label use, not FDA-approved for this purpose) can be used, and postinjection MR images can be obtained for the evaluation of discs.[5,6]

RADIONUCLIDE STUDIES

Various radionuclide agents can be used in the evaluation of spinal disease depending on the clinical scenario. The most commonly used are the 99 m technetium methylene diphosphonate (Tc MDP) bone scan for detection of osseous lesions related to osteolytic or osteoblastic primary and secondary neoplastic lesions, stress fracture, pars defects, degenerative changes with acute component of marrow edema, and so on. In the evaluation of spinal osteomyelitis, 99m technetium MDP and gallium-67 scans can be useful in the evaluation of active osteomyelitis. Radionuclide-labeled whole blood cells (WBCs) can be used in the evaluation of complicating osteomyelitis.[7] FDG-PET (fluoro-deoxy glucose positron emission tomography) is very useful in the evaluation of different types of bone lesions related to infective, neoplastic etiologies, and the like.

The advantages and disadvantages of different imaging modalities are shown in **Table 10-1**.

WHEN AND HOW TO IMAGE THE SPINE

Routine imaging of the spine for nonspecific symptoms in low-risk patients does not improve outcome and can also have deleterious effects, such as exposure to radiation; it may also result in unnecessary invasive treatments. Hence, routine imaging of the spine is not necessary in these patients.[8]

According to the recommendations by different societies such as American College of Physicians, the American Pain Society, and the American College of Radiology, imaging is to be considered based on the clinical presentation, the risk factors for serious condition, and/or if intervention is contemplated.[9,10] These factors are shown in **Table 10-2**.

The criteria for evaluation of neck and thoracic spinal symptoms and signs can be less stringent due to the greater risk for cord compromise and its devastating consequences. Clinical discretion and consultation with spine specialists can help in decision making.

The different types of imaging modalities described here complement each other in the evaluation of spinal disease. Because each modality has its own advantages and disadvantages, it is necessary to use the most cost-effective and accurate modality based on the clinical need.

TABLE 10-2 When to Image the Spine

1. Severe/progressive neurologic deficits
2. Suspicion of serious conditions such as cauda equina syndrome, fracture, infection, or tumor (based on "red flags"); history of recent trauma; unexplained weight loss or fever; immunosuppression; use of corticosteroids; history of known malignancy; IV drug use; osteoporosis
3. Radiculopathy/spinal stenosis and likely candidates for surgery/epidural/facet injections
4. Repeat imaging—only if new/changed clinical diagnosis, features of progression neurologic symptoms/signs, new suspicion for serious condition

Chou R, Qaseem A, Snow B, et al. Diagnosis and treatment of low back pain: a joint clinical practice guideline from the American College of Physicians and the American Pain Society. *Ann Intern Med*. 2007;147:478-491; Davis PA, Wippold II FJ, Cornelius RS, et al. *ACR Appropriateness Criteria for Low Back Pain*. American College of Radiation; 2011.

TABLE 10-3 Indications for Plain Radiographs for Spine Imaging

Plain radiographs	• Osteoporosis and/or age >70 years • Screening study for nonspecific pain • Evaluation of scoliosis • Evaluation of hardware If abnormal/inconclusive ⟶ consider CT/MRI.
Flexion-extension radiographs	To assess latent instability and intersegmental mobility in order to determine the need for intervention Clinical discretion to be used due to potential risk to cord

Chou R, Qaseem A, Snow B, et al. Diagnosis and treatment of low back pain: a joint clinical practice guideline from the American College of Physicians and the American Pain Society. *Ann Intern Med*. 2007;147:478-491; Davis PA, Wippold II FJ, Cornelius RS, et al. *ACR Appropriateness Criteria for Low Back Pain*. American College of Radiation; 2011.

The indications for different types of studies are shown in **Tables 10-3, 10-4,** and **10-5**.

APPROACH TO INTERPRETING SPINE-IMAGING STUDIES

A systematic approach to interpreting spine studies is very important for accurate assessment and to avoid mistakes.

CT STUDIES

It is better to start with sagittal reformations for an overall review and then review the coronal and axial images; appropriate windowing and

TABLE 10-4 Indications for CT Imaging of Spine

CT spine without IV contrast	• Trauma • Evaluate osseous architecture and osseous lesions, degenerative disease, compression fractures, if planning intervention • Evaluate hardware and postsurgery healing
CT spine with IV contrast	• Only if MRI is contraindicated • For assessing soft-tissue abnormalities, e.g., extent of abscess or tumor
CT myelography	• If MRI cannot be performed • To assess the extent of spinal canal stenosis • To assess level and degree of obstruction to CSF flow

Chou R, Qaseem A, Snow B, et al. Diagnosis and treatment of low back pain: a joint clinical practice guideline from the American College of Physicians and the American Pain Society. *Ann Intern Med.* 2007;147:478-491; Davis PA, Wippold II FJ, Cornelius RS, et al. *ACR Appropriateness Criteria for Low Back Pain.* American College of Radiation; 2011.

cross-referencing on picture archiving and communication systems (PACS) are very helpful in accurate localization of abnormalities.

1. Number the vertebrae: This can be one of the most important steps, particularly if there is transitional anatomy. Appropriate and corresponding numbering has to be used when planning any procedure or intervention. Counting from C2 downward is considered as the accurate way of numbering the vertebrae. However, if cervical spine images are not available, counting can be based on morphological identification of sacrum. The location of the ilio-lumbar ligament can be used to identify the level of lumbosacral junction, assuming five lumbar vertebral bodies, which can, however, be a limitation of this method.[11] Note that the ilio-lumbar ligament is not reliably found at the L5 level and cannot be used to help with accurate numbering always.
2. Vertebral bodies: height; alignment by checking the anterior spinal, posterior spinal, and spinolaminar lines on the sagittal plane and C1–C2 alignment in multiple planes; focal lesions.
3. Disc space: height; asymmetric widening; vacuum phenomenon.
4. Uncovertebral processes: degenerative changes.
5. Facet joints: width; alignment; degenerative changes.
6. Posterior elements: focal lesions; degenerative changes.
7. Neural foraminae: narrowing (from disc or osseous changes)/widening (from tumors).
8. Spinal canal: narrowing; occasionally abnormal widening-congenital/tumor.
9. Osseous lesions: fractures, degenerative changes, lytic/sclerotic.
10. Pre- and paravertebral spaces.
11. Vascular structures: stenosis; aneurysm; dissection.
12. Soft-tissue structures and viscera.

TABLE 10-5 Indications for MR Imaging of Spine

MR spine without IV contrast	• Trauma for cord and ligamentous injury • Acuity of traumatic and osteoporotic fractures • For more detailed assessment of spinal pain, radiculopathy, plan for surgery/intervention • Cauda equina syndrome; cord compression
MR spine without and with IV contrast	• Suspicion of infection, tumor, demyelinating disease, vascular lesion • Postsurgery, especially in the lumbar and thoracic spine • Immunosuppression • Pathologic compression fracture; cord compression or cauda equina syndrome due to tumor/infection

Chou R, Qaseem A, Snow B, et al. Diagnosis and treatment of low back pain: a joint clinical practice guideline from the American College of Physicians and the American Pain Society. *Ann Intern Med.* 2007;147:478-491; Davis PA, Wippold II FJ, Cornelius RS, et al. *ACR Appropriateness Criteria for Low Back Pain.* American College of Radiation; 2011.

MR STUDIES

On MR studies, multiple sequences are usually obtained in sagittal and axial planes and sometimes in the coronal plane.

- T1W sequence: sagittal—for numbering of vertebrae, look for alignment and diffuse or focal marrow signal changes.
- T2W sequence: disc dessication; vertebral, spinal cord, neural, and soft-tissue abnormalities; arterial flow voids; spinal canal and foraminal narrowing.
- STIR/water IDEAL sequence: fluid-sensitive sequence that demonstrates most abnormalities as bright or hyperintense, except for purely sclerotic or fibrous lesions.
- Gadolinium-enhanced T1W images: helpful in identifying inflammatory, infective and neoplastic lesions.

IMAGING OF SPINAL DISEASE

DEGENERATIVE DISEASE

Degenerative disease of the spine is one of the most common causes of spinal pain. Degenerative changes can involve different components of the spine and can result in reactive marrow changes, radiculopathy and myelopathy that can produce clinical manifestations. However, it is important to keep in mind that not all degenerative changes seen on imaging are clinically significant. Hence, the importance of imaging findings should be correlated with clinical findings to decide on further management.

Degenerative changes involving the spine can be broadly divided into those involving

1. Intervertebral disc.
2. Vertebral body—spondylosis, uncovertebral joints in cervical spine.
3. Posterior elements such as facets, spinous process, ligamentum flavum.

Intervetebral Disc Degeneration Disc degeneration is multifactorial and can start at an early age. Dehydration and loss of proteoglycans in the nucleus pulposus, fissuring of the annulus fibrosus, and, sometimes, presence of nitrogen gas in the disc (also called vacuum phenomenon) are the main characteristics of disc degeneration.[8] These result in various imaging appearances in the disc and adjacent structures of the vertebra.

Dehydration or disc dessication appears as a low signal of the nucleus pulposus on T2W MRI. Loss of the normal intranuclear cleft and decrease in the height of the disc space are frequently associated with water loss.

Fissuring of the annulus fibrosus (annular fissure) occurs due to disc degeneration, and many believe this, by itself, can cause pain. Annular fissures appear on MRI as hyperintense foci in the dark annulus on fluid-sensitive MR sequences and can sometimes enhance on postcontrast MR sequences. When the integrity of the annulus is weakened or lost, the disc extends outside its normal confines and is classified into different categories depending on the configuration. These categories include (a) disc bulge (b) asymmetric disc bulge (c) disc herniation that can be protrusion or extrusion (d) disc herniation with migration (e) disc herniation with sequestration, based on the standardized nomenclature described by the combined task force. The classifications are depicted in **Figure 10-1**, and MR appearance of disk protrusion and extrusion is shown in **Figure 10-2**.[12]

While annular fissures and disc herniations can be symptomatic, the natural history is spontaneous resolution of symptoms in approximately three-fourths of patients, in particular, those with disc herniations.[13]

Disc degeneration can result in reactive changes in the adjacent end plates and subchondral marrow that are called Modic changes.[14] They are classified into three types and are best characterized on MRI as follows: type 1—due to water accumulation in vascularized fibrous and granulation tissue, hypointense on T1W and hyperintense on T2W images; type 2—due to fatty infiltration of subchondral marrow, hyperintense on T1W and intermediate-hyperintense on T2W images; and type 3—due to bony sclerosis, hypointense on both T1W and T2W images. Type 3 changes related to sclerosis can also be identified on plain radiographs and CT studies (**Fig. 10-3**).[14]

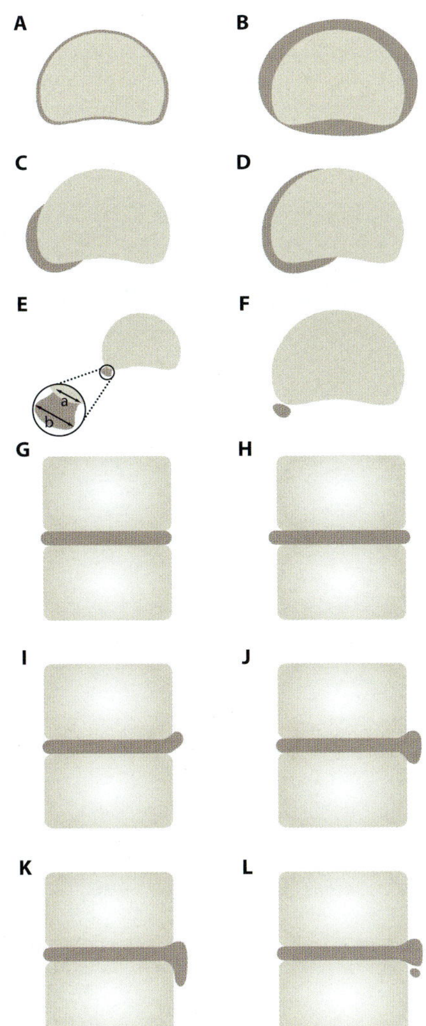

FIGURE 10-1. Diagram depicting disc disease nomenclature in the axial and sagittal planes. A, G: Normal disc outline; B, H: Disc bulge—disc extends outside its normal outline by more than 25% of its circumference; C: Disc herniation—focal displacement of disc material beyond the normal margin of the disc space, less than 25% of disc circumference; can be protrusion or extrusion; D: Asymmetric disc bulge—disc extends more than its normal outline by more than 25% of its circumference, however, more in one section of the periphery than another; E: Disc extrusion—see J; F: Disc sequestration—see L; I: Disc protrusion—type of disc herniation in which the component outside normal disc outline is equal to or lesser than the base of the disc in any plane; J: Disc extrusion—type of disc herniation in which the component outside normal disc outline is longer than the base of the disc in any plane; K: Disc extrusion with migration—part of the extruded disc extends superiorly or inferiorly and remains in continuity with the disc; L: Disc extrusion with sequestration—part of the extruded disc that is separated from and not in continuity with the disc; (Please note that the outline of normal disc is not shown on C,D,E &F to avoid confusion).

Schmorl's nodes, also called "intravertebral disc herniation," are those in which the nucleus pulposus herniates through the end plates into the adjacent portions of the vertebral body (Fig. 10-2C).[15] The different types of Modic changes described earlier can occur with this type of disc herniation as well. While most Schmorl's nodes are asymptomatic and incidentally detected, type 1 Modic changes with enhancement can occur around Schmorl's nodes, and these can be associated with back pain resulting in painful Schmorl's nodes. These need to be differentiated from more serious etiologies such as neoplastic lesion or a focus of infection. Continuity of the disc material from the disc space into the endplate is a helpful clue to establishing the diagnosis on imaging. However, neoplastic or infectious lesions can coexist with Schmorl's nodes and the imaging studies should be carefully interpreted to exclude these.

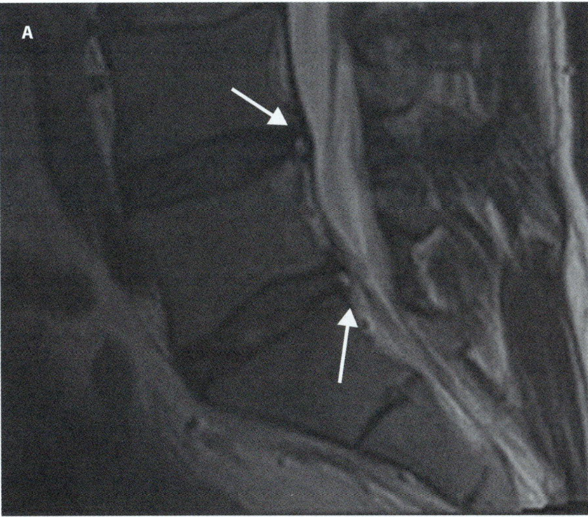

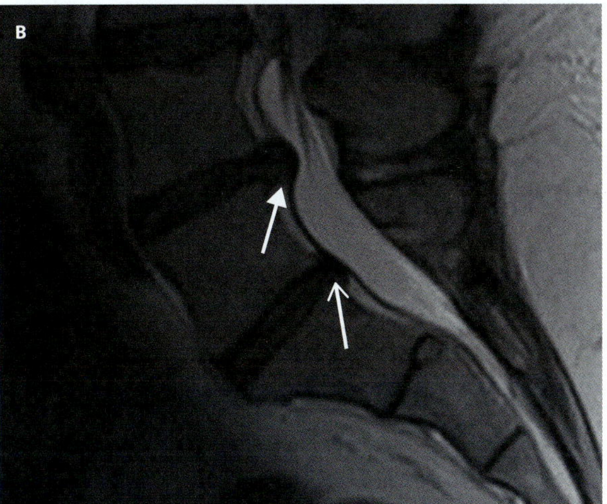

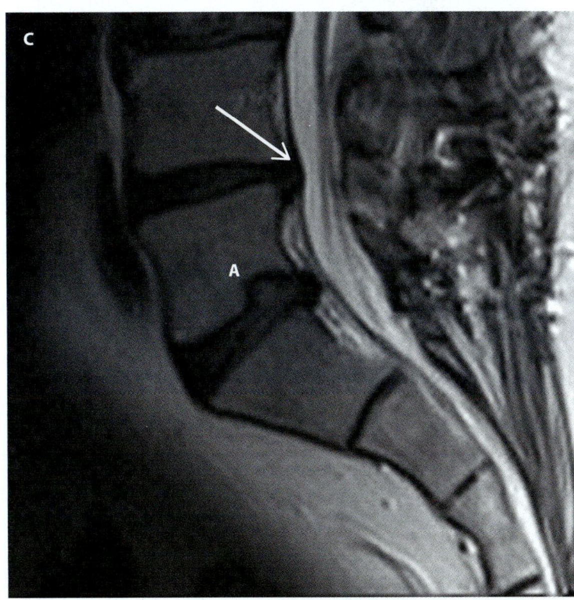

FIGURE 10-2. *Disk disease.* MRI of lumbar spine; sagittal T2W images showing types of disk disease. **A.** Annular fissure. Hyperintense focus in the annulus (closed arrows) indicates annular fissure. **B.** Disc protrusion and extrusion. Disc protrusion (open arrow)—the disk component extending out is smaller than the base of the disk. Disk extrusion (closed arrow)—the disk component extending out is longer than the base of the disk (mushroom cap appearance). **C.** Schmorl's node. Disc component that indents the inferior end plate of vertebral body (A) is the Schmorl's node. There is also a small disk extrusion at superior level (open arrow).

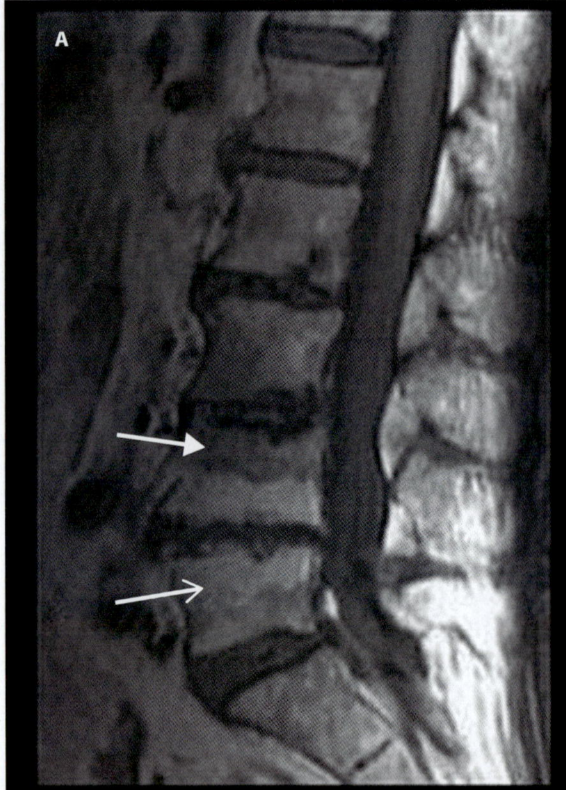

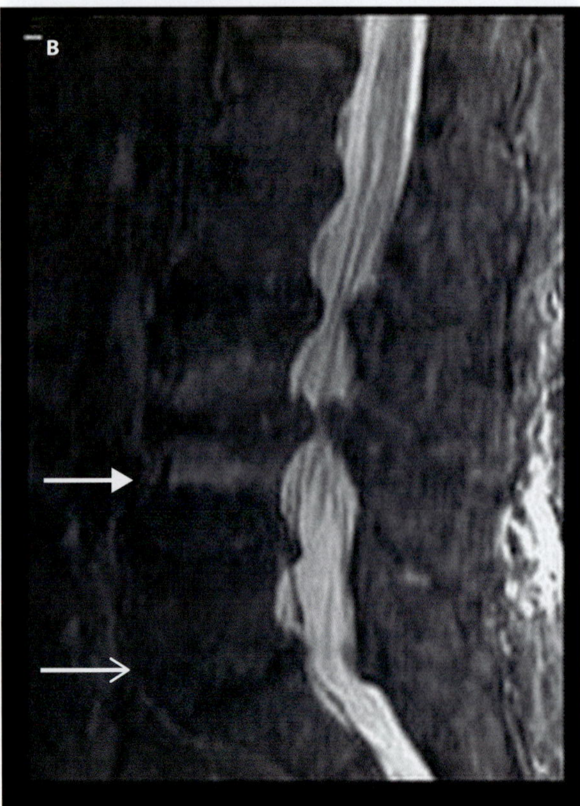

FIGURE 10-3. *Modic changes.* Changes in marrow signal reactive to adjacent degenerative disease. **A.** Sagittal T1W image of MRI lumbar spine. **B.** Sagittal STIR image of MRI lumbar spine. Notations: Closed arrow: Modic type 1 changes—T1 hypointense and STIR hyperintense foci related to edema/water content. Open arrow: Modic type 2 changes—T1 hyperintense and STIR hypointense foci related to fat content; Modic type 3 changes (not shown here): T1 and STIR hypointense foci related to sclerosis—see CT appearance on Fig. 10-4A.

Vertebral Body Degenerative Changes Degenerative changes in the vertebral body usually result in marginal, anterior, or posterior osteophytes and can also occur in uncovertebral processes of the cervical spine. Posterior osteophytes can contribute to spinal canal stenosis; uncovertebral osteophytes can contribute to foraminal narrowing and radiculopathy in the cervical spine (**Figs. 10-4A, 10-4B**).

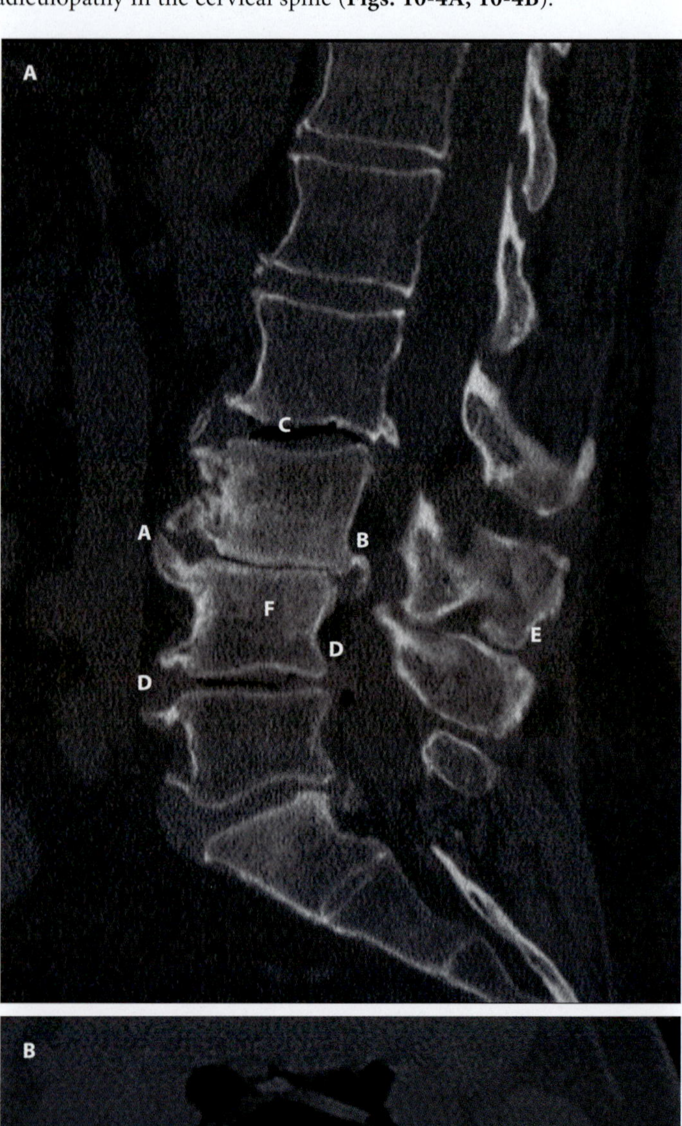

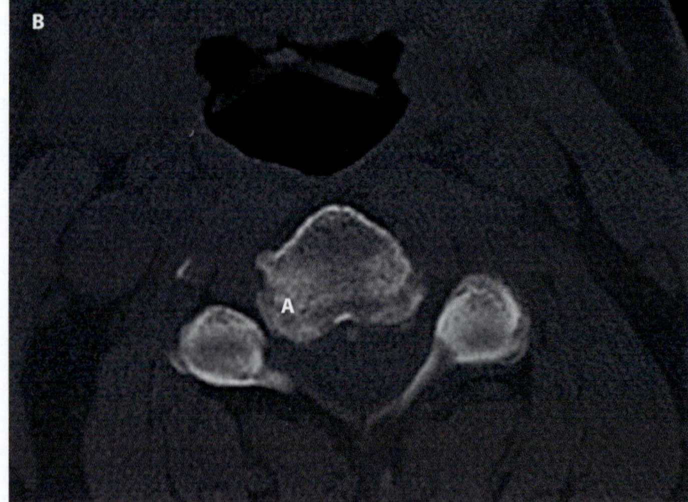

FIGURE 10-4. *CT appearance of degenerative changes.* **A.** CT lumbar spine sagittal bone algorithm reformatted midline image: (A) anterior osteophyte; (B) posterior osteophyte; (C) vacuum phenomenon—gas in disk; (D) disc outline; (E) degenerative changes in spinous process; (F) sclerosis related to Modic type 3 changes. **B.** CT cervical spine, axial bone algorithm image: (A) uncovertebral osteophytes causing right foraminal narrowing.

Transitional anatomy can predispose a patient to degenerative changes due to biomechanical alterations.

Facet Joint Degenerative Changes Degenerative changes in the facet joints can be an important cause of back pain and can involve any of the following components: superior and inferior articular processes, fibrous capsules, and adjacent supporting ligaments. Osteophytes, facet joint space narrowing, sclerosis or widening due to erosions, and synovial cysts are some of the imaging manifestations. These can contribute to spinal canal and foraminal narrowing and deformity on the thecal sac and nerves (**Fig. 10-5**). There can also be reactive inflammatory and synovitis changes with edema and contrast enhancement in the joint capsule and adjacent soft tissues that can result in symptoms. Changes in the subchondral marrow can occur in the articular processes and adjacent pedicles similar to the Modic end-plate changes described earlier.

Degenerative changes in facet joints can also result in spondylolisthesis (usually anterolisthesis of a vertebral body relative to the lower one with increased risk for instability), spinal canal and foraminal stenosis, and nerve impingement. Degenerative spondylolisthesis needs to be differentiated from spondylolytic (isthmic) spondylolisthesis, which is related to pars defects that are usually associated with foraminal narrowing without spinal canal stenosis[16] (**Fig. 10-6**). Sometimes, there can be a combination of the two types of spondylolisthesis. Degenerative disc changes can also cause retrolisthesis of a vertebral body relative to the one below.[8]

Other Posterior Element Degenerative Changes Degenerative changes in the ligamentum flavum usually result in thickening of the ligament with buckling and contribute to spinal canal stenosis.

Degenerative changes in spinous processes can be associated with reactive inflammatory and edematous changes with enhancement on postcontrast MR images in and around the spinous processes and can result in pain, also called Baastrup syndrome.[8]

Spinal Stenosis Spinal stenosis can be categorized as central canal stenosis, lateral recess or subarticular zone stenosis, or foraminal stenosis. These can be congenital/developmental related to congenitally short pedicles that can result in central canal and lateral recess stenosis (**Fig. 10-7A**) or due to pars defects that can result in foraminal stenosis. However, more often, spinal stenosis is acquired due to degenerative changes and soft-tissue and neoplastic abnormalities of the spine and adjacent soft tissues (Figs. 10-4A, **10-7B, 10-7C**). Thecal sac dimension less than 10 mm in antero-posterior (AP) dimension or a dural sac cross-sectional area of less than 100 mm^2 in the lumbar spine is considered to be anatomic stenosis on CT or MRI.[17,18] Although spinal stenosis can be associated with neurogenic claudication due to effects on the cord, cauda equina, and peripheral nerves, it is important to realize that many patients with moderate to severe central canal stenosis can be asymptomatic.[19]

NONDEGENERATIVE DISEASE

Postoperative Spine Imaging Imaging of the postoperative spine is very important in daily practice. Interpreting the imaging studies can be challenging, requiring a systematic approach and knowledge of the surgical details. Different imaging modalities such as plain radiography (static, dynamic flexion and extension views), CT, and MRI complement each other in providing the necessary information to assess the postoperative spine, diagnose complications, and plan further management.

Different types of spinal surgeries that are frequently done are decompressive, stabilization and fusion surgeries, and resection of pathologic lesions, some of which as described here:[20]

1. **Decompressive surgeries**
   a. Percutaneous disc decompression, microdiscectomy, removal of extra-foraminal disc herniation.
   b. Laminotomy, laminectomy with or without facetectomy.

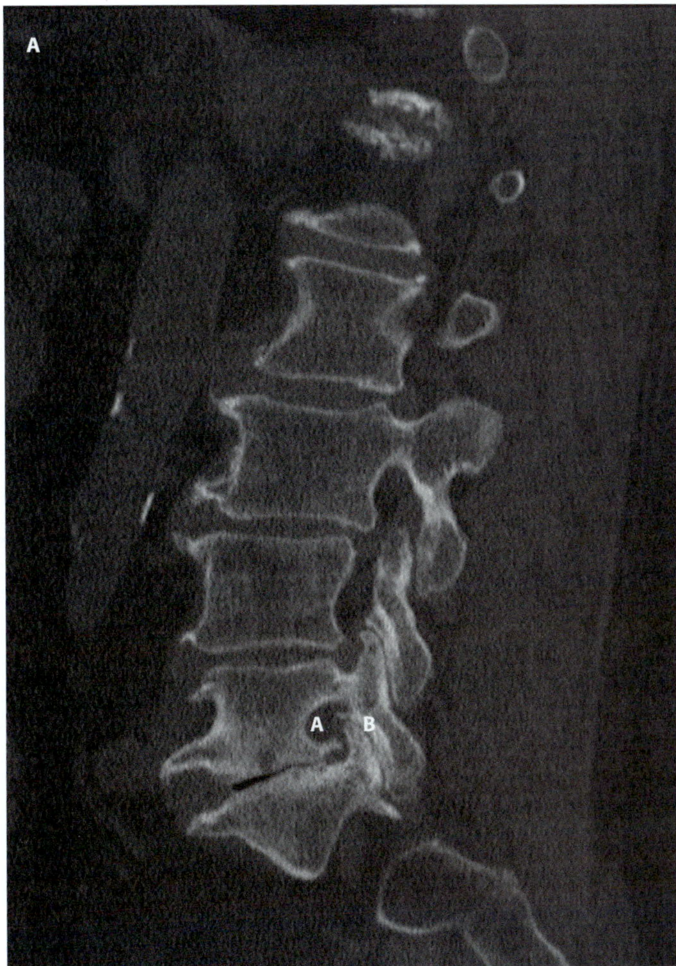

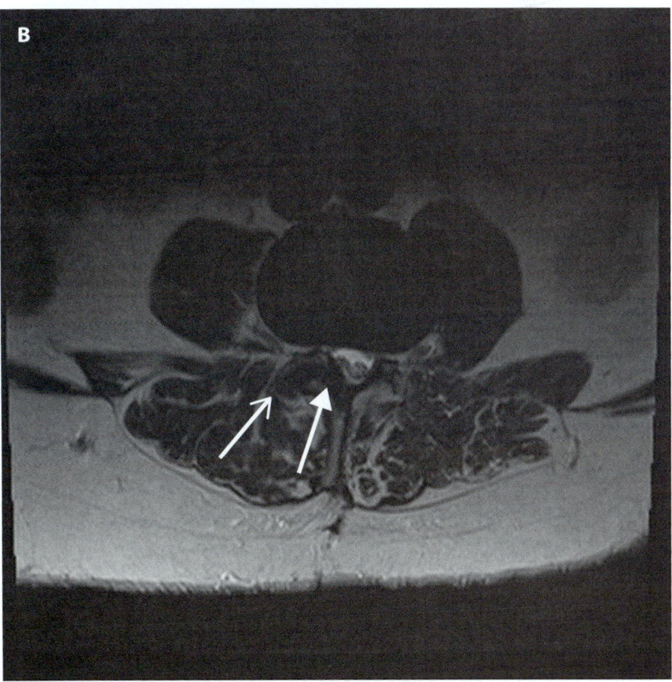

FIGURE 10-5. *Facet degenerative changes.* **A.** CT lumbar spine sagittal bone algorithm reformatted off-midline image: posterior osteophyte (A) and facet osteophyte (B) causing foraminal narrowing. **B.** MRI lumbar spine axial T2W image: facet hypertrophy and degenerative changes (open arrow) and thickened ligamentum flavum (closed arrow) causing deformity on thecal sac and foraminal narrowing.

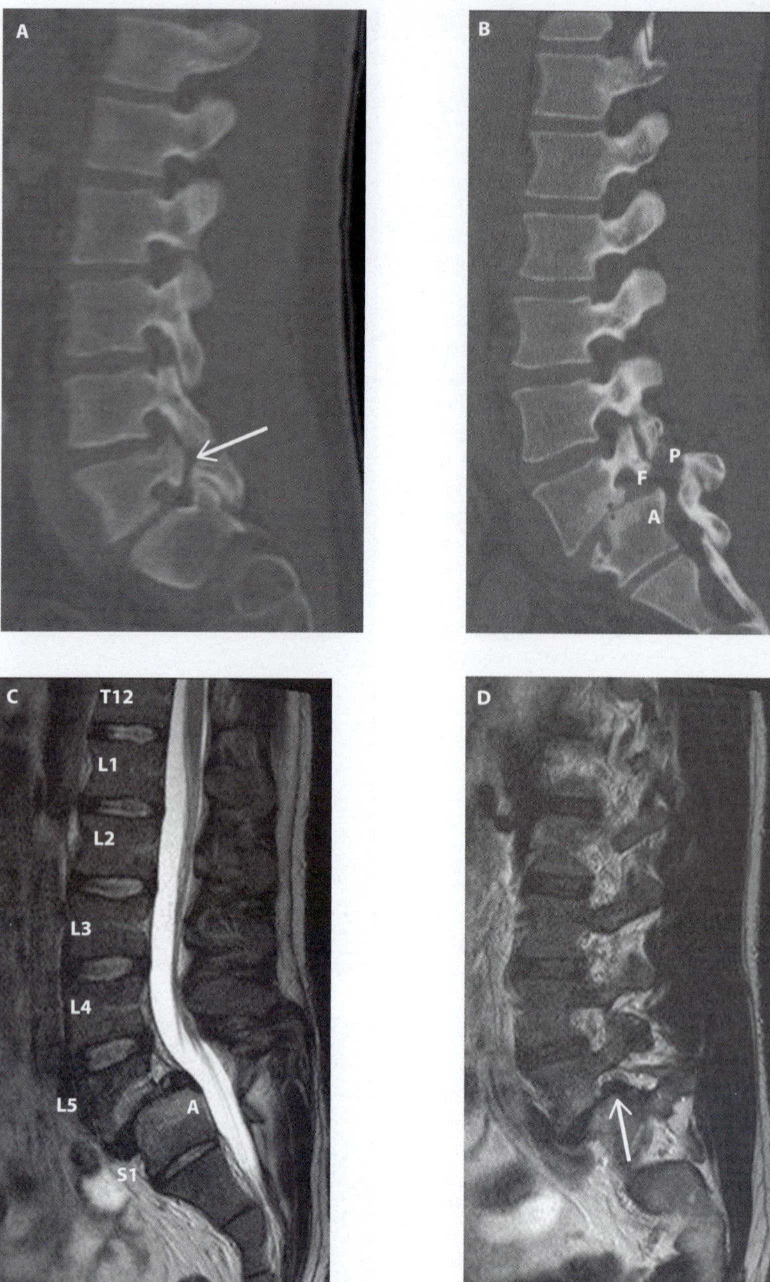

FIGURE 10-6. *Spondylolysis with spondylolisthesis.* **A.** CT Lumbar spine sagittal bone algorithm reformatted off-midline image shows pars defect (arrow) **B.** CT lumbar spine sagittal bone algorithm reformatted off-midline image in a different patient shows part of pars defect (P) with resultant anterolisthesis of L5 vertebra over S1 with sclerosis of adjacent margins (A) and foraminal narrowing (F). **C.** MRI lumbar spine. Sagittal STIR midline image shows anterolisthesis of L5 vertebra over S1 with uncovering of disc without spinal canal stenosis. **D.** MRI lumbar spine. Sagittal STIR off-midline image in the same study shows neural foraminal narrowing (arrow).

2. **Stabilization and fusion surgeries**
   a. Different types of interbody fusion-anterior, lateral, posterior, transforaminal.
   b. Using different types of implants such as rod and plate, transpedicular, translaminar or facet screws, odontoid and lateral mass screws, disc spacers, disc prosthesis, bone grafts, etc.

Certain findings listed below can be seen on imaging during the first few weeks or months of postoperative period and are considered to be normal or expected findings and should not be confused with complications. Sometimes, however differentiation based on imaging alone can be difficult:

1. Asymmetry/edema in the posterior paraspinal muscles.
2. Small seroma.
3. Enhancing vertebral end plates—due to aseptic reaction, up to 6 to 18 months.
4. Postdiscectomy changes—enhancing epidural focus due to granulation tissue; can deform the thecal sac to <25% in extent.
5. Residual or recurrent disc herniation can be seen; however, may not progress.
6. Mild expansion of the dural sac posteriorly due to osseous insufficiency at surgical site, which, however, does not represent a pseudomeningocele.

Postoperative spine complications can be classified into

1. Early or late.
2. Those related to hardware, soft tissues, osseous, intrathecal and neural structures:

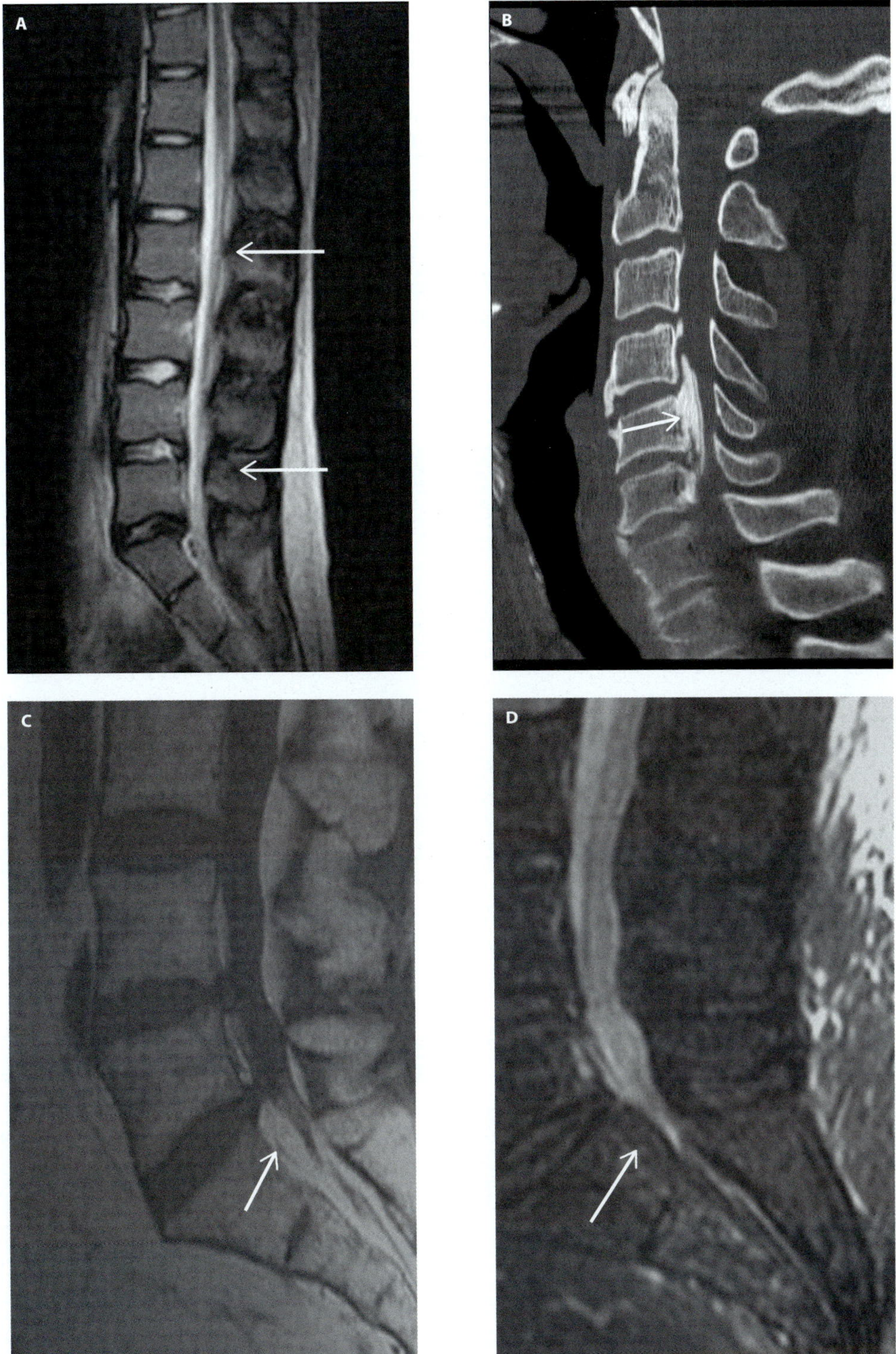

FIGURE 10-7. *Spinal stenosis due to different etiologies.* **A.** Sagittal STIR image showing diffuse narrowing of spinal canal related to congenitally short pedicles (not shown here) without associated disc or facet degenerative changes. **B.** CT cervical spine sagittal bone algorithm reformatted image shows ossification of posterior longitudinal ligament (open arrow), causing severe canal stenosis. **C.** MRI lumbar spine sagittal T1W. **D.** MRI lumbar spine sagittal STIR images show area of high T1W and low STIR signal in the anterior epidural space at S1 level (open arrows), representing epidural fat effacing the CSF space, representing epidural lipomatosis.

a. Hardware-related complications include malalignment, misplacement, loosening, break/fracture, bone graft complications, subsidence, injury to vital structures such as blood vessels, nerves, or cord.

b. Osseous complications include canal or foraminal stenosis, progressive deformity, kyphosis, spondylolisthesis, pseudo-arthrosis, progression of degenerative changes, etc.

c. Other important complications include residual/recurrent disc herniation, scar or epi/peridural fibrosis, infection, hematoma, arachnoiditis, and CSF leak (**Table 10-6**; **Figs. 10-8A, 10-8B, 10-8C**).

Failed back syndrome refers to a condition in which there is persistent low back pain with or without radicular pain after back surgery; it can result from any of the conditions mentioned above.

TABLE 10-6 Imaging Appearance of Certain Postoperative Complications

Disc herniation	Has no enhancement or minimal peripheral enhancement from reactive granulation tissue
Scar (epi/peridural fibrosis)	Has homogeneous mild enhancement; can encase nerves or wrap around disc herniation
Infection	Enhancement in disk, vertebral bodies
	Epidural, pre/paravertebral soft tissues; phlegmon; amorphous relatively uniform enhancement
	Abscess: nonenhancing center filled with pus surrounded by enhancing wall of granulation tissue
Arachnoiditis	Inflammation/infection of the nerves of thecal sac
	Thickened/clumped/peripherally displaced nerves

Role of Imaging in Pain-Relieving Procedures Imaging has an important role in planning, performing, and following up certain pain-relieving procedures such as vertebroplasty (**Fig. 10-9**), epidural and facet joint injections, intrathecal injections, and cord stimulator placement. While fluoroscopic guidance is mostly used for performing these procedures, CT and MRI are used for planning the procedures and evaluating for any complications such as new compression fracture, hematoma, or infectious complications.

Trauma A brief description is given here regarding the role of imaging in patients with trauma because a detailed description of spine trauma is beyond the scope of this chapter.

Plain radiographs are no longer preferred for screening in patients with history of trauma.

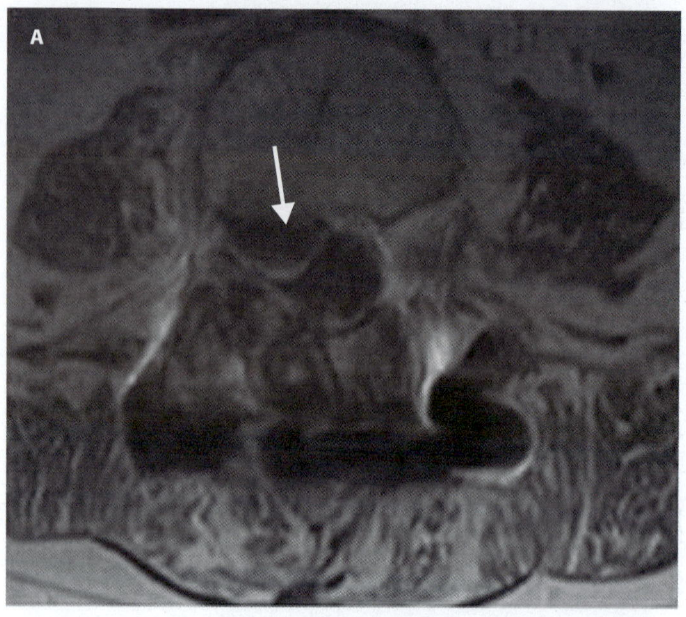

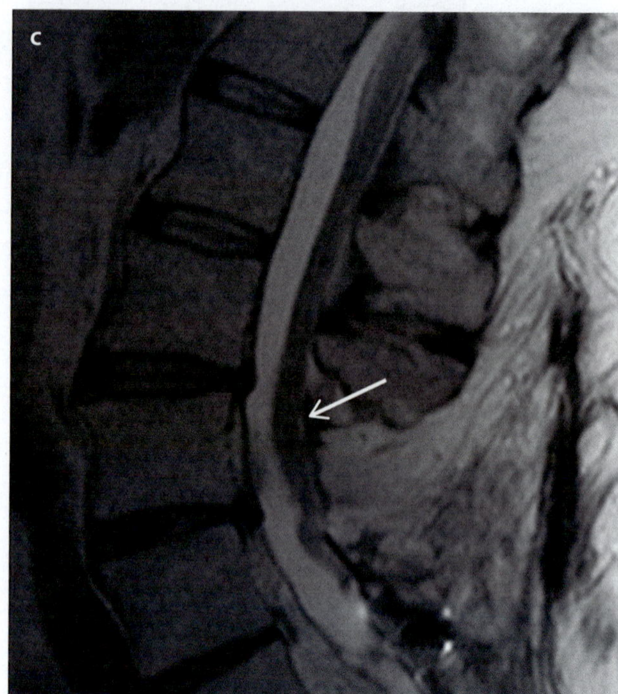

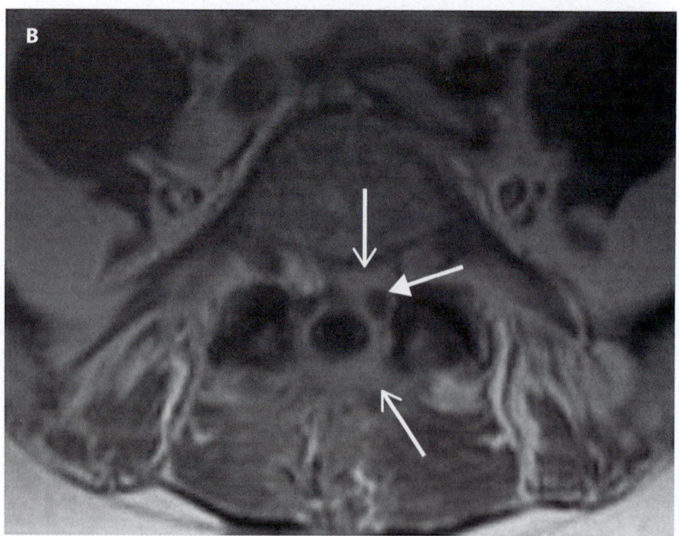

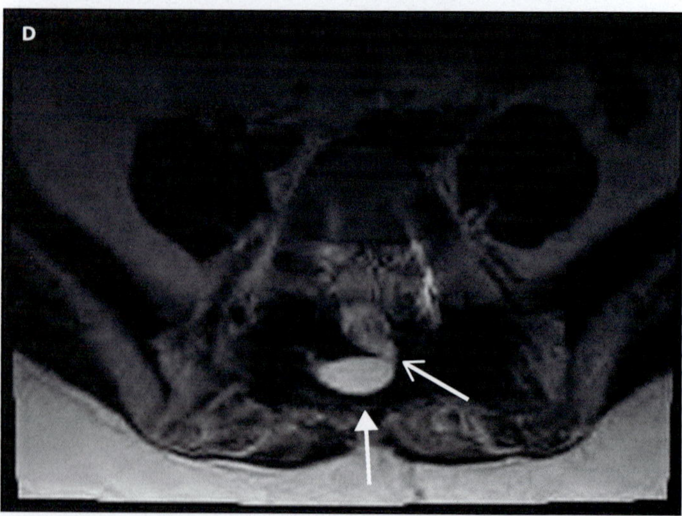

FIGURE 10-8. *Postoperative complications on MRI.* **A.** Recurrent disk herniation; axial T1W postcontrast image shows nonenhancing disc component (closed arrow) deforming the right side of thecal sac. **B.** Scar; axial T1W postcontrast image shows mildly enhancing tissue (open arrows), representing scar tissue surrounding the nerve (closed arrow). **C.** Arachnoiditis; sagittal T2W image shows thickened and clumped cauda equina nerves (open arrow) mimicking cord representing arachnoiditis. **D.** CSF leak; axial T2W image shows a fluid collection in the soft tissues (closed arrow) communicating with CSF in the thecal sac (open arrow), representing a pseudomeningocele related to CSF leak.

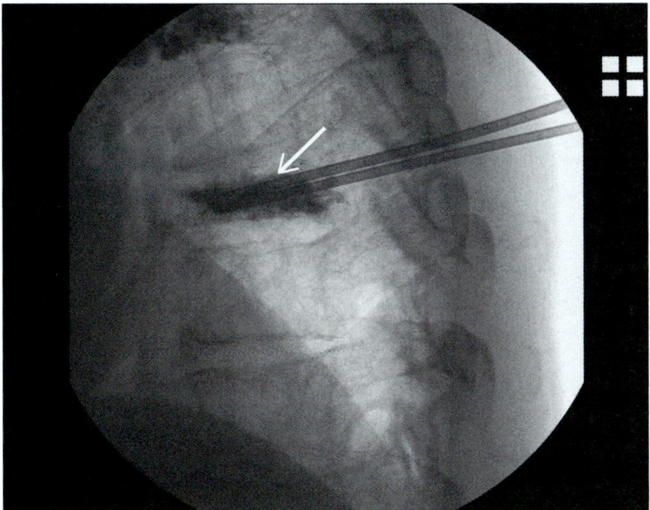

FIGURE 10-9. *Vertebroplasty.* Fluoroscopic image showing injection of cement (open arrow) into a collapsed vertebral body.

CT is far more sensitive, more accurate, faster and generates more reliable evaluation of the spine. Plain radiographs are frequently limited by patient positioning and poor penetration of thicker body parts. Both problems lead to the need for repeat exposures, raising the radiation dose and increasing the time required for these studies. The far lower accuracy of plain radiographs and the time required to perform them has lead to their abandonment for the initial evaluation of spine trauma.

CT is the modality for detailed assessment of fractures, malalignment, and osseous architecture. MRI provides detailed assessment of marrow edema, contusion, focal lesions, ligamentous structures, spinal cord, and nerve and soft-tissue involvement.

Spondylolysis (defects at pars interarticularis) and compression fractures can be an important cause of pain and is better assessed with CT and MRI. Foci of marrow edema around pars defects and in the compressed vertebral bodies indicate an acute component that can result in precipitation/aggravation of symptoms. Imaging also helps in differentiating benign from pathologic compression fractures, in assessment of the extent of disease, and in planning further management.

Pelvic insufficiency fractures can occur in structurally weak bone as in osteoporosis and osteomalacia and related to corticosteroid use, radiation, and the like. Imaging helps in identifying and assessing the acuity of the fractures.

Inflammatory Disease Rheumatoid arthritis and seronegative spondyloarthropathies are the noninfectious inflammatory diseases of spine. Imaging is helpful in localizing, characterizing, and assessing the severity and extent of the disease and complications.

Rheumatoid arthritis involves the cervical spine particularly the atlanto-axial joints. Seronegative spondyloarthropathies include ankylosing spondylitis, psoriatic arthritis, Reiter syndrome, and spondyloarthritis of inflammatory bowel disease.[8] These are characterized by varying degrees of (1) sacroillitis-erosions, sclerosis, and ankylosis; (2) spondylitis-osteitis with sclerosis at anterior corners of vertebral bodies, syndesmophytes, and discovertebral changes; and (3) ankylosis of disc space, facets and costovertebral joints[21] (**Fig. 10-10**).

Differentiating these findings from degenerative disease can be difficult at times based on imaging alone; correlation with clinical and lab findings can be helpful.

Infections Spinal infections include pyogenic and granulomatous infections from various agents. Imaging manifestations include diskitis, osteomyelitis, soft-tissue and epidural phlegmon, abscess, deformities, cord or neural compression, rarely thrombophlebitis, and mycotic aneurysm.

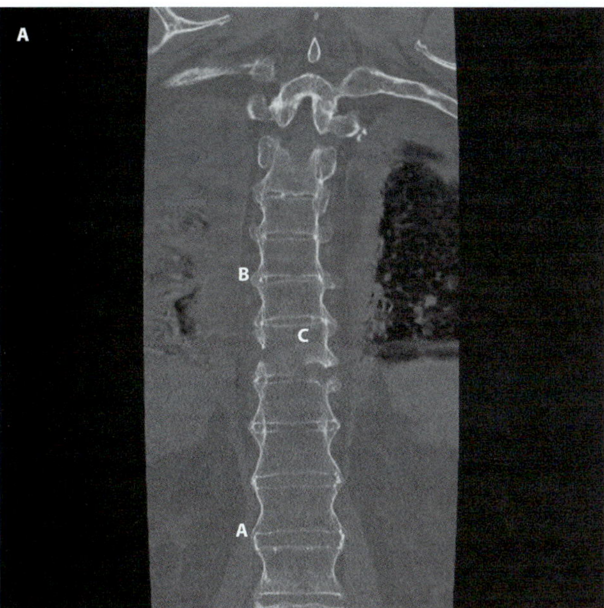

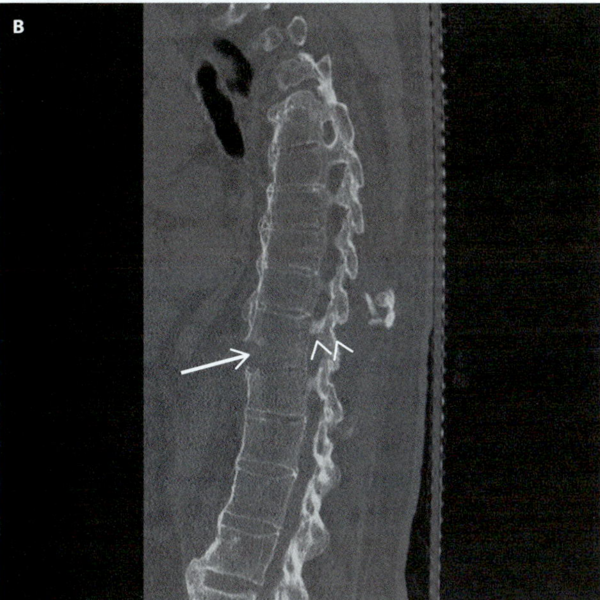

FIGURE 10-10. *Ankylosing spondylitis.* CT thoracic spine sagittal bone algorithm reformatted frontal (**A**) and lateral (**B**) images show syndesmophytes (A), marginal osteophytes (B) along with fracture through ossified anterior longitudinal ligament (open arrow) extending into the vertebral body (C) and posterior elements (double arrow heads).

Imaging with CT and gadolinium-enhanced MRI help in detailed assessment of the abnormalities and complications to plan further management. While MRI can be abnormal even in the early phase of infection, imaging can lag behind the clinical syndrome and response (**Fig. 10-11**).

Though pyogenic and granulomatous infections can have different characteristic features, tissue sampling and culture sensitivity are necessary for definitive diagnosis and management.

Early stages of diskitis and osteomyelitis can mimic degenerative disease. Increased T2 and STIR signals with enhancement in the disc and in the vertebral bodies to a significant extent beyond the end plates, epidural and paraspinal soft-tissue involvement, and follow-up imaging can help to differentiate degenerative disease from infection; however, at times, the distinction can be difficult. Correlation with clinical presentation and lab parameters such as erythrocyte sedimentation rate (ESR) and WBC count and, if necessary, tissue sampling can help in definitive diagnosis.

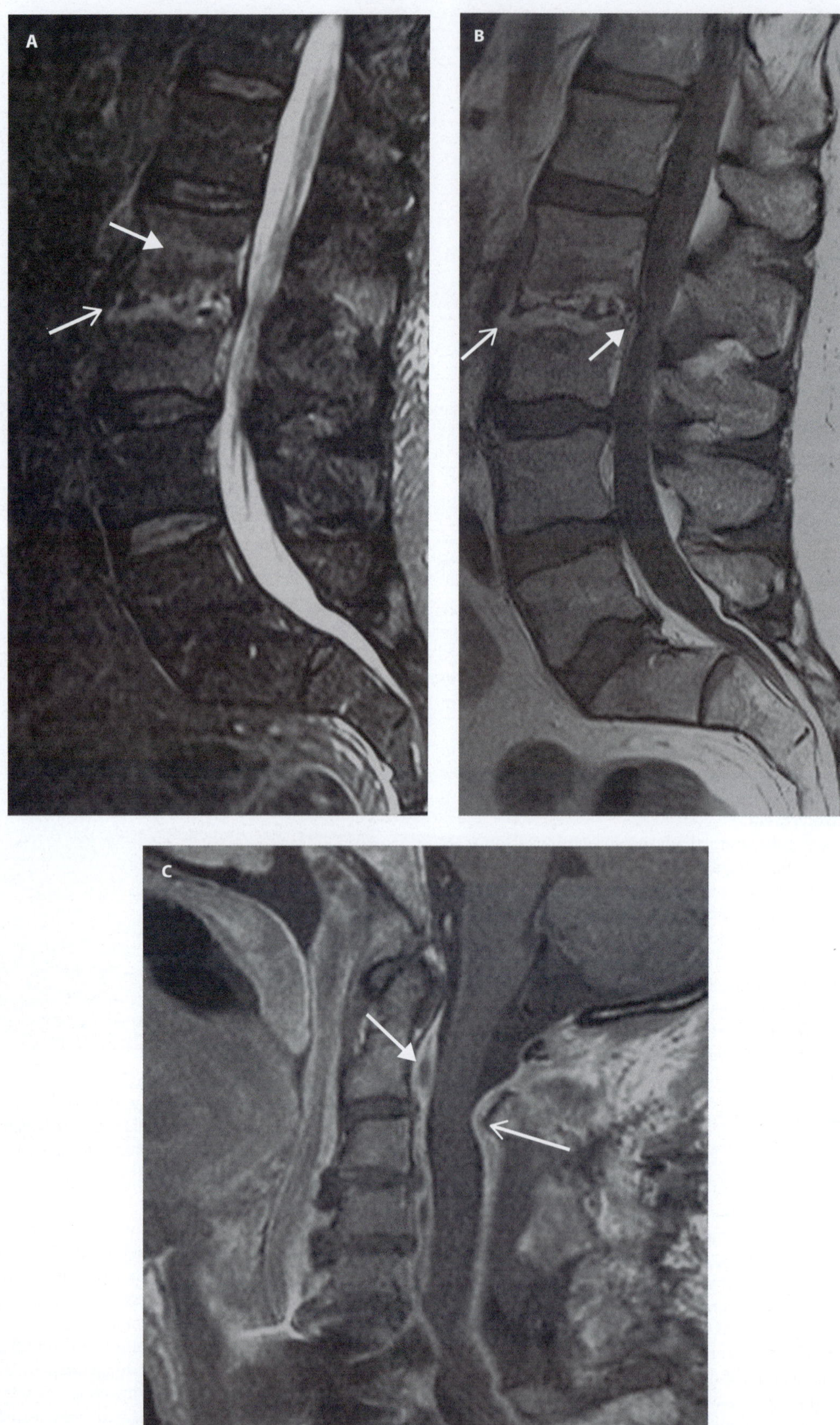

FIGURE 10-11. *Diskitis—osteomyelitis.* **A.** MRI lumbar spine sagittal STIR image shows edema in the disc (open arrow) and vertebral bodies (closed arrow). **B.** MRI lumbar spine sagittal T1W postcontrast image shows enhancement in the disc and adjacent parts of vertebral bodies; there is also small amount of prevertebral (open arrow) and anterior epidural (closed arrow) soft tissue component. **C.** MRI cervical spine sagittal T1W postcontrast image shows abnormal epidural enhancement with nonenhancing central foci (closed arrow), representing epidural abscess; there is also pachymeningeal enhancement posteriorly (open arrow).

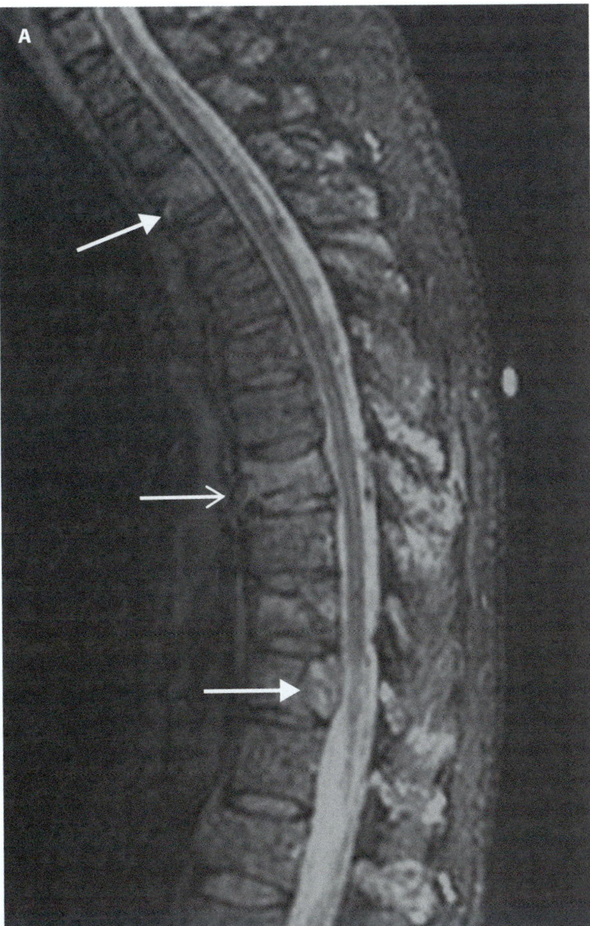

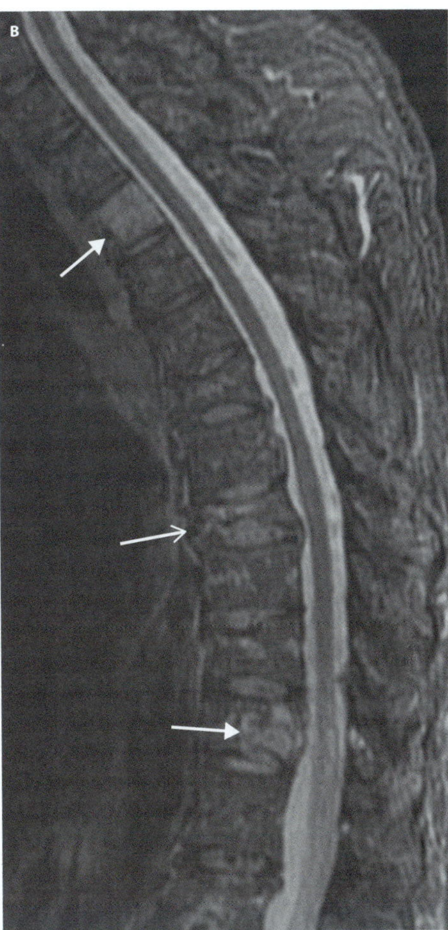

FIGURE 10-12. *Multiple myeloma with vertebral compression fracture.* **A.** MRI thoracic spine sagittal STIR image shows diffusely heterogeneous marrow signal with more focal hyperintense foci related to myeloma deposits (closed arrows); there is also acute compression fracture of mid-thoracic vertebral body with edema (open arrow). **B.** Three months later, MRI shows persistent STIR hyperintense foci related to tumor (closed arrows); interval decrease in the edema of the compressed vertebral body with further decrease in its height (open arrow).

Neoplasms A wide variety of benign and malignant tumors can occur in the spine. Spine neoplasms are classified based on the location and can be (1) extradural, (2) intradural extramedullary, and (3) intramedullary.

Extradural Neoplasms CT helps in the assessment of osseous architecture, while MR is helpful in better characterization of the lesions and extent, including location, paraspinous, and extradural and intraspinal extension.

Most malignant tumors are hypointense or heterogeneously hypointense on T1W sequence and hyperintense on STIR sequence due to the edema. However, sclerotic or cellular metastases can be hypointense on T2W sequence and variable in signal intensity on STIR sequence.

- *Metastases* are the most common extradural spine tumor, mostly from prostate, lung, and breast primary malignancies. The vertebral body is most commonly involved and can be osteoblastic, osteolytic, or mixed.
- *Myeloma* is the most common primary malignant osseous tumor. Reduced bone density, compression fractures, and solitary or multiple focal lytic lesions are the usual imaging findings (**Fig. 10-12**).
- *Osteoid osteoma* can present with back pain. This usually occurs in posterior elements and has a characteristic appearance on imaging with a small lucent nidus surrounded by reactive sclerosis or inflammation; the nidus can enhance on postcontrast MR images and show up as a hot spot on bone scan (**Fig. 10-13**).
- *Hemangioma* is a very common benign tumor of the spine with a characteristic appearance on CT and MRI. On CT, a few trabeculations are noted within a lucent lesion, resulting in stippled or polka-dot appearance without completely lytic appearance. On MRI,

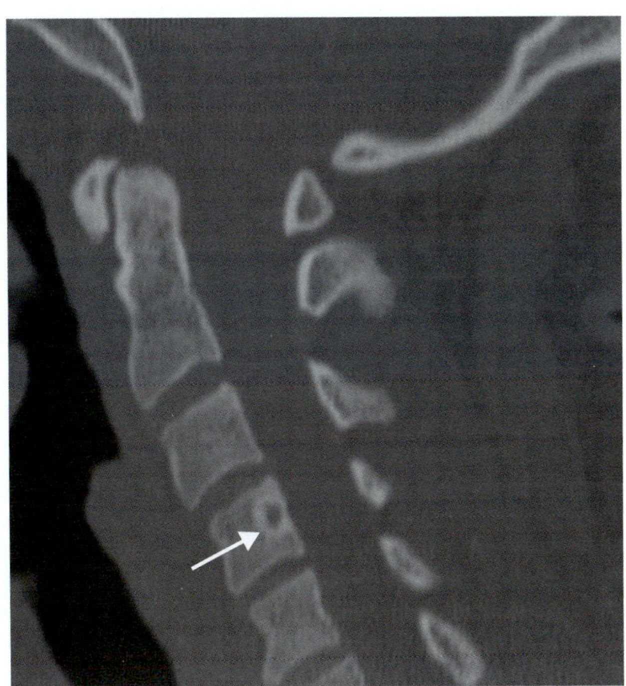

FIGURE 10-13. *Osteoid osteoma.* CT cervical spine sagittal bone algorithm reformatted image shows a focal lesion in the posterior aspect of C4 body with lucent center and surrounding sclerosis representing osteoid osteoma.

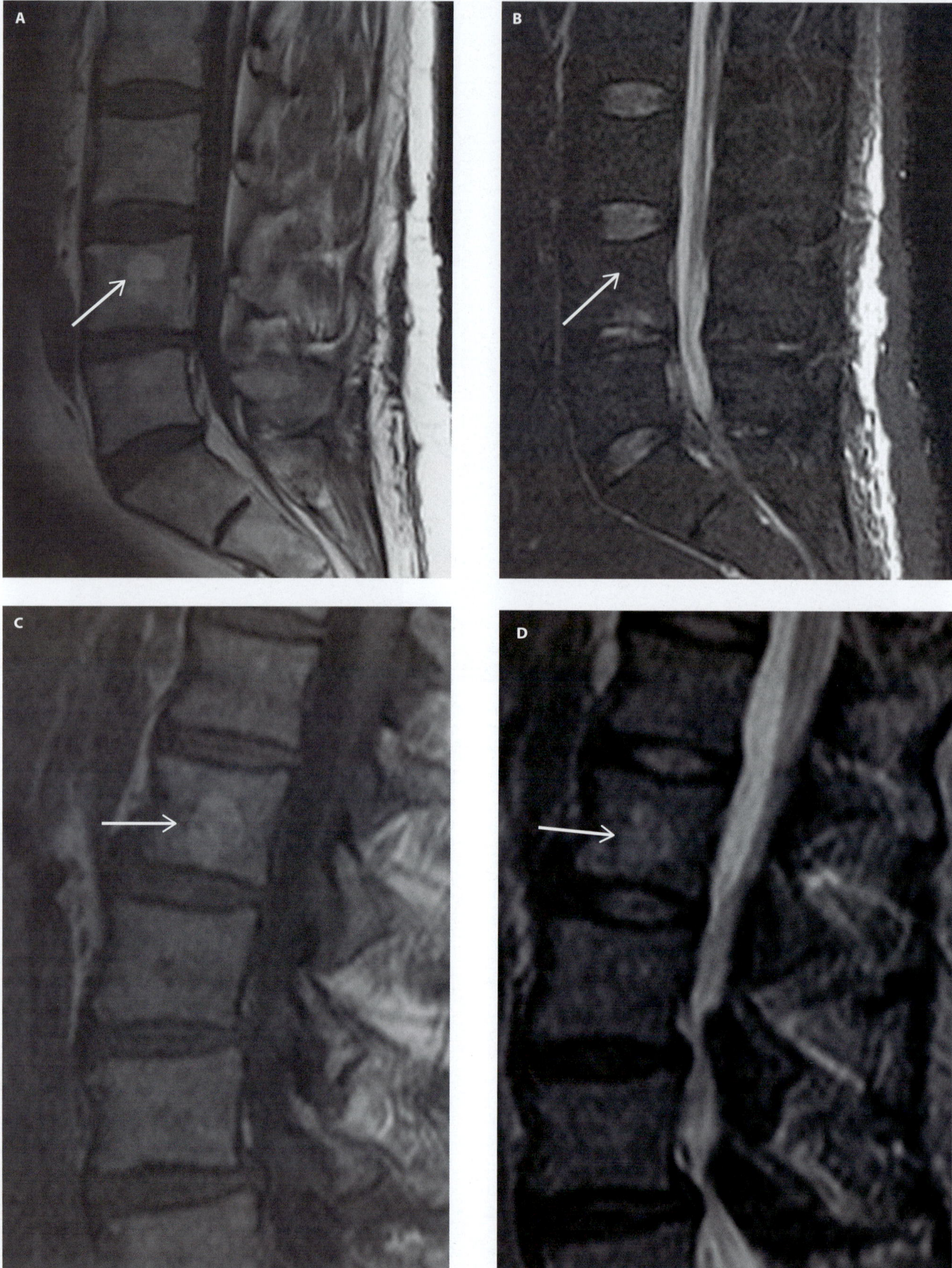

FIGURE 10-14. *Fat deposit.* (**A**) MRI lumbar spine sagittal T1W image shows a T1 hyperintense lesion in L4 vertebral body (arrow). (**B**) MRI lumbar spine sagittal STIR image shows the signal in the lesion is suppressed (arrow), representing fat deposit; there is also incidentally seen fatty filum terminale/lipoma. (Can you identify?) *Typical hemangioma.* (**C**) MRI lumbar spine sagittal T1W image shows a lesion with T1 high signal (open arrow). (**D**) MRI lumbar spine sagittal STIR image shows the lesion has a slightly high signal with a slightly stippled appearance representing hemangioma.

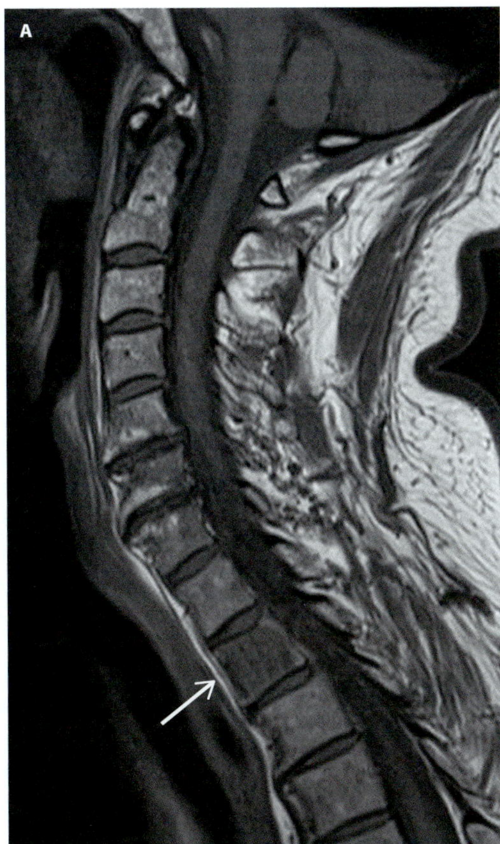

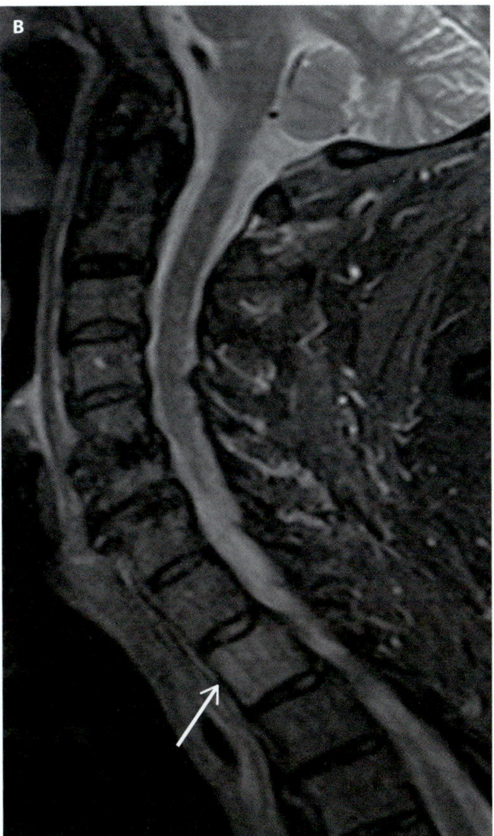

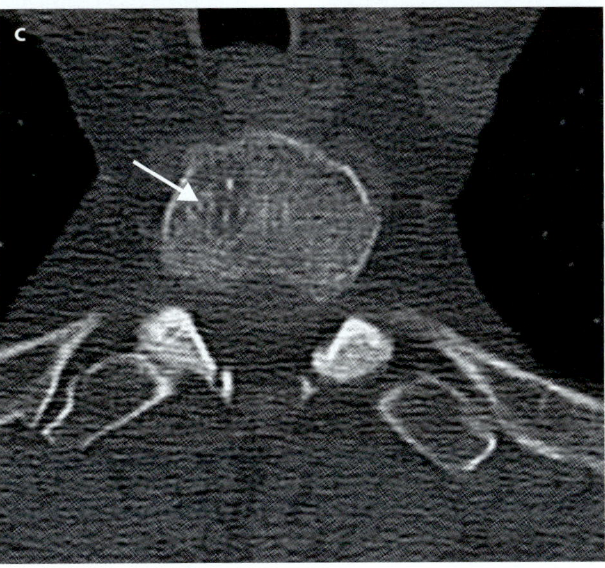

FIGURE 10-15. *Atypical hemangioma.* **A.** MRI cervical spine sagittal T1W image shows a lesion in T2 vertebral body with low signal (open arrow). **B.** MRI cervical spine sagittal STIR image shows high signal in the lesion; differential diagnosis includes atypical hemangioma and metastasis; slight striations related to trabeculations, better seen on CT image, give a clue favoring atypical hemangioma. **C.** CT axial bone algorithm image shows a lucent lesion with trabeculations within and confirms the lesion as hemangioma (a metastatic lesion is lytic with destruction and loss of trabeculations).

the typical hemangioma has a slightly stippled appearance due to intervening low signal trabeculations; there is high T1 signal within, related to adipocytes and vascular stasis, a high signal on T2 and STIR and water IDEAL sequences with some enhancement on fat-suppressed postcontrast images related to the vascularity (**Fig. 10-14**).

Fat-suppressed sequences such as STIR and water IDEAL sequences help differentiate fat deposit from hemangioma because the fat deposit also has a high signal on the T1W sequence but is suppressed on fat-suppressed sequences (Fig. 10-14). Sometimes, a hemangioma can have variable pattern including absence of high signal on T1 related to a less adipose and greater vascular component. This is called "atypical hemangioma" and can resemble other lesions such as metastasis due to high signal on STIR sequence. This can be differentiated based on CT where a metastatic lesion can have a lytic appearance without intact trabeculations (**Fig. 10-15**). According to Matrawy et al, diffusion weighted images can help in differentiating hemangiomas from more aggressive neoplasms such as metastasis; metastasis can have slow diffusion whereas atypical and typical hemangioma do not have slow diffusion.[22]

Sometimes, hemangioma can be extensive and extent into adjacent epidural and paraspinous soft tissues and is called aggressive hemangioma.[8]

Intradural Extramedullary Neoplasms These arise from the dura or nerves and include meningioma, nerve sheath tumor such as schwannoma, and neurofibroma and metastases.

Intramedullary Neoplasms These include cord tumors such as metastases and primary tumors such as astrocytoma, ependymoma, and hemangioblastoma.

SPINAL CORD

Cord lesions related to trauma, demyelinating disease, myelitis, inflammatory or infectious diseases such as tuberculomas, neurosarcoidosis, and metabolic and toxic etiologies can be better assessed with MRI. Vascular conditions such as infarct, AV malformations, and fistulae can be better assessed with MR and conventional angiograms.

CONCLUSIONS

Imaging has a very important role in the evaluation of spinal disease. The different imaging modalities complement each other in the complete assessment of spine disease. While every imaging finding need not be clinically significant, imaging along with clinical correlation and discretion helps in assessing the extent and degree of severity of disease and associated complications to decide on appropriate management.

1. Plain radiography, fluoroscopy, CT, MRI, and radionuclide studies are the different imaging modalities useful in spine imaging and complement each other in the evaluation of spinal disease.
2. Routine imaging of spine for nonspecific symptoms is not necessary because it may not always improve the outcome or be cost-effective, can have deleterious effects such as exposure to radiation, and may result in unnecessary invasive treatment.
3. Imaging should only be considered when clinically appropriate based on clinical presentation, risk factors for systemic or serious disease, or if intervention is contemplated.
4. CT is useful for the evaluation of osseous details of spine. However, assessment of intrathecal and soft-tissue abnormalities is limited.
5. MRI is useful for better characterization of intrathecal and soft-tissue abnormalities and certain osseous lesions.
6. CT and MRI are helpful in the assessment of degenerative changes in spine and the effect on neural structures. However, not all imaging findings are clinically significant.
7. Imaging is very helpful in the evaluation of postoperative and post-procedural spine and associated complications.

REFERENCES

1. American College of Radiology. *Manual on Contrast Media.* Available at: http://www.acr.org/SecondaryMainMenuCategories/quality_safety/contrast_manual.aspx.
2. Sundgren PC, Leander P. Is administration of gadolinium-based contrast media to pregnant women and small children justified? *J Mag Res Imaging.* 2011;34:750-757.
3. Guyer RD, Ohnmeiss DD. Lumbar discography. *Spine J.* May-Jun 2003;3(3 Suppl):11S-27S.
4. Manchikanti L, Glaser ES, Wolfer L, et al. Systematic review of lumbar discography as a diagnostic test for chronic low back pain. *Pain Physician.* 2009;12:541-559.
5. Wagner AL. Gadolinium diskography. *Am J Neuroradiol.* 2004;25:1824-1827.
6. Safriel Y, Ali M, Hayt M, Ang R. Gadolinium use in spine procedures for patients with allergy to iodinated contrast: experience of 127 procedures. *AJNR.* June 2006;27:1194-1197.
7. Pineda C, Espinosa R, Pena A. Radiographic imaging in osteomyelitis: the role of plain radiography, computed tomography, ultrasonography, magnetic resonance imaging, and scintigraphy. *Semin Plast Surg.* May 2009;23(2):80-89.
8. Maus T. Imaging the back pain patient. *Phys Med Rehabil Clin N Am.* 2010;21:725-766.
9. Chou R, Qaseem A, Snow B, et al. Diagnosis and treatment of low back pain: a joint clinical practice guideline from the American College of Physicians and the American Pain Society. *Ann Intern Med.* 2007;147:478-491.
10. Davis PA, Wippold II FJ, Cornelius RS, et al. *ACR Appropriateness Criteria low back pain.* [online publication]. Reston (VA): American College of Radiology (ACR); 2011.
11. Konin GP, Walz DM. Lumbosacral transitional vertebrae: classification, imaging findings, and clinical relevance. *Am J Neuroradiol.* Nov 2010;31(10):1778-1786.
12. Fardon DF, Williams AL, Dohring EJ, et al. Lumbar disc nomenclature: version 2.0 Recommendations of the combined task forces of the North American Spine Society, the American Society of Spine Radiology and the American Society of Neuroradiology. *The Spine J.* 2014;2525-2545.
13. Bush K, Cowan N, Katz D, et al. The natural history of sciatica associated with disc pathology: a prospective study with clinical and independent radiologic follow-up. *Spine.* 1992;17:1205-1212.
14. Modic M, Steinberg P, Ross J, et al. Degenerative disk disease: assessment of changes in vertebral body marrow with MR imaging. *Radiology.* 1988;166:193-199.
15. Mattei TA, Rehman AA. Schmorl's nodes: current pathophysiological, diagnostic, and therapeutic paradigms. *Neurosurg Rev.* 2014;37:39-46.
16. Tehranzadeh J, Andrews C, Wong E. Imaging of low back pain 1. Lumbar spine imaging: normal variants, imaging pitfalls, and artifacts. *Radiologic Clinics of North America.* 2000;38(6):1207-1253.
17. Geisser M, Haig TH, et al. Spinal canal size and clinical symptoms among persons diagnosed with lumbar spinal stenosis. *Clin J Pain.* 2007;23(9):780-785.
18. White A, Panjabi M. *Clinical Biomechanics of the Spine.* 2nd ed. Philadelphia, Pa: Lippincott-Raven; 1990.
19. Jarvik JJ, Hollingworth W, Heagerty P, et al. The longitudinal assessment of imaging and disbility of the back (LAID back) study. *Spine (Phil Pa 1976).* 2001;26(10):1158-1166.
20. Thakkar RS, Malloy IV JP, Thakkar SC, et al. Imaging the postoperative spine. *Radiol Cli N Am.* 2012;50:731-747.
21. Ross JS, Brant-Zawadzki M, Moore KR, et al. *Diagnostic Imaging Spine.* Salt Lake City, Ut: Amirsys; 2007.
22. Matrawy KA, El-Nekeidy AA, El-Sheridy HG. Atypical hemangioma and malignant lesions of spine: can diffusion weighted magnetic resonance imaging help to differentiate? *The Egyptian Journal of Radiology and Nuclear Medicine.* 2013;44(2):259-263.

Role of Electrodiagnostics in Pain Assessment

John C. Keel
Nicholas K. Muraoka
Seward B. Rutkove

INTRODUCTION

Electrodiagnosis (EDx) can play a crucial role in identifying the underlying problem in a patient presenting with a pain disorder. In contrast with radiologic modalities such as magnetic resonance imaging (MRI), EDx provides unique functional information about the integrity of both the central and peripheral nervous systems. In addition to localizing the problem, EDx can give insight into chronicity, severity, and prognosis. For example, disc abnormalities of uncertain clinical significance are routinely found at multiple levels on MRI studies of the lumbar spine. EDx has the unique ability to determine whether one of these disc abnormalities is actually producing nerve damage. Moreover, such testing may also demonstrate abnormalities in patients with inflammatory lesions, where neuroimaging is often normal.

In general, EDx encompasses nerve conduction studies (NCSs) and electromyography (EMG), which together provide information about the peripheral nerves and muscles and evoked potentials, which are used predominantly for evaluation of the central nervous system. Emerging techniques are briefly mentioned, including electrical impedance myography and neuromuscular ultrasound. Other EDx tests—including intraoperative monitoring, autonomic function testing, repetitive nerve stimulation, and analysis of movement disorders—generally have a limited role in the evaluation of pain disorders and are not included in detail here.

In the first part of this chapter, we review the methodology and interpretation of EDx. In the second part, we examine the electrophysiologic testing in specific disorders associated with pain. Additional information regarding this complex topic may be obtained from several excellent texts.[1-4]

ELECTRODIAGNOSIS: METHODS AND INTERPRETATION

NERVE CONDUCTION STUDIES

NCSs and EMG are usually performed at the same session because the procedures are complementary, each providing unique information about the peripheral nerves and muscles. Generally, NCSs are performed before EMG, with the results of the NCS used to guide the needle electrode examination. NCSs provide quantitative information, whereas EMG, as performed in its standard fashion, is more subjective.

NCSs assess large myelinated peripheral nerves, and can provide information about the function of myelination, number of axons, function of motor units, and function of the neuromuscular junction.[5] Only a few nerves are routinely studied. In the arms, these nerves include the median, radial, and ulnar, and in the legs, posterior tibial, deep peroneal, and sural. The facial and trigeminal nerves can also be studied. All of these nerves are easily accessible to stimulation and are commonly involved in neurogenic illness. A number of additional nerves—including musculocutaneous, superficial peroneal, and saphenous—are studied less often but are sometimes helpful in localizing a lesion.

Orthodromic studies record impulses propagated in the same direction as physiologic conduction, while antidromic studies record impulses propagated in the opposite direction of physiologic conduction. Stimulation is achieved by depolarizing a nerve under a negatively charged cathode. The propagated wave is recorded with a standard differential technique via two electrodes: an "active" and a "reference."

Motor Nerve Conduction Studies When performing motor studies, an active recording electrode is placed over a muscle belly and a referential recording electrode is placed over the tendon insertion of that muscle. The nerve is then stimulated at a fixed distance from the muscle (**Fig. 11-1**). The electrical response represents the depolarization of the muscle beneath the active electrode relative to the referential electrode (**Fig. 11-2**). Stimulus intensity is gradually increased until the motor response (the compound motor action potential [CMAP]) no longer increases in amplitude. Stimulation is then performed at a second, more proximal site. Key measurements of the CMAP waveform include distal latency, which is the time from stimulus to the onset of the CMAP, and amplitude, measured from baseline to peak for CMAPs.

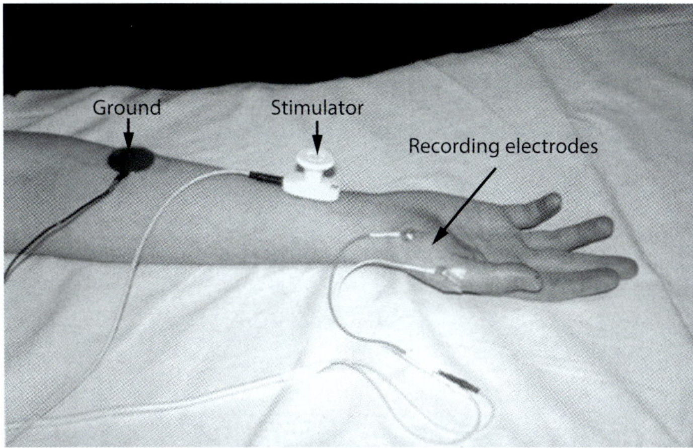

FIGURE 11-1. Standard setup for median motor nerve conduction study, with stimulator at the wrist and recording electrodes over abductor pollicis brevis.

Distal latencies and amplitudes are identified for each stimulation site. Motor conduction velocity for a segment between stimulation sites is the distance between those sites divided by the difference in distal latencies of those sites (see Fig. 11-2). Motor conduction velocity for the distal segment (between most distal stimulation site and muscle) cannot be obtained accurately because of delays inherent to the neuromuscular junction and the depolarization of the muscle fibers.

F responses are also recorded during motor studies. F responses (named for the foot, where they were first identified) are after-discharges that occur normally in motor nerves. When the nerve is stimulated as described earlier, depolarization of the axon actually progresses both distally and proximally. Whereas the distal depolarization produces the motor response described earlier, the proximal depolarization reaches the spinal cord, producing a backfiring of a few motor neurons and resulting in a new descending nerve depolarization. Eventually, this small depolarization reaches the muscle, producing the F response. F-response testing allows for the integrity of the entire motor nerve to be evaluated.

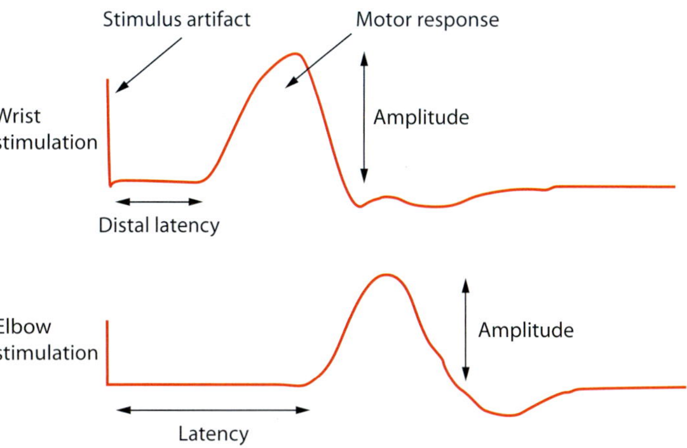

FIGURE 11-2. Median motor responses recording from both wrist and elbow.

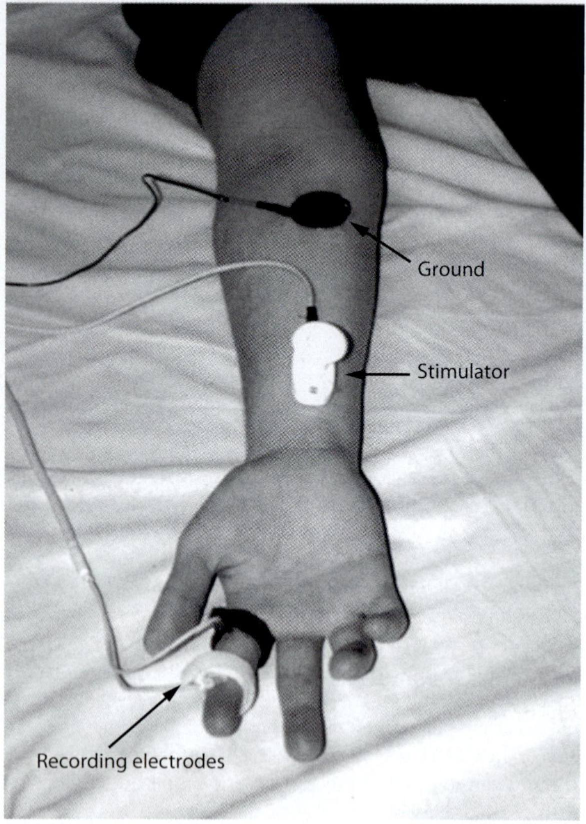

FIGURE 11-3. Standard setup for median antidromic sensory conduction study, with stimulator at the wrist and recording electrodes on digit 2.

Sensory Nerve Conduction Studies Antidromic sensory studies are performed with active and reference electrodes placed over a distal nerve segment and the nerve is stimulated proximally (**Fig. 11-3**). Alternatively, the distal portion of the nerve may be stimulated with proximal recording (orthodromic sensory studies). Similar to motor recordings, stimulation intensity is gradually increased until maximal sensory response amplitude is obtained. The key measurement for the waveform obtained, or sensory nerve action potential (SNAP), is the peak latency, which is the time from stimulus to SNAP peak (**Fig. 11-4**). Sensory amplitude is obtained measuring peak to trough or baseline to peak. Unlike motor studies, stimulation at a second site is not usually performed because a distal conduction velocity can be calculated using the first site alone, by dividing distance from stimulus to recording site by the peak latency time. Also, for complex reasons, when recording over longer segments of nerve, sensory response amplitudes decrease profoundly, making them difficult to record with proximal stimulation. Even with distal stimulation only, sensory responses are about 100 to 1000 times smaller than motor responses, necessitating the use of digital averaging.

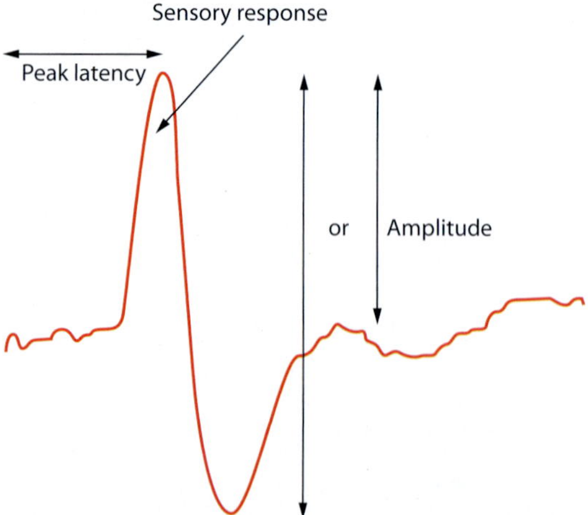

FIGURE 11-4. Antidromic median sensory response recording from digit 2.

Reflex Studies Reflex studies refer to electrical tests in which sensory nerve fibers are stimulated and motor responses are recorded. The two most frequently performed are the soleus H-reflex and the blink reflex. The soleus H-reflex (named after Hoffman, who first described it) is essentially the electrical equivalent of the ankle jerk. To obtain this reflex, *sub*maximal stimulation in the popliteal fossa is used to depolarize selectively the large IA afferent fibers of the posterior tibial nerve. The sensory neurons depolarize to the level of the dorsal horn, which, in turn, produce a depolarization in the motor neurons of the anterior horn and a contraction of the soleus muscle that is recorded.

In the blink reflex, stimulation of the first division of the trigeminal nerve (supraorbital nerve) is performed while recording simultaneously from bilateral orbicularis oculi muscles. Two responses are recorded: a local monosynaptic one and, later, one produced through more diffuse, bilateral polysynaptic connections. This test allows for the integrity of the fifth and seventh cranial nerves, including their central connections, to be evaluated.

ELECTROMYOGRAPHY

As with NCSs, EMG requires reference and active electrodes to record electrical signals. In the case of concentric needles, the active electrode is at the tip while the barrel makes up the reference. Monopolar needles, in which the active tip of the needle is referenced against a separate skin electrode, are also used. Both are usually of small diameter, corresponding to about a 27-gauge phlebotomy needle. The needle is attached to an oscilloscope with an amplifier, allowing the electromyographer to evaluate the muscle by both observing waveforms and listening to their characteristic sounds.

There are two basic parts to EMG: evaluation of spontaneous activity and evaluation of the motor unit action potentials (MUAPs). To evaluate spontaneous activity, the patient is asked to keep the limb as relaxed as possible. The physician then makes small movements with the needle. Normal muscle should remain stable and silent after needle movement. If the muscle fiber membrane is electrically unstable, fibrillation potentials or positive sharp waves may be present (**Fig. 11-5**). Occasionally, other abnormal discharges may be identified.

After evaluating for spontaneous activity, the patient is asked to perform a gentle isometric muscle contraction. The electromyographer observes and listens to the MUAPs, which are produced by the electrical firing of groups of muscle fibers innervated by single motor axons (motor units). Abnormally enlarged MUAPs suggest chronic neurogenic disease, whereas small ones most frequently suggest a primary muscle disorder (**Fig. 11-6**). In addition to these basic abnormalities, the electromyographer evaluates the "recruitment" of motor units. Normally, with increasing effort, additional motor units are "recruited" into the contraction until the oscilloscope screen fills up with dozens of motor units (**Fig. 11-7**). In patients with neurogenic disease, fewer motor units are present so that, with increasing effort, the functioning units fire

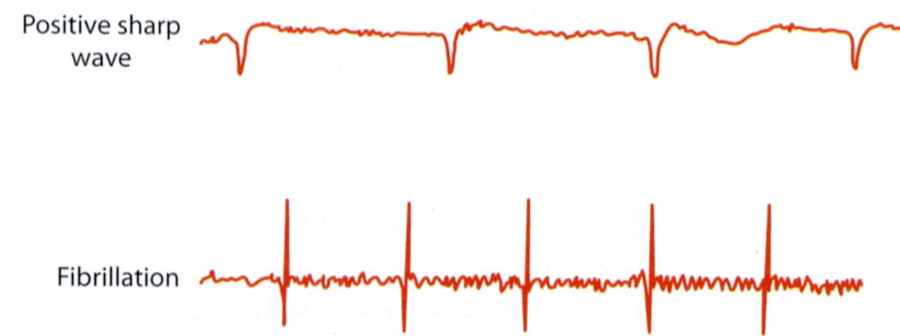

FIGURE 11-5. Positive sharp waves and fibrillations.

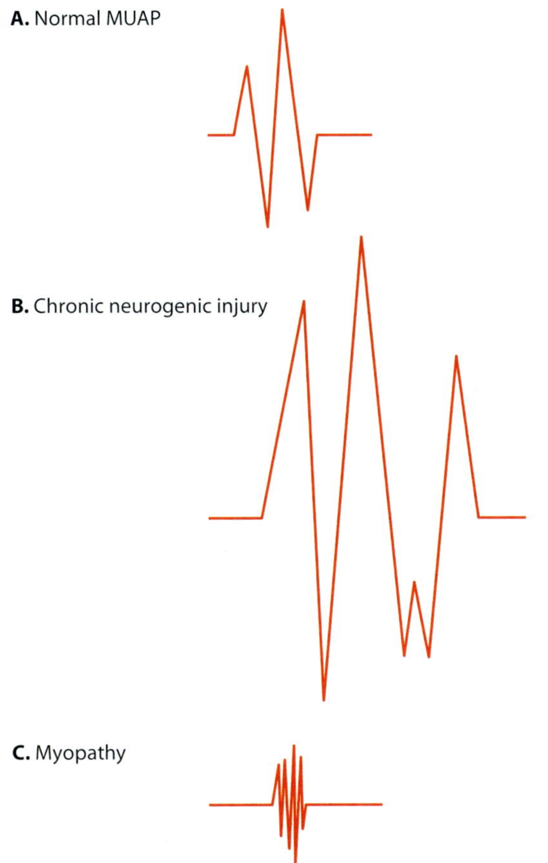

FIGURE 11-6. Motor unit action potential (MUAP) morphology. **A.** Normal MUAP. **B.** Loss of neighboring motor neurons resulting from neurogenic injury has caused the remaining MUAPs to increase in size over normal, with increased amplitude, duration, and phases. **C.** Loss and injury to muscle fibers in a myopathy produces MUAPs with reduced amplitude, duration, and increases phases.

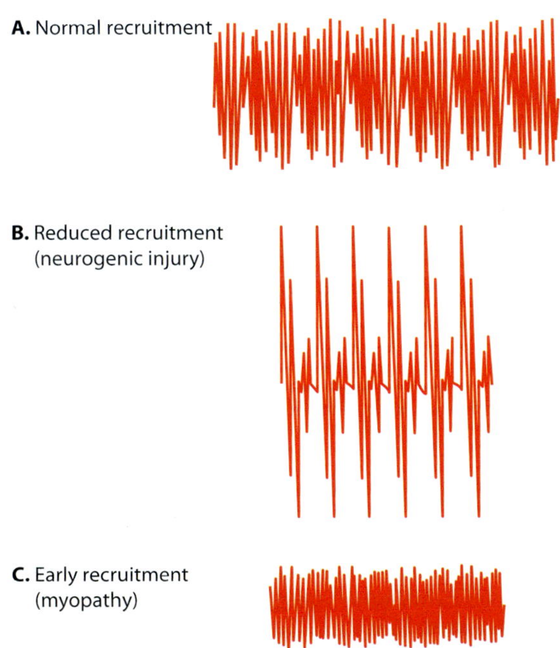

FIGURE 11-7. Recruitment of MUAPs. **A.** Normal recruitment. **B.** Reduced recruitment, as seen in neurogenic injury. Because fewer motor units are present, to produce a muscle contraction with the greatest force, the remaining motor units muscle fire more rapidly. In this case, two motor units remain. **C.** Early recruitment. In this example, the patient's muscles are minimally contracting, yet many small motor units are brought into the contraction to produce some force.

faster than normal, compensating for their missing counterparts. This is described as reduced recruitment. In extreme cases, only one motor unit may remain, firing up to five times as fast as normal. In patients with a primary muscle disease, the opposite occurs because the number of motor units is relatively normal, but their size is reduced as a result of muscle fiber loss. Hence, with only minimal effort, many motor units fire.

Finally, activation is also examined. *Activation* is the term used to describe the central nervous system drive involved in contracting a muscle. This drive, whether reduced by true central pathology or simply poor effort, will look identical on EMG: Only a few motor units fire no matter how hard the patient seems to try. Unlike reduced recruitment, however, the firing rate for a given motor unit does not increase above normal.

EVOKED POTENTIALS

Somatosensory evoked potentials (SSEPs) are one of several electrophysiologic tests that can be used to evaluate central nervous system function. Brainstem auditory evoked potentials and visual evoked potentials are the other two routine studies, but they have minimal relevance in the evaluation of pain disorders.

With the advent of MRI over the past few decades, the utility of SSEPs has decreased significantly. Before MRI, SSEPs may have been the only means for detecting a cervical cord abnormality, for example, in a patient with multiple sclerosis. Today, however, MRI scanning is so sensitive that even small areas of demyelination can be detected within the spinal cord (and although quite sensitive, MRI is very nonspecific in this regard).

SSEPs are performed by electrically stimulating nerves in the upper or lower limbs (generally median or ulnar nerves in the arm and tibial nerve in the leg) and recording responses over the lumbar spine, cervical spine, Erb's point, and over the scalp (**Fig. 11-8**). Because the responses are very small, hundreds of individual recordings are digitally averaged. Generally, these responses should have relatively known and fixed latencies and intervals, as in Figure 11-8. If the expected latency or interval is prolonged significantly, a structural or demyelinating lesion may be present within that segment. Amplitudes may also decrease if abnormalities are severe.[6]

Related to evoked potentials are the less common techniques of motor cortex stimulation. Examples include transcranial magnetic stimulation (TMS) and transcranial direct current stimulation (tDCS). Both techniques have been used to study corticospinal conduction in pain disorders.[7,8]

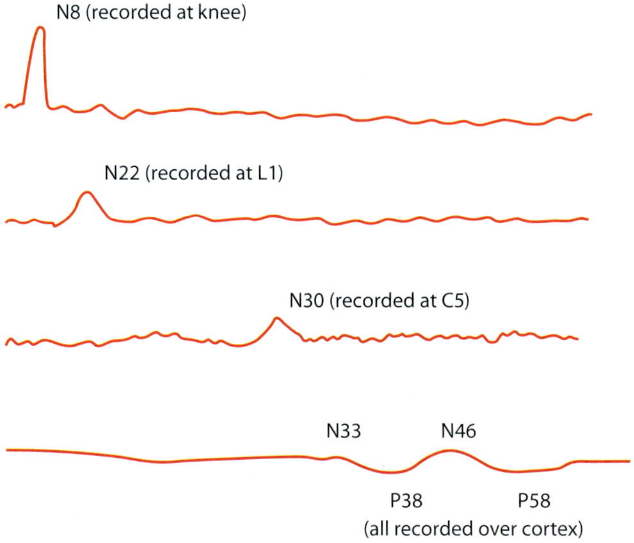

FIGURE 11-8. Tibial somatosensory evoked potentials, recording from popliteal fossa, lumbar spine, cervical spine, and brain.

EMERGING TECHNIQUES

Electrical impedance myography is a noninvasive EDx technique in which a high-frequency, low-intensity electrical current is applied and resulting voltage patterns are measured, all via four surface electrodes on the skin overlying the muscle to be tested. Early studies are promising regarding utility of this fast and painless technique in the diagnosis and status monitoring of neuromuscular disorders, including radiculopathy.[9,10]

Neuromuscular ultrasound, while not an EDx technique itself, is increasingly used as a complementary test during a neuromuscular evaluation. Abnormalities of morphology in nerve and nerve pathways can be detected by ultrasound imaging. For example, in mononeuropathies, the involved nerve at location of entrapment may exhibit a cross-sectional area 1.5 times the size of the adjacent nerve. Nerves in polyneuropathy may show diffuse or variable enlargement.[11,12]

ELECTRODIAGNOSIS OF SPECIFIC DISORDERS

RADICULOPATHY

One of the most frequent reasons for referring a patient to the EDx laboratory is for the evaluation of radiculopathy. In addition to identifying which root or roots are the most likely involved, EDx testing will also provide insight into the severity and chronicity of the lesion (**Table 11-1**). Although the sensitivity of EMG in the diagnosis of radiculopathy is less than that of MRI, its specificity is significantly better.[13-16] EMG may predict MRI abnormalities but also may be especially useful when there is clinical suspicion for radiculopathy but there is no severe nerve pathway compression on MRI.[17]

In general, NCSs play a limited role in the electrodiagnosis of radiculopathy. Rather, they are used to exclude other processes, such as compression mononeuropathy or plexopathy. In most radiculopathy, sensory NCS are normal, as compression of the nerve root occurs proximal to the dorsal root ganglion. Although motor NCS may show mild reductions in response amplitude and distal conduction velocity if radiculopathy is severe, these studies are often normal as well because a given muscle contains contributions from multiple roots, obscuring disease at only one level. F-response prolongation and, in S1 radiculopathy, H-reflex prolongation are also helpful, though nonspecific, findings.

The diagnosis of radiculopathy relies primarily on the electromyographic examination. In a subacute, single nerve root lesion, fibrillations and positive waves will be present in multiple muscles of that myotome. Sampling of additional muscles both proximally and distally in the limb, as well as those innervated by other nerve roots, is also performed in order to "frame" the lesion while excluding other possible etiologies, such as mononeuropathy or polyneuropathy. Paraspinal muscles are also routinely examined; abnormalities in these muscles help confirm the presence of a root lesion.

There is a well-described time course for the development of abnormalities after a root injury. Immediately at the time of injury, the only abnormality identifiable on EMG is reduced recruitment of motor units in muscles innervated by that root. By the end of the first week after injury, positive waves and fibrillations will begin to appear in adjacent paraspinal muscles. It may take 3 to 4 more weeks before fibrillation potentials and positive waves are identified in the most distal limb muscles. Once present, these abnormalities will persist until reinnervation is complete, which can take up to 2 years.

There are a number of important limitations to the electrophysiologic evaluation of radiculopathy. Firstly, not all muscles may be equally affected by a nerve root compression; if the electromyographer happens to study one or two that are relatively uninvolved, the lesion may be missed. Another limitation occurs from the fact that myotomes often overlap in muscles, preventing exact localization of the nerve root level. For example, it may be difficult to differentiate a C5 radiculopathy from a C6, given that most of the muscles typically studied, including deltoid and biceps, are supplied by both nerve roots. In addition, preferential compression and inflammation of the dorsal root with associated pain may produce few EMG abnormalities because the diagnosis of radiculopathy depends on loss of motor neurons in the ventral root. This is sometimes the case in patients who present with exquisitely painful diabetic radiculopathies. Finally, in very mild radiculopathy where there is no axonal loss and only demyelination at the level of the root, few abnormalities will be identified.

Several excellent reviews are provided for further reading on EDx and radiculopathy.[18-21]

POLYNEUROPATHY

EDx testing, especially NCS, is especially helpful in accurately diagnosing polyneuropathy. These studies can help determine the pathology of the process, whether both sensory and motor nerves are involved, and its severity and chronicity (see Table 11-1). However, EDx and NCSs may not be needed in cases of polyneuropathy of known cause, such as in diabetes.[5]

The electrical abnormalities generally fall into two broad categories: axonal and demyelinating injury. They may be further described as

TABLE 11-1 Summary of Abnormalities on Nerve Conduction Studies and Electromyography in Some Common Disorders

Disorder	Motor Studies	F and H Responses	Sensory Studies	EMG
Radiculopathy	Usually normal; occasional reduction in amplitude if severe and muscle studied is derived from affected root	Mild to moderate prolongation of F-and H-response latencies	Normal	Reinnervation and PSWs and fibrillations in muscles supplied by that root
Axonal polyneuropathy	Reduced amplitude in distal muscles of feet	Mild to moderate prolongation of F and H responses	Reduced amplitude of distal nerves (e.g., sural)	Reinnervation and PSWs and fibrillations in distal muscles
Demyelinating polyneuropathy	Variable amplitude reduction; severe slowing of conduction velocity; prolongation of distal latency	Severe prolongation; absence of F and H responses from multiple nerves	Reduced amplitude and conduction velocity	Variable degrees of chronic reinnervation and fibrillations and PSWs; reduced recruitment of motor units
Compression neuropathy	Focal conduction velocity slowing across affected segment if mild; reduction in amplitude if severe	Mild prolongation in F responses	Slowing of conduction velocity across affected segment; reduction in amplitude if severe	Reinnervation and PSWs and fibrillations in muscles supplied by that nerve
Plexopathy	Reduced amplitude in muscles supplied by affected fibers	Mild to moderate prolongation of F-and H-response latencies	Reduced amplitude in sensory nerves traversing affected part of plexus	Reinnervation and PSWs and fibrillations in muscles supplied by affected fibers
Mononeuropathy multiplex	Focal "axonal" lesions of multiple nerves with markedly decreased amplitude	Mild prolongation or absence of F and H responses	Reduced or absent responses in affected nerves	Marked abnormalities in muscles supplied by affected nerve

EMG, electromyography; PSWs, positive sharp waves.

motor versus sensory and diffuse versus multifocal.[22] Demyelination reduces the effectiveness of saltatory conduction, prolonging distal latencies and F responses and causing profound slowing of conduction velocity. Temporal dispersion, the abnormal broadening of the responses, also occurs as the conduction velocity of individual fibers variably slows. In addition, with severe demyelination, neuronal conduction may actually be completely impeded. Termed *conduction block*, this finding represents the ultimate result of myelin injury. Although demyelinating polyneuropathies are uncommon and pain more mild, these disorders are usually treatable with immune-modulating therapies.

Axonal polyneuropathy occurs when there is primary injury to the axon itself, rather than the myelin sheath. In this situation, the predominant abnormality on NCS is reduction in response amplitudes. Nerves of the lower limbs tend to be preferentially affected in most axonal polyneuropathies given the length-dependent nature of the process.[23] Because the fastest conducting fibers are often lost, there is usually a mild prolongation of distal latency and slowing of conduction velocity, although not to the degree of that seen with demyelinating injury. With increasing severity of axonal injury, the response can become undetectable. This process is often more prominent in sensory conduction studies than motor because sensory amplitudes are much smaller than motor responses at baseline. Axonal polyneuropathies are often associated with diabetes mellitus, alcohol use, late-stage human immunodeficiency virus (HIV) infection, and chemotherapy.[24]

On EMG examination of an axonal polyneuropathy, a gradient of abnormalities, with distal musculature being more affected than proximal, is usually found. EMG may show fibrillations and positive waves as well as enlarged motor units, depending on its time course. In demyelinating polyneuropathies, abnormalities may be present in many muscles, and a distal-to-proximal gradient is usually less evident.

Although EDx testing is extremely important in the evaluation of polyneuropathy, it has limitations. First, a specific etiology for the process cannot be identified; instead, only the type of process (i.e., axonal versus demyelinating) can be described. In addition, standard NCSs only examine the largest, myelinated nerve fibers. Patients with painful neuropathies that affect predominantly small, thinly myelinated and unmyelinated fibers may have entirely normal NCSs. The sympathetic skin response can get at this problem by measuring autonomic function in the hand and foot.[25] Unfortunately, however, this is a rather crude test that is not well quantified. Additional autonomic testing, including the quantitative sudomotor axon reflex test (QSART), may be helpful but may not be routinely available. Increasingly, intraepidermal nerve fiber counts (punch biopsy) have become available to also evaluate these small neurons.

COMPRESSION NEUROPATHY

Compression neuropathies occur when a segment of nerve is compressed at an anatomically vulnerable site, producing focal demyelination and, if severe enough, axonal degeneration. These nerve lesions are usually accompanied by pain, with symptoms that may be severe despite only mild nerve irritation. NCSs and EMG are generally extremely effective in characterizing this form of nerve injury (see Table 11-1).

Carpal tunnel syndrome, caused by entrapment of the median nerve as it traverses through a bony tunnel in the wrist, is by far the most common compression neuropathy. The predominant abnormalities in this disorder include slowing of the sensory conduction velocity and prolongation of the distal motor latency. When these results are not clearly abnormal, studying a shorter segment of median nerve across the wrist, only, and comparing it with the same region of ulnar nerve can be extremely helpful. This approach helps eliminate other variables that may slow velocity, such as mild polyneuropathy or reduced hand temperature (even slightly cool limbs are a major source of error on NCSs).[5] EMG of the limb can be very helpful in both assessing severity of the lesion (by looking for abnormalities in abductor pollicis brevis) and excluding a superimposed cervical radiculopathy.[26,27]

Ulnar neuropathy usually occurs at the elbow, with focal demyelination at either the humeral epicondylar groove or slightly more distally in the cubital tunnel, as the nerve passes through the flexor carpi ulnaris muscle. The ulnar motor nerve conduction study is the most important part of this investigation because focal slowing of motor conduction velocity across the elbow segment, occasionally with conduction block, may be demonstrated. In more severe cases, a reduction in distal ulnar sensory and motor response amplitudes may also occur as axonal loss ensues. Identifying the exact area of entrapment within the elbow segment is usually difficult and, because the treatments are similar, not generally attempted. EMG of ulnar-innervated muscles may show fibrillations and positive waves, as well as enlarged motor units. As with carpal tunnel syndrome, in very mild cases all studies may be normal, often disproportionate to the patient's symptoms. Near-nerve studies, incorporating the use of needle electrodes proximal and distal to the presumed site of compression, can demonstrate abnormalities when standard surface studies are entirely normal.[28] Ultrasound imaging may also play a role in avoiding false-negative ulnar NCSs.[29]

The two most common sites of entrapment of the radial nerve occur at the spiral groove of the humerus and in the upper forearm at the arcade of Frohse ("Saturday night palsy" and the posterior interosseous syndrome, respectively).[30] Compression at the spiral groove produces wrist drop, weakness of finger extension, and sensory loss over the dorsum of the hand. NCSs may demonstrate conduction velocity slowing with or without associated conduction block across the spiral groove. Entrapment of the posterior interosseous nerve at the arcade of Frohse is often accompanied by prominent, poorly localized forearm pain. If the lesion is severe enough, slowing of conduction velocity across the arcade can be demonstrated.

In the lower limb, the most common compression neuropathy is a peroneal neuropathy at the fibular head, usually presenting as foot drop and numbness or paresthesias in the dermatomal distribution of the peroneal nerve. Motor NCSs generally reveal slowing of conduction velocity with or without conduction block across the fibular neck. EMG helps to localize the process by excluding L5 radiculopathy or sciatic neuropathy as the source of symptoms.[31]

In patients with foot pain, especially when associated with plantar paresthesias and sensory loss, the possibility of tarsal tunnel syndrome is often raised. This rarely diagnosed malady occurs when the tibial nerve is compressed under the flexor retinaculum at the medial malleolus. Electrophysiologic evaluation includes demonstration of a prolonged tibial motor distal latency and slowing of conduction velocity on additional studies, such as recording at the ankle when stimulating the medial and lateral plantar nerves in the midsole.[32] If only one foot is affected, comparisons can be made with the unaffected side. If pain is present in both feet, convincingly identifying entrapment at the tarsal tunnel becomes much more difficult because mild polyneuropathy may also produce similar electrophysiologic abnormalities. EMG in the affected foot musculature is useful only when compared with the unaffected side because enlargement of motor units and positive sharp waves are present even in most normal feet. Extensive metanalysis of EDx for tarsal tunnel found a paucity of evidence of validity.[33]

A controversial cause of pain, the piriformis syndrome, may be considered in patients presenting with complaints of pain and paresthesias in the gluteal region that radiate in a sciatic distribution.[34] Pain can be reproduced by applying pressure over the sciatic notch, where the nerve is thought to be compressed by the piriformis muscle. H-reflex latency has been found to be prolonged in some individuals with this disorder;[35] however, definite electrophysiologic abnormalities are rare. EMG is helpful in excluding other processes (namely, L5 or S1 radiculopathies).

PLEXOPATHY

Common causes of plexopathy include compression due to mass lesion, inflammation, radiation-induced injury, and, in the upper limbs, traction injury. EDx can be especially helpful in localizing the lesion to a particular region of the plexus and assessing its severity and chronicity[36] (see Table 11-1).

In evaluation of a plexus injury, intimate knowledge of the anatomy of myotomes, dermatomes, and peripheral nerve distribution is required to exclude other processes, such as a radiculopathy or proximal neuropathy.[37] In an investigation of brachial plexopathy, a combination of NCS and EMG is performed to localize the lesion to a particular cord or trunk. Although motor response amplitudes may drop in plexopathy, reductions in sensory response amplitudes are especially helpful because they demonstrate that the lesion is distal to the dorsal root ganglion, hence, helping to exclude a root lesion. Both routine and less commonly performed studies can help localize a lesion. For example, in an upper trunk lesion, the musculocutaneous sensory nerve response may have reduced amplitude, whereas in a lower trunk injury, reduction in the ulnar and medial antebrachial cutaneous sensory responses is common. Careful comparisons to the contralateral, uninvolved arm are also extremely helpful because amplitudes should remain at least 40% to 50% of the normal side. When evaluating the lumbosacral plexus, along with routine studies, the saphenous and superficial peroneal sensory nerves are studied.

EMG further localizes the lesion by looking for abnormalities in muscles supplied by a particular branch or cord of the plexus. Needle examination can exclude a distal peripheral nerve injury by documenting abnormalities in muscles supplied by more than one nerve. In addition, evaluation of shoulder muscles can be very helpful in distinguishing an upper trunk or lateral cord injury from a C5–C6 radiculopathy. In some situations, such as a stretch injury with root avulsion, the findings may support simultaneous radiculopathy and plexopathy. Severity of the lesion can also be judged by the profusion of fibrillation potentials and positive sharp waves and the number of motor units that can be recruited. Finally, an unusual spontaneous discharge on EMG, called a myokymic discharge, may help support the diagnosis of a radiation-induced injury.[38]

Although SSEPs can be used in the evaluation of plexopathy, as with radiculopathy, the combination of NCS with EMG generally is more helpful.

One special case of brachial plexopathy is thoracic outlet syndrome. In neurogenic thoracic outlet syndrome, a fibrous band from a cervical rib to the first thoracic rib impinges on the lower trunk of the plexus. This produces an unusual constellation of abnormalities, including reduced ulnar sensory and median and ulnar motor responses.[39] A prospective study suggests NCSs of medial antebrachial cutaneous nerve and C8 root may be used.[40] EMG generally demonstrates abnormalities most severe in abductor pollicis brevis. In patients with vascular thoracic outlet syndrome (generally diagnosed in patients with chronic arm and shoulder pain, reduced radial pulse with external rotation, and abduction of the arm [Wright maneuver], with or without a cervical rib, but no neurologic signs), electrophysiologic testing is normal. However, physical exam maneuvers have been shown in a prospective study to have a very high false-positive rate, and even more so in patients with carpal tunnel syndrome.[41]

MONONEUROPATHY MULTIPLEX

This disorder, which is usually associated with vasculitic conditions such as Churg-Strauss syndrome and polyarteritis nodosa, is associated with multiple acute painful mononeuropathies. In addition to weakness and sensory loss, pain can be severe in affected limbs. NCSs and EMG generally demonstrate abnormalities consistent with multiple severe axonal mononeuropathies (see Table 11-1). Rather than slowing across a site of entrapment, complete loss of the motor and sensory responses for that nerve with marked fibrillation potentials and positive waves in affected muscles is usually found.[42] In long-standing cases, multiple mononeuropathies in the legs may become confluent, producing the picture of a severe axonal polyneuropathy.

MYOPATHY

Most muscle diseases have only limited pain associated with them.[43] However, in some disorders, such as the metabolic myopathies (including McArdle's disease and phosphofructokinase deficiency), pain can be brought on with exercise. Generally, NCSs reveal minimal abnormalities in myopathies. Occasionally, if severe, reductions in motor response amplitude may occur. On EMG, short-duration, low-amplitude motor units with early recruitment are observed. Spontaneous activity, including fibrillation potentials and positive waves, is also common in many inflammatory, toxic, and congenital myopathies.[44] Finally, the presence of myotonia can limit the diagnostic possibilities to one of the myotonic disorders, such as myotonic dystrophy.

DISORDERS OF THE PERINEAL REGION

Occasionally, patients present with neuropathic pain involving the perineal region. A number of possible diagnoses are often raised, including lumbar radiculopathy, with pain referred into the distribution of the ilioinguinal nerve; ilioinguinal or genitofemoral neuropathies; S2 to S4 radiculopathy, with pain referred to the genitalia; and pudendal neuropathy, occasionally secondary to trauma (such as repeated bike riding in men).[45,46]

Although not often pursued, neurophysiologic testing in this region can be helpful in reaching a diagnosis. Standard studies of the lower limbs can help identify a lumbar or S1–S2 radiculopathy; in a low sacral radiculopathy (e.g., S2–S4), fibrillation potentials in the associated paraspinal muscles and in the anal sphincter may be found. Unfortunately, ilioinguinal and genitofemoral neuropathies are extremely difficult to evaluate. Pudendal nerve integrity can be examined using the electrical bulbocavernosus reflex.[47,48] In this uncomfortable study, the glans of the penis in men or the clitoris in women is electrically stimulated while recording with needle electrodes placed in the external anal and urethral sphincters. Prolonged latency of this reflex, with normal paraspinal muscle EMG, suggests pudendal neuropathy. An extensive battery of tests has been described to evaluate anorectal disorders, including sphincter EMG, anal NCS and evoked potentials, electrophysiologic sacral anal reflex, and autonomic and sensory threshold tests.[49]

DISORDERS OF THE THORACIC AND ABDOMINAL REGIONS

Unfortunately, neurophysiologic tests have a limited role in the evaluation of thoracic or abdominal pain. In these regions, most neurologic problems stem from spinal nerve root or intercostal nerve compression, trauma, or inflammation. Although intercostal NCSs can be performed,[50] they are technically difficult, have few good normal controls, and are unlikely to be definitively diagnostic. Needle EMG of paraspinal muscles can help determine if a problem is occurring at the root level. EMG of intercostal muscles is usually not performed secondary to the potential for pneumothorax. Needle examination of the rectus abdominis muscle is generally safe, providing information about the T8 to T11 intercostal nerves. SSEPs can also be helpful in evaluating the thoracic spinal cord itself (see later discussion).

HERPES ZOSTER

The painful recrudescence of varicella zoster with associated rash in a limited dermatomal distribution produces herpes zoster (shingles). Although pain is the predominant complaint, on careful examination some sensory loss in the region of the rash may also be identified. If zoster occurs in a dermatome of either the leg or arm, sensory NCSs of that involved segment may demonstrate reduced sensory response amplitudes secondary to destruction of sensory nerve cell bodies in the dorsal root ganglia.[51] In some patients, the associated radiculitis is so widespread as to involve the anterior motor root as well, producing reductions in motor response amplitude and abnormalities on needle EMG.[51,52] Peripheral involvement and conduction block on NCS has been described.[53,54]

SYNDROMES OF EXCESSIVE MUSCLE ACTIVITY

Several painful neurologic disorders are associated with generalized or focal excess muscle activity. These unusual disorders include cramps and fasciculation syndrome, stiff-person syndrome, tetanus, and Isaac's syndrome.

Cramps and Fasciculation Syndrome The syndrome of cramps and fasciculations is an unusual neuromuscular disorder in which patients complain of painful cramping in the legs with associated muscle twitching.[55] Exercise and caffeine may worsen symptoms. Repetitive stimulation at 5 Hz can produce cramping in these individuals, with associated muscle contraction that can be measured with surface electrodes.[55,56] Cramp potentials (rapidly firing motor units) may also be observed on EMG. Also, isolated fasciculation potentials are prominent in affected muscles.

Stiff-Person Syndrome In stiff-person syndrome, patients develop intermittent painful stiffness of one or more limbs. Serum antibodies to glutamic acid decarboxylase (one of the enzymes participating in the synthesis of gamma-aminobutyric acid [GABA]) may be identified, suggesting an autoimmune disorder. Generally, the stiffness is episodic, but it can progress over time to become protracted and generalized. Although EMG will only demonstrate normally firing motor units without any other pathology, blink reflex studies may be abnormal in some of these patients.[57]

Tetanus In tetanus, the organism *Clostridium tetani* produces tetanus toxin, which interferes with the inhibitory synapses in the spinal cord and brain, producing excessive muscular activity. Although the diagnosis can usually be reached historically and clinically, electrophysiologic testing may reveal subtle abnormalities using specialized tests.[58]

Isaac's Syndrome In Isaac's syndrome, often a paraneoplastic phenomenon, antibodies are produced against ion channels in motor neurons, producing spontaneous firing of motor units. Unique discharges (termed *neuromyotonic*) are identified on EMG in this disorder.[59] Isaac's syndrome may manifest years before the underlying neoplasm.[60]

Dystonia Patients with dystonia occasionally present with pain as the predominant complaint rather than incoordination of movement. NCSs can be helpful in excluding an underlying nerve lesion, whereas EMG of dystonic muscles, usually normal in idiopathic dystonia, can demonstrate reinnervation if nerve damage has occurred.

COMPLEX REGIONAL PAIN SYNDROME

Complex regional pain syndrome (CRPS), formerly known as reflex sympathetic dystrophy, is a syndrome characterized by skin changes, bone loss, and pain; it may occur after trauma to a limb, with or without associated nerve damage. Sympathetic nerve dysfunction has been suggested as causative. This causation is supported by the fact that patients may show improvement with sympathetic blockade or neurolysis. Despite the presumed involvement of the sympathetic nerves, electrophysiologic studies do not reveal specific abnormalities in this disorder unless an associated nerve injury (e.g., compression neuropathy) can be identified. One study has suggested relative reductions in the amplitude of this response in the affected as compared with the unaffected limb.[61] Sympathetic nerve fiber function itself is difficult to test because it is variable in normal and neuropathic conditions and is limited to the skin sympathetic nerves, which may not be involved in the condition being tested.[62]

Transcranial magnetic stimulation has been used to discover and alter cortical transmission abnormalities in CRPS.[63,64] Quantitative sensory testing is routinely used in research studies of CRPS.[65] EMG and NCSs demonstrate abnormalities more commonly in CRPS type 2, as expected.[66]

FIBROMYALGIA AND MYOFASCIAL PAIN SYNDROMES

Although presumably a disease of muscle, this disorder also has no definite electrophysiologic correlate. As noted earlier, muscle diseases may have pain components, including polymyositis and metabolic myopathies. However, generally, these disorders have limited pain associated with them, and weakness and other symptoms are prominent. In patients in whom the complaint of painful muscles is widespread, a diagnosis of fibromyalgia and myofascial pain may be considered. Increased insertional activity at trigger points has been suggested,[67] and although other studies have not confirmed any abnormality in multiple aspects of muscle function and electrophysiology in trigger points or fibromyalgia,[68-70] the search continues.[71-74] Ultimately, the diagnoses of fibromyalgia and myofascial pain syndromes remain clinical ones.

POLYMYALGIA RHEUMATICA

A sometimes overlooked diagnosis, polymyalgia rheumatica often is associated with complaints of proximal pain and aching in the arms and legs, especially in the morning, with improvement in symptoms as the day progresses. Although there have been reported cases of EMG abnormalities suggestive of inflammatory myopathy,[75,76] in general, electrophysiologic studies are normal. This leaves the overall clinical picture and an associated elevation in sedimentation rate as the usual diagnostic modalities.

FACIAL AND CRANIAL PAIN

In idiopathic trigeminal neuralgia, electrophysiologic testing is usually normal. However, in patients with trigeminal nerve pain secondary to another process, such as that associated with brainstem demyelination or infarcts, blink reflex testing will be abnormal.[77] In addition, brainstem evoked potentials may show prolongation of latencies or reductions in response amplitudes.

Other forms of facial or cranial pain, including glossopharyngeal neuralgia and occipital neuralgia, cannot be readily assessed with electrophysiologic testing. In patients with retroorbital pain secondary to optic neuritis, visual evoked potentials may be helpful in diagnosis.

CENTRAL PAIN SYNDROMES

Again, since the advent of MRI, the utility of EDx testing in the evaluation of central pain has been greatly reduced. Nonetheless, in certain situations, evoked potentials can be helpful in finding the site of a lesion. For example, in a patient presenting with pain affecting a specific limb and in whom peripheral electrophysiologic testing is normal, SSEPs can be used to localize the problem to a region of the central nervous system. In such a case, testing may reveal a prolonged latency in the thoracic cord, hence localizing the problem to that region. Directed MRI scanning of that region may then reveal the cause of the problem.

REFERENCES

1. Aminoff MJ. *Electrodiagnosis in Clinical Neurology*. 6th ed. New York, NY: Churchill-Livingstone; 2012.
2. Kimura J. *Electrodiagnosis in Diseases of Nerve and Muscle: Principles and Practice*. 4th ed. Philadelphia, Pa: FA Davis; 2013.
3. Preston DC, Shapiro BE. *Electromyography and Neuromuscular Disorders: Clinical-Electrophysiologic Correlations*. 3rd ed. Boston, Mass: Butterworth-Heinemann; 2012.
4. Dumitru D, Amato AA, Zwarts MJ, eds. *Electrodiagnostic medicine*. 2nd ed. Philadelphia, Pa: Hanley & Belfus; 2002.
5. Kane NM, Oware A. Nerve conduction and electromyography studies. *J Neurol*. 2012 Jul;259(7):1502-1508.
6. Yamada T, Yeh M, Kimura J. Fundamental principles of somatosensory evoked potentials. *Phys Med Rehabil Clin N Am*. 2004 Feb;15(1):19-42.
7. Currà A, Madungo N, Inghilleri M, et al. Transcranial magnetic stimulation techniques in clinical investigation. *Neurology*. 2002;59:1851-1859.
8. Lima MC, Fregni F. Motor cortex stimulation for chronic pain: systematic review and meta-analysis of the literature. *Neurology*. 2008;70:2329-2337.
9. Rutkove SB, Esper GJ, Lee KS, et al. Electrical impedance myography in the detection of radiculopathy. *Muscle Nerve*. 2005 Sep;32(3):335-341.
10. Spieker AJ, Narayanaswami P, Fleming L, Keel JC, Muzin SC, Rutkove SB. Electrical impedance myography in the diagnosis radiculopathy. *Muscle Nerve*. 2013;48(5):800-805.

11. Chahal PS, Sohail W, Cartwright MS. Neuromuscular ultrasound in the diagnosis of focal neuropathies superimposed on polyneuropathy: a case report. *Clin Neurophysiol.* 2012 March;123(3): 626-627.
12. Cartwright MS, Hobson-Webb LD, Boon AJ, et al. Evidence-based guideline: neuromuscular ultrasound for the diagnosis of carpal tunnel syndrome. *Muscle Nerve.* 2012 Aug;46(2):287-293.
13. Dvorák J. Neurophysiologic tests in diagnosis of nerve root compression caused by disc herniation. *Spine.* 1996;21:39S-44S.
14. Robinson LR. Electromyography, magnetic resonance imaging, and radiculopathy: it's time to focus on specificity. *Muscle Nerve.* 1999;22:149-150.
15. Nardin RA, Patel MR, Gudas TF, et al. Electromyography and magnetic resonance imaging in the evaluation of radiculopathy. *Muscle Nerve.* 1999;22:151-155.
16. Chiodo A, Haig AJ, Yamakawa KS, et al. Needle EMG has a lower false positive rate than MRI in asymptomatic older adults being evaluated for lumbar spinal stenosis. *Clin Neurophysiol.* 2007 Apr;118(4):751-756.
17. Coster S, de Bruijn SF, Tavy DL. Diagnostic value of history, physical examination and needle electromyography in diagnosing lumbosacral radiculopathy. *J Neurol.* 2010 Mar;257(3):332-337.
18. Plastaras CT, Joshi AB. The electrodiagnostic evaluation of radiculopathy. *Phys Med Rehabil Clin N Am.* 2011 Feb;22(1):59-74.
19. Tsao B. The electrodiagnosis of cervical and lumbosacral radiculopathy. *Neurol Clin.* 2007 May;25(2):473-494.
20. Hakimi K, Spanier D. Electrodiagnosis of cervical radiculopathy. *Phys Med Rehabil Clin N Am.* 2013 Feb;24(1):1-12.
21. Cho SC, Ferrante MA, Levin KH, et al. Utility of electrodiagnostic testing in evaluating patients with lumbosacral radiculopathy: an evidence-based review. *Muscle Nerve.* 2010 Aug;42(2):276-282.
22. Craig AS, Richardson JK. Acquired peripheral neuropathy. *Phys Med Rehabil Clin N Am.* 2003 May;14(2):365-386.
23. Albers JW. Clinical neurophysiology of generalized polyneuropathy. *J Clin Neurophysiol.* 1993;10:149-166.
24. Chalk CH. Acquired peripheral neuropathy. *Neurol Clin.* 1997;15:501-528.
25. Shahani BT, Halperin JJ, Boulu P, Cohen J. Sympathetic skin response: a method of assessing unmyelinated axon dysfunction in peripheral neuropathies. *J Neurol Neurosurg Psychiatry.* 1984;47:542-546.
26. Gnatz SM. The role of needle electromyography in the evaluation of patients with carpal tunnel syndrome: needle EMG is important. *Muscle Nerve.* 1999;22:282-283.
27. CTS Task Force. Practice parameter for electrodiagnostic studies in carpal tunnel syndrome: summary statement. *Muscle Nerve.* 2002:25: 918-922.
28. Rosenfalck A. Early recognition of nerve disorders by near-nerve recording of sensory action potentials. *Muscle Nerve.* 1978;1: 360-367.
29. Won SJ, Yoon JS, Kim JY, et al. Avoiding false-negative nerve conduction study in ulnar neuropathy at the elbow. *Muscle Nerve.* 2011 Oct;44(4):583-586.
30. Freedman M, Helber G, Pothast J, et al. Electrodiagnostic evaluation of compressive nerve injuries of the upper extremities. *Orthop Clin North Am.* 2012 Oct;43(4):409-416.
31. Marciniak C, Armon C, Wilson J, et al. Practice parameter: utility of electrodiagnostic techniques in evaluating patients with suspected peroneal neuropathy: an evidence-based review. *Muscle Nerve.* 2005 Apr;31(4):520-527.
32. Oh SJ, Sarala PK, Kuba T, et al. Tarsal tunnel syndrome: electrophysiological study. *Ann Neurol.* 1979;5:327-330.
33. Patel AT, Gaines K, Malamut R, et al.. Usefulness of electrodiagnostic techniques in the evaluation of suspected tarsal tunnel syndrome: an evidence-based review. *Muscle Nerve.* 2005 Aug;32(2):236-240.
34. Kirschner JS, Foye PM, Cole JL. Piriformis syndrome, diagnosis and treatment. *Muscle Nerve.* 2009 Jul;40(1):10-18.
35. Fishman LM, Zybert PA. Electrophysiologic evidence of piriformis syndrome. *Arch Phys Med Rehab.* 1992;73:359-364.
36. Parry GJ. Electrodiagnostic studies in the evaluation of peripheral nerve and brachial plexus injuries. *Neurol Clin.* 1992;4:921-934.
37. Ferrante MA. Electrodiagnostic assessment of the brachial plexus. *Neurol Clin.* 2012 May;30(2):551-580.
38. Albers JW, Alan AA, Bastron JA, et al. Limb myokymia. *Muscle Nerve.* 1981;4:494-504.
39. Forestier N Le, Moulonguet A, Maisonobe T, et al. True neurogenic thoracic outlet syndrome: electrophysiological diagnosis in six cases. *Muscle Nerve.* 1998;21:1129-1134.
40. Machanic BI, Sanders RJ. Medial antebrachial cutaneous nerve measurements to diagnose neurogenic thoracic outlet syndrome. *Ann Vasc Surg.* 2008 Mar;22(2):248-254.
41. Nord KM, Kapoor P, Fisher J, et al. False positive rate of thoracic outlet syndrome diagnostic maneuvers. *Electromyogr Clin Neurophysiol.* 2008 Mar;48(2):67-74.
42. Parry GJG. AAEM case report #11: mononeuropathy multiplex. *Muscle Nerve.* 1985;8:493-498.
43. Griggs RC, Mendell JR, Miller RG. *Evaluation and Treatment of Myopathies.* Philadelphia, Pa: FA Davis; 1995.
44. Paganoni S, Amato A. Electrodiagnostic evaluation of myopathies. *Phys Med Rehabil Clin N Am.* 2013 Feb;24(1):193-207.
45. Oberpenning F, Roth S, Leusmann DB, et al. The Alcock syndrome: temporary penile insensitivity due to compression of the pudendal nerve within the Alcock canal. *J Urol.* 1994;151:423-425.
46. Silbert PL, Dunne JW, Edis RH, et al. Bicycling induced pudendal nerve pressure neuropathy. *Clin Exp Neurol.* 1991;28:191-196.
47. Bilkey WJ, Awad EA, Smith AD. Clinical application of sacral reflex latency. *J Urol.* 1983;129:1187-1189.
48. Tackmann W, Porst H, Ahlen HV. Bulbocavernosus reflex latencies and somatosensory evoked potentials after pudendal nerve stimulation in the diagnosis of impotence. *J Neurol.* 1988;235:219-225.
49. Lefaucheur JP. Neurophysiological testing in anorectal disorders. *Muscle Nerve.* 2006 Mar;33(3):324-333.
50. Pradham S, Taly A. Intercostal nerve conduction study in man. *J Neurol Neurosurg Psychiatry.* 1989;52:763-766.
51. Merchut MP, Gruener G. Segmental zoster paresis of limbs. *Electromyogr Clin Neurophysiol.* 1996;36:369-375.
52. Sachs GM. Segmental zoster paresis: An electrophysiological study. *Muscle Nerve.* 1996;19:784-786.
53. Murakami T, Shibazaki K, Kurokawa K, et al. *Neurology.* 2003:61(8):1153-1154.
54. Reda H, Watson JC, Jones LK Jr. Zoster-associated mononeuropathies (ZAMs): a retrospective series. *Muscle Nerve.* 2012 May;45(5):734-739.
55. Tahmoush AJ, Alonso RJ, Tahmoush GP, et al. Cramp-fasciculation syndrome: a treatable hyperexcitable peripheral nerve disorder. *Neurology.* 1991;41:1021-1024.
56. Harrison TB, Benatar M. Accuracy of repetitive nerve stimulation for diagnosis of the cramp-fasciculation syndrome. *Muscle Nerve.* 2007 Jun;35(6):776-780.

57. Meinck H-M, Ricker K, Conrad B. The stiff-man syndrome: new pathophysiological aspects from abnormal exteroceptive reflexes and the response to clomipramine, clonidine, and tizanidine. *J Neurol Neurosurg Psychiatry*. 1984;47:280-287.
58. Struppler A, Struppler E, Adams RD. Local tetanus in man: its clinical and neurophysiological characteristics. *Arch Neurol*. 1963;8:162-178.
59. Lütschg J, Jerusalem F, Ludin HP. The syndrome of "continuous muscle fiber activity." *Arch Neurol*. 1978;35:198-205.
60. Rana SS, Ramanathan RS, Small G, et al. Paraneoplastic Isaacs' syndrome: a case series and review of the literature. *J Clin Neuromuscul Dis*. 2012 Jun;13(4):228-233.
61. Drory VE, Korczyn AD. The sympathetic skin response in reflex sympathetic dystrophy. *J Neurol Sci*. 1995;128:92-95.
62. Vetrugno R, Liguori R, Cortelli P, et al. Sympathetic skin response: basic mechanisms and clinical applications. *Clin Auton Res*. 2003 Aug;13(4):256-270.
63. Schwenkreis P, Janssen F, Rommel O. Bilateral motor cortex disinhibition in complex regional pain syndrome (CRPS) type I of the hand. *Neurology*. August 26, 2003;61(4):515-519.
64. Lefaucheur JP, Drouot X, Menard-Lefaucheur I. Motor cortex rTMS restores defective intracortical inhibition in chronic neuropathic pain. *Neurology*. November 14, 2006;67(9):1568-1574.
65. Rolke R, Baron R, Maier C, et al. Quantitative sensory testing in the German Research Network on Neuropathic Pain (DFNS): standardized protocol and reference values. *Pain*. 2006;123:231-243.
66. Bruehl S, Harden RN, Galer BS, et al. Complex regional pain syndrome: are there distinct subtypes and sequential stages of the syndrome? *Pain*. 2002 Jan;95(1-2):119-124.
67. Hubbard DR, Berkoff GM. Myofascial trigger points show spontaneous needle EMG activity. *Spine*. 1993;18:1803-1807.
68. Durette MR, Rodriquez AA, Agre JC, et al. Needle electromyographic evaluation of patients with myofascial or fibromyalgic pain. *Am J Phys Med Rehabil*. 1991;70:154-156.
69. Simms RW. Is there muscle pathology in fibromyalgia syndrome? *Rheum Dis Clin North Am*. 1996;22:245-266.
70. Zidar J, Backman E, Bengtsson A, et al. Quantitative EMG and muscle tension in painful muscles in fibromyalgia. *Pain*. 1990;40: 249-254.
71. Ge HY, Arendt-Nielsen L, Madeleine P. Accelerated muscle fatigability of latent myofascial trigger points in humans. *Pain Medicine*. 2012 July;13(7):957-964.
72. Casale R, Rainoldi A. Fatigue and fibromyalgia syndrome: clinical and neurophysiologic pattern. *Best Pract Res Clin Rheumatol*. 2011 Apr;25(2):241-247.
73. Gerdle B, Grönlund C, Karlsson SJ, et al. Altered neuromuscular control mechanisms of the trapezius muscle in fibromyalgia. *BMC Musculoskelet Disord*. 2010 Mar 5;11:42.
74. Bazzichi L, Dini M, Rossi A, et al. Muscle modifications in fibromyalgic patients revealed by surface electromyography (SEMG) analysis. *BMC Musculoskelet Disord*. 2009 Apr 15;10:36.
75. Bromberg MB, Donofrio PD, Segal BM. Steroid-responsive electromyographic abnormalities in polymyalgia rheumatica. *Muscle Nerve*. 1990;13:138-141.
76. Radhamanohar M. An unusual presentation of polymyalgia rheumatica with severe muscle weakness. *Br J Clin Pract*. 1992 Autumn;46(3):213-214.
77. Cruccu G, Biasiotta A, Galeotti F, et al. Diagnostic accuracy of trigeminal reflex testing in trigeminal neuralgia. *Neurology*. 2006 Jan 10;66(1):139-141.

Imaging Pain

Steven J. Scrivani
David Borsook

INTRODUCTION

Chronic pain is an extremely complex and debilitating problem that presents itself in many ways in modern-day society. While there is clearly a biological substrate to chronic pain, there are also societal, psychosocial, financial, political, and public health components that bring far-reaching implications to research, diagnosis, and treatment of chronic pain disorders.

Remarkable advances in understanding pain and providing improved treatments have come through scientific discoveries, improved training and access to specialized clinics, organizations, national agendas, and industry and advocacy groups. However, our clinical armamentarium is relatively limited in providing relief in chronic pain conditions. In the past, the basic therapy has included, for the most part, (1) drugs, mostly belonging to three classes—opioids, nonsteroidal anti-inflammatory drugs, and local anesthetics; (2) interventional treatments; (3) psychological biobehavioral therapy; and (4) some adjuvant medications, as well as complementary and alternative therapies. For all of these efforts, the number of outcome studies of nonpharmacological trials is limited, and most pharmacological studies show poor efficacy of treatment in chronic pain.[1] Pain researchers, pharmaceutical companies, and clinicians have struggled to break the barriers of finding treatments for pain that are both specific and efficient and have limited side effects.

Part of the problem we have faced is a new realization that chronic pain is a disease of the brain. Until recently, there has been a lack of ability to measure changes in the brain that are a consequence of chronic pain. Anatomic, functional, and chemical neuroimaging have opened the door to new vistas and new opportunities for a better understanding of chronic pain, better diagnostic possibilities, and, perhaps, better drug treatments to be developed. Although genetic and other molecular approaches in the pain field have shown tremendous advances, only in recent years has brain imaging contributed to the revolution in understanding pain, greatly changing the field of pain research.

The major insight that emerged from neuroimaging studies is that chronic pain is a disease of the brain, and, thus, all therapeutic modalities will need to take this into consideration. The ability to explore the human brain in human volunteers or patients has dramatically changed our understanding of pain. Imaging has the ability to define theoretical constructs of numerous thinkers in the field of brain processing in chronic pain in the human condition. Imaging has allowed unprecedented interrogation of brain systems in terms of brain circuitry, the effects of analgesics on neural networks, transition of acute into chronic pain, definition of brain regions that heretofore may not have been considered important (e.g., nucleus accumbens, striatal regions), brain plasticity including functional and morphological changes, networks that are involved in the placebo response, and alterations in neurochemistry in chronic pain (**Fig. 12-1**).

It is now increasingly understood that pain represents a multifaceted process shaped by a multitude of factors (somatosensory, emotional, cognitive, genetic) and, in turn, affecting behavioral responses as well as producing an altered brain state. Functional brain imaging may allow us to provide an objective measure of pain—one that may be complex and require taking into account sensory, emotional, and modulatory processes in the context of expectations and life experiences. Imaging pain has already produced far-reaching changes in the way we think about chronic pain[2-5] and define a signature of changes in the brain that contribute or are part of the chronic pain syndrome, which will eventually result in better pain treatments.

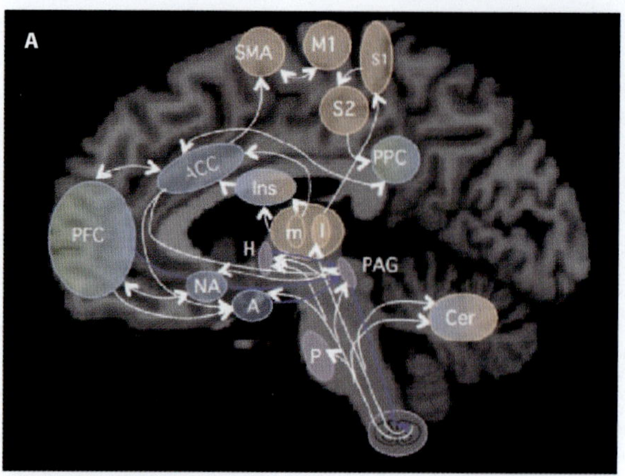

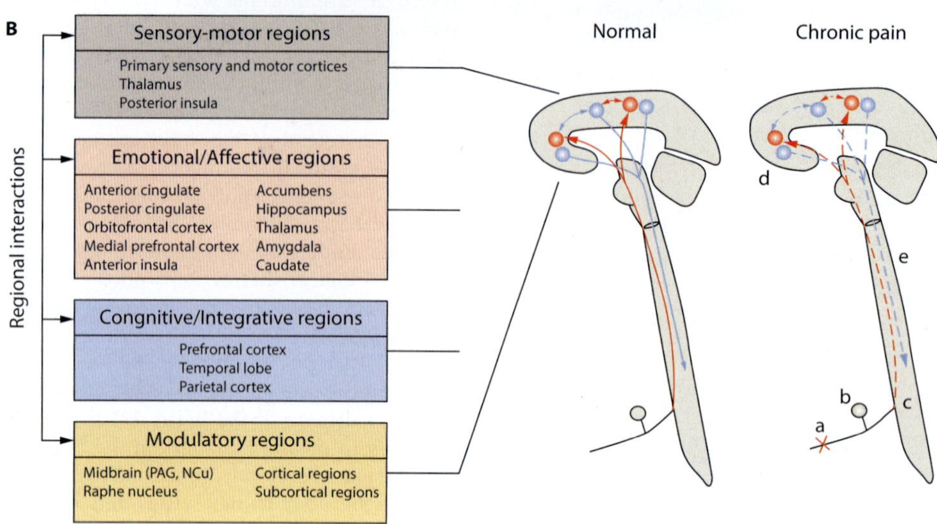

FIGURE 12-1. Placebo response and alterations in neurochemistry in chronic pain. (From Sava et al., The pain imaging revolution: advancing pain into the 21st century. *Neuroscientist*. 2010;16:171-185.)

IMAGING MODALITIES

The development of a number of noninvasive magnetic resonance imaging (MRI) methods, including morphological/anatomical imaging of gray matter (voxel-based morphometry [VBM]), white matter tract connectivity (diffusion tensor imaging [DTI]), functional magnetic resonance imaging (fMRI), and magnetic resonance spectroscopy (MRS), has paved the way to an unprecedented boom in brain research (**Fig. 12-2**). MRI methods, as well as other techniques like magnetic encephalography (MEG) and near-infrared spectroscopy (NIRS), are

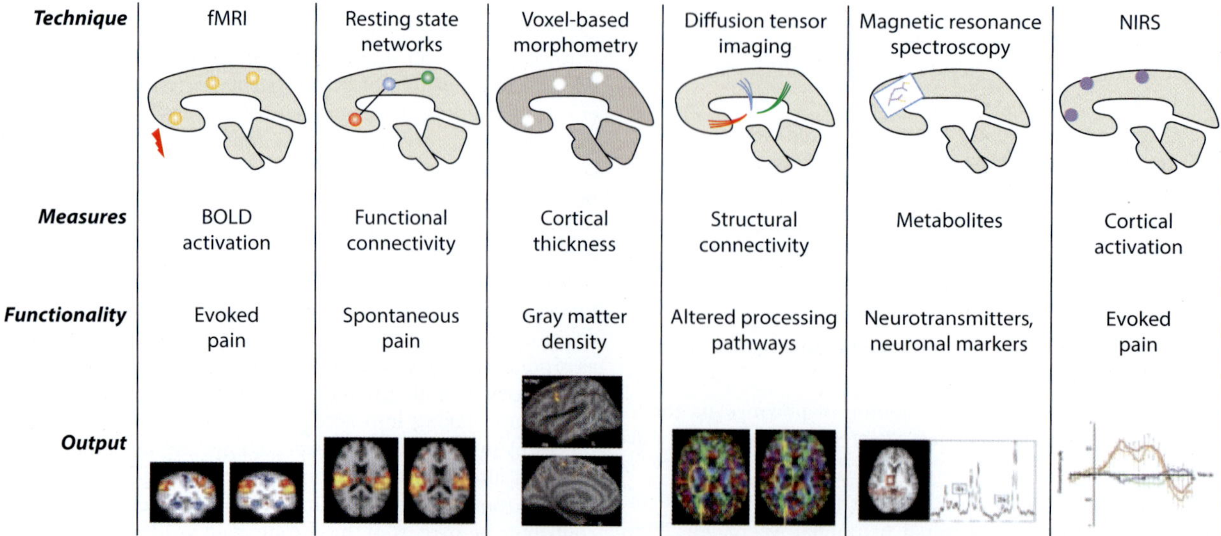

FIGURE 12-2. Imaging modalities. (From Sava et al., The pain imaging revolution: advancing pain into the 21st century. *Neuroscientist*. 2010;16:171-185.)

rapidly evolving as novel analytical methods and more sophisticated equipment become available. Because their noninvasive nature allows *in vivo* longitudinal studies of the dynamic structural and functional changes in the brain as a result of pain, these approaches (described in Fig. 12-2) have produced a shift in our understanding of chronic pain.

From the original definition as an "unpleasant sensory and emotional condition," *chronic pain* is now understood to be a multidimensional "disease affecting the central nervous system," influenced by a variety of biological and psychosocial factors, such as genetics, hormones, emotions, memories, or social expectations.[6,7]

VOXEL-BASED MORPHOMETRY

VBM measures the local concentration of gray matter in different brain voxels. In the pain field, VBM has been used to measure changes in the volume of subcortical structures, including the hippocampus, basal ganglia, thalamus, and amygdale.[8] Most recently, techniques that allow measurement of small changes in cortical thickness have been developed (http://surfer.nmr.mgh.harvard.edu). These techniques will allow documentation of alterations of gray matter that occur in chronic pain conditions.

DIFFUSION TENSOR IMAGING

DTI investigates white matter tract integrity by measuring microstructural changes in directional water diffusion in the brain.[9,10] In the pain field, the technique has been used in fibromyalgia to document alterations in the brain's microcircuitry in the thalamus, insula, amygdala, hippocampus, and frontal and anterior cingulate cortex.[11] By overlaying DTI and fMRI brain maps, future studies may help advance our understanding of functional anatomical mapping in chronic pain conditions.

FUNCTIONAL IMAGING

Blood oxygen level–dependent (BOLD) fMRI measures changes in the local concentration of deoxyhemoglobin and provides an indirect index of neuronal activity. Several BOLD methods have been applied to pain research and have revealed the neural correlates of pain perception and modulation by characterizing the brain response to evoked stimuli (e.g., pain, allodynia), task-driven responses, or drugs (phMRI).

EVOKED-STIMULI fMRI

Evoked-stimuli fMRI has been commonly used in the pain field because of the relative ease of presenting well-characterized objective stimuli during the imaging session (i.e., cold and hot temperatures, somatosensory stimulation). Functional imaging has helped uncover the neural circuitry involved in pain processing and modulation and described the brain areas that reflect sensory, cognitive, and affective dimensions of pain.[12]

RESTING STATE NETWORKS AND FUNCTIONAL CONNECTIVITY

This approach uses low-frequency BOLD signal fluctuations to evaluate the functional brain connectivity during resting states as opposed to task performance. These default mode networks are consistent across healthy subjects[13] and can be used to define disease phenotypes by differentiating disease states (i.e., chronic back pain);[14] from healthy states. Simultaneous imaging of structural and functional connectivity may provide a better understanding of pathological processes by uncovering changes in specific brain networks as a result of disease.

PHARMACOLOGICAL MRI

Pharmacological MRI (phMRI) investigates the functional effects of drugs on the brain and links levels of drug exposure to the changes in evoked responses or RSN activity. More recently, arterial spin labeling (ASL) methodology, which measures blood flow changes with improved contrast and signal-to-noise ratio through magnetization of the blood, has been used to measure the regional dose-related effects of drugs on brain function.[15] These measures can be used to monitor the functional effects of drug receptor binding and the dose relationship of central responses and to provide objective indices of therapeutic efficacy in pain conditions.

CHEMICAL CENTRAL NERVOIS SYSTEM MEASURES

Magenetic Resonance Spectroscopy MRS is used to noninvasively assess different metabolites and neurotransmitters in the brain,[16] to characterize the composition of neuronal and synaptic markers (e.g., glutamate, glutamine, and g-aminobutyric acid [GABA]) in different brain regions and to identify relationships between disease states and changes in the brain metabolic or chemical composition. MRS techniques have been widely applied in the study of psychiatric diseases as well as pain syndromes.[17] Recently, analytic technologies such as 13C-based flux analysis have been developed. This fluxometric method allows real-time analysis of metabolic changes in brain networks. Although this technology has so far been applied to mammalian cells grown in tissue culture but not to the human brain *in vivo*, it represents a potentially promising technique that, in the future, could aid the understanding of the disease-associated metabolic changes in the brain.

Brain Receptor Mapping A novel approach that could aid the localization of functionally activated brain regions in the brain is mapping of multiple neurotransmitter receptors sites.[18] Although not yet applied to pain conditions, this approach may provide a better understanding of the underlying basis of neurotransmission in healthy and disease states by correlating brain data obtained through different techniques (anatomical, functional) with cytoarchitectonical and molecular brain maps.

Near-Infrared Spectrometry NIRS or diffuse optical tomography (DOT) is a noninvasive technique that can detect changes in blood hemoglobin concentrations associated with neural activity and, therefore, assess the brain function through an intact skull in human subjects.[19] NIRS has a great potential in measuring pain effects on the brain. Recent research has shown that it is possible to record a pain-specific signal using NIRS, and this signal was similar to that observed in previous fMRI studies.[20]

Magenetic Encephalography MEG is a noninvasive imaging technique that measures the magnetic field produced by synchronized synaptic currents in the brain. Similar to electroencephalography (EEG), MEG measures parameters of neuronal activity directly. A rich literature exists that describes the correlation between neuronal oscillations as recorded by MEG and different brain functions, including attention, visual processing, or motor planning.[21] Recently, a growing number of studies have employed both MEG and fMRI, taking advantage of the strengths of each method (i.e., excellent spatial resolution of fMRI and the millisecond temporal resolution of MEG) to help uncover the mechanisms of cortical processing.[22]

IMAGING PAIN IN HEALTH

The early pain imaging studies used positron emission tomography (PET) and reported on pain responses to noxious heat. Since then, functional imaging studies in healthy volunteers have either confirmed brain regions involved in pain processing (thalamus, somatosensory cortex, anterior cingulate cortex) or added important new components of pain processing (e.g., nucleus accumbens, insula, dorsolateral prefrontal cortex, basal ganglia, and cerebellum). Thus, there is a new complexity in understanding brain function in pain that allows for sensory, emotional/affective, modulatory, and cognitive responses to pain.

Functional imaging research in healthy subjects has provided new insights into these regions and their possible role in pain. As such, these studies have been invaluable in providing a basis to explore changes in the clinical condition and evaluation of analgesic drugs on brain function. (See **Fig. 12-3**.)

BRAIN REGIONS AND PAIN FUNCTION

In the first imaging study of pain, "Multiple Representations of Pain in the Human Cerebral Cortex," Talbot and colleagues reported on activation in several brain regions in response to noxious heat, including the contralateral anterior cingulate cortex and primary and sensory somatosensory cortices.[23] This study opened up the path for brain imaging of pain, which initially focused on "expected areas" such as the thalamus.

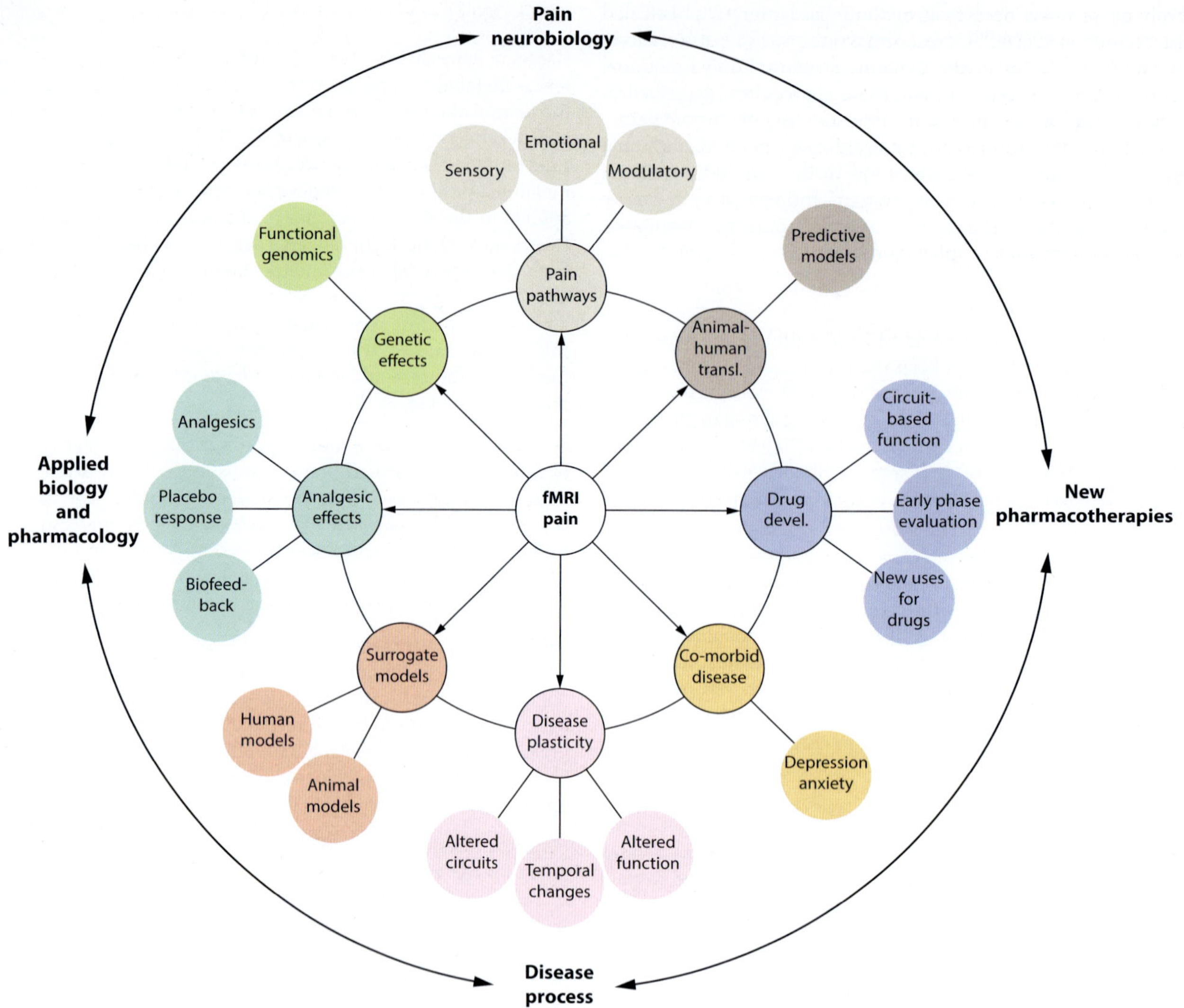

FIGURE 12-3. Imaging of chronic pain. (From Borsook and Becerra, Phenotyping central nervous system circuitry in chronic pain using functional MRI: considerations and potential implications in the clinic. *Current Pain and Headache*. 2007;11(3):201-207.)

What these studies did is raise issues of pain processing in regions beyond the primary somatosensory cortex.[24,25] Subsequently, numerous cortical regions have been shown across pain imaging studies to be activated by painful stimuli (reviewed in Treede et al., Peyron et al., and Apkarian et al.[26-28]).

Overall, these meta-analyses reported that pain produced activation in the primary and secondary somatosensory, insular, anterior cingulate and prefrontal cortices and the thalamus. Some regions such as the cerebellum,[29] the anterior cingulate, and insular cortices, are consistently activated across most functional imaging pain studies but have remained an enigma as to a specific role in pain processing. More recent studies have begun to dissect the pain-induced brain activation as it relates to specific functions, such as sensory processing, emotional/affective and cognitive processing, and pain modulatory processing. The more focused studies have allowed for a better understanding of these regions in pain function.

Imaging Somatosensory Pain Processing Somatosensory processing of pain stimuli classically includes the thalamus and somatosensory cortices. Other studies have used imaging to trace a pain pathway (trigeminal) from the periphery (ganglion) to the dorsal horn (trigeminal nucleus in the brainstem) and traditional sensory pathways through the thalamus and to the cortex.[30,31] Insula is a recent addition to brain regions involved in the evaluation of pain intensity, and imaging studies have uncovered the somatosensory representation of pain in the insular cortex.[32] Still, investigations of the insular functions warrant a broader look at the potential involvement in sensory and emotional evaluative components, as well as interoception (i.e., sensing the physiological condition of the body). As it turns out, this region is intricately involved in complex pain and analgesic processing.

Imaging Emotional Pain Processing The notion that pain is not only a sensory but also an emotional experience required neuroimaging to help define an underlying brain circuitry that contributes to the emotional processing of pain. Generally, greater acute and chronic pain intensity is associated with higher negative emotional state. The experience of pain is able to trigger emotional responses, and the emotional state can also affect the perception of pain. Studies indicated that the classic reward circuitry, which includes regions such as the amygdala, nucleus accumbens, and orbitofrontal lobe, were all activated by noxious heat.[33] Specific connectivity between entorhinal cortex and cingulate regions involved in anxiety and anticipation of pain was also described.[34] Such studies contributed to the characterization of a brain network that could underlie, in addition to emotional responses to pain, the placebo and nocebo responses,[35,36] as well as empathy of pain in others.[37]

This network has also been involved in the development of comorbid symptoms (e.g., depression, anxiety) frequently associated with pain.[38] A recent review suggested that the reciprocal effects of pain on emotional state could be explained by the common anatomical brain network shared by these two processes.[39]

Many brain regions have been discussed in previous reviews.[40] Perhaps the dorsolateral prefrontal (DLPFC) and medioprefrontal (mPFC) cortices, the cingulate cortex (CC), and basal ganglia are worthy of further mention because of their relative importance in understanding chronic pain.

Besides their role in the emotional pain processing, the DLPFC, mPFC, and the CC are also part of the modulatory networks that can alter pain perception, as well as networks involved in cognitive processing (discusses in the next section). The anatomical overlap of these neuronal networks and the known roles of the frontal cortical regions in emotion and cognition may explain the wide effects that pain has on multiple brain functions.

Pain and analgesia are at opposite ends of the reward aversion spectrum. However, the neural circuits that support these functions are similar.[41] Endogenous systems, including opioidergic and dopaminergic, may provide useful models for evaluating these opponent processes in chronic pain and nocebo and placebo responses.[36]

COGNITIVE PROCESSING AND PAIN

Pain can affect cognitive processing, but the neural substrates of this interaction are not well elucidated. Given that acute pain has an adaptive role of signaling injury to the body, it represents a stimulus that can induce rapid emotional learning involving the prefrontal-limbic circuitry (amygdala, insula, the anterior cingulate, and orbitofrontal cortex).[42] Patients with chronic pain, however, often complain of attention and memory deficits. It has been postulated that pain modulates an attention-specific network that includes the DLPFC, anterior and posterior cingulate cortices (ACC and PCC), posterior parietal cortex, and medial frontal cortex.[43]

Imaging Modulatory Circuits Understanding modulatory pain processing (both pro- and antinociceptive effects) has enormous implications for evaluating alterations in disease state and analgesic drug effects.[44] The basic neurobiology of modulatory circuits had been defined previously.[45] A network of subcortical and cortical regions (predominantly frontal areas) has been involved in endogenous pain modulation. Functional imaging studies have been able to evaluate descending modulatory processes in experimental pain and have shown a direct participation of well-described regions such as the periaqueductal gray (PAG) and less well understood regions such as the nucleus cuneiformis (NCF) in pain processing.

Among cortical areas, the mPFC exerts an inhibitory effect on the perception of pain.[46] The DLPFC, orbitofrontal cortex (OFC), and cingulate cortex were also found to have key roles in cortical mechanisms of pain modulation. The pain-modulating roles of the frontal cortices might be mediated by cognitive interference during nociceptive stimulation,[47] inasmuch as patients with chronic pain show increased "vigilance" toward pain and pain-related information. Recent studies have proposed that an altered interaction of pain-inhibitory and pain-facilitatory mechanisms may contribute to the development or maintenance of chronic pain states.[48]

Imaging Analgesic Effect in Healthy Volunteers with phMRI Although many drugs used as analgesics influence central nervous system (CNS) function, little is known about the direct effects of these agents on the brain or the mechanisms through which they provide analgesia in humans. Pharmaocological MRI studies use two approaches: evaluating the brain regions that show activation by the drug and the drug effect on the modulation of pain processing in the brain. In healthy volunteers, studies have evaluated opioids, including morphine[49] and remifentanil;[50] naloxone;[51] ketamine;[52,53] local anesthetics;[47] cox inhibitors;[54] and drugs used in neuropathic pain, including gabapentin and imipramine.[55-57] Overall, these types of studies have provided a basis to investigate pharmacological effects on brain systems as provided by the following three examples:

1. Morphine, a well-characterized drug behaviorally, affects neural circuits that are expected to define these behavioral features of the drug (e.g., sedation, reward, analgesia).
2. Gabapentin, although having a measurable antinociceptive effect on activation patterns, has a more profound antihyperalgesic effect, suggesting that the drug may be more effective in modulating pain when central sensitization is present.[56]
3. Activation patterns in specific brain regions such as mPFC were shown to inversely correlate with individual extent of central hyperalgesia and predict individual pharmacological antihyperalgesic treatment response.[46]

Although remarkable progress has been made, the real advances are still to come in using fMRI on drug development to evaluate new drugs.[58]

Imaging Gender Differences Given that many chronic pain conditions predominantly affect women (e.g., complex regional pain syndrome [CRPS],[59] fibromyalgia,[60] temporomandibular disease,[61] irritable bowel syndrome,[62] and headache[63]), it is possible that gender differences exist in pain processing. Although some of the gender variability in pain thresholds and pain may result from genetic differences at loci on the sex chromosomes, current data on pain sensitivity in women[64,65] and brain activation studies suggest a hormonal contribution as well, supported by the finding that differences in the response to pain are found during the follicular and luteal phase.[66] Still, many pain-imaging studies do not account for the menstrual phase in women who are selected as part of a cohort. In addition, menstrual phase alters reward-related functions[67] as well as chemistry in cortical regions[68] that may have an impact in chronic pain conditions where there is a hedonic deficit syndrome. Importantly, the data suggest that differences in pain responses in women as a result of the modulatory effects of sex hormones may have important implications for therapy.

Imaging and Surrogate Pain Models One of the big questions in pain research is the translation of surrogate models to the clinical condition. Because brain circuits can be measured in both the surrogate model (e.g., capsaicin-induced central sensitization) as well as in human models, imaging may help define the utility of such models for testing analgesic efficacy or understanding brain processes that contribute to the chronic pain condition.

Imaging the Placebo Response Imaging has allowed for a better understanding of the biological mechanism systems that determine the placebo response.[69,70] The placebo response in pain is based on beliefs, expectations, and anticipation of pain. The neural mechanisms of this effect relate to brain regions involved in expectancies (cognitive processing) and also reward related functions that include dopaminergic[71] and opioidergic systems.[72] Both improvement (placebo/therapeutic response) or worsening (nocebo/adverse response) of pain may result from altered brain processing. Functional imaging has focused on a few approaches that investigate the placebo response as provided by the three examples that follow:

1. *Altered expectations in the response to painful stimuli:* Functional MRI experiments using manipulation of expectations in healthy volunteers showed that placebo analgesia resulted in a decrease in activation in thalamus, insula, and ACC, with a corresponding increase in activity in the prefrontal cortex in anticipation of pain. Studies such as this one provided evidence for the involvement of pain-related structures in the placebo response.
2. *Alterations related to opioidergic and dopaminergic function:* Prior studies evaluated the role of endogenous opioid systems in the placebo response using PET.[73] The data indicated that both opioid and placebo analgesia are associated with increased activity in the rostral ACC and in the brainstem, suggesting that placebo-induced analgesia affects the pain circuitry. More recently, this approach has been extended to include evaluation of underlying endogenous chemical processes. Two neurotransmitter systems—one involved in analgesia (opioidergic) and another in reward (dopaminergic)—were examined for their potential role in placebo and nocebo responses.[35] The results of this study are highly significant

in furthering our understanding of these responses. Consistent with the Petrovic study, opioid neurotransmission was increased in the ACC, insular cortex, nucleus accumbens (NAc), amygdala, and PAG, whereas dopaminergic neurotransmission was increased in the basal ganglia with the placebo response. Placebo effects correlated with increased opioidergic and dopaminergic responses in the NAc, whereas nocebo effects were associated with decreased response of both neurotransmitters.

3. *Placebo responses in diseases where expectations may be altered:* In patient populations, the study of the placebo responses and how they may be affected by disease has enormous implications for treatments and clinical trials because the loss of expectation makes analgesic therapies less effective.[68]

Acupuncture Imaging has advanced acupuncture from "a difficult to understand" process to a more plausible process that has scientific underpinnings. Although the basis for neural systems involved in acupuncture has not clearly been differentiated from placebo response, some new data add important information on the underlying CNS processes involved in acupuncture-induced pain control. One such study, using PET, differentiates traditional acupuncture from sham acupuncture based on differences in effects on opioid receptors,[72] suggesting a basis for mediation of analgesic effects in real acupuncture. In a similar vein, differentiation of acupuncture analgesia and expectancy-evoked placebo analgesia seems to involve different brain networks.[73]

IMAGING CHRONIC PAIN

Imaging patients with chronic pain has been a greater challenge than imaging healthy volunteers, owing to a number of confounding factors such as current treatments and duration of disease. Nevertheless, advances have been made in the imaging of several chronic pain conditions, including chronic back pain,[2] complex regional pain syndrome,[74] neuropathic pain,[57,75] fibromyalgia, and gastrointestinal disease.[76] Such studies are attempting to define specific brain phenotypes for different chronic pain conditions, and they could greatly advance diagnostic methods and therapy, with the final goal of developing disease-modifying treatments. Several important and novel insights related to pain processing and treatment effects have been described in these patient populations. (See Fig. 12-3.)

Functional reorganization and chronic pain was most clearly defined in a report on patients with upper extremity amputation and pain.[77] Since then, several articles have described how plasticity occurs in neural circuits in several chronic pain conditions, including complex regional pain syndrome. Most important, it seems as if appropriate treatments "reconstitute" or normalize brain activation patterns concomitant with remission of pain.[78]

Chronic pain patients may have decreased opioid receptor availability,[79] as well as enhanced pain responses or impairment of antinociceptive modulatory processes.[80,81] An alteration in the tone of inhibitory versus facilitatory systems may underlie the unmasking or exacerbation of chronic pain syndromes. In this type of data, imaging has helped define specific regions that show abnormal activation patterns and provided a method to determine if effective therapies alter these abnormal patterns.

In recent years, several laboratories have reported on decreased cortical and subcortical gray matter (using voxel-based morphometry) in chronic pain in a variety of conditions, including chronic back pain, neuropathic pain,[82] and fibromyalgia.[83] These changes in brain structure seem to be related to the chronicity of the pain and have redefined chronic pain as a degenerative disorder. Although the precise mechanism of altered brain volume is not fully described, some studies have pointed to the potential loss of neurons and dendritic spines as potential contributors.[84] As such, our treatment approaches to chronic pain should be radically redefined to include methods of preventing neuronal degeneration and promoting neuronal survival.

Chemical measures using MRS have shown altered neurotransmitters in chronic back pain,[17,85] migraine, complex regional pain syndrome,[86] and fibromyalgia.[87]

The spontaneous component of chronic pain is a critical component of pain symptomatology, and neuroimaging is exploring CNS circuits that are involved in spontaneous or ongoing pain.

A few reports have evaluated spontaneous pain in diabetic neuropathy[88] and treatment effects of ketamine.[17] Default mode resting states are disrupted in chronic pain.[14] Although still early, this approach holds the promise of defining new evaluative processes for disease state and therapeutic effect.

CONCLUSION

Brain imaging of pain has advanced our appreciation of the complexity of brain systems biology in chronic pain. Continued advances will most likely allow us to use this approach as an addendum to clinical diagnosis (including the severity of the disease) and objective measures of therapeutic outcome.

REFERENCES

1. Deyo RA, Mirza SK, Turner JA, Martin BI. Overtreating chronic back pain: time to back off? *J Am Board Fam Med.* 2009;22(1):62-68.
2. Apkarian AV, Krauss BR, Fredrickson BE, Szeverenyi NM. Imaging the pain of low back pain: functional magnetic resonance imaging in combination with monitoring subjective pain perception allows the study of clinical pain states. *Neurosci Lett.* 2001;299(1-2):57-60.
3. Borsook D, Becerra L. Phenotyping central nervous system circuitry in chronic pain using functional MRI: considerations and potential implications in the clinic. *Curr Pain Headache Rep.* 2007;11(3):201-207.
4. Tracey I, Mantyh PW. The cerebral signature for pain perception and its modulation. *Neuron.* 2007;55(3):377-391.
5. Tracey I. Imaging pain. *Br J Anaesth.* 2008;101(1):32-39.
6. Borsook D, Becerra LR. Breaking down the barriers: fMRI applications in pain, analgesia and analgesics. *Mol Pain.* 2006;2:30.
7. Borsook D, Moulton EA, Schmidt KF, Becerra LR. Neuroimaging revolutionizes therapeutic approaches to chronic pain. *Mol Pain.* 2007b;3:25.
8. Jovicich J, Czanner S, Han X, Salat D, van der Kouwe A, Quinn B, et al. MRI-derived measurements of human subcortical, ventricular and intracranial brain volumes: reliability effects of scan sessions, acquisition sequences, data analyses, scanner upgrade, scanner vendors and field strengths. *Neuroimage.* 2009;46(1):177-192.
9. Alexander AL, Lee JE, Lazar M, Field AS. Diffusion tensor imaging of the brain. *Neurotherapeutics.* Jul 2007;4(3):316-329. Review.
10. Mukherjee P, Berman JI, Chung SW, Hess CP, Henry RG. Diffusion tensor MR imaging and fiber tractography: theoretic underpinnings. *AJNR Am J Neuroradiol.* 2008;29(4):631-641.
11. Lutz J, Jager L, de Quervain D, Krauseneck T, Padberg F, Wichnalek M, et al. White and gray matter abnormalities in the brain of patients with fibromyalgia: a diffusion-tensor and volumetric imaging study. *Arthritis Rheum.* 2008;58(12):3960-3909.
12. May A. Neuroimaging: visualizing the brain in pain. *Neurol Sci.* 2007;28(Suppl 2):S101-S107.
13. Damoiseaux JS, Rombouts SA, Barkhof F, Scheltens P, Stam CJ, Smith SM, et al. 2006. Consistent resting-state networks across healthy subjects. *Proc Natl Acad Sci USA.* 103(37):13848-13853.

14. Baliki MN, Geha PY, Apkarian AV, Chialvo DR. Beyond feeling: chronic pain hurts the brain, disrupting the default mode network dynamics. *J Neurosci.* 2008;28(6):1398-1403.
15. Detre JA, Wang J, Wang Z, Rao H. Arterial spin-labeled perfusion MRI in basic and clinical neuroscience. *Curr Opin Neurol.* 2009;22(4):348-355.
16. Soares DP, Law M. Magnetic resonance spectroscopy of the brain: review of metabolites and clinical applications. *Clin Radiol.* 2009;64(1):12-21.
17. Prescot A, Becerra L, Pendse G, Tully S, Jensen E, Hargreaves R, et al. Excitatory neurotransmitters in brain regions in interictal migraine patients. *Mol Pain.* 2009;5:34.
18. Zilles K, Amunts K. Receptor mapping: architecture of the human cerebral cortex. *Curr Opin Neurol.* 2009;22(4):331-339.
19. Boas DA, Dale AM, Franceschini MA. Diffuse optical imaging of brain activation: approaches to optimizing image sensitivity, resolution, and accuracy. *Neuroimage.* 2004;23(Suppl 1):S275-S288.
20. Becerra L, Harris W, Joseph D, Huppert T, Boas DA, Borsook D. Diffuse optical tomography of pain and tactile stimulation: activation in cortical sensory and emotional systems. *Neuroimage.* 2008;41(2):252-259.
21. Bandettini PA. What's new in neuroimaging methods? *Ann NY Acad Sci.* 2009;1156:260-293.
22. Auranen T, Nummenmaa A, Vanni S, Vehtari A, Hamalainen MS, Lampinen J, et al. Automatic fMRI-guided MEG multidipole localization for visual responses. *Hum Brain Mapp.* 2009;30(4): 1087-1099.
23. Talbot JD, Marrett S, Evans AC, Meyer E, Bushnell MC, Duncan GH. Multiple representations of pain in human cerebral cortex. *Science.* 1991;251(4999):1355-1358.
24. Bushnell MC, Duncan GH, Hofbauer RK, Ha B, Chen JI, Carrier B. Pain perception: is there a role for primary somatosensory cortex? *Proc Natl Acad Sci USA.* 1999;96(14):7705-7709.
25. Treede RD, Apkarian AV, Bromm B, Greenspan JD, Lenz FA. Cortical representation of pain: functional characterization of nociceptive areas near the lateral sulcus. *Pain.* 2000;87(2):113-119.
26. Treede RD, Kenshalo DR, Gracely RH, Jones AK. The cortical representation of pain. *Pain.* 1999;79(2-3):105-111.
27. Peyron R, Laurent B, Garcia-Larrea L. Functional imaging of brain responses to pain: a review and meta-analysis. *Neurophysiol Clin.* 2000;30(5):263-288.
28. Apkarian AV, Bushnell MC, Treede RD, Zubieta JK. Human brain mechanisms of pain perception and regulation in health and disease. *Eur J Pain.* 2005;9(4):463-484.
29. Borsook D, Moulton EA, Tully S, Schmahmann JD, Becerra L. Human cerebellar responses to brush and heat stimuli in healthy and neuropathic pain subjects. *Cerebellum.* 2008;7(3): 252-272.
30. DaSilva AF, Becerra L, Makris N, Strassman AM, Gonzalez RG, Geatrakis N, et al. Somatotopic activation in the human trigeminal pain pathway. *J Neurosci.* 2002;22(18):8183-8192.
31. Borsook D, DaSilva AF, Ploghaus A, Becerra L. Specific and somatotopic functional magnetic resonance imaging activation in the trigeminal ganglion by brush and noxious heat. *J Neurosci.* 2003;23(21):7897-7903.
32. Borsook D, Becerra L. Functional imaging of pain and analgesi: a valid diagnostic tool? *Pain.* 2005;117(3):247-250.
33. Becerra L, Breiter HC, Wise R, Gonzalez RG, Borsook D. Reward circuitry activation by noxious thermal stimuli. *Neuron.* 2001;32(5):927-946.
34. Ploghaus A, Narain C, Beckmann CF, Clare S, Bantick S, Wise R, et al. Exacerbation of pain by anxiety is associated with activity in a hippocampal network. *J Neurosci.* 2001;21(24):9896-9903.
35. Scott DJ, Stohler CS, Egnatuk CM, Wang H, Koeppe RA, Zubieta JK. Placebo and nocebo effects are defined by opposite opioid and dopaminergic responses. *Arch Gen Psychiatry.* 2008; 65(2):220-231.
36. Danziger N, Faillenot I, Peyron R. Can we share a pain we never felt? Neural correlates of empathy in patients with congenital insensitivity to pain. *Neuron.* 2009;61(2):203-212.
37. Borsook D, Becerra L, Carlezon WA Jr, Shaw M, Renshaw P, Elman I, et al. Reward-aversion circuitry in analgesia and pain: implications for psychiatric disorders. *Eur J Pain.* 2007a; 11(1):7-20.
38. Duquette M, Roy M, Lepore F, Peretz I, Rainville P. Cerebral mechanisms involved in the interaction between pain and emotion. *Rev Neurol (Paris).* 2007;163(2):169-179.
39. Bruehl S, Burns JW, Chung OY, Chont M. Pain-related effects of trait anger expression: neural substrates and the role of endogenous opioid mechanisms. *Neurosci Biobehav Rev.* 2009;33(3): 475-491.
40. Leknes S, Tracey I. A common neurobiology for pain and pleasure. *Nat Rev Neurosci.* 2008;9(4):314-320.
41. Sehlmeyer C, Schoning S, Zwitserlood P, Pfleiderer B, Kircher T, Arolt V, et al. Human fear conditioning and extinction in neuroimaging: a systematic review. *PLoS ONE.* 2009;4(6):e5865.
42. Seminowicz DA, Davis KD. Pain enhances functional connectivity of a brain network evoked by performance of a cognitive task. *J Neurophysiol.* 2007;97(5):3651-3659.
43. Porreca F, Ossipov MH, Gebhart GF. Chronic pain and medullary descending facilitation. *Trends Neurosci.* 2002;25(6): 319-325.
44. Basbaum AI, Fields HL. Endogenous pain control systems: brainstem spinal pathways and endorphin circuitry. *Annu Rev Neurosci.* 1984;7:309-338.
45. Seifert F, Bschorer K, De Col R, Filitz J, Peltz E, Koppert W, et al. Medial prefrontal cortex activity is predictive for hyperalgesia and pharmacological antihyperalgesia. *J Neurosci.* 2009a;29(19): 6167-6175.
46. Wager TD, Rilling JK, Smith EE, Sokolik A, Casey KL, Davidson RJ, et al. Placebo-induced changes in FMRI in the anticipation and experience of pain. *Science.* 2004;303(5661): 1162-1167.
47. Bingel U, Schoell E, Buchel C. Imaging pain modulation in health and disease. *Curr Opin Neurol.* 2007;20(4):424-431.
48. Becerra L, Harter K, Gonzalez RG, Borsook D. Functional magnetic resonance imaging measures of the effects of morphine on central nervous system circuitry in opioid naivehealthy volunteers. *Anesth Analg.* 2006a;103(1):208-216.
49. Wise RG, Rogers R, Painter D, Bantick S, Ploghaus A, Williams P, et al. Combining fMRI with a pharmacokinetic model to determine which brain areas activated by painful stimulation are specifically modulated by remifentanil. *Neuroimage.* 2002;16(4): 999-1014.
50. Wagner KJ, Sprenger T, Kochs EF, Tolle TR, Valet M, Willoch F. Imaging human cerebral pain modulation by dose-dependent opioid analgesia: a positron emission tomography activation study using remifentanil. *Anesthesiology.* 2007;106(3):548-556.
51. Borras MC, Becerra L, Ploghaus A, Gostic JM, DaSilva A, Gonzalez RG, et al. fMRI measurement of CNS responses to naloxone infusion

and subsequent mild noxious thermal stimuli in healthy volunteers. *J Neurophysiol.* 2004;91(6):2723-2733.

52. Rogers R, Wise RG, Painter DJ, Longe SE, Tracey I. An investigation to dissociate the analgesic and anesthetic properties of ketamine using functional magnetic resonance imaging. *Anesthesiology.* 2004;100(2):292-301.
53. Sprenger T, Valet M, Woltmann R, Zimmer C, Freynhagen R, Kochs EF, et al. Imaging pain modulation by subanesthetic S-(+)-ketamine. *Anesth Analg.* 2006;103(3):729-737.
54. Maihofner C, Ringler R, Herrndobler F, Koppert W. Brain imaging of analgesic and antihyperalgesic effects of cyclooxygenase inhibition in an experimental human pain model: a functional MRI study. *Eur J Neurosci.* 2007b;26(5):1344-1356.
55. Iannetti GD, Zambreanu L, Wise RG, Buchanan TJ, Huggins JP, Smart TS, et al. Pharmacological modulation of pain-related brain activity during normal and central sensitization states in humans. *Proc Natl Acad Sci USA.* 2005;102(50):18195-18200.
56. Borsook D, Becerra L, Hargreaves R. A role for fMRI in optimizing CNS drug development. *Nat Rev Drug Discov.* 2006;5(5):411-424.
57. Scrivani S, Wallin D, Moulton EA, Cole S, Wasan AD, Lockerman L, et al. *A fMRI evaluation of lamotrigine for the treatment of trigeminal neuropathic pain: pilot study. Pain Med.* Jun 2010;11(6):920-941.
58. Wise RG, Tracey I. The role of fMRI in drug discovery. *J Magn Reson Imaging.* 2006;23(6):862-876.
59. Birklein F, Riedl B, Sieweke N, Weber M, Neundorfer B. Neurological findings in complex regional pain syndromes: analysis of 145 cases. *Acta Neurol Scand.* 2000;101(4):262-269.
60. Hooten WM, Townsend CO, Decker PA. Gender differences among patients with fibromyalgia undergoing multidisciplinary pain rehabilitation. *Pain Med.* 2007;8(8):624-632.
61. Dao TT, LeResche L. Gender differences in pain. *J Orofac Pain.* 2000;14(3):169-184; discussion 184-195.
62. Chial HJ, Camilleri M. Gender differences in irritable bowel syndrome. *J Gend Specif Med.* 2002;5(3):37-45.
63. Silberstein SD. The role of sex hormones in headache. *Neurology.* 1992;42(3 Suppl 2):37-42.
64. Fillingim RB, King CD, Ribeiro-Dasilva MC, Rahim-Williams B, Riley JL 3rd. Sex, gender, and pain: a review of recent clinical and experimental findings. *J Pain.* 2009;10(5):447-485.
65. Choi JC, Park SK, Kim YH, Shin YW, Kwon JS, Kim JS, et al. Different brain activation patterns to pain and pain-related unpleasantness during the menstrual cycle. *Anesthesiology.* 2006;105(1):120-127.
66. Dreher JC, Schmidt PJ, Kohn P, Furman D, Rubinow D, Berman KF. Menstrual cycle phase modulates reward-related neural function in women. *Proc Natl Acad Sci USA.* 2007;104(7):2465-2470.
67. Epperson CN, Haga K, Mason GF, Sellers E, Gueorguieva R, Zhang W, et al. Cortical gamma-aminobutyric acid levels across the menstrual cycle in healthy women and those with premenstrual dysphoric disorder: a proton magnetic resonance spectroscopy study. *Arch Gen Psychiatry.* 2002;59(9):851-858.
68. Benedetti F, Mayberg HS, Wager TD, Stohler CS, Zubieta JK. Neurobiological mechanisms of the placebo effect. *J Neurosci.* 2005;25(45):10390-10402.
69. Zubieta JK, Stohler CS. Neurobiological mechanisms of placebo responses. *Ann NY Acad Sci.* 2009;1156:198-210.
70. Wise RA. Dopamine, learning and motivation. *Nat Rev Neurosci.* 2004;5(6):483-494.
71. Petrovic P, Kalso E, Petersson KM, Ingvar M. Placebo and opioid analgesia: imaging a shared neuronal network. *Science.* 2002;295(5560):1737-1740.
72. Harris RE, Zubieta JK, Scott DJ, Napadow V, Gracely RH, Clauw DJ. Traditional Chinese acupuncture and placebo (sham) acupuncture are differentiated by their effects on mu-opioid receptors (MORs). *Neuroimage.* 2009;47(3):1077-1085.
73. Kong J, Kaptchuk TJ, Polich G, Kirsch I, Vangel M, Zyloney C, et al. Expectancy and treatment interactions: a dissociation between acupuncture analgesia and expectancy evoked placebo analgesia. *Neuroimage.* 2009;45(3):940-949.
74. Lebel A, Becerra L, Wallin D, Moulton EA, Morris S, Pendse G, et al. fMRI reveals distinct CNS processing during symptomatic and recovered complex regional pain syndrome in children. *Brain.* 2008;131(Pt 7):1854-1879.
75. Geha PY, Apkarian AV. Brain imaging findings in neuropathic pain. *Curr Pain Headache Rep.* 2005;9(3):184-188.
76. Kwan CL, Diamant NE, Pope G, Mikula K, Mikulis DJ, Davis KD. Abnormal forebrain activity in functional bowel disorder patients with chronic pain. *Neurology.* 2005;65(8):1268-1277.
77. Flor H, Elbert T, Knecht S, Wienbruch C, Pantev C, Birbaumer N, et al. Phantom-limb pain as a perceptual correlate of cortical reorganization following arm amputation. *Nature.* 1995;375(6531):482-484.
78. Flor H. Cortical reorganisation and chronic pain: implications for rehabilitation. *J Rehabil Med.* 2003;41(Suppl):66-72.
79. Harris RE, Clauw DJ, Scott DJ, McLean SA, Gracely RH, Zubieta JK. Decreased central mu-opioid receptor availability in fibromyalgia. *J Neurosci.* 2007;27(37):10000-10006.
80. Jensen KB, Kosek E, Petzke F, Carville S, Fransson P, Marcus H, et al. Evidence of dysfunctional pain inhibition in fibromyalgia reflected in rACC during provoked pain. *Pain.* 2009;144(1-2):95-100.
81. Seifert F, Kiefer G, DeCol R, Schmelz M, Maihofner C. Differential endogenous pain modulation in complexregional pain syndrome. *Brain.* 2009b;132(Pt 3):788-800.
82. DaSilva AF, Becerra L, Pendse G, Chizh B, Tully S, Borsook D. Colocalized structural and functional changes in the cortex of patients with trigeminal neuropathic pain. *PLoS ONE.* 2008; 3(10):e3396.
83. Kuchinad A, Schweinhardt P, Seminowicz DA, Wood PB, Chizh BA, Bushnell MC. Accelerated brain gray matter loss in fibromyalgia patients: premature aging of the brain? *J Neurosci.* 2007;27(15):4004-4007.
84. Metz AE, Yau HJ, Centeno MV, Apkarian AV, Martina M. Morphological and functional reorganization of rat medial prefrontal cortex in neuropathic pain. *Proc Natl Acad Sci USA.* 2009;106(7):2423-2428.
85. Grachev ID, Fredrickson BE, Apkarian AV. Abnormal brain chemistry in chronic back pain: an in vivo proton magnetic resonance spectroscopy study. *Pain.* 2000;89(1):7-18.
86. Grachev ID, Thomas PS, Ramachandran TS. Decreased levels of N-acetylaspartate in dorsolateral prefrontal cortex in a case of intractable severe sympathetically mediated chronic pain (complex regional pain syndrome, type I). *Brain Cogn.* 2002;49(1):102-113.
87. Harris RE, Sundgren PC, Pang Y, Hsu M, Petrou M, Kim SH, et al. Dynamic levels of glutamate within the insula are associated with improvements in multiple pain domains in fibromyalgia. *Arthritis Rheum.* 2008;58(3):903-907.
88. Cauda F, Sacco K, Duca S, Cocito D, D'Agata F, Geminiani GC, et al. Altered resting state in diabetic neuropathic pain. *PLoS ONE.* 2009;4(2):e4542.

CHAPTER 13

Diagnostic Injections for Spine Pain

Mohamed Elkersh

INTRODUCTION

Discography is a diagnostic test in which radiographic contrast is injected into the nucleus pulposus of the intervertebral disc. Although originally developed for the study of disc herniation, discography is now used most commonly to identify symptomatic disc degeneration. There are two components of discography: (1) the anatomic appearance of contrast spread within the disc (using plain radiographs and/or computed tomography [CT]) and (2) the presence or absence of typical pain during contrast injection within the disc (pain provocation).

Discography was first described by Lindblom in 1948. He used the technique to demonstrate disc ruptures and to determine if patients' pain symptoms originated from the abnormal disc. Although the procedure was initially performed more than 60 years ago, discography still remains controversial largely because of validity concerns. In 1968, Holt (cited later) reported that discography was falsely positive in 37% of an asymptomatic population. However, much subsequent work supports the validity of provocative discography in identifying symptomatic disc abnormalities.

Identifying the specific pathology responsible for spinal pain is often difficult. This is particularly true given the high incidence of anatomic abnormalities in asymptomatic individuals and the presence of normal anatomy in some painful individuals, at least as demonstrated on conventional imaging studies.[1,2] The primary purpose of diagnostic injections for chronic spinal pain is to identify which anatomic structure of the spine is causing pain and what the pathologic disorder is that affects it. Discography remains the only test available that attempts to correlate pain response from the patient during provocation with abnormal discs identified on imaging studies.

Whether or not it is important to make an anatomic diagnosis in patients with spinal pain is a matter of some debate.[3,4] While some would argue that in the majority of patients, attempts at making an anatomic diagnosis are contraindicated, others feel that, at a minimum, making a diagnosis will help patients to heal by providing them with a clear understanding of their problem.[5] The most important reason to make an anatomic diagnosis, however, is if there are treatments that can be directed toward specific pathology, leading to good outcomes. Many patients with spinal pain can be treated with interventional pain management procedures. The success of these procedures may depend on an accurate anatomic diagnosis; however, typically, little harm will come to the patient if the procedure fails. Traditionally, the indications for surgery have been felt to be neurologic loss. Increasingly, however, surgery is being performed for pain without neurologic loss, essentially becoming a pain management procedure. Although surgery may help some patients with chronic pain, the tissue injury that necessarily accompanies surgery may potentially lead to devastating consequences. If surgery is being considered for patients with chronic pain, an accurate diagnosis is essential. In this chapter, we focus on the role of diagnostic injections in presurgical decision making.

SPINAL PAIN

There are two types of spinal pain: radicular pain and axial pain.[6] Radicular pain results from mechanical compression or chemical irritation of a nerve root, or both. Establishing an anatomic diagnosis for patients with radicular pain is important, as surgical treatments have excellent outcomes in well-selected patients. The source of radicular pain, typically either a herniated nucleus pulposus or spinal stenosis, can be definitively diagnosed at surgery; therefore, there is a gold standard that can be used to assess the validity of diagnostic studies. Consequently, the ability of both clinical findings and imaging studies to diagnose the site of pathology is well defined. A diagnostic injection may be indicated when imaging studies suggest that more than one nerve root may be responsible for a patient's symptoms. In that circumstance, a selective epidural injection may be useful.

In contrast to radicular pain, the relationship between spinal pathology and axial pain is uncertain. There are a number of anatomic structures that are potential sources of pain, including myofascial tissues, synovial joints, and the intervertebral discs. Although discogenic pain is felt by many to be an indication for surgical fusion, outcome studies have demonstrated variable results.[7-16] Because there is no gold standard for diagnosing the tissue source of axial pain, it is not possible to rigorously validate diagnostic studies.[17] Discography is frequently performed on patients with axial pain, but its use remains controversial.[18,19]

Complicating the diagnosis and treatment of spinal pain is the influence of psychosocial factors on pain. Pain is a complex phenomenon, with components secondary to both tissue injury and the emotional reaction to tissue injury. Although there is considerable controversy regarding the relative importance of psychosocial and biologic factors in causing spinal pain,[20-22] there is evidence to suggest that the level of psychological distress can affect the results from diagnostic injections[23] as well as the outcomes from treatment.[24] It is important to recognize the potential importance of psychosocial factors in diagnosing and treating patients with spinal pain.

If surgery is being considered for a patient with spinal pain—and the source of pain is unclear despite a clinical evaluation, imaging studies, and, potentially, electrodiagnostics—a diagnostic injection may be indicated. Either discography or a selective epidural injection may be considered, depending on whether the patient has radicular pain or axial pain.

LUMBAR DISCOGRAPHY

OVERVIEW

The lumbar intervertebral disc can be injected with contrast, local anesthetic, or other substances.

In addition to provoking pain that can be compared with the patient's clinical symptoms, injecting contrast into the disc may demonstrate pathology that is not otherwise revealed on conventional imaging studies. Practitioners did not stipulate how strongly discs should be stimulated when tested, nor did they stipulate how severe the evoked pain should be in order for the test to be considered positive. Several studies have confirmed the accuracy of lumbar discography as a radiologic test in demonstrating both disc herniations and disc degeneration.[2,26-31] With the advent of MRI scanning, and, in particular, the use of gadolinium enhancement in evaluating postoperative patients, the utility of lumbar discography purely as a radiologic study has diminished. However, clinical studies have demonstrated that discography is more sensitive than MRI in detecting disc degeneration, particularly when postdiscography CT scanning is added.[2,28,31-33]

The purpose of discography is to determine whether the intervertebral disc is a source of clinical symptoms. Although interpretation of the radiologic images obtained at the time of discography is important, in contemporary practice, discography is primarily a provocative clinical test, rather than a radiologic imaging procedure.

The functional anesthetic discography test involves the assessment of the effect of an injection of local anesthetic into one or more discs of the lumbar spine during the generation of a patient's typical pain by a usually provocative position or activity. The injection is accomplished via a catheter that is inserted into the discs in question under fluoroscopic guidance. Without a clear "gold standard" to which the results of testing for discogenic pain can be compared, it is difficult to know how to critically examine the results of the test. Studies have shown negative results using the functional anesthetic discography in patients with positive provocative discography results.

Although observing the effect of a local anesthetic injection on pain and function (analgesic discography) can potentially provide useful information, the clinical utility of this has not been well defined.

PROVOCATIVE DISCOGRAPHY

The primary indication for provocative discography is to determine whether a patient with chronic spinal pain, who has failed aggressive efforts at conservative care, can be helped with spinal fusion.

A variety of pathologic processes affect the intervertebral disc, potentially causing noxious stimulation of nerve endings. A precision injection of contrast dye into the disc nucleus also stimulates nerve endings. The stimulus applied with discography has two components: a chemical stimulus resulting from contact between contrast dye and sensitized tissues and a mechanical stimulus resulting from a fluid-distending stress. The underlying premise of discography is that this applied stimulus replicates the clinical noxious stimulus responsible for the patient's symptoms and that reproduction of the patient's clinical symptoms during the injection confirms the disc as the source of pain.

False Negative and False Positive As with any diagnostic test, it is important to know the false-positive and false-negative rates associated with provocative discography, which are used to calculate sensitivity and specificity. Defining the false-positive and false-negative rates requires comparing the test results against a gold standard.[17,34,35] A gold standard is a method for definitively establishing a diagnosis and is typically obtained from biopsy, surgery, or long-term follow-up.[17] Unfortunately, in contrast to radicular pain, there is no absolute method to determine the tissue origin of lumbar axial pain and, therefore, no way to determine the sensitivity and specificity of discography.

For the provocative discography construct to be valid, the injection must selectively affect the nerve endings in the annulus of the disc being studied, which is the presumed site of the clinical noxious stimulus. A number of authors have suggested alternate sources for the pain of discography, other than stimulation of annular nerve endings.[36] Postulated pain mechanisms include increased pressure at the end plates or within the vertebral body,[37] increased substance P and VIP in the dorsal root ganglion,[38] or transmission of mechanical stimulation to the facet joints. Despite these hypotheses, there is good evidence that the provocative response resulting from discography is related to stimulation of nerve endings in the outer annulus, rather than other factors.[39-41] Although relatively unusual, painful end-plate disruptions can also occur.[42]

The complex nature of anatomic structures can also lead to inaccurate results from discography. Anatomic structures are typically composed of several different types of tissues. A pathologic process can potentially affect just one component of a structure, which may not be the same component targeted by a precision injection. For example, discogenic pain is commonly felt to be a result of annular fissures originating in the nucleus and extending to the outer annulus, which is where the majority of the disc nerve endings reside. During discography, contrast is injected into the nucleus. If there are not fissures, the contrast will be confined to the nucleus. However, histologic studies have demonstrated that there can be middle or outer annular abnormalities that are not contiguous with the nucleus.[28] In such cases, an injection into the nucleus could lead to a false-negative result.

Another potential source of inaccurate results from discography is the change in central nervous system (CNS) nociceptive processing that occurs with chronic pain. The neuroanatomic pathways mediating acute pain behave as a hard-wired system, with a pure stimulus-response relationship.[43] However, these neuroanatomic pathways are plastic, and they change with the development of chronic pain. With chronic pain, central sensitization occurs and dorsal horn cell activity no longer depends on peripheral tissue injury.[43,44] A pure stimulus-response relationship no longer exists. Both previously innocuous stimuli to the dorsal horn and stimuli from outside the original receptive field cause pain. As a result, the interpretation of diagnostic injections based on an acute pain paradigm may be inaccurate.[44] In the presence of chronic pain, it is possible that an anesthetic injection of an injured nerve or structure may not produce complete pain relief, anesthetizing an adjacent normal nerve or structure may relieve pain, and provoking a normal structure or nerve may reproduce a patient's clinical pain.

Finally, psychological factors are important sources of false-positive results with discography. There are two components to pain. The first is the nociceptive process initiated by tissue injury, and the second is the psychological and emotional reaction to nociception. The pain response that is amplified in patients with issues of chronic pain, social stressors (such as secondary gain or litigation claims), or psychological distress disorder increases the false-positive results injection. A patient with chronic pain should always be seen in the context of these interacting factors. Measuring the response to a diagnostic injection, and in particular to provocative discography, always relies, to some extent, on patients' self-reports of pain. Therefore, psychological factors can clearly affect the measurement of the response to a diagnostic injection. As a result, when assessing patients' responses to diagnostic injections, the relative contribution of nociception and psychological factors should be considered and the reliability of patients' self-reports of pain estimated.

Clearly, there are a number of potential sources of both false-positive and false-negative responses with discography. In an effort to study the potential for false-positive results, several studies have investigated the ability of discography to provoke back pain in asymptomatic subjects.

Holt, in 1968, reported a 36% rate of positive discography in asymptomatic subjects, leading him to discredit the use of the test.[45] However, there were several methodologic flaws with this study. The most notable flaws were that all of the subjects were prisoners, a highly irritating contrast medium was used, and, most importantly, Holt did not include a positive pain response as a criterion for a positive injection (i.e., the criteria for a positive result were based primarily on radiologic images).

Holt's findings were subsequently refuted in a well-designed study by Walsh and colleagues, who demonstrated a 0% rate of positive discography in asymptomatic volunteers.[46] Walsh and colleagues studied ten asymptomatic subjects and seven patients with chronic low back pain. The criteria for a positive result differed between the two groups. For both groups, a positive result required a 3-out-of-5 pain intensity (using a pain thermometer), two types of pain behavior (as assessed by videotape review), and structural degeneration. For the patients with chronic low back pain, a positive result also required that the provoked pain be similar to their usual pain. Obviously, it was not possible to evaluate the similarity of pain in asymptomatic subjects because they had no pain prior to the injection. Among the asymptomatic subjects, five of ten had at least one structurally abnormal disc; however, none satisfied the criteria for a positive test. Thus, the false-positive rate in these asymptomatic volunteers was 0%. Among the chronic low back pain patients, all seven had at least one structurally abnormal disc, and six of seven patients had at least one disc that satisfied the criteria for a positive result. Overall, 13 discs were structurally abnormal, with seven being positive and six negative. Of note, two of the seven had at least one disc that was structurally abnormal and was associated with intense, but atypical, provoked pain, as well as pain behaviors. In each case, the test result was considered to be negative, given that the provoked pain was different from the patient's typical pain.

The Walsh study was important for several reasons. First, using strict criteria for a positive test, including postinjection review of videotaped responses, there was excellent interrater reliability. Diagnostic tests that rely on an observer's interpretation are not clinically useful unless there is good interobserver reliability (i.e., the same test applied to the same patient should always produce the same result).[47] Thus, Walsh and colleagues' study established reproducible criteria for a positive result from discography. Second, by demonstrating a 0% false-positive rate in asymptomatic subjects, Walsh and colleagues effectively refuted Holt's assertion that the false-positive rate of discography was so high as to make it useless. Third, Walsh and colleagues demonstrated that patients suffering from chronic low back pain were capable of developing different types of pain in response to provocation discography. According to their criteria, only provoked pain that was similar to the patient's typical symptoms constituted a positive test. Atypical provoked pain, even if intense and accompanied by pain behaviors, constituted a negative test.

The asymptomatic subjects studied by Walsh and colleagues were all healthy volunteers, with an average age of 23. Caragee and colleagues recently expanded on the Walsh study of asymptomatic subjects by studying a cohort of subjects who did not have low back pain, but whose clinical characteristics more closely matched those of patients with low back pain who typically present for discography.[23] Thirty subjects with no history of low back pain were recruited: Ten had previous cervical surgery with good results, ten had the same surgery but had persistent chronic pain, and ten had primary somatization disorders. Lumbar discography was performed and interpreted according to the Walsh protocol. Four somatization patients dropped out before beginning the study and two stopped the study after only one or two discs were injected, and, therefore, were not included in the study analysis.

Among the subjects with good results from previous cervical surgery, seven of ten had at least one disc that had an outer annular rupture (10 of 30 discs, total), while only one of ten had a positive result. The patient with a positive test had a high Zung depression score. Of the subjects with chronic pain, five of ten patients had at least one disc that had an outer annular rupture (11 of 32 discs, total), with four of ten having at least one positive disc. Of the 11 discs with significant structural abnormalities, seven were positive and four were negative. Among the subjects with somatization disorder, three-quarters had at least one disc that had an outer annular rupture (6 of 13 discs, total), with three-quarters having at least one positive disc. Of the six discs with significant structural abnormalities, two were positive and four were negative. Based on these data, Caragee and colleagues concluded that in individuals with normal psychometrics and without chronic pain, the rate of false-positives is very low if strict criteria are applied, and that the false-positive rate increases with increased annular disruption.

The study by Caragee and colleagues is important for a number of reasons. Firstly, it confirms the finding by Walsh and colleagues that in subjects without a history of low back pain, and without psychosocial risk factors, provocation of a significant pain response with discography is unusual, with an incidence of 0% in the Walsh study and 10% in the Caragee study. It also confirms the Walsh finding that although discs in this population are often structurally abnormal (combining the studies, 12 of 20 subjects had at least one structurally abnormal disc), they are no more likely to be positive than a structurally normal disc. More importantly, the Caragee study reveals that in subjects without a history of low back pain, but with a history of chronic pain or a somatization disorder, provocation of a significant pain response with discography is common, with an incidence of 40% in the chronic pain group and 75% in the somatization disorder group. Furthermore, the more disrupted the annulus, the greater is the chance of a positive response.

Caragee and colleagues' study is a powerful reminder of the importance of psychosocial factors in modulating pain, while also demonstrating the potential of false-positive responses with discography. However, in assessing the importance of this information, it is necessary to reconsider the premise of discography.

The premise of discography is that reproduction of a patients' clinical symptoms during the injection identifies the disc as the source of pain. The rationale for its use is that the results can help discriminate among the various structures that may be responsible for axial pain. Therefore, to establish its validity, the criteria for a true positive disc must be determined in the relevant population, which is back pain sufferers. The Walsh data on patients with chronic low back pain demonstrated that it is common for patients undergoing discography to have intense pain that is very different in location and character from their clinical symptoms. In the Walsh study, the criteria for a positive test in the chronic low back pain population required that provoked pain be similar to the patient's clinical symptoms. Unfortunately, without a gold standard for axial pain, the validity of incorporating measures of familiarity of pain into the criteria for a positive test cannot be precisely defined.[17]

Caragee and colleagues clearly demonstrated the potential for false-positive responses with discography. However, given the premise of discography and the fact that patients with chronic low back pain frequently have intense but atypical pain during discography, it is difficult to know the significance of any pain response in an asymptomatic subject.

Although the sensitivity and specificity of provocative discography cannot be precisely defined, it is important to remember that the ultimate criterion for a diagnostic test is whether the patient is better off as a result. If a test can predict the response to treatment, and is reliable and reproducible, then it may be clinically useful,[17,34,35] even without a defined sensitivity and specificity.

In individuals with disc degeneration and annular defects, discography may elicit low back pain (LBP) with injection whether the patient is symptomatic with serious LBP or not. The ability of an individual to differentiate the true site of LBP by the quality of sensation with disc injection (concordancy) of pain produced by the injected disc also may not be reliable. In fact, individuals may not have the neural discrimination to differentiate pain originating from different sites in the low back and pelvis.

In contrast to the surgical treatment of radiculopathy, the surgical treatment of axial pain is controversial, as studies have demonstrated a wide disparity in outcomes.[7-15,48] This disparity has been attributed to a number of factors, including type of fusion (interbody versus intertransverse, instrumented versus noninstrumented), approach (anterior versus posterior versus 360°), surgeon variability, and methodologic differences. The results from discography have been an important part of the preoperative evaluation in most of these studies, but, typically, the criteria for a positive test have not been strictly defined. The validity of the criteria used to define a positive discogram is another variable that could potentially affect surgical outcome.

PRESSURE-CONTROLLED DISCOGRAPHY

In an effort to develop criteria for discography that can be used to predict surgical outcome, Derby and colleagues reported on a cohort of patients who underwent provocative discography under pressure monitoring.[39] Although the pathophysiology of lumbar discogenic pain is still uncertain, there is presumptive evidence that it results from both mechanical stimulation of nociceptors in the annulus as well as by chemical irritation by enzymes and breakdown products involved in the degradative process.[39]

Physiologic loading of the disc creates horizontal and vertical stresses within the nucleus, annulus, and end plates of the disc that are directly related to the weight of the body above the segment and any added moment stresses resulting from body position. The relationship between intradiscal pressure and body position has been quantified by several investigators.[19,49] Derby and colleagues hypothesized that some discs were more sensitive to chemical stimuli than mechanical stimuli. Pain at discography that occurred at low pressures, below the typical weighted values, would result from chemical stimulation of the outer annulus by contact with contrast dye. Pain occurring at higher pressures would result from mechanical stimulation of the annulus by the fluid-distending stress of discography.

In order to establish the criteria for chemical and mechanical stimulation, Derby and colleagues used data from a preliminary study on disc pressure measurements at the time of discography.[39] In a preliminary study, they combined provocative discography with measurement of intradiscal pressure, comparing results from discography performed in the lying position with results from discography performed in the sitting position. The criterion for a positive result was 6-out-of-10 concordant pain. In normal discs, the average opening pressure, representing the intrinsic pressure of the disc, was 27 pounds per square inch (psi) in the side-lying position and 85 psi in the sitting position. As the degree of degeneration increased, the opening pressure decreased in both positions. However, the threefold difference between the opening pressure in the sitting position versus the lying position was maintained between equally degenerated discs. In the majority of discs, concordant pain provocation occurred when contrast first reached the outer annulus, with the maximal pain response usually occurring at pressures only 10 to 30 psi above the opening pressure. From these findings, Derby and colleagues concluded that in degenerated discs with annular disruption, pain provocation during discography is usually caused by low-pressure stimulation of an irritable outer annulus by a chemical stimulus.

Based on this information, the authors created a protocol for grading the sensitivity of the disc annulus that could be used to predict surgical outcome. Four categories of discs were defined. In chemical discs, pain is provoked at minimal pressure; 15 psi above opening pressure was chosen as the threshold for a chemical disc because this is well below the mechanical load resulting from sitting. In mechanical discs, pain is provoked at pressures between standing and lying; that is, between 15 and 50 psi above opening pressure. In indeterminate discs, pain occurs between 51 and 90 psi above opening pressure, and, in normal discs, there is no pain.

This classification system was applied to a consecutive series of patients referred for lumbar discography prior to potential fusion surgery. Following discography, patients were returned to the care of their referring surgeons, who independently decided whether surgery was indicated, and if so, whether it should be an intertransverse or interbody fusion. The disc classification was not reported to the surgeon.

The subjects were contacted at two follow-up intervals, at a mean time of 16 and 32 months, with the overall outcome classified as favorable or unfavorable depending on the results from three different outcome tools. Looking at all surgical cases combined, there was no significant difference in outcome between patients undergoing interbody versus intertransverse fusion, with both groups having approximately a 50% favorable outcome.

However, among patients classified as having a chemically sensitive disc, there was a highly significant difference in outcome between patients undergoing interbody versus intertransverse fusion. Within that group, 89% of the interbody fusion patients had a favorable outcome, while only 20% of the intertransverse fusion patients had a favorable outcome. Patients with chemically sensitive discs who did not have surgery of any kind had an 88% unfavorable outcome. There was no significant difference in patient demographics, including the percentage of patients with workers' compensation claims, between the patients with favorable outcomes and unfavorable outcomes. Other than workers' compensation status, psychosocial risk factors were not assessed.

Until now, the clinical significance of degenerative disc disease in a patient with axial pain was uncertain because treatments directed specifically at the disc (i.e., fusion) led to variable outcomes. Based on the data of Derby and colleagues, it now appears that there is a subset of patients with degenerative disc disease who have chemically sensitive discs and who have outcomes with surgery that rival those of patients undergoing partial disc excision for herniated nucleus pulposus. The surgery performed must be an interbody fusion, presumably because the disc is completely excised, therefore removing the source of the noxious stimulus. If these results stand up to long-term follow-up—and are replicated by other investigators—then the use of pressure-controlled discography as a diagnostic test to predict patients who will benefit from surgical fusion will be validated.

In addition to potentially having the ability to predict outcome, adding pressure monitoring to provocative discography improves interobserver reliability and, therefore, reproducibility. Assessing the response to discography requires measuring pain before and after the injection. There are three components to pain: its intensity, location, and character. If the location and character of the pain provoked at discography is similar to or exactly the same as the patient's clinical symptoms, it satisfies the criteria for concordant pain. The intensity of pain is measured both by the patient's self-report (e.g., using a numerical rating) and by observed pain behaviors. However, the intensity of provoked pain is dependent on the intensity of the stimulus. In simple terms, the harder one pushes on the syringe, the more likely the disc is to hurt. By measuring intradiscal pressures, the intensity of the stimulus can be quantified, allowing more reliable comparisons between patients and discographers. Although it is possible to estimate injection pressures manually, using a controlled inflation syringe with digital pressure readout provides a precise value.

TECHNIQUE

There are two approaches to the lumbar disc: posterior and lateral.[50] The posterior approach necessitates a dural puncture and, therefore, should be avoided. (Disc puncture is typically performed with a 22- or 25-gauge needle.) There is some evidence that using an introducer needle can reduce the risk of infection, although this is not a universal practice.[51] Although rarely encountered, a variety of complications are possible with discography, including neural injury, bleeding, and intradural leakage of injected substances.[36,52,53] There have been case reports of disc herniations resulting from discography.[54,55] Canine studies have had conflicting results on the potential for disc injury during discography; however, the weight of evidence in humans suggests that this is not a significant problem.[55-58]

The most significant risk associated with discography is infection. The rate of discitis reported in the literature is as high as 1.3% per disc, and serious morbidity has resulted.[51,59,60] However, practice audits at centers performing a large volume of discography have demonstrated infection rates as low as 0 out of 10,000 (R. Derby, personal communication). There is experimental evidence that prophylactic antibiotics, both intravenous and intradiscal, can prevent discitis.[61-64] As a result, many practitioners routinely administer prophylactic antibiotics, particularly to high-risk patients such as diabetics.

SUMMARY OF LUMBAR DISCOGRAPHY

The primary utility of discography is as a provocative clinical test for the evaluation of axial spinal pain. The usefulness of any diagnostic study is critically dependent on the critical diagnosis and the pretest probability that a particular disorder is present.[17,34,35] Therefore, the results from discography must always be interpreted in the context of the patient's clinical presentation. In particular, prior to discography there should be a careful assessment of psychosocial risk factors.

An underlying assumption of the rationale for diagnostic injections, including provocative discography, is that it is possible to accurately measure pain. Measuring the change in pain after an injection relies, to a large extent, on a patient's self-report. Psychosocial factors affect the reaction to changes in nociceptive input and, therefore, self-reports of pain. If patients are psychologically distressed, the rationale for the injection may be invalid. This can potentially lead to both false-positive and false-negative responses. In assessing patients' responses to diagnostic injections, the relative contribution of nociception and psychological factors should be considered, and the reliability of patients' self-reports of pain estimated. Caragee and associates demonstrated the potential for psychological factors to affect the results from discography. Although more study is needed in this area, at a minimum, it is important to be aware of psychosocial risk factors and understand how they might affect interpretation of the results from diagnostic injections. Moreover, the implications of psychosocial risk factors on eventual treatment, regardless of any results on diagnostic injections, should be considered. As an example, patients with somatization disorders are probably not good candidates for spinal fusion for axial pain. Therefore, discography is not a clinically useful test in those individuals and should only be performed in exceptional circumstances.

If a patient is being considered for surgical fusion for axial pain, pressure-controlled discography is indicated to determine whether they have chemically sensitized discs, in which case the data of Derby and colleagues suggests a high likelihood of success with an anterior interbody fusion.[39] At present, it is not clear what the appropriate treatment should be for discs falling into either the mechanically sensitive or the indeterminate category. Preliminary information suggests that intertransverse fusion alone may be effective for mechanically sensitive discs.[39] Future research should focus on validating the disc classification system proposed by Derby and colleagues and, in particular, further studying the predictive value of the mechanically sensitive and indeterminate categories.

Although not the primary focus of discography, it is important to assess the radiologic findings. The images should be reviewed to confirm that the needle was placed into the nucleus and that the subsequent dye injection fills the nucleus. Annular injections, injections into the space between the annulus and the nuclear cavity, and venous uptake are all possible and may invalidate the results.[65,66]

Several classification schemes have been developed to describe annular pathology as visualized by discography.[25,33,67-70] Regardless of the exact classification scheme used, it is important to note the degree of annular degeneration, the presence of annular fissures, and whether the annulus is competent or incompetent. If a patient has a convincing pain response but no evidence of a radial annular fissure on discography, postdiscography CT scanning should be considered because some discs that appear normal on discography are found to be disrupted on CT discography.[33] In addition to annular pathology, both Schmorl's nodes and end-plate disruptions should be noted, as they may be clinically significant.[41,71]

If a patient has at least one disc that is both normal structurally and does not elicit a pain response, that is considered by some surgeons to serve as a control disc. A control injection may be helpful in deciding whether a pain response at another disc is a true positive result or reflects an exaggerated reaction to nociception. However, a more valid control would probably be a structurally abnormal disc. Although the significance of the results from control injections has not been formally validated, clinical experience suggests that if at least one structurally abnormal disc does not hurt, then pain provoked at another disc is more likely to be a true positive.

As a final note, there are some surgeons who do not believe that discography is necessary prior to fusion, as they feel that the diagnosis of discogenic pain can be made by clinical and radiographic criteria. There are substantial data suggesting that the clinical examination is of minimal use in discriminating between potential axial pain generators.[72,73] A possible exception to this is a McKenzie mechanical assessment, which may be able to predict the results from discography.[74] There have been several studies demonstrating that MRI cannot reliably predict which discs are painful on discography, at least to the level of confidence required to rely solely on MRI for surgical decision making.[2,31,75] A high-intensity zone in the posterior annulus, as visualized on MRI, has recently been proposed as a marker for painful discs.[76,77] Although highly specific, the sensitivity of this finding is only 26%, which limits the usefulness of the high-intensity zone in selecting patients for surgery.[33] If a patient undergoes a fusion for lumbar axial pain without preoperative discography, both the patient and the surgeon should be aware that the level adjacent to the planned fusion may be a source of clinical symptoms, regardless of the findings on MRI scan.

LUMBAR SELECTIVE EPIDURAL INJECTION

As is the case with the intervertebral disc, spinal nerves can be injected with contrast, local anesthetic, or other substances. Both the provocative response (pain occurring in response to a mechanical or chemical stimulus, or both) and the analgesic response provide clinically useful information.

Nerve root blocks were first developed to diagnose the source of radicular pain when imaging studies suggested possible compression of several roots.[20,47,78-84] Early studies on selective nerve root injections described an extraforaminal approach, in which a needle is advanced at right angles to the spinal nerve outside the neural foramen. Localization of the needle adjacent to the nerve relies on leg pain provocation, presumably resulting from penetration of the nerve by the needle.[20,81,82,84]

A selective epidural injection is a variation of the selective nerve root injection. As the nerve roots leave the dura to enter the foramen and form the spinal nerve, they carry an extension of the dura with them, which becomes the epineurium of the spinal nerve. The epineurium is, in turn, enveloped by an epiradicular membrane, which is an extension of the anterior and posterior epidural membranes.[85] Injection of contrast into the epiradicular membrane will outline the nerve root, dorsal root ganglion, spinal nerve, and ventral ramus. Proximally, contrast will flow around the dural sac at the takeoff of the nerve root. If injected outside the epiradicular membrane, contrast will spread diffusely in the epidural fat and, therefore, be of limited diagnostic value.

A selective epidural injection differs from a selective nerve root injection in that the goal is to inject into the epiradicular tissues. The spread of injected solutions will depend on the anatomy of the epiradicular membrane, which is an extension of the epidural space, leading to the term *selective epidural injection*. There are two major advantages of a selective epidural technique over a selective nerve root technique. (1) With a selective epidural injection, a foraminal approach is used and contact with the nerve is avoided, minimizing the potential for neural injury. Rather than relying on leg pain provocation from needle contact, needle localization is confirmed with contrast-enhanced images demonstrating an outline of the nerve. (2) A selective epidural approach ensures that the injection incorporates all the sites where pathology can affect the nerve, from the disc level in the subarticular zone out lateral to the extraforaminal zone. If the pathology causing a patient's symptoms is a paramedian disc herniation, but the nerve is injected in the extraforaminal zone (as with a classic selective nerve root injection), the portion of the nerve from which the pain is coming may not be anesthetized, potentially leading to a false-negative result.

A selective epidural injection anesthetizes not only the spinal nerve itself, but also all its branches. Two important branches of the spinal nerve are the sinuvertebral nerve and the medial branch of the dorsal primary ramus. The sinuvertebral nerve forms just lateral to the foramen from the ventral ramus and the grey ramus communicans.[6] Once formed, the nerve reenters the foramen, where it runs across the back of the vertebral body just below the upper pedicle. Two branches arise from the nerve—one ascending branch, supplying the posterior longitudinal ligament (PLL) and the next higher disc, and one descending, innervating the disc and PLL at the level of entry of the parent nerve.[6] Each sinuvertebral nerve is also distributed to the dura mater, with descending branches up to two segments caudally and an ascending branch up to one segment. The dorsal primary ramus from each spinal nerve divides into three branches: the medial, lateral, and intermediate (except at L5, which has only a medial and a lateral branch).[6] The most important of these branches is the medial branch, which hooks medially around the base of the superior articular process (SAP) at the inferior-most aspect of the intervertebral foramen, supplying the Z joints just above and below its course. Thus, a selective epidural injection will partially anesthetize the dura (including the dural nerve root sleeves) up to two segments caudally and one segment rostrally, the PLL and intervertebral disc at the same level as the nerve and one segment rostrally, and the Z joints at the same level of the nerve and one segment below.

If a selective epidural injection is being performed for radicular pain, the fact that these structures are also anesthetized is irrelevant because they are sources of axial pain, not radicular pain. However, if an injection is being performed for axial pain, it is important to realize that pain relief after an injection can occur with pathology in any of the structures innervated by the nerve.

A selective epidural injection can potentially be helpful in diagnosing axial pain.[86] Any lesion that affects a nerve root also necessarily affects its dural sleeve and, therefore, is a potential cause of axial pain. In the case of herniated nucleus pulposus, disc material in the epidural space has been demonstrated to elicit an inflammatory response not only in the nerve root but also the dura. Relief of both axial and radicular pain with a selective epidural injection suggests that the same lesion is responsible for both. However, it is difficult to be certain that the axial component of the pain is arising from structures above or below the injected level. In patients with predominantly axial pain, fully characterizing the source of pain may require synovial joint or disc injections, or both, depending on the clinical situation.

A selective epidural injection has two components: (1) the provocative pain response resulting from contrast injection and (2) the analgesic response resulting from injection of local anesthetic or corticosteroid, or both. In evaluating provoked pain, it is important to compare the location and character of the provoked response to the patient's typical symptoms. Furthermore, the onset of provoked pain should be related to the location of the leading edge of the contrast solution when pain begins.[86] Normal epidural tissue is not painful when gently stimulated by contrast solution. In the absence of scar tissue, pain provocation indicates that the tissue being stimulated is irritated. For example, early provocation of pain, when contrast is still in the foramen, suggests foraminal stenosis or a foraminal disc herniation. Late pain provocation when the contrast approaches the disc above is consistent with a paramedian disc herniation.

Immediately after the injection, the effect of the local anesthetic injected on the patient's symptoms should be assessed, both at rest and in response to mechanical stimulation. Studies on selective nerve root injections have used the criterion for a positive analgesic response to be from 80% to 100% relief.[47,86] The significance of lesser degrees of pain relief in response to an injection is uncertain. If corticosteroid is included in the injection, the patient should be reevaluated 1 week afterward because the degree of pain relief at that interval can provide important information (see later discussion).

As is the case with provocative discography, a number of factors can lead to both false-positive and false-negative results from selective epidural injections. These factors include changes in CNS nociceptive processing that occur with chronic pain, psychological factors, and placebo responses.[43,44] However, in contrast to provocative discography, selective epidural injections are performed primarily for radicular pain. Therefore, there is a well-established gold standard—surgical exploration—against which diagnostic tests can be compared.

Several studies have evaluated the clinical utility of selective epidural and selective nerve root injections. Individual studies have investigated the predictive value of pain provocation, immediate pain relief from local anesthetic injection, and prolonged pain relief from corticosteroid in evaluating patients with radiculopathy.[47,83,86,87] A synthesis of the results from the studies on clinical utility suggests that the following protocol should be used to interpret the response to selective nerve root injections:

- If a patient has concordant or exact provoked pain in response to injection of contrast, complete pain relief following injection of local anesthetic, and a prolonged steroid response (>1 week), the injected nerve root is mediating the patient's symptoms, and a good result can be expected from surgical decompression, assuming a correctable lesion is demonstrated on imaging studies.
- If a patient has discordant pain, incomplete immediate pain relief, and no prolonged steroid response, the injected nerve is probably not mediating the patient's symptoms, and an alternate pain generator should be searched for.
- If an intermediate response occurs, a number of different possibilities exist. The patient may still have symptoms arising from a single nerve root, he or she may have symptoms from multiple roots, or he or she may not have radicular pain. If the clinical situation is highly suggestive of radiculopathy, it may be reasonable to repeat the selective nerve root injection, potentially with a control injection at an adjacent nerve. If the control injection is negative, the result from the active injection is more likely to be a true positive, particularly if there are multiple factors supporting a clinical significant response. If the control injection is positive or intermediate, and there is evidence of nerve root compression at both levels, it may be reasonable to perform a multilevel decompression, depending, of course, on the many clinical variables that may exist.

As with any diagnostic injection, if patients are psychologically distressed, the criteria used to interpret the test may be invalid. Recent data from Caragee and colleagues on lumbar discography reinforces the effect that psychosocial risk factors have on pain responses. Although more study is needed in this area, at a minimum it is important to note these risk factors and understand how they might affect interpretation of the result.

The usefulness of a selective epidural injection is primarily related to the associated provocative and analgesic pain responses. However, the contrast-enhanced images from the injection can reveal pathologic findings.[47,86] Two examples of this are a perpendicular nerve root sign, resulting from up-down foraminal stenosis, and obstruction to proximal flow of contrast, which can occur with foraminal stenosis, disc herniations, and scar tissue. The primary utility of findings such as these is to confirm findings evident on advanced imaging studies.

THORACIC DISCOGRAPHY

OVERVIEW

Thoracic spinal pain, while less common, is as disabling as low back pain. Thoracic disc pathology can produce a pain pattern mimicking visceral pain in the absence of true visceral pathology. Musculoskeletal pathology of the thoracolumbar junction can be mistaken for a gynecological problem with pain referred to the pelvic region. Similarly, disc pathology in the mid-thoracic region can present as chronic abdominal pain. The pain from the lower thoracic area can be confused with renal or ureteral pain.

Thoracic discography is performed much less frequently than either cervical or lumbar discography because of the relative infrequency of symptomatic thoracic disc pathology.

Clinicians are less likely to ascribe thoracic pain to discogenic disease of the thoracic spine than to other more common etiologies, such as facet joint pain, muscle pain, skeletal pain, or visceral pain. The role of facet joints has been implicated in 48% of patients with chronic thoracic spinal pain without clinical or radiologic evidence of disc involvement. A comprehensive evaluation for pain is necessary prior to performing or recommending a thoracic discogram.

Mechanically, mid-thoracic discs are subject to greater axial compression and bending due to their location in the apex of the thoracic kyphotic curve of the adult.

TECHNIQUE

The presence of the head of a rib and the attachment to the transverse process, the narrow disc space, and the proximity of the pleura pose difficulty in the visualization and accessing of the disc space. The disc space narrowing may be severe enough to preclude the safe performance of the procedure.

In the thoracic spine, the processes face posteriorly, while, in the lumbar spine, they face medially. The angles of inclination of the thoracic facet joints are 60°, which make the procedure more challenging. Accurate needle placement in thoracic discography requires different needle angulation and more skill by the interventionist for a safe procedure.

Using oblique fluoroscopy, with the patient prone, the x-ray beam is angled 30° to 45° lateromedially to the thoracic spine. The beam is also angled craniocaudally so that it is tangential to the intervertebral disc being studied. A down-the-barrel approach is used with a 25-gauge spinal needle. On oblique fluoroscopy, the target is a "box"-like image on the fluoroscopic image. The vertical sides of this box are formed medially by a line joining the pedicles and laterally by a line joining the head of the ribs. The horizontal margins of this box are the superior and inferior vertebral end plates.

Using an aseptic technique, intermittent fluoroscopy is used to guide a 25-gauge needle toward the box-like image just described. The needle passes between the superior articular facet medially and the head of the rib laterally and enters the intervertebral disc at its posterolateral aspect.

SUMMARY OF THORACIC DISCOGRAPHY

Thoracic discography is indicated when conventional radiologic imaging does not disclose an etiology for thoracic pain. Referred visceral pain and musculoskeletal pain complicate the diagnosis of thoracic pain, often mimicking thoracic spinal pain or obscuring its origin. Like lumbar and cervical discography, thoracic discography is not a screening procedure but rather a confirmatory one, especially when conventional radiologic imaging has not described or disclosed pathology responsible for symptoms.

Pneumothorax has been mentioned as a possible severe complication. By using a meticulous technique and a carefully directed needle advancement, this can be avoided. Immediate recognition of pneumothorax is essential because this condition may not develop until the patient is in recovery.

Thoracic discography is considered a safe procedure when done by an expert spine interventionalist.

CERVICAL DISCOGRAPHY

OVERVIEW

Cervical discography is comparable in many ways to the thoracic and lumbar discography. The underlying premise is the same: Injection of the disc replicates the clinical noxious stimulus responsible for the patient's symptoms, and reproduction of the patients clinical symptoms during the injection confirms the disc as the source of pain.

A major difference between lumbar and cervical discography is the relationship between pain provocation and disc morphology. In the lumbar spine, discs have varying degrees of disruption of the outer annulus. The pain resulting from lumbar discography has been shown to be directly related to the degree of fissuring of the outer annulus.[40,42] This finding provides a link between disc pathology and provoked pain, supporting circumstantial evidence suggesting that internal disc disruption is an important cause of axial low back pain.[6] Obviously, it would not have been possible to make this observation if all lumbar discs had the same degree of annular disruption.

Morphologically, cervical discs are very different from lumbar discs. Although both have a peripheral annulus fibrosus and a central nucleus, the cervical disc also has posterolateral uncovertebral joints. These are not true joints but are clefts in the annulus that communicate with the nucleus in the majority of individuals by early adulthood.[88] As a result of these clefts, if contrast is injected into cervical discs, the majority of them will demonstrate "annular tears."[89] Some cervical discs hurt when injected; others do not. Because they all have annular disruption, however, it is not possible to correlate provoked pain with underlying pathology.[89]

At present, the mechanisms responsible for cervical discogenic pain are unknown. Therefore, although a positive discogram in the lumbar spine can be used to diagnose a specific pathologic syndrome, a positive discogram in the cervical spine cannot. Ideally, a diagnostic test will reveal the underlying target disorder that is responsible for pain.[17] The fact that cervical discography cannot do so compromises its clinical utility and constitutes a significant difference between cervical and lumbar discography.

VALIDITY OF CERVICAL DISCOGRAPHY

Several studies have cast doubt on the validity of cervical discography.[90-92] Holt, in 1964, reported a 100% rate of positive discography in asymptomatic subjects. As in his study on lumbar discography, all the subjects were prisoners, and he used a highly irritating contrast medium. In contrast to his lumbar study, a positive pain response, rather than a radiologic abnormality, was the criterion for a positive result.[91] Shinomaya and colleagues reported a 50% rate of positive discography in patients without neck pain. However, this was a group of patients with spondylitic myelopathy, thus constituting a very different group than the one in which the test is typically performed.[92]

Bogduk and Aprill studied patients who had axial neck pain, only (i.e., without neurologic symptoms), with both Z-joint injections and discography. Using 100% pain relief as the criteria for a positive Z joint, they discovered that 41% had a positive disc and a positive Z joint at the same level. If Z-joint blocks were both highly sensitive and specific, this result would be an indication that there is a high false-positive rate associated with discography; that is, if the Z-joint block is a true positive, the disc must be a false positive. However, the Z-joint blocks in this study were not controlled, which in other studies has been shown to have a false-positive rate of 27%.[93] This would suggest a 14% false-positive rate for discography if the response to Z-joint blocks was used as the gold standard by which to judge discography.[90]

Schellhas and colleagues, in a well-designated study, used a nonirritating contrast medium to perform cervical discography on a group of volunteers recruited from the community as well as on a series of patients with chronic neck pain. They found that the majority of discs in both subjects and patients, including those that appeared normal on MRI, had annular tears on discography. However, discs from asymptomatic subjects, even if morphologically abnormal, were associated with low-level pain responses. Among patients with chronic neck pain, however, there was a group that had intense pain with disc injection.[89]

The results from this study refute the findings of Holt and Shimomaya, which suggested that the degree of pain provocation with discography was unrelated to whether or not the patient had neck pain. The Schellhas findings demonstrated that most cervical discs are morphologically abnormal and are associated with some discomfort on injection, but there is a definite, severe, concordant pain response in symptomatic patients that does not occur in asymptomatic subjects. The Schellhas study complements the Walsh study in the lumbar spine, demonstrating that although pain can occur during injection of discs in asymptomatic subjects, it occurs at low levels of intensity. Schellhas and colleagues evaluated interobserver reliability for the morphologic evaluation of MRI and discograms but did not assess the interobserver reliability of the pain response, as did Walsh. The importance of psychosocial factors was not addressed in the Schellhas study, but presumably they are as important with cervical discography as in lumbar discography.

Regardless of these studies on the sensitivity and specificity of cervical discography, it is important to remember that the ultimate criterion for a diagnostic test is whether the patient is better off as a result.[17] The primary indication for provocative discography is to determine whether a patient with chronic spinal pain, who has failed aggressive efforts at conservative care, can be helped with spinal fusion. As in the lumbar spine, the surgical treatment of axial neck pain is controversial. However, there is evidence that patients selected for anterior spinal fusion on the basis of discography can achieve outcomes in some studies ranging from 70% to 80%.[94-96]

Although the results from discography played an important part in surgical decision making in these studies, the criteria for a positive test were not strictly defined. Unlike the lumbar spine, pressure-controlled discography has not been used in the cervical spine. There is abundant evidence regarding the role of mechanical and chemical factors in causing lumbar spinal pain; however, there is little equivalent information in the cervical spine. While there is some information on the normative values for intradiscal pressures in the cervical spine,[97] for technical reasons, it is difficult to measure pressures accurately at the time of cervical discography. Therefore, at present, there is no way to reproducibly measure the stimulus applied to the cervical disc.

TECHNIQUE

Cervical discography is a technique in which proficiency and expertise are essential. The precise detailed knowledge of the anatomy of the cervical spine and the vital structures in the anterior cervical region is of utmost importance. The procedure is performed with the patient in the supine position and with support under the shoulders and the head and neck slightly hyperextended. The disc cannot be entered posteriorly due to the spinal cord or anteriorly because of the trachea. Therefore, entry into the cervical disc is usually done from the right anterolateral approach.

As a result, a number of potential complications can occur.[98-101] As the needle is advanced to the disc, puncture of the carotid artery or deeper vessels of the neck can lead to bleeding complications and possible airway compromise. If the needle is advanced too far in a posterior direction, it may puncture vessels in the anterior epidural space, potentially resulting in hematoma formation and spinal cord compression. Puncture of the spinal cord itself is possible, with obvious consequences, particularly if contrast is injected into the cord. Acute quadriplegia has been reported following cervical discography, presumably related to posterior displacement of disc tissue with injection and resultant spinal cord compression.[99]

In addition to the risks associated with needle placement, infectious complications related to cervical discography are potentially devastating. In addition to the risk of introduction of skin organisms, there is a potential for enteric organisms to be introduced into the disc if the needle passes through the hypopharynx or esophagus. Discitis may lead to epidural abscess, with resultant quadriplegia.[97] Because of the potentially catastrophic adverse effects associated with discitis in the cervical spine, some consider diabetes mellitus to be an absolute contraindication to cervical discography. Prophylactic antibiotics, either intravenous or intradiscal, should be strongly considered for all patients.

SUMMARY OF CERVICAL DISCOGRAPHY

At this time, cervical discography must be considered primarily an art rather than a science. We do not really know the underlying disorder we are diagnosing with this test, nor can we predict with confidence the results from surgery. Given the potential complications associated with cervical discography, it should only be performed by individuals who have a detailed understanding of the anatomy of the cervical spine and are skilled in performing and interpreting diagnostic spinal injections of other structures, most notably the lumbar disc. Because virtually all cervical discs contain annular tears, the role of CT discography in the cervical spine is limited. There are no published data suggesting that postdiscography CT provides clinically useful information.

Retrospective studies suggest that anterior interbody fusion may be an effective treatment for discogenic neck pain; however, at present, there are no discographic criteria that can be used reliably to predict outcome from surgery. Understanding that clinically useful criteria for interpreting cervical provocative discography have not been defined, experienced discographers consider the following characteristics to suggest a symptomatic disc: concordant or exact pain (exact more significant), intensity greater than 6-out-of-10, pain 1 minute after injection at least 50% of the maximum intensity, two or more pain behaviors in response to injection, low intradiscal pressure at pain provocation (as estimated by manual pressure), and a negative control injection.

CERVICAL SELECTIVE EPIDURAL STEROID INJECTION

As in the lumbar spine, the epineurium of each cervical spinal nerve root is enveloped by an epiradicular membrane, which is an extension of the anterior and posterior epidural membranes.[84] As a result, selective epidural injections may be performed in the cervical spine and, given the analogous innervation of the cervical and lumbar spines,[30] may be used to accomplish the same goal; that is, to determine the nerve root responsible for radicular pain.

Cervical selective nerve root injections are performed using an anterolateral approach, with the radiologic landmark being the base of the superior articular process as viewed in an oblique projection of the spine and the midpoint of the lateral mass as viewed in the anteroposterior projection. Care must be taken to keep the needle tip posterior to the vertebral artery at all times during insertion.

Unlike the lumbar spine, there is no information on the predictive value of pain provocation, immediate pain relief from local anesthetic injection, and prolonged pain relief from corticosteroid in evaluating patients with cervical radiculopathy. Nonetheless, the responses to these injections are commonly interpreted using the same criteria as in the lumbar spine. There have been no studies correlating pathology with the contrast-enhanced images from selective cervical epidural injections; therefore, the primary clinical utility of these images is to ensure that injectate is confined to the target nerve root.

There are multiple reports of serious complications stemming from central nervous system (CNS) infarctions, including anterior spinal artery syndrome, quadriplegia, ischemic stroke, and death. The incidence of these severe complications is unknown, but they are probably rare because none have been recorded in any of the large published series. Several different mechanisms have been postulated to explain the observed infarcts common to these various complications. Needle-induced vessel trauma or spasm has been suggested, and arterial dissection was directly observed in the postmortem examination in one case. However, in most of the reported cases, the cause appeared to be arterial embolization caused by accidental intraarterial injection of the particulate corticosteroids. The transient symptoms resulting from intraarterial injection of local anesthetics into the CNS may be shocking to the patient and physician but may prevent accidental intraarterial injection of corticosteroids.

DISCITIS

Potential complications from discography include discitis, injury to nerve roots, disc herniation, intravascular uptake, bleeding, epidural abscess, subarachnoid puncture, and infectious or chemical meningitis. The incidence of discitis, which is the most feared and serious complication, is actually quite low, approximately 1 in 1,000. Discitis occurs with a reported incidence from 0% to 4.9% per patient or 0% to 1.3% per disc investigated.

Once a patient develops discitis, pain is often severe and can last for months with frequent debilitating effects and prolonged physical recovery.

Intervertebral discs are largely avascular and derive their nutrition from the vertebral end plates and through the cartilaginous end plates by diffusion from capillary plexuses. The avascular nature of the disc leaves it vulnerable to iatrogenic introduction of bacteria during interventional disc procedures.

The most common etiology of discitis is the direct iatrogenic inoculation of the disc during intervertebral disc procedures with Staphylococcus aureus, Staphylococcus epidermidis, a Streptococcal species, or less likely gram-negative and antibiotic-resistant organisms.

Although it is controversial, the use of a double-needle technique with stylets has been shown to decrease the risk of discitis. The stylet prevents tissue from collecting within the needle and entering the disc. In the double-needle technique, a smaller needle is inserted through a larger gauge needle to puncture the disc, thereby avoiding contact with surface tissue.

Infection of an intervertebral disc can result in an inflammatory response with possible end-plate rupture and infection into the vertebral body with resultant vertebritis. Because the avascular nature of intervertebral discs makes treatment of discitis difficult, further complications arising from the infection—such as osteomyelitis, meningitis, and arachnoiditis—may necessitate surgery. Well-established techniques to prevent infection include wearing both sterile gowns and gloves, increased operator experience, and decreased procedure time.

Controversy remains as to whether intravenous or intradiscal antibiotics factor into the prevention of discitis.

Early studies into the penetration of antibiotics into healthy human intervertebral discs after IV administration failed to demonstrate therapeutic levels. Despite giving IV antibiotics at high levels, studies were unable to assay antibiotics within the intervertebral discs. By mixing cefazolin with contrast medium just before disc injection, it was found that intradiscal antibiotics were equally effective as preemptive IV antibiotics in preventing discitis in animal models. Studies determined that low concentrations of cefazolin, clindamycin, and gentamicin remained effective in the presence of contrast medium. In fact, the use of iohexol alone resulted in the inhibition of bacterial growth, which led the authors to conclude that mixing intradiscal antibiotics with contrast might be an alluring alternative to systemic administration.

After discography, increasing back pain or a new febrile illness necessitates a diagnostic evaluation that includes a thorough history, physical examination, and a full panel of investigative laboratory studies, including C-reactive protein, erythrocyte sedimentation rate, and white blood cell count to exclude the development of discitis.

Patients with discitis present mainly with intractable back pain 2 to 4 weeks after the procedure and, in some cases, a few month after the procedure. In one study, the mean interval was 21.3 days between the onset of the surgery and the development of discitis. The delay in diagnosis may be because the treating physician attributes these symptoms to recurrent disc herniation or psychoneurotic disorders. The early and accurate diagnosis frequently depends on a combination of clinical, laboratory, and imaging findings. The diagnosis is strongly suggested by a persistently elevated Sed. Rate (ESR), C-Reactive Protein (CRP) values, and by typical changes on MRI. Although elevation of the ESR and CRP is almost uniformly present in discitis, they are supportive but not confirmatory of the diagnosis. However, these are very useful parameters for following the response to therapy. During the course of antibiotic, all patients had a steady decline, and the values returned to preoperative baseline values within 8 to 30 days (mean was 21 days). The decline of ESR and CRP values significantly correlated with the clinical improvement.

MRI is the most specific and sensitive diagnostic test for discitis. T1-weighted images show narrowing of the disk space and low signals consistent with edema in the marrow of adjacent vertebral bodies. T2-weighted images show increased signals in both the disk space and the surrounding vertebral bodies. MRI with intravenous contrast is a good diagnostic tool to rule out the presence of epidural or soft tissue abscess.

Bone scans are not specific for infection over inflammation; therefore, they are ineffective.

Needle or trocar placement into the infected area is a minimally invasive test used to obtain histologic confirmation of the disease and tissue samples for culture.

While some surgeons prefer to combine open biopsy with surgical debridement, no difference has been found between antibiotics and debridement when compared with antibiotics alone in cases of early discitis.

CONCLUSION

Although there is no clear evidence to support antibiotic use or one route over another for discitis prophylaxis after discography, Centers for Disease Control and Prevention guidelines for prevention of surgical site infection need to be followed for all spinal procedures and in discography in particular. Because prophylactic antibiotic use decreases and possibly eliminates iatrogenic infection of intervertebral discs in animal models, although no prophylaxis results in devastating consequences, strong considerations for the use of either IV or intradiscal antibiotics or both need to be made by the individual practitioner. Although antibiotics are not the standard of care, do not improve results, or offer protection for the patient beyond standard sterile technique, the risk of potential, albeit rare, debilitating effects of discitis should be weighed against potential complications from prophylactic antibiotic use until further evidence is available.

SUMMARY

There is currently no clear definition of presumably painful disc and no reliable means exist for its diagnosis and treatment. With new evidence signifying the risk of accelerated disc degeneration and disc herniation in patients after discography, assuming the shift in risk–benefit ratio, with the lack of clear benefits from the treatments provided and the aforementioned complications of the disc puncture, it is probable that even the established standards for the diagnosis of presumed discogenic pain may be in question. There is a strong need for future work in this area and a need to rethink the entire paradigm being applied to discogenic pain. The spine community needs to develop standardized practice approach for the treatment and diagnosis of this disorder.

REFERENCES

1. Boden SD, Davis DO, Dina TS, et al. Abnormal magnetic-resonance scans of the lumbar spine. In: Asymptomatic subjects: a prospective investigation. *J Bone Joint Surg Am* 1990;72A:403-408.
2. Zucherman J, Derby R, Hsu K, et al. Normal magnetic resonance imaging with abnormal discography. *Spine*. 1988;13:1355-1359.
3. Borkan JM, Koes B, Reis S, et al. A report from the Second International Forum for Primary Care Research on Low Back Pain: reexamining priorities. *Spine*. 1998;23:1992-1996.
4. Hadler NM. Back pain in the workplace: what you lift or how you lift matters far less than whether you lift or when [editorial]. *Spine*. 1997;22:935-940.
5. Cherkin DC. Primary care research on low back pain: the state of the science. *Spine*. 1998;23:1997-2002.
6. Bogduk N. *Clinical Anatomy of the Lumbar Spine and Sacrum*. 3rd ed. New York, NY: Churchill Livingstone; 1997.
7. Colhoun E, McCall IW, Williams L, et al. Provocation discography as a guide to planning operations on the spine. *J Bone Joint Surg Br*. 1988;70B:267-271.
8. Gill K, Blumenthal S. Functional results after anterior lumbar fusion at L5-S1 in patients with normal and abnormal MRI scans. *Spine*. 1992;17:940-942.
9. Greenough C, Peterson M, Taylor L, et al. Lumbar spinal fusion: a comparison of anterior and instrumented posterolateral technique. In: International Society for the Study of the Lumbar Spine; June 1996; Vermont; Abstracts.
10. Knox BD, Chapman TM. Anterior lumbar interbody fusion for discogram concordant pain. *J Spinal Disord*. 1993;6:242-244.
11. Lee CK, Vessa P, Lee JK. Chronic disabling low back pain syndrome caused by internal disc derangements: the results of disc excision and posterior lumbar interbody fusion. *Spine*. 1995;20:356-361.
12. Newman MH, Grinstead GL. Anterior lumbar interbody fusion for internal disc disruption. *Spine*. 1992;17:831-833.
13. Parker LM, Murrell SE, Boden S, et al. The outcome of posterolateral fusion in highly selected patients with discogenic low back pain. *Spine*. 1996;21:1909-1916; discussion 1916-1917.
14. Simmons EH, Segil CM. An evaluation of discography in the localization of symptomatic levels in discogenic disease of the spine. *Clin Orthop*. 1975;108:57-69.
15. Vamvanji V, Fredrickson BE, Thorpe JM, et al. Outcome and intertransverse fusion in internal disc disruption. In: International Society for the Study of the Lumbar Spine; June 25–29, 1996; Burlington, Vermont; Abstracts.
16. Wetzel FT, LaRocca SH, Lowery GL, et al. The treatment of lumbar spinal pain syndromes diagnosed by discography: lumbar arthrodesis [see comments]. *Spine*. 1994;19:792-800.
17. Sackett D. *Clinical Epidemiology. A Basic Science for Clinical Medicine*. 2nd ed. Boston, Ma: Little Brown; 1991.
18. Caragee E, Vittum D, Tanner C, et al. The deceptive discogram: Positive provocative discography as a misleading finding in the evaluation of back pain. In: North American Spine Society, 12th annual meeting; October 22–25, 1997; New York, NY.
19. Nachemson A. Lumbar discography—where are we today? [see comments]. *Spine*. 1989;14:555-557.
20. Hansen FR, Biering-Sorensen F, Schroll M. Minnesota Multiphasic Personality Inventory profiles in persons with or without low back pain: a 20-year follow-up study [see comments]. *Spine*. 1995;20:2716-2720.
21. Sullivan M. The problem of pain in the clinicopathological method. *Clin J Pain*. 1998;14:197-201.
22. Wallis BJ, Lord SM, Barnsley L, et al. Pain and psychologic symptoms of Australian patients with whiplash [see comments]. *Spine*. 1996;21:804-810.
23. Caragee EJ, Tanner CM, Khurana S, et al. The rates of false positive lumbar discography in select patients without low back symptoms. *Spine*. 2000;25:1373-1381.

24. Schofferman J, Anderson D, Hines R, et al. Childhood psychological trauma correlates with unsuccessful lumbar spine surgery. *Spine*. 1992;17:138-144.
25. Lindblom K. Diagnostic puncture of intervertebral disks in sciatica. *Acta Orthop Scand*. 1948;17:237-238.
26. Bernard TN Jr. Using computed tomography/discography and enhanced magnetic resonance imaging to distinguish between scar tissue and recurrent lumbar disc herniation. *Spine*. 1994;19:2826-2832.
27. Brodsky AE, Binder WF. Lumbar discography: its value in diagnosis and treatment of lumbar disc lesions. *Spine*. 1979;4:110-120.
28. Gunzburg R, Parkinson R, Moore R, et al. A cadaveric study comparing discography, magnetic resonance imaging, histology, and mechanical behavior of the human lumbar disc. *Spine*. 1992;17:417-426.
29. Jackson RP, Glah JJ. Foraminal and extraforaminal lumbar disc herniation: diagnosis and treatment. *Spine*. 1987;12:577-585.
30. Mendel T, Wink CS, Zimny ML. Neural elements in human cervical intervertebral discs. *Spine*. 1992;17:132-135.
31. Simmons JW, Emery SF, McMillin JN, et al. Awake discography: a comparison study with magnetic resonance imaging. *Spine*. 1991;16(suppl):S216-S221.
32. Bernard TN Jr. Lumbar discography followed by computed tomography: refining the diagnosis of low-back pain. *Spine*. 1990;15:690-707.
33. Sachs BL, Vanharanta H, Spivey MA, et al. Dallas discogram description: a new classification of CT/discography in low-back disorders. *Spine*. 1987;12:287-294.
34. Jaeschke R, Guyatt G, Sackett DL. Users' guides to the medical literature. III. How to use an article about a diagnostic test. A. Are the results of the study valid? The Evidence-Based Medicine Working Group. *JAMA*. 1994;271:389-391.
35. Jaeschke R, Guyatt GH, Sackett DL. Users' guides to the medical literature. III. How to use an article about a diagnostic test. B. What are the results and will they help me in caring for my patients? The Evidence-Based Medicine Working Group. *JAMA*. 1994;271:703-707.
36. Guyer RD, Ohnmeiss DD. Lumbar discography: position statement from the North American Spine Society Diagnostic and Therapeutic Committee [see comments]. *Spine*. 1995;20:2048-2059.
37. Heggeness MH, Doherty BJ. Discography causes end plate deflection. *Spine*. 1993;18:1050-1053.
38. Weinstein J, Claverie W, Gibson S. The pain of discography. *Spine*. 1988;13:1344-1348.
39. Derby R, Howard M, Grant J, et al. The ability of pressure controlled discography to predict surgical and non-surgical outcome. *Spine*. 1999;24:364-371.
40. Moneta GB, Videman T, Kaivanto K, et al. Reported pain during lumbar discography as a function of anular ruptures and disc degeneration: a re-analysis of 833 discograms. *Spine*. 1994;19:1968-1974.
41. Hsu KY, Zucherman JF, Derby R, Goldthwaite N, Wynne G. Painful lumbar endplate disruptions: a significant discographic finding. *Spine*. 1988;13:76-78.
42. Vanharanta H, Sachs BL, Spivey MA, et al. The relationship of pain provocation to lumbar disc deterioration as seen by CT/discography. *Spine*. 1987;12:295-298.
43. Siddall PJ, Cousins MJ. Spinal pain mechanisms. *Spine*. 1997;22:98-104.
44. North RB, Kidd DH, Zahurak M, et al. Specificity of diagnostic nerve blocks: a prospective, randomized study of sciatica due to lumbosacral spine disease. *Pain*. 1996;65:77-85.
45. Holt EP Jr. The question of lumbar discography. *J Bone Joint Surg Am*. 1968;50:720-726.
46. Walsh TR, Weinstein JN, Spratt KF, et al. Lumbar discography in normal subjects: a controlled, prospective study. *J Bone Joint Surg Am*. 1990;72:1081-1088.
47. Dooley JF, McBroom RJ, Taguchi T, et al. Nerve root infiltration in the diagnosis of radicular pain. *Spine*. 1988;13:79-83.
48. Fluke MM. The treatment of lumbar spine pain syndromes diagnosed by discography: lumbar arthrodesis [letter; comment]. *Spine*. 1995;20:501-504.
49. Quinnell RC, Stockdale HR, Willis DS. Observations of pressures within normal discs in the lumbar spine. *Spine*. 1983;8:166-169.
50. Aprill C. Diagnostic disc injection. In: Fyrmoyer JW, ed. *The Adult Spine*. New York, NY: Raven; 1991:403-442.
51. Fraser RD, Osti OL, Vernon-Roberts B. Discitis after discography. *J Bone Joint Surg Br*. 1987;69B:26-35.
52. MacMillan J, Schaffer JL, Kambin P. Routes and incidence of communication of lumbar discs with surrounding neural structures. *Spine*. 1991;16:167-171.
53. Troisier O. An accurate method for lumbar disc puncture using a single channel intensifier. *Spine*. 1990;15:222-228.
54. Gill K. New-onset sciatica after automated percutaneous discetomy. *Spine*. 1994;19:466-467.
55. Grubb S, Lipscomb H, Guilford W. The relative value of lumbar roentgenograms metrizamide myelography, and discography in the assessment of patients with chronic low-back syndrome. *Spine*. 1987;12:282-286.
56. Inufusa A, Hasegawa T, Fuse K, et al. Effect of annular puncture on the adolescent canine intervertebral disc. In: North American Spine Society, 12th annual meeting; October 22–25, 1997; New York, NY.
57. Johnson RG. Does discography injure normal discs? An analysis of repeat discograms. *Spine*. 1989;14:424-426.
58. Kahanovitz N, Arnoczky SP, Sissons HA, et al. The effect of discography on the canine intervertebral disc. *Spine*. 1986;11:26-27.
59. Guyer RD, Collier R, Stith WJ, et al. Discitis after discography. *Spine*. 1988;13:1352-1354.
60. Junila J, Niinimaki T, Tervonen O. Epidural abscess after lumbar discography—a case report. *Spine*. 1997;22:2191–2193.
61. Fraser RD, Osti OL, Vernon-Roberts B. Iatrogenic discitis: the role of intravenous antibiotics in prevention and treatment: an experimental study. *Spine*. 1989;14:1025-1032.
62. Jamrich E, Fabian H, Raabe T. Antibiotic penetration into the adult human nucleus pulposus. In: North American Spine Society, 12th annual meeting; October 22–25, 1997; New York, NY.
63. Lang R, Folman Y, Ravid M, et al. Penetration of ceftriaxome into the intervertebral disc. *J Bone Joint Surg Br*. 1994;76A:689-691.
64. Osti OL, Fraser RD, Vernon-Roberts B. Discitis after discography—the role of prophylactic antibiotics. *J Bone Joint Surg Br*. 1990;72:271-274.
65. Quinnell RC, Stockdale HR. An investigation of artefacts in lumbar discography. *Br J Radiol*. 1980;53:831-839.
66. Schellhas K. Venous opacification during discography: therapeutic implications. In: International Spinal Injection Society, 4th annual meeting; August 16, 1996; Vancouver, Canada.
67. McCutcheon ME, Thompson WC. CT scanning of lumbar dicography. A useful diagnostic adjunct. *Spine*. 1986;11:257-259.
68. Ninomiya M, Muro T. Pathoanatomy of lumbar disc herniation as demonstrated by computed tomography/discography. *Spine*. 1992;17:1316-1322.

69. Quinnell RC, Stockdale HR. The use of in vivo lumbar discography to assess the clinical significance of the position of the intercrestal line. *Spine*. 1983;8:305-307.
70. Videman T, Malmivaara A, Mooney V. The value of the axial view in assessing discograms: an experimental study with cadavers. *Spine*. 1987;12:299-304.
71. Malmivaara A, Videman T, Kuosma E, et al. Plain radiographic, discographic, and direct observations of Schmorl's nodes in the thoracolumbar junctional region of the cadaveric spine. *Spine*. 1987;12:453-457.
72. Schwarzer AC, Aprill CN, Bodguk N. The sacroiliac joint in chronic low back pain. *Spine*. 1995;20:31-37.
73. Schwarzer AC, Aprill CN, Derby R, et al. The relative contributions of the disc and zygapophyseal joint in chronic low back pain. *Spine*. 1994;19:801-806.
74. Donelson R, Aprill C, Medcalf R, et al. A prospective study of centralization of lumbar and referred pain. A predictor of symptomatic discs and anular competence. *Spine*. 1997;22:1115-1122.
75. Osti OL, Fraser RD. MRI and discography of annular tears and intervertebral disc degeneration: a prospective clinical comparison [published erratum appears in *J Bone Joint Surg Br* 1992;74:793] [see comments]. *J Bone Joint Surg Br*. 1992;74:431-435.
76. Aprill C, Bodguk N. High-intensity zone: a diagnostic sign of painful lumbar disc on magnetic resonance imaging. *Br J Radiol*. 1992;65:361-369.
77. Schellhaus K, Heithoff K, Pollei S. Lumbar disc high intensity zone: Pain managment with intradiscal steroids. In: North American Spine Society, 11th annual meeting; October 23–26, 1996; Vancouver, Canada.
78. Haueisen DC, Smith BS, Myers SR, et al. The diagnostic accuracy of spinal nerve injection studies: their role in the evaluation of recurrent sciatica. *Clin Orthop*. 1985;198:179-183.
79. Herron LD. Selective nerve root block in patient selection for lumbar surgery: surgical results. *J Spinel Disord*. 1989;2:75-79.
80. Hoppenstein R. A new approach to the failed back syndrome. *Spine*. 1980;5:371-379.
81. Kikuchi S, Hasue M, Nishiyama K, et al. Anatomic and clinical studies of radicular symptoms. *Spine*. 1984;9:23-30.
82. Krempen JF, Smith BS. Nerve-root injection: a method for evaluating the etiology of sciatica. *J Bone Joint Surg Am*. 1974;56:1435-1444.
83. Stanley D, McLaren MI, Euinton HA, et al. A prospective study of nerve root infiltration in the diagnosis of sciatica: a comparison with radiculography, computed tomography, and operative findings. *Spine*. 1990;15:540-543.
84. Tajima K. [Selective radiculography and block (author's translation)]. *Nippon Seikeigeka Gakkai Zasshi*. 1982;56:71-90.
85. Kikuchi S. Anatomical and experimental studies of nerve root infiltration. *Nippon Seikeigeka Gakkai Zasshi*. 1982;56:605-614.
86. Derby R, Kine G, Saal J, et al. Precision percutaneous blocking procedures for localizing spinal pain. Part 2: The lumbar neuraxial compartment. *Pain Digest*. 1993;3:175-188.
87. Derby R, Kine G, Saal JA, et al. Response to steroid and duration of radicular pain as predictors of surgical outcome. *Spine*. 1992;17(suppl):S176-S183.
88. Oda J, Tanaka H, Tsuzuki N. Intervertebral disc changes with aging of human cervical vertebra: from the neonate to the eighties. *Spine*. 1988;13:1205-1211.
89. Schellhas KP, Smith MD, Gundry CR, et al. Cervical discogenic pain: prospective correlation of magnetic resonance imaging and discography in asymptomatic subjects and pain sufferers. *Spine*. 1996;21:300-311, discussion 311-312.
90. Bogduk N, Aprill C. On the nature of neck pain, discography, and cervical zygapophysial joint blocks. *Pain*. 1993;54:213-217.
91. Holt E Jr. Fallacy of cervical discography. *JAMA*. 1964;188:799-801.
92. Shinomiya K, Nakao K, Shindoh S, et al. Evaluation of cervical diskography in pain origin and provocation. *J Spinal Disord*. 1993;6:422-426.
93. Lord SM, Barnsley L, Bogduk N. The utility of comparative local anesthetic blocks versus placebo-controlled blocks for the diagnosis of cervical zygapophysial joint pain. *Clin J Pain*. 1995;11:208-213.
94. Kikuchi S, Macnab I, Moreau P. Localisation of the level of sympatomatic cervical disc degeneration. *J Bone Joint Surg Br*. 1981;63B:272-277.
95. Riley LH Jr, Robinson RA, Johnson KA, et al. The results of anterior interbody fusion of the cervical spine. Review of ninety-three consecutive cases. *J Neurosurg*. 1969;30:127-133.
96. Whitecloud TSD, Seago RA. Cervical discogenic syndrome. Results of operative intervention in patients with positive discography. *Spine*. 1987;12:313-316.
97. Pospiech J, Stolke D, Wilke HJ, et al. Intradiscal pressure recordings in the cervical spine. *Neurosurgery*. 1999;44:379-384.
98. Connor PM, Darden BVD. Cervical discography complications and clinical efficacy. *Spine*. 1993;18:2035-2038.
99. Guyer RD, Ohnmeiss DD, Mason SL, et al. Complications of cervical discography: findings in a large series. *J Spinal Disord*. 1997;10:95-101.
100. Laun A, Lorenz R, Agnoli AL. Complications of cervical discography. *J Neurosurg Sci*. 1981;25:17-20.
101. Zeidman SM, Thompson K, Ducker TB. Complications of cervical discography: analysis of 4400 diagnostic disc injections. *Neurosurgery*. 1995;37:414-417.

PART 3

Psychological Evaluation and Treatment of Chronic Pain

CHAPTER 14

Psychological Aspects of Chronic Pain

Dennis C. Turk
Akiko Okifuji

Pain is a complex, perceptual experience, defined as an "unpleasant sensory and emotional experience associated with actual or potential tissue damage, or described in terms of such damage."[1] One of the critical developments in the past several decades in pain research is the progress in our understanding of the multifactorial, biobehavioral mechanisms involved with chronic pain.[2] Research has consistently shown the importance of using multimodal approaches to treat patients with chronic pain[3] because monotherapies appear to provide less than optimal relief.[4] These developments have pointed to various psychological factors—cognitive, emotional, and behavioral—as significant contributors for pain modulation and pain-related disability.[5]

The main objective of this chapter is to review the various psychological factors relevant to the experience of pain. As a background, it is important to consider how we conceptualize pain. Our view of pain will influence our evaluations of patients who report pain and the nature of the interventions that we use to treat them. The way we conceptualize pain depends largely on the nature of the information acquired and the models that we were exposed to during our training. In the first section of this chapter, we review the historical models of how we conceptualized pain. We will argue that although these models are not necessarily inaccurate, they are incomplete. We then suggest that a broader, multidimensional perspective is required to understand pain and to treat patients appropriately. We describe the role of behavioral, cognitive, and affective factors that have been shown to be relevant to the experience of pain, disability, and response to treatment. We provide data demonstrating that these psychological factors may have an effect both on patients' behavior and physiology. Finally, we raise the issue of the "patient uniformity myth" and describe the subgroups of pain patients based on psychosocial and behavioral characteristics. We provide data suggesting that knowledge of such patient subgroups may serve as a basis for matching patients to treatments based on their characteristics.

UNIDIMENSIONAL SENSORY "SOMATOGENIC" MODEL

Historically, pain has been understood from the perspective of Cartesian dualism in which pain was viewed as purely sensory, reflecting the degrees of incoming noxious sensory stimuli. This perspective assumes that there are two ends to a pain pathway. At the periphery, there are sensory receptors (*nociceptors*), where noxious information is received and, at the other end, regions located in the brain where information is registered passively. From this perspective, noxious stimulation inevitably results in the sensation of pain, as if pulling a string at the periphery activates a bell located in the brain. Variations of this model have been prominent since first proposed by Descartes in 1644.

A central belief of sensory models is that the amount of pain experienced is a direct result of the amount, degree, or nature of sensory input or physical damage and is explained in terms of specific neuro physiological mechanisms. Clinically, it is expected that the report of pain will be directly proportional to the amount of pathology. This model dictates that assessment should focus on identifying the cause of the pain. Once identified, treatment should involve removal of the cause or severing or blocking the specific pain pathways by surgical or pharmacological means.

Sensory models continued to maintain a prominent position in medicine despite this model's inability to account for a number of observations. For example,

- Patients with equivalent degrees and types of objectively-determined tissue pathology vary widely in their reports of pain severity.
- Patients with only minimal, objectively determined pathology may report severe pain.
- Asymptomatic individuals often reveal significant amounts of physical pathology on imaging.
- Procedures that might be expected to produce pain sometimes do not. For example, surgical procedures designed to inhibit pain transmission by severing neurological pathways believed to be underlying the reported pain may fail to alleviate pain.
- Patients with equivalent degrees of tissue pathology who are treated with identical treatments respond in widely differently ways.
- There are only modest associations among impairment, pain, and disability.

Thus, we see a number of paradoxes in clinical practice. There are patients who report severe pain with limited physical pathology and, conversely, patients who have significant physical pathology but no pain; pain pathways can be ablated but pain can persist; and identical treatments provided for the same diagnosis can result in different outcomes.

Unfortunately, for many with chronic pain, the underlying causes of pain frequently remain unknown, despite the development and use of sophisticated diagnostic imaging procedures such as CT (computed tomography) scan or MRI (magnetic resonance imaging). For example, objective evidence of physical pathology is only identified in about 15% of the cases of back pain.[6] In knee osteoarthritis (OA), physical findings such as cartilage loss and bone marrow edema are considered to reflect the progression of the disease and clinical presentations. However, when the grading of pathology by the imaging (MRI) was evaluated, neither bone marrow edema nor cartilage abnormality were linearly related to pain severity.[7] Similarly, an MRI study of a total of 256 hips has shown that the large number of hips with no pain showed various degrees of peritrochanteric MRI abnormalities, when compared to those hips with pain.[8]

How can such paradoxes be understood? As is frequently the case in medicine, when objective physical evidence and explanations prove inadequate to explain symptoms, psychological alternatives are proposed. If the pain reported by a patient is believed to be *disproportionate* to objectively determined physical pathology or if the complaint is recalcitrant to "appropriate" treatment, then it is assumed that psychological factors must be involved, even if not causal. Thus, there appears to be a somatogenic–psychogenic dichotomy in how the report of pain is construed.

PSYCHOGENIC PERSPECTIVE

It is important to realize that determination of whether the reported pain is *disproportionate* is subjective. There is no objective way to determine how much pain is *proportionate* to the underlying condition. How much should a given amount of tissue pathology hurt? Similarly, determination of appropriate treatment is not totally objective. Different health care providers might recommend widely different treatments for patients with the same presenting symptoms.[4] For example, treatments for patients with temporomandibular disorders range from surgery to psychotherapy and, for fibromyalgia, from electroconvulsive therapy to sulfur mud baths.

The somatogenic–psychogenic dichotomy forms the basis for the distinction underlying attempts to identify "functional" versus "organic" pain, as well as references to a "functional overlay." The American Psychiatric Association[9] created two psychiatric diagnoses associated with pain in the fourth edition of the *Diagnostic and Statistical Manual of Mental Disorders*—pain associated with psychological factors either with or without a diagnosed medical condition. The specific diagnosis of "pain disorder associated with psychological factors and a general medical condition" is characterized by the fact that both psychological factors and a general medical condition have important roles in the onset, severity, exacerbation, and maintenance of pain. This set of diagnoses is so broadly defined, however, that virtually all patients who have persistent pain may be diagnosed as suffering from a psychiatric disorder.

MOTIVATIONAL VIEW

A variation of the dichotomous somatic–psychogenic views is a conceptualization that may be ascribed to by many insurance companies and other third-party payers. They suggest that if physical pathology is insufficient to support the claim of pain, then the complaint is suspect. Pain is assumed to result from symptom exaggeration to achieve some benefit (e.g., prescription medication, avoidance of undesirable activity, attention) or outright malingering (i.e., financial compensation). The assumption is that reports of pain without adequate biomedical evidence are motivated primarily by desire for some type of reinforcement. This belief has resulted in a number of attempts to *catch* malingerers using surreptitious observational methods (e.g., surveillance, video recording) and the use of sophisticated biomechanical machines geared toward identifying inconsistencies in functional performance. There is, however, very little empirical support for this belief. No studies, for example, have demonstrated dramatic improvement in pain reports subsequent to receiving disability awards (i.e., no further need to exaggerate symptoms).

The conceptualizations described here view physical and psychological factors as if they are mutually exclusive. Before examining models that attempt to integrate psychological factors with somatic factors, let us examine the nature of the psychological processes and factors that have been demonstrated to play an important role in pain perception, disability, and response to treatment.

PSYCHOLOGICAL FACTORS AFFECTING PAIN EXPERIENCE

A number of psychological principles based in learning theory have been extended to pain. These principles provide helpful explanations for many clinical observations. Moreover, a number of cognitive and affective factors have been demonstrated to influence expressions of pain and participation in rehabilitation. We can consider the major psychological, sociocultural, and behavioral principles and factors studied and then consider how they can be integrated to create a comprehensive, integrated model of pain that can serve as a guide for assessment and ultimately treatment.

OPERANT LEARNING MECHANISMS

As long ago as the mid-20th century, the effects of environmental factors in shaping the experience of pain were acknowledged. A new era in thinking about pain began in 1976, when Fordyce[10] extended the principles of "operant conditioning" to chronic pain and disability.

In the operant conditioning formulation, behavioral manifestations of pain rather than pain *per se* are central. When a person experiences a noxious sensation, the initial response is a withdrawal or escape response. This may be accomplished by avoidance of the activity believed to cause or exacerbate pain, seeking help to reduce symptoms, and so forth. These behaviors are observable and, consequently, subject to the principles of operant conditioning—namely, reinforcement and avoidance learning.

The operant view proposes that pain behaviors such as avoidance of activity to protect an injured body part from producing additional noxious input may come under the control of external contingencies of reinforcement (responses increase or decrease as a function of their reinforcing consequences). It is these reinforcement contingencies that contribute to the maintenance of the problems associated with chronic pain and disability. Pain behaviors (e.g., limping, grimacing, and inactivity) are conceptualized as overt expressions of pain, distress, and suffering. These behaviors may be positively reinforced directly, for example, by attention from family or health care providers. Pain behaviors may also be maintained by the escape from noxious stimulation provided by the use of drugs or rest or the avoidance of undesirable activities such as work. In addition "well behaviors" (e.g., activity, working) may not be positively reinforcing and the more rewarding pain behaviors may, therefore, be maintained.

In an experimental study,[11] healthy volunteers' facial expressions in response to noxious stimulation could readily be operantly conditioned by a simple reinforcement method either toward a greater or lesser degree of behavioral exhibition. We can also illustrate the role of operant factors in a case of chronic back pain. When a woman with painful back has a flare up, she may lie down on the floor and hold her back. Her husband may notice these dramatic behaviors and infer that she is experiencing pain. The husband's behavioral response is influenced by his observation of her behavior. He typically responds to her pain displays by spending extra time with her and massaging her back. In this case, the woman's lying down has resulted in receiving attention from her significant other, a positive consequence. According to the laws of operant learning, behaviors resulting in a positive consequence increase their chances of recurring.

Another powerful way the husband might reinforce his wife's pain behaviors is by permitting her to avoid undesirable activities. When observing his wife lying on the floor, the husband suggests that they cancel the evening plans with his brother. If the person experiencing pain would prefer not to spend time with her husband's brother, then the avoidance of the undesirable activity is reinforced and may contribute to reports of pain whenever activities with her husband's brother are planned. In this situation, her pain reports and other behaviors are rewarded both by her husband providing her with extra attention and support and the opportunity to avoid an undesirable social obligation.

Whether operantly conditioned pain behaviors contribute to worsening of pain is somewhat controversial. Based upon the "facial feedback hypothesis" that asserts that overt behaviors affect internal sensory-emotional experience,[12] we may expect that as people's pain behaviors are reinforced, their pain complaints increase. Salomons and colleagues[13] trained their subjects to pain-related and relaxed facial expression. Unpleasantness rating of the noxious heat stimulus was greater when they were told to make a "pain" face than a "relaxed" face, providing some support for the facial feedback theory. However, in this experiment, the facial expressions were not subjected to any reinforcement schedules. On the other hand, in the aforementioned study by Kunz and colleagues,[11] the reinforced facial expression did not increase pain rating. When operant reinforcement is directly applied to a pain task in which contingent stimulus levels change, however, the prolonged sensitization to the noxious heat stimulus was enhanced, with the proportion linearly related to the level of reinforcement.[14]

Operant conditioning seems to have a consistent impact on disability. Particularly, postural guarding may be instrumental in acute to chronic disability of injured workers.[15] A systematic review[16] indicates that operant-based physical therapy significantly improves pain-related disability in chronic back pain patients.

It is important to clarify that the operant learning does not require a person with pain's intentional and conscious efforts to elicit a desirable outcome. It results from a gradual learning process that neither the individual nor others tends to recognize as it unfolds. It should not, however, be assumed that pain behaviors are synonymous with malingering. Malingering involves the consciously and purposeful faking of symptoms such as pain for some gain, usually financial. In the case of pain behaviors, there is no suggestion of conscious deception but rather the unintended performance of pain behaviors resulting from laws of learning based on environmental reinforcement contingencies. The pain behavior in response to initial injury may encounter reinforcing events, thereby determining probability of that behavior recurring in the future; but, once the behavior is learned, the presence of initial pain is no longer needed for that behavior to recur.

The operant conditioning formulation does not concern itself with the initial cause of pain. Rather, it considers pain an internal subjective experience that can only be indirectly assessed and may be maintained even after an initial physical basis of pain has resolved. Because of the consequences of specific behavioral responses, it is proposed that pain behaviors may persist long after the initial cause of the pain is resolved or greatly reduced. Thus, in one sense, the operant conditioning model can be viewed as analogous to the psychogenic models described earlier. That is, psychological factors are treated as secondary reactions to sensory stimulation, rather than directly involved in the perception of pain *per se*.

The operant view has generated what has proven to be an effective treatment for select samples of chronic pain patients.[17] Treatment focuses on eliminating pain behaviors by withdrawal of attention and increasing "well behaviors" (e.g., activity) by positive reinforcement. Although operant factors undoubtedly play a role in the maintenance of disability, exclusive reliance on the operant conditioning model to explain the experience of pain may not be appropriate. It has been criticized for its exclusive focus on motor pain behaviors, failure to consider the emotional and cognitive aspects of pain, and failure to treat the subjective experience of pain.[18]

RESPONDENT LEARNING MECHANISMS

Factors contributing to chronicity that have previously been conceptualized in terms of operant learning may also be initiated and maintained by classical or "respondent conditioning."[19] If an aversive stimulus is paired with a neutral stimulus for a number of times, the neutral stimulus will come to elicit aversive experiences in the individual. The patient learns to anticipate negative consequences even in the absence of the noxious stimulus. This process has been frequently observed in cancer patients receiving chemotherapy. Patients have been observed to report nausea when they enter the room where they have received the chemotherapy even before any cytotoxic medication has been administered. Similarly, a back pain patient who received a painful treatment from a physical therapist may become conditioned to experience a negative emotional response to the presence of the physical therapist, to a treatment room, and to any stimulus associated with the nociceptive stimulus (e.g., exercise equipment). The negative emotional reaction may lead to tensing of muscles, and this, in turn, may exacerbate pain, thereby reinforcing the association between the presence of the physical therapist and pain.

Probably, the most relevant emotional conditioning in pain is anxiety. Anxiety is often the affect underlying avoidance of activities. Pain patients often experience temporary aggravation of pain following physical activities. Avoiding such activities leads to no pain exacerbation, thus reinforcing inactivity and maintaining anxiety for activity. In other words, continuing to avoid specific activities will reduce disconfirmations that could provide corrective feedback.[20] Insofar as avoidance does not produce disconfirmation, the behaviors will persist.[21] By contrast, when an anticipated consequence does not occur (disconfirmation), modification of learning also takes place. Thus, the physical therapist may have to encourage the patient to exercise to provide disconfirmation that, just because exercise may hurt, it will not automatically lead to increased injury. The therapist will have to emphasize that hurt and harm are not eqivalent. Both respondent conditioning and operant learning may contribute to the development and maintenance of dysfunctional behavioral patterns in chronic pain patients. Over time, more and more activities, people, and physical locations may be seen as eliciting or exacerbating pain and may be avoided (stimulus generalization). Fear of pain and avoidance may become conditioned to an expanding number of situations (response generalization). In addition to avoidance learning, pain may be exacerbated and maintained in these encounters with potentially pain-increasing situations because of the anxiety-related sympathetic activation and muscle tension increases that may occur in anticipation of pain and also as a consequence of pain. Thus, as we emphasize later, psychological factors may directly affect nociceptive stimulation and need not be viewed as only reactions to pain.

SOCIAL LEARNING MECHANISMS

Social learning has received some attention in acute pain and in the development and maintenance of chronic pain states. From this perspective, how we experience pain is shaped and influenced by "observational learning"; that is, individuals can acquire responses that were not previously in their behavioral repertoire by watching others perform these activities. Children acquire attitudes about health, health care, and the perceptive style for recognizing and understanding bodily symptoms from their parents and the social environment. They also learn how injuries and diseases should be regarded and addressed. As they grow older, this learning emerges as their tendency to ignore or over-respond to symptoms they experience—the culturally acquired interpretations of symptoms influence how people deal with illness.

There is ample experimental evidence of the role of social learning from controlled laboratory pain studies and some evidence based on observations of patients' behaviors in field and clinical settings. Physiological responses to pain stimuli may be conditioned during observation of others in pain. For example, patients on a burn unit have sufficient opportunity to observe the responses of other burn patients.[22] Each patient's response is affected by his or her observations of other patients. In one study, children of chronic pain patients chose more pain-related responses to scenarios presented to them than did children with pain-free or diabetic parents. Moreover, teachers rated the pain patients' children as displaying more illness behaviors (e.g., complaining, days absent, visits to school nurse) than children of pain-free controls.[23] Expectancies as well as actual behavioral responses to noxious stimuli are based, at least partially, on prior social learning history. This may contribute to the marked variability in response to objectively similar degrees of physical pathology noted by health care providers.

ROLE OF COGNITIVE FACTORS IN PAIN

A great deal of research has been directed toward explicating the role of cognitive factors in pain. These studies have consistently demonstrated that patients' attitudes, beliefs, and expectancies about their plight, themselves, their coping resources, and the health care system affect the reports of pain, activity, disability, and response to treatment.[24,25]

BELIEFS ABOUT PAIN

Clinicians working with chronic pain patients are aware that patients having similar pain histories and expressions of pain may differ greatly in their beliefs about their pain.[26] Behavior and emotion are influenced by how a person interprets events, rather than by objective characteristics of the events. When pain is interpreted as signifying ongoing tissue damage or a progressive disease, such belief often leads to activity avoidance and deactivation in general and is significantly related to greater pain and disability.[27] Even for pain-free individuals, belief that the pain is threatening reduces pain tolerance.[28] For example, very different responses would be expected of a patient if he attributed his headache to excessive alcohol consumption the night before as opposed to his interpretation that the headache signaled a brain tumor. Thus, although the amount of nociceptive input in the two cases may be equivalent, the emotional and behavioral responses would vary in nature and intensity.

Certain beliefs may lead to maladaptive coping, increased suffering, and greater disability. Patients who believe that there is nothing they can do to control pain may be passive in their coping efforts and fail to make use of available resources to cope with pain. Patients who consider their pain to be an unexplainable mystery feel helpless and clueless as to how to cope with the situation. The sense of helplessness contributes to negative evaluations of patients' own abilities and coping strategies as effective in controlling and decreasing pain.[29] Once beliefs and expectations about a disease are formed, they become stable and are very difficult to modify. Patients tend to avoid experiences that might invalidate their beliefs (disconfirmation), and they tend to guide their behavior in accordance with these beliefs (confirmation), even when the beliefs are no longer valid. A part of the treatment needs to focus on modifying such maladaptive thought processes. For example, therapists may point out that muscular pain following activity may be caused by lack of muscle strength and general deconditioning and not by additional tissue damage. Modification of maladaptive beliefs about their pain seems to predict changes in pain and disability via treatment.[30]

Chronic low back pain patients generally demonstrate poor behavioral persistence in various exercise tasks, with their performance on these tasks being independent of physical exertion or actual self-reports of pain, but instead related to previous pain reports.[31] These patients appear to have a negative view of their abilities and expected their pain to increase if they perform physical exercises. Thus, the rationale for their avoidance of exercise was not the presence of pain but their learned expectation of heightened pain and accompanying physical arousal that might exacerbate pain and reinforce their beliefs regarding the pervasiveness of their disability. If patients view disability as an expected consequence of their pain, if they believe that activity is dangerous and that their pain is an acceptable excuse for neglecting responsibilities, they are likely to experience prolonged disability. Patients' negative perceptions of their capabilities for physical performance form a vicious circle, with the failure to perform activities reinforcing the perception of helplessness and incapacity. Once again, avoidance of activity prevents disconfirmation.

In addition to beliefs about capabilities to function despite pain, beliefs about pain *per se* appear to be of importance in understanding response to treatment, adherence to self-management activities, and disability.[29] When successful rehabilitation occurs, there appears to be an important cognitive shift from beliefs about helplessness and passivity to resourcefulness and ability to function regardless of pain.[24,25]

Clearly, it is essential for patients with chronic and recurrent pain to develop adaptive beliefs and to deemphasize the importance of maintaining functionality despite pain. In fact, changes in pain levels do not necessarily parallel changes in other variables of interest, including activity level, medication use, return to work, rated ability to cope with pain, and pursuit of further treatment.[32]

SELF-EFFICACY

Another important cognitive factor related to beliefs about pain is the belief about our ability to cope with pain, referred to as "self-efficacy."[33] A self-efficacy expectation is defined as a personal conviction that we can successfully execute a course of action (perform required behaviors) to produce a desired outcome in a given situation. This variable has been demonstrated as a major mediator of therapeutic change. Given sufficient motivation to engage in a behavior, it is a person's self-efficacy beliefs that determine the choice of activities he or she will initiate, the amount of effort he or she will expend, and how long he or she will persist in the face of obstacles and aversive experiences. Efficacy judgments are based on four sources of information regarding a person's capabilities, listed in descending order of impact:

- His or her own past performance at the task or similar tasks.
- The performance accomplishments of others who are perceived to be similar to the person.
- Verbal persuasion by others that he or she is capable.
- Perception of his or her own state of physiological arousal, which is, in turn, partly determined by prior efficacy estimation.[33]

A low level of self-efficacy belief is related to disability[34,35] and mediates the relationship between pain and physical and psychological functioning[36,37] in chronic pain. Furthermore, longitudinal studies suggest that poor self-efficacy belief is a risk factor for the development of disability associated with chronic pain[38] and work absenteeism.[39]

Whereas low self-efficacy beliefs are related to more severe pain and dysfunction, improvement in self-efficacy is one of the best predictors for successful rehabilitation for pain patients. Elevated levels of self-efficacy beliefs at pretreatment tend to predict better outcomes.[40,41] However, even when the initial level of self-efficacy belief is low, evidence suggests that improved self-efficacy leads to facilitation of healthful practices in chronic pain patients.[42]

Experience of performance mastery is critical in developing adequate self-efficacy belief. It can be achieved by starting patients at a modest level with graded activities added gradually. From this perspective, the occurrence of coping behaviors is conceptualized as being mediated by people's beliefs that situation demands do not exceed their coping resources. Council and his colleagues[43] asked patients to rate their self-efficacy, as well as expected levels of pain related to performing movement tasks. Patients' performance levels were highly related to their self-efficacy expectations, which, in turn, appeared to be determined by their expectancy of pain levels.

CATASTROPHIZING

"Catastrophizing"—spontaneously developing extremely negative thoughts about your plight such that even minor problems are interpreted as major catastrophes—appears to be a particularly potent way of thinking that greatly influences pain and disability. Several lines of research, including experimental laboratory studies of acute pain with normal volunteers and field studies with clinical patients suffering clinical pain, have indicated that catastrophizing and adaptive coping strategies are important in determining reactions to pain.[44] Individuals who spontaneously utilize catastrophizing self-statements reported more pain than those who did not catastrophize in several acute and chronic pain studies. Turk et al.[45] concluded that "what appears to distinguish low from high pain tolerant individuals in their cognitive processing, catastrophizing thoughts and feelings that precede, accompany, and follow aversive stimulation…" (p. 197).

Catastrophizing has been found to be related to higher sensitivity to experimentally induced pain in pain-free children[46] and adults,[47] as well as people with acute and chronic pain.[48-51] For people undergoing a surgery, catastrophizing predicts time to hospital discharge,[52] postoperative pain severity, and poor quality of life, as well as later development of chronic pain.[53] It also is a significant predictor of pain-related disability[54] in chronic pain. The degree to which catastrophizing exerts its influence may depend on the personality factor; catastrophizing seems to influence pain experience among people with higher degrees of anxiety sensitivity in response to physical exertion.[55] Evidence also suggests that catastrophizing seems to worsen the pain experience via attenuation of diffuse noxious inhibitory control (most recently referred to as conditioned pain modulation).[56]

INDIRECT EFFECTS OF COGNITIVE FACTORS ON PAIN

Cognitive factors may act indirectly on pain and disability by reducing physical activity and, consequently reducing muscle flexibility, strength, and tone. Fear of re-injury, fear of losing disability compensation, and a low level of job dissatisfaction can also adversely influence return to work.

People experiencing pain can develop ways of coping that, in the short run, seem adaptive but, in the long run, serve to maintain the chronic pain condition and result in greater disability. As noted earlier, one of these ways of coping is avoidance of activities because of the fear of pain or injury. For example, following an accident in which an individual hurt his back, he learned that certain movements made his pain worse. In response, he stopped engaging in activities that exacerbated his pain and restricted his movements in an attempt to avoid pain. As a result, he lost muscle strength, flexibility, and endurance. Here, a vicious circle began, for as the muscles became weaker, more and more activities caused pain. As the individual remains inactive and becomes more physically deconditioned, he may not allow himself the opportunity to recover and rehabilitate by identifying the activities that build flexibility, endurance, and strength without the risk of pain or injury. In addition, the distorted movements and postures he may use to protect himself from pain may contribute to further pain unrelated to his initial injury. For example, when the patient limps, he protects muscles on one side of his back, but the muscles on the other side may become overactive and can develop painful conditions of their own. Thus, avoidance of activity, although it is a seemingly rational way to manage a pain problem, can actually play a large role in maintaining the chronic pain condition and increasing disability. In addition to contributing to the maintenance of the pain condition, the use of avoidant-coping strategies has other negative consequences.

After having limited success in controlling pain, the person with chronic pain may perceive pain and the factors that influence the pain to be outside of his or her personal control. Individuals who feel pain is uncontrollable are not likely to attempt new strategies to manage their pain. Instead, pain sufferers feel increasingly frustrated and demoralized when *uncontrollable* pain interferes with participation in rewarding recreational, occupational, and social activities. It is not uncommon for pain sufferers to resort to passive coping strategies such as inactivity, self-medication, or alcohol to reduce emotional distress and pain.

Individuals who feel little personal control over their pain are also likely to *catastrophize* about the impact of situations that trigger or exacerbate their pain and catastrophize about pain flare-ups. In contrast, individuals who believe their ability to control the situations contributing to flares are more resourceful and are more likely to develop self-management strategies that are effective in limiting the impact of the pain episodes or flare-ups and, thus, are able to limit the impact of the pain problem.

Whereas maladaptive cognition can worsen pain, adaptive cognition can have a positive effect. Individuals who feel they have a number of successful methods for coping with pain may suffer less than those who feel helpless and hopeless. Psychological interventions such as relaxation, contingency management, and coping skills training have been shown to be effective in helping people with persistent pain to either eliminate their pain or, if pain cannot be eliminated, reduce their pain, distress, and suffering. These interventions are designed not only to decrease pain, but also to improve physical and psychological functioning.

DIRECT EFFECTS OF PSYCHOLOGICAL FACTORS ON PAIN

Several studies have suggested that psychological factors may actually have a direct effect on physiological parameters associated more directly with the production or exacerbation of nociception.[57] Cognitive interpretations and relevant arousal may have a direct effect on physiology by increasing sympathetic tones, endogenous opioid (endorphins) production, and as noted elevated levels of muscle tension.

EFFECTS OF THOUGHTS ON AUTONOMIC AROUSAL

Circumstances that are appraised as potentially threatening to safety or comfort are likely to generate strong physiological reactions. In a sample of patients with recurrent migraine headaches, Jamner and Tursky[58] observed increases in skin conductance, indicating autonomic arousal, in response to seeing words describing migraine headaches simply displayed on a screen. For those with migraine, even thoughts of a migraine can prove autonomically affecting and potentially dysregulating.

Chronic increases in sympathetic nervous system activation are known to increase skeletal muscle tone and thus may set the stage for hyperactive muscle contraction and possibly for the persistence of a contraction following conscious muscle activation. Excessive sympathetic arousal is viewed as the immediate precursor of muscle hypertonicity, hyperactivity, and persistence, which, in turn, are the proximate causes of muscle spasm and pain. It is not unusual for someone in pain to amplify the significance of his or her problem and activate or *turn on* his or her sympathetic nervous system. In this way, thought processes may influence sympathetic arousal and predispose the individual to further injury or otherwise complicate the process of recovery.

In an early study, the direct effect of thoughts on muscle tension response was demonstrated by Flor and colleagues.[57] These investigators interviewed patients with back pain and other pain disorders, as well as pain-free individuals. Muscle tension sensors were placed on the surface of the lower back, forearm, and forehead. During the monitoring of muscle activity, patients were then asked to recall and describe in as much detail as possible the last time they experienced extreme pain and the last time they experienced severe stress. The study found that when discussing their pain or stress, the back pain patients had significantly elevated muscle tension in their backs, but not in their foreheads or forearms. However, when these back pain patients were resting and not discussing their pain or stress, their back muscle tension level was no higher than the non–back pain patients or the healthy individuals. Neither the pain patients without back pain nor the pain-free individuals showed elevations in muscle tension when discussing severe stresses. Thus, back pain patients showed pain-site specific muscular arousal simply by talking about their pain and stress. Similar results have been observed in studies with patients who had chronic arm and shoulder pain,[59] as well as patients with temporomandibular disorders.[60]

EFFECTS OF THOUGHTS ON BIOCHEMISTRY

Bandura and his colleagues[61] directly examined the role of central opioid activity in the cognitive control of pain. They taught their subjects to use various coping strategies for alleviating experimentally produced pain, including attention diversion from pain sensations to other matters, engaging imagery, imaginal separation (dissociation) of the limb in pain from the rest of the body, transformation of pain as nonpain sensations, and self-encouragement of coping efforts. They demonstrated that (1) self-efficacy increased with cognitive training, (2) self-efficacy predicted pain tolerance, and, importantly, (3) naloxone (an opioid antagonist) blocked the effects of cognitive coping. The latter result directly implicates the direct effects of thoughts on endogenous opioids. Bandura and colleagues concluded that the physical mechanism by which self-efficacy influences pain perception might at least be partially mediated by the endogenous opioid system.

O'Leary et al.[62] provided stress management treatment to rheumatoid arthritis (RA) patients. Degree of self-efficacy (expectations about the ability to control pain and disability) enhancement was correlated with treatment effectiveness. Those with higher self-efficacy and greater self-efficacy enhancement displayed greater numbers of suppressor T cells. Significant effects were also obtained for self-efficacy, pain, and joint impairment. Increased self-efficacy for functioning was associated with decreased disability and joint impairment.

EFFECTS OF THOUGHTS ON CENTRAL PROCESSING

Recent brain imaging studies may offer additional insight into how catastrophizing thoughts may influence pain perception. Seminowicz and Davis[63] examined functional MRI (fMRI) images while their pain-free subjects underwent laboratory pain testing and found that the effect of catastrophizing on neural response to painful stimulation may depend on the stimulus intensity levels. Neural responses to mild pain were seen in the regions representing attention, vigilance, and emotion, whereas the relationship is reversed with the moderate pain level, suggesting that catastrophizing attenuates the descending inhibitory system to more intense stimuli, making it more difficult to disengage from pain. Similar results have been reported in an imaging study of fibromyalgia patients in which catastrophizing, independent of depression, was related to the activation in the brain areas reflecting the attentional, anticipatory, and emotional activities in response to pain.[64] These studies suggest that catastrophizing adversely impacts pain experience via increased attention and negative anticipation of pain.

EFFECTS OF AFFECTIVE FACTORS ON PAIN

The International Association for the Study of Pain specifies that "[Pain] is unquestionably a sensation in a part or parts of the body but it is also always unpleasant and therefore also an emotional experience."[1] The affective factors associated with pain include many different emotions, but they are primarily negative in quality. Anxiety and depression have received the greatest amount of attention in chronic pain patients;

however anger has recently received considerable interest as an important emotion in chronic pain patients.

DEPRESSION

The prevalence of depression in chronic pain varies greatly from 5% to 100%, depending on how and where patients were assessed and the criteria for depression used, but it is estimated as at least 50% for the patients in specialized pain centers.[65] Depression adds a significant burden to chronic pain patients and is one of the principal determinants of pain-related disability.[66] Depression in chronic pain also drives the costs associated with disability and health care utilization upward.[67]

Historically, there has been much debate about the causal relationship between pain and depression. The literature typically supports the hypothesis that depression follows the development of chronic pain.[68] Some studies also suggest that the pain-depression relationship is not linear but rather is mediated by how patients view their plight. Turk et al.[69] have demonstrated that the relationship is mediated by a sense of control and life-interference appraisal of patients. The interaction between cognition and mood in chronic pain makes sense given the presence of individual differences in depression among patients with same diagnoses at the comparable pain and physical findings.[70]

This is not to say that depression does not exert any contribution to pain. It is well established that depressed people tend to have an elevated degree of pain complaints.[71] Longitudinal studies[72,73] suggest that depression is a risk factor for developing chronic pain. However, these results do not necessarily indicate that depression is the sole cause of pain. Regardless of the causal priority, both pain and depression require treatment in chronic pain patients.

Depression in chronic pain presents a particularly difficult concern for clinicians given the recent increase in misuse of potent opioid analgesics and unintentional as well as intentional poisoning from them. Fatalistic thoughts and wishes are common in chronic pain patients. Almost a quarter of treatment-seeking chronic pain patients acknowledge a history of suicidal ideation.[74] Thus, the assessment of depression in chronic pain should also be linked to the screening of medication misuse-abuse, as well as suicidal or overdosing history, and proper referral should be made to address this potentially dangerous condition.[75]

FEAR AND ANXIETY

Anxiety and fear-related problems are more prevalent in chronic pain patients than in the general public. The prevalence of any anxiety disorder may be twice as much (35% compared with 18%).[76] Although fear and anxiety are often treated as a single-unit mood condition, they are likely distinct entities with different types of physiological and emotional experiences. In relation to pain experience, they may also lead to differential results. When fear and anxiety states were experimentally induced (fear with exposure to shock, anxiety with threat of shock), people experiencing anxiety had greater pain reactivity than those who were in the low fear group.[77]

Pain is a naturally fear-producing state (i.e., unconditioned stimulus), thus being easily subjected to the behavioral principles to develop conditioned responses. Pain-related avoidance and escape behaviors in pain patients have been known to be integrated into the dysfunctional circle of pain maintenance.[78] Pain-related fear avoidance is significantly associated with functional limitation in various life domains and perceived disability in acute and chronic pain patients.[79,80]

ANGER

Anger has been widely observed in individuals with chronic pain. Pilowsky and Spence[81] reported an incidence of "bottled-up anger" in 53% of chronic pain patients. Of recent interest, trait anger-out, a personal tendency to express anger directly, whether verbally or physically, seems to be related to subjects' reports of greater pain in response to experimentally induced noxious stimulation in healthy and clinical pain populations, as well as greater clinical pain report in chronic pain patients.[82]

It has been suggested that the dysregulation in the endogenous opioid function may mediate the relationship between trait anger-out and pain. Expressed anger seems to attenuate the endogenous opioid activation to experimentally induced pain.[83] Reduced release of beta endorphin in response to pain has also been observed in those with a high degree of anger-out.[84]

Anger also seems to have an adverse impact on pain if it is suppressed; Kerns and colleagues[85] noted that the internalization of anger was strongly related to pain, perceived interference, and reported frequency of pain behaviors. Inhibition of anger expression in particular has been found to be related to depression, especially for those with severe pain.[86] Similarly, a study[87] showed effort to suppress provoked anger-attenuated blood pressure response to pain and was positively related to reports of greater pain.

Anger is not necessarily maladaptive. Anger can be a reasonable emotional response to the injustice that patients perceive. However, the accumulation of research suggests that poorly managed anger exacerbates pain and disability and interferes with treatment efforts. Effective self-management of anger may be essential for the successful rehabilitative effort of pain patients. Psychoeducational approaches help patients to better understand the concept and how poorly managed anger may contribute to their pain. Fernandez[88] suggests several approaches to help patients acquire better anger coping skills via cognitive reappraisal, behavioral modification, and appropriate affective disclosure. There has been a proliferation of research demonstrating the salient effects of poorly managed anger on pain experience in the past decade. By contrast, however, very little has been done to test the efficacy of anger management in improving pain therapy outcomes. Future research is warranted to evaluate the enhancement effects of such approaches for pain rehabilitation.

PATIENT UNIFORMITY MYTH

The importance of psychological factors in chronic pain has been widely recognized, and many pain treatment programs include interventions designed to address cognitive, affective, and behavioral components of the pain experience. One consistent finding, however, is that each treatment seems to work for some patients but that no treatment works for everyone.[4] Thus, we must be careful not to be trapped in the "patient homogeneity myth." Although characterization of patient populations may help us classify patients and direct treatment plans, research has shown that any populations that are defined by pain diagnoses demonstrate heterogeneity in their cognitive-affective-behavioral dimensions.

In order to address the heterogeneity of pain patients, Kerns and colleagues[89] developed a comprehensive inventory, the Multidimensional Pain Inventory (MPI). The MPI was designed to assess chronic pain patients' cognitive, affective, and behavioral responses to their symptoms. The MPI focuses on patients' interpretations of their plight, its effects on interpersonal relationships, and the resulting functional limitations. Using a statistical procedure (i.e., cluster analysis), Turk and colleagues[90] identified three distinct profiles of patients with chronic pain. They were labeled as: (1) *dysfunctional* (DYS), characterized by high levels of pain, life interference, emotional distress, and functional limitations; (2) *interpersonally distressed* (ID), similar to the DYS but further characterized by low level of support from their significant others; and (3) *adaptive copers* (AC), characterized by low levels of pain, functional limitations, and emotional distress. The classification system has been replicated in several studies conducted in Finland,[91] the Netherlands,[92] and in a large, multicentered study in the United States.[93] Recent studies have demonstrated that this subgroup's classification predicted future sickness absence in a working population with neck and back pain[94] and compensation following rehabilitation.[95]

Research using the MPI has demonstrated that the majority of patients with diverse chronic pain disorders (e.g., low back pain, temporomandibular disorder, headaches, fibromyalgia, neck pain, metastatic disease) can be classified into one of the three empirically derived profiles.[4,90,96,97,98] Although the percentage of patients classified within each of the profiles varies across pain disorders, patients' styles of adaptation to pain are very consistent within a profile regardless of their medical diagnosis, suggesting the relative independence of the psychosocial dimension of chronic pain from biomedical factors (see **Fig. 14-1**). The results from these studies further suggest that a dual-diagnostic approach may be useful, whereby two diagnoses are assigned concurrently—physical and psychosocial-behavioral—and treatment plans can be developed within each of the diagnostic frames.[98,99]

EXAMPLE OF TREATMENTS MATCHED TO PSYCHOSOCIAL AND BEHAVIORAL CHARACTERISTICS

We would hypothesize that providing a treatment plan that specifically addresses the psychosocial needs of each profile would show superior outcome to unmatched treatment. A basic cognitive-behavioral approach, including cognitive restructuring and behavioral skill training for pain management, is the most widely practiced method by pain psychologists.[4,99] Our previous trials showed that, although as a group, chronic pain patients show significant treatment gains from this approach, the three profile groups differentially responded to the treatment.[100] Most notably, patients who fit into the interpersonally distressed profile did not show significant improvement, with similar results being found in a Swedish study.[101]

Instead of the "one-size-fits-all" method, we need to address the "what-treatment-works-for-whom" question.[98,102] One example can be seen in **Table 14-1**. Three specific plans may be developed on the basis of the profile characteristics of the MPI classification. In this matrix,

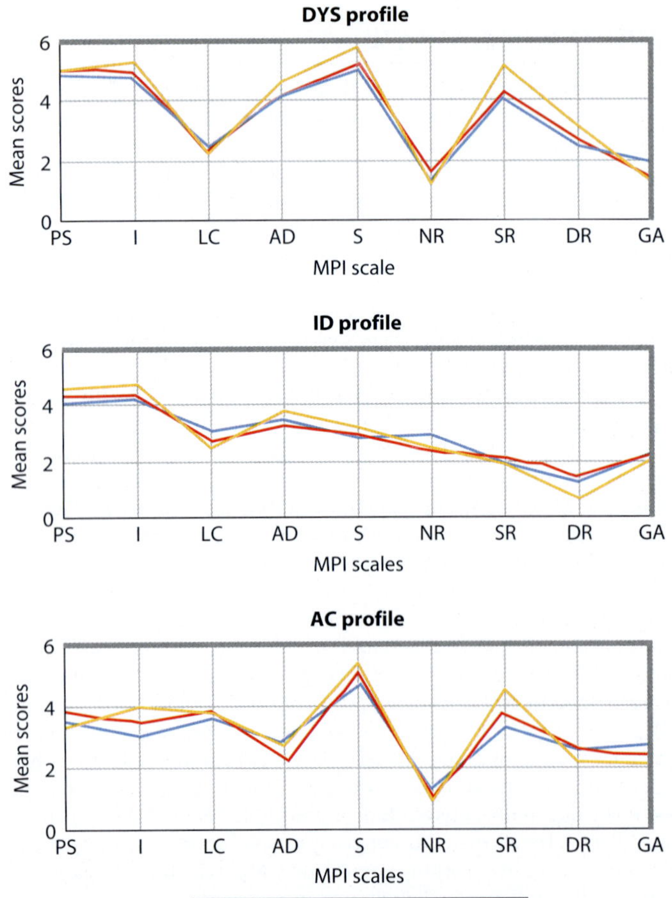

FIGURE 14-1. Mean MPI Scale Scores in Three Groups of Pain Patients—by MPI Profile.

TABLE 14-1 Sample Treatment-Matching Chart

	DYS	ID	AC
Treatment 1: Focusing on maladaptive thoughts and coping skills	Matched treatment	Undertreatment	Potential "overtreatment"
Treatment 2: Focusing interpersonal and communication skills	Undertreatment	Matched treatment	Potential "overtreatment"
Treatment 3: Focusing on supportive counseling	Undertreatment	Undertreatment	Matched treatment

Matched treatment
Potential "overtreatment"
Undertreatment

dysfunctional patients should benefit most from treatment 1, whereas interpersonally distressed patients should show improvement when they undergo treatment 2, over and beyond the improvement expected from the nonspecific effects of treatment. Treatment 3 may be considered as minimal psychological intervention—because adaptive copers are adjusting reasonably well, this minimal approach may be sufficient for these patients to achieve beneficial effects from the overall therapy. Elimination of inappropriate treatment components should save cost, as well as time, effort, and frustration for patients and treating clinicians.

SUMMARY AND CONCLUDING COMMENTS

Understanding the role of psychological factors in the development and maintenance of chronic pain has greatly increased since the first edition of this volume was published. Research efforts have confirmed that pain is a multifactoral phenomenon. A broad array of psychological factors, learning principles, cognitive factors, and affective components have been found to significantly influence how people experience pain, cope with pain, and recover from pain. In this chapter, we described different perspectives on pain and suggested that the unidimensional models (biomedical, psychogenic, motivational, behavioral) are inadequate to explain chronic pain or to serve as the basis for treatment. We examined the range of inter-related psychological factors that play an intricate role in pain perception, disability, and response to treatment. We raised a concern about the patient homogeneity myth and described one effort to subdivide patients based on a set of psychosocial and behavioral factors. Finally, we provided some preliminary evidence demonstrating that patients with different characteristics respond quite differently to the same treatment. Additional studies are needed to confirm these results, just as studies are needed to evaluate the potential of a specific treatment matching strategy.

Although we focused in this chapter on the role of psychological factors in chronic pain, we believe that these same factors may play a role in acute pain states as well. We believe that physical, psychosocial, and behavioral factors are all important in the experience of pain *per se*. The relative weight of these factors may vary, however, with physical factors making a larger contribution in acute pain states than chronic pain states and psychological factors making a more significant contribution in chronic pain than acute pain. In each of these instances, however, attention should be given to the range of factors that contributes to the total experience of pain.

REFERENCES

1. Mersky H, Bogduk N. eds. International Association for the Study of Pain: classification of chronic pain. Descriptions of chronic pain syndromes and definitions of pain terms. *Pain*. 1986;3:S1-S226.
2. Flor H, Turk DC. *Chronic Pain: An Integrated Biobehavioral Approach*. Seattle, Wash: IASP Press, 2012.
3. McCracken LM, Turk DC. Behavioral and cognitive-behavioral treatment for chronic pain: outcome, predictors of outcome, and treatment process. *Spine*. 2002;27(22):2564-2573.

4. Turk DC, Wilson HD, Cahana A. Treatment of chronic non-cancer pain. *Lancet.* 2011;377(9784):2226-2235.
5. Gatchel RJ, Peng YB, Peters ML, Fuchs PN, Turk DC. The biopsychosocial approach to chronic pain: scientific advances and future directions. *Psychol Bull.* 2007;133(4):581-624.
6. Deyo RA. Early diagnostic evaluation of low back pain. *J Gen Intern Med.* 1986;1(5):328-338.
7. Link TM, Steinbach LS, Ghosh S, et al. Osteoarthritis: MR imaging findings in different stages of disease and correlation with clinical findings. *Radiology.* 2003; 226(2):373-381.
8. Blankenbaker DG, Ullrick SR, Davis KW, De Smet AA, Haaland B, Fine JP. Correlation of MRI findings with clinical findings of trochanteric pain syndrome. *Skeletal Radiol.* 2008;37(10):903-909.
9. *American Psychiatric Association: Diagnostic and Statistical Manual of Mental Disorders.* 4th ed. Washington DC: American Psychiatric Press, 1994.
10. Fordyce W. *Behavioral Methods in Chronic Pain and Illness.* St. Louis, Mo: CV Mosby, 1976.
11. Kunz M, Rainville P, Lautenbacher S. Operant conditioning of facial displays of pain. *Psychosom Med.* 2011;73(5): 422-431.
12. Buck R. Nonverbal behavior and the theory of emotion: the facial feedback hypothesis. *J Pers Soc Psychol.* 1980;38(5):811-824.
13. Salomons TV, Coan JA, Hunt SM, Backonja MM, Davidson RJ. Voluntary facial displays of pain increase suffering in response to nociceptive stimulation. *J Pain.* 2008;9(5):443-448.
14. Becker S, Kleinbohl D, Klossika I, Holzl R. Operant conditioning of enhanced pain sensitivity by heat-pain titration. *Pain.* 2008;140(1):104-114.
15. Prkachin KM, Schultz IZ, Hughes E. Pain behavior and the development of pain-related disability: the importance of guarding. *Clin J Pain.* 2007;23(3):270-277.
16. Bunzli S, Gillham D, Esterman A. Physiotherapy-provided operant conditioning in the management of low back pain disability: a systematic review. *Physiother Res Int.* 2011;16(1): 4-19.
17. Vlaeyen JW, Haazen IW, Schuerman JA, Kole-Snijders AM, van Eek H. Behavioural rehabilitation of chronic low back pain: comparison of an operant treatment, an operant-cognitive treatment and an operant-respondent treatment. *Br J Clin Psychol.* 1995;34(Pt 1):95-118.
18. Turk DC, Flor H. Pain greater than pain behaviors: the utility and limitations of the pain behavior construct. *Pain.* 1987;31(3):277-295.
19. Turk D, Flor H. Chronic pain: a biobehavioral perspective. In: Gatchel R, Turk D, eds. *Psychological Factors in Pain.* New York, NY: Guilford, 1999.
20. Schmidt A, Brands A. Persistence behavior of chronic low back pain patients in an acute pain situation. *J Psychosom Res.* 1986; 30:339-346.
21. Arntz A, Vaneck M, DeJong P. Avoidance of pain of unpredictable intensity. *Behav Res Ther.* 1991;29:29:197-202.
22. Fagerhaugh S, Fagerhaugh S. Pain expression and control on a burn care unit. *Nursing Outlook.* 1974;22:645-650.
23. Richard K. The occurrence of maladaptive health-related behaviors and teacher-related conduct problems in children of chronic low back pain patients. *J Behav Med.* 1988;11:107-116.
24. Jensen MP, Turner JA, Romano JM, Karoly P. Coping with chronic pain: a critical review of the literature. *Pain.* 1991;47(3):249-283.
25. Tota-Faucette ME, Gil KM, Williams DA, Keefe FJ, Goli V. Predictors of response to pain management treatment: the role of family environment and changes in cognitive processes. *Clin J Pain.* 1993;9(2):115-123.
26. DeGood D, Shutty M. Assessment of pain beliefs, coping and self-efficacy. In: Turk D, Melzack R, eds. *Handbook of Pain Assessment.* New York, NY: Guilford, 1992.
27. Turner JA, Jensen MP, Romano JM. Do beliefs, coping, and catastrophizing independently predict functioning in patients with chronic pain? *Pain.* 2000;85(1-2):115-125.
28. Jackson T, Pope L, Nagasaka T, Fritch A, Iezzi T, Chen H. The impact of threatening information about pain on coping and pain tolerance. *Br J Health Psychol.* 2005;10(Pt 3):441-451.
29. Williams D, Thorn B. An empirical assessment of pain beliefs. *Pain.* 1989;36:185-190.
30. Nieto R, Raichle KA, Jensen MP, Miro J. Changes in pain-related beliefs, coping, and catastrophizing predict changes in pain intensity, pain interference, and psychological functioning in individuals with myotonic muscular dystrophy and facioscapulohumeral dystrophy. *Clin J Pain.* 2012;28:47-54.
31. Arntz A, Peters M. Chronic low back pain and inaccurate predictions of pain: is being too tough a risk factor for the development and maintenance of chronic pain? *Behav Res Ther.* 1995;33(1):49-53.
32. Turk D, Okifuji A, Sinclair J, Starz T. Interdisciplinary treatment for fibromyalgia syndrome: clinical and statistical significance. *Arthritis Care Res.* 1998;11(3):186-195.
33. Bandura A, Cioffi D, Taylor CB, Brouillard ME. Perceived self-efficacy in coping with cognitive stressors and opioid activation. *J Pers Soc Psychol.* 1988;55(3):479-488.
34. Sarda J, Jr., Nicholas MK, Asghari A, Pimenta CA. The contribution of self-efficacy and depression to disability and work status in chronic pain patients: a comparison between Australian and Brazilian samples. *Eur J Pain.* 2009;13(2):189-195.
35. Benyon K, Hill S, Zadurian N, Mallen C. Coping strategies and self-efficacy as predictors of outcome in osteoarthritis: a systematic review. *Musculoskeletal Care.* 2010;8(4):224-236.
36. Arnstein P, Caudill M, Mandle CL, Norris A, Beasley R. Self efficacy as a mediator of the relationship between pain intensity, disability and depression in chronic pain patients. *Pain.* 1999;80(3):483-491.
37. Arnstein P. The mediation of disability by self efficacy in different samples of chronic pain patients. *Disabil Rehabil.* 2000;22(17):794-801.
38. Costa LC, Maher CG, McAuley JH, Hancock MJ, Smeets RJ. Self-efficacy is more important than fear of movement in mediating the relationship between pain and disability in chronic low back pain. *Eur J Pain.* 2011;15(2):213-219.
39. Busch H, Goransson S, Melin B. Self-efficacy beliefs predict sustained long-term sick absenteeism in individuals with chronic musculoskeletal pain. *Pain Pract.* 2007;7(3):234-240.
40. Buckelew SP, Huyser B, Hewett JE, et al. Self-efficacy predicting outcome among fibromyalgia subjects. *Arthritis Care Res.* 1996;9(2):97-104.
41. Kores RC, Murphy WD, Rosenthal TL, Elias DB, North WC. Predicting outcome of chronic pain treatment via a modified self-efficacy scale. *Behav Res Ther.* 1990;28(2):165-169.
42. Beal CC, Stuifbergen AK, Brown A. Predictors of a health promoting lifestyle in women with fibromyalgia syndrome. *Psychol Health Med.* 2009;14(3):343-353.
43. Council J, Ahern D, Follick M, Kline C. Expectancies and functional impairment in chronic low back pain. *Pain.* 1988;33:323-331.
44. Keefe FJ, Brown GK, Wallston KA, Caldwell DS. Coping with rheumatoid arthritis pain: catastrophizing as a maladaptive strategy. *Pain.* 1989;37(1):51-56.

45. Turk D, Meichenbaum M. *Genest: Pain and Behavioral Medicine: A Cognitive-Behavioral Perspective*. New York, NY: Guilford, 1983.
46. Lu Q, Tsao JC, Myers CD, Kim SC, Zeltzer LK. Coping predictors of children's laboratory-induced pain tolerance, intensity, and unpleasantness. *J Pain*. 2007;8(9):708-717.
47. Edwards RR, Smith MT, Stonerock G, Haythornthwaite JA. Pain-related catastrophizing in healthy women is associated with greater temporal summation of and reduced habituation to thermal pain. *Clin J Pain*. 2006;22(8):730-737.
48. Sterling M, Hodkinson E, Pettiford C, Souvlis T, Curatolo M. Psychologic factors are related to some sensory pain thresholds but not nociceptive flexion reflex threshold in chronic whiplash. *Clin J Pain*. 2008;24(2):124-130.
49. Somers TJ, Keefe FJ, Carson JW, Pells JJ, Lacaille L. Pain catastrophizing in borderline morbidly obese and morbidly obese individuals with osteoarthritic knee pain. *Pain Res Manag*. 2008;13(5):401-406.
50. Geisser ME, Casey KL, Brucksch CB, Ribbens CM, Appleton BB, Crofford LJ. Perception of noxious and innocuous heat stimulation among healthy women and women with fibromyalgia: association with mood, somatic focus, and catastrophizing. *Pain*. 2003;102(3):243-250.
51. George SZ, Wallace MR, Wright TW, et al. Evidence for a biopsychosocial influence on shoulder pain: pain catastrophizing and catechol-O-methyltransferase (COMT) diplotype predict clinical pain ratings. *Pain*. 2008;136(1-2):53-61.
52. Pavlin DJ, Rapp SE, Polissar NL, Malmgren JA, Koerschgen M, Keyes H. Factors affecting discharge time in adult outpatients. *Anesth Analg*. 1998;87(4):816-826.
53. Khan RS, Ahmed K, Blakeway E, et al. Catastrophizing: a predictive factor for postoperative pain. *Am J Surg*. 2011;201(1):122-131.
54. Arnow BA, Blasey CM, Constantino MJ, et al. Catastrophizing, depression and pain-related disability. *Gen Hosp Psychiatry*. 2011;33(2):150-156.
55. Goodin BR, McGuire LM, Stapleton LM, et al. Pain catastrophizing mediates the relationship between self-reported strenuous exercise involvement and pain ratings: moderating role of anxiety sensitivity. *Psychosom Med*. 2009;71(9):1018-1025.
56. Weissman-Fogel I, Sprecher E, Pud D. Effects of catastrophizing on pain perception and pain modulation. *Exp Brain Res*. 2008;186(1):79-85.
57. Flor H, Turk DC, Birbaumer N. Assessment of stress-related psychophysiological reactions in chronic back pain patients. *J Consult Clin Psychol*. 1985;53(3):354-364.
58. Jamner L, Tursky B. Discrimination between intensity and affective pain descriptors: a psychophysiological evaluation. *Pain*. 1987;30(2):271-283.
59. Moulton B, Spence S. Site-specific muscle hyper-reactivity in musicians with occupational upper limb pain. *Behav Res Ther*. 1992;30(4):375-386.
60. Flor H, Birbaumer N, Schugens MM, Lutzenberger W. Symptom-specific psychophysiological responses in chronic pain patients. *Psychophysiology*. 1992;29(4):452-460.
61. Bandura A, O'Leary A, Taylor CB, Gauthier J, Gossard D. Perceived self-efficacy and pain control: opioid and nonopioid mechanisms. *J Pers Soc Psychol*. 1987;53(3):563-571.
62. O'Leary A, Shoor S, Lorig K, Holman H. A cognitive-behavioral treatment for rheumatoid arthritis. *Health Psychol*. 1988;7(6):527-544.
63. Seminowicz DA, Davis KD. Cortical responses to pain in healthy individuals depends on pain catastrophizing. *Pain*. 2006;120(3):297-306.
64. Gracely RH, Geisser ME, Giesecke T, et al. Pain catastrophizing and neural responses to pain among persons with fibromyalgia. *Brain*. 2004;127(Pt 4):835-843.
65. Bair MJ, Robinson RL, Katon W, Kroenke K. Depression and pain comorbidity: a literature review. *Arch Intern Med*. 2003; 163(20):2433-2445.
66. Tripp DA, VanDenKerkhof EG, McAlister M. Prevalence and determinants of pain and pain-related disability in urban and rural settings in southeastern Ontario. *Pain Res Manag*. 2006;11(4):225-233.
67. Katon W. The impact of depression on workplace functioning and disability costs. *Am J Manag Care*. 2009;15(11 suppl):S322-S327.
68. Brown GK. A causal analysis of chronic pain and depression. *J Abnorm Psychol*. 1990;99(2):127-137.
69. Turk DC, Okifuji A, Scharff L. Chronic pain and depression: role of perceived impact and perceived control in different age cohorts. *Pain*. 1995;61(1):93-101.
70. Okifuji A, Turk DC, Sherman JJ. Evaluation of the relationship between depression and fibromyalgia syndrome: why aren't all patients depressed? *J Rheumatol*. 2000;27(1):212-219.
71. Stahl SM. Does depression hurt? *J Clin Psychiatry*. 2002;63(4): 273-274.
72. Dworkin RH, Hartstein G, Rosner HL, Walther RR, Sweeney EW, Brand L. A high-risk method for studying psychosocial antecedents of chronic pain: the prospective investigation of herpes zoster. *J Abnorm Psychol*. 1992;101(1):200-205.
73. Jarvik JG, Hollingworth W, Heagerty PJ, Haynor DR, Boyko EJ, Deyo RA. Three-year incidence of low back pain in an initially asymptomatic cohort: clinical and imaging risk factors. *Spine (Phila Pa 1976)*. 2005;30(13):1541-1548; discussion 1549.
74. Smith MT, Perlis ML, Haythornthwaite JA. Suicidal ideation in outpatients with chronic musculoskeletal pain: an exploratory study of the role of sleep onset insomnia and pain intensity. *Clin J Pain*. 2004;20(2):111-118.
75. Cheatle MD. Depression, chronic pain, and suicide by overdose: on the edge. *Pain Med*. 2011;12(Suppl 2):S43-S48.
76. McWilliams LA, Cox BJ, Enns MW. Mood and anxiety disorders associated with chronic pain: an examination in a nationally representative sample. *Pain*. 2003;106(1-2):127-133.
77. Rhudy JL, Meagher MW. Fear and anxiety: divergent effects on human pain thresholds. *Pain*. 2000;84(1):65-75.
78. Vlaeyen JW, Linton SJ. Fear-avoidance and its consequences in chronic musculoskeletal pain: a state of the art. *Pain*. 2000; 85(3):317-332.
79. Gheldof EL, Vinck J, Van den Bussche E, Vlaeyen JW, Hidding A, Crombez G. Pain and pain-related fear are associated with functional and social disability in an occupational setting: evidence of mediation by pain-related fear. *Eur J Pain*. 2006;10(6):513-525.
80. Swinkels-Meewisse EJ, Swinkels RA, Verbeek AL, Vlaeyen JW, Oostendorp RA. Psychometric properties of the Tampa Scale for kinesiophobia and the fear-avoidance beliefs questionnaire in acute low back pain. *Man Ther*. 2003;8(1):29-36.
81. Pilowsky I, Spence N. Pain, anger, and illness behaviour. *J Psychosom Res*. 1976;20:411-416.
82. Bruehl S, Burns JW, Chung OY, Chont M. Pain-related effects of trait anger expression: neural substrates and the role of endogenous opioid mechanisms. *Neurosci Biobehav Rev*. 2009;33(3):475-491.
83. Bruehl S, Burns JW, Chung OY, Ward P, Johnson B. Anger and pain sensitivity in chronic low back pain patients and pain-free controls: the role of endogenous opioids. *Pain*. 2002;99(1-2):223-233.

84. Bruehl S, Chung OY, Burns JW, Diedrich L. Trait anger expressiveness and pain-induced beta-endorphin release: support for the opioid dysfunction hypothesis. *Pain*. 2007;130(3):208-215.

85. Kerns R, Rosenberg R, Jacob M. Anger expression and chronic pain. *J Behav Med*. 1994;17:57-67.

86. Estlander AM, Knaster P, Karlsson H, Kaprio J, Kalso E. Pain intensity influences the relationship between anger management style and depression. *Pain*. 2008;140(2):387-392.

87. Quartana PJ, Bounds S, Yoon KL, Goodin BR, Burns JW. Anger suppression predicts pain, emotional, and cardiovascular responses to the cold pressor. *Ann Behav Med*. 2010;39(3):211-221.

88. Fernandez E. *Anxiety, Depression, and Anger in Pain*. Toronto, Ontario, Canada: University of Toronto Press, 2002.

89. Kerns RD, Turk DC, Rudy TE. The West Haven-Yale Multidimensional Pain Inventory (WHYMPI). *Pain*. 1985;23(4):345-356.

90. Turk DC, Rudy TE. Toward an empirically derived taxonomy of chronic pain patients: integration of psychological assessment data. *J Consult Clin Psychol*. 1988;56(2):233-238.

91. Talo S, Rytokoski U, Puukka P. Patient classification, a key to evaluate pain treatment: a psychological study in chronic low back pain patients. *Spine*. 1992;17(9):998-1011.

92. Lousberg R, Schmidt AJM, Groenman NH, Vendrig L, Dijkman-Caes CIM. Validating the MPI-DVL using experience sampling data. *J Behav Med*. 1997;20:195-206.

93. Jamison RN, Rudy TE, Penzien DB, Mosley TH, Jr. Cognitive-behavioral classifications of chronic pain: replication and extension of empirically derived patient profiles. *Pain*. 1994;57(3):277-292.

94. Bergstrom C, Hagberg J, Bodin L, Jensen I, Bergstrom G. Using a psychosocial subgroup assignment to predict sickness absence in a working popualtion with neck and back pain. *BMC Musculoskel Dis*. 2011;12:81.

95. Nyberg VE, Novo M, Sjolund BH. Do Multidimensional Pain Inventory score chanes indiate risk of receiving sick leave benefits 1 year after a pain rehabilitation program? *Disabil Rehabil*. 2011;33:1548-1556.

96. Turk DC, Okifuji A, Sinclair JD, Starz TW. Pain, disability, and physical functioning in subgroups of patients with fibromyalgia. *J Rheumatol*. 1996;23(7):1255-1262.

97. Turk DC, Sist TC, Okifuji A, et al. Adaptation to metastatic cancer pain, regional/local cancer pain and non-cancer pain: role of psychological and behavioral factors. *Pain*. 1998;74(2-3):247-256.

98. Turk DC. Customizing treatment for chronic pain patients: who, what, and why. *Clin J Pain*. 1990;6(4):255-270.

99. Turk D, Okifuji A. A cognitive-behavioral approach to pain management. In: Wall P, Melzack R, eds. *Textbook of Pain*. London: Churchill Livingstone, 1999;1431-1444.

100. Turk D, Okifuji A, Starz T, Sinclair J. Differential responses by psychosocial subgroups of fibromyalgia syndrome patients to an interdisciplinary treatment. *Arthritis Care Res*. 1998;11(5):397-404.

101. Bergstrom C, Jensen I, Hagberg J, Busch H, Bergstrom G. Effectiveness of different interventions using a psychosocial subgroup assignment in chronic neck and back pain patients: a 10-year follow -up. *Disabil Rehabil*. 2012;34:110-118.

102. Rusu A, Boersma K, Turk DC. Subgroups of pain patients: the potential of customizing treatments. In: Hasenbring M, Rusu A, Turk DC, eds. *From Acute to Chronic Back Pain: Risk Factors, Mechanisms, and Clinical Implications*. London: Oxford University Press; 2012:485-511.

Psychosocial Assessment of Chronic Pain

Jonathan M. Borkum
R. Joshua Wootton

Why does one patient develop chronic pain and face disability, while another—with seemingly the same injuries, extent of tissue damage, and quality of medical care—recovers and returns to normal activity following a brief convalescence? Arguably, there may be biologic variables between the two that are difficult to discern medically, but a comparison, in most cases, is likely to reveal that the greater portion of the variance consists of psychosocial differences. When pain physicians wonder why a patient fails to respond to procedures and medications that have proven efficacious for many others with the same medical presentation, it is frequently the pain psychologist who can offer the most reasonable and, more importantly, functional set of hypotheses.

Although nociceptive or purely physiologic factors may instigate pain, how it is expressed by the individual, over time, suggests that what might have begun as a simple picture can become considerably more complicated and intricate through the influence of psychological and social factors. Melzack and Wall's gate control theory emphasizes that pain cannot be fully understood without an assessment of the motivational-affective, sensory-discriminative, and cognitive-evaluative processes of the individual.[1] Adherents to the biopsychosocial, mind-body, and behavioral medicine approaches to pain all affirm that, while the origin of pain may not be psychological, how a person *responds* to it is. Assessing this response expediently and accurately may redirect the focus of a patient's treatment, highlighting the psychosocial dimension of the patient's experience as essential to diagnosis and successful outcome. Chronic pain may not lead to adjustment difficulties, mental disorder, and disability, but when it does, psychosocial assessment may offer the only helpful perspective on why, as well as the best hope for recovery.

The principal goal of psychosocial assessment in chronic pain is not, as some patients fear, to determine whether or how much pain can be attributed to psychological sources but rather to identify the emotional, behavioral, and social factors that may be rendering it less tractable to treatment and moving the patient toward physical and psychological disability. The development of a successful plan for treatment often depends on identifying these influences and strategizing how to address them expediently, sensitively, and thoroughly.

RECORD REVIEW

It is helpful, early in the assessment process, to have access to the patient's previous medical records. The records can help in understanding the nature and severity of the underlying medical condition, the suspected peripheral pain generators, the response to previous medical treatments and the rationale for those that are planned, and the expected natural history of the disorder. This background, as it is understood and misunderstood by the patient, becomes highly influential in framing the challenges of treatment. Knowing the biomedical context can be a helpful bridge for conceptualizing and explaining, both to the patient and to other members of the treatment team, what role psychological factors may play. Discrepancies between the medical record and how a patient views his or her pain, as well as between expected and actual outcomes of past treatments, can sometimes indicate areas where psychological factors are central. Discussion with the referral source can be helpful in interpreting the records, hearing observations of the patient that may have been left out of the record, and understanding the concerns and goals behind the referral.

INTERVIEW AND PSYCHOMETRICS

In the interview, we seek to understand in depth the quality, intensity, and patterns of pain; patients' current coping strategies; their life stories before they ever imagined they would be patients; and their current psychological profiles. It is from the dynamic interplay among pain, current psychological makeup, and life stories that the foundations of treatment arise.

PAIN INTENSITY AND CHARACTERISTICS

Almost invariably, patients have been referred because of their pain specifically, and so it is here that our interview should begin. A high pain intensity is generally a given in treatment programs, but the patterns can vary widely. Continuous, high-intensity pain imposes a heavier burden than pain that can be relieved temporarily with a certain posture, position, stretch, or form of counterstimulation. The predictability of the pain is likewise important, as is the degree to which the triggers are controllable. Particularly useful for treatment are triggers in the behavioral (such as overactivity), sympathetic nervous system (such as startle), or emotional realms (such as loss, sorrow, or guilt).

Knowing the qualitative characteristics of the pain is helpful, as well. It is an entrance to the subjective world of the patient and hints at how the pain is encoded. The pain may be described in neutral sensory terms (e.g., sharp, squeezing), as an affective experience (e.g., punishing, vicious), as a judgment (e.g., unbearable), or as a vivid description of tissue damage. Changing the encoding may be part of the challenge of treatment. On a purely sensory level, the pain description may hint at the types of imagery that will be most useful for pain control. Moreover, the pain's qualities and triggers may shed some light on underlying mechanisms. For example, a burning pain that improves with a cool stimulus may turn out to be inflammatory, even if the circumstances of onset did not at first point in this direction.

Patients vary in the range of their vocabularies for pain. It is helpful to have the McGill Pain Questionnaire available (described later in this chapter) for people who have trouble putting their pain into words.

COGNITIVE AND EMOTIONAL FACTORS IN PAIN AND DISABILITY

Especially important are those cognitive and affective variables that are likely to influence how the pain is experienced and whether it follows a benign or deteriorating course. Here, we will discuss the most important of these variables, why they matter, and how they are typically assessed. For some patients, psychoeducation—explaining the relevance of the psychological variables to pain—will be necessary at the outset for the interview to make sense to them.

Depression, Loss, and Attachment

Depression The prevalence of depressive disorders in people with chronic pain is approximately 20% in community samples and 50% in the clinic.[2,3] The impact is significant: Depression is not merely noxious to functioning and quality of life; it is intertwined with pain and its outcome on sensory and affective levels.

Thus, major depressive disorder often involves pain, much as does the flu,[4] through a lowering of thresholds for pain from within the body.[5] Depression increases the probability of the onset,[6] chronicity,[7] and increasing frequency of pain.[8] Moreover, depression is a strong risk factor for poor outcome from lumbar surgery and may interfere with the efficacy of spinal cord stimulation, medial branch nerve blocks, and opiate medications[9-11] (although perhaps not cognitive-behavioral pain treatment, in which depression is addressed directly[12]). In headaches, depression predicts the development of allodynia, a marker of central sensitization and itself a risk factor for migraine chronification.[8]

In the body, the connections between depression and pain are several and strong: In major depressive disorder, much as in physical illness, blood levels of cortisol and proinflammatory cytokines, particularly interleukin 1-β, are elevated.[13] These, in turn, can induce a proinflammatory state in the central nervous system, facilitating pain transmission and presumably contributing over time to pain sensitization.[14]

Moreover, dysphoria and pain-distress activate overlapping structures: the dorsal anterior cingulate cortex, anterior insula, and the amygdala.[15,16] Conversely, pain-distress is modulated by such "reward centers" as the nucleus accumbens and the ventral tegmentum,[17] which are generally underactive in depression.[18]

More generally, depression and pain are inhibited by the same brain regions—dorsolateral, ventral lateral, and orbital prefrontal cortex and rostral anterior cingulate cortex.[19,20] Deficient recruitment of these top-down regulatory circuits likely participates in both disorders.[21,22]

Not only current but also past depression may be relevant: Depression during childhood or adolescence predicts the development of osteoarthritis in adulthood, especially between the ages of 35 and 70, presumably because of the bias toward inflammation.[23]

While we are always interested in knowing the presence and severity of depression, this is particularly true in cases of poor treatment response to medical interventions and signs of erosion of pain thresholds—localized, regional, or whole-body mechanical allodynia or circumscribed pain and tenderness that have spread over time. The erosion of pain thresholds can have many sources; severe depression, when present, may be among them.

The gold standard for diagnosis of a depressive disorder is a structured clinical interview schedule such as the SCID[24,25] or, more briefly, the MINI-Plus.[26] However, both of these are likely too lengthy for an interview focused on pain coping.

People are usually, although not invariably, aware of when they are depressed and will report it during the interview. Most often, they describe depression as a consequence of the pain, and an additional burden, but a few report that depression causes an aching or heavy pain or that guilt triggers a migraine. Sometimes, blunted affect, psychomotor slowing, and/or pessimistic and joyless thought content are the only indicators of depression. Inquiring about the DSM-5 (Diagnostic and Statistical Manual of Mental Disorders, 5th ed.) diagnostic criteria, especially the cognitive and affective elements, can be helpful for clarifying whether the severity rises to the level of a clinical disorder. Items that were endorsed on the psychometrics can be a useful starting point.

Psychometrics are used for screening or as measures of severity. The Beck Depression Inventory (BDI),[27] Centers for Epidemiological Studies—Depression Scale (CES-D),[28] the PHQ-9,[29] and the QIDS-SR[30] have all been studied psychometrically in chronic pain. Because endorsements of somatic symptoms and performance interference on depression inventories can reflect pain rather than mood, modified cutoff scores have been derived, as given in **Table 15-1**.

Loss The feeling of grief, rejection, and social loss is described in terms of physical injury (e.g., feeling "crushed," "burned," or "heartbroken") not only in English and its Indo-European relatives, but in such diverse languages as Mandarin, Bhutanese, Inuktitut, Armenian, Hungarian, and Hebrew.[31] This seems to reflect an overlapping neural architecture representing the hurt from social loss and distress from physical pain: The intensity of both is positively correlated with activation in the dorsal anterior cingulate cortex and negatively correlated with activation in the right ventral prefrontal cortex, an area involved in descending pain control.[32] Not surprisingly, then, distress from social exclusion may potentiate sensitivity to heat-pain.[33]

Not only social inclusion, with its implicit access to social resources, is relevant to pain; so, too, is its symbolic embodiment in money. In the laboratory, when people think about having money, their heat-pain ratings are lower. Conversely, when people are asked to write about their recent expenditures, they feel weaker, and their heat-pain ratings are higher than in a neutral control condition.[34] Conversely, acute physical pain and social rejection seem to increase the desire for money as a compensating social resource.

Chronic pain often entails loss of work with its sense of community, exclusion from activities with family and friends, withdrawal, and isolation. Because it is likely that all of these can intensify pain severity and pain-distress, the evaluation should help gauge their magnitude. For patients still working, the quality of their interactions with supervisors and coworkers, and their sense of job security, are important.

TABLE 15-1 Self-Report Instruments Relevant to Chronic Pain

Construct	Scale	Properties	Comments	References
Acceptance	Chronic Pain Acceptance Questionnaire	20 Items, 2 Subscales $\alpha \approx 0.85$ (full scale) ≈ 0.82 (Activity Engagement) ≈ 0.78 (Pain Willingness)		McCracken et al.[197] Nicholas & Asghari[198]
Coping/ Catastrophizing	Chronic Pain Coping Inventory	65 Items, 8 Subscales $\alpha \approx 0.74$ (Guarding) ≈ 0.75 (Resting) ≈ 0.85 (Asking for Assistance) ≈ 0.73 (Relaxation) ≈ 0.78 (Task Persistence) ≈ 0.89 (Exercise/Stretch) ≈ 0.87 (Coping Self-Statements) ≈ 0.82 (Seeking Social Support) Also: $\alpha \approx 0.79$ (Pacing)	There is also a 42-item version. The Pacing subscale is available only in the 65-item version.	Ersek et al.[276] Jensen et al.[277]
	Coping Strategies Questionnaire	42 Items, 7 Subscales $\alpha \approx 0.84$ (Diverting Attention) ≈ 0.89 (Reinterpreting Pain Sensations) ≈ 0.82 (Coping Self-Statements) ≈ 0.78 (Ignoring Pain Sensations) ≈ 0.80 (Praying and Hoping) ≈ 0.78 (Increasing Activity Level) ≈ 0.74 (Catastrophizing)		Keefe et al.[185] Rosenstiel & Keefe[87]
	Pain Catastrophizing Scale	13 Items, 3 Factors $\alpha \approx 0.94$ (full scale) ≈ 0.89 (Helplessness) ≈ 0.78 (Magnification) ≈ 0.87 (Rumination)		Chibnall & Tait[278] Sullivan et al.[88]
	Vanderbilt Pain Management Inventory	18 Items, 2 Subscales $\alpha \approx 0.71$ (Active Coping) $\alpha \approx 0.81$ (Passive Coping)	An 11-item version is also available ($\alpha \approx 0.71$ active coping; $\alpha \approx 0.71$ passive coping).	Brown & Nicassio[279] Smith et al.[280]
Depression	Beck Depression Inventory (BDI-IA)	21 Items, 1 Scale $\alpha \approx 0.86$ (psychiatric samples) ≈ 0.81 (non-psychiatric)	Modified cutoff of 12, 15, or 20 has been suggested for pain patients.	Beck et al.[27] Geisser et al.[281] Love[282] Wong et al.[283]
	Beck Depression Inventory-II	21 Items, 1 Scale $\alpha \approx 0.91$ (psychiatric and non-psychiatric)	Modified cutoff of 22 has been suggested for pain patients. Appropriate for ages 13–80. Excellent validity.	Beck et al.[233] Dozois & Covin[284] Poole et al.[285]
	Center for Epidemiological Studies—Depression Scale (CES-D)	20 Items, 1 Scale $\alpha \approx 0.87$	Modified cutoff of 26 has been suggested for pain patients.	Geisser et al.[281] Radloff[28] Wong et al.[283]
	PHQ-9	Coefficient $\alpha = 0.89$ Sensitivity ≈ 0.80 Specificity ≈ 0.92 (For cutoff ≥ 10)	Very quick to complete and score.	Gilbody et al.[286] Spitzer et al.[287]
	QIDS-SR$_{16}$	Coefficient $\alpha \approx 0.87$	Designed as a severity (vs. screening) measure.	Rush et al.[288]

(*Continued*)

TABLE 15-1 Self-Report Instruments Relevant to Chronic Pain (*Continued*)

Construct	Scale	Properties	Comments	References
Disability	Oswestry Disability Index	10 Items α ≈ 0.86	Designed for low back pain but good psychometric properties for general pain after substituting "pain" for "back pain" in the instructions.	Fairbank et al.[289] Wittink et al.[290]
	Pain Disability Index	7 Items, 2 Subscales α ≈ 0.92 (Voluntary Activities) ≈ 0.80 (Obligatory Activities)	Validated also for telephone administration.	Tait & Chibnall[291]
Fear of Pain	Fear of Pain Questionnaire – III	30 Items, 3 Subscales α ≈ 0.92 (full scale) ≈ 0.88 (Severe Pain) ≈ 0.87 (Minor Pain) ≈ 0.92 (Medical Pain)	The subscales can be used individually. A 20-item version is also available.	McNeil et al.[68] Asmundson et al.[292]
	Pain Anxiety Symptoms Scale (PASS-20)	20 Items, 4 Subscales α ≈ 0.91 (full scale) ≈ 0.86 (Cognitive) ≈ 0.75 (Escape/Avoidance) ≈ 0.82 (Fear) ≈ 0.81 (Physiological Anxiety)	A 40-item version is also available and has been extensively studied.	McCracken & Dhingra[293]
Kinesiophobia	Tampa Scale for Kinesiophobia	17 Items, 2 Subscales α ≈ 0.68 (osteoarthritis) to 0.76 (chronic LBP)	Extensively normed.	Heuts et al.[294] Roelofs et al.[107,295]
	Fear Avoidance Beliefs Questionnaire	16 Items, 2 Subscales α ≈ 0.90 (full scale) ≈ 0.72 (Physical Activity) ≈ 0.82 (Work)	Also in Chinese, French, German, Portugese, Spanish, and Turkish.	Lee, Chiu, & Lam[110] Swinkels-Meewisse[109]
Multidimensional	West Haven-Yale Multidimensional Pain Inventory	52 Items, 12 Subscales α ≈ 0.78 (Pain Severity) ≈ 0.92 (Life Interference) ≈ 0.78 (Life Control) ≈ 0.64 (Affective Distress) ≈ 0.84 (Support) ≈ 0.82 (Punishing Responses) ≈ 0.81 (Solicitous Responses) ≈ 0.71 (Distracting Responses) ≈ 0.86 (Household Chores) ≈ 0.77 (Outdoor Work) ≈ 0.70 (Activities Away from Home) ≈ 0.74 (Social Activities) ≈ 0.87 (General Activities)	Three-cluster solution used in treatment matching. Reliabilities here are from Nicholas et al.,[188] (first 8 subscales) and Kerns et al.[190] (last 4 subscales). Extensive norms are available in Nicholas et al.[188] General Activities Scale is a combination of the four preceding subscales.	Kerns et al.[190] Nicholas et al.[188] Wittink et al.[290]
Pain Quality and Intensity	McGill Pain Questionnaire-Short-Form, Revised (SF-MPQ-2)	22 Items, 4 Subscales α ≈ 0.95 (full scale) ≈ 0.87 (Continuous Pain) ≈ 0.87 (Intermittent Pain) ≈ 0.83 (Neuropathic Pain) ≈ 0.86 (Affective Descriptors)		Dworkin et al.[268]
	Multidimensional Affect and Pain Survey (101-MAPS)	101 Items, 30 Subclusters, 3 Superclusters α ≈ 0.97 (Somatosensory Pain) ≈ 0.94 (Emotional Pain) ≈ 0.94 (Well-being)	Interval-level scales Free of ethnic and gender bias. Relatively long.	Clark et al.[296] Griswold & Clark[297]

(*Continued*)

TABLE 15-1 Self-Report Instruments Relevant to Chronic Pain (*Continued*)

Construct	Scale	Properties	Comments	References
Posttraumatic Stress Disorder	Impact of Events Scale	15 Items, 2 Components $\alpha \approx 0.80$	Cutoff (≈ 26) does not need adjustment for pain.	Horowitz et al.[117]
	PTSD Symptom Scale – Self-Report	17 Items, 3 Subscales $\alpha \approx 0.95$ (full scale) ≈ 0.92 (Re-experiencing) ≈ 0.88 (Avoidance) ≈ 0.86 (Hyperarousal)	Cutoff does not need adjustment for pain. Scale may not distinguish well between PTSD and other anxiety disorders.	Engelhard et al.[298] Foa et al.[118]
Self-Efficacy	Pain Self-Efficacy Questionnaire	10 Items, No Subscales $\alpha \approx 0.93$	Good convergent and divergent validity. Extensive norms are available in Nicholas et al.[188]	Nicholas[187] Nicholas et al.[188]
Sleep Quality	Chronic Pain Sleep Inventory	5 Items, 1 Overall Index Score $\alpha \approx 0.93$	Pain-related sleep problems. Only 3 items participate in the index score.	Kosinski et al.[174]
	Insomnia Severity Index	7 Items, 1 Scale $\alpha \approx 0.91$	Validated in clinical and community samples. Scores ≥ 11 indicate sleep problems.	Bastien et al.[299] Morin et al.[300]
	Medical Outcomes Study Sleep Scale	12 Items, 6 Domains, 1 Overall Index Score $\alpha \approx 0.78$	General sleep scale, validated in pain. Only 9 items participate in the overall index score.	Hays et al.[173] Rejas et al.[175]
Stages of Change	Pain Stages of Change Quesionnaire	30 Items, 4 Subscales $\alpha \approx 0.77$ (Precontemplation) ≈ 0.82 (Contemplation) ≈ 0.86 (Action) ≈ 0.86 (Maintenance)	Here, the Contemplation subscale subsumes also the preparation stage.	Kerns et al.[217]
Substance Abuse Potential	Opioid Risk Tool	10 Items PPV ≈ 0.91, NPV ≈ 0.94 Concordance ≈ 0.85 female, 0.82 male	Cutoff < 4 vs. ≥ 8. Low sensitivity in the few attempts to cross-validate.	Webster & Webster[238] Moore et al.[240]
	Screener and Opioid Assessment For Patients with Pain—Revised (SOAPP-R)	24 Items $\alpha \approx 0.88$	For cutoff ≥ 18, sensitivity ≈ 0.81 specificity ≈ 0.68. Local norms will likely be helpful.	Butler et al.[237]
Suicidality	Beck Hopelessness Scale	Sensitivity ≈ 0.80; Specificity ≈ 0.42	Low specificity reflects low base rate of suicide.	Beck et al.[230] McMillan et al.[301]
Trauma History	Childhood Trauma Questionnaire – Short Form	28 Items, 6 Subscales $\alpha \approx 0.92$ (Full Scale) ≈ 0.87 (Emotional Abuse) ≈ 0.84 (Physical Abuse) ≈ 0.94 (Sexual Abuse) ≈ 0.88 (Emotional Neglect) ≈ 0.69 (Physical Neglect) ≈ 0.82 (Minimization/Denial)	The five main subscales are highly intercorrelated.	Bernstein et al.[54] Gerdner & Allgulander[302]
Values Orientation	Chronic Pain Values Inventory	12 Items, 2 Subscales $\alpha \approx 0.82$ (Success) ≈ 0.82 (Discrepancy)	Subscales: Success at living in accord with values. Discrepancy between importance of a value and success.	McCracken & Yang[201]

We should be particularly attentive to recent, acute losses that might intensify distress to the point that risk of suicide is increased.

Although questionnaire measures of trait sensitivity to rejection[35] and current social support[36] exist, the simplest and most flexible assessment is through the interview. The perceived support of one's partner specifically is covered in the West Haven-Yale Multidimensional Pain Inventory, discussed later in this chapter. The assessment should also cover economic insecurity, not only for its potential effect on pain, but because some patients may require social work intervention along with their pain treatment.

Insecure Attachment Closely related to vulnerability to rejection is attachment theory, in which individuals are posited to develop in infancy a sense of the dependability of others and the trustworthiness of their own coping ability. These overarching appraisals are thought to have a stable, traitlike character throughout life.[37] In particular, insecure attachment is thought to result when the child's caregiver is inconsistent or unreliable and can be subdivided into an avoidant subtype, in which the individual has difficulty in trusting and being close, and an anxious subtype, in which the individual wishes to merge completely with others to overcome a sense of isolation.[38] In this theory, individuals with insecure attachment are more likely to respond to pain in anxious, depressive, and catastrophic terms and more likely to use emotion-based, ineffective coping strategies. Support seeking (including treatment seeking) may be excessive, avoidant, or ambivalent, depending on the subtype of insecure attachment.[39] It is also possible that insecure attachment is a risk factor for pain because of lifelong vulnerability to stress and/or to maladaptive coping behaviors such as smoking, drinking, or overeating.[40]

A number of studies have indeed shown insecure attachment to be related to depression, catastrophizing, fear of pain, disability, and, in some cases, pain intensity. However, the studies have nearly all been cross-sectional and so, theory aside, it is not yet clear whether insecure attachment is a cause or consequence of how the pain is experienced.[40] This is significant because people may be more vulnerable physically and economically—and have less support available—on account of the pain. It is also not clear whether insecure attachment is a more useful construct in chronic pain than the various forms of distress to which it is related.[38]

Because psychological pain treatment is generally focused on coping skills for reducing pain and its consequences, and is time-limited, the amelioration of broad personality traits is generally outside of its scope. Insecure attachment would be dealt with on a practical level through its effects on mood and coping resources. Nonetheless, it is helpful to observe a patient's preferred way of relating to health care providers, their vulnerability to loss, their sources of resentment, and their sense of boundaries so that treatment can be presented in a way that remains focused and constructive. Sometimes, formal personality assessment, integrated with the medical background to explain the patient's presentation, can be a source of helpful feedback to patient and physician alike.[41] Patients may be perplexed by their symptoms and appreciate someone trying to explain them in depth. However, if personality factors are the overriding feature of presentation (as may occur, for example, in factitious disorder or some expressions of somatoform disorder), then they will generally need to be treated by a therapist who specializes in that field before pain treatment can be successful.

History of Abuse or Other Traumas Traumatic life events in childhood are a risk factor for localized pain syndromes and for chronic widespread pain.[42] A traumatic childhood seems to induce changes in the immune system that persist into adulthood, including elevated levels of such inflammatory mediators as C-reactive protein,[43,44] fibrinogen, interleukin-6,[45] and white blood cell count.[46] Taken together, these suggest a shift to a proinflammatory state, as if the body were permanently preparing itself for injury.[47] A proinflammatory state, in turn, may predispose the nervous system to pain sensitization.[14]

Trauma may also impair the endorphin system. Childhood adversity shows a dose-response relationship in adulthood, at least among depressed patients, with reduced volume of the rostral anterior cingulate cortex.[48] This general region is active during analgesia from placebo, hypnosis, or distraction,[49] raising the possibility that the capacity for endogenous pain control is curtailed by a traumatic childhood. Thus, for example, childhood abuse and, in particular, emotional abuse, independent of adult depression and anxiety, predicts transformation from episodic to chronic migraine and the development of allodynia.[50]

At the interview, then, we would generally ask about childhood trauma, particularly noting exposure to a wide range of traumas and/or a prevailing sense of fear during childhood. Individuals may come into the interview unaware of the connection to pain thresholds and may find the information quite helpful for making sense of their experiences and shifting to more active coping.

Moreover, some of the effects of previous trauma may lie in the psychological and physical cost of suppressing the feelings associated with it. Patients with rheumatoid arthritis[51] and fibromyalgia[52,53] appear to have improved functioning and emotional quality of life 3 months after disclosing, even anonymously or to themselves, a traumatic event. In this sense, too, the interview may have a therapeutic quality.

Psychometric assessment of adverse childhood events is not usually conducted in pain settings, but, because the effects may depend on the number and types of traumas, there is a logic to doing so. There is support in particular for the validity of the Childhood Trauma Questionnaire.[54]

Pain and Narrative That physical pain and social loss would share an underlying neural substrate suggests that social context is as important in the former as it is in the latter. In fact, in the laboratory, people rate stimuli as more painful and are less likely to habituate to them, when they regard the pain as having been intentionally inflicted.[55] In the clinic, perceived injustice—the feeling that an injury is severe, irreparable, and someone else's fault—predicts ongoing disability and treatment failure.[56] It is hard to accept an injury and move on when it should never have happened in the first place. More generally, depressing or angry thoughts about pain, in which the pain is relevant by virtue of being embedded in a cognitive schema—a network of associations—generate more pain-distress than nonspecific negative mood.[57]

Of course, in real life, pain indeed exists in context—for example, frustration over lax safety at the workplace, carelessness by the other driver in a motor vehicle accident, disappointment over previous failed treatments, or even as existential punishment. Inquiring about the origins and history of the pain and current relationships with family, coworkers, and disability systems provides not only a practical understanding of the nature of the problem, but a way of understanding the narrative, the schema, in which the pain is embedded. This can allow us to discern the emotional meanings that may be stabilizing a pain focus. Changing these meanings, or decreasing the amount of mental energy given to them, may then become an aspect of treatment.

Stress, Fear, and Catastrophic Thinking

Fear of Pain Fear of pain seems to intensify pain on a sensory level. It can lead to self-limiting activity, can interfere with successful rehabilitation, and should be suspected in cases of excessive disability.

In the laboratory, fear of pain has a priming quality: It amplifies the experience of a subsequent noxious input.[58] In part, it seems to do so by triggering anti-endorphinergic, descending, pain-facilitating pathways,[59] intensifying pain transmission on a spinal level.[60] This in turn may derive from increased activity in the dorsal anterior cingulate cortex, which encodes the unpleasantness of pain and is a source of pain facilitating pathways.[61]

Fear of pain is also important in chronic pain when it contributes to profound guarding, as in chronic low back pain and, even more consequentially, in complex regional pain syndrome. Perhaps because voluntary movement elicits endogenous pain control,[62] extreme voluntary disuse of a body part can cause hyperalgesia to cold and pressure.[63] It may also function as a type of functional deafferentation,[64] causing the representation of the affected part in primary somatosensory cortex to shrink, giving rise to phantomlike pain.[65] Moreover, if continued long enough, extreme voluntary disuse can lead to neglect, a loss of inhibitory control from motor cortex, and an inability to use the body part.[66] There is preliminary evidence that fear of pain may have a genetic component.[67]

Inquiries can be made directly about whether the pain ever becomes frightening, in what aspects, and under what circumstances. Sometimes, the fear turns out to be one of losing mobility or that a worsening course of pain will continue indefinitely, culminating in pain that is unendurable. Sometimes, the issue is as simple as a misunderstanding of the diagnosis. A patient learned from her MRI report, for example, that her "neural foramina are patent." Although this is good news—an absence of nerve impingement—for more than a year she had been too frightened to inquire about what she assumed was a dire finding. Moreover, even well-educated patients who are exceedingly rational in other areas of their lives may harbor beliefs that they have a severe undiagnosed condition—that intense pain surely corresponds to catastrophic illness—or even that the pain or sleep deprivation itself might kill them.

Psychometrically, fear of pain is generally measured as a trait using the Fear of Pain Questionnaire, comprised of three 10-item subscales measuring fear of severe pain, minor pain, and pain associated with medical procedures.[68] The subscales have excellent internal consistencies, as does the composite scale, and each can be used individually.

Because of social desirability, however, patients may be reluctant to report a fear of pain. It can be helpful to have the observations of their physical therapist or physician. Very guarded behavior (assuming no acute flare-up, for example, from travel to the interview) may suggest pain-related fear. Conversely, a high level of functioning often, but not invariably, implies relatively little fear of pain.

Catastrophic Thinking First noted by Albert Ellis,[69] catastrophizing is an amalgam of several elements: an appraisal of the pain (extreme overestimation of its threat), an appraisal of a person's own coping resources (feeling helpless and overwhelmed), and prolonged attention to the pain (rumination[70]). It is especially important because it predicts a downward spiral of pain, depression, and disability[71,72] and the future development of chronic pain in people who were initially pain-free.[73,74]

Catastrophizing likely exerts its malignant effects through several mechanisms. Psychologically, coping strategies are more likely to be passive[75] and ineffective,[76] and people who catastrophize have a harder time disengaging attention from pain.[77]

Moreover, anxiety about pain adds to pain-distress and increases the activity in a region of the cortex, the parahippocampal gyrus, that likely encodes aversion and the unpleasantness of pain.[78,79] In turn, this activation may trigger descending pain facilitation.[80]

Further, catastrophizing may impede pain regulation by the dorsolateral prefrontal cortex.[81] With repeated stimulation, catastrophizing disrupts endorphinergic buffering[82] and increases temporal summation.[83] Moreover, the stress caused by catastrophic thinking seems to be reflected in higher levels of cortisol and interleukin-6, a proinflammatory cytokine, in response to pain.[84] These, in turn, might induce glial cell activation, slowing reuptake of glutamate in the pain pathways. All of these effects would set the stage for pain sensitization.

Longer term, catastrophizing is associated with structural changes in the basal ganglia that may contribute to pain sensitivity.[85] Moreover, the unpleasantness of pain, to which catastrophizing surely contributes, correlates with a progressive loss of gray matter density in brain regions involved in registering and inhibiting pain.[85,86]

Asking patients if they feel overwhelmed by pain is not necessarily informative because of the social desirability around appearing weak and because "overwhelmed" is often interpreted matter-of-factly to mean that an activity had to be stopped because of pain. Rather, it is helpful to elicit vignettes from the person's recent experience of a time when he or she was coping well, and vignettes from when not coping well, along with the situations, suspected pain triggers, thoughts, emotions, and behavioral responses. This can be followed up with a structured pain diary, with columns for each of these variables. Of course, if a patient becomes visibly overwhelmed when discussing a symptom, tracing back the thoughts that led to this can shed light on catastrophic thinking.

Psychometrically, catastrophizing is usually assessed with the Pain Catastrophizing Scale (PCS) or the Coping Strategies Questionnaire (CSQ). The CSQ consists of seven subscales of six items each, corresponding to the techniques of diverting attention, reinterpreting pain sensations, ignoring pain sensations, using coping self-statements, increasing activity level, praying and hoping, and catastrophizing.[87] The PCS is a 13-item instrument specific to catastrophic thinking. Factors of the PCS correspond to the rumination, helplessness, and magnification components of catastrophizing.[88] Although these instruments are generally administered as trait measures, they can be readily adapted to capture responses that fluctuate over time. Further details are given in Table 15-1.

Fearful Avoidance of Movement (Kinesiophobia) Closely related to fear of pain is fear of movement/reinjury, also termed *kinesiophobia*, often reflecting a belief that movement will cause further physical damage. The construct has been studied mostly in low back pain where, in longitudinal studies, it seems to confer an increased risk for chronicity[73,89,90] and disability.[73,91,92]

The theory that fear-avoidance beliefs prolong pain through deconditioning, a progressive loss of muscle tone, flexibility, and aerobic capacity, has been mostly disconfirmed,[93,94] but other mechanisms are possible. Pain may be increased by the loss of endorphinergic signaling from motor cortex[62,95,96] or through fearful attention to pain during activity.[97] Moreover, fear of pain induces patterns of activity in the musculature of the low back that increase compressive forces on the spine while reducing protection of the intervertebral disks from shearing forces. This pattern of muscle recruitment is strongly predictive of future low back pain, even among initially pain-free subjects.[98] And, behaviorally, vigorous physical activity may be extinguished by fear, contributing to disability.

Fear of movement is often most apparent to the physical therapist, making interdisciplinary communication helpful in its assessment. Nonetheless, patients may report fear that certain movements will herniate a disk or sever the spine. As with all pain reports, we would seek to understand this on a sensory level, for its hints of pain generating mechanism, as well as the affective and interpretive levels. Occasionally, patients with post-concussion syndrome may confide a fear that mental effort will cause brain damage.

Concerns about the harmfulness of physical activity are generally measured with the Fear Avoidance Beliefs Questionnaire (FABQ),[91] the Tampa Scale for Kinesiophobia (TSK),[99-101] or the Pain and Impairment Rating Scale for patients (PAIRS)[102] or for health care providers (HC-PAIRS).[103,104]

The Tampa Scale for Kinesiophobia[99,100] is a 17-item questionnaire found empirically to comprise two factors:[105] activity avoidance (sample item: "I'm afraid that I might injure myself if I exercise") and somatic focus (e.g., "My body is telling me I have something dangerously wrong"). Because six items do not load selectively on either factor, a shorter, 11-item version has also been developed.[106] An advantage of the TSK is that extensive norms are available for patients with a variety of musculoskeletal diagnoses.[107] This is important because patients with back pain have higher mean scores than those with upper extremity disorders, with fibromyalgia and osteoarthritis patients scoring lower still. Also, patients over the age of 60 tend to have higher scores.

The Fear Avoidance Beliefs Questionnaire[91] consists of 16 items. Conceptually, it is divided into subscales measuring fear associated with physical activity and fear associated with work. The two scales are sometimes used separately.[108] They are intercorrelated, however, and the combined scale appears to have much better reliability.[109,110]

Posttraumatic Stress Disorder In the general community, approximately 7% to 8% of individuals with chronic pain also meet the diagnostic criteria for posttraumatic stress disorder.[111,112] The percentage is likely higher in a clinical population. That the two disorders can influence each other is suggested by longitudinal studies showing that early symptoms of posttraumatic stress disorder predict later maintenance of pain[113] and that, conversely, more severe pain after injury predicts persistent posttraumatic stress disorder.[114] Moreover, very preliminary evidence suggests that successful cognitive-behavioral treatment of PTSD may reduce chronic pain as an incidental benefit.[115]

The nature of the linkage is unclear. In the laboratory, the perception of threat or bodily harm increases responsiveness to nociceptive stimuli at a spinal level, as well as at cortical sites such as primary somatosensory cortex and the insula.[80] Not surprisingly, then, posttraumatic stress disorder—in which nightmares, intrusive memories, and reliving the event represent just such priming—is a risk factor for chronic pain.

Alternatively, psychophysiological mechanisms have been suggested. For example, in whiplash there is evidence that degeneration of the neck extensor muscles over the first few months after injury, measured as fatty infiltrates on MRI, may precede a failure to recover. Posttraumatic stress disorder at baseline predicts the muscle degeneration, perhaps because sympathetic outflow impedes healing or prolongs inflammation.[116]

Inquiries can be made directly about the symptoms of PTSD at the interview, covering all three categories (intrusion, avoidance, and arousal) to distinguish the full disorder from subsyndromal cases. In severe PTSD, the patient may seem subtly dazed or confused, or frozen in time, as if nothing of significance in his or her life could ever happen again.

Two screening instruments for PTSD have been validated in chronic pain samples: the Impact of Events Scale[117] and the PTSD Symptom Scale—Self-Report.[118] For neither instrument did cutoff scores need to be adjusted for chronic pain.[119]

Current Stresses For some conditions such as fibromyalgia, myofascial pain syndrome, complex regional pain syndrome, and tension-type and migraine headaches, stress may be the predominant trigger. For chronic pain in general, stress may tax coping resources and lead to psychopathology. Moreover, it appears that stress can precipitate chronic widespread pain, at least when there is already a dysfunction of the hypothalamic-pituitary-adrenal cortex axis, perhaps from high levels of stress in early childhood or in utero.[120] Similarly, stressful life events show a dose-response relationship to later transformation from episodic to chronic migraine.[121]

In the laboratory, stress is analgesic in the short term. However, this tends to be followed by a longer period of rebound hyperalgesia[122] and proneness to inflammatory pain.[123] Of course, in practice, stress can lead to anxiety and depression—likely triggers in their own right.[124] Also, cortisol may induce pronociceptive changes in glial cells[125] or indicate a loss of endogenous analgesia because the upstream precursor to cortisol—corticotrophin-releasing hormone—plays a role in pain inhibition.[120,126]

Moreover, chronic pain itself is highly stressful, as a noxious physical stimulus; as a loss of physical capacity, social role, and economic security; and as a gateway to frustrating interactions with the legal, disability, and insurance systems. Depending on a person's genetic and cognitive diatheses, coping resources can be overwhelmed, leading to distress and psychopathology.[127]

Thus, it is helpful to know the nature and amount of stressors the patient is dealing with, and has dealt with, particularly in the past year. Major life events tend to sensitize a person to subsequent daily hassles, and thus, in practice, both forms of stress may be important. Stressful reminders of the pain (e.g., a workers' compensation case, poor health in a close family member) may be particularly noxious for pain coping. Increasing intakes of nicotine, alcohol, or marijuana or a sudden request to increase opioid dosage may indicate that coping resources have been overwhelmed. In addition to constituting the targets for stress management training, the stressors may point to larger problems that need to be dealt with separately from pain management.

Anger Pain can be annoying, irritating, or frustrating, suggesting an overlap between proneness to anger and the affective dimension of pain. Moreover, heightened perception of the annoying qualities of pain can increase comprehensive pain intensity ratings[128] and pain behaviors.[129] Severe anger may all but preclude the cognitive flexibility required for navigating the problems posed by chronic pain.

To deal with this therapeutically, it is helpful to know the source of the anger. Two causes seem particularly common: the psychological injury to a person's self-worth and the psychosocial injury of economic or physical insecurity. A sense of injustice in how the pain came about can compound both of these, making acceptance of the pain feel to the patient like a defeat.

Secondary to the degree of anger is how the patient deals with it. Consciously suppressing the expression of anger can intensify the problem by causing a subsequent rebound of angry emotions[130] and of psychophysiological arousal such as, in low back pain, muscle tension of the lumbar paraspinals.[131] In turn, the reactivity of lumbar paraspinal muscle tension correlates with daily pain intensity.[132] Presumably, the increased arousal is relevant to other stress-sensitive conditions such as complex regional pain syndrome, myofascial pain, and tension-type or migraine headaches. Other ineffective anger management strategies such as rumination and submission (as opposed to distraction or reframing[133]) likely also intensify the effects of anger on pain.

Psychometrically, the standard measure of trait anger and of anger suppression is the Anger Expression Inventory,[134] but it is unclear how well this measure correlates with actual anger suppression in pain-relevant situations.[128] More useful is to inquire about anger toward the pain, toward treating providers, and toward the patient him- or herself for having the pain, as well as frustration at pain-imposed limits on activity. When irritability is unusually intense during the interview, it is helpful to understand the patient's expectations or past experiences with psychologists. Posttraumatic stress disorder, acute opiate withdrawal, and cluster B personality disorders may also show up as anger.

Repressive Coping Style A tenet of psychodynamic theories of pain is that negative affect, automatically excluded from consciousness through the defense mechanism of repression, can intensify and prolong physical pain.[135] There is, in fact, experimental support for this.

Individuals prone to use repression can be identified psychometrically by the combination of low scores on measures of trait anxiety and high scores on a scale of social desirability.[136] In theory, this combination could reflect impression management rather than repression—the individuals might be well aware of negative affect but choosing not to disclose it so as to make a favorable impression. However, the pattern—low reports of trait anxiety and high scores on social desirability—is little changed when the questionnaires are anonymous or the respondent is attached to a fake but persuasive lie detector. Instructions that make disclosure of negative affect socially desirable actually seem to intensify its denial among repressors.[137,138] On timed tests, people falling in the repression category show less interference than would be expected from threatening stimuli, suggesting that they are skilled at excluding such material from consciousness.[139] All this suggests that repressors are truly less aware of negative affect. This is only true of self-report, however; under conditions of stress, their behavioral and psychophysiological responding suggests a high level of anxiety.[136]

The underlying mechanism seems to be an attentional bias away from distressing emotional material. This is supported by reaction time studies that suggest that as a painful task continues, people scoring high in repression allocate attention away from the threatening emotional aspects of pain (pain-distress) and toward the emotionally neutral sensory aspects.[140] This may be consequential: Following a cold pressor task, repressors report higher (sensory) pain intensity levels.[140] Moreover, repressors show fewer gains in functional capacity or improvements in pain intensity from multidisciplinary pain treatment.[141]

Classically, repression is assessed by low scores on trait anxiety and high scores on social desirability. However, we might suspect repression from the combination of high pain intensity, very low activity level on the West Haven-Yale Multidimensional Pain Inventory and yet see a relative absence of negative affect.[142] People tend not to be aware of their own emotional defenses, but there are exceptions. A patient may speak frankly, for example, about finding physical pain to be a useful way of converting and confining emotional pain to a particular region of the body.

Activity Pacing Involvement in absorbing non-pain-related activities is the foundation of quality of life, living effectively, and reducing the significance and intensity of the pain. This assumes, however, that the nature of the activities, the manner in which they are approached, and the amount in which they are done are not part of the pain problem. Presumably, activity-induced flare-ups can contribute to an erosion of pain thresholds by exposing the pain system to high levels of input and by making frustration part of the narrative that surrounds the pain. Moreover, laboratory data implies that the pain system can be trained to lower thresholds by following instances of increased sensitivity with the reward of pain reduction.[143] Pacing difficulties, in which maximum pain is followed by rest, heat, and/or analgesics, seems very close to this laboratory paradigm. Further, persisting in an activity to the point of severe pain is often associated with active pain suppression, itself a counterproductive strategy.[144]

At the interview, then, we would ask about the frequency of activity-induced pain flare-ups, their intensity and duration, and any tendency of the pain to increase or thresholds to decrease (as reflected, for example, in the development of allodynia or a decline in activity tolerance) over the course of the day or the workweek. Flare-ups that are frequent, are severe, and last more than a day are of particular concern.

Also important is to understand the factors that motivate overactivity. Guilt at seeing family members work, frustration and a desire to battle the pain, a concern that pacing will mean complete inactivity, situational stresses that compel activity, a manic or hypomanic state, anxiety, and Type A personality are all potential contributors.

So far, the options for psychometric assessment of pacing are limited. The six-item Pacing subscale of the Chronic Pain Coping Inventory has been developed in a fibromyalgia sample.[145] It measures the use of specific techniques such as taking breaks, proceeding more slowly, and dividing tasks into more manageable components. The Pain Persistence Scale (seven items, Cronbach's $\alpha \approx 0.76$) of the Avoidance-Endurance Questionnaire (AEQ) was also developed with pacing difficulties in mind. Preliminary evidence suggests that high scores on this subscale, when combined with high scores on the Thought Suppression Scale of the AEQ, predict a high pain level 6 months later.[146] However, the Pain Persistence Scale has been validated so far only in Germany.[144]

Personality

Alexithymia The term alexithymia (literally, "no words for feelings"[147,148]) suggests a difficulty identifying and discriminating emotions, a difficulty describing a person's emotions to others, and a tendency to focus externally rather than on the person's inner life.[149] It is a normal personality trait with a prevalence of 7% to 12% in the general population.[150] In theory, alexithymia makes emotional self-regulation more difficult and promotes a somatic rather than an affective interpretation of the sensations associated with feelings. Thus, alexithymic individuals appear prone to greater pain intensity along its affective dimension (pain distress) by way of negative affect and fear of physical illness.[151]

At this point, the empirical foundation for the relevance of alexithymia to pain is weak. To date, virtually all studies have used a cross-sectional, correlational design. Thus, we do not know whether alexithymia is a cause of chronic pain or a result of pain or the associated medications and sleep disturbance[152] or whether pain and alexithymia are both due to a third variable, such as a disrupted childhood.[153] Moreover, the effects of alexithymia on pain are wholly mediated by negative affect, suggesting that the latter may be the more relevant variable.[151,154,155] Alexithymia is related to reduced risk of compensated disability, perhaps because alexithymic individuals prefer to avoid the myriad of interpersonal interactions involved in filing a workers' compensation claim.[156] Thus, the decision to assess formally for alexithymia is a matter of clinical judgment rather than a prelude to empirically supported treatment.

If alexithymia is felt relevant, formal assessment is generally with the Toronto Alexithymia Scale (TAS),[157,158] although here, too, there are caveats. The TAS contains items that imply somatization (e.g., "I have physical sensations that even doctors don't understand"), suggesting that the two constructs are not well separated. Also, the Difficulty Describing Feelings subscale seems to correlate, not with observed difficulties in describing emotions, but with shame, suggesting that it measures emotional inhibition of expression and not an actual skills deficit.[159,160]

Despite all the difficulties, alexithymic individuals are encountered in the clinic. Their difficulty describing their feelings may be apparent at the interview, or their depression may be apparent to others and on the psychometrics but not to the patients themselves. These patients seem to have particular difficulty in handling frustration with the pain and with finding activities to take the place of vigorous physical recreation.

Other Personality Traits Normal personality traits may be relevant insofar as they predispose to maladaptive coping. For example, from the cross-sectional studies so far available, neuroticism (proneness to negative affect) may increase pain directly and via passive coping; extraversion may predispose to (successful) active coping; novelty seeking may facilitate the positive, appetitive motivations that tend to inhibit pain; low self-directedness implies poor self-efficacy for specific challenges; and harm avoidance may bias an individual toward fearful avoidance of activity.[161,162] Harm avoidance may be particularly important because it is common in people with chronic pain and because, in psychiatric populations, it predicts a poorer response to antidepressants.[163] In all, then, it can be helpful to understand how an individual copes with stressful circumstances other than pain, as well as his or her premorbid level of functioning.

Personality Disorders In chronic pain, personality disorders may be less often a lifelong problem in the DSM-IV or DSM-5 sense than a pervasive deterioration into ineffective coping in response to the stresses of pain. Nevertheless, characterizing these maladaptive patterns is important for highlighting clinical needs (e.g., behaviors by which the patients may cause themselves further problems) and for understanding the idiosyncratic ways that patients interact with staff.[164] A patient whose occupational or academic aspirations have been blocked by pain may seek out ever more esoteric diagnoses and experimental treatments to restore a sense of uniqueness.

It is helpful to know more about the patient's premorbid adjustment in order to sort out which behaviors can be relieved with more effective stress coping and which will likely require long-term treatment. Thus, a patient whose symptoms have acquired a social, attention-seeking quality likely has a better prognosis if, premorbidly, his or her needs were met by success in the business world, as opposed to, say, intensive overinvolvement with his or her children. Beyond the basic facts of history, fine-grained information seems best obtained from people who knew the patient before the pain[164]—including the primary care provider, with whom a phone conversation can often give useful insights.

Interpersonal Most often, patients relate constructive support from a spouse and/or family members that helps to buffer stress and accomplish household tasks. In some instances, however, the support may go awry. Particularly when the spouse has lost someone to catastrophic illness, the support provided may be intrusive, inhibiting, or foreclosing the patient's own efforts to function. Family members' frustrations or worried concern may mirror and corroborate the patient's own feelings about the pain. They may ask about the pain frequently, inadvertently focusing the patient's attention on it. In younger patients, this can come from friends and high school classmates, giving the pain an unwanted celebrity status. Alternatively, spouses may harbor their own frustrations. There may have been veiled or open and contentious talks about ending the marriage, adding to catastrophic interpretation.

HEALTH BEHAVIORS: SMOKING, SLEEP, AND PAIN

Sleep In addition to its effects on attention and mood, sleep disturbance seems to increase pain sensitivity.[165] The resolution of chronic widespread pain in particular is predicted by good sleep quality at baseline.[166] In depression, sleep deprivation can induce reports of pain even as it reduces depression.[167] Further, sleep deprivation may impair the analgesic response to absorption in a nonpain activity (an effect not mediated by disrupted attention[168]) or, from animal data, to morphine[169] or amitriptyline[170].

At this point, it is self-reported sleep disturbance and not behavioral (actigraphic) or polysomnographic data that best predicts subsequent increased pain.[165] Thus, simply inquiring in the interview about trouble falling asleep, frequent awakening, and early morning awakening may be the most useful approach. More intensive assessment is with a 2-week sleep diary, in which patients record the times at which they go to bed and arise, their sleep onset latency, awakening after sleep onset, early morning awakening, total sleep time, and total wake time. The diary may also include subjective ratings of sleep quality and restorativeness.[171] This approach has been validated in chronic pain specifically.[172]

Psychometrically, three instruments have been studied in chronic pain populations: the Medical Outcomes Study (MOS) Sleep Scale, the Insomnia Severity Index (ISI), and the Chronic Pain Sleep Inventory (CPSI). The 12 MOS scale items are distributed across six domains: sleep disturbance, sleep adequacy (restorativeness), sleep quantity, daytime somnolence, snoring, and shortness of breath or headache. Nine of the items are gathered into a sleep problems index. The ISI is a seven-item, single-domain scale measuring difficulty with sleep onset, sleep maintenance, early morning awakening, satisfaction with sleep, distress over sleep, daytime interference, and the extent to which others have noticed the sleep problems. The CPSI is a five-item scale focused on pain-related sleep problems specifically. Three of the items are gathered into a sleep problems index. Both scales show good reliability and convergent and discriminant validity in a chronic pain setting.[173,174,175] The psychometrics are summarized in Table 15-1.

Smoking In prospective studies, cigarette smoking is a risk factor for later onset of chronic pain,[176] possibly by contributing to conditions such as lumbar disk disease[177] and neuropathy[178] and by facilitating central sensitization in the spinal cord.[178] Smoking may also reduce serum levels of opiates[179], and opiate doses tend to be higher in smokers independent of pain intensity.[180] Thus, there is a direct interest in inquiring about how much patients smoke. Conversely, nicotine appears to have acute analgesic effects,[176] which may impede smoking cessation. On the positive side, smoking does not seem to moderate treatment outcome or successful opioid tapering in cognitive-behavioral treatment of chronic pain.[181]

PROTECTIVE FACTORS IN CHRONIC PAIN

Active Coping In stress, our well-being is endangered by environmental demands that are perceived as taxing or exceeding our coping resources.[182] A reasonable way of reducing stress, therefore, is to increase our coping skills. Particularly effective strategies include use of coping self-statements (in contrast to catastrophizing) and reinterpreting pain sensations (in contrast to attribution to severe medical illness). Ignoring pain sensations sometimes facilitates[183] and sometimes interferes with[184] coping. "Praying and hoping," a passive strategy, does not contribute to control over pain. There is some evidence that having a range of tools available facilitates mastery over pain.[184]

Successful use of active coping strategies seems to guard against catastrophic thinking.[185] Thus, we would also inquire about a person's tools for reducing pain and for managing its impact. Further, at the interview, it is helpful to know the areas in which patients have retained functioning and what strategies and resources they have had available for doing so. In the realm of coping, this involves knowing which skills they are using and their ability to draw flexibly on a range of tools as the situation and pain level require.

Ideally, a patient is active in identifying functional relationships—with activity, stress, diet, mood, ergonomics or other variables—that may underlie fluctuations in his or her pain. Not only is this a strong counterforce to depression and catastrophic thinking, but it can turn up ways of preventing flare-ups that might not be discovered otherwise.

Problem Solving The opposite of difficulties in pacing activities is the active process of finding ways to accomplish them without undue flare-up. This may involve creativity in using different types of equipment and ergonomic modifications, approaching the activities with a different posture or body mechanics, switching between tasks with diverse physical demands, and learning when to insert preventive rest breaks. Even the rest breaks can be an expression of active problem solving—learning to minimize the "pain cost" of an activity much as a contractor would minimize the material, labor, and time costs of a project. Similar problem solving applies to work. In the social realm, skills in communication and problem solving are relevant to maintaining connection with friends and family.

At the interview, we would inquire about level of functioning and about how activities are accomplished, looking for the confidence, flexibility, systematic approach, resilience in the face of setbacks, and the ability to learn from results that underlie effective problem solving. Of course, we would also look for the types of thoughts or emotions that interrupt this process, as well as the circumstances in which they occur.

Self-Efficacy Pain self-efficacy refers to a person's sense of confidence in the ability to control pain and to control the effect of pain on functioning and quality of life.[186] People scoring high in self-efficacy would be expected to harbor less fear or pain, use a greater range of coping skills, and have a higher functional status.

We may gain a sense of self-efficacy by understanding how a patient is handling important problems in his or her life, particularly the pain and functional limitations. To the extent that his or her thinking is confident, systematic, realistic, and focused on the problem, as opposed to exclusively on emotions, self-efficacy is suggested.

A number of scales for measuring pain self-efficacy have been developed,[186] among which the Pain Self-Efficacy Questionnaire (PSEQ) seems to be the furthest along in research support. Its ten items refer to coping and accomplishing generalized activities regardless of pain, for example, "I can live a normal lifestyle, despite the pain." Internal consistency is excellent ($\alpha \approx 0.93$). The self-efficacy measure is correlated only weakly with pain intensity and somatic focus but strongly with work status, pain behaviors, noncompletion of a chronic pain program, and the spouse's observation of interference in daily activities, suggesting divergent and convergent validity.[187]

Because of its brevity, reliability, and practical focus, the PSEQ is a useful process measure and encourages discussion of what is working and not working in treatment. Norms from a large pain clinic sample are available, facilitating interpretation: Among the full range of scores from 0 to 60, 40 corresponds to the 85th percentile and seems to be a threshold above which there tends to be return to work and maintenance of treatment gains.[188,189]

A similar construct, perceived control, can also be assessed. The Life Control Scale of the West Haven-Yale Multidimensional Pain Inventory assesses control over a person's life.[190] The Control Scale of the Survey of Pain Attitudes measures control over pain specifically.[191]

Acceptance Ignoring pain sensations can be a double-edged sword. At its best, it is a temporary strategy that allows a person to become absorbed in meaningful activities. At its worst, it becomes effortful suppression, a cognitive battle to keep pain out of awareness. Generally, suppression is not an effective strategy. In the laboratory, instructions to suppress pain lead to greater anxiety, reduced self-efficacy, and a slower return of pain and unpleasantness to baseline after noxious stimulation.[192] Thus, if coping skills have deteriorated into an attempted mental blockade of pain, an alternative strategy is preferable. In these circumstances, acceptance can be particularly useful.

Acceptance has been defined as the moment-to-moment willingness to experience the pain as it is, without attempting to suppress it, and while continuing to pursue one's goals and values. Acceptance is not a goal in itself, but a way of pursuing a full, meaningful life[193] and is associated with greater tolerance for pain[194] and functional performance.[195] Improvements in emotional distress and psychosocial functioning appear to be reliable side benefits.[196]

For some patients, acceptance goes beyond matter-of-fact acknowledgement to encompass actual gratitude. For a patient who nearly passed away in surgery, the pain may be a reminder that she is still alive and an exhortation to treat each moment as precious.

The level of acceptance can be judged in part by the range of emotional investments, beyond pain reduction, as reflected in the patient's goals and current activities and, inversely, by the emotional intensity with which pain reduction is sought.

Formal measurement is generally with the Chronic Pain Acceptance Questionnaire,[197] a 20-item instrument composed of two subscales: Activity Engagement (functioning regardless of pain) and Pain Willingness (openness to experiencing pain without suppression). Conceptually, activity engagement seems similar to the construct tapped by the Chronic Pain Self-Efficacy Questionnaire (CPEQ), and, in fact, the CPEQ seems reasonably highly correlated with Activity Willingness and the total Acceptance score (r = 0.60 and 0.62, respectively[198]).

Values Orientation One of the most valuable types of knowledge to arise from the psychological assessment of the patient in chronic pain—although not necessarily from the first session—is an understanding of those commitments and values that are more important than the pain. Life lived in accordance with these values will likely be more effective and entail less suffering and will allow the pain less influence over one's thoughts and feelings.

Pain—and its activation in the neuromatrix encoding it—is lower when a person is absorbed in an appetitive motivational state.[80] In the laboratory, this is demonstrated with stimuli as mild as pictures of enjoyable activities.[199] Moreover, attention is automatically allotted to stimuli that are relevant to a person's goals—and to pain, if his or her goal is to escape pain.[200] Thus, it is quite helpful that a person's waking moments be filled with goals whose pursuit is absorbing and enjoyable and against which the pain is comparatively unimportant.

A sense of a patient's deep personal commitments often arises from understanding his or her functioning prior to the development of chronic pain—why a particular course of study or a particular career was chosen, for example—as well as major life events that may have crystalized personal values. We are looking not merely for the statement of values, but for a level of involvement in which the nominal purpose of the assessment, to understand pain, is temporarily forgotten. This is quite rare in a first session but may become more natural later.

The main psychometric in this area, the Chronic Pain Values Inventory,[201] can be used to spark discussion. This instrument measures the importance of values in six domains (family, intimate/close interpersonal relationships, friends, work, health [e.g., as fitness], and growth and learning), success in living in accordance with these values, and the divergence between importance and success.

MULTIDIMENSIONAL PAIN MEASURES

The West Haven-Yale Multidimensional Pain Inventory (MPI, 52 items) and its revised form (61 items) is composed of 12 scales measuring the experience of pain, responses of a person's significant other, and the extent to which participation in common activities is preserved. Here, the experience of pain includes pain severity, the amount of life interference and dissatisfaction due to pain, negative mood (tension, irritability, and low mood), sense of control over the person's life, and the amount of perceived support from his or her significant other. Responses of the significant other to pain are divided into solicitous (attempting to be helpful, such as retrieving the loved one's pain medications), punishing (e.g., ignoring or responding with frustration to expressions of pain), and responses designed to help distract the person from his or her pain. Activities are broadly divided into household chores, activities around the yard, social activities, and leisure activities away from home. Subsequent factor analyses have mostly supported this structure.[202] Notably, however, the activity scales do not include employment, which can lead to spuriously low scores in people whose main activity is work.

Extensive norms and percentile conversions for the MPI, divided by age group and pain site, are available in a report by Nicholas and collegaues.[188]

TREATMENT MATCHING

Understanding the patient's individual experience of pain allows the treatment to be tailored. For example, fearful avoidance of activity and frequent flare-ups from overdoing are at opposite ends of a spectrum. There is evidence for good outcomes when treatments are tailored to the specific skills deficit.[203,204] The assessment of fear-avoidance and pacing deficits has been with the Pain Coping Inventory[205] and the pacing scale of the Chronic Pain Coping Inventory,[145] respectively, although other measures of these constructs would presumably perform as well.

Beliefs may also be important. Patients with kinesiophobia, for example, are presumably less likely to complete an exercise-based rehabilitation program unless their beliefs about reinjury are addressed.[206]

Most likely, intensity is relevant, too. For example, there is support in the literature for graded exposure,[207] educational groups,[208,209] and even a well-designed informational booklet[210] for preventing disability from fear of pain. Presumably, the intensity of fear and the chronicity of the pain indicate whether simple education will be sufficient or more intensive therapy is required.[206]

Also important is affective distress. Thus, *in vivo* exposure seems to cause significant reductions in catastrophizing, fear-avoidance beliefs, emotional distress, and, of note, pain intensity, in comparison with a waiting list control.[211] However, preliminary evidence suggests that the cognitive aspects of treatment may be particularly important when affective distress and poor coping, rather than catastrophization and physical impairment, predominate.[212]

In a more exploratory sense, analyses of the West Haven-Yale MPI have consistently revealed three clusters of patients: adaptive copers, showing low levels of pain intensity, interference, and distress, a strong sense of control over their lives, and a high activity level; dysfunctionals, whose scores are the mirror image of those of the adaptive copers; and the interpersonally distressed, whose profiles are characterized by low levels of perceived support and solicitous attention and a high level of punishing responses to their pain by their significant others. As noted, Burns and colleagues have suggested a fourth category consisting of individuals within the dysfunctional group who are repressing emotional distress.[142]

Most studies that have used the three-part typology have found the strongest responses to cognitive-behavioral treatment to be from the dysfunctional group.[213,214] Depending on the study, the interpersonally distressed may have poor[214] or good outcomes.[215] The investigations are still in their infancy but suggest that interpersonally distressed patients may need more intensive work on assertiveness and social problem solving for pain treatment to be effective.[214]

Stages of Change Thus, patients' readiness to manage pain on a psychological level depends in part on how they think about pain and, as in other areas of behavioral change (such as diet, exercise, or smoking cessation), on their willingness for the project. Under the Transtheoretical Model,[216] readiness for change can be broadly divided into five stages: precontemplation (for pain, holding a purely medical model and viewing pain coping as irrelevant), contemplation (an ambivalent stage of considering the possibility of change), preparation (planning for an imminent change, such as by identifying potential strategies), action (taking steps to implement self-management skills), and maintenance.

A patient's readiness for a behavioral approach is often apparent from the nature of the goals he or she expresses. Some patients are perplexed or insulted by the referral to a psychologist. For them, information on how psychological variables influence physical health may need to be given early in the evaluation. Others are skeptical but just frustrated enough with past treatments to try something different. And some patients, committed to self-management in other areas of their lives, arrive seeking specific tools they can implement.

Psychometrically, the relevant measure is the Pain Stages of Change Questionnaire, which has shown good internal consistency, short-term stability, and convergent and divergent validity.[217]

To the extent that stages of change depend on transition from a medical to a psychological model of pain, they may become less important as the two models merge into a more comprehensive and interdisciplinary understanding of pain neurophysiology. Moreover, it is not clear that the stages of change are predictive for medically oriented approaches such as biofeedback. On the other hand, the Transtheoretical Model has shown utility in coming to grips with other forms of effortful behavioral change (e.g., cigarette smoking) for which the medical relevance is never questioned.

ASSESSMENT OF SUICIDE RISK

Although successful treatment is the designated end of psychosocial assessment, psychologists may be asked to evaluate a range of specific issues, such as level of disability or probability of benefiting from a medical or surgical intervention. Here, we focus on two issues that arise frequently and are of particular importance: risk of suicide and potential for abuse of prescribed medications.

People with chronic pain have a two- to threefold increased risk for suicidal ideation, suicide attempts, and suicide completions.[218] This is not surprising because, in addition to the desire to escape the pain and the hopelessness that can come from feeling that one is at a medical endpoint, chronic pain is associated with advanced age, unemployment, financial distress, loss of career and/or relationships, a traumatic childhood, and sleep disturbance—each of which is a risk factor for suicide in its own right.[218]

Among those with chronic pain, additional risk may be conferred by:

- High pain intensity, severe insomnia, and difficulty functioning during the day because of sleep deprivation.[219]
- Depression, catastrophic thinking about pain, and especially their combination, which show a supra-additive effect.[220]
- A family history of suicide attempts or completions.[221]

Other predictors with empirical support include trait anxiety, life interference resulting from pain (as measured by the MPI), use of praying and hoping as a passive coping strategy,[220] personal history of previous attempts,[218] possibly certain types of pain (abdominal, back, and migraine with aura),[221-225] and female gender.[226] This last finding is the reverse of the risk seen in the nonpain population. The use of coping self-statements may confer a modest degree of protection.[220]

Shame, such as from losing one's career or business may increase the risk (suicide as a way of hiding one's face), as may recent losses, which can intensify the affective dimension of pain to a seemingly intolerable level.[227]

Even well-educated patients may be unaware of straightforward treatments (e.g., the existence of specific medications for neuropathic pain), leading to an unnecessary sense of desperation. The medical model of pain, with its emphasis on external treatments, can inadvertently create a feeling of hopelessness when further treatment is deemed unlikely to help. Hopelessness may be further intensified when an eagerly awaited medical consult has a disappointing outcome.

The presence of risk factors gives added reason to assess for suicidality. Patients can be asked straightforwardly about pessimism, hopelessness, and thoughts of harming themselves to help gauge the presence and strength of a cognitive schema for self-harm.[228] We are also interested in knowing about recent stressors and emotional upheaval that may activate or intensify this schema. And, of course, we seek to understand the degree of risk, from the patient's personal and family history, impulsiveness, commitment to remaining alive, and the specificity, accessibility, and lethality of the means for suicide. Thus, ideally, the topic would not be left to the end of the interview because the answers and follow-up may be lengthy. As a rule, this part of the assessment would not be done in the presence of a spouse because the patient may deny suicidal thoughts so as not to alarm the spouse or significant other. Occasionally, however, an especially anxious patient may prefer to discuss threatening topics with his or her spouse nearby for support. Psychologists working in the pain field can benefit much from monographs on suicide assessment.[228,229]

Psychometrically, propensity to suicide is usually measured with the Beck Hopelessness Scale[230,231] and the Beck Scale of Suicidal Ideation.[232] On the Beck Depression Inventory, endorsement of items reflecting hopelessness, pessimism, or suicidal thoughts should obviously lead to follow-up questions at the interview.[233]

SUBSTANCE ABUSE POTENTIAL

In prospective studies, the risk for misuse of prescribed opiates is higher in those with a history of any form of substance abuse, those with other mental health diagnoses, those taking opioids for a longer period of time (i.e., greater than 201 days in one year), those who are younger, those who are male, and those who are single, divorced, or separated. African Americans may have a lower risk than Caucasians.[234]

Difficulty with substances generally becomes clear over time in lost or stolen prescriptions, emergency phone calls, repeated requests for early refills, a pattern of dose escalations, and a reliance on multiple prescribers and/or the emergency room.[235,236] Multiple unexplained car accidents over the course of treatment calls for further assessment, as would a history of abrupt termination with previous physicians. At the first interview, an insistence on opioids or benzodiazepines, rejection of all other treatment options, and a sense of time urgency raise questions of addiction. Although sleep deprivation is very common in chronic pain, actually nodding off during the interview is almost always the result of a substance. Reports of hoarding medications may be an inverse sign (in substance abuse, the compulsion to use is so great that hoarding becomes impossible) but suggests a fear of pain and absence of coping skills that are of concern in their own right.

The main psychometric instruments for predicting substance abuse are the Screener and Opioid Assessment for Patients with Pain (SOAPP-R)[237] and the Opioid Risk Tool (ORT).[238]

The ORT is composed of ten items covering such risk factors as age (16 to 45 years), family history of substance misuse, preadolescent sexual abuse, and specific mental health concerns such as attention deficit disorder.[238] The initial study was very promising but had methodological shortcomings; attempts to cross-validate have been sparse and suggest low sensitivity, perhaps because the items are relatively transparent.[239,240]

The SOAPP-R consists of 24 items, many of them quite subtle, empirically selected for their ability to predict aberrant drug behaviors while minimizing social desirability and excluding various demographic biases. The sensitivity and specificity in the original sample (0.81 and 0.68, respectively) are quite good for a psychometric.

Nonetheless, the literature at this point is still in its infancy.[239] Despite its highly sophisticated construction, the SOAPP-R correlates with social desirability to approximately the same extent as it does to substance misuse. The sensitivity and specificity leave a margin for false conclusions—and, particularly, a false positive—in the individual case. Moreover, on cross-validation, sensitivity has varied considerably across settings,[241,242] suggesting the value of developing local norms. Thus, the SOAPP-R may be most useful for deciding the level of monitoring for an individual patient, rather than being a deciding factor in whether to prescribe.[237] Of note, the SOAPP-R has only been validated for patients in tertiary care pain clinics being considered for opioid therapy and not, for example, in primary care.[237]

MEASUREMENT OF PAIN INTENSITY AND QUALITY

Visual Analogue and Numerical Rating Scales Arising from techniques in personnel measurement in the early 20th century[243-245] and reinvented in the 1960s,[246-248] visual analog scales (VASs) are a form of cross-modality matching in which patients report their pain as the distance along a 10-cm line between two extremes—for example, "no pain" and "the worst pain imaginable." The scale is scored with a ruler, quantifying pain in millimeters. Alternatively, the patient may complete the scale on a computer, using a mouse to drag the location of a pointer.[249]

Visual analog scales have the advantage of fine gradations of measurement and, therefore, sensitivity to change.[250] In contrast, a 10-point numerical rating scale is coarser of necessity, and a 100-point rating scale tends to become coarse as people cluster their ratings around multiples of 10.[251] Moreover, the specific power-law mathematical function relating VAS scores to stimulus intensity in laboratory studies, and their mathematical relationship to other forms of cross-modality matching, implies that the VAS scores conform to a ratio scale and thus convey information about the absolute intensity of the pain.[252] Note, however, that if descriptors are inserted along the length of the scale (e.g., "mild," "moderate," and "severe"), it becomes a graphical implementation of a categorical rating scale, and landmark effects—choosing points near a descriptor—obscure the ratio-level properties.[250]

Their validity is supported by a large number of laboratory studies showing mathematically lawful relationships between VAS scores and such external variables as physical intensity of the painful stimulus, cortical evoked potentials to the stimuli, rate of neural firing in pain pathways, and, for drug studies, analgesic potency.[253] For clinical pain, validity is supported by correlations with such alternative measures as the type of pain, analgesic potency, progress through rehabilitation, number of swollen joints, or grip strength, for example.[250]

The descriptors anchoring the high and low ends of the scales are crucial. If the high endpoint is too intense, responses will pile up at the low end of the line, reducing discrimination among milder pains. If the high endpoint is too weak, responses will pile up at the high end. The endpoints "no pain" and "worst pain imaginable" give a uniform distribution of responses, seemingly with no end effects, for even very mild and very severe pain.[254,255]

Patients tend to be unfamiliar with visual analog scales and, therefore, benefit from practice with them before using them clinically.[250] Useful instructions are found in Littlejohns and Vere.[256]

Verbal rating scales use a list of pain descriptors, ordered to reflect increasing intensity. Verbal scales are coarser than VAS scales but have advantages in three other areas: They do not require training; they are likely better for discriminating between different qualities of pain (e.g., verbal scales of sensory intensity and affective unpleasantness are not as easily confused[255]); and because the meaning of words is mostly shared in a population, verbal scales are arguably the most natural way of telling absolute magnitude of pain.[257] The verbal scale in widest use is the McGill Pain Questionnaire.

McGill Pain Questionnaire The McGill Pain Questionnaire consists of 78 descriptions of pain organized into 20 categories. The three to five descriptors within each category are ordered by intensity. Thus, the set of descriptors chosen by the patient is a representation and communication of the nature of his or her pain and may provide clues to its source. Moreover, 16 of the 20 subclasses are further combined into three dimensions of pain experience: sensory-discriminative (e.g., "burning"), motivational-affective (e.g., "punishing"), and cognitive-evaluative (e.g., "annoying"). There is also a five-level pain intensity scale, whose descriptor at each step was chosen from scaling studies to be at equal intervals from the descriptors above and below the step.[258]

The degree to which the sensory and affective dimensions are truly separate has been questioned on statistical grounds,[259,260] but the distinction seems worthwhile.[261] These two types of qualities are differentially encoded in the brain[262-264] and relate differently to psychological variables. Negative affect, whether global or pain related, tends to differentially intensify the affective dimension of pain.[265] Similarly, the tendency to suppress anger correlates primarily with the affective intensity of acute laboratory-induced pain.[128] That is, while pain-sensation and pain-distress tend to be correlated with each other and with overall pain intensity, they are differentially affected by psychological state, medication, and instructional set.[253]

In routine clinical use, the MPQ is also more a psychophysical and descriptive instrument than a psychometric. For patients at a loss to describe their pain, it can be a useful window to part of their experience. Formal scoring[258] and norms[188,266] are available, as are validated short forms.[267,268]

PSYCHOPHYSIOLOGY

The stress response may function as a key trigger for migraine headaches[269] and as a contributing factor to myofascial pain[270] and tension myalgia.[271] Sympathetic nervous system activity can shift the immune system to a proinflammatory state[272] while, conversely, the parasympathetic system, acting through nicotinic acetylcholine receptors, may be anti-inflammatory.[273] Thus, it is helpful to know not just how stressed a patient feels subjectively, but the level of autonomic responding. Moreover, psychophysiological assessment can be helpful for selecting a relaxation technique, verifying that a criterion level of relaxation has been achieved, and illustrating the mind-body effect to patients. Such assessment is a science unto itself, outside the scope of this chapter, but it is covered in specialized texts.[269,274] Although assessment is generally conducted with biofeedback equipment, one useful measure—hand temperature—can be readily obtained with an accurate thermometer covering the range from 65–95°F.[269] Relevant norms are given in the text by Blanchard and colleagues.[275]

CONCLUSIONS

Psychosocial assessment of the patient in chronic pain helps bring to light the psychological factors that, additively or in interaction with the nociceptive source, influence pain intensity, distress, and coping and facilitate or impede functioning. A better understanding of the psychological factors influencing a patient's pain enhances decision making, provides a foundation for treatment, and helps the patient and physician alike to understand the sometimes complex path to recovery. And, sometimes, in moments of crisis, it can transform dark mystery into clarity and reassurance.

REFERENCES

1. Melzack R, Wall PD. Pain mechanisms: a new theory. *Science*. 1965;150;971-979.
2. Bair MJ, Robinson RL, Katon W, Kroenke K. Depression and pain comorbidity: a literature review. *Arch Intern Med*. 2003;163:2433-2445.
3. Miller LR, Cano A. Comorbid chronic pain and depression: who is at risk? *J Pain*. 2009;10:619-627.
4. Vaccarino AL, Sills TL, Evans KR, Kalali AH. Prevalence and association of somatic symptoms in patients with Major Depressive Disorder. *J Affect Disord*. 2008;110:270-276.
5. Bär K-J, Brehm S, Boettger MK, et al. Pain perception in major depression depends on pain modality. *Pain*. 2005;117:97-103.
6. McFate T, Scher AI. Chronic pain disorders and headache chronification. *Curr Pain Headache Rep*. 2009;13:308-313.
7. Jenewein J, Moergeli H, Wittmann L, et al. Development of chronic pain following severe accidental injury: results of a 3-year follow-up study. *J Psychosom Res*. 2009;66:119-126.
8. Bigal ME, Ashina S, Burstein R, et al. Prevalence and characteristics of allodynia in headache sufferers. a population study. *Neurology*. 2008;70:1525-1533.
9. Celestin J, Edwards RR, Jamison RN. Pretreatment psychosocial variables as predictors of outcomes following lumbar surgery and spinal cord stimulation: a systematic review and literature synthesis. *Pain Med*. 2009;10:639-653.
10. Wasan AD, Davar G, Jamison R. The association between negative affect and opioid analgesia in patients with discogenic low back pain. *Pain*. 2005;117:450-461.
11. Wasan AD, Jamison RN, Pham L, et al. Psychopathology predicts the outcome of medial branch blocks with corticosteroid for chronic axial low back or cervical pain: a prospective cohort study. *BMC Musculoskelet Disord*. 2009;10:22. doi: 10.1186/1471-2474-10-22.
12. Turner JA, Holtzman S, Mancl, L. Mediators, moderators and predictors of therapeutic change in cognitive-behavioral therapy for chronic pain. *Pain*. 2007;127:276-286.
13. Dinan TG. Inflammatory markers in depression. *Curr Opin Psychiatry*. 2008;22:32-36.
14. Milligan ED, Watkins LR. Pathological and protective roles of glia in chronic pain. *Nat Rev Neurosci*. 2009;10:23-36.
15. Mayberg HS. Modulating dysfunctional limbic-cortical circuits in depression: towards development of brain-based algorithms for diagnosis and optimised treatment. *Br Med Bull*. 2003;65:193-207.
16. Wiech K, Tracey I. The influence of negative emotions on pain: behavioral effects and neural mechanisms. *Neuroimage*. 2009;47:987-994.
17. Zubieta JK, Stohler CS. Neurobiological mechanisms of placebo responses. *Ann N Y Acad Sci*. 2009;1156:198-210.
18. Pizzagalli DA, Holmes AJ, Dillon DG, et al. Reduced caudate and nucleus accumbens response to rewards in unmedicated

individuals with major depressive disorder. *Am J Psychiatry*. 2009;166:702-710.

19. Bantick SJ, Wise, RG, Ploghaus A, et al. Imaging how attention modulates pain in humans using functional MRI. *Brain*. 2002;125:310-319.
20. Brody AL, Saxena S, Stoessel P, et al. Regional brain metabolic changes in patients with major depression treated with either paroxetine or interpersonal therapy. *Arch Gen Psychiatry*. 2001; 58:631-640.
21. Johnstone T, van Reekum CM, Urry HL, et al. Failure to regulate: counterproductive recruitment of top-down prefrontal-subcortical circuitry in major depression. *J Neurosci*. 2007;27:8877-8884.
22. Lorenz J, Minoshima S, Casey KL. Keeping pain out of mind: the role of the dorsolateral prefrontal cortex in pain modulation. *Brain*. 2003;126:1079-1091.
23. Von Korff M, Alonso J, Ormel J, et al. Childhood psychosocial stressors and adult onset arthritis: broad spectrum risk factors and allostatic load. *Pain*. 2009;143:76-83.
24. First MB, Gibbon M. The Structured Clinical Interview for *DSM-IV* Axis I Disorders (SCID-I) and Structured Clinical Interview for *DSM-IV* Axis II Disorders (SCID-II). In: Hilsenroth MJ, Segal DL., eds. *Comprehensive Handbook of Psychological Assessment*. Vol. 2. *Personality Assessment*. Hoboken, NJ: Wiley; 2004:134-143.
25. Spitzer RL, Williams JB, Gibbon M, et al. The Structured Clinical Interview for DSM-III-R (SCID). I. History, rationale and description. *Arch Gen Psychiatry*. 1992;49:624-629.
26. Sheehan DV, Lecrubier Y, Sheehan KH, et al. The Mini-International Neuropsychiatric Interview (M.I.N.I.): the development and validation of a structured diagnostic psychiatric interview for DSM-IV and ICD-10. *J Clin Psychiatry*. 1998;59:22-33.
27. Beck AT, Steer RA, Garbin MG. Psychometric properties of the Beck Depression Inventory: twenty-five years of evaluation. *Clin Psychol Rev*. 1988;8:77-100.
28. Radloff LS. The CES-D scale: a self-report depression scale for research in the general population. *Appl Psychol Meas*. 1977;1: 385-401.
29. Kroenke K, Spitzer RL, Williams JB. The PHQ-9: validity of a brief depression severity measure. *J Gen Intern Med*. 2001;16:606-613.
30. Rush AJ, Trivedi MH, Ibrahim HM, et al. The 16-item Quick Inventory of Depressive Symptomatology (QIDS), clinician rating (QIDS-C), and self-report (QIDS-SR): a psychometric evaluation in patients with chronic major depression. *Biol Psychiatry*. 2003;54:573-583.
31. MacDonald G, Leary MR. Why does social exclusion hurt? The relationship between social and physical pain. *Psychol Bull*. 2005;131:202-223.
32. Eisenberger NI, Lieberman MD, Williams KD. Does rejection hurt? An fMRI study of social exclusion. *Science*. 2003;302:290-292.
33. Eisenberger NI. The neural basis of social pain: findings and implications. In: MacDonald G, Jensen-Campbell LA, eds. *Social Pain: Neuropsychological and Health Implications of Loss and Exclusion*. Washington, DC: American Psychological Association; 2011:53-78.
34. Zhou X, Vohs KD, Baumeister RF. The symbolic power of money: reminders of money alter social distress and physical pain. *Psychol Sci*. 2009;20:700-706.
35. Mehrabian A. Questionnaire measures of affiliative tendency and sensitivity to rejection. *Psychol Rep*. 1976;38:199-209.
36. Seeman TE, Berkman LF. Structural characteristics of support networks and their relationship with social support in the elderly: who provides support? *Soc Sci Med*. 1988;23:737-749.
37. Kolb LC. Attachment behavior and pain complaints. *Psychosomatics*. 1982;23:413-425.
38. McWilliams LA, Bailey SJ. Associations between adult attachment ratings and health conditions: evidence from the National Comorbidity Survey Replication. *Health Psychol*. 2010;29:446-453.
39. Mikail SF, Henderson PR, Tasca GA. An interpersonally based model of chronic pain: an application of attachment theory. *Clin Psychol Rev*. 1994;14:1-16.
40. Meredith P, Ownsworth T, Strong J. A review of the evidence linking adult attachment theory and chronic pain: presenting a conceptual model. *Clin Psychol Rev*. 2008;28:407-429.
41. Skillings JL, Murdoch WJ, Porcerelli JH. "I fired my last doctor for not taking me seriously": collaborating with a difficult medical patient in a multidisciplinary primary care facility. *J Pers Assess*. 2010;92:533-543.
42. Davis DA, Luecken LJ, Zautra AJ. Are reports of childhood abuse related to the experience of chronic pain in adulthood? A meta-analytic review of the literature. *Clin J Pain*. 2005;21:398-405.
43. Danese A, Moffitt TE, Pariante CM, et al. Elevated inflammation levels in depressed adults with a history of childhood maltreatment. *Arch Gen Psychiatry*. 2008;65:409-415.
44. Danese A, Pariante CM, Caspi A, Taylor A, Poulton, R. Childhood maltreatment predicts adult inflammation in a life-course study. *Proc Natl Acad Sci*. 2007;104:1319-1324.
45. Slopen N, Lewis TT, Gruenewald TI, et al. Early life adversity and inflammation in African Americans and whites in the midlife in the United States survey. *Psychosom Med*. 2010;72:694-701.
46. Surtees P, Wainwright N, Day N, Brayne C, Luben R, Khaw KT. Adverse experience in childhood as a developmental risk factor for altered immune status in adulthood. *Int J Behav Med*. 2003;10:251-268.
47. Danese A, McEwen BS. Adverse childhood experiences, allostasis, allostatic load, and age-related disease. *Physiol Behav*. 2012;106:29-39.
48. Treadway MT, Grant MM, Ding Z, et al. Early adverse events, HPA activity and rostral anterior cingulate volume in MDD. *PLoS One*. 2009;4(3):e4887.
49. Petrovic P, Ingvar M. Imaging cognitive modulation of pain processing. *Pain*. 2002;95:1-5.
50. Tietjen GE, Brandes JL, Peterlin BL, et al. Childhood maltreatment and migraine (Part II). Emotional abuse as a risk factor for headache chronification. *Headache*. 2010;50:32-41.
51. Kelley JE, Lumley MA, Leisen JCC. Health effects of emotional disclosure among rheumatoid arthritis patients. *Health Psychol*. 1997;16:331-340.
52. Broderick JE, Junghaenel DU, Schwartz JE. Written emotional expression produces health benefits in fibromyalgia patients. *Psychosom Med*. 2005;67:326-334.
53. Gillis ME, Lumley MA, Mosley-Williams A. The health effects of at-home written emotional disclosure in fibromyalgia: a randomized trial. *Ann Behav Med*. 2006;32:135-146.
54. Bernstein DP, Stein JA, Newcomb MD, et al. Development and validation of a brief screening version of the Childhood Trauma Questionnaire. *Child Abuse Negl*. 2003;27:169-190.
55. Gray K, Wegner DM. The sting of intentional pain. *Psychol Sci*. 2008;19:1260-1262.
56. Sullivan MJL, Adams H, Martel M-O, et al. Catastrophizing and perceived injustice: risk factors for the transition to chronicity after whiplash injury. *Spine*. 2011;36:s244-s249.
57. Rainville P, Bao QV, Chrétien P. Pain-related emotions modulate experimental pain perceptions and autonomic responses. *Pain*. 2005;118:306-318.

58. George SZ, Wittmer VT, Fillingim RB, Robinson ME. Sex and pain-related psychological variables are associated with thermal pain sensitivity for patients with chronic low back pain. *J Pain.* 2007;8:2-10.
59. Colloca L, Benedetti F. Nocebo hyperalgesia: how anxiety is turned into pain. *Curr Opin Anaesthesiol.* 2007;20:435-439.
60. Ruscheweyh R, Kreusch A, Albers C, Sommer J, Marziniak M. The effect of distraction strategies on pain perception and the nociceptive flexor reflex (RIII reflex). *Pain.* 2011;152:2662-2671.
61. Ochsner KN, Ludlow DH, Knierim K, et al. Neural correlates of individual differences in pain-related fear and anxiety. *Pain.* 2006;120:69-77.
62. Le Pera D, Brancucci A, De Armas L, et al. Inhibitory effect of voluntary movement preparation on cutaneous heat pain and laser-evoked potentials. *Eur J Neurosci.* 2007; 25:1900-1907.
63. Terkelsen AJ, Bach FW, Jensen TS. Experimental forearm immobilization in humans induces cold and mechanical hyperalgesia. *Anesthesiology.* 2008;109:297–307.
64. Nishigami T, Osako Y, Tanaka K, et al. Changes in calcitonin gene-related peptide expression following joint immobilization in rats. *Neurosci Lett.* 2009;454:97-100.
65. Lissek S, Wilimzig C, Stude P, et al. Immobilization impairs tactile perception and shrinks somatosensory cortical maps. *Curr Biol.* 2009;19:837-842.
66. Kaneko F, Murakami T, Onari K, Kurumadani H, Kawaguchi K. Decreased cortical excitability during motor imagery after disuse of an upper limb in humans. *Clin Neurophysiol.* 2003;114:2397-2403.
67. Binkley CJ, Beacham A, Neace W, et al. Genetic variations associated with red hair color and fear of dental pain, anxiety regarding dental care and avoidance of dental care. *J Am Dent Assoc.* 2009;140:896-905.
68. McNeil DW, Rainwater AJ III. Development of the Fear of Pain Questionnaire—III. *J Behav Med.* 1998;21:389-410.
69. Ellis A. *Reason and Emotion in Psychotherapy.* Secaucus, NJ: Citadel Press; 1962.
70. Sullivan MJL, Thorn B, Haythornthwaite JA, et al. Theoretical perspectives on the relation between catastrophizing and pain. *Clin J Pain.* 2001;17:52-64.
71. Keefe FJ, Brown GK, Wallston KA, Caldwell DS. Coping with rheumatoid arthritis pain: Catastrophizing as a maladaptive strategy. *Pain.* 1989;37:51-56.
72. Sullivan MJ, Adams A, Horan S, et al. The role of perceived injustice in the experience of chronic pain and disability: scale development and validation. *J Occup Rehabil.* 2008;18:249-261.
73. Picavet HSJ, Vlaeyen JWS, Schouten JSAG. Pain catastrophizing and kinesiophobia: predictors of chronic low back pain. *Am J Epidemiol.* 2002;156:1028 1034.
74. Severeijns R, Vlaeyen JWS, van den Hout MA, Picavet HSJ. Pain catastrophizing and consequences of musculoskeletal pain: a prospective study in the Dutch community. *J Pain.* 2005;6:125-132.
75. Verbunt JA, Sieben J, Vlaeyen JW, et al. A new episode of low back pain: who relies on bed rest? *Eur J Pain.* 2008;12:508-516.
76. Heyneman NE, Fremouw WJ, Gano D, et al. Individual differences and the effectiveness of different coping strategies for pain. *Cog Ther Res.* 1990;14:63-77.
77. Van Damme S, Crombez G, Eccleston C. Disengagement from pain: the role of catastrophic thinking about pain. *Pain.* 2004;107: 70-76.
78. Gündel H, Valet M, Sorg C, et al. Altered cerebral response to noxious heat stimulation in patients with somatoform pain disorder. *Pain.* 2008;137:413-421.
79. Ploghaus A, Narain C, Beckmann CF, et al. Exacerbation of pain by anxiety is associated with activity in a hippocampal network. *J Neurosci.* 2001;21:9896-9903.
80. Roy M, Piché M, Chen J-I, Peretz I, Rainville P. Cerebral and spinal modulation of pain by emotions. *Proc Natl Acad Sci.* 2009;106:20900-20905.
81. Seminowicz DA, Davis KD. Cortical responses to pain in healthy individuals depends on pain catastrophizing. *Pain.* 2006;120:297-306.
82. Weissman-Fogel I, Sprecher E, Pud D. Effects of catastrophizing on pain perception and pain modulation. *Exp Brain Res.* 2008;186:79-85.
83. Edwards RR, Smith MT, Stonerock G, Haythornthwaite JA. Pain-related catastrophizing in healthy women is associated with greater temporal summation of and reduced habituation to thermal pain. *Clin J Pain.* 2006;22:730-737.
84. Edwards RR, Kronfli T, Haythornthwaite JA, et al. Association of catastrophizing with interleukin-6 responses to acute pain. *Pain.* 2008;140:135-144.
85. Schweinhardt P, Kuchinad A, Pukall CF, Bushnell MC. Increased gray matter density in young women with chronic vulvar pain. *Pain.* 2008;140:411-419.
86. Schmidt-Wilcke T, Leinisch E, Gänßbauer S, et al. Affective components and intensity of pain correlate with structural differences in gray matter in chronic back pain patients. *Pain.* 2006;125:89-97.
87. Rosenstiel AK, Keefe FJ. The use of coping strategies in chronic low back pain patients: relationship to patient characteristics and current adjustment. *Pain.* 1983;17:33-40.
88. Sullivan MJL, Bishop SR, Pivik J. The Pain Catastrophizing Scale: development and validation. *Psychol Assess.* 1995;7:524-532.
89. Linton SJ, Buer N, Vlaeyen J, Hellsing A-L. Are fear-avoidance beliefs related to the inception of an episode of back pain? A prospective study. *Psychol Health.* 2000;14:1051-1059.
90. Van Nieuwenhuyse A, Somville PR, Crombez G. The role of physical workload and pain related fear in the development of low back pain in young workers: evidence from the BelCoBack Study: results after one year of follow-up. *Occup Environ Med.* 2006;63:45-52.
91. Waddell G, Newton M, Henderson I, Somerville D, Main CJ. A fear-avoidance beliefs questionnaire (FABQ) and the role of fear-avoidance beliefs in chronic low back pain and disability. *Pain.* 1993;52:157-168.
92. Fritz JM, George SZ. Identifying psychosocial variables in patients with acute work-related low back pain: the importance of fear-avoidance beliefs. *Phys Ther.* 2002;82:973-983.
93. Bousema EJ, Verbunt JA., Seelen HAM, Vlaeyen JWS, Knottnerus JA. Disuse and physical deconditioning in the first year after the onset of back pain. *Pain.* 2007; 130: 279 286.
94. Smeets RJEM, Wade D, Hidding A, et al. The association of physical deconditioning and chronic low back pain: A hypothesis-oriented systematic review. *Disabil Rehabil.* 2006;28:673-693.
95. Leo RJ, Latif T. Repetitive transcranial magnetic stimulation (rTMS) in experimentally induced and chronic neuropathic pain: a review. *J Pain.* 2007;8:453-459.
96. Nuti C, Peyron R, Gracia-Larrea L. Motor cortex stimulation for refractory neuropathic pain: four year outcome and predictors of efficacy. *Pain.* 2005;118:43-52.
97. Leeuw M, Peters ML, Wiers RW, Vlaeyen JW. Measuring fear of movement/(re)injury in chronic low back pain using implicit measures. *Cogn Behav Ther.* 2007;36:52-64.
98. Moseley GL, Nicholas MK, Hodges PW. Does anticipation of back pain predispose to back trouble? *Brain.* 2004;127:2339-2347.

99. Kori SH, Miller RP, Todd DD. Kinesiophobia: a new view of chronic pain behavior. *Pain Manag.* 1990;3:35-43.
100. Miller RP, Kori S, Todd D. The Tampa Scale: a measure of kinesiophobia. *Clin J Pain.* 1991;7:51-52.
101. French DJ, France CR, Vigneau F, French JA, Evans RT. Fear of movement/(re)injury in chronic pain: a psychometric assessment of the original English version of the Tampa Scale for Kinesiophobia (TSK). *Pain.* 2007;127:42-51.
102. Riley JF, Ahern DK, Follick MJ. Chronic pain and functional impairment: assessing beliefs about their relationship. *Arch Phys Med Rehabil.* 1988;59:579-582.
103. Houben RMA, Vlaeyen JWS, Peterse M, Ostelo RWJG, Wolters PMJC, Stomp-van den Berg SGM. Health care providers' attitudes and beliefs towards common low back pain: factor structure and psychometric properties of the HC-PAIRS. *Clin J Pain.* 2004;20:37-44.
104. Rainville J, Bagnall D, Phalen L. Health care providers' attitudes and beliefs about functional impairments and chronic back pain. *Clin J Pain.* 1995;11:287-295.
105. Roelofs J, Sluiter J, Frings-Dresen MHW, et al. Fear of movement and (re)injury in chronic musculoskeletal pain: Evidence for an invariant two-factor model of the Tampa Scale for Kinesiophobia across pain diagnoses and Dutch, Swedish, and Canadian samples. *Pain.* 2007;131:181-190.
106. Woby SR, Roach NK, Urmston M, Watson P. Psychometric properties of the TSK-11: a shortened version of the Tampa Scale for Kinesiophobia. *Pain.* 2005;117:137-144.
107. Roelofs J, van Breukelen G, Sluiter J, et al. Norming of the Tampa Scale for Kinesiophobia across pain diagnoses and various countries. *Pain.* 2011;152:1090-1095.
108. George SZ, Calley D, Valencia C, Beneciuk JM. Clinical investigation of pain-related fear and pain catastrophizing for patients with low back pain. *Clin J Pain.* 2011;27:108-115.
109. Swinkels-Meewisse EJCM, Swinkels RAHM, Verbeek ALM, Vlaeyen JWS, Oostendorp RAB. Psychometric properties of the Tampa Scale for Kinesiophobia and the Fear Avoidance Beliefs Questionnaire in acute low back pain. *Man Ther.* 2003;8:29-36.
110. Lee K-C, Chiu TTW, Lam T-H. Psychometric properties of the Fear-Avoidance Beliefs Questionnaire in patients with neck pain. *Clin Rehabil.* 2006;20:909-920.
111. Beck JG, Clapp JD. A different kind of comorbidity: understanding posttraumatic stress disorder and chronic pain. *Psychol Trauma.* 2011;3:101-108.
112. Von Korff M, Crane P, Lane M, et al. Chronic spinal pain and physical-mental co-morbidity in the United States: results from the National Co-Morbidity Survey replication. *Pain.* 2005;113:331-339.
113. Mayou R, Bryant B. Outcome in consecutive emergency department attenders following a road traffic accident. *Br J Psychiatry.* 2001;179:528-534.
114. Sterling M, Kenardy J. The relationship between sensory and sympathetic nervous system changes and posttraumatic stress reaction following whiplash injury: a prospective study. *J Psychosom Res.* 2006;60:387-393.
115. Beck JG, Coffrey SF, Foy DW, Keane TM, Blanchard EG. Group cognitive behavior therapy for chronic posttraumatic stress disorder: an initial randomized pilot study. *Behav Ther.* 2009;40:82-92.
116. Elliott J, Pedler A, Kenardy J, et al. The temporal development of fatty infiltrates in the neck muscles following whiplash injury: an association with pain and posttraumatic stress. *PLoS One.* 2011;6(6):e21194.
117. Horowitz M, Wilner N, Alvarez W. Impact of events scale: a measure of subjective stress. *Psychosom Med.* 1979;41:209-218.
118. Foa EB, Riggs DS, Dancu CV, Rothbaum BO. Reliability and validity of a brief instrument for assessing post-traumatic stress disorder. *J Trauma Stress.* 1993;6:459-473.
119. Coffrey SF, Gudmundsdottir B, Beck JG, Palyo SA, Miller L. Screening for PTSD in motor vehicle accident survivors using the PSS-SR and IES. *J Trauma Stress.* 2006;19:119-128.
120. McBeth J, Silman AJ, Gupta A, et al. Moderation of psychosocial risk factors through dysfunction of the hypothalamic-pituitary-adrenal stress axis in the onset of chronic widespread musculoskeletal pain. *Arthritis Rheum.* 2007;56:360-371.
121. Scher AI, Stewart WF, Buse D, et al. Major life changes before and after the onset of chronic daily headache: a population-based study. *Cephalalgia.* 2008;28:868-876.
122. Quintero L, Moreno M, Avila C, et al. Long-lasting delayed hyperalgesia after subchronic swim stress. *Pharmacol Biochem Behav.* 2000;67:449-458.
123. Le Roy C, Laboureyras E, Gavello-Baudy S, et al. Endogenous opioids released during non-nociceptive environmental stress induce latent pain sensitization via a NMDA-dependent process. *J Pain.* 2011;12:1069-1079.
124. Urry HL, van Rekum CM, Johnstone T, et al. Amygdala and ventromedial prefrontal cortex are inversely coupled during regulation of negative affect and predict the diurnal pattern of cortisol secretion among older adults. *J Neurosci.* 2006;26:4415-4425.
125. García-Bueno B, Caso JR, Leza JC. Stress as a neuroinflammatory condition in brain: damaging and protective mechanisms. *Neurosci Biobehav Rev.* 2008;32:1136-1151.
126. Price DD, Staud R. Neurobiology of fibromyalgia syndrome. *J Rheumatol Suppl.* 2005;75:22-28.
127. Banks SM, Kerns RD. Explaining the high rates of depression in chronic pain: a diathesis-stress framework. *Psychol Bull.* 1996;119:95-110.
128. Burns JW, Quartana PJ, Bruehl S. Anger inhibition and pain: conceptualizations, evidence and new directions. *J Behav Med.* 2008;31:259-279.
129. Burns JW, Quartana PJ, Gilliam W, et al. Effects of anger suppression on pain severity and pain behaviors among chronic pain patients: evaluation of an ironic process model. *Health Psychol.* 2008;27:645-652.
130. Quartana PJ, Yoon KL, Burns JW. Anger suppression, ironic processes, and pain. *J Behav Med.* 2007;30:455-469.
131. Burns JW. The role of attentional strategies in moderating links between acute pain induction and subsequent emotional stress: evidence for symptom specific reactivity among chronic pain patients versus healthy nonpatients. *Emotion.* 2006;6:180-192.
132. Burns JW. Arousal of negative emotions and symptom-specific reactivity in chronic low back pain patients. *Emotion.* 2006;6:309-319.
133. Weber H. Explorations in the social construction of anger. *Motiv Emot.* 2004;28:197-219.
134. Spielberger CD, Johnson EH, Russell SF, et al. The experience and expression of anger: construction and validation of an anger expression scale. In: Chesney MA, Rosenman RH, eds. *Anger and Hostility in Cardiovascular and Behavioral Disorders.* Washington, DC: Hemisphere Publishing Corporation; 1985:5-30.
135. Breuer J, Freud S. *Studies on hysteria (J. Strachey, Trans.).* New York, NY: Basic Books; 1893-1895/1957.
136. Weinberger DA, Schwartz GE, Davidson JR. Low-anxious, high-anxious, and repressive coping styles: psychometric patterns and behavioral and physiological responses to stress. *J Abnorm Psychol.* 1979;88:369-380.

137. Derakshan N, Eysenck MW. Are repressors self-deceivers or other-deceivers? *Cogn Emot*. 1999;13:1-17.

138. Weinberger DA. The construct validity of the repressive coping style. In: Singer JL, eds. *Repression and Dissociation: Implications for Personality Theory, Psychopathology, and Health*. Chicago, Ill: University of Chicago Press; 1990.

139. Newman LS, McKinney LC. Repressive coping and threat avoidance: an idiographic Stroop study. *Pers Soc Psychol Bull*. 2002;28:409-422.

140. Burns JW, Quartana PJ, Elfant E, Matsuura J, Gilliam W, Nappi C, et al. Shifts in attention biases in response to acute pain induction: examination of a model of "conversion" among repressors. *Emotion*. 2010;10:755-766.

141. Burns JW. Repression predicts outcome following multidisciplinary treatment for chronic pain. *Health Psychol*. 2000;19:75-84.

142. Burns JW, Kubilus A, Bruehl S, Harden RN. A fourth empirically-derived cluster of chronic pain patients based on the Multidimensional Pain Inventory: Evidence for repression within the dysfunctional group. *J Consult Clin Psychol*. 2001;69:663-673.

143. Hölzl R, Kleinböhl D, Huse E. Implicit operant learning of pain sensitization. *Pain*. 2005;115:12-20.

144. Hasenbring MI, Hallner D, Rusu AC. Fear-avoidance- and endurance-related responses to pain: development and validation of the Avoidance-Endurance Questionnaire (AEQ). *Eur J Pain*. 2009; 13:620-628.

145. Nielson WR, Jensen MP, Hill ML. An activity pacing scale for the Chronic Pain Coping Inventory: development in a sample of patients with fibromyalgia syndrome. *Pain*. 2001;89:111-115.

146. Hasenbring MI, Hallner D, Klasen B, et al. Pain-related avoidance versus endurance in primary care patients with subacute back pain: psychological characteristics and outcome at a 6-month follow-up. *Pain*. 2012;153:211-217.

147. Sifneos PE. *Short-term Psychotherapy and Emotional Crisis*. Cambridge, Mass: Harvard University Press; 1972.

148. Sifneos PE. The prevalence of "alexithymic" characteristics in psychosomatic patients. *Psychother Psychosom*. 1973;22:255-262.

149. Taylor GJ, Bagby RM, Parker JDA. The alexithymia construct: a potential paradigm for psychosomatic medicine. *Psychosomatics*. 1991;32:153-164.

150. Salminen JK, Saarijärvis S, Äärelä E, et al. Prevalence of alexithymia and its association with sociodemographic variables in the general population of Finland. *J Psychosom Res*. 1999;46:75-82.

151. Huber A, Suman AL, Biasi G, Carli G. Alexithymia in fibromyalgia syndrome: Associations with ongoing pain, experimental pain sensitivity and illness behavior. *J Psychosom Res*. 2009;66: 425-433.

152. Lumley MA, Stettner L, Wehmer F. How are alexithymia and physical illness linked? A review and critique of pathways. *J Psychosom Res*. 1996;41:505-518.

153. Berenbaum H. Childhood abuse, alexithymia and personality disorder. *J Psychosom Res*. 1996;41:585-595.

154. Hosoi M, Molton IR, Jensen MP, et al. Relationships among alexithymia and pain intensity, pain interference, and vitality in persons with neuromuscular disease: considering the effect of negative affectivity. *Pain*. 2010;149:273-277.

155. Saarijiarvi S, Salminen JK, Toikka TB. Alexithymia and depression: a 1-year follow-up study in outpatients with major depression. *J Psychosom Res*. 2001;51:729-733.

156. Mehling WE, Krause N. Alexithymia and 7.5-year incidence of compensated low back pain in 1207 urban public transit operators. *J Psychosom Res*. 2007;62:667-674.

157. Bagby RM, Parker JD, Taylor GJ. The twenty-item Toronto Alexithymia Scale—I. Item selection and cross-validation of the factor structure. *J Psychosom Res*. 1994;38:23-32.

158. Bagby RM, Taylor GJ, Parker JD. The twenty-item Toronto Alexithymia Scale—II. Convergent, discriminant, and concurrent validity. *J Psychosom Res*. 1994;38:33-40.

159. Subic-Wrana C, Bruder S, Thomas W, Lane RD, Kohle K. Emotional awareness deficits in inpatients of a psychosomatic ward: a comparison of two different measures of alexithymia. *Psychosom Med*. 2005;67:483-489.

160. Suslow T, Donges US, Kersting A, Arolt V. 20-item Toronto Alexithymia Scale: do difficulties describing feelings assess proneness to shame instead of difficulties symbolizing emotions? *Scand J Psychol*. 2000;41:329-334.

161. Conrad R, Schilling G, Bausch C, et al. Temperament and character personality profiles and personality disorders in chronic pain patients. *Pain*. 2007;133:197-209.

162. Ramírez-Maestre C, López Martínez AE, Zarazaga RE. Personality characteristics as differential variables of the pain experience. *J Behav Med*. 2004;27:147-165.

163. Mulder RT, Joyce PR, Frampton CM, et al. Six months of treatment for depression: Outcome and predictors of the course of illness. *Am J Psychiatry*. 2006;163:95-100.

164. Weisberg JN. Personality and personality disorders in chronic pain. *Curr Rev Pain*. 2000;4:60-70.

165. Okifuji A, Hare BD. Do sleep disorders contribute to pain sensitivity? *Curr Rheumatol Rep*. 2011;13:528-534.

166. Davies, KA, Macfarlane GJ, Nicholl BI, et al. Restorative sleep predicts the resolution of chronic widespread pain: results from the EPIFUND study. *Rheumatology*. 2008;47:1809-1813.

167. Kundermann B, Hemmeter-Spernal J, Huber MT, Krieg JC, Lautenbacher S. Effects of total sleep deprivation in major depression: overnight improvement of mood is accompanied by increased pain sensitivity and augmented pain complaints. *Psychosom Med*. 2008;70:92-101.

168. Campbell CM, Bounds SC, Simango MB, et al. Self-reported sleep duration associated with distraction analgesia, hyperemia, and secondary hyperalgesia in the heat-capsaicin nociceptive model. *Eur J Pain*. 2011;15:561-567.

169. Nascimento DC, Andersen ML, Hipolide DC, Nobrega JN, Tufik S. Pain hypersensitivity induced by paradoxical sleep deprivation is not due to altered binding to brain mu-opioid receptors. *Behav Brain Res*. 2007;178:216-220.

170. Damasceno F, Skinner GO, Gomes A, Araujo PC, de Almeida OM. Systemic amitriptyline administration does not prevent the increased thermal response induced by paradoxical sleep deprivation. *Pharmacol Biochem Behav*. 2009;94:51-55,

171. Chung K-F, Tso K-C. Relationship between insomnia and pain in major depressive disorder: a sleep diary and actigraphy study. *Sleep Med*. 2010;11:752-758.

172. Haythornthwaite JA, Hegel MT, Kerns RD. Development of a sleep diary for chronic pain patients. *J Pain Symptom Manage*. 1991;6:65-72.

173. Hays RD, Martin SA, Sesti AM, Spritzer KL. Psychometric properties of the Medical Outcomes Study Sleep measure. *Sleep Med*. 2005;6:41-44.

174. Kosinski M, Janagap CC, Gajria K, Schein J. Psychometric testing and validation of the Chronic Pain Sleep Inventory. *Clin Ther*. 2007;29:2562-2577.

175. Rejas J, Ribera MV, Ruiz M, Masrramón X. Psychometric properties of the MOS (Medical Outcomes Study) Sleep Scale in patients with neuropathic pain. *Eur J. Pain*. 2007;11:329-340.

176. Shi Y, Weingarten TN, Maqntilla CB, Hooten WM, Warner DO. Smoking and pain: pathophysiology and clinical implications. *Anesthesiology*. 2010;113:977-992.
177. Cong L, Pang H, Xuan D, Tuu, G. The interaction between aggrecan gene VNTR polymorphism and cigarette smoking in predicting incident symptomatic intervertebral disc degeneration. *Connect Tissue Res*. 2010;51:397-403.
178. Brett K, Parker R, Wittenauer S, et al. Impact of chronic nicotine on sciatic nerve injury in the rat. *J Neuroimmunol*. 2007;186:37-44.
179. Ackerman WE III, Ahmad M. Effect of cigarette smoking on serum hydrocodone levels in chronic pain patients. *J Ark Med Soc*. 2007;104:19-21.
180. Hooten WM, Shi Y, Gazelka HM, Warner DO. The effects of depression and smoking on pain severity and opioid use in patients with chronic pain. *Pain*. 2011;152:223–229.
181. Hooten WM, Townsend CO, Bruce BK, et al. Effect of smoking status on immediate treatment outcomes of multidisciplinary pain rehabilitation. *Pain Med*. 2009;10:347-355.
182. Lazarus RS, Folkman S. *Stress, Appraisal, and Coping*. New York, NY: Springer; 1984.
183. Keefe FJ, Kashikar-Zuck S, Robinson E, et al. Pain coping strategies that predict patients' and spouses' ratings of patients' self-efficacy. *Pain*. 1997;73:191-199.
184. Haythornthwaite JA, Menefee LA, Heinberg LJ, Clark MR. Pain coping strategies predict perceived control over pain. *Pain*. 1998;77:33-39.
185. Keefe FJ, Caldwell DS, Queen KT, et al. Pain coping strategies in osteoarthritis patients. *J Consult Clin Psychol*. 1987;55:208-212.
186. Miles CL, Pincus T, Carnes D, Taylor SJC, Underwood M. Measuring pain self-efficacy. *Clin J Pain*. 2011;27:461-470.
187. Nicholas MK. The Pain Self-efficacy Questionnaire: taking pain into account. *Eur J Pain*. 2007;11:153-163.
188. Nicholas MK, Asghari A, Blyth FM. What do the numbers mean? Normative data in chronic pain measures. *Pain*. 2008;134:158-173.
189. Tonkin L. The Pain Self-Efficacy Questionnaire. *Aust J Physiother*. 2008;54:77.
190. Kerns RD, Turk DC, Rudy TE. The West Haven-Yale Multidimensional Pain Inventory (WHYMPII). *Pain*. 1985;23:345-356.
191. Jensen MP, Turner JA, Romano JM, Lawler BK. Relationship of pain-specific beliefs to chronic pain adjustment. *Pain*. 1994;57:301-309.
192. Cioffi D, Holloway J. Delayed costs of suppressed pain. *J Pers Soc Psychol*. 1993;64:274-282.
193. Thompson M, McCracken LM. Acceptance and related processes in adjustment to chronic pain. *Curr Pain Headache Rep*. 2011;15:144-151.
194. Feldner MT, Hekmat H, Zvolensky MJ, et al. The role of experiential avoidance in acute pain tolerance: a laboratory test. *J Behav Ther Exp Psychiatry*. 2006;37:146-158.
195. Vowles KE, McNeil DW, Gross RT, et al. Effects of pain acceptance and pain control strategies on physical impairment in individuals with chronic low back pain. *Behav Ther*. 2007;38:412-425.
196. Vowles KE, McCracken LM, O'Brien JZ. Acceptance and values-based action in chronic pain: A three-year follow-up analysis of treatment effectiveness and process. *Behav Res Ther*. 2011;49:748-755.
197. McCracken LM, Vowles KE, Eccleston C. Acceptance of chronic pain: component analysis and a revised assessment method. *Pain*. 2004;107:159-166.
198. Nicholas MK, Asghari A. Investigating acceptance in adjustment to chronic pain: is acceptance broader than we thought? *Pain*. 2006;124:269-279.
199. Rhudy JL, Williams AE, McCabe KM, Nguyen MATV, Rambo P. Affective modulation of nociception at spinal and supraspinal levels. *Psychophysiology*. 2005;42:579-587.
200. Legrain V, Van Damme S, Eccleston C, et al. A neurocognitive model of attention to pain: behavioral and neuroimaging evidence. *Pain*. 2009;144:230-232.
201. McCracken LM, Yang S. The role of values in a contextual cognitive-behavioral approach to chronic pain. *Pain*. 2006;123:137-145.
202. Riley JL III, Zawacki TM, Robinson ME, Geisser ME. Empirical test of the factor structure of the West Haven-Yale Multidimensional Pain Inventory. *Clin J Pain*. 1999;15:24-30.
203. Van Koulil S, Kraaimaat FW, Van Lankveld W, et al. Cognitive-behavioral mechanisms in a pain-avoidance and a pain-persistence treatment for high risk fibromyalgia patients. *Arthritis Care Res*. 2011;63:800-807.
204. Van Koulil S, Van Lankveld W, Kraaimaat FW, et al. Tailored cognitive-behavioral therapy and exercise training for high-risk patients with fibromyalgia. *Arthritis Care Res*. 2010;62:1377-1385.
205. Kraaimaat FW, Evers AW. Pain-coping strategies in chronic pain patients: psychometric characteristics of the Pain-Coping Inventory (PCI). *Int J Behav Med*. 2003;10:343-363.
206. Turk DC, Wilson HD. Fear of pain as a prognostic factor in chronic pain: conceptual models, assessment, and treatment implications. *Curr Pain Headache Rep*. 2010;14:88-95.
207. Vlaeyen JW, Linton SJ. Fear-avoidance and its consequences in chronic musculoskeletal pain: a state of the art. *Pain*. 2000; 85:317-332.
208. Linton SJ, Andersson T. Can chronic disability be prevented? A randomized trail of a cognitive-behavior intervention and two forms of information for patients with spinal pain. *Spine*. 2000;25:2825-2831.
209. Linton SJ, Nordin E. A 5-year follow-up evaluation of the health and economic consequences of an early cognitive behavioral intervention for back pain: a randomized, controlled trial. *Spine*. 2006;31:853-858.
210. Coudeyre E, Givron P, Vanbiervliet W, et al. The role of an information booklet or oral information about back pain in reducing disability and fear-avoidance beliefs among patients with subacute and chronic low back pain: a randomized controlled trial in a rehabilitation unit. *Ann Readapt Med Phys*. 2006;49:600-608.
211. Woods MP, Asmundson GJG. Evaluating the efficacy of graded in vivo exposure for the treatment of fear in patients with chronic back pain: a randomized controlled clinical trial. *Pain*. 2008;136:271-280.
212. Thieme K, Turk DC, Flor H. Responder criteria for operant and cognitive-behavioral treatment of fibromyalgia syndrome. *Arthritis Rheum*. 2007;57:830-836.
213. Verra ML, Angst F, Staal JB, et al. Differences in pain, function and coping in Multidimensional Pain Inventory subgroups of chronic back pain: a one-group pretest-posttest study. *BMC Musculoskelet Disord*. 2011;12:145. doi: 10.1186/1471-2474-12-145
214. Turk DC. The potential of treatment matching for subgroups of patients with chronic pain: lumping versus splitting. *Clin J Pain*. 2005;21:44-55.
215. van der Hulst M, Vollenbroek-Hutten MM, Ijzerman MJ. A systematic review of sociodemographic, physical, and psychological predictors of multidisciplinary rehabilitation or, back school treatment outcome in patients with chronic low back pain. *Spine*. 2005;30:813-825.
216. Prochaska JO, DiClemente CC. Stages and processes of self-change of smoking: toward an integrative model of change. *J Consult Clin Psychol*. 1983;51:390-395.

217. Kerns RD, Rosenberg R, Jamison RN, Caudill MA, Haythornthwaite J. Readiness to adopt a self-management approach to chronic pain: the Pain Stages of Change Questionnaire (PSOCQ). *Pain.* 1997;72:227-234.

218. Tang NKY, Crane C. Suicidality in chronic pain: a review of the prevalence, risk factors and psychological links. *Psychol Med.* 2006;36:575-586.

219. Smith MT, Perlis ML, Haythornthwaite JA. Suicidal ideation in outpatients with chronic musculoskeletal pain: an exploratory study of the role of sleep onset insomnia and pain intensity. *Clin J Pain.* 2004;20:111-118.

220. Edwards, RR, Smith MT, Kudel I, Haythornthwaite J. Pain-related catastrophizing as a risk factor for suicidal ideation in chronic pain. *Pain.* 2006;126:272-279.

221. Smith MT, Edwards RR, Robinson RC, Dworkin RH. Suicidal ideation, plans, and attempts in chronic pain patients: factors associated with increased risk. *Pain.* 2004;111:201-208.

222. Breslau N. Migraine, suicidal ideation, and suicide attempts. *Neurology.* 1992;42:392-395.

223. Macfarlane GJ, McBeth J, Silman AJ. Widespread body pain and mortality: prospective population based study. *BMJ.* 2001;323:1-5.

224. Magni G, Rigatti-Luchini S, Fracca F, Merskey H. Suicidality in chronic abdominal pain: an analysis of the Hispanic Health and Nutrition Examination Survey (HHANES). *Pain.* 1998;76:137-144.

225. Penttinen, J. Back pain and risk of suicide among Finnish farmers. *Am J Public Health.* 1995;85:1452-1453.

226. Timonen M, Viilo K, Hakko H, et al. Suicides in persons suffering from rheumatoid arthritis. *Rheumatology.* 2003;42:287-291.

227. Klõves K, Ide N, De Leo D. Suicidal ideation and behaviour in the aftermath of marital separation: gender differences. *J Affect Disord.* 2010;120:48-53.

228. Bryan CJ, Rudd MD. Advances in the assessment of suicide risk. *J Clin Psychol: In Session.* 2006;62:185-200.

229. American Psychiatric Association. Practice guideline for the assessment and treatment of patients with suicidal behaviors. *Am J Psychiatry.* 2003;160(Suppl. 11):1-60.

230. Beck AT, Weissman, A, Lester D, Trexler L. The measurement of pessimism: the Hopelessness Scale. *J Consult Clin Psychol.* 1974;42:861-865.

231. Beck A, Kovacs M, Weissman A. Hopelessness and suicidal behavior: an overview. *JAMA.* 1975;234:1146-1149.

232. Beck AT, Kovacs M, Weissman A. Assessment of suicidal ideation: the scale for suicidal ideation. *J Consult Clin Psychol.* 1979;47:343-352.

233. Beck AT, Steer RA, Brown GK. *Beck Depression Inventory Manual.* 2nd ed. San Antonio, TX: Psychological Corporation; 1996.

234. Edlund MJ, Steffick D, Hudson T, Harris KM, Sullivan M. Risk factors for clinically recognized opioid abuse and dependence among veterans using opioids for chronic non-cancer pain. *Pain.* 2007;129:355-362.

235. Chabal C, Erjavec MK, Jacobson L, et al. Prescription opiate abuse in chronic pain patients: Clinical criteria, incidence, and predictors. *Clin J Pain.* 1997;13:150-155.

236. White AG, Birnbaum HG, Schiller M, Tang J, Katz NP. Analytic models to identify patients at risk for prescription opioid abuse. *Am J Manag Care.* 2009;15:897-906.

237. Butler SF, Fernandez K, Benoit C, Budman SH, Jamison RN. Validation of the revised Screener and Opioid Assessment for Patients with Pain (SOAPP-R). *J Pain.* 2008;9:360-372.

238. Webster LR, Webster RM. Predicting aberrant behaviors in opioid-treated patients: preliminary validation of the Opioid Risk Tool. *Pain Med.* 2005;6:432-442.

239. Chou R, Fanciullo GJ, Fine PG, et al. Opioids for chronic noncancer pain: prediction and identification of aberrant drug-related behaviors: a review of the evidence for an American Pain Society and American Academy of Pain Medicine clinical practice guideline. *J Pain.* 2009;10:131-146.

240. Moore TM, Jones T, Browder, JH, et al. A comparison of common screening methods for predicting aberrant drug-related behavior among patients receiving opioids for chronic pain management. *Pain Med.* 2009;10:1426-1433.

241. Butler SF, Budman SH, Fernandez KC, et al. Cross-validation of a screener to predict opioid misuse in chronic pain patients (SAOPP-R). *J Addict Med.* 2009;3:66-73.

242. Jones T, Moore T, Levy JL, et al. A comparison of various risk screening methods in predicting discharge from opioid treatment. *Clin J Pain.* 2012;28:93-100.

243. Freyd M. The graphic rating scale. *J Educ Psychol.* 1923;14:83-102.

244. Hayes MHS, Patterson DG. Experimental development of the graphic rating method. *Psychol Bull.* 1921;18:98-99.

245. Miner JB. The evaluation of a method for finely graduated estimates of abilities. *J Appl Psychol.* 1917;1:123-133.

246. Aitken RCB, Ferres HM, Gedye JL. Distraction from flashing lights. *Aerosp Med.* 1963;34:302-306.

247. Bond MR, Pilowsky I. Subjective assessment of pain and its relationship to the administration of analgesics in patients with advanced cancer. *J Psychosom Res.* 1966;10:203-208.

248. Clarke PRF, Spear FG. Reliability and sensitivity in the self-assessment of well-being. *Bull Br Psychol Soc.* 1964;17:55.

249. Provenzano DA, Fanciullo GJ, Jamison RN, McHugo GJ, Baird JC. Computer assessment and diagnostic classification of chronic pain patients. *Pain Med.* 2007;8(S3):s167-s175.

250. Scott J, Huskinsson EC. Graphic representation of pain. *Pain.* 1976;2:175–184.

251. Jensen MP, Turner JA, Romano JM. What is the maximum number of levels needed in pain intensity measurement? *Pain.* 1994;58:387-392.

252. Price DD, McGrath PA, Rafii A, Buckingham B. The validation of visual analogue scales as ratio scale measures for chronic and experimental pain. *Pain.* 1983;17:45–56.

253. Price DD. *Psychological and Neural Mechanisms of Pain.* NY: Raven Press. 1988.

254. Seymour RA, Simpson JM, Charlton JE, Philips ME. An evaluation of the length and end-phrase of visual analogue scales in dental pain. *Pain.* 1985;21:177–185.

255. Duncan GH, Bushnell C, Lavigne GJ. Comparison of verbal and visual analogue scales for measuring the intensity and unpleasantness of experimental pain. *Pain.* 1989;37:295-303.

256. Littlejohns DW, Vere DW. The clinical measurement of analgesic drugs. *Br J Clin Pharmacol.* 1981;11:319-332.

257. Ellermeier W, Westphal W, Heidenfelder M. On the "absoluteness" of category and magnitude scales of pain. *Percept Psychophys.* 1991;49:159-166.

258. Melzack R. The McGill Pain Questionnaire: major properties and scoring methods. *Pain.* 1975;1:277-299.

259. Holroyd KA, Holm JE, Keefe FJ, et al. A multi-center evaluation of the McGill Pain Questionnaire: results from more than 1700 chronic pain patients. *Pain.* 1992;48:301-311.

260. Turk DC, Rudy TE, Salovey P. The McGill Pain Questionnaire reconsidered: confirming the factor structure and examining appropriate uses. *Pain.* 1985;21:385-397.

261. Gracely RH. Evaluation of multi-dimensional pain scales editorial. *Pain*. 1992;48:297-300.

262. Price DD. *Psychological Mechanisms of Pain and Analgesia*. Seattle, Wash: IASP Press; 1999.

263. Price DD. Psychological and neural mechanisms of the affective dimension of pain. *Science*. 2000;288:1769-1772.

264. Rainville P, Duncan GH, Price DD, Carrier B, Bushnell MC. Pain affect encoded in human anterior cingulate but not somatosensory cortex. *Science*. 1997;277:968-971.

265. Sist TC, Florio GA, Miner MF, Lema MJ, Zevon MA. The relationship between depression and pain language in cancer and chronic noncancer pain patients. *J Pain Symptom Manage*.1998;15:350-358.

266. Wilkie DJ, Savedra MC, Holzemer WL, Tesler MD, Paul SM. Use of the McGill Pain Questionnaire to measure pain: a meta-analysis. *Nurs Res*. 1990;39:36-41.

267. Melzack R. The Short-Form McGill Pain Questionnaire. *Pain*. 1987;30:191-197.

268. Dworkin RH, Turk DC, Revicki DA, et al. Development and initial validation of an expanded and revised version of the Short-form McGill Pain Questionnaire (SF-MPQ-2). *Pain*. 2009;144:35-42.

269. Borkum JM. *Chronic Headaches: Biology, Psychology, and Behavioral Treatment*. Mahwah, NJ: Lawrence Erlbaum Associates; 2007

270. Ge HY, Fernndez-de-lasPeas C, Arendt-Nielsen L. Sympathetic facilitation of hyperalgesia evoked from myofascial tender and trigger points in patients with unilateral shoulder pain. *Clin Neurophysiol*. 2006;117:1545-1550.

271. Lundberg U, Dohns I.E., Melin B, et al. psychophysiological stress responses, muscle tension, and neck and shoulder pain among supermarket cashiers. *J Occup Health Psychol*. 1999;4:245-255.

272. Bierhaus A, Wolf J, Andrassy M, et al. A mechanism converting psychosocial stress into mononuclear cell activation. *Proc Natl Acad Sci*. 2003;100:1920-1925.

273. Koopman FA, Stoof SP, Straub RH, et al. Restoring the balance of the autonomic nervous system as an innovative approach to the treatment of rheumatoid arthritis. *Mol Med*. 2011;17:937-948.

274. Andreassi JL. *Psychophysiology: Human Behavior and Physiological Response*. 5th ed. Mahwah, NJ: Erlbaum; 2006.

275. Blanchard EB, Morrill B, Wittrock DA, Scharff L, Jaccard J. Hand temperature norms for headache, hypertension, and irritable bowel syndrome. *Biofeedback Self Regul*. 1989;14:319-331.

276. Ersek M, Turner JA, Kemp CA. Use of the Chronic Pain Coping Inventory to assess older adults' pain coping strategies. *J Pain*. 2006;7:833-842.

277. Jensen MP, Turner JA, Romano JM, Strom SE. The Chronic Pain Coping Inventory: development and preliminary validation. *Pain*. 1995;60:203-216.

278. Chibnall JT, Tait RC. Confirmatory factor analysis of the Pain Catastrophizing Scale in African American and Caucasian workers' compensation claimants with low back injuries. *Pain*. 2005;113:369-375.

279. Brown GK, Nicassio PM. Development of a questionnaire for the assessment of active and passive coping strategies in chronic pain patients. *Pain*. 1987;31:53-63.

280. Smith CA, Wallston KA, Dwyer KA, Dowdy SW. Beyond good and bad coping: A multidimensional examination of coping with pain in persons with rheumatoid arthritis. *Ann Behav Med*. 1997;19:11-21.

281. Geisser ME, Roth RS, Robinson ME. Assessing depression among persons with chronic pain using the Center for Epidemiological Studies and the Beck Depression Inventory: a comparative analysis. *Clin J Pain*. 1997;13:163-170.

282. Love AW. Depression in chronic low back pain patients: diagnostic efficiency of three self-report questionnaires. *J Clin Psychol*. 1987;43:84-89.

283. Wong WS, Chen PP, Yap J, et al. Assessing depression in patients with chronic pain: a comparison of three rating scales. *J Affect Disord*. 2011;133:179-187.

284. Dozois DJA, Covin R. The Beck Depression Inventory-II (BDI-II), Beck Hopelessness Scale (BHS), and Beck Scale for Suicide Ideation (BSS). In: Hilsenroth MJ, Segal DL, eds. *Comprehensive Handbook of Psychological Assessment*. Vol. 2. Personality Assessment. Hoboken, NJ: Wiley; 2004:50-69.

285. Poole H, White S, Blake C, Murphy P, Bramwell R. Depression in chronic pain patients: prevalence and measurement. *Pain Pract*. 2009;9:173-180.

286. Gilbody S, Richards D, Brealey S, Hewitt C. Screening for depression in medical settings with the Patient Health Questionnaire (PHQ): a diagnostic meta-analysis. *J Gen Intern Med*. 2007;22:1596–1602.

287. Spitzer RL, Kroenke K, Williams JB. Validation and utility of a self-report version of PRIME-MD: the PHQ primary care study. Primary Care Evaluation of Mental Disorders. Patient Health Questionnaire. *JAMA*. 1999;282:1737–1744.

288. Rush AJ, Bernstein IH, Trivedi MH, et al. An evaluation of the Quick Inventory of Depressive Symptomatology and the Hamilton Rating Scale for Depression: a sequenced treatment alternative to relieve depression trial report. *Biol Psychiatry*. 2006;59:493-501.

289. Fairbank J, Couper J, Davies J, et al. The Oswestry Low Back Pain Disability Questionnaire. *Physiotherapy*. 1980;66:271-273.

290. Wittink H, Turk DC, Carr DB, Sukiennik A, Rogers W. Comparison of the redundancy, reliability, and responsiveness to change among SF-36, Oswestry Disability Index, and Multidimensional Pain Inventory. *Clin J Pain*. 2004;20:133-142.

291. Tait RC, Chibnall JT. Factor structure of the Pain Disability Index in workers' compensation claimants with low back injuries. *Arch Phys Med Rehabil*. 2005;86:1141-1146.

292. Asmundson GJG, Bovell CV, Carleton RN, McWilliams LA. The Fear of Pain Questionnaire—Short Form (FPQ-SF): factorial validity and psychometric properties. *Pain*. 2008;134:51-58.

293. McCracken LM, Dhingra L. A short version of the Pain Anxiety Symptoms Scale (PASS-20): preliminary development and validity. *Pain Res Manage*. 2002;7:45-50.

294. Heuts PHTG, Vlaeyen JWS, Roelofs J, et al. Pain-related fear and daily functioning in patients with osteoarthritis. *Pain*. 2004;110:228-235.

295. Roelofs J, Goubert L, Peters ML, Vlaeyen JWS, Crombez G. The Tampa Scale for Kinesiophobia: further examination of psychometric properties in patients with chronic low back pain and fibromyalgia. *Eur J Pain*. 2004;8:495-502.

296. Clark WC, Kuhl JP, Keohan ML, et al. Factor analysis validates the cluster structure of the dendrogram underlying the Multidimensional Affect and Pain Survey (MAPS) and challenges the a priori classification of the descriptors in the McGill Pain Questionnaire (MPQ). *Pain*. 2003;106:357-363.

297. Griswold GA, Clark WC. Item analysis of cancer patient responses to the Multidimensional Affect and Pain Survey demonstrates high inter-item consistency and discriminability and determines the content of a short form. *J Pain*. 2005;6:67-74.

298. Engelhard IM, Arntz A, van den Hout MA. Low specificity of symptoms on the post-traumatic stress disorder (PTSD) symptom scale: a comparison of individuals with PTSD, individuals with

other anxiety disorders and individuals without psychopathology. *Br J Clin Psychol.* 2007;46:449-456.

299. Bastien CH, Vallières A, Morin CM. Validation of the Insomnia Severity Index as an outcome measure for insomnia research. *Sleep Med.* 2001;2:297-307.
300. Morin CM, Belleville G, Bélanger L, Ivers H. The Insomnia Severity Index: psychometric indicators to detect insomnia cases and evaluate treatment response. *Sleep.* 2011;34:601-608.
301. McMillan D, Gilbody S, Beresford E, Neilly L. Can we predict suicide and non-fatal self-harm with the Beck Hopelessness Scale? A meta-analysis. *Psychol Med.* 2007;37:769-778.
302. Gerdner A, Allgulander C. Psychometric properties of the Swedish version of the Childhood Trauma Questionnaire—Short Form (CTQ-SF). *Nord J Psychiatry.* 2009;63:160-170.

CHAPTER 16

Gender and Ethnicity*

Donald B. Giddon
Robert R. Edwards

INTRODUCTION

The Lord planned to save us from this assigned task by saying, "… Behold, the people is one, and they have all one language; … and now nothing will be restrained from them …," later in response to perceived arrogance, He said, "… let us go down, and there confound their language, that they may not understand one another's speech. So the Lord scattered them abroad from thence upon the face of all the earth" [Genesis 11:6-8[1]], which is why it is necessary to write this chapter on ethnocultural and gender differences in the pain experience. Since the destruction of the Tower of Babel, clinicians have come to accept that there is a tremendous range of ethnocultural differences in sensitivities expressed in spoken language and behaviors. Also, as will be discussed, there are differences between the genders, with women continuing to struggle for parity with men while appropriately expecting recognition of their differences from men in cognition, affect, and behavior. We hope that the new knowledge and insight provided by this chapter will enable us to advance beyond stereotypes to an increased probability of being able to provide a more accurate diagnosis and prognosis for a given patient. The objective of practitioners of pain medicine is to reduce pain and restore pleasure, consistent with the views of many philosophies, including hedonism and utilitarianism. As noted recently by Greenblatt, "The highest goal of human life is the achievement of pleasure and the reduction of pain."[2] Although pain is thought by many to be on a continuum with pleasure, some continue the ancient tradition of rejoicing in the pain of others, with vestiges still vicariously available in modern pornography.

Pain, particularly chronic pain (which persists for more than 6 months or beyond the expected time for recovery from trauma or surgery), is associated with a decline in quality of life and increases the likelihood of physical or mental disability and excessive health care utilization.[3] A broad array of factors, from genotype to sociocultural forces, contributes to individual pain response.[4] Although the primary objective of this chapter is to describe the role of ethnicity and gender in the pain experience of patients, the reciprocal influence of health care providers' ethnocultural backgrounds and genders on their perception of their patients' pain plus the related attitudes, beliefs, and behaviors that they bring to treating their patients should not be overlooked.[5,6] Such differences can have a significant impact on the quality and appropriateness of pain relief strategies and ethno-specific stereotypical clinical judgments, resulting in overmedication of more emotionally expressive patients or undermedication of less expressive or stoic patients.

A related issue is the large differences among ethnocultural groups in access to care, one example of which was shown by a first-year medical resident who presented the case of a 55-year-old black woman with diabetes. However, on reviewing the patient's chart, it was noted that the resident had written that the patient was a 55-year-old white female patient. When the resident was asked if he needed to see an ophthalmologist, he responded that from concern for his patient that she was not likely to receive the highest level of care as a black woman, he noted that she was white.

With the increasing multicultural pool of both patients and providers, the need for providers to be culturally competent and to have an appreciation of health literacy becomes critical for successful pain management. The diversity in languages and comprehension now requires that clinicians ensure that they understand the depth and breadth of their patients' chief complaints and conversely that the patients comprehend clinicians' instructions and whether patients have sufficient self-efficacy to carry out their instructions. This chapter, therefore, primarily focuses on the ethnocultural and gender differences in clinically observed pain along with the results of studies of experimentally induced pain on self-reported thresholds of awareness and tolerance while noting the behaviors associated with the various quantitative parameters of intensity, duration, and so on.

SEX AND GENDER DIFFERENCES

A growing body of research on sex differences demonstrates that men and women perceive and cope with pain differently, including responses to specific classes of analgesic and other psychoactive medications. Although often used interchangeably, sex and gender are separate constructs. This distinction is consistent with the Institute of Medicine's definition of sex as "the classification of living things as male or female according to their reproductive organs" and chromosomes, with gender consisting of a person's masculine or feminine self-representations and role behaviors.[7] Therefore, in further discussion, the term "gender" will be considered as a cultural variable as distinct from the biologically based classification as male or female sex.

Epidemiologically, women are more likely than men to report acute and chronic pain,[8,9] and they use pain-relieving medications significantly more often than men.[10,11] These findings are highly consistent across time and place, with women reporting more frequent, severe, and disabling pain involving multiple body sites than men. As noted in a recent review, the female-to-male ratio for many types of headache and orofacial pain is approximately two to one, with women also having more widespread musculoskeletal pain.[12] Moreover, the greater analgesic use by women is not simply a function of their greater willingness to report actual increased frequency and severity of pain because when pain frequency and severity are controlled, women are still 40% to 50% more likely than men to report using analgesics.[13] Women are also more likely than men to use a variety of nonpharmacologic treatments for orofacial pain, low back pain, and other painful conditions.[12]

Obviously, biological, cultural, psychological, and social factors all contribute in various ways to ethnocultural differences in willingness to report and exhibit pain behavior. Experimental studies help to elucidate the mechanisms accounting for these gender and other cultural differences, for example, that women are more sensitive than men, as measured by subjective thresholds of pain awareness and subsequent tolerance of standardized noxious stimuli.[9,14] There are also more objective indices, such as electromyographically measured thresholds

*Thanks to Christine Cahalan and George Mensing for their extraordinary valuable assistance with the literature review and manuscript preparation. We also gratefully acknowledge the contribution of Caroline Rains, without whose tireless and devoted efforts the challenge of writing this chapter could not have been met.

for muscle reflexes and pupillary dilation or galvanic skin response as manifestations of associated autonomic nervous system activity.[15] Although experimental pain studies provide different information from clinical or epidemiologic reports, these quantitative measures, singly or in combination, do account for the significant amount of the variability observed in clinical pain.[16-18]

Social Factors Pain tolerance has been shown to be significantly greater in both genders when the experimenters are female rather than male.[19] Gender as a cultural variable includes attitudes, beliefs, and behavioral role expectations for a given ethnocultural group. Differentiation by gender begins in early childhood, with boys and girls receiving different cues to interpret and express themselves in response to environmental adversities such as pain. Sanford and colleagues reported that the higher the femininity score, the lower the pain tolerance.[20] Robinson and colleagues found that both men and women consider females more sensitive and less tolerant of pain and more willing to report pain than males.[21] Moreover, when controlling for willingness to report pain, females were still significantly less tolerant of experimental pain than males. In a recent meta-analysis, moderate to highly significant relationships were found between pain-specific gender roles (measured using the Gender Role Expectations of Pain Questionnaire,[21] which asks respondents to indicate, for example, how sensitive to pain "the typical woman" is relative to "the typical man") while obtaining laboratory indices of pain tolerance thresholds.[22]

In fact, fear of pain predicted a lower tolerance for experimental heat and cold pain in men than women.[23] In clinical studies, symptoms may vary as a function of the age, gender, and ethnocultural background of the health care provider, highlighting the importance of the interpersonal context of verbal reports of pain.[24] In addition to classifying actual or potential patients as being worried and sick, worried but well, not worried but sick, and not worried and not sick, Barsky and colleagues[24,25] have subclassified anxious medical patients (who often have pain complaints) into hypochondriacs, who are more unconsciously motivated by preoccupations with illness, and malingerers, who deliberately feign illness, perhaps consciously seeking secondary gain. Although more women than men engage in these behaviors, both of these groups of patients overuse the health care system, regardless of gender. In European studies, both male and female physicians tended to prescribe more drugs for female than male patients with neck pain and ordered additional diagnostic work for the female patients.[26] The same group also reported that female physicians rated written reports by women as more "accurate, trustworthy, relevant and interesting" than those of male patients.[27] As described elsewhere, catastrophizing and anxiety related to fear of pain are greater in females.[28]

Psychological Factors Gender differences in relation to pain prevention and tolerance have been found in psychopathology, including personality disorders, anxiety, depression, catastrophizing, attentional processes, and maladaptive pain-coping strategies. Catastrophizing is associated with negative cognitive and affective and related psychopathological responses to pain, which include feelings of helplessness, pessimism, magnification, and rumination.[29] Anxiety and depression (as well as other negative emotional states) often accompany pain as the chief complaint and potentially confound evaluation and treatment because they are associated with increased pain severity, particularly among women;[30] "anxiety influences pain perception more in men than women ... findings suggest that pain-related anxiety constructs [including state anxiety], but not trait anxiety, are associated with pain perception ... these constructs are associated with pain intensity ratings in men and pain tolerance levels in women."[31]

Conversely, positive emotions have also been shown to reduce pain perception in the laboratory.[30] Clinical pain, however, is often reported to be more intense or prolonged in depressed patients when focusing ordinarily on nonthreatening internal stimuli; that is, ordinary sensory input such as that associated with normal bodily function would not reach the threshold of awareness in nondepressed individuals but will reach the level of awareness in depressed patients.

Experimental Pain Models of noxious stimulation used to evoke pain include pressure, thermal, mechanical, electrical, and cold pressor stimulation. The magnitude of the sex or gender differences may be a function of the method for inducing pain, including the type of the stimulus, anatomic location and duration of the stimulation, size of the area stimulated, number of stimulus repetitions, and so on.[9,32] Observed differences may also be related to how the pain-rating scales are anchored[33] and whether they are based on rating, ranking, or ratio, raising questions about the reliability and validity of subjective responses of men and women to noxious stimuli. Moreover, there may be gender differences in what is considered the endpoints of a painrating scale such as "most intense pain imaginable" or "most intense pain ever experienced." Similarly, evaluating other "objective" or "involuntary" responses to noxious stimulation revealed that women exhibited significantly lower nociceptive flexion reflex thresholds than men.[34] Differences have also been reported in pain-related facial expressions among newborn infants, with female infants demonstrating more frequent and intense facial expressions of pain during and immediately after venipuncture.[35] Positive mood, pleasant meditation, and relaxation all help to reduce pain sensitivity. In laboratory studies, for example, Marchand and Arsenault found that positive mood-inducing odors reduced pain in women but not men, highlighting the possibility that, not surprisingly, emotional processes play a greater role in the experience of pain among women than men.[36]

Thus, it is reasonable to expect that perceived ethnocultural congruity among the beliefs, attitudes, and behaviors related to the pain of the patient and provider will attenuate the pain experience. These observations undoubtedly support the clinical tenet that the relief provided by many integrative medicine procedures relies in part on this alliance with the patient made possible by the greater amount of time spent with patients. Although placebos are generally positive, there are occasional examples of their facilitating negative nocebo outcomes. Placebo effectiveness appears to be based on several factors, not the least of which are the ethnocultural-based beliefs of the patient that they will work. In fact, some placebo effects appear to be quantitatively dose related,[37] averaging approximately one-third the effectiveness of the active agents, particularly for pain relief.[38] In a surprising number of psychophysiological and even pathophysiological processes, placebos' effectiveness may be observed. Many of these processes involve neurohormonal systems, which in turn are influenced by the ethnocultural differences in beliefs, attitudes, and behaviors. Unfortunately, evidence-based research specific to ethnocultural differences may be difficult to obtain, as noted by Williams.[39]

Although not included as a therapeutic intervention elsewhere in this chapter, acupuncture had been historically used as an ethno-specific method of pain relief. Its original success in the Western world was attributed to the unique techniques of Asian providers most likely caused by a placebo effect. In more recent evidence-based research, however, there has been increasing support for a biological basis for the effectiveness of acupuncture.[40] In fact, there does not appear to be any significant difference in perceived relief of pain among various ethnic groups receiving acupuncture.[41]

There is in fact little in the literature suggesting gender or ethnic differences in the magnitude of placebo analgesia, although there are occasional reports of difference in levels of effectiveness for other than pain problems. For example, Latino patients were found to be more likely to respond to placebo in an antidepressant trial than were patients from other ethnic backgrounds,[42] possibly related to differences in suggestibility.

Gender differences in the use of pain-coping strategies have been found in children, adolescents, and adults.[12,43] In general, whereas boys and men report using more behavioral distraction to manage pain, girls and women rely more on social support and positive self-statements.[44] Women catastrophize about pain more than men, substantiating the observation that catastrophizing may account for many of the differences between genders in reporting of clinical pain.[28]

NEUROPHYSIOLOGIC AND NEUROPHARMACOLOGIC FACTORS

Central Nervous System Processing of Pain In addition to quantitative sensory testing (QST), which repeatedly demonstrates sex and gender differences,[9] neuroimaging research now provides better understanding of the underlying neurophysiologic mechanisms of pain responses. Functional magnetic resonance imaging (fMRI) studies using blood oxygen level–dependent (BOLD) and connectivity techniques identify areas responsible for pain perception in both men and women. In both sexes and genders, whereas BOLD activation occurs in the insula, anterior cingulate cortex, and dorsolateral prefrontal cortex,[45,46] connectivity is found between the periaqueductal gray (PAG) and the prefrontal cortex, insula, and uncus.[47,48]

Consistent with gender-related behavior being a cultural phenomenon, the brain is organized and functions to accommodate the evolutionary-based dichotomous, hunter/gatherer tasks, with the brains of males being primarily interconnected during activation from anterior to cephalocaudal posterior and the female brain with its larger corpus callosum having more interhemispheric connections.[49]

Brain imaging research also indicates sex and gender differences in the affective brain regions associated with emotion in response to pain. Henderson and colleagues[46] found increased midcingulate cortex, cerebellar cortex, and hippocampus activation in women experiencing evoked pain from hypertonic saline injections. Similarly, whereas women had more connectivity between the PAG and midcingulate cortex,[47] men show greater PAG to amygdala connectivity.[48] The medial prefrontal cortex, an area thought to process inner-directed (or contemplative) information, is significantly more activated during electrical stimulation at high pain thresholds in females than in males.[50]

In a recent biopsychological study, men with left-lateralized spinal pain reported greater psychopathology and quality of life factors concerns than women with left- or right-lateralized spinal pain, which together were greater than patients with right-lateralized pain.[51] These differences are congruent with research by Symonds et al., who administered experimental pain stimuli to healthy men and women volunteers while recording fMRI changes, finding that the right hemisphere was more activated in men than women.[52] The findings are also consistent with earlier work of Unruh and Merskey in which depressed patients had more pain on the left than the right side.[53,54]

Analgesic and Anesthetic Mechanisms Opioids are among our most potent analgesic medications, with three opioid receptors—μ, κ, and δ—being significantly implicated in modulating pain in humans and animals. Clinically, the μ opioid receptor is often considered the most relevant receptor because morphine and most other opioid agonists act preferentially at that site. Human experiments consistently show that μ opioid agonists have increased potency in females relative to males.[55] Interestingly, the pharmacokinetics of opioids do not necessarily explain these sex differences in analgesic efficacy, with most studies reporting no sex differences in plasma levels of morphine.[56] In general, females appear to have greater concentrations of opioid receptors, which may partially account for μ opioid agonists being found in some human studies to provide greater analgesia for women.[11] The analgesic effects of opioids appear to operate at the genotype level, with sex differences in the distribution of some of the polymorphisms that impact opioid responses. For example, women who have red hair and fair skin, caused by variants of the human melanocortin-1 receptor (*Mc1r*) gene, demonstrated significantly greater analgesic effect from pentazocine, a κ opioid, than did men or women without these variants. In addition, redheads with a nonfunctional *Mc1r* variant showed greater analgesic response to morphine-6-glucuronide and reduced sensitivity to noxious stimuli.[57] However, there are other reports that larger amounts of some anesthetics are required by redheads.[58]

Neuroendocrine Factors The finding that differences between boys and girls in the experience of pain are minimal before puberty but increase thereafter has led to more detailed examination of hormonal contributions to sex-related variability in pain.[12] Some studies have reported menstrual cycle–related changes in the pain responses in women based on a meta-analysis more than a decade ago that sensitivity to noxious stimuli varied in part as a function of cycle phase, with greater pain sensitivity generally noted in the late luteal phase.[59] In addition, Kuba and Quinones-Jenab found that women reported higher rates of back and head pain at the end of the luteal phase of the menstrual cycle.[60] Several reports have also directly evaluated the effects of hormone administration in women, finding that exogenous estrogen is associated with a significant increase in reports of orofacial pain (e.g., temporomandibular joint disorder) in cycling women receiving oral contraceptives.[12] Although men most likely have as yet unknown cycles, few studies have focused on the relationship between men and pain and gonadal hormones. However, one report of low-dose testosterone administration among men with angina showed an analgesic effect of testosterone.[61]

Related information has become available from the outcome of transgender procedures in which individuals undergoing male-to-female surgery and supportive endocrine manipulation reported increased pain after the procedures, but female-to-male transitions resulted in decreases in pain. In a 2007 study of female-to-male transsexual patients who had chronic pain, more than half showed reduced headache pain with testosterone treatment.[62] In the same study, about one-third of the transsexual male-to-female patients who were given hormone treatment (e.g., estrogen) developed chronic pain.

Because the literature on sex and gender differences in pain and analgesic responses is inconsistent, there is always the potential for idiosyncratic treatments for a variety of pain conditions. Despite the fact that opioids increased the likelihood of hypogonadal states in men and women,[63] they continue to be used for patients with chronic pain. Alternatively, for patients whose symptoms vary as a function of hormonal fluctuations, such as during the menstrual cycle, it may be possible to modify treatments accordingly. Also emerging with some renewed emphasis is the relationship between pain and inflammation, which differs by sex and possibly gender.[64] Thus, health care providers need to be aware of the social context of and gender differences in the pain experience from onset through therapeutic intervention, with recognition of the differences between men and women, including awareness of the subtle cues that may influence patients' perceptions, expectations, and behaviors associated with disparities in pain relief.[65]

RACE, ETHNICITY, AND CULTURE DIFFERENCES

As noted in the introduction, both patients and providers bring their ethnocultural backgrounds, behaviors, experiences, attitudes, and beliefs to the examining room. With the increasing multicultural pool of providers, the need, as noted throughout this chapter, for cultural sensitivity and competence has become more critical for pain management clinicians. Although the terms "race," "ethnicity," and "culture" are frequently used interchangeably, they are conceptually quite different. Whereas "race" distinguishes groups of people according to physical characteristics, biology, or ancestry, "ethnicity" focuses on the distinction among groups of people who share a certain social background, culture and traditions, behaviors, and so on. Although skin color may be a useful distinction, largely for the cosmetic and fashion industry, race is rarely used in scientific research as a biological marker, especially with evidence of more genetic variability within than between racial groups. "Culture" typically refers to behavioral and attitudinal norms, acquired knowledge, beliefs, values, and ideas transmitted and reinforced by members of the group.[66,67] Culture thus shapes many aspects of the experience of pain, including pain expression, expectations, perceptions of the health care system, and resulting health care–seeking behavior.

Pain Sensitivity Differences in physiologic responses such as those associated with expressivity among minority groups have been proposed as an explanatory variable for ethnic differences in response to clinical pain,[68] although this variable is only one among many other contributory factors. To minimize confounding in clinical pain reports, several parameters have been generally agreed upon, such as intensity, duration, health care overutilization, average pain, worst pain, most pain, and utilization in controlled laboratory pain testing both in healthy and diseased individuals, as well as indicators of personality and other psychological disorders, to elucidate the bases of ethnic differences. Indeed, beyond the work of Tursky and Sternbach (referred to later), ethnic differences in self-concept, meaning, and location of pain have been shown to partially account for differences observed in experimental pain responses.[69]

When controlling for location in the United States, differences between African Americans and non-Hispanic whites were noted, with African Americans reporting greater sensitivity or a lower pain threshold and reduced tolerance to a variety of quantitative sensory testing methods using noxious stimuli such as heat, cold pressor, ischemic pain, and electrical stimulation.[70] In addition, greater increased temporal summation of pain and reduced endogenous pain-inhibitory activity have been reported among ethnic minorities compared with non-Hispanic whites.[70] Other ethnic differences in experimental pain include a lower threshold with greater pain unpleasantness among South Asians in the United Kingdom than in white British participants.[71] In a Danish study, capsaicin injection of the forehead in healthy volunteers evoked pain responses resembling migraine, which were greater in South Indian participants than in whites,[72] suggesting ethno-specific patterns of pain sensitivity and behaviors related to the stress of readjustment to geographic translocation.

Self-Report of Pain Ethnic differences in pain reports have been documented for a variety of clinically observed chronic complaints. For example, African Americans report greater HIV–related neuropathic pain than whites, as well as greater pain associated with headache, the orofacial area, myofascial origin, angina pectoris, and arthritis, than whites.[67] Recently, American Indians and Alaska Natives were reported to have a higher prevalence of pain symptoms than the U.S. population in general. In Singapore, the pain severity of older adults of Malaysian descent was less than that of Chinese participants; however, Indian participants reported greater pain severity than both Malay and Chinese participants,[73] possibly related to differences in orofacial morphology. However, the prevalence of temporomandibular disorders in German young women was found to be less than for Chinese women.[74]

Neurophysiologic Factors Although there are undoubtedly ethnocultural differences in sensory motor and autonomic nervous system responses to pain, little consideration has been given to how culturally mediated behavior actually affects the brain. In fact, there is considerable evidence and some speculation that beyond the birth trauma ideas of Otto Rank,[75] early childhood pain even before language skills have developed does negatively impact the developing brain. A prime example is circumcision, which was historically an ethnocultural religious rite of both Muslims and Jews but is now favored predominantly for reasons of hygiene. This early trauma for Jewish neonates and later for Muslim boys has significant permanent effects on the developing hippocampus, amygdala, and other stress-related hormonal responses.[76,77] There is much support for the idea that intensely painful early-life experiences (e.g., circumcision) can sensitize children to pain later in life, with one potential mechanism involving the effects of stress hormones on the brain.[78] Similarly, Anand and Scalzo (2000) proposed that repetitive pain in early life damages developing neurons, leading to changes in pain sensitivity.[79] In support of this hypothesis, Taddio et al. (1995) reported that circumcised infants evinced a greater pain response to vaccinations 4 to 6 months post-circumcision, compared with non-circumcised infants.[80]

Compared with non-Hispanic whites, African Americans have reduced nociceptive flexion reflex (NFR) thresholds.[81] The NFR is an electrophysiological, spinally mediated reflex that is not amenable to voluntary control or subject to response bias. In a novel series of studies, Mechlin and colleagues further examined ethnic differences in pain-related biomarkers,[82-84] finding that stress-induced pain changes in blood pressure, norepinephrine, and cortisol returned to homeostatic levels more rapidly in whites than African Americans. Also documented are significant ethnic differences in levels of oxytocin, a neuropeptide associated with social affiliation that also has been linked to functioning of the endogenous opioid and sympathetic nervous systems. Specifically, lower plasma oxytocin levels were found among African American than white women, and lower oxytocin levels were associated with greater sensitivity to pain.[84,85] These studies thus suggest that endogenous, psychoneurohormonal pain-regulatory systems differ across ethnic groups, with some of these systems functioning less efficiently among African Americans than other ethnic groups.

Another interesting facet of this neurocultural interaction involves the recent revelation of the importance of the mirror neuron system,[86,87] which has been implicated in pain-related cortical plasticity, for example, in the use of mirror box therapy for relief of phantom limb pain.[88] The mirror neuron system may also have a role in ethnocultural differences in the function of the somatic nervous system, including the innervations of the muscles of facial expression. Heretofore cultural transmission of knowledge and behavior was based on principles of variation and selection that underlie biologic evolution, which has now shifted from replicating genes as units of biological information to epigenetic replication of units of cultural information or "memes" as the most likely explanation for intergenerational transmission of simple imitation learning of ethnocultural differences in attitudes, beliefs, and pain-related behaviors.

Examples of other neurocultural connection are experiments using fMRI to measure activity of the medial prefrontal cortex (mPFC); self-reference judgments relative to the subjects' mothers resulted in substantially increased activation in the mPFC among Chinese subjects (i.e., individuals from a more "collectivist" cultural background) compared with non-Asians, who tend to have a more "individualistic" response repertoire.[89] Such observations seem to be consistent with the type of stoicism observed in Chinese and other Asians, in whom responses to physical or psychological pain are mostly private in order not to disturb the welfare of others. Pain is accepted as part of suffering and therefore something to be endured. Asians in general try to deal with their pain quietly to appear strong in the face of adversity.[90]

In a recent report by Kitayama,[91] further details on neurocultural interaction and the role of the mPFC in the differences between the expressive Western and more controlled Asian cultures in response to emotion-provoking stimuli were noted. Related differences were also found in the activities of the temporal parietal junction between self-referent subjects and those more concerned with the perspective of others.[89]

There is also new evidence for neuroplasticity from the changes in patterns of brain activation in response to culturally or occupationally specific tasks, for example, in the amount of gamma waves "typically associated with extremely high mental concentration," such as during meditation by Tibetan monks.

The dopamine D4 receptor gene (*DRD4*), which regulates the "brain's capacity to transmit dopamine signals," has geocultural variants that influence the continuum of cultural differences from risk-seeking to avoidance behavior.[91]

Psychosocial Factors Prominent among the psychosocial factors associated with ethnocultural differences in the experience of pain are family, societal traditions, and religious beliefs related to the meaning of pain and coping strategies. For example, African Americans have been shown to have greater pain severity, depression, and disability with a more emotionally based coping style and pain behaviors than non-Hispanic whites.[5] The psychosocial bases of stoic behavior vary considerably among other cultural groups, as demonstrated in a recent study of cancer pain among American Indians for whom, similar to Asians, privacy as a manifestation of stoicism was preferred.[92]

In contrast to Middle Eastern or Mediterranean cultures in which patients exhibit more expressive responses to pain, Asian stoicism reflects an interdependent reliance on the social support system of family privacy about pain, suffering, and mental illness. For comparison, the coping style of white Anglo-Saxon Protestants ("WASPs") is exemplified by stoic determination: "I'm going to do it myself," that is, pride in independent accomplishments. In contrast, those of African descent stereotypically exhibit a stern coping style of courage in the face of adversity or in response to ritualistic infliction of pain, for example, by scarification. Nonblack Hispanics have often been characterized as manifesting a "macho" toughness in response to environmental and social problems.[93] As an example of how culture is transmitted through generations, almost through "inheritance" of the social environment, Sternbach and Tursky[94,95] and Tursky and colleagues[96] found that Jews and Italians were similar in being stereotypically overly expressive but differed in the meaning and related responses to pain.

The concern of the stereotypically anxious Jewish patients was, "While I am in the hospital, who is minding the store?" but the typical concern of Italian patients was more centered on immediate relief of pain, with many of these behaviors found in the follow-up studies of the next generation. Although Jewish patients wanted to know what the meaning of the pain was, Italians were more interested in dealing with the pain itself.[94-96] To the extent that cultures differ in attribution of the source of pain for religious and other reasons, it is extremely important to consider the influence of locus of control.[97]

Aside from unwitting discrimination by providers, the type and frequency of ethnically diverse coping strategies obviously have a profound influence on disparities in health care. Multiple studies have documented lower rates of participation in health-promoting behaviors such as mammography among African Americans, who, similar to other minorities, appear to fear and mistrust the U.S. health care system.[98] Similarly, clinic-based studies report elevated levels of pain-related catastrophizing among ethnic minorities, with follow-up analyses suggesting that catastrophizing and pain-related distress are major drivers of the expression of pain complaints and pain behaviors.[70]

Provider Factors Ethnic differences in health care disparities are widely documented, with studies reporting that minorities receive inadequate care, including being less likely to receive adequate pain medications, and have longer wait times in emergency departments.[5,99] As pointed out by Mossey,[100] racial and ethnic disparities in pain management certainly exist and may be partly attributable to subliminal stereotypes (e.g., expectations or even anticipations of patient perceptions of pain and related behavior). Although most health care providers possess the necessary knowledge, training, and experience, their lack of adequate time to ensure effective communication with their patients may reduce health literacy, thereby impairing their ability to elicit essential important medical and social information essential for at least adequate if not holistic treatment. Spending preoperative time with patients as a covenant of patient management was originally pointed out by Egbert and colleagues at the Massachusetts General Hospital and revalidated many times since, that when the anesthetist or surgeon explained what he or she was going to do and why to patients, the amount of postoperative analgesics needed was significantly reduced and led to earlier hospital discharge.[101]

Not to be overlooked is that health literacy is a two-way process; particularly with ethnic minorities, the clinician should make every effort to ensure that patients understand what is expected of them for a successful treatment outcome by asking patients to tell the clinician in their own words what they think they have been told to do to relieve their pain and then for the provider to be satisfied that the patient is able and willing to comply (i.e., health self-efficacy, which can be determined psychometrically). Unfortunately, some studies suggest that for ethnic minority patients, medical visits are less patient centered, without much discussion of psychosocial issues, and include fewer rapport-building interactions.[102-104] It may be most important for health care providers, therefore, to pay extra attention to interpersonal interactions in visits with patients of differing ethnic and cultural backgrounds.

As stated by Weisse et al.,[105] "the ability to empathize with the pain of others varies considerably across the ethnocultural groups of both patients and providers, with greater empathy between those of the same skin color and/or those perceived as possessing similar ethnocultural identification"; the greater the empathy, the more likely a satisfactory patient alliance. In addition to being a basis for treating phantom pain,[88] mirror neurons also may have a role in explaining the capacity for empathy.[106]

The occasional exception to this usually positive relationship is when a clinician does not want to be identified as having a minority status by being foreign born or by physical appearance, which would negatively affect his or her career and therefore consciously or unconsciously resist demonstrating empathy for patients of a similar ethnic background. This reactivity can be modulated by racial bias and stereotypes.[107] Further evidence for how these factors influence disparity or who gets treated was recently provided in a multicenter study of pain treatment in an emergency department, where nonwhite physicians were more likely to report a reduction in pain intensity among their patients (regardless of patient race) than white physicians.[108] Although nonwhite physicians ordered the same amount of analgesics as white physicians, they reported a greater reduction in pain intensity than their white counterparts. As another example, when Jewish clinicians treated Jewish and Bedouin women in Israel, where ethnicity had a major influence on the estimates of labor pain,[109] there was no difference in self-assessment. However, ratings of the same two patient groups by the medical staff, almost all of whom were Jewish, revealed that the Bedouin women were perceived to experience less pain than the Jewish women, with no evidence, however, that the Bedouin women received more inferior treatment.

In a series of studies, Cleeland and colleagues found that ethnic minority patients seeking care at community oncology centers often were undertreated for pain relief, being three times more likely to be undermedicated than patients seen in other hospital settings less frequented by minorities.[6,110] Disparity in opioid prescribing for severe pain has also been noted, with non-Hispanic whites more likely to receive pain medications than African American, Hispanic, and Asian patients. Remarkably, this underutilization of opioid analgesics, whether provider prescription or patient requested, among ethnic minority patients has persisted despite evidence from large-scale, national databases that adverse events such as lethal overdose are actually more frequent among white patients than ethnic minorities.[111] Thus, there seems to be little doubt that having an ethnocultural background in common with patients would facilitate treatment outcome and enhance the doctor–patient relationship.

Geoclimatic Factors Given that ethnicity and culture are intrinsically related to geography and climate, the influence of climate on local anesthetic effectiveness was investigated by Giddon and Clark,[112] who found that the duration of soft tissue anesthesia of the orofacial area was shorter in patients treated in relatively warmer than those treated in colder climates. This decrease was believed to be related to thermally induced vasodilation facilitating the removal of the vasoconstrictor component of the anesthetic from the injection site.

Other geocultural differences such as between countries have been observed with local anesthetics administered in a double-blind study to approximately 10,000 patients in the United Kingdom and the United States who received one of three different local dental anesthetics. No difference was found in effectiveness of the three anesthetics. A major difference was found in the reported side effects between the United States and United Kingdom for all agents; that is, for the United States, where a checklist of possible side effects was used, there were 10 times the number of side effects checked off compared with the United Kingdom study, in which an open-ended question asked the patient to answer yes or no to having side effects, and if they had any, to please specify which. It remains to be determined whether the observations were due to the differences in the format of the inquiry used by the United States and the United Kingdom to elicit complains or to more underlying differences, that is, the stereotype of the so-called "stiff upper lip" or stoicism of the U.K. patients, who responded to open-ended questions, compared with the U.S. patients,[113] who responded to a checklist of all possible side effects.

Treatment Decisions Recent research has revealed differences among methods of administration and rates of usage of various analgesic treatments, whether clinician prescribed, administered by health care personnel, or self-administered (patient-controlled analgesia [PCA]). In a Singaporean study, Tan and colleagues[114] found differences in PCA (morphine) usage, with Indians having greater pain severity scores and need for morphine than Chinese and Malay patients when controlling for demographic and operational variables. Anderson et al. found that although African and Hispanic Americans were prescribed fewer analgesics than non-Hispanic white patients, they also reported taking their analgesics less frequently than prescribed, thus limiting their pain relief from analgesics.[6] Some of these differences, however, may be explained by the fact that over the past 3 decades of research, substantial pharmacogenetic differences were found among ethnic groups in the metabolism, clinical effectiveness, and side effect profiles of many drugs.[115]

Health Care System Factors Recent studies have suggested that the health care system itself is responsible in part for treatment disparities. It is unfortunate that despite universal access to care in more socialistic societies,[99] the lower the socioeconomic status (SES), the greater the inequities. In the United States, financial status is inversely related to morbidity and mortality, particularly among ethnic minorities. For example, African Americans and Hispanic Americans have uninsured rates that are double or triple those of non-Hispanic whites.[116] Even when controlling for underlying SES, minority patients remain at risk for inadequate or inappropriate pain relief. Low SES area pharmacies, for example, may be less likely to carry potent analgesics, and access to health insurance benefits may be limited.[5] With the prospect of universal health care, there are still cultural differences in ethical and other behaviors related to seeking care, such as the intentional or unintentional abuse of the health care system.[117] In countries with socialized medicine, such as The Netherlands, some patients with low back pain suspected of being of psychogenic origin may abuse the health care system by their overutilization, often seeking compensation for lost wages during their "illness" or disability.[118]

SUMMARY

In summary, ethnocultural differences in pain perception, verbal and motor behaviors, and management have been described. Unfortunately, despite advances in pain care, minorities remain at greater risk for inadequate pain control. A number of complex interactions among variables have been noted that help to explain these differences in pain perception behaviors and treatment strategies. Moreover, as our society becomes more ethnoculturally diverse, the disparities among groups increase. Although retrospective studies have been very helpful, more prospective studies that take advantage of the large intragroup variability are needed, together with research directed toward elucidating the neurocultural mechanisms underlying these differences. Finally, more attention must be directed to ensure that present and future health care providers obtain or maintain cultural competence and are continually updated on the ever-changing physical and mental health care needs of ethnocultural minorities.

REFERENCES

1. *The Holy Bible, King James Version*. Oxford Edition; 1769.
2. Greenblatt S. *The Swerve: How the World Became Modern*. WW Norton & Company. New York City, NY; 2011.
3. Committee on Advancing Pain Research Care and Education, Board on Health Sciences Policy, Institute of Medicine. A call for cultural transformation of attitudes toward pain and its prevention and management. *J Pain Palliat Care Pharmacother*. 2011;25(4):365-369.
4. Gatchel RJ, Peng YB, Peters ML, et al. The biopsychosocial approach to chronic pain: scientific advances and future directions. *PsyB*. 2007;133(4):581-624.
5. Shavers VL, Bakos A, Sheppard VB. Race, ethnicity, and pain among the U.S. adult population. *J Health Care Poor Underserved*. 2010;21(1):177-220.
6. Anderson KO, Mendoza TR, Valero V, et al. Minority cancer patients and their providers: pain management attitudes and practice. *Cancer*. 2000;88(8):1929-1938.
7. Pardue ML, Wizemann TM, eds. *Exploring the Biological Contributions to Human Health: Does Sex Matter?* Washington, DC: National Academies Press; 2001.
8. Unruh AM. Gender variations in clinical pain experience. *Pain*. 1996;65:123-167.
9. Racine M, Tousignant-Laflamme Y, Kloda LA, et al. A systematic literature review of 10 years of research on sex/gender and experimental pain perception—part 1: are there really differences between women and men? *Pain*. 2012;153(3):602-618.
10. Cornally N, McCarthy G. Help-seeking behaviour for the treatment of chronic pain. *Br J Community Nurs*. 2011;16(2):90-98.
11. Olsen MB, Jacobsen LM, Schistad EI, et al. Pain intensity the first year after lumbar disc herniation is associated with the A118G polymorphism in the opioid receptor mu 1 gene: evidence of a sex and genotype interaction. *J Neurosci*. 2012;32(29):9831-9834.
12. LeResche L. Defining gender disparities in pain management. *Clin Orthop Relat Res*. 2011;469(7):1871-1877.
13. Isacson D, Bingefors K. Epidemiology of analgesic use: a gender perspective. *Eur J Anaesthesiol Suppl*. 2002;26:5-15.
14. Fillingim RB. Sex, gender, and pain: women and men really are different. *Curr Rev Pain*. 2000;4(1):24-30.
15. Ellermeier W, Westphal W. Gender differences in pain ratings and pupil reactions to painful pressure stimuli. *Pain*. 1995;61:435-439.
16. Edwards RR, Sarlani E, Wesselmann U, Fillingim RB. Quantitative assessment of experimental pain perception: multiple domains of clinical relevance. *Pain*. 2005;114(3):315-319.
17. Arendt-Nielsen L, Yarnitsky D. Experimental and clinical applications of quantitative sensory testing applied to skin, muscles and viscera. *J Pain*. 2009;10(6):556-572.
18. Paller CJ, Campbell CM, Edwards RR, Dobs AS. Sex-based differences in pain perception and treatment. *Pain Med*. 2009;10(2):289-299.
19. Kallai I, Barke A, Voss U. The effects of experimenter characteristics on pain reports in women and men. *Pain*. 2004;112(1-2):142-147.
20. Sanford SD, Kersh BC, Thorn BE, et al. Psychosocial mediators of sex differences in pain responsivity. *J Pain*. 2002;3(1):58-64.
21. Robinson ME, Riley JL, III, Myers CD, et al. Gender role expectations of pain: relationship to sex differences in pain. *J Pain*. 2001;2(5):251-257.
22. Alabas OA, Tashani OA, Tabasam G, Johnson MI. Gender role affects experimental pain responses: a systematic review with meta-analysis. *Eur J Pain*. 2012;16(9):1211-1223.
23. Fillingim RB. Complex associations among sex, anxiety and pain. *Pain*. 2013;154(3):332-333.
24. Barsky AJ, Peekna HM, Borus JF. Somatic symptom reporting in women and men. *J Gen Intern Med*. 2001;16(4):266-275.
25. Barsky AJ. *Worried Sick: Our Troubled Quest for Wellness*. 1st ed. Boston: Little, Brown; 1988.

26. Hamberg K, Risberg G, Johansson EE, Westman G. Gender bias in physicians' management of neck pain: a study of the answers in a Swedish national examination. *J Womens Health Gend Based Med.* 2002;11(7):653-666.
27. Johansson EE, Risberg G, Hamberg K, Westman G. Gender bias in female physician assessments. Women considered better suited for qualitative research. *Scand J Prim Health Care.* 2002; 20(2):79-84.
28. Edwards RR, Bingham CO, III, Bathon J, Haythornthwaite JA. Catastrophizing and pain in arthritis, fibromyalgia, and other rheumatic diseases. *Arthritis Rheum.* 2006;55(2):325-332.
29. Edwards RR, Calahan C, Mensing G, et al. Pain, catastrophizing, and depression in the rheumatic diseases. *Nat Rev Rheumatol.* 2011;7(4):216-224.
30. Racine M, Tousignant-Laflamme Y, Kloda LA, et al. A systematic literature review of 10 years of research on sex/gender and pain perception—part 2: do biopsychosocial factors alter pain sensitivity differently in women and men? *Pain.* 2012;153(3):619-635.
31. Thibodeau MA, Welch PG, Katz J, Asmundson GJ. Pain-related anxiety influences pain perception differently in men and women: a quantitative sensory test across thermal pain modalities. *Pain.* 2013;154(3):419-426.
32. Mogil JS, Bailey AL. Sex and gender differences in pain and analgesia. *Prog Brain Res.* 2010;186:141-157.
33. Robinson ME, George SZ, Dannecker EA, et al. Sex differences in pain anchors revisited: further investigation of "most intense" and common pain events. *Eur J Pain.* 2004;8(4):299-305.
34. France CR, Suchowiecki S. A comparison of diffuse noxious inhibitory controls in men and women. *Pain.* 1999;81(1-2):77-84.
35. Guinsburg R, de Araujo PC, Branco de Almeida MF, et al. Differences in pain expression between male and female newborn infants. *Pain.* 2000;85(1-2):127-133.
36. Marchand S, Arsenault P. Odors modulate pain perception: a gender-specific effect. *Physiol Behav.* 2002;76(2):251-256.
37. Nakamura Y, Donaldson GW, Kuhn R, et al. Investigating dose-dependent effects of placebo analgesia: a psychophysiological approach. *Pain.* 2012;153(1):227-237.
38. Benedetti F, Carlino E, Pollo A. How placebos change the patient's brain. *Neuropsychopharmacology.* 2011;36(1):339-354.
39. Williams BA. Perils of evidence-based medicine. *Perspect Biol Med.* 2010;Winter:106-120.
40. Saey TH. Enzyme shot may top acupuncture. *Sci News.* 2012; (June 12):16.
41. LaRiccia PJ, McMurphy S, Gallo JJ, et al. Perceived effectiveness of acupuncture: findings from the National Health Interview Survey. *Medical Acupuncture.* 2008;20(4):239-244.
42. Wagner GJ, Maguen S, Rabkin JG. Ethnic differences in response to fluoxetine in a controlled trial with depressed HIV-positive patients. *Psychiatr Serv.* 1998;49(2):239-240.
43. Unruh AM, Ritchie J, Merskey H. Does gender affect appraisal of pain and pain coping strategies? *Clin J Pain.* 1999;15(1):31-40.
44. Lynch AM, Kashikar-Zuck S, Goldschneider KR, Jones BA. Sex and age differences in coping styles among children with chronic pain. *J Pain Symptom Manage.* 2007;33(2):208-216.
45. Moulton EA, Keaser ML, Gullapalli RP, et al. Sex differences in the cerebral BOLD signal response to painful heat stimuli. *Am J Physiol Regul Integr Comp Physiol.* 2006;291(2):R257-R267.
46. Henderson LA, Gandevia SC, Macefield VG. Gender differences in brain activity evoked by muscle and cutaneous pain: a retrospective study of single-trial fMRI data. *Neuroimage.* 2008;39(4): 1867-1876.
47. Kong J, Tu PC, Zyloney C, Su TP. Intrinsic functional connectivity of the periaqueductal gray, a resting fMRI study. *Behav Brain Res.* 2010;211(2):215-219.
48. Linnman C, Beucke JC, Jensen KB, et al. Sex similarities and differences in pain-related periaqueductal gray connectivity. *Pain.* 2012;153(2):444-454.
49. Ingalhalikar M, Smith AS, Parker DP, et al. Sex differences in the structural connectome of the human brain. *Proc Natl Acad Sci U S A.* 2014;111(2):823-828.
50. Straube T, Schmidt S, Weiss T, et al. Sex differences in brain activation to anticipated and experienced pain in the medial prefrontal cortex. *Hum Brain Mapp.* 2009;30(2):689-698.
51. Wasan AD, Anderson NK, Giddon DB. Differences in pain, psychological symptoms, and gender distribution among patients with left- vs right-sided chronic spinal pain. *Pain Med.* 2010;11(9): 1373-1380.
52. Symonds LL, Gordon NS, Bixby JC, Mande MM. Right-lateralized pain processing in the human cortex: an FMRI study. *J Neurophysiol.* 2006;95(6):3823-3830.
53. Hall W, Hayward L, Chapman CR. On "the lateralization of pain." *Pain.* 1981;10:337-351.
54. Pauli P, Wiedemann G, Nickola M. Pain sensitivity, cerebral laterality, and negative affect. *Pain.* 1999;80(1-2):359-364.
55. Greenspan JD, Craft RM, LeResche L, et al. Studying sex and gender differences in pain and analgesia: a consensus report. *Pain.* 2007;132(Suppl 1):S26-S45.
56. Craft RM, Mogil JS, Aloisi AM. Sex differences in pain and analgesia: the role of gonadal hormones. *Eur J Pain.* 2004;8 (5):397-411.
57. Mogil JS, Ritchie J, Smith SB, et al. Melanocortin-1 receptor gene variants affect pain and mu-opioid analgesia in mice and humans. *J Med Genet.* 2005;42(7):583-587.
58. Liem EB, Lin CM, Suleman MI, et al. Anesthetic requirement is increased in redheads. *Anesthesiology.* 2004;101(2):279-283.
59. Riley JLI, Robinson ME, Wise EA, Price DD. A meta-analytic review of pain perception across the menstrual cycle. *Pain.* 1999;81:225-235.
60. Kuba T, Quinones-Jenab V. The role of female gonadal hormones in behavioral sex differences in persistent and chronic pain: clinical versus preclinical studies. *Brain Res Bull.* 2005;66(3):179-188.
61. English KM, Steeds RP, Jones TH, et al. Low-dose transdermal testosterone therapy improves angina threshold in men with chronic stable angina: a randomized, double-blind, placebo-controlled study. *Circulation.* 2000;102(16):1906-1911.
62. Aloisi AM, Bachiocco V, Costantino A, et al. Cross-sex hormone administration changes pain in transsexual women and men. *Pain.* 2007;132(Suppl 1):S60-S67.
63. Aloisi AM, Aurilio C, Bachiocco V, et al. Endocrine consequences of opioid therapy. *Psychoneuroendocrinol.* 2009;34(Suppl 1): S162-S168.
64. Berkley KJ, Zalcman SS, Simon VR. Sex and gender differences in pain and inflammation: a rapidly maturing field. *Am J Physiol Regul Integr Comp Physiol.* 2006;291(2):R241-R244.
65. Gallagher RM. Gender differences in the affective processing of pain: brain neuroscience and training in "biopsychosocial" pain medicine. *Pain Med.* 2010;11(9):1311-1312.
66. Lasch KE. Culture, pain, and culturally sensitive pain care. *Pain Manag Nurs.* 2000;1(3 Suppl 1):16-22.
67. Green CR, Anderson KO, Baker TA, et al. The unequal burden of pain: confronting racial and ethnic disparities in pain. *Pain Med.* 2003;4(3):277-294.

68. Edwards RR, Doleys DM, Fillingim RB, Lowery D. Ethnic differences in pain tolerance: clinical implications in a chronic pain population. *Psychosom Med.* 2001;63:316-323.
69. Rahim-Williams FB, Riley JL, III, Herrera D, et al. Ethnic identity predicts experimental pain sensitivity in African Americans and Hispanics. *Pain.* 2007;129(1-2):177-184.
70. Rahim-Williams B, Riley JL, III, Williams AK, Fillingim RB. A quantitative review of ethnic group differences in experimental pain response: do biology, psychology, and culture matter? *Pain Med.* 2012;13(4):522-540.
71. Watson PJ, Latif RK, Rowbotham DJ. Ethnic differences in thermal pain responses: a comparison of South Asian and White British healthy males. *Pain.* 2005;118(1-2):194-200.
72. Gazerani P, Arendt-Nielsen L. The impact of ethnic differences in response to capsaicin-induced trigeminal sensitization. *Pain.* 2005;117(1-2):223-229.
73. Chan A, Malhotra C, Do YK, et al. Self reported pain severity among multiethnic older Singaporeans: does adjusting for reporting heterogeneity matter? *Eur J Pain.* 2011;15(10):1094-1099.
74. Wu N, Hirsch C. Temporomandibular disorders in German and Chinese adolescents. *J Orofac Orthop.* 2010;71(3):187-198.
75. Rank O. The trauma of birth in its importance for psychoanalytic therapy. *Psychoanal Rev.* 1924;11:224-241.
76. Boyle GJ, Goldman R, Svoboda JS, Fernandez E. Male circumcision: pain, trauma and psychosexual sequelae. *J Health Psychol.* 2002;7(3):329-343.
77. Boyle GJ, Bensley GA. Adverse sexual and psychological effects of male infant circumcision. *Psychol Rep.* 2001;88(3 Pt 2):1105-1106.
78. Prescott JW. Genital pain vs. genital pleasure: Why the one and not the other? *Truth Seeker.* 1989;1:14-21.
79. Anand KJ, Scalzo FM. Can adverse neonatal experiences alter brain development and subsequent behavior? *Biol Neonate.* 2000;77(2):69-82.
80. Taddio A, Goldbach M, Ipp M, Stevens B, Koren G. Effect of neonatal circumcision on pain responses during vaccination in boys. *Lancet.* 1995;345(8945):291-292.
81. Campbell CM, France CR, Robinson ME, et al. Ethnic differences in the nociceptive flexion reflex (NFR). *Pain.* 2008;134(1-2):91-96.
82. Mechlin B, Heymen S, Edwards CL, Girdler SS. Ethnic differences in cardiovascular-somatosensory interactions and in the central processing of noxious stimuli. *Psychophysiol.* 2011;48(6):762-773.
83. Mechlin B, Morrow AL, Maixner W, Girdler SS. The relationship of allopregnanolone immunoreactivity and HPA-axis measures to experimental pain sensitivity: evidence for ethnic differences. *Pain.* 2007;131(1-2):142-152.
84. Mechlin MB, Maixner W, Light KC, et al. African Americans show alterations in endogenous pain regulatory mechanisms and reduced pain tolerance to experimental pain procedures. *Psychosom Med.* 2005;67(6):948-956.
85. Grewen KM, Light KC, Mechlin B, Girdler SS. Ethnicity is associated with alterations in oxytocin relationships to pain sensitivity in women. *Ethn Health.* 2008;13(3):219-241.
86. Rizzolatti G, Fadiga L, Gallese V, Fogassi L. Premotor cortex and the recognition of motor actions. *Brain Res Cogn Brain Res.* 1996;3(2):131-141.
87. Bonini L, Ferrari PF. Evolution of mirror systems: a simple mechanism for complex cognitive functions. *Ann N Y Acad Sci.* 2011;1225:166-175.
88. Subedi B, Grossberg GT. Phantom limb pain: mechanisms and treatment approaches. *Pain Res Treat.* 2011;2011:864605. doi: 10.1155/2011/864605. Epub 2011 Aug 14.
89. Kitayama S, Uskul AK. Culture, mind, and the brain: current evidence and future directions. In: Fiske ST, Schacter DL, Taylor SE, eds. *Annual Review of Psychology 2011.* Vol. 62. Palo Alto, CA: Annual Reviews; 2011:419-449.
90. Nilchaikovit T, Hill JM, Holland JC. The effects of culture on illness behavior and medical care. Asian and American differences. *Gen Hosp Psychiatry.* 1993;15(1):41-50.
91. Kitayama S. Mapping mindsets: the world of cultural neuroscience. *Observer.* 2013;26(10):21-23.
92. Haozous EA, Knobf MT, Brant JM. Understanding the cancer pain experience in American Indians of the Northern Plains. *Psychooncology.* 2011;20(4):404-410.
93. Torres JB. Masculinity and gender roles among Puerto Rican men: machismo on the U.S. mainland. *Am J Orthopsychiatry.* 1998;68(1):16-26.
94. Sternbach RA, Tursky B. Ethnic differences among housewives in psychophysical and skin potential responses to electric shock. *Psychophysiol.* 1965;1:241-246.
95. Tursky B, Sternbach RA. Further physiological correlates of ethnic differences in responses to shock. *Psychophysiology.* 1967;4(1):67-74.
96. Tursky B, Lodge M, Reeder R. Psychophysical and psychophysiological evaluation of the direction, intensity, and meaning of race-related stimuli. *Psychophysiol.* 1979;16(5):452-462.
97. Logan HL, Baron RS, Keeley K, et al. Desired control and felt control as mediators of stress in a dental setting. *Health Psychol.* 1991;10(5):352-359.
98. Schueler KM, Chu PW, Smith-Bindman R. Factors associated with mammography utilization: a systematic quantitative review of the literature. *J Womens Health (Larchmt).* 2008;17(9):1477-1498.
99. Cintron A, Morrison RS. Pain and ethnicity in the United States: a systematic review. *J Palliat Med.* 2006;9(6):1454-1473.
100. Mossey JM. Defining racial and ethnic disparities in pain management. *Clin Orthop Relat Res.* 2011;469(7):1859-1870.
101. Egbert LD, Battit GE, Welch CE, Bartlett MK. Reduction of postoperative pain by encouragement and instruction of patients. a study of doctor-patient rapport. *N Engl J Med.* 1964;270:825-827.
102. Johnson RL, Roter D, Powe NR, Cooper LA. Patient race/ethnicity and quality of patient-physician communication during medical visits. *Am J Public Health.* 2004;94(12):2084-2090.
103. Cooper LA, Roter DL, Johnson RL, et al. Patient-centered communication, ratings of care, and concordance of patient and physician race. *Ann Intern Med.* 2003;139(11):907-915.
104. Roter DL. Observations on methodological and measurement challenges in the assessment of communication during medical exchanges. *Patient Educ Couns.* 2003;50(1):17-21.
105. Weisse CS, Sorum PC, Sanders KN, Syat BL. Do gender and race affect decisions about pain management? *J Gen Intern Med.* 2001;16(4):211-217.
106. Kaplan JT, Iacoboni M. Getting a grip on other minds: mirror neurons, intention understanding, and cognitive empathy. *Social Neuroscience.* 2006;1(3-4):175-183.
107. Avenanti A, Sirigu A, Aglioti SM. Racial bias reduces empathic sensorimotor resonance with other-race pain. *Curr Biol.* 2010; 20(11):1018-1022.
108. Heins A, Homel P, Safdar B, Todd K. Physician race/ethnicity predicts successful emergency department analgesia. *J Pain.* 2010; 11(7):692-697.
109. Sheiner EK, Sheiner E, Shoham-Vardi I, et al. Ethnic differences influence care giver's estimates of pain during labour. *Pain.* 1999;81(3):299-305.

110. Cleeland CS, Gonin R, Baez L, et al. Pain and treatment of pain in minority patients with cancer. The Eastern Cooperative Oncology Group Minority Outpatient Pain Study. *Ann Intern Med.* 1997;127(9):813-816.

111. Bohnert AS, Valenstein M, Bair MJ, et al. Association between opioid prescribing patterns and opioid overdose-related deaths. *JAMA.* 2011;305(13):1315-1321.

112. Giddon DB, Clark RE. Climatological variables and duration of dental anesthesia [abstract]. *Annual meeting of the International Association of Dental Research.* 1969;47:211.

113. Cowan A. Further clinical evaluation of prilocaine (Citanest), with and without epinephrine. *Oral Surg Oral Med Oral Pathol.* 1968;26(3):304-311.

114. Tan EC, Lim Y, Teo YY, et al. Ethnic differences in pain perception and patient-controlled analgesia usage for postoperative pain. *J Pain.* 2008;9(9):849-855.

115. Burroughs VJ, Maxey RW, Levy RA. Racial and ethnic differences in response to medicines: towards individualized pharmaceutical treatment. *J Natl Med Assoc.* 2002;94(10 Suppl):1-26.

116. DeNavas-Walt C, Proctor BD, Smith JC. *Income, Poverty, and Health Insurance Coverage in the United States: 2009. Current Population Reports (Consumer Income).* Washington, DC: US Census Bureau; 2010.

117. Williams ERL, Guthrie E, Mackway-Jones K, et al. Psychiatric status, somatisation, and health care utilization of frequent attenders at the emergency department: a comparison with routine attenders. *J Psychosom Res.* 2001;50:161-167.

118. van Doorn JW. Low back disability among self-employed dentists, veterinarians, physicians and physical therapists in The Netherlands. A retrospective study over a 13-year period (N = 1,119) and an early intervention program with 1-year follow-up (N = 134). *Acta Orthop Scand Suppl.* 1995;263:1-64.

CHAPTER 17

Psychological Evaluation of Patients for Spinal Cord Stimulator Implantation

R. Joshua Wootton

More than 45 years ago, Shealy and colleagues introduced the concept of spinal cord stimulation (SCS) as a means of electrically inhibiting pain that was consonant with Melzack and Wall's gate-control theory of pain.[1-3] SCS, or neuromodulation, is now a widely used technique that delivers pulsed electrical signals, principally to the dorsal column of the spinal cord, for indications that include failed back surgery syndrome, traumatic nerve injury, postherpetic neuralgia, complex regional pain syndrome, refractory angina pectoris, peripheral vascular disease, neuropathic pain, and visceral pain.[4,5] The technique is minimally invasive and reversible; electrodes can frequently be placed percutaneously under local anesthesia during outpatient surgery; and, unlike more invasive surgical approaches, it does not ablate pain pathways or alter anatomy.[6,7] Although the exact mechanism of action is variously described, it is generally held that pain reduction is achieved by inhibiting the conduction of primary neural pathways through the stimulation of large nerve fibers that override the transmission of smaller nerve fibers more directly involved in pain sensation.[6,8-10]

WHEN SPINAL CORD STIMULATION IS INDICATED

When indicated, SCS is generally a safe means of ameliorating chronic and otherwise poorly tractable pain and, when successful, can reduce patients' dependence on medication—including opioid medication—while returning a fair degree of mobility and quality of life. It is no wonder, then, that the technique has proliferated in recent years to annual estimates in the 10,000 to 20,000 range worldwide for permanent implantation.[4,6,10,11] In general, a trial of SCS is considered successful if the patient reports at least a 50% reduction in pain in the affected area,[12] with initial success rates for achieving this threshold varying widely, from as low as 20% to as high as 80%, depending on the group studied, the particular pain syndrome targeted, the hospital or clinic reporting, and the patient selection criteria used.[4,13,14]

Despite ongoing improvements in the technology of SCS and improved discrimination regarding the diagnoses most likely to respond favorably to the therapy, some studies suggest a significant loss of analgesia in 25% to 50% of patients within 12 to 24 months of implantation.[15-17] Although some of the variation can be attributed to operational factors—lead migration and erosion, electrical complications and malfunctions, and clinical misjudgment[10,18]—an increasing amount of attention has been directed toward psychological variables, especially as these may be revealed and addressed through screening procedures during the patient selection process.[4,6,8,10,11,14,19-22]

There is an ever-accumulating body of evidence that psychosocial variables are among the most predictive factors in the outcome of medical interventions and especially the outcome of invasive procedures, such as spinal surgeries.[23] Given the high variability in long-term treatment outcome for SCS, it certainly makes sense—from the perspectives of patients, providers, health care carriers, and industry—to try to narrow the field as accurately as possible to candidates for implantation who are best suited and most likely to benefit from the therapy. For this reason, many carriers, as well as many providers, independently, require psychological evaluation for their patients before proceeding with a trial of SCS.[4,8]

PSYCHOLOGICAL SELECTION CRITERIA

At the Arnold-Warfield Pain Center at Beth Israel Deaconess Medical Center in Boston, Massachusetts, psychological evaluation of the candidate for spinal cord stimulator implantation involves assessment of the patient across three broad dimensions: (1) will his or her intellectual and cognitive capacity prove an obstacle to mastering the device and its ongoing operation; (2) is the patient motivated to collaborate in the management of his or her own pain; and, (3) is there any psychopathology that may inhibit or impair the patient's postimplant adjustment to the device and its ongoing performance? We will look at the process through which these dimensions are examined in further detail, but, first, some consideration of the development and evolution of psychological selection criteria may prove illuminating.

BACKGROUND OF SELECTION CRITERIA

Shealy, who pioneered electrical neuromodulation for pain management, was also the first to suggest that psychological factors may affect the outcome of a patient's experience.[24] He observed that personality variables appeared to be at least as salient as technical and physiologic issues, where outcome was concerned, and began administering the Minnesota Multiphasic Personality Inventory (MMPI-2) to his patients.[19,20,24] He noted that elevations on the first three clinical scales of the MMPI-2—Hypochondriasis (Hs), Depression (D), and Hysteria (Hy)—are common to many patients with chronic pain and did not appear to dispose them toward a poor outcome but that more florid elevations on additional scales may suggest poor stability. His short list of selection criteria included (1) emotional stability, while recognizing that problems with adjustment are nevertheless understandable among patients with chronic pain; (2) elevation of the depression scale (D) within an appropriate range, indicative of an expectable depressive reaction to the development of chronic pain and subsequent changes in circumstance; and (3) cooperation with a rehabilitation program, suggesting that motivation and collaboration are indicative of emotional stability and maturity.[19,20,24]

Shealy was well aware that most patients with chronic pain are likely to present with symptoms of depression and anxiety, a certain preoccupation with their physical problems and pain, and difficulties adjusting to the consequences of their pain. *From the outset of our application of psychological selection criteria to choosing candidates for neuromodulation, then, it was less a question of who is an ideal fit than who can potentially benefit and how can we prepare them to succeed as well as possible.* Most candidates will exhibit a combination of depression and anxiety, somatic preoccupation, and reactivity to stress. As Doleys has rightly pointed out, psychological factors can be mediators, modulators, or maintainers of pain, and they can certainly vary in magnitude and the extent to which they may complicate a particular patient's pain picture.[19,25,26] The question is this: What is the degree and complexity of the psychopathology? Just as important, can we address and remediate these problems psychotherapeutically, psychopharmacologically, and through other psychologically indicated multidisciplinary interventions?

Approach Through Exclusion Criteria In the years following Shealy's initial suggestion of psychological selection criteria, there was considerable disagreement regarding the utility—in some cases, discussion regarding the complicated ethics—of evaluating patients for neuromodulation based on psychological factors.[20,27] Nelson and colleagues[20] were among the first to propose a functional list of exclusionary screening criteria based on a synthesis of a careful historical review and their own experience of evaluating candidates for spinal cord stimulator implantation. The list, including nine items, may be summarized as follows:

1. Active psychosis
2. Active suicidality
3. Active homicidality
4. Untreated or poorly treated major mood disturbance
5. Somatization disorder or other somatoform disorder
6. Alcohol or other drug dependency, excessive drug-seeking behavior, or uncontrolled escalation of either prescribed or nonprescribed substance use
7. Compensation of litigation resolution, including long-term disability determination, dependent on SCS outcome
8. Lack of appropriate social support
9. Neurobehavioral cognitive deficits sufficient to severely compromise reasoning, judgment, and memory

The first six of these criteria are clearly descriptive of symptoms or clusters of symptoms that would greatly compromise an individual's chances of making a good psychological adjustment postimplant. The seventh suggests that an individual's decisions and even his or her subjective experience—at least, in the short run—may be unduly influenced by considerations of livelihood and economics. The eighth recognizes that even the most self-reliant of patients cannot do everything for themselves postsurgically and may not be the best monitors of their own mood and level of functioning. The ninth simply acknowledges that a sophisticated piece of equipment requires a certain degree of cognitive acuity to operate well and that memory and good judgment are essential components of collaborative health care. Individuals with intellectual limitations, such as patients with dementia, for example, pose special challenges to the successful use of a spinal cord stimulator.

Nelson and colleagues[20] did recommend that information regarding these criteria be obtained through observation, interviews, and psychological testing, with clinicians from appropriate disciplines being involved, and they suggested a flexible approach to integrating and weighting the data to arrive at a particular judgment regarding each candidate's fitness to proceed. The screening criteria, although useful as a starting point, however, were in no way standardized or empirically validated, and no particular weights or scores on any measures were suggested as thresholds.

Approach Through Inclusion Criteria Doleys[19] later took a different approach to assembling a list of screening criteria, outlining 15 characteristics of patients that he believed were associated with positive outcome:

1. General psychological stability
2. Effective defensiveness
3. Moderate levels of self-confidence and self-efficacy
4. Realistic concern regarding illness and proposed therapy
5. Mild depression appropriate to the situation
6. General optimism regarding outcome
7. Ability to cope with flare-ups, complications, and side effects appropriately
8. Appropriately educated regarding the procedure and the device
9. Supportive and educated family
10. History of compliance or cooperation
11. Behavior and symptoms consistent with identifiable pathological condition
12. Behavioral or psychological evaluation consistent with symptoms and reported psychosocial status
13. Comprehension of instruction
14. Appropriate expectation by patient and significant other
15. Ability and willingness to tolerate paresthesias

Doleys acknowledged that, as with Nelson's and others' attempts to identify salient psychological selection criteria to include or exclude candidates from proceeding with SCS implantation, his own efforts represented a general apprehension of what has emerged from clinical observation and research and did not represent a clear, evidence-based attempt to delineate a template for selection. Rather, as with many other researchers in the field, he was attempting to map the terrain of consideration: What exactly are the psychological traits, states, features, and symptoms we need to be thinking about, as we consider candidates for SCS?

Arguably, Doleys was laying down a broad, general set of guidelines, allowing psychiatric clinicians—and, here, we will take this to mean any specially trained and licensed clinician, including psychiatrists, clinical psychologists, clinical social workers, and psychiatric nurse practitioners—to observe, interview, and take a history; possibly integrate the results of a battery of psychological tests and inventories; and develop a set of conclusions and recommendations. Because no clear algorithm for psychological selection has yet emerged[4] and no clear approach to psychological screening has yet to demonstrate consistent efficacy in the selection of candidates for neuromodulation,[10,11,18,21] much is left to the clinical acuity and judgment of the individual psychiatric clinician.

Most of Doleys's inclusion criteria are general enough to allow the psychiatric clinician broad scope in his or her consideration of the patient, and this is likely intended, given that each criterion may encompass a multitude of moderating factors. The suggestion, for example, that a certain degree of depression is expectable, appropriate to the situation of chronic pain, gives the clinician appropriate latitude in the assessment of the candidate's mood. It is certainly accurate to say that moderate to severe depression has been identified in a number of studies as reducing the efficacy of neuromodulation, but mild to moderate depression may also be reactive to pain and not a significant factor in a patient's premorbid personality. Additionally, it would be unusual to encounter an individual who does not react with some degree of depressive symptomatology, given the onset of chronic pain and accompanying deterioration in circumstances in his or her life.[4,10,11]

Other criteria, such as realistic concern, general optimism, and ability to cope with complications, require not only that the psychiatric clinician be able to establish a good working alliance and rapport with the candidate in a comparatively brief time but also to be able to draw complicated inferences and make reasonably complex judgments about individuals with a fairly small sampling of data—usually no more than 1 or 2 hours, divided between direct contact with the patient and review of his or her chart and medical records. When you add to this mix the expectation that the clinician will also assess the patient's ideas with regard to outcome, his or her comprehension of the educational materials, the degree to which he or she has adequate psychosocial support from family and other sources, and whether he or she has a history of having been a cooperative and collaborative participant in his or her own care, suddenly the bar has indeed risen to a remarkable height for any psychological evaluation.

PSYCHOLOGICAL ASSESSMENT OF CANDIDATES

Reviewing the literature of the psychological assessment of candidates for SCS, two points become clear: Neither the absence of a precise empirically derived template for psychological screening nor the difficulty of the task should dissuade or discourage those involved in the process from the importance of attempting to gauge the influence of psychological factors in the success of the procedure. Quite apart from research considerations, physicians owe it to their patients to propose and plan treatments that will meet with a reasonable likelihood of success, which includes the patient's ability to adjust well psychologically to benefit from the intervention in both the short and long terms.

In some research settings, patients may undergo several hours of interviews, take an extensive battery of psychological tests and inventories, and be reviewed in one or more multidisciplinary rounds before being accepted for the study.[10,11] In most private medical settings and even hospital clinics, where research is not being conducted, the reality of the situation is closer to this: On occasions when a mental health professional is involved at all in the preparation or vetting of candidates for neuromodulation, the evaluation is usually limited to an hour of clinical contact and perhaps one or two brief scales or instruments presented to the patient for self-administration.

Most psychiatric clinicians in the setting of pain clinics and centers do not have the benefit of having the results of an MMPI-2, let alone a battery of screening instruments for psychopathology, or more than perhaps one or two brief screening tools or scales for the assessment of functioning or coping—not the least reason being that seeking reimbursement for these measures is frequently an arduous and convoluted process. In many cases, the psychiatric consultant may actually be an outside provider who may have only limited exposure to patients in the setting of chronic pain, much less the specialized situation of implantable devices. Psychiatric clinicians are nevertheless expected to comment and render clinical judgments regarding the patient's ability to benefit from and adjust in the short and longer term to a highly sophisticated and expensive piece of implantable hardware.

It is frankly rare that, by the time a candidate is actually referred to us—usually after a number of encounters in the medical setting—we reach an unequivocal conclusion that he or she is *not* appropriate, and this usually occurs only when the level of psychopathology is quite severe or the patient is manifestly uncooperative or combative or has expressed such unrealistic ideas about outcome that one wonders why he or she was referred in the first place. Even so, although the second of these is frequently a pernicious and difficult problem to address, the first and third can sometimes be successfully remediated over time and with concerted multidisciplinary efforts.

The Clinical Interview and Anamnesis The point of a psychiatric clinician's taking a history—*anamnesis*—and performing a clinical interview with candidates for neuromodulation is to gather as much information as expediently as possible in an attempt to discern whether psychological risk factors may prove influential in the patient's successful adjustment to the intervention. There are no standardized or structured interviews tailored to this task, but a general psychiatric interview, specifically directed to the situation of chronic pain, can provide a basic foundation for the psychological evaluation. One example of this may be seen in **Table 17-1**.[28]

As Nelson, Doleys, and others have suggested,[4,19,20] the more specific situation of evaluating a patient's candidacy for spinal cord stimulator implantation will necessarily involve additional questions regarding more pertinent and specialized risk factors. At the Arnold-Warfield Pain Center, we endeavor to assess the following criteria, as well, in our evaluation of candidates for neuromodulation:

- *Motivation:* Is the patient motivated to learn about the procedure? Has he or she reviewed the educational materials and developed appropriate questions? Is he or she compliant and collaborative with medical directives?
- *Readiness for change:* Has the patient reached the preparation and action stages of the transtheoretical model[29,30] in which he or she is capable of collaborating with providers and motivated to contribute toward the development and execution of a plan of managing his or her pain?
- *Cognitive and intellectual capacity:* Does the patient possess the capacity to operate the unit effectively?
- *Adequate psychosocial support:* Has the patient involved family, friends, or other social resources in his or her preparation for the procedure, as well as his or her ongoing pain management?
- *Level of psychological adjustment:* Is the patient reasonably or sufficiently well-adjusted, such that any psychiatric symptomatology is not likely to pose an inordinate complication or jeopardize the functioning of the spinal cord stimulator?
- *History of substance abuse:* Is there a history of substance abuse involving either prescription or illicit substances that may complicate the patient's short- or long-term adjustment to the procedure?
- *Level of stress-reactivity:* Is the patient able to manage stress reasonably well, including unexpected complications? Does he or she exhibit tendencies toward somatization, and how well have these been managed historically?
- *History of trauma:* Is there a history of trauma that may complicate the patient's short- or long-term response to an invasive procedure?
- *Grounded etiology (meaning) and presentation of pain:* Does the patient's pain make sense to him or her, as well as to his or her providers? Is there an identifiable and understandable pathological condition, consonant with the patient's personal philosophy or cosmology?
- *Reasonable expectations regarding outcome:* Has the patient developed a reasonable and realistic set of expectations with regard to how the stimulator will perform and what sort of improvement in quality of life he or she can expect?

Depending on the degree of severity or level of complication, a positive response or red flag on any one of these criteria may result in removing a candidate from consideration of spinal cord stimulator implantation, but it is also the case that expressed concerns even on multiple criteria may not result in permanent rejection of a patient's candidacy, depending on whether the risks and difficulties revealed during the interview and *anamnesis* can be addressed educationally, psychotherapeutically, or by other therapeutic means. This is not always immediately easy to discern, of course, and the revelation of initial concerns may lead to an extended evaluation and even a course of treatment before eventual approval for the procedure.

Psychological Testing Although the clinical interview and *anamnesis* are indispensable features of the psychological evaluation, developing prognostic impressions and a treatment plan based solely on the encounter with the patient and his or her verbal self-report can prove limiting and even misleading. Even in casual conversation, people are likely to forget, editorialize, distort, and defensively censor themselves, whether consciously or unconsciously, and the situation of the clinical interview, with its attendant stress, is no exception.[31] Patients who wish to appear socially conventional, for example, will likely downplay any feelings or symptoms of depression or anxiety they may have while emphasizing and even amplifying their experience and symptoms of pain.[32] Although it is not feasible to test the veracity of every statement, it is nevertheless possible to arrive at an accurate appreciation of an individual patient's experience and level of psychological adjustment by comparing data gathered by other providers, reviewing available records, interviewing family members when appropriate, and administering one or more psychometric instruments.[31]

TABLE 17-1 A Concise Guide to a Psychosocially Based Clinical Pain Interview

Presenting Pain Complaint. What are the origin, nature, and duration of the pain? What previous attempts have been made at treating the pain? Are there current medications and ongoing treatments and therapies? What exacerbates and what tends to relieve the pain? What are the patient's beliefs about his or her pain, including why it continues? Why does the patient come for treatment, here and now, and with what expectations?
Current Level of Functioning. How has the pain changed the patient's life, including changes of status at work, socially, and within the family? What is the patient's current level of activity? Does he or she need assistance with activities of daily living, such as bathing, dressing, and household chores? Has his or her pain interfered with sexual intimacy? Has the patient had to give up activities, pastimes, and recreational pursuits?
Current Identifiable Stressors. What related and unrelated problems, worries, anxieties, and conflicts is the patient aware of, including stressors at work and at home? Has the patient's financial status or ability to provide for his or her family been affected? Has he or she applied for worker's compensation or disability, and, if so, what has the process been like? Has litigation been considered or undertaken around the original source of injury?
Medical History. Has the patient experienced previous episodes of chronic pain, work-related injuries, or extended illnesses? Are there concurrent or previous unrelated medical problems? Is the patient taking medications for any other symptoms or problems? Does he or she have any surgical history or history of hospital admissions for other reasons? Who is his or her primary care physician and for how long? Does the patient exercise or take any over-the-counter remedies, vitamins, or homeopathic or herbal remedies? How does the patient describe his or her diet, eating behaviors, and attitudes toward nutrition? Is there a family history of significant illness or chronic pain?
Psychiatric History. Has the patient ever consulted with a psychologist, psychiatrist, or psychotherapist, and is he or she currently in any form of psychiatric treatment? Has he or she ever taken psychotropic medications or been admitted to a psychiatric facility or hospital for any reason? Are there psychological symptoms or problems for which he or she would now like consultation or treatment (e.g., family or marital conflicts, sleep disturbance, anxiety, or depression)? Is there any family psychiatric history?
Substance Abuse History. Has the patient ever been treated for substance abuse or been referred to a detox or 12-step program? Does he or she have any experience with "recreational" substances, other than alcohol? Have substances, including alcohol, ever proved to be a problem or to cause problems in his or her work or social life? What is his or her current level of consumption of alcohol, caffeine, and nicotine? Is he or she aware of the effects of stimulants and depressants on his or her body and mental status? Has the patient ever had problems modulating the use of prescribed medications, especially opioids and anxiolytics? Is there any family history of substance abuse?
Developmental and Social History. Where was the patient raised, and what were his or her family's circumstances? How would he or she characterize his or her childhood and adolescence, schooling, and relationships with parents and siblings? Has the patient suffered important losses through death, estrangement, or loss of contact? Is there a history of emotional, physical, or sexual abuse? Is there a history of other emotional or physical trauma? What is the patient's significant relational history, including his or her relationships with his or her spouse and children? What is his or her sexual history, and how would he or she characterize his or her current sexual relationship? What is the parents' education and work history; military and legal history? What are his or her interests and pursuits outside of work? Does he or she have a network of friends and social supports? To whom does the patient turn when he or she needs to discuss problems, needs a favor, or has to ask for help?
Mental Status Examination. Questions included in this section are meant to enhance and systematize the clinician's observations about the patient's appearance, attitude, and behaviors, especially the presence or absence of pain behaviors, as well as his or her affect, mood, speech, perception, quality of thinking and reality testing, judgment, and cognitive and intellectual functioning. It also may be helpful to ask about the effects of chronic pain on his or her mental status. Has he or she ever felt suicidal or felt moved to violence because of the pain? How does the pain affect his or her mood, and what was it like before the onset of pain? How has the patient's medication regimen affected his or her mental status? How has the burden of treatment affected his or her mental status?
Psychological Testing. If the results of psychological testing are available, it is often helpful to review them, in brief, with the patient. When the results are at variance with the patient's interview, it is frequently a good idea to point this out and to see what sense the patient is able to make of it. Patients sometimes deny feeling depressed during the interview, for example, but may have indicated considerable mood and neurovegetative disturbance on the Beck Depression Inventory or the Minnesota Multiphasic Personality Inventory.
Patient's Questions and Goals for Treatment. Is there anything the patient has not talked about that he or she believes is important for the interviewer to know? Does he or she come today with specific expectations or questions about what can be done for his or her pain? Does the patient think that the physician who referred him or her had any specific recommendations in mind? Is he or she open to learning new ways of managing his or her pain, apart from procedures and medications? Does the patient feel that he or she has a role in helping to control his or her pain? What are the patient's goals for treatment, and how does he or she envision the next month of treatment? The next 6 months?

Adapted from Wootton RJ. Psychological evaluation of chronic pain. In: Warfield CA, Fausett HJ, eds. *Manual of Pain Management, 2nd ed.* Philadelphia: Lippincott Williams & Wilkins;2002;25–31(p.28).

Cross-validating the information obtained during the clinical interview becomes an essential step toward understanding the patient and evaluating his or her candidacy for implantation. The point is not to catch patients in the act of consciously or unconsciously misleading their providers but to gain as accurate an assessment as possible of the likelihood that a particular patient will make a successful psychological adjustment postsurgically to the implantable device.[31] The addition of psychological testing elicits one more sampling of the patient's behavior for consideration, and patients frequently do react differently to the situation of completing a questionnaire or inventory than they do to questions put to them directly in an interview. Also, because the methods of test construction sometimes obscure the intention of certain questions, the point or interpretation of any particular item or trend is not always immediately discernible, sometimes resulting in a less defensive response.

Although there are no standardized psychometric instruments designed specifically to assess a patient's candidacy for spinal cord stimulator implantation, and no psychological test or battery of tests has been shown to predict outcome reliably,[33] there are many instruments designed to assess various dimensions of psychological adjustment, coping and beliefs about pain, pain intensity, and functional capacity. A wide variety of these are reviewed in Chapter 15: Psychosocial Assessment of Chronic Pain, by Borkum and Wootton; but the cost and time involved in extensive testing makes the careful selection of instruments of critical importance. As previously mentioned, many psychiatric clinicians are unable to integrate more than one or two brief questionnaires into their evaluations, factoring in the constraints of time, the limitations placed on billing by health care carriers, and the availability of clinical training in the scoring and interpretation of more empirically developed tests such as the MMPI-2.

Doleys suggests a battery of four tests, including the McGill Pain Questionnaire (MPQ), Beck Depression Inventory (BDI), MMPI-2, and Oswestry Disability Index (ODI),[33] reporting a typical cost of $500 for administration and interpretation and a time commitment for the patient of between 3 and 4 hours. Each of these tests has pencil-and-paper, as well as computer versions, and each comes with easy instructions in a self-administration format. The MPQ is a measure of quality and intensity of pain; the BDI, of mood; the MMPI-2, of personality and psychological adjustment; and the ODI, of disability and functional capacity. Taken together, they offer excellent amplification of many of the criteria for evaluating candidates for neuromodulation, and, when the results are available before the clinical interview, they tend to ensure that inconsistencies in presentation, whether conscious or unconscious, come to light and can be explored. When a patient states during the interview, for example, that he or she is "not very depressed" but scores in the severely depressed range on the BDI, this is an inconsistency worth investigating and reconciling before proceeding.

FUNCTIONAL SUMMARY

What it means to administer a psychological evaluation directed toward clearing or approving a patient for spinal cord stimulator implantation remains poorly defined, but at this stage in the evolution of the technology, there is no disagreement in the mainstream literature that psychological screening is important.[10,11,18,19,21] The existence of so many approaches to defining a functional set of selection criteria, as well as such a broad array of psychometrics applied to the task, is compelling evidence of the complexity of the problem. The intervention of an implantable spinal cord stimulator is technologically elegant in its simplicity but also potentially complicated in its psychological impact on the patient, and, as previously stated, it makes sense to try to narrow the field as accurately as possible to candidates for implantation who are best suited and most likely to benefit from the therapy.

At the Arnold-Warfield Pain Center, we find that patients typically fall into three broad categories: (1) those who present with psychological resources and a sustained level of reasonable adjustment sufficient to ensure the likelihood of a good response; (2) those who possess some resources but also one or more risk factors of concern, who may nevertheless respond to therapeutic remediation, eventually increasing their chances of responding favorably; and (3) those who reflect risk factors so numerous or so severe that they cannot be considered appropriate candidates for the procedure.

Written evaluations, in the first case, typically conclude in this manner:

> *Where the patient's candidacy for spinal cord stimulator implantation is concerned, he had reviewed the educational materials we provided, asked insightful questions, and demonstrated a good understanding of the device and procedure. He exhibited no significant risk factors to successful postimplant psychological adjustment, and he appears to have developed a reasonable set of expectations with regard to outcome.*
>
> *At this time, we see no psychological contraindication to proceeding with a trial phase of neuromodulation.*

A written evaluation, in the second case, might conclude in this manner:

> *Where the patient's candidacy for spinal cord stimulator implantation is concerned, she had reviewed the educational materials we provided and demonstrated a good understanding of the device and procedure.*
>
> *She has struggled with severe depression in the past year, as well as the modulation of her prescription medications. To her credit, she has sought treatment on her own and is currently in psychotherapy and psychopharmacological management. She is also back on track where her medication management is concerned. The patient has given me permission to contact her outside psychiatric providers to coordinate care, and she has agreed to participate in a brief, structured program of cognitive-behavioral therapy with the goal of improved impulse control and mood management.*
>
> *We have agreed to reassess her candidacy for neuromodulation after another 3 to 6 months of comprehensive care.*

A written evaluation, in the third case, might conclude as follows:

> *Where the patient's candidacy for spinal cord stimulator implantation is concerned, he showed little motivation to learn about the procedure and, in fact, had not reviewed the educational materials we had provided. When asked why he had not read the instruction booklet, he replied, "I don't care how it works. I just want to be fixed."*
>
> *When we discussed his psychiatric history, a similar trend emerged, as he disclosed that he frequently switches providers and medications, always seeking a psychotherapist who will "make me feel better faster" or "a pill that will take the pain away."*
>
> *I did let the patient know that, despite his expectations, no one in my experience achieves complete pain relief with a stimulator and that, more usually, the expectation is 50% relief and sometimes, less. It was at this point that we concluded together: neuromodulation is not a good option for him.*

In this last case, unreasonable expectations regarding outcome—supported by a problematic personality disorder—represented a sufficient reason to stop the process. The patient was simply unmotivated to collaborate in his own care and in the management of his own pain. Other reasons, as previously mentioned, that might potentially rule out a patient would include chronic and poorly tractable mental disorder or substance abuse or dependence—any psychopathology that might inhibit or impair the patient's postimplant adjustment to the device and its ongoing performance—and dementia, mental retardation, or other problems with cognitive impairment. Even with the last of these, however, there are exceptions, with reported cases of family members ably assisting dementing and cognitively compromised patients in the successful and effective use of stimulators.

So complicated is the relationship between the patient in chronic pain and the implantable device that many researchers are now advocating improving the chances of successful postsurgical adjustment to the stimulator with a recommended preimplant course of cognitive-behavioral and psychoeducational treatment, as well as, in some cases, postimplant courses of supportive psychotherapy and psychoeducation.[21,22,34] Given that we have little empirical definition of how exactly to decide who is the best candidate, as the technology of spinal cord stimulators continues to advance, ongoing support for patients who opt for neuromodulation may prove the best way to insure the efficacy of our evaluations.

REFERENCES

1. Shealy CN, Mortimer JT, Reswick JB. Electrical inhibition of pain by stimulation of the dorsal columns: preliminary report. *Anesth Analg*. 1967;46:489-491.
2. Shealy CN, Taslitz N, Mortimer JT, Becker DP. Electrical inhibition of pain: experimental evaluation. *Anesth Analg*. 1967;46:299-305.
3. Melzack R, Wall PD. Pain mechanisms: a new theory. *Science*. 1965;150:971-979.
4. Campbell CM, Jamison RN, Edwards RR. Psychological screening/phenotyping as predictors for spinal cord stimulation. *Curr Pain Headache Rep*. 2013;17:307.
5. Guttman OT, Hammer A, Korsharsky B. Spinal cord stimulation as a novel approach to the treatment of refractory neuropathic mediastinal pain. *Pain Pract*. 2009;9:308-311.
6. Atkinson L, Sundaraj SR, Brooker C, et al. Recommendations for patient selection in spinal cord stimulation. *J Clin Neurosci*. 2011;18:1295-1302.
7. North R, Shipley J, Prager J, et al. Practice parameters for the use of spinal cord stimulation in the treatment of chronic neuropathic pain. *Pain Med*. 2007;8(Suppl):S200-S275.
8. Deer T, Masone RJ. Selection of spinal cord stimulation candidates for the treatment of chronic pain. *Pain Med*. 2008;9(Suppl):S82-S92.
9. North RB, Linderoth B. Spinal cord stimulation. In: Fishman SM, Ballantyne JC, Rathmell JP, eds. *Bonica's Management of Pain*. 4th ed. Philadelphia: Kluwer: Lippincott Williams & Wilkins; 2010:1379-1392.

10. Sparkes E, Raphael JH, Duarte RV, et al. A systematic literature review of psychological characteristics as determinants of outcome for spinal cord stimulation therapy. *Pain*. 2010;150:284-289.
11. Celestin J, Edwards RR, Jamison RN. Pretreatment psychosocial variable as predictors of outcomes following lumbar surgery and spinal cord stimulation: a systematic review and literature synthesis. *Pain Med*. 2009;10:639-653.
12. Burton AW, Phan PC. Spinal cord stimulation for pain management. In: Dilorenzo DJ, Bronzino JD, eds. *Neuroengineering*. Boca Raton, FL: CRC Press; 2008:7:1-16.
13. Kemler MA, Barendse GA, van Kleef M, et al. Spinal cord stimulation in patients with chronic reflex sympathetic dystrophy. *N Engl J Med*. 2000;343:618-624.
14. Monsalve V, de Andres JA, Valia JC. Application of a psychological decision algorithm for the selection of patients susceptible to implantation of neuromodulation systems for the treatment of chronic pain: a protocol. *Neuromodulation*. 2000;4:191-200.
15. Cameron T. Safety and efficacy of spinal cord stimulation for the treatment of chronic pain: 20-year literature review. *J Neurosurg*. 2004;100(3 Suppl):254-267.
16. May MS, Banks C, Thompson SJ. A retrospective, long-term, third-party follow-up of patients considered for spinal cord stimulation. *Neuromodulation*. 2002;5:137-144.
17. Taylor RS, Van Buyten JP, Buchser E. Spinal cord stimulation for chronic back and leg pain and failed back surgery syndrome: a systematic review and analysis of prognostic factors. *Spine*. 2005;30:152-160.
18. Beltrutti D, Lambert A, Barolat G, et al. Expert panel report: the psychological assessment of candidates for spinal cord stimulation for chronic pain management. *Pain Pract*. 2004;4:204-221.
19. Doleys DM. Psychological factors in spinal cord stimulation therapy: brief review and discussion. *Neurosurg Focus*. 2006;21:E1-E6.
20. Nelson DV, Kennington M, Novy DM, et al. Psychological selection criteria for implantable spinal cord stimulators. *Pain Forum*. 1996;5:93-103.
21. Sparkes E, Duarte RV, Raphael JH, et al. Qualitative exploration of psychological factors associated with spinal cord stimulation outcome. *Chronic Illn*. 2012;8:239-251.
22. Van Dorsten B. Psychological considerations for preparing patients for implantation procedures. *Pain Med*. 2006;7:S47-S57.
23. Bruns D, Disorbia JM. Assessment of biopsychosocial risk factors for medical treatment: a collaborative approach. *J Clin Psychol Med Settings*. 2009;16:127-147.
24. Shealy CN. Dorsal column stimulation: optimization of application. *Surg Neurol*. 1975;4:142-145.
25. Doleys DM. Psychological assessment for implantable therapies. *Pain Digest*. 2000;10:16-23.
26. Doleys DM. Preparing patients for implantable technology. In: Turk DR, Gatchel R, eds. *Psychological Aspects of Pain Management*. New York: Guilford Press; 2002:334-347.
27. Taylor ML. Ethical issues for psychologists in pain management. *Pain Med*. 2001;2:147-154.
28. Wootton RJ. Psychological evaluation of chronic pain. In: Warfield CA, Fausett HJ, eds. *Manual of Pain Management*. 2nd ed. Philadelphia: Lippincott Williams & Wilkins; 2002:25-31.
29. Jensen MP, Nielsen WR, Kerns RD. Toward the development of a motivational model of pain self-management. *J Pain*. 2003;4:477-492.
30. Prochaska JO. Transtheoretical model of behavior change. In: Gellman MD, Turner JR, eds. *Encyclopedia of Behavioral Medicine*. New York: Springer; 2013:1997-2000.
31. Wootton RJ. Psychosocial assessment of chronic pain. In: Warfield CA, Bajwa ZH, eds. *Principles and Practice of Pain Medicine, 2nd ed*. New York: McGraw-Hill; 2004;148-156.
32. Deshields TL, Tait RC, Gfeller JD, et al. Relationship between social desirability and self-report in chronic pain patients. *Clin J Pain*. 1995;11:189-193.
33. Doleys DM. Psychological issues and evaluation for patients undergoing implantable technology. In: Krames ES, Peckham PH, Rezai AR, eds. *Neuromodulation*. London: Elsevier; 2009:69-80.
34. Molloy AR, Nicholas MK, Asghari A, et al. Does a combination of intensive cognitive-behavioral pain management and a spinal cord implantable device confer any advantage? A preliminary examination. *Pain Practice*. 2006;6:96-103.

CHAPTER 18 The Placebo Effect in the Clinical Setting: Considerations for the Pain Practitioner

Chantal Berna Renella
Sean R. Zion
John M. Kelley

"The desire to take medicine is perhaps the greatest feature which distinguishes man from animals."
—Sir William Osler

BACKGROUND

Henry Beecher's classic 1955 study "The Powerful Placebo" first attracted attention to the therapeutic effectiveness of placebo treatments in different painful conditions.[1] Although the impressive effect size he attributed to the placebo effect was subsequently questioned given a lack of controls for natural history and regression to the mean, his article initiated a paradigm shift and opened up a new field of research. Further groundbreaking work demonstrated that placebo analgesia could be blocked by naloxone, which implied that endorphins were involved in this context.[2] This work opened the path to a progressively greater understanding of what is now considered *a psychobiological phenomenon*. This chapter aims to review briefly the current knowledge of the psychology and neurophysiology underlying the placebo effect and then to focus on three main questions: (1) why the placebo effect is important in the practice of pain management; (2) what ethical considerations are raised by the clinical use of the placebo effect; and (3) how best to use the placebo effect for therapeutic purposes.

The term *placebo* is derived from the Latin for "I shall please" and originates from its use as an intervention aimed primarily at pleasing, rather than treating, the patient. Today, the word *placebo* is used in multiple contexts to refer to different but related concepts. Consequently, it has been extremely difficult for researchers to reach consensus on terminology in placebo studies, with even the term "the placebo effect" being raised as problematic (i.e., the placebo effect is the effect of something that has no effect). In this chapter, specific definitions are proposed and used (Box 18-1).

PSYCHOLOGICAL MECHANISMS

Placebo effects are recruited through different mechanisms, which can essentially be grouped into two categories: (1) creating positive expectations and (2) learning through classical conditioning is an important form.[3,4] These processes are detailed below. However, it should be emphasized that the placebo effect is often elicited by a combination of the two mechanisms, and disentangling them has been a topic of debate.[5] Considerable evidence suggests that conditioning

BOX 18-1

Key Terms

Placebo Treatment

- "Pure placebo treatments" are inert substances (e.g., sugar pills or saline injections) or inactive physical interventions (e.g., sham surgical procedures or sham acupuncture).
- "Impure placebo treatments" are active substances that do not provide any known benefit for the condition being treated (e.g., vitamin C for pain).

Placebo treatments can be used for two purposes:

1. To control for an active treatment in a randomized clinical trial
2. To elicit a physiological response known as the placebo effect

Placebo and Nocebo Effects

Positive or negative effects after administration of a placebo treatment that are independent of the natural course of the disorder.

- Placebo effect ⟶ Improvement of the disorder
- Nocebo effect ⟶ Worsening of the disorder or negative side effects

Placebo Analgesia

Decrease in pain after placebo treatment

Nonspecific Treatment Effects or Placebo-Related Effects

- Effects elicited by an active treatment that are not attributable to the pharmacologic or physiological properties of a drug or intervention nor to the natural course of the disorder.
- They are also referred to as "placebo-related effects" because these effects meet the criteria for a placebo effect but without the involvement of an actual placebo.
- Placebo arms in clinical trials are meant to control for nonspecific treatment effects. However, in the clinical setting, the goal is to enhance these effects (see Box 18-2).

procedures lead to more robust placebo analgesia than verbally induced expectancy.[6,7] Yet it is almost impossible to condition a human being without some manipulation of expectations.[8,9] In fact, it has been suggested the two processes could lead to a "virtuous cycle": a patient who experiences a positive first encounter has increased expectations of therapeutic benefit, which leads to enhanced conditioning effects associated with treatment and subsequent heightened overall placebo effect.[3]

EXPECTATIONS

Expectancy theory is based on the notion that the expectation of a positive outcome may elicit certain cognitive, emotional, and behavioral changes that increase the likelihood of that outcome occurring.[10,11] Positive expectations in the context of the therapeutic encounter may lead to a reduction in anxiety,[12] a decrease in self-defeating thoughts,[5] or the resumption of a normal daily schedule.[13] In fact, when expecting a painful stimulation, the brain shows patterns of activity in areas relevant to pain inhibition, such as the anterior cingulate cortex (ACC) and brainstem.[14,15] Furthermore, when participants in an experimental pain task are told to expect a higher or a lower painful stimulus, not only does this lead to increased or decreased reports of pain for stimuli that are actually of identical intensity, but it also elicits corresponding changes in the intensity of cerebral activity in areas relevant to pain perception.[16,17] Hence, the degree to which a patient expects a procedure to be painful can have an important impact on the actual perception of pain.[18] Finally, expectations about treatment benefits can also alter the experience of a given stimulus in patient populations.[19]

Expectations regarding a particular treatment may exist prior to the initial contact with a health care provider (e.g., expectancy induced by past experience, advertisement, media, social interaction). These expectations can then be modified by a health care provider through information; suggestions; and other forms of communication, including nonverbal cues.[20]

LEARNING

Classical conditioning is an important form of implicit learning in which an initially *neutral stimulus* is repeatedly paired with a biologically active stimulus (the *unconditioned stimulus*), which reliably elicits a response. After repeating pairings of the two stimuli, when the initially neutral stimulus is presented alone, it evokes a response (the *conditioned response*) by itself. At this point, the originally neutral stimulus is now referred to as a *conditioned stimulus*. For example, morphine is an unconditioned stimulus that reliably elicits analgesia (the unconditioned response). If morphine is repeatedly delivered via a blue pill (the neutral stimulus), eventually a blue pill containing no morphine (the conditioned stimulus) will elicit an analgesic effect (the conditioned response). In clinical settings, conditioning may arise from repeated positive experiences with a specific ritual or attribution of relief to a specific yet potentially noncausal factor. For example, patients frequently attribute a reduction in pain to resting. This attribution can lead certain patients to become fully sedentary over time or develop specific fears of movement,[21] with an important negative impact on their general health.

The study of immune functioning in rodents provided early evidence for a link between classical conditioning and the placebo effect. After a conditioning procedure in which a saccharin-flavored beverage was paired with the immunosuppressant cyclophosphamide, rats who continued to receive a saccharin-flavored placebo beverage showed persistent suppression of immune functioning.[22] Similar effects have been obtained in humans.[23] In the case of experimentally induced placebo analgesia, conditioning mostly consists of pairing a placebo treatment with the surreptitious reduction of stimuli. This procedure leads to placebo analgesia that can last up to 4-7 days, with some reduction in analgesia over time.[24] Interestingly, when first treated with a placebo, subsequent conditioning with an active medication is less efficient than if conditioning with active medication is performed without an initial placebo treatment.[24]

Although classical conditioning is an important form of learning that can produce placebo effects, other types of learning are starting to be investigated. For example, social observation, has been shown to lead to placebo effects: individuals experienced placebo analgesia after simply observing a confederate reporting relief from the same placebo treatment.[25]

NEUROPHYSIOLOGY OF PLACEBO ANALGESIA

The current understanding of the neurobiological underpinnings of placebo analgesia was initiated by a pharmacological study of postoperative pain, which demonstrated that the opioid antagonist naloxone could dampen the analgesic response elicited by a placebo intervention.[2] In parallel, animal models have shown that spinal excitability can be modulated by descending information originating from the brain.[26] This led to the description of a descending pain inhibition system also in humans and set the stage for an understanding of the neuroanatomical correlates of placebo analgesia.[27]

NEUROTRANSMITTERS INVOLVED IN PLACEBO ANALGESIA

Opioids

Following the groundbreaking work of Levine et al.,[2] subsequent studies, including more recent neuroimaging research, have further underlined the role of endogenous opioids in placebo analgesia. For example, a study using positron emission tomography (PET) has shown that placebo analgesia is associated with increased μ-opioid–mediated neurotransmission in prefrontal and subcortical regions.[28] Furthermore, PET imaging has revealed similar patterns of activity in the ACC and the brainstem—two key structures of the descending inhibitory pain system—during both placebo analgesia and opioid induced analgesia.[29] These findings suggest that these two routes to pain reduction share overlapping neural mechanisms. Interestingly, activity in areas known for μ-opioid activity, such as the prefrontal cortex (PFC), periacqueductal gray matter (PAG), and amygdala, is correlated with change in pain perception in placebo analgesia trials.[28,30] Finally, high doses of naloxone, which inhibits endorphin binding, suppress the functional correlation between the ACC and the PAG, with a correlated reduction in the magnitude of the placebo effect.[31]

Non-opioid Neurotransmitters

Cholecystokinin The neurohormone cholecystokinin (CCK) has anti-opioid properties and can both inhibit placebo-induced analgesia and promote nocebo-induced hyperalgesia.[32] Congruently, the blockade of CCK with the antagonist proglumide can enhance the magnitude of placebo analgesia[33] and reduce the magnitude of nocebo-induced hyperalgesia.[34]

Dopamine Dopamine is a neurotransmitter involved in reward, motivation, and goal-directed behavior. It is released in the nucleus accumbens and the striatum upon expectation of analgesia and during the experience of pain relief, both of which can be conceptualized as inherent rewards.[35] The release of dopamine by the nucleus accumbens during placebo analgesia has been demonstrated by PET imaging, with a correlation between the magnitude of neurotransmitter activity and the degree of both the expected and actual analgesia.[36]

Endocannabinoids As noted previously, conditioning with opioids elicits placebo effects that are reversible by naloxone. In contrast, conditioning with nonsteroidal anti-inflammatory drugs results in placebo effects that are *not* reversible by naloxone, suggesting a different mechanism for these effects.[7] Yet, the endocannabinoid CB1 receptor antagonist rimonabant specifically blocks placebo analgesia produced by ketorolac conditioning,[37] suggesting that endocannabinoids act as mediators of placebo analgesia in this context.

NEUROANATOMICAL UNDERPINNINGS OF PLACEBO ANALGESIA

The descending pain inhibitory system has central relays, including the ventrolateral PFC, dorsolateral PFC, ACC, PAG, and thalamus, and it exerts its effect on the posterior horn of the spinal cord, partially through endorphins.[27] Imaging studies have demonstrated that key areas of this system are involved in placebo analgesia, starting at the PFC and descending to the spinal cord, establishing that the descending pain inhibitory system is the likely neuroanatomical underpinning of placebo analgesia.[29,31,38,39] In fact, there is overlap between the neural correlates of placebo analgesia and those underlying other cognitive modulations of pain perception.[40,41,42] Interestingly, cognitive interventions that show potential for the treatment of chronic pain, such as mindfulness meditation and cognitive-behavioral therapy, also recruit similar prefrontal areas.[41,43]

WHY DISCUSS THE PLACEBO EFFECT SPECIFICALLY IN THE SETTING OF PAIN MANAGEMENT?

Pain is defined as a subjective symptom (International Association for the Study of Pain), which is particularly susceptible to the placebo effect and to the nonspecific treatment effects. A large literature suggests that these effects are quite important in the field of pain medicine, with studies performed using several different designs (**Fig. 18-1**).

Figure 18-1A illustrates how a placebo treatment can be used as a control for an active treatment for example in the context of a randomized controlled trial (RCT) of an analgesic medication. The placebo group can demonstrate a significant amount of analgesia. In a meta-analysis of placebo-controlled RCTs of analgesia for postoperative pain, 7% to 37% of patients in the placebo condition reported a 50% reduction in pain versus 5% to 63% of patients in the active treatment conditions.[44] It is interesting to note that some RCTs for analgesic interventions report no difference between the placebo and active treatment conditions, with significant improvement noted in both groups. For example, two trials of vertebroplasty versus a sham

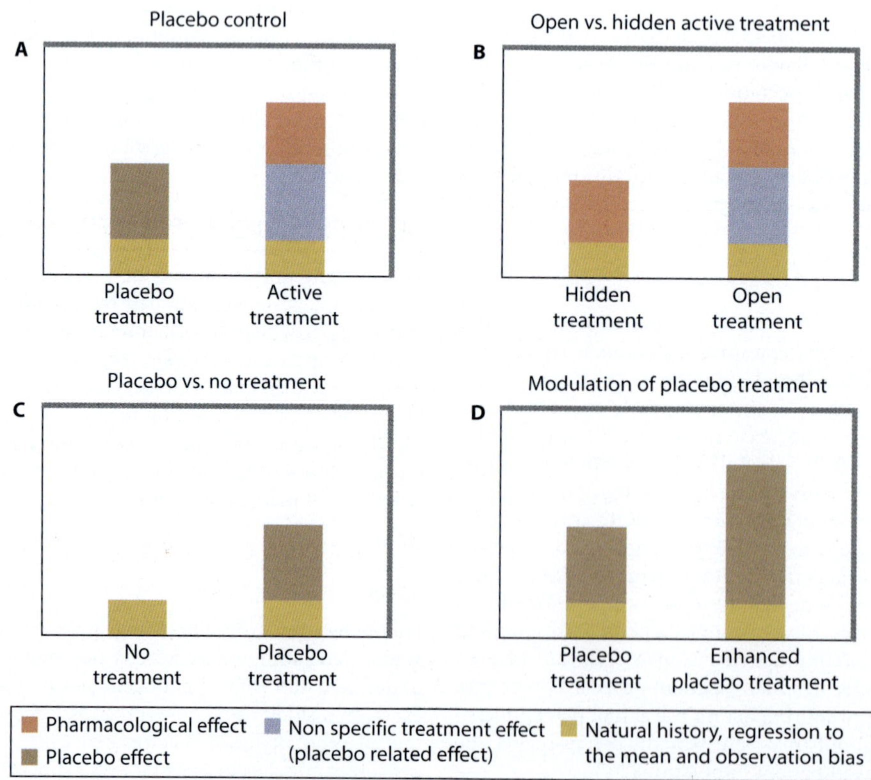

FIGURE 18-1. Trial designs used to identify the various components of placebo and active treatments. Note: The size of these effects is variable among studies and is shown here as a consistent proportion of the medication effect for illustrative purposes.

procedure showed equal clinical improvements with both interventions. However, because the studies did not include a 'no intervention' control group, it is unclear whether the benefits from vertebroplasty are attributable to a placebo effect or to the natural course of the illness or regression to the mean.[45,46]

In an open versus hidden trial design (Fig. 18-1B), active medication can be delivered with or without the subject's awareness. This allows for the nonspecific treatment effects to be teased apart from the overall treatment benefits in both experimentally induced pain in healthy subjects,[47,48] as well as in clinically relevant pain in patients.[49,50] This research suggests that an open injection of a saline solution with the verbal suggestion of analgesia may be as potent as a hidden injection of 6 to 8 mg of morphine.[51,52]

More generally, when compared with the absence of treatment (Fig. 18-1C), placebo analgesia is estimated to produce a two point improvement on a 10-point visual analogue scale.[47,53] This effect size is considered clinically relevant.[54]

Finally, Fig. 18-1D illustrates how placebo treatments can be used to study the response to nonspecific treatment effects. For example, patients with irritable bowel syndrome (IBS) were randomized to one of three conditions: (1) a wait list, (2) sham acupuncture delivered by a practitioner who treated the patient in a business-like way with very little interpersonal interaction, or (3) sham acupuncture delivered by a practitioner who treated the patient in a warm and empathic manner.[55] Interestingly, the patients with the placebo treatment and limited interaction had more improvement than the natural course group yet less than the group with placebo treatment and enhanced relationship. In parallel, the importance of medication labeling was highlighted in a clinical trial with oral medication for patients with migraine. Labeling a placebo as an active medication ("rizatriptan") increased the placebo analgesic effect compared with uncertain labeling ("placebo or rizatriptan"), and in turn, uncertain labeling produced a greater placebo effect than open labeling ("placebo"). Finally, the open label placebo treatment was significantly more effective than no treatment at all.[49] In addition, a group of studies examined the impact of offering participants the choice between two different placebo treatments (presented as different analgesic creams) compared with being randomly allocated to one of the treatments. Volunteers who preferred a high degree of control (compared with those with a lesser need for control) experienced greater placebo analgesia when they were able to choose their treatment.[56] A final example of such designs is a study in which a placebo pill presented as an expensive analgesic drug elicited higher placebo analgesia than the same pill presented as an inexpensive analgesic.[57]

Although clinicians have a number of treatments at their disposal, current therapies provide inadequate relief for many patients with chronic pain and can have significant, use-limiting side effects. Enhancing placebo-related effects is therefore a very interesting target for future research. Furthermore, patients with chronic pain can demonstrate problematic solution seeking,[58] which can lead to requests for further interventional or surgical approaches. These additional interventions can sometimes be harmful. Relief of symptoms and suffering might be better indicated in these situations, which can be achieved through cognitive or behavioral change.[59] Therefore, harnessing the power of the placebo effect might decrease suffering and improve current treatments for patients with chronic pain.

PLACEBO EFFECT AND TREATMENT IN THE CLINICAL CONTEXT

IS IT ETHICAL TO DISPENSE A PLACEBO TREATMENT?

A discussion of benevolent deception Several large surveys suggest that physicians frequently prescribe placebo medication, most often in the form of "impure placebos," such as multivitamins, sedatives, and antibiotics, and only rarely in the form of "pure placebos," such as saline injections or sugar pills.[60–62] This practice has important ethical implications. The use of placebo treatments has been justified in the past by the principle of benevolent deception (a form of paternalism).

Interestingly, the German Medical Association has issued guidelines allowing the deceptive use of placebo treatment as long as the therapy is consistent with the principle of beneficence.[67] In accordance with a recent publication, placebo treatment is deemed ethically acceptable provided that the condition is minor; the placebo is not given in place of a more effective treatment; the placebo treatment seems likely to succeed, as supported by empirical research; and an appropriate explanation is given to the patient if it is requested.[68] This practice could be considered as paternalistic. The American Medical Association (AMA) has issued more restrictive guidelines, which reject the deceptive use of placebo treatments in clinical practice because it may undermine the trust essential to a therapeutic patient–physician relationship.[63,64] Although the AMA rejects the deceptive use of placebo treatments, the guidelines do explicitly approve of the use of authorized concealment, in which the prescriber obtains consent in advance from a patient to surreptitiously reduce the dosage of an active medication without further information about the exact timing and magnitude of dose reduction.[63] After a period of conditioning with active treatment, authorized concealment of a dose reduction has the potential to harness the placebo effect to maintain therapeutic benefits while diminishing side effects and costs. Both deceptive use of placebo treatments and authorized concealment require a careful weighing of the anticipated benefits against the risks of harm either to the patient or to the therapeutic alliance. Such a risk-versus-benefit assessment is best done in a long-term therapeutic relationship.

Scientifically unproven treatments Scientifically unproven treatments (e.g., homeopathy[65]) as well as impure placebo treatments present an interesting case for practitioners. Some patients have high expectations for relief from unproven remedies or, more generally, wish there could be some medication to take for their symptoms. If the physician does not believe in the purported mechanisms of such treatments, what should he or she say when asked about it? In such a scenario, there are several important considerations.[66] Two of them are key: (1) Is there a risk of harm? and (2) Will this treatment prevent the patient from receiving a more effective and validated one? If the answer to either of these questions is yes, then the use of such treatments should be discouraged. However, if the answer to both questions is no, then it becomes a personal choice for the provider. The physician could, for example, say that although he or she does not understand the mechanisms of action of the treatment, some people have found it effective, or that the patient's beliefs about the treatment's efficacy might help him or her to experience a positive outcome. Such a course of action should not prevent the provider from continuing to track the evolution of the symptoms and reassessing the need for further treatment.

Harnessing the placebo effect without deception Recently, several studies involving the use of open-label placebo treatments have challenged the notion that deception or concealment is essential to obtain placebo analgesia. For example, in an RCT, patients with IBS showed substantial improvements in symptoms when they were prescribed an open-label placebo along with a rationale for how this treatment might help.[69] Further work supports the efficacy of nondeceptive placebo treatments in symptomatic conditions such as IBS,[19] migraine,[49] childhood attention deficit hyperactivity disorder,[70] and possibly depression.[71] Collectively, these studies suggest that informing patients about the mechanisms of action of placebos may be an effective method for using nondeceptive placebos in clinical practice. The use of open-label placebo treatments offers the advantage of having less risk and fewer side effects than many traditional therapies.

Finally, beyond dispensing placebo treatments, research suggests that enhancing nonspecific effects of active treatments, such as the ritual of the therapeutic encounter or providing verbal suggestions to expect improvement, leads to similar effects.[72] Therefore, enhancing nonspecific treatment effects presents fewer ethical issues and represents an exciting field of research in a time when transparency and shared decision making have become core ethical values in medical care.[73]

HOW CAN THE PLACEBO EFFECT BE ENHANCED IN THE THERAPEUTIC ENCOUNTER?

Although a placebo treatment may be inert, the context in which medication and interventions are delivered is not. Medical rituals and the therapeutic encounter both carry substantial symbolic weight. The above-mentioned research with patients with IBS shows that, compared with a wait list control group, the therapeutic ritual and a warm and empathic patient–clinician relationship *independently* confer significant benefits to patients.[55] The therapeutic relationship provides the context within which positive expectations can be enhanced and is central to improving treatment outcomes through placebo-related effects. The beneficial effects of the therapeutic encounter can be consciously enhanced through the words and actions of a practitioner (detailed in Box 18-2), as well as through factors that are less conscious, as described below.

BOX 18-2

How to Enhance Nonspecific Treatment Effects

Foster a relationship built on openness and mutual trust

- Treat each therapeutic encounter as an opportunity to build a collaborative and trusting relationship with the patient.
- Show interest and respect for the patient's values and beliefs regarding treatment and care.
- Provide an environment in which the patient feels free to express his or her anxieties and concerns.
- Strive to be genuinely curious about the patient's life, focusing not only his or her experiences of illness but also on his or her resources.
- Be warm and empathic and offer realistic reassurance.
- Foster positive expectations that treatment will be effective.

Know your patient: support his or her strengths and assess ways to palliate his or her limitations

- Explore past experiences with pain and pain management.
- Understand the patient's expectations. Does the patient seem encouraged and excited about a new treatment, or is he or she dismissive, skeptical, or anxious? Use this as an opportunity to counter negative expectations and reduce anxiety.
- Encourage healthy coping strategies and explore opportunities to change unhealthy or counterproductive ones.
- Identify unhelpful thoughts or behaviors that can be addressed over time.
- Assess support system (e.g., family, friends, community, patient support group). Encourage the patient to rely on this system or help the patient identify options to rebuild or expand it (e.g., family therapy if indicated, seeking new activities such as volunteering).
- How ready is the patient to make lifestyle changes toward health maintenance or improvement? Work with the patient at whatever stage of change he or she currently exhibits. For example, lecturing a patient who is not ready to change is less effective at increasing motivation than exploring the reasons *why* that patient finds it so hard to contemplate change.[74]

Maximize verbal communication

- The patient should be encouraged to take ownership of his or her treatment and participate in decision making. Some patients may prefer that the physician take a more authoritative role, which should be acknowledged and accommodated as much as reasonable.
- Evaluate and address the emotional components of chronic pain in addition to the physical issues that need attention.
- Express genuine concern about the patient's symptoms and complaints and share optimism that they can be progressively managed.[75]
- Frame negative outcomes in a positive light. For example, "In 80% of cases similar to yours, people have a good experience with this medication" versus "20% of people taking this medication report adverse outcomes"
- Avoid lecturing, blocking, depending on a routine, collusion, or premature reassurance.[76]

Maximize nonverbal communication

- Shake hands, sit down at the level of the patient, use an open and inviting posture, and make appropriate eye contact when talking with the patient.
- Focus on the patient during the consultation. Limit external interruptions from computers, pagers, or phones.
- Listen. On average, physicians interrupt patients 23 seconds into the visit.[77] Allow the patient to tell his or her story first before asking further questions, offering reassurance, or suggesting options.
- Show signs of caring for the patient. If socially appropriate, touch the patient's arm or shoulder when providing reassurance or expressing empathy.

End the encounter well

- Conclude the therapeutic encounter with a summary and a treatment plan.
- Invite the patient to ask questions. Confirm the patient's understanding by asking him or her to summarize key elements of the discussion.
- Invite the patient to express any wishes for modifications to the treatment plan.
- Provide reassuring comments and express appropriate optimism.
- Clarify when and how you could be available if contact is needed before the next appointment.
- Follow through on any plan that is made.

Elements Under the Practitioner's Conscious Control Expectations directly affect treatment outcomes, as demonstrated by the substantial decrease in medication effects that occurs when treatment is hidden (treatment without expectation) compared with when it is delivered openly (treatment with expectation).[47,48,78] This is also readily apparent in disorders characterized by impaired cognitive abilities, such as Alzheimer's disease, in which expectations cannot be easily enhanced, and consequently treatment effects are reduced.[79] In addition, there is evidence that more invasive treatments have the potential to elicit greater expectations and larger placebo responses than minimally invasive ones.[80,81] In one study, the success of radiofrequency ablation for the treatment of low back pain was best predicted by a combination of factors including the patient's expectations.[82] Furthermore, as described earlier, the benefits of some invasive procedures, such as vertebroplasty for the treatment of painful vertebral fractures, may rely on high expectations, as suggested by the similar rates of improvement between genuine and sham vertebroplasty.[45,46] The clinician should therefore bear in mind that although invasive therapies are typically associated with larger placebo-related effects, they also carry higher risks than noninvasive approaches.

Inducing positive treatment expectations is one of the keys to enhancing placebo-related effects. However, *managing* expectations is complex in the context of specialized pain management. Patients with chronic pain often have already failed multiple treatments, and recruiting any hope can be challenging. Furthermore, when multiple treatment failures have occurred, it is rare to find a simple solution to the patient's suffering. Thus, engendering unrealistic hope might actually lead to intense disappointment and may come perilously close to deception as described earlier in the ethics section.

Social or observational learning may elicit placebo analgesia in certain situations.[25] When considered from a clinical perspective, this finding has important implications for the use of certain psychosocial interventions in the treatment of pain. Support groups in which patients who have improved can provide testimonials and encouragement to those currently undergoing treatment, potentially complementing the information provided by a health care provider.

Enhancing communication and the ritual aspects of the consultation can have powerful effects by making patients feel cared for.[55] There is substantial evidence that the ritual and meaning of the therapeutic encounter, as well as effective, compassionate communication regarding diagnosis and treatment have a positive impact on health outcomes.[83,84] Attending closely to the affective aspects of communication can facilitate emotional disclosure. This form of interaction can also help the clinician to identify and modify any false or maladaptive beliefs about the disease that may be held by the patient.

Nonconscious Cues Recent research has demonstrated that both placebo analgesia and nocebo hyperalgesia can result from conditioning with nonconscious cues.[85] The fact that cues of which the patient is not consciously aware could shape subsequent experiences is not surprising, yet this experimental proof of concept does open exciting new avenues of therapeutic research. This research has the potential to identify subtle environmental or interactive aspects of the therapeutic encounter that influence health outcomes. These could be subsequently modified to promote positive evolutions in patients. To date, there have been very few good empirical studies in this field. Yet factors such as what a physician wears,[86] the number of diplomas in a therapist's office,[87] or the physical properties of a medical center[88] have all been shown to affect how much trust patients place in a health care provider or facility. Furthermore, implicit information about medication such as the size, color, and price can have an impact on placebo analgesia.[89-91] Hence, further studies in environmental psychology[92] and other nonconscious aspects of the therapeutic encounter, such as sounds, smells, and lighting, might prove helpful in designing a health care environment that is optimized for healing.

Are Some Patients More Likely to Experience a Placebo Effect? Experimental data suggest differences in response rates in individuals with certain personality profiles, neuroanatomical characteristics, or clinically relevant conditions. Personality characteristics may explain a portion of the variance in placebo analgesic responses.[93] Factors such as optimism,[94] extroversion,[95] and empathy[25] have all been associated with the propensity to exhibit placebo analgesic responses. Furthermore, an association between certain neuroanatomical characteristics, such as increased gray matter in dopamine-rich brain regions such as the ventral striatum, insula and PFC may also be associated with increased placebo responsiveness.[96] In the clinical context, a study on individuals with chronic low back pain correlated higher levels of psychopathology (e.g., anxiety and depression) with higher placebo analgesia in response to a saline injection.[97] This is consistent with earlier findings of increased placebo responsiveness in highly anxious and compliant patients.[12]

However, propensity to respond to placebo treatment might depend more on the situation rather than patients' psychological characteristics.[98,99] For instance, patients who hold positive beliefs about alternative medicine would be more likely to respond to sham acupuncture than those who hold negative views about such treatments. Therefore, although there may be certain characteristics that are common to individuals who respond to placebo treatment, these traits may simply be a proxy for other situational factors, such as the ability to hold positive expectations about a specific treatment or the desire for relief from suffering, which are known to contribute to the placebo effect.[19]

It is important to note that responding to a placebo treatment does not provide any inference about the cause or source of pain because nearly any patient with any type of pain can respond to a placebo treatment. A notable exception are individuals with prefrontal disorders or dementia, such as Alzheimer's disease, who cannot form treatment-related expectations and hence demonstrate decreased response to placebo interventions.[79] This finding has important implications in the treatment of individuals with comorbid pain and neurodegeneration because the non-specific treatment effects are greatly reduced and increased doses of analgesics might be necessary to address pain.

HOW CAN THE NOCEBO EFFECT BE MINIMIZED IN THE THERAPEUTIC ENCOUNTER?

The nocebo effect may contribute to a wide variety of therapeutic issues, such as medication nonadherence, treatment failure, and the need for additional treatments.[100,101] Verbal communication used during the therapeutic encounter plays an important role in eliciting or preventing nocebo effects.[102] For example, describing an injection of a local anesthetic without any reference to pain ("We are going to give you a local anesthetic that will numb the area, and you will be comfortable during the procedure") led to lower pain reports than when a minimal painful sensation was mentioned.[18] Similarly, including a statement about the possibility of gastrointestinal side effects in a study of aspirin for unstable angina increased their incidence sixfold.[103] Furthermore, information presented to patients may not only alter the perceived effects of a medication but also modulate pharmacokinetic factors such as the rate and degree of absorption. For example, when the muscle relaxant Carisoprodol was administered and described as a stimulant, subjects reported greater tension and metabolized the drug less efficiently (as measured by serum concentration of the major metabolite) than when the drug was described as having relaxing qualities.[104] Finally, nocebo effects, similar to placebo effects, can result from social learning, either by direct observation[105,106] or through the spreading of negative information.[107]

The likelihood of a patient experiencing a nocebo effect depends on a complex combination of both interpersonal and contextual factors, with negative expectations, suggestibility, increased anxiety, and prior experience of adverse symptoms being key elements.[101,108] As such, there is often significant overlap between the profile of a patient with chronic pain and the profile of a nocebo responder. Therefore, it is critical not only to consider the factors that increase placebo analgesia but also to simultaneously use techniques to reduce nocebo hyperalgesia in patients with chronic pain. Nocebo effects may be modulated by both an affective-cognitive pain pathway[109] and the hypothalamic–pituitary–adrenal axis.[34]

Because communicating the potential negative effects of a treatment can increase the likelihood that these effects will actually occur, the use of *contextualized informed consent*[100] may present a means of balancing the importance of transparency and informed consent with the goal of reducing the nocebo effect. Thus, many nonspecific side effects that are common to nearly all medications, such as dizziness, headache, or insomnia, might not be mentioned when discussing a new treatment with a patient, and instead the patient could be told to contact the practitioner about any new or unusual symptom. This avoids the possibility of inducing a nocebo effect by verbal suggestion. Furthermore, in the context of a strong and long-standing relationship, if it has become increasingly clear that any mention of side effects leads to the experience of new symptoms, permission to omit minor side effects from the discussion of potential negative effects of treatment can be sought from the patient. This is, thus, a form of authorized concealment. Additionally, some patients may prefer that their physicians adopt a more authoritative role in the therapeutic relationship. Having an open conversation about the degree of autonomy a patient is most comfortable with may be useful for both the patient and the practitioner, possibly fostering a closer, more trusting relationship and thereby decreasing the anxiety about treatment that may be the root of the nocebo effects.

FINAL CONSIDERATIONS

The placebo effect is a psychobiological phenomenon rooted in expectancy and learned associations. Placebo analgesia relies on a central pain inhibitory pathway, which involves endorphins and other neurotransmitters. Placebo effects are not only observed after the administration of an inert treatment; they also reflect the nonspecific treatment effects involved in an active therapy, such as communication and the ritual of the therapeutic encounter. Novel approaches to the use of placebo treatment, such as open-label placebo, and the enhancement of nonspecific aspects of treatment are harnessing the placebo effect to improve clinical outcomes while respecting patients' autonomy. These therapeutic options are especially relevant in pain management, given the significance of placebo analgesia in various trials and the important limitations in pain practitioners' therapeutic arsenal. In fact, it is proposed here that enhancing the placebo effect and minimizing nocebo effects should be the cornerstone of optimal pain management.

REFERENCES

1. Beecher HK. The powerful placebo. *JAMA*. 1955;159(17):1602-1606.
2. Levine JD, Gordon NC, Fields HL. The mechanism of placebo analgesia. *Lancet*. 1978;312(8091):654-657.
3. Finniss DG, Kaptchuk TJ, Miller FG, Benedetti F. Biological, clinical, and ethical advances of placebo effects. *Lancet*. 2010;375(9715): 686-695.
4. Price DD, Milling LS, Kirsch I, et al. An analysis of factors that contribute to the magnitude of placebo analgesia in an experimental paradigm. *Pain*. 1999;83(2):147-156.
5. Stewart-Williams S, Podd J. The placebo effect: dissolving the expectancy versus conditioning debate. *Psychol Bull*. 2004; 130(2):324.
6. Voudouris NJ, Peck CL, Coleman G. The role of conditioning and verbal expectancy in the placebo response. *Pain*. 1990;43(1): 121-128.
7. Amanzio M, Benedetti F. Neuropharmacological dissection of placebo analgesia: expectation-activated opioid systems versus conditioning-activated specific subsystems. *J Neurosci*. 1999;19(1):484-494.
8. Benedetti F, Pollo A, Lopiano L, et al. Conscious expectation and unconscious conditioning in analgesia, motor, and hormonal placebo/nocebo responses. *J Neurosci*. 2003;23(10): 4315-4323.
9. Montgomery GH, Kirsch I. Classical conditioning and the placebo effect. *Pain*. 1997;72(1-2):107-113.
10. Kirsch I. Response expectancy as a determinant of experience and behavior. *Am Psychologist*. 1985;40(11):1189.
11. Kirsch I. Response expectancy theory and application: a decennial review. *Appl Prevent Psychol*. 1997;6(2):69-79.
12. Turner JA, Deyo RA, Loeser JD, et al. The importance of placebo effects in pain treatment and research. *JAMA*. 1994;271(20):1609-1614.
13. Bandura A. Self-efficacy: toward a unifying theory of behavioral change. *Psychol Rev*. 1977;84(2):191-215.
14. Fairhurst M, Wiech K, Dunckley P, Tracey I. Anticipatory brainstem activity predicts neural processing of pain in humans. *Pain*. 2007;128(1-2):101-110.
15. Ploghaus A, Tracey I, Gati JS, et al. Dissociating pain from its anticipation in the human brain. *Science*. 1999;284(5422): 1979-1981.
16. Atlas LY, Bolger N, Lindquist MA, Wager TD. Brain mediators of predictive cue effects on perceived pain. *J Neurosci*. 2010;30(39): 12964-12977.
17. Koyama T, McHaffie JG, Laurienti PJ, Coghill RC. The subjective experience of pain: where expectations become reality. *Proc Natl Acad Sci U S A*. 2005;102(36):12950-12955.
18. Varelmann D, Pancaro C, Cappiello EC, Camann WR. Nocebo-induced hyperalgesia during local anesthetic injection. *Anesth Analg*. 2010;110(3):868-870.
19. Vase L, Robinson ME, Verne GN, Price DD. The contributions of suggestion, desire, and expectation to placebo effects in irritable bowel syndrome patients. An empirical investigation. *Pain*. 2003; 105(1-2):17-25.
20. Kirsch I, Weixen LJ. Double-blind versus deceptive administration of a placebo. *Behav Neurosci*. 1988;102(2);319-323.
21. Cook AJ, Brawer PA, Vowles KE. The fear-avoidance model of chronic pain: validation and age analysis using structural equation modeling. *Pain*. 2006;121(3):195-206.
22. Ader R, Cohen N. Behaviorally conditioned immunosupression. *Psychosom Med*. 1975;37(4):333-340.
23. Goebel MU, Trebst AE, Steiner J, et al. Behavioral conditioning of immunosuppression is possible in humans. *FASEB J*. 2002; 16(14):1869-1873.
24. Colloca L, Benedetti F. How prior experience shapes placebo analgesia. *Pain*. 2006;124(1):126-133.
25. Colloca L, Benedetti F. Placebo analgesia induced by social observational learning. *Pain*. 2009;144(1):28-34.
26. Basbaum AI, Fields HL. Endogenous pain control systems: brainstem spinal pathways and endorphin circuitry. *Ann Rev Neurosci*. 1984;7:309-338.
27. Tracey I, Mantyh PW. The cerebral signature for pain perception and its modulation. *Neuron*. 2007;55(3):377-391.
28. Zubieta JK, Bueller JA, Jackson LR, et al. Placebo effects mediated by endogenous opioid activity on mu-opioid receptors. *J Neurosci*. 2005;25(34):7754-7762.
29. Petrovic P, Kalso E, Petersson KM, Ingvar M. Placebo and opioid analgesia: imaging a shared neuronal network. *Science*. 2002;295(5560):1737-1740.
30. Wager TD, Scott DJ, Zubieta JK. Placebo effects on human mu-opioid activity during pain. *Proc Natl Acad Sci U S A*. 2007;104(26):11056-11061.
31. Eippert F, Bingel U, Schoell ED, et al. Activation of the opioidergic descending pain control system underlies placebo analgesia. *Neuron*. 2009; 63(4):533-543.
32. Benedetti F. Cholecystokinin type A and Type B receptors and their modulation of opioid analgesia. *News Physiol Sci*. 1997;12: 263-268.
33. Benedetti F, Amanzio M, Maggi G. Potentiation of placebo analgesia by proglumide. *Lancet*. 1995;346(8984):1231.
34. Benedetti F, Amanzio M, Vighetti S, Asteggiano G. The biochemical and neuroendocrine bases of the hyperalgesic nocebo effect. *J Neurosci*. 2006;26(46):12014-12022.
35. Leknes S, Tracey I. A common neurobiology for pain and pleasure. *Nat Rev Neurosci*. 2008;9(4):314-320.
36. Scott DJ, Stohler CS, Egnatuk CM, et al. Placebo and nocebo effects are defined by opposite opioid and dopaminergic responses. *Arch Gen Psychiatry*. 2008;65(2):220-231.
37. Benedetti F, Amanzio M, Rosato R, Blanchard C. Nonopioid placebo analgesia is mediated by CB1 cannabinoid receptors. *Nature Medicine*. 2011;17(10):1228-1230.
38. Wager TD, Rillings JK, Smith EE, et al. Placebo-induced changes in fMRI in the anticipation and experience of pain. *Science*. 2004;303(5661):1162-1167.

39. Eippert F, Finsterbusch J, Bingel U, Buchel C. Direct evidence for spinal cord involvement in placebo analgesia. *Science*. 2009;326(5951):404.
40. Wiech K, Ploner M, Tracey I. Neurocognitive aspects of pain perception. *Trends Cogn Sci*. 2008;12(8):306-313.
41. Jensen KB, Kosek E, Wicksell R, et al. Cognitive behavioral therapy increases pain-evoked activation of the prefrontal cortex in patients with fibromyalgia. *Pain*. 2012;153(7):1495-1503.
42. Petrovic P, Kalso E, Petersson KM, et al. A prefrontal non-opioid mechanism in placebo analgesia. *Pain*. 2010;150(1):59-65.
43. Zeidan F, Martucci KT, Kraft RA, et al. Brain mechanisms supporting the modulation of pain by mindfulness meditation. *J Neurosci*. 2011;31(14):5540-5548.
44. McQuay H, Carroll D, Moore A. Variation in the placebo effect in randomised controlled trials of analgesics: all is as blind as it seems. *Pain*. 1996;64(2):331-335.
45. Buchbinder R, Osborne RH, Ebeling PR, et al. A randomized trial of vertebroplasty for painful osteoporotic vertebral fractures. *N Engl J Med*. 2009;361(6):557-568.
46. Kallmes DF, Comstock BA, Heagerty PJ, et al. A randomized trial of vertebroplasty for osteoporotic spinal fractures. *N Engl J Med*. 2009;361(6):569-579.
47. Amanzio M, Pollo A, Maggi G, Benedetti F. Response variability to analgesics: a role for non-specifc activation of endogenous opioids. *Pain*. 2001;90:205-215.
48. Bingel U, Wanigasekera V, Wiech K, et al. The effect of treatment expectation on drug efficacy: imaging the analgesic benefit of the opioid remifentanil. *Sci Transl Med*. 2011;3(70):70ra14.
49. Kam-Hansen S, Jakubowski M, Kelley JM, et al. Altered placebo and drug labeling changes the outcome of episodic migraine attacks. *Sci Transl Med*. 2014;6(218):218ra215.
50. Pollo A, Amanzio M, Arslanian A, et al. Response expectancies in placebo analgesia and their clinical relevance. *Pain*. 2001;93(1):77-84.
51. Levine JD, Gordon NC. Influence of the method of drug administration on analgesic response. *Nature*. 1984;312(5996):755-756.
52. Levine JD, Gordon NC, Smith R, Fields HL. Analgesic responses to morphine and placebo in individuals with postoperative pain. *Pain*. 1981;10(3):379-389.
53. Gracely RH, Dubner R, Wolskee PJ, Deeter WR. Placebo and naloxone can alter post-surgical pain by separate mechanisms. *Nature*. 1983;306:264-265.
54. Farrar JT, Portenoy RK, Berlin JA, et al. Defining the clinically important difference in pain outcome measures. *Pain*. 2000;88(3):287-294.
55. Kaptchuk TJ, Kelley JM, Conboy LA, et al. Components of placebo effect: randomised controlled trial in patients with irritable bowel syndrome. *BMJ*. 2008;336(7651):999-1003.
56. Geers AL, Rose JP, Fowler SL, et al. Why does choice enhance treatment effectiveness? Using placebo treatments to demonstrate the role of personal control. *J Pers Soc Psychol*. 2013;105(4):549-566.
57. Waber RL, Shiv B, Carmon Z, Ariely D. Commercial features of placebo and therapeutic efficacy. *JAMA*. 2008;299(9):1016-1017.
58. Eccleston C, Crombez G. Worry and chronic pain: a misdirected problem solving model. *Pain*. 2007;132(3):233-236.
59. Barsky AJ. Palliation and symptomatic relief. *Arch Intern Med*. 1986;146(5):905-909.
60. Howick J, Bishop FL, Heneghan C, et al. Placebo use in the United kingdom: results from a national survey of primary care practitioners. *PLoS One*. 2013;8(3):e58247.
61. Meissner K, Höfner L, Fässler M, Linde K. Widespread use of pure and impure placebo interventions by GPs in Germany. *Fam Pract*. 2012;29(1):79-85.
62. Tilburt JC, Emanuel EJ, Kaptchuk TJ, et al. Prescribing "placebo treatments": results of national survey of US internists and rheumatologists. *BMJ*. 2008;337:a1938.
63. Bostick NA, Sade R, Levine MA, Stewart DM. Placebo use in clinical practice: report of the American Medical Association Council on Ethical and Judicial Affairs. *J Clin Ethics*. 2008;19(1):58.
64. Bok S. The ethics of giving placebos. *Sci Am*. 1974;231(5):17-23.
65. Shang A, Huwiler-Müntener K, Nartey L, et al. Are the clinical effects of homoeopathy placebo effects? Comparative study of placebo-controlled trials of homoeopathy and allopathy. *Lancet*. 2005;366(9487):726-732.
66. Renella R, Fanconi S. Decision-making in pediatrics: a practical algorithm to evaluate complementary and alternative medicine for children. *Eur J Pediatr*. 2006;165(7):437-441.
67. Kupferschmidt K. More placebo use promoted in Germany. *Can Med Assoc J*. 2011;183(10):E633-E634.
68. Gold A, Lichtenberg P. The moral case for the clinical placebo. *J Med Ethics*. 2014;40(4):219-224.
69. Kaptchuk TJ, Friedlander E, Kelley JM, et al. Placebos without deception: a randomized controlled trial in irritable bowel syndrome. *PLoS One*. 2010;5(12):e15591.
70. Sandler AD, Bodfish JW. Open-label use of placebos in the treatment of ADHD: a pilot study. *Child: Care, Health and Development*. 2008;34(1):104-110.
71. Kelley JM, Kaptchuk TJ, Cusin C, et al. Open-label placebo for major depressive disorder: a pilot randomized controlled trial. *Psychother Psychosom*. 2012;81(5):312-314.
72. Benedetti F. Mechanisms of placebo and placebo-related effects across diseases and treatments. *Ann Rev Pharmacol Toxicol*. 2008;48:3-60.
73. Blease C. The principle of parity: the "placebo effect" and physician communication. *M Med Ethics*. 2012;38(4):199-203.
74. Prochaska JO, DiClemente CC. Transtheoretical therapy: toward a more integrative model of change. *Psychother Theory Res Pract*. 1982;19(3):276-288.
75. Barrett B, Muller D, Rakel D, et al. Placebo, meaning, and health. *Perspect Biol Med*. 2006;49(2):178-198.
76. Back AL, Arnold RM, Baile WF, et al. Approaching difficult communication tasks in oncology. *CA Cancer J Clin*. 2005;55(3):164-177.
77. Marvel MK, Epstein RM, Flowers K, Beckman HB. Soliciting the patient's agenda: have we improved? *JAMA*. 1999;281(3):283-287.
78. Colloca L, Lopiano L, Lanotte M, Benedetti F. Overt versus covert treatment for pain, anxiety, and Parkinson's disease. *Lancet Neurol*. 2004;3(11):679-684.
79. Benedetti F, Arduino C, Costa S, et al. Loss of expectation-related mechanisms in Alzheimer's disease makes analgesic therapies less effective. *Pain*. 2006;121(1-2):133-144.
80. Kaptchuk TJ, Goldman P, Stone DA, Stason WB. Do medical devices have enhanced placebo effects? *J Clin Epidemiol*. 2000; 53(8):786-792.
81. Kaptchuk TJ, Stason WB, Davis RB, et al. Sham Device versus inert pill: randomised controlled trial of two placebo treatments. *BMJ*. 2006;332(7538):391-394.
82. Van Wijk RM, Geurts JWM, Lousberg R, et al. Psychological predictors of substantial pain reduction after minimally invasive radiofrequency and injection treatments for chronic low back pain. *Pain Med*. 2008;9(2):212-221

83. Moerman DE, Jonas WB. Deconstructing the placebo effect and finding the meaning response. *Ann Intern Med.* 2002; 136(6):471-476.

84. Van Dulmen AM, Bensing JM. Health promoting effects of the physician–patient encounter. *Psychol Health Med.* 2002;7(3):289-300.

85. Jensen KB, Kaptchuk TJ, Kirsch I, et al. Nonconscious activation of placebo and nocebo pain responses. *PNAS.* 2012;109(39): 15959-15964.

86. Rehman SU, Nietert PJ, Cope DW, Kilpatrick AO. What to wear today? Effect of doctor's attire on the trust and confidence of patients. *Am J Med.* 2005;118(11):1279-1286.

87. Devlin AS, Donovan S, Nicolov A, et al. "Impressive?" Credentials, family photographs, and the perception of therapist qualities. *J Environ Psychol.* 2009;29(4):503-512.

88. Devlin AS. Judging a book by its cover medical building facades and judgments of care. *Environ Behav.* 2008;40(3):307-329.

89. Buckalew LW, Coffield KE. An investigation of drug expectancy as a function of capsule color and size and preparation form. *J Clin Psychopharmacol.* 1982;2(4):245-248.

90. Buckalew LW, Ross S. Relationship of perceptual characteristics to efficacy of placebos. *Psychol Rep.* 1981;49(3):955-961.

91. de Craen AJ, Roos PJ, Leonard de Vries A, Kleijnen J. Effect of colour of drugs: systematic review of perceived effect of drugs and of their effectiveness. *BMJ.* 1996;313(7072):1624-1626.

92. Gifford R. Environmental psychology matters. *Ann Rev Psychol.* 2014;65(1):541-579.

93. Peciña M, Azhar H, Love TM, et al. Personality trait predictors of placebo analgesia and neurobiological correlates. *Neuropsychopharmacology.* 2012;38(4):639-646.

94. Geers AL, Wellman JA, Fowler SL, et al. Dispositional Optimism Predicts Placebo Analgesia. *The Journal of Pain.* 2010;11(11):1165-1171.

95. Kelley JM, Lembo AJ, Ablon JS, et al. Patient and practitioner influences on the placebo effect in irritable bowel syndrome. *Psychosom Med.* 2009;71(7):789.

96. Schweinhardt P, Seminowicz DA, Jaeger E, et al. The anatomy of the mesolimbic reward system: a link between personality and the placebo analgesic response. *J Neurosci.* 2009;29(15):4882-4887.

97. Wasan AD, Kaptchuk TJ, Davar G, Jamison RN. The association between psychopathology and placebo analgesia in patients with discogenic low back pain. *Pain Med.* 2006;7(3):217-228.

98. Hoffman GA, Harrington A, Fields HL. Pain and the placebo: what we have learned. *Perspect Biol Med.* 2005;48(2):248-265.

99. Liberman R. An experimental study of the placebo response under three different situations of pain. *J Psychiatr Res.* 1964;2(4):233-246.

100. Wells RE, Kaptchuk TJ. To tell the truth, the whole truth, may do patients harm: the problem of the nocebo effect for informed consent. *Am J Bioethics.* 2012;12(3).

101. Barsky AJ, Saintfort R, Rogers MP, Borus JF. Nonspecific medication side effects and the nocebo phenomenon. *JAMA.* 2002;287(5):622-627.

102. Bingel U, Enck P, Rief W, Schedlowski M. Avoiding nocebo effects to optimize treatment outcome. *JAMA.* 2014;312(7):693-694.

103. Myers MG, Cairns JA, Singer J. The consent form as a possible cause of side effects. *Clin Pharmacol Ther.* 1987;42(3):250-253.

104. Flaten MA, Simonsen T, Olsen H. Drug-related information generates placebo and nocebo responses that modify the drug response. *Psychosom Med.* 1999;61(2):250-255.

105. Vögtle E, Barke A, Kröner-Herwig B. Nocebo hyperalgesia induced by social observational learning. *Pain.* 2013;154(8):1427-1433.

106. Swider K, Babel P. The effect of the sex of a model on nocebo hyperalgesia induced by social observational learning. *Pain.* 2013;154(8):1312-1317.

107. Benedetti F, Durando J, Vighetti S. Nocebo and placebo modulation of hypobaric hypoxia headache involves the cyclooxygenase-prostaglandins pathway. *Pain.* 2014;155(5):921-928.

108. Spiegel H. Nocebo: the power of suggestibility. *Prev Med.* 1997;26(5):616-621.

109. Kong J, Gollub RL, Polich G, et al. A functional magnetic resonance imaging study on the neural mechanisms of hyperalgesic nocebo effect. *J Neurosci.* 2008;28(49):13354-13362.

Evaluation for Opioid Management in Chronic Pain

Robert N. Jamison
Edgar L. Ross

ABSTRACT

Opioid analgesics provide effective treatment for noncancer pain, but many physicians have concerns about adverse effects, tolerance, and addiction. Misuse of opioids is prominent in patients with chronic pain, and early recognition of misuse risk could help physicians offer adequate patient care while implementing appropriate levels of monitoring to reduce aberrant drug-related behaviors. This is a brief review of opioid abuse and misuse issues that often arise in the treatment of patients with chronic noncancer pain and an overview of assessment and treatment strategies that can be effective in improving compliance with the use of prescription opioids for pain. Many persons with chronic pain have significant medical, psychiatric, and substance use comorbidities that affect treatment decisions, and a comprehensive evaluation that includes a detailed history, physical, and mental health evaluation is essential. Although there is no "gold standard" for opioid misuse risk assessment, several validated measures have been shown to be useful. Medical practitioners should regularly use urine drug screens to monitor adherence to long-term opioid therapy. Controlled substance agreements, regular urine drug screens, and interventions such as motivational counseling have been shown to help improve patient compliance with opioids and to minimize aberrant drug-related behavior. Finally, a discussion is presented of the future of abuse-deterrent opioids and other potential strategies for pain management.

INTRODUCTION

Chronic pain negatively impacts every facet of daily living. Chronic pain has been seen to interfere with quality of life by interrupting sleep, employment, social functioning, and many other daily activities. Patients with chronic pain typically report feelings of depression, anxiety, irritability, sexual dysfunction, and decreased energy. Often chronic pain adversely affects family roles and contributes to worry about financial limitations and future disability.[1-5]

Studies analyzing factors affecting health and illness have shown that chronic pain is a widespread international problem.[6-8] More than 90 million Americans show symptoms of chronic pain, which is approximately one-third of the U.S. population. In the United States, chronic pain accounts for 21% of emergency department visits and 25% of annual missed workdays. Chronic pain is also responsible for up to $100 billion in annual direct and indirect costs, making it the most financially challenging condition to date.[9-12]

Opioid analgesics have been used to help manage acute as well as cancer-related pain.[13] This class of prescription medication is also used as a treatment for individuals with chronic noncancer pain; however, many physicians are reluctant to prescribe opioids for these patients because these medications contribute to adverse effects, tolerance, and addiction.[14]

The National Comorbidity Survey of Psychiatric Disorders collected epidemiologic data indicating a lifetime prevalence of 7.5% for drug dependence (illicit or prescription drugs) and 14.1% for alcohol dependence for individuals in the United States.[15] *Diagnostic and Statistical Manual of Mental Disorders,* fourth edition, text revision (DSM-IV) results showed that approximately 3% of U.S. citizens 18 years or older met the criteria for illicit drug abuse or dependence.[16] Another study that used a sample of 363 inpatients between the ages of 18 and 49 years found that 21.8% of the participants had a current addiction to alcohol or illicit drugs.[17]

There has been a steady increase in the use of opioids in the United States.[18] This has been the result of increasing pain awareness, support from pain organizations, changes in treatment guidelines, increasing patient understanding of pain, new formulations, and industry pressure. It is estimated that 235 million opioid prescriptions were written in the United States in 2004 alone.[19] The nonmedical use of prescription opioids has also continually increased among all ages, and now prescription opioid analgesics are reported to be the most frequently abused drugs in the United States.[20] Misuse of opioids is also prominent in patients with chronic pain, and unintentional drug overdose of prescription opioids has continued to increase since 1970 (http://www.cdc.gov/HomeandRecreationalSafety/pdf/poision-issue-brief.pdf). A literature review done by Strain[21] reported that 15% to 23% of patients with chronic pain met the criteria for a substance abuse disorder, suggesting that this continues to be a problem.

The pain literature suggests that physicians are better able to provide suitable treatment and care to patients with chronic pain when substance misuse causes are recognized.[22] Misuse behaviors of prescribed opioid medication are determined by assessment and treatment protocols. These protocols help to identify patients who show signs of opioid misuse, providing clinicians with an overview of the patient's background and behavior.

Reviewing opioid abuse and misuse issues that often arise in the treatment of patients with chronic noncancer pain facilitates a discussion of assessment and treatment strategies that can be effective in improving compliance with the use of prescription opioids for pain.

DEFINITION OF TERMS

A clear definition of terms helps to minimize confusion and to clarify the objectives of therapy for patients taking opioid analgesics for pain (**Table 19-1**). Whereas *substance misuse* is the use of any drug in a manner other than how it is indicated or prescribed, *substance abuse* is defined as the use of any substance when such use is unlawful or when such use is detrimental to the user or others. *Addiction* is a behavioral pattern of substance abuse characterized by overwhelming involvement with the use of a drug. Addiction is generally understood to be a chronic condition from which recovery is possible; however, the underlying neurobiologic dysfunction, after it has manifested, is believed to persist.[16,23] Addiction focuses on compulsive use of the drug that results in physical, psychological, and social harm to the user. An individual who has an addiction to a drug continues to use it despite harm. *Physical dependence* is a common phenomenon of all mammals taking opioids, characterized by physical withdrawal symptoms when an opioid is discontinued. *Tolerance* is also a commonly observed phenomenon when taking opioids over time, in which the individual becomes used to the drug and has a need for increasing doses to maintain the same effect. Both physical dependence and tolerance are typically found among patients who use opioids for chronic pain and are unrelated to true addiction. *Aberrant drug-related behavior* is behavior suggestive of a substance abuse or addiction disorder. Examples are selling prescription drugs, prescription forgery, stealing or "borrowing" drugs from others, injecting oral formulations, obtaining prescription drugs from nonmedical sources, multiple episodes of prescription "loss," repeatedly seeking prescriptions from other clinicians, evidence of deterioration in function (work, home, family), and repeated resistance to therapeutic change despite evidence of physical and psychological problems.

TABLE 19-1 Definition of Terms

Substance misuse: The use of any drug in a manner other than how it is indicated or prescribed.
Substance abuse: The use of any substance when such use is unlawful or when such use is detrimental to the user or others.
Addiction: A primary, chronic, neurobiologic disease that is characterized by behaviors that include one or more of the following: impaired control over drug use, compulsive use, continued use despite harm, and craving. Addiction is generally understood to be a chronic condition from which recovery is possible; however, the underlying neurobiologic dysfunction, after it has manifested, is believed to persist.
Physical dependence: A state of adaptation that is manifested by a drug class-specific withdrawal syndrome that can be produced by abrupt cessation, rapid dose reduction, or decreasing blood levels of the drug or by administration of an antagonist.
Tolerance: A state of adaptation in which exposure to a drug induces changes that result in diminution of one or more of the drug's effects over time.
Aberrant drug-related behavior: Behavior suggestive of a substance abuse or addiction disorder. Examples are selling prescription drugs, prescription forgery, stealing or "borrowing" drugs from others, injecting oral formulations, obtaining prescription drugs from nonmedical sources, multiple episodes of prescription "loss," repeatedly seeking prescriptions from other clinicians, evidence of deterioration in function (work, home, family), and repeated resistance to change therapy despite evidence of physical and psychological problems.

Several authors have shown that the majority of those taking opioids for the treatment of pain typically do not develop addiction or substance use disorders,[24] although most patients on long-term opioid therapy develop physical dependence and tolerance to the medication. Those who are undermedicated may demonstrate drug-seeking behaviors or try to self-manage with unauthorized dosage increases in an attempt to find relief. Among many of these patients, when adequate relief from the pain is obtained, the drug-seeking behaviors, otherwise known as pseudoaddiction, tend to disappear.[25] However, the long-term efficacy of opioid therapy has been questioned, and it is estimated that fewer than 40% reach a 35% improvement in pain intensity.[26]

ADVERSE EFFECTS OF OPIOID THERAPY

A number of adverse effects are associated with chronic opioid therapy, including nausea, sedation, and opioid-induced bowel dysfunction. There has also been a suspected relationship between opioid therapy and a number of other conditions, such as endocrine deficiencies,[27] dose-related cardiac arrhythmia[28] and disordered breathing, possibly contributing to unexplained deaths.[29] It has been observed that some patients become psychologically dependent after long-term opioid use,[30,31] and other patients who are chronically maintained on high doses of opioids manifest impaired cognition, problems with psychomotor performance, and opioid-induced hyperalgesia.[32] Studies also suggest that a relationship exists between early misuse of opioids and addiction. This relationship emphasizes the need for early detection of risk, close monitoring, and direct interventions when needed.

MEDICAL COMORBIDITY AMONG PAIN PATIENTS

Many patients with chronic pain may present with several significant medical comorbidities that can affect the course of treatment. Some of the most common comorbidities include asthma; chronic obstructive pulmonary disease; diabetes mellitus; coronary artery disease; hypertension; ulcers; kidney, bladder, and liver problems; or cancer. When patients are asked to rate their levels of pain, comorbid conditions may contribute to this rating.

Some individuals with chronic pain have a history of unhealthy behaviors, including minimal exercise, poor diet, and smoking cigarettes. Over time they experience weight gain and deconditioning. Many chronic pain patients take multiple medications prescribed by multiple providers, which include blood thinners, blood pressure and heart disease medications, inhalers, and antidepressants. Some patients with chronic pain have allergies and reactions to some medications. They may also have medical devices implanted and wear prostheses. It is essential for clinicians to assess and identify current and past medical conditions to avoid any complications.

INITIAL MEDICAL ASSESSMENT

It should be required for all patients considered for opioid therapy to undergo an extensive initial evaluation, including a thorough medical history, review of past medical records, urine toxicology screen, and physical examination. For most patients, a psychological evaluation should be conducted as well, including completion of screening questionnaires. The comprehensive evaluation process should involve identifying other controlled substance prescribers. Opioid prescriptions should only rarely be prescribed to patients on their first visit, and it is important for patients to be informed of the comprehensive assessment process and the policy not to prescribe opioids until all information is obtained.

A urine toxicology screen should be obtained at the first visit and compared with the patient's recent medication intake to identify any opioid misuse. A diagnosis of the patient's pain should be documented to provide clinicians with the primary pain site and probable cause of pain. It is essential for all of the patient's providers to communicate with one another to properly and effectively manage the patient's care. It is also important for clinicians to examine several factors, including the patient's gender, to provide the best clinical assessment and treatment for the patient. One recent study of gender differences and opioid misuse suggested that whereas women are at greater risk for misusing opioids because of emotional issues and affective distress, men tend to misuse opioids because of legal and problematic behavioral issues.[33] Assessment of levels of emotionality is important, frequently making a psychological evaluation invaluable.

PSYCHIATRIC COMORBIDITY

Many chronic pain patients report feelings of depression, anxiety, and irritability and have a history of physical or sexual abuse or a past history of a mood disorder.[34,35] Close to 50% of patients with chronic pain have a comorbid psychiatric condition, and 35% of patients with chronic back and neck pain have a comorbid depression or anxiety disorder.[36-38] In surveys of chronic pain clinic populations, 50% to 80% of patients with chronic pain had signs of psychopathology, making this the most prevalent comorbidity in these patients.[39-42] Studies suggest that most patients with chronic pain present with some psychiatric symptoms.

One study conducted by Arkinstall and colleagues found a 50% prevalence of mood disorder in patients who were prescribed opioids, showing this to be a common diagnosis for chronic pain patients.[43] Another study found that physicians are more likely to prescribe opioids for noncancer-related pain on the basis of increased affective distress and pain behavior rather than the patient's pain severity or objective physical pathology.[39] It has been found that patients who have chronic pain with psychopathology are more likely to report greater pain intensity, more pain-related disability, and a larger affective component to their pain than those who do not have evidence of psychopathology.[44,45]

Patients with chronic pain and psychopathology, especially those with chronic low back pain, typically have poorer pain and disability outcome from treatments.[46-49] In studies of patients with both chronic pain and anxiety or depression, there was a significantly worse return to work rate 1 year after injury compared with those without any psychopathology.[50,51] Patients who had chronic pain with low psychopathology had a 40% greater reduction in pain with intravenous morphine than those in a high-psychopathology group.[52] It becomes apparent that patients with a high degree of negative affect benefit less from opioids in an attempt to try to control their pain.

Many patients with substance use disorders also have affective disorders. Attempting to manage a comorbid affective disorder may result in decreased substance abuse behaviors for many patients, although some patients may be at risk for relapse.[53-56] Hasin and colleagues found that some patients abuse their pain medication as a way to alleviate their psychiatric symptoms.[57] From this finding and other reviews, there is a strong suggestion that individuals with mood disorders who self-medicate for negative affect are at increased risk for substance abuse.[58] Because many patients with chronic pain frequently report mood swings and prominent anxiety and depression symptoms, it remains important to carefully monitor all patients for psychiatric comorbidity. This way, individuals who self-medicate with opioids for mood fluctuations have a greater chance of being identified and directed toward more appropriate treatment.

SUBSTANCE ABUSE ASSESSMENT

The U.S. Department of Justice has recommended efforts to improve identification of abuse and diversion of controlled substances by health care providers.[59] Physicians continue to struggle with providing the appropriate pain relief for patients while minimizing the misuse of opioid analgesics.[60] Misuse of pain medications includes selling and diverting prescription drugs, seeking prescriptions from multiple providers, using illicit drugs, snorting or injecting medications, and using drugs in a manner other than intended.

A variety of assessment measures can be used to help identify patients who are prone to misuse their pain medications.[61] Structured interview measures have been published for assessment of alcoholism and drug abuse based on DSM-IV criteria,[62] but these measures have not been validated in individuals with chronic pain. Some substance abuse measures, including the CAGE Questionnaire, Michigan Alcoholism Screening Test, and Self-Administered Alcoholism Screening Test were initially designed for other patient populations.[63-65] Using traditional substance abuse assessment tools may be beneficial for patients with a severe substance abuse disorder; however, these assessments may not be useful for individuals with chronic pain because there is a greater chance of a false-positive result with these measures. In general, there is a risk that medication abuse using traditional substance abuse measures will be identified based on reports of tolerance and dependence when, in fact, no abuse exists. Validated measures most appropriate for persons with chronic pain are presented in **Table 19-2**.

The Screener and Opioid Assessment for Patients with Pain—Revised (SOAPP-R) is a 24-item self-administered screening tool developed and validated for persons with chronic pain who are being considered for long-term opioid therapy. The SOAPP-R is designed to predict aberrant medication-related behaviors.[66,67] This questionnaire includes subtle items that encourage the patient to admit to certain factors that are positively correlated with opioid misuse yet outwardly are not perceived to lead to reprisals. Any individual who scores more than an 18 on the SOAPP-R is rated as being at risk for opioid misuse. This screening tool has been found to identify 90% of those who will eventually misuse opioids. It has been cross-validated in more than 600 patients across the

TABLE 19-2 List of Opioid Risk Screening Tools

- Screener and Opioid Assessment for Patients in Pain-Revised (SOAPP-R)
- Current Opioid Misuse Measure (COMM)
- Opioid Risk Tool (ORT)
- Diagnosis, Intractability, Risk, and Efficacy (DIRE)
- Screening Instrument for Substance Abuse Potential (SISAP)
- The Pain Assessment and Documentation Tool (PADT)

United States. The reliability and predictive validity of the SOAPP-R, as measured by the area under the curve (AUC), were found to be highly significant (test–retest reliability, 0.91; coefficient α, 0.86; AUC, 0.74) and were sufficiently similar to values found with the initial sample. A cut-off score of 18 revealed a sensitivity of 0.80 and specificity of 0.52. Results of a cross-validation suggest that the psychometric parameters of the SOAPP-R are not based solely on the unique characteristics of the initial validation sample.[68]

The Current Opioid Misuse Measure (COMM) is a 17-item questionnaire developed and validated for patients who have already been prescribed opioids for chronic pain.[69] The COMM helps to identify patients who are currently misusing their prescribed opioid medication. The COMM is different from other measures that were created to predict misuse behaviors in patients before being prescribed opioids. Rather, the COMM was created to repeatedly document opioid compliance and improve clinicians' sense of appropriateness of opioid therapy. The COMM has been determined to be a brief but useful self-report measure of current aberrant drug-related behavior. The reliability and predictive validity in this cross-validation, as measured by the AUC, were found to be highly significant (AUC, 0.79) and not significantly different from the AUC obtained in the original validation study (AUC, 0.81). Reliability (coefficient α) was 0.83, which is comparable to the 0.86 obtained in the original sample.[69] Results of a cross-validation suggest that the psychometric parameters of the COMM are not based solely on unique characteristics of the initial validation sample.[70] Both the SOAPP-R and COMM include subtle items that are correlated with opioid misuse and that patients appear willing to answer honestly.

Other validated measures have also been developed to screen patients with pain for addiction risk potential. The five-item Opioid Risk Tool (ORT), a brief checklist completed by the clinician, is a validated questionnaire that predicts which patients will display aberrant drug-related behaviors.[65,71] Scores of 8 or higher suggest high risk for opioid medication abuse. A similar rating tool, the DIRE (standing for diagnosis, intractability, risk, and efficacy), is a clinician rating scale used to predict suitability for long-term opioid treatment for noncancer pain.[72] Scores higher than 14 on the DIRE suggest a greater suitability of opioid therapy for patients with pain. The Pain Assessment and Documentation Tool is yet another scale completed by the clinician, which provides a detailed documentation of the patient's progress, and it also facilitates an objective record of a patient's care.[71,73] The Screening Instrument for Substance Abuse Potential (SISAP) is a self-report screening questionnaire for substance abuse potential based mostly on the alcohol literature.[74] Unfortunately, this and other similar measures lack cross-validation studies. When using any tools to assess risk of opioid misuse, it is important to have background information about the patient.

It is also important to note that scores of any clinical assessment tool used to determine abuse risk are not necessarily sufficient reason to deny opioids but rather provide an estimate of the level of appropriate monitoring for the patient. Thus, although these clinical assessments are useful to estimate the risk of noncompliant opioid use, the results are most useful as an aid to determining how closely to monitor patients during opioid therapy.

Patients who are typically at lower risk for misusing opioids include those who are older, generally compliant, have a record of rarely misusing any medication, show stable mood, are thoughtful and responsible, and generally have an easygoing personality. Risk factors for opioid misuse include (1) family or personal history of substance abuse; (2) young age; (3) history of criminal activity or legal problems (e.g., charged driving under the influence); (4) frequent contact with high-risk individuals or environments; (5) history of previous problems with employers, family, and friends; (6) history of risk-taking or thrill-seeking behavior; (7) smoking cigarettes; (8) history of severe depression or anxiety; (9) multiple psychosocial stressors; and (10) previous drug or alcohol rehabilitation (**Table 19-3**). Patients for whom opioids are prescribed should be monitored regularly and should be examined for experiencing any adverse effects. Appropriate follow-up care should include repeated psychological evaluations.

TABLE 19-3 Risk Factors for Opioid Misuse

- Family history of substance abuse
- Personal history of substance abuse
- Young age
- History of criminal activity or legal problems including driving under the influence
- Regular contact with high-risk people or high-risk environments
- Problems with past employers, family members, and friends (mental disorder)
- Risk-taking or thrill-seeking behavior
- Heavy tobacco use
- History of severe depression or anxiety
- Psychosocial stressors
- Prior drug or alcohol rehabilitation

URINE TOXICOLOGY SCREENS

Clinicians use urine drug screens in order to closely monitor patients' adherence to their prescribed opioid medication. Highly sensitive and specific urine screens (e.g., gas chromatography/mass spectrometry [GC/MS]) help to identify the presence and quantities of prescription medications, the presence of illegal substances, and the absence of prescribed medications. Even though many patients for whom opioids are prescribed do not misuse their medications, it still is important to document compliance for all patients on chronic opioid therapy by obtaining a urine screen at least yearly.

The combination of urine screens, self-report questionnaires, and behavioral observation methods has allowed physicians to properly identify which patients are misusing their prescribed opioids. One study gathered urine toxicology results among 122 patients who were prescribed opioids for pain and found abnormal results in 43% of this sample.[75] Another study found that 21% of the study patients with no obvious behavioral issues to have either a positive urine screen result for an illicit drug or a nonprescribed controlled medication. These results imply that some risk factors for opioid misuse may not always properly identify patients who do misuse their pain medication. An additional study of 226 patients with chronic pain surprisingly found 46.5% of the sample to have abnormal urine toxicology screen results.[76] In a retrospective study of 470 patients, four of 10 patients prescribed opioids also had abnormal urine toxicology screen results.[77] These studies underscore the importance of urine toxicology screens along with behavioral observation and self-report measures to help identify aberrant drug-related behavior. Although immunoassay urine screens are often used as the first line of analysis, GC/MS urine screens provide useful results in being able to quantify the extent of illicit and prescription drug use. This type of urine toxicology screen is also able to detect drug metabolites, as well as determine whether the patient has attempted to adulterate the urine sample.

Increasingly, patients with chronic pain are using marijuana for the treatment of their symptoms, and evidence of THC (tetrahydrocannabinol) in the urine has become more prevalent.[78] There is an ongoing debate about the use of medical marijuana and specifically its use among pain patients prescribed opioids for pain.[79] Some clinicians believe that in order to be prescribed opioids, there needs to be a record of clean urine toxicology screens and that use of marijuana is unacceptable when a patient is taking prescription opioids because of its association with abuse of other illicit substances. Others believe that the use of marijuana is not grounds for discontinuation of opioid therapy, although legal implications may need to be considered. Nonetheless, the regular use of urine toxicology screens is important in identifying opioid misuse, and doctor–patient discussions about how the responsible use of opioids is defined are essential.

OPIOID THERAPY AGREEMENT

Controlled substance agreements are frequently used in clinics to clarify the roles of the patients and providers and to ultimately improve patient compliance with their opioid medications. These documented agreements provide education and mutual consent among patients and providers and inform patients of their responsibilities when using prescribed pain medication.

A controlled substance agreement should state that patients are allowed to remain in the program only if they adhere to the termed conditions (**Table 19-4**). The following are sample conditions: (1) patients should use their prescribed medications only as directed by their physicians; (2) they will be unable to receive replacement medications if their medications are lost or stolen; (3) they agree to receive prescription pain medication from only one physician; (4) they will not receive additional medication if their prescription runs out early; (5) they will accept generic brands of prescription medication; (6) if daily function has not improved with their prescription pain medication, then the physician has the right to taper the patient off the medication; (7) they agree to submit to urine and blood screens to detect use of nonprescribed medications and verify the presence of prescribed medications at any time with the use of pill counts; (8) they agree to participate in all aspects of treatment (e.g., physical therapy, psychotherapy, and behavioral medicine); (9) they will use only one pharmacy to fill prescriptions and agree to count pills from that pharmacy; and (10) they will be responsible for maintaining their appointments.

The core elements to the controlled substances agreement should be made clear so that patients know exactly what is expected of them. When patients sign these agreements, they are acknowledging their consent to the proposed treatment plan and agree to adhere to the specific conditions and responsibilities set by the clinic. It is imperative for all individuals placed on chronic opioid therapy to read and sign an opioid therapy agreement. This way, patients can be informed of their responsibilities and work to remain compliant with their prescribed medication while avoiding complications. Physicians should periodically request that the patients complete an opioid compliance checklist, which serves to remind patients of their responsibilities for using opioids for pain (**Table 19-5**).

TABLE 19-4 Example of a Controlled Substance Agreement

CONTROLLED SUBSTANCE AGREEMENT

This agreement relates to my use of controlled substances for chronic pain prescribed by a physician. I have been informed and understand the policies regarding the use of controlled substances. I understand that I will be provided controlled substances while actively participating in this program only if I adhere to the following conditions:

1. I will use the substances only as directed by my physician.
2. I will not expect to receive replacement medications for any medications that I have lost or have been stolen. A police report must be produced for any consideration of replacement of any lost or stolen medication.
3. I will receive controlled substances only from one physician. Information that I have obtained controlled substances from another physician without prior knowledge will lead to discontinuation of treatment.
4. I will not expect to receive additional medication before the time of my next scheduled refill even if my prescription runs out.
5. I will accept generic brands of my prescription medication when determined appropriate by my physician.
6. If it appears to the physician that there are no demonstrable benefits to my daily function or quality of life from the controlled substance, I will gradually taper my medication as directed by my prescribing physician.
7. I agree to submit to urine and blood screens to detect the use of nonprescribed controlled medications (including "street" drugs) and verify the presence of my prescribed medications at any time.
8. I recognize that my chronic pain represents a complex problem, which may benefit from physical therapy, psychotherapy, and behavioral medicine strategies. I also recognize that my active participation in the management of my pain is extremely important. I agree to actively participate in all aspects of my treatment to maximize functioning and improve coping with my condition.
9. I agree to schedule and keep scheduled follow-up appointments with my physician at recommended intervals. I understand that failure to keep appointments may lead to discontinuation of treatment.
10. I am responsible for keeping track of the amount of medication that I have left and to plan ahead for arranging the refill of my prescriptions in a timely manner so I will not run out of medications.
11. I agree to use one pharmacy for filling all my prescriptions except in case of emergency.
12. I will agree to count my pills that I receive from pharmacy and will ensure that the correct amount is received. I understand that I will not expect my physician to cover me for any shortage of medication. Any shortage found must be discussed immediately upon my receiving the prescription with the pharmacist.
13. If I violate any of the above conditions, my obtaining prescriptions or treatment may be terminated.
14. If I violate any of the above conditions and the violation involves obtaining controlled substances or any prescription for my pain condition from another individual or if I engage in any illegal activity such as altering a prescription, I understand that the incident may be reported by my physician. As deemed appropriate for the violation, my physician may report my violations to other physicians caring for me, local medical facilities, pharmacies, local police departments, or drug enforcement agencies.
15. I can designate up to two other people to pick up my prescriptions. I understand that I must notify my physician in advance each and every time a prescription is refilled if an alternate person will be picking up the prescription. Failure to do this could result in the prescription not being released. The names of these people must be entered at the bottom of this contract.
16. This Controlled Substances Contract will become part of my permanent medical record.

THIS AGREEMENT WILL SUPERSEDE ALL OTHER AGREEMENTS.

BY SIGNING BELOW, I INDICATE THAT I UNDERSTAND AND AGREE TO ALL THE TERMS OF THE ABOVE AGREEMENT. I HAVE RECEIVED A COPY OF THIS FOR MY OWN RECORDS.

____________________ ____________________

Patient Date and time

____________________ ____________________

Physician Date and time

Names of the people that I designated to pick up my prescriptions

#1 ____________________ #2 ____________________

TABLE 19-5 Opioid Compliance Checklist

Print name: ______________________ Date: __________

Please answer the following questions as honestly as possible:

Over the past month, have you:

1. Taken your opioid medication other than the way they were prescribed?	Yes	No
2. Used more than one pharmacy to fill your opioid prescriptions?	Yes	No
3. Received opioid prescriptions from more than one provider?	Yes	No
4. Lost or misplaced your opioid medication?	Yes	No
5. Run out of your pain medication early?	Yes	No
6. Missed any scheduled medical appointments?	Yes	No
7. Borrowed opioid medication from others?	Yes	No
8. Used any illegal or unauthorized substances?	Yes	No
9. Taken the highest possible degree of care of your prescription medication?	Yes	No
10. Taken any unauthorized substance that might be found in your urine?	Yes	No
11. Been involved in any activity that may be dangerous to you or someone else if you felt drowsy or were not clear thinking?	Yes	No
12. Been completely honest about your personal drug use?	Yes	No

Please explain anything further below. Thank you.

______________________ __________

Signed Date

Gourlay and colleagues created a rational approach to opioid therapy for the treatment of chronic pain using universal precautions,[80] borrowing the concept from infectious disease paradigms. This approach includes a means of identifying and monitoring patients who may be at risk for misusing physician-prescribed medication. To properly assess if patients should be considered for long-term opioid therapy, they suggest the following recommended steps: (1) diagnosis with the appropriate differential; (2) psychological assessment, including risk potential for addictive disorder; (3) informed consent and treatment agreement; (4) pain and function assessment; (5) opioid therapy trial; (6) reassessment of pain, function, and behavior (e.g., analgesia, activities of daily living, adverse events); (7) periodic urine screens; (8) review of diagnosis and comorbidities; and (9) detailed documentation. A comprehensive pain management center may provide additional assessment and input for patients who were referred by their physicians. Some pain management specialists offer a trilateral agreement with the patient's primary care physician. After it is determined that patients have been compliant and stable with their opioids, they can be referred back to their primary care physicians for management of their pain. The pain specialist can provide periodic reevaluations and supporting documentation, if necessary.

ABUSE-DETERRENT OPIOIDS

Several new opioid formulations that are designed to prevent or deter the abuse of opioids are currently in development, and two have been approved for marketing (morphine sulfate co-formulated with naltrexone hydrochloride [Embeda] and a new formulation of extended-release oxycodone [OxyContin]) (**Table 19-6**). Abuse-deterrent formulations are those that do not necessarily resist tampering but contain substances that are designed to make the formulation less attractive to abusers. Examples of these formulations are Suboxone (buprenorphine co-formulated with the opioid antagonist naloxone), Embeda (an extended-release morphine co-formulated with the opioid antagonist naltrexone), ELI-216 (an extended-release oxycodone co-formulated with naltrexone), and Acurox (an immediate-release oxycodone co-formulated with an aversive agent [niacin]). Tamper-resistant formulations are not co-formulated with an antagonist or aversive agent but are designed to be very difficult to crush or dissolve and thus would prevent chewing, snorting, or injecting the medication. Examples include Remoxy, COL-003, TQ-1017, and the reformulation of OxyContin, all of which are extended-release formulations of oxycodone. There are still many issues

TABLE 19-6 Abuse-Deterrent Opioids

Current Name	Active Drug	Type of Formulation	Manufacturer
Remoxy	Oxycodone (extended release)	Gelatin capsule containing highly viscous liquid	Pain Therapeutics King Pharmaceuticals
COL-003	Oxycodone (extended release)	Multiparticulate matrix with particles in waxy excipient base	Collegium Pharmaceutical
ELI-216	Oxycodone (extended release)	Capsule containing separate oxycodone and naltrexone pellets	Elite Pharmaceuticals
Unknown (reformulation of OxyContin)	Oxycodone (extended release)	Hard polymer that transforms into a viscous gel with hydration	Purdue Pharma
Embeda (ALO-01)	Morphine (extended release)	Pellets of morphine surrounding an inner core of naltrexone	King Pharmaceuticals
TQ-1017	Tramadol (extended release)	Transforms into viscous substance in the presence of solvents	TheraQuest Biosciences
Acurox	Oxycodone (immediate release)	Co-formulated with subtherapeutic doses of niacin	Acura Pharmaceuticals King Pharmaceuticals

yet to be addressed about their integration into clinical practice, as well as their true abuse liability in real-world scenarios. The cost of these new preparations will likely present a challenge, particularly for insurance carriers and pharmacy managers attempting to justify their use based on cost–benefit analyses. The only substantial real-world experience with these types of formulations is with Suboxone even though this combination of buprenorphine and naltrexone is not approved for the treatment of pain. A study has suggested that introduction of Suboxone did not reduce buprenorphine injection in Malaysian substance abusers.[81] Recent findings suggest that Suboxone, which is used by 170,000 people in the United States on a daily basis, is still occasionally crushed and injected by abusers (http://www.choosehelp.com/news/getting-high-on-suboxone-the-fda-says-its-happening-ex-nida-director-blames-doctors.html).

Yet even with a certain level of abuse, Suboxone therapy is still considered the safest treatment for opioid addiction. The Suboxone example suggests that abuse-deterrent or tamper-resistant formulations are not likely to completely prevent or deter abuse but that the reductions in abuse they provide may be an important incremental step toward safer treatments and safer communities.

INTERVENTIONS FOR HIGH-RISK PATIENTS

Chronic pain patients who show aberrant drug-related behavior often are discontinued from treatment when they are noncompliant with their use of opioids for pain. A randomized trial of patients prescribed opioids for noncancer back pain who showed risk potential for or demonstration of opioid misuse was conducted to see if close monitoring and cognitive behavioral substance misuse counseling could increase overall compliance with opioids.[82] Forty-two patients meeting criteria for high risk for opioid misuse were randomized to either standard control (high-risk control; $n = 21$) or experimental compliance treatment consisting of monthly urine screens, compliance checklists, and individual and group motivational counseling (high-risk experimental; $n = 21$). Twenty patients who met criteria indicating low potential for misuse were recruited to a low-risk control group (low-risk control). Patients were followed for 6 months and completed pre- and poststudy questionnaires and monthly electronic diaries. Outcomes consisted of the percent with a positive Drug Misuse Index (DMI), which was a composite score of self-reported drug misuse (Prescription Drug Use Questionnaire), physician-reported abuse behavior (Addiction Behavior Checklist), and abnormal urine toxicology results. After 6 months, significant differences were found between groups with 73.7% of the high-risk control patients demonstrating positive scores on the DMI compared with 26.3% from the high-risk experimental group and 25.0% from the low-risk controls ($P < 0.05$). The results of this study demonstrate support for the benefits of a brief behavioral intervention in the management of opioid compliance among patients with chronic back pain at high risk for prescription opioid misuse. At follow-up, none of the subjects was dismissed from the clinic because of aberrant drug behavior, which was possibly a partial effect of the attention from being in a study and completing monthly electronic diaries. On the whole, this study demonstrated a positive effect of improving opioid compliance, particularly among those patients at high risk for misuse of opioids. The results of this study are encouraging and suggest that compliance training and very careful monitoring of those patients determined to be at high risk for opioid misuse can be incorporated as part of an anesthesia-based multidisciplinary pain program to help improve compliance with opioids and reduce the number of individuals who are discharged from treatment because of aberrant drug-related behavior. Although further research is needed, this trial demonstrates that substantial improvement in compliance with prescription opioids for many high-risk pain patients is possible within a pain management center.

FUTURE CONSIDERATIONS

As the world population ages and life expectancy increases, greater attention will be given to managing medical comorbidities, including chronic pain. The practice of pain management will likely be changing within the next 5 to 10 years in a number of ways. First, opioids will continue to be prescribed as a treatment for pain; however, a balance will likely be reached in effectively managing pain while also addressing the problems with addiction, overdose, and death that these medications can cause. In line with this change, new formulas of abuse-deterrent opioids will continue to be developed, and greater attention will be given to educating physicians and patients about proper dispensing, storing, and disposing practices associated with the use of opioids. Also, health care practitioners will be encouraged to have specialty training and certification in the proper dispensation of opioids. Second, software programs with interactive, dynamic education for prescribers, pharmacists, and patients will continue to be developed and made available to the general public. Greater attention will also be given to outcome studies on the risk factors that predict misuse of opioids.

Third, many other fruitful and exciting areas of study will improve the way pain is managed. Genetics testing holds much promise for the identification of markers for potential opioid misuse. Our understanding of opioid-induced hyperalgesia and craving within certain individuals will also contribute to the identification of sensitive markers for opioid misuse. In particular, complex endogenous chemical reactive systems that affect tolerance and potential opioid misuse will likely be reliably identified. Also, longitudinal investigations on demographic factors such as gender, ethnic origin, and personality predispositions that influence the use of opioids will improve practice guidelines. Fourth, additional studies on other treatments for pain such as the use of cannabinoids and their role in symptom reduction could add to the current pain management armamentarium. Also, the development of other delivery systems such as topical preparations will offer a wider array of treatment options. The exciting area of nanotechnology to deliver a drug to a particular area should also greatly enhance treatment options. Finally, a greater understanding of how an acute pain problem develops into a chronic pain syndrome with subtle effects that this process has on centralized mechanisms will open up interventions that are currently not available. Although the management of chronic pain will always be a challenge, the future will likely hold answers for improved treatment for individuals with chronic pain.

CONCLUSIONS

Comprehensive assessment and monitoring is recommended for all patients who are on long-term opioid therapy for chronic pain. The close monitoring of patients who are at greatest risk for misuse of their prescribed medication should contain a treatment protocol that includes an opioid agreement; regular urine toxicology screens; compliance checklists; pill counts; and, if indicated, motivational counseling. Careful monitoring and use of abuse-deterrent opioids will hopefully decrease the abuse potential of prescribed opioids; however, risk of opioid misuse and addiction will remain, and close attention to screening and documentation of treatment outcomes will continue to be the gold standard of opioid therapy.

ACKNOWLEDGMENTS

This work was supported in part by a grant from the National Institute on Drug Abuse (NIDA) of the National Institutes of Health, Bethesda, MD (R21 DA024298, Jamison, PI). There are no conflicts of interest to declare associated with this study.

REFERENCES

1. Chapman SL, Jamison RN, Sanders SH. Treatment helpfulness questionnaire: a measure of patient satisfaction with treatment modalities provided in chronic pain management programs. *Pain.* 1996;68:349-361.
2. Linton S. The socioeconomic impact of chronic back pain: is anyone benefiting? *Pain.* 1998;75:163-168.
3. Ohman M, Soderberg S, Lundman B. Hovering between suffering and enduring: the meaning of living with serious chronic illness. *Qual Health Res.* 2003;13(4):528-542.

4. Soderberg S, Strand M, Haapala M, Lundman B. Living with a woman with fibromyalgia from the perspective of the husband. *J Adv Nurs*. 2003;42:143-150.
5. Otis JD, Cardella LA, Kerns RD. The influence of family and culture on pain. In: Dworkin RH, Breitbart WS, eds. *Psychosocial Aspects of Pain: A Handbook for Health Care Providers*. Seattle: IASP Press; 2004:29-45.
6. Garofalo JP, Polatin P. Low back pain: an epidemic in industrialized countries. In: Gatchel RJ, Turk DC, eds. *Psychosocial Factors in Pain: Clinical Perspectives*. New York: The Guilford Press; 1999.
7. Fordyce WE. *Back Pain in the Workplace: Management of Disability in Nonspecific Conditions*. Seattle: IASP Press; 1995.
8. Ehrlich GE. Back pain. *J Rheumatol Suppl*. 2003;67:26-31.
9. Frymoyer JW, Cats-Baril WL. An overview of the incidences and costs of low back pain. *Orthop Clin North Am*. 1991;22:263-271.
10. Maniadakis N, Gray A. The economic burden of back pain in the UK. *Pain*. 2000;84:95-103.
11. Ferrari R, Russell AS. Regional musculoskeletal conditions: neck pain. *Best Pract Res Clin Rheumatol*. 2003;17:57-70.
12. Stewart WF, Ricci JA, Chee E, Morganstein D, Lipton R. Lost productive time and cost due to common pain conditions in the US workforce. *JAMA*. 2003;290:2443-2454.
13. American Academy of Pain Medicine, The American Pain Society, The American Society of Addiction Medicine. Definitions related to the use of opioids for the treatment of pain: a consensus document from the American Academy of Pain Medicine, the American Pain Society, and the American Society of Addiction Medicine. ASAM. Chevy Chase, MD 2001.
14. Chou R, Fanciullo GJ, Fine P, Adler J, Ballantyne J, Davies P, et al. Clinical guidelines for the use of chronic opioid therapy in non-cancer pain. *J Pain*. 2009;10:113-130.
15. Kessler RC, McGonagle KA, Zhao S, Nelson CB, Hughes M, Eshleman S, et al. Lifetime and 12-month prevalence of DSM-III-R psychiatric disorders in the United States. Results from the National Comorbidity Survey. *Arch Gen Psychiatry*. 1994;51(1):8-19.
16. *American Psychiatric Association Diagnostic and Statistical Manual of Mental Disorders*. 4 ed. Washington, DC: American Psychiatric Association; 1994.
17. Brown RL, Leonard T, Saunders LA, Papasouliotis O. The prevalence and detection of substance use disorders among inpatients ages 18-49: an opportunity for prevention. *Prevent Med*. 1998;27(1):101-110.
18. Olsen Y, Daumit GL, Ford DE. Opioid prescriptions by U.S. primary care physicians from 1992 to 2001. *J Pain*. 2006;7:225-235.
19. Kuehn BM. Opioid prescriptions soar: increase in legitimate use as well as abuse. *JAMA*. 2007;297:249-51.
20. Administration. SAaMHS. 2006 National Survey on Drug Use and Health; 2007.
21. Strain EC. Assessment and treatment of comorbid psychiatric disorders in opioid-dependent patients. *Clin J Pain*. Jul-Aug 2002; 18(4 Suppl):S14-S27.
22. Gilson AM, Ryan KM, Joranson DE, Dahl JL. A reassessment of trends in the medical use and abuse of opioid analgesics and implications for diversion control: 1997-2002. *J Pain Symptom Manage*. 2004;28(2):176-188.
23. Leshner A. What does it mean that addiction is a brain disease? *Monitor Psychol*. 2001;32:19.
24. Sees KL, Clark HW. Opioid use in the treatment of chronic pain: assessment of addiction. *J Pain Sym Manage*. 1993;8:257-264.
25. Weissman DE, Haddox JD. Opioid pseudoaddiction: an iatrogenic syndrome. *Pain*. 1989;36:363-366.
26. Noble M, Tregear SJ, Treadwell JR, Schoelles K. Long-term opioid therapy for chronic noncancer pain: a systematic review and meta-analysis of efficacy and safety. *J Pain Symptom Manage*. 2008; 35:214-228.
27. Daniell HW. Hypogonadism in men consuming sustained-action oral opioids. *J Pain*. 2002;3:377-384.
28. Krantz MJ. Heterogeneous impact of methadone on the QTc interval: what are the practical implications? *J Addict Dis*. 2008;27:5-9.
29. Webster LR, Choi Y, Desai H, Webster L, Grant BJ. Sleep-disordered breathing and chronic opioid therapy. *Pain Med*. 2008;9:425-432.
30. McNairy SL, Maruta T, Ivnik RJ, Swanson DW, Ilstrup DW. Prescription medication dependence and neuropsychologic function. *Pain*. 1984;18:169-177.
31. Darton LA, Dilts SL. Opioids. In: Frances RJ, Miller SL, eds. *Clinical Textbook of Addictive Disorders*. 2nd ed. New York: The Guilford Press; 1998.
32. Savage SR. Addiction in the treatment of pain: significance, recognition, and management. *J Pain Symptom Manage*. 1993;8:265-278.
33. Jamison RN, Butler SF, Budman SH, Edwards RR, Wasan AD. Gender differences in risk factors for aberrant prescription opioid use. *J Pain*. 2010;11:321-329.
34. Andersson GB. Epidemiological features of low back pain. *Lancet*. 1999;354:581-585.
35. Bair M, Robinson R, Katon W, Kroenke K. Depression and pain comorbidity: a literature review. *Arch Int Med*. 2003;163: 2433-2445.
36. Peloso PM, Bellamy N, Bensen W, Thomson GTD, Harsanyl Z, Babul N, et al. Double blind randomized placebo control trial of controlled release codeine in the treatment of osteoarthritis of the hip or knee. *J Rheumatol Suppl*. 2000;27(3):764-771.
37. Katz JN, Stucki G, Lipson SJ, Fossel AH, Grobler LJ, Weinstein JN. Predictors of surgical outcome in degenerative lumbar spinal stenosis. *Spine*. 1999;24(21):2229-2233.
38. Katz JN, Lipson SJ, Lew RA, Grobler LJ, Weinstein JN, Brick GW, et al. Lumbar laminectomy alone or with instrumented or non-instrumented arthrodesis in degenerative lumbar spinal stenosis. Patient selection, costs, and surgical outcomes. *Spine*. 1997;22(10): 1123-1131.
39. Caldwell J, Hale M, Boyd R, Hague J, Iwan T, Shi M, et al. Treatment of osteoarthritis pain with controlled release oxyco done or fixed combination oxycodone plus acetaminophen added to nonsteroidal antiinflammatory drugs: a double blind, randomized, multicenter, placebo controlled trial. *J Rheum*. 1999;26(4): 862-869.
40. Maier C, Hildebrandt J, Klinger R, Henrich Eberl C, Lindena G. Morphine responsiveness, efficacy and tolerability in patients with chronic non-tumor pain—results of a double-blind placebo-controlled trial (MONTAS). *Pain*. 2002;97(3):223-233.
41. Kalso E, Edwards JE, Moore RA, McQuay HJ. Opioids in chronic non-cancer pain: systematic review of efficacy and safety. *Pain*. 2004;112(3):372-380.
42. von Korff M, Deyo RA. Potent opioids for chronic musculoskeletal pain: flying blind? *Pain*. 2004;109(3):207-209.
43. Arkinstall W, Sandler A, Goughnour B, Babul N, Harsanyl Z, Darke AC. Efficacy of controlled-release codeine in chronic non-malignant pain: a randomized, placebo-controlled clinical trial. *Pain*. 1995;62(2):169-178.
44. Moulin DE, Iezzi A, Amireh R, Sharpe WKJ, Boyd D, Merskey H. Randomised trial of oral morphine for chronic non-cancer pain. *Lancet*. 1996;347:143-147.

45. Breckenridge J, Clark J. Patient characteristics associated with opioid vs. nonsteroidal anti-inflammatory drug management of chronic low back pain. *J Pain.* 2003;4(6):344-350.

46. Rivest C, Katz JN, Ferrante FM, Jamison RN. Effects of epidural steroid injection on pain due to lumbar spinal stenosis or herniated disks: a prospective study. *Arthritis Care Res.* Aug 1998;11(4): 291-297.

47. Rooks DS, Huang J, Bierbaum BE, Bolus S, Rubano AJ, Connelly CE, et al. The effect of preoperative exercise on measures of functional status in men and women undergoing total hip and knee arthroplasty. *Arthritis Care Res.* 2006;55(5):700-708.

48. Rakvag TT, Klepstad P, Baar C, Kvam TM, Dale O, Kaasa S, et al. The Val 158Met polymorphism of the human catechol-O-methyltransferase (COMT) gene may influence morphine requirements in cancer pain patients. *Pain.* 2005;116:73-78.

49. Wasan AD, Kaptchuk TJ, Davar G, Jamison RN. The association between psychopathology and placebo analgesia in patients with discogenic low back pain. *Pain Med.* May-Jun 2006;7(3):217-228.

50. Boersma K, Linton SJ. Screening to identify patients at risk: profiles of psychological risk factors for early intervention. *Clin J Pain.* 2005;21(1):38-43.

51. Fishbain D. Approaches to treatment decisions for psychiatric comorbidity in the management of the chronic pain patient. *Med Clin North Amer.* 1999;83(3):737-759.

52. Wasan AD, Gudarz D, Jamison RN. The association between negative affect and opioid analgesia in patients with discogenic low back pain. *Pain.* 2005;117:450-461.

53. Kessler R, McGonagle K, Zhao S. Lifetime and 12-month prevalence of DSM-III-R psychiatric disorders in the United States: results from the National Comorbidity Survey. *Arch Gen Psychiatry.* 1994;51:8-19.

54. Cornelius J, Salloum I, Ehler J. Fluoxetine in depressed alcoholics: a double-blind, placebo-controlled trial. *Arch Gen Psychiatry.* 1997; 54:700-705.

55. Sonne S, Brady K. Substance abuse and bipolar comorbidity. *Psychiatry Clin North Am.* 1999;22:609-627.

56. Wasan AD, Ross EL, Michna E, et al. Characterizing craving of prescription opioids in patients with chronic pain: a longitudinal outcomes trial. *J Pain.* 2012;13:146-154.

57. Hasin D, Liu X, Nunes E. Effects of major depression on remission and relapse of substance dependence. *Arch Gen Psychiatry.* 2002;59:375-380.

58. Quello S, Brady K, Sonne S. Mood disorders and substance use disorder: a complex comorbidity. *NIDA Science Pract Prespect.* 2005;3:13-24.

59. Department of Justice. Sept 6, 2006. Dispensing controlled substances for the treatment of pain. *Federal Register Notices.* www.deadiversion.usdoj.gov. Accessed Jan 4, 2015.

60. Hampton T. Experts point to lessons learned from controversy over rofecoxib safety. *JAMA.* 2005;293:413-414.

61. Robinson RC, Gatchel RJ, Polatin P, Deschner M, Noe C, Gajraj N. Screening for problematic prescription opioid use. *Clin J Pain.* 2001;17:220-228.

62. Helzer JE, Robins LN. The diagnostic interview schedule: its development, evaluations, and use. *Soc Psychiatry Psychiatric Epidemiol.* 1988;23:6-16.

63. Mayfield D, Mcleod G, Hall P. The CAGE questionnaire: validation of a new alcoholism screening instrument. *AM J Psychiatry.* 1974;131:1121-1123.

64. Selzer M. The Michigan alcoholism screening test: the quest for a new diagnostic instrument. *Am J Psychiatry.* 1971;127:1653-1658.

65. Webster LR, Webster RM. Predicting aberrant behaviors in opioid-treated patients: preliminary validation of the Opioid Risk Tool. *Pain Med.* 2005;6(6):432-442.

66. Butler SF, Budman SH, Fernandez K, Jamison RN. Validation of a screener and opioid assessment measure for patients with chronic pain. *Pain.* 2004;112(1-2):65-75.

67. Butler SF, Fernandez K, Benoit C, Budman SH, Jamison RN. Validation of the revised Screener and Opioid Assessment for Patients with Pain (SOAPP-R). *J Pain.* 2008;9(4):360-372.

68. Butler SF, Budman SH, Fernandez KC, Fanciullo GJ, Jamison RN. Cross-validation of a screener to predict opioid misuse in chronic pain patients. *J Addict Med.* 2009;3:66-73.

69. Butler SF, Budman SH, Fernandez KC, Houle B, Benoit C, Katz N, et al. Development and validation of the Current Opioid Misuse Measure. *Pain.* 2007;130(1-2):144-156.

70. Butler SF, Budman SH, Fanciullo GJ, Jamison R. Cross-validation of the Current Opioid Misuse Measure (COMM) to monitor chronic pain patients on opioid therapy. *Clin J Pain.* 2010;26(9):770-776.

71. Webster LR, Dove B. *Avoiding Opioid Abuse While Managing Pain: A Guide for Practitioners.* North Branch, MN: Sunrise River Press; 2007.

72. Belgrade M. The DIRE score: predicting outcomes of opioid prescribing for chronic pain. *J Pain.* 2006;7:671-681.

73. Passik SD, Kirsch KL, Whitcomb RK, Portenoy RK, Katz NP, Kleinman L, et al. A new tool to assess and document pain outcomes in chronic pain patients receiving opioid therapy. *Clin Ther.* 2004;26(4):552-561.

74. Coambs RB, Jarry JL, Santhiapillai AS, Abrahamsohn RV, Atance CM. The SISAP: a new screening instrument for identifying potential opioid abusers in the management of chronic malignant pain within general medical practice. *Pain Res Manage.* 1996;1:155-162.

75. Fishbain DA, Cutler RB, Rosomoff HL, Rosomoff RS. Validity of self-reported drug use in chronic pain patients. *Clin J Pain.* 1999;15(3):184-191.

76. Michna E, Jamison RN, Pham LD, Ross EL, Janfaza D, Nedeljkovic SS, et al. Urine toxicology screening among chronic pain patients on opioid therapy: frequency and predictability of abnormal findings. *Clin J Pain.* Feb 2007;23(2):173-179.

77. Katz NP, Fanciullo GJ. Role of urine toxicology testing in the management of chronic opioid therapy. *Clin J Pain.* 2002;18(4 Suppl): S76-S82.

78. Reisfield GM, Wasan AD, Jamison RN. The prevalence and significance of cannabis use in patients prescribed chronic opioid therapy: a review of the extant literature. *Pain Med.* 2009;10: 1434-1441.

79. Munsey C. Medicine or menace: psychologists' research can inform the growing debate over legalizing marijuana. *Monitor Psychol.* 2010;41(6):50-55.

80. Gourlay D, Heit H, Almahrezi A. Universal precautions in pain medicine: a rational approach to the treatment of chronic pain. *Pain Med.* 2005;6:107-112.

81. Bruce RD, Govindasamy S, Sylla L, Kamarulzaman A, Altice FL. Lack of reduction in buprenorphine injection after introduction of co-formulated buprenorphine/naloxone to the Malaysian market. *Am J Drug Alcohol Abuse.* 2009;35:68-72.

82. Jamison RN, Ross EL, Michna E, Chen LQ, Holcomb C, Wasan AD. Substance misuse treatment for high-risk chronic pain patients on opioid therapy: a randomized trial. *Pain.* 2010; 150:390-400.

CHAPTER 20

When Psychotherapy Is Indicated in the Management of Pain

R. Joshua Wootton
Margaret A. Caudill-Slosberg
Jillian B. Frank

When the International Association for the Study of Pain (IASP) arrived at a definition of pain that included the "emotional experience," as well as the "unpleasant sensory experience associated with actual or potential tissue damage,"[1] it was acknowledging the impact of pain on our human capacity for sentience and reflection and, by extension, suffering. By the time pain has become chronic in an individual's life, it has almost certainly achieved the status of a major source of stress. More than merely an unpleasant sensory stimulus, chronic pain can come to affect the whole individual by becoming, itself, the source of a broad range of psychosocial stressors. The following case report illustrates the extent to which this is possible.

***Case* 1** A 42-year-old married man was referred to a pain management center, 8 months after sustaining a work-related, crush-type injury to his hand. His pain, which had been diagnosed as complex regional pain syndrome, type 1 (CRPS-1), had remained intractable to conservative measures and surgical intervention. According to the patient, several trials of medications had left him with uncomfortable mental status changes, and a reparative surgery and several procedures had exacerbated his pain considerably. He reported his distress as "worse than ever" and indicated that he was unable to work or pursue any of his previous recreational outlets. Although his primary care physician and surgeon supported his claim to disability, his worker's compensation carrier's representatives insisted that he should be able to return to light duty at his previous job. As a result, the patient had entered a lengthy and frustrating process of litigation, which had proved exhausting and overwhelming. As his anxiety escalated concerning his loss of income, mounting legal fees, and inability to resume work and provide for his family, he became increasingly withdrawn, irritable, and depressed. His marriage and relationships with his children and friends suffered, and by the time he arrived at the pain management center, he reported feeling angry, helpless, hopeless, and suicidal.

Cases such as this are familiar to everyone who specializes in the treatment of patients with chronic pain. The challenge, where successful medical resolution is concerned, is to maintain the focus on the whole of the individual's experience, both sensory and affective, because the development and course of chronic pain represents a progressive series of complex interactions among the biologic, psychological, and social dimensions of an individual's life. Purely physiologic explanations cannot account for its impact.[2] Nor can an exclusive reliance on the interventions that spring from such a limited understanding ordinarily bring the enduring relief and solace sought by many patients with chronic pain.[3]

The quality, intensity, and duration of pain are influenced by a myriad of psychological and social factors, which—although they may have arisen in the context of pain—are by no means less influential or consequential than the unpleasant sensory experience arising from actual or potential tissue damage.[4] Such factors may, indeed, play a critical role in the etiology, severity, exacerbation, and maintenance of pain, suffering, and disability.[5] The experience of chronic pain ultimately comes to be the product of conflict between a sensory stimulus and the entire individual. It will always require some level of adaptation and adjustment, but it can, in many cases, interfere with one's work and livelihood, recreational pursuits, relationships with family and friends, and even sexual intimacy. Through the introduction of more enduring affective changes, it can also influence one's self-esteem and the ways in which one views oneself as a man or woman, husband or wife, father or mother, friend, member of society, and spiritual being.

WHY A MULTIDISCIPLINARY APPROACH IS NEEDED

With so much at stake for patients with chronic pain, it is not surprising that psychological evaluation is a required or highly recommended feature of comprehensive evaluation in many pain management centers.[6] For many patients, some form of psychological intervention is also recommended as part of the comprehensive treatment plan. Such interventions are usually prescribed to run concurrently with medical treatment and other therapies and may include one or more of many available modes of individual or group psychotherapy. When offered as part of a multidisciplinary package, psychotherapeutic approaches to managing chronic pain have demonstrated their efficacy repeatedly, and there is considerable evidence to suggest that the more effectively such interventions are integrated into a comprehensive or team approach, the greater are the chances of improvement for health and quality of life.[7]

With the IASP reporting an incidence of chronic pain in the United States of 70 million and with more than 50 million being partially or totally disabled for periods ranging from a few days to a few months, a concerted multidisciplinary effort becomes even more critical to the effective marshaling of available medical resources.[8] Especially for patients whose chronic pain has remained initially intractable to medical and surgical interventions, a careful plan of treatment coordinated by a team of providers can ultimately result in greatly reducing the costs of health care, as well as raising the quality of that care—improving patients' response to treatment, level of functioning, and satisfaction—and enhancing the morale of all the providers concerned.[9] Psychotherapeutic management, in this context, necessarily involves not only a multidisciplinary approach but also an interdisciplinary effort in which the interventions of each member of the team—physicians, nurses, physical therapists, medical and complementary specialists, and mental health providers—can be seen as having a synergistic therapeutic impact on the patient and must be directed toward having a complementary effect on the interventions of all other members of the team.

PSYCHOLOGICAL FACTORS IN CHRONIC PAIN

It is, by now, a generally accepted, if not always carefully considered, tenet that stress is influential in the development, expression, and tractability of chronic pain.[10] Because stress is also influential in the development and expression of somatization and other psychological symptoms, associations among chronic pain, stress, and psychiatric disorder are frequently observed and well documented in the literature of both pain and psychiatry.[11] Attempting to parse or separate these influences prematurely for the sake of treatment is frequently tantamount to disregarding the often volatile interactions among these factors and the cyclically reinforcing relationship between chronic pain and stress.

When such a unilateral approach is taken, it often represents the attempt of physicians adhering to too strict a medical model to establish the extent to which a patient's problem may be *mental* as opposed to *physical*. As a result, both the physician and patient may be left wondering why a clearly prescribed nerve block or medication has not achieved the expected relief. It may also lead to the premature and potentially harmful conclusion by the physician and the patient's health insurance carrier that nothing further can be done medically or surgically to assuage the patient's pain and that the problem is no longer a medical one but strictly a psychological one, now unrelated to a precipitating injury or historical tissue damage. What is being overlooked is the individual patient's stress reactivity and the enduring influence of the pain–stress cycle on the development and maintenance of chronic pain.

Stress Reactivity and the Pain–Stress Cycle The term *stress reactive* is suggestive of a continuum of the degree to which any individual reacts to external or internal stressors, including the stressors of pain and its psychosocial sequelae. We are all on this continuum, but highly stress-reactive individuals are likely to develop a broader spectrum of more severe psychological and social concomitants or consequences, as well as to experience their pain with greater affective involvement and suffering. Less stress-reactive individuals may still experience the need to accommodate to their pain, psychologically, socially, and occupationally, but their adjustment to living with chronic pain is typically more successful, and their adaptation to their limitations is more enduring.

The term *pain–stress cycle* is indicative of the unfolding neuropsychosocial matrix in which (1) pain tends to amplify the impact of stress while (2) stress magnifies the subjective experience of suffering associated with pain. The former occurs when a patient's experience of pain facilitates the development of new and secondary psychosocial stressors, as in Case 1, but it may also be evident in the patient's tendency to rely on or resort to maladaptive coping strategies, such as self-medication; social withdrawal; and the development of generalized, reactive pain behaviors. The latter refers more specifically to the contributions of heightened autonomic arousal and musculoskeletal tension in the maintenance and intensity of the experience of pain.

We have only an inchoate appreciation of how these mechanisms work and interact, but advances in our understanding of the neurophysiology and molecular biology of our perception and experience of pain strongly suggest that the influence of psychosocial factors and emotions is translated neurophysiologically into the realm of perception and behavior.[12] Stress, regardless of its origin, can result in physiologic deterioration and the exacerbated experience of pain through a variety of mechanisms. Neurosignature patterns can be modulated or altered destructively by stress of psychological origin, no less than by sensory input. Because any stressor, whether external or internal, physical or psychological, can affect stress-regulation systems adversely, the resulting lesions or tissue damage can influence the neurosignature patterns that originate and maintain chronic pain.[13]

Seen from this perspective, the distinction between stresses of psychological versus physical origin tends to assume less importance, and a multidisciplinary or comprehensive approach to treatment becomes paramount. All models of chronic pain acknowledge the neuropsychosocial relationship and interaction between stress and pain; however, it is yet a further step to begin to understand and appreciate how this works in the life of a particular patient or how to incorporate this approach into a successful plan of treatment. In a multidisciplinary approach to treating chronic pain, therefore, making an assessment of the degree to which any patient is stress reactive and addressing the nature of his or her unique expression of the pain–stress cycle become primary objectives of intervention in pain management.

There is a tendency to regard this as the special province or purview of the psychologist, psychiatrist, clinical social worker, mental health counselor, or psychiatric nurse practitioner, but in a team approach, all interventions may be seen as having a psychotherapeutic action. The reassurances of the physician or nurse that a patient's pain is being taken seriously; the verbal reinforcement to the patient by all providers that progress in pain relief and management can be achieved; and even the comforting touch of physicians, nurses, and physical therapists during examinations, procedures, or exercises may all possess a powerful psychotherapeutic dimension. What is shared in team meetings and clinical rounds can also prove critical to all providers in assessing a patient's progress and determining the extent to which he or she remains stress reactive, as well as how the pain–stress cycle continues to unfold in the context of his or her family, social relationships, work, and livelihood.

Influence of Psychopathology As the ongoing evaluation and treatment of chronic pain proceeds, one area in which psychologists, psychiatrists, and clinical social workers can be especially valuable lies in determining the extent to which psychopathology is present and influential. As psychological intervention begins, the first important consideration—one that will likely have implications for both prognosis and treatment—concerns the juxtaposition of psychological factors affecting the patient's pain experience, especially with regard to the order, magnitude, and relative duration of influence. In some cases, psychopathology occurs as a complicating feature in the diagnosis and treatment of chronic pain and existed before the development of the pain syndrome. In these instances, some delineation of the premorbid or existing psychopathology becomes critical to understanding the role and meaning of pain from the patient's perspective. In other cases, psychopathology is reactive to and arises within the context of the patient's experience of pain, and special care may be needed to introduce the idea of and address the disorder without the patient's feeling that the focus has been removed from his or her pain.

Chronic pain is far more prevalent among psychiatrically disordered individuals than in the general population, and there is considerable evidence that alterations in the experience of pain occur in conjunction with some psychiatric disorders, including mood disorders, anxiety disorders, and psychotic disorders.[5,14] Prevalence rates for depression among individuals with chronic pain in clinic-based samples vary in the literature from 30% to 54%,[15] with significant depressive symptoms ranging from 60% to as high as 100% in some samples.[16] The question of which came first—the depression or the pain—remains controversial as an issue but is often made more complicated and even confusing when considered in the context of an individual case.[17] Clinical evaluation can certainly reveal depressive symptomatology to be a premorbid or disposing influence in the development of chronic pain, as well as a comorbid one. That depression might be a consequence of chronic pain is acknowledged by many patients, but that pain might constitute the somatized expression of premorbid but unacknowledged depression or intrapsychic conflict typically meets with resistance from some patients and their families, who may find a psychiatric diagnosis both less accessible and less acceptable than a medical one.

Case 2 A 52-year-old married woman with a previous lumbar laminectomy and a well-documented history of mild and episodic but well-managed low back pain developed an exacerbation shortly after the last of her three children left home to enter college. Her pain did not resolve as easily as it had in the past, and 2 months later, she presented to a pain management center, tearful, agitated, and in obvious distress, having exhausted her primary care physician's ordinarily effective armamentarium of conservative treatments. Her husband reported that she had become increasingly withdrawn from her friends and previously busy schedule and now stayed mostly in bed, watching television or sleeping. With a diagnostic workup and clinical examination devoid of any findings except a few mild trigger points, the patient's pain physicians prescribed an antidepressant, which they were careful to explain is also considered a "pain medication," and referred her to a structured group psychotherapy program, emphasizing the importance of learning techniques for greater musculoskeletal relaxation. One month later, the patient presented for follow up, excitedly discussing her cognitive-behavioral assignments for stress management from her group and chatting with the nurses about the success of her children, with whom she had developed a frequent e-mail correspondence. She complained of occasional, mild residual pain but was not allowing this to impede the gradual resumption of her daily schedule.

In this case, the patient had little insight into the development of her reactive depression or its relationship to her worsening pain. Considering her history of surgery and episodic low back pain, it is difficult to ascribe her distress solely to somatization, but instances of pure somatization are usually difficult to document convincingly. As in most cases, this woman's exacerbation of pain appears to stem from both physiologic and psychological factors, and especially when discussing her experience with the patient herself, it is important not to become distracted by questions of primacy. When there is a clear, established history of a premorbid psychiatric disorder, it becomes critical to understand how such psychological factors may have contributed to the development of chronic pain and how they shape the patient's experience of chronic pain. When there is little to suggest premorbid psychiatric influences, however, it is far more important to maintain a clinical focus on the relationship between psychological and physical factors as a whole, as well as their ongoing interaction.

For this reason, a model reflecting the influence of stress reactivity and the pain–stress cycle is probably more versatile and more efficacious in such cases because it promotes a view of health that takes into account the interaction of psychological and physical factors without the need or presumptive burden of trying to establish causal direction—an enterprise that, despite our best efforts and intentions, might easily result in harm to the patient. With such a model, psychological factors can be viewed as both amplifying pain and inhibiting successful adjustment to it, but chronic pain itself can be viewed as a potent psychological stressor in its own right and one that can easily give rise to other psychosocial stressors.[18]

The disposing premorbidity, for example, of personality disorders, depression, and posttraumatic stress in the development of chronic pain is often accepted uncritically in the clinical arena. That they are found in significantly greater proportion comorbidly is indisputable.[19,20] Yet when viewed according to a diathesis-stress model, even personality-disordered and posttraumatic stress–disordered behaviors may emerge for the first time and coalesce around chronic pain.[21] So the question becomes less a chicken-or-egg issue of, "Which came first, the chronic pain or the psychiatric disorder?" but rather, "What approach is more helpful to the patient in understanding and assisting in the resolution, both psychologically and physically, of his or her pain?"

Somatization, according to this model, can be seen as an immature psychological defense capable either of giving rise to pain in the apparent absence of organic pathology or of complicating and magnifying pain in the established presence of organic pathology. As a defense, it simply represents the symbolic displacement of intrapsychic conflict onto the somatic sphere in an unconscious attempt to avoid distressing affects associated with psychosocial stress. All stress-reactive individuals tend to somatize, when under sustained or escalating stress, and because we are all on a stress-reactive continuum, we all tend to express affects through our bodies to some degree. Highly stress-reactive patients may have well-documented histories of somatization and physical complaints at many sites, but any tendency toward somatization can magnify a patient's suffering well beyond what is expectable, given the nature and extent of actual tissue damage.

Alexithymia—a subclinical inability to identify and describe one's emotions—can be a predisposing, complicating, and exacerbating feature of somatization[22] because patients who are unable to articulate their emotions and affective states in words may have few outlets, other than bodily expression, for their intrapsychic pain and discomfort. For those who have come to regard the experience of psychological distress or displays of affect as signs of weakness or occasions for shame, displacing intrapsychic conflict onto the body may also allow them to feel that they have more legitimate claims to others' attention and the fulfillment of their needs—a phenomenon or symptom also known as *secondary gain*. Such constructs as alexithymia and secondary gain, in turn, raise the question of whether the phenomenologic focus of the interaction between pain and stress is more appropriately placed on psychiatric disorder or on temperament, personality traits, coping attributes, and even environmental factors such as availability of support.[23] Again, shifting the clinical focus too quickly to that of psychiatric disorder can discourage the patient further or even lead to the termination of treatment.

The dangers of prematurely settling on a psychiatric diagnosis were addressed with the promulgation of the category of somatic symptom and related disorders of the *Diagnostic and Statistical Manual of Mental Disorders,* fifth edition (DSM-5), the common feature of which is the prominence of somatic symptoms associated with significant distress and impairment.[24] In the previous nomenclature of the DSM-IV, the emphasis of the somatoform disorders was on their medically unexplained nature. All too frequently, such diagnoses heralded the closing of the door to continued medical attention and intervention. According to the new criteria, somatic symptom disorders can occur concurrently with diagnosed medical disorders, acknowledging our limitations on declaring pain and other somatic symptoms to be medically unexplained.[24] So, too, the coincidence of mood, anxiety, and personality disorders should not be considered a medical end point but rather should highlight the need for multidisciplinary approaches to the treatment of chronic pain. Psychiatric diagnosis in chronic pain is valuable only insofar as it develops a deeper and richer understanding of the patient and promotes multidisciplinary options for treatment, including that of psychotherapeutic intervention.

PREPARING FOR PSYCHOTHERAPEUTIC INTERVENTION

Not all patients with chronic pain exhibit significant psychopathology, of course, or experience the complicating influences of the range of psychological factors that can affect the course of physical symptoms. Many individuals adjust well to the limitations imposed by their pain and continue to work productively and to enjoy satisfying relationships and rewarding personal interests. Most of them have no histories of premorbid psychopathology, and by virtue of resilient temperaments, adaptive personality traits, and successful coping skills, they manage to avoid the comorbid development of psychological distress and psychiatric symptoms that can become associated with chronic pain.

Those who are less fortunate, however, include among them the most memorable and challenging patients in any primary care practice or pain management center. Their suffering is often dramatic and, even when their numbers are few, their drain on resources is considerable when calculated in terms of time, money, and the morale of staff. Their families, other physicians, employers, and even health insurance carriers frequently become demanding agents in their behalf even as their pain remains puzzling and intractable to an ever-lengthening list of interventions, and their escalating sense of urgency continually reminds us of our limitations as health care providers. When all else appears to have failed and all available resources have been tapped, it is a small step toward collusion with the patient's own escalating sense of urgency to make one more referral to yet another specialist or to raise the level of pain medication, one more time; to consider one more improbable intervention; or, as is often the case, to simply close the door, abandoning the patient to begin the process all over again.

It is under such circumstances that psychologists and psychiatrists frequently find patients with chronic pain at their doors. Having been told that there is nothing further that can be done, that there is no hope of further surgical or medical palliation, patients can be left to begin the process of psychologically adjusting to their pain and its sequelae in the most angry, anxious, and despairing of states. For these individuals, pain may already have become an organizing principle, and the enterprise of psychotherapeutic management is no longer only that of addressing transiently reactive mood or anxiety or difficulties with adjustment but that of attempting to alter a way of life or effecting change at the level of personality and identity. Chronic pain of this nature continues to call for a multidisciplinary approach, often just at a time when patients are most discouraged by or disillusioned with their medical care, and it is often a long road back to successful pain management, made far more arduous for having been consigned to being undertaken in pieces.

When psychological factors are influential in the development or maintenance of chronic pain, the greatest progress is likely to be achieved most expediently when there is not only interdisciplinary cooperation but also an integrated, comprehensive plan of treatment in which all providers work together with the same goals in sight. Undertaking medical and psychotherapeutic approaches to chronic pain separately—or worse, sequentially—greatly reduces the chances of making global progress in patients' adjustment to their pain, and increasing the chances that interventions from different disciplines may compete or contradict one another, leaving patients feeling confused and helpless. It can also leave physicians and psychotherapists feeling alone and unassisted in their attempts to help their patients and more likely, as a result, to communicate their own anxiety and sense of helplessness about the slowness or lack of progress back to the patient.

The patient's developing stability and success with managing chronic pain may well depend on an abiding trust that his or her physicians are doing everything possible to offer appropriate relief and comfort through medical means, and his or her psychotherapist is doing everything possible to assist with the adjustment to what the patient sees as the emotional impact and consequences of pain. This does not mean that there is a strict division of labor, however, and patients often turn to their physicians and nurses for emotional support and ask their psychotherapists for reassurance about medical decisions. Patients with chronic pain often ask their providers, without respect to discipline, for *validation*—the reassurance that their physicians, nurses, physical therapists, and psychotherapists have heard their concerns and understand their experience. Many have gone from provider to provider, encountering repeated disappointments in their search for answers, and their often challenging and sometimes provocative presentations may reflect the defensiveness, hypersensitivity, and hypervigilance of the scars, both physical and psychological, they have sustained in their search for relief and solace.

Establishing a good working *alliance* is, therefore, critical for all members of a multidisciplinary team. Patients' compliance with directives and interventions and their cooperation with a plan of treatment often depend on their perception that all members of the team are working together on their behalf. When patients lose trust in their providers or sense that providers are not fully engaged in the process of helping them in their search for answers and relief, the alliance deteriorates, sometimes irredeemably. Patients' complaints of feeling rushed, dismissed, or devalued may result, not surprisingly, in an increase in pain behaviors and dependency, as well as tendencies toward the expression of retaliatory impulses. In a multidisciplinary approach to treatment, the responsibility for maintaining the integrity of the alliance is shared among all providers, with the result that the patient's urgency is experienced by all as less demanding or overwhelming.

When the psychologist, psychiatrist, clinical social worker, mental health counselor, or psychiatric nurse practitioner enters the scene, patients frequently need the reassurance of the rest of the team that their pain has not suddenly been relegated to the uncertain status of being purely psychological in origin or "all in the head." Especially in the initial psychological interview, it is reassuring to patients to be able to focus on what they know best—namely, the emotional impact of pain on their lives—and not to feel as if their beliefs and psychological defenses are being challenged or threatened. When the patient feels secure that his or her story has been heard and fully appreciated, the direction of the psychotherapist's inquiry can turn toward a consideration of the psychological and behavioral antecedents, correlates, and sequelae of pain—all of the factors influencing the pain–stress cycle. When the patient is willing to acknowledge and discuss the possibility that stress may contribute to his or her subjective experience of pain, the way is prepared for psychotherapeutic intervention.

Nevertheless, it is critical not to presume too much or too quickly here. A final, essential question to consider in preparing for psychotherapeutic intervention concerns the range of variables in individual temperament and personality that make psychological adjustment possible: Is the patient disposed toward making the changes necessary to facilitate more adaptive coping? Because patients vary widely in their receptiveness to making the behavioral changes that lead to more successful adjustment, their readiness for change[20,25] may require continual monitoring and nurturing in psychotherapy (see Chapters 14, 15, 18, and 22). Suggesting to a patient, for example, who is waiting for his or her physician to "fix the problem" that relaxation exercises might assist in the management of pain is unlikely to result in anything but frustration. Accurately assessing and nurturing the patient's readiness for change, therefore, becomes one of the principal prerequisites for the successful psychotherapeutic management of chronic pain.

INDIVIDUAL PSYCHOTHERAPY

The psychotherapeutic treatment of chronic pain accompanying other psychiatric disorders may have more than one goal, including the relief of pain itself, the decrease of disability and illness-related or "pain behaviors," the restoration of activity and the increase in functional quality of life, as well as the decrease in reliance on opioid and other analgesic or anxiolytic medications.[26] Individual psychotherapy may prove to be of great benefit in achieving these goals, but it must be noted from the outset that structured group programs, whether inpatient or outpatient, have been studied more widely and demonstrated to be of greater efficacy in their application to chronic pain populations.[27]

The hallmark of such programs has been the successful integration of multidisciplinary approaches into a unified interdisciplinary perspective, with greater coordination of services and frequent communication among all providers. Progress in individual psychotherapy, by itself, is frequently hamstrung by a less unified, more piecemeal approach to the patient's concerns, which may change from session to session. As a result, more structured forms of individual treatment, such as cognitive-behavioral therapy (CBT), have been developed specifically for pain patients. But individual treatment, whether combined with structured group psychotherapy or undertaken on its own, tends to work best when its approach is eclectic and includes a number of components,[20] each of which may appeal to a different or succeeding stage in the patient's receptivity or readiness for change.[25]

Keeping in mind that psychotherapeutic management is the concern of the entire treatment team, any intervention may, broadly speaking, have a psychotherapeutic impact on the patient. The beginning of formal psychotherapeutic intervention, however, is usually marked by a clinical interview and anamnesis administered by a mental health professional. Psychological testing may also be included as a means of evaluating the current level of functioning; symptoms of psychopathology; presence of psychosocial risk factors affecting prognosis; and other cultural, educational, and attitudinal indicators warranting consideration in the planning of treatment. Psychopharmacologic evaluation may be included at this stage as well, but many pain physicians are conversant with the use of psychotropics in pain management, and referral to a specialist is often considered redundant unless the initial interventions have proven unsuccessful. After a picture of the patient's presenting baseline of coping and functioning emerges, ongoing and longitudinal assessments provide a measure of psychotherapeutic progress, as well as indications for appropriate changes in the treatment plan.

PSYCHODYNAMIC PSYCHOTHERAPY

Psychodynamic or insight-oriented and supportive psychotherapies are not usually considered treatments of choice for patients with chronic pain, precisely because their approach is less structured and more patient directed, but they may be the logical starting point for patients whose pain and disability are sustained or exacerbated by intrapsychic conflict or unconscious motives, such as trauma or secondary gain.[28,29] The high correlation between the history of physical or sexual abuse and the subsequent development of chronic pain is well documented in the literatures of psychiatry and pain.[30-32] In patients who have suffered abuse as children or as adults or who have experienced or witnessed situations in which either death or serious injury was real or threatened, chronic pain may come to represent a means of psychologically symbolizing and organizing an unbearable traumatic event or series of events. Nor is the situation of childhood or adult abuse the only form of trauma associated with chronic pain and disability. The development of comorbid posttraumatic stress disorder is also prevalent in work-related injuries and motor vehicle accidents.[33,34]

Whether premorbid or comorbid, posttraumatic stress disorder remains a powerful confounding factor in many cases of chronic pain, and for patients with such a background, a frequently necessary step in the development of their readiness for change is the experience of making a conscious connection between their trauma and their pain. In cases in which premorbid psychopathology has contributed to the development of chronic pain and disability, an understanding of the relationship between the patient's history and the development of his or her symptoms may prove essential in assisting him or her toward a more active role in treatment.

***Case* 3** A 28-year-old, recently married woman was referred to a pain management center with a 6-month history of chronic abdominal and pelvic pain of uncertain etiology. She reported having a history of episodically severe "stomach aches and cramps" as a child but felt that these had long since been resolved. Although similar to these early episodes, her current pain had become more intense and urgent, even to the point where walking was sometimes difficult, literally necessitating her husband's support to get down the stairs in their home. Her anxiety had also escalated, interfering with the couple's sexual intimacy, despite her husband's obvious concern and willingness to assist her in whatever ways she asked. The patient agreed to enter psychotherapy but denied the impact of any stress in her life, beyond that of her pain. During the course of treatment, she disclosed to her psychotherapist that she had endured sexual abuse from her father as a child but, again, placed no significance on its enduring influence. When asked how and when the abuse stopped, she indicated that her father typically became more solicitous of her and less likely to molest her when she became ill. Over time, she made the connection that her pain had begun in the weeks immediately after her wedding, when the couple's sexual intimacy had greatly increased in frequency. Wondering whether there might be a relationship between her pain and her feelings and attitudes about sex, she eventually came to the realization that her developing sexual relationship with her husband was, through no fault of her own or her husband's, recapitulating her childhood trauma. After she recognized that this recapitulation might have contributed to the onset of her pain, she became motivated to address the complete range of issues both influencing and influenced by her pain. Several months later, after the addition of couples therapy and a cognitive-behavioral component to her individual treatment, her pain was largely resolved, and she and her husband were reporting the mutually satisfying reintroduction of sexual intimacy to their relationship.

This case illustrates how an instance of primary somatization can become a defensive process around which a personality can coalesce unconsciously. If the impact of such a process goes unacknowledged and its possible influence unrecognized, then the motivation for change is likely to remain insufficient. In this patient's case, not only did she need to examine her immediate situation, but she also had to recognize and accept the connections between her emotional experience and her chronic pain before she could accept a more active role in her own recovery and rehabilitation. Similarly, when the trauma of a work-related injury or motor vehicle accident triggers and recapitulates an earlier, unresolved emotional trauma, such as childhood abuse, then what appears to be a straightforward physical injury can easily become complicated by premorbid psychological factors, making pain more tenacious and less tractable. It is not unreasonable to think that many individuals sustaining such injuries but without a history of trauma in their backgrounds might experience a few days or weeks of discomfort but otherwise emerge essentially unscathed, having put the experience behind them.

Another problem often adversely affecting a patient's adjustment to and recovery from injury and pain is that of *secondary gain*, an unconscious motivation to maintain a symptom in order to gain some advantage.[11] In secondary gain, the advantage is derived from symptoms that have already formed and so could not have been foreseen or sought, even unconsciously, at the time of the original injury and development of pain and other symptoms. The gain did not contribute to the formation of the symptoms, therefore, but now contributes to the maintenance of the illness and potentially to resistance toward treatment. In psychoanalytic theory, *primary gain*, by contrast, relates to the intrapsychic motivation that led to symptom formation in the first place, such as the need or wish to assume the sick role and to feel both cared for and taken care of, thereby keeping an internal conflict, such as fear of inadequacy or failure, out of awareness.[11]

Secondary gain refers to interpersonal gratifications that, when enjoyed through the sick role, make recovery less appealing. The sympathy and concern of family and friends, preferential treatment, disability benefits, drugs, interpersonal domination, the increased comfort of a socially sanctioned change in role, and the avoidance of certain activities may all be considered forms of secondary gain. Whereas primary gain unfolds intrapsychically, secondary gain tends to manifest in an interpersonal context. A third complication is frequently the presence of *tertiary gain*, which is wholly external to the patient but consists of the benefits derived by family or other caretakers from reinforcing the patient's pain behaviors.[35] The suppression of marital or familial conflict, material benefit, and the reallocation of power within the family are among the more frequently cited tertiary gains in the economy of family dynamics. Because these unconscious motives on the part of family members can have a huge impact on the treatment of the patient and because family members can often be enlisted as allies in treatment, family meetings or, in some cases, ongoing family therapy may prove necessary to the successful psychotherapeutic management of the patient with chronic pain.[36]

According to the strict psychoanalytic scheme, secondary gain follows primary gain, which makes it more accurately applied to instances of somatoform disorders, such as conversion and somatization. In reality, the individual obtains certain gains with any illness, and unconscious secondary gain can develop in the aftermath of actual physical injury or disease just as easily. Identifying what a patient gains and loses—secondary losses, such as loss of a satisfying job, livelihood, and prestige—can be critical, both to the diagnosis and to treatment and recovery.[11] For this reason, the medical and legal scrutiny of secondary gain is frequently given great emphasis in cases of chronic pain, and it is frequently left to a psychiatric evaluation and a psychodynamic approach to treatment to attempt to discern conscious from unconscious motivations and to distinguish instances of malingering, factitious disorder, and primary somatization from the more expectable somatizing complications occurring around physical injury or illness.[37]

Where the medical and legal determination of disability is concerned, strong evidence of primary gain can, nevertheless, point toward a disabling condition but may change the focus of diagnosis and treatment from medical to psychological. In some cases, the effect of this shift is to exculpate employers, insurance carriers, and other litigants from any legal responsibility for compensation or even treatment. For this reason, evidence of premorbid psychopathology is often of as great an interest, legally, as whether the sum total of secondary gains outweighs the apparent secondary losses. As with the problem of measuring pain itself, there is no empirically verifiable method of accurately and reliably determining the presence or influence of primary or secondary gain in any individual's case, but the domain of inquiry can often be approached only through psychodynamic and supportive interventions when the patient's welfare is the prime concern.

A number of difficulties with the traditional concept of secondary gain have called both the concept and its utility into question. Given the obvious problem of trying to discern what is conscious from what is unconscious, some clinical researchers favor definitions of secondary gain that do away with the distinction and focus instead on behaviors that *appear* as if the patient is seeking some expression of gain.[35] This promotes a more operational definition and opens the way to empirical investigation, but it begs the clinical question of how to approach secondary gain that is genuinely unconsciously motivated. For patients who cannot seem to make significant progress in managing their pain through behavioral and cognitive-behavioral psychotherapy and techniques, an insight-oriented approach may prove the only avenue open to influencing their level of motivation.

SUPPORTIVE PSYCHOTHERAPY

Although psychodynamic psychotherapy tends to place the reward on insight and interpretation of unconscious conflicts, the emphasis in supportive psychotherapy is on the strengthening of ego functions and improved adaptation.[38] The psychotherapist's understanding of the patient remains psychodynamic, but the interventions are crafted to improve the patient's level of functioning in at least two critical dimensions: first, to enhance the patient's capacity for reality testing—in effect, to anticipate what others see, when they encounter him or her, and to develop a self-observing capacity for monitoring his or her own reactions and motivations—and, second, to bolster the patient's healthiest psychological defenses and emotional and intellectual resources in the service of adjusting to a new set of circumstances.

The first and often necessary step in this process for many patients with chronic pain is the experience of feeling understood, usually achieved through the opportunity to tell their story to a sympathetic listener whom they perceive to be in the helping role. What patients know best and typically wish to discuss most urgently is the social, emotional, and behavioral impact of their pain on their lives. Even when they make no connection or outright deny any influence of these factors on the development and maintenance of their physical symptoms, patients need to feel that their suffering is validated and the circumstances of their misfortune are fully appreciated by their providers. When the patient begins to trust this inchoate alliance, often made possible by the supportive efforts of psychotherapeutic management by the entire team, the collaborative development of a rationale for psychotherapy may ensue.[39]

The major shift enabled by supportive psychotherapy and the reason why it is frequently a necessary prerequisite step to any other psychotherapeutic intervention lies in its approach to moving patients from a purely mechanistic understanding of their dilemma to one in which they can consider assuming an active role in their own recovery and rehabilitation. Patients whose explanatory models of pain are deterministic or who are unaware of the influence of secondary gain often insist on medical interventions in which they may remain passive. By enhancing their capacity for reality testing, supportive psychotherapists can assist patients in coming to see their own stress reactivity and toward beginning to appreciate their involvement in the pain–stress cycle.

Few patients would deny that their pain is *one* of, if not *the* greatest source of stress in their lives, and this simple acknowledgment is often the beginning of a psychoeducational breakthrough. For many patients, this shift heralds their becoming more sophisticated in their understanding of the physiology and psychology of pain and in their appreciation of the differences between pain and injury, hurt and harm. At that point, many are willing to move ahead by working with a psychotherapist toward developing strategies to make the most of their own strengths and resources for coping with stress and managing pain.

OPERANT-BEHAVIORAL THERAPY

Operant-behavioral therapy (OBT), which has its origins in learning theory, refers to the group of interventions focused principally on the observed behavior of the patient. In the operant model of pain, the reinforcing role of social and environmental factors in the development and maintenance of pain through observed pain behaviors is identified, with the behaviors themselves being targeted for intervention. This approach may prove most effective when patients demonstrate little understanding of the relationship between their pain behaviors and the underlying physiologic damage or disease,[40] and it is especially useful in cases in which the subjective experience of pain appears to go well beyond any established organic basis to the point where secondary gain has become an obvious issue and persistent, often dramatic, pain behaviors have emerged.

The goal of OBT is to encourage the development and practice of more adaptive pain management strategies by establishing and reinforcing new "wellness" behaviors while discouraging or reducing the expression or reinforcement of "illness" or pain behaviors.[7] Thus, increased self-reliance, activity, and socialization are encouraged, and repetitive verbal complaints, grimacing, social isolation, and overreliance on family and caretakers are discouraged. As a form of psychotherapeutic management, OBT is not limited to the setting of individual or group psychotherapy but is usually most effective when supported by the entire team of providers, whether in the setting of office visits, physical therapy sessions, telephone contacts, or walk-in encounters.

The basis of OBT suggests that both wellness and pain behaviors can be shaped—developed, increased, reduced, or extinguished—according to the principles of operant conditioning. Whereas reinforcement increases the likelihood that behaviors will occur, punishment or the withdrawal of reinforcement decreases the likelihood of their occurrence. When attention from a provider or family member, for example, is offered solicitously in response to the patient's facial grimacing, there is immediate reinforcement, ensuring that this pain behavior will recur and possibly become habitual. When reinforcement is withdrawn—when the behavior no longer elicits the sought-after attention—it will decrease and possibly extinguish.

Similarly, when the patient experiences an exacerbation of pain after an increase in activity, the exacerbation itself can serve to punish any motivation toward self-reliance and the development of wellness behaviors. Finding reinforcements that can modulate or offset the negative consequences of increased activity can encourage the patient to adopt wellness behaviors even at the cost of some discomfort. Again, because what occurs at the clinic or psychotherapist's office is a comparatively small sampling of behavior, encouraging the patient's consistency of motivation—through supportive interventions and his or her family's participation in family meetings—will result in the most successful outcome. In severe or poorly tractable cases—in which it is apparent that setting limits and assisting the patient in the development of more adaptive responses on an outpatient basis is failing—an inpatient pain program, in which the highest level of operant control is possible, may become necessary.

Whether outpatient or inpatient, individual or group, informal or structured, a variety of OBT techniques can be adapted to the patient's particular situation, including (1) pacing and graduated activity, (2) scheduling and tapering of pain medications, and (3) social reinforcement.[7] Because these techniques of operant conditioning are common to the interventions of a broad range of behavioral and psychotherapeutic approaches to the management of pain, they can be used as a milieu therapy or as an adjunct to supportive and cognitive-behavioral interventions. On the minutest of levels, no physician, nurse, or psychotherapist can sit with a patient for long without reinforcing some responses and discouraging others with as small an intervention as a facial expression, gesture, or well- or poorly chosen word.[41]

COGNITIVE-BEHAVIORAL THERAPY

Of all the psychological therapies applied to the problem of chronic pain, none has received more attention or been more thoroughly researched than CBT, the treatment introduced by Aaron Beck in the 1960s.[42,43] Because of this—as well as its strong evidence-based efficacy for a variety of pain conditions, such as low back pain, headaches, arthritis, orofacial pain, and fibromyalgia—it is sometimes referred to as the "gold standard" of psychotherapeutic care for patients with chronic pain.[44]

Whereas OBT may be considered a core behavioral therapy, basic to all programs of pain management, CBT has more specific psychotherapeutic goals and is usually undertaken in the formal setting of individual or group psychotherapy, whether outpatient or inpatient. CBT is directed toward changing patients' maladaptive responses to chronic pain by examining and posing alternatives to the thoughts, attitudes, and beliefs underlying them, as well as by encouraging the acquisition of new coping skills and techniques to take their place. CBT usually includes a range of behavioral components, most notably, relaxation training and keeping a pain diary; however, the emphasis is placed on modifying emotional and behavioral responses, those that tend to affect the patient's level of functioning adversely, by challenging and restructuring their cognitive underpinnings.

The focus of CBT, therefore, is on the development of self-control and self-regulation.[45] The work of treatment is often undertaken in a threefold stepwise progression, including (1) a psychoeducational phase, (2) a skills-building phase, and (3) an application phase,[7] with each phase roughly corresponding to a new milestone in self-regulation and a new stage in the patient's readiness for change.[25] In CBT, the goal is the establishment of a higher level of functioning, which the patient is now motivated to sustain and has developed the skills to maintain. In the process, the patient becomes more resilient to the comorbid development of anxiety and depression, increasing his or her perception of pain as a controllable or manageable experience.

The first or psychoeducational phase of CBT is designed to enlist the patient's efforts as an active participant in his or her own recovery and rehabilitation. It is here that what is often referred to as the *mind–body* model of understanding pain is introduced to the patient. Concepts such as stress reactivity and the pain–stress cycle are presented in such a way as to assist the patient in the identification of thoughts, attitudes, and beliefs that tend to make his or her pain less tractable and his or her suffering more severe. These self-defeating cognitions typically develop under the influence of anxiety, misinformation, secondary gain, and poorly resolved intrapsychic conflicts and often lead to depression and feelings of worthlessness, hopelessness, and helplessness. When a patient believes, "I'll never be able to work or provide for my family or have a normal life with this pain," despair cannot be far behind. Yet most patients come to treatment with a personalized array of such poorly examined and unchallenged cognitions.

The second, or skills-building, phase of CBT is designed to develop cognitive strategies enabling the patient to recognize the negative impact of his or her self-defeating cognitions and replace them with self-affirming statements, emphasizing control and adaptive coping. When a patient believes, "I have faced many problems, and I can handle this one, too," or, "I may not be able to do everything I want, but I can do much more than I previously thought," the motivation for rejecting pain behaviors, nurturing wellness behaviors, and raising the level of activity and social interaction becomes apparent. The cognitive restructuring techniques used in CBT not only help patients to recognize those thoughts, attitudes, and beliefs about their pain that make them feel stuck but also encourage the systematic substitution of more stable and positive ones that are likely to facilitate treatment across all modalities, from medications and procedures to physical and complementary therapies.

Part of the skills-building phase may also be devoted to the acquisition of other supportive coping strategies, such as stress management, anger management, assertiveness training, relaxation training, and pacing. Most of these techniques are used in the service of identifying and modifying the patient's response to those environmental, interpersonal, and intrapsychic triggers that increase autonomic arousal and musculoskeletal tension and adversely affect the subjective experience of pain. Relaxation training, in particular, offers a broad range of behavioral techniques designed to quiet the autonomic nervous system and relieve musculoskeletal rigidity and tension. Various forms of meditation, autogenic training, guided imagery and visualization, and self-hypnosis, as well as yoga and even Tai Chi, have been used successfully in pain management programs, with the National Institutes of Health favorably reviewing the empirical data in support of the efficacy of relaxation techniques in the treatment of chronic pain.[46,47]

Biofeedback is another psychoeducational and training device that allows the patient to monitor his or her ongoing progress at developing an effective regimen of relaxation techniques. During a biofeedback session, the patient is connected by surface (skin) electrodes or receptors to an electronic or computerized instrument designed to measure, amplify, and *feed back* physiologic information to the patient and psychotherapist or technician.[48,49] The latter, in turn, assists the patient to refine and increase the efficacy of one or more relaxation techniques to counteract the effects of dysponesis (i.e., maladaptive compensatory bracing in response to pain) and autonomic overarousal.[50] By monitoring the level of musculoskeletal tension through surface electromyographic leads and the level of autonomic activity through measures of heart rate, blood pressure, blood-volume pulse wave amplitude, skin temperature, oxygen saturation, and electrodermographic response, patients can see firsthand the extent to which they are having success at gaining control through the practice of regular and disciplined relaxation over processes that they previously thought were unmanageable. There is sufficient and still growing evidence, including multiple meta-analyses, to suggest that biofeedback monitoring in conjunction with behavioral therapy is an effective treatment in a number of chronic pain conditions, including migraine headache, tension-type headache, disorders of intestinal motility, musculoskeletal pain (including low back pain), and Raynaud's disease.[44,48,51]

There is also growing interest in its application as a psychoeducational tool applied to nociceptive desensitization in patients who have become so highly sensitized to pain and other noxious sensations that their pain perception appears to have an augmented affective component or heightened emotional intensity.[52] In this category, we find patients who are suffering from what may represent limbically augmented pain syndromes (the LAPS hypothesis) characterized by pain that is frequently out of proportion to clinical findings and associated with neurovegetative problems and disturbances of mood.[44,53] This group includes patients who have fibromyalgia, chronic fatigue syndrome, certain types of visceral and headache pain, chronic regional pain syndromes, and phantom pain. In a Cochrane review of psychotherapeutic treatments for chronic orofacial pain, for example, CBT alone or in combination with biofeedback training was shown to be useful, in some cases, by assisting patients to countercondition sensations of pain with sensations of relaxation, warmth, and well-being, thereby ameliorating pain intensity and depression and pain-related interference with activity.[54]

Biofeedback can also help patients to move toward the third or application phase of CBT in which their newly acquired collection of cognitive skills, behavioral techniques, and coping strategies develops into a more enduring and adaptive approach to pain management. CBT concludes, then, as patients learn to apply their skills and maintain their new outlook in progressively more challenging situations.[7] In this way, it becomes not merely a collection of tools or techniques, but also a template for successfully adjusting to the ongoing intrusion of chronic pain. Patients who have successfully completed courses of CBT often refer to it as though they have undergone a change in lifestyle in which relaxation exercises and pacing have become as second nature as eating breakfast and brushing one's teeth.

COMPLEMENTARY TECHNIQUES

Three additional techniques or therapeutic approaches are often undertaken in the attempt to enhance pain management, whether applied on their own or combined with other individual psychotherapies in an eclectic treatment. These are (1) hypnosis; (2) eye movement desensitization and reprocessing (EMDR); and, of more recent origin, (3) contextual cognitive-behavioral therapy (CCBT), the last of which includes acceptance and commitment therapy (ACT) and mindfulness-based therapies.

Whether hypnosis can play an effective first-line role in the management of chronic pain remains controversial, largely owing to the lack of standardization of hypnotic interventions and the typically small size of the clinical trials.[55,56] As a technique for inducing genuine analgesia, it is applied far more often in the management of acute and surgical pain, and many practitioners see its principal worth in addressing chronic pain as simply that of evoking the relaxation response. For patients who cannot master meditative techniques or comfortably use progressive muscle relaxation, self-hypnosis can become an essential skill in the management of musculoskeletal tension and autonomic overarousal. In the case of patients with chronic pain who have used hypnosis—whether hypnotherapy with a practitioner or self-hypnosis—to achieve analgesic relief from exacerbations or flare-ups or who use it regularly for time-limited relief or respite, additional and better designed studies are needed to discern the generalizability and applicability of the techniques used.[57]

Eye Movement Desensitization and Reprocessing (EMDR) is a comparatively new addition to the panoply of psychotherapeutic approaches to the management of pain, but its role in facilitating the cognitive processing of physical and emotional trauma associated with the origin of chronic pain is already promising. EMDR was developed as a precise technique, which, similar to hypnosis, requires specialized training for the practitioner.[58] Although compatible with psychodynamic and cognitive-behavioral approaches, its techniques are directed toward the evocation of the patient's capacity for rapid information processing to facilitate the processing of traumatic or dysfunctional thoughts and feelings.

The goal of this approach is to disengage affective memories that may be linked to pain through remembered or associated experience but not to the specific situation giving rise to pain in the present. By detaching or releasing these affective memories, EMDR restores the affective dimension of pain to a level more consonant with the actual situation giving rise to the pain. In effect, similar to the goal of psychodynamic psychotherapy, the result of EMDR is to separate past from present trauma, allowing the patient to process what were heretofore overwhelming emotions, focus on his or her present dilemma, and move forward in his or her recovery and rehabilitation.[58-60] A recent review concluded that patients with chronic pain who were treated with EMDR reported significant improvement in pain intensity, reduced disability, and improvement in depressive symptoms, although the comparatively small number of studies selected for inclusion provided insufficient evidence for treatment recommendations.[61] The possible applications of EMDR to limbically augmented pain syndromes are nevertheless compelling, but as with hypnosis, additional study is needed to discern the generalizability and criteria for applying the technique in cases of chronic pain.

Acceptance and Commitment Therapy (ACT), dialectical behavior therapy (DBT), functional analytic psychotherapy, and mindfulness-based cognitive therapy are approaches to treatment under the broad umbrella of CBT and are sometimes referred to as contextual cognitive behavioral therapies or the "third wave" of behavioral therapies.[62] Each poses a variant set of guiding principles, where the relationship between thinking and feeling is concerned, as well as a template for achieving improved psychological adjustment. A recent meta-analytic review of some of these approaches to treatment suggested that mindfulness-based stress reduction programs and ACT are not superior to CBT but can offer a good alternative.[63] In so doing, the emphasis has turned, more recently, toward a shift in the process of development—one toward facilitating the introduction of new treatment methods guided by process and theory while paring away the approaches that have ceased to be useful.[64] This trend, in turn, is lending vitality and infusing a spirit of exploration to CBT, which has not seen much innovation in recent years despite the continual replication of positive but comparatively modest treatment effects.

GROUP PSYCHOTHERAPY

The formal practice of conducting group psychotherapy with medically ill patients is nearly a century old.[65] In the first recorded groups of this nature, the leaders—usually medical personnel—instructed patients on the medical aspects of their illnesses and encouraged them to present weekly reports to groups regarding their medical and spiritual progress.[66] The goal of these groups was to help patients cope more adaptively with their illnesses by addressing issues of self-confidence, self-esteem, and physical well-being,[67] and what began with patients with tuberculosis was soon extended to groups for patients with other illnesses, including asthma, cancer, irritable bowel syndrome, skin disorders, and chronic pain.

Participation in groups offers a variety of advantages for patients with chronic pain. Group psychotherapy tends to be more affordable than individual treatment for both patients and health insurance carriers, and there is increasing evidence that participation in a group reduces the number of visits and telephone calls to physicians, further relieving strain on the medical care system.[68] Far more important, however, the effectiveness of group psychotherapy in the reduction of the psychological and physical distress accompanying chronic medical illness is well documented,[67,69] and patients with a broad range of medical illnesses demonstrate improved compliance, decreased physical symptoms, decreased symptoms of anxiety and depression, and increased self-esteem.[70,71]

In the treatment of patients with chronic pain, three approaches have emerged as dominant: support groups, psychodynamic groups, and structured cognitive-behavioral or behavioral medicine groups.[72] Considerable evidence suggests that groups with a strong CBT or behavioral medicine component are the most effective,[7,67] but despite their differences in theory of approach and intervention, all three models share a range of common goals for treatment. Group psychotherapy can offer patients with chronic pain (1) validation of their experience, (2) increased self-esteem, (3) decreased social isolation, (4) opportunities to express frustration appropriately and practice assertiveness, (5) enhanced reality testing through opportunities to compare experiences with others, (6) a sense of satisfaction from helping others, (7) education about the pain–stress cycle and other psychosocial and medical factors involved in chronic pain, (8) the acquisition of a new set of coping skills, (9) encouragement for the development of more adaptive strategies for stress and pain management, and (10) reduction in symptoms.

SUPPORT GROUPS

The most popular and numerous groups for patients with chronic pain are support groups, which are frequently led by patients themselves and are often affiliated with patient- and volunteer-staffed organizations, as opposed to medical clinics, hospitals, or professional personnel. Many of the virtual support groups, electronic bulletin boards, and chat rooms of the various online services may be included in this category. Their emphasis is on providing social and emotional support for their members, as well as a forum for sharing medical information, but they often lack the specific goals of acquiring new coping skills and developing more adaptive stress and pain management strategies. In certain situations, they can also promote the spread of misinformation and lend uncritical endorsement to maladaptive strategies for pain management.

Although support groups can be effective for many patients who would otherwise have little opportunity to compare their experiences with those of others and seek validation, the cohesiveness and continuity of these groups may suffer from a lack of direction or supervision. A number of factors can spark disagreements among members and lead to fragmentation of the group, including erratic attendance by some members; differences in need, level of functioning, and interpersonal skills; dominance of the discussion by stronger personalities; and differences in perceived goals. Having an assigned lay leader or even a skilled professional leader may not rule out all of these pitfalls, but it will likely ensure greater cohesion and longevity of purpose and direction.

PSYCHODYNAMIC GROUPS

Less structured than cognitive-behavioral groups, psychodynamic group psychotherapy in the setting of chronic pain has as its goal the creation of an interpersonal laboratory in which communications among the members can be examined within the dynamics of the group.[73] By observing, analyzing, and interpreting how each member relates to the group, the group's leader—always a professional mental health specialist—can assist each member, as well as enlist each member's help in assisting the others, to come to a better understanding of how chronic pain is affecting his or her relationships, social and occupational functioning, outlook on the world, and self-esteem. As with individual psychodynamic psychotherapy, the goal is to make the unconscious basis of conflicts and maladaptive defensive strategies more accessible to each member by examining the interpersonal impact that each member has on the group.

The psychotherapist in the psychodynamic group uses interventions designed to foster connections among the members and facilitate the give and take of the members' reactions to one another. The use of maladaptive defenses or the adoption by one of the members of self-defeating or interpersonally destructive choices are examples of behaviors that are typically challenged by the psychotherapist and other group members. To consolidate these insights and therapeutic gains, the psychotherapist often articulates the themes and shared struggles of the group in an effort to move the members toward (1) a more realistic appreciation of their situations and the impact of their communications on others; (2) a greater reliance on their own natural resources and strengths; and (3) the acquisition of new behaviors and patterns of communication, reflecting more adaptive strategies for coping and more functional and health-affirming choices.

COGNITIVE-BEHAVIORAL MEDICINE GROUPS

Behavioral medicine and *mind-body medicine* are terms often used to describe a model of care that addresses the effects of stress on a disease or symptom, as well as the stress of chronic illness on the individual patient. Treatment according to this model addresses the biologic, psychological, and social issues, not just the biomedical ones, with the mode of intervention being CBT. In effect, behavioral medicine groups are highly structured, time-limited CBT groups directed toward specific populations of medical patients, such as patients with chronic pain. The varieties of intervention can include any or all of the techniques one would find in individual CBT, including relaxation training—meditation, autogenic training, hypnosis, self-hypnosis, guided imagery and visualization, and even yoga or Tai Chi—cognitive therapy, pacing activities, and keeping a pain diary.

Behavioral medicine has traditionally involved a multidisciplinary effort that recognized and supported the synergy created by bringing together professionals in *both* mind *and* body to focus their expertise on the treatment of medical problems, such as cardiovascular disease, cancer, and chronic pain. Such collaboration has produced considerable research in the clinical efficacy of these combined treatments and in the cost effectiveness of offering them to patients.[74] Behavioral medicine distinguishes itself from psychiatry and psychology by attending principally to the physical symptoms of patients and their effects on stress, coping, and emotions, as well as the effects of stress, coping, and emotions on the experience of physical symptoms. If psychopathology proves to be a determining factor in a particular patient's expression of physical symptoms, then that patient is referred to psychiatric providers; however, many depressed, anxious, and even personality-disordered patients with chronic pain nevertheless benefit from participation in behavioral medicine groups along with their psychiatric care.

Applications of Behavioral Medicine Groups to Chronic Pain In October 1995, the National Institutes of Health convened a Technology Assessment Conference to consider the integration of behavioral and relaxation approaches into the treatment of chronic pain and insomnia.[46] The consensus panel concluded that there were sufficient data to recommend the inclusion of CBTs in the treatment of chronic pain. In a review of the relevant research, the panel cited a range of findings—including that all six of six factors identified in the correlation of treatment failures of low back pain are psychosocial—and recommended the integration of relaxation techniques with conventional medical procedures as a *necessary* step in the successful treatment of chronic pain.

Cognitive-behavioral skills can benefit the majority of patients experiencing chronic pain because the emphasis is on the pain–stress cycle—both the stressful effects of pain and the effects of stress on pain. Groups can, therefore, be composed of patients with different diagnoses or etiologies of pain if there are not sufficient members for a single diagnostic group. Mixing diagnoses, furthermore, may actually have advantages because patients come to realize that the experience of pain has universal features, qualities, and consequences. This realization frequently leads, in turn, to the inevitable comparisons patients make between their circumstances, often accompanied by the observation, "Things could be worse!" One of the principal advantages of group over individual psychotherapy is the power of the experience of validation that comes from sharing a common crisis in one's life with others who have similar experiences. That experience of psychosocial support has been shown repeatedly to have a significant positive influence on patients' coping and the course and outcome of disease.[75]

A further advantage is that the format of the behavioral medicine group can be adapted to small or large numbers of patients, depending on whether the model is largely psychoeducational or more psychotherapeutic. Whereas psychoeducational models can accommodate groups of up to 25 or 30 patients, psychotherapy groups are generally limited to 6 to 10. The format of behavioral medicine groups is flexible enough, in most cases, to adjust to the needs of the setting, the credentials of the providers or leaders, and the mechanism of reimbursement. Some models even incorporate the use of patients who have previously "graduated" from the group—or who have received special training—as assistant facilitators or, with ongoing professional supervision, even as lay providers, conducting groups largely on their own.[76]

Goals and General Format of Behavioral Medicine Groups Behavioral medicine groups are applied to the problem of chronic pain with three specific goals: to assist patients with (1) mastering skills for both stress and pain management, (2) mobilizing those skills routinely but especially during periods of increased stress and pain, and (3) developing self-efficacy—the belief and attitude that engaging in certain behaviors will reach a desired outcome. Encouraging patients to set and discuss the goals they hope to achieve in the group can help them to identify unrealistic expectations and engage them in taking the first steps toward the development of self-efficacy.

Ideally, the recommendation to participate in a cognitive-behavioral group is part of a coordinated multidisciplinary treatment plan formulated after a comprehensive evaluation of the patient. There have been many attempts to predict the attributes associated with the successful completion of behavioral medicine groups, but only a few trends—and multifactorial ones, at that—have been identified.[77] In general, patients who are psychologically or cognitively impaired or who exhibit disruptive behaviors or who are nonambulatory are at greatest risk for failing to enter treatment or for attrition from a group they have begun, but patients who demonstrate high motivation and a collaborative approach to their own medical care tend to have a high rate of completion.

Group leaders or providers may come from a variety of disciplines, including physicians, psychologists, social workers, nurses, and physical therapists, but essential criteria for their success tend to be that they (1) enjoy working with the chronic pain population, (2) have training in group therapy and group dynamics, and (3) recognize the strong influence of learned helplessness on patient compliance. A setting with pleasant surroundings and comfortable chairs, as well as mats for exercising and lying down, is most conducive to learning when patients are in pain, and a schedule of weekly meetings that last 1½ to 2 hours does not overtax most patients' capacity for attention and endurance even if reduced by the presence of pain. Most behavioral medicine groups run for 8 to 10 weeks, which appears to cover the critical period necessary for the three phases of successful CBT: (1) psychoeducation, (2) skills building, and (3) application and maintenance.[7]

There is considerable latitude in the content of sessions, the order of presentation, and the forms of presentation. In most sessions, the time will be divided into several components, with periods allocated for (1) presentation of new instruction; (2) supervised practice of developing skills, such as relaxation techniques; (3) presentation and discussion of homework, such as pain diaries and checklists of daily relaxation exercises; and (4) stretching and mild exercise or yoga. There are many curricula designed specifically for behavioral medicine groups with chronic pain patients available in commercially published workbooks.[78,79] A brief description of the content proposed by one of

TABLE 20-1 Format of a Schedule of Sessions in a Behavioral Medicine Group

Session 1	
Understanding	Pain psychoeducation on the pathophysiology of pain, presentation of a rationale for acute and chronic pain therapies, and review of the program's content
	Members may invite a guest to this initial session.
Session 2	
Mind–Body Connection	Instruction on relaxation techniques and breathing exercises
	Pain puts stress on the body, and many people in pain experience multiple symptoms of stress, as well as pain. Relaxation techniques assuage the harmful effects of prolonged stress on the body and mind. Techniques specific to pain management are introduced during succeeding sessions.
Session 3	
Body–Mind Connection	Instruction on exercise, pleasurable activities, pacing, and body awareness
	Patients with chronic pain make two frequent errors: (1) they cut off awareness of body sensations and become "numb" to signals that might allow them to pace themselves adequately, and (2) they stop "moving" so that deconditioning contributes to dysfunction.
Session 4	
Body–Mind Connection and Nutrition	Review of patients' observations on pacing and exercise and instruction in the role of nutrition in chronic pain
	Good nutrition promotes good health and may assist in the management of pain.
Session 5	
Power of the Mind	Introduction to basic cognitive therapy strategies: (1) identification of negative automatic thoughts and the cognitive distortions behind them and (2) reframing them into more realistic thoughts and attitudes
	Many patients with chronic pain find their coping skills challenged to the point of being overwhelmed. Cognitive restructuring offers them greater flexibility and a way out of their anxiety, anger, and depression.
Session 6	
Adopting Healthy Attitudes	Instruction in the uses of empathy and humor, as well as the adoption of "stress-hardy" attitudes
	Patients' negative thoughts come from old cognitive-behavioral "tapes" applied inappropriately to new situations. Through the adoption of healthy attitudes, they need not suffer twice—with pain and negative emotional responses.
Session 7	
Effective Communication I	Review and role play of effective communication skills
	People frequently do not say what they mean, with the result that conflicts emerge that were often never intended. Patients are encouraged to understand what their intentions are when they see their health care providers and to make their internal conflicts, expectations, and assumptions more consciously accessible.
Session 8	
Effective Communication II	Instruction on making statements match intent and review of the three styles of communication: passive, aggressive, and assertive
	When patients know what they want and begin to repair their self-esteem from the damaging effects of chronic pain, adopting an appropriate style of communication can support their new attitudes and help them to resolve previous conflicts.
Session 9	
Effective Problem Solving	Instruction in problem solving as an aid to setting goals
	Many people are ineffective at setting goals, especially when an emotional "hook" is in conflict with the goal. The goal of losing weight, for example, may be in conflict with the feeling that food is the only means of comforting oneself. Patients in pain have difficulty accomplishing goals because the wish to be able to do what they used to do gets in the way. Learning to separate goals from hooks is the first step toward problem solving more adaptively and effectively.
Session 10	
The End of the Beginning	Review of all the new coping skills acquired and how to use them during exacerbations of pain
	The final discussion focuses on relapse prevention and how patients can consolidate and maintain their new, more adaptive strategies for stress and pain management.

Adapted Data from Caudill MA. *Managing Pain Before It Manages You.* 3rd ed. New York: Guilford Press; 2008.

these workbooks for 10 sessions of a group for patients with chronic pain is presented in **Table 20-1**.[78]

Research has demonstrated that patients with chronic pain who participate in multidisciplinary programs with behavioral medicine groups feel less anxious, less depressed, and less pain while simultaneously experiencing greater control, increased socialization, and a heightened sense of self-efficacy.[80,81] Patients exposed to CBT programs also appear to rely on the medical system more appropriately, reducing the number of clinic visits and telephone contacts made out of frustration and fear.[8,68,76,82-84] One patient summarized her experience of her participation in a behavioral medicine group, capturing the essence of the therapeutic goals, when she said, "I know it's going to be a good day because *I know how to make it a good day.*"[78]

SUMMARY

The goal of psychotherapeutic management of chronic pain is not merely the reduction of pain but the restoration of functioning. The patient with chronic pain will always face limitations, but assisting him or her toward more successful adjustment and more adaptive strategies for coping is the role of psychotherapy in the multidisciplinary approach to pain. Successful psychotherapeutic management involves not only a multidisciplinary approach but also an interdisciplinary effort in which the interventions of each member of the team of providers can be seen as having a psychotherapeutic impact on the patient, as well as a complementary effect on the interventions of the other providers. Assessing the degree to which any patient is stress reactive and addressing his or her own unique expression of the pain–stress cycle may involve the application of one or more types of individual or group psychotherapy. An eclectic approach tends to offer the greatest versatility, but CBTs, whether individual or group, have demonstrated the greatest efficacy with the chronic pain population.

REFERENCES

1. Merskey A, Bogduk N. Task Force on Taxonomy of the International Association for the Study of Pain. *Classification of chronic pain: descriptions of chronic pain syndromes and definition of pain terms.* Seattle: IASP; 1994.
2. Turk DC, Flor H. Chronic pain: a biobehavioral perspective. In: Gatchel RJ, Turk DC, eds. *Psychosocial Factors in Pain: Critical Perspectives*. New York: Guilford Press; 1999:18-34.
3. Jacobson L, Mariano AJ, Chabal C, et al. Beyond the needle: expanding the role of anesthesiologists in the management of chronic non-malignant pain. *Anesthesiology*. 1997;87:1210-1218.
4. American Medical Association. Pain. In: Cocchiarella L, Andersson GB, eds. *Guides to the Evaluation of Permanent Impairment*. 5th ed. Chicago: American Medical Association; 2000:565-592.
5. Gatchel RJ, Peng YB, Peters ML, et al. The biopsychosocial approach to chronic pain: scientific advances and future directions. *Psychol Bull*. 2007;133:581-624.
6. Ashburn MA, Staats PS. Management of chronic pain. *Lancet*. 1999;353:1865-1869.
7. Scascighini L, Toma V, Dober-Spielmann S, et al. Multidisciplinary treatment for chronic pain: a systematic review of interventions and outcomes. *Rheumatology*. 2008;47:670-678.
8. Gatchel RJ, Okifuji A. Evidence-based scientific data documenting the treatment and cost-effectiveness of comprehensive pain programs for chronic non-malignant pain. *J Pain*. 2006;7:779-793.
9. Giordano J, Schatman ME, Hover G. Ethical insights to rapprochement in pain care: bringing stakeholders together in the best interest(s) of the patient. *Pain Physician*. 2009;12:E265-275.
10. Weiner R. Chronic pain and stress. In: Margoles MS, Weiner R, eds. *Chronic Pain: Assessment, Diagnosis, and Management*. Boca Raton, FL: CRC Press; 1999:203-208.
11. Eisendrath SJ. Psychiatric aspects of chronic pain. *Neurology*. 1995;45(Suppl):26-34.
12. Gallagher RM. Treatment planning in pain medicine. *Med Clin North Am*. 1999;83:823-849.
13. Melzack R. Pain and stress: a new perspective. In: Gatchel RJ, Turk DC, eds. *Psychosocial Factors in Pain: Critical Perspectives*. New York: Guilford Press; 1999:89-106.
14. Gatchel RJ, Dersh J. Psychological disorders and chronic pain: are there cause-and-effect relationships. In: Turk DC, Gatchel RJ, eds. *Psychological Approaches to Pain Management: A Practitioner's Handbook*. 2nd ed. New York: Guilford Press; 2002:30-51.
15. Arnow BA, Hunkeler EM, Blasey CM, et al. Comorbid depression, chronic pain, and disability in primary care. *Psychosom Med*. 2006; 68:262-268.
16. Sadock BJ, Sadock VA. *Kaplan and Sadock's Synopsis of Psychiatry: Behavioral Sciences/Clinical Psychiatry*. 10th ed. Baltimore: Lippincott Williams & Wilkins; 2007.
17. Bair MJ, Robinson RL, Katon W, et al. Depression and pain comorbidity: a literature review. *Arch Intern Med*. 2003;163:2433-2445.
18. Miller LR, Cano A. Comorbid chronic pain and depression: who is at risk? *J Pain*. 2009;10:619-627.
19. Vaccarino AL, Sills TL, Evans KR, et al. Prevalence and association of somatic symptoms in patients with major depressive disorder. *J Affect Disord*. 2008;110:270-276.
20. Eimer BN, Freeman A. *Pain Management Psychotherapy: A Practical Guide*. New York: John Wiley & Sons; 1998.
21. Weisberg JN. Personality and personality disorders in chronic pain. *Curr Rev Pain*. 2000;4:60-70.
22. Lumley MA, Asselin LA, Norman S. Alexithymia in chronic pain patients. *Compr Psychiatry*. 1997;38:160-165.
23. Clays E, De Bacquer D, Leynen F, et al. The impact of psychosocial factors on low back pain: longitudinal results from the Belstress study. *Spine*. 2007;32:262-268.
24. American Psychiatric Association. *Diagnostic and Statistical Manual of Mental Disorders*. 5th ed (DSM-5). Washington, DC: American Psychiatric Association; 2013.
25. Prochaska JO, Norcross JC, DiClemente CC. *Changing for Good*. New York: William Morrow; 1994.
26. Kroenke K, Krebs EE, Bair MJ. Pharmacotherapy of chronic pain: a synthesis of recommendations from systematic reviews. *Gen Hosp Psychiatry*. 2009;31:206-219.
27. Gatchel RJ, Turk DC. Interdisciplinary treatment of chronic pain patients. In: Gatchel RJ, Turk DC, eds. *Psychosocial Factors in Pain: Critical Perspectives*. New York: Guilford Press; 1999:435-444.
28. Grzesiak RC, Ury GM, Dworkin RH. Psychodynamic psychotherapy and chronic pain patients. In: Gatchel RJ, Turk DC, eds. *Psychological Approaches to Pain Management: A Practitioner's Handbook*. New York: Guilford Press; 1996:148-178.
29. Sollner W, Schussler G. Psychodynamic therapy in chronic pain patients: a systematic review. *Z Psychosom Med Psychother*. 2001;47:115-139.
30. Danese A, Moffitt TE, Pariante CM, et al. Elevated inflammation levels in depressed adults with a history of childhood maltreatment. *Arch Gen Psychiatry*. 2008;65:409-415.
31. Davis DA, Luecken LJ, Zautra AJ. Are reports of childhood abuse related to the experience of chronic pain in adulthood? A meta-analytic review of the literature. *Clin J Pain*. 2005;21:398-405.
32. Taylor GJ. The challenge of chronic pain: a psychoanalytic approach. *J Am Acad Psychoanal Dyn Psychiatry*. 2008;36:49-68.
33. Beck JG, Clapp JD. A different kind of comorbidity: understanding posttraumatic stress disorder and chronic pain. *Psychol Trauma*. 2011;3:101-108.
34. Mayou R, Bryant B. Outcome in consecutive emergency department attenders following a road traffic accident. *Br J Psychiatry*. 2001;179:528-534.
35. Fishbain DA. Secondary gain concept: definition problems and its abuse in medical practice. *APS J*. 1994;3:264-273.
36. Margoles MS. Chronic pain is a family problem. In: Margoles MS, Weiner R, eds. *Chronic Pain: Assessment, Diagnosis, and Management*. Boca Raton, FL: CRC Press; 1999:65-81.
37. Fishbain DA, Rosomoff HL, Cutler RB, et al. Secondary gain concept: a review of the scientific evidence. *Clin J Pain*. 1995; 11:6-21.
38. Rockland LH. *Supportive Therapy: A Psychodynamic Approach*. New York: Basic Books; 1989.
39. Wootton RJ. Supportive dynamic and existential psychotherapy. *J Cancer Pain Symptom Palliation*. 2005;1:73-78.

40. Sanders SH. Operant conditioning with chronic pain. In: Gatchel RJ, Turk DC, eds. *Psychological Approaches to Pain Management: A Practitioner's Handbook*. New York: Guilford Press; 1996:112-130.
41. Birk L. Cognitive behavior therapy and systemic behavioral psychotherapy. In: Nicholi AM Jr, ed. *The Harvard Guide to Psychiatry*. 3rd ed. Cambridge, MA: Belknap Press of Harvard University; 1999:497-524.
42. Wootton J, Warfield C. Cognitive therapy for chronic pain. In: Smith H, ed. *Current Therapy in Pain*. Philadelphia: Saunders Elsevier; 2008:521-525.
43. Winterowd C, Beck AT, Gruener D. *Cognitive Therapy with Chronic Pain Patients*. New York: Springer; 2003.
44. Ehde DM, Dillworth TM, Turner JA. Cognitive-behavioral therapy for individuals with chronic pain. *Am Psychol*. 2014;69:153-166.
45. Bradley LA. Cognitive-behavioral therapy for chronic pain. In: Gatchel RJ, Turk DC, eds. *Psychological Approaches to Pain Management: A Practitioner's Handbook*. New York: Guilford Press; 1996:131-147.
46. National Institutes of Health Assessment Panel. Integration of behavioral and relaxation approaches into the treatment of chronic pain and insomnia. *JAMA*. 1996;276:313-318.
47. Wootton RJ. Meditation and chronic pain. In: Audette J, Bailey A, eds. *Integrative Pain Medicine: The Science and Practice of Complementary and Alternative Medicine in Pain Management*. Totowa, NJ: Humana Press; 2008:195-209.
48. Turk DC, Swanson KS, Tunks ER. Psychological approaches in the treatment of chronic pain patients—when pills, scalpels, and needles are not enough. *Can J Psychiatry*. 2008;53:213-223.
49. AAPB Web site Public Information Area. About Biofeedback. Available at: http://www.aapb.org/i4a/pages/index.cfm?pageid=3463. Accessed April 11, 2014.
50. Devine DA. Psychological and behavioral management approaches to chronic pain. In: Margoles MA, Weiner R, eds. *Chronic Pain: Assessment, Diagnosis, and Management*. Boca Raton, FL: CRC Press; 1999:195-202.
51. AAPB Web site Public Information Area. Disorders and Treatment. Available at: http://www.aapb.org/i4a/pages/index.cfm?pageid=3404. Accessed April 11, 2014.
52. Danforth DA. Biofeedback. In: Warfield CA, Fausett HJ, eds. *Manual of Pain Management*. 2nd ed. Philadelphia: Lippincott Williams & Wilkins; 2002:334-339.
53. Rome H, Rome J. Limbically augmented pain syndrome (LAPS): kindling, corticolimbic sensitization, and convergence of affective and sensory symptoms in chronic pain disorders. *Pain Med*. 2000;1:7-23.
54. Aggarwal VR, Lovell K, Peters S, et al. Psychosocial interventions for the management of chronic orofacial pain. *Cochrane Database of Systematic Reviews*. 2011;11;Art. No. CD008456;DOI:10.1002/14651858CD008456.pub2.
55. Schoenberger NE. Research on hypnosis as an adjunct to cognitive-behavioral psychotherapy. *Int J Clin Exp Hypn*. 2000;48:154-169.
56. Elkins G, Jensen MP, Patterson DR. Hypnotherapy for the management of chronic pain. *Int J Clin Exp Hypn*. 2007;55:275-287.
57. Webb AN, Kukuruzovic R, Catto-Smith AG, et al. Hypnotherapy for treatment of irritable bowel syndrome. *Cochrane Database of Systematic Reviews*. 2007;4; Art No. CD005110;DOI:10.1002/14651858.CD005110.pub2.
58. Shapiro F. *Eye Movement Desensitization and Reprocessing (EMDR): Basic Principles, Protocols, and Procedures*. 2nd ed. New York: Guilford Press; 2001.
59. New York Times Blog. Expert Answers on EMDR. Available at http://consults.blogs.nytimes.com/2012/03/16/expert-answers-on-e-m-d-r/. Accessed April 9, 2014.
60. EMDR Institute, Inc. EMDR Evaluated Clinical Applications. Available at http://www.emdr.com/general-information/clinical-applications.html. Accessed April 9, 2014.
61. Tesarz J, Leisner S, Gerhardt A, et al. Effects of eye movement desensitization and reprocessing (EMDR) treatment in chronic pain patients: a systematic review. *Pain Med*. 2014;15:247-263.
62. Ost LG. Efficacy of the third wave of behavior therapies: a systematic review and meta-analysis. *Behav Res Ther*. 2008;46:296-321.
63. Veehof MM, Oskam MJ, Schreurs KM, et al. Acceptance-based interventions for the treatment of chronic pain: a systematic review and meta-analysis. *Pain*. 2011;152:533-542.
64. McCracken LM, Vowles KE. Acceptance and commitment therapy and mindfulness for chronic pain. *Am Psychol*. 2014;69:178-187.
65. Lonergan EC. *Group Intervention: How to Begin and Maintain Groups in Medical and Psychiatric Settings*. New York: Jason Aronson; 1982.
66. Stern MJ. Group therapy with medically ill patients. In: Alonso A, Swiller HI, eds. *Group Therapy in Clinical Practice*. Washington, DC: American Psychiatric Press; 1993:185-199.
67. Spira J. Understanding and developing psychotherapy groups for medically ill patients. In: Spira J, ed. *Group Therapy for Medically Ill Patients*. New York: Guilford Press; 1997:3-51.
68. Hellman CJ, Budd M, Borysenko J, et al. A study of the effectiveness of two group behavioral medicine interventions for patients with psychosomatic complaints. *Behav Med*. 1990;16:165-173.
69. Locke SE, Chan PP, Morley DS, et al. Behavioural medicine group interventions for high-utilising somatising patients. *Dis Manage Health Outcomes*. 1999;6:387-404.
70. Goodman B. Group therapy for medically ill patients. In: Halperin DA, ed. *Group Psychodynamics: New Paradigms and New Perspectives*. Chicago: Year Book Medical; 1989:107-124.
71. Compton A. Emotional distress in chronic medical illness: treatment with time-limited group therapy. *Mil Med*. 1992;157:533-535.
72. Keefe FJ, Beaupre PM, Gil K. Group therapy for patients with chronic pain. In: Gatchel RJ, Turk DC, eds. *Psychological Approaches to Pain Management: A Practitioner's Handbook*. New York: Guilford Press; 1996:259-282.
73. Levine JB, Irving KK, Brooks JD, et al. Group therapy and the somatoform patient: an integration. *Psychotherapy*. 1993;30:625-634.
74. Friedman R, Sobel D, Myers P, et al. Behavioral medicine, clinical health psychology, and cost offset. *Health Psychol*. 1995;14:509-518.
75. Hafen B, Frandsaen K, Karen K, et al. *The Health Effects of Attitudes, Emotions and Relationships*. Provo, UT: EMS Associates; 1992.
76. Lorig KR, Mazonson PD, Holman HR. Evidence suggesting that health education for self-management in patients with chronic arthritis has sustained health benefits while reducing health-care costs. *Arthritis Rheum*. 1993;36:439-446.
77. Turk DC, Rudy TE. Neglected factors in chronic pain treatment outcome studies—referral patterns, failure to enter treatment, and attrition. *Pain*. 1990;43:7-25.
78. Caudill MA. *Managing Pain Before It Manages You*. 3rd ed. New York: Guilford Press; 2008.
79. Thorn BE. *Cognitive Therapy for Chronic Pain*. New York: Guilford Press; 2002.

80. Thorn BE, Kuhajda MC. Group cognitive therapy for chronic pain. *J Clin Psychol.* 2006;62:1355-1366.

81. Guzman J, Esmail R, Karjalainen K, et al. Multidisciplinary bio-psycho-social rehabilitation for chronic low back pain. *Cochrane Database of Systematic Reviews.* 2002;1;Art. No. CD000963;doi:10.1002/14651858.CD000963.

82. Caudill MA, Schnable R, Zuttermeister P, et al. Decreased clinic use by chronic pain patients: response to behavioral medicine intervention. *Clin J Pain.* 1991;7:305-310.

83. Chou R, Huffman LH. Nonpharmacologic therapies for acute and chronic low back pain: a review of the evidence for an American Pain Society/American College of Physicians clinical practice guideline. *Ann Intern Med.* 2007;147:492-504.

84. Young LD, Bradley LA, Turner RA. Decreases in health care resource utilization in patients with rheumatoid arthritis following a cognitive behavioral intervention. *Biofeedback Self Regul.* 1995;20:259-268.

Mind/Body Interventions in the Management of Chronic Pain

Daniel Rockers

SCIENCE

MECHANISMS OF MIND–BODY THERAPIES

In the field of Western medicine, we still do not fully grasp how and why many pain conditions develop—why a scanner gun dropped on a foot caused complex regional pain syndrome (CRPS) or why an imaging study failed to show structural evidence of lumbar pain. We also do not fully grasp why some develop a pain condition and others do not—surely many scanner guns have been dropped on many feet without the development of CRPS, and there exist many lumbar imaging studies that show deformation with no experienced pain condition.

There remains much that we do not know about many pain conditions, suggesting that there are portions of our explanatory medical model that are either not adequate or not yet clarified. The expanding interest and research findings in mind–body therapies speak to some of the gaps in the model of Western medicine.

To its credit, inductive experimentalism has yielded quite a number of cures and treatments. But the cost of this advancement was a necessary split in conceptualizing body as separate from the mind. In the scientific age, the mind has been considered a source of error for empirical studies, that is, the effects are contaminants to the "real" findings and must be parceled out. But we are beginning to see a reintegration of the mind into experimentalism—the mind as an independent variable in research studies. Whether it is research in the modulation of gene expression by psychosocial cues,[1] children learning to voluntarily increase oxygen perfusion in tissue,[2] or knowledge of how state-bound memories and experiences manifest somatically,[3,4] it is clear that mind–body therapies represent something real and progressive, even if not completely understood.

In this chapter, we examine some current mind–body therapies that are being used in the treatment of chronic pain. Some are well researched in terms of their efficacy and effects; some are hardly understood in their mechanisms of action. They mark a departure from the norm of medical treatments, and it may be for this reason that they are becoming increasingly popular. More and more, patients are rejecting modern pharmacologic approaches in favor of naturalistic treatments. They are seeking therapies that are holistic and self-empowering.

MIND–BODY THERAPY DEFINED

The National Center for Complementary and Alternative Medicine (NCCAM) defines mind and body medicine as focusing on the interaction among the mind, body, brain, and behavior, with the intent of using the mind to help establish health. Here we are concerned with therapies that can be used to help deal with pain conditions, including hypnosis, biofeedback, meditation, and relaxation, as well as some Eastern therapies such as Tai Chi and Qi Gong.

AVENUES OF ACTION

Mind–body therapies are thought to produce effect in a number of ways. Here we classify three main groupings for understanding the mechanism of dealing with pain: (1) analgesia, (2) psychological healing, and (3) physical healing. We will consider each in turn.

Analgesia Analgesia is probably the most used and recognized method of dealing with pain in the mind–body approach. The ultimate goal is to decrease sensations of pain. Whatever structural abnormalities that might perpetuate the pain problem will remain, but the task in the therapy is to alter conscious perception in some way or another.

One way this can be accomplished is through the psychological process of dissociation, or splitting off, of streams of consciousness. Hilgard and colleagues[5-7] in a series of interesting hypnosis studies discovered the existence of a "hidden observer" in his subjects. When hypnotized and given suggestions of analgesia, there remained a nonconscious pain-experiencing aspect that could be communicated with. So although the conscious aspect of the individual reported analgesia, the nonconscious part indicated a pain level. This finding also correlated with the physical body showing signs of distress when pain was applied, such as increased heart rate.

Another avenue of decreasing pain sensation is what happens in various forms of relaxation. By inducing a general state of relaxation—a "good" feeling—the organism is less susceptible to the experience of pain. Another way of stating this is that whereas positive states decrease pain perception, negative mood states increase pain perception. Neuroanatomically, this ability is related to descending inhibitory tracts from brainstem to spinal junctures, modulated by serotonin and noradrenaline. This is the "pain gate"; in terms of "mind–body," it is the "body" part.

Psychological Healing This area deals with pain caused by what are called psychosomatic issues. Freud called it conversion; others call it somatization. Regardless of the name, in this section, we are concerned with how emotions, stress, and conflicts have been transduced into physical symptoms of pain. Here we will refer to it as psychosomatic.

"Psychosomatic" has acquired something of a pejorative tone in medicine, probably because it is poorly understood as an entity. Psychosomatic pain is no less real (to the experiencer) than pain of physical deformation, neuropathology, or inflammation. But in psychosomatic cases, the "pain generator" is not viewable through any of our current imaging technologies, which makes it difficult to diagnose. In addition, there is somehow less nobility attached to pain that is rooted in psychological conflict. Finally, patients are often resentful if a professional suggests that the pain may have psychological origins; it is easily interpreted as "it's all in your head." Yet it is nonetheless real as a pain experience.

Case 1 Jeremy presented with a lack of mobility bilaterally in his arms, in concert with generalized pain and episodic worsening, seemingly at random. Jeremy also had posttraumatic stress. Two years earlier, the crane he operated had tipped over; the outriggers failed while the crane boom was extended with load. In relaxation training, he noticed the pain increasing in his arms and was encouraged to attend to it. As he paid more attention to the specific sensations, he went back in time to the actual moments of the fall and crash. He recalled raising his arms to block his fall as the crane tipped. After the relaxation, he remembered his bracing against a part of the cab. He realized how his apparently random worsening of the pain was connected with stress and fears surrounding the incident. Remaining therapy consisted of working through unprocessed emotions connected to his pain. For example, his loss of bowel control during the incident did not fit with the "strong" culture of crane operators. With his memory brought to consciousness and the education that loss of bowel and bladder control was a common reaction in trauma, he was able to regain some of his mobility and to find relief from his pain.

For Jeremy, his pain was inextricably bound within a physiological state connected with the extreme of the trauma situation. In such instances, the memories are encoded within the state itself; the biological milieu *is* the memory and the state. Rossi explains how state-bound memories—memories and experiences encoded in a particular physiological state—exert influence in a number of ways, including pain. Because these state-dependent memories exist in an environment that is not the same as the conscious mind in everyday life, they therefore cannot ordinarily be addressed by the conscious mind. Mind–body therapies can provide access to such states, thereby opening a door for healing.

Physical Changes A growing body of evidence supports the idea that actual physical healing occurs from the mind and that changes in consciousness make alterations at the physical level. The most basic route includes making outward behavioral changes such as exercising, doing yoga, or changing one's diet. Stress often equates with negative health behaviors, such as increased alcohol and drug intake, decreased exercise, and so on. This is a behavioral level of mind–body healing. Although dismissed by many, engaging in such behaviors is very important in patients with chronic pain who suffer from the stress of loss of autonomy, loss of efficacy, depression, and so on. Making positive change—that is, getting better sleep, exercise, making healthier choices, and so on—is related to immunologic changes.[8]

At a more intricate level than basic behavioral changes, making physiological changes includes skeletal muscle relaxation, peripheral vasodilation, or reductions in blood pressure. These are frequently done in the mind–body therapies of biofeedback and relaxation training. They also can occur in hypnosis through suggestion and metaphor, as well as in meditation, yoga, and Tai Chi.

The most involved level of mind–body healing (at the current state of our knowledge) is exemplified by remarkable healing case studies such as Norman Cousins self-healing from ankylosing spondylitis[9] or Klopfer's 1957 account of the case of Mr. Wright. This account describes a man diagnosed with terminal lymphosarcoma and tumor masses the size of oranges. In an incredible account, after injection of an inert substance, the masses "melted" within days, and he became ambulatory and energetic.

We recognize these changes in a phenotypical manner, and it may seem that the morphologic changes themselves are the "miracle." But the real miracle—the basis of such changes—occurs in a genotypical fashion: at the molecular and genetic levels.

AN EXPANDED VIEW OF MIND–BODY HEALING

At present, we do not understand such mechanisms of mind-body healing well enough to know how to reproduce them at will (from intention to manifestation), but we are beginning to understand them, some in rough outline form and others in more detail. Much work has been done in the area of psychoneuroimmunology (PNI), for example. Studies of the effects of "allostatic load"—the cumulative effects of long-term exposure to stress, along with the body's ability to respond—demonstrate changes in hypothalamic–pituitary–adrenal (HPA) axis and immune functioning.[10] Negative emotions, such as stress, anxiety, and depression, can up- or downregulate the production of proinflammatory cytokines implicated in chronic pain conditions such as arthritis.[11,12] In addition, this dysregulation then further inhibits immune responses. The loop feeds on itself, so disrupting such cycles is important for the pain practitioner and patient.

Going beyond PNI, Ernest Rossi,[4] in *The Psychobiology of Mind-Body Healing,* outlines routes of mind–body healing, including the autonomic nervous system, endocrine system, and neuropeptide system.

TABLE 21-1 Mind–Body Healing by Physiological System

Physiological System	Messenger Molecules	Function
Autonomic nervous	Neurotransmitters	Regulates SNS and PNS
Endocrine	Hormones	Metabolic processes
Immune	Cytokines	Signals white blood cells, mood, motivation
Neuropeptide	Neuropeptides	Modulates CNS, PNS, and sense organs

CNS, central nervous system; PNS, peripheral nervous system; SNS, sympathetic nervous system.

He emphasizes that all of these are avenues of information transfer, and although some of it is via nervous system, all of it involves messenger molecules such as neurotransmitters, hormones, cytokines, or peptides. In other words, according to this paradigm, all biologic, psychological, and physiological processes are essentially information processing systems, interacting with and influencing the others (**Table 21-1**).

The importance of these findings is that collectively they present the picture that psychology and physiology are tightly bound together, and the dividing line is less clear than was once thought. Event perception and meaning is traceable on the path through the HPA axis, distress or depression regulates production of cytokines, and emotions and stress are expressed through changes in gene regulation.[4,13] More than ever before, the picture that begins to emerge—and this is one of the highlights of mind–body therapies—is that there is much that can be done of personal accord, which has significant health effects.

PRACTICE

HYPNOSIS (TABLE 21-2)

***Case* 2** Lydia's search for medical relief of her pelvic pain of 12 years' duration had left her bitter and resentful. In the initial interview, she was suspicious of the pain psychologist and answered few questions herself, letting her husband field most of them. She was depressed and anxious, stayed inside most of the day, and had no friends. Her only pain relief was her husband massaging her perineal area for 30 minutes every night. Many physicians had tried to help her with her pain, but the outcome was always the same. Lydia was introduced to hypnosis through basic relaxation methods, a cautious approach. In this way, she developed a skill of being able to find hypnotic trance easily. Her hypnotic treatment included posthypnotic suggestions, as well as ideomotor signaling. Soon she brought into treatment her realization of the beginning of her pelvic pain: after a prior relationship in which she had been anally raped on a repeated basis. She had accepted this abuse in exchange for financial security for herself and her son. She was able to exit the relationship and moved across the country in order to begin again. However, the move was disruptive for her son, and he took up drugs; left behind the idea of responsibility; and blamed her, her past relationship, and the cross-country move. As she brought up these conscious realizations, her talking through this helped her to recognize the no-win situation she was in and the connection between her trauma and her pain. She also acknowledged her guilt for moving, which (she believed) caused her son's difficulties. Over a period of weeks, her pain began to subside. Not long after, when she terminated therapy, she was getting involved in community activities, making new friends, and considering returning to work.

TABLE 21-2 Mind–Body Therapies—Hypnosis

Hypnosis			
Therapy	Key Concept	Method	Note
Hypnosis	Uses unconscious processes for physiological or perceptual change	Uses linguistic structures, metaphors, and suggestion to reach unconscious mind	Deep "trance" is not required for success in hypnosis

In the clinical vignette, Lydia was first trained in methods of relaxation, and she became adept at developing deep relaxation. Because of this, her attention, or focus, could be guided fairly easily through metaphors and suggestions. Building the relationship over time and going slow allowed her to build trust in the therapist, which meant that she no longer felt the excessive need to defend through suspicion (judging and monitoring). Still, prior abusive experiences were never directly asked about but were indirectly referenced through posthypnotic suggestions as something that might be helpful in therapy. In this way, she was able to develop a sense of control (the root of her problem) yet was also able to bring it up for the necessary processing.

Common Elements of Hypnosis Hypnosis is a unique mind–body therapy in that it can provide a route for the therapist to communicate with deeper, unconscious structures of the mind of the patient. Although there exists great debate about exactly what hypnosis is, for purposes of the current discussion we adhere to the following common elements reported by Don Price:[14]

1. Sense of relaxation
2. Sustained and absorbed focus
3. Absence of judging, monitoring, and censoring
4. Suspension of usual orientation to time and place
5. Automaticity of response

In the development of hypnotic trance, the above steps each tend to lead to the next. We generally start by some kind of relaxation, which provides an important background for becoming focused. Sustained focus helps lead to a decrease of conscious judging and monitoring. This judging, monitoring, and censoring is a hallmark of conscious mind and includes psychological defense mechanisms. Although these function as personality and protective mechanisms, they also can contribute to an individual's pain problem. One of the goals in hypnosis is to bypass this defended, censoring capacity. The first three steps combined lead to a suspension of orientation in time and location, as well as automaticity of response. Suspension and automaticity contribute to the sense of hypnotic depth.

Response Automaticity as a Critical Element Automaticity in response can occur in patients in a number of different ways, including physical automaticity of response (ideomotor, e.g., fingers move by themselves, or ideosensory, e.g., physical sensations occur, cognitive, or imagery). In Case 2, Lydia experienced ideosensory automaticity through a reduction in her pain symptoms acutely in response to each of the hypnosis sessions.

One aspect of automaticity is that it provides an opening for the introduction of suggestion: usually some kind of analgesia, sensory substitution, or some alteration of sensation. As it is suggested, the patient can experience it as being "automatically" carried out within the body. Another important aspect is that it can provide a means of communicating with unconscious aspects of the individual through ideomotor signaling.

Ideomotor Signals from the Unconscious Ideomotor signaling is the use of a patient's unconscious stereotyped movement patterns to communicate with the unconscious. This can include nervous mannerisms, or everyday movements such as nodding one's head in agreement. Probably the simplest is to use finger signals for yes and no. Ideomotor signals are a good example of the automaticity, noted earlier in the list of characteristics of hypnosis. They are not conscious volitional movements; the patient experiences them as coming from "somewhere else." The value of ideomotor signaling in pain control is that it can be used to uncover and work with intrapsychic conflicts that have somatized, or it can be used as a means of requesting help from the unconscious mind with analgesia.[3] Other related methods include ideosensory signaling—the development of sensations instead of motor signals—and automatic writing, which is the ability of the subject to use the stereotyped movements of writing as an unconscious communication process.

BIOFEEDBACK (TABLE 21-3)

Biofeedback means self-regulation of physiology. The most common modalities include skin temperature, heart rate, electroencephalography, breathing, and sudomotor response. Some of these are the same as what is used in a traditional "lie detector" test because these physiological measures are quite responsive to psychological states. In this section, we review a specific type of feedback, heart rate variability (HRV), but the general principles apply to all types.

Learning Self-Regulation To learn how to self-regulate physiology in biofeedback, we usually use a sensitive instrument to measure the physiological aspect of interest. There are sensors for measuring sweat from eccrine glands in the glabrous skin of the palms, temperature sensors for thermal biofeedback, heart rate monitors, and so on. A computer usually reports the feedback to the patient in an audio or visual format. Through this feedback, control is learned (i.e., the patient tries out different ways of breathing or thinking about certain things). Although autonomic functions are not normally thought to be volitionally controllable, most are, with practice. In fact, surprising levels of control are possible; in electromyographic (EMG) feedback, for instance, it is possible to learn to control the firing of a single motor unit—one single nerve fiber within a bundle of nerve fibers.[15,16] This type of mind–body control typically is beyond what we usually think is possible.

Because no instrument exists to measure pain levels, there is no way to directly operate on pain through biofeedback. What we do instead is to operate on physiological parameters which, when activated, tend to reduce levels of suffering and tension. We create an environment that is incompatible with pain.

Normal Sinus Arrhythmia as Biofeedback A specific type of biofeedback, HRV is concerned with the oscillation in the interval between consecutive heartbeats. Although cardiac automaticity is specific to the heart's pacemaker tissues, the rate is under sympathetic and parasympathetic influence.[17] Central in mind–body therapy is the connection between emotions, thoughts, and the nervous system; HRV is sensitive to emotions and thoughts as shown in this case study.

***Case* 3** The anxiety of daily life was too much for Vasily. Although he had a good job in real estate, he worried all the time—would he still have a job tomorrow, was his girlfriend true to him, and so on. His worries and anxiety consumed him so much that his telephone time was taking away from his work, his girlfriend was feeling smothered by his incessant checking and suspicion, and his back pain was now making it difficult to drive for more than 15 minutes without stopping to stretch. Vasily was taught about the connection between tension and pain and how anxiety and excessive thoughts affected pain conditions. He was trained in HRV biofeedback. Especially helpful was the day when he was doing well in relaxation, but then jealous concerns about his girlfriend crept into his mind, and he saw how the graphing function immediately changed. He understood the mind–body connection at that point.

Biofeedback Is a Tool, Not a Treatment Often the value of biofeedback resides as much in the process as in the direct changes to physiology. This is exemplified in Vasily's case as well as in the case of Lydia in the hypnosis vignette. With respect to Vasily, biofeedback was able to demonstrate undeniably that his thoughts affected his physiology and helped with progress checkpoints. When patients are able to see and experience

TABLE 21-3 Mind–Body Therapies—Biofeedback

Biofeedback			
Therapy	**Key Concept**	**Method**	**Note**
Biofeedback	Conscious control of involuntary physiology	Present ongoing physiological parameter (e.g., heart rate or temperature); information to conscious mind	No instrument can measure pain directly; all biofeedback processes work indirectly for pain

for themselves that they can voluntarily effect changes in their physiological (thought to be outside of conscious control) body, they become believers.

Becoming a believer means developing a sense of agency (self-efficacy). In doing so, the individual establishes a sense of control (information control), which is helpful when facing an ongoing stressor such as chronic pain.[18] An additional benefit is that with this sense of control and belief, the individual is likely to persist in efforts now that he or she knows that change is possible. This is important in learning new skills such as self-regulation, meditation, or self-hypnosis.

Because the value of biofeedback is at least twofold in the above-mentioned senses, the goal to be obtained by biofeedback is important. This means that the clinician must understand what is to be done and generate the mechanism. In addition, the practitioner must possess adequate knowledge of any medications the patient might be taking because they often affect autonomic functions. For example, beta-blockers and calcium channel blockers regulate the heart rate so that HRV biofeedback becomes meaningless; there is very little variability to work with. Opiates and benzodiazepines can decrease emotional reactivity, synonymous with physiological reactivity.

RELAXATION (TABLE 21-4)

While studying hypnosis in the early part of the 20th century, the German psychiatrist Johannes Heinrich Schultz was studying hypnotic depth when he found that in deep relaxation, patients typically reported two sensations: heaviness and warmth. From there he developed "autogenic training," which is a set of suggestions designed to elicit the feelings of heaviness and warmth, thereby achieving deep relaxation without the need for any hypnotic induction. Schultz, along with Wolfgang Luthe, authored a set of volumes covering autogenic therapy in detail.[19-24]

Elmer Greene, in the 1960s, studied autogenics and biofeedback at the Menninger Institute in Topeka, Kansas.[15] He wrote a fascinating account of their research studies and provided examples of different relaxation strategies and approaches. For his studies, he created a "short form" of autogenics, which is quite brief and easy to use.

Autogenic Training Example

1. My feet feel heavy and relaxed.
2. The backs of my legs and the joints of my hips are relaxed and quiet.
3. The whole central portion of my body is relaxed, relaxed, and warm.
4. My hands feel warm.
5. My arms and hands feel heavy and warm.
6. My shoulders feel heavy and relaxed. They droop from my body.
7. My forehead is cool.

Sensations in Autogenics and Other Relaxation Modalities The heaviness that patients often experience results from the deep muscle relaxation. This is the same sensation that results from a long massage or after sitting in the hot tub. When measured with EMG, the muscles at this point can actually be electrically silent.[15] The warmth that is experienced in autogenics and other forms of relaxation is the effect of peripheral vasodilation and is most commonly experienced in the hands. This is probably because of the extensive enervation in the hands (consider the sensory homunculus), which allows for better control.

The effects of relaxation are generally not limited to just pain but occur systemically. For example, a meta-analysis showed positive effects of autogenics for tension headache, migraine headaches, somatoform pain disorder (unspecified type), and Raynaud's disease, anxiety, and mild to moderate depression.[25]

Jacobsonian Relaxation Is Progressive Progressive muscle relaxation (PMR), also known as Jacobsonian relaxation, is a type of relaxation in which muscle groups are progressively (and gently) tensed and relaxed. The subject is instructed to focus minutely on the sensations of muscle tension, and on the resulting sensations of muscle relaxation. The subject learns slight sensations of muscle contractions, as well as healthy relaxed muscle sensations.[26] PMR is fairly widely used and has shown effect for different kinds of pain, including osteoarthritis[27] and cancer pain.[28]

Breathing as Relaxation Breathing is a relaxation modality. It is an integral part of mind–body therapies, including meditation, Qi Gong, Tai Chi, yoga, and biofeedback. It is referred to as deep breathing, diaphragmatic breathing, and effortless breathing.[29] Although easy to dismiss as a therapeutic modality—"I think I know how to breathe; I've been doing it all my life"—specific techniques are used. Common to all is attention to depth; rate; and coordination of intercostal, chest, neck, and shoulder muscles. Breathing is unique in that it is both a voluntary and involuntary function. As an involuntary function, it signals to the conscious mind the state of organismic affairs—consider the short gasps of a panic attack. But breathing can also be used as a voluntary function. For example, in Qi Gong, breathing is to be "deep, slender, long, and soft" to help regulate one's energy.

MEDITATION: CALMING THE MONKEY MIND (TABLE 21-5)

***Case* 4** With the removal of a spinal abscess resulting in ongoing neuropathic pain bilaterally in the lower extremities, 35-year-old Gene was interested in learning meditation to help deal with his pain. He noted that when he was first detoxing from alcohol in the past, his mind was "going a thousand directions at once," and it still seemed that way. He needed pain control so he could resume working, and he wanted to take some trips (by car or plane) with his wife, something he had not been able to do since his surgery 4 years ago. We began with some basic relaxation skills so he could first experience some of the sensations of how it feels to have a calm mind. He was educated in ego processes and in ways of working with the mind (i.e., to gently move it in a direction without force). In addition, he learned ways of developing his awareness by doing small mental exercises throughout the day. After a few months of regular practicing, Gene took his first extended car trip with his wife, planned and took a 4-hour plane trip, and finally took an overseas vacation with his wife. At termination of therapy, he stated that he "had great success with dealing with his pain from practicing meditation." In a follow-up interview 6 months after termination of treatment, Gene had returned to work part time and was planning an even longer overseas vacation.

Meditation deals directly with the mind and consciousness. As shown in Case 4 the idea of ego is also an important part; this concept reflects the sense of autonomy so prevalent in consciousness.

TABLE 21-4 Mind–Body Therapies—Relaxation

Relaxation			
Therapy	**Key Concept**	**Method**	**Note**
Relaxation	Calm the body by direct intention and "passive" action (letting go)	Bring attention to body parts, and "allow" (not force) a letting go of tension	Simple and effective; techniques can be done almost anywhere, anytime

TABLE 21-5 Mind–Body Therapies—Meditation

Meditation			
Therapy	**Key Concept**	**Method**	**Note**
Meditation	Calm the body by calming the mind	Train patient to focus attention; notice when mind "jumps track" and refocus, persistently	Meditation is simple in explanation but quite challenging in execution

This sense of autonomy is also what makes dealing with the mind so challenging. Consider: is the autonomous a part of me, or is it me? In meditation, this issue is central as self-awareness and control of cognitive activity is developed. In addition, the moving meditations of Tai Chi and Qi Gong emphasize the detection, movement, and balance of internal energies.

Important in nearly all mind–body therapies but especially in meditation is the idea of progress through incremental steps. In Case 4, the patient was cautioned early in the treatment that small progress steps should be considered significant. This is important because many people mistakenly think that they can simply change brain–mind processes quickly and easily. This generally is not the case. Mind processes should be thought of as a strong habit that has been practiced for many years. Changing such a habit takes time and effort.

How to Let Go of the Monkey Meditation is known mostly from religion and spiritual circles. Each of the major world religions provides direction on some type of meditative approach. Meditative techniques, whether mindfulness or concentrative, help to quiet cognitive discursiveness and strengthen awareness. Transcendence of the ego (not being reflexively compelled, self-identified) is then possible. In spiritual circles, the ego is considered to be the self-created barrier between the self and the divine (whether it is God, Allah, Buddha nature, the Force, and so on). Through meditative techniques, one can go beyond that barrier. How to do it? It is simple. From a Taoist text:

> Let this monkey go.
> Let the senses go.
> Let desires go.
> Let conflicts go.
> Let ideas go.
> Let the fiction of life and death go.
> Just remain in the center, watching.[30]

However, the simplicity of the approach is deceptive because the execution is challenging, and as noted earlier, it takes regular practice. The essence of meditation is cessation of thought (cognitive, discursive process) and maintenance of awareness. Essentially, it is achieved through a disciplining of the mind. Individuals without a pain condition find this difficult enough, but a pain condition that continually sets off an alarm for attention adds to the challenge.

Mindfulness Probably the best known mindfulness meditative treatment for chronic pain is the Mindfulness Based Stress Reduction (MBSR) program by Jon Kabat-Zinn. MBSR emphasizes the development of present-moment awareness, as well as looking directly into one's own thoughts and thought processes. The spiraling causation cycle of thoughts, breath, body sensations, and emotions is detected, and by playing the role of observer, one can break from the cycle. The program is well known and widely practiced and has been implemented successfully in a number of pain management programs. It has demonstrated positive results in individuals with pain.[31,32]

Relaxation Response Herbert Benson developed the Relaxation Response from investigating a number of Eastern meditation styles. He distilled four basic elements of meditation: the use of a "mental device," a quiet place, a passive attitude, and a comfortable position. Benson's Relaxation Response has been shown helpful for a variety of conditions, including arthritis, chronic pain, and headache.

Tai Chi and Qi Gong In Western medical conceptions, it is the physiological disruption that is diagnosed as an illness. For example, we see depression as a deficit of serotonin or norepinephrine. Another conceptualization might view the physiological disruption as a symptom and the root cause being generated from another system. This is the model that is adhered to in traditional Chinese medicine, for example (**Table 21-6**).

TABLE 21-6 Mind–Body Therapies—Traditional Chinese Medicine

Traditional Chinese Medicine			
Therapy	**Key Concept**	**Method**	**Note**
Tai chi	Balance qi energy through movement and focus	Moving meditation through a set of postures and movements	Well suited for chronic pain because movements are slow, and balance is developed
Qi Gong	Balance qi energy through meditation	Meditation	

In traditional Chinese medicine, there are 12 main channels of qi energy that run through the body. Physical disease is a manifestation of blockage or imbalance of such energies. Diagnosis is made by the examination of certain parts of the body—the eyes, the skin, and pulse—looking for signs of energy disruption. Treatments are methods of rebalancing the energy and include acupuncture, acupressure, massage, herbal treatments, meditation, and Qi Gong. In acupuncture, fine-gauge needles are used to inhibit or facilitate flow of energy; acupressure is the application of pressure to certain areas of the body to accomplish the same purpose.

Qi Gong is the intentional development and manipulation of one's energy field; this energy field is affected by thoughts, feelings, activities, food, and lifestyle.[34] With respect to treating pain, it usually refers to a meditative type of energy manipulation. This manipulation can be internal—done singularly—or it can be external—performed on the patient by an experienced practitioner.

A review of internal (self-directed) Qi Gong pain management studies failed to show significant results but also noted that randomized controlled trials (RCTs) were few and lacked quality controls.[35]

In contrast, a systematic review of external Qi Gong (i.e., not self-directed, meaning they were applied by another) showed significant effect.[36] It is important to keep in mind that not many RCTs exist for such treatments, and they are usually applied without stratified or selected pain conditions. Not enough comprehensive quality studies exist at this point to suggest efficacy.

Tai chi, as popularly known in the West, is a type of moving meditation consisting of forms of sets of postures and movements. Often characterized by slow movement, Tai Chi emphasizes the development and balancing of qi. Tai chi is considered a martial art and can be learned for either self-defense or for health. Tai chi is a good form of exercise for those with chronic pain because it can help develop strength and balance and includes gentle movements. Positive effects are noted for fibromyalgia[37] and musculoskeletal pain.[38] More studies are needed for Tai Chi as well.

MOVING FORWARD

The history of medicine begins with shamanistic or religion-based approaches that view disease pathogenesis from the perspective of animated energies and spirits and was often causal in terms of the individual's actions. Because of this, treatments were associated with certain beliefs, rituals, and customs; they were embedded within a cultural context.

The context of modern medicine is much less personal; the focus is on the physiological disruption in the individual, and causal factors are seen in the biology of the individual. Current sentiment, however, is seeking some type of more personal aspect; witness the growth of complementary and alternative medicines. In some ways, mind–body medicine represents a positive return to causality in terms of an individual's actions. That is, the patient wants to know "what can I do about this?" This parallels the current trend toward self-empowerment and holistic approaches.

As mind–body approaches become more popular, more research and understanding are needed for each of the therapies. We know little about alternative conceptualizations of disease and disease processes, hardly realizing that our medical approaches are in some ways ethnocentric. In itself, that is not a problem. But there remain a number of pain conditions that we do not fully understand, and for which we do not have solid, efficacious treatments. Perhaps this is because the conditions straddle the line between mind and body, psyche and soma, and psychology and medicine. Maybe what is needed is an updated conceptualization that incorporates both, explains symptoms, and directs treatment. Regardless, mind–body therapies are gaining in popularity. The increased use of such therapies benefits both physicians and patients.

REFERENCES

1. LLoyd D, Rossi E. *Ultradian Rhythms in Life Processes: A Fundamental Inquiry Into Chronobiology and Psychobiology*. New York: Springer Verlag; 1992.
2. Olness K, Conroy M. A pilot study of voluntary control of transcutaneous PO2 by children. *Int J Clin Exp Hypn*. 1985;33(1):1-5.
3. Rossi E, Cheek D. *Mind-Body Therapy: Methods of Ideodynamic Healing in Hypnosis*. New York: WW Norton & Company; 1988.
4. Rossi E. *The Psychobiology of Mind-Body Healing*. New York: WW Norton & Company; 1993.
5. Hilgard ER, Morgan AH, MacDonald H. Pain and dissociation in the cold pressor test: a study of hypnotic analgesia with "hidden reports" through automatic key pressing and automatic talking. *J Abnorm Psychol*. 1975;87:17-31.
6. Hilgard ER. *Divided Consciousness: Multiple Controls in Human Thought and Action*. New York: John Wiley & Sons; 1977.
7. Hilgard ER, Hilgard JR. *Hypnosis in the Relief of Pain*. New York: Brunner/Mazel; 1994.
8. Kiecolt-Glaser JK, Glaser R. Methodological issues in behavioral immunology research with humans. *Brain, Behavior, and Immunity*. 1988;2:67-78.
9. Cousins N. *Anatomy of an Illness*. New York: WW Norton & Company; 1979.
10. McEwen B. Protective and damaging effects of stress mediators. *N Engl J Med*. 1998;338(3):171-179.
11. Kiecolt-Glaser JK, McGuire L, Robles T, et al. Psychoneuroimmunology: psychological influences on immune function and health. *J Consult Clin Psychol*. 2002;70(3):537-547.
12. Dentino AN, Pieper CF, Rao KMK, et al. Association of interleukin-6 and other biologic variables with depression in older people living in the community. *J Am Geriatr Soc*. 1999;47:6-11.
13. Glaser R, Kenedy S, Lafuse W, et al. Psychological stress-induced modulation of interleukin 2 receptor gene expression and interleukin 2 production in peripheral blood leukocytes. *Arch Gen Psychiatry*. 1990;47:707-712.
14. Price D, Barrell J. An experiential approach with quantitative method: a research paradigm. *J Hum Psychol*. 1980;20:75-95.
15. Green E, Green A. *Beyond Biofeedback*. Delacorte Press/Seymour Lawrence. New York City, NY; 1977.
16. Basmajian J. *Muscles Alive: Their Functions Revealed by Electromyography*. Baltimore: Williams & Wilkins; 1962.
17. Malik M, Bigger JT, Camm AJ, et al. et al. Heart rate variability: Standards of measurement, physiological interpretation, and clinical use. *European Heart J*. 1996;17:354-381.
18. Thompson S. Will it hurt less if I can control it? A complex answer to a simple question. *Psychol Bull*. 1981;90(1):89-101.
19. Luthe W, Schultz J. *Autogenic Therapy*. Autogenic Therapy. Vol. 1. *Autogenic Methods*. New York: Grune & Stratton; 1969.
20. Luthe W, Schultz J. *Autogenic Therapy*. Autogenic Therapy. Vol. 2. *Medical Applications*. New York: Grune & Stratton; 1969.
21. Luthe W, Schultz J. *Autogenic Therapy*. Autogenic Therapy. Vol. 6. *Treatment with Autogenic Neutralisation*. New York: Grune & Stratton; 1969.
22. Luthe W, Schultz J. *Autogenic Therapy*. Autogenic Therapy. Vol. 3. *Applications in Psychotherapy*. New York: Grune & Stratton; 1969.
23. Luthe W, Schultz J. *Autogenic Therapy*. Autogenic Therapy. Vol. 4. *Research and Theory*. New York: Grune & Stratton; 1969.
24. Luthe W, Schultz J. *Autogenic Therapy*. Autogenic Therapy. Vol. 5. *Dynamics of Autogenic Neutralisation*. New York: Grune & Stratton; 1969.
25. Stetter F, Kupper S. Autogenic training: a meta-analysis of clinical outcome studies. *Appl Psychophysiol Biofeedback*. 2002;27(1):45-98.
26. Jacobson E. *You Must Relax: Practical Methods for Reducing the Tension of Modern Living*. New York: McGraw-Hill; 1978.
27. Baird CL, Sands L. A pilot study of the effectiveness of guided imagery with progressive muscle relaxation to reduce chronic pain and mobility difficulties of osteoarthritis. *Pain Manag Nurse*. 2004;5(3):97-104.
28. Kwekkeboom K, Wanta B, Bumpus M. Individual difference variables and the effects of progressive muscle relaxation and analgesic imagery interentions on cancer pain. *J Pain Symptom Manage*. 2008;36(6):604-615.
29. Bakal D. *Minding the Body: Clinical Uses of Somatic Awareness*. New York: The Guilford Press; 1999.
30. Walker B. *Hua Hu Ching: The Unknown Teachings of Lao Tzu on the Attainment of Enlightenment and Mastery*. Clark City Press. Livingston, MT; 1992.
31. Kabat-Zinn J. An out-patient program in behavioral medicine for chronic pain patients based on the practice of mindfulness meditation: theoretical considerations and preliminary results. *Gen Hosp Psychiatry*. 1982;4:33-47.
32. Kabat-Zinn J, Lipworth L, Burney R. The clinical use of mindfulness meditation for the self-regulation of chronic pain. *J Behav Med*. 1985;8:163-190.
33. Kabat-Zinn, J, Lipworth L, Burney R, Sellers W. Four year follow-up of a meditation-base program for the self-regulation of chronic pain: treatment outcomes and compliance. *Clin J Pain*. 2000;2:159-173.
34. Yang J-M. *Back Pain: Chinese Qigong for Healing and Prevention*. Boston: YMAA Publication Center; 1997.
35. Lee M, Pittler M, Ernst E. Internal Qi Gong for pain conditions: a systematic review. *J Pain*. 2009;11:1121-1127.
36. Lee M, Pittler M, Ernst E. External Qi Gong for pain conditions: a systematic review of randomized clinical trials. *J Pain*. 2007; 11:827-831.
37. Taggart H, Arsianian C, Bae S, et al. Effects of t'ai chi exercise on fibromyalgia symptoms and health-related quality of life. *Orthop Nurs*. 2003;22:353-360.
38. Hall A, Maher C, Latimer J, et al. The effectiveness of Tai Chi for chronic musculoskeletal pain conditions: a systematic review and meta-analysis. *Arthritis Rheum*. 2009;61:717-724.

CHAPTER 22

Management of Difficult Patients in the Chronic Pain Setting

Nina K. Anderson
Robert N. Jamison
Ajay Wasan

WHO ARE DIFFICULT PATIENTS?

There are patients in every practice who give the doctor and staff a feeling of "heartsink" every time their names are seen on the day's appointment list and evoke feelings of exasperation, defeat, guilt, negativity, and sometimes active dislike.[1] Important factors in the assessment of difficult patients include identifying past or current history of abuse, depression, psychosocial stress, occupational stress, and not having sufficient coping skills. Patients whom physicians find to be difficult are also high users of health care services, and they may be dissatisfied with the care they receive.

Difficult patients often fail to respond to nerve blocks, medications, or physical therapy, and they may be noncompliant with treatment, harbor objections to their physicians' approaches to their care, or be resistant to forming an effective alliance with their medical providers. Individuals with chronic pain may be difficult because of the psychosocial stressors that arise from having chronic pain, and these psychological symptoms, in turn, may lead to a preoccupation with physical symptoms, feelings of worthlessness, loneliness, fear of abandonment, and becoming socially isolated.

Particularly in Western societies, being sick implies certain expectations, including rights and duties.[2] The perceived "rights" of being sick include being temporarily exempt from "normal" social roles, with the more severe the sickness, the greater the exemption, and that the sick person is not held responsible for his or her condition (beyond the patient's control or absence of blame). The duties of a patient, which are quite applicable to those in pain, include the obligation to try to "get well," to seek help from a professional, and to cooperate in the process of "trying to recover." Patients with chronic pain who do not fulfill or comply with the social expectations of the sick role run the risk of being perceived as malingering or difficult by their clinicians and becoming isolated from friends and families.[3]

Because physicians are under increasing time pressures, patients with pain who exhibit vague symptoms and who are unresponsive to many different interventions for pain can be particularly frustrating, especially when the burden of providing treatment is shouldered by a lone individual rather than by an interdisciplinary team. Not all patients with difficult behavior exhibit significant psychopathology, such as major depression, anxiety, or a personality disorder. Patients who are otherwise "normal" can also be perceived as difficult when they arrive at a pain center for treatment with unrealistic expectations. They may have had problems in previous health care settings in which they were accused of exaggerating their pain and may suffer from a lack of sleep, poor eating habits, and long commutes on public transportation to their appointments, which can also contribute to outbursts, hostility, and unstable behavior. They may feel that their physicians are dismissive or skeptical of their pain rather than understanding and sympathetic. Even comparatively well-adjusted patients can have the idea that their pain physicians should be able to eliminate all of their pain and that failure to do so is tantamount to withholding treatment.

WHAT IS THE EFFECT OF DIFFICULT PATIENTS ON CLINIC PRACTICE AND STAFF?

Difficult patients drain clinic time and financial resources. They tax staff relationships and deplete emotional energy. Staff members report feeling "beat up" after interacting with these patients, which leads to low morale and high staff turnover. Difficult patients can keep staff members on edge for fear of an outburst, and staff members report feeling helpless and vengeful in the wake of such encounters. The fears of clinic staff may be justified because epidemiologic evidence indicates that health care workers are at a higher risk than other occupations for becoming victims of assaults by their patients.[4,5] Gerberich and colleagues[4] and Bruns and colleagues[5] determined that the primary risk factor for being assaulted at work was "working with unstable or volatile persons in health care, social service, or criminal justice settings."

According to the National Institute of Occupational Safety and Health, 51% of all reported nonfatal workplace assaults were of individuals who worked in a medical setting.[6]

The figures do not reflect verbal, passive aggressive behaviors; bullying; harassment; and implied threats, which are more pervasive than actual assaults. A true estimate of the number of difficult patient–clinician encounters is impossible because many of the incidents go unreported by the clinical staff for fear of retribution or being perceived as weak or incompetent by their peers or supervisors.

Patient-perpetrated violence against physicians or violent ideations is also associated with psychopathologies (e.g., antisocial and narcissistic personality traits), situational variables (litigation, workmen's compensation), and the perception of the patients' relationship to their physicians.[7-9]

HOW CAN I IDENTIFY AND CATEGORIZE DIFFICULT PATIENTS?

Not all providers view the same patient as difficult, but difficult patients in general tend to have similar things in common. Hahn et al. developed a 30-item Difficult Doctor-Patient Relationship Questionnaire (DDPRQ) for quantifying the characteristics of difficult patients.[10] In the original 30-item DDPRQ, physicians classified up to 20.6% of patient encounters as "difficult," or evoking a level of physician distress that "transcends the expected and accepted level of difficulty" with patients described as "hateful," "heartsink," "problem," or "difficult." Half of the physicians "secretly hoped" that difficult patients would not return.

The DDPRQ-10 (**Fig. 22-1**) requires less than 1 minute to complete, has an R^2 of 0.96 with the original 30-item instrument (indicating that responses on the short 10-item form are almost perfectly correlated to the original 30-item form), and has an internal consistency reliability (Cronbach a) of 0.88.[11] Using the 10-item DDPRQ, a constellation of three characteristics has been associated with patients being perceived as difficult. Compared with not-difficult patients, difficult patients have twice the prevalence of significant psychopathologic disorders (67% vs. 35%; P <0.001). Second, 90% of difficult patients have an abrasive personality style or personality disorder. Third, difficult patients are more likely to have one or more of 16 physical (often somatoform) symptoms as shown in **Table 22-1**.

Some difficult patients have a history of victimization or abuse, which is associated with significantly greater health care use, levels of depression, somatization, negative temperament, and catastrophizing.[12] For women, having a history of physical or sexual abuse increases the risk of experiencing difficulty in the physician–patient relationship and increases self-reported pain four- to fivefold versus those without a history of abuse.[12]

The role that physical and somatoform symptoms play in the generation of practitioner-experienced difficulty has implications for clinical management. First, clinicians should recognize the need to assess patients with many physical symptoms for common mental disorders by using structured methods. Second, clinicians should strive to understand their patients' experience of illness and to address their symptom-related concerns.[13] A patient-centered approach that validates the patient's experience and enlists the patient's active participation in setting treatment objectives is critical. Third, health care providers should assess the role that symptoms play in the patient's family system and should acquire skills in redirecting patients' attention to underlying psychosocial issues so that the patients can be effectively referred for further therapy when indicated.[14] Understanding that caring for

DDPRQ-10	Not at all					A great deal
1. How much are you looking forward to this patient's next visit after seeing this patient today?	○	○	○	○	○	○
2. How "frustrating" do you find this patient?	○	○	○	○	○	○
3. How manipulative is this patient?	○	○	○	○	○	○
4. To what extent are you frustrated by this patient's vague complaints?	○	○	○	○	○	○
5. How self-destructive is this patient?	○	○	○	○	○	○
6. Do you find yourself secretly hoping this patient will not return?	○	○	○	○	○	○
7. How at ease did you feel when you were with this patient today?	○	○	○	○	○	○
8. How time consuming is caring for this patient?	○	○	○	○	○	○
9. How enthusiastic do you feel about caring for this patient?	○	○	○	○	○	○
10. How difficult is it to communicate with this patient?	○	○	○	○	○	○

FIGURE 22-1. Difficult doctor–patient relationship 10-item questionnaire. Each item is scored from 1 (not at all) to 6 (a great deal) except items 1, 7, and 9, which are reverse scored from 6 (not at all) to 1 (a great deal). The score is the sum of all items.

TABLE 22-1 Physical Symptoms Associated with Being Difficult

Stomach Pain	Nausea or Gas	Sleep Problems	Loose Stools or Diarrhea
Being worried about serious disease	Pain/problems with sexual intercourse	Shortness of breath	Palpitations
Back pain	Fainting	Dizziness	Chest pain
Joint pain	Headache	Tired/low energy	Menstrual pain

patients experienced as "difficult" can be understood in terms of these three components is a first step in rendering the experience less difficult.

HOW DO I ADDRESS THE PATIENT'S EXPECTATION TO BE FIXED?

Patients prone to difficult behavior who perceive that the pain physician's role is to cure them completely tend to react with frustration when pain persists. Difficult pain patients may see themselves as "broken" by pain, and although treatments may lead to partial relief of pain and some improvement in function, pain and disability often persist. Some of the primary tasks a pain clinician may face are to foster realistic expectations for treatment success, to convey that patients are not "broken" by pain, and to encourage patients to appreciate that improvements in their pain allow them to carry on satisfying lives.

Difficult patients have very different coping styles. In a correlational study of lower back and neck pain to coping styles, Carroll et al. found that the highest levels of self-reported disabling pain were seven times more highly associated with those having high passive coping (e.g., remaining inactive and not using self-management strategies for pain control) regardless of the level of active coping.[15] High active coping was more associated with higher education and better general health.[15] In other smaller studies of clinic patients, coping styles that have been identified with more disabling pain include passive coping, catastrophizing, and adversarial attitudes.[12]

James Groves was one of the first clinicians to describe types of difficult patients. He classified these patients as falling into one of four groups: (1) dependent clingers, (2) entitled demanders, (3) manipulative help rejecters, and (4) self-destructive deniers. He recommended treatment strategies for each of these patient types as shown in **Table 22-2**.[16]

WHAT IS THE RELEVANCE OF MOTIVATIONAL INTERVIEWING?

The concept of motivational interviewing evolved from the experience of treating alcoholism.[17] Further refinement defines motivational interviewing as "a collaborative, person-centered form of guiding to elicit and strengthen motivation for change."[17,18] The fundamentals of motivational interviewing are based on the assumption that people generally have the skill set to adopt change but vary in the degree to which they are ready to engage in new behaviors.

In the precontemplation stage of change, people with chronic pain have not yet begun to consider changing, owing to a purely physical view of their pain. They assume a passive role and rely on the physician to provide the appropriate treatment. The clinician's role is fostering acknowledgment of risks and problems owing to passivity and inactivity—problems such as increased pain and physical deconditioning. In the contemplation stage, people with chronic pain acknowledge the risks associated with inactivity and passivity. The clinical goal at this stage is to assist the patient to realize that the risks of inactivity outweigh the perceived benefits.

When the patient is ready to become more active (preparation stage), the clinician helps the patient outline appropriate structured physical activities in which the individual is willing to participate. Finally, in the action stage, the clinician helps the individual increase activity. This is followed by maintenance, geared toward the individual's ongoing motivation and commitment (**Table 22-3**).

Motivational interviewing is a framework for preparing individuals for treatment, not the treatment itself.[19] From the clinicians' perspective, the five strategies to follow for effective motivational interviewing are (1) express empathy, (2) develop discrepancy, (3) avoid argumentation, (4) roll with resistance, and (5) support self-efficacy. Clinicians can encourage progression throughout the stages of change by providing

TABLE 22-2 Grove's Summary of Difficult Patient Types

I. Dependant clinger		
1. Initial mild or appropriate requests 2. Secondary escalation to repeated demands 3. Ultimate perception that physician is inexhaustible	1. Early feeling of being special 2. Progression to weary aversion 3. Final sense of exhaustion and depletion	1. Recognize that sense of "superman" is occurring 2. Begin to limit visits to regular office hours or specific times 3. Continue to remind patient or parent that their child's health will be monitored but less frequently as he or she improves
II. Entitled demander		
1. Early in visit patient or parent may use intimidation, devaluation, and blame 2. Patient or parent may act smug, self-important, and superior 3. Unable to recognize that hostility is a reflection of his or her "terror of abandonment" by physician 4. Does not acknowledge his or her fear and lack of control surrounding their child's illness	1. Preliminary desire to engage in conflict with patient or parent 2. Secondary reaction may be rage and frustration 3. Final response is for physician to "second guess" or doubt the effectiveness of his or her care of the patient and then order more tests or interventions than he or she normally would have done	1. Resist urge to enter into conflict; use personal radar or "early warning system" 2. Support efforts of patient or parent to ensure that he or she are getting best care 3. Reassure patient or parent that he or she will not be "abandoned" 4. Discuss case or get feedback from previous physicians and current physician colleagues
III. Manipulative help rejecter		
1. Immediately reject the possibility that any treatment can help 2. Act self-assured at return visits he or she was right and physician wrong (e.g., symptoms persist) 3. Continue to show up at appointments angry at everyone in the clinic	1. Initial response that physician may have overlooked something, that a diagnosis was missed 2. Secondary sense of trying to win over patient or parent that he or she will be the only one that can "fix it" 3. Ultimate implication that physician is a failure	1. Stop and listen to patient or parent 2. Reflect back to patient or parent that previously he or she may not have a partnership with treatment team 3. Recognize that his or her own response may be a reflection of his or her own exhaustion or burnout 4. Take a break; suggest another colleague
IV. Self-destructive denier		
1. Unconscious self-destructive health behaviors 2. Helpless and hopeless endeavors to defeat physician attempts at improving health	1. Physician may feel loathing and even disgust 2. Ultimately come up with excuses to not see patient or parent; become unavailable and unconsciously provide substandard care	1. Recognize feelings; self-monitor and disengage 2. Understand that the patient or parent may have significant mental health needs 3. Discuss case with colleagues 4. Elicit assistance from mental health professionals to help provide the care of the patient or parent

Adapted with permission from Groves JE. Taking care of the hateful patient. *N Engl J Med*. 1978;288(16):883-887.

patients with motivational statements, listening with empathy, asking open-ended questions, providing feedback and affirmation, and handling resistance by rolling not arguing. Examples of the types of open-ended questions used in motivational interviewing include:

What changes would you most like to talk about?
What have you noticed about . . . ?
How important is it for you to change . . . ?
How confident do you feel about changing . . . ?
How do you see the benefits of . . . ?
How do you see the drawback of . . . ?
What will make the most sense to you?
How might things be different if you . . . ?
In what way . . . ?
Where does this leave you now?

TABLE 22-3 Stages of Change and Therapist Tasks

Patient's Stage	Clinician's Motivational Tasks
Precontemplation	Raise doubt—increase the patient's perception of the risks and problems associated with the current behavior.
Contemplation	Tip the balance—evoke reasons to change, risks of not changing; strengthen the patients' self-efficacy for change of current behavior.
Preparation	Help the patient to determine the best course of action to take in seeking change.
Action	Help the patient to take steps toward change.
Maintenance	Review progress; renew motivation and commitment as needed.
Relapse	Help the patient review the processes of contemplation, determination, and action without becoming stuck or demoralized because of relapse.

By using a guiding rather than directing style, clinicians can develop strategies to elicit the patient's own motivation to change and eliciting or encouraging change talk from the patient. The following are examples of directing versus guiding styles:

Directing style: "Your weight is putting your health at serious risk and contributing to your lower back pain. You need to exercise more frequently and to try to lose weight." (*Patient replies with a "yes, but . . ." argument.*)

Guiding style: "Let's have a look at this together and see what you think. From my perspective, losing some weight and getting more exercise will help your health, but what feels right for you? (*Patient often expresses ambivalence at this point.*) . . . . So you can see the value of trying these things, but you don't see how you can attempt to do it at this point in time. OK. It's up to you to decide when and how to make any changes. I wonder, what sort of small changes might make sense to you?" (*Patient says how small change might be possible.*)

HOW IMPORTANT IS THE DOCTOR–PATIENT RELATIONSHIP?

Historically, difficult encounters focused on the patient. More recently, however, the importance of the physicians' attributes has been recognized. Jackson and Kroenke found that the greatest predictor of difficult patient encounters was not the patient but the physician.[20] The results from their study revealed that physicians with poorer attitudes toward approaching psychosocial issues averaged almost three times as many (23% vs. 8%) "difficult" encounters than physicians with positive attitudes.[20]

The *Field Guide to the Difficult Patient Interview*[21] states that the strongest predictor of patient adherence is the doctor–patient relationship itself. Having a healthy relationship based on trust, empathy, and confidence in the physician is the first step in preventing patients from becoming difficult. Patients often become difficult because of perceived deficiencies or inequities in the relationships with their physicians, and the physicians become suspicious and perceive patients as difficult when the patients benefit from being ill and when biomedical explanations do not match patients' experience.[22]

Failure to improve may fuel a patient's frustration, but it seldom proves to be the sole reason for the development of difficult behaviors and interactions. A number of factors can be addressed in an effort to foster a relationship in which the physician is seen as a healer, ally, and guide to improved health, not merely a service provider. Learning to say no in a way that makes the patient believe that he or she is still involved in the decision-making process can make patient encounters less difficult.[23] The physicians' attributes associated with malpractice suits do not appear to be related to the quality of the medical care.[24,25] The amount of time spent with a patient, having good communication skills, using humor, and even a physician's tone of voice are all associated with not having a malpractice claim history.[23,24,26] Bruns and Disorbio found that worker's compensation patients have a higher frequency of violent ideation than other insured patients.[5] The patient reports being "disabled" by the pain, but when medical evidence suggests otherwise, the relationship may become adversarial, made worse by the fact that the patient cannot leave this physician's care because of a loss of disability benefits.

WHAT IF MY PERSONALITY DOES NOT MIX WELL WITH DIFFICULT PATIENTS?

Feelings of job dissatisfaction and job stress are problems shared by providers in many countries. A lack of time and heavy workload are cited as the main causes of these feelings of discontent and stress, which in the long term may lead to burnout. Burnout is a syndrome of emotional exhaustion, depersonalization, and reduced personal accomplishment that can occur among individuals who work with people in some capacity.[27] Emotional exhaustion is a key factor in burnout and may evoke feelings of reduced personal accomplishment and depersonalization. Depersonalization is expressed as a negative, cynical, and distant attitude toward others, including patients.

Granek et al. interviewed oncologists to determine if they experienced grief at the loss of their patients.[28] The results of their interviews revealed that half of the oncologists struggled to manage their feelings of grief, failure, self-doubt, and powerlessness. Even though the oncologists were grieving, they reportedly hid these emotions from colleagues so as to not be considered weak and unprofessional. Their discomfort over their grief led them to recommend more aggressive treatment strategies when palliative care would be a better option. When evaluated for burnout, the most consistent finding was the use of compartmentalization of their grief from other aspects of their lives as a coping strategy to prevent burnout.[28]

One of the perspectives to explain burnout is found in equity theory. When job demands are high or rewards are low, people may experience an imbalance between their investment and reward. Clinicians who deal with difficult patients are at great risk of experiencing an imbalance between their investment and rewards and which may eventually lead to burnout. Zantinge et al. hypothesized that physicians who were emotionally exhausted and burned out would invest less in their patient contacts; have shorter consultations; be less inclined to encourage their patients to discuss their problems; and behave in a cynical, negative manner toward patients than other physicians.[29] Contrary to their expectations, exhausted and burned out physicians had longer consults and discussed more psychosocial or biomedical issues with their patients than other physicians. The exception to these results were the physicians who felt "incompetent" or had feelings of reduced accomplishment.

Gillette recommends that health care professionals continually assess and understand their own strengths and weaknesses and strive to improve their communication skills.[30] In fact, self-assessment and lifelong learning were adopted by the American Board of Medical Specialties explicitly as one of four elements in its Maintenance of Certification program.[31] The American Board of Internal Medicine requires the "capacity of physicians to self-assess" in diplomates who choose to recertify.[32]

To determine how accurately physicians self-assess compared with external observations of their competence, Davis et al. (2006) conducted a systematic review of 725 articles, 17 of which met inclusion criteria. Across studies, weak or no associations were found between physicians' self-rated assessments and external assessments.[33] A number of the 17 studies found that the worst accuracy in self-assessment was among physicians who performed the least well by external assessment, independent of level of training, specialty, or manner of assessment and comparison.

Providing physicians a framework to effectively evaluate their own behavior and emotions and understand how these can affect the outcomes of encounters with difficult patients is important. Physicians also benefit from hiring support staff that are pleasant and adept at dealing with interpersonal problems. Perceived rude, insensitive, and crude behaviors of physicians and the support staff have the potential to complicate care.[34]

Being conscious of verbal communications, such as properly introducing oneself, speaking without medical jargon, and using a discourse tempo that is not rushed, also helps to create a positive environment for consults. Attention to aspects of verbal and nonverbal communication in the training of medical students or inexperienced clinicians may improve care and draw attention to the physician attributes in the interactions with difficult patients, particularly those with mental health problems.

HOW ELSE CAN I IMPROVE MY EMPATHIC LISTENING SKILLS?

Not all clinicians are adept at handling difficult patients, but this ability can be improved. Every practitioner faces difficult patients, and a conscious attempt at being empathic will help to avoid personality conflicts. For some patients, scheduling regular visits, encouraging the patient to take an active part in his or her care, and working with the patient's family may avoid difficult encounters, irrespective of a physician's unease in dealing with difficult patients. Regular visits convey the message that the patient should deal with pain flares and not respond to them as crises. Such visits establish a set period when the physician will be most available to them, which reassures patients that their physicians care about their progress. Using a guided versus directed interviewing style to encourage change and motivation to participate in their care (e.g., physical rehabilitation) can shift the burden of improvement from being solely on the physician. A patient's family can reinforce this idea and help monitor compliance.

Intrinsic to the healing process is the perception by patients that their health care providers are listening and genuinely appreciate their suffering. As outlined earlier, difficult patients are often those who have difficulty not only with the level of their pain but also with their pain physician. Coulehan et al. identified ways for a clinician to build empathy and, in turn, defuse problematic encounters with difficult patients. Asking questions such as "Is there anything else?"; using clarifying statements such as "Let me see if I have this right"; and responding with feeling statements such as "I can imagine how this might feel" can be helpful.[35]

Simple questions can be powerful tools in conveying a physician's empathy for and appreciation of a patient's suffering. Questions such as "Is having chronic pain a lot of work for you?", "How is your life changed because of the pain?", and "What have you lost as a result of having chronic pain?" acknowledge that the patient is experiencing extreme difficulty and loss and that the patient is trying his or her best to cope effectively. Haas et al. lists specific communication techniques that may help physicians in communicating with difficult patients (**Table 22-4**).[36]

TABLE 22-4 Communication techniques for physicians

Goal	Activity	Suggested Phrases
Improve listening and understanding.	Summarize the patient's chief concerns. Interrupt less. Offer regular, brief summaries of what you are hearing from the patient. Reconcile conflicting views of the diagnosis or the seriousness of the condition.	"What I hear from you is that .... Did I get that right?"
Improve partnership with patient.	Discuss the fact that the relationship is less than ideal; offer ways to improve care.	"How do you feel about the care you are receiving from me? It seems to me that we sometimes don't work together very well."
Improve skills at expressing negative emotions.	Decrease blaming statements. Increase "I" messages. Example: "I feel ..." as opposed to "You make me feel ..."	"It's difficult for me to listen to you when you use that kind of language."
Increase empathy; ensure understanding of patient's emotional responses to condition and care.	Attempt to name the patient's emotional state; check for accuracy and express concern.	"You seem quite upset. Could you help me understand what you are going through right now?"
Negotiate the process of care.	Clarify the reason for the patient seeking care. Indicate what part the patient must play in caring for his or her health. Revise expectations if they are unrealistic.	"What's your understanding of what I am recommending, and how does that fit with your ideas about how to solve your problems?" "I wish I (or a medical miracle) could solve this problem for you, but the power to make the important changes is really yours."

Drawing from the principles of medical ethics consultation and mediation services may also be useful.[37] For example, (1) Reframe the problem as bilateral and refer to the situation rather than the patient as "difficult." (2) Express curiosity about the patient. "Why would a reasonable person behave this way?", "What do they hope for from the medical team, and what do they fear?", or "What can our team do to help them through this?" (3) Affirm and accept frustrations regarding circumstances over which the provider has no control, such as lack of insurance, social support, or transportation to get to appointments.

HOW DOES PSYCHIATRIC COMORBIDITY AFFECT DIFFICULT PATIENTS?

Despite a physician's best efforts, significant psychopathology may make patients unavoidably difficult. The main areas of psychopathology associated with chronic pain patients include personality, affective, somatoform, and substance abuse disorders.

Psychopathology affects between 30% and 50% of patients seen in academic and community pain centers.[38,39] Recently, Knaster and colleagues found that more than half of the patients seeking treatment for chronic pain fulfilled the criteria for at least one psychiatric disorder during the past 12 months. The diagnoses included a wide range of psychiatric disorders; mood disorder was diagnosed in 45% and an anxiety disorder in 25% of the patients. The lifetime prevalence of any psychiatric disorder was 75%.[40] Among patients attending pain clinics, 30% to 50% have a major depressive or anxiety disorder.[41-43] Common symptoms are low mood, increased worry, and irritability. Although such symptoms are most apparent to the spouse or family members, they may emerge in the clinician–patient encounter.

Goral et al. found that two-thirds of chronic pain patients with depression and anxiety disorders had sleep problems compared with one-third of chronic pain patients with no comorbid psychiatric disorders.[44] Longer duration and higher severity of pain were also significantly associated with having depressive or anxiety disorders.[44] Gerrits et al. found that patients having a high number of reported pain sites, pain of the joints and longer duration of joint pain (90+ days), daily use of prescription medication, and more severe pain at baseline were at a significantly increased risk of still having a depressive or anxiety disorder at a 2-year posttreatment follow-up.[45] Arthritis or reported pain in the joints in particular has been associated with psychiatric disorders, including depression and anxiety.[45,46] In their review of the prevalence of major depression in patients with chronic pain, those with pain lasting longer than 6 months were more than four times as likely to have a depressive disorder as those without chronic pain; 65% of patients with depression experienced one or more pain complaints, and depression was present in 5% to 85% of patients.[47] At least 75% of primary care patients with depression present with physical complaints only. However, pain symptoms are rarely attributed to depression or other psychiatric illness. These physical complaints may be due to amplification of chronic physical disease and remain medically unexplained after extensive workup. As a result, patients with depression who present with physical symptoms such as pain are particularly likely to receive an inaccurate diagnosis.

Screening chronic pain patients for psychiatric comorbidity in secondary care is important because psychopathology may have serious consequences for prognosis, outcome, and health care utilization. Untreated or undertreated psychopathology is the single most important factor in poor pain treatment outcome regardless of the treatment modality.[48,49] Pain patients with comorbid psychiatric disorders report higher pain ratings and show greater pain-related disability than do other patients. Furthermore, patients with psychiatric comorbidities more often have a poor response to pain medications, neural blocks, and physical rehabilitation than do those without psychopathology. The evidence suggests that a reciprocal relationship may exist; the presence of persistent pain significantly increases the risk of future depression or major depression or anxiety and vice versa.[12] Depressed or anxious patients may "lash out" at their pain physicians, blaming them for overwhelming pain and failure of treatment. Although a patient may be adjusting to pain and making reasonable attempts at functional improvement when first evaluated, the development of an affective disorder may manifest as poor motivation to remain active and a perceived intensification of pain in the absence of changes in pain pathology. Suggestions by the pain physician that the patient's pain cannot be "cured" may be met by frustration and anguish over the anticipation of a life with unbearable pain.

Individuals with personality disorders may present with a pattern of maladaptive emotional and cognitive reactions to daily events or challenging circumstances. Patients who appear odd or eccentric may meet the criteria for paranoid, schizoid, or schizotypal disorders. Patients who appear dramatic, emotional, or erratic may have an antisocial, borderline, histrionic, or narcissistic personality disorder. Patients who appear to be extremely anxious or fearful may have an avoidant, dependent, or obsessive-compulsive personality disorder.

A personality disorder, as described in the *Diagnostic and Statistical Manual of Mental Disorders*, fourth edition, text revision (DSM-IV-TR),[50] is "an enduring pattern of inner experience and behavior that deviates markedly from the expectations of the individual's culture."

Polantin et al.[51] and others[2,52,53] find consistently higher prevalence of psychiatric disorders among chronic pain patients compared with the general population as seen across 17 countries. More recently, evidence indicates that anxiety disorders occur as frequently as depressive disorders in chronic pain patient populations.[54-57] A high percentage of patients with chronic pain receiving treatment in a pain center have some form of a personality disturbance that manifests in a general tendency to respond to stress with negative emotions, such as fear, anxiety, sadness, anger, and impatience, also termed neuroticism. These personality or character vulnerabilities worsen in times of stress, such as enduring chronic pain. For example, when a person with a dependent personality type fears abandonment, increased anxiety and demands for attention may lead to inconsiderate behaviors. When an obsessive individual is uncertain about her long-term treatment plans, the response to a threat of her lack of control may include rude behavior. When a histrionic patient fears an attack on his masculinity, lewd or provocative interactions happen. When a masochistic patient believes his or her efforts are underappreciated, rude responses may result. When a paranoid person perceives an impending assault, aggressive behaviors may follow. When a narcissistic individual senses that he is not receiving the full attention of a health care provider, hostile interactions may ensue.

The combination of psychotropic medications and psychotherapy yields the best treatment success for both depression and anxiety disorders. Epstein et al. recommend that to avoid blaming the patient, the clinician should embrace a biopsychosocial perspective and attempt to understand the patient's experience of illness.[58] They suggest that the clinician explore the patient's life context (things that led up to and perpetuate the presenting problem), find mutually meaningful language (use language that the patient can understand), and normalize the patient's bodily experience of distress (help explain the physical and emotional reactions to the condition).

Anxiety disorders share common symptoms such as fear, avoidance, and arousal. However, anxiety disorders are clinically heterogenous, and thus, the type of a comorbid anxiety disorder affects the pain experience and treatment differently depending on the core presenting anxiety symptoms. Generalized anxiety disorder and panic disorder share common physical features with pain, such as muscle tension and autonomic arousal symptoms. On the other hand, social phobia and obsessive-compulsive disorder (OCD) are characterized by obsessions, avoidance, and control. The cognitive and social rigidity associated with these two disorders can influence the response to treatment, and a treatment plan that encourages and supports patients to verbalize their pain-related fears and disabilities can be helpful.

Obsessive-compulsive disorder is defined as a "pervasive pattern of preoccupation with orderliness, perfectionism, and mental and interpersonal control, at the expense of flexibility, openness, and efficiency, beginning by early adulthood and present in a variety of contexts."

The prevalence of OCD in chronic pain patients ranges between 1.1% and 8.2%.[57] The excessive rituals or habits that are characteristic of OCD are performed to obtain relief, suppress the intrusive thoughts, or prevent an outcome such as contamination. Although the symptoms of people with anxiety disorders are generally apparent, people with OCD are often ashamed of their rituals or habits and are secretive, which are two of the ten characteristics of Gerard and Ridell's difficult patient encounters.[59] Obsessiveness may be of relevance to treating chronic pain because a number of case reports have described patients who "overvalue" their pain experience to the point of its being an obsession.

Anxiety disorders are the most prevalent type of mental disorder, and they frequently occur with various medical conditions, including chronic pain. Santana and Fontenelle found that anxiety disorders are two to seven times more prevalent in the population of people with chronic pain and migraines than in the general population.[60]

Financial incentives are known to influence outcomes in chronic pain, and their presence introduces the potential for malingering. Malingering is defined as "the intentional production of false or grossly exaggerated physical or psychological symptoms, motivated by external incentives such as avoiding military duty, avoiding work, obtaining financial compensation, evading criminal prosecution, or obtaining drugs" (DSM-IV-TR). One study suggests that the prevalence of malingering in chronic pain patients with financial incentives in the midst of a legal determination of disability status and benefits may be between 20% and 50%.[61] A nationwide survey found that 20% of Americans believed that purposeful misrepresentation of claims in the compensation system was acceptable.[62] The DSM-IV-TR further suggests that malingering should be strongly suspected with any combination of the following: medicolegal context of presentation (as in disability evaluations), marked discrepancies between claims and objective findings, lack of cooperation with evaluations or treatment, or presence of antisocial personality disorder. A number of strategies have been developed to detect malingering of cognitive symptoms, including forced-choice symptom validity tests. (For reviews of symptom validity tests, see Bianchini et al.[63] and Grote and Hook.[64])

HOW DO I DEAL WITH A BORDERLINE PERSONALITY DISORDER?

Perhaps the most difficult personality disorder a clinician faces in a pain practice is borderline personality disorder (BPD). The diagnostic criteria of BPD include a pervasive pattern of instability of interpersonal relationships, self-image, and affect, with marked impulsivity.[20]

Patients with BPD have an intense desire to be valued and to idealize authority figures, such as their pain physicians. Upon interview, childhood antecedents emerge such as family conflicts as well as physical and sexual abuse.[65] Patients with BPD tend to distort reality and succumb easily to rage and despair, feeling abandoned and depressed, and may even become psychotic. Patients with BPD exhibit suicidal tendencies and may have a history of suicide attempts. Intentional self-injury occurs in 70% to 80% of patients[66] with the majority of patients claiming that their injuries are not painful. Although there are more similarities than differences between male and female BPD patients, men tend toward substance abuse and schizotypic, narcissistic, and antisocial personality traits, but women are more prone to having posttraumatic stress disorder (PTSD), eating disorders, or borderline identity disturbance.[67]

Patients with BPD have specific psychodynamics and behaviors that can potentially compromise overall psychosocial and occupational functioning. For example, Kroll describes the theme of victimization in these patients and emphasized that this victim theme is critical to understanding the psychopathology of patients with BPD.[68] Individuals with BPD engage others to ". . . act upon [them], usually in a negative, rejecting, or aggressive way, but sometimes in a caretaking ... way" and that the behaviors of helplessness and incompetence are intended to coerce others to "take over ordinary adult functions and decision-making activities." This underlying theme of victimization can readily lead to chronic "medical victimization" and medical disability.[68] Patients with BPD have long been known to have poor compliance to treatment, and the therapeutic relationship is often "stormy."[69,70]

Using the Personality Diagnostic Questionnaire, Self-Harm Inventory, and diagnostic interviews, Sansone et al. found that 18% of pain patients scored positively on all three measures for BPD.[67,71] The authors suggested that the emotional self-regulatory disturbances in these patients either amplify the nociceptive components of chronic pain or are, by themselves, the basis for a purely somatoform pain syndrome. BPD encompasses a pattern of poor regulation of powerful emotions.[20]

Medications can be useful, along with types of cognitive-behavioral therapy (CBT). The most effective CBT for this type of disorder is dialectical behavioral therapy (DBT). DBT emphasizes the idea that patients will always have powerful emotions, and the key to improvement is not to react in familiar, maladaptive patterns to such emotions. Although early recognition of BPD helps to minimize the occurrence of difficult situations, avoiding the use of invasive procedures with these patients may also prevent difficulties. Because the level of affective distress is high in patients with BPD, the nociceptive or neuropathic components of a pain syndrome that could possibly respond to an interventional procedure are much less likely to be effective. In addition, procedures may temporarily worsen pain, and if a patient with BPD is prone to self-mutilation or suicidal behavior in the face of distress, an elevated risk of self-harm may occur after a procedure.

HOW DO I TREAT WOUNDED MILITARY PATIENTS?

Chronic musculoskeletal pain disorders are rising because of combat injuries and the physical demands of military deployments such as wearing heavy body armor, carrying backpacks weighing more than 70 lb, and treading on uneven and soft ground (sand) under harsh conditions. Pain disorders in the U.S. Armed Forces account for 53% of all Army discharges, with musculoskeletal system pain being the leading cause of hospitalization in the Marine Corps (28%), Navy (22%), Army (18%), and Air Force (14%).[72] Army women are approximately 67% more likely than Army men to be discharged for musculoskeletal conditions (e.g., back pain).

Changes in wounding patterns associated with technological advances in body armor and improvised explosive devices have resulted in an increased survival but with multiple injuries and disabilities in today's military. For example, in cases of limb loss, burns involving the residual stump or limb present in nearly 75% of cases, and 21% of injured soldiers require amputations solely because of the severity of their burns. The average burn size is 40% of total-body surface area. Injuries to the ear are the single most common injury type, accounting for 23% of all injuries, 72% of which include hearing loss.

Polytrauma, chronic pain presenting with PTSD and traumatic brain injury (TBI), occurs in 42% of military personnel returning from deployments in Iraq and Afghanistan.[73] Patients having comorbid pain, PTSD, and TBI present a challenge in that the overlapping symptoms that characterize these conditions (e.g., headache, irritability, sleep disturbance, memory impairments) can make accurate and differential diagnosis difficult.

From 2005 to 2009, there was a 64% increase in the number of veterans who were forced to leave the military because of mental health conditions. Currently, more soldiers are hospitalized because of mental health issues than from physical injuries (including war wounds).[74] Furthermore, although all honorably discharged veterans are eligible for Veterans Administration (VA) medical benefits, since January 2003, veterans with income or net worth over certain limits are limited or not eligible to enroll in the VA benefits systems and may be forced to seek care outside of the VA system. Based on the increasing number of wounded warriors with limited access to health care, civilian pain centers may see an increase in numbers of military patients with polytrauma.

Military patients seeking treatment for polytrauma outside the VA health care system are often treated by medical professional who are not familiar with the unique aspects of military culture and how to treat military combat–related disorders. Military personnel are unique in that service members tend to ignore injuries or try to manage them on their own to avoid the stigma associated with perceived weakness and loss of status and degradation of their identity as a "strong soldier." Soldiers with combat-related injuries are at fivefold increased risk of developing PTSD (e.g., survivor guilt) than those with noncombat injuries.

Identification of polytrauma is the first step, but the critical question remains, "How can we best treat these military individuals?"

One program with promise, the Functional and Occupational Rehabilitation Treatment (FORT) Program,[75] is based on a sports medicine approach. The integral components of functional restoration involve tertiary treatment, the objective and physical-based evaluation of physical and functional capacity, psychosocial assessment, the identification of potential socioeconomic barriers to recovery, physician-directed treatment, an interdisciplinary treatment team approach, and an intense focus on returning the patient to activity and function without focus being placed on the patient's current symptoms of pain.

The FORT program has been shown to be effective with participants being six times less likely to seek high levels of treatment for pain at 1-year follow-up, 3.6 times less likely to rely on multiple pain medications, and two times more likely to remain on active duty than patients treated using traditional pain management methods. The fact that it has been shown to be effective not only in the United States but also in other countries (Canada, Denmark, France, Germany, Japan, and The Netherlands) demonstrates the potential of the FORT program.[76]

HOW DO I TREAT A PATIENT I BELIEVE TO BE SOMATICIZING?

Barsky and Borus used the term "functional somatic syndrome" to characterize individuals with a perceived serious medical problem with self-perpetuating somatic symptoms in the absence of organic pathology.[77] These individuals believe that they have a serious disease that will likely get worse. They often have psychiatric comorbidity and portray their conditions as catastrophic and disabling. They present with a "sick role" and significant disability despite a lack of anatomic or functional pathology. From a "systems perspective," somatization often alters the patient's entire family system, which enhances the "gain" for the patient.[24,78]

Historically, patients with chronic back pain are by some regarded to be somatizing patients who express psychological and social distress through persistent subjective health complaints.[51,52,79] On the other hand, Reme and colleagues found that only 16% of patients with chronic lower back pain were diagnosed with a somatoform pain disorder.[80]

Righter and Sansone (1999) suggest a number of treatment strategies for difficult patients who show normal results from physical examination and diagnostic tests yet have multiple unexplained symptoms, patterns of high health care utilization, and problematic family and social history.[78] To offset continued problematic behavior and failed treatments, they recommend honest discussions, behavior management strategies, CBT, antidepressant medication, and psychiatric consultation.

Dominick et al. investigated the association of chronic pain with physical and mental comorbidity in the general population by measuring chronic pain status independent of comorbid conditions.[81] A significant relationship was found between 15 medical conditions (e.g., asthma, prostate problems) and reported chronic pain ranging from 26% to 49.2% (**Table 22-5**). Patients having osteoporosis (49.2%), arthritis (45.2%), and bronchitis or emphysema (41.4%) had the highest proportions as shown in Table 22-5.

WHAT ARE THE BEST WAYS TO HANDLE A HOSTILE PATIENT?

A risk management article produced by Princeton Insurance[82] recommended the following steps when facing a hostile patient. First, remain calm and collected. By maintaining a relaxed posture and respecting the patient's personal space, you can set the stage to defuse a difficult situation. Second, handle the problem in private. Gently redirect the patient into a room away from the reception area. This action will be less disturbing to others and can reduce the chances of a hostile outburst. Third, listen actively to the patient's complaints.

TABLE 22-5 Prevalence of Chronic Conditions with Chronic Pain

Frequency and Percentage of Adult Population Reporting Doctor-Diagnosed Chronic Condition				Percentage of Those with Chronic Condition also Reporting Chronic Pain		
Chronic Condition (ever diagnosed)	**Weighted Frequency (NZ pop.)**	**Percent (NZ pop.)**	**95% CI**	**Percent Reporting Chronic Pain**	**95% CI**	***P* Value**
Neck or back disorder[a]	755,142	24.2	(23.2-25.2)	36.8	(34.7-38.9)	<0.0001
Arthritis	460,027	14.7	(14-15.5)	45.2	(42.5-47.9)	<0.0001
Heart disease[b]	328,225	10.5	(9.9-11.2)	34.3	(31.2-37 3)	<0.0001
Migraine	296,021	9.5	(8.8-10.1)	28.9	(25.6-32.2)	<0.0001
Recent asthma[c]	216,736	6.9	(6.3-7.5)	26 0	(22.6-29.5)	<0.0001
Eczema or dermatitis	204,772	6.6	(6.0-7.1)	19.7	(16.6-22.9)	0.0568
Cancer	202,775	6.5	(6.0-7.0)	28.8	(25.1-32.6)	<0.0001
Bowel disease[d]	157,006	5.0	(4.6-5.5)	34.1	(29.6-38.5)	<0.0001
Diabetes	157,121	5.0	(4.6-5.5)	30.3	(26.2-34.4)	<0.0001
Gallbladder disease or gallstone	118,830	3.8	(3.4-4.2)	31.4	(26.5-36.3)	<0.0001
Thyroid condition	113,109	3.6	(3.2-4.0)	28.1	(23 3-32.9)	<0.0001
Stomach or gastric ulcers	102,833	3.3	(2.9-3.7)	34.0	(28.7-39 3)	<0.0001
Osteoporosis	89,967	2.9	(2.6-3.2)	49.2	(43.6-54.8)	<0.0001
Stroke	57,658	1.8	(1.6-2.1)	34.6	(27.8-41.3)	<0.0001
Endometriosis	51,760	N/A	(N/A)	31.7	(24.2-39.3)	<0.0001
Bronchitis, emphysema, or COPD[f]	95,860	N/A	(N/A)	41.4	(35.7-47.1)	<0.0001
Prostate problems[g]	72,870	N/A	(N/A)	21.0	(15.8–26.3)	0.0387
Mental health condition[h]	432,015	13.8	(13.1-146)	29.6	(27.0-32.3)	<0.0001

[a]This condition is not entirely independent of chronic pain because the survey question wording was "disorder of the neck or back. This includes lumbago, sciatica, chronic back or neck pain, vertebrae or disk problems. It can be injury related or something you were born with. . . ."

[b]Includes those ever diagnosed with a heart attack, angina, heart failure, or other heart disease (excludes high blood pressure and high cholesterol).

[c]Includes those who have experienced asthma attack or been woken by an attack or shortness of breath in the past 12 months.

[d]Includes irritable bowel syndrome, inflammatory bowel disease, Crohn disease, ulcerative colitis, celiac disease, diverticular disease, and other bowel problems.

[e]This condition relates to women only.

[f]The question was asked only of those age 45 years and older.

[g]This condition relates to men only.

[h]Long-term diagnosed mental health condition that has lasted or is expected to last 6 months or more; the symptoms may be present all the time or be intermittent.

CI, confidence interval; COPD, chronic obstructive pulmonary disease; N/A, not applicable; NZ, New Zealand; pop, population.

Pay attention, maintain eye contact, and let the patient vent to create a greater likelihood that some resolution will be reached. Fourth, convey kindness and reassurance. Although this response may be extremely difficult, acknowledge the patient's feelings and let the patient know that you want to help. Fifth, try to reach some solution and conclude the meeting with willingness to follow up on any recommended action. Sixth, document any hostile encounter. You may not need to include this information in the patient's record, but a detailed description of what happened may prove valuable at a later date. Remembering these steps as the five A's for dealing with hostile patients, as shown in **Table 22-6**, may be helpful. Unfortunately, sometimes a satisfactory solution cannot be reached, and assistance from security is needed. If the physician or staff members feel threatened by a hostile patient and think the patient may become violent, security should be called to escort him or her from the clinic. Only in situations of imminent self-harm or harm to others should clinic staff attempt to restrain the patient themselves.

TABLE 22-6 Five A's for Dealing with Hostile Patients

Acknowledge the problem.
Allow the patient to vent uninterrupted in a private place.
Agree on what the problem is.
Affirm what can be done.
Assure follow-through.

Hostile and violent ideation is present in 9% to as high as 27% of rehabilitation patients and is associated with substance abuse, lack of trust in the physician, and presence of litigation.

WHAT IF THE PATIENT IS SUICIDAL?

Suicidal ideation and suicide attempts are common among patients with chronic pain. In fact, the presence of pain has been added to the list of "suicide risk factors."[83] Fishbain et al. found that the suicide completion rate in their chronic pain patients was two to three times that of the general population.[84] Pain catastrophizing and pain avoidance are two psychological responses to pain that may be associated with an increased risk of suicidality. Pain-related catastrophizing has been found to be one of two most consistent predictors for the presence and degree of suicide ideations, the other being magnitude of depressive symptoms. Pain-catastrophizing chronic pain patients are at five times greater risk than

TABLE 22-7 Evaluation and Treatment Planning for Suicidal Patients

Evaluate suicidal intent and lethality.
Establish existence and feasibility of a suicide plan.
Identify evidence of self-destructive behavior and past suicide attempts.
Attempt to establish an alliance with the patient.
Consider an agreement for safety.
Refer to mental health specialist with training in suicidal evaluation and treatment or escort to a hospital emergency department for psychiatric evaluation.
Document communication with patient and treatment strategies.

healthy nonpain patients for killing themselves. Heavy smoking and having problems with alcohol,[85] depression,[86] hopelessness,[87] headaches,[88,89] head pain,[90] nonback or non-neck pain,[88,91] history of suicide attempt or having a suicide plan, and elevated pain scores[90] have been shown to be associated with increased patient risk for suicidal ideation.[84,92,93]

It is clinically and ethically appropriate to address suicidality. Providers should not hesitate to ask patients about possible suicidal ideation and for clarification of intent. Such questioning will not increase the chances of self-harm. Most patients appreciate knowing that their providers are concerned about their lives and well-being, and this knowledge in itself can decrease the chances of attempted suicide.

Distinctions should be drawn among patients who wish they were dead (passive death wish), who actively want to end their lives (suicidal intent), and who have a specific plan to do so (suicidal intent with a plan). Suicidal intent should be taken seriously despite any suspicion that the patient is engaged in attention-seeking behavior (see **Table 22-7** for evaluation guidelines).

Coordination with a licensed mental health professional who has training in managing suicidal patients is essential. Suicide attempts should be discussed openly with patients, and in some cases, a written comprehensive treatment plan and an agreement with the patient to guarantee his or her safety may be needed. All encounters and behaviors should be well documented. Although difficult patients who progress to a suicidal crisis may present the greatest challenge to a health care provider, patients in crisis should not be abandoned. Rather, seeking coordination with mental health professionals and establishing a comprehensive treatment team become essential. Patients should be informed that hospitalization may be considered in emergency situations and can become an integral part of a comprehensive pain treatment plan. Treatment recommendations must be clear, and careful monitoring of prescription medications should be a regular part of follow-up visits. Patients must be informed of the specific limits of confidentiality and the necessity of active consultation with colleagues.

WHAT SHOULD I DO WITH A PATIENT WHO HAS A SUBSTANCE-ABUSE DISORDER?

Patients with chronic pain have a high risk of substance abuse, and determining an individual's potential for substance abuse is important.[94,95] According to the Centers for Disease Control and Prevention, the number of drug-related fatalities in 2008 exceeded the number of motor vehicle traffic deaths for the first time since 1980. There were more than 41,000 poisoning deaths compared with 38,000 motor vehicle traffic deaths. Multiple drugs were listed in 72% of deaths classified as "opioid-related fatality," including antidepressants (32%), illicit drugs (22%), and benzodiazepines (21%).[96]

Opioid abuse is characterized by an overwhelming focus on opioid issues in combination with problematic behaviors such as a pattern of early refills, lost prescriptions, and illicit substance use. Addicted patients often report a craving for opioids and take more medication than prescribed.[94,95] Studies indicate that 10% to 16% of patients treated in a general practice and 25% to 40% of hospitalized patients have prior problems related to drug or alcohol addiction.[97] All patients should be asked about a substance abuse history as part of their initial evaluation, even among those who appear at the outset to be at a low risk for opioid addiction. If opioids are being considered, a more detailed assessment of the risk of opioid abuse should be performed.

TABLE 22-8 Portenoy's Risk Factors and Aberrant Behaviors

Representative Aberrant Drug-Related Behaviors
Selling prescription drugs
Prescription forgery
Stealing or "borrowing" drugs from others
Injecting oral formulations
Obtaining prescription drugs from nonmedical sources
Concurrent abuse of alcohol or illicit drugs
Multiple dose escalations or other noncompliance with therapy despite warnings
Multiple episodes of prescription "loss"
Repeatedly seeking prescriptions from other clinicians or from emergency departments without informing prescriber or after warnings to desist
Evidence of deterioration in the ability to function at work, in the family, or socially that appear to be related to drug use
Repeated resistance to changes in therapy despite clear evidence of adverse physical or psychological effects from the drug
Less Predictive Aberrant Drug-Related Behaviors
Aggressive complaining about the need for more drugs
Drug hoarding during periods of reduced symptoms
Requesting specific drugs
Openly acquiring similar drugs from other medical sources
Unsanctioned dose escalation or other noncompliance with therapy on one or two occasions
Unapproved use of the drug to treat another symptom
Reporting psychic effects not intended by the clinician
Resistance to change in therapy associated with "tolerable" adverse effects with expressions of anxiety related to the return of severe symptoms

Fitzcharles and colleagues recommend that patients be categorized as drug-seeking if they exhibit any of the following: altered medical or pharmacy records, documented repeated inappropriate requests for opioids from multiple physicians, or use of multiple pharmacies.[98] Portenoy[99] identified additional risk factors and aberrant behaviors that are more predictive and less predictive of a substance abuse problem (**Table 22-8**).

Chou et al. concluded that although several screening instruments may be useful, the predictive ability or identification of aberrant drug-related behaviors is still limited.[100] A summary of screening tools is shown in **Table 22-9**.

For patients who may be at a high risk for opioid abuse, either not prescribing opioids or careful monitoring consisting of biweekly prescriptions, regular physician visits, and random urine toxicology screens should be instituted. Recent guidelines for patient assessment and use of opioids for chronic nonmalignant pain include the American Pain Society and Academy of Pain Medicine,[101] Washington State (http://www.agencymeddirectors.wa.gov/Files/OpioidGdline.pdf),[102] and the Royal Australasian College of Physicians.[103] Physicians and patients also demonstrate a potent reciprocal relationship of reinforcement that can influence each other's behaviors. Studies have shown that physicians are influenced by patients' behaviors, including emotional distress and nonverbal expressions.[104,105] Conversely, patients observe the responses of their physicians. If patients with a substance abuse problem perceive that medications are increased when they are more demonstrative (e.g., complain more, appear more distressed), at the next consult, they may present as even more extreme to obtain further treatment.[19]

TABLE 22-9 Screening tools for prediction of substance abuse. Based on a review of the literature and a consensus of the advisory committee, the first three highlighted tools are recommended for their clinical utility in screening opioid therapy patients

	To screen for			To monitor	Tool characteristics			
	Risk of opioid addiction	Current or past substance abuse	Depression, mental or behavioral health	Opioid therapy	Administration	Time to complete (min)	Length	Available for public use (cost)
Opioid Risk Tool (ORT)	X				Clinician or patient self-report	5 min	5 (yes/no) questions	X (Free)
CAGE Adapted to Include Drugs (CAGE-AID)		X			Clinician	<5 min	4 (yes/no) questions	X (Free)
Patient Health Questionnaire 9 (PHQ-9)			X		Patient self-report	<5 min	10 items	X (Free)
Screener and Opioid Assessment for Patients with Pain (SOAPP-R) www.painedu.org/soapp.asp	X				Patient self-report	<10 min	24 items	X (Free, with licensing agreement)
Alcohol Use Disorders Identification Test (AUDIT)		X			Clinician or patient self-report	<5 min	10 items	X (Free)
Center for Epidemiologic Studies Depression Scale (CES-D)			X		Patient self-report	5 min	20 items	X (Free)
Global Appraisal of Individual Needs Short Screener (GAIN-SS)			X		Staff or patient self-report	5 min	15 (yes/no) questions	X (Free)
Current Opioid Misuse Measure (COMM) www.painedu.org/soapp.asp				X	Patient self-report	<10 min	17 items	X (Free, with licensing agreement)

The tools listed in this table have demonstrated good content, face, and construct validity in screening for risk of addiction and monitoring opioid therapy. Further validation studies and prospective outcome studies are needed to determine how the use of these tools predicts and affects clinical outcomes.

HOW DO I HANDLE NONCOMPLIANCE AND NONADHERENCE?

Noncompliance generally denotes failure to follow an order, policy, or law. The implication is that the party whose behavior is in question has a legal or contractual obligation to conform. Medical patients do not necessarily have this obligation. They have the prerogative to accept or reject medical recommendations for medical treatment, surgery, or changes in habits or behaviors.

Often, difficult patients may reject prescribed treatments through noncompliance with medications, physical rehabilitation, or lifestyle modifications. These patients may not be ready to make the changes necessary for improvement and may express their unwillingness to accept the treatment plan through noncompliance and maladaptive behaviors.

Noncompliance or nonadherence has been associated with greater levels of mistrust in the prescribing doctor, concerns about the side effects of medications, and concern about withdrawal from medications. Rosser et al. found that 28.5% of patients reported concerns that their doctor was not adequately educating them on the nature of the medication, resulting in greater mistrust toward that doctor and subsequent over or underuse of prescribed medications.[106] These results demonstrate the importance of the patient–doctor relationship in compliance. Moreover, patients underusing or overusing their medication may have different reasons for doing so.[107]

The first step to solving nonadherence problems is to modify the treatment plan. Perhaps the estimation of their abilities and motivation was overly optimistic, or perhaps the patient has good reasons for noncompliance. Modifying the prescription of medication, physical rehabilitation, and recommended lifestyle changes may coax patients into complying. If this attempt fails, motivation may be elicited by guiding patients to understand that adherence to treatment plans is a necessary condition for the continuation of treatment and instrumental to their improvement. Although patient preferences for treatment should generally be respected, for some pain patients, this indulgence can be countertherapeutic. An insistence on following the treatment plan can be justified by underlining the importance of mutual respect and patient cooperation. If patients are ready to adopt the changes or willing to comply, it may be necessary to inform them that additional appointments will be scheduled only when they are ready to accept the recommended treatment plan. In these cases, detailed documentation is always important in a decision to discontinue treatment, even if it is temporary.

WHAT ARE MY LEGAL OBLIGATIONS IN DISMISSING A DIFFICULT PATIENT?

After a patient–physician relationship is begun, a physician generally is under both an ethical and a legal obligation to provide services as long as the patient needs them.[108] Even a difficult patient will rarely have to be dismissed or "fired" from a practice. There may be times, however, when it is no longer possible to provide care (e.g., opioid-addicted patient who refuses treatment for his or her addiction and continues to ask for prescriptions or a patient who is repeatedly hostile), and "firing" a patient is the only option.

Regardless of the situation, to avoid a claim of "patient abandonment," a physician must follow appropriate steps to terminate the patient–physician relationship. Patient abandonment is defined as "the termination of a professional relationship between physician and patient at an unreasonable time and without giving the patient the chance to find an equally qualified replacement."[108]

According to the American Medical Association's Council on Ethical and Judicial Affairs, a physician may not discontinue treatment of a patient as long as further treatment is medically indicated, without giving the patient reasonable notice and sufficient opportunity to make alternative arrangements for care. Physicians have the option of terminating the patient–physician relationship, but they must give sufficient notice of withdrawal to the patient to allow another physician to be found.

Appropriate steps to terminate the patient–physician relationship typically include:

1. Giving the patient written notice, preferably by certified mail, with a return receipt requested
2. Providing the patient with a brief explanation for terminating the relationship (this should be a valid reason, e.g., noncompliance, failure to keep appointments)
3. Agreeing to continue to provide treatment and access to services for a reasonable period of time, such as 30 days, to allow a patient to secure care from another person (a physician may want to extend the period for emergency services)
4. Providing resources or recommendations to help a patient locate another physician of similar specialty
5. Offering to transfer records to a newly designated physician upon signed patient authorization to do so

Actual negligence appears to be poorly correlated with the incidence of lawsuits.[109] In a study of 100 medicolegal cases, Neale found that in lawsuits in which no negligence was found (44%), reasons for filing the lawsuit were inability to come to terms with the disease or its end results (21%); lack of understanding of the disease process (16%); and unreasonable medicolegal action (7%), indicating that patients who are dissatisfied with their care for reasons other than that of alleged negligence may initiate legal action against their physicians.[109]

Fishbain et al. found that patients with chronic pain are at greater risk than acute pain and other rehabilitation patients for wishing to bring legal actions against their physicians.[110] Using the BH 2, significant associations were found among patient factors and the "Sue MD Wish"—i.e., the patient's wish to sue his or her physician (**Table 22-10**). Overall, Fishbain's clinical portraits of a patient who contemplates suing his or her physician include the following characteristics: he or she is nonwhite, has a higher educational level, is a workers' compensation patient, and has an attorney. The patient has cynical beliefs about physicians in general and is angry with the physician who he or she may have been forced to see. He or she may also have significant psychiatric problems, such as addiction, depression or suicidal ideation, violent ideation, or PTSD symptoms, and is from a dysfunctional family with a history of abuse in childhood. Finally, this patient also has feelings of entitlement and is focused on compensation. A wide variety of inciting factors may be implicated, including the physician's perceived interest in the patient, his or her demeanor, and even his or her mode of dress.[111-121]

Using a sequential logistical regression model, the odds of reporting a desire to sue a physician were decreased by 35% for lower levels of education and by 78% if the patient did not have an attorney involved who was involved in health care issues. The probability of wanting to sue a physician was increased by a factor of 3.63 if the subject was of a race other than white.[110]

TABLE 22-10 Significant BH 2 Items Associated with Patients' Wish to Litigate

Angry with physician	Fear of dying
Harmful treatment	Flashbacks
Forced to see physician; do not trust physician	Severe childhood punishments
Physician only want money	Thinking about killing
Physicians never help	Feeling dangerous
Same old treatment	Many violent thoughts
Physicians do not listen	Thinking about killing physician
Some physicians are idiots	Suicidal ideation
Reason to mistrust physician	History of suicide attempt
Hearing voices	My concerns more important than others
Nothing seems real	Expects special attention
Addiction to prescription medications	Somebody owes me for pain and suffering
History of substance treatment	I should be paid for the rest of my life

CONCLUSIONS

The "difficulty" with difficult patients has less to do with such patients' behaviors themselves and more to do with the feelings their behaviors evoke in their providers. Frustration, anxiety, guilt, or dislike on the part of patient or provider can inhibit or even damage the doctor–patient relationship, and effective management of such emotions is critical to the successful treatment of pain. Effectively managing difficult patients depends on the physician's willingness to understand the reasons behind the behaviors that give rise to difficult feelings, as well as his or her ability to intervene in these behaviors in a way that is likely to defuse their negative impact and encourage both compliance and a greater sense of safety and efficacy on the part of the patient. Understanding the experience of chronic pain is important in evaluating any patient but is crucial in treating difficult patients. Demonstrating empathy, helping the patient to feel heard and understood, and guiding him or her to participate in treatment form the bases of successful care of difficult patients. Acquiring a greater sensitivity toward comorbid psychopathology and certain patterns of problematic behavior, such as hostility, suicidality, aberrant drug behavior, and chronic noncompliance, and developing the skills necessary to address them with greater confidence can improve the experience of difficult patients and yield the greatest chance of success.

REFERENCES

1. O'Dowd TC. Five years of heartsink patients in general practice. *BMJ*. Aug 20-27, 1988;297(6647):528-530.
2. Parsons T. *The Social System New York*. Glencoe, IL: The Free Press of Glencoe; 1951.
3. Koekkoek B, van Meijel B, van Ommen J, et al. Ambivalent connections: a qualitative study of the care experiences of non-psychotic chronic patients who are perceived as 'difficult' by professionals. *BMC Psychiatry*. 2010;10(96):1-11.
4. Gerberich SG, Church TR, McGovern PM, et al. An epidemiological study of the magnitude and consequences of work related violence: the Minnesota Nurses' Study. *Occup Environ Med*. Jun 2004;61:495-503.
5. Bruns D, Fishbain DA, Disorbio JM, Lewis JE. What variables are associated with an expressed wish to kill a doctor in community and injured patient samples? *J Clin Psychol Med Settings*. 2010;17:87-97.
6. National Institute for Occupational Safety and Health. Current Intelligence Bulletin 57, Violence in the workplace: risk factors and prevention strategies. DHHS (NIOSH) Publication No. 96-100. Washington, DC: US Department of Health and Human Services, Public Health Service, Centers for Disease Control and Prevention, 1996.
7. Richard-Devantoy S, Olie JP, Gourevitch R. Risk of homicide and major mental disorders: a critical review. *L'Encephale*. 2009;35:521-530.
8. Bruns D, Disorbio JM, Hanks R. Chronic pain and violent ideation: testing a model of patient violence. *Pain Med*. 2007;8:207-215.

9. Fishbain DA, Cutler RB, Rosomoff HL, Steele-Rosomoff R. Risk for violent behavior in patients with chronic pain: evaluation and management in the pain facility setting. *Pain Med.* 2000;1:140-155.
10. Hahn SR, Kroenke K, Spitzer RL, et al. The difficult patient: prevalence, psychopathology, and functional impairment. *J Gen Intern Med.* 1996;11:1-8.
11. Hahn SR. Physical symptoms and physician-experienced difficulty in the physician–patient relationship. *Ann Intern Med.* 2001;134:897-904.
12. Tunks ER, Weir R, Crook J. Epidemiologic perspective on chronic pain treatment. *Can J Psychiatry.* 2008;53(4):235-242.
13. Dworkin R, Richlin D, Handelin D, Brandt L. Predicting treatment response in depresssed and non-depressed chronic pain patients. *Pain.* 1986;24:343-353.
14. Righter EL, Sansone RA. Managing somatic preoccupation. *Am Fam Phys.* 1999;59:3113-3120.
15. Carroll L, Mercado AC, Cassidy JD, et al. A population-based study of factors associated with combinations of active and passive coping with neck and low back pain. *J Rehabil Med.* 2002;34:67–72.
16. Groves JE. Taking care of the hateful patient. *N Engl J Med.* 1978;298:883-887.
17. Miller WR. Motivational interviewing with problem drinkers. *Behav Psychother.* 1983;11:147-172.
18. Miller WR, Rollnick S. *Motivational Interviewing, Preparing People to Change Addictive Behavior.* New York: The Guildford Press, 1991.
19. Turk DC, Swanson KS, Tunks ER. Psychological approaches in the treatment of chronic pain patients—when pills, scalpels, and needles are not enough. *Can J Psych.* 2008;53(4):213-223.
20. Jackson JL, Kroenke K. Difficult patient encounters in the ambulatory clinic: clinical predictors and outcomes. *Arch Intern Med.* 1999;159(10):1069-1075.
21. Platt FW, Gordon GH. *Field Guide to the Difficult Patient Interview.* Philadelphia: Lippincott Williams & Wilkins, 1999.
22. Kristiansson MH, Brorsson A, Wachtler C, Troein M. Pain power and patience—a narrative study of general practitioners' relations with chronic pain patients. *BMC Fam Prac.* 2011;12:1-8.
23. Levinson W, Roter DL, Mullooly JP, Dull VT, Frankel RM. Physician-patient communication. The relationship with malpractice claims among primary care physicians and surgeons. *JAMA.* 1997;277:553-559.
24. Ambady N, Laplante D, Nguyen T, et al. Surgeons' tone of voice: a clue to malpractice history. *Surgery.* 2002;132(1):5-9.
25. Entman SS, Glass CA, Hickson GB, et al. The relationship between malpractice claims history and subsequent obstetric care. *JAMA.* 1994;272:1588-1591.
26. Oliver D. Teaching medical learners how to appreciate "difficult" patients. *Can Fam Phys.* 2011;57:506-508.
27. Maslach C, Jackson S, Leiter M. *Maslach Burnout Inventory Manual.* Palo Alto, Calif, CA: Consulting Psychologists Press; 1996.
28. Granek L, Tozer R, Mazzotta P, et al. Nature and impact of grief over patient loss on oncologists' personal and professional lives. *Arch Intern Med.* 2012;172(12):964-966.
29. Zantinge EM, Verhaak PFM, deBakker DH et al. Does burnout among doctors affect their involvement in patients' mental health problems? A study of videotaped consultations. *BMC Family Practice.* 2009;10:1-10.
30 Gillette RD. 'Problem patients': a fresh look at an old vexation. *Fam Pract Manag.* 2000;7(7):57-62. PMID: 11010611.
31. American Board of Medical Specialties. Approved initiatives for maintenance of certification for the ABMS board members. Available at: http://www.abms.org%20for%20MOC.pdf. Accessed June 9, 2012.
32. Wasserman SI, Kimball HR, Duffy FD. Task force on recertification. Recertification in internal medicine: a program of continuous professional development. *Ann Intern Med.* 2000;133:202-208.
33. Davis DA, Mazmanian PE, Fordis M, et al. Accuracy of physician self-assessment compared with observed measures of competence. *JAMA.* 2006;296:1094-1102.
34. Kahn MW. Etiquette-based medicine. *N Engl J Med.* 2008;358:1988-1989.
35. Coulehan JL, Platt FW, Egener B, et al. "Let me see if I have this right": words that help build empathy. *Ann Intern Med.* 2001;135:221-227.
36. Haas LJ, Leiser JP, Magill MK. Management of the difficult patient. *Am Fam Physician.* 2005;72:2063-2068.
37. Abbott J. Difficult patients, difficult doctors: can consultants interrupt the "blame game"? *Am J Bioeth.* 2012;12:18-20.
38. Fishbain DA. The association of chronic pain and suicide. *Semin Clin Neuropsychiatry.* 1999;4:221-227.
39. Wasan AD, Gallagher RM. Psychopharmacology for pain medicine. In: Benzon HT, Raja SN, Malloy RE, Liu S, Fishman SM, eds. *Essentials of Pain Medicine and Regional Anesthesia, Ed 2.* New York: WB Saunders; 2004:124-133.
40. Knaster P, Karlsson H, Estlander AM, Kalso E. Psychiatric disorders as assessed with SCID in chronic pain patients: the anxiety disorders precede the onset of pain. *Gen Hosp Psychiatry.* 2012;34:46-52.
41. Fishbain DA, Cutler RB, Rosomoff HL, et al. Chronic pain-associated depression: antecedent or consequence of chronic pain? A review. *Clin J Pain.* 1997;13:116-137.
42. Fishbain DA. Approaches to treatment decisions for psychiatric comorbidity in the management of the chronic pain patient. *Med Clin North Am.* 1999;83:737-760.
43. McWilliams LA, Cox BJ, Enns MW. Mood and anxiety disorders associated with chronic pain: an examination in a nationally representative sample. *Pain.* 2003;106:127-133.
44. Goral A, Lipsitz JD, Gross R. The relationship of chronic pain with and without comorbid psychiatric disorder to sleep disturbance and health care utilization: results from the Israel National Health Survey. *J Psychosom Res.* 2010;69:449-457.
45. Gerrits MMJG, Vogelzangs N, van Oppen P, et al. Impact of pain on the course of depressive and anxiety disorders. *Pain.* 2012;153:429-436.
46. Wells KB, Golding JM, Burnam M. Psychiatric disorder in a sample of the general population with and without medical conditions. *Am J Psychiatry.* 1988;145:976-981.
47. Blair MJ, Robinson RL, Katon W, Kroenke K. Depression and pain comorbidity: a literature review. *Arch Intern Med.* 2003;163:2433-2445.
48. Linton S. A review of psychological risk factors in back and neck pain. *Spine.* 2000;25:1148-1156.
49. Dworkin R, Richlin D, Handelin D, Brandt L. Predicting treatment response in depresssed and non-depressed chronic pain patients. *Pain.* 1986;24:343-353.
50. *Diagnostic and Statistical Manual of Mental Disorders,* ed 4. Washington, DC: American Psychiatric Association, 2000.
51. Polatin P, Kinney RK, Gatchel RJ, et al. Psychiatric illness and chronic low-back pain. The mind and the spine—which goes first? *Spine.* 1993;18(1):66-71.
52. Gatchel RJ, Polatin PB, Kinney RK. Predicting outcome of chronic back pain using clinical predictors of psychopathology: a prospective analysis. *Health Psychol.* 1995;14(5):415-420.
53. Reich J, Tupin JP, Abramowitz SI. Psychiatric diagnosis of chronic pain patients. *Am J Psychiatry.* 1983;140(11):1495-1498.

54. McWilliams L, Cox B, Enns M. Mood and anxiety disorders associated with chronic pain: an examination in a nationally representative sample. *Pain*. 2003;106:127-133.

55. Stang P, Brandenburg N, Lane M, et al. Mental and physical comorbid conditions and days in role among persons with arthritis. *Psychosom Med*. 2006;68(1):152-158.

56. von Korff M, Crane P, Lane M, et al. Chronic spinal pain and physical-mental comorbidity in the United States: results from the national comorbidity survey replication. *Pain*. 2005;113:331-339.

57. Gerhardt A, Hartmann M, Schuller-Roma B, et al. The prevalence and type of axis-I and axis-II mental disorders in subjects with non-specific chronic back pain: results from a population-based study. *Pain Med*. 2011;12:1231-1240.

58. Epstein RM, Quill TE, McWhinney IR. Somatization reconsidered: incorporating the patient's experience of illness. *Arch Intern Med*. 1999;159:215-222.

59. Gerrard TJ, Riddell JD. Difficult patients: black holes and secrets. *BMJ*. 1988;297:20-27.

60. Santana L, Fontenelle LF. A review of studies concerning treatment adherence of patients with anxiety disorders. *Patient Prefer Adherence*. 2011;5:427-439.

61. Greve KW, Ord JS, Bianchini KJ, Curtis KL. Prevalence of malingering in patients with chronic pain referred for psychologic evaluation in a medico-legal context. *Arch Phys Med Rehabil*. 2009;90:1117-1126.

62. Samuel RZ, Mittenberg W. Determination of malingering in disability evaluations. *Primary Psychiatry*. 2005;12:60-68.

63. Bianchini KJ, Mathias CW, Greve KW. Symptom validity testing: a critical review. *The Clin Neuropsych*. 2004;15:19-45.

64. Grote CL, Hook JN. Forced-choice recognition tests of malingering. In: Larrabee GJ ed. *Assessment of Malingered Neuropsychological Deficits*. New York: Oxford University Press; 2007:44-79.

65. Friedman S, Chernen L. Discriminating the panic disorder patient from patients with borderline personality disorder. *J Anxiety Disord*. 1994;8:49-61.

66. Magerl W, Burkart D, Fernandez A, Schmidt LG, Treede RD. Persistent antinociception through repeated self-injury in patients with borderline personality disorder. *Pain*. 2011;153(3):575-584.

67. Sansone RA, Sinclair DJ, Wiederman MW. Disability and borderline personality disorder in chronic pain patients. *Pain Res Manage*. 2010;15:369-370.

68. Kroll J. *The Challenge of the Borderline Patient*. New York: WW Norton & Company, 1988.

69. Horwitz L. Indications for group psychotherapy with borderline and narcissistic patients. *B Menninger Clin*. 1987;51(3):248-260.

70. Stone MH. Psychotherapy of borderline patients in light of long-term follow-up. *B Menninger Clin*. 1987;51(3):231-247.

71. Sansone RA, Whitecar P, Meier BP, Murry A. The prevalence of borderline personality among primary care patients with chronic pain. *Gen Hosp Psychiatry*. 2001;23:193-197.

72. Gardner JW, Amoroso PJ, Grayson JK, Helmkamp J, Jones BH. Hospitalizations due to injury: inpatient medical records data. *Mil Med*. 1999;164(8 Suppl):1-143.

73. Lew HL, Otis JD, Tun C, et al. Prevalence of chronic pain, posttraumatic stress disorder, and persistent postconcussive syndrome in OIF/OEF veterans: polytrauma clinical triad. *J Rehabil Res Devel*. 2009;46:697-702.

74. US Department of Defense. Available at http://www.defense.gov/pubs/. Bethesda, MD. Accessed April 2012.

75. Wilford Hall Medical Center Lackland Airforce Base. Available at http://www.whasc.af.mil/. San Antonio, TX. Accessed March 2012.

76. Gatchel RJ, Okifuji A. Evidence-based scientific data documenting the treatment and cost-effectiveness of comprehensive pain programs for chronic nonmalignant pain. *J Pain*. Nov 2006;7(11):779-793.

77. Barsky AJ, Borus JF. Functional somatic syndromes. *Ann Intern Med*. June 1, 1999;130(11):910-921.

78. Righter EL, Sansone RA. Managing somatic preoccupation. *Am Fam Phys*. 1999;59:3113-3120.

79. Ford CV. *The Somatizing Disorders: Illness as a Way of Life*. New York: Elsevier Science; 1983.

80. Reme SE, Tangen T, Moe T, Eriksen HR. Prevalence of psychiatric disorders in sick listed chronic low back pain patients. *Eur J Pain*. 2011;15:1075-1080.

81. Dominick CH, Blyth FM, Nicolas MK. Unpacking the burden: understanding the relationships between chronic pain and comorbidity in the general population. *Pain*. 2012;153:293-304.

82. Princeton Insurance. Six steps for dealing with angry patients. www.riskreviewonline.com. 2002.

83. Jacobs DG, Baldessarini RJ, Conwell Y, et al. Practice guideline for the assessment and treatment of patients with suicidal behaviors. Work group on suicidal behaviors. American Psychiatric Association. 2003;1-184.

84. Fishbain DA, Bruns D, Disorbio JM, Lewis JE. Risk for five forms of suicidality in acute pain patients and chronic pain patients vs pain-free community controls. *Pain Med*. 2009;10:1095-1105.

85. Fishbain DA, Lewis JE, Gao J, Cole B, Rosonoff RS. Are chronic low back pain patients who smoke at greater risk for suicide ideation? *Pain Med*. 2009;10:340-348.

86. Edwards RE, Smith MT, Kudel I, Haythorthwaite JH. Pain-related catastrophizing as a risk factor for suicidal behavior in chronic pain. *Pain*. 2006;126:272-279.

87. Campbell LC, Clauw DJ, Keefe FJ. Persistent pain and depression: a biopsychosocial perspective. *Biol Psychiatry*. 2003;54(3):399-409.

88. Morriss RK, Ahmed M, Wearden AJ, et al. The role of depression in pain, psychophysiological syndromes and medically unexplained symptoms associated with chronic fatigue syndrome. *J Affect Disord*. 1999;55:143-148.

89. Evans DL, Charney DS, Lewis L, et al. Mood disorders in the medically ill: scientific review and recommendations. *Biol Psychiatry*. 2005;58:175-189.

90. Chellappa P, Ramaraj R. Depression, homocysteine concentration, and cardiovascular events. *JAMA*. 2009;301(15):1541-1542.

91. Fava M, Rush AJ, Alpert JE, et al. What clinical and symptom features and comorbid disorders characterize outpatients with anxious major depressive disorder: a replication and extension. *Can J Psychiatry*. 2006;51(13):823-835.

92. Tang NK, Crane C. Suicidality in chronic pain: a review of the prevalence, risk factors and psychological links. *Psychol Med*. 2006;36:575-586.

93. Fishbain DA, Lewis JE, Bruns D, Gao J, Disorbio JM, Meyer L. Patient predictor variables for six forms of suicidality. *Eur J Pain*. 2011;16(5):706-717.

94. Nedeljkovic SS, Wasan A, Jamison RN. Assessment of efficacy of long-term opioid therapy in pain patients with substance abuse potential. *Clin J Pain*. 2002;18(suppl):S39-S51.

95. Savage SR. Assessment for addiction in pain treatment settings. *Clin J Pain*. 2002;18(suppl):S28-S38.

96. NCHS Data Brief #81. Available at: http://www.slideshare.net/UnitB166ER/drug-poisoning-deaths-in-the-united-states-1980-to-2008-by-margaret-warner-ph-d-li-hui-chen-phd-diane-m-makuc-dr-ph-robert-n-anderson-phd-and-arialdi-m-minio-mph. Atlanta, GA. Accessed June 10, 2012.

97. Kissen B. Medical management of alcoholic patients. In: Kissen B, Begleiter H, eds. *The Biology of Alcoholism, Vol. 5, Treatment*

and Rehabilitation of the Chronic Alcoholic. New York: Plenum; 1997:53-103.

98. Fitzcharles MA, Ste-Marie PA, Gansa A, Ware MA, Shir Y. Opioid use, misuse, and abuse in patients labeled as fibromyalgia. *Am J Med*. 2011;124:955-960.
99. Portenoy RK. Opioid therapy for chronic nonmalignant pain: a review of the critical issues. *J Pain Symptom Manage*. 1996;11(4):203-217.
100. Chou R. Prediction and identification of aberrant drug-related behaviors: a review of the evidence for an American Pain Society and American Academy of Pain Medicine Clinical Practice Guideline," Appendix B. Clinical guidelines from the APS/AAPM on the use of chronic opioid therapy in chronic noncancer pain: what are the key messages for clinical practice? *Pol Arch Med*. 2009;119:469-477.
101. Butler SF, Fernandez K, Benoit C, Budman SH, Jamison RN. Validation of the revised screener and opioid assessment for patients with pain (SOAPP-R). *J Pain*. 2008;9:360-372.
102. Agency Medical Directors Group. Available at: http://www.agencymeddirectors.wa.gov/Files/OpioidGdline.pdf. Washington. Accessed May 20, 2012.
103. The Royal Australasian College of Physicians. Prescription opioid policy: improving management of chronic nonmalignant pain and prevention of problems associated with prescription opioid use. Available at: http://www.racp.edu.au/index.cfm?objectid=EA87198D-CA47-AB21-072D9B2F26FD4AA3. Sydney, Australia. Accessed June 1, 2012.
104. Martell BA, O'Connor PG, Kerns RD, et al. Systematic review: opioid treatment for chronic back pain: prevalence, efficacy, and association with addiction. *Ann Intern Med*. 2007;146:116-127.
105. Turk DC, Okifuji A. Evaluating the role of physical, operant, cognitive, and affective factors in the pain behaviors of chronic pain patients. *Behav Modif*. 1997;21:259-280.
106. Rosser BA, McCracken LM, Velleman SC, Boichat C, Eccleston C. Concerns about medication and medication adherence in patients with chronic pain recruited from general practice. *Pain*. 2011;152:1201-1205.
107. Broekmans S, Dobbels F, Milisen K, Morlion B, Vanderschueren S. Determinants of medication underuse and medication overuse in patients with chronic non-malignant pain: a multicenter study. *Int J Nurs Stud*. 2010;47(11):1408-1417.
108. American Medical Association. Available at: http://www.amaassn.org/ama/pub/physician-resources/medical-ethics/code-medical-ethics/opinion8115.page. Chicago, IL. Accessed May 24, 2012.
109. Neale G. Clinical analysis of 100 medicolegal cases. *BMJ*. 1993;307:1483-1487.
110. Fishbain DA, Bruns D, Lewis JE, et al. Predictors of homicide-suicide affirmation in acute and chronic pain patients. *Pain Med*. 2011;12:127-137.
111. Cline RJW, Haynes KM. Consumer health information seeking on the Internet: the state of the art. *Health Ed Res*. 2001;61(6):671-692.
112. Stilwell NA, Wallick MM, Thal SE, Burleson JA. Meyers-Briggs type and medical specialty choice: a new look at an old question. *Teach Learn Med*. 2000;12(1):14-20.
113. Roback HB, Strassberg D, Iannelli RJ, et al. Problematic physicians: a comparison of personality profiles by offence type. *Can J Psychiatry*. 2007;52:315-322.
114. Silverman BC, Stern TW, Gross AF. Lewd, crude, and rude behavior: the impact of manners and etiquette in the general hospital. *Psychosomatics*. 2012;53:13-20.
115. Rabkin MT. Etiquette: preaching and teaching. *JAMA*. 1988;260:2562-2563.
116. Dunn JJ, Lee TH, Percelay JM, et al. Patient and house officer attitudes on physician attire and etiquette. *JAMA*. 1987;257:65-68.
117. Rehman SU, Nietert PJ, Cope DW, et al. What to wear today? Effect of doctor's attire on the trust and confidence of patients. *Am J Med*. 2005;118:1279-1286.
118. Lill MM, Wilkinson TJ. Judging a book by its cover: descriptive survey of patients' preferences for doctors' appearance and mode of address. *BMJ*. 2005;331:1524-1527.
119. Nihalani ND, Kunwar A, Staller K, et al. How should psychiatrists dress?—A survey. *Community Ment Health J*. 2006;42:291-302.
120. Kinney RK, Gatchel RJ, Polatin P, Fogarty WT, Mayer TG. Prevalence of psychopathology in acute and chronic low back pain patients. *J Occup Rehabil*. 1993;3(2):5-103.
121. Jacobson JA. The effect of patients' noncompliance on their surgeons' obligations. *Surg Clin North Am*. 2007;87:937-948.

New Prospects for Alleviation of Anger in the Context of Chronic Pain

Ephrem Fernandez
Robert D. Kerns

CONCEPTUALIZATION OF ANGER

WHAT IS ANGER?

Anger has been defined with different shades of emphasis, but in psychology, there is general agreement that anger is a subjective feeling rooted in an attribution or appraisal of wrongdoing and coupled with an action tendency to undo that wrongdoing in ways that may range from resistance to retaliation. This is consistent with the cognitive-motivational view of all emotions.[1] It also reflects Smedslund's[2] depiction of the lay perspective on anger.

Similar to fear and sadness, anger can assume any one of three forms: emotion, mood, or temperament.[3] Emotion is a momentary episode, mood is relatively prolonged in duration, and temperament is a proneness to the particular feeling or emotion so that it recurs. These three forms are reflected in the varied and nuanced vocabulary of anger. As an emotion, anger can range in intensity from annoyance to rage; as a mood, it is tonic rather than phasic as implied by the words *irritability* or *irascibility*; as temperament, it is a propensity to frequent anger as captured in the word *hostility*, which, in affect science, is reserved for dispositional or attitudinal rather than situational anger.[4,5]

Some of these lexical boundaries may be ignored in common parlance. However, for scientists and professionals, proper classification and terminology facilitate comparisons across studies, integration of findings, and scholarly discourse. Hence, there is interest in choosing the right words and (when necessary) coining new terms for different phenomena. Along such lines, anger is further distinguishable from two other terms, aggression and violence. *Aggression*, in social psychology, refers to behavior (physical or verbal) that is intended to hurt. *Violence* is behavior that intentionally and actually culminates in physical injury or damage.

WHEN IS ANGER A PROBLEM?

According to the *Diagnostic and Statistical Manual of Mental Disorders*, fifth edition (DSM-5),[6] a mental disorder is "a syndrome characterized by clinically significant disturbance in an individual's cognition, emotion regulation, or behavior that reflects a dysfunction in the psychological, biological, or developmental processes underlying mental functioning" (p. 20). A conspicuous departure from the earlier version of the DSM has been the omission of the statement about significantly increased risk of "pain, disability, death, or important loss of freedom"[7] (p. xxxi). By the new rule, a heightened risk of pain or other catastrophic consequences does not signal a mental disorder. However, aggressive or violent anger would almost certainly be regarded as a disorder inasmuch as it represents a marked disturbance in actions, thoughts, or emotional control. Yet, at present there are no DSM diagnostic labels for anger disorders. One exception is intermittent explosive disorder (IED), which is grouped under "Disruptive, Impulse-Control and Conduct Disorders" along with conditions such as pyromania, kleptomania, and oppositional defiant disorder. A diagnosis of IED refers to recurrently uncontrolled anger culminating in physical or verbal aggression that is very disproportionate to provocation. Nevertheless, the risks and deleterious effects of anger are increasingly well documented and extend beyond aggression and violence to a range of medical health problems. Prominent among these health problems are cardiovascular disease[8,9] and pain.[10,11]

ANGER AND PAIN

A relatively large and growing body of research has documented important associations between the experiences of anger and pain.[12] Persons with chronic pain are more likely than others without pain to report high levels of anger. Among those with chronic pain, those who appear to readily express anger toward others and possibly those who seem to suppress anger report relatively higher levels of pain intensity and even pain-related disability.[13] Ongoing research is investigating the hypothesis that endogenous opioid systems[13] and other physiological mechanisms[14] may play a role in determining the impact of anger and its expression on the experience of pain.

EXPERIENCE OF ANGER

ANGER IN THE PATIENTS WITH PAIN

A recent article by Wootton[15] offers an incisive review of the etiology of anger in pain; it also describes various psychological instruments for the assessment of anger. To complement that review, the present chapter explores the experience of anger in patients with pain and then expands on how to treat anger in the context of chronic pain.

Although underresearched compared with depression and anxiety, anger has been recognized as a problem that merits attention in individuals with chronic pain and one that is closely related to pain severity as well as depression.[16] The scarcity of epidemiologic data in this area is partly due to an underdeveloped psychiatric nosology. IED has been reported by about 10% of pain patients assessed in an early study by Fishbain and colleagues.[17] Interestingly, this exceeds the 12-month prevalence rate of IED in the community, which is about 4% according to the National Comorbidity Survey Replication study of U.S. households.[18] Other than these data on IED, the co-prevalence of anger-related "disorder" and chronic pain is undeterminable.

Directing attention to emotions rather than psychiatric disorders, Fernandez and Milburn (1994) found that chronic pain patients rated their anger higher than sadness, fear, or any one of seven other basic emotions. In a study of 2400 school children in Iceland, Kristjansdottir[19] found that anger was the most common concern in 76.5% of those with weekly back pain, 76.9% of those with weekly headache, and 78.3% of those with weekly stomach pain. This was higher than the prevalence of anxiety or sadness in pain. The relationship of anger to pain became further evident in a survey by Fernandez and collegues,[20] which revealed that patients attributed the bulk of their anger to the pain itself rather than to circumstances extraneous to pain. In a data mining study across all geographical zones of the United States, Fishbain et al.[21] found that anger was affirmed at a significantly higher frequency in chronic pain patients (37.5%) than community patients (28.5%); furthermore, chronic pain patients reported chronic anger at a rate (19.7%) that was much higher than that in acute pain patients or patients without pain.

This brings us to the question: "What is it about chronic pain that makes it highly comorbid with anger?" There are several possible answers. First, it should be noted that comorbidity simply means co-occurrence of diagnoses. Expressed in percentages, proportions, or odds ratios, it represents the relationship in static terms. Alternatively, the conditions may be dynamically related.[22,23] For example, one condition may covary as a function of the other, as indexed in a correlation coefficient. Unfortunately, correlations do not permit inferences about causation. To overcome that limitation, there are experimental or prospective studies that can test for temporal succession—whether A preceded B or vice versa. However, this so-called "chicken versus egg conundrum" is itself an oversimplification.[23] Indeed, anger may be a precipitant that suddenly triggers the onset of pain or an immediate consequence of pain. Furthermore, anger may be a predisposing factor that increases the probability of pain in the long run, anger may be an exacerbating factor that intensifies preexisting pain, and anger may be a perpetuating factor that prolongs the duration of preexisting pain. These represent additional possibilities in the dynamic interaction between pain and anger just as they have characterized other interactions between psyche and soma.

So far, no single study has appeared in which all of the above interactions are pitted against one another much like separate hypotheses of the relationships between anger and pain. However, as in the literature on depression and pain, trends appear across multiple studies. One particularly interesting model suggests that anger as a "trait" combined with a characteristic style of anger inhibition may predispose persons to the development of chronic pain, and emerging research offers some support.[24] The weight of evidence favors a strong role of anger as a consequence of pain. This does not necessarily mean that the anger is hardwired as in a neurophysiological reflex arc. Neither should the anger be viewed as occurring in a vacuum or emerging mysteriously out of a "black box." Although classical conditioning theory can partly account for the quick annoyance in response to toothache, the pain from a punch, or other types of acute pain, it is limited in explaining the anger of chronic pain. This is because chronic pain occurs within a broad psychosocial context, which can drive anger through various cognitive appraisal pathways.[25] In other words, anger in chronic pain patients is the product of multiple and elaborate interpretations of the many entities and activities within the psychosocial context.

THE PSYCHOSOCIAL CONTEXT

Encompassed within the psychosocial arena of chronic pain are a number of possible agents whose actions are construed (by the individual with pain) as wrongdoings. Each of these agent–action complexes can be viewed as an instantiation of the earlier stated definition of anger. The doctor's failure to cure is perceived as an act of incompetence, the insurance company's denial of coverage is viewed as a breach of agreement, and the lack of emotional support from a family member is often viewed as neglect or abandonment. Accordingly, clinicians may venture beyond the basic question: "Is the patient angry?" to the two questions: "Why is the pain patient angry?" and "Toward whom is the anger directed?" An instrument called the Targets and Reasons for Anger in Pain Sufferers[26] (TRAPS) lists 10 common targets of anger in patients as broached by Fernandez and Turk:[10]

1. Person causing an injury or illness
2. Physicians and medical care providers
3. Psychologists and mental health professionals
4. Attorneys and the legal system
5. Insurance and third-party payers
6. Employers
7. Significant others
8. God, higher being, destiny
9. Whole world
10. Other

Using a 0 to 10 numerical scale, the patient rates his or her anger toward each of the above targets. Then, using a checkbox format, the patient identifies and ranks the reasons for his or her anger toward each target, with reference to the following:

1. Pain
2. Diagnostic or treatment difficulties
3. Implication that pain is psychogenic
4. Dispute, scrutiny, or arbitration
5. Inadequate coverage or compensation
6. Loss of employment or retraining
7. Lack of interpersonal support
8. Predetermined event; ill fate
9. Decline in functioning or appearance
10. Regarded as different or unimportant
11. Other

Okifuji, Turk, and Curran (1999) adapted the TRAPS for self-administration by 96 chronic pain patients, most of whom had low back or leg pain. They found that 65% of male and 71% of female patients reported some level of anger. The percentages of patients with anger toward targets were 60% toward health care providers, 20% toward attorneys, 30% toward insurance companies, 26% toward employers, and 39% toward significant others. Additionally, the vast majority, 70%, were angry at themselves. When actual anger ratings were averaged after a TRAPS interview of chronic pain patients, these patients were found to be angriest toward insurance companies and least angry toward psychologists.[10] Results from the TRAPS reveal the scope of the psychosocial context of anger in chronic pain patients.

Clinical anecdotes of anger are common in case conferences on patients with pain. Such anecdotes can also be found in published work. For example, Roy describes a pain patient's anger over loss of employment:

"When Mrs. Abrams resigned her position, she lost . . . a vital element of her sense of self. She lost her place . . . as a valued member of a helping profession. Above all, she lost a simple, yet a core, component of her identity. Redefinition of the self was called for, but the answer was far from acceptable. The answer in her case was that of a chronic patient. This radical change in identity extracts an enormous psychological cost. Some patients may experience relief, but not Mrs. Abrams, who took exceptional pride in her profession. She felt humiliated, unfairly treated by the world, sad, and even grief-struck and very angry." (Roy, 2002, p. 4).

Graham, Lobel, Glass & Lokshina (2008) provide excerpts of written accounts of anger from two pain patients: "I am in constant pain due to your negligence. I wish I could make you understand what it feels like. . . . I feel so mad. . . . I hope you never have another good night's sleep in your life. I know I won't." "I can't believe that after all this I have to listen to a druggist [who] has no idea how I feel. . . . You make me feel like a criminal and a drug addict" (p. 201).

A single individual may harbor anger at multiple targets for a variety of perceived wrongdoings. This is illustrated in the following anecdote from a victim of a major industrial accident:

"Lured by their promise of jobs, the government gave them a permit to develop their industry. With the bare minimum staff, we worked longer and harder as management kept cutting corners, and then—Disaster!. Now, the jobs are gone, the factory has changed hands, they've taken the heap of profits, and left us with pain, unimaginable health problems, and a toxic environment. Where's the justice? My wife gave birth to a baby who died after 4 weeks, then she died of cancer or depression, I'm not sure which. I'm stuck with pain every day—pain in the stomach and chest and difficulty breathing. I know I'm the next to go, because there is no cure and the pain only gets worse. The doctors don't have all the answers and just keep giving me pain killers and steroids. Health insurance won't pay for anything else. We need money just to stay alive but no one will give us even a basic job as long as they suspect we're sick. We filed for compensation but that will take years and who knows what we'll get after the sharks take their bite. The corporation is already talking about an out-of-court settlement so they can escape future liability while the CEO and upper managers still live it up; can you believe it? Now you know why I'm so angry and don't trust any official working for the system; they're not there to help us. Every time I feel the pain, the anger returns as I remember what happened that dreadful day. I remember my family members . . . I couldn't even afford a proper funeral for them after using all my life savings to pay for fees and expenses. I cannot bring them back, and I may not stop sliding downhill, but I'll stomach the poison and keep going as long as I can to get those criminals to pay. I don't want to see any decent human being go through what we go through; I just want to see those responsible pay in some way. And many of us are hanging on just to see that day."

Similar to this, there are many narratives of anger from people whose pain originated in the context of work, combat, crime, or even recreation. The unifying theme is that the anger evolves in a psychosocial environment where there are many agents, some active and some passive, each blamed for some kind of transgression, ineptitude, or negligence.[27] Chronic pain is aversive in and of itself, but it can also become a powerful reminder of the grievances, thus generating recurrent anger. In fact, pain can become a cue for everything that has gone awry in the individual's life.

TREATMENT OF ANGER

COGNITIVE-BEHAVIORAL THERAPY

Because chronic pain is, by definition, intractable, recurrent anger in this patient population would be more fruitfully handled by turning attention to the psychosocial context of anger. If what has transpired cannot be reversed, then what can be changed is the way the individual construes it. Cognitive-behavioral therapies (CBTs) are designed to do just that. They help the patient reappraise circumstances and cope with unpleasant realities, apart from also countering anger arousal with relaxation. In a meta-analysis of CBT for anger, Beck and Fernandez[28] found a grand weighted mean effect size of +0.70, meaning that the average subject receiving CBT was better off than 76% of no-treatment control participants in terms of dependent measures of anger. A subsequent meta-analysis by Di Giuseppe and Tafrate (2003) has replicated this effect. With this evidence base in hand, there is good reason to apply the same approach to anger in chronic pain patients.

COGNITIVE-BEHAVIORAL AFFECTIVE THERAPY

Cognitive-behavioral therapy for anger may be enriched by the inclusion of affective techniques that directly target the (distressing) feeling inherent in anger. With origins in experiential psychotherapy, these techniques have undergone a revival under the label of emotion-focused therapies.[29,30] Such techniques are not incompatible with cognitive or behavioral techniques as long as they are meaningfully sequenced within an integrative program for anger regulation. Recently, Fernandez[31] developed an integrative psychotherapy that incorporates affective therapies in addition to enhanced cognitive and behavioral techniques for treating anger. The resulting cognitive-behavioral affective therapy (CBAT) can serve as a model for integrative treatment of anger in the context of chronic pain. Following is a brief explication of CBAT and its principles and techniques as applicable to patients with pain.

One myth to be dispelled at the outset is the proposition that ignoring anger will make it go away. This may stem, in part, from a simplistic behavioral extinction approach to temper tantrums in children and from the widely publicized accounts of how solicitude can reinforce illness behavior in children and adults alike. Indeed, angry outbursts can be manipulative and readily reinforced by contingent attention. However, to make that a blanket assumption for all is a risky proposition. So, anger may be feigned to achieve concessions from others, but genuine anger, if ignored or stifled, may further deteriorate into deep resentment. Barring any obvious signs of secondary gain from the patient's anger, it behooves the clinician to take anger at face value. After all, anger is a function of

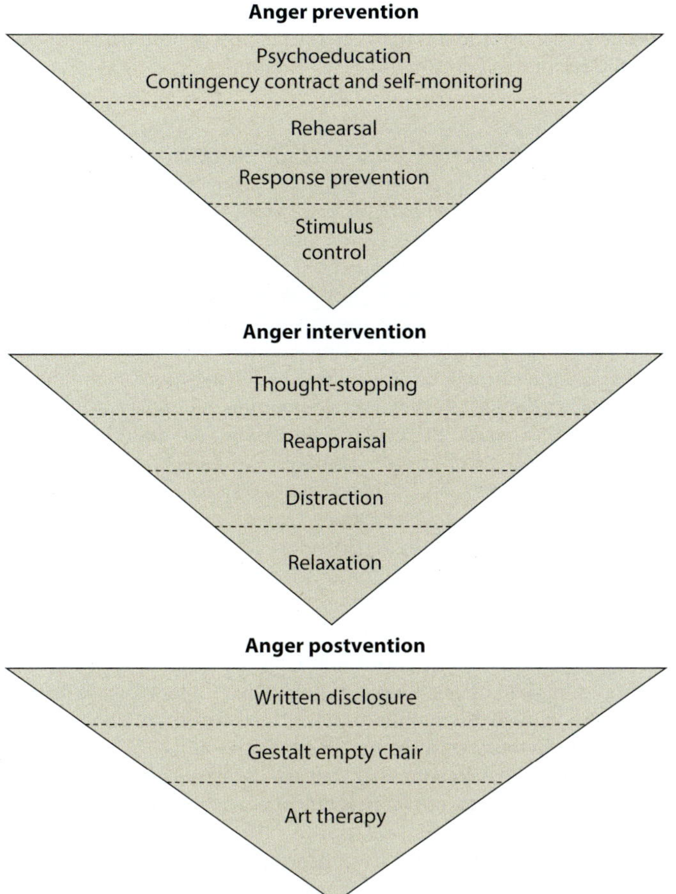

FIGURE 23-1. Successive filters of anger through cognitive-behavioral affective therapy.

perceived wrongdoing, and individual differences abound in what we interpret as wrongdoing; it is not the clinician's place to adjudicate as in a court of law. At least in a self-referred patient who is motivated to control his or her anger, a productive starting point is to ascertain the degree of anger-related dysfunction. Where impairment is evident, anger is not to be discounted as a natural feature of a person's emotional repertoire but better recognized as a disorder worthy of clinical attention.

Cognitive-behavioral affective therapy, as outlined by Fernandez,[31,32] is premised on the notion that anger is a process, with three main phases: onset, progression, and offset. Treatment, therefore, comprises prevention or preparation for potential anger-provoking events, intervention upon outbursts or other experiences of anger, and postvention on the residual traces of anger. As shown in **Figure 23-1**, reappraisal and relaxation remain key features of this approach but are enhanced by several other cognitive and behavioral strategies plus affective techniques for filtering anger through successive phases. The prevention phase is essentially behavioral, the intervention phase is predominantly cognitive, and the affective phase is primarily experiential.

PREVENTION

The customary starting point is psychoeducation. This involves defining anger and acknowledging its ramifications for health, including its hypertensive effect, risks posed for coronary heart disease, possible aggravation of pain, and its pivotal role in interpersonal conflict. In this way, a rationale for anger reduction is put in place. This paves the way for a formal commitment to reduce anger. As in many standard behavioral treatment programs, a contingency contract is prepared by the therapist in consultation with the patient. This spells out the treatment goals and the rewarding consequences for attainment of such goals. Participants are then trained to self-monitor their anger on a regular basis. This provides a source of outcome measures from the naturalistic settings where anger is likely to occur while also generating relevant data to ascertain the extent to which the contract has been fulfilled. Self-monitoring also engenders a certain "reactivity" that is responsible for changing behavior in the desired direction (as often observed in the self-monitoring of eating, smoking, exercise levels, and so on). The gains thus obtained do not compare with gains from treatment per se,[33] but they do promote awareness of anger and create a momentum toward the goal of anger reduction.

Response prevention is an option in case anger erupts. This entails self-inhibitory strategies such as reducing vocal amplitude and motor agitation. Much as in cue-controlled relaxation, the patient implements these strategies upon detecting the earliest signs of anger. This curbs afferent feedback of anger-related arousal while also reducing the risk of escalating anger in other parties involved in the interaction.

If rehearsal and response prevention fail repeatedly, stimulus control would be a preventive option of last resort. If an environment has certain discriminative properties that inevitably elicit uncontrollable anger, then stimulus control offers a way of extricating the individual from that situation. Just as a pathological gambler is well advised to stay away from casinos and an overeater is persuaded to keep certain "problem foods" out of sight, a patient with pain who "loses it" whenever she or he meets with a particular service provider is better off finding an alternative. This does happen in the clinical context where patients, already frustrated by many obstacles, show profound "knee-jerk" antagonism to some clinicians but not to others. The idea of stimulus control is not to offer an easy way out for the patient or to disengage the patient altogether but, as far as possible, to find acceptable alternatives in such extreme irrevocable anger-triggering situations.

INTERVENTION

If attempts to prevent anger prove futile or just impracticable, the next wave of options comes from intervention. Anger, after it has been ignited, can still be brought under control through cognitive techniques such as thought-stopping and reappraisal as well as a host of time-honored relaxation techniques.

Thought stopping is the silent repetition of a word or phrase that runs counter to the abjured thought, in this case, the thought of anger. The idea is to automatize the procedure so that as soon as angry ideation begins, it is met with the thought stopper. Repeated practice is designed to achieve this as long as the individual's anger has not reached obsessive-compulsive proportions.[34]

Reappraisal, by contrast, is a far more elaborate intervention and is the centerpiece of cognitive therapy for emotional disturbance. It entails challenging beliefs on empirical and logical grounds. Given that anger is perceived wrongdoing or mistreatment, one stock retort that is part and parcel of rational emotive therapy is, "Where is the evidence?" The patient may reply with many suppositions of deliberate provocation that led to harm or grievance. Because intentional harm or neglect by the offender has been shown to be central to the belief system of the offended individual, reappraisal would entail a challenge of interpretations about intentionality or harm. In the psychosocial context of chronic pain, the patient may hold that the pain persists because of errors of commission or omission on the part of health professionals. Inasmuch as pain rehabilitation involves tapering of analgesic medications, setting exercise quotas, and refraining from overattending or overnurturing the patient, a misperception may arise that the health care providers are uncaring or (worse still) mistreating the patient. To dispute these ideas, the patient may be reminded of the state of science in pain management techniques, that all others in the same condition are treated equitably, and that it is not in the interest of the health care providers to see the patient suffer. Most important, the often mistaken beliefs about chronic pain may be corrected to make the patient realize that although there is no cure for such pain, neither is there imminent harm, and hence the emphasis is on reduction of functional impairment. In short, the patient is trained to address misattributions about intentionality and harm through empirical evidence and logical reasoning. Such reappraisal has been recently found to reduce anger while also being correlated with neural changes in the brain.[35]

Reappraisal may consume a lot of attentional resources without redirecting the patient away from the pain. In such circumstances, attention diversion may offer a simpler way out. This may take the form of passive distraction or active performance of tasks that can reallocate attention away from the pain and negative affect.[36]

Relaxation has become a cornerstone not only in pain management but also in anger management. Anger subserves the fight response that is mobilized by sympathetic nervous system arousal. Relaxation counters that very arousal, in turn producing afferent feedback that ultimately allows the individual to relabel his or her state in a manner that is inconsistent with anger.[37]

Historically, progressive muscle relaxation has become a technique of choice for stress management, but in the reduction of anger arousal, it has taken a back seat to autogenic relaxation and diaphragmatic breathing. This is largely because Jacobsonian relaxation demands alternations between flexing and releasing of tension in many muscle groups from the head to the feet; this would be contraindicated if the individual wants to continue interacting with others during the anger-eliciting situation. The two alternative relaxation techniques, however, allow the individual to remain relatively engaged in the situation while unobtrusively maintaining his or her efforts to relax.

Autogenic relaxation can follow the same sequence of muscle groups as in Jacobsonian relaxation, but the method of reducing arousal is essentially by self-suggestion. The patient is trained to imagine the release of tension from the muscles of the neck, back, hands, and so on. Additionally, sensations of pleasant warmth and a general slowing down of autonomic activity are self-suggested. These may be supplemented with imagery, including sensory imagery as well as emotive imagery.[36] Imaginal though it is, autogenic relaxation has been shown to diminish sympathetic arousal (Stemmler, Aue & Wacker, 2007) and thereby regulate the physiological component of anger. Diaphragmatic breathing shares the same advantage of reducing the arousal aspect of anger without requiring the individual to totally disconnect from the interpersonal context of anger.

POSTVENTION

If anger persists despite intervention, it may be addressed in one last phase in which the residual flow of anger is filtered out well after the provoking event or stimulus has passed. Rather than targeting cognitions at intermediate points in the emergence of anger, postvention is directed at the subjective feeling of anger that can endure over time. This affective approach, as it is called, relies on emotion-focused therapies, including some drawn from Gestalt therapy.

Let us consider a pain patient who continues to harbor resentment toward perceived wrongdoers. This patient may be asked to participate in an "empty chair" role play. As in Gestalt therapy, the patient would sit opposite an empty chair with an imaginary person in it—the offending individual. What proceeds is a verbal communication of the anger in the "here and now." This is particularly appropriate if actual interactions with the "offending person" are no longer possible. In the safety of the therapeutic situation, whatever pent up anger the patient has may be communicated. This should not be confused with a stirring up of anger or an unrestrained catharsis of emotion. Rather, it is a means of safely alleviating the burden of unresolved angry feelings.

Another technique of the same genre is writing a letter. The pain patient is granted license to transfer emotions in all their richness and depth onto paper without any attention to grammar or such; this becomes a channel for confession or disclosure of private feelings (Pennebaker & Seagal, 1999; Pennebaker & Stone, 2004). Variations of this technique (e.g., White and Epston 1989) include the disposal of the letter or the invitation of a confidante to read the letter.

Postvention may also incorporate elements of art therapy, especially when language is not a preferred medium of expression. Art allows for affective expression with many degrees of freedom. In her observations of art therapy for anger, Liebmann (2008) has relied mainly on drawing and sketches. Other options include sculpture, sketching, and even musical performance. A pain patient with residual anger that is too cumbersome for verbalization or writing may find in these affective approaches a convenient way to convey feelings of both pain and anger, as in the celebrated paintings of Frida Kahlo.

OUTCOME

In review, CBAT and CBT share common elements of reappraisal and relaxation but differ largely in scope and sequence. CBAT uses about a dozen techniques drawn from behavioral, cognitive, and affective domains. These techniques are not presented like a menu to choose from at will but are carefully sequenced for use in a contingent fashion, for example, stimulus control becomes a meaningful option only if rehearsal and response prevention fail; if thought stopping fails, then reappraisal is applicable; if composing a written letter is too demanding, then expression through art is encouraged. Furthermore, techniques are grouped according to prevention, intervention, and postvention, which are designed to handle the onset, progression, and residual aspects of anger, respectively. Preliminary findings show that the effect size for anger reduction after CBAT is between +0.80 and +0.99.[38] In principle, there is no reason why this treatment program would not be applicable to the anger of chronic pain patients, too, although more research will be needed to determine its outcome efficacy in this specific population.

FURTHER ALTERNATIVES

One characteristic of both CBAT and CBT for anger is the skills training format. Instead of engaging in extended psychotherapeutic dialogue, participants actually learn skills, much as in a workshop. These skills are meant to equip them with the means to regulate anger if it occurs (as it often does) in everyday naturalistic settings. By implication, anger is handled primarily as an intrapsychic problem amenable to self-regulation.

Yet, as has been emphasized in this chapter, the anger of chronic pain patients arises within a psychosocial context rife with perceived wrongdoings and interpersonal conflict. In fact, there is a relational aspect that is ubiquitous in anger, as emphasized by Laughlin and Warner.[39] The solution may reside not only in intrapsychic regulation but also in addressing important interpersonal dynamics. Traditionally, this has been handled by psychodynamic therapy, which as pointed out by Wootton,[15] is applicable to the anger of pain patients. Also recruited may be strategies well entrenched in the conflict resolution literature. Here, participants are trained to negotiate, compromise, and ultimately reach mutually acceptable settlements on key issues that have previously kept them locked in disputes with others. Problem solving is also well aligned with the relational approach. Here, the patient is encouraged to brainstorm for options to resolve a dilemma, select a suitable option, implement that option in vivo, review the result, and then use that as feedback in an iterative process of approaching the optimal outcome.

In keeping with the idea of sequencing techniques in a contingent fashion, one last perspective on anger regulation merits mention. This is the outlook that promotes forgiveness and acceptance. With roots in many theological and philosophical traditions (especially Buddhism, Sufism, Hinduism, and Christianity), this outlook is hardly new but is now attracting increasing research interest.[40] In a study of pain patients, Carson et al.[41] found a significant (inverse) correlation between forgiveness and anger related to chronic low back pain. Therefore, a patient with chronic pain who is angry at so much but finds so little relief from either pain or anger may still be open to a major philosophical shift or change in outlook, one that holds a bit of promise especially when the self-regulatory skills prove insufficient and the interpersonal conflicts are beyond resolution.

CONCLUSION

Anger is one of the key presenting problems in medical patients, especially those with chronic pain.[11,21] In the past, this has been largely overlooked as a secondary issue or a problem that diminishes or vanishes with the patient's recovery from the somatic disturbance. However, recent research has shown that anger interferes with the very alliance between patient and doctor, thereby undermining adherence to treatment. Moreover, it can exacerbate pain, and when chronic, it is also a risk factor for cardiovascular disease. Hence, it is a problem that warrants clinical attention. In doing so, special emphasis is paid to the psychosocial context of anger. In other words, the anger of pain patients does not occur in a vacuum or emanate from a black box but derives from a myriad of attributions of wrongdoing. It is this context that needs to be specially addressed when attempting to alleviate anger. Fortunately, CBT offers some tried and tested techniques for this purpose.[32] These center around reappraisal, relaxation, and coping. A new development in the anger regulation literature shows that CBT can be enriched into a new hybrid termed CBAT, which incorporates many more cognitive and behavioral strategies as well as techniques from the affective domain of experiential therapy. However, CBAT techniques are most usable and effective when sequenced in a contingent fashion so that the patient is first trained to prevent the onset of anger, then intervene on the progression of anger, and finally resort to postvention to diminish any residual anger. Preliminary outcome data are supportive of this approach. Although there is no reason to suspect that it could be contraindicated for some patients with chronic pain, further research will be necessary to determine its efficacy in this population. The frontier of anger regulation extends beyond the self-regulation paradigm of CBT or CBAT into the relational features of conflict resolution and problem solving. Finally, there is a revival of interest in certain theologically and philosophically inspired approaches that encourage acceptance and forgiveness. In conclusion, we may continue to draw from self-regulation techniques while also exploring interpersonal dynamics as well as fundamental characterologic issues in our attempts to reduce anger in individuals with pain and the burden of such anger on health care professionals and caregivers.

REFERENCES

1. Lazarus RS. Cognitive-motivational-relational theory of emotion. In: Hanin YL, ed. *Emotions in Sport*. Champaign, IL: Human Kinetics; 2000:39-63.
2. Smedslund J. How shall the concept of anger be defined? *Theory Psychol*. 1992;3:5-34.
3. Fernandez E, Kerns RD. Anxiety, depression, and anger: the core of negative affect in medical populations. In: Boyle GJ, Matthews D, Saklofske D, eds. *International Handbook of Personality Theory and Testing: Vol. 1: Personality Theories and Models*. London: Sage; 2008;659-676.
4. Buss AH. *Aggression, Anger, and Hostility*. Hoboken, NJ: John Wiley & Sons; 1961.
5. Ramírez JM, Andreu JM. Aggression, and some related psychological constructs (anger, hostility, and impulsivity): some comments from a research project. *Neurosci Biobehav Rev*. 2006;30:276-291.
6. American Psychiatric Association. *Diagnostic and Statistical Manual of Mental Disorders*. 5th ed (DSM-5). Washington, DC: American Psychiatric Publishing; 2013.
7. American Psychiatric Association. *Diagnostic and Statistical Manual of Mental Disorders*. 4th ed. text rev. Washington, DC: American Psychiatric Publishing; 2000.
8. Miller TQ, Smith TW, Turner CW, et al. A meta-analytic review of research on hostility and physical health. *Psychol Bull*. 1996;119:322-348.
9. Williams JE. Anger/hostility and cardiovascular disease. In: Potegal M, Stemmler G, Spielberger C, eds. *The International Handbook of Anger: Constituent and Concomitant Biological, Psychological, and Social Processes*. New York: Springer; 2010;435-447.
10. Fernandez E, Turk DC. The scope and significance of anger in the experience of chronic pain. *Pain*. 1995;61:165-175.
11. Kerns RD, Rosenberg R, Jacob MC. Anger expression and chronic pain. *J Behav Med*. 1994;17:57-67.
12. Bruehl S, Chung OY, Burns JW. Anger expression and pain: an overview of findings and possible mechanisms (invited). *J Behav Med*. 2006;29:593-606.
13. Bruehl S, Burns JW, Chung OY, Chont M. Interacting effects of trait anger and acute anger arousal on pain: the role of endogenous opioids. *Psychosom Med*. 2011;73:612-619.
14. Burns JW, Quartana PJ, Gilliam W, et al. Suppression of anger and subsequent pain intensity and behavior among CLBP patients: the role of symptom-specific physiological reactivity. *J Behav Med*. 2012;35:103-114.
15. Wootton J. Anger and pain. In: Ballantyne JC, Rathmell JP, Fishman SM, eds. *Bonica's Management of Pain*. 4th ed. Philadelphia: Lippincott, Williams & Wilkins; 2009:1208-1220.
16. Tan G, Jensen MP, Thornby J, Sloan PA. Negative emotions, pain, and functioning. *Psychol Serv*. 2008;5(1):26-35.
17. Fishbain DA, Goldberg M, Meagher BR, Steele R. Male and female chronic pain categorized by DSM-III psychiatric diagnostic criteria. *Pain*. 1986;26:181-197.
18. Kessler R, Coccaro E, Maurizio F. The prevalence and correlates of DSM-IV intermittent explosive disorders. *Directions Psychiatry*. 2007;27:221-229.
19. Kristjansdottir GK. The relationships between pains and various discomforts in schoolchildren. *Childhood*. 1997;4:491-504.
20. Fernandez E, Clark TS, Rudick-Davis D. A framework for conceptualization and assessment of affective disturbance in pain. In: Block AR, Kremer EF, Fernandez E, eds. *Handbook of Pain Syndromes: Biopsychosocial Perspectives*. Mahwah, NJ: Erlbaum; 1999:123-147.
21. Fishbain DA, Lewis JE, Bruns D, et al. Exploration of anger constructs in acute and chronic pain patients vs. community patients. *Pain Pract*. 2011;11:240-251.
22. Fernandez E. *Anxiety, Depression, and Anger in Pain: Research Findings and Clinical Options*. Dallas, TX: Advanced Psychological Resources; 2002.
23. Fernandez E, Kerns RD. Pain and affective disorders: looking beyond the "chicken and egg" conundrum. In: Giamberardino MA, Jensen T, eds. *Pain Comorbidities: Understanding and Treating the Complex Patient*. Seattle: IASP Press; 2012:279-296.
24. Burns JW, Bruehl S, Caceres C. Anger management style, blood pressure reactivity and acute pain sensitivity: evidence for a "trait x situation" model. *Ann Behav Med*. 2004;27:195-204.
25. Fernandez E, Wasan A. The anger of pain sufferers: attributions to agents and appraisals of wrongdoing. In: Potegal M, Stemmler G, Spielberger C, eds. *The International Handbook of Anger: Constituent and Concomitant Biological, Psychological, and Social Processes*. New York: Springer; 2010:449-464.
26. Fernandez E, Salinas N, Swift P, et al. *Psychosocial factors that predict anger in chronic pain sufferers*. Sixteenth Annual Scientific Meeting of the Society of Behavioral Medicine, San Diego; 1995.
27. Trost Z, Vangronsveld K, Linton SJ, et al. Cognitive dimensions of anger in chronic pain. *Pain*. 2012;153(3):515-517.
28. Beck R, Fernandez E. Cognitive-behavioral therapy in the treatment of anger: a meta-analysis. *Cogn Ther Res*. 1998;22:63-74.
29. Greenberg LS, Goldman RN. *Emotion-Focused Couples Therapy: The Dynamics of Emotion, Love, and Power*. Washington, DC, US: American Psychological Association; 2008:351-364.
30. Paivio SC, Pascual-Leone A. *Emotion-Focused Therapy for Complex Trauma: An Integrative Approach*. Washington, DC: American Psychological Association; 2010.
31. Fernandez E. Toward an integrative psychotherapy for maladaptive anger. In: Potegal M, Stemmler G, Spielberger C, eds. *The International Handbook of Anger: Constituent and Concomitant Biological, Psychological, and Social Processes*. New York: Springer; 2010:499-514.

32. Fernandez E, ed. *Treatments for Anger in Specific Populations: Theory, Application, and Outcome*. New York: Oxford University Press; 2013.
33. Fernandez E, Beck R. Cognitive-behavioral self-intervention versus self-monitoring of anger: effects on anger frequency, duration, and intensity. *Behav Cogn Psychother*. 2001;29:345-356.
34. Bakker GM. In defence of thought stopping. *Clin Psychologist*. 2009;13(2):59-68.
35. Fabiansson EC, Denson TF, Moulds ML, et al. Don't look back in anger: neural correlates of reappraisal, analytical rumination, and angry rumination during recall of an anger-inducing autobiographical memory. *NeuroImage*. 2011;59(3):2974-2981.
36. Fernandez E. A classification system of cognitive coping strategies for pain. *Pain*. 1986;26:141-151.
37. Deffenbacher JL, McKay M. *Overcoming Situational and General Anger: A Protocol for the Treatment of Anger Based on Relaxation, Cognitive Restructuring, and Coping Skills Training*. Oakland, CA: New Harbinger Publications; 2000.
38. Fernandez E, Scott S. Anger treatment in chemically-dependent inpatients: evaluation of phase effects and gender. *Behav Cogn Psychother*. 2009;37:431-447.
39. Laughlin MA, Warner KW. A relational approach to anger: a case study. *J Syst Ther*. 2005;24:75-89.
40. Day A, Howells K. The development of CBT programmes for anger: the role of interventions to promote perspective-taking skills. *Behav Cogn Psychother*. 2005;36:299-312.
41. Carson JW, Keefe FJ, Goli V, et al. Forgiveness and chronic low back pain: a preliminary study examining the relationship of forgiveness to pain, anger, and psychological distress. *J Pain*. 2005;6:84-91.

BIBLIOGRAPHY AND ADDITIONAL RESOURCES

Di Giuseppe R, Tafrate RC. Anger treatment for adults: a meta-analytic review. *Clinical Psychology: Science and Practice*. 2003;10:70-84.

Fernandez E, Milburn TW. Sensory and affective predictors of overall pain and emotions with affective pain. *Clinical J Pain*. 1994;10:3-9.

Graham JE, Lobel M, Glass P, et al. Effects of written anger expression in chronic pain patients: making meaning from pain. *J Beh Med*. 2008;31:201-212.

Kinder BN, Curtiss G. *Assessment of anxiety, depression, and anger in chronic pain patients: Conceptual and methodological issues. Advances in Personality Assessment*. Hillsdale, NJ: Lawrence Erlbaum; 1988.

Liebmann M. Art *Therapy and Anger*. London: Jessica Kingsley; 2008.

Okifuji A, Turk DC, Curran SL. Anger in chronic pain: investogations of anger targets and intensity. *J Psychosomatic Research*. 1999;47:1-12.

Pennebaker JW, Seagal JD. Forming a story: the health benefits of narrative. *J of Clinical Psychology*. 1999;55:1243-1254.

Pennebaker JW, Stone LD. Translating traumatic experiences into language: implications for child abuse and longterm health. In: Koenig LJ, Doll LS, O'Leary A, eds. *From Child Sexual Abuse to Adult Sexual Risk: Trauma, Revictimization, and Intervention*. Washington, DC: American Psychological Association; 2004;201-216.

Roy R. Nature of social dislocation for chronic pain sufferers. In: *Social Relations and Chronic Pain*. New York: Springer;2002;1-13.

Schwartz L, Slater MA, Birchler GR, et al. Depression in spouses of chronic pain patients: the role of patient pain and anger, and marital satisfaction. *Pain*. 1991;44:61-67.

Stemmler G, Aue T, Wacker J. Anger and fear: separable effects of emotion and motivational direction on somatovisceral responses. *International J of Psychophysiology*. 2007;66:141-153.

Wasan AD, Wootton J, Jamison RN. Dealing with difficult patients in your pain practice. *Reg Anesth Pain Med*. 2005;30:184-192.

White M, Epston D. *Literate Means to Therapeutic Ends*. Adelaide, Australia: Dulwich Centre Publications; 1989.

Chronic Pain, Disability, and Interdisciplinary Rehabilitation

Michael R. Clark

INTERDISCIPLINARY CHRONIC PAIN REHABILITATION

Patients with chronic pain suffer dramatic reductions in physical, psychological, and social well-being with health-related quality of life rated lower than those with almost all other medical conditions.[1] Evidence-based practice guidelines emphasize interdisciplinary rehabilitation, integrated treatment, and patient selection criteria.[2] Interdisciplinary pain rehabilitation programs provide the full range of treatments for the most difficult pain syndromes within a framework of collaborative ongoing communication among team members, the patient, and other interested parties.[3] Unfortunately, there is considerable variability in the type of practitioners and scope of practice of "multidisciplinary" pain clinics.[4] A recent survey in North Carolina found that only 7% met the criteria of having a medical physician, registered nurse, physical therapist, and mental health specialist.[5]

There is substantial evidence that interdisciplinary pain rehabilitation programs improve patient functioning in a number of areas for patients with a number of chronic pain syndromes, even the severely disabled.[6-9] In a seminal review, a meta-analysis of 65 studies evaluated the efficacy of treatments in patients who attended multidisciplinary pain clinics.[10] Although there were limitations, the study concluded that multidisciplinary pain clinics are efficacious. Combination treatments were superior to unimodal treatments or no treatment; treatment effects were maintained over a period of up to 7 years; and improvements were found, not only on subjective but also objective measures of effectiveness, on such variables as return to work and decreased health care utilization. More recent analyses of interdisciplinary programs that use comprehensive assessments, severity-adapted or stepped-care treatments, and rehabilitation goals demonstrate significant reductions in pain along with functional and quality of life improvements.[11,12]

The goal of treating patients with chronic pain is to end disability and return people to work or other productive activities. Multidisciplinary interventions do show efficacy in returning patients to work.[13] In a long-term follow-up study, only half of the patients remained unemployed after treatment in an inpatient pain management program.[14] In a 30-month follow-up study of patients with chronic pain receiving multidisciplinary treatment, employment status was predicted by the patient's desire to return to work, the perception of a job's dangerousness, and the patient's education level.[15] Patients not intending to return to work were more likely to complain of their job's excessive physical demands and reported more job dissatisfaction and feelings of disability. Individualized subjective quality of life (ISQoL) is defined as the appraisal of quality of life based on personal values, desired goal attainment, and life priorities.[16] Poorer ISQoL was not predicted by work status but by higher levels of distress, pain intensity, and perceived disability.

THE PAIN TREATMENT PROGRAM AT THE JOHNS HOPKINS HOSPITAL

The Pain Treatment Program (PTP) at The Johns Hopkins Hospital is a patient-centered, systematic, organized, and rational approach for restoring the benefits of health and alleviating the consequences of sickness for patients with chronic pain. The service is dedicated to rehabilitation with three guiding principles: (1) a restorative (not curative) model, (2) an active (not passive) role for the patient, and (3) an emphasis on function and independence (not comfort). The founder of the PTP, Donlin M. Long, MD, PhD, emphasized in 1972 that patients with chronic pain should receive an accurate physical diagnosis, an accurate and comprehensive psychiatric and psychosocial evaluation, and an individualization of therapy in an eclectic mode.

The critical therapeutic components of the PTP are organized around a methodology, structure, and rationale for care. The methodology includes a standardized evaluation, case formulation, and individualized treatment plan. The structure of the program exists not only within the physical environment but also a therapeutic milieu with implementation of operationalized general principles and delivery of therapies. The rationale is manifested in the design of individualized treatment plans, the applied components of the structure, and the explicit expectations for patients and staff. The overall goal is to promote rehabilitation for patients disabled by chronic pain. This focus is accomplished by providing the patient with a predictable world, avoiding distractions, gaining experience with healthy behaviors, learning from mistakes, practicing independent problem solving, and setting personal goals.

COMPREHENSIVE EVALUATION AND CASE FORMULATION

When patients with chronic pain are in need of interdisciplinary rehabilitation, they want to know the generative nature of their conditions and how to differentiate them for the sake of receiving specific and effective treatments.[17,18] The biopsychosocial approach offers only the ingredients and end products but not the recipes and processes for improvement. Multidisciplinary pain treatment functions with the same limitations.[19,20] Without the method to determine a set of unique causes and direct specific treatments, the patient receives symptomatic treatments with the expected "partial" response. Despite the involvement of more disciplines, the message is clear—cures for "organic" problems and management for "functional" problems. True interdisciplinary treatment is needed.

The cause of disability cannot be found until the investigation expands to include not only the diseases of the body but also the disruptions of the motivational rhythms of behavior, the psychological constitution of the individual, and the personal chronicle of desire and encounters.[21] All chronic pain disorders are expressions of life under altered circumstances that affect characteristic functional capacities and generate particular behavioral expressions of disability.[22,23] The clinical distinctions allow for independently informed perspectives about the nature of chronic pain disorders and what may have happened to generate the disability. Four perspectives—diseases, behaviors, dimensions, and life stories—represent classes of disorders, and each has a common essence and logical implications for causation and treatment.[24,25] In this approach to patient care, diseases are what people *have*, behaviors are what people *do*, dimensions are what people *are*, and life stories are what people *encounter*. The formulation of a plan for a patient with chronic pain should address the contributions from each perspective to the overall presentation and inform the design of a treatment plan that can address each component of the patient's illness.

Diseases of the brain manifest psychologically. The psychological faculties of the brain include but are not limited to consciousness, cognition, memory, language, affect, and executive functions. Abnormalities in the structures or their associated functions of these faculties are expressed in the criteria that describe the common diagnoses such as delirium, dementia, panic disorder, and major depression. However, the patient may describe deficits in these faculties with difficulty and rely on somatic symptoms (e.g., pain) as incomplete proxies for these criteria. The physical symptoms occur because the brain is malfunctioning and suggesting pathology in the body. The unifying feature of diseases is a broken part within the individual that is causing pathology.[25,26] The pathology causes the characteristic signs and symptoms typically manifested by the affliction.[23] For the patient, there is no meaningful interpretation to be understood, no individual deficiency to be addressed, and no goal that is trying to be achieved. Finding a cure may repair the broken part, prevent the initial damage from progressing, or compensate for the pathology through secondary compensatory measures.

The perspective of *behavior* encompasses a wide range of actions and activities. The complex behaviors of human beings are designed with purpose to achieve goals. Human consciousness is characterized by the regular, rhythmic alterations of attention and perception produced by internal drives that increase a person's motivation toward a particular activity.[25,26] The drive pushes the individual into action. Then, after the actions, the drive is satisfied, and a state of satiety emerges. Over time, drives reemerge with subsequent effects on the individual's perceptual attitude toward his or her setting. In addition, personal assumptions or external opportunities increase the likelihood of certain behaviors. These present a choice to the person, who must decide what action to take. After the choice is made and the behavior completed, external consequences emerge from the outcome and influence future actions. The person learns which choices are most effective. When aspects of choice and control over behavior become disrupted, physicians are asked to address the distorted goals, excessive demands, damaging consequences, and lack of responsiveness to negative feedback.[27,28] Treatment of behavioral disorders begins with regaining temporary control of the situation by stopping the behavior.[20,29] Restricting the patient's actions and preventing these problematic behaviors eventually limit the chaos of destructive actions. This stable foundation is required for the patient to gain insight about and motivation toward appropriate choices that will result in less distress and more satisfaction.[30]

In contrast, many mental disorders emerge not from a disease of the brain or some form of abnormal illness behavior but from a patient's personal affective or cognitive constitution.[25,26] Each individual possesses a set of personal *dimensions* such as intelligence, extraversion, and neuroticism. These traits describe who a person is and are carried into the world as a set of innate capabilities of their psychological makeup. Which traits are relied upon and how much of them a person possesses will determine his or her potential to cope with different situations. Some circumstances are overwhelming and provoke a person's vulnerability to distress. The patient cannot manage the situation and what is required because of who he or she is. Treatment for disorders of the dimensional type focuses on remediation of specific deficiencies and guidance about overcoming potential vulnerabilities through adaptations such as education about, assistance with, or modification of the particular stressors.[20,29]

The *life story* perspective uses a narrative composed of a series of events that a person encounters and determines to be personally meaningful.[25,26] These self-reflections are the means by which a person judges the value of his or her life as a whole. They impart a sense of self as the agent of a life plan unfolding in a social setting, as well as the reflective subject experiencing and interpreting the outcome of such plans and commitments. If events are occurring as planned, then the person feels on track and successful. However, if the sequence of events results in an unexpected or disappointing outcome, the person will feel a sense of distress about this failure. Life story disorders are interpretive responses to life encounters such as grief from loss or anxiety resulting from expected threats.[27,31,32] Treatment begins with the expectation to forge a narrative of setting and sequence that suggests some role for the patient in his or her life and that illuminates the troubled state of mind as the outcome of that role and course of events.[20,29] The effective treatment of life story disorders requires reframing and reinterpreting to remoralize the patient by transforming the story into one with the potential for success and fulfillment.

The four perspectives provide a comprehensive yet flexible formulation for the evaluation of a patient disabled with chronic pain.[20,25,26,33] The treatments prescribed are now designed from the individual formulation and relevant perspectives. If a patient's symptoms and disability continue, the physician must consider other factors that may have been overlooked. Usually these factors are within one of the perspectives initially thought to be less important. A new combination of therapies is then required to treat the patient successfully.

THE PATIENT'S EXPERIENCE: BELIEFS AND MEANINGS

The success of the PTP emanates from understanding and articulating the illness experience of chronic pain. A patient who has suffered with chronic pain for years may present with disability as a result of the failure to make choices to successfully navigate the challenge and accept the burden of suffering. As the patient becomes more ill, the meaning of life is lost, and he or she begins to seek immediate relief or comfort. As this approach is adopted, the patient may acquire the means to have enough to live by but nothing to live for. As a result, if suffering does not have some meaning, then ultimately there is no meaning to survival. And if survival becomes the only goal of living, then life is really not worth living at all. The conclusion for the patient is that life is hopeless. Patients exhibit this approach to living by demonstrating that they have nothing more to expect from life. However, for a successful rehabilitation, patients must believe that life is still expecting something from them.

Beliefs are conceptualized as the thoughts of an individual about his or her personal pain problem.[34] The success of interdisciplinary chronic pain rehabilitation treatment has led to focused attention on many elements of the chronic pain experience, including psychological resilience and illness adaptation.[35] Adjustment is defined as the ability to carry out normal physical and psychosocial activities.[36] Cognitive variables derived from social learning theory associated with chronic pain include self-efficacy, outcome expectancies, and locus of control.[37] Whereas a self-efficacy expectancy is a belief about one's ability to perform a specific behavior, an outcome expectancy is a belief about the consequences of performing a behavior. Individuals are considered more likely to engage in coping efforts they believe are both within their capabilities and will result in a positive outcome. Acceptance of chronic pain is associated with multiple domains of the experience of chronic pain. Acceptance of pain was also found to be associated with reports of lower pain intensity, less pain-related anxiety and avoidance, less depression, less physical and psychosocial disability, more daily uptime, and better work status.[38] One's acceptance of chronic pain predicts one's adjustment to the illness and is independent from catastrophizing, coping skills, and pain-related beliefs and cognitions.[39-41]

Patients with disabling chronic pain pursue comfort to avoid distress. In other words, they want to find relief for their suffering. However, a rehabilitation model essentially attempts to persuade the patient to change his or her behavior and stop being disabled. The expectation of making changes in daily life is a significant paradigm shift, and patients are not easily accepting of this approach. The process of making this paradigm shift begins with focusing on the patient's suffering. Instead of simply enduring pain, the patient has to understand that suffering is a task. The task is unique to that individual patient and isolating because no one person can actually relieve him or her of this suffering. No one can suffer in his or her place.

The inherent optimism of rehabilitation lies in recognizing the potential for the patient to improve his or her level of functioning. There is a tension between what the patient has already achieved and what he or she still ought to accomplish. Explaining to patients that they can do more than they might think may be a difficult message to deliver but one that begins to combat the hopelessness each patient feels about his or her own case. Then the patient is oriented toward striving for a worthwhile goal of becoming something more instead of just struggling to tolerate an unbearable existence. The next step for the patient is to begin accepting responsibility for making changes. If the patient can understand that, even though change seems impossible, there is at least a possibility of this change being realizable. If the patient's world could be different, he or she will spontaneously start taking the responsibility to search for answers to his or her problems. The patient will then attempt to overcome challenges in everyday life, appreciating them as tasks to be completed.

The patient's first choice is to change his or her attitude and believe in the benefits of change. Rather than accepting a role of powerlessness, the patient can recognize that there are always choices to be made. Therefore, the patient can determine his or her own existence. Making choices means taking action. As the patient takes those actions, he or she is implicitly admitting that to be sick and disabled is not enough and that there is a better existence to which one must eventually proceed. And so, the paradigm shift moves the patient from "It can't be" to "I will do it." A patient who is able to navigate this process in treatment may have accepted that failure before admission but must now accept that the way he or she has been living needs to change and that change is possible because the alternative reality is one that might include increased function and decreased suffering. Now, the possibility of success is much more desirable than the existing reality of failure. Most important, the patient now has a role to play in creating this new reality of health.

COGNITIVE-BEHAVIORAL MODELS OF CHRONIC PAIN TREATMENT

Psychological treatment for chronic pain was pioneered by Fordyce using an operant conditioning behavioral model.[42] The behavioral approach is based on an understanding of pain occurring in a social context. The behaviors of patients with chronic pain are reinforced by others. In a study of medical practice patterns, observed pain behaviors were predictive of whether opioid medications were prescribed to patients with chronic pain.[43] If pain behaviors are reinforced, the behavioral model assumes pain and disability will persist. In treatment, healthy behaviors are targeted for reinforcement to replace extinguished pain behaviors.

The cognitive-behavioral model of chronic pain assumes individual beliefs, attitudes, and expectations affect emotional and behavioral reactions to life experiences. If patients believe pain, depression, and disability are inevitable and uncontrollable, then they will likely experience more negative affective responses, increased pain, and even more impaired physical and psychosocial functioning. The components of cognitive-behavioral therapy (CBT) such as relaxation, guided imagery, biofeedback, meditation, hypnosis, motivational interviewing, external reinforcement, cognitive restructuring, and coping self-statement training all tend to interrupt this cycle of disability. Patients are taught to become active participants in the management of their pain through the utilization of methods that minimize distressing thoughts and feelings. The goals of CBT focus on self-control and self-management to increase activity, independence, and resourcefulness.[44] Outcome studies of CBT in patients with a variety of chronic pain syndromes have demonstrated significant improvements in pain intensity, pain behaviors, distress, depression, and coping.[44-46] The benefits of CBT have been found to continue up to 6 months after the completion of active treatment sessions.

THE TREATMENT PROGRAM

Although the concepts and research outlined in this chapter are certainly rational, the patient requires concrete activities and the environment in which to perform them, hence, the structured milieu and schedule of the PTP. The elements of the structure provide an organized routine for the day. The patient has an hour-by-hour schedule of events to follow. The expectations for his or her behavior are explicit and not conditional on how he or she feels. Even the simplest actions of getting dressed in the morning, eating meals at regular times, and going to bed at night are scripted. Every discipline is part of the schedule, reiterating to the patient that he or she should actively execute these tasks. In contrast to activities of daily living, specific therapies are incorporated into the patient's day. These include educational classes, grief and loss seminars, physical therapy, coping skills training, interpersonal group therapy, and occupational therapy. The principles of cognitive-behavioral psychotherapy and social psychology are thematic foundations for these therapeutic modalities. The patient's transition from disability to function must include practice in catastrophizing less and coping better to master the therapies provided in order to experience their benefits.

Catastrophic thinking about pain involves the amplification of threatening information and interference with the attentional focus needed to facilitate patients remaining involved with productive instead of pain-related activities.[47] In one study, high levels of catastrophizing combined with lower levels of active pain coping to predict higher levels of depressive symptoms and disability.[48] The use of adaptive coping skills decreased pain and disability when patients perceived an increase in the effectiveness of their new skills and reduced their use of maladaptive coping strategies, such as catastrophic thinking.

Coping is "a person's cognitive and behavioral efforts to manage the internal and external demands of the person-environment transaction that is appraised as taxing or exceeding the person's resources."[49] Higher levels of disability were found in persons who remain passive or use maladaptive coping strategies of catastrophizing, ignoring or reinterpreting pain sensations, diverting attention from pain, and praying or hoping for relief. In a 6-month follow-up study of patients completing an inpatient pain rehabilitation program, improvement was associated with decreases in the use of passive coping strategies and changing beliefs about pain being an incurable illness.[50]

Although the specific content of these therapies will not be discussed, the logic of each modality will be presented as to how it fits into the framework of interdisciplinary rehabilitation. Educational classes simply present material about a range of pain-related topics. The purpose of these classes from the perspective of promoting change is to address patients' resistance that emerges from their assertion that the staff are coercing them to do more than they can do and that the staff does not really know what it is like to suffer with pain. The expectation of the PTP imbedded in education of the patient is that the staff do possess the expertise to help him or her get better. The conflict with the patient is indirectly resolved by putting this expertise on display in a lecture demonstration and showing the content's relevance to their pain. Seminars dealing with grief and loss are more actively engaging of the patient and involve exercises supervised by staff. Patients with chronic pain suffer tremendous losses, and much of their daily energy is spent on trying to acquire resources that will address those perceived needs. Often, the patient will express that sense of having lost so much that he or she needs more than the average person. Getting patients to begin addressing their losses in more productive ways begins with them engaging in treatment in the PTP instead of resisting it. The unspoken expectation is that being admitted to this program is truly a scarce opportunity to get better. Conflicts with patients are resolved as they begin to use the resources of the program. Now they are not just possessing the admission but also gaining from it.

The need for physical therapy in the treatment of patients with chronic pain is obvious given their deactivation, weakness, and abnormal body mechanics. However, the rehabilitative purpose of physical therapy sessions is to address the assertion of the patient that the PTP should commit to fixing him or her. This passive orientation of the patient undermines rehabilitation and the expectation of the staff that it is now time to commit to change and build a new consistency in daily life. As patients participate in physical therapy without catastrophe, they learn that small changes are possible and that to continue their previous ways of living would be an example of maintaining an unproductive consistency. Similarly, occupational therapy is aimed at increasing function and problem solving in each patient's unique environment. The patient's resistance to these changes often emerges as feelings of being criticized by staff for what they cannot do and results in the avoidance of therapy sessions. Occupational therapy spends time with the patient learning about his or her unique needs and designing solutions. The underlying message is that the staff are engaged with the patient and expect the patient to cooperate with them. And the conflict with the patient is resolved by demonstrating to the patient that the staff have something of value to offer him or her.

Group therapies offer the additional support of other patients who have been through similar stresses and can offer a different perspective based on their own progress in rehabilitation. Coping skills training addresses the patient's concern that many people are sick and never get better. The staff are trying to change the patient's view by emphasizing that many people are not perfectly healthy but still functional and that sick individuals generally try to get well. As patients practice coping skills and gain proficiency, the conflict is resolved because the patient experiences firsthand that he or she can get better and just lacked the skills to achieve that goal. Interpersonal group therapy addresses similar issues about the patient's obligations to be healthy and contribute to the lives of others. The patient usually feels that someone or some entity has an obligation to enable the sick role and provide associated resources. As the patient's experiences of interpersonal relationships are discussed and the value of them exposed, the patient learns that rehabilitation is not an exploitation of the sick but a pathway back to health.

CONCLUSION

Chronic pain is a significant public health problem and is frustrating to everyone affected by it, especially the patients who believe the health care system has failed them. Interdisciplinary rehabilitation programs emphasize an active role for patients in their treatment. These programs offer expertise with pharmacologic and psychological treatments now recognized as effective in the management of chronic pain. Recent advances in the treatment of chronic pain include the diagnosis and treatment of psychiatric comorbidity, the application of psychiatric treatments to chronic pain, and the development of integrated efforts to provide comprehensive health care to patients suffering with disabling and refractory chronic pain syndromes. Specifically, the interdisciplinary rehabilitation approach provides the framework for treating diseases, as well as examining mental life and behavior in the context of understanding the individual person and the systems in which he or she functions.

REFERENCES

1. O'Connor AB. Neuropathic pain: quality-of-life impact, costs and cost effectiveness of therapy. *Pharmacoeconomics.* 2009;27:95-112.
2. Sanders SH, Harden RN, Vicente PJ. Evidence-based clinical practice guidelines for interdisciplinary rehabilitation of chronic nonmalignant pain syndrome patients. *Pain Pract.* 2005;5:303-315.
3. Stanos S, Houle TT. Multidisciplinary and interdisciplinary management of chronic pain. *Phys Med Rehabil Clin North Am.* 2006;17:435-450.
4. Peng P, Stinson JN, Choiniere M, et al. STOPPAIN Investigators Group. Role of health care professionals in multidisciplinary pain treatment facilities in Canada. *Pain Res Manag.* 2008;13:484-488.
5. Castel LD, Freburger JK, Holmes GM, et al. Spine and pain clinics serving North Carolina patients with back and neck pain: what do they do, and are they multidisciplinary? *Spine.* 2009;34:615-622.
6. Angst F, Brioschi R, Main CJ, et al. Interdisciplinary rehabilitation in fibromyalgia and chronic back pain: a prospective outcome study. *J Pain.* 2006;7:807-815.
7. Lake AE 3rd, Saper JR, Hamel RL. Comprehensive inpatient treatment of refractory chronic daily headache. *Headache.* 2009;49:555-562.
8. McCracken LM, MacKichan F, Eccleston C. Contextual cognitive-behavioral therapy for severely disabled chronic pain sufferers: effectiveness and clinically significant change. *Eur J Pain.* 2007;11: 314-322.
9. Van Wilgen CP, Dijkstra PU, Versteegen GJ, et al. Chronic pain and severe disuse syndrome: long-term outcome of an inpatient multidisciplinary cognitive behavioural programme. *J Rehabil Med.* 2009;41:122-128.
10. Flor H, Fydrich T, Turk DC. Efficacy of multidisciplinary pain treatment centers: a meta-analytic review. *Pain.* 1992;49:221-230.
11. Kainz B, Gulich M, Engel EM, et al. Comparison of three outpatient therapy forms for treatment of chronic low back pain-findings of a multicentre, cluster randomized study. *Rehabilitation.* 2006;45:65-77.

12. Marnitz U, Weh L, Muller G, et al. Multimodal integrated assessment and treatment of patients with back pain. Pain related results and ability to work. *Schmerz*. 2008;22:415-423.
13. Norlund A, Ropponen A, Alexanderson K. Multidisciplinary interventions: review of studies of return to work after rehabilitation for low back pain. *J Rehabil Med*. 2009;41:115-121.
14. Maruta T, Malinchoc M, Offord KP, et al. Status of patients with chronic pain 13 years after treatment in a pain management center. *Pain*. 1998;74:199-204.
15. Fishbain DA, Cutler RB, Rosomoff HL, et al. Impact of chronic pain patients' job perception variables on actual return to work. *Clin J Pain*. 1997;13:197-206.
16. Moliner CE, Durand MJ, Desrosiers J, et al. Subjective quality of life according to work status following interdisciplinary work rehabilitation consequent to musculoskeletal disability. *J Occup Rehabil*. 2007;17:667-682.
17. McHugh PR, Slavney PR. Methods of reasoning in psychopathology: conflict and resolution. *Comprehensive Psychiatry*. 1982;23:197-215.
18. McHugh PR, Clark MR. Diagnostic and classificatory dilemmas. In: Blumenfield M, Strain JJ, eds. *Psychosomatic Medicine in the 21st Century*. Baltimore: Lippincott Williams & Wilkins; 2006:39-45.
19. Clark MR, Chodynicki MP. Pain management. In: Levenson JL, ed. *Textbook of Psychosomatic Medicine*. Arlington, VA: American Psychiatric Publishing; 2005:827-867.
20. Clark MR, Cox TS. Refractory chronic pain. *Psychiatr Clin North Am*. 2002;25:71-88.
21. Kirmayer LJ, Groleau D, Looper KJ, Dao MD. Explaining medically unexplained symptoms. *Can J Psychiatry*. 2004;49:663-672.
22. Brown RJ. Psychological mechanisms of medically unexplained symptoms: an integrative conceptual model. *Psychol Bull*. 2004;130:793-812.
23. Rief W, Barsky AJ. Psychobiological perspectives on somatoform disorders. *Psychoneuroendocrinology*. 2005;30:996-1002.
24. McHugh PR. A structure for psychiatry at the century's turn—the view from Johns Hopkins. *J R Soc Med*. 1992;85:483-487.
25. McHugh PR, Slavney PR. *Perspectives of Psychiatry*. 2nd ed. Baltimore: The Johns Hopkins University Press; 1998.
26. Slavney PR. *Perspectives on "Hysteria"*. Baltimore: The Johns Hopkins University Press; 1990.
27. Ford CV. Somatization and fashionable diagnoses: illness as a way of life. *Scand J Work Environ Health*. 1997;23(Suppl 3):7-16.
28. Reuber M, Mitchell AJ, Howlett SJ, et al. Functional symptoms in neurology: questions and answers. *J Neurol Neurosurg Psychiatry*. 2005;76:307-314.
29. Clark MR, Treisman GJ. Perspectives on pain and depression. *Adv Psychosom Med*. 2004;25:1-27.
30. Stone J, Carson A, Sharpe M. Functional symptoms and signs in neurology: management. *J Neurol Neurosurg Psychiatry*. 2005;76(Suppl 1):i13-i21.
31. Kirmayer LJ, Robbins JM. Three forms of somatization in primary care: prevalence, co-occurrence, and sociodemographic characteristics. *J Nervous Ment Dis*. 1991;179:647-655.
32. Rief W, Nanke A. Somatoform disorders in primary care and inpatient settings. *Adv Psychosom Med*. 2004;26:144-158.
33. Clark MR, Swartz KL. A conceptual structure and methodology for the systematic approach to the evaluation and treatment of patients with chronic dizziness. *J Anxiety Disord*. 2001;15:95-106.
34. Morley S, Wilkinson L. The pain beliefs and perception inventory: a British replication. *Pain*. 1995;61:427-433.
35. Karoly P, Ruehlman LS. Psychological "resilience" and its correlates in chronic pain: findings from a national community sample. *Pain*. 2006;123:90-97.
36. Lazarus RA, Folkman S. *Stress, Appraisal, and Coping*. New York: Springer; 1984.
37. Solberg Nes L, Roach AR, Segerstrom SC. Executive functions, self-regulation, and chronic pain: a review. *Ann Behav Med*. 2009;37:173-183.
38. McCracken LM. Learning to live with the pain: acceptance of pain predicts adjustment in persons with chronic pain. *Pain*. 1998;74:21-27.
39. Vowles KE, McCracken LM, Eccleston C. Processes of change in treatment for chronic pain: the contributions of pain, acceptance, and catastrophizing. *Eur J Pain*. 2007;11:779-787.
40. Vowles KE, McCracken LM, Eccleston C. Patient functioning and catastrophizing in chronic pain: the mediating effects of acceptance. *Health Psychol*. 2008;27(2 Suppl):S136-S143.
41. Esteve R, Ramirez-Maestre C, Lopez-Marinez AE. Adjustment to chronic pain: the role of pain acceptance, coping strategies, and pain-related cognitions. *Ann Behav Med*. 2007;33:179-188.
42. Fordyce W, Fowler R, Lehmann J, et al. Operant conditioning in the treatment of chronic pain. *Arch Phys Med Rehab*. 1973;54:399-408.
43. Turk DC, Okifuji A. What factors affect physicians' decisions to prescribe opioids for chronic noncancer pain patients? *Clin J Pain*. 1997;13:330-336.
44. Turk DC, Swanson KS, Tunks ER. Psychological approaches in the treatment of chronic pain patients—when pills, scalpels, and needles are not enough. *Can J Psychiatry*. 2008;53:213-223.
45. Eccleston C, Williams AC, Morley S. Psychological therapies for the management of chronic pain (excluding headache) in adults. *Cochrane Database Syst Rev*. 2009;2:CD007407.
46. Molton IR, Graham C, Stoelb BL, et al. Current psychological approaches to the management of chronic pain. *Curr Opin Anaesthesiol*. 2007;20:485-489.
47. Crombez G, Eccleston C, Baeyens F, et al. When somatic information threatens, catastrophic thinking enhances attentional interference. *Pain*. 1998;75:187-198.
48. Buenaver LF, Edwards RR, Smith MT, et al. Catastrophizing and pain-coping in young adults: associations with depressive symptoms and headache pain. *J Pain*. 2008;9:311-319.
49. Folkman S, Lazarus RS, Gruen RJ, et al. Appraisal, coping, health status, and psychological symptoms. *J Per Soc Psychol*. 1986;50:571-579.
50. Jensen MP, Turner JA, Romano JM, et al. Relationship of pain-specific beliefs to chronic pain adjustment. *Pain*. 1994;57:301-309.

Work Disability and Chronic Pain: A Review of Psychosocial and Environmental Factors

Melissa T. Stone
Ronald J. Kulich

Disability and chronic pain commonly co-occur, particularly in the case of diagnoses with controversial etiologies. When disability impacts work, the contributory factors become even more complex, with occupational disability bearing scant relationship to a patient's specific clinical state. Given the weak relationship between medical diagnosis, clinical severity, and work disability, investigators have championed the decade of "yellow flags," outlining a series of proposed predictors of work disability, including psychosocial, economic, and environmental factors. Identification of these factors in the individual patient can assist the clinician in achieving a better outcome. Conversely, failure to adequately assess can contribute to unnecessary or inappropriate treatment and chronic disability.

Recent studies note that about 17% of people in the United States have a disability, or 54 million American people.[1] Notwithstanding measurement difficulties, studies consistently reveal that people with disabilities are less likely to be employed than people without disabilities (21% vs. 59%), are more likely to live in poverty (34% vs. 15% as defined by less than $15,000 annually), are more likely to not have graduated high school (17% vs. 11%), and are more likely to have a significantly lower quality of life (34% vs. 61%).[2] The problem is worldwide, although estimates across countries vary widely, largely because of the variability in the operational definition of disability. In addition, social factors and practice patterns of health care providers result in response bias.

Even within a given state, work disability rates may show considerable variability over time based on economic conditions or local laws that reinforce changes in behavior. State law may eliminate benefits after a specified time, resulting in dramatically increased work return rates. Some states restrict access to subspecialists, another factor that may directly impact work disability.[3] The U.S. Federal Social Security Disability Insurance (SSDI) program reported return-to-work rates that hovered at less than 1% for 25 years, with more recent changes resulting in financial incentives that encourage a return to part-time employment. In many cases, a patient's disability may have little relationship to diagnosis or any "objective" measure of physical impairment.

Many studies report higher rates of physical disability in underdeveloped countries, particularly when more objective measurements are used.[4] Not surprisingly, many individuals may work despite physical disabilities or pain, particularly if the government fails to provide a financial safety net. Conversely, the percentage of people who report chronic pain is significantly lower in developing countries (2.9%); the United States has a rate of 15.5%.[5] Patients in developed countries may also expect that they should not or cannot work with chronic pain conditions, a belief system often shared by treating physicians.[6] Chronic pain remains one of the leading factors contributing to disability in the United States, regardless of diagnosis or physical impairment.[5,7–12]

Clinicians who care for patients with chronic pain are often fully aware of the high rates of disability. Lacking knowledge, tools, or an incentive to address work disability, some may simply ignore the issue and instead focus on what they know best: treatment approaches that narrowly target impairment, nociception, or some underlying pathological etiology. If frustrating questions arise with respect to the patient's functional status or return-to-work goals, they are commonly ignored. In other cases, return-to-work issues may be addressed by asking the patient to return to his or her primary care physician "because our office doesn't do disability forms." When psychological factors are readily apparent, a referral may be made to a mental health clinician. A general mental health practitioner would typically address immediate psychiatric comorbidities, often ignoring or failing to understand risk factors associated with chronic work disability.

This vacuum of care with respect to return-to-work assessment is often filled with commercial disability assessment specialists, a field populated by independent medical examination and functional and work capacity experts. These "independent" physicians often work in concert with insurance carriers or government-funded assessment panels, relationships that may not always favor the patient. In this setting, the patient's disability is typically addressed from a medical standpoint, with a preference for "objective" medicolegal measures of impairment. There often is an expectation that the evaluation results would provide an objective basis for compensation. Failure to find and identify sufficient underlying physical pathology, as in the case with many chronic pain patients, may result in conclusions about "symptom magnification" or even malingering. Despite lack of validity, there are examples in which Waddell signs or functional capacity assessments are used to assess the patient's credibility, with the authors of these tests decrying such uses.[13,14] All of the above approaches typically ignore the body of evidence that underscores the complexity of the work-related factors, often to the peril of the patient.

The role of pain physicians in work-related disability cases is widely debated, and failure to understand the ramifications of the physician's responsibilities may greatly compromise the patient's status.[15] Kosny and his colleagues[7,16] found that practitioners unwittingly play a "key role in complicating and prolonging compensation claims"(p. 583).[17] This is in part due to limited understanding of the compensation system and requirements, as well as confusion about decision making with respect to patient care. The results of a study by Lotters et al.[8,18] are even more damning, with the authors concluding that regardless of the severity of the pain disorder, merely visiting a subspecialist was associated with a failure to fully return to work. Although the claim that physicians may promote disability is nothing new, the tendency to disable our patients may go largely unrecognized even by the most diligent and empathic clinician.

Despite these findings, there are some bright spots. Dasinger and his colleagues[9,19] found that the direct advice from a physician to return to work was associated with a 34% decrease in disability benefit status compared with patients who were not encouraged by physicians to return to work. Other investigations suggest that choice of active interventions by the clinician, such as self-directed exercise, may significantly improve return-to-work rates over the selection of passive treatments, such as massage or aquatherapy.[10,20] Underscoring the importance of active approaches in management of chronic pain and disability, others report that a return to "full active duty" may be better than suggesting "light duty." The limited "light duty" responsibilities may perpetuate an image of an underperforming disabled worker and contribute to the development of a worker sick role at the work site.[11]

DISABILITY: MEDICAL AND SOCIAL APPROACHES

Disability is a complex concept that is continually being redefined. The definition differs greatly based on who, what, where, and why one is asking. The social and medical models are often seen in conflict, with the medical model of disability closely related to the construct of "impairment."[16] *Impairment* is a loss or abnormality of body structure or of a physiological or psychological function, such as a loss of a limb or a loss of vision. Because of its narrow focus, impairment can be more objectively defined and reliably measured. In contrast, the construct of *disability* typically refers to an inability to carry out necessary tasks in any important domain of life because of a medical (or psychiatric) condition.[17] The American Medical Association (AMA) defines disability as "an alteration of an individual's capacity to meet personal, social, or occupational demands or statutory or regulatory requirements because of an impairment"[17] (p. 2). Those espousing a social model seek to further broaden this definition, with reasonable support from empirical studies. Combining both the social and medical aspects of disability but keeping the construct of impairment, the United Nations Convention on the Rights of People with Disabilities (CPD) offered the following: "Persons with disabilities include those who have long-term physical, mental, intellectual or sensory impairments which in interaction with various barriers may hinder their full and effective participation in society on an equal basis with others."[18] Although 101 of 149 countries from the United Nations have ratified this text of the CPD as of 2011, controversies persist with respect to operational definitions and strategies for assessing disability. Some academics and leaders in the disability rights movement who advocate exclusive use of a social model have taken the position in the extreme, affirming, "The body has nothing to do with disability."[19]

DIAGNOSTIC COMORBIDITIES

There are various strategies for classifying psychological factors that impact on disability. Nicholas and his colleagues[21] proposed a five-color nomenclature that uses warning "flags," each with a different type of risk factor (**Table 25-1**). Most factors overlap, and a patient may easily fall into several categories. No single psychological factor controls most of the variance in predicting to work disability, and there are conflicting data for some. However, all appear to be better predictors than more "objective" physical parameters. Most of the work has been conducted with chronic low back pain populations, but other persistent pain populations have been widely studied. These include neck pain, chronic headache, fibromyalgia, complex regional syndrome, and various other persistent myofascial and neuropathic pain syndromes.[22–27]

TABLE 25-1 Predictor Variables for Work-Related Disability

Biological	Red flags	• Cauda equina syndrome, fracture, tumor • Serious psychiatric pathology, substance use • Comorbidity
Psychosocial	Orange flags	• Depression • PTSD • Somatoform disorder
	Yellow flags	• Avoidant coping strategies • Emotional distress • Passive role
	Blue flags	• Perceived low support at work • Perceived unpleasant work • Low job satisfaction • Perception of excessive demands
Environmental	Black flags	• Legislative criteria for compensation • Nature of workplace • Threats to financial security

PTSD, posttraumatic stress disorder.

Data from Nicholas et al. (2011).[20]

It is unremarkable that patients with chronic pain and severe psychiatric factors tend to have problems with work-related disability, in contrast to patients who have fewer psychiatric comorbidities. The typical predictive comorbid psychiatric disorders include depression, anxiety (including posttraumatic stress disorder [PTSD]), somatoform disorders, and substance use disorders. Not surprisingly, the presence of severe psychopathology not only predicts to work disability but also various adverse health outcomes, poor medical adherence, and a poor response to many types of treatment.[28,29] They are often missed by the physician or minimized by the patient during initial assessment, partly because of the singular focus on the pain complaints.

Bair and colleagues[30] addressed the relationships among anxiety, depression, pain intensity, pain-related disability, and quality of life. They replicated the work of numerous other investigators who demonstrated the relationship between depression and anxiety in patients with chronic pain and its association to increased levels of disability. As expected, depression and anxiety also predicted to overall poorer health-related quality of life.[31,32] The impact also appears to have a lasting effect. Brage and his associates found that severe emotional distress was a predictor of work disability in a 12-year follow-up study of patients with low back pain.[33] It can be argued that low levels of distress or dissatisfaction with disability may motivate the patient to improve function and return to work, although more severe psychiatric symptoms may be a different matter. Again, adequate patient assessment and treatment may help, including efforts to provide the patient with avenues for rapid return to employment.

Although active substance abuse has been shown to be a predictor of work disability through decades of research, patients with chronic pain may even have a greater risk. Substance abuse disorders in the general population range from 3% to 16%,[34] and substance abusers are two to six times more likely to appear in chronic pain populations.[35] Issues of iatrogenic addiction also can occur with chronic opioid therapies.[36] Although screening for addiction is often considered a minimum standard of care for all medical patients, the need is particularly relevant with chronic pain populations. Most attention to substance abuse occurs within the context of risk stratification for opioid therapy, with the opportunity for substance abuse screening being missed with the majority of the other patients.

Somatoform disorders, particularly somatization disorder, are often overlooked when addressing work-related disability. In part, the patient meeting criteria for this disorder may obtain a more palatable multiple co-occurring medical diagnosis such as fibromyalgia, diffuse myofascial pain, chronic headache, and so on. Commonly missed by mental health clinicians and subspecialists, patients with somatoform disorders usually present with chronic pain conditions as a component of their full set of symptoms, seek out multiple physicians, and experience long-standing work disability. Fear avoidance of activity is common, with many patients developing iatrogenic complications from multiple surgical, interventional, or pharmacologic approaches aimed at treating their supposed underlying disease.[12] Patients commonly underestimate their ability to function. Barsky et al. (2005)[37] estimate that $256 billion is spent per year on medical care costs attributable to the incremental effects of somatization alone.[37] Many of these patients report disablement in all areas of functioning and often seek out work disability. As with the other psychiatric conditions, overlay with anxiety and affective disorders is quite common. For patients with marked oversomatization, the best practice includes avoiding unnecessary subspecialists and coordinating through primary care. Although some data support interdisciplinary pain care and cognitive therapy as adjunctive approaches, studies are few.[37] In most cases, the patient benefits from the focus and distraction of employment, and time off for symptoms should be avoided.

Although fibromyalgia has been accepted as a medical disorder and there appears to be a growing body of research suggesting biological markers, the overlap with psychiatric disorders remains significant. Patients with fibromyalgia have a prevalence rate of 20% for PTSD.[38] Similarly, back pain, headaches, pelvic pain, chronic abdominal pain, irritable bowel syndrome, and temporomandibular joint disorder have been correlated with psychological trauma, and each one commonly co-occurs with fibromyalgia.[39] All have been shown to contribute to work disability. Indeed, many argue that these are "spectrum disorders" closely overlapping in etiology. In each case, evidence-based treatment recommendations include reinforcement of activity, cognitive therapy approaches, and early return to work when possible.

Consistent with many diffuse chronic pain diagnoses, the number of pain sites appears to be a significant factor that impacts disability. In contrast, the severity, intensity, and frequency of pain do not appear directly related to the level of work disability.[40] A prospective study conducted over 14 years demonstrated that 80% of the variance in disability related to chronic pain was accounted for by the number of pain sites.[41] Again, these are likely to be patients with diffuse pain diagnoses as noted earlier. Each subspecialist may chase the patient's changing symptoms with new diagnostics and peripheral treatments and perhaps forget that the patient is at great risk for chronic work disability. Being aware of patients who present with multiple pain sites may give the practitioner an opportunity to intervene early and identify sources for return to work.

COGNITIVE AND BELIEF FACTORS

Cognitive constructs or belief factors with chronic pain are some of the most studied psychological factors related to a person's functioning, quality of life, and work-related disability. These include the constructs of "acceptance," "catastrophizing," "fear avoidance," "pain perception," "disease or disability conviction," and "self-efficacy." Each has been shown to be predictive to general disability measures and work disability in particular.

McCracken and his colleagues[42] found that acceptance of pain predicted better adjustment on all measures of pain function independent of pain intensity.[43] Thus, a person's ability to adapt to new (and often stressful) situations is a relevant factor in the response to treatment. Acceptance has often been misunderstood as satisfaction with a situation, which may not be the case. Hence, a patient with pain may not be happy or even satisfied with a situation, but he or she can still "accept" the facts of the moment and respond to the situation effectively.[44] Examples of positive acceptance might include statements such as "I know the pain sometimes will get worse, but I won't injure myself if I work, or if I walk to the store."

Relating to the construct of acceptance, Gross et al.[6] found that those who believed that a *reduction* in pain is necessary for resumption in functioning showed a greater likelihood of obtaining disability claims. Patients who took the most time off from work were most likely to agree with the premise that *if you have back pain, you should rest until it gets better.* Rather than "accept" the typical variability in pain level common with chronic pain conditions, the work-disabled patient may wait until the clinician offers a "fix" or "a cure" or at least "gets better" in terms of pain level. Unfortunately, the pain returns, often unrelated to work activity, and the patient becomes fearful of injury, withdrawing again from work.

Casey and colleagues[27] found that there were several factors related to the formation of chronic pain and disability after an acute back injury, with the most predictive factor being negative pain beliefs. Patients who felt that pain would be *permanent* had higher rates of disability at a 3-month follow up. Other studies have demonstrated that results consistent with these findings, (e.g., "learned helplessness" and pessimistic views about the future) predict higher levels of work disability.[45,46]

Fear avoidance and catastrophizing have also been shown to be strong predictors of disability and work status. In particular, fear avoidance describes a person's beliefs that certain physical activities are more harmful and would end up causing more pain. Prior studies have evaluated the effect of fear avoidance in patients with low back pain and found that fear-avoidant beliefs predict both disability status and work status after 1 month.[47] This appeared to be the case despite level of pain and level of "objective" impairment. Although other reviews on fear avoidance are mixed with respect to the amount of impact on return to work, fear avoidance remains an important component of chronic disability behavior.[48]

Similar to many of the dysfunctional cognitions discussed, fear avoidance and catastrophizing are interrelated constructs. Catastrophizing can be thought of as an exaggerated and overly negative perception of pain, worry related to injury, or related belief.[77] Negative thoughts about work activity are reinforced as activity is avoided, and the patient feels transiently better with a reduction in anxiety after terminating work. The cycle continues, leading to increased disability and further fear-avoidance behaviors, culminating in more extensive catastrophizing thoughts, actions, and behaviors. Buer and Linton[22] compared patients with back pain with the general population, finding that fear avoidance and catastrophizing were related to reduced activities of daily living and reports of pain among patients with persistent pain. Although both cognitions were present in the general population during the beginning stages of pain, these negative thoughts did not persist with the nonpain patients.

Although fear avoidance and catastrophizing are interrelated, there may be differences with respect to predicting longer term work disability. In a prospective study of 202 patients with pain, Wideman and Sullivan found that whereas catastrophizing was most related to long-term pain intensity, fear was most related to long-term work disability.[48,49] In either case, the pain clinician may query the patient with respect to specific fears and worries about activities, fears related to return to work, or other barriers that might be preventing success. Although it is common to assess the patient's objective behaviors with respect to work activities such as lifting and carrying, we often fail to assess the patient's fears about these activities and their perceived consequences.

The construct of "self-efficacy" has also received attention as a predictor of disability. Similar to the other cognitive constructs, self-efficacy is defined as a person's beliefs about his or her capabilities to produce a certain level of performance in order to influence events that affect his or her life. For example, an individual may have a belief that he or she can control or manage activities of daily living despite pain.[49] With respect to work, a belief in one's ability to return to work has been shown to be a better indicator of return to work than other measures such as control over health status.[50] Overall, general cognitive measures that are not work specific tend to be less predictive of work disability, although they may be predictive of other health behaviors.[24] From a clinical standpoint, this underscores the need to modify the assessment to address work barriers specific to the patient. General psychological questionnaires have a place in the assessment, but they do not replace a thorough review of the patient's beliefs and concerns about his or her work setting.

ENVIRONMENTAL AND OCCUPATIONAL FACTORS

Job-specific psychosocial variables directly impact work-related disability. These include constructs such as job "burnout," job security, job satisfaction, supervisor satisfaction, social supports at work, job control, and work history.[9] Over the past 20 years, investigators have consistently found that these occupational variables are more predictive in work disability than measures of physical functioning, physical pathology, or general psychological variables.[51,52]

Job satisfaction and supervisor satisfaction appear to have a particular impact on work disability, factors that have been studied for more than 25 years. The classic Boeing studies of aircraft employees by Bigos et al. (1991) found that those responding "yes" to a single item ("I hardly enjoy the tasks involved in my job") were 2.5 times more likely to incur a back injury than those who responded "no."[53]

A recent prospective study followed 1704 healthy participants for 3 years, finding that changes in level of "burnout" predicted the onset of pain complaints and work disability.[54] The author defined "burnout" as a "unique affective response to chronic exposure to stress" (p. 1).[54] Although "burnout" is clearly related to work disability, it is also interrelated with other variables of supervisor support and satisfaction.

Although job and supervisor satisfaction can be changed, other work-related variables cannot be easily rectified. Risk of job loss or financial hardship may impact complaints of pain and pain-related disability. In fact, some studies suggest that patients with pain may be more likely to continue to work if there is a risk of job loss in the absence of a financial safety net.[55] Other financial factors also can have an impact. For example, a patient may choose to continue work despite pain to maintain his or her health insurance plan. In contrast, a patient receiving SSDI may elect to avoid returning to work because his or her Medicare coverage would terminate.

Compensation issues and work disability are not unique to the United States. **Table 25-2** reveals the relative contribution of various medically related conditions to work disability from a Rand Labor and Population working paper (2005).[56] Although level of pain appears to contribute to most of the variance when contrasted with other medical conditions, the most striking comparison appears between the Dutch and U.S. samples. One can assume that the Dutch do not have a constitutionally lower pain threshold than the U.S. population, yet pain is a greater contribution to work disability among the Dutch sample. Assuming response bias and other methodological issues are not contributory, the difference may be due to the financial compensation available within the Dutch disability system because it may be more tolerant to work disability than the U.S. system.[56]

TABLE 25-2 Relative Impact of Pain on Work Disability by Percentage: Holland Versus United States

Variables	Holland	United States
"Objective" health conditions	2.14	3.85
Heart problems	2.29	2.55
Emotion	3.33	2.50
Arthritis	2.23	3.97
Pain	**15.49**	**7.66**
Demographics	2.73	2.82

Data from Smith JP. Unraveling the SES-Health Connection. *Rand Labor and Population Working Paper*. 2005.

MEDICOLEGAL ISSUES

The mere presence of litigation should not lead a practitioner to assume a poor outcome with respect to return to work. As noted previously, few patients receiving SSDI return to work, possibly because of financial compensation and the health care benefit provided by this entitlement. Similarly, the adversarial nature of occupational injury cases often complicates return to work, factors over which the clinician and patient have minimal control. **Table 25-3** illustrates the variability across types of injury, identifying the percentages of people who returned to work after injury as well as the number of studies reviewed for that group.

TABLE 25-3 Comparison of Median Return-to-Work Rates Across Studies[56,57]

Group	Studies (*n*)	Median RTW Rate (%)
Back injury	51	65
Whiplash	8	95
Motor vehicle accident	4	96
Work related	30	71
Compensation	27	63
Social Security Disability Insurance: <1% RTW		

RTW, return to work.

Data from Athanasou JA. *Return to Work Following Whiplash and Back Injury*. Sydney, Australia: OVAL Research, University of Technology; 2007.

Whiplash injuries typically involve civil litigation, a condition in which the patient has no financial safety net. The patient is often required to continue working. In contrast, entitlement programs provide compensation for injuries that commonly occur in a work setting, such as back injury. The clinician's understanding of the compensation system can provide the best vehicle for encouraging return to work despite these barriers. Sadly, the likelihood of return to work may still be poor with some types of compensation systems in place.[15,58]

PRACTICAL SELF-REPORT QUESTIONNAIRES

Similar to the dispute of how to define a disability, there are controversies with respect to the best strategies for measurement. Disability measurement instruments typically fall into two categories: impairment screening and functional screening. Impairment can be defined as a problem in the body structure or body function.[59] The most popular impairment assessment screening involves the AMA's Guide to Permanent Impairment Ratings.[60] Although currently undergoing revision, this assessment paradigm offers minimal value with respect to predicting work-related disability or measuring treatment outcomes. This assessment model serves mainly as a vehicle for determining financial awards based on loss of a body part or limitation in a discrete area of physical functioning. Any physician can pursue a certification course or training for use of this instrument, but it offers little utility in the care of patients with chronic pain.

In contrast to impairment screening, a social model includes not only bodily function or impairment but also addresses level of activities and ability to participate in various domains of life. Multiple disability screening and outcome questionnaires have been developed for this purpose over the past 30 years. **Table 25-4** offers a sample of brief clinician-friendly instruments, and there are supportive studies on reliability and validity with respect to work-injured patients. Some were designed to specifically address general disability such as the World Health Organization Disability Assessment (WHODAS), and others have been widely studied with respect to predicting work-related disability.

TABLE 25-4 Brief Screening and Outcome Measures for Work-Related Disability

Questionnaire	Reference	Notes
Oswestry Disability Index	Fairbank and Pynsent (2000)[61] Copay et al. (2009)[62]	Brief; used in assessment of spine-related disability; multiple studies for use in screening and outcome
Neck Disability Index	Carreon et al. (2010)[63]	Brief; specific to upper extremity disorders and neck pain
Roland-Morris Disability Questionnaire	Shiphorst et al. (2007)[64]	General disability questionnaire but used in multiple RTW studies as screening and outcome measure; weak psychosocial measures
Migraine Disability Assessment (MIDAS) and HIT-6	Sauro et al. (2009)[65]	Most widely used screening for disability and headache; limited data on work disability versus general disability
Disability of the Arm, Shoulder, and Hand Scale (DASH)	Bot et al. (2004)[66]	Addresses self-reported limitations with upper extremities, areas of disability underrepresented in general disability and other spine questionnaires
Pain Disability Questionnaire	Anagnostis et al. (2004)[67]	Brief, most widely studied short self-report questionnaire; used with prediction of RTW
Fibromyalgia Impact Questionnaire	Bennet (2005)[68]	Used as disability screening for fibromyalgia, covering a range of symptoms, limited data related to work disability
Fear-Avoidance Beliefs Questionnaire	Waddell et al. 1993[12,36]	Multiple studies chronic pain and general disability; used with several studies for prediction of work disability
Short Form 36 (SF-36) Health Survey	Ware and Sherbourne (1992)[69]	Widely used to estimate disease burden with general population norms; studied with many disease populations, including back pain, arthritis, depression, migraine headaches, IBS, and musculoskeletal conditions

IBS, irritable bowel syndrome; RTW, return to work.

More global quality of life questionnaires such as the Short Form 36 or Sickness Impact Profile provide less utility for specific work-related issues, although they may have value for addressing a wide range of disability domains unrelated to work.[70] In a comprehensive review, Copay et al. (2010)[62,71] assert that there are still numerous inconsistencies and psychometric problems with most work-specific instruments. In particular, no single measure can cover all domains of work function, and thus it is imperative that clinicians carefully select questionnaires to address the myriad of psychosocial and other factors impacting the patient's outcome. From a practical standpoint, these may assist clinicians in targeting specific patient barriers, but they should not be used to determine whether the patient is "disabled" or "work ready." Recent developments in real-time digital activity monitoring devices may provide an improved measure of the patient's physical functioning status. Additionally, these devices may potentially reinforce improvements in physical activity.[86–88]

MANAGEMENT AND TREATMENT CONSIDERATIONS

With the majority of chronic pain conditions, reduction of work disability and return to work remain admirable outcome goals. As discussed earlier, efforts to "fix" or address underlying medical issues often do not result in a return to work with patients who have chronic pain. Conversely, specific approaches may maximize success.

Assuming the clinician has assessed "flags" as outlined in Table 25-1, in most cases, a rapid return to work appears to be one of the best strategies for minimizing the likelihood of chronicity. Early reports from Linton (1991) clearly demonstrate that the "risk zone" is within the first 12 weeks of leaving the job after a work injury.[71,72] After 6 months of being out of work, chances of return to work range from 40% to 55%, with the chance of returning to work after 2 years almost nil.[72,73] Hence, a return to work regardless of pain may be the most important factor in predicting the best outcome.[6,74] If a disability specialist or rehabilitation consultant is involved, cross-communication among clinicians is paramount, and time is of the essence.

The selection of treatment approaches can play a significant role in work-related disability. In general, active treatment approaches instead of passive approaches show better return-to-work rates and lower risk of disability. Again, patients may prefer passive approaches in which treatment is done "to them," a factor that may be reinforced by medically oriented clinicians. Encouragement of both independent exercise and return to work often predicts the best results across a range of chronic pain conditions. Houben et al. (2005)[74] note that therapists with a "biomedical orientation" typically view daily activities as "harmful," a major predictor of continued work disability. Approaches that target quota-based activity offer a more successful alternative because patients learn to function despite the level of pain.[75-77]

Formal functional restoration programs offer an alternative to passive therapies, with the best success seen in programs that have a multidisciplinary focus.[75] However, all "multidisciplinary" treatments are not equal. Although some programs effectively integrate multidisciplinary rehabilitative treatments, others incorporate numerous passive treatments that may occupy the patient's time without providing effective results. The American Pain Society collected commentary on tertiary care pain services, with one managed care executive commenting, "Being totally candid, there's a lot of suspicion among physician executives that there's chicanery in the field. We not long ago found that we were sending a patient to a pain center and he was getting magnet therapy." In the same series, another medical director commented that a local interdisciplinary program "never saw a discipline they didn't like."[78] Caution and knowledge of the rehabilitation program are critical factors in effective patient treatment, particularly if return to work remains the primary goal.

Even when the ideal, work-focused multidisciplinary program is found, prognosis may be guarded as the patient typically spent previous months or years involved in passive, symptom-based treatments. Kapural et al. (2010)[79] found that the average time for referral to multidisciplinary pain centers was 43.1 months. Again, early intervention may greatly improve results.[79]

Selection of time-limited, activity-based therapies is not enough to ensure an optimal recovery. In addition, there must be recognition that some therapeutic approaches target only pain symptoms and offer little in the way of return-to-work assistance. This is not meant to denigrate the potential value of these treatments. For example, spinal column stimulation is often a reasonable option for reduction of neuropathic pain. However, studies have not supported spinal column stimulation as a strategy that offers an improved likelihood of return to work. Similarly, chronic opioid therapy may have a place in the care of chronic pain. Although evidence-based studies support the use of opioids for pain and patient satisfaction, reduced disability behavior and return to work have not been realized as likely outcomes.[80,81] Many interventions appear to have an effect with pain, but others have a better effect with disability. Judicious clinicians should consider return to work and pain reduction as independent goals, with different interventions selectively targeting toward each.

Assuming a patient with persistent pain is ready to return to work, a question always arises with respect to the consideration of "light duty," work restrictions, part-time work, or work accommodations. Studies have suggested that returning patients to work on light duty rather than normal duty often results in poorer outcomes.[82] The "light duty" approach is contrasted with efforts to permanently "accommodate" the patient within the American for Disabilities Act (ADA) guidelines. The latter approach has been shown to be effective in successfully integrating people into work settings, perhaps because it requires clear modification of work tasks with defined employer obligations. Although most pain physicians lack familiarity with the ADA, resources are available to assist patients and clinicians.[83]

Even if the clinician chooses an effective multidisciplinary rehabilitation program and rapidly attempts to return the patient to the work setting, employer support and onsite treatment at the worksite remain the most effective strategies for success. Pomaki (2011)[14,57,69,84] found that workplace-based high-intensity psychological interventions were most effective in improving work functioning and overall quality of life for patients with chronic pain. The program also reduces costs. Again, the data appear to reflect the theme that treatment should directly address the goal of return to work, and the possibility of integrating care at the worksite might offer the best hope for gainful employment.

A comprehensive assessment addressing the risks and barriers for work disability should be undertaken, and Table 25-1 offers the common factors. There are always patient-specific barriers, and the treating physician should explore those with the same energy as underlying medical pathology is explored. **Table 25-5** provides a template for managing at-risk patients. Indeed, most patients with chronic pain could be deemed at risk.

TABLE 25-5 Management Recommendations for the Worker at Risk for Disability

1	Identify psychosocial and nonmedical risk factor "flags."
2	Identify and discuss RTW barriers with the patient.
3	Delay work disability and consider onsite treatment options or accommodations.
4	Discuss an RTW timeline from the onset of treatment.
5	Discuss and address fears, irrational thoughts and beliefs (e.g., catastrophizing), and irrational fears (e.g., increased pain resulting in reinjury, the patient cannot work with pain).
6	Consider treatments that have high success rates for RTW instead of passive treatments that reinforce disability and somatic concern.
7	Refer for interdisciplinary rehabilitation treatment, particularly programs that emphasize RTW issues.
8	Consider for adjunctive behavioral treatment with specialists who have knowledge of RTW issues.
9	Contact the patient's resources to help facilitate rapid return to work (e.g., rehabilitation nurses and rehabilitation counselors, co-treating clinicians).

RTW, return to work.

CONCLUSIONS

Work-related disability is a complicated phenomenon. Although the role of physical factors cannot be discounted when one is targeting illness or impairment, these factors likely have a limited role when return to work is considered a goal. Although measures of impairment may be easily quantified, their predictive value for disability remains suspect.

Clinicians have a unique role in the evaluation and assessment of patients with chronic pain and must not abrogate their responsibilities when the issue of return to work arises. By identifying patients with at-risk factors, one can intervene and provide a more comprehensive and efficacious treatment. Early intervention leads to better outcomes, less financial burden, and reduced frustration on the part of clinicians and patients.

REFERENCES

1. Lezzoni L. Eliminating health and health care disparities among the growing population of people with disabilities. *Health Aff.* 2011;30(12):1947-1954.
2. Kessler Foundation and National Organization on Disabilities. The ADA, 20 years later: 2010. New York.
3. Kominski GF, Pourat N, Roby DH, Cameron ME. Return to work and degree of recovery among injured workers in California's workers' compensation system. *J Occup Environ Med.* 2008;50(3):296-305.
4. Palmer M. Disability and poverty: a conceptual review. *J Disabil Policy Studies.* 2011;21(4):210-218.
5. Macor JE. *Annual Reports in Medicinal Chemistry.* Vol. 42. San Diego: Academic Press; 2007.
6. Gross DP, Ferrari R, Russel AS, et al. A population-based survey of back pain beliefs in Canada. *Spine.* 2006;31(18):2142-2145.
7. Kosny A, MacEachen E, Ferrier S, Chambers L. The role of health care providers in long term and complicated workers' compensation claims. *J Occup Rehabil.* 2011;21(4):582-590.
8. Lotters FJB, Foets M, Burdorf A. Work and health, a blind spot in curative healthcare? A pilot study. *J Occup Rehabil.* 2011;21:304-312.
9. Dasinger L, Krause N, Thompson P, et al. Doctor proactive communication, return to work recommendations, and duration of disability after a workers' compensation low back injury. *J Occup Environ Med.* 2001;43(6):515-525.
10. Verhagen AP, Scholten-Peeters GGM, Wijngaarden SV, et al. Conservative treatments for whiplash. *Cochrane Database Syst Rev.* 2007;2:CD003338.
11. Turner JA, Franklin G, Fulton-Kehoe D, et al. Early predictors of chronic disability: a prospective, population-based study of workers with back injuries. *Spine.* 2008;33(5):2809-2818.
12. Waddell G, Newton M, Henderson L, et al. A fear-avoidance beliefs questionnaire (FABQ) and the role of fear-avoidance beliefs in chronic low back pain and disability. *Pain.* 1993;52(2):157-168.
13. Abbema R, van Lakke SE, Reneman MF, et al. Factors associated with functional capacity test results in patients with non-specific chronic low back pain: a systematic review. *J Occup Rehabil.* 2011;21(4):455-473.
14. Kulich RJ, Driscoll J, Prescott J, et al. The Daubert standard: a primer for pain specialists. *Pain Medicine.* 2004;4(1):1-7.
15. Kulich RJ, Driscoll S, Scrivani S, Mehta N. A survey of medico-legal practice patterns among pain specialists. *Pain Med.* 2004;5(1):98-103.
16. Palmer M, Harley D. Models and measurement in disability: an international review. *Health Policy Plan.* 2012;27(5):357-364.
17. Talmage JB, Melhorn JM, Hyman MH. *AMA Guides to the Evaluation of Work Ability and Return to Work.* Second ed. Washington DC: American Medical Association; 2011.
18. United Nations. Convention on the Rights of Persons with Disabilities: Conventional and Optional Protocol Signatories and Ratification. Available at: http://www.un.org/disabilities/default.asp?navid=14&pid=150. Accessed December 16, 2011.
19. Oliver M. *Understanding Disability: From Theory to Practice.* London: Macmillan; 1996.
20. Nicholas MK, Linton SJ, Watson PJ, et al. Early identification and management of psychological risk factors ("yellow flags") in patients with low back pain: A reappraisal. *Physical Therapy.* 2011;91:1-17.
21. Shaw WS, van der Windt DA, Main CJ, et al. "Decade of the Flags" working group. Early patient screening and intervention to address individual-level occupational factors (blue flags) in back disability. *J Occup Rehabil.* 2009;19(1):64-80.
22. Buer N, Linton S. Fear avoidance beliefs and catastrophizing: occurrence and risk factor in back pain and ADL in the general population. *Pain.* 2002;99:485-491.
23. Brage S, Sandanger I, Nygard J. Emotional distress as a predictor for low back disability: a prospective 12-year population-based study. *Spine.* 2007;32:269-274.
24. Foster N, Thomas E, Bishop A, et al. Distinctiveness of psychological obstacles to recovery in low back pain patients in primary care. *Pain.* 2010;148:398-406.
25. Fritz J, George S, Delitto A. The role of fear-avoidance beliefs in acute low back pain: relationships with current and future disability and work status. *Pain.* 2001;94(1):7-15.
26. McCracken L, Vowles K. Psychological flexibility and traditional pain management strategies in relation to patient functioning with chronic pain: an examination of a revised instrument. *J Pain.* 2007;8:339-349.
27. Casey C, Greenberg M, Nicassio P, et al. Transition from acute to chronic pain and disability: a model including cognitive, affective, and trauma factors. *Pain.* 2008;134:69-79.
28. Kroenke K, Bair M, Damush T, et al. Stepped care for affective disorders and musculoskeletal pain (SCAMP) study: design and practical implications of an intervention for comorbid pain and depression. *Gen Hosp Psychiatry.* 2007;29(6):506-517.
29. Bair M, Wu J, Damush T, et al. Association of depression and anxiety alone and in combination with chronic musculoskeletal pain in primary care patients. *Psychosom Medicine.* 2008;70:890-897.
30. Bair M, Robinson R, Katon W, Kroenke K. Depression and pain comorbidity—a literature review. *Arch Intern Med.* 2003;163:2433-2445.
31. Miller LR, Cano A. Comorbid chronic pain and depression: who is at risk? *J Pain.* 2009;0(6):619-627.
32. Keefe FJ, Rumble ME, Scipio CD, et al. Psychological aspects of persistent pain: currents state of science. *J Pain.* 2004;5(4):195-211.
33. Brage S, Sandanger I, Nygard JF. Emotional distress as a predictor for low back disability: a prospective 12-year population-based study. *Spine.* 2007;32(2):269-274.
34. NIDA. *Overview of Findings from the 2002 National Survey on Drug Use and Health.* Report DHHS publication No. SMA 03-3774. Rockville, MD: Substance Abuse and Mental Health Services Administration; 2003.
35. Jamison RN, Ross EL, Michna E, et al. Substance misuse treatment for high risk chronic pain patients on opioid therapy: a randomized trial. *Pain.* 2010;150(3):390-400.
36. Parks PD, Pransky GS, Stefanos K. Case reports iatrogenic disability and narcotics addiction after lumbar fusion in a worker's compensation claimant. *Spine.* 2010;35(12):549-552.
37. Barsky AJ, Orav EJ, Bates DW. Somatization increases medical utilization and costs independent o psychiatric and medical comorbidities. *Arch Gen Psychiatry.* 2005;62:903-910.
38. Wolfe F, Ross K, Anderson J. The prevalence and characteristics of fibromyalgia in the general population. *Arthritis Rheum.* 1995;38:19-28.

39. Campbell SM, Clark S, Tindeall EA. Clinical characteristics of fibromyalgia. A "blinded" controlled study of symptoms and tender points. *Arthritis Rheum.* 1983;26:817-824.
40. Kamaleri Y, Natvig B, Ihlebaek CM, et al. Number of pain sites is associated with demographic, lifestyle, and health-related factors in the general population. *Eur J Pain.* 2008;12(6):742-748.
41. Kamaleri Y, Natvig B, Ihlebaek CM, Bruusgaard D. Does the number of musculoskeletal pain sites predict work disability? A 14-year prospective study. *Eur J Pain.* 2009;13(4):426-430.
42. McCracken L, Vowles KE, Eccleston C. Acceptance of chronic pain: component analysis and a revised assessment method. *Pain.* 2004;107(1-2):159-166.
43. Vowles K, McCracken L. Acceptance and values-based action in chronic pain: a study of effectiveness and treatment process. *J Consult Clin Psychol.* 2008;76:397-407.
44. Hayes S, Luoma J, Bond F, et al. Acceptance and commitment therapy: model, processes and outcomes. *Behav Res Ther.* 2006;44(1):1-25.
45. Wells N. Perceived control over pain: relation to distress and disability. *Res Nurs Health.* 1994;17:295-302.
46. Pincus T, Burton AK, Vogel S, Field AP. A systematic review of psychological factors as predictors of chronic/disability in prospective cohorts of low back pain. *Spine.* 2002;27(5):109-120.
47. Fritz JM, George SZ, Delitto A. The role of fear-avoidance beliefs in acute low back pain: relationships with current and future disability and work status. *Pain.* 2001;94(1):7-15.
48. Rainville J, Rob JEM, Smeets, et al. Fear-avoidance beliefs and pain avoidance in low back pain—translating research into clinical practice. *Spine J.* 2011;11(9):895-903.
49. Wideman TH, Sullivan MJK. Reducing catastrophic thinking associated with pain. *Pain Manag.* 2011;1(3):249-256.
50. Richard S, Dionne CE, Nouwen A. Self-efficacy and health locus of control: relationship to occupational disability among workers with back pain. *J Occup Rehabil.* 2011;21(3):421-430.
51. Waddell G, Burton K. Concepts of rehabilitation for the management of low back pain. *Best Pract Res Clin Rheumatol.* 2005;19(4):655-670.
52. Pransky GS, Louisel P, Anema JR. Work disability prevention research: current and future prospects. *J Occup Rehabil.* 2011;287-292.
53. Bigos SJ, Battie MC, Spengler DM, et al. A prospective study of work perceptions and psychosocial factors affecting the report of back injury. *Spine.* 1991;16(1):1-6.
54. Melamed S. Burnout and risk of regional musculoskeletal pain—a prospective study of apparently healthy employed adults. *Stress Health.* 2009;25:313-321.
55. Rios R, Zautra AJ. Socioeconomic disparities in pain: the role of economic hardship and daily financial worry. *Health Psychol* 2011;30(1):58-66.
56. Smith JP. Unraveling the SES-Health Connection. *Rand Labor and Population Working Paper.* 2005.
57. Athanasou JA. *Return to Work Following Whiplash and Back Injury.* Sydney, Australia: OVAL Research, University of Technology; 2007.
58. Kulich RJ, Kreis PG, Fishman SM, et al. Forensic issues in pain: review of current practice. *Pain Pract.* 2001;1(2):119-135.
59. Barbotte E, Gullemin F, Chau N; Lorhandicap Group. Prevalence of impairments, disabilities, handicaps and quality of life in the general population: a review of recent literature. *Bull World Health Organ.* 2001;79(11).
60. American Medical Association. *Guides to the Evaluation of Permanent Impairment.* 6th ed. Washington DC: American Medical Association; 2008.
61. Fairbank JC, Pynsent PB. The Oswestry disability index. *Spine* (2000):25;2940-2953.
62. Copay AG, Glassman SD, Subach BR, Berven S, Schuler TC, Carreon LY. Minimum clinically important difference in lumbar spine surgery patients: a choice of methods using the Oswestry Disability Index, Medical Outcomes Study questionnaire Short Form 36, and pain scales. *Spine J* (2008):8;968-974.
63. Carreon LY, Glassman SD, Campbell MJ, Anderson PA. Neck Disability Index, short-form-36 physical component summary, and pain scales for neck and arm pain: the minimum clinically important difference and substantial clinical benefit after cervical spine fusion. *Spine J* (2010):10;469-474.
64. Schiphorst Preuper HR, Reneman MF, Boonstra AM, Dijkstra PU, Versteegen GJ, Geertzen JHB. The relationship between psychophysical distress and disability assessed by the Symptom Checklist-90-Revised and Roland Morris Disability Questionnaire in patients with chronic low back pain. *Spine J* (2007):7; 525-530.
65. Sauro KM, Rose MS, Becker WJ, et al. HIT-6 and MIDAS as measures of headache disability in a headache referral population. *Headache* (2010):50;383-395.
66. Bot SD, Terwee CB, van der Windt DA, Bouter LM, Dekker J, de Vet HC. Clinimetric evaluation of shoulder disability questionnaires: a systematic review of the literature. *Ann Rheum Dis* (2004):63;335-341.
67. Anagnostic C, Gatchel RJ, Mayer TG. The pain disability questionnaire: a new psychometrically sound measure for chronic musculoskeletal disorders. *Spine* (2004): 29;2290-2302.
68. Bennett, R. The Fibromyalgia Impact Questionnaire (FIQ): a review of its development, current version, operating characteristics and uses. *Clin Exp Rheumatol* (2005) 23;S154.
69. Ware JE, Sherbourne CD. The MOS 36-item Short-Form Health Survey (SF-36): I. Conceptual framework and item selection. *Medical Care.* 1992;30(6):473-483.
70. Ware JE, Gandek B. Overview of the SF-36 Health Survey and the International Questionnaire of Life Assessment (IQOLA) Project. *J Clin Epidemiol.* 1998;51(11):903-912.
71. Linton SJ. The manager's role in employees' successful return to work following back injury. *Work Stress.* 1991;5(3).
72. Waddell G. Clinical model for the treatment of low-back pain. *Spine.* 1987;12:632-644.
73. Woolf AD, Pfleger B. Burden of major musculoskeletal conditions. *Bull World Health Organ.* 2003;81(9).
74. Houben RMA, Ostelo RWJG, Vlaeyen JWS, et al. Stomp-van den Berg SGM. Health care providers' orientations towards common low back pain predict perceived harmfulness of physical activities and recommendations regarding return to normal activity. *J Pain.* 2005;9(2):173-183.
75. Rainville J, Vouve CA, Hartigan C, et al. Comparison of short and long term outcomes for aggressive spine rehabilitation delivered two versus three times per week. *Spine J.* 2002;2(6): 402-407.
76. Malmivaara AMC, Koes BW, Bouter LM, van Tulder MW. Applicability and clinical relevance of results in randomized controlled trials: the Cochrane Review on exercise therapy for low back pain as an example. *Spine.* 2006;31(13):1405-1409.
77. Guzman J, Esmail R, Kargalainen K, et al. Multidisciplinary bio-psycho-social rehabilitation for chronic low back pain. *Cochrane Database Syst Rev.* 2007;(2):CD000963.
78. Kulich RJ, Loeser JD. The business of pain medicine: the present mirrors antiquity. *Pain Med.* 2011;12:1063-1095.

79. Kapural L, Deer T, Yakovlev A, et al. Technical aspects of spinal cord stimulation for managing chronic visceral abdominal pain: the results from the national survey. *Pain Med.* 2010;11:685-691.

80. MacLaren JE, Gross RT, Sperry JA, Boggess JT. Impact of opioid use on outcomes of functional restoration. *Clin J Pain.* 2006;22(4): 392-398.

81. Kidner CL, Mayer TG, Gatchel RJ. Higher opioid doses predict poorer functional outcome in patients with chronic disabling occupational musculoskeletal disorders. *J Bone Joint Surg Am.* 2009;91(4):919-927.

82. Slater MA, Weickgenant AL, Greenberg MA, et al. Preventing progression to chronicity in first onset, subacute low back pain: an exploratory study. *Arch Phys Med Rehabil.* 2009;90(4):545-552.

83. U.S. Department of Justice Civil Rights Division. American with Disabilities Act Questions and Answers. Available at: http://www.ada.gov/q%26aeng02.htm. Last accessed: December 17, 2011.

84. Pomaki G, Franche RL, Murray E, et al. Workplace-based work disability prevention interventions for workers with mental health conditions: a review of literature. *J Occup Rehabil.* 2011.

85. Gatchel RJ, McGeary DD, McGeary CA, Lippe B. Interdisciplinary chronic pain management: Past, present, and future. *Am Psychol.* 2014;69:119-130.

86. Munguía-Izquierdo D, Santalla A, Legaz-Arrese A. Evaluation of a wearable body monitoring device during treadmill walking and jogging in patients with fibromyalgia syndrome. *Arch Phys Med Rehabil.* 2012;93(1):115-122.

87. Whybrow S, Ritz P, Horgan GW, Stubbs RJ. An evaluation of the IDEEA™ activity monitor for estimating energy expenditure. *Br J Nutr.* 2013;109(1):173-183.

PART 4

Pain by Anatomic Location

SECTION A
Head and Neck

Approach to the Patient with Headache

Paul G. Mathew
Huma Sheikh

INTRODUCTION

Among the complaints from patients presenting to outpatient practices, headache is one of the most common. Even the most experienced providers often have a difficult time formulating a diagnosis and effective treatment plan. The authors of this chapter evaluate some of the imperative concepts of headache diagnosis, including headache-specific history, physical examination, warning signs of secondary headache disorders, and when to contemplate further diagnostic studies. The criteria used in making a specific diagnosis are located in the International Headache Society's International Classification of Headache Disorders, second edition (ICHD-2).[1]

EVALUATION

A thorough headache evaluation should begin with the determination of whether a headache is a primary or secondary headache disorder. Primary headache disorders lack an underlying cause, but secondary headaches are attributable to an identifiable pathologic cause. Treatment of underlying pathology can at times lead to a cessation of headaches in the case of secondary headaches.

HISTORY

The most important tool in formulating a headache diagnosis is a proper history, which should include past medical history; surgical history; medications; allergies; and family history, including headaches. A thorough medication history should include previous medications that have been used for the abortive and preventive treatment of headache. To ensure adequate trials of these headache medications, dose, duration of treatment, effectiveness, and side effects should be recorded for each medication.

A headache history should begin with the genesis of the headache. For many patients with primary headache disorders, headaches can begin during adolescence or even childhood. In patients with a long history of headaches, recall can often be an issue, but recalling any events that may have precipitated the headaches, such as head trauma, infections, or surgery, is crucial. The features of individual headaches should also be recorded. These features should include intensity, quality, location, radiation, and duration of individual headaches.

Pain intensity can be difficult to assess, but it is an important headache feature in terms of establishing a diagnosis and monitoring improvement with treatment. Although helpful, a visual analog pain scale of 0 to 10 with zero being no pain and 10 being the worst pain imaginable can often lead to an exaggeration of pain. In clinical practice, it is common for a patient to complain of a 9 of 10 pain in the office while being able to converse while sitting comfortably in no clear distress. As such, associating disability ratings to this scale may help correct for this subjective exaggeration. Below is a combined pain and disability scale that can be used to assess headache intensity.[2]

COMBINED PAIN AND DISABILITY SCALE

- 1 to 3 of 10 indicates mild pain with no significant impairment of function.
- 4 to 6 of 10 indicates moderate pain with some impairment of function.
- 7 to 10 of 10 indicates severe pain with complete impairment of function.

When addressing frequency, it should be made clear that total number headache days per month is being assessed rather than just severe headache days. It is useful to confirm this number by asking the number of headache-free days per month. For example, if the patient responds to headache frequency questioning by claiming to have 15 headache days in a 28-day month, the patient should be asked if he or she has 13 headache-free days per month for confirmation.

Some other headache features that should routinely be assessed include the presence of photophobia, phonophobia, osmophobia, nausea, vomiting, and cutaneous allodynia. Although some patients may deny these features, asking questions regarding pain behaviors can at times provide a clearer establishment of associated features. For example, a patient may initially deny photophobia and phonophobia on direct questioning. When asked specifically during a severe headache, the same patient may prefer to rest in a dark, quiet room.

In addition, the presence of autonomic features such as unilateral conjunctival injection, lacrimation, nasal congestion, rhinorrhea, ptosis, miosis, and forehead or facial sweating should be assessed. Although these autonomic features can be appreciated in various headache syndromes, their presence on the ipsilateral side of unilateral headache is suggestive of a trigeminal autonomic cephalgia, such as cluster headache. In female patients, assessing headache pattern changes caused by menstruation, pregnancy, hormone therapy, and menopause can help establish a diagnosis, as well as steer therapeutic decision making.

Auras are neurologic symptoms that occur before the onset of a migraine or during the early headache phase. Migraine auras can present as visual, sensory, language, or motor disturbances that last less than 60 minutes. Discriminating migraine aura from other neurologic symptoms can at times be difficult. Classic visual auras include scintillating scotomas and fortification spectrums. Most visual auras start in one area of the visual field and slowly progress over minutes. Blurry vision can be appreciated during the peak phase of a headache and should not be confused with visual aura. In addition, ophthalmologic pathology should be ruled out when atypical visual disturbances are present or when vision does not return to baseline with resolution of the headache. Sensory aura typically involves tingling and numbness that starts in an extremity or the face and gradually radiates over minutes. In the case of sensory aura, ruling out radiculopathy, plexopathy, and peripheral neuropathy is important in labeling a sensory disturbance as a sensory aura. Although sensory aura usually remains unilateral, bilateral sensory auras can also occur. Speech aura usually presents as expressive aphasia and should not be confused with the concentration difficulties that can occur with a migraine. Motor aura refers to focal weakness that can occur with a subtype of migraine known as hemiplegic migraine. This focal weakness should not be confused with the generalized weakness that can occur with any type of migraine or the clumsiness that can occur in the setting of a sensory aura. A simple way to delineate motor aura from sensory aura clumsiness is to ask the patient about his or her ability to bear weight on the affected leg or raise his or her arm above the head on the affected side. If the patient is able to perform these tasks but has problems walking or grasping objects, he or she likely has a sensory aura rather than focal weakness suggestive of hemiplegic migraine.

When recording a headache history, lifestyle features should be scrutinized because they can serve as primary headache triggers or causes of secondary headache. For example, inadequate or poor-quality sleep can serve as a migraine trigger. On the other hand, sleep apnea can be a cause of secondary headache.[1] Some other lifestyle features that should be assessed include caffeine intake, drug and alcohol use, and stress (professional, academic, and home).

Headaches that tend to have a positional component are suggestive of a secondary headache. For example, headaches that tend to be the worse upon awakening and improve with progression of the day while upright are suggestive of elevated intracranial pressure (ICP). This can be attributable to a brain tumor or idiopathic intracranial hypertension (pseudotumor cerebri). Elevated ICP tends to involve projectile vomiting, which can at times improve the headache. Conversely, low ICP, which can occur in the setting of a cerebrospinal fluid (CSF) leak, can cause headaches that improve with lying flat and worsen while upright.

Some other "red flags" in a patient history suggestive of a secondary headache disorder include the onset of headache after the age of 50 years, neurologic symptoms that are inconsistent with typical aura, fever, weight loss, a history of cancer, intractable headache in a solitary location, a sudden worsening of frequency or intensity, and a history of systemic disease that can manifest as headache (e.g., HIV).[3]

PHYSICAL EXAMINATION AND DIAGNOSTIC TESTING

In the evaluation of patients with headache, a thorough physical examination, including a neurologic examination, should be performed. A vital and often overlooked portion of the neurologic examination is the funduscopic examination. Funduscopy can reveal ophthalmic pathology, including papilledema, which is indicative of elevated ICP. In addition, several headache-specific assessments can be helpful in arriving at the diagnosis. Palpation of the temporomandibular joint (TMJ) with opening and closing of the jaw can produce popping and clicking of the joint. TMJ disorders commonly occur in the setting of headache disorders, and adequate treatment can lead to improvement of headache frequency and intensity. Palpation of the scalp can reveal cutaneous allodynia, temporal artery prominence or tenderness, and surface lesions. Active and passive range of motion assessments of the neck can trigger headache in the setting of cervicogenic headache and occipital neuralgia, and neck stiffness can be suggestive of meningismus. For occipital neuralgia, an occipital Tinel's sign may be performed by tapping over the bilateral occiput, which can produce painful jolts of pain radiating toward the apex, as well as areas posterior and superior to the ipsilateral ear. In cases of suspected low-ICP headache, assessing the patient's headache pain intensity before and after 5- to minutes of lying supine can be helpful.

In general, imaging studies are not warranted in most cases. A long history of headaches that meet criteria for a primary headache disorder, a nonfocal neurologic examination, and a strong family history of primary headaches are usually present in most patients who present for headache evaluation. In such cases, it is reasonable to proceed with treatment and to reconsider imaging studies if the patient is not responding to treatment. The decision to proceed with imaging studies should be made on a case-by-case basis.

In the emergency department, patients often present with the worst headaches of their live, new-onset headaches, or headaches with associated neurologic symptoms. In such cases, computed tomography (CT) imaging is the study of choice given the short duration of the test, availability of CT scanners in most hospitals, and CT sensitivity for detecting blood. With headaches that present in a less urgent manner, magnetic resonance imaging is the imaging modality of choice.

According to American Academy of Neurology Practice Parameters, the following symptoms significantly increase the odds of finding a significant abnormality on neuroimaging in patients with nonacute headache:[4]

- Rapidly increasing headache frequency
- History of lack of coordination
- History of localized neurologic signs
- History of headache causing awakening from sleep (although this can occur with migraine and cluster headache)

Contrast administration should be considered in cases such as those involving suspected mass lesions or low ICP to look for brain sag. Arteriograms and venograms should also be considered based on index of suspicion. For example, patients with exertional headaches, suspected sentinel bleeding, or a family history of aneurysms should have magnetic resonance angiography. Magnetic resonance venography should be considered to rule out sinus thrombosis during pregnancy and other situations involving potential hypercoagulable states.

In addition to imaging modalities, other studies can also be performed based on clinical suspicion. Lumbar punctures (LPs) are usually performed for diagnostic purposes but can also be therapeutic in the evaluation of patients with idiopathic intracranial hypertension. Although controversial, the author believes that LPs should not be performed in patients with suspected low-ICP headaches. In such cases, a normal opening pressure does not rule out this diagnosis, and the LP itself creates another source for a CSF leak, which may potentially worsen any underlying brain sag.

Brain imaging should always be performed before proceeding with a LP. To get a more accurate opening pressure, this procedure should be performed in the sidelying position. Routine CSF analysis should be performed in addition to any specific testing based on clinical suspicion such as polymerase chain reaction testing for suspected herpes encephalitis. Although there are no CSF or serum markers for primary headache disorders, blood tests should be ordered based on suspicion of secondary headache disorders. For example, in patients older than 50 years of age with new-onset headaches, the erythrocyte sedimentation rate should be checked for evaluation of temporal arteritis. Likewise, patients in wooded areas should be evaluated for Lyme disease.

CONCLUSION

The evaluation and diagnosis of headaches in the outpatient setting can be challenging. A thorough history and physical examination can often yield enough clues to formulate a diagnosis. As such, imaging studies and other tests are often unnecessary. Such testing can be expensive, invasive, and a wasteful use of resources and the patient's time. In addition, such studies often uncover incidental findings, which can compound any baseline patient anxiety regarding the diagnosis. As such, a reasonable approach would be to proceed with treatment if there are no clear red flags suggestive of a secondary headache disorder and order additional testing in cases that are refractory treatment.

REFERENCES

1. Headache Classification Subcommittee of the International Headache Society. The International Classification of Headache Disorders. 2nd ed. *Cephalalgia*. 2004;24(Suppl 1):9-160.
2. Mathew PG, Mathew T. Taking care of the challenging tension headache patient. *Curr Pain Headache Rep*. 2011;15(6):444-450.
3. Mathew PG, Garza I. Headache. *Semin Neurol*. 2011;31(1):5-17.
4. Silberstein, SD. Practice parameter: Evidence-based guidelines for migraine headache (an evidence-based review). *Neurology*. 2000;55(6):754-762.

CHAPTER 27

Epidemiology of Headaches

Daniel P. Schwartz
Mark Sollars
Brian M. Grosberg

INTRODUCTION

Headache is a common pain symptom that inflicts a substantial burden on individuals and on society. Headache has many causes; a range of headache diagnoses was defined for the first time by the International Headache Society (IHS) in 1988 in the first edition of the International Classification of Headache Disorders (ICHD-1).[1] The second edition of the International Classification of Headache Disorders (ICHD-2) was published by the IHS in 2004, and the third edition (ICHD-3 beta version) was published in 2013.[2,3] The ICHD-3 beta version classifies headache disorders into three major categories: (1) primary headaches; (2) secondary headaches; and (3) painful cranial neuropathies, other facial pains, and other headaches. Secondary headache disorders result from an underlying condition, such as a sinus infection or brain tumor. In primary headache disorders, the headache disorder is the fundamental problem. The primary headaches include four categories: migraine, tension-type headache (TTH), trigeminal autonomic cephalalgias (TACs), and other primary headache disorders. The two most common types of primary headache disorders are episodic tension-type headache (ETTH) and migraine.

The epidemiology of headache varies by headache type and demographics. ETTH, the most common headache type, affects slightly more women than men.[4-9] Between the ages of 18 and 65 years, about 36% of men and 42% of women have ETTH.[10] In contrast, migraine occurs approximately three times more often in women than in men: approximately 18% of women and 6% of men between 12 and 80 years of age have migraine.[11,12]

Episodic tension-type headache exerts a modest impact on the individual; however, the aggregate societal impact is high because the disorder is so prevalent. Although migraine is less common, individual attacks are considerably more painful and disabling and often result in lost work time. Because the societal impact of both ETTH and migraine is significant, this chapter focuses on the epidemiology of the two disorders. This chapter does not cover secondary headaches because the epidemiology of the underlying condition is an important determinant of the epidemiology of the related headaches. This chapter begins with a review of the diagnostic criteria for migraine and TTH followed by a review of migraine epidemiology, including incidence, prevalence, and public health impact. The chapter closes with a review of the epidemiology of TTH.

DIAGNOSTIC CRITERIA

Migraine is characterized by various combinations of neurologic, gastrointestinal, and autonomic changes that occur during different phases of the migraine attack. Although the ICHD-3 beta version defines five major categories of migraine, by far the two most important are *migraine without aura* (1.1) and *migraine with aura* (1.2). The ICHD-3 beta version definitions for migraine with and without aura are found in **Tables 27-1** and **27-2**. The revised diagnostic criteria for 1.3, *chronic migraine*, as published by the IHS in the ICHD-3 beta version, are found in **Table 27-3**.

Migraine is both a diagnosis of inclusion because specific diagnostic features are required and a diagnosis of exclusion because secondary headache disorders have to be eliminated based on the history, physical examination, or laboratory studies.

The features of the migraine attack can be divided into four phases: premonitory phase, aura, headache phase, and resolution phase. None of these phases is obligatory for diagnosis, and most people with migraine do not have all four phases. The premonitory phase (prodrome) occurs in approximately 60% of individuals with migraine, with

TABLE 27-1 International Headache Society Diagnostic Criteria for Migraine Without Aura

Migraine without aura

Description: Recurrent headache disorder manifesting in attacks lasting 4-72 hours. Typical characteristics of the headache are unilateral location, pulsating quality, moderate or severe intensity, aggravation by routine physical activity and association with nausea and/or photophobia and phonophobia.

Diagnostic criteria

- A. At least five attacks fulfilling criteria B-D
- B. Headache attacks lasting 4-72 hours (untreated or unsuccessfully treated)
- C. Headache has at least two of the following four characteristics:
  1. unilateral location
  2. pulsating quality
  3. moderate or severe pain intensity
  4. aggravation by or causing avoidance of routine physical activity (e.g. walking or climbing stairs)
- D. During headache at least one of the following:
  1. nausea and/or vomiting
  2. photophobia and phonophobia
- E. Not better accounted for by another ICHD-3 diagnosis

Data from Classification and diagnostic criteria for headache disorders, cranial neuralgias and facial pain. Headache Classification Committee of the International Headache Society. *Cephalalgia*. 1988;8:1-96, by permission of Scandinavian University Press.

TABLE 27-2 International Headache Society Diagnostic Criteria for Migraine with Aura

Migraine with aura

Description: Recurrent attacks, lasting minutes of unilateral fully reversible visual, sensory or other central nervous system symptoms that usually develop gradually and are usually followed by headache and associated migraine symptoms.

Diagnostic criteria

- A. At least two attacks fulfilling criteria B and C
- B. One or more of the following fully reversible aura symptoms:
  1. visual
  2. sensory
  3. speech and/or language
  4. motor
  5. brainstem
  6. retinal
- C. At least two of the following four characteristics:
  1. at least one aura symptom spreads gradually over >5 minutes, and/or two or more symptoms occur in succession
  2. each individual aura symptom lasts 5-60 minutes
  3. at least one aura symptom is unilateral
  4. the aura is accompanied, or followed within 60 minutes, by headache
- D. Not better accounted for by another ICHD-3 diagnosis, and transient ischaemic attack has been excluded

Data from Classification and diagnostic criteria for headache disorders, cranial neuralgias and facial pain. Headache Classification Committee of the International Headache Society. *Cephalalgia*. 1988;8:1-96, by permission of Scandinavian University Press.

TABLE 27-3 International Headache Study Diagnostic Criteria for Episodic Tension-Type Headache

1. Episodic tension-type headache

Description: Recurrent episodes of headache, typically bilateral, pressing or tightening in quality and of mild to moderate intensity, lasting minutes to days. The pain does not worsen with routine physical activity and is not associated with nausea, but photophobia or phonophobia may be present. Infrequent episodic tension-type headache occurs on <1 day per month on average (<12 days per year). Frequent episodic tension-type headache occurs on 1-14 days per month on average for >3 months (>12 and <180 days per year).

Diagnostic criteria

- A. At least 10 episodes of headache fulfilling criteria B-D.
- B. Lasting from 30 minutes to 7 days
- C. At least two of the following four characteristics:
  1. bilateral location
  2. pressing or tightening (non-pulsating) quality
  3. mild or moderate intensity
  4. not aggravated by routine physical activity such as walking or climbing stairs
- D. Both of the following:
  1. no nausea or vomiting
  2. no more than one of photophobia or phonophobia
- E. Not better accounted for by another ICHD-3 diagnosis

Data from Classification and diagnostic criteria for headache disorders, cranial neuralgias and facial pain. Headache Classification Committee of the International Headache Society. *Cephalalgia*. 1988;8:1-96, by permission of Scandinavian University Press.

equal frequency in both migraine with and without aura.[13] It usually begins hours to days before headache onset. Symptoms that may occur during the prodrome include depression, hyperactivity, yawning, food cravings, and thirst.[13]

In migraine with aura, various focal neurologic symptoms precede or accompany the attack. The aura usually develops over a period of 5 to 20 minutes and typically lasts less than 1 hour. It is most often characterized by visual phenomena but may also involve other secondary features such as sensory, speech or language, motor, brainstem, or retinal disturbances. The aura is usually, but not always, followed by a headache. Approximately 20% to 25% of individuals have migraine with aura, but even in these individuals, most attacks are migraine without aura.[14]

The third phase is the headache phase. The headache of migraine is typically unilateral, pulsating, of moderate to severe intensity, and aggravated by routine physical activity. Other features, including photophobia, phonophobia, nausea, and vomiting, also occur during the headache phase.

During the final resolution phase, the pain and accompanying symptoms subside. Although some individuals with migraine feel euphoric and energetic, others feel lethargic and tired.

The clinical diagnosis of TTH is also based on a characteristic symptom profile and the exclusion of secondary headache. Unlike migraine, there is no prodrome or aura in TTH. The headache is usually bilateral, dull, nonpulsating, and of mild to moderate intensity. Although associated features are not required for diagnosis, various symptoms are compatible with the diagnosis.

The diagnostic category TTH (ICHD-3, beta version) includes three main subtypes: *infrequent episodic TTH* (2.1) (headache episodes on <1 day per month), *frequent episodic TTH* (2.2) (headache episodes on 1-14 days per month), and *chronic TTH* (CTTH) (2.3) (headache on ≥15 days per month, perhaps without recognizable episodes). The primary difference between these disorders is the frequency with which the headaches occur. Whereas TTHs that occur less than 15 days per month are classified as ETTH, those that occur more than 15 days per month are classified as CTTH. In addition, for ETTH, nausea is not permitted, but either photophobia or phonophobia is permitted. For CTTH, any one of nausea, photophobia, or phonophobia is permitted. The diagnostic criteria for ETTH and CTTH are presented in **Tables 27-4** and **27-5**.

TABLE 27-4 International Headache Society Diagnostic Criteria for Chronic Tension-Type Headache

Chronic tension-type headache

Description: A disorder evolving from frequent episodic tension-type headache, with daily or very frequent episodes of headache, typically bilateral, pressing or tightening in quality and of mild to moderate intensity, lasting hours to days, or unremitting. The pain does not worsen with routine physical activity, but may be associated with mild nausea, photophobia or phonophobia.

Diagnostic criteria:

A. Headache occurring on >15 days per month on average for >3 months (>180 days per year), fulfilling criteria B-D
B. Lasting hours to days, or unremitting
C. At least two of the following four characteristics:
   1. bilateral location
   2. pressing or tightening (non-pulsating) quality
   3. mild or moderate intensity
   4. not aggravated by routine physical activity such as walking or climbing stairs
D. Both of the following:
   1. no more than one of photophobia, phonophobia or mild nausea
   2. neither moderate or severe nausea nor vomiting
E. Not better accounted for by another ICHD-3 diagnosis

Data from Classification and diagnostic criteria for headache disorders, cranial neuralgias and facial pain. Headache Classification Committee of the International Headache Society. *Cephalalgia.* 1988;8:1-96, by permission of Scandinavian University Press.

MIGRAINE EPIDEMIOLOGY AND DISEASE BURDEN

INCIDENCE

Incidence is defined as the rate of onset of new cases of disease in a defined population. Estimating the incidence of migraine is challenging because the disease affects individuals of all ages, and the incidence rate varies substantially by age. To accurately describe incidence requires a large cohort study of individuals ranging in age from 4 to 60 years. There have been few studies of migraine incidence.

Breslau and colleagues[15] conducted a prospective study to estimate the incidence of migraine. The investigators interviewed 1007 members of a health maintenance organization who were between the ages of 21 and 30 years. Approximately 98% (972 of 1007) of the participants completed a follow-up interview 3.5 and 5.5 years later. The at-risk population was composed of 848 participants who did not meet the criteria for migraine at baseline. The 5.5-year cumulative incidence was 8.4% (71 of 848; women 60; men, 11), or a rate of 17.0 per 1000 person years (24.0, women, 6.0, men).

Two population-based studies estimated the incidence of migraine using the reported age of migraine onset. Stewart and colleagues[16] conducted telephone interviews among 10,169 residents of Washington County, Maryland, who were between the ages of 12 and 29 years. In this study, 392 men and 1018 women interviewees were identified as having migraine. As shown in **Figure 27-1**, in both mens and womens, the incidence rate of migraine with aura peaks 3 to 5 years earlier than migraine without aura. In addition, the onset of migraine in womens occurs at a later age than in mens. An important strength of this study is that it adjusted for telescoping. Telescoping is the tendency to report the occurrence of past events at times closer to the present.[17] Thus, studies estimating the age-specific incidence of migraine based on recall would likely be biased toward older ages of headache onset.[17,18] To minimize the effect of telescoping, Stewart and colleagues[16] estimated the age-specific incidence rates, adjusted for the time interval between the reported age of onset and the age at interview. However, because of the limited age range of the participants, the generalizability of the results is limited.

The second population-based study, conducted by Rasmussen,[19] reported that the age-adjusted annual incidence of migraine was 3.7 per 1000 person years (womens, 5.8; mens, 1.6). Neither age-specific incidence nor incidence by migraine subtypes was reported.

One study, conducted in Olmstead County, Minnesota, used linked medical records to estimate the incidence of migraine.[20] Of the 6400 patient records reviewed, 629 fulfilled the criteria for migraine. The overall age-adjusted incidence rate was 1.37 per 1000 person years for mens and 2.94 per 1000 person years for womens. The incidence rates in this study are lower than those reported in the aforementioned studies, probably because only individuals who consulted a health care provider for headache were included.

Lyngberg and colleagues published a population-based study of the incidence of migraine in a Danish population. This study was a follow-up to a cross-sectional epidemiology study from 1989. Of the 453 subjects ranging in age from 25 to 64 years who did not have migraine in 1989, 42 developed migraine during the study period, resulting in an annual incidence of 0.8%. The annual incidence in womens was 1.5% and in mens was 0.3%.[21]

Khil and colleagues published a population-based study of the incidence of migraine based on data from the German Migraine and Headache Society (DMKG). Incidences were assessed in the general population in Germany via standardized headache questions using ICHD-2 criteria. The population was drawn from a 5-year age group–stratified and gender-stratified random sample from the population register. Of the 1122 participants in three different populations at risk, the incidence of migraine ranged between 0% and 3.3%.[22]

Key Points: Migraine Incidence from the American Migraine Prevalence and Prevention (AMPP) Study[23]

- The cumulative migraine incidence is 43% in women and 18% in men.
- Migraine incidence peaks between 20 and 24 years of age for women and between 15 and 19 years of age for men.

TABLE 27-5 Gender- and Age-Specific Migraine Prevalence as Reported in Population-Based Studies of Migraine That Used International Headache Society Diagnostic Criteria[19]

Author	Age Range (yr)	Women	Men	Author	Age Range (yr)	Women	Men
Abu-Arefeh and Russell[38]	5–15	11.5	9.7	O'Brien et al.[39]	18–24	18.3	10.9
Alders[76,†]	5–15	4.4	2.6	O'Brien et al.[39]	25–34	23.0	9.1
Alders[76]	16–25	11.3	8.1	O'Brien et al.[39]	35–44	33.3	8.7
Alders[76]	26–35	11.5	6.7	O'Brien et al.[39]	45–54	32.3	5.9
Alders[76]	36–45	20.3	17.7	O'Brien et al.[39]	55–64	28.7	5.4
Alders[76]	46–55	22.7	7.7	O'Brien et al.[39]	65–74	11.7	1.9
Alders[76]	56–65	6.7	0.0	Rasmussen[19]	45–54	12.0	6.0
Alders[76]	66–87	5.3	0.0	Rasmussen[19]	55–64	19.0	7.0
Arregui[77]	0–9	0.0	0.8	Sakai[83,†]	15–19	11.5	2.0
Arregui[77]	10–19	3.7	1.5	Sakai[83]	20–29	13.0	7.0
Arregui[77]	20–29	8.8	0.0	Sakai[83]	30–39	20.0	6.0
Arregui[77]	30–39	8.5	0.0	Sakai[83]	40–49	18.0	2.5
Arregui[77]	40–49	18.0	2.3	Sakai[83]	50–59	11.0	3.0
Arregui[77]	50–59	8.1	3.1	Sakai[83]	60–69	9.0	0.5
Arregui[77]	60–69	4.0	0.0	Sakai[83]	70–79	3.0	0.0
Arregui[77]	0–9	4.8	0.7	Stewart[33,‡]	18–25	22.7	10.0
Arregui[77]	10–19	20.1	8.1	Stewart[33]	26–30	22.1	11.5
Arregui[77]	20–29	16.8	5.0	Stewart[33]	31–35	19.0	8.2
Arregui[77]	30–39	22.1	10.0	Stewart[33]	36–40	21.2	9.8
Arregui[77]	40–49	21.5	16.1	Stewart[33]	41–45	21.0	9.1
Arregui[77]	50–59	38.1	12.0	Stewart[33]	46–55	20.9	6.5
Arregui[77]	60–69	15.4	0.0	Stewart[33]	56–65	9.8	3.2
Barea et al.[6]	10–18	10.2	9.6	Stewart[11,‡]	12–19	8.1	4.3
Breslau et al.[15]	21–30	12.9	3.4	Stewart[11]	20–29	19.8	7.1
Cruz[78]	0–9	1.4	1.5	Stewart[11]	30–39	28.7	8.9
Cruz[78]	10–19	8.2	8.4	Stewart[11]	40–49	24.4	7.4
Cruz[78]	20–29	9.7	6.2	Stewart[11]	50–59	18.7	6.0
Cruz[78]	30–39	10.1	5.8	Stewart[11]	60–69	10.5	3.4
Cruz[78]	40–49	13.0	6.6	Stewart[11]	70–85	6.6	2.5
Cruz[78]	50–59	10.3	7.1	Tekle-Haimanot et al.[72]	20–29	4.8	1.1
Cruz[78]	60–69	8.1	6.5	Tekle-Haimanot et al.[72]	30–39	5.6	4.3
Franceschi[79]	65–84	2.0	0.0	Tekle-Haimanot et al.[72]	40–49	3.8	1.4
Henry[80,‡]	15–24	6.0	2.0	Tekle-Haimanot et al.[72]	50–59	3.4	1.6
Henry[80]	25–34	12.0	3.9	Tekle-Haimanot et al.[72]	60–69	1.9	0.6
Henry[80]	35–49	12.0	2.4	Tekle-Haimanot et al.[72]	70–79	0.6	0.6
Henry[80]	50–64	6.7	2.2	Tekle-Haimanot et al.[72]	80–89	0.0	0.0
Henry[80]	65–75	2.8	0.9	Thomson[84,†]	17–29	15.5	13.4
Launer[81]	20–24	17.0	3.0	Thomson[84]	30–49	14.4	10.7
Launer[81]	25–29	24.1	3.8	Thomson[84]	50–70	12.1	5.3
Launer[81]	30–34	21.4	4.4	Wong et al.[5]	15–24	0.8	0.4
Launer[81]	35–39	33.2	8.8	Wong et al.[5]	25–34	2.6	0.9
Launer[81]	40–44	27.5	6.5	Wong et al.[5]	35–44	2.7	1.0
Launer[81]	45–49	27.4	8.3	Wong et al.[5]	45–54	1.4	0.2
Launer[81]	50–54	24.0	15.7	Wong et al.[5]	55–64	0.6	0.4
Launer[81]	≥55	20.4	5.6	Wong et al.[5]	65–74	0.4	0.2
Linet[82,‡]	12–17	10.2	5.4				
Linet[82]	18–23	13.1	5.2				
Linet[82]	24–29	18.8	5.4				

†Data were estimated from published information.

‡Data were obtained from the author.

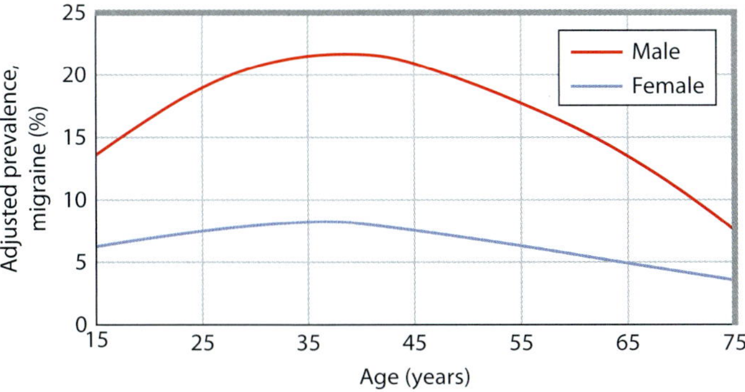

FIGURE 27-1. Sex- and age-specific incidence of migraine headache with and without aura among 10,131 survey respondents age 12 to 29 years: Washington County, Maryland, 1987. (Used with permission from Stewart WF, Linet MS, Celentano DD, et al. Age- and sex-specific incidence rates of migraine with and without visual aura. *Am J Epi-demiol* 1991;134:1111-1120.)

- The median age of onset is 25 years among women and 24 years among men.
- The onset occurs before age 25 years in 50% of cases.
- The onset occurs before age 35 years in 75% of cases.

PREVALENCE

In contrast to the limited number of studies of migraine incidence, there have been many studies of the prevalence of migraine. *Prevalence* is defined as the proportion of a given population that has migraine over a defined period of time. *Lifetime prevalence* refers to the proportion of individuals who have ever had the disease. *Period prevalence* refers to the proportion of individuals who have experienced at least one attack within a defined interval, usually within 1 year of the survey. Prevalence is a function of both the incidence and duration of a disease.

The prevalence of migraine has been assessed in numerous studies using a variety of case definitions and methods. Estimates became much less variable after standard diagnostic criteria were developed and applied. Most large studies generate estimates in the 15% to 20% range for women and 4% to 7% range for men. In the United States, there have been three large-scale studies in nationally representative samples of the U.S. population conducted in 1989 (American Migraine Study 1 [AMS-1]),[24] in 1999 (American Migraine Study 2 [AMS-2]),[25,26] and in 2004 (American Migraine Prevalence and Prevention Study [AMPP]).[27]

In AMS-1, 15,000 households received mailed questionnaires, and each household member who had severe headache was asked to respond to detailed questions about symptoms, frequency, and severity of the headaches. After a single mailing, 20,468 subjects between 12 and 80 years of age responded to the survey. The prevalence of migraine was 17.6% in womens and 5.7% in mens.

To identify shifting patterns in epidemiology, the same research team conducted a study 10 years later that was methodologically identical. In this study, AMS-2, validated questionnaires were mailed to 20,000 households, generating responses from about 30,000 individual respondents. Results were virtually identical to the previous study in terms of prevalence, although rates of diagnosis and treatment had improved. In 2004, the largest migraine epidemiology study, the AMPP, was conducted. In the survey, Lipton and colleagues screened a representative sample of 120,000 households for data on 162,576 people age 12 years and older. It provided results identical to AMS-1 and AMS-2, indicating that the prevalence of migraine had been stable in the United States at least over the prior 15-year period.

Key Points: U.S. Migraine Prevalence and Preventive Therapy[27]

- At least one in four individuals with migraine are candidates for preventive medications, yet many do not receive them.
- The 1-year period U.S. prevalence of migraine is 11.7% (17.1% in women and 5.6% in men).
- A total of 25.7% individuals meet the criteria for preventive medications.
- In 13.1% of individuals, prevention medications should be considered.
- A total of 13% of individuals report current use of daily migraine preventives.

As part of the Global Campaign to Reduce the Burden of Headache, organized by the World Health Organization (WHO), Stovner and colleagues recently reviewed population studies and estimated that the worldwide prevalence of ongoing migraine was 10%, and the lifetime prevalence of migraine was 14%.[28]

The majority of studies estimate the prevalence of chronic migraine (CM) worldwide to be 1% to 3%.[29-31] Natoli and colleagues conducted a systematic literature search to estimate CM prevalence.[29] Sixteen publications representing 12 population-based studies of CM prevalence were reviewed, and estimates were subdivided based on the criteria used in each study. The prevalence of CM was 0.5% to 1%, with estimates typically in the range of 1.4% to 2.2%. Seven studies used Silberstein-Lipton criteria (or equivalent), with prevalence ranging from 0.9% to 5.1%. Three estimates used migraine that occurred 15 days or more per month, with prevalence ranging from 0% to 0.7%.

Prevalence by Age and Gender Migraine prevalence varies by age and gender. Most studies find that migraine prevalence is higher among womens than mens. As depicted in **Figure 27-2**, the prevalence of migraine is higher among womens than mens and varies considerably with age, with a peak between 25 and 55 years. In the adult population, in every region of the world, and in every racial and ethnic group studied, migraine is two to three times more common among womens than mens. In the AMS-1 and -2, as well as in the AMPP study, the average women-to-men migraine prevalence ratio is around 2.8, with a peak of 3.3 between ages 40 and 45 years. The ratio remains above 2.0 even after the age of menopause.

Key Points: Sex Differences in Migraine and Probable Migraine and Other Severe Headaches[32]

- Migraine and probable migraine are more common among women than men.
- No sex differences exist in the prevalence of other severe headaches.
- Women with migraine and probable migraine exhibit higher rates of migraine symptoms, aura, and impairment than men.
- No sex differences exist in symptoms, aura, and impairment in other severe headaches.

Prevalence by Race and Geographic Region Migraine prevalence appears to vary by race and geographic region, two factors that are associated with each other. Stewart and colleagues[33] conducted a population-based study to compare the prevalence of migraine among whites, African Americans, and Asian Americans in the United States. Both before and after adjusting for sociodemographic covariates, other than race, they found the lowest prevalence in Asian Americans (women, 9.2%; men, 4.2%) and the highest prevalence among whites (women, 20.4%; men, 8.6%). Similarly, a meta-analysis[34] found the lowest prevalence in Asia and Africa and considerably higher prevalence in Europe, Central and South America, and North America.

The international variation in migraine prevalence may be explained in several ways. The variation may be caused by regional differences in genetic susceptibility. This hypothesis is supported by the evidence of lower migraine prevalence in Africa and Asia, as well as among African Americans and Asian Americans in the United States.[33] However, because the prevalence of migraine in Asia is considerably lower than the prevalence among Asian Americans in the United States, it suggests that a role for environmental or cultural factors is likely. A limitation in evaluating the role of genetic and environmental factors in race

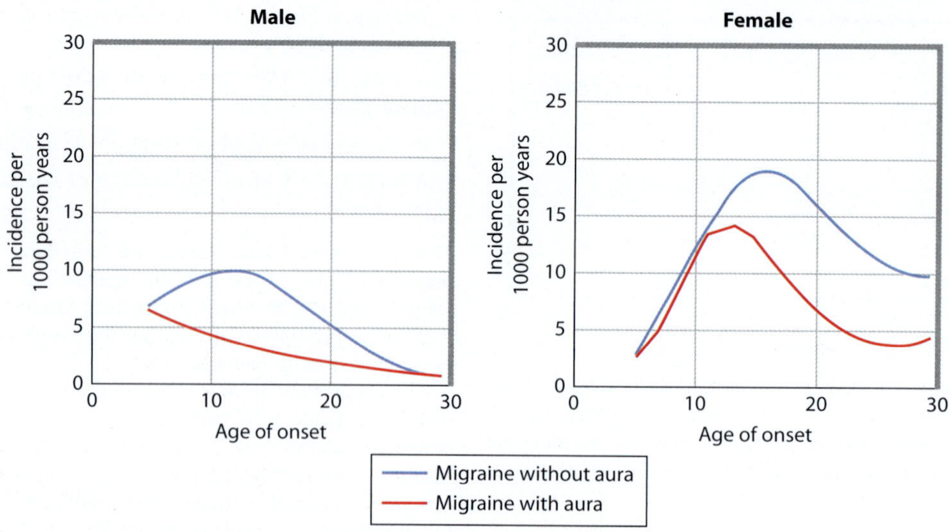

FIGURE 27-2. Gender- and age-specific estimates of migraine prevalence (North America) based on 18 population studies that used International Headache Society (IHS) diagnostic criteria. (Used with permission from Scher A, Stewart W, Lipton R. Migraine and headache: a meta-analytic approach. In: Crombie I, ed. *Epidemiology of Pain.* Seattle, Wa: IASP Press; 1999:159-170.)

differences is that the exact same methods have not been used in studies conducted in different countries and race groups.

Prevalence by Socioeconomic Status In the past, migraine was thought to be a disease of the affluent. However, population-based studies conducted in North America indicate that, in the community, migraine prevalence is inversely related to household income or education.[11,12,33,35] That is, as income or education increases, migraine prevalence declines. Prior beliefs regarding the apparent direct relationship between migraine prevalence and income may be explained by patterns of health care utilization. Migraine may appear to be a disease of high income in the physician's office because medical diagnosis of migraine is more common among high-income groups.[36] The contrasting finding of the National Health Interview Survey (NHIS)[37] supports the inverse association and the role of access to care shaping physicians' perceptions about this condition. In the NHIS study, prevalence was lower in the low-income compared with the middle-income group and was highest in the high-income group. Because the NHIS relied on self-reported medical diagnosis, the higher prevalence among the high-income group is likely to be the result of an increased likelihood of diagnosis of migraine as income rises. Interestingly, studies outside the United States have generally not reported the inverse relationship between migraine prevalence and income.[38-41] It is unclear what accounts for the international variation in these findings.

Key Points: Headache Disorders World Prevalence[28]

- Forty-six percent of the adult population has an active headache disorder.
- Eleven percent of the adult population has migraine.
- Forty-two percent of the adult population has TTH.
- Three percent of the adult population has chronic daily headache.
- Disability, worldwide, is greater because of TTH than migraine.
- The WHO ranks headache disorders in the top ten most disabling conditions for both genders and in the top five for women.

Key Points: U.S. Chronic Migraine Prevalence[42]

- A total of 0.91% of individuals meet the criteria for chronic migraine (1.29% of women; 0.48% of men).
- Chronic migraine represents 7.68% of cases of overall migraine.
- Chronic migraine prevalence peaks in middle age (1.89% for women and 0.79% for men).
- Lower income groups have higher rates of chronic migraine.
- People with chronic migraine have higher rates of disability relative to those with episodic migraine (EM).
- Headache-related disability is higher among women with chronic migraine than men.

PUBLIC HEALTH SIGNIFICANCE

Migraine is a disabling disorder that exerts an impact on both the individual and society. The individual impact of migraine is measured by quantifying the frequency and severity of attacks, as well as through quality-of-life studies. The societal impact is measured in economic terms, which include direct costs, such as health care utilization, as well as indirect costs resulting from lost productivity at work.

Individual Impact: Frequency and Severity of Attacks The individual impact of migraine is measured by the level of pain intensity, the presence and severity of associated symptoms (nausea, vomiting, photophobia, phonophobia), and the frequency and duration of attacks. The individual impact of migraine has been evaluated in several studies.[11,12,33,43]

In the AMS-2, 80% of those with migraine reported pain that was severe or very severe. The remaining subjects reported mild to moderate pain. In addition to pain, associated symptoms, such as photophobia (81.9%) and phonophobia (77.9%), were common. Approximately 60% reported that nausea accompanied their migraine headache more than half of the time. Vomiting was uncommon.[26]

Stewart and colleagues[33] reported the migraine characteristics of 1748 people with migraine residing in Baltimore County, Maryland. The majority of subjects reported one to two migraine attacks per month. The duration of an untreated attack varies considerably by gender. Among womens, approximately 71% of attacks last longer than 24 hours. In contrast, 48% of mens reported attacks that last longer than 24 hours. The results reported by Stewart and colleagues[33] were comparable to those reported in previous studies.[11,12,43]

Quality-of-Life Studies Measures of quality of life provide a broad-based assessment of the specific and global impact of a condition such as migraine. However, most studies of the impact of migraine have been conducted in clinic-based samples. As such, the quality-of-life impact is likely to be overestimated by these studies. Nonetheless, using the generic health-related quality-of-life (HRQoL) instrument from the Medical Outcomes Study,[44] these studies demonstrate that people with migraine have lower quality of life than control participants in the U.S. population.[45,46]

One study[46] found that individuals with migraine have quality-of-life scores similar to those of patients with osteoarthritis, hypertension, or diabetes. However, quality of life as measured in clinic-based samples may differ from that of people with migraine in the community. In addition, many studies conducted using clinic-based samples lack a contemporaneous control group. The lack of a control group can lead to an overestimation of treatment benefits because of regression toward the mean.

At least three population-based studies of quality of life in migraine cases versus control participants have been conducted.[47–49] In these studies, individuals with migraine had substantially lower HRQoL relative to population controls. In addition, quality of life and frequency of attacks were inversely correlated; as the frequency of attacks increased, quality of life decreased.[47] Lower quality-of-life scores were associated with higher levels of headache-related disability.[49]

Lofland and colleagues[50] assessed the outcomes of individuals with migraine enrolled in a mixed-model staff/independent practice association–managed care organization. The study enrolled patients with migraine when they received their first prescription for sumatriptan. After 6 months of sumatriptan therapy, four of the HRQoL dimensions and the physical component summary score of the Short-Form Health Survey (SF-36) showed significant improvement.[44,51] Furthermore, the Migraine-Specific Quality of Life Questionnaire (MSQ),[52] a disease-specific quality-of-life instrument, showed significant improvement at both 3 and 6 months after initiation of sumatriptan therapy. Despite these striking findings, results are limited by the lack of a control group, leading to a possible overestimation of treatment benefits resulting from apparent improvements that can be explained by regression toward the mean.

Key Points: Diagnosis and Disability[25]

- The diagnosis of migraine continues to increase (38% in 1989; 48% in 1999).
- The proportion of patients with migraine using prescription medications has shown a modest increase (37% in 1989; 41% in 1999).
- About half of those with migraine remain undiagnosed.
- With or without a diagnosis, migraine causes significant disability: 38% of diagnosed and 24% of undiagnosed migraineurs missed at least 1 day of work or school in the previous 3 months.

SOCIETAL IMPACT

Direct Costs Direct costs related to health care include outpatient visits, hospitalization, the use of emergency department (ED) services, the cost of prescriptions, and other treatments. For migraine, most of the direct costs were the result of outpatient visits and the cost of prescription medications. Hospitalization[37,53] and the use of ED services[53–55] are uncommon among individuals with migraine.

According to the AMS-1,[56] 68% of womens and 57% of mens have ever consulted a physician for migraine. The study also found that certain demographic and headache characteristics are associated with consultation. For example, womens and older adults are more likely to consult physicians for migraine. In addition, higher pain intensity, the number of migraine symptoms, attack duration, and disability were all associated with an increased likelihood of physician consultation.

Individuals with migraine are more likely to consult their physicians for medical care than individuals in the general population who do not have migraine. Clouse and colleagues[53] compared the health care utilization patterns of individuals with migraine and those without migraine enrolled in a United Healthcare Corporation–affiliated plan. A total of 1336 individuals with migraine were compared with a matched sample (i.e., matched on the basis of age, sex, duration of enrollment, and subscriber or dependent status) of individuals without migraine. During the 18-month study period, individuals with migraine made 22,587 physician visits, of which, 2616 were for migraine. In contrast, individuals without migraine made a total of 13,072 visits during the same period. Interestingly, a small proportion of the individuals with migraine accounts for the majority of physician visits among individuals with migraine. Although most individuals with migraine reported only one to four visits per year, 7.6% reported more than 12 visits.

Few studies have translated use of medical care into direct monetary estimates. Hu and colleagues[57] estimated the annual treatment costs of migraine in a population-based sample. They found that the annual treatment costs for migraine were over $1 billion, about $100 per individuals with migraine per year. These are likely to be underestimates because the figures were derived from 1994 data. Consultation and medication use have increased substantially since then.[58] Clouse and Osterhaus[53] reported similar, although slightly higher, average claim costs per member per month ($145). The costs reported by Clouse and colleagues differ from those of Hu and colleagues because they were not separated by diagnosis. Individuals with migraine are likely to have comorbid conditions; thus, the increased costs may reflect the costs resulting from the treatment of migraine as well as other medical conditions. Edmeads and Mackell[59] estimated total direct medical costs, including physician visits, ED visits, and hospitalization, in matched migraine and migraine-free control populations. Over a 6-month period, total direct medical costs were significantly higher in the migraine group ($522) than the control population ($415). The costs of physician and ED visits were strong drivers behind the significant difference in total direct medical care costs. The cost of outpatient physician visits was $221 for the migraine group and $177 for the comparison group. ED visits were also significantly higher in the migraine group ($33) versus the control population ($18).

Insinga and colleagues[60] estimated direct migraine-related health care costs associated with outpatient and ER visits and inpatient hospitalizations in the United States. Costs were retrospectively estimated from the 2007 Medstat MarketScan Commercial Claims & Encounters database and were adjusted to 2010 U.S. dollars. The estimated mean cost for migraine-related care per outpatient visit was $140, per ED visit was $775, and per inpatient hospitalization was $7317. Estimated annual U.S. health care costs in 2010 for migraine associated with outpatient visits were $3.2 billion, ED visits were $700 million, and inpatient hospitalizations were $375 million.

Stokes and colleagues[61] estimated direct health care costs associated with CM and EM in the United States and Canada. Data were based on cross-sectional survey results and included sociodemographic and clinical characteristics and medical resource use for headache. The analysis included data from respondents with migraine in the United States and Canada and presented estimated costs in 2010 U.S. and Canadian dollars. Total mean headache-related costs for participants with CM in the United States were $1036 over 3 months compared with $383 for persons with EM. In Canada, total mean headache-related costs among CM patients were $471 compared with $172 for EM patients.

Indirect Costs The indirect economic impact of migraine is primarily a consequence of lost productivity at work. Because many individuals with migraine continue to work, even while suffering from a migraine attack, it is important to account not only for lost workdays caused by migraine but also reduced productivity while at work when estimating indirect costs.

The early studies of migraine-associated disability had limitations. For example, some studies examined selected populations such as clinical trial participants or individuals with a self-reported diagnosis of migraine.[37,62] Other studies used designs that were limited by uncertainties regarding the accuracy of recall over a period of up to 1 year.[63–65]

Von Korff and colleagues[66] conducted a population-based diary study as one approach to addressing the limitations of previous studies. They estimated the amount of lost work time among individuals with migraine who completed a daily diary for 3 months. During this 3-month period, individuals with migraine missed an average of 1.1 days per month because of headache. Participants who worked during migraine attacks reported work effectiveness that was reduced by an average of 41%.

Some studies combine lost workdays and reduced effectiveness days into an overall measure, termed lost workday equivalent (LWDE). The LWDE equals actual days of missed work plus days at work with headache times 1 minus percent effectiveness while at work with headache.[63] In the study reported by Stewart and colleagues,[63] subjects experienced an average of three LWDEs during the study period. The majority of the lost workdays and LWDEs were the result of migraine rather than any other headache type.

The missed workday and LWDE estimates reported by Von Korff and colleagues[66] are higher than those reported in other population-based studies.[37,62,63,67] The use of a daily diary may have improved the accuracy of reporting that is inherently limited by asking people to recall events over the past 3 to 12 months.

In the study reported by Von Korff and colleagues,[66] a relatively small percentage of individuals with migraine accounts for the majority of lost work time. In this study, the most disabled 20% of the participants accounted for 77% of the missed workdays, and 40% of subjects accounted for 75% of the total LWDEs. Similarly, Stewart and colleagues[63] found that 51% of women and 38% of men reported six or more LWDEs per year, which accounted for more than 90% of all lost workdays.

The early studies that attempted to quantify the monetary cost of the lost work also had significant limitations. One study was based on self-identified individuals with migraine;[37] thus, it probably underestimated the cost because it excluded those who did not know they had migraine. Another study[62] probably overestimated the cost because it included a population of clinical trial participants who were likely to be more disabled than those with migraine in the community.

Using the human capital method, Hu and colleagues[57] estimated the indirect costs of migraine. Human capital studies assume that the economic value of a missed day of work is equivalent to the wages for that day. According to the results of this population-based study, Hu estimated that migraine costs American employers $13 billion per year as a result of absenteeism and reduced effectiveness at work. Approximately 62% of the cost was a result of absenteeism. Importantly, the greatest indirect costs were found among middle-aged individuals (30–49 years). Although this study provided important information, the human capital method values the indirect costs of the disease according to the salaries of the individuals with migraine. A lost workday is valued by the individual's wages for that day. This is a reasonable approach, but it may be an overestimate if the worker makes up for lost time or coworkers effectively cover for his or her absence. However, if an individual with migraine makes an error while at work, it may be an underestimate. In addition, the impact of the disease in a laborer or homemaker would be valued at a lower rate than that of a business executive with a high salary. A limitation of all studies reported to date is that reduced productivity while at work when having a migraine is based on self-report. No studies to date have actually quantified reductions in productivity.

Edmeads and Mackell[59] calculated the number of days missed from both employment and household activities over a 6-month period after matching individuals with migraine with a migraine-free control group. Among full- and part-time workers, the individuals with migraine missed 5 days of work, and the control group missed only 3 days. The individuals with migraine who were not employed missed more days of household duties than their counterparts.

Stewart and colleagues[68] used data from the American Productivity Audit to estimate the pain-related lost productive time (LPT) and the associated costs due to headache and other conditions in the U.S. workforce. Overall, 5.4% of the workforce reported LPT due to headache. The mean LPT for headache was 3.5 hours per week. LPT due to headache was much more common than absenteeism. The total cost of LPT due to headache in the U.S. workforce was calculated to be approximately $20 billion per year, most of which is in the form of reduced productivity while at work.

More recently, Stewart and colleagues[69] used published estimates of migraine epidemiology and related LPT to model the impact of migraine on two typical U.S. workforce scenarios. In a simulated service sector workforce of 10,000 individuals, the migraine-related LPT was $2.9 million annually compared with $2.1 million for a manufacturing workforce. Individuals with moderate-frequency EM accounted for 42% of the cost. Individuals with high-frequency EM and CM comprised 10% of all individuals with migraine and accounted for 22% of the LPT.

In the AMPP study, data indicated that those with CM were less likely to be employed full time (CM, 37.8%; EM, 52.3%) and almost twice as likely to be disabled (CM, 20.0%; EM, 11.1%).[70] The Migraine Disability Assessment Scale (MIDAS) captures lost days in three domains: paid work or school, household work, and nonwork activities. The mean MIDAS score in a population with CM is 63.4 compared with a mean score of 10 for people with EM. For EM, severe disability scores 20 or higher. Thus, the mean MIDAS score for chronic migraineurs is three times higher than for those with EM.[71]

TENSION-TYPE HEADACHE EPIDEMIOLOGY AND DISEASE BURDEN

PREVALENCE

The prevalence of TTH has not been widely studied. Among published studies of TTH, the 1-year period prevalence ranges between 14.3[7] and 93.0[4] for ETTH and 0.0[7,72] and 8.1[72] for CTTH (**Table 27-6**). Variation in prevalence estimates may be due, in part, to differences in study methodology. Lifetime prevalences are higher than 1-year period prevalences. The age distribution of the population studied influences prevalence estimates. Case definition also plays a role. Studies of the epidemiology of TTH use various levels of diagnostic specificity. Although some studies group all TTH (ICHD-2, 2.0) subjects together, other studies distinguish between subjects with ETTH (ICHD-2, 2.1 and 2.2) and CTTH (ICHD-2, 2.3). Prevalence estimates may also vary because of differences in the diagnostic sensitivity and specificity of the methods used to collect symptom data. Methods of data collection (e.g., self-administered questionnaires, telephone interviews, and clinical examinations) as well as the quality of data collection may influence levels of diagnostic accuracy. Finally, the source of the study population, community based or clinic based, is likely to cause varying prevalence estimates. A meta-analysis might help explain how much each of these factors contributes to the variation in prevalence among studies. Following is a summary of several TTH studies.

Schwartz and colleagues[10] conducted the only large-scale population survey in the United States describing the epidemiology of ETTH and CTTH, as defined by the IHS criteria. These investigators used data from a telephone survey of 13,345 residents of the Baltimore County, Maryland, area[33] to estimate the 1-year period prevalence of ETTH and CTTH by sex, age, education, and race. They found that the overall prevalence of ETTH in the past year was 38.3%.

Lavados and Tenhamm[7] interviewed a representative sample of 1385 adults (>14 years old) in Santiago, Chile, using an in-person interview. Subjects reported details about the type of headache they had most often. The 1-year prevalence of ETTH was 24.3%. The lower prevalence in this study compared with that of Schwartz and colleagues[10] may be explained by the case definition used by Lavados and Tenhamm. Cases were only identified if TTH was the most common headache. When Schwartz and colleagues[10] used similar criteria, they found an ETTH prevalence of 25.3% compared with 38.3% after the second headache type was classified.

Rasmussen and colleagues,[4] on the other hand, reported ETTH prevalence estimates that are higher than those of most other studies (see Table 27-5). In this study, potential participants were identified from the Danish National Central Person Registry and invited to a general health examination, with an emphasis on headache. Of the 1000 potential study subjects, 740 mens and womens participated in the study. The 1-year period prevalence of ETTH was estimated to be 74.0%. The prevalence of ETTH may be higher in this study because of the way in which the invitation was worded. Because potential subjects were invited to a health examination with an emphasis on headache, individuals who had headaches may have been more likely to participate. Thus, there may have been an overrepresentation of individuals with headache among the participants.

As part of the Global Campaign to Reduce the Burden of Headache organized by WHO, Stovner and colleagues recently reviewed population studies for TTH. They estimated that the worldwide prevalence was 38% for current TTH and that the lifetime prevalence was 46%.[28]

The prevalence of CTTH is markedly lower than that of ETTH. Schwartz and colleagues[10] found that the overall prevalence of CTTH was 2.2%. Tekle-Haimanot and colleagues,[72] Lavados and Tenhamm,[7]

TABLE 27-6 Prevalence of Episodic Tension-Type Headache (ETTH) and Chronic Tension-Type Headache (CTTH) as Reported in 18 Population-Based Studies That Used International Headache Society (IHS) Criteria

Author, Country	Population Type	Response Method	Sample Size	Headache Type	Prevalence Period	Age Range (yr)*	Women
Abu-Arefah and Russell[38] (United Kingdom)	Community	Mail SAQ; clinical examination	2165	Unspecified	1 year	5–15	—
Barea et al.[6] (Brazil)	School survey	In-person interview; clinical examination	538	2.1, 2.2, 2.3	1 year	5th–8th grade	76.7
					1 week	5th–8th grade	35.3
					24 hours	5th–8th grade	10.1
Castillo et al.[30] (Spain)	Community	SAQ; clinical examination	1883	CTTH	1 month	18–89	2.0
Franceschi[79] (Italy)	Community	In-person interview; clinical examination	312	Unspecified	Lifetime	"Elderly"	4.0
					1 year	"Elderly"	4.0
Gobel et al.[40] (Germany)	Community	Mail SAQ	4,061	ETTH	Lifetime	18–35	
						36–55	
						≥56	
						All ages (≥18)	13.0
				CTTH	Lifetime	18–35	
						36–55	
						≥56	
						All ages (≥18)	1.0
Tekle-Haimanot et al.[72] (Ethiopia)	Community	In-person interview	15,000	CTTH	1 year	20–29	0.0
						30–39	0.7
						40–49	4.3
						50–59	8.1
						60–69	3.9
						70–79	0.0
						80–89	1.7
						All ages (20–89)	2.3
Jabbar[5] (Saudi Arabia)	Community	In-person interview	5891	Unspecified	Lifetime	16–19	
						20–29	
						30–39	
						40–49	
						50–59	
						≥60	
						All ages (≥16)	
Lavados Tenhamm[7] (Chile)	Community	In-person interview	1385	ETTH	1 year	15–29	30.5
						30–39	34.8
						40–49	33.0
						50–59	32.1
						≥60	23.2
						All ages (≥15)	
				CTTH	1 year	15–29	1.6
						30–39	2.6
						40–49	7.3
						50–59	5.9
						≥60	6.2

(*Continued*)

TABLE 27-6 Prevalence of Episodic Tension-Type Headache (ETTH) and Chronic Tension-Type Headache (CTTH) as Reported in 18 Population-Based Studies That Used International Headache Society (IHS) Criteria (*Continued*)

Author, Country	Population Type	Response Method	Sample Size	Headache Type	Prevalence Period	Age Range (yr)*	Women
						All ages (≥15)	
Merikangas[86] (Switzerland)	Community	In-person interview	379	ETTH + CTTH	1 year	28–29	18.0
				ETTH	1 year	28–29	
				CTTH	1 year	28–29	
Mitsikostas[87] (Greece)	Monks	SAQ; clinical examination	449	ETTH	Lifetime	>50	
				CTTH	Lifetime	>50	
Pereira Monteiro[88] (Portugal)	Medical school students	In-person SAQ	491	ETTH + CTTH	Unknown	18–32	
				ETTH			
				CTTH			
Pryse-Phillips et al.[8] (Canada)	Community	Telephone interview	1,573	ETTH + CTTH	Unspecified	15–24	
						25–34	
						25–44	
						45–54	
						55–65	
						>65	
						All ages (≥15)	64.0
Rasmussen[4] (Denmark)	Community	Clinical examination	740	ETTH	1 year	25–34	93.0
						35–44	92.0
						45–54	82.0
						55–64	74.0
						All ages (25–64)	86.0
					Lifetime	All ages (25–64)	88.0
				CTTH	1 year	All ages (25–64)	
Roh[88] (South Korea)	Community	Telephone interview; mail SAQ	2500	2.1, 2.2, 2.3	1 year	0–9	
						10–19	
						20–29	
						30–39	
						40–49	
						50–59	
						≥60	
						All ages	14.7
Schwartz et al.[10] (USA)	Community	Telephone interview	13,345	ETTH	1 year	18–29	40.8
						30–39	46.9
						40–49	46.5
						50–59	40.6
						60–65	27.1
						All ages (18–65)	
				CTTH	1 year	18–29	2.6
						30–39	2.5
						40–49	2.9
						50–59	4.2
						60–65	2.7
						All ages (18–65)	

(*Continued*)

TABLE 27-6 Prevalence of Episodic Tension-Type Headache (ETTH) and Chronic Tension-Type Headache (CTTH) as Reported in 18 Population-Based Studies That Used International Headache Society (IHS) Criteria (*Continued*)

Author, Country	Population Type	Response Method	Sample Size	Headache Type	Prevalence Period	Age Range (yr)*	Women
Srikiatkhachorn[90] (Thailand)	Old age home	In-person interview	241	ETTH	1 year	61–98	
				CTTH	1 year	61–98	
Wang et al.[9] (China)	Community	In-person interview; clinical examination	1533	2.1, 2.2, 2.3	1 year	65–69	45.0
						70–74	44.0
						75–79	47.0
						≥80	48.0
						All ages (≥65)	46.0
				ETTH	1 year	All ages (≥65)	
				CTTH	1 year	All ages (≥65)	
				2.3	1 year	All ages (≥65)	
Wong et al.[5] (Hong Kong)	Community	Telephone interview	7356	2.1, 2.2, 2.3	1 year	15–24	1.82
						25–34	2.96
						35–44	5.78
						45–54	2.33
						55–64	2.11
						≥65	0.73
						All ages (≥15)	

*In years, unless otherwise specified.

SAQ, self-administered questionnaire.

and Castillo and colleagues[30] reported similar estimates of 1.7%, 2.6%, and 2.2%, respectively, among the subjects they studied.

Prevalence by Demographic Features The prevalences of both ETTH and CTTH vary by age, gender, race, and educational level. TTH is slightly more common among womens than mens. Schwartz and colleagues[10] found that women had a higher prevalence of ETTH than men (men, 36.3%; women, 42.0%), with an overall prevalence ratio of 1.16 to 1.0. The women preponderance occurred at all age, race, and educational levels. Several other studies also report a higher prevalence of TTH among women,[4–9] with women-to-men gender ratios ranging from 1.25[4] to 1.9.[7]

Similarly, the prevalence of CTTH is also higher among women than men. In the study published by Schwartz and colleagues,[10] the prevalence was 2.8 in women and 1.4 in men, with an overall prevalence ratio of 2.0. Studies reported by Tekle-Haimanot and colleagues,[72] Lavados and Tenhamm,[7] and Castillo and colleagues[30] also reported higher prevalence among women than men.

Prevalence by Age The prevalence of TTH varies by age. Prevalence peaks in the 30s and 40s, with a decline thereafter.[5,7,10] Pryse-Philips and colleagues[8] reported a similar, although slightly earlier, peak prevalence in the 25- to 34-year-old age group. Rasmussen and colleagues,[4] on the other hand, found that the prevalence of TTH decreased with increasing age, and Gobel and colleagues[40] found no difference in prevalence by age. The lack of association reported by Gobel and colleagues may be attributed to the use of very wide age intervals; in most studies, age is categorized into 10-year intervals,[4,5,7,8,10] Gobel and colleagues used 20-year age groupings.

Tekle-Haimanot and colleagues,[72] Lavados and Tenhamm,[7] and Schwartz and colleagues[10] all reported an increase in the prevalence of CTTH with increasing age. This may be explained by the hypothesis that in some individuals, ETTH develops into a chronic form over a prolonged period of time.[19,73] Gobel and colleagues[40] did not find any difference in the prevalence of CTTH by age, but again, this may be attributed to the use of very wide age intervals.

Prevalence by Geographic Region and Race Some of the observed variation in the prevalence of TTH among studies may be the result of racial or ethnic differences. Each of the reported studies of the epidemiology of TTH using the IHS criteria was conducted in a different country, and based on these results, prevalence appears to be highest in the Western Hemisphere[7,8,10] and Denmark[4] and lowest in the Asian countries.[5]

The only published study of TTH using the IHS criteria that reported the prevalence of TTH by race was that of Schwartz and colleagues.[10] In this study, the prevalence of ETTH was significantly higher in whites than in African Americans in both men (40.1% vs. 22.8%) and in women (46.8% vs. 30.9%). The prevalence of CTTH by race paralleled that observed for ETTH: prevalence was higher in whites than in African Americans in both men (1.6% vs. 1.0%) and women (3.0% vs. 2.2%).

Prevalence by Socioeconomic Status The evidence regarding the relationship between socioeconomic status (SES) and the prevalence of ETTH is mixed. Schwartz and colleagues[10] reported that the prevalence of ETTH increases with increasing educational level, a measure of SES. Prevalence peaked among those with a graduate level education (men, 48.5%; women, 48.9%). Lavados and Tenhamm[7] found a similar direct correlation between ETTH prevalence and SES. Other studies have not found this direct association.[8,40] Gobel and colleagues[40] reported no significant differences by education; however, their study used only two educational categories (i.e., basic and secondary) and, as such, may simply lack the sensitivity to detect patterns observed in other studies that used a greater number of educational or income categories. It is also possible that the influence of SES varies by country.

The relationship between SES and migraine may differ for CTTH. Schwartz and colleagues[10] and Lavados and Tenhamm[7] reported that the prevalence of CTTH declines with increasing educational level, especially among women. Gobel and colleagues[40] found no association between CTTH prevalence and educational level. Schwartz and colleagues[10] suggested that the epidemiology of CTTH, with its higher risk in women and strong relationship to SES, is intermediate between that of ETTH and migraine and may reflect the progression of both headache types to a chronic form.

Key Points: Prevalence of Tension-Type Headache

- The 1-year prevalence of TTH in 2001 was 86.5%.[74]
- In a population-based study of Koreans, Chu et al.,[91] found:

  A 29.1% 1-year prevalence in women

  A 32.5% 1-year prevalence in men

  College education is associated with lower prevalence of TTH in women.

  Living in rural areas is associated with lower prevalence of TTH in women.

  Among men, there was no significant difference in prevalence by socioeconomic variables.
- Seven percent of people with TTH reported being substantially or severely impacted by headache.[75]

HEADACHE CHARACTERISTICS

More than 90% of subjects with ETTH report mild to moderate headache pain intensity; attacks typically occur three times per month.[4,10,40] Lavados and Tenhamm[7] found that more than 86% of people with TTH report mild to moderate pain that occurs three to four times per month. The headache frequency reported by Lavados and Tenhamm is slightly higher than those reported by Schwartz,[10] Gobel,[40] and Rasmussen and their colleagues[4] because the Lavados and Tenhamm sample included both people with ETTH and CTTH.

Chronic tension-type headache, on the other hand, is typically associated with higher pain intensity and more frequent attacks. In one study, 86% of subjects reported moderate or severe pain (moderate, 44%; severe, 42%).[40] Using a 10-point scale, Schwartz and colleagues[10] found significantly higher pain intensity scores among CTTH subjects than ETTH subjects (CTTH, 5.55; ETTH, 4.98; $P < 0.001$). For CTTH, headache frequency ranges from 15 to 30 headaches per month.[10,40]

Certain clinical characteristics occur more frequently among those with TTH, and these characteristics often differ by gender. Lavados and Tenhamm[7] reported that bilateral pain occurs in the majority of individuals with TTH but occurs with even greater frequency among women than men (men, 87.9%; women, 61.1%; $P < 0.01$). Throbbing pain occurs approximately equally in 66.4% of men and 56.8% of women; this feature, often viewed as a hallmark of migraine, does not discriminate the two disorders. These investigators also found that many TTH subjects report pain that is exacerbated with movement (men, 69.8%, women, 75.5%; $P = 0.4$), which is surprising because pain that is exacerbated by movement is normally associated with migraine rather than TTH. Pressing pain, photophobia, and phonophobia were also frequently reported; each of these characteristics occurred significantly more often among women than men. Nausea was not commonly reported by any of the study participants.

DISABILITY

Rasmussen and colleageus[64] reported the first population-based study to examine work loss data in ETTH. Of the employed participants with ETTH, 12% reported being absent from work at least once during the previous year because of ETTH. Among those who reported lost workdays, the majority (68%) were absent from 1 to 7 days during the previous year, 25% were absent between 8 and 14 days during the year, and only 16% were absent more than 14 days during the previous year.

In their survey of Baltimore County residents,[10] Schwartz and colleagues also measured the impact of headache in the workplace.[65] In this study, reduced ability to function and an inability to function (actual missed work) were measured separately. Of the lost work time associated with headache, 19% of the missed workdays and 22% of the reduced effectiveness days were specifically the result of ETTH.[65]

Schwartz and colleagues[10] also reported that among subjects with ETTH, 8.3% reported missed workdays, but 43.6% reported reduced effectiveness days because of headache. Among those with missed workdays, an average of 8.9 missed workdays were reported, but subjects with reduced effectiveness days reported approximately 5.0 reduced effectiveness days per person.

Lavados and Tenhamm[7] found higher levels of missed work among their sample of individuals with TTH: 25% of men and 38.9% of women reported missed work because of their headaches. They also found that individuals with TTH were likely to miss family and social activities as a result of their headaches. Approximately 27.6% of men and 25.3% of women missed family or social activities because of their headaches.

In the Schwartz[10] study, the proportions of CTTH subjects reporting lost and reduced effectiveness days were similar to those reported by ETTH subjects: 11.8% of individuals with CTTH reported lost workdays, and 46.5% reported reduced effectiveness days. However, in contrast with the individuals with ETTH, those with CTTH reported more frequent lost workdays and reduced effectiveness days. Whereas subjects with lost workdays reported an average of 27.4 lost workdays per person, subjects with reduced effectiveness days reported approximately 20.4 reduced effectiveness days per person.

CONCLUSION

Headache is a very common condition; approximately 36% of men and 42% of women have ETTH,[10] and 18% of women and 6% of men have migraine.[11,12] These disorders impose a burden on the individual, his or her family, and society.

Individuals with migraine report frequent and painful attacks that inhibit their ability to carry out their usual activities. In several population-based studies, individuals with migraine reported notable impairments in quality of life.[47–49] In addition, Hu and colleagues[57] estimated that the annual treatment costs for migraine were more than $1 billion, about $100 per person with migraine per year. Furthermore, Hu and colleagues reported that migraine costs American employers $13 billion per year because of absenteeism and reduced effectiveness at work.

Compared with migraine, the impact of ETTH is more modest. ETTH is generally less painful and has a smaller impact on daily functioning.[10,65] However, the aggregate societal impact is large because the disorder is highly prevalent. The individual impact of CTTH is greater than that of ETTH, but the disorder is relatively rare; thus, the societal impact is relatively small.

There have been many studies of the epidemiology of migraine; however, TTH has been studied less often. Future research should seek to expand understanding of the variation in TTH prevalence among certain subgroups, as well as heighten awareness of the impact of TTH on the individual and society. This information will enhance understanding about the relative impact of both migraine and TTH.

ACKNOWLEDGMENT

BMG acknowledges the generous support of the Heffer Family Foundation, who underwrote the preparation of this chapter.

REFERENCES

1. Headache Classification Committee of the International Headache Society. Classification and diagnostic criteria for headache disorders, cranial neuralgias and facial pain. *Cephalalgia*. 1988;8 (Suppl 7):1-96.
2. Headache Classification Committee of the International Headache Society. The International Classification of Headache Disorders 2nd ed. *Cephalalgia*. 2004;24:1-160.
3. Headache Classification Committee of the International Headache Society. The International Classification of Headache Disorders 3rd ed. (beta version). Cephalalgia. 2013;33(9):627-808.
4. Rasmussen B, Jensen R, Schroll M, Olesen J. Epidemiology of headache in a general population: a prevalence study. *J Clin Epidemiol*. 1991;44:1147-1157.
5. Wong T, Wong K, Yu T, Kay R. Prevalence of migraine and other headaches in Hong Kong. *Neuroepidemiology*. 1995;14:82-91.

6. Barea L, Tannhauser M, Rotta N. An epidemiologic study of headache among children and adolescents of southern Brazil. *Cephalalagia*. 1996;16:545-549.
7. Lavados P, Tenhamm E. Epidemiology of tension-type headache in Santiago, Chile: a prevalence study. *Cephalalgia*. 1998;18:552-558.
8. Pryse-Phillips W, Findlay H, Tugwell P, et al. A Canadian population survey on the clinical, epidemiologic and societal impact of migraine and tension-type headache. *Can J Neurol Sci*. 1992;19:333-339.
9. Wang S, Liu H, Fuh J, et al. Prevalence of headaches in a Chinese elderly population in Kinmen: age and gender effect and cross-cultural comparisons. *Neurology*. 1997;49:195-200.
10. Schwartz BS, Stewart WF, Simon D, Lipton RB. Epidemiology of tension-type headache. *JAMA*. 1998;279:381-383.
11. Stewart WF, Lipton RB, Celentano DD, Reed ML. Prevalence of migraine headache in the United States: relation to age, income, race, and other sociodemographic factors. *JAMA*. 1992;267:64-69.
12. Lipton RB, Stewart WF. Migraine in the United States: a review of epidemiology and health care use. *Neurology*. 1993;43(Suppl):S6-S10.
13. Silberstein S, Lipton R, Goadsby P. *Headache in Clinical Practice*. Oxford, England: Isis Medical Media Ltd; 1998.
14. Johannes C, Linet M, Stewart W, et al. Relationship of headache to phase of the menstrual cycle among young women: a daily diary study. *Neurology*. 1995;45:1076-1082.
15. Breslau N, Chilcoat H, Andreski P. Further evidence on the link between migraine and neuroticism. *Neurology*. 1996;47:663-667.
16. Stewart WF, Linet M, Celentano D, et al. Age- and sex-specific incidence rates of migraine with and without visual aura. *Am J Epidemil*. 1991;134:1111-1120.
17. Brown N, Rips L, Shevell S. The subjective dates of natural events in very long-term memory. *Cognit Psychol*. 1985;17:139-177.
18. Cummings R, Kelsey J, Nevitt M. Methologic issues in the study of frequent and recurrent health problems. *Ann Epidemiol*. 1990;1:49-56.
19. Rasmussen B. Epidemiology of headache. *Cephalalgia*. 1995;15:45-68.
20. Stang P, Yanagihara T, Swanson J, et al. Incidence of migraine headache: a population-based study in Olmstead County, Minnesota. *Neurology*. 1992;42:1657-1662.
21. Lyngberg AC, Rasmussen BK, Jørgensen T, Jensen R. Incidence of primary headache: a Danish epidemiologic follow-up study. *Am J Epidemiol*. 2005;161:1066-1073.
22. Khil L, Pfaffenrath V, Straube A, et al. Incidence of migraine and tension-type headache in three different populations at risk within the German DMKG headache study. *Cephalalgia*. 2012;32:328-336.
23. Stewart WF, Wood C, Reed ML, et al. Cumulative lifetime migraine incidence in women and men. *Cephalalgia*. 2008;28:1170-1178.
24. Stewart WF, Lipton RB, Celentano DD, Reed ML. Prevalence of migraine headache in the United States: relation to age, income, race, and other sociodemographic factors. *JAMA*. 1992;267:64-69.
25. Lipton RB, Diamond S, Reed M, et al. Migraine diagnosis and treatment: results from the American Migraine Study II. *Headache*. 2001;41:638-645.
26. Lipton RB, Stewart WF, Diamond S, et al. Prevalence and burden of migraine in the United States: data from the American Migraine Study II. *Headache*. 2001;41:646-657.
27. Lipton RB, Bigal ME, Diamond M, et al. Migraine prevalence, disease burden, and the need for preventive therapy. *Neurology*. 2007;68:343-349.
28. Stovner L, Hagen K, Jensen R, et al. The global burden of headache: a documentation of headache prevalence and disability worldwide. *Cephalalgia*. 2007;27:193-210.
29. Natoli JL, Manack A, Dean B, et al. Global prevalence of chronic migraine: a systematic review. *Cephalalgia*. 2010;30:599-609.
30. Castillo J, Muñoz P, Guitera V, Pascual J. Epidemiology of chronic daily headache in the general population. *Headache*. 1999;39:190-196.
31. Scher AI, Stewart WF, Liberman J, Lipton RB. Prevalence of frequent headache in a population sample. *Headache*. 1998;38:497-506.
32. Buse DC, Loder EW, Gorman JA, et al. Sex differences in the prevalence, symptoms, and associated features of migraine, probable migraine and other severe headache: results of the American Migraine Prevalence and Prevention (AMPP) Study. *Headache*. 2013;53:1278-1299.
33. Stewart WF, Lipton RB, Liberman J. Variation in migraine prevalence by race. *Neurology*. 1996;16:231-238.
34. Scher A, Stewart W, Lipton R. Migraine and headache: a meta-analytic approach. In: Crombie I, ed. *Epidemiology of Pain*. Seattle: IASP Press; 1999:159-170.
35. Kryst S, Scherl E. A population-based survey of the social and personal impact of migraine. *Headache*. 1994;34:344-350.
36. Lipton R, Stewart W, Celentano D, Reed M. Undiagnosed migraine headaches: a comparison of symptom-based and reported physician diagnosis. *Arch Intern Med*. 1992;152:1273-1278.
37. Stang P, Osterhaus J. Impact of migraine in the United States: data from the National Health Interview Survey. *Headache*. 1993;33:29-35.
38. Abu-Arefeh I, Russell G. Prevalence of headache and migraine in schoolchildren. *BMJ*. 1994;309:765-769.
39. O'Brien B, Goeree R, Streiner D. Prevalence of migraine headache in Canada: a population-based survey. *Int J Epidemiol*. 1994;23:1020-1026.
40. Gobel H, Petersen-Braun M, Soyka D. The epidemiology of headache in Germany: a nationwide survey of a representative sample on the basis of the headache classification of the International Headache Society. *Cephalalgia*. 1994;14:97-106.
41. Rasmussen B. Migraine and tension-type headache in a general population: psychosocial factors. *Int J Epidemiol*. 1992;21:1138-1143.
42. Buse DC, Manack AN, Fanning KM, et al. Chronic migraine prevalence, disability, and sociodemographic factors: results from the American Migraine Prevalence and Prevention Study. *Headache*. 2012;52:1456-1470.
43. Stewart W, Schechter A, Lipton R. Migraine heterogeneity: disability, pain intensity, and attack frequency and duration. *Neurology*. 1994;44(Suppl):S24-S39.
44. Tarlov A, Ware J, Greenfield S, et al. The Medical Outcomes Study: an application of methods for monitoring the results of medical care. *JAMA*. 1989;262:925-930.
45. Solomon G, Skobieranda F, Gragg L. Quality of life and well-being of headache patients: measurement by the medical outcomes study instrument. *Headache*. 1993;33:351-358.
46. Osterhaus J, Townsend R, Gandek B, Ware J. Measuring functional status and well-being of patients with migraine headache. *Headache*. 1994;34:337-343.
47. Terwindt G, Launer L, Ferrari M. The impact of migraine on quality of life in the general population: the GEM study. *Neurology*. 1998;50(Suppl):A434.
48. Steiner TJ, Lipton RB, Liberman JN, et al. Work and family impact of migraine: a population-based case-control study. *Neurology*. 1999;52(Suppl):A470-A471.
49. Lipton R, Liberman J, Kolodner K, et al. Migraine headache disability and quality-of-life: a population-based case-control study. *Headache*. 1999;39:365.
50. Lofland JH, Johnson NE, Batenhorst AS, Nash DB. Changes in resource use and outcomes for patients with migraine treated with sumatriptan. *Arch Intern Med*. 1999;159:857-863.
51. Lofland J, Johnson N, Nash D, Batenhorst A. Improvements in managed care patients' health-related quality of life after sumatriptan (Imitrex). *Headache*. 1998;38:391.
52. Jhingran P, Osterhaus J, Miller D, et al. Development and validation of the Migraine-Specific Quality of Life Questionnaire. *Headache*. 1998;38:295-302.

53. Clouse J, Osterhaus J. Healthcare resource use and costs associated with migraine in a managed healthcare setting. *Ann Pharmacother*. 1994;28:659-664.
54. Edmeads J, Findlay H, Tugwell P, et al. Impact of migraine and tension-type headache on life-style, consulting behavior, and medication use: a Canadian population survey. *Can J Neurol Sci*. 1993;20:131-137.
55. Celentano D, Stewart W, Lipton R, Reed M. Medication use and disability among migraineurs: a national probability sample survey. *Headache*. 1992;32:223-228.
56. Lipton R, Stewart W, Simon D. Medical consultation for migraine: results of the American migraine study. *Headache*. 1998;38:87-90.
57. Hu X, Markson L, Lipton R, et al. Burden of migraine in the United States: disability and economic costs. *Arch Int Med*. 1999;159:813-818.
58. Lipton R, Stewart W, Kolodner K, Liberman J. Epidemiology and patterns of health care use for migraine in the United States. *Headache*. 1999;39:363-364.
59. Edmeads J, Mackell JA. The economic impact of migraine: an analysis of direct and indirect costs. *Headache*. 2002;42:501-509.
60. Insinga RP, Ng-Mak DS, Hanson ME. Costs associated with outpatient, emergency room and inpatient care for migraine in the USA. *Cephalalgia*. 2011;31:1570-1575.
61. Stokes M, Becker WJ, Lipton RB, et al. Cost of health care among patients with chronic and episodic migraine in Canada and the USA: results from the International Burden of Migraine Study (IBMS). *Headache*. 2011;51:1058-1077.
62. Osterhaus JT, Gutterman DL, Plachetka JR. Healthcare resource and lost labour costs of migraine headache in the US. *PharmacoEconomics*. 1992;1:67-76.
63. Stewart W, Lipton R, Simon D. Work-related disability: results from the American Migraine Study. *Cephalalgia*. 1996;16:231-238.
64. Rasmussen B, Jensen R, Olesen J. Impact of headache on sickness absence and utilisation of medical services: a Danish population study. *J Epidemiol Community Health*. 1992;46:443-446.
65. Schwartz B, Stewart W, Lipton R. Lost workdays and decreased work effectiveness associated with headache in the workplace. *J Occup Environ Med*. 1997;39:320-327.
66. Von Korff M, Stewart WF, Simon DS, Lipton RB. Migraine and reduced work performance: a population-based diary study. *Neurology*. 1998;50:1741-1745.
67. van Roijen L, Essink-Bot M, Koopmanschap M, et al. Societal perspective on the burden of migraine in the Netherlands. *PharmacoEconomics*. 1995;7:170-179.
68. Stewart WF, Ricci JA, Chee E, et al. Lost productive time and cost due to common pain conditions in the US workforce. *JAMA*. 2003;290:2443-2454.
69. Stewart WF, Bruce C, Manack A, et al. A case study for calculating employer costs for lost productive time in episodic migraine and chronic migraine: results of the American Migraine Prevalence and Prevention Study. *J Occup Environ Med*. 2011;53:1161-1171.
70. Buse DC, Manack A, Serrano D, et al. Sociodemographic and comorbidity profiles of chronic migraine and episodic migraine sufferers. *J Neurol Neurosurg Psychiatry*. 2010;81:428-432.
71. Lipton RB. Chronic migraine epidemiology, classification, and differential diagnosis. Presented at Decoding Chronic Migraine: Translating Clinical Trial Data Into Optimal Outcomes with Novel Therapies; June 25, 2010; Los Angeles, CA.
72. Tekle-Haimanot R, Seraw B, Forsgren L, et al. Migraine, chronic tension-type headache, and cluster headache in an Ethiopian rural community. *Cephalalgia*. 1995;15:482-488.
73. Langemark M, Olesen J, Poulsen D, Bech P. Clinical characterization of patients with chronic tension headache. *Headache*. 1988;28:590-596.
74. Lynberg A, Jensen R, Rasmussen BK, Jorgensen T. Is there a change in prevalence of migraine and tension-type headache? *Cephalalgia*. 2003;23:594.
75. Kim BK, Chu MK, Lee TG, et al. Prevalence and impact of migraine and tension-type headache in Korea. *J Clin Neurol*. 2012;8:204-211.
76. Alders EE, Hentzen A, Tan CT. A community-based prevalence study on headache in Malaysia. *Headache*. 1996 Jun;36(6):379-384.
77. Arregui A, Cabrera J, Leon-Velarde F, Paredes S, Viscarra D, Arbaiza D. High prevalence of migraine in a high-altitude population. *Neurology*. 1991 Oct;41(10):1668-1669.
78. Cruz ME, Cruz I, Preux PM, Schantz P, Dumas M. Headache and cysticercosis in Ecuador, South America. *Headache*. 1995 Feb;35(2):93-97.
79. Franceschi M, Colombo B, Rossi P, Canal N. Headache in a population-based elderly cohort. An ancillary study to the Italian Longitudinal Study of Aging (ILSA). *Headache*. 1997 Feb;37(2):79-82.
80. Henry P, Auray JP, Gaudin AF, et al. Prevalence and clinical characteristics of migraine in France. *Neurology*. 2002 Jul 23;59(2):232-237.
81. Launer LJ, Terwindt GM, Ferrari MD. The prevalence and characteristics of migraine in a population-based cohort: the GEM study. *Neurology*. 1999 Aug 11;53(3):537-542.
82. Linet MS, Stewart WF, Celentano DD, Ziegler D, Sprecher M. An epidemiologic study of headache among adolescents and young adults. *JAMA*. 1989 Apr 21;261(15):2211-2216.
83. Sakai F, Igarashi H. Prevalence of migraine in Japan: a nationwide survey. *Cephalalgia*. 1997 Feb;17(1):15-22.
84. Thomson AN, White GE, West R. The prevalence of bad headaches including migraine in a multiethnic community. *N Z Med J*. 1993 Nov 10;106(967):477-480.
85. Abdul Jabbar M, Ogunniyi A. Sociodemographic factors and primary headache syndromes in a Saudi community. *Neuroepidemiology*. 1997;16(1):48-52.
86. Merikangas KR, Whitaker AE, Isler H, et al. The Zurich study: XXIII. Epidemiology of headache syndromes in the Zurich cohort study of young adults. *Eur Arch Psychiatry Clin Neuroscience*. 1994;244:145-152.
87. Mitsikostas DD, Thomas A, Gatzonis S, Ilias A, Papageorgiou C. An epidemiological study of headache among the Monks of Athos (Greece). *Headache*. 1994 Oct;34(9):539-541.
88. Pereira Monteiro JM, Matos E, Calheiros JM. Headaches in medical school students. *Neuroepidemiology*. 1994 May-Jun; 13(3):103-107.
89. Roh JK, Kim JS, Ahn YO. Epidemiologic and clinical characteristics of migraine and tension-type headache in Korea. *Headache*. 1998 May;38(5):356-365.
90. Srikiatkhachorn A. Epidemiology of headache in the Thai elderly: a study in the Bangkae Home for the Aged. *Headache*. 1991 Nov;31(10):677-681.
91. Chu MK, Kim DW, Kim BK, Kim JM, Jang TW, Park JW, Lee KS, Cho SJ. Gender-specific influence of socioeconomic status on the prevalence of migraine and tension-type headache: the results from the Korean Headache Survey. *J Headache Pain*. 2013 Oct 4;14:82.

CHAPTER 28

Historical Features in Primary Headache Syndromes

Gerald W. Smetana

INTRODUCTION

Headache is a nearly universal symptom. As an example of the prevalence of headache, a study of 410 patients who had visited a primary care internal medicine practice found that headache was the fourth most common symptom and was exceeded only by fatigue, back pain, and dyspnea.[1] In an early study of more than 1 million unselected individuals from the general population, headache was the single most common current symptom and was reported by 39% of men and 56% of women.[2] As physicians, nearly all of us have had personal experience with headache and can understand the headache descriptions that we hear from our patients. Chapter 27 elegantly details the prevalence of this common symptom and of common primary headache syndromes. Primary headaches are those without a pathologic basis.[3–5] These are benign recurring headaches of unknown cause. The most common primary headache syndromes are migraine, tension-type headache (TTH), and cluster headache. Secondary headaches are caused by an underlying pathologic cause.

When faced with the large numbers of patients who seek medical evaluation for headache, clinicians seek to identify the rare patient with a serious headache from the rest whose headaches are benign in nature. Two general approaches assist this effort. First, one must learn the warning symptoms and signs that suggest a pathologic cause for headache. Many published reviews have offered such advice.[3,6,7] A complementary approach is to learn to confidently diagnose benign primary headache syndromes through careful history taking and the systematic application of established diagnostic criteria. Primary headaches are clinical diagnoses that are based on history taking alone. With the exception of the occasional persistence of a partial Horner's syndrome among asymptomatic patients with a history of cluster headaches, the physical examination of a patient with primary headaches is normal during headache-free intervals.

The most commonly used criteria are the International Classification of Headache Disorders, second edition (ICHD-2). The use of these criteria, most recently updated in 2004, helps to identify uniform populations of patients for research and epidemiologic studies. The criteria themselves are, however, complicated, not easily committed to memory, and may be unnecessarily restrictive in the daily clinical care of patients.

When evaluating individual patients with headache, clinicians will benefit from understanding which historical features are most useful in establishing or excluding a particular primary headache diagnosis. This chapter reviews and summarizes published clinical series of patients with migraine, TTH, and cluster headache, to determine the sensitivity, specificity, and likelihood ratios of individual historical features.

IS THIS AN OLD OR NEW HEADACHE?

Clinicians may initially classify all headaches as either old or new. Old headaches are similar to those that have occurred repeatedly over time. Primary headaches are old headaches. New headaches are either headaches of recent onset or those that represent a change in the character or pattern of an old headache. A new headache may ultimately prove to be the first instance of a primary headache syndrome, but clinicians cannot reach this conclusion with certainty until a pattern of similar headaches emerges over time.

A change in the intensity or frequency of an old headache is still an old headache. In this case, the physician must establish the precipitant for the increase in the severity of the old headache. A change in the quality, character, or descriptors of the headache, however, is a new headache. As an example, if a patient's headaches are typically unilateral and throbbing, a headache that is bilateral, constant, and progressive is a new headache. Most old headaches are benign, and the longer a headache syndrome has been present, the more likely it is to be benign.

MIGRAINE

Migraine headaches are common. Buse and colleagues performed a survey study of 162,756 U.S. individuals age 12 years old or greater and used the ICHD-2 definitions to determine migraine prevalence.[8] Migraine prevalence was 6% among men and 17% among women. The initial onset of migraine headaches most commonly occurs during between ages 10 and 25 years. Migraine headaches occur for the first time after age 40 years uncommonly. In one incidence study, for example, 77% of all patients with migraine first sought medical attention for migraine before age 40 years.[9] The new appearance of a migraine-like headache in a person older than age 40 years should prompt consideration of other possible diagnoses. Hamelsky and colleagues characterize migraine prevalence in more detail in Chapter 27.

In practice, clinicians most commonly entertain the diagnoses of migraine and TTH for patients with long-standing recurring headaches. Although less common than TTH, individuals with migraine are more likely to be disabled by their headaches and to seek medical attention for their symptoms.[10]

CLINICAL FEATURES

Tables 28-1 and **28-2** list the ICHD-2 for the diagnosis of migraine without aura and migraine with aura, respectively. The principal historical

TABLE 28-1 International Classification of Headache Disorders, 2nd Edition Criteria for the Diagnosis of Migraine Without Aura

A. At least five attacks fulfilling B–D
B. Headache attacks lasting 4–72 hours (untreated or unsuccessfully treated)
C. Headache has at least two of the following characteristics:
   1. Unilateral location
   2. Pulsating quality
   3. Moderate or severe intensity that inhibits or prohibits daily activities
   4. Aggravation by or causing avoidance of routine physical activity (e.g., walking or climbing stairs)
D. During headache, at least one of the following occurs:
   1. Nausea or vomiting
   2. Photophobia and phonophobia
   3. Not attributed to another disorder

Adapted from Headache Classification Subcommittee of the International Headache Society. The International Classification of Headache Disorders: 2nd edition. *Cephalalgia*. 2004;24(Suppl)1:9-160; with permission from SAGE journals.

TABLE 28-2 International Classification of Headache Disorders, 2nd Edition Criteria for the Diagnosis of Migraine with Aura

A. At least two attacks fulfilling criterion B
B. Migraine aura fulfilling criteria for one of the six subforms
C. Not attributed to another disorder

The six subforms are:*

1. Typical aura with migraine headache
   a. Aura consisting of at least one of the following but no motor weakness
      i. Fully reversible visual symptoms, including positive features (e.g., flickering lights, spots, or lines) or negative features (i.e., loss of vision)
      ii. Fully reversible sensory symptoms, including positive features (i.e., pins and needles) or negative features (i.e., numbness)
      iii. Fully reversible dysphasic speech disturbance
   b. At least two of the following:
      i. Homonymous visual symptoms or unilateral sensory symptoms
      ii. At least one aura symptom develops gradually over ≥5 minutes or different aura symptoms occur in succession over ≥5 minutes
      iii. Each symptom lasts ≥5 and ≤60 minutes
   c. Headache fulfilling criteria for migraine without aura begins during the aura or follows aura within 60 minutes
   d. Not attributed to another disorder
2. Typical aura with nonmigraine headache
3. Typical aura without headache
4. Familial hemiplegic migraine
5. Sporadic hemiplegic migraine
6. Basilar-type migraine

*See reference above for Table 28-1 for detailed definitions of the subforms 2-6.

Adapted from Headache Classification Subcommittee of the International Headache Society. The International Classification of Headache Disorders: 2nd edition. *Cephalalgia*. 2004;24(Suppl)1:9-160; with permission from SAGE journals.

TABLE 28-3 Headache Features in Migraine with or Without Aura Versus Tension-Type Headache

Clinical Feature*	Study Selection†	References	Sensitivity for Diagnosis of Migraine % (total number of patients)	Specificity for Diagnosis of Migraine Compared with TTH % (total number of patients)	Positive Likelihood Ratio for the Diagnosis of Migraine (CI)‡	Negative Likelihood Ratio for the Diagnosis of Migraine (CI)
Nausea	HIS	28,39,52–63	82 (5531)	96 (1443)	23.2 (17.7–30.4)	0.19 (0.18–0.20)
	All		81 (7780)	96 (1474)	19.2 (15.0–24.5)	0.20 (0.19–0.21)
Photophobia	HIS	28,39,52,55–63	79 (5182)	87 (1443)	6.0 (5.2–6.8)	0.24 (0.23–0.26)
	All		79 (6524)	86 (1474)	5.8 (5.1–6.6)	0.25 (0.24–0.26)
Phonophobia	HIS	28,39,56,57,59,61–63	69 (2188)			
	All		67 (3632)	87 (1443)	5.2 (4.5–5.9)	0.38 (0.36–0.40)
Exacerbation by physical activity	All	28,56,58,59,61,62,64	81 (3032)	78 (1843)	3.7 (3.4–4.0)	0.24 (0.23–0.26)
Unilateral	HIS	28,52–54,56–66	66 (5925)	78 (1874)	3.1 (2.8–3.3)	0.43 (0.41–0.45)
	All		65 (8832)	82 (2874)	3.7 (3.4.9)	0.43 (0.41–0.44)
Throbbing or pulsating	HIS	28,54,56–66	76 (5925)	77 (1874)	3.3 (3.1–3.6)	0.32 (0.30–0.33)
	All		73 (7832)	75 (2874)	2.9 (2.7–3.1)	0.36 (0.34–0.37)
Duration 4–24 hours	All	28,52,66,67	57 (785)	67 (499)	1.7 (1.5–2.0)	0.64 (0.58–0.71)
Duration 24–72 hours	All	28,66,67	13 (497)	91 (499)	1.4 (1.0–2.0)	0.96 (0.92–1.0)
Duration <4 hours	All	28,67	26 (628)	51 (499)	0.52 (0.44–0.61)	1.5 (1.3–1.6)

*In descending order of positive likelihood ratios using data from all studies.

†The International Headache Society (IHS) indicates pooled data from only those studies that used the IHS criteria as the reference standard.

‡95% confidence interval (CI).

IHS, International Headache Society; TTH, tension-type headache.

Adapted from Smetana GW. The diagnostic value of historical features in primary headache syndromes: a comprehensive review. *Arch Intern Med*. 2000;160(18):2729-2737.

features are headaches that are unilateral; throbbing; moderate to severe in intensity; worse with ordinary physical activity; lasting from 4 to 72 hours; are associated with nausea, photophobia, and phonophobia. All of these features are, however, not equally useful to clinicians in establishing a diagnosis of migraine. **Table 28-3** summarizes reported clinical series that detailed the frequency of particular clinical features in patients with migraine and TTH. These data were pooled from multiple series published from 1960 to 2000. All studies were classified as to their use of the International Headache Society (IHS) diagnostic criteria (first edition) or other criteria. Sensitivity, specificity, and likelihood ratios were calculated for the diagnosis of migraine compared with TTH. A positive likelihood ratio indicates the increase in the odds of the diagnosis of migraine if the particular feature is present. A negative likelihood ratio indicates the decrease in the odds of the diagnosis of migraine if the feature is absent.

Nausea, exacerbation by physical activity, photophobia, and throbbing headache are the most sensitive features for the diagnosis of migraine. Sensitivities are 81%, 81%, 79%, and 73%, respectively. Despite the origin of the word migraine from "hemicrania," only 65% of migraines are unilateral, and this is the least sensitive of the major clinical criteria. Compared with patients with TTH, the most specific features for migraine are nausea, phonophobia, photophobia, and unilateral headache, with specificities of 96%, 87%, 86%, and 82%, respectively.

The features with the best overall predictive value are nausea, photophobia, phonophobia, and exacerbation by physical activity. The particularly high positive predictive value of nausea results in part from the inclusion of large numbers of patients who were classified according to the IHS criteria. The IHS criteria for the diagnosis of TTH require the absence of nausea. However, questionnaire studies that have used less restrictive criteria for the diagnosis of TTH have also found nausea to be highly specific.[11,12] Headache duration is less useful to distinguish between the two diagnoses with the exception that headaches lasting less than 4 hours are less likely to be migraine.

Authors used many different diagnostic criteria for migraine and TTH in the pre-IHS era. Despite these varied definitions, the likelihood ratios for all pooled studies are not substantially different than those restricted to studies using the IHS criteria. The data suggest that the pre-IHS studies also included fairly uniform populations of patients.

Migraine Aura Features Among patients with migraine, one-third experience migraine with aura. In a study of 4000 randomly selected 40-year-old patients in a Danish population, the lifetime prevalence of migraine without aura was 11.8%; that of migraine with aura was 5.5%.[13] The migraine aura is sufficiently characteristic that a carefully obtained history of an aura substantially increases confidence in the diagnosis of migraine. Both the subjective aura elements and the duration of the aura are important features. **Table 28-4** summarizes the sensitivity of various aura features among pooled series of patients with migraine with aura.

Visual aurae are most common; 84% of patients with migraine with aura experience a visual aura. Positive visual phenomena occur slightly more frequently than negative visual phenomena. Positive phenomena include zigzags (fortification spectra), stars, or flashes. Many eloquent descriptions of visual aurae exist in the medical literature. In an early review of migrainous visual aura, Alvarez described his personal experience of fortification spectra:[14] "Another time I saw a fine zigzag line running up and down and a coarse one running below it, horizontally. Later, the two ran together, end to end, and bowed out to the right. The line resembles a snake fence, or an old-style fortification with projecting angles. In some spells, the line is so brilliant one can see it easily with the eyes open."*

*Reprinted from Ref. 14; Copyright 1960, with permission from Elsevier Science.

TABLE 28-4 Sensitivity of Aura Features Among Patients with Migraine with Aura

Feature	References	Sensitivity % (total number of patients)
Any visual aura	17,18,58,64,68	84 (1477)
Positive visual phenomena		
• Any	17,64,68	74 (390)
• Zigzags (fortification spectra)	18,68,69	56 (340)
• Stars or flashes	18,68	83 (263)
Negative visual phenomena		
• Any	17,68,70	56 (383)
• Scotoma	18,68,69	40 (340)
• Hemianopsia	68,69	7 (177)
Disturbance of visual perception	17,64,68,70	20 (490)
Duration of visual aura		
• <30 minutes	17,18,68	70 (400)
• 30–60 minutes	17,18,68	18 (400)
• >60 minutes	17,18,68	7 (369)
Visual aura without headache	14,18	12 (781)
Sensory aura	17,18,58,64,69	20 (1454)
Aphasia	17,18,58,64	11 (1377)
Motor aura	17,18,58,69	4 (1325)

Adapted from Smetana GW. The diagnostic value of historical features in primary headache syndromes: a comprehensive review. *Arch Intern Med*. 2000;160(18):2729-2737.

Negative visual phenomena include scotoma and hemianopsia. The presence of hemianopsia is one of the features that establish a diagnosis of migraine with typical aura (previously referred to as complicated migraine). Disturbances of visual perception are least common. In a study by Queiroz and colleagues,[15] aura features that occurred in at least 20% of patients were, in descending order of frequency, foggy vision, stars, zigzags, flashes, blind spots, flickering, waves, hemianopsia, white spots, colored spots, corona phenomena, curved lines, black, dots, and C-shaped forms. Lewis Carroll, the author of *Alice in Wonderland*, was known to have migraine with aura; some authors have speculated that Alice's visual distortions in his novel may have paralleled complex visual hallucinations that he himself experienced during migrainous aurae.[16]

The duration of the aura is also characteristic. ICHD-2 criteria require that each aura feature last from 5 to 60 minutes. In practice, the most common aura duration is 20 minutes, and 70% of visual aurae last less than 30 minutes (Table 28-4). Aurae that last a few seconds or minutes are distinctly uncommon in migraine and should raise the possibility of seizure phenomena.

Nonvisual aurae nearly always occur in conjunction with visual aura rather than as isolated events. In one study, only 4% of all aurae were complex nonvisual aurae that occurred in isolation without accompanying visual aurae.[17] Among nonvisual aurae, sensory aurae are most common followed by aphasia and motor aurae. The sensitivities are 20%, 11%, and 4%, respectively. Sensory aurae are unilateral and usually begin in the hand and then progresses to the arm, face, and tongue.[18] Aphasic aura symptoms include paraphasia, impaired production of language, and impaired comprehension of language. Motor aurae usually occur in conjunction with sensory aurae rather than in isolation.

HISTORICAL FEATURES OF INDIVIDUALS WITH MIGRAINE

Individuals with migraine are more likely to have a family history of migraine and a childhood history of vomiting attacks or motion sickness. Although these factors by themselves are insufficient to establish a diagnosis of migraine, they can be useful in the evaluation of an individual patient if the type of primary headache remains uncertain after taking a careful history.

Of these features, the familial tendency is the least controversial. In a review of more than 2500 patients with data on family history, 58% of individuals with migraine had a family history of migraine compared with 12% of unselected individuals without headache.[19] In a case control study, Stewart and colleagues reported a relative risk of 1.50 among family members of probands with migraine.[20] A positive family history was more often present among patients with severe migraine and disability. Russell and coworkers noted different family histories among patients with migraine without aura and those with migraine with aura.[21] In their study of 183 patients, migraine without aura was associated with a 2.9 relative risk of family history of migraine without aura but no increase in risk of migraine with aura. Patients with migraine with aura were twice as likely to have family histories of both migraine with and without aura than expected. In a survey of 18,714 adolescents, those with a parent with migraine were two to four times more likely to have migraine that those without a family history.[22]

Neither childhood vomiting attacks nor motion sickness are criteria for the diagnosis of migraine in the ICHD-2 classification. However, each of these features is more common in patients destined to develop migraine than those without migraine. Thirty-two percent of patients with migraine report a history of childhood vomiting attacks as compared with only 14% of individuals without headaches.[19] Data for a history of motion sickness are similar. Children who develop disabling headaches by age 5 years are 2.8 times more likely to report motion sickness than those without disabling headaches.[23] In addition, children with migraines score significantly higher on a motion sickness susceptibility questionnaire than children without migraines.[24]

CLINICAL DECISION TOOL

In the rational clinical examination in series in *The Journal of the American Medical Association*, Detsky and colleagues extracted data from a 2000 review[19] and updated the summary with more recent studies through 2005 of clinical features of migraine.[25] Their purpose was to develop a clinical decision tool that would accurately discriminate migraine from other causes of headache. They performed a systematic review of studies that assessed the performance characteristics of screening questions to diagnose migraine. They identified five features with good discriminating ability. The authors developed a mnemonic: POUND, which stands for **p**ulsating, 4 to 72 h**o**urs, **u**nilateral, **n**ausea, a**n**d **d**isabling. The positive likelihood ratios for the diagnosis of migraine if one or two, three, or more than four features were present are 0.41, 3.5, and 24, respectively.

TENSION-TYPE HEADACHE

Tension-type headache is considerably more common than migraine. Thirty-six percent of men and 46% of women have episodic TTH (see Chapter 27). Chronic TTH occurs uncommonly; in one study, 3.3% of Europeans were affected.[26] The lifetime prevalence is 78%.[27] Patients with TTH are, however, less likely to seek medical attention than are those with migraine because their headaches are less frequently disabling.

The ICHD-2 criteria define TTH largely as a chronic recurring headache with few or no migrainous features (**Table 28-5**). TTH is diagnosed based as much on the absence of particular features as the presence of specific historical features. The principal features are headaches that are pressing or tightening, mild or moderate (not severe) in intensity, and bilateral and are not associated with nausea, photophobia, phonophobia, or aggravation by ordinary physical activity. Table 28-3 summarizes the prevalence of these features (1-specificity) based on pooled data from clinical series. The ICHD-2 criteria are restrictive and do not permit the diagnosis of TTH if nausea is present or if both phonophobia and photophobia are present. As such, published series that report the frequency of particular clinical features run the risk of circular reasoning. Few series precede the publication of the IHS criteria (first edition), so it is difficult to determine if specific clinical features would be equally frequent using less restrictive criteria.

TABLE 28-5 International Classification of Headache Disorders, 2nd Edition Criteria for the Diagnosis of Frequent, Episodic Tension-Type Headache

A. At least 10 episodes occurring on ≥1 but <15 days per month for at least 3 months and fulfilling criteria B–D
B. Headache lasting from 30 minutes to 7 days
C. Headache has at least two of the following characteristics:
  a. Bilateral location
  b. Pressing or tightening (nonpulsating) quality
  c. Mild or moderate intensity
  d. Not aggravated by routine physical activity such as walking or climbing stairs
D. Both of the following:
  a. No nausea or vomiting (anorexia may occur)
  b. No more than one of photophobia or phonophobia
E. Not attributable to another disorder

Adapted from Headache Classification Subcommittee of the International Headache Society. The International Classification of Headache Disorders: 2nd edition. *Cephalalgia*. 2004;24(Suppl)1:9-160; with permission from SAGE journals.

Although the ICHD-2 criteria allow TTHs to last from 30 minutes to 7 days, Ulrich and colleagues studied 499 patients with TTH and found that 82% of patients reported headache duration of less than 24 hours.[28] Chronic recurring headaches that usually last more than 72 hours are more likely to be TTH than migraine, but this occurrence is rare. In general, the duration of headache episodes is not useful as a distinguishing feature between the two diagnoses.

The differential diagnosis of TTH includes several secondary causes for headache. Cervicogenic headache, temporomandibular joint (TMJ) dysfunction, and temporal arteritis may occasionally be confused with TTH. Cervicogenic headache is suggested by a predominantly occipital and occasionally frontal location in addition to neck pain. This headache is more commonly daily as opposed to episodic and may occur for the first time in an older individual older than age 50 years. In contrast, the peak prevalence of TTH is in individuals age 30 to 39 years,[29] and the first occurrence is most commonly in the teens or twenties.

Temporomandibular joint dysfunction is suggested by a temporal location of pain, morning headaches, bruxism with excessive dental wear, and jaw pain. These features help to distinguish it from TTH. Symptoms of TMJ dysfunction are common among patients with headache. In one report, 73% patients with TMJ related symptoms report headache compared with 38% of patients without TMJ symptoms.[27]

The headache of temporal arteritis is variable but, similar to that of TTH, is commonly pressing and bilateral without migrainous features.[30] In a systematic review, 32% of patients with biopsy-proven temporal arteritis report headache, but only 8% report temporal headache.[31] The most important factor that distinguishes the headache of temporal arteritis from that of TTH is the later age at onset. In addition, associated symptoms of temporal arteritis may be present, including polymyalgia rheumatica symptoms, fatigue, anorexia, jaw claudication, scalp tenderness, and visual symptoms. Physicians should consider this possibility in any patient with a new onset headache after age 50 years.

CLUSTER HEADACHE

Cluster headache is a distinct syndrome that is easily recognized by clinicians familiar with its historical features. It is the least common primary headache syndrome. The prevalence is less than 1%; the estimates have ranged from 0.09% to 0.33%.[26] Given the mean age of onset of this disorder at age 30 years,[32–34] the actual prevalence is probably higher and may be as high as 0.4% to 1.0% among men.[35] **Table 28-6** lists the ICHD-2 criteria for the diagnosis of cluster headache. The principal features are headaches that are severe, unilateral, supraorbital, or temporal, lasting from 15 to 180 minutes and associated with autonomic symptoms on the involved side.

Table 28-7 outlines the sensitivity of particular clinical features of cluster headaches and was derived by pooling data from published clinical series. With one exception, all of the large clinical series of patients

TABLE 28-6 International Classification of Headache Disorders, 2nd Edition Criteria for the Diagnosis of Cluster Headache

A. At least five attacks fulfilling B–D
B. Severe or very severe unilateral orbital, supraorbital, or temporal pain lasting 15–180 minutes if untreated
C. Headache is accompanied by at least one of the following ipsilateral features:
  1. Conjunctival injection or lacrimation
  2. Nasal congestion or rhinorrhea
  3. Eyelid edema
  4. Forehead and facial sweating
  5. Miosis or ptosis
  6. Or a sense of restlessness or agitation
D. Frequency of attacks: from 1 every other day to 8 per day
E. Not attributable to another disorder

Adapted from Headache Classification Subcommittee of the International Headache Society. The International Classification of Headache Disorders: 2nd edition. *Cephalalgia*. 2004;24(Suppl)1:9-160; with permission from SAGE journals.

TABLE 28-7 Sensitivity of Clinical Features Among Patients with Cluster Headache

Clinical Feature	References	Sensitivity % (total number of patients)
Male gender	32–34,71–76	86 (1634)
Family history of primary headache	34,37,72,73,75,77–79	26 (1131)
Location of pain		
• Ocular	37,72,73,77,78,80	80 (952)
• Temporal	34,37,72,73,77,78	72 (846)
• Frontal	34,37,72,73	69 (768)
• Maxillary	34,37,72,78	30 (766)
Laterality of pain		
• Right	34,37,72,73,78	48 (826)
• Left	34,37,72,73,78	38 (826)
• Either	34,37,72,73,78	14 (826)
Duration of headache		
• <30 minutes	37,73,78,80,81	11 (795)
• 30–60 minutes	37,73,80,81	43 (741)
• 1–2 hours	37,73,80,81	32 (741)
• 2–3 hours	37,73,78,80,81	10 (795)
Cluster duration of 4–8 weeks	34,37,73,76,81	57 (733)
Cluster frequency of 1–2 per year	34,37,73,76,81	66 (807)
Nocturnal headaches	34,73,77,81	54 (395)
Headache triggers:		
• Alcohol	34,73,75–78	32 (446)
• Stress	34,37,75,77,78	30 (769)
Character of pain		
• Throbbing	34,72,73,77	30 (395)
• Neuralgic	34,72,77	30 (335)
Ipsilateral lacrimation	34,37,72,73,77,78	76 (503)
Rhinorrhea	34,37,72,73,77,78	51 (503)
Nausea	34,37,72,73,76–78	35 (554)
Partial Horner's syndrome	34,37,72,73,78	37 (453)

Adapted from Smetana GW. The diagnostic value of historical features in primary headache syndromes: a comprehensive review. *Arch Intern Med*. 2000;160(18):2729-2737.

with cluster headache precede the development of the IHS criteria. The most commonly used criteria for these series were the ad hoc criteria,[36] which were published in 1962.

Cluster headache is the only primary headache syndrome that is more common in men than in women; the male:female ratio is 6:1. In contrast to patients with migraine, a family history of migraine or other primary headache syndrome is no more common among patients with cluster headache than among individuals without headache. The pain is ocular in 80% of patients; the next most common locations are temporal, frontal, and maxillary. The pain is, by definition, strictly unilateral. Interestingly, in individual patients, the headache commonly always occurs on the same side.[34,37] In the pooled data, 48% of patients experience their headaches exclusively on the right side, 38% exclusively on the left side, and only 14% of patients on both sides over their lifetimes. In contrast, this "side-locked" feature is distinctly uncommon among patients with migraine. The onset of cluster headaches is rapid, and the most common duration of each headache is 30 to 60 minutes. This is an important distinguishing characteristic from migraine headaches, which nearly always last for at least 4 hours.

These headaches are called cluster headaches because of their tendency to cluster over the lifetime of each patient. In between each cluster, patients are completely asymptomatic. In 57% of patients, each cluster lasts from 1 to 2 months, and the most common cluster frequency is one to two per year. A patient with cluster headache will often report that during a cluster each headache occurs at the same time of the day. Nocturnal headaches are most common and are reported by 54% of patients.

The character of the pain is variable and is less helpful to clinicians who seek to make a diagnosis of cluster headache. Tradition holds that cluster headaches are piercing or neuralgic. However, the pooled data indicate that only 30% of patients describe their headaches in such a fashion; this is identical to the percentage of patients that report their cluster headaches as throbbing. The pain is excruciating and sufficiently distracting that most patients cannot continue their daily routine during an episode. Patients commonly pace the room and appear restless and agitated to observers.[38] This is in contrast to patients with migraine, who usually prefer to rest in a dark, quiet room.

Among ipsilateral autonomic symptoms, 76% of patients experience lacrimation. Next most common are rhinorrhea and a partial Horner's syndrome (miosis and ptosis). The partial Horner's syndrome may persist after resolution of the headache. The differential diagnosis of cluster headache includes trigeminal neuralgia. Clinicians may distinguish trigeminal neuralgia from cluster headache by its briefer duration of seconds to several minutes, the absence of autonomic features, and the lack of periodicity.

HEADACHE PRECIPITANTS

Many patients with recurring primary headaches recognize that certain triggers often precipitate their headaches. Clinicians may be tempted to use these triggers as clues to particular headache diagnoses. **Table 28-8** summarizes the published experience on the sensitivity of particular headache precipitants among patients with migraine and TTH. The only triggers that are significantly more frequent among patients with migraine are chocolate, cheese, and any food. Using pooled data from all series, the positive likelihood ratios for these findings are 7.1, 4.9, and 3.6, respectively. Other precipitants that are present in at least 30% of patients with migraine include stress, alcohol, weather change, menses, missing a meal, lack of sleep, and perfume or odors. However, none of these triggers is significantly more common among patients with migraine than those with TTH.

TABLE 28-8 Headache Precipitants in Migraine with or Without Aura Versus Tension-Type Headache

Precipitant*	Study Selection†	References	Sensitivity for Diagnosis of Migraine	Specificity for Diagnosis of Migraine when Compared with TTH	Positive Likelihood Ratio for the Diagnosis of Migraine (CI)‡	Negative Likelihood Ratio for the Diagnosis of Migraine (CI)
			% (total number of patients)			
Chocolate	HIS	28,82–85	22 (69)	95 (384)	4.6 (2.5–8.8)	0.82 (0.73–0.93)
	All		33 (3252)	95 (384)	7.1 (4.5–11.2)	0.70 (0.68–0.73)
Cheese	All	82–85	38 (3252)	92 (52)	4.9 (1.9–12.5)	0.68 (0.62–0.73)
Any food	HIS	39,52,82,83,86,87,45,60,88	24 (1157)	86 (407)	1.7 (1.3–2.3)	0.88 (0.84–0.93)
	All		49 (5020)	86 (407)	3.6 (2.8–4.6)	0.59 (0.56–0.62)
Stress	HIS	28,39,45,60,83,85–87	50 (797)	57 (751)	1.2 (1.0–1.3)	0.88 (0.80–0.97)
	All		60 (2008)	57 (751)	1.4 (1.3–1.5)	0.70 (0.65–0.76)
Alcohol	HIS	28,60,75,82,83,85,86,88	30 (778)	77 (622)	1.3 (1.1–1.6)	0.91 (0.85–0.97)
	All		29 (3710)	77 (678)	1.3 (1.1–1.5)	0.92 (0.88–0.96)
Weather change	HIS	39,45,83,85–87	31 (554)	74 (388)	1.2 (1.0–1.5)	0.93 (0.86–1.0)
	All		35 (1765)	74 (388)	1.4 (1.1–1.6)	0.87 (0.82–0.94)
Menses	HIS	39,40,52,53,60,75,83–87,89	44 (374)	56 (165)	1.0 (0.80–1.2)	1.0 (0.86–1.2)
	All		56 (4008)	54 (221)	1.2 (1.0–1.4)	0.82 (0.72–0.93)
Missing a meal	All	82,85,87	62 (2876)	46 (32)	1.1 (0.89–1.8)	0.83 (0.61–1.1)
Lack of sleep	All	28,39,45,83,85,87	31 (1646)	62 (553)	0.83 (0.73–0.94)	1.1 (1.0–1.2)
Perfume or odors	All	85,87	32 (563)	44 (52)	0.58 (0.44–0.76)	1.5 (1.1–2.1)

*In descending order of positive likelihood ratios using data from all studies.

†The International Headache Society (IHS) indicates pooled data from only those studies that used the IHS criteria as the reference standard.

‡95% confidence interval (CI).

IHS, International Headache Society; TTH, tension-type headache.

Adapted from Smetana GW. The diagnostic value of historical features in primary headache syndromes: a comprehensive review. *Arch Intern Med*. 2000;160(18):2729-2737.

These data, however, are limited by the relatively small numbers of patients with TTH for whom there are reports of trigger frequency.

The observation that menstrual variation of headache is no more common among patients with migraine than TTH is particularly surprising but is based on observations of only 221 women with TTH. Most clinicians find this clinical feature to be useful to suggest a diagnosis of migraine. Migraines occur most commonly in the 1 or 2 days before the onset of menses and the first 1 or 2 days of menses.[39,40]

In a more recent study of a large number of subjects ($n = 327$), triggers that occurred in at least 20% of patients were, in descending order of frequency, sick days, smoking, disturbing air condition, white wine, beer, menses, spirits, oversleeping, red wine, and odors.[41] Triggers that occurred significantly more often among patients with migraine with aura than among headache without aura included smoking, menses, bright lights, odors, noise, tiredness, hunger, and stress.

Caffeine withdrawal may precipitate headaches both in patients with and without a history of primary headaches, but they occur more commonly in patients with a background of primary headaches.[42–44] No data suggest that the development of caffeine withdrawal headaches distinguishes patients with migraine from those with TTH.

One study compared the frequency of precipitating factors for 366 patients with IHS-diagnosed migraine with 169 people without migraine.[45] Presumably, the individuals without migraine had TTHs, but they were not required to meet the IHS definition for TTH. Fatigue, stress, certain foods or drinks, menstruation, and weather were all significantly more common triggers for patients with migraine than those without migraine. The stronger association of these factors with migraine than in the pooled data of Table 28-8 may reflect a more heterogeneous population of patients in the nonmigraine category that included patients who would not meet the IHS definition for TTH.

The most common triggers for cluster headache are alcohol and stress. These occur in 32% and 30% of patients, respectively (Table 28-7). These values are similar to those reported for TTH and migraine headache and are not helpful in differential diagnosis. From a review of these data, one can conclude that the decision not to include headache triggers in the ICHD-2 criteria was appropriate. Obtaining a careful history of headache triggers is most useful to guide subsequent advice to patients related to lifestyle changes that may decrease headache frequency. With the exception of chocolate, cheese, and any food, this information does not make a particular headache diagnosis more or less likely.

VALUE OF HISTORY TAKING TO MINIMIZE DIAGNOSTIC IMAGING

In a cost-constrained environment, physicians must minimize the unnecessary use of diagnostic imaging in the evaluation of patients with headache. Neuroimaging is, by definition, normal or unhelpful (nondiagnostic) in patients with primary headaches. A carefully obtained history of migraine, TTH, or cluster headache will minimize the need for such testing. Several studies have confirmed the low yield of diagnostic imaging among patients with clinical diagnoses of primary headache syndromes.

The history and physical examination may identify patients who need no further diagnostic evaluation. A retrospective study evaluated 592 patients with headache and normal neurologic examinations who had been referred for cranial computed tomography (CT) studies.[46] There were no cases of intracranial pathology sufficient to explain headache in this entire group. Mitchell and coworkers studied 350 patients with headache who were referred by their clinicians for head CT studies.[47] Among the 320 patients with normal neurologic examinations, there were only three clinically significant CT abnormalities. Each of these three patients had a headache of recent onset with worrisome atypical features.

In 1994, the American Academy of Neurology reviewed the role of neuroimaging in the evaluation of patients with headache and normal neurologic examinations.[48] The incidences of clinically important pathologic findings among patients with normal neurologic examination results and migraine or unspecified headache were 0.4% and 2.4%, respectively. They recommended no routine imaging for patients with typical migraine who had no recent change in pattern, seizures, or focal neurologic signs. They acknowledged insufficient evidence but suggested that neuroimaging may be indicated for patients with atypical headache patterns, seizures, or focal neurologic signs or symptoms.

TABLE 28-9 Clinical Features That Increase or Decrease the Likelihood of Abnormal Neuroimaging

Clinical Feature	LR+ (95% CI)	LR− (95% CI)
Cluster-type headache	11 (2.2–52)	0.95 (0.84–1.1)
Abnormal findings on neurologic examination	5.3 (2.4–12)	0.71 (0.60–0.85)
"Undefined" headache	3.8 (2.0–7.1)	0.66 (0.44–0.97)
Headache with aura	3.2 (1.6–6.6)	0.51 (0.24–1.1)
Headache with focal symptoms	3.1 (0.37–25)	0.79 (0.51–1.2)
Headache aggravated by exertion or Valsalva	2.3 (1.4–3.8)	0.70 (0.56–0.88)
Headache with vomiting	1.8 (1.2–2.6)	0.47 (0.29–0.76)
Worsening headache	1.6 (0.23–10)	1.0 (0.78–1.2)
Male sex	1.3 (0.89–1.8)	0.86 (0.68–1.1)
Quick-onset headache	1.3 (0.33–5.1)	0.79 (0.14–4.4)
New-onset headache	1.2 (0.74–2.0)	0.89 (0.63–1.3)
Headache with nausea	1.1 (0.87–1.3)	0.86 (0.63–1.2)
Increased headache severity	0.83 (0.54–1.3)	1.2 (0.91–1.4)
Migraine-type headache	0.55 (0.28–1.1)	1.2 (0.84–1.7)

CI, confidence interval; LR+, positive likelihood ratio, LR−, negative likelihood ratio.

Data from Detsky ME, McDonald DR, Baerlocher MO, et al. Does this patient with headache have a migraine or need neuroimaging? *JAMA*. 2006;296(10):1274-1283.

In 2000, the U.S. Headache Consortium reviewed the incidence of significant intracranial abnormalities in patients with migraine or TTH and normal neurologic examination results.[49] They found only two abnormal imaging studies among 1086 patients with migraine and no abnormal studies among 83 patients with TTH. In contrast, among patients with unspecified types of headaches and normal neurologic examination results, the prevalence of significant intracranial abnormalities on imaging studies varied from 0% to 6.7%. These reports confirm the importance of careful history taking to identify patients for whom the yield of imaging is sufficiently low that clinicians can establish a clinical diagnosis without further study.

In the 2006 rational clinical examination study, the authors identified 11 eligible studies of the value of the clinical examination to predict significant intracranial abnormality (i.e., to exclude a diagnosis of a primary headache syndrome).[25] **Table 28-9** summarizes the 15 clinical features that significantly changed the likelihood of abnormal neuroimaging when faced with a patient with headache. Surprisingly, cluster-type headache and headache with aura each increased the likelihood of abnormal neuroimaging. The remaining factors with a positive likelihood ratio substantially greater than one are features that are not characteristic of primary headache syndromes.

When neuroimaging is indicated, magnetic resonance imaging is preferred over CT because of a higher detection rate of clinically meaningful abnormalities.[50,51] In the case of a patient with a probable primary headache syndrome who develops new features that raise the possibility of an alternative diagnosis, the principal diagnoses to exclude are a mass lesion and an arteriovenous malformation.

SUMMARY

Nausea, photophobia, phonophobia, and exacerbation by physical activity confer the highest positive likelihood ratio for the diagnosis of migraine compared with TTH. Nausea, exacerbation by physical activity, photophobia, and throbbing headache confer the highest negative likelihood ratio, and their absence makes the diagnosis of migraine significantly less likely. Headache duration may be a useful distinguishing feature.

Among the one-third of patients with migraine who experience an aura, visual symptoms are most common and occur in 84% of patients. Positive visual phenomena, including zigzags and stars or flashes, are more common than negative visual phenomena. Sensory, aphasic, and motor aurae are each less common and nearly always occur in conjunction with a visual aura rather than in isolation.

Headache precipitants are helpful when counseling individual patients about nonpharmacologic approaches to headache management. Only chocolate, cheese, and any food significantly increase the odds that a particular headache is migraine. Other commonly reported triggers, including menses, stress, alcohol, missing a meal, fatigue, and weather change are equally common among patients with TTH and migraine headache. Alcohol and stress are the most common triggers of cluster headache but are not helpful in establishing this diagnosis.

Cluster headache is a distinct headache syndrome that is easy to distinguish from the other two primary headache syndromes. It is strictly unilateral and periorbital; lasts most commonly less than 2 hours; occurs primarily in men; and is associated with ipsilateral lacrimation, rhinorrhea, ptosis, and miosis. The most common cluster duration is 1 to 2 months, and affected patients have symptom-free intervals that average 6 to 9 months.

The use of the ICHD-2 criteria for diagnosing patients with suspected primary headache syndromes ensures homogeneous populations of patients for inclusion in studies. Practicing clinicians, however, may find these criteria too complicated and restrictive. This chapter identifies clinical features that are most useful to suggest or exclude particular primary headache diagnoses.

REFERENCES

1. Kroenke K, Arrington ME, Mangelsdorff AD. The prevalence of symptoms in medical outpatients and the adequacy of therapy. *Arch Intern Med.* 1990;150:1685-1689.
2. Hammond EC. Some preliminary findings on physical complaints from a prospective study of 1,064,004 men and women. *Am J Publ Health.* 1964;54:11-23.
3. Dalessio DJ. Diagnosing the severe headache. *Neurology.* 1994;44(Suppl 3):S6-S12.
4. Marks DR, Rapoport AM. Practical evaluation and diagnosis of headache. *Semin Neurol.* 1997;17(4):307-312.
5. Solomon GD, Cady RK, Klapper JA, Ryan RE. National Headache Foundation: standards of care for treating headache in primary care practice. *Cleve Clin J Med.* 1997;64(7):373-383.
6. Dodick D. Headache as a symptom of ominous disease. What are the warning signals? *Postgrad Med.* 1997;101(5):46-64.
7. Couch JR. Headache to worry about. *Med Clin N Amer.* 1993;77(1):141-167.
8. Buse DC, Manack AN, Fanning KM, et al. Chronic migraine prevalence, disability, and sociodemographic factors: results from the American Migraine Prevalence and Prevention Study. *Headache.* 2012;52(10):1456-1470.
9. Stang PE, Yanagihara T, Swanson JW, et al. Incidence of migraine headache: a population-based study in Olmsted County, Minnesota. *Neurology.* 1992;42:1657-1662.
10. Silberstein SB, Lipton RB. Headache epidemiology: emphasis on migraine. *Neurol Clin.* 1996;14(2):421-434.
11. Gervil M, Ulrich V, Olesen J, Russell MB. Screening for migraine in the general population: validation of a simple questionnaire. *Cephalalgia.* 1998;18:342-348.
12. Michel P, Henry P, Letenneur L, et al. Diagnostic screen for assessment of the IHS criteria for migraine by general practitioners. *Cephalalgia.* 1993;13(Suppl 12):54-59.
13. Russell MB, Rasmussen BK, Thorvaldsen P, Olesen J. Prevalence and sex-ratio of the subtypes of migraine. *Int J Epidemiol.* 1995;24:612-618.
14. Alvarez WC. The migrainous scotoma as studied in 618 persons. *Am J Ophthalmol.* 1960;49:489-504.
15. Queiroz LP, Friedman DI, Rapoport AM, Purdy RA. Characteristics of migraine visual aura in Southern Brazil and Northern USA. *Cephalalgia.* 2011;31(16):1652-1658.
16. Rolak LA. Literary neurologic syndromes: Alice in Wonderland. *Arch Neurol.* 1991;48:649-651.
17. Bana DS, Graham JR. Observations on prodromes of classic migraine in a headache clinic population. *Headache.* 1986;26(5):216-219.
18. Russell MB, Olesen J. A nosographic analysis of the migraine aura in a general population. *Brain.* 1996;119:355-361.
19. Smetana GW. The diagnostic value of historical features in primary headache syndromes: a comprehensive review. *Arch Intern Med.* 2000;160(18):2729-2737.
20. Stewart WF, Staffa J, Lipton RB, Ottman R. Familial risk of migraine: a population-based study. *Ann Neurol.* 1997;41:166-172.
21. Russell MB, Hilden J, Sorensen SA, Olesen J. Familial occurrence of migraine without aura and migraine with aura. *Neurology.* 1993;43:1369-1373.
22. Bigal ME, Lipton RB, Winner P, et al. Migraine in adolescents: association with socioeconomic status and family history. *Neurology.* 2007;69(1):16-25.
23. Aromaa M, Rautava P, Helenius H, Sillanpaa ML. Factors if early life as predictors in children at school entry. *Headache.* 1998;38:23-30.
24. Golding JF. Motion sickness susceptibility questionnaire revised and its relationship to other forms of sickness. *Brain Res Bull.* 1998;47:207-516.
25. Detsky ME, McDonald DR, Baerlocher MO, et al. Does this patient with headache have a migraine or need neuroimaging? *JAMA.* 2006;296(10):1274-1283.
26. Stovner LJ, Andree C. Prevalence of headache in Europe: a review for the Eurolight project. *J Headache Pain.* 2010;11(4):289-299.
27. Crystal SC, Robbins MS. Epidemiology of tension-type headache. *Curr Pain Headache Rep.* 2010;14(6):449-454.
28. Ulrich V, Russell MB, Jensen R, Olesen J. A comparison of tension-type headache in migraineurs and in non-migraineurs: a population-based study. *Pain.* 1996;67:501-506.
29. Schwartz BS, Stewart WF, Simon D, Lipton R. Epidemiology of tension-type headache. *JAMA.* 1998;279:381-383.
30. Reich KA, Giansiracusa DF, Strongwater SL. Neurologic manifestations of giant cell arteritis. *Am J Med.* 1990;89:67-72.
31. Smetana GW, Shmerling RH. Does this patient have temporal arteritis? *JAMA.* 2002;287(1):92-101.
32. Ekbom K. Clinical aspects of cluster headache. *Headache.* 1974;13:176-180.
33. Kudrow L. Cluster headache: diagnosis and management. *Headache.* 1979;19:142-150.
34. Manzoni GC, Terzano MG, Bono G, et al. Cluster headache—clinical findings in 180 patients. *Cephalalgia.* 1983;3(1):21-30.
35. Kudrow L. Clinical symptomatology and differential diagnosis of cluster headache. In: Tollison CD, Kunkel RS, eds. *Headache Diagnosis and Treatment.* Baltimore: Williams & Wilkins; 1993:185-189.
36. Ad hoc committee on classification of headache. Classification of headache. *JAMA.* 1962;179:717-718.

37. Kudrow L. *Cluster Headache, Mechanism and Management.* New York: Oxford University Press; 1980.
38. Sjaastad O. *Cluster Headache Syndrome.* Vol 23. London: W.B. Saunders; 1992.
39. Silberstein SB. Migraine symptoms: results of a survey of self-reported migraineurs. *Headache.* 1995;35:387-396.
40. Granella F, Sances G, Zanferrari C, et al. Migraine without aura and reproductive life events: a clinical epidemiological study in 1300 women. *Headache.* 1993;33:385-389.
41. Salhofer-Polanyi S, Frantal S, Brannath W, et al. Prospective Analysis of Factors Related to Migraine Aura—The PAMINA Study. *Headache.* Jun 1, 2012.
42. Mosek A, Korczyn AD. Yom Kippur headache. *Neurology.* 1995;45(11):1953-1955.
43. Weber JG, Ereth MH, Danielson DR. Perioperative ingestion of caffeine and postoperative headache. *Mayo Clin Proc.* 1993;68(9):842-845.
44. Silverman K, Evans SM, Strain EC, Griffiths RR. Withdrawal syndrome after the double-blind cessation of caffeine consumption. *N Engl J Med.* 1992;327(16):1109-1114.
45. Chabriat H, Danchot J, Michel P, et al. Precipitating factors of headache. A prospective study in a national control-matched survey in migraineurs and nonmigraineurs. *Headache.* 1999;39:335-338.
46. Akpek S, Arac M, Atilla S, et al. Cost-effectiveness of computed tomography in the evaluation of patients with headache. *Headache.* 1995;35:228-230.
47. Mitchell CS, Osborn RE, Grosskreutz SR. Computed tomography in the headache patient: is routine evaluation really necessary? *Headache.* 1993;33:82-86.
48. Quality standards subcommittee of the American Academy of Neurology. Practice parameter: the utility of neuroimaging in the evaluation of headache in patients with normal neurologic examinations (summary statement). *Neurology.* 1994;44:1353-1354.
49. Frishberg BM, Rosenberg JH, Matchar DB, et al. US Headache Consortium. Evidence-based guidelines in the primary care setting: neuroimaging in patients with nonacute headache. 2000; http://www.aan.com/cgi-bin/whatsnewlink.pl?loc=/public/practiceguidelines/headache_gl.htm.
50. American College of Radiology. ACR appropriateness criteria: headache. 2009; http://www.acr.org/~/media/ACR/Documents/AppCriteria/Diagnostic/Headache.pdf. Accessed August 19, 2012.
51. Evans RW. Diagnostic testing for migraine and other primary headaches. *Neurol Clin.* 2009;27(2):393-415.
52. Selby G, Lance JW. Observations on 500 cases of migraine and allied vascular headache. *J Neurol Neurosurg Psychiatry.* 1960;23:23-32.
53. Lance JW, Anthony M. Some clinical aspects of migraine. A prospective survey of 500 patients. *Arch Neurol.* 1966;15:356-361.
54. Olesen J. Some clinical features of the acute migraine attack. An analysis of 750 patients. *Headache.* 1978;18(5):268-271.
55. Manzoni GC, Farina S, Lanfranchi M, Solari A. Classic migraine—clinical findings in 164 patients. *Eur Neurol.* 1985;24(3):163-169.
56. Rasmussen BK, Jensen R, Olesen J. A population-based analysis of the diagnostic criteria of the International Headache Society. *Cephalalgia.* 1991;11:129-134.
57. Lipton RB, Stewart WF, Celentano DD, Reed ML. Undiagnosed migraine headaches: a comparison of symptom-based and reported physician diagnoses. *Arch Intern Med.* 1992;152:1273-1278.
58. Dahlof C, Riman E. How does the International Headache Society classification perform in a European headache clinic? In: Olesen J, ed. *Headache Classification and Epidemiology.* Vol 4. New York: Raven Press; 1994:77-86.
59. Wober-Bingol C, Wober C, Karwautz A, et al. Diagnosis of headache in childhood and adolescence: a study in 437 patients. *Cephalalgia.* 1995;15:13-21.
60. Rothrock J, Patel M, Lyden P, Jackson C. Demographic and clinical characteristics of patients with episodic migraine versus chronic daily headache. *Cephalalgia.* 1996;16(1):44-49; discussion 44.
61. Wober-Bingol C, Wober C, Karwautz A, et al. Tension-type headache in different age groups at two headache centers. *Pain.* 1996;67:53-58.
62. Lavados PM, Tenhamm E. Epidemiology of migraine headache in Santiago, Chile: a prevalence study. *Cephalalgia.* 1997;17:770-777.
63. Lipton RB, Stewart WF, Simon D. Medical consultation for migraine: results from the American Migraine Study. *Headache.* 1998;38:87-96.
64. Roh JK, Kim JS, Ahn YO. Epidemiologic and clinical characteristics of migraine and tension-type headache in Korea. *Headache.* 1998;38:256-265.
65. Friedman AP, von Storch TJC, Merritt HH. Migraine and tension headaches. A clinical study of two thousand cases. *Neurology.* 1954;4:773-788.
66. Phanthumchinda K, Sithi-Amorn C. Prevalence and clinical features of migraine: a community survey in Bangkok, Thailand. *Headache.* 1989;29:594-597.
67. Henry P, Michel P, Brochet B, et al. A nationwide survey of migraine in France: prevalence and clinical features in adults. *Cephalalgia.* 1992;12:229-237.
68. Queiroz LP, Rapoport AM, Weeks RE, et al. Characteristics of migraine visual aura. *Headache.* 1997;37:137-141.
69. Gherpelli JLD, Nagae Poetscher LM, Souza AMMH, et al. Migraine in childhood and adolescence: a critical study of the diagnostic criteria and of the influence of age on clinical findings. *Cephalalgia.* 1998;18:333-341.
70. Hachinski VC, Porchawka J, Steele JC. Visual symptoms in the migraine syndrome. *Neurology.* 1973;23:570-579.
71. Lovshin LL. Clinical caprices of histaminic cephalalgia. *Headache.* 1961;1:7-10.
72. Ekbom K. A clinical comparison of cluster headache and migraine. *Acta Neurol Scand.* 1970;46(Suppl 41):1-48.
73. Lance JW, Anthony M. Migrainous neuralgia or cluster headache? *J Neurol Sci.* 1971;13:401-414.
74. Graham JR. Cluster headache. *Headache.* 1972;11:175-185.
75. Drummond PD. Predisposing, precipitating and relieving factors in different categories of headache. *Headache.* 1985;25:16-22.
76. Riess CM, Becker WJ, Robertson M. Episodic cluster headache in a community: clinical features and treatment. *Can J Neurol Sci.* 1998;25(2):141-145.
77. Friedman AF, Midropoulos HE. Cluster headaches. *Neurology.* 1958;8:653-663.
78. Sutherland JM, Eadie MJ. Cluster headache. *Res Clin Stud Headache.* 1972;3:92-115.
79. Andersson PG. Migraine in patients with cluster headache. *Cephalalgia.* 1985;5:11-16.
80. Manzoni GC, Terzano MG, Moretti G, Cocchi M. Clinical observations on 76 cluster headache cases. *Eur Neurol.* 1981;20:88-94.
81. Ekbom K. Patterns of cluster headache with a note on the relations to angina pectoris and peptic ulcer. *Acta Neurol Scand.* 1970;46:225-237.
82. Dalton K. Food intake prior to a migraine attack: study of 2,313 spontaneous attacks. *Headache.* 1975;15:188-193.

83. Van den Bergh V, Amery WK, Waelkens J. Trigger factors in migraine: a study conducted by the Belgian Migraine Society. *Headache*. 1987;27:191-196.
84. Davies PT, Peatfield RC, Steiner TJ, et al. Some clinical comparisons between common and classical migraine: a questionnaire-based study. *Cephalalgia*. 1991;11(5):223-227.
85. Scharff L, Turk DC, Marcus DA. Triggers of headache episodes and coping response of headache diagnostic groups. *Headache*. 1995;35:397-403.
86. Rasmussen BK. Migraine and tension-type headache in a general population: precipitating factors, female hormones, and relation to lifestyle. *Pain*. 1993;53:65-72.
87. Robbins L. Precipitating factors in migraine: a retrospective review of 494 patients. *Headache*. 1994;34:214-216.
88. Peatfield RC. Relationship between food, wine, and beer-precipitated migrainous headaches. *Headache*. 1995;35:355-357.
89. Epstein MT, Hockaday JM, Hockaday TDR. Migraine and reproductive hormones throughout the menstrual cycle. *Lancet*. 1975;1: 543-547.

CHAPTER 29

Pathophysiology of Headaches

F. Michael Cutrer
Paul G. Mathew

Headaches are estimated to affect more than 90% of the general population at some point in their lives[1] and may be encountered by physicians in a wide variety of clinical settings. Headaches can be divided into two major categories. The overwhelming majority of recurrent headaches are *primary headache disorders,* in which no identifiable underlying cause can be found. *Secondary headache disorders* are symptomatic of an underlying pathological cause. Secondary headaches can be due to causes such as transient viral illness, intracranial tumor, aneurysm, or drug withdrawal (for differential diagnosis of secondary headache disorder, see Cutrer[2]). Prevalence studies indicate that a benign process, such as a mild febrile illness or alcohol withdrawal, usually causes secondary headaches and that the lifetime prevalence of headache resulting from more ominous intracranial structural lesions is less than 2%.[3]

Head pain occurs when nociceptive neurons within the trigeminal, vagus, or glossopharyngeal cranial nerves or within the upper cervical roots become depolarized. Information from procedures involving intracerebral electrode implantation suggests that direct electrical or mechanical activation of areas within the brain involved in pain processing may also cause head pain.[4] The causes of head pain vary widely and include not only direct mechanical, chemical, or inflammatory stimulation of pain-generating structures but also less well-characterized events that occur in primary headache disorders. After being initiated, the transmission and processing of the painful information is likely to be quite similar regardless of the inciting cause. This chapter reviews the anatomy involved in generating generic head pain and then discusses current theories of the pathophysiology of the major primary headache disorders, including migraine, cluster headache, and tension-type headache (TTH).

ANATOMY OF HEAD PAIN

Under normal physiologic conditions, the brain is largely insensate. This has been demonstrated in neurosurgical procedures in which stimulation of the brain parenchyma in awake patients caused no pain.[5,6] Head pain is mediated by projections from the trigeminal and upper cervical dorsal root ganglia, which innervate the pial, dural, and extracranial blood vessels. In general, these pseudounipolar neurons innervate the vessels on the same side, which can explain the unilateral distribution of pain in certain headache types, but some of the cells project bilaterally to innervate midline vessels. On activation, these unmyelinated C fibers transmit nociceptive information from perivascular terminals through the trigeminal ganglia[7] to project centrally to synapses on second-order neurons within the trigeminal nucleus caudalis. The primary neurotransmitter for the C fibers is glutamate, but the primary afferents also co-store substance P, calcitonin gene–related peptide (CGRP), and neurokinin A, as well as other neurotransmitters and neuromodulators, in their central and peripheral (e.g., meningeal) axons.

Activity in the trigeminal nucleus caudalis can be modulated by projections from rostral trigeminal nuclei,[8] the periaqueductal gray matter, and the nucleus raphe magnus,[9] as well as by descending cortical inhibitory systems.[9,10] From the trigeminal nucleus caudalis, second-order neurons transmit the nociceptive information, projecting to numerous subcortical sites, including the more rostral portions of the trigeminal complex,[11] the reticular formation of the brainstem,[12] midbrain and pontine parabrachial nuclei,[13,14] and the cerebellum,[15,16] as well as to the ventrobasal thalamus,[11,16-18] the posterior thalamus,[19,20] and the medial thalamus.[21] From the rostral brainstem, nociceptive information is transmitted to other areas of the brain (e.g., limbic areas) involved in the emotional and vegetative responses to pain.[13] From the ventrobasal thalamus, projections are sent to the somatosensory cortex, where discrimination and localization of pain are thought to occur. The medial thalamus projects to frontal cortex, where the affective and motivational responses to pain are thought to be mediated. In addition, evidence from positron emission tomography (PET) studies indicates that the medial thalamus may participate in the transmission of both discriminative and affective components of pain.[22]

PATHOPHYSIOLOGY OF MIGRAINE

Migraine is one of the most common primary headache disorders and is characterized by throbbing headaches associated with nausea, vomiting, photophobia, and phonophobia. Before the onset or during the early phase of a headache, some individuals with migraine experience transient focal neurologic symptoms, which may include visual disturbances, unilateral numbness, unilateral weakness, and language dysfunction. These neurologic symptoms are collectively known as migraine aura. At the most basic level, migraine for most people is a complex genetic disorder with susceptibility arising from one or more variants in their genetic code. The details of how the susceptibility activates the migraine attacks are still incompletely understood. Because of the neurologic symptoms of migraine aura, the prevalence of migraine, and the intensity the headache, the research and speculation surrounding the pathophysiology of migraine has been the most intensive of all primary headache disorders. The speculation that has arisen around migraine has greatly influenced the discussion of pathophysiology of other headache syndromes. Traditional theories of migraine pathogenesis fall into two categories, vasogenic and neurogenic.

VASOGENIC THEORY

In the late 1930s, Dr. Harold Wolff[23] and coworkers observed that (1) extracranial vessels became distended and pulsated during migraine attacks in many patients, implying that dilation of cranial vessels might be important in migraine; (2) stimulation of intracranial vessels in awake patients resulted in an ipsilateral headache; and (3) vasoconstricting substances, such as ergotamine, could abort headaches, and vasodilatory substances, such as nitrates, could trigger migraine attacks. Based on these observations, it was theorized that intracranial vasoconstriction was responsible for the aura of migraine and that the subsequent headache resulted from a rebound dilation and distention of cranial vessels and activation of inflamed perivascular sensory neurons.

NEUROGENIC THEORY

The competing neurogenic theory held that migraine is a brain disorder based on an altered cerebral susceptibility to migraine attacks and that the vascular changes occurring during a migraine were the result rather than the cause of the attack. Advocates of the neurogenic theory pointed to the neurologic symptoms, both focal (in the aura) and vegetative (in the prodrome), that are often prominent components of migraine attacks, which cannot be explained on the basis of vasoconstriction within a single neurovascular territory. The expanding nature of the visual and sensory symptoms during migraine aura has led to speculation that the phenomenon of spreading depression might underlie the aura.[24] Spreading depression is a wave of neuronal hyperexcitation followed by suppression that is observed to move across areas of contiguous cortex in experimental animals after chemical or mechanical perturbation.[25] The speculation that spreading depression might be important in migraine aura was reawakened when Olesen, Lauritizen, and their colleagues used intraarterial xenon 133 (^{133}Xe) blood flow techniques to investigate the hemodynamic changes occurring during aura-like symptoms induced during carotid angiography. Olesen and coworkers reported that aura symptoms were accompanied by reductions in cerebral blood flow, usually in posterior regions of the brain.[26,27] Some studies reported a transient increase in blood flow before the blood flow reductions as well as an apparent anterior spread of the blood flow decrements, which moved across neurovascular boundaries.[27] The estimated rate of the spread was about 2 to 3 mm/min,[27] although the accuracy of this rate has been questioned because of the convoluted nature of the human cerebral cortex. The estimated reductions in blood flow observed in these ^{133}Xe blood flow studies ranged from 17%[28] to 35%,[26] which is well above the threshold (i.e., >75%) for frank ischemia and were therefore termed *spreading oligemia*. However, some researchers have speculated that the artifact of Compton scattering might account for both an underestimation of the magnitude of blood flow reduction and the apparent spreading pattern of the blood flow change.[29]

If applied rigidly, neither of these traditional theories completely explains the clinical symptomatology of migraine. It is likely that migraine is not a disease per se but rather a syndrome in which acute attacks occur when one or more triggering environmental events interact with a vulnerable nervous system. The reasons why certain individuals possess this vulnerability to migraine attacks are not fully understood but are likely a result of a combination of genetic and acquired factors. There is great variability among the environmental triggers that are potentially capable of inciting a migraine attack. Most individuals with migraine are aware of several to which they are sensitive. The triggers most commonly reported include exposure to certain foods or food additives, certain types of physical exertion, alteration of usual sleep patterns, increased personal or professional stress, hormonal fluctuation, unaccustomed fasting, exposure to glaring or flickering lights, strong smells, and changes in weather patterns or barometric pressure. The triggers for attacks vary widely from one individual to another, and may change with time for an individual person with migraine. The mechanisms by which these provocative factors initiate a migraine are not well understood. Neither the biochemical nature nor the exact site of migraine initiation is known, but recent advances in functional neuroimaging are beginning to yield some clues.

Initiation One study performed during the first 6 hours of nine spontaneous attacks of migraine without aura using PET has led to speculation that a so-called migraine generator may exist in the proximal brainstem.[30] In this study, a significant increase in regional cerebral blood flow (rCBF) was observed in the anterocaudal cingulate cortex, as well as the visual and auditory associative cortices. In addition, an 11% increase in rCBF was noted in medial brainstem structures over several planes slightly contralateral to the headache side. Activation in the medial brainstem but not the cingulate and auditory association cortices persisted even after effective treatment of the headache with 6 mg of subcutaneous sumatriptan. Activation within the medial brainstem was not observed during a subsequent study during a headache-free interval nor was it observed in another series after subcutaneous injection of capsaicin in the forehead.[31] Although this pattern of activation in the brainstem takes place in a region important in nociceptive and vascular control (locus ceruleus and dorsal raphe nucleus), the persistence of the increase in rCBF after relief of symptoms has been interpreted to suggest the presence of a migraine generator. In contrast, other information based on molecular genetic investigations of familial hemiplegic migraine has suggested that altered activation thresholds within cortical neurons may be important in the initiation of migraine attacks in some patients.[32]

Aura Approximately 25% of individuals with migraine experience attacks in which the headache is preceded by auras that persist for up to 1 hour. These transient symptoms are characterized by an unexpected onset and a slow expansion of the area affected by the dysfunction followed by gradual resolution. Functional neuroimaging in humans during the opening minutes of spontaneous migraine attacks has demonstrated that decreases in relative cerebral blood flow occur in areas of the occipital cortex. In one case, the beginning of a migraine attack was fortuitously captured using PET and ^{15}O-labeled water. A bilateral spreading area of decreased blood flow was observed that started in visual associative cortex (Brodmann's areas 18 and 19) within a few minutes after the onset of a bioccipital throbbing headache. The hypoperfusion progressed anteriorly with time across vascular and anatomic boundaries.[33] Although the subject's difficulty in focusing on a visual target during a part of the study has been interpreted as an atypical migraine aura, it is difficult to draw conclusions about more typical auras because neither scintillations nor a scotoma were reported and because the subject had previously only attacks of migraine without aura.

Additional studies using functional magnetic resonance imaging (fMRI) techniques, such as perfusion and diffusion-weighted imaging, to study patients during spontaneous migraine visual auras have demonstrated that during the visual symptoms, there are increases in mean transit time, the amount of time required for a given amount of blood to move through a set volume of brain parenchyma, of 10% to 54% in the occipital cortex contralateral to the reported visual field symptoms. These studies have also demonstrated decreases in both relative cerebral blood flow (15%–53%) and relative cerebral blood volume (6%–33%) in the same region.[34] In between attacks, perfusion-weighted imaging and T2-weighted anatomic images in all of the subjects studied (eight thus far) were normal. In one subject, in whom multiple perfusion images were obtained during the same aura, the margin of the perfusion defect appeared to be more anterior in the second image than in the first, suggesting a spread reminiscent of Olesen's findings.

Diffusion-weighted imaging was also performed in subjects during acute migraine with visual auras. Diffusion-weighted imaging, based on the mobility of water molecules, reflects the ability of neurons to maintain normal osmotic membrane gradients. Changes in diffusion-weighted imaging can indicate a loss of this very basic cell function, which can be seen very early in the evolution of ischemic neuronal injury[35] and in the cortex of experimental animals after the induction of spreading depression.[36] Of the subjects for whom diffusion-weighted images were obtained during visual symptoms, none demonstrated any evidence of regional hyperintensity to suggest the loss of the ability to regulate water mobility. No changes in apparent diffusion coefficient were seen even in areas of the occipital lobe that had perfusion decrements of up to 52%.[34] Based on earlier studies of human stroke, the absence of measurable diffusion abnormalities suggests that the threshold for ischemia is not crossed during the migraine aura.[35] Negative diffusion data also suggest that the abnormality that underlies migraine aura in humans, although possibly analogous, is not identical to spreading depression as it occurs in experimental animals. Most recently, fMRI studies using blood oxygen level–dependent imaging (BOLD) during both spontaneous and physiologically inducible migraine have confirmed the occurrence of changes within the occipital cortex consistent with a primarily neuronal process similar to the phenomenon of cortical spreading depression.[37]

In general, recent information from functional neuroimaging tends to favor a primarily neuronal rather than vascular origin for the symptoms of migraine aura. The apparent spread across vascular territories and the moderate blood flow reductions seen in both PET[33] and fMRI[34,37] investigations of spontaneous migraine aura symptoms are more suggestive of primary neuronal dysfunction than frank ischemia as the basis for the aura. It is interesting to note that the findings from PET and fMRI (neither of which is vulnerable to Compton scattering) are consistent with the earlier observations using ^{133}Xe blood flow techniques. Whether the characteristics of the neuronal dysfunction prove to be consistent with a human analogue of spreading depression is not clear.

Headache Several lines of evidence are consistent with functional neuroimaging findings suggesting that dysfunction within the brain is related to the aura and may provoke head pain. For example, vegetative and affective prodromal symptoms, such as alteration of mood, appetite, and fluid balance, may precede the onset of the headache by up to 24 hours. Furthermore, the majority of patients with aura report that the headache is more severe on the side of the brain hemisphere to which the aura symptoms localize. In addition, the possibility that events intrinsic to the cerebral cortex may be capable of activating meningeal nociceptive neurons is suggested by the fact that seizures are followed by headache in many patients, and that repeated spreading depressions in experimental animals result in the induction of c-fos immunoreactivity (a marker of activation) in second-order nociceptive neurons within the trigeminal nucleus caudalis.[38] After depolarization, perivascular and meningeal C fibers transmit nociceptive information via the trigeminal nerve and upper cervical nerve roots to areas of pain processing within the trigeminal nucleus caudalis in the distal medulla and dorsal horn of the upper cervical segments.

The gradual intensification and prolongation of headache that occur during migraine may be governed by a series of events that result in peripheral and central sensitization of the trigeminal system. Information from animal studies indicates that after activation, C fibers release neuropeptides such as substance P, neurokinin A, and CGRP.[39] Similar increases in neuropeptides have been observed during acute migraine attacks in humans.[40] These neuropeptides generate a neurogenic inflammatory response within the meninges consisting of increased plasma leakage from meningeal vessels, vasodilation, and activation of mast cells and endothelial cells.

After being set into motion, this process is thought to lower the threshold of the C fibers to further activation, resulting in the prolongation and intensification of the headache attack. Drugs known to be effective in ending a migraine attack, such as dihydroergotamine or sumatriptan, act at serotonin 5-HT_{1B} and 5-HT_{1D} receptor subtypes to cause constriction of vascular smooth muscle and to block the release of neuropeptides that mediate the development of neurogenic inflammation. Animal studies have confirmed that after stimulation of the meningeal pain system there is a reduction in activation thresholds. After chemical stimulation of the meninges, nociceptive neuronal responses and pain-induced changes in blood pressure were evoked by much smaller levels of dural mechanical stimulation and by previously innocuous cutaneous stimulation, indicating the generation of both central sensitization and cutaneous allodynia.[41]

Generation of an Acute Attack A possible scenario for the generation of an acute attack in some forms of migraine is as follows:

1. Endogenous neurophysiologic events in the neocortex generate the observed neurologic symptoms of aura and promote the release of nociceptive substances (e.g., H^+ and K^+ ions, arachidonic acid metabolites) from the neocortex into the interstitial space.
2. Within the Virchow-Robin spaces, the released substances accumulate to levels sufficient to activate or sensitize trigeminovascular fibers that surround pial vessels supplying the neocortex.
3. Substances that discharge or sensitize small, unmyelinated fibers that transmit pain accumulate in proximity to trigeminovascular fibers and may possibly provide the trigger for headache or sensitize perivascular afferents to bloodborne or other as yet unidentified factors. The headache latency (20–40 minutes) may reflect the time needed for extracellular levels to reach a threshold for depolarization.
4. Upon activation, the trigeminal nociceptive neurons transmit the nociceptive information through the trigeminal ganglia to synapse on second-order neurons within the trigeminal nucleus caudalis.
5. Numerous projections from the trigeminal nucleus caudalis then transmit the nociceptive information to various brain areas that underlie various aspects of pain (see the earlier section Anatomy of Head Pain).

In this scenario, the brain of migraine-susceptible individuals acts as a transducer, interfacing with the environment. Triggering events, such as those associated with emotional stress, glaring lights, or interrupted sleep, modulate activity within brain regions physically contiguous to the meningeal vessels innervated by the trigeminal nerve. In susceptible individuals, these events may be sufficient to initiate neurophysiologic events leading to chemical activation of meningeal fibers. The photophobia, nausea, and vomiting are probably not specific to migraine but are related to meningeal irritation because similar symptoms are seen with infection or when blood enters the subarachnoid space. This proposed cascade provides a pathogenetic framework for further investigation of migraine and is based on currently understood principles of neurobiology and the physiology of pain. However, the details will need revision as new data emerge from experimental studies in humans and animals.

PATHOPHYSIOLOGY OF CLUSTER HEADACHE

In the past, very little was known about the pathophysiology of cluster headaches, but recent observations have given rise to new speculation about the origins of this primary headache disorder. Similar to other vascular headaches (e.g., migraine), cluster headaches are presumed to develop from pathophysiologic events that ultimately activate the trigeminovascular system.

In the complete form of the syndrome, patients with cluster headache manifest pain in the first and second trigeminal divisions, sympathetic activation (sweating of the forehead and face), sympathetic dysfunction (Horner's syndrome), and parasympathetic activation (lacrimation and nasal congestion). This constellation of symptoms and signs can best be explained as the consequence of an abnormality at the point at which fibers from the ophthalmic and maxillary trigeminal division converge with projections from the superior cervical and the sphenopalatine ganglia. This plexus is contained within the cavernous sinus, and narrowing of the cavernous carotid artery has been observed in selected cases of cluster headache. Although a subject of some controversy, changes in the drainage pattern of the cavernous sinus have also been reported in patients with this condition.[42] A history of trauma and variations in the anatomical structure of the cavernous sinus may provide additional clues to the pathophysiologic features of cluster headache. In one study, external craniometric measurements in a group of 25 patients with cluster headache revealed an apparent narrowing of the anterior-middle cranial fossa when compared with age-matched healthy volunteers ($n = 21$) and individuals with migraine ($n = 20$).[43] Intraorbital lesions and lesions at remote sites in the middle fossa should be investigated in patients with only a partial set of signs and symptoms.

The circadian rhythmicity of this syndrome is another striking clinical feature that has led to speculation that the hypothalamus or a related structure may be involved in the generation of this headache.[44–46] In a recent PET study of nine patients with acute cluster attacks, investigators observed brain activation in areas known to be involved in pain processing, such as the bilateral anterior cingulate cortex, the contralateral posterior thalamus, and the insular cortex. They also observed activation in the hypothalamic gray matter.[47] This appears to be specific for cluster headache because it has not been observed in migraine[48] or in head pain induced by capsaicin injection.[49] When trigeminal pain fibers are activated, many of the processes associated with the prolongation and intensification of the pain in migraine may apply in cluster headache as well (see the earlier discussion of headache in the section Pathophysiology of Migraine).

PATHOPHYSIOLOGY OF TENSION-TYPE HEADACHE

It is ironic that the pathophysiology of the most common of the primary headache disorders is the least well understood. TTH continues to defy a single or simple pathophysiologic explanation, although the importance of muscular and myofascial structures is acknowledged in many, but not all, cases.[50,51] In one of the more widely accepted paradigms, headache pain is viewed as the sum of nociceptive input from vascular structures, similar input from myofascial and muscular sources, as well as descending supraspinal modulation.[52] The relative importance of these three factors varies among patients and among attacks in the same patient. In TTH, myofascial input may predominate, but in migraine, cerebrovascular and meningeal nociceptive stimulation may predominate. Whereas peripheral factors are very important in episodic headaches, chronic headaches seem to be strongly influenced by changes in the supraspinal modulation of pain. This view of TTH may explain the frequent overlap with migraine.

CONCLUSION

The details of the pathophysiology of the various primary and secondary headache disorders undoubtedly differ, especially those pertaining to initiation of the attack. However, the basic biologic principles governing the development, modulation, and prolongation of head pain are likely to be the same regardless of the underlying cause of the headache. As our understanding of these principles increases, so too will the effectiveness and tolerability of new acute therapies. Improvements in prophylactic therapy will require a better knowledge of the factors involved in headache initiation.

REFERENCES

1. Rasmussen BK, Jensen R, Schroll M, Olesen J. Epidemiology of headache in a general population: a prevalence study. *J Clin Epidemiol.* 1991;44:1147-1157.
2. Cutrer FM. Headache. In: Borsook D, LeBel A, McPeek B, eds. *The Massachusetts General Hospital Handbook of Pain Management.* Boston, MA: Little, Brown; 1996:270-302.
3. Rasmussen BK, Olesen J. Symptomatic and non-symptomatic headaches in general population. *Neurology.* 1992;42:1225-1231.
4. Raskin NH, Hosobuchi Y, Lamb SA. Headache may arise from perturbation of brain. *Headache.* 1987;27:416-420.
5. Ray BS, Wolff HG. Experimental studies on headache. Pain-sensitive structures of the head and their significance in headache. *Arch Surg.* 1940;41:813-856.
6. Penfield W. A contribution to the mechanism of intracranial pain. *Assoc Res Nerv Ment Dis.* 1935;15:399-416.
7. Mayberg MR, Zervas NT, Moskowitz MA. Trigeminal projections to supratentorial pial and dural blood vessels in cats demonstrated by horseradish peroxidase histochemistry. *J Comp Neurol.* 1984;223:46-56.
8. Kruger L, Young RF. Specialized features of the trigeminal nerve and its central connections. In: Samii M, Janetta PJ, eds. *The Cranial Nerves.* Berlin, Germany: Springer-Verlag; 1981:273-301.
9. Sessle BJ, Hu JW, Dubner R, Lucier GE. Functional properties of neurons in trigeminal subnucleus caudalis of the cat, II. Modulation of responses to noxious and non-noxious stimulation by periaqueductal gray, nucleus raphe magnus, cerebral cortex and afferent influences, and effect of naloxone. *J Neurophysiol.* 1981;45:193-207.
10. Wise SP, Jones EG. Cells of origin and trigeminal distribution of descending projections of the rat somatic sensory cortex. *J Comp Neurol.* 1977;175:129-158.
11. Jacquin MF, Chiaia NL, Haring JH, Rhoades RW. Intersub-nuclear connections within the rat trigeminal brainstem complex. *Somatosen Motor Res.* 1990;7:399-420.
12. Renehan WE, Jacquin MF, Mooney RD, Rhoades RW. Structure-function relationship in rat medullary and cervical dorsal horns. II. Medullary dorsal horn cells. *J Neurophysiol.* 1986;55:1187-1201.
13. Bernard JF, Peschanski M, Besson JM. A possible spino-(trigemino)-ponto amygdaloid pathway for pain. *Neurosci Lett.* 1989;100:83-88.
14. Hayashi H, Tabata T. Pulpal and cutaneous inputs to somatosensory neurons in the parabrachial area of the cat. *Brain Res.* 1990;511:177-179.
15. Huerta MF, Frankfurter A, Harting JK. Studies of the principal sensory and spinal trigeminal nuclei of the rat: projections to the superior colliculus, inferior olive, and cerebellum. *J Comp Neurol.* 1983;220:147-167.
16. Mantle St John LA, Tracey DJ. Somatosensory nuclei in the brainstem of the rat: independent projections to the thalamus and cerebellum. *J Comp Neurol.* 1987;255:259-271.
17. Huang L-YM. Origin of thalamically projecting somatosensory relay neurons in the immature rat. *Brain Res.* 1989;495:108-114.
18. Kemplay S, Webster KE. A quantitative study of the projections of the gracile, cuneate, and trigeminal nuclei and of the medullary reticular formation to the thalamus in the rat. *Neuroscience.* 1989;32:153-167.
19. Peschanski M, Roudier F, Ralston HJ III, Besson JM. Ultrastructural analysis of the terminals of various somatosensory pathways in the ventrobasal complex of the rat thalamus: an electron-microscopic study using wheatgerm agglutinin conjugated to horseradish peroxidase as an axonal tracer. *Somatosens Res.* 1985;3:75-87.
20. Shigenaga Y, Nakatani A, Nishimori T, et al. The cells of origin of cat trigeminothalamic projections: especially in the caudal medulla. *Brain Res.* 1983;277:201-222.
21. Craig AD Jr, Burton H. Spinal and medullary lamina I projection to nucleus submedius in medial thalamus: a possible pain center. *J Neurophysiol.* 1981;45:443-466.
22. Bushnell MC, Duncan GH. Sensory and affective aspects of pain perception: is medial thalamus restricted to emotional issues? *Exp Brain Res.* 1989;78:415-418.
23. Wolff HG, Tunis MM, Goodell H. Studies on headache: evidence of tissue damage and changes in pain sensitivity in subjects with vascular headaches of the migraine type. *Trans Assoc Am Physicians.* 1953;66:332-341.
24. Milner P. Note on a possible correspondence between the scotomas of migraine and spreading depression of Leao. *EEG Clin Neurophysiol.* 1958;10:705.
25. Leao AAP. Spreading depression of activity in the cerebral cortex. *J Neurophysiol.* 1944;8:379-390.
26. Olesen J, Larsen B, Lauritzen M. Focal hyperemia followed by spreading oligemia and impaired activation of rCBF in classic migraine. *Ann Neurol.* 1981;9:344-352.
27. Lauritzen M, Skyhoj Olsen T, Lassen NA, Paulson OB. Changes of regional cerebral blood flow during the course of classical migraine attacks. *Ann Neurol.* 1983;13:633-641.
28. Lauritzen M, Olesen J. Regional cerebral blood flow during migraine attacks by xenon-133 inhalation and emission tomography. *Brain.* 1984;107:447-461.
29. Skyhoj Olsen T, Friberg L, Lassen NA. Ischemia may be the primary cause of neurologic deficits in classical migraine. *Arch Neurol.* 1987;44:156-161.
30. Weiller C, May A, Limmroth V, et al. Brain stem activation in spontaneous human migraine attacks. *Nat Med.* 1995;1:658-660.
31. May A, Kaube H, Buchel C, et al. Experimental cranial pain elicited by capsaicin: a PET study. *Pain.* 1998;74:61-66.
32. Ferrari MD. Migraine. *Lancet.* 1998;351:1043-1051.
33. Woods RP, Iacoboni M, Mazziotta JC. Bilateral spreading cerebral hypoperfusion during spontaneous migraine headache. *N Eng J Med.* 1994;331:1689-1692.
34. Cutrer FM, Sorenson AG, Weisskoff RM, et al. Perfusion-weighted imaging defects during spontaneous migrainous aura. *Ann Neurol.* 1998;43:25-31.

35. Warach S, Gaa J, Siewert B, et al. Acute human stroke studied by whole brain echo planar diffusion-weighted magnetic resonance imaging. *Ann Neurol.* 1995;37:231-241.
36. Hasegawa Y, Latour LL, Sotak C, et al. Spreading waves of reduced diffusion coefficient of water in the rat brain. *Neurology.* 1994;44 (Suppl):A341.
37. Hadjikhani N, Sanchez Del Rio M, Wu O, et al. Mechanisms of migraine aura revealed by functional MRI in human visual cortex. *Proc Natl Acad Sci U S A.* 2001;10:98(8):4687-4692.
38. Moskowitz MA, Nozaki K, Kraig RP. Neocortical spreading depression provokes the expression of c-fos protein-like immunoreactivity within trigeminal nucleus caudalis via trigeminovascular mechanisms. *J Neurosci.* 1993;13:1167-1177.
39. Dimitriadou V, Buzzi MG, Theoharides TC, Moskowitz MA. Ultrastructural evidence for neurogenically mediated changes in blood vessels of the rat dura mater and tongue following antidromic trigeminal stimulation. *Neuroscience.* 1992;48:187-203.
40. Goadsby PH, Edvinsson L, Ekman R. Vasoactive peptide release in the extracerebral circulation of humans during migraine headache. *Ann Neurol.* 1990;28:183-187.
41. Yamamura H, Makick A, Chamberlin NL, Burstein R. Cardiovascular and neuronal responses to head stimulation reflect central sensitization and cutaneous allodynia in a rat model of migraine. *J Neurophysiol.* 1999;81:479-493.
42. Hannerz J. Orbital phlebography and signs of inflammation in episodic and chronic cluster headache. *Headache.* 1991;31:540-542.
43. Afra J, Cecchini AP, Schoenen J. Craniometric measures in cluster headache patients. *Cephalalgia.* 1998;18:143-145.
44. Ekbom K. Patterns of cluster headache with a note on the relations to angina pectoris and peptide ulcer. *Acta Neurol Scand.* 1970;46:225-237.
45. Kudrow L. The cyclic relationship of natural illumination to cluster period frequency. *Cephalgia.* 1987;7:76-78.
46. Strittmater M, Hamann GF, Grauer M, et al. Altered activity of the sympathetic nervous system and changes in the balance of hypophyseal, pituitary and adrenal hormones in patients with cluster headache. *Neuroreport.* 1996;7:1229-1234.
47. May A, Bahra A, Büchel C, et al. First direct evidence for hypothalamic activation in cluster headache attacks. *Lancet.* 1998;352:275-278.
48. Weiller C, May A, Limmroth V, et al. Brain stem activation in spontaneous human migraine attacks. *Nat Med.* 1995;1:658-660.
49. May A, Kaube H, Buchel C, et al. Experimental cranial pain elicited by capsaicin: a PET study. *Pain.* 1998;74:61-66.
50. Jensen R, Rasmussen BK, Pedersen B, Olesen J. Cephalic muscle tenderness and pressure pain threshold in headache. *Pain.* 1993;52:193-199.
51. Langemark M, Olesen J. Pericranial tenderness in tension headache. *Cephalalgia.* 1987;7:249-255.
52. Olesen J. Clinical and pathophysiological observations in migraine and tension-type headache explained by integration of vascular, supraspinal and myofascial inputs. *Pain.* 1991;46:125-132.

Common Headache Syndromes

Sarah E. Vollbracht
Alan M. Rapoport

INTRODUCTION

Headache is one of the most common pain syndromes for which patients consult physicians. Surveys indicate that in any given year, more than 90% of American adults will have some kind of headache or head pain.[1] A wide variety of conditions can present with headache. The first step in treating a patient with a primary complaint of headache is to determine whether there is a primary or a secondary headache disorder. Then it is important to make a specific, accurate diagnosis. Secondary headache disorders have an underlying cause, which can usually be determined, such as infection, eye or jaw dysfunction, tumor, aneurysm, dissection or other vascular problems, meningitis, and trauma. Fortunately, very few headaches are caused by serious organic conditions, and most of them are actually primary headache disorders, idiopathic conditions that are benign and tend to recur. The great majority of patients that present to a physician with bad headaches are diagnosed with migraine. The pathophysiology of primary headache disorders is complex and probably involves, among other things, the activation of the trigeminovascular system, meningeal inflammation, and involvement of the cortex, brainstem, and thalamus (see Chapter 29 for a discussion on the pathophysiology of headaches). Chapter 28 presents the historical features in primary headache syndromes and describes the diagnostic criteria for the three most common primary headache disorders, which are migraine, tension-type headache (TTH), and cluster headache. This chapter discusses the differential diagnosis, diagnostic testing, and management of patients with these common primary headache disorders.

MIGRAINE

Migraine is a chronic neurologic disorder with episodic manifestations. The two most common patterns of migraine are migraine without aura and migraine with aura, formerly called *common migraine* and *classic migraine,* respectively. Migraine prevalence in the United States has remained stable, reported to be 12% in the general population. There is a female predominance; migraine affects approximately 18% of women compared with 6% of men.[2] Migraine can be extremely disabling, with more than 50% of individuals with migraine reporting severe impairment or the need for bed rest during a migraine attack compared with only 7.2% reporting no attack-related disability.[3]

CLINICAL FEATURES

A migraine attack is best looked at as being divided into four phases: the prodrome, the aura, the headache phase, and the postdrome. All four phases are not always present, and no single phase is necessary in order to diagnose migraine in a specific patient.[4,5]

The first phase, or prodrome, consists of various combinations of psychological, neurologic, autonomic, and constitutional symptoms that precede the headache phase of the migraine attack by several hours or even days. The reported prevalence of this phase has been variable, but more than 80% of patients have reported at least one prodromal symptom.[6] Symptoms may include altered mood, irritability, depression or euphoria, fatigue, yawning, excessive sleepiness, food cravings, dizziness, pale face, stiff neck, photophobia, phonophobia, blurry vision, sensitive skin, frequent urination, nausea, excessive thirst, concentration difficulties, speech difficulties, reading or writing difficulties, or other vegetative symptoms. The prodromal phase of a migraine attack indicates that changes in the central nervous system (CNS), possibly involving the hypothalamus and altered dopamine regulation, begin well before the onset of the headache phase. Prodromal symptoms are variable among individuals but are often consistent within the same individual, and astute individuals with migraine can predict with relative accuracy that a migraine attack has begun when these symptoms are present.[6–8] Many physicians are unaware of these symptoms if they do not ask about them, and the patient often does not mention them.

The second phase of migraine is the aura, which consists of either visual or sensory phenomena (the two most common aura symptoms), or motor weakness, incoordination, or dysphasic symptoms (e.g., word-finding difficulties). As many as 38% of patients with migraine may experience aura with at least some of their attacks, but migraine with aura remains infrequent compared with migraine without aura. Approximately 60% to 80% of patients who experience migraine with aura also experience migraine without aura, but more than one-third of patients report migraine headache attacks exclusively with aura. In patients reporting aura, however, aura occurs with an average of only 20% of migraine headache attacks. The aura symptoms usually precede the headache phase of the migraine attack, but they occasionally occur simultaneously and rarely after the headache. Up to one-third of patients have experienced aura without headache at some point.[9,10] The occurrence of aura without headache becomes more common as individuals with migraine grow older than 50 years of age.

The aura symptoms appear gradually over 5 to 20 minutes and usually last less than 60 minutes, subsiding just before the onset of the headache phase, which usually occurs within 30 minutes. A typical aura lasts about 20 minutes and is followed fairly quickly by headache. Visual aura is by far the most common, occurring in more than 90% of patients with aura. It is often the only aura symptom, and nonvisual aura symptoms are rarely present without the presence of a visual aura, suggesting that the occipital cortex is especially susceptible to cortical-spreading depression. The visual aura is often described as a series of both positive and negative phenomena. One commonly described aura begins as a flickering, zig-zag line beginning in the center of the visual field and enlarging as it migrates toward the periphery in a hemianopic distribution, often leaving a scotoma in its wake. Many other positive and negative symptoms occur, including seeing small dots that move, flashes of light, blind spots, homonymous hemianopsias, and various types of distortion of vision. Sensory auras in the form of paresthesias are the second most common type of aura symptom, occurring in approximately one-third of patients with aura. The typical sensory aura is unilateral, beginning in the hand and moving up the arm to affect the face and tongue in a cheiro-oral or digitolingual distribution. The leg is rarely but sometimes involved in sensory auras. As with visual aura, positive phenomena (paresthesias) are often followed by negative phenomena (numbness). Motor symptoms have been reported in up to 18% of patients and almost always occur in association with both visual and sensory auras. True weakness, however, is rare, and it is essential not to confuse sensory ataxia with weakness, an error that has both diagnostic and therapeutic implications. The most common motor aura is strictly unilateral weakness of the hand and arm. Unlike other aura symptoms, which usually last less than 60 minutes, motor auras are often prolonged, lasting a mean of 13 hours. Aphasic auras can take the form of paraphasia, impaired production of language, or impaired comprehension of language. Aphasic aura has been reported to occur in approximately 20% of patients[4,5,9–13]

When examining a patient who has recently experienced only one or two such attacks for the first time, the clinician must determine whether these focal neurologic symptoms represent migrainous aura or are manifestations of a transient ischemic attack (TIA) or even a focal sensory seizure. Passage of time, repeated identical attacks, and diagnostic testing may be required to obtain certainty, but certain features are more typical of migraine aura. First, whereas visual and sensory symptoms of TIA and seizures usually develop abruptly, a migrainous aura gradually progresses over 5 to 20 minutes. Second, migraine aura is characterized by a combination of both negative and positive symptoms; the individual with migraine experiences a visual scotoma or hole in the vision (negative symptoms) *and* dazzling, glimmering, scintillating lights (positive symptoms). The sensory aura of migraine usually consists of numbness (negative symptoms) *and* tingling or paresthesias (positive symptoms). TIA, such as amaurosis fugax or hemianopic scotoma, usually manifests as a black or blank negative visual loss.

Sometimes, especially in those older than 50 years of age, the visual aura occurs repeatedly without any headache. C.M. Fisher described these features as "late life migraine accompaniments."[14] Sometimes these patients experienced more typical migraine in youth, with the migraine subsiding for many years only to recur as migraine aura without headache in later life. In this setting, the clinician may be more secure in the diagnosis. However, these late-life migraine accompaniments often develop with no previous history of migraine. Patients with new late-life migraine symptoms must be carefully evaluated to rule out cerebrovascular disease, structural hemispheric disease, or even retinal detachments.

The aura phase is usually, although not always, followed by the headache phase, which is the third phase of the migraine attack and usually the most dramatic. It is the headache phase of migraine for which most patients consult a physician. The International Classification of Headache Disorders, Third Edition (beta version) (ICHD-3 beta) defines a migraine attack as lasting from 4 to 72 hours and characterized by at least two of the following four pain characteristics: unilateral location, throbbing quality, moderate or severe in intensity, and aggravated by or causing avoidance of routine physical activity. Additionally, either nausea or vomiting or both photophobia and phonophobia must be present.[15] It is important to remember that these strict criteria were designed chiefly for purposes of finding a uniform population of migraine patients to be entered into investigational drug trials and epidemiologic studies. The experienced clinician uses the ICHD-3 beta as a guide but is not rigidly bound by them. Often a patient may be missing one or more component of the ICHD-3 beta criteria (**Table 30-1**), at which time a diagnosis of probable or possible migraine can be made. Furthermore, both migraine and TTH are very common, and when patients report symptoms of both, there may be overlapping features that may make it difficult to differentiate between probable migraine and episodic or chronic TTH.

The headache of migraine is unilateral in 60% of cases and usually alternates sides from one attack to the next.[5] Often, patients state that the headache is always on one side but when pressed recall that rarely, perhaps 10% of the time, the headache occurs on the opposite side. This alternating hemicrania, however infrequent, makes the clinician more secure in the diagnosis of migraine. Some individuals with migraine report that the headache is bilateral but worse on one side. Others report that an attack may start on one side and subsequently spread to other areas of the head or neck to become more generalized. The headache usually builds over a period of 30 minutes to several hours but may occur with sudden intensity, sometimes resembling a thunderclap headache. Although possibly attributed to migraine, a thunderclap headache must always be thoroughly investigated because an underlying secondary cause is often found. Although the pain of migraine is usually moderate to severe, many patients report milder headaches, which they refer to as "sinus headaches" or "regular headaches" and that, in reality, are probably milder migraine attacks. A migraine attack may occur at any time of day but happens most often in the morning hours between 5 AM and noon.[5,16]

Contributing to the disability of a migraine attack are the associated features that accompany the pain of the headache phase. The ICHD-3 beta mandates that either nausea or vomiting or both light and sound sensitivity be present, but other features are also frequently present. The individual with migraine frequently reports a decreased appetite or just a queasy feeling but sometimes may report cravings for specific foods. Other gastrointestinal (GI) disturbances, such as diarrhea, constipation, and gastroparesis, may occur. Gastroparesis is common amongst individuals with migraine and leads to lack of absorption of oral medications from the small bowel, which may prevent optimal treatment

TABLE 30-1 International Classification of Headache Disorders, Third (beta version), Diagnostic Criteria for Migraine Without Aura

A. At least five attacks fulfilling criteria B–D
B. Headache attacks lasting 4–72 hours (untreated or unsuccessfully treated)
C. Headache has at least two of the following four characteristics:
   a. Unilateral location
   b. Pulsating quality
   c. Moderate or severe pain intensity
   d. Aggravation by or causing avoidance of routine physical activity
D. During headache at least one of the following:
   a. Nausea and/or vomiting
   b. Photophobia and phonophobia
E. Not better accounted for by another ICHD-3 diagnosis

by tablet. In addition to light and sound sensitivity, the individual with migraine is often especially sensitive to smells. Many patients report that they feel lightheaded or even vertiginous during an attack or even between attacks. Autonomic symptoms may occur, even unilaterally, such as red eyes and tearing. These autonomic symptoms are more common in cluster headache, invariably unilateral and often diagnostic. Systemic symptoms such as blurred vision, nasal congestion, facial pallor or redness, sweating, sensations of heat or cold, fluid retention, and increased urination have also been reported. There may be neck or sinus pain and discomfort. The individual with migraine is often unable to brush or comb his or her hair and must remove any hats, scarves, earrings, and necklaces and change into loose clothing because of tenderness of the scalp, neck, or limbs due to the allodynia caused by central sensitization. Prodromal symptoms can continue and may even become more prominent in the headache phase of the attack.[4,5,7,17,18]

The duration of a headache attack is approximately 4 to 72 hours in adults when untreated or ineffectively treated. It typically lasts 12 to 36 hours. Sleep, even a brief nap of 1 or 2 hours, is the most common natural method of headache resolution, but biofeedback training and relaxation exercises may train the patient in other beneficial techniques that may help terminate an attack. Pharmacologic treatment, briefly discussed later in this chapter and in more detail in Chapter 33, is the most common medical treatment to terminate an acute migraine attack.

The fourth and final phase of a migraine attack is the postdrome. This phase has been reported in up to 94% of patients, but the symptoms have not been widely studied.[19] Postdromal symptoms may last from several hours to approximately 24 hours or even longer in some patients and range from feeling drained or exhausted to an unusual sense of elation or euphoria. Patients may have trouble functioning, reading, speaking, and thinking. The headache is usually milder but may still be present. Symptoms that occur during the prodromal phase and headache phase of the attack often continue into the postdrome.[7]

DIFFERENTIAL DIAGNOSIS

Clinicians must always be aware of so-called migraine mimics, which are paroxysmal headaches caused by arteriovenous malformations, pheochromocytoma, repeated exposure to carbon monoxide, transient increased spinal fluid pressure resulting from a colloid cyst of the third ventricle, adult-onset of headaches caused by type I or II Arnold-Chiari malformations, or other structural brain disease. In the elderly, especially women older than 55 years with unilateral headaches and tender temples, temporal arteritis (giant cell arteritis) must always be considered. Primary CNS angiitis may manifest as frequent headaches before other symptoms, such as encephalopathy, seizures, or infarctions, occur as a result of the vasculitis.

When evaluating a patient with headaches, it is essential to look for so-called red flags, or danger signals that warn the clinician that a headache may be more serious than migraine (**Table 30-2**).[1,20] The problem is that some of these red flags are prominent symptoms of migraine and can be difficult to differentiate:

1. Headache that is changing or different from previous headaches may herald a brain tumor superimposed on a long-standing primary headache disorder, such as migraine or TTH.
2. Headache with progressive worsening over 24 hours or several days suggests a mass lesion or infectious disease such as meningitis, abscess, subdural or intracerebral hematoma, or vasculitis.
3. Headache precipitated by exertion, bending over, coughing, or sneezing, may result from transient blockage of cerebrospinal fluid (CSF) flow or increased intracranial pressure.
4. Sudden explosive onset of severe headache spontaneously or during exercise or sexual activity can occur with subarachnoid hemorrhage (SAH) or with primary exercise headache, primary headache associated with sexual activity, or primary thunderclap headache. A thunderclap headache reaches maximum intensity within seconds and can be attributable to SAH, arterial dissection, cerebral venous occlusion, and reversible cerebral vasoconstriction syndrome (RCVS).
5. Vomiting may result from a brain tumor or other mass lesion with increased ICP.
6. Early morning headache can occur with obstructive sleep apnea, medication overuse, and hypertension.
7. Any abnormal physical or neurologic finding must be considered suspect: fever, stiff neck, rash, lymphadenopathy, proximal leg weakness suggestive of polymyalgia rheumatica, scalp tenderness, altered sensorium, or focal neurologic signs other than typical visual or sensory aura.
8. Headache in a patient with papilledema may suggest increased intracranial pressure (ICP) related to idiopathic intracranial hypertension, cerebral venous sinus thrombosis, or intracranial mass lesion.
9. New onset of a headache during pregnancy or postpartum may suggest headache secondary to cerebrovascular disease or cerebral venous sinus thrombosis.
10. Headache in a patient with cancer, HIV, or other systemic illness may indicate metastatic disease, a structural lesion, or CNS infection such as meningitis or encephalitis.
11. Headache with an onset after the age of 55 years may suggest temporal arteritis, other cerebrovascular disease, glaucoma, or structural brain disease.

A young, healthy patient with a textbook history of migraine and a normal physical and neurologic examination seldom requires diagnostic investigation. It is often done to rule out secondary disorders. If, however, the patient fails to respond as expected to treatment efforts, diagnostic testing may be wise.

Unsuspected granulomatous inflammations, such as sarcoidosis; meningeal malignancy; and cryptococcal, tuberculous, or Lyme meningitis, can be diagnosed only by CSF examination. Elevated or reduced spinal fluid pressure may confirm the diagnosis of pseudotumor cerebri or spontaneous intracranial hypotension, respectively. Low CSF pressure can usually be noticed on MRI scans with and without gadolinium as the meninges light up with contrast and other structural changes can be seen.

For structural brain lesions, magnetic resonance imaging (MRI) is much more sensitive than computed tomography (CT) scanning and is always preferable unless there is a contraindication to MRI or if bone windows are desired. Whereas CT scanning is more sensitive for demonstrating SAH in the first 24 hours, MRI becomes more sensitive after 48 hours. Unenhanced CT scans made within 24 hours of SAH have a sensitivity of 98%, falling to only 50% within 1 week, stressing the importance of immediate neuroimaging in cases of suspected SAH.[21] If a small SAH, a so-called sentinel bleed, is being considered, CSF examination is essential even when results of the CT are normal. The presence of fresh blood or xanthochromia should prompt angiography. Cerebral

TABLE 30-2 Summary of Red Flags in the Diagnosis of Migraine

- Change in headache pattern
- Headache with progressive worsening over 24 hours or several days
- Headache triggered by exertion, bending over, coughing, or sneezing
- Sudden explosive onset headache
- Headache associated with vomiting
- Early morning headache
- Abnormal physical or neurologic examination findings or abnormal vital signs
- Headache in a patient with papilledema
- New onset headache during pregnancy of postpartum
- Headache in the immunocompromised patient (e.g., cancer, HIV/AIDS)
- Headache onset after age 55 years

angiography is also required if primary CNS granulomatous angiitis is suspected. Magnetic resonance angiography is sensitive for identifying unruptured aneurysms as small as 3 to 4 mm, and conventional angiography would be definitive.[22] CT angiography is another noninvasive technique for detecting intracranial aneurysms.

There is a high familial incidence of aneurysms; unsuspected asymptomatic intracranial aneurysms were found in 9% of 396 persons having a first-degree relative with an aneurysm.[22] A careful family history is, therefore, important if a warning leak is suspected. If two first-degree relatives of a patient have aneurysms, then the patient should be investigated.

As discussed earlier, sinus pressure and pain can be symptoms associated with the headache phase of a migraine attack. Often patients may believe that this represents "sinus headaches" rather than migraine. A thorough history in this case is important, and recurrent benign headaches, even if they involve pain and discomfort over the sinuses or nasal congestion, most likely represent migraine or TTH rather than acute sinusitis or sinus disease. Sometimes radiography is needed to settle the issue and CT scanning of the sinuses is more sensitive than sinus radiography or MRI in diagnosing acute sinusitis.

Clinicians must not omit dental disease or jaw dysfunction as a cause of head or facial pain or localized eye disease, such as glaucoma, which can cause unilateral orbital pain that mimics migraine. Cervical spine disease or lesions at the foramen magnum may cause suboccipital pain, and plain radiography or other imaging modalities (CT or MRI) may be considered.

Certain medications, such as the nonsteroidal anti-inflammatory drug (NSAID) indomethacin, estrogen and estrogen withdrawal, progestins, selective serotonin reuptake inhibitors (SSRIs), certain calcium channel blockers, or certain anticonvulsants, may cause headaches (**Table 30-3**). Because these drugs are often used to treat headaches, sorting out the diagnosis may be difficult, and the temporal pattern of headache development or progression in relation to when the drug in question was initiated is essential in diagnosing a headache secondary to a medication.

MANAGEMENT

The first step in treating a patient with migraine or any other medical condition is to establish an accurate diagnosis. The diagnosis must be conveyed to the patient who, very often, is fearful of a tumor or aneurysm or may erroneously believe he or she has a chronic sinus or psychiatric condition. Many of these patients have been discouraged in the past by physicians who have ignored their complaints of headache. Headache is a common complaint, and many busy physicians are reluctant to take the time or may not have the time required to obtain an adequate headache history, or they may view headache as being a result of nervousness or stress. Busy physicians may choose to direct the brief office visit at management of hypertension, diabetes, or arthritis even if the patient is more troubled by headache.

Headache treatment begins with educating patients about the nature of migraine and setting realistic expectations. Patients should be reassured that migraine is a biological disorder, usually with a hereditary predisposition, that is caused by altered brain biochemistry with secondary vascular, peripheral nervous system, and CNS changes. Patients need to be told that although migraine cannot be cured, treatments are available that can control and reduce the pain and associated symptoms that lead to the severe disability of a migraine attack. Patients often are relieved that at last they have found a physician who is knowledgeable about headaches and who expresses an interest in helping them. Sometimes it is helpful to have the spouse or another family member present and explain that headaches in general, and migraine in particular, are often provoked by hormonal changes, stress, certain food triggers, missing meals, irregular sleep patterns, travel, or specific environmental changes. Visual and sensory stimuli, such as bright lights, excessive noise, cigarette smoke, certain perfumes or smells, or other stimuli, may also act as migraine triggers.[23–27] Some medications, both over-the-counter (OTC) and prescription drugs, can precipitate headache (Table 30-3).[4,28,29] There is also an underlying predisposition for people with migraine to have a biochemical comorbidity of depression, anxiety, or other psychiatric problem.[2]

It is vital to consider behavioral medicine therapies for most patients, whether they think they need it or not (**Table 30-4**). For many patients, this can be more helpful than medication and there are no adverse effects.

In a specialty headache practice, there is usually a nurse, nurse practitioner, or physician's assistant who instructs the patient to keep a headache calendar, watch for repeated food or environmental triggers, and record the amount of medication taken and response to treatment. Having this accurate record enables the physician to alter pharmacologic treatment depending on response. The power of the written word cannot be overemphasized, and publications are available that describe and explain many of these issues for individuals with migraine. Information is available free of charge from the American Headache Society (www.americanheadachesociety.org), American Council for Headache Education (www.achenet.org), National Headache Foundation (www.headaches.org), American Migraine Foundation (www.americanmigrainefoundation.org), Headache Cooperative of New England (www.hacoop.org), ProMyHealth (www.promyhealth.org),

TABLE 30-3 Incomplete List of Commonly Used Medications Associated with Headache

Antibiotics and antimalarials	Tetracyclines, trimethoprim–sulfamethoxazole, metronidazole, nitrofurantoin, rifampin, isoniazid, griseofulvin, amphotericin, linezolid, chloroquine, mefloquine, ethionamide, ampicillin, penicillin, amoxicillin, ciprofloxacin, cephalosporins
Antiplatelet agents	Dipyridamole
Asthmatic agents	Aminophylline, theophylline, pseudoephedrine, terbutaline, zafirlukast
Cardiovascular agents	Nitroglycerin, isosorbide dinitrate, hydralazine, nifedipine, amiodarone, digoxin, quinidine, niacin
CNS agents	Alcohol, barbiturates, benzodiazepines, caffeine, methylphenidate, amantadine, levodopa, bromocriptine, pramipexole, SSRIs, trazodone, lithium, carbamazepine
Endocrinologic agents	Octreotide, thyroxine
GI agents	Cimetidine, ranitidine, famotidine, omeprazole, lansoprazole
Hematologic, oncologic, or immunosuppressant agents	Erythropoietin, tamoxifen, cyclosporine, tacrolimus, sirolimus, everolimus, cytarabine, methotrexate, retinoic acid, corticosteroids, diaziquone, OKT3
Immunologic agents	Interferons, intravenous immunoglobulin, alemtuzumab
NSAIDs	Indomethacin, diclofenac, piroxicam, ibuprofen, naproxen, ketoprofen, salicylates
Reproductive agents	Estrogens, progesterones, oral contraceptives, sildenafil, vardenafil, tadalafil
Vitamins	Vitamin A, isotretinoin
Miscellaneous	Allopurinol, beta-human chorionic gonadotrophic hormone, growth hormone, anabolic steroids

CNS, central nervous system; GI, gastrointestinal; NSAID, nonsteroidal anti-inflammatory drug; SSRI, selective serotonin reuptake inhibitor.

TABLE 30-4 Behavioral Therapies for Migraine with Grade A Evidence

- Relaxation training
- Thermal biofeedback combined with relaxation training
- Electromyographic biofeedback
- Cognitive-behavioral therapy

Canadian Headache Society (headachenetwork.ca), and the Headache Cooperative of the Pacific (www.hcop.com).

Some headache patients express a desire to be treated without "drugs," and others prefer to take natural substances, such as herbal or vitamin supplements. Biofeedback training can be beneficial in conjunction with or without medication.[30,31] Biofeedback training teaches relaxation skills as part of overall headache management. Patients learn to be aware of skeletal muscle status and hand temperature and learn how to relax general and specific muscle contraction and tension, breathing techniques, and how to enhance blood flow to the peripheral vessels producing hand warming. With practice, patients can alter autonomic nervous function to produce measurable temperature changes in the hands. These exercises may reduce afferent sensory volleys from peripheral muscular pain and modulate sensory impulses ascending through cervical segments into the trigeminal nerve complex in the brainstem.

Cognitive behavioral therapy and relaxation techniques can help patients deal with the headache condition in a positive way.[31] If the patient spontaneously asks about stress or if he or she recognizes anxiety or depression as significant problems, consultation with a behavioral psychologist may be very helpful.

Physical therapy with heat or cold applications, ultrasonography, myofascial release, a structured exercise program, and massage therapy are beneficial for many patients. Attention to nutrition and observing for food triggers, especially alcohol, are important. The patient's headache diary can be especially useful in this aspect because the patient can identify food triggers and as a result can avoid the specific foods that may trigger a migraine attack. Correcting irregular eating and sleeping habits may be beneficial.

Some of these measures, such as keeping an accurate headache calendar, practicing biofeedback exercises, daily exercise, and paying attention to diet and lifestyle, have the added benefit of insisting that the patient play an active role in the treatment program. Many patients express a sense of empowerment and satisfaction that they are contributing to the management of their headache disorder and gaining more control over their lives and the condition.

PHARMACOTHERAPY

The U.S. Headache Consortium Guidelines, published in 2000, recognize that migraine is a heterogeneous disorder and that treatment must be tailored to the individual patient.[32] A treatment plan must take into consideration the frequency, severity, and duration of attacks; the associated symptoms; and the degree of disability that the patient experiences. Pharmacotherapy may be divided into three types: (1) acute treatment with nonspecific analgesics; (2) acute treatment with migraine-specific agents that have pharmacologic affinity to bind to certain serotonin and other receptors and alter the neurochemical, inflammatory, and vascular processes of migraine; and (3) the daily use of preventive medications.

Nonspecific analgesics that may be useful for patients with mild to moderate migraine headaches include simple analgesics, such as aspirin and acetaminophen, NSAIDs in low doses (e.g., naproxen sodium), and combination analgesics (e.g., acetaminophen, aspirin, and caffeine). The butalbital-containing combination analgesics, including Fioricet and Fiorinal, are prescription medications that may be beneficial in those with migraine if taken early, but these compounds have a strong potential to cause dependency and analgesic overuse (rebound) headache if taken too frequently (see later discussion). They are not approved for migraine, only for TTH, but they can work and are probably safe to take for migraine attacks that occur three or four times a month or less. Analgesic overuse headache is more likely related to the frequency of dosing of these drugs rather than to the total number of doses that may be taken safely in a day or week. One of the reasons that patients like the butalbital-containing medications is that they treat anxiety as well as pain and make patients feel better in addition to relieving pain. This results in patients taking them more frequently than the number of headache days per month. This leads to dependency and overuse syndromes, and they start losing their effectiveness.

TABLE 30-5 2000 U.S. Headache Consortium Guidelines for the Acute Care of a Migraine Attack

- NSAIDS, simple analgesics, or combination analgesics containing caffeine are appropriate first-line therapy for mild to moderate migraine attacks and for severe attacks that have previously responded to such therapies.
- Migraine-specific medications are appropriate first-line therapy for moderate to severe migraine attacks and for migraine attacks of any severity that do not respond to NSAIDs or combination analgesics.
- Consider a non-oral route of administration if significant nausea or vomiting is present or if the patient fails two oral triptans.

NSAID, nonsteroidal anti-inflammatory drug.

Treatment of acute migraine attacks was revolutionized in the United States in 1993 with the introduction of sumatriptan. There are currently seven triptans approved by the U.S. Food and Drug Administration (FDA). Each of them—sumatriptan, zolmitriptan, naratriptan, rizatriptan, almotriptan, eletriptan, and frovatriptan—can be good therapeutic options. All seven are available in tablet formulation, and rizatriptan and zolmitriptan are also available as orally dissolving tablets (ODT), zolmitriptan and sumatriptan are also available in nasal spray formulation, and sumatriptan is available as a subcutaneous injection (both with a needle and in a needle-free formulation). An iontophoretic transdermal delivery system of symatriptan has been FDA approved, but is not yet available. Sumatriptan also comes in a fixed-dose combination with naproxen sodium under the name Treximet. Dihydroergotamine (DHE) has been available since 1945 as an injection; a nasal spray formulation, Migranal NS, was introduced in 1997. An inhaled formulation of DHE has had a successful phase 3 trial, but issues with the manufacturing of the inhaler has delayed FDA approval.[33]

The 2000 U.S. Headache Consortium Guidelines (**Table 30-5**) consider NSAIDs and combination analgesics that contain caffeine reasonable choices for mild to moderate migraine attacks or for severe migraine attacks that have responded to such agents in the past. Migraine-specific medications such as triptans and ergots such as ergotamine tartrate and DHE are considered appropriate first-line therapy for patients with moderate to severe intensity migraine attacks and for patients who do not respond to nonspecific analgesics.[34,35] One other medication that is migraine specific and approved by the FDA only for acute treatment of migraine with and without aura is Cambia (diclofenac potassium for solution, 50 mg). It probably works both peripherally and centrally as an anti-inflammatory, with a more rapid onset of action than the same medication in a tablet formulation.[36]

All of these migraine specific drugs, except Cambia, are effective because of their specific pharmacologic affinity to bind to serotonin (5-HT) and other receptors and interrupt the neurochemical, inflammatory, and vascular changes that occur in migraine. It is thought that triptans work on both peripheral and central mechanisms by binding to 5-HT_{1B} receptors on vascular smooth muscle cells causing cranial vasoconstriction and binding to 5-HT_{1D} receptors on the presynaptic trigeminovascular nerve terminals in the meninges and within the trigeminal nucleus caudalis in the pons or dorsal horn in the spinal cord. This prevents the release of vasoactive peptides from the perivascular trigeminal neurons peripherally and the presynaptic nerve terminal at the synapse of the first- and second-order neurons in the trigeminal nucleus caudalis in the pons. Peripherally, this prevents mast cell degranulation, neurogenic inflammation, and vasodilation and centrally prevents increased transmission of pain signals heading toward the third-order neurons in the thalamus. This latter action may prevent central sensitization that begins in the brainstem. Through unknown mechanisms, it is theorized that triptans may also facilitate descending pain inhibitory systems, especially in the periaqueductal gray area and rostral ventromedial medulla.[37]

Although the triptans are more similar than different, there are differences in lipophilicity, metabolism, route of administration, and differential therapeutic response of patients. Differences in lipophilicity leads to differential ability to cross the blood–brain barrier. The slight

TABLE 30-6 Pharmacologic Properties of Triptans

Drug	Available Formulations	Bioavailability	Tmax	Half-life	Metabolism	Maximum Daily Dose
Almotriptan (Axert)	Tablet: 6.25 and 12.5 mg	80%	1.4–3.8 h	3.2–3.7 h	Hepatic: P450 CYP3A4 and CYP2D6 and monoamine oxidase (MAO)-mediated	25 mg
Eletriptan (Relpax)	Tablet: 20 and 40 mg	50%	1–2 h	3.6–5.5 h	Hepatic: P450 CYP3A4	80 mg
Frovatriptan (Frova)	Tablet: 2.5 mg	24–30%	2–4 h	26 h	Hepatic: P450 CYP1A2	7.5 mg
Naratriptan (Amerge)	Tablet: 1 and 2.5 mg	63% (men) 74% (women)	2–3 h	5–6.3 h	Hepatic: P450	5 mg
Rizatriptan (Maxalt)	Tablet: 5 and 10 mg Orally dissolving tablet (ODT): 5 and 10 mg	45%	Tablet: 1.2 h ODT: 1.6–2.5 h	2 h	Hepatic: monoamine oxidase-A	30 mg
Sumatriptan (Imitrex)	Tablet: 25, 50, and 100 mg Nasal Spray (NS): 5 and 20 mg Subcutaneous (SC) injection: 4 and 6 mg	Oral: 14% for 50 mg tablet SC: 97%	Tablet: 2–2.5 h NS: 1 h SC: 5–20 min	Tablet: 2 h NS: 2 h SC: 2 h	Hepatic: monoamine oxidase-A	Tablet: 200 mg NS: 40 mg SC: 12 mg
Zolmitriptan (Zomig)	Tablet: 2.5 and 5 mg Orally dissolving tablet (ODT): 2.5 and 5 mg Nasal Spray (NS): 5 mg	40–48%	Tablet: 2 h ZMT: 3.3 h NS: 4 h	Tablet: 2.71–3 h ZMT: 2.5–3 h NS: 2.82 h	Hepatic: monoamine oxidase-A	Oral: 10 mg NS: 10 mg

molecular differences of each triptan confer different pharmacologic properties, such as bioavailability, time to peak concentration, onset of action, metabolic half-life, and excretion, among others (**Table 30-6**).[37,38] Sumitriptan, zolmitriptan, and rizatriptan are metabolized by the enzyme monoamine oxidase-A (MAO-A); therefore, these drugs are contraindicated in patients taking MAO inhibitors or within 2 weeks of their discontinuation. The other four triptans and DHE are not contraindicated with MAO inhibitors. Almotriptan and eletriptan are metabolized by the hepatic enzyme CYP3A4, and thus a reduction in dose of almotriptan to 6.25 mg when used concurrently with drugs that are potent CYP3A4 enzyme inhibitors is appropriate. Eletriptan should not be used concurrently with such drugs because metabolism may be inhibited, resulting in higher blood levels and an increased risk of adverse effects. Propranolol inhibits the metabolism of rizatriptan, and a dose reduction to 5 mg is recommended for patients taking propranolol. Other beta-blockers are not problematic. Of note, sumatriptan contains a sulfonamide group and should not be used in patients with definite sulfa allergies. Almotriptan contains a sulfonyl group, and although structurally different from a sulfonamide, caution should be exercised when prescribing almotriptan to patients with sulfa allergies. Other triptan formulations do not contain a sulfa group.[37,38]

All of the triptans share similar adverse effect profiles. Most effects are mild and transient; however, the primary concern with this class of drugs, as well as with DHE, is that these compounds can cause coronary vasoconstriction. A few serious and life-threatening cardiac events have been reported in patients using triptans, and caution should be exercised in prescribing any of the triptans or DHE for patients with cardiac risk factors. Contraindications to triptan use include known coronary artery disease, Printzmental's angina, history of stroke or myocardial infarction, peripheral vascular disease, uncontrolled high blood pressure, and history of hemiplegic migraine or migraine with brainstem aura (**Table 30-7**). In vitro studies of isolated human coronary artery segments demonstrate that these drugs are unlikely to cause myocardial ischemia at therapeutic concentrations in healthy subjects,[39] and they are safe for young, otherwise healthy patients with migraine. The triptans and DHE have improved the lives of people formerly disabled who have had migraine pain several times a month. Because of the pharmacologic and individual patient genetic differences, one triptan may be very helpful to a patient even if treatment with another triptan has failed.

Most headache specialists, as well as the U.S. Headache Consortium Guidelines, recommend stratified care in the treatment of acute migraine attacks. This method requires the clinician to choose treatment depending on headache severity and patient need. It allows the patient to use analgesics, low-dose NSAIDs, or combination medications for milder migraine attacks but migraine-specific therapy, such as triptans, ergots, or Cambia to treat moderate to severe migraine attacks. It also calls for migraine-specific therapy if the patient has been poorly responsive to analgesics, low-dose NSAIDs, or combination therapy in the treatment of prior attacks, even if those attacks are of mild to moderate severity. An alternative approach, which we dislike but may be required by managed care plans attempting to save money, is step care. Step care, in contrast to stratified care, treats all migraine attacks, regardless of severity, with simple analgesics or low-dose NSAIDs as first-line therapy and reserves triptans, ergots, and Cambia for patients whose headaches do not respond to these measures or to combination medications. Most headache specialists use stratified care, which has been proven to be not only more cost effective than step care but also is more likely to improve headache response, pain-free response, and duration of disability.[34,40]

Back-up treatment consists of repeating the medication used at the start of the migraine attack 2 hours after the first dose. This is sometimes helpful. Rescue treatment refers to using analgesics including potent opioid analgesia or sedatives for an acute attack when specific acute care treatment and back-up treatment has failed. We do not use opiates as back-up, but rather dexamethasone 4mg, DHE, or a sedating antiemetic or rare dose of a benzodiazepine. Markley provides a thorough review of the appropriate use of opioid analgesics and recommends sound guidelines for the use of these drugs.[41] We agree that it is unfair and

TABLE 30-7 Contraindications to Triptan Use

- Coronary artery disease
- Printzmental's angina
- History of stroke
- History of myocardial infarction
- Peripheral vascular disease
- Uncontrolled high blood pressure
- History of hemiplegic or migraine with brainstem aura

possibly unethical to deny patients with intractable pain effective analgesia; however, it may be the most appropriate treatment. Many patients who "require" opiates for their headache end up developing medication-overuse headaches (MOHs), dependency, and a worsening of their headache syndrome. Not starting down that path will prevent such results. Clinicians must assume the responsibility to accurately monitor patient responses to all medication, especially ones that produce dependency. Again, we emphasize the importance of having the patient keep an accurate headache calendar, recording the number, duration, and intensity of headaches and number of and response to acute care medications, including opioids. Keeping track of what medicine is prescribed and ensuring that the patient obtains strong medications from only one prescriber is essential. The use of headache calendars and patient education helps to guard against MOH, which can be brought about by use of almost any acute medications more than 2 to 3 days per week.

Preventive medications should be prescribed daily for individuals with migraine who have frequent attacks and for those who become disabled for 24 hours or more even once or twice per month. Consensus guidelines differ between the U.S. and their European counterparts. The U.S. Headache Consortium recommends starting preventive medication when a patient has six or more headache days per month regardless of impairment, four or more headache days per month with at least some impairment, or three or more headache days per month with severe impairment or requiring bed rest. Additionally, the guidelines recommend considering preventive therapy if a patient has from 4 or 5 migraine days per month with no impairment, 3 migraine days per month with some impairment, and 2 migraine days per month with severe impairment. The guidelines state that prevention is not indicated if there are fewer than 4 headache days per month and no impairment or in patients with less than or equal to 1 headache day per month regardless of impairment.[3] European guidelines, on the other hand, recommend preventive therapy if a patient has two or more attacks per month.[42] Given the differences in U.S. and European guidelines, the importance of treating the individual patient cannot be overemphasized, and patient preference plays a major role in the decision on whether to initiate preventive therapy as well as what type of preventive therapy to use. Only the patient can determine if he or she wishes to take daily preventive medication after hearing the pros and cons and having a discussion with the health care provider.

Some patients express concerns about adverse events or habituation, and clinicians must always monitor continuous medication use in young women of childbearing potential and caution them of potential harm to the fetus. Patients who are reluctant to take daily medication should be reassured that the drug can be discontinued if they experience any adverse reactions or if their migraine symptoms are not reduced after a trial period. We explain that we begin with a low dose, which can gradually be increased to reduce the risk of adverse effects. The patients must be told that at least 4 to 6 weeks of treatment at a therapeutic dose should elapse before deciding on effectiveness. Patients also often ask if they will have to take these medications for the rest of their lives. They should be reassured that migraine is a dynamic disease and that the treatment plan will be constantly reassessed. When the patient is well controlled for 6 months to 1 year, it is reasonable to begin to slowly taper medications with the goal of maintaining the patient on the lowest possible therapeutic dose of preventives or none at all. The most commonly used preventive medications are listed in **Table 30-8**. The exact mechanism of action of these medications is not always known, but a likely common mechanism may be the suppression of cortical-spreading depression.[43]

The choice of preventive medicine should be determined by considering clinical effectiveness, side effect profile, an understanding of previously effective or ineffective treatment trials, the patient's overall medical condition, and especially any comorbid illnesses. For example, a beta-blocker would be a good choice if the patient has mild untreated hypertension, has coexisting essential tremor, or is nervous and excitable. On the other hand, beta-blockers should be avoided if the patient has asthma or depression or is taking other vasoactive antihypertensive drugs. Tricyclic antidepressants (TCAs) might be especially helpful for patients who have sleep disturbance, depression, or loss of appetite.

TABLE 30-8 Common Preventive Therapies in Migraine

Beta-blockers	Propranolol Timolol Nadolol Metoprolol Atenolol
Calcium channel blockers	Verapamil Flunarizine (not available in the United States)
ACE inhibitors and ARBs	Lisinopril Candesartan Cilexetil
Antidepressants	Amitriptyline Nortriptyline Doxepin Venlafaxine
Anticonvulsants	Topiramate Valproate and divalproex sodium Gabapentin
Serotonin agonists	Methysergide (not available in the United States) Methylergonovine maleate Cyproheptadine
Nutraceuticals	Petasites (concern for potential liver toxicity) Riboflavin Coenzyme Q10 Magnesium
Other	Botulinum toxin type A (U.S. FDA approved only for chronic migraine)

ACE, angiotensin-converting enzyme; ARB, angiotensin receptor blockers; FDA, Food and Drug Administration.

Divalproex sodium might be the drug of choice for migraine patients who have obsessive-compulsive traits or bipolar disorder or who have had seizures in the past; however, this drug should be avoided if the patient has known liver or pancreatic disease and in general should be avoided in young women of childbearing potential given its known risk of teratogenicity. The pharmacologic treatment of headache is discussed in more detail in Chapter 33.

TENSION-TYPE HEADACHE

Tension-type headache is the most common primary headache disorder with a lifetime prevalence reported to be as high as 89.4%, suggesting that most people will experience this headache type at some time in their lifetime.[44] Similar to migraine, TTH is more common in women than in men. The age of onset is between 20 and 30 years, and the peak prevalence is between 30 and 39 years for both sexes.[4] Before the publication of the original International Headache Society (HIS) criteria in 1988 and its subsequent revisions, the ICHD-2 in 2004 and the ICHD-3 beta in 2013, TTH was called *tension headache or muscle contraction headache*. It was thought by many that the etiology was related to tense muscles in the head and neck. The ICHD-3 beta names this headache disorder *tension-type headache* and divides it into three different categories: infrequent episodic (less than 1 attack per month), frequent episodic (between 1 and 14 attacks per month for at least 3 months), and chronic (at least 15 attacks per month for at least 3 months) (**Table 30-9**). These three categories are further subdivided to distinguish between patients with or without pericranial muscle tenderness detected by manual palpation.[15] TTH is less intense than migraine and is seldom disabling. Unlike migraine, which is defined by the presence of distinctive characteristics, TTH is defined by the absence of these characteristics, and it is often considered a featureless disorder. The most common subtype by far is the infrequent episodic subtype.[45–47] Most people

TABLE 30-9 International Classification of Headache Disorders, Third Edition Beta Version (ICHD-3) Diagnostic Criteria for Tension-Type Headache
ICHD-2 Diagnostic Criteria for Infrequent Episodic Tension-Type Headache
A. At least 10 episodes occurring on <1 days/month (<12 days/year) and fulfilling criteria B–D
B. Headache lasting from 30 minutes to 7 days
C. Headache has two or more of the following characteristics:
a. Bilateral location
b. Pressing or tightening (nonpulsating) quality
c. Mild or moderate intensity
d. Not aggravated by routine physical activity
D. Both of the following:
a. No nausea or vomiting
b. No more than one of photophobia or phonophobia
E. Not better accounted for by another ICHD-3 diagnosis
ICHD-3 beta version Diagnostic Criteria for Frequent Episodic Tension-Type Headache
A. At least 10 episodes occurring on more than 1 but <15 days/month for ≥3 months (≥12 and <180/year) and fulfilling criteria B–D
B. Headache lasting from 30 minutes to 7 days
C. Headache has two or more of the following characteristics:
a. Bilateral location
b. Pressing or tightening (nonpulsating) quality
c. Mild or moderate intensity
d. Not aggravated by routine physical activity
D. Both of the following:
a. No nausea or vomiting
b. No more than one of photophobia or phonophobia
E. Not better accounted for by another ICHD-3 diagnosis
ICHD-3 beta Diagnostic Criteria for Chronic Tension-Type Headache
A. Headache occurring on 15 or more days/month (≥180 days/year) for >3 months and fulfilling criteria B–D
B. Headache lasting hours or days
C. Headache has two or more of the following characteristics:
a. Bilateral location
b. Pressing or tightening (nonpulsating) quality
c. Mild or moderate intensity
d. Not aggravated by routine physical activity
D. Both of the following:
a. Not more than one of photophobia, phonophobia, mild nausea
b. Neither moderate or severe nausea nor vomiting
E. Not better accounted for by another ICHD-3 diagnosis

who experience this headache type take OTC acute care medication occasionally and never consult a physician.

CLINICAL FEATURES

Tension-type headache attacks can be of variable duration, lasting between 30 minutes and 7 days for episodic TTH, but attacks may be continuous in chronic TTH. Attacks contain at least two of the following four pain characteristics: pressing or tightening (nonpulsating) quality, mild or moderate intensity, bilateral location, and no aggravation by routine physical activity. Additionally, for both the infrequent and frequent episodic subtype, they must include both of the following: no nausea or vomiting, although anorexia may occur, and either photophobia or phonophobia may be present but not both. For chronic TTH (CTTH), attacks must also include both of the following in addition to the pain characteristics previously described: no more than one of photophobia, phonophobia, or mild nausea and neither moderate or severe nausea nor vomiting (Table 30-9).[15] We commonly see patients whose symptoms begin with frontal or occipital pressure or suboccipital tightness or nuchal pressure; these mild headaches can often be relieved with simple analgesics, physical therapy, or just physical activity or relaxation. If not treated early, however, this TTH may progress to assume some characteristics of migraine.

Distinguishing between TTH and probable migraine often presents a diagnostic challenge. Although usually bilateral, TTH attacks can be unilateral in up to 20% of patients. Some patients also describe throbbing or pulsating pain and associated photophobia, phonophonia, osmophobia, or nausea.[48,49] These associated symptoms, as well as the severity of head pain, increase with increasing frequency of TTH attacks, making distinguishing between these two disorders especially difficult in patients with CTTH, a disorder in which one of the distinguishing characteristics of migraine (photophobia, phonophobia, or nausea) can be present to a mild but not moderate or severe extent. Distinguishing between TTH and probable migraine in patients with coexisting migraine is also difficult. So when an individual with migraine has a mild headache, it is usually impossible to tell if it will stay as a mild TTH or progress to a severe migraine. Although the prevalence of TTH is not significantly different in individuals with and without migraine, TTH in patients with migraine is more frequent and more severe than those in individuals without migraine.[50,51] Despite this occasional overlap of symptoms, associated symptoms of a TTH attack, when present, are always mild to moderate and almost never severe, but in migraine attacks, the associated symptoms are often rated by the patient as severe.[48] Perhaps the best pain criterion to distinguish between migraine and TTH is the lack of aggravation by physical activity for TTH attacks.[52]

Prior headache history is essential in distinguishing between the patient with chronic TTH and chronic migraine because CTTH is thought to evolve from ETTH and CM is thought to evolve from episodic migraine. Complicating this picture is that patients with CM may lose migrainous features and develop more mild headaches as they progress to chronic daily headache.[53] The overlapping features have led some headache experts to argue for the existence of a headache spectrum rather than TTH and migraine being distinct disorders. Supporting this view is the Spectrum study, which showed that TTH attacks respond to sumatriptan in patients with a history of migraine, but there is no clinical effect of sumatriptan on TTH attacks in those without migraine.[54,55] Perhaps two different biological profiles exist for TTH in that patients with both ETTH and migraine may have a biological profile similar to migraine, but patients with pure ETTH may have a different one.[56]

Not supporting the spectrum argument are the findings that the brains of patients with CTTH are different from those of patients with MOH and healthy control participants. Patients with CTTH were demonstrated to have a significant decrease in the gray matter in certain areas of the brain involved in pain processing and that this decrease was positively correlated with increasing duration of headache. Similar changes were not seen in the brains of patients with MOH, all of whom had a history of episodic migraine, or in the brains of patients with no personal history of headache.[57] Patients with chronic migraine with MOH have been demonstrated to have functional MRI (fMRI) changes in the areas of the pain matrix that reversed with medication withdrawal.[58,59] The additional finding that there are no structural differences between patients with migraine and healthy control participants[60] allows extrapolation to suggest that this decrease in gray matter is specific to CTTH. The current view of the pathophysiology of TTH is that the sensitization of peripheral nociceptors in myofascial tissues is important for the development of ETTH, but the evolution to CTTH reflexts central sensitization at the level of the spinal dorsal horn or trigeminal spinal nucleus and supraspinally at third-order neurons in the thalamus and higher somatosensory cortex.[61,62]

DIFFERENTIAL DIAGNOSIS

Because TTH is often considered a featureless disorder, one must be alert to potential secondary mimics. The history, physical, and neurologic examination are essential to tease out any red flags that may be present to suggest an alternative diagnosis. Potential secondary causes of TTH include intracranial mass lesions, subdural hematomas, hemorrhagic or ischemic stroke, subacute or chronic meningitis, cervicogenic headache, giant cell arteritis, obstructive sleep apnea, hypothyroidism, major depression, temporomandibular disorders, intracranial hypertension, intracranial hypotension, chronic sinusitis, head trauma, MOH, and others.[53,63] After secondary disorders are excluded, it is essential to distinguish ETTH from probable migraine and CTTH from other causes of chronic daily headache (CDH), such as chronic ("transformed") migraine, hemicrania continua, and new daily persistent headache. Prior headache history is essential in confirming the diagnosis, and an accurate diagnosis is essential to guide therapy.

MANAGEMENT

Adequate acute therapy is the cornerstone of treatment of ETTH, but when TTH attacks become frequent or progress to CTTH, preventive pharmacotherapy and nonpharmacologic management are essential to reduce patient disability and prevent the development of MOH. Needless to say, the treatment of patients with chronic headache is more difficult than that of patients with straightforward, infrequent, and uncomplicated episodic migraine or ETTH. The patient–physician relationship, described by Rapoport and Sheftell as having mutuality of input and shared decision making, is essential in these and other situations.[1]

Pharmacotherapy begins with being able to distinguish TTH from migraine. Early treatment of TTH may afford complete relief. Low-dose NSAIDs are the first-line drugs of choice in the acute treatment of TTH attacks. Although generally more effective than simple analgesics, there is little evidence suggesting the efficacy of one NSAID over another. Also used are aspirin, acetaminophen, and cyclooxygenase-2 inhibitors. The addition of caffeine or barbiturates, such as is seen in combination medications, such as Excedrin, Fioricet, or Fiorinal, to these simple analgesics may be more effective in some patients. Opiates may be helpful for patients with severe TTH but must be used sparingly. Given the typically mild to moderate pain seen in TTH, opiate therapy should not be necessary. The use of acute therapy should be limited to an average of 2 days weekly to avoid medication overuse.[4,63–65] If use approaches or exceeds these limitations, preventive therapy should be used.

Adequate studies assessing the efficacy of preventive pharmacotherapy for TTH are lacking. Tricyclic antidepressants (TCAs) are considered the first-line therapy for prevention of CTTH and frequent ETTH (more than 2 attacks weekly on average). Amitriptyline is the most commonly used, but other TCAs such as nortriptyline, clomipramine, doxepin, and protriptyline may also be used. Tetracyclic antidepressants, such as maprotiline, and mirtazapine are sometimes used. Mirtazapine has demonstrated efficacy at a dose of 15 to 30 mg/day, usually given at bedtime. SSRIs are generally thought to be ineffective for the treatment of TTH. Muscle relaxants have no proven role in the acute therapy of TTH, but the centrally acting muscle relaxant tizanidine has some evidence for its efficacy as daily preventive therapy. The evidence for antiepileptic drugs is lacking, but topiramate was effective in an open-label study. Onabotulinum toxin A is not effective in CTTH or ETTH.[4,64–68]

For a difficult patient with chronic headache, behavioral modification techniques are important, and a cornerstone of treatment must include the patient becoming an active participant rather than a passive consumer of medication. Behavioral treatment begins with the patient keeping an accurate headache calendar or diary, maintaining good sleep hygiene, identifying and avoiding potential food and environmental triggers, and engaging in nonpharmacologic therapies (e.g., physical therapy, electromyography and temperature biofeedback, stress management, cognitive-behavioral therapy, and relaxation techniques).[4,64] The evidence for spinal manipulation is weak, but acupuncture is used by several headache specialists, and the evidence is slightly stronger.[65,69–71] Confirming the importance of behavioral modification in the treatment of CTTH, a randomized controlled trial demonstrated that although both TCAs and stress management therapy are more effective than placebo in reducing headache activity, analgesic medication use, and headache-related disability, combined therapy is more effective than either therapy alone.[72]

CLUSTER HEADACHE

The symptoms of cluster headache are usually so distinctive that when the clinician is aware of the characteristic presentation (**Table 30-10**), there seldom is any difficulty in making the diagnosis. Of all the headache disorders, cluster headache pain is by far the most excruciating and disabling. Despite its dramatic clinical presentation, however, the diagnosis is often missed, and many patients suffer unnecessarily for years before the proper diagnosis is made. The term *cluster* derives from two characteristics of the condition: (1) a cluster of symptoms accompanies the pain, and (2) the frequent headache attacks are clustered, or grouped, over a period of about 4 to 12 weeks in patients with episodic cluster headache. This is termed the *cluster period,* and it is subsequently followed by long headache-free periods, which can last for months or years, termed the *remission period.* Cluster headaches tend to occur on a regular schedule, often occurring at night; awakening the patient from sleep at precisely the same time every night, most frequently between 12 and 3 AM; and seldom deviating by even 5 minutes.[73] A traditional teaching is that the first attack at night usually occurs with the first REM (rapid eye movement) cycle, about 90 minutes after sleep initiation; however, the relationship between cluster and REM has been called into question with polysomnography of patients during cluster attacks demonstrating no relationship to REM sleep and suggesting that possibly sleep stage transition is more important in generation of a cluster attack.[74] The relationship of cluster headache to sleep stages remains unclear and further studies are needed. Furthermore, the attacks usually have a seasonal periodicity, occurring at the same time every year in an individual patient. Although cluster periods can occur at any time of year, they most often occur in late autumn or springtime, which may be related in part to long and short photoperiods of available light, which occur on either side of June 21 and December 21, the longest and shortest days of the year, respectively.

TABLE 30-10 International Classification of Headache Disorders, 3rd Edition (beta version) Diagnostic Criteria for Cluster Headache

A. At least five attacks fulfilling criteria B-D
B. Severe or very severe unilateral orbital, supraorbital, and/or temporal pain lasting 15-180 minutes (if untreated)
C. Either or both of the following:
    1. At least one of the following symptoms or signs, ipsilateral to the headache:
        a. conjunctival injection and/or lacrimation
        b. nasal congestion and/or rhinorrhea
        c. eyelid edema
        d. forehead and facial sweating
        e. forehead and facial flushing
        f. sensation of fullness in the ear
        g. miosis and/or ptosis
    2. A sense of restlessness or agitation
D. Attacks have a frequency between one every other day and eight per day for more than half of the time when the disorder is active
E. Not better accounted for by another ICHD-3 diagnosis

CLINICAL FEATURES

Cluster attacks often begin as a vague discomfort in the distribution of the first division of the trigeminal nerve, usually centered in or behind one eye, that rapidly escalates, reaching peak intensity within minutes. The patient often describes the pain as boring or searing in quality, feeling as if a "red-hot poker" is being stuck through his or her eye. Although most commonly boring, searing, sharp, and stabbing in quality, the pain of cluster headache can also be throbbing or pressure-like, as though the eye is being pushed out of the orbit.[75] This intense pain is most commonly deep in the eye, but it can also involve the supraorbital area and temple. Although most common in areas innervated by the first division of the trigeminal nerve, pain has been reported to occur in other areas as well, often in the second division distribution but also including the forehead, jaw, cheek, upper and lower teeth, ear, nose, occiput, neck, shoulder, and other areas of the head.[76] The duration of a cluster attack is much shorter than that of migraine, lasting from 15 to 180 minutes, with most attacks being 45 to 90 minutes in duration.[77] Attacks often end as abruptly as they began. Some patients describe a low-level pain in the same distribution as the severe pain, which is present between attacks.

The associated symptoms of cluster headache are often quite dramatic and characteristic of each patient's attack. These symptoms, caused by autonomic dysfunction, include ipsilateral lacrimation, conjunctival injection, nasal congestion, rhinorrhea, eyelid edema, forehead and facial sweating or flushing, sensation of fullness in the ear, ptosis, and miosis. Behavior during the acute cluster headache attack is very different from that of an individual with migraine, who prefers to lie still in a dark, quiet room. During a cluster attack, patients cannot lie still, are up walking or sitting, rocking back and forth with pain, or may beat their head with their fists or bang their head on the wall, sometimes becoming agitated and possibly violent. Although ipsilateral autonomic features are almost universally present, they can occasionally be absent, and the presence of this sense of restlessness or agitation during an attack is sufficient to make the diagnosis of cluster headache in the absence of autonomic features. Although classically considered migrainous features, nausea, photophobia, phonophobia, and osmophobia are not uncommon during a cluster headache attack. Interestingly, rather than being bilateral as in migraine, photophobia and phonophobia are often lateralized to the side of the head pain. Symptoms consistent with migraine aura have also been reported to occur.[76,78,79]

Cluster headache is almost without exception unilateral, and every occurrence over many years is usually on the same side. There are rare reports of the opposite side being involved, with this side shift occurring most commonly in a subsequent cluster period. Although much more rare, side shift within a cluster period has been reported.[76,77] Reports of bilateral cluster headache are extremely rare.[80–82]

The neurovascular and neuropeptide changes that set this painful periodic disorder in motion remain incompletely understood. Vasoactive intestinal peptide and calcitonin gene-related peptide are increased during a cluster headache attack and thus may play a role in the pathogenesis.[83] The location of the headache and the associated autonomic features point to the trigeminal nerve and sphenopalatine ganglion as locations of the pathophysiology. The striking circadian periodicity and circannual rhythmicity, however, suggest higher centers of involvement and the suprachiasmatic nucleus, and the ipsilateral inferior posterior hypothalamic gray area has been proposed to be the generator of cluster headache attacks.[84]

Similar to migraine, which has a strong familial tendency, cluster headache has a hereditary predisposition, with first-degree relatives being 5 to 18 times more likely and second-degree relatives being 1 to 3 times more likely to develop cluster headache compared with the general population. It has recently been reported that 17% of individuals with cluster headache report having a first-degree relative with cluster headache. The mode of inheritance has been suggested to be multimodal, being autosomal dominant with low penetrance in some families and multifactorial or autosomal recessive in other families.[73,85] Approximately 0.07% to 0.1% of the population is affected compared with 12% for migraine.[2] In contrast to migraine, which is more common in women, cluster headache occurs primarily in men. The male-to-female ratio may be diminishing over time, however, with a review of 482 patients finding that the ratio has fallen from 6.2:1 to 2.1:1 for patients with cluster headache onset before the 1960s and in the 1990s, respectively. The International Headache Society (IHS) cites a 3:1 male-to-female ratio in the ICHD-3 beta diagnostic criteria.[15] The reason for the declining ratio is unclear, with some believing that it is due to a prior underrecognition of cluster headache in women and others speculating that the decline represents an increase in the prevalence of cluster headache in women. This may be related to lifestyle factors such as the parallel increases in education, employment, and smoking rates among women over the same time periods.[86]

Men with cluster headache often have a characteristic physiognomy: they are athletic or mesomorphic, with prominent thick facial features, furrowed brows, and deep nasolabial folds. They may have an orange peel–like skin (called peau d'orange) and telangiectasias of the nose and cheeks. They are often intense, busy, dynamic men who manage many people and travel a lot and are heavy smokers and drinkers who have an increased incidence of coronary and GI problems. The incidence of coronary artery disease and GI problems in cluster patients is now thought to be less than previously believed.[73] During a cluster headache period, patients quickly learn that alcohol will trigger a cluster headache attack, but between cluster periods they may drink with impunity.

About 80% to 90% of individuals with cluster headache have episodic cluster headache (ECH), with the cluster period lasting on average 4 to 12 weeks and remission periods lasting an average of 12 months. Chronic cluster headache (CCH), defined as a cluster period of 365 days with no remission period longer than 1 month, exists in the remaining 10% to 20% of individuals. Approximately 10% of patients with CCH have the primary form, in which the attacks are continuous from the onset, and the remainders have the secondary form, having evolved from ECH, when over time cluster periods lengthen in duration, and remission periods shorten until attacks become continuous.[76,77] CCH is more resistant to treatment than ECH, and patients suffer terribly. They sometimes need interventional procedures, such as electrical stimulation of the occipital nerve, sphenopalatine ganglion, or posterior hypothalamus.

DIFFERENTIAL DIAGNOSIS

Before a diagnosis of cluster headache can be confidently made, a history, physical examination, and neurologic examination as well as appropriate neuroimaging studies must be undertaken to distinguish this disorder from primary and secondary headache disorders that can mimic cluster headache. Some believe that given the relative rarity of cluster headache, neuroimaging in the form of MRI should always be performed, but others believe that neuroimaging is unnecessary in patients with a typical history and normal neurologic examination results unless the patient fails to respond to treatment and the condition continually worsens. We believe that one good MRI of the brain is essential to rule out parasellar and other structural pathology and an MRA of the neck to rule out cervical arterial dissection.

The history and examination are sometimes suggestive of secondary headache disorders. Any patient with an abnormal neurologic symptomatology or examination should undergo appropriate neuroimaging. Neuroimaging should also be considered in cases that are atypical, whether they lack the classical periodicity of attacks followed by remission periods or are unresponsive to therapy. Secondary causes of cluster headache that have been reported include vertebral artery dissection or aneurysm; intracranial aneurysms; parasellar mass or other structural lesions; arteriovenous malformations; giant cell arteritis; high cervical meningioma; unilateral cervical cord infarction; lateral medullary infarction; pituitary tumors; intracranial meningiomas; facial trauma; orbitosphenoidal aspergillosis; Tolosa-Hunt syndrome; maxillary sinusitis; head, neck, or trigeminal nerve injury; sinusitis; and glaucoma.[5]

Primary headache disorders that can be confused with cluster headache include migraine, the other trigeminal autonomic cephalalgias (episodic and chronic paroxysmal hemicrania, short-lasting unilateral neuralgiform headache with conjunctival injection and tearing, hemicrania continua), and trigeminal neuralgia. These disorders can be distinguished from cluster headache by taking a careful history because the attack duration and frequency differ among these various primary headache disorders. It is interesting to note that some general physicians and many patients think that a headache in the sinus areas associated with stuffed or running nostrils is caused by sinus headaches. They are not easily convinced otherwise. We have seen patients with facial and dental trauma go on to develop cluster headache.

MANAGEMENT

In cluster headache, unlike migraine, nonpharmacologic treatment is seldom effective. There are three approaches to the management of cluster headache: treatment of the acute attack, transitional or bridge therapy, and preventive pharmacotherapy. Because a cluster attack reaches peak intensity within minutes, acute therapy must use an agent with a rapid onset of action.

Inhalation of 100% oxygen via a nonrebreather face mask at a rate of 7 to 12 L/min for 15 minutes results in rapid pain relief in approximately 75% of attacks. Flow rates as high as 15 L/min may be required in some patients.[87,88] Patients usually rent a D cylinder from an oxygen supply company for the duration of their cluster period. They should be instructed to cover all leaky areas of the mask and to sit leaning forward with their arms on their knees during the oxygen inhalation. The oxygen cylinder is often kept at the bedside, and prompt relief is achieved for evening and nocturnal attacks. Some patients, however, find that rather than aborting an attack, oxygen merely delays the attack onset. Whereas oxygen has no adverse effects, it can be used in conjunction with other therapies, and it can be used multiple times daily, other acute therapies have dosing limitations.

A 6-mg subcutaneous injection of sumatriptan is approved in the United States for cluster headache and is the most effective acute therapy for relief of a cluster attack, with 74% of patients attaining complete pain relief within 15 minutes. Response is usually consistent without tolerance or loss of effectiveness throughout the cluster period.[89] If the patient has more than two attacks in a 24-hour period, the 4-mg dose may be considered to allow for a maximum of three doses rather than two because the maximum daily dose is 12 mg per 24 hours. Although less effective than the subcutaneous route, 20 mg of intranasal sumatriptan is sometimes effective in aborting an acute cluster headache attack.[90] Zolmitriptan 5 and 10 mg in both the oral and intranasal formulation can also be effective.[91–94] Zolmitriptan 5-mg nasal spray is approved for the acute treatment of a cluster attack in the European Union. Migranal nasal spray (DHE) or ergotamine sublingual and oral tablets or suppositories may also be helpful.[95] A viscous solution of 4% lidocaine delivered intranasally may be effective and useful as an adjunctive therapy, but is not a first-line acute care treatment.[96]

As noted previously, patients with cluster headache are usually middle-aged men who are heavy smokers, so potent vasoconstrictor medications must be given with caution and are contraindicated if there is a suspected history of heart disease or poorly controlled hypertension.

The goal of preventive pharmacotherapy is to rapidly suppress attacks and to maintain the patient relatively pain free throughout the anticipated duration of the cluster period. Preventive pharmacotherapy can be divided into transitional or bridge therapy and maintenance phases. Transitional or bridge therapy is used to rapidly suppress attacks, and maintenance prevention becomes effective over a few days. Maintenance prevention is then used throughout the anticipated duration of the cluster period in patients with ECH and is used indefinitely in patients with CCH. Approximately one-third of patients with CCH will revert to the episodic form,[77] so treatment should always be reassessed, and we suggest attempting to slowly taper medication when patients with CCH have been attack free for at least 6 months. If attacks recur, the dose should be increased back to the previous effective dose.

Several options exist for transitional therapy. A brief tapering course of corticosteroids is highly likely to break the headache cycle. Treatment is commonly initiated with prednisone 60 mg/day for 3 days and then decreased by 10 mg every 3 days over an 18-day period. An alternative regimen is dexamethasone 4 mg twice daily for 2 weeks followed by once daily for 1 week. We prefer to limit steroid dosing to 7 to 10 days to increase the chance of preventing complications, which can occur after just 1 to 2 days of high-dose steroids. Greater occipital nerve blockade with local anesthetic and corticosteroid administered ipsilateral to the side of the pain is another safe and effective option for transitional therapy and often provides significant and prolonged relief. Ergotamine tartrate may also be used as a tablet or suppository and DHE as an injection or nasal spray administered daily for 2 to 3 weeks. Both of these medications can be administered in divided doses, not exceeding 4 mg/day of ergotamine tartrate or 3 mg/day of DHE. Although effective, ergots are potent vasoconstrictors and must be used cautiously. Treatment with ergotamine derivatives limits available acute options for breakthrough attacks because the use of triptans is contraindicated within 24 hours of their use.

Verapamil, although used off label without large controlled trials, is considered to be the first-line preventive therapy for both episodic and CCH. Dosing is initiated at 80 mg three times daily for the short-acting tablet formulation, which can then be switched to the 240-mg sustained-release formulation. Higher doses are often required. Most patients do well with 480 mg in divided doses, but doses up to 720 mg/day or sometimes even higher might be needed.[97,98] These are much higher doses than are generally used for cardiac indications. Because of the potential for the development of atrioventricular conduction delay or block, regular electrocardiograms should be monitored on doses higher than 240 mg/day.

Lithium carbonate is often helpful, especially for patients with CCH.[99] The starting dose is 300 mg twice daily or 450 mg sustained release once daily, and the dose is increased slowly if needed. Blood levels of lithium, electrolytes, renal function, and thyroid function tests must be monitored in patients receiving lithium therapy because high doses can be nephrotoxic and lithium has been associated with nephrogenic diabetes insipidus and hypothyroidism. The target therapeutic lithium concentration is 0.4 to 0.8 mEq/L, and the serum lithium level should not exceed 1 mEq/L. A level of 0.6 mEq/L is often effective and is usually achieved with 300 mg of lithium three times a day or less. Lithium levels must be monitored carefully because lithium has an extremely narrow therapeutic window. The level should be a trough level, drawn 8 to 12 hours after the last dose. Concurrent use of lithium with diuretics or carbamazepine should be avoided. Patients should be warned not to get dehydrated in warm weather or when exercising. Given its side effect profile and the relative safety and efficacy of verapamil, lithium is often reserved for refractory cases and for patients with CCH and is not used as first-line treatment.

Often combination therapy is required if patients are unable to tolerate high doses or are unresponsive to first-line therapies. Ergot derivatives, such as ergotamine tartrate and methysergide, are often effective for both ECH and CCH. Methysergide is no longer available in the United States, so we sometimes use a metabolite, methylergonovine (Methergine), starting at 0.2 three times a day and with a maximum dose of 0.6 mg three times a day. Divalproex sodium, topiramate, gabapentin, melatonin, acetazolamide, and intranasal capsaicin have been used successfully and should be considered as add-on therapy in refractory cases. Knowledge of potential toxicity is essential, and side effects must be communicated to the patient.[1,4,5,100]

The pain of cluster headache is intense and disabling, and the fact that 90% of patients can be helped makes treatment of this condition especially gratifying. For the 10% of patients who respond poorly to outpatient medical management, inpatient intensive therapy or surgery may be offered. Before considering surgical treatment options in these patients, it is essential to try to exhaust combination medical therapy because patients may require more than one agent. Successful surgical procedures targeting the sensory trigeminal nerve include radiofrequency trigeminal rhizotomy, retrogasserian glycerol injection, alcohol injection into the supraorbital or infraorbital nerves, gamma-knife radiosurgery, microvascular decompression, and trigeminal root sectioning. Sphenopalatine ganglionectomy has also been used with success.[4,5]

Peripheral neuromodulation has also been used with success for refractory cases of cluster headache. Greater occipital nerve stimulation has emerged as a potential treatment for cluster headache and is also effective in refractory occipital neuralgia.[101–103] Another possible site for stimulation is the vagus nerve.[104] Noninvasive transcutaneous vagal nerve stimulation using the gammaCore device is actively being investigated as a treatment for cluster headache. More recently, sphenopalatine ganglion stimulation using the ATI Neurostimulation system is being studies for the acute treatment of cluster headache attacks in patients with refractory CCH. Early results are very promising in the majority of patients tested, with early data demonstrating pain relief in 67.1% of full stimulation treated attacks compared to 7.4% of sham treated attacks. Many patients also saw attack frequency decrease, suggesting a preventive benefit.[105] Further studies are needed to validate this procedure because this may be a desirable treatment for patients who are unable to tolerate or are unresponsive to other acute medications.

The discovery of the critical role of the ipsilateral posterior inferior hypothalamus in the generation of cluster headache attacks in a positron emission tomography scan study of nine patients led to the investigation of hypothalamic deep brain stimulation as a treatment for refractory cluster headache. The results are promising in some centers, and many studies have shown a positive response.[106–117] Because this is an invasive procedure with serious adverse events in a few patients, it should be reserved for patients who have failed medical management and have not responded to attempts at peripheral neuromodulation. The first group to perform this operation successfully was the Milan group headed by Angelo Franzini, Massimo Leone and Gennaro Bussone. They have done about 23 procedures, two bilaterally, but now always do occipital nerve stimulation first because it is less invasive and often successful.

CONCLUSION

Headache is an extremely common disorder, and this chapter has reviewed the clinical characteristics, differential diagnosis, and management of the three most common headache disorders: migraine, TTH, and cluster headache. The first step in headache management is making an appropriate diagnosis. Although clinical features can sometimes overlap, each headache disorder is distinct, and an understanding of these disorders is essential to the diagnosis and treatment of headache patients. Accurate diagnosis and appropriate treatment can make a dramatic difference in a patient's life, and this difference can be incredibly gratifying for the treating physician.

REFERENCES

1. Rapoport AM, Sheftell FD. *Headache Disorders, A Management Guide for Practitioners*. Philadelphia: WB Saunders; 1996.
2. Robbins MS, Lipton RB. The epidemiology of primary headache disorders. *Semin Neurol*. 2010;30:107-119.
3. Lipton RB, Bigal ME, Diamond M, et al. Migraine prevalence, disease burden, and the need for preventive therapy. *Neurology*. 2007;68:343-349.
4. Silberstein SD, Lipton RB, Dodick DD, eds. *Wolff's Headache and Other Head Pain*. Eighth ed. New York: Oxford University Press; 2008.
5. Silberstein SD, Lipton RB, Goadsby PJ. *Headache in Clinical Practice*. Second ed. London: Martin Dunitz Ltd; 2002.
6. Schoonman GG, Evers DJ, Terwindt GM, et al. The prevalence of premonitory symptoms in migraine: a questionnaire study in 461 patients. *Cephalalgia*. 2006;26:1209-1213.
7. Griffen NJ, Ruggiero L, Lipton RB, et al. Premonitory symptoms in migraine: an electronic diary study. *Neurology*. 2003;60:935-940.
8. Kelman L. The premonitory symptoms (prodrome): a tertiary care study of 893 migraineurs. *Headache*. 2004;44:865-872.
9. Kelman L. The aura: a tertiary care study of 952 migraine patients. *Cephalalgia*. 2004;24:728-734.
10. Queiroz LP, Friedman DI, Rapoport AM, Purdy RA. Characteristics of migraine visual aura in Southern Brazil and Northern USA. *Cephalalgia*. 2011;31:1652-1658.
11. Russell MB, Olesen J. A nosographic analysis of the migraine aura in a general population. *Brain*. 1996;119:355-361.
12. Jensen K, Tfelt-Hansen P, Lauritzen M, Olesen J. Classic migraine: a prospective recording of symptoms. *Acta Neurol Scand*. 1986;73:359-362.
13. Manzoni G, Farina S, Lanfranchi M, Solari A. Classic migraine—clinical findings in 164 patients. *Eur Neurol*. 1985;24:163-169.
14. Fisher CM. Late-life migraine accompaniments as a cause of unexplained transient ischemic attacks. *Can J Neurol Sci*. 1980;7:9-17.
15. Headache Classification Committee of the International Headache Society (IHS). The International Classification of Headache Disorders, 3rd edition (beta version). *Cephalalgia*. 2013;33(9):629-808.
16. Selby G, Lance JW. Observation on 500 cases of migraine and allied vascular headaches. *J Neurol Neurosurg Psychiatry*. 1960;23:23-32.
17. Silberstein SD. Migraine symptoms: results of a survey of self-reported migraineurs. *Headache*. 1995;35:387-396.
18. Boyle R, Behan PO, Sutton JA. A correlation between severity of migraine and delayed gastric emptying measured by an epigastric impedance method. *Br J Clin Pharmac*. 1990;30:405-409.
19. Blau JN. *Migraine: Clinical and Research Aspects*. Baltimore: Johns Hopkins University Press; 1987.
20. Bigal ME, Lipton RB. The differential diagnosis of chronic daily headaches: an algorithm-based approach. *J Headache Pain*. 2007;8:263-272.
21. Morgenstern LB, Luma-Gonzalez H, Huber JCJ, et al. Worst headache and subarachnoid hemorrhage: prospective, modern computed tomography and spinal fluid analysis. *Ann Emerg Med*. 1998;32:297-304.
22. Schieving WI. Intracranial aneurysms. *N Engl J Med*. 1997;336:28-40.
23. Wober C, Holzhammer J, Zeitlhofer J, et al. Trigger factors of migraine and tension-type headache: experience and knowledge of the patients. *J Headache Pain*. 2006;7:188-195.
24. Karli N, Zarifoglu M, Calisir N, Akgoz S. Comparison of pre-headache phases and trigger factors of migraine and episodic tension-type headache: do they share similar clinical pathophysiology? *Cephalalgia*. 2005;25:44-451.
25. Zivadinov R, Willheim K, Sepic-Grahovac D, et al. Migraine and tension-type headache in Croatia: a population-based survey of precipitating factors. *Cephalalgia*. 2003;23:336-343.
26. Chabriat H, Danchot J, Michel P, et al. Precipitating factors of headache. A prospective study in a national control-matched survey in migraineurs and nonmigraineurs. *Headache*. 1999;39:335-338.
27. Hauge AW, Kirchmann M, Olesen J. Trigger factors in migraine with aura. *Cephalalgia*. 2010;30:346-353.
28. Toth C. Medications and substances as a cause of headache: a systematic review of the literature. *Clin Neuropharmacol*. 2003;26:122-136.
29. Evans RW, Kruuse C. Phosphodiesterase-5 inhibitors and migraine. *Headache*. 2004;44:925-926.
30. Rains JC, Penzien DB, McCrory DC, Gray RN. Behavioural headache treatment: history, review of the empirical literature, and methodological critique. *Headache*. 2005;45(Suppl 2):S92-S109.
31. Buse DC, Andrasik F. Behavioral medicine for migraine. *Neurol Clin*. 2009;27:445-465.
32. Silberstein SD, Rosenberg J. Multispecialty consensus on diagnosis and treatment of headache. *Neurology*. 2000;54:1553-1554.
33. Tepper SJ, Kori SH, Borland SW, et al. Efficacy and safety of MAP0004, orally inhaled DHE in treating migraine with and without allodynia. *Headache*. 2012;52:37-47.
34. Lipton RB, Silberstein SD. The role of headache-related disability in migraine management. *Neurology*. 2001;56(Suppl 1):S35-S42.
35. Silberstein SD. Practice parameter: evidence-based guidelines for migraine headache (an evidence-based review): report of the Quality Standards Subcommittee of the American Academy of Neurology. *Neurology*. 2000;55:754-762.
36. Diener H-C, Montagna P, Gacs G, et al. Efficacy and tolerability of diclofenac potassium sachets in migraine: a randomized, double-blind, cross-over study in comparison with diclofenac potassium tablets and placebo. *Cephalalgia*. 2006;26:537-547.
37. Loder E. Triptan therapy in migraine. *N Engl J Med*. 2010;363:63-70.
38. Rapoport AM, Tepper SJ, Bigal ME, Sheftell FD. The triptan formulations: how to match patients and products. *CNS Drugs*. 2003;17:431-447.

39. VanDenBrink AM, Reekers M, Bax WA, et al. Coronary side-effect potential of current and prospective antimigraine drugs. *Circulation*. 1998;98:25-30.
40. Lipton RB, Stewart WF, Stone AM, et al. Stratified care vs step care strategies for migraine: results of the Disability in Stratefies of Care (DISC) Study. *JAMA*. 2000;284:2599-2605.
41. Markley HG. Chronic headache: appropriate use of opiate analgesics. *Neurology*. 1994;44(Suppl):518-524.
42. Goadsby PJ, Sprenger T. Current practice and future directions in the prevention and acute management of migraine. *Lancet Neurol*. 2010;9:285-298.
43. Ayata C, Jin H, Kudo C, et al. Suppression of cortical spreading depression in migraine prophylaxis. *Ann Neurol*. 2006;59:652-661.
44. Lyngberg AC, Rasmussen BK, Jorgensen T, Jensen R. Has the prevalence of migraine and tension-type headache changed over a 12-year period? A Danish population survey. *Eur J Epidemiol*. 2005;20(3):243-249.
45. Russell MB, Levi N, Saltyte-Benth J, Fenger K. Tension-type headache in adolescents and adults: a population based study of 33,764 twins. *Eur J Epidemiol*. 2006;21(2):153-160.
46. Russell MB. Tension-type headache in 40-year olds: a Danish population-based sample of 4000. *J Headache Pain*. 2005;6:441-447.
47. Schwartz BS, Stewart WF, Simon D, Lipton RB. Epidemiology of tension-type headache. *JAMA*. 1998;279(5):381-383.
48. Pfaffenrath V, Isler H. Evaluation of the nosology of chronic tension-type headache. *Cephalalgia*. 1993;13(Suppl 12):60-62.
49. Rasmussen BK, Jensen R, Olesen J. A population-based analysis of the diagnostic criteria of the International Headache Society. *Cephalalgia*. 1991;11:129-134.
50. Ulrich V, Russell MB, Jensen R, Olesen J. A comparison of tension-type headache in migraineurs and in non-migraineurs: a population-based study. *Pain*. 1996;67:501-506.
51. Rasmussen BK, Jensen R, Schroll M, Olesen J. Interrelations between migraine and tension-type headache in the general population. *Arch Neurol*. 1992;49:914-918.
52. Iversen HK, Langemark M, Andersson PG, et al. Clinical characteristics of migraine and episodic tension-type headache in relation to old and new diagnostic criteria. *Headache*. 1990;30:514-519.
53. Sacco S. Diagnostic issues in tension-type headache. *Curr Pain Headache Rep*. 2008;12:437-441.
54. Lipton RB, Stewart WF, Cady R, et al. 2000 Wolfe Award. Sumatriptan for the range of headaches in migraine sufferers: results of the spectrum study. *Headache*. 2000;40(10):783-791.
55. Brennum J, Brinck T, Schriver L, et al. Sumatriptan has no clinically relevant effect in the treatment of episodic tension-type headache. *Eur J Neurol*. 1996;3;23-28.
56. Lipton RB, Cady RK, Stewart WF, et al. Diagnostic lessons from the spectrum study. *Neurology*. 2002;58:S27-S31.
57. Schmidt-Wilcke T, Leinisch E, Straube A, et al. Gray matter decrease in patients with chronic tension type headache. *Neurology*. 2005;65:1483-1486.
58. Grazzi L, Chiapparini L, Ferraro S, et al. Chronic migraine with medication overuse pre-post withdrawal of symptomatic medication: clinical results and FMRI correlations. *Headache*. 2010;50(6):998-1004.
59. Ferraro S, Grazzi L, Mandelli ML, et al. Pain processing in medication overuse headache: a functional magnetic resonance imaging (fMRI) study. *Pain Med*. 2012;13(2):255-262.
60. Matharu MS, Good CD, May A, et al. No change in the structure of the brain in migraine: a voxel-based morphometric study. *Eur J Neurol*. 2003;10:53-57.
61. Bendtsen L. Central and peripheral sensitization in tension-type headache. *Curr Pain Headache Rep*. 2003;2:460-465.
62. Ashina S, Bendtsen L, Ashina M. Pathophysiology of tension-type headache. *Curr Pain Headache Rep*. 2005;9:415-422.
63. Kaniecki RG. Tension-type headache in the elderly. *Curr Pain Headache Rep*. 2006;10:448-453.
64. Fumal A, Schoenen J. Tension-type headache: current research and clinical management. *Lancet Neurol*. 2008;7:70-83.
65. Bigal ME, Rapoport AM, Hargreaves R. Advances in the pharmacologic treatment of tension-type headache. *Curr Pain Headache Rep*. 2008;12:442-446.
66. Bendtsen L, Jensen R, Olesen J. A non-selective (amitriptyline), but not a selective (citalopram), serotonin reuptake inhibitor is effective in the prophylactic treatment of chronic tension-type headache. *J Neurol Neurosurg Psychiatry*. 1996;61:285-290.
67. Bendtsen L, Jensen R. Mirtazapine is effective in the prophylactic treatment of chronic tension-type headache. *Neurology*. 2004; 62:1706-1711.
68. Lampl C, Marecek S, May A, Bendtsen L. A prospective, open-label, long-term study of the efficacy and tolerability of topiramate in the prophylaxis of chronic tension-type headache. *Cephalalgia*. 2006;26:1203-1208.
69. Schiapparelli P, Allais G, Rolando S, et al. Acupuncture in primary headache treatment. *Neurol Sci*. 2011;32(Suppl 1):S15-S18.
70. Linde K, Allais G, Brinkhaus B, et al. Acupuncture for migraine prophylaxis. *Cochrane Database Syst Rev*. 2009;(1):CD001218.
71. Li Y, Zheng H, Witt CM, et al. Acupuncture for migraine prophylaxis: a randomized controlled trial. *CMAJ*. 2012;184:401-410.
72. Holroydx KA, O'Donnell FJ, Lipchik GL, et al. Management of chronic tension-type headache with (tricyclic) antidepressant medication, stress-management therapy and their combination: a randomized controlled trial. *Cephalalgia*. 2000;20:433.
73. Rozen TD, Fishman RS. Cluster headache in the United States of America: demographics, clinical characteristics, triggers, suicidality, and personal burden. *Headache*. 2012;52:99-113.
74. Zaremba S, Holle D, Wessendorf TE, et al. Cluster headache shows no association with rapid eye movement sleep. *Cephalalgia*. 2012;32:289-296.
75. Manzoni GC, Terzano MG, Bono G, et al. Cluster headache—clinical findings in 180 patients. *Cephalalgia*. 1983;3:21-30.
76. Bahra A, May A, Goadsby PJ. Cluster headache: a prospective clinical study with diagnostic implications. *Neurology*. 2002;58:354-361.
77. Dodick DW, Rozen TD, Goadsby PJ, Silberstein SD. Cluster headache. *Cephalalgia*. 2000;20:787-803.
78. Silberstein SD, Niknam R, Rozen TD, Young WB. Cluster headache with aura. *Neurology*. 2000;54(1):219-220.
79. Schurks M, Kurth T, de Jesus J, et al. Cluster headache: clinical presentation, lifestyle features, and medical treatment. *Headache*. 2006;46:1246-1254.
80. Torelli P, Cologno D, Cadamartiri C, Manzoni G. Application of the international headache society classification criteria in 652 cluster headache patients. *Cephalalgia*. 2001;21:145-150.
81. Sjaastad O, Saunte C, Fredriksen T. Bilaterality of cluster headache. An hypothesis. *Cephalalgia*. 1985;5:55-58.
82. Young WB, Rozen TD. Bilateral cluster headache: case report and theory of (failed) contralateral suppression. *Cephalalgia*. 1999;19:188-190.
83. Edvinsson L, Goadsby PJ. Neuropeptides in migraine and cluster headache. *Cephalalgia*. 1994;14:320-327.
84. May A, Bahra A, Buchel C, et al. Hypothalamic activation in cluster headache attacks. *Lancet*. 1998;352:275-278.

85. Russell MB. Epidemiology and genetics of cluster headache. *Lancet Neurol.* 2004;3:279-283.

86. Manzoni GC. Gender ratio of cluster headache over the years: a possible role of changes in lifestyle. *Cephalalgia.* 1998;18:138-142.

87. Cohen AS, Burns B, Goadsby PJ. High-flow oxygen for treatment of cluster headache: a randomized trial. *JAMA.* 2009;302(22):2451-2457.

88. Rozen TD. High oxygen flow rates for cluster headache. *Neurology.* 2004;63:593.

89. Ekbom K. The sumatriptan cluster headache study group. Treatment of acute cluster headache with sumatriptan. *New Eng J Med.* 1991; 325(5):322-326.

90. Van Vliet JA, Bahra A, Martin V, et al. Intranasal sumatriptan in cluster headache: randomized placebo-controlled double-blind study. *Neurology.* 2003;60:630-633.

91. Bahra A, Becker WJ, Blau JN. Efficacy of oral zolmitriptan in acute treatment of cluster headache [abstract]. *Cephalalgia.* 1999;19:457.

92. Cittadini E, May A, Straube A, et al. Effectiveness of intranasal zolmitriptan in acute cluster headache: a randomized, placebo-controlled, double-blind crossover study. *Arch Neurol.* 2006;63:1537-1542.

93. Rapoport AM, Mathew NT, Silberstein SD, et al. Zolmitriptan nasal spray in the acute treatment of cluster headache: a double blind study. *Neurology.* 2007;69:821-826.

94. Hedlund C, Rapoport AM, Dodick DD, Goadsby PJ. Zolmitriptan nasal spray in the acute treatment of cluster headache: a meta-analysis of two studies. *Headache.* 2009;49:1315-1323.

95. Anderson PG, Jesperson LT. Dihydroergotamine nasal spray in the treatment of attacks of cluster headache. *Cephalalgia.* 1996;6:51-54.

96. Robbins L. Intranasal lidocaine for cluster headache. *Headache.* 1995;35:83-84.

97. Gabaj IJ, Spierings EHL. Prophylactic treatment of cluster headache with verapamil. *Headache.* 1989;29:167-168.

98. Gobel H, Holzgreve H, Heinze A, et al. Retarded verapamil for cluster headache prophylaxis. *Cephalalgia.* 1999;19:458-459.

99. Ekbom K. Lithium for cluster headache: review of the literature and preliminary results of long-term treatment. *Headache.* 1981;21(4):132-139.

100. Mathew NT. Cluster headache. *Neurology.* 1992;42(Suppl):32-36.

101. Magis D, Allena M, Bolla M, et al. Occipital nerve stimulation for drug-resistant chronic cluster headache. *Lancet Neurol.* 2007;6:314-321.

102. Burns B, Watkins L, Goadsby PJ. Treatment of medically intractable cluster headache by occipital nerve stimulation: long-term follow-up of eight patients. *Lancet.* 2007;369:1099-1106.

103. Schwedt T, Dodick DD, Trentman T, Zimmerman R. Occipital nerve stimulation for chronic cluster headache and hemicrania continua: pain relief and persistence of autonomic features. *Cephalalgia.* 2006;26:1025-1027.

104. Mauskop A. VNS relieves chronic refractory migraine and cluster headache. *Cephalalgia.* 2005;25(2):82-86.

105. Scoehnen J, Jensen RH, Lanteri-Minet M, et al. Stimulation of the sphenopalatine ganglion (SPG) for cluster headache treatment. Pathway CH-1: a randomized, sham-controlled study. Cephalalgia. 2013;33(10):816-830.

106. Ansarinia M, Rezai A, Tepper SJ, et al. Electrical stimulation of sphenopalatine ganglion for acute treatment of cluster headaches. *Headache.* 2010;50:1164-1174.

107. Leone M, Proletti Cecchini A, Franzini A, et al. Lessons from 8 years experience of hypothalamic stimulation in cluster headache. *Cephalalgia.* 2008;28:789-797.

108. Leone M, Franzini A, Broggi G, Bussone G. Hypothalamic stimulation for intractable cluster headache: long-term experience. *Neurology.* 2006;67:150-152.

109. Schoenen J, Di Clemente L, Vandenheede M, et al. Hypothalamic stimulation in chronic cluster headache: a pilot study of efficacy and mode of action. *Brain.* 2005;128:940-947.

110. D'Andrea G, Nordera GP, Piacento M. Effectiveness of hypothalamic stimulation in two patients affected by intractable chronic cluster headache [abstract]. *Neurology.* 2006;(Suppl)2:A140.

111. Starr PA, Barbaro NM, Raskin NH, Ostrem JL. Chronic stimulation of the posterior hypothalamic region for cluster headache: technique and 1-year results in four patients. *J Neurosurg.* 2007;106:999-1005.

112. Bartsch T, Pinsker MO, Rasche D, et al. Hypothalamic deep brain stimulation for cluster headache: experience from a new multicase series. *Cephalalgia.* 2008;28:285-295.

113. Benabid AL, Chabardes S, Seigneuret E, Torres N. Intraventricular stimulation for targets close to the midline: periaqueductal gray, posterior hypothalamus, subcommissural structures [abstract]. *Acta Neurochir (Wein).* 2006;148:I-LXIV.

114. Owen SLF, Green AL, Davies P, et al. Connectivity of an effective hypothalamic surgical target for cluster headache. *J Clin Neurosci.* 2007;14:955-960.

115. Leone M, Franzini A, Bussone G. Stereotactic stimulation of posterior hypothalamic gray matter for intractable cluster headache. *N Engl J Med.* 2001;345:1428-1429.

116. Leone M, Franzini A, Broggi G, et al. Long-term follow up of bilateral hypothalamic stimulation for intractable cluster headache. *Brain.* 2004;127:2259-2264.

117. Franzini A, Ferroli P, Leone M, et al. Hypothalamic deep brain stimulation for the treatment of chronic cluster headache: a series report. *Neuromodulation.* 2004;1:1-8.

Diagnosis and Management of Cervicogenic Headache

David M. Biondi
Zahid H. Bajwa

INTRODUCTION

Neck pain and cervical muscle tightness are common and prominent symptoms of primary headache disorders such as tension-type headache (TTH) and migraine.[1] Conversely, head pain referred from bony structures or soft tissues of the neck is a condition that is commonly called cervicogenic headache.[2] Cervicogenic headache can be a perplexing pain disorder that is often refractory to common headache treatments when it is not recognized. The successful treatment of cervicogenic headache usually requires a multifaceted approach using pharmacologic, nonpharmacologic, anesthetic, and occasionally surgical interventions.

CERVICOGENIC HEADACHE

Cervicogenic headache can be generally defined as a recurring or persistent pain that is referred to the head from bony structures or soft tissues of the neck. Although the condition's pathophysiology and source of pain have been debated,[3-5] pain is believed to be referred to the head or face from one or more muscular, neurogenic, osseous, articular, and vascular structures in the neck through a functional convergence of cervical spinal and trigeminal sensory pathways in the upper cervical spinal cord.[6] It is often a sequela of head or neck injury but may also

TABLE 31-1 The Cervicogenic Headache International Study Group Diagnostic Criteria

Major Criteria of Cervicogenic Headache
(I) Symptoms and signs of neck involvement: (a) Precipitation of head pain, similar to the usually occurring one: (1) By neck movement or sustained awkward head positioning or (2) By external pressure over the upper cervical or occipital region on the symptomatic side (b) Restriction of the range of motion in the neck (c) Ipsilateral neck, shoulder, or arm pain of a rather vague nonradicular nature or, occasionally, arm pain of a radicular nature
Points (I) (a through c) are set forth in a surmised sequence of importance. It is obligatory that one or more of the phenomena in point (I) are present. Point (a) suffices as the sole criterion for positivity within group (I); points (b) and (c) do not. Provisionally, the combination of (I) (b and c) has been set forth as a satisfactory combination within (I). The presence of all three points (a, b, and c) fortifies the diagnosis (but still, point [II] is an additional obligatory point for scientific work).
(II) Confirmatory evidence by diagnostic anesthetic blockades
Point (II) is an obligatory point in scientific works.
(III) Unilaterality of the head pain without sideshift
For scientific work, point (III) should preferably be adhered to.
Head Pain Characteristics
(IV) (a) Moderate to severe, nonthrobbing, and nonlancinating pain, usually starting in the neck (b) Episodes of varying duration or (c) Fluctuating, continuous pain
Other Characteristics of Some Importance
(V) (a) Only marginal effect or lack of effect of indomethacin (b) Only marginal effect or lack of effect of ergotamine and sumatriptan (c) Female sex (d) Not infrequent occurrence of head or indirect neck trauma by history, usually of more than only medium severity
None of the single points under (IV) and (V) are obligatory.
Other Features of Lesser Importance
(VI) Various attack-related phenomena, only occasionally present: (a) Nausea (b) Phonophobia and photophobia (c) Dizziness (d) Ipsilateral "blurred vision" (e) Difficulty in swallowing (f) Ipsilateral edema, mostly in the periocular area

occur in the absence of recognized injury. The clinical features of cervicogenic headache may mimic those commonly associated with primary headache disorders such as TTH, migraine, or hemicrania continua, and as a result, distinguishing the etiology of chronic head pain from among these headache types by medical history alone can be difficult.

DIAGNOSTIC CRITERIA

The Cervicogenic Headache International Study Group developed diagnostic criteria that have provided a detailed, clinically useful description of the condition[7] (**Table 31-1**).

EPIDEMIOLOGY

The prevalence of cervicogenic headache in the general population is estimated to be 0.4% to 4.0% but may be as high as 20% in populations of patients with chronic headache.[8-11] Although there have been no large epidemiologic studies, available information suggest the mean age of patients with cervicogenic headache is 40 to 45 years and the condition is up to four times more prevalent in women. Interestingly, the mean age and gender prevalence of cervicogenic headache are similar to those associated with migraine.

ANATOMIC BASIS

The trigeminocervical nucleus is a region of the upper cervical spinal cord, where sensory nerve fibers in the descending tract of the trigeminal nerve (trigeminal nucleus caudalis) are believed to interact with sensory fibers from the upper cervical roots. This functional convergence of cervical spinal and trigeminal sensory pathways is thought to allow the transfer of painful sensations between anatomic structures of the neck and trigeminal sensory receptive fields of the face and head.[6]

The first three cervical spinal nerves and their rami are the primary peripheral nerve structures thought to be most involved in the referral of pain sensations from the neck to the head:

- The *suboccipital nerve (dorsal ramus of C1)* innervates the atlanto-occipital joint; injury or pathology affecting this bony joint is a potential source for head pain that is referred to the occipital region of the head.
- The *C2 spinal nerve and its dorsal root ganglion* have a close proximity to the lateral capsule of the atlanto-axial (C1–C2) zygapophyseal joint and innervate the atlantoaxial and C2 to C3 zygapophyseal joints; injury or pathology affecting these joints can be potential sources of referred head pain. Pain from C2 neuralgia is typically described as a deep or dull pain that usually radiates from the occipital to the parietal, temporal, frontal, and periorbital regions of the head. A paroxysmal sharp or shocklike pain is often superimposed over the constant pain. Ipsilateral eye lacrimation and conjunctival injection can commonly be associated signs. Arterial or venous compression of the C2 spinal nerve or its dorsal root ganglion has been suggested as a cause for C2 neuralgia in some cases.[12-14]
- The *third occipital nerve (dorsal ramus C3)* has a close anatomical proximity to and innervates the C2 to C3 zygapophyseal joint. This joint and the third occipital nerve appear most vulnerable to trauma from acceleration–deceleration ("whiplash") injuries of the neck.[15] Pain from the C2 to C3 zygapophyseal joint is referred to the occipital region but is also referred to the frontotemporal and periorbital regions of the head; the condition is commonly known as *third occipital headache*. One study found a 27% prevalence of third occipital headache in patients with chronic neck pain after whiplash injury.[16] The majority of cervicogenic headaches occurring after whiplash are believed to resolve within 1 year of the injury.[17]

In general, involvement of the C2 to C3 zygapophyseal joint is believed to be the most frequent source of cervicogenic headache, accounting for up to 70% of cases.[16,18-22] The atlantoaxial joint is likely the second most common pain source, although its true prevalence in cases of cervicogenic headache is not known.[19,22] Uncommon sources

TABLE 31-2 Clinical Characteristics of Cervicogenic Headache

(a) Unilateral head or face pain without sideshift; the pain may occasionally be bilateral
(b) Pain localized to the occipital, frontal, temporal, or orbital regions
(c) Moderate to severe pain intensity
(d) Intermittent attacks of pain lasting hours to days, constant pain, or constant pain with superimposed attacks of pain
(e) Pain is generally deep and nonthrobbing in character; throbbing may occur when migraine attacks are superimposed
(f) Head pain is triggered by neck movement, sustained or awkward neck postures; digital pressure applied to the suboccipital, C2, C3, or C4 regions or over the greater occipital nerve. The Valsalva maneuver, coughing, or sneezing may also trigger head pain
(g) Restricted active and passive neck range of motion; neck stiffness
(h) Associated signs and symptoms are variably present: similar to typical migraine accompaniments such as nausea, vomiting, photophobia, phonophobia, and dizziness; ipsilateral blurred vision, lacrimation, conjunctival injection; ipsilateral neck, shoulder, or arm pain

of cervicogenic headache include the C3 to C4 zygapophyseal joint, upper cervical intervertebral discs, and lower cervical zygapophyseal joints.[18,23-25]

DIAGNOSTIC EVALUATION

A comprehensive and carefully conducted history; review of systems; and physical examination, including a complete neurologic assessment, often identify symptoms and signs that can be considered characteristic of an etiologic structural or systemic disorder for cervicogenic headache.[26] Several historical elements and physical findings obtained from a directed medical history and physical examination can be helpful in the clinical identification of cervicogenic headache (**Table 31-2**).

Diagnostic imaging such as radiography, magnetic resonance imaging (MRI), and computed tomography (CT) myelography cannot confirm the diagnosis of cervicogenic headache but can lend support to its diagnosis.[27,28] Imaging is primarily used to search for secondary causes of pain that may require surgery or other invasive forms of treatment.[29] A laboratory evaluation may be needed to identify systemic diseases that can cause inflammation or pain in muscles, bones, joints, or blood vessels (e.g., rheumatoid arthritis, systemic lupus erythematosus, thyroid or parathyroid disorders, primary muscle disease, Lyme disease).

Distinguishing cervicogenic headache from primary headache disorders, such as TTH, migraine, or hemicrania continua, may occasionally be difficult by medical history and examination alone.[30] An accurate diagnosis has important implications for the selection of treatments that would have the greatest probability of being effective. When a headache diagnosis is indeterminable by medical history and physical, diagnostic anesthetic blockade can confirm the etiology of head pain that is referred from pain sources in the neck.[30] Anesthetic blockade for the evaluation of cervicogenic headache can be directed to several anatomical structures such as the atlanto-occipital joint, atlantoaxial joint, other cervical zygapophyseal joint(s), C2 or C3 spinal nerves, third occipital nerve (dorsal ramus C3), or intervertebral discs based on the location and characteristics of the pain, and findings of the physical examination.[31] Fluoroscopic or interventional MRI–guided blockade can assure accurate and specific targeting of the suspected pain source.[32-34]

DIFFERENTIAL DIAGNOSIS

MIGRAINE AND TENSION-TYPE HEADACHE

Neck pain and muscle tightness are common symptoms of a migraine attack.[1,35-37] In a study of 50 migraine patients, 64% reported neck pain or stiffness associated with their migraine attacks, with 31% experiencing neck symptoms during the prodrome, 93% during the headache phase, and 31% during the recovery phase.[1] In this study, seven patients reported that pain referred into the ipsilateral shoulder, and one patient reported that pain extended from the neck into the low back region. In another study of 144 migraine patients from a university-based headache clinic, 75% of patients reported neck pain associated with migraine attacks.[36] Of these patients, 69% described their pain as "tightness," 17% reported "stiffness," and 5% reported "throbbing." The neck pain was unilateral in 57% of the respondents, 98% of whom reported that it occurred ipsilateral to the side of headache. The neck pain occurred during the prodrome in 61%, the acute headache phase in 92%, and the recovery phase in 41%. In addition, recurrent, unilateral neck pain without headache has been described as a variant of migraine.[38] Careful history gathering in cases of recurrent neck pain discovered that previously overlooked symptoms were either similar or identical to those associated with migraine.

Differences in neck posture, pronounced levels of muscle tenderness, and the presence of myofascial trigger points were observed in subjects with migraine, TTH, or a combination of both but not in a control group of subjects without headache.[1,39,40] A comparison of patients with chronic headache demonstrated no significant differences in myofascial symptoms or signs between headache diagnostic groups, dispelling the common belief that TTH is associated with a greater degree of musculoskeletal involvement (e.g., muscle tightness or spasm) than migraine.[40]

OCCIPITAL NEURALGIA

Occipital neuralgia (ON) is a specific pain disorder characterized by pain that is isolated to the sensory fields of the greater or lesser occipital nerves.[41] The classical description of ON includes the presence of constant deep or burning pain with superimposed paroxysms of shooting or shock-like pain. Paresthesia and numbness over the occipital scalp are often present. It is often difficult to determine the true source of pain in patients with this condition. In its classical description, the pain of ON is believed to arise from trauma to or entrapment of the occipital nerve within the neck or scalp, but similar pain may also arise from the C2 spinal root, C1 to C2 or C2 to C3 zygapophyseal joints, or pathology within the posterior cranial fossa. Occipital nerve blockade, as it is typically performed in a clinic setting, often results in a nonspecific regional blockade rather than a specific nerve blockade, which could result in misidentification of the occipital nerve as the source of pain. This "false localization" might lead to unnecessary interventions aimed at the occipital nerve, such as surgical transection or other neurolytic procedures.[5] Furthermore, there is no anatomic rationale for the use of occipital nerve blockade in the definitive diagnosis or treatment of cervicogenic headache.[22]

REGIONAL MYOFASCIAL PAIN SYNDROME

Regional myofascial pain syndrome (MPS) affecting the cervical, pericranial, or masticatory muscles can be associated with pain that is referred to the head. Sensory afferent nerve fibers from upper cervical regions have been observed to enter the spinal column by way of the spinal accessory nerve before entering the dorsal spinal cord.[42,43] The close anatomic association of sensorimotor fibers of the spinal accessory nerve with upper spinal sensory nerves is believed to allow for a functional exchange of sensory signals originating in the trapezius, sternocleidomastoid, and other cervical muscles with those of the spinal sensory nerves. The spinal sensory signals then converge with trigeminal nerve fibers in the trigeminocervical nucleus and ultimately result in the referral of pain sensation to trigeminal sensory fields of the head and face. Muscular trigger points, a clinical hallmark of MPS, are discreet hyperirritable areas of contracted muscle that have a lower than normal pain threshold and refer pain (spontaneously or when stimulated) to distant sites in predictable and reproducible patterns.[44,45] Anesthetic injections into trigger point regions that by physical examination have been associated with referred head pain can assist in the diagnostic evaluation and therapeutic management of cervicogenic headache referred from pain sources in cervical muscles.[44]

OTHER SYSTEMIC AND STRUCTURAL DISORDERS

Other disorders that may be associated with referral of pain from the neck to the head include posterior fossa tumors, Arnold-Chiari malformation, cervical spondylosis or arthropathy, herniated intervertebral cervical disc, spinal nerve compression, spinal nerve tumor, arteriovenous malformation, vertebral artery dissection, and intramedullary or extramedullary spinal tumors. Of interest, substantial relief of chronic head pain has been reported after discectomy at cervical spine levels as low as C5 to C6.[24,25] A diagnosis other than cervicogenic headache should be considered in cases with clinical presentations atypical for the diagnosis, neurological deficits, or refractoriness to treatments expected to be effective for cervicogenic headache.

TREATMENT

No single treatment has been proven effective for the treatment of cervicogenic headache. The successful treatment of cervicogenic headache usually requires a multifaceted approach using pharmacologic, nonpharmacologic, anesthetic, and occasionally surgical interventions (**Table 31-3**). Medications alone are often ineffective or provide only modest benefit for

TABLE 31-3 Potential Treatment Interventions for Cervicogenic Headache

Pharmacologic*

(a) Monoamine Reuptake Inhibitors
- TCAs (amitriptyline, nortriptyline, doxepin, desipramine, and others)
- SNRIs (duloxetine, venlafaxine)

(b) AEDs (pregabalin, gabapentin, carbamazepine, topiramate, divalproex sodium, and others)
(c) Muscle relaxants (tizanidine, baclofen, cyclobenzaprine, metaxalone, and others)
(d) NSAIDs
- Nonselective COX inhibitors (indomethacin, ibuprofen, naproxen, and others)
- COX-2 selective inhibitor (celecoxib)

(e) Botulinum toxin injections (intramuscular injections)
(f) Opiate and opioid analgesics

Nonpharmacologic

(a) Physical therapy and physical conditioning
(b) Manual or manipulative therapies
(c) Biofeedback or relaxation therapies
(d) Individual psychotherapy

Interventional

(a) Anesthetic blockade
- Spinal roots, nerves, rami, or branches
- Zygapophyseal joints
- Muscular trigger points

(b) Neurotomy
- Percutaneous radiofrequency neurolysis

(c) Occipital nerve stimulator

Surgical

(a) Microvascular decompression
(b) Nerve exploration and "release"
(c) Zygapophyseal joint fusion
(d) Dorsal rhizotomy
(e) Neurectomy

*None of the listed medications has an approved indication for management of cervicogenic headaches. Prescribers should refer to drug references or approved product package inserts for recommended dosages, laboratory monitoring guidelines, and full side effect profiles before prescribing any of the medications or medication classes listed.

AED, antiepileptic drug; COX, cyclooxygenase; NSAID, Nonsteroidal anti-inflammatory drug; SNRI, serotonin–norepinephrine reuptake inhibitor; TCA, tricyclic antidepressant.

this condition. Anesthetic injections directed to the anatomic source or sources of pain can temporarily reduce pain intensity but have their greatest benefit by allowing greater participation in physical treatments or rehabilitation. The success of diagnostic cervical spinal nerve, medial branch, or zygapophyseal joint blockade may help predict response to subsequent percutaneous radiofrequency neurolysis. After the accurate diagnosis of cervicogenic headache, developing an individualized treatment plan tends to enhance the likelihood of a successful outcome.

PHYSICAL AND MANUAL THERAPIES

Physical therapy can provide long-term improvement and is an important therapeutic modality for the rehabilitation of cervicogenic headache.[46-49] The intensity of head pain might initially worsen during or after physical therapy, especially if it is too vigorously applied. Physical treatment is better tolerated when initiated with gentle muscle stretching and manual cervical traction. Therapy can be slowly advanced as tolerated and should include regional muscle strengthening and general aerobic conditioning. Using anesthetic blockade and neurolytic procedures for temporary pain relief may enhance the effectiveness of physical therapy. Cervical manipulation, in particular high-velocity cervical manipulation techniques,have been associated with risks of arterial dissection and stroke in the vertebrobasilar territory.[50] Cervical manipulation should only be performed by a practitioner with expertise and extensive experience in these types of manipulation techniques.

PSYCHOLOGICAL AND BEHAVIORAL TREATMENTS

Psychological and nonpharmacologic interventions such as biofeedback, relaxation, and cognitive-behavioral therapy are important adjunctive treatments in the comprehensive management of chronic pain.[51] Ongoing intensive, individual psychotherapy may be required if the patient has a prominent affective or behavioral component, pain-related disability, or persistent pain despite aggressive treatment.

PHARMACOLOGIC TREATMENT

Pharmacologic treatments for cervicogenic headache include many medications that are used for the preventive management of episodic or chronic migraine, or the palliative management of chronic neuropathic pain syndromes. The medications listed here have neither been approved by the U.S. Food and Drug Administration (FDA) nor rigorously studied in controlled clinical trials specifically for the treatment of cervicogenic headache. Accordingly, the medications are only suggested as potential treatments based on the anecdotal experiences of clinicians who treat this condition or similar pain disorders. Some of these medications have FDA approval for migraine prophylaxis and might be particularly useful for the management of patients with cervicogenic headache who have coexisting migraine. Prescribers should refer to drug references or approved product package inserts for recommended dosages, laboratory monitoring guidelines, and full side effect profiles before prescribing any of the listed medications or medication classes.

Medication, when used alone, does not generally provide substantial pain relief in most cases of cervicogenic headache. As a consequence, many patients with cervicogenic headache overuse or become dependent on analgesics. Despite this observation, the judicious use of medications can provide patients with sufficient pain relief to allow greater participation in a physical therapy and rehabilitation program. To improve medical side effect tolerance and treatment persistence, medications that are to be taken every day for the management of chronic pain are often prescribed at a low initial dose and increased as tolerated over 4 to 8 weeks to a beneficial effect or to the maximum recommended daily dosage. Cautiously combining medications with different or complementary pharmacologic mechanisms of analgesic action (i.e., rational multiple drug therapy) may provide greater effectiveness than using individual drugs alone. Frequent follow-up visits for medication dosage adjustments, monitoring of serum drug levels, and signs of medication toxicity are recommended.

SIMPLE ANALGESICS

Acetaminophen, aspirin, or nonsteroidal anti-inflammatory drugs (NSAIDs) may be used as needed for the treatment of acute pain. NSAIDs may be judiciously used as a regularly scheduled medication for around-the-clock management of chronic pain. The cyclooxygenase-2 inhibitor celecoxib may have less gastrointestinal toxicity than nonselective NSAIDs. Renal toxicity and cardiovascular events with extended use are common risks to all NSAIDS.

ANTIEPILEPTIC DRUGS

Antiepileptic drugs (AEDs) are believed to be modulators or stabilizers of peripheral and central transmission of pain signals and are commonly used for the management of chronic neuropathic pain and face pain syndromes, and migraine prophylaxis. Pregabalin is indicated for the management neuropathic pain associated with postherpetic neuralgia, diabetic peripheral neuropathy, and spinal cord injury. It is also indicated for the management of pain associated with fibromyalgia, and therefore it might be considered in the management of chronic cervicogenic headache. No specific laboratory monitoring is typically needed. Gabapentin is indicated for the management of postherpetic neuralgia and anecdotally has been helpful in the management of other neuropathic pain syndromes and migraine. No specific laboratory monitoring is typically needed. Topiramate is indicated for preventive management of migraine in adults and anecdotally has been helpful in the management of pain associated with diabetic neuropathy and cluster headache prophylaxis. Regular laboratory monitoring (e.g., serum electrolytes) is suggested because of this medication's diuretic effect through carbonic anhydrase inhibition. Carbamazepine has demonstrated effectiveness for the treatment of trigeminal neuralgia and central neuropathic pain syndromes. Serum drug levels are used as a therapeutic dosing guide, and regular laboratory monitoring is recommended. Divalproex sodium is indicated for the preventive management of migraine headache and anecdotally has been helpful for cluster headache prophylaxis and management of neuropathic pain (e.g., trigeminal neuralgia). Serum drug levels are used as a therapeutic dosing guide, and regular laboratory monitoring is recommended. Several of the other AEDs might be considered for use in cases of refractory pain.

MONOAMINE REUPTAKE INHIBITORS (ANTIDEPRESSANTS)

Tricyclic antidepressants, such as amitriptyline and nortriptyline, have demonstrated effectiveness in the management of chronic musculoskeletal pain, migraine, TTH, facial neuralgias, and other neuropathic pain syndromes. Analgesic dosages are typically lower than those used in the treatment of depression. Serotonin–norepinephrine reuptake inhibitors (SNRIs), such as venlafaxine and duloxetine, anecdotally have been helpful in the preventive management of migraine. Duloxetine is indicated for the management of pain associated with diabetic neuropathy and fibromyalgia, and venlafaxine anecdotally has been helpful in these conditions. The selective serotonin reuptake inhibitors (SSRIs) are generally not effective in the management of pain but might improve mood when depression and chronic pain are comorbid.

MUSCLE RELAXANTS AND BOTULINUM TOXIN

Muscle relaxants, particularly those with central activity such as tizanidine and baclofen, might be helpful in the management of chronic pain and muscle spasms associated with cervicogenic headache. Botulinum toxin type A injected into pericranial and cervical muscles is indicated for the management of chronic migraine, and although it anecdotally has been helpful in the management of cervicogenic headache,[52,53] a well-designed clinical study demonstrated no benefit for this condition.[54]

OPIATE AND OPIOID ANALGESICS

Opiate and opioid analgesics may be cautiously prescribed for temporary relief of moderate to severe acute pain. Tapentadol, an opiate analgesic that also inhibits reuptake of norepinephrine, might also be considered for temporary relief of moderate to severe acute pain. Tramadol might be an alternative to the more potent opioid analgesics for temporary relief of moderate acute pain. Opiate and opioid analgesics have generally not demonstrated effectiveness in the long-term management of chronic headache[55] and therefore might only be considered in cases of refractory pain when other reasonable and appropriate treatment options have failed.

MIGRAINE-SPECIFIC TREATMENTS

Migraine-specific abortive medications such as ergot derivatives or triptans are not indicated for the treatment of chronic head pain associated with cervicogenic headache but may be effective in relieving the acute pain of episodic migraine attacks experienced by some patients.

ANESTHETIC BLOCKADE AND NEUROLYSIS

Cervical epidural steroid injections may be considered in cases of multilevel disc or spine degeneration.[56] Anesthetic injections of the lateral atlantoaxial joint, the C2 to C3 zygapophyseal joint, or the C3 to C4 zygapophyseal joint can temporarily reduce or relieve pain. Despite there being no anatomic rationale for occipital nerve blockade in the definitive diagnosis of cervicogenic headache, greater and lesser occipital nerve blockade has reportedly provided temporary pain relief in some cases.[22,57] Small retrospective studies have suggested some relief can be obtained from spinal intraarticular glucocorticoid injections.[58,59] Local anesthetic injections or dry needling of intramuscular trigger points may provide temporary pain relief and relaxation of local muscle spasm. If the directed diagnostic blockade of a cervical nerve, medial branch, or zygapophyseal joint provides substantial but temporary pain relief, consideration can be given to treatment with a neurolytic procedure such as percutaneous radiofrequency neurotomy.[60,61] Although the benefit of this procedure for cervicogenic headache has not been established by adequate randomized controlled trials, clinical studies have demonstrated evidence of benefit in cases of cervicogenic headache when the diagnosis has been confirmed by diagnostic anesthetic nerve blockade.[62-64] A course of physical therapy and rehabilitation is recommended after anesthetic blockade or neurolytic procedures to enhance functional restoration and affect a longer lasting analgesic benefit.

SURGERY

Surgical procedures such as neurectomy, dorsal rhizotomy, and microvascular decompression of nerve roots or peripheral nerves are not generally recommended without compelling radiologic evidence for a surgically correctable pathology and a history of refractoriness to reasonable nonsurgical treatments. A variety of surgical interventions have been performed for presumed cases of cervicogenic headache. Surgical decompression and microsurgical neurolysis of the C2 spinal nerve have reportedly been helpful in cases of cervicogenic headache that were confirmed by diagnostic block of the C2 spinal nerve.[65] Arthrodesis may be a treatment option in cases of chronic neck pain and headache related to osteoarthritis of the lateral atlantoaxial joint.[66-68] Surgical liberation of the occipital nerve from "entrapment" in the trapezius muscle or surrounding connective tissues has been reported to provide temporary pain relief in some cases.[69] Similarly, temporary pain relief has been observed after surgical transection of the greater occipital nerve.[70] Of concern is that ablative or surgical interventions involving peripheral nerves may be associated with risks of worsening of pain intensity, adverse changes in pain quality, or anesthesia dolorosa.

SUMMARY

Cervicogenic headache is a relatively common cause of chronic headache that is often unrecognized or misdiagnosed. Its presenting symptom profile can be similar to that of the more commonly encountered primary headache disorders such as TTH or migraine. Early diagnosis and management that targets the source of the referred pain is essential to reducing the protracted course of disability and costly treatment that is often observed when the condition is not appropriately identified and managed.

Although the underlying pathophysiology and source of pain in cervicogenic headache have been debated, the leading explanation is that the pain in cervicogenic headache is referred to the head from one or more anatomic structures or soft tissues in the neck through a functional convergence of cervical spinal and trigeminal sensory pathways in the trigeminocervical nucleus located in the upper cervical spinal cord.

There is no widely accepted consensus guideline for the diagnosis of cervicogenic headache, but the Cervicogenic Headache International Study Group has developed diagnostic criteria that provide a useful clinical guideline. Comprehensive medical history and physical examination are necessary to identify the historical elements and physical findings that are characteristic of cervicogenic headache and clinically differentiate it from the common primary headache disorders. Complete pain relief after controlled anesthetic blockade of specified cervical structures or their sensory nerve supply can definitively confirm the diagnosis. Other headache diagnoses or etiologies should be considered if the response to diagnostic anesthetic blockade is incomplete.

There is no single treatment that has been proven effective for cervicogenic headache. Using a multidisciplinary treatment program provides the best opportunity for success. Multidisciplinary treatment programs would typically include physical therapy, anesthetic blockade of the involved cervical structure or its sensory nerve supply, palliative medications, and psychological or behavioral therapies as needed. For patients who temporarily respond to anesthetic blockade but are refractory to physical and pharmacologic treatments, percutaneous radiofrequency rhizolysis may be considered. Surgical interventions are not recommended unless the pain is refractory to all reasonable nonsurgical treatments and there is compelling radiologic evidence of a surgically correctable lesion.

REFERENCES

1. Blau JN, MacGregor EA. Migraine and the neck. *Headache.* 1994;34:88-90.
2. Sjaastad O, Saunte C, Hovdahl H, et al. Cervicogenic headache—a hypothesis. *Cephalalgia.* 1983;3:249-256.
3. Edmeads J. The cervical spine and headache. *Neurology.* 1988; 38:1874-1878.
4. Pollmann W, Keidel M, Pfaffenrath V. Headache and the cervical spine: a critical review. *Cephalalgia.* 1997;17:501-516.
5. Leone M, D'Amico D, Grazzi L, et al. Cervicogenic headache: a critical review of the current diagnostic criteria. *Pain.* 1998;78:1-5.
6. Bogduk N. The anatomical basis for cervicogenic headache. *J Manipulative Physiol Ther.* 1992;15:67-70.
7. Sjaastad O, Fredriiksen TA, Pfaffenrath V. Cervicogenic headache: diagnostic criteria. The cervicogenic Headache International Study Group. *Headache.* 1998;38:442-445.
8. Haldeman S, Dagenais S. Cervicogenic headaches: a critical review. *Spine J.* 2001;1:31-46.
9. Sjaastad O. Cervicogenic headache: comparison with migraine without aura; Vågå study. *Cephalalgia.* 2008;28(Suppl 1):18-20.
10. Nilsson N. The prevalence of cervicogenic headache in a random population sample of 20-59 year olds. *Spine.* 1995;20:1884-1888.
11. Sjaastad O, Fredriksen TA. Cervicogenic headache: criteria, classification and epidemiology. *Clin Exp Rheumatol.* 2000;18:S3-S6.
12. Pikus HJ, Phillips JM. Outcome of surgical decompression of the second cervical root for cervicogenic headache. *Neurosurgery.* 1996;39:63-70.
13. Pikus HJ, Phillips JM. Characteristics of patients successfully treated for cervicogenic headache by surgical decompression of the second cervical root. *Headache.* 1995;35:621-629.
14. Jansen J, Bardosi A, Hildebrandt J, Lucke A. Cervicogenic hemicranial attacks associated with vascular irritation or compression of the cervical nerve root C2. Clinical manifestations and morphological findings. *Pain.* 1998;39:203-212.
15. Lord SM, Barnsley L, Wallis BJ, Bogduk N. Chronic cervical zygapophyseal joint pain after whiplash. A placebo controlled prevalence study. *Spine.* 1996;21:1737-1744.
16. Lord SM, Barnsley L, Wallis BJ, Bogduk N. Third occipital nerve headache: a prevalence study. *J Neurol Neurosurg Psychiatry.* 1994;57:1187-1190.
17. Drottning M, Staff PH, Sjaastad O. Cervicogenic headache after whiplash injury. *Cephalalgia.* 2002;22:165-171.
18. Cooper G, Bailey B, Bogduk N. Cervical zygapophysial joint pain maps. *Pain Med.* 2007;8:344-353.
19. Dwyer A, Aprill C, Bogduk N. Cervical zygapophyseal joint pain patterns. A study in normal volunteers. *Spine.* 1990;15:453-457.
20. Bogduk N, Marsland A. The cervical zygapophysial joints as a source of neck pain. *Spine.* 1988;13:610-617.
21. Bogduk N, Marsland A. On the concept of third occipital headache. *J Neurol Neurosurg Psychiatry.* 1986;49:775-780.
22. Bogduk N, Govind J. Cervicogenic headache: an assessment of the evidence on clinical diagnosis, invasive tests, and treatment. *Lancet Neurol.* 2009;8:959-968.
23. Schofferman J, Garges K, Goldthwaite N, et al. Upper cervical anterior diskectomy and fusion improves discogenic cervical headaches. *Spine.* 2002;27:2240-2244.
24. Park SW, Park YS, Nam TK, Cho TG. The effect of radiofrequency neurotomy of lower cervical medial branches on cervicogenic headache. *J Korean Neurosurg Soc.* 2011;50:507-511.
25. Michler RP, Bovim G, Sjaastad O. Disorders in the lower cervical spine. A cause of unilateral headache? A case report. *Headache.* 1991;31:550-551.
26. Pfaffenrath V, Dandekar R, Pollman W. Cervicogenic headache—the clinical picture, radiologic findings and hypothesis of its pathophysiology. *Headache.* 1987;27:495-499.
27. Fredriksen TA, Fougner R, Tangerud A, Sjaastad O. Cervicogenic headache. Radiological investigations concerning head/neck. *Cephalalgia.* 1989;9:139-146.
28. Knackstedt H, Kråkenes J, Bansevicius D, Russell MB. Magnetic resonance imaging of craniovertebral structures: clinical significance in cervicogenic headaches. *J Headache Pain.* 2012;13:39-44.
29. Delfini R, Salvati M, Passacantilli E, Pacciani E. Symptomatic cervicogenic headache. *Clin Exp Rheumatol.* 2000;18:S29-S32.
30. Bogduk, N. Distinguishing primary headache disorders from cervicogenic headache: clinical and therapeutic implications. *Headache Currents.* 2005;2:27-36.
31. Van Suijlekom JA, Weber WE, van Kleef M. Cervicogenic headache: techniques of diagnostic nerve blocks. *Clin Exp Rheumatol.* 2000;18:S39-S44.
32. Stolker RJ, Vervest AC, Groen GJ. The management of chronic spinal pain by blockades: a review. *Pain.* 1994;58:1-20.
33. Schellhas KP. Facet nerve blockade and radiofrequency neurotomy. *Neuroimaging Clin N Am.* 2000;10:493-501.
34. Bovim G, Berg R, Dale LG. Cervicogenic headache: anesthetic blockades of cervical nerves (C2- C5) and facet joint (C2/C3). *Pain.* 1992;49:315-320.
35. Tfelt-Hansen P, Lous I, Olesen J. Prevalence and significance of muscle tenderness during common migraine attacks. *Headache.* 1981;21:49-54.
36. Kaniecki RG. Migraine and tension-type headache: an assessment of challenges in diagnosis. *Neurology.* 2002;58:S15-S20.
37. Waelkens J. Warning symptoms in migraine: characteristics and therapeutic implications. *Cephalalgia.* 1985;5:223-228.
38. De Marinis M, Accornero N. Recurrent neck pain as a variant of migraine: description of four cases. *J Neurol Neurosurg Psychiatry.* 1997;62:669-670.
39. Lebbink J, Spierings EL, Messinger HB. A questionnaire survey of muscular symptoms in chronic headache. An age- and sex-controlled study. *Clin J Pain.* 1991;7:95-101.
40. Marcus DA, Scharff L, Mercer S, Turk DC. Musculoskeletal abnormalities in chronic headache: a controlled comparison of headache diagnostic groups. *Headache.* 1999;39:21-27.
41. Bogduk N. The anatomy of occipital neuralgia. *Clin Exp Neurol.* 1981;17:167-184.
42. Bremner-Smith AT, Unwin AJ, Williams WW. Sensory pathways in the spinal accessory nerve. *J Bone Joint Surg.* 1991;81:226-228.
43. Fitzgerald MJ, Comerford PT, Tuffery AR. Sources of innervation of the neuromuscular spindles in sternomastoid and trapezius. *J Anat.* 1982;134(Pt 3):471-490.
44. Jaeger B. Are "cervicogenic" headaches due to myofascial pain and cervical spine dysfunction? *Cephalalgia.* 1998;9:157-164.

45. Travell J. Referred pain from skeletal muscle; the pectoralis major syndrome of breast pain and soreness and the sternomastoid syndrome of headache and dizziness. New York State *J Med.* 1955;55:331-340.

46. Nilsson N, Christensen HW, Hartvigsen J. The effect of spinal manipulation in the treatment of cervicogenic headache. *J Manipulative Physiol Ther.* 1997;20:326-330.

47. Jull G, Trott P, Potter H, et al. A randomized controlled trial of exercise and manipulative therapy for cervicogenic headache. *Spine.* 2002;27:1835-1843.

48. Hall T, Chan HT, Christensen L, et al. Efficacy of a C1-C2 self-sustained natural apophyseal glide (SNAG) in the management of cervicogenic headache. *J Orthop Sports Phys Ther.* 2007;37:100-107.

49. Kay TM, Gross A, Goldsmith CH, et al. Exercises for mechanical neck disorders. *Cochrane Database Syst Rev.* 2012;8(8):CD004250.

50. Smith WS, Johnston SC, Skalabrin EJ, et al. Spinal manipulative therapy is an independent risk factor for vertebral artery dissection. *Neurology.* 2003;60:1424-1428.

51. Roberts AH, Sternbach RA, Polich J. Behavioral management of chronic pain and excess disability: long-term follow-up of an outpatient program. *Clin J Pain.* 1993;9:41-48.

52. Hobson DE, Gladish DF. Botulinum toxin injection for cervicogenic headache. *Headache.* 1997;37:253-255.

53. Wheeler AH. Botulinum toxin A: adjunctive therapy for refractory headaches associated with pericranial muscle tension. *Headache.* 1998;38:468-471.

54. Linde M, Hagen K, Salvesen Ø, et al. Onabotulinum toxin A treatment of cervicogenic headache: a randomised, double-blind, placebo-controlled crossover study. *Cephalalgia.* 2011;31:797-807.

55. Saper JR, Lake III AE, Hamel RL, et al. Daily scheduled opioids for intractable head pain. Long-term observations of a treatment program. *Neurology.* 2004;62:1687-1694.

56. Reale C, Turkiewicz AM, Reale CA, et al. Epidural steroids as a pharmacological approach. *Clin Exp Rheumatol.* 2000;18:S65-S66.

57. Anthony M. Cervicogenic headache: prevalence and response to local steroid therapy. *Clin Exp Rheumatol.* 2000;18:S59-S64.

58. Slipman CW, Lipetz JS, Plastaras CT, et al. Therapeutic zygapophyseal joint injections for headaches emanating from the C2-3 joint. *Am J Phys Med Rehabil.* 2001;80:182-188.

59. Narouze SN, Casanova J, Mekhail N. The longitudinal effectiveness of lateral atlanto-axial intra-articular steroid injection in the treatment of cervicogenic headache. *Pain Med.* 2007;8:184-188.

60. McDonald GJ, Lord SM, Bogduk N. Long-term follow-up of patients treated with cervical radiofrequency neurotomy for chronic neck pain. *Neurosurgery.* 1999;45:61-67.

61. Lord SM, Barnsley L, Wallis BJ, et al. Percutaneous radio-frequency neurotomy for chronic cervical zygapophyseal joint pain. *N Engl J Med.* 1996;335:1721-1726.

62. Govind J, King W, Bailey B, Bogduk N. Radiofrequency neurotomy for the treatment of third occipital headache. *J Neurol Neurosurg Psychiatry.* 2003;74:88-93.

63. Lord SM, Barnsley L, Wallis BJ, et al. Percutaneous radio-frequency neurotomy for chronic cervical zygapophyseal joint pain. *N Engl J Med.* 1996;335:1721-1726.

64. Stovner LJ, Kolstad F, Helde G. Radiofrequency denervation of facet joints C2-C6 in cervicogenic headache: a randomized, double-blind, sham-controlled study. *Cephalalgia.* 2004;24:821-830.

65. Pikus HJ, Phillips JM. Characteristics of patients successfully treated for cervicogenic headache by surgical decompression of the second cervical root. *Headache.* 1995;35:621-629.

66. Joseph B, Kumar B. Gallie's fusion for atlantoaxial arthrosis with occipital neuralgia. *Spine.* 1994;19:454-455.

67. Ghanayem AJ, Leventhal M, Bohlman HH. Osteoarthrosis of the atlanto-axial joints. Long-term follow-up after treatment with arthrodesis. *J Bone Joint Surg Am.* 1996;78:1300-1307.

68. Schaeren S, Jeanneret B. Atlantoaxial osteoarthritis: case series and review of the literature. *Eur Spine J.* 2005;14:501-506.

69. Sharma RR, Parekh HC, Prabhu S, et al. Compression of the C-2 root by a rare anomalous ectatic vertebral artery. Case report. *J Neurosurg.* 1993;78:669-672.

70. Bovim G, Fredriksen TA, Stolt-Nielsen A, Sjaastad O. Neurolysis of the greater occipital nerve in cervicogenic headache. A follow-up study. *Headache.* 1992;32:175-179.

CHAPTER 32 Chronic Daily Headache

Egilius L.H. Spierings

Chronic daily headache relates to the daily or almost-daily occurrence of headache for a prolonged period of time. However, not all daily or almost-daily headaches fall under this denominator, as is the case with the daily or almost-daily headaches of (chronic) cluster headache and (chronic) paroxysmal hemicrania. These conditions can be referred to as *paroxysmal* daily headaches in which the headaches occur in well-defined attack patterns. In cluster headache, the attack pattern is that of headaches occurring once or twice a day and lasting 1 to 2 hours, whereas in paroxysmal hemicrania, it is that of headaches occurring 5 to 15 times per day and lasting 10 to 30 minutes.

Of the *non*paroxysmal daily headaches, *hemicrania continua* is a condition that does not fall under the denominator of chronic daily headache, either. However, it is discussed in this chapter because it is very difficult, if not impossible, to distinguish from chronic daily headache on the basis of presentation alone. It differs from chronic daily headache in having a somewhat more consistent and less variable intensity of the pain and in an absolute response to preventive treatment with indomethacin.

In *The International Classification of Headache Disorders*, 2nd edition,[1] hemicrania continua is described under 4.7 as a persistent, strictly unilateral headache responsive to indomethacin. The diagnostic criteria are:

A. Headache for more than 3 months fulfilling criteria B through D.

B. All of the following characteristics:

   1. Unilateral pain without side-shift.
   2. Daily and continuous, without pain-free periods.
   3. Moderate intensity but with exacerbations of severe pain.

C. At least one of the following autonomic features occurs during exacerbations and ipsilateral to the side of pain:

   1. Conjunctival injection and/or lacrimation.
   2. Nasal congestion and/or rhinorrhea.
   3. Ptosis and/or miosis.

D. Complete response to therapeutic doses of indomethacin.

E. Not attributed to another disorder.

In terms of the diagnoses listed in *The International Classification of Headache Disorders*, chronic daily headache comprises the following three: chronic migraine (1.5.1), chronic tension-type headache (2.3), and new daily-persistent headache (4.8).

Chronic migraine is described as migraine headache occurring on 15 or more days per month for more than 3 months in the absence of medication overuse. The diagnostic criteria are:

A. Headache fulfilling criteria C and D for 1.1 *Migraine without aura* on 15 or more days per month for more than 3 months.

B. Not attributed to another disorder.

The criteria C and D for 1.1 Migraine without aura are as follows:

C. Headache has at least two of the following characteristics:
   1. Unilateral location.
   2. Pulsating quality.
   3. Moderate or severe pain intensity.
   4. Aggravation by or causing avoidance of routine physical activity.

D. During the headache, at least one of the following:
   1. Nausea and/or vomiting.
   2. Photophobia and phonophobia.

In 2006, the Headache Classification Subcommittee[2] changed the diagnostic criteria for chronic migraine as follows to be more inclusive:

A. Headache on 15 days or more per month for more than 3 months.

B. Occurring in a patient who has had at least five attacks fulfilling criteria for 1.1 *Migraine without aura.*

C. On 8 or more days per month for more than 3 months, headache has fulfilled C1 and/or C2 below, that is, it has fulfilled criteria for pain and associated symptoms of 1.1 *Migraine without aura*
   1. Has at least two of a through d:
      a. Unilateral location.
      b. Pulsating quality.
      c. Moderate or severe intensityc.
      d. Aggravation by or causing avoidance of routine physical activity and has at least one of a or b.
      e. Nausea and/or vomiting.
      f. Photophobia and phonophobia.
   2. Treated and relieved by triptan(s) or ergot before the expected development of C1 above.

D. No medication overuse and not attributed to another causative disorder.

Chronic tension-type headache is described as a disorder evolving from episodic tension-type headache, with daily or very frequent episodes of headache lasting minutes to days. The diagnostic criteria are:

A. Headache occurring on 15 or more days per month on average for more than 3 months (180 or more days per year) and fulfilling criteria B through D.

B. Headache lasts hours or may be continuous.

C. Headache has at least two of the following characteristics:
   1. Bilateral location.
   2. Pressing/tightening (nonpulsating) quality.
   3. Mild or moderate intensity.
   4. Not aggravated by routine physical activity such as walking or climbing stairs.

D. Both of the following:
   1. No more than one of photophobia, phonophobia, or mild nausea.
   2. Neither moderate or severe nausea nor vomiting.

E. Not attributed to another disorder.

New daily-persistent headache is described as headache that is daily and unremitting from very soon after onset (within 3 days at most). The diagnostic criteria are:

A. Headache for more than 3 months fulfilling criteria B through D.

B. Headache is daily and unremitting from onset of within 3 days from onset.

C. At least two of the following pain characteristics:
   1. Bilateral location.
   2. Pressing/tightening (nonpulsating) quality.
   3. Mild or moderate intensity.
   4. Not aggravated by routine physical activity such as walking or climbing stairs.

D. Both of the following:
   1. No more than one of photophobia, phonophobia, or mild nausea.
   2. Neither moderate or severe nausea nor vomiting.

E. Not attributed to another disorder.

Regarding the preceding diagnostic criteria, of the four nonparoxysmal, daily-headache conditions, two remarks should be made: (1) The diagnosis of the condition Sjaastad and I[3] described as hemicrania continua does not require "exacerbations of severe pain" or "autonomic features." (2) The criteria under C and D for the diagnosis of chronic tension-type headache are the same as those under C and D for that of new daily-persistent headache. This suggests that abrupt, as opposed to gradual, onset of daily or almost daily headache is unique to chronic tension-type headache; in my experience, it is not and is also quite common in chronic migraine. In addition, chronic migraine can also develop out of a history of episodic tension-type headache.

PREVALENCE

With regard to the prevalence of *daily* headache in the general population, the most reliable information comes from a non-headache study conducted in the Netherlands in 1975–1976.[4] The study was conducted in two districts of Zoetermeer, a midsize town near Leiden, and involved a random sample of 15,563 subjects. The sample size was 4522 (29% of the population), and the response rate was 77%, generating 2198 subjects who were 20 years of age or older. The respondents were asked to fill out a questionnaire that included the following question: "How often do you have headache?" One of the answer options was "daily." In the study, 6% of the respondents aged 20 years or older (4% of the men, 8% of the women) acknowledged the daily occurrence of headache. The highest prevalence was found in the age groups 20 to 24 years (8%) and older than 64 years (8%), and the lowest prevalence in the age group 35 to 54 years (5%).

The prevalence of frequent headache, that is, headaches occurring at least 180 days per year, in the general population is known from two more recent studies.[5,6] One of the studies was conducted in Baltimore County, Maryland. It involved 13,343 randomly selected subjects 18 to 65 years of age, comprising 77% of the total of 17,237 eligible subjects. Of the respondents, 40% were men and 60% were women, and their median age was 38 years. The 1-year prevalence of frequent headache was 4%: 3% in men and 5% in women. Using the International Headache Society (IHS) criteria for chronic tension-type headache and Silberstein's modified criteria for transformed migraine,[7] the investigators found a prevalence of 2.2% for chronic tension-type headache, 1.3% for frequent headache with migrainous features, and 0.6% for other frequent headaches. They found the prevalence of frequent headache to be highest in the age group 41 to 55 years and lowest in the age group 56 to 65 years.

The other study was conducted in Camargo, Spain. The study involved 1883 subjects older than 14 years of age, which was 84% of the randomly selected sample of 2252. Of the respondents, 47% were men and 53% were women. Participants who indicated that they had headaches 10 days per month or more were requested to keep a headache diary for 1 month. On the basis of the diary, the prevalence of frequent headache—that is, headaches occurring 15 days per month or more—was determined to be 4.7%: 1.0% in men and 8.7% in women. The

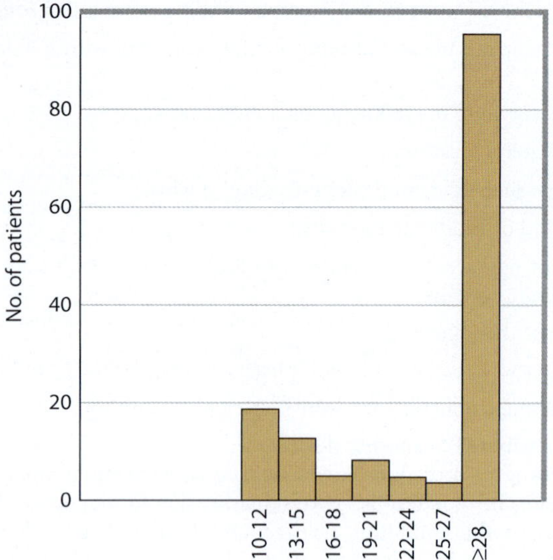

FIGURE 32-1. Distribution of patients according to the number of headache days per month. (Reproduced with permission from Langemark M, Olesen J, Loldrup D, Bech P. Clinical characterization of patients with chronic tension headache. *Headache*. 1988;28:590-596.)

mean age of the subjects with frequent headache was 50 years; the mean age at onset of the frequent headaches was 38 years. Using the criteria presented earlier, the prevalence of chronic tension-type headache was determined to be 2.2% and that of transformed migraine 2.4%. Overuse of abortive medications was found to be the case in (only) 19% of the patients with chronic tension-type headache and in 31% of those with transformed migraine.

With regard to frequent headache, Langemark and colleagues[8] studied the clinical features of 148 patients with chronic tension headache. The patients had to have at least 10 days with headache per month and no more than one migraine attack. Ninety-three percent of them turned out to have at least 28 days with headache per month, that is, daily headaches (**Fig. 32-1**). With regard to headache dynamics, this suggests that once headaches have increased to a frequency of 2 or 3 days per week, they rapidly progress to daily or almost-daily occurrence. The implication of this observation for the diagnostic criteria of chronic daily headache is that there is no need for an arbitrary number such as 15 (or 180). The diagnostic criterion for the condition with regard to frequency of headache could simply be "daily or near/almost daily," and the same simplification could be made for chronic tension-type headache. Everything that falls short of this frequency criterion would be episodic, that is, episodic tension-type headache or (episodic) migraine. This observation also means that the prevalence of frequent headache can be equated with that of daily headache.

On the basis of the preceding epidemiologic studies, and taking the study by Langemark and colleagues into account, it can safely be stated that the prevalence of daily headache in the general population is approximately 5%. About half of these headaches are accounted for by chronic tension-type headache. With regard to age and gender characteristics of chronic daily headache, women are affected two times more often than are men, but age does not seem to have much of an effect on the prevalence of the condition.

The prevalence of chronic tension-type headache in the general population was also separately determined in Denmark.[9] The study included 740 (76%) of 975 randomly selected subjects out of a total population of 325,621. The subjects were interviewed clinically, generating a prevalence number for chronic tension-type headache of 3%: 2% in men and 5% in women. It can, therefore, be safely stated that the prevalence of chronic tension-type headache in the general population is 2% to 3%, which accounts for about half of daily headaches.

PRESENTATION

In a study of chronic daily headache that my colleagues and I conducted,[10-12] we defined the condition as headaches occurring at least 5 days per week for a period of 1 year or longer. We excluded only the patients with paroxysmal daily headaches—that is, cluster headache and paroxysmal hemicrania—in order to capture as much of the presentation, development, and outcome of chronic daily headache as possible. The study was conducted in 258 patients from my private headache practice, 19% men and 81% women, with an average age at consultation of 42 years. The distribution of the age of (any) headache onset for the men and women separately is shown in **Figure 32-2**. Seventy-seven percent of the patients (69% of the men and 79% of the women) experienced the onset of headache before the age of 30 years. The onset of headache occurred in the second decade of life in 36% of the women, compared with 24% of the men. The peak of headache onset in the second decade in women is consistent with the importance of the menstrual cycle in headache occurrence.

With regard to diurnal pattern, the daily headaches were present on awakening or occurred in the course of the morning in 79% of the patients, occurred in the afternoon or evening in 6%, and had a variable time of onset in 15% (**Fig. 32-3**). In 25% of patients, the headaches were worst on awakening or in the course of the morning; in 53%, they were worst in the afternoon or evening, and in 22%, they were worst at a variable time of the day. The results agree with my clinical observation that daily headaches come in two distinct diurnal patterns. In the most common pattern, the headaches gradually increase in intensity as the day progresses, being worst in the afternoon or evening. According to the

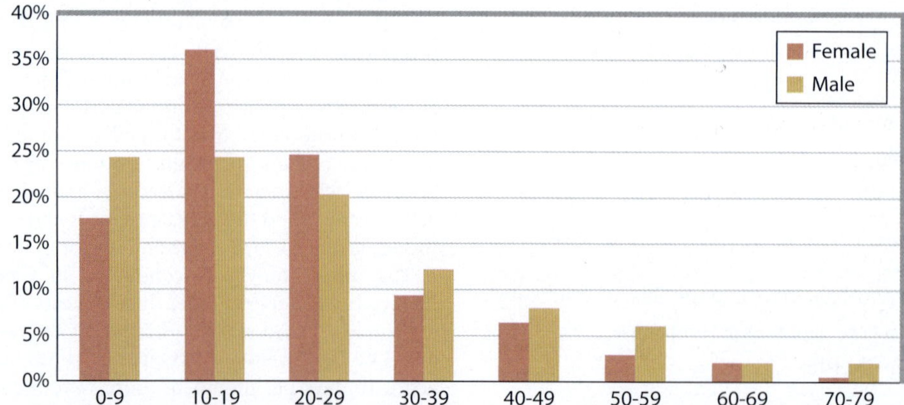

FIGURE 32-2. Distribution of the age of (any) headache onset per gender (n = 251). (Reproduced with permission from Spierings ELH, Schroevers M, Honkoop PC, Sorbi M. Presentation of chronic daily headache: a clinical study. *Headache*. 1998;38:191-196.)

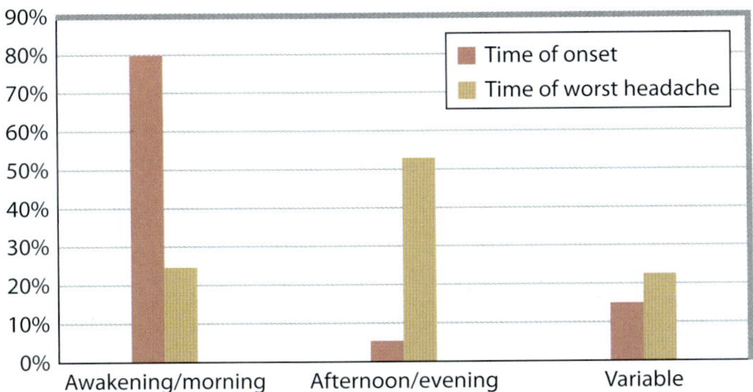

FIGURE 32-3. Diurnal pattern of the daily headaches (n = 214). (Reproduced with permission from Spierings ELH, Schroevers M, Honkoop PC, Sorbi M. Presentation of chronic daily headache: a clinical study. *Headache*. 1998;38:191-196.)

results of the study, this is the pattern in more than half of the patients with chronic daily headache. In the less common pattern, which I have referred to as the *reversed diurnal pattern*, the headaches are worst on awakening in the morning and gradually improve as the day progresses. This was the case in one-quarter of the patients, while in the remaining one-quarter, the diurnal course of the headaches was variable.

The reversed diurnal pattern is, in my experience, particularly associated with the overuse of analgesics, vasoconstrictors, or both, for headache. Overuse in this context is defined as medication intake that is detrimental rather than beneficial to headache. In the reversed diurnal pattern, the severe headaches on awakening in the morning are caused by the withdrawal of medication overnight, and the gradual improvement during the day results from the resumption of medication intake. This scenario also is associated with the most frequent nighttime awakenings with headache. In the study, nocturnal awakening by headache occurred at least once a week in 36% of the patients. Of those patients who were awakened by headache at least once a week, 48% experienced the worst headache on awakening or in the course of the morning, compared with 22% of the patients who were awakened by headache less than once a week.

Ninety-four percent of the patients experienced severe headaches in addition to the daily headaches. The distribution of the frequency of the severe headaches in days per month is shown in **Figure 32-4**. Twenty-six percent of the patients experienced severe headaches more than 15 days per month. Otherwise, they experienced severe headaches mostly 10 days per month or less (63%). The results suggest that the majority of the patients with chronic daily headache who seek specialty care for their headaches have chronic migraine.

In the development of chronic daily headache, medication intake is considered to play an important role—in particular, the intake of

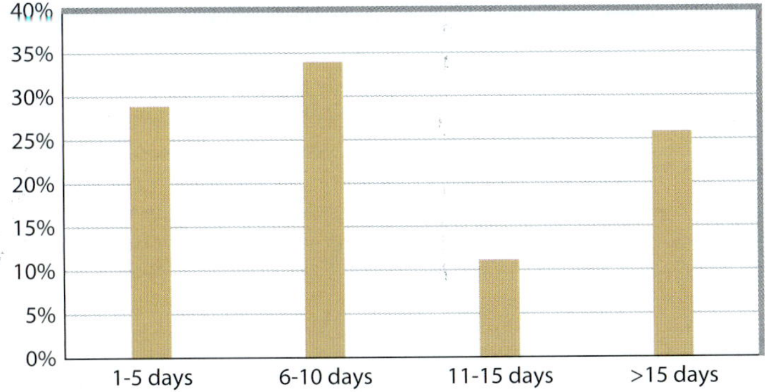

FIGURE 32-4. Frequency of the severe headaches in days per month (n = 197). (Reproduced with permission from Spierings ELH, Schroevers M, Honkoop PC, Sorbi M. Presentation of chronic daily headache: a clinical study. *Headache*. 1998;38:191-196.)

analgesics and vasoconstrictors. A widely used vasoconstrictor for the abortive treatment of headache is caffeine, which is contained in beverages, especially coffee, but also in prescription and nonprescription medications. We determined the caffeine intake in our patients with chronic daily headache by looking at their coffee and medication intake. A cup of coffee was considered to contain 100 mg of caffeine. We found that 43% of the patients used less than 100 mg of caffeine per day, 35% used between 100 and 300 mg, and 22% used more than 300 mg. The average caffeine intake was 170 mg per day, which is approximately the equivalent of two cups of coffee.

With regard to analgesic use, we considered only the nonopioid medications because opioids were hardly used by the patients for the treatment of their headaches. Also, of the barbiturate-containing medications, we did not take into account the barbiturate component because it is not strictly an analgesic. With these limitations, we found that 26% of the patients used less than 500 mg of aspirin equivalents per day and 48% less than 1500 mg. The average analgesic intake was 1860 mg of aspirin equivalents per day.

DEVELOPMENT

Of the 230 patients in the study with known onset of daily headaches, 22% experienced daily headaches from the onset. This could be called *primary* chronic daily headache, in the same way that we speak of primary and secondary chronic cluster headache. The remaining 78% initially experienced intermittent headaches, that is, had *secondary* chronic daily headache. The distribution of the age of onset of the (daily) headaches in the patients with daily headaches from the onset, or primary chronic daily headache, is shown in **Figure 32-5**. Sixty-six percent of the patients experienced onset of daily headaches between the ages of 10 and 39 years.

Of the patients with daily headaches but who initially had intermittent headaches—that is, of those with secondary chronic daily headache—19% experienced an abrupt onset of daily headaches and 81% experienced

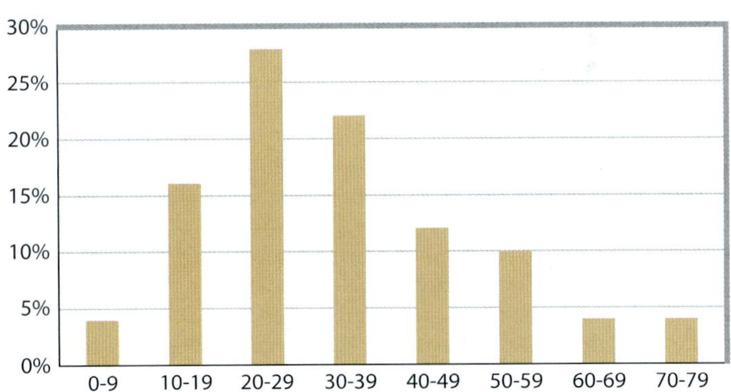

FIGURE 32-5. Distribution of the age of (daily) headache onset in the patients with primary chronic daily headache (n = 50). (Reproduced with permission from Spierings ELH, Schroevers M, Honkoop PC, Sorbi M. Development of chronic daily headache: a clinical study. *Headache*. 1998;38:529-533.)

TABLE 32-1 Circumstances of (Abrupt) Onset of the Daily Headaches[11]

	Primary Chronic Daily Headache (n = 51)	Abrupt-Onset Secondary Chronic Daily Headache (n = 34)	Combined Group (n = 85)
Head/neck/back injury	25%	29%	27%
Flulike illness/sinusitis	12%	18%	14%
Medical illness/ surgical procedure	14%	15%	14%
Miscellaneous	18%	12%	15%
No apparent reason	31%	26%	30%

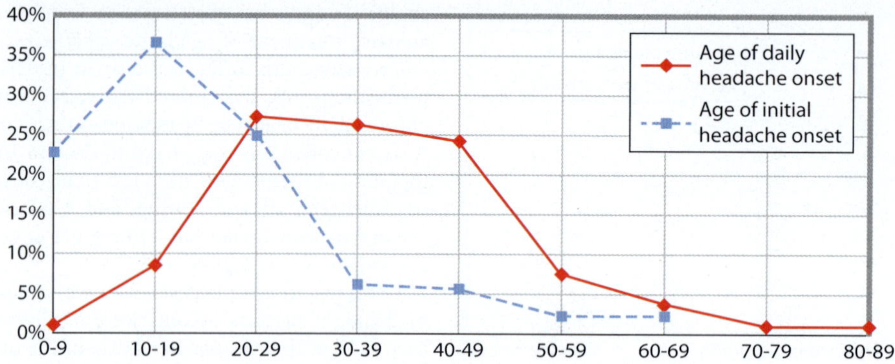

FIGURE 32-6. Distribution of the age of initial and daily headache onset in the patients with gradual-onset secondary chronic daily headache (n = 106 and 145, respectively). (Reproduced with permission from Spierings ELH, Schroevers M, Honkoop PC, Sorbi M. Development of chronic daily headache: a clinical study. *Headache.* 1998;38:529-533.)

a gradual onset. The distribution of the age of onset of daily headaches in the patients with abrupt-onset secondary chronic daily headache was similar to that of the patients with primary chronic daily headache shown in Figure 32-5.

The circumstances related to the onset of daily headaches in the patients with primary chronic daily headache and in those with abrupt-onset secondary chronic daily headache are shown in **Table 32-1**. The table also shows the circumstances of daily headache onset for the two groups combined because there was no difference in distribution of the circumstances between the two groups. The most common circumstance of daily headache onset in the two groups combined was head, neck, or back injury, caused by a motor vehicle accident in 61%. This was followed by flulike illness or sinusitis and medical illness or surgical procedure as causes of daily headache onset. Examples of medical illness associated with the (abrupt) onset of chronic daily headache are colitis, fibromyalgia, vertigo, encephalitis, and meningitis.

There were also no differences between the patients with primary chronic daily headache and those with abrupt-onset secondary chronic daily headache with regard to the following features: gender distribution, time of daily headache occurrence, worst headache time daily, nocturnal headache awakening, laterality of the daily headaches, occurrence and frequency of severe headaches, laterality of the severe headaches, and parental occurrence of headache. The only difference between the two groups was the association of the daily *and* severe headaches with nausea. Nausea was more common in the patients with abrupt-onset secondary chronic daily headache than in those with primary chronic daily headache. The difference probably results from the fact that 57% of the patients in the abrupt-onset group had a prior history of severe headaches, which tend to be associated with gastrointestinal symptoms.

The distribution of the age of onset of the daily headaches in the patients with gradual-onset secondary chronic daily headache is shown in **Figure 32-6** (solid line). Seventy-eight percent of the patients experienced the onset of daily headaches between the ages of 20 and 49 years. The distribution of the age of onset of the initial, intermittent headaches in these patients is also shown in Figure 32-6 (interrupted line). The average duration of the transition of the headaches from intermittent to daily was 11 years, which is reflected in the figure by the separation of the two distributions by approximately a decade.

With regard to parental occurrence, headache in the father or mother, or both, was more common in the patients with gradual-onset secondary chronic daily headache than in the combined group of those with primary chronic daily headache and abrupt-onset secondary chronic daily headache (69% versus 45%). This finding is interesting because conditions that develop abruptly generally have lesser genetic involvement than do those that develop gradually. On the basis of the information gathered on parental headache occurrence, this also seems to be the case in chronic daily headache.

With regard to the intensity of the initial headaches, in the 145 patients with gradual-onset secondary chronic daily headache, the headaches were mild in 33% and severe in 67% (**Table 32-2**). The mild headaches were associated with nausea in 25% and vomiting in 0% compared with the severe headaches, which were associated with nausea in 84% and vomiting in 72%. With regard to the frequency of the initial headaches, there was no difference between the mild and severe headaches. The mild headaches occurred less than twice per week in 88% of the patients and the severe headaches in 91%.

The features of the daily headaches that these patients ultimately developed were the same, whether the initial headaches were mild or severe in intensity. They were the same with regard to age of onset of the (initial) headaches, gender distribution, diurnal headache pattern, nocturnal headache awakening, associated symptoms and laterality of the daily headaches, occurrence of severe headaches, and the frequency, associated symptoms, and laterality of the severe headaches.

From a classification perspective, does it make sense to distinguish between primary and secondary chronic daily headache as we did and, within the latter group, between abrupt- and gradual onset? Judging from the age of onset of the daily headaches, gender distribution, headache presentation, circumstances of headache onset, and parental headache occurrence, there does not seem to be a reason for the distinction between primary and secondary chronic daily headache with *abrupt* onset. The two groups probably should be considered as having the same chronic daily headache condition, which could be referred to as *abrupt-onset chronic daily headache*, representing 37% of our study group. However, this group should probably be distinguished from the group having chronic daily headache with *gradual* onset because of the very different development of the headaches and the difference in parental headache occurrence. The latter group could be referred to as *gradual-onset chronic daily headache,* and future studies are needed to determine whether this distinction is meaningful in terms of predicting treatment or outcome or both.

TABLE 32-2 Features of the Initial Headaches in the Patients with Gradual-Onset Secondary Chronic Daily Headache[12]

	Mild	Severe
Headache intensity (n = 112)	33%	67%
Associated symptoms	(n = 12)	(n = 61)
Nausea	25%	84%
Vomiting	0%	72%
Headache frequency	(n = 25)	(n = 60)
≤4 per month	60%	73%
5–9 per month	28%	18%
10–19 per month	8%	7%
≥20 per month	4%	2%

OUTCOME

Of the 145 patients in our study with gradual-onset (secondary) chronic daily headache, we were able to contact 91 (63%) for follow-up telephone interviews. Seven patients refused to participate in the follow-up interview, and 11 no longer remembered the nature of their initial headaches. One patient was excluded from the analysis because of the absence of headaches at the time of contact, and three patients because of missing data. The remaining 69 patients (77%) were able to provide adequate information to classify their initial and present headaches as tension-type headache or migraine.

Twenty-three of the 69 patients (33%) still had daily headaches, whereas the remaining 46 (67%) again experienced intermittent headaches. Of the latter 46 patients, the initial headaches were classified as (episodic) migraine in 39 (85%) and as (episodic) tension-type headache in 7 (15%). Their present headaches were classified as (episodic) migraine in 34 (74%) and as (episodic) tension-type in 12 (26%). Thus, over time, a slight shift had occurred from migraine to tension-type headache, accomplishing an improvement of the intermittent headaches for the group as a whole.

However, the question that we wanted to address was not whether the patients with intermittent headaches had improved in comparison with their initial headaches but whether patients with gradual-onset chronic daily headache revert back to their initial headache condition once the headaches become intermittent again. In the study, of the 39 patients whose initial headaches were classified as (episodic) migraine, 30 (77%) also had (episodic) migraine at follow-up and 9 (23%) had (episodic) tension-type headache. Of the 7 patients whose initial headaches were classified as (episodic) tension-type headache, 3 (43%) had (episodic) tension-type headache at follow-up and 4 (57%) had (episodic) migraine. Therefore, it seems that after experiencing daily headaches, migraine patients as a rule revert back to (episodic) migraine, although some find their headaches improved to the extent that they are now classified as (episodic) tension-type headache. However, the situation is different for those patients who initially had (episodic) tension-type headache. They seem to be worse after having experienced daily headaches, with some patients experiencing headaches that have features and associated symptoms categorized as migraine.

TREATMENT

The first step in the treatment of chronic daily headache is the accurate establishment of the use of analgesics and vasoconstrictors, both prescription and nonprescription. It is important to establish their use in terms of the number of tablets or capsules taken per day and the number of days of use per week or month. Patients tend to be notoriously vague about the intake of medications they use "as needed only." They also often have to be reminded specifically to include nonprescription medications in their tally. Once the exact intake of analgesics and vasoconstrictors has been established, the clinician must determine whether overuse has occurred. As previously mentioned, *overuse* is defined as medication intake that is detrimental rather than beneficial to headache. It is use that promotes the occurrence of headache long term rather than providing headache relief. Analgesics and vasoconstrictors promote headache when they are taken for headache at time intervals shorter than their duration of action. This dosing schedule allows them to accumulate in the system, with a return of headache whenever their effect wears off, a phenomenon known as *rebound.*

Rebound headache generally occurs when analgesics or vasoconstrictors are taken more often than 2 days per week on the average. This is particularly true for caffeine-containing medications because of the prolonged vasoconstrictor effect of caffeine, which can last for up to 2 or 3 days. A higher frequency of intake of analgesics or vasoconstrictors can be permitted for simple analgesics and the shorter-acting triptans, such as sumatriptan. A lower frequency of intake should be considered with the longer-acting ergots, ergotamine and dihydroergotamine. However, it must be kept in mind that the rebound threshold has not been determined for any medication or group of medications. Furthermore, the diagnosis of rebound headache can only be made retrospectively, after withdrawal from analgesics and vasoconstrictors has been accomplished and improvement of headaches has occurred. A *suspicion* of rebound headache can be based not only on the frequency of medication intake, but also on increased medication usage over time with decreasing efficacy (**Fig. 32-7**). The decreasing efficacy is often attributed to the development of tolerance, but, in my opinion, it is more likely a manifestation of worsening of the headaches and an indication that use has become overuse.

If it is suspected that medication overuse and rebound headache are present, this situation needs to be addressed next. However, it can only be addressed after the patient has been given insight into the situation. With regard to vasoconstrictors, reference can be made to the vascular mechanism of headache. The vascular mechanism is antagonized by the vasoconstrictors, resulting in rebound vasodilation and headache recurrence when the vasoconstrictor effect wears off. Analgesics address only the pain of the headache and not the underlying mechanisms. Consequently—and as with symptomatic treatment in general—the underlying mechanisms deteriorate, resulting in worsening of headaches.

The withdrawal of analgesics or vasoconstrictors is generally best accomplished abruptly. However, whether that is possible also depends on the kind and quantity of the medications taken. When specific quantities of barbiturate-containing or opioid medications are involved, withdrawal may require hospitalization for close monitoring of withdrawal symptoms and intravenous administration of medications. The withdrawal of

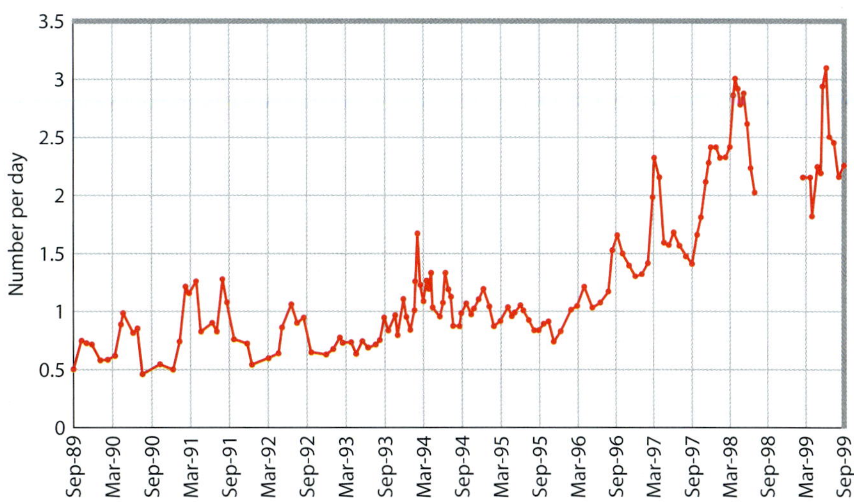

FIGURE 32-7. Example of increase in the intake of an analgesic for headache, as shown by the number of tablets per day over a period of 10 years.

a significant amount of barbiturate-containing medication also requires a barbiturate taper to prevent seizure. The withdrawal of a significant amount of opioid medication requires expertise in addiction medicine and may have to be carried out in a detoxification center. Otherwise, it can often be accomplished on an outpatient basis, and several protocols have been developed to assist the patient with the withdrawal.

An outpatient protocol that I have used successfully to withdraw patients with daily headaches from daily or almost-daily use of abortive medications uses a short course of prednisone. Depending on the kind and quantity of the medications from which the patient has to be withdrawn, I give the prednisone for 3 or 6 days. The 3-day schedule consists of 15 mg prednisone four times per day for 1 day, 10 mg four times per day for 1 day, and 5 mg four times per day for 1 day; the days are doubled in the 6-day schedule. If the patient exhibits prominent muscular symptoms—that is, complains of tight or sore neck and shoulder muscles—I add diazepam to the schedule in a dose of 1 to 5 mg four times per day to help to relax the muscles.

I have used a similar schedule for patients admitted to the hospital when outpatient withdrawal was unsuccessful because of inability of the patient to tolerate the withdrawal headache or its association with severe nausea or vomiting. Under these circumstances, I add metoclopramide as an antinausea medication, given intravenously in a dose of 10 mg four times per day. It is important to start the metoclopramide immediately—that is, before the patient becomes sick—because once vomiting has developed, it is difficult to control even with intravenous administration of the medication. Instead of prednisone orally, dexamethasone can be given intravenously, in a dose of 4 mg four times per day, for several consecutive days. Diazepam can then be given every 6 hours, but only as needed for severe headache, and can also be given intravenously. An alternative to diazepam intravenously is lorazepam intramuscularly in a dose of 1 or 2 mg as needed every 6 hours.

An alternative to the preceding inpatient protocol with metoclopramide, dexamethasone, and diazepam or lorazepam is a regimen using metoclopramide and dihydroergotamine. In this protocol, both medications are given intravenously on a regular, generally 8-hour, schedule with the metoclopramide administered *before* the dihydroergotamine. This sequence is important to prevent the occurrence of nausea or vomiting as a result of the intravenous administration of dihydroergotamine. The dose of metoclopramide is usually 10 mg and that of dihydroergotamine is gradually increased from 0.25 to 1 mg, depending on the ability of the patient to tolerate the medication, especially in terms of its gastrointestinal side effects. A long-term follow-up study of 50 consecutive patients with chronic daily headache treated with an intravenous dihydroergotamine protocol showed 44% to have good or excellent results after 3 months and 59% after 2 years.[13]

After withdrawal from analgesics and vasoconstrictors, headaches may improve for up to 3 months. Often, preventive pharmacologic treatment is initiated immediately after the withdrawal, but generally I do not do that. An exception is when the patient has problems sleeping at night, for which I will prescribe amitriptyline, doxepin, or trazodone. These are sedating tricyclic or tetracyclic antidepressants, of which the first two have also been shown to be effective in the preventive treatment of chronic tension headache. However, I do recommend that patients immediately begin nonpharmacologic treatments, such as using a heating pad daily on the neck and shoulders, to help decrease the muscle tightness that many of these patients have developed over time. At a later stage, I may prescribe more formal physical therapy—consisting of massage, ultrasound, stretching exercises, and so forth—or use trigger-point or botulinum-toxin injections to further relax the muscles.

For the daily headaches, I allow patients to use fast- and short-acting muscle relaxants, such as metaxalone or carisoprodol. For the severe headaches, promethazine, 50-mg suppositories, can be helpful as long as it is judged better for the patient not to use analgesics or vasoconstrictors. Once the headaches have become intermittent, I focus with my abortive treatment on the severe headaches, for which I try to find effective treatment, relying as much as possible on specific antimigraine medications. I define *effective treatment* as treatment that provides *full* relief of headache and associated symptoms within 2 hours of initiation. It is important for this treatment to be *consistently* effective as well, which would allow the patient to wait until the headache is severe before initiating it. This is the only way that patients can be prevented from falling back, over time, into the pattern of frequent intake of analgesics or vasoconstrictors.

With regard to preventive pharmacologic treatment, a particularly useful combination in those patients with frequent and severe headaches is that of a tricyclic and a beta blocker. The tricyclics that I prefer to use are amitriptyline, doxepin, and imipramine. I prescribe the first two when sedation is needed to help the patient fall asleep or sleep through the night. If sleep is not an issue, I prefer imipramine because it has fewer side effects—in particular, a reduced likelihood of increased appetite and weight gain.

With regard to the beta blockers, six medications have been shown in randomized, double-blind, placebo-controlled studies to be effective in migraine prevention. These beta blockers are atenolol, bisoprolol, metoprolol, nadolol, propranolol, and timolol. In the patients with chronic daily headache, they are often effective in decreasing the intensity of headaches, whereas the tricyclics tend to have more of an effect on headache frequency. I have found the calcium-entry blockers—in particular, verapamil—helpful if, after analgesic or vasoconstrictor withdrawal, the headaches continue to awaken the patient regularly from sleep at night (nocturnal migraine).

Kudrow determined the effect of analgesic withdrawal and preventive treatment with amitriptyline in 200 patients with chronic muscle-contraction headache who used analgesics daily, as documented by 1-month pretrial records.[14] Patients were randomly divided into two groups and four subgroups. Half of the patients were prescribed amitriptyline (25 mg per day for 1 week and 50 mg per day thereafter). In each group, half of the patients were allowed to continue taking analgesics without restriction, while the other half was instructed to discontinue these medications. The percentage of headache improvement observed in the four groups is shown in **Table 32-3**. Analgesic withdrawal, by itself, resulted in a 43% improvement in headache as determined 1 month after initiation of treatment. The addition of amitriptyline to the analgesic withdrawal increased the headache improvement to 72%.

Our study suggests that, with the previously outlined treatment approach, two-thirds of patients who have daily headaches can be improved to intermittent headaches. Preventive treatment in these patients may reduce the symptoms of the intermittent headaches somewhat, as suggested by the shift from (episodic) migraine to (episodic) tension-type headache observed in our study, when the present headaches were compared with those that occurred initially.

What should be done with the patients who continue to have frequent and severe headaches, despite being taken off analgesics and vasoconstrictors and despite efforts at preventive treatment? This situation may be an indication for the use of long-acting opioids to relieve the pain sufficiently to allow these patients to function in their personal and professional lives.[15] The long-acting opioids that I have used in such patients are fentanyl patch, oxycodone, and morphine sulfate. I have found these medications to be effective for a shorter period than manufacturers indicate and, therefore, use the fentanyl patch every 2, rather than 3, days

TABLE 32-3 Headache Improvement 1 Month After Initiation of Treatment in 200 Patients with Chronic Muscle-Contraction Headache Who Used Analgesics Daily[14]

Treatment Protocol	Improvement
Treated with amitriptyline	
Analgesics continued (n = 50)	30%
Analgesics withdrawn (n = 50)	72%
Not treated with amitriptyline	
Analgesics continued (n = 50)	18%
Analgesics withdrawn (n = 50)	43%

and long-acting oxycodone every 6 or 8, rather than 12, hours. I gradually increase the dose of the medication until *satisfactory* pain control is achieved and the patient has returned to a relatively normal level of functioning. I prefer the use of long-acting to short-acting opioids because of the reduced likelihood that patients will develop tolerance and addiction. For some reason, rebound headache does not seem to develop with the long-acting opioids, although it is a routine consequence of short-acting analgesics, including opioids. The development of tolerance *and* rebound headache increases the use of opioid analgesics over time and makes it very difficult, if not impossible, to accomplish adequate pain control.

HEMICRANIA CONTINUA[3]

As far as its presentation is concerned, hemicrania continua can be looked on as a form of chronic daily headache. It is a nonparoxysmal daily headache, present continuously throughout the day, and limited to one side of the head. However, it is different from chronic daily headache in its treatment. Hemicrania continua is treated with indomethacin to which it has an absolute response, similar to paroxysmal hemicrania. The different treatment suggests a different etiology, which would preclude the condition from being grouped together with chronic daily headache.

It has been suggested that there is a form of hemicrania continua resistant to preventive treatment with indomethacin. Resistance to treatment with indomethacin, however, by definition, means that it is *not* hemicrania continua. This does not mean that there are not numerous patients who have continuous unilateral headaches with fixed lateralization that do not respond preventively to indomethacin. These patients have chronic daily headache and should be treated accordingly. The key to look for in the history is a response to aspirin, which seems to predict the responsiveness of the headaches to indomethacin. This is also the feature that ultimately led to the identification of both paroxysmal hemicrania and hemicrania continua as indomethacin-responsive headache syndromes.

REFERENCES

1. Headache Classification Subcommittee of the International Headache Society. The International Classification of Headache Disorders, 2nd ed. *Cephalalgia*. 2004;24(Suppl 1):1-160.
2. Headache Classification Subcommittee of the International Headache Society. New appendix criteria open for a broader concept of chronic migraine. *Cephalalgia*. 2006;26:742-746.
3. Sjaastad O, Spierings ELH. "Hemicrania continua": another headache absolutely responsive to indomethacin. *Cephalalgia*. 1984;4:65-70.
4. Instituut Epidemiologie. *Epidemiologisch Preventief Onderzoek Zoetermeer (EPOZ): Tweede en Derde Voortgangsverslag*. Rotterdam, The Netherlands: Erasmus University; 1976.
5. Scher AI, Stewart WF, Liberman J, Lipton RB. Prevalence of frequent headache in a population sample. *Headache*. 1998;38:497-506.
6. Castillo J, Muñoz P, Guitera V, Pascual J. Epidemiology of chronic daily headache in the general population. *Headache*. 1999;39:190-196.
7. Silberstein SD, Lipton RB, Solomon S, Mathew NT. Classification of daily and near-daily headaches: proposed revisions of the IHS criteria. *Headache*. 1994;34:1-7.
8. Langemark M, Olesen J, Loldrup D, Bech P. Clinical characterization of patients with chronic tension headache. *Headache*. 1988;28:590-596.
9. Rasmussen BK, Jensen R, Schroll M, Olesen J. Epidemiology of headache in a general population: a prevalence study. *J Clin Epidemiol*. 1991;44:1147-1157.
10. Spierings ELH, Schroevers M, Honkoop PC, Sorbi M. Presentation of chronic daily headache: a clinical study. *Headache*. 1998;38:191-196.
11. Spierings ELH, Schroevers M, Honkoop PC, Sorbi M. Development of chronic daily headache: a clinical study. *Headache*. 1998;38:529-533.
12. Spierings ELH, Ranke AH, Schroevers M, Honkoop PC. Chronic daily headache: a time perspective. *Headache*. 2000;40:306-310.
13. Silberstein SD, Silberstein JR. Chronic daily headache: long-term prognosis following inpatient treatment with repetitive iv DHE. *Headache*. 1992;32:439-445.
14. Kudrow L. Paradoxical effects of frequent analgesic use. *Adv Neurol*. 1982;33:335-341.
15. Piekos K, Spierings ELH. Management of daily headache unresponsive to preventive treatment: daily triptans versus daily opioids. *Rev Neurol Dis*. 2009;6:E121-E130.

Headache Therapeutics

Melissa L. Rayhill
Paul G. Mathew

INTRODUCTION TO HEADACHE THERAPEUTICS

Headache is one of the most common complaints among patients presenting to an outpatient practice. Once secondary causes of headache are excluded and a primary headache diagnosis has been established, selecting appropriate pharmacotherapy can be a very complex process. Medications must be tailored to each patient's unique combination of comorbidities and lifestyle considerations. In this chapter, treatment strategies for some of the more common primary headache disorders are reviewed. This discussion will focus on migraine, tension-type headache (TTH), and the trigeminal autonomic cephalalgias (TACs). Our discussion of TACs will include cluster headache, paroxysmal hemicrania, short-lasting unilateral neuralgiform headaches with conjunctival injection and tearing or autonomic features (SUNCT/SUNA), and hemicrania continua.

MIGRAINE HEADACHE TREATMENT

ABORTIVE MIGRAINE TREATMENT

Nonsteroidal anti-inflammatory medications (NSAIDs), triptans, dihydroergotamine, and antiemetics are the mainstays of abortive treatment for migraine headaches. Other commonly used, nonspecific analgesics include acetaminophen, aspirin, cyclooxygenase-2 inhibitors, opiates, and combination analgesics. In general, opiates and most combination analgesics are avoided due to the high potential for medication overuse headaches.

NSAIDs are some of the most commonly used and effective first-line agents for abortive migraine treatment. They can be used as monotherapy or in combination with other medications.[2,3] Commonly used NSAIDs include ibuprofen, naproxen sodium, diclofenac, ketoprofen, and ketorolac. These drugs are relatively inexpensive, readily available, and are available in a variety of administration routes. For example, intravenous ketorolac is often used in the emergency department setting, but it is also available in tablet form and as an intranasal spray. Renal toxicity is an important side effect with any NSAID, but extra caution should be exercised with ketorolac use. Diclofenac is available in tablet form, but it also comes in a powdered form for oral solution that has proven efficacy in acute migraine.[4] In addition to nephrotoxicity, NSAIDs as a class are associated with dyspepsia and fluid retention. It is important to note that NSAIDs carry U.S. Food and Drug Administration Black Box warnings for cardiovascular risks, gastrointestinal ulceration, and bleeding risks. Despite these risks, moderate NSAID use is generally quite well tolerated.

Several different triptans are available for the treatment of migraines (**Table 33-1**). As a class of medications, the differences between oral triptans are relatively small, but the effects can vary among individual patients.[5] When choosing a triptan, it is important to consider the formulary coverage and costs associated with an individual's insurance plan. Sumatriptan, naratriptan, zolmitriptan, and rizatriptan are currently the only generic triptans on the market. Sumatriptan has been

TABLE 33-1 Formulations and Half-Lives of Triptan Medications

Generic Name	Brand Name	Half-Life (hours)	Administration/Dose
Almotriptan	Axert®	3–4	Oral 6.25, 12.5 mg
Eletriptan	Relpax®	4	Oral 20, 40 mg
Frovatriptan	Frova®	26	Oral 2.5 mg
Naratriptan	Amerge®	6	Oral 1, 2.5 mg
Rizatriptan	Maxalt®	2–3	Oral 5, 10 mg ODT 5, 10 mg
Sumatriptan	Imitrex®	2.5	Oral 25, 50, 100 mg Intranasal 5, 20 mg Subcutaneous 4, 6 mg
Zolmitriptan	Zomig®	3	Oral 2.5, 5 mg ODT 2.5, 5 mg Intranasal 5 mg

Data from Ferrari MD, Goadsby PJ. Triptans (serotonin, 5-$HT_{1B/1D}$ agonists) in migraine: detailed results and methods of a meta-analysis of 53 trials. *Cephalalgia*. 2002;22(8):633-658.

a generic medication longer than any other triptan and is almost universally the preferred triptan from an insurance coverage standpoint. Studies have demonstrated that triptan use decreases as copayment increases. In addition, demand for pharmaceuticals was relatively unchanged with copayment increases.[6]

If a triptan is tolerated, but only somewhat beneficial, this may be due to delayed administration. It has clearly been established that triptans tend to be more effective when taken during the early phase of migraine, and delays in administration can lead to significant reductions in efficacy.[7] In clinical practice, some patients may report complete ineffectiveness of a triptan if administration is delayed for an excessive period of time. The ability of a triptan to terminate a headache can be enhanced by coadministration with an NSAID and/or an antiemetic. In addition to oral formulations, triptans are available in orally dissolving, intranasal, injectable, and needle-free subcutaneous delivery systems. These routes of administration may be particularly useful for migraine patients with early and prominent vomiting. In cases where sumatriptan is ineffective, switching to a different triptan or different formulation would be a reasonable approach.[8]

It is essential to warn patients that triptans often induce transient side effects, including chest or throat tightness, flushing, a hot sensation, dizziness, nausea, drowsiness, and tingling. Warning patients of these transient side effects can prevent patient anxiety related to future triptan use and may even prevent emergency department visits for what patients erroneously perceive to be an anaphylactic reaction. Triptans should be avoided in patients with a history of coronary artery disease, stroke, transient ischemic attack (TIA), and peripheral vascular disease. Other relative contraindications include uncontrolled blood pressure, smoking, hormone replacement, pregnancy, and breast-feeding (though some triptans, like eletriptan, are only minimally excreted in breast milk and may still be considered in the appropriate clinical setting). Triptans carry a very low risk of serotonin syndrome when used concomitantly with selective norepinephrine reuptake inhibitors (SNRIs), selective serotonin reuptake inhibitors (SSRIs), and/or tricyclic antidepressants. The use of these medications should not prevent appropriate patients from receiving treatment with triptans.[9] However, patients should be warned of the symptoms of serotonin syndrome and should seek medical attention immediately if those symptoms occur.

In patients who fail to respond to NSAIDs and triptans, dihydroergotamine (DHE) is a reasonable option. DHE has similar contraindications to triptans, and pregnancy is an absolute contraindication to dihydroergotamine use. Due to poor bioavailability, DHE is not available in an oral form. It is, instead, available in intranasal, injectable, and intravenous formulations. Intravenous DHE is often used in the emergency department and inpatient settings for the treatment of status migrainosis. It commonly causes nausea, so most patients are pretreated with an antiemetic prior to dosing. Intravenous DHE administration requires close monitoring as rare, but serious,side effects include arterial spasm (sometimes resulting in limb necrosis) and myocardial infarction.

Antiemetics and neuroleptics have long been used alone or in combination with other drugs to treat acute migraine. Like NSAIDs, neuroleptics/antiemetics come in multiple different administration routes, enabling parenteral use in the emergency department as well as at home with oral or suppository formulations. The mechanism of action for most of these medications is primarily the dopamine D2 receptor antagonism, though other neurotransmitter systems are thought to be involved. This D2 receptor activity can help relieve migraine-associated nausea in addition to relieving the headache itself.[10,11] Orthostatic hypotension and sedation are potential side effects of the D2 antagonists. Extrapyramidal symptoms may also occur, including akathisia, parkinsonism, and acute dystonic reactions. With long-term use, tardive dyskinesia may also occur. Prochlorperazine, metoclopramide, and chlorpromazine are commonly used dopamine antagonists used in the treatment of acute migraine. Prochlorperazine is available in tablet, suppository, and parenteral forms. Metoclopramide is available in tablet and oral suspension. Chlorpromazine is available in tablet and parenteral forms. Promethazine is an antihistamine that is quite effective for the treatment of migraine-associated nausea, but little evidence supports its use in the treatment of migraine pain.[12] Although ondansetron has no pain-specific effect, it may be helpful in conjunction with other therapies.

PREVENTIVE MIGRAINE TREATMENT

Preventive medications should be considered in cases in which migraines occur with high frequency or significantly interfere with the patient's level of function. Preventives should also be considered when abortive treatments are contraindicated, ineffective, poorly tolerated, or overused. There are several different classes of drugs used to prevent migraines (**Table 33-2**), which include beta-blockers (propranolol, atenolol, nadolol, metoprolol, timolol), calcium-channel blockers (verapamil), anticonvulsants (topiramate, divalproex sodium, gabapentin), and tricyclic antidepressants (amitriptyline, nortriptyline).

There are several factors to consider when choosing a preventive medication. Importantly, the medication should have proven efficacy. For this reason, propranolol, topiramate, divalproex sodium, and amitriptyline are considered first-line medications (all except amitriptyline are FDA approved for migraine). Onabotulinum toxin type A is also FDA approved for chronic migraine, but this treatment modality will be covered in detail in a separate chapter.

The presence of comorbid conditions should influence preventive medication choices because treating more than one condition with a single medication would be ideal from compliance and side-effect standpoints. Beta blockers or calcium channel blockers should be considered in patients with hypertension. In patients with sleep dysfunction, tricyclic antidepressants or gabapentin would be reasonable choices given their sedating effects. Topiramate is a good first choice when deciding on therapies for obese patients, given its effect on appetite suppression and weight loss. For patients with seizure disorders, topiramate, divalproex sodium, or gabapentin should be considered to raise the threshold for both seizure and migraine. In some cases, a preventive medication may be initiated primarily to address a poorly controlled comorbid condition. For example, a patient with poorly controlled hypertension with infrequent, moderate severity migraines could be started on atenolol. As a general guideline, all preventive medications should be started at low doses and titrated slowly until the minimum effective dose is reached.

A reasonable goal of prophylaxis should be to decrease headache frequency and intensity. Total elimination of headache is a common patient treatment expectation that is usually unrealistic. All preventive medication trials should be at least 2 to 3 months in duration at a therapeutic dose before a decision regarding efficacy can be made. It is important to be mindful of patient and provider expectations of medication efficacy. Adequate dose and duration of medication may cause only mild improvements in headache frequency and intensity, and these

TABLE 33-2 Commonly Used Prophylactic Migraine Medications

Level A: established as effective
(Should be offered to patients requiring migraine prophylaxis)

Drug	Examples of Studied Doses
Divalproex/sodium valproate	400–1000 mg/day
Metoprolol	50–200 mg/day
Petasites (butterbur)*	50–75 mg bid
Propranolol	80–240 mg/day
Timolol	5–15 mg bid
Topiramate	25–200 mg/day

*Serious hepatotoxicity limits the use of this agent

Level B: probably effective
(Should be considered for patients requiring migraine prophylaxis)

Drug	Examples of Studied Doses
Amitriptyline	25–150 mg/day
Fenoprofen	200–600 mg tid
Feverfew	50–300 mg bid; 2.08–18.75 mg tid for MIG-99 preparation
Histamine	1–10 ng subcutaneously twice a week
Ibuprofen	200 mg bid
Ketoprofen	50 mg tid
Magnesium	600 mg magnesium dicitrate qd
Naproxen/naproxen sodium	500–1000 mg/day for naproxen; 550 mg bid for naproxen sodium
Riboflavin	400 mg/day
Atenolol	50–100 mg/day
Venlafaxine	150 mg extended release/day

Level C: possibly effective
(May be considered for patients requiring migraine prophylaxis)

Drug	Examples of Studied Doses
Candesartan	16 mg/day
Carbamazepine	600 mg/day
Clonidine	0.1–0.25 mg/day; patch formulations also studied
Guanfacine	0.5–1 mg/day
Lisinopril	10–20 mg/day
Nebivolol	5 mg/day
Pindolol	10 mg/day
Flurbiprofen	200 mg/day
Mefenamic acid	500 mg tid
Coenzyme Q10	100 mg tid
Cyproheptadine	4 mg/day

Adapted from: Loder E, Burch R, Rizzoli P. The 2012 AHS/AAN Guidelines for Prevention of Episodic Migraine: A Summary and Comparison With Other Recent Clinical Practice Guidelines. *Headache.* 2012;52:930-945.

small improvements could be overlooked if preexisting expectations are impractical. A preventive medication should be considered successful if it decreases headache frequency by 50%. Although monotherapy is preferred, in clinical practice, some patients with refractory headaches may receive additive benefit from combinations of preventive treatments.[13]

Many women have an association between their migraines and menstruation. Specific prophylactic strategies can be applied around the time of menstrual periods, and these strategies can be used in addition to more continuous preventive treatment. This concept can be applied to both pure menstrual migraine (migraines occur only around menses), as well as menstrually related migraine (increased frequency and/or intensity of migraines around menses, but migraines also occur outside of this period) as described in the ICHD-IIIb.[1] For example, longer-acting triptans such as frovatriptan or naratriptan can be used twice a day on a standing basis, starting 1-2 days prior to the onset of menses and continuing for 3 days into menses.[14,15] A similar strategy for menstrual migraine involves administration of an NSAID such as naproxen sodium twice a day on a standing basis, starting 1-2 days prior to the onset of menses and continuing for 3 days into menses.[16,17]

TENSION-TYPE HEADACHE TREATMENT

ABORTIVE TENSION-TYPE HEADACHE TREATMENT

Aspirin, acetaminophen, naproxen sodium, and diclofenac have all demonstrated efficacy as abortive treatments for TTH in clinical trials.[18-21] Most of these medications are available over the counter, which in addition to TTH being mild to moderate in severity by definition, may explain why patients with episodic tension-type headaches often do not present to the doctor's office. Triptans are generally not effective for the abortive treatment of pure TTH.[22]

PREVENTIVE TENSION-TYPE HEADACHE TREATMENT

Due to the mild/moderate intensity of TTH headache, either high frequency or high levels of headache-related disability are two reasons to consider prophylactic treatment. The mainstays of preventive treatment for TTH are tricyclic antidepressants. Among the tricyclic antidepressants, amitriptyline has the most data to support its efficacy in TTH.[23-25] For patients who benefit from amitriptyline but cannot tolerate side effects, nortriptyline or protriptyline may be reasonable alternatives with better side-effect profiles. Other options with proven efficacy in TTH include mirtazapine and tizanidine.[26-28] Tricyclic antidepressants are considered to be superior to both SSRIs and SNRIs for the prevention of TTH.[29] The use of botulinum toxin injections for chronic TTH has not been well supported in double-blind clinical trials.[30,31] Some studies suggest that in TTH involving myofascial trigger points, injecting directly into the trigger points may provide relief, though this is controversial.[32]

THE TRIGEMINAL AUTONOMIC CEPHALGIAS

ABORTIVE CLUSTER HEADACHE TREATMENT

Acute cluster headache attacks require a swift therapeutic response. High-flow oxygen using a non-rebreather mask is one of the mainstays of treatment for an acute cluster attack. Regular administration of oxygen by nasal cannula is insufficient. Oxygen should be given at 100% fraction of inspired oxygen (FiO_2), at a rate of 12 to 15 liters per minute. Some therapeutic effect is typically achieved by 15 minutes.[33] Rapid administration of triptans can offer relief in the event of an acute cluster attack as well. The only FDA-approved therapy for acute cluster is subcutaneous injection of 6 mg sumatriptan.[34] Triptans administered via nasal spray may also provide some relief if administered immediately after headache symptoms occur.

PREVENTIVE CLUSTER HEADACHE TREATMENT

Two major categories of preventive treatments are used for cluster headaches: transitional preventives and maintenance preventives. *Transitional preventives* are medications that are used for days to weeks, with the primary goal of stopping a cluster period and inducing remission. *Maintenance preventives* are used continuously to maintain remission from cluster periods, though many clinicians stop these preventives in between cluster periods. Steroid tapers and occipital nerve blocks are transitional preventive treatments that can be employed to terminate a cluster period. Steroid tapers have proven to be effective in helping terminate cluster periods but are limited by relapses and side effects. There is no standardized corticosteroid treatment strategy. The type of corticosteroid and taper schedules vary among headache specialists. In clinical practice, oral prednisone tapers can be started at doses of up to 80 mg and patients are typically tapered over 7-56 days, though much variability exists. Alternatively, studies have demonstrated the efficacy of dexamethasone at 4 mg twice a day for 1 week followed by 4 mg daily for 1 week.[35] Occipital nerve blocks may be effective in treating cluster periods in some patients, but the techniques vary widely among studies. Techniques for occipital nerve blocks are discussed in detail in another chapter.

Commonly used maintenance preventive treatments for cluster headache include verapamil, lithium, divalproex sodium, and topiramate. Verapamil is the first-line treatment for cluster headaches due to its efficacy and tolerability. It is typically started at doses of 40 to 80 mg daily and titrated up by 40 to 80 mg per week as needed. The usual goal dose is 240 mg daily, though occasionally doses as high as 960 mg daily are required. The titration should be slow because many patients may find benefit at lower doses. Routine electrocardiograms (ECGs) should be checked while titrating verapamil to monitor for atrioventricular block and bradycardia, especially when doses of verapamil exceed 240 mg per day.[36] Constipation and extremity swelling can also occur on lower doses of verapamil.

Lithium is an effective treatment for chronic cluster headaches, but it is limited by its side-effect profile and the need for monitoring blood levels. Lithium does not appear to be as effective for episodic cluster as it is for chronic cluster. Lithium is typically dosed at 600 to 1200 mg daily with a target serum concentration of 0.4 to 0.8 mEq/L. Side effects include weakness, nausea, thirst, tremor, slurred speech, and blurred vision. Lithium toxicity may manifest as nausea, vomiting, anorexia, diarrhea, confusion, nystagmus, ataxia, extrapyramidal signs, and seizures. Lithium can also affect thyroid and kidney function; therefore, baseline tests are necessary prior to initiation of this medication. Lithium drug levels, creatinine, sodium, TSH, and ECG should be performed periodically while on lithium.[35]

In patients refractory to a single medication, combinations of preventive medications are often required. Verapamil is usually administered with other agents such as topiramate, lithium, or divalproex sodium.

In patients who fail to respond adequately to oral medications for long-term prophylaxis, surgical interventions, peripheral nerve stimulation, and transcranial magnetic stimulation could be considered. In general, neurostimulation for medically refractory cluster headache tends to have fewer side effects than destructive nerve procedures. Any procedures for medically refractory cluster headache should be performed at a center with expertise in these procedures. These topics are discussed in detail in another chapter.

HEMICRANIA TREATMENTS

Paroxysmal hemicrania and hemicrania continua are both defined by their response to indomethacin. Some patients with hemicrania develop intolerance to indomethacin, which is usually related to its gastrointestinal side effects. Some patients may have response to cyclooxygenase-2 inhibitors, but the side-effect profile of these medications raises serious concerns with cardiovascular risk—so much so that the risk may outweigh any potential benefit. Topiramate appears to be effective in case reports of paroxysmal hemicrania and hemicrania continua when patients are no longer able to take indomethacin.[37,38] Occipital nerve blocks and neurostimulators may also show some promise if other options are exhausted.[39]

SUNCT/SUNA TREATMENT

Lamotrigine is the treatment of choice for short-lasting unilateral neuralgiform headache attacks with conjunctival injection and tearing or with cranial autonomic symptoms (SUNCT/SUNA). Unfortunately, only two-thirds of patients are reported to be responders.[40] There is very limited evidence to support the role of topiramate in these rare headache syndromes, given most studies include very small sample sizes and report only modest effects.[41] Parenteral lidocaine provides another option for patients. In one study, 20% of patients responded by going into remission after 10 days of intravenous lidocaine.[42] Overall, evidence-based treatment options are quite limited given the low prevalence of these conditions.

SUMMARY

The effective treatment of headache requires accurate diagnosis of primary versus secondary headache, as well as the headache type based on ICHD-II criteria. Once a diagnosis is established, the best medications for acute and preventive therapy can best be determined by a discussion with the patient. Side-effect profiles of these medications, along with patient preferences and lifestyle, can usually help to select a well-tolerated and successful therapeutic regimen.

REFERENCES

1. Headache Classification Subcommittee of the International Headache Society. The International Classification of Headache Disorders. 2nd ed. *Cephalalgia*. 2004;24(Suppl 1):9-160.
2. Rabbie R, Derry S, Moore RA, McQuay HJ. Ibuprofen with or without an antiemetic for acute migraine headaches in adults. *Cochrane Database Syst Rev*. 2010;(10):CD008039.
3. Magis D, Schoenen J. Treatment of migraine: update on new therapies. *Curr Opin Neurol*. 2011;24(3):203-210.
4. Lipton RB, Grosberg B, Singer RP, et al. Efficacy and tolerability of a new powdered formulation of diclofenac potassium for oral solution for the acute treatment of migraine: results from the International Migraine Pain Assessment Clinical Trial (IMPACT). *Cephalalgia*. 2010;30(11):1336-1345.
5. Ferrari MD, Goadsby PJ, Roon KI, Lipton RB. Triptans (serotonin, 5-HT1B/1D agonists) in migraine: detailed results and methods of a meta-analysis of 53 trials. *Cephalalgia*. 2002;22(8):633–658.
6. Landsman PB, Yu W, Liu X, Teutsch SM, Berger ML. Impact of 3-tier pharmacy benefit design and increased consumer cost-sharing on drug utilization. *Am J Manag Care*. 2005 Oct;11(10):621-628.
7. Lantéri-Minet M, Mick G, Allaf B. Early dosing and efficacy of triptans in acute migraine treatment: the TEMPO study. *Cephalalgia*. 2012 Feb;32(3):226-35. doi:10.1177/0333102411433042. Epub 2012 Jan 10.
8. Mathew PG, Garza I. Headache. *Semin Neurol*. 2011 Feb;31(1):5-17.
9. Wenzel RG, Tepper S, Korab WE, Freitag F. Serotonin syndrome risks when combining SSRI/SNRI drugs and triptans: is the FDA's alert warranted? *Ann Pharmacother*. 2008;42(11):1692-1696.
10. Jones J, Sklar D, Dougherty J, White W. Randomized double-blind trial of intravenous prochlorperazine for the treatment of acute headache. *JAMA*. 1989;261(8):1174-1176.
11. Marmura MJ. Use of dopamine antagonists in treatment of migraine. *Curr Treat Options Neurol*. 2012;14(1)27-35.
12. Rizzoli PB. Acute and preventive treatment of migraine. *Continuum Lifelong Learning Neurol*. 2012;18(4):764-782.
13. Pascual J, Leira R, Lainez JM. Combined therapy for migraine prevention? Clinical experience with a beta-blocker plus sodium valproate in 52 resistant migraine patients. *Cephalalgia*. 2003;23(10):961-962.
14. Newman L, Mannix LK, Landy S, et al. Naratriptan as short-term prophylaxis of menstrually associated migraine: a randomized, double-blind, placebo-controlled study. *Headache*. 2001;41(3):248-256.
15. MacGregor EA, Brandes JL, Silberstein S, et al. Safety and tolerability of short-term preventive frovatriptan: a combined analysis. *Headache*. 2009;49(9):1298-1314.
16. Garza I, Swanson JW. Prophylaxis of migraine. *Neuropsychiatr Dis Treat*. 2006;3(1):281-291.
17. Rothrock JF. Menstrual migraine. *Headache*. 2009;49(9):1399-1400.

18. Steiner TJ, Lange R, Voelker M. Aspirin in episodic tension-type headache: placebo-controlled dose-ranging comparison with paracetamol. *Cephalalgia*. 2003;23(1):59-66.
19. Prior MJ, Cooper KM, May LG, Bowen DL. Efficacy and safety of acetaminophen and naproxen in the treatment of tension-type headache: a randomized, double-blind, placebo-controlled trial. *Cephalalgia*. 2002;22(9):740-748.
20. Kubitzek F, Ziegler G, Gold MS, Liu JM, Ionescu E. Low-dose diclofenac potassium in the treatment of episodic tension-type headache. *Eur J Pain*. 2003;7(2):155-162.
21. Brennum J, Brinck T, Schriver L, et al. Sumatriptan has no clinically relevant effect in the treatment of episodic tension-type headache. *Eur J Neurol*. 1996;3:23-28.
22. Cady RK, Gutterman D, Saiers JA, Beach ME. Responsiveness of non-IHS migraine and tension-type headache to sumatriptan. *Cephalalgia*. 1997;17(5):588-590.
23. Mathew P, Peterlin B. Tension-type headache. In: Jay GW ed. *Clinician's Guide to Chronic Headache and Facial Pain*. New York: Informa Healthcare; 2010:16-26.
24. Bendtsen L, Jensen R. Amitriptyline reduces myofascial tenderness in patients with chronic tension-type headache. *Cephalalgia*. 2000;20(6):603-610.
25. Goadsby T, Silberstein S, Dodick D. *Chronic Daily Headache for Clinicians*. Hamilton: BC Decker Inc; 2005:57-64.
26. Saper JR, Lake AE III, Cantrell DT, Winner PK, White JR. Chronic daily headache prophylaxis with tizanidine: a double-blind, placebo-controlled, multicenter outcome study. *Headache*. 2002;42(6):470-482.
27. Fogelholm R, Murros K. Tizanidine in chronic tension-type headache: a placebo controlled double-blind cross-over study. *Headache*. 1992;32(10):509-513.
28. Bendtsen L, Jensen R. Mirtazapine is effective in the prophylactic treatment of chronic tension-type headache. *Neurology*. 2004;62(10):1706-1711.
29. Holroyd KA, Labus JS, O'Donnell FJ, Cordingley GE. Treating chronic tension-type headache not responding to amitriptyline hydrochloride with paroxetine hydrochloride: a pilot evaluation. *Headache*. 2003;43(9):999-1004.
30. Padberg M, de Bruijn SF, de Haan RJ, Tavy DL. Treatment of chronic tension-type headache with botulinum toxin: a double-blind, placebo-controlled clinical trial. *Cephalalgia*. 2004;24(8):675-680.
31. Rozen D, Sharma J. Treatment of tension-type headache with botox: a review of the literature. *Mt Sinai J Med*. 2006;73(1):493-498.
32. Harden RN, Cottrill J, Gagnon CM, et al. Botulinum toxin a in the treatment of chronic tension-type headache with cervical myofascial trigger points: a randomized, double- blind, placebo-controlled pilot study. *Headache*. 2009;49(5):732-743.
33. Cohen AS, Burns B, Goadsby PJ. High-flow oxygen for treatment of cluster headache: a randomized trial. *JAMA*. 2009;302(22):2451-2457.
34. The Sumatriptan Cluster Headache Study Group.Treatment of acute cluster headache with sumatriptan. *N Engl J Med*. 1991;325(5):322-326.
35. Matharu MS, Goadsby PJ. Trigeminal autonomic cephalalgias: diagnosis and management. In: Silberstein SD, Lipton RB, Dodick DW eds. *Wolff's Headache and Other Head Pain*. 8th ed. New York: Oxford University Press; 2008:379-402.
36. Cohen AS, Matharu MS, Goadsby PJ. Electrocardiographic abnormalities in patients with cluster headache on verapamil therapy. *Neurology*. 2007;69(7):668-675.
37. Cohen AS, Goadsby PJ. Paroxysmal hemicrania responding to topiramate. *J Neurol Neurosurg Psychiatry*. 2007;78(1):96-97.
38. Brighina F, Palermo A, Cosentino G, Fierro B. Prophylaxis of hemicrania continua: two new cases effectively treated with topiramate. *Headache*. 2007;47(3):441-443.
39. Burns B, Watkins L, Goadsby PJ. Treatment of hemicrania continua by occipital nerve stimulation with a novel bion device: long-term follow-up of a crossover study. *Lancet Neurol*. 2008;7(11):1001-1012.
40. Goadsby, PJ. Trigeminal autonomic cephalgias. *Continuum Lifelong Learning Neurol*. 2012;18(4):883-895.
41. Cohen A, Matharu MS, Goadsby PJ. Double-blind placebo-controlled trial of topiramate in SUNCT. *Cephalalgia*. 2007;27:758.
42. Matharu MS, Cohen AS, Goadsby PJ. Intravenous lidocaine is effective in the treatment of SUNCT syndrome. *Cephalalgia*. 2003;23:738.

Botulinum Toxins for the Treatment of Headaches

Atif B. Malik
Maaz Sohail
Zahid H. Bajwa

Since the 1980s, botulinum toxins (BTXs) have been used for many putative conditions that cause pain. The U.S. Food and Drug Administration (FDA) has approved BTX type A as a prophylactic treatment for headaches due to chronic migraines and approved both BTX type A and B for other medical conditions associated with pain and discomfort. Although BTX is currently not approved for any other headache disorders, it continues to be used successfully by a range of specialists to address pain control.

Although there are many case reports and open-label studies on the effectiveness of BTX in treating painful conditions, a dearth of double-blind, placebo-controlled, randomized clinical trials exist that directly addresses its use for pain management. Some double-blind, placebo-controlled, randomized clinical studies show that botulinum toxin type A (BTX-A) injections are effective in treating various headache disorders (**Table 34-1**). However, so far, an open study has shown BTX is ineffective for patients with episodic cluster headaches.[13]

All of the data presented in this chapter, and most of the published experience in headache management, is from BTX-A studies, but botulinum toxin type B (BTX-B) also may be effective, given the similarity of the two serotypes.

HEADACHE DEFINITIONS

Headache is one of the most common types of pain disorder, responsible for more than 10 million physician visits annually in the United States. Although the terminology of various types of headaches may be confusing, we limit our discussion here to mostly primary headaches, for which BTX data are available. More research continues, with the largest chronic migraine study to date done in 2010, leading to FDA approval of BTX. Other large, double-blind, randomized, placebo-controlled trials are coming forward for other types of headaches.

Migraine is a neurologic disorder that features recurrent attacks of headache, most often occurring unilaterally. It accompanies various combinations of symptoms, such as nausea, vomiting, and sensitivity to light, sound, and other stimuli. Migraine attacks can occur at any time of day or night. Episodes may last from several hours to days, 4 to 72 hours by International Headache Society (IHS) criteria, and are often disabling. Even routine activity or slight head movement can exacerbate the pain. Pain can migrate from one part of the head to another and may radiate down the neck or shoulder. The majority of patients also experience scalp tenderness during or after an attack.

Tension-type headache has two subcategories: episodic and chronic. The episodic tension-type headache (ETTH) is defined by the IHS[14] as headache frequency of greater than 10 lifetime attacks, but fewer than 15 attacks per month; with an average attack duration of 30 minutes to

TABLE 34-1 Summary of Results from Clinical Trials

Type/Subtype	Authors/Year	Study Type	N	Results
Migraine headache	Silberstein, 2000[1]	Double-blind vehicle-controlled	123	Effective prophylaxis
	Binder, 2000[2]	Open-label	77	Effective with acute attacks and prophylaxis
	Binder, 1998[3]	Retrospective review	96	Effective
Tension-type headache				
ETTH or CTTH	Rollnik, 2002[4]	Double-blind, placebo-controlled	21	No difference with Dysport
CTTH	Relja and Korsic, 1999[5]	Double-blind, placebo-controlled	16	Effective
CTTH and migraines	Smuts, 1999[6]	Double-blind, placebo-controlled	37	Effective
ETTH or CTTH	Schulte-Mattler et al., 1999[7]	Open-label	9	Effective in 8 of 9 patients
CTTH	Wheeler, 1998[8]	Open-label	4	Effective in 4 patients
CTTH	Relja, 1997[9]	Open-label	10	Effective in all 10 patients
CTTH	Zwart et al, 1994[10]	Open-label	6	Unilateral temporal injection not effective
Chronic daily headache				
Secondary to whiplash injury	Klapper and Klapper, 1999[11]	Case studies	5	Effective in 4 of 5 patients
	Freund and Schwartz, 2000[12]	Randomized, double-blind, placebo-controlled patients	26	Effective in 11 of 14

CTTH, chronic tension-type headache; ETTH, episodic tension-type headache.

7 days; and at least two features that may include mild to moderate pain intensity, pressing, tightening, a bandlike sensation bilaterally, nonpulsatile quality, and no exercise-induced exacerbation.

The IHS chronic tension-type headache (CTTH) criteria are identical to those for ETTH except that the attack frequency is 15 or more attacks per month for at least 6 months. The CTTH definition permits one migraine-associated symptom of nausea, photophobia, or phonophobia, in contrast to that of ETTH. Patients who have two different headaches that both meet criteria for ETTH are defined as having CTTH if the sum of the attack frequencies for the two headaches is 15 or more attacks per month.

Chronic daily headache has not been satisfactorily characterized by the IHS but Silberstein and colleagues[15] have proposed that this condition represents a group of disorders that includes CTTH, transformed migraine, new daily persistent headache, and hemicrania continua. Chronic daily headaches usually evolve over a period of months or years but can be of sudden onset. The chronic daily headache spectrum may include transformed migraines that occur more than 4 hours per day and 15 days per month. There is usually a slow increase in tension-type headache and a concomitant decrease in migraine features. Chronic daily headaches often are associated with analgesic abuse or overuse in many patients.

Although not a primary headache, new research has shed light on BTX for the treatment of a nummular headache. According to the IHS, a *nummular headache* is defined as pain coming from a small circumscribed area of the head where there is no sign of any lesion of the underlying structures. Mild to moderate pain can be felt and is confined to a rounded area usually ranging from 2 to 6 cm, and the affected area may present with paraesthesia, hypesthesia, dysesthesia, and/or tenderness. The area of pain in a nummular headache is usually found in the parietal region and is slightly more predominant in females.

HISTORY OF BOTULINUM TOXIN

The existence of BTX has been known for centuries, but its positive effects have only recently been realized. Justinus Kerner, a German physician and poet (1786–1862), coined the term "sausage poison," later called "botulism" for the Latin form *botulus*, which means sausage. Professor Emile Pierre van Ermengem, of Ellezelles, Belgium, identified the bacterium *Bacillus botulinus* in 1885 that was later renamed Clostridium botulinum. In 1944, Edward Schantz cultured C. botulinum and isolated the neurotoxin. In 1949, Burgen and associates discovered that BTX blocks neuromuscular transmission. Dr. Vernon Brooks, in the 1950s, discovered that BTX-A could be injected into hyperactive muscle, causing temporary "paralysis" by blocking the release of acetylcholine at the motor nerve ending.

In 1973, Alan B. Scott, MD, of Smith-Kettlewell Eye Research Institute, used BTX-A in monkey experiments, and, in 1980, he was the first to use BTX-A to treat strabismus in humans. In 1988, Allergan acquired the rights to distribute Scott's BTX-A product, Oculinum, and the responsibilities to conduct clinical trials of the drug's effectiveness for other indications, including cervical dystonia. In 1989, the FDA approved Oculinum (renamed Botox in the United States and Dysport in Europe) as an orphan drug to treat strabismus and blepharospasm associated with dystonia, including benign essential blepharospasm or eighth cranial nerve disorder (hemifacial spasms) in patients 12 years of age and older. BTX-A received FDA approval in 2000 for cervical dystonia and for improvement in the appearance of glabellar lines in 2002. The newest form of the botulinum toxin, BTX-B, was studied recently, and several products currently are available commercially (MyoBloc in the United States; NeuroBloc in Europe). BTX-B (MyoBloc) was approved by the FDA in 2000 for treatment of cervical dystonia to reduce the severity of abnormal head position and neck pain. Clinicians are also using BTX-B when patients become immunologically resistant to serotype A. Recently, the FDA has approved BTX-A for therapeutic use in patients with moderate to severe glabellar lines (2002) and for the prophylactic treatment of chronic migraine in adults (2010).

BIOCHEMISTRY AND MECHANISM OF ACTION

The BTX molecule is produced by C. botulinum, which is a gram-positive anaerobic bacterium. BTX can be divided into seven neurotoxins (labeled as types A, B, C [C1, C2], D, E, F, and G) that are antigenically and serologically distinct but structurally similar. BTX-A, -B, -E, and, -F (rarely) can cause the clinical syndrome of "botulism," which may occur following ingestion of contaminated food, from colonization of the infant gastrointestinal tract, or from an infected wound. BTX-C and -D cause toxicity only in animals.

BTX is synthesized as a single chain (150 kDa) and cleaved to form a dichain molecule with a disulfide bridge. The light chain (~50 kDa) acts as a zinc (Zn^{2+}) endopeptidase similar to tetanus toxin with proteolytic activity located at the N-terminal end. The heavy chain (~100 kDa) provides cholinergic specificity and binding to the presynaptic receptors. This promotes light chain translocation across the endosomal membrane.

BTX acts by binding presynaptically on the cholinergic nerve terminals, thus decreasing the release of acetylcholine and causing a neuromuscular blocking effect. This effect is temporary, and recovery occurs through proximal axonal sprouting and muscle reinnervation by the formation of new neuromuscular junctions. BTX-A and -E cleave synaptosome-associated protein (SNAP-25), a presynaptic membrane protein required for fusion of neurotransmitter-containing vesicles. BTX-B, -D, and -F cleave a vesicle-associated membrane protein (VAMP), also known as synaptobrevin. BTX-C acts by cleaving syntaxin, a target membrane protein.

Recent work has shown that BTX-A inhibits the release of several nociceptive mediators. These include substance P, glutamate, and calcitonin gene-related peptide, from the primary afferents (peripheral terminals).[16-24] Blocking of these mediators decreases neurogenic inflammation and, therefore, reduces pain sensation in the periphery. There are fewer signals from the peripheral nociceptors to the central nervous system, and this leads to a reduction in central sensitization.[16,17,22-24]

CLINICAL EVIDENCE OF BOTULINUM TOXIN AS AN ANTIHEADACHE AGENT

Clinicians began using BTX with the prospect of reducing pericranial muscular tension and contractions that are thought to contribute to headaches. BTX may reduce muscle spindle activity, and this, in turn, may decrease the sensory feedback. BTX may also directly affect sensory nerves by possibly inhibiting the neuropeptide-containing fibers. Although large multicenter, double-blind, randomized data are lacking, the evidence so far shows that BTX is an effective antiheadache medication when certain criteria are met.

Although there are numerous case studies focusing on use of BTX-A for treating migraines,[1,3] chronic daily headaches with migraine features,[11] and chronic tension-type headache,[4–6,8,9,25] there is no uniformity with the injection techniques or dosages. The studies use two general injection paradigms for treating headaches. In the fixed-site paradigm (**Fig. 34-1**), BTX is injected in sites that are predetermined and the same for everyone in the study. In the follow-the-pain paradigm, BTX is injected into or around the tender points that are reported by the patients and confirmed on physical examination.

Recent double-blind, placebo-controlled studies have shown consistency and homogeny with injection technique and dosage, allowing better comparative data analysis. An upcoming wave of large multicenter, double-blind, randomized placebo-controlled trials will further clarify the role of BTX in the prophylactic treatment of a variety of headache disorders.

MIGRAINE STUDIES

Silberstein and colleagues, in 2000,[1] reported a double-blind, placebo-controlled study in which 123 patients were randomly assigned into three groups, as follows: placebo (n = 42); BTX-A, 25 units (n = 42); and BTX-A, 75 units (n = 40). Patients who had two to eight moderate to severe, IHS-defined migraine attacks per months were enrolled. BTX-A injection sites were fixed site and included frontalis, glabellar, and bilateral temporalis muscles. BTX-A decreased the frequency of moderate to severe migraines per month but failed to reach statistical significance. This study also showed a decrease in the number of days of acute medication usage. All treatment-related adverse events were transient and were more commonly associated with the 75-unit dose.

Binder, also in 2000,[2] reported an open-label study that included 77 patients with migraine. Results confirmed the efficacy of BTX-A in reducing the number and severity of acute attacks per month.

In 1998, Binder and colleagues[3] performed a retrospective review of 96 patients who had chronic migraines but were treated with BTX-A for their movement disorder or were seen in the cosmetic surgery clinics. This study evaluated patients who received BTX-A injections into glabellar, temporalis, and occipitalis regions. The mean total dosage of BTX-A was 26 ± 14 units. This study reported that 51% of the 96 patients had complete elimination of their headaches, while 28% of the subjects had more than 50% reduction in the frequency or severity of their headaches. The remaining 21% of the 96 patients either had less than 50% response in headache frequency and severity or were lost to follow-up. The duration of benefit in the complete responders group was 3.6 ± 2.4 months. The partial responders group (≥50% decrease in headache frequency or severity) was 2.9 ± 1.6 months. Adverse effects reported were ecchymosis and transient, local pain at the injection site.

In 2010, Aurora and colleagues[26] showed promising results in their phase III study. The Phase III Research Evaluating Migraine Prophylaxis Therapy 1 (PREEMPT 1) consisted of a 24-week placebo-controlled, double-blind, parallel-group phase leading to a 32-week open-label phase. Injections of BTX of 155–195 U (n = 341) or a placebo (n = 338) were given every 12 weeks. Diener and colleagues[27] conducted PREEMPT 2 under the same parameters, with the BTX group (n = 347) and the placebo group (n = 358) and found positive results. The pooled results[28] from the two studies showed BTX as significantly superior to the placebo in the reduction of the symptoms. Significant reduction from baseline of headache days and the frequency of the headaches were noticed after 24 weeks in both studies.

Mathew and colleagues[29] in 2009 compared Onabotulinumtoxin A and Topimarate (approved by the FDA for migraine prophylaxis). Topimarate is recommended at a daily dose of 100 mg or 200 mg by the FDA. Their study included 60 people who were suffering from chronic migraine with or without aura occurring at least 15 days per month for at least 3 months. Over 9 months, 30 people were given injections of Onabotulinumtoxin A of approximately 143 U at month 1 and month 3.The dosage of Topimarate at approximately 100 mg over the 9-month period continued throughout the study to the 30 other people. The study concluded no remarkable difference between the injections of Onabotulinumtoxin A and Topimarate in preventing chronic migraines because both had at least a moderate positive response in a majority of the people.

TENSION-TYPE HEADACHES

The first reported study, by Zwart and colleagues in 1994,[10] showed no effect in six patients with tension-type headache, not using the IHS criteria. This study was carried out using the follow-the-pain paradigm, with BTX-A injected unilaterally into the temporal muscle.

Since then, Rollnik and colleagues,[4] in 2000, conducted a double-blind, placebo-controlled study involving 21 patients with CTTH or ETTH. The injection sites were specified as follows: "pericranial muscles

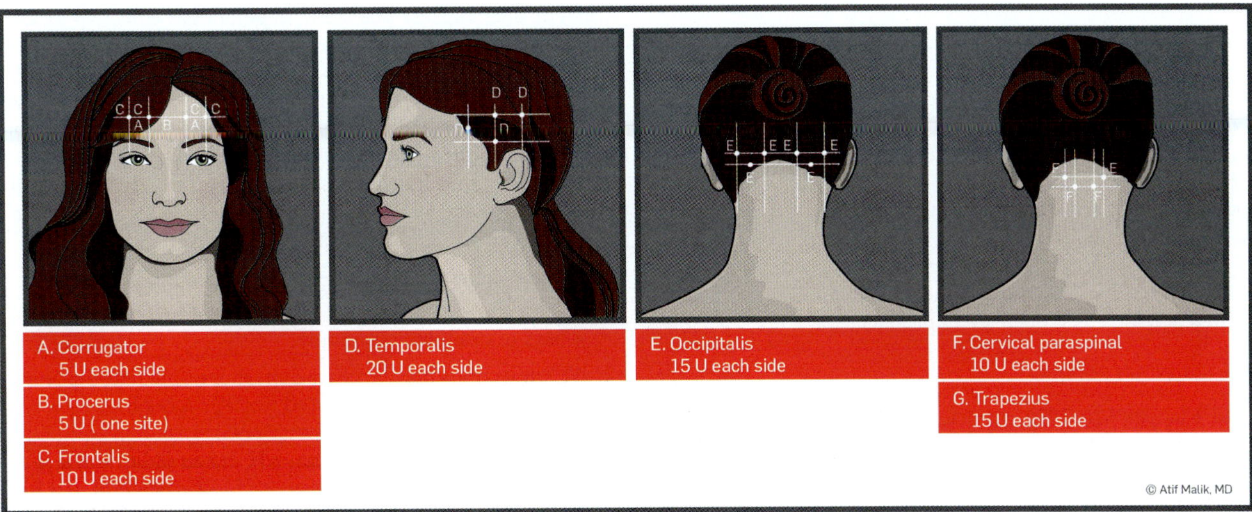

FIGURE 34-1. Fixed-site, fixed-dose injection site locations: the (A) corrugators, (B) procerus, (C) frontalis, (D) temporalis, (E) occipitalis, (F) cervical paraspinal, and (G) trapezius muscle injection sites.

around the head (2 injections into the fronto-occipital muscle and 3 into the temporal muscles bilaterally)." This study used BTX-A (Dysport) from Ipsen. The total dose used was 200 units. These investigators found no significant difference ($P > 0.5$) between the BTX-A and saline-treated groups. The study evaluated the pain intensity (visual analog scale), clinical global impression, headache frequency, and consumption of analgesics. Both groups tended to improve on several measures. The authors of this study suggest that given that Dysport is freeze dried and susceptible to breakdown, in contrast to the Botox (an American BTX-A), which is vacuum dried, a higher dose of Dysport may be needed to obtain a successful outcome.

Smuts and colleagues,[6] in 1999, reported a double-blind, placebo-controlled study in which 37 patients with CTTH were randomized into one of two groups: placebo (n = 15) or BTX-A (n = 22). Of the 37 patients, 38% also had history of migraines. The BTX-A injection sites were fixed and included 100 units into bilateral trapezius, splenius capitis, and temporalis muscles. At 3 months, 59% of the patients in the BTX-A group had at least a 25% improvement in their headache severity score and number of headache-free days, whereas only 13% of the placebo had the same response.

Schulte-Mattler and colleagues,[7] in an open-label prospective study also in 1999, injected nine patients who had ETTH and CTTH with BTX-A. They reported that eight of the nine patients showed improvement of their headache symptoms.

In 1998, Wheeler[8] reported four case studies of patients with CTTH for whom previous multiple therapies had been unsuccessful. BTX-A was injected in a follow-the-pain paradigm, using variable doses (20 units to 100 units) at the tender sites. All four patients had subjective pain relief.

Relja,[9] in 1997, did a preliminary open-label study in which 10 patients with CTTH were injected with 15 to 35 units of BTX-A in up to six sites based on local tenderness. All of the patients were refractory to previous pain medications, and all reported elimination or reduction in severity and duration of headaches at 2 weeks.

In 1999, Relja and Korsic[5] enrolled 16 CTTH patients in a double-blind, placebo-controlled, crossover study. The 35 to 80 units of BTX-A or placebo were injected in up to six sites into bilateral frontalis, trapezius, or sternocleidomastoid muscles based on local tenderness. The patients were followed 1, 2, 4, and 8 weeks postinjection. BTX-A significantly decreased tenderness scores, as recorded in patient diaries, and also decreased severity and duration of attacks (probability values not listed). Adverse events included local pain at the injection site, which occurred in some patients (number not specified) following BTX-A and saline.

A randomized, single-blind, placebo-controlled study done by Hamdy and colleagues[30] in 2009 was done on 28 Egyptian patients with chronic tension-type headaches. Following the fixed-site and follow-the-pain approach, results showed significant improvement within 1 month of the BTX-A injection.

In 2004, Padberg and colleagues[31] used a maximum dose of 100 U of BTX in 19 patients and a placebo in 21 patients. The patients from this double-blind, placebo-controlled parallel study did not show any significant improvement at the checkup dates at weeks 4, 8, and 12.

In 2006, Silberstein and colleagues[32] also found negative results in their multicenter, double-blind, placebo-controlled, randomized, and parallel-group study. Doses at 0 U, 50 U, 100 U, and 150 U were tested at five different sites in patients (total n = 279) with chronic tension-type headaches. Results showed no significant difference between the placebo groups; however, in the BTX groups, some patients in three of the BTX groups showed at least a 50% decrease in headache days.

CHRONIC DAILY HEADACHES

Klapper and Klapper,[11] in 1999, reported five case studies of patients who had chronic daily headache (CDH) with migrainous features. All five received 75 units of BTX-A at 11 fixed injection sites into the frontalis, glabellar, and temporalis muscles. Three of the five patients showed more than 75% subjective improvement. One patient had no response, and one showed only 35% subjective improvement.

Freund and Schwartz,[12] in 2000, reported a double-blind, placebo-controlled study in which 26 patients (n = 14 BTX-A; n = 12 placebo) with daily headaches secondary to cervical whiplash injuries were randomly assigned to one of two groups. The inclusion criteria included neck pain with musculoskeletal signs for more than 6 months. All of the patients were 2 years postinjury and had failed conservative therapy. BTX-A injection involved fixed doses of 100 units and the follow-the-pain paradigm. After 4 weeks, 11 of 14 patients showed a significant decrease in pain, and there was significant improvement in neck pain and range of motion. No adverse effects were reported.

Ondo and colleagues[33] in 2004 conducted a double-blind, placebo-controlled study for 12 weeks with 60 patients and saw a positive result with a moderate difference between the placebo and the injection of botulinum toxin type A (BTX-A) at 200 U. They then conducted an open-label study for another 12 weeks offering patients a dose of 200 U of BTX-A. The patients receiving two injections over the total 24-week period (n = 26 completed) reported fewer headache days overall than the group receiving only the one injection in the latter 12 weeks (n = 25 completed). The result was 40 ± 26 compared with 26 ± 19, respectively, and suggests that multiple injections may help increase the effectiveness of the treatment.

In 2005, Mathew and colleagues[34] conducted a single-blind study with 355 patients enrolled. The patient criteria was age 18 to 65 with at least 16 headaches over a 30-day period. The study was conducted over 9 months, with injections every 3 months, and showed a significant number of people who reported at least a 50% decrease in the frequency of their headaches by the end of the study.

In the same year, Dodick and colleagues[35] enrolled 355 patients in a double-blind, placebo-controlled study. They showed that botulinum toxin type A is a significant reducer in headache frequency and severity in people with chronic daily headaches who are not on other prophylactic headache medications.

In 2006, Farinelli and colleagues[36] conducted a 5-year long study with 1347 patients suffering from CDH. A dose of 100 U along with the fixed sites–fixed doses (FSFD) protocol was used, and the study showed that the best results were observed after 12 months of treatment. This resulted in patients having 23 headache-free days per month.

NUMMULAR HEADACHES

Mathew and colleagues[37] in 2008 showed positive results with four female patients aged 35 to 58 years. The patients were given 25 U injections over 10 different sites around affected areas. Two sets of injections were given about 14 weeks apart. Patients reported a decrease in the number of headaches.

CONCLUSION

Current data suggest that BTX is potentially effective as an agent for treating severe headaches. It has been successfully used to treat not only myofascial pain syndrome but also headaches and is now FDA approved for use in preventive treatment for chronic migraines. BTX appears to work primarily at the neuromuscular junction by binding presynaptically to the cholinergic nerve terminals, causing a neuromuscular blocking effect. The exact mechanism of BTX on nociceptors continues to be studied, but new data have shown that it reduces nociceptive signaling through several neurotransmitters.

1. BTX should be considered in treating migraines that are moderate to severe, resistant to conventional treatments, or cause more than 4 days of disability per month.
2. BTX injections may be efficacious in treating chronic severe tension-type headaches causing missed work or school.
3. BTX may potentially be the most efficacious agent in patients with chronic daily headaches.
4. BTX may be effective in patients with cervicogenic headaches and cervicothoracic myofascial pain syndromes associated with frequent headaches.

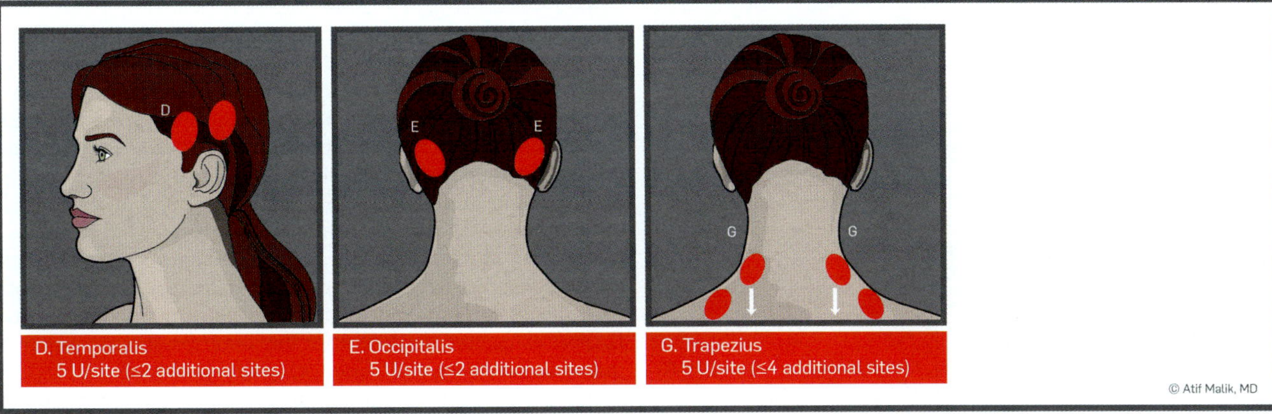

FIGURE 34-2. Follow-the-pain injection site locations: optional injections are distributed between the right and left (D) temporalis, (E) occipitalis, and (G) trapezius muscles in areas of maximal tenderness and/or pain.

All of the headache studies carried out thus far have shown that BTX is a safe drug. The adverse effects are limited to localized pain at the injection site, muscle weakness, and flulike symptoms. There is a possibility of developing immunity to BTX-A, in which case this form of the toxin could be replaced with BTX-B. Current data suggest that headaches can be treated using a relatively low dose, thus further decreasing the potential for developing antibodies. BTX-A doses closer to 100 units show more favorable results in reducing headache frequency and intensity. Data also suggest that the fixed-site injection (Figure 34-1) may be more effective than follow-the-pain paradigm (**Fig. 34-2**), and it appears to be gaining popularity among headache specialists.

REFERENCES

1. Silberstein S, Mathew N, Saper J. Botulinum toxin type A as a migraine preventive treatment. For the BOTOX Migraine Clinical Research Group. *Headache*. 2000;40:445-450.
2. Binder WJ, Brin MF, Blitzer A, et al. Botulinum toxin type A (BOTOX) for treatment of migraine headaches: an open-label study. *Otolaryngol Head Neck Surg*. 2000;123:669-676.
3. Binder WJ, Blitzer A, Brin MF. Treatment of hyperfunctional lines of the face with botulinum toxin A. *Dermatol Surg*. 1998;123:1198-1205.
4. Rollnik JD, Tanneberger O, Schubert M. Treatment of tension-type headache with botulinum toxin type A: a double-blind, placebo-controlled study. *Headache*. 2000;40:300-305.
5. Relja MA, Korsic M. Treatment of tension-type headache by injections of botulinum toxin type A: double-blind placebo-controlled study. *Neurology*. 1999;52:A203. (Abstract)
6. Smuts JA, et al. Prophylactic treatment of chronic tension-type headache using botulinum toxin type A. *Europ J Neurol*. 1999;6:S99-S102.
7. Schulte-Mattler WJ, Wieser T, Zierz S. Treatment of tension-type headache with botulinum toxin: a pilot study. *Eur J Med Res*. 1999;4:183-186.
8. Wheeler AH. Botulinum toxin A, adjunctive therapy for refractory headaches associated with pericranial muscle tension. *Headache*. 1998;38:468-471.
9. Relja M. Treatment of tension-type headache by local injection of botulinum toxin. *Europ J Neurol*. 1997;4:S71-S73.
10. Zwart JA, Bovim G, Sand T. Tension headache: botulinum toxin paralysis of temporal muscles. *Headache*. 1994;34:458-462.
11. Klapper J, Klapper JA. Use of botulinum toxin in chronic daily headaches associated with migraine. *Headache*. 1999;10:141-143.
12. Freund BJ, Schwartz M. Treatment of whiplash associated with neck pain with botulinum toxin-A: a pilot study. *J Rheumatol*. 2000;27:481-484.
13. Sostak P, Krause P, Förderreuther S, Reinisch V, Straube A. Botulinum toxin type-A therapy in cluster headache: an open study. *Journal of Headache and Pain* [serial online]. September 2007;8(4):236-241.
14. Headache Classification Committee of the International Headache Society. Classification and diagnostic criteria for headache disorders, cranial neuralgias, and facial pain. *Cephalalgia*. 1988;8(Suppl):1-96.
15. Silberstein SD, Lipton RB, Solomon S, Mathew NT. Classification of daily and near-daily headaches: proposed revisions to the HIS criteria. *Headache*. 1994;34:1-7.
16. Aoki KR. Review of a proposed mechanism for the antinociceptive action of botulinum toxin type A. *Neurotoxicology*. 2005;26:785-793.
17. Aoki KR. Evidence for antinociceptive activity of botulinum toxin type A in pain management. *Headache*. 2003;43(Suppl 1):S9-S15.
18. Cui M, Khanijou S, Rubino J, Aoki KR. Subcutaneous administration of botulinum toxin A reduces formalin-induced pain. *Pain*. 2004;107:125-133.
19. Durham PL, Cady R, Cady R. Regulation of calcitonin gene-related peptide secretion from trigeminal nerve cells by botulinum toxin type A: implications for migraine therapy. *Headache*. 2004;44:35-42.
20. Purkiss J, Welch M, Doward S, Foster K. Capsaicin stimulated release of substance P from cultured dorsal root ganglion neurons: involvement of two distinct mechanisms. *Biochem Pharmacol*. 2000;59:1403-1406.
21. Welch MJ, Purkiss JR, Foster KA. Sensitivity of embryonic rat dorsal root ganglia neurons to Clostridium botulinum neurotoxins. *Toxicon*. 2000;38:245-258.
22. Gazerani P, Staahl C, Drewes AM, Arendt-Nielsen L. The effects of botulinum toxin type A on capsaicin-evoked pain, flare, and secondary hyperalgesia in an experimental human model of trigeminal sensitization. *Pain*. 2006;122:315-325.
23. Gazerani P, Pedersen NS, Staahl C, Drewes AM, Arendt-Nielsen L. Subcutaneous botulinum toxin type A reduces capsaicin-induced trigeminal pain and vasomotor reactions in human skin. *Pain*. 2009;141:60-69.
24. Blumenfeld A, Silberstein S, Dodick D, Aurora S, Turkel C, Binder W. Method of injection of onabotulinumtoxinA for chronic migraine: a safe, well-tolerated, and effective treatment paradigm based on the PREEMPT clinical program. *Headache*.
25. Freund BJ, Schwartz M. Treatment of chronic cervical-associated headache with botulinum toxin A: a pilot study. *Headache*. 2000;40:231-236.

26. Aurora SK, Dodick DW, Turkel CC, et al. Onabotulinum toxin A for treatment of chronic migraine: results from the double-blind, randomized placebo controlled phase of the PREEMPT 1 trial. *Cephalalgia*. Published 2010.
27. Diener HC, Dodick DW, Aurora SK, et al. Onabotulinum toxin A for treatment of chronic migraine: Results from the double-blind, randomized, placebo-controlled phase of the PREEMPT 2 trial. *Cephalalgia*. Published 2010.
28. Dodick D, Turkel C, Brin M, et al. Onabotulinum toxin A for treatment of chronic migraine: pooled results from the double-blind, randomized, placebo-controlled phases of the PREEMPT clinical program. *Headache* [serial online]. June 2010;50(6):921-936.
29. Mathew N, Jaffri S. A double-blind comparison of botulinum toxin A (BOTOX) and topiramate (TOPAMAX) for the prophylactic treatment of chronic migraine: a pilot study. *Headache* [serial online]. November 2009;49(10):1466-1478.
30. Hamdy S, Samir H, El-Sayed M, Adel N, Hasan R. Botulinum toxin: could it be an effective treatment for chronic tension-type headache? *Journal of Headache and Pain* [serial online]. February 2009;10(1):27-34.
31. Padberg M, de Bruijn S, de Haan R, Tavy D. Treatment of chronic tension-type headache with botulinum toxin: a double-blind, placebo-controlled clinical trial. *Cephalalgia* [serial online]. August 2004;24(8):675-680.
32. Silberstein S, Göbel H, Turkel C, et al. Botulinum toxin type A in the prophylactic treatment of chronic tension-type headache: a multicentre, double-blind, randomized, placebo-controlled, parallel-group study. *Cephalalgia* [serial online]. July 2006;26(7):790-800.
33. Ondo WG, Vuong KD, Derman HS. Botulinum toxin A for chronic daily headache: a randomized, placebo-controlled, parallel design study. *Cephalalgia*. 2004;24(1):60-65.
34. Mathew NT, Frishberg BM, Gawel M, Dimitrova R, Gibson J, Turkel C, Botox CDH Study Group. Botulinum toxin type A (Botox) for the prophylactic treatment of chronic daily headache: a randomized, double-blind, placebo-controlled trial. *Headache*. 2005;45(4):293-307.
35. Dodick DW, Mauskop A, Elkind AH, DeGryse R, Brin M, Silberstein S, Botox CDH Study Group. Botulinum toxin type A for the prophylaxis of chronic daily headache: subgroup analysis of patients not receiving other prophylactic medications: a randomized double-blind, placebo-controlled study. *Headache*. 2005;45(4):315-324.
36. Farinelli I, Coloprisco G, De Filippis S, Martelletti P. Long-term benefits of botulinum toxin type A (BOTOX) in chronic daily headache: a five-year long experience. *J Headache Pain*. 2006;7:407-412.
37. Mathew N, Kailasam J, Meadors L. Botulinum toxin type A for the treatment of nummular headache: four case studies. *Headache* [serial online]. March 2008;48(3):442-447.

Facial Pain

Thomas N. Ward
Morris Levin

The diagnosis and management of patients with facial pain can be daunting even to experienced physicians. The causes are myriad, ranging from the mundane (sinus and dental disease) to the exotic (short-lasting unilateral neuralgiform headache with conjunctival injection and tearing, or SUNCT). Misdiagnosis and mismanagement are common. The goal of this chapter is to discuss some of the more important causes of facial pain and to guide proper identification and treatment.

Simply because pain is felt in the face does not imply that it necessarily originates in facial structures. As elsewhere in the body, pain may be local in origin, or *referred*. The role of the trigeminovascular system and the spinal trigeminal nucleus as a point of anatomic and physiologic convergence is discussed in Chapter 19. Suffice it to say that the location of the pain may not be so important diagnostically as other features.

The approach to the evaluation of facial pain requires careful attention to detail. In the patient history, it is essential to obtain an accurate description of the nature of the pain, or pains, what may have incited it, and what currently provokes and ameliorates it. Are there associated phenomena, such as autonomic changes? Past medical history, including trauma and surgical or dental procedures, may provide essential clues. Is there associated depression or any other psychiatric problem? What therapies have been tried, and with what outcomes?

After obtaining a detailed history, a thorough examination is necessary. In addition to the general physical examination, a thorough neurologic examination is essential. The examiner looks for signs of raised intracranial pressure (papilledema, diminished up gaze, sixth cranial nerve palsies) and cranial nerve dysfunction (particularly oculosympathetic paresis). The head and neck require careful attention. Are there trigger points? Is there dental or sinus tenderness? Auscultation for bruits and palpation of the carotid artery are sometimes informative maneuvers.

Finally, the results of prior diagnostic studies are reviewed, noting the timing of the studies. Were the appropriate studies performed? If the situation has changed, perhaps an imaging study should be repeated. Sometimes a diagnosis may become apparent only after serial clinical examinations or diagnostic studies, or both.

After a careful history, examination, and review of the data, a tentative diagnosis may be rendered. Often, further consultation is required. Treatment is offered based on the tentative diagnosis and may, in itself, sometimes be diagnostic. The thoughtful physician should always be willing to reconsider the diagnosis.

Facial pain clearly represents a diagnostic challenge. With attention to the fundamental approach outlined in the preceding paragraphs, the vast majority of patients may achieve a satisfying outcome.

NEURALGIAS

Neuralgias are paroxysmal pain in the distribution of a particular nerve. The pain is typically *maximal at onset and lancinating and may be described as "electric shocks" or "jabbing."* There may be a single, sharp pain or repetitive pains in succession. The pain may be so brief as to last but an instant, or it may last several seconds. There is usually a refractory period after the severe pain, during which pain does not occur. Some neuralgic conditions have trigger zones (areas that, when stimulated, provoke an attack) or other triggers. Careful history taking often reveals other pain occurring as well, such as continuous aching, burning, or throbbing. Inquiry must be made about all the sensations that occur because some patients mention only the severe exacerbations. Response to treatment may provide a clue to diagnosis but can also be misleading. "Diagnostic blocks" in the setting of facial pain do not necessarily define the site from which the pain arises because of overlap of cranial nerves V, IX, and X (which converge on the spinal trigeminal nucleus and the tractus solitarius). Facial and cranial neuralgias are classified in the *International Classification of Headache Disorders*, 2nd edition (ICHD-II) by the presumed nerve of origin (**Table 35-1**).

The best-known facial neuralgia is trigeminal neuralgia, which is discussed in detail in this chapter and, in many ways, serves as a model for understanding other neuralgias causing facial pain.

TRIGEMINAL NEURALGIA

Trigeminal neuralgia is a severe, (usually) unilateral facial pain, characterized by lancinating pains in the distribution of one or more divisions of the trigeminal nerve. Although onset may occur in the second and

TABLE 35-1 Cranial Neuralgias and Central Causes of Facial Pain

International Classification of Headache Disorders, 1st revision (ICHD-II)
13.1 Trigeminal neuralgia
13.1.1 Classical trigeminal neuralgia
13.1.2 Symptomatic trigeminal neuralgia
13.2 Glossopharyngeal neuralgia
13.2.1 Classical glossopharyngeal neuralgia
13.2.2 Symptomatic glossopharyngeal neuralgia
13.3 Nervus intermedius neuralgia
13.4 Superior laryngeal neuralgia
13.5 Nasociliary neuralgia
13.6 Supraorbital neuralgia
13.7 Other terminal branch neuralgias
13.8 Occipital neuralgia
13.9 Neck-tongue syndrome
13.10 External compression headache
13.11 Cold-stimulus headache
13.11.1 Headache attributed to external application of a cold stimulus
13.11.2 Headache attributed to ingestion or inhalation of a cold stimulus
13.12 Constant pain caused by compression, irritation or distortion of cranial nerves or upper cervical roots by structural lesions
13.13 Optic neuritis
13.14 Ocular diabetic neuropathy
13.15 Head or facial pain attributed to herpes zoster
13.15.1 Head or facial pain attributed to acute herpes zoster
13.15.2 Postherpetic neuralgia
13.16 Tolosa-Hunt syndrome
13.17 Ophthalmoplegic "migraine"
13.18 Central causes of facial pain
13.18.1 Anaesthesia dolorosa
13.18.2 Central poststroke pain
13.18.3 Facial pain attributed to multiple sclerosis
13.18.4 Persistent idiopathic facial pain
13.18.5 Burning mouth syndrome
13.19 Other cranial neuralgia or other centrally mediated facial pain

third decades, the majority of cases begin in middle and old age. With an annual incidence rate of 4 to 5 per 100,000, it is one of the most frequently seen neuralgias in the elderly.[1] The pain may be so excruciating that facial muscle spasms can be seen—hence, the older term, tic douloureux. Hemifacial spasm, which can be seen with trigeminal neuralgia, can look similar to these spasms and, while rapid and involuntary—as opposed to the reactive spasms of tic douloureux—can be difficult to differentiate.

The facial pain tends to occur in paroxysms and is maximal at or near onset. The severe exacerbations tend to last from one to several seconds but may occur in volleys. There may also be a coexisting continual deep or dull pain. Patients may or may not, therefore, have pain-free periods.

Trigeminal neuralgia most often involves the second and third divisions of the trigeminal nerve (V_2 and V_3) but can include or be limited to the first division as well. Trigger zones may be present. Often, lightly touching these areas will trigger a paroxysm, and patients tend to protect these areas. Other triggers may include chewing, talking, brushing teeth, cold air, or smiling and grimacing. A refractory period of several minutes typically follows an episode, during which a paroxysm cannot be provoked. In occasional patients, the pain may be bilateral, but not on both sides simultaneously.

This condition may be idiopathic (primary) or symptomatic (secondary). Idiopathic implies no known underlying condition, but many idiopathic cases are probably the result of vascular compression of the trigeminal nerve near its entry into the pons. Symptomatic causes include multiple sclerosis, tumors, and basilar artery aneurysm or ectasia.[2-4]

Unlike some other facial pain conditions, trigeminal neuralgia typically does not awaken patients at night. Some patients have a history of so-called pretrigeminal neuralgia, which is said to be dull, continuous, aching pain in the jaw, evolving eventually into trigeminal neuralgia. This brief, milder pain is sometimes wrongly suspected to have a dental origin, and dental procedures are performed. Because trigeminal neuralgia is sometimes precipitated by dental procedures (e.g., dental extraction), confusion about etiology has resulted.[5]

The pathophysiology of trigeminal neuralgia is not fully elucidated. Demyelinative lesions of trigeminal fibers appear to set up ectopic impulses and ephapses. This alteration of afferent input may disinhibit pain pathways in the spinal trigeminal nucleus. Evidence for a role of central pain mechanisms includes the presence of refractory periods after a triggered episode, trains of painful sensations after a single stimulus, and some latency from the time of stimulation to the onset of pain.[6]

Clinically, certain features of the history help in making the diagnosis. Paroxysms of pain in the distribution of the trigeminal nerve, especially if trigger points are present, are typical. The examination may reveal these trigger zones, which often are near the midline. If sensory loss is present, a mass lesion is more likely. In younger patients (20 to 40 years old) with trigeminal neuralgia, multiple sclerosis should be considered. A demyelinative lesion in the pons would explain bilateral symptoms.

Once the diagnosis is suspected on clinical grounds, a careful search for ipsilateral dental pathology should be undertaken (oral surgery consultation should be considered). Magnetic resonance imaging (MRI) and magnetic resonance angiography (MRA) should be performed to look for evidence of demyelinating lesions, a mass lesion in the cerebellopontine angle, or an ectatic blood vessel (rarely seen with MRA). The differential diagnosis includes SUNCT/SUNA (discussed later in the section, "SUNCT/SUNA"), cluster-tic syndrome, jabs and jolts syndrome, and other neuralgias—all of which are discussed later in this chapter.

Trigeminal neuralgia is usually successfully treated with medication (**Table 35-2**). The American Academy of Neurology has published evidence-based guidelines.[7] Carbamazepine is felt to be the most effective medication. Oxcarbazepine has somewhat less evidence but is the second choice. Baclofen, phenytoin, valproate, pimozide, and clonazepam may have utility as well, alone or in various combinations, but this is anecdotal information and does not have the same level of evidence-based support. Baclofen may be synergistic with carbamzepaine.[8]

TABLE 35-2 Medications for Trigeminal Neuralgia

Acute
Phenytoin or fosphenytoin intravenously
Chronic
Carbamazepine*
Oxcarbazepine*
Baclofen (may be added to carbamazepine for "synergy")
Valproate
Clonazepam
Pimozide
Gabapentin
Lamotrigine
Topiramate
Perphenazine
Olanzapine
Tizanidine

*Evidence-based support, American Academy of Neurology Practice Parameter, reference 7.

See Chapters 48, 49, and 52 for details on the use of these agents.

Misoprostol, a prostaglandin E analogue, has been reported as effective in trigeminal neuralgia caused by multiple sclerosis.[9] Gabapentin and lamotrigine have also been reported to be useful, although there is less clinical experience with these agent.[10,11]

Neuroleptic medications, including chlorpromazine and perphenazine, have been used successfully in intractable cases, and novel neuroleptics such as olanzapine and quetiapine have been tried as well. Tizanidine has been used in selected cases. Topiramate has been suggested, because other anticonvulsant medication has been effective.

We have found carbamazepine to be the most useful of all the available drugs. If doses are started low, especially in the elderly (e.g., 50 mg b.i.d. or less) and advanced gradually, the drug is highly efficacious with few side effects, and few patients develop tolerance. If pain control is insufficient, baclofen may be added. With both carbamazepine and oxcarbazepine, the occasional development of hyponatremia needs to be monitored by laboratory evaluation. If the patient is desperate for immediate pain relief, intravenous infusion of phenytoin or fosphenytoin (250 to 500 mg at no more than 50 mg/min, monitoring pulse and blood pressure) may be rapidly effective, although many patients quickly develop tolerance to the drug. Nonetheless, intravenous phenytoin may afford immediate temporary relief while oral carbamazepine therapy is begun. This maneuver may also enable the physician to better examine the patient with a sensitive face.[12] Details of the use of these medications may be found elsewhere in this book (see Chapters 62, 63, and 64). Rarely, there are spontaneous permanent remissions of trigeminal neuralgia. More often, the illness tends to wax and wane in terms of severity and frequency of exacerbations. Therefore, in patients achieving good relief of pain with medications, periodic attempts to gradually withdraw these drugs are warranted.

For patients refractory to therapy with drugs, various surgical procedures may have efficacy. Janetta has popularized microvascular decompression, the dissection away from the trigeminal nerve of various vascular structures, often an ectatic superior cerebellar artery.[13] Long-term outcome is good (more than 80% pain-free), but this procedure does involve an intracranial approach with some morbidity and mortality risk. Other procedures directed against the trigeminal nerve include percutaneous radiofrequency rhizotomy, glycerol rhizolysis, and balloon compression. Complications include anesthesia dolorosa (a central pain disorder resulting from hypersensitization of the second-order spinal trigeminal nucleus neuron) and keratitis, as well as facial weakness caused by injury of the facial nerve. More recently, excellent results with minimal morbidity have been reported with gamma knife therapy.[14] For patients unable or unwilling to tolerate more aggressive surgical procedures, peripheral nerve root avulsion may provide relief. Although often temporarily effective, nerves often regenerate and pain recurs.

Tenser has noted that, after surgery for trigeminal neuralgia, herpes simplex virus reactivation occurs in 17% to 94% of patients. The speculation is that altered function of cranial nerve V (CNV) underlies the beneficial response to the various surgical manipulations (injury to the trigeminal root ganglion).[15]

In summary, patients suffering from trigeminal neuralgia deserve a careful evaluation, especially to exclude symptomatic causes such as multiple sclerosis or a cerebellopontine angle mass. Ipsilateral dental pathology should be sought. Pain relief can usually be achieved through aggressive pharmacologic therapy, surgery, or both.

CLUSTER-TIC SYNDROME

It has been reported that the pains of trigeminal neuralgia and cluster headache may coexist.[16] In the cluster-tic syndrome, there are three types of pain. One component of the pain resembles trigeminal neuralgia—paroxysmal, extremely brief, and severe. The second component is more similar to cluster headache, although of variable length, with autonomic phenomena (lacrimation, rhinorrhea). The third type of pain is a mixture of the first two. This pain may be provoked by trigger points or moving the neck.

Cluster-tic syndrome usually afflicts patients between 20 and 70 years old. It may exist in chronic or episodic forms (remissions and recurrences). Medical therapy is usually unsuccessful, although when surgery (microvascular decompression or trigeminal rhizotomy) relieves the neuralgia, the clusterlike pain may be lessened and become more responsive to therapy.

The differential diagnosis includes SUNCT/SUNA, which is discussed later in this chapter. Secondary (symptomatic) SUNCT has been reported as a result of arteriovenous malformation in the cerebellopontine angle, and secondary cluster-tic syndrome has been associated with an ectatic basilar artery running deep into the cerebellopontine cistern.[17,18] We feel it is possible that so-called cluster-tic syndrome and SUNCT may actually be the same condition, at least in some cases.

GLOSSOPHARYNGEAL NEURALGIA

Glossopharyngeal neuralgia is defined as paroxysmal pain in areas supplied by cranial nerves IX and X (CN IX, X). There are numerous analogies to trigeminal neuralgia, with which it occasionally coexists.

This entity is much less common than trigeminal neuralgia. While probably underdiagnosed, it is rare with an annual incidence in the range of 0.2 to 0.7 cases/100,000.[19] Age of onset ranges from childhood to old age, although middle age is most frequent. This condition usually occurs as paroxysmal, severe, unilateral pain involving the ear, larynx, tonsil, or tongue. It is almost never bilateral. Triggers include chewing, swallowing, coughing, speaking, yawning, certain tastes, and touching the neck or external auditory canal (rarely the pre- or postauricular areas).[20]

The pain typically radiates upward from the oropharynx toward the ear. The duration of the severe paroxysms is seconds to minutes, but there may also be a low-grade, constant, dull background pain. Up to several dozen attacks may occur each day, some of which awaken the patient from sleep. Some episodes are associated with strenuous coughing or hoarseness.

Similar to trigeminal neuralgia, glossopharyngeal neuralgia may occur in a pattern of bouts lasting weeks to months, alternating with longer periods of remission. Severe attacks may be associated with bradycardia and asystole, resulting in syncope.[21] Pacemaker placement may be necessary.[22] Presumably, in these cases, input from CN IX into the tractus solitarius has an effect on the dorsal motor nucleus of X.

Also, similar to trigeminal neuralgia, there are idiopathic and secondary (symptomatic) forms. Presumably, in the idiopathic form, peripheral demyelinization results in brainstem discharges. Alternatively, vascular compression of CN IX and X may occur at the nerve root entry zone by the vertebral artery, posterior inferior cerebellar artery, or, infrequently, the anterior inferior cerebellar artery.[23] Symptomatic causes include cerebellopontine angle tumor, brainstem demyelinative lesions, peritonsillar abscess, carotid aneurysm, multiple sclerosis, metastatic cancer, Chiari I malformation, arachnoiditis, direct carotid puncture, Paget's disease, and Eagle's syndrome (in which CN IX is compressed laterally against an ossified stylohyoid ligament).[23]

The evaluation of a patient suspected of suffering from glossopharyngeal neuralgia includes a careful history, especially inquiring about the presence of trigger factors and nocturnal awakening. All aspects of an attack need to be recorded. MRI and MRA are appropriate because approximately 25% of cases of glossopharyngeal neuralgia result from secondary causes, such as brainstem mass lesions. Plain skull films might reveal an ossified stylohyoid ligament in Eagle's syndrome.

Medical therapy of glossopharyngeal neuralgia is essentially the same as for trigeminal neuralgia, but because of its relative rarity, there is no strong evidence base (see Table 35-1). Additionally, the application or injection of local anesthetics to the oropharynx may be both diagnostic and therapeutic.[24] Injection of local anesthetic into the region of the stylohyoid ligament can be diagnostic if Eagle's syndrome is strongly considered. Patients failing drug therapy may be candidates for surgical treatment. Procedures include intracranial sectioning of CN IX along with the upper three to four rootlets of CN X at the jugular foramen, or vascular decompression.[23,25] Imaging such as high-resolution MRI may show ninth nerve compression. Patients may have coexistent trigeminal neuralgia and symptomatic vagal nerve compression.[19]

The differential diagnosis of glossopharyngeal neuralgia includes so-called geniculate neuralgia (nervus intermedius neuralgia of Hunt), which is discussed later in this chapter. The obvious overlap of clinical features between the two conditions fosters suspicions that they may actually be variations of the same condition.

SUPERIOR LARYNGEAL NEURALGIA

The superior laryngeal nerve is a branch of CN X that runs adjacent to the carotid bifurcation and supplies the cricothyroid muscle of the larynx. A lesion of this nerve produces a weak, hoarse voice. The nerve may be involved by local disease of the carotid or injured by carotid endarterectomy.[26]

Clinically, the patient suffers paroxysmal pain that radiates from the throat to the ear or eye, similar to the pain of glossopharyngeal neuralgia. There is generally hoarseness. The episodes last seconds to minutes and may occur spontaneously or be triggered by coughing, swallowing, or speaking. During severe paroxysms, the patient temporarily may be rendered mute.

On examination, hoarseness of speech and a trigger point superolateral to the thyroid cartilage may be noted. The differential diagnosis includes glossopharyngeal neuralgia, geniculate neuralgia, and carotidynia (all discussed elsewhere in this chapter). Local blockade of the nerve is diagnostic. Some patients respond to carbamazepine and possibly other drugs used for neuralgias. Neurectomy may be curative.[26]

POSTHERPETIC NEURALGIA

Acute herpes zoster (shingles) often causes facial pain, especially affecting V_1. The varicella zoster virus persists in sensory nerve ganglia and may cause a painful rash. Postherpetic neuralgia (PHN) is variably defined as pain that persists (anywhere from 1 to 6 months) after the rash has healed. Although treatment of acute zoster with acyclovir, valacyclovir, famciclovir, steroids, pain medications, and even sympathetic nerve blocks may shorten the duration and alleviate the immediate pain, none has been clearly proven to prevent the occurrence of postherpetic neuralgia. Age is the major risk factor. Patients younger than 40 years of age rarely develop postherpetic neuralgia, whereas more than 75% of patients older than age 70 years are afflicted.[27] Lesser risk factors include diabetes mellitus, V_1 involvement, and other immunologic compromise.

Clinically, there is usually scarring and pigmentary changes in the affected dermatome. The pain is constant and variably aching, burning, lancinating, or itchy. The mechanism of the pain is likely deafferentation pain. Pathologically, there are degenerative changes in the involved axons, dorsal ganglion, and even the dorsal horn of the spinal cord. Patients complain of allodynia (pain with non-noxious stimulus) in the affected area.[28]

Because this condition preferentially affects the elderly, treatment can be difficult. Unlike trigeminal neuralgia, anticonvulsants are usually ineffective. Amitriptyline is the single most useful agent, although the anticholinergic side effects may be troublesome. Beginning with a low dose (e.g., 10 mg) and slowly escalating toward 75 mg at bedtime may improve tolerance. If side effects are troublesome, either nortriptyline or doxepin, which have fewer anticholinergic side effects, may be substituted (both are available in liquid form, allowing very gradual dose titration if necessary). Approximately 60% of patients obtain significant relief with these agents.[29,30]

Both pregabalin (Lyrica®) and gabapentin (Neurontin®) have also been shown to be effective for PHN (both approved by FDA for PHN) and, in some patients, may be better tolerated than cyclic antidepressants. Dosage of pregabalin is 75 to 150 mg twice daily or 50 to 100 mg three times daily. Dosage of gabapentin should begin at 300 mg daily and be increased as tolerated and necessary to a dose as high as 3600 mg daily, generally divided into three doses. A recent study showed that the combination of amitriptyline and gabapentin was even more effective than either alone in the treatment of neuropathic pain.

Many other agents have been anecdotally reported[31] to benefit patients with postherpetic neuralgia. These include controlled-release oxycodone, capsaicin cream, topical lidocaine gel, EMLA cream, and other anticonvulsants.[8] With persistence, pain relief can usually be achieved. Fortunately, for most patients, the pain eventually spontaneously remits, for the majority in less than 3 years. Prevention is worth considering as there is now a vaccine available.

OTHER NEURALGIAS

Numerous neuralgias have been described as causes of facial pain. However, some share many features with other conditions, and it is likely that some of these conditions simply share several names. Of these, Raeder's paratrigeminal syndrome is the best recognized.

Raeder's syndrome consists of constant, unilateral, burning facial pain with hypesthesia or dysesthesia, or both, in the distribution of the trigeminal nerve, most often V_1, plus oculosympathetic paresis (ptosis and miosis). This syndrome may be caused by carotid artery dissection. It may also occur with trauma, mass or lesion of the middle cranial fossa, syphilis, and sinusitis. In the absence of these underlying conditions, it is generally a self-limited process, remitting in weeks to month.[32]

Supraorbital neuralgia is defined by the International Headache Society as paroxysmal or constant pain in the region of the supraorbital notch and medial aspect of the forehead in the area supplied by the supraorbital nerve, with tenderness over the nerve in the supraorbital notch. The definition requires that pain is abolished by local anaesthetic blockade or ablation of the supraorbital nerve. This neuralgia is commonly the sequel of trauma to the supraorbital nerve (see "Posttraumatic Facial Pain").

Sphenopalatine neuralgia (with numerous other synonyms, including greater superficial petrosal neuralgia) is described as unilateral, episodic, perinasal facial pain with nasal congestion.[33] Most of these cases closely resemble cluster headache, and the existence of this neuralgia as a separate diagnostic entity is questionable.

The same may be said for geniculate neuralgia (or nervus intermedius neuralgia of Hunt). This condition has been described as lancinating pains deep in the ear with a trigger zone in the external auditory canal.[34] The existence of geniculate neuralgia as a separate entity also has been called into question. The similarities with the better-accepted diagnosis—glossopharyngeal neuralgia—are obvious.

CAROTID ARTERY PAIN

The carotid artery, like most arteries of its caliber, is sensitive to pain. Distention or inflammation of nociceptive fibers in its walls tends to produce pain, which can seem localized to the neck or, quite commonly, be referred to a number of areas including the jaw, face and periorbital regions, and sinus areas.

CAROTIDYNIA

Carotidynia is pain that appears to emanate from the carotid artery. Raskin has described two types: acute and chronic recurrent carotidynia.[35]

The acute form seems to be a self-limited problem. The patient suffers from unilateral or, less often, bilateral neck, jaw, and facial pain that may be provoked by swallowing, coughing, or moving the neck. The pain may be pounding, sharp, or dull. The duration is from a few days to (rarely) several months. Corticosteroids have been advocated for relief. The differential diagnosis includes giant cell arteritis and carotid dissection. The evaluation of such complaints should include an erythrocyte sedimentation rate (ESR) and MRI or MRA to evaluate the anatomy of the carotid arteries.

Chronic recurrent carotidynia is felt to be a manifestation of migraine. This condition, like migraine, seems to be more common in women. Pain occurs in the jaw, cheek, or periorbitally. The frequency of attacks is quite variable. Pain may be dull and continuous, or sharp, or throbbing. An association with dental extraction has been speculated. Drugs effective in the prophylaxis of migraine are effective in this condition. Examples include propranolol, methysergide, and amitriptyline. It should be noted that if one examines a migraineur during an attack, the carotid artery is usually found to be tender.

CAROTID ARTERY DISSECTION

Arterial dissection is caused by penetration of blood into the arterial wall with resultant narrowing of the vascular lumen, sometimes even leading to complete occlusion. Carotid artery dissection may be spontaneous (no discernible inciting event), posttraumatic, or the result of underlying disease of the vessel (such as fibromuscular dysplasia, Marfan's syndrome, or cystic medial necrosis).

Carotid dissection is a frequently recognized cause of stroke in the young, especially in migraineurs.[36] Clinically, patients complain of neck pain radiating to the cheek or periorbitally. The pain may be dull, sharp, or throbbing. Uncommonly, the headache is bilateral. Focal ischemic symptoms (transient ischemic attack or stroke) may ensue as a result of loss of blood flow or embolization from the tip of the clot. There may be an ipsilateral oculosympathetic paresis (ptosis, miosis) resulting from involvement of the internal carotid plexus. Bruits may be appreciated, either subjective or objective, or both.[37] MRI and MRA may, in some cases, be as sensitive as angiography for the detection of this lesion.[38] Carotid ultrasound and transcranial Doppler, although less effective for initial detection, are excellent noninvasive methods for studying the resolution of the dissection, which may occur over weeks to months.[39] Treatment may involve antiplatelet agents, heparin, or warfarin. An urgent neurologic consultation is indicated.

POSTTRAUMATIC FACIAL PAIN

Facial pain may occur after trauma. Although bullet wounds and other head injuries may trigger pain, surgery is also a cause. Facial pain may occur after maxillofacial surgery, orbital enucleations, sinus procedures, and dental procedures. Dental procedures may trigger a variety of syndromes, including neuralgia and facial migraine.

In all cases of posttraumatic facial pain, a careful search should be made for underlying pathology, especially dental. Some patients manifest constant burning pain, occasionally with tingling and intermittent stabbing. With trophic changes, edema, and redness, reflex sympathetic dystrophy (complex regional pain syndrome, type 1) should be suspected.[40] In patients who complain of significant burning pain, sympathetic blockade of the stellate ganglion may be effective, even without obvious complex regional pain syndrome.

Treatment of posttraumatic facial pain can be challenging. Brief lancinating pains may respond to agents used in treatment of neuralgias (see Table 35-2). Amitriptyline may reduce pain and lessen associated depression. Other agents useful for treating migraine headaches have been employed empirically for symptomatic benefit. Fortunately, posttraumatic facial pain is a self-limited condition, generally resolving spontaneously within, at most, several years.

In some cases, direct trauma to superficial facial nerves, such as the supraorbital and supratrochlear nerves, can lead to persistent lancinating or, less typically, aching pain. Neuroma formation is a postulated mechanism, and local nerve block with lidocaine or bupivacaine can be both diagnostic and therapeutic. We have found percussion tenderness over the nerve in question to be particularly helpful in predicting response to local nerve block.

SINUS DISEASE

Acute sinusitis—maxillary sinusitis being the most common—may cause facial pain. The pain may be felt in the cheeks, upper teeth, or bifrontally. The discomfort may be dull and continuous, throbbing, or sharp. The differential diagnosis includes migraine, which is often misdiagnosed as "sinus headaches."

To make a diagnosis of acute sinusitis as a cause of facial pain, positive findings should be present. On examination, there is tenderness to percussion, often with a purulent nasal discharge, and fever. Laboratory evaluation may show an elevated ESR and elevated white blood count. Sinus imaging (x-rays or computed tomography scan) should be abnormal. Without these findings, alternate diagnoses should be sought.

TABLE 35-3 Mucosal Contact Point Headache

International Classification of Headache Disorders, 1st revision (ICHD-II)—Appendix
Diagnostic criteria:
A. Intermittent pain localized to the periorbital and medial canthal or temporozygomatic regions and fulfilling criteria C and D
B. Clinical, nasal endoscopic, and/or CT imaging evidence of mucosal contact points without acute rhinosinusitis
C. Evidence that the pain can be attributed to mucosal contact based on at least one of the following:
a. Pain corresponds to gravitational variations in mucosal congestion as the patient moves between upright and recumbent postures.
b. Abolition of pain within 5 minutes after diagnostic topical application of local anaesthesia to the middle turbinate using placebo- or other controls[1]
D. Pain resolves within 7 days, and does not recur, after surgical removal of mucosal contact points.

Sphenoid sinusitis can be less obvious, and referred pain can include periorbital and maxillary regions.

The acute condition often responds to decongestants and simple analgesics. More severe, progressive cases require antibiotics. Refractory cases are candidates for ear, nose, and throat (ENT) consultation for surgery. Chronic sinusitis is rarely a cause of headaches and facial pain.

"Mucosal contact point headache" is speculated to occur when there is contact between the nasal septum and lateral nasal structures. It is a controversial entity and not yet validated according to the International Headache Society's classification, where it appears in the Appendix (ICHD-II) (**Table 35-3**).[41] Abolition of pain by application of local anesthetic may assist in diagnosis.

DENTAL PAIN

Oromandibular conditions as a cause of pain are discussed in detail in Chapter 26. Dental pains are an extremely common cause of facial pain. Specific inquiry regarding prior dental procedures should be made of all patients. Trigeminal neuralgia has been associated with ipsilateral dental pathology. The presence of provocative factors, such as chewing, or the effect of hot or cold liquids may provide useful clues. The teeth and temporomandibular joints should be carefully evaluated in cases of facial pain. Temporomandibular joint syndrome (limitation of jaw movement, crepitus in the joint, and pain with chewing) may cause pain in the temple, jaw, and neck. Dental or oral surgical consultation may be extremely useful.

Before declaring a diagnosis of dental or sinus disease as the etiology of facial pain, positive evidence must be sought. Many patients with primary headache syndromes have been subjected to numerous dental or surgical procedures because of where their pain was located, not because of truly local disease.

PERSISTENT IDIOPATHIC FACIAL PAIN

"Persistent idiopathic facial pain" is the term used by the ICHD-II to replace the outdated term "atypical facial pain,"[42] and refers to facial pain that does not meet diagnostic criteria for neuralgias. ICHD-II defines it as facial pain present for all or most of the day, poorly localized, not associated with sensory loss nor other physical signs, and no abnormality found on imaging. It is said to often begin unilaterally near the nasolabial fold or chin, but it may spread. Patients, usually women, present with unremitting facial pain, usually unilateral at onset, sometimes spreading bilaterally. The neurologic examination is, by definition, normal.

In some cases of persistent idiopathic facial pain, serious underlying pathology may not declare itself initially.[43] For example, nasopharyngeal carcinoma and other cancers have eventually been implicated in some cases. Only when a neurologic deficit appears (e.g., cranial nerve palsies) may the real diagnosis become evident. Lung cancer has been another reported cause (due to referred pain presumably via CN X).[44] Occult dental pathology, such as infected cavities of maxillary and mandibular bones at the sites of previous extractions, is another consideration. Dental evaluation with injection of anesthetic followed, when effective, by curettage and antibiotics has cured some sufferers.[45]

Many cases have been labeled psychogenic. This may be appropriate if there is evidence for somatization disorder, conversion disorder, or somatic delusions, but "psychogenic" is probably an overused label. Certainly, many patients have concomitant depression, which should be addressed.

All patients presenting with idiopathic facial pain require a careful history and examination. Dental consultation to rule out occult pathology is important. An MRI scan of the head, with attention to the base of the brain, is indicated. A chest x-ray, perhaps with a chest CT scan, may help rule out lung cancer, especially in smokers. Serial examinations may be required as the clinician looks for an occult process to declare itself.

The treatment of idiopathic facial pain is extremely challenging. Burning pain may respond to stellate ganglion blocks. Heterocyclic antidepressants may lessen pain as well as help coexistent depression. Behavioral medicine measures, such as biofeedback and cognitive behavioral therapy, may be tried.

(Clearly, "idiopathic facial pain" is a more appropriate designation than "psychogenic" or "atypical." A multidisciplinary approach to both diagnosis and treatment yields the best results.)

OTHER FACIAL PAIN

PRIMARY (FACIAL) HEADACHE

It should be remembered that migraine, cluster headache, and other so-called headaches (such as chronic paroxysmal hemicrania) may present mainly in the face. Many patients diagnosed with "sinus headaches" are, in fact, migraineurs. Careful attention to details of the history and examination should clarify the diagnosis. Patient reports revealing a family history, trigger factors, or the presence of an aura point toward migraine as the etiology.

Likewise, cluster headache and other short-lasting headaches may present with pain mainly in the face rather than peri- or retro-orbitally. The clarification of the duration of the episodes, plus associated autonomic features (ptosis, rhinorrhea, lacrimation), is diagnostically helpful.

JABS AND JOLTS

This head pain syndrome has many names; the International Headache Society terms it *primary stabbing headache* unless there is a secondary/underlying cause. Other authors refer to it as ice-pick headache. This is a primary headache syndrome with paroxysmal pain lasting up to 10 seconds, but usually less than 2 seconds. Like trigeminal neuralgia, it may occur in volleys.[46] Pain is generally multifocal and can involve the face as well as the head, with the orbital region most commonly affected. The frequency of these sudden brief pains is quite variable—from rare isolated jolts to 50 or more per day.

These pains may occur as a separate, primary head pain condition or in association with other disorders, including migraine, giant cell arteritis, cluster headache, chronic paroxysmal hemicrania, or even tension-type headache. The differential diagnosis of jabs and jolts syndrome includes SUNCT/SUNA (see following section) and trigeminal neuralgia. Jabs and jolts syndrome usually responds to treatment with indomethacin. Trigeminal neuralgia often has trigger points and responds much more readily to carbamazepine or other appropriate therapies (see Table 35-2).

SUNCT/SUNA

Short-lasting unilateral neuralgiform headache with conjunctival injection and tearing (SUNCT), and SUNA (the "A" stands for autonomic symptoms)

TABLE 35-4 Short-Lasting Unilateral Neuralgiform Headache Attacks with Conjunctival Injection and Tearing (SUNCT)

International Classification of Headache Disorders, 1st revision (ICHD-II)
Diagnostic criteria:
A. At least 20 attacks fulfilling criteria B, C, and D.
B. Attacks of unilateral orbital, supraorbital, or temporal stabbing or pulsating pain lasting 5 to 240 seconds.
C. Pain is accompanied by ipsilateral conjunctival injection and lacrimation.
D. Attacks occur with a frequency from 3 to 200 per day.
E. Not attributed to another disorder.

TABLE 35-5 Short-Lasting Unilateral Neuralgiform Headache Attacks with Cranial Autonomic Symptoms (SUNA)

International Classification of Headache Disorders, 1st revision (ICHD-II)—Appendix
Diagnostic criteria:
A. At least 20 attacks fulfilling criteria B through E.
B. Attacks of unilateral orbital, supraorbital or temporal stabbing or pulsating pain lasting from 2 seconds to 10 minutes.
C. Pain is accompanied by one of:
1. Conjunctival injection and/or lacrimation.
2. Nasal congestion and/or rhinorrhoea.
3. Eyelid oedema.
D. Attacks occur with a frequency of ≥1 per day for more than half of the time.
E. No refractory period follows attacks triggered from trigger areas.
F. Not attributed to another disorder.

are rare syndromes. SUNA is not yet fully validated in ICHD-II, so it is found in the Appendix of that publication[47] (**Tables 35-4** and **35-5**). The brief pain (usually 15 to 120 seconds in duration) is typically near the eye but may occur in the temple or face. Multiple (up to 100) episodes occur daily, sometimes with other autonomic associations (ptosis, rhinorrhea).

The pain is almost always unilateral and is far more common in men. Neck movements trigger the pain in some patients. There are primary and secondary (symptomatic) forms.[48] Secondary causes of SUNCT include cerebellopontine angle lesions. Clinical similarities with trigeminal neuralgia and cluster-tic syndrome are apparent. Because secondary trigeminal neuralgia and SUNCT can be caused by cerebellopontine angle arteriovenous malformations, it may be that microvascular decompression could alleviate other SUNCT cases. MRI is indicated in the evaluation of SUNCT. Medical treatment is difficult but lamotrigine may be the most effective therapy. Topiaramate, gabapentine, and intravenous lidocaine have also been utilized.[49]

SUMMARY

Patients presenting with facial pain are often challenging, diagnostically as well as therapeutically. The number of pain-sensitive structures in the face is impressive, and many different entities share similar presenting symptoms. However, close attention to the fundamentals of thorough history taking and examination maximize diagnostic accuracy, the foundation upon which rational treatment rests.

REFERENCES

1. Kateric S, Williams DB, Beard CM, et al. Epidemiology and clinical features of idiopathic trigeminal neuralgia and glossopharyngeal neuralgia: similarities and differences. *Neuroepidemiology*. 1991;10: 276-281.
2. Gass A, Kitchen N, MacManus DG, et al. Trigeminal neuralgia in patients with multiple sclerosis: lesion localization with magnetic resonance imaging. *Neurology*. 1997;49:1142-1144.

3. Cheng TM, Cascino TL, Onofrio BM. Comprehensive study of diagnosis and treatment of trigeminal neuralgia secondary tumors. *Neurology*. 1993;43:2298-2302.
4. Linskey ME, Jho HD, Janetta PJ. Microvascular decompression for trigeminal neuralgia caused by vertebrobasilar compression. *J Neurosurg*. 1994;81:1-9.
5. Fromm GH, Graff-Radford SB, Terrence CF, et al. Pre-trigeminal neuralgia. *Neurology*. 1990;40:1493-1495.
6. Fromm GH, Terrence CF, Maroon JC. Trigeminal neuralgia: current concepts regarding etiology and pathogenesis. *Arch Neurol*. 1984;41:1204-1207.
7. Gronseth G, Cruccu J, Alksne C, et al. Practice parameter: the diagnostic evaluation and treatment of trigeminal neuralgia (an evidence-based review): report of the Quality Standards Subcommittee of the American Academy of Neurology and the European Federation of Neurological Societies. *Neurology*. 2008;71:1183-1190.
8. Cruccu G, Bonamico LH, Zakrzewska JM. Cranial neuralgias. *Handbook of Clinical Neurology*. 2011;97:Chapter 56, 663-678.
9. Reder AT, Arnason BG. Trigeminal neuralgia in multiple sclerosis relieved by a prostaglandin E analogue. *Neurology*. 1995;45:1097-1100.
10. Khan OA. Gabapentin relieves trigeminal neuralgia in multiple sclerosis patients. *Neurology*. 1998;51:611-614.
11. Lunardi G, Leandri M, Albano C, et al. Clinical effectiveness of lamotrigine and plasma levels in essential and symptomatic trigeminal neuralgia. *Neurology*. 1997;48:1714-1717.
12. Raskin NH. *Headache*. 2nd ed. New York, NY: Churchill Livingstone; 1988:343-344.
13. Janetta PJ. Microsurgical management of trigeminal neuralgia. *Arch Neurol*. 1985;42:800.
14. Young RF, Vermeulen SS, Grimm P, et al. Gamma knife radio surgery for treatment of trigeminal neuralgia: idiopathic and tumor related. *Neurology*. 1997;48:603-614.
15. Tenser RB. Trigeminal neuralgia: mechanisms of treatment. *Neurology*. 1998;51:17-19.
16. Watson P, Evans R. Cluster-tic syndrome. *Headache*. 1985;25:123-126.
17. Bussone G, Leone M, Volta GD, et al. Short-lasting unilateral neuralgiform headache attacks with tearing and conjunctival injection: the first symptomatic case. *Cephalalgia*. 1991;11:123-127.
18. Ochoa JJ, Alberca R, Canadillar F, et al. Cluster-tic syndrome and basilar artery ectasia: a case report. *Headache*. 1993;33:512-513.
19. Gaul, C, Hastreiter P, Duncker A, Naraghi R. Diagnosis and neurosurgical treatment of glossopharyngeal neauralgia: clinical findings and 3-D visualization of neurovascular compression in 19 cases. *J headache Pain*. 2011;12:527-534.
20. Bohm E, Strang RR. Glossopharyngeal neuralgia. *Brain*. 1962; 85:371-388.
21. Rushton JG, Stevens JC, Miller RH. Glossopharyngeal (vasoglossopharyngeal) neuralgia. *Arch Neurol*. 1981;38:201-205.
22. Kim SH, Han KR, Kim DW, et al. Severe pain attack associated with neurocardiogenic syncope induced by glossopharyngeal neuralgia: successful treatment with carbamazepine and a permanent pacemaker. *Korean J Pain*. 2010;23(3):215-218.
23. Bryun GW. Glossopharyngeal neuralgia. In: Vinken PJ, Gruyn GW, Klawans HL, eds. *Handbook of Clinical Neurology*. Amsterdam, Holland: Elsevier; 1985:459-473.
24. Isbir CA. Treatment of a patient with glossopharyngeal neuralgia by the Anterior Tonsillar Pillar Method. *Case Rep Neurol*. 2011;3:27-31.
25. Kandan SR, Khan S, Jeyaretna DS, et al. Neuralgia of the glossopharyngeal and vagal nerves: long-term outcome following surgical treatment and literature review. *Brit Jour Neurosurg*. 2010;24(4): 441-446.
26. Bruyn GW. Superior laryngeal neuralgia. *Cephalalgia*. 1983;3:235-240.
27. Kost RG, Straus SE. Postherpetic neuralgia-pathogenesis, treatment, and prevention. *N Engl J Med*. 1996;335:32-42.
28. Nurmikko T. Clinical features and pathophysiologic mechanisms of postherpetic neuralgia. *Neurology*. 1995;45(Suppl):554-555.
29. Watson CP. The treatment of postherpetic neuralgia. *Neurology*. 1995;45(Suppl):558-560.
30. Watson CPN, Vernick L, Chipman M, et al. Nortriptyline versus amitriptyline in postherpetic neuralgia. *Neurology*. 1998;51:1166-1171.
31. Gilron I, Bailey JM, Tu D, Holden RR, Jackson AC, Houlden RL. Nortriptyline and gabapentin, alone and in combination for neuropathic pain: a double-blind, randomised controlled crossover trial. *Lancet*. Oct 10 2009;374(9697):1252-1261.
32. Mokri B. Raeder's paratrigeminal syndrome: original concept and subsequent deviations. *Arch Neurol*. 1982;39:395-399.
33. Bruyn G. Sphenopalatine neuralgia (Slyder). In: Vinken PJ, Bruyn GW, Klawanus HC, Rose FC, eds. *Handbook of Clinical Neurology*. Amsterdam, Holland: Elsevier; 1986:475-482.
34. Bruyn GW. Nervus intermedius neuralgia (Hunt). *Cephalalgia*. 1984;4:71-78.
35. Raskin NH. *Headache*. 2nd ed. New York, NY: Churchill Livingstone; 1988:353-357.
36. Ganesan V, Kirkham FJ. Carotid dissection causing stroke in a child with migraine. *BMJ*. 1997;314:291-292.
37. Mokri B, Sundt TM, Houser W, et al. Spontaneous dissection of the cervical internal carotid artery. *Ann Neurol*. 1986;19:126-138.
38. Nguyen BL, Grant-Zawadzki M, Verghese P, et al. Magnetic resonance angiography of cervicocranial dissection. *Stroke*. 1993;24:126-131.
39. Sturzenegger M, Mattle HP, Rivoir A, et al. Ultrasound findings in carotid artery dissection: analysis of 43 patients. *Neurology*. 1995;45:691-698.
40. Jaeger B, Singer E, Kroening R. Reflex sympathetic dystrophy of the face: report of two cases and a review of the literature. *Arch Neurol*. 1986;43:693-695.
41. Headache Classification Committee of the International Headache Society 2004. The International Classification of Headache Disorders: 2nd ed. *Cephalalgia*. 24(Suppl 1):146.
42. Headache Classification Committee of the International Headache Society 2004. The International Classification of Headache Disorders: 2nd ed. *Cephalalgia*. 24(Suppl 1):133.
43. Raskin NH. *Headache*. 2nd ed. New York, NY: Churchill Livingstone; 1998:366-367.
44. Copobianco DJ. Facial pain as a symptom of nonmetastatic lung cancer. *Headache*. 1995;35:581-585.
45. Ratner EJ, Person P, Kleinman DJ, et al. Jawbone cavities and trigeminal and atypical facial neuralgias. *Oral Surg*. 1979;48:3-20.
46. Pareja JA, Ruiz J, de Isla C, et al. Idiopathic stabbing headache (jabs and jolts syndrome). *Cephalalgia*. 1996;16:93-96.
47. Headache Classification Committee of the International Headache Society 2004. The International Classification of Headache Disorders: 2nd ed. *Cephalalgia*. 24(Suppl 1):141-142.
48. Pareja JA, Sjaastad O. SUNCT syndrome: a clinical review. *Headache*. 1997;37:195-202.
49. Silberstein SD, Lipton RB, Dodick DW, eds. *Wolff's Headache and Other Head Pain*. 8th ed. New York, NY: Oxford University Press; 2008:413-416.

CHAPTER 36

Temporomandibular Disorders

Noshir R. Mehta
Steven J. Scrivani

INTRODUCTION

Pain syndromes that involve the face are very common in clinical practice. Many facial pain syndromes are also unique, given the complex anatomy and specialized sensory innervation of the head, face, and neck. These syndromes represent a clinical diagnostic challenge and deserve special attention. The common descriptive terms for facial pain complaints are frequently misleading. To avoid confusion, pain clinicians should be familiar with the International Headache Society's Diagnostic Classification for Head, Face, and Neck Pain Disorders[1] (**Table 36-1**). Clinicians should be comfortable distinguishing painful conditions that arise from structural pathology, headache syndromes, oral and facial structures, temporomandibular joint disorders, myofascial pain disorders, and primary cranial neuralgias.

Temporomandibular disorders are defined as a subgroup of craniofacial pain problems that involve the temporomandibular joint (TMJ), masticatory muscles, and associated head and neck musculoskeletal structures.[2] Patients with temporomandibular disorders most frequently present with complaints of pain, limited or asymmetric mandibular motion, and TMJ sounds.[3,4] The pain or discomfort is often localized to the jaw, TMJ, and muscles of mastication. Common associated symptoms include ear pain and stuffiness, tinnitus, dizziness, neck pain, and headache. In some cases, the onset is acute and symptoms are mild and self-limiting. Other patients develop a chronic temporomandibular disorder with persistent pain in association with physical, behavioral, psychological, and psychosocial symptoms similar to those of patients with chronic pain syndromes in other areas of the body[5-7] (e.g., arthritis, low back pain, chronic headache, fibromyalgia, and chronic regional pain syndrome), all requiring a coordinated interdisciplinary diagnostic and treatment approach.

Temporomandibular disorders are classified as one subtype of secondary headache disorder by the International Headache Society (IHS), Classification of Headache Disorders II (2004).[1] The American Academy of Orofacial Pain has expanded upon this IHS classification, as shown in **Tables 36-2** and **36-3**.[2]

TABLE 36-1 International Headache Society: International Classification of Headache Disorders II, *Cephalalgia*, 2004

14 CATEGORIES
• The Primary Headaches: 1–4
• The Secondary Headaches: 5–12
• Cranial Neuralgias (central and primary facial pain and other headache disorders): 13–14
The Primary Headaches (1–4)
1. Migraine
Without aura
With aura
2. Tension-type headache
3. Cluster headache and other trigeminal autonomic cephalalgias
4. Other primary headaches
The Secondary Headaches (5–12)
5. Attributed to head and/or neck trauma
6. Attributed to cranial or cervical vascular disorder
7. Attributed to nonvascular intracranial disorder
8. Attributed to a substance or its withdrawal
9. Attributed to infection
10. Attributed to disorder of homeostasis
11. HA or facial pain attributed to disorder of cranium, neck, eyes, ears, nose, sinuses, teeth, mouth, or other facial or cranial structures
12. Attributed to psychiatric disorder
Headache or facial pain attributed to disorders of cranium, neck, eyes, ears, nose, sinuses, teeth, mouth or other facial or cranial structures (11.1–11.8)
11.1 Cranial bones
11.2 Neck
11.3 Eyes
11.4 Ears
11.5 Rhinosinusitis (sinus disorders)
11.6 Teeth, jaws or related structures
11.7 TMJ disorders (TMD)
11.8 Other
Cranial Neuralgias (central and primary facial pain and other headache disorders) (13–14)

TABLE 36-2 Temporomandibular Joint Articular Disorders

- Congenital or developmental
  - Aplasia
  - Hypoplasia
  - Hyperplasia
  - Neoplasia
- Disc derangement disorders
  - Disc displacement with reduction
  - Disc displacement without reduction
- Temporomandibular joint dislocation
- Inflammatory disorders
  - Capsulitis/synovitis
  - Polyarthridites
- Osteoarthritis (noninflammatory)
  - Primary osteoarthritis
  - Secondary osteoarthritis
- Ankylosis
- Fracture

TABLE 36-3 Masticatory Muscle Disorders

11.7.2.1	Local myalgia
11.7.2.2	Myofascial pain
11.7.2.3	Centrally mediated myalgia
11.7.2.4	Myospasm
11.7.2.5	Myositis
11.7.2.6	Myofibrotic contracture
11.7.2.7	Neoplasia

TMD: A TRIAD OF DYSFUNCTIONS

There are at least three distinct and separate dysfunctions that create or affect the symptoms described by the TMD patient.[8] These are as follows:

I. Muscle disorder (myofascial pain dysfunction, MPD)

   MPD is related to muscle dysfunction, often leading to muscle spasms, pain, and dysfunction. This type of dysfunction can occur in any skeletal muscle. The triggering area lies in the fascial coverings and attachment zones of the muscles—thus the term *myofascial*. This syndrome is sometimes incorrectly referred to as myofascial pain dysfunction.

II. Temporomandibular joint articular disorder (TMJD)

   TMJD is related to specific problems in the temporomandibular joints. These problems may range from joint sounds to locking, pain, and degenerative changes of the joints themselves. Invariably, muscle dysfunction is a secondary effect of true TMJD.

III. Cervical spinal dysfunction (CSD)

This syndrome is related to the spinal column, the vertebrae, the ligaments, and the muscles related to them. The majority of symptoms not directly related to the jaw muscles are triggered or affected by the CSD syndrome.

The prevalence among adults in the United States of at least one sign of temporomandibular disorders is reported as 40% to 75%, and those with at least one symptom, as 33%.[7,9,10] TMJ sounds and deviation on opening the jaw occur in approximately 50% of otherwise asymptomatic persons and are considered within the range of normal and do not require treatment.[10] Other signs, such as decreased mouth opening and occlusal changes, occur in fewer than 5% of the general population.[11] Temporomandibular disorders are most commonly reported in young to middle-aged adults (age 20–50). The female-to-male ratio of patients seeking care has been reported to be from 3:1 to as high as 9:1.[10,12] Despite the high prevalence of temporomandibular disorders, signs and symptoms, only 5% to 10% of symptomatic people require treatment, given the wide spectrum of symptoms and the fact that the natural history of this disorder suggests that many patients (up to 40%) undergo spontaneous resolution of their symptoms.[7,13]

ETIOLOGY

In 1934, Costen, an otolaryngologist, evaluated 13 patients who presented with pain in or near the ear, tinnitus, dizziness, a sensation of ear fullness, and difficulty swallowing.[14] He observed that these patients had many missing teeth, and, as a result, their mandibles were overclosed. The patients seemed to improve when their missing teeth were replaced and the proper vertical dimension of the occlusion was restored. The malocclusion and improper jaw position was perceived to be the cause both of "disturbed function of the temporomandibular joint" and the associated facial pain. Thereafter, the emphasis of treatment was on altering the affected patient's occlusion.

More recently, advances in the understanding of joint biomechanics, neuromuscular physiology, autoimmune and musculoskeletal disorders, and pain mechanisms have resulted in changing concepts of the etiology of temporomandibular disorders. These disorders are now considered multifactorial in etiology, with biologic, behavioral, environmental, social, emotional, and cognitive factors alone or in combination contributing to the development of signs and symptoms of temporomandibular disorders.[2,15]

Various forms of trauma to the TMJ structures (ligaments, articular cartilage, articular disc, bone) can lead to intraarticular biochemical alterations that have been demonstrated to produce oxidative stress and the generation of free radicals. Subsequent inflammatory changes in synovial fluid with the production of a variety of proinflammatory cytokines can then lead to alteration in the functioning of normal tissues and degenerative disease in the TMJ.[16-20]

Genetic marker studies involving catecholamine metabolism and adrenergic receptors suggest that certain gene polymorphisms (e.g., in the catechol-O-methyl transferase [COMT] gene) might be associated with changes seen in pain responsiveness and pain processing in patients with chronic temporomandibular disorders.[21-23]

Differences in pain modulation have been reported between women and men with temporomandibular disorders; women have been observed to demonstrate decreased thresholds to noxious stimuli and more hyperalgesia. In addition, in women with temporomandibular disorders, some studies suggest that the affective component of pain may be enhanced during the low-estrogen phase of the menstrual cycle.[24-27]

Functional brain imaging studies demonstrating changes in cortical circuitry support the concept that temporomandibular disorders are very similar to other chronic pain disorders and may be related to abnormal pain processing in the trigeminal system.[28,29] In particular, muscle pain disorders appear to have little, if any, abnormality of the muscles or peripheral tissues and may represent a central sensitization pain producing process.

Lastly, numerous biobehavioral studies support a connection between chronic temporomandibular disorders and comorbid psychopathology (anxiety and depression disorders; posttraumatic stress disorder; and childhood physical, sexual, and psychological abuse).[29-36]

CLINICAL EVALUATION

Although temporomandibular disorders are a common cause of craniofacial pain, it is imperative for the health care provider to obtain a comprehensive history, perform a careful physical examination, and obtain appropriate diagnostic studies to exclude other potentially serious disorders. The differential diagnosis should include odontogenic (caries, periodontal disease) and nonodontogenic causes of facial pain, primary or metastatic jaw tumors, intracranial tumors and skull base tumors, disorders of other facial structures (including the salivary glands), primary and secondary headache syndromes, trigeminal neuropathic pain disorders, and systemic disease (cardiac, viral, autoimmune, diabetes, temporal arteritis).

The most common complaint of patients with temporomandibular disorders is unilateral facial pain. The pain may radiate into the ear, to the temporal and periorbital regions, to the angle of the mandible, and, frequently, to the posterior neck. The pain is usually reported as a dull, constant ache that is worse at certain times during the day. There can be bouts of more severe, sharp pain typically triggered by movements of the mandible. The pain may be present daily or intermittently, but many patients have pain-free intervals. Mandibular motion is usually limited, and attempts at active motion (chewing, talking, yawning) increase the pain. Patients frequently describe "locking" of the jaw, either in the closed-mouth position with inability to open (most common) or in the open-mouth position with inability to close the jaw. These complaints are often worse in the morning, particularly in patients who clench or grind their teeth during sleep. Clenching, grinding of the teeth, and other nonfunctional, involuntary mandibular compensatory movements (so-called oral parafunctional habits) are common.

Along with limitation of motion, there is often deviation to the affected side of the mandible on opening and a "clicking" or "popping" noise in the joint. While some of the preceding differential diagnoses can present with facial pain, temporomandibular disorders often have a stereotypical presentation (as described earlier), which helps in the diagnostic process. It is well appreciated that pain of cardiac origin (ischemia or myocardial infarction) may present with neck, jaw, and face pain, but cardiac pain is generally acute in nature with very different associated signs and symptoms.[37]

Other commonly associated symptoms of TMD are discussed in the following sections.

Headache Symptoms of bilateral head and face pain involve multiple postural muscles and/or the muscles of mastication. The pain is typically moderate in intensity, dull and aching in quality, and usually described as deep and constant.[38-42] Pain exacerbations are often provoked by functional use of the affected muscles. Morning headaches may be related to nocturnal bruxism and or sleep disorders,[43] while increasing pain during the day may be related to masticatory muscle use or head posture.[44]

A. **Front of Head**

Patients complaining of pain in the front of the head often refer to it as "sinus headache." There is usually accompanying pressure along the upper anterior teeth, bridge of the nose, and pressure behind the eyes. Chronic front-of-the-head pain and facial pain are generally not due to chronic sinus disease but are a primary headache disorder. This can also be due to a reduction in posterior occlusal dimension causing heavy incisal contact, resulting in pain of pressure in the anterior vortex of the face. A bandlike feeling of the front of the head can also be brought about by posterior neck muscle contractions or muscle tension of the frontalis muscle.

B. **Side of Head**

Temporal headaches are mainly related to muscle contraction and fiber spasm of the temporalis muscle. The temporalis muscle has three groups of muscle fibers: anterior, middle, and posterior. The anterior fibers function to bring the lower jaw up and forward, while the middle and posterior fibers swing the jaw to full closure and retract the mandible.

Clenching, grinding, or biting on objects while the jaw is in an anterior displaced position (edge-to-edge) generally creates pain in the anterior temporal group—that is, the patient has pain in the "temple" area. Individuals who work at desk jobs where the head is forward and down tend to clench and grind in this forward position due to gravity affecting the mandible. This would be further aggravated by habits such as pencil or pen biting, pipe smoking, or gum chewing.

Clenching or grinding during sleep or clenching in a posterior position tends to tire the middle and posterior group of fibers, and the pain is more posteriorly located. Generally, the temporalis is affected in any dysfunction of the lower jaw.

C. **Back of Head**

Deep dull pain, constant and aggravating in the back of the head, is usually a result of fiber spasms within the trapezius and sternocleidomastoid muscles. These muscles have strong large bodies that, when under tension, pull on their bony attachments to the sill—the occiput and mastoid areas. This leads to soreness in the bone and deep, dull pain radiating up the back of the head and down the neck. The muscle tension may be independent of, or secondarily related to, vertebral displacement in the cervical and upper thoracic region.

Face Pain Pain in the sides of the face, or pain described by the patient as "sinus" pain in the zygomatic or orbital area, may also have a musculoskeletal origin.[8] Clenching; acute or chronic stress; reduction of dental vertical dimension (height) related to loss of posterior teeth, combined with daytime tooth clenching; and acute or chronic stress can create muscle trigger points or muscle fatigue. This is particularly noticed by the patient after meals and is reported as "a heavy and tired feeling" in the jaw muscles. Face pain related to sinuses and other pathologies are discussed separately in this chapter.

Eye Pain Orbital pain symptoms are often described as unilateral and constant and "boring." This is frequently seen in patients with TMD complaints, which include pain symptoms involving the eye and periorbital region.[8,45-47] Patients with a history of trauma or chronic upper cervical vertebral subluxations or nerve root impingements related to the occiput and the atlantoaxial region may present with orbital symptoms. In addition, entrapment of the greater occipital nerve at the occiput level can also produce this type of pain, which is often diagnosed as occipital neuralgia. This is frequently amenable to physical medicine, along with changes in head posture and mandibular position through the use of dental bite appliances.

Ear Symptoms Pain, stuffiness, and tinnitus may have a musculoskeletal etiology.[48,49] Mandibular posture related to the maxilla affects the masticatory elevator muscles. The medial pterygoid muscles help stabilize the left-to-right balance of the mandible on tooth closure. Innervation from the nerve to the medial pterygoid also supplies the middle ear muscles. The tensor tympani and tensor palati are actually one muscle with a raphe that wraps around the hamulus notch of the maxilla. Growth and development problems related to the proper expansion of the maxilla can affect Eustachian tube function and have been known to precipitate middle ear infections in children as well as ear stuffiness with changes in pressure in the ear in adults. Maxillary and mandibular dysfunctions aid in the development and maintenance of such symptoms.

Tinnitus and other types of ear sounds may also have a peripheral musculoskeletal etiology. Specifically, cervical factors and mandibular postural factors have been seen in subjects with tinnitus. A combination of physical medicine and dental jaw appliance therapy has been effective in some cases where there has been a history of trauma or childhood growth and development affecting the proper expansion of the maxilla.

Ear pain that is sharp and jabbing upon movement of the mandible is frequently seen in patients who have an internal derangement of the temporomandibular joint. Usually, it presents unilaterally and ipsilateral to the joint in question.

Ear pain and symptoms such as stuffiness in the absence of positive otologic findings are among the most common reasons to evaluate the patient for dental and maxillo mandibular imbalance. Treatment can often alleviate the symptoms completely or reduce the impact on the patient in conjunction with standard medical intervention.[50-54]

Neck Pain Neck stiffness and pain are commonly part of the TMD complex.[55-57] Trauma, habitual posturing, and musculoskeletal tension will chronically affect the cervical area, creating pain, stiffness, and trigger point flare-up in the muscles of the head and neck. It is well documented that the trigeminal and cervical nerve systems are interactive in the maintenance of head neck and jaw posture.[58] The act of mastication and jaw function relies on all the anterior and posterior cervical muscles to interact with the jaw closing and opening muscles. In addition, mandibular and head posture interacts to maintain the airway space during function and in sleep.

Studies on the relationship between the maxillo-mandibular position and the cervical spine have shown that loss of vertical dimension of the teeth and a deep bite can adversely affect cervical muscle function, leading to chronic stiffness, pain, and reduction of range of motion.[59] It is, therefore, important to assess the dental factors in patients with chronic neck pain.

Arm and Back Symptoms Patients presenting with TMD may also commonly present with shoulder pain or pain radiating down the arm that may or may not be accompanied by tingling and/or numbness. Physical medicine assessments frequently are positive for thoracic outlet syndrome, costoclavicular syndrome, vertebral subluxations or nerve impingement of the brachial plexus of nerves, and even rotator cuff injuries previously undiagnosed.[60]

Physical examination should include observation and measurement of mandibular motion (maximal interincisal opening, lateral movements, and protrusion), palpation of the muscles of mastication (masseter, temporalis, medial and lateral pterygoids) and the cervical musculature, and palpation and/or auscultation of the TMJ, as well as examination of the oral cavity, dentition, occlusion and salivary glands, and inspection and palpation of the anterior and posterior neck. Auscultation of the carotids and examination of the cranial nerves, with special attention to the trigeminal system, should also be part of the physical examination.

As already noted, noise in the TMJ on mandibular movement is frequently present in patients with temporomandibular disorders. However, noise alone is also a very common finding in completely asymptomatic people and may represent a range of normal rather than intraarticular pathology. Muscle tenderness, producing pain or discomfort, is generally found on both extraoral and intraoral palpation of the masticatory muscles. Tenderness may also be present in the anterior neck muscles (suprahyoid muscles and sternocleidomastoid muscles), posterior cervical paraspinal muscles (semispinalis capitus, splenius capitus, and suboccipital muscles), and upper shoulder muscles (trapezius and levator scapulae). There may be mandibular hypomobility and deviation on opening. Finally, the neurological examination is typically normal, without any objective neurosensory or motor deficits of the trigeminal nerve or other focal cranial nerve abnormalities.

Diagnostic studies are designed to rule out other disorders and may include blood and serum inflammatory markers (to rule out autoimmune disorders and vasculitides), imaging, diagnostic nerve blocks, muscle trigger point injections, and dental models for maxillomandibular analysis.

The most important diagnostic advances during the past 30 years have occurred in imaging techniques for the TMJ. The panoramic radiograph (a single-cut tomogram of the entire jaw) remains the most useful screening tool. Plain radiographs have been almost completely replaced by computerized tomography (CT) for evaluation of bony morphology and pathology of the joint, mandibular ramus, and condyle. Cone beam maxillofacial CT is a newer and faster technique, with a lower radiation dose, than that of conventional, whole-body CT scans.[61] This technique provides thin slice images in the axial, coronal, and sagittal planes that can be modified with an interactive viewing program to study all details of the maxillofacial skeleton. There is also a three-dimensional program for analysis prior to potential surgical procedures. CT images provide fine, three-dimensional, anatomic detail of the TMJ and surrounding skeleton.

Magnetic resonance imaging (MRI) has replaced other imaging modalities for evaluation of soft-tissue abnormalities of the joint and surrounding region. The anatomy of the joint and the position and structure of the intraarticular disc may be accurately visualized both at rest and in motion. The blood supply and vascularity of the condyle can be analyzed on the MRI, and pathologic accumulations of fluid within and around the joint may be detected. Continuous cine-MRI allows evaluation of the joint structures during mandibular movement. In addition, investigators have demonstrated that in intraarticular disc derangement disorders, there is poor correlation between signs and symptoms and displacement of the articular disk based on solely imaging studies alone.[62]

Skeletal scintigraphy is useful for evaluating developmental or growth abnormalities of the mandible but is not particularly helpful for diagnosis of temporomandibular disorders.[63-66]

Diagnostic arthroscopy is a minimally invasive surgical technique that allows direct visualization of the anatomy of the TMJ. Patients who have had nonsurgical therapies for 3 to 6 months and continue to have persistent pain in the joint, decreased range of mandibular movement, and interference with normal daily activities (talking, chewing) may benefit from diagnostic and/or therapeutic arthroscopy.[67-71] Synovitis, adhesions, cartilage degeneration, cartilage tears, loose bodies, disc degeneration, perforations, and capsular attachment tears can all be documented using arthroscopy.[67,68] Therapeutic surgical arthroscopy of the TMJ (like other joints) can eliminate cartilage and bony pathology, correct articular disc and ligament abnormalities, and remove true joint pathology (synovial chondromatosis, osteoarthritis).

Despite the improvements in diagnostic techniques and new insights into the pathology of the temporomandibular joint, the specific pathophysiology of temporomandibular disorders is not completely understood.

MANAGEMENT

Currently, management of temporomandibular disorders consists of a combination of home self-care, counseling, physiotherapy, pharmacotherapy, jaw appliance therapy, physical medicine, behavioral medicine, and surgery (**Table 36-4**). Surgery is performed only to treat structural anatomic pathology that is producing pain and dysfunction. Surgical procedures include arthrocentesis, arthroscopy, open arthrotomy, and combined joint and reconstructive jaw procedures.

The vast majority of temporomandibular disorders (approximately 85%–90%), whether articular or muscular, can be treated by noninvasive, nonsurgical, and reversible interventions.[2,70,71] For patients with intraarticular disorders that do not respond to a reasonable course of nonsurgical interventions, generally 3 to 6 months in length, surgical therapy may be considered if the pain is substantial and the limitation of function severe enough to interfere with activities of daily living.

COMMON CLINICAL DISORDERS

MYOFASCIAL PAIN DISORDER

Myofascial pain disorder of the masticatory muscle system is the most common of all temporomandibular disorders. The vast majority of patients present with facial pain, limitation of jaw motion, muscle tenderness, and stiffness, along with any number of associated complaints in the head, face, and neck region (described earlier). Imaging studies of the TMJs most commonly show no evidence of anatomic pathology.

Patients with myofascial pain disorder generally will respond to simple, noninvasive treatments that are described next.

Reassurance/Counseling It is important that the patient be counseled on the natural history and course of temporomandibular disorders, the role of stress and parafunctional habits such as clenching and grinding of the teeth, frequency of the problem in the population, and self-limiting nature of the disorder. As a health care professional, it is

TABLE 36-4 Temporomandibular Disorders

Diagnosis	TMJ Articular Disorders	Muscle Disorders	Myofascial Disorders
Diagnostic features	Pain localized in the pre-auricular area during jaw function. Usually presence of painful click or crepitus during mouth opening. Limited opening (<35 mm), deviated or painful jaw movements.	Tenderness of the masticatory muscles. Dull, aching pain exacerbated by jaw function or palpation.	Diffused dull or aching pain affecting multiple groups of muscles of the head and neck region, as well as other parts of the body.
Diagnostic evaluation	Internal derangement of the TMJ with abnormal function of the disc-condyle complex, and/or degeneration of the joint surface. Palpation is painful. Possible joint swelling in acute phases. MRI, CT, etc. of the joint may rule out tumors and advanced degenerative stages.	Tenderness during palpation of the masticatory muscles and tendons. Possible limited range of jaw movement and during passive stretching exam. Can be associated with a para-functional habit (bruxism-early morning pain).	Presence of trigger or tender points in one or more groups of muscles. Pain can radiate to distant areas with stimulation or not of the trigger points. Rule out presence of lupus erythematosus.
Treatment	Patient education and self-care Medication: NSAID, nonopiate analgesics. Physical Therapy: excersise program. Occlusal splints Oral maxillofacial surgery: arthrocentesis, arthroscopic surgery, open surgery.	Patient education and self-care. Medication: topical and systemic NSAIDs., nonopiate analgesics, muscle-relaxants, antideppressants (usually TCAs), anxiolytics, anticonvulsants, BTX, trigger point injections, and vapoicoolant spray. Physical therapy: TENS, massage, exercise program. Occlusal splints Cognitive-behavior: biofeedback, relaxation, coping skills.	Same as muscle disorders

important to let the patient know that both the physical and emotional suffering associated with temporomandibular disorders is understood.

Rest Although it is not prudent to immobilize the mandible, the patient should be instructed to avoid extremes of mechanical movements (yawning, laughing, jaw clenching). Certain habits that may affect jaw function, such as chewing gum, and biting fingernails or pencils should be eliminated.

Heat The application of heat to the sides of the face by means of a heating pad, hot towel, or hot water bottle will be comforting and will help to relieve muscle pain. More vigorous treatment may be achieved with ultrasound or short-wave diathermy heat treatments, which are widely available in physical therapy offices.[72,73]

Medications Nonsteroidal anti-inflammatory agents are often of value in the acute stage.[74-78] Initial treatment is usually administered for 10 to 14 days, at which time the patient should be reevaluated. Muscle relaxants are frequently used for acute episodes of pain but have not been proven efficacious in chronic conditions.[74,79,80] Chronic opioid analgesic use should be avoided, if at all possible.[74,78] Antidepressants have a long history of effectiveness for the treatment of chronic pain. Their use is often justified, especially when the pain and dysfunction is part of the complex of generalized muscle pain with signs and symptoms of depression.[81-87] Tricyclic antidepressants are the most widely used, and a bedtime-only schedule of 10–50 mg of nortriptyline, desiprimine, or doxepin can be expected to alleviate symptoms in 2 to 4 weeks.[81] Treatment, if successful, is maintained for 2 to 4 months and then tapered to a low maintenance dose. Recently, serotonin selective reuptake inhibitors (SSRIs) have also been employed as part of the treatment regimen.[74,78] However, some of these agents (fluoxetine and paroxetine) have now been implicated in producing increased masticatory muscle activity (bruxism), especially during sleep, and are generally not recommended.[88-91] The tricyclic antidepressants and some of the newer selective norepinephrine reuptake inhibitor antidepressants (e.g., duloxetine) can be recommended and show some efficacy. Anxiolytic agents, such as the benzodiazepines, are also commonly used.[74,78-80,92] Short-term use (a few weeks) of the long-acting benzodiazepines in low dose, typically at night are recommended (diazepam, 2.5–5 mg; clonazepam, 0.5 mg). It is important that benzodiazepine use be limited and patients followed frequently because of the potential for dependency.

Jaw Appliance Therapy Many types of intraoral occlusal orthotic appliances exist for the treatment of temporomandibular disorders, and their multiplicity suggests that the optimum design has yet to be discovered. These devices are worn on the teeth like a "retainer" or a removable denture and are usually made of processed, hard acrylic. They are designed to improve TMJ function by altering joint mechanics and increasing potential mobility, to improve the function of the masticatory motor system while reducing abnormal muscle function, and to protect the teeth from jaw clenching and potential tooth fracture or attrition. It has been hypothesized that these devices may make patients more conscious of their oral parafunctional habits, altering proprioceptive input and central motor system areas that initiate and regulate masticatory function ("oral central pattern generator").[93-95]

The most common appliance is one that is custom-made of hard acrylic and that fits over all the teeth in the dental arch (either upper or lower). The patient's dentist should be able to construct and supervise the use of such an appliance. Due to the difficulty in controlling for a study utilizing any type of appliance that is placed in the mouth, there have been few good randomized, controlled, and blinded studies of the long-term efficacy of these oral orthotic appliances.[96] In a recent Cochrane database review (2004), it was reported that there is insufficient evidence either for or against the use of oral appliance therapy.[97] However, with appropriate adjuvant therapies (as outlined earlier), these devices may play a role in alleviating the pain and dysfunction of temporomandibular disorders in 70% to 90% of patients.[97-100]

Malocclusion, loss of teeth, and tooth-to-tooth occlusal interferences as a primary cause of temporomandibular joint and muscle symptoms are not well supported by the evidence.[101-104] However, as a general principle, maxillomandibular tooth-to-tooth interferences and anterior–posterior jaw position discrepancies (a bad bite) should be eliminated and missing teeth replaced in an effort to achieve optimum dental occlusion and masticatory function. In addition, the long-term efficacy of repositioning adult, nongrowing jaws with occlusal splints or functional appliances has not been proven by the available data.

Behavioral Approaches Counseling, relaxation techniques, stress management, work pacing, guided-imaging, biofeedback, cognitive therapy, and other behavioral modalities have all been reported as helpful.[105-109] A 1996 National Institutes of Health Consensus Conference on Behavioral Medicine in the Management of Chronic Pain outlined techniques that are considered effective and the indications for using them.[110] The most important factor, however, is the therapeutic interaction (context effect) of the practitioner with the patient.

Physical Medicine Manual manipulation, massage, ultrasound, and iontophoresis are helpful in reconditioning and retraining the masticatory and the other craniocervical muscles that are usually involved in temporomandibular disorders.[111-115] Passive motion has also been reported as effective in rehabilitating some of the biochemical and biomechanical changes that occur in injured synovial joints, muscles, and periarticular tissues.[116,117] Several commercial jaw passive-motion devices (similar to those used for the knee) are currently in use for temporomandibular disorders.

Intraarticular Disc Derangement Disorder Disc derangement disorder is defined as a temporomandibular disorder resulting from displacement of the TMJ disk from its normal position or deformation of the disk. This may lead to synovitis, pain, and limitation of motion.[2] The diagnosis is confirmed by history, clinical examination, and MRI scan in the open- and closed-mouth positions. Diagnostic/therapeutic arthroscopy (as described earlier) may also be helpful in confirming the diagnosis and providing minimally invasive surgical manipulation, if necessary.[118,119]

Internal derangements may include anterior displacement of the disk with reduction and anterior displacement without reduction.[2] Anterior displacement with reduction is defined as disc displacement in the closed-mouth position that reduces (with a click) to the normal relationship at some time during opening. Reduction implies that, to some extent, the disc is gliding normally with opening and translational movement. In these circumstances, the patient complains of a click with a variable amount of pain on opening. Often, patients have no pain with this condition. The mandible deviates to the affected side on opening until the click occurs and then returns to the midline. This situation may worsen, and there may be intermittent locking of the disk.

Intermittent locking may progress over time to anterior disk displacement without reduction (closed lock).[2] This implies that the dislocated disk acts as a mechanical obstruction to opening and translation of the condyle. These patients have a marked decrease in mandibular opening on the affected side and with a variable amount of pain. They feel that there is a mechanical obstruction to opening in the joint. Maximal opening may be limited to 20 to 25 mm (normal range of maximal interincisal opening ranges from 35 to 55 mm with a mean of 40–43 mm) with restricted movement to the contralateral side. There may also be a prior history of clicking with intermittent locking. MRI demonstrates a displaced disc without reduction on opening (closed lock) and may also demonstrate degenerative changes in the condyle. In such cases, the signs and symptoms of degenerative joint disease may also be present.[120]

Initial treatment for internal derangement consists of the same noninvasive therapies used for myofascial pain dysfunction syndrome: behavioral medicine, occlusal appliances, heat, muscle relaxants, nonsteroidal anti-inflammatory agents, physical therapy, and so forth. These strategies are often successful for patients with an anteriorly displaced disk with reduction (intermittent locking). In contrast, patients with a closed lock, especially one that is long standing, will most often require interventions such as intraarticular injection with steroids, arthrocentesis, or arthroscopy.[121,122]

Osteoarthritis Osteoarthritis of the TMJ may result from trauma (acute or chronic), infection, metabolic disturbances, and previous joint surgery.[9] The patient complains of pain on moving the mandible, limited motion, and deviation of the jaw to the affected side. There may be acute tenderness to palpation of the joint. Joint sounds are described as grating, grinding, or crunching but not as clicking or popping. Imaging studies typically reveal degenerative changes and remodeling and a loss of joint space.[123]

The features of degenerative disease of the TMJ are different from those of most other joints in the body. There is a strong predilection for females in the third or fourth decade. Only a few patients have generalized osteoarthritis. The natural course of the disease suggests that the pain and limitation may "burn themselves out" after as little as several months in some patients.[2,119,120] The majority of patients can be kept comfortable until remission with the noninvasive techniques outlined previously. In the acute phase, patients may require intraarticular injection of a long-acting corticosteroid such as beclomethasone or hyaluronic acid.[121] Neither corticosteroids nor hyaluronic acid are recommended for long-term use and have equivocal data. These injection treatments are generally reserved for older patients and are limited to two or three injections separated by 4 to 6 weeks. In patients who are refractory to these techniques, surgery may be indicated to remove the loose fragments of bone (so-called joint mice) and reshape the condyle.

Rheumatoid Arthritis Adults and children with rheumatoid arthritis may exhibit involvement of the TMJ. Fifty percent of children with juvenile rheumatoid arthritis (JRA) present with TMJ pain, swelling, and/or limitation of motion.[124] There may be associated growth restriction of the jaw, resulting in micrognathia and ankylosis. Adults with long-standing rheumatoid arthritis may develop TMJ symptoms late in the course of the disease and may only complain when they have marked limitation of jaw motion. Other stigmata of rheumatoid arthritis will be evident. TMJ imaging varies, depending on the stage of the disease, but, ultimately, there is resorption of the condyle with shortening of the mandibular ramus-condyle unit and potential reduction of joint space and hypomobility. Medical management along with altering TMJ biomechanics with the same modalities listed earlier (physical medicine, jaw appliance, biobehavioral therapy) may be initially helpful. If medical management is not effective, surgical treatment may be necessary, similar to other joints in the body.

CONCLUSION

Temporomandibular disorders remain a frequent cause of visits to dental practitioners/specialists, primary care physicians, internists, and pediatricians. Some approaches to understanding the basic etiologies of these conditions may prove to be promising as much of the fundamental pathophysiology remains poorly understood. Substantial improvements have been made in our diagnostic and imaging capabilities, and some treatment advances have been helpful in the long-term management of these common disorders. Future directions in the field of genetics, pain research, and arthritis offer the possibility of better defining this heterogeneous group of disorders and providing more focused and effective treatment strategies.

REFERENCES

1. Oleson J. The International Classification of Headache Disorders. *Cephalalgia*. 24(Suppl 7), Blackwell Publishing; 2004.
2. de Leeuw R. *Orofacial Pain: Guiedelines for Assessment, Diagnosis and Management*. 4th ed. Quintessence Publishing, Co., 2008.
3. Okeson JP. *Bell's Orofacial Pains: The Clinical Management of Orofacial Pains*. 6th ed. Chicago, Ill: Quintessence; 2004.
4. Dworkin SF, Burgess JA. Orofacial pain of psychogenic origin: current concepts and classification. *JADA*. 1987;115:265-571.
5. Fordyce WE. Pain and suffering: a reappraisal. *Am Psychol*. 1988;43: 276-283.
6. Parker MW, Holmes EK, Terezhalmy GT. Personality characteristics of patients with temporomandibular disorders: diagnostic and therapeutic implications. *J Orofac Pain*. 1993;7:337-334.
7. Solberg WK. Epidemiology, incidence and prevalence of temporomandibular disorders: a review. In: *The President's Conference on the Examination, Diagnosis and Management of Temporomandibular Disorders*. Chicago, Ill: American Dental Association; 1983:30-39.
8. Mehta NR, Forgione AG, Rosenbaum RS, Holmberg R. Temporomandibular disorders: a triad of dysfunctions. *J Mass Dental Soc*. 1984;33(4).
9. Schiffman E, Fricton JR. Epidemiology of TMJ and craniofacial pains. In: Fricton JR, Kroening RJ, Hathaway KM eds. *TMJ and Craniofacial Pain*. St. Louis, Mo: Ishiro Euro America; 1988:1-10.
10. Dworkin SF, Huggins KH, LeResche L, et al. Epidemiology of signs and symptoms of temporomandibular disorders: clinical signs in cases and controls. *JADA*. 1990;120:273-281.
11. Wabeke KB, Spruijt RJ. *On Temporomandibular Joint Sounds: Dental and Psychological Studies [Thesis]*. Amsterdam: University of Amsterdam; 1994:91-103.
12. Huber NU, Hall EH. A comparison of the signs of temporomandibular joint dysfunction and occlusal discrepancies in a symptom-free population of men and women. *Oral Surg Oral Med Oral Path Oral Rad and Endo*. 1990;70:180-183.
13. Levitt SR, McKinney MW. Validating the TMJ scale in a national sample of 10,000 patients: demographic and epidemiologic characteristics. *J Orofac Pain*. 1994;8:25-34.
14. Costen JB. A syndrome of ear and sinus symptoms dependent upon disturbed function of the temporomandibular joint. *Ann Otol Rhin Laryng*. 1934;43:1-15.
15. Laskin DM. Temporomandibular disorders: a term past its time? Guest editorial. *JADA*. 2008;139:124-128.
16. Milam SB, Zardeneta G, Schmitz JP. Oxidative stress and degenerative temporomandibular joint disease: a proposed hypothesis. *J Oral Maxillofac Surg*. 1998;56(2):214-223.
17. Milam SB, Schmitz JP. Molecular biology of temporomandibular joint disorders: proposed mechanisms of disease. *J Oral Maxillofac Surg*. 1995;53(12):1448-1454.
18. Zardeneta G, Milam SB, Schmitz JP. Presence of denatured hemoglobin deposits in diseased temporomandibular joints. *J Oral Maxillofac Surg*. 1997;55(11):1242-1248; discussion 1249.
19. Israel HA, Langevin CJ, Singer MD, Behrman DA. The relationship between temporomandibular joint synovitis and adhesions: pathogenic mechanisms and clinical implications for surgical management. *J Oral Maxillofac Surg*. 2006;64(7):1066-1074.
20. Ratcliffe A, Israel HA, Saed-Nejad F, Diamond B. Proteoglycans in the synovial fluid of the temporomandibular joint as an indicator of changes in cartilage metabolism during primary and secondary osteoarthritis. *J Oral Maxillofac Surg*. 1998;56(2):204-208.
21. Nackley AG, Tan KS, Fecho K, Flood P, Diatchenko L, Maixner W. Catechol-O-methyltransferase inhibition increases pain sensitivity through activation of both beta2- and beta3-adrenergic receptors. *Pain*. 2007;128(3):199-208.
22. Diatchenko L, Nackley AG, Slade GD, Bhalang K, Belfer I, Max MB, Goldman D, Maixner W. Catechol-O-methyltransferase gene

polymorphisms are associated with multiple pain-evoking stimuli. *Pain*. 2006;125(3):216-224.

23. Diatchenko L, Anderson AD, Slade GD, Fillingim RB, Shabalina SA, Higgins TJ, Sama S, Belfer I, Goldman D, Max MB, Weir BS, Maixner W. Three major haplotypes of the beta2 adrenergic receptor define psychological profile, blood pressure, and the risk for development of a common musculoskeletal pain disorder. *Am J Med Genetics. Part B, Neuropsychiatric Genetics: The Official Publication of the International Society of Psychiatric Genetics*. 2006; 141(5):449-462.
24. Bhalang K, Sigurdsson A, Slade GD, Maixner W. Associations among four modalities of experimental pain in women. *J Pain*. 2005;6(9):604-611.
25. Diatchenko L, Slade GD, Nackley AG, Bhalang K, Sigurdsson A, Belfer I, Goldman D, Xu K, Shabalina SA, Shagin D, Max MB, Makarov SS, Maixner W. Genetic basis for individual variations in pain perception and the development of a chronic pain condition. *Human Molecular Genetics*. 2005;14(1):135-143.
26. Bragdon EE, Light KC, Costello NL, Sigurdsson A, Bunting S, Bhalang K, Maixner W. Group differences in pain modulation: pain-free women compared to pain-free men and to women with TMD. *Pain*. 2002;96(3):227-237.
27. de Leeuw R, Albuquerque RJ, Andersen AH, Carlson CR. Influence of estrogen on brain activation during stimulation with painful heat. *J Oral Maxillofac Surg*. 2006;64(2):158-166.
28. de Leeuw R, Albuquerque R, Okeson J, Carlson C. The contribution of neuroimaging techniques to the understanding of supraspinal pain circuits: implications for orofacial pain. *[Review] [65 refs] c.* 2005;100(3):308-314.
29. de Leeuw R, Bertoli E, Schmidt JE, Carlson CR. Prevalence of post-traumatic stress disorder symptoms in orofacial pain patients. *Oral Surg Oral Med Oral Path Oral Rad and Endo*. 2005;99(5):558-568.
30. Ferrando M, Andreu Y, Galdon MJ, Dura E, Poveda R, Bagan JV. Psychological variables and temporomandibular disorders: distress, coping, and personality. *Oral Surg Oral Med Oral Path Oral Rad and Endo*. 2004;98(2):153-160.
31. Manfredini D, di Poggio AB, Romagnoli M, Dell'Osso L, Bosco M. Mood spectrum in patients with different painful temporomandibular disorders. *Cranio*. 2004;22(3):234-240.
32. Dworkin SF, Sherman J, Mancl L, Ohrbach R, LeResche L, Truelove E. Reliability, validity, and clinical utility of the research diagnostic criteria for Temporomandibular Disorders Axis II Scales: depression, non-specific physical symptoms, and graded chronic pain. *J Orofac Pain*. 2002;16(3):207-220.
33. Auerbach SM, Laskin DM, Frantsve LM, Orr T. Depression, pain, exposure to stressful life events, and long-term outcomes in temporomandibular disorder patients. *J Oral Maxillofac Surg*. 2001;59(6):628-633; discussion 634.
34. Turner JA, Dworkin SF, Mancl L, Huggins KH, Truelove EL. The roles of beliefs, catastrophizing, and coping in the functioning of patients with temporomandibular disorders. *Pain*. 2001; 92(1-2):41-51.
35. Campbell LC, Riley JL 3rd, Kashikar-Zuck S, Gremillion H, Robinson ME. Somatic, affective, and pain characteristics of chronic TMD patients with sexual versus physical abuse histories. *J Orofac Pain*. 2000;14(2):112-119.
36. Fillingim RB, Maixner W, Sigurdsson A, Kincaid S. Sexual and physical abuse history in subjects with temporomandibular disorders: relationship to clinical variables, pain sensitivity, and psychologic factors. *J Orofac Pain*. 1997;11(1):48-57.
37. Patel H, Rosengren A, Ekman I. Symptoms in acute coronary syndromes: does sex make a difference? *Am Heart J*. 2004;148:27-33.
38. Kapur N, Kamel IR, Herlich A. Oral and craniofacial pain: diagnosis, pathophysiology, and treatment. *Int Anesthesiol Clin*. 2003;41:115-150.
39. Egermark I, Magnusson T, Carlsson GE. A 20-year follow-up of signs and symptoms of temporomandibular disorders and malocclusions in subjects with and without orthodontic treatment in childhood. *Angle Orthod*. 2003;73:109-115.
40. Sipila K, Zitting P, Siira P, Laukkanen P, Jarvelin MR, Oikarinen KS, Raustia AM. Temporomandibular disorders, occlusion, and neck pain in subjects with facial pain: a case-control study. *Cranio*. 2002;20:158-164.
41. Nassif NJ, Talic YF. Classic symptoms in temporomandibular disorder patients: a comparative study. *Cranio*. 2001;19:33-41.
42. Johansson A, Unell L, Carlsson GE, Soderfeldt B, Halling A. Gender difference in symptoms related to temporomandibular disorders in a population of 50-year-old subjects. *J Orofac Pain*. 2003;17:29-35.
43. Macfarlane TV, Blinkhorn AS, Davies RM, Kincey J, Worthington HV. Oro-facial pain in the community: prevalence and associated impact. *Community Dent Oral Epidemiol*. 2002;30:52-60.
44. Rasmussen P. Facial pain. IV. A prospective study of 1052 patients with a view of: precipitating factors, associated symptoms, objective psychiatric and neurological symptoms. *Acta Neurochir (Wien)*. 1991;108:100-109.
45. de las Penas CF, Cuadrado ML, Gerwin RD, Pareja JA. Referred pain from the trochlear region in tension-type headache: a myofascial trigger point from the superior oblique muscle. *Headache*. 2005;45: 731-737.
46. Kalina R, Orcutt J. Ocular and periocular pain. In: Bonica JJ, ed. *The Management of Pain*. Philadelphia, Pa: Lee and Ferbiger; 1990: 759-768.
47. Curtis AW. Myofascial pain-dysfunction syndrome: the role of nonmasticatory muscles in 91 patients. *Otolaryngol Head Neck Surg*. 1980;88:361-367.
48. Alvarez DJ, Rockwell PG. Trigger points: diagnosis and management. *Am Fam Physician*. 2002;65:653-660.
49. Kuttila S, Kuttila M, Le BY, Alanen P, Suonpaa J. Characteristics of subjects with secondary otalgia. *J Orofac Pain*. 2004;18:226-234.
50. Kuttila M, Le BY, Savolainen-Niemi E, Kuttila S, Alanen P. Efficiency of occlusal appliance therapy in secondary otalgia and temporomandibular disorders. *Acta Odontol Scand*. 2002; 60:248-254.
51. Kuttila SJ, Kuttila MH, Niemi PM, Le Bell YB, Alanen PJ, Suonpaa JT. Secondary otalgia in an adult population. *Arch Otolaryngol Head Neck Surg*. 2001;127:401-405.
52. Wright EF, Syms CA III, Bifano SL. Tinnitus, dizziness, and nonotologic otalgia improvement through temporomandibular disorder therapy. *Mil Med*. 2000;165:733-736.
53. Bush FM, Harkins SW, Harrington WG. Otalgia and aversive symptoms in temporomandibular disorders. *Ann Otol Rhinol Laryngol*. 1999;108:884-892.
54. Wazen JJ. Referred otalgia. *Otolaryngol Clin North Am*. 1989; 1205-1215.
55. Fink M, Wahling K, Stiesch-Scholz M, Tschernitschek H. The functional relationship between the craniomandibular system, cervical spine, and the sacroiliac joint: a preliminary investigation. *Cranio*. 2003;21:202-208.
56. Ciancaglini R, Testa M, Radaelli G. Association of neck pain with symptoms of temporomandibular dysfunction in the general adult population. *Scand J Rehabil Med*. 1999;31:17-22.
57. Svensson P, Wang K, Sessle BJ, Arendt-Nielsen L. Associations between pain and neuromuscular activity in the human jaw and neck muscles. *Pain*. 2004;109:225-232.

58. Kushida CA, Morgenthaler TI, Littner MR, Alessi CA, Bailey D, Coleman J Jr., Friedman L, Hirshkowitz M, Kapen S, Kramer M, Lee-Chiong T, Owens J, Pancer JP. Practice parameters for the treatment of snoring and Obstructive Sleep Apnea with oral appliances: an update for 2005. *Sleep*. 2006;29:240-243.
59. Chakfa AM, Mehta NR, Forgione AG, Al-Badawi EA, Lobo SL, Zawawi KH. The effect of stepwise increases in vertical dimension of occlusion on isometric strength of cervical flexors and deltoid muscles in nonsymptomatic females. *Cranio*. 2002;20:264-273.
60. Abduljabbar T, Mehta NR, Forgione AG, Clark RE, Kronman JH, Munsat TL, George P. Effect of increased maxillo-mandibular relationship on isometric strength in TMD patients with loss of vertical dimension of occlusion. *Cranio*. 1997;15:57-67.
61. Hashimoto K, Kawashima S, Kameoka S, Akiyam Y, Honjoya T, Ejima K, Sawada K. Comparison of image validity between cone beam computed tomography for dental use and multidetector row helical computed tomography. *Dentomaxillofac Radiol*. 2007;36:465-471.
62. Israel HA, Diamond B, Saed-Nejad F, Ratcliffe A. The relationship between parafunctional masticatory activity and arthroscopically diagnosed temporomandibular joint pathology. *J Oral Maxillofac Surg*. 1999;57(9):1034-1039.
63. Cisneros GJ, Kaban LB. Computerized skeletal scintigraphy for assessment of mandibular asymmetry. *J Oral Maxillofac Surg*. 1984;42(8):513-520.
64. Kaban LB, Cisneros GJ, Heyman S, Treves S. Assessment of mandibular growth by skeletal scintigraphy. *J Oral Maxillofac Surg*. 1982;40(1):18-22.
65. Cisneros G, Kaban LB. Computerized skeletal scintigraphy for assessment of mandibular asymmetry. *J Oral Maxillofac Surg*. 1984;42:513-520.
66. Pogrel MA. Quantitative assessment of isotope activity in the temporomandibular joint regions as a means of assessing unilateral condylar hypertrophy. *J Oral Maxillofac Surg*. 1985;60:15-17.
67. McCain JP, de la Rua H, Le Blanc WG. Correlation of clinical, radiographic, and arthroscopic findings in internal derangements of the TMJ. *J Oral Maxillofac Surg*. 1989;47(9):913-921.
68. Perrott DH, Alborzi A, Kaban LB, Helms CA. A prospective evaluation of the effectiveness of temporomandibular joint arthroscopy. *J Oral Maxillofac Surg*. 1990;48(10):1029-1032.
69. Nitzan DW, Dolwick MF, Heft MW. Arthroscopic lavage and lysis of the temporomandibular joint: a change in perspective. *J Oral Maxillofac Surg*. 1990;48(8):798-801; discussion 802.
70. McCain JP, Sanders B, Koslin MG, Quinn JH, Peters PB, Indresano AT. Temporomandibular joint arthroscopy: a 6-year multicenter retrospective study of 4,831 joints. *J Oral Maxillofac Surg*. 1992;50(9):926-930.
71. Israel HA. Part I: The use of arthroscopic surgery for treatment of temporomandibular joint disorders. *J Oral Maxillofac Surg*. 1999;57(5):579-582.
72. Truelove E, Huggins KH, Mancl L, Dworkin SF. The efficacy of traditional, low-cost and nonsplint therapies for temporomandibular disorder: a randomized controlled trial. *J Am Dental Assoc*. 2006;137(8):1099-1107.
73. De Laat A, Stappaerts K, Papy S. Counseling and physical therapy as treatment for myofascial pain of the masticatory system. *J Orofac Pain*. 2003;17(1):42-49.
74. Dionne RA. Pharmacologic treatments for temporomandibular disorders. *Oral Surg Oral Med Oral Path Oral Rad and Endo*. 1997;83(1):134-142.
75. Schutz TC, Andersen ML, Tufik S. Effects of COX-2 inhibitor in temporomandibular joint acute inflammation. *J Dental Res*. 2007;86(5):475-479.
76. Ta LE, Dionne RA. Treatment of painful temporomandibular joints with a cyclooxygenase-2 inhibitor: a randomized placebo-controlled comparison of celecoxib to naproxen. *Pain*. 2004;111(1-2):13-21.
77. Kerins C, Carlson D, McIntosh J, Bellinger L. A role for cyclooxygenase II inhibitors in modulating temporomandibular joint inflammation from a meal pattern analysis perspective. *J Oral Maxillofac Surg*. 2004;62(8):989-995.
78. List T, Axelsson S, Leijon G. Pharmacologic interventions in the treatment of temporomandibular disorders, atypical facial pain, and burning mouth syndrome. A qualitative systematic review. *J Orofac Pain*. 2003;17(4):301-310.
79. Rizzatti-Barbosa CM, Martinelli DA, Ambrosano GM, de Albergaria-Barbosa JR. Therapeutic response of benzodiazepine, orphenadrine citrate and occlusal splint association in TMD pain. *Cranio*. 2003;21(2):116-120.
80. Herman CR, Schiffman EL, Look JO, Rindal DB. The effectiveness of adding pharmacologic treatment with clonazepam or cyclobenzaprine to patient education and self-care for the treatment of jaw pain upon awakening: a randomized clinical trial. *J Orofac Pain*. 2002;16(1):64-70.
81. Onghena P, Van Houdenhove B. Antidepressant-induced analgesia in chronic nonmalignant pain: a meta-analysis of 39 placebo-controlled studies. *Pain*. 1992;49:205-219.
82. Max MB, Lynch SA, Muir J, et al. Effects of desiprimine, amitriptyline and fluoxetine on pain in diabetic neruopathy. *N Engl J Med*. 1992;326:1250-1256.
83. Sullivan MD, Robinson JP. Antidepressant and anticonvulsant medication for chronic pain. In: Robinson JP, ed. *Pain Rehabilitation. Phys Med Rehabil Clin N Am*. 2006;17:381-400.
84. Rowbotham MC, Goli V, Kunz NR, et al. Venlafaxine extended release in the treatment of painful diabetic neuropathy: a double-blind, placebo-contolled study. *Pain*. 2004;110:697-706.
85. Sindrup SH, Bach FW, Madsen C, et al. Venlafaxine versus imipramine in painful polyneuropathy: a randomized, controlled trial. *Neurology*. 2003;60:1284-1289.
86. Goldstein DJ, Lu Y, Detke MJ, et al. Duloxetine versus placebo in patients with painful diabetic neuropathy. *Pain*. 2005;116:109-118.
87. Denucci DJ, Dionne RA, Dubner R. Identifying a neurobiologic basis for drug therapy in TMDs. *J Am Dental Assoc*. 1996;127(5):581-593.
88. Kishi Y. Paroxetine-induced bruxism effectively treated with tandospirone. *J Neuropsych Clin Neurosci*. 2007;19(1):90-91.
89. Malki GA, Zawawi KH, Melis M, Hughes CV. Prevalence of bruxism in children receiving treatment for attention deficit hyperactivity disorder: a pilot study. *J Clin Ped Dentistry*. 2004;29(1):63-67.
90. Lobbezoo F, van Denderen RJ, Verheij JG, Naeije M. Reports of SSRI-associated bruxism in the family physician's office. *J Orofac Pain*. 2001;15(4):340-346.
91. Romanelli F, Adler DA, Bungay KM. Possible paroxetine-induced bruxism. *Ann Pharmacotherapy*. 1996;30(11):1246-1248.
92. Singer E, Dionne R. A controlled evaluation of ibuprofen and diazepam for chronic orofacial muscle pain. *J Orofac Pain*. 1997;11(2):139-146.
93. Dao TT, Lavigne GJ. Oral splints: the crutches for temporomandibular disorders and bruxism? *Crit Rev Oral Biol Med*. 1998;9(3):345-361.
94. Fricton J. Myogenous temporomandibular disorders: diagnostic and management considerations. *Dental Clin N Am*. 2007;51(1):61-83.
95. Fricton J. Current evidence providing clarity in management of temporomandibular disorders: summary of a systematic review of randomized clinical trials for intra-oral appliances and occlusal therapies. *J Evidencebased Dental Prac*. 2006;6(1):48-52.

96. Fricton J, Look JO, Wright E, Alencar FGP, Chen H, Lang M, Ouyang W, Velly AM. Systematic review and meta-analysis of randomized controlled trials evaluating intraoral orthopedic appliances for temporomandibular disorders. *J Orofac Pain*. 2010;24:237-254.

97. Al-ani, et al. Stabilization splint therapy for temporomandibular pain dysfunction, *Cochrane Database of Systematic Reviews*, issue 1, CD002778, 2004.

98. Ekberg E, Nilner M. Treatment outcome of appliance therapy in temporomandibular disorder patients with myofascial pain after 6 and 12 months. *Acta odontologica Scandinavica*. 2004;62(6):343-349.

99. Wassell RW, Adams N, Kelly PJ. The treatment of temporomandibular disorders with stabilizing splints in general dental practice: one-year follow-up. *J Am Dental Assoc*. 2006;137(8):1089-1098; quiz 1168-9.

100. Al-Ani Z, Gray RJ, Davies SJ, Sloan P, Glenny AM. Stabilization splint therapy for the treatment of temporomandibular myofascial pain: a systematic review. *J Dental Educ*. 2005;69(11):1242-1250.

101. Seligman DA, Pullinger AG. Analysis of occlusal variables, dental attrition, and age for distinguishing healthy controls from female patients with intracapsular temporomandibular disorders. *J Prosthetic Dentistry*. 2000;83(1):76-82.

102. Pullinger AG, Seligman DA. Quantification and validation of predictive values of occlusal variables in temporomandibular disorders using a multifactorial analysis.[see comment]. *J Prosthetic Dentistry*. 2000;83(1):66-75.

103. Tsukiyama Y, Baba K, Clark GT. An evidence-based assessment of occlusal adjustment as a treatment for temporomandibular disorders. *J Prosthetic Dentistry*. 2001;86(1):57-66.

104. Koh H, Robinson PG. Occlusal adjustment for treating and preventing temporomandibular joint disorders. *Cochrane Database of Systematic Reviews*. 2007;2.

105. Dworkin SF. The case for incorporating biobehavioral treatment into TMD management. *J Am Dental Assoc*. 1996;127(11):1607-1610.

106. Turk DC. Psychosocial and behavioral assessment of patients with temporomandibular disorders: diagnostic and treatment implications. *Cochrane Database of Systematic Reviews*. 1997;83(1):65-71.

107. Raphael KG, Klausner JJ, Nayak S, Marbach JJ. Complementary and alternative therapy use by patients with myofascial temporomandibular disorders. *J Orofac Pain*. 2003;17(1):36-41.

108. Crider A, Glaros AG, Gevirtz RN. Efficacy of biofeedback-based treatments for temporomandibular disorders. *Appl Psychophysiol Biofeed*. 2005;30(4):333-345.

109. Stowell AW, Gatchel RJ, Wildenstein L. Cost-effectiveness of treatments for temporomandibular disorders: biopsychosocial intervention versus treatment as usual. *J Am Dental Assoc*. 2007;138(2):202-208.

110. NIH Technology Assessment panel. Integration of behavioral and relaxation approaches into the treatment of chronic pain and insomnia: special communication. *JAMA*. 1996;276:313-318.

111. De Laat A, Stappaerts K, Papy S. Counseling and physical therapy as treatment for myofascial pain of the masticatory system. *J Orofac Pain*. 2003;17(1):42-49.

112. Venancio Rde A, Camparis CM, Lizarelli Rde F. Low intensity laser therapy in the treatment of temporomandibular disorders: a double-blind study. *J Oral Rehab*. 2005;32(11):800-807.

113. McNeely ML, Armijo Olivo S, Magee DJ. A systematic review of the effectiveness of physical therapy interventions for temporomandibular disorders. *Phys Ther*. 2006;86(5):710-725.

114. Medlicott MS, Harris SR. A systematic review of the effectiveness of exercise, manual therapy, electrotherapy, relaxation training, and biofeedback in the management of temporomandibular disorder. *Phys Ther*. 2006;86(7):955-973.

115. Craane B, De Laat A, Dijkstra PU, Stappaerts K, Stegenga B. Physical therapy for the management of patients with temporomandibular disorders and related pain. *Cochrane Database of Systematic Reviews*. 2007;2.

116. Israel HA, Syrop SB. The important role of motion in the rehabilitation of patients with mandibular hypomobility: a review of the literature. *Cranio*. 1997;15(1):74-83.

117. Horrell BM, Vogel LD, Israel HA. Passive motion therapy in temporomandibular joint disorders: the use of a new hydraulic device and case reports. *Compend Cont Educ Dentistry*. 1997;18(1):73-76.

118. Israel HA. Part 1: The use of arthroscopic surgery for the treatment of temporomandibular joint disorders. *J Oral Maxillofac Surg*. 1999;57:579-582.

119. Israel HA, Diamond B, Saed-Nejad F, Ratcliffe A. Osteoarthritis and synovitis as major pathoses of the temporomandibular joint: comparison of clinical diagnosis with arthroscopic morphology. *J Oral Maxillofac Surg*. 1998;56:1023-1027.

120. Dimitroulis G. The prevalence of osteoarthrosis in cases of advanced internal derangement of the temporomandibular joint: a clinical, surgical and histological study. *Int J Oral Maxillofac Surg*. 2005;34:345-349.

121. Bjornland T, Gjaerum AA, Moystad O. Osteoarthritis of the temporomandibular joint: an evaluation of the effects and complications of corticosteroid injections compared with injection with sodium hyaluronate. *J Oral Rehab*. 2007;34:583-589.

122. Koslin MG. Advanced arthroscopic surgery. *Oral Maxillofac Surg Clin N Am*. 2006;18:329-343.

123. Limchaichana N, Petersson A, Rohlin M. The efficacy of magnetic resonance imaging in the diagnosis of degenerative and inflammatory temporomandibular joint disorders: a systematic literature review. *Oral Surg Oral Med Oral Path Oral Rad and Endo*. 2006;102:521-536.

124. Kaban LB. Acquired abnormalities of the temporomandibular joint, juvenile rheumatoid arthritis. In: Kaban LB, Troulis MJ, eds. *Ped Oral Maxillofac Surg*. Philadelphia, Pa: Saunders; 2004:372-375.

CHAPTER 37 Neck Pain

Thomas T. Simopoulos

Neck pain is a common complaint. The prevalence is approximately between 75% and 80% in the U.S. population. Fortunately, acute neck pain has a very favorable prognosis, with 80% of cases resolved within 2 years.[1] But 20% of cases are estimated not to improve and of these, 5% are characterized by severe disabling chronic neck pain.[2] The International Association for the Study of Pain (IASP) describes chronic cervical spine pain as follows: Pain perceived as arising from anywhere within the region bounded superiorly by the superior nuchal line, inferiorly by an imaginary transverse line through the tip of the first thoracic spinous process, and laterally by sagittal planes tangential to the lateral borders of the neck.[3] The potential sources of neck pain are derived from those structures that have abundant nociceptive innervation, which include the cervical zygapophysial (facet) joints (including atlantoaxial and atlanto-occipital), posterior neck muscles, cervical intervertebral discs, vertebral bodies, anterior and posterior ligaments, dura mater of cervical spine, prevertebral muscles, carotid and vertebral arteries, and the transverse ligament.[4] The paucity of nociceptors in ligamentous structures makes them less likely to cause pain. The neck is a very mobile structure and is, therefore, susceptible to trauma in addition to wear and tear. It is further burdened by the weight of the head and rests on a relatively fixed thorax.

DIAGNOSIS

The evaluation of neck pain is based upon history, physical examination, radiologic, and laboratory tests. In the assessment of acute pain, history is of paramount importance in that it offers clues to potentially rare but serious disorders (**Table 37-1**).

TABLE 37-1 Classification of Neck Pain

Classification of Neck Pain
Neck Pain Without Stiffness
Enhanced by Swallowing
Carotid artery (carotidynia,[5] carotid body tumor, inflamed thyroglossal duct)
Esophagus (inflamed diverticulum, peptic esophagitis, radiation esophagitis)
Mediastinum (spontaneous pneumomediastinum)[6]
Pharynx (pharyngitis or Ludwig's angina)
Salivary gland (mumps, suppurative parotidits)
Thyroid gland (acute suppurative parotiditis, subacute thyroiditis with pain radiating to ear, hemorrhage, thyroid cystadenoma)
Tongue (ulcers, neoplasm)
Tonsils (tonsillitis, neoplasm)
Neck pain enhanced by chewing
Mandible (fracture, osteomyelitis, periodontitis)
Salivary gland (mumps, suppurative parotiditis)
Temporomandibular joint (associated with myofascial pain syndrome in neck)
Neck pain enhanced by head movement
Cervical spine (whiplash, acute or subacute fracture, dislocation, ligamentous damage, herniated inververtebral disk, rheumatoid neck,[7] facet joint syndrome,[8] occipital neuralgia with C1 to C2 arthrosis syndrome[9])
Nuchal muscles or trapezius muscles (viral myalgia, myofascial pain syndrome)[10]
Sternocleidomastoid (torticollis, hematoma, myofascial pain)
Neck pain enhanced by shoulder movement
Cervical rib
Costoclavicular syndrome
Scalenus anticus syndrome
Pectoralis minor syndrome
Neck pain not enhanced by movement
Branchial cleft remnant (inflamed pharyngeal cyst)
Lymph node, acute (adenitis) or chronic (Hodgkin's disease, scrofula, gummas, actinomycosis, carcinomatous metastatsis)
Nervous system (cervical herpes zoster, postherpetic neuralgia, spinal cord neoplasm, Arnold-Chairi malformation, syringomyelia, epidural abscess or hematoma, poliomyelitis)
Salivary gland (calculus in duct)
Skin and subcutaoneous tissue (furuncle, carbuncle, erysipelas)
Soft-tissue calcium deposit at first and second cervical vertebrae[11]

(*Continued*)

TABLE 37-1 Classification of Neck Pain (*Continued*)

Classification of Neck Pain
Spinal vertebrae (primary metastatic neoplasm, infectious osteomyelitis, tuberculosis, herniated intervertebral disk)
Subclavian artery (aneurysm)
Referred neck pain
Angina
Brochus (bronchial tumor)
Pain from sixth cervical dermatomal band
Pancoast's (superior sulcus lung) tumor
Stiff Neck, Neck Pain, and Limitation of Motion
Acquired (spasmodic torticollis)
Acute infections
Epidural abscess
Fibrositis (transient stiff neck)
Reflex spasm (meningitis or adenitis from acute pharyngitis)
Torticollis
Acute traumatic
Epidural hematoma
Cervical spina strain
Dislocations
Facet dislocation
Fractures
Herniated disk (herniated nucleus pulposus)
Ligamentous (strain whiplash, rupture)
Subluxation
Chronic infection
Infectious arthritis
Intramuscular gummas
Tuberculous spondylitis
Chronic posttraumatic
Contracture from burns
Nerve injury
Untreated acute injuries
Congenital (congenital torticollis)
Degenerative
Cervical spondylosis with fibrositis
Fibromyalgia, myofascial pain syndrome
Inflammatory bone lesions
Calcific tendinitis of the longus colli
Subluxation of atlas

HISTORY

The key elements of history include elucidation of the onset, mechanism, neurological symptoms, and psychosocial setting. Therefore, these features include:

1. Precipitating and associated events (trauma, infection, emotional stress).
2. Duration (acute versus chronic).
3. Characteristics of pain (sharp, burning, dull, throbbing).

4. Point of origin (axial neck with or without appendicular radiation).
5. Aggravating and alleviating factors.
6. Topographical regions of maximal pain.
7. Co-existing neurologic symptoms (weakness, numbness, clumsiness, bowel and bladder dysfunction, and disturbances of balance).
8. Associated medical symptoms and conditions (fever, night sweats, weight loss, dysphagia, immunosuppression, illicit drug use, infections).
9. Previous treatment (surgery, manipulation).
10. Pending litigation or workers' compensation.

Acute neck pain as defined by neck pain of less than 3 months is often in the setting of trauma. The main concern is cervical spine instability that can compromise the long tracts of the spinal cord. Progressive weakness of the upper extremity, lower extremities, or bowel and/or bladder dysfunction warrants radiographic evaluation and spine surgical referral. Additionally, undiagnosed tumors, infections, epidural hematomas, and autoimmune disorders (e.g., rheumatoid arthritis) are rare causes with a prevalence of less than 0.4%.[4]

The risk factors for developing neck pain commonly seen in clinical practice are not structural as would be expected. Degenerative intervertebral discs as well as zygapophysial joints do not seem to imply that a patient is at risk for neck pain.[12] Interestingly, educational level, previous injuries, motor vehicle accident that causes whiplash, and occupation factors are presently the key risk factors.[13,14] While operating machinery is linked to the development of neck pain, there has been no clear ergonometric pattern of work-related physical stress that can be modified in a positive manner.[15] Higher levels of education and the lack of previous injuries to the neck decrease the probability of developing neck pain. While there are no apparent psychological factors contributing to the onset of neck pain, psychosocial stress in the work place is felt play a role in symptom complaint.[16] As expected, high work demands, time pressure, and lack of support are at the root of an unfavorable work environment that may precipitate pain in the neck region.

While there have been risk factors identified for the development of neck pain, there is very little the literature offers to the clinician to aid in prognosticating long-term outcome. Aside from most acute neck pain improving as already discussed, there are no validated prognostic risk factors for neck pain—with the exception of whiplash. Patient with complaints of a high level of pain and disability following a whiplash injury carry a long-term unfavorable probability of recovery.[17] These patients are characterized by diffuse hyperalgesia, greater work interference by pain, and reduced activity.[18] The additional factor of litigation is weaker but seems to be a definite factor in trending toward poor recovery. Taken together, our understanding of neck pain in the acute setting will improve, but it is unclear as to why it has such a favorable outcome.

PHYSICAL EXAMINATION

The examination of the neck has several overall elements as listed:

- Anterior and posterior inspection and palpation.
- Range of motion.
- Neurological examination.

Inspection of the neck begins when first encountering the patient and during the interview process. A clinician can gain insight into the range of motion and usual posture. The general medical exam includes inspection for masses, muscular asymmetries, scars, discolorations, and cutaneous lesions. The thyroid gland should be assessed for tenderness, enlargement, and nodules. The presence of cervical lymphadenopathy may signify the presence of malignancy or infection. Lymphadenitis may present as torticollis. Similarly the supraclavicular fossa must be assessed for masses that could be related to lymphadenopathy, aneurysm of the subclavian artery, or an outflow obstruction from a superior vena cava syndrome. Tenderness over the bifurcation of the carotid artery is the hallmark of carotidynia. Horner's syndrome raises concern for

TABLE 37-2 Motor and Reflex Distribution of Cervical Roots

Disk	Reflex	Muscles
C4, C5, and root C5	Biceps	Deltoid or biceps
C5, C6, and root C6	Brachioradialis	Wrist extensors or biceps
C6, C7, and root C7	Triceps	Wrist flexors, finger extensors, or triceps
C7, T1, and root C8	—	Finger flexors or hand intrinsic muscles
T1, T2, and root T1	—	Hand intrinsic muscles

carotid artery dissection. Finally, in an ill-appearing patient with severe headache and neck pain, passive forward flexion of the neck triggers significant pain (Kernig's sign) secondary to meningeal inflammation. Unfortunately, with respect to diagnosing the musculoskeletal disorder responsible for a patient's neck pain (whether acute or chronic), the physical exam has limited utility. Documentation of the range of motion is important to gage the benefit of future therapies, but this does not give insight as to the cause of pain. Palpation of the base of the occiput may reveal tenderness in the territory of the greater occipital nerves but is a nonspecific finding as this can be seen in primary headache disorders such as migraine in addition to occipital nerve entrapment. Tenderness of the muscles overlying the cervical zygapophysial joints raises suspicion for facetogenic pain. But, again, sensitivity over the cervical facets is not diagnostic of the cause of pain. Finally, tenderness over a taut band of muscle that causes referred pain may signify the presence of trigger points. Muscles such as the trapezius and semispinalis cervicis may have such entities and can be a primary or a secondary (e.g., underlying facetogenic pain) myofascial pain syndrome.

The neurological examination serves as a screen for potential nerve root involvement but does not diagnose the cause of a patient's neck pain. The extent of neurological deficit (motor weakness, hyporeflexia, and sensory loss) of the upper extremities is of significant importance and can be assessed via the information in **Table 37-2** and **Figure 37-1**.

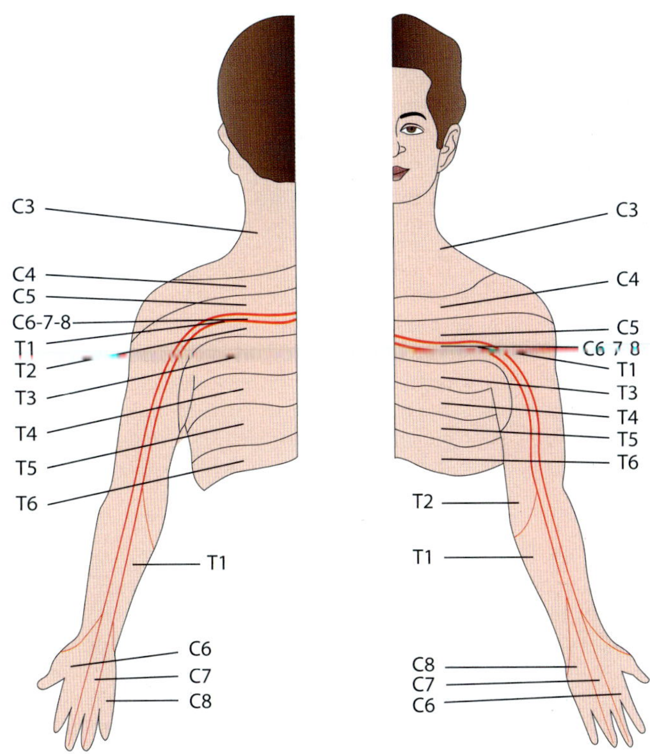

FIGURE 37-1. Dermatomes of the chest and upper extremities.

TABLE 37-3 Specialized Physical Examination Maneuvers for Eliciting Cervical Radicular Symptoms

Test	Physical Description	Sensitivity/Specificity
L'hermitte Sign	Passive anterior flexion of the neck causing radiating pain down the spine or extremities	<28%/high[19]
Neck Distraction Test	Axial traction is applied vertically after grasping the occiput and chin in order to reduce radicular symptoms	40%/100%[20]
Shoulder Abduction (relief) Sign	The patient abducts the shoulder on the symptomatic side placing the hand on the head. Symptoms are then alleviated	43-50%/80-100%[20]
Neck Compression (Spurling) Test	Radicular symptoms are reproduced or exacerbated with the passive lateral flexion of the neck and compression of the head	40-60%/92-100%[20]

The lower extremities should be screened for myelopathy, which can present with sensory loss, spastic weakness, clonus, or impaired vibratory or position sense. Other specialized examination maneuvers for provoking symptoms of cervical radiculopathy are summarized in **Table 37-3**. The basic trend in the literature suggests these tests have a low sensitivity, high specificity, and reasonable inter-examiner reliability.

CERVICAL TRAUMA

WHIPLASH-ASSOCIATED DISORDERS

Neck pain from a traumatic origin includes many injuries ranging from self-limited acute cervical strain to cervical fracture with paralysis. The Quebec Task Force proposed a theoretical classification of whiplash-associated disorders (WADs) in order to allow comparative research on an international basis.[21,22] The following grading system is presently in use:

- Grade 0: No complaints in the neck. No physical signs.
- Grade I: Neck pain without symptoms indicating serious pathology and minimal influence on daily activities.
- Grade II: Neck pain without symptoms indicating serious pathology but having an impact on activities of daily living.
- Grade III: Neck pain with no symptoms indicating serious pathology but with the presence of neurologic dysfunction that includes weakness, sensory loss, or decreased reflexes.
- Grade IV: Neck pain that involves serious underlying pathology, which may include fracture, myelopathy, hemorrhage, or neoplasm.

The patients typically presenting in the outpatient setting fall into WAD I and II, and, therefore, these categories will be discussed. Reports indicate that 85% of neck disorders result from acute or repetitive neck injuries or chronic stresses and strain.[23] Minor trauma resulting in acute cervical pain is often secondary to musculoskeletal injury and, most frequently, is self-limited using conservative treatment. Indeed the prognosis for WAD I remains favorable, with 85% returning to baseline activities within 6 months post-accident while at least 15% to 26% develop chronic symptoms.[21,24]

MECHANISMS OF INJURY

The term *whiplash* classically describes the resultant injury caused by an abrupt hyperextension of the neck from an indirect force. When forward flexion of the neck is produced by acceleration or deceleration, the forward flexion of the head is limited by the chin touching the chest.[25] Lateral flexion movement stops when the ear hits the shoulder. These movements are within the physiologic range of motion of the cervical spine. By contrast, backward extension of the head stops when the occiput hits the posterior thorax. This is beyond the physiologic range of motion. In a rear-end collision, the body is propelled in a linear horizontal direction.[26] The head abruptly moves backward, necessitating acute hyperextension of the cervical spine. This is followed by recoil of the head with severe cervical neck flexion and, finally, a return to the neutral position. The opposite sequence occurs in head-on collisions.

Modern studies have recently begun to refute the flexion-extension injury or acceleration-deceleration injury model. High-speed photography has allowed researchers to determine that the trunk is forced upward into the cervical spine, causing compression from below.[27] The cervical spine is forced into a sigmoid deformation, during which the posterior neck structures are impacted while the anterior elements are distracted.[28] To be specific, the cervical zygapophysial joints are found to have intra-articular hemorrhages, meniscoid contusions, articular subchondral fracture, and articular pillar fracture, while the cervical discs have annular tears.[29] Chronic pain in WAD I or II is thought to be a result of traumatic arthritis to the cervical zygapophysial joints and/or annular tears of the cervical discs. While alar ligaments can also be damaged by whiplash trauma, the contributions of these structures to chronic pain are uncertain.[30]

SYMPTOM COMPLEX

It is important to note that symptoms may not occur for 12 to 24 hours after a whiplash injury because muscular hemorrhage and edema may need to evolve prior to inciting a nociceptive response. The cervical flexor muscles—specifically, the sternocleidomastoid, the scalene muscles, and the longus colli—undergo an acute stretch reflex, which can disrupt muscle fibers.[31] One study reported characteristic symptoms of patients after a motor vehicle accident.[32] This author followed 146 walk-in patients for 5 years after motor vehicle accidents that caused soft-tissue neck injury without fractures or dislocations. Seventy percent of these accidents were rear-end collisions. Loss of consciousness occurred in 10% of patients. Almost all patients complained of neck pain and stiffness. Two-thirds of patients had headaches, and one-third had shoulder or intrascapular pain. Ten percent had arm and hand pain or arm and hand numbness. Only 3% had a focal neurologic deficit.

The primary complaint of WAD is pain typically perceived on the back of the neck that is dull and/or achy accompanied by exacerbations on movement. Persistent suboccipital pain does not necessarily involve a local lesion at the atlantoaxial region but may be referred pain from a damaged cervical segment.[33] In specific, the C2-3 facet joint may account for up to 53% of cervicogenic headache post-whiplash.[34] As indicated earlier, transverse and alar ligaments and the atlantoaxial joint may produce cervical pain with headache, but the contribution and confirmation remains to be determined. Although pain and numbness radiating down the arm are prognostic indicators of chronicity of symptoms, they do not necessarily indicate nerve root pressure.[35] Non-neurogenic radiation of pain and numbness may be caused by chronic irritation of the musculoligamentous joint and intervertebral disk rather than by organic nerve pressure. These radicular symptoms are non-neurogenic; therefore, they follow no specific nerve pathway. They are not well defined by the patient in contradistinction to the well-defined dermatomal pattern of neurogenic symptoms. Subjective numbness in the ulnar distribution may represent anterior scalenus spasm and entrapment of the brachial plexus; this scenario is amenable to injection of the muscle with a local anesthetic and corticosteroid (see "Thoracic Outlet Syndrome"). Radicular-type symptoms (across the back, shoulders, and into the arms) may be caused by damage to the posterior scapular muscles.[36] History taking usually allows the provider to rule out WAD III and IV.

In addition to pain, WAD commonly presents with associated symptoms, which include dizziness, paresthesia, tinnitus, weakness, cognitive impairment, visual disturbances, and back pain.[37] However, temporomandibular joint abnormalities are not associated with whiplash syndrome.[38] None of these lesser symptoms have been adequately studied, but suggested explanations are as follows:

- Dizziness: Speculative damage to vestibular apparatus.
- Paresthesia: Proposed myogenic thoracic outlet syndrome.

- Tinnitus: No attractive explanation.
- Cognitive impairment: No conclusive evidence to support traumatic brain damage, though still believed to be the primary mechanism.
- Visual disturbances: Most common report is difficulty focusing thought to relate to disturbances in the spinociliary reflex. Persistent pain in the neck can therefore affect sympathetic outflow to the eye.
- Weakness: Often a global complaint and thought to relate to reflex inhibition of muscle groups secondary to persistent neck pain.
- Back pain: A common report but unclear as to the mechanism or actual prevalence.

Psychosomatic reactions may occur after soft-tissue neck injuries. Psychological factors have not been found to consistently predict the persistence of pain and disability post-whiplash injury. A randomized, double-blind, placebo-controlled trial demonstrated resolution of psychological distress with radiofrequency neurotomy of the nerves to a single cervical zygapophysial joint.[39] In addition to WAD being dismissed on a psychological basis, symptoms have also been attributed primarily to ongoing litigation. One study evaluated the effects of pending litigation on patients with persistent symptoms after a motor vehicle accident.[40] If litigation claims were settled within 6 months, 83% were symptom free at 5 years. However, if litigation settlement did not occur until 18 months after the accident, then follow-up at 5 years revealed that only 38% were symptom free. Two other studies have found persistent symptoms in 12% to 45% of patients after litigation settlements.[41,42] As would be expected from the underlying anatomic pathology, in many cases, patients are not "cured by a verdict," as is commonly thought.

DIAGNOSIS

The physical examination is first used to confirm the absence of significant neurological deficit. The clinical examination of the neck often reveals localized muscle spasm, tenderness, and reduced range of motion (usually rotation, lateral bending, and extension). No definitive diagnosis is derived from the clinical exam in WAD I and II.

The patient with neck trauma is classically evaluated with a plain-film x-ray study, which includes (1) anteroposterior (AP) view of the atlanto-axial articulation (open mouth), (2) AP view of the lower cervical spine, (3) lateral view, and (4) each oblique view.[43] While this approach is used as the initial imaging evaluation for cervical spine instability, there is no evidence of utility in WAD I and II.[44] Advanced studies with magnetic resonance imaging (MRI), which are agreed upon as a helpful screening tool for occult fractures, infections, and tumors, also fail to determine the cause of WAD I and II. Electrophysiologic studies do not help target the cause or assist in the treatment of WAD I or II. Thus, a clinician is often left short as to the cause of pain in a whiplash case even after careful review of the history, physical exam, and imaging data.

TREATMENT

The initial treatment is conservative and is largely confined to the symptomatic treatment of the pain and range of motion. Most authors recommend a soft cervical collar, nonsteroidal anti-inflammatory agents (NSAIDs), analgesics, and limited bed rest with gradual increase in activity for the first 1 to 2 weeks. Some suggest physical therapy, such as Greenfield isometric neck exercises, heat, and traction.[41] Transcutaneous electrical nerve stimulation (TENS) has been found to be useful for acute cervical train; it hastens pain relief and the return or range of motion.[40]

Despite improvement in most patients' symptoms, a substantial number of patients with whiplash have chronic symptoms. Forty-three percent of patients assessed 5 years after an automobile accident reported persistent symptoms.[40] Interventional strategies are often used in the chronic stage, after 3 to 6 months. These have included epidural steroid injections, trigger points, medial branch or facet injections, botulinum toxin intramuscular injections, and radiofrequency neurotomy of medial branches supplying the cervical facet joints. The effectiveness of epidural injections for the axial complaints of WAD I and II categories has not been established. Intra-articular facet injections have not proven effective in whiplash patients.[45] Trigger-point injections have comparable effects to ultrasound and physical therapy, and the addition of botulinum toxin has not proven to be effective.[46,47]

The analgesic effects of radiofrequency treatment of the cervical facet joints are well documented. Both a randomized, double-blind study and a prospective observation study find that between 58% and 70% of patients with WAD thought to stem from cervical facets derived substantial improvement with reduction in neck disability.[48,49] The analgesic effects following this treatment can endure for more than 1 year.[50] The lack of relief or partial improvement suggests additional pain generators may coexist. Studies have found that it is not always possible to determine the exact source of neck pain and that it is not uncommonly multifactorial.[51,52] Cervical discography has been utilized to assist in the diagnosis of discogenic pain following WAD, and anterior cervical discectomy and fusion have been proposed by some authors as the treatment, though this remains contentious.[53]

CERVICAL SOFT-TISSUE PAIN SYNDROMES

MYOFASCIAL PAIN SYNDROME

One of the most common and frequently overlooked causes of neck pain is the myofascial pain syndrome (MFPS). A myofascial trigger point is a hyperirritable locus that is palpable as an exquisitely tender taut band or knot in a skeletal muscle. Active trigger points are tender, prevent full lengthening of the muscle, weaken the muscle, and can mediate a local twitch response if stimulated adequately. Digital compression causes a characteristic pain reproduction, often with a distal site referral and autonomic phenomena (sweating, vasoconstriction, and pilomotor activity).[54] The pain pattern may not be limited to a specific dermatome or peripheral nerve segment. Many times, this pattern may superficially mimic other pathology (i.e., herniated nucleus pulposus, radiculopathy), and, therefore, the diagnosis of myofascial pain syndrome is not entertained.

A myofascial pain syndrome may coexist with other cervical disorders. These other pathologic conditions must be evaluated and treated as well. Myofascial pain is often abrupt in onset, and patients may remember a specific precipitating event, often traumatic—for example, a whiplash injury. However, the pain may be more gradual in onset from a chronically overused muscle. Myofascial pain may develop after, or be worsened by, psychogenic stress, viral illness, visceral disease, exposure to cold or damp weather, and strenuous exercise or prolonged tensing of the involved muscle.[55] The patient often describes pain that is steady, deep, and aching in quality. Although the pain may follow a dermatomal myotomal pattern, it does not follow a characteristic nerve root pattern nor is there usually dysesthesia or paresthesia, which often is present with nerve root irritation.

Diagnosis There remains a lack of consensus in the literature on the validity and reliability of diagnostic criteria for MFPS with associated trigger points.[56] However, most would agree that in neck pain of myofascial origin, the muscles of the shoulder and neck are often tense with spasm. Palpation of a taut, bandlike trigger point that reproduces the patient's pain pattern is pathognomonic for a myofascial pain syndrome. There may be associated weakness but not atrophy of the involved muscles.[57] Trigger points commonly responsible for pain referred to the cervical area are located in several muscles (**Table 37-4**). Many patients exhibit a sleep disturbance.

Management There is considerable clinical overlap among myofascial pain, fibromyalgia, and tension-type headaches, and, as a result, the pharmacological, nonpharmacological, as well as the interventional approaches tend to be similar—even if the evidence is only in one of the three aforementioned syndromes (**Table 37-5**). Nonsteroidal anti-inflammatory drugs have limited literature supporting their use in MFPS but are considered helpful in fibromyalgia.[58] The strong evidence supporting the use of tricyclic antidepressants in tension-type headache and dual reuptake inhibitors in the fibromyalgia syndrome

TABLE 37-4 Cervical Myofascial Trigger Points*

Muscle	Area of Referred Pain
Trapezius	Neck, shoulder, or temporal region
Splenius capitis or cervicis	Head, occiput, shoulder, or neck (there may be blurred vision)
Posterior neck muscles (semispinalis *capitis*, cervicis, or multifidi)	Suboccipital area, neck, or shoulders
Levator scapulae	Angle of neck or along vertebral border of scapula
Scalene muscles (anterior, medial)	Chest, upper central border of scapula, or along arm
Infraspinatus	Posterior neck, suboccipital area, deltoid, deep in shoulder joint, or front and lateral aspects of arm and forearm

*Adapted from Travell JG, Simons DG. *Myofascial Pain and Dysfunction. The Trigger Point Manual.* Vol 1. Baltimore, Md: Williams & Wilkins; 1983.[10]

have led to their common use in MFPS of the neck.[59-61] The safety and ease of use of the gabapentinoids—especially pregabalin—coupled with its proven efficacy in fibromyalgia has led to its common use in muscle pain.[62] Lastly, numerous clinical studies demonstrate the effectiveness of skeletal muscle relaxants—particularly cyclobenzaprine and tizanidine—in cervical muscle pain.[63,64]

Treatment of the myofascial pain syndrome and eradication of acute myofascial trigger points may be achieved by passive stretching with augmentation by trigger-point injections, ultrasound or laser therapy. Trigger-point injections safely augment the treatment outcomes of muscle stretches.[65] The involved muscles can be sprayed with vapocoolant coupled with passive stretching of the muscle. A stream of vapocoolant is sprayed in parallel sweeps in the direction of the referred pain over the skin of the involved muscle. The muscle then is stretched passively and slowly to the normal full muscle length in an effort to inactivate the trigger point. For refractory cases, botulinum toxin injections have proven to be beneficial overall; however, the duration of the effect may not be significantly different than trigger-point injections with local anesthetic in many cases.[66]

Because many conditions of daily living contribute to the formation and exacerbation of myofascial trigger points, therapy must incorporate a multifaceted approach. Biofeedback and relaxation techniques are useful in diminishing the psychogenic stress that can cause and exacerbate pain from myofascial trigger points. Driving, typing, heavy shoulder bags, exposure to cold drafts, and improper sleeping positions are a few conditions that contribute to and exacerbate myofascial trigger points and result in cervical pain. Practices and activities that lead to prolonged overutilization, strain, or tensing of the shoulder and neck muscles should be avoided. In addition, a formal physical therapy program often is beneficial. A program that encompasses stretch-and-spray techniques, strengthening exercises, and use of moist heat, ultrasound, and electrical stimulation is useful.[67] The patient also can institute a program of passive stretching while taking a hot shower or with application of moist hot packs.

TABLE 37-5 Treatment of Myofascial Pain Syndrome of the Neck

Treatment	Comment
Nonsteroidal Anti-inflammatory Drugs	Helpful in fibromyalgia and tension-type headache
Antidepressants	Tricyclics and dual uptake inhibitors effective in fibromyalgia, tension-type headache
Anticonvulsants	Gabapentinoids exert an analgesic effect in soft-tissue syndromes of fibromyalgia
Muscle Relaxants	Cyclobenzaprine and tizanidine effective in muscle-based neck pain
Trigger-Point Injections	Safe and augments stretching exercises
Botulinum Toxin Injection	Safe and of similar effectiveness to conventional trigger points

TORTICOLLIS

Torticollis is a severe state of neck muscle sustained contractions, giving rise to repetitive twisting movements or abnormal postures. Most commonly, the sternocleidomastoid and trapezius muscles are involved. Other muscles that may be associated are the so-called cervical strap muscles. The contracture is sometimes spasmodic but usually is tonic. It is almost always unilateral: The head often is twisted painfully to one side, with the chin directed to the opposite side because of contraction of the sternocleidomastoid. Torticollis results from disease or injury to the central nervous system (CNS) or the musculoskeletal tissues of the neck.[68] It may be congenital or acquired (**Table 37-6**). Long-standing torticollis can produce permanent contracture of the cervical muscles, fibrotic changes in the tissue, and degeneration of the cervical spine. There may be variable degrees of pain associated with the course of the disease.[68]

Diagnosis Evaluation of the patient with torticollis should include the history (e.g., trauma, drugs, familial tendencies, and infection), physical findings (including careful neurologic examination and evaluation

TABLE 37-6 Causes of Torticollis

Congenital Torticollis	Acquired Torticollis
Muscular and postural torticollis	**Traumatic**
Muscle trauma	Fracture
Tumor	Subluxation of the odontoid, C1, C2, or C3
Inflammation	Atlantoaxial instability
C1 to C2 articulations	Trauma to the clavicle, scapula, or cervical ligaments
Atlantoaxial dislocation	Neck muscle injuries
Anomalies of the cervical vertebrae	**Infectious**
Klippel-Feil syndrome	Cervical abscess
Absence of cervical muscles	Osteomyelitis
Neurogenic	Fascitis
Arnold-Chiari malformations	Nasopharyngeal torticollis associated with upper respiratory tract infection
Spina bifida	Cervical adenitis: viral, bacterial, tubercular
Hydrocephalus	**Post-infectious**
Syringomyelia	Influenza
Syringobulbia	Diphtheria
Colloid cyst	Scarlet fever[7]
	Neoplastic
	Bone: multiple myloma, metastasis
	Muscle: rhabdomyosarcoma
	Lymphatic: lymphoma
	Vascular
	Scar formation
	Vascular abnormalities
	Anterior scalenus syndrome
	Pharmacologic
	Phenothiazines (dystonic reactions)
	Neurologic
	Syringomyelia
	Dystonic syndrome
	Posterior fossae disease: acoustic neuroma
	Herniated cervical disk
	Hydrocephalus
	Postencephalitis
	Spasmodic torticollis

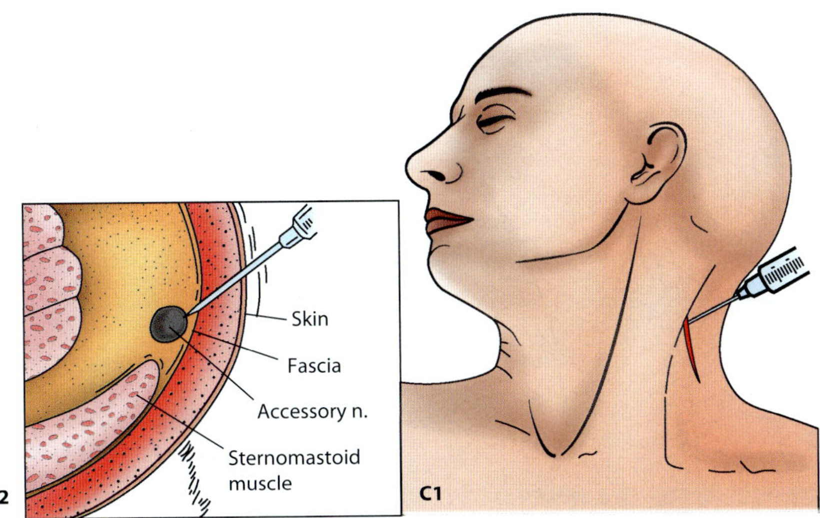

FIGURE 37-2. Diagram of a spinal accessory nerve block. (Used by permission. Romanoff ME. Somatic nerve blocks of the head and neck. In: Raj P, ed. *Practical Management of Pain*. 3rd ed. St. Louis: Mosby Inc.; 2000).

of the cervical spine), and x-ray findings (including cervical spine films of the odontoid and AP, lateral, and oblique views of the neck). This information enables the clinician to classify torticollis as acquired or congenital, traumatic origin, or involving musculoskeletal or neurologic structures. When torticollis is associated with a neurologic deficit, additional radiographic investigations are warranted, including CT or MRI scan with and without contrast or myelography.[69] Based on the lack of specific diagnostic tests, in order to make a final and accurate diagnosis, referral to a movement disorder expert is recommended.[70]

Treatment Pharmacologic therapy of spasmodic torticollis has been somewhat effective. Therapies manipulating the dopaminergic, cholinergic, adrenergic, and serotonergic systems, and the use of γ-aminobutyric acid (GABA) agonists have had varying degrees of success. Anticholinergics have been recommended for mild symptoms of torticollis, including trihexyphenidyl (2–4 mg/day) or benztropine (1–3 mg/day). Diazepam (5–15 mg/day) or amantadine (100–300 mg/day) has been used for patients with mild to moderate symptoms. Moderate to severe symptoms can be treated with haloperidol (1–8 mg/day). With the exception of levodopa, which is the treatment of choice for dopamine-sensitive dystonia, there is a dearth of evidence to support efficacy of any particular pharmaceutical agent in the symptom management of dystonia.[69] Psychological approaches such as psychotherapy, hypnosis, behavior modification, and biofeedback also have been advocated.

The spinal accessory nerve innervates the sternocleidomastoid and trapezius muscles. Traditionally, spinal accessory nerve block was used to relax the trapezius and sternocleidomastoid muscles in torticollis (**Fig. 37-2**). Alternatively, local anesthetic may be injected diffusely into the muscle belly similar to a trigger-point injection. When other neck muscles are involved, a superficial or deep cervical plexus block is required to relieve the spasm (**Figs. 37-3** and **37-4**). But, experience over the past decade has shown injection of botulinum toxin complex A (Botox 100–200 unit injections) to be effective and has now become first-line treatment.[71] If injection therapies including botulinum toxin prove ineffective, selective peripheral denervation of the aforementioned nerves is safe with minimal side effects.[69,72]

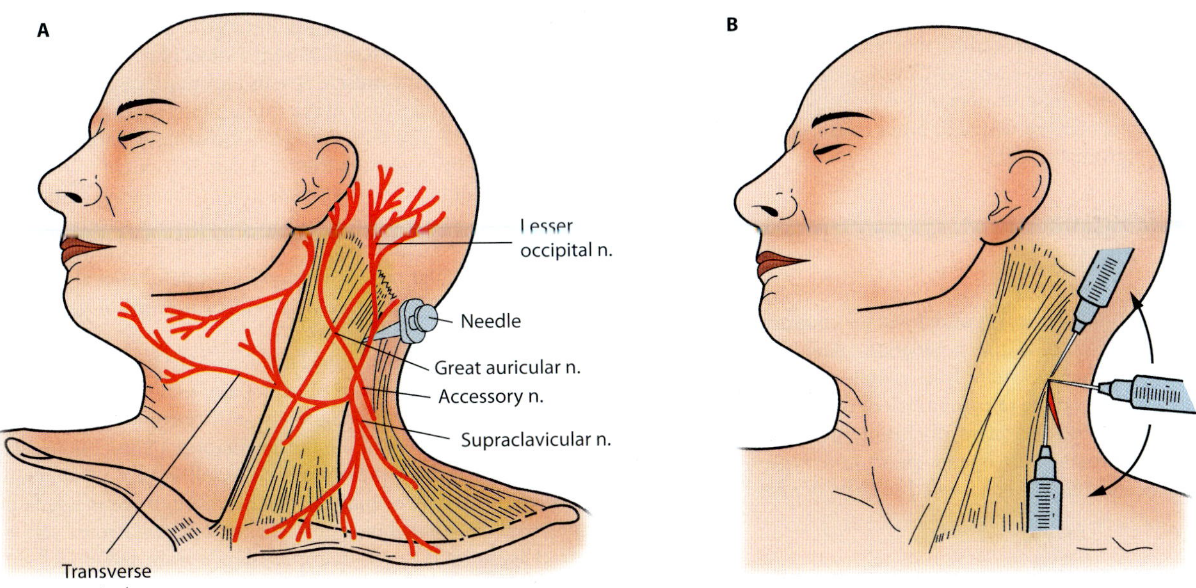

FIGURE 37-3. Diagram of a superficial cervical nerve block. (Used by permission. Romanoff ME. Somatic nerve blocks of the head and neck. In: Raj P, ed. *Practical Management of Pain*. 3rd ed. St. Louis: Mosby Inc.; 2000).

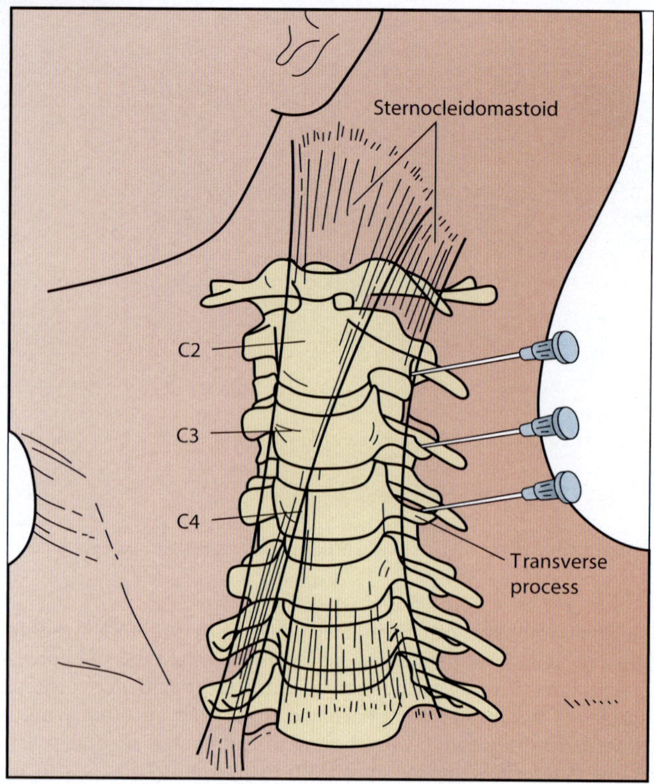

FIGURE 37-4. Diagram of multiple cervical nerve root blocks or deep cervical plexus block. (Used by permission. Romanoff ME. Somatic nerve blocks of the head and neck. In: Raj P, ed. *Practical Management of Pain*. 3rd ed. St. Louis: Mosby Inc.; 2000).

Neurosurgical options for severe refractory cases include cervical rhizotomy, selective excision of the hyperkinetic cervical muscles, and stereotactic ablative and deep brain stimulation (DBS). These surgical approaches have had varied degrees of success.[73] DBS of the globus pallidus has been thought especially beneficial in cervical torticollis, and it is noted that the tremulous and myoclonic features improve within days after surgery, while abnormal postures may take months to appreciate results.[74,75] Cervical rhizotomy, radiofrequency stereotactic ablations, and microvascular decompressions are no longer recommended because of lack of effect and/or postprocedure morbidity.[69] Surgical management of the underlying condition (Arnold-Chiari malformation, syringomyelia, colloid cysts, etc.) may be considered in patients with neurogenic torticollis if medical management and other conservative measures have not provided symptomatic relief.

CERVICAL SPONDYLOSIS

CERVICAL DISC DEGENERATION

Disk degeneration and cervical spondylosis are common causes of neck pain. Approximately 50% of the population older than 50 years and 75% of those older than 65 years have radiologic evidence of cervical spondylosis.[76] However, there remains a lack of consensus in the literature regarding the causes and treatment of chronic neck pain. Cervical disc herniation, radiculopathy, discogenic pain, and zygapophysial joints (discussed later) are commonly accepted sources of pain.[77,78]

PATHOPHYSIOLOGIC FINDINGS

As a consequence of aging, the vascular supply to the disk is diminished, resulting in disk degeneration. The annulus dehydrates, leading to approximation of the vertebrae. These changes, which can lead to disk bulging, glycoprotein leakage, inflammation, and fibrosis, may be related

TABLE 37-7 Symptoms of Cervical Spondylosis

Symptoms	Incidence
Headache, brachial radiculopathy	30%
Vertigo, myelopathy, neck pain	15%
Vertebral-basilar insufficiency Loss of consciousness "Drop Attacks"	5%

to phospholipase A_2 activity.[79] Cervical intervertebral discs can produce metalloproteinases, nitric oxide, prostaglandin E2, and interleukin-6, which can all cause inflammation at the level of the segmental spinal nerve.[80] Ultimately, this process can result in calcification and osteophyte formation. The resultant bone formation can lead to narrowing of the spinal canal, with subsequent cord compression or narrowing of the intervertebral foramina, resulting in nerve root compression. Cervical radiculopathy is most commonly (up to 75%) a result of combined degenerative changes of discs, uncovertebral joints, and zygapophysial joints.[81] Thus, radiculitis as a result from stenosis and/or nerve irritation, disc herniation, internal disc disruption (discogenic pain), and zygapophysial joints can result in axial neck pain. The exact mechanisms remain elusive to this date.

The nerve roots most often involved in spondylo-radiculopathy are C6 and C7 because of the increased mobility, angulation, and degeneration that can occur in the midcervical region.[81] Presenting symptoms in patients with radiographic evidence of cervical spondylosis are summarized in **Table 37-7.**[82] In the chronic phase, cervical radiculopathy can persist because of a combination of chronic inflammation, mechanical stenosis, or neuroplasticity, perpetuating a neuropathic pain state.

AXIAL NECK PAIN

Neck pain from cervical disc degeneration can be classified into two distinct subtypes: radicular pain and cervical internal disc disruption. In the majority of cases involving the cervical root, pain is caused by acute intermittent nerve irritation, generally as a result of nerve impingement in narrowed intervertebral foramen.[83] The pain may occur insidiously, as in cervical spondylosis, but can be precipitated or exacerbated by minor trauma. Alternatively, more acute severe neck pain may occur with a herniated cervical intervertebral disk in the setting of a degenerated spondylitic spine. The neck pain often is poorly localized, worsens with movement, and is associated with muscular spasm.[76] Ill-defined intrascapular pain with muscle spasm and tenderness as a result of anterior disk disease rather than nerve root irritation has been described for quite some time.[76,84] The pain pattern is indistinguishable from zygapophysial pain clinically. Although the C2/3 disc is thought to refer pain primarily into the occiput, recent disc stimulation mapping demonstrates discs as low as C6/7 can refer pain suboccipitally with referral down the arms, so as to mimic radicular pain.[85,86] Interestingly, pain in the neck, trapezius, and interscapular region were common pain referral patterns for C3/4 to C6/7 discal levels. This pain can occur months or years before evidence of root entrapment is seen.

Cervical spine x-rays and a CT or MRI scan of the neck are helpful in excluding other causes of neck pain, including primary osteomyelitis, tuberculous osteitis, malignancy, and retropharyngeal abscess.[4,87] Bone scans also are helpful in the evaluation of infectious causes of neck pain. However, all radiographic modalities are incapable identifying a degenerative disc as painful; furthermore, there is a lack of correlation between disc morphology on MRI and pain. Chronic cervical pain from discs is thought to range in prevalence from 16% to 41%. Cervical discography remains a valuable tool to determine the presence of cervical discogenic pain when there is a lack of disc herniation or radiculitis.[88] To reduce the false positives from a disc stimulation study, authors have proposed that cervical zygapophysial joint pain be excluded first, that four discs be evaluated at a minimum during a provocation study, and that the positive disc replicates the patient's pain with an intensity of at least 7 on a 10-point visual analogue or equivalent scale.[4] A final note is that it is critical that adjacent discs fail to reproduce the patient's pain in order for a study to determine the presence of discogenic pain.

CERVICAL RADICULOPATHY

There are no universally accepted criteria for diagnosis, but the following symptoms and exam findings are thought to be sufficient. The symptom of cervical nerve root impingement at the level of the intervertebral foremen usually is shooting or burning pain, originating in the posterior neck, with radiation across the shoulder and down the outer arm to the elbow or hand.[89] Persistent nerve root impingement leads to a characteristic sensory loss (hypesthesia or anesthesia), motor loss (weakness or atrophy), and diminished reflexes. Radicular pain is sometimes the only presenting symptom.[81] Patients may not recognize the associated mild triceps weakness because of compensation. They may first become aware of this weakness during the neurologic examination.

An acute protruded disk is associated with more severe pain, occurring acutely after trauma or violent moment, with symptoms radiating down the arm. Neurologic deficits soon appear. Other conditions that may produce symptoms similar to brachial radiculopathy include myofascial pain syndrome, apical lung tumors (Pancoast), and shoulder disorders (including capsulitis, rotator cuff injuries, bursitis, and thoracic outlet compression of the brachial plexus nerves or subclavian artery). Imaging studies such as a cervical CT or MRI scan may demonstrate significant disk herniation and nerve root impingement because of foraminal narrowing. Nerve conduction studies can help distinguish a radiculopathy from plexopathies as well as distal neuropathies. Many elderly patients have some degree of spondylosis and degenerative disk disease, and these findings are not necessarily the cause of the symptoms. One study evaluated the MRI findings in asymptomatic patients.[90] This study revealed that the prevalence of degenerative disc disease was approximately equal to the patient's age in years. That is, a 65-year-old patient has a 65% chance of having degenerative disc disease. The prevalence of a bulging disk was approximately one-half of this percentage, and the finding of spinal stenosis was approximately one-third.

CERVICAL MYELOPATHY

Cervical myelopathy can be a result of compression of the spinal cord by ligaments or protruded disks, trauma, radiation therapy, or compromise of the blood supply. If compression originates anteriorly by an osteophyte or a central disk protrusion, a predominately motor deficit is seen. However, posterior compression from a hypertrophied ligament causes dorsal column dysfunction and sensory loss. The limited mobility of the spinal cord in the cervical area associated with cervical spondylosis magnifies the effect of movement because it contributes to spinal cord compression. Spinal cord compression often is painless, although, in the early stages, the patient may complain of foot numbness and an unsteady gait.[76] It is essential to perform a thorough neurologic examination to identify lower motor deficits of the upper extremities and associated long tract signs affecting the lower extremities.

Other disorders that may mimic cervical spondylitic myelopathy include dorsal column loss from subacute combined degenerative disease (e.g., vitamin B_{12} deficiency), multiple sclerosis (although, often, other evidence of CNS plaques and deficits are present), motor neuron disease (e.g., amyotrophic lateral sclerosis), and syringomyelia.[76] Other causes of cord compression (including spinal cord tumors, metastatic disease, infectious processes, and Arnold-Chiari syndrome) can be excluded by more specific radiographic investigations. Progressive neurologic deficit or signs of cord compression are indications for the patient to undergo spinal myelography, MRI or CT scanning, or evaluation by an orthopedist or neurosurgeon.

A patient with neck pain or cervical radicular symptoms of less than 2 to 4 weeks' duration and with a normal neurologic examination and insignificant radiographic abnormalities may be treated conservatively. Treatment includes a soft collar for up to 2 weeks, NSAIDs, analgesics, and possibly traction. Cervical traction appears to aggravate symptoms in approximately 10% of patients.[91] Any myofascial pain syndrome is treated as mentioned previously.

For symptoms greater than 4 weeks in duration, conservative management includes cervical isometric exercises to increase cervical muscle strength.[92] In addition, TENS, tricyclic antidepressants (TCAs), anticonvulsants (gabapentin, clonazepam), muscle relaxants (baclofen, tizanidine), and local heat or ice can be used. Other conservative approaches to cervical discogenic pain with or without associated radicular pain such as patient education ("neck school"), stress reduction, traction, and heat remain as anecdotal.[93,94]

In a systematic review, cervical epidural corticosteroid injections (CESIs) were determined to be effective for chronic neck pain and cervical radicular symptoms.[95] Indications for injection include cervical spinal stenosis, degenerative disc pain, and radiculopathy.[96-98] The interlaminar approach for CESI has proven to be relatively safe.[99] Minor complications resolve rapidly and include increased neck pain, headache, and vasovagal reactions. Major complications involving neurological injury to the nerve roots and spinal cord are, fortunately, rare. This is in contrast to the transforaminal approach, which is considered to pose a greater probability of neurological injury via introduction of particulate steroid into deep cervical arteries that supply the spinal cord.[100] Nonetheless, there have been case reports of intrinsic cervical cord damage after interlaminar CESI in sedated patients.[101] It may be prudent to perform these injections with a responsive patient so any spinal cord irritation can be detected prior to injection. Finally, for patients with chronic cervical radicular pain, both pulsed and conventional radiofrequency treatments of the cervical dorsal root ganglion (DRG) have been advocated.[102] Though multiple clinical trials support the safety and efficacy of radiofrequency treatments of the cervical DRG, this mode of treatment is less commonly practiced in the United States because of reimbursement issues.

Surgery usually is reserved for progressive neurologic deficits or signs of cord compression. Minor neurologic deficits that do not seem to interfere with function can be managed nonsurgically. Neurologic deficits that interfere with important functions should be managed surgically.[92] Prospective observational data following patients for 2 years demonstrate that 75% of patients have marked improvement in pain and numbness as well as a lessening of weakness.[83] Lastly, patients with inadequate response to surgery and chronic refractory symptoms may respond to spinal cord stimulation, but large prospective trials validating this approach in chronic cervical radiculopathy are lacking.[103,104]

OCCIPITAL NEURALGIA

Cervicogenic headache may result from occipital neuralgia. The greater occipital nerve arises from the posterior primary ramus of C2 and C3 and supplies the skin overlying the occiput and scalp. The splenius capitis inferior syndrome is a form of greater occipital neuralgia secondary to a myofascial pain syndrome involving that muscle. Chronic spasm may cause inflammation or direct compression of the nerve. Typically, the pain is in the sensory fields of the greater and or lesser occipital nerves. Paroxysmal sharp shooting pain may become continuous. Degenerative atlanto-occipital disorders must be excluded radiographically. One author suggests that, in children, suboccipital neuralgia must be investigated by a pediatric neurologist or neurosurgeon.[76] Additional known causes include trauma and tumors, but in the vast majority of occipital neuralgia cases, the cause is unknown.

Diagnosis The International Headache Society (IHS) has defined occipital neuralgia as paroxysms of sharp shooting pain in the territories of the greater or lesser occipital nerves.[105] Palpation of the greater occipital nerve often reveals tenderness and may reproduce the patient's symptoms. Dysesthesias or hypesthesias can also be present in some patients. Finally, temporary improvement of symptoms following a local anesthetic block of the greater or lesser occipital nerve(s) can further support the diagnosis. Radiographic imaging of the craniocervical junction by MRI is performed to exclude neoplasm or severe cervical spine degeneration.[106]

Treatment Conservative treatment may include the following measures: NSAIDs, TCAs, muscle relaxants, antiepileptic drugs, physical therapy, and massage therapy. The efficacy of conservative management has not been formally evaluated in prospective randomized controlled trials. More commonly greater/lesser occipital nerve blocks are usually performed using bupivacaine 0.25% (2–5 ml) with or without a corticosteroid. Several small studies indicate that, for most patients, the effect is short lived.[107,108] Botulinum toxin infiltration has yielded mixed results but may render greater than 50% reduction on the visual analog scale for up to 4 months.[109,110]

Neuromodulation using either pulsed radiofrequency or implanted occipital nerve stimulators is evolving as a potential treatment option for patients with recalcitrant occipital neuralgia. Pulsed radiofrequency (PRF), which is an isothermal nondestructive form of radiofrequency, seems to offer appreciable relief for up to 4 months.[111] In a prospective observational trial, PRF was applied to the peripheral nerves in patients with occipital neuralgia; 68.4%, 57.9%, and 52.6% reported at least 50% improvement in pain intensity at 1, 2, and 6 months post-PRF treatment, respectively.[112] Patients who cease to respond or fail to derive appreciable benefit from the preceding modalities may be candidates for occipital nerve stimulation (ONS). The effectiveness of this therapy has been described for more than 15 years in the form of both small prospective and retrospective observational trials in multiple centers around the world.[113] Outcomes have tended to be very favorable in terms of reduced headache frequency, intensity, duration, and medication consumption. So far, no major complications have been reported but lead displacement tended to be by far the most common adverse event followed by an occasional infection.

Resistant cases have been treated by neuroablative procedures but have fallen out of favor or been used as a very last resort because of short-term effects, potential for deafferentation pain, and neuritis. A neurolytic greater occipital nerve block with phenol can be performed. Alternatively, radiofrequency thermocoagulation or cryoablation of the greater occipital nerve can be performed. The analgesic effects of all three ablative modalities are limited in duration to 3 to 6 months. Neuritis is a complication of all procedures (least with cryoablation); skin irritation and skin sloughing have occurred only with phenol. Surgical treatment includes greater occipital neurectomy or a C2-to-C3 rhizotomy. Postoperative neuritis appears to be more common after surgery than with neuroablative percutaneous procedures.

CERVICAL FACET JOINT SYNDROME

Cervical facet joint, or zygapophyseal, syndrome can cause both local and radicular symptoms that often are indistinguishable from cervical disk disease.[114,115] Often, cervical facet and disk disorders, leading to cervical pain, occur together. The radiating pain from facets rarely passes the shoulder level, however.

Each posterior facet joint has a dual nerve supply, with one branch arising from the posterior primary ramus at the same level and the other from the posterior primary ramus from above. Therefore, to block the C4-to-C5 facet joint, for example, the nerves from C4 and C5 must be blocked. Acute facet joint irritation may occur from local trauma or excessive movement. More commonly, facet joint irritation arises from chronic changes of facet joint thickening and hypertrophy initiated by disk degeneration, trauma, or excessive load-bearing stress.[114] The low and middle cervical levels (C4 to C7) are most commonly affected.

Upper cervical facet joint degeneration (most commonly C2/3) with muscle spasm may be responsible for symptoms of upper neck pain, with radiation to the occipital region and ipsilateral frontal area.[115] Occipital and vascular headaches may also coexist with facet arthropathy.[8] Low cervical facet pain may coexist with radicular symptoms to the shoulder and arms and may be caused by discogenic nerve root irritation. The degeneration and consequent hypertrophy of the facet joint may also contribute to radiculitis. It is important to remember that facet joint disease—in particular, at the C5/6 and C6/7—may produce axial neck pain and/or radicular symptoms.[115] The absence of neurologic symptoms and pain on the dorsolateral aspect of the neck increases the suspicion for cervical facet disease. Unlike in the lumbar spine, cervical facet pain may account for up to 50% of chronic axial neck pain presenting to pain clinics.[116]

Diagnosis Extension and rotation of the neck stresses the facet joints and exacerbates symptoms. Specifically, rotation after flexion of the neck assesses the range of motion of the upper facet joints. Rotation after positioning the neck in extension evaluates the lower facet joints. Facet joint tenderness may be seen with palpation 3 to 4 cm laterally from the midline. While local pressure on the facets is felt to favorably predict radiofrequency treatments, of itself it has no diagnostic value.[117,118] As discussed previously with degenerative disc disease, many patients have at CT- or MRI-documented abnormality involving the cervical spine up to 75% by age 70.[119] Radiographic findings (x-rays of the cervical spine, CT, MRI) often reveal degenerative changes of the facet joint (hypertrophy and thickening). In many cases, these are incidental findings and cannot establish the presence or absence of cervical zygapophysial pain.

Presently, the only method to establish the diagnosis of cervical facet pain is using comparative cervical medial branch blocks. These blocks have been validated for diagnostic purposes in chronic neck pain.[120] Evidence from properly conducted randomized control trials utilizing controlled comparative blocks has demonstrated a sensitivity of 86% and a specificity of 65%.[121,122] There remains no consensus on the definition of a positive block. The accepted minimum degree of pain intensity reduction is 50%, which is considered positive in a recent review.[123] Reducing cervical medial branch block volume to as little as 0.25 ml may improve diagnostic accuracy.[124]

Treatment The initial therapy is conservative. Similar to facet syndrome in the lumbar region, patients often respond to NSAIDs, TCAs, physical therapy, TENS, and exercises to strengthen the cervical musculature. For patients who are unsuccessfully managed by conservative measures, interventional approaches consist of intra-articular steroid injections, local infiltration of the medial branches, and radiofrequency treatment of the medial branches. There remains a paucity of literature on the therapeutic value of intra-articular facet joint injections.[122] Therefore, no significant conclusions can be drawn on the safety, effectiveness, and predictive value for radiofrequency therapy.

In contrast, blockade of the medial branches supplying the cervical facet joint—in addition to being a diagnostic aid—can offer therapeutic value. Patients who derive at least 80% pain reduction on the first medial branch block are likely to respond well to serial blocks (pain relief >50%) for up to 16 weeks.[125] In this well-designed randomized control trial, the effect of medial branch blocks with bupivacaine alone was compared with bupivacaine and steroid. The safety and efficacy was equal in both groups. Finally, any infectious and neurological complications are thought to be rare.

Multiple observational studies support the effectiveness of radiofrequency (RF) lesioning of the cervical medial branches for degenerative cervical facet pain.[117,126,127] The RF denervation procedure is well tolerated, and occasional short-lived burning with associated numbness may present postprocedure and dissipate after 3 to 6 weeks. There are no data on the incidence of complications following RF of cervical facets, but the clinical impression is that the procedure is felt to be safe. One retrospective study determined that the mean duration of relief is 12.5 months following the cervical facet RF denervation and that up to 90% of patients respond to serial treatments (up to six additional interventions) with the duration of analgesic response ranging from 8 to 12 months.[128] Finally, if RF should not render relief for chronic degenerative cervical facet pain, it remains unclear what the long-term outcomes are from anterior cervical discectomy and fusion or from other ablative modalities such as cryoanalgesia.

THORACIC OUTLET SYNDROME

ANATOMY

Compression of the neurovascular bundle in the area of the cervical thoracic dorsal outlet can produce symptoms that mimic the neck pain and extremity dysesthesia and numbness found in cervical radiculopathy. Thoracis outlet syndrome (TOS) should be suspected in the patient who has cervical pain and associated extremity symptoms, which may be reproduced by appropriate positioning of the arms and neck. In most scenarios, TOS is a controversial clinical entity without uniform diagnostic or treatment strategies.[129] Therefore, it is absolutely necessary to exclude other causes, including cervical disk disease, degenerative joint disease, cervical facet joint arthropathy, carpal tunnel syndrome, multiple sclerosis, nerve sheath tumor, ulnar nerve entrapment, syrinx, Raynaud's, rotator cuff injuries, coronary artery disease, and complex regional pain syndrome. Disorders of the apical thorax—including Pancoast's tumor, subclavian artery aneurysm, or other supraclavicular fossa or axillary disease—also may mimic compression syndromes.

The brachial plexus is formed by the anterior primary rami of C5, C6, C7, C8, and T1. These roots emerge from the intervertebral foramina and become sandwiched between the scalenus anticus and medius. At this point, the roots unite to form three trunks: an upper trunk (C5 and C6), a middle trunk (C7), and a lower trunk (C8 to T1). The three trunks are grouped closely and emerge laterally and between the anterior and middle scalene muscles and across the first rib to pass through the interscalene triangle. At the lateral portion of the first rib and posterior to the clavicle, each trunk separates into an anterior and posterior division. These six divisions descend into the axilla.

In the apex of the axilla, the divisions join to form three cords. Grouped around the axillary artery are (1) the lateral cord, composed of the anterior division of the upper (CS to C6) and middle (C7) trunk; (2) the medial cord, a continuation of the anterior division of the lower trunk (C8 to T1); and (3) the posterior cord, the posterior division of all three trunks (upper, middle, and lower). Behind the pectoralis minor, the cords orient around the axillary artery according to their names. They continue and form the peripheral nerves and branches of the upper extremity. The lateral and medial cords comprise the median nerve, the medial cord gives rise to the ulnar nerve, and the posterior cord becomes the radial nerve.

The subclavian artery arches over the first rib and joins the brachial plexus immediately behind where the anterior scalenus inserts into the first rib. The subclavian vein runs over the first rib, but usually it is anterior to the anterior scalenus muscle.

The sites of irritation/compression are summarized in **Table 37-8**. The vast majority of cases of TOS are thought to involve neural and or vascular structures within the interscalene triangle.[130] Each site of potential impingement has been described as a syndrome, but all are presently labeled as TOS.

Furthermore, TOS itself can be subdivided into three categories: (1) neurogenic TOS in which there is actual compression of the brachial plexus; (2) vascular TOS with compression of the subclavian artery or vein; and (3) nonspecific or disputed TOS, which is a chronic pain syndrome that is thought to involve the brachial plexus. Nonspecific TOS is, by far, the most common and usually follows a whiplash injury, repetitive work injury, or neck trauma, or it lacks a precipitating cause. The main anatomic factors associated with nonspecific TOS are anomalous cervical bands, congenital narrow scalene triangle, and fibrosis of the scalene muscles.[131]

TABLE 37-8 Sites of Compression of the Brachial Plexus in Thoracic Outlet Syndrome

Anatomic Space	Syndrome (presently all syndromes are bundled under thoracic outlet syndrome)
Interscalene triangle formed by the scalenus anticus and medius, and the first rib	Anterior scalene syndrome
Clavicle and first rib	Costoclavicular syndrome
Pectoralis minor and rib cage	Pectoralis minor or hyperabduction syndrome

DIAGNOSIS

Neurovascular entrapment at the level of the anterior scalene may involve the nerve and artery and possibly the vein or lymphatic vessels. Vascular TOS is felt to be rare, but is easy to suspect. Venous TOS can be acute or chronic and is often associated with thrombosis of the subclavian/axillary vein. Hand edema and finger stiffness may be present because the subclavian vein is compressed between the first rib and clavicle secondary to a taut anterior scalene.[132] In arterial TOS, an elongated C7 transverse process narrows the subclavian artery, and there can be associated thrombosis. This entity is suspected with ischemia to the hand. The diagnosis is reached with a combination of duplex ultrasonography, magnetic resonance arteriography, and CT angiography.[130]

Most often, irritation of the brachial plexus is felt to occur with symptoms of numbness, tingling, and hypesthesia in the arms and hands, chiefly in the ulnar distribution. The pain is often dull and aching in quality and may include the neck, shoulders, arm, or hand. Symptoms may occur during the early morning, awakening the patient from sleep, or after prolonged activity using the hands. They occur primarily in young to middle-aged women. It is very rare for symptoms to progress to actual severe sensory and motor deficits involving the median- and ulnar-innervated forearm and intrinsic hand muscles. The diagnosis of true neurogenic TOS is supported by nerve conduction/electromyographic studies, cervical MRI, and x-rays. The cervical x-rays invariably reveal an elongated C7 transverse process often referred to as a rudimentary cervical rib, which compresses the brachial plexus.

By contrast, nonspecific/disputed (sometimes confusingly referred to as neurogenic) TOS lacks objective findings. These patients may have mild hypesthesia to light touch and pinprick, although other findings often are absent. Maneuvers that are used to stress the brachial plexus exacerbate the pain. The Addison test (tensing the scalenus and elevating the first rib) reproduces the patient's symptoms. This test is performed with the examiner abducting and extending the involved arm while monitoring the radial pulse. The patient faces the involved side, extends the neck, and takes a deep breath. Reproduction of the symptoms and obliteration of the pulse constitute a positive result. Normal subjects may have obliteration of the radial pulse with this maneuver, but they do not have the characteristic symptoms; therefore, the test is unreliable with low sensitivity and specificity.[133] Finally, diagnostic studies including nerve conduction studies, duplex ultrasonography of the subclavian vessels, MRI (cervical brachial plexus), and cervical x-rays are normal.[130]

Spasm of the anterior scalene muscle (myofascial syndrome) generally is believed to be the most likely cause. One histologic study suggests that fibrosis of the scalene muscles causes compression/irritation of the brachial plexus.[134] Scalene muscle injections have been reported to confirm the diagnosis of TOS independent of whether the brachial plexus is anesthetized or not.[135] The injection is done with 2 to 3 ml of local anesthetic blindly or with the aid of ultrasound, EMG, or CT.[135-137] The optimal volume of injection is not known, and the degree of relief is generally accepted as a 50% reduction in pain intensity or better.

TREATMENT

Because of the controversial nature of TOS, conservative treatment is the basis of the majority of cases regardless of the etiology. It commonly consists of a soft collar and strengthening, stretching, and posture exercises to decrease the cervical lordosis and increase shoulder girdle strength. There is general agreement in the literature that both vascular and true neurogenic TOS should be treated surgically if conservative measures fail. The supraclavicular approach is favored whereby any cervical rib, congenital bands, and the first rib may be resected.[130] Long-term follow-up documents alleviation of pain, stabilization of neurologic symptoms, but persistence of deficits.[138]

The interventional treatment for disputed TOS is less clear. The anterior scalene muscle and associated trigger points may be injected with a local anesthetic with or without corticosteroid to diminish spasms and relax trigger points. Without adjuvant therapies, local anesthetic injections in chronic are likely short-lived relief.[135] Botulinum toxin has emerged recently as a minimally invasive option for some patients, rendering symptomatic relief for 3 to 4 months.[137,139] Finally, refractory cases treated with scalenectomy and first rib resection report 90% success rates.[140] However, complication rates range from 1% to 30%.[141] Thus, the optimal management of disputed TOS remains elusive.

SUMMARY

The causes of neck pain are many and varied. They may be self-limited, requiring little intervention, or life-threatening, requiring immediate invasive action. A working knowledge of the anatomy of the neck is invaluable to the clinician who diagnoses and treats painful cervical conditions. Although the neck may be the source of the patient's pathology, symptoms may involve the neck, head, shoulder, or upper extremities. A thorough history and physical examination—along with carefully chosen ancillary studies (radiographs, CT, MRI, electromyography, nerve conduction velocities, bone scan)—often can identify serious causes of neck pain. The source of chronic neck pain may not always be determined, and, likewise, the optimal treatment may not be feasible in all cases.

REFERENCES

1. Radavov BP, Sturzenegger M, Di Stefano G. Long-term outcome after whiplash injury: a two-year follow up considering features of injury mechanism and somatic, radiologic, and psychosocial findings. *Medicine*. 1995;74:281-297.
2. Gore DR, Sepic SB, Gardner GM, Murray MP. Neck pain: a long-term follow-up of 205 patients. *Spine*. 1987;12:1-5.
3. Merskey H, Bogduk N, eds. *Classification of Chronic Pain. Descriptions of Chronic Pain Syndromes and Definitions of Pain Terms*. 2nd ed. Seattle, Wash: IASP Press; 1994:11.
4. Bogduk N, McGuirk B. Sources and causes of neck pain. In: *Management of Acute and Chronic Neck Pain: An Evidence Based Approach*. Philadelphia, Pa: Elsevier; 2006:10.
5. Roseman DM. Carotidynia: A distinct syndrome. *Arch Otolaryngol*. 1967;85:81-84.
6. Rose VP, Veach JS, Tehranzdeh J. Spontaneous pseudomediatinum as a cause of neck pain, dysphagia, and chest pain. *Arch Intern Med*. 1984;144:392-393.
7. March JS. Rheumatoid neck. *Br J Med*. 1985;33:96-100.
8. Sluijter ME, Koetsveld-Baart CC. Interruption of pain pathways in the treatment of the cervical syndrome. *Anaesthesia*. 1980;35:302-307.
9. Ehni G, Benner B. Occipital neuralgia and the C1-2 arthrosis syndrome. *J Neurosurg*. 1984;61:961-965.
10. Travell JG, Simons DG. *Myofascial Pain and Dysfunction. The Trigger Point Manual*. Vol 1. Baltimore, Md: Williams & Wilkins; 1983.
11. Bernstein SA. Acute cervical pain associated with soft tissue calcium deposition anterior to the interspace of the first and second cervical vertebrae. *J Bone Joint Surg*. 1975.
12. Van der donk J, Schouten JSAG, Passchier J, van Romunde LKJ, Valkenburg HA. The associations of neck pain with radiological abnormalities of the cervical spine and personality traits in the general population. *J Rheumatol*. 1991;18:1884-1889.
13. Borghouts JAJ, Koes BW, Bounter LM. The clinical course and prognostic factors of non-specific neck pain: a systematic review. *Pain*. 1998;77:1-13.
14. Berglund A, Alfredsson L, Cassidy JD, Jensen I, Nygren A. The association between exposure to a rear-end collision and future neck or shoulder pain: a cohort study. *J Clin Epidemiol*. 2000;35:1089-1094.
15. Kamwendo K, Linton SJ, Moritz, U. Neck and shoulder pain disorders in medical secretaries. Part II. Ergonomical work environment and symptom profile. *Scand J Rehab Med*. 1991;23:135-142.
16. Cote P, Cassidy JD, Carroll L. The factors associated with neck pain and its related disability in the Saskatchewan population. *Spine*. 2000;25:1109-1117.
17. Sterling M, Jull G, Vicenzino B, Kennedy J, Darnell R. Physical and psychological factors predict outcome following whiplash injury. *Pain*. 2005;21:141-148.
18. Cassidy JK, Carrol LJ, Cote P, Lemstra M, Berglund A, Nygren A. Effect of eliminating compensation for pain and suffering on the outcome of insurance claims for whiplash injury. *New Engl J Med*. 2000;342:1179-1186.
19. Viikari-Juntura E, Porras M, Laasonen EM. Validity of clinical tests in the diagnosis of root compression in cervical disease. *Spine*. 1989;14:253.
20. Uchihara T, Furukawa J. Compression of brachial plexus a diagnostic test of cervical cord lesion. *Spine*. 1994;19:2170.
21. Spitzer WO, Skovron MI, Salmi IR, et al. Scientific monograph of the Quebec Task Force on whiplash-associated disorders: redefining "whiplash" and its management. *Spine*. 1995;20:1S-73S.
22. Halderman S, Carroll L, Cassidy JD, et al. The bone and joint decade 2000-2010 task force on neck pain and its associated disorders: executive summary. *Spine*. 2008;33:S5-S7.
23. Ellis H, Feldman S. *Anatomy for the Anaesthetist*. Boston, Mass: Blackwell Scientific Publications; 1983:164-170.
24. Bogduk N, Lord SM. Cervical spine disorders. *Curr Opin Rheumatol*. 1998;10:110-115.
25. MacNab I. The whiplash syndrome in symposium on disease of the intervertebral disk. *Orthop Clin North Am*. 1971;2:389-403.
26. Hohl M. Soft issue injuries of the neck in automobile accidents. *J Bone Joint Surg Am*. 1974;56:1675-1681.
27. McConnel WE, Howard RP, Guzman HM, et al. Analysis of human test subject kinematic responses to low velocity rear end impacts. Proceedings of the 37th Stapp Car Crash Conference, San Antonio, Tex, 1993:21-30.
28. Panjabi MM, Pearson AM, Ito S, Ivancic PC, Wang JL. Cervical spine curvature during simulated whiplash. *Clin Biomech*. 2004;19:1-9.
29. Taylor JR, Taylor MM. Cervical spine injuries: an autopsy study of 109 blunt injuries. *J Musculoskelet Pain*. 1996;4:61-79.
30. Krakenes J, Kacile BR. Magnetic resonance imaging assessment of craniovertebral ligaments and membranes after whiplash trauma. *Spine*. 2006;31(24):2820-2826.
31. Silverman JL, Rodrigues AA, Agre Jc. Quantitiative cervical flexor strength in health subjects and in subjects with mechanical neck pain. *Arch Phys Med Rehabil*. 1991;72:679-681.
32. Hohl M. Soft issue injuries of the neck in automobile accidents. *J Bone Joint Surg Am*. 1974;56:1675-1681.
33. Iida H, Tachibana S, Kitahara T, et al. Association of head trauma with cervical spine injury, spinal cord injury, or both. *J Trauma*. 1999;46:450-452.
34. Lord SM, Barnsley L, Wallis BJ, Bogduk N. Third occipital headache: a prevalence study. *J Neurol Neurosurg Psychiat*. 1994;57(10):1187-1190.

35. Nordemar R, Thorner C. Treatment of acute cervical pain-comparative group study. *Pain*. 1981;10:93-101.
36. Cloward R. Acute cervical spine injuries. *Clin Symp*. 1980;32:4.
37. Barnsley L, Lord S, Bogduk N. Whiplash injury. *Pain*. 1994;58: 283-307.
38. McKay DC, Christensen LV. Whiplash injuries of the temporomandibular joint in motor vehicle accidents: speculations and facts. *J Oral Rehabil*. 1998;25:731-746.
39. Wallis BJ, Lord SM, Bogduk N. Resolution of psychological distress of whiplash patients following treatment by radiofrequency neurotomy: a randomized, double-blind, placebo-controlled trial. *Pain*. 1997;73:15-22.
40. Nordemar R, Thorner C. Treatment of acute cervical pain-comparative group study. *Pain*. 1981;10:93-101.
41. Iida H, Tachibana S, Kitahara T, et al. Association of head trauma with cervical spine injury, spinal cord injury, or both. *J Trauma*. 1999;46:450-452.
42. Gotten N. Survey of 100 cases of whiplash injury after settlement of litigation. *JAMA*. 1956;162:865-867.
43. Harris JH Jr. Radiographic evaluation of spinal trauma. *Orthop Clin North Am*. 1986;17:75-86.
44. Suijlekom HV, Mekhail N, Patel N, Van Zundert J, Van Kleef, M, Patijn J. Whiplash-associated disorders. *Pain Prac*. 2010;10(2): 131-136.
45. Barnsley L, Lord SM, Wallis BJ, et al. Lack of effect of intraarticular corticosteroid for chronic pain in the cervical zygapophysial joints. *N Eng J Med*. 1994;3(30):1047-1050.
46. Esenyel M, Caglar N, Aldemir T. Treatment of myofascial pain. *Am J Phys Med Rehabil*. 2000;79:48-52.
47. Wheeler AH, Goolkasian P, Gretz SS. Botulinum toxin A for the treatment of chronic neck pain. *Pain*. 2001;94:255-260.
48. Lord SM, Barnsley L, Wallis BJ. Percutaneous radiofrequency neurotomy in the treatment of cervical zygapophysial joint pain. *N Eng J Med*. 1996;335:1727-1726.
49. Prushansky T, Pevzner E, Gordon C, et al. Cervical radiofrequency neurotomy in patient with chronic whiplash: a study of multiple outcome measures. *J Neurosurgery*. 2006;4:365-373.
50. McDonald GJ, Lord SM, Bogduk N. Long-term follow-up of patients treated with cervical radiofrequency neurotomy for chronic neck pain. *Neurosurgery*. 1999;45:61-67.
51. Bogduk N, April C. On the nature of neck pain, discography, and cervical zygapophysial joints. *Pain*. 1993;54:213-217.
52. Yin W, Bogduk N. The nature of neck pain in a private clinic in the United States. *Pain Med*. 2008;9(2):196-203.
53. Garvey T, Transfeldt EE, Malcolm JR, Kos P. Outcome of anterior discectomy and fusion as perceived by patients treated for dominant axial mechanical cervical spine pain. *Spine*. 2002;27(17):1887-1895.
54. Simons DG, Travell JG, Simons LS. *Travell & Simmons' Myofascial Pain and Dysfunction: The Trigger Point Manual, Vol. I, Upper Half of Body*. Baltimore, Md: Williams & Wilkins; 1999.
55. Cloward R. Acute cervical spine injuries. *Clin Symp*. 1980;32:4.
56. Tough E, White AR, Richards S, Campbell J. Variability of criteria used to diagnose myofascial trigger point pain syndrome-evidence from a review of the literature. *Clin J Pain*. 2007;23(3):278-286.
57. Borg-Stein J, Simons DG. Myofascial pain. *Arch Phys Med Rehab*. 2002;83:S40-S47.
58. Wolfe F, Zhao S, Lane N. Preference for nonsteroidal anti-inflammatory drugs over acetaminophen by rheumatic disease patients: a survey of 1799 patients with osteoarthritis, rheumatoid arthritis, and fibromyalgia. *Arthritis Rheum*. 2000;43:378-385.
59. Bendtsen L, Jensen R. Amitriptyline reduces myofascial tenderness in patients with chronic tension-type headache. *Cephalalgia*. 2000; 20:603-610.
60. Arnold LM, Lu Y, Crofford LJ, et al. A double-blind, multicenter trial comparing duloxetine with placebo in the treatment of fibromyalgia patients with or without major depressive disorder. *Arthritis Rheum*. 2004;50(9):2974–2984.
61. Offenbaecher M, Ackenheil M. Current trends in neuropathic pain treatments with special reference to fibromyalgia. *CNS Spectr*. 2005;10(4):285–297.
62. Crofford LJ, Rowbotham MC, Mease PJ, et al. Pregabalin for the treatment of fibromyalgia syndrome: results of a randomized, double-blind, placebo-controlled trial. *Arthritis Rheum*. 2005;52(4): 1264–1273.
63. Cohen SP, Mullings R, Abdi S. The pharmacologic treatment of muscle pain. *Anesthesiology*. 2004;101:495-526.
64. Malanga GA, Gwynn MW, Smith R, Miller D. Tizanidine is effective in the treatment of myofascial pain syndrome. *Pain Phys*. 2002;5(4):422-432.
65. Scott NA, Guo B, Barton PM, Gerwin RD. Trigger-point injections for non-malignant pain musculoskeletal pain: a systematic review. *Pain Med*. 2009;10(1):54-69.
66. Jeynes LC, Gauci CA. Evidence for the use of botulinum toxin in the chronic pain setting: a review of the literature. *Pain Prac*. 2008;8(4):269-276.
67. Foley-Nolan D, Barry C, Coughlan RJ, O'Conner P, Roden D. Pulsed high frequency (27MJz) electromagnetic therapy for persistent neck pain: a double blind, placebo-controlled study of 20 patients. *Orthopedics*. 1990;13:445-451.
68. Maxwell R. Surgical management of torticollis. *Postgrad Med*. 1984;75:147-155.
69. Albanese A, Barnes MP, Bhatia KP, Fernandez-Alvarez E, Filippini G, Gasser T, et al. A systematic review on the diagnosis and treatment of primary (idiopathic) dystonia and dystonia plus syndromes: report of an EFNS/MDS-ES task force. *Eur J Neurol*. 2006;13:433-444.
70. Logroscino G, Liverea P, Anaclerio D, Aniello MS, Benedetto G, Cazzato G, et al. Agreement among neurologists on the clinical diagnosis of dystonia at different body sites. *J Neurol, Neursurg, and Psych*. 2003;74:348-350.
71. Costa J, Borges A, Espirito-Santo C, Ferreira J, Coelho M, Moore P, et al. Botulinum toxin type A versus bot- ulinum toxin type B for cervical dystonia. *Cochrane Database Systems Review*. 2005;1: CD004314.
72. Bertrand CM. Selective peripheral denervation for spasmodic torticollis: surgical technique, results, and observations in 260 cases. *Surgical Neurology*. 1993;40:96-103
73. Maxwell R. Surgical management of torticollis. *Postgrad Med*. 1984;75:147-155.
74. Krause M, Fogel W, Kloss M, Rasche D, Volkmann J, Tronnier V. Pallidal stimulation for dystonia. *Neurosurgery*. 2004;55: 1361-1370.
75. Eltahawy HA, Saint-Cyr J, Poon YY, Moro E, Lang AE, Lozano AM. Pallidal deep brain stimulation in cervical dystonia: clinical outcome in four cases. *Can J Neurol Sci*. 2004;31:328-332.
76. Jeffries RV. Cervical spondylosis in persistent pain. In: Lipton S, ed. *Modern Methods of Treatment*. 2nd ed. New York, NY: Grune & Stratton; 1980:115.
77. Manchikanti L, Dunbar EE, Wargo BW, Shah RV, Derby R, Cohen SP. Systematic review of cervical discography as a diagnostic test for chronic spinal pain. *Pain Physician*. 2009;12:305-321.

78. Falco FJE, Erhart S, Wargo BW, et al. Systematic review of diagnostic utility and therapeutic effectiveness of cervical facet joint injections. *Pain Phys*. 2009;12:323-344.
79. Lee HM, Weinstein JN, Meller ST, et al. The role of steroids and their effects on phospholipase A2. An animal model of radiculopathy. *Spine*. 1998;23:1191-1196.
80. Kang JD, Georgescu HI, McIntyre-Larkin I, et al. Herniated cervical intervertebral discs spontaneously produce metalloproteinases, nitric oxide, interleukin-6 and prostaglandin E2. *Spine*. 1995;22: 2373-2375.
81. Cailliet R. *Neck and Arm Pain*. Philadelphia, Pa: FA Davis Co; 1981.
82. Brain L. Some unresolved problems of cervical spondylosis. *Br Med J*. 1963;1:771-777.
83. Carette S, Fehlings MG. Cervical radiculopathy. *N Eng J Med*. 2005;353:392-399.
84. Schellhas KP, Smith M, Gundry C, Pollei, SR. Cervical discogenic pain: prospective correlation of magnetic resonance imaging and discography in asymptomatic subjects and pain sufferers. *Spine*. 1996;21(3):300-311.
85. Grubb SA, Kelly CK. Cervical discography: clinical implications from 12 years experience. *Spine*. 2000;25(11):1382-1389.
86. Slipman CW, Plastaras C, Patel R, et al. Provocative cervical discography symptom mapping. *Spine J*. 2005;5:381-388.
87. Manchikanti L, Boswell MV, Singh V, et al. Comprehensive review of neurophysiologic basis and diagnostic interventions in managing chronic spinal pain. *Pain Phys*. 2009;12:E71-E121.
88. Manchikanti L, Dunbar EE, Wargo BW, Shah RV, Derby R, Cohen SP. Systematic review of cervical discography as a diagnostic test for chronic spinal pain. *Pain Phys*. 2009;12:305-321.
89. Kelsey JL, Githens PB, Walter SD, et al. An epidemiologic study of acute prolapsed cervical intervertebral disc. *J Bone Joint Surg Am*. 1984;66:907-914.
90. Matsumoto M, Fujimura Y, Suzuki N, et al. MRI of cervical intervertebral discs in asymptomatic sujects. *J Bone Joint Surg Br*. 1998;80:19-24.
91. Swezey RL, Swezey AM, Warner K. Efficacy of home cervical traction therapy. *Am J Physical Med Rehabil*. 1999;78:30-32.
92. Rothman R. The acute cervical disc. *Clin Orthop*. 1975;109:59-68.
93. Haines T, Gross A, Burnie SJ, Goldsmith CH, Perry L. Patient education for neck pain with or without radiculpathy. *Cochrane Database Syst Rev*. 2009;1:CD005106.
94. Graham N, Gross A, Goldsmith CH, et al. Mechanical traction for neck pain with or without radiculopathy. *Cochrane Database Syst Rev*. 2008;3:CD006408.
95. Ramsin B, Singh V, Parr AT, Conn A, Diwan S, Abdi S. Systematic review of the effectivenss of cervical epidurals in the management of chronic neck pain. *Pain Phys*. 2009;12:137-157.
96. Manchikanti L, Malla, Y, Cash, KA, McManus CD, Pampati V. Fluoroscopic epidural injections in cervical spinal stenosis: Preliminary results of a randomized, double-blinded, active control trial. *Pain Phys*. 2012;15:E59-E70.
97. Manchikanti, L, Cash KA, Pampati V, Wargo BW, Malla Y. Cervical epidural injections in chronic discogenic neck pain without disc herniation or radiculitys: preliminary results of a randomized, double-blinded, controlled trial. *Pain Phys*. 2010;13:E265-E278.
98. Manchikanti, L, Cash KA, Pampati V, Wargo BW, Malla Y. The effectiveness of fluoroscopic cervical epidural injections in managing chronic cervical disc herniation and radiculitis: preliminary results of a randomized, double-blinded, controlled trial. *Pain Phys*. 2010;13: 223-236.
99. Abbasi A, Malhotra G, Malanga G, Elovic EP, Kahn S. Complications of interlaminar cervical epidural steroid injections: a review of the literature. *Spine*. 2007;32:2144-2151.
100. Scanlon GC, Moeller-Bertram T, Romanowsky SM, Wallace MS. Cervical transforaminal epidural steroid injections: more dangerous than we think? *Spine*. 2007;32:1249-1256.
101. Rathmell JP, Michna E, Fitzgibbon D, Stephens LS, Posner KL, Domino K. Injury and liability associated with cervical procedures for chronic pain. *Anesthesiology*. 2011;114(4):918-926.
102. Van Zundert J, Huntoon M, Patijn J, Lataster A, Mikhail N, Van Kleef M. Cervical radicular pain. *Pain Prac*. 2009;10(1):1-17.
103. Wolter T, Kiesel K. Cervical spinal cord stimulation: an analysis of 23 patients with long-term follow-up. *Pain Phys*. 2012;15:203-212.
104. Vallejo R, Kramer J, Benyamin R. Neuro-modulation of the cervical spinal cord in the treatment of chronic intractable neck and upper extremity pain: a case series and review of the literature. *Pain Phys*. 2007;10:305-311.
105. IHC, IHSCS. International Classification of Headache Disorders. The international classification of headache disorders: 2nd edition. *Cephalalgia*. 2004;24:1-160.
106. Vanelderen P, Lataster A, Levy R, Mekhail N, van Kleef M, Van Zundert J. Occipital neuralgia. *Pain Prac*. 2010;10(2):137-144.
107. Kuhn WF, Kuhn SC, Gilberstadt H. Occipital neuralgias: clinical recognition of complicated headache: a case series and review of the literature. *J Orofac Pain*. 1997;11:158-165.
108. Hammond SR, Danta G. Occipital neuralgia. *Clin Exp Neuol*. 1978;15:258-270.
109. Taylor M, Silva S, Cottrel C. Botulinum toxin in the treatment of occipital neuralgia: a pilot study. *Headache*. 2008;48:1476-1481.
110. Kapural L, Stillman M, Kapural M, et al. Botulinum toxin occipital nerve block for the treatment of severe occipital neuralgia: a case series. *Pain Pract*. 2007;7:337-340.
111. Navani A, Mahajan G, Kreis P, Fishman SM. A case of pulsed radiofrequency lesioning for occipital neuralgia. *Pain Med*. 2006;7: 453-456.
112. Vanelderen P, Rouwette T, Devooght P, et al. Pulsed radiofrequency for the treatment of occipital neuralgia: a prospective study with 6 month follow-up. *Reg Anesth Pain Med*. 2010;35(2):148-151.
113. Jasper J, Hayek S. Implanted occipital nerve stimulators. *Pain Phys*. 2008;11:187-200.
114. Aprill C, Dwyer A, Bogduk N. Cervical zygapophyseal joint pain patterns, II: a clinical evaluation. *Spine*. 1990;15:458-461.
115. Cooper G, Bailey B, Bogduk N. Cervical zygapohysial joint pain maps. *Pain Med*. 2007;8(4):344-353.
116. Yin W, Bogduk N. The nature of neck pain in a private pain clinic in the United States. *Pain Med*. 2008;9:196-203.
117. Cohen SP, Bajwa ZH, Kraemer JJ, et al. Factors predicting success and failure for cervical facet radiofrequency denervation: a multi-center analysis. *Reg Anesth Pain Med*. 2007;32:495-503.
118. Siegenthaler A, Eichenberger U, Schmidlin K, Arendt-Nielsen L, Curatolo M. What does local tenderness say about the origin of pain? An investigation of cervical zygaposhysial joint pain. *Anesth Analg*. 2010;110(3):923-927.
119. Friedenberg ZB, Miller WT. Degenerative disc disease of the cervical spine. *J Bone Joint Surg Am*. 1963;45:1171-1178.
120. Falco FJE, Manchikanti L, Datta S, Wargo BW, Geffert S, Bryce DA, Atluri S, et al. Systematic review of the therapeutic effectiveness of cervical facet joint interventions: An Update *Pain Phys*. 2012; 15(6):E839-E868.

121. Lord SM, Barnsley L, Bogduck N. The utility of comparative local anesthetic blocks versus placebo-controlled blocks for the diagnosis of cervical zygapophysial joint pain. *Clin J Pain*. 1995;11: 208-213.

122. Falco FJE, Erhart S, Wargo BW, et al. Systematic review of diagnostic utility and therapeutic effectiveness of cervical facet joint interventions. *Pain Phys*. 2009;12:323-344.

123. Van Eerd M, Patijn J, Lataster A, et al. Cervical facet pain. *Pain Prac*. 2010;10(2):113-123.

124. Cohen SP, Strassels SA, Kurihara C, et al. Randomized study assessing the accuracy of cervical facet joint nerve (medial branch) blocks using different injectate volumes. *Anesthesiology*. 2010;112:14-52.

125. Manchikanti L, Damron K, Cash K, Manchukondia R, Pampati V. Therapeutic cervical medial branch blocks in managing chronic neck pain: a preliminary report of a randomized, double-blind, controlled trial: clinical trial NCT0033272. *Pain Phys*. 2006;9:333-346.

126. McDonald GJ, Lord SM, Bogduk N. Long-term follow-up of patients treated with cervical radiofrequency neurotomy for chronic neck pain. *Neurosurgery*. 1999;45:61-67.

127. Barnsley L. Percutaneous radiofrequency neurotomy for chronic neck pain; outcomes in a series of consecutive patients. *Pain Med*. 2005;6:282-286.

128. Husted DS, Orton D, Schofferman J, et al. Effectiveness of repeated radiofrequency neurotomy for cervical facet joint pain. *J Spinal Disord Tech*. 2008;21:406-408.

129. Mackinnon SE, Novak CB. Thoracic outlet syndrome. *Curr Probl Surg*. 2002;39(11):1070-1145.

130. Huang JH, Zager EL. Thoracic outlet syndrome. *Neurosurg*. 2004;55(4):897-902.

131. Sanders RJ, Hammond SL, Rao NM. Thoracic outlet syndrome. A review. *The Neurologist*. 2008;14:365-373.

132. Urschel JD, Hameed MS, Grewal RP. Neurogenic thoracic outlet syndromes. *Post Med J*. 1994;70:785-789.

133. Sanders RJ, Hammond SH, Rao NM. Diagnosis of thoracic outlet syndrome. *J Vasc Surg*. 2007;46:601-604.

134. Sanders RJ, Jackson CG, Banchero N, Pearce WH. Scalene muscle abnormalities in traumatic thoracic outlet syndrome. *Am J Surg*. 1990;159:231-236.

135. Benxon HT, Rodes ME, Chekka K, Malik K, Pearce WH. Scalene muscle injection for neurogenic thoracic outlet syndrome: case series. *Pain Prac*. 2011;12(1):66-70.

136. Jordan SE, Machleder HI. Diagnosis of thoracic outlet syndrome using electrophysiologically guided anterior scalene blocks. *Ann Vasc Surg*. 1998;12:260-264.

137. Christo PJ, Christo DK, Carinci AJ, Freischlag JA. Single CT-guided chemodenervation of the anterior scalene muscle with botulinum toxin for neurogenic thoracic outlet syndrome. *Pain Med*. 2010;11:504-511.

138. Roos DB. The thoracic outlet syndrome is underrated. *Arch Neurol*. 1990;47:327-328.

139. Jordan SE, Ahn SS, Gelabert HA. Combining ultrasonography and electromyography for botulinum chemodenervation treatment of thoracic outlet syndrome: comparison with fluoroscopy and electromyographic guidance. *Pain Phys*. 2007;10:541-546.

140. Roos DB. Thoracic outlet syndrome is underdiagnosed. *Muscle Nerve*. 1999;22:126-129.

141. Franklin GM, Fulton-Kehoe D, Bradley C, Smith-Weller T. Outcome of surgery for thoracic outlet syndrome in Washington state workers' compensation. *Neurology*. 2000;54(6):1252-1257.

SECTION B
Spine

CHAPTER 38 Low Back Pain

Anthony C. Lee
Steven P. Cohen
Salahadin Abdi

EPIDEMIOLOGY

Low back pain (LBP) is the leading cause of disability in adults under 45 years of age, the second most common cause of missed work days after upper respiratory conditions, and the fifth most common reason for all visits to a physician. It is the number-one most common pain condition, the second being headaches. Jobs that are thought to increase the risk of low back pain include nursing, construction, factory work, farm work, law enforcement, firefighting, sanitation, sedentary office work, nursery school teaching, and occupational driving. Low back pain is the leading cause of expenditures for workers' compensation. The economic burden for low back pain to American society is up to $200 billion annually, with one-third of this total occurring as direct medical costs and the remainder from lost productivity. Approximately 5% of low back pain patients account for 75% of these costs. Chronic pain of all types, including low back pain, costs American society up to $635 billion annually in both medical costs and lost productivity.

About 70% to 80% of all people will experience low back pain in their lives. Of these, approximately 70% will resolve in 6 to 12 weeks. Approximately 85% will have recurrences of low back pain. Approximately 7% will go on to have significant chronic pain.

The prevalence of back pain is highest in the age groups of 45 to 64 years old, yet people under 45 experience the most activity limitations. The majority of younger patients are men, while the majority of patients over 60 years old are women. Return-to-work rates for back pain are dismal for pain lasting 6 months or longer. For those out of work for 6 months, the return-to-work rate is 50%, and for those out of work for 1 year, the return-to-work rate is 25%. After 2 years of unemployment due to back pain, the return-to-work rate is nearly zero.

The literature demonstrates a higher prevalence of chronic back pain in those with depression, anxiety, substance abuse, somatization, and personality disorders. Major depression was found in 30% to 65% of chronic low back pain patients compared to the rate of depression in the general population of 5% to 17%. The relationship between obesity and the prevalence of back pain continues to be controversial. One study found that a BMI higher than 30 (obese) increased the risk for chronic low back pain by 20% but that this risk is reduced with exercise. A systematic review involving 56 studies found, at best, a very weak correlation between obesity and low back pain. On the other hand, exercise has been shown to reduce the risk of low back pain regardless of weight, while lack of exercise increases the risk for low back pain. Smoking has been independently linked in some studies to an increased risk of chronic low back pain.

ETIOLOGIES

Table 38-1 shows ranks the etiological sources of back pain.

TABLE 38-1 Final Diagnosis in 2374 Chronic Low Back Pain Patients Participating in the National Low Back Pain Study

Diagnosis	Percentage
Herniated disc	36.7
Myofascial pain	19.6
Spinal stenosis	14.0
Lumbar spondylosis	12.2
Osteoarthritis root compression	8.7
Unknown etiology	8.5
Spondylolisthesis	7.3
Discogenic pain	6.1
Facet arthropathy	4.8
Lumbar instability	3.6
Spondylolysis	3.1
Scoliosis	3.1
Pain with psychiatric component	2.2
Compression fracture	1.9
Epidural fibrosis	1.3
Epineural fibrosis	0.8
Arachnoiditis	0.6
Spina bifida	0.5
Other diagnoses	5.1

HERNIATED NUCLEUS PULPOSUS

In herniated nucleus pulposus (HNP), patients present with low back pain that is typically worsened with increasing pressure on the disc, such as when the patient coughs or sneezes, or strains on the toilet (Valsalva maneuvers). MRIs often show protruded or extruded discs. In more than 95% of cases, HNP occurs at either the L4–5 or L5–S1 levels. Approximately 50% of HNP found on MRIs is asymptomatic. MRIs may show multiple herniations, not all of which have clinical relevance. It is not uncommon to have a poor correlation between patient complaints and MRI findings. In this case, an experienced clinician can formulate diagnoses and treatment planning on the comprehensive collection of data, possibly including electromyography, which may offer additional information.

A recent study measuring *in vivo* intradiscal pressures allows for comparison of intradiscal pressure with different positions and conditions:

- Standing relaxed: defined at 100%.
- Lying prone: 20%.
- Sitting unsupported: 92%.
- Standing and flexing forward: 220%.
- Sitting and flexing forward: 166%.
- Lifting a 45-lb weight with rounded flexed back: 460%.
- Lifting a 45-lb weight with flexed knee: 340%.
- Lifting a 45-lb weight with flexed knee and weight close to body: 220%.
- Nighttime lying down: 96%.

The preceding list demonstrates that lifting objects the "correct" way reduces intradiscal pressures. Despite this, most disc herniations do not occur from lifting heavy objects. One study found that 62% of all herniated discs have no particular inciting event, with an additional 25% due to activities such as tying shoes or releasing a handbrake on a car.

Only 6.5% of herniated discs are due to heavy lifting, 2% are due to light lifting, and 1.3% are due to trauma. Thus, disc herniations occur during routine activities that are generally unavoidable, such as sitting, bending to unplug an appliance, or putting on a winter coat. The most likely reason discs herniate is simply from degenerating discs, as studies have found an inverse relationship between the force required to herniate a nucleus pulposus and the degree of degeneration. The term *age-appropriate degeneration* can be applied to most patients, and this phenomenon seen on MRI should not warrant excessive concern or invasive procedures. Instead, patients' complaints and concerns should be met with appropriate treatment, education, and reassurance.

Interestingly, evidence has shown that lifting crates while keeping the crate's center of gravity close to the body but allowing the actual work to be done by the back muscles, rather than the leg muscles, in a therapeutic regimen under supervision can, in fact, benefit back pain sufferers of most etiologies in terms of pain and function. Inclusion of this particular exercise in a therapeutic regimen along with use of a Roman Chair and back extension weight machines do not seem to increase the incidence of HNP.

Whereas the outer annulus of the disc is recognized as "self" by the body's immunological system, the herniated portion of the disc is not recognized, resulting in an immune-mediated inflammatory response to this "foreign body." This inflammatory process recruits cells, proteins, and fluid that serve to increase the mass effect. A large immunogenic reaction to even a small herniation can cause well-defined radiculopathy, but because this inflammation is not well visualized on MRI, the actual disc pathology may be visually underappreciated. This is often referred to as a "chemical radiculopathy." Over 4 to 6 weeks, but often up to 6 months, this inflammation subsides, and most patients with an acute herniated disc will improve spontaneously without medical intervention. Improvement involves immunogenic removal of the herniated disc material, potentially leading to resolution of symptoms. Therefore, observation is often appropriate care for acute disc herniations. Patients should be encouraged to stay active during this process.

Some patients experience intense pain that affects their ability to work and enjoy a high quality of life. In these individuals, conservative medical treatments are recommended. They range from nonsteroidal anti-inflammatory drugs (NSAIDs) and acetaminophen to intravenous or oral Prednisone. The latter should be of a moderately high dose and tapered quickly to temper the inflammatory response thought to be responsible for acute pain. Although there are no studies that define effective and appropriate steroid dosing, in our clinic, we typically prescribe Prednisone 60 mg for 2 days followed by 40 mg for 2 days, and finally 20 mg for 2 days. At least anecdotally, this has been shown to be effective and safe for back pain and, particularly, radiculopathy. This seems especially true for a chemical radiculopathy when the MRI is unimpressive. Other clinics have used Medrol dosepaks with reported efficacy for their patients, although the Prednisone taper used by our clinic seems to be more effective. Patients should be warned of the potential side effects from oral steroids, including increased hunger, sleep disturbance if taken near bed time, agitation, psychosis, and increased blood glucose in diabetics. Serious side effects include avascular necrosis, especially of the hip, and glaucoma exacerbation. These can occur with prolonged duration of oral steroids. Our office limits the use of oral Prednisone to a maximum of two 6-day tapering courses. Typically, the efficacy of oral steroids is the greatest within the first 6 weeks of low back pain when inflammation is thought to be maximal.

Great care should be taken in prescribing opioids for long-term use as this may lead to progressive opioid-induced hyperalgesia, escalating opioid dosages due to tolerance, and aberrant behaviors. Studies have also shown that patients prescribed high-dose opioids as initial treatment can lead to increased work days lost, increased physician visits, and increased surgical and interventional procedures without satisfactory relief of pain. Although opioids clearly provide some benefit for acute back pain episodes compared to placebo, there is scant evidence to support their use for chronic back pain. For many patients, a weak opioid agonist with dual functions such as Tramadol or Tapentadol can provide a safe and effective alternative.

Interventional procedures such as epidural steroid injections can be employed to place steroids in the area where the inflammation is believed to be occurring. It has been shown that while both particulate and nonparticulate steroids provide statistical benefit compared to controls, particulate steroids result in better and longer-lasting pain relief. It is often advised to choose a level below the area of herniation where the epidural space is larger as this is thought to minimize complications during the procedure, but there is no evidence to support this. However, the Artery of Adamkiewicz lies above L2, and epidural injection above the L2–3 level increases the risks for spinal cord injury. A small number of patients have this artery at a level lower, so care must be taken to avoid complications, especially with particulate steroids.

Exercise has long been shown to be an important way to treat chronic back pain. However, for acute disc herniation, there is little evidence for its efficacy. Exercise does not accelerate the healing process for an acute herniated disc. It can be expensive for both patients with copays and for insurance companies that, in turn, pass these expenses on to the general public. Along with medications (nonopiates) and ice, observation is an appropriate course of action for an acute herniated disc. Exercise can become beneficial if back pain persists longer than the acute phase, typically 6 weeks or more, with increasing symptoms but with a benign MRI. Systematic reviews almost universally support the efficacy of exercise for chronic low back pain.

Surgery for herniated discs is indicated in a minority of cases. The conditions widely acknowledged to be indications for emergent surgery include bowel or bladder incontinence with accidents that occur generally without the patient being aware during the episode, only to discover its occurrence after the accident. This is in distinction to overflow or stress incontinence when a patient senses leakage while it happens. Other emergent indications include new onset of urinary retention, new sexual dysfunction, cauda equina, or saddle anesthesia. An indication for urgent surgery includes physical exam findings of progressive weakness occurring over the course of weeks. Manual muscle testing and atrophy can be measured at the initial visit and remeasured at a follow-up visit 2 to 3 weeks later. Historical evidence such as progressive difficulty climbing stairs or foot drop can also be helpful in making a decision for surgical referral. Surgery for intractable pain, failure of conservative treatments, and poor quality of life due to pain is elective and dependent on patient choices, keeping in mind that discogenic pain can resolve spontaneously without any intervention. In clinical trials comparing surgical decompression to conservative management for neuropathic low back pain, where all studies demonstrate a benefit for surgery at 6 months, most show no statistically significant benefit after 2 years.

Finally, a note about bed rest as a course of treatment. Studies have shown that bed rest has, at best, a neutral effect, and, at worse, it is detrimental. Patients should, therefore, be encouraged to stay active regardless of treatment course. Extreme physical activity, on the other hand, should be avoided during the first 4 to 6 weeks of herniation.

Table 38-2 lists favorable and unfavorable prognosticators for HNP with nonoperative care.

MYOFASCIAL PAIN

Myofascial pain is a common cause of LBP, with one study conducted by spine surgeons finding its prevalence to be almost 20%, second only to herniated discs. In addition, some studies have found LBP to be associated with elevated levels of paraspinal muscle tension. Myofascial LBP often presents as a deep, achy pain that is aggravated by activity and position changes. It may be localized to the low back or radiate into the buttock, sacrum, thigh, abdominal wall, or even calf, depending on the affected muscle(s). Pain-induced weakness or paresthesias, or both, may be present but are nonmyotomal and nondermatomal in distribution. On physical examination, a tender, taut band of muscle may be noted (trigger point) that, when palpated, results in a characteristic referral pattern, but, often, a discrete trigger point cannot be appreciated in the

TABLE 38-2 Prognostic Factors of Positive and Negative Outcomes with Nonoperative Care for Lumbar Disc Herniation

Favorable Factors	Unfavorable Factors
Absence of crossed straight-leg raising (SLR)	Positive crossed SLR
Absence of leg pain during spinal extension	Reproduction of leg pain during spinal extension
Large extrusion or sequestration	Subligamentous contained lumbar disc herniation
>50% reduction in leg pain within first 6 weeks of onset	<50% reduction in leg pain within 6 weeks of onset
Positive response to corticosteroids	Poor response to corticosteroids
Limited psychosocial issues	Overbearing psychosocial issues
Self-employed	Receiving workers' compensation
Educational level >12 years	Educational level <12 years
Good fitness level	Poor fitness level
Absence of spinal stenosis	Presence of spinal stenosis
Progressive return of neurologic deficits within first 12 weeks	Progressive neurologic deficits and cauda equina syndrome

deeper muscle layers. When a trigger point is appreciated, deep, traverse "snapping" palpation or needle insertion often elicits the characteristic local twitch response. In severe cases, decreased lumbar lordosis, or if the muscle spasm is unilateral, functional scoliosis—or "listing"—may be noted. Patients may present with significant concern because their posture has changed suddenly, listing to one side or the other. Patients should be reassured that this condition will likely resolve spontaneously as their back pain resolves.

The treatment of myofascial LBP is mainly conservative. Some of the therapies used for myofascial pain include ischemic compression massage, the so-called spray-and-stretch technique, iontophoresis, and physical therapy. Ice applied to the low back slows the metabolism required for muscle contraction and subsequently reduces painful spasms. Ice also decreases the conduction velocity of pain fibers, thereby decreasing pain and, debatably, also floods the central neurologic gateway with temperature signals that override pain signal transmission. Ice should be applied 20 minutes at a time with 1 hour in between applications. Ice should not be in direct contact with the skin, and a towel barrier is recommended.

A large, randomized controlled trial compared osteopathic manipulation with conventional noninvasive therapy in patients with axial LBP of less than 6 months' duration. The osteopathic treatment group required less pain medication than the conventional treatment group but had similar outcomes. When trigger points are identified, trigger-point injections using local anesthetic can be helpful. A recent, randomized, double-blind study in patients with chronic LBP found injections with botulinum toxin A to be an effective treatment. When myofascial pain is associated with other pathology of the lumbar spine, as is often the case, these problems need to be treated as well.

SPINAL STENOSIS

This is a common occurrence as people age. Spinal stenosis can refer to central canal narrowing, foraminal narrowing, or lateral recess stenosis. Axial and/or radiating pain is often provoked with hyperextension, walking, and descending stairways or hills. It is often relieved by leaning over a shopping cart, counter, or walker. Disc protrusions, hypertrophied ligamentum flava, enlarged facet joints, facet cysts, osteophytosis, and spondylolisthesis can all contribute to central canal stenosis. Patients may present with unilateral or bilateral neuropathic symptoms of pain, numbness, tingling, or weakness that often extends to multiple dermatomes. In addition, they may also have signs such as lower extremity hyperreflexia compared to the upper extremities, clonus, and a positive Babinski, especially if significant stenosis occurs in the high lumbar or thoracic regions. MRI findings of myelomalacia are concerning, but, often, surgery is not required. Aggressive physical therapy may improve pain scores and quality of life, especially if pain is movement induced (so-called dynamic pain, see the later section on chronic back pain), or if the patient has kinesiophobia, fear-avoidance beliefs, pain behaviors or is deconditioned. However, these patients should be closely monitored for symptomatic progression, and if this is observed over time, a surgical referral is warranted. Surgical referral is also warranted if conservative treatments fail to improve pain or quality of life. While facet blocks or radiofrequency denervation may relieve axial pain, it is thought by some that facet blocks, in particular, may cause inflamed and hypertrophic facet joints to reduce in size, thereby relieving the stenosis and radicular pain. This has anecdotally been observed frequently in our office, although the exact mechanism remains unknown.

Decreased disc height from desiccation or herniation, as well as bony changes and osteophyte complexes, may cause foraminal stenosis or lateral recess stenosis, and these changes are usually detected on an MRI. These usually affect a single nerve root or multiple nerve roots at different levels, causing pain, radiculopathy, dermatomal numbness and tingling, and myotomal weakness as the lower motor neurons are affected. Deep tendon reflexes can be hyporeflexic. Epidural steroid injections that allow for steroid and local anesthetic dispersion through multiple levels may provide relief to those who are symptomatic at these levels, though the duration of effect tends to be shorter than that achieved for a herniated disc. A transforaminal approach may benefit those with unilateral pain in a well-delineated dermatomal distribution.

As with lumbar disc herniations, treatments to avoid if possible are bed rest and opioids. Bed rest tends to cause deconditioning and reinforce fear-avoidance beliefs, while opioids increase the risk of falling, especially in seniors, and increase the risk of continued use and long-term hyperalgesia. Neuropathic medications such as gabapentin have been shown to increase walking distances and reduce pain.

For spinal stenosis unrelated to spondylolisthesis, treatment outcomes, whether surgical or nonsurgical, are poorer for those patients with duration of symptoms longer than 12 months. This is not true for degenerative spondylolisthesis. Therefore, an MRI should be ordered early, and nonoperative treatments should be exhausted promptly to remain within the window of surgical efficacy. In a randomized, multicenter study comparing surgery to conservative care for spinal stenosis without spondylolisthesis, the surgical group did better through 2-year follow-up in the "as treated" analysis.

DEGENERATIVE DISC DISEASE AND DISCOGENIC PAIN

The intervertebral disc over time loses proteoglycans and chondroitin, which are molecules that attract and retain water. Losing these molecules means that the disc loses its water content. Loss of water translates to loss of compressive strength of the disc. This water is then replaced with collagen, which makes the disc less compliant under pressure and more susceptible to tears. With significant loss of water, the disc is less likely to herniate, but disc space is reduced, possibly narrowing the foramina through which nerve roots exit.

The annulus fibrosus is innervated anteriorly by the ventral rami and gray rami communicans. The posterior part of the annulus is innervated by the sinuvertebral nerves. Therefore, tears within the lamellae of the disc without herniation can produce back pain without radiation. An MRI may show a zone of high intensity. With decreased lamellae, the integrity of the disc is reduced and the stress increases, especially with activities that are associated with increased pressure such as prolonged sitting. Over time, chemical sensitization may occur that can lead to axial pain with even normal activities, which did not produce pain previously. Desensitization may occur chemically at the level of the disc. Alternatively, regional or generalized nonchemical desensitization usually occurs over time in most people, resulting in a recalibrated and electrically stable neurophysiological pain system. When these desensitization processes or systems fail, pain continues and becomes chronic.

Patients with low back pain often have degenerative disc disease (DDD). According to many studies, DDD is the most common cause of nonradicular chronic low back pain. Similar to HNP, a majority of patients, 85% in one study, with DDD on MRI are asymptomatic, and this percentage increases with age.

Discogenic pain can present with back pain radiating into the buttock, hip, groin, or even the lower limb. It is typically worsened by prolonged sitting. Often, this pain mimics HNP, and it is sometimes difficult to discriminate between HNP and discogenic pain. However, there should be an absence of focal neurologic findings, and the radiation pattern tends to be nondermatomal.

Treatment for acute discogenic pain involves NSAIDs, acetaminophen, Tramadol, and the passage of time. For the aforementioned reasons, prescribing opioids should be done with great care. Discograms are usually not indicated and can produce false positives, especially in those with abnormal psychometric testing, multiple somatic complaints, and previous back surgery. The results of the few studies conducted yield mixed evidence as to whether they improve fusion outcomes. The use of Intradiscal Electrothermal Annuloplasty (IDET) has been shown in uncontrolled studies to provide moderate pain relief. However, for chronic discogenic pain, IDET has been shown to be of benefit only in the short term. Only one of four randomized studies demonstrated significant improvement of fusion compared to conservative care, and the benefit experienced with fusion tends to be modest. Fusing the spine may also be associated with juxtafusional degenerative changes such as accelerated disc and facet joint degeneration, spondylolisthesis and scoliosis. Disc replacement may be considered for patients with no significant radicular or facetogenic component to their pain and may be as effective as fusion for one- or two-segment disease. The advantages of disc replacement include more rapid recovery and better preservation of spinal motion. As mentioned in the chronic back pain section, desensitization through aggressive physical therapy or cognitive interventions are viable options should the patient choose to exhaust nonsurgical options before deciding on surgery.

DDD is thought to facilitate facet arthropathy from redistribution of load forces from the disc to the facet joints (loads are normally shared when both discs and facets are healthy).

FACET ARTHROPATHY

Facet joints (also called zygapophysial joints or Z-joints) are estimated to be involved in up to 40% of all back pain sufferers. Facet joints are paired, true synovial joints that connect adjacent vertebrae posterolaterally. The function of facet joints in the lumbar spine (as opposed to the function in the cervical spine) is to limit rotation and assist the intervertebral discs in resisting compressive forces during lordotic postures, such that maximal stress on the facet joints occurs during lumbar extension and rotation.

The mechanism of how facet arthropathy develops is unclear. Kirkaldy-Willis described the three-joint complex at a given level and how the deterioration of this complex occurs in three phases. In the dysfunctional phase, circumferential and radial tears occur in the disc, and synovitis and hypomobility occur in the facet joints. This results in disc herniations and dysfunction of the three-joint complex. In the instability phase, disc herniations and resorption of the disc material, combined with facet capsular laxity and subluxation, cause instability and lateral nerve entrapment. In the stabilization phase, osteophytes form and facet enlargement occurs, causing stenosis at that particular level. The three phases collectively describe the process of *spondylosis*. Multilevel spondylosis results in multilevel stenosis.

The degenerative changes observed in facet arthropathy include microtrauma, capsular tears, synovial inflammation (seen on MRI as fluid in the joints), chondromalacia, microhemorrhage, and meniscoid entrapment. Facet joint degeneration can also involve outpouching of the synovium, forming a synovial cyst. Rupture of synovial cysts by fluoroscopic-guided, contrast-enhanced cystic distention has been shown to have potential for safe, long-term pain relief of back pain.

Similar to other forms of arthritis, the prevalence of facet joint pain increases with age. Facet pain is often described as back pain that does not radiate. It is often worse with hyperextension and with rotation, such as when swinging a golf club. Facet pain may also radiate down the buttocks and thighs unilaterally or bilaterally, but weakness and paresthesias are usually not present. This pain rarely radiates distal to the knees, except when facet hypertrophy results in clinically significant foraminal stenosis. Facet joints share similar anatomical features to nonaxial joints such as knuckles, knees, and hips. They are encapsulated with joint fluid, their articular surfaces are lined with cartilage, and the periosteum is innervated. As people age, these joints degenerate, resulting in loss of cartilage, irregularity of articulating surfaces, and joint pain. Joints at each level are innervated by medial branches of the dorsal rami at that level and the one above. For example, at the L4–5 articulation, the superior aspect of the facet is innervated by the L3 medial branch, while the inferior aspect of the facet is innervated by the L4 medial branch.

Facet pain can also be treated with aggressive quota-based, non-pain-contingent therapy if pain is movement induced. Alternatively, facet blocks can quiet inflammation within the joint. Fluid in the joint may be present on an MRI, but this is not always the case. Studies suggest that there is little difference whether the steroid/local anesthetic is actually deposited within the joint capsule or merely in the vicinity of the joint. That is, good efficacy can be achieved in either instances, although this remains controversial. Medial branch blocks that reduce pain by 80% are diagnostic, and medial branch radiofrequency ablation (often called "rhizotomy") may then be beneficial. On the other hand, it is believed by some that if facet blocks do not relieve pain, medial branch blocks may not be warranted. It is also believed by some that medial branch blocks should be performed instead of facet blocks, but this is also controversial.

SACROILIAC JOINT PAIN

The sacroiliac (SI) joint is a large joint connecting the sacrum to the iliac bones. The joint is heterogeneous in that while the anterior surface of the articulation between the sacrum and ilium is a true diarthrodial joint, the dorsal surface is mostly comprised of an intricate network of ligamentous and muscular connections. It functions to dissipate shock forces from the upper trunk to the lower extremities. SI pain can present as unilateral buttock pain, but it is also known to cause pain radiation down to the feet bilaterally. It can also present as groin pain or as clicking or popping in the posterior pelvis. There should be no associated weakness or paresthesias in SI joint pain.

SI joint pain as a cause of low back pain is controversial for many reasons. Many believe that its relative lack of movement; the complex force distribution among the SI joint, hips, pubic symphysis, and spine; and overlapping symptoms of other more common and identifiable pathologies make it difficult to define the SI joint as a definite pain generator in a patient's complaints of back pain. Furthermore, while there are many physical exam maneuvers to evaluate for SI joint pathology, no single test has been shown to be very sensitive or specific, including tenderness to palpation over the joint itself. Similar to facet joint pain, the only way to diagnose a painful SI joint is by diagnostic blocks. Imaging such as CT and MRIs is usually not helpful in evaluating SI joint pain but could be ordered to rule out other concerning pathologies.

Several conditions may be associated with a higher risk of SI joint pain that include ankylosing spondylitis, pregnancy (which involves hormonal-induced ligamentous laxity and exaggerated hyperlordosis), true or apparent leg length discrepancies, and, rarely, infection or tumors. Among patients with axial low back pain predominantly below L5, the estimated prevalence is between 20% and 35%.

Other sources of pain should be investigated before concluding that a patient has pure SI joint pain. Treatments for SI joint pain ranges from ice and NSAIDs in the acute phase (1–3 days) and physical therapy for muscle balancing in the recovery phase (3 days–8 weeks). Maladaptations of movement due to pain should be addressed during this time. Functional leg length discrepancies (measured from the umbilicus to the medial malleoli) in the absence of actual leg length discrepancies (measured from the Anterior Superior Iliac Spine (ASIS) to the medial malleoli) should be addressed with muscle balancing and not with shoe lifts. One study showed that 32% of Army recruits had actual leg length discrepancies of up to three-fifths of an inch (15 mm) without symptoms. The subsequent recommendations are to address leg length discrepancies only for values exceeding this.

In any event, while many may attribute pain to mechanical abnormalities such as leg length discrepancy or pelvic malrotation, it should be pointed out that these abnormalities likely persisted long before the patient's development of back pain and that the patients' neurophysiologic pain system had, up to the point of an exacerbating event, suppressed pain signal transmission. The exacerbating event then pushed the stimulus beyond the pain threshold of transmission, resulting in a new onset of pain perception. Retraining of the pain system to increase the pain threshold (through aggressive physical therapy) is a reasonable first-line treatment option associated with less adverse side effects than fixing the anatomic abnormality. Muscular stretching, strengthening, and balancing can also be performed as part of the therapy.

In terms of interventional procedures, both intraarticular and periarticular injections have been shown to provide benefit. In those who respond with only short-term relief to injections, the use of radiofrequency ablation of the L4 and L5 dorsal rami and lateral branches of S1 to S3 may provide pain relief lasting up to 1 year.

PIRIFORMIS SYNDROME

The piriformis is a flat, pyramidal muscle extending from the anterior sacrum, greater sciatic foramen, and sacrotuberous ligament to the greater trochanter of the femur. The major function of the piriformis is to abduct and externally rotate the femur. The possibility that sciatic symptoms may stem from the piriformis muscle dates back to 1928, when Yeoman examined the relationship of the sacroiliac joint, sciatic nerve, and piriformis muscle. Although six anatomic variations between the sciatic nerve and piriformis muscle have been described, in the large majority of cases, the sciatic nerve passes anterior to the muscle. Any process that causes the piriformis to hypertrophy, spasm, or contract inappropriately can cause sciatic nerve impingement, leading to piriformis syndrome.

The typical presentation of piriformis syndrome is buttock pain, sciatica, or both, exacerbated by activities that necessitate hip adduction and internal rotation, such as cross-country skiing or prolonged sitting. Pain that accompanies bowel movements may be present and, for women, dyspareunia. Physical examination may reveal tenderness in the buttock extending from the lateral border of the sciatic foramen to the greater trochanter. Both pelvic and rectal examinations may reproduce the pain pattern. Pain is also elicited during resistance to hip flexion, adduction, and internal rotation (FADIR test), otherwise known as the Freiberg's sign. The neurologic examination is usually nonfocal, with most patients having a negative straight-leg raising test. Although CT, MRI, and electrodiagnostic studies may be helpful, by themselves, these tests are insufficient to make the diagnosis. Imaging should be used with caution as they may lead to misdiagnoses. For example, an L5-S1 herniation seen on imaging, a very common finding that is commonly non-painful, may be assumed to be the cause for leg pain, when the actual cause may be from the piriformis muscle. This may result in a series of invasive treatments for the wrong target.

For most patients with piriformis syndrome, conservative treatment is sufficient. This includes physical therapy and correction of leg-length discrepancies, pelvic obliquity, abnormalities in gait or posture mechanics, and associated back or leg problems. Medications such as NSAIDs and muscle relaxants can sometimes be helpful. Other treatments that have been advocated include transrectal massage, vapocoolant spray coupled with soft-tissue stretching maneuvers, and Transcutaneous Electrical Nerve Stimulation (TENS) therapy. When conservative treatment fails, injection of the piriformis with local anesthetic and corticosteroids can relieve muscle spasm and pain. This treatment should be done using either a nerve stimulator to locate the sciatic nerve or fluoroscopy with contrast. In instances in which relief is short term, piriformis injections can be repeated with botulinum toxin. In rare instances, surgical sectioning of the piriformis muscle may be necessary.

One disorder that is easily mistaken for piriformis syndrome is ischiogluteal bursitis. Patients with ischiogluteal bursitis usually complain of severe pain in the center of the buttock, which is worse with sitting or walking. This pain may radiate into the thigh, but rarely extends below the knee. Tests involving motion at the hip joint, such as the straight-leg raise and Patrick's tests, are often positive. Pressure applied on the lateral rectal wall during a digital rectal examination can elicit excruciating pain. Conservative treatment includes NSAIDs and soft pillows or so-called doughnuts for sitting. For patients with severe pain, bursa injections performed with corticosteroids and local anesthetic are indicated.

SCOLIOSIS

It has been shown that patients with progression of congenital scoliosis or idiopathic juvenile scoliosis have a higher incidence of herniated discs and back pain. On the other hand, those with degenerative scoliosis are not more likely to have back pain compared with the general population. One study showed the presence of scoliosis in 68% of elderly patients (mean age 70.5) without significant correlation to pain. Another study following patients (ages 50–84) over a 12-year period showed *de novo* development of scoliosis in more than 36% of patients. Patients should not attribute their pain primarily to scoliosis, though it is thought by some that the asymmetric loading present in scoliosis may predispose patients to other abnormalities such as facet and disc degeneration. Potential sources of back pain in the setting of scoliosis include facet pain, discogenic pain, disc herniations and degeneration, and stenosis. These conditions should be treated the same way as they would in the absence of scoliosis.

CHRONIC BACK PAIN AND EXERCISE TREATMENT

Chronic pain is usually defined as pain that has persisted beyond the expected duration of an acute pain event. In discogenic back pain for example, this is usually 4 to 6 weeks. However, as noted earlier, pain from disc herniations may take as long as 6 months to resolve. Chronic back pain occurs when the neurophysiologic pain response from acute changes in the spinal column continues to transmit pain signals to the brain. In theory, most neurophysiologic systems continue to adjust and adapt to these changes, increasing the threshold to which stimulus input produces pain. This may explain why older people are not in excruciating pain despite having significantly degenerated spines seen on an MRI. This may also explain why patients "get better" despite showing a persistent disc herniation on a follow-up MRI. Another example is when a microdiscectomy is performed. While 23% of patients reherniate the same disc postoperatively, only 56% of these patients are symptomatic.

When this threshold is increased sufficiently, the neurophysiologic system is said to have adjusted to the anatomic change (e.g., disc herniation) that previously occurred. The patient does not feel pain despite the fact that the spinal column is permanently changed. These changes occur throughout our adult lives, and our neurophysiologic system continuously adjusts and adapts; hence, back pain often appears in episodes that resolve spontaneously in most cases. It is overwhelmingly common to have significant anatomic changes in the spine without significant pain. On the other hand, some patients have relatively mild changes in their spines seen on MRI, yet have significant pain. Practitioners should be cautious in correlating pain to anatomic changes because, often, these correlations are poor.

When threshold fails to adjust, *pathologic pain* ensues. Pathologic pain serves no functional purpose. This is in contrast to *physiologic* or *"Darwinistic" pain*, which serves to protect the body and prevent injury. Patients should be educated that while they may have significant degenerative changes, resuming all the activities that they enjoy doing without fear of injury may improve long-term outcomes because their chronic pain is pathologic and not physiologic.

When the pain threshold is kept low, pain is recreated intermittently or constantly. Pain provoked with movement is called *dynamic pain* and is the most common type of pain associated with mechanical, nociceptive pain (e.g., facet arthropathy, SI joint pain, discogenic pain). Dynamic pain is produced when the pain threshold is low to the point where a small stimulus produced by benign movement activates pain fibers. In patients with normal or adequately adjusted pain thresholds, pain fibers do not activate with normal movements.

It is important to distinguish to patients the difference between "pain threshold" and "pain tolerance." *Threshold* is the amount of stimulus necessary to activate pain fibers. If the stimulus fails to activate pain fibers, the event goes unnoticed by the patient. On the other hand, *tolerance* describes what the patient chooses to do after the pain threshold is exceeded, that is, what the patient does when he or she feels pain. Thus, a low-threshold, high-tolerant patient may feel pain with the slightest of movements but choose to go to work despite the pain because of the fear of lost income. The low-threshold, low-tolerant patient may choose to minimize movements by staying in bed or purchasing a wheelchair.

A decrease in pain threshold is thought to be facilitated by chronic use of narcotic medication, hypervigilence to avoid activities that are thought to provoke the pain (known as fear-avoidance beliefs or kinesiophobia), depression and anxiety, personality disorders, and other psychosocial phenomena such as compensation. Compensation can be in the form of financial or other compensation, such as having family members perform the daily chores that the patient would normally have done but is now excused from doing because of perceived disability. This may explain opioid-induced hyperalgesia, higher prevalence of back pain with psychiatric or personality disorders, and the failure to improve when compensated financially, for example. Studies have shown that return-to-work rates are significantly lower when patients are financially compensated compared with those who are not compensated. Additionally, attorney involvement further decreases return-to-work rates. When threshold- or tolerance-lowering factors are present, chronic pain is likely to continue despite aggressive physical therapy, interventional procedures, and even surgery.

Even in those with a fully adjusted neurophysiologic system, high thresholds can be overcome with a large stimulus. This may explain why a pain-free patient with a large osteophyte complex from an old disc herniation may be painfully symptomatic after a fall—because the subsequent inflammatory reaction stimulated pain fibers that exceeded the threshold. These patients improve over time with resolution of said inflammation with or often without treatment.

Dynamic chronic pain from a lowered pain threshold is often amenable to aggressive physical therapy combined with a cognitive behavioral component. Many studies have shown profound effectiveness with this approach. Fear-avoidance beliefs are dispelled and kinesiophobia is remedied. Constant exposure to the familiar pain by repetition of pain-provoking movements increases the threshold to which these movements induce pain. This is written on a physical therapy order as "quota-based, non-pain-contingent" exercises. The prescription should also contain "no *passive* modalities" because most have no proven long-term benefit and therapy time is better allocated to *active* physical exercises. Therapy should be twice weekly for 6 weeks because one study has shown that thrice-weekly physical therapy has no added benefit. While MRIs should not be routinely ordered for chronic back pain unless concerning signs or symptoms are reported, or if a procedure is planned, patients often present to the pain specialist with a recent MRI. In this case, and if the results are benign, health care providers should provide reassurance that there is nothing concerning about their back anatomy other than age-appropriate degeneration. Again, it should be explained to patients that age-appropriate degeneration is common in all people of that particular age group but typically produces no pain. Finally, patients need to be instructed to continue their exercises in their own gym twice a week because complete resolution of pain takes longer than 6 weeks, often up to 6 months. They should be told that the main reason for aggressive physical therapy is for desensitization (increasing the pain threshold), and that the secondary benefits are a stronger core, increased cardiovascular fitness and health, confidence in returning to activities that they enjoy, reduction in pain behaviors and fear avoidance, cessation of catastrophic thinking patterns, and a better sense of well-being.

Static pain—that is, pain with sitting or lying in bed, but improved with standing or moving around—is often more challenging to manage. It is important to note that static pain may fail to respond to aggressive physical therapy and other methods of treatment should be prescribed, usually interventional procedures.

Pain in the setting of depression may be improved with simple aerobic exercise. Babyak showed that aerobic exercise three times per week for 10 months treated depression better than antidepressants and better than antidepressants plus exercises. For those patients unable to or who decline exercise as a treatment plan, antidepressants have been FDA approved for chronic back pain. The antidepressant Duloxetine is FDA approved for musculoskeletal pain, including low back pain, and systematic reviews have generally found that tricyclic antidepressants may provide a slightly greater beneficial effect (compared with newer antidepressants) in some individuals with LBP regardless of the etiology. The fact that serotonin- and norepinephrine-specific reuptake inhibitors are weakly effective analgesic agents suggests that both neurotransmitters are involved in the pain modulatory effects. When antidepressants are used to treat pain, the dosing regimen, total dosage, and onset are all lower or shorter than when they are used to treat depression. For nortripytline, a dose range of 25 to 75 mg at night is often therapeutic.

In addition to exercise treatment for chronic low back pain, chiropractic manipulation, acupuncture, interventional procedures, and surgery have been shown to benefit many patients. Ergonomic evaluation of the workplace or home can be of benefit. Many patients will ask a physician for a recommendation for a particular bed or mattress that will alleviate back pain. One study showed reduced back pain with a "medium-firm" mattress versus "soft" or "firm" mattresses, but these terms are ill-defined. In the absence of compelling evidence, practitioners should be wary of making a recommendation because mattresses, especially those that are advertised to be therapeutic, tend to be expensive.

FAILED BACK SURGERY SYNDROME

The definition of failed back surgery syndrome (FBSS) is the persistence or development of low back or leg pain following surgery on the lumbosacral spine. Two statistics highlight the magnitude of FBSS as a pain problem in the United States. First, approximately 300,000 lumbosacral spine procedures are performed each year in the United States as a treatment for chronic LBP. Second, depending on the definition of failure, the incidence of FBSS can be as high as 60%.

The reasons patients continue to have pain following spine surgery can be broadly categorized as follows: (1) poor patient selection (e.g., patients with threshold lowering factors); (2) surgery was performed on a structure that was incorrectly thought to be the primary pain generator (e.g., a patient thought to have an L4–5 discogenic radiculopathy because it was seen on an MRI, but actually had a piriformis syndrome as the primary cause of pain); (3) clear indication for surgery, but the procedure did not correct the original problem; (4) complication from surgery (e.g., discitis, pseudomeningocele, or a pars defect, especially from far lateral discectomies); (5) recurrent disc herniation; (6) secondary instability or degenerative changes occurring as a consequence of surgery (e.g., adjacent level discogenic pain, facetogenic pain, sacroiliac joint pain developing after a spinal fusion, spondylolisthesis following laminectomy, or pain that develops over the site of a donor graft); (7) persistent or established neural injury (e.g., arachnoiditis or epidural scarring); and (8) an intercurrent diagnosis, such as cancer.

The workup of patients with FBSS begins with a detailed history and physical examination. Of particular importance is determining whether the patient's pain is of the same character and quality as before the surgery or if it represents a new symptom that has arisen. For instance, a new pain complaint might indicate a surgical complication. Equally crucial is determining whether or not, and for how long, the patient experienced a pain-free interval. The three most common scenarios are as follows:

1. No relief or the worsening of pain shortly after surgery. This category includes a retained disc fragment, failure to remove the offending disc, and certain iatrogenic infections. No relief following

surgery might also indicate an incorrect diagnosis or poor patient selection.

2. Initial relief followed shortly thereafter by pain, numbness, or weakness. Examples of this group of disorders are arachnoiditis, epidural fibrosis, and battered-root syndrome with perineural scarring. Note that this pattern can also occur as the patient is weaned off of their post-op pain medications.
3. Excellent relief after the surgery followed by development of pain months or years later. This group includes a recurrent disc at the same or different level, pseudoarthrosis, juxtafusional degeneration, and lumbar instability.

Overall, the most frequent causes of pain in patients with FBSS syndrome are recurrent disc herniation, spinal stenosis, epidural scarring, and arachnoiditis. **Table 38-3** lists the most frequent diagnoses conferred at one pain management center in patients with failed back surgery syndrome.

After obtaining a detailed history, the physician should arrive at a reasonable differential diagnosis. At this point, diagnostic studies are usually necessary. If a recurrent herniated disc or spinal stenosis is suspected, an MRI scan is indicated. Because scar tissue is relatively vascular, a gadolinium-enhanced MRI or contrast CT scan is usually necessary to detect epidural fibrosis. This diagnosis can be confirmed with epidural mapping by the injection of contrast media through the caudal canal. In patients with epidural fibrosis, a filling defect is present. When arachnoiditis is suspected, myelography is the diagnostic imaging study of choice. Additional accuracy can be obtained when a myelogram is followed by a CT scan. For osteomyelitis, a bone scan is the preferred test.

The treatment of FBSS is aimed at the underlying cause. Depending on the diagnosis, nerve blocks—including epidural corticosteroid injections, sacroiliac joint blocks, and facet blocks—can sometimes be of benefit. In patients with radicular symptoms, neuropathic pain medications may provide relief. Some clinicians report good results with epidural lysis of adhesions (i.e., Racz procedure) in FBSS patients with epidural fibrosis, although, in our experience, the analgesia conferred by this procedure tends to be short-lived. Causes of FBSS that may be amenable to surgery include a recurrent disc herniation, postlaminectomy instability, recurrent spinal stenosis, nonunion, and a host of surgical complications. However, in a study by North and colleagues that followed 102 patients who underwent repeat back surgery, only 34% had a successful outcome. In patients who do not respond to nerve blocks, repeat surgery, or other medications, opioids are indicated. Finally, spinal cord stimulation may be of benefit for patients with FBSS who have intractable pain, especially those for whom leg pain is the predominant complaint.

TABLE 38-3 Pain Center Diagnosis in 78 Patients with Failed Back Surgery Syndrome

Diagnosis	Number of Cases
Normal	16
Minor spondylitic/expected postoperative changes	16
Epidural fibrosis	11
Arachnoiditis	10
Traumatic neuritis	5
Severe spondylosis	4
Spinal stenosis	4
Cancer	3
Musculoskeletal abnormality only	2
Compression fracture	1
Traumatic meningocele	1
Lateral foraminal stenosis	1
Tarsal tunnel syndrome	1
Fractured hip	1
Scoliosis	1
Disc herniation	1

RARE CAUSES

In addition to the usual causes of LBP, the astute clinician must also consider the unusual. Because of their effects on the musculoskeletal system, a host of different metabolic and endocrine disorders can result in LBP, including hyperthyroidism, hyperparathyroidism, and Cushing's disease. For similar reasons, virtually any rheumatologic disorder can present as LBP. Visceral pain emanating from internal organs can be referred to the back secondary to convergence in the spinal cord. These sources of visceral pain include genitourinary organs, the kidneys, gallbladder, bowel, liver, and pancreas. Vascular disease can manifest as LBP, which, if not detected, can be catastrophic. Not only is the spine a common site of metastatic tumors, but primary tumors may originate there as well. In some patients, hematologic disorders such as mastocytosis and hemoglobinopathies can lead to low back pain, as can diseases such as sarcoidosis, Paget's disease, and infectious endocarditis. Finally, psychiatric and functional disorders can manifest as chronic back pain, which can be extremely difficult to treat.

CONCERNING PATHOLOGIES

Back pain that is constant or worse at night, night sweats or fever, unintentional weight loss, or a history of cancer warrants an MRI or CT scan if an MRI is contraindicated.

Infection of the Lumbosacral Spine Infectious causes of LBP include vertebral osteomyelitis, epidural abscess, and discitis. Vertebral osteomyelitis accounts for between 2% and 4% of all cases of osteomyelitis, with males being affected more than females and the elderly more than young people. In descending order, the most common sources of infection are the genitourinary system, skin, respiratory tract, and spine surgery. Risk factors include intravenous drug abuse, immune suppression, and rectosigmoid disease. Although vertebral osteomyelitis may sometimes begin abruptly, more often, the presentation is insidious. Back pain typically is described as sharp, persistent, and exacerbated with movement. Fever may be minimal or absent. On physical examination, there is usually marked tenderness over the affected vertebra, guarding, and paraspinal muscle spasm. Treatment involves antibiotics and immobilization.

Because of its poor blood supply, most cases of discitis either are iatrogenic or occur secondary to direct spread from an infected vertebra. Classically, patients report the onset of intense, spasmodic pain appearing 1 to 2 weeks after spine instrumentation. Fever is usually absent. In patients without previous surgery, the diagnosis may take months or even years to make. Pain from discitis may be referred into the groin, flanks, hips, abdomen, or lower extremities. It usually is exacerbated by movement and relieved by rest. In one study, 3 of 13 patients with discitis had neurologic deficits at diagnosis. Physical examination of the spine reveals localized tenderness and restricted range of motion. Treatment is supportive, with antibiotics and pain medication being the mainstays of therapy. Although the treatment course is usually prolonged, surgical debridement is rarely necessary. Some studies have shown discitis to be associated with an increased incidence of chronic LBP.

Epidural abscesses account for approximately 1 in 10,000 hospital admissions. Predisposing factors include intravenous drug abuse, cirrhosis, and alcoholism, with men being affected at a greater rate than women. Although severe back pain that follows a spinal procedure should arouse suspicion, spinal instrumentation is usually not the cause of an epidural abscess. In a review of 39 cases of spinal epidural abscess over 27 years at Massachusetts General Hospital, only one was secondary to epidural placement.

The four cardinal signs of an epidural abscess are back pain, tenderness, leukocytosis, and fever. Interestingly, although it is the most common symptom of epidural abscess, back pain itself is not universal. If left untreated, symptoms progress over a period of hours to weeks. Generally, the order of progression proceeds from localized back pain to radicular pain, weakness, incontinence, and paralysis. An epidural abscess is a surgical emergency. In one study, in which patients diagnosed within 36 hours of the onset of symptoms had minimal residual weakness, no recovery was observed in patients paralyzed longer than 48 hours. Other infections that can result in back pain include herpes zoster, Lyme disease, and infectious sacroiliitis.

Vertebral Fractures and Spondylolysis As the life expectancy of the U.S. population has continued to increase, so, too, has the incidence of spinal fractures. There are two main reasons for this: increasing disability with age and a higher incidence of osteoporosis. In clinical practice, only 30% of vertebral fractures come to the attention of physicians, primarily because lack of severe back pain in many patients does not trigger obtaining radiologic studies. However, the prevalence of radiographically demonstrated vertebral deformities rises from 5% of individuals between the ages of 50 and 54, to 50% in women over 80 years. The most common locations for vertebral fractures are at the thoracolumbar junction, the mid-thoracic spine (T7–8), and the lumbar vertebral column. The prevalence of spinal fractures is highest in Caucasian and Asian women, owing to their increased incidence of osteoporosis. Aside from the increased propensity for vertebral fractures, some experts believe osteoporosis in and of itself can cause spinal pain.

The patient with a vertebral fracture typically presents with acute pain overlying the fracture site. For sacral fractures, pain may radiate into the buttocks or leg. The precise incidence of neurologic deficit depends on the extent, type, and location of injury but is usually cited as being greater than 30%. One fact that distinguishes spinal fractures from those with other types of fractures or other acute pain conditions is the fact that more than half of all patients with severe vertebral fractures go on to develop chronic pain. Physical examination of the patient with a vertebral fracture(s) usually reveals marked tenderness on palpation. In patients with lumbar fractures who develop radiculopathy, straight-leg-raising tests may be positive.

Exercise programs for elderly patients suffering from spinal fractures have been shown to increase bone density, decrease the use of analgesics, and improve quality of life. Because patients with vertebral fractures are at increased risk to develop hip and other fractures, walking programs, fall-prevention courses, and even Tai Chi may be beneficial. One study showed that Tai Chi may reduce the risk falls by up to 55% in the elderly. Tai Chi also helps protect stroke survivors from falls and improve balance and motor control in those with Parkinson's disease.

In most patients with isolated spinal fractures, NSAIDs and/or short-acting opioids are sufficient for pain relief. In those with constant pain, sustained release opioids may be necessary. For patients whose main symptoms are consistent with radiculopathy, an epidural steroid injection(s) or trial with neuropathic pain medications may be a worthwhile endeavor. Two treatments that have been shown to both reduce subsequent fractures and provide analgesia for fracture patients are bisphosphonates and salmon calcitonin. In patients with focal pain and limited acute spinal fractures who do not respond to conservative measures, vertebroplasty or kyphoplasty can be considered. Finally, surgical intervention may be necessary in patients with unrelenting pain, spinal instability, or worsening neurologic deficit. In many patients, analgesics and activity modifications are sufficient treatment.

One particular type of vertebral fracture is spondylolysis, also known as pars interarticularis. For the Caucasian adult population, the incidence of spondylolysis has been reported to range between 3% and 6%. There is general agreement that most pars defects occur during childhood, with the large majority of cases being asymptomatic. Risk factors for pars fractures include spondylolisthesis, involvement in sports, and genetics. In active adolescents, spondylolysis can be a significant cause of LBP.

Patients with pars interarticularis usually present with focal LBP, although radiation into the buttock or thigh can occur. This pain may be increased during activities that require extension or rotation of the spine. On physical examination, many patients are noted to have a hyperlordotic posture with tight hamstrings. Diagnosis can be confirmed with plain radiographs, CT, or MRI.

The treatment of patients with symptomatic spondylolysis includes analgesics, bracing, cessation of sports activities, hamstring stretching, and strengthening of the abdominal muscles. In patients who require further pain management, pars injections may be helpful. In some cases, surgery may be necessary.

Metastatic Spinal Tumors Bone is the third most common location of tumor metastases after the lungs and liver. In patients with metastatic cancer, tumor invades bone in 60% to 84% of cases, with the vertebral column and pelvis being the most frequently affected sites. In one study, 39% of all skeletal metastases were to the spine. The pain associated with spinal metastases develops slowly over weeks or months, gradually becoming more intense. Frequently, it can be localized to the involved vertebral bodies. Patients typically characterize it as a dull, but constant, pain. Aggravating factors may include weight bearing, activity, and nighttime, when the patient is trying to sleep. Besides back pain, other signs of spinal metastases include fever, chills, weight loss, and generalized fatigue. Pain treatment includes NSAIDs, neuropathic pain medications, opioids, orthotics, and activity modification. In patients with neurologic deficits, surgical decompression may be necessary. As an adjunct to conventional modalities, chemotherapy, hormone treatment, corticosteroids, bisphosphonates, salmon calcitonin, radioisotopes, and radiotherapy can be helpful.

Kidney Stones Kidney stones, which can be identified by imaging, may be the source of low back pain, and, in these cases, medical referral is the best course of action. Pyelonephritis should also be considered with costovertebral angle tenderness and fever.

HISTORY AND PHYSICAL

Table 38-4 shows the typical associated pattern of pain, numbness, weakness, and atrophy by lumbar disc level.

HISTORY

The initial visit to a spine or pain specialist should be comprehensive. The magnitude of pain (0–10 on a 10-point scale or other descriptors as "mild," "moderate," or "severe"), location ("in the middle," "off to the right/left side," "in the buttock"), radiation pattern (medial, lateral, anterior, or posterior thigh; medial, lateral, or posterior lower leg; lateral, dorsal, or plantar foot; and medial or lateral toes), whether the patient is experiencing more back pain than leg pain or vice versa, and aggravating and remitting factors should be noted. Worsening pain with Valsalva maneuvers that increase intradiscal pressure (coughing, sneezing, bearing down when defecating) or prolonged sitting suggests disc pathology with or without radiculopathy. Pain with standing or walking with pain relief while leaning forward (on a shopping cart, counter, or walker) or sitting may indicate stenosis or facet arthropathy. Sacroiliac joint pain is typically worsened when arising from sitting. Other information to note are changes pain with lying down and changes in relation to the time of day or with particular activities such as swinging a golf club or driving. Pain with swinging a golf club ("the golf sign" should be reproducible on a physical exam) could indicate facet joint pain. Pain that is aggravated more with driving than just sitting can imply increased tension through the sciatic nerve because the knee is held in extension for an extended period of time.

Leg pain experienced going up stairs is often due to vascular claudication because plantar flexors are oxygen depleted due to significant vascular disease. Pain typically decreases when a patient stands still either upright or seated. In contrast, leg pain that occurs while descending stairs or walking down a hill may indicate neurogenic claudication because patients are usually leaning backward slightly as they descend (in order to shift their

TABLE 38-4 Level of Disc Herniation as Differentiated by History and Physical Examination

L2–3 Disc (L3 nerve root)
Pain: low back, upper buttock to anterior thigh, anterior knee, medial lower leg Numbness: anterior thigh, knee (may be absent) Weakness: hip flexion, hip adduction, knee extension Atrophy: iliopsoas, quadriceps femoris, sartorius, hip adductors Associated reflex: patellar
L3–4 Disc (L4 nerve root)
Pain: low back, hip, thigh, anterior leg, inner leg to medial portion of foot Numbness: anteromedial thigh, medial aspect of lower leg (may be absent) Weakness: knee extension, sometimes dorsiflexion of foot Atrophy: quadriceps femoris, tibialis anterior, gluteus medius, gluteus minimus, tensor fasciae latae Associated reflex: patellar, gluteal
L4–5 Disc (L5 nerve root)
Pain: low back, buttock, hip, posterolateral thigh, lateral aspect of lower leg, dorsum of foot, first two toes Numbness: lateral leg, dorsum of foot, first two toes Weakness: dorsiflexion of foot and great toe, difficulty walking on heels, possible foot drop Atrophy: hamstrings, tibialis posterior, extensor hallucis longus, extensor digitorum brevis, sometimes gluteals Associated reflex: tibialis posterior, gluteal
L5–S1 Disc (S1 nerve root)
Pain: sacroiliac joint, hip, buttock, posterolateral thigh and leg, lateral edge of foot, heel, sole Numbness: calf, lateral border of foot, heel, sole, sometimes fourth and fifth toes Weakness: gastrocnemius, soleus, gluteus maximus, hamstrings, peroneus Associated reflex: ankle jerk, hamstring

center of gravity posteriorly to minimize falling forward), which narrows the neuroforamina. Standing upright at the bottom of the stairway or hill does not relieve pain, but it is relieved by leaning forward or sitting. The "shopping cart sign" describes the behavior of leaning over a shopping cart in the grocery store to relieve pain. Alternatively, patients say that they lean on the bathroom sink while performing activities of daily living (ADLs) that relieves the pain. Note that while this behavior may classically be associated with spinal stenosis, it may also relieve discogenic pain by providing traction, so the "cart sign" should be used in the proper context. Note the presence of numbness, tingling, or subjective weakness, with examples for the latter often described as difficulty climbing stairs or subjective knee buckling. It is important to try to distinguish between pain-induced weakness and true neurological weakness, which may be associated with muscle atrophy or hyporeflexia. Difficulty putting on socks or shoes may indicate hip pathology.

A review of back-related symptoms should include questions regarding bowel or bladder incontinence, recent fevers, unintentional weight loss, or falling. Red flags to keep in mind include gait ataxia/upper motor neuron complaints that could indicate myelopathy. Bowel, bladder, or sexual dysfunction could indicate cauda equina syndrome. Night pain, fevers, chills, or unintentional weight loss could indicate infection or cancer. In order to better identify these conditions, a detailed history should include questions directed toward previous drug abuse (for infection) and family history (for cancer). Frequent falling is a dangerous condition particularly in seniors or in patients on anticoagulation. These red flags may require urgent or emergent medical care. A general review of systems should always be performed when evaluating a new patient with back pain (discussed later).

The evaluator should note the date and the activity or event that the patient associates with the onset of pain and whether there has been an increase or decrease in symptoms since the event. Sacroiliac joint pain is more likely to be associated with a specific inciting event than facet joint or discogenic pain, as is radicular pain from a herniated disc more likely to have a distinct onset than spinal stenosis. The course of pain may have been altered by therapeutic interventions prescribed by prior health care providers, including opioid medications, oral Prednisone, "muscle relaxers," antiepileptics, antidepressants, aspirin or other anti-inflammatories, acetaminophen, or other medications, including herbal remedies. Prior interventional procedures should be listed, such as epidural steroid injections, facet blocks, nerve blocks, medial branch blocks, radiofrequency ablations, SI joint injections, and the like and whether they were performed under fluoroscopy. The percentage of relief from these procedures, as well as duration of effect, should be noted because this information can guide future treatments. Previous physical therapy courses should include details such as the number of sessions, whether modalities were used, stretching and methods of strengthening that were employed, and whether the patient is continuing a home exercise program after the completion of the therapy prescription. Other forms of therapy such as acupuncture, chiropractic manipulation, and cognitive behavioral therapy should be documented.

Dose and duration of opioid use should be noted, as well as changes in use over time (increasing, decreasing, or relatively constant) and conversion to stronger opioids, such as going from oral Oxycodone to Fentanyl patches. Recent studies have shown that chronic opioid use is associated with chronic opioid-induced hyperalgesia and effectively lowers pain threshold such that susceptibility to pain is increased. Evidence suggests that patients on high doses of opioids are more likely to fail procedural interventions, such as radiofrequency denervation and surgery. One study showed that patient treated for acute low back pain with a morphine equivalent amount (MEA) of 450 mg or more over the first 15 days are out of work 69 days longer, are three times more likely to have surgery, and are six times more likely to continue on opioids than those who were not treated with opioids. Finally, another study showed that patients with compensable back injuries on long-term opioids tend to increase opioid dosages without significant improvement of pain. It also concluded that the dosages used to treat acute low back pain predict long-term usage.

A careful medical, surgical, family, and social history should be done. Studies have shown that smoking increases susceptibility to chronic pain. Return to work was approximately 70% more likely in married workers than unmarried workers. A poor social support system has been linked to a higher risk of low back pain. Family history offers clues and may be a useful prognosticator. In patients with painful herniated disc, 35% of them had a first-degree relative with a history of a painful herniated disc compared with 12% for controls. Five percent of herniated disc patients had a family member who had back surgery for a herniated disc compared with 1% for controls.

The patient's relationship to work should be assessed. Patients who "hardly ever enjoyed their job" were 2.5 times more likely to report back pain than those who "almost always enjoyed their job." Many studies have shown a decreased return-to-work rate with higher compensation in the form of workers' compensation, disability insurance, and other forms of financial compensation. Financially compensated low back pain lasted, on average, 12 months in one study compared with 1 week on average for uncompensated low back pain. Low back injuries that occurred at work were associated with up to four times longer "out-of-work" duration than injuries that did not occur at work. Assessment should include whether an attorney is involved in the patient's case of back pain and whether it is in the setting of workers' compensation, a motor vehicle accident, or other settings that may involve litigation. One study showed that when an attorney is involved in a workers' compensation case, the return-to-work rate decreased by approximately 50% compared with cases without attorney involvement. Other studies show similar trends. Recommendations to employers to reduce work injury claims should not only include safety and ergonomic optimization, but also improve employee satisfaction, fitness for specific job tasks, and relationships among fellow employees and supervisors.

The patient's attitude toward exercise and details of their routine exercise regimen should be assessed. Patients who exercise regularly tend to have fewer episodes of back pain and recover more quickly. Monitoring of progressive return to their normal exercise routine is a positive prognosticator. If physical therapy is prescribed, knowledge of their normal exercise routine could allow for better integration of their therapeutic regimen.

A general medical evaluation should be performed, which includes listing the patient's medications and allergies and a general review of systems. Each of the patient's medical conditions should be surveyed to determine if they are controlled medically, in quiescence, or otherwise being followed by the patient's primary care physician or a particular specialist. If not, recommendations can be made to the patient and his or her primary care physician to get the issue(s) addressed.

PHYSICAL EXAMINATION

The physical exam is a key component of the complete evaluation of the spinal pain patient. However, it is important to understand that a definitive diagnosis can rarely be conferred based on physical examination alone. Each part of the comprehensive patient visit represents one piece of a complex puzzle that includes history, psychosocial and family history, physical exam, imaging, and ancillary tests as deemed necessary (e.g., electromyography/nerve conduction studies). In some respects, the main value of the physical examination is to identify those patients who may benefit from advanced diagnostic testing (e.g., MRI) and/or for referral to an interventional pain specialist for injections or to a spine surgeon for surgical evaluation.

General Appearance Look for open wounds, rashes, skin lesions, signs of infection, edema, or other issues that should be addressed. Port wine or other birth marks or doughy lipomata may indicate spina bifida. An unusual patch of hair on the spine can signify underlying bony abnormalities. Patients may present in the examination room unable to sit, pacing back and forth, leaning over the exam table, lying down as means to minimize back pain, or otherwise express and demonstrate the physical and emotional content of their pain experience, which may include these and other behaviors.

Gait and Movement Abnormal gait can indicate pain-associated movement, muscle weakness that may indicate level of pathology (e.g., foot slap for L4 pathology), or fear-avoidance beliefs (FABs). Scissoring gait, where the legs cross when walking, can be observed after cerebrovascular events, spinal cord injury or syringomyelia, or cervical myelopathy. Steppage gait often accompanies foot drop and can occur with a herniated disc, with peroneal neuropathy or polyneuropathy, and after spinal cord injury. Waddling gait often ensues with muscular dystrophies, gluteus medius weakness, spinal muscle atrophy, and hip problems.

FABs are maladaptations from misinformation regarding the potential for physical injury of the low back stemming from generalized or specific activities. They involve avoidance of repeating the emotional content of the pain experience. FABs can stem not only from the patient, but also from misinformation, misinterpretation of information, and transference of these fears from health care providers or the Internet. It has been shown that excessive FABs result in hypervigilence in monitoring a patient's own pain and represent a significant obstacle for recovery from low back pain. It has also been shown that those who confront their pain and are able to increase physical and social activities over time have improved recovery rates, while those who respond to their pain with avoidance are more likely to develop chronic pain, increased impairment, and eventual disability.

Pain behavior, on the other hand, refers to the cognitive and emotional expression of pain such as limping, grimacing, moaning, crying, and asking for more pain medications. It has been suggested that these behaviors, through perceived validation, are reinforced with positive rewards by family, friends, and even health care providers; they also reinforce patient identity as being disabled. Further reinforcement comes in the form of financial rewards and excuses from returning to work and doing household chores. Ultimately, pain behaviors, through multiple studies, have been shown to be a significant barrier to recovery, and they enhance the perception of pain. When positive reinforcement ceases, the behavior is vulnerable to extinction, and the barrier to recovery is removed.

Lumbosacral Range of Motion, Including Flexion, Extension, Side Bending, and Rotation It is not practical to try to isolate lumbar motion, and it has been shown that lumbosacral motion is an equivalent measure of function of the lumbar spine. If any motion causes pain, it should be documented. These quantitative measures can be monitored in subsequent follow-up visits to track progress. Pain with movement may indicate a potentially greater benefit from aggressive physical therapy as opposed to pain while sitting, lying down, or otherwise not moving. Normal ranges for lumbosacral spinal flexion are commonly between 70° and 100°; for extension, between 20° and 35°; for lateral bending, between 15° and 25°; and for axial rotation, between 20° and 30°.

Sit-to-Stand Test The sit-to-stand test is 50% to 54% sensitive and 77% to 81% specific for L3/L4 nerve root impingement, respectively, and possibly the best test for this. The patient stands from a seated position on one leg while the examiner maintains patient's balance if needed.

Great Toe Extensor Strength The great toe extensor strength test is 61% sensitive and 86% specific for an L5 nerve root impingement. Results are best if performed in isolation with foot flat on step stool with the great toe extending beyond edge of step stool and with examiner applying resistance.

Hip Abductor Strength The hip abductor strength test is 29% sensitive and 97% specific for an L5 nerve root impingement. Results are best if performed with the patient lying on his or her side with the hip slightly flexed. The test is performed when the patient abducts the hip against examiner's resistance. The test may differentiate between Tensor Fascia Lata (TFL) and gluteal weakness if first performed with the hip in slight flexion and then in extension, keeping the knee fully extended at all times. If there is a difference, a nerve root impingement is unlikely.

Plantar Flexor Strength Plantar flexor strength is 4% sensitive and 86% specific for an L2, L3, and/or L4 impingement but does not differentiate among these levels. Likewise, this test is 14% sensitive and 96% specific for an L5 and/or S1 nerve root impingement. The patient is asked to stand on one foot and plantar flex his or her weight maximally 10 times. The test is then repeated on the contralateral foot.

Heel Walking The heel walking test is 20% sensitive and 86% specific for an L2, L3, and/or L4 impingement but does not differentiate among these levels. Likewise, this test is 14% sensitive and 80% specific for an L5 and/or S1 nerve root impingement.

Dorsiflexor Strength The dorsiflexor strength test is for L4–L5, but it may not be specific for a particular root. Results are best when performed with the patient's ankles in firm contact on a step stool and dorsiflexed against examiner's resistance.

The hip flexors and adductors should also be tested.

Anterior Thigh Pinprick In comparing different modes of sensory testing, it can be generally agreed that vibration is the first to be affected by radiculopathy and, therefore, would be the most sensitive but least specific test for radiculopathy at a given level. On the other hand, it is also known that light touch, pin prick, and temperature dermatomes do not overlap precisely. The quantitative findings in detecting levels in radiculopathy were performed using pinprick and so they are presented here. Anterior thigh pinprick is 50% sensitive and 96% specific for an L2 nerve root impingement.

Medial Ankle Pinprick This test is 61% sensitive and 86% specific for an L4 nerve root impingement.

Medial Knee Pinprick This test is 17% sensitive and 96% specific for an L2, L3, and/or L4 impingement but does not differentiate among these levels. Likewise, this test is 4% sensitive and 83% specific for an L5 and/or S1 nerve root impingement.

Dorsal Great Toe Pinprick This test is 13% sensitive and 82% specific for an L2, L3, and/or L4 impingement but does not differentiate among these levels. Likewise, this test is 18% sensitive and 87% specific for an L5 and/or S1 nerve root impingement.

Lateral Foot Pinprick This test is 8% sensitive and 79% specific for an L2, L3, and/or L4 impingement but does not differentiate among these levels. Likewise, this test is 21% sensitive and 92% specific for an L5 and/or S1 nerve root impingement. This test is best performed at the most distal areas of the lateral foot.

Patellar Reflex Abnormality Patellar reflex abnormality test is 39% sensitive and 95% specific for an L4 nerve root impingement. Together with an abnormal medial ankle pinprick, it is 62% sensitive and 95% specific for an L4 nerve root impingement.

Achilles Reflex Abnormality Achilles reflex abnormality test is 33% sensitive and 91% specific for an L5 nerve root impingement. Together with a weak hip abduction, it is 61% sensitive and 89% specific for an L5 nerve root impingement.

Ipsilateral Straight Leg Raise The ipsilateral straight-lef raise test is 67% sensitive and 67% specific for an L5 nerve root impingement. It is 73% sensitive and 63% specific for an S1 nerve root impingement. It is 69% sensitive and 84% specific for either an L5 or S1 nerve root impingement. Reproduction of the patient's radiating pain pattern when hip is passively flexed between 30° and 70° is a positive result.

Contralateral Straight Leg Raise The contralateral straight-leg raise test is 7% sensitive and 96% specific for either an L5 or S1 nerve root impingement. Reproduction of the patient's radiating pain pattern when contralateral hip is passively flexed between 30° and 70° is a positive result.

Ipsilateral Femoral Stretch Test The ipsilateral femoral stretch test is 70% sensitive and 88% specific for an L3 nerve root impingement. It is 50% sensitive and 100% specific for an L2, L3, and/or L4 impingement, but does not differentiate among these levels. Reproduction of the patient's radiating pain pattern is a positive result.

Contralateral Femoral Stretch Test The contralateral femoral stretch test is 9% sensitive and 100% specific for an L4 nerve root impingement. Reproduction of the patient's radiating pain pattern is a positive result.

Babinski and Clonus Babinksi and Clonus tests evaluate for upper motor neuron involvement.

FABER/FADIR/Hip Grind/Hip External/Internal Rotation These tests are used to evaluate hip pain and limited ROM due to degenerative joint disease in the hip or labral tear. The majority of pain should be in the groin, but patients may complain of lateral hip pain from these maneuvers. Applying pressure to the SI joint while in FABRE may indicate SI joint pain, but this is nonspecific. Applying pressure to the piriformis while in the FADIR position with reproduction of radiating symptoms may indicate piriformis syndrome, especially if the patient's hip rests in external rotation compared to the contralateral hip or if the patient has difficulty in active hip internal rotation. In practice, however, this is also nonspecific.

Applying Pressure to Spinous Processes at Midline When testing in this manner, tenderness may indicate a fracture, interspinous ligamentous sprain, or underlying disc pathology.

Applying Pressure Paraspinally When applying pressure of this kind, tenderness may indicate primary muscular spasm or strain (i.e. trigger point) or may occur secondarily in response to other pathology, such as with facetogenic or sacroiliac joint pain. Identifying the primary source of pain by palpation is controversial. Because the facet joint lies as much as 7 cm below the skin, it is not likely that a particular painful facet joint can be palpated with specificity. Multiple studies have demonstrated increased levels of myoelectric activity during electromyography (EMG) testing.

Waddell's Signs Arguably antiquated, Wadell's Signs were originally described more than 30 years ago. The presence of signs from the following five categories has been the subject of widespread misinterpretation and misuse over the ensuing decades. A review by Fishbain and colleagues found either negative or conflicting evidence for an association between Waddell's signs and psychological stress or secondary gain and their ability to reliably distinguish organic from nonorganic pathology. However, the authors concluded that the presence of signs in three of the five categories was positively associated with greater baseline pain and disability and poorer treatment outcomes. During the physical exam, there should be ample opportunities to observe these physical signs in five categories that may caution the examiner when considering invasive procedures, and may prompt a more detailed psychological evaluation:

1. Overreaction: Excessive pain behaviors and verbal expressions while doing maneuvers that require patient to move either actively or passively.
2. Tenderness: Pain behaviors with light touching or pinching of skin in a nonanatomic pattern.
3. Nonanatomic findings: Patients with signs and symptoms that do not correlate well with known anatomy. Examples include discord between myotomal findings and dermatomal findings or findings that include parts of dermatomes but exclude other parts of the same dermatomes. An example of this would be entire right foot pain without pain above the right ankle or numbness of the entire leg but not the foot.
4. Distraction: Tests that are abnormal but become normal when patient is distracted or that stay abnormal without following through with the test. An example is a patient who shows marked weakness in the plantar flexors or quads in isolation but is later climbing stairs without difficulty alongside the examiner who is carrying on a conversation about a distracting topic. Another example is when a patient is hyperreflexic at the patellae and also hyperreflexic when the examiner stops the hammer before striking the patellar tendon.
5. Simulation: Low back pain exacerbation by pushing down on the top of the patient's head or shoulders.

Other physical exam maneuvers are performed as deemed necessary. Patients with complaints of balance problems or exam findings of clonus should receive a full neurological exam, including cranial nerve evaluation, tightrope walking, Rhomberg test, heel-to-toe walking, and so forth. Patients with hip, knee, or foot pain should receive appropriate examinations to rule in or rule out nonspinal causes of pain. Often, these are the reasons for referral to a pain or spine physician to help determine whether the pain is coming from the hip, knee, or foot or from the spine. For example, it would be a mistake for surgeons to perform hip surgery for groin pain that is referred from the spine.

See the Chapter Addendum for other exam maneuvers that may be useful in a physical exam.

RADIOLOGIC IMAGING

With the advent of new procedures, neuroimaging has taken on a greater role in recent years for the diagnosis of LBP. Conventional radiographs are frequently used during an initial evaluation of LBP, especially in patients with known musculoskeletal disease, or when a fracture is suspected. Disorders likely to be picked up on plain x-rays include spondylolisthesis, pars interarticularis defects, scoliosis, ankylosing spondylitis, Scheuermann's disease, spinal stenosis, and osteoporosis. However, because of the low yield with radiographs, their utility in patients with LBP is controversial.

Magnetic resonance imaging is the diagnostic test of choice for evaluating patients with radiculopathy. Other disorders in which MRI is the preferred imaging tool include myelomalacia, syringomyelia, intramedullary tumors of the spinal cord, spinal cord infarction, traumatic injury, and multiple sclerosis. In a study by Jensen et al. published in the *New England Journal of Medicine*, 64% of individuals without LBP were found to have abnormal intervertebral disks on MRI scans of their lumbar spine. The results of this study have been confirmed by numerous other investigators, with the prevalence of abnormalities increasing with age. Currently, the American College of Physicians recommends an MRI only for serious or progressive neurological deficits or when referring patients for surgical evaluation or epidural steroid injections.

The strength of computed tomography in evaluating patients with LBP lies not in its resolution but in its ability to define spatial relationships between anatomic structures. As such, CT is helpful in patients with spinal stenosis, spinal infections, primary metastatic tumors of the spine, and spinal cord injuries. Because CT provides better images of bone than does MRI, it is preferred for patients with suspected bony abnormalities. Frequently, CT is used in conjunction with myelograms for the evaluation of radiculopathy and following discography to better delineate disk disease.

Radionuclide bone scanning is the procedure of choice for detecting a variety of bone disorders. Bone scanning is the primary modality used to diagnose and follow skeletal metastases. Whereas osteomyelitis may not be detectable radiographically for more than a week after onset, a bone scan usually shows areas of enhancement within hours of onset. Other indications for bone scanning include occult vertebral fractures, bone disease associated with metabolic disorders, and spondyloarthropathies.

CONCLUSION

The complexity of low back pain and radiation can be daunting to the unfamiliar practitioner. In any given patient, the number of pain generators can range from a single source (such as a herniated disc) to multiple sources (such as multilevel disc herniations, facet arthropathy, and stenosis) plus pain generated from remote sources (such as the hip, sacroiliac joint, or piriformis muscle). In addition, psychosocial factors are likely to affect the diagnosis, treatment, or prognosis of any given patient. Finally, there is often no single piece of historical information, no particular physical exam finding, nor a particular MRI result that can reliably result in a definitive diagnosis or prognosis. It often takes a well-informed and experienced practitioner, as well as a motivated patient, to arrive at a meaningful diagnosis, prescribe viable treatment options, and improve patient outcomes. A patient visit of at least 30 minutes is often required to gather all pertinent information from the patient, formulate treatment options, and provide meaningful education and reassurance to the patient.

It is also important to closely monitor patient progress in the form of follow-up visits. Often during these visits, a patient may report increased pain from a particular treatment course, and the experienced practitioner should understand the side effects of these treatments and also the natural course of the particular etiology being treated. Increased pain is expected in the early course of any effective physical therapy and it is rarely is a cause to cease therapy. Injections can also cause transient increases in pain. Finally, some etiologies, such as disc herniations, most often have a natural course of waxing and subsequently waning regardless of whether treatment has been prescribed or not. The experienced practitioner should be able to rule out very rare but concerning processes, such as a new vertebral fracture or more commonly a painful reherniation. Most often, however, increased pain is benign. The practitioner should be comfortable with complaints of increased pain and also with reassuring the patient that his or her increased pain is part of the neurologic or muscular pathology and does not indicate harmful anatomic events.

ADDENDUM: SPECIAL TESTS BY CATEGORY FOR LOW BACK PAIN WITH OR WITHOUT RADICULOPATHY

TESTS FOR RADICULOPATHY

Bow String Sign. The patient is seated with the body bent forward and knee flexed to 70°, a position that lengthens the course of the sciatic nerve. The examiner then applies pressure on the sciatic nerve by pressing the fingers into the popliteal fossa. An increase in leg pain signifies a radiculopathy.

Brudzinski's Test. With the patient supine, the head is passively flexed to the chest. Reproduction of the patient's leg pain signifies nerve root irritation.

Kernig's Test. The patient lies supine with the hip flexed 90°. The patient is then asked to extend the knee. Back pain may be a sign of nerve root irritation.

Lasegue's Test. The patient lies supine with the hip flexed 90°. The patient is then asked to slowly extend the knee. A positive test occurs with the elicitation of sciatic pain.

Milgram's Test. The patient, lying supine, is asked to elevate both extended legs approximately 2 inches off the examining table. If the patient can hold this position for 30 seconds without pain, it aids the examiner in eliminating intrathecal pathology as a cause of pain. If the patient experiences pain during this maneuver or cannot hold the position, intrathecal pathology, such as a herniated disk, must not be ruled out.

Stoop Test. The patient is asked to walk briskly for several minutes. When back, posterior thigh, and leg pain appear, the patient sits and flexes forward. Disappearance of the pain suggests neurogenic claudication. During this time, reflexes may be diminished.

Valsalva's Test. The patient is asked to bear down, as during a bowel movement or coughing, thus increasing intrathecal pressure. A positive test suggests intrathecal pathology.

TESTS FOR SACROILIAC JOINT DYSFUNCTION

Cranial Shear Test. With the patient prone and the pelvis immobilized through the hip, pressure is applied to the coccygeal end of the sacrum. This test may be positive in patients with sacroiliac joint pain.

Extension Test. The patient is placed in the prone position, with one hand of the examiner on the thigh of the affected side and other hand over the opposite iliac crest. Downward pressure is exerted on the iliac crest, while pulling slightly on the anterior thigh, to elicit sacroiliac joint pain.

Flamingo Test. The patient is asked to stand on the involved leg and hop. Pain in the sacroiliac region may be indicative of sacroiliac joint dysfunction.

Gaenslen's Test. The patient lies supine on the examining table with both knees drawn to the chest. The patient is then asked to shift over to the edge of the table, so that the leg being tested hovers over the edge. The examiner presses down on the affected side, hyperextending the hip. A positive Gaenslen's test is generally considered a sign of sacroiliac joint pain but may indicate hip pathology as well.

Gillet's Test. While the patient stands with the feet approximately 12 inches apart, the examiner sits behind the patient and palpates the S2 spinous process with one thumb and the posterior superior iliac spine with the other. As if taking a large marching step, the patient then flexes the knee and hip of the side being tested. If the posterior superior iliac spine fails to move posteroinferiorly with respect to S2, the test is positive. This may be indicative of sacroiliac joint dysfunction.

Patrick's Test. The patient is positioned supine with the foot of the involved side against the opposite knee. The sacroiliac joint is then stressed by pressing simultaneously against the flexed knee and contralateral anterior superior iliac supine. The Patrick's test is used to assess both sacroiliac joint dysfunction as well as hip pathology when, in the latter, pain is elicited in the inguinal or hip area. Because this test involves flexion, abduction, and external rotation of the hip, it is also called the FABER test.

Pelvic Compression Test. This test compresses the pelvis by the application of lateral pressure to the uppermost iliac crest, directed toward the opposite iliac crest. It is believed to stretch the posterior sacroiliac ligaments and compress the anterior part of the joint.

Pelvic Distraction Test. For this test, the examiner applies pressure to both anterior superior iliac spines, directed posteriorly and laterally. This test is alleged to stretch the anterior sacroiliac ligaments.

Pelvic Rock Test. The patient lies supine, and the examiner cups both hands around the iliac crests with the thumbs on the anterior superior iliac spine and the palms on the iliac tubercles. The examiner then forcibly compresses the patient's pelvis toward the midline of the body. Complaints of pain may indicate pathology in the sacroiliac joint.

Sacroiliac Shear Test. With the patient lying prone, the examiner crosses both hands over the sacrum. The overlying hand delivers a postero-anterior thrust, while the underlying hand is used to detect motion in the joint.

Shift Test. Patient stands with feet 12 inches apart and is asked to shift his or her weight from foot to foot, back and forth. Transient pain is felt on the offloading side with each shift. Again as with all SI joint testing, this test is nonspecific for SI joint pathology.

Thigh Thrust Test. This test applies a posterior shearing stress to the sacroiliac joint through the femur.

TESTS FOR PIRIFORMIS SYNDROME

Beatty's Maneuver. From the lateral decubitus position with the nonpainful side dependent, the patient is asked to abduct the thigh by moving the nonpainful leg off the table. Contraction of the piriformis muscle elicits pain in patients with piriformis syndrome.

Freiberg's Sign. Recreation of buttock or leg pain, or both, occurs during internal rotation of the hip. This test may be positive in patients with piriformis syndrome.

Pace Sign. An indicator of piriformis syndrome, this test is positive when the patient experiences weakness during resisted abduction and external rotation of the leg.

TESTS FOR MUSCLE PATHOLOGY

Beevor's Sign. While the examiner observes the patient's umbilicus, the patient is asked to do a quarter sit-up with the arms crossed over the chest. Normally, the umbilicus should not move. If the umbilicus is drawn up, down, or over to one side (the stronger side), weakness, atrophy, or asymmetry of the anterior abdominal or paraspinal muscles may be present. This sign is frequently positive in patients with meningomyelocele or poliomyelitis.

Sit-up Test. Patient's with severe discogenic pain or paraspinal muscle spasm have difficulty sitting up unassisted when flexed at their lumbar spine. They have a tendency to push up with their arms for support.

Tripod Sign. As the patient sits with legs dangling and hips flexed 90°, the knees are passively extended. Patients with hamstring muscle tightness will extend the trunk to relieve the pressure.

TESTS FOR NONORGANIC COMPONENTS TO DYSFUNCTION

Hoover's Test. This test should be performed in conjunction with the straight-leg raise test. A patient who is making a genuine effort to raise the affected leg will automatically put pressure on the calcaneus of his opposite leg in order to gain leverage. By placing one hand under the patient's heel, the examiner can determine whether or not the patient is making a concerted effort.

Ratcheting versus Smooth Strength Testing. When attempting a sustained muscle contraction such as dorsiflexion at the ankle, patients with nonorganic components to dysfunction exhibit ratcheting and jerking movements and, eventually, breakaway weakness. In contrast, patients with isolated myotomal weakness are overcome in a smooth fashion.

TESTS FOR UPPER MOTOR LESIONS

Babinski's Reflex. Stimulation is applied to the plantar surface of the foot with a dull object. When the lateral four toes flex and fan and the large toe extends, an upper motor lesion is suspected.

Chaddock Reflex. This test is similar to the Babinski's reflex test, except that the lateral aspect of the foot beneath the lateral malleolus is stimulated.

Oppenheim's Test. A dull object is run down the anterior portion of the tibia. A positive response is similar to Babinski's reflex.

MISCELLANEOUS TESTS

Schober's Test. This test measures the flexibility of the lumbar spine. The patient's back is marked twice, once at the level of the sacroiliac dimples and again 10 cm above this point. As the patient flexes forward, the distance between the two points should increase by at least 4 cm. An abnormal test may indicate spondyloarthropathy.

BIBLIOGRAPHY

Allen TL, Tatli Y, Lutz GE. Fluoroscopic percutaneous lumbar zygapophyseal joint cyst rupture: a clinical outcome study. *Spine J.* 2009 May;9(5):387-395. Epub 2008 Sep 21.

American Academy of Orthopedic Surgeons website: www.aaos.org

Anderson GBJ. Epidemiological features of chronic low-back pain. *Lancet.* 1999;354:581-585.

Andersson GBJ, Lucente T, Davis AM, et al. A comparison of osteopathic spinal manipulation with standard care for patients with low back pain. *N Engl J Med.* 1999;341:1426-1431. [PMID: 10547405].

Angst MS, Clark DJ. Opioid-induced hyperalgesia: a qualitative systematic review. *Anesthesiology.* 2006;104:570-587.

Babyak M, Blumenthal J, Herman S, Khatri P, Doraiswami M, Moore K, Craighead E, Baldewicz T, Krishnan KR. Exercise treatment for major depression: maintenance of therapeutic benefit at 10 months. *Psychosomatic Med.* 2000;62:633-638.

Baker AS, Ojemann RG, Swartz MN, Richardson EP Jr. Spinal epidural abscess. *N Engl J Med.* 1975;293:463-468. [PMID: 1152860]

Bigos SJ, Battié MC, Spengler DM, Fisher LD, Fordyce WE, Hansson TH, Nachemson AL, Wortley MD. A prospective study of work perceptions and psychosocial factors affecting the report of back injury. *Spine.* 1991 Jan;16(1):1-6.

Blackwell TL, Leierer S, Haupt S, Kampotsis A. Predictors of vocational rehabilitation return to work outcomes in workers compensation. *Rehabilitation Counseling Bulletin.* Winter 2003;46(108).

Bloomfield DJ. Should bisphosphonates be part of the standard therapy of patients with multiple myeloma or bone metastases from other cancers? An evidence-based review. *J Clin Oncol.* 1978;16:1218-1225. [PMID: 9508210]

Boos N, et al. 1995 Volvo Award in clinical science: the diagnostic accuracy of MRI, work perception, and psychosocial factors in identifying symptomatic disc herniations. *Spine.* 1995;20:2613-2625.

Carey TS, Garrett J, Jackman A, McLaughlin C, Fryer J, Smucker DR. The outcomes and costs of care for acute low back pain among patients seen by primary care practitioners, chriropracters, and orthopedic surgesons: the North Carolina Back Pain Project. *N Engl J Med.* 1995;333(14):913-917.

Cayi SR, Koçak A, Alkan A, Kirimlioğclu H. Is there a clinical correlate to the histological and radiological evidence of inflammation in trans-ligamentous extruded and sequestered lumbar disc herniaton? *Br J Neurosurg.* 2004 Dec;18(6):576-583.

Celerier E, Laulin J-P, Corcuff J-B, Le Moal M, Simonnet G. Progressive enhancement of delayed hyperalgesia induced by repeated heroin administration: A sensitization process. *J Neurosci.* 2001;21:4074-4080.

Centers for Disease Control and Prevention. Prevalence of disabilities and associated health conditions among adults—United States, 1999. *JAMA*. 2001;285(12):1571-1572.

Cohen I, Rainville J. Aggressive exercise as treatment for chronic low back pain. *Sports Med*. 2002;32(1):75-82.

Cohen SP, Dawson T, Abdi S. Lateral branch blocks as a treatment for sacroiliac joint pain: a pilot study. *Reg Anesth Pain Med*. 2003;28:113-119. [PMID: 12677621]

DePalma AF, Rothman RH. *The Intervetebral Disc*. Philadelphia, Pa: WB Saunders; 1970.

Dreyer SJ, Dreyfuss PH. Low back pain and the zygapophysial (facet) joints. *Arch Phys Med Rehabil*. 1996;77:290-300. [PMID: 8600875]

Dreyfuss P, Michaelsen M, Pauza K, et al. The value of medical history and physical examination in diagnosing sacroiliac joint pain. *Spine*. 1996;21:2594-2602. [PMID: 8961447]

Dreyfuss P, Schwarzer AC, Lau P, Bogduk N. Specificity of lumbar medial branch and L5 dorsal ramus blocks. *Spine*. 1997;22:895-902. [PMID: 9127924]

Eismont FJ, Montero C. Infections of the spine. In: Davidoff RA, ed. *Handbook of the Spinal Cord*. New York, NY: Marcel Dekker; 1987:411-449.

Fishbain DA, Cutler RB, Rosomoff HL, Rosomoff RS. Is there a relationship between nonorganic physical findings (Waddell signs) and secondary gain/malingering? *Clin J Pain*. 2004 Nov-Dec;20(6):399-408.

Foster L, Clapp L, Erickson M, Jabbari B. Botulinum toxin A and chronic low back pain: a randomized, double-blind study. *Neurology*. 2001;56: 1290-1293. [PMID: 11376175]

Franklin GM. Opioid use for chronic low back pain: a prospective, population-based study among injured workers in Washington state, 2002-2005. *Clin J Pain*. 2009;25:743-751.

Freburger JK, Holmes GM, Agans, RP, et al. The rising prevalence of chronic low back pain. *Arch Intern Med*. Feb 2009;169(3):251-258.

Freedman BA, Cohen SP, Kuklo TR, Lehman RA, Larkin P, Giuliani JR. Intradiscal electrothermal therapy (IDET) for chronic low back pain in active-duty soldiers: 2-year follow-up. *Spine J*. 2003;3:502-509.

Frymoyer, JW, Cats-Baril, WL. An overview of the incidences and costs of low back pain. *Orthop Clin North A*. 1991;22:263-271.

Goldberg MS, Scott SC, Mayo NE. A review of the association between cigarette smoking and the development of nonspecific back pain and related outcomes. *Spine*. 2000;25:995-1014. [PMID: 10767814]

Goldthwait JE. The lumbosacral articulation: an explanation of many cases of lumbago, sciatica and paraplegia. *Boston Med Surg J*. 1911;164:365-372.

Gordon W, McCulloch J, Kummel Ed, Venner R. Nonorganic physical signs in low-back pain. *Spine*. March/April 1980;5(2):117-125.

Hagen KB, Hilde G, Jamtvedt G, Winnem MF. The Cochrane review of bed rest for acute low back pain and sciatica. *Spine*. 2000;25:2932-2939. [PMID: 11074682]

Hart, LG, Deyo RA, Cherkin DC. Physician office visits for low back pain: frequency, clinical evaluation, and treatment patterns from a U.S. national survey. *Spine*. 1995;20:11-9.

Hoppenfeld S. *Physical Examination of the Spine and Extremities*. Norwalk, Conn: Appleton-Century-Crofts; 1976.

Institute of Medicine Report from the Committee on Advancing Pain Research, Care, and Education: Relieving Pain in America. *A Blueprint for Transforming Prevention, Care, Education and Research*. Washington, DC: The National Academies Press; 2011.

Jensen MC, Brant-Zawadzki MN, Obuchowski N, et al. Magnetic resonance imaging of the lumbar spine in people without back pain. *N Engl J Med*. 1994;331:69-73. [PMID: 8208267]

Katz JN. Lumbar disc disorders and low-back pain: socioeconomic factors and consequences. *J Bone Joint Surg Am*. 2006;88(Suppl 2):21-24.

Kirkady-Willis WH, Burton CV, eds. *Managing Low Back Pain*. 3rd ed. New York, NY: Churchill Livingstone; 1992.

Kobayashi T, Atsuta Y, Takemitsu M, Matsuno T, Takeda N. A prospective study of de novo scoliosis in a community based cohort. *Spine (Phila Pa 1976)*. 2006 Jan 15;31(2):178-182.

Kovacs FM, Abraira V, Pena A, et al. Effect of firmness of mattress on chronic non-specific low-back pain: randomised, double-blind, controlled, multicentre trial. *Lancet*. 2003 Nov 15;362(9396):1599-1604.

Kraft GH. A physiological approach to the evaluation of lumbosacral spinal stenosis. *Phys Med Rehabil Clin N Am*. 1998;9:381-389. [PMID: 9894123]

Laslett M, Williams M. The reliability of selected pain provocation tests for sacroiliac joint pathology. *Spine*. 1994;19:1243-1249. [PMID: 8073316]

Leboeuf-Yde C. Body weight and low back pain. A systematic literature review of 56 journal articles reporting on 65 epidemiologic studies. *Spine (Phila Pa 1976)*. 2000 Jan 15;25(2):226-237.

Leboeuf-Yde C. Body weight and low back pain: a systematic literature review of 56 journal articles reporting on 65 epidemiologic studies. *Spine*. 2000;25:226-237. [PMID: 10685488]

Lebow RL, Adogwa O, Parker SL, Sharma A. Asymptomatic same-site recurrent disc hernation after lumbar discectomy: results of a prospective longitudinal study with 2-year serial imaging. *Spine*. 36(25): 2147-2151.

Lethem J, Slade PD, Troup JDG, Bently G. Outline of a fear-avoidance model of exaggerated pain perception. *Behav Res Ther*. 1983;21:401-408.

Li F, Harmer P, Fisher KJ, et al. Tai Chi and fall reductions in older adults: a randomized controlled trial. *J Gerontol A Biol Sci Med Sci*. 2005 Feb;60(2):187-194.

Li F, Harmer P, Fitzgerald K, et al. Tai chi and postural stability in patients with Parkinson's disease. *N Engl J Med*. 2012;366:511-519.

Long DM, BenDebba M, Torgerson WS, et al. Persistent back pain and sciatica in the United States: patient characteristics. *J Spinal Disord*. 1996;9:40-58. [PMID: 8727456]

Long DM, Filtzer DL, BenDebba M, Hendler NH. Clinical features of the failed-back syndrome. *J Neurosurg*. 1998;69:61-71. [PMID: 2967891]

Lysgaard AP, Fonager K, Nielsen CV. Effect of financial compensation on vocational rehabilitation. *J Rehabil Med*. 2005 Nov;37(6):388-391.

Maigne JY, Aivaliklis A, Pfefer F. Results of sacroiliac joint double block and value of sacroiliac pain provocation tests in 54 patients with low back pain. *Spine*. 1996;21:1889-1892.

Malmivaara A, Hakkinen V, Aro T, et al. Treatment of acute low back pain: bed rest, exercises, or ordinary activity? *N Engl J Med*. 1995;332:351.

Mao J. Opioid-induced abnormal pain sensitivity: implications in clinical opioid therapy. *Pain*. 2002;100:213-217.

Mayer HM, Wiechert K, Korge A, Qose I. Minimally invasive total disc replacement: surgical technique and preliminary clinical results. *Eur Spine J*. 2002:11(Suppl 2):S124-S130.

Mercadante S. Malignant bone pain. *Pain*. 1997;69:1–18. [PMID: 9060007]

Mulleman D, Mammou S, Griffoul I, Watier H, Goupille P. Pathophysiology of disk-related sciatica. I.—Evidence supporting a chemical component. *Joint Bone Spine*. 2006;73:151-158.

National Centers for Health Statistics, Chartbook on Trends in the Health of Americans 2006, Special Feature: Pain. http://www.cdc.gov/nchs/data/hus/hus06.pdf

Nilsen TIL, Holtermann A, Mork PJ. Physical exercise, body mass index, and risk of chronic pain in the low back and neck/shoulders: longitudinal data from the Nord-Trøndelag health study. *Am J Epidemiol*. 2011;174(3):267-273.

North RB, Campbell JN, James CS, et al. Failed back surgery syndrome: 5-year follow-up in 102 patients undergoing repeated operation. *Neurosurgery*. 1991;28:685-690.

North RB, Kidd DH, Piantadosi S. Spinal cord stimulation versus reoperation for failed back surgery syndrome: a prospective, randomized study design. *Acta Neurochir Suppl (Wien)*. 1995;64:106-108.

Onofrio BM. Intervertebral discitis: incidence, diagnosis, and management. *Clin Neurosurg*. 1980;27:481-516. [PMID: 7273569]

Papaioannou A, Watts NB, Kendler DL, et al. Diagnosis and management of vertebral fractures in elderly adults. *Am J Med*. 2002;113:220-228. [PMID: 12208381]

Parziale JR, Hudgins TH, Fishman LM. The piriformis syndrome. *Am J Orthop*. 1996;25:819-823. [PMID: 9001677]

Postacchini F, Lami R, Pugliese O. Familial predisposition to discogenic low-back pain: an epidemiologic and immunogenetic study. *Spine (Phila Pa 1976)*. 1988 Dec;13(12):1403-1406.

Prather H. Sacroiliac joint pain: practical management. *Clinical Journal of Sport Medicine*. 13:252-255.

Radcliff KE, Rihn J, Hilibrand A, et al. Does the duration of symptoms in patients with spinal stenosis and degenerative spondylolistheis affect outcomes? *Spine*. 36(25): 2197-2210.

Rainville J, Hartigan C, Martinez E, et al. Exercise as a treatment for chronic low back pain. *The Spine Journal*. 2004;4:106-115.

Rainville J, Jouve C, Finno M, Limke J. Comparison of four tests of quadriceps strength in L3 or L4 radiculopathies. *Spine (Phila Pa 1976)*. 2003 Nov 1; 28(21):2466-2471.

Rainville J, Smeets RJEM, Bendix T, Tveito TH, Poiraudeau S, Indahl AJ. Fear-avoidance beliefs and pain avoidance in low back pain—translating research into clinical practice. *Spine J*. 2011;11:895-903.

Rainville J, Sobel JB, Hartigan C. Comparison of total lumbosacral flexion and true lumbar flexion measured by a dual inclinometer technique. *Spine (Phila Pa 1976)*. 1994 Dec 1;19(23):2698-2701.

Rubin, DI. Epidemiology and risk factors for spine pain. *Neuro Clin*. 2007;25(2):353-371.

Saal JA. Natural history of nonoperative treatment of lumbar disc herniation. *Spine*. 1996;21:2S-9S. [PMID: 9112320]

Sakura S, Sumi M, Yamada Y, Saito Y, Kosaka Y. Quantitative and selective assessment of sensory blocks during lumbar epidural anaesthesia with 1% or 2% lidocaine. *Brit J Anesth*. 1998;81:718-722.

Schwab F, Dubey A, Gamez L, et al. Adult scoliosis: prevalence, SF-36, and nutritional parameters in an elderly volunteer population. *Spine*. 1 May 2005;30(9):1082-1085.

Schwarzer AC, Aprill CN, Derby R, et al. The prevalence and clinical features of internal disc disruption in patients with chronic low back pain. *Spine*. 1995;20:1878-1883. [PMID: 8560335]

Sehgal N, Fortin JD. Internal disc disruption and low back pain. *Pain Physician*. 2000;3(2):143-157.

Sinaki M, Mokri B. Low back pain and disorders of the lumbar spine. In: Braddom RL, ed. *Physical Medicine and Rehabilitation*. 2nd ed. Philadelphia, Pa: WB Saunders; 2000:853-893.

Speed C. Low back pain. *BMJ*. 2004;328:1119-1121.

Standaert CJ, Herring SA, Halpern B, King O. Spondylolysis. *Phys Med Rehabil Clin N Am*. 2000;11:785-803. [PMID: 11092019]

Stevens CS, Dubois RW, Larequi-Lauber T. Efficacy of lumbar discectomy and percutaneous treatments for lumbar disc herniation. *Soz Praventivmed*. 1997;42:367-379.

Suni JH, Oja P, Miilunpalo SI, Pasanen ME, Vuori IM, Bos K. Health related fitness test battery for adults: associations with perceived health, mobility, and back function and symptoms. *Arch Phys Med Rehabil*. 1998;79:559-569.

Suri P, Hunter DJ, Jouve C, et al. Inciting events associated with lumber disc herniation. *Spine J*. 2010;10:388-395.

Suri P, Rainville J, Katz JN, et al. The accuracy of the physical examination for the diagnosis of midlumbar and low lumbar nerve root impingement. *Spine (Phila Pa 1976)*. 2011 Jan 1;36(1):63-73.

Taylor-Piliae RE, Haskell WL. Tai Chi exercise and stroke rehabilitation. *Top Stroke Rehabil*. 2007 Jul-Aug;14(4):9-22.

Thomas E, Silman AJ, Croft PR, et al. Predicting who develops chronic low back pain in primary care: a prospective study. *BMJ*. 1999; 318:1662-1667. [PMID: 10373170]

Van Tulder, M, Koes B, Bombardier C. Low back pain. *Best Pract Res Clin Rheumatol*. 2002;16(5):761-775.

Wargo E. Back Pain and Operant Conditioning, http://www.nyu.edu/classes/keefer/therapy/therapy1.html with references to studies by Fordyce, Premarck, Catania, and others.

Webster BS, Verma SK, Gatchel RJ. Relationship between early opioid prescribing for acute occupational low back pain and disability duration, medical costs, subsequent surgery and late opioid use. *Spine (Phila Pa 1976)*. 2007 Sep 1;32(19):2127-2132.

Weingarten TN, Shi Y, Mantilla CB, Hooten WM, Warner DO. Smoking and chronic pain: a real-but-puzzling relationship. *Minn Med*. 2011 Mar;94(3):35-37.

Weinstein JN, Tosteson TD, Lurie JD, et al. Surgical versus nonsurgical therapy for lumbar spinal stenosis. *N Engl J Med*. 2008;358:794-810.

Weishaupt D et al. MRI of the lumbar spine: prevalence of intervertebral disc extrusion and sequestration, nerve root compression and plate abnormalities, and osteoarthritis of the fact joints in asymptomatic volunteers. *Radiology*. 1998;209:661-666.

Whitten C, Donovan M, Cristobal K. Treating chronic pain: new knowledge, more choices. clinical contributions. *Permanente J*. Fall 2005;9(4).

Wilke HJ, Neef P, Caimi M, Hoogland T, Claes LE. New in vivo measurements of pressures in the intervertebral disc in daily life. *Spine (Phila Pa 1976)*. 1999 Apr 15;24(8):755-762.

Wood KB, et al. Magnetic resonance imaging of the thoracic spine. Evaluation of asymptomatic individual's. *J Bone Joint Surg Am*. 1995 Nov;77(11):1631-1638.

Yaksi A, Özgönenel L, Özgönenel B. The efficiency of gabapentin therapy in patients with lumbar spinal stenosis. *Spine*. 2007;32(9):939-942.

Yeoman W. The relation of arthritis of the sacroiliac joint to sciatica. *Lancet*. 1928;2:1119-1122.

Zeidman SM, Long DM. Failed back surgery syndrome. In: Menezes AH, Sonntag VKH, eds. *Principles of Spinal Surgery*. Vol. 1. New York, NY: McGraw-Hill; 1996:657-679.

Facetogenic Pain

Daniel P. Gray
Thomas T. Simopoulos

More than 60% of people in developed countries will experience spinal pain at some time in their lives. Back pain is the most common complaint of patients referred to pain clinics. The pain is nonspecific in about 85% of the cases, and onset of symptoms is most often between the ages of 35 and 55 years. According to some sources, 15% to 45% of all adults experience lower back pain, and 1 in 20 people present with a new episode annually. In 2008, 3.7 million workplace injuries were reported, and of these, 65% were attributed to the low back. In 2012, state workers' compensation programs provided almost $60 billion in cash and medical care benefits.

Risk factors for spinal pain include trauma, heavy physical labor, frequent twisting, bending, vibrations, pulling and pushing, and repetitive motion, especially that involving static postures. Psychological features such as anxiety, depression, job dissatisfaction, and stress also can play an important role.

ANATOMIC CONSIDERATIONS

The spine consists of 7 cervical, 12 thoracic, and 5 lumbar vertebrae in addition to the sacrum and coccyx. They articulate anteriorly through the disks and posteriorly through the left and right synovial facet joints. Anterior to the ligamentum flavum and covering the facet (apophyseal) joint is a variable amount of vascularized adipose tissue, which directly contacts the dural sleeve of the nerve root. The sleeve is located so close to the facet that it is possible, inadvertently, to inject medication directly into the cerebrospinal fluid. The articular surfaces of the facets are covered by cartilage. Joints are lined by synovium and contain variable amounts of fluid. The fibrous joint capsule forms superior and inferior joint recesses and blends anteromedially with the ligamentum flavum. It is located close to the neural foramen and the nerve root. Enlarged and osteophytic joints can contribute to significant narrowing of the neuroforaminal opening and can cause radicular symptoms.

Computed tomography (CT), magnetic resonance imaging (MRI), and intraarticular contrast medium can be used to demonstrate these anatomic features. The volume of injectate that can be accommodated by the facet joints varies as follows: cervical, up to 1.0 ml; thoracic, 1.0 ml to perhaps 1.5 ml; and lumbar, 1.0 ml to perhaps 1.5 ml.

In the upper lumbar spine, approximately 80% of the facet joints are curved and 20% are flat. This situation is reversed in the lower lumbar spine, where approximately 80% of the joints are flat. The upper lumbar facets are oriented more strongly in the sagittal plane, and, by the L5 to Sl level, they rotate obliquely. The lumbar facet joints are oriented 45 degrees from the sagittal plane, but because of the curvature of the joints, the posterior part of the joint is close to the sagittal plane. Lumbar facet syndrome has been considered to be a significant source of lower back pain, with a prevalence from 15% to 45% using strict diagnostic interventional criteria.

The thoracic facet joints are almost parallel to the coronal plane. They extend superiorly and inferiorly from the junctions of the laminae and pedicles and are oriented approximately 20 degrees from the coronal plane. Thoracic facet syndrome is less clearly established as a cause of spinal pain. However, recent limited, good-quality investigations have suggested a prevalence as high as 40%.

The anatomy of the cervical facets is significantly different from that of the lumbar ones. The cervical facets extend laterally from the junction of the laminae and pedicles and are oriented in the coronal plane to permit extension, flexion, and lateral bending. The atlanto-occipital and atlantoaxial joints are the C0–1 and C1–2 facet joints. Their structure, function, and innervation are unique. The C2–3 through C5–6 joints are angled 35 degrees from the coronal plane. The C6–7 apophyseal joint is tipped 22 degrees from the coronal plane. All of the cervical facet joints from C2–3 to C7–T1 are angled 110 degrees from the midline posterior sagittal plane, which makes their orientation similar to that of the thoracic facets. The cervical facets play a larger role, physically, in the spinal articular tripod structure and are commonly described as the superior and inferior ends of articular pillars. The vertebral artery, which passes through the transverse foramen of the transverse processes of the C1 to C6 vertebrae, is a landmark of the cervical spine. The prevalence of pain in the cervical spine may even be higher than that of the lumbar spine, using strict interventional diagnostic criteria.

The facet joints appear to function to protect the spine from excessive mobility and distribute axial loading over a broad area. The orientation and shape of the facets are specifically designed to accommodate the stresses and movements expected at each spinal level.

NEUROANATOMY OF THE FACET JOINTS

The nonspecific localization of facet joint pain is explained by profuse overlapping of sensory innervation. The medial branch nerve supplies the lower facet at its own level as well as the upper part of the joint below (the L4–5 joint is supplied by the L3 and L4 medial branch nerves). Therefore, each of the facet joints receives innervation from a medial branch nerve of two posterior primary rami. These branches also innervate the paraspinal muscles, ligaments, and periosteum, with significant dermatomal sensory overlapping.

In the lumbar region (**Fig. 39-1**), the medial branch nerve lies in a groove on the base of the superior articular process and passes under the mammilo-accessory ligament. It then runs in a posterior and inferior direction, first sending fibers to innervate the adjacent joint capsule before sending fibers to the next lower level. The course of the L5 medial

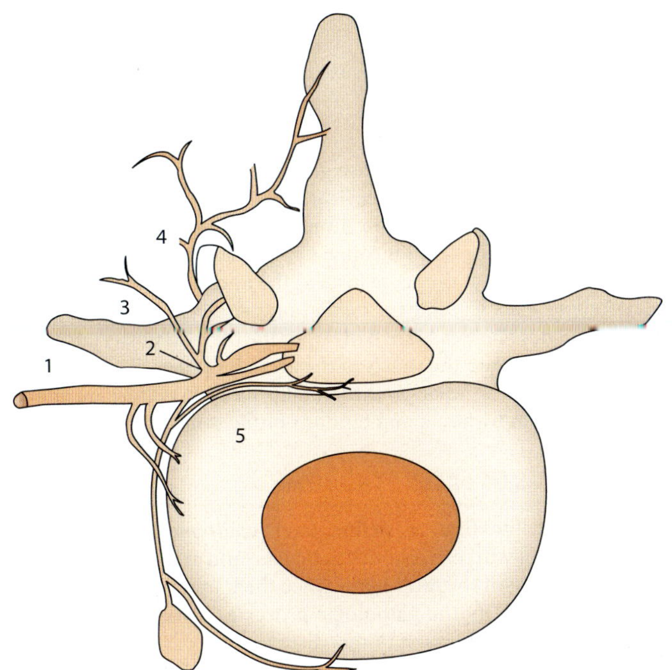

A. Tranverse view

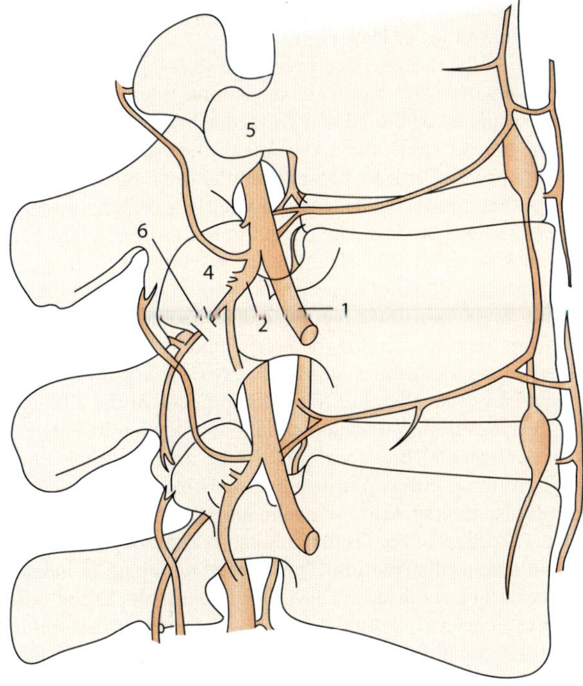

B. Lateral view

FIGURE 39-1. Lumbar spine anatomy: **1.** spinal nerve; **2.** posterior primary ramus; **3.** lateral branch; **4.** medial branch; **5.** sinu-vertebral nerve (innervation to the disc annulus).

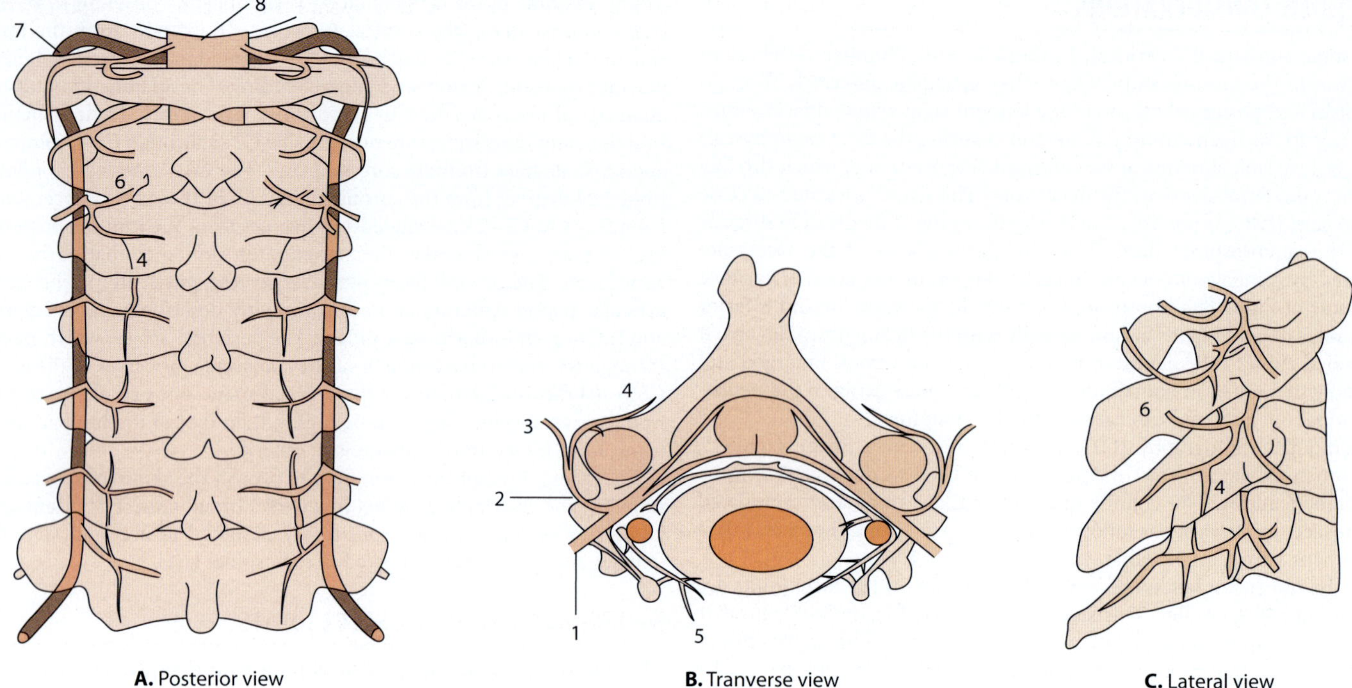

FIGURE 39-2. Illustration of the cervical zygapophyseal (facet joint) anatomy: **1.** segmental nerve root; **2.** posterior primary ramus; **3.** lateral branch.

branch is different because the transverse process is replaced by the ala of the sacrum. The L5 medial branch is actually the L5 dorsal ramus proper. The L5–S1 facet joint may have additional innervation from the S1 nerve root branch. Because of the dual nerve innervation, each joint must be blocked at two segments, both at and above the level of the involved joint. The lumbosacral facet joint should be blocked at two, and perhaps even three, levels.

There is evidence of multilevel innervation of the lumbar facet joints, which includes not only the posterior primary rami, but also the sympathetic and parasympathetic ganglia. The sympathetic fibers have been reported to regulate the activity of sensory neurons and may contribute to the experience of lower back pain.

Innervation of the thoracic facets is similar to that of the lumbar spine. Medial branches from two segmental levels innervate each joint (i.e., the T4–5 joint is supplied by the T3 and T4 medial branch nerves). However, unlike in the lumbar spine, the nerve crosses the superolateral corner of the transverse process (at least 12 mm lateral to the root of the transverse process) and then passes medially and inferiorly across the posterio surface of the transverse process. The exception to this description occurs at the midthoracic level (T5–T8). Here, the nerves assume a course parallel to the typical levels but does not reliably make bony contact with the superolateral corner of the transverse process and, as they turn medialy, remain separated from the surface of the transverse process. The T11 branch also has different anatomic features and runs across the lateral surface of the root of the relatively smaller T12 transverse process. At the T12 level, the medial branch localization is analogous to that of the lumbar spine.

The cervical medial branches (**Fig. 39-2**) mainly supply the facet joints, with minimal innervations of the following posterior neck muscles: multifidus, interspinalis, semispinalis cervicis, and semispinalis capitis. The C3 dorsal branch is the only cervical dorsal ramus below C2 that has a cutaneous distribution. Therefore, if neck pain or headache is caused by cervical facet disease, cervical facet joint blocks can relieve it.

The upper cervical synovial joints—the atlanto-occipital and lateral atlantoaxial joints—are innervated by cervical ventral rami (**Fig. 39-3**). The only suitable procedure to relieve pain at these joints is an intraarticular injection. The C2–3 facet joint is innervated mainly by the third occipital nerve and sometimes by the C2 dorsal rami (the greater occipital nerve). There are eight cervical nerves and seven cervical vertebrae. The first seven cervical nerve roots exit the spine above the vertebral body, and they are numbered according to the vertebral body below them. The C3–4 through C7–T1 facet joints are supplied by the medial branches at the same level as the joint and from the segmental level above (i.e., C5 and C6 medial branch nerves supply the C5–6 facet joint). These nerves branch off from the cervical posterior primary rami and wrap around the waists of the articular pillars (viewed as "centroid" of the articular pillar on the lateral projection). They are attached to the periosteum by fascia and tendons of the semispinalis capitis.

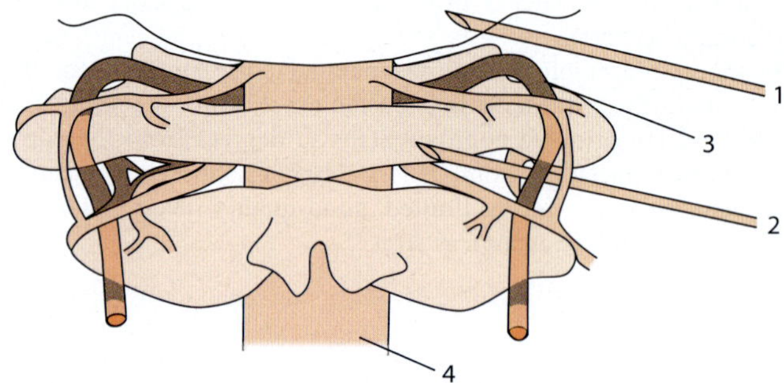

FIGURE 39-3. Illustration of **1.** atlanto-occipital joint injection; **2.** atlantoaxial joint injection;**3.** vertebral artery; **4.** spinal cord.

PATHOGENESIS OF FACET SYNDROME

Ghormley was the first to define *facet syndrome*, describing it as lumbosacral pain with or without sciatic pain and associated with sprain or violent twisting of the facet joint. Since then, much research has been carried out to identify the pathologic processes involved and to find a specific therapeutic approach to this disease.

Neurophysiologic studies have shown that the medial branch nerves transmit nociceptive and proprioceptive signals from the facet joints, which are triggered by inflammatory and mechanical factors. Researchers have identified multiple mechanosensitive somatosensory

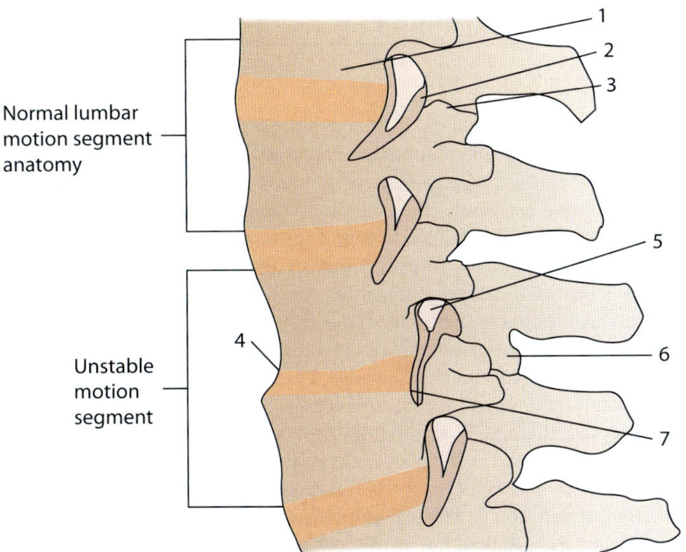

FIGURE 39-4. Anatomy of normal and degenerative zygopophyseal joints explaining possible mechanisms of facet syndrome: **1.** vertebrae; **2.** spinal nerve; **3.** normal facet joint; **4.** retrolisthesis; **5.** narrowing of intervertebral foramen with compression of adjacent nerve root; **6.** subluxation;**7.** intervetebral disk narrowing due to degeneration.

receptors and neuromodulators of nociception within the facet capsule, including calcitonin gene-related peptide, substance P, and vasoactive intestinal peptide. Chronic inflammation—with consecutive joint hypertrophy, degeneration, and osteophyte formation—may contribute to neuroforaminal narrowing and compression of the nerve roots. On occasion, this causes referred pain to the extremities, as well as abnormal joint stress with possible subluxation and muscle spasm (**Fig. 39-4**). Pain originating from the apophyseal joints can be attributed to a synovitis, degenerative arthritis, and segmental instability.

The pathophysiology of thoracic and cervical facet syndrome can be explained by the same factors that are exhibited in the lumbar spine. There is also growing evidence that cervical facet syndrome can contribute to the etiology of cervicogenic headaches.

FACET BLOCKING: INDICATIONS AND CONTRAINDICATIONS

The clinical picture of facet joint syndrome could easily be considered to be almost intuitive. Making the diagnosis is one of exclusion starting with a careful history and physical examination. There are classic, unreliable features of lumbar facet pain, which include the following (**Fig. 39-5A**):

- Pain located in the lower back with occasional (unilateral or bilateral) radiation to the buttock, groin, hip, and lower extremities, usually above level of the knee.
- Pain that is dull, deep, and difficult to describe.
- No evidence of neurologic deficits.
- Paralumbar tenderness with or without muscle spasm.
- Onset of symptoms associated with twisting, bending, or rotation.
- Deterioration by lateral bending, extension, sitting, and forward flexion in the standing position.
- Symptoms improved by walking.
- No aggravation on Valsalva's maneuver or during walking.
- Evidence of degenerative changes on radiologic studies.
- An increased uptake during technetium Tc 99 scanning.

The manifestations of thoracic pain syndrome are thought to be similar to those of lumbar pain syndrome, but data are limited on this subject (**Fig. 39-5B**).

Patients with cervicalgia (**Figs. 39-5C** and **39-6**) can be diagnosed on the basis of the initiating factors. People with prior trauma may have whiplash syndrome and possible cervicogenic headaches. Pathophysiology of this syndrome includes:

- Facet joints sprain with muscle and ligament involvement.
- Nerve root irritation.
- Muscle spasm.
- Periosteum tearing.

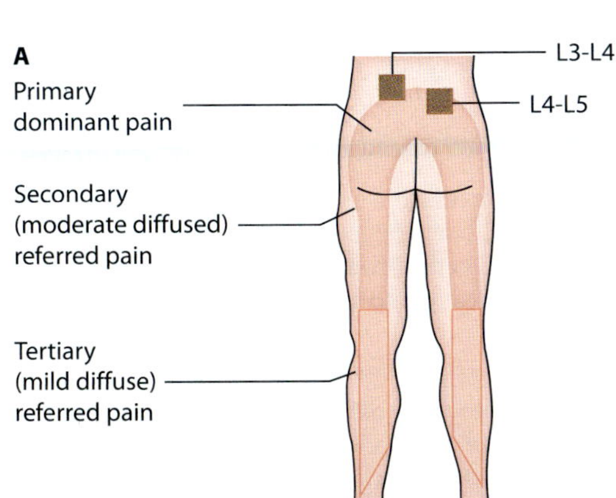

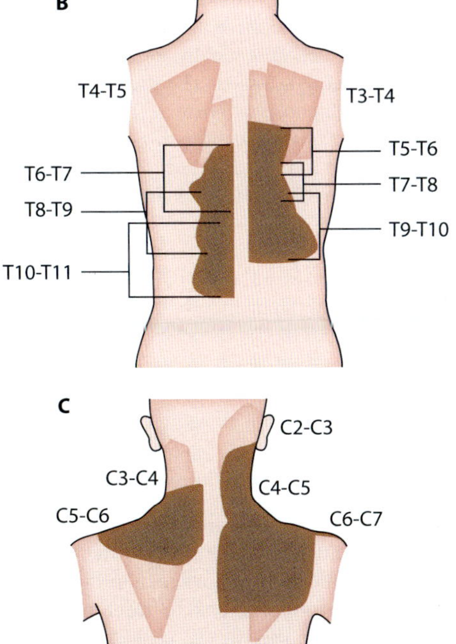

FIGURE 39-5. **(A)** Sketch of the lumbar facet joint pain distribution. Primary pain relates to the distribution of the segmental nerve supply at each facet level. Secondary pain demonstrates caudad distribution of posterior branches. Tertiary pain mimicks referred pain from anterior division of the segmental nerve. **(B)** Sketch of thoracic facet joint pain distribution. **(C)** Sketch of cervical facet joint pain distribution.

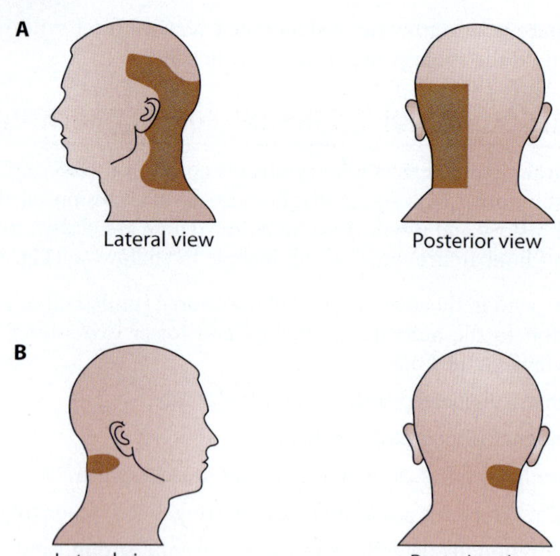

FIGURE 39-6. (A) Atlanto-occipital joint. (B) Atlantoaxial (C1-C2) joint.

Patients without a history of trauma may have degenerative disease as a primary diagnosis.

Radiographic facet joint changes are common and nonspecific in adults. Routine lumbar radiographs may be normal or may reveal facet degeneration with or without changes in the discs. Arthrography is an additional study that may provide some limited data based on the spread of the dye. CT and MRI do not provide specific information, although some studies have suggested that CT and single photon emission computed topography (SPECT) have some value as tools to assess clinically significant facet joint disease. Nevertheless, it seems that a radiographically normal joint is unlikely to be a significant pain generator except in the case of whiplash syndrome.

The clinical criteria for making the diagnosis of facet syndrome are unfortunately nonspecific and unreliable. The only reliable method of diagnosing facet pain is by double diagnostic interventional blocks. It is important to recognize that a single diagnostic block is falsely positive in about 30% of cases and falsely negative in about 8%. A true positive block requires a minimum of 50% and, ideally, greater than 75% reduction in pain from the joint being assessed. The greater the pain reduction, the more reliable the diagnosis is correct. The standard for the diagnostic block is blocking the medial branch nerve of the cervical-(excluding C0–1 to C2–3) and lumbar-affected joints. There is limited, but promising, research of thoracic facet joints for diagnostic injections of the medial branch nerves.

Interventional procedures should be offered to patients without neurologic deficits or other causes for their pain who have exhausted conservative treatment measures (analgesics, bed rest, physical therapy). Interventional techniques consist of:

- Intraarticular or periarticular injections of local anesthetics and corticosteroids.
- Medial branch nerve blocks.
- Neuroablative facet denervation with radiofrequency and cryotherapy.

In the thoracic and cervical spine, the joints to be injected should be selected based on clinical evaluation in conjunction with the presence of radiologic abnormalities analogous to those seen in the lumbar spine.

There are no absolute contraindications to facet injections other than those for any regional block; specifically, coagulopathies, systemic or local infection at the site of the injection, and possible pregnancy. Allergy to contrast media is a relative contraindication, because the procedure can be performed without dye under fluoroscopic guidance or with nonionic contrast agents.

FACET BLOCKING TECHNIQUES

LUMBAR FACET BLOCKS

For this procedure, the patient is placed in the prone position, with the back slightly flexed and the hips supported by pillows. The injection is performed under sterile conditions and with continuous vital sign monitoring. The oblique fluoroscopic view reveals a typical facet joint picture reminiscent of a "Scottie dog." The back of the Scottie dog's head is formed by the inferior articular process, and the front feet outline the superior articular process that is adjacent to the inferior articular process of the vertebra below. Local anesthetic is injected at the point where an imaginary line from the center of the image intensifier intersects the skin on the way toward the facet joint. The clinician advances a 22-gauge, 10-cm spinal needle, or a radiofrequency cannula designed for neuroablation, to the desired position under fluoroscopic guidance. A small amount of radiologic dye (0.1 to 0.3 ml) may be injected to visualize placement of the needle tip prior to instilling 1.0 to 1.5 ml of injectate (i.e., 2-4% lidocaine with 20 mg of triamcinolone or methylprednisolone). The feel of the needle "walking off" the bone into the joint can also confirm the proper position.

Medial branch blocks are performed using a similar technique, but the final needle placement is different. The medial branch is blocked at the junction of the dorsal surface of the transverse process and superior articular process, just caudal to the most medial end of the superior edge of the transverse process. At the lumbosacral level, the posterior primary ramus of L5 is blocked in the groove between the ala of the sacrum and the superior articular process of the sacrum. Blocking a single joint requires that the two medial branch nerves be injected. At the L5–S1 level, the S1 nerve branch may also need to be blocked. It is located cephalad to the S1 posterior opening in a line between the S1 opening and the L5–S1 facet joint. To make a precise injection, the use of a small volume of local anesthetic (0.5–1.0 ml) is mandatory.

For therapeutic purposes, a less specific periarticular injection can be performed using a larger volume of injectate.

THORACIC FACET BLOCK

There is still very limited research on thoracic facet blocks. A technique for an intraarticular injection has been described but not yet validated. This procedure is conducted with the patient in the prone position, using the ribs as the main landmark. The joint lies posterior to the foramina. The steep angle of the joints requires that the skin entry point overlie the distal pedicle located one or two segments caudally to the intended joint. A 25-gauge, 10-cm spinal needle is directed into the joint, and this is confirmed by an arthrogram of 0.1 to 0.3 ml of contrast. A total of 1.0 to 1.5 ml of local anesthetic plus contrast may be injected into the joint.

The diagnostic block for thoracic facet pain has been described and looks promising, but the evidence is limited (three studies) and comes from one group of authors. In the prone position with a posterior approach, a 25-gauge, 10-cm spinal needle is advanced to the superolateral corner of the transverse process for the T1–4 and T9 and T10 nerves. The target point for the T5–8 nerves is analogous but is in the intertransverse space slightly cephalad to the superolateral corner of the transverse process. It is opposite the upper border of the rib at the target level and at the same depth as the transverse process. The location of the T11 and T12 nerves is analogous to the lumbar spine. Once the target point is reached, 0.5 to 1.0 ml of local anesthetic is injected.

CERVICAL FACET BLOCK

To perform blockade of the C3 through C7 medial branches, the patient is placed in a lateral position with the painful side facing the clinician. A 25-gauge, 10-cm spinal needle is inserted using a posterolateral approach. In slim individuals, it may be possible to use a 25-gauge, 1½-inch needle. The target point is the periosteum at the centroid of the projection of the articular pillar as seen on the lateral fluoroscopic image. After a negative aspiration of blood or cerebrospinal fluid, 0.5 ml of local anesthetic is injected very slowly. The medial branch of the

C8 nerve crosses the T1 transverse process and runs medially onto the lamina of T1, where it should be blocked.

Intraarticular blockade of cervical facets C3–4 through C7–T1 is performed using a 25-gauge, 10-cm spinal needle (or, again, a 25-gauge, 1½-inch needle). The needle is inserted from lateral to medial into the joint. It is essential to have the image of the articular pillars and joints from the right and left sides perfectly overlap. As the needle is being advanced, the image intensifier beam needs to be rotated 90 degrees to the needle to make sure the needle only enters the joint and does not pass completely through it into the spinal canal. A maximum of 0.5 to 1.0 ml of injectate (including the dye) should be administered to avoid rupture of the facet joint.

Blockade of the C2–3 facet joint requires location of the third occipital nerve. The target points are located along a vertical line that bisects the articular pillar of C3. Injections should be made immediately above the subchondral plate of the C2 inferior articular process and below the subchondral plate of the C3 superior articular process, as well as at a point between these two. At each of these three sites, 0.5 ml of local anesthetic is injected.

The atlantoaxial joint is usually blocked via a posterolateral approach with the patient in the lateral decubitus position. The patient's head should be slightly flexed and rotated 45 degrees toward the table. The lateral half of the posterior capsule is the final target for a 25-gauge needle. The mastoid process, the occipital prominence, and, located between them, the occipital brim are bony landmarks. With oblique imaging, the C-arm of the fluoroscope and head are moved until the occipital brim is located over the superior, posterior, and lateral aspect of the joint (the destination point). This procedure is complex and should only be done by an individual with considerable experience at other interventional procedures. The needle is advanced slowly along this path. This position is confirmed regularly with posteroanterior, open mouth, lateral, and oblique views. The final needle placement is visualized using arthrography. Aspiration for blood or cerebrospinal fluid should precede the administration of dye and medication (total volume of 1 ml).

NEUROABLATION OF THE FACET JOINTS

Facet denervation is performed on the medial branch nerves with radiofrequency (heat lesion or pulsed), and perhaps even cryotherapy lesioning, using the same technique to locate the nerves as for the medial branch blocks. Antero-posterior and lateral imaging prior to lesioning is essential to safely confirm the needle tip position. Previous double diagnostic blocks determine which facets should be neuroablated. To reliably lesion the nerve, the needle tip should be adjusted slightly where it crosses the path of the nerve to produce two or three separate lesions per nerve. A single lumbar facet denervation requires that two nerves be treated, and possibly three, in the case of the L5–S1 facet joint. Two nerves also are denervated for each of the cervical facets, C3–4 to C7–T1. The technique of denervation of the cervical facets should carefully avoid advancing the needle anterior to the level of the foraminal opening. This will minimize the risk to the nerve root or vertebral artery. The C2–3 facet joint requires three-point lesioning, as in the technique described earlier, plus lesioning posterior to where the medial branch nerve exits the foraminal opening like for the other cervical medial branch nerves. Because denervation is obviously a destructive procedure and carries some risk of deafferentation pain and neurologic deficits, there must be clear indications for this treatment.

Thoracic medial branch denervation is not recommended because of the lack of a validated technique for medial branch blocks in this region of the spine.

ADVERSE EFFECTS

Complications secondary to interventions on the facet joints are rare and usually transient. They include:

- Exacerbation of pain.
- Failure to relieve pain.
- Spinal or epidural anesthesia with or without transient motor and sensory blocks.
- Infection and abscess formation.
- Chemical meningitis.
- Puncture of the vessel, including vertebral artery, with possible local anesthetic toxicity.
- Transient ataxia caused by partial blockade of the third occipital nerve and proprioceptive afferents.
- Persistent motor or sensory deficits (neuroablative procedures).
- Allergic reactions.

EFFICACY OF FACET JOINT BLOCKS

The reported success of facet joint injections and neuroablation varies widely, with positive outcomes cited that range from 16% to 83%. The success rate will be at the high end of the range by using the strict criteria of two positive diagnostic blocks that produce greater than 75% reduction of pain from the affected joint being blocked. The best diagnostic block is of the medial branch nerve rather than from an intraarticular injection. Accurate clinical diagnosis and careful patient selection are essential to ensure a good outcome. Other causes of low back pain—such as neoplasm, myofascial pain, degenerative disk disease, infection, and spondylolysis—must be excluded.

CONCLUSION

In the assessment of patients with spinal pain, it is essential to rule out serious pathology that requires neurologic or surgical evaluation. Interventions should always be integrated with a well-tailored treatment program that is individually designed for each patient. A one-size-fits-all approach to the problem of spinal pain is neither efficient nor prudent. Facet syndrome remains a diagnosis of exclusion that cannot be confirmed definitively by any specific laboratory, radiologic, or clinical findings. Conservative management should always be offered before scheduling interventional procedures. It is well known that about 80% of people with acute low back pain of a mechanical nature and without a radicular component will recover spontaneously within 6 weeks (with help of simple analgesic and physical therapy), often without any complications or absenteeism from work.

The patient who was screened for other causes of spinal pain and who has a clinical picture of facet pain correlating with radiologic evidence of facet abnormalities usually responds to facet injections. The success rate is significantly reduced in patients with a history of spinal surgery, especially fusion. However, some of these patients have benefited from the procedure, and, for those who have exhausted other conventional therapies, the risk is very small and may be worth trying.

BIBLIOGRAPHY

Anderson GBJ. The epidemiology of spinal disorders. In: Frymoyer JW, ed. *The Adult Spine: Principles and Practice*. 2nd ed. New York, NY: Raven Press; 1997:93-141.

Bland JH, Boushey DR. Anatomy and physiology of the cervical spine. *Semin Arthritis Rheum*. 1990;20:1-20.

Bogduk N. The innervation of the lumbar spine. *Spine*. 1983;8:286-293.

Bogduk N. International Spine Injection Society Guidelines for the performance of spinal injection procedures. Part 1: zygapophysial joint blocks. *The Clinical Journal of Pain*. 1997;13(4):286-302.

Bogduk N, Anat D. The clinical anatomy of the cervical dorsal rami. *Spine*. 1982;7:319-330.

Bogduk N, Marsland A. The cervical zygapophysial joints as a source of the neck pain. *Spine*. 1988;13:610-617.

Cavanaugh JM. Lumbar facet pain: biomechanics, neuroanatomy and neurophysiology. *J Biomech*. 1996:29:1117-1129.

Cho J, Park YG, Chung SS. Percutaneous radiofrequency lumbar rhizotomy in mechanical low back pain syndrome. *Stereotact Func Neurosurg*. 1997;68;212-217.

Chua WH, Bogduk N. The surgical anatomy of thoracic facet denervation. *Acta Neurochir*. 1995;136:140-144.

Deyo RA, Rainville J, Kent DL. What can the history and physical examination tell us about low back pain? *JAMA*. 1992;268:760-765.

Dreyfuss P, Michaelsen M, Fletcher D. Atlanto-occipital and lateral atlanto-axial joint pain patterns. *Spine*. 1994;19:1125-1131.

Dreyfuss P, Tibiletti C, Dreyer S. Thoracic zygapophyseal joint pain patterns. *Spine*. 1994;19:807-811.

Dweyer A, Aprill C, Bogduk N. Cervical zygapophyseal joint pain patterns I: a study in normal volunteers. *Spine*. 1990;15:453-457.

Dweyer A, Aprill C, Bogduk N. Cervical zygapophyseal joint pain patterns II: a clinical evaluation. *Spine*. 1990;15:458-461.

Falco FJ. Lumbar spine injection procedures in the management of low back pain. *Occup Med*. 1998;13:121-149.

Ghormley RK. Low back pain with special reference to the articular facet with presentation of an operative procedure. *JAMA*. 1993;101: 1773-1777.

Grob D. Surgery in the degenerative cervical spine. *Spine*. 1998;23: 2674-2683.

Hourigan CL, Bassett JM. Facet syndrome: clinical signs, symptoms, diagnosis, and treatment. *J Manipulative Physiol Ther*. 1989;12: 293-297.

International Association for the Study of Pain. *Classification of Chronic Pain*. 2nd ed. Revised, 2011. www.iasp-pain.org/Content/NavigationMenu/Publications/Freebooks/Classification_of_Chronic_Pain.

Jerosch J, Castro WHM, Liljenqvist U. Percutaneous facet coagulation: indication, technique, results, and complications. *Neurosurg Clin North Am*. 1999;7(1):119-139.

Kaplan M, Dreyfuss P, Halbrook B, et al. The ability of lumbar medial branch blocks to anesthetize the zygapophyseal joint: a physiologic challenge. *Spine*. 1998;23:1847-1852.

Lovely TY, Rastogi P. The value of provocative facet blocking as a predictor of success in lumbar spinal fusion. *J Spinal Disord*. 1997;10:512-517.

Manchikanti L. Facet joint pain and the role of neural blockade in its management. *Curr Rev Pain*. 1999;3:348-358.

Manchikanti L. An update of comprehensive evidence-based guidelines for interventional techniques in chronic spinal pain. Part II: guidance and recommendations. *Pain Physician*. 2013;16:S49-283.

Nelemans PJ, deBie RA, DeVet HC, Sturmans AF. Injection therapy for subacute and chronic benign low back pain. *Spine*. 2001;26: 501-515.

North RB, Han M, Zahurak M, Kidd DH. Radiofrequency lumbar facet denervation: analysis of prognostic factors. *Pain*. 1994;57:77-83.

Savage RA. The relationship between the magnetic resonance imaging appearance of the lumbar spine and low back pain, age, and occupation in males. *Eur Spine J*. 1997;6:106-114.

Schwarzer AC, Derby R, Aprill CN, et al. The value of the provocation response in lumbar zygapophyseal joint injections. *Clin J Pain*. 1994;10:309-313.

Tzaan WC, Tasker RR. Percutaneous radiofrequency facet rhizotomy-experience with 118 procedures and reappraisal of its value. *Can J Neurol Sci*. 2000;27:125-130.

Failed Back Surgery

Jerome Schofferman

INTRODUCTION

Failed back surgery syndrome (FBSS) is a nonspecific term that has probably outlived its usefulness as we learned more about the problem, but the phrase remains embedded in the vernacular of the pain and spine worlds. One useful definition of FBSS is that the outcome of surgery did not meet the expectations of *both* the patient and the surgeon.[1-4] This implies that the patient and surgeon had the same reasonable expectations for the outcome of surgery. It does not and should not mean the patient failed to get total pain relief or return to full function.

The structural cause of FBSS might have been present prior to surgery and not recognized or recognized but inadequately treated. On the other hand, the problem could have arisen after the surgery as a consequence of the surgery or might have nothing to do with the surgery itself.

The evaluation of the patient with FBSS must include the same careful history and physical examination that would be performed in any patient with chronic low back pain (CLBP). The history, which is most important, will help generate the likely differential diagnosis and form the basis for the subsequent diagnostic testing. As with all patients with CLBP, it is necessary to know the location of the pain, its intensity, and the effect on function. The response of the pain with changes in body position and basic functions such as standing, walking, and sitting provide clues to the diagnosis.[5-10] In addition to patients with no surgery and CLBP, there are other important pain-related facts that are specific to those patients with FBSS.[1,2] It is important to note whether the pain ever improved after surgery and, if so, for how long. It is necessary to know if the pain location, quality, and referral patterns are the same or different compared to before surgery. Needless to say, it is important to review past imaging studies, the operative report, and the preoperative notes to know the actual goals of the surgeon. Finally, it is important to consider that patients with FBSS can have an extraspinal source of pain that was overlooked prior to surgery or arose afterward.[11-16]

There are many causes of FBSS, but it is useful to keep in mind that "common things occur commonly." The physician who is very familiar with the most common causes of FBSS will be able to arrive at the proper diagnoses for most patients.

There are many treatment options for patients with FBSS. We assume that the best patient outcomes will be obtained when the treatment is the one most appropriate for the patient's structural disorder. In order to arrive at the proper diagnosis, physicians must know the common structural causes of FBSS.

STRUCTURAL CAUSES OF *AXIAL* LOW BACK PAIN AFTER SURGERY

Many of the common structural causes of FBSS are the same as the structural disorders responsible for CLBP in patients who have not had surgery. For patients with LBP significantly greater than leg pain, the most common sources of pain are disc(s), facet joint(s), and sacroiliac joint(s) (SIJ).[5-10,17-24] After surgery, the common causes of LBP expand to include pain from instability (e.g., spondylolisthesis), pseudarthrosis, and the tissues surrounding the "hardware" used for internal fixation[25-27] (**Tables 40-1** and **40-2**).

DISCOGENIC PAIN

Discogenic pain arises from the disc itself absent extrinsic nerve root compression. One or more painful discs were the cause of FBSS in about 21% of patients[17-19] in three older studies. More recently, discogenic pain was the problem identified in patients after fusion[21] and in a remarkable 82% of patients after discectomy without fusion.[20]

TABLE 40-1 Some of the More Common Structural Causes of Failed Back Surgery

Mostly Low Back Pain	Mostly Leg Pain
Painful disc(s)	Foraminal stenosis
Facet joint pain	Disc herniation with neural compression
Sacroiliac joint pain	Neuropathic pain
Spondylolisthesis (instability)	
Extraspinal sources	

The general principle in the surgical treatment of discogenic pain is that fusion is necessary, although the type of fusion might be less important. Therefore, if there is a painful disc but no fusion, the problem may not have been properly addressed. When there is a painful disc at an adjacent segment, it was either present prior to surgery and not included in the surgery or the disc degenerated after surgery.

Painful discs can occur at the level of prior surgery or at an adjacent motion segment. When there is a residual painful disc at the surgical level, there are several possible explanations. Quite often, the patient had a partial discectomy for disc herniation or decompression without fusion, thereby leaving the painful disc untreated. Another scenario is that the patient had several abnormal discs on MRI before surgery, the surgeon addressed only the most abnormal, and the others were also contributing to the pain. Rarely, a painful disc can occur at the surgery level, even in the presence of prior posterolateral fusion.[22]

A disc can degenerate and become painful well after surgery due to the natural history of disc degeneration, the effects of fusion putting increased load on the adjacent disc, or some combination of both. This type of discogenic pain is referred to as adjacent segment disease (ASD) or breakdown.[28]

The time course of pain occurrence/recurrence provides some information. When a painful disc was present before surgery, the patient never gets meaningful relief. Patients with adjacent segment degeneration usually experience significant relief after surgery for months or years before recurrence of pain. MRI and radiographs will usually reveal the problem.

There is no discogenic pain syndrome—that is, no set of symptoms or signs that have high specificity and sensitivity for the diagnosis.[8-10] However, extrapolating from studies of patients with CLBP, there are some clues.[5-8,10] A dominance of midline pain may be expected, although pain often radiates more distally into the gluteal region and/or to the left and right of the midline. The absence of midline pain speaks strongly against the diagnosis of discogenic pain. Pain is usually worse sitting and during transition from sitting to standing, and pain might improve with standing or walking. Physical examination is nonspecific. There may be decreased flexion in standing. There may be tenderness over the spinous processes of the involved levels.

MRI scan is very useful. Most painful discs appear abnormal on MRI. However, because painless discs can look abnormal, it is important to correlate the MRI with the patient's description of pain. MRI findings of high intensity zone, end-plate changes, and disc degeneration correlate with discogenic pain, using provocation disc injection as the reference standard.[9] If there is no abnormal disc on MRI, it is far less likely that the problem is discogenic pain. Until recently, provocative disc injection (discography) was used frequently to determine if a suspicious disc on MRI was painful.[29] However, a recent study suggested that disc injection can cause accelerated degeneration in a small, but important, number of patients, so this procedure is being used less often.[30] When it is clinically important to use disc injection, only the suspicious discs are injected, not normal appearing ones, which is a change from prior recommendations.

FACET JOINT PAIN

One or more facet joints can be the cause of FBSS in at least 3% to 16% of patients.[17,19,20,21,23] Facet pain may have been present before surgery, alone or in combination with the structural pathology that led to the surgery. Facet pain can develop after surgery as part of the ASD or injury to the joint during surgery.

There is no "facet joint syndrome." Extrapolating from data in patients with CLBP, there are clues.[5,6,8-10] Dominance of midline LBP speaks against facet joint pain. Patients with facet joint pain almost always identify their worst pain just off to the left and/or right of midline. Young and colleagues found that patients with facet joint pain did not have increased pain when rising from sit to stand.[8] A panel of physical therapist and physician experts arrived at consensus regarding features of symptoms and signs that were suggestive of facet joint pain.[31] These included localized unilateral back pain, replication or aggravation of pain by unilateral pressure over the facet joint or transverse process, lack of pain below the knee, pain eased in flexion (sitting), pain in extension, and pain in extension plus side bending or rotation to the ipsilateral side.

There is no reliable correlation between MRI or x-ray and facet joint pain.[32,33] The diagnosis is made by medial branch block. In patients with

TABLE 40-2 Differential Diagnosis of Some of the Most Common Causes of Failed Back Surgery According to Symptoms, Signs, Imaging, and Injections

Diagnosis	Symptoms	Signs	Radiology	Injections
Painful disc	LBP? worse with sitting	Restricted flexion while standing	MRI: degenerated disc(s)	Not helpful
Facet joint pain	Left and/or right sided LBP	? Facet tenderness	Not specific	Medial branch block relieves pain
SIJ pain	Gluteal pain; often referred to groin or leg	May have + provocative testing	Not helpful	SIJ injection relieves pain
Foraminal stenosis	Leg pain dominance Relief with sitting	Loss of lumbar lordosis	MRI: foraminal stenosis	Relief with transforaminal epidural
Neuropathic pain	Leg pain Burning Dysesthesia	Hypoalgesia Allodynia Often none	To exclude other diagnoses	To exclude other diagnoses
Disc herniation with radiculopathy	Leg pain greater than LBP	Variable	Herniation on MRI	Epidural may provide temporary relief

LBP = low back pain

+/− = may be helpful

SIJ = sacroiliac joint pain

MRI = magnetic resonance imaging scan

FBSS, the choice of segment to inject is dependent on the pain topography and referral pattern, possibly location of tenderness, and whether the segment is abnormal in any way on imaging.

SACROILIAC JOINT PAIN

SIJ pain after surgery is being recognized with increasing frequency.[24,34] Once again, SIJ pain might have been present before surgery and not recognized; may have occurred after fusion to S1 or sometimes L5; or, less often in the modern surgical era, after violation of the joint during surgery. Older studies have placed the prevalence of SIJ pain in patients with FBSS at 2% to 3%,[18,19] while more recent studies have found SIJ can be the major source of pain in as many as 43% of patients with prior fusion.[21]

Again, there are no specific signs or symptoms specific for SIJ pain, but there are definite clues to the diagnosis.[8-10,35,36] Virtually all patients have pain distal to the posterior iliac crest and lateral to the midline spine. Some patients will point directly over the SIJ when asked to show where the pain is centered. Pain is frequently referred to the groin and can also be referred to the thigh, calf, and occasionally the foot—patterns that might suggest radiculopathy or even hip joint pathology. Pain may increase with single leg weight bearing.

Most often, there is tenderness directly over the SIJ. Although other signs are not specific, the diagnosis is probable when tenderness and three or four other provocative tests are present.[8] Plain radiographs, MRI, and CT are not really very helpful. The confirmation of SIJ pain requires relief of the target pain after fluoroscopically guided local anesthetic SIJ injection.[36]

SPONDYLOLISTHESIS AND INSTABILITY

Spondylolisthesis after surgery is an interesting problem. Once again, it may have been present before surgery and not recognized or addressed, it can occur as a result of wide decompression, or it could be part of the patient's natural history of spine degeneration. In some patients, the spondylolisthesis is not present when the person is lying down for an MRI and may only become visible when standing plain radiographs with flexion and extension are viewed.[27]

PSEUDARTHROSIS

It might be argued that pseudarthrosis itself is not a cause of pain, but the nonunion creates a mechanical situation that allows other things to hurt. Most nonunions are not painful. In fact, there are data that show no significant differences in outcome after fusion in patients with versus without pseudarthrosis, but other studies have found differences in long-term outcome.[27] Of course, the reference standard for the diagnosis is exploration of the fusion mass. However, the diagnosis can be straightforward if there is motion on flexion-extension radiographs. High-quality computed tomography is quite reliable for the diagnosis.[37]

In the patient with pseudarthrosis, it is necessary to evaluate the adjacent segments with MRI scan, facet joints with medial branch blocks, and—when pain has the appropriate location and mechanics—the SIJ before the pain can be attributed to the nonunion.

STRUCTURAL CAUSES OF LEG PAIN AFTER SURGERY

For patients with a dominance of leg pain with or without prior surgery, the common causes are foraminal stenosis, central stenosis, and disc herniation with neural compression. Leg pain can also be referred from SIJ or a disc and can also be from the hip or knee. After surgery, additional causes of leg pain include neuropathic pain, arachnoiditis, and misplaced internal fixation screws.

FORAMINAL STENOSIS

Foraminal stenosis was found in 12% to 29% of FBSS patients in the Slipman and Waguespack studies, half of what was seen by Burton 20 years earlier.[17-19] The lower prevalence may be due to increased awareness of the problem, improved imaging studies, and/or better understanding of the need for meticulous decompression. Patients with foraminal stenosis have pain that is predominantly in the leg or buttock, often in the distribution of a single dermatome. Pain is usually worsened by standing and walking and relieved by sitting. MRI or CT scan shows narrowing of the canal at the index level or an adjacent segment. Potential confirmation that the stenosis is the cause of pain is at least temporary relief of leg pain after transforaminal epidural injection around the suspected nerve.[38,39] There may be longer relief if corticosteroids are administered.[40] Foraminal stenosis must be differentiated from neuropathic pain and mixed pain syndrome, which have similar presentations.

DISC HERNIATION WITH RADICULOPATHY

Recurrent or residual disc herniation was seen in 7% to 12% of patients with FBSS.[17-19] There are two common presentations of pain from a disc herniation—radicular and axial. The topography of the pain is primarily due to the location of the herniation. A posterolateral herniation is more likely to compress or irritate a nerve root and therefore present with predominant leg pain. A midline herniation, unless very large, does not compress neural elements and presents with predominant LBP and must be treated like discogenic pain. A degenerated disc with a herniation can cause both leg and LBP. In the presence of epidural or perineural fibrosis, a disc herniation may cause more leg pain than expected if there were no fibrosis.

Diagnosis of recurrent or residual disc herniation is inferred from the history and physical examination and confirmed by MRI. There is no useful advantage to using gadopentate 6 months or more after surgery.

NEUROPATHIC PAIN

Neuropathic pain is defined as pain due to injury or physiological dysfunction of the peripheral or central nervous system (CNS). Neuropathic pain was the predominant problem in 5% to 9% of FBSS patients.[17-19] It is likely that there is an increased awareness and, therefore, recognition of neuropathic pain rather than an increased prevalence.

There are several potential mechanisms for neuropathic pain after spine surgery. A nerve root could have been damaged prior to surgery due to either acute disc herniation or prolonged compression from foraminal stenosis or chronic disc herniation. In these examples, radicular-type pain continues despite technically successful surgery.

Alternatively, a nerve could be damaged during the surgery itself, which is sometimes referred to as a "battered nerve." The incidence of new cases of arachnoiditis has probably decreased, perhaps because oil-based myelography is no longer performed.

By definition, in pure and uncomplicated neuropathic pain, there is no evidence of nerve root compression on imaging studies. It is important to distinguish neuropathic pain from what might be called neurogenic pain, which implies that a nerve is being compressed or irritated rather than it being permanently damaged. To further complicate matters, some patients have both neuropathic pain plus ongoing neural compression (neurogenic), a condition referred to as a mixed pain syndrome.

EPIDURAL FIBROSIS

Epidural fibrosis occurs after most, if not all, posterior lumbar surgeries. There is one school of thought that considers fibrosis to be responsible for many failures of lumbar spine surgery.[41] The other view is that, in most instances, fibrosis is an innocent and incidental finding that does not cause pain but has the potential to make other problems—such as radiculopathy due to disc herniation or spinal stenosis—worse.[42] The disagreement is not resolved.

MISCELLANEOUS CAUSES

EXTRASPINAL CAUSES

Disorders of the hip can mimic and/or coexist with lumbar spine disorders.[11,12] The prevalence of hip pain lasting longer than 1 month in persons aged 65 to 74 years is 19%, so it is not surprising that in older patients, disorders of the hip (most often osteoarthritis) and spine (particularly spinal stenosis) may coexist.[11,13] To complicate matters, there is overlap between their respective symptoms and signs. Sembrano and Polly evaluated the source of LBP in 200 patients referred to a tertiary spine center. Sixty-five percent had only a spinal disorder, 17% had a combination of spine and hip and/or SIJ pathology, and 8% had hip and/or SIJ pathology without a spine disorder.[11]

Brown and colleagues studied a referral population with leg pain to determine if there were signs or symptoms that might differentiate between osteoarthritis of the hip and a spinal disorder.[13] The factors that were strongly suggestive of primary hip pathology were the presence of a limp, groin pain, or limited internal rotation of the hip. Factors more suggestive of spinal stenosis were lateral thigh pain, buttock pain, and pain below the knee, particularly in the absence of groin pain.

Weight-bearing radiographs of the hip are the standard for diagnosing hip pathology. A single, weight-bearing anterior-posterior pelvis view can serve as a screening tool in patients felt to be a risk for hip osteoarthritis. The classic four radiographic signs of osteoarthritis are subchondral sclerosis, loss of joint space, subchondral cysts, and osteophyte formation. When hip pathology is suspected and x-rays are nondiagnostic, MRI may be useful for the diagnosis of osteonecrosis of the femoral head; labral pathology; lesions of soft tissue, bone, and cartilage; and impending or occult fractures. Injections under fluoroscopy of local anesthesia are frequently helpful.

Greater trochanteric pain is a common problem that may be confused with or coexist with spine pain referred to the leg.[12,16] Patients typically complain of pain in the proximal lateral thigh, often with radiation to the distal thigh. It is common for pain to be increased by lying on the affected side. Pain is usually worsened by walking, running, and activities that necessitate internal or external rotation of the hip. On exam, there is tenderness over the bursa. There is excellent relief after the injection of local anesthetic and steroids into the bursa and surrounding muscles.

COMPLICATIONS OF SURGERY

Many of the true complications of spinal surgery occur early in the postoperative period. Therefore, it is less likely the pain specialist will be evaluating these patients. Such complications include misplaced pedicle screws, wrong surgical level and facet or pedicle fracture.

TECHNICAL FAILURE

Despite the fact that the surgery was appropriate for the symptoms and pathology, the surgeon may not have been able to accomplish the technical goals. Technical failure is usually apparent to the surgeon and can usually be diagnosed on good-quality imaging studies. There may be inadequate decompression of a foramen, incomplete removal of a disc herniation, especially if it was a far lateral herniation, or misplacement of fixation screws.

DECONDITIONING

Deconditioning has long been considered to be at least partially responsible for the persistent pain and pain-related impairment and disability in some patients with FBSS.[43,44] There are three deconditioning models. The pure physical deconditioning model holds that loss of muscle strength and endurance is responsible for pain, reduced activity, impairment, and disability. The cognitive-behavioral model emphasizes fear avoidance, which holds that some patients avoid activities out of pain-related fear. They might believe that attempts to increase their function will result in increased pain and progressive structural damage. As a result, they markedly curtail their activity. The third model is a combination of the two in which patients have both the maladaptive fear avoidance and true physical deconditioning. As a result of the fear-avoidant decreased activity, there is disuse (perhaps better termed *underuse*) with progressive loss of muscle strength and endurance. No matter what the full explanation, there is evidence that exercise is effective in reducing impairment and disability.[45,46] Many, but not all, studies also show decreases in LBP.

TABLE 40-3 Catagories of Psychological Status in FBSS Patients

DSM[50]	Descriptive[54]
Depression	Adaptive coping
Anxiety disorder	Dysfunctional
PTSD	
Substance abuse disorder	
Character disorders	
Cognitive-Behavioral[51-53]	**Gains[55,56]**
Fear and fear avoidance	Primary
Catastrophic thinking	Secondary
Passive coping	Tertiary

PSYCHOLOGICAL RESPONSES

Most patients with FBSS have some form of psychological response (see Table 40-2). In general, psychological conditions are more likely to adversely affect function than they are to cause pain. Most often in CLBP patients, the common psychological disorders develop after back pain began and, as such, would have been present prior to surgery.[47] It appears that spine surgeons and conservative care specialists are not very good at detecting psychological illness unless it is very obvious, and formal psychological testing fares better.[48] In patients who had fusion spine surgery, a systematic review suggested, although the evidence was somewhat weak, that patients with personality disorder, neuroticism, or depression did worse after fusion.[49]

I have found it useful to use four broad categories when thinking about FBSS patients[50-56] (**Table 40-3**). The psychological illnesses such as depression, anxiety disorder, posttraumatic stress disorder, substance abuse, and character disorders are familiar. However, there may be less familiarity with other types of psychological problems such as fear avoidance and catastrophizing, both of which can have significant impact on function. The common fears are that increased activity will cause increased pain or further spine damage and that something serious might have been missed. Although the role of secondary gain is often discussed, recent reviews of a whiplash model show the evidence does not support the negative impact of personal injury litigation, at least in whiplash injury, which serves as a good model.[56] It is clear, however, that injured workers do not do as well as patients with similar structural problem who are not part of the workers' compensation system.

ESTABLISHING THE MOST LIKELY DIFFERENTIAL DIAGNOSIS

In order to plan further testing for the patient with FBSS, the physician needs to establish a differential diagnosis in the approximate order of likelihood. The history is probably the most important part of that task. It is useful to divide FBSS patients into those with predominantly low back pain versus those with primarily leg pain. As discussed earlier, the differential diagnosis for each condition is quite different.

By reviewing the history and medical records, it is often straightforward to determine if the surgery performed was appropriate for the preoperative type of pain, and such a review will give a clue as to whether the current problem was present before surgery and not fully addressed. Generally speaking, there are surgeries for back pain versus surgeries for leg pain. Surgery for low back pain usually requires fusion or total disc replacement, while surgery for leg pain requires direct or indirect decompression of the involved nerve root(s) and, when there is a disc herniation, discectomy. Fusion might be necessary as well if there is preoperative instability (spondylolisthesis) or if there is need for a very wide decompression that results in instability.

Consider the time course of the (re)appearance of pain. Pain that never improved suggests a structural problem that was present before surgery and either not recognized or inadequately addressed. Pain that appeared in the immediate postoperative period and was not present before surgery suggests an intraoperative complication such as nerve injury, pars or facet fracture, or misplaced internal fixation screw(s). Severe low back pain that begins days or a week after surgery can be due to infection. Pain that improves for months or even years and then recurs can be due to ASD and resultant disc and/or facet joint pain. Patients who had fusion with hardware are still vulnerable to pseudarthrosis and to pain from the internal fixation. The usual course is improvement for months followed by recurrence of a different type of back pain.

Determine whether the pain after surgery has approximately the same qualities and topography as the preoperative pain. If so, again this might suggest that the original structural problem was not adequately addressed.

By combining these models with knowledge of the presentations and evaluations of the various structural causes of low back and leg pain, the physician will be able to arrive at the proper diagnosis in a high percentage of patients.

TREATMENT OF PATIENTS WITH FAILED BACK SURGERY

NONSPECIFIC TREATMENTS

There are many treatment options that include, among other things, rehabilitation, medications, psychotherapy, interventions (e.g., injections, radiofrequency neurotomy), neuromodulation, and further surgery. Each is discussed in detail elsewhere in this text. It is important to mention that, even in a pain medicine setting, there are patients for whom additional spine surgery is the best treatment.

Rehabilitation Rehabilitation is often the first line of treatment for patients with FBSS regardless of the structural cause. There can be no doubt that exercise is effective treatment for many patients.[57,58] It serves to improve physical impairments and to help overcome the catastrophic thinking and fear avoidance. There are a wide variety of program types, intensities, and duration. For patients with FBSS after discectomy, Brox and colleagues reported improvements in pain and function from a program that was 25 hours per week for 3 weeks and included cognitive-behavioral therapy and lectures by physicians.[45] Miller and colleagues compared the outcomes of CLBP and FBSS patients in an interdisciplinary functional restoration program.[46] Both groups did well. The no-surgery CLBP patients had greater reductions in pain and disability, but the FBSS patients were significantly more improved in strength and endurance measures, activities of daily living, and fear of exercise. Kernan and Rainville demonstrated clinically important improvements in pain, function, and kinesiophobia in a 6-week, two sessions per week program plus independent exercise but no specific cognitive-behavioral treatment.[59]

Medications There are no specific studies of the efficacy of medications for patients with FBSS. However, there are multiple studies with reasonable levels of evidence that demonstrated the efficacy of opioid analgesics for moderate to severe refractory CLBP.[60] Many of these studies included some patients with FBSS. In general, about one-third of patients get good relief, one-third fair, and one-third minimal or no improvement. Other categories of medications that can be useful in this patient population are anticonvulsants and antidepressants. Medication management is detailed elsewhere in this text.

SPECIFIC TREATMENTS (TABLE 40-4)

Discogenic Pain FBSS caused by one or more painful discs can be difficult to treat. Only rehabilitation and fusion surgery have been evaluated in this patient population. For patients with mild to moderate pain after discectomy, a 3-week intensive interdisciplinary functional rehabilitation program was shown to be equal to fusion surgery.[45] This is consistent with several studies comparing intensive rehabilitation with fusion in mixed populations of idiopathic CLBP that included some patients with prior back surgery.[61,62] It appears that most of these studies excluded patients with severe pain and severe functional impairment. These studies did not subgroup patients by the source of their pain.

TABLE 40-4 Commonly Used treatment Options for Some of the Structural Causes of Failed Back Surgery

Problem	Preferred Treatment	Other Options
Painful disc	Severe pain: fusion; moderate pain: rehabilitation fusion	Opioid analgesics
Facet joint pain	RFN	
SIJ pain	Corticosteroid injections	Rehabilitation RFN SIJ fusion
Recurrent disc herniation with radiculopathy	Discectomy for radiculopathy Fusion if mostly LBP	Functional restoration
Foraminal stenosis	Decompression	TFE? anticonvulsants
Spondylolisthesis	Fusion	RFN if facets are source of pain TFE if mostly leg pain
Neuropathic pain	Medications	SCS

TFE = transforaminal epidural corticosteroid injection

RFN = radiofrequency neurotomy

SIJ = sacroiliac joint

SCS = spinal cord stimulation

Medications might be useful, but most studies showing efficacy evaluated nonspecific CLBP and were not limited to discogenic pain. There is no specific evidence that injections are helpful for discogenic pain in FBSS patients. When rehabilitation and medications are not sufficient, total discectomy with fusion can help a significant number of patients, although the issue remains controversial.[60]

Facet Joint Pain There is high-quality evidence to support the efficacy of properly performed radiofrequency neurotomy (RFN) for facet joint pain in patients with no prior surgery.[63,64] Successful RFN relieves pain to a meaningful degree for about 9 to 12 months.[64,65] When pain recurs, RFN can be repeated. Repeat RFN is usually successful unless there has been disease progression or technical failure of the procedure itself.[65]

Sacroiliac Joint Pain The treatment options for SIJ pain include systemic and topical medications, repeated SIJ corticosteroid injections, radiofrequency neurotomy, and SIJ fusion.[66-70] The duration of relief after steroid injection varies greatly. Some patients achieve long-lasting relief after one to three injections, but others require several injections each year.[68] For patients who do not respond to these treatments, SIJ radiofrequency neurotomy has been useful in a limited number of patients.[64,69] Finally, for patients with severe and refractory pain, SIJ fusion has been reported to be helpful.[70]

Spinal Stenosis Foraminal stenosis is more common than central stenosis in patients with FBSS. Successful treatment for central stenosis has been reported with medications (anticonvulsants), rehabilitation, and epidural corticosteroid injections.[71-74] Patients who fail medical treatment and rehabilitation usually do well with surgery.[75] The same paradigm seems appropriate for foraminal stenosis. If stenosis is severe and extensive decompression is needed, fusion may be required. For mixed pain syndromes, if decompression is not sufficient, medications and/or spinal cord stimulation may be useful.

Neuropathic Pain Neuropathic pain is best treated sequentially. Medications are usually the first line of treatment, and opioids are often added. If there is limited success, spinal cord stimulation (SCS) can be useful. Kumar and colleagues randomized 100 patients with FBSS and predominant leg pain to receive either SCS plus conventional medical management or medical management alone.[76] The primary outcome measure was 50% reduction in leg pain, which was achieved in 48% of the SCS plus medication group versus only 9% of the medication only group. In addition, the SCS plus medication group had improved low back pain, quality of life, and function as well as greater treatment satisfaction.

REFERENCES

1. Schofferman J. Failed back surgery. In: Fishman S, Ballantyne J, Rathmell J, eds. *Bonica's Management of Pain*. Lippincott, Baltimore, MD, Williams & Wilkins; 2010.
2. Chan C, Peng P. Failed back surgery syndrome. *Pain Med.* 2011;12:577-606.
3. Guyer R, Patterson M, Ohnmeiss D. Failed back surgery syndrome: diagnostic evaluation. *J Am Acad Orthop Surg.* 2006;14:534-543.
4. Arts M, Kols N, Onderwater S, Peul W. Clinical outcome of instrumented fusion for the treatment of failed back surgery syndrome: a case series of 100 patients. *Acta Neurochir.* 2012;154:1213-1217.
5. DePalma M, Ketchum J, Trussell B, et al. Does the location of low back pain predict its source? *PM R.* 2011;3:33-39.
6. DePalma M, Ketchum J, Saullo T. What is the source of chronic low back pain and does age play a role? *Pain Med.* 2011;12:224-233.
7. Laplante BL, Ketchum JM, Saullo TR, DePalma MJ. Multivariable analysis of the relationship between pain referral patterns and the source of chronic low back pain. *Pain Phys.* 2012;15:171-178.
8. Young S, Aprill C, Laslett M. Correlation of clinical examination characteristics with three sources of chronic low back pain. *Spine J.* 2003;3:460-465.
9. Hancock M, Maher C, Latimer J, et al. Systematic review of tests to identify the disc, SIJ or facet joint as the source of low back pain. *Eur Spine J.* 2007;16:1539-1550.
10. Schwarzer AC, Aprill CN, Derby R, et al. Clinical features of patients with pain stemming from the lumbar zygapophysial joints: is the lumbar facet syndrome a clinical entity? *Spine.* 1994;19:1132-1137.
11. Sembrano J, Polly C. How often is low back pain not coming from the hip. *Spine.* 2008;34:E27-E32.
12. Bolt P, Wahl M, Schofferman J. The roles of the hip, spine, sacroiliac joint and other structures in patients with persistent pain after back surgery. *Seminars in Spine Surgery.* 2008;20:14-19.
13. Brown MD, Gomez-Marin O, Brookfield KF, et al. Differential diagnosis of hip disease versus spine disease. *Clin Orthop Rel Res.* 2004;419:280-284.
14. Saal J, Dillingham M, Gamburd R, Fanton G. The pseudoradicular syndrome: lower extremity peripheral nerve entrapment masquerading as lumbar radiculopathy. *Spine.* 1988;13:926-930.
15. Harney D, Patijn J. Meralgia paresthetica: diagnosis and management strategies. *Pain Med.* 2007;8:669-677.
16. Tortolani P, Carbone J, Quartararo L. Greater trochanteric pain syndrome in patients referred to orthopedic spine specialists. *Spine J.* 2002;2:251-254.
17. Burton C, Kirkaldy-Willis W, Yong-Hing K, Heithoff KB. Causes of failure of surgery on the lumbar spine. *Clin Orthop.* 1981;157:191-199.
18. Waguespack A, Schofferman J, Slosar P, Reynolds J. Etiology of long-term failures of lumbar spine surgery. *Pain Med.* 2002;3:18-22.
19. Slipman CW, Shin CH, Patel RK, et al. Etiologies of failed back surgery syndrome. *Pain Med.* 2002;3:200-214.
20. DePalma M, Ketchum J, Saullo T, Laplante B. Is the history of a surgical discectomy related to the source of chronic low back pain? *Pain Phys.* 2012;15:E53-E58.
21. DePalma M, Ketchum J, Sullo T. Etiology of chronic low back pain in patients having undergone lumbar fusion. *Pain Med.* 2011;12:732-739.
22. Barrick W, Schofferman J, Reynolds J, et al. Anterior fusion improves discogenic pain at levels of posterolateral fusion. *Spine.* 2000;25:853-857.
23. Manchikanti L, Manchukonda R, Pampati V, et al. Prevalence of facet joint pain in chronic low back pain in postsurgical patients by controlled comparative local anesthetic blocks. *Arch Phys Med Rehabil.* 2007;88:449-455.
24. Katz V, Schofferman J, Reynolds J. The sacroiliac joint: a potential cause of pain after lumbar fusion. *J Spinal Disorders and Tech.* 2003;16:96-99.
25. Lee Y, Sclafani J, Garfin S. Lumbar pseudarthrosis: diagnosis and treatment. *Semin Spine Surg.* 2011;23:275-281.
26. Bhargava A. Fusion hardware mediated low back pain. In: DePalma M, ed. *ISpine evidence based interventional spine care*. New York, NY: Demos Publishing, 2011; 151-155.
27. Kizilkilic O, Yalcin O, Sen O, et al. The role of standing flexion-extension radiographs for spondylolisthesis following single level disk surgery. *Neurol Res.* 2007;29:540-543.
28. Malveaux W, Sharan A. Adjacent segment disease after lumbar spinal fusion: a systematic review of the current literature. *Sem Spine Surg.* 2011;23:266-274.
29. Manchikanti L, Glaser S, et al. Systematic review of lumbar discography as a diagnostic test for chronic low back pain. *Pain Phys.* 2009;12:541-559.
30. Carragee E, Angus D, Hurwitz E, et al. Does discography cause accelerated progression of degeneration changes in the lumbar disc: a ten-year matched cohort study. *Spine.* 2009;34:2338-2345.
31. Laslett M, McDonald D, Aprill CN, et al. Clinical predictors of screening lumbar zygapophyseal joint blocks: development of clinical prediction rules. *Spine J.* 2006;6(4):370-379.
32. Schwarzer AC, Wang SC, O'Driscoll D, et al. The ability of computed tomography to identify a painful zygapophysial joint in patients with chronic low back pain. *Spine.* 1995;20:907-912.
33. Stojanovic MP, Sethee J, Mohiuddin M. MRI analysis of the lumbar spine: can it predict response to diagnostic and therapeutic facet procedures? *Clin J Pain.* 2010;26:110-115.
34. Yoshihara H. Sacroiliac joint pain after lumbar/lumbosacral fusion: current knowledge. *Eur Spine J.* 2012;21:1788-1796.
35. Schwarzer A, Aprill C, Bogduk N. The sacroiliac joint in chronic low back pain. *Spine.* 1995;20:31-37.
36. Dreyfuss P, Dreyer S, Cole A, Mayo K. Sacroiliac joint pain. *J Am Acad Orthop Surg.* 2004;12:255-265.
37. Herzog RJ, Marcotte PJ. Assessment of spinal fusion: critical evaluation of imaging techniques. *Spine.* 1996;21:1114-1118.
38. Slosar P, White A, Wetzel F. The use of selective nerve root blocks: diagnostic, therapeutic, or placebo? *Spine.* 1998;20:2253-2256.
39. van Akkerveeken P. The diagnostic value of nerve root sheath infiltration. *Acta Orthop Scand.* 1993;64:61-63.
40. Derby R, Kine G, Saal JA, et al. Response to steroid and duration of radicular pain as predictors of surgical outcome. *Spine.* 1992;17:S176-S183.
41. Coskun E, Süzer T, Topuz O, et al. Relationships between epidural fibrosis, pain, disability, and psychological factors after lumbar disc surgery. *Eur Spine J.* 2000;9:218-223.
42. Annertz M, Jonsson B, Stromquist B, Holtas S. No relationship between epidural fibrosis and sciatica in lumbar postdiscectomy syndrome. A study with contrast-enhanced MRI in symptomaic and asymptomatic individuals. *Spine.* 1995;20:449-453.

43. Verbunt J, Seelen H, Vlaeyen J, et al. Disuse and deconditioning in chronic low back pain: concepts and hypotheses on contributing mechanisms. *Eur J Pain*. 2003;7:9-21.
44. Smeets R, Wade D, Hidding A, et al. The association of physical deconditioning and chronic low back pain: a hypothesis-oriented systematic review. *Disab Rehab*. 2006;28:673-693.
45. Brox J, Reikeras O, Nygaard, et al. Lumbar instrumented fusion compared with a cognitive intervention and exercises in patients with chronic back pain after previous surgery for disc herniation: a prospective randomized controlled study. *Pain*. 2006;122:145-155.
46. Miller B, Gatchel R, Lou L, et al. Interdisciplinary treatment of failed back surgery syndrome (FBSS): a comparison of FBSS and non-FBSS patients. *Pain Pract*. 2005;5:190-202.
47. Dersh J, Mayer T, Theodore B, et al. Do psychiatric disorders first appear preinjury or postinjury in chronic disabling occupational spinal disorders? *Spine*. 2007;32:1045-1051.
48. Daubs MD, Patel AA, Willick SE, et al. Clinical impression versus standardized questionnaire: the spinal surgeon's ability to assess psychological distress. *J Bone Joint Surg Am*. 2010;92:2878-2883.
49. Daubs M, Norvell DC, McGuire R, et al. Fusion versus nonoperative care for chronic low back pain: do psychological factors affect outcomes? *Spine*. 2011;36(Suppl):S96-S109.
50. Dersh J, Gatchel R, Mayer T, et al. Prevalence of psychiatric disorders in patients with chronic disabling occupational spinal disorders. *Spine*. 2006;31:56-62.
51. Crombez G, Vlaeyen J, Heuts P, Lysens R. Pain-related fear is more disabling than pain itself: evidence on the role of pain-related fear in chronic back pain disability. *Pain*. 1999;80:329-339.
52. Leeuw M, Goossens ME, Linton SJ, et al. The fear-avoidance model of musculoskeletal pain: current state of scientific evidence. *J Behav Med*. 2007;30:77-94.
53. Hasenbring M, Plaas H, Bischbein B, Willburger R. The relationship between activity and pain in patients 6 months after lumbar disc surgery: do pain-related coping modes act as moderator variables. *Eur J Pain*. 2006;10:701-709.
54. Kerns RD, Turk DC, Rudy TE. The West Haven-Yale Multidimensional Pain Inventory (WHYMPI). *Pain*. 1985;23:345-356.
55. Dersh J, Polatin PB, Leeman G, Gatchel RJ. The management of secondary gain and loss in medicolegal settings: strengths and weaknesses. *J Occup Rehabil*. 2004 Dec;14(4):267-279.
56. Spearing N, Connelly L. Whiplash and the compensation hypothesis. *Spine*. 2011;36:S303-S308.
57. Mayer T, McMahon M, Gatchel R, et al. Socioeconomic outcomes of combined spine surgery and functional restoration in workers' compensation spinal disorders with matched controls. *Spine*. 1998;23: 598-605.
58. Smeets R, Vlaeven J, Hidding A, et al. Chronic low back pain: physical training, graded activity with problem solving training, or both? The one-year post-treatment results of a randomized controlled trial. *Pain*. 2008;134:263-276.
59. Kernan T, Rainville J. Observed outcomes associated with a quota-based exercise approach on measures of kinesiophobia in patients with chronic low back pain. *J Ortho Sports Phys Ther*. 2007;11:679-667.
60. Schofferman J, Mazanec D. Evidence-informed management of chronic low back pain with opioid analgesics. *Spine J*. 2008;8:185-194.
61. Mirza S, Deyo R. Systematic review of randomized trials comparing lumbar fusion surgery to nonoperative care for the treatment of chronic low back pain. *Spine*. 2007;32:816-823.
62. Fairbank J, Frost H, Wilson-MacDonald J, et al. Randomised controlled trial to compare surgical stabilization of the lumbar spine withan intensive rehabilitation programme for patients with chronic low back pain: the MRC spine stabilization trial. *BMJ*. 2005;330:1233-1239.
63. Dreyfuss P, Halbrook B, Pauza K, Joshi A, McLarty J, Bogduk N. Efficacy and validity of radiofrequency neurotomy for chronic lumbar zygapophysial joint pain. *Spine*. 2000;25:1270-1277.
64. Speldewinde GC. Outcomes of percutaneous zygapophysial and sacroiliac joint neurotomy in a community setting. *Pain Med*. 2011 Feb;12:209-218.
65. Schofferman J, Kine G. The effectiveness of repeated radiofrequency neurotomy for lumbar facet pain. *Spine*. 2004;29:2471-2473.
66. Foley B, Buschbacher R. Sacroiliac joint pian: anatomy, biomechanics, diagnosis and treatment. *Am J Phys Med Rehabil*. 2006;85:997-1006.
67. Slipman CW, Lipetz JS, Vresilovic EJ, et al. Fluoroscopically guided therapeutic sacroiliac joint injections for sacroiliac joint syndrome. *Am J Phys Med Rehab*. 2001;80:425-432.
68. Hawkins J, Schofferman J. Serial sacroiliac joint injections: a practice audit. *Pain Med*. 2009;10:850-853.
69. Patel N, Gross A, Brown L, Gekht G. A randomized, placebo-controlled study to assess the efficacy of lateral branch neurotomy for chronic sacroiliac joint pain. *Pain Med*. 2012;13:383-398.
70. Buchowski J, Kebaish K, Sinkov V, et al. Functional and radiographic outcome of sacroiliac arthrodesis for the disorders of the sacrioilac joint. *Spine J*. 2005;5:520-528.
71. White A, Arnold P, Norvell D, et al. Pharmacologic management of chronic low back pain: synthesis of the evidence. *Spine*. 2011;36:S131-S143.
72. Yaksi A, Ozgonenel L, Ozgonenel B. The efficacy of gabapentin therapy in patients with lumbar spinal stenosis. *Spine*. 2007;32:939-942.
73. Khoromi S, Patsalides A, Parada S, et al. Topiramate in chronic lumbar radicular pain. *J Pain*. 2005;6:829-836.
74. Smith C, Booker T, Schaufele M, Weiss P. Interlaminar versus transforaminal epidural steroid injections for the treatment of symptomatic lumbar spinal stenosis. *Pain Med*. 2010;11:1511-1515.
75. Weinstein JN, Tosteson TD, Lurie JD, et al. Surgical versus nonoperative treatment for lumbar spinal stenosis four-year results of the Spine Patient Outcomes Research Trial. *Spine*. 2010;15(35):1329-1338.
76. Kumar K, Taylor R, Eidabe S, et al. Spinal cord stimulation versus conventional medical management for neuropathic pain: a multicentre randomised controlled trial in patients with failed back surgery syndrome. *Pain*. 2007;132:179-188.

SECTION C
Extremities and Joints

Pain Management in Medical Rheumatologic Diseases

Fadi Badlissi

"When a patient with arthritis walks in the front door, I feel like leaving out the back door."

—Sir William Osler

INTRODUCTION

Pain is the most common presenting symptom in rheumatologic diseases. Pain is what brings patients to seek medical attention. It interferes with their mental and physical wellness as well as their quality of life.

A study of the U.S. adult population estimated the prevalence of "self-reported doctors-diagnosed arthritis" to be at 21% (46.4 million persons). Among those, 27 million were estimated to have osteoarthritis, 3 million to have gout, and 1.3 million to have rheumatoid arthritis.[1,2]

There are certain principles that will help guide clinicians in the general management of arthritis pain:

1. Diagnose correctly the underlying etiology of the pain such as rheumatoid arthritis (RA) versus osteoarthritis (OA), and distinguish rheumatic diseases from nonmusculoskeletal sources of pain such as neuropathies or somatic etiologies. Recognize that there could be an overlap among different disorders at times, and pain could be of multifactorial etiology. This will influence which approaches to choose to treat the underlying diseases and the ensuing pain.
2. Almost always treat the underlying disease first and consider consulting a rheumatologist. For example, starting a disease-modifying anti-rheumatic drug (DMARD) in rheumatoid arthritis will alleviate the inflammation and, thus, the pain.
3. When the underlying disease is amenable to treatment with other long-term measures, employ pain management as a bridge therapy until achieving long-term disease control (i.e., controlling the activity of RA with DMARDs or preventing gout attacks with uric acid–lowering agents).
4. Consider nonpharmacological interventions such as physical therapy; orthotics, if indicated; and safe, potentially effective, alternative therapies, and address other comorbidities such as obesity.[3-7]
5. Keep in mind the potential treatment side effects, consider the individual risk factors, and thrive to prevent those side effects.
6. Pay more attention to potential treatment-related complications in the elderly population.[8] Always ask the question, "Do the benefits really outweigh the risks?"
7. Consider starting with milder agents and low doses initially, as patients respond differently to medications. (See **Table 41-1**.)

While this chapter will focus on the management of pain in OA and RA, the same concepts apply for joint pain in other rheumatic diseases.

TABLE 41-1 General Principles of Management of Arthritic Pain

- Accurate diagnosis
- Treat the underlying disease
- Consider nonpharmacological therapies
- Balance risks and benefits of treatment
- Start with milder medication at a smaller dose

The administration and management for narcotics and treatment of pain in fibromyalgia are beyond the scope of this chapter and are covered elsewhere in this textbook.

NONPHARMACOLOGIC THERAPY IN OSTEOARTHRITIS AND RHEUMATOID ARTHRITIS

Nonpharmacologic approaches depend on the site of OA and include patient education, self-management and exercise programs, physical and occupational therapy, quadriceps-strengthening exercises,[9,10] knee braces, correct footwear, lateral wedged insole (for medial knee OA), and patellar bracing or taping for patellofemoral pain and knee OA. Proper use of a cane in the contralateral hand to the affected hip or knee can also reduce pain and improve function.[3,7,11] Nonpharmacological therapies such as education and occupational physical therapy and joint protection techniques have a role in RA as well.

Glucosamine and chondroitin sulfate (GCS) are dietary supplements commonly used in knee OA. However, their use is considered controversial; while certain guidelines recommend GCS, others recommend against them.[3,7] As dietary supplements, GCS products are not controlled by the Food and Drug Administration (FDA). The largest randomized placebo-controlled study of chondroitin sulfate and glucosamine did not reduce pain in knee OA.[12] A meta-analysis from 2010 also did not show clinically significant reduction in pain or progression of joint space narrowing in knee OA.[13] The updated Osteoarthritis Research Society International (OARSI) 2010 guidelines also revised downward the effect size of GCS on pain in knee OA compared to its 2008 guidelines.[14] Potential explanations of the heterogeneity and variability among the studies could be related to a different brand or regimen of glucosamine used (i.e., glucosamine sulfate), industry bias, and failed concealment of allocation during the randomization process of the trials subjects.[15]

If patients inquire about the use of GCS for knee OA, it is reasonable if they wish to try them for a period of 3 to 6 months to see if they gain any benefit—assuming they recognize the evidence of the lack of effectiveness of CGS, their cost, and the lack of monitoring or control of those supplements by a governmental agency.

Acupuncture may benefit some patients, but it is operator dependent; a meta-analysis suggested benefits compared to sham acupuncture. It is a reasonable option considering its safety profiles in expert hands.[3,7,16,17] Financial constraints are a limiting factor because most insurers do not reimburse for acupuncture.

NONSTEROIDAL ANTI-INFLAMMATORY DRUGS

Nonsteroidal anti-inflammatory drugs (NSAIDs) include the traditional, nonselective NSAIDs such as naproxen and ibuprofen and the selective NSAIDs, which are the cyclooxygenase-2 (cox-2) inhibitors. Only celecoxib is available in the U.S. market; the other two—rofecoxib and valdecoxib—were withdrawn from the market due to the association with increased cardiovascular risks.[18]

EFFICACY

There is evidence that selective and nonselective NSAIDs are modestly effective in reducing pain in osteoarthritis and rheumatoid arthritis. There is no evidence from clinical trials that either selective or nonselective NSAIDs are more effective than each other,[19-21] or that a particular NSAID is more potent than others, although the individual response to one agent versus the other does vary.[22-24] On the other hand, analysis of multiple studies suggested that nonselective NSAIDs might be more effective, compared with selective NSAIDs, in severe OA.[18]

NSAIDs in RA are almost always used in combination with DMARDs and are often used with corticosteroids. This complicates interpreting the effects of NSAIDs on pain in subjects with RA. In any case, the goal of treatment in RA is to reduce the disease activity to enable discontinuing pain medications, including NSAIDs, when feasible.

CARDIOVASCULAR RISKS

Most nonselective and selective NSAIDs seem to be associated with a small to moderate increased risk of cardiovascular diseases (CVDs). However, several patients' characteristics may be associated with increased CVD risk when using NSAIDs, such as patient age over 80, history of cardiovascular disease, RA, chronic obstructive pulmonary disease (COPD), renal disease, and hypertension.[25] There is no evidence, though, from placebo-controlled trials that nonselective NSAIDs are associated with cardiovascular risk; otherwise, this could be due to the relatively short duration of those trials. A meta-analysis suggested that rofecoxib, diclofenac, and ibuprofen were associated with increased cardiovascular risk, while naproxen and celecoxib were not.[26] This could be explained by the cox-2 selectivity of diclofenac and the relatively weak cox-2 selectivity of celecoxib as compared with rofecoxib. Ibuprofen may interfere with the protective role of low-dose aspirin; hence, it might be associated with increased cardiovascular risks.[27,28] There are no adequate data regarding other NSAIDs, but one study suggested a similar role to naproxen in blocking the effect of aspirin.[29] (See **Table 41-2**.)

GASTROINTESTINAL RISKS AND PREVENTIVE STRATEGIES

NSAIDs are associated with gastrointestinal (GI) side effects including gastritis, ulcers, and their complications such as perforation, bleeding, and obstruction. Nonselective NSAIDs are associated with a 2.7- to 5.4-fold increase in GI side effects.[30-32] The relationship between endoscopic ulcers and clinically significant GI events is not well established.[33] Thus, studies looking at peptic ulcer–related complications might be more clinically relevant.

There is a higher risk of GI complications in subjects with RA; other risk factors for NSAIDs and related GI complications include patient age over 75, previous history of GI bleed, female gender, concomitant corticosteroid use or anticoagulants, and cardiovascular disease.[30-32,34,35]

Nonacetylated salicylate seems to be associated with a better GI safety profile, but it is less effective compared with other NSAIDs.[18,36]

Lumiracoxib and rofecoxib, both selective NSAIDs and not available in the United States, were associated with decreased GI serious complications compared with naproxen and ibuprofen.[37,38] Although the decrease in the GI-related complications disappeared in aspirin users in the lumiracoxib study,[37] being on low-dose aspirin seems to wipe out the benefit from cox-2 inhibitors in regard to GI-related complications. High-dose celecoxib (400 mg twice daily) did not decrease the risk of serious ulcers compared with ibuprofen or diclofenac at 6 and 12 months.[19,39] For the secondary outcomes of symptomatic ulcers, high-dose celecoxib was better than ibuprofen but not diclofenac. However, there was no significant difference with celecoxib in aspirin users compared with nonselective NSAIDs.[19]

Other strategies for GI protection are proton pump inhibitors (PPIs) and misoprostol, which are more effective than the regular dosing of antihistamine-2 in preventing peptic ulcer disease in patients on NSAIDs.[40-43]

TABLE 41-2 Risk Factors for NSAIDs—Cardiovascular Risk

- Age >80
- Presence of cardiovascular disease
- Chronic obstructive pulmonary disease (COPD)
- Rheumatoid arthritis
- Hypertension
- Renal disease

TABLE 41-3 Risk Factors for NSAIDs—Gastrointestinal Complications

- Age >75
- Previous history of GI bleed
- Female gender
- Rheumatoid arthritis
- Concomitant corticosteroid use or anticoagulants
- Presence of cardiovascular disease

One trial compared celecoxib 200 mg twice daily with and without esmoprazole in high-risk subjects who had recent peptic ulcer disease. The study found that the combination with a PPI was more effective in reducing the risk of recurrent ulcers. There was no control arm with nonselective NSAIDs and PPIs.[44]

Looking at serious lower and upper GI side effects, 4484 subjects were randomly allocated to receive celecoxib 200 mg twice daily versus diclofenac 75 mg twice daily with omeprazole 20 mg daily. In this trial, 0.9% in the celecoxib group versus 3.8% in the diclofenac plus omeprazole group developed a serious lower or upper GI event (hazard ratio 4.3, 95% CI 2.6–7.0; $p < 0.0001$).[45]

When used in patients with a high risk for GI complications, NSAIDs should be combined with misoprostol or a PPI. Celecoxib might have a modest decrease in GI side effects compared with nonselective NSAIDs but not in patients who are on low-dose aspirin. In those patients, using nonselective NSAIDs with PPIs or misoprostol is probably more cost effective. In patients with a previous history of serious GI complications, NSAIDs should be avoided completely; however, if they have to be on NSAIDs, then selective NSAIDs combined with PPI might provide better protection. More data are needed to evaluate the safety of nonselective NSAIDs combined with PPI for that population. (See **Table 41-3.**)

In the choice of NSAIDs, balancing the GI and cardiovascular risks and patient's response, should be considered on an individual basis. In addition, NSAIDs should be used with caution in subjects with mild renal insufficiency (glomerular filtration rate [GFR] 60–90 ml/min), and they should be, preferably, avoided altogether in moderate to severe renal insufficiency (GFR <60).

TOPICAL NSAIDs AND CAPSAICIN

Topical NSAIDs and capsaicin are recommended for hand and knee OA in existing guidelines.[3,7,14] Topical NSAIDs have a modest effect in reducing pain in OA based on a meta-analysis of 13 trials.[46] There is evidence, though, of publication bias, which might overestimate the effect of NSAIDs. Topical diclofenac was effective in reducing pain and improving function in knee OA.[47-49] Topical NSAIDs seem overall to be as effective and safer than oral NSAIDs; they are well tolerated overall but have more local skin reactions, such as itching or redness.[49-51] Nonetheless, topical NSAIDs could have systemic side effects; an FDA warning recommended checking liver function tests for topical and oral diclofenac due to reported cases of liver toxicity, including failure.[52]

Capsaicin cream is extracted from chili peppers; it activates and sensitizes peripheral c-nocireceptors.[3] There is evidence based on a meta-analysis that capsaicin 0.025% cream when applied four times a day on painful joints has a mild to modest effect on pain in knee and hand OA.[53] It is important to point out, though, that blinding in randomized controlled trials is not possible with capsaicin because it causes skin burning, which is a common side effect.

ACETAMINOPHEN

Acetaminophen is an alternative to NSAIDs for mild to moderate OA.[3,7] It has a better safety profile, especially regarding the GI tract and renal function. If it is used in high doses (more than 4 grams daily), it is associated with liver toxicity. The long-term use of high doses of acetaminophen could be associated with GI and liver toxicity, especially in the elderly.[54,55] Hence, it is necessary to keep the daily dose of acetaminophen lower than 4 grams—and probably at 3 grams or lower in the elderly.

Acetaminophen is less potent than NSAIDs, based on multiple trials and a Cochrane review.[56,57] In addition, acetaminophen seems to be less effective than NSAIDs in inflammatory arthritis such as RA.[58]

ORAL CORTICOSTEROIDS

Prednisone, even in small doses for RA, such as 5 to 10 mg, is effective in reducing pain. It is often used initially in RA as a bridge therapy in conjunction with DMARDs until they take effect. The corticosteroid side effects preclude their use for a prolonged period of time; those side effects in a smaller dose of 5 mg or less are minimal. A small study of 31 subjects with RA showed that 1 to 4 mg of prednisone was effective; more subjects withdrew in the placebo arm compared to the prednisone-treated ones.[59]

TRAMADOL

Tramadol is another alternative to NSAIDs for the treatment of osteoarthritis. Tramadol is a mild opioid but has a distinct effect on serotonin and norepinephrine as well.

A meta-analysis showed that Tramadol had a modest effect on reducing pain and improvement in function.[60] Tramadol was well tolerated overall.

Randomized controlled trials of extended-release Tramadol showed modest effects on reducing pain and improving global function in hip and knee OA; it was comparable in efficacy to diclofenac.[61,62] In one randomized controlled trial, though, the controlled-release Tramadol failed to improve pain and physical function on the Western Ontario and McMaster Universities Osteoarthritis (WOMAC) Index compared to the placebo, while the other active comparator, celecoxib, did meet the primary end point and was statistically better than the placebo. Only high-dose Tramadol of 300 mg improved patient global assessment in that study.[63]

Tramadol combined with acetaminophen could allow reducing the dose of NSAIDs and add efficacy to cox-2 inhibitors in reducing pain in subjects with knee and hip OA with inadequate response.[64,65]

Tramadol seems to be effective and safe in the elderly population with OA. Low-dose Tramadol combined with acetaminophen (37.5 mg/325) was effective in reducing pain in subjects over age 65 with OA when added to cox-2 inhibitors or nonselective NSAIDs.[66] A post hoc analysis also showed Tramadol to be effective and well tolerated overall in subjects over age 65.[67]

Common side effects mostly include GI side effects such as nausea, vomiting, and constipation in addition to dizziness and headaches.[60,61,66,67] A special caution is needed in subjects who are on antidepressants, in particular, serotonin reuptake inhibitors because, in combination with Tramadol, there is a risk of serotonin syndrome and seizures. In those instances, lower dosages of Tramadol should be employed.

Tramadol is a mild opioid and an alternative treatment for joint pain studied mostly in OA. It differs from classic opioids by affecting the serotonin and norepinephrine pathways; it has a modest effect but does not have the GI and renal toxicity associated with NSAIDs.

OPIOIDS

Short-acting and long-acting opioids could be considered in subjects with OA or RA with inadequate pain control, despite maximizing other pharmacological and nonpharmacological therapies, who are not candidates for surgical interventions.[7,14]

There are available guidelines for the management of noncancer pain with opioids published by the American Pain Society and the American Academy of Pain Medicine.[68]

INTRAARTICULAR CORTICOSTEROID INJECTIONS

Intraarticular (IA) corticosteroids are helpful in joint pain exacerbation or when the pain is not well controlled with other measures. They could be used in different types of arthritis, including OA, RA, and crystal-induced arthropathies such as gout or pseudogout.

IA corticosteroids seem to be effective in reducing pain but not in improving function in knee OA based on a Cochrane systematic review.[69] The effect size is large initially at 1 week at 0.72 (95% CI 0.42–1.01), but it declines to 0.28 (95% CI 0.17–0.73) 4 weeks after the injection.[69]

There is no adequate head-to-head comparison data to show if one intraarticular corticosteroid is superior to another.[3] Methylprednisolone and triamcinolone are commonly used. It is not clear at what frequency it is safe to administer IA corticosteroids. Most experts recommend against using them more than four times per year.[3]

A randomized controlled trial for IA corticosteroid injections in subjects with hip OA awaiting hip replacement showed that triamcinolone was not more effective than local anesthetics.[70] Another study of IA triamcinolone injections in severe hip OA showed an improvement in pain and mobility at 3 weeks and 3 months.[71]

IA corticosteroids are well tolerated. Complications such as bleeding and infections are rare. Corticosteroid-induced cartilage atrophy is a concern with frequent injections. There is systemic absorption of corticosteroids even with IA injection, which could lead to systemic side effects. There is evidence of higher glucose levels in diabetics for 2 weeks post–IA corticosteroid injections.[72] It is important to place the corticosteroid injections accurately to maximize efficacy and minimize adverse events.

INTRAARTICULAR VISCOSUPPLEMENTATION

Viscosupplementation with intraarticular hyaluronic acid (HA) derivatives is classified under instrumental therapy. HA is a large molecular weight glycosaminoglycan that is a constituent in synovial fluid. It is not clear what the mechanism of action is, particularly as the compounds have a relatively short half-life (hours in some cases) in synovial fluid, yet there could be a prolonged benefit in some patients. HA injections are an attractive alternative to NSAIDs, considering the potential adverse reactions of NSAIDs; however, their effectiveness is controversial at a high cost.[3,14]

A randomized controlled trial of 337 subjects with moderate to severe OA that compared five injections of sodium hyalorunate (hyalgan) to placebo saline injections showed no benefits from the HA injections in knee OA.[73] Another study comparing four intraarticular hyalgan injections with saline injections showed no significant difference in treatment benefits between the two groups.[74] A meta-analysis of nine randomized controlled trials comparing HA with saline IA injections showed no improvement in pain or joint function.[75]

A meta-analysis of HA injections in knee OA showed a modest effect on pain reduction but significant heterogeneity among the studies and the possibility of publication bias that might overestimate the effect size. The study concluded that the highest molecular weight HA may be more efficacious than the lower molecular weight treating knee OA, but the heterogeneity of these studies limited any definitive conclusion.[76] A 2007 meta-analysis of 13 RCTs compared outcomes following IA injections of high molecular weight with standard HA products in 2085 subjects with knee OA. The analysis showed that high molecular weight IA HA was not more effective in relieving pain, but there was a high degree of heterogeneity among trials as well.[77]

The largest industry-sponsored Cochrane review showed IA HA injections to reduce pain and improve physical function with pooled effect size (ES) versus placebo at 1 to 4 weeks of 0.60 (95% CI 0.37–0.83) and 0.61 (95% CI 0.35–0.87), respectively.[78] But, there was a possibility of publication bias and considerable heterogeneity of outcomes among trials. In addition, when the analysis was restricted to high-quality studies, there was no evidence for significant pain relief.

The same meta-analysis compared IA HA with corticosteroid injection in 10 trials. It found no difference in effects between 1 and 4 weeks postinjection but more improvement with IA HA injection in weeks 5 through 13.[78] This was further confirmed with a systematic review that showed that at baseline to week 4, IA corticosteroids were relatively more effective for pain relief than IA HA; by week 4, the two approached

TABLE 41-4 Intraarticular Corticosteroid and Hyaluronic Acid Injections

- Corticosteroids effect declines after 4 weeks
- No evidence if one corticosteroid is more effective
- Hyalorunic acid injections might have more prolonged effects than corticosteroids
- Hyalorunic acid injections is more effective in mild to moderate OA

equal efficacy, but beyond week 8, HA had greater efficacy.[79] There were no significant safety issues with IA HA injections. Transient joint pain and swelling following the HA injections were more common with the high molecular weight HA.[78]

Single IA injection of 6 ml HA is now an available alternative to multiple injections. A placebo-controlled study demonstrated that a single 6-ml IA injection of hylan G-F 20 had a modest effect on pain relief over 26 weeks compared to placebo in moderate knee OA.[80]

In summary, IA hyaluronic acid injections have modest effects in mild to moderate knee OA. There is contradictory evidence concerning their effectiveness. They seem to have more lasting effects than IA corticosteroids. They could play a role in mild to moderate knee OA, where other pain management options are contraindicated or inadequate or if the patient has a limited response to corticosteroid injections. IA HA injections could play a role in patients with symptomatic knee OA who are not surgical candidates, though at that stage of OA, they may have limited response to such injections. The accuracy of HA injections is important for better efficacy and fewer complications. In the case of no or limited response to IA HA injections, it is sensible not to repeat them. The cost of IA HA injections is an issue to consider. (See **Table 41-4**.)

A general approach for managing musculoskeletal pain is depicted in **Figure 41-1**.

EMERGING THERAPIES IN OSTEOARTHRITIS

TANEZUMAB

Tanezumab is a humanized monoclonal antibody that binds to and inhibits nerve growth factor; tanezumab is administered intravenously. In a proof-of-concept study, tanezumab showed promising results in reducing pain and improving function in moderate to severe knee OA.[81] After the completion of the study, 16 participants in the phase III trial developed rapidly progressive OA with radiographic evidence of avascular necrosis that required joint replacement.[81] Hence, the FDA put the osteoarthritis program for tanezumab on hold for further evaluation. But in February 2012, an FDA advisory committee did not find the rapid progression of OA and osteonecrosis to be drug related. The advisory committee recommended resuming clinical trials for tanezumab in OA.[82]

Tanezumab was associated with significant reduction in pain and improvement in function in a Japanese population with moderate to severe OA. Peripheral sensory abnormalities such as paresthesia and allodynia were common side effects.[83]

ZOLIDRONIC ACID

Zolidronic acid (ZA) is an intravenous bisphosphonate antiresorptive drug used for osteoporosis treatment. A randomized clinical trial of 59 subjects with moderate to severe OA showed improvement in pain visual analogue scores at 6 months in the ZA group but not at 3 and 12 months postinfusion compared with a placebo. The study followed knee magnetic resonance imaging (MRI) at the beginning and at 6 and 12 months. It did show statistically significant improvement in bone

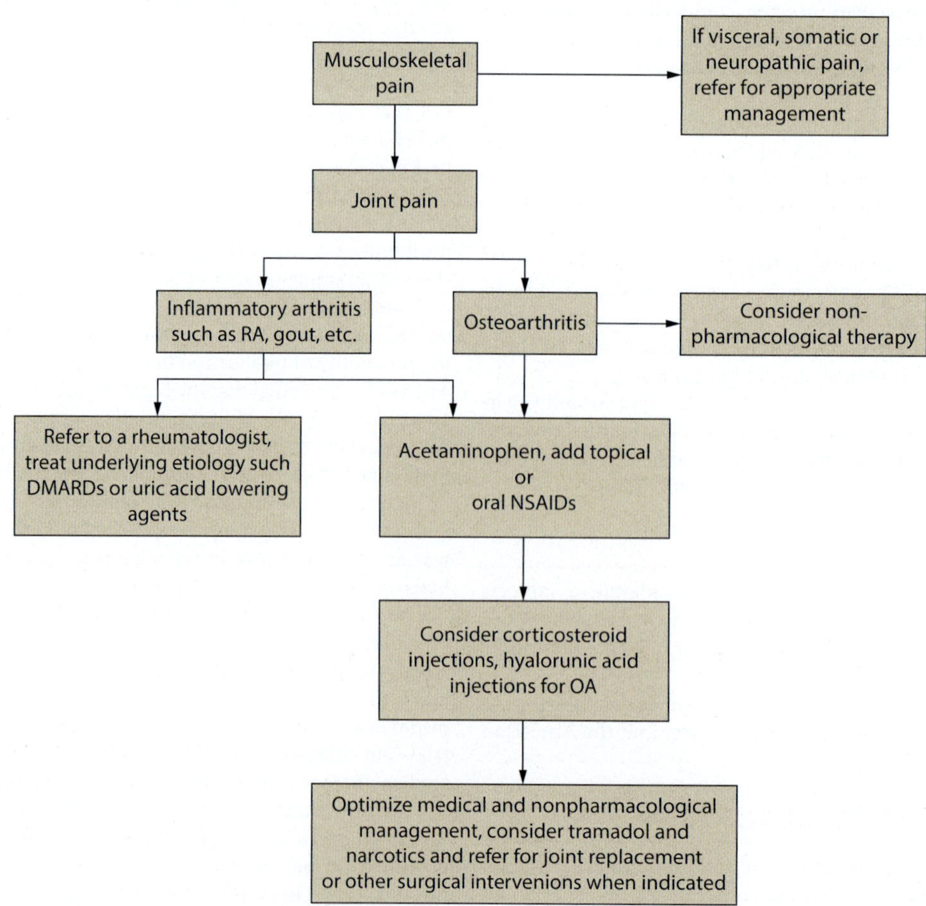

FIGURE 41-1. General approach for the management of musculoskeletal pain.

marrow lesions in the ZA group compared with a placebo at 6 months but only a trend of improvement at 12 months.[84]

GOUT

Gout is a syndrome defined by hyperuricemia and deposition of uric acid crystals associated with acute inflammatory arthritis. Gout could also lead to the accumulation of urate crystals in the form of tophus (tophaceous gout), destructive arthritis, and urate nephrolithiasis.

The treatment of acute gout arthropathy should target the inflammatory process; it includes NSAIDs, colchicine, and intraarticular or parenteral corticosteroids.[85]

NSAIDs are commonly used for acute gout attack. Many randomized controlled studies showed their effectiveness in controlling acute gout attacks,[86-89] although the quality of the trials is variable and there are very few placebo-controlled studies.[85,90] Indomethacin is used frequently for gout. However, it does not have a greater advantage compared with other NSAIDs and might be associated with more toxicity; most studies did not show any superiority for one NSAID compared to others.[89]

There is a dearth of data regarding the use of corticosteroids and gout. Intraarticular (IA) corticosteroids are commonly used for acute gout attack. One small, uncontrolled study showed that a small dose (10 mg) of IA triamcinolone reduced pain significantly in acute gouty arthritis.[91]

Oral or intramuscular systemic corticosteroids and adrenocorticotropic hormone (ACTH) are commonly used for acute gout attacks, especially when they are oligo or polyarticular and particularly when NSAIDs and colchicine are contraindicated.[92-94]

Colchicine has been used for gout for many years. A study showed that low-dose oral colchicine was as effective as high-dose colchicine and was associated with fewer GI side effects.[95] (See **Table 41-5**.). Although only 37.8% in the low-dose, compared to 32.7% in the high-dose group, it had 50% or more improvement in pain at 24 hours.

In general, gout attack responds better to treatment as long as it is initiated as soon as the attack starts. If the patient is experiencing more than two attacks per year, destructive arthropathy, tophaceous gout, polyarticular attack, or urate nephrolithiasis, he or she should be considered for uric acid–lowering agents. This will prevent future gout attacks and provide long-term control of the disease.

SERONEGATIVE SPONDYLOARTHROPATHIES

Seronegative spondyloarthropathies (SSps) include ankylosing spondylitis, psoriatic arthritis, reactive arthritis, and arthropathies associated with inflammatory bowel disease (IBD). The specific treatment of this family of diseases is beyond the scope of this chapter.

NSAIDs are an important part of the pain management for SSp except for IBD-associated arthropathies because they could exacerbate the bowel disease. NSAIDs and cox-2 inhibitors are recommended in symptomatic patients with ankylosing spondylitis, and they do improve pain and function.[96,97] There is evidence that continuous treatment with NSAIDs, including celecoxib, might delay the radiographic progression in ankylosing spondylitis (AS).[98]

While treating arthritis is still challenging at times, we have therapeutic options now; hopefully, then, we don't have to leave out the back door as Sir William Osler wanted to do.

TABLE 41-5 Treatment of Acute Gout

- NSAIDs
- Colchicine
- Intraarticular corticosteroids
- Parenteral corticosteroids and adrenocorticotropic hormone (ACTH)

REFERENCES

1. Helmick CG, Felson DT, Lawrence RC, et al. Estimates of the prevalence of arthritis and other rheumatic conditions in the United States. Part I. *Arthritis Rheum*. Jan 2008;58(1):15-25.
2. Lawrence RC, Felson DT, Helmick CG, et al. Estimates of the prevalence of arthritis and other rheumatic conditions in the United States. Part II. *Arthritis Rheum*. Jan 2008;58(1):26-35.
3. Zhang W, Moskowitz RW, Nuki G, et al. OARSI recommendations for the management of hip and knee osteoarthritis, Part II: OARSI evidence-based, expert consensus guidelines. *Osteoarthritis and Cartilage/OARS, Osteoarthritis Research Society*. Feb 2008;16(2):137-162.
4. Luqmani R, Hennell S, Estrach C, et al. British Society for Rheumatology and British health professionals in rheumatology guideline for the management of rheumatoid arthritis (the first two years). *Rheumatol (Oxford)*. Sep 2006;45(9):1167-1169.
5. Luqmani R, Hennell S, Estrach C, et al. British Society for Rheumatology and British Health Professionals in Rheumatology guideline for the management of rheumatoid arthritis (after the first 2 years). *Rheumatol (Oxford)*. Apr 2009;48(4):436-439.
6. Gossec L, Pavy S, Pham T, et al. Nonpharmacological treatments in early rheumatoid arthritis: clinical practice guidelines based on published evidence and expert opinion. *Joint, Bone, Spine: Revue du rhumatisme*. Jul 2006;73(4):396-402.
7. Hochberg MC, Altman RD, April KT, et al. American College of Rheumatology 2012 recommendations for the use of nonpharmacologic and pharmacologic therapies in osteoarthritis of the hand, hip, and knee. *Arthritis Care Res*. Apr 2012;64(4):455-474.
8. American Geriatrics Society Panel on Pharmacological management of persistent pain in older persons. *J Am Geriat Soc*. Aug 2009;57(8):1331-1346.
9. McKnight PE, Kasle S, Going S, et al. A comparison of strength training, self-management, and the combination for early osteoarthritis of the knee. *Arthritis Care Res*. Jan 15 2010;62(1):45-53.
10. Jenkinson CM, Doherty M, Avery AJ, et al. Effects of dietary intervention and quadriceps strengthening exercises on pain and function in overweight people with knee pain: randomised controlled trial. *BMJ*. 2009;339:b3170.
11. Felson DT. Clinical practice. Osteoarthritis of the knee. *N Engl J Med*. Feb 23 2006;354(8):841-848.
12. Clegg DO, Reda DJ, Harris CL, et al. Glucosamine, chondroitin sulfate, and the two in combination for painful knee osteoarthritis. *N Engl J Med*. Feb 23 2006;354(8):795-808.
13. Wandel S, Juni P, Tendal B, et al. Effects of glucosamine, chondroitin, or placebo in patients with osteoarthritis of hip or knee: network meta-analysis. *BMJ*. 2010;341:c4675.
14. Zhang W, Nuki G, Moskowitz RW, et al. OARSI recommendations for the management of hip and knee osteoarthritis: part III:Changes in evidence following systematic cumulative update of research published through January 2009. *Osteoarthritis and Cartilage/OARS, Osteoarthritis Research Society*. Apr 2010;18(4):476-499.
15. Vlad SC, LaValley MP, McAlindon TE, Felson DT. Glucosamine for pain in osteoarthritis: why do trial results differ? *Arthritis Rheum*. Jul 2007;56(7):2267-2277.
16. Kwon YD, Pittler MH, Ernst E. Acupuncture for peripheral joint osteoarthritis: a systematic review and meta-analysis. *Rheumatol (Oxford)*. Nov 2006;45(11):1331-1337.
17. Suarez-Almazor ME, Looney C, Liu Y, et al. A randomized controlled trial of acupuncture for osteoarthritis of the knee: effects of patient-provider communication. *Arthritis Care Res*. Sep 2010;62(9):1229-1236.

18. Desai SP, Solomon DH, Abramson SB. American College of Rheumatology Ad Hoc Group on Use of Selective and Nonselecetive Nonsteroidal Antiinflammatory Drugs. Recommendations for use of selective and non-selective anti-inflammatory drugs: an American College of Rheumatolkogy white paper. *Arthritis Rheum.* 2008;59:1058-1073.
19. Silverstein FE, Faich G, Goldstein JL, et al. Gastrointestinal toxicity with celecoxib vs nonsteroidal anti-inflammatory drugs for osteoarthritis and rheumatoid arthritis: the CLASS study: a randomized controlled trial. Celecoxib Long-term Arthritis Safety Study. *JAMA.* Sep 13 2000;284(10):1247-1255.
20. Deeks JJ, Smith LA, Bradley MD. Efficacy, tolerability, and upper gastrointestinal safety of celecoxib for treatment of osteoarthritis and rheumatoid arthritis: systematic review of randomised controlled trials. *BMJ.* Sep 21 2002;325(7365):619.
21. Singh G, Fort JG, Goldstein JL, et al. Celecoxib versus naproxen and diclofenac in osteoarthritis patients: SUCCESS-I Study. *Am J Med.* Mar 2006;119(3):255-266.
22. Huskisson EC, Woolf DL, Balme HW, Scott J, Franklin S. Four new anti-inflammatory drugs: responses and variations. *BMJ.* May 1 1976;1(6017):1048-1049.
23. Simpson J, Golding DN, Freeman AM, et al. A large multicentre, parallel group, double-blind study comparing tenoxicam and piroxicam in the treatment of osteoarthritis and rheumatoid arthritis. *Brit J Clin Prac.* Sep 1989;43(9):328-333.
24. Krug H, Broadwell LK, Berry M, DeLapp R, Palmer RH, Mahowald M. Tolerability and efficacy of nabumetone and naproxen in the treatment of rheumatoid arthritis. *Clin Therap.* Jan 2000;22(1):40-52.
25. Solomon DH, Glynn RJ, Rothman KJ, et al. Subgroup analyses to determine cardiovascular risk associated with nonsteroidal antiinflammatory drugs and coxibs in specific patient groups. *Arthritis Rheum.* Aug 15 2008;59(8):1097-1104.
26. Antman EM, DeMets D, Loscalzo J. Cyclooxygenase inhibition and cardiovascular risk. *Circulation.* Aug 2 2005;112(5):759-770.
27. concomitant use of ibuprofen and aspirin: potential of attenuation of the anti-platelet effect of aspirin. 2006; http://www.fda.gov/cder/drug/infopage/ibuprofen/science_paper.htm.
28. Ellison J, Dager W. Recent FDA warning of the concomitant use of aspirin and ibuprofen and the effects on platelet aggregation. *Prev Cardiol.* Spring 2007;10(2):61-63.
29. Capone ML, Sciulli MG, Tacconelli S, et al. Pharmacodynamic interaction of naproxen with low-dose aspirin in healthy subjects. *J Am Coll Cardiol.* Apr 19 2005;45(8):1295-1301.
30. Ofman JJ, MacLean CH, Straus WL, et al. A metaanalysis of severe upper gastrointestinal complications of nonsteroidal antiinflammatory drugs. *J Rheumatol.* Apr 2002;29(4):804-812.
31. Bollini P, Garcia Rodriguez LA, Perez Gutthann S, Walker AM. The impact of research quality and study design on epidemiologic estimates of the effect of nonsteroidal anti-inflammatory drugs on upper gastrointestinal tract disease. *Arch Int Med.* Jun 1992;152(6):1289-1295.
32. Gabriel SE, Jaakkimainen L, Bombardier C. Risk for serious gastrointestinal complications related to use of nonsteroidal anti-inflammatory drugs. A meta-analysis. *Ann Int Med.* Nov 15 1991;115(10):787-796.
33. Singh G, Triadafilopoulos G. Epidemiology of NSAID induced gastrointestinal complications. *J Rheumatol. Suppl.* Apr 1999;56:18-24.
34. Hernandez-Diaz S, Rodriguez LA. Association between nonsteroidal anti-inflammatory drugs and upper gastrointestinal tract bleeding/perforation: an overview of epidemiologic studies published in the 1990s. *Arch Int Med.* Jul 24 2000;160(14):2093-2099.
35. Silverstein FE, Graham DY, Senior JR, et al. Misoprostol reduces serious gastrointestinal complications in patients with rheumatoid arthritis receiving nonsteroidal anti-inflammatory drugs. A randomized, double-blind, placebo-controlled trial. *Ann Int Med.* Aug 15 1995;123(4):241-249.
36. Lanza F, Rack MF, Doucette M, Ekholm B, Goldlust B, Wilson R. An endoscopic comparison of the gastroduodenal injury seen with salsalate and naproxen. *J Rheumatol.* Dec 1989;16(12):1570-1574.
37. Schnitzer TJ, Burmester GR, Mysler E, et al. Comparison of lumiracoxib with naproxen and ibuprofen in the Therapeutic Arthritis Research and Gastrointestinal Event Trial (TARGET), reduction in ulcer complications: randomised controlled trial. *Lancet.* Aug 21-27 2004;364(9435):665-674.
38. Bombardier C, Laine L, Reicin A, et al. Comparison of upper gastrointestinal toxicity of rofecoxib and naproxen in patients with rheumatoid arthritis. VIGOR Study Group. *N Engl J Med.* Nov 23 2000;343(21):1520-1528, 1522 p following 1528.
39. Hrachovec JB, Mora M. Reporting of 6-month vs 12-month data in a clinical trial of celecoxib. *JAMA.* Nov 21 2001;286(19):2398; author reply 2399-2400.
40. Massimo Claar G, Monaco S, Del Veccho Blanco C, Capurso L, Fusillo M, Annibale B. Omeprazole 20 or 40 mg daily for healing gastroduodenal ulcers in patients receiving non-steroidal anti-inflammatory drugs. *Alim Pharmacol Therap.* May 1998;12(5):463-468.
41. Bianchi Porro G, Lazzaroni M, Petrillo M. Double-blind, double-dummy endoscopic comparison of the mucosal protective effects of misoprostol versus ranitidine on naproxen-induced mucosal injury to the stomach and duodenum in rheumatic patients. *Am J Gastroenterol.* Apr 1997;92(4):663-667.
42. Taha AS, Hudson N, Hawkey CJ, et al. Famotidine for the prevention of gastric and duodenal ulcers caused by nonsteroidal antiinflammatory drugs. *N Engl J Med.* May 30 1996;334(22):1435-1439.
43. Yeomans ND, Tulassay Z, Juhasz L, et al. A comparison of omeprazole with ranitidine for ulcers associated with nonsteroidal antiinflammatory drugs. Acid suppression trial: ranitidine versus omeprazole for NSAID-associated ulcer treatment (ASTRONAUT) Study Group. *N Engl J Med.* Mar 12 1998;338(11):719-726.
44. Chan FK, Wong VW, Suen BY, et al. Combination of a cyclooxygenase-2 inhibitor and a proton-pump inhibitor for prevention of recurrent ulcer bleeding in patients at very high risk: a double-blind, randomised trial. *Lancet.* May 12 2007;369(9573):1621-1626.
45. Chan FK, Lanas A, Scheiman J, Berger MF, Nguyen H, Goldstein JL. Celecoxib versus omeprazole and diclofenac in patients with osteoarthritis and rheumatoid arthritis (CONDOR): a randomised trial. *Lancet.* Jul 17 2010;376(9736):173-179.
46. Lin J, Zhang W, Jones A, Doherty M. Efficacy of topical non-steroidal anti-inflammatory drugs in the treatment of osteoarthritis: meta-analysis of randomised controlled trials. *BMJ.* Aug 7 2004;329(7461):324.
47. Baer PA, Thomas LM, Shainhouse Z. Treatment of osteoarthritis of the knee with a topical diclofenac solution: a randomised controlled, 6-week trial [ISRCTN53366886]. *BMC Musculoskel Disord.* 2005;6:44.
48. Roth SH, Shainhouse JZ. Efficacy and safety of a topical diclofenac solution (pennsaid) in the treatment of primary osteoarthritis of the knee: a randomized, double-blind, vehicle-controlled clinical trial. *Arch Int Med.* Oct 11 2004;164(18):2017-2023.
49. Tugwell PS, Wells GA, Shainhouse JZ. Equivalence study of a topical diclofenac solution (pennsaid) compared with oral diclofenac in symptomatic treatment of osteoarthritis of the knee: a randomized controlled trial. *J Rheumatol.* Oct 2004;31(10):2002-2012.
50. Evans JM, MacDonald TM. Tolerability of topical NSAIDs in the elderly: do they really convey a safety advantage? *Drugs Aging.* Aug 1996;9(2):101-108.
51. Evans JM, McMahon AD, McGilchrist MM, et al. Topical non-steroidal anti-inflammatory drugs and admission to hospital for upper gastrointestinal bleeding and perforation: a record linkage case-control study. *BMJ.* Jul 1 1995;311(6996):22-26.

52. Voltaren gel (diclofenac sodium topical gel) 1%: hepatic effects labeling changes. 2009; http://www.fda.gov/Safety/MedWatch/SafetyInformation/SafetyAlertsforHumanMedicalProducts/ucm193047.htm.
53. Zhang WY, Li Wan Po A. The effectiveness of topically applied capsaicin: a meta-analysis. *Eur J Clin Pharmacol.* 1994;46(6):517-522.
54. Rahme E, Pettitt D, LeLorier J. Determinants and sequelae associated with utilization of acetaminophen versus traditional nonsteroidal antiinflammatory drugs in an elderly population. *Arthritis Rheum.* Nov 2002;46(11):3046-3054.
55. Garcia Rodriguez LA, Hernandez-Diaz S. Relative risk of upper gastrointestinal complications among users of acetaminophen and nonsteroidal anti-inflammatory drugs. *Epidemiol.* Sep 2001;12(5):570-576.
56. Towheed TE, Maxwell L, Judd MG, Catton M, Hochberg MC, Wells G. Acetaminophen for osteoarthritis. *Cochrane Database Syst Rev.* 2006(1):CD004257.
57. Zhang W, Jones A, Doherty M. Does paracetamol (acetaminophen) reduce the pain of osteoarthritis? A meta-analysis of randomised controlled trials. *Ann Rheum Dis.* Aug 2004;63(8):901-907.
58. Wienecke T, Gotzsche PC. Paracetamol versus nonsteroidal anti-inflammatory drugs for rheumatoid arthritis. *Cochrane Database Syst Rev.* 2004;(1):CD003789.
59. Pincus T, Swearingen CJ, Luta G, Sokka T. Efficacy of prednisone 1-4 mg/day in patients with rheumatoid arthritis: a randomised, double-blind, placebo controlled withdrawal clinical trial. *Ann Rheum Dis.* Nov 2009;68(11):1715-1720.
60. Cepeda MS, Camargo F, Zea C, Valencia L. Tramadol for osteoarthritis: a systematic review and metaanalysis. *J Rheumatol.* Mar 2007;34(3):543-555.
61. Beaulieu AD, Peloso PM, Haraoui B, et al. Once-daily, controlled-release tramadol and sustained-release diclofenac relieve chronic pain due to osteoarthritis: a randomized controlled trial. *Pain Res Manage.* Mar-Apr 2008;13(2):103-110.
62. Babul N, Noveck R, Chipman H, Roth SH, Gana T, Albert K. Efficacy and safety of extended-release, once-daily tramadol in chronic pain: a randomized 12-week clinical trial in osteoarthritis of the knee. *J Pain Symp Manage.* Jul 2004;28(1):59-71.
63. DeLemos BP, Xiang J, Benson C, et al. Tramadol hydrochloride extended-release once-daily in the treatment of osteoarthritis of the knee and/or hip: a double-blind, randomized, dose-ranging trial. *Am J Therap.* May 2011;18(3):216-226.
64. Schnitzer TJ, Kamin M, Olson WH. Tramadol allows reduction of naproxen dose among patients with naproxen-responsive osteoarthritis pain: a randomized, double-blind, placebo-controlled study. *Arthritis Rheum.* Jul 1999;42(7):1370-1377.
65. Emkey R, Rosenthal N, Wu SC, Jordan D, Kamin M. Efficacy and safety of tramadol/acetaminophen tablets (Ultracet) as add-on therapy for osteoarthritis pain in subjects receiving a COX-2 nonsteroidal antiinflammatory drug: a multicenter, randomized, double-blind, placebo-controlled trial. *J Rheumatol.* Jan 2004;31(1):150-156.
66. Rosenthal NR, Silverfield JC, Wu SC, Jordan D, Kamin M. Tramadol/acetaminophen combination tablets for the treatment of pain associated with osteoarthritis flare in an elderly patient population. *J Am Geriat Soc.* Mar 2004;52(3):374-380.
67. Vorsanger G, Xiang J, Jordan D, Farrell J. Post hoc analysis of a randomized, double-blind, placebo-controlled efficacy and tolerability study of tramadol extended release for the treatment of osteoarthritis pain in geriatric patients. *Clin Therap.* 2007;29(Suppl):2520-2535.
68. Chou R, Fanciullo GJ, Fine PG, et al. Clinical guidelines for the use of chronic opioid therapy in chronic noncancer pain. *J Pain.* Feb 2009;10(2):113-130.
69. Bellamy N, Campbell J, Robinson V, Gee T, Bourne R, Wells G. Intraarticular corticosteroid for treatment of osteoarthritis of the knee. *Cochrane Database Syst Rev.* 2006;(2):CD005328.
70. Flanagan J, Casale FF, Thomas TL, Desai KB. Intra-articular injection for pain relief in patients awaiting hip replacement. *Ann Royal Coll Surg Engl.* May 1988;70(3):156-157.
71. Kullenberg B, Runesson R, Tuvhag R, Olsson C, Resch S. Intraarticular corticosteroid injection: pain relief in osteoarthritis of the hip? *J Rheumatol.* Nov 2004;31(11):2265-2268.
72. Habib GS. Systemic effects of intra-articular corticosteroids. *Clin Rheumatol.* Jul 2009;28(7):749-756.
73. Jorgensen A, Stengaard-Pedersen K, Simonsen O, et al. Intra-articular hyaluronan is without clinical effect in knee osteoarthritis: a multicentre, randomised, placebo-controlled, double-blind study of 337 patients followed for 1 year. *Ann Rheum Dis.* Jun 2010;69(6):1097-1102.
74. Lundsgaard C, Dufour N, Fallentin E, Winkel P, Gluud C. Intra-articular sodium hyaluronate 2 mL versus physiological saline 20 mL versus physiological saline 2 mL for painful knee osteoarthritis: a randomized clinical trial. *Scand J Rheumatol.* Mar-Apr 2008;37(2):142-150.
75. Arrich J, Piribauer F, Mad P, Schmid D, Klaushofer K, Mullner M. Intra-articular hyaluronic acid for the treatment of osteoarthritis of the knee: systematic review and meta-analysis. *CMAJ.* Apr 12 2005;172(8):1039-1043.
76. Lo GH, LaValley M, McAlindon T, Felson DT. Intra-articular hyaluronic acid in treatment of knee osteoarthritis: a meta-analysis. *JAMA.* Dec 17 2003;290(23):3115-3121.
77. Reichenbach S, Blank S, Rutjes AW, et al. Hylan versus hyaluronic acid for osteoarthritis of the knee: a systematic review and meta-analysis. *Arthritis Rheum.* Dec 15 2007;57(8):1410-1418.
78. Bellamy N, Campbell J, Robinson V, Gee T, Bourne R, Wells G. Viscosupplementation for the treatment of osteoarthritis of the knee. *Cochrane Database Syst Rev.* 2006;(2):CD005321.
79. Bannuru RR, Natov NS, Obadan IE, Price LL, Schmid CH, McAlindon TE. Therapeutic trajectory of hyaluronic acid versus corticosteroids in the treatment of knee osteoarthritis: a systematic review and meta-analysis. *Arthritis Rheum.* Dec 15 2009;61(12):1704-1711.
80. Chevalier X, Jerosch J, Goupille P, et al. Single, intra-articular treatment with 6 ml hylan G-F 20 in patients with symptomatic primary osteoarthritis of the knee: a randomised, multicentre, double-blind, placebo controlled trial. *Ann Rheum Dis.* Jan 2010;69(1):113-119.
81. Lane NE, Schnitzer TJ, Birbara CA, et al. Tanezumab for the treatment of pain from osteoarthritis of the knee. *NE J Med.* Oct 14 2010;363(16):1521-1531.
82. Tanezumab, Arthritis Advisory Committee Briefing Document. 2012; http://www.fda.gov/downloads/AdvisoryCommittees/CommitteesMeetingMaterials/Drugs/ArthritisAdvisoryCommittee/UCM295205.pdf.
83. Nagashima H, Suzuki M, Araki S, Yamabe T, Muto C. Preliminary assessment of the safety and efficacy of tanezumab in Japanese patients with moderate to severe osteoarthritis of the knee: a randomized, double-blind, dose-escalation, placebo-controlled study. *Osteoarthritis and Cartilage/OARS, Osteoarthritis Research Society.* Dec 2011;19(12):1405-1412.
84. Laslett LL, Dore DA, Quinn SJ, et al. Zoledronic acid reduces knee pain and bone marrow lesions over 1 year: a randomised controlled trial. *Ann Rheum Dis.* Feb 21 2012.
85. Zhang W, Doherty M, Bardin T, et al. EULAR evidence based recommendations for gout. Part II: Management. Report of a task force of the EULAR Standing Committee for International Clinical Studies Including Therapeutics (ESCISIT). *Ann Rheum Dis.* Oct 2006;65(10):1312-1324.

86. Maccagno A, Di Giorgio E, Romanowicz A. Effectiveness of etodolac ('Lodine') compared with naproxen in patients with acute gout. *Curr Med Res Opin*. 1991;12(7):423-429.

87. Shrestha M, Morgan DL, Moreden JM, Singh R, Nelson M, Hayes JE. Randomized double-blind comparison of the analgesic efficacy of intramuscular ketorolac and oral indomethacin in the treatment of acute gouty arthritis. *Ann Emerg Med*. Dec 1995;26(6):682-686.

88. Schumacher HR, Jr., Boice JA, Daikh DI, et al. Randomised double blind trial of etoricoxib and indometacin in treatment of acute gouty arthritis. *BMJ*. Jun 22 2002;324(7352):1488-1492.

89. Altman RD, Honig S, Levin JM, Lightfoot RW. Ketoprofen versus indomethacin in patients with acute gouty arthritis: a multicenter, double blind comparative study. *J Rheumatol*. Sep 1988;15(9):1422-1426.

90. Sutaria S, Katbamna R, Underwood M. Effectiveness of interventions for the treatment of acute and prevention of recurrent gout—a systematic review. *Rheumatol (Oxford)*. Nov 2006;45(11):1422-1431.

91. Fernandez C, Noguera R, Gonzalez JA, Pascual E. Treatment of acute attacks of gout with a small dose of intraarticular triamcinolone acetonide. *J Rheumatol*. Oct 1999;26(10):2285-2286.

92. Groff GD, Franck WA, Raddatz DA. Systemic steroid therapy for acute gout: a clinical trial and review of the literature. *Sem Arthritis Rheum*. Jun 1990;19(6):329-336.

93. Siegel LB, Alloway JA, Nashel DJ. Comparison of adrenocorticotropic hormone and triamcinolone acetonide in the treatment of acute gouty arthritis. *J Rheumatol*. Jul 1994;21(7):1325-1327.

94. Werlen D, Gabay C, Vischer TL. Corticosteroid therapy for the treatment of acute attacks of crystal-induced arthritis: an effective alternative to nonsteroidal antiinflammatory drugs. *Rev Rhum Engl Ed*. Apr 1996;63(4):248-254.

95. Terkeltaub RA, Furst DE, Bennett K, Kook KA, Crockett RS, Davis MW. High versus low dosing of oral colchicine for early acute gout flare: twenty-four-hour outcome of the first multicenter, randomized, double-blind, placebo-controlled, parallel-group, dose-comparison colchicine study. *Arthritis Rheum*. Apr 2010;62(4):1060-1068.

96. Sieper J, Klopsch T, Richter M, et al. Comparison of two different dosages of celecoxib with diclofenac for the treatment of active ankylosing spondylitis: results of a 12-week randomised, double-blind, controlled study. *Ann Rheum Dis*. Mar 2008;67(3):323-329.

97. Braun J, van den Berg R, Baraliakos X, et al. 2010 update of the ASAS/EULAR recommendations for the management of ankylosing spondylitis. *Ann Rheum Dis*. Jun 2011;70(6):896-904.

98. Wanders A, Heijde D, Landewe R, et al. Nonsteroidal antiinflammatory drugs reduce radiographic progression in patients with ankylosing spondylitis: a randomized clinical trial. *Arthritis Rheum*. Jun 2005; 52(6):1756-1765.

CHAPTER 42 Osteoarthritis of the Major Joints

Ayesha Abdeen

INTRODUCTION

Osteoarthritis (OA) is the most common form of arthritis. Also known as degenerative joint disease, OA is characterized by loss of articular cartilage within a joint resulting in chronic pain, stiffness, deformity, and subsequent functional disability. Osteoarthritis may be classified as *primary/idiopathic*, for which the cause is unknown, or *secondary osteoarthritis*, which occurs as a result of trauma, infection, neuropathy, bone ischemia, congenital abnormality, chronic inflammatory arthropathy, or other cause.

EPIDEMIOLOGY

It is estimated that, in the United States, symptomatic osteoarthritis afflicts 13.9% of adults age 25 and older and 33.6% of those above the age of 65. The prevalence of the disease has been increasing in recent years: an estimated 21 million suffered from the disease in 1990 compared with 26.9 million in 2005.[1] The incidence of osteoarthritis increases with age; however, there has been a recent increase in patients presenting with symptoms earlier in adulthood, prior to the age of 65. The precise etiology of osteoarthritis is unknown. A number of biomechanical and biochemical causes have been implicated to suggest that the etiology is multifactorial. The risk factors for OA can be classified into modifiable and nonmodifiable. *Modifiable* risk factors include obesity, joint trauma, occupations that involve repetitive loading of the joint, and muscle weakness. *Nonmodifiable* risk factors include older age, gender (women are at higher risk in most joints), race (possible lower risk in some Asian populations), and congenital deformity or ligamentous laxity. A genetic predisposition to OA is speculated; however, this has not yet been well defined.[2]

PATHOPHYSIOLOGY

Although older age is associated with OA, the changes in osteoarthritic cartilage are pathologic and distinct from those of normal senescence.[3-5] In healthy cartilage, the chondrocytes maintain a balance between synthesis and regeneration of hyaline cartilage by producing the proteoglycans and collagen that form the matrix. In OA, this balance is interrupted and chondrocytes do not synthesize a sufficient matrix. As a result, clefts and fissures occur in the hyaline cartilage. In the early stages of OA, the cartilage softens, and, with more advanced disease, portions of full thickness cartilage are lost. Some of these cartilage fragments may become free within the joint space as loose bodies. *Loose bodies* within a joint can cause pain and mechanical symptoms such as locking of the joint. Once the matrix fails mechanically, the underlying bone is exposed. New bone forms in the subchondral region, resulting in sclerosis. This sclerotic subchondral bone is more apt to fissure, allowing synovial fluid to extrude into the bone, creating subchondral cysts. As the bone attempts to repair itself, bone spurs—or osteophytes—occur inside and at the margins of the joint. These changes within the articular cartilage surface and surrounding bone then manifest as pain and deformity of the joint.

DIAGNOSIS

CLINICAL PRESENTATION

The symptoms of OA include activity-related joint pain, joint stiffness, and subsequent progressive disability. Pain typically begins gradually—this reflects the pathophysiology of the disease, whereby articular cartilage degeneration occurs over a prolonged period of time. However, in many patients, there is a history of a mild traumatic inciting event after which they may experience either an exacerbation of their pain or, in some cases, the first onset of pain, which often prompts the patient to seek medical advice. The joint pain is typically activity related. As the disease progresses, those afflicted may develop difficulty with activities of daily living, including walking, sitting, or standing for prolonged periods. Impairment of fine and gross motor function and overhead activities occurs when joints of the upper extremity are involved. In addition to pain, patients with osteoarthritis complain of joint stiffness, swelling, and impaired range of motion. Unlike inflammatory arthropathy, which is characterized by morning joint pain, stiffness, and swelling, which improves during the day, symptoms of osteoarthritis tend to worsen as the day progresses.

The clinical features and treatment modalities in osteoarthritis specific to the joint involved are outlined in the following sections with respect to the major joints, including hip, knee, shoulder, and elbow.

Hip Osteoarthritis of the femoro-acetabular joint causes pain localizing to the groin, lateral hip, and/or buttock. The pain frequently radiates down the thigh to the knee. In some situations, the pain is referred exclusively to the knee; for this reason, OA of the hip should always be considered when evaluating a patient with isolated knee pain. It is important that a hip examination is routinely performed when evaluating knee pain to rule out the possibility of referred pain from the hip to the knee. Conversely, radicular pain or spinal stenosis can mimic osteoarthritic pain of the hip. It is prudent to perform a spine examination when assessing patients who present with hip pain.

Features on physical examination that occur with hip OA include an antalgic (painful) or Trendelenburg gait. A Trendelenburg gait is a lurching gait due to hip abductor weakness that occurs as a result of long-standing hip pain/pathology. Leg length discrepancy can occur, resulting in shortening on the affected side in cases of very advanced disease as a result of cartilage loss. A hip flexion contracture and/or adductor contracture may be present; this may cause an apparent, rather than a true, leg length difference. Pain with log-rolling the lower extremity, limited range of motion of the hip, and pain with hip range of motion (particularly in maximal flexion with internal rotation) are the hallmarks of the clinical examination in patients with OA of the hip. In some patients with severe stiffness due to a very prominent femoral head osteophyte, there may be obligate external rotation of the hip upon attempted flexion. Crepitus may be noted with range of motion as well.

Knee Patients with osteoarthritis of the knee present with activity-related knee pain that worsens as the day progresses. They may experience locking or "catching" of the knee, which can occur due to loose bodies within the knee joint or to a degenerative tear of the medial or lateral meniscus. As with OA of the hip, pain is typically of gradual onset but, in many cases, may present with an inciting minor traumatic event; following such an event, pain and disability are either initiated for the first time, or mild, occasional pain abruptly worsens in severity and/or frequency. Pain usually localizes to the medial or lateral joint line or to the anterior aspect of the knee, depending upon whether the arthritis localizes primarily to the medial, lateral, or patellofemoral compartments, respectively.

In osteoarthritis of the knee, the joint is usually affected asymmetrically such that one compartment out of the three compartments (medial, lateral, or patellofemoral) is affected primarily. As the disease progresses, the remaining compartments become involved such that end-stage knee OA is often *tricompartmental*. The most common pattern of osteoarthritis of the knee affects predominantly the medial compartment (**Fig. 42-1**). With time, this causes erosion of the cartilage and bone of the proximal medial tibia, and the medial soft tissues (capsule and medial collateral ligament [MCL]) become contracted and tightened. As a result, the knee develops a varus or "bow-leg" deformity. In severe cases, this deformity can manifest as a *varus thrust* during gait: a dynamic bowing out of the knee laterally during stance phase, following which the lower leg thrusts into a less varus position during the swing phase. Examination of the collateral ligaments in a varus knee reveals a phenomenon called *pseudolaxity* on the medial side: When a valgus force is applied to the knee with a preexisting varus deformity, there is apparent laxity of the MCL as the knee opens medially and corrects into a valgus position. The joint appears loose on the medial side when, in fact, it has collapsed on the tight medial side due to medial tibial bone loss and contractures of the MCL and medial joint capsule. The applied valgus force creates a false sensation of MCL laxity as the knee is moved to a neutral position.

While the majority of patients with osteoarthritis of the knee have a varus deformity owing to primary involvement of the medial compartment of the joint, less than 20% have a valgus deformity due to preferential involvement of the lateral compartment of the knee (**Fig. 42-2**). On examination, patients will have a "knock-knee" deformity. The valgus deformity is caused by progressive erosion of bone in the lateral compartment—typically, the lateral femoral condyle. As the disease progresses, the lateral soft-tissue structures—including the lateral collateral ligament (LCL), popliteus, and lateral joint capsule—become contracted. The MCL subsequently becomes lax with progressive disease and deformity, and, in severe cases, the MCL may rupture.

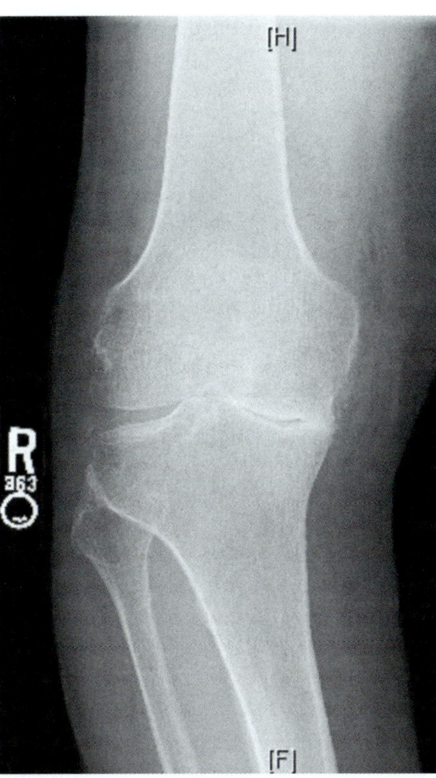

FIGURE 42-1. The most common form of OA of the knee affects the medial compartment preferentially, resulting in varus malalignment.

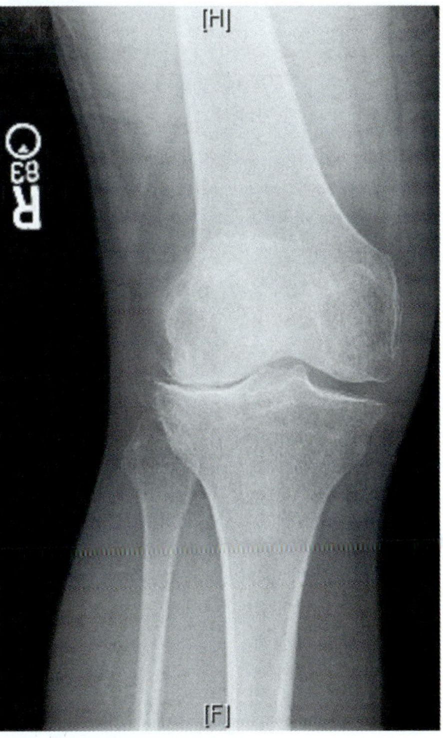

FIGURE 42-2. Preferential involvement of the lateral compartment of the knee with valgus deformity is less commonly found in OA.

In addition to examination of the alignment of the lower extremity, the clinical examination of patients with osteoarthritis of the knee should include an evaluation of gait, which may show an antalgic (painful) gait or a varus thrust as described earlier. Upon inspection and palpation, the knee may demonstrate an effusion. Palpation of the osteoarthritic knee may also reveal a popliteal or *Baker's cyst* due to accumulation of synovial fluid in the posterior aspect of the knee. The knee should be palpated for areas of tenderness. Tenderness commonly occurs at the joint line. An acutely swollen knee with a large effusion, warmth, erythema, and exquisite tenderness should alert the clinician to the possibility of an inflammatory or infectious etiology rather than osteoarthritis. Fever would further support a diagnosis of septic arthritis and would require urgent management.

Crepitus is often present in OA due to loss of cartilage and loose bodies within the joint. Range of motion of the knee may be limited due to pain or soft-tissue contracture. The posterior capsule of the joint may be contracted, resulting in a *flexion contracture* or the inability to fully extend/straighten the knee. Flexion also becomes limited as the disease progresses due to cartilage loss and pain. McMurray's test may be positive, indicating a degenerative meniscal tear. In cases of predominantly patellofemoral arthritis, the patella may track laterally (rather than centrally) within the femoral sulcus. This patellar maltracking is often due to a soft-tissue imbalance that occurs congenitally or in childhood or adolescence that predisposes the patient to developing patellofemoral osteoarthritis later in life.

Shoulder Osteoarthritis of the glenohumeral joint is one of the most common causes of shoulder pain. It is more common in women, and the incidence increases with advanced age. Clinical features include gradual onset of activity-related shoulder pain, stiffness, nocturnal pain, and decreased functional ability, particularly with overhead activities. Pain is typically vague and diffuse rather than sharp or localized.

Examination of the shoulder should include examination of the cervical spine because pathology of the cervical spine can lead to referred shoulder pain. Muscle atrophy of the shoulder girdle occurs in shoulder OA due to disuse. Strength testing should include evaluation of the rotator cuff, scapulothoracic musculature, biceps, and deltoid. Decreased shoulder range of motion and crepitus are common physical examination findings. During the clinical history and physical examination, it is important to rule out other sources of pain such as subacromial bursitis, rotator cuff tear, or labral pathology.

Elbow Primary OA of the elbow is relatively rare in comparison to that of other joints and affects approximately 2% of the population. The average age of onset is 50 years, which is also younger than OA of other joints. It is more common in men than in women, also contrary to OA of other joints. A history of strenuous manual labor and the use of pneumatic drills are considered to be a predisposing factor.[6] Secondary OA of the elbow occurs as a result of trauma, osteochondritis dissecans, and synovial chondromatosis. Patients often report pain at the extremes of motion rather than in mid-range. This pain occurs primarily with terminal elbow extension due to osteophyte impingement. Nocturnal pain and inflammation are often not a component and suggest an inflammatory condition such as rheumatoid arthritis.

On examination there may be an intraarticular effusion seen in the lateral aspect of the elbow. Crepitus is commonly present throughout the arc of motion. There is often global loss of range of motion in flexion, extension, supination, and pronation. Neurovascular examination may reveal evidence of ulnar neuropathy.

RADIOGRAPHIC FEATURES

The diagnosis of osteoarthritis is confirmed with plain radiographs. The four cardinal radiographic features of OA include asymmetric joint space narrowing, osteophyte (bone spur) formation, subchondral sclerosis, and subchondral cysts. Osteoarthritis tends to affect the joint asymmetrically or focally. This is in contradistinction to that found in inflammatory arthropathy, such as rheumatoid arthritis, which typically affects the joint symmetrically.

The radiographic evaluation of patients with osteoarthritis should include at least two views (antero-posterior and lateral views) of the affected joint. For weight-bearing joints such as the hip and knee, the radiographs must be taken during weight bearing to fully assess the degree to which the joint is affected during physiologic loading of the joint. Non-weight-bearing/supine views of the hip and knee can be misleading because they may underestimate the amount of joint space narrowing that occurs when the patient is bearing weight.

In the hip, osteoarthritis often preferentially affects the superior lateral portion of the joint (**Fig. 42-3**). There are often osteophytes involving the femoral head and acetabulum. Subchondral sclerosis and cysts occur in the acetabulum and femoral head. Cartilage and bone

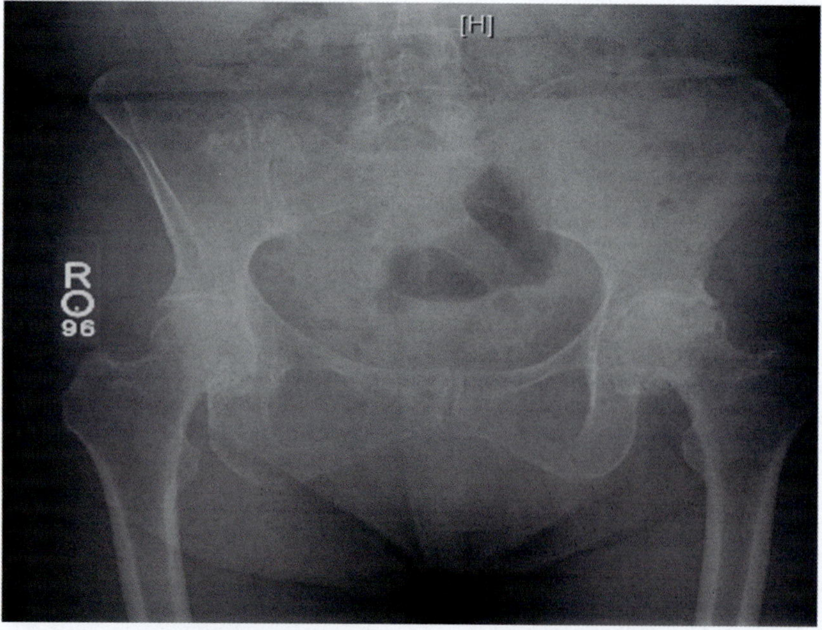

FIGURE 42-3. Severe OA of the hip is characterized by joint space narrowing, subchondral sclerosis, subchondral cysts, and osteophyte formation. The joint is affected asymmetrically, typically involving predominantly the superior lateral portion of the joint as seen in this patient's LEFT hip.

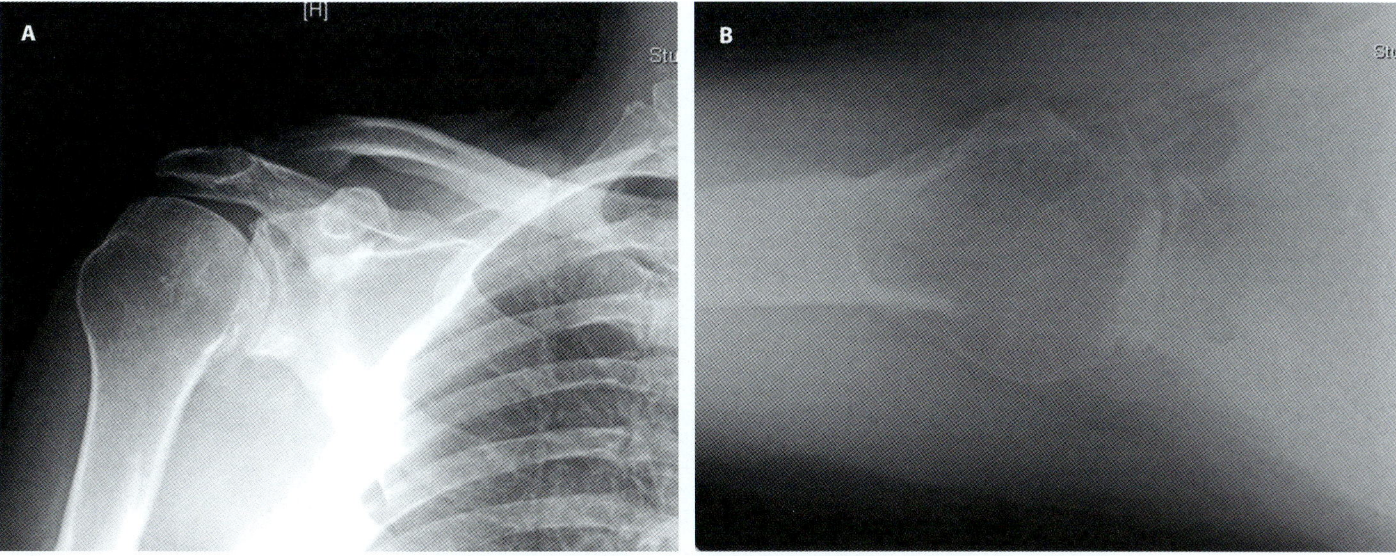

FIGURE 42-4. **A:** Radiograph demonstrating glenohumeral OA with joint space narrowing, subchondral sclerosis, subchondral cysts, and osteophyte formation. **B:** Axillary view reveals posterior glenoid erosion.

destruction within the joint can result in a leg length discrepancy on the affected side that can be measured radiographically.

Glenohumeral osteoarthritis is characterized by a prominent osteophyte at the inferior margin of the humeral head or glenoid. There may be asymmetric posterior wear of the glenoid, which is best visualized on an axillary view of the shoulder (**Figs. 42-4A** and **42-4B**).

Radiographs of the elbow with primary OA typically reveal an anterior and medial osteophyte involving the coronoid process and a posteromedial osteophyte on the olecranon process (**Fig. 42-5**). There is commonly preservation of the ulnohumeral and radiocapitellar joint spaces. Conversely, severe joint space narrowing without large marginal osteophytes is more characteristic of inflammatory arthritis of the elbow.

In the osteoarthritic knee, 3-foot standing films that image the hip, knee, and ankle on one film can further characterize and measure the amount of coronal plane deformity. Normal *anatomic* alignment of the lower extremity is such that the coronal angle contended by the femur and tibia creates an angle of 5 to 7 degrees. In the early stages of OA, neutral alignment will be maintained. In severe osteoarthritis, there is malalignment of this anatomic axis, whereby the angle is less than 5 to 7 degrees, causing varus ("bow-leg") malalignment, or greater than 5 to 7 degrees, causing valgus ("knock-knee") malalignment (**Figs. 42-6A** and **42-6B**).

A variety of grading systems have been used to evaluate the severity of OA of the knee, including the Kellgren & Lawrence system and Ahlbäck system.[7,8] The Ahlbäck system focuses primarily on joint space narrowing as a surrogate measure for cartilage loss; the more widely used Kellgren & Lawrence system evaluates osteophyte formation and joint space narrowing. The two systems have been shown to correlate with one another. A comparison of the two grading systems is outlined in **Table 42-1**.[9]

Advanced imaging is rarely indicated in the setting of osteoarthritis. If a patient has evidence of OA on plain radiographs, an MRI will also demonstrate cartilage abnormalities; therefore, routine MRI is not indicated for the evaluation of OA. In the case of very mild arthritis and pain

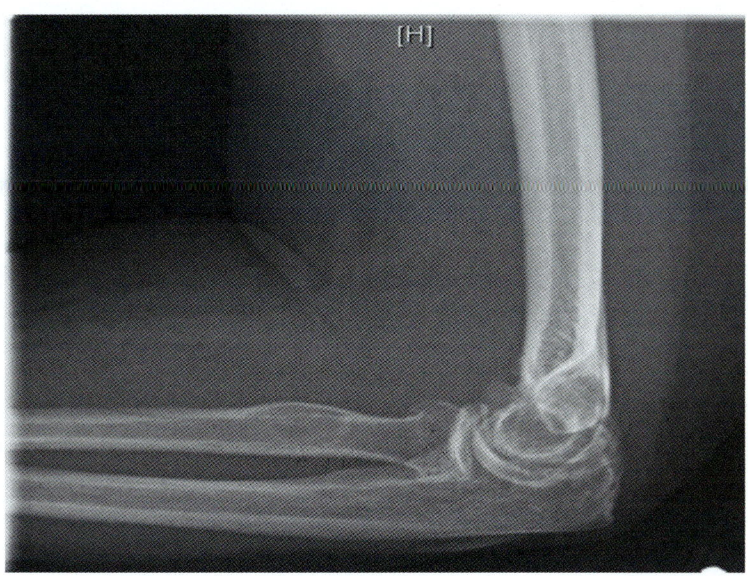

FIGURE 42-5. Lateral view of the elbow reveals osteophytes of the coronoid and olecranon fossa.

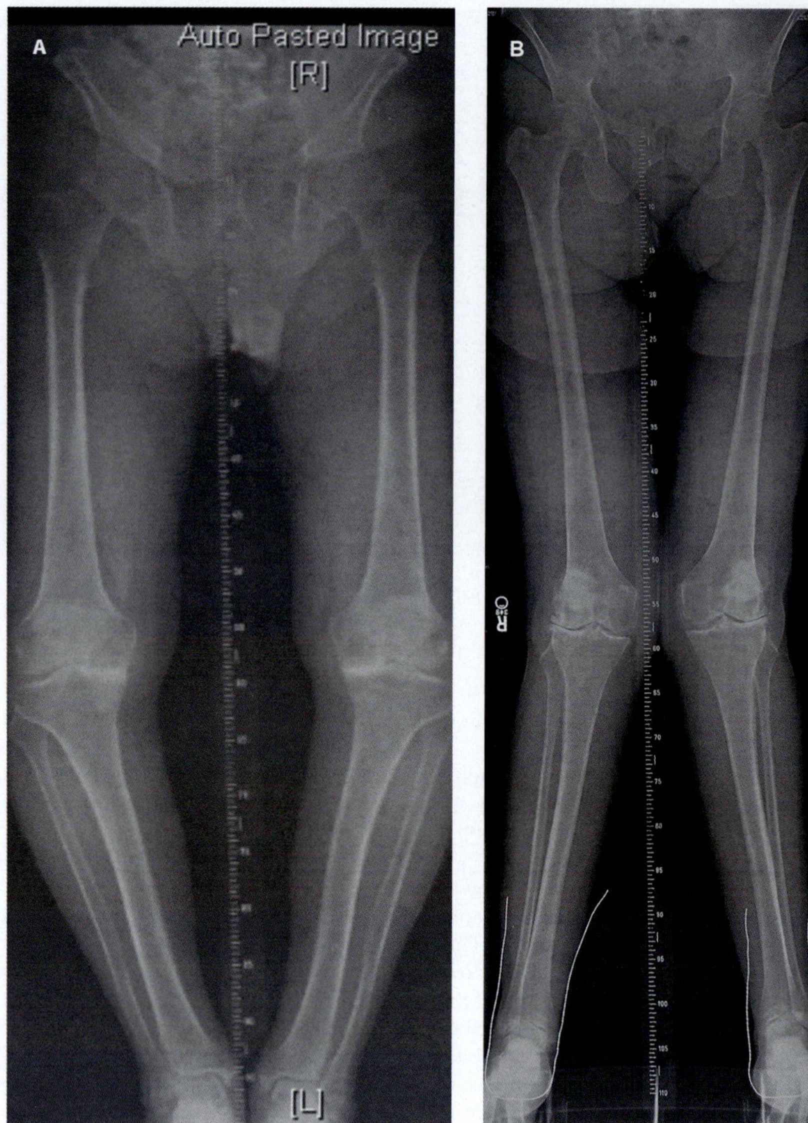

FIGURE 42-6. **A:** Three-foot standing film with severe OA of the medial compartment of the knee results in varus ("bow-leg") deformity (3A). **B:** Three-foot standing film with severe OA of the lateral compartment of the knee results in valgus ("knock-knee") deformity.

TABLE 42-1 The Ahlbäck and Kellgren & Lawrence Radiographic Classification Systems for Osteoarthritis of the Knee[7-9]

Ahlbäck Grade	Ahlbäck Definition	Kellgren & Lawrence Grade	Kellgren & Lawrence Definition
		Grade 1—Doubtful	Minute osteophyte, doubtful significance
		Grade 2—Minimal	Definite osteophyte, unimpaired joint space
Grade I	Joint space narrowing (joint space <3 mm)	Grade 3—Moderate	Moderate diminution of joint space
Grade II	Joint space obliteration	Grade 4—Severe	Joint space greatly impaired with sclerosis of subchondral bone
Grade III	Minor bone attrition (0–5 mm)	Grade 4—Severe	Joint space greatly impaired with sclerosis of subchondral bone
Grade IV	Moderate bone attrition (5–10 mm)	Grade 4—Severe	Joint space greatly impaired with sclerosis of subchondral bone
Grade V	Severe bone attrition (>10 mm)	Grade 4—Severe	Joint space greatly impaired with sclerosis of subchondral bone

that is out of proportion to the radiographic findings, cross-sectional imaging may be performed to rule out other structural abnormalities and evaluate the surrounding soft tissue structures. If given a history to suggest an acute meniscal tear of the knee (mechanical locking of the knee in the setting of a twisting injury), an MRI may be indicated. MRI is not necessary to evaluate degenerative meniscal tears in the context of OA of the knee because this will not alter the indicated treatment plan.

PRINCIPLES OF NONSURGICAL TREATMENT

PHYSICAL TREATMENT MODALITIES

There are a number of nonpharmacologic, or physical treatment modalities that can help to alleviate pain in osteoarthritis. Activity modification is recommended for patients with osteoarthritis. This involves elimination of high-impact activities such as running and jumping activities that excessively load the joint. Low-impact activities such as walking, swimming, or cycling are encouraged. Periodic daily rest is recommended; however, prolonged bed rest can cause muscle atrophy, general de-conditioning, and other comorbidities and should be avoided.

Patients who are overweight (BMI >25) should start a weight loss program with dietary modification and exercise with a goal weight reduction of at least 5% of body weight.

For lower extremity OA, the use of an assistive device for walking such as a cane or walker will provide pain relief by distributing forces away from the affected joint.

Physical therapy with a program directed toward increasing periarticular muscle strength, reducing joint contractures, and maintaining range of motion can be of benefit. Application of local heat or ice may adequately relieve joint pain before and after exercise. If an activity exacerbates pain or causes pain lasting more than 15 minutes following therapy, the activity/exercise should be discontinued.

In patients with predominantly medial compartment knee OA with varus deformity, a lateral shoe wedge can redistribute forces away from the painful medial compartment and subsequently provide some relief of pain. The use of a knee unloader brace to transfer load away from the affected compartment has been used with reported benefit; however, the level of evidence to support the use of such braces is poor.

PHARMACOLOGIC AGENTS

Unless otherwise contraindicated, an analgesic regimen for the treatment of OA should include acetaminophen to address the mechanical pain of osteoarthritis and a nonsteroidal anti-inflammatory drug (NSAID) to address the secondary inflammatory component of OA. The most common side effects of NSAIDs are gastric irritation or bleeding. Increased risk for GI bleeding includes patient age over 60, history of peptic ulcer disease, smoking, prior GI bleed, and concurrent use of corticosteroids and/or anticoagulants. Acetaminophen, topical NSAIDs, a nonselective oral NSAID with a gastroprotective agent, or a cyclooxygenase-2 (COX-2) inhibitor should be selected as an alternative to oral (COX-1) NSAIDs in patients with increased risk of GI bleeding.

Topical analgesics such as capsaicin creams may also provide pain relief of arthritic pain.

There has been widespread use of nutritional and herbal supplements, including glucosamine and/or chondroitin sulfate for the treatment of arthritic pain. These are oral agents designed with the intent to stimulate formation of aggrecan (the primary proteoglycan in cartilage) and hyaluronic acid (the molecule to which aggrecan binds) within the joint. Both glucosamine and chondroitin sulfate have been shown to stimulate formation of proteoglycans, glycosaminoglycans, and collagen *in vitro*; however, this has not been demonstrated *in vivo*. Furthermore, subsequent randomized control trials and systematic reviews on the use of these supplements suggest there is no clinical benefit of these nutraceuticals. An evidence-based report on the "Treatment of Primary and Secondary Osteoarthritis of the Knee" prepared by the Agency for Healthcare Research and Quality (AHRQ) evaluated one randomized controlled trial and six systematic reviews on the use of glucosamine and/or chondroitin sulfate or hydrochloride in patients with symptomatic OA of the knee. The AHRQ concluded that "the best available evidence found that glucosamine hydrochloride, chondroitin sulfate or their combination did not have any clinical benefit in patients with primary OA of the knee."[10] The American Academy of Orthopaedic Surgeons (AAOS) guidelines for the treatment of OA of the knee concurs with this statement and does not support the prescribing of glucosamine and/or chondroitin supplements for knee OA.[11]

Viscosupplementation—the intraarticular injection of hyaluronic acid—has been reported to be of benefit for temporary relief of osteoarthritis of the knee. A variety of preparations are available including Synvisc® (Biomatrix, Richfield, NJ), Hyalgan® (New York, NY), and Euflexxa® (Parsippany, NJ). The AHRQ report states that "viscosupplementation generally shows positive effects."[10] However, the AHRQ report also noted that the "pooled effects from poor-quality trials were as much as twice those obtained from higher ones (trials)."[10] On this basis, the AAOS guidelines for the treatment of osteoarthritis of the knee graded the evidence as "inconclusive" and concluded that the true clinical utility of viscosupplementation is unclear.[11]

Viscosupplementation was designed for use in the knee and has yet to be approved for use in other joints by the U.S. Food and Drug Administration. However, hyaluronic acid injections have been reported in a number of clinical trials to be a safe and effective treatment modality for shoulder OA.[12,13] There are reports of its use in the hip; however, the evidence is less clear with respect to the benefit of viscosupplementation for OA of hip.[14] Viscosupplementation has not been established as a recommended treatment for OA of the elbow.

If arthritic pain persists despite NSAID and/or acetaminophen use, local intraarticular injections may be used for short-term symptomatic relief. Pain relief varies among patients and can last for a duration of 1 week to up to 24 weeks.[15] Serious risks of repeated corticosteroid injections into the joint space include further cartilage damage or infection/joint sepsis, and, therefore, these should not be performed more than two or three times annually. Intraarticular injections of the hip are best performed with image guidance such as fluoroscopy.

Narcotic medications should not be used in the long-term treatment of osteoarthritis. Pain that persists despite physical treatments and non-narcotic analgesics may respond to intraarticular corticosteroid injections. In very advanced OA, these injections may provide only short-term or partial relief of pain and, therefore, may be performed as a temporizing measure prior to definitive surgical treatment.

PRINCIPLES OF SURGICAL TREATMENT

Surgical intervention for OA is reserved for recalcitrant cases in which joint pain persists despite a comprehensive, nonoperative treatment program. Prior to surgery, it is important to evaluate the patient to elucidate the precise problem—whether it is capsular contracture; ligamentous contracture; or laxity, tendon contracture, or osseous deformity. Patient goals and expectations vary tremendously among patients and must be clarified preoperatively. **Table 42-2** summarizes common surgical procedures for the treatment of osteoarthritis of the major joints.[16]

HIP

The definitive treatment of severe, symptomatic hip osteoarthritis is a total hip replacement (THR) (**Fig. 42-7**). Long-term outcome studies have revealed excellent functional outcomes and an implant survival rate of more than 90% at 20 years.[17] Other indications for THR include osteonecrosis of the femoral head, inflammatory arthritis of the hip, hip fractures with preexisting severe OA, nonunion following hip fractures, and posttraumatic arthritis. There are also a number of congenital or developmental deformities of the hip that may result in secondary osteoarthritis of the hip, including developmental dysplasia of the hip, Legg-Calvé-Perthes disease, slipped capital femoral epiphysis, and other childhood conditions that may result in end stage degenerative joint disease later in the patient's life.

Absolute contraindications to THR include active infection. Relative contraindications include multiple medical comorbidities; movement disorders (e.g., Parkinson's disease) that can increase hip prosthetic dislocation risk; any disorder that impairs the patient's ability to comply with postoperative restrictions, thus increasing the risk of dislocation (alcohol/drug abuse, dementia); as well as the young age of a patient. Patients under the age of 40 present a challenge due to their increased functional demands, as well as their increased life expectancy, which exceeds that of the implant, thus potentially requiring multiple revision procedures in the patient's lifetime. Historically, joint fusion (arthrodesis), rather than prosthetic joint replacement, was the standard of care for young patients with severe unilateral hip arthritis. However, in the setting of bilateral disease, fusion is contraindicated. With advances in prosthetic design and bearing surfaces

TABLE 42-2 Surgical Treatment Options for Osteoarthritis of the Major Joints

Joint	Surgical Procedure	Indication	Expected Results	Limitations and Potential Complications
Hip	Arthroplasty (total hip replacement)	Severe OA of the hip; failure of nonoperative treatment	Relief of pain; improved range of motion; improved ambulation	Aseptic loosening of prosthesis at 20 years; prosthetic joint infection (PJI)* <1%
	Arthrodesis (rarely performed)	Young patient with severe OA; prior joint sepsis; failed THR	Relief of pain; complete loss of hip ROM	Ipsilateral joint pain and DJD in spine or knee; disability due to loss of hip ROM
Knee	Microfracture, OAT, ACI	Young patient with traumatic focal cartilage injury	Relief of pain; improved function	Recurrence of pain; progression of OA despite procedure
	Osteotomy	Unicompartmental OA in young patient/high functional demand patient	Relief of pain; improved function; delayed need for prosthetic replacement	Persistent limitation of function; progression of disease in other compartments
	Unicompartmental joint replacement	Unicompartmental disease in older/lower functional demand patient	Relief of pain; improved function	Wear/loosening of prosthesis at 10–15 years; PJI (<1%)
	Total knee replacement	Severe symptomatic knee OA; bi- or tricompartmental disease	Relief of pain; restoration of function Correction of malalignment and soft tissue contracture can be performed simultaneously	Wear/loosening at 15–20 years; PJI (<1%)
Shoulder	Shoulder arthroplasty (hemi-arthroplasty or total shoulder replacement)	Severe pain; failure of nonoperative treatment	Relief of pain	Limited ROM; wear/loosening; PJI (<1%)
	Arthrodesis (rarely performed)	Severe pain; prior septic arthritis, salvage procedure for failed arthroplasty	Relief of pain; scapulothoracic motion maintained; loss of glenohumeral ROM	Functional disability due to loss of glenohumeral ROM
Elbow	Capsular release and joint débridement	Severe pain; failed nonoperative treatment; preservation of joint space	Relief of pain; improved elbow motion	Recurrent contracture; ulnar neuropathy
	Arthroscopic débridement	Same as above	Same as above	Technically demanding procedure; risk of radial/median/ulnar nerve injury
	Distraction interposition	Pain; decreased elbow ROM; posttraumatic OA; younger patient who is not a candidate for TEA due to higher functional demand	Relief of pain; improved motion	Pin site infection; neuropathy
	Arthroplasty Total elbow arthroplasty	Elderly patients with low demand who have failed nonoperative treatment and débridement and capsular release	Relief of pain; improved motion	Periprosthetic fracture; implant loosening, PJI

*PJI = prosthetic joint infection

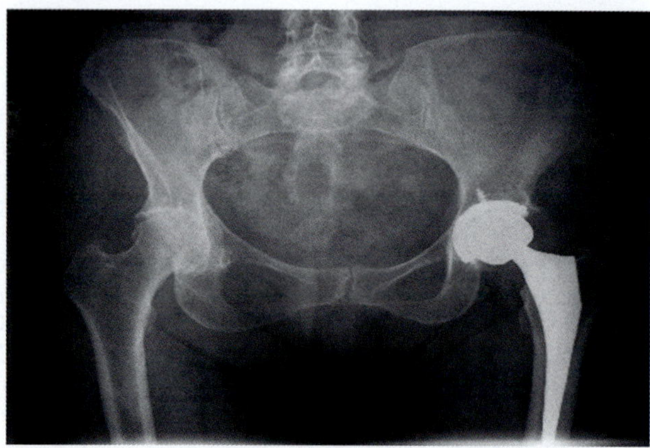

FIGURE 42-7. Total hip replacement performed for severe OA of the hip.

used in total hip replacement, prosthetic replacement is increasingly used in younger patients with severe OA of the hip.

Total hip replacement involves removal of the native femoral head and replacement with a metal or ceramic femoral head attached to a metal stem that is either cemented (with polymethylmethacrylate bone cement) or uncemented ("press-fit," whereby bone grows directly into the stem) into the medullary canal of the femur. The decision to use cemented versus uncemented fixation techniques is largely based upon surgeon preference; however, in general, the cemented technique is often recommended in very poor quality bone to improve stem fixation. The cement is pressurized into the femoral medullary canal. In rare cases, cementing of the femoral component can result in life-threatening cardiopulmonary compromise.

On the pelvic/acetabular side, a total hip replacement involves using a series of hemispheric reamers to remove any remaining cartilage and create a smooth surface into which a metal acetabular cup is placed. The articulation between the head and the socket is made either of polyethylene or ceramic. The conventional bearing surface between the metal head and socket is a plastic (polyethylene) liner. Historically, the use of conventional polyethylene liners has led to the accumulation of polyethylene debris in the joint, which, in turn, incites a cell-mediated response resulting in recruitment of macrophages. These macrophages cause bone loss surrounding the implant, resulting in a phenomenon known as *osteolysis* that leads to *aseptic loosening* of the implant, which is the primary cause of failure of total hip replacement surgery. In order to circumvent this phenomenon, particularly in the younger patient in whom the issue of implant longevity is paramount, a number of alternate bearing surfaces have been developed, including highly cross-linked polyethylene, ceramics, and metal-on-medal devices. Each of these novel bearing surfaces have demonstrated improved wear characteristics in the lab setting using wear simulators and in short- to mid-term clinical studies. The optimal bearing surface for the young patient with degenerative joint disease of the hip remains an issue of ongoing debate.

In the postoperative period following THR, patients are encouraged to ambulate and start physical therapy starting immediately following surgery. The precise postoperative protocol varies based upon surgeon preference; however, patients are typically permitted to be weight bearing as tolerated on the operative leg with an assistive device such as crutches or a walker for support for the first 2 to 6 weeks following surgery. Depending upon surgical approach and surgeon preference, there may be a period of restricted range of motion (ROM) to reduce the risk of dislocation in the first 6 to 12 weeks. Following an inpatient stay of 2 to 3 days, most patients are discharged to home. A portion of patients in whom multiple medical comorbidities or severe limitations in their ambulatory status perioperatively preclude discharge to home are transferred to a longer-term facility or rehabilitation center for a period of time until they are able to ambulate and perform activities of daily living independently. A combination of NSAIDs, acetaminophen, and low-dose narcotic medications are recommended for postoperative pain control. Analgesics are typically required for the first 1 to 2 weeks. This is variable among patients; those who have been taking opiate medications for a longer duration prior to surgery may require an extended postoperative regimen. Venous thromboembolic prophylaxis is recommended from 10 to 35 days postoperatively and include a combination of mechanical prophylaxis (sequential compression devices, compressive stockings) and pharmacoprophylaxis, including low molecular weight heparin (LMWH), or warfarin treatment.[18,19]

KNEE

Surgical management for osteoarthritis of the knee is recommended for patients in whom pain persists despite nonoperative treatment modalities. Knee arthroscopy with débridement or lavage was historically performed for OA of the knee; however, this has since been shown to be of no clinical benefit and should not be performed in patients with a primary diagnosis of symptomatic knee OA.[11,20] Only in cases in which the patient has concomitant mechanical locking of the knee caused by a loose body or meniscal tear may arthroscopic débridement be beneficial in the context of knee OA.[11]

In young patients with focal, traumatic cartilage defects, there are a variety of techniques aimed at cartilage regeneration that may be performed. Arthroscopic microfracture is a procedure in which an awl is used in the region of a full-thickness cartilage defect to penetrate the exposed bone and incite a healing process, which results in a fibrocartilaginous scar. Unlike normal hyaline cartilage which is formed by type II cartilage, this scar is formed by type I cartilage. A systematic literature review of this technique concluded that there was an improvement in knee function for 24 months, but results were inconclusive beyond 1 year.[21]

Other techniques aimed at repair and regeneration of cartilage include osteochondral autograft transplantation (OAT), or mosaicplasty, in which bone plugs are removed from a region of the knee joint that bears less load and transplanted to the region of cartilage loss typically measuring <10 mm. Autologous chondrocyte implantation (ACI) involves harvest of chondrocytes from a nonessential region of the knee, culture and expansion of the chondrocytes *in vitro*, and then reimplantation of the cells into the cartilage defect during a second surgical procedure, whereby the cells are protected and covered by a segment of periosteum. Current evidence has not demonstrated the results of ACI to be superior to those of microfracture. There is evidence to support the notion that OAT may provide some functional benefit over microfracture when performed in young, active patients.[22] Microfracture, OAT, and ACI are indicated in the treatment of isolated, focal cartilaginous lesions and are not recommended in the context of osteoarthritis that affects the joint globally. It remains to be proven as to whether these procedures alter the natural history of the development of osteoarthritis in patients with focal traumatic cartilaginous lesions of the knee.

For young, active patients (physiologically less than 60 years in age) who have symptomatic, isolated, unicompartmental knee OA and malalignment (varus or valgus deformity) of the knee, a periarticular osteotomy is a surgical option that preserves the native joint. Pain is alleviated by altering the mechanical axis of weight bearing. The osteotomy involves cutting the periarticular bone and correcting the alignment of the lower extremity such that the forces are directed away from the area of the joint affected by the arthritis. In patients with medial sided disease with varus deformity, alignment can be corrected with a proximal tibial osteotomy. Conversely, for lateral sided disease with valgus deformity, alignment can be corrected with a distal femoral osteotomy. For an osteotomy to be successful, the remaining two compartments must demonstrate preservation of the articular cartilage.

In low-demand patients over the age of 60 with severe knee pain due to isolated unicompartmental knee OA, a unicompartmental knee replacement is a surgical option. Criteria for a unicompartmental knee replacement include intact cruciate and collateral ligaments and absence of fixed flexion contracture. Unicompartmental knee replacement can be performed for either the medial, lateral, or patellofemoral joints.

The gold standard surgical procedure for severe symptomatic knee arthritis remains total knee replacement/arthroplasty (TKR) (**Figs. 42-8A** and **42-8B**). Malalignment, joint contracture, and ligament insufficiency

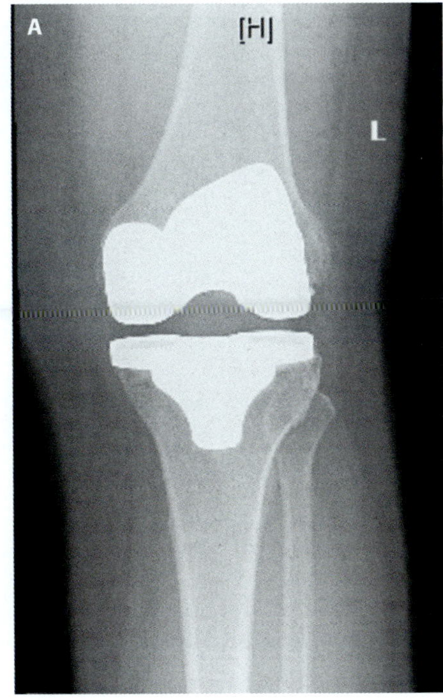

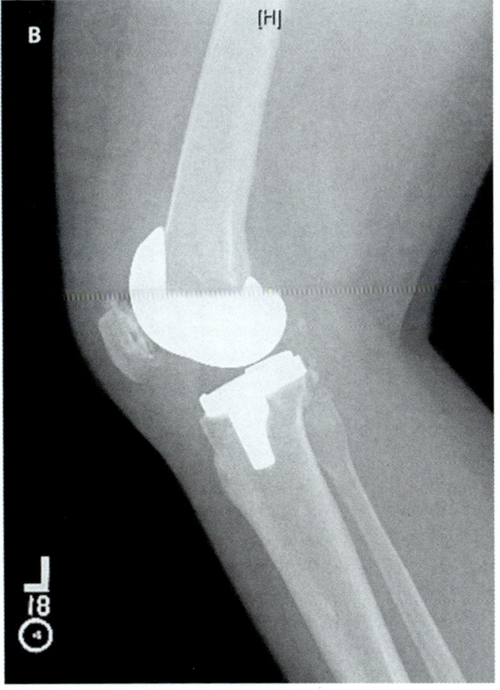

FIGURE 42-8. Total knee arthroplasty.

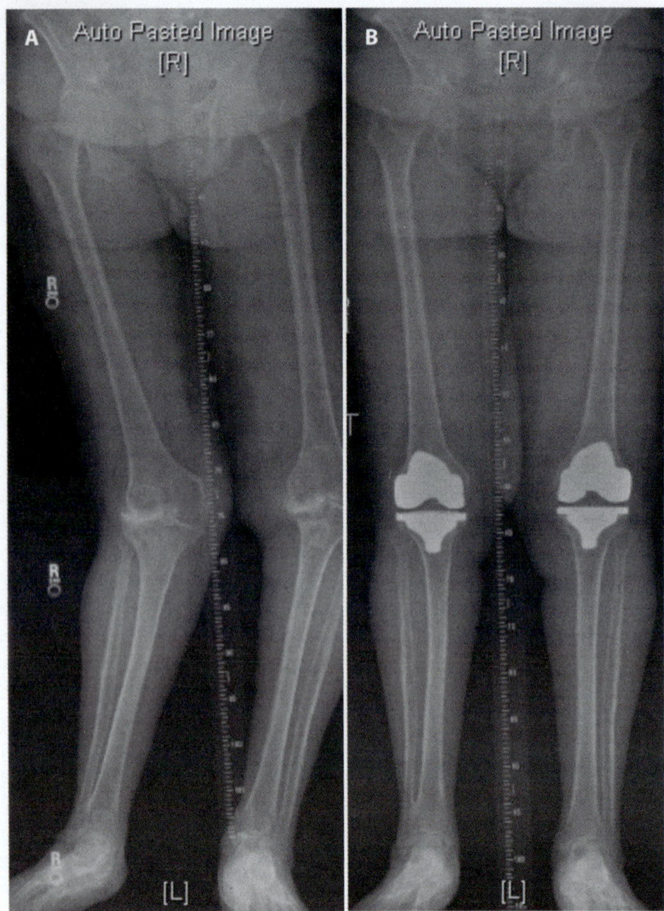

FIGURE 42-9. A: Preoperative 3-foot standing radiograph in a patient with a *wind-swept* knee deformity with one knee in varus malalignment and the contralateral knee in valgus malalignment. **B:** Postoperative radiograph of the patient in Figure 42-8A demonstrates correction of malalignment following bilateral total knee replacement.

can be corrected at the time of TKR (**Figs. 42-9A** and **42-9B**). The survival rate for TKR at 15 to 20 years is greater than 90%.[23,24] Functional outcome studies have revealed significant improvements in pain and function in patients who undergo TKR.

TKR is performed under either general anesthetic and/or a combination of regional anesthetic techniques, including epidural/spinal anesthesia or femoral and/or sciatic nerve block. In the postoperative course, a combination of narcotic and non-narcotic analgesics is used. Prophylactic anticoagulants in the form of Coumadin or low-molecular-weight heparin are used for a duration of 10 to 35 days following surgery.[18,19] Intensive physical therapy is necessary in the postoperative period to maintain knee range of motion, improve gait, and prevent flexion contracture.

SHOULDER

The shoulder is, after the knee and hip, the third most common joint to require surgical reconstruction/replacement. Adults over the age of 60 tolerate shoulder OA better than hip or knee OA. Those with lower functional demands can adapt their lifestyle to avoid activities that elicit the pain. For elderly patients with low functional demand in whom severe pain persists despite nonoperative measures, partial replacement (hemi-arthroplasty) of the shoulder and total shoulder replacement have demonstrated excellent long-term results and improvement in functional outcome. Whether partial (hemi-arthroplasty) or total shoulder replacement is the optimal surgical treatment is an issue of ongoing debate.

In younger patients with glenohumeral arthritis, arthroplasty outcomes are less predictable. Higher functional demands as well as the need for implant longevity pose significant challenges in this patient population. In younger patients, the etiology of shoulder arthropathy is typically more complex than in older patients in whom primary OA is the most common pathology. Secondary degenerative joint disease due to trauma, osteonecrosis, or rotator cuff pathology is more common in younger patients with glenohumeral arthritis. Functional outcome for patients with these diagnoses following shoulder arthroplasty tends to be worse than for patients with primary OA.

Nonprosthetic surgical treatment options for glenohumeral arthritis in the young patient are somewhat limited: Arthroscopic débridement can be of benefit in patients with mild shoulder arthritis. Methods of cartilage repair and reconstruction are emerging techniques; however, the role of such procedures is not yet well defined. Arthrodesis (fusion) of the glenohumeral joint is a salvage technique indicated in patients with failed arthroplasty, chronic infection, or massive rotator cuff tear with an insufficient deltoid.[25] The selected treatment should be tailored to each specific case, taking into consideration the etiology, functional demands of the patient, prior shoulder surgery, infection, and patient goals.

ELBOW

Elbow joint débridement, capsular release, and removal of osteophytes is a joint-preserving procedure termed *ulnohumeral arthroplasty* that is indicated in patients with OA of the elbow who have loss of range of motion, have pain at terminal flexion and/or extension, and have preservation of the joint space radiographically. Young patients with high functional demands who have had pain despite nonoperative treatment modalities are good candidates for this procedure. Results have demonstrated good functional outcomes despite recurrence of osteophyte formation radiographically. Recurrent joint contracture and ulnar neuropathy are potential complications of this procedure. Decompression or transposition of the ulnar nerve may be performed at the time of ulnohumeral arthroplasty in patients in whom there is a severe flexion contracture or preexisting ulnar nerve symptoms.[6]

Arthroscopic debridement with capsular release has been introduced in order to reduce morbidity associated with large open incisions. Other potential benefits of an arthroscopic technique are reduced postoperative pain and bleeding. Its indications are similar to that of open

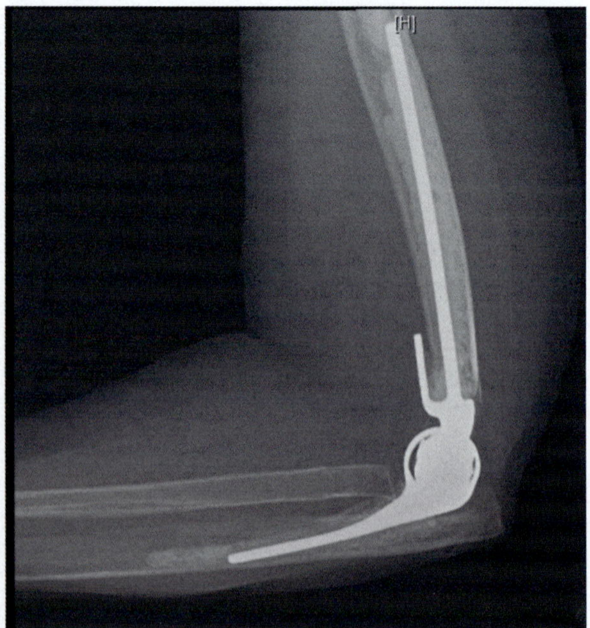

FIGURE 42-10. Total elbow arthroplasty.

ulnohumeral arthroplasty. Possible complications include transient of permanent nerve injury of the radial nerve (at risk due to proximity to the anterior capsule), median nerve (can be transected in rare cases), or ulnar nerve (minimized by placement of medial portal anterior to the medial intermuscular septum).

Distraction interposition arthroplasty is a technique whereby the articular surface is reshaped and resurfaced with the interposition of autograft fascia lata, dermis, or Achilles tendon allograft. A hinged external fixator is placed to hold the elbow in a distracted position during the healing period of approximately 4 weeks. This technique has shown satisfactory results in patients with posttraumatic arthritis. Although results have not been published in patients with primary elbow OA, the technique is a reasonable option in younger patients with pain that persists despite other interventions. Potential complications include nerve injury, donor site morbidity of the autograft fascia lata (muscle herniation), and superficial pin-site infection at the site of the external fixator.[26]

Total elbow replacement/arthroplasty (TEA) is rarely indicated for primary OA of the elbow, primarily because it is a disease that occurs in young or middle age male laborers in whom high functional demands preclude joint replacement due to issues of durability and expected longevity of the implant. Total elbow arthroplasty (**Fig. 42-10**) is indicated for lower-demand patients over the age of 65 in whom nonoperative treatment and joint-preserving techniques (capsular release and osteophyte débridement) have failed.[6]

REFERENCES

1. Lawrence RC, Felson DT, Helmick CG, et al. Estimates of the prevalence of arthritis and other rheumatic conditions in the United States. Part II. *Arthritis Rheum.* Jan 2008;58(1):26-35.
2. Jordan JM, Helmick CG, Renner JB, et al. Prevalence of knee symptoms and radiographic and symptomatic knee osteoarthritis in African Americans and Caucasians: the Johnston County Osteoarthritis Project. *J Rheumatol.* Jan 2007;34(1):172-180.
3. Felson DT. Risk factors for osteoarthritis: understanding joint vulnerability. *Clin Orthop Relat Res.* Oct 2004;(427 Suppl):S16-S21.
4. Felson DT, Zhang Y. An update on the epidemiology of knee and hip osteoarthritis with a view to prevention. *Arthritis Rheum.* Aug 1998;41(8):1343-1355.
5. Rossignol M, Leclerc A, Allaert FA, et al. Primary osteoarthritis of hip, knee, and hand in relation to occupational exposure. *Occup Environ Med.* Nov 2005;62(11):772-777.
6. Gramstad GD, Galatz LM. Management of elbow osteoarthritis. *J Bone Joint Surg Am.* Feb 2006;88(2):421-430.
7. Ball J, Jeffrey MR, Kellgren JH. The Epidemiology of Chronic Rheumatism; Volume 2: Atlas of Standard Radiographs of Arthritis. Oxford: Blackwell Scientific; 1963.
8. Ahlback S. Osteoarthrosis of the knee: a radiographic investigation. *Acta Radiol Diagn (Stockh).* 1968;Suppl 277.7-72.
9. Petersson IF, Boegard T, Saxne T, Silman AJ, Svensson B. Radiographic osteoarthritis of the knee classified by the Ahlback and Kellgren & Lawrence systems for the tibiofemoral joint in people aged 35-54 years with chronic knee pain. *Ann Rheum Dis.* Aug 1997;56(8):493-496.
10. Samson DJ, Grant MD, Ratko TA, et al. Treatment of primary and secondary osteoarthritis of the knee. Rockville, MD: Agency for Healthcare Research and Quality; 2007 Sep 1 (No. 157). Report.
11. Richmond J, Hunter D, Irrgang J, et al. Treatment of osteoarthritis of the knee (nonarthroplasty). *J Am Acad Orthop Surg.* Sep 2009;17(9):591-600.
12. Saito S, Furuya T, Kotake S. Therapeutic effects of hyaluronate injections in patients with chronic painful shoulder: a meta-analysis of randomized controlled trials. *Arthritis Care Res (Hoboken).* Jul;62(7):1009-1018.
13. Izquierdo R, Voloshin I, Edwards S, et al. Treatment of glenohumeral osteoarthritis. *J Am Acad Orthop Surg.* Jun;18(6):375-382.
14. Zhang W, Nuki G, Moskowitz RW, et al. OARSI recommendations for the management of hip and knee osteoarthritis. Part III: changes in evidence following systematic cumulative update of research published through January 2009. *Osteoarthritis Cartilage.* Apr;18(4):476-499.
15. Arroll B, Goodyear-Smith F. Corticosteroid injections for osteoarthritis of the knee: meta-analysis. *BMJ.* Apr 10 2004;328(7444):869.
16. Juan J, Rodrigo MEG. *Management of the Arthritic Joint.* Vol 3. 3rd ed. Philadelphia, Pa: Lippincott Williams & Williams; 2001.
17. Glassman AH, Lachiewicz PF, Tanzer M. *Orthopaedic Knowledge Update Hip and Knee Reconstruction.* Vol 4. American Academy of Orthopaedic Surgeons; 2011.
18. Hirsh J, Guyatt G, Albers GW, et al. Antithrombotic and thrombolytic therapy: American College of Chest Physicians evidence-based clinical practice guidelines. *CHEST Journal.* 2008 Jun 1;133(6 suppl): 110S-112S.
19. Johanson NA, Lachiewicz PF, Lieberman JR, et al. Prevention of symptomatic pulmonary embolism in patients undergoing total hip or knee arthroplasty. *J Am Acad Orthop Surg.* Mar 2009;17(3):183-196.
20. Kirkley A, Birmingham TB, Litchfield RB, et al. A randomized trial of arthroscopic surgery for osteoarthritis of the knee. *N Engl J Med.* Sep 11 2008;359(11):1097-1107.
21. Mithoefer K, McAdams T, Williams RJ, Kreuz PC, Mandelbaum BR. Clinical efficacy of the microfracture technique for articular cartilage repair in the knee: an evidence-based systematic analysis. *Am J Sports Med.* Oct 2009;37(10):2053-2063.
22. Safran MR, Seiber K. The evidence for surgical repair of articular cartilage in the knee. *J Am Acad Orthop Surg.* May;18(5):259-266.
23. Abdeen AR, Collen SR, Vince KG. Fifteen-year to 19-year follow-up of the Insall-Burstein-1 total knee arthroplasty. *J Arthroplasty.* Feb;25(2):173-178.
24. Gill GS, Joshi AB, Mills DM. Total condylar knee arthroplasty. 16- to 21-year results. *Clin Orthop Relat Res.* Oct 1999;(367):210-215.
25. Denard PJ, Wirth MA, Orfaly RM. Management of glenohumeral arthritis in the young adult. *J Bone Joint Surg Am.* May 4;93(9): 885-892.
26. Cheung EV, Adams R, Morrey BF. Primary osteoarthritis of the elbow: current treatment options. *J Am Acad Orthop Surg.* Feb 2008; 16(2):77-87.

CHAPTER 43

Foot and Ankle Pain

Brant McCartan
Thanh Dinh

In this chapter, we examine the common causes of foot pain, evaluate the appropriate laboratory and imaging modalities used in diagnosis, review the relevant clinical examination, and detail the effectiveness of current treatments.

INTRODUCTION

Foot pain, not unlike pain experienced in other areas of the body, can be debilitating. One aspect separating it from other areas is that the entire weight of the body rests on the feet. It is difficult to ambulate while maintaining a non-weight-bearing position and almost impossible without assistive devices. Although the geographic region of foot pain may be visible, palpable, or reproducible, its etiology is more difficult to determine, and a definitive treatment may not exist.

This chapter examines the common causes of foot pain, evaluating the appropriate laboratory and imaging modalities used to diagnose foot pain. Coupled with a review of the relevant clinical examination, the effectiveness of current treatments is detailed for regularly encountered foot pathologies.

The following six sections guide the clinician in diagnosis and treatment of foot pain, beginning with the most commonly seen painful pathologies. The remaining sections review pain caused by overuse injuries, trauma, and neurologic, metabolic, and iatrogenic causes.

COMMON FOOT DEFORMITIES

The diagnosis of distal extremity pain is usually not difficult in that there is often either a visible malformation or the pain has a trigger point and is reproducible. In this section, the most common pathologies seen in the foot are discussed in detail. The cause of deformity is addressed along with clinical, laboratory, and imaging tools that aid in the diagnosis. Treatment modalities are discussed for the following pathologies: onychocryptosis, hyperkeratosis, soft-tissue tumors, tinea pedis, hammertoes, hallux valgus, pes plano valgus, neuroma, gout, and plantar fasciitis.

ONYCHOCRYPTOSIS/INGROWN NAIL

The normal appearance of the nail is a translucent nail plate with an underlying nail bed; the matrix is deep and proximal with surrounding periungual tissue medially and laterally. Discomfort presents when external pressures such as tight shoe gear, a misshapen nail, or a thickened nail from a fungal infection of the nail (onychomycosis) impinge on the nail plate that has been driven into the periungual tissue. Internal pressure from abnormal bone growth (subungual exostosis) may also cause an ingrown toenail. Pain is a result of inflammation or resulting soft-tissue infection caused by a break in the skin, allowing the entry of bacteria (see **Table 43-1**).

The diagnosis is based on clinical examination, noting the ingrown nail with erythema, or edema to the surrounding soft tissue. If the nail plate is misshapen, an x-ray is beneficial to help rule out an underlying deformity such as a subungual exostosis. Treatment involves removal of the ingrown border followed by twice daily diluted salt or warm water foot soaks for up to 7 days to help drain and dry the wound. If there is a local infection, a short course of antibiotics is recommended.[1] Prevention of recurrence requires addressing the underlying cause such as removal of the subungual exostosis when present, surgical matrixectomy, or treatment of onychomycosis with antifungal medications (see **Fig. 43-1**).

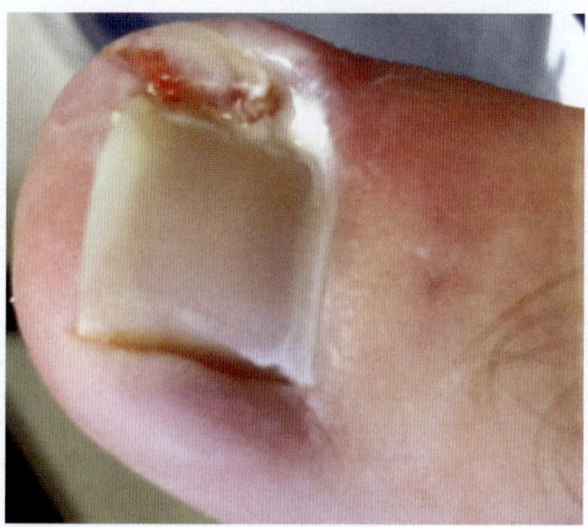

FIGURE 43-1. Picture of an ingrown nail with worsening paronychia: The rolled borders can be appreciated as well as the erythema and drainage. A partial nail avulsion is recommended for relief of the patients' symptoms.

HYPERKERATOSIS/CORNS AND CALLUSES

Corns and calluses are a result of pressure over a bony deformity. A "corn" is seen on the dorsal surface of the digits and is usually a result of a joint buckling. The head of the proximal or middle phalanx becomes more prominent and, combined with superficial pressure of shoes, irritates the epidermis, resulting in increased keratinization and a resultant corn.[2] A callous is the result of abnormal plantar pressures from either a biomechanical disturbance or bony malalignment. Shear forces between the plantar foot and ground reactive forces create a thickening of the skin, resulting in point tenderness. Corns and calluses are sometimes confused with other skin lesions such as verruca, porokeratoma, or intractable plantar keratomas. Diagnosis is clinical evaluation of the hyperkeratotic lesion and radiographs to detect any osseous abnormalities. Treatment consists of debridement of the lesion followed by padding and a topical emollient to soften the corn or callus. In intractable lesions, surgical correction of the underlying bone deformity (exostosis, hammertoe, etc.) may be necessary (see **Fig. 43-2**).

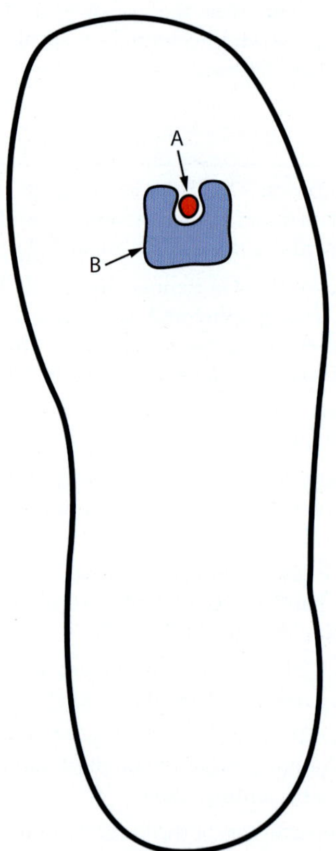

FIGURE 43-2. Image of a common off-loading technique. These can be incorporated into orthotics or dispensed over-the-counter and in-office in various shapes and sizes. **A:** Indicates the painful area, typically a callous. **B:** Indicates the pad or off-loading material that is built up to take on more pressure, with a central cut-out over the painful region to reduce contact.

TABLE 43-1 Common Causes of Onychocryptosis

Etiology of Nail Pathology
Genetic
Improper maintenance
Tight shoe gear
Trauma to matrix
Fungal infection
Subungual exostosis

TABLE 43-2 Characteristic Differences of a Wart and Callus Differentiate the Lesions and Help the Clinician with Diagnosis and Treatment

Verruca	Callus
Pain with lateral compression	Pain with direct pressure
Breaks through skin lines	Contains skin lines
No location predilection	Weight-bearing surfaces
Soft center, pinpoint bleeding	Hard center
Common in children	Common in adults

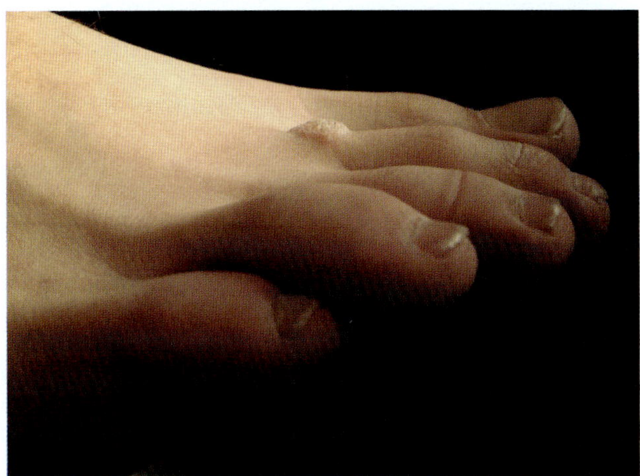

FIGURE 43-3. Picture of a wart on the dorsal surface of the toe; this is different from a corn, which would be atop the joint, and different from a callus, which would be on the bottom or side of the foot atop a weight-bearing area or bony prominence. Though difficult to visualize, the lesion has dark spots on close inspection, showing the capillary ingrowths. It is also soft and spongy on palpation, as opposed to a callus, which has a hard center.

Verruca, or a plantar wart, can be mistaken for a corn or callus. On clinical examination, verruca appears different from a callus in that it has dark spots, which represent capillary ingrowths and result in pinpoint bleeding on debridement. Additionally, plantar warts demonstrate obliteration of skin lines and are painful with side-to-side compression or a pinching of the lesion compared to direct compression. Warts can appear on non-weight-bearing areas as opposed to a callus, which results from plantar pressures. There are countless treatments for verruca, primarily involving paring of the lesion to pinpoint bleeding followed by desiccation of the lesion with topical preparations.[3] Topical preparations commonly used include salicylic acids, cantharidin, cryotherapy, and electrodesiccation, though numerous other topical treatments are often employed (see **Table 43-2** and **Fig. 43-3**).

SOFT-TISSUE TUMORS/CYSTS

Common soft-tissue tumors of the foot include cysts and fibromas. Various forms of cysts exist, but ganglionic, synovial, and mucinous are seen most commonly in the foot.[4] Trauma or excessive stretching creates an out-pouching similar to an aneurismal sac or cyst, which is found along the course of a tendon near the joint. Clinical exam reveals a firm mass that can be tender to palpation. Transillumination of the mass with a pen light will demonstrate an orange glow consistent with a fluid-filled mass. Initial treatment consists of aspiration with or without the administration of a steroid. In the event of recurrence, surgical intervention can be performed to excise the cystic sac and its stalk (see **Fig. 43-4**).

Plantar fibromas are benign, solid, soft-tissue tumors deep to the subcutaneous tissue and present as a painful bump or raised area. Commonly originating from the plantar fascial ligament, imaging studies such as MRI help determine the location of the mass and its characteristics. Soft-tissue biopsy is necessary for definitive diagnosis along with evaluation of malignant potential. These masses can be treated with pressure off-loading and custom orthotics, and topical preparations have shown relief, though some require surgical excision.

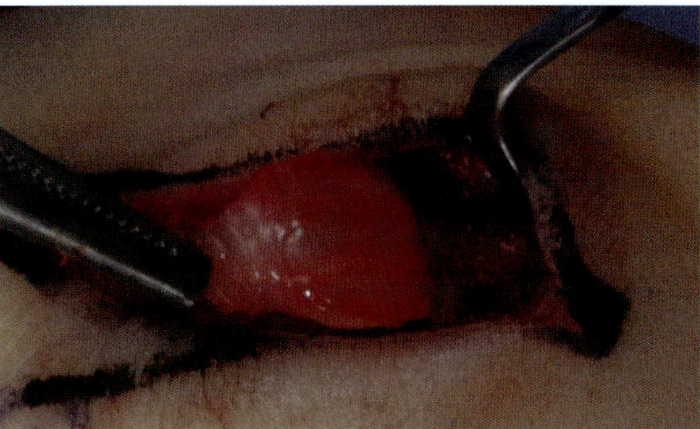

FIGURE 43-4. Picture of a cyst being excised intraoperatively; its fluid-filled appearance can be appreciated as it is being removed in toto.

TINEA PEDIS/ATHLETE'S FOOT

Tinea pedis, more commonly referred to as "athlete's foot," is a condition that begins with an itchy rash and scaling of the skin. On clinical examination, the rash can involve the webspaces or the entire foot in a slipper-like distribution. The itching can result in excoriation of the skin, which can then become very painful. Breaks in the skin from the rash and scratching may lead to a soft-tissue infection or cellulitis. The fungus is typically caused by the dermatophyte trichophyton rubrum, though others can be isolated and identified with potassium hydroxide testing and periodic acid-Schiff staining. Treatment typically consists of topical as well as systemic antifungal therapies.[5]

HAMMERTOES

Hammertoes involve a flexion deformity of the proximal and/or distal toe joint. There are different terms to describe this deformity, depending on the plane of the deformity and the combination of deformities: mallet toe, hammer toe, curly or claw toe, and overlapping toe.[6] Painful hyperkeratotic lesions may develop as a result of the pressure from shoes and activity on the underlying digital deformity.

Hammertoes and callus/corns can be appreciated during the clinical exam with occasional soft-tissue inflammation. Radiographic evaluation will demonstrate the flexion deformity at the involved joint and are helpful in preoperative planning when surgery is required. Conservative care consists of off-loading of the digital deformities with wider shoes and larger toe boxes. Padding and off-loading devices can also reduce pressure on the prominent areas or space out the digits. These are temporary treatments, which do not correct the underlying osseous deformities (see **Fig. 43-5**).

Surgical correction of hammertoe deformities includes realigning the joint with arthroplasty or arthrodesis procedures. Skin plasties are also helpful for angular deformities and straightening the toe in long-standing deformities. Digital vessels and nerves are small in caliber and thus can be severed during surgery. Swelling and edema are usually expected postoperatively and can take more than 6 months to fully resolve.

HALLUX VALGUS/BUNIONS

Classically, bunions (hallux valgus) present with pain on the medial, or inside, aspect of the first metatarsal-phalangeal joint (MTPJ). There may

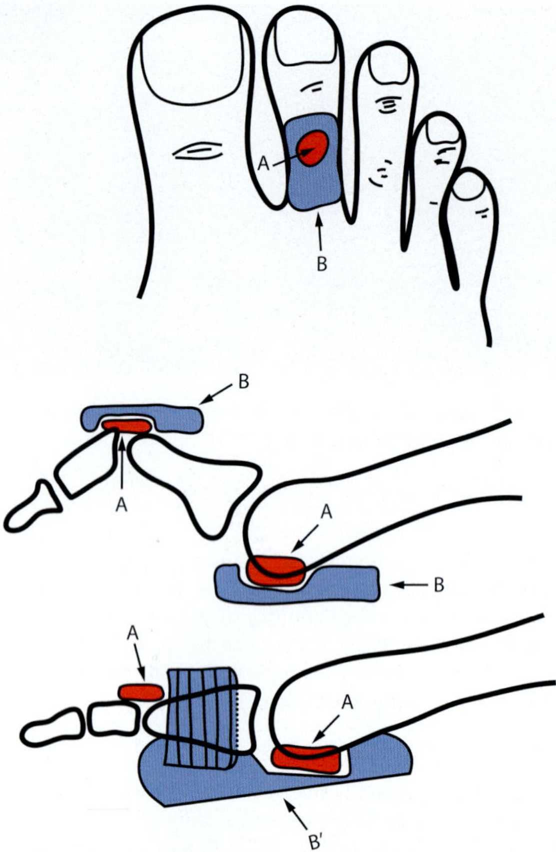

FIGURE 43-5. Hammertoe deformities cause pain due to a dorsal callous and retrograde pressure on the metatarsal. **A:** Indicates the painful area, typically a corn or callous. **B:** Indicates the pad or off-loading material that is built up. This helps to relieve pressure on the lesion directly and disperse weight over a greater area. **B′:** Metatarsal pad modification with loop around the phalanx helps to decrease MPJ extension and retrograde buckling as well as padding plantar to the metatarsal.

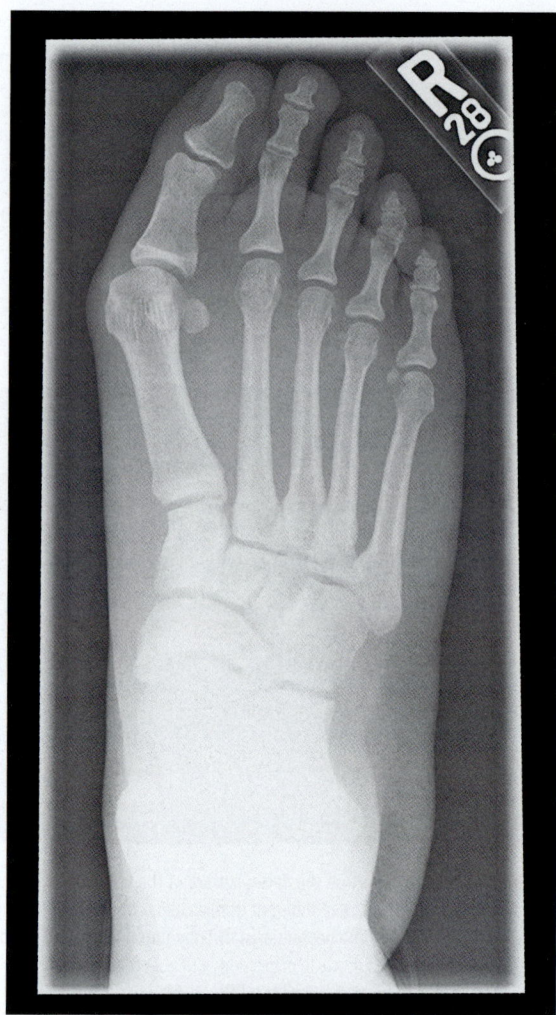

FIGURE 43-6. Radiograph depicting a bunion deformity. There is a prominent medial eminence off of the first metatarsal. Also, the sesamoid apparatus is lateral to the metatarsophalangeal joint. The proximal phalanx is deviated in an abducuted and valgus position compared to the metatarsal.

be surrounding redness and swelling with a possible underlying bursitis. Clinically, there is a "bump" on the medial aspect of the first metatarsal with lateral deviation and valgus rotation of the big toe (see **Fig. 43-6**).

There have been a number of postulated etiologies for the development of bunions, with the prevailing theory indicating that they are caused by a biomechanical abnormality; there is, however, a genetic component. These deformities are progressive and pain is exacerbated with tight shoes such as high heels or athletic cleats. Clinically, the medial column of the foot should be evaluated for hypermobility or decreased range of motion (hallux limitus). If the bunion is severely worse on one side, there may be a limb length discrepancy, which can be measured during the biomechanical exam. Orthotics, padding, and splints may help to relieve the pain from pressure on the boney prominence, but surgery correction is often indicated.

PES PLANO VALGUS/FLAT FOOT

Flat feet can result from a number of different etiologies. If seen in children, it is usually genetic or resulting from a coalition, or inappropriate differentiation, of a joint. In adults, it is generally biomechanical in origin, where there is overpronation of the talus. Usually, flat-footed patients complain of "tired feet" with aching joints and arch pain. Arthritis can develop, and the foot accommodates, resulting in joint contractures and soft-tissue attenuation.

If a unilateral flat foot occurs suddenly, it may be the result of a tendon rupture or insufficiency of the tibialis posterior. Clinically, the deformity involves collapse of the midfoot along with heel valgus. Tenderness may be elicited with palpation along the course of the posterior tibial tendon in addition to associated weakness during muscle testing. The single heel raise, in which patients are asked to raise their heel off the ground and "stand on their toes," is highly suggestive of posterior tibial tendon dysfunction when the patient is unable to perform this maneuver.[7] Plain radiographs will reveal the collapse of the midfoot joints, while MR imaging will assist in evaluation of tendon integrity. Depending on the severity of the deformity, treatment consists of conservative care with orthoses and bracing with surgical intervention warranted in more advanced deformities (see **Fig. 43-7**).

MORTON'S NEUROMA

Originally described in 1876, the third webspace is the most common location for a neuroma to occur because the medial and lateral plantar nerve branches join together via a communicating branch to form the third common plantar digital nerve, making this nerve enlarged compared with its medial and lateral counterparts.[8] The patient will commonly describe the pain as a "burning" sensation to the forefoot, though it may also be described as "knifelike" and "electric." The pain can radiate distally, with numbness experienced to the toes. Another common description is a feeling of walking on a pebble or a wrinkled sock. The pain is relieved when the shoe gear is removed and activity is stopped, but it can be reproduced by squeezing the forefoot together, essentially

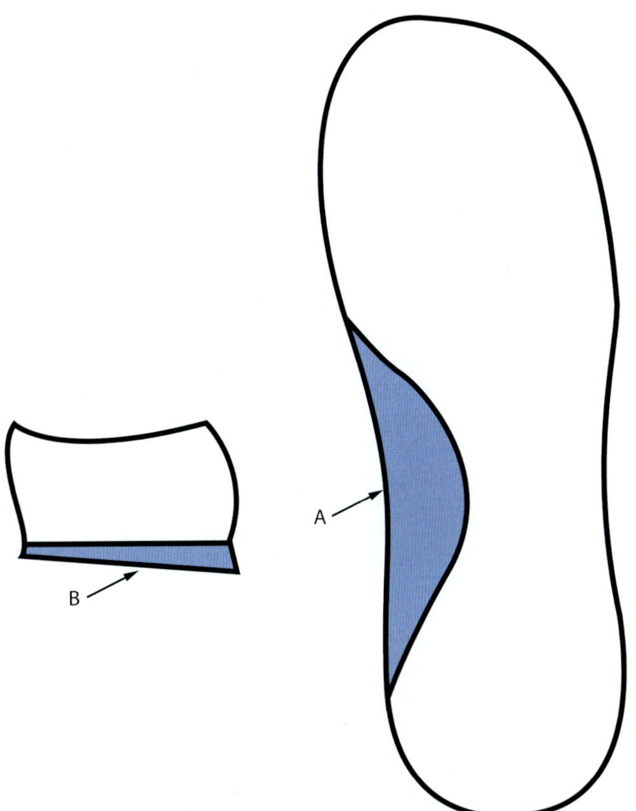

FIGURE 43-7. A: Within the shoe, a functional orthotic can be molded to help build up the arch and control pronation. **B:** A medial heel skive can also transfer pressure and invert the rearfoot.

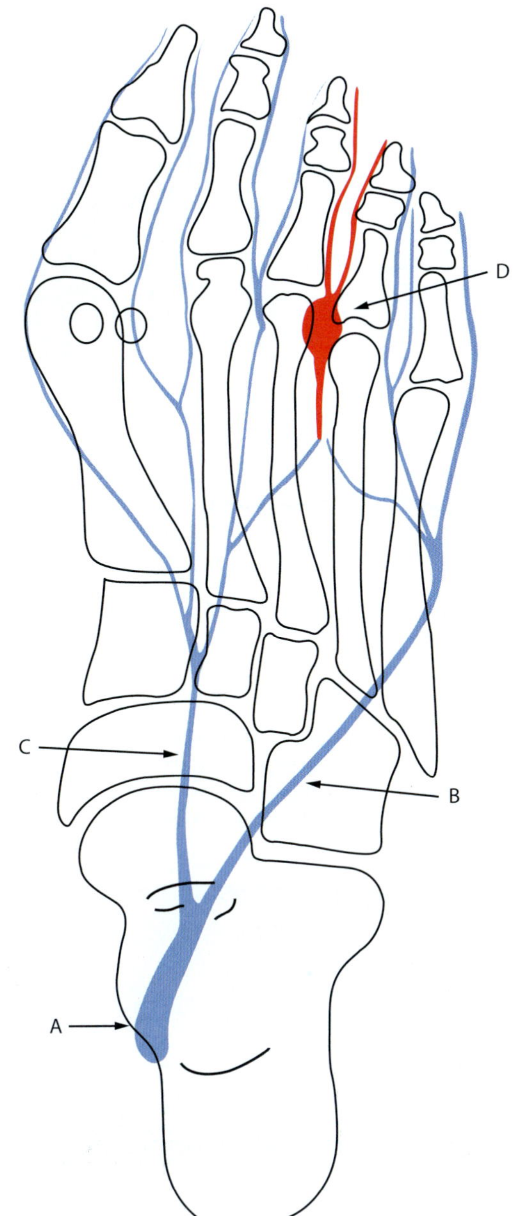

FIGURE 43-8. Image of the plantar nerve distribution to the foot. A represents the tibial nerve. **B** represents the lateral plantar nerve. C represents the medial plantar nerve. D represents a Morton's neuroma – commonly found between the third webspace, between the third and forth metatarsal heads.

compressing the metatarsal heads together against the neuroma. On physical exam, a silent "click" may be felt when the neuroma is manually compressed, shifting between the metatarsal heads[9] (see **Fig. 43-8**).

Radiographs may be used to rule out other pathologies such as stress fractures or other bony abnormalities. However, the most sensitive imaging study is an MRI, which typically shows nerve thickening and edema surrounding the nerve. Treatment consists of injections with corticosteroids, diluted alcohol, or other analgesics. These can help confirm the diagnosis as well as be therapeutic. Sclerosing injections of ~4% diluted alcohol solution have been described to cause chemical neurolysis and nerve dehydration (Wallerian degeneration).[10] Off-loading the neuroma with orthotics or a metatarsal pad may help reduce pressure on the metatarsal and the neuroma. If conservative care is unsuccessful, surgical decompression of the nerve or neurolysis may be necessary (see **Figs. 43-9** and **43-10**).

GOUT

Gout involves the deposition of uric acid in a joint and most commonly manifests in the first MTPJ of the foot due to a cooler temperature gradient, which results in crystal formation. Gout is the result of overproduction or underexcretion of uric acid. Gout was originally titled the "disease of kings" because it was seen most frequently in wealthy citizens who could afford more expensive foods such as wines, red meats, and cheeses, which are rich in purines.[11] Uric acid is the end product of purine metabolism, and when present in excess, crystal formation results (see **Table 43-3**).

On clinic examination, the first MTPJ is red, hot, swollen, and exquisitely painful to the touch. There is also pain on range of motion, and allodynia is present where even light percussion is barely tolerable. Other pathologies that present similarly are a septic joint or inflammatory arthritis. To adequately diagnose gout, blood work is used to assess for an elevated uric acid concentration (above 6 mg/dl in women and 7 mg/dl in men).[11] Joint aspiration with crystal analysis remains the gold standard for diagnosis, with negatively birefringent, needle-shaped gold crystals noted.

Treatment of acute gout consists of addressing the inflammation with a strong anti-inflammatory agent. Additionally, monotherapy with colchicine—a natural plant product derived from the autumn crocus—is often employed. For chronic gout, medicinal therapy should be directed on the overproduction or underexcretion of uric acid. The majority of chronic gout (90%) is the result of underexcretion of uric acid. In this instance, inhibition of uric acid reabsorption in the proximal renal tubules with probenecid is recommended along with avoidance of foods high in purines. If overproduction is the cause, allopurinol, a xanthine oxidase inhibitor, blocks uric acid synthesis. Gout can destroy the joint, and radiographs may reveal joint destructions and a "rat-bitten" appearance termed "Martel's sign."[12]

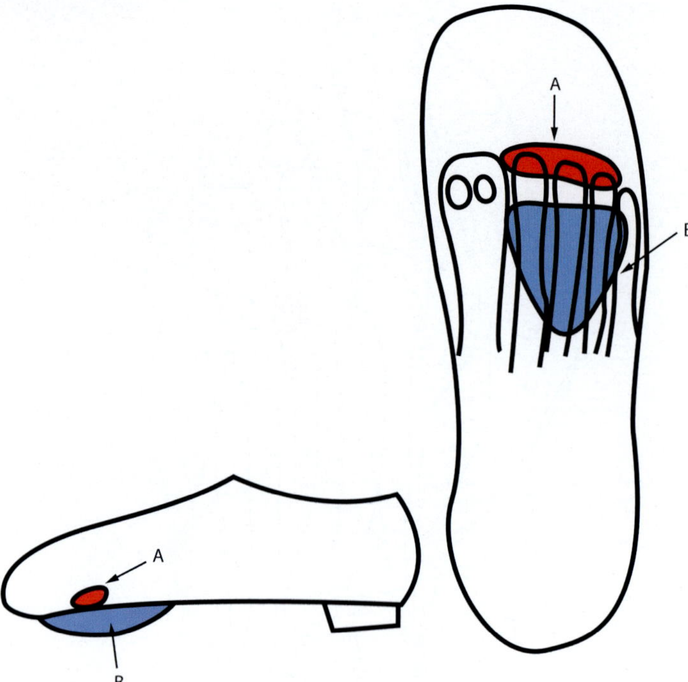

FIGURE 43-9. Metatarsal pads help alter the biomechanics when the patient is weight-bearing and cushion the painful area. Rocker bottom shoes help with metatarsalgia. **A:** Represents the painful area. **B:** Represents the metatarsal pad and rocker bottom area of the shoe. Both ultimately disperse the pressure more evenly off of the metatarsal head.

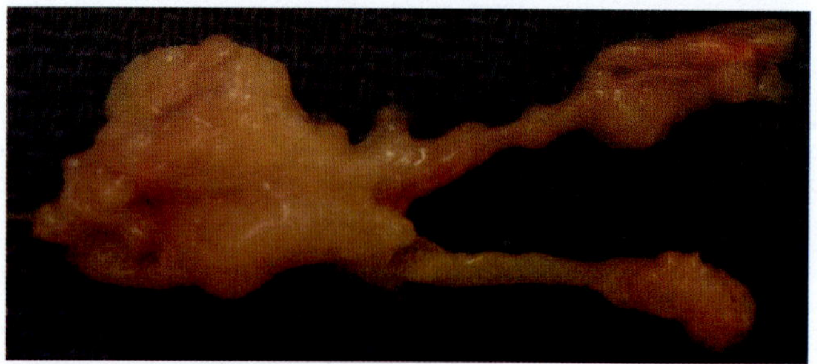

FIGURE 43-10. Gross image of a neuroma surgically removed. The medial and lateral distal branches and the bulbous neuroma proximally that was irritated by the metatarsal heads can be seen.

PLANTAR FASCIITIS/HEEL PAIN

Plantar fasciitis, a common cause of heel pain, is a condition in which the plantar fascia becomes irritated due to microtearing of the ligament. The patient will classically describe pain with the first step in the morning when getting out of bed or with the first step after sitting due to a sudden pulling of the tight ligament, or poststatic dyskinesia. Pain improves with use but feels sharp and "knife-like" on initial presentation. On clinical exam, direct palpation to the origin or insertion of the fascia at the heel reproduces the symptoms.

While diagnosis is primarily based on the history and physical exam, imaging modalities may help exclude differential etiologies of heel pain not limited to stress fractures. Plain radiographs often reveal a plantar spurring of the calcaneus as a result of the inflammation to the ligament; however, this is rarely the cause of the pain. Other diagnostic modalities include ultrasound and MRI, which may reveal thickening of the plantar fascia ligament consistent with chronic inflammation or microtears.

Treatments should begin conservatively with a course of stretching to include the Achilles tendon and plantar fascial ligaments. Reduction of increased strain to the plantar fascia ligament with orthoses, strappings, and supportive shoes helps by maintaining the longitudinal arch of the foot and thus relaxing the pull on the plantar fascia. Addressing the inflammation of the ligament with oral non-steroidal inflammatory medications (NSAIDs), ice, and corticosteroid injections is also beneficial. A night-splint can be worn to keep the tendon and fascia stretched throughout the night when not ambulating. Plantar fasciitis is a self-limiting condition, but it is very disabilitating, and surgical intervention (fasciotomy) may be warranted if daily functions are lost.

TABLE 43-3 Two Etiologies of Gout: Overproduction Versus Underexcretion

Etiology of Gout	
Overproducer	**Underexcreter**
10% of cases	90% of cases
Genetic deficit, metabolic, diet	Increased uric acid, renal
Treated with allopurinol	Treated with probenecid

Though the acute treatment is similar, chronic prevention must be directed toward the cause.

OVERUSE INJURIES

Overuse injuries are most commonly seen in athletes but are also present in previously sedentary individuals beginning a new activity. Excessive repetitive trauma causes inflammation, adaptation, and tissue disorganization that can lead to rupture or fracture. Soft-tissue structures involved in the foot and ankle are tendons, ligaments, and fascia. Overuse injuries to the bone can result in bone contusions and stress fractures.

Tendonitis involves inflammation of a tendon that has been stretched or pulled with individual collagen fibers subsequently disrupted. The Achilles tendon is often involved and can be painful at its insertion into the calcaneus or midsubstance behind the ankle. Pain can be reproduced with direct palpation of the tendon or when the joint is brought through range of motion, but there is also, occasionally, a palpable thickening of the tendon and swelling. An MRI is useful in evaluation of partial tears and surrounding edema or bursal formations.

The usual treatment regimen is highlighted by the acronym PRICE, which stands for: protection (with bracing), rest from activity or activity modification, ice, compression of swelling if present, and elevation to help minimize the edema. NSAIDs can also be used to help decrease the swelling and pain. Steroid injection around this major tendon is typically avoided given the increased incidence of tendon rupture.

It is important to distinguish tendonitis from tendinosis, which involves degeneration of the tendon without inflammation.[13] Tendinosis is likely the more common condition and is seen in athletes due to repetitive microtrauma and disorganization of the collagen tissues. Where tendonitis should resolve in a short amount of time by decreasing inflammation, tendinosis is more refractory to PRICE, and the opposite treatment algorithm should be applied—with eccentric stretching and emphasis on strengthening the tissues. It typically takes longer for the pain associated with tendinosis to resolve compared to tendonitis (see **Table 43-4**).

TABLE 43-4 Tendonitis Versus Tendinosis

Tendonitis	Tendinosis
Less common	More common
Inflammatory cells within/around tendon	Collagen disorganization
Weeks to recovery (2–6)	Months to recovery (2–6)
Treated with stretching and strengthening, emphasizing reorganization	Treatment by controlling inflammation

It is important to think of tendinosis when the patient is reluctant to improve with PRICE. Aggressive physical therapy, if started early, can be therapeutic.

Bursitis can occur in any area of the foot where a bursa is found anatomically that helps cushion the tendon's insertion from the bone. Adventitious bursa can occur as a result of shearing or direct force atop a bony deformity. This can present as a raised area over the protuberance. The adventitious bursa initially acts as an area of extra padding, but it becomes painful when it results in swelling and when combined with tight shoe gear. A common location of an adventitious bursitis is on the lateral aspect of the fifth metatarsal head caused from tight shoe gear. The correction is off-loading with accommodative shoes, padding, or surgical excision (see **Fig. 43-11**).

Stress fractures are a result of increased pressure on an area of bone. This is more commonly seen after repetitive stress on one area as opposed to an isolated incident. Common areas for stress fractures in the foot include the lesser metatarsals and the calcaneus as a result of increased biomechanical load during a normal walking heel-toe gait cycle. This can be aggravated by poorly supportive shoe wear or in a foot with biomechanical abnormalities such as overpronation or oversupination.

On clinical examination of stress fracture, pain is reproducible with direct palpation of the involved area. Calcaneal stress fractures often demonstrate pain with direct percussion to the bottom of the heel with the clinician's palm as well as lateral compression of the calcaneus. Radiographs may be helpful, revealing periosteal reaction or a healing bone callous to the affected bone. However, these radiographic signs may lag 3 to 4 weeks following the injury. MRI is more sensitive, often revealing increased fluid to the area of injury (see **Fig. 43-12**).

Treatment consists of rest and immobilization to facilitate bone healing. Immobilization can be performed with casting, walking boots, stiff-soled shoes, and assistive devices such as crutches or a walker. The type of immobilization employed and length of time will vary with the individual fracture location and pattern, but it is usually patient-driven and based on comfort.

Sesamoiditis is another common overuse injury seen in runners and dancers where there is irritation to the sesamoid apparatus of the foot. The sesamoids articulate with the plantar aspect of the first metatarsal and, with repetitive trauma, become inflamed. The diagnosis is made by reproduction of the pain symptoms with direct palpation of the sesamoids. Imaging studies such as radiographs, MRI, and bone scans may help with the diagnosis in addition to ruling out the possibility of a fractured sesamoid. Treatment consists of off-loading with padding and orthotics, rest, NSAIDs, and ice. Injections can also be of benefit to locally reduce inflammation with an analgesic or corticosteroid (see **Fig. 43-13**).

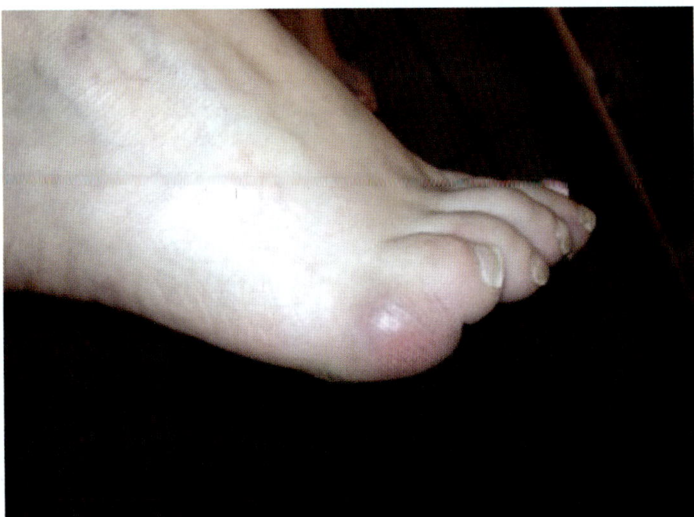

FIGURE 43-11. Clinical presentation of adventitious bursitis on the lateral aspect of the fifth metatarsophalangeal joint; erythema as a result of direct pressure from too tight of shoes is appreciated.

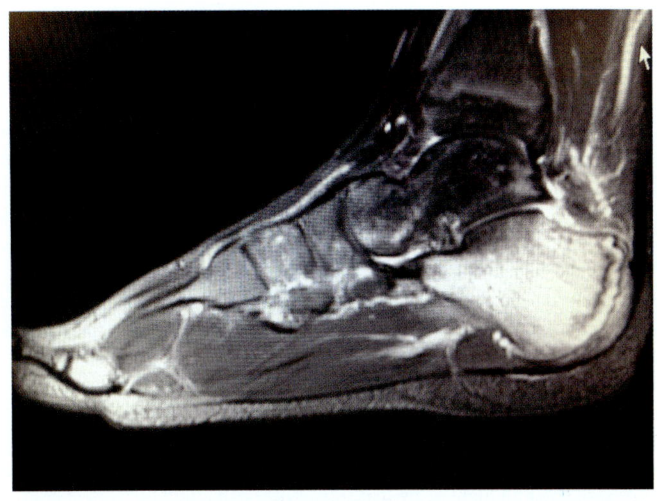

FIGURE 43-12. T2-saggital MRI of the foot. The calcaneal stress fracture almost jumps out where the increased fluid accumulation is appreciated from the resultant inflammation within the calcaneus.

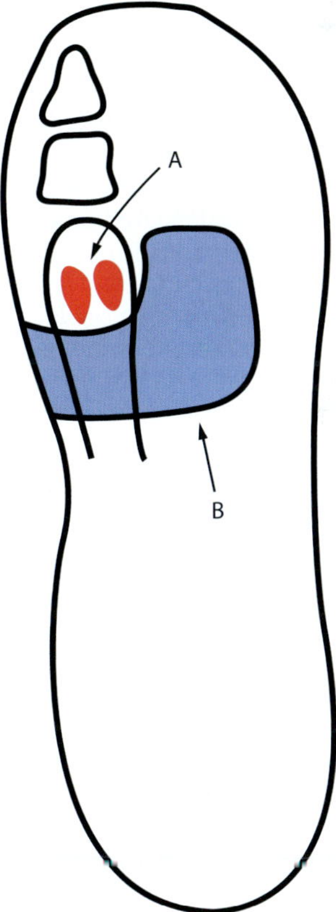

FIGURE 43-13. Sesamoids (A) may become irritated and cause a trigger point. These can be off-loaded with moleskin (B) to take pressure off of the "hot spot".

TRAUMA

Blunt, sharp, and penetrating trauma can affect any area of the body. The foot is a common place for sprains and fractures, although high-velocity injuries can also be seen. Common soft-tissue traumas of the foot and ankle include subungual hematomas, strains, sprains, tendon and ligament ruptures, and compartment syndrome. Traumatic injuries to the bone are contusions, fractures, and dislocations.

Diagnosis of foot trauma is achieved with a thorough history and physical examination of the affected extremity. The mechanism of injury, as well as direct visualization and palpation of the injury, may help guide imaging of the involved foot. Imaging should begin with radiographs followed by more advanced studies to further evaluate soft-tissue or joint structures. Most traumatic conditions of the foot are initially treated with PRICE (protection/protected weight bearing, rest/activity modification, ice, compression and elevation).

A subungual hematoma is usually caused by a direct blow to the nail plate from dropping a heavy object. If more than 25% of the nail bed shows hematoma, the nail should be removed to assess for a nail bed laceration. The pain is often described as throbbing and worsens in a dependent position. Radiographs can be taken to assess for fracture of the distal phalanx, which is treated similarly to an open fracture if the nail bed is violated. Pain is relieved by draining the hematoma—either by complete removal of the nail plate or by drilling a hole with a needle or heat cautery.

Sprains are a result of excess force on a joint with subsequent stretching of the ligaments, muscle, or tendons. *Sprain* is typically reserved to describe the stretching and partial tearing of ligamentous fibers, while *strain* is used to describe the stretching and possible partial tearing of muscle fibers and/or tendinous fibers. Clinically, bruising and ecchymosis are visualized to the injured area and are indicative of the severity. If the injury is chronic and instability is present, stress radiographic views may reveal opening of the joint and increased motion compared with the contralateral or unaffected side. The medial ankle ligaments are dense and stable, collectively grouped together, and called the deltoid ligaments. They are substantially stronger than the lateral ankle ligaments and, thus, are less commonly affected than the lateral ligaments, which are affected 85% of the time.[14] The anterior talofibular ligament is the most commonly affected ankle ligament involved, and injury to this ligament is tested with the anterior drawer test, whereby the foot is pulled in an anterior direction away from the leg a greater distance compared to the unaffected side.[15]

In more severe strain or sprain injuries, the ligaments may be ruptured. This is seen in conjunction with excessive ecchymosis and loss of function and joint stability. The patient may also report a snapping sound—for instance, with an Achilles tendon rupture, which is often described as the feeling of someone striking the back of the heel with a racket. Clinical evaluation for Achilles tendon ruptures may employ the Thompson test, in which the patient lies prone on a table and the calf is squeezed.[16] If the foot does not plantarflex, the Achilles tendon is thought to be disrupted. Radiographs may also reveal disruption of Kager's fat triangle, a normally dark-appearing area between the calcaneus and Achilles tendon.[17] MRI is sensitive in identifying the level and severity of the injury.

Compartment syndrome is a severe sequela of trauma resulting from increased foot compartment pressures and the potential for injury to muscle and nerve structures. Typically, the patient presents with pain out of proportion with the symptoms clinically described as the five P's: pain out of proportion, pallor, paresthesia, paralysis, and pulselessness. If pulselessness is found, there is likely already irreversible damage to muscle and other tissues. Some surgeons elect to forgo compartment pressure, instead measuring with a Wick catheter (normal range is <10 mm Hg, affected range is >30 mm Hg at rest) and bringing the patient to the operating room for immediate fasciotomies, opening up all potentially involved compartments.[18]

Bone injuries may range from direct trauma resulting in contusions of bone to more severe fracture patterns. A history of the mechanism of injury—in addition to baseline radiographs to evaluate acute osseous injury—usually suffices in establishing the diagnosis. Fractures of the foot commonly involve the digits, metatarsals, and calcaneus. The "bedpost fracture" is a classic example in which the patient reports accidently catching or kicking the bedpost in the middle of the night, resulting in a digital fracture. When the fracture demonstrates minimal displacement, treatment with buddy taping (to the next digit) along with a stiff-soled shoe is the appropriate treatment for central digits two, three, and four.

Metatarsal fractures may result from dropping a heavy object on top of the foot where the neck may be fractured or from excessive twisting where the base can be disrupted. The MTPJ may be affected as well with forced hyperextension of the joint, commonly termed "turf toe." Calcaneal fractures typically result from falling from a height with an associated injury to the lumbar spine. A clinical sign of severe heel pain, swelling, and a specific distribution of ecchymosis extending from the ankle to the sole of the foot is termed "Mondor's sign."

Baseline radiographs of the foot and ankle are essential in the initial diagnosis as well as suggestive for more advanced imaging studies such as CT (computed tomography) and MRI to evaluate for soft-tissue and intraarticular fracture patterns. Depending on the extent of displacement and intraarticular involvement, conservative management with immobilization or surgical reduction followed by a period of immobilization is often the recommended treatment course.

NEUROLOGIC

Complex regional pain syndrome (CRPS), previously referred to as RSD (reflex sympathetic dystrophy), can be seen following surgery or with both mild and severe trauma. The pain experienced is typically out of proportion to the injury described, and the patient is often unable to bear weight on the affected extremity. Furthermore, the affected area may exhibit changes in color, temperature, and hydration regulation (see **Figure 43-15**). Treatment of this complex process is multifactorial, including injections, antidepressants, antiseizure medications, ketamine hydrochloride, physical therapy, nerve transmission interference, and psychotherapy. The key to effective treatment is early diagnosis and aggressive and early intervention. Should this condition fail to be treated in a timely manner, muscle atrophy and loss of limb function result.[19]

There are several systemic neuropathies that can present primarily as foot pain. One prime example is pain associated with peripheral neuropathy commonly seen in patients with poorly controlled diabetes, but it is also seen in alcoholics. Other neuropathies that may present with painful feet include inflammatory, vasculitic, sarcoid, renal disease associated, viral, parasitic, tumor associated, radiation, cold-induced, drug/nutrition related (alcohol, B12), and entrapment. The diagnosis of these neuropathies may be performed with laboratory testing and nerve conduction velocities. Treatment is focused on identifying the cause and removing the negative stimulus or supplementing the deficiency. Other treatments may include non-narcotic analgesics, antidepressants, anticonvulsants, local blocks, topical agents, vitamins, and antipsychotics.

Nerve entrapments can occur in a number of different locations in the foot as a result of anatomical variation. The reported complaint may include symptoms of pain associated with numbness, burning, and tingling. Advanced imaging studies with ultrasound and MRI may reveal fluid surrounding the affected nerve suggestive of inflammation. The gold standard remains nerve conduction and EMG (electromyography) testing. Treatment often involves conservative removal of the pressure on the nerve with padding and orthotic management, NSAIDs to reduce local inflammation, and surgical decompression of the nerve when conservative management fails (see **Table 43-5**).

Tarsal tunnel syndrome involves entrapment of the posterior tibial nerve in the sulcus just inferior to the medial malleolus of the ankle.

TABLE 43-5 Neuroma Nicknames Based on Forefoot Location

Neuroma	Plantar Location
Joplin	Medial 1st MPJ
Heuter's	1st interspace (1st common digital nerve)
Hauser's	2nd interspace (2nd common digital nerve)
Morton's	3rd interspace (3rd common digital nerve)
Islen's	4th interspace (4th common digital nerve)

Compression of the nerve leads to pain, numbness, and burning symptoms. This pain can also feel like pins and needles and can radiate both proximally and distally along the foot or leg.[20] Causes of tarsal tunnel syndrome include space-occupying lesions, biomechanical faults such as overpronation, trauma, and inflammatory conditions. Examples of space-occupying lesions that cause tarsal tunnel syndrome include varicosities, ganglions, lipomas, and edema. Biomechanical faults usually involve excess stretch on the tibial nerve from overpronation. No matter the lesion, pain is caused from an entrapment or compression of the tibial nerve or its branches: medial and lateral plantar nerves and the medial calcaneal nerve. Upon clinical examination, symptoms can be reproduced by maximally everting the foot, thus stretching the tibial nerve and compressing the tarsal tunnel. Tapping on the medial aspect of the tarsal tunnel may also reveal a shooting electrical pain sensation toward the toes (Tinel's sign) or proximally up the foot (Valleix's sign). Treatment includes NSAIDs, local nerve blocks, physical therapy, and orthotic management to address biomechanical etiologies. Surgical treatment consists of decompressing the nerve by releasing the flexor retinaculum or removing the space-occupying lesion and freeing up the tibial nerve and its branches (see **Figure 43-16**).

METABOLIC

Metabolic conditions can manifest in the feet, with gout as one of the most common conditions. Other metabolic conditions include pseudogout, chondrocalcinosis, and calcium pyrophosphate dehydrate (CPPD), which is an acute or chronic inflammatory arthritis. It typically runs a longer course than gout and affects larger joints like the ankle as opposed to the big toe joint seen in classic gout. Laboratory tests can be of benefit to rule out increased uric acid levels. An arthrocentesis and microscopic examination show rhomboid-shaped crystals. Treatment of pseudogout typically involves immobilization and oral pain control during acute flares (see **Table 43-6**).

Rheumatoid arthritis (RA) is an inflammatory arthritis that affects the entire body. In the foot, pain is described as an insidious aching with reports of morning stiffness. Multiple joints are involved, and the pain and swelling often improve with motion. Painful rheumatoid nodules may also arise, affecting the small joints of the digits. Located in the subcutaneous tissue, these nodules are comprised of fibrous tissue and commonly located over bony prominences.

In contrast, osteoarthritis (OA) is a degeneration of the articular joint surfaces secondary to excessive "wear and tear." The cartilage is damaged, and, once the subchondral bone is exposed, it becomes sclerotic. Pain is asymmetric and worsens during activity, with changes in weather aggravating symptoms. There is usually subsequent decreased range of motion, classically seen in the first MTPJ, coined *hallux limitus* or *rigidus* if severe. It can also be seen in the midfoot following a trauma or in the anterior ankle joint with decreased ankle range of motion. Diagnosis is made clinically, though severity can be depicted radiographically with loose bodies and uneven joint disruption. Treatments include NSAIDs, joint injections, orthotic therapy, and physical therapy to ease the pain symptoms. If surgery is indicated, the joint is usually remodeled, replaced, or fused (see **Table 43-7**).

TABLE 43-6 Gout Versus Pseudogout

Gout	Pseudogout
Uric acid	Calcium pyrophosphate dihydrate
Smaller joints—MPJ	Larger joints—ankle, knee
Negative birefringent crystals	Positive birefringent crystals
Gold, needle-shaped crystals	Blue, rhomboid-shaped crystals
Short course	Long course
Low-grade fever	High-grade fever

TABLE 43-7 Osteoarthritis Versus Rheumatoid Arthritis

OA	RA
Asymmetrical destruction	Symmetrical destruction
Pain worse at end of day, worse with motion	Pain worse in morning, improves with motion
Larger joints (MPJ, knees, hips)	Small joints (IPJs, MPJs)
No swelling, noninflammatory	Soft-tissue swelling, inflammation
Osteosclerosis	Osteopenia
Treated with joint replacement or fusion	Treated with corticosteroids, NSAIDs

IATROGENIC

Iatrogenic causes of foot pain can be as simple as a surgical scar. Both hypertrophic and keloid formation, when the scar extends beyond the incision line, can be uncomfortable physically and emotionally to the patient. Hypertrophic scars can be excised, and the underlying tissue can be freed up and better approximated. Keloid treatment is more controversial, but steroid injections can be utilized to help with the pain.[21] Physical therapy, massage, therapeutic heat, stretching, paraffin wax, and ultrasound treatments have also been recommended to assist in releasing the adhered tissues.

During surgery, or trauma, there may be injury to the nerve, leading to compression, entrapment, or complete severance. Compression can result from a tight dressing and cast or even if the nerve is retracted too aggressively during the procedure. The nerve may be bruised with pain, and numbness may result following the removal of the inciting trauma and the decrease in inflammation. If the nerve axon is injured and subsequent Wallerian degeneration occurs, it may take months to repair. If the nerve is completely severed, it is usually irreversible[22,23] (see **Table 43-8**).

Nerve conduction tests can be used to determine the distribution of deficit, and, if possible, an end-to-end repair is recommended. The consulted chronic pain medicine physician can expect the lesion to be located near the incisional scar. Gabapentin, pregabalin, and other anticonvulsant medications may help diminish the symptoms. It is important to appreciate the sensory distribution and spinal nerve root in cases where a local nerve block or proximal nerve stimulator is indicated (see **Figs. 43-14** and **43-15**).

Bone healing complications, as a result of trauma or operative in origin, can also cause foot pain. Bone healing complications include delayed union, nonunion, and pseudoarthrosis. Differentiation of each bone healing complication primarily involves the length of time from the attempted arthrodesis procedure. In delayed union (3–6 months to heal), there may be swelling and pain secondary to continued motion and further non-weight-bearing may be required to allow the bone to heal. If there is a nonunion—defined as up to 9 months without fusion or absence of healing—the addition of a bone stimulator in addition to immobilization is necessary.[24] In the case of pseudoarthrosis,

TABLE 43-8 Nerve Trauma Describing Severity, If Axonal Involvement or Complete Transection of the Nerve

Nerve Trauma Classification		
Seddon	**Sunderland**	**Deficit**
Neurapraxia	1st degree	Bruised nerve, axon unaffected, reversible
Axonotmesis	2nd degree	Injured axon, Wallerian degeneration, regeneration possible
	3rd degree	Axon injured, with irregular regeneration
	4th degree	Axon destroyed but nerve trunk remains intact
Neurotmesis	5th degree	Nerve completely severed; irreversible numbness

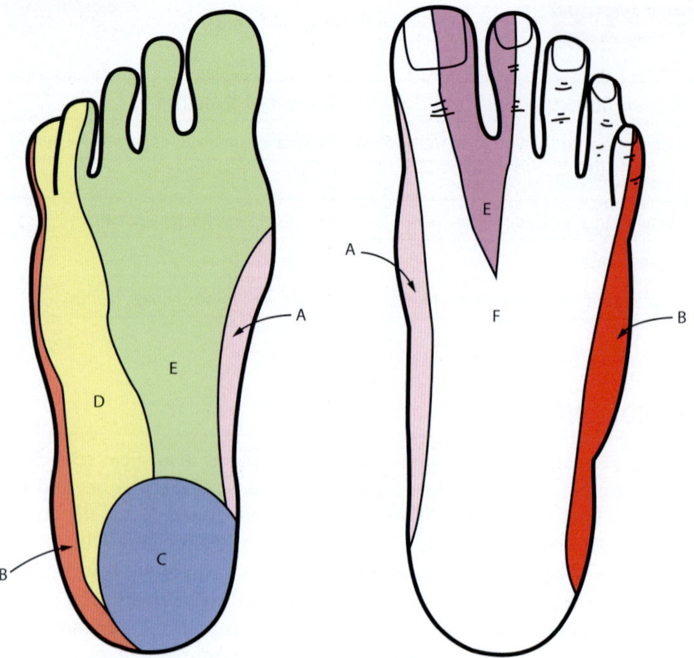

FIGURE 43-14. **A:** Saphenous nerve distribution (L3,4). **B:** Sural nerve distribution (S1,2). **C:** Medial calcaneal nerve distribution (S1,2). **D:** Lateral plantar nerve distribution (S1,2). **E:** Medial plantar nerve distribution (L4,5). **F:** Superficial peroneal nerve distribution (L5, S1);. **G:** Deep peroneal nerve distribution (L4,5).

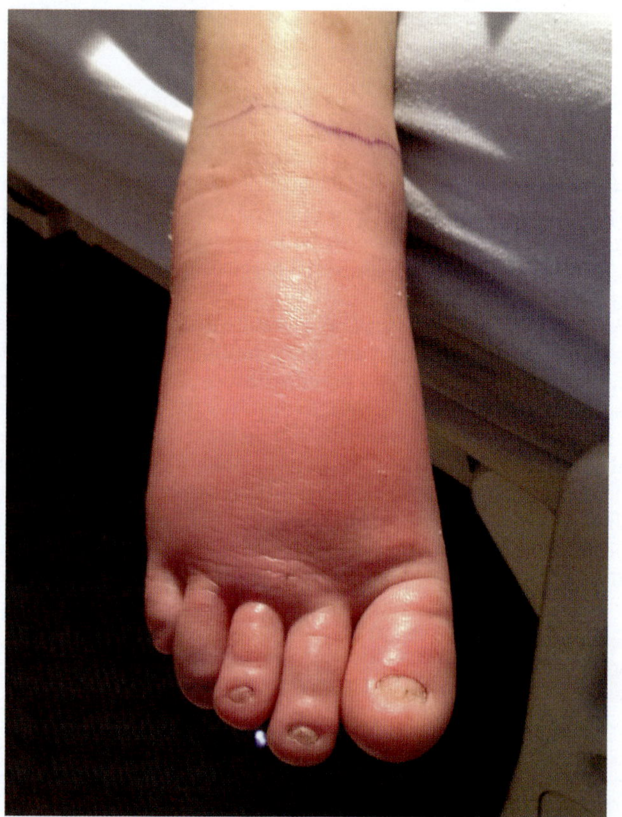

FIGURE 43-15. Clinical presentation of a patient with chronic CRPS already treated with Transcutaneous Electrical Nerve Stimulator and several oral medications. This limb has lost its function due to pain, swelling, and resultant disuse atrophy.

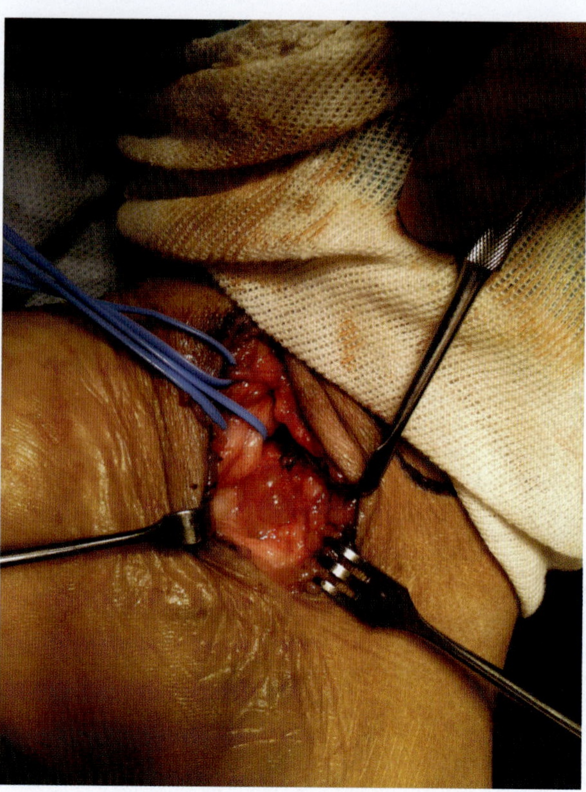

FIGURE 43-16. Intraoperative picture of a tarsal tunnel release; the space-occupying lesion was discovered and evacuated with further release of the nerve branches.

reoperation with removal of the nonunion and bone graft is often indicated to stimulate osteogenesis and eventual healing (see **Fig. 43-16**).

CONCLUSION

As depicted in this chapter, the origins of foot pain are varied, originating from several anatomic, physiologic, and mechanical etiologies. The medical history and physical examination are essential to finding the etiology of foot pain. Coupled with appropriate diagnostic laboratory and radiographic tests, the diagnosis is made, and treatment typically addresses the underlying cause. For complicated and chronic pain situations, a multidisciplinary team approach is necessary to adequately treat the pain symptoms fully.

REFERENCES

1. Rigopoulos D, Larios G, Gregoriou S, Alevizos A. Acute and chronic paronychia. *Amer Fam Physician*. Feb 1, 2008;77(3):339-346.
2. Freeman DM. Corns and calluses resulting from mechanical hyperkeratosis. *Amer Fam Physician*. Jun 1, 2002;65(11):2277-2280.
3. Bavinck JN, Eekhof JA, Bruggink SC. Treatments for common and plantar warts. *BJM*. Jun 7, 2011;342:d3119.
4. Walter JH, Goss LR. How to detect soft tissue tumors. *Podiat Today*. Jun 2003;16(6):50-54.
5. Gianni C. Update on antifungal therapy with terbinafine. Giornale italiano di dermatologia e venereologia: organo ufficiale, Societa italiana di dermatologia e sifilografia. Jun 2010;145(3):415-424.
6. Hofbauer, MH Shane-Reeves AM. Lesser digital surgery: arthroplasty, arthrodesis, and flexor tendon transfer. In: Chang TJ, eds. *Master Techniques in Podiatric Surgery: The Foot and Ankle*. Philadelphia, Pa: Lippincott Williams & Wilkins; 2005:35-48.

7. Johnson KA. Tibialis posterior tendon rupture. *Clin Orthop Rel Res.* Jul-Aug 1983;(177):140-147.
8. Morton TG. A peculiar and painful affection of the fourth metatarsophalangeal articulation. *Amer J Med Sci.* Jan 1876;71:141; American Periodicals pg 37.
9. Mulder JD. The causative mechanism in morton's Metatarsalgia. *J Bone Joint Surg.* Feb 1951;33B(1):94-95.
10. Bennett GL, Graham CE, Mauldin DM. Morton's interdigital neuroma: a comprehensive treatment protocol. *Foot Ankle Int.* Dec 1995;16(12):760-763.
11. Terkeltaub R, Edwards NL. Disease definition and overview of pathogenesis of hyperuricemia and gouty inflammation. In: *Gout: Diagnosis and Management of Gouty Arthritis and Hyperuricemia.* 2nd ed. West Islip, NY: Professional Communications, Inc.;2011: 15-46.
12. Martel W. The overhanging margin of bone: roentgenologic manifestations of gout. *Radiol.* 1968;91:755-756.
13. Khan KM, Cook JL, Kannus P, Maffulli N, Bonar SF. Time to abandon the tendinitis myth: painful, overuse tendon conditions have a non-inflammatory pathology. *BJM.* Mar 2002;324(16): 626-627.
14. Gerver JP, Williams GN, Scoville CR, et al. Persistent disability associated with ankle sprains: a prospective examination of an athletic population. *Foot Ankle Int.* 1998;19:653-660.
15. Landeros O, Frost HM, Higgins CC. Post-traumatic anterior ankle instability. *Clin Orthop Rel Res.* Jan-Feb 1968;56:169-178.
16. Thompson IC, Doherty JG. Spontaneous rupture of the tendon of Achilles: a new clinical diagnostic test. *J Trauma.* 1962;2:126-131.
17. Cetti R, Andersen I. Roentgenographic diagnosis of ruptured Achilles tendons. *Clin Orthop Rel Res.* 1993;286:215-221.
18. Whitesides TE, Henry TC, Morimoto R, et al. Tissue pressure measurements as a determinant for the need of fasciotomy. *Clin Orthop Rel Res.* 1975;113(4):3-51.
19. Borg AA. Reflex sympathetic dystrophy syndrome: diagnosis and treatment. *Disabil Rehabil.* 1996;18(4):174-180.
20. Schon LC, Mann RA. Diseases of the nerves. In: Coughlin MJ, Mann RA, Saltzman CL, eds. *Surgery of the Foot and Ankle.* 8th ed. Philadelphia, Pa: Mosby Elsevier; 2007:613-685.
21. Juckett G, Hartman-Adams H. Management of keloids and hypertrophic scars. *Amer Fam Physician.* Aug 2009;1:80(3):253-260.
22. Seddon HJ. A classification of nerve injuries. *BJM.* August 29, 1942;2(4260):237-239.
23. Sunderland S. *Nerves and Nerve Injuries.* 2nd ed. New York, NY: Churchill Livingston; 1978.
24. Downey MS, Bernstein SA. Augmentation of bone growth and healing. In: Banks AS, Downey MS, Martin DE, Miller SJ, eds. *Foot and Ankle Surgery.* 3rd ed. Philadelphia, Pa: Lippincott Williams & Wilkins; 2001:2051-2064.

SECTION D

Abdomen, Pelvis, and Genitalia

Pelvic and Abdominal Pain

Harrison Kibe
Jessica B. Jameson
Jyotsna V. Nagda

INTRODUCTION

Pelvic and abdominal pain is a common diagnostic and management dilemma that spans a wide diversity of clinical settings. One of the most significant challenges in the diagnosis and management of these conditions is the lack of consensus for diagnostic criteria.

PELVIC PAIN

Pelvic pain refers to pain primarily in the anatomic pelvis, anterior abdominal wall at or below the umbilicus. It is a common presenting symptom in women and, occasionally, in men, both as an acute or a chronic symptom. Chronic pelvic pain is noncyclic pain of a duration of at least 6 months in the pelvis, anterior abdominal wall at or below umbilicus, lumbosacral back, or buttock that is severe enough to cause functional disability requiring medical evaluation.

ABDOMINAL PAIN

Abdominal pain is a generic term for focal or general discomfort localized to the abdominal region. Recurrent abdominal pain is defined as at least three separate episodes of abdominal pain that occur in a 3-month period. Despite recent technologic advances, the diagnosis and treatment of chronic, recurrent abdominal pain has remained a challenge.

Pain is a subjective sensation that patients often find difficult to describe. In contrast to other areas of the body, the abdominal and pelvic organs have a poorly developed sensory system, which contributes to the patients' difficulty in describing and localizing the pain.

Both pelvic and abdominal pain can be of visceral or somatic etiology.

VISCERAL PAIN

Visceral pain results from activation of visceral nociceptors. Visceral structures are highly sensitive to stretch, distension, ischemia, and inflammation but are relatively insensitive to other stimuli such as cutting or burning. Visceral pain is diffuse, poorly localized, often referred to other structures, and associated with autonomic and somatosensory reflexes and strong negative affective symptoms.

Visceral abdominal pain is transmitted from nociceptors found on the walls of the abdominal viscera via sympathetic (thoracic branches and lumbar splanchnic nerves synapsing in subsidiary plexuses: celiac, splenic, hepatic, aorticorenal, superior mesenteric, adrenal) and parasympathetic (vagus and nervi erigentes S2–4; motor and sensory) pathways. Visceral nociceptors are polymodal—activated by mechanical, thermal, and chemical stimuli—and sensitize after tissue insult. Some visceral nociceptors are silent, which can be recruited in certain disease states like inflammation. Visceral pain is nonspecific because of wide divergence and a relatively small number of afferent fibers innervating a large area with extensive ramifications. Patients usually have difficulty localizing the source of pain and will describe it as aching, cramping, or burning that fluctuates in intensity. Visceral pain usually is paroxysmal, colicky, deep, squeezing, and diffuse, and it may be referred to other structures. Functional visceral disorders like irritable bowel disorders and functional dyspepsia are characterized by hypersensitivity, often in the absence of pathological explanation for the discomfort and pain.

Viscero-somatic convergence and viscero-visceral convergence of sensory pathways play an important role in the manifestation of acute and chronic visceral pain syndromes.

The phenomenon of referred pain is secondary to viscero-somatic convergence, which is the convergence of visceral afferent nerve fibers entering the spinal cord at the same level as the superficial, somatic structures entering the spinal cord.

Visceral pain syndromes affecting different organ systems often coexist due to viscero-visceral convergence—that is, a visceral afferent from different organs converging on the same spinal segments. Cross-organ sensitization between the lower gut and pelvic gynecologic and urinary organs leads to a major challenge in the diagnosis and clinical management of abdominal and pelvic pain. Patients with functional bowel disorders often also complain of pelvic pain or symptoms consistent with interstitial cystitis. Conversely, many patients with interstitial cystitis also suffer from functional bowel disorders. Both peripheral and central mechanisms are involved in the generation and maintenance of cross-organ sensitization.

PELVIC PAIN

CLASSIFICATION OF PELVIC PAIN

Pelvic pain has a number of classifications (**Table 44-1**).

Prevalence Approximately 9 million women in the United States have pelvic pain: 10% of all gynecologic office visits are for pelvic pain; 44% of all gynecologic laparoscopies and 10% to 15% of hysterectomies are for chronic pelvic pain; 30% of women presenting to a pain clinic have already undergone hysterectomy. The male pelvic pain syndrome comprises 8% of all urologic visits and 1% of all visits to primary care physicians.

The economic impact is enormous, with medical costs of $1.2 billion per year and missed work and productivity totaling more than $15 billion per year.[1,2]

Pelvic Anatomy Any discussion of pelvic pain requires an appreciation of the spatial relations of the pelvic viscera, along with their vascular supply and innervations.

The bony pelvis serves as the wall of the pelvis, and the pelvic diaphragm acts as its floor. The pelvis is lined by an intricate vascular tree and traversed by sympathetic and parasympathetic afferent, visceral afferent, and efferent nerves from the lumbar and sacral plexus.

The bony pelvis includes two hip bones formed from the fusion of the ischium, ilium and pubis, sacrum, and coccyx. The two innominate bones form the sides of the pelvis. They are joined in front at the symphysis pubis and articulate with the sacrum and coccyx in back.

The pelvis is divided into a major pelvis and a minor pelvis and is separated by the pelvic brim, which also serves as the boundary between the abdominal and pelvic cavities (**Fig. 44-1**). The pelvis contains the bladder and the paravesical fossae anteriorly, the rectum and the

TABLE 44-1 Classifications of Pelvic Pain

Etiology	Pain Pathway	Organ System
Traumatic	Visceral	Genitourinary
Mechanical	Somatic	Gastrointestinal
Psychological		Neurologic
		Musculoskeletal

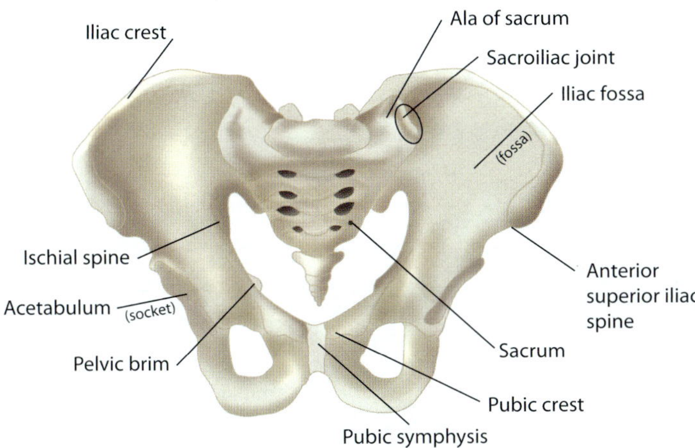

FIGURE 44-1. Anatomy of the bony pelvis.

para-rectal fossae posteriorly, and the internal genital organs in the middle (**Fig. 44-2**).

The pelvic diaphragm, or floor of the pelvis, arises anteriorly from the body of the pubis and continues posteriorly to the coccyx. It includes the levator ani muscles and the coccygeus muscles, holds the lower part of the rectum, and supports the bladder and vagina or prostate by maintaining sufficient intraabdominal pressure. Beneath the diaphragm is the perineum, with the external genitalia.

The pelvic vasculature resembles a woven lining composed of large, thin-walled veins through which the arteries thread their way.

The veins are divided into vesicle, uterine and vaginal or prostatic, and rectal venous plexuses, which drain into the internal iliac vein and into the inferior mesenteric veins via the superior rectal (hemorrhoidal) vein, eventually reaching the portal vein. The middle rectal vein emerges from the lower part of the side of the rectum, passes to the internal iliac vein, and anastomoses with the superior and inferior rectal veins and with the other plexuses of pelvic veins (**Fig. 44-3**).

The arteries of the pelvis arise from the internal iliac artery, which runs retroperitoneally, is posterior to the ureter, and is divided into anterior and posterior divisions. The anterior division has seven branches, and the posterior division has three. Collateral circulation is abundant (**Fig. 44-4**).

The major afferent pathways for nociception from the female pelvic organs travel with the sympathetic nerve bundles and have cell bodies in the thoracolumbar distribution.

The suprapubic region is innervated by the iliohypogastric nerve (L1, L2). The inguinal area and the base of scrotum or labia are supplied by the ilioinguinal nerve (L1, L2). The skin of the penis is supplied by the two dorsal nerves of the penis, which are branches of pudendal nerves. The skin of the scrotum and perineal skin are supplied by the posterior scrotal nerves (S2, S3, and S4). The skin between the anus and coccyx is innervated by the lower sacral and coccygeal plexus. The lower third of the vagina is supplied by the pudendal nerve. The genital branch of the genitofemoral nerve supplies the lateral side of the scrotum, the vulva, and the cremasteric muscles (**Fig. 44-5**).

There are sympathetic, parasympathetic, and visceral somatic afferent nerves to the pelvic viscera. The sympathetic nerves cause muscular contraction and vasoconstriction, whereas the parasympathetic nerves cause relaxation and vasodilation.

Most of the autonomic fibers enter the pelvis through the superior hypogastric plexus, which is located bilaterally at the lower third of the fifth vertebral body and the upper third of the first sacral vertebra at the sacral promontory. This plexus is primarily sympathetic and is formed by the confluence of lumbar sympathetic chains and branches of the aortic plexus containing fibers that traverse the celiac and

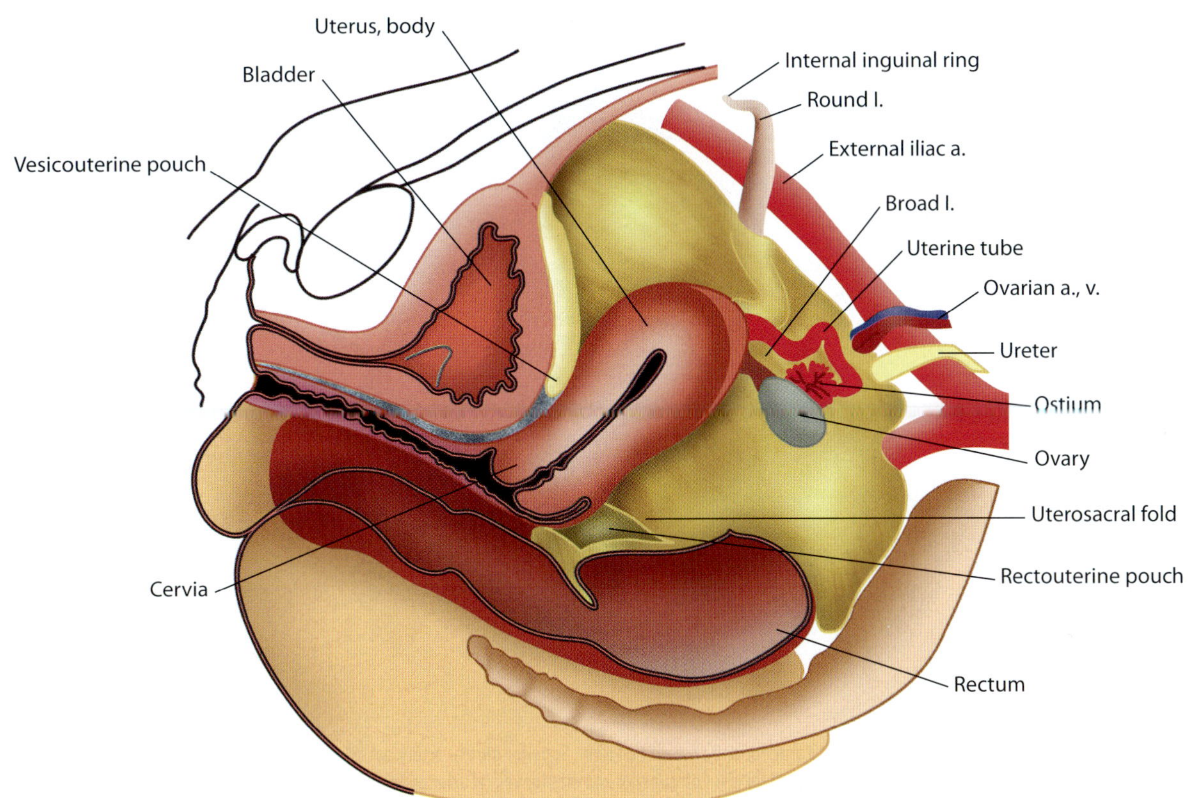

FIGURE 44-2. Peritoneal relationships in the female. (Reproduced with permission from Hinman F Jr. *Atlas of Urosurgical Anatomy*. Philadelphia, Pa: WB Saunders, 1993.)

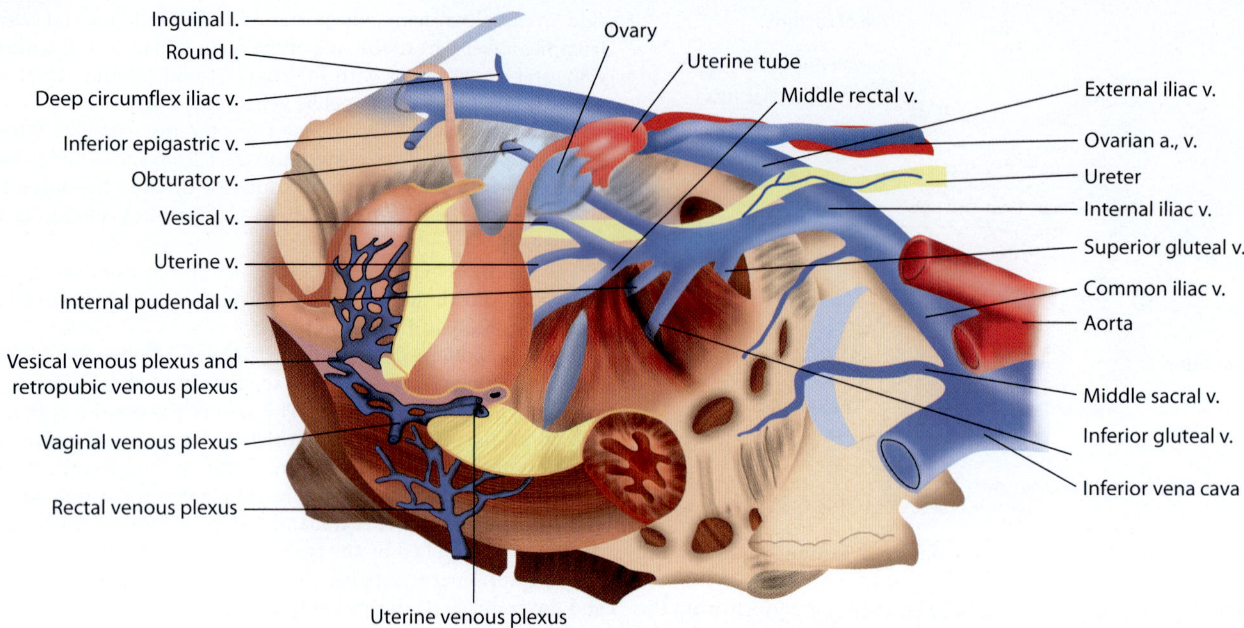

FIGURE 44-3. Veins of female pelvis. (Reproduced with permission from Hinman F Jr. *Atlas of Urosurgical Anatomy*. Philadelphia, Pa: WB Saunders, 1993.)

inferior mesenteric plexus. The superior hypogastric plexus divides into the right and the left hypogastric nerves, which descend laterally to the sigmoid colon to reach the inferior hypogastric plexus.

The inferior hypogastric plexus is located against the inside of the pelvis, lateral to the uterovaginal junction and the rectum. It is the major neuronal integrative center in the pelvis. It innervates multiple pelvic organs, including the urinary bladder, proximal urethra, distal ureter, rectum, and internal anal sphincter, as well as genital and reproductive structures via communication through the uterovaginal plexus and the vesical and the inferior rectal plexus.

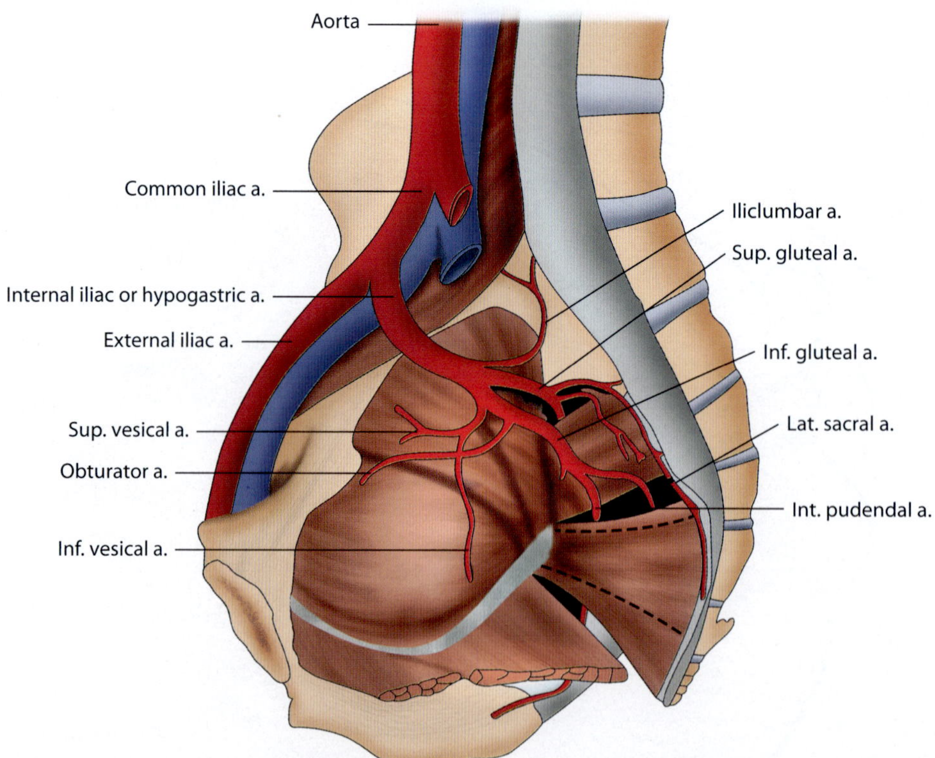

FIGURE 44-4. Internal iliac (hypogastric) artery branches into anterior and posterior division. Superior gluteal artery passes through superior portion of greater sciatic foramen. Inferior gluteal artery enters foramen below piriformis muscle. Inferior gluteal artery gives off superior and inferior vesical arteries and obturator artery before entering foramen. (Two unpaired arteries in the pelvis, the median sacral and superior rectal, are not shown.) All these arteries enter the pelvis extraperitoneally and may be ligated with impunity. (Modified from Skandalakis LJ, Gadacz TR, Mansberger AR Jr, Mitchell WE Jr, Colborn GL, Skandalakis JE. *Modern Hernia Repair*. Pearl River, NY: Parthenon, 1996; with permission.)

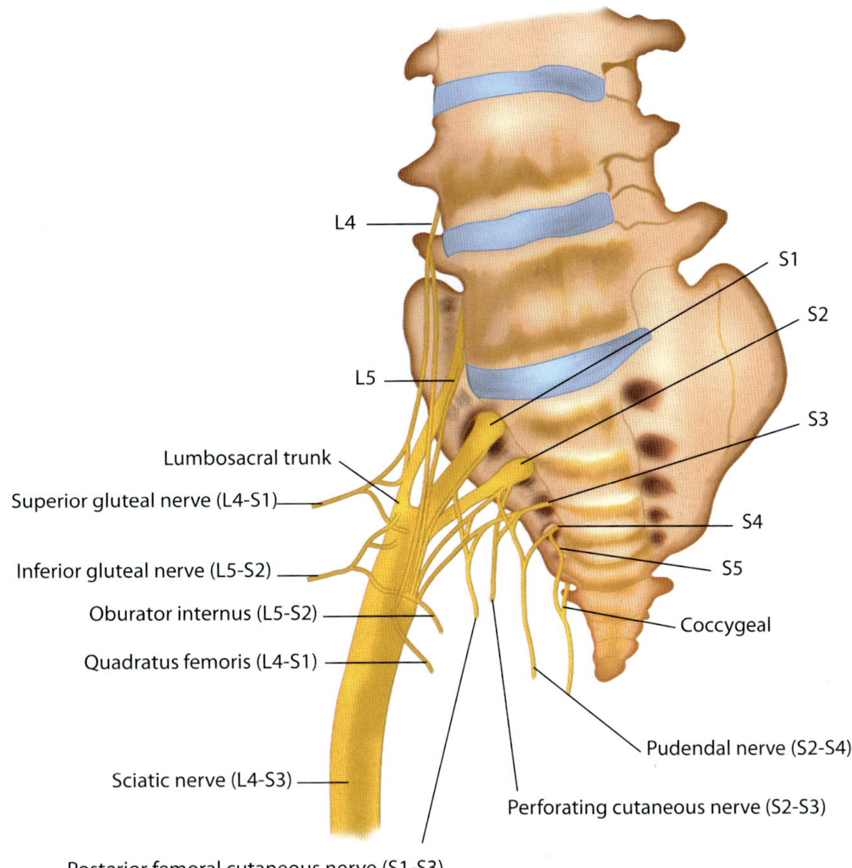

FIGURE 44-5. Formation of lumbosacral trunk and further formation of sciatic and pudendal nerves (highly diagrammatic).

The parasympathetic nerves, which are branches of anterior rami of the S2, S3, and S4 nerve roots, traverse the inferior hypogastric plexus, in contrast to the superior hypogastric plexus, which is situated predominantly in the extending tissue postero-anteriorly and parallel to the pelvic floor. The location and configuration of the inferior hypogastric plexus does not lend itself to surgical or chemical extirpation (**Fig. 44-6**).

The sensory nerves from the uterus accompany the sympathetic nerves and enter the spinal cord at the T11 and T12 level, and refer pain to the abdomen. The S2, S3, and S4 afferents from the cervix are referred to the lower back and lumbosacral area.[1,2]

The ganglion impar (also known as the ganglion of Walther) is a solitary retroperitoneal structure located at the level of the sacrococcygeal junction that marks the termination of the paired paravertebral chains. It receives fibers from the lumbar and sacral portions of the sympathetic and parasympathetic nervous system and provides sympathetic innervation to portions of the perineum, rectum, and genitalia.

Acute Pelvic Pain Acute pelvic pain refers to pelvic pain that has been present for less than 6 months. It is caused by structural disruption or physiologic dysfunction. The etiology of acute pelvic pain is presented in **Table 44-2**.

Ninety-eight percent of women with ectopic pregnancy experience unilateral pain, which may be accompanied by light or missed menses. Symptoms of pregnancy such as nausea and breast tenderness may be present.[3]

The pain of ovarian cysts may be dull and aching, localized to the side of the abscess, and accompanied by pelvic tenderness. An ovarian cyst with a twisted pedicle can cause acute pain, which becomes intermittent when the pedicle untwists. Other symptoms include nausea and vomiting, diarrhea or constipation, and leukocytosis.

Symptoms of a palpable mass, delayed menses, and pelvic tenderness also occur with corpus luteum cysts, which can bleed into the peritoneum and mimic pelvic inflammatory disease.

Pelvic inflammatory disease (PID) is defined as a spectrum of upper genital tract inflammatory disorders that may include endometritis, salpingitis, tubo-overian abscess, and pelvic peritonitis. The diagnosis should not be considered conclusive without a positive cervical culture. The primary pathogens are *Neisseria gonorrhea* and *Chlamydia trachomatis*. Cervical cultures for *Chlamydia* can detect up to 80% of cervical infections, and antibody testing, enzyme-linked immunosorbent assay, and DNA probe testing can detect 60% to 90% of infections. Because of this wide range in positive findings, specimen cultures from the urethra and anus should also be considered.

Tubo-ovarian abscesses may occur as a complication of PID, in postpartum and postoperative patients, and in women with implanted intrauterine devices. Bacteria present in tubo-ovarian abscesses occur in the lower genital tract and may not be the same agents involved in PID.[4]

Chronic Pelvic Pain Pelvic pain is considered chronic when it has been present for at least six months. It may initially be an acute episode, transition into episodic pain, and then persist for 6 months or longer. Several causes for chronic pelvic pain exist on both female and male patients.

Female Chronic Pelvic Pain

Differential Diagnosis of Female Chronic Pelvic Pain

- Endometriosis
- Adenomyosis
- Uterine leiomyomas
- Cervical/endometrial/ovarian cancer

- Ovarian remnant syndrome
- Primary and secondary dysmenorrhea
- Premenstrual syndrome
- Pelvic congestion syndrome
- Sympathetic pelvic syndrome
- Focal vulvitis
- Irritable bowel syndrome
- Inflammatory bowel disease
- Interstitial cystitis/painful bladder syndrome
- Infectious cystitis
- Musculoskeletal and myofascial pain
- Chronic pelvic pain without obvious pathology
- Psychogenic pelvic pain

Endometriosis Endometriosis is the presence of ectopic endometrial glands and stroma outside the uterine cavity. In addition to persistent pelvic pain, patients with endometriosis may have dysmenorrhea, dyspareunia, back pain, and rectal discomfort. The symptoms are related to the site of the endometrial implant. However, the intensity of the pain may not correlate with the size of the implant.[5] The incidence of endometriosis is 1% to 2% of the general female population and 15% to 25% of infertile women. Some patients may remain asymptomatic until they are evaluated for infertility. Definitive diagnosis can only be made by gynecologic laparoscopy, although elevated serum CA-125 levels correlate with severity and reflect the course of the disease. Treatment includes medical and surgical options. Medical options include oral contraceptives, Medroxy-progesterone acetate, danazol, and gonadotrophin-releasing analogues. The goals of surgery are to restore normal pelvic anatomy and to resect, coagulate, or vaporize all endometrial implants.

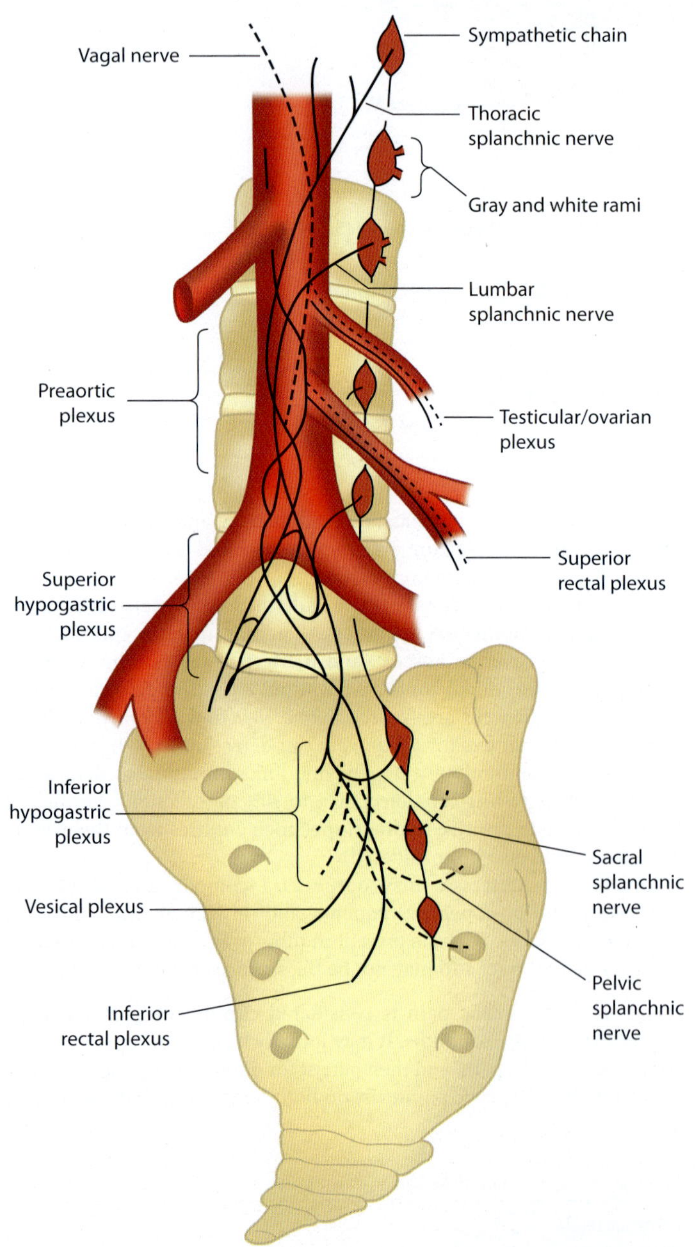

FIGURE 44-6. Neuroanatomy of visceral pelvic pain. (Reproduced with permission from Boscher H. Blockade of the superior hypogastric plexus block for pelvic pain. *Pain Practice* 2001; 1:165.)

TABLE 44-2 Differential Diagnosis of Acute Pelvic Pain

Differential Diagnosis of Acute Pelvic Pain
Ectopic pregnancy
Complications of pregnancy
Ruptured cysts
Ovarian and adnexal torsion
Uterine fibroids
Pelvic inflammatory diseases

Adenomyosis Adenomyosis is a benign invasion of the wall of the uterus by endometrial tissue. Most patients are 35 to 50 years of age and have had a prior pregnancy. Additional presenting symptoms include dysmenorrhea and menorrhagia.

Uterine Leiomyomas Uterine leiomyomas (fibroids) are painful when they press on, or become entangled in, other structures and cause discomfort when they grow. Dyspareunia, dysmenorrhea, and pelvic pressure are frequent symptoms, along with intermenstrual, post-menstrual, and heavy menstrual bleeding. A degenerating leiomyoma may cause only episodic pain in the initial phase and then cause fever, increased pain, and leukocytosis with a left shift in the later phase. Leaking purulent material can cause peritonitis. Leiomyomas undergo malignant transformation in 2 to 3 per 100,000 women, but grow slowly. Surgical intervention is typically utilized in the management of heavy bleeding, growths of large size, and additional symptoms.[6]

Cervical/Endometrial/Ovarian Cancer Cervical cancer may be a cause of pelvic pain as it metastasizes. Ovarian cancer may be asymptomatic until later stages, after which it causes vague and nonspecific symptoms. In 90% of cases, endometrial cancer presents with vaginal bleeding or discharge. Pelvic pressure or discomfort occurs from uterine enlargement and then spread of the tumor into extrauterine structures. Any tumor that compresses the bladder or rectum can cause pressure, pain, or dyspareunia.[7]

Ovarian Remnant Syndrome Women with ovarian remnant syndrome present with unilateral constant or cyclical pain, postcoital ache, post-micturition pain, or postdefecation pain. Patients may have a history of removal of one or both residual ovaries for pain associated with pelvic adhesions or endometriosis. Although localized abdominal pain is a constant feature of the syndrome, no mass is often found on pelvic examination. Ultrasound examination is usually diagnostic, revealing a mass that must be distinguished from accessory ovaries, an embryologic variant of normal development. Treatment is surgical removal of the remnant.[8]

Primary and Secondary Dysmenorrhea Women with major gynecologic diseases can have pelvic pain in the form of dysmenorrhea. This term is applied to severe cramping in the lower abdomen, lower back, and upper thighs that occurs during menstruation. Primary dysmenorrhea is the most prevalent source of chronic episodic pain in premenopausal women. It is primarily caused by prostaglandin release from the endometrium at menses, in particular prostaglandins F_2 alpha and E_2. Cramping pelvic pain is often accompanied by nausea, vomiting, headache, diarrhea, and fatigue. Secondary dysmenorrhea and atypical cyclic pain are caused by underlying intrauterine or extrauterine pathology, such as endometriosis, adenomyosis, and other pathology that alters blood flow, increases pressure, or causes irritation of the pelvic organs.

The treatment of primary dysmenorrhea includes nonsteroidal anti-inflammatory drugs (NSAIDs) and oral contraceptive pills. NSAIDs are effective in up to 80% of cases. Other modes of menstrual hormonal suppression are recommended for patients who obtain no relief with NSAIDs and oral contraceptives. Secondary dysmenorrhea requires a thorough evaluation and treatment of the underlying cause.

Premenstrual Syndrome Premenstrual syndrome (PMS) includes mood, behavioral, and physical changes that occur during the luteal phase of most menstrual cycles. Studies suggest that about one-third of premenopausal women experience some degree of PMS. As in the treatment of dysmenorrhea, underlying illnesses, such as endometriosis and leiomyomas, should be ruled out. Treatment includes NSAIDs for pain, diuretics such as spironolactone for fluid retention, and antidepressants for dysphoria.

Pelvic Congestion Syndrome Pelvic congestion syndrome is usually seen in premenopausal women, thus suggesting that there are hormonal factors involved in pelvic venous dilation.[9] The capacity of pelvic veins to increase in size 60-fold by the end of pregnancy makes them, in the nonpregnant state, vulnerable to chronic dilation and stasis. Weakened fascial support during parturition and the vasodilating effects of cyclically fluctuating hormones augment the tendency to dilation.[10] The most common symptom is a dull, aching pain in the pelvic area that worsens on standing, walking, and lifting and is relieved by lying down. Deep dyspareunia is one of the most consistent symptoms of pelvic congestion syndrome, with an incidence ranging from 71% to 78%. The severity of the pain is determined by the extent of the venous stasis, which leads to hypoxemia and local tissue damage followed by the release of pain-producing substances. The presence of dilated veins in the infundibulo pelvic ligament, ovarian hilum, or broad ligament—combined with polycystic changes in the ovary, which may be apparent only on close inspection—is diagnostic of pelvic congestion. Imaging via ultrasound and computed tomography is important for identifying polycystic changes in the ovaries and dilated veins in the broad ligament and uterus. Medical therapy consists of oral contraceptives to suppress ovarian function and intermittent courses of anti-inflammatory agents and antibiotics when inflammation occurs secondary to local infection.[11] Surgical management includes hysterectomy and ligation of the ovarian vein. Radiologic transcatheter embolization of the ovarian veins has been used with varying success.

Sympathetic Pelvic Syndrome Sympathetic pelvic syndrome is assumed to be secondary to visceral illness being transmitted to a corresponding cutaneous region. The area of innervation includes the cervix and vagina (with innervation from the pudendal nerves, having derivation from S2 through S4), along with the uterus, fallopian tubes, and ovaries (with innervation from the sympathetic pelvic branches of T10 through T12). Repeat local anesthetic sympathetic nerve blocks are recommended in addition to the medications used in patients with chronic pain.

Focal Vulvitis Another chronic pelvic pain syndrome is focal vulvitis, characterized by burning vulvar pain and superficial dyspareunia. One study found that a majority of patients continued to have symptoms of vulvitis after Woodruff perineoplasty. The authors concluded that surgery was not the best treatment. They noted that these women often had insufficient lubrication or hypertonia of the pelvic floor, or both, during sexual intercourse. Thus, an integrated approach was recommended, including protection of the vulvar skin, relaxation of pelvic muscles, and treatment of psychosexual and relational aspects of the disorder.[12]

Irritable Bowel Syndrome One study of women with chronic pelvic pain found that more than 75% had irritable bowel syndrome. Among women referred to a gynecologic clinic for dysmenorrhea, dyspareunia, and abdominal pain, half had significantly more symptoms of irritable bowel syndrome than did those referred for symptoms other than pain. Irritable bowel syndrome is a functional bowel disorder of uncertain etiology characterized by a chronic relapsing pattern of abdomino pelvic pain and bowel dysfunction with constipation or diarrhea, or both. It affects 10% to 15% of the population. Symptoms include abdominal pain, bloating, belching, excessive flatus, diarrhea and constipation, passage of mucus, and painful defecation with a sense of incomplete evacuation. Symptoms are often worse during periods of increased stress—and the premenstrual phase of the cycle—and may accompany anxiety and depression.

The pathophysiology of irritable bowel syndrome is multifactorial, involving altered bowel motility, visceral hypersensitivity, intestinal inflammation, alteration in gut flora, and genetic and psychosocial factors. Other contributing factors include diet and prior infection. Therapeutic options range from education, reassurance, dietary modifications, psychotherapy, and hypnotherapy to adjunctive pharmacological agents, which include antidepressants, antispasmodics, 5 hydroxytryptamine (serotonin) receptor 4 agonists for constipation, 5 hydroxytryptamine (serotonin) receptor 3 antagonists for diarrhea-prone irritable bowel syndrome, and probiotics.[13] The diagnosis of irritable bowel syndrome is made by taking a careful history and by use of colonoscopy or barium enema to exclude other conditions.

Inflammatory Bowel Disease Inflammatory bowel disease may manifest the same symptoms as irritable bowel syndrome. More than 50% of patients with Crohn's disease and ulcerative colitis present with abdominal and/or pelvic pain. Ulcerative colitis is a chronic inflammatory condition characterized by relapsing and remitting episodes of inflammation of the colonic mucosa, which invariably involves the rectum and extends proximally to the other portions of the colon. Crohn's disease is characterized by transmural inflammation and by skip lesions. About 90% of patients with Crohn's disease have bloody diarrhea, whereas patients with ulcerative colitis have moderate cramping that resolves with defecation. In one study, chronic pelvic pain was reported in 35% of patients with irritable bowel syndrome and in 13.8% of those with inflammatory bowel disease.[14] Although the pathogenesis of inflammatory bowel disease remains unclear, a number of risk factors—including age, racial ethnicity, genetic susceptibility, smoking, dietary allergens, and infections of the gut with antibiotic use—have been identified.

At present, available therapies mainly rely on the control of inflammation and alleviation of abdominal pain. Pharmacotherapy is used in remission and exacerbations and the surgical options are used in severe cases. Pharmacotherapy includes aminosalicylates, corticosteroids, immunosuppressants, antibiotics, and biological agents targeted against certain inflammatory markers.[15]

Interstitial Cystitis/Painful Bladder Syndrome Interstitial cystitis/painful bladder syndrome is a chronic, progressive, severely debilitating, heterogeneous syndrome that affects the urinary bladder. It is characterized by urgency, frequency, and pain. Its etiology is poorly understood; current hypotheses focus on occult or resistant microorganisms, urothelial hyper-permeability from a defective glycosaminoglycan mucus layer, neurogenic or hormonal dysfunction, mast cell activation, and genetic susceptibility as possible causative factors. The diagnosis is made clinically, by cystoscopy with hydro-distention, and sometimes by biopsy when other pathology has been excluded.[16] This condition is underdiagnosed in women with pelvic pain. Symptoms of urinary frequency and urgency, dysuria, hematuria, and nocturia occur along with the pelvic pain. Patients have often been treated for recurrent urinary tract infections. Urinalysis results may be normal, but microscopic hematuria without white blood cells is sometimes noted. Patients must have at least two of the following symptoms: pain in the suprapubic, perineal, and urethral region; pain on bladder filling that is relieved by emptying; decreased compliance on cystometrogram; and glomerulations on endoscopy. When these criteria are not met, patients are considered to have urgency-frequency syndrome.

Treatment approaches include use of systemic agents, instillation therapy, and surgical management. Trials of systemic agents—including antihistamines, azathioprine, corticosteroids, Heparin, pentosan polysulfate, and tricyclic compounds—have shown inconsistent results. Dimethyl sulfoxide (DMSO) has been used for intravesical therapy, with varying response rates. Surgical treatments include urinary diversion procedures and augmentation cystoplasty. Denervation procedures are reserved for patients with severe, intractable disease. Hypogastric plexus blocks and neuromodulatory procedures have been used with some success.

Infectious Cystitis Infectious cystitis manifests with symptoms of suprapubic pain, dysuria, and frequency and urgency, along with pyuria and a positive urine culture. These symptoms respond to antibiotics. In about 25% of women with irritant urinary symptoms and pyuria, *C. trachomatis* is found in the urethra. Urethral syndrome occurs when the urinary bacterial count is low, urinalysis is negative, and *Chlamydia* is negative. The etiology of this syndrome is unclear, but it may be caused by chronic inflammation of the peri-urethral glands or urethral spasticity with peri-urethral muscle fatigue. Treatment is similar to that of interstitial cystitis and urgency-frequency syndrome and consists of a combination of medication, biofeedback, and reeducation of voiding habits.[17]

Musculoskeletal and Myofascial Pain Evolving lumbar disk disease and intradural neoplasms in the upper lumbar spine produce symptoms that may be interpreted as pelvic pain. Symptoms consistent with radiculopathy occur late in the course of these diseases. Musculoskeletal pain can be the result of decreased abdominal and pelvic muscle strength, decreased range of motion of the hip, and limb-length discrepancy. Trigger points for this pain may be near surgical incisions.

Surgical procedures can lead to significant postoperative pain that develops months to years afterward. An example is the Pfannenstiel incision, a horizontal incision across the lower pelvis, which can lead to pulling along the pathway of the ilioinguinal and iliohypogastric nerves. The stretching and trauma arising from labor and delivery also can lead to pelvic pain from the lower pelvis, although it may be experienced as visceral in origin.[18] Pelvic pain during pregnancy has been associated with pubic symphyseal distention. However, the degree of pain is not proportional to the degree of distention. Studies of pain in pregnancy have attempted to correlate pain with elevated hormones, such as serum concentrations of relaxin and the propeptide of Type III Pro-collagen measured in early pregnancy.[19,20]

Similar pain symptoms may occur with adhesions, which may be responsible for pelvic pain as sequelae of past infection, chronic active inflammatory state, endometriosis, and postoperative adhesions. Colposcopy is the key diagnostic procedure after history taking and physical examination. There is no systematic relation between the clinical picture and anatomic findings. A diagnosis of chronic pelvic pain is recommended in the absence of any macroscopic, histologic, and bacteriologic lesions.[21]

In laparoscopic studies, about 25% of cases of acute pain and 35% of cases of chronic pain have been attributed to adhesions. The primary sources for the adhesions are in the bowel and omentum. It has been suggested that this pain develops when adhesions fix the pelvic organs in place, hampering their motility. The pain of adhesions can be aggravated by activity. Lysis of adhesions can reduce symptoms of pain, but the duration of relief cannot be predicted. There is no strong scientific evidence that using crystalloids, macromolecular solutions, intraperitoneal heparin, corticosteroids, mechanical barriers such as intercede and Gore-Tex, or biodegradable barriers to reduce adhesions.[22]

A study of laxity of the posterior ligament support of the uterus suggests that concurrent pelvic pain is attributable to parasympathetic pain at the T12 to L1 level. The pain may result from gravitational pull on nerves that are not being supported by the lax uterosacral ligaments.[23]

Vulvar vestibulitis refers to pain that occurs during sexual intercourse. The diagnosis is based on the presence of dyspareunia that lasts for at least 6 months and red areas in the vestibulum that are extremely sensitive to touch. The etiology is multifactorial and includes repeated use of antibiotics, local treatment of *Candida* and human papillomavirus infections, use of hormonal contraceptives, frequent use of local substances that may be irritative, lack of arousal, vaginismus, and tense pelvic floor muscles. There is increased intraepithelial innervation and no inflammation. Treatment includes biofeedback, tricyclic antidepressants, psychotherapy, and surgery.[24]

Pudendal nerve entrapment should be considered as a differential diagnosis in patients with anoperineal pain. The idea that pudendal nerve entrapment is the cause of some pelvic pain syndromes has gained momentum in the past 15 years.[25,26] The pudendal nerve navigates along a tortuous path, supplying sensation to virtually the entire pelvic area, including the penis, scrotum, perineum, and rectum, as well as motor function to the pelvic floor musculature and urethral sphincter. The two major areas of entrapment include the junction of the sacrotuberous and sacrospinous ligaments and the pudendal canal of Alcock. Also, scar tissue from previous trauma or surgery in the surrounding structures can be a cause of entrapment. Evaluation includes reproduction of pain on application of rectal digital pressure at the ischial spine. In addition, rectal stimulation of the pudendal nerve trunk and a recording response in the bulbospongiosus muscle with distal motor latency longer than 5.0 msec is suggestive of pudendal neuropathy. Treatment includes fluoroscopic, computed tomography-guided, or ultrasound-guided local anesthetic and corticosteroid injections at the ischial spine[27] or the canal of Alcock; physical therapy; and neuropathic agents. Other modalities include surgical pudendal nerve decompression, radiofrequency stimulation, and spinal cord stimulation.

Coccygodynia is a common problem, characterized by pain and tenderness at the tip of the spine or in the coccyx. The pain frequently radiates to the perineal, gluteal, and posterior sacral areas; worsens on sitting; and is eased on standing. The common causes are trauma, abnormal mobility of coccyx, disc degeneration at the sacrococcygeal and intercoccygeal segments, coccygeal spicules, osteomyelitis, and tumors. Treatment includes conservative methods such as physical therapy, local heat, anti-inflammatory agents, use of cushion, injection of the sacrococcygeal joint with local anesthetic and corticosteroid, and radiofrequency ablation. Some patients—especially those with abnormal mobility of coccyx and who are refractory to conservative treatment—may benefit from coccygectomy.

Tension myalgia refers to spasm of the involved muscles, which can be the levator ani, the piriformis, or the coccygeus muscle groups. Treatment includes heat and massage, local anesthetic injection of the muscles, and follow-up exercises.[28]

Pelvic joint instability and persistent pelvic pain can occur in instances of precocious puberty and use of oral contraceptives prior to the age of reproduction. Diagnosis is based on a history of early onset of menarche. Osteoporotic sacral fractures are associated with pelvic pain.

Sports-related injuries leading to pelvic pain include pyramidal muscle hematoma, osteitis pubis, and adductor tendonitis.

Pyramidal hematomas can cause impingement of the sciatic, inferior gluteal, and pudendal nerves when the nerves are compressed between the muscle and the iliac spine.

Osteitis pubis, considered to be the most common inflammatory disease of the pubic symphysis, is a self-limiting inflammation secondary to trauma, pelvic surgery, childbirth, or overuse. It occurs more often in men during the third and fourth decades of life, causing pain in the pubic area, in one or both groins, and in the lower rectus abdominis muscle. The pain may be exacerbated by exercise or by specific movements, such as running, kicking, or pivoting on one leg, and is relieved with rest.

During physical examination, pain can be elicited by resisted long and flexed adductor contraction. A waddling antalgic gait and symphysis tenderness also can occur. Initial therapy should focus on decreasing inflammation with active rest, ice, nonsteroidal anti-inflammatory agents, and physical therapy. In selected cases, local injections with steroids are helpful. In refractory cases, surgical options are sometimes considered to excise the inflamed tissue with or without fusion of the joint.

Chronic Pelvic Pain Without Obvious Pathology Studies indicate that between 10% and 50% of chronic pelvic pain patients experience pelvic pain without pathology. The wide incidence range cited suggests there may be some ambiguity in the definition of chronic pain and in the procedures used to evaluate patients with pelvic symptoms.[29,30]

For a group of chronic pelvic pain patients, no physiologic mechanisms have been elucidated. Some of these patients have pelvic pain that is considered a somatoform disorder similar to irritable bowel syndrome, the prevalence of which is comparable to that of asthma and back pain.[31]

A syndrome of chronic pelvic pain without obvious pathology (CPPWOP) has been described, but it is unclear whether it exists because pathology that may be present has been overlooked or the pathology typically found in specific diseases is not present, thus possibly excluding damage to ligaments and smooth and striated muscle. Patients with CPPWOP have a constellation of symptoms that include intermittent pain that can vary with the menstrual cycle and is localized to the low abdomen and back and dyspareunia. Patients are typically aged 20 to 30 years of age and usually have a history of childhood sexual abuse or abuse in their present relationships.[32]

Treatment of CPPWOP is similar to that of other chronic pelvic pain syndromes and includes NSAIDs and antidepressants. Psychological intervention also plays a major role in the treatment of patients with these syndromes and may include cognitive behavioral therapy.

Psychogenic Pelvic Pain Psychobiological factors, including anxiety, depression, and possible history of sexual trauma, may play a role in patients presenting with chronic pelvic pain, particularly in patients with no obvious pathology. Studies of patients with chronic pelvic pain syndrome and chronic vulvar pain syndrome have shown a significantly higher incidence of sexual abuse compared with women who do not have a history of abuse. In addition to physical and emotional trauma, there is a significant association between sexual victimization before age 15 years and chronic pelvic pain. Sexual abuse and somatization are highly predictive factors for chronic pain. There is a higher incidence of depressive symptoms in this group of patients as well.

The association of sexual abuse and pelvic pain was the basis for psychoanalytic studies of personality development throughout the past century. The first case studies were women with the diagnosis of hysteria. The term *hysterus* is Greek for uterus, and the concept of hysteria, derived from a theory of a "wandering womb" as the root of inexplicable symptoms in women, was the basis for treatments that reflected sociocultural values about the status of women. Hysteria is no longer considered a valid diagnosis; it has been replaced in current practice by the diagnoses of conversion and somatoform disorders, which may affect both men and women. Nevertheless, the legacy of hysteria as a medical condition persists.

Hysterical conversion has been defined as somatization in which physical symptoms express a psychological conflict (often sexual) that includes affects that were not sufficiently expressed at the time of the incident and are now represented symbolically. In classical psychotherapy, after elucidating the traumatic precipitant, the next step was to clarify how affects were not expressed directly and were converted into physical symptoms. Patients were said to be using the defenses of repression, denial, and somatization to deal with their feelings. Because women were under social pressure to limit their direct expression of aggression and their vulnerability to sexual abuse, it was postulated that they were more likely to have chronic pain and to express themselves somatically.[33,34]

An alternative explanation has been sought for pelvic pain that occurs in the absence of confirmed laparoscopic and imaging findings—because not all women with chronic pelvic pain have been previously abused. The bio-psycho-social model attempts to integrate physiologic and psychological causes of pain, suggesting the existence of a mind–body dualism between psychological factors and physical symptoms. However, given newer theories on central pain mechanisms focusing on neurotransmitters and neural networks that express affective and cognitive functions, a major deconstruction of studies for chronic pelvic pain needs to be carried out before the diagnosis of hysteria can be considered obsolete.

Male Chronic Pelvic Pain Evaluation and treatment of male chronic pelvic pain is complicated by the lack of objective diagnostic criteria (**Table 44-3**).

Chronic Prostatitis Chronic prostatitis is poorly understood. The diagnosis is based on symptoms, with no measurable parameter to define the presence of the disease, its severity, or etiology. A National Institutes of Health (NIH) classification system indicates that 38% of men with chronic prostatitis have chronic bacterial prostatitis, with 7% of cases resulting from inflammatory chronic pain syndrome and 55% from noninflammatory chronic pelvic pain syndrome.[35]

The objectives of current studies include refining and standardizing the evaluation of symptoms of chronic prostatitis. Some men have elevated levels of tumor necrosis factor-α and interleukin-1β proinflammatory cytokines. Seminal cytokine levels may provide an objective measure of disease in these patients and suggest specific therapeutic strategies.[36] Patients with prostatitis report more perineal, lower abdominal, testicular, penile, and ejaculatory pain than patients with benign prostatic hypertrophy and sexual dysfunction.

Another attempt at determining objective criteria is to look for evidence of T-cell reactivity with normal prostatic proteins in autoimmune prostatitis. In one study, the CD4 T-cell proliferative response to seminal plasma was found to be statistically significant in men with a history of chronic prostatitis and chronic pelvic pain syndrome, but it was not statistically significant in normal men.[37] In studies using color Doppler ultrasonography, chronic prostatitis was associated with abnormal prostate blood flow in men with and without inflammation in comparison with controls.[38]

In a study of men with pelvic pain, the reported locations of the pain were the prostate or perineal region, or both, in 45.6% of cases; the scrotum or bladder in 38.8% of cases; the penis in 5.8%; the bladder in 5.8%; and the lower abdomen and back in 1.9%.[39] Regardless of the location, most subjects had increased urethral sensitivity, suggesting an apparent association of pelvic floor dysfunction with pelvic pain. Treatment was aimed at modulating the pelvic floor with biofeedback, medication like alpha blockers, antibiotics, 5 alpha reductase inhibitors, and sacral anterior root stimulation.[40]

Pelvic Floor Tension Myalgia Pelvic floor tension myalgia may also contribute to the symptoms in men with chronic pelvic pain syndrome. The presence of detrusor instability, hypersensitivity to filling, or bladder-sphincter pseudodyssynergia on pretreatment urodynamic studies is not predictive of treatment results. Treatment recommendations include a formalized program of neuromuscular reeducation of the pelvic floor muscles plus interval bladder training to improve

TABLE 44-3 Differential Diagnosis of Chronic Pelvic Pain in Men
Chronic prostatitis
Pelvic floor tension myalgia
Pelvic varicocele
Seminal vesicle dystrophy
Irritable bowel syndrome
Inflammatory bowel disease
Interstitial cystitis
Infectious cystitis

objective measures of pain, urgency, and frequency in patients with chronic pelvic pain syndrome.[41]

Pelvic Varicocele and Seminal Vesicle Dystrophy Pelvic varicocele and seminal vesicle dystrophy are other causes of pelvic pain. In men, diagnosis of varicocele is based on clinical findings (in contrast with women, in whom instrument evaluation is needed to identify causes such as incontinence of ovarian veins or development of adnexal varicosities). Treatment of male varicocele involves percutaneous sclerotization, surgical excision, or therapeutic embolization.[42]

TREATMENT APPROACHES

Medical Therapy NSAIDs have been studied extensively in the treatment of primary dysmennorrhea and have proven efficacy in various causes of pelvic pain. Combination estrogen-progestin oral contraceptives, danazol, and gonadotropin-releasing hormone agonist are used in a stepwise sequence in the management of pelvic pain secondary to endometriosis. Other adjuvant medications, such as tricyclic antidepressants, have a role in some chronic pelvic pain conditions.

Neural Blockade Superior Hypogastric Plexus Block This block modulates pain that results from a sympathetic mechanism originating in the pelvic viscera. Several techniques have been described for performing it. Needle placement with fluoroscopy from the posterior approach, using landmarks and coaxial imaging technique, is commonly used. A transdiscal approach through the L5–S1 disk using fluoroscopy or CT guidance has been reported. An anterior approach under CT guidance may be used in selected cases. Neurolytic hypogastric plexus is quite effective in relieving pelvic pain in patients with gynecologic, colorectal, or genitourinary cancer[43] (**Fig. 44-7**).

Ganglion Impar Block This block is used to evaluate and manage pain of sympathetic origin that has its root in the perineum, rectum, or genitalia. There are various techniques for performing this block. One technique uses fluoroscopic guidance and an approach via the trans-sacrococcygeal with a straight needle.[44] Another technique involves entering at the level of the anococcygeal ligament with a curved needle.[45] Neurolysis of ganglion impar is used for refractory cases of perineal pain. Neurolysis can be achieved by using chemicals such as phenol or by cryoablation or radiofrequency lesioning (**Fig. 44-8**).

Pudendal Nerve Blockade Pudendal nerve block is an effective diagnostic and/or therapeutic modality for perineal pain. Various approaches such as transperineal, transvaginal, computerized tomography (CT) guided, fluoroscopy guided, and sono guided have been well described.

In women, the block can be performed transvaginally with the patient in the lithotomy position. The needle tip must be advanced through the sacrospinous ligament just past the ischial spine. The transperineal approach is used in men. CT-guided pudendal nerve block has also been reported as a very effective technique in the treatment of pudendal neuralgia.[46] The fluoroscopy-guided approach is now one of the most commonly practiced approaches. With the patient in prone position, the C-arm is tilted in the ipsilateral oblique angle to visualize the ischial spine. The needle is then guided toward the ischial spine.[47] The ultrasound-guided technique has also been described for blocking the pudendal nerve as it passes between the sacrospinous and sacrotuberous ligaments.

Neuromodulation Several different techniques of neuromodulation—including spinal cord stimulation, sacral root stimulation, pudendal nerve stimulation, and even tibial nerve stimulation—have been described for pelvic pain. Sacral neuromodulation, which involves insertion of sacral nerve stimulators, has been performed for patients with voiding disorders, including urinary urge continence, urgency-frequency, and nonobstructive urinary retention; for patients with intractable interstitial cystitis; and for those with chronic intractable pelvic pain.[47] This technique is especially beneficial in patients with bladder sphincter dysfunction because it restores balance between the sacral reflexes. Electrical stimulation of the S3 nerve activates the pelvic floor and modulates innervations of the bladder, sphincter, and pelvic floor. Neuromodulation has also been described as beneficial in male chronic pelvic pain syndrome.

Neuraxial Drug Delivery Delivery of an analgesic into the epidural or subarachnoid space is used most often in the management of patients with pain secondary to malignancy. Opioids remain the most commonly used drugs for this therapy; however, several other agents, such as local anesthetics and clonidine, can be used in conjunction.

Neuroablation In patients with unilateral pelvic pain secondary to malignancy, cordotomy or rhizotomy can be used in selected patients. The side effects include paresis, ataxia, and bladder dysfunction.

Surgical Therapy

Laparoscopy In a review of 1524 gynecologic laparoscopies performed for chronic pelvic pain, endometriosis was the most commonly diagnosed disorder (33%), followed by adhesive disease (24%), chronic PID (5%), ovarian cysts (3%), pelvic varicosities (<1%), leiomyomata (<1%), and a variety of other diagnoses (4%). No visible pathology was detected in 35% of patients.[12] Resection and ablation of the endometriotic lesions and lysis of adhesions are the two therapeutic approaches commonly employed laparoscopically.

Nerve Transection Laparoscopic uterosacral nerve ablation involves the destruction of the uterine nerve fibers that exit the uterus through the uterosacral ligaments. There seems to be little evidence to support the performance of this procedure.[48]

Presacral neurectomy is a procedure designed to interrupt the sympathetic innervation of the uterus at the level of superior hypogastric plexus. It is performed by incising the pelvic peritoneum over the sacrum and then identifying and transecting the sacral nerve plexus.

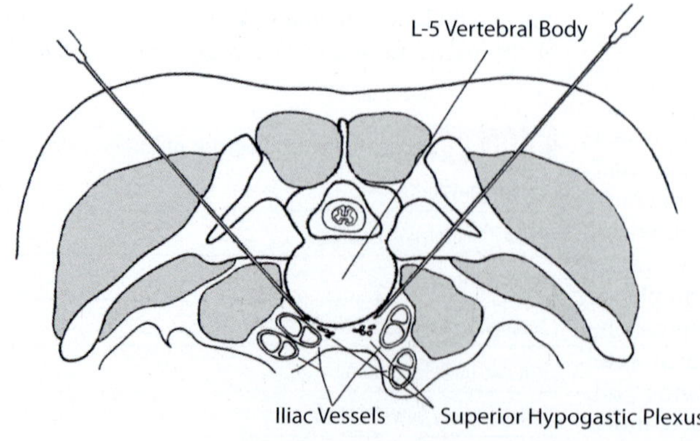

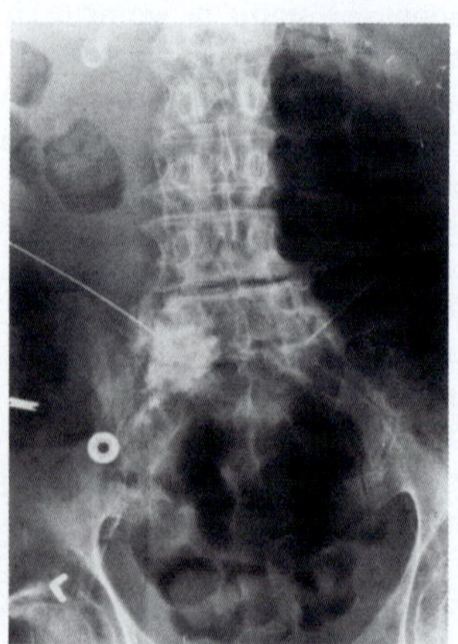

FIGURE 44-7. Superior hypogastric plexus block: transverse section illustrating proper needle placement. Superior hypogastric plexus block: AP radiograph illustrating proper needle placement and contrast spread.

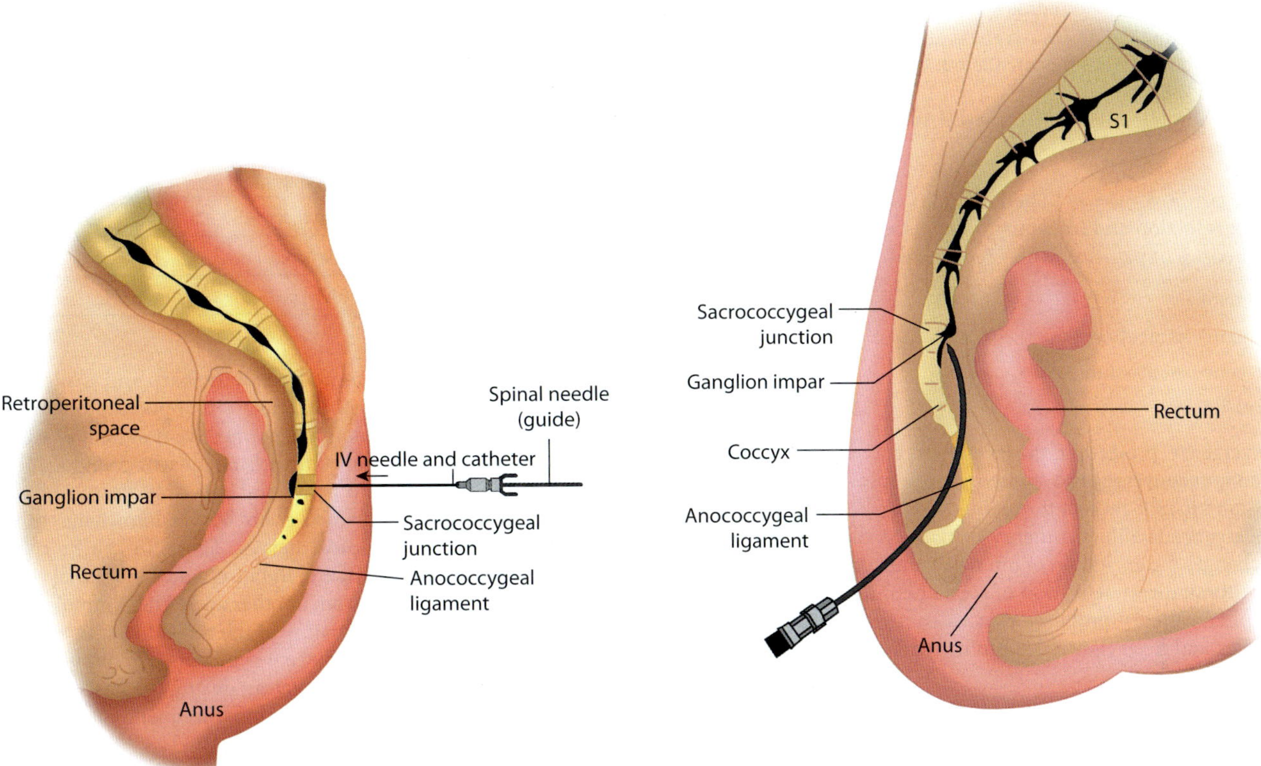

FIGURE 44-8. A 22-gauge, 7-inch spinal needle (passed through a 10-gauge, 5-inch intravenous needle and angiocath) is percutaneously advanced to the anterior border of the sacrococcygeal disc. Diagrammatic lateral view of the proper placement of curved needle for blockade of the ganglion impar.

This procedure is helpful in the management of patients with persistent midline pelvic pain.

Gonadectomy and Hysterectomy Bilateral oophorectomy with or without hysterectomy is the most effective procedure for women who have recurrent symptomatic endometriosis and who have no desire to retain reproductive function.

Physical Therapy Pelvic floor manual therapy, which involves decreasing the pelvic floor hypertonicity, may ameliorate the symptoms of urgency-frequency syndrome and interstitial cystitis.[49] Other physical therapy modalities, including heat, electrical stimulation, deep ultrasound, and massage, may be used depending on the individual need of the patient.

Botox Injections Intra-levator injection of Botulinum toxin type A (Botox) injections for refractory myofascial pelvic pain with short tight pelvic floor may provide significant relief with few self-limiting adverse effects.[50,51]

Psychological Treatment The various psychological modalities of treatment should be selected based on individual need, which can vary dramatically among patients. Behavioral therapy, progressive relaxation training, guided imagery, self-hypnosis, breathing exercises, and biofeedback are some of the techniques employed. Other options that may be more useful in the setting of chronic pelvic pain include group therapy, couples therapy, and sex therapy.

Alternative Medicine Alternative or complementary medicine is receiving greater interest from both patients and health care providers. Yoga, meditation, chiropractic treatment, acupuncture, and magnet therapies are some of the common forms of these modalities.

Multidisciplinary Management Pelvic pain is the end result of disease-initiated stimuli and the interpretation of these stimuli by the central nervous system. It is a complex interaction that involves sensory, psychological, and environmental factors. Hence, applying a multidisciplinary approach that involves employing an integrative approach to the psycho-social-mind-body paradigm is the most effective strategy in the management of patients with chronic pain states. This approach integrates medical intervention with identification and management of socioenvironmental problems, cognitive behavioral pain strategies, and treatment of concurrent psychological morbidity. Available evidence suggests that outcomes—including pain severity, general health, and functional status and disability—improve more significantly after this approach than after isolated medical or surgical interventions.

ABDOMINAL PAIN

Abdominal pain is one of the most common presenting complaints in the primary care physician's office and is often a diagnostic dilemma for surgeons. Frequently, it is a benign complaint; however, it can also herald serious acute pathology. The prevalence of abdominal pain is consistently high across diverse geographic regions and age groups.

By contrast with other areas of the body, the abdominal organs have poorly developed sensory systems that also may contribute to the patient's difficulty when trying to describe and localize the pain. For a patient to perceive pain, the autonomic nervous system must be intact.[51] The abdominal viscera are relatively insensitive to many stimuli compared with a more sensitive organ such as the epidermis. In addition to the relative paucity of sensory nerve endings, the same group of nerves may innervate several viscera. There are a few well-known nociceptive triggers in the abdominal cavity. These include abnormal distention or contraction of hollow organ walls; ischemia of the visceral musculature; direct action of chemical substances on the mucosa; formation of allogenic mediators; and traction or compression of ligaments, vessels, or mesentery.[52,53]

The location and cause of pain patterns are not well differentiated. Nevertheless, there are some recognizable pain patterns, and a careful history often can lead to the correct diagnosis. The history and physical examination provide diagnosis in approximately two-thirds of clinical presentations. Laboratory and radiologic tests are important adjuncts for investigative workup.[54-57] The invasiveness and cost-effectiveness of the proposed tests should always be considered.

CLASSIFICATIONS OF ABDOMINAL PAIN (TABLE 44-4)

Visceral Pain

Theories of Abdominal Pain Transduction There remains only a theoretical explanation for transduction and transmission of visceral pain.[58] Central and peripheral theories of pain are widely recognized.

- Central Theory
  - Convergence projection
  - Convergence facilitation
- Peripheral Theory

The convergence projection theory states that visceral fibers with nociceptive input converge onto somatosensory spinal neurons and that the viscerosomatic cells project through nociceptive pathways.

The convergence facilitation theory focuses on the fact that visceral activation changes the excitation of multiple spinal units (including pain pathways) without direct activation of spinal neurons.

The peripheral theory proposes that vasoactive substances released into cutaneous and deep tissues lead to hyperalgesia and referred pain from these structures.

Somatic and Referred Pain Differentiating somatic from referred pain can typically be accomplished by a combination of history and selective blocks.

TABLE 44-4 Classifications of Abdominal Pain

Etiology	Pain Pathway	Organ System
Physical (organic)	Nociceptive (visceral or somatic)	Genitourinary
Psychogenic (nonorganic)		Gastrointestinal
	Neuropathic	Neurologic
Duration	Psychogenic	Musculoskeletal
Acute < 6 months	Referred	
Chronic > 6 months		

Somatic pain tends to be more intense or sharp and is aggravated by movement. It is produced by the stimulation of nociceptors in the parietal peritoneum and intraabdominal connective tissues. It is usually well localized and described as constant, aching, gnawing, and throbbing. It can be relieved by opiates and peripheral nerve blocks.

Referred pain can be explained easily by our knowledge of the segmental distribution of the spinal nerves. The pain can be referred to remote areas of the body if visceral impulses enter the spinal cord at the same level as afferent nerves from another area. These impulses are mistakenly interpreted as pain initiating at the second site. In addition, the pain may spread cranially to adjacent segments. Diaphragmatic irritation as a result of abdominal insufflation during laparoscopy frequently presents as shoulder pain. This is the most frequently used example of referred pain (**Fig. 44-9**).

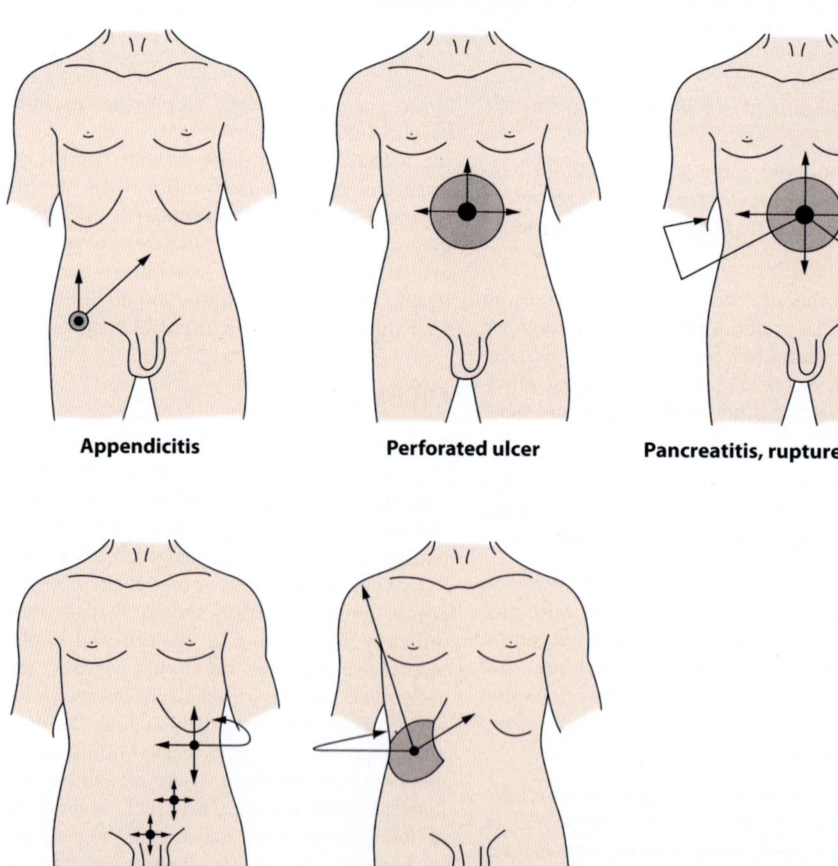

FIGURE 44-9. Examples of referred pain.

Diagnosis It is important to have an organized approach to the examination of the patient with abdominal pain. Description of current and previous disease (including psychiatric treatment) in conjunction with a social and family history will create a picture of the pain and possibly provide a presumptive diagnosis. A history of allergies and current medications must also be elicited. Knowledge of the pain pattern and character is also important. Following this, the patient should be carefully examined.[58,59] A useful algorithm is presented in **Figures 44-10** and **44-11**.

Frequently, it is easy for the patient to differentiate superficial abdominal pain from deep abdominal pain.

The more common deep abdominal pain is, by definition, either somatic or visceral (autonomic: sympathetic and parasympathetic). Somatic pain originates in the parietal peritoneum, the root of the mesentery, and near the nociceptive source. It is intense, sharp, precisely localized, associated with external stimuli, and represented at the cortical levels. Severity is related to the intensity of the stimulus. Visceral pain is often described as a poorly localized, vague (can be colicky, cramping, squeezing, dull, aching) pain associated with internal factors. Sometimes, the pain can be referred to another part of the body. It can also present as diffuse midabdominal discomfort. The intensity of the stimulus is as essential as its quality (i.e., cutting or coagulating the bowels is painless, but distention will cause pain). This pain is primarily reflexive and can be represented at the cord levels. Sometimes, severe visceral pain can generate a secondary physiologic reaction mediated by the autonomic nervous system and manifested by nausea, vomiting, sweating, lightheadedness, and salivation.

The pain from the stomach, pancreas, and hepatobiliary tree is referred to the epigastrium. Periumbilical localization occurs from the small bowel and right colon; the rest of the colon and the genitourinary organs cause pain that presents in the epigastrium. The common midline pain location is a result of the bilateral innervation of the abdominal organs from both sides of the spinal cord (**Fig. 44-12**).

To determine the source of the pain, it is important to assess its intensity, location, and character. It is also important to note its onset, whether acute or insidious, and its temporal profile. The circumstances that intensify or alleviate the pain are significant. Relief with eating or antacids suggests ulcer disease or gastroesophageal reflux. Postprandial pain—depending on its location, character, and timing—could be biliary, ischemic, or associated with a more benign condition, such as lactose intolerance or irritable bowel syndrome. Seasonal patterns are frequently seen in ulcer disease and, occasionally, with regional enteritis. The pain of inflammatory bowel disease and irritable bowel syndrome may be relieved by defecation, whereas heat usually relieves pain of musculoskeletal origin. Posture, sudden movement, coughing, straining, and sneezing may worsen the pain from peritoneal irritation or of spinal origin. The abdomen is not exempt from psychogenic pain. This may be manifested as a component of irritable bowel syndrome. Although common, psychological pain should and does remain a diagnosis of exclusion.

PHYSIOLOGICAL CAUSES OF ABDOMINAL PAIN

Esophagus Functional esophageal disorders comprise a group of conditions that present with symptoms presumed to originate from the esophagus (chest pain, heartburn, dysphagia, and globus sensation). The exact etiology is unclear; however, the different proposed underlying mechanisms include esophageal hypersensitivity due to peripheral and/or central sensitization, altered central processing of stimuli, and altered autonomic activity. Primary esophageal motility disorders such as achalasia and diffuse esophageal spasm and gastroesophageal reflux disease have to be ruled out. Heartburn is the most common symptom attributable to the esophagus. It is a burning or warm substernal discomfort that frequently migrates toward the neck. It may also be localized to the epigastrium. Eating, bending, lying down after eating, and, occasionally, vigorous exercise may precipitate it. It is not entirely clear whether heartburn is caused by the chemical irritation of acid or bile, or if secondary muscle spasm plays a role. Occasionally, the pain is described as a heaviness or tightness in the chest, with secondary restricted respiration and subsequent shortness of breath, simulating myocardial ischemia. The shortness of breath may be caused by an intercostal muscle spasm mediated by spinal reflex arcs.

Typically, esophageal pain is felt at the level of the irritation. In some patients, however, pain caused by a lesion in the lower third of the esophagus is felt in the throat or in the superior retrosternal area. The opposite is uncommon. When heartburn is severe, such as that associated with an ulcerating or infiltrating process, esophageal pain can radiate into the back, between the shoulder blades.

Pain modulators such as antidepressants, antiepileptic agents, and adenosine antagonists are often used in the treatment of functional esophageal disorders.

Stomach and Duodenum The character of pain from ulcer disease varies widely. Typically, it is located in the epigastrium. It may be a sharply localized burning or gnawing pain or a vague discomfort occurring from ½ to 2 hours after eating. Occasionally, it occurs shortly before meals or on an empty stomach, and it may wake the patient up in the early hours of the morning. Food or antacids tend to relieve it. The pain may, at times, be more localized to the right or left upper quadrant. When the pain bores through into the back, it may indicate a posterior duodenal wall ulcer with secondary irritation of, or penetration into, the pancreas. This pain is typically deep, persistent, poorly localized, and does not respond well to treatment. Unlike heartburn,

Clinical approach to chronic abdominal pain

Diagnostic workup
History
Physical exam
Psychological evaluation
Laboratory results
Radiological tests

Interdisciplinary discussion
Primary care physician
Gastroenterologist
Surgeon
Psychologist/Psychiatrist

Medical therapy
Pharmacological (Tx relevant to disease)
Enzymes replacement
Dietary restrictions

Surgical options
Diagnostic
- Laparoscopy
- Laparotomy
Definitive
(e.g. mass resection, Pancreatojunostomy, lysis of adhesions)

Analgesic/Anesthetic management
Diagnostic regional blocks (local anesthetics)
Definitive curative blocks (e.g. neurolitic)
- Celiac
- Splanchnic
- Hypogastric
- Intercostal

FIGURE 44-10. Clinical approach to abdominal pain.

General principles of diagnosis and treatment of acute abdominal pain

History	**Physical exam**	**Clinical testing**
Duration	Inspection	Blood tests*
Onset	Palpation	Urinalysis, stool exam
Mode of progression	- Guarding	Endoscopy, biopsy
character	- Rigidity	Radiography, ultrasound
- Nature	- Costal and costovertebral tenderness	Paracentesis
- Severity	Percussion	Culdocentesis
- Periodicity	Auscultation	
Differential diagnosis	Rectal/Pelvic exam	

Analgesia and respiratory therapy	**Consultation**
	Primary care physician
	specialist

Hospitalization indicated	**Hospitalization not indicated**
Nonsurgical treatment	Hydration
- Conservative measures	Analgesia
- Electrolyte balance	
- Pharmacological approach	
- Observation	
- Further investigational studies**	

Surgical treatment

Analgesic/Anesthetic options

Regional	**Parenteral**	**Alternatives**
Nerve blocks	IM/IV Narcotics/NSAIDs.	PO analgesics
- Intercostal	IV PCA	Acupuncture
- Ilioinguinal	Transdermal (fentanyl)	Tens
- Splanchnic		
- Pudendal		
- Intrapleural		
Wound infiltration		
Neuroaxial blocks		
- Epidural		
- Intrathecal		

***Routine baseline screening blood tests**

Blood count (CBC)
Electrolytes, creatinine, urea (SMA-7)
Calcium
Glucose
Liver function tests (LFT's)
Erythrocyte sedimentation rate (ESR)
C-reactive protein

****Further investigative studies**

GI tract	Gastroduodenoscopy, biopsy (gastroduodenoscopy, colonoscopy, proctosigmoidoscopy, ERCP); Barium swallow test; Abdominal x-ray
Pancreas and hepatobiliary system	Ultrasonogram ERCP Choloangiography CT with/without contrast
Abdominal vasculature	Angiogram Radionuclide scan
Genitourinary	Abdominal x-ray Ultrasonogram Cystoscopy, ureteroscopy, hysterescopy

FIGURE 44-11. Diagnosis and treatment of acute abdominal pain.

ulcer pain frequently occurs in clusters; several weeks of daily pain may be followed by variably long pain-free intervals. There may be seasonal variation with the symptoms as well.

Pain from gastritis tends to be more persistent and may be difficult to abolish. The associated nausea and vomiting may be particularly troublesome. As in heartburn, it is not known whether the pain is produced by acid irritation of the nerve endings in the ulcer bed or secondary to a spasm of antral or duodenal smooth muscle.

Epigastric pain occurring soon after eating, unrelieved by antacids, and with lack of periodicity does not necessarily exclude ulcer disease.

Differential diagnosis of abdominal pain based on localization

Epigastrium

Right upper quadrant	**Left upper quadrant**
Acute cholecystitis	Spleen disease (infarct, rupture, distention)
Biliary colic	Disease of colon splenic flexure
Duodenal peptic ulcer disease	
Liver disease (hepatitis, acute hepatic distention, abscess, carcinoma)	

Mesogastrium

Gastroenteritis
Peptic ulcer disease
Pancreatitis (acute, chronic)
Small intestine and stomach pathology

Hypogastrium

Right upper quadrant	**Left upper quadrant**
Acute and chronic appendicitis	Acute and chronic diverticulitis
Pyogenic sacroiliitis	Pyogenic sacroiliitis
Large and small bowel disease	Large and small bowel disease
Renal disease (calculus, pyelonephritis)	Renal disease
Acute rheumatic fever	
Ob-Gyn (can be bilateral) (Tubo-ovarian disease, ectopic pregnancy)	
Mesenteric lymphadenitis	

FIGURE 44-12. Differential diagnosis of abdominal pain based on location.

Pyloric channel ulcers may present in such a manner, and, unless there is associated postprandial vomiting, the diagnosis may not be made until frank gastric outlet obstruction occurs.

Small Intestine As a rule, pain originating in the small intestine is periumbilical in location and crampy or colicky in nature. Jejunal lesions tend to be associated with pain in the left upper quadrant. Ileal pain tends to localize in the right lower quadrant, and it may result from abnormal bowel motility patterns. A low threshold for the pain of bowel distention or contraction can also contribute. A lesion obstructing the lumen of the bowel, such as regional enteritis or a malignant process, may be the precipitating factor.

The pain of irritable bowel syndrome frequently is chronic and, at times, can be incapacitating. The pain is frequently located in the lower abdomen, in either the right or left lower quadrants. Its description ranges from burning, sharp, and stabbing to dull and achy. Most commonly, it is intermittent, but it may be constant, with superimposed acute attacks. The pain may remain localized or may migrate with time. Eating usually precipitates it; defecation or fasting tends to relieve it. Nausea, bloating, and dyspepsia frequently occur and may simulate peptic ulcer or biliary tract disease. A change in bowel habits is not a universal finding, but, classically, diarrhea alternates with constipation. Predominant diarrhea or constipation, however, can be part of the syndrome.

Pain from partial small bowel obstruction also occurs after meals. The closer the lesion is to the stomach, the earlier the pain occurs. Moreover, nausea and vomiting are more likely to occur when the lesion is close to the stomach. The pain is frequently described as crampy and comes in waves. Regional enteritis is suggested by localization of the discomfort to the right lower quadrant and associated diarrhea, fever, weight loss, or extraintestinal manifestations, such as arthritis and mouth ulcers. Significant weight loss and cachexia may suggest an underlying lymphoma or metastatic disease to the bowel. It may be several months before complete obstruction occurs. At this time, the diagnosis becomes more evident. As in appendicitis, the initial pain may be a nonspecific discomfort, but as the underlying process develops and eventually involves the overlying peritoneum, the pain localizes and approximates the site of the underlying disease.

Postoperative adhesions are frequently blamed for chronic or recurrent abdominal pain. Before exploration is considered, definitive evidence of bowel obstruction using plain abdominal x-rays or angulation and proximal dilation of the bowel using a barium study should be documented.

Colon Pain from the colon is typically poorly localized to the lower abdomen. However, an adenocarcinoma of the colon or diverticula of the colon with secondary microperforation and abscess formation may have localized symptoms overlying the area of disease. Pain from the rectosigmoid area, in addition to being in the left lower quadrant, may be located in the sacral region as well.

Pancreas, Liver, and Biliary Tract Because the pancreas, liver, biliary tract, stomach, and duodenum share some of the same afferent neuropathways, it is easy to understand some of the difficulties involved in the differential diagnosis of chronic epigastric pain. Diseases of the pancreas—in particular, pancreatic cancer—are some of the most difficult to diagnose. Pain resulting from pancreatic cancer usually signifies infiltration of the retroperitoneal region or celiac axis or spread to surrounding organs. Some of the pain may be a result of pancreatic duct obstruction and surrounding pancreatitis. Tumors in the head of the pancreas cause pain that is more localized to the epigastrium or right upper quadrant. Those in the tail tend to cause pain in the left upper quadrant. Lesions in the body of the pancreas can cause the pain to radiate into the back. Back pain, alone, can also be a presenting symptom.

The pain of chronic pancreatitis, which is often a result of alcohol abuse, can be constant and debilitating and can frequently lead to drug abuse. The persistent inflammation of the pancreas causes some of the pain, as does the ductal distention secondary to ductal obstruction by creation of strictures. The pain may be dull or sharp, burning, and steady. It commonly radiates into the back. Superimposed, more acute attacks last from days to several weeks. Eating, moving, or lying down may aggravate the pain; sitting up or leaning forward may relieve it.

Mechanisms of pain generation in pancreatic cancer and pancreatitis have not been completely understood. In the past, pain in these two conditions was attributed to various causes such as increased intraductal pressure, ductal strictures, and increased parenchymal pressures. It is now widely accepted that pain sensation in both pancreatic cancer and chronic pancreatitis has been identified as neuropathic due to the prominent neuroplastic changes in the form of neural hypertrophy, increased neural density, perineural invasion of inflammatory cells in pancreatitis, and cancer cells in pancreatic cancer.[53]

In patients who are not surgical candidates, the pain specialist may be asked to intervene. Neurolytic celiac plexus block has been used to treat patients who have not responded to conservative or surgical therapies.

Placement of stents during endoscopic retrograde cholangiopancreatography was used initially to decompress a dilated biliary tree. Recently, however, this technique has been used to decompress the pancreatic duct. Relief may occur if the dilated biliary (or pancreatic) duct was the cause of the pain. Both benign and malignant lesions are amenable to this technique.

Biliary pain may be due to a calculus or biliary tree dilation secondary to an obstruction. Contrary to the commonly used term *biliary colic*, the pain tends to have a gradual onset. After it peaks, it tends to reach a plateau until again, hours later, it diminishes. An attack can last from several hours to a day or more. The pain is characteristically localized in the right upper quadrant and may radiate to the right shoulder and shoulder blade, but it is also commonly felt in the epigastrium, with radiation into the back. Vomiting occurs in most patients and may provide some relief. After an acute attack, residual soreness may persist for several days to weeks. Commonly, these symptoms occur after eating, but they may become constant if the common bile duct is impacted by a stone or infiltrated by a malignant process. Associated dyspepsia is common and occurs in approximately one-quarter of all patients. It responds to antacids, further confusing its cause. The appearance of complicating cholangitis (with symptoms of fever and jaundice) usually leads quickly to the correct diagnosis.

The liver parenchyma is insensitive to pain, but relatively rapid distention of the liver capsule will initiate well-localized right upper quadrant pain. Acute processes such as viral hepatitis, alcoholic hepatitis, and cardiac decompensation with secondary liver congestion may infrequently present as right upper quadrant pain, but this pain does not evolve into a chronic complaint. Chronic, active hepatitis may follow a course of recurrent attacks of right upper quadrant pain. The pain is frequently well localized and accompanied by worsening liver function tests.

Benign focal nodular hyperplasia or adenomas associated with the use of birth control pills may cause recurrent right upper quadrant discomfort or, occasionally, a dramatic crisis of severe abdominal pain and hypotension from a hemorrhage into the capsule or peritoneum. The recurrent warning pains are likely caused by small bleeding episodes into the lesions. Bleeding into or necrosis of malignant lesions in the liver causes similar pain, but this usually is accompanied by fever and jaundice. The pain may be well localized, sharp, and steady. Any movement producing friction between the liver surface and the ribs may exacerbate this pain. When sought, a bruit over the lesion may be identified in approximately 25% of patients.

VASCULAR DISEASES OF THE BOWEL

Although mainly asymptomatic, occlusive vascular disease may be associated with chronic, recurrent, dull periumbilical, or epigastric pain. The pain of intestinal angina begins approximately 1½ hours after eating and lasts throughout digestion and absorption of the meal. Typically, at least two of the three major splanchnic vessels are affected by significant obstruction from atherosclerotic changes. It is postulated that the collateral supply is insufficient to meet the increased need during digestion, and this state of relative ischemia creates subsequent pain. Classically, this recurrent pain may create a fear of eating and can lead to severe weight loss. When patients with acute ischemia are questioned carefully, they often will report postprandial abdominal discomfort preceding the acute event by weeks to months.

Superior mesenteric artery syndrome and celiac compression syndrome are frequently mentioned in the differential diagnosis of chronic abdominal pain, but their validity is controversial. Superior mesenteric artery syndrome is described as occurring in so-called asthenic patients or patients with significant weight loss. The postprandial epigastric pain, vomiting, and distention are believed to be caused by compression of the duodenum by the superior mesenteric artery. The pain of celiac compression syndrome is not necessarily related to meals. The celiac axis frequently has a high take-off and may be compressed by the median arcuate ligament of the diaphragm or by the tissue of the celiac ganglion. Whether bowel ischemia is the cause of the pain or whether the pain originates from the celiac ganglion is also unclear.

An abdominal aortic aneurysm usually presents more acutely, but a slowly expanding or leaking aneurysm may be associated with recurrent, dull midepigastric or back pain over several months. As with pancreatic pain, sitting up or leaning forward may occasionally relieve this pain. The pulsating, sometimes tender, mass can be palpated, and a bruit may be heard.

Peritoneum The parietal peritoneum is well innervated by the branches of the spinal nerves, and, consequently, the pain perceived is well localized. Such pain is frequently associated with secondary muscle spasm of the overlying abdominal wall. The visceral peritoneum, however, has no pain receptors, and any pain that is generated is poorly defined. A malignant process most often causes chronic pain originating in the peritoneal cavity. Metastatic bowel or ovarian tumors and lymphoma are common. Mesothelioma is the most common primary tumor. Teratoma, carcinoid, or sarcoma is much less common. The abdominal discomfort is often compounded by the presence of ascites, which distends the peritoneum further and causes more pain.

In young patients of Mediterranean descent who have chronic recurrent attacks of sudden diffuse or localized peritoneal pain, familial Mediterranean fever should be considered. Abdominal tenderness, fever, and arthritis are common. Despite feeling very ill, the patient recovers in several days and is well until the next attack.

Mesentery and Omentum Recurrent localized or generalized abdominal pain in an older patient associated with the displacement of the stomach or bowel on x-ray studies should suggest a mesenteric or omental lesion. Fever, weight loss, nausea, vomiting, and a palpable tender mass may be associated with mesenteric panniculitis or retractile mesenteritis. Metastatic tumors to the mesentery are more common than primary lesions. The latter usually are fibromas, myomas, histiocytic, or lipomatous tumors. Leiomyomas and leiomyosarcomas tend to involve the omentum.

Genitourinary System The acute pain of renal colic or pyelonephritis is classic. The triad of hematuria, flank pain, and a palpable mass suggests renal cell carcinoma, but this triad occurs infrequently. The tumor is often diagnosed as a result of systemic complaints (dull upper abdominal or flank pain may be included). Perinephric abscess, although uncommon, should be considered in a patient with a history of urinary tract infections or pyelonephritis. Typically, dull upper quadrant or flank discomfort is present, accompanied by malaise and low-grade fevers.

Gynecologic problems usually cause acute pain. Depending on the patient's age, chronic lower abdominal pain, usually more localized to one of the lower quadrants, could be a presenting symptom of chronic pelvic inflammatory disease or uterine or ovarian cancer. The pain can be dull, steady, or crampy. The local irritation by the mass or inflammatory process can cause changes in the urine or bowel patterns.

MUSCULOSKELETAL CAUSES OF ABDOMINAL PAIN

Chronic Abdominal Wall Pain Chronic abdominal wall pain (CAWP) has been recognized for more than 75 years but remains a frequently overlooked diagnosis. This can lead to extensive diagnostic testing before an accurate diagnosis is achieved.[60-63] It occurs in about 10% to 30% of patients with chronic abdominal pain.

A variety of causes such as myofascial pain, thoracic radiculopathy, abdominal wall lesions including nerve entrapment, and referred pain secondary to neural convergence from abdominal or thoracic viscera have been discussed in literature.

Anterior cutaneous nerve entrapment syndrome (ACNES) is the most common cause of abdominal wall pain. This is thought to be caused by entrapment of the anterior branch of the T7 to T11 intercostal nerves as they pass through the lateral border of the rectus abdominis.[64,65] The diagnosis can typically be established via history and physical examination. The pain is often sharp, and the patient is usually able to point with one or two fingers to the exact location. A positive Carnett's sign with increased pain during muscle tensing is diagnostic. A study by Greenbaum and colleagues showed a sensitivity of 85% and a specificity of 97%.[64] False positives may result from visceral causes of pain that affect the peritoneum. Local injections of anesthetic/steroid under ultrasound guidance are the treatment of choice for patients with moderate to severe pain resulting from the abdominal wall. Pain relief is achieved in anywhere from 60% to 90% of patients and assists in confirming the diagnosis.[66-68] In some patients, neurolysis may be a possible option. In refractory cases, surgical explorations and neurectomy may be considered.

Xiphoidalgia (Xiphodynia) Xiphoidalgia is a relatively rare syndrome that presents with localized discomfort and tenderness to palpation over the xiphoid process. This can occasionally cause nausea and vomiting with pressure on the area and can be exacerbated by eating a heavy meal or by bending or twisting movements. Anti-inflammatory medications or injections of anesthetics/steroids into the area often provide a cure for the condition.[69,70]

Lower Rib Syndromes Pain syndromes involving the lower ribs have been given many names over the years, including rib-tip syndrome, slipping rib, twelfth rib, and clicking rib. The syndrome itself is characterized by reproducible pain in the lower chest or upper abdomen and a tender area located on the costal margin. In slipping rib syndrome, the rib intermittently slips out of place, causing a stretching of the ligamentous support of the ribs in the front and back. Without muscles to hold the ribs in place, loose ligaments allow extended rib movements that can cause further stretching of the ligaments, manifested as periodic episodes of severe pain and underlying chronic chest, upper abdominal, and/or upper back pain. The mobile ribs may also irritate intercostal nerves, resulting in excruciating pain around the chest into the back. Many practitioners recommend a diagnostic test called the "hooking maneuver," in which the examiner's curled fingers are hooked under the ribs at the costal margin and then gently pulled forward. A positive test may reproduce pain and may cause a click. The majority of patients with this condition are female, with a mean age of 40.[71,72]

In mild cases, simple oral analgesics, topical ice packs, and transient reduction of physical activity may be recommended. For moderately severe cases, intercostals block with local anesthetic agents and steroids may provide temporary relief. If conservative management fails or for those cases interfering with regular activities, resection of the anterior end of the rib and costal cartilage may be performed with many reports of successful outcomes.

Neuralgias Ilioinguinal, iliohypogastric, and genitofemoral neuralgias are among the common causes of lower abdominal and pelvic pain. All three nerves overlap in their pattern of innervations, which may lead to confusion in the diagnosis. The most common cause of these neuralgia is injury to the nerve induced by trauma, including direct blunt trauma to the nerve and damage during inguinal or pelvic surgery.

Ilioinguinal neuralgia is caused by compression of the ilioinguinal nerve as it passes through the transverse abdominis muscle at the level of the anterior superior iliac spine. Ilioinguinal neuralgia presents as paresthesias, burning pain, and occasionally numbness over the lower abdomen that radiates into the scrotum or labia and occasionally into the inner upper thigh.

Iliohypogastric neuralgia is caused by compression of the iliohypogastric nerve as it passes through the transverse abdominis muscle. It presents as paresthesias, burning pain, and occasionally numbness of the abdominal skin above the pubis.

Genitofemoral neuralgia presents as paresthesias, burning pain, and occasionally numbness over the lower abdomen, which radiate into the inner thigh in men and women and into the labia majora in women and the bottom of the scrotum and cremasteric muscles in men.

Treatment of these neuralgias includes simple analgesics, neuropathic agents, and nerve blocks with local anesthetic steroids. In some cases, neuromodulatory and neurolytic blocks with radiofrequency and cryoablation may be useful. Advanced therapies include surgical options to relieve entrapment and neuromodulation by using peripheral stimulation.

METABOLIC CAUSES OF ABDOMINAL PAIN

Metabolic causes of chronic abdominal pain are rare but should be considered when the usual diagnostic avenues have been exhausted. The hepatic porphyrias have many features in common, including their clinical presentation. Abdominal pain is the most prominent symptom. It is thought to result from autonomic neuropathy, which causes disturbances in gastrointestinal motility. Spasm and dilation of the bowel can cause severe pain. The frequent association of fever and leukocytosis mimics an inflammatory process. Although vomiting and constipation are frequently present, the abdomen is soft, without marked tenderness. These attacks may last from days to weeks. Fasting, infections, the menstrual cycle, and drugs whose metabolism involves the hemoproteins of cytochrome P-450 are often the precipitating factors. Such drugs include alcohol, barbiturates, anticonvulsants, estrogens, and contraceptives. Knowledge of so-called safe or probably safe drugs may be useful to the clinician treating the pain. Drugs that are considered safe include morphine and related opiates, which may be required to treat the pain in an acute attack.

In the United States, lead poisoning is primarily encountered in children. Although anemia, peripheral neuritis, and encephalopathy complete the picture, the young patient may have only lead colic, sometimes called painter's cramps. Severe, migrating, poorly localized guarding and rigidity of the abdominal wall should raise the suspicion of an acute intraabdominal event that may accompany crampy abdominal pain.

When in a hemolytic crisis, a patient with paroxysmal nocturnal hemoglobinuria may have substernal, lumbar, or abdominal pain, in addition to generalized weakness. The pain may be colicky and last for several days. The abdomen may be tender, with some guarding and even a rebound phenomenon. Venous thrombosis occurs with increased frequency in these patients. It should be considered if a sudden increase in liver size accompanies these attacks, suggesting thrombosis involving the portal system.

Hyperparathyroidism has been called the syndrome of bones, stones, and groans. Associated peptic ulcer disease or pancreatitis usually causes the abdominal pain.

The lightening-sharp abdominal pain of tabes is associated with syphilis, but it may occur with diabetes and meningeal tumors. This is a radicular syndrome resulting from damage to the large posterior lumbosacral roots.

The diagnosis of chronic recurrent abdominal pain can be a challenge to both diagnose and subsequently treat. Unfortunately, many patients with this type of pain undergo multiple surgical procedures without any significant findings. Good knowledge of the underlying anatomy and pain patterns can improve the diagnosis and subsequent treatment (**Fig. 44-13**).

PSYCHOSOMATIC CAUSES OF ABDOMINAL PAIN

The abdomen is the third most common site of pain in psychiatric patients. Diagnosis of psychological pain can be made based on exclusion criteria. There are some signs that can be helpful or supportive. Suspicion is raised when location, timing, quality, and distribution of symptoms do not relate to pathophysiologic patterns. There is often marked discrepancy between reported severity of pain and presented behavior. The patient sometimes reports pain in other parts of the body and may have a history of many negative diagnostic workups for various complaints. The onset of pain may have an obvious relationship to a stressful event.

MANAGEMENT OF ABDOMINAL PAIN

When a treatable disorder is identified, appropriate therapy should be instituted. Unfortunately, in many patients with chronic abdominal pain, a specific diagnosis is not identified despite an extensive workup. In other patients, a condition is diagnosed, but conventional methods fail to treat the disease and pain.

Medical management in most cases of chronic abdominal pain requires a multidisciplinary approach including identification of risk factors associated with disease progression and appropriate modification.

A systematic evaluation of the exact cause of pain and complications followed by appropriate treatments is essential in all patients. Analgesics are typically titrated according to the World Health Organizatin ladder principle, but, in some situations, a top-down approach may be useful to control pain and avoid sensitization of central pain pathways. Also, adjuvant analgesics should be considered at an early stage and combinations of drugs are often used.

Modification of diet, nonencapsulated enzyme therapy, somatostatin-analogues, and antioxidants can be considered as supplements to conventional analgesics in special situations. Nerve blocks can be helpful

Classification of pain (pain patterns)	
Intraabdominal disease	**Disease of diaphragm and pelvic viscera**
Parietal peritoneal disease Generalized peritonitis Primary bacterial infection Secondary bacterial infection (perforated viscera, ruptured abdominal abscess) Localized peritonitis Appendicitis, hepatitis, peptic ulcer DX, colitis, abscess, gastroenteritis, pancreatitis, distention, traction, torsion of omentum **Acute and chronic ischemia** Mesenteric embolism, thrombosis, nonorganic venous thrombosis Abdominal angina, celiac band compression Jogger's pain (? acute splanchnic ischemia) **Rapid extention of solid viscus or hollow viscera** **Obstruction of hollow viscera**	Diaphragmatic hernia, tumors, rupture Genitourinary disorders Ureteral and renal colic Pyelonephritis and cystis Renal infarct or abscess Gynecological disease Endometriosis Dysmenorrhea Salpingitis Ectopic pregnancy **Metabolic disease** Endocrinologic abnormalities *Diabetes mellitus, addisonian crisis and other* Acute intermittent porphyria Uremia Acute hyperlipoproteinemia Hereditary mediterranean fever Carbohydrate maldigestion and malabsorption *Hypolactasia, hyposucrasia, stagnant loop syndrome*
Extraabdominal pathology	**Hematologic disease**
Thoracic organ disorders Lung DX (pneumonia, embolism, pneumothorax) Heart disease (CAD, acute MI, myocarditis) Esophagus pathology (spasm, rupture, infection, inflammation) **Neruologic and musculoskeletal diseases** Disorders of brain and brain stem Spine cord compression Thoracic radiculopathy due to degenerative DX of Spine/infectious process/tumors (e.g. compression fracture, degenerative disc DX, herpes zoster infection, and postherpetic neuralgia) Myofascial pain Rib fracture and intercostal neuralgia Costochondroitis and rib/costal cartilages dislocation (slipping rib syndrome) Xiphoidalgia Traumatic hematoma Cicatrices and subcutaneous neuromas **Systemic infectious and inflammatory disorders** Tabes dorsalis Acute rheumatic disease, polyarteritis nodosa, SLE Henoch-schonlein purpura Herpes zoster Tuberculosis	Sickle cell anemia Acute and chronic hemolytic anemia Acute leukemia **Toxins and poisons and certain medications** Lead and other heavy metal digestion Spider bites (e.g. black widow) Opiate withdrawal **Pain of psychologic origin** Somatoform (psychophysiologic) Irritable bowel syndrome, peptic ulcer disease, crohn's DX, ulcerative disease Hypochondria Hysteria Conversion DX Delusional or hallucinatory pain Depression and anxiety DX

FIGURE 44-13. Classification of pain (pain patterns).

in treating acute and chronic abdominal pain. Nonspecific methods, such as antidepressants, stress reduction techniques, and behavioral approaches, often are useful in treating these difficult presentations. Nonoperative treatment for functional abdominal pain syndromes includes cognitive, behavioral, physical, occupational, recreational, and medical therapies. Detailed discussion about the role of cognitive and behavioral therapies is beyond the scope of this chapter.

Celiac plexus block and splanchnic nerve block are interventional techniques utilized for diagnostic and therapeutic purposes in the treatment of abdominovisceral pain. The richly innervated celiac plexus provides sensory input about pathologic processes in the liver, pancreas, spleen, omentum, alimentary tract to the mid-transverse colon, adrenal glands, and kidney. Chronic pancreatitis and chronic pain from pancreatic cancer have been treated with celiac plexus block to theoretically decrease the side effects of opioid medications and to enhance analgesia from medications. Fluoroscopy, CT guidance, and endoscopic ultrasound assistance may be utilized to aid the practitioner in performing the blockade of the celiac plexus.

The celiac plexus innervates the abdominal viscera with fibers arising from preganglionic splanchnic nerves, preganglionic parasympathetic vagus nerve fibers, sensory nerve contribution from the phrenic and vagus nerves, and postganglionic sympathetic fibers. Sympathetic innervation is derived from the anterolateral horn of the spinal cord as axons from T5 to T12 leave the spinal cord with ventral nerve roots to join white rami communicans (WRC) en route to the sympathetic chain. The greater, lesser, and least splanchnic nerves provide the major preganglionic contribution to the celiac plexus and transmit the majority of nociceptive information from the viscera. The splanchnic nerves are contained in a narrow compartment made up by the vertebral body and the pleural laterally, the posterior mediastinum ventrally, and the pleural attachment to the vertebra dorsally.

Although celiac and splanchnic nerve blocks share common risks, the rates of pneumothorax, thoracic duct injury, and inadvertent spread of the injected drug to the somatic nerve roots are higher for splanchnic nerve block than for celiac plexus block.

Neurolysis with alcohol, phenol, and radiofrequency techniques have been well described.

Video-assisted thoracoscopic splanchnicectomy has also been used in the treatment of chronic pancreatitis pain and in pancreatic cancer pain.[73]

CONCLUSION

Pelvic and abdominal pain remains a diagnostic and therapeutic challenge for the health care provider. Patients presenting with this are best assessed and treated using a multidisciplinary approach. Close collaboration among gynecologists, urologists, proctologists, neurologists, pain specialists, gastroenterologists, psychiatrists, psychologists, physiatrists, and neurologists is needed. Special emphasis should be placed on preventive strategies, such as screening and treatment of avoidable causes.

REFERENCES

1. Kumazawa T. Sensory innervation of reproductive organs. In: Cervero F, Morrison J, eds. *Visceral Sensation*. New York, NY: Elsevier; 1986:115-131.
2. McDonald JS. Chronic pelvic pain. In: Copeland LJ, Jarrell JF, eds. *Textbook of Gynecology*. New York, NY: WB Saunders; 2000: 741-758.
3. Bjorklund K, Bergstrom S. Is pelvic pain in pregnancy a welfare complaint? *Acta Obstet Gynecol Scand*. 2000;79:24-30.
4. Weiner SL. Acute right iliac pain. In: Weiner SL, ed. *Differential Diagnosis of Acute Pain by Body Regions*. New York, NY: McGraw-Hill; 1993:274-276.
5. Vercellini P, Trespidi L, De Giorgi O, Cortesi I, Parazzini F, Crosignani PG. Endometriosis and pelvic pain: relation to disease stage and localization. *Fertil Steril*. 1996;65:299-304.
6. Hillard PA. Benign diseases of the female reproductive tract: symptoms and signs. In: Berek JS, Adaski EY, Hilard PA, eds. *Novak's Gynecology*. 12th ed. Baltimore, Md: Williams & Wilkins; 1996:331-397.
7. Rigor BM. Pelvic cancer pain. *J Surg Oncol*. 2000;75:280-300.
8. Orford VP, Kuhn RJ. Management of ovarian remnant syndrome. *Aust N Z J Obstet Gynaecol*. 1996;36:468-471.
9. MacKay HT. Gynecology. In: Tierney LM, McPhee SJ, Papadakis MA, eds. *Current Medical Diagnosis and Treatment*. New York, NY: Lange/McGraw Hill; 2003;42:699-733.
10. Foong LC, Gamble J, Sutherland IA, Beard RW. Altered peripheral vascular response of women with and without pelvic pain due to congestion. *Br J Obstet Gynaecol*. 2000;107:157-164.
11. Charles G. Congestive pelvic syndromes. *Rev Fr Gynecol Obstet*. 1995;90:84-90.
12. DeJong JM, van Lunsen RH, Robertson EA, Stam LN, Lammes FB. Focal vulvitis: a psychosexual problem for which surgery is not the answer. *J Psychosom Obstet Gynecol*. 1995;16:85-91.
13. Camilleri M, Heading RC, Thompson WG. Consensus report: clinical perspectives, mechanisms, diagnosis and management of irritable bowel syndrome. *Alim Pharmacol Ther*. 2002;16:1407-1430.
14. Rapkin AJ, Mayer EA. Gastroenterological causes of chronic pelvic pain. *Obstet Gynecol Clin North Am*. 1993;20:663-683.
15. Sobcjak M, Fabisiak A, Murawska N, Wesolowska E, Woccjikowsk M, Zatorski H, Zwolinska M, Fichna J. Current overview of extrinsic and intrinsic factors in etiology and progression of inflammatory bowel diseases. *Pharmacol Rep*. 2014 Oct;66(5):766-775.
16. Oberpenning F, van Ophoven A, Hertle L. Interstitial cystitis: an update. *Curr Opin Urol*. 2002;12:321-332.
17. Yoon SM, Jung JK, Lee SB. Treatment of female urethral syndrome refractory to antibiotics. *Yonsei Med J*. 2002;43:644-651.
18. McDonald JS. Chronic pelvic pain. In: Copeland LJ, Jarrell JF, eds. *Textbook of Gynecology*. New York, NY: WB Saunders; 2000: 741-758.
19. Kristiansson P, Svardsudd K, von Schoultz B. Reproductive hormones and aminoterminal propeptide of type III procollagen in serum as early markers of pelvic pain during late pregnancy. *Am J Obstet Gynecol*. 1999;180:128-134.
20. Bjorklund K, Bergstrom S, Nordstrom ML, Ulmsten U. Symphyseal distention in relation to serum relaxin levels and pelvic pain in pregnancy. *Acta Obstet Gynecol Scand*. 2000;79:269-275.
21. D'Ercole C, Bretelle F, Heckenroth H, Cravello L, Boubli L, Blanc B. Painful pelvic adhesion syndrome. *Rev Fr Gynecol Obstet*. 1995;90:73-76.
22. Saravelos HG, Li TC, Cooke ID. An analysis of the outcome of microsurgical and laparoscopic adhesiolysis for chronic pelvic pain. *Hum Reprod*. 1995;10:2895-2901.
23. Petros PP. Severe chronic pelvic pain in women may be caused by ligamental laxity in the posterior fornix of the vagina. *Aust N Z J Obstet Gynecol*. 1996;36:351-354.
24. Bohn-Starke N, Rylander F. Vulvar-vestibulitis is a condition with diffuse etiology. *Lakartidningen*. 2000;97:483222-483226.
25. Robert R, Prat-Pradal D, Labat JJ, et al. Anatomic basis of chronic perineal pain: role of the pudendal nerve. *Surg Radiol Anat*. 1998;20(2):93-98.
26. Thoumas D, Leroi AM, Mauillon J, et al. Pudendal neuralgia: CT-guided pudendal nerve block technique. *Abdom Imaging*. 1999;24(3):309-312.
27. Roche B, Marti MC. Pelvic pain of proctological origin. *Schweiz Med Wochenschr*. 1996;126:316-321.
28. Meyers WC, Foley DP, Garrett WE, Lohnes JH, Mandlebaum BR. Management of severe lower abdominal or inguinal pain in high performance athletes. *Am J Sports Med*. 2000;28:2-8.
29. Howard FM. The role of laparoscopy as a diagnostic tool in chronic pelvic pain. *Ballieres Best Pract Res Clin Obstet Gynecol*. 2000;14:467-494.
30. Zondervan K, Barlow DH. Epidemiology of chronic pelvic pain. *Ballieres Best Pract Res Clin Obstet Gynecol*. 2000;14:403-414.
31. Jamieson DJ, Steege JF. The prevalence of dysmenorrhea, dyspareunia, pelvic pain, and irritable bowel syndrome in primary care practices. *Obstet Gynecol*. 1996;87:55-58.
32. Badura AS, Reiter RC, Altmaier EM, Rhomberg A, Elas D. Dissociation, somatization, substance abuse and coping in women with chronic pelvic pain. *Obstet Gynecol*. 1997;90:405-410.
33. Lipsett DR. The painful woman: complaints, symptoms and illness. In: Notman MT, Nadelson CC, eds. *The Woman Patient*. Vol. III. New York, NY: Plenum Press; 1982:147-171.
34. Nadelson CC, Notman MK, Miller JB, Zilbach J. Aggression in women: conceptual issues and clinical implications. In: Notman MT, Nadelson CC, eds. *The Woman Patient*. Vol. III. New York, NY: Plenum Press; 1982:17-29.
35. Strohmaier WL, Bichler KH. Comparison of symptoms, morphological, microbiological and urodynamic findings in patients with chronic prostatitis/pelvic pain syndrome: is it possible to differentiate separate categories? *Urol Int*. 2000;65:112-116.
36. Alexander RB, Ponniah S, Hasday J, Hebel JR. Elevated levels of proinflammatory cytokines in the semen of patients with chronic prostatitis/chronic pelvic pain syndrome. *Urology*. 1998;52:744-749.
37. Alexander RB, Brady F, Ponniah S. Autoimmune prostatitis: evidence of T cell reactivity with normal prostatic proteins. *Urology*. 1997;50:893-899.
38. Cho IR, Keener TS, Nghiem HV, Winter T, Krieger JN. Prostate blood flow characteristics in the chronic prostatitis/pelvic pain syndrome. *J Urol*. 2000;163:1130-1133.

39. Krieger JN, Egan KJ, Ross SO, Jacobs R, Berger RE. Chronic pelvic pains represent the most prominent urogenital symptoms of "chronic prostatitis." *Urology*. 1996;48:715-721.

40. Zermann DH, Ishigooka M, Doggweiler R, Schmidt RA. Neurological insights into the etiology of genitourinary pain in men. *J Urol*. 1999;161:903-908.

41. Clemens JQ, Nadler RB, Schaeffer AJ, Belani J, Albaugh J, Bushman W. Biofeedback, pelvic floor re-education, and bladder training for male chronic pelvic pain syndrome. *Urology*. 2000;56:951-955.

42. Bitker MO, Delcourt A, Yonneau L, Barrow B, Richard F. Seminal vesicle dystrophy as the cause of chronic unilateral pelvic pain in a 20-year-old male. *Prog Urol*. 2000;10:461-464.

43. PlanCarte R, De Leon Casasola OA. Neurolytic superior hypogastric plexus block for chronic pelvic pain associated with cancer. *Region Anesthesia*. 1997;22:562-568.

44. Loev M, Varklet V, Wilsey B, et al. Cryoablation A novel approach to the neurolysis of the ganglion impar. *Anesthesiology*. 1998;88:1391-1393.

45. Nebab E, Florence I. An alternative needle geometry for interruption of the ganglion impar. *Anesthesiology*. 1997;86:1213-1214.

46. Calvillo O, Skaribas IM, Rockett C. Computed tomography guided pudendal nerve block. A new diagnostic approach to long term anoperineal pain: a report of two cases. *Region Anesth Pain Med*. 2000;25:420-423.

47. Abdi S, Shenouda P, Patel N, Saini B, Bharat Y, Calvillo O. A novel technique for pudendal nerve block. *Pain Physician*. 2004, July;7(3)327-331.

48. Siegel S, Paszkiewicz E, Kirkpatrick C, Hinkel B, Oleson K. Sacral nerve stimulation in patients with chronic intractable pelvic pain. *J Urol*. 2001;166:1742-1745.

49. Weiss JM. Pelvic floor myofascial trigger points: manual therapy for interstitial cystitis and the urgency-frequency syndrome. *J Urol*. 2001;166:2226-2231.

50. Adelowo A, Hacker MR, Shapiro A, Modest AM, Elkadry E. Botulinum toxin type A (BOTOX) for refractory myofascial pelvic pain. *Female Pelvic Med Reconstr Surg*. 2013 Sep-Oct;19(5): 288-292.

51. Doherty G, Boey J. The acute abdomen. In: Way L, Doherty G, eds. *Current Surgical Diagnosis and Treatment*. 7th ed. New York: Lange Medical Books/McGraw-Hill; 2003:503-516.

52. Dominitz J, Sekijima J, Watts M. Abdominal pain. In: Kearney DJ, ed. *Gastroenterology and Hepatology for the Primary Care Provider. Principles, Practice, and Guidelines for Referral*. University of Washington Medical Center, Division of Gastroenterology; 2000.

53. Demir IE, Ceyhan GO, Rauch U, Altintas B, Klotz M, Müller MW, Büchler MW, Friess H, Schäfer KH. The microenvironment in chronic pancreatitis and pancreatic cancer induces neuronal plasticity. *Neurogastroenterol Motil*. 2010;22:480-490, e112-113.

54. Gallegos NC, Hobsley M. Abdominal wall pain: an alternative diagnosis. *Br J Surgery*. 1990;77:1167.

55. Haubrich W. Abdominal pain. In: Haubrich W, Schaffner F, Berk J, eds. *Gastroenterology*. Philadelphia, Pa: W.B. Saunders Company; 1995.

56. Kearny D. Approach to the patient with gastrointestinal disorders. In: Friedman S, McQuaid K, Grendell J, eds. *Current Diagnosis and Treatment in Gastroenterology*. 2nd ed. New York, NY: Lange Medical Book/McGraw-Hill; 2003;1-33.

57. Klein KB. Approach to the patient with abdominal pain. In: Yamada T, ed. *Textbook of Gastroenterology*. 2nd ed. Philadelphia, Pa: JB Lippincott Co.; 1995;750-771.

58. Thompson WG, Creed F, Drossman DA, et al. Functional bowel disease and functional abdominal pain. *Gastroenterol Int*. 1992;5:75.

59. Wolf S. Eliciting and interpreting symptoms and signs. In: Haubrich W, Schaffner J, eds. *Gastroneterology*. Philadelphia, Pa: WB Saunders Company; 1995.

60. Olesen SS, Juel J, Graversen C, Kolesnikov Y, Wilder-Smith OH, Drewes AM. Pharmacological pain management in chronic pancreatitis. *World J Gastroenterol*. Nov 14, 2013;19(42):7292-7301.

61. Srinivasan R, Greenbaum DS. Chronic abdominal wall pain: a frequently overlooked problem. Practical approach to diagnosis and management. *Am J Gastroenterol*. 2002;97:824.

62. Hershfield NB. The abdominal wall: a frequently overlooked source of abdominal pain. *J Clin Gastroenterol*. 1992;14:199.

63. Carnett JB. Intercostal neuralgia as a cause of abdominal pain and tenderness. *SGO Surg Gynecol Obstet*. 1926;42:625.

64. Greenbaum DS, Greenbaum RB, Joseph JG, Natale JE. Chronic abdominal wall pain. Diagnostic validity and costs. *Dig Dis Sci*. 1994;39:1935.

65. McGrady EM, Marks RL. Treatment of abdominal nerve entrapment syndrome using a nerve stimulator. *Ann R Coll Surg Engl*. 1988;70:120.

66. Gallegos NC, Hobsley M. Recognition and treatment of abdominal wall pain. *J R Soc Med*. 1989;82:343.

67. Tung AS, Tenicela R, Giovanitti J. Rectus abdominis nerve entrapment syndrome. *JAMA*. 1978;240:738.

68. Nazareno J, Ponich T, Gregor J. Long-term follow-up of trigger point injections for abdominal wall pain. *Can J Gastroenterol*. 2005; 19:561.

69. Lipkin M, Fulton LA, Wolfson EA. The syndrome of the hypersensitive xiphoid. *N Engl J Med*. 1955;253:591.

70. Howell JM. Xiphodynia: a report of three cases. *J Emerg Med*. 1992; 10:435.

71. Scott EM, Scott BB. Painful rib syndrome: a review of 76 cases. *Gut*. 1993;34:1006.

72. Heinz GJ, Zavala DC. Slipping rib syndrome. *JAMA*. 1977;237:794.

73. Noble M, Gress FG. Techniques and results of neurolysis for chronic pancreatitis and pancreatic cancer pain. *Curr Gastroenterol Rep*. 2006 Apr;8(2):99-103.

BIBLIOGRAPHY

Boescher H. Blockade of the superior hypogastric plexus block for visceral pelvic pain. *Pain Practice*. 2001;1:162-170.

Chrousos GP, Gold PW. The concepts of stress and stress system disorders. *JAMA*. 1992;267:1244.

Heim C, Ehlert U, Hellhammer DH. The potential role of hypocortisolism in the pathophysiology of stress-related bodily disorders. *Psychoneuroendocrinology*. 2000;25:1.

Johnson N, Wilson M, Farquhar C. Surgical pelvic neuroablation for chronic pelvic pain: a systematic review. *Gynaecol Endosc*. 2000;9:351-361.

Lampe A, Soder E, Ennemoser A, et al. Chronic pelvic pain and previous sexual abuse. *Obstet Gynecol*. 2000;96(6):929-933.

Nader A, Candido KD. Pelvic pain. *Pain Practice*. 2001;1:187-196.

Neuroanatomy of visceral pelvic pain. From Boscher H. Blockade of the superior hypogastric plexus block for pelvic pain. *Pain Practice*. 2001;1:165.

Walker EA, Roy-Byrne PP, Katon WJ, Jemelka R. An open trial of nortriptyline in women with chronic pelvic pain. *Int J Psychiatry Med*. 1991;21:245-252.

Perineal Pain

Ursula Wesselmann
Andrew P. Baranowski
Peter P. Czakanski

Chronic, nonmalignant pain syndromes of the perineal area have been well described in the medical literature dating back more than 100 years. However, the etiology of these focal pain syndromes is poorly understood. The patient who is experiencing pain in the perineal area is often embarrassed because these areas of the body are considered taboo in our society. These pain syndromes are frequently underreported and underrecognized.

Patients with these pain syndromes often have seen a variety of specialists in different subspecialties—including urologists, gynecologists, gastroenterologists, proctologists, and internists—and, despite an extensive evaluation, no specific etiology has been found in the majority of cases. Not surprisingly, many of these patients are frustrated because they have suffered from chronic pain for many years, but the disease has not been "given a name" and the pain is not controlled. It is important to recognize that these focal chronic pain syndromes of the perineal area do exist. The etiology of these pain syndromes is not known, and a specific secondary cause can be identified in a minority of patients only. Although these patients often are depressed, rarely are these pain syndromes the only manifestation of a psychiatric disease. Currently available treatment strategies are empirical only. Although complete cures are uncommon, effective treatment modalities exist to lessen the impact of pain and offer reasonable expectations of an improved functional status.

The intent of this chapter is to first give a brief overview of the current taxonomy of perineal pain in the context of pelvic pain and of the neurobiology of the perineal area and then to review the clinical characteristics and treatment strategies of the different perineal pain syndromes.

DEFINITION OF PERINEAL PAIN

Similar to other areas in the health sciences, where multiple disciplines are involved, developing a uniform and comprehensive terminology that improves clinical communication and enhances research efforts into the etiology of perineal pain remains a challenge. The International Association for the Study of Pain (IASP) appointed a Task Force in Taxonomy early on to develop descriptions of pain syndromes and detailed pain definitions.[1] This pain terminology has been recently updated[2] by PUGO's Classification Committee (PUGO is IASPs Special Interest Group for Urogenital and Pelvic Pain; PUGO has recently been renamed as the IASP Special Interest Group on Abdominal and Pelvic Pain) to reflect the emerging and multidisciplinary field of pelvic and urogenital pain. This taxonomy has been used in this chapter and reflects the multifactorial nature of perineal pain, requiring a multidisciplinary approach, as well as the multisystem aspects of the perineal pain complaint. To briefly review the concept of this 2012 taxonomy, perineal pain is presented under the umbrella term *chronic pelvic pain*. Chronic pelvic pain is chronic or persistent pain perceived in structures related to the pelvis of either men or women. Here, *perceived* indicates that the patient and clinician, to the best of their ability from the history, examination, and investigations (where appropriate) have localized the pain as being perceived in the specified anatomical pelvic area. Such pain is often associated with negative cognitive, behavioral, sexual, and emotional consequences, as well as with symptoms suggestive of lower urinary tract, sexual, bowel, pelvic floor, or gynecologic dysfunction. In the case of documented nociceptive pain that becomes chronic/persistent through time, pain must have been continuous or recurrent for at least 6 months. That is, it can be cyclical over a 6-month period, such as the cyclical pain of dysmenorrhea. Six months is arbitrary; however, 6 months was chosen because 3 months was not considered long enough if cyclical pain conditions are included. If nonacute and central sensitization pain mechanisms are well documented, then the pain may be regarded as chronic, irrespective of the time period.

Chronic pelvic pain may be subdivided into those conditions with well-defined classical pathology (such as infection or cancer) and those where no obvious pathology is found. For the purpose of this classification, the term *specific disease-associated pelvic pain* is proposed for the former and *chronic pelvic pain syndrome* for the latter. Chronic pelvic pain syndrome (CPPS) is the occurrence of chronic pelvic pain where there is no proven infection or other obvious local pathology that may account for the pain. CPPS is a subdivision of chronic pelvic pain (as described earlier). Pain perceived in the pelvis in CPPSs might be focused within a single organ, more than one pelvic organ, or even associated with systemic symptoms such as chronic fatigue syndrome, fibromyalgia, or Sjögren's syndrome.

Many CPPSs are associated with a range of concurrent negative psychological, behavioral, and sexual consequences that must be described and assessed. Examples are depression, anxiety, fears about pain or its implications, unhelpful coping strategies, and distress in relationships—all of which need to be considered. Both anxiety and depression can be significant, important concomitants that are relevant with respect to pain, disability, and a poorer quality of life. Catastrophic interpretations of pain have been shown to be particularly salient variables, predicting patients' reports of pain, disability, and poorer quality of life—over and above psychosocial variables such as depression or behavioral factors such as self-reported sexual dysfunction. It is suggested that CPPS symptoms sometimes create a sense of helplessness that can be reported as overwhelming in patients, which may be associated with the refractory nature of their symptoms. It is important to note that many of these biopsychosocial consequences are common to other persistent pain problems but may show varying degrees of salience for any one individual suffering from CPPS. In all patients with CPPS, these consequences must be clearly described as a part of the phenotype (where the term *phenotype* is used to indicate the observable characteristics of the syndrome).

It is well recognized that the end organ where the pain is perceived may not be the center of pain generation (e.g., the prostate in perineal pain in men). This classification is based upon the most effective accepted method of classifying and identifying different pains—that is, by site of presentation. It is argued that keeping the end organ name in the classification is inappropriate because, in most cases, there are multisystem causes and effects with the result that symptoms are perceived in multiple areas. This is a field where discussions are ongoing, and, despite there being strong arguments for both keeping and dispensing with an end organ classification, the IASP taxonomy has not taken the umbrella approach of referring to all pains perceived in the pelvis as being chronic pelvic pain syndrome.

NEUROBIOLOGY OF PERINEAL PAIN

The perineum is a highly specialized area of the body, responsible for carrying out a host of basic biologic functions, including defecation, micturition, copulation, and reproduction. The display of these diverse functions relies on precise nervous system control, coordinated with endocrine and other local control mechanisms. Compared with other areas of the body, there has been fairly little research on the neuroanatomy, neurophysiology, and neuropharmacology of the perineum.[3] The complexity of the perineum in carrying out many different specialized functions has largely been considered to account for the slow progress in our understanding of the neurobiology of this area. The fact that these areas of the body often are considered taboo in our society also may account for the scarcity of research on this topic.

A detailed review of the neurobiology of the pelvic floor is provided by Burnett and Wesselmann.[4] Briefly, the innervation of the perineum is served by both components of the autonomic nervous system—the sympathetic and parasympathetic divisions—as well as by the somatic

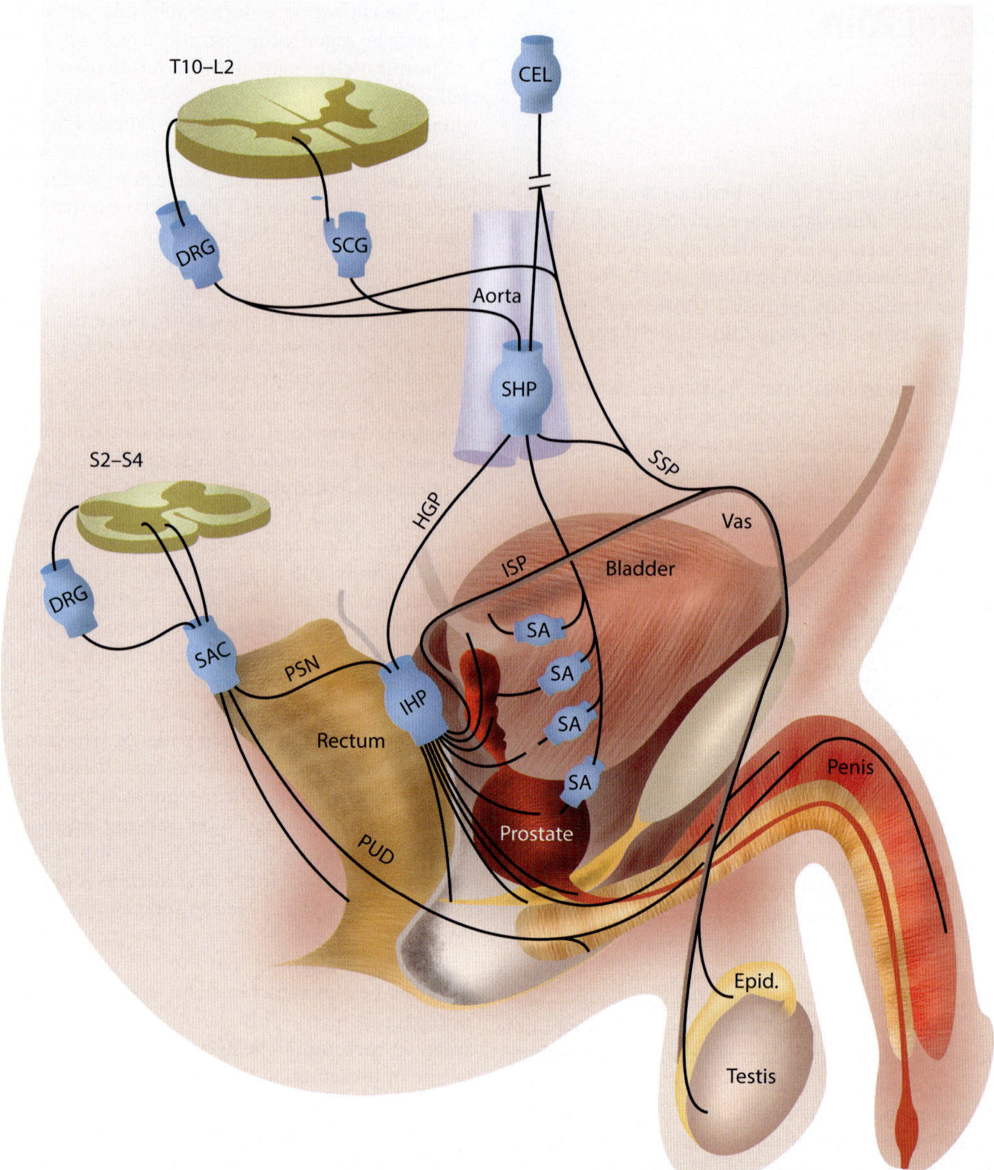

FIGURE 45-1. Schematic drawing showing the innervation of the pelvic floor in males. Although this diagram attempts to show the innervation in humans, much of the anatomic information is derived from animal data. CEL, celiac plexus; DRG, dorsal root ganglion; HGP, hypogastric plexus; IHP, inferior hypogastric plexus; ISP, inferior spermatic plexus; PSN, pelvic splanchnic nerve; PUD, pudendal nerve; Epid., epididymis; SA, short adrenergic projections; SAC, sacral plexus; SCG, sympathetic chain ganglion; SHP, superior hypogastric plexus; SSP, superior spermatic plexus. (Reproduced with permission from Wesselmann U, Burnett AL, Heinberg LJ. The urogenital and rectal pain syndromes. *Pain* 1997;73:269-294.)

nervous systems[5,6] (**Figs. 45-1** and **45-2**). Sensations from the pelvic floor are mainly conveyed via the sacral afferent parasympathetic system, with a far lesser afferent supply from afferents traveling with the thoracolumbar sympathetics.[7] However, sensations of the testis and epididymis may predominantly involve thoracolumbar afferents.[7] Somatic efferent and afferent innervation to the perineum originates from sacral spinal cord levels S2 to S4. Sacral nerve roots emerge from the spinal cord to form the sacral plexus, from which arises the pudendal nerve.[8] The pudendal nerve also receives postganglionic axons from the caudal sympathetic chain ganglia.[6] The pudendal nerve runs medial to the internal pudendal vessels along the lateral wall of the ischiorectal fossa dorsal to the sacrospinous ligament. First, a branch splits off to become the dorsal nerve of the penis (or clitoris); then, the remaining pudendal nerve fibers distribute a medial branch to the anal canal, dorsal branches to the urethral sphincter, and dorsolateral branches to the anterior perineal musculature. The posterior perineal musculature is supplied by nerves originating predominantly from sacral level S4. Branches of the S4–S5 nerve roots form the coccygeal plexus, distributing fibers to the perineal, perianal, and scrotal (labial) skin.[9]

Neuropeptide release appears to account for perineal sensations.[7] Numerous peptides have been associated with afferent pathways of the pelvic floor, although a preponderance of evidence supports the roles of substance P and calcitonin gene–related peptide (CGRP) as the primary chemicals released from these sensory neurons.[10-12]

CLINICAL CHARACTERISTICS AND TREATMENT STRATEGIES

VULVODYNIA (IASP CLASSIFICATION: VULVAR PAIN SYNDROME)

The term *vulvodynia* (Latin: *vulva*; Greek: *-odynia*, or pain) is a modern word for an age-old pain condition. Historically, vulvar pain cannot be separated from the earlier description of painful intercourse: dyspareunia.[3] The first recorded reference to vulvar pain is embedded in the ancient Egyptian Ramesseum Papyrus more than 2000 years ago.[13]

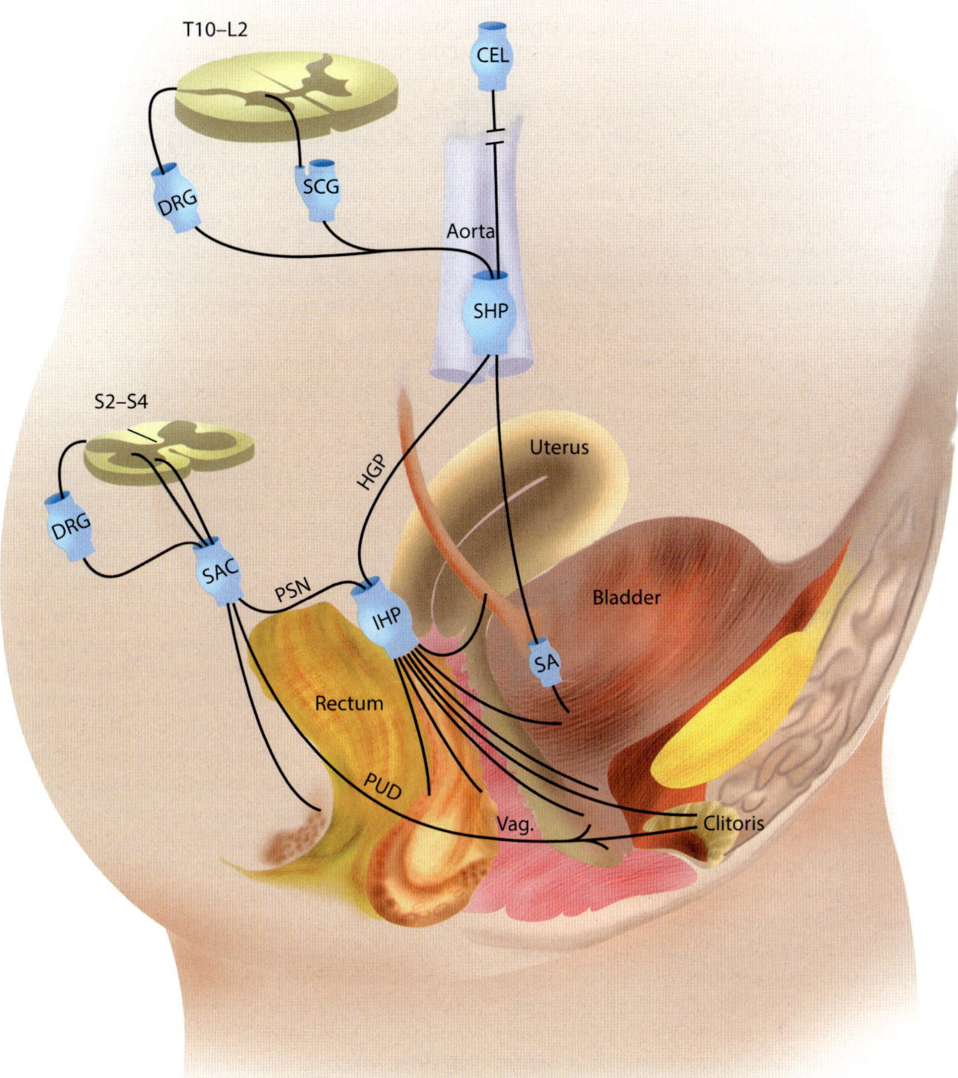

FIGURE 45-2. Schematic drawing showing the innervation of the pelvic floor in females. Although this diagram attempts to show the innervation in humans, much of the anatomic information is derived from animal data. CEL, celiac plexus; DRG, dorsal root ganglion; HGP, hypogastric plexus; IHP, inferior hypogastric plexus; PSN, pelvic splanchnic nerve; PUD, pudendal nerve; SA, short adrenergic projections; SAC, sacral plexus; SCG, sympathetic chain ganglion; SHP, superior hypogastric plexus; Vag., vagina. (Reproduced with permission from Wesselmann U, Burnett AL, Heinberg LJ. The urogenital and rectal pain syndromes. *Pain* 1997;73: 269-294.)

Detailed descriptions of hyperesthesia of the vulva can be found in U.S. and European textbooks of gynecology from the last century.[14,15] Surprisingly, despite these early reports, the medical literature did not mention vulvar pain again until the early 1980s, when a new awareness of this chronic pain syndrome developed. In 1984, the International Society for the Study of Vulvar Disease (ISSVD) Task Force defined vulvodynia as chronic vulvar discomfort, characterized by the patient's complaint of a burning and sometimes stinging sensation in the vulvar area.[16,17]

The ISSVD stated that vulvodynia was a symptom rather than a diagnosis and that multiple etiologies might be possible. Subsequently, two subsets of vulvodynia were identified. One subgroup of patients complained about entrance dyspareunia (pain with tampon insertion and pain at vaginal penetration during sexual intercourse), rather than diffuse vulvar pain. The term *vulvar vestibulitis* was introduced for this subset of vulvodynia, and the following diagnostic criteria were established: (1) presence of severe pain on vestibular touch or attempted vaginal entry, (2) tenderness to pressure localized within the vulvar vestibule, and (3) physical findings confined to vestibular erythema of various degrees.[18] The other main subgroup of patients with vulvodynia presented with generalized, spontaneous vulvar pain occurring in the absence of physical findings. The term *dysesthetic (or essential) vulvodynia* was suggested for this symptom complex. Clinically, two different groups of patients with vulvar vestibulitis have been described: *Primary vulvar vestibulitis* is defined as dyspareunia from the first attempt of sexual intercourse, whereas, in *secondary vulvar vestibulitis*, the dyspareunia appears after a period of pain-free sexual intercourse. It has been suggested that these two subgroups differ in etiological, clinical, and genetic variables.[19-23] Based on the concern that the suffix "-itis" in vulvar vestibulitis incorrectly implies an inflammatory etiology, the term *vestibulodynia* has been suggested.[17] The most recent revision of the ISSVD of the terminology of vulvodynia was published in 2004.[17] This classification suggests categorizing a generalized and a localized (vestibulodynia, clitorodynia, hemivulvodynia, etc.) form of vulvodynia and to differentiate subgroups within those two categories based on the observation of whether the vulvar pain is provoked, unprovoked, or mixed (provoked and unprovoked). Vulvodynia has a significant impact on patient's psychological well-being and quality of life. Because of the location of the pain complaint, this pain condition has a significant effect on the patient's sexual functioning. The *Diagnosis and Statistical Manual of Mental Disorders-V* suggests a single diagnostic entity called genito-pelvic pain/penetration disorder, which includes vulvodynia in the context of sexual pain disorders.[24]

Community studies suggest that vulvar pain is common, but the prevalence rates vary widely from 3% to 18%.[25-29] A survey of sexual dysfunction, analyzing data from the National Health and Social Life Survey, reported that 16% of women between the ages of 18 and 59 years living in households throughout the United States experience pain during sex.[30] When these data were analyzed by age group, the highest number of women reporting pain during sex was in the age group of 18 to 29 years old. The location and etiology of pain was not analyzed in this study. Goetsch[31] reported that 15% of all patients seen in her general gynecologic private practice fulfilled the definition of vulvar vestibulitis—a major subgroup of vulvodynia. It is important to point out that these patients had not come for a gynecologic evaluation because of vulvar pain but for a routine gynecologic checkup. Fifty percent of these patients had always experienced entry dyspareunia and pain with inserting tampons, and most of these had experienced pain since their teenage years. Epidemiological studies have confirmed that localized provoked vulvodynia is the most common vulvodynia subtype in premenopausal women.[25,26] Initial reports postulated that vulvodynia affects primarily women of Caucasian origin;[24,31] however, a survey in the United States of ethnically diverse women showed that Hispanic women were 80% more likely to experience chronic vulvar pain than were white and African American women.[26] A small study done in Ghana in 2005 revealed a prevalence rate of 20% in an all-black population.[32] Vulvodynia affects women of all age groups. The incident of symptom onset is highest between ages 18 and 25, decreases through age 44, and then remains fairly constant.[26] Several widely divergent estimates have been postulated for the lifetime cumulative incidence of vulvar pain syndrome, ranging between 200,000 and 14 million women in the United States.[26]

The etiology of vulvodynia is considered multifactorial. Systemic factors that facilitate abnormal inflammatory processes have been considered. It has been hypothesized that a subgroup of women experience vulvodynia of an inflammatory origin, yet the existence of such a subgroup has not been confirmed or rejected by clinical phenotyping efforts. Foster and Hasday found elevated tissue levels of interleukin I-ß (IL-1) and tumor necrosis factor alpha in vulvar tissue of patients with vulvodynia, but these proinflammatory mediators were actually at higher levels in the surrounding vulvar tissue than in the area of inflammation, confirming the clinical finding of a wider area of involvement beyond the area of erythema.[33] However, these results were not supported in a subsequent study by Eva and colleagues.[34] There is increasing evidence of genetic polymorphisms that are found more often in women with localized provoked vulvodynia, indicating that, in some women, the over- or underexpression of certain proinflammatory cytokines could underlie abnormal physiological mechanisms driving vulvar pain.[35] However, equivocal findings of occasional redness and inflammatory infiltrate in vulvar biopsy tissue of women with provoked vulvar pain have called this inflammatory hypothesis into question.[36]

A possible etiological correlation between oral contraceptives (OCs) and provoked localized vulvodynia has been investigated in epidemiologic studies. In a clinic-based study from 2002, the results showed an increased relative risk of vulvar vestibulitis for users compared to nonusers.[37] These findings were, however, not confirmed by a population-based case-control study from 2008.[38] More data are urgently needed, and it has been recommended by European researchers to continue to prescribe the pill when it is needed, but both users and prescribers should be aware of side effects such as dryness, soreness, and pain;[39] however, no practice guidelines have been established.

Women with vulvodynia have lower touch detection and mechanical pain thresholds in the genital area compared to age-matched controls,[40] as well as heightened pain sensitivity at nongenital body sites,[40-42] indicating that vulvar pain may not simply be a local sensory phenomenon but that central pain modulatory mechanisms might be involved. Notably, some evidence suggests symptomatic overlap between vulvodynia and systemic pain disorders such as fibromyalgia.[43] MRI studies of the brain indicated that women with vulvodynia exhibit an augmentation of genital sensory processing that is similar to that observed for a variety of syndromes causing hypersensitivity, including fibromyalgia, irritable bowel syndrome, and neuropathic pain.[44]

As in other pelvic pain syndromes, increased prevalence of comorbid psychopathology has been reported in women with vulvodynia,[3] including higher rates of depression and anxiety. These findings might be considered either a cause or a consequence for different women. Personality characteristics in women with provoked vulvodynia include higher levels of trait anxiety, shyness, hysterical personality, perfectionism, reward dependency, low self-esteem, fear of negative evaluation, and harm avoidance, as compared to healthy female controls. Although women with vulvodynia, not surprisingly, report negative feelings about sexual contact with their partner, their relationship satisfaction regarding nonsexual aspects did not differ from controls.

Vulvodynia is a diagnosis of exclusion and is established largely through history and clinical examination.[3,45] On physical examination, patients with vulvodynia usually present with no visible abnormalities. Other causes of burning and irritation must be ruled out, including genital infections (candidiasis, human papillomavirus, herpes simplex virus, bacterial vaginosis), vulvar dermatoses, vulvar dysplasia, and urogenital atrophy. Local agents applied to the vulvar region can cause irritant reactions, which resolve after discontinuation of the irritant agent. Depending on the location of the pain, a diagnosis of generalized or localized vulvar dysesthesia is made. In patients with localized vulvar pain, pain can easily be elicited or exacerbated by a simple "Q-tip test," where touching the dysesthetic area with a moist cotton swab results in sharp, burning pain. The natural history of vulvodynia over a woman's life span is not well known. Approximately half of the patients with clinical symptoms of vulvar vestibulitis eventually seem to experience spontaneous remission.[46] Because the pathophysiologic mechanisms of vulvodynia are not yet known, targeted therapy is not available at present. Treatment approaches are empirical only. Multiple treatments have been used for vulvodynia, including vulvar care measures; topical, oral, and injectable medications, which have been used for other chronic pain conditions; biofeedback; physical therapy; low oxalate diet and calcium citrate supplements; surgery (perineoplasty and pudendal nerve release); implantable sacral nerve stimulation; and acupuncture, nitroglycerin, hypnotherapy, and botulinum toxin injections. Haefner and colleagues[47] reviewed the literature and provided guidelines based on expert opinion regarding the treatment of vulvodynia. A recent trial assessing the efficacy of oral desipramine and topical lidocaine, as monotherapy or in combination, failed to reduce vulvodynia pain more than placebo.[48] A randomized comparison of vaginal biofeedback, group cognitive behavioral therapy, and vestibulectomy found similar treatment outcomes for all modalities.[49]

In summary, vulvodynia (vulvar pain syndrome) is a recognized disease entity, and an emerging body of literature is reporting on several different etiologic factors, attesting to the multifactorial aspects of this disease.[50] For the treating physician, it is important to realize that many women with vulvodynia are in their reproductive ages and previously had satisfying sexual relationships. In contrast to many other chronic pain syndromes, vulvodynia may only interfere to a moderate extent with the daily activities of a woman, but the disease usually interferes 100% with her sexual life. To confirm the diagnosis of vulvodynia (vulvar pain syndrome)—excluding secondary causes such as dermatitis or gynecologic infections—and to design a treatment plan, a multidisciplinary approach involving collaborations of gynecologists, dermatologists, neurologists, pain specialists, psychologists, psychiatrists, and sexologists is necessary.

IASP CLASSIFICATION (CLITORAL PAIN SYNDROME)

In contrast to the large body of literature that has emerged over the past 30 years on vulvodynia, few reports exist on clitoral pain. In the most recent revision of the ISSVD of the terminology of vulvodynia (vulvar pain syndrome),[17] clitoral pain has been considered within the category of localized vulvodynia as clitorodynia, similar to other localized forms of vulvodynia such as vestibulodynia, hemivulvodynia, and the like. In clinical practice, clitoral pain occasionally is also seen in women presenting with generalized vulvodynia if the pain is extending throughout the whole perineum, and the ongoing pain (often a burning, stinging sensation) is usually exacerbated by mechanical stimuli such as tight clothing and sexual contact. Chronic pain is reported as one of the complications of female circumcision.[51] This procedure involves excision of the clitoris and the labia minora and is still performed on young females in many parts of the world.[52-54] As mobility is increasing, some of these women have moved to Western countries; for example, it is estimated that 2000 young women living in the United Kingdom undergo this ritual per year.[53] Few of these women seem to seek medical attention, and the incidence of chronic pain in this group is not known. Reconstructive surgery after female genital mutilation has been reported to result in improvement of pain.[51]

URETHRAL PAIN SYNDROME AND SPECIFIC, DISEASE-ASSOCIATED URETHRAL PAIN

Many women present to the urologist, gynecologist, or family physician with painful micturition without evidence of organic disease. The urine culture is negative by standard techniques. Gallagher and colleagues[55] in 1965 coined the term *urethral syndrome* to describe this problem. Both the European Association for Urology and the International Association for Pain use the term *urethral pain syndrome*.[2,56] It has been estimated that urethral pain syndrome accounts for as many as 5 million medical office visits a year in the United States.[57] This syndrome is defined as a disease entity characterized by urinary urgency, frequency, dysuria, and, at times, suprapubic and back pain and urinary hesitance in the absence of objective urologic findings. Urethral pain syndrome typically occurs in women during their reproductive years, but it has also been reported in children and men.[58,59] In contrast to other chronic perineal syndromes involving nonmalignant pain, the rates of spontaneous remission are very high in this patient population.[60,61]

Several different theories have been proposed to explain the etiology of urethral pain syndrome, most, however, with little supporting evidence. It has been suggested that symptoms are caused by urethral obstruction and, thus, are surgically treatable.[62,63] It is important to note that rarely is there evidence to support an anatomically obstructive etiology. Although surgical procedures aimed at relieving a urethral obstruction claim excellent results, it must be cautioned that long-term follow-up rarely is provided. These procedures involve some risk of incontinence and are of uncertain and usually temporary efficacy.[64,65] Urinary hesitance, which often is reported by patients with urethral syndrome, might be the result of spasms of the external urethral sphincter, rather than an anatomic obstruction. Several studies reported a staccato or prolonged flow phase during uroflowmetry and increased external sphincter tone detected on urethral pressure profilometry in patients with urethral syndrome.[59] However, these urodynamic findings may also be produced voluntarily in a neurologically intact person and are, therefore, difficult to interpret.[66] To date, an inflammatory or infectious etiology of the urethral syndrome has not been supported,[66] and controlled studies using molecular techniques to assess for infection are necessary to further clarify whether an occult infection is maintaining the chronic pain syndrome.

A thorough diagnostic evaluation is very important because the symptoms of urethral syndrome are indistinguishable from those caused by urinary infections, tumors, stones, interstitial cystitis/bladder pain syndrome, and many other urologic diseases. Urethral syndrome is a diagnosis of exclusion. The urologic evaluation includes urine analysis, culture, and cytology. Radiographic studies, urodynamic studies, and cystoscopy are indicated in selected patients.[66] Systemic diseases affecting the innervation of the urogenital area, including multiple sclerosis, collagen diseases, and diabetes mellitus, have to be included in the differential diagnosis. In female patients, a gynecologic examination is necessary to rule out symptoms that may be secondary to a gynecologic cause. As in other chronic pain syndromes, a psychological evaluation should be part of the multidisciplinary evaluation to assess for emotional symptoms that may be associated with the chronic pain problem. A sexual history is also required because secondary sexual issues will often arise and the patient may need advice and management of these issues.

Various invasive and medical treatment options have been suggested for patients with urethral syndrome;[66] most are anecdotal clinical reports, and controlled clinical studies are urgently needed to assess which approach might be most successful for this painful disorder. Endoscopic and open surgical procedures have been suggested to eliminate a presumed urethral stenosis. Fulguration, scarification, resection, or cryosurgery has been considered to obliterate cystoscopically apparent urethritis. Bladder instillations with a variety of anti-inflammatory or cauterizing agents and systemic therapy with anticholinergics, α-adrenergic blockers, and muscle relaxants have been advocated. High rates of success were found with skeletal muscle relaxants or electrostimulation combined with biofeedback techniques.[58,65] Realizing the different surgical and nonsurgical treatment options discussed in the literature, a conservative treatment approach has been recommended as the first choice because this usually is as effective as surgery, less expensive, and, most importantly, less subject to risk.[61,67] A comprehensive multidisciplinary approach may be required.

TESTICULAR PAIN SYNDROME AND SPECIFIC, DISEASE-ASSOCIATED TESTICULAR PAIN

Similar to women who suffer from pain syndromes of the reproductive organs, men with chronic testicular pain are usually embarrassed to talk about it. Many patients cannot recall any precipitating event that led to the onset of the chronic pain syndrome. Specific disease-associated testicular pains include infection, tumor, testicular torsion, varicocele, hydrocele, spermatocele, trauma (bicycle accident), and previous surgical interventions.[68,69] The differential diagnosis includes referred pain from the ureter or the hip or lumbar facet joints (particularly the thoraco-lumbar area) and entrapment neuropathies of the ilioinguinal or genitofemoral nerve (such as with psoas muscle pathology, as well as groin pathology). Chronic testicular pain has been reported as a complication of vasectomy.[70] This chronic genital pain syndrome is usually not associated with erectile or ejaculatory dysfunction.[68]

A careful history, physical examination, and urologic evaluation reveal most of the specific disease causes of chronic testicular pain. In selected patients, a gastroenterologic evaluation might be indicated to rule out referred pain from the lower pelvic organs or herniography to evaluate for an occult hernia. The functional role of such hernias is debatable. The neurologic evaluation is directed toward the lumbosacral roots, the ilioinguinal, genitofemoral, and pudendal nerves, and the autonomic nerve supply to the testis. Referral from trigger points within the pelvic floor muscles has been associated with testicular pain (as well as referral to the penis and other areas).[71] Furthermore, the possible role of the pelvic floor is supported by investigations of its tone.[72] Treatment of chronic testicular pain is directed toward the underlying etiology if such an underlying etiology can be identified. A hydrocele, varicocele, or spermatocele are rarely the cause of chronic testicular pain, but rather are coincidental findings.[73]

Traditionally, pain management for chronic testicular pain in the urology clinics consisted of a trial of antibiotics and nonsteroidal anti-inflammatory drugs (NSAIDs), with the aim of treating a possible occult inflammatory process. Case reports suggest that medical management—including medications used for other chronic pain syndromes such as low-dose antidepressants, anticonvulsants, membrane-stabilizing agents, and opiates—often are effective for treatment of chronic testicular pain;[69,74,75] however, no placebo-controlled studies have been published yet. Transcutaneous electrical nerve stimulation (TENS) might be helpful.[74] Repeated lumbar sympathetic blocks with local anesthetic and oral sympatholytic drugs have been reported to result in marked pain relief in selected patients in whom a sympathetic component is suspected in the maintenance of chronic testicular pain.[76] In the past, drastic surgical procedures have been recommended for the treatment of chronic testicular pain, such as epididymectomy and orchiectomy. As an alternative to surgical removal of these organs, microsurgical denervation has been suggested.[77] Such surgery may result in chronic pain in its own right.[78] As with all pelvic pain syndromes, psychological interventions and sexual support and advice may be required.

PROSTATE PAIN SYNDROME (PREVIOUS TERMS HAVE INCLUDED PROSTATITIS AND PROSTATODYNIA[56,79,80])

Prostatitis is a diagnosis that is often given to patients presenting with unexplained symptoms or condition that might possibly originate from the prostate gland.[81] In many cases, the term is incorrect. It is recommended to use either the term *chronic pelvic pain syndrome* (CPPS), if the pain is nonspecific, or *prostate pain syndrome*, if the pain is truly localized to the prostate.[56,79,80] In the United States, approximately 25% of men presenting with genitourinary tract problems are diagnosed with prostatitis.[82,83] Drach and colleagues[84] defined four categories of prostatitis: (1) acute bacterial prostatitis, (2) chronic bacterial prostatitis, (3) nonbacterial prostatitis (including nonbacterial infections, allergic and autoimmune prostatitis), and (4) prostatodynia. They defined *prostatodynia* as persistent complaints of urinary urgency, dysuria, poor urinary flow, and perineal discomfort and pain, without evidence of bacteria or purulence in the prostatic fluid.[84] The definition is similar to the new IASP and EAU definition of prostate pain syndrome.[2,56] In addition to the perineal pain, patients often report that the pain is radiating to the lower back, suprapubic area, and groin. In contrast to patients with chronic testicular pain, patients with prostate pain syndrome often complain about pain with ejaculation. Prostate pain syndrome is said to account for approximately 30% of patients presenting with prostatitis, though this may be an underestimate; the age range is from 20 to 60 years of age.[85,86]

Physical examination of the prostate is typically normal in CPPS and, by definition, should be tender in prostate pain syndrome. A thorough urologic evaluation is indicated, including urinalysis, urine culture, urine cytology, and urethral cultures.[87] Referred pain from the colon or rectum needs to be ruled out. Prostate pain syndrome is a diagnosis of exclusion in which it is assumed that the chronic pain syndrome is related to the prostate but no inflammatory prostatic process can be identified. Pelvic floor muscle assessment looking for trigger points and referred pain is an essential part of the examination.[71,88-93] The most frequently advocated treatment is antibiotics despite the fact that usually no infectious etiology can be found. The urodynamic abnormalities observed in some patients with prostatodynia suggest that there is increased sympathetic tone. Oral α-adrenergic blockers have been shown to improve the voiding abnormalities as well as lessen pain; however, their use is often limited by side effects, most frequently hypotension.[94] It has been suggested that there is an increase in pelvic floor muscle tone in patients presenting with prostatodynia, and pelvic floor relaxation techniques, "hands on" physical therapy, and muscle-relaxing agents have been reported to result in marked improvement of the symptomatology.[91,92,95]

COCCYGODYNIA (IASP CLASSIFICATION: COCCYX PAIN SYNDROME)

Pain localized to the coccyx is a common perineal pain syndrome. The term *coccygodynia* was first used by Simpson[96] to describe a chronic pain syndrome characterized by tenderness and pain in the area of the coccyx and is most severe with sitting. This chronic pain syndrome occurs more frequently in women and among elderly, debilitated patients.[97,98] Some patients can remember a history of acute trauma to the coccyx—either a fall in the sitting position or birth trauma. Chronic trauma to the coccyx might result from poor sitting positions in which continued pressure occurs on the coccyx. Although one series related 70% of all cases of coccygodynia to a traumatic etiology,[99] others have suggested that trauma is an unlikely cause of coccygodynia, and, instead, a rheumatic etiology should be considered.[100] Currently, a traumatic and an idiopathic form are differentiated, based on the patient's history, but the precise incidence and prevalence figures for both forms of this condition are not known.[101]

On physical examination the coccyx is usually tender on palpation. Because pain can be referred to the coccyx from the lumbosacral spine, sacrum, anus, rectum, pelvis, and genitourinary tract, a thorough history is important, including questions regarding a precipitating cause. In addition to a standard physical and neurological examination, it is important to evaluate for anal fissures, hemorrhoids, anorectal or gynecologic infections, or rare causes such as space-occupying lesions, including tumors. As in many other perineal pain syndromes, despite a thorough evaluation, no cause can be found in many patients with coccygodynia. Additional radiological tests recommended include lateral images of the coccyx and, in selected cases, dynamic radiological studies and MRI (to rule out infections, pre-coccygeal cysts, and malignancies).[101]

The first step in the treatment of coccygodynia is protection of the painful coccyx from further irritation by sitting in such a position that no pressure occurs on the coccyx.[98] This measure alone often results in significant pain improvement after a few weeks. Nonsteroidal anti-inflammatory drugs have been advocated.[101,102] Physical therapy interventions—including hot sitz baths, pelvic relaxation techniques, and pelvic massages—have been reported to result in pain relief.[95,103] Local infiltrations with local anesthetic of the painful area, coccygeal nerve blocks, and caudal injections with local anesthetic, alone or in combination with corticosteroids, often are helpful.[103,104] Wray and coworkers[104] reported that manipulations of the coccyx under anesthesia resulted in marked pain relief. In these manipulations, the coccyx is repeatedly flexed and extended with the aim of stretching ligaments so that the ordinary ranges of motion are no longer painful. In patients with intractable pain who experience significant temporary pain relief with caudal local anesthetic injections, cryoanalgesia of the posterior rami of the lower sacral nerve roots and the coccygeal nerve should be considered.[105] Surgical removal of the coccyx, the treatment of choice during the 19th and early 20th centuries, is rarely necessary today because conservative measures are usually sufficient.[98,101,104] In selected patients whose pain is clearly related to the coccyx and in whom conservative measures have failed, coccygectomy is indicated and has a high success rate.[104,106,107] However, before considering this irreversible surgical procedure, it is important to first make use of conservative measures. Selective neuromodulation of the sacral nerve roots has also been suggested[102] and is gaining popularity.

RECTAL PAIN SYNDROMES

Pain in the rectal-anal area can occur as constant pain—*chronic proctalgia*—or as paroxysms of pain—*proctalgia fugax*. To provide greater consistency in the labeling of anorectal pain syndromes, the Rome III criteria define chronic proctalgia as chronic or recurrent rectal pain or aching lasting at least 20 minutes, in the absence of structural or systemic disease explanations for these syndromes.[108] Pain duration of at least 20 minutes is a key feature because shorter episodes of pain are suggestive of proctalgia fugax, which is defined as a sudden, severe pain in the anorectal region lasting less than 20 minutes and then disappearing completely.[108]

Chronic proctalgia is often caused by local disease of the anus or rectum, or it can be referred from the urogenital tract or the lumbosacral spine. The diagnosis is based on clinical symptoms and exclusion of alternative explanations for these symptoms.[109] A comprehensive workup is indicated because, in most cases of chronic proctalgia, and in contrast to many of the other perineal pain syndromes, the underlying etiology can be found. Digital massage of the puborectalis sling, intended to relax tense muscles, was one of the first treatments proposed for chronic proctalgia.[110] Intractable rectal pain has been associated with pudendal neuralgia in 24% of the cases in one study and has been treated successfully with neuropathic pain medications.[111] A pudendal nerve block with local anesthetic might be helpful to assess the contribution of the pudendal nerve to the chronic pain syndrome. Chronic idiopathic anal pain has been associated with abnormal anorectal manometric profiles, probably resulting from a dysfunction of the striated external anal sphincter. Biofeedback training has been shown to be effective in these cases.[112] Importantly, there is no evidence that surgery can improve pain in patients suffering from proctalgia, and invasive interventions should be avoided in the absence of a clearer etiologic understanding of proctalgia patients who do not respond to noninvasive therapies.[109,113]

Proctalgia fugax is characterized by sudden attacks of intense pain of short duration in the region of the internal anal sphincter and the anorectal ring. The incidence of proctalgia fugax has been reported to be as high as 14% in the general population and as high as 33% in patients with gastrointestinal disease.[114,115] Familial forms of proctalgia fugax have been described, and it is important to take a family history. The immediate cause of proctalgia fugax seems to be muscle spasms, but the etiology of this syndrome remains unclear.[116] A consistent phenomenon in all studies seems to be gastrointestinal smooth muscle dysfunction. In the majority of patients with proctalgia fugax, the physical examination is normal, and common anorectal diseases such as hemorrhoids and anal fissures seem to be unrelated to the paroxysmal pain problem, in contrast to patients with constant rectal pain (proctodynia).

Simple and effective remedies have been suggested to end the acute pain attack associated with proctalgia fugax:[117] immediate taking of food or drink, dilation of the anorectum (by digital dilation, attempting a bowel movement, or inserting a tap-water enema), hot sitz baths, and firm pressure to the perineum.[118-120] A variety of drugs have been suggested in anecdotal reports: antispasmodics, nitroglycerin, nifedipine, carbamazepine, diltiazem, and salbutamol.[121] Eckhardt and colleagues[122] showed, in a controlled crossover trial, that salbutamol inhalation significantly shortened the duration of the severe pain. Because this is an easy-to-use medication during the acute attack, and given that this is the only controlled study on medications for proctalgia fugax, salbutamol should be the first choice if a decision is made to use medications to abort pain attacks. It is important to reassure the patient that the symptoms, although quite troublesome (the pain often reaches an intensity of 10/10 on a visual analog scale), are not signs of a life-threatening disease and may improve with time. Psychological assessment is important to rule out a depressive symptomatology contributing to the chronic pain syndrome.

PERINEAL PAIN SYNDROME AND SPECIFIC, DISEASE-ASSOCIATED PERINEAL PAIN

Perineal pain can be localized to a specific area of the perineum, as previously discussed. In some cases, the perineal pain syndrome starts at a specific area and, over time, extends to the whole perineum. In other cases, perineal pain starts as a diffuse discomfort involving, from the beginning, most of the perineum and gradually increases in intensity—this is chronic generalized perineal pain syndrome.

The differential diagnosis is complex: Gastrointestinal, proctologic, urologic, gynecologic, and neurologic etiologies have to be excluded. Systemic diseases associated with painful peripheral neuropathies such as diabetes mellitus and acquired immunodeficiency syndrome (AIDS), have to be considered. Pudendal nerve entrapment is a recognized cause of chronic perineal pain,[123] a diagnosis initially pioneered by French physicians.[124] The pudendal nerve arises from the S2, S3, and S4 nerve roots. Its course and branches may be variable, and this can cause diagnostic confusion.[125-128] Essentially, it has three main branches that contain motor, sensory, and autonomic nerves in variable amounts: inferior anal/rectal nerve, deep perineal nerve that ends as the dorsal nerve of the penis/vulvar, and the posterior scrotal/labial nerves. Injury to the nerve from prolonged pressure, accidents, surgery, and cancer[129] may result in the symptoms and signs of nerve injury, including pain, in the distribution of the branches affected. In the buttock region, the pudendal is close to a number of other nerves, including the sciatic nerve, and injury at that site may also cause leg symptoms. Diagnosis of pudendal neuralgia can be difficult. MRI (including MRI neurography, nerve conduction, and EMGs) and sensory testing have been advocated, though systematic diagnostic blocks may be the most useful approach and may also be therapeutic.

It is important to consider the other nerves in that area that may cause pain (e.g., the cluneal) and other causes of perineal pain, especially referral from the pelvic muscles.[130-141] If patients do not respond to injection treatments, surgical neurolysis-transposition has been recommended, with best results obtained in patients in whom pudendal nerve entrapment was diagnosed early.[124,142] The approach for the surgery probably depends upon the site of injury, although there are strong advocates for different techniques.[143] There are also advocates for short applications of pulsed radiofrequency neuromodulation and various types of implant neuromodulation devices.[144-147] In patients presenting with perineal pain and sacral meningeal cysts (Tarlov cysts), surgical resection of the cysts has been reported to result in pain relief;[148,149] however, all published series are small. The findings have raised controversy because such cysts are not thought to be associated with pain in the majority of cases.[150] If previous surgery has resulted in nerve damage, reexploration of the area may benefit the patient.[93,138,147,151] Perineal pain has been reported in the context of movement disorders. Chronic perineal pain occurred as a complication of neuroleptic drug exposure. Catecholamine depletors resulted in complete resolution of the painful sensations.[152] In addition, chronic perineal pain has been reported in the context of Parkinson's disease, and excellent pain relief was achieved using medications regularly used for Parkinson's disease.[153]

PSYCHOLOGICAL ASPECTS OF CHRONIC PERINEAL PAIN

The literature examining psychological factors in chronic perineal pain has been reviewed in detail.[3,121] No sex effects were found on measures of pain, pain-related disability, or symptoms of depression in men and women presenting with chronic pelvic/urogenital pain.[154] As with other chronic pain syndromes, in the absence of obvious organic pathology, many etiologies regarding a purely psychogenic origin of perineal pain have been entertained. Many of these studies have neglected to examine whether the psychological findings were likely to be preexisting or reactive. It would not be surprising, or necessarily indicative of psychopathology, if a patient with a chronic perineal pain syndrome were depressed. The critical issue is whether this patient was depressed before the chronic pain syndrome started and whether his or her mood returned to normal after successful therapy for the chronic pain syndrome. Even a patient with a premorbid psychological state can develop chronic pain and a potential worsening of their psychology. A history of negative sexual encounters (rape, abuse, sexual torture) does not necessarily mean that the pain is psychological and unreal.[155-160] This group of patients will need specialist support as well as pain management strategies.

It is important that health care providers treating patients with chronic perineal pain realize that these patients are often embarrassed to talk about their chronic pain syndrome.[161] In addition, they often are afraid of being labeled as not really suffering from a pain syndrome but as having a psychosomatic or psychiatric illness or of being hypochondriacs. They also may be afraid that conclusions about their sexual life will be drawn (because the genitalia are either directly affected by the chronic pain syndrome or are close to the painful area), which might further isolate them. The difficulties that many of these patients have in talking about their chronic perineal pain syndrome become more obvious in relation to two situations in which a patient is in so much pain that he or she cannot come to work: In the first scenario, someone takes a day off from work, telling coworkers that he or she has really bad back pain; in the second scenario, a patient has to take sick leave because of an exacerbation of chronic perineal pain. The patient with perineal pain might invent an excuse, a more legitimate and accepted disease, to prevent any gossip among the coworkers.

Location of pain may be a significant predictor for appraisals of pain and disclosure of pain complaints. Klonoff and colleagues[162] demonstrated that subjects asked to imagine pain in their genitals appraised themselves as more ill than if they were asked to imagine chest, stomach, head, and mouth pain. Further, subjects reported that they would be least likely to disclose genital pain and would be more worried, depressed, and embarrassed by pain in the genitals than in all other areas of the body.

Given these social implications of chronic pelvic pain, it should not be surprising that this group of patients needs a lot of support within their personal relationships and sexual intimacy.[3] Sexual dysfunction is common in the normal population and is associated with distress.[163-169] This group is at a greater risk.

Mental distress is very common with catastrophizing around the pain being a major determinant of depression and other emotional disorders that significantly affect the patient's quality of life. Fear around activity may result in inappropriate rest and inactivity with the consequence that the pain problem escalates. Support from family and friends and a multidisciplinary approach to pain management are important.[170-174] It is for this reason that, all patients require assessment of their emotional, cognitive, and behavioral response to their pain, and that management—especially of the more complex patients—should occur in a multidisciplinary setting with input from a range of specialties as appropriate (urology, gynecology, urogynecology, neurology, pain medicine, colorectal, etc.) and disciplines (medical, nursing, psychology, physiotherapy).[3,56,175-180]

SUMMARY

Although the chronic perineal pain syndromes discussed in this chapter are quite frequent, and although some were described in detail more than 100 years ago, many of the patients suffering from these pain syndromes do not receive adequate pain management, and some patients do not receive any pain treatment at all. In many cases, the focus is on finding and possibly treating the underlying etiology, and patients go from physician to physician in different subspecialties and, after extensive evaluation, hear that nothing abnormal can be found. However, the pain persists, and many patients who have suffered for many years from chronic perineal pain without finding a cure are quite frustrated and angry.

As a first step, it is important to acknowledge that these chronic perineal pain syndromes do exist and that they are well described but poorly understood. A thorough workup is mandatory, often including several medical subspecialties. Perineal pain can be a symptom of a malignant or nonmalignant disease, for which specific treatment is available, and the diagnosis of a chronic perineal pain syndrome is a diagnosis of exclusion.

In many patients who present with chronic perineal pain, the workup does not reveal any underlying pathology. In the future, novel treatment strategies might become available, targeted specifically against the pathophysiologic mechanisms of the chronic pain syndromes discussed here. Although these developments are still on the horizon, it is very important to realize what can be done now for patients who suffer from chronic perineal pain. Most currently available treatment options for these pain syndromes are empirical only. Although these pain syndromes can rarely be cured, some pain relief can be provided to almost all patients using a multidisciplinary approach that includes pain medications, local treatment regimens, nerve blocks, selected surgical procedures, physical therapy, and psychological and psychosexual support.

REFERENCES

1. Merskey H, Bogduk N. *Classification of Chronic Pain: Descriptions of Chronic Pain Syndromes and Definitions of Pain Terms*. 2nd ed. IASP Press; 1994:240.
2. Baranowski AP, et al. IASP visceral /pelvic pain classification (http://www.iasp-pain.org), 2012.
3. van Lankveld JJ, Granot M, Weijmar Schultz WC, Binik YM, Wesselmann U, et al. Women's sexual pain disorders. *J Sex Med*. 2010;(7):615-631.
4. Burnett AL, Wesselmann U. Neurobiology of the pelvis and perineum: principles for a practical approach. *J Pelvic Surgery*. 1999;(5):224-232.
5. de Groat WC, Booth AM, Yoshimura N. Neurophysiology of micturition and its modification in animal models of human disease. In *Nervous Control of the Urogenital System*. Chur, Switzerland: Hardwood Academic Pub; 1993:227-290.
6. de Groat WC. Neurophysiology of the pelvic organs. In *Handbook of Neuro-Urology*. New York, NY: Marcel Dekker; 1994:55-93.
7. Jänig W, Koltzenburg M. Pain arising from the urogenital tract. In *Nervous Control of the Urogenital System*. Chur, Switzerland: Hardwood Academic Pub; 1993:525-578.
8. Elbadawi A. Functional anatomy of the organs of micturition. *Urol Clin North Am*. 1996;23(2):177-210.
9. Matzel KE, Schmidt RA, Tanagho EA. Neuroanatomy of the striated muscular anal continence mechanism: implications for the use of neurostimulation. *Dis Colon Rectum*. 1990; 33(8):666-673.
10. de Groat WC. Neuropeptides in pelvic afferent pathways. *Experientia*. 1987;43(7):801-813.
11. Bohm-Starke N, Hilliges M, Falconer C, Rylander E. Neurochemical characterization of the vestibular nerves in women with vulvar vestibulitis syndrome. *Gynecol Obstet Invest*. 1999;(48):270-275.
12. Aughton KL, Hamilton-Smith K, Gupta J, Morton JS, Wayman CP, et al. Pharmacological profiling of neuropeptides on rabbit vaginal wall and vaginal artery smooth muscle in vitro. *Br J Pharmacol*. 2008;155(2):236-243.
13. Farmer MA, Kukkonen T, Binik YM. Female genital pain and its treatment. In *Handbook of Sexual and Identity Disorders*. Hoboken, NJ: John Wiley & Sons, Inc; 2008:220-250.
14. Thomas TG. *Practical Treatise on the Diseases of Woman*. Philadelphia, Pa: Henry C Lea's Son; 1880:145-147.
15. Pozzi SJ. *Traite de gynecologie clinique et operatoire*. Paris, France: Masson; 1897.
16. McKay M. Burning vulva syndrome. *J Reprod Med*. 1984;(29):457.
17. Moyal-Barracco M, Lynch PJ. 2003 ISSVD terminology and classification of vulvodynia: a historical perspective. *J Reprod Med*. 2004;49(10):772-777.
18. Friedrich EG. Vulvar vestibulitis syndrome. *J Reprod Med*. 1987; 32(2):110-114.
19. Zolnoun D, Park EM, Moore CG, Liebert CA, Tu FF. Somatization and psychological distress among women with vulvar vestibulitis syndrome. *Int J Gynaecol Obstet*. 2008;103(1):38-43.
20. Babula O, Linhares IM, Bongiovanni AM, Ledger WJ, Witkin SS. Association between primary vulvar vestibulitis syndrome, defective induction of tumor necrosis factor-alpha, and carriage of the mannose-binding lectin codon 54 gene polymorphism. *Am J Obstet Gynecol*. 2008;198(1):101, e101-04.
21. Witkin SS, Gerber S, Ledger WJ. Differential characterization of women with vulvar vestibulitis syndrome. *Am J Obstet Gynecol*. 2002;187(3):589-594.
22. Bornstein J, Maman M, Abramovici H. "Primary" versus "secondary" vulvar vestibulitis: one disease, two variants. *Am J Obstet Gynecol*. 2001;184(2):28-31.
23. Granot M, Friedman M, Yarnitsky D, Tamir A, Zimmer EZ. Primary and secondary vulvar vestibulitis syndrome: systemic pain perception and psychophysical characteristics. *Am J Obstet Gynecol*. 2004;191(1):138-142.
24. Bergeron S, Rosen NO, Morin M. Genital pain in women: beyond interference with intercourse. *Pain*. 2011;152(6):1223-1225.
25. Harlow BL, Wise LA, Stewart EG. Prevalence and predictors of chronic lower genital tract discomfort. *Am J Obstet Gynecol*. 2001;185(3):545-550.

26. Harlow BL, Stewart EG. A population-based assessment of chronic unexplained vulvar pain: have we underestimated the prevalence of vulvodynia? *J Am Med Womens Assoc*. 2003;58(2):82-88.

27. Paavonen J. Diagnosis and treatment of vulvodynia. *Ann Med*. 1995;27(2):175-181.

28. Arnold LD, Bachmann GA, Rosen R, Rhoads GG. Assessment of vulvodynia symptoms in a sample of US women: a prevalence survey with a nested case control study. *Am J Obstet Gynecol*. 2007;196(2):128; e121-26.

29. Reed BD, Crawford S, Couper M, Cave C, Haefner HK. Pain at the vulvar vestibule: a web-based survey. *J Low Genit Tract Dis*. 2004;8(1):48-57.

30. Laumann EO, Paik A, Rosen RC. Sexual dysfunction in the United States: prevalence and predictors. *JAMA*. 1999;281(6):537-544.

31. Goetsch MF. Vulvar vestibulitis: prevalence and historic features in a general gynecologic practice population. *Am J Obstet Gynecol*. 1991;164(6 Pt 1):1609-1614; discussion 1614-1616.

32. Adanu RM, Haefner HK, Reed BD. Vulvar pain in women attending a general medical clinic in Accra, Ghana. *J Reprod Med*. 2005;50(2):130-134.

33. Foster DC, Hasday JD. Elevated tissue levels of interleukin-1 beta and tumor necrosis factor-alpha in vulvar vestibulitis. *Obstet Gynecol*. 1997;89(2):291-296.

34. Eva LJ, Rolfe KJ, MacLean AB, et al. Is localized, provoked vulvodynia an inflammatory condition? *J Reprod Med*. 2007;52(5):379-384.

35. Gerber S, Witkin SS, Stucki D. Immunological and genetic characterization of women with vulvodynia. *J Med Life*. 2008;1(4):432-438.

36. Bohm-Starke N. Medical and physical predictors of localized provoked vulvodynia. *Acta Obstet Gynecol Scand*. 2010;89(12):1504-1510.

37. Bouchard C, Brisson J, Fortier M, Morin C, Blanchette C. Use of oral contraceptive pills and vulvar vestibulitis: a case-control study. *Am J Epidemiol*. 2002;156(3):254-261.

38. Harlow BL, Vitonis AF, Stewart EG. Influence of oral contraceptive use on the risk of adult-onset vulvodynia. *J Reprod Med*. 2008;53(2):102-110.

39. Johannesson U, Blomgren B, Hilliges M, Rylander E, Bohm-Starke N. The vulval vestibular mucosa-morphological effects of oral contraceptives and menstrual cycle. *Br J Dermatol*. 2007;157(3):487-493.

40. Pukall CF, Binik YM, Khalife S, Amsel R, Abbott FV. Vestibular tactile and pain thresholds in women with vulvar vestibulitis syndrome. *Pain*. 2002;96(1-2):163-175.

41. Giesecke J, Reed BD, Haefner HK, Giesecke T, Clauw DJ, Gracely RH. Quantitative sensory testing in vulvodynia patients and increased peripheral pressure pain sensitivity. *Obstet Gynecol*. 2004; 104(1):126-133.

42. Granot M, Friedman M, Yarnitsky D, Zimmer EZ. Enhancement of the perception of systemic pain in women with vulvar vestibulitis. *BJOG*. 2002;109(8):863-866.

43. Pukall CF, Baron M, Amsel R, Khalife S, Binik YM. Tender point examination in women with vulvar vestibulitis syndrome. *Clin J Pain*. 2006;22(7):601-609.

44. Pukall CF, Strigo IA, Binik YM, et al. Neural correlates of painful genital touch in women with vulvar vestibulitis syndrome. *Pain*. 2005;115(1-2):118-127.

45. Edwards L. New concepts in vulvodynia. *Am J Obstet Gynecol*. 2003;189(3 Suppl):S24-S30.

46. Peckham BM, Maki DG, Patterson JJ, Hafez GR. Focal vulvitis: a characteristic syndrome and cause of dyspareunia. Features, natural history, and management. *Am J Obstet Gynecol*. 1986; 154(4):855-864.

47. Haefner HK, Collins ME, Davis GD, et al. The vulvodynia guideline. *J Low Genit Tract Dis*. 2005;9(1):40-51.

48. Foster DC, Kotok MB, Huang LS, et al. Oral desipramine and topical lidocaine for vulvodynia: a randomized controlled trial. *Obstet Gynecol*. 2010;116(3):583-593.

49. Bergeron S, Binik YM, Khalife S, et al. A randomized comparison of group cognitive: behavioral therapy, surface electromyographic biofeedback, and vestibulectomy in the treatment of dyspareunia resulting from vulvar vestibulitis. *Pain*. 2001;91(3):297-306.

50. Bachmann GA, Rosen R, Pinn VW, et al. Vulvodynia: a state-of-the-art consensus on definitions, diagnosis and management. *J Reprod Med*. 2006;51(6):447-456.

51. Foldes P, Cuzin B, Andro A. Reconstructive surgery after female genital mutilation: a prospective cohort study. *Lancet*. 2012;14:380(9837):134-141.

52. Dirie MA, Lindmark G. The risk of medical complications after female circumcision. *East Afr Med J*. 1992;69(9):479-482.

53. Hanly MG, Ojeda VJ. Epidermal inclusion cysts of the clitoris as a complication of female circumcision and pharaonic infibulation. *Cent Afr J Med*. 1995;41(1):22-24.

54. Briggs LA. Female circumcision in Nigeria—is it not time for government intervention? *Health Care Anal*. 1998;6:14-23.

55. Gallagher DJ, Montgomerie JZ, North JD. Acute infections of the urinary tract and the urethral syndrome in general practice. *Br Med J*. 1965;1(5435):622-626.

56. Fall M, Baranowski AP, Elneil S, et al. EAU guidelines on chronic pelvic pain. *Eur Urol*. 2010;57(1):35-48.

57. Peters-Gee JM. Bladder and urethral syndromes. In *Chronic Pelvic Pain*. Philadelphia, Pa: W.B. Saunders; 1998:197-204.

58. Kaplan WE, Firlit CF, Schoenberg HW. The female urethral syndrome: external sphincter spasm as etiology. *J Urol*. 1980;124(1):48-49.

59. Barbalias GA. Prostatodynia or painful male urethral syndrome? *Urology*. Aug 1990;36(2):146-153.

60. Zufall R. Ineffectiveness of treatment of urethral syndrome in women. *Urology*. 1978;12(3):337-339.

61. Carson CC, Segura JW, Osborne DM. Evaluation and treatment of the female urethral syndrome. *J Urol*. 1980;124(5):609-610.

62. Bergman A, Karram M, Bhatia NN. Urethral syndrome: a comparison of different treatment modalities. *J Reprod Med*. 1989;34(2):157-160.

63. Sand PK, Bowen LW, Ostergard DR, Bent A, Panganiban R. Cryosurgery versus dilation and massage for the treatment of recurrent urethral syndrome. *J Reprod Med*. 1989;34(8):499-504.

64. Mabry EW, Carson CC, Older RA. Evaluation of women with chronic voiding discomfort. *Urology*. 1981;18(3):244-246.

65. Schmidt RA, Tanagho EA. Urethral syndrome or urinary tract infection? *Urology*. 1981;18(4):424-427.

66. Messinger EM. *Urethral syndrome. Campbell's Urology*. 6th ed. Philadelphia, Pa: W.B. Saunders; 1992:997-1005.

67. Bodner DR. The urethral syndrome. *Urol Clin North Am*. 1988;15(4):699-704.

68. Davis BE, Noble MJ, Weigel JW, Foret JD, Mebust WK. Analysis and management of chronic testicular pain. *J Urol*. 1990;143(5):936-939.

69. Costabile RA, Hahn M, McLeod DG. Chronic orchialgia in the pain prone patient: the clinical perspective. *J Urol*. 1991;146(6):1571-1574.

70. McMahon AJ, Buckley J, Taylor A, et al. Chronic testicular pain following vasectomy. *Br J Urol*. 1992;69(2):188-191.

71. Anderson RU, Sawyer T, Wise D, Morey A, Nathanson BH. Painful myofascial trigger points and pain sites in men with

chronic prostatitis/chronic pelvic pain syndrome. *J Urol.* 2009;182(6):2753-2758.

72. Planken E, Voorham-van der Zalm PJ, Lycklama ANAA, Elzevier HW. Chronic testicular pain as a symptom of pelvic floor dysfunction. *J Urol.* 2010;183(1):177-181.
73. Holland JM, Feldman JL, Gilbert HC. Phantom orchalgia. *J Urol.* 1994;152(6 Pt 2):2291-2293.
74. Hayden LJ. Chronic testicular pain. *Aust Fam Physician.* 1993;22(8):1357-1365.
75. Wesselmann U, Burnett AL. Treatment of neuropathic testicular pain. *Neurology.* 1996;46(suppl):206.
76. Wesselmann U, Burnett AL, Campbell JN. The role of the sympathetic nervous system in chronic visceral pain. *Soc Neurosci Abstr.* 1995;21:1157.
77. Levine LA, Matkov TG, Lubenow TR. Microsurgical denervation of the spermatic cord: a surgical alternative in the treatment of chronic orchialgia. *J Urol.* 1996;155(3):1005-1007.
78. Puhse G, Wachsmuth JU, Kemper S, et al. Phantom testis syndrome: prevalence, phenomenology and putative mechanisms. *Int J Androl.* 2010;33(1):e216-e220.
79. Abrams P, Baranowski A, Berger RE, et al. A new classification is needed for pelvic pain syndromes: are existing terminologies of spurious diagnostic authority bad for patients? *J Urol.* 2006;175(6):1989-1990.
80. Baranowski AP, Abrams P, Berger RE, et al. Urogenital pain: time to accept a new approach to phenotyping and, as a consequence, management. *Eur Urol.* 2008;53(1):33-36.
81. Nickel JC. Prostatitis: myths and realities. *Urology.* 1998;51(3):362-366.
82. Lipsky BA. Urinary tract infections in men: epidemiology, pathophysiology, diagnosis, and treatment. *Ann Intern Med.* 1989;110(2):138-150.
83. Meares EMJ. Prostatitis and related disorders. In *Campbell's Urology.* 6th ed. Philadelphia, Pa: W.B. Saunders; 1992:807-822.
84. Drach GW, Fair WR, Meares EM, Stamey TA. Classification of benign diseases associated with prostatic pain: prostatitis or prostatodynia? *J Urol.* 1978;120(2):266.
85. Brunner H, Weidner W, Schiefer HG. Studies on the role of Ureaplasma urealyticum and Mycoplasma hominis in prostatitis. *J Infect Dis.* 1983;147(5):807-813.
86. Moul JW. Prostatitis: sorting out the different causes. *Postgrad Med.* 1993;94(5):191-194.
87. de la Rosette JJ, Hubregtse MR, Karthaus HF, Debruyne FM. Results of a questionnaire among Dutch urologists and general practitioners concerning diagnostics and treatment of patients with prostatitis syndromes. *Eur Urol.* 1992;22(1):14-19.
88. Clemens JQ, Nadler RB, Schaeffer AJ, et al. Biofeedback, pelvic floor re-education, and bladder training for male chronic pelvic pain syndrome. *Urology.* 2000;56(6):951-955.
89. Langford CF, Udvari Nagy S, Ghoniem GM. Levator ani trigger point injections: an underutilized treatment for chronic pelvic pain. *Neurourol Urodyn.* 2007;26(1):59-62.
90. Tu FF, Fitzgerald CM, Kuiken T, Farrell T, Harden RN. Comparative measurement of pelvic floor pain sensitivity in chronic pelvic pain. *Obstet Gynecol.* 2007;110(6):1244-1248.
91. Rosenbaum TY, Owens A. The role of pelvic floor physical therapy in the treatment of pelvic and genital pain-related sexual dysfunction (CME). *J Sex Med.* 2008;5(3):513-523.
92. Van Alstyne LS, Harrington KL, Haskvitz EM. Physical therapist management of chronic prostatitis/chronic pelvic pain syndrome. *Phys Ther.* 2010;90(12):1795-1806.
93. Fisher HW, Lotze PM. Nerve injury locations during retropubic sling procedures. *Int Urogynecol J.* 2011;22(4):439-441.
94. Barbalias GA, Nikiforidis G, Liatsikos EN. Alpha-blockers for the treatment of chronic prostatitis in combination with antibiotics. *J Urol.* 1998;159(3):883-887.
95. Segura JW, Opitz JL, Greene LF. Prostatosis, prostatitis or pelvic floor tension myalgia? *J Urol.* 1979;122(2):168-169.
96. Simpson JY. Coccygodynia and diseases and deformities of the coccyx. *Med Times Gazette.* 1859;861:1.
97. Stern FH. Coccygodynia among the geriatric population. *J Am Geriatr Soc.* 1967;15(1):100-102.
98. Johnson PH. Coccygodynia. *J Ark Med Soc.* 1981;77(10):421-424.
99. Torok G. Coccygodynia. *J Bone Joint Surg Br.* 1974;56B:386-392.
100. Nutz V, Stelzner F. Der glomustumor als ursache einer coccygodynie. *Chirurgie.* 1985;56:243-246.
101. Patijn J, Janssen M, Hayek S, et al. Coccygodynia. *Pain Pract.* 2010;10(6):554-559.
102. De Andres J, Chaves S. Coccygodynia: a proposal for an algorithm for treatment. *J Pain.* 2003;4(5):257-266.
103. Bonica JJ. Pelvic and perineal pain caused by other disorders. In *The Management of Pain.* 2nd ed. Philadelphia, Pa: Lea and Febiger; 1990:1384-1385.
104. Wray CC, Easom S, Hoskinson J. Coccydynia. Aetiology and treatment. *J Bone Joint Surg Br.* 1991;73(2):335-338.
105. Evans PJ, Lloyd JW, Jack TM. Cryoanalgesia for intractable perineal pain. *J R Soc Med.* 1981;74(11):804-809.
106. Grosso NP, van Dam BE. Total coccygectomy for the relief of coccygodynia: a retrospective review. *J Spinal Disord.* 1995;8(4):328-330.
107. Kerr EE, Benson D, Schrot RJ. Coccygectomy for chronic refractory coccygodynia: clinical case series and literature review. *J Neurosurg Spine.* 2011;14(5):654-663.
108. Wald AB, Bharucha AE, Enck P, Rao S. *The Functional Gastrointestinal Disorders.* Vol 1. 3rd ed. ROME III; 2006.
109. Chiarioni G, Asteria C, Whitehead WE. Chronic proctalgia and chronic pelvic pain syndromes: new etiologic insights and treatment options. *World J Gastroenterol.* 2011;17(40):4447-4455.
110. Salvati EP. The levator syndrome and its variant. *Gastroenterol Clin North Am.* 1987;16(1):71-78.
111. Ger GC, Wexner SD, Jorge JM, et al. Evaluation and treatment of chronic intractable rectal pain: a frustrating endeavor. *Dis Colon Rectum.* 1993;36(2):139-145.
112. Grimaud JC, Bouvier M, Naudy B, Guien C, Salducci J. Manometric and radiologic investigations and biofeedback treatment of chronic idiopathic anal pain. *Dis Colon Rectum.* 1991;34(8):690-695.
113. Andromanakos NP, Kouraklis G, Alkiviadis K. Chronic perineal pain: current pathophysiological aspects, diagnostic approaches and treatment. *Eur J Gastroenterol Hepatol.* 2011;23(1):2-7.
114. Thompson WG, Heaton KW. Proctalgia fugax. *J R Coll Physicians Lond.* 1980;14(4):247-248.
115. Thompson WG. Proctalgia fugax in patients with the irritable bowel, peptic ulcer, or inflammatory bowel disease. *Am J Gastroenterol.* 1984;79(6):450-452.
116. Karras JD, Angelo G. Proctalgia fugax. *Am J Surg.* 1951;82(5):616-625.
117. Jeyarajah S, Chow A, Ziprin P, Tilney H, Purkayastha S. Proctalgia fugax, an evidence-based management pathway. *Int J Colorectal Dis.* 2010;25(9):1037-1046.
118. Ewing MR. Proctalgia fugax. *Br Med J.* 1953;1(4819):1083-1085.
119. Penny RW. The doctor's disease: proctalgia fugax. *Practitioner.* 1970;204(224):843-845.

120. Rockefeller R. Digital dilatation for relief of proctalgia fugax. *Am Fam Physician*. 1996;54(1):72.

121. Wesselmann U, Burnett AL, Heinberg LJ. The urogenital and rectal pain syndromes. *Pain*. 1997;73(3):269-294.

122. Eckardt VF, Dodt O, Kanzler G, Bernhard G. Treatment of proctalgia fugax with salbutamol inhalation. *Am J Gastroenterol*. 1996;91(4):686-689.

123. Hibner M, Desai N, Robertson LJ, Nour M. Pudendal neuralgia. *J Minim Invasive Gynecol*. 2010;(17):148-153.

124. Robert R, Brunet C, Faure A, et al. La chirurgie du nerf pudental lors de certaines algies perineales: Evolution et resultats. *Chirurgie*. 1993;119:535-539.

125. Robert R, Prat-Pradal D, Labat JJ, et al. Anatomic basis of chronic perineal pain: role of the pudendal nerve. *Surg Radiol Anat*. 1998;20(2):93-98.

126. Kirici Y, Yazar F, Ozan H. The neurovascular and muscular anomalies of the gluteal region: an atypical pudendal nerve. *Surg Radiol Anat*. 1999;21(6):393-396.

127. Antolak SJ, Jr., Hough DM, Pawlina W, Spinner RJ. Anatomical basis of chronic pelvic pain syndrome: the ischial spine and pudendal nerve entrapment. *Med Hypotheses*. 2002;59(3):349-353.

128. Mahakkanukrauh P, Surin P, Vaidhayakarn P. Anatomical study of the pudendal nerve adjacent to the sacrospinous ligament. *Clin Anat*. 2005;18(3):200-205.

129. Moszkowicz D, Alsaid B, Bessede T, et al. Where does pelvic nerve injury occur during rectal surgery for cancer? *Colorectal Dis*. 2011;13(12):1326-1334.

130. Amarenco G, Ismael SS, Bayle B, Denys P, Kerdraon J. Electrophysiological analysis of pudendal neuropathy following traction. *Muscle Nerve*. 2001;24(1):116-119.

131. Kovacs P, Gruber H, Piegger J, Bodner G. New, simple, ultrasound-guided infiltration of the pudendal nerve: ultrasonographic technique. *Dis Colon Rectum*. 2001;44(9):1381-1385.

132. Naja MZ, Al-Tannir MA, Maaliki H, et al. Nerve-stimulator-guided repeated pudendal nerve block for treatment of pudendal neuralgia. *Eur J Anaesthesiol*. 2006;23(5):442-444.

133. Lefaucheur JP, Labat JJ, Amarenco G, et al. What is the place of electroneuromyographic studies in the diagnosis and management of pudendal neuralgia related to entrapment syndrome? *Neurophysiol Clin*. 2007;37(4):223-228.

134. Labat JJ, Riant T, Robert R, et al. Diagnostic criteria for pudendal neuralgia by pudendal nerve entrapment (Nantes criteria). *Neurourol Urodyn*. 2008;27(4):306-310.

135. Antolak SJ, Jr., Antolak CM. Therapeutic pudendal nerve blocks using corticosteroids cure pelvic pain after failure of sacral neuromodulation. *Pain Med*. 2009;10(1):186-189.

136. Fanucci E, Manenti G, Ursone A, et al. Role of interventional radiology in pudendal neuralgia: a description of techniques and review of the literature. *Radiol Med*. 2009;114(3):425-436.

137. Labat JJ, Delavierre D, Sibert L, Rigaud J. Electrophysiological studies of chronic pelvic and perineal pain. *Prog Urol*. 2010;20(12):905-910.

138. Rigaud J, Delavierre D, Sibert L, Labat JJ. Management of chronic pelvic and perineal pain after suburethral tape placement for urinary incontinence. *Prog Urol*. 2010;20(12):1166-1174.

139. Romanzi L. Techniques of pudendal nerve block. *J Sex Med*. 2010;7(5):1716-1719.

140. Filippiadis DK, Velonakis G, Mazioti A, et al. CT-guided percutaneous infiltration for the treatment of Alcock's neuralgia. *Pain Physician*. 2011;14(2):211-215.

141. Kim S, Song S, Paek O, et al. Nerve-stimulator-guided pudendal nerve block by pararectal approach. *Colorectal Dis*. 2012;14(5):611-615

142. Bensignor MF, Labat JJ, Robert R, Ducrot P. Diagnostic and therapeutic pudendal nerve blocks for patients with perineal non-malignant pain. Abstract presented at the 8th World Congress on Pain; Vancouver, Canada. 1996:56.

143. Robert R, Labat JJ, Khalfallah M, et al. Pudendal nerve surgery in the management of chronic pelvic and perineal pain. *Prog Urol*. 2010;20(12):1084-1088.

144. Carmel M, Lebel M, Tu le M. Pudendal nerve neuromodulation with neurophysiology guidance: a potential treatment option for refractory chronic pelvi-perineal pain. *Int Urogynecol J*. 2010;21(5):613-616.

145. Marcelissen T, Van Kerrebroeck P, de Wachter S. Sacral neuromodulation as a treatment for neuropathic clitoral pain after abdominal hysterectomy. *Int Urogynecol J*. 2010;21(10):1305-1307.

146. Peters KM, Killinger KA, Boguslawski BM, Boura JA. Chronic pudendal neuromodulation: expanding available treatment options for refractory urologic symptoms. *Neurourol Urodyn*. 2010;29(7):1267-1271.

147. Bondili A, Cooper J. Pudendal neuralgia: a rare cause of pain after tension free vaginal tape. *J Obstet Gynaecol*. 2011;31(5):454-455.

148. Van de Kelft E, Van Vyve M. Sacral meningeal cysts and perineal pain. *Lancet*. 1993;341(8843):500-501.

149. Hiers RH, Long D, North RB, Oaklander AL. Hiding in plain sight: a case of Tarlov perineural cysts. *J Pain*. 2010;(11):833-837.

150. Lucantoni C, Than KD, Wang AC, Valdivia-Valdivia JM, Maher CO, et al. Tarlov cysts: a controversial lesion of the sacral spine. *Neurosurg Focus*. 2011;(31):E14.

151. Shafik A, El Sibai O, Shafik IA, Shafik AA. Role of sacral ligament clamp in the pudendal neuropathy (pudendal canal syndrome): results of clamp release. *Int Surg*. 2007;92(1):54-59.

152. Ford B, Greene P, Fahn S. Oral and genital tardive pain syndromes. *Neurology*. 1994; 44(11):2115-2119.

153. Ford B, Louis ED, Greene P, Fahn S. Oral and genital pain syndromes in Parkinson's disease. *Mov Disord*. 1996;11(4):421-426.

154. Heinberg LJ, Fisher BJ, Wesselmann U, Reed J, Haythornthwaite JA. Psychological factors in pelvic/urogenital pain: the influence of site of pain versus sex. *Pain*. 2004;108(1-2):88-94.

155. Williams AC, Pena CR, Rice AS. Persistent pain in survivors of torture: a cohort study. *J Pain Symptom Manage*. 2010;40(5):715-722.

156. Chandler HK, Ciccone DS, Raphael KG. Localization of pain and self-reported rape in a female community sample. *Pain Med*. 2006;7(4):344-352.

157. Raphael KG, Widom CS, Lange G. Childhood victimization and pain in adulthood: a prospective investigation. *Pain*. 2001;92(1-2):283-293.

158. Raphael KG. Childhood abuse and pain in adulthood: more than a modest relationship? *Clin J Pain*. 2005;21(5):371-373.

159. Anda RF, Felitti VJ, Bremner JD, et al. The enduring effects of abuse and related adverse experiences in childhood: a convergence of evidence from neurobiology and epidemiology. *Eur Arch Psychiatry Clin Neurosci*. 2006;256(3):174-186.

160. Wuest J, Merritt-Gray M, Ford-Gilboe M, et al. Chronic pain in women survivors of intimate partner violence. *J Pain*. 2008;9(11):1049-1057.

161. Nguyen RH, MacLehose RF, Veasley C, et al. Comfort in discussing vulvar pain in social relationships among women with vulvodynia. *J Reprod Med*. 2012;57(3-4):109-114.

162. Klonoff EA, Landrine H, Brown M. Appraisal and response to pain may be a function of its bodily location. *J Psychosom Res.* 1993;37(6):661-670.

163. Althof SE, Buvat J, Gutkin SW, et al. Sexual satisfaction in men with erectile dysfunction: correlates and potential predictors. *J Sex Med.* 2010;7(1 Pt 1):203-215.

164. Corona G, Ricca V, Boddi V, et al. Autoeroticism, mental health, and organic disturbances in patients with erectile dysfunction. *J Sex Med.* 2010;7(1 Pt 1):182-191.

165. Hirshfield S, Chiasson MA, Wagmiller RL, Jr., et al. Sexual dysfunction in an Internet sample of U.S. men who have sex with men. *J Sex Med.* 2010;7(9):3104-3114.

166. Nickel JC, Tripp DA, Pontari M, et al. Psychosocial phenotyping in women with interstitial cystitis/painful bladder syndrome: a case control study. *J Urol.* 2010;183(1):167-172.

167. Traeen B, Stigum H. Sexual problems in 18-67-year-old Norwegians. *Scand J Public Health.* 2010;38(5):445-456.

168. Christensen BS, Gronbaek M, Osler M, et al. Sexual dysfunctions and difficulties in Denmark: prevalence and associated sociodemographic factors. *Arch Sex Behav.* 2011;40(1):121-132.

169. Serefoglu EC, Yaman O, Cayan S, et al. Prevalence of the complaint of ejaculating prematurely and the four premature ejaculation syndromes: results from the Turkish Society of Andrology Sexual Health Survey. *J Sex Med.* 2011;8(2):540-548.

170. Nickel JC, Baranowski AP, Pontari M, Berger RE, Tripp DA. Management of men diagnosed with chronic prostatitis/chronic pelvic pain syndrome who have failed traditional management. *Rev Urol.* 2007;9(2):63-72.

171. Nickel JC, Shoskes D, Irvine-Bird K. Clinical phenotyping of women with interstitial cystitis/painful bladder syndrome: a key to classification and potentially improved management. *J Urol.* 2009;182(1):155-160.

172. Tripp DA, Nickel JC, Fitzgerald MP, et al. Sexual functioning, catastrophizing, depression, and pain, as predictors of quality of life in women with interstitial cystitis/painful bladder syndrome. *Urology.* 2009;73(5):987-992.

173. Ginting JV, Tripp DA, Nickel JC. Self-reported spousal support modifies the negative impact of pain on disability in men with chronic prostatitis/chronic pelvic pain syndrome. *Urology.* 2011;78(5):1136-1141.

174. Tripp DA, Nickel JC, Katz L. A feasibility trial of a cognitive-behavioural symptom management program for chronic pelvic pain for men with refractory chronic prostatitis/chronic pelvic pain syndrome. *Can Urol Assoc J.* 2011;5(5):328-332.

175. Hedelin HH. Evaluation of a modification of the UPOINT clinical phenotype system for the chronic pelvic pain syndrome. *Scand J Urol Nephrol.* 2009;43(5):373-376.

176. Nickel JC. Chronic prostatitis/chronic pelvic pain: the syndrome. *J Urol.* 2009;182(1):18-19.

177. Shoskes DA, Nickel JC, Dolinga R, Prots D. Clinical phenotyping of patients with chronic prostatitis/chronic pelvic pain syndrome and correlation with symptom severity. *Urology.* 2009;73(3):538-542; discussion 542-543.

178. Shoskes DA, Nickel JC, Kattan MW. Phenotypically directed multimodal therapy for chronic prostatitis/chronic pelvic pain syndrome: a prospective study using UPOINT. *Urology.* 2010; 75(6):1249-1253.

179. Nickel JC, Shoskes DA. Phenotypic approach to the management of the chronic prostatitis/chronic pelvic pain syndrome. *BJU Int.* 2010;106(9):1252-1263.

180. Magri V, Wagenlehner F, Perletti G, et al. Use of the UPOINT chronic prostatitis/chronic pelvic pain syndrome classification in European patient cohorts: sexual function domain improves correlations. *J Urol.* 2010;184(6):2339-2345.

PART 5

Pain Syndromes

SECTION A

Neuropathic Pain

CHAPTER 46 Peripheral Neuropathies

Edison H. Wong
Zahid H. Bajwa

Painful polyneuropathy (PN) is a debilitating neurologic problem and frequently a challenging therapeutic management issue. Difficulties in managing patients are too often the result of poor understanding of their problem on the part of the treating physician. Many physicians assume that there is no need to work up neuropathy because the final outcome is likely to be an idiopathic, axonal disorder for which there is no effective therapy. In fact, many neuropathies are responsive to immunosuppressive and other conservative therapies. Although responses to such therapy constitute the minority, they should be vigorously sought before telling patients there is no treatment for their progressive disorder. In many cases, treatment of the PN also leads to improved pain control; however, pain is often a primary issue in and of itself and must be treated irrespective of the potential for improvement of the underlying PN. In these cases, pain management specialists may work in concert with neurologists to provide a comprehensive treatment approach.

CLINICAL ISSUES IN POLYNEUROPATHY

INTRODUCTION

The first step in developing a rational approach to patient management is obtaining a working knowledge of the underlying disorders that fall under the category of neuropathy. Although it is often used loosely to refer to PN, the term *neuropathy* is actually not specific and implies any peripheral nerve lesion, focal or diffuse. Classification schemes used widely among peripheral neurologists are based on anatomic and physiologic characteristics of the various disorders affecting peripheral nerves. The use of these classifications is not just an academic exercise but creates a basis for rational decision making in the evaluation and management of patients. The workup and treatment of individual patients with neuropathy must be approached with a basic understanding of the clinical behavior, including the anatomic and pathophysiologic characteristics, of the various neuropathic disorders.

CLASSIFICATION AND CLINICAL COURSE

The term *polyneuropathy* is used to describe a condition that is fairly symmetric and generalized, as opposed to focal neuropathy (mononeuropathy) or multifocal neuropathy (mononeuropathy multiplex [MM]). This chapter focuses on the diffuse disorders, including PN and multifocal mononeuropathies. These two groups of disorders may be indistinguishable clinically and are frequently accompanied by severe and disabling pain.

When a disorder of peripheral nerves is suspected, an attempt should be made to characterize the clinical features based on the time course, anatomic distribution, and physiology. Using this information, a reasonable differential diagnosis can be developed, which will determine appropriate further workup and management. This section further discusses the clinical and physiologic features of the diffuse neuropathies; their diagnostic evaluation is covered in the next section.

Polyneuropathy

Time Course An important clue as to the etiology of a particular PN is its time course. Generally accepted guidelines classify a neuropathy as acute (<3 weeks), subacute (weeks to months), or chronic (>4–6 months). Notably, neuropathies in each of these categories may be associated with debilitating pain. The typical clinic patient presenting with chronic, insidious PN is probably the most easily diagnosed; the more acute neuropathies may be difficult to differentiate from central nervous system (CNS) disease, particularly spinal cord compression.

Fiber Type and Distribution Polyneuropathy may involve motor, sensory, or autonomic fibers. There is a tendency in some neuropathies for selective involvement of fibers of the same general size distribution. Thus, a neuropathy may involve predominantly large-diameter sensory fibers (mediating vibration and proprioception) in addition to intermediate-sized motor fibers. Conversely, PN may primarily involve small-diameter sensory fibers (mediating pain and temperature) with or without involvement of autonomic fibers. Typically, pain is a prominent feature of these so-called small-fiber neuropathies. Certainly, a neuropathy may be generalized in terms of the fiber type involvement (as commonly seen in diabetes); however, careful examination often reveals a predominance of one group of fibers over another.

Pathophysiology A detailed description of the pathophysiologic mechanisms underlying PN in various disorders is beyond the scope of this chapter; instead, we focus on the relevant clinical-pathologic correlates as well as the electrodiagnostic characteristics of the different neuropathies, depending on the primary site of pathologic change.

The two primary sites of pathologic involvement in neuropathy are the axon and the myelin sheath, or Schwann cell, the former being more common in PN. In general, in axonopathies, the longest and larger diameter fibers tend to be involved first, with degeneration originating in distal portions of individual axons and proceeding proximally. This creates a length-dependent pattern, which can be demonstrated both clinically and electrophysiologically. This generalized "dying back" is theorized to result from metabolic derangement in the cell bodies or diffusely within axons. Axonopathies tend to be quite symmetric in terms of side-to-side involvement, a feature that distinguishes them from the multiple mononeuropathies. These are the most common type of PN; almost all toxic and metabolic insults to the peripheral nervous system (PNS) result in axonal degeneration.

Less frequently, the axon is largely spared, and demyelination is the primary pathologic change. Although myelinopathies may be the result of abnormal Schwann cell development or metabolism, these situations are rare, and the most frequent clinical situation is one in which segmental demyelination, or loss of myelin between the nodes of Ranvier, occurs. Segmental demyelination usually is the result of an autoimmune attack on peripheral nerves and nerve roots (as in Guillain-Barré syndrome), with the clinical pattern being somewhat variable; the limbs are involved proximally as well as distally but are usually fairly symmetric side to side.

Etiology and Prognosis **Tables 46-1** and **46-2** list the most common causes of PN based on their physiology (axonal vs. demyelinating) and time course.

Although the clinical course of various neuropathies is highly variable, depending on etiology, there are a few generalizable rules regarding prognosis. Patients with any disorder involving significant axonal injury will be less likely to recover than patients with disorders in which the primary physiology is segmental demyelination. Thus, the differentiation between these two is of practical importance for the clinician. In a disorder characterized purely by the latter, recovery occurs by remyelination and usually occurs over 6 to 8 weeks. In generalized neuropathies, even of primary demyelinating type (e.g., Guillain-Barré syndrome), there is nearly always some accompanying axonal injury and, ultimately,

TABLE 46-1 Common Causes of Axonal Polyneuropathy

Acute–Subacute	Chronic
Toxins	Toxins
Drugs (see Table 46-5)	Metabolic disorders
Alcohol	
Lead	Hypothyroidism
Arsenic	Acromegaly
Thallium	Chronic liver disease
Organophosphates	Autoimmune disorder
Pyridoxine (vitamin B_6)	Lupus
Overdose	Rheumatoid arthritis
Acrylamide	Sarcoidosis
	Sjögren's syndrome
Metabolic Disorders	
Diabetes	Paraneoplastic
Uremia	Multiple myeloma
Porphyria	Paraproteinemia
Nutritional deficiency	Inherited (Charcot-Marie-Tooth, type II)
Malabsorption	Lyme disease
Amyloidosis	HIV related
Paraneoplastic (rare)	
Carcinoma	
Lymphoma	
Guillain-Barré syndrome, axonal form	
Lyme disease	
Cryoglobulinemia	

HIV, human immunodeficiency syndrome.

the prognosis depends on its severity. Thus, recovery may be complete but take months or even years.

In primary axonal neuropathies, the prognosis depends on the nature and severity of the axonal injury. For example, in typical MM, in which nerve injury results from ischemic insult, recovery occurs largely through axonal regrowth. Individual regrowth of axons occurs from the proximal nerve stump at a rate of about 1 inch per month. This form of recovery is very slow and nearly always incomplete. In neuropathies characterized by a dying-back type of physiologic change, there usually is very little regrowth of individual axons. Instead, functional recovery occurs through reinnervation of muscle fibers by nearby healthy axons, a mechanism that probably only limits the severity of the deficit related to axonal loss rather than allowing any improvement in function.

Mononeuropathy Multiplex

Clinical Course Mononeuropathy multiplex is a diffuse neuropathic disorder, similar to PN, but it is distinguished by involvement of multiple individual nerves. MM may be impossible to distinguish from PN based on history and examination alone because the cumulative involvement of multiple nerves can produce a generalized and fairly symmetric picture. A high index of suspicion for MM is important in the appropriate clinical setting. MM is almost invariably the result of ischemic insult to nerves, the most common etiology being small- and medium-vessel vasculitis. MM occurs in the majority of cases of systemic vasculitis and may be its presenting symptom; in rare cases, vasculitis is restricted to the PNS (nonsystemic vasculitic neuropathy).[1]

Regardless of etiology, MM typically presents with an acute onset of severe pain and numbness in the involved limb; motor and sensory deficits develop over days. Nerves that are often involved early are those at so-called watershed zones of the vascular tree (e.g., the sciatic nerve in the thigh, the ulnar nerve in the forearm). Progression to other nerves eventually produces a picture suggestive of severe, axonal PN; the progression may be subacute or, rarely, chronic. In all cases, pain remains a prominent feature of the disorder.

The prognosis depends on the underlying etiology of the MM. In vasculitic neuropathy, aggressive treatment of the underlying disease is aimed at preventing further ischemia. Recovery of existing lesions occurs by means of axonal regrowth at a pace of about 1 inch per month from the site of the injury. An aggressive therapeutic approach to pain is appropriate, particularly early in the course of the disorder, when immunosuppressive therapy has not reached maximum effectiveness. Over time, if the vasculitis can be adequately treated, it may be possible to reduce or withdraw pain therapies.

Etiology **Table 46-3** lists the most common etiologies of MM based on time course.

DIAGNOSTIC EVALUATION

History and Physical Examination

History The first step in the diagnostic evaluation of any neuropathy is the history and physical examination of the patient. Several important historical points should be reviewed. One should determine the time course of the illness—acute, subacute, or chronic. Next, involvement of nerve fiber types should be ascertained—sensory, motor, and autonomic, with regard to both *positive* and *negative* symptoms. Specific inquiry should be made regarding the presence or absence of pain. Whereas positive symptoms refer to abnormal spontaneous sensory or motor phenomena (e.g., pins and needles, fasciculations), negative symptoms describe a loss of function (e.g., weakness, numbness). Inquiry should be made regarding the symptom distribution and symmetry (i.e., stocking glove vs. individual nerve territories), as well as the progression (i.e., slow and insidious vs. acute onset deficits with plateaus).

Past medical history obviously factors into the diagnostics, especially because hyperglycemic disorders are in a spectrum and increased

TABLE 46-2 Common Causes of Demyelinating Polyneuropathy

Acute–Subacute	Chronic
Guillain-Barré syndrome Diphtheria (rare) Multifocal motor neuropathy with conduction block	Chronic inflammatory demyelinating polyneuropathy Metabolic disorders Diabetes mellitus Uremia Hypothyroidism Myeloma (osteosclerotic) Paraproteinemia Cryoglobulinemia Hepatitis C Inherited (Charcot-Marie-Tooth and others)

TABLE 46-3 Mononeuropathy Multiplex—Common Etiologies

Vasculitis
- Polyarteritis nodosa
- Rheumatoid arthritis
- HIV associated

Diabetes
Sarcoidosis
Lyme disease
Leprosy (rare in United States)

HIV, human immunodeficiency syndrome.

incidence of diabetic PN in prediabetes correlates with impaired glucose tolerance rather than fasting hyperglycemia.[2] A remote cancer history can also include chemotherapy. Nutritional deficiencies of the B vitamins may accompany gastric and other gastrointestinal disorders with malabsorption through one or another mechanism (treatment of gastroesophageal reflux disease, peptic ulcer disease, and other conditions can involve chronic acid suppression and resultant decreased absorption of nutrients;[3,4] gastric bypass, banding, and other gastric function alteration surgeries;[5,6] short gut syndrome from surgical resection of small or large bowel;[7] and gluten enteropathy).[8] Social and work history can also impact diagnostics (exposure as a child or adult to old residences with lead paint; work exposure to toxic chemicals or heavy metals; substance abuse history may be direct through heavy alcohol use or indirect through concomitant poor nutrition and infection such as hepatitis C and HIV; hunting, fishing, and other recreational activities as well as residence location may give exposure to Lyme disease; pet dogs with Lyme disease may be the best predictor of their owners contracting Lyme disease).[9] Finally, one should obtain a family history, with an eye to excluding a congenital form of neuropathy.

Characteristic features of neuropathic pain are useful in differentiating it from pain from any other source. It is vital that these symptoms and signs are sought during the history and physical examination because they are often primary evidence for a diagnosis of PN. In some neuropathies, such as those limited to involvement of small fibers, normal laboratory studies are the rule, and the diagnosis is based on clinical grounds alone. The presence of positive symptoms is typical of the neuropathic disorders.

Positive symptoms that are typical of PN include (1) *paresthesias*—nonpainful, spontaneous sensory phenomena such as pins and needles or tingling; (2) *dysesthesias*—unpleasant spontaneous or evoked sensory phenomena such as burning; (3) *hyperesthesia*—increased sensitivity to stimuli, often with an unpleasant quality; (4) *allodynia*—pain created by a normally nonpainful stimulus, such as the bedcovers; and (5) *hyperpathia* or *hyperalgesia*—exaggerated pain response created by a normally painful stimulus.

The presence of these symptoms should be sought specifically in addition to allowing the patient to describe the precise nature of his or her pain. Also, the effect of pain on quality of life and functional status is extremely important. Specific pain measures, such as the Neuropathic Pain Scale,[10] may be used to quantify the patient's pain and its effect on the quality of life. Such scales are particularly helpful for patients involved in clinical therapeutic trials and may be used to assess efficacy of treatment regimens outside of experimental trials. However, neuropathic pain symptoms may also be found in musculoskeletal and other nonneuropathic conditions, so they are not pathognomonic by themselves.

Physical Examination The physical examination should be guided by the patient history. For example, the suggestion of asymmetric onset of symptoms should prompt a careful search for evidence of individual nerve involvement as opposed to a stocking-glove distribution of sensory loss.

A complete neurologic examination is required. One cannot adequately localize the problem to the peripheral nerve without a careful physical examination to rule out myelopathy, polyradiculopathy, or myopathy, which may mimic or complicate PN. The details of the neurologic examination are not reviewed here, but a few points are worth emphasizing. The goal of the physical examination is to characterize the pattern, symmetry, and distribution of abnormalities and to determine which modalities are involved (motor, sensory, autonomic); the distribution with regard to fiber type should also be demonstrable. The typical pattern to look for is bilaterally symmetric, usually distally predominant. The proximal lower extremities tend to be involved before the distal upper extremities, although this is variable; the anterior thoracic region is often involved in more severe cases. However, there may be proximal predominance, and the upper extremities may be involved disproportionately. In MM, the pattern is usually multiple nerve involvement, although it may likely be impossible to differentiate from PN, other than subtle asymmetry in an otherwise stocking-glove distribution. The deep tendon reflexes are part of the overall pattern as well and are typically reduced or absent in a distribution consistent with the underlying pathophysiology. For example, whereas patients with distal axonopathies typically have absent ankle jerks, those with chronic demyelinating neuropathies are areflexic.

In patients with painful positive symptoms, correlative signs may often be found in the physical examination. Allodynia may be elicited by lightly stroking the involved area (mechanical stimulus) or by testing with a cold instrument (thermal stimulus). Hyperalgesia or hyperpathia may be elicited during pinprick testing. A single, painful stimulus may be reported as a sensory deficit, but repeated stimuli in the same area produce an exaggerated pain; this phenomenon is called *summation*.[11] Abnormal sensations may last for several seconds or minutes after discontinuation of the stimulus, a phenomenon called *after sensations*.[11] These examination findings are important because they are unique to patients with neuropathic pain.

Clinical Neurophysiology

Electrophysiologic Studies The second logical step in the diagnostic evaluation is the electrodiagnostic examination, specifically, nerve conduction studies (NCS) and electromyography (EMG). The utility of these studies is several. First, they usually clarify the diagnosis of PN. Although important, there is a limit to the localizing value of physical examination, even when carefully performed. For example, a detailed physical examination cannot differentiate multiple root involvement from PN or MM in most cases; coexisting neurologic problems may also significantly alter the physical examination. It is important to note that NCS cannot assess the integrity of small-diameter sensory fibers (i.e., those mediating pain and temperature), so results will be normal in patients with pure small-fiber neuropathies. However, these neuropathies are rare, and in patients with involvement of larger fibers, NCS are more sensitive than physical examination for diagnosing PN.

In addition to establishing a diagnosis with accuracy, electrodiagnostic studies provide several other types of information, including the predominant pathophysiology (i.e., axonal or demyelinating), the time course and severity of the disorder, and whether motor or sensory fibers (or both) are involved. NCS can differentiate hereditary from acquired forms of PN and is much more sensitive than physical examination for identifying MM. Chapter 11 discusses the use of electrodiagnostic testing in detail. After the underlying pathophysiology and the time course are understood, the differential diagnostic possibilities are narrowed considerably.

Quantitative Sensory Testing Quantitative sensory testing (QST) is a specialized technique for measuring the intensity of a given stimulus required to elicit specific sensory perceptions.[12] Specifically, QST assesses a sensory detection threshold to various stimuli, including touch pressure, vibration, heat, and coolness. QST, when properly performed, provides a quantitative, noninvasive means of assessing sensory function. One major advantage is that QST for thermal thresholds allows some quantifiable measure of small-fiber function, which is not possible with routine NCS. Several commercial systems exist for QST. However, a major problem with QST is that it is not widely available for clinical use, and its reliability is highly operator dependent. Notably, its sensitivity in patients with pure small-fiber neuropathies, the group in whom it is potentially of the greatest diagnostic importance, has been reported in several studies to be around 60%.[13,14] Nonetheless, it can be quite helpful in confirming the physical examination findings and substantiating the clinical suspicion of neuropathy. In small-fiber neuropathies, in particular, QST is recommended because it may provide the only objective means for establishing a diagnosis and can be used to measure efficacy of various therapeutic modalities.[12] QST is typically pursued in the evaluation of PN if the routine NCS are nondiagnostic.

Laboratory Studies The differential diagnostic considerations in any given neuropathy depend on the physiologic characteristics and time course of the underlying disorder (Tables 46-1 to 46-3). Thus, the diagnostic evaluation should proceed initially with electrophysiologic studies, as discussed earlier, and laboratory workup should be guided by the differential diagnostic considerations raised by these findings. The laboratory

TABLE 46-4 Laboratory Investigation of Diffuse Neuropathies

Routine studies		
Complete blood count, differential		
Liver function studies		
Fasting serum glucose		
Erythrocyte sedimentation rate, antinuclear antibodies, rheumatoid factor		
Lyme titer		
Thyroid-stimulating hormone		
Vitamin B_{12} level		
Serum protein electrophoresis, immunoelectrophoresis, urine protein electrophoresis		
	Special Studies Based on Physiology	
Axonal	**Demyelinating**	**Mononeuropathy Multiplex**
Heavy metal screen	HIV titer, if appropriate	HIV titer, if appropriate
Cryoglobulins	Cryoglobulins	Cryoglobulins
HIV titer, if appropriate	Anti-MAG, GM1 antibody	Angiotensin-converting enzyme
dsDNA	CSF evaluation (acute forms)	ANCA
Vitamin levels, if appropriate		Nerve biopsy
Consider CSF evaluation		Consider CSF evaluation
Consider nerve biopsy		

ANCA, Anti-neutrophil cytoplasmic antibodies; CSF, cerebrospinal fluid; HIV, human immunodeficiency virus.

workup will nearly always include blood studies and occasionally urine studies. Cerebrospinal fluid (CSF) evaluation is no longer routinely necessary; it is most commonly obtained in fairly acute neuropathies in which Guillain-Barré syndrome is suspected.

Table 46-4 outlines the appropriate laboratory workup for PN and MM based on time course and electrophysiology.

Biopsy

Nerve and Muscle Nerve biopsy is required in a small proportion of patients with neuropathy and should be performed only in situations in which the indication is clearly defined. Only rarely is biopsy necessary to establish a diagnosis of PN. Nerve biopsy is most useful in patients with MM as a means of determining the causative disorder, which is usually inflammatory in nature and has a high morbidity and mortality if untreated. Other disorders appropriately diagnosed by nerve biopsy include sarcoidosis, amyloidosis, and (rarely) leprosy. In the cases of vasculitis and sarcoidosis, a muscle biopsy is usually obtained simultaneously. Nerve biopsy is infrequently performed in cases of progressive PN in which exhaustive workup has failed to reveal an underlying diagnosis. In these cases, the aim of the biopsy is to determine the presence or absence of a potentially treatable disorder.

Skin In recent years, a technique has been developed for quantitative assessment of cutaneous innervation in punch biopsies of the skin. The epidermis contains free nerve endings, which are the terminals of small-caliber, unmyelinated fibers. Using control values obtained from a healthy cohort, investigators have been able to identify abnormal patterns of intraepidermal nerve fiber (IENF) density in patients with small-fiber sensory neuropathies (SFSNs).[13,15] Examination of patients with idiopathic, human immunodeficiency virus (HIV)–associated, and diabetic painful sensory neuropathies indicates a correlation between IENF density and clinical estimates of small-fiber sensory dysfunction.[15] Studies of patients with idiopathic SFSNs suggest that IENF is a more sensitive diagnostic indicator of pure, small-fiber neuropathies than either QST or sural nerve biopsy.[13] Although IENF density is still available only in specialized centers, it holds promise as an important tool for routine use in patients with painful sensory neuropathies whose routine workup results may be entirely normal, especially when small-fiber involvement predominates.

TABLE 46-5 Neuropathies with Pain As a Prominent Feature

Polyneuropathies	Mononeuropathy Multiplex
Toxic	Diabetic syndromes (see section III)
Arsenic	Idiopathic brachial neuritis
Thallium	Idiopathic lumbosacral plexopathy
Drugs	Paraneoplastic
Cisplatinum	Infection
Disulfiram	Lyme
Isoniazid	Cytomegalovirus (HIV related)
Nitrofurantoin	Vasculitis
Thallium	
Vincristine	
Generalized small fiber	
Neuropathies	
Acute pandysautonomia	
Amyloidosis	

NEUROPATHIES WITH PAIN AS A PROMINENT FEATURE

OVERVIEW

The painful neuropathies are clinically heterogeneous. Even if one restricts analysis to the diffuse neuropathies, the frequency with which pain will occur in a given setting is impossible to predict based on etiology or physiology. Pain may be present early or late in the clinical course of a given neuropathy. It is important for the clinician to evaluate pain issues in an individual patient with knowledge of the underlying disorder and its clinical course, understanding that the course of the pain may be independent of the disease. To that end, it is worth reviewing the neuropathies most commonly associated with pain.

The most commonly encountered painful PN syndromes occur in the setting of diabetes, HIV and acquired immunodeficiency syndrome (AIDS), and toxic-metabolic disorders. Aside from these, Guillain-Barré syndrome is probably seen most frequently. These disorders are discussed individually in the following sections. **Table 46-5** lists diffuse neuropathies commonly associated with pain as a prominent feature. MM syndromes, although significantly less frequent, are worth noting as they are almost invariably associated with pain. MM is usually the result of ischemic vascular injury, regardless of the underlying etiology (see Table 46-3). Pure SFSNs are classically painful as well, although they are a rare form of neuropathy.

DIABETIC NEUROPATHIES

The diabetic neuropathies are clinically diverse and involve focal, multifocal, and diffuse disorders of varying types. Pain, although not universal, is a characteristic feature of neuropathy in patients with diabetes, and the most common cause of painful PN is diabetes. It is worth noting that the majority of patients with diabetes have chronic, distal, predominantly sensory PN with involvement of all fiber types; this syndrome is frequently painless for much of its course. However, small sensory fibers may be involved disproportionately or exclusively in diabetes mellitus, and in these syndromes, pain is invariably a feature. Painful diabetic neuropathies include several clinical syndromes, including PN. The acute syndromes include lumbar radiculoplexopathy (i.e., diabetic amyotrophy), acute thoracic radiculopathy, and acute distal sensory PN. Rarely, patients may develop an acute, distal sensory PN shortly after initiation of insulin therapy; this has been termed *insulin neuritis*.

The PN syndromes encountered in diabetics include acute–subacute and chronic forms. Typical, chronic, axonal PN may be associated with pain at any point during its course, usually in proportion to the severity of the overall neuropathy; however, the most important factor appears to be the severity of small-fiber injury, and this may be disproportionate in an otherwise typical axonal PN. Diabetes is the most common etiology underlying pure SFSN, in which small-diameter sensory fibers are almost exclusively involved. These patients typically present with distal lower extremity burning pain as the chief complaint. Clinically, pain and temperature sensation are reduced, with sparing of large-fiber sensory modalities (vibration, proprioception); reflexes are usually intact. Autonomic dysfunction may be prominent in these patients. Nerve biopsies demonstrate a predominant loss of small fibers.[16] The clinical course in these patients is variable, and pain may be a chronic problem.

Acute diabetic PN, although less common, is much more likely to be associated with neuropathic pain. The SFSNs associated with diabetes may be acute; in some of these cases, there may be a mixed pattern of involvement, with large fibers being less affected than small fibers. In rare cases, the onset follows the initiation of insulin therapy (so-called insulin neuritis). A similar picture may be seen after precipitous weight loss in patients with diabetes (so-called diabetic cachexia). The relationship to glycemic control is unclear; a similar syndrome has been reported after episodes of ketoacidosis as well as establishment of tight control. These cases appear to be largely self-limited, with slow resolution of symptoms as glycemic control and normal weight are established and appropriately maintained.[16]

HIV/AIDS-RELATED NEUROPATHIES

The neuropathies associated with HIV manifest a wide spectrum of disorders, both clinically and pathophysiologically. The most common HIV-associated neuropathy in which pain is a characteristic feature is distal, primarily sensory, symmetric polyneuropathy (DSPN). Other painful polyneuropathies include those produced by toxins (particularly antiretroviral agents) and Guillain-Barré syndrome. Painful MM occurs in this population but is relatively rare.

DSPN is the most common HIV-related form of neuropathy. A predominantly sensory neuropathy, it has been estimated to affect 10% to 30% of patients with AIDS.[17,18] Although DSPN is a relatively uncommon entity in early HIV infection, electrophysiologic studies have shown that up to one-third of patients with AIDS have DSPN.[19] As immunologic status worsens, clinical manifestations of DSPN increase in incidence. Clinical features include symmetric numbness; burning paresthesias and dysesthesias in the distal lower extremities, with decreased pinprick, temperature, and vibratory sense in a stocking distribution; and depressed ankle reflexes.

Several of the antiretroviral medications have dose-dependent peripheral nerve toxicities, resulting in a clinical syndrome identical to HIV-associated DSPN. These include the nucleoside analogues didanosine (ddI), zalcitabine (ddC), and the pyrimidine analogue stavudine (d4T). Didanosine is now a well-known cause of a painful peripheral neuropathy. Early clinical trials found that 8 of 37 patients receiving ddI developed a dose-related painful neuropathic syndrome, which resolved within 8 weeks of the removal of the drug.[20] Likewise, ddC and d4T have been clearly shown to cause dose-dependent neurotoxicity, which improves with drug withdrawal.[21-23] Notably, when the offending agent is removed, intensified neuropathic symptoms may persist for several weeks, a phenomenon known as coasting.[21] DSPN is the most important side effect limiting the use of thalidomide in the treatment of painful aphthous ulcers in patients with AIDS.[24] PN is also a well-described complication of therapy with isoniazid, an antituberculous agent used in patients with AIDS.[25] Chemotherapeutic agents such as vincristine and paclitaxel, used in the treatment of Kaposi's sarcoma and lymphoma, also have been associated with DSPN.

Rarely, in early HIV disease, patients may develop MM involving cranial as well as peripheral nerves, which responds either spontaneously or with immunomodulating therapy.[26] In late HIV disease, a more fulminant, progressive MM may develop. In both cases, pain is a prominent feature. Etiologic agents identified include toxoplasmosis, herpes zoster, cryptococcus,[27] cryoglobulinemia,[28] and lymphoma. However, the most prevalent etiologic agent is cytomegalovirus; in these cases, marked improvement in symptoms is expected with ganciclovir or foscarnet therapy.[29] MM in HIV patients also has been associated with vasculitis; in these patients, pain is a presenting symptom and may take months to abate.[30]

Diffuse infiltrative lymphocytosis syndrome (DILS) has been recognized as a rare complication of HIV disease for more than a decade; only recently has it been found to be associated with a characteristic peripheral neuropathy. DILS-associated neuropathy is a painful, symmetric, axonal sensorimotor PN of acute–subacute onset.[31] Immunosuppressive and antiviral therapy are helpful in improving symptoms of the neuropathy.[32]

Otherwise-typical Guillain-Barré syndrome (see later discussion) may occur in patients with early HIV, particularly at the time of seroconversion.[33]

GUILLAIN-BARRÉ SYNDROME

Acute inflammatory demyelinating polyradiculoneuropathy, or Guillain-Barré syndrome, is the most common cause of acute–subacute PN. Guillain-Barré syndrome is an immune-mediated PN, which is characterized physiologically by segmental demyelination. The typical clinical picture develops over days to weeks, with limb paresthesias developing in a distal to proximal fashion accompanied by weakness and loss of tendon reflexes in a similar distribution. Weakness may spread to involve craniobulbar and respiratory muscles. A classic laboratory finding is a CSF protein with relatively few white blood cells (albuminocytologic dissociation). Electrophysiologic studies reveal evidence of primary demyelination with conduction block. Spontaneous recovery, in variable degrees, occurs over weeks to months. Death from respiratory complications occurs in a small number of patients. Pain has been a relatively underappreciated aspect of the disease but is actually a prominent feature in the majority of cases, as pointed out by Ropper and colleagues.[34]

Patients with Guillain-Barré syndrome describe deep, aching muscular pain involving large muscles of the thighs, buttocks, and back and, less often, sciatica or painful distal limb paresthesias. Pain is usually worst at night and interferes with sleep. Some patients may respond to simple analgesic agents. There is no published experience regarding the use of tramadol, a non-narcotic analgesic, in Guillain-Barré syndrome, but its use should be considered before resorting to narcotic analgesic agents. The pain, even dysesthetic limb pain, generally responds poorly to antidepressants and anticonvulsants, therapeutic agents that are considered first-line therapy in chronic PN.[34] The experience to date indicates that narcotics have been the most effective treatment and should be used appropriately to control pain, particularly when it is interfering with sleep. In patients whose respiratory status is so marginal that there is a concern of decompensation with the use of narcotics, intubation should be considered.[34]

TOXIC NEUROPATHIES

The largest number of toxic neuropathies is related to the use of pharmaceutical agents in appropriate clinical situations. Environmental and occupational toxins are much less frequently seen. **Table 46-6** lists pharmaceutical agents that are commonly associated with neuropathy. The typical clinical scenario is a distal axonopathy that develops after sustained use of the medication, although the time course to onset of symptoms is highly variable. Sensory and motor symptoms and signs develop in a length-dependent fashion, in a time course ranging from weeks to months or even years, depending on the dose and neurotoxic properties of the drug. Painful paresthesias and dysesthesias are common complaints. The prognosis is variable, but in most cases, significant resolution of clinical signs and symptoms occurs with drug withdrawal; however, recovery is variable and related to the severity of the underlying axonal injury.

TABLE 46-6 Drugs Commonly Associated with Toxic Neuropathy

Antiarrhythmics	Antineoplastic Agents
Amiodarone	Cis-platinum
Antibiotics and Antituberculous Agents	Doxorubicin
Chloramphenicol	Misonidazole
Dapsone	Vincristine
Ethambutol	Taxol
Isoniazid (INH)	Antiretroviral Agents
Metronidazole	Didanosine (ddI)
Nitrofurantoin	Stavudine (d4T)
Anticonvulsants	Zalcitabine (ddC)
Phenytoin	Other
Antihypertensives	Gold
Hydralazine	Disulfiram
	Nitrous oxide (chronic abuse)
	Pyridoxine
	Thalidomide

PATHOPHYSIOLOGY: PAIN IN THE NEUROPATHIC DISORDERS

PROPOSED MECHANISMS OF PAIN IN POLYNEUROPATHY

Peripheral Mechanisms

Anatomic and Physiologic Considerations The perception of pain is the result of a complex interplay among cells at multiple levels of the nervous system. When an insult results in damage to a peripheral nerve, the transmission and sensation of pain involves the axon, the dorsal root ganglion, and the CNS as well. In this section, we review theories concerned with the role of the PNS in the generation and propagation of pain. These include a number of possible pathophysiologic mechanisms, such as ectopic generation, afferent sensitization and hyperexcitability, amplification of neural pacemakers, and electrical cross-talk. We also focus on the pathophysiology of neuronal damage in common illnesses associated with peripheral neuropathies, including diabetes mellitus and HIV infection.

Neuroma Formation and Ectopic Generation When an axon is injured and disconnected from its cell body, it undergoes wallerian degeneration, or so-called dying back. Subsequently, nerve regeneration occurs through axonal sprouting and elongation from the proximal terminal. If there is some obstacle to forward progress, the axonal sprouts grow in a disorganized fashion and may form a neuroma, a mass of tangled neuronal tissue.[35] Several studies have found the neuroma to function as the nerve's sensory terminal,[36,37] as well as being a source of ectopic discharge in both myelinated and unmyelinated axons.[35] Thus, axonal injury may result in positive symptoms (e.g., paresthesias), as well as negative symptoms (e.g., numbness).

The function of a sensory axon is to propagate information from the sensory receptors to the CNS. In normal nerve, a temporary noxious stimulus results in transient pain because the axon ceases its firing when the stimulus is removed.[38] The development of ongoing pain and paresthesias after the removal of an external stimulus implies a fundamental change in the properties of the axon. Instead of functioning purely as an impulse conductor, it has become an impulse generator.[35] It has been proposed that this metamorphosis after nerve injury results from the formation of a neuroma that has spontaneous pacemaker activity. The neuroma can depolarize and fire continuously in response to various different types of stimulation and may depolarize in the absence of a stimulus; this phenomenon is termed *ectopic generation*.[35] An electrically active neuroma is demonstrated in **Figure 46-1**.

The development of electrogenetic potential in nerve fibers is one of the key changes that underlie the generation of neuropathic pain. After an ectopic generator has been established, various stimuli affecting membrane excitability can induce repeated nerve depolarization. Examples of such stimuli include ischemia; mechanical stimuli; and neuroactive substances, including histamines, prostaglandins, and catecholamines.[39]

Unlike peripheral afferents, which develop pacemaker capability as a result of injury, there are a small number of cells in the dorsal root ganglia (DRG) that normally discharge spontaneously. This intrinsic rhythmogenicity is amplified by chronic nerve damage.[40] It has been postulated that enhanced pacemaker activity in the DRG, as well as changes in central pathways, might explain why peripheral nerve blocks may fail to relieve sensory symptoms associated with peripheral nerve lesions.[35] **Figure 46-2** demonstrates a prolonged afterdischarge of an afferent axon after mechanical stimulation of the DRG.

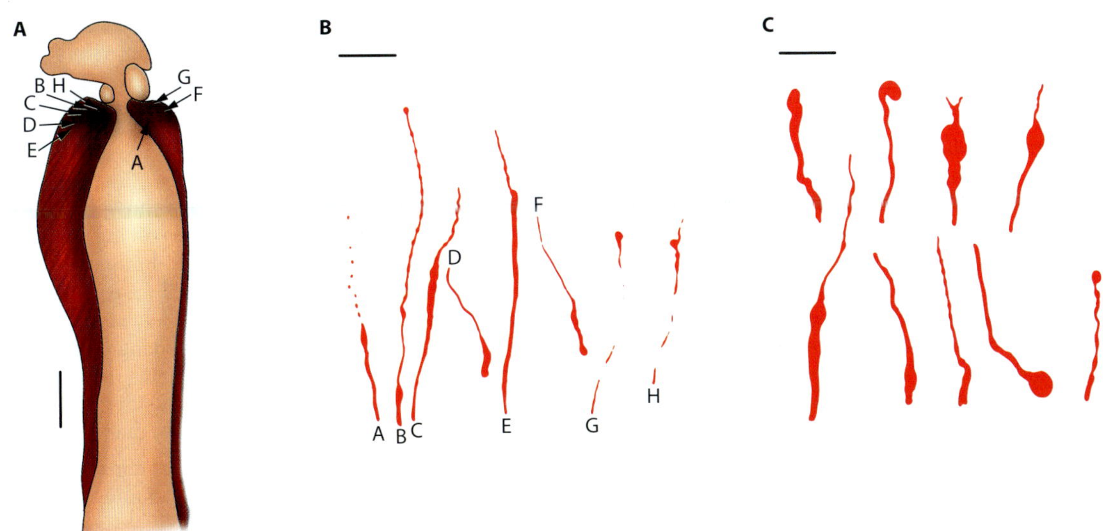

FIGURE 46-1. (**A**) Structure of an electrically active rat nerve-end neuroma (15 days postinjury). (**B**) End-structure of individual sensory axons (A–H). (**C**) High-magnification of individual end-structures. Such end bulbs are the probable source of spontaneous and evoked ectopic neuroma discharge. (Reproduced with permission from Fried K, Devor M. End structure of afferent axons injured in the peripheral and central nervous system. *Somatosens Mot Res.* 1988;6:79-99.)

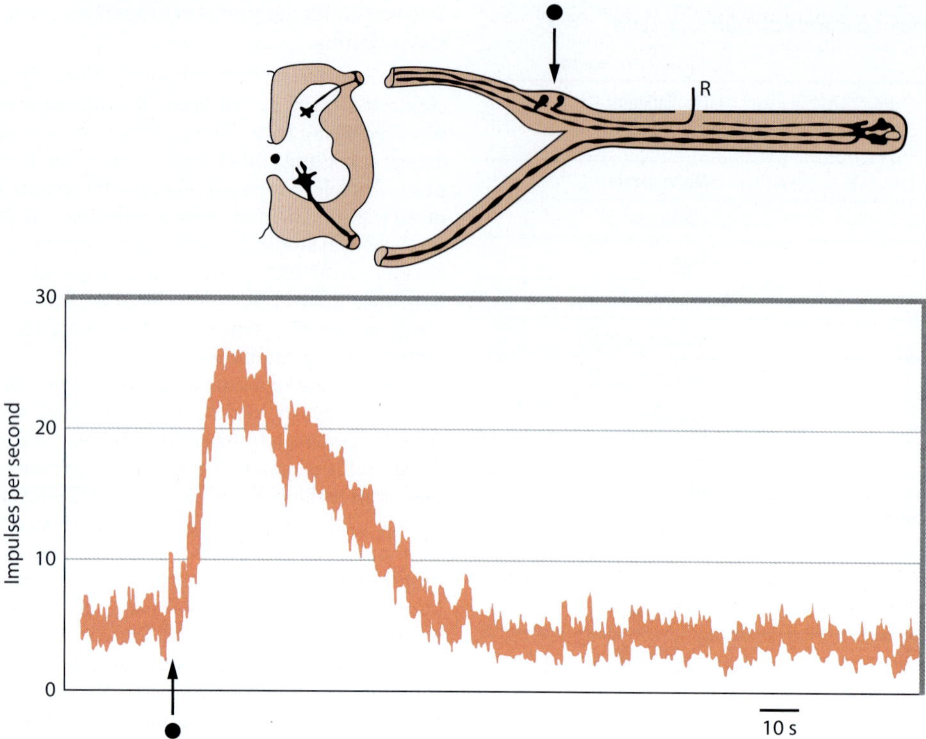

FIGURE 46-2. Prolonged afterdischarge of an afferent axon following mechanical disturbance of the dorsal root ganglia using a 150-mg von Frey hair (*arrow*). The sciatic nerve had been cut 11 days previously. (Reproduced with permission from Devor M. The pathophysiology of damaged nerves. In: Wall P, Melzack R, eds. *Textbook of Pain*. Edinburgh: Churchill Livingstone, 1994:79-99.)

Sensitization and Hyperexcitability Several studies have shown that after injury, intact nerve fiber endings adjacent to injured nerve fibers start to grow and exhibit collateral sprouting. It appears that nociceptive afferent fibers proliferate preferentially. Thus, after nerve injury, an area of denervation may become surrounded by an area that is partially reinnervated but has increased sensitivity to noxious stimuli.[41]

Other changes that take place as a result of nerve injury include axonal membrane remodeling, with an accumulation of voltage-sensitive sodium channels in the end bulb of the axon.[42] These channels are normally in a constant state of turnover, and there is continuous transport of sodium channels downstream.[43] However, if the axon is disrupted, the sodium channels accumulate in the end bulb and render the cell membrane hyperexcitable. Even minor injury, resulting in the loss of myelin without any damage to the axon, triggers the deposition of sodium channels in areas of the axon where they are not usually present.[44]

Amplification Initiation of an action potential by an undamaged neuron is an all-or-none phenomenon, which occurs when a threshold potential is reached. However, the attainment of a certain threshold potential by a damaged neuron can result in *amplification*, or repetitive firing. For example, ectopic neuronal pacemakers that are depolarized to their threshold potentials will fire repetitively despite a single stimulus. A further increase in the intensity of a stimulus can cause a linear, proportional increase in the rate of firing. Because ectopic neuronal pacemakers and DRG pacemaker cells have resting membrane potentials near the repetitive-firing threshold potential, even a weak stimulus may initiate repetitive firing, resulting in symptoms of ongoing pain or paresthesias.[45]

Electrical Cross-Talk Experiments performed in the 1940s by Granit and Skoglund[46] suggest that if the glial insulation between adjacent axons is disrupted, current may flow from severed axons to neighboring fibers. This electrical cross-talk initially subsides after acute injury but may reappear during the process of nerve regeneration and neuroma formation. Because different fiber types lie adjacent to one another (e.g., large, myelinated IA afferent fibers next to nociceptive C fibers), a low-threshold large fiber may be stimulated distally, but because of electrical cross-talk at the site of nerve damage, current might be transferred to a proximal nociceptive afferent.[47]

Central Mechanisms Individuals with pain syndromes associated with both PNS and CNS lesions may have altered firing in thalamic neurons, changes in the somatotopic organization of the ventrobasal complex of the thalamus, and altered responses to electrical stimulation of the CNS.[48] Thus, both the PNS and CNS play important pathophysiologic roles with respect to pain in peripheral nerve disorders.

MECHANISMS OF NERVE INJURY IN SPECIFIC DISORDERS

The two disorders most commonly associated with painful PN are diabetes and HIV/AIDS. Although mechanisms of pain in these specific disorders are not well studied, the pathophysiology of nerve injury in these diseases may shed light on the underlying process that ultimately leads to some of the peripheral mechanisms discussed in the previous section.

Diabetes The diabetic neuropathies are clinically heterogeneous. Pain related to diabetic neuropathies occurs in several clinical syndromes, including DSPN (predominantly involving small fibers), diabetic amyotrophy, truncal radiculopathy, and mononeuritis multiplex.

Several theories have been proposed to explain the pathophysiology of diabetic neuropathies; the most widely accepted are those invoking either metabolic derangement or microangiopathy as primary mechanisms. Despite intensive study, it remains unclear how metabolic and vascular abnormalities affect the excitability of nerve cell membranes to result in the clinical manifestations of diabetic PN, including pain.

Metabolic Theories It is generally agreed that chronic hyperglycemia plays a key role in complications of diabetes, including neuropathy. In 1993, the Diabetes Control and Complications Trial (DCCT) provided evidence that intensive glycemic control delayed the onset and slowed the progression of the long-term complications of insulin-dependent diabetes mellitus, including neuropathy.[49,50] Additionally, several studies have shown improvement of diabetic PN after pancreatic or pancreatic–renal transplants.[51-53] Two proposed mechanisms for the induction of neuropathy by hyperglycemia are the aldose reductase–sorbitol model and the glycation model.

In the first model, investigators note that in the setting of hyperglycemia, glucose is converted to sorbitol by aldose reductase within the nerve. Sorbitol competitively inhibits myoinositol uptake into nerve cells; theoretically, reduced uptake of myoinositol into nerve results in decreased Na^+/K^+-ATPase activity at the nodes of Ranvier. Ultimately, sodium accumulates within the axon, leading to loss of sodium channels and potassium current leak.[54] Loss of sodium channels is, in turn, associated with disruption of the junctional complexes between myelin and axons in the paranodal region. Subsequent paranodal demyelination and axonal shrinkage are the predecessors to clinical neuropathy.

Although attractive, this hypothesis has been challenged based on incomplete metabolic, electrophysiologic, and morphometric evidence.[55,56] Additionally, aldose reductase inhibitors and supplementation with myoinositol have failed to demonstrate therapeutic efficacy in clinical trials of patients with diabetic neuropathy.[57]

According to the glycation model, the presence of excessive glucose in the extracellular matrix results in the formation of so-called advanced glycation end products (AGE). Theoretically, these compounds interfere with several cell functions; DNA and nuclear proteins also may be modified by AGE.[56] In animal studies, diabetic complications have been reduced by the administration of aminoguanidine, an inhibitor of AGE formation.[58,59]

Vascular Theory Another putative mechanism for the development of painful diabetic neuropathy is through microangiopathic changes in the vasi nervorum. Theoretically, nerve injury results directly from ischemia or from ischemia and inflammation associated with immune-mediated vasculitis. Various studies have demonstrated pathologic evidence in nerve biopsy samples for both inflammation and immune complex deposition in vessel walls in patients with various painful forms of diabetic neuropathy.[60,61]

In addition, significant structural changes are seen in the blood vessels of patients with diabetes, including basement membrane thickening and deposition of cellular debris. A significant increase in vascular mural area resulting from deposition of cellular debris is described in diabetes, even in the absence of clinical neuropathy.[62] These microvascular changes appear to precede the development of clinical neuropathy, and their severity correlates with the duration of diabetes and with the severity of the neuropathy.[63] These pathologic findings, although well described, are of unclear significance in the development of neuropathy in diabetes.

Nitric Oxide Endoneurial blood flow has been shown to be reduced in experimental animal models of diabetes.[64] The pathogenesis of this is unclear; however, it appears that the endothelium-derived relaxing factor nitric oxide (NO) may be involved. Depletion of NO or reduced smooth muscle sensitivity to NO is thought to decrease endothelium-dependent relaxation of smooth muscle, a function that has been found to be reduced in diabetic animal models and humans.[64-66] Alternatively, NO may act indirectly on endoneurial blood by modulating sympathetic tone; depletion of NO may result in nerve ischemia as the result of increased vasoconstriction.[67-69]

The metabolic and vascular mechanisms proposed as underlying diabetic neuropathy may converge with the NO theory.[70] Studies have demonstrated a metabolic competition for NADPH by aldose reductase, the enzyme that converts glucose to sorbitol, and NO synthetase, the enzyme that converts L-arginine to NO. It has been shown that aldose reductase inhibitors improve nerve blood flow and restore endothelium-dependent relaxation to normal.[71,72] **Figure 46-3** demonstrates the theoretical mechanism by which this metabolic defect might lead to endoneurial ischemia and abnormalities in nerve conduction.

HIV/AIDS-Related Neuropathies The HIV-associated neuropathies manifest a wide spectrum of disorders, both clinically and pathophysiologically. The most common HIV-associated neuropathy in which pain is a characteristic feature is DSPN. Of the HIV-related neuropathies, this one is the best studied with regard to pathophysiology. The leading theories that have undergone rigorous investigation propose either direct HIV infection or immune-mediated nerve injury as the primary mechanisms underlying DSPN.

Several studies have demonstrated perivascular inflammatory infiltrates in peripheral nerves of patients with HIV-associated DSPN consisting of macrophages and T lymphocytes, suggesting an immune mechanism underlying the disorder.[18,73,74] It appears unlikely that immune complex deposition is involved in the pathogenesis of this neuropathy based on the absence of electron microscopic evidence for immune globulin or complement deposition in nerves.[73,75] However, HIV could lead to a cell-mediated immune attack on the nerves, with resultant demyelination and axonal degeneration.[73] Evidence of cytokine activation and T cells and macrophages at all levels in the PNS suggests that the damage to the PNS in AIDS is a multifocal, immunologic process.[18,74]

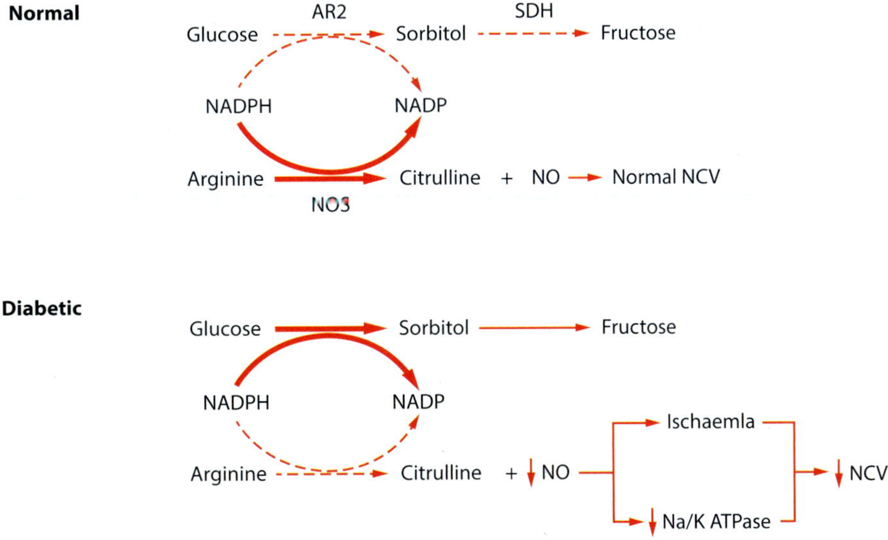

FIGURE 46-3. Metabolic competition for NADPH by aldose reductase and nitric oxide synthase in normal and diabetic state. AR2, aldose reductase; NO, nitric oxide; NOS, nitric oxide synthase; NCV, nerve conduction velocity; SDH, sorbitol dehydrogenase. (Reproduced with permission from Stevens MJ, Feldman EL, Greene DA. The aetiology of diabetic neuropathy: the combined roles of metabolic and vascular defects. *Diabet Med.* 1995;12:566-579.)

The isolation of HIV, HIV-like particles, and HIV-associated mRNA in the peripheral nerves of patients with DSPN led some investigators to postulate that neuropathy results from direct invasion of peripheral nerve by the virus.[75,76] Others have suggested direct infection by the virus of lumbosacral dorsal root ganglion cells, with subsequent central–peripheral distal axonal degeneration as a possible mechanism of DSPN.[77] Subsequent pathologic studies have not been able to confirm HIV particles or antigens in peripheral nerves, nerve roots, or DRG cells.[77,78] Furthermore, in patients in whom HIV was isolated from peripheral nerve in the original studies, the diagnosis of DSPN was subsequently revised to other types of neuropathy.

THERAPEUTICS OF PAIN IN POLYNEUROPATHY

APPROACH TO PAIN IN POLYNEUROPATHY

The pharmacologic approach to patients with PN who have positive symptoms, particularly pain, is the same regardless of the underlying cause of the neuropathy. To date, most clinical studies looking at pharmacologic efficacy in painful neuropathy have been done in patients with diabetic neuropathies, and only a limited number of studies have used double-blind, controlled methodology. Nonetheless, management of pain in patients with PN is often successful using standard agents, particularly when the appropriate principles are considered. Often, patients fail to achieve pain control because of inadequate dosing rather than inefficacy of a particular agent.

In neuropathy, amelioration of pain may be achieved with the use of agents that block pain transmission centrally or peripherally; the role of agents that act on the sympathetic nervous system is less clear. Certainly, some patients with PN may have an element of sympathetically maintained pain. Often, patients require trials with various agents and dosages before optimal therapeutic effect is achieved. The choice of therapy must be tailored to the individual patient (i.e., with regard to age, medical illnesses, previous medication record, and concomitant medications). Drug dosages must be titrated slowly to achieve relief of pain without intolerable side effects. One of the primary principles of pharmacologic management should be the use of single drug therapy whenever possible.

Several classes of drugs are currently used to treat patients with painful peripheral neuropathies. These include tricyclic antidepressants (TCAs), anticonvulsants, antiarrhythmics, analgesics, and narcotic agents. For an extensive discussion of pharmacologic therapies for pain, including specific pharmacologic agents, see Part VI (Chapters 67 to 79). A brief review of the efficacy of the most commonly used agents for painful PN is presented next.

PHARMACOLOGIC AGENTS

Antidepressants The TCAs have been shown to be safe and effective in alleviating the pain of peripheral neuropathy. Commonly used agents include amitriptyline, nortriptyline, imipramine, and desipramine. These agents have been studied in double-blind, randomized controlled trials (RCTs) with results suggesting that each of them reduces pain independent of its effect on depression.[79-82] In one study, 74% of patients who received 75 to 150 mg of amitriptyline attained moderate or greater relief of their pain compared with 41% of patients receiving placebo.[79] Similar results were seen with desipramine.

The TCAs are thought to exert their analgesic effect by inhibiting norepinephrine and serotonin reuptake in the CNS. They also affect cholinergic, histaminergic, and adrenergic transmission, resulting in some limiting side effects. These include sedation, orthostasis, cardiac arrhythmia, and urinary retention. Nortriptyline and desipramine, secondary amine tricyclics, tend to have fewer of these adverse effects, which is preferable for many patients, especially elderly adults. Side effects may be minimized by slow titration, starting with 10 to 25 mg at night and increasing the dose by 10 to 25 mg once or twice weekly. There is no specific target dose; however, the dose usually associated with pain relief is between 50 and 150 mg/day.[83,84]

Anticonvulsants The classic anticonvulsant agents phenytoin and carbamazepine have been used in treating neuropathic pain since the 1960s. It is postulated that anticonvulsants modulate pain by suppressing neuronal firing.[85] These agents have been examined in controlled trials and found to be efficacious in treating pain associated with diabetic neuropathy. A systematic review of these agents found them to be efficacious in treating some neuropathic pain syndromes, including trigeminal neuralgia and diabetic neuropathy, but noted that the risk of adverse effects was equal to the likelihood of significant benefit.[86] Other agents such as clonazepam and valproate have been used anecdotally without much success in pain relief. Overall, the clinical experience suggests that these older anticonvulsant agents are less beneficial in treatment of pain in PN than TCAs or the newer anticonvulsants.[11]

In 1994, gabapentin was approved for use in the United States as an anticonvulsant. It has subsequently enjoyed broad use, including off-label use in the treatment of neuropathic pain. A recent RCT of gabapentin for treatment of pain in diabetic neuropathy found that patients treated with gabapentin had clinically significant alleviation of daily pain severity and improvement of quality-of-life measures.[87] Patients were started on 900 mg/day, and the dose increased by 900 mg/day every week for a total of 4 weeks. Sixty-seven percent of patients achieved the maximum dose of 3600 mg/day, although patients reported therapeutic effect at doses of 900 to 1800 mg/day. Reported side effects included mild dizziness and somnolence. It was concluded that gabapentin monotherapy was efficacious and safe in treating the pain of diabetic neuropathy.

Antiarrhythmics Studies in animal models have shown that antiarrhythmic agents modulate pain pathways by decreasing spontaneous discharges associated with pain generation in injured nerves.[88] Oral mexiletine has been evaluated in several controlled studies; the general consensus is that mexiletine is safe and effective in treating neuropathic pain.[89-91] The dosage found to be efficacious in the studies has been 450 to 675 mg/day. It is recommended that the drug be started at 150 mg/day and titrated upward for effective pain relief. Side effects in the studies were mild and included nausea and dizziness. Electrocardiographic changes were not demonstrable in patients without cardiac disease.

Analgesics

Non-narcotic Agents Another recent addition to the pain therapy armamentarium is tramadol, a centrally acting, synthetic, non-narcotic analgesic that has been available in the United States since 1995. Its two mechanisms of action are (1) low-affinity binding to μ-opioid receptors and (2) weak inhibition of norepinephrine and serotonin reuptake.[92] A recent double-blind, randomized, placebo-controlled trial of patients with painful diabetic neuropathy found that patients receiving an average dose of 210 mg/day of tramadol had significant pain relief with better physical and social functioning compared with patients receiving placebo.[93] The most frequently occurring side effects were headache, constipation, nausea, and somnolence.

Narcotic Agents Clinicians often prescribe narcotics when other therapies have failed. As with other therapeutic agents, it is recommended that a low dose be begun initially and titrated upward to achieve either effective pain relief or intolerable side effects. Patients should be informed of the risk of tolerance. When prescribing an opiate for painful neuropathies, it is recommended that a long-acting agent, such as extended-release morphine, oxycodone, or methadone, be used.[11] In 2012, tapentadol, a novel narcotic with norepinephrine reuptake inhibitor properties, was approved for use in painful diabetic PN. It is available in both short- and long-acting formats, but there is a therapeutic ceiling for dosages.

Topical Agents Capsaicin is an alkaloid found in capsicum peppers. When applied topically, it produces desensitization to noxious stimuli.[94] It has been studied in patients with painful diabetic neuropathies with mixed results. One double-blind comparison of topical capsaicin and oral amitriptyline found topical capsaicin to be equally efficacious as amitriptyline but without any systemic side effects.[95] Another RCT of the drug in painful diabetic neuropathy found it to be of no benefit.[96] Although the literature appeared optimistic originally, clinical experience has been disappointing. Patients find the drug difficult to use because care must be taken not to allow contamination of unaffected body parts. Even in affected body parts, the drug causes significant burning pain on application, which most patients find an intolerable side effect. The mechanism of action of capsaicin is believed to be depletion of substance P. Proper usage requires frequent application (three or four times a day) for at least 1 week to obtain benefit; premature termination of treatment after 3 or 4 days results in a flood of substance P into nerve terminals but insufficient time to appreciate the depleted levels in the axons. Capsaicin is available topically over the counter, but a much more potent formulation is available only as a prescription administered by a physician.

Other Agents Dextromethorphan, a low-affinity *N*-methyl-D-aspartate (NMDA) receptor antagonist and dextro isomer of the codeine analogue levorphanol, has been studied in a randomized, double-blind, placebo-controlled crossover trial of patients with a painful diabetic neuropathy and patients with postherpetic neuralgia.[97] In diabetic neuropathy, patients who received dextromethorphan had their pain decrease by an average of 24% relative to patients who received placebo. Dextromethorphan did not alleviate pain for patients with postherpetic neuralgia. The average dose received by the patients with diabetes was 381 mg/day. The limiting side effects of treatment with dextromethorphan include ataxia and sedation. Although this study suggests that NMDA receptor antagonists may be useful in the treatment of painful neuropathies, the clinical experience has been disappointing.[11]

REFERENCES

1. Dyck PJ, Benstead TJ, Conn DL, et al. Nonsystemic vasculitic neuropathy. *Brain*. 1987;110:843-853.
2. Dobretsov M, Romanovsky D, Stimers JR. Early diabetic neuropathy: triggers and mechanisms. *World J Gastroenterol*. 2007;13(2):175-191.
3. Ruscin JM, Page RL 2nd, Valuck RJ. Vitamin B(12) deficiency associated with histamine(2)-receptor antagonists and a proton-pump inhibitor. *Ann Pharmacother*. 2002;36(5):812-816.
4. Termanini B, Gibril F, Sutliff VE, et al. Effect of long-term gastric acid suppressive therapy on serum vitamin B12 levels in patients with Zollinger-Ellison syndrome. *Am J Med*. 1998;104(5):422-430.
5. Carvaho IR, Loscalzo IT, Reitas MF, et al. Incidence of vitamin B deficiency in patients submitted to Fobi-Capella Roux-en-Y bariatric surgery. *Arq Bras Cir Dig*. 2012;25(1):36-40.
6. Xanthakos SA. Nutritional deficiencies in obesity and after bariatric surgery. *Pediatr Clin North Am*. 2009;56(5):1105-1121.
7. Sentongo TA, Azzam R, Charrow J. Vitamin B12 status, methylmalonic acidemia, and bacterial overgrowth in short bowel syndrome. *J Pediatr Gastroenterol Nutr*. 2009;48(4):495-497.
8. Wierdsma NJ, van Bokhorst-de van der Schueren MA, Berkenpas M, et al. Vitamin and mineral deficiencies are highly prevalent in newly diagnosed celiac disease patients. *Nutrients*. 2013;5(10):3975-3992.
9. Mead P, Goel R, Kugeler K. Canine serology as adjunct to human Lyme disease surveillance. *Emerg Infect Dis*. 2011;17(9): 1710-1712.
10. Galer BS, Jensen MP. Development and preliminary validation of a pain measure specific to neuropathic pain: the Neuropathic Pain Scale. *Neurology*. 1997;48:332-338.
11. Galer B. Painful polyneuropathy. *Neurol Clin*. 1998;16:791-812.
12. Peripheral Neuropathy Association. Quantitative sensory testing: a consensus report from the Peripheral Neuropathy Association. *Neurology*. 1993;43:1050-1052.
13. Holland NR, Crawford TO, Hauer P, et al. Small-fiber sensory neuropathies: clinical course and neuropathology of idiopathic cases. *Ann Neurol*. 1998;44:47-59.
14. Giuliani M, Tobin K. Small-fiber neuropathy: evaluation recommendations. *Neurology*. 1996;46(Suppl):A312.
15. McCarthy BG, Hsieh ST, Stocks A, et al. Cutaneous innervation in sensory neuropathies: evaluation by skin biopsy. *Neurology*. 1995;45:1848-1855.
16. Thomas P, Tomlinson D. Diabetic and hypoglycemic neuropathy. In: Dyck P, Thomas P, Griffin J, et al, eds. *Peripheral Neuropathy*. Philadelphia: WB Saunders; 1993:1222-1250.
17. Cornblath D, McArthur J. Predominantly sensory neuropathy in patients with AIDS and AIDS-related complex. *Neurology*. 1988;38:794-796.
18. Rizzuto N, Cavallaro T, Monaco S, et al. Role of HIV in the pathogenesis of distal symmetrical peripheral neuropathy. *Acta Neuropathol (Berl)*. 1995;90:244-250.
19. So Y, Holtzman D, Abrams D, et al. Peripheral neuropathy associated with acquired immunodeficiency syndrome: prevalence and clinical features from a population based survey. *Arch Neurol*. 1988;45:945-948.
20. Lambert J, Seidlin M, Reichman R, et al. 2′,39′-dideoxyinosine (ddI) in patients with the acquired immunodeficiency syndrome or AIDS-related complex. A phase I trial. *N Engl J Med*. 1990;322:1333-1340.
21. Berger A, Arezzo J, Schaumburg H, et al. 2′,3′-dideoxycytidine (ddC) toxic neuropathy: a study of 52 patients. *Neurology*. 1993;43:358-362.
22. Simpson D, Tagliati M. Nucleoside analogue-associated peripheral neuropathy in human immunodeficiency virus infection. *J Acquir Immune Defic Syndr Hum Retrovirol*. 1995;9:153-161.
23. Browne M, Mayer K, Chafee S, et al. 2′,3′-didehydro-3′-deoxythymidine (d4t) in patients with AIDS or AIDS-related complex: a phase I trial. *J Infect Dis*. 1993;167:21-29.
24. Ochonisky S, Vernoust J, Bastuji-Garin S, et al. Thalidomide neuropathy incidence and clinicoelectrophysiologic findings in 42 patients. *Arch Dermatol*. 1992;130:66-69.
25. Figg W. Peripheral neuropathy in HIV patients after isoniazid therapy initiated. *DICP*. 1991;25:100-101.
26. So Y, Olney R. The natural history of mononeuritis multiplex and simplex in patients with HIV infection. *Neurology*. 1991;41(Suppl 1):375.
27. Engstrom J, Lewis E, McGuire D. Cranial neuropathy and the acquired immunodeficiency syndrome. *Neurology*. 1991;41(Suppl 1):374.
28. Stricker R, Sanders K, Owen W, et al. Mononeuritis multiplex associated with cryoglobulinemia in HIV infection. *Neurology*. 1992;42:2103-2105.
29. Roullet E, Assuerus V, Gozlan J, et al. Cytomegalovirus multifocal neuropathy in AIDS: analysis of 15 consecutive cases. *Neurology*. 1994;44:2174-2182.
30. Said G, Lacroix-Ciaudo C, Fujimura H, et al. The peripheral neuropathy of necrotizing arteritis: a clinicopathological study. *Ann Neurol*. 1988;23:461-465.
31. Moulignier A, Authier F, Baudrimont M, et al. Peripheral neuropathy in human immunodeficiency virus–infected patients with the diffuse infiltrative lymphocytosis syndrome. *Ann Neurol*. 1997;41:438-445.
32. Price R. Neuropathy complicating diffuse infiltrative lymphocytosis. *Lancet*. 1998;352:592-594.

33. Vendrell J, Heredia C, Pujol M, et al. Guillain-Barré syndrome associated with seroconversion for anti-HTLV-III. *Neurology.* 1987;37:544.
34. Ropper A, Wijdicks E, Truax B. *Guillain-Barre Syndrome.* Philadelphia: FA Davis; 1991.
35. Devor M, Rappaport Z. Pain and the pathophysiology of damaged nerve. In: Fields H, ed. *Pain Syndromes in Neurology.* London: Butterworth & Co; 1990:42-83.
36. Gouvrin-Lippmann R, Devor M. Ongoing activity in severed nerves: source and variation with time. *Brain Res.* 1978;159:406-410.
37. Blumberg H, Janig W. Discharge pattern of afferent fibers from a neuroma. *Pain.* 1984;20:335-353.
38. Ruiz J, Kocsis J, Preson R. *Repetitive Firing Characteristics of Mammalian Myelinated Axons: An Intra-axonal Analysis.* Vol. 7. Bethesda, MD: Society for Neuroscience; 1981.
39. Devor M, White D, Goetzl E, et al. Eicosanoids, but not tachykinins, excite C-fiber endings in rat sciatic nerve-end neuromas. *Neuroreport.* 1992;3:21-24.
40. Kajander K, Wakisaka S, Bennet G. Spontaneous discharge originates in the dorsal root ganglion at the onset of a painful peripheral neuropathy in the rat. *Neurosci Lett.* 1992;138:225-228.
41. Inbal R, Rousso M, Ashur H, et al. Collateral sprouting and sensory recovery after nerve injury in man. *Pain.* 1987;28:141-154.
42. Devor M, Gouvrin-Lippmann R, Angelides K. Na+ channel immunolocalization in peripheral mammalian axons and changes following nerve injury and neuroma formation. *J Neurosci.* 1993;13:1976-1992.
43. Matzner O, Devor M. Na+ conductance and the threshold for repetitive neuronal firing. *Brain Res.* 1992;597:92-98.
44. Devor M. The pathophysiology of damaged nerves. In: Wall P, Melzack R, eds. *Textbook of Pain.* Edinburgh: Churchill Livingstone; 1994:79-99.
45. Lisney S, Devor M. Afterdischarge and interactions among fibers in damaged peripheral nerve in the rat. *Brain Res.* 1987;415:122-136.
46. Granit R, Skoglund C. Facilitation, inhibition, and depression at the "artificial synapse" formed by the cut end of a mammalian nerve. *J Physiol.* 1945;103:435-448.
47. Bernstein J, Pagnarelli D. Long-term axonal opposition in rat sciatic nerve neuroma. *J Neurosurg.* 1982;57:682-684.
48. Willner C, Low P. Approaches to neuropathic pain. In: Dyck P, ed. *Peripheral Neuropathy.* Vol 2. Philadelphia: WB Saunders; 1993:1709-1720.
49. Diabetes Control and Complications Trial and Research Group. The effect of intensive treatment of diabetes on the development and progression of long-term complications in insulin-dependent diabetes mellitus. *N Engl J Med.* 1993;329:977-986.
50. Diabetes Control and Complications Trial and Research Group. Effect of intensive diabetes treatment on nerve conduction in the diabetes control and complications trial. *Ann Neurol.* 1995;88:869-880.
51. Kennedy W, Navarro X, Goetz F. Effects of pancreatic transplantation on diabetic neuropathy. *N Engl J Med.* 1990;322:1031-1037.
52. Orloff M, Greenfield G, Gerard B. Reversal of diabetic somatic neuropathy by whole pancreas transplantation. *Surgery.* 1990;108:179-190.
53. Navarro X, Sutherland D, Kennedy D. Long-term effects of pancreatic transplantation on diabetic neuropathy. *Ann Neurol.* 1997;42:727-736.
54. Greene D, Lattimer S, Sima A. Sorbitol, phosphoinositodes, and sodium-potassium ATPase in the pathogenesis of diabetic complications. *N Engl J Med.* 1987;316:599-605.
55. Dyck P, Giannini C. Pathologic alterations in the diabetic neuropathies of humans: a review. *J Neuropathol Exp Neurol.* 1996;55:1181-1193.
56. Brownlee M. Glycation products and the pathogenesis of diabetic complications. *Diabetes Care.* 1992;15:1835-1845.
57. Krentz A, Honigsberger L, Ellis S. A 12-month randomized controlled study of the aldose reductase inhibitor ponalrestat in patients with chronic symptomatic diabetic neuropathy. *Diabet Med.* 1992;9:463-468.
58. Hammes H, Martin S, Federlin K, et al. Aminoguanidine treatment inhibits the development of experimental diabetic retinopathy. *Proc Natl Acad Sci U S A.* 1991;88:11555-11558.
59. Yagihashi S, Kamijo M, Baba M, et al. Effect of aminoguanidine on functional and structural abnormalities in peripheral nerve of STZ-induced diabetic rats. *Diabetes.* 1992;41:47-52.
60. Said G, Goulon-Goeau C, Lacroix C, et al. Nerve biopsy findings in different patterns of proximal diabetic neuropathy. *Ann Neurol.* 1994;35:559-569.
61. Younger D, Rosoklija G, Hays A, et al. Diabetic peripheral neuropathy: a clinicopathologic and immunohistochemical analysis of sural nerve biopsies. *Muscle Nerve.* 1996;19:722-727.
62. Yasuda H, Dyck P. Abnormalities of endoneurial microvessels and sural nerve pathology in diabetic neuropathy. *Neurology.* 1987;37:20-28.
63. Giannini C, Dyck P. Basement membrane reduplication and pericyte degeneration precede development of diabetic polyneuropathy and are associated with its severity. *Ann Neurol.* 1995;37:498-504.
64. Mayhan WG, Simmons LK, Sharpe GM. Mechanism of impaired responses of cerebral arterioles during diabetes mellitus. *Am J Physiol.* 1991;260:H319-H326.
65. Vallance P, Collier J, Moncada S. Effects of endothelium-derived nitric oxide on peripheral arteriolar tone in man [see comments]. *Lancet.* 1989;2:997-1000.
66. Calver A, Collier J, Vallance P. Inhibition and stimulation of nitric oxide synthesis in the human forearm arterial bed of patients with insulin-dependent diabetes. *J Clin Invest.* 1992;90:2548-2554.
67. Greene DA, Sima AA, Stevens MJ, et al. Complications: neuropathy, pathogenetic considerations. *Diabetes Care.* 1992;15:1902-1925.
68. Bult H, Boeckxstaens GE, Pelckmans PA, et al. Nitric oxide as an inhibitory nonadrenergic non-cholinergic neurotransmitter [see comments]. *Nature.* 1990;345:346-347.
69. Cameron NE, Cotter MA, Low PA. Nerve blood flow in early experimental diabetes in rats: relation to conduction deficits. *Am J Physiol.* 1991;261:E1-E8.
70. Stevens MJ, Dananberg J, Feldman EL, et al. The linked roles of nitric oxide, aldose reductase and, (Na+, K+)-ATPase in the slowing of nerve conduction in the streptozotocin diabetic rat. *J Clin Invest.* 1994;94:853-859.
71. Yasuda H, Sonobe M, Yamashita M, et al. Effect of prostaglandin E1 analogue TFC 612 on diabetic neuropathy in streptozocin-induced diabetic rats. Comparison with aldose reductase inhibitor ONO 2235. *Diabetes.* 1989;38:832-838.
72. Cameron NE, Cotter MA. Impaired contraction and relaxation in aorta from streptozotocin-diabetic rats: role of polyol pathway. *Diabetologia.* 1992;35:1011-1019.
73. de la Monte S, Gabuzda D, Ho D, et al. Peripheral neuropathy in the acquired immunodeficiency syndrome. *Ann Neurol.* 1988;23:485-492.
74. Bradley W, Shapshak P, Delgado S, et al. Morphometric analysis of the peripheral neuropathy of AIDS. *Muscle Nerve.* 1998;21:1188-1195.
75. Bailey R, Baltch A, Venkatesh R, et al. Sensory motor neuropathy associated with AIDS. *Neurology.* 1988;38:886-891.

76. Ho D, Rota T, Schooley R, et al. Isolation of HTLV-III from cerebrospinal fluid and neural tissues of patients with neurologic syndromes related to the acquired immunodeficiency syndrome. *N Engl J Med*. 1985;313:1493-1497.

77. Rance N, McArthur J, Cornblath D. Gracile tract degeneration in patients with sensory neuropathy and AIDS. *Neurology*. 1988;38:265-271.

78. Grafe M, Wiley C. Spinal cord and peripheral nerve pathology in AIDS: the roles of cytomegalovirus and human immunodeficiency virus. *Ann Neurol*. 1989;25:561-566.

79. Max M, Lynch S, Muir J, et al. Effects of desipramine, amitriptyline, and fluoxetine on pain in diabetic neuropathy. *N Engl J Med*. 1992;326:1250-1256.

80. Gomez-Perez F, Rull J, Dies H, et al. Nortriptyline and fluphenazine in the symptomatic treatment of diabetic neuropathy: a double blind cross-over study. *Pain*. 1985;23:395-397.

81. Max M, Kishore-Kumar R, Schafer S, et al. Efficacy of desipramine in painful diabetic neuropathy: a placebo-controlled trial. *Pain*. 1991;45:3-9.

82. Kurnsdahl B, Molin J, Froland A, et al. Imipramine treatment of painful diabetic neuropathy. *JAMA*. 1984;251:1727-1730.

83. Portenoy R. Painful polyneuropathy. *Neurol Clin*. 1989;7:265-288.

84. Bajwa ZH, Simopoulos TT, Pal J, et al. Low and therapeutic doses of antidepressants are associated with similar response in the context of multimodal treatment of pain. *Pain Physician*. 2009;12(5):893-900.

85. Maciewicz R, Bouckoms A, Martin J. Drug therapy of neuropathic pain. *Clin J Pain*. 1985;1:39-49.

86. McQuay H, Carroll D, Jadad A, et al. Anticonvulsant drugs for management of pain: a systematic review. *BMJ*. 1995;311:1047-1052.

87. Backonja M, Beydoun A, Edwards K, et al. Gabapentin for the symptomatic treatment of painful neuropathy in patients with diabetes mellitus: a randomized controlled trial. *JAMA*. 1998;280:1831-1836.

88. Chabal C, Jacobson L, Russell L, et al. Pain response to perineuromal injection of normal saline, epinephrine, and lidocaine in humans. *Pain*. 1989;38:333-338.

89. Oskarsson P, Ljunggren J, Lins P. Efficacy and safety of mexiletine in the treatment of painful diabetic neuropathy. The Mexiletine Study Group. *Diabetes Care*. 1997;20:1594-1597.

90. Dejgard A, Petersen P, Kastrup J. Mexiletine for treatment of chronic painful diabetic neuropathy. *Lancet*. 1988;1:9-11.

91. Stracke H, Meyer U, Schumacher H, et al. Mexiletine in the treatment of diabetic neuropathy. *Diabetes Care*. 1992;15:1550-1555.

92. Raffa R, Friderichs E, Reimann W, et al. Opioid and nonopioid components independently contribute to the mechanism of action of tramadol, an "atypical" opioid analgesic. *J Pharmacol Exp Ther*. 1992;260:275-285.

93. Harati Y, Gooch C, Swenson M, et al. Double-blind randomized trial of tramadol for the treatment of the pain of diabetic neuropathy. *Neurology*. 1998;50:1842-1846.

94. Tandan R, Lewis GA, Krusinski PB, et al. Topical capsaicin in painful diabetic neuropathy. Controlled study with long-term follow-up [see comments]. *Diabetes Care*. 1992;15:8-14.

95. Biesbroek R, Bril V, Hollander P, et al. A double-blind comparison of topical capsaicin and oral amitriptyline in painful diabetic neuropathy. *Adv Ther*. 1995;12:111-120.

96. Chad DA, Aronin N, Lundstrum R, et al. Does capsaicin relieve the pain of diabetic neuropathy? [letter]. *Pain*. 1990;42:387-388.

97. Nelson K, Park K, Robinovitz E, et al. High-dose oral dextromethorphan versus placebo in painful diabetic neuropathy and postherpetic neuralgia. *Neurology*. 1997;48:1212-1218.

Central Neuropathic Pain Following Spinal Cord Injury

Christine N. Sang
Rodrigo Benavides

INTRODUCTION

The development of debilitating central neuropathic pain (CNP), defined as pain caused by a lesion or dysfunction of the central nervous system (CNS),[1,2] can occur after any lesion of the CNS, including demyelinating, vascular, infectious, inflammatory, and traumatic events. In contrast to CNP after stroke (including thalamic stroke resulting in Dejerine-Roussy syndrome), multiple sclerosis, and tumors,[3,4] the prevalence of CNP after spinal cord injury (SCI) is high; most cite a prevalence ranging from 50% to 66%.[5-8] With the number of individuals in the United States who have SCIs estimated to be as high as 1,275,000 and estimated lifetime costs from SCI ranging from $681,843 to more than $3 million if the injury is sustained at age 25 years,[9] CNP after SCI has become a growing public health concern.

Lesions of the spinal cord, particularly those caused by trauma, are also associated with lesions of adjacent nerve roots, including the cauda equina; therefore, CNP is typically associated with peripheral neuropathic pain (PNP). CNP may also be associated with visceral pain through sympathetic and vagal nerve input and pain secondary to musculoskeletal overuse, muscle spasms, or mechanical instability of the spine.[10] The primary insult to the somatosensory pathway may be limited, with only mild sensory loss on clinical examination, or extensive, with complete anesthesia on clinical examination. Notably, refractory deafferentation pain may be associated with only mild sensory loss on examination.

Traumatic SCIs account for 65% of CNP, and other causes include iatrogenic (12%), inflammatory (9%), neoplastic (6%), skeletal (2%), and vascular (2%).[11,12] At the time of injury, typical symptoms of CNP are often not present but may appear during the rehabilitation phase. The distribution of these lesions is 42% in the cervical spine, 21% in T1 to T9, and 37% in T10 to L2.[12,13]

CLINICAL CHARACTERISTICS OF CENTRAL NEUROPATHIC PAIN AFTER SPINAL CORD INJURY

Although several different heterogeneous pain syndromes may develop after SCI, CNP is potentially the most problematic. CNP is characterized as spontaneous pain (e.g., allodynia and hyperalgesia with temporal and spatial summation) in a distribution from which spinal and supraspinal mechanisms may be inferred. Moreover, negative or positive sensory signs are present at or below the level of injury or in the distribution of the area of pain. Therefore, in 2000, the International Association for the Study of Pain proposed a classification based on the distribution of pain relative to the level of injury: (1) at-level pain, distributed segmentally at the border of normal and interrupted sensory innervation, and (2) below-level pain, distributed diffusely below the level of injury.[13] At-level pain typically presents within two to three segments above and below the level of injury[13] and often involves a lesion to the spinothalamic tract or changes in the spinal cord dorsal horn, producing hyperexcitability in the pain pathways. Nerve root injuries contribute to an increased impulse generation.[14-16] Below-level pain involves sensory hypersensitivity and neuronal hyperactivity at the level of injury;[17,18] pathophysiologic changes at supraspinal levels may include spinothalamic tract lesions, such as a spinothalamic dysrhythmia, or thalamic structural reorganization.[19,20] A longitudinal study suggests that the onset of at-level pain may precede that of below-level pain.[5] Above-level pain has been typically associated with compressive mononeuropathies and other lesions and syndromes not directly caused by cord damage at the level of injury; however, animal models of CNP after thoracic spinal cord lesions show behavioral changes above the level of injury that are associated with peripheral and central sensitization and reactive glia in the uninjured cervical cord.[21-23]

Syringomyelia may also be an important source of neuropathic pain and often presents long after the initial injury.[24-26] It involves the dilation of the central canal (termed *cyst*) within the spinal cord that expands and damages the center cord. Patient may present initially with a small injury and later develops progressively worsening painful symptoms.[25,26]

MECHANISMS OF CENTRAL NEUROPATHIC PAIN AFTER SPINAL CORD INJURY

Experimental rodent models of CNP after SCI have contributed to our understanding of pathophysiological mechanisms (**Figs. 47-1** and **47-2**). Models include ischemic, traumatic (hemisection, contusion, compression, anterolateral cut, electrolytic), and neurotoxic (quisqualate).[22] Behavioral assays include measures of evoked hyperalgesia and allodynia, such as mechanical and thermal withdrawal thresholds; however, the development of central spasticity in these models is a potential confounder.[27] Excitatory amino acids such as glutamate are briefly released in and around the site of injury, resulting in neuronal hyperexcitability.[28,29] Data also suggest that the dysfunction of descending inhibitory control mechanisms after lesions of the dorsal or dorsolateral quadrant of the spinal cord results in a component of spontaneous pain that is associated with CNP.[30,31] Inhibitory neurons containing γ-aminobutyric acid (GABA) are highly susceptible to hypoxia, and the loss of tonic central inhibitory actions and their participation in descending inhibitory tracts may also contribute to an increased responsiveness of neurons in pain pathways.[32,33]

Functional changes of receptor and ion channels include the altered expression of sodium channels in the spinal cord and thalamus[34] and the upregulation of voltage-gated calcium channel $\alpha 2\delta$-1 subunit protein in the spinal cord.[35] Other neurochemical changes with a possible role in SCI pain include elevation of intracellular calcium, calcium activation of phospholipase A2, protein kinase C activation, and changes in nitric oxide and peptides such as substance P and dynorphin.[36] Neuroinflammation involving the activation of a complex network of neuroimmune processes also contributes to regeneration and degeneration of the injured tissue after SCI; glial (astrocytes and microglia) cells are inherently involved in the activation and dysfunction of central neurons in the spinal cord[36-42] and contribute to the development of "gliopathy," which results in sensory dysfunction. Structural and functional abnormalities in several brain regions are also associated with nociceptive processing.[43-45]

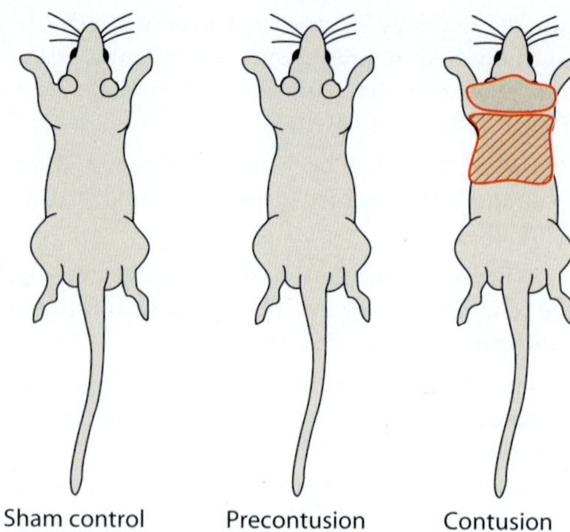

FIGURE 47-1. Mechanical allodynia in a rat with a T13 spinal cord injury (contusion model). Red: Touch-evoked allodynia; area determined using von Frey filament to determine vocalization threshold to graded mechanical allodynia. (Courtesy of Claire Hulsebosch, PhD.)

TREATMENTS FOR CENTRAL NEUROPATHIC PAIN AFTER SPINAL CORD INJURY

Given the range of molecular mechanisms involved in CNP, combination therapy is typically prescribed; however, clinically available treatments for neuropathic pain are associated with unacceptable side effects that can interfere with activities of daily living, such as cognitive, anticholinergic, or motor dysfunction in an ambulating patient.[46-49]

Among the tricyclic antidepressants, only amitriptyline has been studied in CNP after SCI, with one positive clinical trial evaluating

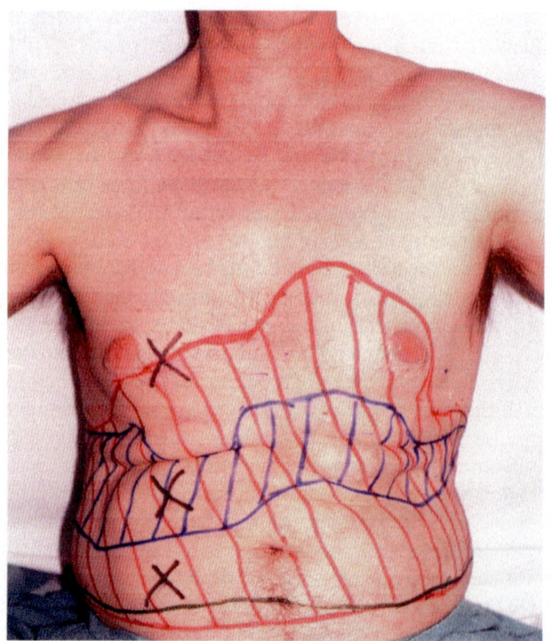

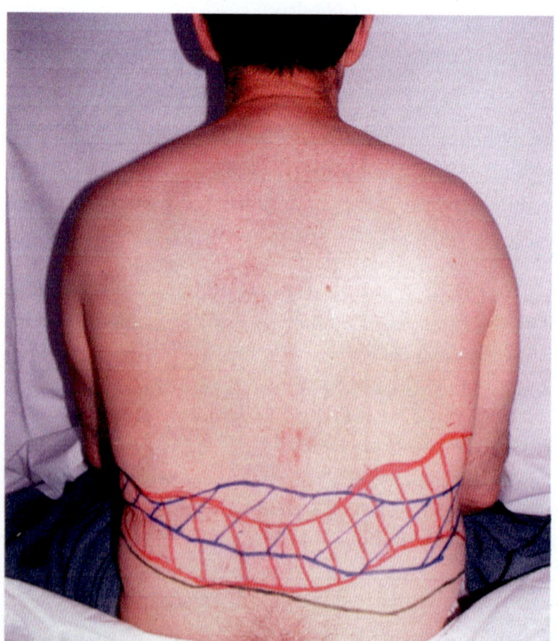

FIGURE 47-2. T7 complete spinal cord injury (SCI) in a patient with central neuropathic pain after SCI. Red: Touch-evoked allodynia. Blue: Pin prick hyperalgesia.

150 mg/day ($n = 38$)[50] and one negative clinical trial at 125 mg/day ($n = 84$).[51] Duloxetine is the only serotonin norepinephrine reuptake inhibitor to have been evaluated in CNP to date; Vranken et al.[52] failed to show an analgesic effect in 48 subjects at a daily dose of 120 mg versus placebo, although the clinical trial was likely to have been underpowered.

The α2δ ligand gabapentin, considered first-line treatment for neuropathic pain, has been evaluated in three clinical trials in CNP.[50,53,54] Only Levendoglu was able to show an analgesic effect in 20 subjects at 3600 mg/day. Pregabalin, also an α2δ ligand, has been shown to have an analgesic effect in two large clinical trials in CNP, resulting in its Food and Drug Administration approval specifically for CNP. Siddall et al.[55] showed an analgesic effect of 150 to 600 mg/day (mean, 460 mg/day) in 137 patients, and Cardenas et al.[56] showed an analgesic effect of 150 to 600 mg/day (mean, 410 mg/day) in 220 patients with below-level CNP. Pregabalin has anxiolytic effects in patients with generalized anxiety disorders and may be preferable to gabapentin in patients with concurrent anxiety.[57] Gabapentin has consistently been shown to relieve central spasticity in SCI,[58,59] confirming preclinical studies that gabapentin is associated with motor dysfunction at analgesic doses.[60-62] There are few reports of pregabalin's effect on central spasticity and hence the potential for motor dysfunction in individuals with SCI; they include one retrospective case series[63] showing an effect of pregabalin on spasticity and one prospective case series[64] showing that pregabalin withdrawal results in self-reports of increased spasticity without a concomitant increase in pain. Therefore, gabapentin and pregabalin are to be used with caution in ambulating patients because at least some spasticity is required to ambulate. Sodium channel antagonists such as lamotrigine are considered adjunctive therapy primarily in patients with incomplete SCI with evoked pain, although evidence for this is limited.[65,66]

Oral opioids, including tramadol, have not been broadly studied in CNP, in part because of side effects that may impact on comorbidities such as neurogenic bowel and bladder. However, in patients with severe refractory neuropathic pain, intrathecal drug administration with morphine in combination with clonidine or baclofen may be an effective alternative, although the evidence is limited.[64-68]

Intravenous (IV) administration of lidocaine, 5 mg/kg over 30 minutes, reduces spontaneous pain and evoked allodynia in CNP.[69] Other IV analgesics such as ketamine and propofol may also relieve CNP but are generally not suitable for long-term management.[70,71] There are thus far no data to show an effect of early treatment with IV agents after acute injury to reduce the risk or severity of CNP.[69]

Cognitive-behavioral therapy for the treatment of concomitant anxiety, depression, and psychological distress may also serve as adjuncts for the treatment of CNP. Specific management of other associated conditions, such as sleeping disorders, cognitive impairment, limitations in daily activity, and social relations, may also present challenges in the management of individuals with chronic SCI.[72,73]

Physical therapy, with strengthening and stretching exercises as well as recommendations for optimized movement techniques, upper extremity weight-bearing techniques, and wheelchair propulsion are recommended for associated musculoskeletal pain.[74] Acupuncture, transcutaneous electrical nerve stimulation, and spinal cord stimulation may be effective in some patients with incomplete lesions and in cases of painful spasms or at the level pain, but results for long-term efficacy are limited.

Surgical techniques on the spinal cord including percutaneous radiofrequency rhizotomy, cordotomies, and dorsal root entry zone lesions have been described for use in CNP, but clear evidence is lacking. Published reports suggest that different pain characteristics may respond differently to different destructive procedures.[75-77] Dorsal column stimulation may be used, although results are disappointing;[78] placement can be challenging because of the anatomical distortion or scar tissue, and the dorsal columns may degenerate after complete lesions.[77] In contrast to dorsal column stimulation, deep brain stimulation has been used to treat CNP but also with disappointing results.[79]

CONCLUSION

Central neuropathic pain remains a great unmet need after SCI, with a prevalence that exceeds that after isolated peripheral nerve injury. Supraspinal and spinal mechanisms, even distant from the level of injury, are implicated; therefore, pharmacologic interventions may be necessary. Pregabalin is thus far the only treatment approved for the treatment of CNP; however, similar to gabapentin, its use is limited by dose-limiting side effects, including motor dysfunction, which is problematic in ambulating SCI patients. A greater investment in the discovery of new drugs for the treatment of CNP is warranted.

REFERENCES

1. Tasker RR. Central pain states. In: Warfield C, Bajwa Z (eds.) *Principles and Practice of Pain Medicine.* 2nd ed. NewYork: McGraw Hill; 2004:432-453.
2. Mersky H, Bogduk N. *Classification of Chronic Pain.* Seattle: IASP Press; 1994:1-222.
3. Yezierski RP. Pain following spinal cord injury: pathophysiology and central mechanisms. *Prog Brain Res.* 2000;129:429-449.
4. Boivie J. Central pain. In: McMahon, Koltzenburg, eds. *Wall and Melzack's Textbook of Pain.* Oxford: Churchill Livingstone; 2005:1057-1074.
5. Siddall PJ, McClelland JM, Rutkowski SB, Cousins MJ. A longitudinal study of the prevalence and characteristics of pain in the first 5 years following spinal cord injury. *Pain.* 2003;103(3):249-257.
6. Woolsley RM. Chronic pain following spinal cord injury. *J Am Paraplegia Soc.* 1986;9(3-4):39-41.
7. Nepomuceno C, Fine PR, Richards JS, et al. Pain in patients with spinal cord injury. *Arch Phys Med Rehabil.* 1979;60(12):605-609.
8. Störmer S, Gerner HJ, Grüninger W, et al. Chronic pain/dysaesthesiae in spinal cord injury patients: results of a multicentre study. *Spinal Cord.* 1997;35(7):446-455.
9. Christopher and Dana Reeve Foundation. Spinal Cord Injury Paralysis Resource Center: paralysis facts & figures. http://www.christopherreeve.org/site/c.mtKZKgMWKwG/b.5184189/k.5587/Paralysis_Facts__Figures.htm.
10. Finnerup NB, Baastrup C. Spinal cord injury pain: mechanisms and management. *Curr Pain Headache Rep.* 2012;16(3):207-216.
11. Eide PK. Pathophysiological mechanisms of central neuropathic pain after spinal cord injury. *Spinal Cord.* 1998;36:601-612.
12. Tasker RR, De Carvalho GTC. Intractable pain of spinal cord origin: clinical features and implications for surgery. *J Neurosurg.* 1992;77:373-378.
13. Siddall PJ, Yezierski RP. Pain following spinal cord injury: clinical features, prevalence and taxonomy. *IASP Newsletter.* 2000.
14. Siddall PJ, Middleton JW. A proposed algorithm for the management of pain following spinal cord injury. *Spinal Cord.* 2006;44(2):67-77.
15. Yezierky RP, Park SH. The mechanosensitivity of spinal sensory neurons following intraspinal injections of quisqualic acid in the rat. *Neurosci Lett.* 1993;157(1):115-119.
16. Drew GM, Siddall PJ. Responses of spinal neurons to cutaneous and dorsal root stimuli in rats with mechanical allodynia after contusive spinal cord injury. *Brain Res.* 2001;893(1-2):59-69.
17. Finnerup NB, Jensen TS. Spinal cord injury pain—mechanisms and treatment. *European Journal of Neurology.* 2004;11:73-82.
18. Siddall PJ. Pain following spinal cord injury. In: *Wall and Melzack's Textbook of Pain.* 5th ed. St. Louis: Elsevier Churchill Livingstone; 2006:1043-1055.
19. Lenz FA, Weiss N. The role of the thalamus in pain. *Suppl Clin Neurophysiol.* 2004;54:50-61.

20. Craig A. A new version of the thalamic disinhibition hypothesis of central plain. *Pain Forum*. 1998;7:1-14.
21. Carlton SM, Du J, Tan HY, et al. Peripheral and central sensitization in remote spinal cord regions contribute to central neuropathic pain after spinal cord injury. *Pain*. 2009;147(1-3):265-276.
22. Gwak YS, Hulsebosch CE. Spatial and temporal activation of spinal glial cells: role of gliopathy in central neuropathic pain following spinal cord injury in rats. *Exp Neurol*. 2012;234(2):362-372.
23. Redondo-Castro, García-Alías G, Navarro X. Plastic changes in lumbar segments after thoracic spinal cord injuries in adult rats: an integrative view of spinal nociceptive dysfunctions. *Restor Neurol Neurosci*. 2013;31:411-430.
24. Nicholson B. Evaluation and treatment of central pain syndromes. *Neurology*. 2004;62:30-36.
25. Todor DR, Mu HT. Pain and syringomyelia: a review. *Neurosurg Focus*. 2000;8(3):E11.
26. Milhorat TH, Kotzen RM. Dysesthetic pain in patients with syringomyelia. *Neurosurgery*. 1996;38(5):940-946.
27. Baastrup C, Maersk-Moller CC, Nyengaard JR, et al. Spinal-, brainstem- and cerebrally mediated responses at- and below-level of a spinal cord contusion in rats: evaluation of pain-like behavior. *Pain*. 2010;151(3):670-679.
28. Leem JW, Kim HK, Hulsebosch CE, Gwak YS. Ionotropic glutamate receptors contribute to maintained neuronal hyperexcitability following spinal cord injury in rats. *Exp Neurol*. 2010;224:321-324.
29. McAdoo DJ, Xu GY. Changes in amino acid concentrations over time and space around an impact injury and their diffusion through the rat spinal cord. *Exp Neurol*. 1999;159:538-544.
30. Vierck CJ, Light AR. Effects of combined hemotoxic and anterolateral spinal lesions on nociceptive sensitivity. *Pain*. 1999;83:447-457.
31. Vierck CJ, Light AR. Allodynia and hyperalgesia within dermatomes caudal to a spinal cord injury in primates and rodents. *Prog Brain Res*. 2000;129:411-428.
32. Wiesenfeld-Hallin Z, Aldskogius H. Central inhibitory dysfunctions: mechanisms and clinical implications. *Behav Brain Sci*. 1997;20:420-425.
33. Zhang AL, Hao JX. Decreased GABA immunoreactivity in spinal cord dorsal horn neurons after transient spinal cord ischemia in the rat. *Brain Res*. 1994;656:187-190.
34. Hains BC, Waxman SG. Sodium channel expression and the molecular pathophysiology of pain after SCI. *Prog Brain Res*. 2007;161:195-203.
35. Boroujerdi A, Zeng J, Sharp K, et al. Calcium channel alpha-2-delta-1 protein upregulation in dorsal spinal cord mediates spinal cord injury-induced neuropathic pain states. *Pain*. 2011;152(3):649-655.
36. DeLeo JA, Yezierski RP. The role of neuroinflammation and neuroimmune activation in persistent pain. *Pain*. 2001;90:1-6.
37. Ramer MS, Harper GP. Progress in spinal cord research—a refined strategy for the International. *Spinal Cord*. 2000;38:449-472.
38. Gwak YS, Hulsebosch CE. Remote astrocytic and microglial activation modulates neuronal hyperexcitability and below-level neuropathic pain after spinal injury in rat. *Neuroscience*. 2009;161(3):895-903.
39. Fitch MT, Doller C, Combs CK, et al. Cellular and molecular mechanisms of glial scarring and progressive cavitation: in vivo and in vitro analysis of inflammation-induced secondary injury after CNS trauma. *J Neurosci*. 1999;19(19):8182-8198.
40. Kyrkanides S, Olschowka JA, Williams JP, et al. TNF alpha and IL-1beta mediate intercellular adhesion molecule-1 induction via microglia-astrocyte interaction in CNS radiation injury. *J Neuroimmunol*. 1999;95(1-2):95-106.
41. Knerlich-Lukoschus F, von der Ropp-Brenner B, et al. Chemokine expression in the white matter spinal cord precursor niche after force-defined spinal cord contusion injuries in adult rats. *Glia*. 2010;58(8):916-931.
42. Nesic O, Lee J, Johnson KM, et al. Transcriptional profiling of spinal cord injury-induced central neuropathic pain. *J Neurochem*. 2005;95(4):998-1014.
43. Yoon, et al. *Brain Res*. in press.
44. Nardone R, Höller Y, Brigo F, et al. Functional brain reorganization after spinal cord injury: systematic review of animal and human studies. *Brain Res*. 2013;1504:58-73.
45. Jurkiewicz MT, Mikulis DJ, McIlroy WE, et al. Sensorimotor cortical plasticity during recovery following spinal cord injury: a longitudinal fMRI study. *Neurorehabil Neural Repair*. 2007;21(6):527-538.
46. Attal N, Cruccu G, Baron R, et al. EFNS guidelines on the pharmacological treatment of neuropathic pain: 2010 revision. *Eur J Neurol*. 2010;17(9):1113.
47. Dworkin RH, O'Connor AB, Audette J, et al. Recommendations for the pharmacological management of neuropathic pain: an overview and literature update. *Mayo Clin Proc*. 2010;85(3):S3-S14.
48. Widerstrom-Noga EG, Turk DC. Types and effectiveness of treatments used by people with chronic pain associated with spinal cord injuries: influence of pain and psychosocial characteristics. *Spinal Cord*. 2003;41:600-609.
49. Cardenas DD, Jensen MP. Treatments for chronic pain in persons with spinal cord injury: a survey study. *J Spinal Cord Med*. 2006;29:109-117.
50. Rintala DH, Holmes SA, Courtade D, et al. Comparison of the effectiveness of amitriptyline and gabapentin on chronic neuropathic pain in persons with spinal cord injury. *Arch Phys Med Rehab*. 2007;88(12):1547-1560.
51. Cardenas DD, Warms CA, Turner JA, et al. Efficacy of amitriptyline for relief of pain in spinal cord injury: results of a randomized controlled trial. *Pain*. 2002;96(3):365-373.
52. Vranken JH, Hollmann MW, van der Vegt MH, et al. Duloxetine in patients with central neuropathic pain caused by spinal cord injury or stroke: a randomized, double-blind, placebo-controlled trial. *Pain*. 2011;152(2):267-273.
53. Tai Q, Kirshblum S. Gabapentin in the treatment of neuropathic pain after spinal cord injury: a prospective, randomized, double-blind, crossover trial. *J Spinal Cord Med*. 2002;25:100-105.
54. Levendoglu F, Ogun CO, Ozerbil O, et al. Gabapentin is a first line drug for the treatment of neuropathic pain in spinal cord injury. *Spine*. 2004;29(7):743-751.
55. Siddall PJ, Cousins MJ, Otte A, et al. Pregabalin in central neuropathic pain associated with spinal cord injury: a placebo-controlled trial. *Neurology*. 2006;67(10):1792-1800.
56. Cardenas DD, Nieshoff EC, Suda K, et al. A randomized trial of pregabalin in patients with neuropathic pain due to spinal cord injury. *Neurology*. 2013;80(6):533-539.
57. Frampton JE, Foster RH. Pregabalin: in the treatment of generalized anxiety disorder. *CNS Drugs*. 2006;20(8):685-693.
58. Gruenthal M, Mueller M. Gabapentin for the treatment of spasticity in patients with spinal cord injury. *Spinal Cord*. 1997;35:686-689.
59. Priebe MM, Sherwood AM, Graves DE, et al. Effectiveness of gabapentin in controlling spasticity: a quantitative study. *Spinal Cord*. 1997;35(3):171-175.
60. Hulsebosch CE, Xu GY, Perez-Polo JR, et al. Rodent model of chronic central pain after spinal cord contusion injury and effects of gabapentin. *J Neurotrauma*. 2000;17(12):1205-1217.

61. Kitzman PH, Uhl TL, Dwyer MK. Gabapentin suppresses spasticity in the spinal cord-injured rat. *Neuroscience*. 2007;149(4):813-821.

62. Rabchevsky AG, Patel SP, Duale H, et al. Gabapentin for spasticity and autonomic dysreflexia after severe spinal cord injury. *Spinal Cord*. 2011;49(1):99-105.

63. Bradley LJ, Kirker SG. Pregabalin in the treatment of spasticity: a retrospective case series. *Disabil Rehabil*. 2008;30(16):1230-1232.

64. Braid JJ, Kirker SG, Baguley IJ. Spasticity increases during pregabalin withdrawal. *Brain Inj*. 2013;27(1):120-124.

65. Finnerup NB, Sindrup SH. Lamotrigine in spinal cord injury pain: a randomized controlled trial. *Pain*. 2002;96:375-383.

66. Eisenberg E, Lurie Y. Lamotrigine reduces painful diabetic neuropathy: a randomized, controlled study. *Neurology*. 2001;57:505-509.

67. Siddall PJ, Molloy AR. The efficacy of intrathecal morphine and clonidine in the treatment of pain after spinal cord injury. *Anesth Analg*. 2000;91(6):1493-1498.

68. Saulino M. Simultaneous treatment of intractable pain and spasticity: observations of combined intrathecal baclofen-morphine therapy over a 10-year clinical experience. *Eur J Phys Rehabil Med*. 2012;48(1):39-45.

69. Attal N, Gaude V. Intravenous lidocaine in central pain: a double-blind, placebo-controlled, psychophysical study. *Neurology*. 2000;54(3):564-574.

70. Kvarnstrom A, Karlsten R. The analgesic effect of intravenous ketamine and lidocaine on pain after spinal cord injury. *Acta Anaesthesiol Scand*. 2004;48(4):498-506.

71. Canavero S, Bonicalzi V. Intravenous subhypnotic propofol in central pain: a double-blind, placebo-controlled, crossover study. *Clin Neuropharmacol*. 2004;27(4):182-186.

72. Norrbrink BC, Kowalski J. A comprehensive pain management programme comprising educational, cognitive and behavioural interventions for neuropathic pain following spinal cord injury. *J Rehabil Med*. 2006;38(3):172-180.

73. Perry KN, Nicholas MK. Multidisciplinary cognitive behavioural pain management programmes for people with a spinal cord injury: design and implementation. *Disabil Rehabil*. 2011;33:1272-1280.

74. Mulroy SJ, Thompson L. Strengthening and optimal movements for painful shoulders (STOMPS) in chronic spinal cord injury: a randomized controlled trial. *Phys Ther*. 2011;91:305-324.

75. Falci S, Best L. Dorsal root entry zone microcoagulation for spinal cord injury-related central pain: operative intramedullary electrophysiological guidance and clinical outcome. *J Neurosurg*. 2002;97:193-200.

76. Chun HJ, Kim YS. A modified microsurgical DREZotomy procedure for refractory neuropathic pain. *World Neurosurg*. 2011;75:551-557.

77. Tasker RR, DeCarvalho GT, Dolan EJ. Intractable pain of spinal cord origin: clinical features and implications for surgery. *J Neurosurg*. 1992;77:373-378.

78. American Society of Anesthesiologists Task Force on Chronic Pain Management; American Society of Regional Anesthesia and Pain Medicine. Practice guidelines for chronic pain management: an updated report by the American Society of Anesthesiologists Task Force on Chronic Pain Management and the American Society of Regional Anesthesia and Pain Medicine. *Anesthesiology*. 2010;112(4):810-833.

79. Bendok B, Levy RM. Brain stimulation for persistent pain management. In: Gildenberg PL, Tasker RR, eds. *Textbook of Stereotactic and Functional Neurosurgery*. New York: McGraw-Hill; 1998:1539-1546.

Complex Regional Pain Syndrome

Michael Stanton-Hicks
Salahadin Abdi

Ever since Claude Bernard implicated the sympathetic nervous system in sensation, its role in nociception has been the subject of debate.[1] No one would argue with the fact that the sympathetic nervous system is intimately involved with the preservation of homeostasis and noxious challenges in humans, although the manner in which it influences the sensation of pain has, until recently, escaped explanation.[2] Anatomically, the sympathetic nervous system constitutes a highly complex arrangement of preganglionic and postganglionic neurons that subserve specific and diverse functions of target organs, including enteric neurons, smooth muscle, syncytial muscle, and striated muscle.[3] Physiologically, the sympathetic nervous system is associated in some way with both systemic and specific local reactions, which are expressed by supratentorial and confrontational aspects that are represented in the periaqueductal gray matter of the midbrain (e.g., nonopioid analgesia).[4,5] In contrast, rest and quiescence are represented in the ventrolateral periaqueductal gray matter, being associated with endogenous opioid analgesia.

The stress response described by Selye,[6] "fight or flight," involves both spinal levels of integration, with hypothalamo-mesencephalic centers, but is associated with adrenocortical and hypothalamo-hypophyseal responses designed to protect the organism under normal biologic conditions. A secondary set of responses to sympathetic activity that can be considered pathophysiologic and occur with or without obvious nerve injury are changes in blood flow, sudomotor and muscle activity, with subsequent trophic changes and abnormal sensation long after the noxious event.[7,8] Sensory changes include allodynia, hypoalgesia, hyperalgesia, hyperesthesia, and hyperpathia. Why, and in what manner, the sympathetic nervous system is involved in these changes that occur in a small but readily identifiable group of patients is still unclear. However, recent research has clarified some of the previous misconceptions with regard to levels of sympathetic activity, involvement of the central nervous system (CNS), and the possibility of preexisting immunologic factors. Interestingly, similarities in the characteristics of complex regional pain syndrome (CRPS) are seen in other chronic pain states, such as irritable bowel syndrome, interstitial cystitis, nonulcer dyspepsia, and certain cases of angina pectoris.

During the Civil War, Weir Mitchell[9] drew attention to the exaggerated response to nerve injury that was distinct from the neurogenic inflammation that is associated with most nerve injuries. These patients typically sustained a penetrating injury in the vicinity of a major nerve, in most cases without disruption, and typically caused by a musket shot. Mitchell called this *causalgia* because of the bizarre swelling, heat (*causa*), and pain (*algia*), which were out of all proportion to the signs and symptoms of most nerve injuries. Leriche,[10] a French surgeon, also described similar syndromes in the lower extremities for which he developed the surgical procedure of stripping the sympathetic nervous plexus from the large vessels in the lower extremities. Sudeck, in a series of articles, provided similar descriptions with detailed observations of the bony and trophic changes after injury that came to be described in German-speaking countries as "morbus Sudeck" or "Sudeck's atrophy."[11]

Perhaps Livingston, more than any other individual, influenced contemporary thinking with regard to these CRPSs. Livingston[12] proposed the concept of a vicious circle that involved the spinal cord at the level of sensory interneurons, which are maintained in a state of abnormal repetitive firing from the periphery (**Fig. 48-1**). In other words, Livingston proposed that a linkage existed between afferent nociception, and the efferent responses generated by spinal neurons in some manner contributed to an exaggeration of the nociceptive signals in the local injured tissue. This so-called sympathosomatic coupling suggested the genesis of a reflex mechanism that was fundamental to these disorders.

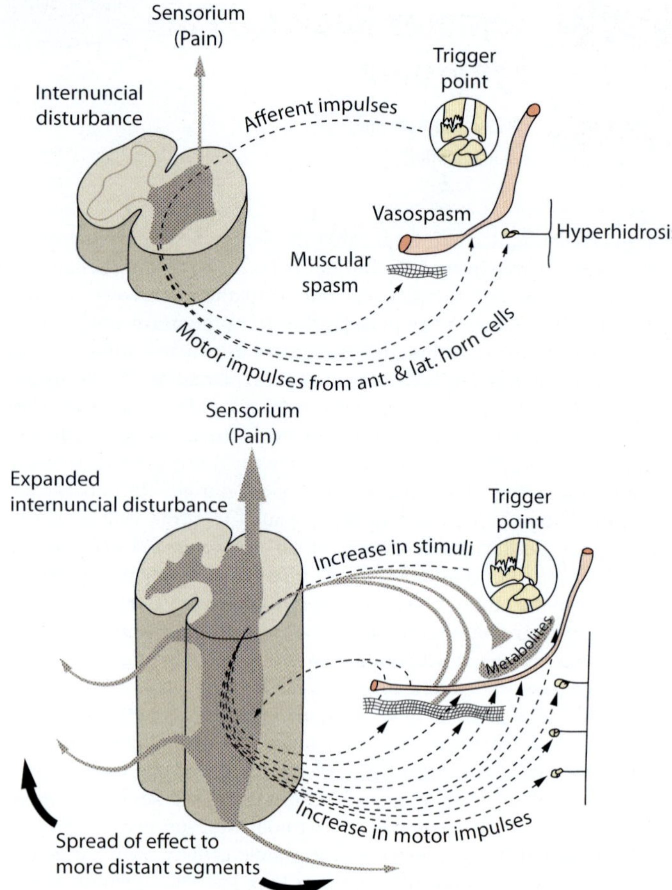

FIGURE 48-1. Figure illustrates the concept of a vicious circle involving the spinal cord both at the level of the sensory disturbance and the temporal and spatial expansion that was proposed by Livingston in 1943. (Used with permission from Livingston WK. *Pain Mechanisms: A Physiological Interpretation of Causalgia and Its related States*. New York: Plenum; 1976.)

Obviously influenced by Livingston's thinking, Evans[13] coined the term *reflex sympathetic dystrophy* in a single stroke implying a mechanism that had not yet been scientifically validated. It is interesting to note that Lewis,[14] also a contemporary, made the suggestion that secretory dysfunction might be responsible for the dystrophic changes and atrophy that are seen in integumentary structures, although he did not specifically imply that there was a disturbance of autonomic function. He suggested that the nocifensor nerves actually became irritated in causalgic states, thereby potentiating the clinical process.

Experiments by Walker and Nulsen,[15] who were interested in autonomic physiology, determined that stimulation of the sympathetic trunk in patients who had undergone a thoracic sympathectomy for causalgia elicited burning and tingling paresthesias in the affected extremity. Twenty years later, these observations were confirmed by White and Sweet,[16] who contended that a *sympathetically dependent* mechanism is responsible for the disturbance that is seen in patients with causalgia and reflex sympathetic dystrophy. Other clinical observations that support a role of the sympathetic nervous system in pain are the relief that frequently attends interruption of the paravertebral ganglia with local anesthetics, chemical or physical modalities, and surgery, as well as intravenous (IV) regional application of guanethidine, bretylium, and systemic IV phentolamine.[17-20]

Observations by Jänig and McLachlan,[21] Blumberg and Jänig,[22] Häbler and colleagues,[23] Jänig and Koltzenburg,[24] and Price and colleagues[25] provide evidence in favor of a role for the sympathetic nervous system in the generation of pain in such patients. Likewise, Torebjörk and coworkers[26] have demonstrated that α-adrenoceptor agonists that are applied by injection or iontophoresis in a previously affected extremity rekindle symptoms in patients who had been in remission for periods exceeding 15 years. Similar responses have been elicited by injection of epinephrine into a chronic neuroma.

In 1986, Roberts[27] introduced the concept of sympathetically maintained pain (SMP), which he postulated accompanies CRPS at some point in the natural history of the condition. His suggestion that low-threshold mechanoreceptors types I and II (Aβ fibers) are induced by postganglionic sympathetic activity that, in turn, induces chronic firing in wide-dynamic-range (WDR) multireceptive neurons (lamina 5, dorsal horn), thereby maintain the status quo (**Fig. 48-2**). The hypothesis is supported by animal experiments that demonstrate an activation of mechanoreceptors by sympathetic postganglionic sympathetic efferents. Although there is a qualitative difference from the proposal by Livingston[12] some 40 years earlier, there are striking parallels between the two hypotheses. Indeed, Torebjörk and Hallin[28] were unable to demonstrate any lowering of nociceptor mechanical threshold nor the relief of pain by C-fiber block but did demonstrate analgesia by pressure (differential) ischemic block induced by tourniquet in patients who exhibited hyperalgesia after nerve injury (i.e., hyperalgesia was in this instance mediated by large, myelinated afferents).

Campbell and coworkers[29] and Raja and coworkers[30] believe that the genesis of SMP results from an expression of additional α_1-adrenoreceptors on primary afferent nociceptors that, in turn, are stimulated by postganglionic sympathetic efferents (i.e., physiologic and not a result of sympathetic dysfunction). This theory would imply a peripheral and not central cause for the clinical syndrome.

In fact, the studies already referred to by Torebjörk, using microneurography in the 1970s, and an analysis of catecholamine levels in affected extremities have never reflected any increase in sympathetic activity. To the contrary, in many cases, sympathetic activity in patients with CRPS was actually found to be less than normal.[31] However, studies by McLachlan and colleagues[32] in rats have demonstrated adrenergic sprouting at dorsal root ganglia within 2 weeks after complete sciatic nerve transection, suggesting functional adrenergic change in response to injury. These investigators were able to demonstrate evoked activity in primary sensory neurons that were blocked by α-receptor antagonists when the postganglionic sympathetic fibers were stimulated. Using the Chung model[33] of neuropathic pain (spinal nerve ligation), they found accelerated sympathetic sprouting at the dorsal root ganglion of segmental nerves within 4 days of this injury. They noted a reduction in mechanosensory threshold that preceded changes in the thermal threshold. These authors believed that the more rapid manifestation of changes in the sympathetic nervous system could be attributed to the influence of nerve growth factor expressed by the damaged axon. Drummond et al. had produced evidence that increased density of α_1-adrenoceptors are found in the epidermis of hyperalgesic skin of patients with CRPS.[34]

All of the foregoing observations do not support the previously held opinion that sympathetic hyperactivity is necessary to explain the clinical features of CRPS. In fact, an alternate theory, and one whose origins go back to Sudeck, suggests that local inflammatory mediators with changes in vascular hydrostatic pressure resulting from dorsal root reflexes may amplify inflammatory responses and pain in the periphery. Wall,[35] in a recent editorial, has drawn attention to the current understanding of neuropathic pain mechanisms and relationship, if it exists and in what manner, by which the sympathetic nervous system might be involved. Two recent important communications underscore a possible central origin for the expression of CRPS, whether of clinical nerve injury or tissue damage. Sieweke and colleagues[36] showed that hyperalgesia in association with SMP is mechanical (brush evoked), but thermal hyperalgesia is not present. This finding, together with the ineffectiveness of acetylsalicylic acid in treatment, strongly supports a major central component that contributes to pain, at least in the late stages of CRPS. The second study, by Schürmann and colleagues[37] using laser

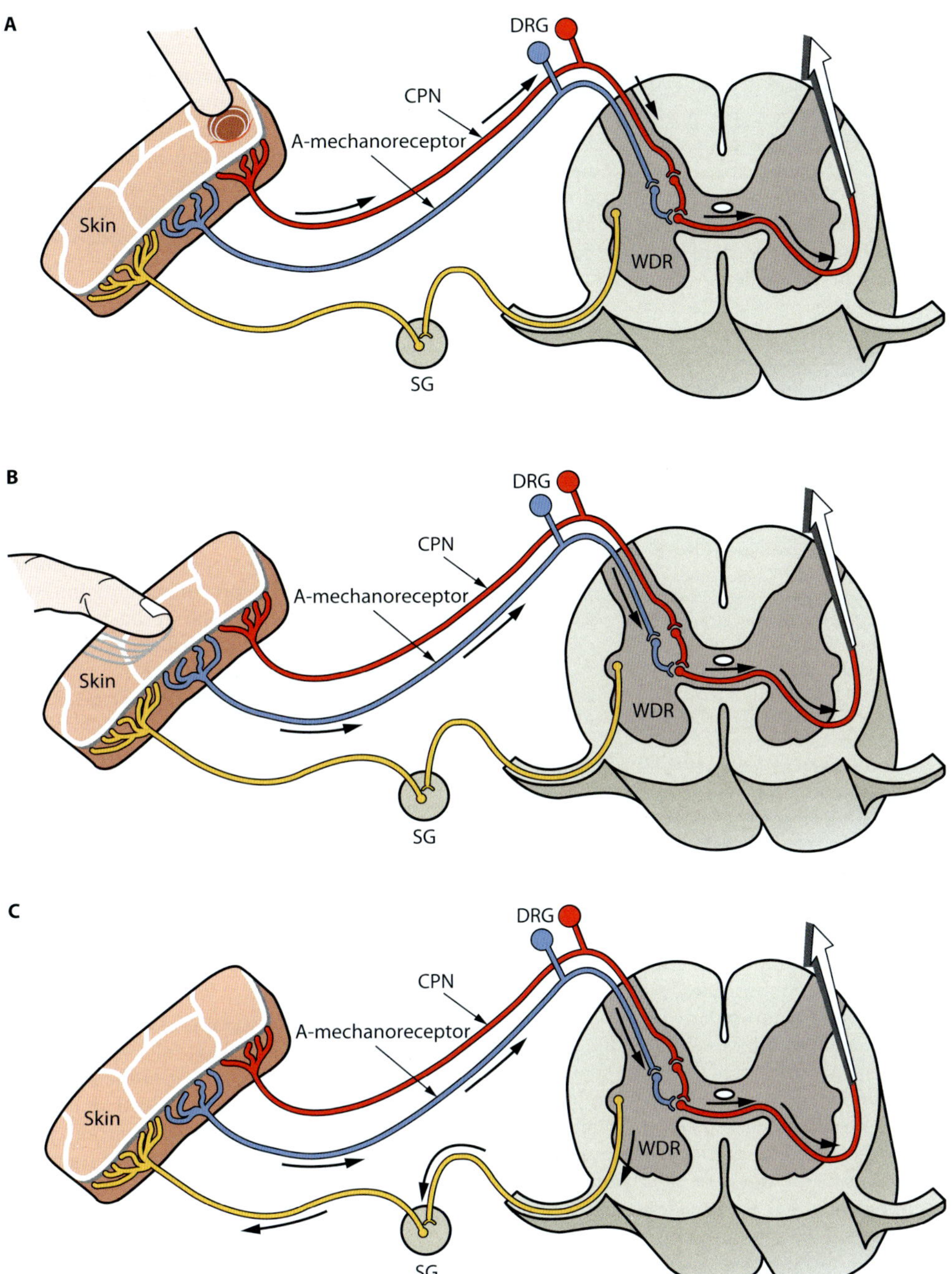

FIGURE 48-2. This figure illustrates the hypothesis of Roberts, introduced in 1986, to explain the phenomenon of sympathetically maintained pain (SMP). (**A**) Initiation of C nociceptor response to injury with excitation of the wide-dynamic-range (WDR) neurons and spinothalamic transmission. (**B**) WDR neurons now become sensitized to activity in large-diameter A-mechanoreceptors, which respond to light touch (allodynia). (**C**) Increased WDR response to A-mechanoreceptor activity resulting from sympathetic efferent action at the nociceptor. *Note:* This last phase represents SMP and requires no further cutaneous stimulation. DRG, dorsal root ganglion; CPN, C-polymodal nociceptor; SG, sympathetic ganglion. (Used with permission from Torebjork HE, Wahren LK, Wallin G, et al. Noradrenalin-evoked pain in neuralgia. *Pain.* 1995;63:11-20.)

Doppler flowmetry found that a loss of the normal sympathetic control of the microcirculation in an ipsilateral extremity of patients with CRPS was also a systemic-wide phenomenon, a finding that strongly supports a central foundation for CRPS. In fact, this study corroborates earlier observations by Schwartzman and McClellen.[38] Although predisposing psychological characteristics have not found support in numerous studies, there has been some suggestion that patients who developed CRPS may acquire an excessive preoccupation with or hypervigilance about their disease.[39] In this regard, positron emission tomographic studies reveal extensive cortical and subcortical activity in several neuropathic pain states.[40] Rommel and colleagues determined that 24 patients with CRPS-1 were found to have hemisensory and motor impairment suggestive of supratentorial areas of central processing.[41] Likewise, it has not been possible to distinguish between the protective response behavior that occurs in association with these diseases as being merely a response to the excessive pain or an abnormal psychological response that is seen only in patients with these syndromes.[42]

In sum, the pathophysiology of CRPS remains unclear; however, recent advances in both preclinical and clinical research, particularly, research in genetics and in biochemical as well as biophysical changes in the peripheral nervous system (PNS) and CNS, help to enrich our understanding that multiple mechanisms might be involved in the pathogenesis of CRPS. Currently, it is widely accepted that there are three concepts that define the pathogenesis of CRPS, namely, neurogenic inflammation, abnormal efferent sympathetic and afferent sensory nerve coupling, and neuroplasticity of the CNS.[43] Additionally, it is believed that genetic factors might be involved in the pathogenesis of CRPS based on a small number of studies.

DEVELOPMENT OF A NEW TAXONOMY

The foundations for a new taxonomy had their origins in a meeting that was held in 1988 at Schloss-Rettershof, Germany.[44] A consensus statement describing reflex sympathetic dystrophy in the following terms was presented at a meeting of the Special Interest Group (SIG), Pain and the Sympathetic Nervous System of the International Association for the Study of Pain (IASP) at the Sixth World Congress on Pain in Adelaide, Australia, in 1990. This statement read:

> Reflex Sympathetic Dystrophy is a descriptive term meaning a complex disorder or group of disorders that may develop as a consequence of trauma affecting the limbs, with or without an obvious nerve lesion. RSD may also develop after visceral disease, central nervous system lesions, or rarely without an obvious antecedent event. RSD consists of pain and sensory abnormalities, abnormal blood flow, decreased or increased sweating, abnormalities of the motor system, and changes in the structure of both superficial and deep tissues (trophic changes). It is not necessary that all components be present. The name "Reflex Sympathetic Dystrophy" is used in a descriptive sense and does not imply any specific underlying mechanisms.[5]

As would be expected, making a change in concepts that had been introduced to characterize certain aspects of reflex sympathetic dystrophy and causalgia such as SMP and sympathetically independent pain tended to complicate rather than improve the level of understanding, at least by practitioners of whichever discipline who are faced with the diagnosis and treatment of these syndromes.

In November, 1993, under the auspices of the SIG, Pain and the Sympathetic Nervous System, another closed workshop convened in association with the annual scientific meeting of the American Pain Society in Orlando, resulting in the development of a strict set of clinical descriptors to characterize features of these medical entities to distinguish them from other diseases, the mechanism for which, or their pathophysiology, is well known. These recommendations were made to the Committee on Taxonomy of Chronic Pain Conditions of the International Association for the Study of Pain and formed the basis for the term *complex regional pain syndromes* that was published in the second edition of the *Classification of Chronic Pain: Description of Chronic Pain Syndromes and Definition of Pain Terms*, published by the IASP Press in 1994.[46,47]

REQUIREMENTS FOR A NEW TAXONOMY

1. Any new taxonomy for reflex sympathetic dystrophy should suggest areas of basic research and development of animal models that identify how the sympathetic nervous system is involved and should promote clinical investigation or corroborate hypotheses born out of the basic research.
2. A new taxonomy should improve the differential diagnosis from other medical entities that have features that are similar but not identical to those found in reflex sympathetic dystrophy.
3. A new taxonomy should suggest tests in support of a diagnosis of reflex sympathetic dystrophy.

NEW TAXONOMY

The term *complex regional pain syndrome* was chosen to replace the former terminology of reflex sympathetic dystrophy and causalgia.[47] Acknowledging that at the time, no mechanism was available to explain the clinical features of these disorders and using a linguistic convention adopted by the Subcommittee on Taxonomy for inclusion in the classification of chronic pain, the term allows for the later inclusion of a variety of painful conditions that may occur after injury. These conditions are manifested regionally, mostly in an extremity, predominantly distal, and with findings that exceed in magnitude and duration the expected course after such an inciting event. The taxonomy also acknowledges that in some cases, these disorders may occur on the trunk or face and spread to other body areas. Frequently, there is impairment of motor function (especially as the disease progresses), which is evident as tremor, weakness, dystonia, or muscle atrophy. Because a temporal sequence is variable, the terms *complex* and *regional* were used to distinguish this from other syndromes. The taxonomy emphasizes that the clinical features tend to commence in the distal part of an extremity and tend to extend proximally, involving the musculature of the shoulder or pelvic girdles, respectively, but in a small percentage of cases, the syndrome may emanate proximally.

The order of classifying these conditions was changed, with the term *CRPS type I (RSD)* being the generic disease and *CRPS type II (causalgia)* being applied to conditions in which there is obvious nerve injury. The previous listing in the first edition of the IASP classification was historical in deference to the description by Mitchell.[9] Causalgia is well described by both Richards[48] and Bonica[49] and requires no elaboration here.

The terminology for CRPS types I and II acknowledges that both spontaneous and touch-evoked (allodynia or hyperalgesia) pain may be concurrent in the affected region. Pain of either nature is regarded as a cardinal symptom in these medical disorders, although in rare cases, pain in association with all other clinical features that satisfy the diagnosis may be absent.

In patients who do not fulfill the criteria for a diagnosis of CRPS type I or II, allowance was made in the taxonomy for a third type of CRPS, not otherwise specified (NOS). With this instrument, the taxonomy encourages the clinician to identify specific types or subgroups of CRPS types I and II. For example, one patient group may meet all the criteria specified for CRPS type I but uniformly have in addition another specific symptom or clinical finding. The temporal course of their disease process follows a uniformly different course or their response differs from that of the main type I group, in which case the classification could be changed to include this as a specific subgroup within the main CRPS type I group. Bonica[50] introduced the concept of staging, which he believed was important to the description of these diseases, but experience has questioned the utility of this in diagnosis or treatment and, as a consequence, it was eliminated from the taxonomy. As a result of internal and external validation studies, a statistically derived revision of CRPS criteria was achieved. For research purposes, the criteria were tightened to achieve a sensitivity of 0.70 and specificity of 0.96. In 2004 at a closed-consensus workshop in Budapest, the foregoing criteria were codified and formally adopted by the IASP Committee for Classification of Chronic Pain in 2012, to be subsequently included as the "Budapest criteria" in the next revision of the Taxonomy of Chronic Pain Terms.[51]

The epidemiology of CRPS has now been systematically studied in one prospective and two retrospective studies.[52-54] The earlier publications in relation to Colles fracture[38] and statistics from Sweden (T. Gordh, 1998, personal communication) suggest a prevalence of about 10%. Also, a clinical study by Mailis and Wade[55] concerning the development of CRPS types I and II in white women suggests genetically similar profiles, but Devor and Raber[56] and Bhatia and colleagues,[57] in two separate studies, demonstrated the predisposition for neuropathic pain behavior in genetically selected laboratory animals, providing support for this concept.

Motor symptoms and signs are frequently reported (>75%) in patients with CRPS types I and II. During preparation of the new taxonomy, a lack of scientific evidence in support of this being a specific movement disorder resulted in the exclusion of these findings from the standard clinical criteria, but they are now formally a part of the "Budapest criteria."[54] Likewise, the response to sympathetic blockade (SNB) is also removed from the taxonomy of CRPS types I and II but receives attention in the discussion of SMP and other neuralgias.

Specific exclusion criteria for the definition of CRPS types I and II were necessary to prevent the inclusion of other clinical entities and syndromes in which the findings are consistent with a particular injury but resemble those of CRPS types I and II. One example might be a patient who met the criteria for causalgia but whose signs and symptoms lie outside of the territory of the injured nerve. If the clinical findings were to occur within the regional territory of that nerve, however, they would then satisfy inclusion criteria under this definition. Another exception might be a patient in whom the clinical findings are localized to the trunk or face but are not associated with a particular injured nerve. Although these entities might be classified as a subset within the main definition, similar to the primary classification, they must have signs and symptoms that are completely disproportionate in both nature and severity to the injury.

Signs of vasomotor instability may not be present at the time of clinical examination. However, a patient history of swelling, sweating, color, and temperature changes, if presenting with motor weakness and dystrophic features, would, of necessity, satisfy the new diagnostic criteria for CRPS.

SYMPATHETICALLY MAINTAINED PAIN

Sympathetically maintained pain is defined as *pain that is maintained by sympathetic efferent innervation or by circulating catecholamines.*[46] A positive response to sympatholysis (sympathetic block) historically is necessary before a diagnosis of CRPS can be made. Given the current ignorance of the manner in which the sympathetic nervous system is involved in the pathophysiology of these conditions and the contradictory literature in this regard, it has been necessary to abandon the convention that only after a positive response to sympatholysis can a diagnosis of CRPS be made. The concept of sympathetically independent pain was introduced to explain cases in which sympatholysis (either pharmacologic or nerve blockade) provides no pain relief. This concept[4] is illustrated in **Figure 48-3**.

In this figure, a symbolic patient (A) may be seen at one time in the course of his or her disease in which most of the patient's pain is sympathetically maintained (i.e., it responds to sympatholysis) but temporarily becomes less responsive to blockade and ultimately is composed mostly of sympathetically independent pain. Similarly, A and B may be two separate patients who, at the time of their physical examination, exhibit

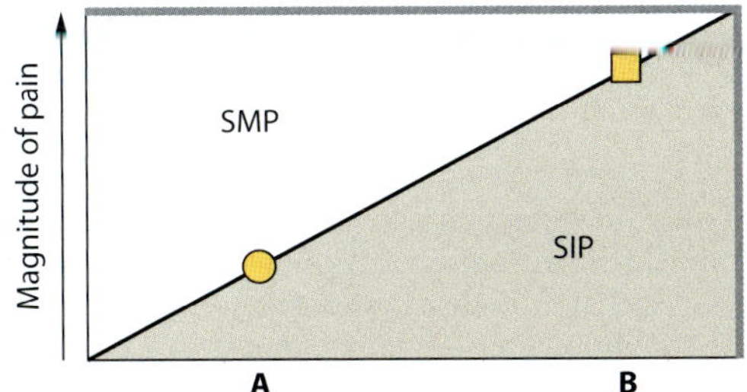

FIGURE 48-3. Illustration of the relative contribution of sympathetically maintained pain (SMP) to overall pain. Whereas the symbolic patient A would demonstrate maximum response to sympatholysis (i.e., demonstrating a large component of SMP), patient B would have almost no response to sympathetic block, therefore exhibiting sympathetically independent pain. It should be noted that points A and B may also represent the same patients at different times in the course of these patients' diseases.

these distinguishing characteristics of pain by their response to SNB. This example illustrates the poor diagnostic specificity when SNB is used for this purpose and is the reason for which a positive response to sympathetic block is no longer regarded as being necessary for a diagnosis of CRPS to be sustained.

However, the response to sympatholysis may contribute to other clinical signs and symptoms that support the diagnostic criteria for CRPS. This and other tests, including temperature measurement, sudomotor function, skin blood flow, and skin resistance, have been developed to assess sympathetic activity.[58-60] The hypothesis for SMP already discussed may be as important to treatment as it is to diagnosis. The sensitization of C-polymodal nociceptors and sensitization of WDR neurons in lamina-5 fibers of the dorsal horn may, as a response to sympatholysis, subside but can only be regarded as a contributory phenomenon or symptom in CRPS or, for that matter, in many other conditions (**Fig. 48-4**).

MUSCULOSKELETAL DISORDERS AND PAIN DYSFUNCTION SYNDROMES

Those medical entities that do not satisfy specific diagnostic criteria for a specific condition are described in the International Classification of Diseases (ICD-10) as NOS codes. The diagnostic criteria for CRPS types I and II use a similar device. As an example, pain in a limb without the other characteristics of CRPS is defined as limb pain, NOS type III. The IASP classification of chronic limb pain conditions provides a code for such instances: X1.19 pain in the limbs, NOS: upper limb (S) 2XX. XXZ, and lower limb (S) 6XX. XXZ. Pain in the hand (musculoskeletal disorder) that does not meet the criteria for CRPS might be diagnosed as pain dysfunction syndrome (a nonstandard classification)[61] (see the discussion of differential diagnosis later in this chapter). Several medical conditions that have been described using nonstandard terminology, including cumulative trauma disorder, repetitive strain injury, overuse syndrome, and tennis elbow,[62-65] are included under the umbrella term *pain dysfunction syndrome*. The International Coding Diseases Manual classification of such conditions is musculoskeletal disorders, which includes a large number of diseases and syndromes such as carpal tunnel syndrome. Many of these conditions that are associated with mechanical hyperalgesia, pain that is out of the ordinary, temperature changes, and myofascial pain syndrome might be considered as CRPS type III. However, the differential diagnosis, depending on tenderness and hyperalgesia that is found specifically over a particular muscle group or epicondylar region, would favor occupational overuse, bursitis, a nerve entrapment, or tennis elbow, for example. Often a long antecedent history of fibromyalgia with hyperresponsiveness, associated headache, fatigue, sleeplessness, depression, and other subjective symptoms may occur in conjunction with CRPS or these musculoskeletal entities.[65]

It also should not be forgotten that the specialty of the physician may influence the primary or secondary diagnosis, particularly its differential, if sufficiently stringent criteria do not satisfy a diagnosis of CRPS.

DIFFERENTIAL DIAGNOSIS

Many medical entities have characteristics that are similar to the clinical features of CRPS. Although many of these conditions are frequently found in the distal part of an extremity, they must be distinguished from other musculoskeletal and neuropathic pain conditions. As already discussed, their clinical presentation may suggest SMP; however, its interpretation, at least early in the course of the disease, must be circumspect. Pain relief after sympatholysis is not specific for reflex CRPS (see Fig. 48-3) but may merely reflect an altered response to physiologic sympathetic activity.

Patients with myofascial dysfunction, a frequent accompaniment, may present with regional temperature differences and mechanical hyperalgesia yet still not satisfy all of the criteria for a diagnosis of CRPS. The broad group of musculoskeletal disorders that have been described

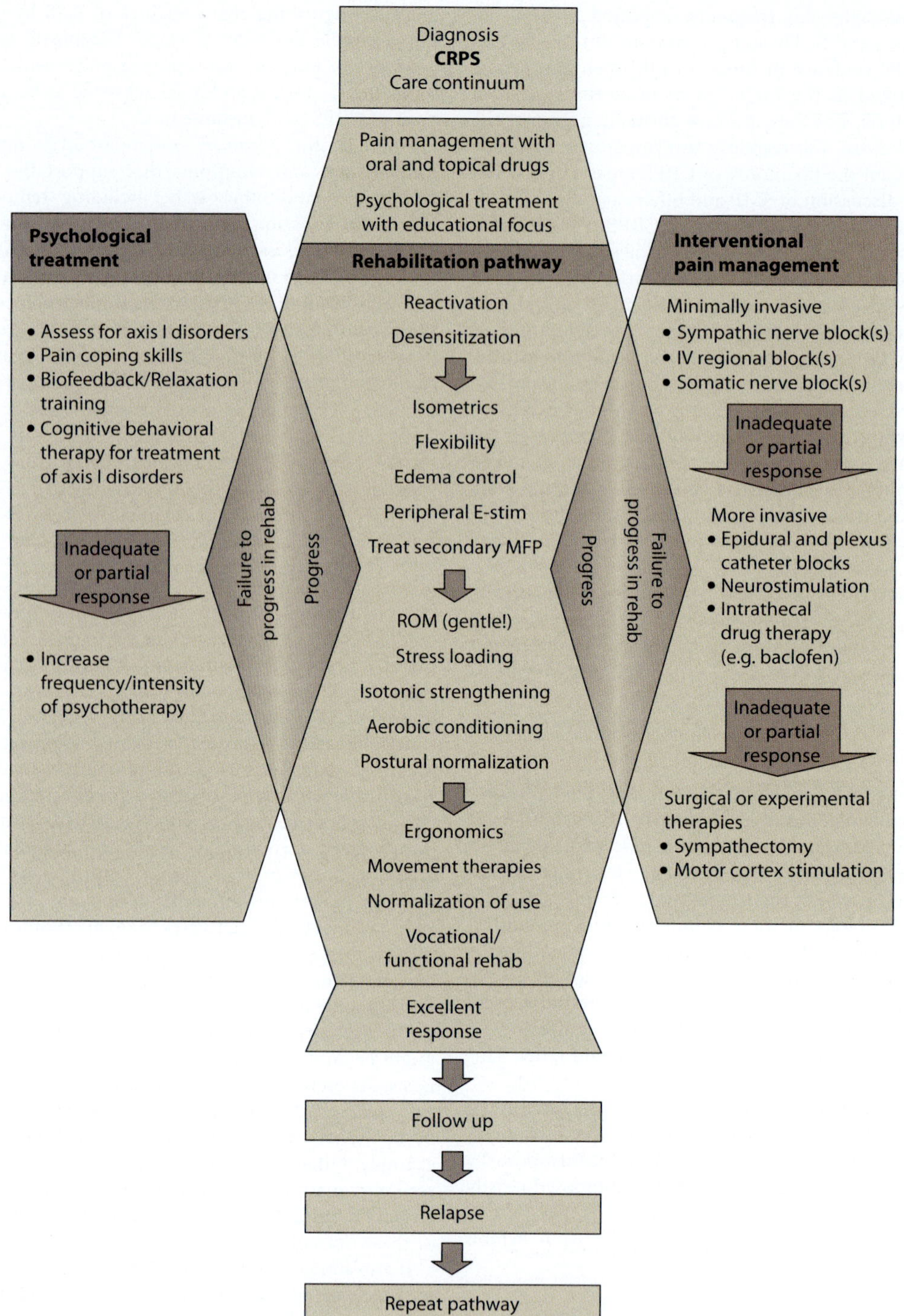

FIGURE 48-4. Revised therapeutic pathway with emphasis on the therapeutic modalities that are used in response to the patient's clinical progress in the rehabilitation algorithm. Adapted from the 1998 guidelines. (Used with permission from Swerdlow M. Anticonvulsants in the therapy of neuralgia pain. *Pain Clin.* 1986;1:9-19.)

as pain dysfunction syndromes may have some clinical signs and symptoms but are insufficient in number or character to satisfy a diagnosis of CRPS. **Table 48-1** is a list of conditions that should be considered in the diagnosis of CRPS.

Myofascial pain dysfunction (MFD), a frequent association with CRPS, must be distinguished from primary MFD that may have been present before the onset of CRPS. Because of its prevalence, its recognition is essential not only as a diagnostic sign but also as a target for therapy.[66-68] Dystonia, limitation of movement, and weakness must be carefully distinguished from a lack of voluntary effort or dystrophic changes in joint components.

The differential diagnosis of CRPS II can be distinguished from a nerve injury in which neurogenic inflammation is associated with pain and by symptoms that are out of proportion, as described in the new taxonomy. The additional criteria are edema, skin temperature, color changes, and sudomotor changes that also are out of proportion to those that would be found in association with a painful nerve injury. Although one or more of these signs and symptoms may dominate, all should be found at some time during the course of the disease. The pain, including allodynia and hyperalgesia, without vasomotor changes by itself would not satisfy the criteria for CRPS. Only rarely do patients present with all or most of the clinical features of CRPS but without pain. Although the

TABLE 48-1 Conditions to Be Considered in the Differential Diagnosis of Complex Regional Pain Syndrome
Musculoskeletal disorders
Pain dysfunction syndrome
Cumulative trauma disorder
Repetitive strain injury
Overuse syndrome
Tennis elbow
Shoulder–hand syndrome
Nonspecific thoracic outlet syndrome
Fibromyalgia
Posttraumatic vasoconstriction
Undetected fracture
Peripheral vascular disease

temporal course and response to treatment modalities may be identical with that of CRPS, the taxonomy requires that such patients should remain outside the CRPS umbrella.

A few patients with CRPS types I and II may have premorbid psychological or psychiatric disturbances, the occurrence of which does not exclude their primary diagnosis. Likewise, malingering and factitious disease are well-recognized clinical entities that are separate from a diagnosis of CRPS but must be included in the differential diagnosis. Conversion disorders and somatization, well recognized in association with chronic pain, have their own specific criteria and may occur independently or in association with CRPS types I and II.[69] Occasionally, the diagnosis of these conditions is difficult and may only be determined after medical treatment is instituted. In the final analysis, pain that is neuropathic and out of proportion to that occurring as a symptom of many other medical conditions is required for a diagnosis of CRPS. SMP is neuropathic pain that is associated with many conditions, for example, postherpetic neuralgia, diabetic neuropathy, and most cases of CRPS types I and II early in the course of the disease.

DIAGNOSTIC TESTS

Although no diagnostic tests specifically support a diagnosis of CRPS, a number of measurements and laboratory tests may contribute to the clinical diagnosis.

Temperature Measurement Temperature change that is reflective of changes in the cutaneous blood flow[70] may be measured by thermometry, telethermometry, passive infrared methods, or thermography. For these measurements to have any relevance, they should also be taken on corresponding sites or areas of the contralateral extremity. At least 1.5°C is required for the difference to be significant. Thermography in conjunction with cold physiologic stress testing of an unaffected independent extremity is a useful test of autonomic function in the ipsilateral extremity. This test should be undertaken only in a thermostable and preferably comfortable—about 22°C—environment. Either the failure to respond to cold stress or the delay in rewarming, particularly when the contralateral temperature side differences are 1.5°C or greater, may indicate dysfunction of the autonomic nervous system.

Caution is necessary when interpreting temperature changes as has been demonstrated by Wasner et al.[31] When whole-body temperature changes were induced, three distinct vascular patterns were identified, namely inhibition of cutaneous sympathetic vasoconstrictor neurons as characterized by a warmer affected limb early in the disease. In chronic CRPS, sympathetic vasoconstrictor neurons are still inhibited, but secondary changes in neurovascular transmission caused the skin changes to remain cold, and an intermediate change characterizes the dynamic vascular abnormalities that depend on the specific activity of sympathetic vasoconstrictor neurons at the time. These authors noted that the maximal difference in skin temperature during induced thermoregulatory changes is a reliable means of distinguishing CRPS from other extremity pain syndromes.[71]

Peripheral Blood Flow This measurement may be made by laser Doppler flowmetry. As already mentioned, Schürmann and colleagues have clearly demonstrated that this test is an early predictor of sympathetic dysfunction and therefore supportive of a diagnosis of CRPS.[37,38]

Quantitative Sweat Testing The quantitative sudomotor axon reflex test (QSART) is another clinical laboratory test that focuses on abnormalities of evoked sweat production. Taken together with the resting sweat output (RSO) and alteration in vasomotor activity, QSART provides a good laboratory correlation with the clinical features of CRPS.[70,72]

Quantitative Sensory Testing This test is a useful evaluation of vibratory, thermal, and cold responses that, although not specific for CRPS, may contribute to the clinical picture and support a differential diagnosis of CRPS.[73]

Sympathetic Skin Response This response may be used to identify increased conductance when comparing the ipsilateral with the contralateral extremity.[59]

Bone Scan Three-phase bone scintigraphy with technetium diphosphonate usually demonstrates a reduction in flow during the early phase of CRPS but increased periarticular uptake during the third phase. Sensitivity is approximately 60%, and specificity of 86% has been claimed, but many reports describe 30% false-positive and 30% false-negative responses.[74] The recent paper by Wüppenhorst et al.[74] suggests that its sensitivity and specificity have improved with early application.

Muscle Strength and Joint Testing The measurement of muscle strength depends on patient cooperation, psychological factors, and pain. Nevertheless, grip strength with thumb adduction and opposition, along with pinch testing and goniometry, may be important measurements both as baseline and as prognostic indicators. Joint mobility, including range of motion (ROM), although subjective, may be obtained most reliably by a therapist who works frequently with orthopedic patients.

Psychological Tests It is not uncommon to encounter psychiatric abnormalities in patients with CRPS. Disorders such as somatoform disorders, malingering, and conversion disorders have been shown to be associated with CRPS. Further, depression and anxiety are shown to be associated with chronic CRPS. The most useful instruments for psychological testing are the Beck Depression Inventory and the McGill Pain Questionnaire.

TREATMENT

PHYSICAL THERAPEUTIC ALGORITHM

If early diagnosis is crucial to the institution of an appropriate treatment plan, incorporating a graduated and stepwise approach to treatment using modalities that experience has shown to be most effective is a natural corollary.

Until a clear mechanism for CRPS is established, functional restoration using physiotherapeutic methods is regarded as essential to providing a remission in most cases. Three requirements are necessary if physical therapy is to be successful:

1. Pain control
2. "Turning off" the disturbance
3. Development of patient rapport and confidence in the requirements of a treatment program

Depending on the complexity or fulminant nature of the disease in a particular patient, it may be necessary to increase the proposed time for each step in the physical therapeutic algorithm.[75] This point is arbitrary and serves two purposes: (1) to prevent the patient who, because of symptoms, may no longer progress with a particular treatment modality and (2) to reassess the disease process and introduce measures of symptom control that will permit exercise therapy to continue.

Initially, it is important to gain rapport with the patient so that he or she will develop confidence in the planned investment of effort and time using the various therapeutic modalities that will be necessary, in most cases, to achieve a remission. After each patient buys into this approach, the business of motivation, mobilization, and desensitization is introduced. It is important at each step to rapidly achieve increments of symptomatic improvement using non-narcotic or narcotic analgesics[76] while at the same time addressing the disturbances of sleep, anxiety, depression, and motor dysfunction.[77,78] Some patients with recent onset of CRPS may respond well with a reduction in pain to anticonvulsants or antiarrhythmic medications.[79-83] Unacceptable side effects, together with the length of time (3–4 weeks) to realize any efficacy, may preclude their use. Further deterioration in functional integrity, failure to improve, or an increase in symptoms should trigger the use of a therapeutic and prognostic sympathetic block.

Figure 48-4 is an updated clinical pathway illustrating the main domains of rehabilitation, pain management, and psychological treatment that are fundamental to regaining function and, ultimately, a remission of CRPS.[71,84] The new clinical pathway (guideline) emphasizes an intradisciplinary, time-contingent guidance that incorporates the recently published treatment options. These are addressed simultaneously and vary according to the patient's response to treatment. Important to the use of this clinical guideline is the recommendation to use whichever treatment modality works, when a patient fails to respond to whatever level of treatment after 12 to 16 weeks. The clinical pathway focuses on quality of life as well as function.

A word should be said about joint movement, particularly ROM, in patients with these syndromes. Orthopedic experience in particular has shown that the use of aggressive ROM, passive ROM, or both may be deleterious to progress or worse because mechanoreceptor stimulation in the joint, ligamentous, and tendon structures can cause a dramatic worsening of both pain and the inflammatory response.[85] This is evident by immediate increase in edema, allodynia or hyperalgesia, and hyperpathia.

The technique of so-called *stress loading* with isometric exercises and gentle ROM has been found most effective.[85] It may be necessary to use cognitive-behavioral methods to assist the patient against pain avoidance, kinesophobia, bracing, and overprotection, all of which may develop in a patient in whom previously *inappropriate* exercise therapy may have been used.[86-88] Treatment of the nociceptive and neuropathic generators is required using the following pharmacologic, regional anesthetic, and neuromodulation techniques. In fact, a combination or sequence of these modalities may, in some cases, be required to ultimately achieve a return of function.

PHARMACOLOGIC MANAGEMENT

The following section summarizes drugs that have been found useful in the treatment of CRPS. Although none is specific for the disease, each has a place in managing an aspect of the clinical presentation.

Nonsteroidal Anti-inflammatory Drugs These agents are most successful in the treatment of early or very late CRPS type I or II. Their use should be tempered by the development of gastrointestinal or renal side effects.[75] If one member is without effect, then others with a better side effect profile should be chosen. It may also be worth using one of the cyclooxygenase-2 (COX-2) agents. Topical use of these drugs has also been suggested. It should be remembered that these agents have a tendency to cause water retention with edema, a side effect that may interfere with rehabilitation.

Opioids Although opioids are more effective in the treatment of nociceptive pain, they have a place in the treatment of pain of a neuropathic nature.[76] If tolerated by the patient, the use of slow-release opioids on a round-the-clock basis is preferable to as-needed dosing. The side effects of one class of opioid do not preclude use of another class. It is important to remember that abrupt discontinuation of opioids may lead to an extreme exacerbation of a patient's symptoms, as well as other signs and symptoms of withdrawal. It should be noted that although there is a greater acceptance in the use of opioids for neuropathic pain, such as CRPS, prolonged use may be contraindicated because of the development of tolerance. They may be excellent, however, for the management of pain during early therapy. It is worth noting that among opioids, methadone seems to play a special role because it has a dual mechanistic effect, namely, μ-agonist and NMDA (*N*-methyl-D-aspartate) antagonist activity.

KETAMINE

In recent years, ketamine, which is an NMDA receptor antagonist, has experienced a resurgence as an analgesic agent in subanesthetic doses. It has successfully been used especially for intractable neuropathic pain such as CRPS via IV infusions over several days for both outpatients and inpatients. Its side effects such as hallucination and dysphoria, which could happen even at small doses, normally respond to the use of benzodiazepines.[89]

Anticonvulsants and Antiarrhythmics Agents generally classified as so-called membrane stabilizers include anticonvulsants, local anesthetics, and antiarrhythmic agents. Drugs that are the most effective for neuropathic pain are carbamazepine, gabapentin, pregabalin, lamotrigine, topiramate, zonisamide, and Gabitril.[79-83] Recent studies with gabapentin, a selective voltage-gated Na^{2+} channel blocker, have demonstrated some efficacy in the treatment of CRPS pain. The oral antiarrhythmic lidocaine analogue mexiletine may prove quite effective in a small but significant number of patients with CRPS.[82] The drug has been found effective in the treatment of diabetic neuropathy in a dose of 10 mg/kg. In general, an IV bolus and infusion of lidocaine, the so-called lidocaine test, can be used to predict the response to oral analogues.[90] However, in some cases, those who have not responded to the lidocaine test might still respond to its oral analogue, such as mexiletine. In addition, transdermal lidocaine, which has been shown to be quite effective in the treatment of postherpetic neuralgia, can in some patients reduce the touch-evoked allodynia of CRPS.[91] The conotoxin SNX-111 (ziconotide), infused intrathecally, may be successful in the treatment of long-standing CRPS that has proved refractory to all other treatment.[92]

Tricyclic Antidepressants The serotonin and norepinephrine reuptake blocking agents (amitriptyline, nortriptyline, desipramine, and maprotiline) have all demonstrated efficacy in the treatment of neuropathic pain syndromes, including CRPS.[93-95] These agents are much more effective than the selective serotonin reuptake inhibitors (SSRIs), suggesting that it is the catecholaminergic aspect of the former three agents that is therapeutic. These agents are also particularly useful in providing sedation and reducing nocturnal symptoms. They should, therefore, be prescribed for use at night.

Adrenergic Drugs The α_1-adrenoceptor blocking agents (terazosin, prazosin, and phenoxybenzamine) may be strikingly effective in patients with SMP.[96] They do, however, have a poor side effect profile, with tachycardia; chest pain; gastric symptoms; and, in some cases, sedation that preclude their use. However, more than 30% of patients with SMP respond dramatically to these agents. The α_2 agonist clonidine may be effective when introduced by the epidural or intrathecal (IT) route of administration.[97] Its use is not supported by systematic review, level 1 evidence. It may be tried topically, and in some cases, it may be dramatically effective when applied to a discrete area of hyperalgesia.[98,99]

Corticosteroids Corticosteroids have been successful in the treatment of early CRPS when the acute inflammatory response may be most pronounced.[100,101] It is during this phase that intraosseous plasma extravasation can be demonstrated scintigraphically by labeled immunoglobulins. It should be noted that corticosteroids are most successful when sympathetic blocks are completely effective in relieving the continuous pain.

Other Drugs Other agents that are sometimes used include calcitonin, bisphosphonates, and topical agents such as capsaicin and dimethylsulfoxide (DMSO). There is level 1 evidence for the use of calcitonin when given early.[102] It is, however, poorly tolerated. There are now three randomized controlled trials (RCTs) supporting the use of bisphosphonates, the most recent[103] claiming a greater than 75% remission when administered in early CRPS, level 2 evidence. Free radical scavengers such as topical DMSO were shown to be effective in a small RCT.[104]

Prophylactic vitamin C can prevent the incidence of CRPS in Colles fracture of the wrist. This is supported by three RCTs and a review and could become a standard of practice.[105] The foregoing agents demonstrate their antioxidant properties and role in tissue inflammatory responses during acute CRPS, level 1 evidence.

Immunoglobulins Emergent treatment with immune-modulating agents is receiving a lot of attention because of the identification of autoantibodies to a number of tissues (muscarinic-2 receptor, β_2 adrenergic receptor, α1 adrenoceptor) in CRPS. In a small cohort (RCT) with intravenous immunoglobulin (IVIG), a significant reduction in pain was demonstrated.[106]

HYPERBARIC OXYGEN THERAPY

The use of hyperbaric oxygen (HBO) treatment in patients with CRPS is supported by one RCT in which 71 patients were selected to receive either HBO or pressurized room air.

Hyperbaric oxygen is always a consideration when skin breakdown with ulceration supervenes. This physical modality can be valuable as an adjunct to wound healing. In the foregoing study, which was only undertaken in upper extremity CRPS, the authors observed significant improvement in wrist flexion and edema. As an alternative therapy, HBO may be effective when the patient has exhausted other treatments and in particular is having slow or nonhealing cutaneous lesions. Frequently, 25 to 30 sessions may be required to achieve the maximum effect.[107]

REGIONAL ANESTHESIA

Regional anesthetic techniques have two purposes: (1) the relief of symptoms otherwise not controlled by pharmacologic means and (2) the demonstration of pain that is sympathetically maintained (SMP).[29,70] Traditionally, this approach has been used in the treatment of CRPS involving both the upper and lower extremities. Significantly, when used early in the course of the disease, pain relief that is either partial or complete, depending on the degree of SMP, may be realized. Blocks of the sympathetic nervous system interrupt efferent vasomotor, sudomotor, and visceromotor fibers as well as visceral afferents, somatic afferents, and nociceptor fibers.

For sympatholysis in the upper extremity, the paratracheal technique of stellate ganglion block at the level of C6, with the development of Horner's syndrome (myosis, ptosis, and enophthalmos), has been a standard approach for many years. However, as has been pointed out by many authors, including Bonica, Kuntz, and others, the anatomic position of the stellate ganglion anterior to the costovertebral articulation and neck of the first rib makes it more amenable to block at the lower portion of the C7 vertebral body.[108,109] In addition, the local anesthetic has a greater chance of diffusing on the longus colli muscle to reach the T2 through T4 ganglia, thereby providing a more effective SNB to the upper extremity. In 2004, Abdi et al. described a new and easy oblique technique to do stellate ganglion block that seems to be a safe technique.[110] Signs of a successful sympathetic block include a temperature rise to 34°C, measured at the finger pulp. A temperature of 34°C implies greater than 90% sympatholysis in the region. Supplementary tests of sympathetic function are the sympathetic skin response using a modified electrocardiogram and cold pressor test to demonstrate that this response has been disabled when an unaffected extremity is placed in ice-cold water. Laser Doppler flowmetry is an excellent noninvasive measurement of changes in skin blood flow, the loss of which is clearly evident.

In the same manner, lumbar SNB can be realized using a single needle under fluoroscopic guidance at the lower third of the body of L2 or L3.[111] The correct anatomic site is clearly demonstrated by the flow of radiocontrast in the gutter formed by the fascia overlying the psoas muscle and its continuation as the periosteum overlying the vertebral bodies of L2 through L4. Verification of effective sympatholysis can be demonstrated by using one of the previously described measurements.

When SNB completely eliminates the patient's symptoms, prolonged sympatholysis for a few weeks may be achieved by pulsed radiofrequency (pRFA).[112] There is little support for repeated sympathetic blocks that last a few hours or days. A good response demonstrating SMP would suggest that an α-adrenoceptor blocking agent such as terazosin or prazosin could be tried. A good pharmacologic response with these agents might preclude further SNB. Apart from the number of patients who do have a prolonged (i.e., months) response to SNBs, knowledge that a patient has SMP is helpful in determining his or her expected responses to immune therapy and neurostimulation.

Mixed conduction blocks of peripheral nerves of the brachial or lumbar plexus, or in the form of a central neural block, are useful to facilitate physiotherapy. They should be used only when analgesia by pharmacologic means is insufficient to support exercise therapy. Although intermittent blocks are helpful to initiate therapy, in some cases, it is necessary to use continuous conduction analgesia.[113] A catheter implanted in the brachial or lumbosacral plexus allows infusions for 1 to 2 weeks but is subject to technical failure or infection when used for longer periods. The epidural route with a tunneled catheter offers the greatest utility and enables the long-term administration of local anesthetics and adjuncts for many months. Although this technique is useful to promote exercise therapy,[114,115] it is also prone to failure from dislodgment, breakage, or infection, mostly at the skin entry site but less frequently in the deeper tissues (7%), requiring its removal, treatment, and ultimately, replacement of the catheter.

A word of caution with regard to implanted catheters is in order. Because these devices may be used for long durations, they should be treated as minor surgical procedures and can only successfully achieve their purpose if placement is made under strict asepsis using fluoroscopic guidance to ensure that the epidural infusion is ipsilateral, or if the contralateral extremity is also involved, that bilateral spread can be assured.

In a few cases, a long-acting local anesthetic such as bupivacaine or ropivacaine may be sufficient to provide analgesia commensurate with exercise therapy. However, it is common to add an opiate, such as fentanyl, or other agents, including morphine, hydromorphone, fentanyl, or sufentanil, to achieve an adequate level of "working" analgesia. Occasionally, it may be necessary to consider the use of an α_2-adrenoceptor agonist, clonidine, when hyperalgesia or allodynia prevents effective physical therapy. A short, 2- to 5-day hospital admission is required to determine the clinically most effective infusion in each case.

From this account, it should be clear to the reader that although once regional anesthetic techniques such as SNB were necessary to support a diagnosis of CRPS, their conventional application is primarily to determine whether pain is modified by sympathetic block (i.e., SMP) and whether its response alone will support exercise therapy and other treatment modalities that will ensure a return of function.

NEUROMODULATION

Neuromodulation incorporating either spinal cord stimulation or peripheral nerve stimulation aims to enhance or modify the inhibitory components of the CNS and/or PNS. Although neurostimulation has been in use since its introduction by Shealy and colleagues[116] in 1967, it is the past 10 years that have seen such a dramatic increase in its use for the treatment of neuropathic and vasculopathic pain.[117-120] Although the posterior columns were thought to be the primary target for spinal cord stimulation, stimulation of the descending inhibitory pathways and the dorsal root fibers is now recognized as being equally important for modulating nociception.[121]

Computer modeling of spinal cord stimulation has helped to determine the putative clinical response that could be achieved by electrode geometry and the ratio of dorsal column to dorsal root fibers.[122] The pain in CRPS tends to be more global than dermatomal, and electrodes that have a longitudinal and central disposition tend to have greater spatial selectivity and are likely to be more efficient in providing pain relief to the affected extremity.

If, as has already been mentioned, CRPS is a neurologic disease, it should be amenable to treatment by neurostimulation. Perhaps one of the best indications for either spinal cord or peripheral nerve stimulation is injury to a peripheral nerve. Similarly, CRPS with its altered cutaneous sensibility, tactile allodynia to cold, and mechanical stimuli, is also likely to respond well to spinal cord stimulation. The autonomic effects of spinal cord stimulation, with improvement in both the micro- and macrocirculation in the stimulated region, appear to be a result of preganglionic modification of the autonomic nervous system function.[123]

Although there have only been two prospective studies describing the successful use of neuromodulation in the treatment of pain resulting from CRPS, a number of clinical retrospective case studies support use of the modality.[124-126] Functional restoration is central to the treatment of CRPS, and adequate relief of pain and correction of the autonomic disturbance position this modality well among other modalities in achieving this end.

Because time is of the essence in the treatment of CRPS, any failure to progress through the therapeutic algorithm must be regarded as a trigger to introduce regional anesthetic or neuromodulatory methods to support progressive rehabilitation. The temporal introduction of the different treatment modalities must be seen only as a guide, and their order does not constitute priority. For patients with CRPS of either an upper or lower extremity, a single octapolar lead may be adequate. In bilateral CRPS or when some degree of stimulation instability is experienced during trial stimulation, a second electrode should be added. Similarly, if difficulty in obtaining appropriate topographic paresthesia is experienced at the target site, a second electrode should be added. Although it is beyond the scope of this chapter to discuss in detail the technical aspects of neurostimulation, there are a number of systems from different manufacturers, each of which has specific characteristics from which it is possible to choose a system that is most appropriate for each individual clinical situation. For CRPS II in a distal extremity, selection of a peripheral nerve stimulator is more likely to provide stable and specific control of symptoms than can spinal cord stimulation relative to the injured nerve.

INTRATHECAL THERAPY

When all conservative measures, including pharmacotherapy and physical, psychological, and neurostimulation, have not yielded any symptomatic or functional improvement, consideration of IT therapy is necessary. Intraspinal opioids have been used for years to treat refractory chronic pain. Unfortunately tolerance, particularly in patients younger than 50 years of age, frequently interferes with long-term administration. Although morphine is approved for IT use, fentanyl and hydromorphone are often substituted because of their higher lipophilicity and comparatively more manageable side effect profiles.[127]

Bupivacaine and ropivacaine are frequent adjuncts to opioid IT solutions because of their different site of action and opioid-sparing properties.

Baclofen can be administered alone or together with an opioid for severe spasticity unresponsive to oral intake.[128]

Ziconotide, an n-calcium channel blocking agent, is proving to be a very potent agent for managing neuropathic and mixed pain. Although its side effect profile precludes its use in many patients, it is well tolerated with a greater than 50% reduction of pain in about 35% of patients. As with many centrally acting medications (anticonvulsants), the side effect profile is broad, but because the half-life of ziconotide is short (one cerebrospinal fluid circulation time), the effects rapidly disappear. Ziconotide has no withdrawal propensity.[129] Trialing IT ziconotide can be achieved by an indwelling (small 24-guage) IT catheter for several days or by serial bolus injections.

All patients considered suitable for neuromodulation must first satisfy behavioral criteria and undergo a structured psychological examination.[75,130] Self-report tests such as the Beck Depression Inventory and McGill Pain Questionnaire are suitable instruments.

It can be concluded that for cases characterized by failure to progress through the physiotherapeutic algorithm or an exacerbation of the patient's symptoms, a trial of spinal cord stimulation may prove to be a most effective tool when other modalities have failed.

PSYCHOLOGICAL ASPECTS

Most studies in patients with CRPS have failed to show any correlation with a preexisting psychological disorder.[131,132] However, a significant percentage of these patients develop behavioral abnormalities and require psychological support during treatment. Commonly, 6 months into their disease, patients demonstrate varying degrees of depression manifested by disturbed sleep, anxiety, and despair that their disease is not improving. Measures such as biofeedback, relaxation, temperature control, and reduction in muscle tension are indicated. Group therapy, in which a spouse or family member is present, is sometimes helpful for CRPS patients, as for other patients with chronic pain. Use of a single antidepressant, particularly a tricyclic such as amitriptyline, is preferable to a combination of different antidepressants or the newer SSRIs.

COMPLEX REGIONAL PAIN SYNDROME IN CHILDREN

It can be categorically stated that CRPS in children, particularly before puberty and in adolescence, is a different disease from that in adults.[133,134] Although the same signs and symptoms constituting the clinical entity are present, the course of the disease and its response to treatment suggests early behavioral and psychological aspects that may require special skills in cognitive management. Because of their dependence on their parents, children exhibit more behavioral aspects, reflecting problems of enmeshment and bizarre responses to the slightest degree of family dysfunction.[135] In fact, in many cases, one sees a parallel in an adult with a conversion disorder.

Usually, children do not require the use of interventions and respond appropriately to pharmacologic measures and good psychological support.[84] Physical therapy should be presented either as a challenge or as a game, with goals being set to win and overcome the disability. Transcutaneous electrical nerve stimulation often provides sufficient analgesia (in more than half of patients) to allow for their participation in physical therapy.[84] It is preferable to avoid invasive therapies; however, a lumbar sympathetic block or an epidural catheter should not be withheld if there is failure to progress in exercise therapy or the disease process has remained refractory to conservative treatment. In rare cases, it may actually be necessary to use a spinal cord stimulator or even a peripheral nerve stimulator, which in either case may be subsequently removed when the disease process is in remission. In principle, at least 85% of children will respond well to physical therapeutic measures and pharmacologic therapy, but almost all require strong support with these or whichever additional psychological measures are used to gain confidence in and increase compliance with their therapy.

SUMMARY

Complex regional pain syndrome is a disease, the exact pathophysiology and mechanism of which remain unknown. The disease is complex and generally commences in a particular region of the body, usually the distal aspect of an extremity. Sometimes it occurs in other parts of the body, and it may also spread to other areas. Pain is the *sine qua non* of CRPS but, in rare cases, may actually be minimal or absent. The diagnosis is one of exclusion after having eliminated, in the differential diagnosis, other conditions for which the pathophysiology is well categorized. However, what is now known is that the pathophysiology of CRPS is multifactorial, including neurogenic or hypoxic changes in the affected region; dysfunction of CNS and PNS; or changes in the immune system, particularly cytokines and autoimmunologic responses to different tissues. The treatment plan should be orderly and use a structured physiotherapeutic approach facilitated by pharmacologic, interventional, and behavioral components.[136] Time is of the essence, and any delay or failure to progress with exercise therapy after 2 to 3 weeks of treatment should prompt the introduction of modalities that at the time seem most appropriate (e.g., immune modulators, IVIG) and more likely to facilitate therapy and achieve a remission. It frequently is necessary to make continuous adjustments in physical therapy commensurate with the clinical response. Such therapy, in each case, must be individualized to be successful.

REFERENCES

1. Bernard C. Influence du grand sympathique sur la sensibilit et sur la calorification. *CR Soc Biol (Paris)*. 1851;3:163-164.
2. Hess WR, Brhgger M. Das subcorticale Zentrum der affecktiven Abwehreaktion. *Helv Physiol Acta*. 1943;1:33-52.
3. Jänig W. Organization of the lumbar sympathetic outflow to skeletal muscle and skin of the cat hind limb and tail. *Rev Physiol Biochem Pharmacol*. 1985;102:119-213.
4. Treede RD. Pathophysiology and diagnosis in patients with sympathetically independent pain. *Schmerz*. Aug 27, 1998;12(4):250-260.
5. Jänig W. The sympathetic nervous system in pain. *Eur J Anesthesiol*. 1995;12(suppl 10):53-60.
6. Selye H. *The Stress of Life*. New York: McGraw-Hill; 1957.
7. Jänig W, Schmidt FR, eds. *Reflex Sympathetic Dystrophy: Pathophysiological Mechanisms and Clinical Implications*. Weinheim, Germany: VCH Verlags Gesell Schaft; 1992.
8. Jänig W, Koltzenburg M. What is the interaction between the sympathetic terminal and the primary afferent fiber? In: Basbaum AI, Besson, JM, eds. *Towards a New Pharmacotherapy of Pain*. Chichester, England: Dahlen Workshop Reports, Wiley; 1991:331-352.
9. Mitchell SW. *Injuries of Nerves and Their Consequences*. Philadelphia: JB Lippincott; 1872.
10. Leriche R. *La Chiurgie del la Douleur*. Paris: Masson & Cie; 1939.
11. Sudeck D. Über die akute entzundliche Knochenatropie. *Arch Klin Chir*. 1962:147-156.
12. Livingston WK. *Pain Mechanisms: A Physiological Interpretation of Causalgia and Its Related States*. New York: Plenum; 1976.
13. Evans JA. Reflex sympathetic dystrophy. *Surg Clin North Am*. 1946;26:780-790.
14. Lewis T. *Pain*. London: MacMillan; 1942.
15. Walker AE, Nulsen F. Electrical stimulation of the supper thoracic portion of the sympathetic chain in man. *Arch Neurol Psychiatr*. 1948;59:559-560.
16. White JC, Sweet WH. *Pain and the Neurosurgeon*. Springfield, IL: Charles C Thomas; 1969.
17. Bonica JJ. Causalgia and other reflex sympathetic dystrophies. In: Bonica JJ, Lieberskiend JC, Albe-Fessard, DG, eds. *Advances in Pain Research and Therapy*. Vol 3. New York: Raven; 1979:141-166.
18. Casale R, Glynn CJ, Buonocore M. The role of ischemia in the analgesia which follows Bier's block technique. *Pain*. 1992;50:169-175.
19. Jadad AR, Carroll D, Glynn CJ, et al. Intravenous regional sympathetic blockade for pain relief in reflex sympathetic dystrophy: a systematic review and a randomized double-blind crossover study. *J Pain Symptom Manage*. 1995;10:1313-1320.
20. Ramamurthy S, Hoffman J, The Guanethidine Study Group. Intravenous regional guanethidine in the treatment of reflex sympathetic dystrophy/causalgia: a randomized double-blind study. *Anesth Analg*. 1995;81:718-723.
21. Jänig W, McLachlan E. The role of modifications in noradrenergic peripheral pathways after nerve lesions in the generation of pain. In: Fields HC, Liebeskind JC, eds. *Pharmacological Approaches to the Treatment of Chronic Pain: New Concepts and Critical Issues, Progress in Pain Research and Management*. Vol 1. Seattle: IASP Press; 1994:101-129.
22. Blumburg H, Jänig W. Clinical manifestations of reflex sympathetic dystrophy and sympathetically-maintained pain. In: Wall PD, Melzack R, eds. *Textbook of Pain*. 3rd ed. Edinburgh: Churchill Livinstone; 1994:685-697.
23. Häbler HJ, Jänig W, Koltzenburg M. Activation of unmyelinated efferents and chronically lesioned nerves by adrenalin and excitation of sympathetic efferents in the cat. *Neurosci Lett*. 1987;82:35-40.
24. Jänig W, Koltzenburg M. Sympathetic reflex activity in neuroeffector transmission change after chronic nerve lesions. In: Bond MR, Charlton JE, Woolf CJ, eds. *Proceedings of the Sixth World Congress on Pain, Pain Research and Clinical Management*. Vol 4. Amsterdam: Elsevier; 1991:365-371.
25. Price DD, Long S, Huitt C. Sensory testing of pathophysiological mechanisms of pain in patients with reflex sympathetic dystrophy. *Pain*. 1992;49:163-173.
26. Torebjörk HE, Wahren LK, Wallin G, et al. Noradrenalin-evoked pain in neuralgia. *Pain*. 1995;63:11-20.
27. Roberts WJ. A hypothesis on the physiological basis for causalgia and related pains. *Pain*. 1986;124:297-311.
28. Torebjörk HE, Hallin RG. Microneurographic studies of peripheral pain mechanisms in man. In: Bonica JJ, Lieberskind JC, Alb-Fessard DG, eds. *Advances in Pain Research and Therapy*. Vol 3. New York: Raven; 1979:121-131.
29. Campbell JN, Meyer RA, Raja SN. Is nociceptor activation by alpha-1 adrenoceptors the culprit in sympathetically-maintained pain? *APS J*. 1992;1:3-11.
30. Raja SN, Treede RD, Davis KD, et al. Systemic alpha-adrenergic blockade with phentolamine: a diagnostic test for sympathetically-maintained pain. *Anesthesiology*. 1991;74:691-698.
31. Wasner G, Heckmann K, Maier C, et al. Vascular abnormalities in acute reflex sympathetic dystrophy (CRPS I)—complete inhibition of sympathetic nerve activity with recovery. *Arch Neurol*. 1999;56:613-620.
32. McLachlan EM, Jänig W, Devore M, et al. Peripheral nerve injury triggers noradrenergic sprouting within dorsal root ganglia. *Nature*. 1993;363:543-545.
33. Carlton SM, Lekan HA, Kim SH, et al. Behavioral manifestation of an experimental model for peripheral neuropathy produced by spinal nerve ligation in the primate. *Pain*. 1994;56:155-166.
34. Drummond PD, Skipworth S, Finch PM. Alpha-1 adrenoceptors in normal and hyperalgesic skin. *Clin Sci*. 1996;91:73-77.
35. Wall PD. Inflammatory and neurogenic pain: new molecules, new mechanisms. *Br J Anesth*. 1995;75:123-124.
36. Sieweke N, Birklein F, Riedl B, et al. Patterns in hyperalgesia in complex regional pain syndrome. *Pain*. 1999;80:171-177.
37. Schürmann M, Grad LG, Andress HJ, et al. Assessment of peripheral sympathetic nervous function for diagnosing early post-traumatic complex regional pain syndrome type I. *Pain*. 1999;88:149-159.
38. Schwartzman RJ, McLellan TL. Reflex sympathetic dystrophy: a review. *Arch Neurol*. 1987;44:555-561.

39. Eccleston C, Crombez G, Aldrich S, et al. Attention and somatic awareness in chronic pain. *Pain*. 1997;72:209-215.
40. Darbyshire SW, Jones AK, Davani P, et al. Cerebral responses to pain in patients with atypical facial pain, measured by positron emission tomography. *J Neurol Neurosurg Psychiatry*. 1994;57:1166-1172.
41. Rommel O, Gehling M, Dertwinkel R, et al. Hemisensory impairment in patients with complex regional pain syndrome. *Pain*. 1999;80:95-101.
42. Vlaeyen JWS, Kole-Snijders AMJ, Boern RGB, et al. Fear of movement/re-injury in chronic low back pain and its relation to behavioral performance. *Pain*. 1995;62:363-372.
43. Maihoefner C. Komplex regionals Schmerzsyndrom. *Schmerz*. 2014;28:319-338.
44. Stanton-Hicks M, Jänig W, Boas RA. *Reflex Sympathetic Dystrophy*. Boston: Kluwer; 1990.
45. Jänig W, Blumburg H, Boas RA, et al. The reflex sympathetic dystrophy syndrome: consensus statement and general recommendations for diagnosis and clinical research. In: Bond MR, Charlton JE, Woolf CJ, eds. *Proceedings of the Sixth World Congress on Pain, Pain Research and Clinical Management*. Vol 4. Amsterdam, Holland: Elsevier; 1991:372-375.
46. Stanton-Hicks M, Jänig W, Hassenbusch S, et al. Reflex sympathetic dystrophy: changing concepts and taxonomy. *Pain*. 1995;63: 127-133.
47. Merskey H, Bogduk N, eds. *Classification of Chronic Pain: Descriptions of Chronic Pain Syndromes and Definitions of Pain Terms*. 2nd ed. Seattle: IASP Press; 1994.
48. Richards RK. Causalgia: a centennial review. *Arch Neurol*. 1967;16:339-350.
49. Bonica JJ. Causalgia and other reflex sympathetic dystrophies. In: Bonica JJ, Lieberskiend JC, Albe-Fessard, DG, eds. *Advances in Pain Research and Therapy*. Vol 3. New York: Raven; 1979:141-166.
50. Bonica JJ. *The Management of Pain*. Philadelphia: Lea & Febiger; 1953.
51. Sandroni P, Benrud-Larson LM, McClelland RI, Low PA. Complex regional pain syndrome type 1: incidence and prevalence in Olmsted county, a population-based study. *Pain*. 2003;103:199-207.
52. de Mos M, de Bruijn AG, Huygen FJ, et al. The incidence of complex regional pain syndrome: a population-based study. *Pain*. 2007;129:12-20.
53. Beerthuizen A, Stronks DL, Van't Spijker A, et al. Demographic and medical parameters in the development of complex regional pain syndrome type 1 (CRPS1): prospective study on 596 patients with a fracture. *Pain*. 2102;153(6):1187-1192.
54. Harden RN, Bruehl S, Perez RS, et al. Validation of proposed diagnostic criteria (the "Budapest Criteria") for complex regional pain syndrome. *Pain*. 2010;150:268-274.
55. Mailis A, Wade J. Profile of Caucasian women with possible genetic predisposition to reflex sympathetic dystrophy: a pilot study. *Clin J Pain*. 1994;10:210-217.
56. Devor M, Raber P. Heritability of symptoms in an experimental model of neuropathic pain. *Pain*. 1990;42:51-67.
57. Bhatia KP, Bhatt MH, Masden CD. The causalgia-dystonia syndrome. *Brain*. 1993;116:843-851.
58. Low PA, Caskey PE, Tuck RR, et al. Quantitative sudomotor axon reflex test in normal and neuropathic subjects. *Ann Neurol*. 1983;14:573-580.
59. Knezevic W, Bajada S. Peripheral autonomic surface potential: quantitative technique for recording autonomic neural function in man. *Clin Exper Neurol*. 1985;21:201-210.
60. Glynn C, Walsh JA, Basedow RW, et al. A model for investigating the effect of drugs in the peripheral sympathetic nervous system in man. *J Auton Nerv Syst*. 1982;5:195-205.
61. McCain GA, Scudds RA. The concept of primary fibromyalgia (fibrositis): clinical value, relation and significance to other chronic musculoskeletal pain syndromes. *Pain*. 1988;33:273-287.
62. Browne CD, Nolan BM, Faithfull DK. Occupational repetition strain injuries: guideline for diagnosis and management. *Med J Aust*. 1984;140:329-332.
63. Frye HJH. Overuse syndrome in musicians: prevention and management. *Lancet*. 1986;11:728-731.
64. Punett L, Robbins JM, Wegman DH, et al. Soft tissue disorders in the upper limbs of female garment workers. *Scan J Work Environ Health*. 1985;11:417-425.
65. Lautenbacher S, Rolman GB, McCain GA. Multi-method assessment of experimental and clinical pain in patients with fibromyalgia. *Pain*. 1994;59:45-53.
66. Deuschl G, Blumburg H, Lückling CH. Tremor in reflex sympathetic dystrophy. *Arch Neurol*. 1991;48:1247-1258.
67. Schott G. Clinical features of algodystrophy: is the sympathetic nervous system involved? *Funct Neurol*. 1989;4:131-134.
68. Jancovic J, van der Linden C. Dystonia and tremor induced by peripheral trauma: predisposing factors. *J Neurol Neurosurg Psychiatry*. 1988;51:1512-1519.
69. American Psychiatric Association. *Diagnostic and Statistical Manual of Mental Disorders: DSM IV-TR*. Washington, DC: American Psychiatric Association; 2000.
70. Stanton-Hicks M, Raj PP, Racz GB. Use of regional anesthetics for diagnosis of reflex sympathetic dystrophy and sympathetically-maintained pain: a critical evaluation. In: Janig W, Stanton-Hicks M, eds. *Reflex Sympathetic Dystrophy: A Reappraisal, Progress in Pain Research and Management*. Vol 6. Seattle: IASP Press; 1996:217-237.
71. Birklein F, Sittl R, Spitzer A, et al. Susomotor function in sympathetic reflex dystrophy. *Pain*. 1997;69:49-54.
72. Sandroni P, Low PA, Ferrer T, et al. Complex Regional Pain Syndrome I (CRPS I): prospective study and laboratory evaluation. *Clin J Pain*. 1998;14:282-289.
73. Gracely RH, Price DD, Roberts WJ, et al. Quantitative sensory testing in patients with complex regional pain syndrome (CRPS) I and II. In: Janig W, Stanton-Hicks M, eds. *Reflex Sympathetic Dystrophy: A Reappraisal, Progress in Pain Research and Management*. Vol 6. Seattle IASP Press; 1996:151-172.
74. Wüppenhorst N, Maier C, Frettlöh J, et al. Sensitivity and specificity of 3-phase bone scintigraphy in the diagnosis of complex regional pain syndrome of the upper extremity. *Clin J Pain*. Mar-Apr 2010;26(3):182-189.
75. Stanton-Hicks M, Baron R, Boas R, et al. Complex regional pain syndromes: guidelines for therapy. *Clin J Pain*. 1998;14:155-166.
76. Portenoy RK, Foley KM, Inturrisi CE. The nature of opioid responsiveness and its implications for neuropathic pain: a new hypothesis derived from studies of opioid infusions. *Pain*. 1990;43:273-286.
77. Max MB, Schafer SC, Culnane M, et al. Amitriptyline relieves diabetic neuropathy pain in patients with normal or depressed mood. *Neurology*. 1987;37:589.
78. Macks MB, Kisore-Kumar R, Schafer SC, et al. Efficacy of desipramine in painful diabetic neuropathy: a placebo-controlled trial. *Pain*. 1991;45:69-73.
79. Swerdlow M. Anticonvulsants in the therapy of neuralgia pain. *Pain Clin*. 1986;1:9-19.
80. Chaturvedi SK. Phenytoin in reflex sympathetic dystrophy. *Pain*. 1989;36:379-380.

81. Mellick GA, Mellick LB. Gabapentin in the management of reflex sympathetic dystrophy. *J Pain Symptom Manage.* 1995;10: 265-266.

82. Dajgard A, Petersen P, Kastrup J. Mexiletine for treatment of chronic painful diabetic neuropathy. *Lancet.* 1988;1:9-11.

83. Kastrup J, Angelo HR, Peterson P, et al. Treatment of chronic painful diabetic neuropathy with intravenous lidocaine infusion. *Br Med J.* 1985;292:173.

84. Kessler RW, Saulsbury FT, Miller LT, et al. Reflex sympathetic treatment with transcutaneous nerve stimulation. *Pediatrics.* 1988;82:728-732.

85. Carlson LK, Watson HK. Treatment of reflex sympathetic dystrophy using the stress-loading program. *J Hand Ther.* 1988;1: 149-154.

86. Egle UT, Hoffman SO. Psychosomatic aspects of reflex sympathetic dystrophy. In: Stanton-Hicks M, Janig W, Boas RA, eds. *Reflex Sympathetic Dystrophy.* Boston: Kluwer; 1990:26-36.

87. Geertzen JB, DeBruyn H, DeBruyn-Kofman AT, et al. Reflex sympathetic dystrophy: early treatment and psychological aspects. *Arch Phys Med Rehabil.* 1994;75:442-446.

88. Wilder RT, Wolohan M, Vieyra MA, et al. Reflex sympathetic dystrophy in children. *J Bone Joint Surg.* 1992;74:910-919.

89. Schwartzman RJ, Alexander GM, Grothusen JR, et al. Outpatient intravenous ketamine for the treatment of complex regional pain syndrome: a double-blind placebo controlled study. *Pain.* 2009;147:107-115.

90. Boas RA, Covino BG, Shahnarian A. Analgesic responses to lidocaine. *Br J Anaesth.* 1982;54:501.

91. Rowbotham MC, Davies PS, Galer BS. Multicenter, double-blind vehicle controlled trial of long-term use of lidocaine patches for postherpetic neuralgia. Paper presented at the 8th World Congress on Pain, IASP; August 17-22, 1996; Vancouver, Canada.

92. Pope JE, Deer TR. Ziconotide: a clinical update and pharmacologic review. *Expert Opin Pharmacother.* 2013;14(7):957-966.

93. Kishore Kumar R, Schafer SC, et al. Efficacy of desipramine in painful diabetic neuropathy: a placebo-controlled trial. *Pain.* 1991;45:69-73.

94. Watson CP, Evans RJ, Reed K, et al. Amitriptyline vs. placebo in postherpetic neuralgia. *Neurology.* 1981;32;671-673.

95. Watson CP, Chipman M, Reed K, et al. Amitriptyline in postherpetic neuralgia: a randomized, double-blind crossover trial. *Pain.* 1991;48;29-36.

96. Ghostine SY, Comair YG, Turner DM. Phenoxybenzamine in the treatment of causalgia: report of 40 cases. *J Neurosurg.* 1984;6;1263-1268.

97. Rauck RI, Eisenach JC, Jackson K, et al. Epidural clonidine treatment for refractory reflex sympathetic dystrophy. *Anesthesiology.* 1993;79:1163-1169.

98. Byas-Smith MG, Max MB, Muir J, et al. Transdermal clonidine compared to placebo in painful diabetic neuropathy using a 2-stage enriched enrollment design. *Pain.* 1995;60:267-274.

99. Davis KD, Treede RD, Raja SM, et al. Topical application of clonidine relieves hyperalgesia in patients with sympathetically-maintained pain. *Pain.* 1991;47:309-317.

100. Christiansen K, Jensen EN, Noer I. The reflex sympathetic dystrophy syndrome: response to treatment with corticosteroids. *Acta Chir Scand.* 1982;148:653-1985.

101. Oyen WJ, Arntz I, Claessens RM, et al. Reflex sympathetic dystrophy of the hand: an excessive inflammatory response. *Pain.* 1993;59:151-157.

102. Forouzanfar T, Koke AJ, van Kleef M, Weber WE. Treatment of complex regional pain syndrome type 1. *E J Pain.* 2002;6:105-122.

103. Varenna M, Adami S, Rossini M, et al. Treatment of complex regional pain syndrome type 1 with neridronate: a randomized, double-blind placebo-controlled study. *Rheumatology (Oxford).* 2013;52:534-542.

104. Zuurmond WW, Langdendijk PN, Bezemer PD, et al. Treatment of acute reflex sympathetic dystrophy with DMSO 50% in a fatty cream. *Acta Anaesthesiol Scand.* 1996;410:364-367.

105. Shibuya N, Humphers JM, Agarwal MR, Jupiter DC. Efficacy and safety of high-dose vitamin C on complex regional pain syndrome in extremity trauma and surgery—systematic review and meta-analysis. *J Foot Ankle Surg.* 2013;52(1):62-66.

106. Goebel A, et al. Intravenous immunoglobulin treatment of the complex regional pain syndrome: a randomized trial. *Ann Intern Med.* 2010;2:152-158.

107. Kiralp MZ, Yildiz S, Vural D, et al. Effectiveness of hyperbaric oxygen therapy in the treatment of complex regional pain syndrome. *J Int Med Res.* 2004;32(3):258-262.

108. Racz G, Stanton-Hicks M. Radiofrequency (RFA) sympatholysis for CRPS. *Pain Practice.* 2002;2:250-256.

109. Moore DC. Anterior (paratracheal) approach for block of the stellate ganglion. In: Moore DC, ed. *Regional Block: A Handbook for Use in the Clinical Practice of Medicine and Surgery.* 4th ed. Springfield, IL: Charles C Thomas; 1975:123-137.

110. Abdi S, Zhou Y, Patel N, et al. A new and easy technique to block the stellate ganglion. *Pain Physician.* 2004;7:327-331.

111. Hatangdi DS, Boas RA. Lumbar sympathectomy: a single needle technique. *Br J Anesth.* 1985;57:285-289.

112. Pernak J. Percutaneous radiofrequency thermolumbar sympathectomy. *Pain Clinic.* 1995;80:99-106.

113. Raj PP. Continuous epidural infusion and patient-controlled epidural analgesia in the management of pain. In: Waldman S, Winnie A, eds. *Interventional Pain Management.* Philadelphia: WB Saunders; 1996:333-338.

114. Raj PP, Denson DD. Prolonged analgesia technique with local anesthetics. In: Raj PP, ed. *Practical Management of Pain.* Chicago: Yearbook Medical Pub; 1986:687-700.

115. DuPen S, Williams A. Management of patients receiving combined epidural morphine and bupivacaine for the treatment of cancer pain. *J Pain Symptom Manage.* 1992;7:56-58.

116. Shealy CN, Mortimer JT, Hagfors NR. Dorsal column electroanalgesia. *J Neurosurg.* 1970;32:560-564.

117. Simpson EL, Duenas A, Holmes MW, et al. Spinal cord stimulation for chronic pain of neuropathic or ischaemic origin: systematic review and economic evaluation. *Health Technol Assess.* 2009;13(17):iii, ix-x, 1-154.

118. Kumar K, Rizvi S, Bnurs SB. Spinal cord stimulation is effective in management of complex regional pain syndrome I: fact or fiction. *Neurosurgery.* 2011;69(3):566-578.

119. Augusinsson L, Linderoth B, Mannheimer C. Spinal cord stimulation in various ischemic conditions. In: Illis L, ed. *Spinal Cord Dysfunction.* Vol 3. *Functional Stimulation.* Oxford, England: Oxford Medical Pub; 1992.

120. Hassenbusch SJ, Stanton-Hicks M, Schoppa D, et al. Long-term results of peripheral nerve stimulation for reflex sympathetic dystrophy. *J Neurosurg.* 1996;84:415-423.

121. Alo KM, Yland MJ, Redko V, et al. Lumbar and sacral nerve root stimulation (NRS) in the treatment of chronic pain: a novel anatomic approach and neurostimulation technique. *Neuromodulation.* 1999;2(1):23-31.

122. Holsheimer J, Struijk JJ, Tas NR. Effects of electrogeometry and combinational nerve fiber selectivity in spinal cord stimulation. *Med Biol Eng Comput*. 1995;33:676-682.

123. Linderoth B. Neurophysiological mechanism involved in vasodilatation and ischemic pain relief by spinal cord stimulation. In: Galley D, Illis SL, Krainick M, et al., eds. *First Congress of the International Neuromodulation Society*. Bologna, Italy: Monduzzi Editore; 1993:27-40.

124. Kemler MA, Barendse GA, van Kleef M, et al. Spinal cord stimulation in patients with chronic reflex sympathetic dystrophy. *N Engl J Med*. 2000;343:618-624.

125. Oakley JC, Weiner RL. Spinal cord stimulation for complex regional pain syndrome. A prospective study in 19 patients. *Neuromodulation*. 1999;2:47-50.

126. Kumar K, Caraway DL, Rizvi S, Bishop S. Current challenges in spinal cord stimulation. *Neuromodulation*. 2014;17(suppl 1):22-35.

127. Carrillo-Ruiz JD, Andrade P, Godinez-Cubillos N, et al. Polyanalgesic Consensus Conference 2012: recommendations for the management of pain by intrathecal (intraspinal) drug delivery: report of an interdisciplinary expert panel. *Neuromodulation*. 2013;16(4):387.

128. van Hilten JJ, Vander Plass AA, Van Rijn MA, et al. Efficacy of intrathecal baclofen on different pain qualities in complex regional pain syndrome. *Anesth Analg*. 2013;116(1):211-215.

129. Kapural L, Lokey K, Leong MS, et al. Intrathecal ziconotide for complex regional pain syndrome: seven case reports. *Pain Pract*. 2009;9(4):296-303.

130. Burchiel KJ, Anderson VC, Wilson BJ, et al. Prognostic factors of spinal cord stimulation for chronic back and leg pain. *Neurosurgery*. 1995;36:1101-1111.

131. Bruehl S, Carlson CR. Predisposing psychologic factors in the development of reflex sympathetic dystrophy: a review of the empirical evidence. *Clin J Pain*. 1992;8:287-299.

132. Haddox JD. Psychological aspects of reflex sympathetic dystrophy. In: Stanton-Hicks M, ed. *Pain and the Sympathetic Nervous System*. Boston: Kluwer; 1990:207-224.

133. Stanton-Hicks M. Plasticity of complex regional pain syndrome (CRPS) in children. *Pain Med*. Aug 2010;11(8):1216-1223.

134. Wilder RT, Berde CB, Wolohan M, et al. Reflex sympathetic dystrophy in children: clinical characteristics in follow up of 70 patients. *J Bone Surg Am*. 1992;74A:910-919.

135. Stanton RP, Malcolm JR, Wersdock KA, et al. Reflex sympathetic dystrophy in children: an orthopedic perspective. *Orthopedics*. 1993;16:773-779.

136. Stanton-Hicks M, Burton AW, Bruehl SP, et al. An updated interdisciplinary clinical pathway for CRPS: report of an expert panel. *Pain Practice*. 2002;2:1-16.

Shingles, Postherpetic Neuralgia, and Postherpetic Itch

Mohamed Elkersh
Steve C. Lee
Zahid H. Bajwa

Shingles is caused by the varicella-zoster virus (VZV), which primarily affects the dorsal root ganglia (DRG) of the spinal nerves or trigeminal nerve. A single DRG is commonly affected, but a small number of adjacent DRGs may be affected, usually on the same side.

DEFINITIONS

Acute herpetic neuralgia is defined as pain during the first 30 days after the eruption of the rash. If the pain resolves within the next 4 months, it is defined as subacute herpetic neuralgia. Pain persisting beyond this time frame is called postherpetic neuralgia (PHN). Although spontaneous resolution of herpes zoster may be expected in many patients, a significant number of patients develop chronic intractable pain of PHN.

ETIOLOGY

Herpes zoster most frequently occurs in adults who previously have had chickenpox. The virus remains dormant in the DRG until, many years later, it is reactivated, producing herpes zoster because of decreased cell-mediated immunity. The decrease in immunity that permits the reactivation may be caused by infection or malignancy, or it may be iatrogenic. Persistent stress and untreated depression are thought to lower immunity, hence increasing the likelihood of shingles with severe pain, increasing the risk of chronic PHN.[1,2]

Although the DRGs of the spinal and cranial nerves are involved most commonly, any part of the central nervous system (CNS) can be affected. For example, the anterior motor horn may be involved, or the patient may have myelitis or encephalomyelitis. It has been suggested that T-cell recognition of VZV proteins is a likely mechanism involved in the control of reactivation of the virus from latency.[3–5]

INCIDENCE

The incidence of herpes zoster in the U.S. population indicates a steep increase in the general population over the past 30 years.[6] The incidence of herpes zoster is low in immunocompetent children[7] but is higher in immunosuppressed children.[8] The disease is more common in elderly adults, and the risk increases proportionately with age. The best incidence data for PHN in older patients come from the placebo arm of a large randomized trial that evaluated vaccination against VZV.[9] In 334 patients from 60 to 69 years of age who developed herpes zoster, PHN occurred in 6.9%. In contrast, among 308 patients age 70 years or older who developed herpes zoster, PHN occurred in 18.5%.

DIAGNOSIS

The virus may be recovered from early vesicles and has been recovered from blood, lung, liver, and cerebrospinal fluid (CSF) but only occasionally from the oropharynx. Scrapings also provide cellular material containing multinuclear giant cells. Acidophilic intranuclear inclusions can be seen in the Tzanck smear stained with hematoxylin and eosin, Giemsa, Papanicolaou, or Paragon multiple stain. A punch biopsy for electron microscopic examination provides even more reliable material; the more reliable material may permit a diagnosis before the vesicular stage develops (**Table 49-1**).

ACUTE HERPES ZOSTER

The diagnosis of herpes zoster is difficult to make before the rash develops. After the lesions appear, the clinical features are so typical that the diagnosis is easy. Before eruption, herpes zoster often is mistaken for other pain-causing conditions, such as trigeminal neuralgia, cluster headache, coronary artery disease, pleurisy, cholecystitis, and painful spine conditions.

Epithelial cells with eosinophilic intranuclear inclusions and multinucleated giant cells can be identified in material scraped from the base of a vesicle. The leukocyte count is normal in uncomplicated herpes zoster. Mononuclear pleocytosis is present in the CSF of patients with herpes zoster, particularly those with cranial nerve involvement.

Acute herpes usually has pain that is localized to the dermatomal distribution of one or more affected DRGs. Typically, herpes zoster occurs in one or two adjacent dermatomes, usually in the thoracic area. The

TABLE 49-1 Laboratory Diagnosis of Acute Herpes Zoster

Techniques	Comments
Virus recovery from	Rapid diagnostic tests allow for early diagnosis
Vesicles	
Blood	
Lung	
Liver	
Cerebrospinal fluid	
Oropharynx (only occasionally)	
Scrapings from the vesicles contain cellular material with multinucleated giant cells	Show acidophilic intranuclear inclusions
Tzanck smear	
Hematoxylin and eosin stain	
Giemsa stain	
Papanicolaou stain	
Paragon multiple stain	
Punch biopsy for electron microscopy	More reliable and provides diagnosis before vesicular stage develops
Culture tests (in human epithelioids or fibroblasts) Virus specifically identified in culture by intranuclear inclusions after staining and by gel-precipitation techniques	Focal lesion with swollen refractile cells in 3–4 days
Staining of cellular material with direct fluorescent antibody of Tzanck smear	Readily identifies infected cells

Data from Raj P. Pain due to herpes zoster. In: Raj P, ed. *Practical Management of Pain*. 2nd ed. Chicago: Mosby-Year Book; 1992.

ophthalmic division of the trigeminal nerve is the most common single nerve affected. The pain may be accompanied by fever and malaise. It may be mild at onset, becoming severe over the next few days. It can be dull, sharp, burning, aching, or shooting with paresthesia.

It starts with redness and swelling followed by red papules that become vesicles, blebs, and pustules and then to the crusting stage over 2 to 3 weeks. The lesions typically are unilateral, appearing along a dermatome. In mild cases, the skin lesions may not affect the whole dermatome, but sensory involvement of the whole dermatome usually is present. In severe cases, larger blebs usually cover the entire dermatome and tend to coalesce.

The lesions appear in thoracic dermatomes in more than 50% of patients. The next region where they commonly are seen is the trigeminal distribution, with an incidence of 3% to 20%. The ophthalmic division is involved in 75% of these patients. Lumbar and cervical eruptions occur in 10% to 20% of patients, with a sacral distribution being much less common. With advancing age, the incidence of trigeminal (ophthalmic) zoster increases, and that of spinal zoster declines. Bilateral zoster occurs in less than 1% of patients. Recurrent zoster is reported in a small percentage of patients usually in the same or adjacent dermatomes.

If the trigeminal (gasserian) ganglion is affected, the symptoms usually include pain in the nerve distribution, headache, and weakness of the eyelid muscles. Lesions may appear on the face, cornea, mouth, and tongue. Scarring and anesthesia of the cornea may occur. The first division of the trigeminal nerve most often is affected. If there is involvement of the geniculate ganglion, the patient may develop Bell's palsy, vertigo, disorders of hearing, and lesions of the external ear and canal and the anterior portion of the tongue. Pink scars eventually become hypopigmented, with persistent pain despite sensory loss.

Risk factors for severe, persistent pain associated with acute herpes zoster include prodromal symptoms, age greater than 50 years, and moderate to severe pain at presentation.[10] The duration of pain has been shown to correlate with severity of lesions at worst phase and the involved region, with age over 60 years and those with trigeminal involvement most likely to have significantly longer durations of pain.[11]

POSTHERPETIC NEURALGIA

Postherpetic neuralgia also can be confused with other problems, but the patient usually has a history of a previous unilateral skin eruption, and there may be residual scarring of the skin. Hyperesthesia, dysesthesia, and anesthesia also may be present in the affected areas. Skin eruption may be minimal in some cases, and few or even no scars may be present with PHN (zoster *sine herpete*). In these patients, the CNS was damaged by the original infection, resulting in neuralgia without producing any scars to the skin. A rising zoster antibody titer in the acute stage confirms the infectious agent.

POSTHERPETIC ITCH

In 10% to 50% of patients with herpes zoster, pain and hyperesthesia persist after the lesions are healed. Herpes zoster–related pain (HZRP) ranges in severity from a mild, bothersome discomfort to a debilitating and agonizing condition. Severe HZRP is commonly described as aching, burning, and lancinating. It may occur spontaneously, continuously without stimulation, and intermittently with stimulation. Itch that arises from disease located at any point along the afferent pathway is called neuropathic itch. Patients may experience a deep aching or burning pain, unbearable itching, a paresthesia that may be painful (dysesthesia), an exaggerated response to stimuli (hyperalgesia), or electric shock–like pains. These abnormal sensations may resolve or persist unpredictably.

Relief usually is found during sleep. In chronic PHN, the patient commonly has hyperpathia, often associated with damage to a peripheral nerve, the spinothalamic tract, or the thalamus. It may be caused by a reduction in the number and proportion of conducting nerve fibers.

Dysesthesia often is interpreted as pain. Uncomfortable unpleasant sensations make the patient unable to bear the lightest contact with the skin. Some patients even cut holes in their clothing to minimize the problem. A slight breath of wind can incite a paroxysm of pain. Curiously, most patients can tolerate firm pressure on the affected area but not light pressure. They may wear especially tight clothing or keep their hands pressed over the painful region. Patients may complain about a feeling of worms under the skin or of ants crawling over the skin (formication).

Itch can be present as well. Theoretically, it is possible that the few remaining cutaneous neurons may have been itch fibers from adjacent unaffected dermatomes. This possible discriminatory preservation of peripheral itch fibers that have unusually large innervation territories can become sensitized by ongoing tissue inflammation. The products of chronic inflammation perpetuate sensitization of itch fibers.

Another possible explanation independent of peripheral inflammation is that itch could also be generated by central itch neurons firing excessively when deprived of afferent input (phantom itch). Centrally mediated herpes zoster–related itch may include electrical hyperactivity of deafferented central itch–specific neurons, imbalances between excitation, and inhibition of second-order sensory neurons. Preservation of a few scattered sensory neurons after a herpes zoster eruption may have allowed activation of occasional second-order neurons without concomitant recruitment of inhibitory interneurons.

PREVENTION

Clinical trials have demonstrated that zoster vaccine reduces the incidence of zoster and PHN. Specifically, a 2012 meta-analysis evaluated the efficacy of the zoster vaccine in eight randomized trials that included 52,269 individuals 60 years of age or older, the majority of whom came from the Shingles Prevention Study (SPS), a placebo-controlled clinical trial of 38,546 adults 60 years of age or older, using a live attenuated Oka/Merck VZV vaccine.[12] A similar reduction in herpes zoster was observed as was seen in the SPS. Thus, individuals who are 60 years of age or older are strongly recommended to receive zoster vaccination to decrease the risk of zoster and PHN. Preliminary data also suggest that zoster vaccine is effective in reducing the incidence of zoster and preventing PHN in persons 50 to 59 years of age.[13]

TREATMENT

ACUTE HERPES ZOSTER

The goals are aggressive treatment of acute zoster and prevention of PHN, which is shown to reduce the incidence and severity of PHN.[14] Pain should be treated aggressively, especially in elderly and immunosuppressed patients, who are prone to PHN.[15,16]

Drug Therapy The various drugs used in the treatment of the acute stage of herpes zoster are summarized in **Table 49-2**.

Antiviral Agents Antiviral agents are now the standard preferred therapy for acute herpes zoster infections. The VZV, similar to all viruses, is a parasite that takes over healthy cells and uses their DNA to reproduce itself. It is believed that if viral DNA synthesis can be slowed or inhibited, then specific host immune systems might have more time to help control the viral infection. Some substances that grossly inhibit DNA synthesis were developed as possible anticancer drugs and have been found to have more significant antiviral than anticancer activity. Theoretically, these agents could either kill the virus or alter its replication. To be effective, the agents must be given before significant tissue damage occurs. Such agents include acyclovir, cytarabine, vidarabine, idoxuridine, sorivudine, famciclovir, valaciclovir, and brivudine. The nucleoside analogues acyclovir, famciclovir, and valacyclovir are the current preferred antivirals.

Acyclovir masquerades as one of the building blocks of the DNA needed by the herpesvirus to reproduce itself. This stops the chain, and the virus ceases to replicate. Although acyclovir accelerates cutaneous changes in herpes zoster, the intensity and duration of acute herpetic neuralgia appear to be directly related to time of therapy initiation (not later than 6 days after onset).[14] The author of a meta-analysis of 30 clinical trials in immunocompetent patients found five homogeneous, randomized, placebo-controlled trials that showed that oral acyclovir, 800 mg/day within 72 hours of rash onset, may reduce the incidence of residual pain at 6 months by 46%.[17]

Although acyclovir has been shown to be effective in shortening the duration of zoster pain, other newer agents may offer some advantages. Sorivudine has compared favorably with acyclovir in terms of accelerating cutaneous healing[18] and preventing recurrences and new episodes.[19]

Famciclovir has been shown to be efficacious in treating herpes zoster.[20–22] A placebo-controlled clinical trial was conducted in 419 immunocompetent adults (mean age, 50 years) with uncomplicated zoster to evaluate the efficacy of standard dose famciclovir (500 mg three times daily) or high-dose famciclovir (750 mg three times daily) for the treatment of acute zoster and prevention of PHN.[21] All patients were initiated on the intervention or placebo within 72 hours of rash and were treated for 7 days. After 5 months of monthly follow-up, the intention-to-treat analysis demonstrated that famciclovir was associated with modest improvement in lesion healing rates (median, 5–6 days with low- and high-dose famciclovir) compared with placebo (median, 7 days). In addition, compared with placebo, the median duration of PHN was reduced by approximately 2 months with famciclovir therapy, regardless of dose (62 and 55 days with low- and high-dose famciclovir, respectively, compared with 119 days with placebo). In addition, famciclovir may be as or more effective than acyclovir in prevention of reactivation from latency for genital herpes.[23]

Valacyclovir may be even more efficacious in treating herpes zoster than acyclovir, shortening the time to complete resolution of herpes zoster–associated pain.[24,25] It may even offer cost benefits.[26] In a randomized, double-blind study of 1141 immunocompetent adults with herpes zoster (mean age, 68 years), the efficacy and safety of valacyclovir (1000 mg orally three times daily for 7 or 14 days) were compared with acyclovir (800 mg orally five times daily for 7 days) over 6 months of follow-up.[27] An intent-to-treat analysis demonstrated that valacyclovir for 7 or 14 days accelerated the resolution of acute neuritis (median duration of pain, 38 and 44 days, respectively) compared with acyclovir (median, 51 days). The proportion of patients with pain persisting for 6 months was modestly lower in the combined valacyclovir arms (19%) than the acyclovir arm (26%). No additional benefit was observed with a longer duration of valacyclovir.

Anti-inflammatory Agents The effects of oral steroids on herpes zoster are not clear. Recent studies suggest that prednisone is well tolerated and may significantly reduce the duration of acute herpetic neuralgia and improve quality of life.[28] Inflammation and scarring are reduced with anti-inflammatory agents. Despite limited data, we recommend the use of steroids for cases with severe acute herpetic neuralgia.

A mixture of long-acting local anesthetic with a small amount of depot steroids has been administered via intralesional injection. Anecdotal reports claim excellent success in treating acute herpes zoster, with a rapid resolution of pain and diminished incidence of PHN.

Antidepressants The tricyclic antidepressants (TCAs) are known to block serotonin and norepinephrine reuptake among other analgesic effects. The serotonin-norepinephrine reuptake inhibitors (SNRIs) are a class of newer antidepressants with dual reuptake inhibition as analgesic mechanisms.

TCAs are commonly used, although depression is not common in acute herpes zoster, many patients experience anxiety along with severe pain. Amitriptyline has been shown to significantly reduce pain

TABLE 49-2 Drug Therapy for Acute Herpes Zoster

Antiviral Agents
Acyclovir
Cytarabine
Vidarabine
Idoxuridine
Thymidine analogues
Sorivudine
Famciclovir
Valaciclovir
Brivudine
Interferon
Zoster immune globulin
Adenosine monophosphate
Analgesics
Anti-inflammatory agents
Prednisone
Antidepressants and Tranquilizers
Amitriptyline and fluphenazine
Doxepin
Other
Vitamin B_{12}
B-complex vitamins
L-tryptophan

by more than half, making a strong argument for its use with an antiviral in this group of patients.[29] In addition to their antidepressant and analgesic properties, the TCAs enable these patients to sleep at night when PHN pain is usually worse.

Amitriptyline and Doxepin may improve sleep onset, frequent awakenings, and the early morning awakening that are common in severe chronic pain states. The adverse side effects of the TCAs include hypotension, hypertension, tachycardia, arrhythmias, drowsiness, confusion, disorientation, dry mouth, blurred vision, increased intraocular pressure, urinary retention, and constipation.

Nerve Blocks Because nerve root involvement is suspected in acute herpes zoster, somatic nerve blocks have been used in its treatment. These include brachial plexus, epidural, paravertebral, intercostal, and sciatic blocks. As understanding of the pathology of herpes zoster developed, attention was directed toward the sympathetic ganglia. Sympathetic blocks have been used to relieve the vasospasm that was thought to cause the pain and nerve damage.

Epidural blocks using local anesthetic have been successful in treating acute herpes zoster pain.[30] The duration of the infection is shorter, the lesions dry faster, and the pain is relieved. Spinal blocks usually are not indicated because they are not as specific as epidural blocks. The use of lumbar plexus blockade has been reported to relieve pain in an elderly patient for whom other approaches were contraindicated.[31]

POSTHERPETIC NEURALGIA

Drug Therapy (Table 49-3) A threefold purpose governs the role of drug therapy in the patient with PHN: (1) to provide analgesia for pain, (2) to reduce depression and anxiety, and (3) to decrease insomnia. Because a considerable degree of depression, anxiety, and insomnia accompany all chronic pain syndromes, hypnotics, tranquilizers, antidepressants, and anticonvulsants frequently have been used as analgesic adjuvants in the management of PHN.

It is important to warn the patient of the potential side effects of any drug. The patient is less likely to stop taking the prescribed medication if he or she knows that certain unpleasant effects are expected as a normal occurrence and that they usually are not permanent.

Opioids A number of trials support the efficacy of opioid analgesics for PHN.[32,33] In theory, opioids are attractive adjuncts to the treatment of neuropathic pain because of their central mechanism of action on μ receptors at the spinal and supraspinal level. The extent and site of the lesion may also be an important determinant of therapeutic success. In practice, the use of opioids for relief of neuropathic pain is considered controversial because of increased risk for tolerance, dependence, and overdose. Thus, opioids remain second- or third-line treatment options for PHN.[34]

Antidepressants The TCAs and SNRIs, as mentioned earlier, have been used effectively in the management of PHN. Amitriptyline and doxepin are preferred agents when insomnia is a major problem. Nortriptyline and desipramine are preferred in high-risk patients. Venlafaxine and duloxetine have also been used successfully in treating PHN.

TABLE 49-3 Drug Therapy for Postherpetic Neuralgia
Analgesics
Antidepressants and tranquilizers
Anticonvulsants
Phenytoin
Carbamazepine
Sodium valproate and amitriptyline
Topical capsaicin
Oral antiarrhythmics

Anticonvulsants Anticonvulsants can also be very helpful in optimizing pain control in patients with PHN. Drugs that have been evaluated in randomized trials include gabapentin,[35,36] pregabalin,[37] and valproic acid.[38]

A 2011 systematic review[35] identified four placebo-controlled randomized trials, with two trials evaluating immediate-release gabapentin[39,40] and two trials evaluating extended-release gabapentin.[41,42] In the pooled analysis, gabapentin at doses between 1800 and 3600 mg/day was beneficial for PHN compared with placebo for the outcome of "much or very much improved" (38% vs. 20%; risk ratio, 1.9; 95% confidence interval, 1.5–2.3; number needed to treat, 5.5).[35]

The gastroretentive extended-release formulation of gabapentin is typically administered with the evening meal. In a trial of 452 patients with PHN, the group assigned to extended-release gabapentin (1800 mg) taken once daily had a statistically significant reduction in mean pain scores compared with placebo, leading to regulatory approval of the drug in the United States as once-daily treatment for PHN.[43,44]

Another extended-release gabapentin formulation is gabapentin enacarbil, the prodrug of gabapentin. In two small randomized controlled trials (RCTs), this formulation showed some evidence of benefit for reducing average pain intensity scores in PHN.[45,46]

Pregabalin is a structural analog of GABA and is similar to gabapentin, binding to the α2-δ subunit of calcium channels to reduce neurotransmitter release. Randomized studies in patients with PHN have shown improvement in sleep and decrease in pain at doses of 150 to 600 mg/day.[47,48] Common side effects are dizziness, somnolence, dry mouth, peripheral edema, and weight gain. It is designated as a schedule V controlled substance in the United States because it has been reported to cause euphoria. The recommended starting dose is 150 mg divided into two or three doses daily and increased to a total daily dose of 300 mg. When stopping the drug, it should be tapered over 1 week because withdrawal symptoms may occur.[49]

Divalproex sodium is another anticonvulsant that has been shown to be helpful in the treatment of PHN. In an 8-week study of 48 patients with PHN, treatment with divalproex sodium (1000 mg/day) led to significantly greater pain relief than placebo.[38] More patients treated with divalproex sodium had at least moderate improvement in pain (58% vs. 15%).

Carbamazepine, oxcarbazepine, lamotrigine, and topiramate are particularly helpful for neuralgic pain in PHN patients.

Topical Medications The application of a topical medication has the potential benefit of less systemic absorption with less potential for side effects. With these advantages, the topical application of compounded pain creams has grown in popularity. Reports have been positive; however, given the paucity of evidence and trials, no firm conclusions can be made regarding the efficacy of topical compounded pain creams for the treatment of PHN.

Capsaicin Topical application of standard concentration capsaicin may be effective for PHN. However, capsaicin can cause burning, stinging, and erythema, making application of capsaicin intolerable in up to one-third of patients. Another approach is the use of a single 60-minute application of a high-concentration capsaicin patch (8%) rather than the multiple daily applications needed for standard concentration capsaicin cream (0.025%–0.075%). A one-time office application of this high-concentration capsaicin patch to the area of pain can confer up to 3 months of neuropathic pain management before reapplication is needed.

The mechanism of action is thought to be through increased conductance of sodium and calcium into the nerve axon upon activation of the C nerve fiber. The increased calcium that becomes sequestered in various organelles within the nerve fiber may disrupt its microtubular and neurofilament organization, resulting in decreased axoplasmic transport of cellular components. Ultimately, this results in desensitization of the C nerve fibers. Substance P depletion appears to be a secondary effect.

In a meta-analysis of the Qutenza Clinical Trials Database, seven studies were performed with the high-dose 8% capsaicin Qutenza patch and a 0.04% low-dose control patch. Response was defined as a greater than or equal to 30% decrease in mean pain intensity score during weeks 2 to 12. The superiority of the 8% capsaicin patch to the low-dose patch was demonstrated.[50]

Botulinum Toxin Subcutaneous botulinum toxin injection for PHN is not well studied, but the available evidence suggests it is effective. One double-blind RCT evaluated 30 adults with PHN who had persistent pain for at least 3 months. Compared with placebo injections, botulinum toxin type A (onabotulinumtoxinA) injections were beneficial for pain reduction at 2 weeks; the number of responders (i.e., patients achieving at least a 50% reduction in pain score) was significantly greater for the active treatment group (13 of 15 patients [87%] vs. none of 15 in the placebo group), and the benefit persisted for a median of 16 weeks.[51] Treatment was well tolerated.

NMDA Receptor Antagonists Animal data suggest a role for excitatory amino acid neurotransmitters in the maintenance of chronic pain caused by nerve injury.[52] Antagonists of the *N*-methyl-D-aspartate (NMDA) receptor have been shown to relieve neuropathic pain in humans. The most widely available NMDA receptor antagonists are ketamine and dextromethorphan. Intravenous ketamine induces modest pain relief in patients with PHN but at doses that cause sedation, dysphoria, and dissociative episodes.[53] However, in a randomized, double-blind, crossover trial that compared 6 weeks of treatment with dextromethorphan versus placebo, no significant relief was demonstrated.[54]

Antiarrhythmics Intravenous lidocaine has been advocated for the treatment of many types of chronic neurogenic pain, including PHN. The oral antiarrhythmics (e.g., mexiletine) have been tried, and reports are encouraging.[55] However, definitive studies on the efficacy of oral antiarrhythmics for the treatment of PHN are lacking.

Epidural Clonidine Epidural clonidine has been used in relieving neuropathic itch and pain in a patient with PHN in the distribution of the ophthalmic division of the trigeminal nerve.[56] A continuous high thoracic epidural infusion of 1 μg/mL of clonidine and 0.05% bupivacaine successfully treated postherpetic itch and decreased the frequency and intensity of lancinating attacks.

Cryotherapy Freezing peripheral nerves has also been used as a means of producing long-term neural blockade. A small, unblinded study of cryotherapy for facial pain was unable to show a significant benefit in patients with PHN. The authors did not provide inclusion criteria, concomitant therapies, or information on how the response was assessed. In contrast, a second trial reported "considerable" relief in 11 of 14 patients with cryotherapy to the intercostal nerves for PHN.[57] In most cases, however, the duration of relief was less than 2 weeks as assessed by questionnaire.

Spinal Cord Stimulation Spinal cord stimulation (SCS) has been used in the management of PHN.[58,59] Possible mechanisms by which SCS may alleviate pain from PHN include attenuating one of three pain-generating mechanisms: (1) damage to A-δ and C fibers with collateral sprouting occurring from A-β sensory fibers to nociceptors causing hyperalgesia and allodynia; (2) loss of both large and small neural fibers causing anesthesia dolorosa, resulting in hyperpathia and an absence of sensation; and (3) peripheral sensitization with hyperactive primary sensory fibers, causing allodynia with primarily intact sensation.

The mechanism of action for SCS is still unclear. Studies have demonstrated that the release of γ-aminobutyric acid (GABA) and the activation of the GABA-B and adenosine A-1 receptors by SCS may inhibit the release of the excitatory amino acids glutamate and aspartate in the dorsal horn, thus suppressing neuronal pain transmission and sympathetic outflow.[65] Although the role of the sympathetic nervous system in the development and maintenance of PHN is uncertain, there is evidence to link sympathetic activity and pain. Patients may develop allodynia secondary to an impaired balance between excitatory and inhibitory mechanisms.[63] Dorsal column stimulation resulting in decreased sympathetic outflow may result in enhanced pain relief.

Management of PHN with SCS can be challenging not only because the location of pain in the patients' perception may expand into surrounding unaffected regions but also because SCS effects are necessarily dependent on anatomically intact pathways. Early treatment of PHN with SCS is essential to the success of the therapy. SCS may offer the possibility of normalizing the neuronally perturbed transmitter levels and the inhibitory system, attenuating the sympathetic activities in the dorsal horn and DRG.

A literature review, however, showed that the response of PHN to SCS was less predictable than other pain conditions. Success rates from 27% to 60% have been reported. A major predicting factor for a successful SCS outcome is the achievement of an ideal distribution of paresthesia covering the painful area and affected neuronal structures. Verbal communication with the patient during the SCS placement process is essential for optimal paresthesia coverage.

Patients with pain as well as allodynia have preserved neuronal and dorsal column function and tend to respond well to SCS. However, there are patients with marked sensory loss in the affected dermatomes who are in constant pain without allodynia. These patients have anesthesia dolorosa secondary to the deafferentation and degeneration of dorsal column fibers and would experience no change in pain with SCS.

Peripheral Nerve Stimulation Peripheral nerve stimulation (PNS), which is the stimulation of the distal sensory fibers, has been used successfully to treat cases of PHN. Although controversial, PNS is an emerging area of neuromodulation technique that has been gaining interest. Subcutaneous placement of leads in the region of the cranial nerves of the head and neck for intractable headaches has been more recently adapted to the placement of stimulator leads subcutaneously in the trunk. Similar to dorsal column stimulation, the exact mechanism of action of PNS is unknown. The most likely mechanism of action by which PNS alleviates pain is by stimulation of A-β fibers in the dermis and hypodermis with subsequent inhibition of A-δ and C fibers. Electrical stimulation in the subcutaneous region may increase the concentration of local endorphins, affect blood flow, alter neurotransmitters, and inhibit cell membrane depolarization, with the end result of inhibiting nociception. There are several case reports to suggest the effectiveness of PNS when placing subcutaneous leads near the affected distal sensory nerves.

Lead placement with conventional spinal cord stimulator leads along the lateral recess of the spinal canal to stimulate the dorsal roots has also been reported for truncal PHN with mixed results. In fact, some practitioners have evolved their approach for PHN to consist of a hybrid system with a single eight-contact cylindrical SCS lead placed at the lateral recess of the spinal canal corresponding to the dermatome of involvement and two four-contact subcutaneous leads bordering the area of pain in the posterior trunk to maximize chances of a successful trial.

Dorsal Root Ganglion Stimulation Spinal cord stimulation of the DRG is emerging as a new therapy for treating chronic neuropathic pain, which may be adapted to treat PHN and possibly alleviate truncal pain from PHN significantly. Previous work has demonstrated the effectiveness of DRG SCS for pain associated with other neuropathic pain syndromes, including failed back surgery syndrome, complex regional pain syndrome, and chronic postsurgical pain.[60]

Intrathecal Infusion Therapy In one study, the efficacy of intrathecal opioids in selected patients with PHN who were refractory to conventional agents for neuropathic pain was examined. All patients initially reported a dramatic improvement in pain after a trial dose of intrathecal or epidural morphine and during initial titration. Patients reported that intrathecal opioids appeared to help both the deep and allodynic pain with a lesser benefit in patients with anesthesia dolorosa. The study was also consistent with the observation of others that opioid efficacy appears dose responsive. In one case report, a high thoracic epidural catheter was placed in a patient with metastatic malignant melanoma who developed acute herpes zoster–related pain and itching unresponsive to conventional oral medications.[56] The patient described severe and frequent attacks of lancinating pain occurring in a dermatomal distribution within the left ophthalmic division of the trigeminal nerve along with a disturbing itch in the same distribution as her pain. The patient had significant reduction in the frequency and intensity of the lancinating attacks after placement of a thoracic epidural catheter with continuous infusion of 1 μg/mL of clonidine.

The central itch–specific neurons may be responsive to clonidine's central inhibitory action. Clonidine's analgesic activity is mediated through pre- and postsynaptic$_2$ receptors localized in the superficial layers of the spinal dorsal horn.[61-62] Inhibitory effects of epidural clonidine include its ability to increase potassium conductance and hyperpolarize dorsal horn neurons. Also, stimulation of α-2 receptors increases acetylcholine in the dorsal horn, leading to further cell inhibition.[64] When epidural clonidine is given as a continuous infusion, prolonged inhibition of central itch–specific neurons may occur.

Behavioral Interventions It is important to remind the clinician to treat the whole patient and not just an area of the skin. The emotional stability of the patient almost always is affected, and the stresses involved for the patient and all members of the household require thoughtful management.[66-69]

Severe depression is seen in more than 50% of these patients, and suicide commonly is considered by those with long-term intractable pain. Counseling by a psychologist or clinical social worker who is experienced in pain management is a valuable adjunct to drug therapy. Training the patient in stress management and relaxation techniques is important. Anxiety and stress can exacerbate and prolong the pain. By practicing these techniques, the patient may be able to control pain to some degree.

In some patients, the pain–tension–anxiety cycle can convert acute pain symptoms into a chronic condition. Often, no matter what is done to treat these patients, the pain is not relieved unless the stress factors also are removed. Basically, two types of persons are susceptible to chronicity: the tense, hard-driving, conscientious perfectionist and the dependent individual unable to cope with life but burdened with repressed anger and hostility. Reinforcement of the patient's response to pain (e.g., moaning, grimacing, asking for medication, remaining in bed) or favorable consequences of the pain (e.g., attention and expressions of sympathy, perhaps also the occasion to manipulate others) may lead to chronic behavior that, eventually, is independent of the original underlying pathologic condition.

The most important guideline in preventing chronicity is complete honesty. Make patients aware of the relationship between the psyche and pain and relieve them of the fear of organic disease. After the patient fully accepts the emotional causes of pain, he or she can learn to relieve the pain by controlling anxiety and tension.

Family and friends should be included in counseling sessions. They, too, must cope with the pain a loved one is experiencing. The counselor not only can ease their anxiety but also can teach them how to provide effective emotional support to help the patient endure an extremely difficult period. Concentrating on the special needs of families may require extra effort on the part of the staff, but it should result in a greater number of patients who recover with the physical and emotional well-being of the family intact.

Many patients are elderly and live alone. They are unable to turn to family and friends to provide the assistance they need for routine daily tasks. The counselor should contact appropriate social service agencies to provide transportation and other necessities (e.g., prepared meals, grocery shopping, housework, regular contact with the patient to check on his or her well-being).

Other Therapies Because many patients continue to have some residual pain of varying degrees that can be aggravating, they may require management with other techniques. The following techniques are used when all others fail (**Table 49-4**).

The effectiveness of narrow band ultraviolet B therapy in attenuating PHN was recently demonstrated. Similarly, the use of transcutaneous electrical nerve stimulation (TENS) units may significantly reduce the pain associated with PHN.[70]

TABLE 49-4 Other Therapies for Postherpetic Neuralgia
Transcutaneous electrical nerve stimulation
Cold therapies
Ice
Ethyl chloride
Cryocautery with dry ice
Acupuncture
Hypnosis
Surgery and neurosurgery

Acupuncture Significant pain relief is anecdotally reported in patients with PHN treated with acupuncture. More RCTs are necessary to establish its efficacy.

Neurosurgery Surgery may be the last resort for severe medically intractable PHN. Surgery usually attacks the pain pathway in stages at progressively higher divisions. Because the origin of pain was linked to the scar and peripheral receptors, wide excision and skin grafting were tried but are rarely used.

Rhizotomy of the somatic afferents and DRG had poor outcomes, leading to the recommendation that ablation include several segments above and below the affected area. Sympathectomy has not been successful in treating PHN.

Cordotomy has been used with good results. In most cases, however, the pain returns. Early recurrence has been blamed on failure to ablate all the nerves in the pathway, which resume function after the swelling has decreased. Stereotactic ablation of the conducting paths in the thalamus and mesencephalon and frontal lobotomy has been used. These should be tried only in patients with short life expectancies who have not had success with any other methods.

Because of the high risk and unpredictable results, neuroablation has mostly been replaced by neuromodulation. These include peripheral and dorsal column stimulators discussed elsewhere in this chapter. Deep brain stimulators and motor cortical stimulators have also been used with variable success when other therapies fail.

REFERENCES

1. Irwin M, Costlow C, Williams H, et al. Cellular immunity to varicella-zoster virus in patients with major depression. *J Infect Dis*. 1998;178(Suppl 1):S104-S108.
2. Fields HL, Rowbotham MC. Pathophysiology of postherpetic neuralgia. Presented at the Herpes Zoster and Postherpetic Neuralgia Satellite Symposium; August 13 and 14, 1996; Whistler Mountain, British Columbia.
3. Terada K, Tanaka H, Kawano S, et al. Specific cellular immunity in immunocompetent children with herpes zoster. *Acta Paediatr*. 1998;87:692-694.
4. Glaser R, Jones JF, eds. *Herpes Virus Infections*. New York: Marcel Dekker; 1994.
5. Sadzot-Delvaux C, Arvin AM, et al. Varicella-zoster virus IE63, a virion component expressed during latency and acute infection, elicits humoral and cellular immunity. *J Infect Dis*. 1998;178(Suppl 1):S43-S47.
6. Donahue JG, Choo PW, Manson JE, et al. The incidence of herpes zoster. *Arch Intern Med*. 1995;155:1605-1609.
7. Petursson G, Gelgason S, Gudmundsson S, et al. Herpes zoster in children and adolescents. *Pediatr Infect Dis J*. 1998;17:905-908.

8. Broyer M, Tete MJ, Guest G, et al. Varicella and zoster in children after kidney transplantation: long-term results of vaccination. *Pediatrics*. 1997;99:35-39.
9. Oxman MN, Levin MJ, Johnson GR, et al. A vaccine to prevent herpes zoster and postherpetic neuralgia in older adults. *N Engl J Med*. 2005;352:2271.
10. Whitley RJ, Shukla S, Crooks RJ. The identification of risk factors associated with persistent pain following herpes zoster. *J Infect Dis*. 1998;178(Suppl 1):S71-S75.
11. Higa K, Mori M, Hirata K, et al. Severity of skin lesions of herpes zoster at the worst phase rather than age and involved region most influences the duration of acute herpetic pain. *Pain*. 1997;69:245-253.
12. Gagliardi AM, Gomes Silva BN, Torloni MR, Soares BG. Vaccines for preventing herpes zoster in older adults. *Cochrane Database Syst Rev*. 2012;(10):CD008858.
13. Schmader KE, Levin MJ, Gnann JW Jr, et al. Efficacy, safety, and tolerability of herpes zoster vaccine in persons aged 50-59 years. *Clin Infect Dis*. 2012;54:922.
14. Jovanovic J, Cvjetkovic D, Pobor M, et al. Herpes zoster—treatment with acyclovir. *Med Pregl*. 199;50:305-308.
15. Bennett GJ. Animal models and their relation to neuropathic pain: particularly HZ and PHN. Presented at the Herpes Zoster and Postherpetic Neuralgia Satellite Symposium; August 13 and 14, 1996; Whistler Mountain, British Columbia.
16. Bennett GJ. Hypotheses on the pathogenesis of herpes zoster-associated pain. *Ann Neurol*. 1994;35:538-541.
17. Jackson JL, Gibbons R, Meyer G, et al. The effect of treating herpes zoster with oral acyclovir in preventing postherpetic neuralgia. A meta-analysis. *Arch Intern Med*. 1997;157:909-912.
18. Gnann JW Jr, Crumpacker CS, Lalezari JP, et al. Sorivudine versus acyclovir for treatment of dermatomal herpes zoster in human immunodeficiency virus–infected patients: results from a randomized, controlled clinical trial. Collaborative Antiviral Study Group/AIDS Clinical Trials Group, Herpes Zoster Study Group. *Antimicrob Agents Chemother*. 1998;42:1139-1145.
19. Bodsworth NJ, Boag F, Burdge D, et al. Evaluation of sorivudine (BV-araU) versus acyclovir in the treatment of acute localized herpes zoster in human immunodeficiency virus–infected adults. The Multinational Sorivudine Study Group. *J Infect Dis*. 1997;176:103-111.
20. Stott GA. Famciclovir: a new systemic antiviral agent for herpesvirus. *Am Fam Physician*. 1997;55:2501-2504.
21. Tyring S, Barbarash RA, Nahlik JE, et al. Famciclovir for the treatment of acute herpes zoster: effects on acute disease and postherpetic neuralgia. A randomized, double-blind, placebo-controlled trial. *Ann Intern Med*. 1995;123:89-96.
22. Degreef H, Famciclovir Herpes Zoster Clinical Study Group. Famciclovir, a new oral drug: results of the first controlled clinical study demonstrating its efficacy and safety in the treatment of uncomplicated herpes zoster in immune-competent patients. *Int J Antimicrob Agents*. 1994;4:241-246.
23. Loveless M, Sacks SL, Harris JRW. Famciclovir in the management of first-episode genital herpes. *Infect Dis Clin Pract*. 1997;6(Suppl 1):S12-S16.
24. Wood MJ, Shukla S, Fiddian AP, et al. Treatment of acute herpes zoster: effect of early (< 48 h) versus late (48–72 h) therapy with acyclovir and valaciclovir on prolonged pain. *J Infect Dis*. 1998;178(Suppl 1):S81-S84.
25. Stein GE. Pharmacology of new antiherpes agents: famciclovir and valacyclovir. *J Am Pharm Assoc*. 1997;NS37:157-163.
26. Grant DM, Mauskopf JA, Bell L, et al. Comparison of valaciclovir and acyclovir for the treatment of herpes zoster in immunocompetent patients over 50 years of age: a cost-consequence model. *Pharmacotherapy*. 1997;17:333-341.
27. Beutner KR, Friedman DJ, Forszpaniak C, et al. Valaciclovir compared with acyclovir for improved therapy for herpes zoster in immunocompetent adults. *Antimicrob Agents Chemother*. 1995;39:1546.
28. Ernst ME, Santee JA, Klepser TB. Oral corticosteroids for pain associated with herpes zoster. *Ann Pharmacother*. 1998;32:1099-1103.
29. Bowsher D. The effects of pre-emptive treatment of postherpetic neuralgia with amitriptyline: a randomized, double-blind, placebo-controlled trial. *J Pain Symptom Manage*. 1997;13:327-331.
30. Higa K, Hori K, Harasawa I, et al. High thoracic epidural block relieves acute herpetic pain involving the trigeminal and cervical regions: comparison with effects for stellate ganglion block. *Reg Anesth Pain Med*. 1998;23:25-29.
31. Hadzic A, Vloka JD, Saff GN, et al. The "three-in-one block" for treatment of pain in a patient with acute herpes zoster infection. *Reg Anesth*. 1997;22:575-578.
32. Boureau F, Legallicier P, Kabir-Ahmadi M. Tramadol in postherpetic neuralgia: a randomized, double-blind, placebo-controlled trial. *Pain*. 2003;104:323.
33. Raja SN, Haythornthwaite JA, Pappagallo M, et al. Opioids versus antidepressants in postherpetic neuralgia: a randomized, placebo-controlled trial. *Neurology*. 2002;59:1015.
34. Johnson RW, Rice AS. Clinical practice. Postherpetic neuralgia. *N Engl J Med*. 2014;371:1526.
35. Moore RA, Wiffen PJ, Derry S, McQuay HJ. Gabapentin for chronic neuropathic pain and fibromyalgia in adults. *Cochrane Database Syst Rev*. 2011;(4):CD007938.
36. Edelsberg JS, Lord C, Oster G. Systematic review and meta-analysis of efficacy, safety, and tolerability data from randomized controlled trials of drugs used to treat postherpetic neuralgia. *Ann Pharmacother*. 2011;45:1483.
37. Dubinsky RM, Kabbani H, El-Chami Z, et al. Practice parameter: treatment of postherpetic neuralgia: an evidence-based report of the Quality Standards Subcommittee of the American Academy of Neurology. *Neurology*. 2004;63:959.
38. Kochar DK, Garg P, Bumb RA, et al. Divalproex sodium in the management of post-herpetic neuralgia: a randomized double-blind placebo-controlled study. *QJM*. 2005;98:29.
39. Rowbotham M, Harden N, Stacey B, et al. Gabapentin for the treatment of postherpetic neuralgia: a randomized controlled trial. *JAMA*. 1998;280:1837.
40. Rice AS, Maton S, Postherpetic Neuralgia Study Group. Gabapentin in postherpetic neuralgia: a randomised, double blind, placebo controlled study. *Pain*. 2001;94:215.
41. Irving G, Jensen M, Cramer M, et al. Efficacy and tolerability of gastric-retentive gabapentin for the treatment of postherpetic neuralgia: results of a double-blind, randomized, placebo-controlled clinical trial. *Clin J Pain*. 2009;25:185.
42. Wallace MS, Irving G, Cowles VE. Gabapentin extended-release tablets for the treatment of patients with postherpetic neuralgia: a randomized, double-blind, placebo-controlled, multicentre study. *Clin Drug Investig*. 2010;30:765.
43. Medical Letter. Once-daily gabapentin (Gralise) for postherpetic neuralgia. *Med Lett Drugs Ther*. 2011;53:94.
44. Sang CN, Sathyanarayana R, Sweeney M, DM-1796 Study Investigators. Gastroretentive gabapentin (G-GR) formulation reduces intensity of pain associated with postherpetic neuralgia (PHN). *Clin J Pain*. 2013;29:281.

45. Backonja MM, Canafax DM, Cundy KC. Efficacy of gabapentin enacarbil vs placebo in patients with postherpetic neuralgia and a pharmacokinetic comparison with oral gabapentin. *Pain Med.* 2011;12:1098.
46. Zhang L, Rainka M, Freeman R, et al. A randomized, double-blind, placebo-controlled trial to assess the efficacy and safety of gabapentin enacarbil in subjects with neuropathic pain associated with postherpetic neuralgia (PXN110748). *J Pain.* 2013;14:590.
47. Dworkin RH, Corbin AE, Young JP Jr, et al. Pregabalin for the treatment of postherpetic neuralgia: a randomized, placebo-controlled trial. *Neurology.* 2003;60:1274.
48. Sabatowski R, Gálvez R, Cherry DA, et al. Pregabalin reduces pain and improves sleep and mood disturbances in patients with postherpetic neuralgia: results of a randomised, placebo-controlled clinical trial. *Pain.* 2004;109:26.
49. Pregabalin (Lyrica) for neuropathic pain and epilepsy. *Med Lett Drugs Ther.* 2005;47:75.
50. Derry S, Sven-Rice A, Cole P, et al. Topical capsaicin (high concentration) for chronic neuropathic pain in adults. *Cochrane Database Syst Rev.* 2013;(2):CD007393.
51. Apalla Z, Sotiriou E, Lallas A, et al. Botulinum toxin A in postherpetic neuralgia: a parallel, randomized, double-blind, single-dose, placebo-controlled trial. *Clin J Pain.* 2013;29:857.
52. Chizh BA, Headley PM. NMDA antagonists and neuropathic pain—multiple drug targets and multiple uses. *Curr Pharm Des.* 2005;11:2977.
53. Eide PK, Jørum E, Stubhaug A, et al. Relief of post-herpetic neuralgia with the N-methyl-D-aspartic acid receptor antagonist ketamine: a double-blind, cross-over comparison with morphine and placebo. *Pain.* 1994;58:347.
54. Nelson KA, Park KM, Robinovitz E, et al. High-dose oral dextromethorphan versus placebo in painful diabetic neuropathy and postherpetic neuralgia. *Neurology.* 1997;48:1212.
55. Baranowski AP, De Courcey J, Bonello E. A trial of intravenous lidocaine on the pain and allodynia of postherpetic neuralgia. *J Pain Symptom Manage.* 1999;17:429.
56. Elkersh MA, Simopoulos T, Malik AB, et al. Epidural clonidine relieves intractable neuropathic itch associated with herpes zoster-related pain. *Reg Anesth Pain Med.* 2003;28(4):344-346.
57. Jones MJ, Murrin KR. Intercostal block with cryotherapy. *Ann R Coll Surg Engl.* 1987;69:261.
58. Harke H, Gretenkort P, Ladleif HU, et al. Spinal cord stimulation in postherpetic neuralgia and in acute herpes zoster pain. *Anesth Analg.* 2002;94(3):694-700; table of contents.
59. Tamimi MA, Davids HR, Langston MM, et al. Successful treatment of chronic neuropathic pain with subcutaneous peripheral nerve stimulation: four case reports. *Neuromodulation.* 2009;12(3):210-214.
60. Liem L, Russo M, Huygen FJ, et al. One-year outcomes of spinal cord stimulation of the dorsal root ganglion in the treatment of chronic neuropathic pain. *Neuromodulation.* August 21 2014, Epub ahead of print.
61. Yi JY, Kim TY, Shim JH, et al. Histopathological findings, viral DNA distribution and lymphocytic immunophenotypes in vesicular and papular types of herpes zoster. *Acta Derm Venereol.* 1997;77:194-197.
62. Worrell JT, Cockerell CJ. Histopathology of peripheral nerves in cutaneous herpesvirus infection. *Am J Dermatopathol.* 1997;19:133-137.
63. Nurmikko T, Wells C, Bowsher D. Sensory dysfunction in postherpetic neuralgia. In: Boivie J, Hansson P, Lindblom U, eds. *Touch, Temperature and Pain in Health and Disease: Mechanisms and Assessments.* Vol 3. Seattle: IASP Press; 1994:133-141.
64. Fields HL, Rowbotham MC. Multiple mechanisms of neuropathic pain: A clinical perspective. In: Gebhart GF, Hammond DL, Jensen TS, eds. *Proceedings of the 7th World Congress on Pain.* Vol 2. Seattle: IASP Press; 1994:437-454.
65. Haanpaa M, Dastidar P, Weinberg A, et al. CSF and MRI findings in patients with acute herpes zoster. *Neurology.* 1998;51:1405-1411.
66. Applegate KL, Cacioppo TJ, Keicolt-Glaser JK, et al. The effects of stress on the immune system: implications for reactivation of latent herpesviruses. Presented at the Herpes Zoster and Postherpetic Neuralgia Satellite Symposium; August 13 and 14, 1996; Whistler Mountain, British Columbia.
67. Lutgendorf S, Antoni MH, Jumar M, et al. Changes in cognitive copying strategies predict EEBV-antibody titre following a stressor disclosure induction. *J Psychosom Res.* 1994;38:63-78.
68. Esterling BA, Antoni MH, Fletcher MA, et al. Emotional disclosure through writing or speaking modulates latent Epstein-Barr virus antibody titers. *J Consult Clin Psychol.* 1994;62:130-140.
69. Tyring SK. Advances in the treatment of herpesvirus infection: the role of famciclovir. *Clin Ther.* 1998;20:661-670.
70. Ahmed HE, Craig WF, White PF, et al. Percutaneous electrical nerve stimulation: an alternative to antiviral drugs for acute herpes zoster. *Anesth Analg.* 1998;87:911-914.

SECTION B
Acute and Perioperative Pain

CHAPTER 50 Preemptive Analgesia

Amar Parikh
Thomas T. Simopoulos

The understanding of postoperative pain has evolved greatly during the past half century. Many laboratory investigations have established that peripheral tissue injury during surgery can trigger a prolonged state of spinal cord excitation. A reduction in neuronal thresholds in the central nervous system (CNS) is thought to amplify pain in postsurgical patients. Preemptive analgesia is an antinociceptive treatment targeted to block CNS hyperexcitability and leads to a reduced postoperative pain state. This treatment also has the long-term goals of facilitating rapid return to usual baseline function as well as decreasing the risk of chronic pain. However, despite numerous investigations, the clinical relevance of such treatment remains in controversy.

HISTORY AND BACKGROUND

The modern concept of preemptive analgesia was based on experimental animal studies demonstrating CNS plasticity and sensitization after nociception. It was theorized that postoperative pain is amplified by continuous processing of afferent input. The preemptive administration of antinociceptive treatments aims to alter the processing of this afferent input and in turn reduce postoperative pain.[1]

An editorial in the 1980s postulated that (1) a reduction in massive small-fiber input into the CNS during surgery would prevent a central sensitization, and (2) analgesia that is present preoperatively has the potential to render prolonged effects, well beyond the known time frame of drug action.[2] Consistent with this proposal were experimental data by Woolf and Wall demonstrating that low doses of opioids, given before a painful stimulus, can effectively prevent central sensitization.[3] In contrast, much higher doses of opioids are required to suppress an already sensitized spinal cord. Since Wall's editorial, a large number of investigations have been carried out with overall equivocal results. There has been an appreciation for the multiple variables that influence postoperative pain as well as short-term and long-term goals of preemptive analgesia. In the short term, a reduction in pain scores, analgesic consumption (usually opioids) is sought, and in the long run, a quicker return to function and reduction in chronic pain is desired. In the absence of significant preoperative pain, the surgical incision does remain the key stimulus of central sensitization in most operations that triggers multiple mediators, which serve to extend a peripheral and central excited neural state into the postoperative period. Therefore, in the majority of preemptive studies, the preincisional therapy is not continued into the postoperative period.

PATHOPHYSIOLOGY OF POSTINJURY PAIN

PERIPHERAL SENSITIZATION

The establishment of sensitization in the periphery involves the transition of high-threshold nociceptors into ones of low threshold, as induced by the release of various chemicals soon after surgical incision.[4] At the site of damage, a complex array of inflammatory mediators, as outlined in **Table 50-1**, is mobilized from injured tissue, and others are delivered by the circulation.[5] Small-diameter primary afferent neurons, Aδ and C fibers innervating the region of insult, subsequently enter a state characterized by ongoing discharge and excitation elicited by suprathreshold stimulation (hyperalgesia).[6] On a molecular level, it is suggested that the phosphorylation of voltage-gated sodium and potassium channels works to reduce the action potential threshold and refractory period while enhancing repetitive firing.[7] The center of a surgical wound, which is the primary zone of injury, would be expected to demonstrate static mechanical hyperalgesia.

TABLE 50-1 Biochemical Mediators That Induce Peripheral Sensitization

Hydrogen ions	Purines
Noradrenaline	Cytokines
Bradykinin	Serotonin
Potassium ions	Leukotrienes
Histamine	Nerve growth factor
Prostaglandins	Neuropeptides

Immediately surrounding the primary zone is an area of erythema, edema, and hyperalgesia initiated by axon reflexes.[8] Activation of C fibers lead to neurogenic inflammation as a result of antidromic release of neuropeptides (e.g., substance P) from collateral axons.[9] Substance P release degranulates histamine and serotonin and causes vasodilation to further fuel peripheral sensitization. The skin, muscle, tendons, and other deep somatic structures become sore, achy, and tender. Clinically, patients refrain from movement and deep breathing and guard their surgical sites. With ensuing healing, inflammatory mediators decrease and primary afferent neurons resume their usual high threshold state, emphasizing the normal reversibility of peripheral sensitization.

CENTRAL SENSITIZATION

Peripheral sensitization provoked by surgical incision leads to massive and prolonged afferent nociceptor input into the CNS, particularly the spinal cord.[10] C fibers release neuropeptides (substance P, neurokinin A, calcitonin gene-related peptide) and excitatory amino acids (glutamate, aspartate) on second-order neurons (nociceptive specific and wide dynamic range) in the dorsal horn.[11] Second-order neurons enter a state of increased spontaneous firing, prolonged cell discharge ("windup"), reduced thresholds, and expansion of peripheral receptive fields.[12] This process is central sensitization at the level of the spinal cord, which now abnormally amplifies future incoming impulses (**Table 50-2**).

Sensitized wide-dynamic-range (WDR) neurons receive input not only from Aδ and C fibers but also from low-threshold Aβ fibers (mediating light touch). Such convergence results in an innocuous stimulus being perceived as painful (allodynia).[13] Receptive fields are expanded to involve normal-appearing areas surrounding the primary site of tissue injury. Such secondary hyperalgesic zones are characteristically painful to light

TABLE 50-2 Terms Indicating Sensitization or Facilitation of the Dorsal Horn

Term	Description
Central sensitization	Persistent changes in second-order neuron processing caused by lower thresholds, which result in amplified peripheral receptive fields
Windup	Increased and prolonged discharge of dorsal horn cells
Central hyperexcitability	Exaggerated and prolonged responsiveness of second-order neurons to normal stimulation
Long-term potentiation	Cellular memory for pain, giving rise to enhanced response to noxious stimulation

touch, indicating that large Aβ fibers are transmitting impulses to a spinal cord that is sensitized.[14] Dynamic allodynia is established through the convergence of Aβ and C fibers on hyperexcitable WDR cells. It should be noted that peripheral sensitization also causes Aδ and C fibers to respond to low-intensity stimuli. Central sensitization alters dorsal horn cell processing such that impulses from large-diameter, low-threshold, mechanoreceptive afferents fibers (Aβ) produce pain. Under physiologic conditions, central sensitization, similar to peripheral, is reversible.

The persistence of central sensitization has clinical correlation with regards to chronic pain. For example, evidence suggests that patients with fibromyalgia have a dysfunction in the central nociceptive system with extensive disinhibition. Regional blood flow studies, levels of substance P, and NMDA (*N*-methyl-D-aspartate) receptor activity have all been shown to be altered in those suspected to have fibromyalgia. The ongoing research supports the importance of central sensitization, but the pain mechanisms in this syndrome are still a matter of ongoing study.[15]

CELLULAR AND BIOCHEMICAL MECHANISMS OF CENTRAL SENSITIZATION

The prevention of central sensitization forms the basis of preemptive analgesia. Central changes produced by tissue damage and noxious stimulation associated with surgery have been the focus of intense investigation because of the potential to result in prolonged recovery and possibly chronic pain. There is a fair degree of confidence concerning molecular physiology underlying central neuroplasticity deserving of further discussion.

As indicated previously, neuropeptide and excitatory amino acid release in the dorsal horn initiates central sensitization. Both types of ligands lead to increases in intracellular calcium.[16] Neuropeptides bind to neurokinin-G protein–coupled receptors that activate voltage-gated calcium channels to enhance the flux of calcium ion into the dorsal horn cells. Similarly, aspartate interaction with the NMDA receptor leads to increases in intracellular calcium, which is thought to be the predominant mechanism responsible for persistent abnormal neuronal hypersensitivity after noxious stimulation.[17]

In addition, glutamate interacts with metabotropic receptors to activate phospholipase C (PLC), a common second messenger system.[18] Receptor-triggered activation of PLC results in hydrolysis of polyphosphatidylinositol (a cell membrane phospholipid) into two intracellular messengers, inositol triphosphate (IP_3) and diacylglycerol (DAG). Whereas IP_3 stimulates the release of calcium from internal cellular stores, DAG activates protein kinase C (PKC). PKC is enzymatically active only in the presence of calcium. Increased calcium concentrations, together with PKC, result in increased expression of proto-oncogenes, such as c-fos and c-jun.[19] The gene products of c-fos and c-jun regulate the encoding of dynorphin and enkephalin peptides. These peptides are then thought to mediate long-term changes in cellular function.[20,21] Finally, PKC itself can phosphorylate NMDA receptors, leading to sustained alterations in cell membrane conduction[22] (**Table 50-3**). Cellular memory for pain (long-term potentiation) results in enhanced response to noxious stimulation.

TABLE 50-3 Summary of the Biochemical Basis of Central Sensitization

Biochemical Mediator	Effect
Excitatory amino acid (e.g., glutamate) and neuropeptides (e.g., substance P)	Neurotransmitters that initiate an increase in intracellular Ca^{2+} of second-order neurons
N-methyl-D-aspartate (NMDA) receptor	Key role in windup, allowing large influx of Ca^{2+} after binding excitatory amino acids
Second messengers (e.g., G proteins and phosphor-inositol cascade)	Further enhance the increase in Ca^{2+} and activate protein kinase C
Proto-oncogenes (e.g., c-fos, c-jun)	Regulate mRNA encoding of dynorphin and enkephalin peptides
Dynorphin, enkephalin peptides	Enhanced excitability and long-term alternations in cell function

PEVENTION OF CENTRAL SENSITIZATION

NMDA ANTAGONISTS

The concept of preemptive analgesia makes ketamine a very suitable candidate for investigation of postoperative pain reduction. Ketamine is a noncompetitive antagonist of the NMDA receptor and thereby reduces associated ion channel conduction.[23] The NMDA receptor is thought to be considerably involved in central pain processing and spinal cord neural plasticity. Preclinical models strongly suggest the importance of administering specific NMDA antagonists before noxious stimulation to effectively block central sensitization.[24] Clinical trials have shown significant benefit in the management of acute postoperative pain even when administered after surgical insult.[25] Unlike other more selective NMDA antagonists (e.g., MK-801), ketamine does not lead to reduced spinal Fos protein.[26,27]

Mechanistically, the neuropharmacology of ketamine is complex. Ketamine may inhibit sodium and L-type calcium channels, a-amino-hydroxy-5-methyl-4-isoxazole-proprionic acid (AMPA), kainate receptors, neuronal uptake of norepinephrine as well as exert agonistic properties at the opioid receptors.[28] Ketamine also inhibits the NMDA receptor when the channel is in an open state.[29,30] This latter point may help explain the clinical findings that ketamine is effective not only in reducing central facilitation after an acute noxious input but also in chronic painful conditions (e.g., postherpetic neuralgia).[30,31]

A large meta-analysis in 2004 by Subramaniam and colleagues summarized that ketamine certainly has a role as an effective adjuvant to narcotics in postoperative pain control. Intravenous (IV) ketamine infusions decreased IV and opioid requirements in 6 of 11 studies. A majority of studies also demonstrated that bolus ketamine and epidural ketamine have beneficial effects.[32] IV ketamine (0.5 mg/kg bolus with 0/25 mg/kg/hr) has also been shown to be an effective complement to traditional epidural analgesia in patients undergoing major digestive surgery.[33]

However, ketamine use alone has not consistently been shown to reduce postoperative pain scores or analgesic usage. A preemptive effect would consist of a reduction of secondary hyperalgesia by diminishing or ablating central sensitization. Prolonged analgesic effects would then be appreciated. Tverskoy and colleagues administered preincisional ketamine intravenously and demonstrated a reduction in wound hyperalgesia compared with control participants, by measuring pain threshold to pressure.[34] Despite profound reductions in wound hyperalgesia after abdominal hysterectomy, there was no significant effect on postoperative pain or opioid consumption. Similar results in kidney donors have been reported later by Stubhaug and coworkers, which have led investigators to question the relevance of central sensitization in postoperative pain.[35]

However, studies not assessing secondary hyperalgesia have been able to show a moderate reduction in postoperative opioid consumption lasting between 24 and 48 hours with early administration of low-dose ketamine (0.15 mg/kg).[36] Recent attention focused on the effect of preoperative ketamine for patients undergoing laparoscopic procedures. Kwok and colleagues randomized 135 patients to receive 0.15 mg/kg of ketamine bolus preincision versus postclosure bolus and placebo for gynecologic laparoscopic surgery. When assessed postoperatively, the preincision group had lower mean morphine consumption with no change in hemodynamic variables or side effects ($P < 0.04$).[37] The extended benefits of ketamine suggest a preemptive effect, yet diminution of secondary hyperalgesia has not correlated with pain reduction. Noncompetitive interaction of ketamine at the NMDA receptor may limit the development of acute opioid tolerance.[38] This may offer a partial explanation for the observed decrease in postoperative opioid consumption.

Similarly, epidural ketamine can result in prolongation to first analgesic request, and reduction in postoperative analgesic needs in patients after total knee replacement and hysterectomy.[39] These beneficial effects appear to be independent of whether ketamine is administered before or after incision.[40] Both studies administered generous doses (30–60 mg) and may still be adequate to ablate central sensitization even after it has been initiated. Reduction of wound hyperalgesia was not assessed in either study. Epidural ketamine has also been assessed in patients undergoing lower limb amputation procedures. Postoperative pain was reduced in all patients receiving epidural analgesia preoperatively. However, immediate postoperative pain and mechanical stump sensitivity were lower in a group receiving epidural ketamine. Long-term effects of ketamine at 1-year follow-up were inconclusive.[41]

The search for other NMDA antagonists has also recently gained attention. Limited studies using preincisional dextromethorphan showed promise. Helmy and Bali found a statistically significant reduction in postoperative meperidine patient-controlled analgesia (PCA) use in patients undergoing elective upper abdominal surgeries who had received 120 mg of preincisional intramuscular dextromethorphan.[42] Further research into the efficacy of dextromethorphan in this setting is needed.

OPIOIDS

Preclinical studies have evaluated both systemically and spinally administered opioids in their ability to prevent central facilitation. Neuraxial opioids are known to yield significant dose-dependent analgesia via modulation at the dorsal horn of the spinal cord. Opioids render analgesia at the level of the spinal cord by two distinct mechanisms: (1) preventing the release of excitatory neurotransmitters from small, primary afferent fibers and (2) hyperpolarization of second-order neurons.[43] Intraspinal opioids would be reasonable to investigate as agents that may produce preemptive analgesia. Systemically administered opioids are believed to have a more complex mechanism of action that is not fully understood.[44] Supraspinal sites have been implicated in studies of animals with high-spinal transections. Supraspinal opioid targets activate descending inhibitory pathways, which lead to dorsal horn modulation.[45] Unknown is the impact of this descending inhibition on the release of excitatory neurotransmitter from primary afferent fibers or the response of dorsal horn cells. CNS modulation is agreed to be the main mechanism of the action of opioids, but peripheral opioid receptors may contribute to analgesia. Aside from intraarticular application, opioid interaction with peripheral receptors does not appear to manifest in clinically significant pain reduction[45] and would indicate that peripheral sensitization may be modestly affected by systemically or neuraxially administered opioids. Limited new research has been conducted in this area.

At the present time, both spinally and systemically administered opioids have given inconsistent results in preemptive trials. Postinjury facilitation of dorsal horn cells using subcutaneous formalin has been shown to be routinely blocked by intrathecal μ agonists. Interestingly, Yamamoto and Yaksh demonstrated that central facilitation (phase II of the formalin test) may be suppressed even if intrathecal morphine is given after noxious stimulation (phase I of the formalin test, corresponding to acute C fiber–evoked activity in spinal neurons).[46] Previous studies had stressed the failure of postinjury administration of intrathecal μ agonists to entirely ablate central sensitization.[47] Other animal models, which involve the generation of more intense peripheral inflammation by either deep tissue injury with 5% formalin (e.g., into a knee joint) or a plantar incision of the hind paw, have identified that ongoing input from the periphery may be adequate to sustain central sensitization long after injury.[48] Actual incisional pain with associated hyperalgesia may progress during the surgery and actually peak shortly after. It is not surprising that these latter studies inflicting an intense and prolonged inflammatory injury were unable to document a significant difference in pain behavior between subjects administered intrathecal opioids before and after injury.

Systemic opioids have produced mixed results in experimental animal models. Abram and Olson used the rat formalin test to show that high doses of morphine or alfentanil, administered systemically, were unable to prevent central sensitization.[49] Even at high IV doses, morphine concentrations achieved in the subarachnoid space remained an order of magnitude lower than those achieved by direct subarachnoid injection. In contrast, Lascelles and colleagues using a model of ovariohysterectomy in rats were able to prevent surgically induced hyperalgesia by early administration of meperidine.[50] Applying the same rat ovariohysterectomy model, Gonzalez and coworkers reported a preemptive effect with subcutaneous morphine before surgical incision.[51] The conflicting experimental results involving preemptive analgesia reflect the different animal models studied. It is of critical importance that a model parallels as much as possible the usual human intraoperative and postoperative pain state. It remains unclear if typical doses of systemically administered opioids are capable of suppressing dorsal horn activity.

Clinical trials have evaluated both systemic and spinal opioids, given pre- and postincision, to determine whether a preemptive effect generates appreciable postoperative pain reduction. Initial trials with systemic opioids appeared to reduce wound hyperalgesia. Richmond and colleagues reported reductions in visual analog scale (VAS) scores and postoperative opioid consumption when pretreating women undergoing abdominal hysterectomy with 10 mg of morphine before incision,[52] as well as an associated decrease in secondary hyperalgesia. In a follow-up study, Collis and colleagues reported similar findings in women undergoing abdominal hysterectomy but found no advantage with increasing the preemptive dose of morphine to 20 mg.[53] Tverskoy and colleagues demonstrated a decline of secondary hyperalgesia in women after abdominal hysterectomy with early administration of fentanyl, but without significant impact on VAS or opioid use.[54] Griffin and coworkers demonstrated less morphine consumption in posthysterectomy patients at 48 and 72 hours with preincisional high-dose alfentanil (70 μg/kg),[55] but VAS pain scores did not differ significantly between pre- and postincisional groups. Several other investigators, using the hysterectomy model, have not shown a difference with presurgical versus postsurgical administration of systemic opods.[56] Given the experimental uncertainty of systemic opioids to affect central sensitization in animal models, it should be expected that human studies would generate inconsistent results. Moreover, data suggest that tolerance can develop rapidly in both rats and humans.[57] Large preincisional doses of opioids may potentially increase the dose requirements of analgesics postoperatively because of acute opioid tolerance.

Studies of epidural opioids, alone or in combination with epidural or systemic ketamine, have demonstrated consistent differences between pre- and postincisional groups. Clinical studies evaluating the value of epidural opioids in thoracotomy, lumbar laminectomy, and prostatectomy have shown a significant reduction in postoperative pain scores, as well as analgesic consumption, in preemptive groups compared with control participants.[58] Katz and coworkers studied 141 patients undergoing gynecologic laparotomy. Preincisional administration of epidural lidocaine with fentanyl (4 mcg/kg) led to lower postoperative morphine consumption and secondary hyperalgesia. This effect was not noted in those who received the same epidural medication regimen in the intraoperative period.[59] Similarly, Gottschalk and colleagues found that preemptive epidural fentanyl for radical prostatectomy can decrease postoperative pain at 9.5 weeks and increase function after hospital discharge.[60]

Enhanced blockade of dorsal horn cell excitation offered by ketamine, when added to epidural opioids, has consistently been shown to decrease postoperative pain and analgesic requirements. As previously noted, ketamine may also reduce acute opioid tolerances, making reduced postoperative opioid consumption a possibly less valid measure of preemptive analgesia. The degree of diminution of secondary wound hyperalgesia was not evaluated using this combination of analgesics. Choe and coworkers showed that epidural ketamine (60 mg) plus morphine (2 mg) for upper abdominal surgery, given preincisionally, provided longer analgesia than postincisional treatment.[61] Similarly, Wong and colleagues found that administration of preincisional epidural ketamine and morphine for total knee replacement, performed under epidural lidocaine anesthesia, was more effective than postincisional administration.[62] More recently, Aida and colleagues concluded in a randomized, double-blind study that a combination of epidural morphine (0.06 mg/kg followed by infusion of 0.02 mg/kg per hour) and IV ketamine (1 mg/kg) was more definitive in reducing VAS scores and morphine consumption than either agent alone for patients undergoing gastrectomy.[63] These research studies offer reasonable support for using preincisional epidural opioids to decrease postoperative pain and opioid consumption. These effects can be boosted by ketamine given before surgical trauma. This clinical impression would be consistent with laboratory work described earlier. However, the researchers did not attempt to directly correlate a decrease of secondary wound hyperalgesia with a decline in postoperative pain and thus the need for decreased analgesic administration. The studies simply suggest that the reduction of dorsal horn activity decreases postoperative pain.

NONSTEROIDAL ANTI-INFLAMMATORY DRUGS

Nonsteroidal anti-inflammatory drugs (NSAIDs) have both peripheral and central effects. Indeed, C fiber–evoked activity in dorsal horn cells may be reduced by intrathecal NSAIDs.[64] Furthermore, case reports have shown that prolonged relief was achieved when these drugs were given epidurally.[65] Cyclooxygenase inhibition in second-order neurons results in decreased excitation of the dorsal horn.[66]

However, the predominant mechanism of parenteral or oral NSAIDs is thought to be peripheral reduction in prostaglandin synthesis.[67] Subsequently, inflammation is reduced followed by pain. This is the mechanism thought to account for the reduction in postoperative pain scores in patients receiving preincisional ketorolac, celecoxib, and rofecoxib. Norman and colleagues demonstrated that 30 mg of IV ketorolac before tourniquet inflation has preemptive analgesic effects on patients undergoing ankle surgery.[68] Oral celecoxib has been shown to improve analgesia in postthoracotomy patients with thoracic epidural analgesia.[69] Similarly, rofecoxib has been shown to be efficacious when given as a preemptive oral dose before arthroscopic knee surgery.[70]

One potential drawback to preemptive analgesia with NSAIDs has been the concern for perioperative bleeding complications. Existing data regarding this matter have given conflicting results. Moiniche and colleagues conducted a systematic review on the incidence of perioperative bleeding when NSAIDs were administered for tonsillectomy and found results to be ambiguous at best.[71] These findings, sound clinical judgment as well as preoperative discussion with surgical professionals about NSAID use, should be employed before the administration of such medications.

LOCAL ANESTHETICS

Local anesthetics prevent impulse generation and propagation by blocking initiation of an action potential.[72] The predominant mechanism is "plugging" of transmembrane sodium channels that allow for the intracytoplasmic increase in the concentration of sodium ions. Thus, local anesthetics allow a clinically reliable method for preventing afferent input into the spinal cord during noxious stimulation. In both preemptive preclinical and clinical studies; neuraxial, local infiltration, and peripheral nerve blockades by these agents have been evaluated. Direct infiltration of local anesthetics into the wound can abolish the axon reflex, thereby reducing the spread of inflammation.[73] A central or peripheral nerve blockage is less likely to interfere with peripheral sensitization and can more appropriately be used to assess the value of preemptive analgesia.

Laboratory investigations modeling the inflammatory generating nature of surgery have not demonstrated a clear advantage of preadministration versus postadministration use of local anesthetic. Brennan and colleagues characterized a rat model of surgical pain, with an incision on the plantar aspect of the hindpaw.[74] Skin, fascia, and muscle were cut, yielding mechanical hyperalgesia with an expected duration. Preincisional treatment with intrathecal bupivacaine did not differ from postincisional treatment using measures of hyperalgesia in this model.[75] Yashpal and coworkers demonstrated the declining value of preemptive intrathecal lidocaine as peripheral sensitization (induced by escalating doses of formalin injection) becomes more intense and sustained.[76] They speculated that peripheral inflammation must fall below a certain level for preemptive treatment to become appreciated. Kissin and colleagues demonstrated that paw hyperalgesia induced by carrageenan injection in rats is preventable by administration of a nerve block, either before or after injury.[77] Long-lasting, effective peripheral nerve blockade (tonicaine, 16-hour duration), administered 5 hours after injury, reversed secondary hyperalgesia almost entirely. Trials comparing pre–nerve block versus post–nerve block by local anesthetics run a high probability of showing no significant difference.

Human trials have generated varied results depending on the duration of analgesia provided. For example, analgesic requirements for patients undergoing abdominal hysterectomy did not differ whether they received spinal bupivacaine before or after surgery.[78] Comparable results were obtained when evaluating pre- and postincisional epidural bupivacaine in a similar population posthysterectomy.[79] Multiple investigations found no apparent difference between pre- and postincision caudal block on postoperative analgesic consumption for patients undergoing hypospadias repair, herniorrhaphy, orchidopexy, and circumcision.[80] In all of these studies, secondary hyperalgesia was not assessed between groups. Central sensitization was probably reestablished after the block (spinal or caudal) wore off, given that there is adequate tissue injury during these procedures. Dahl and colleagues examined the difference between epidural analgesia with bupivacaine and morphine initiated before and after colonic surgery and total knee arthroplasty.[81] After either surgery, a continuous infusion of bupivacaine and morphine was administered for 48 hours in the knee arthroplasty group and for 72 hours in the postcolectomy patients. There was no significant difference in requests for additional analgesics or VAS pain scores for either group of patients. The results of these trials parallel the results of Kissin and colleagues' laboratory findings, discussed earlier, whereby central sensitization can be reversed by late neural blockade and prevented from returning by intense postoperative analgesia. Ilioinguinal and iliohypogastric nerve blocks together with spinal anesthesia in patients postinguinal hernia repair provided better pain control up to 48 hours after the surgery than did spinal anesthesia alone.[82] Dahl and colleagues' study illustrates the importance of ongoing afferent blockage while peripheral sensitization declines. The authors then appreciated a prolonged analgesic effect.

In contrast to laboratory investigations, Carr and colleagues were able to show that individuals receiving interscalene block with 0.5% levobupivacaine before shoulder surgery, rather than after, had a lower incidence of requests for analgesic medication as well as lower pain scores for the first 8 hours after surgery.[83] Use of opioids and VAS scores approximated each other by 24 hours after shoulder surgery. Katz and coworkers demonstrated a more pronounced effect with early administration of 15 mL of 0.5% bupivacaine, given epidurally, in patients undergoing lower abdominal procedures.[84] Postoperative pain was controlled by PCA. There was an average reduction of morphine consumption by 25% for up to 72 hours after the procedure, as well as McGill Pain Questionnaire ratings, in those receiving preincisional treatment compared with the postincisional group. Likewise, Gottshalk and colleagues, with preemptive use of epidural fentanyl, found comparable results using epidural bupivacaine in the recovery of patients after radical prostatectomy.[85] Here investigations showed not only benefit in the immediate postoperative period but also increased activity and function long after discharge from the hospital. Reuben and colleagues supplemented intraarticular bupivacaine with morphine in the preincision period and noted a decrease in postoperative analgesic requirements and increase in the time to first opiate use (defined as the analgesic duration).[86] These later studies hint at the potential benefit of preemptive treatment, but it is difficult to reconcile all the incongruities among the various studies.

THE COMPLEXITY OF DEMONSTRATING PREEMPTIVE ANALGESIA

The overall clinical expectation of preemptive analgesia was the reduction of subsequent postoperative pain that could be measured by VAS, postoperative analgesic consumption, or both. Unfortunately, the effect of preemptive analgesia may not be so apparent. The complexity of clearly demonstrating preemptive analgesia has been evolving in the literature during the past decade. Multiple variables continue to be identified and require adequate control or defining, as pointed out in an editorial by Kissin.[87] It is evident that high-intensity noxious stimuli are not only present during surgical incision but also persist well into the postoperative period in the form of peripheral sensitization. Neglecting to block immense small-fiber afferent input during the postoperative period may certainly establish central sensitization even if there was adequate block of peripheral input throughout the surgery and immediately postoperatively.[88] Very painful operations, such as a thoracotomy or total knee arthroplasty, certainly mandate ongoing intense analgesia during the postoperative period even with a sufficient afferent blockade during the procedure. By the same token, the nature of the surgery must generate enough noxious signals to induce central sensitization so that preemptive analgesia has the opportunity to alter the postoperative pain state.

To prevent central sensitization, one must ensure that the treatments provide adequate disruption of the afferent barrage on dorsal horn cells. In addition, Ong and colleagues cite that the nature of pain along with its inflammatory component determines the efficacy of an analgesic intervention. The analgesic intervention should have a sufficiently dense and long-lasting block to impede the transmission of the noxious stimuli. This suggests why epidural analgesia has been shown to be more effective than parenteral opiates.[89] However, the determination of the appropriate doses of drug necessary to achieve this end is more challenging in the clinical setting. Performing highly noxious surgery under regional anesthesia (e.g., epidural) with ongoing interruption of afferent central input is likely the most practical method of ensuring that central hyperexcitability is avoided.

Complicating matters further is the concern of many investigators of inadequate controls. Opioids are commonly given to both the control group and preemptive group on induction, as is nitrous oxide for maintenance. The analgesic properties of nitrous oxide may lead to a preemptive effect.[90] Potent inhaled anesthetics are also known to suppress spinal cord sensitization, and the degree of this effect varies among the inhaled agents.[91] Furthermore, early studies investigating preemptive analgesia had no control group. There was no comparison of preincisional analgesic treatment with the same therapy instituted postoperatively.

Opioid consumption as a measure of outcome is not without its problems. Multiple confounding factors influence any patient's analgesic usage. Anxiety, depression, perception of the surgical course, and overall care may contribute to opioid use. Kissin further added that pain intensity and analgesic requirements have not been demonstrated to consistently correlate.[87] Despite multiple confounding factors and shortcomings, total opioid consumption delivered via PCA devices has been most commonly used to assess preemptive analgesia.

THE EVOLUTION OF PREEMPTIVE ANALGESIA INTO PREVENTIVE ANALGESIA

As can be deduced from the earlier discussion, preemptive analgesia has led too much confusion and controversy regarding how to evaluate, define, and administer this antinociceptive treatment. Evaluations have focused on two groups whereby one group receives a treatment before incision and the other after incision or at the conclusion of surgery. One large flaw of such studies has been that the main afferent input, which establishes central sensitization, is during surgery and that postoperative afferent barrage contributes very little.[92] A preventive analgesic effect is present when there is a reduction in pain intensity or analgesic requirements beyond the pharmacologic activity of the drug (more than 5.5 half-lives).[93] In addition, preventive analgesic strategies have focused beyond the immediate perioperative period addressing the reduction in pain months after surgery as well as the transition of acute into chronic pain. For example, two recent studies using pregabalin, a calcium channel modulator, demonstrated reduced pain months after surgery. Burke et al. demonstrated that patients who received perioperative pregabalin were with less pain and disability 3 months after lumbar discectomy.[94] Buvanendran et al. found that a 2-week course of pregabalin initiated preoperatively resulted in less chronic neuropathic pain at 3 and 6 months after total knee replacement.[95] The ability of present-day multimodal therapies to prevent chronic pain via the blockade of peripheral and central sensitization remains equivocal.[96] Katz et al. in a recent review of preventive analgesia point out future directions of this therapy and at the same time summarize our knowledge gaps that new research must address[92]:

- Preventive analgesia fails to work for everyone. Perhaps genetic differences and an inability to adequately control pain in all three perioperative phases may account in part for this observation. Further characterizing the patients who fail to benefit from this therapy is essential.
- There is a lack of full understanding of the exact mechanisms that contribute most to the transition of acute to chronic pain. For example, if preoperative pain (pain memory), intraoperative pain (inflammation), and postoperative pain (ectopic activity, inflammation) are the major causative factors, then blockade of the afferent barrage at all of these phases will prevent chronic pain. But if coexisting psychopathology and other factors play a more important role, then blockade of perioperative pain will have a modest effect.

CONCLUSION

Despite a significant number of clinical studies throughout the past decade, the contribution of central sensitization to the overall postoperative pain state remains unclear. To what degree central facilitation amplifies pain after surgery is unknown in humans. Although modern studies have attempted to address the impact of preemptive techniques on secondary wound hyperalgesia, more is yet to be learned. The preemptive trials comparing pre- with postincisional treatment groups are now regarded by many authors to be too simplistic and narrow focused. As mentioned earlier, many of the postinjury interventions are adequate to reverse central sensitization. Furthermore, when adequate afferent blockade to the spinal cord is lost, postsurgical inflammatory injury may establish central facilitation. Thus, any preemptive treatment is unlikely to render any benefits. Investigators now agree that the initial postoperative period must be covered.[97]

Even with these shortcomings, several studies have documented modest benefit comparing patients' preincisional interventions with those administered postoperatively. Meta-analyses suggest that the clearest benefit has been seen with epidural analgesia, preincisional wound infiltration, and systemic NSAID administration. Aggressive control of postoperative pain may manifest more of its beneficial effects not in the immediate postsurgical time frame but weeks later. Improved functional restoration, marked by more rapid return to the usual activity level and use postprocedure, may be an outcome of preemptive analgesia (now preventive analgesia). Last, reduction of chronic pain after surgery may be another benefit of preventing central sensitization.

REFERENCES

1. Ong CKS, Lirk P, Seymour RA, Jenkins BJ. The efficacy of preemptive analgesia for acute postoperative pain management: a meta-analysis. *Anesth Analg*. 2005;100:757-773.
2. Wall PD. The prevention of postoperative pain. *Pain*. 1988;33: 289-290.

3. Woolf CJ, Wall PD. A dissociation between the analgesic and antinociceptive effects of morphine. *Neurosci Lett*. 1986;64:238.
4. Woolf CJ, Chong M-S. Preemptive analgesia-treating postoperative pain by preventing the establishment of central sensitization. *Anesth Analg*. 1993;77:362-789.
5. Levine J, Taiwo Y. Inflammatory pain. In: Wall PD, Melzack R, eds. *Textbook of Pain*. 3rd ed. London: Churchill Livingstone; 1994:45-56.
6. Fields HL, Rowbotham M, Baron R. Postherpetic neuralgia: irritable nociceptors and deafferentation. *Neurobiol Dis*. 1998;5: 209-227.
7. Bhave G, Gereau RW. Posttranslational mechanisms of peripheral sensitization. *J Neurobiol*. 2004;61:88-106.
8. Chapman LF. Mechanisms of the flare reaction in human skin. *J Invest Dermatol*. 1977;69:88-97.
9. Lembeck F. Mediators of vasodilation in the skin. *Br J Dermatol*. 1983;109(Suppl 25):1-9.
10. Cook AJ, Woolf CJ, Wall PD, McMahon SB. Dynamic receptive field plasticity in the rat spinal cord dorsal horn following C-primary afferent inputs. *Nature*. 1987;325:151-153.
11. Nagy I, Maggi CA, Dray A, et al. The role of neurokinin and N-methyl-d-aspartate receptors in synaptic transmission from capsaicin sensitive primary afferents in the rat spinal cord in vitro. *Neuroscience*. 1993;52:1029-1037.
12. Coderee TJ, Katz J, Vaccarino AL, Melzack R. Contribution of central neuroplasticity to pathologic pain: review of clinical and experimental evidence. *Pain*. 1993;52:259-285.
13. Woolf CJ, King AK. Dynamic alterations in the cutaneous mechanosensitive receptive field of dorsal horn neurons in the rat spinal cord. *J Neurosci*. 1990;10:2717-2726.
14. Simone DA, Sorkin LS, Oh U, et al. Neurogenic hyperalgesia: central neural correlates in responses of spinothalamic tract neurons. *J Neurophysiol*. 1991;66:228-246.
15. Desmueles JA, Cedraschi C, Rapiti E, et al. Neurophysiologic evidence for central sensitization in patients with fibromyalgia. *Arthritis Rheum*. 2003;1420-1429.
16. MacDermott AB, Mayer ML, Westbrook GL, et al. NMDA-receptor activation increases cytoplasmic calcium concentration in cultured spinal cord neurons. *Nature*. 1986;321:519-522.
17. Womack MD, MacDermott AB, Jessell TM. Sensory transmitters regulate intracellular calcium in dorsal horn neurons. *Nature*. 1988;334:351-353.
18. Woolf CJ, Thompson SWN. The induction and maintenance of central sensitization is dependent on N-methyl-d-aspartic acid receptor activation; implications for the treatment of post-injury pain hypersensitivity states. *Pain*. 1991;44:293-299.
19. Sugiyama H, Ito I, Hirono C. A new type of glutamate receptor linked to inositol phospholipid metabolism. *Nature*. 1987;325:531-533.
20. Naranjo JR, Mellstrom B, Achaval M, Sassone-Corsi P. Molecular pathways of pain: Fos/Jun-mediated activation of a noncanonical AP-1 site in the prodynorphin gene. *Neuron*. 1991;6:607-617.
21. Iadorola MJ, Sanders SR, Draisci G. Differential activation of spinal cord dynorphin and enkephalin neurons during hyperalgesia: evidence using cDNA hybridization. *Brain Res*. 1988;455: 205-212.
22. Dubner R, Ruda MA. Activity-dependent neuronal plasticity following tissue injury and inflammation. *Trends Neurosci*. 1992;15: 96-103.
23. Naranjo JR, Mellstrom B, Achaval M, Sassone-Corsi P. Molecular pathways of pain: Fos/Jun-mediated activation of a noncanonical AP-1 site in the prodynorphin gene. *Neuron*. 1991;6:607-617.
24. Yamamura T, Harada K, Okamura A, Kemmotsu O. Is the site of action of ketamine anesthesia the N-methyl-d-aspartate receptor? *Anesthesiology*. 1990;72:704-710.
25. Yamamoto T, Yaksh TL. Comparison of the antinociceptive effects of pre- and posttreatment with intrathecal morphine and MK801, and NMDA antagonist, on the formalin test in the rat. *Anesthesiology*. 1992;77:757-763.
26. Schmid RL, Sandler AN, Katz J. Use and efficacy of low-dose ketamine in the management of acute postoperative pain: a review of current techniques and outcome. *Pain*. 1999;82:111-125.
27. Gilron I, Quirion R, Coderre TJ. Pre-versus postformalin effects of ketamine or large-dose alfentanil in the rat: discordance between pain behavior and spinal fos-like immunoreactivity. *Anest Analg*. 1999:89:128-135.
28. Kohrs R, Durieux ME. Ketamine: teaching an old drug new tricks. *Anesth Analg*. 1998;87:1186-1193.
29. Eide PK, Strubhaug A, Oye I. The NMDA-antagonist ketamine for prevention and treatment of acute and chronic post-operative pain. *Baillieres Clin Anesthesiol*. 1995;9:539-540.
30. Eide PK, Stubhaug A, Oye I, Breivik H. Continuous subcutaneous administration of the N-methyl-d-aspartic acid (NMDA) receptor antagonist ketamine in the treatment of post-herpetic neuralgia. *Pain*. 1995;61:221-228.
31. Eide PK, Jorum E, Strubhaug A, et al. Relief of post-herpetic neuralgia with N-methyl-d-aspartic acid (NMDA) antagonist: a double-blind, cross-over comparison with morphine and placebo. *Pain*. 1994;58:347-354.
32. Subramaniam K, Subramaniam B, Steinbrook R. Ketamine and adjuvant analgesic to opioids: a quantitative and qualitative systemic review. *Anesth Analg*. 2004;99:482-495.
33. Lavand'homme P, DeKock M, Waterloos H. Intraoperative epidural analgesia combined with ketamine provides effective analgesia in patients undergoing major digestive surgery. *Anesthesiology*. 2005;103:813-820.
34. Tverskoy M, Oz Y, Isakson A, et al. Preemptive effect of fentanyl and ketamine on postoperative pain and wound hyperalgesia. *Anesth Analg*. 1994;78:205-209.
35. Stubhaug A, Breivik H, Eide PK, et al. Mapping of punctuate hyperalgesia around a surgical incision demonstrates that ketamine is a powerful suppressor of central sensitization to pain following surgery. *Act Anaesthesiol Scand*. 1997;41:1124-1132.
36. Fu ES, Miguel R, Scharf JE. Preemptive ketamine decreases postoperative narcotic requirements in patients undergoing abdominal surgery. *Anesth Analg*. 1997;84:1086-1090.
37. Kwok RF, Lim J, Chan MTV, et al. Preoperative ketamine improves postoperative analgesia after gynecologic laparoscopic surgery. *Anesth Analg*. 2004;98:1044-1049.
38. Eisenach JC. Preemptive hyperalgesia, not analgesia? *Anesthesiology*. 2000;92:465-472.
39. Wong CS, Lu CC, Cherng CH, Ho ST. Preemptive analgesia with ketamine, morphine, and lidocaine prior to total knee replacement. *Can J Anaesth*. 1997;44:31-37.
40. Abdel-Ghaffar ME, Abdulatif M, Al-Ghamdi A, et al. Epidural ketamine reduces post-operative epidural PCA consumption of fentanyl/bupivacaine. *Can J Anaesth*. 1198;45:103-109.
41. Wilson JA, Nimmo JF, Fleetwood-Walker SM, Colvin LA. A randomized double blind trial of the effect of preemptive epidural ketamine on persistent pain after lower limb amputation. *Pain*. 2008;108-118.
42. Helmy SAK, Bali A. The effect of preemptive use of NMDA receptor antagonist dextromethorphan on postoperative analgesic requirements. *Anesth Analg*. 2001;92:739-744.

43. Dickinson AH. Mechanisms of the analgesic actions of opiates and opioids. *Br Med Bull.* 1992;47:690-702.

44. Advokat C, Burton P. Antinociceptive effects of systemic and intrathecal morphine in spinally transected rats. *Eur J Pharmacol.* 1987;139:335-343.

45. Stein C. The control of pain in peripheral tissue by opioids. *N Engl J Med.* 1995;332:1685-1690.

46. Yamamoto T, Yaksh TL. Comparison of the antinociceptive effects of pre- and posttreatment with intrathecal morphine and MK801, and NMDA antagonist, on the formalin test in the rat. *Anesthesiology.* 1992;77:757-763.

47. Dickerson AG, Sullivan AF. Subcutaneous formalin-induced activity of dorsal horn neurons in the rat: differential response to an intrathecal opiate administered pre or post formalin. *Pain.* 1987;30:349-360.

48. Yashpal K, Katz J, Coderre TJ. Effects of preemptive or postinjury intrathecal local anesthesia on persistent nociceptive response in rats. *Anesthesiology.* 1996;84:1119-1128.

49. Abram SE, Olson EE. Systemic opioids do not suppress spinal sensitization after subcutaneous formalin in rats. *Anesthesiology.* 1994;80:1114-1119.

50. Lascelles BDX, Waterman AE, Cripps PJ, et al. Central sensitization as a result of surgical pain: investigation of the pre-emptive value of pethidine for ovariohysterectomy in the rat. *Pain.* 1995;62:201-212.

51. Gonzalez MI, Field MJ, Bramwell S, et al. Ovariohysterectomy in the rat: a model of surgical pain for evaluation of preemptive analgesia? *Pain.* 2000;88:79-88.

52. Richmond CE, Bromley LM, Woolf CJ. Preoperative morphine preempts postoperative pain. *Lancet.* 1993;342:73-753.

53. Collis R, Bradner B, Bromley LM, Woolf CJ. Is there any clinical advantage of increasing the pre-emptive dose of morphine or combining pre-incisional with postoperative morphine administration? *Br J Anaesth.* 1995;74:396-399.

54. Tverskoy M, Oz Y, Isakson A, et al. Preemptive effect of dentanyl and ketamine on postoperative pain and wound hyperalgesia. *Anesth Analg.* 1994;78:205-209.

55. Griffin MJ, Hughes D, Knaggs A, et al. Late onset preemptive analgesia associated with preincisional large-dose alfentanil. *Anesth Analg.* 1997;85:1317-1321.

56. Mansfield M, Meikle R, Miller C. A trial of pre-emptive analgesia: influence of timing of preoperative alfentanil on postoperative pain and analgesic requirements. *Anaesthesia.* 1994;49:1091-1093.

57. Kissin I, Bright CA, Bradley EL. Acute tolerance to continuously infused alfentanil: the role of cholecystokinin and N-methyl-d-aspartate-nitric oxide systems. *Anest Analg.* 2000;91:110-116.

58. Katz J, Kavanagh BP, Sandler AN, et al. Preemptive analgesia: clinical evidence of neuroplasticity contributing to postoperative pain. *Anesthesiology.* 1992;77;439-446.

59. Katz J, Cohen L, Schmid R, et al. Postoperative morphine use and hyperalgesia are reduced by preoperative but not intraoperative epidural analgesia. *Anesthesiology.* 2003;98:1449-1460.

60. Gottschalk A, Smith DS, Jobes DR, et al. Preemptive epidural analgesia and recovery from radical prostatectomy. *JAMA.* 1998;279:1076-1082.

61. Choe H, Choi Y-S, Kim Y-H, et al. Epidural morphine plus ketamine for upper abdominal surgery: improved analgesia from preincisional versus postincisional administration. *Anesth Analg.* 1997;84:560-563.

62. Wong CS, Lu CC, Cherng CH, Ho ST. Preemptive analgesia with ketamine, morphine, and lidocaine prior to total knee replacement. *Can J Anaesth.* 1997;44:31-37.

63. Aida S, Yamakura T, Baba H, et al. Preemptive analgesia by intravenous low-dose ketamine and epidural morphine in gastrectomy. *Anesthesiology.* 2009;92:527-541.

64. Malmberg AB, Yaksh TL. Hyperalgesia mediated by spinal glutamate or substance P receptor blockade by spinal cyclooxygenase inhabitation. *Science.* 1992;257:1276-1279.

65. Lauretti GR, Reis MP, Mattos AL, et al. Epidural nonsteroidal anti-inflammatory drugs for cancer pain. *Anesth Analg.* 1998; 86:117-118.

66. Saito Y, Kaneko M, Kirihara Y, et al. Intrathecal prostaglandin E1 produces a long-lasting allodynic state. *Pain.* 1995;63: 303-311.

67. Crile GW. The kinetic theory of shock and its prevention through anociassociation. *Lancet.* 1913;185:7-16.

68. Norman PH, Daley MD, Lindsey RW. Preemptive analgesic effects of ketorolac in ankle fracture surgery. *Anesthesiology.* 2001;94:599-603.

69. Senard M, Deflandre EP, Ledoux D, et al. Effect of celecoxib combined with thoracic epidural analgesia of pain after thoracotomy. *Brit J Anesth.* 2010;105:196-200.

70. Reuben SS, Bhopatkar S, Maciolek H, et al. The preemptive analgesic effect of rofecoxib after ambulatory arthroscopic knee surgery. *Anesth Analg.* 2002;94:55-59.

71. Moiniche S, Romsing J, Dahl JB, Tramer MR. NSAIDs and the risk of operative site bleeding after tonsillectomy: a quantitative systematic review. *Anesth Analg.* 2003;96:68-77.

72. de Jong RH. Nerve impulse blockade. In: de Jong RH, ed. *Local Anesthetics.* St Louis: Mosby; 1994:45-63.

73. Meyer Ra, Campbell JN, Raja SN. Peripheral neural mechanisms of nociception. In: Wall PD, Lelzak R, Bonica JJ, eds. *Textbook of Pain.* 3rd ed. Edinburgh, Scotland: Churchill Livingstone; 1994:13-44.

74. Brennan TJ, Vandermeulen EP, Gebhart GF. Characterization of a rat model of incisional pain. *Pain.* 1996;64:493-501.

75. Brennan TJ, Umali EF, Zahn PK. Comparison of pre- versus post-incision administration of intrathecal bupivacaine and intrathecal morphine in a rat model of postoperative pain. *Anesthesiology.* 1997;87:1518-1528.

76. Yashpal K, Katz J, Coderre TJ. Effects of preemptive or postinjury intrathecal local anesthesia on persistent nociceptive responses in rats. *Anesthesiology.* 1996; 84:1119-1128.

77. Kissin I, Lee SS, Bradley EL. Effect of prolonged nerve block on inflammatory hyperalgesia in rats: prevention of late hyperalgesia. *Anesthesiology.* 1998;88:224-232.

78. Dakin MJ, Oinubi OYO, Carli F. Preoperative spinal bupivaine does not reduce postoperative morphine requirement in women undergoing total abdominal hysterectomy. *Reg Anesth.* 1996;21: 99-102.

79. Pryle BJ, Vanner RG, Enriquez N, Reynolds F. Can pre-emptive lumbar epidural blockade reduce postoperative pain following lower abdominal surgery? *Anaesthesia.* 1993;48:120-123.

80. Ho JWS, Khambatta HJ, Pang LM, et al. Preemptive analgesia in children. *Reg Anesth.* 1996;22:125-130.

81. Dahl JB, Hansen NC, Jortso NC, et al. Influence of timing on the effect of continuous extradural analgesia with bupivacaine and morphine after major abdominal surgery. *Br J Anaesth.* 1992; 69:4-8.

82. Bugedo G, Carcamo CS, Mertens RA, et al. Preoperative percutaneous ilioinguinal and iliohypogastric nerve block with 0.5% bupivacaine for post-herniorrhaphy pain management in adults. *Reg Anesth*. 1990;15:130-132.
83. Carr DB, Sternlicht A, Carabuena JM, et al. Efficacy and safety of preemptive levobupivacaine in elective shoulder surgery. *Reg Anesth Pain Med*. 2000;25S:20.
84. Katz J, Caliroux M, Kavanagh BP, et al. Pre-emptive lumbar anesthesia reduces postoperative pain and patient-controlled morphine consumption after lower abdominal surgery. *Pain*. 1994;59: 395-403.
85. Gottschalk A, Smith DS, Jobes DR, et al. Preemptive epidural analgesia and recovery from radical prostatectomy. *JAMA*. 1998;279:1076-1082.
86. Reuben SS, Sklar J, Mansouri ME. The preemptive analgesic effect of intra-articular bupivacaine and morphine after ambulatory arthroscopic knee surgery. *Anesth Analg*. 2001;92:923-926.
87. Kissin I. Preemptive analgesia: why its effect is not always obvious. *Anesthesiology*. 1996;84:1015-1019.
88. Kissin I. Preemptive analgesia. *Anesthesiology*. 2000;93:1138-1143.
89. Ong CKS, Lirk P, Seymour RA, Jenkins BJ. The efficacy of preemptive analgesia for acute postoperative pain management: a meta-analysis. *Anesth Analg*. 2005;100:757-773.
90. Goto T, Marota JJA, Crosby G. Nitrous oxide induces preemptive analgesia in the rat that is antagonized by halothane. *Anesthesiology*. 1994;80:409-416.
91. O'Connor TC, Abram SE. Inhibition of nociceptive-induced spinal sensitization by anesthetic agents. *Anesthesiology*. 1995;82:259-266.
92. Katz J, Clarke H, Seltzer Z. Preventive analgesia: quo vadimus? *Anesth Analg*. 2011;113:1242-1253.
93. Katz J, Clarke H. Preventive analgesia and beyond: current statues, evidence, and future directions. In: Macintyre PE, Walker SM, Rowbotham DJ, eds. *Clinical Pain Management: Acute Pain*. 2nd ed. London: Hordder Arnold; 2008:154-198.
94. Burke SM, Shorten GD. Perioperative pregabalin improves pain and function outcomes 3 months after lumbar discectomy. *Anesth Analg*. 2010;110:1180-1185.
95. Buvanendran A, Kroin JS, Della Valle CJ, et al. Perioperative oral pregabalin reduces chronic pain after total knee arthroplasty: a prospective, randomized, controlled trial. *Anesth Analg*. 2010;110:199-207.
96. Rathmell JP, Kehlet H. Do we have the tools to prevent phantom limb pain? *Anesthesiology*. 2011;114:1021-1024.
97. Goto T, Marota JJA, Crosby G. Nitrous oxide induces preemptive analgesia in the rat that is antagonized by halothane. *Anesthesiology*. 1994;80:409-416.

Acute Pain Management in Adults

Abhilasha Solanki
Vimal K. Akhouri

Pain relief in an acute pain situation, besides having a humane value, has an important bearing in the well-being of an individual. Although it may not be possible to achieve total relief in all situations, a serious effort should be made.

Since the discovery of opioid receptors in 1978, efforts have been made to improve the delivery of analgesic drugs in a more effective way. Thanks to these advances in basic science on the clinical front, the past few decades have witnessed major strides in postoperative analgesia with the creation of acute pain services, the increased use of regional and epidural techniques, and the introduction of the concept of multimodal approach.

The tissue damage produced by surgery is similar to that of acute injury. It causes local and systemic noxious stimuli that initiate nociceptive impulses, relays, and reflexes throughout the nervous system. In addition to the disturbances associated with the conscious interpretation of these impulses, there are autonomic effects generated that may disrupt the healing and recovery process. The deleterious physiologic side effects of acute pain are well recognized. In a patient who is breathing spontaneously, muscle splinting (seen in conjunction with discomfort of chest or abdominal origin) may result in decreased vital capacity, decreased functional residual capacity, and ultimately decreased alveolar ventilation. Atelectasis is a frequent postoperative complication. Discomfort experienced during coughing may result in retention of secretions and subsequent pneumonia. The sympathetic response to pain may cause increased cardiovascular demands. This may be apparent clinically by signs of tachycardia, increased peripheral resistance, and hypertension; these signs are associated with increased cardiac work and myocardial oxygen consumption. The potential for myocardial ischemia and infarction is obvious. Muscle spasm produced by segmental and suprasegmental reflex motor activity may perpetuate pain. In the chest wall and abdomen, pain and muscle spasm may compromise respiratory function. The gastrointestinal (GI) tract similarly is affected by increased sympathetic activity. Pain increases intestinal secretions and smooth muscle sphincter tone and decreases intestinal motility. By similar mechanisms, pain may produce urinary retention. Acute injury also has an impact on the endocrine system, causing sodium and water retention and hyperglycemia. Immobility from acute postoperative pain may predispose the patient to deep vein thrombosis and pulmonary embolism as a result of venostasis and platelet aggregation. In a complex intertwined relationship, psychological alterations may occur concomitantly with the physiologic ones.[1]

Numerous guidelines have been published about the management of postoperative pain. First, the Agency for Health Care Policy and Research (AHCPR) took the lead in educating caregivers as well as the public. The American Pain Society and the American Society of Anesthesia then followed suit, and the Joint Commission on Accreditation of Healthcare Organizations (JCAHO; now The Joint Commission) published "Standards for Pain Management in Hospital Settings," which were implemented in 2001.[2,3] In 2012, the American Society of Anesthesia published its updated guidelines on acute pain management.[4]

PAIN AS THE FIFTH VITAL SIGN

The guidelines from The Joint Commission incorporate pain measurements in the bedside chart in addition to tracking the patient's temperature, blood pressure, heart rate, and respiratory rate, thus making pain rating the fifth vital sign.

However, a simple numerical assessment of pain on the visual analog scale or verbal rating scale does not differentiate between pain at rest and pain with movement or incident pain, which is usually more challenging to manage.

Also, to effectively adjust the analgesic regimen, one needs to track sedation and other possible adverse effects associated with the administration of analgesics such as nausea and vomiting, respiratory depression, and cognitive impairment.

The importance of good postoperative analgesia and its impact on favorable postsurgical outcomes are undeniable. Pain in the postoperative period may contribute to adverse outcomes, including thromboembolic and pulmonary complications.

Many factors influence our perception of postoperative pain. Determinants of the intensity, quality, and duration of postoperative pain include:

1. The site, nature, and duration of the operation, including the type of incision and the amount of intraoperative trauma
2. The physiologic and psychological makeup of the patient
3. The preoperative psychological, physical, and pharmacologic preparation of the patient
4. The presence of serious related complications
5. The anesthetic management
6. The quality of postoperative care. Some of the ineffectiveness of current medical analgesic therapy can be attributed to inadequate understanding by nurses of the pharmacology of narcotics.

Inadequate understanding by physicians of the nature of pain also has been demonstrated. A structured interview of 37 medical inpatients showed that 32% had severe distress despite a narcotic analgesic regimen; an additional 41% declared themselves to be in moderate distress. As part of the study, a questionnaire survey of 102 staff physicians showed an underestimation of effective dose ranges, an overestimation of the duration of action, and an exaggerated concern with the addictive potential of meperidine in a therapeutic dosing range. It is thought that the development of addiction in patients with no previous addictive history is rare. Children, perhaps the most dependent group in the hospital population, also bear the burden of postoperative suffering. As a reaction to discomfort, many children withdraw and vegetate. This may be misinterpreted as coping with the pain. Many immature patients fear injection, deny pain, and are unable to realize that a short-term discomfort may grant a longer period of analgesia.[5,6] Postoperative pain management is still undermanaged, and the reason is multifactorial, although there is increased awareness, and more studies are being performed in this area.[7]

In summary, few major factors contribute to the inadequacy of traditional analgesic therapy. Foremost is the incomplete comprehension by medical personnel of analgesic pharmacodynamics. This lack of knowledge coupled with overconcern about respiratory depression and addiction liability leads to the administration of inadequate doses. Second is the inadequate use of interventional techniques (regional and neuraxial) along with systemic analgesics in the postoperative period. There are system deficiencies of structured pain management, such as protocols for assessment and management and education of caregivers. Logistics and the cost of administering pain management protocols in resource-deficient countries are common reasons. Another barrier to adequate analgesia is a common hospital community attitude that stoicism is a virtue. A suffering patient may sense such an attitude and, rather than attacking this formidable barrier, refrain from requesting appropriate medication.[8]

PHYSIOLOGIC RESPONSE TO ACUTE PAIN

The perioperative physiologic changes that occur after surgery affect all organ systems.

CARDIOVASCULAR SYSTEM

Approximately 5% of the worldwide surgical population will develop some type of perioperative cardiac morbidity. An imbalance between myocardial oxygen supply and demand contributes to this. Uncontrolled pain causes an increase in sympathetic tone and a resetting of baroreceptors that cause an increase in heart rate and blood pressure. This in turn translates into increased work for the myocardium. In the presence of coronary artery disease, this predisposes the myocardium to ischemia and arrhythmias. Stress per se is also arrhythmogenic in a nonischemic myocardium.

Neural outflow also causes redistribution of blood to and within various organs. Besides the increase in catecholamines and sympathetic neural outflow, there is a reflex decrease in parasympathetic outflow caused by pain. This imbalance in the autonomic nervous system alters baroreceptor settings. Although individual randomized controlled trials might seem equivocal on whether postoperative pain management might affect perioperative outcomes, two meta-analyses suggest that thoracic epidural analgesia might be associated with an improvement in perioperative cardiac outcomes.[9,10]

PULMONARY SYSTEM

Pulmonary dysfunction is commonly seen after thoracic and upper abdominal surgery. It is a significant problem affecting up to 10% patients undergoing elective abdominal surgery. The pathophysiology is multifactorial and includes disruption of normal respiratory muscle activity; reflex inhibition of diaphragmatic function; and reflex increased spinal arc activity, causing increased intercostal and abdominal muscle tone and pain. All of these factors cause voluntary inhibition of respiratory activity, which manifests clinically as a decrease in functional residual capacity and tidal volume. Preexisting pulmonary disease or respiratory depression caused by opioids may compound these problems. Multiple meta-analyses suggest that postoperative pain management may decrease the risk of postoperative pulmonary complications.[9,11,12]

ENDOCRINE AND METABOLIC RESPONSE

Any injury provokes a neurohumoral response involving the hypothalamic–pituitary–adrenal axis, activation of sympathetic nervous system, and an increase in glucagon secretion.[1] Surgery leads to a similar reproducible response, which causes hyperglycemia, increased lipolysis, lipid oxidation, accelerated protein breakdown, and nitrogen loss.[2,3]

These responses begin during surgery and may last for many days, especially after major abdominal or thoracic surgery. The stress response peaks in the postoperative period.[4] Clinically, this presents as hypertension, tachycardia, arrhythmias, myocardial ischemia, protein catabolism, immune system suppression, and impaired renal excretory function. Suppression of the stress response is possible but not complete. The intensity of the stress response depends on the site of surgery (extremities vs. thoracic or abdominal), pain control modality, (neuraxial vs. systemic), medication used (local anesthetic vs. opioid), and initiation and maintenance of treatment (intraoperative vs. postoperative). Studies have shown that stress response and morbidity in the first 24 hours are lower in patients receiving epidural analgesia with local anesthetics with or without opioids.[13,14]

GASTROINTESTINAL SYSTEM

A combination of surgery and anesthesia in addition to pain produces a decrease in gastric motility, especially in the colon. Whereas the stomach and small intestines recover within 12 to 24 hours after abdominal surgery, the colon recovers in 48 to 72 hours. The pathophysiology of postoperative ileus and decreased GI motility is multifactorial. It includes neurogenic (spinal, supraspinal, adrenergic) pathways, local inflammatory responses that initiate neurogenic inhibitory pathways, and pharmacologic mechanisms. Analgesic agents differ in their effects on GI motility.[15] Epidural opioids inhibit GI motility less than systemic opioids.[16]

IMMUNE SYSTEM

A large amount of clinical evidence shows suppression of both humoral and cellular mechanisms of the immune system after trauma and surgery. These mechanisms include a decrease in responsiveness to antigen and mitogen, delayed hypersensitivity, natural killer cell activity, and antibody response.[17] The exact causative mechanism is not known. Increased release of glucocorticoids is seen as one of the reasons, but other stress response hormones may also cause immune modulation.[18]

COAGULATION SYSTEM

The incidence of fatal pulmonary embolism in the absence of thromboembolic prophylaxis is about 0.1% to 0.8% after general surgery, 0.3% to 0.7% after elective hip surgery, and 4% to 7% after emergency hip surgery. Surgery causes activation of the coagulation cascade, increased platelet activity, and decreased fibrinolytic activity, leading to increased coagulability. It is believed that intraoperative neuraxial anesthesia may attenuate perioperative hypercoagulability and increased extremity blood flow, both of which may contribute to a decrease in perioperative coagulation-related complications. However, it is unclear if postoperative analgesia continues to provide the same benefits as those conferred by intraoperative neuraxial anesthesia. It has been found to produce less platelet activity and improved fibrinolysis, which may be related to the systemic effects of local anesthetics.[19]

COGNITIVE DYSFUNCTION

Postoperatively, 10% to 50% of patients develop transient cognitive impairment, which is worse on the second day, but they usually recover within 1 week. Elderly patients may take up to 3 months to recover baseline cognitive function. Exact mechanisms are not clear, and there are no conclusive data to suggest a particular choice of anesthetic technique. Delirium occurs in about 10% of patients undergoing noncardiac surgery after age 50 years. Electrolyte abnormality, sleep apnea, history of alcohol abuse, and benzodiazepines and meperidine intake are risk factors for delirium. Studies have found that high levels of postoperative pain can cause delirium, and vice versa, delirium can impair cognition and cause exacerbation of pain.

POSTOPERATIVE PAIN

A surgical incision cuts through a variety of tissues, including nerve endings, and activates specific nociceptors (pain receptors) as well as free nerve endings. It is associated with the release of inflammatory mediators such as bradykinin, serotonin, and histamine, contributing to peripheral sensitization. Clinically, this phenomenon is manifested by hyperalgesia, which is an amplification of noxious pain signals. These painful signals are transmitted to the dorsal horn of the spinal cord in an amplified fashion and are increased in duration.

The nociceptor information is transmitted to the cord via the A-δ (myelinated) fibers and the C (unmyelinated) fibers. When peripheral sensitization occurs, painful information can also be carried by A-α and A-β fibers. This is manifested by allodynia, a pain state in which non-noxious stimuli are transformed and expressed as painful. Signals entering the central nervous system from the periphery are increased in amplitude and duration. This is the phenomenon of "wind up" or central sensitization.[20]

Analgesic techniques, to be effective, need to counteract these activations of nociceptors at the periphery as well as centrally, thus the need for a multimodal or "balanced" analgesia. Multimodal technique of using more than one group of analgesics or technique provides additive or synergistic effects while minimizing individual side effects.[21]

Poorly controlled acute pain can result in increased catabolism, increased cardiorespiratory work, immunosuppression, and coagulation disturbances. Higher levels of postoperative pain can result in poor patient satisfaction, impaired quality of recovery, and increased health care costs.

STRATEGIES OF POSTOPERATIVE PAIN MANAGEMENT

The American Society of Anesthesiologists Task Force on Acute Pain Management describes pain management in the perioperative setting as actions taken before, during, and after a procedure that are induced to reduce or eliminate postoperative pain before discharge. Several clinical studies support the notion that an approach based on the use of multimodal techniques to manage postsurgical pain is the most effective strategy for achieving optimal analgesia.

PHARMACOLOGIC APPROACH

Opioids Opioids remain the mainstay of postoperative analgesia and have demonstrated their efficacy in the management of severe pain. Their efficacy is limited by side effects such as nausea, vomiting, ileus, biliary spasms, respiratory depression, and the potential for abuse (although in the immediate postoperative period, abuse is rarely an issue). Opioids can be administered intramuscularly, subcutaneously, or intravenously.

The administration of opioids by intravascular injections prescribed on an as-needed basis provides fluctuating opioid levels, resulting in sedation and other adverse effects when levels are high and inadequate analgesia when levels are low. A better method of administration of opioids is via a microprocessor-controlled infusion pump or patient-controlled analgesia (PCA).[22,23]

A preset dose of opioids is delivered to the patient when activating the demand switch, given that a predetermined time has elapsed since the previous dose; this is the "lockout" time. An upper limit per hour or per 4 hours is predetermined and set in the program as an additional safety device. Numerous studies have demonstrated the safety and opioid-sparing effect of PCA (**Table 51-1**). PCA technique is also associated with multiple errors that could be a result of:

- Improper patient selection
- Improper patient education
- Inadequate staff education
- Errors in prescription
- Errors in dispensing
- Errors in programming the PCA pump
- Inadequate monitoring

A paradoxical response of hyperalgesia instead of analgesia is seen in some patients—opioid-induced hyperalgesia (OIH)—and is attributed to the upregulation of the nociceptive pathways.[24] It is different from tolerance in which a downregulation to response is seen and is difficult to differentiate in a clinical setting. Different medications have been used to modulate this effect, and work done in this area is mostly with NMDA (*N*-methyl-D-aspartate) receptor antagonists.

Patients taking opioids preoperatively will show some tolerance intraoperatively and postoperatively. One can safely assume that patients taking two tablets of combination analgesics such as Percocet (5-mg oxycodone/tablet) or Vicodin (5 or 7.5-mg hydrocodone) four times daily require 1 mg of morphine per hour postoperatively to replace their regular opioids.

NONOPIOID ANALGESICS

With opioids alone, intramuscularly or intravenously, the analgesia may be marginal and side effects intolerable (nausea, vomiting,

TABLE 51-1 Patient-Controlled Analgesia (PCA) Suggested Dosing

	PCA Dose	Lockout Time	1-Hour Limit	Basal Rate†
Morphine 1 mg/mL	0.5–3 mg	5–10 min	10–20 min	0.5–2 mg/1 h
Hydromorphone 0.2 mg/mL	0.1–0.5 mg	5–10 min	1–2 mg	0.1–0.2 mg/h
Fentanyl	25–50 μg	5–10 min	250 μg	25–50 μg/h
Meperidine 10 mg/mL	10–20 mg	5–10 min	100 mg*	100–200 mg/h

*Toxic metabolite normeperidine may accumulate rapidly if patient is getting more than 1000 mg/day.

†Basal rates should not be used routinely and can be reserved for nighttime when indicated.

sedation), thus the need for synergy, choosing drug classes that will overlap for analgesia but not for side effects. Drug classes that fit these requirements are cyclooxygenase inhibitors, α_2 agonists, nitric oxide synthetase inhibitors, NMDA receptor blockers, and local anesthetics when delivered by thoracic epidural catheters. This balanced analgesia or delivery of different classes of analgesics will result in effective pain relief by synergistic or additive effect with reduced incidence of side effects.[25]

Acetaminophen (Paracetamol) Paracetamol is an effective analgesic for mild to moderate pain. It has been proven to be a good adjuvant to opioid analgesia and has shown to reduce the requirement of opioid analgesia by 20% to 30% when given regularly.[26] Currently, it is available in intravenous form in the United States and extensively used perioperatively.

NONSTEROIDAL ANTI-INFLAMMATORY DRUGS

Nonsteroidal anti-inflammatory drugs (NSAIDs) produce their effect by inhibiting the prostaglandin synthesis and releasing at the level of cyclooxygenase. These drugs have proven efficacy as the sole analgesic agent for management of mild to moderate pain in minor surgical procedures. See Table 51-1 for PCA suggested dosing and **Table 51-2** for epidural catheter insertion sites.

Ketorolac, the only parenteral NSAID presently available, is a nonspecific inhibitor of both cyclooxygenase isoenzymes (COX-1 and COX-2). The COX-1 isoenzyme is normally found in blood vessels, platelets, the GI tract, and the kidneys. On the other hand, the COX-2 isoenzyme is induced by inflammation in peripheral tissues. The inhibition of the COX-1 isoenzyme is responsible for the gastric and renal side effects of NSAIDs and for its inhibitory effect on platelet function.[27,28]

One should be cautious when using NSAIDs in the immediate postoperative period and must take into consideration risk factors such as a history of bleeding peptic ulcers; volume depletion (for NSAID-induced acute renal failure), especially in elderly patients; or when the risk of hemorrhage is considerable and the surgical site involves the airway. The usual dose of ketorolac is 15 mg intravenously every 6 hours for 24 to 48 hours. COX-2 inhibitors appear to be safer, but parenteral forms of these molecules are not yet available.

Tramadol Tramadol is a synthetic centrally acting analgesic with weak agonist activity at opioid receptors. Unlike other opioids, it lacks the respiratory depressant effects and exhibits lower risk of bowel dysfunction at conventional doses. The combination of paracetamol and tramadol provides superior analgesia without additional toxicity.[29]

ANALGESIC ADJUVANTS

Other classes of drugs may enhance the effects of opioids or may have independent analgesic effects. Most of these drugs are not available in parenteral form and are usually reserved for patients not responding to more routine therapies. The addition of an α_2 agonist may be beneficial and opioid sparing. Clonidine, dexmedetomidine, and tizanidine are representative of that class, but only clonidine is approved by the Food and Drug Administration and may contribute to hypotension in the perioperative period.

Antihyperalgesic drugs, which block the effect of the transmitter release, include nitric oxide synthetase inhibitors and NMDA receptor blockers. There is no available pure nitric oxide synthetase inhibitor. However, there is some evidence that acetaminophen exerts its action by inhibition of nitric oxide production. For this reason, acetaminophen administered around the clock in the immediate postoperative period may be very useful. Proparacetamol, the precursor of acetaminophen, is being clinically investigated in a parenteral form. Otherwise, acetaminophen is available orally (pill form and elixir) and rectally. The only concern may be that acetaminophen, because of its antipyretic properties, will mask febrile states in the immediate postoperative period.

Dextromethorphan is the most readily available NMDA blocker, although it is often used in combination with other drugs such as cough suppressants.[30] The clinically useful dosage appears to be 30 to 60 mg every 4 to 6 hours. Ketamine in low doses (up to 10 mg per hour intravenously) may also be a useful NMDA blocker for postoperative pain.[31]

Gabapentin, an antiepileptic, binds to the voltage-gated calcium channel and inhibits neurotransmitter release. When used perioperatively, it reduces pain and opioid consumption but does cause sedation.[32,33]

NEURAXIAL ANALGESIA

Opioids and local anesthetics can be provided by the epidural or intrathecal route. Of these, the epidural catheter infusion is the most commonly used method and, recently, a cumulative meta-analysis of various postoperative therapies has shown that epidural opioids and epidural local anesthetics with or without opioids decrease the incidence of pulmonary complications as opposed to systemic opioids. Epidural analgesia is also associated with a lower incidence of cardiovascular events and provides a decreased stress response to surgery, earlier ambulation, rapid return of bowel function, shortened hospitalization, reduced costs, and overall a lower mortality rate.

Large surveys show that the most effective placement of the epidural catheter for infusion of local anesthetic (bupivacaine or ropivacaine in dilute concentration) with a lipophilic opioid such as fentanyl is the upper thoracic region (T3) for thoracic surgery, the midthoracic region (T6) for upper abdominal surgery, and the lower thoracic region (T9) for lower abdominal surgery (see **Table 51-2**).

The amount of opioids needed by the neuraxial route to provide effective analgesia is less than by the systemic route, especially when combined with local anesthetics. This is definitely the case with morphine and to a lesser degree with fentanyl and hydromorphone.

When using a combination of local anesthetic and opioids, an infusion technique is required. The advantages of the combination are a synergistic effect with lower opioid doses and overall fewer side effects. However, with an infusion technique, there is a risk of local anesthetic

TABLE 51-2 Epidural Catheter Insertion Sites

Cord Segment	Target For	Central Bony Location	Landmark
Upper thoracic cord	Thoracotomy	T3	Root of scapular spine
Lower thoracic cord	Upper abdominal surgery	T6	Scapular tip
Lumbosacral cord	Lower abdominal surgery	T11–T12	12th rib
	Lower extremity surgery above the knee	L1–L2	12th rib
	Perineal surgery	L3–L4	Tuffier's line L4–L5
	Lower extremity surgery below the knee	L3–L4	Tuffier's line L4–L5
		L4–L5	

toxicity, catheter migration, potential sympathetic block, and orthostatic hypotension (**Table 51-3**).[34-36]

A large recent study shows an incidence of respiratory depression of 0.07%, nausea and vomiting of 22%, and pruritus of 22%. Another equally large study showed an overall rate of complications of 3% associated with the placement of thoracic epidural catheters. The complications included dural perforation (0.7%); unsuccessful catheter placement (1.1%); postoperative radicular type of pain (0.2%); responsive to catheter withdrawal in all cases; and peripheral nerve lesions (0.6%), 0.3% of which were peroneal nerve palsies probably related to surgical positioning and other transient peripheral nerve lesions (0.2%).[37] See Table 51-3.

Coagulopathy and systemic infection associated with bacteremia are definite contraindications to neuraxial techniques. Anticoagulation is a relative contraindication. The American Society of Regional Anesthesia recently published a concern statement on neuraxial anesthesia and anticoagulation.[38] For postoperative analgesia, the timing of the epidural catheter removal is important because most case reports of epidural hematomas have been documented on removal of the epidural catheter.

Patients receiving low-dose warfarin therapy during epidural analgesia should have their prothrombin times and internationalized normalized ratios (INRs) monitored on a daily basis and checked before catheter removal if the initial dose was more than 36 hours earlier. Initial studies evaluating the safety of epidural analgesia in association with oral anticoagulation using low-dose warfarin may require more intensive monitoring of the coagulation status.

Neurologic testing of sensory and motor function should be performed routinely on patients on anticoagulation with epidural analgesia and continued for at least 24 hours afterward. An INR above 3 should prompt the physician to withhold or reduce the warfarin dose in patients with indwelling neuraxial catheters.

The use of antiplatelet drugs alone does not create a level of risk that will interfere with the performance of neuraxial blockade. When used in combination with other anticoagulant regimens, there may be an increased chance of hematoma formation.

It is recommended that indwelling catheters be removed before initiation of low-molecular-weight heparin (LMWH) thromboprophylaxis. If a continuous technique is selected, the epidural catheter may be left indwelling overnight and removed the following day, with the first dose of LMWH administered 2 hours after catheter removal.

For any LMWH prophylaxis regimen, catheter removal should be delayed for at least 10 to 12 hours after a dose of LMWH.

TABLE 51-3 Epidural Local Anesthetic and Opioids*

Local Anesthetic		Opioid
Bupivacaine	0.0625%–0.125%	Fentanyl 1–10 μg/mL
Ropivacaine	0.05%–0.2%	Hydromorphone 0.1–0.3 mg/mL

*Usual rate is 4 to 16 mL/h.

A single intrathecal opioid injection can also be used either alone or in combination with epidural infusion and other methods for pain control. However, the pain relief achieved with this method usually lasts no longer than 12 to 18 hours, and the need for monitoring for possible respiratory depression is the same as for epidural opioid administration.[39]

With the use of neuraxial opioids, it is paramount to adequately educate the nursing and support staff to the monitoring and possible side effects of the techniques. Policies and protocols need to be in place to ensure patient safety, and it has been demonstrated that an organized acute pain service provides superior postoperative analgesia care than standard delivery of analgesics.

PERIPHERAL NERVE BLOCKS

Peripheral nerve blocks provide excellent short-term pain relief when placed appropriately. These days with the use of ultrasound, nerve blocks are placed under direct visualization, resulting in a high success rate of blocks. Several studies have been done to show the advantages of using peripheral nerve blocks in the pain management of a surgical patient. These patients require fewer opioids and hence have a much lower risk of opioid-related side effects. These patients also have a decrease in duration of hospital stay and costs, decreased incidence of postoperative nausea and vomiting, lower rates of hospital readmission after surgery, and much greater patient satisfaction.

A continuous peripheral nerve catheter technique has been used for acute pain management, including continuous femoral nerve block, thoracic paravertebral block, and continuous brachial plexus catheter techniques. Although some of these techniques can be extremely useful (especially in certain circumstances), most continuous catheter techniques remain underused, potentially because of fears of complications, unfamiliarity, time constraints, and possibly reimbursement issues.

For both PCA and epidural analgesia, standard orders for monitoring and for medications such as antiemetics (e.g., droperidol) and antipruritic agents (e.g., diphenhydramine), as well as orders for small titrations greatly facilitate the delivery of postoperative care.

NONPHARMACOLOGIC APPROACH

Nonpharmacologic methods of pain management and stimulation-induced analgesia can be used in the postoperative period with either acupuncture or transcutaneous electrical nerve stimulation (TENS). With TENS, a small electrical current presumably stimulates the touch pressure and proprioception fiber (A-β) to release endogenous opiates and closes the "gate" of pain transmission at the spinal level. The TENS technique is considered safe but does not reliably provide analgesia in all cases.[40] It is best used for amputations, back surgery, and after cesarean sections. Sterile electrodes are available to be placed close to surgical sites. TENS is contraindicated for patients with demand pacemakers and may interfere with electrocardiogram monitoring.

Behavioral techniques such as relaxation therapy and hypnosis have also been successfully used in the treatment of postoperative pain, but these techniques require postoperative preparation and motivation on the part of the patient to be effective in the immediate postoperative period.

This approach can be used alongside a traditional pharmacologic approach. It helps to reduce the total amount of analgesic needed and hence helps reduce the incidence of side effects related to analgesics.

REFERENCES

1. Sinatra RS. Acute pain management and acute pain services. In: Cousins MJ, Bridenbaugh PO, eds. *Neural Blockade in Clinical Anesthesia and Management of Pain*. 2nd ed. Philadelphia: Lippincott-Raven; 1988:793-836.
2. Acute Pain Management Guidelines Panel. Acute Pain Management: Operative or Medical Procedures and Trauma. Clinical Practice Guideline. Rockville, MD: US Dept of Health and Human Services, Agency for Health Care Policy and Research; 1992. AHCPR publication 92–0032.
3. Practice guidelines for acute pain management in the perioperative setting. ASA Task Force on Pain Management. *Anesthesiology*. 1995; 82:1071.
4. Practice guidelines for acute pain management in the perioperative setting. ASA Task Force on Pain Management. *Anesthesiology*. 2012; 116:248-273.
5. Cohen FL. Post surgical pain relief: patient status and nurses' medication choices. *Pain*. 1980;9:265.
6. Houck C, Berde C, Anand K. Pediatric pain management. In: Gregory G. ed. *Pediatric Anesthesia*. New York: Churchill Livingstone; 1994:743-771.
7. Wu CL, Raja SN. Treatment of acute post operative pain. *Lancet*. 2011;2215:2225.
8. Marks RM, Sachar EJ. Undertreatment of medical inpatients with narcotic analgesics. *Ann Intern Med*. 1973;78:173.
9. Liu SS, Block BM, Wu CL. Effects of perioperative central neuraxial analgesia on outcome after coronary artery bypass surgery: a meta-analysis. *Anesthesiology*. 2004;101:153-161.
10. Beattie WS, Badner NH, Choi P. Epidural analgesia reduces postoperative myocardial infarction: a meta-analysis. *Anesth Analg*. 2001;93:853-858.
11. Walder B, Schafer M, Henzi I, Tramer MR. Efficacy and safety of patient-controlled opioid analgesia for acute postoperative pain: a quantitative systematic review. *Acta Anaesthesiol Scand*. 2001;45:795-804.
12. Ballantyne JC, Carr DB, deFerranti S, et al. The comparative effects of postoperative analgesic therapies on pulmonary outcome: cumulative meta-analyses of randomized, controlled trials. *Anesth Analg*. 1998;86:598-612.
13. Kehlet H. Modification responses to surgery by neural blockade. In: Cousins MJ, Bridenbaugh PO, eds. *Neural Blockade in Clinical Anesthesia and Management of Pain*. 2nd ed. Philadelphia: Lippincott-Raven; 1998:129-175.
14. Basbaum AI. Spinal mechanisms of acute and persistent pain. *Reg Anesth Pain Med*. 1999;24:59.
15. Bardram L, Funch-Jensen P, Jensen P, et al. Recovery after laparoscopic surgery with epidural analgesia, and early oral nutrition and mobilization. *Lancet*. 1995;345:763.
16. Kehlet H. Acute pain control and accelerated postoperative surgical recovery. *Surg Clin North Am*. 1999;79:431-443.
17. Dantzer R, Kelly KW. Stress and immunity: an integrated view of the relationship between the brain and the immune system. *Life Sci*. 1998;44:1995.
18. Liebeskind JC. Pain can kill [editorial]. *Pain*. 1991;44:3.
19. Kehlet H. Multimodal approach to control postoperative pathophysiology and rehabilitation. *Br J Anaesth*. 1997;78:606.
20. Woolf CJ, Chong M. Preemptive analgesia—treating postoperative pain by preventing the establishment of central sensitization. *Anesth Analg*. 1993;77:362.
21. Buvanendran A, Kroin JS. Multimodal analgesia for controlling acute postoperative pain. *Curr Opin Anesthesiol*. 2009;22: 588-593.
22. Momeni M, Crucetti M, de Kock M. Patient-controlled analgesia in the management of postoperative pain. *Drugs*. 2006;18:2321-2337.
23. Ballantyne JC, Carr DB, Chalmers TC, et al. Postoperative patient-controlled analgesia: meta-analyses of initial randomized control trials. *J Clin Anesth*. 1993;5:182.
24. Angst MS, Clark JD. Opioid-induced hyperalgesia: a qualitative systematic review. *Anesthesiology*. 2006;104:570-587.
25. Power I, Barratt S. Analgesic agents for the postoperative period. *Surg Clin North Am*. 1999;79:275-295.
26. Cobby F, Crighton IM, Kyriakides K, Hobbs GJ. Rectal paracetamol has a significant morphine sparing effect after hysterectomy. *Br J Anaesth*. 1999;83(2):253-256.
27. Shen Q, Sinatra R, Luther M. Preoperative rofecoxib 25 mg and 50 mg: effects on postsurgical morphine consumption and effort-dependent pain. *Anesthesiology*. 2001;95:A961.
28. Camu F, Beecher T, Recker DP, Verburg KM. Valdecoxib, a COX-2 specific inhibitor, is an efficacious, opioid-sparing analgesic in patients undergoing hip arthroplasty. *Am J Therap*. 2002;9:43.
29. McQuay H, Edwards J. Meta analysis of single dose oral tramadol plus acetaminophen in acute post operative pain. *Eur J Anaesthesiol*. 2003;18(Suppl):19-22.
30. Grace RF, Power I, Umedaly H, et al. Preoperative dextromethorphan reduces intraoperative but not postoperative morphine requirements after laparotomy. *Anesth Analg*. 1998;87:1135.
31. Kohrs R, Durieux ME. Ketamine: teaching an old drug new tricks. *Anesth Analg*. 1998;87:1186.
32. Peng PW, Wijeysundera DN, Li CC. Use of gabapentin for perioperative pain control—a meta-analysis. *Pain Res Manag*. 2007;12: 85-92.
33. Hurley RW, Cohen SP, Williams KA, et al. The analgesic effects of perioperative gabapentin on post operative pain: a meta-analysis. *Reg Anesth Pain Med*. 2006;31:237-247.
34. Yeager MP, Glass DD, Neff RK, Brinck-Johnsen T. The safety and efficacy of intrathecal opioid analgesia for acute postoperative pain: seven years' experience with 5969 surgical patients at Indiana University Hospital. *Anesth Analg*. 1999;88:599.
35. Liu S, Carpenter RL, Neal JM. Epidural anesthesia and analgesia. *Anesthesiology*. 1995;76:342.
36. Bylon JF, Katz J, Kavanagh BP, et al. Epidural bupivacaine-morphine analgesia versus patient-controlled analgesia following abdominal aortic surgery. *Anesthesiology*. 1998;89:585.
37. Wang LP, Hauerberg J, Schmidt JF. Incidence of spinal epidural abscess after epidural analgesia. *Anesthesiology*. 1999;91:1928-1936.
38. Consensus on anticoagulation and neuraxial anesthesia. American Society of Regional Anesthesia and Pain Medicine. Available at http://www.asra.com
39. Ready LB. Acute perioperative pain. In: Miller RD, ed. *Anesthesia*. Philadelphia: Churchill Livingstone; 2000;2323-2350.
40. Carrol D, Tramèr M, McQuay H, Nye B, Moore A. Randomisation is important in studies with pain outcome: systematic review of TENS in acute post operative pain. *Br J Anaesth*. 1996;77(6):798-803.

Ultrasound-Guided Peripheral Nerve Blockade

Nicholas R. Wasson
Lauren J. Fisher

OVERVIEW

GENERAL DATA AND INFORMATION

Regional anesthesia (often called peripheral nerve blockade) involves injecting a volume of local anesthetic in specific locations around nerves that supply various parts of the body, rendering them insensate to a surgical stimulus and allowing for pain relief postoperatively. It can be combined with general anesthesia or sedation for surgical procedures or may be the sole anesthetic of a surgical procedure. These techniques can also be used in the treatment of patients with chronic pain syndromes. For the purposes of this chapter, neuraxial techniques (e.g., spinal and epidural anesthesia) will not be mentioned because they are discussed elsewhere in this text.

The benefits of regional anesthesia include faster discharge times at ambulatory surgical centers along with improved early pain postoperative control,[1] reduction in opioid use in the immediate postoperative period, and less nausea and vomiting postoperatively.[2] Another advantage is the potential to avoid general anesthesia, particularly in higher-risk patients with significant comorbidities.

For these reasons, the use of regional anesthesia techniques may translate to higher patient satisfaction rates, overall lower health care costs, and improved patient outcomes and quality. The role of regional anesthesia will likely continue to expand because there continues to be tremendous growth in ambulatory surgical procedures, as well as continually evolving changes in reimbursement coupled with the safety, effectiveness, portability, and affordability of ultrasound techniques. Its use will likely only continue to rise, and the authors believe it should be an important part of any anesthesiologist's armamentarium.

GENERAL INDICATIONS AND PATIENT SELECTION

Indications for regional anesthesia are multifactorial. It is most dependent on the type of procedure performed; preexisting patient comorbidities; and the preferences of the patient, surgeon, and anesthesiologist. It is useful when the discussion of the type of anesthesia starts with the surgeon in the office in order to set patient expectations for the day of surgery to include a regional anesthetic.

For indications for each specific type of block, please refer to each individual block.

GENERAL CONTRAINDICATIONS

Absolute There are very few absolute contraindications to a regional anesthetic block. These include the following:

- Patient refusal
- Active infection at the site where injection of the local anesthetic is to be performed
- Presence of a history of true allergy or anaphylactic reaction to the medications to be injected (e.g., local anesthetic)

Relative Several relative contraindications to regional anesthesia are often related to patient factors. Some of these include:

- Inability to perform the block because of poor patient tolerance or cooperation (e.g., an awake young child)
- Preexisting neurologic deficit or need for immediate neurologic examination after the procedure
- Preexisting comorbidities that may worsen with peripheral blockade (e.g., prior respiratory dysfunction would preclude the placement of an interscalene nerve block because of the high incidence of ipsilateral phrenic nerve paralysis)
- Surgeon preference for a specific technique (e.g., general anesthesia)
- Expertise of the anesthesiologist and available equipment for nerve block

Anticoagulation The presence of systemic anticoagulation in a patient presenting for a regional anesthetic is one of intense debate and is continuously evolving as newer medications continue to be brought to the market and more evidence emerges regarding existing anticoagulation medications and regional anesthesia. The American Society of Regional Anesthesia (ASRA) has released three versions of its guidelines for neuraxial and peripheral nerve blockade in patients receiving systemic anticoagulation and antithrombotic therapy, most recently in January 2010.[3] These guidelines are generally accepted as the gold standard in the United States in assessing the risk of neuraxial and peripheral anesthesia for complications caused by systemic anticoagulation. These complications include mainly hemorrhage and clinically significant hematoma. However, despite these guidelines, many of the data regarding risk remain incomplete or unknown, and often it is left to a discussion among the surgeon, patient, and anesthesiologist to determine the risk versus benefit of performing a regional anesthetic in the presence of systemic anticoagulation.

Few investigations have examined the frequency and severity of hemorrhagic complications after plexus or peripheral blockade in anticoagulated patients. Despite this, a summary of the current recommendations for peripheral nerve blockade is given in this chapter with discussion of several commonly used anticoagulants.

Aspirin and Nonsteroidal Anti-Inflammatory Drugs

- In general, peripheral nerve blockade in patients receiving systemic aspirin or nonsteroidal anti-inflammatory medications is deemed safe.

Clopidogrel and Ticlopidine

- Current recommendations suggest waiting 5 to 7 days after the last dose before the performance of a peripheral nerve blockade and 10 to 14 days for ticlopidine, given the half-lives of these drugs and prolonged platelet-altering effect.

Low-Dose Prophylactic Subcutaneous Unfractionated Heparin (e.g., 5000 units)

- Twice-daily dosing: This is *generally considered safe* because of its widespread use, no change in clotting parameters, and lack of widespread complications directly related to peripheral nerve blockade.
- Thrice-daily dosing or higher doses: *Unknown safety*. This is mainly attributable to a lack of data of complications involving this dosing. Per the ASRA consensus statement, "A review of relevant literature shows that there are reports that document an increased risk of minor and major bleeding in surgical and in nonsurgical patients receiving thrice-daily subcutaneous unfractionated heparin" (UFH). Also, it is recommended to not check the activated thromboplastin time or platelet count unless there is concern about changes in these values after "prolonged administration" or in patients with "many comorbidities that might influence the pharmacology of subcutaneous UFH." Therefore, it is left to the discretion of the practitioner and the type of block to be performed, such as a superficial versus a deeper blockade, and it is recommended to closely follow these patients for potential complications.

Low-Molecular-Weight Heparin

- In patients receiving prophylactic dosing with low-molecular-weight heparin (LMWH) without any other hemostatic-modifying drugs, it is recommended to wait approximately 10 to 12 hours after the last dose before the performance of regional anesthesia. In patients receiving a full anticoagulation dose, 24 hours should elapse after the last dose of LMWH before performance of regional anesthesia.

Oral Anticoagulation (e.g., Warfarin)

- In patients receiving systemic oral warfarin therapy, it is recommended to stop warfarin 4 or 5 days earlier, and the international normalized ratio should be normalized (<1.5) before placement of a nerve block

The above recommendations are for patients undergoing so-called "deep" versus "superficial" peripheral nerve blocks. These include deep plexus blocks (e.g., lumbar plexus, lumbar sympathetic, paravertebral) and deep peripheral nerve blocks when hematoma formation and hemorrhage may not be readily apparent after peripheral blockade.

For further recommendations regarding systemic anticoagulation and regional anesthesia, refer to the general ASRA evidence-based guidelines.

PREOPERATIVE ASSESSMENT AND PREPARATION

Before the performance of any peripheral nerve block, as in any anesthetic procedure, several things must take place. First, a review of the patient's history and physical examination findings, including vital signs, height and weight, medications, and functional capacity, is crucial before the placement in order to elicit any potential complications or contraindications of performing this procedure. (For specific complications regarding each individual block, refer to the section discussing the individual block.) It is also important to discuss with the surgeon the procedure, including the location and length of the procedure, as well as postoperative pain control options, in order to choose a proper peripheral blockade site and technique and the desired local anesthetic volume and concentration.

It is helpful to gather all of the materials needed for the block to facilitate efficiency. These include the following:

- Local anesthetic for skin infiltration
- Syringes and needles
- Local anesthetic choices
- Ultrasound machine and probe or nerve stimulator
- Chlorhexidine/Betadine skin preparation
- Intravenous (IV) line placement before block
- Availability of intralipid in the event of local anesthetic systemic toxicity[4]
- Gloves and appropriate sterile attire
- Sedation (e.g., midazolam IV) before the block to ease patient anxiety
- Marking of the correct side and site

MONITORING DURING BLOCK

Monitoring of a patient during regional anesthesia should proceed in accordance with American Society of Anesthesiology's guidelines.[5] The basic principles used in monitoring for general anesthesia should be assessed during performance of regional anesthetics. Oxygen and resuscitation equipment should be readily available in the event of any adverse reaction or complication of the block occurs.

TYPES OF BLOCKS

INTERSCALENE NERVE BLOCK

Surgical Indications This block is used for any procedure from the shoulder through the upper arm. Coverage of the inferior trunk is not reliable with this block, so it is generally not the preferred nerve block for coverage for procedures below the elbow.

Anatomic Coverage Blockade at the interscalene groove targets the brachial plexus at the trunks, blocking the superior trunk composed of C5 and C6 nerve roots, the middle trunk composed of the nerve root from C7, and the inferior trunk composed of the C8 and T1 nerve root. The suprascapular nerve arises from fibers from the superior trunk and exits the brachial plexus to travel posteriorly through the suprascapular notch traveling between the supraspinatus and infraspinatus muscles. The superficial cervical plexus arises from the ventral rami of C2 to C4 and provides sensation to the skin overlying the shoulder and clavicle.

Technique A landmark-guided approach traditionally describes needle insertion at the level of the cricoid cartilage, or C6, locating the groove between the anterior and middle scalene muscles at the posterior border of the clavicular head of the sternocleidomastoid muscle.[6]

An ultrasound-guided approach favors the location of a vascular structure, either tracing the nerve bundle in a superior direction from the supraclavicular location or locating the carotid or internal jugular vein and moving the probe laterally to locate the plexus as it runs between the anterior and middle scalene muscles (**Fig. 52-1**).

There is much debate in the regional anesthesia community regarding optimal needle placement for this block. Many experts in the field advocate for keeping needle placement as far away from the neural structures as possible while still obtaining adequate spread of local anesthetic to minimize the risk of needle–nerve trauma.[7] Extra-sheath injection (local anesthetic spread between the anterior and middle scalene muscles) compared with intra-sheath injection (needle placement between the trunks) results in comparable block onset and quality of sensorimotor block, although intra-sheath injection results in a modestly prolonged duration of blockade.[8]

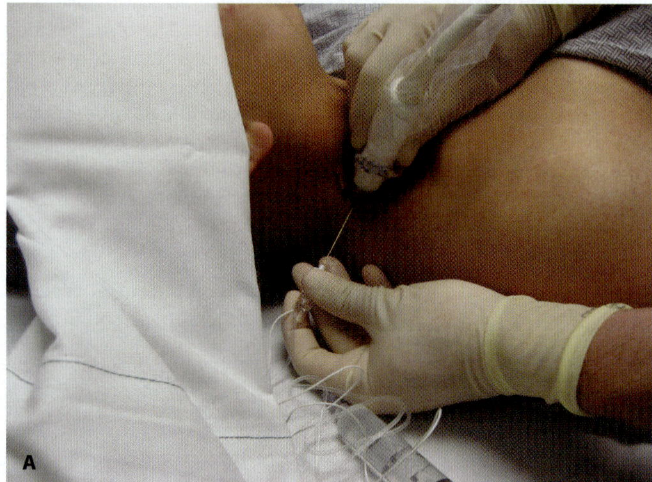

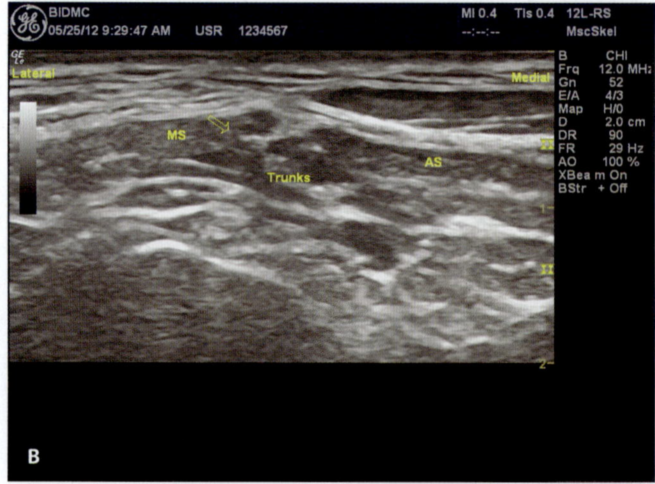

FIGURE 52-1. **A** and **B**, Interscalene nerve block. AS, anterior scalene; MS, middle scalene. The arrow indicates the needle trajectory.

Choice of Local Anesthetic and Volume An interscalene nerve block is typically used for postoperative analgesia, so longer-acting anesthetics, such as ropivacaine and bupivacaine, are usually favored. Minimizing the volume of local anesthetic results in a lower incidence of phrenic nerve paralysis (13% to 45% as opposed to 100% in traditional nerve stimulator techniques), so most practitioners use a volume of between 5 and 10 mL of 0.75% ropivacaine or bupivacaine 0.5%.[9–11]

Contraindications The traditional nerve stimulator technique has been found to result in a 100% incidence of ipsilateral phrenic nerve paralysis,[12] so an advantage of ultrasound-guided blockade is the ability to reduce the incidence to 13% to 45% by using a lower volume of local anesthetic.[13–15] Unilateral hemidiaphragmatic paresis decreases the forced vital capacity and forced expiratory volume by approximately 20%, so significant underlying pulmonary pathology is considered a contraindication to interscalene blockade.[16,17] Additionally, patients with contralateral phrenic nerve paralysis should not have this type of nerve block because complete diaphragmatic paralysis would result in respiratory failure and a need for intubation and ventilator support until resolution of blockade. The interscalene nerve block is also associated with a remote incidence of recurrent laryngeal nerve block, so the presence of a contralateral laryngeal nerve block would make this blockade contraindicated.[18]

Complications Possible complications include infection, hematoma, nerve injury, pneumothorax, total spinal, Horner's syndrome (blockade of the stellate ganglion resulting in ptosis, miosis, and anhydrosis), recurrent laryngeal nerve paralysis, and diaphragmatic paralysis.

SUPRACLAVICULAR NERVE BLOCK

Surgical Indications This block is used for any upper extremity procedure from the shoulder to the hand.

Anatomic Coverage Blockade at the supraclavicular location blocks the divisions of the brachial plexus. The suprascapular nerve and supraclavicular nerve have already left the plexus by this location, so they must be blocked separately if coverage is desired for the top of the shoulder.

Technique An ultrasound-guided technique favors the location of the subclavian artery and corresponding reliable location of the plexus at approximately the 2 o'clock position. When performed correctly, the supraclavicular block is considered the "spinal block of the upper extremity" because it anesthetizes the entire upper extremity. The technique, described as "eight ball corner pocket" in which the needle is advanced under from a lateral to medial approach to deposit local anesthetic between the subclavian artery, first rib, and divisions of the brachial plexus, is described as providing a fast-onset full blockade with as little as 15 mL of local anesthetic[19] (**Fig. 52-2**). Obviously, close ultrasound tracking of the needle tip is essential to stay above the first rib and avoid contacting pleura, with the consequence of pneumothorax.[20] Fifteen to 20 mL of local anesthetic is an adequate volume to block the plexus in this location.

Contraindications This block has similar contraindications to those for the interscalene nerve block. Some practitioners advocate for the supraclavicular block because of a lower incidence of phrenic nerve palsy caused by a more distal injection point. The supraclavicular block performed via traditional nerve stimulation techniques is reported to cause a 50% incidence of hemidiaphragmatic paralysis[21] compared with a 0% incidence in the ultrasound-guided group using identical volumes of 20 mL of 0.75% ropivacaine.[22] Although this decreased incidence is reassuring, this block would still be considered contraindicated in patients who would be unable to tolerate hemidiaphragmatic paralysis and the resulting 20% decrement in pulmonary function.

Complications Possible complications include infection, hematoma, nerve injury, pneumothorax, total spinal, Horner's syndrome (blockade of the stellate ganglion resulting in ptosis, miosis, and anhydrosis), recurrent laryngeal nerve paralysis, and diaphragmatic paralysis.

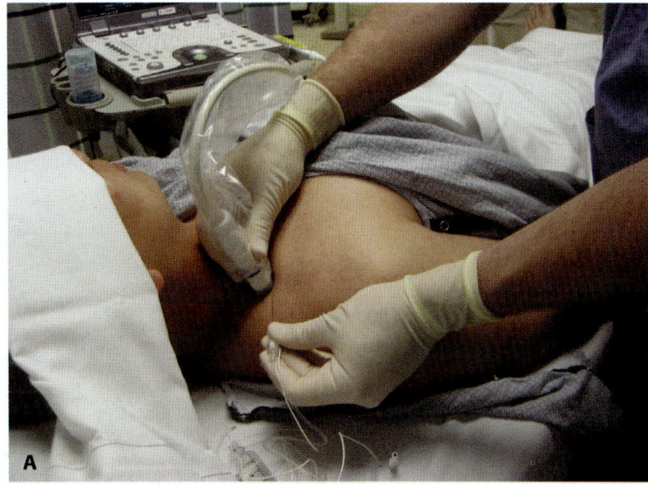

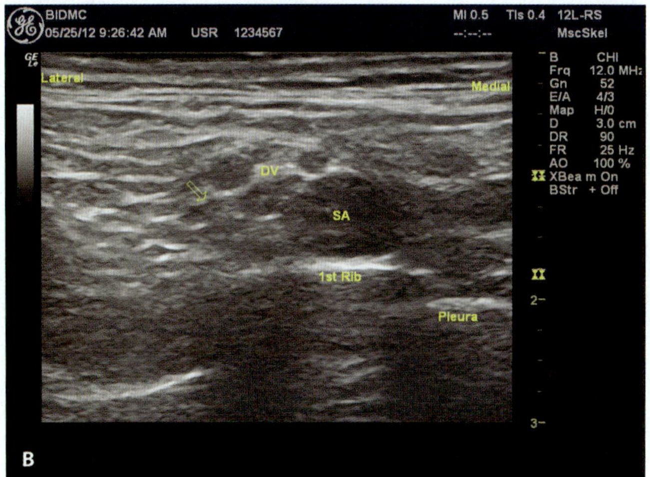

FIGURE 52-2. **A** and **B,** Supraclavicular nerve block. DV, divisions; SA, subclavian artery. The arrow indicates the needle trajectory.

INFRACLAVICULAR NERVE BLOCK

This block is done for elbow, forearm, and hand procedures. The infraclavicular block has been shown in some studies to provide enhanced blood flow in arteriovenous fistula procedures.[23] Infraclavicular blockade has a similar area of anesthesia as axillary blockade but can be performed with fewer needle passes; hence, it is the block of choice for some providers for hand surgery.[24] It tends to have a faster onset than the supraclavicular block.[25] In patients at either weight extreme, either very obese or cachectic, it can be difficult to visualize or plan a safe needle trajectory, so for these patients, an alternative block may be a better option. Abduction of the arm may pull the artery into a more superficial location, easing the performance of this block.[26]

Anatomic Coverage The infraclavicular nerve block blocks the brachial plexus at the level of the cords. The musculocutaneous nerve is closely applied to the lateral cord in this location, so it is blocked with an infraclavicular block.

Technique The ultrasound probe is placed in a sagittal orientation in the deltopectoral groove to cut the subclavian artery and cords in cross-section (**Fig. 52-3**). It is prudent to stay as lateral as possible to avoid puncture of the pleura with the block needle. It is crucial to

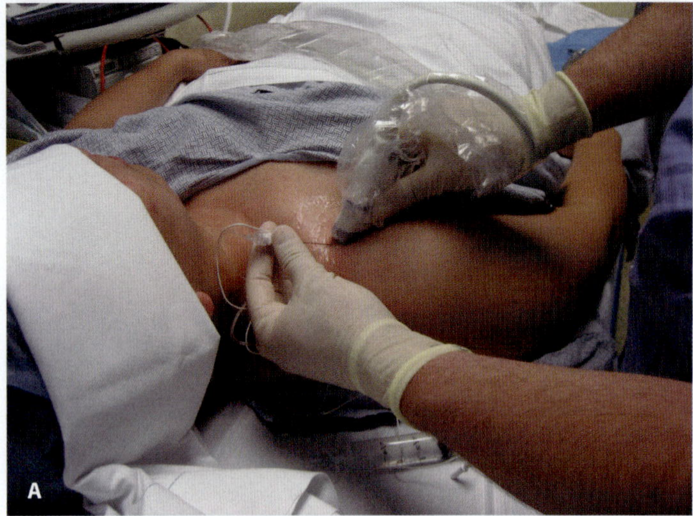

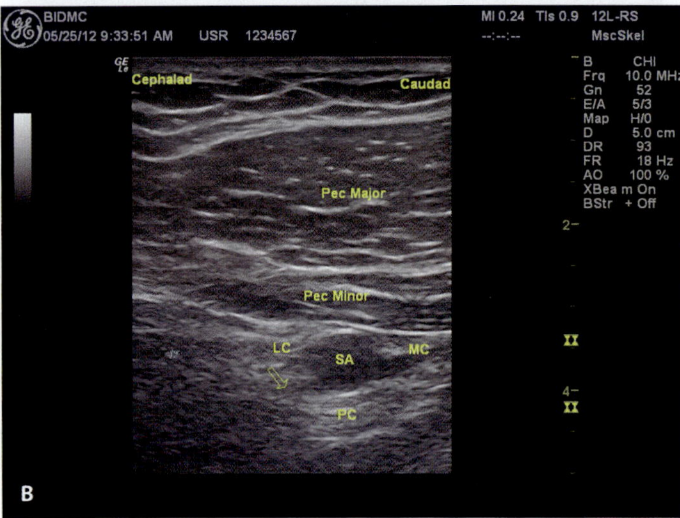

FIGURE 52-3. **A** and **B**, Infraclavicular nerve block. SA, subclavian artery; LC, lateral cord; PC, posterior cord; MC, medial cord. The arrow indicates the needle trajectory.

use color Doppler for blockade in this location to visualize and avoid potential anomalous vasculature. Much debate has occurred regarding a single injection versus a triple injection technique around all three cords, but the single injection technique of 20 to 30 mL of local anesthetic posterior to the artery has been shown to be an effective technique with an optimal procedural time.[27]

Contraindications This block is considered a deeper block in a noncompressible area, so caution is advised in performing this block in a coagulopathic patient. Although a lateral approach is advised to avoid pleural puncture, bullous emphysematous disease is a relative contraindication.

Complications Possible complications include infection, hematoma, nerve injury, and pneumothorax, especially when performed from a more medial approach.

AXILLARY NERVE BLOCK

Surgical Indications This block is used for surgery at the elbow and below, including the hand.

Anatomic Coverage Axillary blockade provides coverage of the brachial plexus at the terminal branches. The musculocutaneous nerve has already left the plexus and travels in the body of the coracobrachialis muscle, so it must be localized separately to anesthetize the lateral, cutaneous aspect of the forearm. The intercostobrachial nerve providing sensation to the medial aspect of the upper arm travels separately from the thoracic region, so separate blockade would be necessary in any brachial plexus block.

Technique The orienting structure is the axillary artery. The patient is positioned with the arm abducted and the hand resting 90 degrees from the elbow or behind the head while lying supine. The axillary artery is then palpated in the axilla, and the area is prepped in standard fashion using aseptic technique. The artery can then be visualized in short axis by placing the ultrasound probe parallel to the pectoralis major muscle in the anterior axillary fold (**Fig. 52-4A**). When the axillary artery and vein are identified in this probe orientation, the nerves of the brachial plexus may be visualized. Using this probe orientation, the median nerve is often first visualized superoanterior to the artery, with the radial nerve located inferolateral to the artery and the ulnar nerve located more inferior to the artery. The musculocutaneous nerve is located within the coracobrachialis muscles and is more superior to the artery; it appears very hyperechoic and bright relative to the surrounding muscle (**Fig. 52-4B**).

The needle is inserted in an in-line approach at a shallow angle from the cephalad aspect of the probe and directed inferiorly and posteriorly toward the nerves. Upon placement of the needle next to the target nerve, approximately 3 to 5 mL of local anesthetic is injected after negative aspiration, with spread observed with each injection around the target nerve. Then the needle is redirected to each target nerve, with care taken to avoid any vascular structures. Often multiple passes are needed to block each separate nerve, and often anywhere from 20 to 40 mL of local anesthetic is used in the performance of this portion of the block.

In blocking the musculocutaneous nerve, the same insertion site for the other axillary brachial plexus nerves is used, only with the needle at a steeper angle toward the nerve. Five to 10 mL of local anesthetic is then used in blockade of this nerve.

Contraindications In general, this block is performed away from the pleura and neuraxis and therefore can be performed with relative safety.

Complications Possible complications include infection, hematoma, and nerve injury. The intercostobrachial block is performed in this location starting at the skin insertion site from the axillary block. A superficial skin wheal is injected using 5 to 10 mL of local anesthetic on the interior aspect of the arm to the groove between the biceps and triceps muscles (see Fig. 52-4C).

UPPER EXTREMITY PERIPHERAL NERVE BLOCKADE

These blocks may be used in conjunction with each other for sensory blockade of the distal upper extremity for hand surgery or for supplementation of the aforementioned brachial plexus blocks in the event of incomplete sensory blockade. These are superficial blocks, and they carry the standard complications of infection, hematoma, and nerve injury.

RADIAL

The radial nerve provides sensation to the majority of the dorsal aspect of the hand involving the first, second, and third and lateral fourth digits. With the patient supine, the arm is placed across the chest, with the ultrasound probe at a perpendicular angle to the arm near the lateral epicondyle (**Fig. 52-5A**). The radial nerve visualized next to the radial artery above the humerus (**Fig. 52-5B**). A needle is advanced in plane from the lateral probe end, and 3 to 5 mL of local anesthetic is injected, with care taken to avoid the artery.

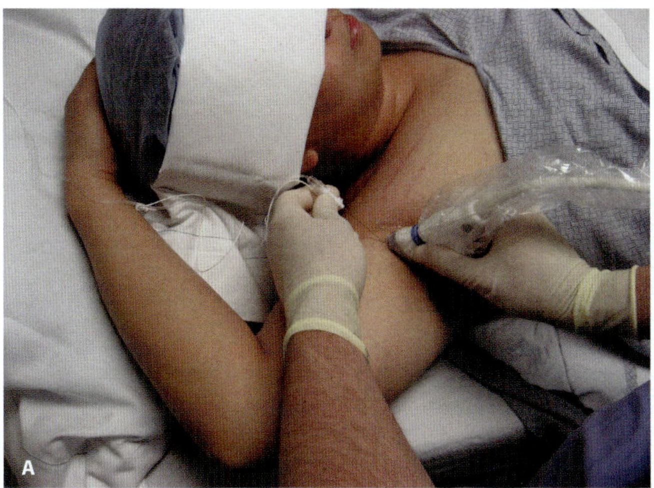

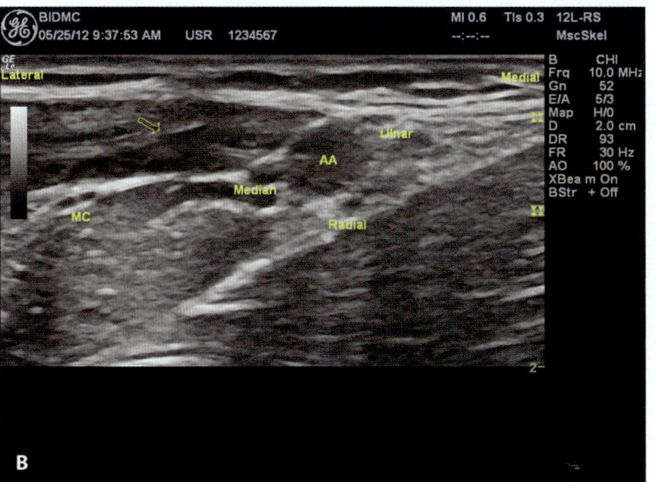

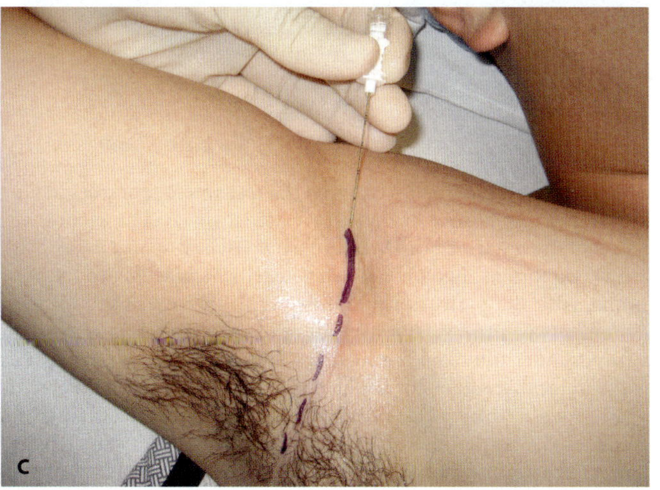

FIGURE 52-4. **A** and **B**, Axillary nerve block. **C**, Intercostobrachial nerve block. AA, axillary artery; MC, musculocutaneous nerve. The arrow indicates the needle trajectory.

ULNAR

The ulnar nerve provides sensation to the medial aspect of the hand, both palmar and dorsal sides, as well as sensation to the medial portion of the fourth and entire fifth digits. For this block, the patient is placed supine with the arm extended and abducted. The probe is then placed in a perpendicular axis on the medial aspect of the forearm approximately

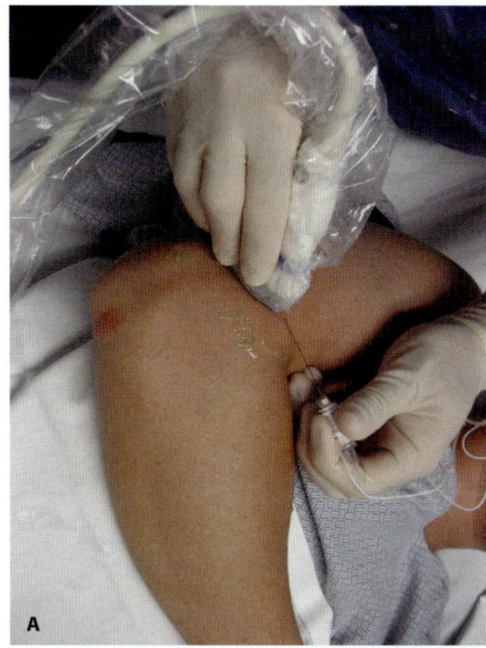

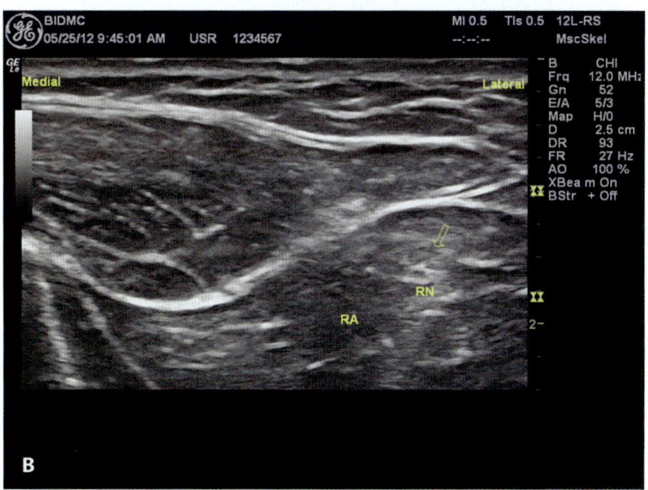

FIGURE 52-5. **A** and **B**, Radial nerve block. RA, radial artery; RN, radial nerve. The arrow indicates the needle trajectory.

half the distance between the hand and the elbow (**Fig. 52-6A**). The ulnar nerve is visualized next to the ulnar artery (**Fig. 52-6B**). The needle is advanced from the lateral portion of the probe and directed medially, and 3 to 5 mL of local anesthetic is injected around the nerve, again with care taken to avoid the surrounding vasculature.

MEDIAN

The median nerve provides sensory innervation of the palm of the hand, including the palmar surfaces of the first, second, and third and the lateral portion of the fourth digits. For this block, the patient is placed supine with the arm abducted and the arm turned in supination. The pulse of the brachial artery is felt, and the probe is placed in a perpendicular axis over the distal humerus closer to the medial aspect of the arm (**Fig. 52-7A**). The median nerve is located medial relative to the artery, and its course may be followed until it separates from the artery more distally (**Fig. 52-7B**). The needle trajectory is from the medial aspect of the probe and is directed laterally to inject 3 to 5 mL of local anesthetic.

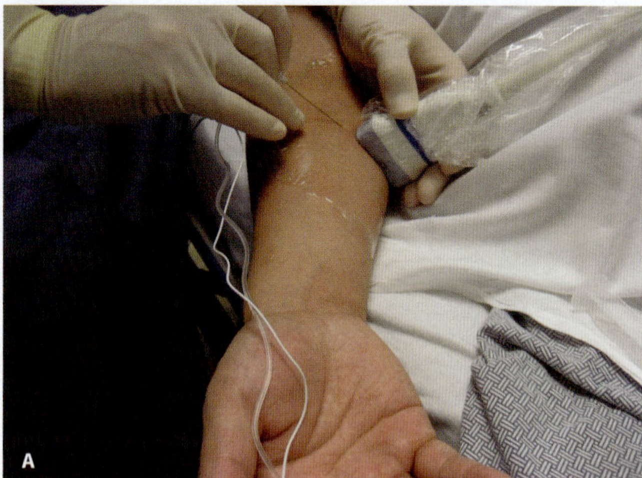

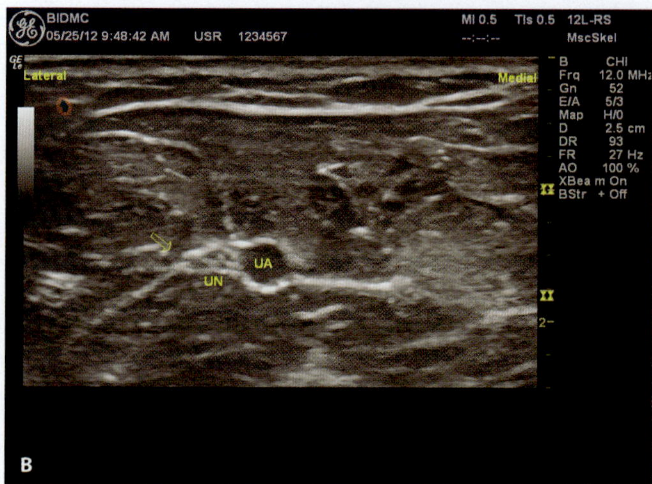

FIGURE 52-6. **A** and **B**, Ulnar nerve block. UA, ulnar artery; UN, ulnar nerve. The arrow indicates the needle trajectory.

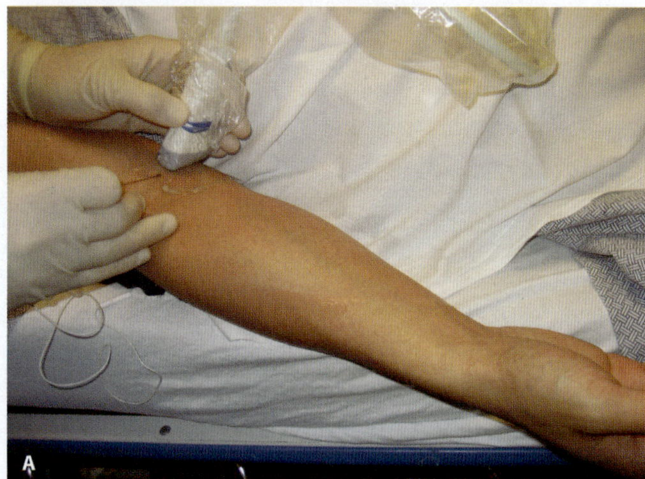

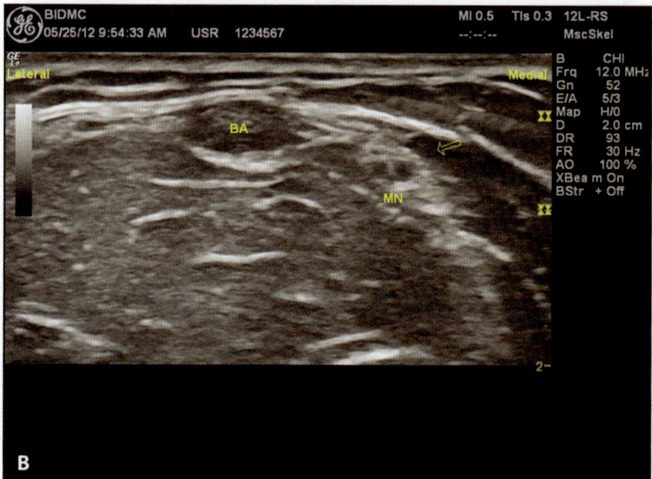

FIGURE 52-7. **A** and **B**, Median nerve block. BA, brachial artery; MN, median nerve. The arrow indicates the needle trajectory.

ABDOMINAL AND TRUNK

PARAVERTEBRAL NERVE BLOCK

Surgical Indications This block is used for surgery of the thorax or trunk, breast procedures, thoracic procedures (thoracotomy and thoracoscopy), chest tube pain, and rib fractures.[28] It has also been used with success in inguinal hernia repair.[29]

Anatomic Coverage The paravertebral nerve block refers to blockade of spinal nerves immediately after they traverse the intervertebral foramina. It provides unilateral dermatomal coverage of the desired spinal nerve levels. However, because of significant overlap of innervation near the midline from the opposite side, one-sided blocks may not be adequate for procedures located near the midline. Also, often the dermatome above and below the desired spinal levels must be blocked because of overlap in innervation.

Technique The patient may be positioned sitting, prone, or lateral based on physician preference. With a deep (low-frequency) ultrasound probe orientated vertically so that the anatomy is viewed in the sagittal plane, midline spinous processes are identified. Moving the probe laterally and at a slight oblique angle, the transverse processes are identified (**Fig. 52-8A**). The superior costotransverse ligament is identified as the brighter band that travels between the transverse processes, delineating the posterior border of the paravertebral space. The pleura, which consists of the anterior border of the paravertebral space, is easily identified by the bright, hyperechoic structure, which seems to "shimmer" or move with the patient's respiration. With the top of the transducer oriented between the two transverse processes, the tip of the needle is advanced under ultrasound guidance through the costotransverse ligament, and local anesthetic is injected (**Fig. 52-8B**).[30] The pleura is noted to "move down" on the live ultrasound image as the local anesthetic is administered. The number of levels blocked varies according to practice: some prefer to administer a single injection of 15 to 20 mL at one level, and others prefer to administer a lower volume (3–5 mL) at multiple levels to maximize dermatomal coverage.[31–33]

Contraindications In addition to the general contraindications, this block is considered to be a deeper block in a noncompressible area, so caution is advised in performing this block in a coagulopathic patient.

Complications Possible complications include infection, hematoma, and nerve injury, as with other peripheral nerve blocks. *Hypotension* is also a concern (4% incidence in one study).[34] The posterior border of the paravertebral space is the pleura, so great care is taken with needle advancement to avoid pleural puncture and resultant pneumothorax. Epidural spread is also a concern, and spinal spread is possible if the

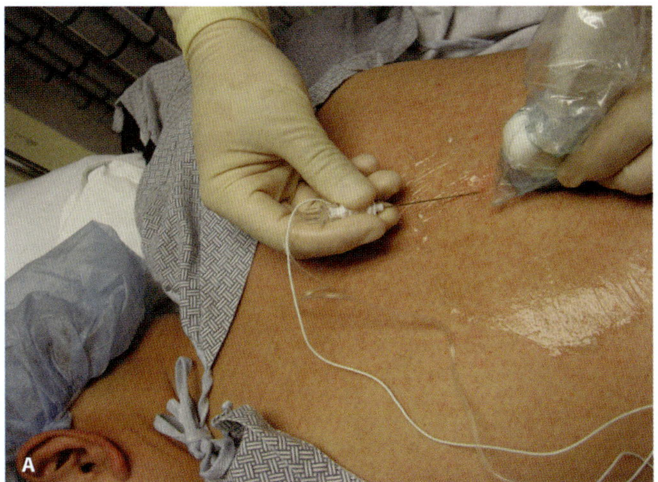

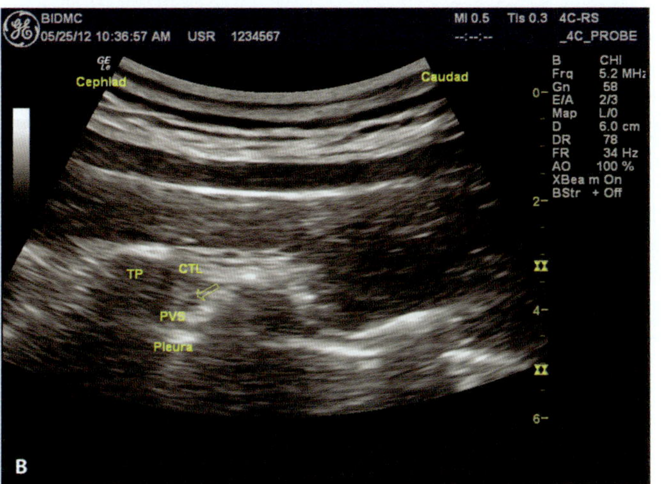

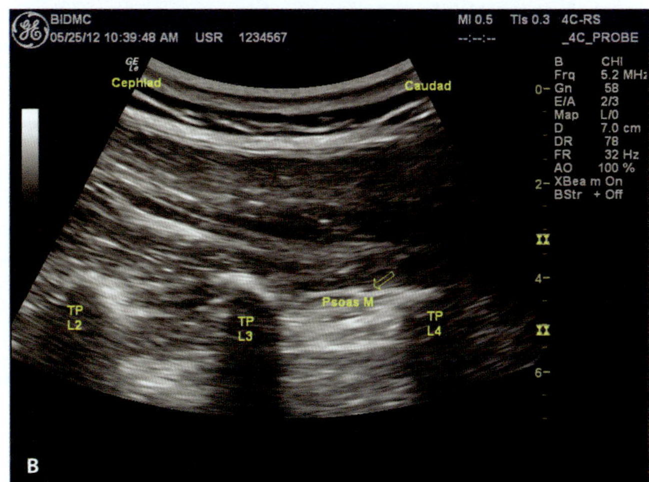

FIGURE 52-8. **A** and **B**, Paravertebral nerve block. TP, transverse process; CTL, costotransverse ligament; PVS, paravertebral space. The arrow indicates the needle trajectory.

FIGURE 52-9. **A** and **B**, Lumbar plexus nerve block. TP, transverse process. The arrow indicates the needle trajectory.

needle punctures the dural sheath that extends from the intervertebral foramen. *Systemic toxicity* of local anesthetic may be caused by more rapid absorption of local anesthetic and the larger volumes that are often used for performance of this block.[35]

LUMBAR PLEXUS NERVE BLOCK

Surgical Indications This block is used for hip, thigh, and knee procedures.

Anatomic Coverage This block covers the lumbar plexus arising from nerve roots L1 to L4 as well as the subcostal branch of T12, passing through the psoas. It gives innervation to the hip and anterior and medial thigh and sensory innervation to the medial aspect of the foot as the terminal branch of the saphenous nerve.

Technique Using a deep (low-frequency) ultrasound probe, the ultrasound is oriented in a sagittal direction, starting with the junction of L5 and the sacrum. The ultrasound probe is then moved cranially to count up and visualize the transverse processes of L2, L3, and L4 (**Fig. 52-9A**). This is considered the "trident sign," and the psoas muscle is seen between the bony shadows of the transverse processes in this location (**Fig. 52-9B**).[36] The nerve roots of the lumbar plexus are occasionally seen depending on patient anatomy, appearing as hyperechoic structures. The block needle is inserted in plane to rest between the transverse processes of L3 and L4 in the posterior portion of the psoas muscle. After negative aspiration, 20 to 25 mL of local anesthetic is deposited in an incremental fashion.

Contraindications Contraindications include infection, hematoma, and nerve injury. This block is considered a deeper block in a noncompressible area, so caution is advised in performing this block in a coagulopathic patient. Reports of retroperitoneal hemorrhage have been reported.

Complications Possible complications include retroperitoneal hemorrhage.[37,38] This block results in significant motor weakness to the thigh and leg, rendering the patient at risk for falls for the duration of the block.[39,40]

TRANSVERSUS ABDOMINIS PLANE BLOCK

Surgical Indications This block is used for abdominal surgery, including midline, oblique, and transverse incisions. The use of the transversus abdominis plane (TAP) block has shown the ability to decrease postoperative pain ratings as well as postoperative opiate consumption in patients undergoing abdominal surgery.[41] This block is particularly useful in patients who cannot receive epidural anesthesia for postoperative pain control.

Anatomic Coverage This block covers the parietal peritoneum as well as the skin and musculature of the abdominal wall.

Technique The ultrasound probe is oriented transversely over the anterolateral abdominal wall, where the three muscle layers from superficial to deep are imaged (external oblique, internal oblique, and transversus abdominis). The probe is moved posterolaterally to lie across the midaxillary line just superior to the iliac crest (over the triangle of petit) (**Fig. 52-10A**). The needle is inserted from anterior to posterior in direct view of the ultrasound beam, with the end point in the plane between the internal oblique and the transversus abdominis muscles to block the lateral nerve branches (**Fig. 52-10B**).[42] There is a trend toward superior analgesia when 15 mL or more of local anesthetic is used per side,[43] so a larger volume (~20 mL) of a lower concentration (bupivacaine 0.25% or ropivacaine 0.2%) is our preferred solution of choice.

Contraindications Contraindications include infection or surgical intervention (i.e., colostomy stoma) over the planned insertion site. Also, morbid obesity can make technical performance of this block either difficult or impossible depending on the ability to visualize the abdominal musculature via ultrasonography.

Complications To date, there have been no case reports of toxicity arising from TAP blocks.[44] There is potential for entering the peritoneal cavity and subsequent damage to visceral structures. There have been several accounts of liver laceration from right-sided TAP blocks, including one ultrasound-guided block, which was probably attributable to failure to fully visualize the needle tip before advancement.[45]

LOWER EXTREMITY

FEMORAL NERVE BLOCK

Surgical Indications This block is used for thigh and knee procedures.

Anatomic Coverage The femoral nerve, arising from the second, third, and fourth lumbar nerves, makes up the largest branch of the lumbar plexus. It supplies sensory and motor innervation to the anterior thigh and knee; therefore, blockade results in anesthesia of these areas.

Technique The orienting structure is the femoral artery at the level of the inguinal ligament. The patient is placed supine, and the inguinal area of the desired side is prepped in sterile fashion. The probe is held in a coronal orientation in the inguinal crease to obtain images of the nerve, artery, and vein in cross-section, listed in lateral to medial orientation (**Fig. 52-11**). The needle is advanced from lateral to medial direction to inject 20 to 30 mL of local anesthetic circumferentially around the nerve. Care is taken to note the surrounding vasculature and avoid inadvertent puncture with needle advancement.

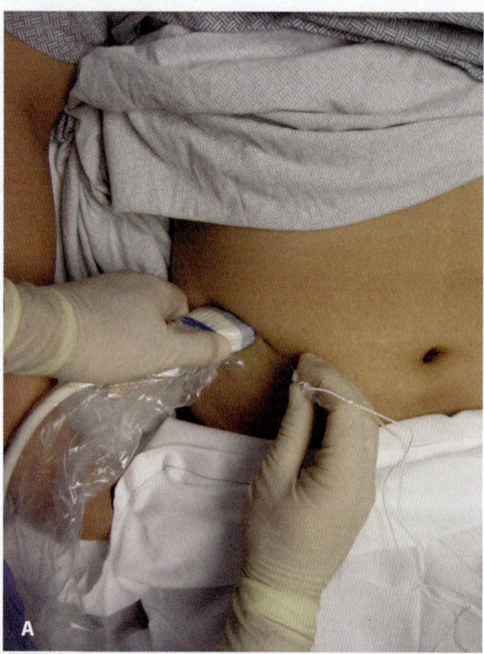

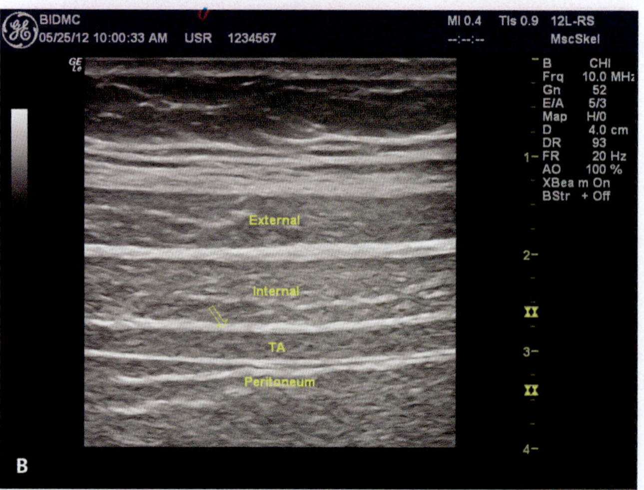

FIGURE 52-10. **A** and **B**, Transversus abdominis plane block. TA, transversus abdominis. The arrow indicates the needle trajectory.

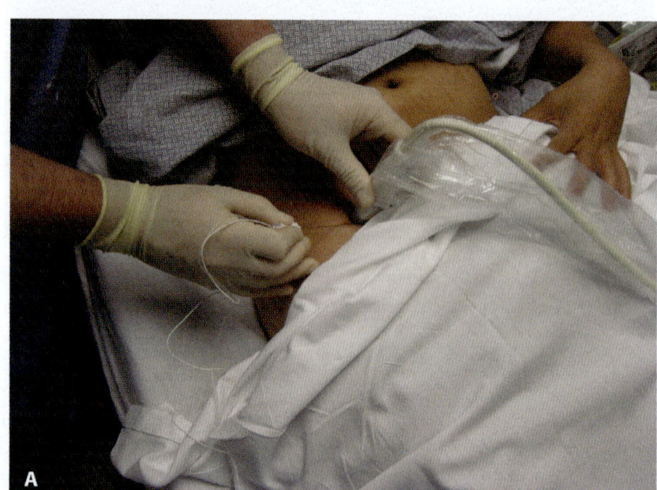

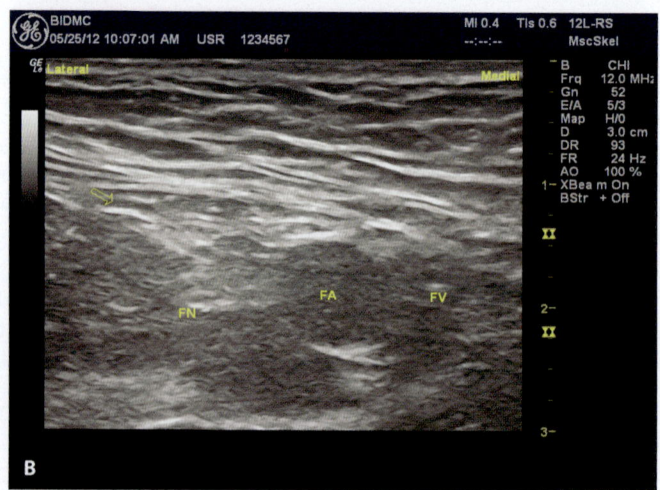

FIGURE 52-11. **A** and **B**, Femoral nerve (FN) block. The arrow indicates the needle trajectory. FA, femoral artery; FV, femoral vein; FN, femoral nerve.

Contraindications Underlying weakness or balance disturbance may be considered a relative contraindication given the fall risk inherent to femoral nerve blockade.

Complications Possible complications include infection, hematoma, and nerve injury. Quadriceps weakness is inherent in this blockade, so it is important to educate patients that they have a significant risk for falls until full motor strength has returned.[46–48]

SCIATIC NERVE BLOCK

Surgical Indications This block is used for procedures on the posterior aspect of the leg and any procedure below the knee.

Anatomic Coverage The sciatic nerve is formed from branches of the lumbar plexus, specifically L4 to S3. It travels in the posterior thigh until reaching the popliteal fossa, where it divides into the tibial (medial) and common peroneal nerves (lateral). It supplies sensory motor innervation to the posterior leg, ankle, and foot, with the exception of the medial portions of the distal leg, ankle, and foot (which are supplied by the saphenous nerve, a sensory branch of the femoral nerve).

Technique The orienting structure in the subgluteal approach is the bony landmark of the greater trochanter. The patient is positioned laterally with the side to be blocked up. Using a lower-frequency abdominal probe, the greater trochanter is located on the lateral thigh, and the probe is slid posteriorly to rest in the subgluteal fossa, locating the thick sciatic nerve traveling between the greater trochanter and the ischial tuberosity (**Fig. 52-12**).[49]

Contraindications Contraindications include infection, hematoma, and nerve injury. Underlying weakness or balance disturbance may be considered a relative contraindication given the fall risk inherent to sciatic nerve blockade.

Complications Given the motor weakness of the hamstring muscles, foot, and ankle inherent to this block, the patient is considered to be at risk for falls until full resolution.[50]

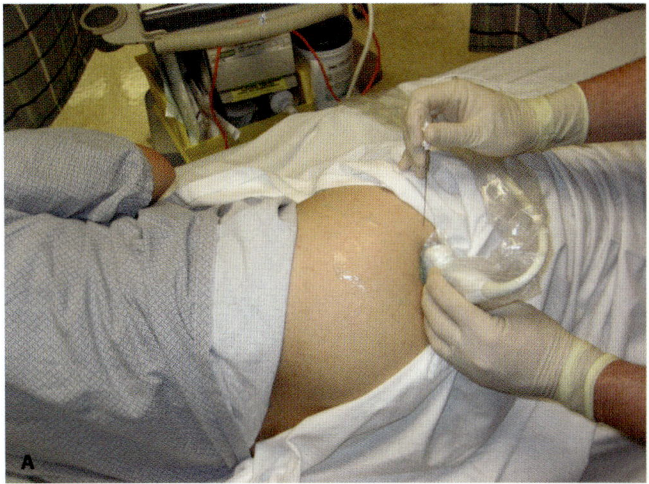

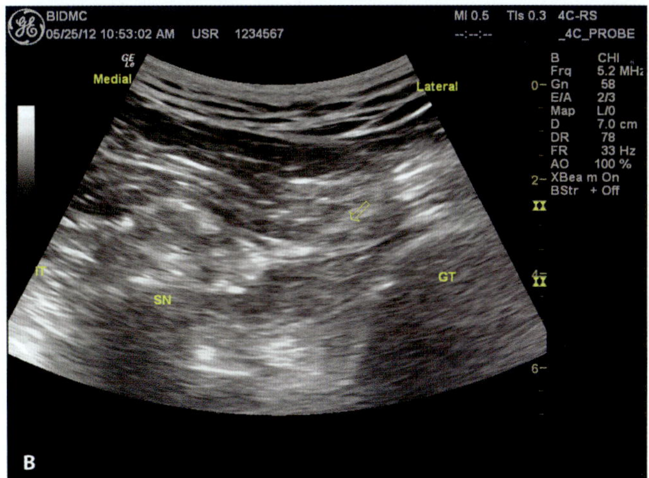

FIGURE 52-12. **A** and **B**, Sciatic nerve (SN) block. The arrow indicates the needle trajectory. GT, greater trochanter; IT, ischial tuberosity.

POPLITEAL NERVE BLOCK

Surgical Indications This block is used for surgical procedures of the leg, ankle, and foot.

Anatomic Coverage The popliteal nerve block is blockade of the sciatic nerve in the popliteal fossa, encompassing the tibial and common peroneal components of the sciatic nerve. This block requires supplementation when the surgical site includes the medial portion of the distal leg, ankle, and foot (supplied by the saphenous nerve, a sensory branch of the femoral nerve).

Technique Most practitioners position the patient either laterally with the affected leg up or prone to access the posterior aspect of the leg. The orienting structures are the popliteal vascular structures at the level of the popliteal fossa. The tibial component of the sciatic nerve can be reliably located slightly lateral and posterior to the vascular component (**Figs. 52-13A** and **52-13B**). The tibial component of the nerve is traced in a superior fashion up the leg (**Fig. 52-13C**) until the common peroneal component is observed joining it (**Figs. 52-13D** and **52-13E**).

Contraindications Contraindications include infection, hematoma, and nerve injury. Care must be taken to note any preexisting neurologic deficit of the leg, ankle, and foot, which may be worsened with the motor blockade achieved by this block.

Complications A well-placed popliteal block renders the patient with foot drop as well as lack of proprioception of the foot on the blocked side, so the patient is considered to be at risk for falls until full resolution of the block.

SAPHENOUS NERVE BLOCK

Surgical Indications This block is used for the medial aspect of the leg below the knee, ankle, and foot.

Anatomic Coverage The saphenous nerve is the sensory portion of the femoral nerve extending below the knee, innervating the medial aspects of the leg, ankle, and foot. This block is often required as a supplement to a popliteal and sciatic block when coverage of the medial aspect of the lower leg is required. This area can also be covered with a femoral nerve block if the anterior thigh and knee are to be anesthetized as well.

Technique The saphenous nerve can be blocked at multiple levels in the leg. The authors most often use a transsartorial approach. This involves placing the patient supine with the operative leg rotated externally. The ultrasound probe is placed transversely on the medial aspect of the distal thigh, with the femur being visualized. The probe is then moved proximally until the vastus medialis is viewed and continues proximal until the sartorius muscle is viewed. At the intersection of these two muscles, the hyperechoic saphenous nerve is located (**Fig. 52-14**). The needle is advanced from lateral to medial to approach the target nerve. When it is adjacent to the nerve, after negative aspiration, 5 to 10 mL of local anesthetic is deposited around the nerve, with care taken to not puncture the descending genicular artery, which can travel with the nerve in this location.

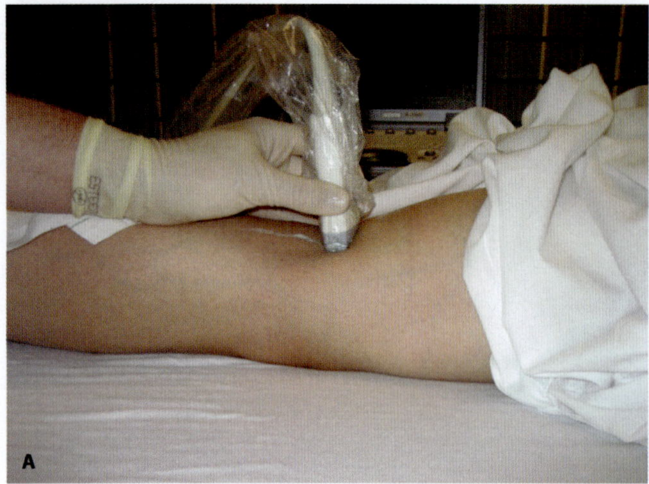

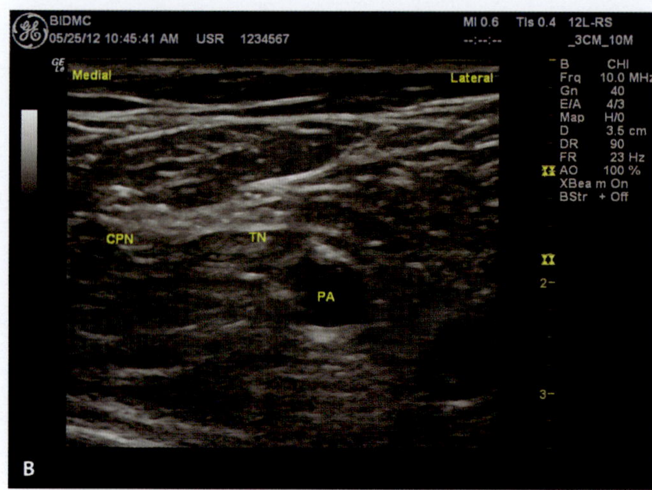

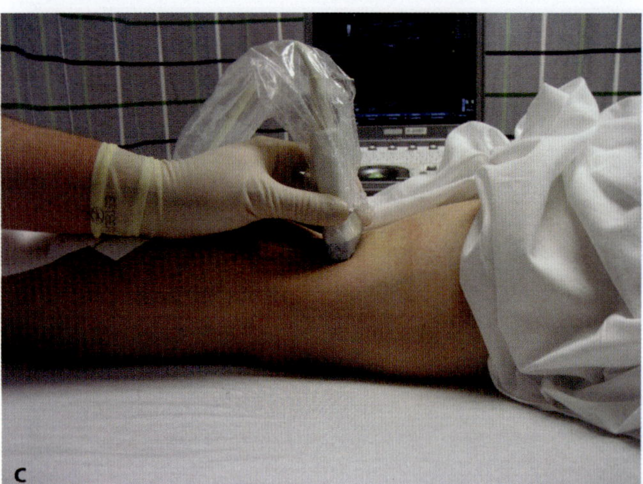

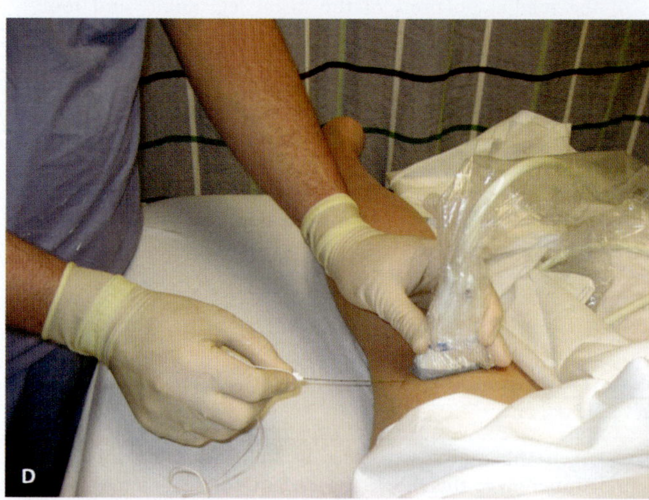

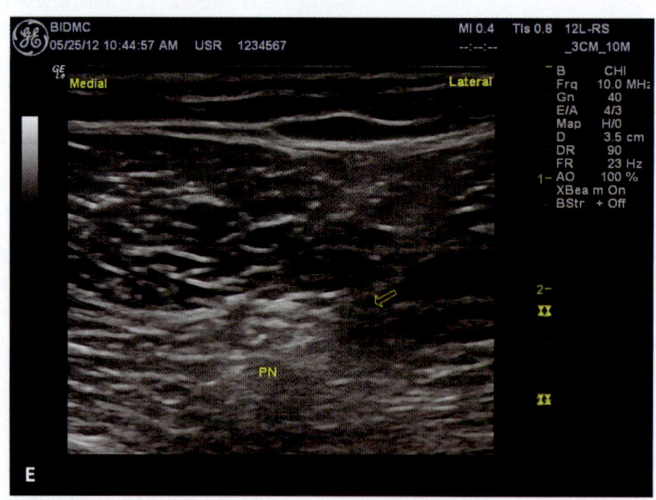

FIGURE 52-13. **A**, Popliteal nerve block; the probe is placed in the popliteal fossa initially. **B**, CPN, common peroneal nerve; PA, popliteal artery; TN, tibial nerve. **C**, The probe is moved from the popliteal fossa cephalad following the courses of the common peroneal nerve and tibial nerve until they join to form the sciatic nerve. **D**, Location of needle insertion. **E**, PN, popliteal nerve. The arrow indicates the needle trajectory.

Contraindications Contraindications include infection and skin breakdown over the needle insertion site.

Complications Possible complications include infection, hematoma, and nerve injury.

ANKLE BLOCK

Surgical Indications This block is used for foot or toe surgery.

Anatomic Coverage This block covers the five nerves that innervate the foot—four derived from the sciatic (posterior tibial, deep peroneal,

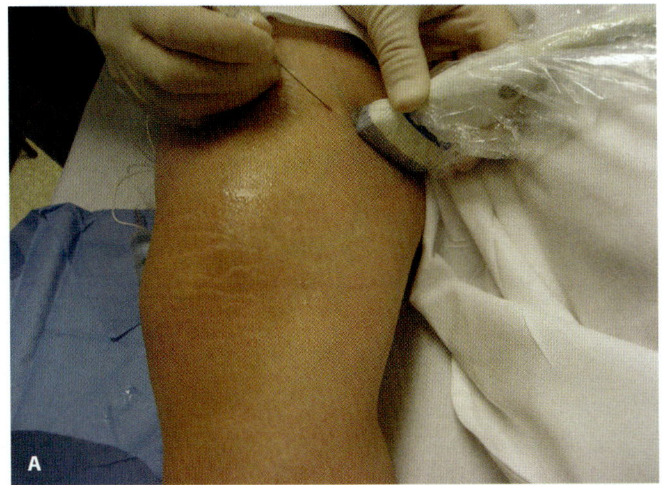

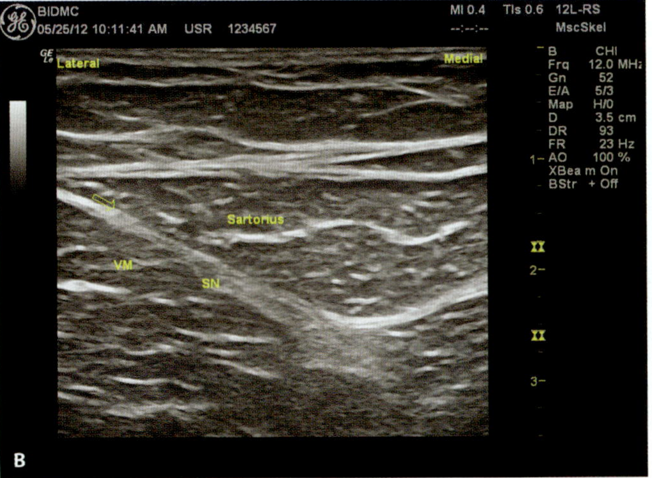

FIGURE 52-14. A and B, Saphenous nerve (SN) block. VM, vastus medialis. The arrow indicates the needle trajectory.

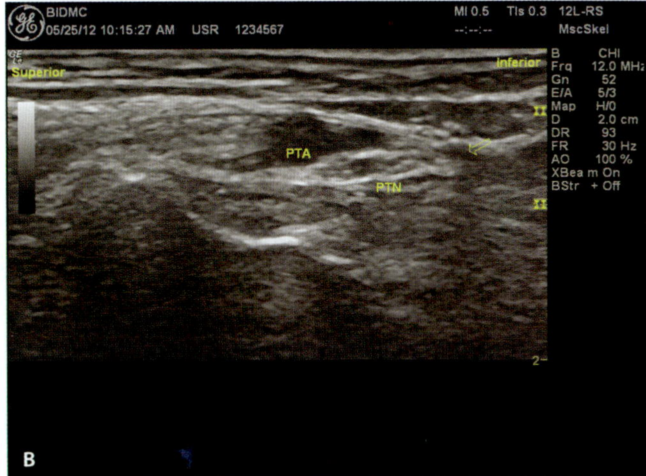

FIGURE 52-15. A, Posterior tibial nerve block. B, PTA, posterior tibial artery; PTN, posterior tibial nerve block. The arrow indicates the needle trajectory.

superficial peroneal, and sural) and one derived from the femoral (the saphenous nerve).

Technique The two deep nerves (posterior tibial and deep peroneal) are blocked by injection under the superficial fascia while the three superficial nerves (saphenous, sural, and superficial peroneal) are blocked by a subcutaneous skin infiltration. Described here are techniques using ultrasound guidance to locate the posterior tibial, deep peroneal, and sural nerves.

Posterior Tibial Nerve Block In performing an ankle block for foot surgery, the posterior tibial nerve should be blocked first because this nerve provides the majority of the sensation to the bottom of foot, including the deeper bony structures. This nerve courses between the Achilles tendon and medial malleolus, traveling slightly posterior and deep to the posterior tibial artery as it travels inferior to the medial malleolus (**Fig. 52-15**). The flexor hallucis longus tendon also travels with the neurovascular structures at this level, distinguished from the nerve by showing tendon movement with great toe flexion while the nerve is stationary. Using ultrasound to locate the nerve and injecting 5 mL of local anesthetic results in a greater success rate and quality of block compared with the traditional landmark technique.[51]

The saphenous nerve block is accomplished by infiltrating a subcutaneous ring of local anesthetic on the medial aspect of the ankle, from the medial malleolus to the Achilles tendon. To minimize the number of needle punctures, after placement of the posterior tibial block, subcutaneous infiltration of this area is achieved while the needle is withdrawn (**Fig. 52-16**).

Deep Peroneal Nerve Block It is possible to identify the deep peroneal nerve just lateral to the anterior tibial artery at the anterior aspect of the ankle at the level of the medial malleolus (**Fig. 52-17**).[52] However, this is compared with the traditional landmark technique consisting of injection between the tendons of the tibialis anterior and the extensor hallucis longus, contacting bone, and then injecting an equivalent volume of 5 mL of local anesthetic upon withdrawal of the needle by 1 to 2 mm. The ultrasound technique results in a denser motor block at 10 minutes compared with the landmark technique, but the overall success rate of the block was equivocal.[53]

For the superficial peroneal nerve block, on withdrawal of the needle after deep peroneal block, a subcutaneous ring infiltration of local anesthetic is administered in a fanlike distribution across the anterior surface of the ankle (**Fig. 52-18**).

The sural nerve is consistently located slightly medial to the lesser saphenous vein anterolateral to the Achilles tendon at the lateral malleolus. Use of ultrasound to locate the lesser saphenous vein (potentially using a tourniquet to distend the vessel) and the performance of a perivascular technique with 5 mL of local anesthetic results in a greater success rate and quality of block compared with the traditional landmark technique (**Fig. 52-19**).[54]

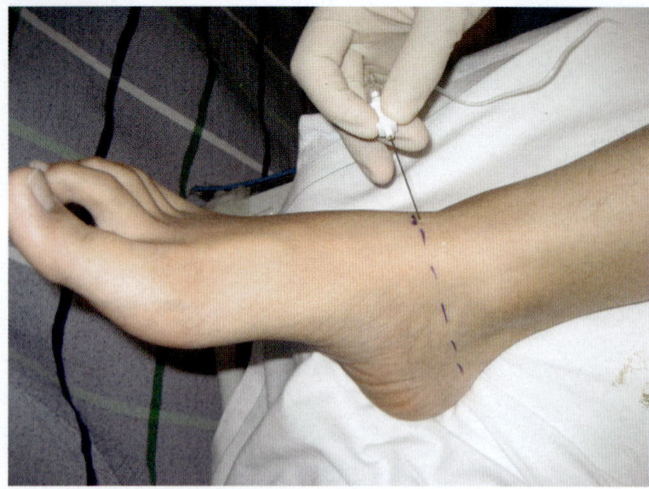

FIGURE 52-16. Saphenous nerve block at the ankle performed by injecting a subcutaneous skin ring of local anesthetic around the medial aspect of the ankle in the area shown.

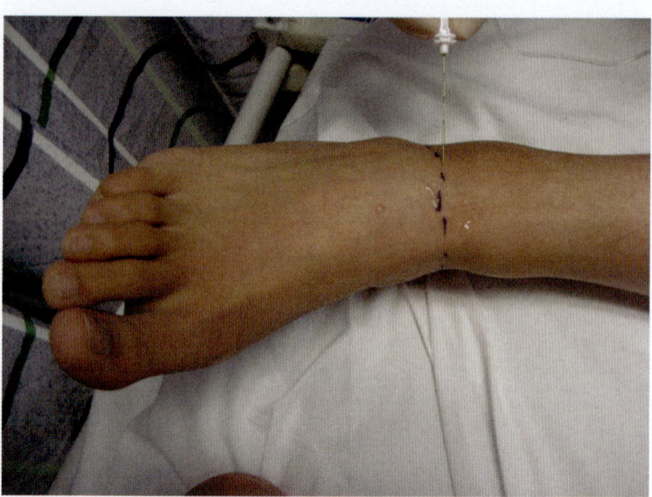

FIGURE 52-18. Superficial peroneal nerve block; upon withdrawal of the needle for the deep peroneal nerve block, a subcutaneous ring of local anesthetic is injected across the anterior surface of the ankle in the area shown.

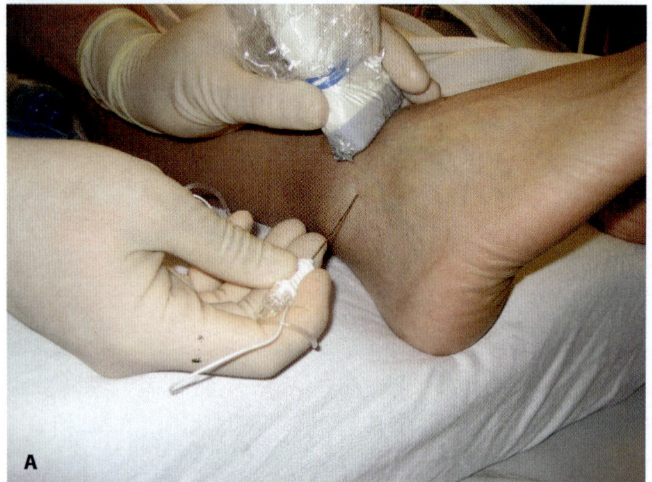

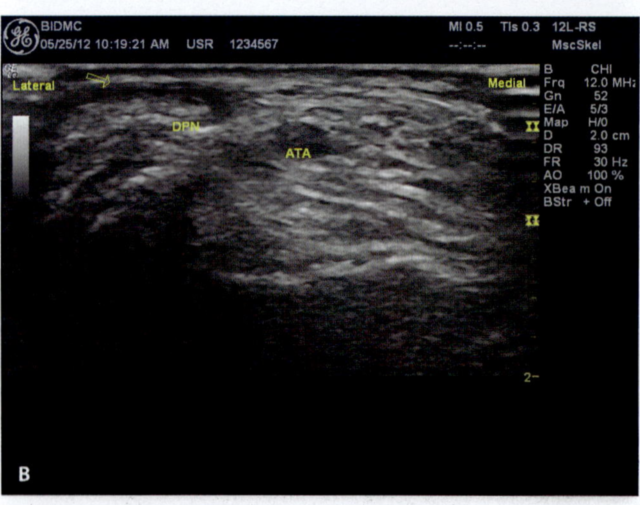

FIGURE 52-17. **A** and **B**, Deep peroneal nerve block. ATA, anterior tibial artery; DPN, deep peroneal nerve. The arrow indicates the needle trajectory.

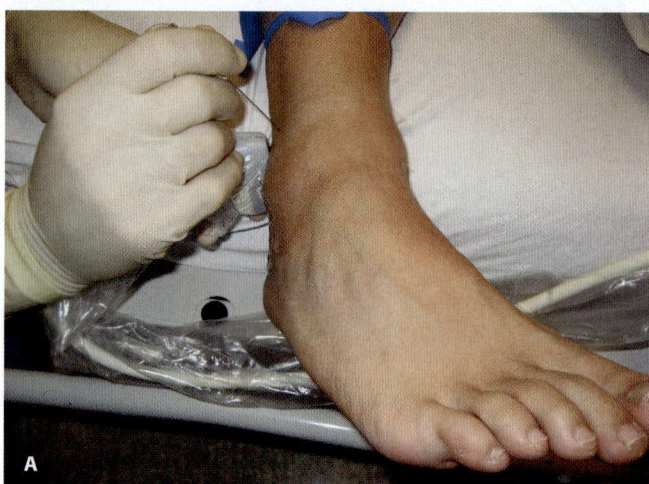

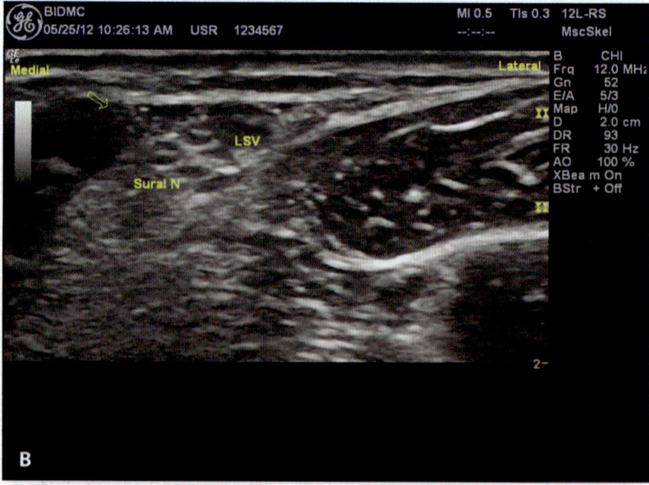

FIGURE 52-19. **A** and **B**, Sural nerve block (note tourniquet use to aid in identification of lesser saphenous vein). The arrow indicates the needle trajectory. LSV, lesser saphenous vein; Sural N, sural nerve.

Local anesthetic choice is determined by the required duration of action. For significant postoperative pain relief, 0.5% ropivacaine is a typically used agent. Duration also appears to be a function of local anesthetic volume, so total volumes of 16 mL of 0.5% ropivacaine show significantly inferior analgesia during the first 24 hours after foot surgery compared with blocks using 30 mL of 0.5% ropivacaine.[55] Traditionally, epinephrine-containing solutions are avoided in foot and ankle blocks because of a fear of ischemia in a distal site.

Contraindications Contraindications include infection or skin breakdown over the needle insertion site and coagulopathy.

Complications Possible complications include infection (rare), hematoma, intravascular injection into the smaller veins of the foot, and nerve injury.

REFERENCES

1. McCartney, CJ, Brull, R, Chan, VW. Early but no long-term benefits of regional compared with general anesthesia for ambulatory hand surgery. *Anesthesiology*. 2004;101:461-467.
2. Jacob, AK, Walsh, MT, Dilger, JA. Role of regional anesthesia in the ambulatory environment. *Anesthesiol Clin*. 2010;28(2):252-256.
3. Horlocker, TT, Wedel DJ, Rowlingson JC, et al. Regional anesthesia in the patient receiving antithrombotic or thrombolytic therapy. *Reg Anesth Pain Med*. 2010;35(1):64-101.
4. Neal JM, Bernards CM, Butterworth JF, et al. ASRA Practice advisory on local anesthetic toxicity. *Reg Anesth Pain Med*. 2010;35(2):152-193.
5. American Society of Anesthesiologists. Monitoring standards. Available at: http://www.asahq.org/For-Members/Standards-Guidelines-and-Statements.aspx. Park Ridge, IL.
6. Winnie AP. Interscalene brachial plexus block. *Anesth Analg*. 1970;49:455-466.
7. Neal JM, Hebl JR, Gerancher JC, et al. Brachial plexus anesthesia: essentials of our current understanding. *Reg Anesth Pain Med*. 2002;27:402-428.
8. Spence BC, Beach ML, Gallagher JD, et al. Ultrasound-guided interscalene blocks: understanding where to inject the local anaesthetic. *Anaesthesia*. 2011;66(6):509-514.
9. Renes SH, Rettig HC, Gielen MJ, et al. Ultrasound-guided low-dose interscalene brachial plexus block reduces the incidence of hemidiaphragmatic paresis. *Reg Anesth Pain Med*. 2009;34(5):498-502.
10. Riazi S, Carmichael N, Awad I, et al. Effect of local anaesthetic volume (20 vs 5 ml) on the efficacy and respiratory consequences of ultrasound-guided interscalene brachial plexus block. *Br J Anaesth*. 2008;101(4):549-556.
11. Lee JH, Cho SH, Kim SH, et al. Ropivacaine for ultrasound-guided interscalene block: 5 mL provides similar analgesia but less phrenic nerve paralysis than 10 mL. *Can J Anaesth*. 2011;58(11):1001-1006.
12. Urmey WF, Talts KH, Sharrock NE. One hundred percent incidence of hemi-diaphragmatic paresis associated with interscalene brachial plexus anesthesia as diagnosed by ultrasonography. *Anesth Analg*. 1991;91:498-503.
13. Renes SH, Rettig HC, Gielen MJ, et al. Ultrasound-guided low-dose interscalene brachial plexus block reduces the incidence of hemidiaphragmatic paresis. *Reg Anesth Pain Med*. 2009;34(5):498-502.
14. Riazi S, Carmichael N, Awad I, et al. Effect of local anaesthetic volume (20 vs 5 mL) on the efficacy and respiratory consequences of ultrasound-guided interscalene brachial plexus block. *Br J Anaesth*. 2008;101(4):549-556.
15. Lee JH, Cho SH, Kim SH, et al. Ropivacaine for ultrasound-guided interscalene block: 5 mL provides similar analgesia but less phrenic nerve paralysis than 10 mL. *Can J Anaesth*. 2011;58(11):1001-1006.
16. Urmey WF, McDonald M. Hemidiaphragmatic paresis during interscalene brachial plexus block: effects on pulmonary function and chest wall mechanics. *Anesth Analg*. 1992;74:352-357.
17. Hortense A, Perez MV, Amaral JL, et al. Interscalene brachial plexus block: effects on pulmonary function. *Rev Bras Anestesiol*. 2010;60(2):130-137, 74-78.
18. Seltzer JL. Hoarseness and Horner's syndrome after interscalene brachial plexus block. *Anesth Analg*. 1977;56(4):585-586.
19. Soares LG, Brull R, Lai J, et al. Eight ball, corner pocket: the optimal needle position for ultrasound-guided supraclavicular block. *Reg Anesth Pain Med*. 2007;32(1):94-95.
20. Macfarlane AJ, Perlas A, Chan V, et al. Eight ball, corner pocket ultrasound-guided supraclavicular block: avoiding a scratch. *Reg Anesth Pain Med*. 2008;33(5):502-503; author reply 504.
21. Neal JM, Moore JM, Kopacz DJ, et al. Quantitative analysis of respiratory, motor, and sensory function after supraclavicular block. *Anesth Analg*. 1998;86:1239-44
22. Renes SH, Spoormans HH, Gielen MJ, et al. Hemidiaphragmatic paresis can be avoided in ultrasound-guided supraclavicular brachial plexus block. *Reg Anesth Pain Med*. 2009;34(6):595-599.
23. Sahin L, Gul R, Mizrak A, et al. Ultrasound-guided infraclavicular brachial plexus block enhances postoperative blood flow in arteriovenous fistulas. *J Vasc Surg*. 2011;54(3):749-753.
24. Trande QH, Russo G, Muñoz L, et al. A prospective, randomized comparison between ultrasound-guided supraclavicular, infraclavicular, and axillary brachial plexus blocks. *Reg Anesth Pain Med*. 2009;34(4):366-371.
25. Koscielniak-Nielsen ZJ, Frederiksen BS, Rasmussen H, et al. A comparison of ultrasound-guided supraclavicular and infraclavicular blocks for upper extremity surgery. *Acta Anaesthesiol Scand*. May 2009;53(5):620-626.
26. Ruíz A, Sala X, Bargalló X, et al. The influence of arm abduction on the anatomic relations of infraclavicular brachial plexus: an ultrasound study. *Anesth Analg*. Jan 2009;108(1):364-366.
27. Fredrickson MJ, Wolstencroft P, Kejriwal R, et al. Single versus triple injection ultrasound-guided infraclavicular block: confirmation of the effectiveness of the single injection technique. *Anesth Analg*. 2010;111(5):1325-1327.
28. Davies, RG, Myles PS, Graham JM. A comparison of analgesic efficacy and side-effects of paravertebral vs. epidural blockade for thoracotomy—a systematic review and meta-analysis of randomized trials. *Br J Anaesth*. 2006;96(4):418-426.
29. Hadzic A, Kerimoglu B, Loreio D, et al. Paravertebral blocks provide superior same-day recovery over general anesthesia for patients undergoing inguinal hernia repair. *Anesthesia Analgesia*. 2006;102(4):1076-1081.
30. O Riain SC, Donnell BO, Cuffe T, et al. Thoracic paravertebral block using real-time ultrasound guidance. *Anesth Analg*. 2010;110(1):248-251.
31. Hara K, Sakura S, Nomura T, et al. Ultrasound guided thoracic paravertebral block in breast surgery. *Anaesthesia*. 2009;64(2):223-225.
32. Das S, Bhattacharya P, Mandal MC, et al. Multiple-injection thoracic paravertebral block as an alternative to general anaesthesia for elective breast surgeries: a randomised controlled trial. *Indian J Anaesth*. 2012;56(1):27-33.
33. Kaya FN, Turker G, Mogol EB, et al. Thoracic paravertebral block for video-assisted thoracoscopic surgery: single injection versus multiple injections. *J Cardiothorac Vasc Anesth*. 2012;26(1):90-94.
34. Naja Z, Lonnqvist PA. Somatic paravertebral nerve blockade. Incidence of failed block and complications. *Anesthesia*. 2001;56(12):1184-1188.

35. Karmarkar MK, Ho AM, Law BK, et al. Arterial and venous pharmacokinetics of ropivacaine with and without epinephrine after thoracic paravertebral block. *Anesthesiology* 2005;103(4):704-711.

36. Karmaker MK, Ho AM-H, Li X, et al. Ultrasound-guided lumbar plexus block through the acoustic window of the lumbar ultrasound trident. *Br J Anaesth.* 2008;100(4):533-537.

37. Weller RS, Gerancher JC, Crews JC, et al. Extensive retroperitoneal hematoma without neurologic deficit in two patients who underwent lumbar plexus block and were later anticoagulated. *Anesthesiology.* 2003;98(2):581-585.

38. Aveline C, Bonnet F. Delayed retroperitoneal haematoma after failed lumbar plexus block. *Br J Anaesth.* 2004;93(4):589-591.

39. Muraskin SI, Conrad B, Zheng N, et al. Falls associated with lower extremity blocks: a pilot investigation of mechanisms. *Reg Anesth Pain Med.* 2007;32(1):67-72.

40. Atkinson HD, Hamid I, Gupte CM, et al. Postoperative fall after the use of the 3-in-1 femoral nerve block for knee surgery: a report of four cases. *J Orthop Surg (Hong Kong).* 2008;16(3):381-384.

41. Charlton S, Cyna AM, Middleton P, et al. Perioperative transversus abdominis plane (TAP) blocks for analgesia after abdominal surgery. *Cochrane Database Syst Rev.* 2010;8. Article ID CD007705.

42. Hebbard P, Fujiwara Y, Shibata Y, et al. Ultrasound-guided transversus abdominis plane (TAP) block. *Anaesth Intensive Care.* 2007;35(4):616-617.

43. Abdallah FW, Chan VW, Brull R. Transversus abdominis plane block: a systematic review. *Reg Anesth Pain Med.* 2012;37(2):193-209.

44. Young MJ, Gorlin AW, Modest VE, et al. Clinical implications of the transversus abdominis plane block in adults. *Anesthesiol Res Pract.* 2012;2012:731645.

45. Lancaster P, Chadwick M. Liver trauma secondary to ultrasound-guided transversus abdominis plane block. *Br J Anaesth.* 2010;104(4):509–510.

46. Muraskin SI, Conrad B, Zheng N, et al. Falls associated with lower extremity blocks: a pilot investigation of mechanisms. *Reg Anesth Pain Med.* 2007;32(1):67-72.

47. Sharma S, Iorio R, Specht LM, et al. Complications of femoral nerve block for total knee arthroplasty. *Clin Orthop Relat Res.* 2010;468(1):135-140.

48. Kandasami M, Kinninmonth AW, Sarungi M, et al. Femoral nerve block for total knee replacement—a word of caution. *Knee.* 2009;16(2):98-100.

49. Karmakar MK, Kwok WH, Ho AM, et al. Ultrasound-guided sciatic nerve block: description of a new approach at the subgluteal space. *Br J Anaesth.* 2007;98(3):390-395.

50. Muraskin SI, Conrad B, Zheng N, et al. Falls associated with lower extremity blocks: a pilot investigation of mechanisms. *Reg Anesth Pain Med.* Jan-Feb 2007;32(1):67-72.

51. Redborg KE, Antonakakis JG, Beach ML, et al. Ultrasound improves the success rate of a tibial nerve block at the ankle. *Reg Anesth Pain Med.* 2009;34(3):256-260.

52. Benzon HT, Sekhadia M, Benzon HA, et al. Ultrasound-assisted and evoked motor response stimulation of the deep peroneal nerve. *Anesth Analg.* 2009;109(6):2022-2024.

53. Antonakakis JG, Scalzo DC, Jorgenson AS, et al. Ultrasound does not improve the success rate of a deep peroneal nerve block at the ankle. *Reg Anesth Pain Med.* 2010;35(2):217-221.

54. Redborg KE, Sites BD, Chinn CD, et al. Ultrasound improves the success rate of a sural nerve block at the ankle. *Reg Anesth Pain Med.* 2009;34(1):24-28.

55. Fredrickson MJ, White R, Danesh-Clough TK. Low-volume ultrasound-guided nerve block provides inferior postoperative analgesia compared to a higher-volume landmark technique. *Reg Anesth Pain Med.* 2011;36(4):393-398.

Assessment and Treatment of Pain in Sports Injuries

Joanne Borg-Stein
Jennifer Luz
Anna Serels

OVERVIEW

As our knowledge increases regarding the health benefits of exercise, more and more people attempt to stay healthy and physically fit with sports-related activities. As a result, sports injuries are no longer confined to a small group of competitive athletes but affect an ever-growing segment of the population. Improper training techniques, overambitious routines, and the use of faulty equipment have led to an increase in sports injuries (especially overuse injuries) and result in pain. In the pediatric population, children engage in highly competitive sports with training schedules that put them at increased risk for injury. Elite athletes, under the pressure of commercial interests and more widely applied knowledge about exercise physiology and training methods, are driven to greater extremes in order to gain small but significant advantages over the competition. This has led to overambitious workouts with inadequate rest periods. Many athletes suffer from chronic pain and injury as a result.

This chapter presents a review of the essential elements of bone, joint, tendon, ligament, and muscle physiology to lay the foundation for understanding both acute and repetitive stress injuries that are commonly seen in athletics. We will provide treatment strategies for both acute and more chronic pain syndromes.

BASIC PHYSIOLOGY

BONE

Bone is composed of organic proteins, matrix, and cells. The organic component of bone is 90% collagen type I and provides the tensile strength. The mineral phase of bone matrix accounts for 50% of the volume and 65% of the weight of bone and is composed of highly structured hydroxyapatite crystals and amorphous calcium phosphates. Bone cells account for only 3% of bone volume and include osteoblasts, osteoclasts, and osteocytes. Bone remodeling is ongoing throughout life and occurs predominantly at the trabecular part of the skeleton. Wolff's law of adaptation states that mechanical remodeling of bone occurs in response to deforming strain. Both osteoclasts (responsible for bone resorption) and osteoblasts (responsible for bone formation and remodeling) are involved. The exact mechanism of how mechanical strain activates osteocytes to initiate remodeling is still unknown, but both chemical messengers (dependent on the prostaglandins PGI_2 and PGE_2, insulin like growth factor 1 [IGF-1], and parathyroid hormone) and piezoelectric effects are believed to be involved.[1]

High levels of physical activity and stress loading in athletes increase bone density. The degree of increase in bone density is proportional to the level of stress loading accomplished in the athletic activity. For example, the bone mineral density (BMD) of the distal femur is found to be highest in world-class weightlifters followed by throwers, runners, soccer players, and then swimmers. This positive effect on BMD from mechanical loading is also observed in young women skaters and may counter some of the adverse estrogen-deficient effects on bone density seen in woman who are thin and amenorrheic.

Studies on both the elderly and the young confirm that strength training at higher loads increases BMD more compared with endurance training at low weights with high repetitions.[2]

JOINTS

Diarthrodial or synovial joints are capable of large degrees of motion and, under normal circumstances, tolerate high levels of friction, shear, and wear with little deterioration throughout a normal life span. A typical knee

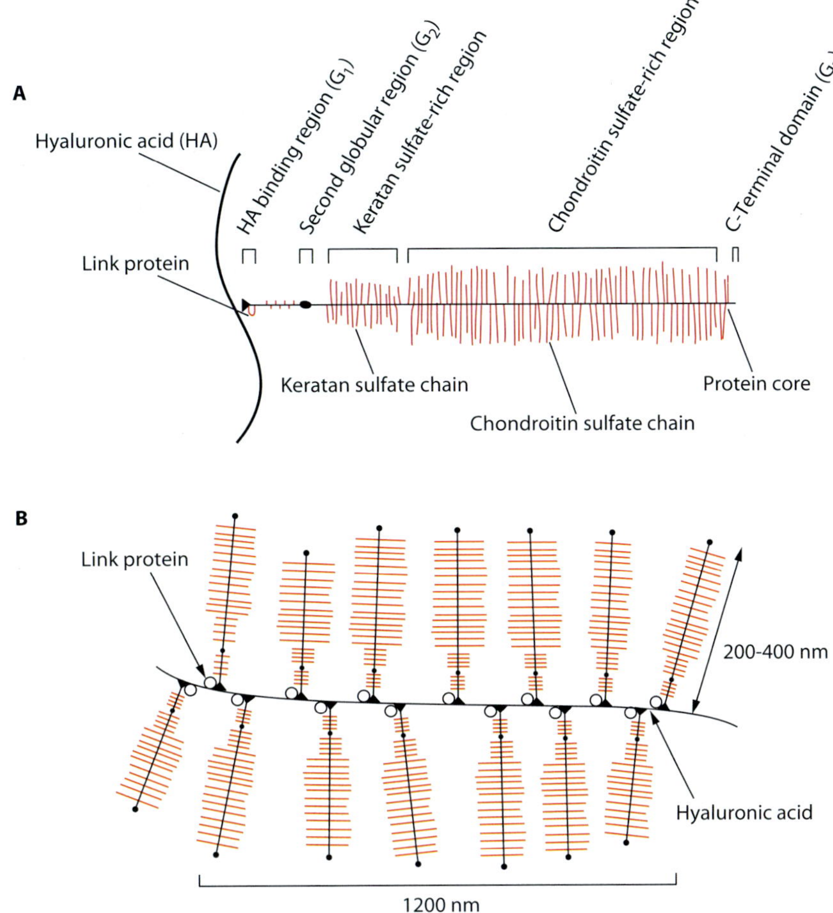

FIGURE 53-1. **(A)** Schematic depiction of the molecular arrangement of the PG monomer. **(B)** The PG aggregates along a hyaluronate chain. (Reproduced with permission from Zimmerman JR, et al. In Chapter 8: Downey JA, Myers SJ, et al, eds. *The Physiological Basis of Rehabilitation Medicine*. 2nd ed. Boston, MA: Butterworth-Heinemann, 1994.)

or hip joint may withstand loads up to six times body weight on a repetitive basis for up to a million times a year.[3] Synovial fluid and soft connective tissue are common to all diarthrodial joints. The soft connective tissue includes the articular cartilage, joint capsule, meniscal cartilage, and ligaments. The primary load-bearing structure of the joint is the articular cartilage. Cartilage is primarily made up of type II collagen with up to 150 proteoglycan (PG) monomers linked to a central core of hyaluronic acid (**Fig. 53-1**). The link between PG and hyaluronic acid is essential for the structural integrity of cartilage. These macromolecules are highly hydrophilic but, because they are confined in the semirigid collagen matrix, reach only 20% of their theoretical swell volume. The absorbent effects caused by the embedded PG are resisted by the tension that develops in the collagen matrix, and it is this balance of forces that is essential for modulating the compressibility of the structure under various loads.

Immobilization of a joint for prolonged periods causes significant loss of PGs in the articular cartilage, which results in a loss of resistance to compression. In the recovery process after injury, both joint range of motion (ROM) and stress loading are necessary to reverse these changes.

TENDONS AND LIGAMENTS

Tendons and ligaments are made up of highly organized collagen fibers (predominantly type I) arranged in a linear fashion. Tendons transmit the force generated by muscle actions to bones and generate movement about a joint. Ligaments are capsular if they extend off the joint capsule or accessory when extending between bones. In contrast to tendons, ligaments prevent excessive movement and contribute to joint stability. Both tendons and ligaments are made up of collagen fascicles that spiral on each other with successive folds or crimps that permit stretch and buffer elongation. The blood supply to tendons and ligaments is sparse compared with joints, muscle, and bone. For example, avascular regions are found in the central region of the anterior cruciate ligament (ACL) of the knee and the supraspinatus tendon of the shoulder.

Tendons are often surrounded by synovial sheaths when there is a significant pulley action present (e.g., the digit flexor tendons of the hand). At the junction with the bone, or enthesis, small synovial bursa are often present to prevent friction (e.g., greater trochanter bursa, retrocalcaneal bursa, and subacromial bursa).

Golgi and Pancinian organs lie at the myotendinous junction and transmit information to the central nervous system (CNS) about muscle tension and pressure. Tendons demonstrate nonlinear deformation in response to stress. In the first phase, collagen fibers straighten and elastic fibers elongate. The second phase requires much greater force and is characterized by breaking of collagen cross-links and disruption of smaller collagen fibers. Finally, increased forces result in tendon rupture, and failure occurs when a tendon is stretched 5% to 8% beyond its resting length (**Fig. 53-2**).

Changes in activity significantly affect tendons and ligaments. Physical training increases the weight and size of tendons and ligaments and increases the cross-links between collagen fibers. Immobilization decreases these cross-links and thus diminishes the tensile strength.

MUSCLE

Skeletal muscle makes up approximately 40% to 45% of the total body weight. There are two major types of muscle fibers (type I and II), which

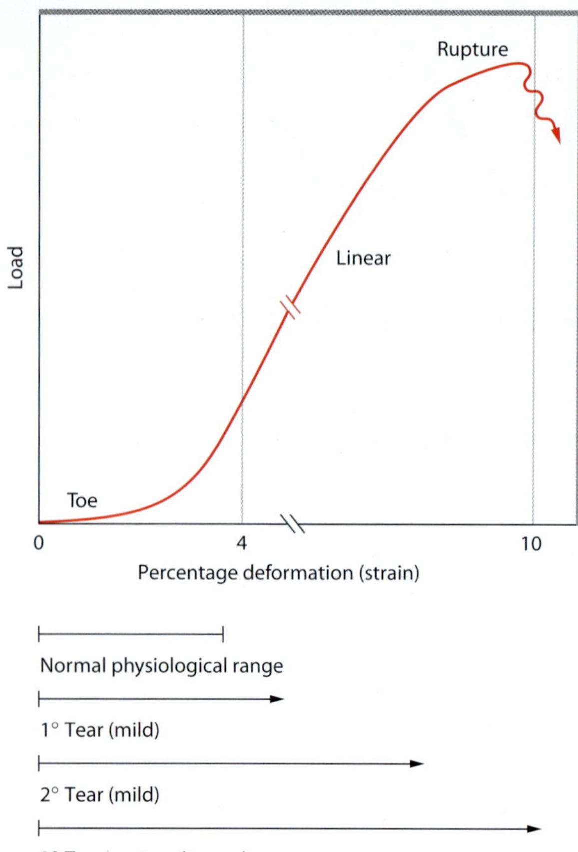

FIGURE 53-2. Load-deformation (strain) curve for ligaments and tendons. The "toe" region of the curve is within the normal physiologic range. Greater than 4% strain causes tissue damage. (Reproduced with permission from Oxford Textbook of Sports Medicine 2nd Edition edited by Harris (1998) Fig. from Chp.4.4.3 "Tendon/Ligament Basic Science" by Oakes p. 584. By permission of Oxford University Press.)

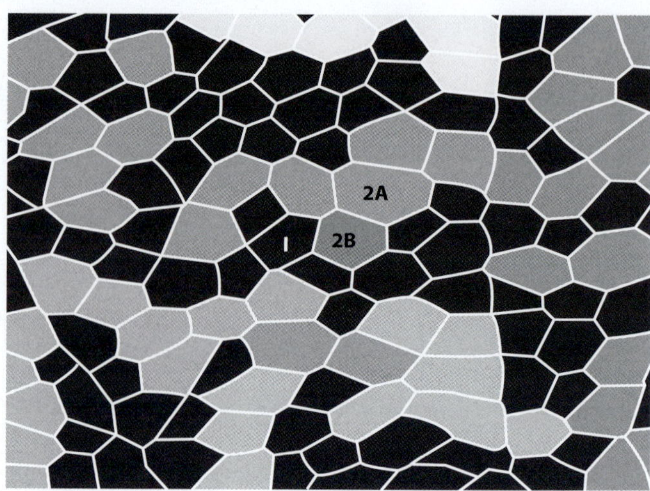

FIGURE 53-3. Photomicrograph of vastus lateralis from a 21-year-old man stained for ATPase at pH 4.6 showing type I, type IIA, and type IIB fibers. (Reproduced with permission from Lieberman JS, et al. Skeletal muscle: structure, chemistry, and function. In: Downey JA, Myers SJ, et al, eds. *The Physiological Basis of Rehabilitation Medicine*. 2nd ed. Boston, MA: Butterworth-Heinemann, 1994: 88.)

were originally identified with basic histochemical staining techniques (**Fig. 53-3**). These staining differences correlate with underlying differences in structural, contractile, and biochemical properties. Subtypes of type I and II have been characterized as well, and **Table 53-1** summarizes the differences among fiber types.

The response of muscle to changes in levels of physical activity can be profound. There are two basic forms of muscle actions: static (or isometric), in which there is no joint movement, and dynamic, in which there is a change in the length of the muscle and joint movement occurs. Dynamic actions can be further divided into concentric, in which the muscle shortens during the increased load (triceps in a shot put hurl), and eccentric, in which the muscle lengthens during the increased load (quadriceps when landing from a jump). Eccentric actions demand a lower metabolic expenditure compared with concentric actions but carry an increased risk of muscle damage and tearing because of higher forces.

Increases in muscle mass with resistance training are primarily brought about by type II fiber hypertrophy (with a contribution from type I hypertrophy) rather than by muscle fiber proliferation. It has been found in animal models that repetitive stretching of muscle fibers alone is sufficient to cause massive increases in gene expression of contractile proteins, causing muscle hypertrophy. The resistance to fatigue that develops with endurance training results from a number of factors, including increases in capillary supply and mitochondrial content (i.e., increase in oxidative capacity) of the muscle fibers and metabolic adaptations favoring fat metabolism and glycogen sparing. It is still a contested question whether transformation of fiber types contributes to the adaptation of muscle to various training stimuli. The predominance of type I fibers in distance runners probably results from genetic influences, environmental factors such as training, and the interaction between the two. Some studies have shown changes in type IIB to type I with high-intensity interval training, but others did not show such changes or have shown only a shift from type IIB to type IIA with endurance training. In disuse atrophy, the reduction of muscle bulk can be profound, with up to 30% reduction in cross-sectional area after 1 month of immobilization. Both type I and type II fibers are reduced in size to varying degrees depending on the individual.[4]

Aging alone has been thought to lead to the loss of muscle mass and strength. There is a loss of both cross-sectional area and total number of muscle fibers with age, predominantly affecting type II. This loss in muscle mass coincides with loss of bone density. However, recent studies have supported the idea that many of the changes seen are not inevitable but are the result of decreased activity. The positive training effects seen on muscles in young people also occur in elderly adults. Even in the 10th decade of life, an elderly person can make significant increases in muscle mass and strength if given a progressive resistance-training program. Similar positive changes in muscle respiratory capacity seen in young people can occur with endurance training in elderly adults.[5]

Finally, the CNS also changes with training. This is evidenced by the marked improvement in performance that can occur with training in a

TABLE 53-1 Muscle Fiber Type Classification

	Type I	Type IIA	Type IIB
Glycogen content	Low	High	High
Mitochondria	Many	Many	Few
Oxidative enzymes	High	Intermediate	Low
Contraction speed	Slow	Fast	Fast
Fatigue resistance	High	High	Low
Aerobic capacity	High	Medium	Low
Anaerobic capacity	Low	Medium	High
Strength	Low	High	High

specific activity over time, with much less dramatic changes in peripheral muscle strength. For example, during a 12-week period of training that included lifting boxes from the floor to the waist by knee extension, a 200% increase in weight was achieved with only a 15% increase in absolute isometric strength of the quadriceps muscle group. Also, the untrained contralateral limb will show an improvement in performance when the ipsilateral limb is repetitively trained, suggesting that the central mechanism plays a role. These changes are felt to result from neural adaptations, including synchronization of motor units in the trained activity with a more advantageous balance of agonist versus antagonist muscle activation.

NERVE

After an acute injury, there is a release of molecules, creating an "inflammatory soup" at the cellular level, including nerve growth factor, bradykinin, serotonin, and prostaglandins. These molecules excite nociceptors, thereby stimulating afferent pain signaling and neurogenic inflammation. Neurogenic inflammation is the process by which active nociceptors release neurotransmitters such as substance P to induce vasodilation, leak proteins and fluids into the extracellular space near the end of the nociceptor, and stimulate immune cells which perpetuate the inflammatory soup.[6]

These processes are evident in acute injuries throughout the musculoskeletal system. For example, human synovial joints are richly innervated in type IVa free nerve endings. These are found in joint capsules, tendons, retinacula, fat pads, synovium, subchondral bone, and surrounding ligaments. They detect pressure and mediate proprioception during joint movement. Muscle and fascia are rich in free nerve endings which detect substance P and mediate nociception. Cadaver studies have shown that substance P and calcitonin gene-related peptide (CGRP) are increasingly expressed in degenerative knees versus healthy subjects. Anatomic studies demonstrate that periosteum is rich in myelinated and unmyelinated sensory fibers, CGRP, and sympathetic nerve fibers expressing tropomyosin receptor kinase A. Hyaline cartilage is avascular and aneural, but cartilage tears initiate local inflammation, which triggers a nociceptive response in adjacent tissue.[7]

The neurogenic inflammation produced after tendon injury includes molecules such as catecholamines, acetylcholine, and glutamate. In addition to its production by nerves, increased levels of glutamate in damaged tendons have been linked to local tenocyte production as well. Substance P may signal tenocytes to modulate their expression of growth factors, proteinases, and proteinase inhibitors. There are more mast cells in tendinopathic tissue as well. Neuropeptides may stimulate mast cells to degranulate and release histamine. Histamine promotes axonal stimulation and neuropeptide release, thereby perpetuating the neurogenic inflammation.[8–10]

A normal tendon is sparsely innervated. However, paratendinous tissue is well supplied with nerves as they run in proximity with the vascular bundle. Most of these nerves are sensory, responding to substance P and CGRP. There is evidence that tendon injury encourages paratendon nerve sprouting and penetration of repairing scar tissue within the tendon body. This is an example of the "failed healing response" that has been demonstrated in tendinopathy. The degeneration and abnormal regeneration includes an aberrant increase in microvessels and nerves, abnormal quality and accelerated remodeling of extracellular matrix (ECM), and increased local metabolism, all within damaged tendons.[8–14]

In a retrospective study by Sanchis-Alfonso and colleagues,[11] the nerve morphologies at the patellar tendon–bone junction of 17 surgical specimens collected during tendon repair were examined. Small nerve fibers discovered in the patellar osteotendinous junction, with increased density at Hoffa's fat pad, led to the hypothesis of "nerve sprouting." This process is similar to that of regeneration after sectioning a nerve. At the osteotendinous junction, there are small nerve fibers which leave the main nerve and disseminate into fibrous tissue. Hoffa's fat pad and the osteotendinous junction are potential sources of nociception resulting from chronic repetitive impingement and compressive forces on the tendon. The samples also revealed neuromatous changes. Nerves were disorganized at the osteotendinous zone with bundles of small nerve fibers immersed in fibrous stroma.[8,11] Similarly, nerve sprouting has been observed in Achilles tendinopathy. The abnormal nerve endings discovered in the Achilles tendon were positive for substance P.[9]

In conjunction with aberrant nerve growth, there is also evidence of altered blood supply to the damaged tendon. Tendon innervation is crucial to normal healing. There is an increase in sensory nerves 2 to 6 weeks after an acute injury; sympathetic nerves are abundant 8 weeks later in areas of repair. Sensory neuropeptides increase blood flow by vasodilation and angiogenesis, and then later sympathetic neuropeptides downregulate blood flow as healing progresses and the metabolic requirement lessens. However, in a damaged tendon, there is increased blood flow.[8,9,11]

For example, increased vascular innervation is most prominent at Hoffa's fat pad adjacent to the inferior pole of the patella in patellar tendinopathy. An increased number of microvessels are associated with the abnormal nerve supply to damaged Achilles tendons as well. Particularly, studies have found a reduced number of sympathetic nerves which modulate blood supply. Perhaps the loss of sympathetic control explains an observed increased blood flow on Doppler ultrasound of tendinopathy.[10]

Neuropathic pain has been studied as a mechanism of chronic tendinopathy. A study by van Wilgen and Keizer[15] examined the presence of "sensitization" by testing for the presence of allodynia with light touch and pressure application to the injury site compared with the contralateral side. There is statistical significance in the fact that sensitized patients suffer more frequently from chronic injury. Frequent injuries promote functional and structural changes within the nervous system that in turn aggravate pain and disability. The authors state that if sensitization is present, antineuropathic medications such as tricyclic antidepressants (TCAs) and anticonvulsants may be effective treatment. Also, treatments that focus on improving functionality, such as eccentric training, instead of pain relief may desensitize the CNS.[15]

INJURY IN SPORTS

Injuries in sports can be caused by a sudden overload to structural components of the bones, joints, and soft tissue or from chronic overuse. The forces that various structures must withstand during athletic activity are enormous. For example, a runner weighing 165 lb will absorb a total of nearly 500,000 lb of force on each foot during a 1.6-km run. Various extrinsic and intrinsic factors influence the type and severity of injury listed in **Table 53-2**. In the majority of injuries that are not traumatic, there has usually been a sudden change in the training routine that underlies the onset of pain. Typically, either there was a recent initiation of a new sport activity or there was a recent marked increase in training load involving changes in frequency, duration, and intensity.

BONE AND JOINT

Bone injury can occur with the extremes of repetitive forces seen in athletics and is characterized by the formation of stress fractures. The

TABLE 53-2 Factors That Influence Injuries in Healthy Athletes

Extrinsic Factors	Intrinsic Factors
Excessive loads	Structural malalignment
Training errors	Muscle weakness or imbalances
Adverse environment (e.g., training surface)	Decreased flexibility
Poor equipment	Joint laxity
Sport rules	Gender or age

incidence of stress fractures in athletic populations of men is approximately 2% and of women from 3.8% to 10%. Up to 49% of women track runners with fewer than five menstrual periods a year develop stress fractures, suggesting that a hypoestrogenic state increases the risk. In runners, stress fractures account for nearly 25% of all injuries.[16] Stress fractures are seen more commonly in different bones depending on the athletic endeavor[17] (**Table 53-3**).

The most common joints injured in sports are the shoulder and the knee. The shoulder is the most unstable joint in the body and depends almost exclusively on ligaments and the tendons of the intrinsic muscles to maintain a balance between the extremes of ROM and stability. As a result, these ligamentous and tendinous structures are commonly injured in sports when this tenuous balance is tested to achieve optimal performance. Both acute and chronic repetitive injuries are seen. **Table 53-4** lists some less common shoulder injuries in the athletic population.[18]

The knee is typically injured acutely because of sudden forces that overwhelm the supporting ligaments. Often, if the loads are sufficient to disrupt the relatively tough intrinsic ligaments of the knee, the cartilaginous structures such as the menisci will also be torn. Common causes of knee pain in athletes include meniscal tears, patellofemoral pain syndrome, ligamentous injuries, patellar tendinitis, and osteochondral injury. In the juvenile population, apophysitis of the tibia (Osgood-Schlatter's syndrome) is often seen. **Table 53-5** lists some less common injuries to the knee in the athletic population.[19]

TABLE 53-3 Stress Fracture Sites

Fracture Site	Return to Sport	Comments
Lower Extremity		
Femoral neck	7–12 weeks	High incidence of late nonunions and avascular necrosis Surgical management often necessary
Femoral shaft	8–14 weeks	Vague thigh or groin pain often only clue
Tibia	Prolonged	Common in runners, dancers, and jumping sports; casting may be necessary, most common stress fracture in the LE
Fibula	6 weeks	Differential diagnosis includes compartment syndrome and peroneal nerve entrapment
Tarsal navicular	16–20 weeks	Commonly missed; 6 weeks of casting, followed by semirigid shoe with medical arch necessary
Metatarsal	4–6 weeks	March fracture; second and third rays most common; rigid shoe recommended to promote healing
Upper Extremity		
Ribs	6–8 weeks	Rare; seen in rowers and baseball players
Clavicle	8 weeks	Rare; found typically with throwing activity
Scapula	6–8 weeks	Rare; intense weightlifting is common etiology
Humerus	10–16 weeks	Seen in adolescent athletes
Olecranon	8–12 weeks	Seen in throwers and gymnasts
Ulna	4–6 weeks	More common; seen in a variety of sports
Radius	12–16 weeks	Commonly seen in gymnasts
Metacarpals	4 weeks	Tennis racquet gripping or ball gripping underlie injuries

LE, lower extremity.

Data from Brukner P. Stress fractures of the upper limb. *Sports Med.* 1998;26:415.

TABLE 53-4 Uncommon Causes of Shoulder Injuries in Athletes

Causes	Comments
Neurovascular	
Suprascapular nerve compression	Commonly caused by traction or blunt trauma; seen in volleyball players
Long thoracic nerve palsy	Scapular winging caused by serratus anterior, weakness
Axillary nerve compression	Seen in throwing athletes
Spinal accessory nerve injury	Trapezius weakness with shoulder sagging after trauma
Thoracic outlet syndrome	Brachial plexus compression; often seen after clavicle fracture
Effort thrombosis	Axillary vein injury commonly with repetitive throwing
Soft Tissue	
SLAP lesions	Deceleration injury to anterior glenoid labrum transmitted by biceps
Posterior-superior impingement	Injury to posterior-superior labrum in throwing sports
Tendon ruptures	Biceps, pectoralis major, subscapularis, coracobrachialis, and serratus
Snapping scapula syndrome	Usually myofascial in origin

SLAP, Superior Labrum, Anterior to Posterior.

SPINE

Just as in the occupational arena, low back pain (LBP) is common in sports. Pain can develop as a result of any of the causes seen in nonathletes. Of particular interest to adolescent athletes is the development of symptomatic spondylolysis with pars interarticularis defects. Spondylolisthesis can occur with bilateral pars defects. Excessive loading of spinal elements during growth in adolescence is believed to be harmful and puts athletes in this age group at greater risk for developing LBP than sedentary control participants. The cumulative prevalence of LBP in juveniles is 30% with only 8% having more chronic or recurrent

TABLE 53-5 Less Common Causes of Knee Injuries in Athletes

Causes	Comments
Neurovascular	
Saphenous nerve entrapment	Fascia of sartorius and vastus medialis 10 cm proximal to medial condyle of femur
Soft Tissue	
Iliotibial band syndrome	Pain at site of friction over lateral femoral condyle; common in runners and cyclists
Popliteus tendinitis	Commonly seen with downhill walking or running
Hoffa's disease	Infrapatellar fat pad syndrome; injured during repetitive extension
Semimembranosus tendinitis	Pain at posteromedial corner of knee; more common with runners
Pes anserinus tendinitis	Common insertion of sartorius, gracilis, and semitendinosus
Tibial collateral ligament bursitis	Deep to medial collateral ligament; pain without locking or instability to valgus stress

problems.[20] Among adolescent athletes referred for evaluation of LBP, up to 47% have been found to have spondylolysis. Stress loading in extension and rotation is thought to be particularly problematic, and as a result, there is a higher prevalence of spondylolysis in sports such as soccer, tennis, wrestling, gymnastics, football, volleyball, and rugby. The level most frequently involved is L5 (88.6%) with L4 seen less often.[21] Spina bifida occulta has been found to be more prevalent in patients with spondylolysis.

SOFT TISSUE

Tendons Tendinitis and muscle strains account for 30% to 50% of all sports injuries. A recent review of the literature on the etiology and treatment of tendinitis suggests that there are few well-controlled prospective studies that can guide care.[22] Nevertheless, some basic concepts are generally accepted. The forces that injure a tendon can be either extrinsic to the tendon itself, causing an impingement on the tendon, or intrinsic, related to excessive stretch forces on the tendon during activity. A common example of an extrinsic tendinitis is *shoulder impingement syndrome*, in which there is inadequate space between the humeral head and the acromion for free passage of the rotator cuff tendons during overhead activity (throwing and swimming), leading to direct tendon trauma. Intrinsic tendinitis commonly results from repetitive overuse or sudden excessive loading as is seen with weightlifting. Eccentric loading of the tendon applies greater forces and under many circumstances can be more traumatic. This occurs when the muscle–tendon complex is lengthening during an action. An example of acute eccentric loading to the patellar tendon occurs when landing from a jump as the knee bends and the quadriceps muscle lengthens to absorb the shock. In addition, a lengthening of the muscle to maximize force generation briefly precedes most concentric actions. This puts the maximum force on the tendon when the tendon is elongated, potentially causing damage.

Acute tendinitis usually is due to a traumatic event and may cause partial or complete rupture of the tendon. In this case, inflammation leads to healing and repair. In contrast, repetitive loading may cause chronic tendon injury or tendinosis. Histologically, there is little inflammation but instead angiofibroblastic changes. The "failed healing response" was discussed previously. The process of acute healing is normally dominated by the growth of type 1 collagen. In contrast, type 3 collagen dominates, producing a thinner, weaker structure in the process of chronic healing. Ultrasound findings include thickened tendon, local hypoechoic areas, irregular fiber structure, and neovascularization. The tendon has a 7.5 times lower oxygen consumption rate than muscle. This gives the advantage of allowing anaerobic metabolism to bear high loads for long periods of time. However, this also puts the tendon at a disadvantage because of slow healing.[12–14,23]

As the tendon's structure becomes disrupted, it loses the ability to absorb forces. Risk factors for the development of tendinosis include age over 35 years, frequency of training more than three times per week, duration of training longer than 30 minutes per session, "demanding" training intensity, and female gender. With advancing age, tendons lose strength, elasticity, and the ability to repair. An aggressive training regimen does not allow time for microtrauma to repair. There is also the observation that the healing responses in load bearing, such as Achilles and patellar tendons versus non–load-bearing tendons, such as the wrist extensors, are different and possible because of varied mechanical stimulation.[12,24]

Ligaments Ligament injuries, or sprains, commonly occur in the knees and ankles of athletes. The etiology of such injuries is almost always the result of a sudden excessive force on the ligament. Examples include a sudden valgus stress to the knee with a football tackle at the knees causing disruption of the medial collateral ligament and a sudden change in direction on a tennis court or football field with the foot firmly planted, which can lead to ACL injury. Joint stability may be significantly impaired with serious ligamentous injury and, if improperly treated, can lead to chronic stresses to the joint and supporting muscles and tendons.

Muscles Muscle injuries occur either from an acute excessive load or from excessive chronic use. Myotendinous failure is a function of the force applied and the strength and level of fatigue of the muscle. The myotendinous junction is highly infolded, increasing the contact surface area by 20 times to provide added strength. As a result, tears occur near but not at the true histologic junction. If severe enough, muscle and tendon tears can occur and be associated with hematomas. Muscles that cross two joints or have a higher percentage of type II fibers are more prone to strain patterns. Examples of such muscles include the hamstrings, the rectus femoris, and the gastrocnemius.

Eccentric actions put muscles at greater risk for strain and can cause the disruption of contractile elements at the Z lines. Delayed onset of muscle soreness is more common after eccentric loading.[25] This condition usually appears 24 to 48 hours after an exercise bout and is associated with high serum levels of intramuscular enzymes such as creatine kinase.

Other causes of muscle pain in sports include muscular contusions by blunt trauma. Myositis ossificans is a complication of muscle contusion characterized by intramuscular calcifications. Exertional rhabdomyolysis can also occur, with or without direct trauma, and is potentially fatal. Complications include compartment syndrome in the affected limb caused by excessive muscle swelling and renal failure.[26] Compartment syndrome can also occur in chronic situations and results from repetitive injury to a muscle group, leading to swelling and increased pressures in the muscle with exertion (often seen in the lower extremities of runners).

NERVE

The differential diagnosis of acute or chronic sports injury should include neurologic processes. In fact, the five most common causes of chronic lower extremity pain are medial tibial stress syndrome; stress fracture; chronic exertional compartment syndrome; popliteal artery entrapment syndrome; and importantly, nerve entrapment. Burning pain during activity, exacerbated by exercise, with regional motor and/or sensory symptoms should include a differential of nerve entrapment. Trauma is a primary cause. Electromyography and nerve conduction studies are helpful in diagnosis.[27–29]

An example of nerve entrapment in the upper extremity is carpal tunnel syndrome. This is also a common injury in nonathletes. In athletes, it is caused by repetitive wrist motion, at times with prolonged dorsi- or palmar flexion. It is most often observed in those participating in racket sports, cycling, or gripping sports. It usually presents with paresthesias at the thumb, index, long digit, or forearm. There may also be hypoalgesia in a dermatomal pattern. The history usually includes nocturnal pain. Tinel's and Phalen's signs are less accurate than the observation of weak thumb abduction, diminished grip strength, thenar atrophy, and loss of two-point discrimination.[27,30,31]

An example of nerve entrapment in the lower extremities is tarsal tunnel syndrome. The tibial nerve or its branches become entrapped, usually as a result of trauma associated with a contusion or poorly fitting footwear. It may be caused by compression from a space-occupying lesion such as venous stasis, local ganglion, tenosynovitis, os trigonum, tumors, bone fragments, or accessory calf muscles. The most common cause in sports injury is biomechanical, including excessive hindfoot pronation and joint hypermobility. This may contribute by provoking a tense abductor halluces muscle, which traps the tibial nerve. Patients may relate cramping, burning, or tingling at the medial ankle or plantar foot. Symptoms worsen with activity and improve with rest, elevation, and looser footwear. Rest or night pain is common. The examination may reveal abnormalities such as forefoot pronation, claw toe, talipes calcaneus, and calcaneovalgus. Provocative testing entails sustained passive eversion and great toe dorsiflexion to exert tension on the nerve.

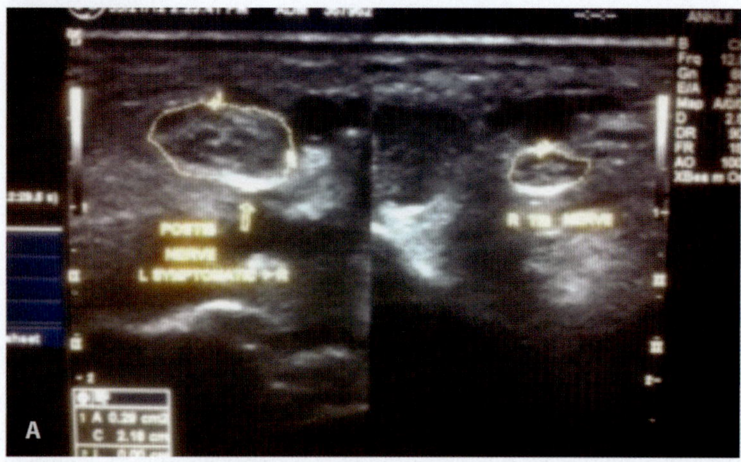

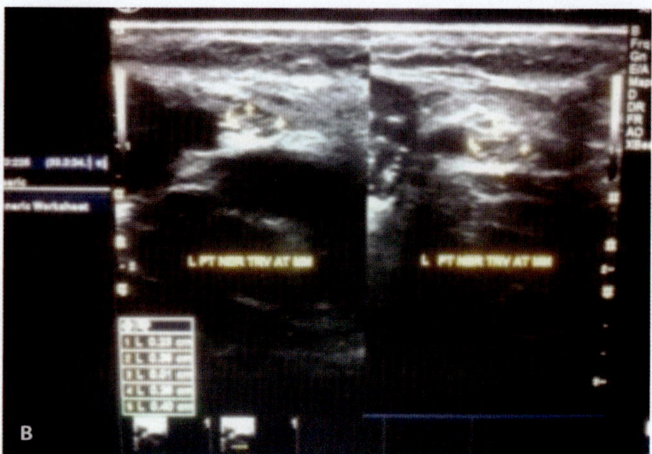

FIGURE 53-4. **A.** Ultrasound examination of the posterior tibial nerve in a speedwalker with tarsal tunnel syndrome. The symptomatic nerve is on the left compared with the asymptomatic nerve on the right. **B.** Posterior tibial nerve 6 months later after resolution of tarsal tunnel syndrome, previously symptomatic nerve on the left; the asymptomatic nerve is on the right.

Diagnostic ultrasound is useful to directly observe compressive mass lesions or focal change in the tibial nerve itself (see **Fig. 53-4**). The diagnosis includes three criteria: (1) foot pain with paresthesias, (2) positive Tinel's sign, and (3) confirmation on electrodiagnostic studies.[27–29,32,33]

ASSESSMENT

HISTORY

Historically, it is important to determine if there has been a recent change in duration, intensity, and frequency of the training regimen. Symptoms usually present 2 to 4 weeks after a training regimen changes. In addition, other common risk factors for new injury include changes in the environment or terrain and changes in equipment such as new running shoes or tennis racquets. The exact mechanism of injury (inversion sprains or decelerating injuries) contributes to establishing a diagnosis. Associated disease states should be looked for, including arthritis, circulation problems, and prior history of injuries. Special considerations for female athletes and athletes in the pediatric and elderly age groups are highlighted later in the chapter.

PHYSICAL EXAMINATION

When examining an athlete, even one with a specific, well-localized pain problem, it is important not to focus too narrowly on the problem. Biomechanical factors that underlie an injury can be determined only by viewing the relationship of the various joints involved at least one level above and below the area of pain, both at rest and dynamically in the sports-related activity. Side-to-side comparisons of muscle strength and mass should be made to get a better understanding of muscle imbalances. In sports that involve the asymmetrical use of an extremity (e.g., tennis), one should expect to find significant differences, but in many cases, large differences can be problematic. Strength testing of antagonist and agonist muscle groups (e.g., hamstrings and quads) should also be made in the injured and noninjured sides to help with future training recommendations. Finally, grading of the ligamentous sprains and overuse injuries is important to help with clinical decision making regarding immobilization, rehabilitation, and the need for surgical interventions (**Tables 53-6** and **53-7**). Assessment of problems in the upper or lower extremities should include a thorough examination of the peripheral vascular and nervous system integrity.

TABLE 53-6 Grading of Acute Ligament Injuries

Injury Grade	Examination Feature	Comments
I	Applied stress meets with distinct endpoint	Minimal swelling, discomfort, and functional loss
II	Soft endpoint with applied stress	More swelling, ecchymosis, and functional loss (i.e., inability to walk)
III	Lack of distinct endpoint	Other structures often involved (i.e., torn cartilage)

TABLE 53-7 Grading of Overuse Injuries

Injury Grade	Symptom	Duration
I	Pain only after activity	2 weeks
II	Pain during and after activity with no functional disability otherwise	>2 weeks
III	Pain during and after activities with significant functional limitations	>6 weeks
IV	Constant pain, unable to train or compete	Impending tissue failure

DIAGNOSTICS

In most injuries, imaging can be delayed until treatment response is assessed. Of particular concern in an athletic population is the increased prevalence of stress fractures. Stress fractures can be observed under ideal circumstances as little as 3 weeks and at times up to 3 months after injury with conventional radiology. Findings on initial plain films will be negative up to 67% of the time. Classic findings include periosteal new bone formation with sclerosis and radiolucent lines called DBLs (dreaded black lines) that are transverse cortical striations. The three-phase bone scan is the gold standard with virtually 100% sensitivity but poor specificity. For example, infection and arthritic conditions also cause positive findings, requiring other tests to provide clinical correlation. Changes in bone scans can be seen as early as 48 to 72 hours after the onset of symptoms and can remain positive for 6 months to 2 years after injury. Only 10% to 25% of bone scan–positive stress fractures show evidence of fracture on plain films. With the use of the technetium 99 methylene diphosphonate three-phase technique (angiogram, blood pool, and delayed image phases), other stress injuries can be observed in addition to stress fractures. For example, stress fractures will be positive in all three phases, whereas medial-tibial stress syndrome (shin splints) will be positive only in the third or delayed image phase. In up to 50% of athletes with positive bone scans, asymptomatic sites of uptake will be seen and are thought to be areas of subclinical bone strain (**Table 53-8**).[34]

TABLE 53-8 Classification of Stress Reactions

Grade	Nomenclature	Examination	Pain with Activity	Bone Scan	Radiograph
0	Normal remodeling	None	–	+	–
I	Mild stress reaction	Pain with activity	+	+	–
II	Moderate stress reaction	Pain with activity	+	+	+
		Mild tenderness			
III	Severe stress reaction	Pain with activity	+	+	+
		Marked tenderness			
		Palpable mass			
IV	Stress fracture	Rest pain	+	+	+
		Palpable mass			

Many advances have been made recently in the use of magnetic resonance imaging (MRI) and musculoskeletal ultrasound for the soft tissue injuries. MRI allows for direct visualization of bone and soft tissue structures such as hyaline cartilage, menisci, ligaments, and tendons. It can help diagnose the severity of bone stress injuries or severity of ligament and tendon injuries. There are different grading systems in place for various injuries (**Table 53-9**).[35]

Magnetic resonance imaging has excellent sensitivity and superior specificity for bone abnormalities. The advantage over CT scanning is in being able to differentiate between stress fractures and bone tumors or infectious processes. Single-photon emission computed tomography (SPECT) is more sensitive for the early detection of spondylotic changes in the spine than bone scan or plain films but may not be effective for detection 3 months after symptomatic onset. Imaging of muscles in athletes is rarely indicated. If there is concern over severe muscle tears or soft tissue masses, MRI is the technique of choice, although there is a growing literature about the positive sensitivity and specificity of diagnostic ultrasound in soft tissue injury.[36]

Magnetic resonance elastography is noninvasive and measures the stiffness of tissue. This method uses MRI equipment plus gradient coupled vibration that causes shear waves. The stiffer the tissue, the longer the wavelengths. This can help in quantifying myofascial taut bands and the presence or absence of trigger points.[35]

Positional MRI is more sensitive and specific than traditional MRI for spondylosis, spondylolisthesis, or disc herniation because these disorders can be highlighted better in different positions such as flexed or extended posturing. Studies have shown that there are posture-dependent differences in the cross-sectional area of the spinal cord. It can help detect even very mild neural compromise.[35]

Magnetic resonance arthrography has been shown to be quite specific and sensitive for analyzing specific anatomy and pathology, especially of the shoulder, hip, and elbow. It looks at capsuloligamentous structures, loose bodies, and small chondral defects. It can be especially beneficial in diagnosing labral tears in shoulder and hip or ligament tears in the ankle.[35]

TABLE 53-9 Magnetic Resonance Imaging Grading of Tendon Injuries

Grade 1: mild to moderate periosteal edema on short tau inversion recovery imaging without marrow changes
Grade 2: moderate to severe periosteal edema with marrow changes seen on T2-weighted images
Grade 3: includes two or more marrow changes seen on T1-weighted imaging
Grade 4: visible fracture line

TABLE 53-10 Ultrasonography in Soft Tissue Injuries

Location	Benefit
Muscle	Loss of the normal muscle fibers can be seen after the first 24 hours.
Muscle-tendon injury	Using dynamic stress at the junction, the operator can visualize partial tears.
Tendon	US can analyze the amount of fluid in the tendon sheath, which is increased in tendinopathy. US can detect earlier changes than via MRI. Color Doppler US can diagnose neovascularization and permit visualization of blood vessels. There is direct visualization of split tendons and partial tears.
Enthesis	US can evaluate cortical irregularities and can display increased vascularity.
Ligament	Partial ruptures and neovascularization caused by repetitive injury can be detected via US.

MRI, magnetic resonance imaging; US, ultrasonography.

Musculoskeletal ultrasonography is a noninvasive and inexpensive but very operator-dependent imaging technique that is revolutionizing our approach to both diagnostics and treatment. It is especially beneficial in diagnosing tendinosis, tendon tears, nerve entrapments, muscle strains, ligament sprains, medial epicondyle pain, and joint effusions. It can also be used to detect acute injury and changes immediately after competing because it can detect early signs of inflammation and overuse injury and aid the athlete in preventing a more serious injury. Ultrasound uses reflected sound waves to evaluate flow in blood vessels and can detect neovascularization, which has been shown to be present in areas of repeated stress. Its use is preferred for imaging tendinopathies involving the hamstring, Achilles, rotator cuff, groin, elbow, ankle, patella, and wrist. It can help diagnose tendon subluxation and shoulder impingement because these structures can be easily visualized during provocative testing. Ultrasound can also be used as a guiding tool for injections (**Table 53-10**).[35]

TREATMENT

THE PHYSIOLOGY OF WOUND HEALING

The normal biological healing pattern of a wound involves three phases: (1) The inflammatory phase happens during the first week after injury and involves recruiting inflammatory mediators and hemostasis. During this phase, cyclooxygenase-2 is activated by tissue injury and causes vasodilation and growth factors attract fibroblasts and macrophages. (2) The proliferative phase occurs in the next 2 weeks and involves the formation of the ECM via contraction, granulation, and epithelialization. (3) The remodeling or repair phase can take as long as 1 year after injury and involves formation of collagen (especially type I) and scar tissue.[37]

The healing of soft tissues and tendons involves cell proliferation, angiogenesis, deposition of the ECM, remodeling, and maturation. During these steps, various growth factors are secreted that are crucial in cell differentiation, proliferation, regulation, chemotaxis, and matrix synthesis. They are most abundant during the repair phase starting 5 to 14 days after injury. This is the basis of some injection therapies, as will be discussed later. The growth factors are secreted by the α granules of platelets and include: insulin like growth factor (IGF-1), platelet-derived growth factor (PDGF), transforming growth factor β (TGF-β), basic fibroblast growth factor (b-FGF), vascular endothelial growth factor (VEGF), epidermal growth factor (EGF), hepatocyte growth factor, chemokines, cytokines, and metabolites. The granules also release various neurotransmitters such as dopamine, serotonin, adenosine, and histamine, which help with immediate pain relief.[37,38] All together, these factors contribute to inducing mitosis,

ECM production, angiogenesis, differentiation, maturation, and finally repair.[37] b-FGF and IGF-1 are especially important in muscle repair and play a role in myoblast differentiation and proliferation. TGF-β, IGF, and PDGF play important roles in cartilage repair in terms of inducting chondrocyte proliferation, differentiation, and proteoglycan synthesis.[37]

TREATMENT GOALS

Treatment of injured athletes has three primary goals: (1) control pain and inflammation, (2) restore normal pain-free ROM, and (3) return individuals to prior levels of strength, endurance, and optimal biomechanical coordination for the sport-specific activity. Many of the therapies involved promote tissue regeneration and healing[35] in the hopes of ultimately restoring full sports performance and preinjury levels of function in the shortest time possible.[39] There have been studies suggesting that highly trained athletes may have a decreased sensitivity to noxious stimuli.[40] Athletes as a group tend to be highly motivated and often overaggressive in the implementation of a treatment plan. Recognition of this phenomenon is important to prevent further injury during the recovery phase. One must also take into account that athletes may not have a normal response to pain during training and fail to appropriately limit activity in response to nociceptive input. There is still debate about the etiology of this phenomenon. Whether training produces sustained effects on raising the pain threshold or whether competitive athletics preselects individuals with high pain thresholds, not enough is currently known to decide. Clearly, the culture of highly competitive athletics is to endorse the notion that without pain there will be no significant gains made in performance. This can engender repetitive injuries, and a balance must be struck between encouraging normal soreness of aggressive conditioning and strengthening routine versus pain caused by a repetitive injury associated with the athletic activity.

In past decade, significant advances have been made in approaches for treating nonsurgical muscle and tendon injuries.[35]

TREATMENT OF ACUTE PAIN VERSUS CHRONIC PAIN

A useful acronym for managing an acute sports-related injury is RICE: rest, ice, compression, and elevation of the injured part. With grade II or III sprains, appropriate immobilization will be necessary. Treatment can be broken up into three phases for grade I and II injuries: acute, subacute, and chronic. Chronic tendon injuries demonstrate a different mechanism of healing than acute injuries. In chronic injuries, the usually neatly arranged and hypocellular ECM becomes disrupted by an increase in the number of cells. In chronic healing, the ECM produces type III collagen, which is thinner and does not form bundles like type I, which is produced in acute healing. This altered structure will then disrupt the tendon and affect its ability to absorb forces.[35]

Briefly, in the acute phase, ice should be applied to the inflamed structure for 15 to 20 minutes several times a day with ROM allowed within the limits of pain. Relative rest is preferred rather than complete lack of activity to avoid severe deconditioning. If the injury involves a weight-bearing structure, crutches should be used when active. This phase can last from a few to several weeks, up to 2 to 5 weeks depending on severity. After the acute inflammatory phase of the injury, ice is not necessary, and heat can be applied to improve circulation to the area of injury and can ease stretching of the affected area to prevent dense scar tissue formation in the injured tissue. During this phase, atrophy is prevented with isometric or static muscle actions. Functional electrical stimulation can also be used to maintain muscle mass. In the subacute phase, gradual increases in ROM and progressive, active strengthening and endurance training of the involved muscles as well as cardiovascular conditioning should be attempted. Finally, in the final phase of rehabilitation, sport-specific training should occur.[41]

Many treatment options are effective for both chronic and acute injuries, such as exercise or and acupuncture. Others are more beneficial for one versus the other. For example, nonsteroidal anti-inflammatory drugs (NSAIDs) or steroid therapy works best in the acute setting, and a newer therapy called prolotherapy, which is discussed later in the chapter, has been found particularly useful in chronic injuries.

TREATMENT OF REPETITIVE INJURIES

In repetitive or overuse injuries, correction of underlying external and internal risk factors is essential. In addition to a careful analysis and correction of the biomechanical factors that may underlie the injury, changes in training routines will also have to be made. Long-term repetitive loading can produce inflammatory mediators (e.g., PGE_2) and degradative enzymes (e.g., matrix metalloproteases).[39] Treatment must be more cautious than in acute traumatic injuries and is often more prolonged, but many of the same principles of treating acute injuries apply. If there is an acute exacerbation of a chronic problem, ice in the first 48 hours can be helpful to reduce inflammation and swelling. Subsequently, heat is likely to be of more benefit. Initially, flexibility training is more important than strength training. When strength training is introduced, the focus should be directed at muscle imbalances observed during the examination. When the pain has subsided, eccentric exercises for chronic tendinitis have been found to be extremely effective to increase the strength of the involved structure and can help prevent reinjury.[42]

The treatment of stress fractures is somewhat different from that outlined earlier for chronic soft tissue injuries. It is also important to keep in mind that there are different treatment strategies depending on the location of the stress fracture itself. Certain stress fractures are high risk and may require special attention or a prolonged treatment plan. Examples of such areas include the tension side of the femoral neck, base of fifth metatarsal and tension side of the tibia, and navicular in the foot. There are two phases to the treatment of stress fractures. Phase I involves modified weight bearing (activities of daily living allowed but not sports) and time to allow the bone to heal. Active treatment includes use of NSAIDs and ice for pain control (ultrasound is contraindicated), with stretching and cross-training to maintain aerobic fitness using a method that avoids stress to the affected limb (upper extremity bicycle if lower extremity is injured). Use of casting or immobilization is not necessary unless there are hormonal or other factors that may lead to late nonunion of the fracture. When the athlete has been pain free for 2 to 3 weeks, percussion tenderness is negative, and plain films show bone healing, phase II can begin. Here the focus is on the gradual reintroduction of the sport with a focus on better controlling any biomechanical and training factors that may have led to the original injury.

Stress fractures of the spine are in general more difficult to treat than those in other bones given the difficulty in isolating the structure for rest. The treatment of spondylolysis of the lumbar spine is focused on limiting extension of the spine to promote healing. If there is a normal plain film but positive bone scan or SPECT, many advocate treatment without bracing of the spine. However, given recent concern over excessive radiation exposure, all attempts are made to diagnose the athlete using MRI rather than plain films or bone scans. The mean time for fracture healing is about 7 months. Specific spine stabilization exercises have been shown to be superior to rest and general conditioning exercises.[43] When braces are used after failure of more conservative measures, they must immobilize the thoracolumbar or the lumbosacral segment (or both), depending on the fracture location.

EXERCISE

Eccentric (lengthening) exercises usually involve five steps: warm up, stretching, eccentric exercise, repeat stretching, and finally icing. These exercises have been shown to be beneficial for many soft tissue injuries, especially chronic tendinopathies such as achillodynia (pain of the Achilles tendon). Studies have also shown that eccentric exercises are effective for chronic tendinopathy.[35] Mechanical loading at certain frequencies and magnitudes has been shown to increase fibroblast stimulation and thus improve tendon repair and remodeling.[39]

MEDICATIONS

The use of medications for controlling pain and inflammation in sports-related injuries is not without controversy. Many injuries seen in sports are associated with swelling and inflammation, and this makes the use of anti-inflammatory medications for pain control an obvious choice. Both NSAIDs and corticosteroids are known to have suppressive effects on the inflammatory response to injury. NSAIDs have been the first-line treatment in sports injuries, especially in the acute setting. They provide antipyretic, anti-inflammatory, and analgesic benefits. Their use is recommended for only 5 to 7 days because they are associated with potentially serious adverse effects such as hypertension, peptic ulceration, poor renal function, and increased rates of myocardial infarction.[35] The mechanism of action begins with tissue injury, which causes the release of cell membrane phospholipids that degrade to arachidonic acid. This in turn leads to a cascade of enzymatic reactions that release proinflammatory substances, including the prostaglandins, thromboxanes, and leukotrienes. Corticosteroids act early in the cascade to inhibit phospholipase A_2. This limits the production of inflammatory mediators by both the cyclooxygenase (COX) and the lipoxygenase pathways and underlies the greater potency of corticosteroids and the adverse effects retarding normal tissue repair. Most NSAIDs inhibit COX-1 and COX-2 nonspecifically, thereby limiting production of both PGE_1 and PGE_2. PGE_1 is a constitutive enzyme involved with normal *housekeeping* activity in the body, including the maintenance of normal renal and gastric function. PGE_2 is an inducible form of the enzyme and is expressed only in inflamed tissue. There has been great interest in the recent marketing of more specific COX-2 inhibitors. It is still unclear whether they will provide any additional safety or benefit when used to control pain and inflammation in sport-related injuries. Both NSAIDs and corticosteroids also have other cellular and noncellular effects on suppressing the response to inflammation.

The controversy with using anti-inflammatory medications revolves around the concern that the inflammatory response to injury is not purely pathologic and that it is necessary to remove necrotic tissue and disrupted connective tissue from the injured area. Studies of the effects of NSAIDs on tissue repair in an acute muscle strain injury animal model have shown a delay in the degradation of damaged tissue and slowed muscle regeneration. The majority of the evidence also shows that corticosteroids inhibit tendon and ligament healing after injury.

Nevertheless, in a recent review of clinical studies addressing the benefit of short-term use of NSAIDs for sports injuries, modest benefits were seen with slight decreases in pain symptoms, disability, and inflammation. No clinical evidence for delaying healing was found. Generally, short-term use of NSAIDs (3 to 5 days) is recommended to control pain, to assist in the reduction of swelling, and to promote early mobilization of the involved structure. Long-term use is not recommended and vastly increases the risk of potentially lethal side effects, including gastric and renal compromise. These side effects can be a serious consequence of overuse of these medications in highly trained athletes during the extremes of competition. Anti-inflammatory medications should not be used to mask a persistent pain problem in an athlete because this will promote further injury and does not address the underlying training or biomechanical issues. There has been no well-controlled study to justify the use of steroids in soft tissue injuries. A list of available NSAIDs and dosing frequency can be found in **Table 53-11**.

Stronger pain medications are generally not encouraged in athletics, and the International Olympic Committee bans most of the opioids. Obviously, use of opioid analgesics in an acute traumatic injury may be appropriate when the pain is severe. However, in the recovery period, strong analgesics should not be used to mask pain while training.

Topical preparations work well for soft tissue injuries and deliver the medication in a local and noninvasive fashion. Examples include capsaicin, lidocaine patches, and salicylates. Diclofenac, a topical NSAID, has been shown to be particularly effective for lateral epicondylitis and shoulder periarthritis. Nitroglycerine (NTG) patches have also been shown to be effective in treating chronic tendinopathies, particularly Achilles tendinopathy, supraspinatus tendinopathy, elbow extensor tendinosis, and lateral epicondylitis. The inhibition of nitric oxide, which normally leads to decreased collagen synthesis and collagen content, is reduced by the NTG patch, thus leading to increased collagen and reduction in pain. Side effects to be mindful of include rash, headache, and hypotension when used concomitantly with phosphodiesterase inhibitors.[35]

Botulinum toxin type A (Botox) is a neurotoxin that inhibits the release of acetylcholine at the neuromuscular junction, thus inhibiting skeletal muscle contraction.[35] Botox is used in attempt to reverse the distortion caused by shortened or damaged muscles that lead to weakness, elongation of adjacent muscles, and tendon distortion.[44] It has been found to be especially useful for chronic whiplash-associated disorder and myofascial pain.[35] When combined with the appropriate physical therapy program, Botox allows for repair and strengthening of the affected structures. Botox works by disrupting exocytosis of cholinergic vesicles, which leads to a temporary chemodenervation. This chemodenervation can, in turn, lead to reduction in clonus, muscle tone, and muscle spasms and the pain associated with these muscular states.[44] It helps reduce muscular spasticity, decrease myofascial pain, and reduce local muscle overactivity in the short term. Adverse effects are usually mild but may include allergic reactions and permanent muscle and tendon injury.[35] The best effects are achieved

TABLE 53-11 Dosages of Currently Available Nonsteroidal Anti-inflammatory Drugs

Generic Name	Brand Name	Common Unit Dose (mg)	Usual Dosing Frequency
Aspirin		325	Q 2–4 h
Diclofenac	Voltaren	75	BID
Diflunisal	Dolobid	500	BID
Etodolac	Lodine	400	BID
Fenoprofen	Nalfon	600	QID
Flurbiprofen	Ansaid	100	TID
Ibuprofen	Motrin	800	QID
Indomethacin	Indocin	25	TID
Ketoprofen	Orudis	75	TID
Ketorolac	Toradol	10	QID
Meclofenamate	Meclomen	100	TID
Nabumetone	Relafen	500	2 QD
Naproxen	Naprosyn	500	BID
Oxaprozin	Daypro	600	2 QD
Piroxicam	Feldene	20	QD
Salicylsalicylic acid	Disalcid	750	QID
Sodium salicylate		650	Q 4 h
Sulindac	Clinoril	200	BID
Tolmetin	Tolectin	400	TID

BID, twice a day; Q, every; QID, four times a day; TID, three times a day.

Data from Leadbetter WB. Anti-inflammatory therapy in sports injury: the role of nonsteroidal drugs and corticosteroid injection. *Clin Sports Med* 1995;14(2):353.

when Botox is used in combination with other treatments such as reconditioning, strengthening, and flexibility programs rather than as a monotherapy. It has been shown that Botox treatment can also decrease the overall cost of medication and need for multiple treatments.[35] There is weak evidence supporting its use for tendon injuries, but some studies have shown that it can help reduce muscle overactivity in the short term. One study found significant improvement in pain and strength in patients with epicondylitis who were treated with Botox injections.[35]

Antidepressants can act on the cholinergic, histaminergic, and adrenergic neurochemical pathways in athletes with chronic pain by modulating serotonin and norepinephrine. For example, selective serotonin reuptake inhibitors such as fluoxetine have been proven to be effective in treating fibromyalgia. TCAs such as nortriptyline, desipramine, and amitriptyline provide relief for fibromyalgia as well as tension-type headaches and painful muscle spasms. Serotonin and neuroepinephrine reuptake inhibitors (SNRIs) such as milnacipran, duloxetine, and venlafaxine also provide benefit for fibromyalgia in addition to chronic regional muscle pain.[35]

Anticonvulsants have been shown to provide benefit for neuropathic pain. For example, carbamazepine, lamotrigine, zonisamide, and gabapentin have been shown to help treat fibromyalgia and perhaps chronic regional muscle pain. However, this application of these medications has not yet been approved by the Food and Drug Administration (FDA). Pregabalin has recently been approved to treat fibromyalgia.[35]

Tramadol is an SNRI in addition to being a weak opioid μ-receptor agonist. It is helpful in nociceptive and neuropathic pain and has been proven to help in fibromyalgia.[35]

INTERVENTIONAL

Appropriate use of injection techniques into joints, tendon sheaths, bursa, muscle trigger points, and other soft tissue structures can be of great benefit both from a diagnostic and therapeutic point of view in athletes. It is often useful before injecting to have the athlete provoke the pain by performing the activity that induces the discomfort. This can help with localization of the inflamed tissue. If in doubt about the pain generator, it can be useful to inject with local anesthetic alone initially and then try to provoke the pain 10 to 20 minutes later to determine whether the location was accurate before infusing corticosteroid (**Table 53-12**).

The risk of tendon rupture with repeated steroid injections is real. The maximum load strength of tendons and ligaments after steroid injection has been demonstrated to be reduced in many animal studies. This effect is particularly predominant immediately after injection. Unfortunately, there is a general lack of well-designed clinical studies to guide the safe use of steroids.[45]

A conservative approach would permit only one or two tendon or tendon sheath injections in 1 year, and some would recommend that no vigorous muscle loading should be performed for at least 2 weeks after injection to avoid complications. Many would advocate, however, never injecting a tendon in an athlete, given the potential for loss in tissue durability. Joints can typically be injected up to three times a year. Bursa can be injected more frequently. With injections into superficial structures such as the epicondyles of the elbow or the pes anserine bursa, avoid depositing the steroid into the skin because this can cause depigmentation. One technique is to pinch the skin and pull away from the deeper structures before inserting the needle to avoid such complications. When injecting into perineural areas such as the carpal tunnel, it is safe to touch the nerve if using a 27-gauge needle and then pull back 1 to 2 mm before injecting. Infection or bleeding can be avoided with proper sterile and hemostatic technique. Other risks of steroid use are summarized in **Table 53-13**.

Corticosteroid injections have been a long-time treatment option for chronic and acute pain. Lately, however, they have been shown to not be as beneficial for chronic tendinopathies as originally thought to be. Their mechanism of action involves preventing lysosomal enzyme release, inhibition of neutrophil accumulation, and thus synthesis of inflammatory mediators. This, in theory, will diminish tissue destruction.[35]

TABLE 53-12 Common Sites of Injection in Athletes

Injection Sites	Needle	Volume (mL)*	Comments
Joints			
Ulnocarpal	#25, 1.5 in	1–3	Steroid volume to anesthetic ratio, 1:1
Radiocarpal			
Carpometacarpal			
Elbow	#25, 1.5 in	2–3	Steroid volume to anesthetic ratio, 1:2
Ankle			
Shoulder	#25, 1.5 in	7–10	Steroid volume to anesthetic ratio, 1:6 to 1:9
Knee			
Sacroiliac joint			
Bone-Tendon			
Medial/lateral epicondyle	#27, 1.25 in	2–3	Steroid volume to anesthetic ratio, 1:1
Plantar fascia			
Pubic symphysis	#25, 1.5 in	3–5	Steroid volume to anesthetic ratio, 1:2 to 1:4
Hamstrings			
Adductors			
Tendon Sheaths			
Thumb extensor	#27, 1.25 in	1–3	Steroid volume to anesthetic ratio, 1:1
Finger flexors			
Posterior tibial	#27, 1.25 in	3–5	Steroid volume to anesthetic ratio, 1:2 to 1:4
Biceps (long head)			
Bursae			If aspirating, will need #18–20 needle first
Prepatellar	#25, 1.5 in	2–3	Steroid volume to anesthetic ratio, 1:1
Pes anserine			
Olecranon			
Subacromial	#25, 1.5 in	7–10	Steroid volume to anesthetic ratio, 1:6 to 9
Greater trochanter			
Perineural			
Carpal tunnel	#27, 1.25 in	2–5	Steroid volume to anesthetic ratio, 2:1
Tarsal tunnel			
Suprascapular notch			
Cubital tunnel			

*Use 1% lidocaine or 0.25% bupivacaine with long-acting, insoluble steroid salts such as triamcinolone acetate or betamethasone acetate.

However, studies have shown that limiting neutrophil and leukocyte numbers and inhibiting fibroblast growth is detrimental to tendon healing, leading to reduced tensile strength and lack of elasticity instead.[39] Even though corticosteroid injections can provide up to 6 to 8 weeks of pain relief, direct intratendinous injections should be avoided for fear

TABLE 53-13 Local and Systemic Complications with Local Injections of Corticosteroids

Local	Systemic
Subcutaneous atrophy	Transient hyperglycemia in diabetics
Pigmentation abnormalities	Vasovagal symptoms with syncope
Tendon or ligament rupture	Cognitive affects "steroid psychosis"
Accelerated joint destruction	Allergic reactions
Local sterile abscess	Systemic infection
Peripheral nerve injury	Suppression of pituitary–adrenal axis
Muscle necrosis or vascular injury	Avascular necrosis of hip

of tendon weakening or rupture. Other potential complications from corticosteroid injections include avascular necrosis, articular cartilage degeneration, and osteonecrosis of the femur and hips. Frequent repeated injections should also be avoided. Although steroid treatment may be a superior short-term pain relief option, in the long term, it has been shown to be less beneficial and does not correct the underlying problem.[35]

Acupuncture was extrapolated from Chinese medicine many decades ago. This form of alternative treatment for both acute and chronic injuries has been a very popular choice, especially since the 1970s, with relatively few side effects. It has been shown in study after study to have superior effects on pain relief over placebo or sham acupuncture, especially for lateral epicondylitis, plantar fasciitis, patellar tendonitis, frozen shoulder, LBP, and osteoarthritis.[46,47] Some trials have shown that acupuncture may even be superior to steroid therapy in lateral epicondylitis.[46]

NEWER INJECTION TREATMENTS

In the past decade or so, there has been a paradigm shift in understanding the pathophysiology and therefore treatment of chronic tendinopathy.[35]

Extracorporeal Shock Wave Therapy Extracorporeal shock wave therapy (ESWT) is a newer treatment method that has been found particularly useful for tendinopathies. An external shock wave generated outside the body is focused on a particular internal structure or area, similar to lithotripsy in renal stone disruption. The repeated shocks cause microtrauma to the affected area, which in turn fosters neovascularization and ultimately promotes healing of tissues. This method is FDA approved for plantar fasciitis with associated calcaneal osteophytes and lateral epicondylitis. However, other studies have shown that ESWT is also effective in treating chronic patellar tendinopathies, rotator cuff calcific tendonitis, and chronic insertional Achilles tendinopathy.[35]

Platelet-Rich Plasma Injections A small amount of the patient's blood is centrifuged to separate the platelets from the rest of the blood. This produces a platelet-rich solution three to eight times the normal platelet concentration that is then injected into the painful area.[37,38] Since platelets contain growth factors such as b-FGF, IGF-1, PDGF, VEGF, EGF, and TGF-β, injecting them to an injured area can promote soft tissue repair in ligaments, tendons, and muscles.[35,37] The growth factors then help increase cell proliferation and maturation and angiogenesis, leading to tendon repair, tissue regeneration, and graft integration. Furthermore, focal bleeding from the needle itself can promote further recruitment of healing mediators.[37] Studies have shown that the best time for platelet-rich plasma (PRP) injection is 3 to 6 months after injury when there is persistent pain. PRP injections have been shown to improve pain, increase activity level, and allow for earlier return to sport or competition (2–3 weeks earlier compared with no PRP injection), especially for patients with lateral epicondylitis, patellar tendinopathy, knee tendinitis, plantar fasciitis, ligament sprains, or even rupture. Please consult **Table 53-14** for an overview on clinical use of PRP injections.

Although this treatment is minimally invasive and has less chance of adverse effects because the patient's own cells are used, it still remains a relatively expensive treatment that is not usually covered by insurance. Of course, the benefits of PRP injections are potentiated if performed in conjunction with other therapy such as acute pain management, physical therapy, flexibility and strengthening exercises, aerobic conditioning, eccentric strengthening (2–3 weeks after a PRP injection), and later sports-specific training. NSAIDs or corticosteroids should not be used in combination with PRP as their effects would negate the proinflammatory effects of PRP.[37,38]

Prolotherapy (Regenerative Injection Therapy) The goal of prolotherapy is to avoid suboptimal healing and to restore an injured area to its full tensile strength and prevent repetitive injury or rupture. It is used in combination with physical therapy, ROM, strengthening, and stretching exercises.[39] A proliferative substance such as hypertonic dextrose, which acts as an osmotic agent, is injected to the injured area (usually

TABLE 53-14 Clinical Use of Platelet-Rich Plasma Injections

CONSIDER PRP IN THE FOLLOWING PATHOLOGIES
Tendinopathy: lateral and medial epicondylitis, rotator cuff tendinosis, hip, peroneal tendon, plantar fasciitis Chronic pain and OA: knee, ankle, foot, shoulder, or hip Chronic ligamentous injury and pain (ankle, knee, hip, sacroiliac joint) Muscle tears
CONSIDER PLATELET-RICH PLASMA IF THE FOLLOWING CONDITIONS ARE MET
Duration of pain >3–6 months and is on average >4 on 0–10 VAS Signs and symptoms consistent with tendinopathy, muscle or ligamentous injury Pain persists despite standard conservative treatments MRI or US evidence of tendinopathy or muscle or ligamentous injury A diagnostic bupivacaine injection was successful Patient is pursuing a nonsurgical solution and has time to be out of play for about 4 weeks No contraindications (e.g., immunocompromised state, coagulopathy, anticoagulation)
CONTRAINDICATIONS TO PLATELET-RICH PLASMA THERAPY
Immunocompromised patient Active infection Inability to comprehend or comply with postprocedure instructions for activity INR >2.5 Patients with prosthetic joints Prosthetic hardware infection Severe cases of advanced OA
RETURN TO ACTIVITY AFTER PLATELET-RICH PLASMA
Immediate activity. No weight bearing or minimal weight bearing except usual activities of daily living. Exercise: No impact to the area of injection and consider cross-training and aerobic exercise. 1–3 weeks: After pain from an injection subsides, safe to do daily stretching and ROM at the area of injection with weight bearing as tolerated. Exercise: Continue cross-training, elliptical, aerobic exercises. For LE injection: No running, jumping, or other impact. 3 weeks: Begin strengthening, isometrics (no ROM strengthening) for 2 weeks; then isotonic with low weight for 1 week. 6–8 weeks: If isometric, isotonic exercise training is well tolerated and pain remains less and tolerable, eccentric exercises may begin around 6 weeks after the procedure. 8–10 weeks: If the previous strengthening step is tolerated, progress strengthening to include polymeric and other sports-specific training. At 10 weeks, if pain remains low, the patient may return to all activities and sports as tolerated. 12 weeks: Reassessment for PRP effect, activity evaluation, and a repeat injection.[37,38]

INR, international normalized ratio; LE, lower extremity; MRI, magnetic resonance imaging; OA, osteoarthritis; PRP, platelet-rich plasma; ROM, range of motion; US, ultrasonography; VAS, visual analog scale.

interligamentous) to induce collagen synthesis and fibroblast proliferation, causing ligament hypertrophy and regeneration of normal cells and tissues. When a cell is exposed to extra dextrose, it begins to produce extra growth factors.[38,39,48] Some studies also mentioned some benefit with injecting phenol, which acts as an irritant, or sodium morrhuate, which acts as a chemotactic agent instead.[48] Studies have shown this therapy to be effective in chronic ligament, joint capsule, fascial, and tendinous injuries; chronic enthesopathies; tendinopathies; and osteoarthritis[35] but not in bone injuries.[39] Examples include Achilles tendon rupture, elbow extensor tendinosis, patellar tendinosis, and bicipital tendinosis.[39] A 10% dextrose solution injected every 2 months for half a year was shown to reduce pain and improve ROM in patients with finger and knee osteoarthritis and ACL laxity.[35]

This treatment is minimally invasive and relatively inexpensive, and its effects can be followed by interval ultrasound imaging.[35,38] Adverse effects include causing a flare-up of a true inflammatory process, usual risks associated with needle injections, stiffness and soreness, allergy, chemical arachnoiditis,[39] and liver function test elevation. Contraindications include patients with systemic inflammation, metastatic cancer, nonmusculoskeletal pain, bleeding disorders, chemical dependency, or whole-body pain.[48]

SPECIAL CONSIDERATIONS

FEMALE ATHLETES

After puberty, significant differences emerge between male and female athletes. Females maintain a higher percentage of body fat, gain less muscle mass, have lower lung capacities, and have lower oxygen-carrying capacity than men. In addition, there are biomechanical differences that may put female athletes at more risk for injury. For example, women have a higher incidence of genu valgus, which can lead to patellar tracking disorders and injury.

Perhaps more important than these differences are the effects that excessive training can have on normal endocrine function in the female population. Recognition of problems related to athletic amenorrhea has improved among trainers and physicians. Up to 28% of women participation in college varsity athletics will be amenorrheic. The prevalence increases to 57% in cross-country runners and is high in dancers, swimmers, and cyclists. The most significant physiologic consequence of this is the effect on bone density; as a result, stress fractures are more common in this group. Special attention must be given to the risk factors for *anorexia athletica*, which can in some cases be fatal (**Table 53-15**).[49]

TABLE 53-15 Diagnostic Criteria for Anorexia Athletica

Symptom	Absolute Criteria	Relative Criteria
Weight loss >5% of IBW	+	
Absence of medical or other psychological illness	+	
Excessive fear of being obese	+	
Excessive restriction of food intake	+	
Delayed puberty (>age 16 years)		
Amenorrhea or other menstrual dysfunction		+
Distorted body image		+
Use of purging methods (vomiting, diuretics, laxatives)		+
Binge eating		+
Compulsive exercise		

IBW, ideal body weight.

ELDERLY ATHLETES

Acute injuries are common in the elderly participating actively in sports. The safety margin of an exercise routine is much narrower and puts this population at greater risk. Changes in the cardiovascular and neurologic system will inevitably compromise aerobic capacity and coordination of elderly athletes and should be taken into account when recommending training regimens. Injury rates vary from 14% to 57% in elderly athletes in different series. Common sites of injuries involve the shoulder or knee and are often caused by preexisting orthopedic problems in those joints. In general, lower extremity injuries are the most common.

Muscle strains occur frequently, and rupture of muscle and tendons is more likely to occur than in younger populations. Acute injuries related to falls are a common scenario seen in this group. Overuse injuries typically involve tendons and muscles rather than bone, and recovery can be extended up to 2 years in some studies. Stress fractures are rare, but it should be noted that the sensitivity of bone scan may decrease to 80% to 95% in patients older than 65 years of age.[50]

PEDIATRIC ATHLETES

In children and adolescents, the muscles and tendons are stronger than the bone, and thus bone avulsions are seen more frequently than in adults. The growth plates at the apophyses in the pelvis and hips are particularly at risk and are common sites of acute avulsion. In addition, skeletal immaturity puts the pediatric population at greater risk for stress fractures if overambitious training routines are followed.

Exercise performance is limited compared with adults partly because of lower anaerobic capacity. During exertion, children use more oxygen per kilogram of body weight and thus experience a higher metabolic cost than adults for an equivalent, absolute exercise level (i.e., walking at a given speed). The response to strength training in children is also different than in adults. In the prepubescent population, the muscles respond to training with central neurogenic adaptations in firing rate and recruitment but not by muscle fiber hypertrophy and increases in lean muscle mass. As a result, aggressive strength training with high weights and low repetitions should not be attempted in this population because it increases the risk of tendon and bone trauma without benefit. However, strength training is safe in children if the program is properly designed and supervised by individuals experienced with this age group. In addition, during growth spurts, the apophyses (the sites of tendon insertion into the bone) are particularly at risk for injury, and training regimens should be reduced (**Table 53-16**).[51]

TABLE 53-16 Common Sites of Apophysitis in Pediatric Athletes

Injury Site	Sport Activity	Comments
Medial epicondyle	Throwing sports	Caused by repetitive valgus stress
Little League elbow		
Tibial tubercle	Football, running, soccer, basketball	Affects 10- to 13-year-old athletes
Osgood-Schlatter disease		
Inferior pole patella	Basketball, jumping sports, running	Affects 10- to 12-year-old boys
Sinding-Larson-Johansson disease (jumper's knee)		
Iliac bone	Running, dancing	Affects 16-year-old athletes
Calcaneus bone	Soccer, hockey, basketball	Seen with tight calf muscles
Sever's disease		

CONCLUSION

Treating pain syndromes in athletes can often present major challenges. Although the group as a whole is highly motivated, the goals of treatment are often more difficult to attain than in the general population. Athletes do not only want to be pain free but to be pain free while performing an extremely stressful activity that requires a high degree of tissue, biomechanical, and psychological integrity. A complex set of intrinsic and extrinsic factors must be taken into account and corrected in order to be successful and prevent chronic reinjury. As a result, a thorough understanding of both the underlying physiology of the structural elements involved and the external factors that are often unique to each sport is essential.

ACKNOWLEDGMENTS

Dr. Walter Frontera, chairman and professor of PM&R, Vanderbilt University, and Joseph F. Audette, MA, MD and chief, Department of Pain Medicine, Harvard Vanguard Medical Associates, Boston, MA, contributed to this chapter in earlier editions.

REFERENCES

1. Smith EL, Gilligan C. Dose response to mechanical loading. *Bone.* 1996;18(1):45S.
2. Kerr DA, Prince RL, et al. Does high resistance weight training have a greater effect on bone mass than low resistance weight training? *J Bone Miner Res.* 1994;9:S152.
3. Zimmerman JR, Mow VC. Physiology of synovial joints and articular cartilage. In: Downey JA, Myers SJ, et al, eds. *The Physiological Basis of Rehabilitation Medicine.* 2nd ed. Boston, MA: Butterworth-Heinemann; 1994:149.
4. McComas AJ. Human neuromuscular adaptations that accompany changes in activity. *Med Sci Sports Exerc.* 1994;26(12):1498.
5. Kirkendall DT, Garrett WE. The effects of aging and training on the skeletal muscle. *Am J Sports Med.* 1998;26(4):598.
6. Garland E. Pain processing in the human nervous system. *Prim Care Clin Office Pract.* 2012;39(3):561-571.
7. Vora A, Borg-Stein J, Nguyen R. Regenerative injection therapy for osteoarthritis: fundamental concepts and evidence-based review. *PM R.* 2012;S104-S109.
8. Scott A, Bahr R. Neuropeptides in tendinopathy. *Front Biosci (Landmark Ed).* 2009;2203-2211.
9. Schubert TE, Weidler C, Lerch K, et al. Achilles tendinosis is associated with sprouting of substance P positive nerve fibres. *Ann Rheum Dis.* 2005;64(7):1083-1086.
10. Lian Ø, Dahl J, Ackermann PW, et al. Pronociceptive and antinociceptive neuromediators in patellar tendinopathy. *Am J Sports Med.* 2006;34(11):1801-1808.
11. Sanchis-Alfonso V, Rosello-Sastre E, Subias-Lopez A. neuroanatomic basis for pain in patellar tendinosis ("jumper's knee"): a neuroimmunohistochemical study. *Am J Knee Surg.* 2001;174-177.
12. Borg-Stein J, Zaremski JL, Hanford MA. New concepts in the assessment and treatment of regional musculoskeletal pain and sports injury. *PM R.* 2009;744-754.
13. Rees JD, Maffulli N, Cook J. Management of tendinopathy. *Am J Sports Med.* 2009;37:1855-1867.
14. Abate M, Silbernagel KG, Siljeholm C, et al. Pathogenesis of tendinopathies: inflammation or degeneration? *Arthritis Res Ther.* 2009;11(3):235.
15. Van Wilgen CP, Keizer D. Neuropathic pain mechanisms in patients with chronic sports injuries: a diagnostic model useful in sports medicine? *Pain Med.* 2011;12(1):110-117.
16. Fredericson M. Common injuries in runners: diagnosis, rehabilitation, and prevention. *Sports Med.* 1996;2:49.
17. Brukner P. Stress fractures of the upper limb. *Sports Med.* 1998;26:415.
18. Schulte KR, Warner JJP. Uncommon causes of shoulder pain in the athlete. *Sports Med.* 1995;26:505.
19. Safran MR, Fu FH. Uncommon causes of knee pain in the athlete. *Orthop Clin North Am.* 1995;26(3):547.
20. Duggleby T, Kumar S. Epidemiology of juvenile low back pain: a review. *Disabil Rehabil.* 1997;19(12):505.
21. Micheli LJ, Wood R. Back pain in young athletes. *Arch Pediatr Adolesc Med.* 1995;149:15.
22. Almekinders LC, Temple JD. Etiology, diagnosis, and treatment of tendinitis: an analysis of the literature. *Med Sci Sports Exerc.* 1998;30(8):1183.
23. Danielson P, Andersson G, Alfredson H, Forsgren S. Marked sympathetic component in the perivascular innervation of the dorsal paratendinous tissue of the patellar tendon in arthroscopically treated tendinosis patients. *Knee Surg Sports Traumatol Arthrosc.* 2008;16:621-626.
24. Mautner K, Colberg RE, Malanga G, et al. Outcomes after ultrasound-guided platelet-rich plasma injections for chronic tendinopathy: a multicenter, retrospective review. *PM R.* 2013;5:169-175.
25. Garrett WE. Muscle strain injuries. *Am J Sports Med.* 1996;24:S2.
26. Arrington ED, Miller MD. Skeletal muscle injuries. *Sports Med.* 1995;26:411.
27. Toth C. Peripheral nerve injuries attributable to sport and recreation. *Neurol Clin.* 2008;89-113.
28. Brewer R, Gregory A. Chronic lower leg pain in athletes: a guide for the differential diagnosis, evaluation, and treatment. *Sports Health.* 2012;121-127.
29. Edwards P, Wright M, Hartman J. A Practical approach for the differential diagnosis of chronic leg pain in the athlete. *Am J Sports Med.* 2005;1241-1249.
30. Neal S, Fields K. Peripheral nerve entrapment and injury in the upper extremity. *Am Fam Physician.* 2010;147-155.
31. Aldridge J, Bruno R, Strauch R, Rosenwasser M. Nerve entrapment in athletes. *Clinics in Sports Medicine.* 2001;95-122.
32. Peck E, Finnoff J, Smith J. Neuropathies in runners. *Clin Sports Med.* 2010;437-457.
33. McCrory P, Bell S, Bradshaw C. Nerve entrapments of the lower leg, ankle and foot in sport. *Sports Med.* 2002;371-391.
34. Monteleon GP. Stress fractures in the athlete. *Orthop Clin North Am.* 1995;26(3):423.
35. Borg-Stein J, Zaremski J, Hanaford MA. New concepts in the assessment and treatment of regional musculoskeletal pain and sports injury. *PM R.* 2009;1:744-754.
36. El-Khoury GY, Brandser EA, Kathol MH, et al. Imaging of muscle injuries. *Skeletal Radiol.* 1996;25(1):3.
37. Nguyen RT, Borg-Stein J, McInnis K. Applications of platelet-rich plasma in musculoskeletal and sports medicine: an evidence based approach. *PM&R.* 2011;3:226-250.
38. Vora A, Borg-Stein J, Nguyen RT. Regenerative injection therapy for osteoarthritis: fundamental concepts and evidence-based review. *PM&R.* 2012;4:S104-S109.

39. Reeves KD, Fullerton BD, Topol G. Evidence-based regenerative injection therapy (prolotherapy) in sports medicine. In: Seidenberg PH, Beutler PI, eds. *The Sports Medicine Resource Manual.* St. Louis: Saunders (Elsevier); 2008:611-619. Chapter 50.
40. O'Connor PJ, Cook DB. Exercise and pain: the neurobiology, measurement, and laboratory study of pain in relation to exercise in humans. *Exerc Sport Sci Rev.* 1999;27:119.
41. Curwin SL. The aetiology and treatment of tendonitis. In: Harries M, Williams C, et al. eds. *Oxford Textbook of Sports Medicine.* 2nd ed. Oxford, England: Oxford University Press; 1998.
42. Renstrom AFH. In Chapter 5: Harries M, Williams C, et al, eds. *Oxford Textbook of Sports Medicine.* 2nd ed. Oxford, England: Oxford University Press; 1998.
43. O'Sullivan PB, Phyty GD, Twomey LT, Allison GT. Evaluation of specific stabilization exercise in the treatment of chronic low back pain with radiologic diagnosis of spondylolysis or spondylolisthesis. *Spine.* 1997;22:2959.
44. Lang AM. Botulinum toxin type A therapy in chronic pain disorders. *Arch Phys Med Rehabil.* 2003;84(1):S69-S73.
45. Leadbetter WB. Anti-inflammatory therapy in sports injury: the role of nonsteroidal drugs and corticosteroid injection. *Clin Sports Med.* 1995;14(2):353.
46. Meleger A, Borg-Stein J. Acupuncture and sports medicine. *Medical Acupuncture.* 1999;11(2):1-7.
47. Berman BM, Langevin HH, Witt CM, Dubner R. Acupuncture for chronic low back pain. *N Engl J Med.* 2010;363(5):454-461.
48. Dagenais S, Mayer J, Haldeman S, Borg-Stein J. Evidence-informed management of chronic low back pain with prolotherapy. *Spine J.* 2008;8:203-212.
49. Beim G, Stone DA. Issues in the female athlete. *Orthop Clin North Am.* 1995;26(3):443.
50. Kallinen M, Markku A. Aging, physical activity, and sports injuries. An overview of common sports injuries in the elderly. *Sports Med.* 1995;20:41.
51. Cook PC, Leit ME. Issues in the pediatric athlete. *Sports Med.* 1995;26:453.

SECTION C

Pain in the Terminally Ill

CHAPTER 54

Cancer Pain Syndromes

Danijela Levačić
Stuart W. Hough
Ronald M. Kanner

OVERVIEW

Pain is a complex symptom experienced by many cancer patients. It affects most aspects of life, and controlling it well can make a great difference in patients' perception of their diagnosis. The etiology of pain in cancer patients is very heterogeneous. Finding the cause directs the treatment and improves the chances of good pain control. In general, cancer pain syndromes can be divided into acute and chronic. Acute ones are usually direct consequence of invasive diagnostic or therapeutic procedures, but they can less commonly be related to cancer itself. Chronic ones are more likely to be caused by the neoplastic process or by antineoplastic therapy.

Metastatic disease may invade bone, obstruct a hollow viscus, and compress nerve or spinal cord. Radiation treatment may cause fibrosis of nerve or spinal cord. Chemotherapeutic agents may cause peripheral neuropathy or aseptic bone necrosis and predispose to painful opportunistic infections. Surgical treatment leads to acute postoperative pain and may cause deafferentation pain if major nerves or nerve plexi are cut. In any given patient, one or more of these factors may be in play, and more than 50% of cancer patients with pain have more than one source of pain.[1]

Primary care physicians and oncologists should be able to recognize and treat most cancer-related pain. They should be able to initiate treatment for the more common causes with opioids and nonopioid analgesics. More than 70% of patients can be treated effectively with simple analgesics and adjuvant drugs. Effective pain relief, without intolerable side effects, is occasionally difficult to obtain with the use of conventional analgesics. When this occurs, consultation with a specialist in pain management may be necessary.

DIMENSIONS OF THE PROBLEM

Based on rates from 2008 to 2010, National Cancer Institute estimates that 40.76% of men and women born today will be diagnosed with cancer of all sites at some time during their lifetimes.[2] About half of cancer patients experience pain, most commonly caused by their primary cancer. Pain severity is at least moderate for most patients experiencing cancer-related pain. Pain may also persist in long-term cancer survivors. Cancer-related pain adds to mood disturbance and disability in cancer patients.[3]

In 1982, Daut and Cleeland found that 36% of 286 patients with nonmetastatic cancer reported pain versus 59% of 381 with metastatic disease.[4] In 1994, Cleeland and colleagues found that 67% of 1308 outpatients with metastatic cancer had pain, and 62% of those had severe pain. Thirty-six percent reported disability from pain, and 42% of those with pain reported inadequate analgesia.[5] Terminal pain, refractory to escalating opioid administration, is a more challenging problem. Depression, uncontrolled pain, the adverse effects of opioids, and fear of pain may precipitate suicidal thoughts or requests for aid in dying.[6,7] Pain also adds to the discomfort experienced by those caring for dying patients.

The likelihood of pain associated with cancer depends on the type and stage of disease. Foley, in a 1-week survey of 540 patients hospitalized at Memorial Sloan-Kettering Cancer Center, showed that the prevalence of pain requiring analgesic drugs varies by cancer type (**Table 54-1**).[8] In contrast, among 1308 outpatients with metastatic cancer, Cleeland and colleagues did not find variation in pain prevalence according to cancer type.[5]

TABLE 54-1 Prevalence of Pain in Hospitalized Cancer Patients

Type of Cancer	Patients with Pain (%)
Bone	85
Oral cavity	80
Male genitourinary	75
Female genitourinary	78
Breast	52
Lung	45
Gastrointestinal	40
Lymphoma	20
Leukemia	5

From Foley KM. Pain syndromes in patients with cancer. In: Bonica JJ, Ventafridda B, eds. *Advances in Pain Research and Therapy*. Vol. 2. New York: Raven Press, 1979:59. Used with permission of Lippincott Williams & Wilkins.

Gutsgel and colleagues conducted a prospective study on 141 palliative medicine patients. Forty-one patient did not have pain within 1 month before enrollment or could not provide reliable history. Of 100 remaining evaluable patients (71%) who reported pain, 95 had cancer. Sixty-eight percent of them had pain directly caused by tumor, 18% caused by cancer treatment, 3% caused by cancer-associated conditions (e.g., postherpetic neuralgia), and the remaining 16% not related to cancer. Pain was somatic in 52%, visceral in 22%, neuropathic in 10%, and of mixed origin in 16%. Usual pain intensity was moderate to severe in 73%, and maximal pain intensity was moderate or greater in 93% of affected patients. This study supported prior observations of most patients experiencing pain at one site (61%) or two sites (27%) and much less frequently at three or more.[9]

Although significant improvements have been seen in understanding pain and the availability of treatment options, there is still a high prevalence of inadequately treated cancer pain. Both patient and practitioner factors contribute to poor cancer pain assessment and management.[10] Two of three doctors feel insufficiently prepared to manage cancer pain.[11] About three of four oncologists and palliative care doctors likewise believe they inadequately assess pain and pain response in their patients.[12] Furthermore, half of doctors are concerned about legal issues related to prescribing opioids for patients with cancer pain, and three of four doctors believe opioid use for cancer pain is associated with high rates of addiction and abuse.[3,11] Patients are often reluctant to report pain. They can have poor treatment adherence, cognitive issues, and affective distress, which can limit reporting, fear of addiction, or developing tolerance and fear of side effects. They often try to be "good patients" by tolerating pain or believe that the doctor should focus on cancer cure rather than pain relief. Some have concerns about negative views of family, friends, and coworkers if they use pain medications.[3,10] There are also considerable gender and ethnic differences in cancer pain reporting and perception, which providers should have in mind when assessing each patient.[13] All ethnic groups believe that cancer pain is taken more seriously when reported by male patients.[3,13] Meta-analysis of cultural differences in Western and Asian patient-perceived barriers to managing cancer pain has shown significantly higher perceived barriers among Asian patients.[3,14]

THE THREE TYPES OF PAIN

Pain can be divided into three pathophysiologic categories—somatic nociceptive, visceral nociceptive, and neuropathic—on the basis of the inferred mechanisms of pain (see Chapter 2). It is useful to characterize pain in this way because the approach to treating each type is somewhat different. However, they are not mutually exclusive, and cancer patients, in particular, may have pain with multiple causes. The mechanisms of each type are the subject of considerable ongoing research.

SOMATIC NOCICEPTIVE PAIN

This is the typical pain that we all have experienced acutely or chronically: the cutaneous burn and arthritic joint are examples. The painful site is tender and corresponds to the site of tissue damage. Somatic pain is described as constant and sometimes throbbing or aching. Bone metastases are the most common malignant cause of somatic pain and, in fact, are the most common source of pain in cancer.[15]

Noxious (potentially tissue-damaging) mechanical, thermal, and chemical stimuli trigger nociceptive ischemia, inflammation, and perhaps substances produced by a nearby tumor may sensitize nociceptors to ordinarily non-noxious stimuli. Pain signals are carried by small, myelinated Aδ fibers (mechanical and thermal stimuli) and unmyelinated C fibers (all three stimulus types) to the dorsal horn of the spinal cord. From there, they ascend in the contralateral spinothalamic and spinoreticular tracts to the thalamus and reticular formation, respectively (see Chapter 2). Although most research into nociceptive mechanisms has focused on cutaneous pain, nociceptors exist in most tissues to varying degrees.

VISCERAL PAIN

Pain originating from the viscera is familiar to many of us; abdominal cramps and the pain of passing a renal stone are examples. It may be less constant than somatic pain, occurring in dull, colicky waves. Visceral pain is poorly localized and often referred to a distant cutaneous site, which may be tender. Unlike somatic pain, it is often associated with nausea and diaphoresis. Cancer patients experience primary and referred visceral pain from pancreatic cancer, bowel obstruction, and other causes.

The noxious stimuli required to trigger visceral pain include ischemia, inflammation, torsion, traction, distension, and impaction. In fact, cutting, crushing, and burning may not be felt as painful.[16]

It took many years to understand that true visceral pain did exist and that somatic tenderness observed during visceral dysfunction was due to convergence of visceral and somatic sensory afferents in the spinal cord, a phenomenon commonly known as "referred pain." The majority of thoracic and abdominal visceral organs, except the pancreas, are dually innervated by parasympathetic (craniosacral) and sympathetic (thoracolumbar) outflows. Thoracic viscera and upper abdominal viscera are primarily innervated by the vagus (cranial nerve X) and spinal thoracolumbar outflows. The lower abdominal viscera, including the small and large intestine and the urogenital organs, are innervated by thoracolumbar (i.e., lumbar splanchnic nerve and hypogastric nerve) and sacral (i.e., pelvic nerve) outflows.

Sensory afferents innervating the visceral organs are not just a homogeneous group of afferents signaling visceral pain to the CNS. It is now a general notion that pain is primarily signaled by spinal afferents, and vagal afferents signal nonpainful sensations such as hunger, satiety, fullness, and nausea.

Considering the fact that afferent nerve sensitization initiates visceral hypersensitivity, attempts have been made to pharmacologically modulate the excitability of the afferents to alleviate visceral sensitivity. The advantage of targeting visceral afferents with a peripherally restricted drug is to avoid unnecessary CNS complications. Among many target receptors, κ-opioid receptors (KOR), P2X purine receptors, 5-HT_3 and 5-HT_4 serotonin receptors, *N*-methyl-D-aspartate (NMDA) receptors (NMDAr), tachykinin (NK1, NK2, and NK3) receptors, TRPV1, and γ-aminobutyric acid B (GABA-B) receptors have been documented to have modulating effects on responses of sensory afferents and spinal processing of pain.[17]

NEUROPATHIC PAIN

In everyday life, chronic neuropathic pain is uncommon. However, acute and transient neuropathic pain is felt whenever the "funny bone" is struck or an extremity "falls asleep" from pressure. Perhaps the most frequent nonmalignant chronic neuropathic pain is that produced by nerve root compression from a herniated intervertebral disk. Neuropathic pain is often described as prolonged, severe, burning, lancinating, and squeezing and is often associated with focal neurologic deficits. It is usually constant but may be interrupted by paroxysms of dramatically increased pain. There may be no area of tenderness or areas of exquisite sensitivity to normally innocuous stimuli (allodynia). Symptoms and signs of autonomic instability may accompany neuropathic pain. The clinical hallmarks of neuropathic pain are spontaneous pains and painful responses to non-noxious stimuli. Neuropathic pain is also characterized by its relative resistance to opioids, making it the most challenging of pain conditions to treat.[18] Cancer patients experience neuropathic pain from a variety of causes. Direct infiltration of neural structures by tumor is the most common, but iatrogenic causes, such as radiation fibrosis and surgical injury, also occur.

Injury to any part of the nervous system, whether central or peripheral, may result in neuropathic pain. A number of theories have been advanced to explain both peripheral and central mechanisms for maintaining the perceived pain. In the periphery, C fibers may become sensitized by direct injury or by ongoing nociception from injured tissues. This sensitization would make them susceptible to stimuli that are not normally perceived as painful, including sympathetic discharges.[19,20] Two other peripheral mechanisms include neuroma formation (in which an injured nerve's attempt to regrow results in an overly sensitive, disordered jumble of fibers) and abnormal foci of sensitivity along the course of a nerve, resulting in ephaptic transmission (cross-talk) or ectopic discharges.[21,22]

Regardless of the initial site of neurologic injury, the central nervous system probably plays a significant role in maintaining the pain syndrome. Increased sensitivity to peripheral stimuli can be demonstrated in the dorsal horn of the spinal cord, as can spontaneous activity. This spinal cord hypersensitivity could explain both the spontaneous pain and the allodynia felt in neuropathic pain syndromes.

CANCER PAIN SYNDROMES

Most pain syndromes in patients with advanced cancer are caused by direct tumor invasion of pain-sensitive structures. The specific pain syndrome depends more on the type of structure involved (e.g., bone pain, visceral pain, mucosal irritation) than on the causative tumor. Similarly, though less commonly, the injury is iatrogenic from diagnostic, surgical, chemotherapeutic, and radiotherapeutic interventions. In many patients, pain has multiple causes. Because increasing pain may signal advancing disease, determining its cause is important.[23] In addition, knowing the cause of pain assists in selecting the most appropriate analgesic approach. The following are several common, recognizable painful conditions that occur in cancer patients. They are grouped according to the type or location of pain.

BONE PAIN

Tumor involvement of bone is the most common cause of cancer pain.[15] Any tumor may involve bone, but the most common include metastatic cancer of the breast, lung, prostate, and thyroid and multiple myeloma.[1,24] This is purely somatic pain unless pathologic fracture or tumor extension disrupts nerve. As such, pain is usually described as focal and constant but may be referred. Typically, patients experience several days or weeks of increasing pain. Acutely increased bone pain may signal fracture or neural impingement. Tumors may activate nociceptors by pressure, ischemia, or secretion of algesic substances (e.g., prostaglandin E_2, osteoclast activating factor).[25] Most pain is probably sensed in periosteum and synovium; these are quite sensitive to surgical manipulation. Common sites of bony metastasis are the vertebral column, skull, humerus, ribs, pelvis, and femur.[8]

Hematologic malignancies can rarely produce painful bone marrow expansion, presumably caused by nests of rapidly growing cells in the marrow.[24,26]

Diagnosis of bony metastases in known cancer patients may be made by plain radiographs when tumor involves the cortex. A computed tomography (CT) scan further defines the morphology of bone lesions that are seen on radiographs. When the radiographs are normal, radionuclide scintigraphy (bone scan) may identify osteoid formation in the marrow before cortical destruction has occurred. Even in predominantly osteolytic tumors, some reactive osteoid formation usually occurs, and the bone scan result is positive (**Table 54-2**).[27] A bone scan, however, is often normal in purely lytic tumors, such as multiple myeloma, and in previously irradiated bone. Furthermore, it lacks the anatomic detail of radiography. Magnetic resonance imaging (MRI) is more sensitive than radiography and bone scan and can identify bony metastases in previously irradiated bone.[8] MRI is not used as the initial diagnostic tool because it is expensive, time consuming, and often not immediately available.

Other forms of bone pain in cancer are iatrogenic; these include avascular necrosis of the femoral and humeral heads from steroid treatment, osteoradionecrosis after radiation treatment, and pseudorheumatism from steroid withdrawal. Radiographs do not confirm avascular necrosis for several weeks or months after the onset of pain; a bone scan is more sensitive.[8] Osteoradionecrosis usually occurs in the mandible and may develop months or years after irradiation. It must always be distinguished from recurrent tumor, radiation-induced sarcoma, and osteomyelitis.[28] Reinstitution of steroid treatment, followed by slow withdrawal, confirms the diagnosis of pseudorheumatism by relieving the arthralgias and myalgias.[8]

To relieve the pain, pathologic fractures of long bones are surgically stabilized when feasible. Vertebral collapse is more often treated conservatively with analgesics or with vertebroplasty or kyphoplasty. Radiation adds to pain control of all pathologic fractures. Local field external-beam radiation therapy is an effective palliative modality for painful bone metastases, with pain relief seen in 80% to 90% of cases.[24] A rare paraneoplastic form of renal phosphate wasting called oncogenic osteomalacia can cause osteomalacia, multifocal bone pain, and fractures.[24,29] This rare syndrome is most often associated with mesenchymal neoplasms, and complete tumor removal can lead to rapid correction of the biochemical derangements, remineralization of bone, and symptom improvement.

BACK PAIN

The vertebral column (particularly the thoracic spine) is the most common site of bony metastases.[30] Although cancer causes less than 1% of back pain in the general population, 98% of known cancer patients who present with back pain have underlying malignancy.[31] Up to one-third of cancer patients develop metastases to the spine, with prostate, breast, thyroid, and lung cancers being most common.[30,32] Because back pain in cancer patients usually signifies bone or epidural metastasis, aggressive investigation to define the presence and extent of tumor is necessary. Left untreated, metastases destabilize the axial skeleton and encroach on the spinal cord or cauda equina.

TABLE 54-2 Primary Bone Response to Some Tumors

Osteoblastic	Osteolytic
Prostate	Thyroid
Breast	Kidney
Carcinoid	Colorectal
	Breast (may be either)
	Non-Hodgkin's lymphoma
Hodgkin's disease	Lung
	Multiple myeloma

Investigation of back pain should begin with a detailed history and physical examination, attending to the presence of rapid pain progression, referral patterns, and neurologic symptoms and findings. Points that should raise the suspicion of epidural disease include failure of pain to resolve with recumbency; point tenderness of the spine on examination; and, of course, any history of bowel or bladder dysfunction or focal neurologic deficit. Vertebral disease at certain levels of the spine may initially have a confusing presentation. High cervical spine metastases may produce only posterior headache, which could be mistaken for tension headache. Involvement of C7 to T1 causes pain in the interscapular region. Lesions of T12 or L1 may refer pain to the flank, iliac crest, or sacroiliac joint. Sacral destruction may refer pain in a saddle pattern.[1] Radiation myelopathy causes local burning pain, which radiates bilaterally, and progressive neurologic deficits.[33]

Stable back pain in cancer patients, without neurologic symptoms or signs, warrants nonurgent radiography of the affected area. Radiographs will detect approximately 70% of vertebral tumors.[31] If plain radiographs are normal, radionuclide bone scan is indicated because it has a higher sensitivity than radiography for early osteoblastic lesions, fractures, and infection. If radiography or bone scan is positive or equivocal, MRI should be performed to detect or define the extent of disease, especially that involving soft tissue.[27] If both radiography and bone scan results are normal, CT or MRI of the paraspinal and retroperitoneal areas is warranted to detect a source of referred or extraaxial soft tissue pain.

Magnetic resonance imaging is always the test of first choice when there is evidence of neural compression and should be completed urgently if cord compression is suspected. MRI is sensitive for early metastases, easily images the entire spine in one scan (unlike CT), and accurately defines the extent of adjacent soft tissue disease.[27] CT with myelography may be used when MRI is not available.

Even when there is no evidence of neural compression by history or physical examination, radiologic evaluation should not be delayed for more than several days if back pain is positional or progressing. Unstable vertebral fractures may lead to acute cord compression and may require prophylactic stabilization or irradiation.[34]

Some patients with back pain due to epidural malignancy do not have vertebral metastases. Tumor may reach the epidural space by hematogenous spread or by direct extension along nerves, through the intervertebral foramina. Neoplastic epidural spinal cord compression (ESCC) is a common complication of cancer that can cause pain and potentially irreversible loss of neurologic function. Most often, ESCC is caused by posterior extension of a vertebral body metastasis into the epidural space. ESCC almost always presents initially as back or neck pain. Because pain usually precedes neurologic impairment by weeks or months, it is crucial to diagnose epidural disease extension in patients when pain is the sole complaint so that effective treatment may be started to prevent or retard the progression of neurologic impairment. For most patients, MRI is the preferred approach to evaluate the epidural space.[24]

For most patients, radiation therapy (RT) represents first-line definitive treatment for ESCC. Glucocorticoid treatment is useful to temporarily improve pain and neurologic functioning, often providing a window of time during which RT can be provided. Surgical decompression is considered if the tumor type is typically radioresistant and the lesion is high grade, the neurologic status is deteriorating during RT, ESCC occurs in a previously irradiated field, the lesion is posterior and can be easily extirpated, or a tissue diagnosis is needed.[24]

Other patients with back pain in the absence of vertebral disease may have leptomeningeal carcinomatosis (LC). They have signs of neurologic dysfunction at several levels and usually complain of headache, nausea, and nuchal rigidity but may also have lumbar radicular pain.[33] Contrast-enhanced MRI of the entire spine and head followed by lumbar puncture is appropriate when LC is detected. LC may require treatment with radiation, steroids, or intrathecal chemotherapy.

Loss of motor function, hyper- or hyporeflexia, and bowel or bladder disturbances are suggestive of myelopathy. Their presence should prompt immediate intervention, even before diagnostic imaging has been obtained, to prevent permanent neurologic impairment (**Fig. 54-1**). Even in the absence of myelopathy, certain situations require urgent radiologic evaluation. Rapidly progressing pain is highly suspect for tumor and should be investigated until the extent of disease is known. Increased pain when supine or erect may signal positional cord compression, which will progress to overt myelopathy unless treated. In these situations, MRI of the entire spine should be performed to define the extent of disease and the threat to neural tissue.[35]

BRACHIAL PLEXOPATHY

Brachial plexopathy is a common neurologic complication of cancer.[33] Metastatic brachial plexopathy (MBP) and radiation-induced brachial plexopathy (RBP) are the most likely culprits when shoulder and arm pain is present in a patient with cancer. The differential diagnosis for arm pain includes cervical radiculopathy, osteoarthritis, bursitis of the shoulder, and myofascial pain. Less common cancer-related causes are iatrogenic plexus injury during surgery or central venous catheter placement, chemotherapeutic neurotoxicity, and secondary plexus tumors after radiation.[36] Primary brachial plexus tumors are uncommon and rarely symptomatic. They are mostly solitary but can be multiple in patients with neurofibromatosis type I. These patients are more likely to present with pain or neurologic deficits.

Metastatic brachial plexopathy, also called Pancoast syndrome and thoracic inlet syndrome, presents in 2% to 9% of patients with lung and breast cancer[37,38] and is also seen in lymphoma, thyroid cancer, and others.[36] Tumor may spread to the plexus from the apex of the lung or from nearby lymph nodes. Differentiating MBP from RBP may be difficult when a patient has received radiation (**Table 54-3**). MBP typically presents with neuropathic pain in the ipsilateral shoulder or arm, which is rapidly progressive. Although both conditions may eventually involve the entire plexus, selective lower plexus involvement implies MBP, and upper plexus involvement occurs with RBP. The time from cancer diagnosis to presentation (3–6 years) is similar for MBP and RBP in patients who have received radiation.[36] Horner's syndrome is much more likely in MBP than RBP and is highly associated with epidural tumor spread, which occurs in 25% of MBP patients, often without abnormalities on radiography, bone scan, or myelogram.[39] MRI is more sensitive than myelography for epidural disease and should be used in the evaluation of patients with cancer and brachial plexopathy (Fig. 54-1).[40,41]

Olsen and colleagues found that 14% of 128 breast cancer patients receiving surgery and radiation developed RBP. The addition of cytotoxic chemotherapy increased the likelihood of RBP. Forty-seven percent of the RBP patients had pain.[42] The dose of radiation may also affect the incidence of RBP, as does treatment technique. RBP is associated with progressive fibrous constriction of nerve bundles, thickening of endoneurium, loss of myelin, and obliteration of small blood vessels. Initial symptoms of RBP are paresthesias, numbness, heaviness, weakness, and swelling. Pain is a presenting symptom in 18% and becomes a major symptom in 35%. Sensory and motor loss progress gradually, eventually rendering the arm useless. Reversible radiation-induced plexopathy has been reported in conjunction with chemotherapy for breast cancer. This entity presents earlier than RBP, rarely causes pain or weakness, and resolves in time.[43]

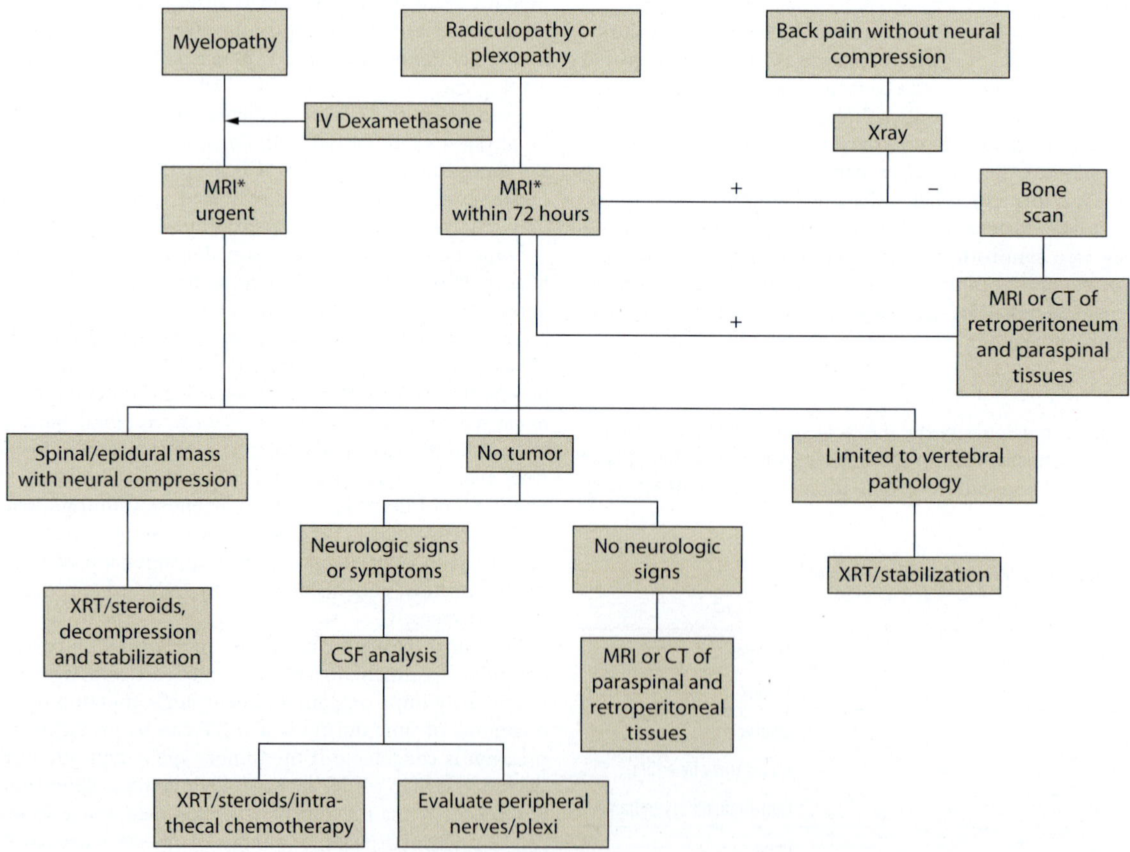

FIGURE 54-1. Diagnostic approach to back pain in the cancer patient. (*Combined computed tomography and myelography may be used in place of magnetic resonance imaging [MRI] if MRI is unavailable or contraindicated.)

TABLE 54-3 Clinical Presentation of Patients with Metastatic Brachial Plexopathy (MBP) Versus Radiation-Induced Brachial Plexopathy (RBP)

	MBP, *n* (%)		
Presenting Symptom	With Prior Radiation (*n* = 44)	Without Prior Radiation (*n* = 34)	RBP (*n* = 22), *n* (%)
Pain	33 (75)	39 (89)	4 (18)
Arm swelling	0 (0)	0 (0)	9 (40)
Dysesthesia	11 (25)	2 (6)	12 (55)
Arm weakness	0 (0)	2 (6)	6 (27)
Horner's syndrome	23 (53)	19 (56)	3 (14)
Lymphedema	6 (13)	5 (15)	16 (73)
Upper trunk (C5–C6)	0 (0)	3 (9)	17 (77)
Lower (C8–T1)	33 (75)	23 (68)	0 (0)
Whole plexus	11 (25)	8 (23)	5 (23)

Magnetic resonance imaging is the best imaging modality to differentiate MBP from RBP.[41] If MRI is not available, however, CT should be performed with intravenous contrast. An electromyelogram (EMG) of the affected arm and shoulder muscles shows fibrillation potentials and myokymia in RBP but not in pure MBP. However, patients with brachial plexus tumor may also have some radiation fibrosis, so EMG cannot rule out MBP. Biopsy also may confirm fibrosis or tumor but cannot rule out either one. When pain presents many years after radiation in a patient who was thought to be free of cancer, MRI and biopsy should be used to rule out radiation-induced secondary neoplasm.[1]

LUMBOSACRAL PLEXOPATHY

Pelvic tumors may invade or compress the lumbar and sacral plexuses to produce pain, bowel and bladder dysfunction, and leg weakness. Jaeckle and colleagues studied 85 patients with pelvic tumor and low back or leg pain.[44] The most common primary tumors were colorectal, uterine, cervical, breast, sarcoma, and lymphoma. Seventy percent presented with pain, and 98% eventually developed pain, which was aching and pressure-like. Pain was local, radicular, or referred, and a combination of local and radicular was common. Two-thirds developed weakness, and half developed sensory symptoms. Twenty-seven percent had bilateral plexopathy. Epidural extension was detected in 35% of patients.

Neoplastic lumbosacral plexopathy is virtually always associated with known malignancy or obvious pelvic metastatic disease. Uncommonly, prostate cancer can present as a lumbosacral plexopathy occurring through direct pelvic spread. There is a report of two cases of lumbosacral radiculoplexopathy from infiltrative prostate cancer without evidence of other pelvic or extraprostatic spread. The authors proposed perineural spread along prostatic nerves as probable etiology of tumor spreading into the lumbosacral plexus.[45]

Radiation-induced lumbosacral plexopathy (LP) is rare, and, as in RBP, sensory and motor symptoms commonly precede pain; approximately half of patients never develop pain. Plexopathy follows radiation by an average of 5 years, but there is a considerable range. Symptoms are usually bilateral but asymmetric.[46]

Diagnosis of LP starts with a history of unilateral or bilateral pain or weakness in the low back, abdomen, perineum, or leg. Bowel and bladder function may be spared when only the upper plexus is involved. Involvement of the lower lumbosacral plexus (sciatic nerve), occurring in one half of patients, resembles sciatica from a herniated intervertebral disk, with a positive straight leg raising test result and tenderness in the sciatic notch. Upper plexus involvement, occurring in one-third of patients, produces tenderness in the lumbar region.[44] Lower (sacral) plexopathy results in urinary incontinence, sexual impotence, and neuropathic perineal and genital pain. Radiologic evaluation of LP begins with MRI or contrast-enhanced CT of the lumbosacral spine. If the results are negative, an extraaxial pain source is sought (see Fig. 54-1). If the history suggests radiation fibrosis of the plexus, EMG to detect fibrillation potentials and myokymic discharges is useful but does not rule out tumor as the cause of LP.[46]

CERVICAL PLEXOPATHY

Injury to the cervical plexus, whether from tumor or surgery, causes pain in and around the ear or in the anterior neck to the clavicle. The phrenic nerve may also be paralyzed. Horner's syndrome is seen if the superior cervical ganglion is affected. The differential includes disease of the upper cervical spine and the base of the skull.[33] In a patient who has had surgery in the area, Horner's syndrome, phrenic nerve paralysis, and signs of cervical myelopathy or contralateral radiculopathy should suggest recurrent tumor. In such patients, and in those who have not had neck surgery, MRI with contrast is indicated to define the extent of the disease.

HEADACHE AND FACIAL PAIN

Headache occurs in about 60% of patients presenting with primary brain tumors and is the presenting symptom in 50% of patients with cerebral metastases (see also Chapter 29, Pathophysiology of Headaches). It is usually of mild or moderate intensity, similar to a tension-type headache. Only 25% of patients have awakening or morning headaches. Cancer patients with new headaches or a change in headache pattern should be investigated for cerebral metastases. Neurologic signs are more common than neurologic symptoms in these patients. Weakness is a presenting symptom in approximately 30%, but a hemiparesis can be found in about 60%.[47] Papilledema is surprisingly uncommon, appearing in only 25%, so its absence should not be taken as reassuring. Investigation of the suspicious headache should include MRI or CT, both with intravenous contrast. MRI is more sensitive, especially for skull base and posterior fossa tumors, and delineates the extent of disease more precisely than CT. Initial management is with corticosteroids followed by antitumor therapy or symptomatic treatment.[48] Brain tumor headache characteristically responds rapidly to the administration of corticosteroids.

Not all headaches in patients with cancer are caused by cerebral metastases. Leptomeningeal metastases cause headaches that are commonly associated with radicular or cranial nerve findings. Multiple metastases, posterior fossa metastases, and LC are the most frequent intracranial causes of head pain. Any solid or hematologic neoplasm can potentially infiltrate the leptomeninges, but the common tumors are lung and breast cancer, lymphoma, and leukemia.[49,50] Cerebrospinal fluid analysis is almost always abnormal, but only a positive cytology or demonstration of intrathecal synthesis of tumor markers is diagnostic. T1-weighted gadolinium-enhanced sequence of the entire neuraxis (brain and spine) plays an important role in supporting the diagnosis, demonstrating the involved sites, and guiding treatment.[50]

Other cancer-related causes include ischemic or hemorrhagic stroke, pseudotumor cerebri from superior vena cava syndrome, and sagittal sinus occlusion by tumor or thrombus.[33] Fever and migraine are the most common noncancer causes of headaches in patients with cancer.

Cancer is a rare cause of facial pain. Extracranial bony or soft tissue metastases may impinge on cranial and upper cervical nerves, causing headache or facial pain. Pain in these cases is usually unilateral and may be accompanied by focal tenderness. Glossopharyngeal neuralgia may be seen in patients with leptomeningeal metastases, jugular foramen invasion, or more peripheral primary head or neck malignancies. Pain occurs in the pharynx and base of the tongue and sometimes around the ear. Pain in the trigeminal distribution has been described with middle and posterior fossa tumors, skull base metastases, and lymphomatous meningitis.[33] Of 2972 patients with a diagnosis of trigeminal neuralgia at the Mayo Clinic, 10% were found to have tumors, the majority of which were benign.[51] Unilateral facial pain has been described as a presenting symptom of ipsilateral nonmetastatic lung cancer. It is typically severe, around the ear and temple, and resolves with radiation of the tumor. It probably occurs when tumor invades the vagus nerve.[52]

Metastases to the base of the skull produce distinct patterns of head and facial pain.[33,48] Breast, lung, prostate, and nasopharyngeal tumors are common primary tumors. A tumor in the orbit produces progressive pain in the supraorbital area, proptosis, and external ophthalmoplegia. A parasellar tumor may present with unilateral supraorbital and frontal headache with diplopia. Middle fossa tumors often present with pain and sensory changes in the mandibular and maxillary trigeminal distributions, which may be followed by headache, diplopia, dysarthria, and dysphagia. Tumor invading the jugular foramen affects the glossopharyngeal, vagus, and accessory nerves to cause throat pain, hoarseness, dysphagia, and weakness of the sternocleidomastoid and trapezius muscles. Involvement of the occipital condyle causes occipital pain and neck stiffness with associated hypoglossal nerve paralysis. Metastasis to the clivus presents with vertex headache, worse with neck flexion, and eventual lower cranial nerve dysfunction. Sphenoid sinus tumor may cause bifrontal headache radiating to the temples and retro-orbital areas, sometimes with abducens nerve palsy. Fracture of the odontoid process (dens), pathologic or not, causes posterior headache with increased pain on neck flexion. The resulting cervical spine instability or mass effect from such a tumor may cause spinal cord or brain stem compression.

PERIPHERAL NEUROPATHIES

Peripheral neuropathies in cancer can be divided into mononeuropathies and more symmetric polyneuropathies. Any nerve may be directly affected by tumor, but radicular pain and intercostal entrapment from rib metastasis are the most common.[33]

The most common symmetric polyneuropathies are paraneoplastic syndromes and those resulting from chemotherapy. One paraneoplastic syndrome associated with oat-cell lung cancer, breast, colon, and ovarian cancers is a painful sensory neuropathy. It is characterized clinically by tingling, burning, and lancinating pains in the extremities. Pathologic examination reveals an inflammatory process in the dorsal root ganglia followed by loss of peripheral myelinated and unmyelinated fibers.[53] This syndrome may be a presenting feature of the cancer. Multiple myeloma is commonly associated with a painful sensorimotor neuropathy that responds to tumor therapy.[33] Ovarian, lung, and breast cancer may also cause sensorimotor neuropathy as they progress.[54,55] In these cases, segmental demyelination and axonal degeneration are seen histologically.[53]

Chemotherapy often produces a painful peripheral neuropathy with dysesthesias. The vinca alkaloids and cisplatinum are most commonly to blame, and symptoms are dose related. Burning in the feet and hands and vibratory and proprioceptive deficits are characteristic.[33,56] Paclitaxel, oxaliplatin, thalidomide, and bortezomib also have a high incidence of polyneuropathy. The onset of pain is most commonly insidious, but it can present acutely (e.g., oxaliplatin-induced pharyngolaryngeal spasm). Chemotherapy-induced neuropathic pain usually gradually improves after the treatment is stopped or the dose is reduced; occasionally, neuropathic pain becomes chronic.[24]

ACUTE ZOSTER AND POSTHERPETIC NEURALGIA

Painful varicella-zoster reactivation causes a dermatomal rash and neuropathic pain. It occurs two to three times as frequently in cancer patients as in the general population. Lymphoma and breast cancers cause a disproportionate number of cases. The dermatome involved is likely to correlate with the site of primary tumor in breast, lung, and gynecologic cancer.[57] Advancing age, the severity of the initial rash and pain, and an ophthalmic distribution predispose to the later development of postherpetic neuralgia. Cancer does not appear to increase the likelihood of postherpetic neuralgia when age is accounted for.[58] A thorough review of zoster and related pain is provided in Chapter 49.

ABDOMINAL AND PELVIC PAIN

In a review of 5675 patients presenting with acute abdominal pain to a group of five European hospitals, 106 (1.9%) were eventually found to have intraabdominal cancer. The risk of cancer for those older than 50 years was 10%.[59] Abdominal pain from cancer is typically visceral in nature. As such, it is poorly localized and often referred to distant sites and is often accompanied by nausea and vomiting. Diaphragmatic irritation and distension of the hepatic capsule produce ipsilateral shoulder pain, retroperitoneal tumor may cause back pain, and pelvic tumor may cause perineal pain. Viscus or duct blockage and distension, peritoneal inflammation or tension, mesenteric torsion, and vascular or lymphatic obstruction typically produce pain. Pelvic cancer pain occurs primarily in patients with malignancies of the rectum and genitourinary tracts. Extraabdominal cancers also often metastasize to the sacrum and pelvis.

Abdominal pain not directly caused by intraperitoneal or retroperitoneal malignancy is also common. Radiation-induced enteritis occurs in acute and chronic forms. Acute injury manifests as abdominal or pelvic pain, diarrhea, or tenesmus in up to half of patients. Chronic injury, occurring in 2% to 5% of patients, presents as stricture, bleeding, perforation, or fistula 6 to 24 months after radiation. Pain may be associated with bowel ischemia, obstruction, or intraabdominal infection in patients with chronic enteritis.[60] Pain may radiate or refer to the abdomen from destructive low thoracic and high lumbar spine disease and nerve root compression. After abdominal surgery for cancer, adhesions may form and cause painful bowel obstruction.

Pain from pancreatic cancer is of particular interest because of its frequency, severity, and amenability to celiac plexus block. Up to 80% of patients with this disease present with significant pain. With advanced disease, the figure rises to 90% and probably represents gastric or retroperitoneal invasion. Most tumors are at the head of the gland and may cause bile duct obstruction early in the disease. Pain from the pancreatic head localizes to the right epigastrium, that from the body of the pancreas is felt in the mid-epigastrium, and tumor in the tail produces pain in the left epigastrium and posterior intercostal space.[61]

Kelsen and colleagues prospectively assessed pain, pain intensity, and pain location in 77 newly diagnosed patients with operable adenocarcinoma of the pancreas. They concluded that even if the patient can undergo resection, the presence of preoperative pain is associated with a poor prognosis. Patients with operable pancreatic cancer who present with pain, even those whose evaluation shows a likelihood of resectability, are at high risk for recurrence with an impaired survival compared with those patients without pain.[62]

MUCOSITIS

In about 70% of patients, chemoradiotherapeutic conditioning for bone marrow or stem cell transplantation causes noninfectious mucositis (stomatitis) by killing cells with high mitotic rates.[63] Several days after conditioning, hemorrhagic degradation and ulceration of the oropharyngeal mucosa begins. Although initially causing constant mild or moderate burning discomfort, the condition progresses to preclude talking, eating, or swallowing. Significant pain requiring opioid use persists in half of patients at 3 weeks after transplant.[64] Mucositis from head and neck radiation usually develops in the second or third week of therapy, affects almost all patients, and is otherwise similar to that from bone marrow conditioning. Normal doses of chemotherapeutic agents also cause mucositis in about 40% of patients.[63] On a molecular pathology level, mucositis is characterized as having five phases: initiation, upregulation with messenger generation, signaling and amplification, ulceration and inflammation, and finally healing.[65] Oral mucositis is a common complication of cancer therapy that may limit the completion of treatment and affect the quality of life of the patient. This problem can be addressed with prevention of infection through good oral hygiene, oral rinses and antibiotic pastilles, prevention of free radical damage via cytoprotectants, targeting the inflammatory process via anti-inflammatories, and promoting reepithelialization via biologic response modifiers. Cryotherapy is most commonly used before administration of 5-fluorouracil bolus.[66]

Pain may be more severe or prolonged when mucosal ulcers become superinfected with bacteria or fungus and when graft-versus-host disease occurs. Reactivation of herpes simplex, cytomegalovirus, or varicella-zoster infections in an immunocompromised cancer patient may present with vesiculo-ulcerative mucositis.

CHRONIC POSTSURGICAL PAIN

Four postsurgical chronic pain syndromes have been identified. They result from injury to nerve or plexus, so the pain is neuropathic in nature.

Mastectomy Burning, aching, and tight constriction of the axilla, medial upper arm, and chest with superimposed lancinations and scar sensitivity are characteristic of postmastectomy pain. Phantom breast pain is also described, and uncomfortable lymphedema of the arm is common. Whereas previously fewer than 10% of mastectomy patients were said to develop chronic pain,[33] half of 467 mastectomy patients recently surveyed went on to develop pain, paresthesias, and phantom sensations.[67] Less extensive surgery was more often associated with pain in the ipsilateral arm. In fact, the radiation and chemotherapy that followed less extensive surgery were probably responsible for much of the arm pain. Progressive pain was more common in patients with recurrent disease.

Maunsell and colleagues studied arm symptoms in 223 women who underwent breast surgery with or without axillary dissection.[68] About half complained of arm pain at 3 months postoperatively and a similar proportion at 15 months. Patients who had axillary dissection were more likely to have arm pain, although this result did not reach statistical significance. Wallace and colleagues also found that breast reconstruction with implants after mastectomy increases the likelihood of chronic pain from about 30% (mastectomy alone or with simple reconstruction) to 50%.[69] Submuscular implant placement may injure the long thoracic, thoracodorsal, lateral pectoral, and medial pectoral nerves. Capsule formation around the implant may entrap the long thoracic and the two pectoral nerves.

Evaluation of chest and arm pain after mastectomy should focus on the nature of the pain and its location, as well as neurologic examination to define the areas of sensory loss and hypersensitivity. A neuroma is sought in the chest wall and axilla. Autonomic changes and limited shoulder motion may be present in the "frozen shoulder" syndrome. Scapular winging is seen when the long thoracic nerve has been disrupted. Pain that is not typical of postmastectomy pain syndrome should prompt evaluation for infection and tumor recurrence.

Neck Dissection During radical neck dissection, the superficial cervical plexus is dissected out. The result is often neuropathic pain and sensory loss in the anterolateral neck and extending to the shoulder. Division of the accessory nerve and removal of the sternocleidomastoid muscle may also lead to chronic pain via postural changes that affect the shoulder girdle and entrap the upper brachial plexus.[33] Loss of trapezius function leads to drooping of the shoulder, mild scapular winging; an inability to abduct the shoulder above 90 degrees; and forward rotation of the scapula, often with sternoclavicular subluxation (**Fig. 54-2**).[70] Frozen shoulder often develops as a result of weakness and pain.[71]

Ewing and Martin described 100 radical neck dissection patients in 1952.[70] Of 89 with unilateral operations, 42 patients had persistent shoulder pain. In two more recent studies, 76 of 100 radical neck dissection patients had shoulder pain and dysfunction when evaluated at least 6 months after surgery.[72,73] In 31, the pain was severe. The deep cervical plexus innervates enough of the trapezius muscle to maintain shoulder mobility and prevent shoulder and arm pain in some patients.[73] Any patient who has increasing pain after neck dissection should be evaluated for infection and tumor recurrence.

Thoracotomy Chronic chest pain after thoracotomy affects up to 55% of patients followed for more than 1 year.[74] Keller and colleagues

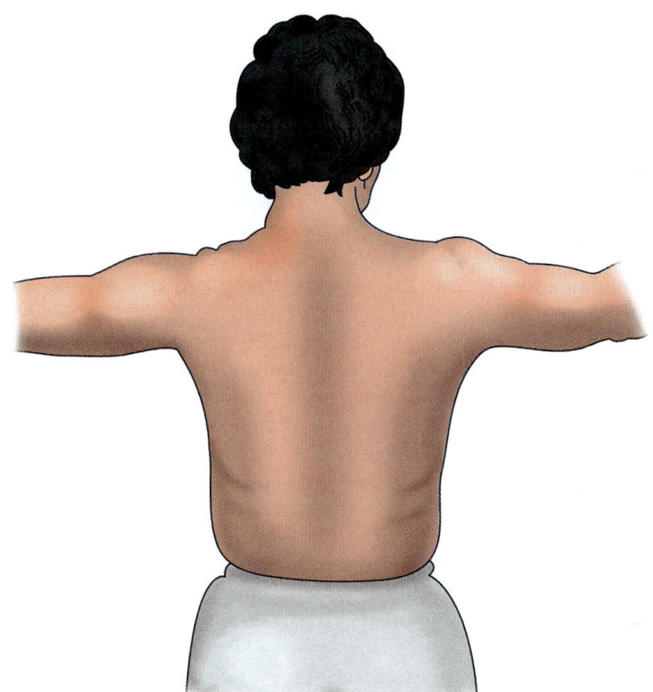

FIGURE 54-2. Posterior view of musculoskeletal changes seen after radical neck dissection. (From Braddom RL, Buschbacher RM, Dumitru D, et al, eds. *Physical Medicine and Rehabilitation*. Philadelphia: WB Saunders; 1996. With permission of Baylor College of Medicine, Houston, TX.)

reviewed the records of 238 consecutive thoracotomy patients.[75] Postthoracotomy pain was defined as that requiring regular use of analgesics beyond 3 months from surgery. Eleven percent of patients met this definition, but half of these used opioid analgesics preoperatively. Chest wall resection and pleurectomy increased the likelihood of chronic pain when compared with pulmonary resection. Importantly, all 20 patients with recurrence of pain after initial control were found to have tumor regrowth. The use of video-assisted thoracic surgery for pulmonary resection may decrease the incidence of chronic pain and disability when compared with thoracotomy.[76]

Mechanisms for chronic pain after thoracotomy are several. The intercostal nerves may be injured during rib resection or compressed with a retractor. Incidental rib fractures may entrap an intercostal nerve during healing. These patients may develop dermatomal chest wall numbness and neuropathic pain complaints, including point tenderness from neuroma formation. Severe rib retraction may also disarticulate the costochondral and costovertebral junctions, resulting in somatic pain and tenderness. Because the latissimus dorsi and serratus anterior muscles are often cut during thoracotomy, ipsilateral shoulder disability is also common. Untreated thoracotomy pain and inadequate rehabilitation may lead to frozen shoulder. Symptomatic myofascial trigger points often develop in chest wall muscles. All patients with increasing or recurrent pain after thoracotomy should be evaluated for tumor and infection.[75]

Koethe and colleagues recently reported a case of a patient with intractable postthoracotomy pain syndrome (PTPS) that was treated with intercostal nerve (ICN) cryoablation under cone-beam CT guidance with software-assisted needle trajectory planning and ablation zone simulation. This procedure provided the patient about 8 weeks of relief. This case demonstrated that ICN cryoablation is feasible under image guidance with device navigation and ablation simulation and may result in a few months of pain relief in cases of intractable PTPS.[77] Percutaneous ICN cryoablation by palpation of surface landmarks can be risky because inaccurate probe placement can lead to hemo- or pneumothorax. This case and the general idea of ever-improving surgical and imaging techniques give hope for more efficient management of surgery-related pain.

Amputation Chronic pain after limb amputation is stump pain, phantom pain, or both. Wartan and colleagues surveyed 590 patients with war-related amputations in England to assess the prevalence of chronic pain.[78] Of these, 55% reported phantom pain, and 56% had stump pain. Sherman and colleagues surveyed 5000 American veterans with amputations.[79] Fifty-five percent responded, and 78% of those reported phantom pain. Stump pain is due to local disease, most commonly infection or neuroma formation. Neuroma formation several weeks after amputation produces exquisite stump tenderness and pain that is either constant or elicited by palpation or movement. An ill-fitting prosthesis, recurrent tumor, infection, or ischemia may also cause local pain and tenderness.[80]

Phantom sensation, the sensory experience that the amputated limb is still present, occurs in most individuals with amputations. Phantom pain is often described as a paroxysmal burning, crushing, and twisting in the missing part. Phantom pain peaks in the first month after surgery and may fade slowly as it "telescopes" toward the stump.[79] It is more common after more proximal amputations.[81] Patients with extremity pain before amputation are more likely to develop immediate postamputation phantom pain,[82] and preemptive analgesia with lumbar epidural blockade may reduce the incidence of phantom pain.[83] In a randomized, double-blind, placebo-controlled, cross-over study completed by 14 patients, Bone and colleagues[84] found that after 6 weeks of treatment, gabapentin monotherapy was better than placebo in relieving postamputation phantom limb pain.

Numerous neurophysiologic explanations for phantom pain have been advanced, from changes at the stump to functional cortical changes. Sensory deafferentation in primates and arm amputation in humans cause cortical somatosensory reorganization.[85] This may explain the elicitation of phantom pain by sensory stimulation at other sites. As with the other postsurgical pain syndromes, an unexpected increase in or recurrence of pain should prompt evaluation for infection, ischemia, or tumor recurrence.[80,81]

PSYCHOLOGICAL ASPECTS OF CANCER PAIN

It is important to recognize that the experience of cancer pain is not merely physical. Cancer patients and those close to them suffer emotionally as well as physically. The way in which a patient and his or her family adjust to the experience of pain and dying markedly influences their perception of physical pain. Conversely, uncontrolled pain causes or contributes to anxiety, depression, and delirium in many cancer patients.[86] Derogatis and colleagues evaluated 215 unselected cancer patients for psychiatric disorders. Forty-seven percent had a DSM-defined (*Diagnostic and Statistical Manual of Mental Disorders*) psychiatric disorder (**Table 54-4**).[87]

Suicide is only slightly more common in cancer patients than the general population, but suicidal ideation is frequent and strongly associated with mood disturbance. Successful suicide typically occurs in patients with uncontrolled pain. Self-destructive personality traits and delirium also contribute to suicide attempts. The degree to which noncompliance and refusal of life-extending treatment represent suicide is not known.[88]

Fear of opioid addiction and abuse in cancer patients is a factor in the ongoing underuse of these medications for cancer pain. Tolerance (the need for increasing doses to achieve the same effect) and physical dependence (the occurrence of withdrawal symptoms when stopping or reducing opioid dosage) are expected with chronic opioid use. Addiction (a behavioral pattern of compulsive drug procurement and use for nonmedical reasons) is quite rare in cancer pain patients and may be less common than in those with nonmalignant pain.[89] Given their utility and safety, the sparing use of opioid analgesics in patients with cancer pain is inappropriate. As mentioned earlier in this chapter, the reasons for poorly treated pain come from both sides, from patients and health care providers. The goal should be to educate patients and to motivate physicians to follow pain management guidelines. Treatment should be escalated from nonopioid medications with or without adjuvant to opioid for mild to moderate pain and finally to opioid for moderate to severe pain[90] until adequate pain control is achieved.

TABLE 54-4 Prevalence of Psychiatric Disorders and Pain in 215 Cancer Patients

Psychiatric Diagnoses	Patients, *n* (%)	Psychiatric Diagnoses (%)	Patients with Significant Pain, *n* (%)
Adjustment disorders	69 (32)	68	—
Major affective disorders	13 (6)	13	—
Organic mental disorders	8 (4)	8	—
Personality disorders	7 (3)	7	—
Anxiety disorders	4 (2)	4	—
Total with psychiatric diagnosis	101 (47)		39 (39)
Total without psychiatric diagnosis	114 (53)		21 (19)
Total patients	215 (100)		60 (28)

Data from Derogatis LR, Morrow GR, Fetting J, et al. The prevalence of psychiatric disorders among cancer patients. *JAMA*. 1983;249:751. © 1983, American Medical Association. As adapted by Breitbard W. Psychiatric management of cancer pain. *Cancer*. 1989;63:2336. © 1989 American Cancer Society. Reprinted by permission of Wiley-Liss, Inc., a subsidiary of John Wiley & Sons.

REFERENCES

1. Portenoy RK. Cancer pain: epidemiology and syndromes. *Cancer*. 1989;63:2298.
2. National Cancer Institute website. Available at http://seer.cancer.gov/statfacts/html/all.html. Accessed August 2013.
3. Marcus DA. Epidemiology of cancer pain. *Curr Pain Headache Rep*. 2011;15(4):231-234.
4. Daut RL, Cleeland CS. The prevalence and severity of pain in cancer. *Cancer*. 1982;50:1913.
5. Cleeland CS, Gonin R, Hatfield AK, et al. Pain and its treatment in outpatients with metastatic cancer. *N Engl J Med*. 1994;330:592.
6. Coyle N, Adelhardt J, Foley KM, Portenoy RK. Character of terminal illness in the advanced cancer patient: pain and other symptoms during the last four weeks of life. *J Pain Symptom Manage*. 1990;5:83.
7. Quill TE. Doctor, I want to die. Will you help me? *JAMA*. 1993;270:870.
8. Foley KM. Pain syndromes in patients with cancer. In: Bonica JJ, Ventafridda B, eds. *Advances in Pain Research and Therapy*. Vol. 2. New York: Raven Press; 1979:59.
9. Gutgsell T, Walsh D, Zhukovsky DS, et al. A prospective study of the pathophysiology and clinical characteristics of pain in a palliative medicine population. *Am J Hosp Palliat Care*. 2003;20(2):140-148.
10. Jacobsen R, Liubarskiene Z, Møldrup C, et al. Barriers to cancer pain management: a review of empirical research. *Medicina (Kaunas)*. 2009;45(6):427-433.
11. Peker L, Celebi N, Canbay O, et al. Doctors' opinions, knowledge and attitudes towards cancer pain management in a university hospital. *Agri*. 2008;20:20-30.
12. MacDonald N, Ayoub J, Farley J, et al. A Quebec survey of issues in cancer pain management. *J Pain Symptom Manage*. 2002;23:39-47.

13. Eun-Ok I, Seung HL, Yi L, et al. A national online forum on ethnic differences in cancer pain experience. *Nurs Res.* 2009;58:86-94.

14. Chen CH, Tang ST, Chen CH. Meta-analysis of cultural differences in Western and Asian patient-perceived barriers to managing cancer pain. *Palliat Med.* 2012;26(3):206-221.

15. Foley KM. The treatment of cancer pain. *N Engl J Med.* 1985; 13:84.

16. Capps JA, Coleman GH. *An Experimental and Clinical Study of Pain in the Pleura, Pericardium, and Peritoneum.* New York: McMillan; 1932.

17. Sengupta JN. Visceral pain: the neurophysiological mechanism. *Handb Exp Pharmacol.* 2009;(194):31-74.

18. Portenoy RK, Foley KM, Inturrisi CE. The nature of opioid responsiveness and its implications for neuropathic pain: new hypotheses derived from studies of opioid infusions. *Pain.* 1990;43:273.

19. Cline MA, Ochoa J, Torebjork HE. Chronic hyperalgesia and skin warming caused by sensitized C nociceptors. *Brain.* 1989;112:621.

20. Hu S, Zhu J. Sympathetic facilitation of sustained discharges of polymodal nociceptors. *Pain.* 1989;38:85.

21. Devor M. Neuropathic pain and injured nerve: peripheral mechanisms. *Br Med Bull.* 1991;47:619.

22. Burchiel KJ. Abnormal impulse generation in focally demyelinated trigeminal roots. *J Neurosurg.* 1980;53:674.

23. Gonzales GR, Elliott KJ, Portenoy RK, Foley KM. The impact of a comprehensive evaluation in the management of cancer pain. *Pain.* 1991;47:141.

24. Portenoy RK, Dhingra LK. Overview of cancer pain syndromes. http://:ww.uptodate.com/store. Topic last updated August 20, 2012.

25. Payne R. Cancer pain: anatomy, physiology, and pharmacology. *Cancer.* 1989;63(suppl):2266.

26. Beckers R, Uyttebroeck A, Demaerel P. Acute lymphoblastic leukaemia presenting with low back pain. *Eur J Paediatr Neurol.* 2002;6(5):285.

27. Tryciecky EW, Gottschalk A, Ludema K. Oncologic imaging: interactions of nuclear medicine with CT and MRI using the bone scan as a model. *Semin Nucl Med.* 1997;27:142.

28. Friedman RB. Osteoradionecrosis: causes and prevention. *NCI Monogr.* 1990;9:145.

29. Jan de Beur SM. Tumor-induced osteomalacia. *JAMA.* 2005;294(10):1260-1267.

30. Posner JB. Back pain and epidural spinal cord compression. *Med Clin North Am.* 1987;71:185.

31. Deyo RA, Diehl AK. Cancer as a cause of back pain: frequency, clinical presentation, and diagnostic strategies. *J Gen Intern Med.* 1988;3:230.

32. Ruff RL, Lanska DJ. Epidural metastases in prospectively evaluated veterans with cancer and back pain. *Cancer.* 1989;63:2234.

33. Elliott K, Foley KM. Neurologic pain syndromes in patients with cancer. *Crit Care Clin.* 1990;6:393.

34. Hoskin PJ. Radiotherapy in the management of bone pain. *Clin Orthop Rel Res.* 1995;312:105.

35. Heldmann U, Myschetzky PS, Thomsen HS. Frequency of unexpected multifocal metastasis in patients with acute spinal cord compression. Evaluation by low-field MR imaging in cancer patients. *Acta Radiol.* 1997;38:372.

36. Kori SH. Diagnosis and management of brachial plexus lesions in cancer patients. *Oncology.* 1995;8:756.

37. Berrino F. Epidemiology of superior pulmonary sulcus syndrome (Pancoast syndrome). In: Bonica JJ, Ventafridda V, Pagni CA, eds. *Advances in Pain Research and Therapy.* Vol. 4. New York: Raven Press; 1982:15.

38. Ampil FL. Radiotherapy for carcinomatous brachial plexopathy. *Cancer.* 1985;56:2185.

39. Kanner RM, Martini N, Foley KM. Epidural spinal cord compression in Pancoast syndrome (superior pulmonary sulcus tumor): clinical presentation and outcome. *Ann Neurol.* 1981;10:77.

40. Sarpel S, Sarpel G, Yu E, et al. Early diagnosis of spinal-epidural metastasis by magnetic resonance imaging. *Cancer.* 1987;59:1112.

41. Thayagarajan D, Cascino T, Harms F. Magnetic resonance imaging in brachial plexopathy of cancer. *Neurology.* 1995;45:421.

42. Olsen NK, Pfeiffer P, Johannsen L, et al. Radiation-induced brachial plexopathy: neurological follow-up in 161 recurrence-free breast cancer patients. *Int J Radiat Oncol Biol Phys.* 1993;26:43.

43. Salner AL, Botnick LE, Herzog AG, et al. Reversible brachial plexopathy following primary radiation therapy for breast cancer. *Cancer Treat Rep.* 1981;65:797.

44. Jaeckle KA, Young DF, Foley KM. The natural history of lumbosacral plexopathy in cancer. *Neurology.* 1985;35:8.

45. Ladha SS, Spinner RJ, Suarez GA, et al. Neoplastic lumbosacral radiculoplexopathy in prostate cancer by direct perineural spread: an unusual entity. *Muscle Nerve.* 2006;34(5):659-665.

46. Thomas JE, Cascino TL, Earl JD, et al. Differential diagnosis between radiation and tumor plexopathy of the pelvis. *Neurology.* 1985;35:1.

47. Cairncross JG. Neurological emergencies in cancer patients. *Prog Clin Biol Res.* 1983;132D:319.

48. Jaeckle KA. Causes and management of headaches in cancer patients. *Oncology (Huntingt).* 1993;7:27.

49. Taillibert S, Laigle-Donadey F, Chodkiewicz C, et al. Leptomeningeal metastases from solid malignancy: a review. *J Neurooncol.* 2005; 75(1):85-99.

50. Nolan CP, Abrey LE. Leptomeningeal metastases from leukemias and lymphomas. *Cancer Treat Res.* 2005;125:53.

51. Cheng TMW, Cascino TL, Onofrio BM. Comprehensive study of diagnosis and treatment of trigeminal neuralgia secondary to tumors. *Neurology.* 1993;43:2298.

52. Capobianco DJ. Facial pain as a symptom of nonmetastatic lung cancer. *Headache.* 1995;35:581.

53. Lamarche J, Vital C. Carcinomatous neuropathy. An ultrastructural study of ten cases. *Ann Pathol.* 1987;7:98.

54. Cavaletti G, Bogliun G, Marzorati L, et al. The incidence and course of paraneoplastic neuropathy in women with epithelial ovarian cancer. *J Neurol.* 1991;238:371.

55. Peterson K, Forsyth PA, Posner JB. Paraneoplastic sensorimotor neuropathy associated with breast cancer. *J Neurooncol.* 1994; 21:159.

56. van der Hoop RG, van der Burg MEL, Huinink WWB, van Houwelingen JC. Incidence of neuropathy in 395 patients with ovarian cancer treated with or without cisplatin. *Cancer.* 1990; 66:1697.

57. Rusthoven JJ, Ahlgren P, Elhakim T, et al. Varicella-zoster infection in adult cancer patients. A population study. *Arch Intern Med.* 1988;148:1561.

58. Choo PW, Galil K, Donahue JG, et al. Risk factors for postherpetic neuralgia. *Arch Intern Med.* 1997;157:1217.

59. deDombal FT, Matharu SS, Staniland JR, et al. Presentation of cancer to hospital as 'acute abdominal pain'. *Br J Surg.* 1980;67:413.

60. Nussbaum ML, Campana TJ, Weese JL. Radiation-induced intestinal injury. *Clin Plast Surg.* 1993;20:573.

61. Alter CL. Palliative and supportive care of patients with pancreatic cancer. *Semin Oncol*. 1996;23:229.
62. Kelsen DP, Portenoy R, Thaler H, Tao Y, Brennan M. Pain as a predictor of outcome in patients with operable pancreatic carcinoma. *Surgery*. 1997;122(1):53.
63. Berger AM, Bartoshuk LM, Duffy VB, Nadoolman W. Capsaicin for the treatment of oral mucositis pain. *PPO Updates*. 1995;9:1.
64. Chapko MK, Syrjala KL, Schilter L, et al. Chemoradiotherapy toxicity during bone marrow transplantation: time course and variation in pain and nausea. *Bone Marrow Transplant*. 1989;4:181.
65. Sonis ST, Elting LS, Keefe D, et al; Mucositis Study Section of the Multinational Association for Supportive Care in Cancer; International Society for Oral Oncology. Perspectives on cancer therapy-induced mucosal injury: pathogenesis, measurement, epidemiology, and consequences for patients. *Cancer*. 2004;100(9 Suppl):1995-2025.
66. Georgiou M, Patapatiou G, Domoxoudis S, et al. Oral mucositis: understanding the pathology and management. *Hippokratia*. 2012;16(3):215-216.
67. Tasmuth T, von Smitten K, Hietanen P, et al. Pain and other symptoms after different treatment modalities of breast cancer. *Ann Oncol*. 1995;6:453.
68. Maunsell E, Brisson J, Deschenes L. Arm problems and psychological distress after surgery for breast cancer. *Can J Surg*. 1993;36:315.
69. Wallace MS, Wallace AM, Dobke MK. Pain after breast surgery: a survey of 282 women. *Pain*. 1996;66:195.
70. Ewing MR, Martin H. Disability following radical neck dissection. *Cancer*. 1952;5:873.
71. Patten C, Hillel AD. The 11th nerve syndrome. Accessory nerve palsy or adhesive capsulitis. *Arch Otolaryngol*. 1993;119:215.
72. Shone GR, Yardley PJ. An audit into the incidence of handicap after unilateral radical neck dissection. *J Laryngol Otol*. 1991;105:760.
73. Krause HR. Shoulder-arm syndrome after radical neck dissection: its relation with the innervation of the trapezius muscle. *Int J Oral Maxillofac Surg*. 1992;21:276.
74. Dajczman E, Gordon A, Dreisman H, Wolkove N. Long-term postthoracotomy pain. *Chest*. 1991;99:270.
75. Keller SM, Carp NZ, Levy MN, Rosen SM. Chronic post thoracotomy pain. *J Cardiovasc Surg*. 1994;35(6 Suppl 1):161.
76. Landreneau RJ, Mack MJ, Hazelrigg SR, et al. Prevalence of chronic pain after pulmonary resection by thoracotomy or video-assisted thoracic surgery. *J Thorac Cardiovasc Surg*. 1994;107:1079.
77. Koethe Y, Mannes AJ, Wood BJ. Image-guided nerve cryoablation for post-thoracotomy. *Pain Syndrome Cardiovasc Intervent Radiol*. 2014;37(3):843-846.
78. Wartan SW, Hanann W, Bedley JR, McColl I. Phantom pain and sensation among British war amputees. *Br J Anaesth*. 1997;78:652.
79. Sherman RA, Sherman CJ, Parker L. Chronic phantom and stump pain among American veterans: results of a survey. *Pain*. 1984;18:83.
80. Weinstein SM. Phantom pain. *Oncology*. 1994;8:65.
81. Sugarbaker PH, Weiss CM, Davidson DD, Roth YF. Increasing phantom limb pain as a symptom of cancer recurrence. *Cancer*. 1984;54:373.
82. Jensen TS, Krebs B, Nielsen J, et al. Immediate and long-term phantom limb pain in amputees: incidence, clinical characteristics, and relationship to pre-amputation limb pain. *Pain*. 1985;21:267.
83. Bach S, Noreng MF, Tjelden NY. Phantom limb pain in amputees during the first 12 months following limb amputation, after preoperative lumbar epidural blockade. *Pain*. 1988;33:297.
84. Bone M, Critchley P, Buggy DJ. Gabapentin in postamputation phantom limb pain: a randomized, double-blind, placebo-controlled, cross-over study. *Reg Anesth Pain Med*. 2002;27(5):481-486.
85. Flor H, Elbert T, Knecht S, et al. Phantom-limb pain as a perceptual correlate of cortical reorganization following arm amputation. *Nature*. 1995;375:482.
86. Breitbart W. Psychiatric management of cancer pain. *Cancer*. 1989;63:2336.
87. Derogatis LR, Morrow GR, Fetting J, et al. The prevalence of psychiatric disorders among cancer patients. *JAMA*. 1983;249:751.
88. Breitbart W. Cancer pain and suicide. In: Foley KM, ed. *Advances in Pain Research and Therapy*. Vol. 16. New York: Raven Press; 1990:399.
89. Kanner RM, Foley KM. Patterns of narcotic use in a cancer pain clinic. *Ann NY Acad Sci*. 1981;362:161.
90. DeAngelis LM, Posner JB. *Neurologic Complications of Cancer*. 2nd ed. New York: Oxford University Press; 2009:122.

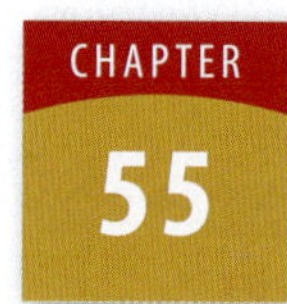

Medical Management of Cancer Pain

Thomas Chai
Stuart W. Hough
Russell K. Portenoy
Dhanalakshmi Koyyalagunta
Larry C. Driver

OVERVIEW

Cancer pain is usually caused directly by neoplastic injury to pain-sensitive structures. For this reason, primary antineoplastic therapy, including radiation, chemotherapy, and palliative surgery, should be considered part of an analgesic strategy in some cases. When therapy directed at the tumor is inappropriate, is not feasible, is ineffective, or causes painful therapy-related syndromes, symptomatic analgesic therapies become the overriding concern. Opioid-based pharmacotherapy is the mainstay approach, but adjunctive anesthetic, surgical, psychiatric, and physical modalities may be essential as well (see Chapter 54, Cancer Pain Syndromes). Pharmacologic approaches may be systemic or regional (anesthetic).

The World Health Organization (WHO) proposed a three-step approach—the analgesic ladder—to the selection of drugs for the treatment of cancer pain (**Fig. 55-1**).[1] Step 1, for mild pain, uses nonopioid analgesics and adjuvant drugs. Adjuvant drugs can be either nontraditional analgesics or drugs added to manage the side effects of the primary analgesics. For more intense pain, an opioid is added. Some opioids are used conventionally for moderate pain, and others are used for severe pain. This approach is designed to be simple to understand and usable around the world. Uncontrolled field testing has found the WHO guidelines effective for 70% to 100% of patients with cancer.[2] The aim of this chapter is to provide an overview of the approach to medical management of cancer pain, particularly covering the use of systemic analgesics recommended by the WHO's analgesic ladder for cancer pain.

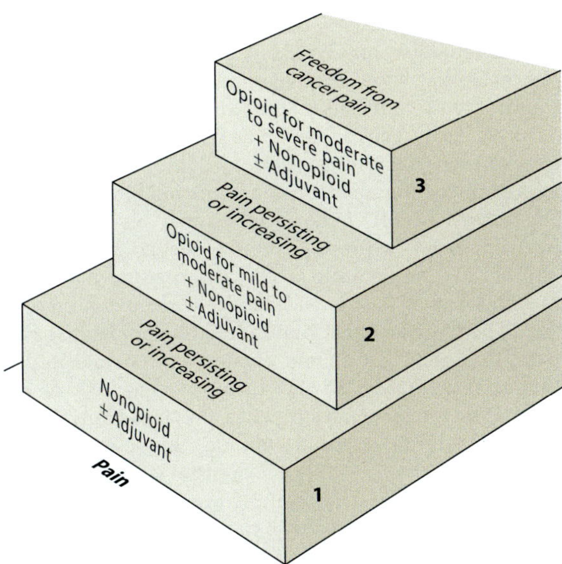

FIGURE 55-1. The three-step analgesic ladder for cancer pain treatment. (Reproduced by permission of World Health Organization. *Cancer Pain Relief,* 2nd ed. Geneva: Author; 1996.)

PAIN ASSESSMENT

Pain is often underrecognized in cancer patients. Cleeland et al.[3] surveyed outpatients with metastatic cancer and physicians from 54 treatment centers. They found that 42% of 597 patients with pain were not receiving adequate analgesia by the WHO guidelines (see **Fig. 55-1**). Insufficient pain relief was particularly common among minorities, women, and elderly adults. An important barrier to effective pain management was a discrepancy between the patient's and the physician's assessment of the extent to which pain was interfering with daily activities. The data underscore the importance of accurate pain assessment in providing adequate cancer pain relief.

The assessment should allow inferences about the pain mechanisms, identification of the pain syndrome (see Chapter 44, Cancer Pain Syndromes), and classification of the relationship between the pain and the disease. The clinician must also assess the functional impact of the pain and psychosocial comorbidities. It is essential to accept the patient's report of pain at face value. Pain should be assessed frequently and systematically, especially when a new pain is reported or a new analgesic treatment is initiated. The location, intensity, and quality of the pain; aggravating and relieving factors; pain impact or interference with daily activities; and the patient's emotional and cognitive response to pain should all be noted.

PAIN MEASUREMENT TOOLS

Although there is no quantitative biochemical or neurophysiologic test for pain, tools have been devised to assess pain intensity[4,5] (see Chapter 6, Evaluating the Patient with Chronic Pain). Categorical scales, such as the verbal rating scale (VRS), which ask patients to rate pain intensity using adjectives such as "mild" and "excruciating," are simple to use but assume an understanding of the adjectives. Pain *relief* may also be rated with a categorical or percentage scale. The numerical rating scale (NRS), rating pain from 0 for "no pain" to 10 for "the worst imaginable pain," is easily implemented and recorded during frequent assessments. The use of numbers removes any linguistic misunderstanding of categorical descriptors. Similarly, a 100-mm visual analog scale (VAS) may be used, with or without intensity descriptors. Although a VAS score may not mean the same thing to different patients, it is reliable on repeated use with the same patient.[6] This permits serial assessments by different clinicians, if necessary, over the course of treatment. Patients must be instructed in the use of these analog scales.

All of the pain scales just described are validated and reliable measures of pain intensity;[7] however, they are unidimensional pain measures, so they do not reflect the complexity of the pain experience.[8,9] Nonetheless, they provide a score that can be recorded, as vital signs are.[10] This is useful for tracking pain intensity and can prompt intervention when pain exceeds an acceptable level. Although there is inconsistency with translating between numerical and categorical scales, a recent systematic review suggested that a numerical score of 0 to 4 should represent mild pain, 5 to 6, moderate pain, and 7 to 10, severe pain.[11]

When the patient cannot communicate, pain must be evaluated by other means. Next of kin are usually able to verify the existence of pain, but they cannot accurately describe its intensity, location, and treatment.[12] Non-English speakers need a translator or a pain scale with instructions in their language. Originally designed for use in children, the Wong-Baker Faces Pain Rating Scale might also be useful in some cognitively impaired adult patients.[13]

Attention to nonverbal pain manifestations is also important. Autonomic changes may be present, including hypertension, tachycardia, and diaphoresis. Patients with organic brain disease may show agitation or confusion, or they may be apathetic, inactive, or irritable. They may also refuse to eat without explanation, protect the painful part, and show facial grimacing. Although these manifestations are not specific for pain, empiric analgesic treatment in such situations, after ruling out more serious acute illness, often confirms the assessment. The Behavioral Pain Scale (BPS) is a clinical tool developed to assess pain in sedated, critically ill patients. The BPS score is calculated as the sum of three observer-based behavioral categories (each rated from 1 to 4): facial expression, upper extremity movement, and compliance with ventilation.[14]

Several multidimensional assessment instruments incorporate pain quality, intensity, location, emotional and functional impact, and effectiveness of coping skills.[15] Among the most well-known of these are the McGill Pain Questionnaire (MPQ)[16] and its short form (MPQ-SF).[17] The MPQ-SF is more appropriate for the time-restricted clinical setting. It consists of 15 descriptors, 11 of which are sensory items (throbbing, shooting, stabbing, sharp, cramping, gnawing, hot-burning, aching, heavy, tender, splitting); the remaining four (tiring-exhausting, sickening, fearful, punishing-cruel) are affective items. These items are rated using a 4-point VRS. The MPQ-SF also contains a VAS and a VRS for intensity of pain. A recent systematic review of the MPQ in the cancer population supported its utility as a valid, reliable, and sensitive measure for cancer pain.[18]

The Brief Pain Inventory (BPI) and its short version (BPI-SF) are scales that assess the severity of pain and its impact on the patient's daily function[19]—the sensory and reactive dimensions of pain, respectively. The BPI-SF is more widely used in the clinic setting because of its brevity. The BPI-SF contains front and back body diagrams for the patient to label the site(s) of pain, four items on pain severity (worst, least, average, and current pain over the past 24 hours), and seven items on pain interference (general activity, mood, walking ability, normal work, relations with other people, sleep, and enjoyment of life). Each item is scored using an NRS. There is also a question regarding pain response to analgesics.

The MD Anderson Symptom Inventory (MDASI)[20] is based on the BPI and is used as a single tool to measure 13 of the most common cancer-related symptoms. The following symptoms are included in the MDASI: pain, fatigue, nausea, disturbed sleep, emotional distress, shortness of breath, lack of appetite, drowsiness, dry mouth, sadness, vomiting, memory difficulties, and numbness/tingling. The patient rates each of these symptoms with an NRS. The MDASI also includes a section on interference caused by pain.

The Edmonton Symptom Assessment System (ESAS) and a recent revision (ESAS-r) assess nine symptoms common in advanced cancer patients.[21] The symptoms are rated using an NRS and are as follows: pain, nausea, tiredness, depression, anxiety, drowsiness, appetite, well-being, and shortness of breath. There is also an optional tenth symptom that the patient may add to the questionnaire. The revised version was designed to improve ease of use by providing definitions for each symptom and by rearranging the order of the symptoms, among other updates.

NONOPIOID ANALGESICS

Nonsteroidal anti-inflammatory drugs (NSAIDs) and acetaminophen are routinely used in the treatment of cancer pain (see Chapter 61, NSAIDs). In general, they should be used on an around-the-clock schedule for patients with mild pain before advancing to Step 2 of the WHO analgesic ladder.[1] At that step and beyond, nonopioid analgesics may be continued in addition to starting opioids. NSAIDs may be especially effective for neoplastic bone pain[22,23] and in cancer patients experiencing arthralgias associated with aromatase inhibitor therapy,[24,25] but they are probably useful in all types of pain because they provide at least additive analgesia. They can act synergistically with opioids in the spinal cord[26] and allow reduction of opioid dose, lessening the likelihood of opioid-related side effects (opioid sparing). When one NSAID is ineffective or poorly tolerated, another NSAID should be tried. When the oral route is not available, as in patients with unremitting nausea, some NSAIDs and acetaminophen may be given rectally. Ketorolac is available for intramuscular and intravenous (IV) use in the United States but is not recommended for prolonged use because of potential renal toxicity (**Table 55-1**).

Before initiating NSAID or acetaminophen therapy, the potential for toxicity must be considered (see Chapter 61, NSAIDs).[27] Nonselective NSAIDs inhibit cyclooxygenase-1 and -2 enzymes (COX-1 and COX-2, respectively) and can produce gastroduodenal irritation and ulceration, renal cortical ischemia from reduced renal blood flow, hepatotoxicity, and platelet dysfunction. These toxicities are believed to be related more so to inhibition of COX-1, the constitutive enzyme.[28] COX-2 is induced by injury or inflammation, and it is therefore likely that analgesia is related mainly to inhibition of this particular enzyme. Certain NSAIDs, including choline magnesium trisalicylate, meloxicam, nabumetone, diclofenac, and etodolac, may be less likely to cause gastrointestinal (GI) toxicity because they show relative selectivity for COX-2.[29] Celecoxib inhibits only COX-2, so it causes less GI toxicity than most NSAIDs.[30]

NSAID-induced dyspepsia is best managed prophylactically by taking the drugs with food. If this is insufficient, addition of a histamine-2 (H_2) receptor blocker, coating agent, proton pump inhibitor (PPI), or antacid may be necessary. NSAID-induced ulcers may be prevented with H_2 blockers, misoprostol (a prostaglandin E analog), or PPIs. Yeomans et al.[31] showed that omeprazole, a PPI, is somewhat more effective in preventing and healing gastric and duodenal ulcers than ranitidine, an H_2 blocker. The same group also found that omeprazole is better than misoprostol in healing gastric and duodenal ulcers and in preventing their reappearance during NSAID therapy.[32] The risk of ulceration during NSAID therapy increases with age, previous NSAID intolerance, history of peptic ulcer disease, and smoking.[33] In these patients, prophylactic use of an H_2 blocker, PPI, or misoprostol is warranted.

Most NSAIDs interfere with platelet aggregation, thereby creating possible bleeding risk associated with their use. For instance, despite its short elimination half-life, aspirin *irreversibly* inhibits platelet aggregation for the lifetime of the platelet (4–7 days). The platelet effect of other NSAIDs lasts about 2 days after the drug is discontinued. Choline magnesium trisalicylate, however, does not prevent normal platelet aggregation, as measured experimentally, and appears to be associated with less occult GI bleeding.[34] COX-2 inhibitors have less or no platelet effect.[30]

The renal side effects of NSAIDs include reversible renal insufficiency, interstitial nephritis, and predisposition to acute tubular necrosis in patients with low renal perfusion. NSAIDs should be prescribed with caution for patients with hypertension, renal insufficiency, or congestive heart failure.

Other toxicities are also possible; both acetaminophen and NSAIDs may cause hepatotoxicity, even at normally recommended doses.[35] Confusion and inability to concentrate are possible central nervous

TABLE 55-1 Doses and Routes of Some Nonopioid Analgesics

Drug	Dose	Frequency	Route	Daily Maximum	Comments
Acetaminophen	500–1000 mg	q4–6h	PO/PR	4000 mg	Liquid available
Aspirin	500–1000 mg	q4–6h	PO/PR	4000 mg	
Diflunisal	500 mg	q8h	PO	1500 mg	First dose: 1000 mg
Choline magnesium trisalicylate	750–1500 mg	q8–12h	PO	3000 mg	Liquid available; less dyspepsia and platelet dysfunction
Ibuprofen	200–600 mg	q4–6h	PO	2400 mg	
Ketoprofen	25–75 mg	q4–8h	PO	300 mg	
Flurbiprofen	50–100 mg	q4–6h	PO	300 mg	
Naproxen	250 mg	q6–8h	PO	1250 mg	Sustained release available
					First dose: 500 mg
Indomethacin	25–50 mg	q8–12h	PO/PR	100 mg	Frequent side effects
Ketorolac	10–30 mg	q6h	PO	40 mg	Lower dose for repeated use
			IV/IM	60 mg	Limit to 5 days (PO/IV)
Etodolac	200–400 mg	q6–8h	PO	1200 mg	
Diclofenac	25–100 mg	q6–12h	PO	200 mg	
Nabumetone	500–1500 mg	q24h	PO	1500 mg	
Oxaprozin	600–1200 mg	q24h	PO	1200 mg	
Celecoxib	100–200 mg	q12	PO	400 mg	COX-2 inhibitor
Rofecoxib	12.5–50 mg	q24h	PO	50 mg	COX-2 inhibitor

COX, cyclooxygenase; IM, intramuscular; IV, intravenous; PO, oral; PR, per rectum; Q, every.

system (CNS) effects of NSAIDs. Patients who are allergic to aspirin or to an NSAID may have a cross-reactive allergy to other NSAIDs.

OPIOIDS

Opioids are indicated for the treatment of cancer pain because of their effectiveness, reliability, safety, and ease of administration (see Chapter 58, Opioid Pharmacology). Although neuropathic pain may be more difficult to treat with opioids, its presence does not preclude a favorable response to opioid-based analgesia.[36]

Steps 2 and 3 of the WHO analgesic ladder advocate the addition of opioids for moderate to severe pain, with or without an adjuvant drug.[1] "Weak" and "strong" opioids are not inherently different in their ability to control pain but are customarily used in amounts appropriate for milder and stronger pain, respectively. The so-called weak opioids (e.g., codeine and hydrocodone) for Step 2 are commonly prepared in combination with co-analgesics (acetaminophen, aspirin, or an NSAID). The co-analgesic limits dose escalation, necessitating a change to another opioid or preparation as pain increases.

THE CONCEPTS OF TOLERANCE, PHYSICAL DEPENDENCE, AND ADDICTION

Opioids can induce tolerance and physical dependence. Addiction—defined as loss of control over drug use, compulsive use, and use despite harm—is rare in cancer pain patients with no history of substance abuse.[37] Although demands for opioids and dramatic pain behavior are commonly interpreted as markers of addiction, undertreatment of pain is an alternative explanation (a phenomenon known as pseudoaddiction).[38]

Although tolerance to opioid analgesia occurs, disease progression is usually to blame for increasing analgesic requirements.[39] Tolerance to adverse effects, such as respiratory depression and somnolence, also occurs and thus allows for dose escalation to satisfactory analgesia. Physical dependence is another pharmacologic effect of opioids and is defined solely by the development of withdrawal symptoms (an "autonomic arousal") after abrupt cessation of therapy or after administration of an opioid partial agonist or antagonist in an opioid-tolerant individual. Physical dependence is not a clinical problem if this aforementioned abstinence syndrome is avoided. It should be mentioned, of note, that many patients confuse the concept of physical dependence with the state of addiction; therefore, the difference should be explained to them for reassurance purposes.

The U.S. Food and Drug Administration (FDA) defines "opioid tolerant" as follows:

> Patients receiving, for one week or longer, at least 60 mg oral morphine/day, 25 mcg transdermal fentanyl/hour, 30 mg oral oxycodone/day, 8 mg oral hydromorphone/day, 25 mg oral oxymorphone/day, or an equianalgesic dose of another opioid.

CHOOSING AN OPIOID

Few comparative clinical trials exist to differentiate opioids according to responsiveness. Hence, they are usually chosen on the basis of familiarity by the prescriber. Other factors to consider are their potency, route of administration, cost, convenience, and availability. Individual patients vary greatly in their response to different opioids, supporting the practice of sequential opioid trials (opioid rotation) to find the most acceptable balance between analgesia and side effects (see the Changing Opioids and Routes of Administration section later in this chapter).[40] There is ongoing research, however, in applying pharmacogenomics testing to patients, with the idea being to identify specific genetic polymorphisms in each patient that could affect response to opioids.[41-43] This information would allow tailored treatment, which in turn could translate to better prediction and monitoring of analgesic response.

In general, the initial opioid should be a short-acting drug when the patient (1) has severe pain and requires rapid dose titration, (2) has intermittent pain, or (3) is opioid naïve and there is concern about delayed toxicity from a long-acting preparation. In other cases in opioid-tolerant patients, however, a long-acting drug or extended-release drug may be the initial opioid. Long-acting opioids include methadone and levorphanol, and extended-release preparations include hydrocodone, morphine, oxycodone, oxymorphone, hydromorphone, tapentadol, and fentanyl.

There are differences among opioids in relative toxicities. Meperidine, for instance, should be avoided for cancer pain treatment, especially in patients with renal failure.[44] Its active metabolite, normeperidine, has a long half-life and causes CNS excitability that can result in seizures. It can accumulate with high doses, prolonged use, and renal dysfunction. Morphine is hepatically biotransformed into its metabolites of morphine-3-glucuronide (M3G) primarily, and morphine-6-glucuronide (M6G), the latter being an active metabolite that is much more potent than the parent compound. These metabolites do not tend to cause problems in patients with normal renal function, but they could accumulate and lead to toxicity in those with renal insufficiency.

Partial opioid receptor agonists (e.g., buprenorphine) and mixed agonist–antagonists (e.g., pentazocine, nalbuphine, and butorphanol) should also be avoided. They may precipitate both withdrawal symptoms and pain in patients who are opioid tolerant. When used alone, increasing amounts provide less incremental analgesia, a phenomenon known as a "ceiling effect." Some of the mixed agonist–antagonists also have relatively greater toxicity than the pure μ agonists.[45]

Combination analgesics, which often contain acetaminophen, should be used with caution because of the possibility of acetaminophen toxicity, as previously mentioned. Daily acetaminophen intake should not exceed 3 g, per recent FDA guidelines. Alcohol use, coexisting hepatic disease, and starvation (which may be present in debilitated cancer patients) predispose to acetaminophen hepatotoxicity at even lower doses.[35]

Methadone and levorphanol have long half-lives and may be considered in place of extended-release preparations for baseline opioid requirements. One advantage of these drugs is that they are absorbed easily by the gut and may be effective in patients with bowel pathology who are unable to completely absorb the aforementioned extended-release preparations[46] or in patients who have feeding tubes that preclude the use of most extended-release pills. Methadone may be difficult to titrate, however, because the initial duration of action (~6 hours) is shorter than its elimination half-life, leading to potentially fatal drug accumulation with repeated dosing over 2 to 5 days.[47] Furthermore, methadone pharmacokinetics are highly variable among patients owing to differences in protein binding, urinary excretion, and induction of metabolism by other drugs.[46-48] Methadone's elimination half-life is usually about 24 hours, but it may be as short as 12 hours or longer than 50 hours.

OPIOID DOSING

The appropriate opioid dose and interval should control pain without end-of-dose failure and unacceptable side effects at peak concentration (i.e., without bolus effects). The required dose varies with the severity of pain, the type of pain, preexisting opioid exposure, psychological distress, and other factors.[36] Elderly adults are more sensitive to opioid-induced analgesia but may also be more susceptible to its side effects.[49] Large doses may be necessary as the disease progresses. Although there is no theoretical limit to the dose, a practical limit is imposed by the occurrence of intolerable side effects, a large injectate volume, numerous pills or suppositories, or excessive skin surface required for transdermal applications.

When initiating opioid therapy, a short-acting drug may be given on an as-needed basis every 2 or 3 hours (**Table 55-2**). After 5 or 6 half-lives (1 day for morphine), the basal daily opioid requirement is determined, and a long-acting opioid preparation may be substituted. Alternatively, a long-acting opioid may be used initially when pain is constant and not severe or progressive. Long-acting opioids should be provided regularly

TABLE 55-2 Equivalent and Recommended Opioid Doses and Routes

	Approximate Equianalgesic Dose		Usual Starting Dose	
Drug	**Oral**	**Parenteral**	**Oral**	**Parenteral**
Morphine[a,c,d]	30 mg q3–4 h	10 mg q3–4 h	20–60 mg q3–4 h	10 mg q3–4 h
Hydromorphone[d]	7.5 mg q3–4 h	1.5 mg q3–4 h	4–8 mg q3–4 h	1–2 mg q3–4 h
Methadone	20 mg q6–8 h	10 mg q6–8 h	20 mg q6–8 h	10 mg q6–8 h
Levorphanol	4 mg q6–8 h	2 mg q6–8 h	2–4 mg q6–8 h	1–2 mg q6–8 h
Meperidine[b]	300 mg q2–3 h	100 mg q3 h	300 mg q2–3 h	100 mg q2–3 h
Codeine	200 mg q3–4 h	130 mg q4 h	30–60 mg q3–4 h[e]	60 mg q2 h[e]
Hydrocodone	30 mg q3–4 h	N/A	5–10 mg q3–4 h[e]	N/A
Oxycodone[c]	30 mg q3–4 h	N/A	5–10 mg q3–4 h[e]	N/A
Fentanyl	N/A	100 μg/h[f]	N/A	25–50 μgh[f]

[a]Doses of morphine shown are for chronic use. Larger doses of oral morphine are needed for equivalent acute analgesia.[36]

[b]Meperidine is not recommended for chronic use.

[c]Morphine and oxycodone are available in controlled-release forms, which are given two or three times per day. The total daily dose is unchanged.

[d]Available as a rectal suppository. Rectal opioids are roughly equianalgesic to oral opioids.[37]

[e]Doses recommended for codeine, hydrocodone, and oxycodone are for milder pain. Usually used in fixed combinations with acetaminophen or nonsteroidal anti-inflammatory drugs.

[f]Provided as a transdermal patch, which is changed every 2 to 3 days. Fever increases drug uptake.

to prevent most pain. An additional short-acting opioid (5%–15% of the basal daily requirement) is made available for breakthrough pain every 1 to 3 hours.[50] If the short-acting opioid is needed more than three times per day, the amount of long-acting opioid is usually increased. It is inconvenient and unnecessary to increase the dosing frequency of long-acting oral preparations when increasing the total daily dose. Dose changes should be in increments of one-third to half of the preceding dose or according to the patient's usage of breakthrough opioid. If side effects prevent dose escalation, switching to another opioid should be considered before changing to another route of administration or abandoning opioids.[40]

Cessation or reduction of opioid use may be appropriate when the patient is pain free after antitumor therapy or after a successful anesthetic or neuroablative procedure. Based on clinical observation, reduction of the daily dose by 50% every 3 days usually prevents symptomatic withdrawal. Withdrawal symptoms include yawning, nausea, vomiting, abdominal cramps, diarrhea, insomnia, anxiety, irritability, temperature instability, diaphoresis, and salivation. It is generally not considered a life-threatening event; however, patients describe the withdrawal syndrome as a severe, flulike experience.

ROUTES OF ADMINISTRATION

The usual route of systemic opioid administration is oral. The peak effect is typically in 20 to 90 minutes, and the duration is 3 to 6 hours.[51] Extended-release oral preparations are available for maintenance of steady analgesia, with the peak effect at 2 to 3 hours and a duration of 8 to 24 hours.[52–54] The clear advantages of oral administration are the numerous drugs available and their ease of use. However, some patients may not be able to use oral medications, including those with oral mucositis, dysphagia, bowel obstruction, and severe nausea.[55]

Fentanyl is a highly lipid-soluble opioid available in transdermal form (a transdermal therapeutic system), which is especially important when the oral route is less preferred.[56] Transdermal fentanyl might also be selected if patient compliance or adherence with oral analgesics is an issue. The onset of analgesia is about 12 hours after initial patch application and continues for 16 to 24 hours after removal. A comparative trial against extended-release morphine suggests that transdermal fentanyl is associated with less constipation.[57] It should be noted that transdermal fentanyl is indicated for pain in patients who are opioid tolerant only. Fentanyl is also available in transmucosal forms (buccal, sublingual, intranasal) for severe breakthrough cancer pain in opioid-tolerant patients. Transmucosal fentanyl is characterized by a more rapid onset compared with oral opioid alternatives,[58–60] partly related to bypassing hepatic first-pass metabolism.

Morphine, oxymorphone, and hydromorphone are manufactured for rectal use. Injectable methadone and sustained-release morphine have also been used rectally.[55,61] A disadvantage of rectal administration is the interpatient variability in absorption and degree of first-pass metabolism. Partial avoidance of the portal circulation may result in slightly increased bioavailability compared with oral opioids. Whereas morphine suppositories are slowly absorbed,[55] morphine microenemas (10 mg in 1 mL) have a more rapid onset and longer duration than the same dose given orally.[62] Mucositis or transmucosal lesions, diarrhea, thrombocytopenia, and neutropenia contraindicate the rectal route.

Injected opioids may be useful for patients who cannot take opioids by the oral, sublingual, or rectal routes; for those who need rapid dose titration; and for those whose high opioid needs cannot be easily met by other routes. IV injection of most opioids provides peak effect in 5 to 15 minutes, with a similarly shortened duration of effect. Subcutaneous injection analgesia peaks at 30 minutes and is preferred over intramuscular injection because the latter is more painful. The usual conversion ratio between subcutaneous and IV is considered 1:1. Continuous infusion (subcutaneous or IV) or frequent redosing is usually necessary to maintain analgesia with injected opioids. Subcutaneous infusion volume should be limited, especially in cachectic patients, to permit stable absorption.[63] Moulin et al.[64] compared subcutaneous with IV opioid infusion in 15 patients with cancer pain in a double-blind, randomized, crossover trial. The mean bioavailability was 78% with subcutaneous infusion, but pain scores and the need for breakthrough medication were no different from IV infusion.

Patient-controlled analgesia (PCA) may be useful for initiation of parenteral opioid therapy, rapid opioid titration with changing pain intensity, and treatment of incident pain.[65] Because the patient controls the delivery of the opioid, individual differences in pain intensity, drug clearance, and effectiveness are less likely to interfere with therapy. In a study of 26 patients with oral mucositis after bone marrow transplantation, psychological dependence was no more likely, total opioid consumption and side effects were less, and analgesia was the same or better with PCA as with nurse-administered opioids.[66] PCA devices are individually programmed for the size of the dose (demand dose), the

TABLE 55-3 Suggested Post–Controlled Analgesia Opioid Programming for an Opioid-Naïve Patient After a Loading Dose of the Opioid Is Given

Drug	Bolus Dose	Lockout Interval	Hourly Maximum
Morphine 1 mg/mL	0.5–2.5 mg	5–15 min	5–15 mg
Hydromorphone 0.25 mg/mL	0.125–0.375 mg	5–15 min	1.25–3 mg
Fentanyl 25 or 50 μg/mL	12.5–50 μg	5–10 min	100–300 μg

minimum time between doses (lockout interval), and the cumulative dose allowed in 1 or 4 hours (several times higher than the anticipated need). In addition, an optional nursing bolus may be allowed. Continuous infusion (a basal rate) may be programmed in addition to the demand doses to allow sleep and to cover baseline pain. An important inherent safety feature of PCA is that the patient cannot self-administer additional medication if he or she is already overly sedated. Those attending to the patient must not circumvent this safety feature by pressing the demand button for the patient.

Recommended PCA settings for morphine, hydromorphone, and fentanyl are shown in **Table 55-3**. Much larger doses may be needed for opioid-tolerant patients. To limit the total volume of injectate, hydromorphone may be chosen over fentanyl and morphine because of its potency and solubility. Whereas fentanyl is commercially available only at 50 μg/mL, morphine and hydromorphone can be compounded to 50 mg/mL for injection.

Patient-controlled analgesia is an efficient means of determining a patient's opioid requirement when initiating or changing opioids. The pump records the amount of drug used, which is then converted to continuous infusion, transdermal fentanyl, or a sustained-release oral preparation. PCA is available for use in the home as well as the hospital. Patients without IV access may use subcutaneous PCA.[65]

CHANGING OPIOIDS AND ROUTES OF ADMINISTRATION

Dose-limiting side effects and the loss of the previous route of administration are the usual reasons for changing drugs or routes. Trials of several opioids should be considered before abandoning systemic opioids for treatment of cancer pain because patients may respond differently to different drugs. Incomplete cross-tolerance between opioids may account for the apparent decrease in required dose when changing analgesic drugs.[40,67] When changing one opioid to another drug or route of administration, conversion is made with the assistance of opioid conversion charts (see Table 55-2).

All opioid doses can be expressed as equianalgesic doses. Typically, 10 mg of parenteral morphine is considered the unit dose, and doses of other drugs for oral or parenteral administration are listed in equianalgesic amounts. The conversion tables (see Table 55-2) contain approximations based largely on short-term use of smaller opioid doses. When converting large opioid doses, caution dictates dose reduction by one-third to half to account for incomplete cross-tolerance.[40,67] When changing to methadone, a 75% to 90% initial dose reduction is indicated because of the greater potential for drug accumulation and the possibility of unexpectedly high potency.[40] If inadequate analgesia necessitates the conversion and there are no significant side effects, the new drug may be started closer to the equianalgesic dose.[50] Additional short-acting opioid is made available while titrating the new drug to achieve stable analgesia. When any change in opioid or route is made, frequent assessments are needed to keep pain controlled and to prevent side effects.

SELECT ADJUVANTS

Optimal therapy may not be achieved in the cancer pain population with opioids alone. Often, opioids combined with nonopioid analgesics and adjuvant analgesics are necessary to achieve satisfactory relief.[68] A number of adjuvant drugs are used in conjunction with opioids, especially to relieve the neuropathic component of the pain state, which is considered at times to be an opioid-resistant type of pain (or only partially responsive to opioids). An additional benefit of adding adjuvants is to provide an opioid-sparing effect, thus lessening opioid-related side effects.

ANTIDEPRESSANTS

The tricyclic antidepressants (TCAs) were used as analgesics shortly after their introduction.[69,70] The mechanism of their analgesic action is not certain, but it probably includes enhancement of monoamine concentrations in the dorsal horn[71] and stimulation of α_2 receptors[72] (see Chapter 62, Adjuvant Analgesics). They are useful in treating neuropathic pain and have been proven analgesic in well-designed trials for postherpetic neuralgia (PHN), diabetic neuropathy, atypical facial pain, migraine headache, fibrositis, and central poststroke pain.[69,70] There have been few controlled trials of TCAs for the treatment of cancer pain, perhaps because cancer pain encompasses so many somatic, visceral, and neuropathic entities (see Chapter 44, Cancer Pain Syndromes). Amitriptyline has been shown effective, however, in a placebo-controlled study of 20 patients with neuropathic postmastectomy pain;[73] however, in another randomized controlled trial (RCT), its effectiveness was not supported.[74] The analgesic effect of the TCAs on neuropathic pain seems to be separate from their antidepressant or sedative effects.[73,75–78]

The TCAs are most appropriate for cancer patients with neuropathic pain, which is often described as burning, searing, aching, or dysesthetic, and occurs in the setting of known or probable nerve injury. The choice of drug is empiric; there is no clearly superior drug. A patient having difficulty with sleep may benefit from a more sedating drug, such as amitriptyline, imipramine, or doxepin. Nortriptyline is less sedating, and desipramine has the fewest side effects.[75,79] Trazodone is not an effective analgesic for neuropathic pain but may be indicated in cancer pain patients with sleep disturbances. Probably fewer than half of patients with neuropathic pain achieve greater than 50% pain relief with an antidepressant,[71] and a lack of complete relief should not be interpreted as treatment failure.

Suggested dosing for the TCAs is shown in **Table 55-4**. Because these drugs are usually sedating, they are best given in the evening. If the initial low dose is not effective, it should be increased every few days to weeks until an effect is seen or side effects become intolerable. As with opioids, greater analgesia is seen with higher doses.[76]

Adverse effects with TCAs are common.[70] They are primarily anticholinergic, including sedation, constipation, urinary retention and overflow incontinence, tachycardia, dry mouth, blurred vision, dysphoria, and agitation. Antihistamine effects are responsible for sedation and weight gain and may exacerbate hypotension. α_1 and α_2 Blockade contributes to orthostatic hypotension and tachycardia. Most of these side effects are not life threatening and diminish with time. Dry mouth tends to persist. The side effects are troubling, however, and often result in discontinuation of the TCA. Cardiac conduction abnormalities and seizures are more concerning effects. A history of seizure is a relative contraindication to TCA use.[80] An electrocardiogram should be obtained before TCA initiation to rule out bundle branch block and bifascicular block, which are also relative contraindications.[81] Dose adjustment according to drug levels may help to prevent these consequences of antidepressant therapy.[80] When a patient experiences unwanted side effects, it is wise to switch to another TCA because patient responses are variable and often idiosyncratic. Persistence in treatment is essential because analgesic response may take several weeks to become evident.[69]

Duloxetine is a serotonin-norepinephrine reuptake inhibitor approved for many indications, such as depression, painful diabetic neuropathy, fibromyalgia, chronic multisite musculoskeletal pain, and others. Matsuoka et al.[82] performed a pilot study to determine the analgesic effects of duloxetine for neuropathic cancer pain. In this study, 15 cancer patients with neuropathic pain were administered duloxetine, and a retrospective analysis of the data revealed that 11 of these

TABLE 55-4 Doses of Some Tricyclic Antidepressants Used for Pain Management

Antidepressant	Dose Range (mg)	Comments
Amitriptyline	10–150	Sedation and hypotension are common; effective for insomnia
Imipramine	10–150	Sedating
Nortriptyline	10–100	Sedating but less so than others tricyclics
Desipramine	10–150	May have an alerting effect; tachycardia
Doxepin	10–150	Very sedating

15 patients benefitted either by a reduction in pain intensity as recorded on NRS or improvement of other symptoms, such as sleepiness and lightheadedness.

ANTICONVULSANTS

Carbamazepine has long been used for treatment of trigeminal neuralgia.[83] Several anticonvulsants are now commonly used to treat lancinating and burning dysesthesias complicating nerve injury (see also Chapter 62, Adjuvant Analgesics). In addition to trigeminal neuralgia, glossopharyngeal neuralgia, tabes dorsalis, diabetic neuropathy, PHN, postamputation pain, migraines, central pain, and other conditions have been reported to respond to anticonvulsants in case reports, case series, and poorly controlled trials.[84] Two randomized, double-blind, placebo-controlled studies support the use of gabapentin for diabetic neuropathy and PHN.[85,86]

Swerdlow studied 200 patients with lancinating pain in an open-label, uncontrolled trial of carbamazepine, phenytoin, valproate, and clonazepam.[84] Patients were switched from one drug to another if they failed to obtain relief. Most patients did respond to one of the drugs, but there was no clearly superior medication in general or for any particular condition. McQuay et al.[87] conducted a systematic review of 20 randomized, controlled anticonvulsant trials. Patients with trigeminal neuralgia responded to carbamazepine, and those with diabetic neuropathy responded to both carbamazepine and phenytoin. Valproate and carbamazepine were effective for migraine prophylaxis.

Although there have been few prospective, controlled trials of anticonvulsants for patients with cancer pain, individual patients may respond dramatically, and these medications should not be withheld from patients in pain pending definitive evidence of their efficacy. Yajnik et al.[88] compared phenytoin with buprenorphine and the combination in three groups of 25 patients with cancer pain resulting from various causes. A low dose of phenytoin (100 mg twice daily) provided greater than 50% pain relief in most patients and enhanced the effect of buprenorphine without increasing side effects.

Carbamazepine is started at 100 mg twice daily and is escalated until toxicity occurs, pain is relieved, or the safe plasma level is exceeded (12 μg/mL). Bone marrow suppression often manifests as mild leukopenia or thrombocytopenia and rarely aplastic anemia. If bone marrow suppression is anticipated from radiation, chemotherapy, or tumor replacement, carbamazepine should be avoided. Patients receiving carbamazepine should have their complete blood counts and hepatic transaminases monitored. Reversible hepatotoxicity, resembling viral hepatitis, occurs rarely, and fatal hepatic necrosis is less common.[89] Cutaneous reactions may also occur and require cessation of the medication. Sedation, vertigo, ataxia, hyponatremia, and nausea are more common effects.[84] Oxcarbazepine is a structural derivative of carbamazepine with a safer side effect profile in that it is less likely to cause the above-mentioned hematologic and hepatic adverse effects. It should be noted, though, that both carbamazepine and oxcarbazepine have not been well studied for cancer-related pain.

Phenytoin and valproate are available in oral and IV forms. A new form of phenytoin, fosphenytoin, may be administered intramuscularly. Treatment with phenytoin begins with an oral loading dose, and maintenance therapy, starting at 100 mg three times daily, is adjusted to control pain with a plasma concentration of less than 20 μg/mL. Side effects may include anemia, anorexia, nausea, somnolence, and ataxia. Bone marrow suppression is less likely with phenytoin than carbamazepine. The potential for hepatotoxicity mandates periodic monitoring of liver function tests.[84] Hypersensitivity to phenytoin is rare but potentially fatal and manifests with rash, fever, and hepatitis. Up to 19% of patients taking phenytoin develop cutaneous reactions, usually without hypersensitivity.[90] Oral valproate therapy is usually started at 125 mg twice daily. The most common side effects are nausea and epigastric pain, which are reduced by taking it with food and with enteric-coated tablets. Hepatotoxicity is rare.[84]

Gabapentin has received considerable attention in pain management, and there is evidence to support its use in diabetic neuropathy and PHN.[85,86] Several studies support the effectiveness of gabapentin as an adjuvant for cancer-related neuropathic pain,[91–93] and a recent literature review corroborates this finding.[94] It is usually started at 300 mg at bedtime and increased as high as 3600 mg/day in divided doses. The dosage should be reduced in patients with renal impairment because it is eliminated unchanged in the urine. Side effects (somnolence, ataxia, peripheral edema, and dizziness) are not life threatening, and plasma concentrations are not monitored, making this an easy anticonvulsant to use.[95]

Pregabalin is a structurally similar anticonvulsant to gabapentin, with similar indications for use. The use of pregabalin for cancer pain has not been extensively studied; however, there is some evidence in the literature to support its use for cancer-related bone and neuropathic pain. For example, Sjolund et al.[96] performed a randomized trial on pregabalin's effect on cancer-induced bone pain. A total of 152 patients enrolled in this study were assigned either to pregabalin or placebo. The endpoint was the duration-adjusted average change from baseline in the daily worst pain. The study had to be discontinued after interim review because of an insufficient sample size to make meaningful statistical analyses, yet descriptive analyses of the data suggested that pregabalin could be helpful in reducing metastatic bone pain. Several studies support pregabalin use in neuropathic cancer pain,[97,98] although a systematic review was not able to draw any conclusions because of the limitations for comparison of the available studies.[99]

SYSTEMIC LOCAL ANESTHETICS

Systemic local anesthetics are often used to treat neuropathic pain (see also Chapter 62, Adjuvant Analgesics). IV lidocaine (5 mg/kg over 30 minutes) has been found effective for PHN and diabetic neuropathy.[100,101] A small number of case reports and higher level evidence in the literature demonstrate the effectiveness of IV lidocaine for refractory cancer pain with a neuropathic component. For instance, Sharma et al.[102] conducted an RCT to evaluate the use of IV lidocaine in cancer pain refractory to opioid therapy. Fifty eligible patients enrolled in this study received both IV lidocaine and IV placebo 2 weeks apart. There was a significant difference in the degree of pain relief after lidocaine infusion, and more patients reported reduced analgesic requirements afterward compared with placebo infusion.

Ketamine is a dissociative anesthetic with a number of pharmacodynamic properties useful for pain, including its antagonism of the *N*-methyl-D-aspartate (NMDA) receptor and its agonist activity at the opioid receptor, among other mechanisms of action. Common side effects of ketamine include sedation, somnolence, sensory illusions, dissociative feelings, and visual disturbance. Transaminitis has been reported in those undergoing continuous ketamine infusion.[103] Ketamine has been shown to be effective in treating refractory cancer pain as supported by a recent systematic review and synthesis of available data by Bredlau et al.[104] One of the studies included in this review, for example, was a randomized, double-blind, crossover trial[105] of IV ketamine at two doses (0.25 or 0.50 mg/kg) or saline as a control performed in ten participants with various cancer diagnoses. Each participant received each intervention, with a 2-day washout between interventions. Compared with saline, ketamine administration provided significantly improved analgesia, and there was no significant difference in pain scores between the two ketamine doses. It should also be noted that ketamine as an infusion is suggested to be no more than 0.5 mg/kg/h. In the oral route, 0.2 to 0.5 mg/kg (maximum, 50 mg/dose) two or three times daily has been suggested.[104]

ORAL TOPICAL ANALGESICS

Several compounded agents are used to create an oral topical solution for mucositis-related pain, which can occur with chemotherapy, radiation therapy, and hematopoietic stem cell transplant. These compounded agents may consist of local anesthetics, antimicrobials, analgesics, anti-inflammatories, adjuvants, and others. A survey was conducted to compare the ingredients used in 40 U.S. institutions' compounded oral solutions (known as "magic mouthwash") for chemotherapy-induced oral mucositis,[106] finding that diphenhydramine, viscous lidocaine, magnesium hydroxide–aluminium hydroxide, nystatin, and steroids were the most commonly used ingredients.

CORTICOSTEROIDS

Corticosteroids are used as co-analgesics when inflammation or the mass effect of vasogenic edema causes pain.[107] They reduce inflammation by inhibiting phospholipase activity and thus prostaglandin synthesis. In addition, they may reduce axonal sprouting and neurokinin concentration in sensory fibers near injured tissue.[108] Regenerating axons in neuromas discharge spontaneously or with minimal tactile stimulation because of high sodium channel expression;[109] locally injected corticosteroids reduce neuroma discharge in animal models and appear to be effective in humans as well. Acute neural compression (e.g., in spinal cord compression), intracranial hypertension (from brain metastases), bony and soft tissue infiltration, and visceral distention cause pain that may respond to steroids.[110] Dexamethasone is probably the most commonly prescribed corticosteroid for cancer-related symptoms, including pain. For bone or neuropathic pain, the typical oral dose of dexamethasone is 4 to 8 mg/day (which can be in divided doses).[111]

Corticosteroids have numerous toxicities when taken chronically.[107] These include fluid retention and electrolyte disturbances, hypertension, proximal myopathy, osteoporosis and aseptic necrosis, insomnia, psychosis, gastritis, hyperglycemia, and impaired cellular immunity. These adverse effects may be undesirable in cancer patients who are expected to survive for more than several months. Mood elevation, antiemesis, and appetite stimulation are often desirable side effects of corticosteroids, but they may diminish with prolonged use.[107]

BISPHOSPHONATES

The term *skeletal-related events (SREs)* describes a constellation of clinical complications from bone metastases, including bone pain, hypercalcemia of malignancy, pathologic fracture that may result in cord compression, need for radiotherapy, or need for surgery. Bone-modifying agents can be used to reduce SREs, and evidence supports the use of bisphosphonates to reduce metastatic bone pain and induce healing of lytic lesions.[112] Body and colleagues[113] studied the effect of oral ibandronate on bone pain and quality of life in patients with metastatic breast cancer to bone. A total of 564 patients enrolled in these two double-blind randomized studies received either oral ibandronate at 50 mg/day or placebo for up to 96 weeks. There was a significant reduction and maintenance of pain scores below baseline in the ibandronate group through the length of the study. There were also improved scores for quality of life in the ibandronate group compared with the placebo group. The authors of this study concluded that the results were suggestive of a clinically useful co-analgesic property of ibandronate.

CLONIDINE

Clonidine, an α_2 receptor agonist, may contribute to analgesia by stimulating presynaptic or postsynaptic receptors in the superficial dorsal horn, decreasing sympathetic outflow, and enhancing noradrenergic inhibitory fibers from the brain stem.[114] These mechanisms may make clonidine a useful analgesic adjuvant for opioids, especially in the setting of neuropathic pain.[115,116] Max et al.[114] found a single dose of oral clonidine (0.2 mg) superior to placebo, ibuprofen (800 mg), and codeine (120 mg) in the treatment of PHN. *Oral* clonidine has not been well studied, however, for cancer pain. The epidural route appears to be more effective than the systemic route for clonidine,[116] and *spinal* delivery of clonidine has demonstrated effectiveness in a number of reports in cancer-related pain.[117,118] Side effects associated with clonidine include orthostatic hypotension, sedation, dry mouth, and constipation. Clonidine does not appear to aggravate opioid-induced respiratory depression.

MANAGEMENT OF ANALGESIC SIDE EFFECTS

Many of the analgesics described in the earlier sections produce dose-limiting side effects, particularly the opioids. Tolerance to opioid side effects generally occurs after repeated use for at least 1 week; however, many patients may continue to experience intolerable side effects, particularly with repeated titration of opioid dosages. Achieving a balance between analgesia and tolerable side effects can be aided by adjuvants as described in the text below.

NAUSEA AND VOMITING

Opioids have three emetogenic mechanisms: a direct effect on the chemoreceptor trigger zone, an enhancing effect on vestibular sensitivity, and a slowing effect on gastric emptying. Although nausea is common with opioids, tolerance to this effect occurs quickly. Treatment is therefore given as needed.[50] When evaluating opioid-induced nausea, refractory constipation and impaction of stool must be considered and treated first. If nausea follows meals or is accompanied by postprandial vomiting, metoclopramide is an appropriate choice to stimulate GI motility. If nausea occurs with movement, meclizine may be more effective as an antihistamine and anticholinergic for vertigo or motion sickness. In the absence of these associations, a phenothiazine, antihistamine, or serotonin antagonist is appropriate (**Table 55-5**). If these are ineffective, a corticosteroid[107] or benzodiazepine may also be useful.

CONSTIPATION

Opioids bind to specific receptors in the CNS as well as in the GI system to produce constipation by direct and anticholinergic effects.[119] An increased GI transit time causes excessive water and electrolyte reabsorption from the feces. Decreased biliary and pancreatic secretion further dehydrates the stool. The TCAs, clonidine, dehydration, surgical procedures, and bowel obstruction by tumor contribute to constipation as well. Elderly patients are particularly susceptible to constipation and impaction of stool.[120]

Opioid-induced constipation is so common that cathartic and stool-softening medications should be routinely initiated alongside around-the-clock opioid orders. The coadministration of docusate (a stool softener) and sennosides (a stimulant laxative) is appropriate for most patients. Adequate hydration, physical activity, and proper nutrition are also helpful. If constipation develops or persists with this bowel regimen, then an osmotic laxative, such as lactulose (15–30 mL) or magnesium citrate (200 mL), is added after ruling out fecal impaction. Bisacodyl suppository or sodium phosphate–biphosphate enemas are used for patients who are too nauseated to take oral cathartics. Disimpaction may be facilitated with mineral oil or saline enemas. Refractory constipation may respond to oral naloxone (1–12 mg), which antagonizes enteric opioid receptors. Because naloxone is only about 3% bioavailable, systemic opioid withdrawal and recrudescence of pain may be avoided with low doses. Oral naloxone should be avoided in patients with bowel obstruction.[121,122] Methylnaltrexone, a *peripherally acting* opioid antagonist, is FDA approved for opioid-induced constipation. The dosage is weight based and administered subcutaneously, and it produces a rapid, robust, and consistent response usually within 4 hours of administration.[123] Caution is suggested in the patient population at

TABLE 55-5 Some Antiemetics

Drug	Dose	Route
Metoclopramide	10 mg QID	PO/IV
Cisapride	10–20 mg BID	PO
Meclizine	12.5–25 mg QID	PO
Prochlorperazine	25 mg BID	PR
	10 mg QID	PO/IV/IM
Promethazine	12.5–25 mg BID–QID	IM/IV
Droperidol	0.625 ng QID	IV
Hydroxyzine	10–50 mg QID	PO
	50–100 mg	IM
Ondansetron	4–32 mg in one to four divided doses	PO/IV

BID, twice a day; IM, intramuscular; IV, intravenous; PO, oral; PR, per rectum; QID, four times a day.

risk for bowel perforation, such as those with history of bowel obstruction or abdominal or pelvic malignancy.

SEDATION

Somnolence and mental clouding are common complaints when opioids are initiated or escalated. Some patients continue to have these problems, especially when certain co-analgesics (antidepressants, anticonvulsants, benzodiazepines, antihistamines, and phenothiazines) with similar drowsiness side effect profile are being used. After ruling out primary CNS abnormalities and metabolic derangement, unnecessary sedative medications should be gradually eliminated. If symptoms persist and analgesia is adequate, the opioid dose may be reduced or the opioid drug may be changed. If analgesia is unsatisfactory, co-analgesics may be initiated or increased to achieve an opioid-sparing effect. An anesthetic or neuroablative procedure may be necessary if the patient finds sedation particularly troubling.[50]

Psychostimulants, such as caffeine (100–200 mg orally per day), dextroamphetamine (2.5–10 mg orally twice daily), and methylphenidate (5–10 mg orally twice daily), are commonly used to offset fatigue or the sedative effects of opioids.[124] Bruera et al.[125] studied the cognitive effects of methylphenidate versus placebo in a double-blind, crossover trial involving 20 patients with cancer pain who were receiving continuous infusions of opioids. Cognitive function was improved by methylphenidate, and most patients preferred it to placebo. Amphetamines, similar to antidepressants, have mood-elevating and analgesic properties.[124]

RESPIRATORY DEPRESSION

Respiratory depression occurs with sedation when opioids are given systemically, and tolerance to this effect occurs quickly. All opioids affect the medullary respiratory center directly. No pure opioid agonist is less likely to cause respiratory depression than another when given at an equianalgesic dose. For most patients, mild respiratory depression (respiratory rate, 8–12 breaths/min) is well tolerated. For those with limited ventilatory or respiratory reserve, it may be problematic. If a low respiratory rate and moderate sedation occur after the expected peak of opioid activity, it is best to withhold further opioids until the respiratory rate rises or pain returns. If necessary, ventilatory support and a small dose of dilute naloxone (20–80 μg intravenously) may be given and repeated as necessary. Because naloxone's reversal effects are shorter than the sedation and respiratory depressant effects of most opioids, continued close monitoring for recurrence of respiratory depression is necessary[50] and may require continuous naloxone infusion.

MYOCLONUS AND HYPERALGESIA

Myoclonus (uncontrollable spasms of certain muscle groups) and hyperalgesia (excessive sensitivity to mildly noxious stimuli) are sometimes seen at very high doses of opioids. Their occurrence, separately or together, may limit the ability of opioids to control pain at the end of life.[126] The mechanisms of these conditions are not certain but may include the inhibition of nonopioid CNS inhibitory systems[127] and the potentiation of glutamate activity at NMDA receptors.[106] A change to another opioid (to take advantage of incomplete cross-tolerance) and the addition of co-analgesics and adjuvants (to exploit opioid dose-sparing effects) may allow a reduction in total opioid dosage, thereby possibly relieving both complications.[67] Clonazepam (0.5–2 mg orally three times daily) and perhaps other anticonvulsants may also be used to suppress myoclonus.[67,128] Finally, an anesthetic or neuroablative procedure may be indicated for refractory cases.

SUMMARY

Refractory pain is a symptom that can lead to a cancer diagnosis and everything that diagnosis entails. Cancer pain relief engenders hope that disease is stabilized or in remission or cured. Recurrent pain may signal recurrent disease. Worsening pain may indicate failure of curative therapy and herald progression of disease and portend the end of life.

Pain experienced by patients with cancer may be from primary or metastatic tumor. It may be an aftereffect of treatments—surgery, chemotherapy, or radiation therapy. Or cancer patients may suffer from pain unrelated to their cancer diagnosis. Similar to many of us, patients with cancer have various acute and chronic pain issues.

Pain in a patient with cancer does not exist in isolation from other problems. Instead, it is part of a complex constellation of concurrent symptoms that burden the patient. These issues can be bothersome enough by themselves. When they are intertwined with each other, they each contribute to suffering individually, and they synergize to yield a potentiated level of discomfort. This gestalt of misery requires multidisciplinary assessment and multimodal management to achieve best outcomes. In addition to various nonmedication approaches, rational polypharmacotherapy is key to a balanced analgesic strategy.

When pharmacotherapy is the basis of treatment, opioids are often the cornerstone of that foundation. Adjuvant co-analgesics serve as the mortar that facilitates the strength of the regimen. Additional help comes from psycho-social-spiritual support, rehabilitation therapy, integrative strategies, and procedural interventions ranging from simple injections to advanced neuromodulation.

In addition, cancer pain may respond to palliative cancer therapies such as surgery, chemotherapy, or radiotherapy. Indeed, a palliative mindset enables the health care team to provide comprehensive care at any stage of the disease experience, even parallel to curative efforts. Palliative care strategies use a team approach to provide patient-centered care focused on relief of pain and symptom distress that negatively impacts the patient and family. This extra layer of support has an ultimate goal to provide patients with the best possible quality of life for as long as they live.

REFERENCES

1. World Health Organization. *Cancer Pain Relief.* Geneva: Author; 1996.
2. Jadad AR, Browman GP. The WHO analgesic ladder for cancer pain management. Stepping up the quality of its evaluation. *JAMA.* 1995;274:1870-1873.
3. Cleeland CS, Gonin R, Hatfield AK, et al. Pain and its treatment in outpatients with metastatic cancer. *N Engl J Med.* 1994;330:592-596.
4. Cleeland CS, Osoba D. Pain assessment in cancer. In: *Effect of Cancer on Quality of Life.* Boca Raton, FL: CRC Press; 1991.
5. Fainsinger RL, Nekolaichuk CL. Cancer pain assessment—can we predict the need for specialist input? *Eur J Cancer.* 2008;44:1072-1077.
6. Revill SI, Robinson JO, Rosen M, Hogg MI. The reliability of a linear analogue for evaluating pain. *Anaesthesia.* 1976;31:1191-1198.

7. Hjermstad MJ, Fayers PM, Haugen DF, et al. Studies comparing Numerical Rating Scales, Verbal Rating Scales, and Visual Analogue Scales for assessment of pain intensity in adults: a systematic literature review. *J Pain Symptom Manage.* 2011;41:1073-1093.
8. Fishman S, Ballantyne J, Rathmell JP, Bonica JJ. *Bonica's Management of Pain.* Baltimore, MD: Lippincott, Williams & Wilkins; 2010.
9. Burton AW, Chai T, Smith LS. Cancer pain assessment. *Curr Opin Support Palliat Care.* 2014;8:112-116.
10. McCaffery M, Pasero CL. Pain ratings: the fifth vital sign. *Am J Nurs.* 1997;97:15-16.
11. Oldenmenger WH, de Raaf PJ, de Klerk C, van der Rijt CC. Cut points on 0-10 numeric rating scales for symptoms included in the Edmonton Symptom Assessment Scale in cancer patients: a systematic review. *J Pain Symptom Manage.* 2013;45:1083-1093.
12. O'Brien J, Francis A. The use of next-of-kin to estimate pain in cancer patients. *Pain.* 1988;35:171-178.
13. Bieri D, Reeve RA, Champion GD, et al. The Faces Pain Scale for the self-assessment of the severity of pain experienced by children: development, initial validation, and preliminary investigation for ratio scale properties. *Pain.* 1990;41:139-150.
14. Aissaoui Y, Zeggwagh AA, Zekraoui A, et al. Validation of a behavioral pain scale in critically ill, sedated, and mechanically ventilated patients. *Anesth Analg.* 2005;101:1470-1476.
15. Bruera E, Watanabe S. New developments in the assessment of pain in cancer patients. *Support Care Cancer.* 1994;2:312-318.
16. Melzack R. The McGill Pain Questionnaire: major properties and scoring methods. *Pain.* 1975;1:277-299.
17. Melzack R. The short-form McGill Pain Questionnaire. *Pain.* 1987;30:191-197.
18. Ngamkham S, Vincent C, Finnegan L, et al. The McGill Pain Questionnaire as a multidimensional measure in people with cancer: an integrative review. *Pain Manag Nurs.* 2012;13:27-51.
19. Cleeland CS, Ryan KM. Pain assessment: global use of the Brief Pain Inventory. *Ann Acad Med Singapore.* 1994;23:129-138.
20. Cleeland CS, Mendoza TR, Wang XS, et al. Assessing symptom distress in cancer patients: the M.D. Anderson Symptom Inventory. *Cancer.* 2000;89:1634-1646.
21. Chang VT, Hwang SS, Feuerman M. Validation of the Edmonton Symptom Assessment Scale. *Cancer.* 2000;88:2164-2171.
22. Stambaugh JE, Jr., Drew J. The combination of ibuprofen and oxycodone/acetaminophen in the management of chronic cancer pain. *Clin Pharmacol Ther.* 1988;44:665-669.
23. Smith HS, Barkin RL. Painful boney metastases. *Am J Ther.* 2014;21:106-130.
24. Presant CA, Bosserman L, Young T, et al. Aromatase inhibitor-associated arthralgia and/or bone pain: frequency and characterization in non-clinical trial patients. *Clin Breast Cancer.* 2007;7:775-778.
25. Coleman RE, Bolten WW, Lansdown M, et al. Aromatase inhibitor-induced arthralgia: clinical experience and treatment recommendations. *Cancer Treat Rev.* 2008;34:275-282.
26. McCormack K. Non-steroidal anti-inflammatory drugs and spinal nociceptive processing. *Pain.* 1994;59:9-43.
27. Amadio P, Jr., Cummings DM, Amadio PB. NSAIDs revisited: selection, monitoring, and safe use. *Postgrad Med.* 1997;101:257-260, 263-257, 270-251.
28. Seibert K, Zhang Y, Leahy K, et al. Distribution of COX-1 and COX-2 in normal and inflamed tissues. *Adv Exp Med Biol.* 1997;400a:167-170.
29. Cryer B, Feldman M. Cyclooxygenase-1 and cyclooxygenase-2 selectivity of widely used nonsteroidal anti-inflammatory drugs. *Am J Med.* 1998;104:413-421.
30. Bombardier C. An evidence-based evaluation of the gastrointestinal safety of coxibs. *Am J Cardiol.* 2002;89:3d-9d.
31. Yeomans ND, Tulassay Z, Juhasz L, et al. A comparison of omeprazole with ranitidine for ulcers associated with nonsteroidal anti-inflammatory drugs. Acid Suppression Trial: Ranitidine versus Omeprazole for NSAID-associated Ulcer Treatment (ASTRONAUT) Study Group. *N Engl J Med.* 1998;338:719-726.
32. Hawkey CJ, Karrasch JA, Szczepanski L, et al. Omeprazole compared with misoprostol for ulcers associated with nonsteroidal antiinflammatory drugs. Omeprazole versus Misoprostol for NSAID-induced Ulcer Management (OMNIUM) Study Group. *N Engl J Med.* 1998;338:727-734.
33. Robinson M, Mills RJ, Euler AR. Ranitidine prevents duodenal ulcers associated with non-steroidal anti-inflammatory drug therapy. *Aliment Pharmacol Ther.* 1991;5:143-150.
34. Stuart JJ, Pisko EJ. Choline magnesium trisalicylate does not impair platelet aggregation. *Pharmatherapeutica.* 1981;2:547-551.
35. Schiodt FV, Rochling FA, Casey DL, Lee WM. Acetaminophen toxicity in an urban county hospital. *N Engl J Med.* 1997;337: 1112-1117.
36. Portenoy RK, Foley KM, Inturrisi CE. The nature of opioid responsiveness and its implications for neuropathic pain: new hypotheses derived from studies of opioid infusions. *Pain.* 1990;43:273-286.
37. Kanner RM, Foley KM. Patterns of narcotic drug use in a cancer pain clinic. *Ann N Y Acad Sci.* 1981;362:161-172.
38. Weissman DE, Haddox JD. Opioid pseudoaddiction—an iatrogenic syndrome. *Pain.* 1989;36:363-366.
39. Gonzales GR, Elliott KJ, Portenoy RK, Foley KM. The impact of a comprehensive evaluation in the management of cancer pain. *Pain.* 1991;47:141-144.
40. Galer BS, Coyle N, Pasternak GW, Portenoy RK. Individual variability in the response to different opioids: report of five cases. *Pain.* 1992;49:87-91.
41. Jannetto PJ, Bratanow NC. Pain management in the 21st century: utilization of pharmacogenomics and therapeutic drug monitoring. *Expert Opin Drug Metab Toxicol.* 2011;7:745-752.
42. Branford R, Droney J, Ross JR. Opioid genetics: the key to personalized pain control? *Clin Genet.* 2012;82:301-310.
43. Droney J, Riley J, Ross J. Opioid genetics in the context of opioid switching. *Curr Opin Support Palliat Care.* 2012;6:10-16.
44. Chan GL, Matzke GR. Effects of renal insufficiency on the pharmacokinetics and pharmacodynamics of opioid analgesics. *Drug Intell Clin Pharm.* 1987;21:773-783.
45. Houde RW. Analgesic effectiveness of the narcotic agonist-antagonists. *Br J Clin Pharmacol.* 1979;7(Suppl 3):297s-308s.
46. Fainsinger R, Schoeller T, Bruera E. Methadone in the management of cancer pain: a review. *Pain.* 1993;52:137-147.
47. Richards-Waugh LL, Primerano DA, Dementieva Y, et al. Fatal methadone toxicity: potential role of CYP3A4 genetic polymorphism. *J Anal Toxicol.* 2014;38:541-547.
48. Plummer JL, Gourlay GK, Cherry DA, Cousins MJ. Estimation of methadone clearance: application in the management of cancer pain. *Pain.* 1988;33:313-322.
49. Kaiko RF, Wallenstein SL, Rogers AG, et al. Narcotics in the elderly. *Med Clin North Am.* 1982;66:1079-1089.
50. Cherny NI. The management of cancer pain. *CA Cancer J Clin.* 2000;50:70-116; quiz 117-120.
51. Sawe J, Dahlstrom B, Rane A. Steady-state kinetics and analgesic effect of oral morphine in cancer patients. *Eur J Clin Pharmacol.* 1983;24:537-542.

52. Shepard K. Review of a controlled-release morphine preparation. In: *Advances in Pain Research and Therapy*. New York: Raven Press; 1990:191-202.
53. Broomhead A, Kerr R, Tester W, et al. Comparison of a once-a-day sustained-release morphine formulation with standard oral morphine treatment for cancer pain. *J Pain Symptom Manage.* 1997;14:63-73.
54. Kaiko RF, Benziger DP, Fitzmartin RD, et al. Pharmacokinetic-pharmacodynamic relationships of controlled-release oxycodone. *Clin Pharmacol Ther.* 1996;59:52-61.
55. Ripamonti C, Zecca E, Brunelli C, et al. Rectal methadone in cancer patients with pain. A preliminary clinical and pharmacokinetic study. *Ann Oncol.* 1995;6:841-843.
56. Grond S, Zech D, Lehmann KA, et al. Transdermal fentanyl in the long-term treatment of cancer pain: a prospective study of 50 patients with advanced cancer of the gastrointestinal tract or the head and neck region. *Pain.* 1997;69:191-198.
57. Ahmedzai S, Brooks D. Transdermal fentanyl versus sustained-release oral morphine in cancer pain: preference, efficacy, and quality of life. The TTS-Fentanyl Comparative Trial Group. *J Pain Symptom Manage.* 1997;13:254-261.
58. Dietrich E, Gums JG. Intranasal fentanyl spray: a novel dosage form for the treatment of breakthrough cancer pain. *Ann Pharmacother.* 2012;46:1382-1391.
59. Portenoy RK, Taylor D, Messina J, Tremmel L. A randomized, placebo-controlled study of fentanyl buccal tablet for breakthrough pain in opioid-treated patients with cancer. *Clin J Pain.* 2006;22:805-811.
60. Weinstein SM, Messina J, Xie F. Fentanyl buccal tablet for the treatment of breakthrough pain in opioid-tolerant patients with chronic cancer pain: a long-term, open-label safety study. *Cancer.* 2009;115:2571-2579.
61. Campbell WI. Rectal controlled-release morphine: plasma levels of morphine and its metabolites following the rectal administration of MST Continus 100 mg. *J Clin Pharm Ther.* 1996;21:65-71.
62. De Conno F, Ripamonti C, Saita L, et al. Role of rectal route in treating cancer pain: a randomized crossover clinical trial of oral versus rectal morphine administration in opioid-naive cancer patients with pain. *J Clin Oncol.* 1995;13:1004-1008.
63. Bruera E, Brenneis C, MacDonald RN. Continuous Sc infusion of narcotics for the treatment of cancer pain: an update. *Cancer Treatment Rep.* 1987;71:953-958.
64. Moulin DE, Kreeft JH, Murray-Parsons N, Bouquillon AI. Comparison of continuous subcutaneous and intravenous hydromorphone infusions for management of cancer pain. *Lancet.* 1991;337:465-468.
65. Ripamonti C, Bruera E. Current status of patient-controlled analgesia in cancer patients. *Oncology (Williston Park).* 1997;11:373-380, 383-374; discussion 384-376.
66. Chapman CR, Hill HF. Prolonged morphine self-administration and addiction liability. Evaluation of two theories in a bone marrow transplant unit. *Cancer.* 1989;63:1636-1644.
67. MacDonald N, Der L, Allan S, Champion P. Opioid hyperexcitability: the application of alternate opioid therapy. *Pain.* 1993; 53:353-355.
68. Swarm R, Anghelescu DL, Benedetti C, et al. Adult cancer pain. *J Natl Compr Canc Netw.* 2007;5:726-751.
69. Magni G. The use of antidepressants in the treatment of chronic pain. A review of the current evidence. *Drugs.* 1991;42:730-748.
70. McQuay HJ, Tramer M, Nye BA, et al. A systematic review of antidepressants in neuropathic pain. *Pain.* 1996;68:217-227.
71. Spiegel K, Kalb R, Pasternak GW. Analgesic activity of tricyclic antidepressants. *Ann Neurol.* 1983;13:462-465.
72. Yaksh TL. Pharmacology of spinal adrenergic systems which modulate spinal nociceptive processing. *Pharmacol Biochem Behav.* 1985;22:845-858.
73. Kalso E, Tasmuth T, Neuvonen PJ. Amitriptyline effectively relieves neuropathic pain following treatment of breast cancer. *Pain.* 1996;64:293-302.
74. Mercadante S, Arcuri E, Tirelli W, et al. Amitriptyline in neuropathic cancer pain in patients on morphine therapy: a randomized placebo-controlled, double-blind crossover study. *Tumori.* 2002;88:239-242.
75. Kishore-Kumar R, Max MB, Schafer SC, et al. Desipramine relieves postherpetic neuralgia. *Clin Pharmacol Ther.* 1990;47:305-312.
76. Max MB, Schafer SC, Culnane M, et al. Amitriptyline, but not lorazepam, relieves postherpetic neuralgia. *Neurology.* 1988;38: 1427-1432.
77. Max MB, Culnane M, Schafer SC, et al. Amitriptyline relieves diabetic neuropathy pain in patients with normal or depressed mood. *Neurology.* 1987;37:589-596.
78. Watson CP, Evans RJ. A comparative trial of amitriptyline and zimelidine in post-herpetic neuralgia. *Pain.* 1985;23:387-394.
79. Max MB, Lynch SA, Muir J, et al. Effects of desipramine, amitriptyline, and fluoxetine on pain in diabetic neuropathy. *N Engl J Med.* 1992;326:1250-1256.
80. Preskorn SH, Fast GA. Tricyclic antidepressant-induced seizures and plasma drug concentration. *J Clin Psychol.* 1992;53:160-162.
81. Dietch JT, Fine M. The effect of nortriptyline in elderly patients with cardiac conduction disease. *J Clin Psychol.* 1990;51:65-67.
82. Matsuoka H, Makimura C, Koyama A, et al. Pilot study of duloxetine for cancer patients with neuropathic pain non-responsive to pregabalin. *Anticancer Res.* 2012;32:1805-1809.
83. Blom S. Tic douloureux treated with new anticonvulsant; experiences with G 32883. *Arch Neurol.* 1963;9:285-290.
84. Swerdlow M. Anticonvulsant drugs and chronic pain. *Clin Neuropharmac.* 1984;7:51-82.
85. Backonja M, Beydoun A, Edwards KR, et al. Gabapentin for the symptomatic treatment of painful neuropathy in patients with diabetes mellitus: a randomized controlled trial. *JAMA.* 1998;280:1831-1836.
86. Rowbotham M, Harden N, Stacey B, et al. Gabapentin for the treatment of postherpetic neuralgia: a randomized controlled trial. *JAMA.* 1998;280:1837-1842.
87. McQuay H, Carroll D, Jadad AR, et al. Anticonvulsant drugs for management of pain: a systematic review. *BMJ.* 1995;311: 1047-1052.
88. Yajnik S, Singh GP, Singh G, Kumar M. Phenytoin as a coanalgesic in cancer pain. *J Pain Symptom Manage.* 1992;7:209-213.
89. Horowitz S, Patwardhan R, Marcus E. Hepatotoxic reactions associated with carbamazepine therapy. *Epilepsia.* 1988;29:149-154.
90. Conger LA, Jr., Grabski WJ. Dilantin hypersensitivity reaction. *Cutis.* 1996;57:223-226.
91. Caraceni A, Zecca E, Bonezzi C, et al. Gabapentin for neuropathic cancer pain: a randomized controlled trial from the Gabapentin Cancer Pain Study Group. *J Clin Oncol.* 2004;22:2909-2917.
92. Bennett MI. Gabapentin significantly improves analgesia in people receiving opioids for neuropathic cancer pain. *Cancer Treat Rev.* 2005;31:58-62.
93. Bar Ad V. Gabapentin for the treatment of cancer-related pain syndromes. *Rev Recent Clin Trials.* 2010;5:174-178.

94. Yan PZ, Butler PM, Kurowski D, Perloff MD. Beyond neuropathic pain: gabapentin use in cancer pain and perioperative pain. *Clin J Pain*. 2014;30:613-629.

95. Ramsay RE. Clinical efficacy and safety of gabapentin. *Neurology*. 1994;44(Suppl):S23-S30; discussion S31-S22.

96. Sjolund KF, Yang R, Lee KH, Resnick M. Randomized study of pregabalin in patients with cancer-induced bone pain. *Pain Ther*. 2013;2:37-48.

97. Manas A, Ciria JP, Fernandez MC, et al. Post hoc analysis of pregabalin vs. non-pregabalin treatment in patients with cancer-related neuropathic pain: better pain relief, sleep and physical health. *Clin Transl Oncol*. 2011;13:656-663.

98. Baba M, Gomyo I. [Retrospective evaluation of pregabalin for cancer-related neuropathic pain]. *Masui*. 2012;61:147-154.

99. Bennett MI, Laird B, van Litsenburg C, Nimour M. Pregabalin for the management of neuropathic pain in adults with cancer: a systematic review of the literature. *Pain Med*. 2013;14:1681-1688.

100. Rowbotham MC, Reisner-Keller LA, Fields HL. Both intravenous lidocaine and morphine reduce the pain of postherpetic neuralgia. *Neurology*. 1991;41:1024-1028.

101. Kastrup J, Angelo H, Petersen P, et al. Treatment of chronic painful diabetic neuropathy with intravenous lidocaine infusion. *Br Med J*. 1986;292:173.

102. Sharma S, Rajagopal MR, Palat G, et al. A phase II pilot study to evaluate use of intravenous lidocaine for opioid-refractory pain in cancer patients. *J Pain Symptom Manage*. 2009;37:85-93.

103. Noppers IM, Niesters M, Aarts LP, et al. Drug-induced liver injury following a repeated course of ketamine treatment for chronic pain in CRPS type 1 patients: a report of 3 cases. *Pain*. 2011;152:2173-2178.

104. Bredlau AL, Thakur R, Korones DN, Dworkin RH. Ketamine for pain in adults and children with cancer: a systematic review and synthesis of the literature. *Pain Med*. 2013;14:1505-1517.

105. Mercadante S, Arcuri E, Tirelli W, Casuccio A. Analgesic effect of intravenous ketamine in cancer patients on morphine therapy: a randomized, controlled, double-blind, crossover, double-dose study. *J Pain Symptom Manage*. 2000;20:246-252.

106. Chan A, Ignoffo RJ. Survey of topical oral solutions for the treatment of chemo-induced oral mucositis. *J Oncol Pharm Pract*. 2005;11:139-143.

107. Twycross R. The risks and benefits of corticosteroids in advanced cancer. *Drug Saf*. 1994;11:163-178.

108. Hong D, Byers MR, Oswald RJ. Dexamethasone treatment reduces sensory neuropeptides and nerve sprouting reactions in injured teeth. *Pain*. 1993;55:171-181.

109. Devor M, Govrin-Lippmann R, Raber P. Corticosteroids suppress ectopic neural discharge originating in experimental neuromas. *Pain*. 1985;22:127-137.

110. Vyvey M. Steroids as pain relief adjuvants. *Can Fam Physician*. 2010;56:1295-1297, e1415.

111. Leppert W, Buss T. The role of corticosteroids in the treatment of pain in cancer patients. *Curr Pain Headache Rep*. 2012;16:307-313.

112. Bloomfield DJ. Should bisphosphonates be part of the standard therapy of patients with multiple myeloma or bone metastases from other cancers? An evidence-based review. *J Clin Oncol*. 1998;16:1218-1225.

113. Body JJ, Diel IJ, Bell R, et al. Oral ibandronate improves bone pain and preserves quality of life in patients with skeletal metastases due to breast cancer. *Pain*. 2004;111:306-312.

114. Max MB, Schafer SC, Culnane M, et al. Association of pain relief with drug side effects in postherpetic neuralgia: a single-dose study of clonidine, codeine, ibuprofen, and placebo. *Clin Pharmacol Ther*. 1988;43:363-371.

115. Ossipov MH, Lopez Y, Bian D, et al. Synergistic antinociceptive interactions of morphine and clonidine in rats with nerve-ligation injury. *Anesthesiology*. 1997;86:196-204.

116. Eisenach JC, De Kock M, Klimscha W. alpha(2)-adrenergic agonists for regional anesthesia. A clinical review of clonidine (1984-1995). *Anesthesiology*. 1996;85:655-674.

117. Tumber PS, Fitzgibbon DR. The control of severe cancer pain by continuous intrathecal infusion and patient controlled intrathecal analgesia with morphine, bupivacaine and clonidine. *Pain*. 1998;78:217-220.

118. Eisenach JC, DuPen S, Dubois M, Miguel R, Allin D. Epidural clonidine analgesia for intractable cancer pain. The Epidural Clonidine Study Group. *Pain*. 1995;61:391-399.

119. Canty SL. Constipation as a side effect of opioids. *Oncol Nurs Forum*. 1994;21:739-745.

120. Portenoy RK. Pain management in the older cancer patient. *Oncology (Williston Park)*. 1992;6:86-98.

121. Culpepper-Morgan JA, Inturrisi CE, Portenoy RK, et al. Treatment of opioid-induced constipation with oral naloxone: a pilot study. *Clin Pharmacol Ther*. 1992;52:90-95.

122. Sykes NP. An investigation of the ability of oral naloxone to correct opioid-related constipation in patients with advanced cancer. *Palliat Med*. 1996;10:135-144.

123. Nalamachu SR, Pergolizzi J, Taylor R Jr, et al. Efficacy and tolerability of subcutaneous methylnaltrexone in patients with advanced illness and opioid-induced constipation: a responder analysis of 2 randomized, placebo-controlled trials. *Pain Pract*. 2014 May 10. doi:10.1111/papr.12218. [Epub ahead of print].

124. Sjogren P. Psychomotor and cognitive functioning in cancer patients. *Acta Anaesthesiol Scand*. 1997;41:159-161.

125. Bruera E, Miller MJ, Macmillan K, Kuehn N. Neuropsychological effects of methylphenidate in patients receiving a continuous infusion of narcotics for cancer pain. *Pain*. 1992;48:163-166.

126. Truog RD, Berde CB, Mitchell C, Grier HE. Barbiturates in the care of the terminally ill. *N Engl J Med*. 1992;327:1678-1682.

127. Dickenson AH. Mechanisms of the analgesic actions of opiates and opioids. *Br Med Bull*. 1991;47:690-702.

128. Eisele JH, Jr., Grigsby EJ, Dea G. Clonazepam treatment of myoclonic contractions associated with high-dose opioids: case report. *Pain*. 1992;49:231-232.

Interventional Cancer Pain Management

Amit Asopa
Moris Aner

OVERVIEW

A substantial proportion of cancer patients have moderate to severe pain. Cancer pain is multifactorial and could be related to the disease process, metastasis, or treatment modalities. The World Health Organization's (WHO's) three-step "analgesic ladder" provides guidelines for pharmacologic management of cancer pain and is probably the most widely used in the clinical setting.[1]

Application of these guidelines provides good pain relief in approximately 80% to 90% of patients with cancer pain.[2] It has been suggested that a fourth step—"interventional techniques"—should be considered in these patients, who do not get adequate pain relief from medication management.[3,4]

With few exceptions, noninvasive analgesic approaches should precede invasive treatments. Among these exceptions are palliative radiotherapy for pain at the site of a long bone metastasis or an isolated brain metastasis and celiac block for a patient with pancreatic or other retroperitoneal tumor who presents with pain. These procedures are designed to improve analgesia or minimize analgesic side effects. Most are intended for pain that is localized to a nerve or plexus distribution. Because of their complexity, risk, and cost, invasive procedures are reserved for patients with intractable pain despite full application of the WHO guidelines[1] and those with intolerable side effects from systemic pharmacologic pain treatment. However, it is important not to delay excessively when conventional pharmacologic management appears inadequate. Referral to a multidisciplinary pain clinic might be considered early in the course of cancer pain management to optimize current pharmacologic, psychological, and physical management techniques and to educate the patient, family, and referring physician about pain progression and future treatment options.

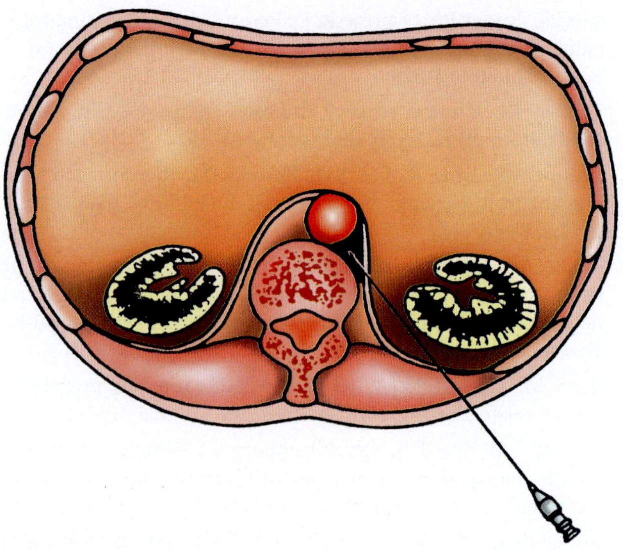

FIGURE 56-1. Celiac plexus block. Classic retrocrural approach, wherein a neurolytic agent is injected bilaterally behind the crus of the diaphragm adjacent to the aorta and vena cava. (Reproduced with permission from Mercadante S, Nicosia F. Celiac plexus block: a reappraisal. *Reg Anesth Pain Med.* 1998;23:37.)

INTERVENTIONAL PAIN MANAGEMENT PROCEDURES

SOMATIC NERVE BLOCKS

Somatic and neuropathic pain localized to a single nerve, plexus, or dermatome distribution is amenable to local anesthetic block of the nerve. Although pain relief is often dramatic, the longest lasting local anesthetics wear off within 1 day. To prolong the effect of local anesthetics, anesthesiologists may insert a catheter for continuous delivery to a nerve or plexus. The brachial plexus and femoral nerve sheath are the usual sites of peripheral catheter placement. Maintenance of peripheral catheters is difficult because movement may easily displace them.

SOMATIC NEUROLYTIC BLOCKS

Neurolytic blocks are often performed after a successful local anesthetic block to extend relief for weeks to months.[5,6] Because neural disruption causes motor, sensory, and autonomic dysfunction, these blocks are reserved for those who cannot get relief by other means. Phenol and ethanol are the most popular agents for chemical neurolysis. Both agents cause extensive damage to the neuron. Subsequent inflammation and fibrosis of the nerve and adjacent tissues may cause secondary neuralgic pain.[7] Radiofrequency neurolysis coagulates nerves by heating a small area around the tip of a needle-shaped probe. The size and shape of the lesion are more controlled than with chemical neurolysis, which may decrease the likelihood of damage to adjacent tissues. Neurolytic blocks are not permanent despite the neural injury they entail.

Ramamurthy et al.[7] published a case series on 28 patients with a variety of pain problems with either phenol or cryoneurolysis. Only 28% of patients had at least 40% relief 4 weeks after treatment. These low success rates further restrict the use of peripheral neurolysis to patients in the last few weeks to months of life.

SYMPATHETIC BLOCKS

Visceral cancer pain, which is difficult to control with opioids and other analgesics, is especially suited for sympathetic plexus and splanchnic nerve blockade. Visceral afferents travel with the autonomic nervous system, permitting their blockade without resulting in somatosensory or motor dysfunction.[8]

Sympathetic blocks are successful and safe enough that they should be offered early in the course of cancer pain, especially if the patient has any difficulty with opioid side effects.[9-11] Neurolytic injections potentially could provide months of visceral pain relief.

Celiac Plexus Block Pain from tumor involvement of the upper abdominal viscera (pancreas, liver, diaphragm, spleen, stomach, small bowel, kidneys, abdominal aorta, adrenals, mesentery, and proximal colon) is treated with celiac plexus block (**Fig. 56-1**). The celiac plexus lies anterior to the aorta at the level of the celiac artery and has contributions from the T5 to T12 preganglionic sympathetic fibers. It contains splanchnic afferents, preganglionic parasympathetic fibers, and postganglionic sympathetic fibers. It can be accessed intraoperatively[12] or percutaneously from a bilateral posterior or midline anterior approach. Fluoroscopic or computed tomography (CT) guidance[13] is used to facilitate proper needle placement, avoid organ puncture, and monitor the spread of neurolytic solutions. More recently, an ultrasound-guided endoscopic approach to celiac plexus neurolysis has been described. Wyse et al.[14] concluded that early endoscopic ultrasound-guided celiac plexus neurolysis (EUS-CPN) reduces pain and may moderate morphine consumption in patients with painful, inoperable pancreatic adenocarcinoma. EUS-CPN can be considered in all such patients at the time of diagnostic and staging EUS.

Erdek et al.[15] did a retrospective analysis of 44 patients with terminal visceral (mostly pancreatic) cancer who failed conservative measures and concluded that celiac plexus neurolysis may provide intermediate pain relief to a significant percentage of patients with cancer. Both careful selections of candidates based on clinical variables and technical factors aimed at enhancing the specificity of blocks may lead to improved outcomes.

A transdiscal approach to splanchnic nerve blockade has been described as an alternative to the celiac plexus block in upper abdominal pain relief.[16]

A meta-analysis of 24 papers on celiac plexus block, including only two randomized and controlled studies, found that 90% of suitable cancer patients had partial to complete analgesia 3 months after the procedure.[17]

About 20% of patients experienced recurrent pain before death. Repeat celiac block should be offered in these cases,[11] although McGreevy et al. have recently demonstrated that repeat celiac plexus neurolysis (CPN) does not provide as much pain relief as the initial CPN.[18]

Intraoperative chemical splanchnicectomy (interrupting the preganglionic sympathetic fibers) has been used prophylactically in patients with pancreatic cancer at the time of surgical exploration and palliation. Compared with placebo in a randomized trial, prophylactic splanchnicectomy delayed the onset of pain or decreased its intensity.[19] Among patients with pain at the time of surgery, splanchnicectomy provided analgesia and appeared to improve survival. By providing constant, prolonged analgesia and limiting side effects, neurolytic celiac plexus block appears to maintain quality of life for patients with pancreatic cancer better than systemic opioid and adjuvant treatment.[9]

Failure of the celiac plexus block to provide analgesia is often due to extension of tumor to the peritoneum or abdominal wall, which are innervated by somatic pain fibers. Hypotension, back pain, and diarrhea are expected outcomes of celiac plexus block.[11,17]

The patient compensates for relative hypovolemia caused by mesenteric vasodilation over a period of about 2 days. Diarrhea is often a desirable outcome for a patient with opioid-induced constipation and is also usually limited to 2 days. Less common complications, such as unilateral paresis from somatic neurolysis, paraplegia from subarachnoid neurolysis or anterior cord infarction, pneumothorax, and retroperitoneal bleeding, are rare.[17] In a 5-year retrospective survey, only four of 2730 neurolytic celiac plexus blocks resulted in paraplegia or loss of sphincter function.[20]

Superior Hypogastric Plexus Block Pain from the pelvic viscera (rectum and sigmoid colon, bladder and ureters, uterus and adnexa) is often responsive to superior hypogastric plexus block.[21]

The superior hypogastric plexus lies in the retroperitoneum and extends from the anterior aspect of L5 to the superior sacrum (**Fig. 56-2**). Afferent fibers from the pelvic viscera pass through the plexus, which also contains sympathetic postganglionic fibers. As with celiac plexus block, only visceral pain responds to superior hypogastric

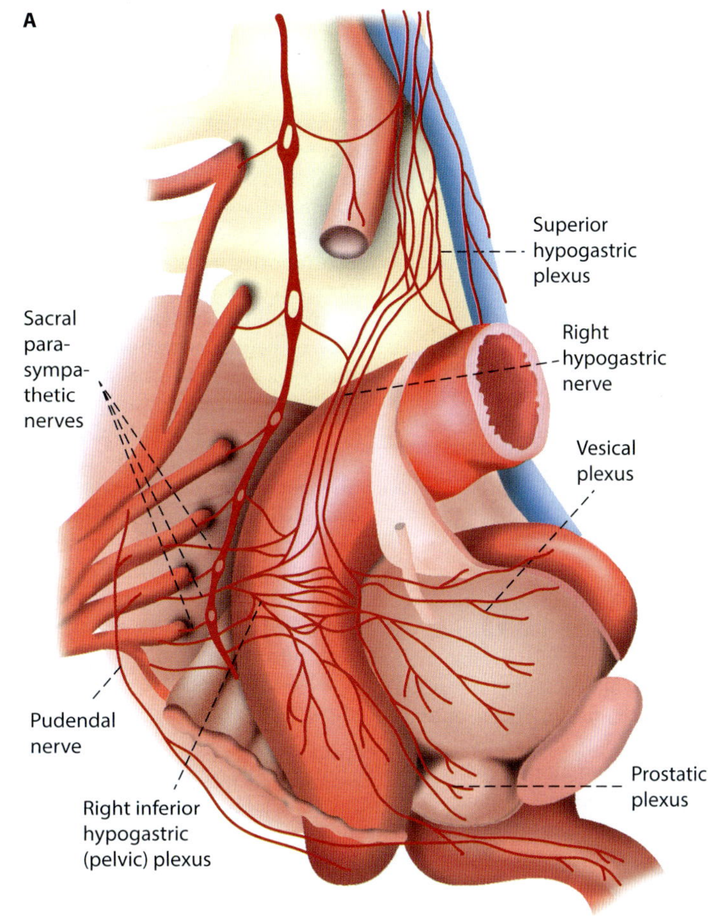

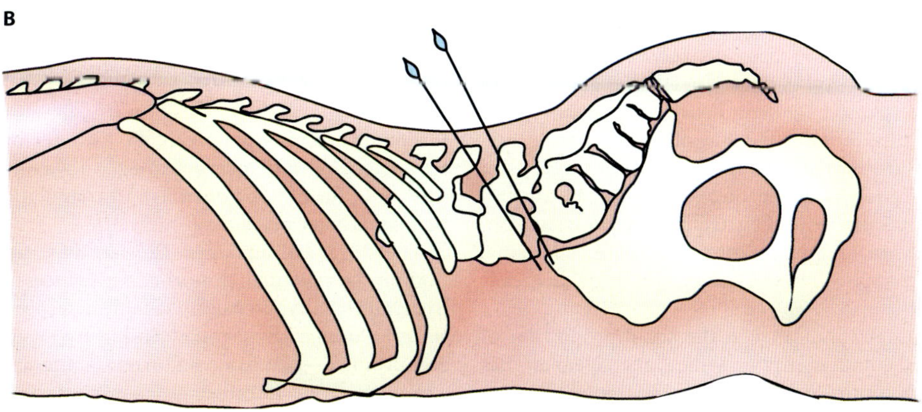

FIGURE 56-2. Superior hypogastric plexus block. **A.** Relevant anatomy. **B.** Needle placement anterior to the L5-S1 interspace. (Reproduced with permission from Lee RB, Stone K, Magelssen D, et al. Presacral neurectomy for chronic pelvic pain. *Obstet Gynecol*. 1986;68(4):517-521.)

plexus block. Somatic pain from sacral or muscle involvement and neuropathic pain from nerve root compression or infiltration do not respond to this block. An initial local anesthetic block is used to predict response to neurolytic phenol block.[21]

The superior hypogastric plexus can be accessed intraoperatively[22,23] or percutaneously via a bilateral posterior approach. Fluoroscopy is used to facilitate needle placement and to confirm appropriate spread of phenol. Plancarte et al. studied 227 patients with pelvic cancer pain who had poor analgesia or intolerable sedation with opioid management.[21] Seventy-nine percent of patients had a favorable response to local anesthetic test block. Visual analog pain scores decreased from greater than 7 of 10 to less than 4 of 10 in 72% of the responders. The other 28% experienced more modest pain reductions. Both groups of responders reduced opioid usage after the neurolytic block. Of 18 patients who were enrolled because of excessive sedation, 16 showed improvement after the procedure. There are no placebo-controlled studies of this block or studies that comprehensively evaluate other outcomes, such as quality of life, complications, and symptoms other than pain.

Because the plexus lies over the sacrum, hypotension, diarrhea, and injury to the aorta or spinal cord are unlikely. Lumbar plexus injury, bladder puncture, and iliac artery puncture with retroperitoneal bleeding or cholesterol plaque embolization might occur. In the Plancarte et al. study, no significant complications were reported.[21]

More recently CT-guided,[24] transdiscal,[25,26] and anterior ultrasound-guided approaches have been described.[27]

Other Sympathetic Blocks Anesthetic blocks are also possible elsewhere along the sympathetic chain. Blockade of the cervicothoracic (stellate), middle, and superior cervical ganglia—stellate ganglion block—affects sympathetic tone and visceral afferent sensation of the head, neck, and arms. These ganglia are easily reached anteriorly at the C6 transverse process. Some patients with cancer pain in the head and neck might benefit from stellate ganglion block.

INTRATHECAL DRUG DELIVERY

Intrathecal (IT) drug delivery is a viable treatment strategy for both neuropathic and nociceptive pain in the cancer population.[28,29]

By delivering opioids closer to their site of action in the substantia gelatinosa of the dorsal horn, IT drug delivery allows reduction in the total opioid dose and possibly decreasing side effects. When opioids and local anesthetics are delivered together, activity-induced pain and side effects are less than when either drug is used alone.[30,31] Because they are synergistic in the dorsal horn, small amounts of each drug may be used to treat regional pain by delivering the mixture at the appropriate spinal level. Taking advantage of drug synergy may reduce sensory and motor block, urinary retention, pruritus, nausea, and respiratory depression.

Comprehensive consensus-based guidelines on IT drug delivery systems in the treatment of pain caused by cancer pain are intended to assist clinicians in identifying the candidacy of patients with cancer-related pain who may benefit from IT drug delivery.[32] The guidelines were a product of a panel of expert clinicians that evaluated and analyzed current available data on IT drug delivery in patients with cancer-related pain, including those at the end of life. In conclusion, with careful consideration of the patient's medical comorbidities and prior therapies, communication with the oncologist, proper psychological evaluation, and appropriate trialing technique, clinicians can effectively optimize the use of IT therapy for cancer pain. The panel advocates for a much wider application of IT therapy to provide meaningful analgesia for patients.

Intrathecal therapy is usually indicated in the small proportion of cancer patients for whom comprehensive medical management has not provided optimal pain control or has caused unacceptable, dose-limiting, analgesic-related toxicity.

Studies have evaluated the efficacy of IT therapy versus comprehensive medical management (CMM) and have largely found IT drug delivery to provide superior relief compared with standard medical management. A 4-week randomized clinical trial by Smith et al. found that 84.5% of patients who received an implantable drug delivery system in addition to CMM achieved clinical success—defined as pain control combined with change of toxicity—compared with 70.8% of patients receiving CMM alone ($P = 0.05$).[29] Patients in the IT therapy cohort also reported greater improvements in fatigue and depressed level of consciousness and were found to have improved survival.

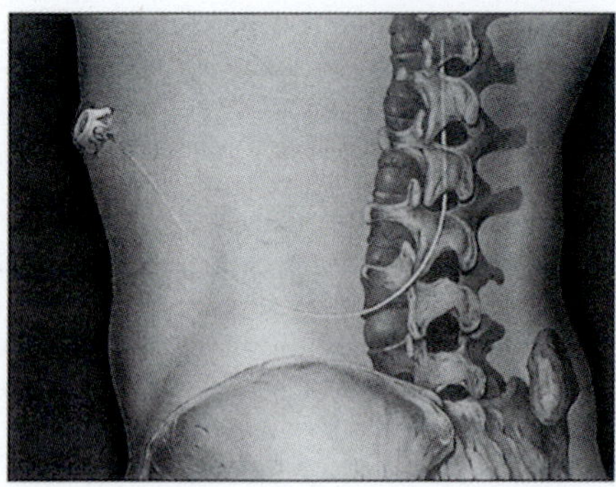

FIGURE 56-3. SynchroMed implantable intrathecal delivery system, including pump and catheter. (Reproduced with permission from Medtronic Neurological, Minneapolis, MN.)

An epidural catheter is usually used for the initial trial to assess efficacy of neuraxial technique to relieve pain.[33] If the infusions provide analgesia, an implanted infusion system is considered. Life expectancy is often taken into consideration. If life expectancy is few days to weeks, an epidural or IT catheter is connected to an external pump. If life expectancy is few months, the catheter can be tunneled and connected to a port, which can be connected to an external pump. Implantable drug delivery systems (IDDS) are usually considered when survival is likely more than 3 to 6 months (**Fig. 56-3**). IDDS uses a small, programmable computerized electronic pump to deliver drug to the IT space through a catheter. Recently, a handheld "remote control" patient-controlled analgesia device, the Patient Therapy Manager (PTM), has been introduced and approved by the Food and Drug Administration. It allows patients to give themselves a controlled bolus from the implanted pump.

Choice of Medications In 2011, the Polyanalgesic Consensus Conference reconvened to update the standard of care for IT therapies to reflect current changes in literature and clinical practice. In an effort to support and standardize IT therapies, the panel of experts had convened in 2000, 2003, and 2007 before this update. The panel reviewed the recent literature from 2007 to 2011 and decided on new algorithmic tracks for neuropathic and nociceptive pain. Although not specific to cancer-related pain, these guidelines serve as important fundamentals in IT drug therapy in cancer pain patients as well.[34] Initial therapy starting with dual agents using opioid and bupivacaine and even with triple agents using opioid with bupivacaine along with clonidine is common in IT drug delivery in cancer pain patients[35] (**Tables 56-1** and **56-2**).

Complications Intraoperatively, IT catheter insertion can be associated with bleeding and nerve damage. To avoid complications, systemic infection, thrombocytopenia, and coagulation defects must be treated before catheter placement.

The 2012 Polyanalgesic Consensus Conference recommendations outline the potential clinical consequences—including opioid-induced hyperalgesia, hypotension, sedation, respiratory depression, catheter-tip granulomas, hypogonadotropic hypogonadism, and immunologic compromise—that can result from IT therapy.[34,36]

When given intrathecally, local anesthetics can block incoming sensory nerves and produce complete anesthesia. The numbness may be unpleasant, and the proprioceptive loss may interfere with motor function. In addition, motor blockade itself may occur, causing

TABLE 56-1 2012 Polyanalgesic Algorithm for Intrathecal Therapies in Neuropathic Pain

Line 1	Morphine	Ziconotide		Morphine + bupivacaine
Line 2	Hydromorphone	Hydromorphone + bupivacaine or Hydromorphone + clonidine		Morphine + clonidine
Line 3	Clonidine	Ziconotide + opioid	Fentanyl	Fentanyl + bupivacaine or Fentanyl + clonidine
Line 4	Opioid + clonidine + bupivacaine		Bupivacaine + clonidine	
Line 5	Baclofen			

Line 1: Morphine and ziconotide are approved by the U.S. Food and Drug Administration for intrathecal therapy and are recommended as first-line therapy for neuropathic pain. The combination of morphine and bupivacaine is recommended for neuropathic pain on the basis of clinical use and apparent safety. **Line 2:** Hydromorphone, alone or in combination with bupivacaine or clonidine, is recommended. Alternatively, the combination of morphine and clonidine may be used. **Line 3:** Third-line recommendations for neuropathic pain include clonidine, ziconotide plus an opioid, and fentanyl alone or in combination with bupivacaine or clonidine. **Line 4:** The combination of bupivacaine and clonidine (with or without an opioid drug) is recommended. **Line 5:** Baclofen is recommended on the basis of safety, although reports of efficacy are limited.

Data from Deer TR, Prager J, Levy R, et al. Polyanalgesic Consensus Conference 2012: recommendations for the management of pain by intrathecal (intraspinal) drug delivery: report of an interdisciplinary expert panel. *Neuromodulation.* 2012;15:436-466.

TABLE 56-2 2012 Polyanalgesic Algorithm for Intrathecal Therapies in Nociceptive Pain

Line 1	Morphine	Hydromorphone	Ziconotide	Fentanyl
Line 2	Morphine + bupivacaine	Ziconotide + opioid	Hydromorphone + bupivacaine	Fentanyl + bupivacaine
Line 3	Opioid (morphine, hydromorphone, or fentanyl) + clonidine			Sufentanil
Line 4	Opioid + clonidine + bupivacaine		Sufentanil + bupivacaine or clonidine	
Line 5	Sufentanil + bupivacaine + clonidine			

Line 1: Morphine and ziconotide are approved by the U.S. Food and Drug Administration for intrathecal therapy and are recommended as first-line therapy for nociceptive pain. Hydromorphone is recommended on the basis of widespread clinical use and apparent safety. Fentanyl has been upgraded to first-line use by the consensus conference. **Line 2:** Bupivacaine in combination with morphine, hydromorphone, or fentanyl is recommended. Alternatively, the combination of ziconotide and an opioid drug can be used. **Line 3:** Recommendations include clonidine plus an opioid (i.e., morphine, hydromorphone, or fentanyl) or sufentanil monotherapy. **Line 4:** The triple combination of an opioid, clonidine, and bupivacaine is recommended. An alternative recommendation is sufentanil in combination with either bupivacaine or clonidine. **Line 5:** The triple combination of sufentanil, bupivacaine, and clonidine is suggested.

Data from Deer TR, Prager J, Levy R, et al. Polyanalgesic Consensus Conference 2012: recommendations for the management of pain by intrathecal (intraspinal) drug delivery: report of an interdisciplinary expert panel. *Neuromodulation.* 2012;15:436-466.

weakness, and sympathetic nervous system blockade may result in hypotension. Serious acute complications of neuraxial infusion are uncommon if initial drug doses are low and titration is carefully performed. The risks are greatest at the start of treatment, and patients must be closely monitored in the first 24 hours for potentially life-threatening respiratory depression, weakness, urinary retention, hypotension, and intraspinal hematoma.

Epidural abscess and meningitis are significant delayed complications of catheter placement. Cerebrospinal fluid (CSF) hygroma and pump pocket seroma may occur after pump placement but are usually self-limited. Catheter migration and blockage are other rare complications.

Chronic continuous infusion of high-concentration opioids at increased daily doses is associated with formation of IT inflammatory masses at the IT catheter tip in a small group of patients. Catheter-tip granulomas have been of great concern because of devastating neurologic sequelae. In a separate publication, the 2012 Polyanalgesic Consensus Panel has recommended use of lowest effective concentration and dose of IT opioid agents, as well as use of bolus dosing instead of continuous infusion.[36]

The panel further recommends IT catheter placement below the conus medullaris, use of nonopioid adjuvants, and switching to ziconotide if there is concern about granuloma formation.

INTRATHECAL AND EPIDURAL NEUROLYSIS

Absolute alcohol (ethanol) and phenol may be used to selectively interrupt dorsal root function when pain is limited to four dermatomes.[37,38]

This anesthetic version of the neurosurgical rhizotomy can be accomplished on an awake patient. It lacks the precision of an open rhizotomy, resulting in damage to Lissauer's tract and the posterior columns in addition to the dorsal roots. This procedure is limited to use for regional somatic pain in the trunk or in a functionless limb. Visceral pain is not affected, and neuropathic pain may not be susceptible inasmuch as it is due to deafferentation and pathologic changes in the spinal cord or brain.

For IT neurolysis, the patient is positioned on his or her side, and a spinal needle is introduced at the appropriate cord level (**Fig. 56-4**).[38] Small aliquots of the neurolytic agent are injected until analgesia develops in the area of pain. Pelvic and perineal pain are also amenable to IT neurolysis with phenol, wherein the patient is seated and the agent is allowed to pool around the sacral roots.[37] Epidural neurolysis has also been described.[39]

Paresis from anterior root or cord injury is possible with any of these procedures, although it is uncommon. In several large studies of IT neurolysis, about three-quarters of patients experienced fair to good relief.[38] As with peripheral neurolytic procedures, pain may recur in weeks to months after the procedure.

SPINAL CORD STIMULATION

Spinal cord stimulation (SCS) is used to treat intractable, regional neuropathic pain.[40,41] A set of electrodes is inserted into the epidural space to deliver electrical stimulation to the appropriate segment of the spinal cord. The electrodes are then connected to an implantable pulse generator, similar to a pacemaker. Primarily used for treatment of pain caused by spinal disease, SCS is rarely used for patients with advanced cancer with neuropathic features. The cost of SCS and the need for patient involvement in its use make it unsuitable for debilitated cancer patients near the end of life.

Radiofrequency Ablation of Painful Bone Metastasis Bone pain caused by metastatic lesions is a common complication of multiple cancer types. This pain is mostly treated with radiation; opioid and nonsteroidal anti-inflammatory drugs; and chemotherapy, bisphosphonates, and corticosteroids. Radiofrequency ablation via image-guided needle placement has been applied to use thermal destruction as a modality to control pain. Goetz et al., in a multicenter study, have treated

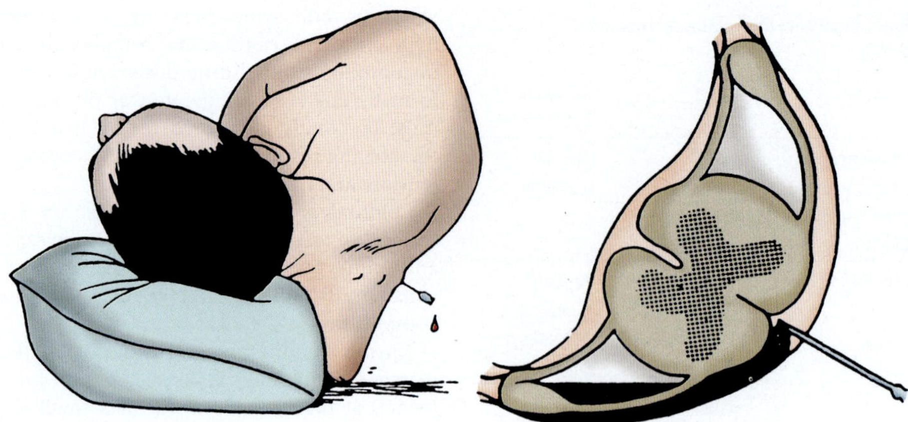

FIGURE 56-4. Intrathecal neurolysis: patient positioning for phenol injection. (From Swerdlow M. Intrathecal neurolysis. *Anaesthesia* 1978;33:733. Reproduced with permission from Blackwell Science.)

43 patients with image-guided radiofrequency ablation (RFA).[42] These patients had failed standard therapy for painful osteolytic metastases. Of these patients, 95% had clinically significant reduction in pain (visual analog scale score decrease of ≥2 on a 10-point scale). Before treatment, the mean worst pain score was 7.9; after treatment, the average worst pain score was 4.5 ($P < 0.0001$) at 4 weeks, 3.0 ($P < 0.0001$) at 12 weeks, and 1.2 ($P < 0.0005$) at 24 weeks. Opioid consumption also improved during the 24 weeks of reported follow-up. Complications were seen in three patients, with one involving an acetabular fracture after RFA.

RADIATION THERAPY

Radiation is an adjunct to pharmacologic pain management. Often used in the treatment of primary cancers, it has a prominent role in palliation of pain caused by bony metastases.[43] Pain from neural compression and soft tissue metastases may also respond, but the liver and kidneys do not tolerate radiation.

Palliative external-beam radiation is prescribed according to the patient's condition, the site to be treated, the tumor type, and previous exposure to radiation.

PALLIATIVE SURGERY

Even when curative surgery is impossible, certain operations may reduce pain and other symptoms. A few common palliative surgeries are mentioned here.

Pathologic fracture stabilization improves function and decreases pain for well over 80% of patients.[44] With improved survival with advanced cancer, patients may now obtain substantial benefit from aggressive surgical management of long bone, pelvic, and vertebral fractures and impending fractures. Metastatic plexopathy may be treated with en bloc resection of tumor and surrounding structures together with radiation and chemotherapy. Palliative tumor resection, ostomy placement, and gastrointestinal bypass may permit continued enteral nutrition and relieve obstruction in patients who have not responded to conservative measures. Spinal decompression and stabilization relieves pain from epidural cord compression and prevents impending paralysis. Extensive vertebral body destruction may leave the spine unstable, and positional changes may be painful.

NEUROSURGERY

Several neurosurgical treatments have been designed to interrupt pain pathways and stimulate modulatory systems. Over the past 2 decades, high-dose opioid treatment has replaced many of these surgeries.[45] The WHO analgesic ladder should be followed before resorting to a neurosurgical pain procedure.

INTRAVENTRICULAR OPIOID DELIVERY

Morphine may be injected into the cerebral ventricles after placement of an Ommaya reservoir or with a continuous infusion pump. It is appropriate for certain patients with pain from head and neck cancer, but no studies have demonstrated superiority of intraventricular over systemic opioid delivery. The relatively small experience with this technique has shown 50% to 90% good to excellent initial relief.[45,46] As with IT and epidural opioid delivery, respiratory depression and bleeding are potential early complications. Infection is the most concerning late complication.

CORDOTOMY

A lesion in the anterolateral quadrant of the spinal cord blocks the spinothalamic tract (**Fig. 56-5**), which carries pain signals from the contralateral body to the thalamus. Cordotomy is most useful for patients with unilateral somatic pain below the C5 dermatome but is useless in cases of deafferentation pain.[37] Lumbosacral plexopathy from tumor invasion is ideally suited to cordotomy. High cervical cordotomy may be used for arm pain. Because corticospinal and reticulospinal tracts are also located in the anterolateral quadrant, voluntary and involuntary respiration may be hampered by high cordotomy. Autonomic fiber disruption may interfere with bowel and bladder function in about 2% of patients. Persistent paresis is seen in 2%. These complications are more likely when bilateral lesions are made. Although initial success with cordotomy is high, recurrence of pain is common months to years later.

DORSAL RHIZOTOMY AND DORSAL ROOT ENTRY ZONE LESIONS

Dorsal rhizotomy is the surgical version of IT neurolysis. Interruption of dorsal roots blocks all regional sensation, including pain. Motor function is impaired if proprioception is blocked, so this procedure is limited to several dermatomes serving the trunk or functionless limbs. Pain sensation may be selectively interrupted without loss of normal sensation or proprioception. As with IT neurolysis, rhizotomy is not effective for purely neuropathic pain. Dorsal root entry zone lesioning destroys Lissauer's tract and the outer laminae of Rexed, preventing the development of deafferentation pain (**Fig. 56-6**).[47]

CRANIAL RHIZOTOMIES

When tumor growth causes somatic or neuralgic orofacial pain, percutaneous and open rhizotomies of the glossopharyngeal and trigeminal nerves may be effective.[48] These procedures may result in pain relief, but neurologic deficit is expected and recurrent pain is not uncommon.

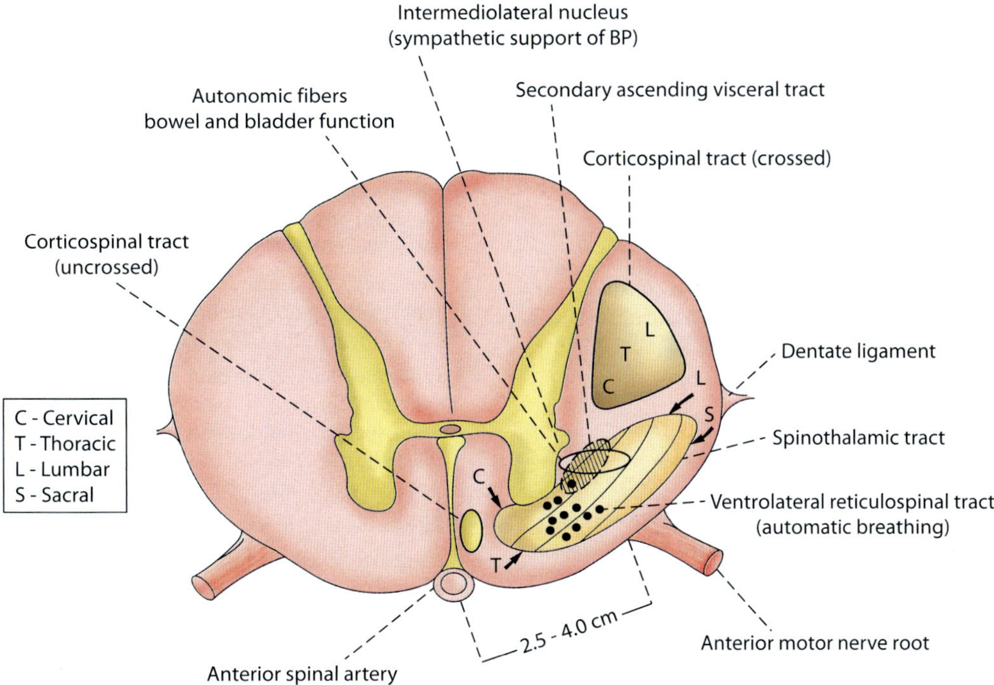

FIGURE 56-5. Cross-section of the spinal cord showing the locations of the spinothalamic, autonomic, reticulospinal (automatic breathing), and corticospinal (motor) tracts. Anterolateral cordotomy interrupts the spinothalamic tract, but complications may occur if surrounding fibers are affected. (Reproduced with permission from Poletti CE. Open cordotomy medullary tractotomy. In: Schmidek HH, Sweet WH, eds. *Operative Neurosurgical Techniques: Indications, Methods, Results.* New York: Grune and Stratton; 1988.)

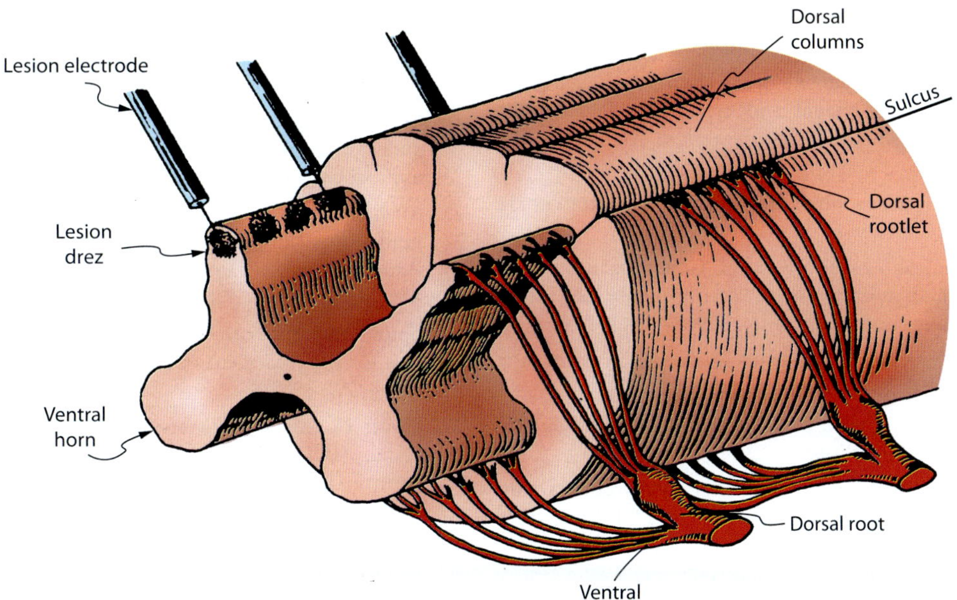

FIGURE 56-6. Radiofrequency dorsal root entry zone lesions as originally described by Nashold and Ostdahl. (Reproduced with permission from Nashold BS, Ostdahl FH. Dorsal root entry zone for pain relief. *J Neurosurg*. 1979;51:59. Used with permission of the American Association of Neurological Surgeons.)

HYPOPHYSECTOMY

Widespread pain from metastases may respond well to ablation of the pituitary. Hypophysectomy was introduced in 1953 for treatment of breast and prostate tumors.[49,50] The analgesic mechanism is still unknown. Most hypophysectomy patients achieve partial or total pain relief that lasts weeks to months and infrequently longer than 1 year. Alcohol instillation via the transsphenoidal route has also been described.[51,52] CSF leakage, infection, coma, and cranial nerve palsies may result. Hypopituitarism is expected but not uniformly with chemical and thermoablation.

NEUROSTIMULATION

Stimulation of thalamic nuclei is useful for some neuropathic pain conditions but requires considerable expertise for lead placement.[53]

The periaqueductal and periventricular gray matter contains receptors for opioids. Deep brain stimulation of these regions produces naloxone-reversible analgesia. Since systemic and neuraxial opioid treatment has become more accepted, these procedures have fallen from favor.

SUMMARY

Pain management is a prominent part of disease management in patients with cancer. Interventional pain therapies can provide good pain relief in selected patients. Pain specialists should be consulted early in the course of the disease process, and these procedures should be considered early in the treatment course as part of the oncology interdisciplinary plan.

REFERENCES

1. Cancer pain relief and palliative care. Report of a WHO Expert Committee. *World Health Organ Tech Rep Ser.* 1990;804:1-75.
2. Quigley C. Opioids in people with cancer-related pain. *Clin Evid (Online).* 2008;2008:2408.
3. Miguel R. Interventional treatment of cancer pain: the fourth step in the World Health Organization analgesic ladder? *Cancer Control.* 2000;7(2):149-156.
4. Krames ES. Interventional pain management. Appropriate when less invasive therapies fail to provide adequate analgesia. *Med Clin North Am.* 1999;83(3):787-808, vii-viii.
5. Ferrer-Brechner T. Anesthetic techniques for the management of cancer pain. *Cancer.* 1989;63(11 Suppl):2343-2347.
6. Kongsgaard UE, Bjorgo S, Hauser M. Neurolytic blocks for cancer pain—still a useful therapeutic strategy. *Tidsskr nor Laegeforen.* 2004;124(4):481-483.
7. Ramamurthy S, Walsh NE, Schoenfeld LS, Hoffman J. Evaluation of neurolytic blocks using phenol and cryogenic block in the management of chronic pain. *J Pain Symptom Manage.* 1989; 4(2):72-75.
8. Bonica JJ. Autonomic innervation of the viscera in relation to nerve block. *Anesthesiology.* 1968;29(4):793-813.
9. Kawamata M, Ishitani K, Ishikawa K, et al. Comparison between celiac plexus block and morphine treatment on quality of life in patients with pancreatic cancer pain. *Pain.* 1996;64(3):597-602.
10. Mercadante S. Celiac plexus block versus analgesics in pancreatic cancer pain. *Pain.* 1993;52(2):187-192.
11. Mercadante S, Nicosia F. Celiac plexus block: a reappraisal. *Reg Anesth Pain Med.* 1998;23(1):37-48.
12. Stefaniak T, Basinski A, Vingerhoets A, et al. A comparison of two invasive techniques in the management of intractable pain due to inoperable pancreatic cancer: neurolytic celiac plexus block and videothoracoscopic splanchnicectomy. *Eur J Surg Oncol.* 2005;31(7):768-773.
13. Kambadakone A, Thabet A, Gervais DA, et al. CT-guided celiac plexus neurolysis: a review of anatomy, indications, technique, and tips for successful treatment. *Radiographics.* 2011;31(6):1599-1621.
14. Wyse JM, Carone M, Paquin SC, et al. Randomized, double-blind, controlled trial of early endoscopic ultrasound-guided celiac plexus neurolysis to prevent pain progression in patients with newly diagnosed, painful, inoperable pancreatic cancer. *J Clin Oncol.* 2011;29(26):3541-3546.
15. Erdek MA, Halpert DE, Gonzalez Fernandez M, Cohen SP. Assessment of celiac plexus block and neurolysis outcomes and technique in the management of refractory visceral cancer pain. *Pain Med.* 2010;11(1):92-100.
16. Plancarte R, Guajardo-Rosas J, Reyes-Chiquete D, et al. Management of chronic upper abdominal pain in cancer: transdiscal blockade of the splanchnic nerves. *Reg Anesth Pain Med.* 2010;35(6): 500-506.
17. Eisenberg E, Carr DB, Chalmers TC. Neurolytic celiac plexus block for treatment of cancer pain: a meta-analysis. *Anesth Analg.* 1995;80(2):290-295.
18. McGreevy K, Hurley RW, Erdek MA, et al. The effectiveness of repeat celiac plexus neurolysis for pancreatic cancer: a pilot study. *Pain Practice.* 2013;2:89-95.
19. Lillemoe KD, Cameron JL, Kaufman HS, et al. Chemical splanchnicectomy in patients with unresectable pancreatic cancer: a prospective randomized trial. *Ann Surg.* 1993;217(5):447-455; discussion 456-457.
20. Davies DD. Incidence of major complications of neurolytic coeliac plexus block. *J R Soc Med.* 1993;86(5):264-266.
21. Plancarte R, de Leon-Casasola OA, El-Helaly M, et al. Neurolytic superior hypogastric plexus block for chronic pelvic pain associated with cancer. *Reg Anesth.* 1997;22(6):562-568.
22. Lee RB, Stone K, Magelssen D, et al. Presacral neurectomy for chronic pelvic pain. *Obstet Gynecol.* 1986;68(4):517-521.
23. Kapetanakis V, Jacob K, Klauschie J, et al. Robotic presacral neurectomy—technique and results. *Int J Med Robot.* 2012;8(1): 73-76.
24. Dooley J, Beadles C, Ho KY, et al. Computed tomography-guided bilateral transdiscal superior hypogastric plexus neurolysis. *Pain Med.* 2008;9(3):345-347.
25. Gamal G, Helaly M, Labib YM. Superior hypogastric block: transdiscal versus classic posterior approach in pelvic cancer pain. *Clin J Pain.* 2006;22(6):544-547.
26. Turker G, Basagan-Mogol E, Gurbet A, et al. A new technique for superior hypogastric plexus block: the posteromedian transdiscal approach. *Tohoku J Exp Med.* 2005;206(3):277-281.
27. Mishra S, Bhatnagar S, Gupta D, Thulkar S. Anterior ultrasound-guided superior hypogastric plexus neurolysis in pelvic cancer pain. *Anaesth Intensive Care.* 2008;36(5):732-735.
28. Rauck RL, Cherry D, Boyer MF, et al. Long-term intrathecal opioid therapy with a patient-activated, implanted delivery system for the treatment of refractory cancer pain. *J Pain.* 2003;4(8): 441-447.
29. Smith TJ, Coyne PJ, Staats PS, et al. An implantable drug delivery system (IDDS) for refractory cancer pain provides sustained pain control, less drug-related toxicity, and possibly better survival compared with comprehensive medical management (CMM). *Ann Oncol.* 2005;16(5):825-833.
30. Penning JP, Yaksh TL. Interaction of intrathecal morphine with bupivacaine and lidocaine in the rat. *Anesthesiology.* 1992;77(6):1186-2000.
31. Dahl JB, Rosenberg J, Hansen BL, et al. Differential analgesic effects of low-dose epidural morphine and morphine-bupivacaine at rest and during mobilization after major abdominal surgery. *Anesth Analg.* 1992;74(3):362-365.
32. Deer TR, Smith HS, Burton AW, et al. Comprehensive consensus based guidelines on intrathecal drug delivery systems in the treatment of pain caused by cancer pain. *Pain Physician.* 2011;14:E283-E312.
33. Deer TR, Prager J, Levy R, et al. Polyanalgesic Consensus Conference—2012: recommendations on trialing for intrathecal

(intraspinal) drug delivery: report of an interdisciplinary expert panel. *Neuromodulation*. 2012;15:420-435.

34. Deer TR, Prager J, Levy R, et al. Polyanalgesic Consensus Conference 2012: recommendations for the management of pain by intrathecal (intraspinal) drug delivery: report of an interdisciplinary expert panel. *Neuromodulation*. 2012;15:436-466.
35. Stearns L, Boortz-Marx R, Du Pen S, et al. Intrathecal drug delivery for the management of cancer pain: a multidisciplinary consensus of best clinical practices. *J Support Oncol*. 2005;3:399-408.
36. Deer TR, Prager J, Levy R, et al. Polyanalgesic Consensus Conference—2012: consensus on diagnosis, detection, and treatment of catheter-tip granulomas (inflammatory masses). *Neuromodulation*. 2012;15:483-495.
37. Ischia S, Luzzani A, Ischia A, et al. Subarachnoid neurolytic block (L5-S1) and unilateral percutaneous cervical cordotomy in the treatment of pain secondary to pelvic malignant disease. *Pain*. 1984;20(2):139-149.
38. Swerdlow M. Intrathecal neurolysis. *Anaesthesia*. 1978;33(8):733-740.
39. Takahashi-Sato K, Hashimoto K, Nakano Y, et al. Two cases of thoracic epidural neurolysis after local anesthetic titration in cancer patients. *Fukushima J Med Sci*. 2011;57(2):66-68.
40. Yakovlev AE, Ellias Y. Spinal cord stimulation as a treatment option for intractable neuropathic cancer pain. *Clin Med Res*. 2008;6(3-4):103-106.
41. Yakovlev AE, Resch BE, Karasev SA. Treatment of cancer-related chest wall pain using spinal cord stimulation. *Am J Hosp Palliat Care*. 2010;27(8):552-556.
42. Goetz MP, Callstrom MR, Charboneau JW, et al. Percutaneous image-guided radiofrequency ablation of painful metastases involving bone: a multicenter study. *J Clin Oncol*. 2004;22:300-306.
43. Arcangeli G, Micheli A, Arcangeli G, et al. The responsiveness of bone metastases to radiotherapy: the effect of site, histology and radiation dose on pain relief. *Radiother Oncol*. 1989;14(2):95-101.
44. Harrington KD. Orthopedic surgical management of skeletal complications of malignancy. *Cancer*. 1997;80(8 Suppl):1614-1627.
45. Sundaresan N, DiGiacinto GV, Hughes JE. Neurosurgery in the treatment of cancer pain. *Cancer*. 1989;63(11 Suppl):2365-2377.
46. Dennis GC, DeWitty RL. Long-term intraventricular infusion of morphine for intractable pain in cancer of the head and neck. *Neurosurgery*. 1990;26(3):404-407; discussion 407-408.
47. Nashold BS Jr, Ostdahl RH. Dorsal root entry zone lesions for pain relief. *J Neurosurg*. 1979;51(1):59-69.
48. Giorgi C, Broggi G. Surgical treatment of glossopharyngeal neuralgia and pain from cancer of the nasopharynx: a 20-year experience. *J Neurosurg*. 1984;61(5):952-955.
49. Hayashi M, Taira T, Chernov M, et al. Gamma knife surgery for cancer pain-pituitary gland-stalk ablation: a multicenter prospective protocol since 2002. *J Neurosurg*. 2002;97(5 Suppl):433-437.
50. Flitsch J, Bernreuther C, Hagel C, Ludecke DK. Hypophysectomy for prostate cancer: a revival of old knowledge? *J Neurosurg*. 2008;109(4):760-764.
51. Levin AB, Katz J, Benson RC, Jones AG. Treatment of pain of diffuse metastatic cancer by stereotactic chemical hypophysectomy: long term results and observations on mechanism of action. *Neurosurgery*. 1980;6(3):258-262.
52. Katz J, Levin AB. Treatment of diffuse metastatic cancer pain by instillation of alcohol into the sella turcica. *Anesthesiology*. 1977;46(2):115-121.
53. Young RF, Brechner T. Electrical stimulation of the brain for relief of intractable pain due to cancer. *Cancer*. 1986;57(6):1266-1272.

Pain Management in End of Life: Palliative Care

Jaya Vijayan
J. Cameron Muir
Matthew G. Kestenbaum

The basic principles of the diagnosis and management of pain syndromes are similar across all clinical settings. Details of the application of these principles, however, can vary significantly depending on the clinical context. One context that is especially important is the care of patients with incurable, progressive, and ultimately fatal illnesses who are in or approaching the terminal phase. This is sometimes referred to in the context of "palliative care," and this term, although not fully satisfactory,[1] is used throughout most of the discussions in this chapter. The range of pain syndromes that arise in these situations includes most of the acute and chronic pain syndromes addressed in detail in other chapters in this text, and their management primarily involves the same diagnostic and therapeutic strategies and skills. Nonetheless, pain management in the palliative care setting often raises clinical and ethical issues that are at least somewhat different from those in other settings. This chapter focuses primarily on those differences.

PAIN MANAGEMENT AND PALLIATIVE CARE: OVERVIEW

"Life cannot simply be put on hold while treatment is endured."
—Ira Byock, MD

The Task Force on Palliative Care of the Last Acts Campaign,[2] formulated by representatives of many leading U.S. professional organizations, states: "Palliative care refers to the comprehensive management of physical, social, spiritual, and existential needs of patients, particularly those with incurable, progressive illnesses. Palliative care affirms life and regards dying as a natural process that is a profoundly personal experience for the individual and family. The goal of palliative care is to achieve the best possible quality of life through relief of suffering, control of symptoms, and restoration of functional capacity while remaining sensitive to personal, cultural and religious values, beliefs, and practices." The Task Force identified five "core precepts" of the evolving field of palliative care:

1. *Respecting patient goals, preferences, and choices:* Identifies and honors the preferences of the patient and family through careful attention to their values, goals, and priorities, as well as their cultural and spiritual perspectives and assists patients in establishing goals of care by facilitating their understanding of their diagnosis and prognosis, clarifying priorities, promoting informed choices, and providing an opportunity for negotiating a care plan with providers
2. *Comprehensive caring:* Places a high priority on physical comfort and functional capacity, including management of pain and other symptoms; diagnosis and treatment of psychological distress and assistance in remaining as independent as possible or desired; and provides physical, psychological, social and spiritual support to help the patient and family adapt to the anticipated decline associated with advanced, progressive, incurable disease
3. *Using the strengths of interdisciplinary resources:* Requires an interdisciplinary approach drawing on the expertise of, among others, physicians, nurses, psychologists, pharmacists, pastoral caregivers, social workers, ancillary staff, volunteers, and family members to address the multidimensional aspects of care; incorporates the full array of interinstitutional and community resources (hospitals, home care, hospice, long-term care, adult day services); and promotes a seamless transition between institutions or settings and services

4. *Acknowledging and addressing caregiver concerns:* Appreciates the substantial physical, emotional, and economic demands placed on families caring for someone at home as they attempt to fulfill caregiving responsibilities and meet their own personal needs; anticipates that some family caregivers may be at high risk for fatigue, physical illness, and emotional distress; and considers the special needs of these caregivers in planning and delivering services
5. *Building systems and mechanisms of support:* Promotes equitable and timely access to the full array of interdisciplinary services necessary to meet the multidimensional needs of patients and caregivers

Palliative care complements other therapies that are available and appropriate to the identified goals of care early in the course of a chronic illness. The intensity and range of palliative interventions may increase as the illness progresses and the complexity of the care and needs of patients and their families increases. The priority of care frequently shifts during this time to focus on end-of-life decision making and care that support comfort and are consistent with the values and expressed desires of the patient. Palliative care guides patients and their families as they make the transition through the changing goals of care. It also helps patients who wish to address issues of life completion and life closure.

For many people who desire ongoing traditional curative care, hospice is not an attractive option. Patients who are averse to the word or concept of hospice or who have difficulty acknowledging that they are facing a terminal illness may benefit from and should be able to receive palliative services. To best prepare patients and families physically, emotionally, and spiritually and to ensure the highest quality of life, "palliative discussions" should begin earlier in the disease trajectory. Palliative care should be considered not as an "alternative" to other types of medical treatment but as an adjunct type of care to allow comprehensive, whole patient–directed, high-quality management. Palliative care services should be provided along the continuum of care from acute care to ambulatory care to long-term care and should include hospice care.[3]

Palliative care discussions should occur at the time of diagnosis of a chronic, progressive disease, providing the patient with full informed consent for all treatment options. If the disease progresses, the focus on curative treatments may decrease as an emphasis on palliative care and relief of suffering (physical, emotional, and spiritual) increases. The patient and family are informed partners in decision making from the beginning and have time to prepare for and respond to physical, psychosocial, and spiritual issues.[3]

PERCEPTIONS ABOUT PALLIATIVE CARE

The 2011 Public Opinion Research on Palliative Care was commissioned by the Center to Advance Palliative Care to explore the awareness and understanding of palliative care among key audiences. Their report found that consumers have concerns about the level of care patients with serious illness receive. The biggest concerns identified were:

1. Doctors might not provide all of the treatment options available (58%).
2. Doctors might not talk and share information with each other (55%).
3. Doctors might not choose the best treatment option for a seriously ill patient's medical condition (54%).
4. Patients with serious illness and their families leave a doctor's office or hospital feeling unsure about what they are supposed to do when they get home (51%).
5. Patients with serious illness and their families do not have enough control over their treatment options (51%).
6. Doctors do not spend enough time talking with and listening to patients and their families (50%).

More than 70% of consumers were not knowledgeable about palliative care.

Physicians tended to equate palliative care with "hospice" or "end-of-life" care and were resistant to believing otherwise. Although the physicians surveyed said that they have referred patients to palliative care services, they admitted they only did so when it was for end-of-life care.

The following revised definition of palliative care based on the qualitative research was found to have a positive effect when defining or describing palliative care for consumers:

> Palliative care is specialized medical care for people with serious illnesses. This type of care is focused on providing patients with relief from the symptoms, pain and stress of a serious illness—whatever the diagnosis. The goal is to improve quality of life for both the patient and the family. Palliative care is provided by a team of doctors, nurses and other specialists who work with a patient's other doctors to provide an extra layer of support. Palliative care is appropriate at any age and any stage in a serious illness, and can be provided together with curative treatment.[4]

PATIENT-CENTERED GOALS: ETHICAL AND PRACTICAL IMPORTANCE

Defining clear patient-centered goals of care is a prerequisite to developing optimal diagnostic and therapeutic strategies. In the medical ethics literature, four core values that physicians are obligated to consider are frequently identified: autonomy, beneficence, justice, and nonmaleficence. The physician's professional integrity is an additional important value. Although cases in which these values are in conflict can pose exceedingly difficult ethical dilemmas, in most cases involving the clinical care of an individual patient, the central question that should be posed about *any* proposed intervention is: *Do the expected benefits outweigh the expected burdens from the patient's perspective?*

If the answer is yes, the intervention should almost always be instituted unless an alternative is even more favorable. If the answer is no, the intervention should never be instituted, and if it is already in place, it should be withdrawn. This assessment applies equally to minor interventions such as phlebotomy or plain radiography and to much more complex interventions such as surgery or a course of radiation therapy.

The simplicity of this framework should not mask the frequent complexity of its application, which requires as full as possible an understanding of what the individual patient considers a "benefit" or a "burden," as well as an assessment of the probability of those benefits and burdens for each intervention under consideration. In this process, there is a natural division of labor between the respective roles of the patient (or his or her surrogate) and the patient's physician or other members of the clinical team, as illustrated in **Figure 57-1**. In developing plans of care, it is therefore vitally important for the clinician to engage the patient (or surrogate) in a careful consideration of the relative priority of a wide range of possible goals of care (**Figs. 57-2** and **57-3**).

One common error in planning care is that discussions of relative priority for various potentially competing goals of care are limited to comfort versus length of life. As described earlier, however, comfort is rarely the most important human life goal but rather the prerequisite to achieving other goals. Furthermore, recent evidence indicates that this presumed notion that the goals of comfort and length of life are mutually exclusive may be an inaccurate representation of this more complex issue. In fact, research has shown that in patients with metastatic non–small cell lung cancer, median survival times were longer in those receiving early palliative care interventions versus those who received standard care; importantly, patients who received early palliative care also reported significantly improved quality of life and mood.[5] **Table 57-1** lists some of the goals of care that are most commonly expressed by patients confronting an ultimately fatal illness.

It is also important to appreciate that the relative priority of various goals of care almost always varies over the course of an illness, either

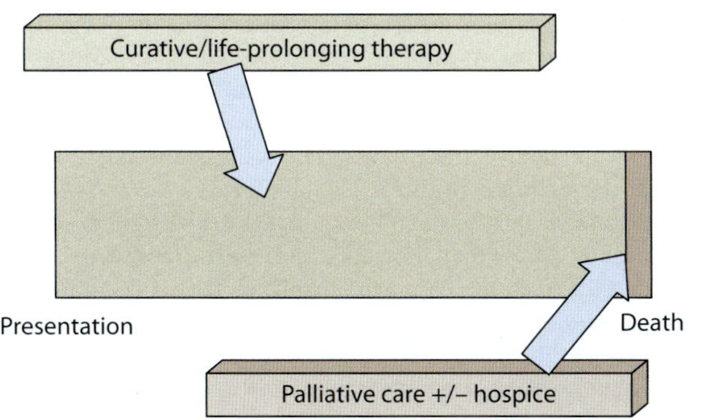

FIGURE 57-1. Common view of the relationship between curative and life-prolonging therapy and palliative care. (Adapted from the EPEC Project. Curriculum Emanuel LL, von Gunten CF, Ferris FD, eds. The Education in Palliative and End-of-life Care (EPEC) Curriculum: © The EPEC Project, 1999, 2003.)

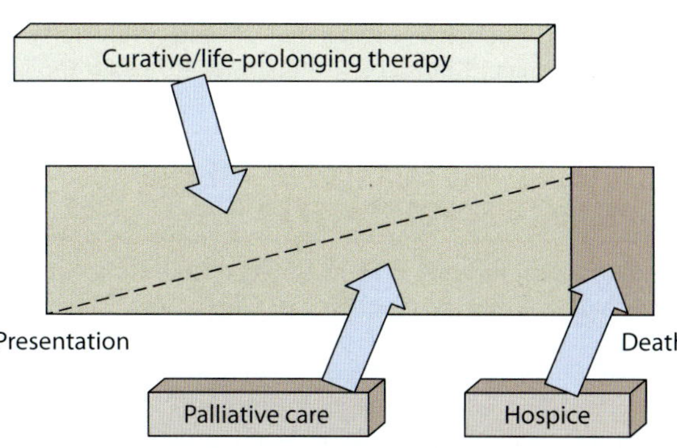

FIGURE 57-2. Preferred model of the relationship between curative and life-prolonging therapy and palliative care efforts. (Adapted from the EPEC Project. Curriculum Emanuel LL, von Gunten CF, Ferris FD, eds. The Education in Palliative and End-of-life Care (EPEC) Curriculum: © The EPEC Project, 1999, 2003.)

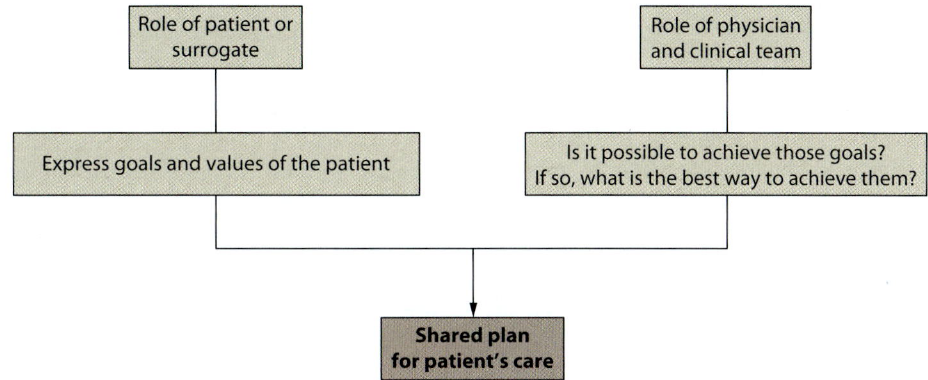

FIGURE 57-3. Shared decision making.

TABLE 57-1 Goals of Care

Examples of Possible Goals of Care
Longer life or living until a particularly important event (e.g., wedding, anniversary)
Relief of symptoms
Spend time at home or at a favorite location
Ability to travel
Maintenance of control
Maintenance or improvement of function
Ability to interact with loved ones
Chance to mend relationships
Minimizing burdens on loved ones
Personal or spiritual growth
"Dignity" (specific meaning will vary)
A good death

as the illness itself progresses or as the person changes during the process of living with the illness. The clinician therefore needs to review regularly with the patient not only how well various goals of care are being achieved but also whether the relative priority of various goals has changed (or whether entirely new goals have been identified).

A second common error in planning care is to confuse the articulation of *goals* of care with the determination of the most appropriate *means* of accomplishing those goals. This is a frequent shortcoming of both written and orally conveyed advance directives, which are often framed in terms of preferences for or against various clinical interventions (e.g., mechanical ventilation, cardiopulmonary resuscitation [CPR], or "feeding tubes"). Many patients who express with great confidence some variant of "I would never want to be kept alive by machines" will, on further discussion, quickly agree that "if a limited period of extremely intensive care in an intensive care unit might restore me to near-normal condition, I would want it." For some patients who have previously adamantly expressed the view that they do not want any further "surgery," the expected benefits of an anatomical pain intervention that includes a relatively minor surgical procedure may far outweigh any likely burdens.[6]

In the opposite direction, patients are frequently asked some variant of "if your heart stops, would you want to be resuscitated?" The common affirmative response leads to a "full code" status that clinical staff may believe is inappropriate. But the desire to be "resuscitated" is an expression of a *goal*, which may not at all reflect a well-informed judgment about whether the expected benefits of administering CPR are likely to outweigh the expected burdens. A discussion that is much more likely to yield a plan of care that optimally serves the patient's most important goals might begin with a conversation about the patient's attitude toward death ("At this point in your illness, is death the enemy?"), as well as what conditions of prolonged life are most hoped for or feared. From an understanding of those parameters, the clinician may offer specific suggestions of the clinical interventions that are most likely to achieve goals that are important to the patient and most likely to avoid burdens or outcomes to which the patient is particularly averse.

PAIN, SUFFERING, AND MEANING AT THE END OF LIFE: PALLIATIVE CARE CONTEXT

As discussed at length elsewhere in this text, pain is a complex phenomenon that includes nociceptive, psychological, behavioral, and social components (see Chapter 4). Pain must also be distinguished from suffering, which is not directly related to the severity of physical symptoms.[7,8] As Cassell suggests, suffering is experienced by *persons*, not bodies, and generally stems from conditions or events that threaten the integrity of the person as a complex psychological and social entity. Absence or loss of affirmative meaning and purpose, absence or loss of control, and absence or loss of hope are major sources of suffering.[9]

In his landmark study *Man's Search for Meaning*, psychiatrist Viktor Frankl analyzed experiences of his fellow concentration camp inmates at Auschwitz, in part to try to understand what distinguished those who survived from those who did not. He quotes Friedrich Nietzsche: "He who has a *why* to live for can put up with almost any *how*."[10] Analogously, for patients confronting serious or even life-threatening illnesses, the *meaning* (or absence thereof) of their continued life is often the strongest determinant of whether symptoms are bearable. A growing number of studies of requests for physician assistance in suicide support this insight: patients who ask for such assistance do not have higher levels of pain or other physical symptoms than those who do not make such requests. Rather, the primary concerns of many (if not most) patients asking for such assistance have more to do with issues of *meaning*, including the loss of a sense of any purpose in continued life, and concerns that the terminal phase of illness will involve a serious loss of personal dignity.

Biomedical efforts to control pain and other symptoms therefore constitute only a limited component of a broader effort to relieve suffering and help patients find affirmative value in the last phase of life. Nonetheless, a failure to achieve consistent control of pain and other symptoms may make achievement of any other goals quite impossible. It is obvious that uncontrolled severe pain or other symptoms can so dominate a person's consciousness that he or she has no energy or capacity to focus on any affirmative goals or meaningful experiences. Even when pain is recently well controlled, fears that severe pain will recur and not be controllable can interfere with or even overwhelm other psychological processes. In addition, a perceived lack of control over pain often interacts synergistically with other perceptions by the patient that he or she has lost control over important parts of life, fueling a downward spiral of increasing depression and hopelessness. Conversely, the demonstrated controllability of pain not only has the direct benefit of relieving important symptoms, it can also help fuel an upward spiral of increasing optimism and hope.

TOLERANCE, PHYSICAL DEPENDENCE, AND ADDICTION IN PALLIATIVE CARE

A comprehensive understanding of these three distinct phenomena is vital in many areas of pain management and is covered in detail elsewhere in this text. In the palliative care setting, misconceptions about these phenomena or a lack of attention to their potential importance can significantly compromise the quality of pain management involving opioids.

TOLERANCE

Tolerance is characterized by the need to use escalating doses of a drug to maintain the same effect. When the underlying disease process is clearly stable and there is no evidence of either addiction or drug "diversion" (see the following section, Addiction), the need for increased doses can with reasonable confidence be attributed to this phenomenon. In some cases, switching to another opioid, for which a patient may have only partial cross-tolerance, can be useful. In actual practice, however, when a chronically effective dose has been well established in the treatment of a stable disease process, it is unusual for subsequent tolerance to be an important clinical problem.

In the palliative care context, however, the underlying disease process is rarely stable, and when increased doses are needed to achieve the same analgesic effect, the clinician's primary suspicion should always be disease progression. If disease progression is in fact the cause, then further increases in the dose of the current opioid may be effective. These increases may be quite large, sometimes as high as 20-fold.[11,12]

PHYSICAL DEPENDENCE

Physical dependence is characterized by symptoms of withdrawal after abrupt discontinuation of the drug and can be a severe problem in the context of chronic use of significant doses of opioids. In the palliative care context, clinicians rarely, if ever, consciously stop chronic opioids abruptly. Nonetheless, serious withdrawal syndromes can become manifest in the terminal phase of illness if the route of administration of chronic opioids is suddenly no longer available, as in the case of a patient taking opioids orally who becomes moribund and unable to swallow. In this situation, it is important to find an alternate route to administer an amount of medication sufficient to achieve both continued pain control and prevention of withdrawal. In the palliative care population, the subcutaneous route is often preferred in this scenario; the efficacy and benefits of the subcutaneous route of administration are discussed later in this chapter.

Palliative care patients and caregivers may confuse physical dependence with addiction; at times, they may bring about withdrawal by abruptly discontinuing an opioid—even if it is effective and free of adverse effects—for "fear of becoming addicted." As discussed in more detail in the next section, a thoughtful discussion about the differences between physical dependence and addiction before the initiation of opioids (or during the initial visit with the palliative care specialist) can often prevent this scenario.

ADDICTION

Addiction is characterized by psychological dependence on the involved drug; compulsive use; loss of control; associated loss of interest in other pleasurable activities; and, most important, continued use despite evident harm. It is rare for this to be a problem in pain management in the setting of terminal illness, and it is virtually unheard of in terminally ill patients with no preexisting history of addiction or substance abuse. For patients with such a preexisting history, the risks of addiction must be carefully assessed and proactively addressed in planning any pain management regimen. Concern about these risks, however, must not lead to plans of care that leave a dying patient with inadequate symptom relief. Furthermore, even when there is an apparent pattern of opioid consumption or "lost prescriptions" suggesting the possibility of substance abuse, anecdotal experience in the care of terminally ill patients suggests that two alternative explanations (neither with a simple solution) must be considered at least as strongly: another household member may be stealing the patient's medication, or the patient him- or herself may be selling the medication to cover other living expenses.

A much more frequent problem than true addiction is the unwarranted concern of patients (or their loved ones) that they will become addicted if they consume significant opioid doses over time. This concern can become a major obstacle to adequate symptom management and should be explicitly addressed with all patients. This can begin by simply inquiring about whether the patient or involved family members have any concerns about addiction to prescribed medications. Any concerns about addiction should be addressed with appropriate information and reassurance, emphasizing that the physical, psychological, and spiritual problems associated with uncontrolled pain take a far, far greater toll on most patients confronting a life-threatening illness.

OPIOIDS, RESPIRATORY SUPPRESSION, AND HASTENING DEATH

When high (or at least increasing) doses of opioids are required for effective pain control, clinicians are often concerned that in administering these doses they may depress a patient's respiratory drive and thereby hasten death. Even clinicians deeply committed to ensuring comfort at the end of life may exercise such caution in opioid administration that they fail to achieve adequate analgesia.

Although it is true that respiratory suppression can be a primary drug effect of opioids, it is in fact far less common than many physicians believe they "know" from their own clinical experience.[13–15] Azoulay et al., in a retrospective observational study conducted in 114 consecutive hospice patients, found that opioid usage, even at high doses (mean opioid dosage, 146 ± 245 mg/day) had no effect on survival among patients with advanced cancer in a hospice setting.[16] Tachypnea is a frequent manifestation both of acute pain and of anxiety, and the decreased respiratory rate that almost always follows administration of an opioid in the setting of intense, acute pain is in most cases a secondary result of the drug's primary analgesic and anxiolytic effects.

Given the widespread belief that administration of opioids in the terminal setting may hasten death, there is a surprising dearth—indeed, a virtual absence—of convincing data that this is a real phenomenon, with the exception of rapid dose escalation in previously opioid-naive patients. Experienced palliative care clinicians are generally adamant that as long as escalations in opioids are carefully titrated on the basis of appropriate symptoms and signs (usually of pain or dyspnea), concerns that death will thereby be hastened are simply unfounded. Twycross argues that "the use of morphine in the relief of cancer pain carries no greater risk than the use of aspirin *when used correctly*" [italics in the original], and far from being the cause of death, "the correct use of morphine is more likely to prolong a patient's life . . . because he is more rested and pain-free."[17] Bakker et al. report that because of their effect of decreasing oxygen demand in patients with cardiorespiratory distress, sedatives and opioids may actually prolong life rather than hasten death.[18] Portenoy and Coyle report that "the development of new respiratory symptoms is virtually never a primary drug effect in patients who have been receiving stable doses or who are undergoing dose increases following substantial prior opioid intake."[19] Foley adds that "respiratory depression is not a significant limiting factor in the management of patients with pain because with repeated doses, tolerance develops to this effect."[20]

Nonetheless, even though it is far less commonly a real clinical issue than is generally perceived, the possibility in a specific case that opioid administration may directly hasten death cannot be completely excluded, particularly for a patient who has had limited previous exposure to opioids. Some clinicians (and some family members) will therefore at least occasionally confront the difficult clinical and ethical challenge of trying simultaneously to fulfill their duty to relieve suffering and their obligation not to knowingly cause a patient's death. The most widely used analytic framework for deciding what to do when a proposed action has two foreseeable effects, one good and one bad, is known as the "doctrine of double effect."

DOCTRINE OF DOUBLE EFFECT

Historically rooted in Roman Catholic theology dating back to Aquinas, the doctrine of double effect states that when an action (e.g., administering escalating doses of opioids to relieve pain in the terminal setting) has the possibility of both a "good" effect (relief of pain) and a "bad" effect (hastening death), the action is ethically permissible if *all* of the following conditions are met:[21,22]

1. The action itself must be morally good or at least indifferent (i.e., not intrinsically evil).

   Administering effective medication to a suffering patient unquestionably qualifies. Most people would agree that killing the patient with a weapon would not.

2. Only the good effect must be intended even though the bad effect is foreseeable.

   The only morally acceptable goal of the clinician is the relief of the patient's symptoms. It is ***not*** *morally acceptable for the clinician to* ***intend****, as a stated or unstated goal of administering the opioid, to shorten the patient's life.*

3. The good effect must not be achieved as a result of the bad effect.

   Relieving suffering ***by*** *causing death (as would be the case if the drug in question were a bolus of intravenous potassium) is not acceptable.*

4. The good effect must outweigh the bad effect.

The benefit to the patient of the relief of suffering must be greater than the harm to the patient of a shortened life. When the administered opioid offers the best available likelihood of relieving suffering, when the length of time by which the patient's life might be shortened is small (minutes, hours, or perhaps a few days), and when that time would add little or no value to the patient's life (e.g., if the patient is permanently incapable of meaningful interaction), this condition is clearly met. In different circumstances (e.g., administering the drug risks greatly shortening a patient's life that has clear ongoing meaning), an opposite conclusion might be reached.

Recent evidence suggests that opioids do not hasten death.[16,18] In a letter to the *British Medical Journal* in 2011, Regnard et al. were of the opinion that when opioids are correctly prescribed, they do not hasten death, and there is no need to invoke the doctrine of double effect to justify their use. Opioid dose requirements cannot be predicted, so to avoid adverse effects, doses should always be titrated to the individual. There are no circumstances in which the prescription of a lethal dose of opioid is necessary to control suffering, and therefore there is no need to invoke the doctrine of double effect.[23]

OTHER OPIOID-RELATED ISSUES IN THE PALLIATIVE CARE CONTEXT

There are several additional important issues related to the use of opioids in the palliative care context. Details of each of these are covered in other chapters in this text, and only major points will be reviewed here.

ROUTES OF ADMINISTRATION

Many routes of administration are available, including oral, intravenous, subcutaneous, rectal (morphine, oxymorphone, hydromorphone, or methadone suppositories), sublingual (concentrated morphine elixir, oxycodone, or hydromorphone), and transdermal and oral transmucosal (fentanyl citrate). The oral route is safe and effective and has been recommended as the first-line approach to cancer pain management by the World Health Organization and the European Association for Palliative Care. However, as patients move closer to the end of life, the need for one or more alternate routes of medication increases.

A systematic review of the literature by Radbruch et al. found no differences in efficacy between the subcutaneous and intravenous routes, confirming that both routes are feasible, effective, and safe. Because the risk of complications is lower with subcutaneous administration, this route should be preferred. For patients with a port system or an indwelling venous line for other therapeutic indications, the intravenous administration route is an alternative. Rectal or transdermal therapy offers a good alternative to the subcutaneous route for a number of patients. The review found no significant differences in efficacy or side among the alternative application routes.[24]

The side effect profile appears to be very similar for the subcutaneous, intravenous, rectal, and transdermal routes, with sedation, nausea, vomiting, and dry mouth being most frequent as typical opioid-related side effects. Local side effects have been reported for rectal application as well as for subcutaneous and transdermal administration, with erythema and pruritus being most frequent.[24]

As new forms of opioid delivery have become available, cost has become an increasing factor. Transdermal preparations of fentanyl citrate, for example, provide stable blood levels in most patients but at far greater cost than slow-release forms (either oral or rectal) of morphine or oxycodone. Similarly, oral transmucosal fentanyl citrate has been shown to be highly effective for breakthrough pain in alert patients but again at far greater cost than other alternatives. Often pharmacy colleagues can be helpful not only in creatively shaping an approach that is well suited to an individual patient's circumstances but also in choosing the most cost-effective approach if there is more than one clinically suitable alternative.

UNDESIRABLE EFFECTS

As discussed in detail elsewhere (see Chapter 60), optimal use of opioids requires careful attention to identifying and treating their undesirable effects and to preventing their occurrence whenever possible. Because the beneficial effects of the opioid can sometimes be adequately achieved at a lower dose, that should always be considered first. Opioid rotation can also be helpful.[25] Other alternatives include using localized routes of administration (e.g., spinal) that do not generate such high circulating drug levels; using nonopioid analgesics, either as adjuvants that allow reduction in the opioid dose or as substitutes; continuing the opioid while adding pharmacologic agents that counteract the undesirable effect(s); and nonpharmacologic approaches (see Chapters 58, 60, and 62).

Common opioid effects that will be addressed briefly here include constipation, nausea, vomiting, sedation, and delirium. For all of these except constipation, tolerance may develop, and patients should be counseled that even if the undesirable effects are significant with initial doses, a trial of at least a few days may be warranted before deciding that an alternative medication should be used or that the dose of the opioid can be reduced. In the meantime, symptoms should be monitored closely and vigorously treated.

Constipation is a predictable effect of chronic opioid use. In the palliative care setting, where patients frequently have markedly reduced levels of physical activity and other serious comorbidities, it is even more significant and can become a cause of significant abdominal discomfort. A proactive bowel regimen designed to prevent constipation, with daily monitoring of its effectiveness, is a mandatory component of chronic opioid therapy in this setting. Bulk-forming agents should generally be avoided unless the patient is physically active because an increase in the volume of stool can pose difficulties for bed-bound patients.

Nausea and vomiting caused by opioids is typically mediated by the chemoreceptor trigger zone or stimulation of the vestibular apparatus.[26] An opioid-related decrease in intestinal peristalsis may also be the culprit. Dopamine antagonists (e.g., prochlorperazine) or anticholinergics (e.g., scopolamine) may be helpful in most situations, and $5HT_3$ antagonists (e.g., ondansetron) may be helpful in more refractory cases. If vertiginous symptoms are noted, an antihistamine may be useful, and a prokinetic agent (e.g., metoclopramide) should be considered in patients with ongoing constipation and nausea or vomiting. If tolerance to these adverse effects does not develop and therapy is ineffective, opioid rotation may be tried.[25] It is important to keep in mind, however, that many palliative care patients have illnesses or are taking other medications that may themselves be the cause of the nausea or vomiting, and the opioid may be only partially to blame or may even be an entirely innocent bystander.

Delirium is a common problem for patients in the terminal setting, with estimated prevalence rates ranging from 25% to 85%.[27-34] Many of these patients are receiving opioids, but even when administration of the opioid is the precipitating factor, the cause is frequently multifactorial,[35] including the contributing factors indicated in **Table 57-2**.

Delirium can take both agitated and nonagitated forms,[36] with the latter more frequently unrecognized. When the delirious state is clearly distressing to the patient, its evaluation and treatment should have the same urgency as that of uncontrolled pain. In some cases, however, it is unclear whether or not the delirious patient is suffering from his or her loss of mental clarity, and some near-death experiences that many would categorize as delirious are reported by patients as extremely peaceful, reassuring, and pleasant.[27,37] Nonetheless, even when the patient is not clearly suffering, the delirious state interferes with his or her ability to have meaningful interactions with loved ones, and it thus warrants close attention.

TABLE 57-2 Risk Factors for Delirium in Terminal Illness

Risk Factors
Impending death
Advanced age
Severity of illness
Limitations on physical mobility
Social isolation
Reduced sensory acuity (vision, hearing)
Underlying neurologic degeneration or injury
Seizures
Brain tumors, abscesses, hemorrhages
Fever or hypothermia
Hypoxia
Severe anemia
Infection
Dehydration
Metabolic imbalances
Low serum albumin
Polypharmacy
Drug withdrawal (e.g., benzodiazepines, alcohol, opiates)
Medications
Opiates (especially meperidine and anileridine)
Anticholinergic agents (e.g., antihistamines)
Corticosteroids
Antiemetics
Psychostimulants
Sedative-hypnotics
Drugs of abuse (including alcohol)

Adapted from Schuster JL. Delirium, confusion, and agitation at the end of life. *J Palliat Med.* 1998;1:177 and Harris D. Delirium in advanced disease. *Postgrad Med J.* 2007;83(982):525.

Because some forms of delirium do not manifest themselves with obvious behavioral abnormalities, it is important to screen all patients at risk, which includes virtually all patients receiving opioids in the terminal phase of illness. The simplest and most commonly used assessment tool is the Mini-Mental State Exam.[38] When evidence of delirium is detected, a comprehensive evaluation of potentially contributing factors is warranted, with efforts to treat the underlying cause(s) whenever the benefits of doing so would outweigh the burdens from the patient's perspective. Although delirium in the terminal care setting may not be reversible in the majority of cases, some authors estimate that up to 33% of cases are.[27,30,32,39,40]

Changing the opioid can be useful.[39] In addition, a variety of pharmacologic agents can be used to treat delirium, and nonpharmacologic approaches can also be useful.[27,41] Haloperidol has generally been considered the drug of choice and has been shown superior to lorazepam and chlorpromazine in a double-blind, controlled study of the treatment of delirium in hospitalized patients with AIDS.[42] In one small series, all four patients who developed delirium while taking an opioid improved after being switched to an alternative opioid supplemented by haloperidol.[43] An alternative agent that may be considered is methotrimeprazine.[44] In some cases of agitated delirium, only sedation is effective.[45–48] If benzodiazepines are used for this purpose, close monitoring for a paradoxical increase in agitation (attributed to the disinhibiting effects of benzodiazepines) is warranted.[27]

Sedation is an effect of opioids that can be either desirable or undesirable in the palliative care setting. If the latter and if dose reduction is not possible without a return of unacceptable symptoms, a psychostimulant such as methylphenidate, caffeine, or amphetamine should be tried unless there is a specific contraindication.[49–51]

Finally, if other efforts to address undesirable side effects have been unsuccessful, careful titration of an extremely low dose of an opioid antagonist (e.g., naloxone via continuous intravenous administration or repeated parenteral boluses of nalmefene, essentially a long-acting form of naloxone) may be a viable option. There is evidence to suggest that opioid antagonists, in extremely low doses, may exhibit the potential to increase analgesia, diminish side effects, and diminish tolerance.[52] The use of larger, conventional bolus doses of an opioid antagonist to attempt to reverse opioid side effects is usually ill-advised in the palliative care setting because of the substantial risk of precipitating recurrent pain or even a withdrawal syndrome.[12,53,54]

OPIOIDS AND RENAL INSUFFICIENCY

In the terminal phase of end-of-life care, end-organ insufficiency is common. There is no clear, prospective evidence for the safe use of any opioid in patients with renal impairment, so all opioids should be used with a degree of caution. It also remains unclear from direct evidence at what level of renal impairment caution is needed. Given the lack of relevant clinical data, stratification of risk needs to be based largely on the activity of metabolites and the potential of the metabolite to accumulate. There is clear evidence for the activity of morphine metabolites and their accumulation in renal impairment. Assumptions are made for a similar potential for toxicity with diamorphine and codeine because the same metabolic pathways are involved.[55]

Clinical experience and some published retrospective data suggest that hydromorphone and tramadol may be safer than morphine in patients with renal impairment. Opioids for which there are thought to be no clinically significant metabolites include fentanyl, alfentanil, and methadone. Adjuvant analgesic medications, appropriately adjusted for renal impairment as needed, should still be used to maximize the control of cancer pain. Opioids remain the key to relieving cancer pain, and the presence of renal failure should not be allowed to delay the appropriate use of an opioid analgesic.[55]

ADDITIONAL SPECIAL ISSUES IN THE TERMINAL PHASE

The management of other symptoms in the palliative care setting is beyond the scope of this text and is well covered in other sources.[56,57] A few remaining issues are covered in this section.

IDENTIFICATION AND TREATMENT OF THE UNDERLYING ETIOLOGY OF PAIN

A cardinal principle of pain management is that an accurate delineation of the pathophysiology of a particular pain syndrome is crucial to the formulation of an optimal plan of management. Although this is more often than not true in the palliative care setting as well, there are clear exceptions, especially in the latter phases of illness. The burdens of diagnostic assessments, including the amount of time spent undergoing them when life expectancy may be measured in days or even hours, may outweigh the sometimes small incremental benefits of more precise pathophysiologic understanding and resulting targeting of analgesic therapies. As always, however, the balancing of burdens and benefits, from the patient's perspective, of attempting more precise definitions of the etiology of a pain syndrome depends on an assessment of the relative priorities of various goals of care.

SYMPTOM ASSESSMENT IN PATIENTS WITH REDUCED LEVELS OF CONSCIOUSNESS

Assessing the adequacy of analgesia in a patient with a reduced level of consciousness can be exceedingly difficult. If increased alertness is either not an important goal or has become impossible to attain (at least without unacceptable symptoms), then even ambiguous signs of discomfort should usually be treated. At the same time, a patient who is actively dying may groan or grunt in ways that cause clinical staff, and especially family members, to have concern that he or she is in pain. Although it is not possible to know with certainty what an incommunicative patient is experiencing, some clues may be useful. Signs of possible discomfort that are accompanied by increases in respiratory rate or heart rate should be taken more seriously. If physical stimulation of the patient elicits signs of discomfort, either during bathing or by deliberate, gentle administration of a noxious stimulus, then increased analgesia may be warranted. Tachypnea by itself may not be a sign of discomfort, especially if it occurs in the setting of metabolic acidosis with respiratory compensation because even conscious patients in those situations infrequently report a sense of dyspnea. Nonetheless, prolonged respiratory rates over 20 breaths/min can be uncomfortable because of muscle fatigue, and it is reasonable to consider treatment.

In the subpopulation of palliative care patients with dementia, the Pain Assessment in Advanced Dementia Scale (PAINAD) (**Table 57-3**) has been endorsed for use by the American Medical Directors Association. Although it is not a definitive tool, it is a useful agent when used in conjunction with other methods of assessment (e.g., family and staff reports, results of analgesic trials, and behavioral changes).[58,59]

NUTRITION AND HYDRATION

Artificial nutrition and hydration (ANH) were originally developed to provide short-term support for patients who were acutely ill. When used in patients near the end of life, the available data suggest that these measures are seldom effective in preventing suffering or prolonging life. Patients with advanced, life-limiting illness often lack interest in foods and fluids, and most ultimately lose the capacity to eat and drink. Ethical issues may arise when patients, families, or caregivers request ANH even if there is no prospect of recovery from the underlying illness.

The American Academy of Hospice and Palliative Medicine's (AAHPM's) approved position statement[60] suggests the following key elements in this situation:

1. Recognize that ANH is a form of medical therapy that, similar to other medical interventions, should be evaluated by weighing its benefits and burdens in light of the patient's goals of care and clinical circumstances.
2. Acknowledge that ANH, similar to other medical interventions, can ethically be withheld or withdrawn, consistent with the patient's wishes and the clinical situation.
3. Establish open communication among patients, families, and caregivers to assure that their concerns are heard and that the natural history of advanced illness is clarified.
4. Respect patients' preferences for treatment after the prognosis and anticipated trajectory with and without ANH have been explained.

PALLIATIVE SEDATION

Palliative care seeks to relieve suffering associated with disease. Unfortunately, not all symptoms associated with advanced illness can be controlled with pharmacologic or other interventions. Patients need and

TABLE 57-3 Pain Assessment in Advanced Dementia Scale

	0	1	2	Score
Breathing independent of vocalization	Normal	Occasional labored breathing Short period of hyperventilation	Noisy, labored breathing Long period of hyperventilation Cheyne-Stokes respirations	
Negative vocalization	None	Occasional moan or groan Low-level speech with a negative or disapproving quality	Repeated troubled calling out Loud moaning or groaning Crying	
Facial expression	Smiling or inexpressive	Sad, frightened, frowning	Facial grimacing	
Body language	Relaxed	Tense Distressed pacing Fidgeting	Rigid; fists clenched Knees pulled up Pulling or pushing away Striking out	
Consolability	No need to console	Distracted or reassured by voice or touch	Unable to console, distract, or reassure	
			TOTAL	

Reproduced with permission from Warden V, et al. Development and psychometric evaluation of the Pain Assessment in Advanced Dementia (PAINAD) scale. *J Am Med Dir Assoc*. 2003;4(1):9-15.

ITEM DEFINITIONS

Breathing

1. *Normal breathing* is characterized by effortless, quiet, rhythmic (smooth) respirations.
2. *Occasional labored breathing* is characterized by episodic bursts of harsh, difficult, or wearing respirations.
3. *Short period of hyperventilation* is characterized by intervals of rapid, deep breaths lasting a short period of time.
4. *Noisy labored breathing* is characterized by negative sounding respirations on inspiration or expiration. They may be loud, gurgling, or wheezing. They appear strenuous or wearing.
5. *Long period of hyperventilation* is characterized by an excessive rate and depth of respirations lasting a considerable time.
6. *Cheyne-Stokes respirations* are characterized by rhythmic waxing and waning of breathing from very deep to shallow respirations with periods of apnea (cessation of breathing).

Negative Vocalization

1. *None* is characterized by speech or vocalization that has a neutral or pleasant quality.
2. *Occasional moan or groan* is characterized by mournful or murmuring sounds, wails, or laments. Groaning is characterized by louder than usual inarticulate involuntary sounds, often abruptly beginning and ending.
3. *Low-level speech with a negative or disapproving quality* is characterized by muttering, mumbling, whining, grumbling, or swearing in a low volume with a complaining, sarcastic, or caustic tone.
4. *Repeated troubled calling out* is characterized by phrases or words being used over and over in a tone that suggests anxiety, uneasiness, or distress.
5. *Loud moaning or groaning* is characterized by mournful or murmuring sounds, wails, or laments in much louder than usual volume. Loud groaning is characterized by louder than usual inarticulate involuntary sounds, often abruptly beginning and ending.
6. *Crying* is characterized by an utterance of emotion accompanied by tears. There may be sobbing or quiet weeping.

Facial Expression

1. *Smiling or inexpressive.* Smiling is characterized by upturned corners of the mouth, brightening of the eyes, and a look of pleasure or contentment. Inexpressive refers to a neutral, at ease, relaxed, or blank look.
2. *Sad* is characterized by an unhappy, lonesome, sorrowful, or dejected look. There may be tears in the eyes.
3. *Frightened* is characterized by a look of fear, alarm, or heightened anxiety. The eyes appear wide open.
4. *Frown* is characterized by a downward turn of the corners of the mouth. Increased facial wrinkling in the forehead and around the mouth may appear.
5. *Facial grimacing* is characterized by a distorted, distressed look. The brow is more wrinkled as is the area around the mouth. Eyes may be squeezed shut.

Body Language

1. *Relaxed* is characterized by a calm, restful, mellow appearance. The person seems to be taking it easy.
2. *Tense* is characterized by a strained, apprehensive, or worried appearance. The jaw may be clenched (exclude any contractures).
3. *Distressed pacing* is characterized by activity that seems unsettled. There may be a fearful, worried, or disturbed element present. The rate may be faster or slower.
4. *Fidgeting* is characterized by restless movement. Squirming about or wiggling in the chair may occur. The person might be hitching a chair across the room. Repetitive touching, tugging, or rubbing body parts can also be observed.
5. *Rigid* is characterized by stiffening of the body. The arms or legs are tight and inflexible. The trunk may appear straight and unyielding (exclude any contractures).
6. *Fists clenched* is characterized by tightly closed hands. They may be opened and closed repeatedly or held tightly shut.
7. *Knees pulled up* is characterized by flexing the legs and drawing the knees up toward the chest. This is an overall troubled appearance (exclude any contractures).
8. *Pulling or pushing away* is characterized by resistiveness upon approach or to care. The person is trying to escape by yanking or wrenching him- or herself free or shoving you away.
9. *Striking out* is characterized by hitting, kicking, grabbing, punching, biting, or other form of personal assault.

Consolability

1. No need to console is characterized by a sense of well-being. The person appears content.
2. Distracted or reassured by voice or touch is characterized by a disruption in the behavior when the person is spoken to or touched. The behavior stops during the period of interaction with no indication that the person is at all distressed.
3. Unable to console, distract, or reassure is characterized by the inability to sooth the person or stop a behavior with words or actions. No amount of comforting, verbal or physical, will alleviate the behavior.

Reprinted with permission from Warden V, et al. Development and psychometric evaluation of the Pain Assessment in Advanced Dementia (PAINAD) scale. *J Am Med Dir Assoc*. 2003;4(1):9-15.

deserve assurance that suffering will be effectively addressed because both the fear of severe suffering and the suffering itself add to the burden of terminal illness.

The AAHPM position statement on palliative sedation (PS) states that health care providers serving patients near the end of life have a responsibility to offer sedatives in appropriate circumstances, usually targeted at specific symptoms (ordinary sedation). PS is occasionally necessary to relieve otherwise intractable suffering, with the degree of sedation proportionate to the severity of the target symptom. PS to unconsciousness should only be considered in the rare circumstance that thorough interdisciplinary assessment and treatment of a patient's suffering have not resulted in sufficient relief (or is associated with unacceptable side effects) and when sedation to unconsciousness is needed to meet the patient's goal of relief from suffering. As with all treatment, the use of PS requires informed consent. Treatment of pain and other symptoms should be continued with PS because sedation may decrease the patient's ability to communicate symptoms. PS should not be considered irreversible; reducing the sedation should be considered if clinical evaluation suggests that the symptom status may have changed.[61]

CARING FOR FAMILIES

Although most of this chapter has focused on the needs of patients, the definitions of palliative care with which this chapter began emphasize the needs and concerns of family members as well. In part, this is because family members are often centrally involved in providing important aspects of care to the patient, and providing these caregivers with adequate education, counseling, and other support can be crucial to ensuring that their care is effective. In addition, however, the impact of terminal care extends far beyond the death of the patient, through the memories and adaptations of bereaved loved ones. Family members often remember vividly the last days of their loved one's life, especially whether he or she seemed comfortable. These family perceptions of the patient's dying process can profoundly influence not only their own bereavement course but also how they approach their own deaths. Simple steps on the part of involved clinicians, both during the terminal phase and after the patient's death, can make a significant difference to involved family.[57-66] The effort and skills (or shortcomings therein) that clinicians bring to the care of dying patients and their families thus not only have frequently profound benefits for patients themselves but also are likely to have positive (or negative) repercussions throughout the lives of surviving loved ones.

REFERENCES

1. Doyle D, Hanks G, MacDonald N. Introduction. In: *Oxford Textbook of Palliative Medicine*. 2nd ed. Oxford, England: Oxford University Press; 1998:3-8.
2. Task Force on Palliative Care, Last Acts Campaign, Robert Wood Johnson Foundation. Precepts of palliative care. *J Palliat Med*. 1998;1(2):109.
3. Schonwetter RS. The emergence of palliative care [editorial]. *Cancer Control*. 2001;8(1).
4. Center to Advance Palliative Care. 2011 *Public Opinion Research on Palliative Care: A Report Based on Research by Public Opinion Strategies*. https://www.capc.org/media/filer_public/18/ab/18ab708c-f835-4380-921d-fbf729702e36/2011-public-opinion-research-on-palliative-care.pdf. Last accessed 5 March, 2015.
5. Temel JS, Greer JA, Muzikansky A, et al. Early palliative care for patients with metastatic non–small-cell lung cancer. *N Engl J Med*. 2010;363(8):733-742.
6. Forrow L. The green eggs and ham phenomena. *Hastings Cent Rep*. 1994;24(6 Suppl):S29.
7. Fishman B. The treatment of suffering in patients with cancer pain: cognitive-behavioral approaches. In: Foley K, Bonica J, eds. *Advances in Pain Research and Therapy*. New York: Raven Press; 1990:310-316.
8. Portenoy RK. Pain and quality of life. *Oncology*. 1990;4:172.
9. Cassell E. *The Nature of Suffering and the Goals of Medicine*. New York: Oxford University Press; 1991.
10. Frankl VE. *Man's Search for Meaning*. New York: Washington Square Press; 1984.
11. Foley KM. Clinical tolerance to opioids. In: Basbaum AL, Besson JM, eds. *Towards a New Pharmacotherapy of Pain*. Chichester, England: John Wiley & Sons, Inc; 1991:181-204.
12. Foley KM. Pain and symptom control. In: Curtis JR, Rubenfeld GD, eds. *Managing Death in the Intensive Care Unit*. New York: Oxford University Press; 2001:103-125.
13. Fohr SA. The double effect of pain medication: separating myth from reality. *J Palliat Med*. 1998;1:315.
14. Walsh TD. Opiates and respiratory function in advanced cancer. *Recent Results Cancer Res*. 1984;89:115.
15. Grond S, Zech D, Schug SA, et al. Validation of the World Health Association guidelines for cancer pain relief during the last days and hours of life. *J Pain Symptom Manage*. 1991;6:411.
16. Azoulay D, Jacobs JM, Cialic R, et al. Opioids, survival, and advanced cancer in the hospice setting. *J Am Med Dir Assoc*. 2011;12(2):129-134.
17. Twycross RG. Ethical and clinical aspects of pain treatment in cancer patients. *Acta Anaesthesiol Scand Suppl*. 1982;74:83.
18. Bakker J, Jansen TC, Lima A, Kompanje EJ. Why opioids and sedatives may prolong life rather than hasten death after ventilator withdrawal in critically ill patients. *Am J Hosp Palliat Care*. 2008;25(2):152-154.
19. Portenoy RK, Coyle N. Controversies in the long-term management of analgesic therapy in patients with advanced cancer. *J Pain Symptom Manage*. 1990;5:307.
20. Foley KM. The relationship of pain and symptom management to patient requests for physician-assisted suicide. *J Pain Symptom Manage*. 1991;6:289.
21. Garcia JLA. Double effect. In: Reich WT, ed. *Encyclopedia of Bioethics*. New York: Simon & Schuster; 1995:636–641.
22. Beauchamp TL, Childress JF. *Principles of Biomedical Ethics*. 3rd ed. New York: Oxford University Press; 1989:128.
23. Regnard C, George R, Grogan E, et al. So, farewell then, doctrine of double effect. *BMJ*. 2011;343:d4512.
24. Radbruch L, Trottenberg P, Elsner F, et al. Systematic review of the role of alternative application routes for opioid treatment for moderate to severe cancer pain: an EPCRC opioid guidelines project. *Palliat Med*. 2011;25:57824.
25. Ashby MA, Martin P, Jackson KA. Opioid substitution to reduce adverse effects in cancer pain management. *Med J Aust*. 1999;170:68.
26. Weissman DE. Fast Fact and Concepts #25: Opioids and Nausea. End-of-Life Physician Education Resource Center; October 2000. http://www.eperc.mcw.edu
27. Shuster JL. Delirium, confusion, and agitation at the end of life. *J Palliat Med*. 1998;1:177.
28. Massie MJ, Holland J, Glass E. Delirium in terminally ill cancer patients. *Am J Psychiatry*. 1983;140:1048.
29. Bruera E, Chadwick S, Weinlick A, MacDonald N. Delirium and severe sedation in patients with terminal cancer. *Cancer Treat Rep*. 1987;71:787.
30. Goodman RM, Goodman H, Gray G, et al. Reversible, narcotic-associated mental status impairment in patients with metastatic cancer. *Pharmacology*. 1987;35:47.
31. Fainsinger R, MacEachern T, Hanson J, et al. Symptom control during the last week of life on a palliative care unit. *J Palliat Care*. 1991;7:5.
32. Bruera E, Miller L, McCallion J, et al. Cognitive failure in patients with terminal cancer: a prospective study. *J Pain Symptom Manage*. 1992;7:192.
33. Minogawa H, Uchitomi Y, Yamawaki S, Ishitani K. Psychiatric morbidity in terminally ill cancer patients: a prospective study. *Cancer*. 1996;78:1131.
34. Conill C, Verger E, Henriquez I, et al. Symptom prevalence in the last week of life. *J Pain Symptom Manage*. 1997;14:328.

35. Caraceni A, Martini C, De Conno F, Ventafridda V. Organic brain syndromes and opioid administration for cancer pain. *J Pain Symptom Manage.* 1994;9:527.

36. Lipowski ZJ. *Delirium: Acute Confusional States.* New York: Oxford University Press; 1990.

37. Callanan M, Kelley P. *Final Gifts: Understanding the Special Awareness, Needs, and Communications of the Dying.* New York: Bantam Books; 1992.

38. Folstein MF, Folstein SE, McHugh PR. Mini-Mental State: a practical method of grading the cognitive state of patients for the clinician. *J Psychiatr Res.* 1975;12:189.

39. Maddocks I, Somogyi A, Abbott F, et al. Attenuation of morphine-induced delirium in palliative care by substitution with infusion of oxycodone. *J Pain Symptom Manage.* 1996:182.

40. de Stoutz ND, Tapper M, Fainsinger RL. Reversible delirium in terminally ill patients. *J Pain Symptom Manage.* 1995;10:249.

41. Breitbart W, Chochinov HM, Passik S. Psychiatric aspects of palliative care. In: Doyle D, Hanks GWC, MacDonald N, eds. *Oxford Textbook of Palliative Medicine.* 2nd ed. Oxford, England: Oxford University Press; 1998:933-954.

42. Breitbart W, Marotta R, Platt MM, et al. A double-blind trial of haloperidol, chlorpromazine, and lorazepam in the treatment of delirium in hospitalized AIDS patients. *Am J Psychiatry.* 1996;153:231.

43. Bruera E, Schoeller T, Montejo G. Organic hallucinosis in patients receiving high doses of opiates for cancer pain. *Pain.* 1992;48:397.

44. Foley KM. Management of cancer pain. In: DeVita VT, Hellman S, Rosenberg SA, eds. *Cancer Principles and Practice of Oncology.* 3rd ed. Philadelphia: JB Lippincott; 1997:2807-2841.

45. Mercadante S, De Conno F, Ripamonti C. Propofol in terminal care. *J Pain Symptom Manage.* 1995;10:639.

46. Moyle J. The use of propofol in palliative medicine. *J Pain Symptom Manage.* 1995;10:643.

47. Truog RD, Berde CB, Mitchell C, Grier HE. Barbiturates in the care of the terminally ill. *N Engl J Med.* 1992;327:1678.

48. Cherny NI, Portenoy RK. Sedation in the management of refractory symptoms: guidelines for evaluation and treatment. *J Palliat Care.* 1994;10:31.

49. Bruera E, Chadwick S, Brenneis C, Hanson J. Methylphenidate associated with narcotics in the treatment of cancer pain. *Cancer Treat Rep.* 1987;71:67.

50. Forrest WH, Brown BW, Brown CR, et al. Dextroamphetamine with morphine for treatment of postoperative pain. *N Engl J Med.* 1977;296:712.

51. Laska EM, Sunshine A, Mueller F, et al. Caffeine as an analgesic adjuvant. *JAMA.* 1984;251:1711.

52. Crain SM, Shen KF. Antagonists of excitatory opioid receptor functions enhance morphine's analgesic potency and attenuate opioid tolerance/dependence liability. *Pain.* 2000;84:121.

53. Fins JJ. Acts of omission and commission in pain management: the ethics of naloxone use. *J Pain Symptom Manage.* 1991;17:1210.

54. Manfredi PL, Ribeiro S, Chandler SW, Payne R. Inappropriate use of naloxone in cancer patients with pain. *J Pain Symptom Manage.* 1996;11:131.

55. King S, Forbes K, Hanks GW et al. A systematic review of the use of opioid medication for those with moderate to severe cancer pain and renal impairment: a European Palliative Care Research Collaborative opioid guidelines project *Palliat Med.* 2011;25:525.

56. Doyle D, Hanks GWC, MacDonald N. *Oxford Textbook of Palliative Medicine.* 2nd ed. Oxford, England: Oxford University Press; 1998.

57. Wrede-Seaman L. *Symptom Management Algorithms. A Handbook for Palliative Care.* 2nd ed. Yakima, WA: Intellicard; 1999. http://www.intelli-card.com.

58. Warden V, et al. Development and psychometric evaluation of the Pain Assessment in Advanced Dementia (PAINAD) scale. *J Am Med Dir Assoc.* 2003;4(1):9-15.

59. Horgas A, Miller L. Pain assessment in people with dementia. *Am J Nurs.* 2008;108(7):62-70.

60. AAHPM Position Statement on Artificial Hydration and Nutrition Near the End of Life; December 2006. http://www.aahpm.org/positions/default/nutrition.html

61. AAHPM Position Statement on Palliative Sedation; September 2006. http://www.aahpm.org/positions/default/sedation.html

62. Tilden V, Tolle S, Garland M, Nelson CA. Decisions about life-sustaining treatment. Impact of physicians' behaviors on the family. *Arch Intern Med.* 1995;155:633.

63. Schulz R, Beach SR, Lind B, et al. Involvement in caregiving and adjustment to death of a spouse: findings from the caregiver health effects study. *JAMA.* 2001;285:3123.

64. Billings JA, Kolton E. Family satisfaction and bereavement care following death in the hospital. *J Palliat Med.* 1999;2:33.

65. Casarett D, Kutner JS, Abrahm J, et al. Life after death: a practical approach to grief and bereavement. *Ann Intern Med.* 2001;134:208.

66. Prigerson HG, Jacobs SC. Caring for bereaved patients. *JAMA.* 2001;286:1369.

Pain in HIV and AIDS

Daniel B. Carr
Preeti Gandhi

RECOVERING FROM A PUBLIC HEALTH CATASTROPHE

The older of the coauthors (DBC) was a medical trainee when five previously healthy young men in Los Angeles were reported to have developed an unusual pneumonia caused by *Pneumocystis carinii* (now termed *Pneumocystis jiroveci*), which was fatal in two. Reported in the June 5, 1981, issue of the Centers for Disease Control and Prevention's (CDC's) *Morbidity and Mortality Weekly Reports*, these are now taken as the index cases of acquired immune deficiency syndrome (AIDS), a worldwide epidemic unequalled in human history. Several years later, after the causative agent was identified as human immunodeficiency virus-1 (HIV-1), banked serologic specimens from a handful of isolated earlier cases of undiagnosed catastrophic acute illness retroactively tested positive for the same agent. However, 1981 is the reference date for the current catastrophe, subsequent voluminous epidemiologic analyses, and recent (2011) reflections on AIDS reaching age 30 years.[1]

More than any other painful condition, HIV/AIDS exemplifies the public health perspective on disease as a population-based interaction among environment, pathogen, and host, as well as the World Health Organization's (WHO's) model of the social determinants of health. When author DBC helped convene a 1994 French–U.S. conference on pain in HIV/AIDS,[2] the modern era of highly active antiretroviral therapy (HAART), also termed combination antiretroviral therapy (cART), was still 2 years away. HIV was then for the most part a rapidly progressive condition without a cure whose sufferers were at risk for a range of secondary infections and cancers along with metabolic disturbances contributing to wasting in the relatively short interval before their deaths. Research on and discussions of pain assessment and treatment in HIV/AIDS often emerged from palliative care services, as did Dr. Lefkowitz's chapter on this topic in the prior edition of this textbook.[3] By 2002, when DBC was next involved in preparing a comprehensive review of pain in HIV/AIDS, it was clear that "[t]here is now a striking disparity between developed and developing nations in the epidemiology and natural history of HIV/AIDS."[4] Whereas those treated with cART in prosperous settings had life expectancies approaching those of HIV-negative individuals,[5] those at the margins of prosperous society and virtually the entire developing world were unable to access effective preventive or maintenance therapies.

Thus, at present, we may be in the third phase of the HIV/AIDS story. The first phase was its explosive entrance worldwide as a fulminant fatal disease. The availability of cART heralded a second phase in prosperous Western nations. HIV/AIDS was transformed into a chronic disease with only a modest effect on life expectancy, particularly as drug therapy has become progressively more effective, less toxic, and easier to adhere to by virtue of once-daily oral formulations.[6,7] Yet during this second phase, developing countries were left behind in what truly seemed like a hopeless pandemic. We are now in a third phase in which the demographics of HIV infection in the developed Western countries are changing (see later discussion) and prospects of a cure worldwide are coming into focus thanks to an unprecedented collaboration involving communities of patients, researchers, policymakers, and public health workers. "In fact, new modelling by UNAIDS [Joint United Nations Programme on HIV/AIDS] suggests that actions taken in the next five to eight years will determine whether we can end the AIDS epidemic by 2030."[6]

This chapter briefly presents the demographics of HIV/AIDS as they have evolved in the United States since the epidemic began using data and graphical figures provided by the CDC. This discussion should help clinicians to understand how these changes are likely to impact clinical practice. **Box 58-1** is a "snapshot" of the epidemiology of HIV/AIDS using current data (often such "big data" require several years to release owing to the time required to gather and validate it).

Next, we will survey the common clinical presentations of pain and pain syndromes identified in HIV/AIDS. We shall next draw connections between the pathophysiology of pain, particularly the characteristic distal symmetric polyneuropathy (DSP, also called HIV-associated sensory neuropathy [HIV-SN]), and efforts to base clinical treatment on a strong evidentiary basis. After presenting the relatively meager evidence for a variety of drug, nondrug, and integrative pain therapies, we will describe a basic approach to the assessment and management of pain and related processes (e.g., leukoencephalopathy) in this often challenging population. Finally, we will end on a hopeful note concerning how the HIV/AIDS epidemic may be brought under control worldwide. Bear in mind, however, that even if that goal is achieved, the use of cART itself contributes to HIV-SN through mitochondrial toxicity,[8,9] and therefore pain treatment will continue to be an essential component of comprehensive HIV/AIDS care in the future.[10,11] For clarity, we remind readers that AIDS is defined as stage 3 of HIV disease according to modifications in the case definition introduced by the CDC in 2008 (**Table 58-1**). This definition refers to AIDS-defining conditions that are presented in **Table 58-2**.

BOX 58-1 U.S. HIV/AIDS Epidemic at a Glance

- 600,000 deaths since first recognized in 1981
- 1.2 million Americans HIV positive in 2008, up 71,000 from 2006
- 20% overall (and 60% in the 13- to 24-year-old age group) are unaware they are HIV positive
- Each year 50,000 newly infected with and 15,000 die of HIV
- Longer survival since cART availability (1996): half of the HIV-positive population in United States is older than 50 years
- Other group of concern: at-risk young men (IDU, MSM) unaware of HIV status
- Currently, declining sense of public urgency
- Prevalence of pain (55%–90%) little changed since advent of cART

cART, combination antiretroviral therapy; IDU, intravenous drug use; MSM, men who have sex with men.

Source: CDC.

TABLE 58-1 Stages of HIV Infection

HIV infection, stage 1
• No AIDS-defining condition* and either a CD4 count of ≥500 cells/μL or a CD4 percentage of total lymphocytes of ≥29
HIV infection, stage 2
• No AIDS-defining condition and either a CD4 count of 200–499 cells/μL or a CD4 percentage of total lymphocytes of 14–28
HIV infection, stage 3 (i.e., AIDS)
• Documentation of an AIDS-defining condition or either a CD4 count of <200 cells/μL or a CD4 percentage of total lymphocytes of <14 • Documentation of an AIDS-defining condition supersedes a CD4 count or percentage that would not, by itself, be the basis for a stage 3 (AIDS) classification
HIV infection, stage unknown
• No reported information on AIDS-defining conditions and no information available on CD4 count or percentage

*An AIDS-defining condition (see Table 58-2) is one of more than two dozen infections or malignancies that are indicative of an acquired deficit in cell-mediated immunity.

Source: Centers for Disease Control and Prevention.

TABLE 58-2 AIDS-Defining Conditions

- Bacterial infections, multiple or recurrent*
- Candidiasis of the bronchi, trachea, or lungs
- Candidiasis of the esophagus†
- Cervical cancer, invasive§
- Coccidioidomycosis, disseminated or extrapulmonary
- Cryptococcosis, extrapulmonary
- Cryptosporidiosis, chronic intestinal (>1 month's duration)
- Cytomegalovirus disease (other than liver, spleen, or nodes), onset at age >1 month
- Cytomegalovirus retinitis (with loss of vision)†
- Encephalopathy, HIV related
- Herpes simplex: chronic ulcers (>1 month's duration) or bronchitis, pneumonitis, or esophagitis (onset at age >1 month)
- Histoplasmosis, disseminated or extrapulmonary
- Isosporiasis, chronic intestinal (>1 month's duration)
- Kaposi's sarcoma†
- Lymphoid interstitial pneumonia or pulmonary lymphoid hyperplasia complex*,†
- Lymphoma, Burkitt (or equivalent term)
- Lymphoma, immunoblastic (or equivalent term)
- Lymphoma, primary, of brain
- *Mycobacterium avium* complex or *Mycobacterium kansasii*, disseminated or extrapulmonary†
- *Mycobacterium tuberculosis* of any site, pulmonary,†,§ disseminated,† or extrapulmonary†
- *Mycobacterium*, other species or unidentified species, disseminated† or extrapulmonary†
- *Pneumocystis jiroveci* (previously termed *Pneumocystis carinii*) pneumonia†
- Pneumonia, recurrent†,§
- Progressive multifocal leukoencephalopathy
- *Salmonella* septicemia, recurrent
- Toxoplasmosis of brain, onset at age >1 month†
- Wasting syndrome attributed to HIV

*Only among children younger than 13 years.

†Condition that might be diagnosed presumptively.

§Only among adults and adolescents older than 13 years.

Source: Centers for Disease Control and Prevention.

WHO GETS HIV/AIDS NOW?

Clinicians should be aware of the changing demographics of HIV/AIDS to maintain suitable vigilance, such as in those age 50 years and older, who constitute an increasing proportion of known and unrecognized HIV-positive persons (see later discussion). The CDC is a source for abundant data on every aspect of HIV/AIDS in the United States and its dependent areas; readers should assume that to avoid repetitive citations, all United States–based data in this chapter derive from the CDC's frequently updated website (http://www.cdc.gov/hiv).

Figure 58-1 depicts the course of diagnoses of AIDS (i.e., stage 3 HIV disease) during most of the course of this epidemic. The CDC points out that "the peak in stage 3 (AIDS) in 1993 can be associated with the expansion of the HIV surveillance case definition implemented in January 1993. The overall declines in stage 3 (AIDS) and deaths of persons with stage 3 (AIDS) are due in part to the success of highly active antiretroviral therapies, introduced in 1996. In recent years, stage 3 (AIDS) classifications and deaths of persons with stage 3 (AIDS) have remained stable."

Although deaths have remained stable in recent years, as shown in **Figure 58-2**, the distribution of HIV infections classified as stage 3 (AIDS) among racial/ethnic groups has changed. The percentage among whites has decreased, "while the percentages among blacks/African Americans and Hispanics/Latinos have increased. Of persons

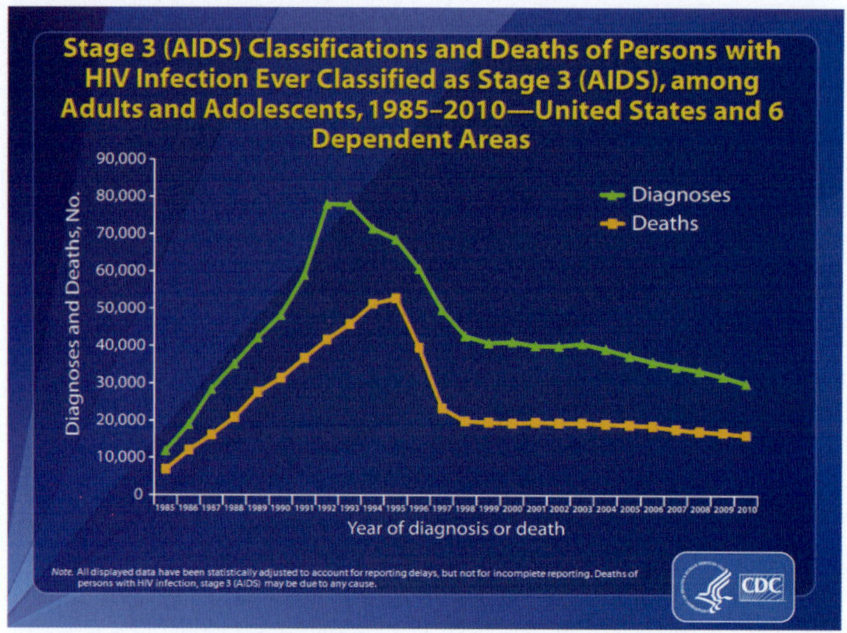

FIGURE 58-1. Stage 3 (AIDS) classifications and deaths of persons with HIV infection ever classified as stage 3 (AIDS) among adults and adolescents, 1985 to 2010—United States and six dependent areas. (From Centers for Disease Control and Prevention. *Slide Sets on HIV/AIDS*. http://www.cdc.gov/hiv/library/slideSets.)

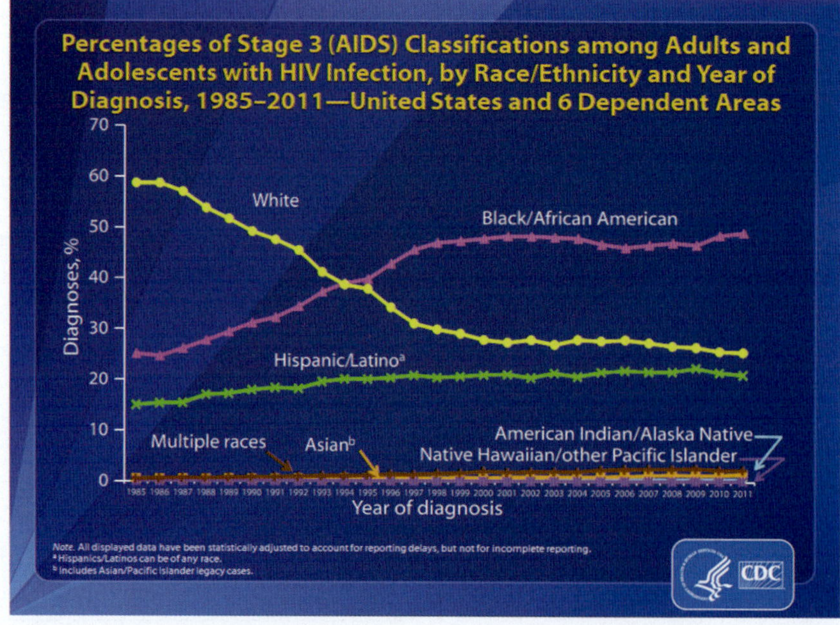

FIGURE 58-2. Percentages of stage 3 (AIDS) classifications among adults and adolescents with HIV infection by race/ethnicity and year of diagnosis, 1985 to 2011—United States and six dependent areas. (From Centers for Disease Control and Prevention. *Slide Sets on HIV/AIDS*. http://www.cdc.gov/hiv/library/slideSets.)

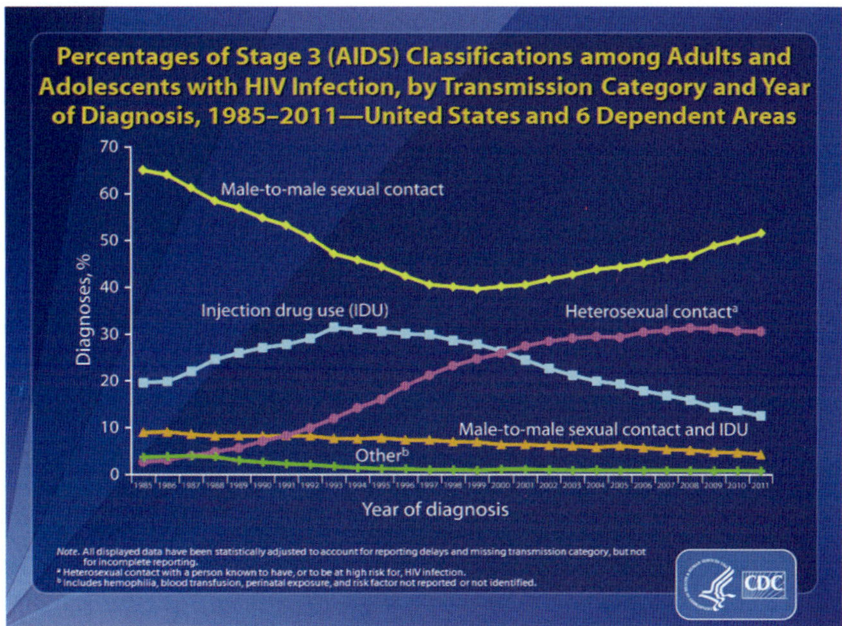

FIGURE 58-3. Percentages of stage 3 (AIDS) classifications among adults and adolescents with HIV infection by transmission category and year of diagnosis, 1985 to 2011—United States and six dependent areas. (From Centers for Disease Control and Prevention. *Slide Sets on HIV/AIDS*. http://www.cdc.gov/hiv/library/slideSets.)

with infection classified as stage 3 (AIDS) in the United States and dependent areas in 2011, 49% were black/African American, 26% were white, 21% were Hispanic/Latino, 2% each were Asian and persons of multiple races, and less than 1% each were American Indian/Alaska Native and Native Hawaiian/other Pacific Islander." Adjusting for the absolute numbers of minority populations, these data indicate an 8-fold greater prevalence of HIV seropositivity in blacks and African Americans and a 2.5-fold greater prevalence in Hispanic and Latinos compared with whites (**Fig. 58-3**).

Of persons with AIDS, the means by which they acquired the HIV-1 virus has shown major shifts over time. During recent years, whereas injection drug use (IDU) has become less prominent as a cause, heterosexual contact has increased (see later discussion). Male-to-male sexual contact remains the most common route of HV transmission. "Other" on this graph refers to hemophilia, blood transfusion, and perinatal exposure. Notably, as the public perception of HIV/AIDS has lost some of its urgency, risk-taking behavior continues, and many persons are unaware that they are HIV positive (**Fig. 58-4**).

In parallel with men with AIDS, the majority (69%) of whom acquired their infection from male-to-male sexual contact, women with AIDS were also most likely (78%) to have acquired HIV infection from men. On a global level, adolescent girls and young women have been

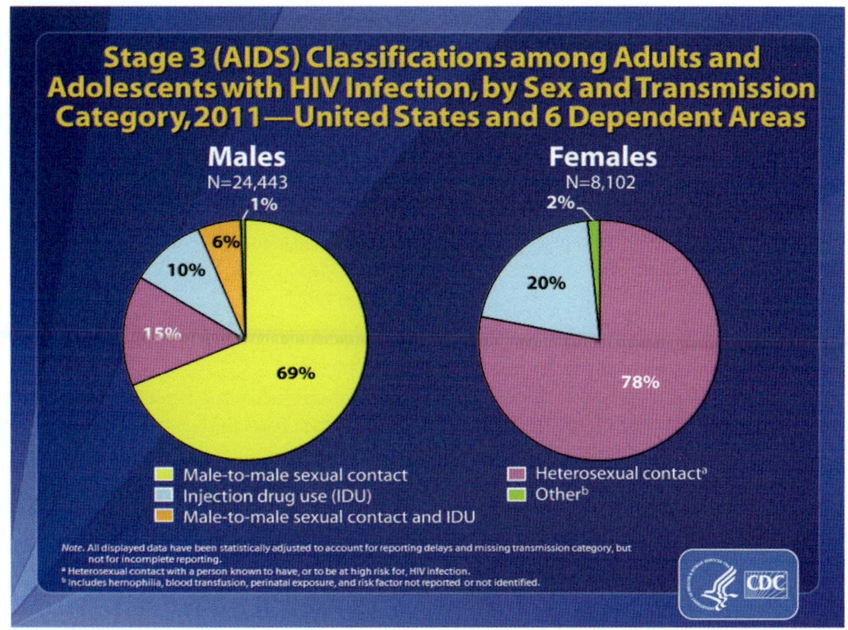

FIGURE 58-4. Stage 3 (AIDS) classifications among adults and adolescents with HIV infection by sex and transmission category, 2011—United States and six dependent areas. (From Centers for Disease Control and Prevention. *Slide Sets on HIV/AIDS*. http://www.cdc.gov/hiv/library/slideSets.)

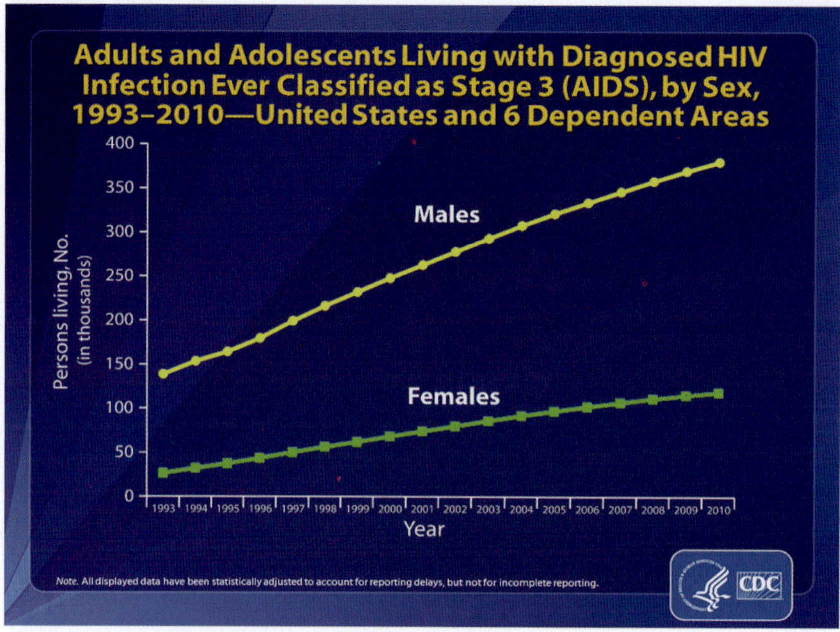

FIGURE 58-5. Adults and adolescents living with diagnosed HIV infection ever classified as stage 3 (AIDS) by sex, 1993 to 2010—United States and six dependent areas. (From Centers for Disease Control and Prevention. *Slide Sets on HIV/AIDS*. http://www.cdc.gov/hiv/library/slideSets.)

identified by UNAIDS as one of 12 groups left behind: "gender-based violence and limited access to healthcare and education, coupled with systems and policies that do not address the needs of young people, are obstacles that block adolescent girls and young women from being able to protect themselves against HIV, particularly as they transition into adulthood"[6] (**Fig. 58-5**).

When originally recognized, AIDS was considered a disease of previously healthy young people. Ongoing improvements in the early diagnosis of HIV disease combined with progressively more effective, less toxic, and more convenient (i.e., once-daily) therapies have led to increasingly longer survival periods. Strikingly, the magazine of the AARP (formerly the American Association of Retired Persons) has declared that "three decades after its emergence, AIDS has a new face: people over 50."[12] This broad statement is confirmed by an in-depth analysis from Massachusetts indicating that "only half of those newly diagnosed individuals over 50 were documented as being aware that they were at risk for HIV."[13] Heterosexual activity represents the largest proportion of HIV acquisition in that state's over-50 population, having increased from 43% to 77%, presumably on the basis of age-related divorce or spousal death, erectile dysfunction medications, and low awareness of HIV risk and prevention methods.[13] It is also true on a global level, with people older than age 50 years identified as one of the groups "left behind" in the 2014 UNAIDS *Gap Report*.[6]

Clinical Presentation of HIV/AIDS and Related Pain The natural history of HIV disease goes through phases. Half or more of persons display an "acute retroviral syndrome" (i.e., a nonspecific viral illness) in the first 6 months after acquiring HIV. A meta-analysis to estimate the sensitivity and specificity of symptoms and signs during that phase for the early diagnosis or ruling out of HIV found "limited clinical utility" of the history and clinical examination for that purpose.[14] Symptoms that increased the likelihood were a history of genital ulcers, weight loss, vomiting, and swollen lymph nodes. The most useful sign was generalized lymphadenopathy. However, none of the symptoms and signs provided strong enough sensitivity and specificity to be recommended for routine use, especially when applied in populations that might be at increased risk for HIV.

After the acute phase, a latent phase of HIV infection may persist for a decade, during which time the patient may be asymptomatic. Reflecting the differing resources available worldwide to treat patients after they are diagnosed as seropositive for HIV, some countries such as the United States initiate long-term cART therapy immediately after seropositivity is established regardless of the CD4 count. Others have policies that delay treatment until CD4 counts fall below a predefined threshold that may be as low as 200 cells/μL in some countries. Yet as CD4 counts decrease in untreated patients, immunodeficiency progresses, and they enter the final phase, during which they may fall victim to a host of AIDS-defining opportunistic infections and malignancies (see Table 58-2). Many of the common pain syndromes, including those associated with AIDS-defining events, were first observed in the pre-cART era (**Table 58-3**).

Reflecting consensus taxonomy,[15] the mechanisms of pain are categorized as nociceptive, neuropathic, inflammatory, or idiopathic and are divided according to location as visceral or somatic (**Box 58-2**).

TABLE 58-3 Common Painful Syndromes in HIV/AIDS First Observed in the Pre–Combination Antiretroviral Therapy Era*

- Abdominal pain
- Peripheral neuropathy
- Throat pain
- HIV-related headaches
- Idiopathic headaches (e.g., tension, migraine)
- AZT-induced headache
- Arthralgia
- Herpes zoster
- Back pain

*AZT, zidovudine.

From Bouhassira D, Lefkowitz M, Meynadier J, Serrie A. Origins of pain in HIV/AIDS. In Carr D, ed. *Pain in HIV/AIDS*. Chicago: France-USA Pain Association; 1994. Reproduced with permission.

BOX 58-2 Operational Taxonomy of HIV/AIDS Pain

- Nociceptive pain: tissue injury signaled through otherwise normal neural pathways
- Neuropathic pain: caused by dysfunction or pathology of peripheral nerves or the central nervous system
- Inflammatory pain: generated or augmented by immune responses; may contribute to nociceptive or neuropathic pain
- Idiopathic pain: occurs without or out of proportion to known organic pathology

Furthermore, pain in HIV/AIDS has been categorized operationally in a similar way as pain caused by cancer: related to the disease, its treatment, or neither, as illustrated in **Table 58-4**.

Long-term treatment from the moment of HIV diagnosis with increasingly effective, less toxic, and more convenient cART medication has become standard practice in the United States and increasingly around the world.[6,7] Accordingly, the CD4 counts of people with HIV disease have remained higher, viral burden lower, quality of life better, and relative importance of secondary sources of nociceptive pain lower. That said, secondary nociceptive sources of pain (**Table 58-5**) remain important in HIV/AIDS and should be diagnosed and removed whenever possible while providing analgesia emphasizing acute-on-chronic pain control, an approach that emphasizes multimodal analgesia using agents (nonsteroidal anti-inflammatory drugs [NSAIDs], acetaminophen, opioids, and local anesthetics all used with care in HIV/AIDS) different from that for neuropathic pain.

Neuropathic Pain in HIV/AIDS From the earliest days of the HIV/AIDS epidemic, even before treatments were available, HIV-SN was evident in about one-third of patients as a frequent source of pain. It presents as a symmetric small-fiber sensory neuropathy in the "stocking" distribution and with reduced or absent ankle-jerk reflexes and lessened vibration sense. Patients may report pain (along with numbness and tingling) in stocking-and-glove distributions. In the pre-cART era, during which deoxynucleoside reverse transcriptase inhibitors (dNRTIs) were the mainstay of therapy, a range of painful neuropathies[4,9] was observed (**Table 58-6**), generally in relation to having more advanced disease (e.g., CD4 count <200 mm³). Other risk factors identified in the pre-cART era included exposure to dNRTIs, older age, and indirect indices of disease progression (e.g., lower weight, hemoglobin, or albumin).

Unfortunately, although the advent of cART has transformed the disease in terms of survival, preserved CD counts, and decreased viral load, it has not decreased the incidence of HIV-SN, primarily DSP. Some studies show an actual rise in the incidence of HIV-SN from pre- to post-cART cohorts.[8-11] Risk factors for HIV-SN in the present cART era include increasing age; greater height; lowest CD4 count and peak viral load (but not current values for either marker); a history of an AIDS-defining illness (see Table 58-2); prior exposure to dNRTIs; and in some studies, race.

The reasons underlying this mild paradox that viral burden can be lowered or suppressed on cART, without an effect on the incidence of HIV-SN, appear several-fold. First, although HIV is a neurotrophic virus, direct injury of neural tissue by HIV is unusual and inadequate by itself to explain most instances of cART-induced HIV-SN. An exception is white matter–associated pathology manifest as mild cognitive dysfunction, particularly in advanced cases of untreated HIV disease,[9] although central nervous system infection by Cryptococcus or tertiary syphilis must be excluded. Much of the neurotoxicity associated with HIV infection is viewed as indirect, resulting from HIV-secreted proteins and inflammatory responses that they trigger. A prime example of the former, implicated in HIV-SN, is the HIV surface glycoprotein gp120.[8,9] This glycoprotein induces neuronal apoptosis directly and activates macrophages that release neurotoxic inflammatory mediators such as tumor necrosis factor-α and interleukin-1. Mitochondrial DNA damage also appears greater in patients with HIV-DSP, providing another mechanism for neuropathy. The observation of greater mitochondrial DNA damage distally than proximally is consistent with patient height being a risk factor for HIV-DSP. HIV-evoked inflammatory responses may be sufficiently robust during an interval of immune reconstitution after the initiation of HIV therapy that "the immune reaction to the antigen may be excessive and pathological" in response to a variety of concurrent infectious agents, an effect first reported in 1992 and termed the "immune reconstitution inflammatory syndrome."[16]

Most important, it is now clear that HIV therapy, from the earlier NRTIs (especially stavudine) to the present cART, leads to antiviral toxic neuropathy that may be synergistically harmful with HIV itself. This insight dictates careful selection of ART in order to minimize

TABLE 58-4 Selected Causes of Pain in Persons with HIV Disease

- Related to HIV/AIDS
  - HIV neuropathy or myelopathy
  - Opportunistic infections
  - Kaposi's sarcoma
- Related to medical care
  - Antiretrovirals (e.g., nucleoside-associated neurotoxicity, pancreatitis)
  - Procedures (biopsies, bronchoscopy)
  - Cancer treatment with radiation, surgery, or chemotherapy
- Unrelated to HIV or its treatment
  - Diabetic neuropathy
  - Tension headache
  - Intervertebral disc disease

Reproduced with permission from Lefkowitz M. Pain in HIV and AIDS. In: Bajwa Z, Warfield CA, eds. *Principles and Practice of Pain Medicine*. 2nd ed. New York: McGraw-Hill; 2004:503-512.

TABLE 58-5 Sources of Nociceptive Pain in HIV/AIDS

- Somatic cutaneous
  - Kaposi's sarcoma
  - Oral cavity pain (e.g., aphthous ulcers, candidiasis)
- Visceral
  - Tumor (e.g., invasive cervical carcinoma)
  - Gastritis
  - Pancreatitis
  - Infection
  - Hepatic and biliary tract disorders
- Deep somatic
  - Rheumatologic (e.g., arthralgia)
  - Back pain
  - Myopathy
- Headache
  - HIV-related (e.g., fungal or bacterial meningitis, encephalitis, neoplasm)
  - HIV-unrelated (e.g., migraine, tension)
  - Iatrogenic (e.g., zidovudine therapy)

Adapted with permission from: Bouhassira D, Lefkowitz M, Meynadier J, Serrie A. Origins of pain in HIV/AIDS. In Carr D, ed. *Pain in HIV/AIDS*. Chicago: France-USA Pain Association; 1994.

TABLE 58-6 Painful Neuropathies by Stage of HIV Infection

- Acute or seroconversion phase
  - Mononeuritides, brachial plexopathy
  - Acute demyelinating polyneuropathy (Guillain-Barré syndrome)
- Latent (asymptomatic) phase (>500 CD4 cells/μL)
  - Acute demyelinating polyneuropathy (Guillain-Barré syndrome)
  - Chronic inflammatory demyelinating polyneuropathy
- Transition phase (200–500 CD4 cells/μL)
  - Herpes zoster (shingles)
  - Mononeuritis multiplex
- Late phase (<200 cells/μL)
  - Predominantly sensory polyneuropathy
  - Autonomic neuropathy
  - Cytomegalovirus polyradiculopathy
  - Mononeuritis multiplex (severe)
  - Mononeuropathies associated with aseptic meningitis
  - Mononeuropathies associated with lymphomatous meningitis
  - Nucleoside (dideoxyinosine, dideoxycytidine) toxicity

Reproduced with permission from: Bouhassira D, Lefkowitz M, Meynadier J, Serrie A. Origins of pain in HIV/AIDS. In Carr D, ed. *Pain in HIV/AIDS*. Chicago: France-USA Pain Association; 1994.

neurotoxicity (e.g., NRTI-sparing regimens) as well as a search for other treatable causes of neuropathy in patients with HIV (e.g., vitamin B_2, B_6, or $B1_2$ or folate deficiency; hypothyroidism; monoclonal gammopathy; lymphoma). When other comorbidities such as diabetes mellitus or alcoholism are present, these must also be addressed and controlled.

Therapies for Pain in HIV/AIDS: Weighing the Evidence Prior reviews of pain control in HIV/AIDS,[3] including several in which the older author participated,[2,4] provided extensive discussions of nondrug, integrative, and drug therapy for pain in HIV/AIDS based on generalization of the WHO's "three-step staircase" for cancer pain relief or previous literature trials evaluating medications for neuropathic pain in patient diagnoses other than HIV. According to the WHO ladder, one begins with a "simple analgesic" such as acetaminophen or an NSAID, adding if necessary an opioid for mild to moderate pain.[28-30] If the latter is not effective, it is switched to an opioid (e.g., morphine) for moderate to severe pain. Adjuvant medications such as anticonvulsants or antidepressants (given to reduce pain or to boost the effects of the other, primary analgesics) may be used at any step of the ladder. As the clinical trial literature has progressed to enroll patients with HIV-SN specifically, however, the results have been discouraging overall (**Table 58-7**).

The apparently negative trials may not all have applied the latest advances and recommendations to ensure the sensitivity of chronic pain clinical trials,[20] particularly those in neuropathic pain.[21] Such recommendations include prestudy stratification of placebo responders, a factor that some have speculated may be important in analgesic trials for HIV/AIDS pain. One potentially important study of duloxetine or methadone individually or given together versus placebo ended inconclusively because of a number of challenges related to patient recruitment and retention.[19,22]

How, then, is the clinician to proceed when the available clinical trial literature suggests few of the available treatments for neuropathic pain have demonstrated their value for HIV-SN? First, we must accept that the variety of etiologies and manifestations of pain in HIV/AIDS, particularly neuropathic pain, may make it unrealistic to hope for a treatment formula that works for the majority or even a plurality of patients at any time. Second, shared decision making, whether with the patient him- or herself or involving significant others if mentation is clouded, is widely accepted to help with formulation of realistic treatment plans and compliance to them. Based on this insight, exploration of patient interest in nondrug therapies, including behavioral therapies, integrative therapies, and traditional drug therapies, should be undertaken and synthesized in a way that considers the patient's social and family setting and living situation.

TABLE 58-7 Controlled Clinical Trials for Painful HIV-Associated Sensory Neuropathy[8,9,17-19]

- Negative results
  - Acetyl-L-carnitine
  - Acupuncture
  - Amitriptyline
  - Capsaicin 0.075%
  - Gabapentin
  - Mexiletine (or amitriptyline)
  - Peptide-T
- Positive results
  - Acupuncture + moxibustion
  - Cannabis (smoked)
  - Capsaicin 8% (one of two trials)
  - Hypnosis
  - Nerve growth factor (recombinant human)
- Inconclusive
  - Duloxetine
  - Methadone

As mentioned, the long-standing WHO method for cancer pain relief has served to anchor prior descriptions of pharmacotherapy for HIV/AIDS, and in the absence of another such framework, it may be taken as the starting point. However, at the outset, there are several important points to emphasize. First, given the prevalence of infections and cancer that coexist with HIV/AIDS, pain relief should always involve a search for an underlying addressable cause for pain ranging from a bacterial abscess, to tuberculous osteomyelitis, to tumor, to mucositis or aphthous ulcers. Concurrent non-HIV infections should always be kept in mind; these include several that involve the liver, such as hepatitis C and cytomegalovirus. Second, in part because of the organ dysfunction just described, great caution must be used in prescribing potentially hepato- or nephrotoxic agents such as acetaminophen or NSAIDs, concerning which little thought is normally given. Third, the pharmacokinetics and pharmacodynamics for many drugs—particularly those metabolized through cytochrome P450 pathways—may be greatly altered in patients with HIV/AIDS and organ dysfunction with or without concurrent infections, both because of such dysfunction and because of many drug–drug interactions involving cART as well as other drugs (e.g., opioids). Ignoring these interactions can undermine the success of cART or raise blood levels of its components to the toxic range. Given how numerous they are, these potential interactions should be evaluated on a case-by-case basis. Drug–drug interactions also should be considered for any folk medicines or traditional Chinese medicines (e.g., herbs) that the patient may be taking. Fourth, the population of patients with HIV/AIDS includes many persons who are intravenous drug users or otherwise have a history of substance abuse or other mental health issues, requiring that opioid analgesia be approached with even greater caution than normally.

With the above in mind, a general approach to the patient with HIV/AIDS and pain is outlined in **Table 58-8**. For specific problems such as pain caused by superficial ulcers, one may use topical agents such as lidocaine impregnated into a gauze to curtail systemic absorption. Other local therapies for oral ulcers include Amlexanox, antibiotic rinse, chlorhexidine, ice chips, and liquid formulation of corticosteroids for oral use. Systemic therapies for recurrent aphthous ulcers include colchicine, dapsone, pentoxifylline, and thalidomide.[23] We refer to other chapters for comprehensive accounts of the history and examination

TABLE 58-8 General Strategies to Control Pain in Patients with HIV/AIDS

- Diagnose and treat any painful syndrome whenever possible.
- Record the pain reported by the patient and monitor function.
- Incorporate nonpharmacologic and integrative approaches early on, guided by patient preferences.
- For pain requiring analgesic drugs:
  - Use noncontrolled substances first.
  - Individualize therapy.
  - Use adequate doses of appropriately potent analgesics but be aware of potential drug interactions, especially with cART.
  - Supplement analgesics with adjuvant analgesics and nonpharmacologic approaches as needed.
  - Prescribe opioids within a consistent, documented framework anchored by an opioid agreement that involves specifics as to how prescriptions will be obtained (frequency, prescriber) and other aspects of care such as ongoing assessment of risk versus benefit, prescription monitoring program participation, and drug testing.
  - Consider alternative routes to oral administration (transdermal, sublingual, intranasal) in the presence of ulcers, malabsorption, diarrhea, or altered stomach acidity.
- Document pain relief and adherence and change treatment as indicated.
- Provide analgesia during diagnosis and treatment of the underlying disease process(es) (e.g., procedures).
- Seek consultants' input when needed (e.g., infectious disease, addiction medicine).

cART, combination antiretroviral therapy.

Modified from Lefkowitz M. Pain in HIV and AIDS. In: Bajwa Z, Warfield CA, eds. *Principles and Practice of Pain Medicine*. 2nd ed. New York: McGraw-Hill; 2004:503-512.

of patients with pain; related morbidities such as depression and their treatment using nondrug and drug therapies; the agents available for neuropathic pain; behavioral and physical measures to improve pain and quality of life; and the complex issues surrounding chronic use of opioids for noncancer pain, particularly in instances of known or suspected substance abuse.

Future Directions for the Epidemic and Its Control As recounted in the introduction, less than a decade ago, the prospects for global recovery from the worst epidemic in recorded history were dim. Yet in the past 5 years, owing to a combination of screening, enhanced access to care, once-daily medications with improved benefit-to-side effect ratios, and aggressive prevention of transmission between adults and from mother to child on a global basis, more and more one hears serious researchers and policymakers speak of the possibility of defeating HIV and AIDS.[24,25] **Box 58-3** summarizes these successes.

Current literature concerning a "cure" for HIV is of two sorts. The first focuses on a tiny handful of index cases such as the Berlin man treated for leukemia with hematopoietic stem cell transplantation and the Mississippi baby born to an HIV-infected mother, treated twice postnatally with ART, and then disease free for long intervals without any further treatment. These individuals may well represent experiments of nature pointing the way toward eradication of HIV on an individual scale.[23]

The second type of cure speaks to the steady reduction of the harmful effects of HIV disease in the populations of nations and also globally, as articulated by UNAIDS: "More than ever before, there is hope that ending AIDS is possible." This hope is embodied in UNAIDS' goals for 2030 of a 90% reduction in each of new HIV infections, stigma and discrimination faced by people with AIDS, and AIDS-related deaths.[6] These goals are achievable if eight global action points, tabulated in **Box 58-4**, are carried out. A corresponding set of high-impact preventive steps tailored to the United States has been prepared by the CDC (**Box 58-5**). Notably, these global action points and domestic high-impact preventive steps do not require development of a vaccine for HIV-1, a goal toward which progress has been very slow.[26] Speaking to the latter, two senior HIV/AIDS scientists have written: "Although it might be possible to control and even end the HIV-AIDS pandemic using existing interventions, in order to reach this goal more quickly and to sustain the success, we believe that a safe and at least moderately effective HIV vaccine is essential."[27] Whether or not a successful vaccine is produced, the natural history of HIV/AIDS may well—after having caused incalculable suffering worldwide and in sub-Saharan Africa, the worst social disaster since slavery—parallel that of other epidemics, from polio to guinea worm, that now are approaching extinction because of laboratory insights applied to prevention and treatment at the community and, ultimately, individual levels.

BOX 58-3 Beginning of the End of the Global AIDS Epidemic

- Fewer new HIV infections: of 82 countries with data sufficient for analysis, 10 had >75% and 27 had >50% declines
- Dramatic progress in stopping HIV infections in children: 58% decrease from 2002 to 2013 (~900,000 new HIV infections averted in children since 2009)
- More people (now almost half) living with HIV know their status and are receiving HIV treatment
- AIDS-related deaths have fallen by 35% since 2005, when deaths peaked
- The number of men who opted for medical male circumcision in priority countries has tripled since 2012

Source: Joint United Nations Programme on HIV/AIDS. *The gap report*. Geneva: Joint United Nations Programme on HIV. AIDS. 2014.

BOX 58-4 Ending the Global AIDS Epidemic: Eight Action Points

1. Protect human rights, embrace the human family, and leave no one behind.
2. Invest in communities.
3. Think big—secure leadership and investments.
4. Focus on local epidemics and populations.
5. Decentralize delivery of HIV services.
6. Expand the choices for HIV prevention and treatment.
7. Integrate HIV programs with other health and development programs.
8. Innovate and invest in science for a cure and vaccine.

Source: Joint United Nations Programme on HIV/AIDS. *The gap report*. Geneva: Joint United Nations Programme on HIV. AIDS. 2014.

BOX 58-5 High-Impact HIV Prevention in the United States

- Testing for HIV
- Antiretroviral therapy
- Condoms, syringes
- Efforts targeting people with HIV-positive partners
- Efforts targeting high-risk groups (e.g., MSM, IDU)
- Substance abuse treatment
- Screening for and treatment of other concurrent diseases (e.g., tuberculosis, hepatitis C)

IDU, injection drug use; MSM, men who have sex with men.

Source: CDC.

REFERENCES

1. Anonymous. The 30 years war: hard pounding is gradually bringing AIDS under control. *Economist*. 2011;399:89-91.
2. Carr D, ed. *Pain in HIV/AIDS*. Chicago: France-USA Pain Association; 1994.
3. Lefkowitz M. Pain in HIV and AIDS. In: Bajwa Z, Warfield CA, eds. *Principles and Practice of Pain Medicine*. 2nd ed. New York: McGraw-Hill; 2004:503-512.
4. Carr DB, Goudas LC. Evaluating and managing pain for patients with HIV/AIDS: an overview. In: Nedeljković SS, ed. *Pain Management, Anesthesia, and HIV/AIDS*. Boston: Butterworth-Heinemann; 2002:119-141.
5. Antiretroviral Therapy Cohort Collaboration. Life expectancy of individuals on combination antiretroviral therapy in high-income countries: a collaborative analysis of 14 cohort studies. *Lancet*. 2008; 372:293-299.
6. Joint United Nations Programme on HIV/AIDS (UNAIDS). *The Gap Report*. (English original, Geneva: UNAIDS, July 2014).
7. Gandhi M, Gandhi RT. Single-pill combination regimens for treatment of HIV-1 infection. *N Engl J Med*. 2014;371:248-258.
8. Schutz SG, Robinson-Papp J. HIV-related neuropathy: current perspectives. *HIV AIDS (Auckl)*. 2013;5:243-251.
9. Phillips TJC, Cherry CL, Moss PJ, Rice ASC. Painful HIV-associated sensory neuropathy. *Pain Clin Updates*. 2010;18:1-8.
10. Miaskowski C, Penko JM, Guzman D, et al. Occurrence and characteristics of chronic pain in a community-based cohort of indigent adults living with HIV infection. *J Pain*. 2011;12:1004-1016.
11. Merlin JS, Cen L, Praestgaard A, et al. Pain and physical and psychological symptoms in ambulatory HIV patients in the current treatment era. *J Pain Symptom Manage*. 2012;43:638-645.

12. Anft M. AIDS at 30. *AARP The Magazine*. 2011;July/August: 66-72.
13. Yates K. *Aging with HIV in Massachusetts: Current Trends in Health Outcomes and Health Services*. Public Health Rounds. Public Health and Professional Degree Programs. Tufts University School of Medicine. 2011;Spring:1-11.
14. Wood E, Kerr T, Rowell G, et al. Does this adult patient have early HIV infection? The rational clinical examination systematic review. *JAMA*. 2014;312:278-285.
15. Eidelman A, Carr DB. Taxonomy of cancer pain. In: de Leon Casasola OA, ed. *Cancer Pain: Pharmacological, Interventional, and Palliative Care Approaches*. Philadelphia: Saunders Elsevier; 2006;3-12.
16. Costello DJ, Gonzalez RG, Frosch MP. Case 18-2011: a 35-year-old woman with headache and altered mental status. *N Engl J Med*. 2011;364:2343-2352.
17. Shlay JC, Chaloner K, Max MB, et al. Acupuncture and amitriptyline for pain due to HIV-related peripheral neuropathy. A randomized controlled trial. *JAMA*. 1998;280:1590-1595.
18. Dorfman D, George MC, Schnur J, et al. Hypnosis for treatment of HIV neuropathic pain: a preliminary report. *Pain Med*. 2013;14:1048-1056.
19. Harrison T, Miyahara S, Lee A, et al. Experience and challenges presented by a multicenter crossover study of combination analgesic therapy for treatment of painful HIV-associated polyneuropathies. *Pain Med*. 2013;14:1039-1047.
20. Dworkin RH, Turk DC, Peirce-Sandner S, et al. Considerations for improving assay sensitivity in chronic pain clinical trials: IMMPACT recommendations. *Pain*. 2012;153:1148-1158.
21. Katz J, Finnerup NB, Dworkin RH. Clinical trial outcome in neuropathic pain. Relationship to study characteristics. *Neurology*. 2008;70:263-272.
22. Walk D, Backonja M. HIV neuropathy pain continues to pose a challenge [editorial]. *Pain Med*. 2013;14:957-958.
23. Fauci AS, Marston HD, Folkers GK. An HIV cure: feasibility, discovery and implementation. *JAMA*. 2014;312:335-336.
24. Farmer PE. Chronic infectious disease and the future of health care delivery. *N Engl J Med*. 2013;369:2424-2436.
25. Mermin J, Fenton JA. The future of HIV prevention in the United States. *JAMA*. 2012;308:347-348.
26. Barouch DH. The quest for an HIV-1 vaccine—moving forward. *N Engl J Med*. 2013;369:2073-2075.
27. Fauci AS, Marston HD. Ending AIDS—is an HIV vaccine necessary? *N Engl J Med*. 2014;370:495-498.
28. Krashin DL, Merrill JO, Trescot AM. Opioids in the management of HIV-related pain. *Pain Physician*. 2012;15(3 Suppl):ES157-ES168.
29. Robinson-Page J, Elliott K, Simpson DM, Morgello S. Problematic prescription opioid use in an HIV-infected cohort. *J Acquir Immune Defic Syndr*. 2012;61:187-193.
30. Wiebe LA, Phillips TJC, Li J-M, et al. Pain in HIV: an evolving epidemic. *J Pain*. 2011;12:619-624.

SECTION D

Pain Associated with Medical Illness

CHAPTER 59

Fibromyalgia

Cristin A. McMurray

Understanding of fibromyalgia syndrome (FMS) has evolved over the past 20 years. Once thought to be related to muscular pain and inflammation, it is now more widely understood to be a largely noninflammatory, soft-tissue pain condition, best separated from the entity of myofascial pain, with which it has traditionally been grouped. FMS also has strong associations with other diseases that are deemed central sensitivity syndromes, suggesting that central sensitization plays an important role in the chronic nature of fibromyalgia.[1] Because of the complexity of the disorder, a multimodal approach has the most success in effectively treating the physical, psychological, and emotional aspects of FMS.

CLINICAL FEATURES

DIAGNOSIS

The hallmarks of FMS are widespread pain, fatigue, sleep disturbances, and cognitive changes, as well as psychological distress. Patients often complain of pain "all over my body." They often report chronic insomnia, either having trouble falling asleep or waking up frequently in the night, leaving them exhausted and stiff in the daytime. They also complain about difficulty with cognition and concentration; the phenomenon of "fibro fog" is frequently mentioned in patient forums and websites. Additionally, patients experience depression; in one study, as many as 40% of patients with FMS were diagnosed with depression at the same time as their FMS was diagnosed.[2] Many features of FMS overlap with other diseases, and, indeed, FMS is often seen in conjunction with other diseases that lack structural pathology, including irritable bowel syndrome (IBS), interstitial cystitis, temporomandibular disorder, tension headache and migraine, chronic fatigue syndrome, posttraumatic stress disorder, and vulvodynia. These disease states all share a common feature of central sensitization and have been named *central sensitivity syndromes* to denote this.[1] Any patient with this broad spectrum of symptoms should be evaluated for FMS.

The diagnosis of FMS is criteria-based rather than a diagnosis of exclusion.[2] The American College of Rheumatology (ACR) developed criteria for FMS research that have been used clinically to diagnose FMS since their publication in 1990.[3] The diagnosis depends on the presence of generalized pain in three or more sites, as well as the physical examination finding of tenderness in at least 11 of 18 defined anatomic locations (**Table 59-1** and **Fig. 59-1**). Patients with FMS have pain with 4 kg of digital pressure; this can be estimated by pressing the examining thumb against the spot in question with enough pressure to blanch the thumbnail about halfway down the nail bed.[2]

Since publication of the ACR criteria, many clinicians have used them but bemoaned the lack of attention given to the other clinically important features of FMS such as fatigue and depression. Multiple other surveys, scales, and questionnaires have been developed to try to follow objectively these very subjective complaints. None has proved universally satisfactory, but consensus in research circles shows relevant aspects of FMS to be pain, fatigue, problems with sleep, diminished global as well as physical functioning, depression, anxiety, and cognitive dysfunction.[4] These domains demonstrate areas that clinicians must investigate and follow in patients with FMS in order to better diagnose the disorder and to assess the results of treatment.

TABLE 59-1 Diagnostic Criteria for Fibromyalgia

Generalized pain in three or more sites for 3 months or longer	
Exclusion of other conditions that may cause similar symptoms	
Reproducible tenderness in 11 of 18 prespecified sites	
Area (Bilateral)	**Site**
Occiput	Suboccipital muscle insertion
Cervical	Anterior aspect of C5–C7
Trapezius	Midpoint of the upper border
Supraspinous muscle	Medial border of the scapular
Second rib	Upper surface of the costochondral junction
Lateral epicondyle	2 cm distal to the epicondyle
Gluteal muscles	Upper outer quadrant of the buttocks
Greater trochanter	Trochanteric prominence
Knee	Medial fat pad

Although FMS is not a diagnosis of exclusion, other causes of reported symptoms should be investigated before concluding that a patient has FMS. FMS occurs frequently as a secondary diagnosis with a host of other rheumatologic diseases such as systemic lupus, rheumatoid arthritis, and Sjögren's syndrome. Conditions such as hypothyroidism, Lyme disease, tuberculosis, and HIV can cause similar findings as well. Conversely, after a patient is diagnosed with FMS, these other disease states can still occur and should not be overlooked.

There is no gold standard of testing for FMS. Rather, the clinician must rely largely on patient history for the diagnosis; there is a relatively minor role for the physical examination. Patients may report hyperalgesia (increased experience of pain to a normally painful stimulus) or allodynia (experience of pain with a nonpainful stimulus). Many clinicians still use the tender point examination, but the importance of this finding in the treatment of FMS is dwindling.

PATHOPHYSIOLOGY

New understanding of central sensitization (discussed elsewhere in this book) has led to useful information in understanding the etiology of FMS. Although the "causes" of FMS have not been discovered, it has proven useful clinically, and with regard to treatment, to view the disorder as one of altered sensory processing. Patients with FMS not only have increased pain with pressure applied to various body parts but also have lower pain thresholds for cold, heat, and electrical stimuli, as well as lower noxious thresholds to auditory stimuli.[4] These findings imply that individuals with FMS experience a biologic amplification of sensory stimuli, which has been likened to an altered "volume control" with respect to their pain and sensory processing. Functional MRI (fMRI) studies of patients with fibromyalgia seem to support this concept. Patients with FMS consistently show increased activity in the so-called "pain matrix" of the primary and secondary somatosensory cortex, the insula, and the anterior cingulate cortex; these areas light up in healthy control participants undergoing painful stimuli, but they light up more often in people with FMS at baseline and light up more actively in people with FMS undergoing pressure stimuli.[4]

There is also a role for peripheral input or nociception. FMS is a soft-tissue pain disease, and many patients report deep aching pain, as well

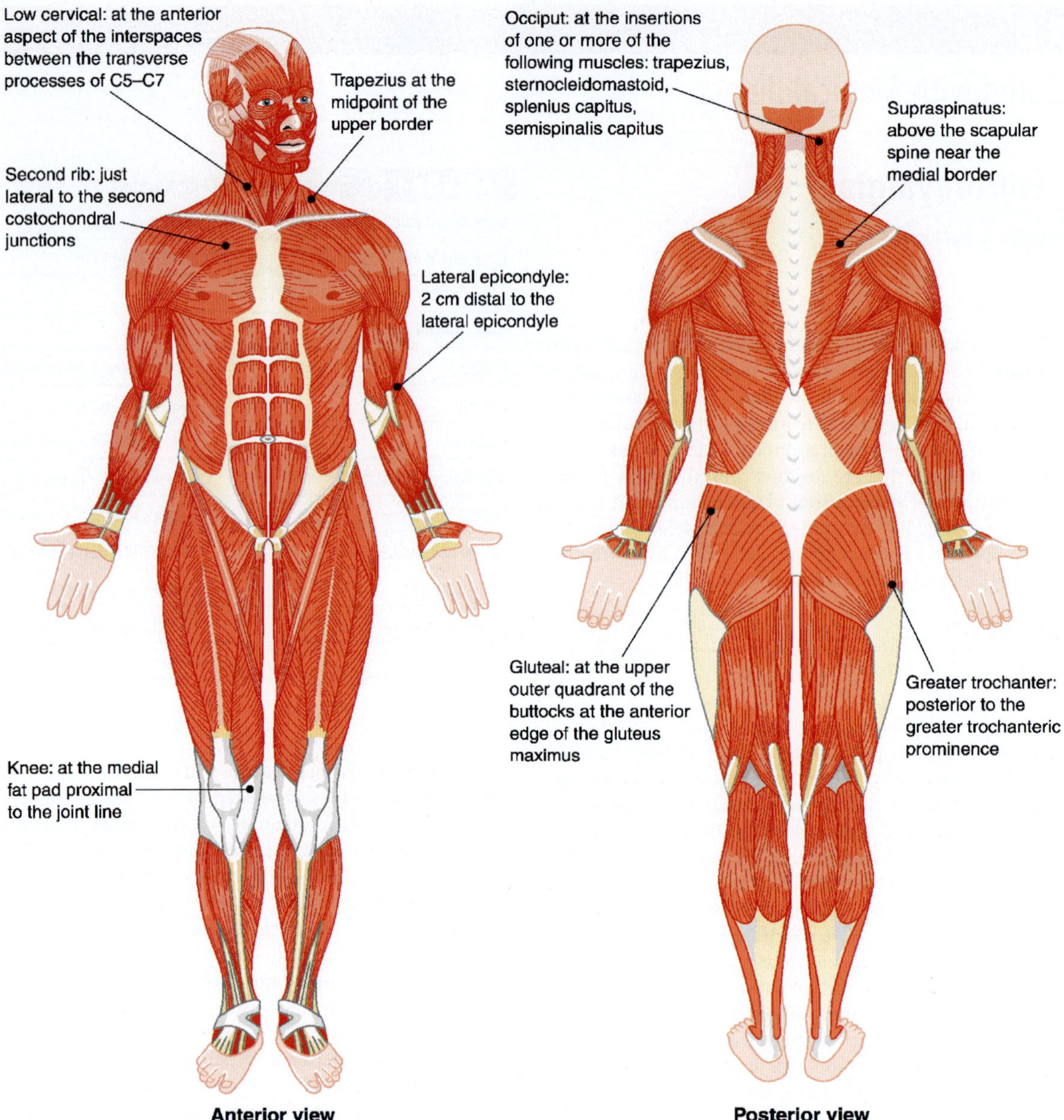

FIGURE 59-1. Typical tender areas in fibromyalgia. Source: Longnecker DE, Brown DL, Newman MF, Zapol WM. *Anesthesiology*: http://www.accessanesthesiology.com.

as increased pain with applied pressure. In attempts to locate structural pathology, multiple muscle biopsy studies of patients with FMS have been done, but none has borne out inherent differences when blinded and matched for inactive normal control participants.[1] Therapeutically, however, trigger point injections into tender muscle spots have had some success in ameliorating FMS pain despite a lack of randomized controlled trials (RCTs).[5] Studies involving lidocaine and saline injection into muscles did show an interesting effect on decreasing heat hyperalgesia at a remote site in patients with FMS, indicating that perhaps there is a role for peripheral input.[6] In some reports, there is a temporal relationship between physical trauma, especially of the trunk, and the development of FMS,[4] implying that potentially some triggering incident provokes the altered processing, a concept widely accepted as the way in which central sensitization occurs.[7] Other stressors such as infections (e.g., hepatitis C, Lyme disease, Epstein-Barr virus), emotional stress, and concomitant diseases (e.g., rheumatoid arthritis, systemic lupus erythematosus) all predispose patients to develop FMS as well.

The role of neurotransmitters and cytokines is less clear, but there are abnormalities in patients with FMS. Cerebrospinal fluid analysis shows higher than normal levels of pronociceptive substances such as substance P,[8] glutamate, and nerve growth factor[9] and low levels of antinociceptive substances such as serotonin, norepinephrine, and dopamine metabolites.[10] The overall effect of these imbalances supports the concept of altered processing of sensory information augmenting pain. Interestingly, the endogenous opioid system in patients with FMS seems increased rather than reduced; some authors suggest that this may explain why opioids often fail to help with the pain of FMS.[4] Many of these findings have pointed in the direction of explaining responses to certain medications and suggest targets for future treatment.

EPIDEMIOLOGY AND PREVALENCE

The symptoms of FMS have a wide overlap with other disease states, making prevalence studies of FMS difficult. However, past studies and present evidence show that women are more likely to be affected than men, with U.S. prevalence rates of 3.4% for women and 0.5% for men and an overall population prevalence of 2%.[11] Patients between 20 and 60 years of age are most likely to have FMS. However, prevalence rates in women are highest between 70 and 79 years of age, with a rate of 7.4%; a smaller peak of 1% occurs in men in their 80s. A 2008 estimate suggested that about 5 million people in the United States are affected by fibromyalgia.[12] These trends are borne out in other surveys, including a 2011 European study that yielded a 2.9% to 4.7% prevalence across Italy, Spain, Portugal, France, and Germany.[13]

A longitudinal Norwegian study showed a 60% to 70% higher risk of FMS in overweight and obese women with body mass indexes of 25 or greater. The risk was greater in overweight women who were also inactive or exercised less than 1 hour per week.[14] Exercise does not exert a wholly protective effect, however, as seen in a 2010 report showing a prevalence of FMS of 2% in competitive athletes.[15]

An interesting review of the health care quality of life impact of FMS showed the impact of FMS on productivity in workers; separated into mild, moderate, and severe symptoms; these individuals with FMS missed an average of 5, 13, and 39 days of work each year, respectively. Caregivers of patients with FMS provided an average of 47, 296, and 460 hours per year of unpaid help with activities of daily living to the mild, moderate, and severe groups of patients, respectively.[16] All of these statistics illustrate the widespread financial, emotional, and physical effects of FMS on patients and their families and communities.

TREATMENT

Recent years have seen Food and Drug Administration (FDA) approval of three medications to treat FMS. Pregabalin, an α_2 ligand and antiepileptic agent, was approved in 2007, followed by duloxetine, a serotonin-norepinephrine reuptake inhibitor (SNRI), in 2008, and milnacipran, also an SNRI, in 2009. Although these have shown great promise, the treatment of FMS must take into account the chronic nature of the disease, including the physiologic and psychological stresses that contribute to its development and perpetuate the disease process. Given the spectrum of symptoms experienced by patients with FMS, there is clearly a role for a strong multidisciplinary approach to successful treatment. A team involving pain medicine physicians, rheumatologists, clinical psychologists, physiatrists, physical therapists, and social workers would be ideal to formulate and carry out a viable and ongoing course of treatment for patients with FMS. Treatment options include pharmacologic management, cognitive-behavioral therapy, exercise, trigger point injections, electrical stimulation, heat application, and massage.

It is important to recall that the mechanism of FMS is altered sensory processing, often triggered or worsened by peripheral input; any other source of pain or discomfort such as degenerative disc disease, cervical or lumbar radiculopathy, dysmenorrhea, temporomandibular disorder, or IBS should also be treated with disease-specific interventions to reduce the impact on FMS symptoms.

Similarly, each of the facets of FMS experienced by a patient should be addressed in developing a treatment strategy. If fatigue is a major symptom presenting in a patient, treatment for that problem must be incorporated into the overall FMS management. Depression often plays a large role in ongoing FMS and must also be assessed and treated if present.

In addition, patient education is extremely important in the treatment of FMS. It is not a disease with a quick fix; successful treatment typically requires major changes in patient lifestyle, exercise, and diet. Clinicians must play a role in helping patients take a crucial active role in their own treatment.

PHARMACOLOGIC MANAGEMENT

ANTIDEPRESSANTS

Alterations in the descending pain inhibitory pathways mediated by serotonin and norepinephrine are thought to play a significant role in the pain of FMS and other central pain states.[17] Antidepressants are widely used in pain medicine, and FMS is no different. Before the creation of SNRIs, tricyclic antidepressants (TCAs) were used to help with neuropathic pain, sleep, and depression. The most used and studied agents have been amitriptyline and cyclobenzaprine. Cyclobenzaprine is a centrally acting muscle relaxant with a chemical structure similar to amitriptyline.[4] A recent study indicated that a low dose of cyclobenzaprine in the evening could decrease fatigue, muscle pain, tenderness, depression, and anxiety, probably through its effects on sleep patterns.[18] The beneficial effects of the TCAs are thought to be attributable to their serotonin and norepinephrine reuptake inhibition; however, the lack of specificity of the medications contributes to the side effects many patients complain about, namely dry mouth and sedation. The sedative side effect may be helpful if the medication is given at bedtime to help with sleep, but daytime use of these drugs is problematic. Starting with low doses of amitriptyline (10 mg) and cyclobenzaprine (5 mg) is advisable to improve patient tolerance and adherence.

Selective serotonin reuptake inhibitors (SSRIs) such as Prozac and Paxil do not seem to be effective for treatment of FMS pain. Duloxetine and milnacipran, both SNRIs, have undergone multicenter, large-scale RCTs demonstrating efficacy in controlling FMS symptoms. Duloxetine has slightly more serotonin reuptake inhibitor selection than norepinephrine; it has been shown to improve pain as well as other global functioning measures in FMS, decrease stiffness, and reduce the number of trigger points.[4,17] Typical dosages are 60 mg one or two times per day. Milnacipran offers slightly more norepinephrine reuptake inhibition activity than serotonin and shows promise in improving fatigue, physical function, and discomfort.[4] Usual effective dosages for milnacipran are 25 to 50 mg twice daily. Side effects of both medications are mild and include nausea, diarrhea, constipation, dry mouth, and anorexia. These usually resolve with continued use.

α_2-δ LIGANDS

The anticonvulsants are thought to raise the threshold for depolarization of pain fibers, much the same way they act centrally to control seizures. The voltage-gated calcium channels mediate some of this activity. Pregabalin, one of three FDA-approved medications for FMS, is a ligand for the α_2-δ subunit of these calcium channels. It has analgesic, anxiolytic, and anticonvulsant properties and reduces the release of pronociceptive neurochemicals such as glutamate and substance P.[19] Studies show improvement in pain, fatigue, and sleep disturbance, as well as improved global measures.[20] Usual effective dosages are 300 to 600 mg/day in two to three divided doses. Side effects such as somnolence and dizziness usually resolve after steady use; many clinicians start at low doses and gradually titrate up to improve tolerance and adherence. Occasionally, weight gain, peripheral edema, or blurry vision occurs but may improve with lower dosing.

Gabapentin is a structurally similar α_2-δ ligand that has shown efficacy in FMS and other neuropathic pain states. It is not FDA approved, but it can be used similarly to pregabalin in treating the symptoms of FMS.

ANALGESICS

Nonsteroidal anti-inflammatory drugs have not shown to be particularly effective in treating the pain of FMS. The role of opioids in treating FMS is controversial and lacks scientific evidence. The general consensus among most clinicians is that these medications are not particularly helpful in treating FMS and have major side effects and problems that outweigh any benefit.

Tramadol is a unique medication with weak μ-receptor activity as well as serotonin and norepinephrine reuptake inhibition. It has shown some benefit in treating pain in FMS, also when combined with acetaminophen.[21] Dosages are typically in the range of 50 to 100 mg three to four times daily. Because of its SNRI activity, there is a risk of serotonin syndrome when combined with TCAs, SSRIs, or SNRIs, so education of the patient is important to assess for early signs of problems.

OTHER MEDICATIONS

One medication that has been used in FMS but has not succeeded in acquiring FDA approval for FMS is sodium oxybate. It is a γ-aminobutyric acid (GABA) metabolite, approved for use in narcolepsy and excessive daytime sleepiness. A small RCT with placebo control in patients with FMS showed increased sleep time, improved quality of sleep, less awakening, and less daytime sleepiness, as well as decreased pain perception and decreased tender points.[19] Dosing requires two divided doses (usually 3–6 g/day) at night, about 2 hours apart; it is well tolerated, with nausea and dizziness usually abating after time.

Pramipexole, a dopamine receptor agonist approved for use in restless leg syndrome, shows some efficacy in FMS. Improvements in pain, fatigue, and global functioning were seen in a small RCT and warrant further investigation.[22] Tizanidine, an α_2 receptor agonist that acts centrally, is a muscle relaxant that may improve similar measures such as pain, sleep, and quality of life.[4]

Some clinicians use benzodiazepines such as clonazepam or alprazolam to help with induction of sleep and to help with anxiety in patients with FMS. Caution is advised when these medications are combined with other sedative medications.

Topical medications have not been widely studied in FMS but may yield some benefit for symptom relief. Over-the-counter menthol preparations may provide some abatement of pain. Compound pharmacies can blend custom-ordered creams, including local anesthetics; muscle relaxants; and neuropathic medications such as ketamine, gabapentin, and amitriptyline. Patients may tolerate these with few side effects; however, their use is limited to the most painful areas because these compounds cannot be spread all over the body at once.

NONPHARMACOLOGIC TREATMENT

The importance of exercise in treatment of FMS has been shown in a large number of studies. The most consistent and widely studied type of exercise is aerobic activity, both land and water based. This type of exercise seems to help with many aspects of FMS symptoms, including pain, fatigue, and depression. Strength exercise also shows benefit, as does a mix of the two. In addition, other types of physical activity, such as Tai Chi, yoga, and Pilates, have shown benefit in reducing FMS symptoms.[15] There is no strong evidence to suggest that one type of activity is better than another, so patient preference should guide any therapeutic program of activity. Typically, patients with FMS should start with low-intensity, low-resistance activity and gradually increase as tolerated so that they do not cause increased pain. Input from a physiatrist or physical therapist can be invaluable in constructing a well-tolerated and beneficial program.

The mechanism for the benefit of exercise in FMS is not completely understood but may relate to the decreased sympathetic output to muscles during exercise, as well as increased blood flow to muscles and heat generation. Additionally, the beneficial effect of exercise on symptoms of depression and stress may improve those FMS domains.[23]

Cognitive-behavioral therapy approaches, including biofeedback, relaxation, and behavior modification, have shown benefit in FMS treatment. Psychotherapy, either individual or group based, also may be useful in helping patients cope and manage their psychological problems.[4]

The role of trigger point injections and Botox in FMS has dwindled in importance, but these modalities may still be helpful in treating specific problems such as painful trigger points in muscle and migraines.

Transcutaneous electrical nerve stimulation (TENS) devices have also been used successfully to help with FMS pain and stiffness; the benefit is temporary, but the side effects are negligible.[24] Heat application, whether through a hot bath or shower, electric heating pads, or microwavable heat packs, can also help temporarily with muscle pain, stiffness, and headache. Massage can also offer relaxation of stiff muscles, but often lighter massage is necessary in those with FMS.[19]

SUMMARY

Fibromyalgia syndrome is a complex disease encompassing symptoms of widespread pain, fatigue, and depression. Often, patients have sought opinions from multiple providers before being diagnosed with FMS, and many are disheartened and skeptical that improvement is possible. Education and awareness are vital to convince patients with FMS that they must commit to changing many of their attitudes toward exercise, sleep, and diet, as well as their attitudes toward their pain and functional limitations. With the advent of newer understandings of the nature of FMS along with newer medications, clinicians now have opportunities to instill patients with optimism that their symptoms can improve. A multidisciplinary and multimodal approach is typically the most effective in treating individuals with FMS.

REFERENCES

1. Yunus M. The prevalence of fibromyalgia in other chronic pain conditions. *Pain Res Treat*. 2012;2012:584573.
2. Russell IJ. Fibromyalgia syndrome: presentation, diagnosis and differential diagnosis. *PrimPsychiatry*. 2006;13(9):40-45.
3. Wolfe F, Smythe HA, Yunus MB, et al. The American College of Rheumatology 1990 criteria for the classification of fibromyalgia: report of the Multicenter Criteria Committee. *Arthritis Rheum*. 1990;33:160-172.
4. Smith HS, Harris R, Clauw D. Fibromyalgia: an afferent processing disorder leading to a complex pain generalized syndrome. *Pain Physician*. 2011;14(2):E217-E245.
5. Goldenberg DL, Burckhardt C, Crofford L. Management of fibromyalgia syndrome. *JAMA*. 2004;292(19):2388-2395.
6. Staud R, Nagel S, Robinson ME, et al. Enhanced central pain processing of fibromyalgia patients is maintained by muscle afferent input: a randomized, double-blind, placebo controlled study. *Pain*. 2009;145(1-2):96-104.
7. Woolf CJ. Central sensitization: implications for the diagnosis and treatment of pain. *Pain*. 2011;152(3 Suppl):S2-S15.
8. Russell IJ, Orr MD, Littman B, et al. Elevated cerebrospinal fluid levels of substance P in patients with the fibromyalgia syndrome. *Arthritis Rheum*. 1994;37(11):1593-1601.
9. Sarchielli P, Mancini ML, Floridi A, et al. Increased levels of neurotrophins are not specific for chronic migraine: evidence from primary fibromyalgia syndrome. *J Pain*. 2007;8(9):737-745.
10. Russell IJ, Vaerøy H, Javors M, et al. Cerebrospinal fluid biogenic amine metabolites in fibromyalgia/fibrositis syndrome and rheumatoid arthritis. *Arthritis Rheum*. 1992;35(5):550-556.
11. Wolfe F, Ross K, Anderson J, et al. The prevalence and characteristics of fibromyalgia in the general population. *Arthritis Rheum*. 1995;38(1):19-28.
12. Lawrence RC, Felson DT, Helmick CG, et al. Estimates of the prevalence of arthritis and other rheumatic conditions in the United States: part II. *Arthritis Rheum*. 2008;58(1):26-35.
13. Branco JC, Bannwarth B, Failde I, et al. Prevalence of fibromyalgia: a survey of five European countries. *Semin Arthritis Rheum*. 2010;39(6):448-453.
14. Mork PJ, Vasseljen O, Nilsen TI. Association between physical exercise, body mass index, and risk of fibromyalgia: longitudinal data from the Norwegian Nord-Trøndelag Health Study. *Arthritis Care Res (Hoboken)*. 2010;62(5):611-617.
15. Busch AJ, Webber SC, Brachaniec M, et al. Exercise therapy for fibromyalgia. *Curr Pain Headache Rep*. 2011;15(5):358-367.
16. Schaefer C, Chandran A, Hufstader M, et al. The comparative burden of mild, moderate and severe fibromyalgia: results from a cross-sectional survey in the United States. *Health Qual Life Outcomes*. 22 2011;9:71.
17. Arnold LM, Clauw DJ, Wohlreich MM, et al. Efficacy of duloxetine in patients with fibromyalgia: pooled analysis of 4 placebo-controlled trials. *Prim Care Companion J Clin Psychiatry*. 2009;11(5):237-234.

18. Moldofsky H, Harris HW, Archambault WT, et al. Effects of bedtime very low dose cyclobenzaprine on symptoms and sleep physiology in patients with fibromyalgia syndrome: a double-blind randomized placebo-controlled study. *J Rheumatol.* 2011;38(12):2653-2663.
19. Russell IJ. Fibromyalgia syndrome: approach to management. *Prim Psychiatry.* 2006;13(9):76-84.
20. Crofford LJ, Rowbotham MC, Mease PJ, et al. Pregabalin for the treatment of fibromyalgia syndrome: results of a randomized, double-blind, placebo controlled trial. *Arthritis Rheum.* 2005;52(4):1264-1273.
21. Russell IJ, Kamin M, Bennett RM, et al. Efficacy of tramadol in treatment of pain in fibromyalgia. *J Clin Rheumatol.* 2000;6(5):250-257.
22. Holman AJ, Myers RR. A randomized, double-blind, placebo controlled trial of pramipexole, a dopamine agonist, in patients with fibromyalgia receiving concomitant medications. *Arthritis Rheum.* 2005;52(8):2495-2505.
23. Vierck C. A mechanism-based approach to prevention of and therapy for fibromyalgia. *Pain Res Treat.* 2012;2012:95135.
24. Löfgren M, Norrbrink C. Pain relief in woman with fibromyalgia: a cross-over study of superficial warmth stimulation and transcutaneous electrical nerve stimulation. *J Rehab Med.* 2009;41(7):557-562.

CHAPTER 60 Muscle Pain: Pathophysiology, Evaluation, and Treatment

Norman J. Marcus
Siegfried Mense

INTRODUCTION AND EPIDEMIOLOGY

INTRODUCTION

Muscles, representing approximately 50% of the body by weight, have long been recognized by clinicians as a source of common pain problems. Various terms have been applied to muscles and soft tissue pain, generally reflecting the prevailing concepts of muscle pain mechanisms or clinical observations of painful muscles. The changing concepts about the nature of muscle pain make it difficult to collect data on the incidence and impact of muscle-related pain. A brief review of the history of these concepts is presented.

DESCRIPTIVE TERMS

The terms *muscular rheumatism*[1] and *nonarticular rheumatism*[2] were used to suggest that pain and stiffness in the region of a joint were caused by soft tissue rather than articular dysfunction. Inflammation as the cause of muscle pain led to the terms *fibrositis* and *myofibrositis*,[3] which were abandoned with the awareness that inflammation could generally not be demonstrated in painful muscles.

The palpable changes in the muscles, revealing increased resilience, ropiness, and nodularity, led to the terms *Myogelosen* (muscle gelling),[4] *Muskelhärten* (hardened muscle),[5] and *Muskelschwiele* (muscle callus). The term *myofascial pain*, suggesting pain originating in muscle and connective tissue, first used by Reynolds in 1952, is now confusingly used interchangeably with *myofascial pain syndrome*, suggested by Travell and Simons,[6] referring to muscle pain originating in myofascial trigger points (TrPs).

PAIN DISTRIBUTION AND PUTATIVE ETIOLOGY AFFECT NOMENCLATURE

Littlejohn[7] suggests that the term *regionalized musculoskeletal disorders* be used for muscle pain when the causes appear to be inflammation, sprain, strain, or degeneration of muscles and tendons. When no obvious etiology is present to account for muscle pain, tenderness, stiffness, and often associated nonanatomic dysesthesias and autonomic disturbances, four overlapping and confusing diagnoses are often used: (1) regional pain syndrome, (2) complex regional pain syndrome, and when muscle pain is widespread, (3) chronic widespread pain (CWP), or (4) fibromyalgia syndrome (FMS). Central nervous system (CNS) dysregulation is generally thought to underlie these diagnoses rather than peripheral muscle pain generators.

MUSCLE PAIN AND NEUROPLASTICITY

When muscle nociceptors (discussed later in the chapter) are sensitized, they stimulate and may sensitize dorsal horn neurons, which may result in opening previously ineffective synaptic pathways, leading to stimulation of neurons at adjacent and distant spinal levels. This mechanism may produce referred muscle pain. Sensitized CNS neurons and primary dysfunction in descending inhibitory pathways may lower the threshold for nociceptive stimulation and result in enhanced muscle pain. Pain from other tissue (nerve, joint, viscera) may refer to muscle and may result in the production of independently self-sustaining muscle pain and a confounded clinical presentation.

MUSCLE PAIN AS A CAUSE OF OR COEXISTING WITH OTHER SUSPECTED PAIN DIAGNOSES

Although diagnoses such as nonspecific low back, neck, and shoulder pain are often thought to be the result of sprains and strains of muscles and other soft tissue,[8,9] they would not show up in an epidemiologic survey as muscle-related pain. (The following discussion alludes to muscle pain as a representative for soft tissue pain, understanding that fascia, ligaments, and tendons are also sources of soft tissue pain.)

A large study showed that 70% or more of patients with acute low back pain (LBP) in an ambulatory setting were diagnosed as having nonspecific LBP, defined as sprains and strains of soft tissue,[8] so it is remarkable that muscles are not considered in the etiology of LBP in guidelines from important national and international organizations.[10] Pain presentations in a region of the body may be incorrectly labeled based on a body part (e.g., epicondylitis) and ignore the surrounding musculature,[11] which may be important in the total pain presentation.[12]

Tension-type headaches (TTHs) may be related to muscle-generated pain.[13] Ten percent of pain complaints in patients with cancer are unrelated to the cancer or treatment and are generally thought to be caused by soft tissue.[14] Therefore, statistics on the incidence and prevalence of muscle pain in the general population are confounded and we believe underestimate the clinical and economic importance of muscles in common pain syndromes.

EPIDEMIOLOGY

Fifty percent of adolescents reported previous lifetime incidence as well as prospectively for 1 to 5 years of LBP, CWP, FMS, shoulder pain, or musculoskeletal pain.[15] Associated significant reductions in health-related quality-of-life scores were noted when pain occurred at least once a week at more than one site.[16] A 2009 European study reported a 1-month period prevalence of LBP of nearly 40% in adolescents.[17]

Twenty-seven percent of adults reported LBP in the preceding 3 months, and 14% reported neck pain in the 2008 National Health Interview Survey Report.[18] A 2009 study showed a rising prevalence of chronic LBP across all age groups during a 14-year period.[19] In the United Kingdom, the lifetime prevalence of chronic LBP in the general population is estimated to be 6.3% to 11.1%.[20]

The 12-month prevalence of neck pain was 30% to 50% in 2008 in The Bone and Joint Decade 2000–2010 Task Force on Neck Pain and Its Associated Disorders.[21] The 1-month period prevalence of shoulder pain is between 20% and 33%.[22]

U.S. and U.K. data for CWP show a 10% to 11% point prevalence, with women affected 1.5 times more often than men.[23-25] Point prevalence for FMS is 0.5% to 4% from the same data, with women affected 10 times more often than men. Data also show that patients with

FMS frequently have a history of work-related neck and shoulder pain, whiplash, LBP, and muscle tension,[26,27] suggesting that many of these patients' diffuse pain problems may have begun in clinically or subclinically damaged muscles.

DIAGNOSIS

HISTORY

Muscles may be the cause of pains mistakenly attributed to other tissue and may contribute to the overall pain presentation in patients who have pain from other sources (e.g., HNP, rotator cuff tear, arthritis). Therefore, unless a muscle assessment is a standard part of the physical examination of the patient in pain, it may not be considered in the pain diagnoses. For example, a detailed work and social history may reveal factors that could produce overt or subclinical muscle injury.

Work-related factors may include recent changes in the physical demands in the work setting, prolonged positioning, repetitive movements, and consistently physically or psychologically demanding labor. Sports-related activity may include changes in activity, type, intensity, frequency, and equipment. Examples are playing tennis for longer than usual, incorporating a new serve, and using a new racket. Upper body activities associated with the initiation or perpetuation of neck and shoulder pain include use of the computer keyboard with an elbow angle of less than 90 degrees, a nonergonomic monitor position, regular use of a phone without using a headset or speaker, and reading or watching television in bed.

SIGNS AND SYMPTOMS

Muscle pain may occur in a discrete area or in multiple regions as an activity-related aching discomfort but at times also at rest. Patients typically complain of a dull, aching sensation that is made worse with more aggressive activity of the painful region and prolonged positioning. If pain occurs with prolonged positioning, movement tends to initially reduce the pain (e.g., standing in one spot causing LBP, which is then diminished with walking). The painful muscle generally has diminished ability for maximal effort (pain inhibition) related to suppressed activity in the painful agonist with associated problems in coordination and diminished flexibility related to increased activity in the antagonist.[28]

Because nerves traveling through or adjacent to contracted muscles may become compressed, the presentation may suggest a neuropathic problem. Piriformis syndrome is only one such example.[29]

BASIC NEUROANATOMY AND NEUROPHYSIOLOGY OF MUSCLE PAIN

NEUROANATOMY OF MUSCLE NOCICEPTORS AND THEIR AFFERENT FIBERS

Small-diameter high-threshold afferent fibers have to be excited in order to elicit muscle pain. Histologically, they consist of thin myelinated (group III) and nonmyelinated (group IV)[30] fibers. The conduction velocity of these fibers is low: group IV fibers conduct at 0.5 to 2.5 m/s in a cat and group III fibers at 2.5 to 30 m/s. Group III fibers correspond to cutaneous Aδ- and group IV to C fibers. Not all of these small-caliber fibers are nociceptive; they also include thermoreceptive and mechanoreceptive fibers with a low threshold in the innocuous range.[31,32]

The typical structure mediating muscle pain is the free nerve ending.[33] The term indicates that in a light microscope, no corpuscular receptive structure can be recognized (**Fig. 60-1**). Free nerve endings, having a high mechanical threshold in the noxious range or responding to pain-producing chemicals, are called *nociceptors* or *nociceptive endings*. They are not excited by light deformation of the muscle or physiological movements. The expression "pain receptor" should be avoided because a nociceptor does not measure pain but the intensity of a painful stimulus. Pain is the sequela of a strong excitation of nociceptors and originates in the cortex.

Whereas group III afferents terminate not only in free nerve endings but also in paciniform corpuscles, group IV fibers supply exclusively free nerve endings. The predominant location of free nerve endings is the adventitia of arterioles and venules. The muscle fibers proper are not supplied by free nerve endings.[35]

The density of free nerve endings in the peritendineum (the connective tissue around a tendon) of the rat calcaneal tendon was several times higher than that in the gastrocnemius-soleus (GS) muscle.[35] The dense innervation of the peritendineum may explain the high prevalence of tenderness or pain in the tissue around tendons and their insertion sites.

NEUROPEPTIDE CONTENT OF NOCICEPTIVE FREE NERVE ENDINGS

There is evidence from studies on dorsal root ganglion (DRG) cells that substance P (SP) and, to a lesser extent, calcitonin gene-related peptide (CGRP) are characteristic of nociceptive units.[36] Other neuropeptides, such as somatostatin (SOM), vasoactive intestinal polypeptide (VIP), and nerve growth factor (NGF), are also present in unmyelinated fibers in muscle[35] but are not as closely related to a nociceptive function as SP

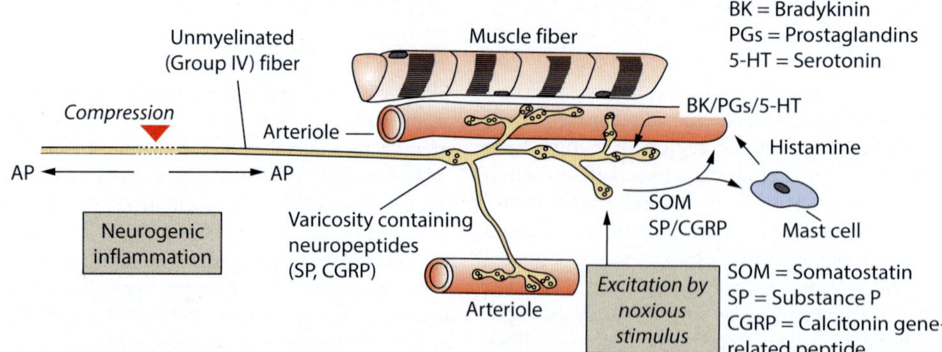

FIGURE 60-1. Structure of a muscle nociceptor and events occurring around the receptor during noxious stimulation. The nociceptor has several branches close to arterioles. The noxious stimulus (upward arrow) excites the nociceptor, leading to the release of neuropeptides from the ending, such as substance P (SP), calcitonin gene-related peptide (CGRP), and somatostatin (SOM). SP and CGRP cause vasodilation and increased capillary permeability in the small blood vessels in the vicinity of the ending. SP also degranulates mast cells; the released histamine is likewise a vasodilator. The release of neuropeptides from nociceptive endings can also occur when action potentials invade the ending retrogradely (against the normal direction of propagation) in neuropathy or radiculopathy (left part of figure). At the site of a nerve compression, action potentials originate in the nociceptive fiber and propagate both anterogradely (to the central nervous system, causing pain) and retrogradely (to the receptive ending, causing neurogenic inflammation through the release of neuropeptides). The neurogenic inflammation is a sterile inflammation around the nociceptive ending caused by an increase in blood vessel permeability followed by plasma extravasation. The plasma extravasation leads to the formation of bradykinin and other agents that sensitize the nociceptor. The result of a neurogenic inflammation is a local edema with sensitized nociceptors. (Modified from Mense and Gerwin.[34] Mense S, Gerwin R. *Muscle Pain: Understanding the Mechanisms. 1st ed*. Heidelberg: Springer; 2010.)

and CGRP. A strong argument supporting a nociceptive function of SP is that noxious stimulation in the body periphery is followed by a release of SP in the dorsal horn of the spinal cord where nociceptive endings terminate. Both SP and CGRP are presumably released together when the afferent fiber is active because they coexist in nociceptive units.

Generally, the neuropeptide content of nerve fibers from muscle is similar to that of cutaneous nerves.[37,38] However, compared with skin nerves, muscle nerves appear to contain less SP. In rats in which a chronic myositis had been induced, the innervation density of the muscle with free nerve endings containing SP and NGF was significantly increased.[35]

In the CNS, neuropeptides function as neuromodulators, substances that enhance or attenuate the action of neurotransmitters. Glutamate is the main neurotransmitter of nociceptive afferents in the spinal cord, and the neuropeptides enhance the central nervous effects of glutamate released by peripheral noxious stimuli.[39]

PHYSIOLOGICAL PROPERTIES OF MUSCLE NOCICEPTORS

Whenever a nociceptor is excited, it releases the neuropeptides stored in its ending into the interstitial tissue. Many of these agents, particularly CGRP and SP, cause vasodilatation and an increase in vascular permeability of the blood vessels around the active ending. The result is a shift of blood plasma from the intravascular to the interstitial space. Here, bradykinin (BKN) is cleaved from plasma proteins, serotonin (5-HT) is released from platelets, and prostaglandin E_2 (PGE_2) is released from endothelial and other tissue cells. All of these substances sensitize nociceptors. Thus, the main tissue alteration induced by a noxious mechanical stimulus is a localized region of vasodilatation, edema, and sensitized nociceptors. These effects can also be evoked by the compression of a peripheral nerve or dorsal root, which triggers action potentials at the compression site. Action potentials traveling to the CNS cause neuropathic pain; those traveling to the body periphery lead to the release of sensitizing substances from the nociceptive ending. The result is a neurogenic inflammation (see Fig. 60-1) which may enhance the pain of patients with neuropathy.

SUBSTANCES EXCITING MUSCLE NOCICEPTORS

The membrane of a nociceptor is equipped with receptor molecules to which sensitizing or stimulating agents bind (**Fig. 60-2**) or that are sensitive to thermal or mechanical stimuli. The following substances are effective stimulants for muscle receptors, most of which are released together in damaged muscle.[40,41]

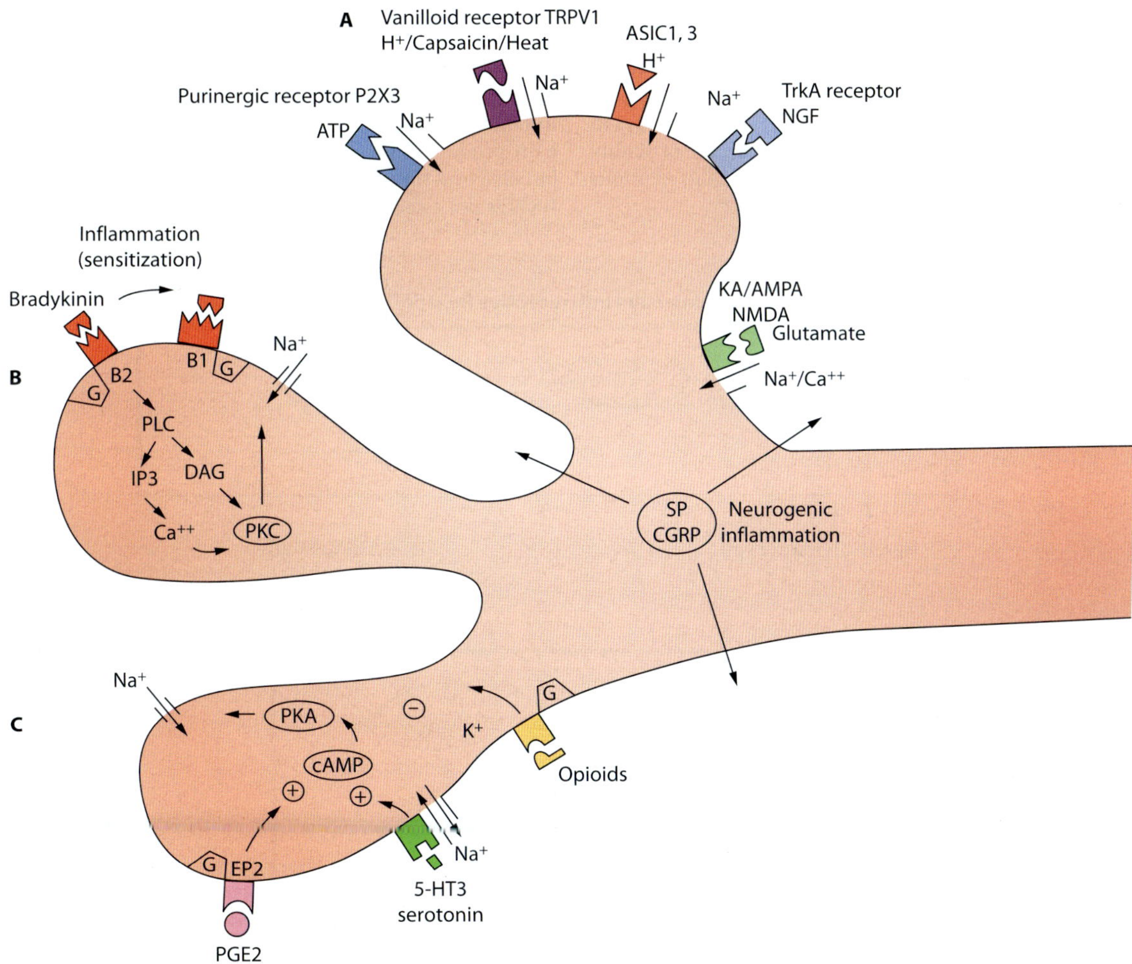

FIGURE 60-2. Receptor molecules in the membrane of a nociceptive ending, which are important for muscle pain. Branch A: Receptor molecules that excite the ending by opening Na^+ channels. Three receptors are sensitive to H^+ ions: the transient receptor potential subtype V1 (TRPV1) and the acid-sensing ion channels (ASIC) 1 and 3. When H^+ binds to the receptor, an Na^+ channel opens, and positively charged ions (mainly Na^+) enter the cell. The purinergic receptor P2X3 binds adenosine triphosphate (ATP) that has a relatively high concentration in muscle cells. Branch B: Inflammation-induced change of the bradykinin receptor molecule. In intact tissue, bradykinin (BKN) excites or sensitizes the ending through the B2 receptor. In inflamed tissue, BKN acts on the B1 receptor. B1 is synthesized in the dorsal root ganglion (DRG), transported to the ending, and built in the membrane. BKN exerts its action by activating a G protein that regulates intracellular second messengers, such as protein kinase C (PKC). PKC increases the permeability of Na^+ channels and thus sensitizes the ending. Branch C: Receptors that mainly sensitize the ending. Prostaglandin E_2 (PGE_2) and serotonin (5-HT) increase the intracellular concentration of the second messengers cAMP and protein kinase A (PKA). PKA increases the permeability of the Na^+ channels and thus allows larger ion currents to enter the ending. This renders the ending more sensitive to external stimuli. The opioid receptor molecule inhibits the sensitization process. (Modified from Mense and Gerwin.[34] Mense S, Gerwin R. *Muscle Pain: Understanding the Mechanisms. 1st ed.* Heidelberg: Springer; 2010.)

CAPSAICIN

Capsaicin, the active ingredient of chili peppers, is the specific stimulant for the transient receptor potential receptor subtype 1 (TRPV1), formerly called VR1.[42] The TRPV1 receptor is one of the most important molecules for the induction of pain; its endogenous ligands are H^+ ions. The receptor is also sensitive to heat. Acidity of the tissue increases this sensitivity. For instance, in tissue with an acidic pH, as occurs after strenuous exercise, the normal body temperature is sufficient for activating the receptor and causing pain.[43] With fever, stimulation of TRPV1 may explain the often accompanying total-body ache. In humans, muscle nociceptors were found that could be activated by injections of capsaicin,[44] indicating the presence of the TRPV1 receptor.

MECHANICAL STIMULI

TRPV4 is a mechanoreceptor that is sensitive to both weak and strong (noxious) intensities of local pressure.[45] It may be the receptor for pain evoked by mechanical stimuli.

PROTONS (H^+)

Protons are a particularly important stimulus for muscle pain because almost all pathologic changes in muscle (e.g., exhausting exercise, ischemia, inflammation) are accompanied by a drop in tissue pH. In these conditions, the pH of the muscle tissue can drop to 5 to 6. Protons bind to acid-sensing ion channels (ASICs), with ASIC3 being particularly important for muscle pain,[46] reacting to small pH changes (e.g., pH 7.4–7.1).[47] Muscle nociceptors respond to pathophysiologic decreases in pH, with the magnitude of response depending on the degree of acidity (**Fig. 60-3**). Repeated intramuscular (IM) injections of acidic solutions have been reported to induce a long-lasting hyperalgesia.[48]

ADENOSINE TRIPHOSPHATE

Adenosine triphosphate (ATP) binds to the purinergic P2X3 receptor.[49] ATP is present in every tissue cell and is released during trauma and other pathologic cell changes. Therefore, ATP has been considered a general signal substance for pain.[50] ATP is particularly important for muscle pain because it is present in muscle cells in high concentrations.[51] The ATP concentration released from a damaged muscle is sufficient to excite muscle nociceptors (see Fig. 60-3). When injected into human muscle, ATP causes pain.[52]

NERVE GROWTH FACTOR

The receptor molecule for NGF is the tyrosine kinase A (TrkA) receptor.[53] NGF has a sensitizing action on peripheral nociceptors and neurons in the CNS. It has a close relationship to muscle: it is synthesized in muscle, and its synthesis is increased during pathophysiologic changes of the muscle (e.g., inflammation).[54] NGF appears to be the only substance that excites nociceptors exclusively without influencing non-nociceptive free nerve endings.[32] However, the excitatory action of NGF is restricted to a special subset of nociceptors that have a strong sensitizing effect on spinal neurons (see later discussion).

BRADYKININ

Bradykinin is cleaved from plasma proteins when blood plasma moves from blood vessels into the interstitium. In intact tissue, BKN excites nerve endings by binding to the receptor molecule B2; however, in inflamed tissues, the receptor B1 is the predominant one.[55] Many of the pain-producing substances, including BKN, excite not only nociceptors but also low-threshold mechanosensitive free nerve endings. Therefore, BKN is not a specific excitant of nociceptors.

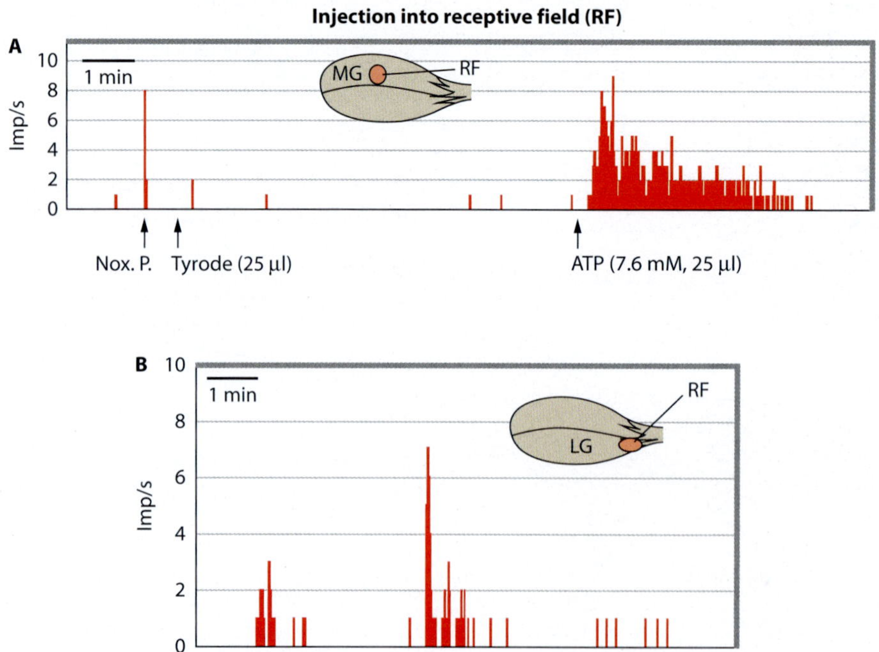

FIGURE 60-3. Electrical activity of single muscle receptors tested with intramuscular injections of adenosine triphosphate (adenosine triphosphate [ATP]; A) and acidic solutions (B), respectively. The activity was recorded from the gastrocnemius-soleus (GS) nerve and transformed to time histograms by a computer. Both receptors also responded to noxious mechanical pressure (Nox.P; see left part of A); they probably were so-called polymodal nociceptors responding to all kinds of noxious stimuli. **A,** Response to ATP injected into the unit's mechanosensitive receptive field (RF) in the medial head of the GS muscle (MG). Note that ATP was injected at a concentration that exists in muscle cells and is released when these cells are damaged. Before the ATP injection, the solvent tyrode solution was injected as a control, without any effect. **B,** Stimulating effect of acidic buffer solutions on another muscle nociceptor. The ending was tested with intramuscular injections of buffer solutions, two acidic ones (pH 6 and 5) and one at a neutral pH (7.4). The unit responded with a larger response to pH 5 than to pH 6, the neutral solution had no effect. (Modified from Mense and Gerwin.[34] Mense S, Gerwin R. *Muscle Pain: Understanding the Mechanisms. 1st ed.* Heidelberg: Springer; 2010.)

SEROTONIN

Serotonin (5-hydroxytryptamine, 5-HT) is released from blood platelets during blood clotting. The action of serotonin on nociceptors in the body periphery is predominantly mediated by the 5-HT_3 receptor. The serotonin concentrations usually released are likely to sensitize nociceptors rather than exciting them.

PROSTAGLANDIN E_2

Prostaglandins are released in a pathologically altered muscle by the action of cyclooxygenases. PGE_2 binds to the prostanoid receptor (EP2) in the membrane of the nociceptive ending. Similar to serotonin, PGE_2 may sensitize nociceptors without exciting them.[56]

GLUTAMATE

Evidence indicates that receptor molecules for glutamate (e.g., *N*-methyl-D-aspartate [NMDA] receptors) exist on nociceptive endings in masticatory muscles.[57] In female rats, the responses of group III/IV muscle receptors to glutamate were greater than in male rats.[58] Thus, gender differences are present even at the level of the nociceptor. The NMDA receptor has been reported to be a mediator of inflammatory pain.[59] Hypertonic NaCl may excite free nerve endings indirectly through glutamate released by Na^+.[60]

SUBSTANCES EXCITING MUSCLE NOCICEPTORS INDEPENDENT OF MEMBRANE RECEPTORS

Hypertonic Saline Hypertonic NaCl solutions (4.5%–6.0%) are often used to elicit pain from muscles in humans[61] (for a review, see Graven-Nielsen[62]). Injections of the hypertonic solution elicit a medium level of pain in healthy control participants. The mechanism of the pain produced by hypertonic saline is still obscure. Two members of the TRP receptor family appear to be sensitive to osmotic stimuli, named TRPV4[45] and TRPA1.[63]

The different behavior of the various functional types of free nerve endings (nociceptors, mechanoreceptors, thermoreceptors) is probably due to the expression of special combinations of receptor molecules in their cell membrane.[64]

Potassium Ions (K^+) K^+ ions can excite nociceptors directly by depolarizing the membrane potential to threshold. This stimulus was used in many studies in the beginning of experimental pain research[65] but is no longer common. Nevertheless, K^+ can be the cause of muscle pain when muscle cells are damaged and the intracellular K^+ ions are set free.

CLINICAL PHENOMENA ASSOCIATED WITH MUSCLE-GENERATED PAIN

Tenderness Pressure to muscles causing discomfort is the most obvious manifestation of common muscle pain. Such tenderness is found in acute muscle pain, for example, after blunt trauma or aggressive physical work or exercise. If additional provocations do not occur, the tenderness disappears.

Peripheral Sensitization The reason for the tenderness is sensitization of the peripheral nociceptor by sensitizing inflammatory substances (the peripheral sensitization is, in most cases, combined with central sensitization; discussed later in the chapter). Many substances that are released from damaged muscle (e.g., BKN, PGE_2, NGF, tumor necrosis factor-α [TNF-α]) increase the mechanical sensitivity of nociceptors.[65,66] In intact tissue, a nociceptor has a high mechanical threshold, but when it is sensitized, it lowers its threshold into the innocuous range and is excited by everyday stimuli, such as weak muscle deformation. This transition from high- to low-threshold mechanosensitivity can be seen when an intact muscle is experimentally inflamed (**Fig. 60-4**). Some of the sensitizing effects are due to intermediate substances (e.g., TNF-α induces sensitization through the release of PGE_2).[67] Another example is the increased excitatory action of BKN after exposure to PGE_2 and serotonin.[56] A combination of BKN and 5-HT injected into the temporalis muscle in humans elicited stronger pain than that caused by each stimulant alone.[68]

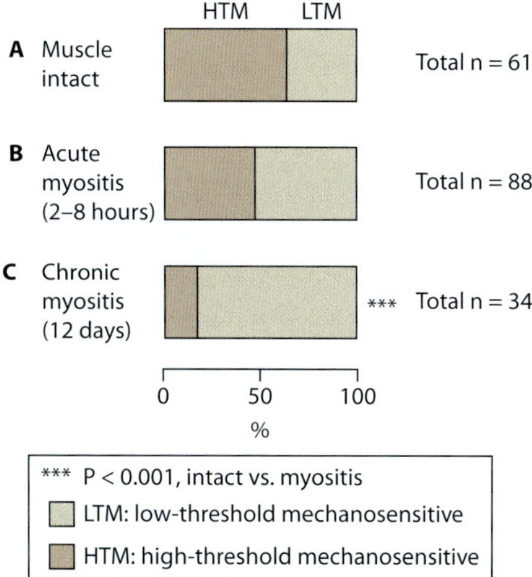

FIGURE 60-4. Myositis-induced change in mechanical responsiveness of mechanosensitive free nerve endings in muscle receptors in the gastrocnemius-soleus (GS) muscle of the rat. In **A** to **C**, the proportion of low-threshold mechanosensitive (LTM, mechanoreceptive) endings relative to high-threshold mechanosensitive (HTM, nociceptive) units is shown. **A,** In intact muscle, the proportion of HTM endings is close to 60%, and that of LTM units is 40%. **B,** In acutely inflamed muscle (2- to 8-hour duration), the proportion of HTM receptors was (nonsignificantly) decreased, presumably because of a beginning sensitization of the nociceptors. **C,** In chronically inflamed muscle, the proportion of HTM receptors had dropped to less than 20%, and that of LTM units was increased to more than 80%. Many of the LTM units in C must have been former HTM receptors that were sensitized and lowered their threshold into the innocuous range. (Modified from Mense and Gerwin.[34] Mense S, Gerwin R. *Muscle Pain: Understanding the Mechanisms. 1st ed.* Heidelberg: Springer; 2010.)

Central Sensitization In the long run, every input from muscle nociceptors to the spinal cord probably sensitizes central nociceptive neurons. The central sensitization is associated with one or several of the following.

Appearance of New Receptive Fields A receptive field (RF) of a central neuron is the body region from which the neuron can be excited or inhibited. In animal experiments, new RFs of a neuron can be induced by injecting a pain-producing agent into a muscle. For instance, a neuron that initially had a single high-threshold mechanosensitive RF in one muscle of the hindlimb acquired additional RFs in other muscles and tissues of that hindlimb.[69]

The appearance of new RFs is probably caused by the opening of formerly ineffective synapses on the neuron.[70] Probably, the newly induced RFs originally had ineffective synaptic connections with the neuron, but after painful stimulation of the muscle sensitized the neuron, these connections became effective.

This unmasking of synaptic connections represents pain-induced changes in the wiring of the dorsal horn. When an entire limb muscle is damaged, many spinal neurons acquire new RFs. The result is that the input from a given muscle excites more neurons in the spinal cord. Thus, the spinal target area in which input from the damaged muscle excites dorsal horn neurons expands. Such an effect can be induced by an experimental muscle inflammation in the rat (**Fig. 60-5**).[71] In these myositis animals, responses were obtained from neurons in the segment L3, where neurons do not normally respond to input from the inflamed GS muscle. The unmasking of ineffective synapses is partly due to neuromodulatory substances in the CNS (e.g., neuropeptides such as SP and CGRP or neurotrophins such as brain-derived neurotrophic factor).[72,73] When the central sensitization has become chronic, it is independent of further input from the damaged muscle.[48]

The expansion of the spinal input area from a given muscle is the basis for the referral of muscle pain. When, for instance, rat neurons in the segment L6 are pathologically excited by input from the GS muscle (the normal target area of that muscle is L4 and L5), they send the signal

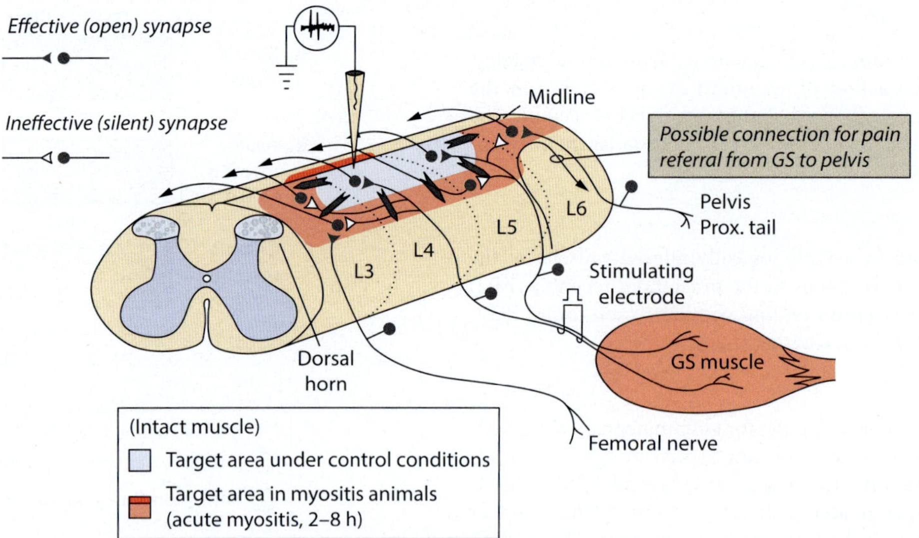

FIGURE 60-5. Reorganization of the wiring in the spinal cord during an acute muscle inflammation. The figure shows the change in the target area of the gastrocnemius-soleus (GS) muscle nerve in the spinal cord. "Target area of a nerve" indicates the regions in the spinal cord where dorsal horn neurons can be excited by a standard electrical stimulus applied to the nerve. The dorsal horn neurons were searched in systematic microelectrode tracks in the segments L3 to L6. Before induction of the myositis, neurons responding to electrical stimulation of the GS nerve were found only in the segments L5, L4, and caudal L3 (gray area). A few hours after induction of the myositis, the target area had expanded and included the entire segment L3 and L6. Apparently, the input from nociceptors in the inflamed GS muscle had opened formerly ineffective synaptic connections with the muscle in these segments. After expansion of the target area (right part of figure), there are effective synaptic connections between the GS muscle and neurons in L6, which supply the pelvic region. This newly opened connection may form the basis for the referral of pain from the GS muscle to the pelvic region. (Modified from Mense and Gerwin.[34] Mense S, Gerwin R. *Muscle Pain: Understanding the Mechanisms. 1st ed.* Heidelberg: Springer; 2010.)

"tissue-damaging stimulus in the pelvis" to higher centers because the neurons in L6 normally process input from the pelvis. Thus in humans, after opening of the formerly ineffective synaptic connections from the GS (triceps surae) muscle to the L5 and S1 segments, a patient may feel referred pain in the pelvis when the GS muscle is pathologically altered.

Central Sensitization by Subthreshold Potentials in Dorsal Horn Neurons Many studies on central sensitization used high-frequency electrical stimulation (e.g., 100 Hz) to elicit the sensitization. However, one of the authors Mense has found that high-frequencies are not required for sensitization because in Mense's laboratory, in chronic pathophysiological muscle lesions, the afferent input does not reach mean frequencies exceeding 1 Hz. Recent data showed that even subthreshold synaptic potentials in dorsal horn neurons are sufficient to cause central sensitization. The subthreshold potentials were evoked by injection of NGF into the GS muscle. In single-fiber recordings, NGF was found to excite a large proportion of rat nociceptors,[32] but the animals did not show any immediate pain reactions. One day after IM injection of NGF, the rats exhibited a marked mechanical allodynia and hyperalgesia. Intracellular recordings from dorsal horn neurons in rats showed that NGF elicited mainly subthreshold synaptic potentials in dorsal horn neurons.[74] The NGF-induced central sensitization involved the activation of NMDA receptors because administration of ketamine (an NMDA antagonist) prevented the NGF-induced allodynia and hyperalgesia. Svensson and colleagues[75] likewise observed the combination of lack of immediate pain followed by allodynia when they injected NGF into the masseter muscle in humans.

Glial Cells and Central Sensitization Approximately 90% of all cells in the CNS are glial cells, but only recently have they been systematically studied in pain mechanisms.[76] Glial cells can be activated by nociceptive input from muscle and, when activated, release substances that sensitize dorsal horn neurons.[73,77] Among the various types of glial cells, microglia appear to be a key factor in the pain-related behavior of rats in which a chronic muscle inflammation has been induced. When the microglial activation was prevented by intrathecal (IT) administration of minocycline, the myositis-induced allodynia (**Fig. 60-6**) and reduction of locomotor activity were largely normalized.[78]

In the clinical setting, it is difficult to distinguish between peripheral and central sensitization. The above animal data suggest that both forms of sensitization usually occur together. Therefore, when a patient presents with chronic muscle tenderness, often peripheral and central sensitization have already occurred.

Conditioned Pain Modulation In contrast to CS, conditioned pain modulation (CPM; formerly known as diffuse noxious inhibitory control) is the phenomenon of one pain suppressing another pain. A painful stimulus can cause an increase in the threshold of spinal cord neurons outside the RF of the primary stimulus, which can result in decreased pain perception to a second potentially painful stimulus.[79] CPM is mediated through a spinal-medullary spinal pathway but appears to be under cortical control.[80] Conceptually, a painful stimulus could be emotionally assessed for its potential harm and then be selectively inhibited. It has been demonstrated that CPM can be impaired in the presence of chronic pain,[81] such as osteoarthritis of the hip, and can be restored to normal after a hip replacement. An impaired CPM response has also been found in fibromyalgia,[82] chronic TTH,[83] and irritable bowel syndrome[84] but not in chronic LBP.[85]

Suboptimal CPM was found to be associated with an increased chance of developing chronic postthoracotomy pain.[86] Therefore, in the future, measurement of CPM could be found to be a useful factor in predicting persistent postprocedure pain.

Clinical Applications Persistent tenderness occurs in muscles whose neurochemical and contractile apparatus is altered. Two common reasons for chronic muscle tenderness are TrPs and FMS (see later discussion). TrPs are tender nodules in the muscle and its attachments with altered neurochemistry that facilitates sensitization of muscle nociceptors. Sensitized nociceptors in the periphery stimulate nociceptive neurons in the dorsal horn and may cause central sensitization. Fibromyalgia, in contrast, is thought to be caused by an altered processing of nociceptive information in the CNS. One possible mechanism is a dysfunction in central pain-modulating pathways, resulting in lowered pain threshold to noxious stimuli with the associated phenomenon of tender points (TPs) in 11 of 18 areas. However, recent studies have shown

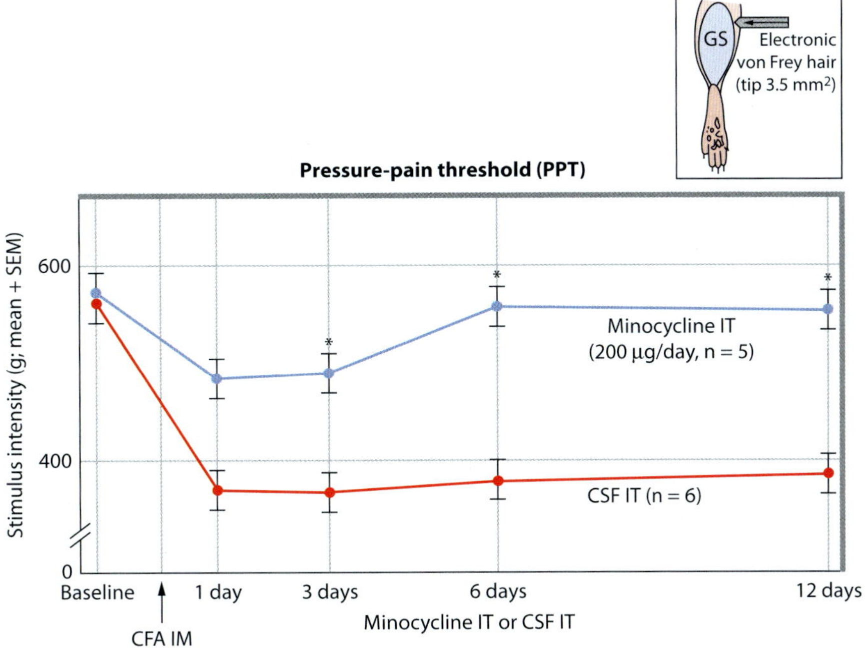

FIGURE 60-6. Effect of a microglia block on the myositis-induced reduction of the pressure-pain threshold (PPT). The PPT was determined by applying pressure to the gastrocnemius-soleus (GS) muscle with an electronic von Frey hair (inset in the upper right). The pressure was increased until a withdrawal reaction of the hindlimb occurred. The mean intensity of pressure that led to withdrawal was defined as PPT. Red line and data points, Animals in which a myositis had been induced by an intramuscular injection of complete Freund's adjuvant (CFA IM; upward arrow). The rats received artificial cerebrospinal fluid (CSF) but no microglia block (control). Blue line and data points, Myositis rats treated with intrathecal (IT) minocycline, a drug that blocks the activation of microglia cells. The drugs were administered continuously through an IT catheter connected to an implanted osmotic pump. Note that in the minocycline-treated animals, the PPT was largely normal 6 and 12 days after onset of the treatment, although the GS muscle was inflamed. Asterisks indicate statistically significant differences between untreated myositis animals and myositis animals treated with minocycline; $^*P < 0.05$. (Modified after Chacur et al.[78])

the importance of peripheral pain generators in the genesis of FMS symptoms.[87]

Digital palpation is generally used to determine tenderness, but its use presents two major problems. First, varying amounts of pressure by the examiner diminish the reliability of the examination and contribute to poor interrater reliability. Use of pressure-recording devices may improve the accuracy of the amount of applied pressure necessary to elicit discomfort in the patient.[88–90] Structured training programs to teach palpation skills may increase interrater reliability in the identification of TPs and TrPs, but the results are inconsistent.[91] Second, palpation to elicit a subjective experience of pain is often performed on a sedentary muscle, but most functional muscle pain is experienced with activity rather than rest. Therefore, an examination of a resting muscle is likely to be less accurate in determining the muscle that is the source of the pain, frequently identifying a referred muscle pain, compared with an examination that is more consistent with a patient's experience, namely, muscle movement[92,93] causing pain (movement or muscle allodynia).

Pain During Contractions Sensitized muscle nociceptors are excited at a lower than normal threshold, producing pain with everyday movement (muscle or mechanical allodynia), which is the usual clinical presentation of patients with painful muscles (vs. rest pain). Electrical stimulation has been reported to be more accurate than palpation in determining if a specific muscle is a source of regional pain.[92] Multiple mechanisms in the muscle and surrounding tissue contribute to the experience of pain. The entire muscle may be involved in pain production, not just TrPs, which are found in the muscle attachments as well as the muscle proper[94] (see later for a discussion of TrPs). Electrical stimulation of a muscle to induce contraction is thought to cause pain by two mechanisms. First is traction on the sensitized nociceptors in the entheses. As pointed out earlier, the peritendineum has been found to have a particularly dense innervation with free nerve endings, including nociceptive ones. A persistent pull at the entheses by a shortened or overloaded muscle or one harboring a TrP probably releases sensitizing substances (a mechanical tissue lesion is generally assumed to be associated with a sterile inflammation caused by sensitizing substances[73]). Second is deformation of the nociceptors in the muscle TrPs. Nociceptors in a TrP are likely to be sensitized because in the TrP, the concentration of sensitizing substances is high.[95] Because of their low mechanical threshold, sensitized nociceptors respond to light deformation of the muscle. The evaluation assumes that if pain is produced by minimal physical contraction of the muscle along its entirety from origin to insertion and not in adjacent suspected muscles, it is the putative source of pain and a target of treatment.[94] In addition, if pain is produced initially but is gone with continued stimulation, it is assumed that the muscle in question is stiff or tense and would respond, as it just did to conservative measures, such as neuromuscular stimulation, to eliminate the cause of pain.

Restricted Range of Motion Muscles that are painful during normal activities typically have diminished flexibility. Muscle flexibility is measured as a function of joint movement. Restrictions in motion can be the result of articular pathology (capsule, bone, ligaments, cartilage), nerve, or muscle–tendon dysfunction. In the absence of articular and nerve dysfunction as causes of pain, active range of motion assessment may reveal the possible source to be tension or stiffness in the related muscles. Other causes are painful alteration of the entheses by persistent muscle pull at the insertion zone or central inhibition of the α-motoneurons supplying the muscles (see discussion later in the chapter).

Simple tests that can be incorporated into the physical examination are, for the lower body, straight leg raising for hamstrings, finger to floor touch with knees locked for the low back and hamstrings, and assessment of the symmetry of the position of the right versus the left knee when one leg is crossed over the other to gauge the stiffness of the hip rotator muscles. For the upper body, tests include forward flexion and abduction of the extended arm and functional internal and external rotation of the shoulder by measuring asymmetry in touching the upper back from above and below (see Fig. 60-10). Findings of stiffness suggest muscle–tendon dysfunction; possible sources of current pain; and in some cases, predictors of pain in the course of physically demanding activity. For example, deficits in functional (scapular–humeral or scapular–thoracic) internal rotation in a patient with shoulder pain suggest that the examiner may find tenderness in the infraspinatus, teres major, or rhomboid muscles; increasing hamstring flexibility in army recruits appears to decrease the incidence of overuse lower extremity injuries;[96] and increased tightness in the hamstrings or quadriceps in elite athletes was associated with an increase in lower extremity muscle injuries.[97]

Weakness Muscle weakness must be differentiated from neurogenic weakness associated with nerve compression or dysfunction. Painful muscles are frequently found to be weakened on muscle strength testing. It is assumed that the inability to perform a maximal contraction protects the "injured" muscle from further harm. Psychological distress also contributes to weakness.[98] The main mechanism underlying the weakness probably is the central inhibition of the α-motoneurons supplying the painful muscles. Because of impaired muscle coordination, weakness may result in damaged joints and thus form a source of additional pain. As early as 1984, Stokes and Young put forward a "vicious cycle" hypothesis of arthrogenous weakness describing reflex inhibition of muscles by joint input.[99] Elimination of the pain in the joint restores normal strength. Weakness over time may also be a function of endurance,[100] and rest in this case will restore strength.

Diminished muscle strength is typically assumed in clinical discussions of common pain syndromes such as LBP (i.e., core weakness), leading to the conclusion that core strengthening exercises would be helpful.[101] However, the construct validity and treatment protocols for core strengthening programs have been questioned.[102] Various nonspecific exercises have been associated with long-term improvement in patients with nonspecific low back pain (NSLBP).[103,104] The absence of subgroupings of patients[105] based on psychosocial variables and specific assessments for level of conditioning (strength and flexibility) may contribute to the failure to find any one exercise protocol superior to another. The muscle fasciae may also be a possible source of nociceptive stimuli resulting in NSLBP.[106]

The clinician will generally not have equipment to measure the strength of postural muscles. Norman J. Marcus uses the KW test, which is a simple means to test for minimal muscle strength and flexibility of key postural trunk muscles.[107] In a large uncontrolled study, elimination of the deficiencies was correlated with improvement in LBP.[108] This is in contrast to a February 2011 Cochrane review showing no relationship between a positive clinical outcome and the putative target of the exercise for chronic NSLBP.[109]

Spasm and Cramp Involuntary long-lasting contraction of striated muscle accompanied by increased electromyography (EMG) activity is defined as spasm, which may or may not be associated with pain. Cramps are brief, self-limiting, and generally painful contractions of a muscle or muscle group, also accompanied by increased EMG activity.

Muscle spasm is often misunderstood because of (1) prior incorrect explanations of its pathophysiology and (2) other conditions that present clinical similarities to spasm. The classical understanding of the pain–spasm–pain cycle has been disproved. Although spasm, present for a long enough time, may result in muscle ischemia and pain, the pain does not in turn produce muscle contraction. On the contrary, painful muscles typically show diminished or absent EMG activity, but an antagonistic muscle typically shows increased EMG activity.[34] This phenomenon is thought to limit movement in an injured region to prevent further damage and facilitate healing.

The pain–spasm–pain concept states that the input from muscle nociceptors excites the homonymous α-motoneurons, causing a tonic (ischemic) contraction of the painful muscle. The ischemic contraction is painful and activates muscle nociceptors, which in turn excite the α-motorneurons.[110] However, in clinical experiments on myofascial LBP, the low back muscle activity was reduced in the phase associated with normally high EMG activity.[111] This finding speaks in favor of an inhibition, rather than activation, of homonymous α-motoneurons. γ-Motoneuron activity was likewise not facilitated during nociceptive input from muscle.[112] Thus, the pain–spasm–pain hypothesis is not supported by recent experimental findings and has to be considered a misconception.

To date, the pain-adaptation model of Lund and colleagues[113] has largely replaced the pain–spasm–pain vicious cycle. The model predicts decreased muscle activity in agonistic contraction phases and increased muscle activity in antagonistic phases of a painful muscle (i.e., contraction to inhibit motion). Collectively, the recent data show that a muscle spasm is not caused by a painful lesion in that muscle but by a lesion somewhere else. The true source of pain may be located in another muscle, a joint that is moved by the muscle, an inflamed nerve, or an internal organ, helping explain the frequent failure to obtain long-term benefit from injections into a muscle with painful spasm. The rigid abdomen that accompanies an inflamed appendix is an example of a spasm caused by a painful internal organ. The examiner has to find the original source of pain; otherwise, the treatment will not be successful.

Physical examination may detect a hardened, stiffened muscle. This may be the result of inappropriate muscle contraction (tension) or neurogenic involuntary muscle contraction (spasm), both associated with increased EMG activity. Tension may respond to a variety of biobehavioral approaches.[114–116] Hardened muscles may also be the result of increases in muscle tone or decreases in elasticity (from stiffness, contractures, or myofascial TrPs) that occur without accompanying increases in EMG activity, presenting a diagnostic and subsequently a treatment challenge. The absence of an animal model to study the various conditions associated with increases in muscle hardness and a testable pathophysiological mechanism further challenges our understanding and interferes in the development of effective treatment. A recent study suggests that an animal model may be possible for FMS.[117]

Because multiple overlapping mechanisms can contribute to spasm-like regional pain, it is understandable that a wide variety of pharmacologic interventions are thought to be possibly effective with as yet no demonstrated superiority between classes of medication[118,119] and no clear evidence of effectiveness for injection and denervation procedures for back pain thought to be related to painful muscles.[120]

Cramps Although cramps generally occur after age 60 years, they have also been observed in young exercisers.[121] In elderly adults, they most often occur at night and involve the lower extremities. Movement of the painful part generally quickly diminishes and then eliminates the cramp. Cramps may be the result of a variety of neurologic diseases, including amyotrophic lateral sclerosis.[122] The majority are from unknown causes but are thought to involve the spinal α-motoneuron, which appears to have a lowered electrical stimulation threshold frequency to produce cramping.[123] Two other possible mechanisms for the cramp pain are (1) not the whole muscle but only parts of it contract at the transition zone between cramping and inactive muscle parts (sheering forces may excite nociceptors), and (2) motor and nociceptive fibers are entrapped in the contracting muscle. The compressed motor fibers maintain the cramp, and the nociceptive fibers elicit pain.

Quinine has been the drug of choice for nonspecific cramping, but the U.S. Food and Drug Administration banned its use for anything but the treatment of malaria because of concerns about serious albeit nonfatal side effects. Comparisons of quinine with other possible treatments still favor quinine.[124] Nonpharmacologic treatments have not been found to be effective,[125] and a recent Cochrane review[126] opines that quinine is still the treatment of choice despite the chance of side effects.

Pain Affects Muscle Function and Patterns of Coordination Painful muscles and joints affect our ability to perform tasks. Maximal effort, ability to sustain the effort, and coordinated movement are all detrimentally affected by pain. As a corollary, some physical activities can produce muscle pain.

Altered patterns of muscle activity may precede or follow the appearance of regional muscle pain (see later discussion). Patients have a decrease of the maximal voluntary contraction of a painful muscle and a variety of changes in the static (contraction without movement), resting, and dynamic activity level of regionally painful muscles compared with normal control participants. Exploring the mechanisms of these alterations may facilitate effective treatment.

Muscle activity may produce movement through a shortening muscle contraction (concentric contraction, e.g., quadriceps contraction going up stairs) or by a lengthening contraction (eccentric contraction, e.g., quadriceps contraction going down stairs). It is actually more demanding of our muscles to go down than upstairs. Prolonged eccentric contractions are often followed by delayed-onset muscle soreness (DOMS) with the pain peaking 1 or 2 days after the exercise.

When a painful muscle is activated, decreased activity in the agonist phase and increased activity in the antagonist phase occur.[113] Such changes reduce the ability of the muscle to produce maximum contractions. It also leads to recruitment of adjacent muscles to substitute for the reduced capacity of the muscle proper to the task. The changes in muscle activation may be adaptive to promote healing by minimizing the work of the painful muscle but may also lead to additional and ongoing pain by using muscles that are inappropriate for a task and creating suboptimal conditions for joint movement and stability.[127]

CHANGED PATTERN OF LOCOMOTION

IMPACT OF MUSCLE PAIN ON LOCOMOTION

The physiologic basis of the influence of muscle pain on locomotion is related to the synaptic connections between (nociceptive) group III and IV muscle afferents and the α-motoneurons in the ventral horn.[128,129] Normally, the activity in the many thousands of synapses on the surface of a single α-motoneuron is predominantly inhibitory, and as such, the motor unit supplied by the neuron is silent (i.e., a normal resting muscle has no EMG activity).

ELECTROMYOGRAPHIC ACTIVITY OF A RESTING PAINFUL MUSCLE

In patients with myofascial pain, both increased and unchanged resting EMG activities have been found. In fibromyalgia, Elert et al.[130] observed an increase in the resting EMG activity. The same finding was reported in temporomandibular pain,[131] neck pain,[132] and LBP.[133,134] DOMS can occur with EMG activity at rest[135] or without any EMG activity.[136,137]

Thus, the overall evidence for increased resting EMG activity in humans during muscle pain is weak. Rather, there is an inhibition of α-motoneurons, which is partly attributable to a facilitated homonymous recurrent inhibition during experimental muscle pain.[138]

However, in animal experiments on masticatory muscles, there was an increase in EMG activity during painful stimulation.[139] In these studies, the jaw-opening muscles showed the strongest activity. These findings cannot be transferred to limb muscles because the central wiring of the masticatory muscles differs from that of muscles supplied by spinal nerves. In the masticatory muscles, opening of the jaw is a protective pain reflex as is the reduced activity in painful limbs.

INFLUENCE OF MUSCLE PAIN ON STATIC CONTRACTIONS

During acute experimental muscle pain, the MVC is significantly lower than in control conditions.[140–142] Likewise, in localized clinical pain conditions such as lateral epicondylalgia, reduced MVC is also found in the sore arm.[143] In fibromyalgia, the reduction in strength is assumed to be caused by impaired central activation of motor units. In these patients, when the ulnar nerve is supramaximally stimulated, there is no reduced MVC of the adductor pollicis muscle.[144] In addition to reduced MVC, patients with muscle pain exhibit a decreased endurance during submaximal contractions.[145,146]

It is worth noting that during static contractions, muscle pain decreases not only the activity of the painful muscle but also that of synergistic muscles.[147,148] Because of the inhibition of the painful muscle, the required force can be achieved only by a changed muscle recruitment pattern and eventual overload of otherwise nonpainful muscles. Spinal motoneurons as well as motor cortex motoneurons may be inhibited by nociceptive input from muscle.[149]

MUSCLE PAIN AND DYNAMIC MUSCLE ACTIVITY

Experimental and clinical low back muscle pain influence muscle activity during gait. Such an influence was found in recordings of the activity of low back muscles on a treadmill. Muscle activity was increased in phases during which there is normally no EMG activity, and there was no or decreased activity in movement phases when pain-free subjects exhibited strong EMG activity.[150] Moreover, when pain is induced in the low back muscles, the feedforward response of the abdominal muscles is reduced. This effect may impair spinal stability.[151]

Muscle pain can also have a strong impact on joints, particularly in the legs. Gait analyses during experimental pain in the vastus medialis muscle showed that the pain resulted in impaired knee joint control and joint instability during walking.[152] The impaired joint control may render the knee joint prone to injury and may perpetuate the chronicity of musculoskeletal pain.

FEAR THAT MOVEMENT WILL BE HARMFUL

Kinesiophobia, defined by Kori et al. as "an excessive, irrational, and debilitating fear of physical movement and activity resulting from a feeling of vulnerability to painful injury or re-injury,"[153] is a major impediment to recovery in patients with persistent pain.[154–156] Patients equate "hurt" with "harm" and avoid fear-producing activities.[157] This affects a patient's capacity to resume social activities after an injury[158] as well as the ability to maximally rehabilitate after surgeries.[159] It has been shown that in patients with negative beliefs about movement and exercise, even the thought of a specific movement can produce pain and swelling.[160]

POSTURE

Posture, defined as the position or bearing of the body, whether characteristic or assumed for a special purpose when deviating from a theoretically healthy stance, has been thought to be a result of and a contributing factor to muscle pain.[161–163] Experimentally induced pain in the muscles surrounding the knee alters postural stability and may be associated with an increased likelihood of falling.[164] Awkward postures are a factor in work-related back, neck, and temporomandibular joint pain.[165,166] Postural changes, such as those observed in patients with an "antalgic" gait, are minimized with programs encouraging movement and use of the painful part.[158,167,168] Based on assuming a relationship between posture and pain, it is surprising that a systematic review of adults and a longitudinal study of children and adolescents did not find any association between posture and the occurrence of LBP,[169,170] and reviews of workplace interventions to diminish neck pain found no evidence of effectiveness on neck pain or sickness absence.[171] Postural dysfunction appears to be related to multiple factors. Inactivity in adolescents was found to be associated with poor posture and the report of LBP.[172] LBP inhibits anticipatory muscle contractions mediated through the anterior cortex.[173,174] Psychosocial factors may be associated with the production of muscle tension patterns resulting in postural changes and pain.[83,175–178] Because no standard of care exists for the physical and psychological examination to describe the patient in pain, identify painful muscles, or provide an accepted exercise routine, it is not surprising that no clear evidence has yet emerged supporting the widespread use of specific interventions to promote healthy postures.

OCCUPATIONAL MUSCLE PAIN (CHRONIC WORK-RELATED MYALGIA, REPETITIVE STRAIN INJURY)

Work-related myalgias (WRMs) contribute to loss in productive work time. In a 2002 U.S. study of more than 20,000 workers, 13% experienced pain-related reduced productivity at an estimated value of $61 billion,[179] representing the largest category of work-related illness in the United States, the Nordic countries, and Japan and accounting for the largest number of work absences and disabilities in the United States, Canada, Finland, Sweden, and England.[180,181]

Physical factors include (1) high-intensity contractions to address jobs requiring high degrees of muscle strength; (2) continuous demands for output with minimal ability to rest, relax, and stretch fatigued muscles; (3) awkward posturing resulting in sustained muscle contraction; and (4) tasks requiring fine motor skills that rely on the coactivation of muscles to stabilize the extremity.[182] Psychological factors are related to both the cognitive demands of the job and the emotional experience working in a particular job setting, both contributing to psychosocial tension and stress and resulting in myalgia-related physiologic effects.

OVERLOAD RELATED TO JOB DEMANDS

STRENUOUS WORK

Overload, subjecting muscle fibers to forces beyond their capacity, can produce pain and damage. This typically occurs in physically demanding jobs in industries such as manufacturing, mining, and agriculture. The muscles of a worker with the strength to manage most job demands may become strained in the event of the need to lift a heavier than usual object or with an awkward movement. A worker is best protected by being able to lift as much as 100% more than is typically demanded by the job task. But muscle strength alone is not sufficient to protect against pain and injuries. In relationship to back pain, the concept that strengthening (core strengthening) certain weakened deep paraspinal muscles could diminish or eliminate back pain has been challenged.[102,183] Repetitive demands on strong muscles without sufficient recovery time can produce muscle fatigue, dysfunction, and pain.

MONOTONOUS WORK AT A LOW WORKLOAD

Workers who perform seemingly nonstrenuous activity may develop muscle pain. Jobs that require repetitious muscle movement in a small range may be associated with a higher incidence of muscle pain and spasm. Hägg[184] observed that all muscle fibers do not contract at the same time. Some fibers may be recruited, and others in the same muscle are quiescent. At a low workload, muscle contraction typically involves recruitment of the type Ia muscle fibers first,[185] and these fibers are also the last to be derecruited, thus overworking the Ia fibers and possibly producing fatigue, dysfunction, and pain. At the suggestion of a colleague Mats Bjurvald, Hägg named his theory the *Cinderella hypothesis*.

NONSPECIFIC LOW BACK PAIN

Nonspecific low back pain is the most costly chronic pain condition facing our health care system.[186] Despite advances in our understanding of pain mechanisms and various treatments, we remain challenged by patients with persistent back pain. The pain generator remains controversial, frequently chosen on the basis of clinician's specialty and mode of practice.[187,188] Because muscle and other soft tissue is presumed to frequently account for NSLBP, it is surprising that the evaluation and treatment of muscular causes of LBP are not addressed in the American or European guidelines.[189,190]

Of the wide variety of treatments commonly used, the most promising seem to be cognitive-behavioral interventions encouraging activity and exercise. Almost all other interventions have not demonstrated clear effectiveness when analyzed in rigorous, systematic reviews.[172,189-209] Of all the putative pain generators that might respond to exercise—remaining active, massage, and relaxation approaches—logic suggests that muscle is a major target of these interventions and thus a source of pain. However, translating the concept of muscle-related NSLBP to successful treatment interventions has been a challenge. Attempts to incorporate proper ergonomic principles to proactively address musculoskeletal disorders in the workplace have not been effective.[210] Even the consensus that remaining active and at work is beneficial for patients with NSLBP has not dissuaded most physicians from advising patients not to work.[211]

Exercise, defined as a "series of movements to promote good physical health," allows almost any activity to be defined as an exercise protocol. Indeed, a systematic review has concluded that various nonspecific exercises have produced long-term results in patients with NSLBP.[212] However, idiosyncratic provision of exercise protocols without patient subclassification may confound outcome data and eliminate the possibility of meta-analyses. Systematic reviews of the effects of published exercise interventions[213,214] revealed that although most were statistically significant, many were not clinically meaningful.[9] A much needed head-to-head study is currently under way to compare the effects of two different exercise protocols.[215]

A suggested reason for the inability to show effectiveness in many exercise programs is the general absence of subgroups of patients[216] based on psychosocial variables and specific assessments for level of conditioning (strength and flexibility). Conversely, another hypothesis is that the effects of exercise are more related to central phenomena, such as improvement in coordination and reductions in kinesiophobia, than to any specific exercise effect.[217]

Nonspecific LBP is assumed to originate in the soft tissues of the low back such as muscles, ligaments, and fascia.[218] Back muscles are relatively well established as a source of NSLBP, for instance, when they harbor myofascial TrPs[219] (see discussion later in the chapter). In contrast, the fascia have attracted much less interest.

THE THORACOLUMBAR FASCIA AS A POSSIBLE CAUSE OF NONSPECIFIC LOW BACK PAIN

The thoracolumbar fascia (TLF) is the largest fascia of the low back and wraps the genuine back muscles with a posterior and anterior lamina. It thus forms a sheath around the muscles which reduces friction during movements. Its role in the biomechanics of the lumbar spine is well established. The TLF transfers loads among the arm, spine, pelvis, and lower limbs. Actually, it links the legs and arms crosswise; that is, it is part of a biomechanical chain between the fascia latae of the leg and the fascia of the contralateral latissimus dorsi muscle that attaches to the upper arm. Moreover, it is the insertion site for the broad abdominal muscles and thus further stabilizes the trunk. The TLF contains myofibroblasts and therefore has contractile properties.[220] It is a plastic structure and adjusts to altered tensions and forces that occur during long-lasting changes in posture and movement patterns.

FASCIA INNERVATION AND NEURONAL DATA PROCESSING OF INPUT FROM THE FASCIA

Little information is available about a possible sensory role of the TLF, particularly in NSLBP. If it really performs such a function, the TLF should have a dense innervation with sensory fibers, including nociceptors. However, the results of existing studies are inconsistent and partly contradictory. The group of Bednar and colleagues[221] did not find any sensory end organs in the TLF of patients with LBP and stated that in these patients, the fascia was "deficiently innervated." In contrast, another group[222] demonstrated that the TLF is innervated. A recent study on the innervation of the fascia in rats and humans presented evidence for a possible contribution of the TLF to NSLBP.[223] The main histologic findings were that (1) the fascia is densely innervated (**Fig. 60-7**); (2) it exhibits SP-containing free nerve endings, which are assumed to be nociceptors; and (3) it has an abundant innervation with efferent sympathetic nerve endings, accounting for more than 30% of all nerve fibers of the fascia. The purpose of this dense innervation with sympathetic fibers is obscure. Because the thickest layer of the fascia is not supplied by blood vessels, these fibers are probably not vasoconstrictors. Possibly, the sympathetic fibers modulate pain sensations from the fascia[224] and may explain why some patients with NSLBP report that their pain is worse when they are under psychological stress.

Sensory endings in fascia have been found in the iliolumbar ligament[225] and the fascia of the arm[226] in addition to the TLF.

In another study of the group of Siegfried Mense,[106] the electrical activity of spinal neurons processing input from sensory endings in the

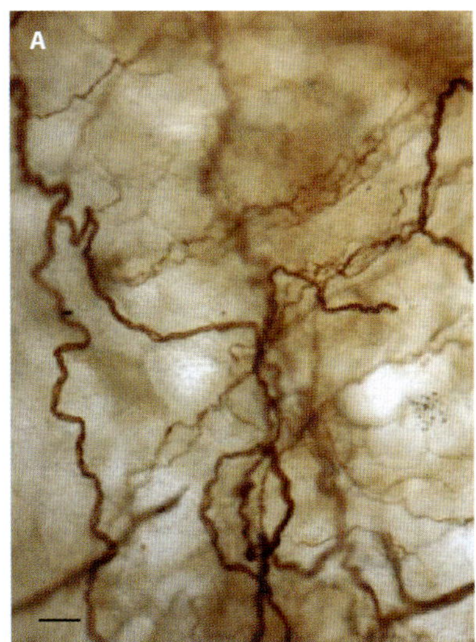

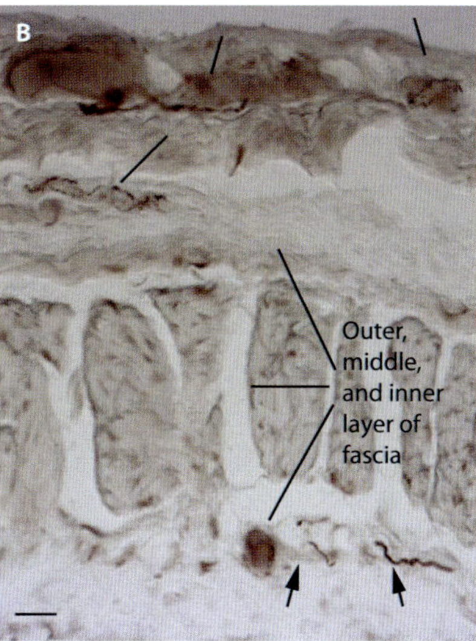

FIGURE 60-7. Innervation of the thoracolumbar fascia of the rat. **A,** Whole-mount preparation of the fascia at the level of the vertebral body L5. The figure shows a dense network of nerve fiber bundles and single fibers, many of which outlined blood vessels (upper half of panel). The fibers were stained with antibodies to protein gene product (PGP) 9.5, which stains all fibers irrespective of their function. **B,** Cross-section in the coronal plane through the fascia at the same level as panel A. The main layer of the fascia consists of massive collagen fiber bundles (cross-sectioned) that appear as bricklike structures in the figure. On both sides, thin layers of connective tissue connect these collagen bundles to the subcutaneous tissue and underlying muscle, respectively. Nerve fibers are mainly present in the subcutaneous tissue and in the layer between the fascia and muscle. A free nerve ending is visible in the upper left of the panel (open arrow). It has a granular structure because of many axonal expansions that contain neuropeptides. Filled arrows indicate small-diameter fibers of passage.

TLF was recorded. Most neurons had no exclusive input from the fascia but showed a marked input convergence from the multifidus muscle and the skin (**Fig. 60-8**). The input from most tissues was dominated by nociceptors; that is, the neurons were excited by painful stimulation of their RFs (pinching, squeezing, injections of hypertonic saline). The neurons behaved like typical wide-dynamic range (WDR) neurons, one of the nociceptive spinal cell types. The input convergence from many tissues and receptor types of the low back may explain why the subjective nature of NSLBP is usually described as diffuse. An interesting finding was that an experimental inflammation of the multifidus muscle increased not only the proportion of neurons responding to stimulation of the inflamed muscle but also the proportion of those neurons that responded to input from the fascia.[106] This finding suggests that the fascia becomes more sensitive even if the original pain source is located in the low back muscles.

Recent human data underpin a nociceptive role of fascia tissue. For instance, DOMS in the lower leg appears to be partly attributable to nociceptors in the fascia of the anterior tibial muscle.[227] In that study, the authors made systematic injections of a painful dose of hypertonic saline into the anterior tibial muscle and the overlying tissues after induction of DOMS in that muscle. When the hypertonic solution was injected directly underneath the fascia, it caused more pain than after injection into the muscle itself. These results show that the fascia of the human anterior tibial muscle is supplied with nociceptors and that these nociceptors are probably involved in DOMS.

PAIN CAUSED BY MYOFASCIAL TRIGGER POINTS

Trigger points are considered by many clinicians to be synonymous with myofascial pain syndrome and to account for most muscle pain, but others believe them to be nonsignificant epiphenomena.[228-231] TrPs are defined as palpable tender nodules in muscles that refer pain or discomfort to adjacent or distant muscles. Treatments are varied but usually involve needle placement (dry needling), the injection of one of a number of substances into the TrP, or both.

HISTORICAL PERSPECTIVE

Kellgren was the first to demonstrate muscle pain referral with his experiments with hypertonic saline,[232-234] but Travell and Simons described

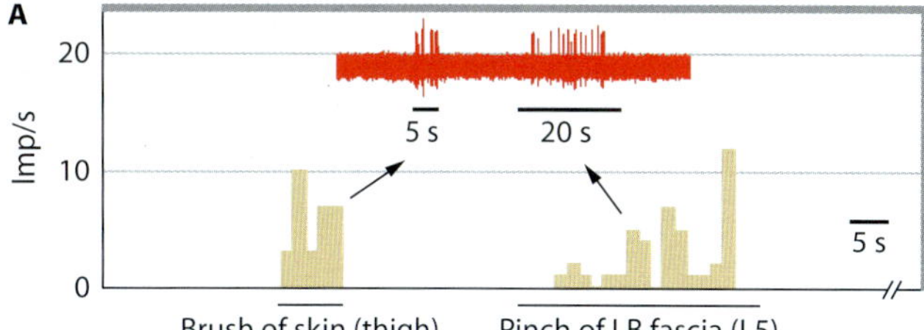

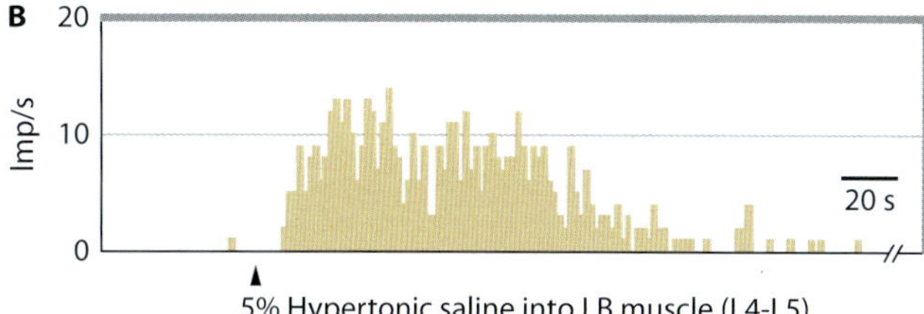

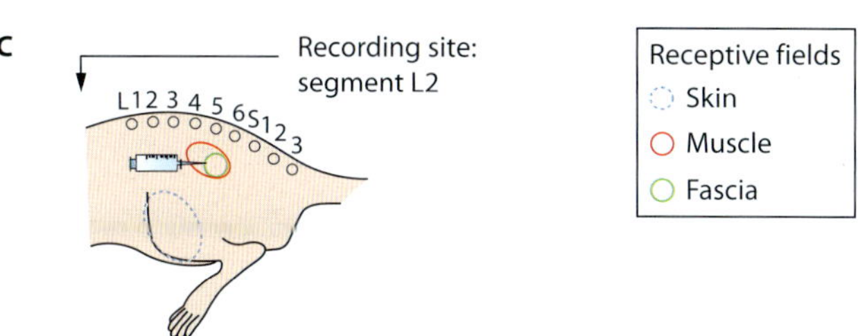

FIGURE 60-8. Electrical activity of a single dorsal horn neuron that had input from the thoracolumbar fascia and other tissues. Recording site: spinal segment L2. **A,** Response to brushing of the skin of the thigh and pinching of the fascia at the level of vertebra L5. LB, low back. **B,** Response to the injection of hypertonic saline (5%, 50 μL) into the erector spinae muscle at the level of vertebrae L4 to L5. The neuron also responded to weak deformation and noxious pressure of the same muscle (not shown). **C,** Approximate location and size of the receptive fields (RFs) of the neuron. Note the marked input convergence of this neuron from many tissues (fascia, skin, muscle) and receptor types (low-threshold mechanoreceptors and nociceptors). The neuron was dominated by input from nociceptors and behaved like a nociceptive wide-dynamic range (WDR) neuron. It may mediate pain from the soft tissues of the low back. (Modified after Taguchi et al.[106])

the typical patterns of referred pain from specific muscles.[235] Shah[236] has found biochemical alterations in the TrP that support the assumption that TrPs are a source of pain.

CURRENT HYPOTHESES OF TRIGGER POINT MORPHOLOGY AND FORMATION

Generally, the palpable myofascial TrP is assumed to consist of several contraction knots surrounded by normal muscle fibers.[237] A contraction knot is a localized (segmental) contraction of only part of an individual muscle fiber. Actually, it is a contracture in the physiological sense (i.e., a contraction of a muscle fiber without electrical activation of the endplate). Therefore, a TrP is silent in the surface EMG. One of the few good histologic figures of a contraction knot was published long ago.[238] The knot was found in the gracile muscle of a dog; it was located in a palpable TrP. The typical histologic feature of the contraction knot was a close packing of the A bands within the contracted region so that no individual A bands can be recognized. In the region of the contraction knot, the affected muscle fibers are swollen and therefore probably compress the accompanying capillaries.

It is unknown if a human TrP exhibits the same features, but evidence points in that direction. One of the few systematic studies on the morphology of human TrPs was performed by Reitinger and colleagues.[239] The biopsy specimen were obtained from fresh cadavers that still exhibited palpable TrPs. Cross-sections showed large muscle fibers, which may have represented contraction knots. In electron microscopic sections, the I-band configuration was missing, which likewise indicates a contraction. The findings indicate that the cross-sectioned large muscle fibers were contracted and therefore had a greater diameter.

To date, there are no data on the TrP histology from living patients. Knowledge about the time course of TrP formation and morphologic differences between latent and active TrPs is completely missing. Large-scale open biopsies of TrPs would allow us to observe their evolution and help refine the understanding of the pathophysiological process. Therefore, the following considerations on the formation of a TrP, which are based on the minimally available scientific data, are largely hypothetical.

From clinical inspection, it appears that the first stage of TrP formation is the taut band, which often exhibits a latent TrP that exists without spontaneous pain but causes local, and sometimes referred, pain when mechanically stimulated. The next stage is the active TrP, which is spontaneously painful. Thus, there may be a sequence from the latent to the active TrP; that is, first there is a muscle lesion that does not cause pain, and then the active TrP develops.[240]

The integrated hypothesis of TrP formation was put forward by Simons[241] and later modified by Gerwin and colleagues.[242] The steps of this hypothesis are still not proven, but to date, there are no better hypotheses (**Fig. 60-9**). The formation of a TrP starts with trauma to the muscle, such as overuse, which mainly damages the endplate region of the neuromuscular junction. The damaged endplate releases excess amounts of acetylcholine (ACh), which release Ca^{++} from the sarcoplasmic reticulum and cause contraction knots in some of the muscle fibers underneath the endplate. The key factor of TrP formation and maintenance appears to be localized ischemia of the muscle, probably caused by capillary compression by the contraction knots. Ischemia is known to release BKN and other inflammatory agents and sensitize muscle nociceptors (see earlier discussion). This explains the pain and tenderness of the TrP. Using a microdialysis needle, Shah[238] has measured the concentration of inflammatory substances and H^+ ions in active and latent TrP and found significantly higher concentrations for most of these agents in active TrPs. The ischemia in the TrP is also important for maintaining the contracture because ischemia results in diminished

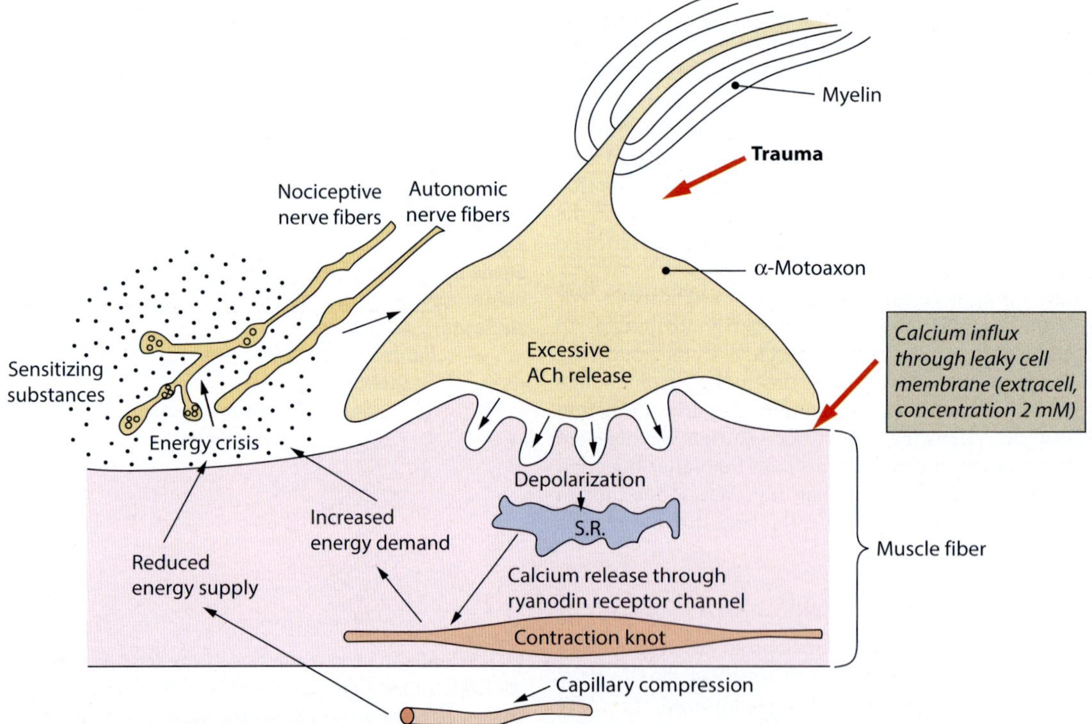

FIGURE 60-9. Integrated hypothesis of trigger point formation by Simons. The hypothesis assumes that a muscle lesion (e.g., overuse) mainly damages the presynaptic portion of the neuromuscular endplate. The result is an excessive release of acetylcholine (ACh), which causes a depolarization of the postsynaptic muscle cell membrane. This leads to the release of calcium ions from the sarcoplasmic reticulum (SR). The calcium ions produce a local contracture (the contraction knot) underneath the endplate. The contraction knot compresses capillaries, and the resulting ischemia together with an increased energy demand by the contraction knot causes an "energy crisis" associated with the release of inflammatory substances that sensitize nociceptors. This is the reason for the tenderness of a trigger point. The ACh release is under the control of autonomic (sympathetic) nerve fibers. The red arrow at the right indicates a speculative alternative mechanism for the formation of the contraction knot, namely, the influx of calcium ions from the interstitial space through lesion-induced leaks in the muscle cell membrane. The interstitial calcium concentration is more than 100 times higher than that needed for the sliding of the myosin and actin filaments. (Modified after Simons and Travell.[93])

production of ATP, which is necessary for the relaxation of the myosin and actin filaments.

There are also ways of releasing Ca^{++} from the intracellular sarcoplasmic reticulum independent of the neuromuscular junction: (1) dysfunctional ryanodine receptor calcium channels that control the release of Ca^{++} from the sarcoplasmic reticulum into the sarcoplasm[243,244] or (2) damage to the muscle cell, which produces small leaks in the membrane. Rhabdomyolysis after strenuous exercise has been described in the literature,[245] and it is conceivable that overuse of a muscle or part of a muscle damages its cell. Small leaks in the cell membrane would allow Ca^{++} ions to enter the cell and cause sliding of the actin and myosin filaments underneath the leaky membrane. The basis of these considerations is that in the interstitial fluid around the muscle cell, the Ca^{++} concentration is approximately 2 mM, but 0.01 mM is sufficient (see Fig. 60-9) for filament sliding to occur. It has to be emphasized that these hypothetical mechanisms have not yet been tested.

Even in healthy normal control participants, the region of the endplate has been found to be particularly sensitive to painful stimuli.[246] This finding suggests a high density of nociceptors in that region and may explain—besides the location of the contraction knots underneath the endplate—why in many muscles, TrP pain is worst in the endplate region.

Even with an enhanced understanding of TrP pathophysiology, clinicians' ability to identify TrPs is inconsistent.[247–252] Although the interrater reliability increases significantly with experienced versus novice clinicians, the experts' intrarater reliability curiously diminishes with repeated assessments.[253] Multiple criteria have been proposed to identify TrPs with palpation, such as finding a taut band, local tenderness,

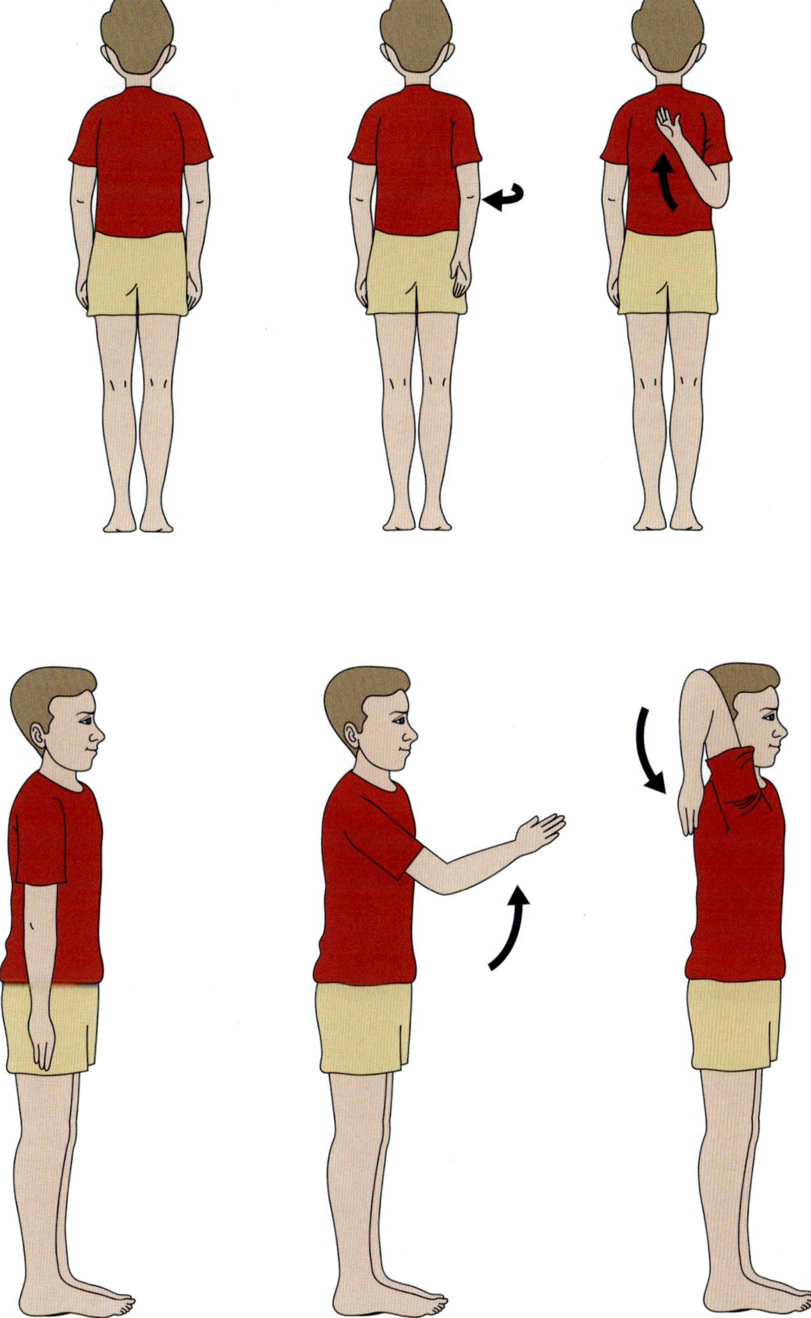

FIGURE 60-10. Assessment of shoulder functional (scapulohumeral and scapulothoracic) internal and external rotation. Compare the points of maximal excursion of the two hands reaching over the shoulder and down the back for external rotation and from below up toward the scapula for internal rotation. The differences represent the relative deficits.

patient pain recognition, pain referral, a local twitch response, and a jump sign. In addition to not being applied uniformly across studies, the interrater identification of the criteria has proved to be generally unreliable.[254] Further confounding the accurate identification of muscles harboring TrPs, Simons noted that TrPs also exist at the muscle attachment sites,[255] but the usual examination for TrPs is solely in the muscle tissue, resulting in overlooking sources of pain and targets for treatment.[94]

Various treatment protocols have been suggested to treat TrPs, including manual techniques, physical therapy modalities, and injections.[237] Trigger point injections (TPIs) are done with a variety of injectates or with none (dry needling). Use of local anesthetics versus dry needling is reasonable because it results in diminished postinjection pain.[256] Although all local anesthetics have been shown to be myotoxic (most profoundly with bupivacaine and chloroprocaine), they do not affect satellite cells. Damaged cells rarely produce clinically significant effects and generally regenerate in 4 to 6 weeks.[257,258] The cell damage from the injectate (and needling) may actually enhance the treatment effect through the elimination of dysfunctional fibers and by allowing the regeneration of normal fibrils. Although some studies suggest that there may be sustained benefit in the treatment of LBP with use of botulinum toxin or corticosteroids, systematic reviews[201,208] cannot support or reject their use. In a Cochrane review of neck pain,[259] botulinum toxin was found to be no better than saline. Considering the cost and potential risks, the routine use of botulinum toxin or corticosteroids for TrPs does not appear to be justified.

It is not surprising that with lack of agreement on criteria for diagnosis, poor interrater reliability to find TrPs, varied treatments, and the absence of any consistent postinjection protocol,[260] the outcomes for the treatment of TrPs do not rise to the level of evidence in the treatment of NSLBP (with or without sciatica).[261] To validate current approaches to assess and treat TrPs, head-to-head studies of competing methods to evaluate and treat muscle pain must be done to establish the most effective standard of care for identification of tender areas of muscles, injection techniques, injectates and their dosages, and postinjection protocols.

Two technologies to image muscles thought to harbor taut bands and TrPs have been suggested as possible means to more objectively identify the presence of pain-generating structures. Magnetic resonance elastography (MRE) allows visualization and identification of tissues with varied elasticity and has been shown to be capable of identifying taut bands that have diminished elasticity compared with normal muscle tissue. MRE appears to offer greater reliability than palpation in identifying taut bands.[262] Visualization of TrPs is more elusive, but recent studies have demonstrated the use of ultrasound in identifying TrPs.[263,264] Both of these techniques may help objectify the identification of taut bands and TrPs but have not yet been clinically tested to determine if they will improve the effectiveness of treatment for muscle pain.

Muscle pain is complicated. It is found as a sole source of common pain presentations and occurs as a result of painful phenomena in other tissue. More attention to the presence of muscle pain will facilitate refinement of our understanding of the initiation and perpetuation of common pain syndromes. It should therefore be included in our routine pain assessments and treatments. Absent a consensus opinion for addressing functional muscle pain, the below plan that incorporates many of the variables necessary to manage muscle pain is suggested by Norman J. Marcus.

Any patients with persistent pain should undergo a thorough examination of all muscles that could possibly contribute to the pain complaint.

A. Distinguish injectable muscle pain from pain related to tension, deficiency (weakness, stiffness, or both), and spasm. The KW test for strength and flexibility of key postural muscles for LBP and lower extremity pain identifies patients who are deconditioned (decreased strength and flexibility of postural muscles). Standard tests of upper body strength, along with assessment of forward elevation, abduction of the arm, and functional internal and external rotation of the shoulder (scapulohumeral and scapulothoracic motion) may find asymmetries of motion in the shoulder girdles, suggesting which muscle(s) may be involved (**Fig. 60-10**).

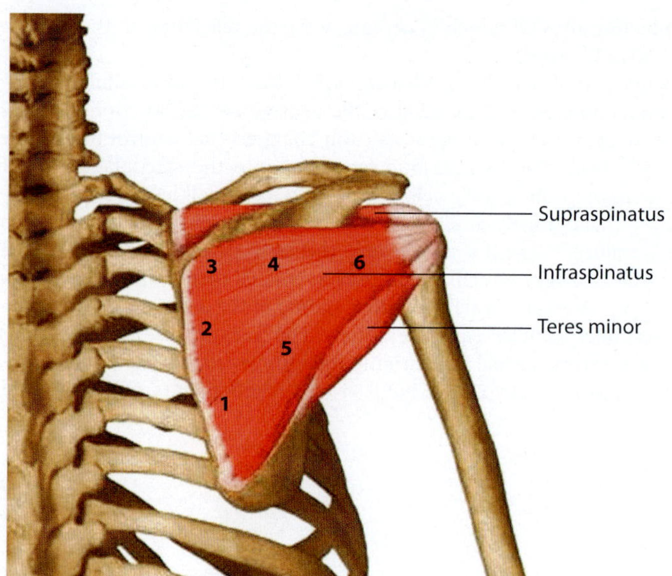

FIGURE 60-11. The numbers represent the suggested sequence of muscle tendon injections into the infraspinatus muscle.

B. Attempt to identify primary versus referred muscle pain. (Identification through muscle stimulation appears to be more accurate than palpation.[265])

C. Use a standardized exercise program to correct muscle deficiencies. Norman J. Marcus provides the Kraus exercises: 8 for the upper body and 21 for the lower body.[266]

D. Suggest conditioning exercises (i.e., all patients, if possible, gradually increase their daily walking up to 2 to 3 miles each day).

E. Marcus identifies a specific muscle as a pain source rather than a TrP, and calls the identified muscle "Muscle Pain Amenable to Injection (MPAI)" and the muscle injection is called "Muscle-Tendon Injection (MTI)" rather than a TPI. When injecting a specific muscle, pay particular attention to the entheses of the identified muscle rather than just TrPs and taut bands. Consider injecting only one muscle during a given injection session (**Fig. 60-11**).

F. If you use an injection procedure (MTI) that targets the entire muscle, 3 days of a postinjection physical therapy protocol will minimize postinjection soreness and stiffness.[267]

G. If more than one MPAI is identified and multiple treatments are planned, reassess the patient for continued presence of MPAI before injecting the next planned muscle. It is possible that changes may have taken place as a result of successful injections. These changes may be related to diminished central sensitization, resulting in the next muscle no longer being painful to manual or electrical stimulation or conversely the ability to discern a new muscle as painful after the previous, most severely painful muscle was successfully treated.

REFERENCES

1. Resnick DK, Choudhri TF, Dailey AT, et al. Guidelines for the performance of fusion procedures for degenerative disease of the lumbar spine. Part 13: injection therapies, low-back pain, and lumbar fusion. *J Neurosurg Spine*. 2005;2(6):707-715.
2. Ellman P, Shaw D. The "chronic rheumatic" and his pains; psychosomatic aspects of chronic non-articular rheumatism. *Ann Rheum Dis*. 1950;9(4):341-357.
3. Reynolds M. The development of the concept of fibrositis. *J Hist Med Allied Sci*. 1983;38(1):5-35.
4. Lange M. *Die Muskelhärten (Myogelosen): Ihre Entstehung und Heilung*. Munich: Lehmann; 1931.

5. Schade H. Untersuchungen in der Erkaltungsfrage. III: Ueber den rheumatismus, insbesondere den muskelrheumatismus (myogelose). *Munch Med Wschr*. 1921;68:418-420.
6. Simons D, Travell J. Myofascial origins of low back pain: principles of diagnosis and treatment. *Postgrad Med*. 1983;73(2):66-73.
7. Littlejohn G. Regional pain syndrome: clinical characteristics, mechanisms and management. *Rheumatology*. 2007;3(9):504-511.
8. Deyo R, Weinstein J. Low back pain. *N Engl J Med*. 2001;344(5): 363-370.
9. Rosomoff HL, Fishbain DA, Goldberg M, et al. Physical findings in patients with chronic intractable benign pain of the neck and/or back. *Pain*. 1989;37(3):279-287.
10. Van Tulder M, Becker A, Bekkering T, et al. European guidelines for the management of acute nonspecific low back pain in primary care. *Eur Spine J*. 2006;15(Suppl 2):S169-S191.
11. Feleus A, Bierma-Zeinstra SMA, Miedema HS, et al. Incidence of non-traumatic complaints of arm, neck and shoulder in general practice. *Man Ther*. 13(5):426-433.
12. Fernández-Carnero J, de la Llave-Rincón AI, Ge H, Arendt-Nielsen L. Prevalence of and referred pain from myofascial trigger points in the forearm muscles in patients with lateral epicondylalgia. *Clin J Pain*. 2007;23(4):353-360.
13. Jensen R, Olesen J. Initiating mechanisms of experimentally induced tension-type headache. *Cephalalgia*. 1996;16(3):175-182.
14. Marcus N. Pain in cancer patients unrelated to the cancer or treatment. *Cancer Investig*. 2005;23(1):84-93.
15. McBeth J, Jones K. Epidemiology of chronic musculoskeletal pain. *Best Prac Res Clin Rheumatol*. 2007;21(3):403-425.
16. Petersen S, Hägglöf BL, Bergström E. Impaired health-related quality of life in children with recurrent pain. *Pediatrics*. 2009;124(4):e759-e767.
17. Pellisé F, Balagué F, Rajmil L, et al. Prevalence of low back pain and its effect on health-related quality of life in adolescents. *Arch Pediatr Adolesc Med*. 2009;163(1):65-71.
18. Pleis J, Lucas J, Ward B. Summary health statistics for U.S. adults: National Health Interview Survey, 2008. *Vital Health Stat 10*. 2009;10(242):6-7.
19. Freburgre J, Homes G, Agans R, et al. The rising prevalence of chronic low back pain. *Arch Int Med*. 2009;169(3):251-258.
20. Juniper M, Le T, Mladsi D. The epidemiology, economic burden, and pharmacological treatment of chronic low back pain in France, Germany, Italy, Spain and the UK: a literature-based review. *Expert Opin Pharmacother*. 2009;10(16):2581-2592.
21. Hogg-Johnson S, van der Velde G, Carroll LJ, et al. The burden and determinants of neck pain in the general population: results of the Bone and Joint Decade 2000-2010 Task Force on Neck Pain and Its Associated Disorders. *Spine*. 2008;33(4 Suppl):S39-S51.
22. Pope D, Croft P, Pritchard C, Silman A. Prevalence of shoulder pain in the community: the influence of case definition. *Ann Rheum Dis*. 1997;56(5):308-312.
23. Croft P, Rigby A, Boswell R, et al. The prevalence of chronic widespread pain in the general population. *J Rheumatol*. 1993;20(4):710-713.
24. Wolfe F, Ross K, Anderson J, et al. The prevalence and characteristics of fibromyalgia in the general population. *Arthritis Rheum*. 1995;38(1):19-28.
25. Weir P, Harlan G, Nkoy F, et al. The incidence of fibromyalgia and its associated comorbidities: a population-based retrospective cohort study based on International Classification of Diseases, 9th Revision codes. *J Clin Rheumatol*. 2006;12(3):124-128.
26. Buskila D, Neumann L. The development of widespread pain after injuries. *J Musculoskelet Pain*. 2002;10:261-267.
27. Littlejohn G. Regional pain syndrome: clinical characteristics, mechanisms and management. *Nat Clin Pract Rheumatol*. 2007;3(9):504-511.
28. Graven-Nielsen T, Arendt-Nielsen L. Sensory and motor manifestations of muscle pain. *J Musculoskelet Pain*. 2008;16(1-2):93-105.
29. Koppell H, Thompson W. *Peripheral Entrapment Neuropathies*. Baltimore: Williams & Wilkins; 1963.
30. Lloyd D. Neuron patterns controlling transmission of ipsilateral hind limb reflexes in cat. *J Neurophysiol*. 1943;6:293-315.
31. Light A, Perl E. Unmyelinated afferent fibers are not only for pain anymore. *J Comp Neurol*. 2003;461(2):137-139.
32. Hoheisel U, Unger T, Mense S. Excitatory and modulatory effects of inflammatory cytokines and neurotrophins on mechanosensitive group IV muscle afferents in the rat. *Pain*. 2005;114:168-176.
33. Stacey M. Free nerve endings in skeletal muscle of the cat. *J Anat*. 1969;105:231-254.
34. Mense S, Gerwin R. *Muscle Pain: Understanding the Mechanisms*. 1st ed. Heidelberg: Springer; 2010.
35. Reinert A, Kaske A, Mense S. Inflammation-induced increase in the density of neuropeptide-immunoreactive nerve endings in rat skeletal muscle. *Exp Brain Res*. 1998;121:174-180.
36. Lawson S, Crepps B, Perl E. Relationship of substance P to afferent characteristics of dorsal root ganglion neurones in guinea-pig. *J Physiol*. 1997;505:177-191.
37. Molander C, Ygge I, Dalsgaard C. Substance P-, somatostatin-, and calcitonin gene-related peptide-like immunoreactivity and fluoride resistant acid phosphatase-activity in relation to retrogradely labeled cutaneous, muscular and visceral primary sensory neurons in the rat. *Neurosci Lett*. 1987;74:37-42.
38. O'Brien C, Woolf CJ, Fitzgerald M, et al. Differences in the chemical expression of rat primary afferent neurons which innervate skin, muscle or joint. *Neuroscience*. 1989;32(2):493-502.
39. Kow L, Pfaff D. Neuromodulatory actions of peptides. *Annu Rev Pharmacol Toxicol*. 1988;28:163-188.
40. Mense S. Muscle nociceptors and their neurochemistry. In: Schmidt R, Willis W, eds. *Encyclopedic Reference of Pain*. Berlin, Heidelberg: Springer; 2007.
41. Light AR, Hughen RW, Zhang J, et al. Dorsal root ganglion neurons innervating skeletal muscle respond to physiological combinations of protons, ATP, and lactate mediated by ASIC, P2X, and TRPV1. *J Neurophysiol*. 2008;100(3):1184-1201.
42. Caterina M, Julius D. The vanilloid receptor: a molecular gateway to the pain pathway. *Annu Rev Neurosci*. 2001;24:487-517.
43. Reeh P, Kress M. Molecular physiology of proton transduction in nociceptors. *Curr Opin Pharmacol*. 2001;1:45-51.
44. Marchettini P, Simone D, Caputi G, Ochoa J. Pain from excitation of identified muscle nociceptors in humans. *Brain Res*. 1996;740:109-116.
45. Liedtke W. TRPV4 plays an evolutionary conserved role in the transduction of osmotic and mechanical stimuli in live animals. *J Physiol*. 2005;567:53-58.
46. Walder R, Gautam M, Wilson S, et al. Selective targeting of ASIC3 using artificial miRNAs inhibits primary and secondary hyperalgesia after muscle inflammation. *Pain*. 2011;152(10):2348-2356.
47. Immke D, McCleskey E. Protons open acid-sensing channels by catalyzing relief of Ca2+ blockade. *Neuron*. 2003;37:75-84.
48. Sluka K, Kalra A, Moore S. Unilateral intramuscular injections of acidic saline produce a bilateral long-lasting hyperalgesia. *Muscle Nerve*. 2001;24:37-46.

49. Burnstock G. Physiology and pathophysiology of purinergic neurotransmission. *Physiol Rev*. 2007;87:659-797.

50. Cook S, McCleskey E. Cell damage excites nociceptors through release of cytosolic ATP. *Pain*. 2002;95:41-47.

51. Stewart LC, Deslauriers R, Kupriyanov VV. Relationships between cytosolic [ATP], [ATP]/[ADP] and ionic fluxes in the perfused rat heart: a 31P, 23Na and 87Rb NMR study. *J Mol Cell Cardiol*. 1994;26(10):1377-1392.

52. Mork H, Ashina M, Bendtsen L, et al. Experimental muscle pain and tenderness following infusion of endogenous substances in humans. *Eur J Pain*. 2003;7(2):145-153.

53. Caterina M, David J. Sense and specificity: a molecular identity for nociceptors. *Curr Opin Neurobiol*. 1999;9:525-530.

54. Pezet S, McMahon S. Neurotrophins: mediators and modulators of pain. *Annu Rev Neurosci*. 2006;29:507-538.

55. Perkins M, Kelly D. Induction of bradykinin-B1 receptors in vivo in a model of ultra-violet irradiation-induced thermal hyperalgesia in the rat. *Br J Pharmacol*. 1993;110:1441-1444.

56. Mense S. Sensitization of group IV muscle receptors to bradykinin by 5-hydroxytryptamine and prostaglandin E2. *Brain Res*. 1981;225:95-105.

57. Cairns B, Svensson P, Wang K, et al. Ketamine attenuates glutamate-induced mechanical sensitization of the masseter muscle in human males. *Exp Brain Res*. 2006;169:467-472.

58. Cairns BE, Hu JW, Arendt-Nielsen L, et al. Sex-related differences in human pain and rat afferent discharge evoked by injection of glutamate into the masseter muscle. *J Neurophysiol*. 2001;86(2):782-791.

59. Bennell K, Wee E, Crossley K, et al. Effects of experimentally-induced anterior knee pain on knee joint position sense in healthy individuals. *J Orthop Res*. 2005;23(1):46-53.

60. Tegeder I, Zimmermann J, Meller ST, Geisslinger G. Release of algesic substances in human experimental muscle pain. *Inflamm Res*. 2002;51(8):393-402.

61. Kellgren J. Observations on referred pain arising from muscle. *Clin Sci*. 1938;3:175-190.

62. Graven-Nielsen T. Fundamentals of muscle pain, referred pain and deep tissue hyperalgesia. *Scand J Rheumatol*. 2006;35:1-43.

63. Zhang X, Chen J, Faltynek C, et al. Transient receptor potential A1 mediates an osmotically activated ion channel. *Eur J Neurosci*. 2008;27:605-611.

64. Cesare P, McNaughton P. Peripheral pain mechanisms. *Curr Opin Neurobiol*. 1997;7:493-499.

65. Mense S, Meyer H. Bradykinin-induced modulation of the response behaviour of different types of feline group III and IV muscle receptors. *J Physiol*. 1988;398:49-63.

66. Mann M, Dong X, Svensson P. Influence of intramuscular nerve growth factor injection on the response properties of rat masseter muscle afferent fibers. *J Orofac Pain*. 2006;20:325-336.

67. Hakim A, Dong X, Cairns B. TNFα mechanically sensitizes masseter muscle nociceptors by increasing prostaglandin E2 levels. *J Neurophysiol*. 2011;105:154-161.

68. Jensen K, Tuxen C, Pedersenbjergaard U, et al. Pain and tenderness in human temporal muscle induced by bradykinin and 5-hydroxytryptamine. *Peptides*. 1990;11(6):1127-1132.

69. Hoheisel U, Mense S, Simons DG, Yu XM. Appearance of new receptive-fields in rat dorsal horn neurons following noxious-stimulation of skeletal-muscle—a model for referral of muscle pain. *Neurosci Lett*. 1993;153(1):9-12.

70. Wall P. The presence of ineffective synapses and circumstances which unmask them. *Phil Trans R Soc Lond B*. 1977;278:361-372.

71. Hoheisel U, Koch K, Mense S. Functional reorganization in the rat dorsal horn during an experimental myositis. *Pain*. 1994;59:111-118.

72. Millan M. The induction of pain: an integrative review. *Prog Neurobiol*. 1999;57:1-164.

73. Marchand F, Perretti M, McMahon S. Role of the immune system in chronic pain. *Nat Rev Neurosci*. 2005;6:521-532.

74. Hoheisel U, Unger T, Mense S. Sensitization of rat dorsal horn neurons by NGF-induced subthreshold potentials and low-frequency activation. A study employing intracellular recordings in vivo. *Brain Res*. 2007;1169:34-43.

75. Svensson P, Cairns BE, Wang K, Arendt-Nielsen L. Injection of nerve growth factor into human masseter muscle evokes long-lasting mechanical allodynia and hyperalgesia. *Pain*. 2003;104(1-2):241-247.

76. Watkins L, Milligan E, Maier S. Spinal cord glia: new players in pain. *Pain*. 2001;93(3):201-205.

77. Hunt S, Mantyh P. The molecular dynamics of pain control. *Nat Rev Neurosci*. 2001;2:83-91.

78. Chacur M, Lambertz D, Hoheisel U, Mense S. Role of spinal microglia in myositis-induced central sensitisation: an immunohistochemical and behavioural study in rats. *Eur J Pain*. 2009;13(9):915-923.

79. Van Wijk G, Veldhuijzen DS. Perspective on diffuse noxious inhibitory controls as a model of endogenous pain modulation in clinical pain syndromes. *J Pain*. 2010;11(5):408-419.

80. Moont R, Crispel Y, Lev R, et al. Temporal changes in cortical activation during conditioned pain modulation (CPM), a LORETA study. *Pain*. 2011;152(7):1469-1477.

81. Kosek E, Ordeberg G. Lack of pressure pain modulation by heterotopic noxious conditioning stimulation in patients with painful osteoarthritis before, but not following, surgical pain relief. *Pain*. 2000;88(1):69-78.

82. Lannersten L, Kosek E. Dysfunction of endogenous pain inhibition during exercise with painful muscles in patients with shoulder myalgia and fibromyalgia. *Pain*. 2010;151(1):77-86.

83. Cathcart S, Petkov J, Winefield A, et al. Central mechanisms of stress-induced headache. *Cephalalgia*. 2010;30(3):285-295.

84. Heymen S, Maixner W, Whitehead WE, et al. Central processing of noxious somatic stimuli in patients with irritable bowel syndrome compared with healthy controls. *Clin J Pain*. 2010;26(2):104-109.

85. Julien N, Goffaux P, Arsenault P, Marchand S. Widespread pain in fibromyalgia is related to a deficit of endogenous pain inhibition. *Pain*. 2005;114(1-2):295-302.

86. Yarnitsky D, Crispel Y, Eisenberg E, et al. Prediction of chronic post-operative pain: pre-operative DNIC testing identifies patients at risk. *Pain*. 2008;138(1):22-28.

87. Affaitati G, Costantini R, Fabrizio A, et al. Effects of treatment of peripheral pain generators in fibromyalgia patients. *Eur J Pain*. 2011;15(1):61-69.

88. Fischer A. Pressure algometry over normal muscles. Standard values, validity and reproducibility of pressure threshold. *Pain*. 1987;30(1):115-126.

89. Jensen K, Andersen H, Olesen J, Lindblom U. Pressure-pain threshold in human temporal region: evaluation of a new pressure algometer. *Pain*. 1986;25(3):313-323.

90. Orbach R, Crow H. Examiner expectancy effects in the measurement of pressure pain thresholds. *Pain*. 1988;74:163-170.

91. Myburgh C, Lauridsen H, Larsen A, Hartvigsen J. Standardized manual palpation of myofascial trigger points in relation to neck/

shoulder pain; the influence of clinical experience on inter-examiner reproducibility. *Man Ther.* 2011;16(2):136-140.

92. Hunter C, Dubois M, Zou S, et al. A new muscle pain detection device to diagnose muscles as a source of back and/or neck pain. *Pain Med.* 2010;11(1):35-43.
93. Simons D, Travell J. Myofascial pain and dysfunction. In: *The Trigger Point Manual.* Vol 5. 2nd ed. Philadelphia: Lippincott, Williams & Wilkins; 1999:37.
94. Marcus N, Gracely E, Keefe K. A comprehensive protocol to diagnose and treat pain of muscular origin may successfully and reliably decrease or eliminate pain in a chronic pain population. *Pain Med.* 2010;11(1):25-34.
95. Shah J, Gilliams E. Uncovering the biochemical milieu of myofascial trigger points using in vivo microdialysis: an application of muscle pain concepts to myofascial pain syndrome. *J Bodywork Movement Ther.* 2008;12(4):371-384.
96. Hartig D, Henderson J. Increasing hamstring flexibility decreases lower extremity overuse injuries in military basic trainees. *Am J Sports Med.* 1999;27(2):173-176.
97. Witvrouw E, Danneels L, Asselman P, et al. Muscle flexibility as a risk factor for developing muscle injuries in male professional soccer players. *Am J Sports Med.* 2003;31(1):41-46.
98. Verbunt J, Seelen H, Vlaeyen J, et al. Pain-related factors contributing to muscle inhibition in patients with chronic low back pain: an experimental investigation based on superimposed electrical stimulation. *Clin J Pain.* 2005;21(3):232-240.
99. Stokes M, Young A. The contribution of reflex inhibition to arthrogenous muscle weakness. *Clin Sci.* 1984;67:7-14.
100. Fitts R. The cross-bridge cycle and skeletal muscle fatigue. *J Appl Physiol.* 2008;104(2):551-558.
101. Jull G, Richardson C. Motor control problems in patients with spinal pain: a new direction for therapeutic exercise. *J Manipulative Physiol Ther.* 2000;23(2):115-117.
102. Lederman E. The myth of core stability. *J Bodyw Mov Ther.* 2010;14(1):84-98.
103. Hayden J, van Tulder MW, Malmivaara A, Koes B. Exercise therapy for treatment of non-specific low back pain. *Cochrane Database Syst Rev.* 2005;(3):CD000335.
104. Abenhaim L, Rossignol M, Valat J-P, et al. The role of activity in the therapeutic management of back pain: report of the International Paris Task Force on Back Pain. *Spine.* 2000;25(Suppl 4):1S-33S.
105. Fersum K, Dankaerts W, O'Sullivan P, et al. Integration of subclassification strategies in RCTs evaluating manual therapy treatment and exercise therapy for non-specific chronic low back pain (NSLBP): a systematic review. *Br J Sports Med.* 2010;44(14).
106. Taguchi T, Hoheisel U, Mense S. Dorsal horn neurons having input from low back structures in rats. *Pain.* 2008;138:119-129.
107. Kraus H. *Diagnosis and Treatment of Muscle Pain.* Chicago: Quintessence Books; 1988.
108. Kraus H, Nagler W, Melleby A. Evaluation of an exercise program for back pain. *Am Fam Physician.* 1983;28(3):153-158.
109. Steiger F, Wirth B, de Bruin E, Mannion A. Is a positive clinical outcome after exercise therapy for chronic non-specific low back pain contingent upon a corresponding improvement in the targeted aspect(s) of performance? A systematic review. *Eur Spine J.* 2011:1-24.
110. Travell J, Rinzler S, Herman M. Pain and disability of the shoulder and arm: treatment by intramuscular infiltration with procaine hydrochloride. *JAMA.* 1942;120:417-422.
111. Arendt-Nielsen L, Graven-Nielsen T, Svarrer H, Svensson P. The influence of low back pain on muscle activity and coordination during gait: a clinical and experimental study. *Pain.* 1996;64(2):231-240.
112. Ro JY, Capra NF. Modulation of jaw muscle spindle afferent activity following intramuscular injections with hypertonic saline. *Pain.* 2001;92(1-2):117-127.
113. Lund J, Donga R, Widmer C, Stohler C. The pain-adaptation model: a discussion of the relationship between chronic musculoskeletal pain and motor activity. *Can J Physiol Pharmacol.* 1991;69(5):683-694.
114. Pluess M, Conrad A, Wilhelm F. Muscle tension in generalized anxiety disorder: a critical review of the literature. *J Anxiety Disord.* 2009;23(1):1-11.
115. Nestoriuc Y, Rief W, Martin A. Meta-analysis of biofeedback for tension-type headache: efficacy, specificity, and treatment moderators. *J Consult Clin Psychol.* 2008;76(3):379-396.
116. Kerns R, Sellinger J, Goodin B. Psychological treatment of chronic pain. *Annu Rev Clin Psychol.* 2011;7(1):411-434.
117. Green PG, Alvarez P, Gear RW, et al. Further validation of a model of fibromyalgia syndrome in the rat. *J Pain.* 2011;12(7):811-818.
118. Chou R, Huffman L. Medications for acute and chronic low back pain: a review of the evidence for an American Pain Society/American College of Physicians clinical practice guideline. *Ann Intern Med.* 2007;147(7):505-514.
119. Malanga G, Wolff E. Evidence-informed management of chronic low back pain with nonsteroidal anti-inflammatory drugs, muscle relaxants, and simple analgesics. *Spine J.* 2008;8(1):173-184.
120. Henschke N, Kuijpers T, Rubinstein S, et al. Injection therapy and denervation procedures for chronic low-back pain: a systematic review. *Eur Spine J.* 2010;19(9):1425-1449.
121. Norris F, Gasteiger E, Chatfield P. An electromyographic study of induced and spontaneous muscle cramps. *Electroencephalogr Clin Neurophysiol.* 1957;9(1):139-147.
122. Miller T, Layzer R. Muscle cramps. *Muscle Nerve.* 2005;32(4):431-442.
123. Miller K, Knight K. Electrical stimulation cramp threshold frequency correlates well with the occurrence of skeletal muscle cramps. *Muscle Nerve.* 2009;39(3):364-368.
124. Katzberg H, Khan A, So Y. Assessment: symptomatic treatment for muscle cramps (an evidence-based review). *Neurology.* 2010;74(8):691-696.
125. Monderer R, Wu W, Thorpy M. Nocturnal leg cramps. *Curr Neurol Neurosci Rep.* 2010;10(1):53-59.
126. El-Tawil S, Musa TA, Valli H, et al. Quinine for muscle cramps. *Cochrane Database Syst Rev.* 2010;(12):CD005044.
127. Henriksen M, Alkjær T, Lund H, et al. Experimental quadriceps muscle pain impairs knee joint control during walking. *J Appl Physiol.* 2007;103(1):132-139.
128. Schomburg E, Steffens H, Kniffki K. Contribution of group III and IV muscle afferents to multisensorial spinal motor control in cats. *Neurosci Res.* 1999;33:195-206.
129. Schomburg E, Steffens H. Only minor spinal motor reflex effects from feline group IV muscle nociceptors. *Neurosci Res.* 2002;44:213-223.
130. Elert J, Dahlqvist S, Almay B, Eisemann M. Muscle endurance, muscle tension and personality traits in patients with muscle or joint pain—a pilot study. *J Rheumatol.* 1993;20:1550-1556.
131. Bodere C, Tea SH, Giroux-Metges MA, Woda A. Activity of masticatory muscles in subjects with different orofacial pain conditions. *Pain.* 2005;116(1-2):33-41.
132. Larsson R, Öberg P, Larsson S-E. Changes of trapezius muscle blood flow and electromyography in chronic neck pain due to trapezius myalgia. *Pain.* 1999;79:45-50.

133. Collins G, Cohen M, Nailboff B, Schandler S. Comparative analysis of paraspinal and frontalis EMG, heart rate and skin conductance in chronic low back pain patients and normals to various postures and stress. *Scand J Rehabil Med.* 1982;14:39-46.

134. Ahern D, Follick M, Council J, et al. Comparison of lumbar paravertebral EMG patterns in chronic low back pain patients and non-patient controls. *Pain.* 1988;34:153-160.

135. DeVries H. Quantitative electromyographic investigation of the spasm theory of muscle pain. *Am J Phys Med.* 1966;45:119-134.

136. Howell J, Chila A, Ford G, et al. An electromyographic study of elbow motion during postexercise muscle soreness. *J Appl Physiol.* 1985;58:1713-1718.

137. Bobbert M, Hollander A, Huijing P. Factors in delayed onset muscular soreness of man. *Med Sci Sports Exerc.* 1986;18:75-81.

138. Rossi A, Mazzocchio R, Decchi B. Effect of chemically activated fine muscle afferents on spinal recurrent inhibition in humans. *Clin Neurophysiol.* 2003;114(2):279-287.

139. Sessle B. Acute and chronic craniofacial pain: brainstem mechanisms of nociceptive transmission and neuroplasticity, and their clinical correlates. *Crit Rev Oral Biol Med.* 2000;11:57-91.

140. Graven-Nielsen T, Lund H, Arendt-Nielsen L, et al. Inhibition of maximal voluntary contraction force by experimental muscle pain: a centrally mediated mechanism. *Muscle Nerve.* 2002;26:708-712.

141. Graven-Nielsen T, Svensson P, Arendt-Nielsen L. Effects of experimental muscle pain on muscle activity and co-ordination during static and dynamic motor function. *Electroencephalogr Clin Neurophysiol.* 1997;105:156-164.

142. Wang K, Arima T, Arendt-Nielsen L, Svensson P. EMG-force relationships are influenced by experimental jaw-muscle pain. *J Oral Rehabil.* 2000;27:394-402.

143. Slater H, Arendt-Nielsen L, Wright A, Graven-Nielsen T. Sensory and motor effects of experimental muscle pain in patients with lateral epicondylalgia and controls with delayed onset muscle soreness. *Pain.* 2005;114(1-2):118-130.

144. Bäckman E, Bengtsson A, Bengtsson M, et al. Skeletal muscle function in primary fibromyalgia. Effect of regional sympathetic blockade with guanethidine. *Acta Neurol Scand.* 1988;77:187-191.

145. Clark G, Beemsterboer P, Jacobson R. The effect of sustained submaximal clenching on maximum bite force in myofascial pain dysfunction patients. *J Oral Rehabil.* 1984;11:387-391.

146. Bengtsson A, Bäckman E, Skogh T. Long term follow-up of fibromyalgia patients: clinical symptoms, muscular function, laboratory test—an eight year comparison study. *J Musculoskelet Pain.* 1994;2:67-80.

147. Ciubotariu A, Arendt-Nielsen L, Graven-Nielsen T. The influence of muscle pain and fatigue on the activity of synergistic muscles of the leg. *Eur J Appl Physiol.* 2004;91(5-6):604-614.

148. Falla D, Farina D, Dahl M, Graven-Nielsen T. Muscle pain induces task-dependent changes in cervical agonist/antagonist activity. *J Appl Physiol.* 2007;102:601-609.

149. Prasartwuth O, Taylor J, Gandevia S. Maximal force, voluntary activation and muscle soreness after eccentric damage to human elbow flexor muscles. *J Physiol.* 2005;567:337-348.

150. Arendt-Nielsen L, Graven-Nielsen T, Svarrer H, Svensson P. The influence of low back pain on muscle activity and coordination during gait: a clinical and experimental study. *Pain.* 1996;64:231-240.

151. Hodges P, Moseley G, Gabrielsson A, Gandevia S. Experimental muscle pain changes feedforward postural responses of the trunk muscles. *Exp Brain Res.* 2003;151:262-271.

152. Henriksen M, Alkjaer T, Lund H, et al. Experimental quadriceps muscle pain impairs knee joint control during walking. *J Appl Physiol.* 2007;103:132-139.

153. Kori SH, Miller RP, Todd DD. Kinisiophobia: a new view of chronic pain behavior. *Pain Management.* 1990;Jan/Feb:35-43.

154. George S, Dover G, Fillingim R. Fear of pain influences outcomes after exercise-induced delayed onset muscle soreness at the shoulder. *Clin J Pain.* 2007;23(1):76-84.

155. Moseley G, Nicholas M, Hodges P. Does anticipation of back pain predispose to back trouble? *Brain.* 2004;127(Pt 10):2339-2347.

156. Roseman I. Appraisals, rather than unpleasantness or muscle movements, are the primary determinants of specific emotions. *Emotion.* 2004;4(2):145-150, discussion 151-155.

157. Vlaeyen JWS, Linton SJ. Fear-avoidance and its consequences in chronic musculoskeletal pain: a state of the art. *Pain.* 2000;85(3):317-332.

158. Koho P, Orenius T, Kautiainen H, et al. Association of fear of movement and leisure-time physical activity among patients with chronic pain. *J Rehabil Med.* 2011;43(9):794-799.

159. Abbott AD, Tyni-Lenne R, Hedlund R. Early rehabilitation targeting cognition, behavior, and motor function after lumbar fusion a randomized controlled trial. *Spine.* 2010;35(8):848-857.

160. Moseley GL, Zalucki N, Birklein F, et al. Thinking about movement hurts: the effect of motor imagery on pain and swelling in people with chronic arm pain. *Arthritis Rheum.* 2008;59(5):623-631.

161. Fernández-de-las-Peñas C, Cuadrado M, Pareja J. Myofascial trigger points, neck mobility and forward head posture in unilateral migraine. *Cephalalgia.* 2006;26(9):1061-1070.

162. Griegel-Morris P, Larson K, Mueller-Klaus K, Oatis CA. Incidence of common postural abnormalities in the cervical, shoulder, and thoracic regions and their association with pain in two age groups of healthy subjects. *Phys Ther.* 1992;72(6):425-431.

163. Murphy S, Buckle P, Stubbs D. Classroom posture and self-reported back and neck pain in schoolchildren. *Appl Ergon.* 2004;35(2):113-120.

164. Hirata RP, Ervilha UF, Arendt-Nielsen L, Graven-Nielsen T. Experimental muscle pain challenges the postural stability during quiet stance and unexpected posture perturbation. *J Pain.* 2011;12(8):911-919.

165. Van Dieen JH, Visser B, Hermans V. The contribution of task-related biomechanical constraints to the development of work-related myalgia. In: Johansson H, Windhorst U, Djupsjobacka M, Passatore M, eds. *Chronic Work-Related Myalgia: Neuromuscular Mechanisms Behind Work-Related Chronic Muscle Pain Syndromes.* Sweden: Gavle University Press; 2003:83-93.

166. Ariens GA, Bongers PM, Douwes M, et al. Are neck flexion, neck rotation, and sitting at work risk factors for neck pain? Results of a prospective cohort study. *Occup Environ Med.* 2001;58(3):200-207.

167. Damsgard E, Dewar A, Roe C, Hamran T. Staying active despite pain: pain beliefs and experiences with activity-related pain in patients with chronic musculoskeletal pain. *Scand J Caring Sci.* 2011;25(1):108-116.

168. Silbernagel KG, Brorsson A, Lundberg M. The majority of patients with Achilles tendinopathy recover fully when treated with exercise alone: a 5-year follow-up. *Am J Sports Med.* 2011;39(3):607-613.

169. Roffey DM, Wai EK, Bishop P, et al. Causal assessment of awkward occupational postures and low back pain: results of a systematic review. *Spine J.* 2010;10(1):89-99.

170. Widhe T. Spine: posture, mobility and pain. A longitudinal study from childhood to adolescence. *Eur Spine J.* 2001;10(2):118-123.

171. Aas R, Tuntland H, Holte K, et al. Workplace interventions for low-back pain in workers (protocol). *Cochrane Database Syst Rev.* 2009(4):CD008160.

172. Kratenova J, Zejglicova K, Maly M, Filipova V. Prevalence and risk factors of poor posture in school children in the Czech Republic. *J Sch Health*. 2007;77(3):131-137.
173. Tsao H, Galea MP, Hodges PW. Reorganization of the motor cortex is associated with postural control deficits in recurrent low back pain. *Brain*. 2008;131(Pt 8):2161-2171.
174. Tsao H, Hodges PW. Persistence of improvements in postural strategies following motor control training in people with recurrent low back pain. *J Electromyogr Kinesiol*. 2008;18(4):559-567.
175. Sarno J. Etiology of neck and back pain. An automatic myoneuralgia? *J Nerv Ment Dis*. 1981;169(1):55-59.
176. Burns J. Arousal of negative emotions and symptom-specific reactivity in chronic low back pain patients. *Emotion*. 2006;6(2):309-319.
177. Asendorpf J, Scherer K. The discrepant repressor: differentiation between low anxiety, high anxiety, and repression of anxiety by autonomic-facial-verbal patterns of behavior. *J Pers Soc Psychol*. 1983;45(6):1334-1346.
178. Blair S, Djupsjobacka M, Johansson H, et al. Neuromuscular mechanisms behind chronic work-related myalgias: an overview. In: Johansson H, Windhorst U, Djupsjobacka M, Passatore M, eds. *Chronic Work-Related Myalgia: Neuromuscular Mechanisms Behind Work-Related Chronic Muscle Pain Syndromes*. Sweden: Gavle University Press; 2003:5-46.
179. Stewart WF, Ricci JA, Chee E, et al. Lost productive time and cost due to common pain conditions in the US workforce. *JAMA*. 2003;290(18):2443-2454.
180. Tanaka S, Petersen M, Cameron L. Prevalence and risk factors of tendinitis and related disorders of the distal upper extremity among U.S. workers: comparison to carpal tunnel syndrome. *Am J Ind Med*. 2001;39(3):328-335.
181. Punnett L. Work-related musculoskeletal disorders: the epidemiologic evidence and the debate. *J Electromyogr Kinesiol*. 2004;14(1):13.
182. Blair S DM, Johansson H, et al. Neuromuscular mechanisms behind chronic work-related myalgias: an overview. In: Johnansson HEA, ed. *Chronic Work-Related Myalgias*. Sweden: Gävle University Press; 2003.
183. Bliss L, Teeple P. Core stability: the centerpiece of any training program. *Curr Sports Med Rep*. 2005;4(3):179-183.
184. Hägg G. Static work loads and occupational myalgia—a new explanation model. In: Anderson P, Hobart D, Danoff J, eds. *Electromyographical Kinesiology*. St. Louis: Elsevier Science; 1991:141-144.
185. Henneman E, Somjen G, Carpenter D. Functional significance of cell size in spinal motoneurons. *J Neurophysiol*. 1965;28:560-580.
186. Martin BI, Deyo RA, Mirza SK, et al. Expenditures and health status among adults with back and neck problems. *JAMA*. 2008;299(6):656-663.
187. Conclusions, recommendations, and research priorities. *Spine*. 1987;12(7 Suppl 1):S37-S39.
188. Diagnosis of the problem (the problem of diagnosis). *Spine*. 1987;12(7 Suppl 1):S16-S21.
189. Chou R, Qaseem A, Snow V, et al. Diagnosis and treatment of low back pain: a joint clinical practice guideline from the American College of Physicians and the American Pain Society. *Ann Intern Med*. 2007;147(7):478-491.
190. Airaksinen O, Brox J, Cedraschi C, et al. Chapter 4 European guidelines for the management of chronic nonspecific low back pain. *Eur Spine J*. 2006;15(0):s192-s300.
191. Roncoroni C, Baillet A, Durand M, et al. Efficacy and tolerance of systemic steroids in sciatica: a systematic review and meta-analysis. *Rheumatology*. 2011;50(9):1603-1611.
192. Henschke N, Kuijpers T, Rubinstein S, et al. Injection therapy and denervation procedures for chronic low-back pain: a systematic review. *Eur Spine J*. 2010;19(9):1425-1449.
193. French S, Cameron M, Walker B, et al. Superficial heat or cold for low back pain. *Cochrane Database Syst Rev*. 2006;(1):CD004750.
194. Van Duijvenbode IC, Jellema P, van Poppel MN, van Tulder MW. Lumbar supports for prevention and treatment of low back pain. *Cochrane Database Syst Rev*. 2008;(2):CD001823.
195. Furlan A, van Tulder MW, Cherkin D, et al. Acupuncture and dry-needling for low back pain. *Cochrane Database Syst Rev*. 2005;(1):CD001351.
196. Dagenais S, Yelland M, Mar CD, Schoene M. Prolotherapy injections for chronic low-back pain. *Cochrane Database Syst Rev*. 2007;(2):CD004059.
197. Rubinstein S, Middelkoop MV, Assendelft W, et al. Spinal manipulative therapy for chronic low-back pain. *Cochrane Database Syst Rev*. 2011;(2):CD008112.
198. Walker B, French S, Grant W, Green S. Combined chiropractic interventions for low-back pain. *Cochrane Database Syst Rev*. 2010;(4):CD005427.
199. Sahar T, Cohen M, Ne'eman V, et al. Insoles for prevention and treatment of back pain. *Cochrane Database Syst Rev*. 2007;(4):CD005275.
200. Hayden J, van Tulder MW, Malmivaara A, Koes B. Exercise therapy for treatment of non-specific low back pain. *Cochrane Database Syst Rev*. 2005;(3):CD000335.
201. Waseem Z, Boulias C, Gordon A, et al. Botulinum toxin injections for low-back pain and sciatica. *Cochrane Database Syst Rev*. 2011;(1)CD008257.
202. Verbeek J, Martimo K, Karppinen J, et al. Manual material handling advice and assistive devices for preventing and treating back pain in workers. *Cochrane Database Syst Rev*. 2011;(6):CD005958.
203. Dahm K, Brurberg K, Jamtvedt G, Hagen K. Advice to rest in bed versus advice to stay active for acute low-back pain and sciatica. *Cochrane Database Syst Rev*. 2010;(6):CD007612.
204. Furlan A, Imamura M, Dryden T, Irvin E. Massage for low-back pain. *Cochrane Database Syst Rev*. 2008;(4):CD001929.
205. Engers A, Jellema P, Wensing M, et al. Individual patient education for low back pain. *Cochrane Database Syst Rev*. 2008;(1):CD004057.
206. Choi B, Verbeek J, Tam W, Jiang J. Exercises for prevention of recurrences of low-back pain. *Cochrane Database Syst Rev*. 2010;(1):CD006555.
207. Karjalainen K, Malmivaara A, van Tulder MW, et al. Multidisciplinary biopsychosocial rehabilitation for subacute low-back pain among working age adults. *Cochrane Database Syst Rev*. 2003;(2):CD002193.
208. Staal J, Bie RD, Vet HD, et al. Injection therapy for subacute and chronic low-back pain. *Cochrane Database Syst Rev*. 2008;(3):CD001824.
209. Heymans M, van Tulder MW, Esmail R, et al. Back schools for non-specific low-back pain. *Cochrane Database Syst Rev*. 2004;(4):CD000261.
210. Palmer KT, Harris EC, Linaker C, et al. Effectiveness of community- and workplace-based interventions to manage musculoskeletal-related sickness absence and job loss—a systematic review. *Rheumatology (Oxford)*. 2012;51(2):230-242.
211. Pincus T, Greenwood L, McHarg E. Advising people with back pain to take time off work: a survey examining the role of private musculoskeletal practitioners in the UK. *Pain*. 2011;152(12):2813-2818.
212. Oesch P, Kool J, Hagen K, Bachmann S. Effectiveness of exercise on work disability in patients with non-acute non-specific low

back pain: systematic review and meta-analysis of randomised controlled trials. *J Rehabil Med.* 2010;42:193-205.

213. Abenhaim L, Rossignol M, Valat JP, et al. The role of activity in the therapeutic management of back pain. Report of the International Paris Task Force on Back Pain. *Spine.* 2000;25(4 Suppl):1S-33S.
214. Hayden JA, van Tulder MW, Malmivaara A, Koes BW. Exercise therapy for treatment of non-specific low back pain. *Cochrane Database Syst Rev.* 2005;(3):CD000335.
215. Saner J, Kool J, Bie RD, et al. Movement control exercise versus general exercise to reduce disability in patients with low back pain and movement control impairment: a randomised controlled trial. *BMC Musculoskelet Disord.* 2011;12:207.
216. Van Tulder M, Malmivaara A, Hayden J, Koes B. Statistical significance versus clinical importance: trials on exercise therapy for chronic low back pain as example. *Spine.* 2007;32(16):1785-1790.
217. Steiger F, Wirth B, de Bruin E, Mannion A. Is a positive clinical outcome after exercise therapy for chronic non-specific low back pain contingent upon a corresponding improvement in the targeted aspect(s) of performance? A systematic review. *Eur Spine J.* 2012;21(4):575-598.
218. Borg-Stein J, Wilkins A. Soft tissue determinants of low back pain. *Curr Pain Headache Rep.* 2006;10:339-344.
219. Malanga G, Wolff E. Evidence-informed management of low back pain with trigger point injections. *Spine J.* 2008;8:243-252.
220. Schleip R, Kingler W, Lehmann-Horn F. Fascia is able to contract in a smooth muscle-like manner and thereby influence musculoskeletal mechanics. In: Findley T, Schleip R, eds. *Fascia Research. Basic Science and Implications for Conventional and Complementary Health Care.* Munich: Urban and Fischer; 2007:76-77.
221. Bednar D, Orr F, Simon G. Observations on the pathomorphology of the thoracolumbar fascia in chronic mechanical back pain. A microscopic study. *Spine.* 1995;20(10):1161-1164.
222. Yahia L, Rhalmi S, Newman N, Isler M. Sensory innervation of human thoracolumbar fascia: an immunohistochemical study. *Acta Orthop Scand.* 1992;63:195-197.
223. Tesarz J, Hoheisel U, Wiedenhöfer B, Mense S. Sensory innervation of the thoracolumbar fascia in rats and humans. *Neuroscience.* 2011;194:302-308.
224. Pertovaara A. Noradrenergic pain modulation. *Prog Neurobiol.* 2006;80:53-83.
225. Kiter E, Karaboyun T, Tufan A, Acar K. Immunohistochemical demonstration of free nerve endings in iliolumbar ligament. *Spine.* 2010;35:E101-E104.
226. Stecco C, Gagey O, Belloni A, et al. Anatomy of the deep fascia of the upper limb. Second part: study of innervation. *Morphologie.* 2007;91:38-43.
227. Gibson W, Arendt-Nielsen L, Taguchi T, et al. Increased pain from muscle fascia following eccentric exercise: animal and human findings. *Exp Brain Res.* 2009;194:299-308.
228. *Bonica's Management of Pain.* 4th ed. Philadelphia: Lippincott Williams & Wilkins; 2009.
229. *Wall and Melzack's Textbook of Pain.* 5th ed. Philadelphia: Elsevier/Churchill Livingstone; 2005.
230. Cohen M, Quintner J. The horse is dead: let myofascial pain syndrome rest in peace. *Pain Med.* 2008;9(4):464-465.
231. Bennett R, Goldenberg D. Fibromyalgia, myofascial pain, tender points and trigger points: splitting or lumping? *Arthritis Res Ther.* 2011;13(3):117.
232. Kellgren J. Observations on referred pain arising from muscle. *Clin Sci.* 1938;3:174-190.
233. Kellgren J. On distribution of pain arising from deep somatic structures with charts of segmental pain areas. *Clin Sci.* 1939;4:35-36.
234. Lewis T, Kellgren J. Observations relating to referred pain, visceromotor reflexes and other associated phenomena. *Clin Sci.* 1939;4:47-71.
235. Simons DG, Travell JG. Myofascial origins of low back pain. 1. Principles of diagnosis and treatment. *Postgrad Med.* 1983;73(2):66.
236. Shah JP, Phillips TM, Danoff JV, Gerber LH. An in vivo microanalytical technique for measuring the local biochemical milieu of human skeletal muscle. *J Appl Physiol.* 2005;99(5):1977-1984.
237. Simons DG, Travell JG, Simons LS. *Travell & Simons' Myofascial Pain and Dysfunction: the Trigger Point Manual.* Vol 1. 2nd ed. Baltimore: Williams & Wilkins; 1999.
238. Simons D, Stolov W. Microscopic features and transient contraction of palpable bands in canine muscle. *Am J Phys Med.* 1976;55:65-88.
239. Reitinger A, Radner H, Tilscher H, et al. Morphologische Untersuchung an Triggerpunkten [Morphologic study of trigger points]. *Man Med.* 1996;34:256-262.
240. Mense S, Gerwin R, eds. *Muscle Pain: Diagnosis and Treatment.* 1st ed. Heidelberg: Springer; 2010.
241. Simons DG. Clinical and etiological update of myofascial pain from trigger points. *J Musculoskelet Pain.* 1996;4(1-2):93-121.
242. Gerwin R, Dommerholt J, Shah J. An expansion of Simons' integrated hypothesis of trigger point formation. *Curr Pain Headache Rep.* 2004;8:468-475.
243. Gerwin R. The taut band and other mysteries of the trigger point: an examination of the mechanisms relevant to the development and maintenance of the trigger point. *J Musculoskelet Pain.* 2008;15(Suppl 13):115-121.
244. McPartland J, Simons D. Myofascial trigger points: translating molecular theory into manual therapy. *J Man Manipulative Ther.* 2006;14(4):232-239.
245. Graves R, Machen M, Zubak J, Warme W. Rhabdomyolysis attributable to severe overuse of the supraspinatus muscle: a report of two cases. *Mil Med.* 2007;172:1306-1309.
246. Qerama E, Fuglsang-Frederiksen A, Kasch H, et al. Evoked pain in the motor endplate region of the brachial biceps muscle: an experimental study. *Muscle Nerve.* 2004;29(3):393-400.
247. Christensen HW, Vach W, Manniche C, et al. Palpation for muscular tenderness in the anterior chest wall: an observer reliability study. *J Manipulative Physiol Ther.* 2003;26(8):469-475.
248. Levoska S. Manual palpation and pain threshold in female office employees with and without neck-shoulder symptoms. *Clin J Pain.* 1993;9(4):236-241.
249. Maher C, Adams R. Reliability of pain and stiffness assessments in clinical manual lumbar spine examination. *Phys Ther.* 1994;74(9):801-809; discussion 809-811.
250. Marcus N, Kraus H, Rachlin E. Comments on K.H. Njoo and E. Van der Does, PAIN, 58 (1994) 317-323. *Pain.* 1995;61(1):159.
251. Njoo KH, Van der Does E. The occurrence and inter-rater reliability of myofascial trigger points in the quadratus lumborum and gluteus medius: a prospective study in non-specific low back pain patients and controls in general practice. *Pain.* 1994;58(3):317-323.
252. Wolfe F. Stop using the American College of Rheumatology criteria in the clinic. *J Rheumatol.* 2003;30(8):1671-1672.
253. Myburgh C, Lauridsen HH, Larsen AH, Hartvigsen J. Standardized manual palpation of myofascial trigger points in relation to neck/shoulder pain; the influence of clinical experience on inter-examiner reproducibility. *Man Ther.* 2011;16(2):136-140.

254. Myburgh C, Larsen AH, Hartvigsen J. A systematic, critical review of manual palpation for identifying myofascial trigger points: evidence and clinical significance. *Arch Phys Med Rehabil.* 2008;89(6):1169-1176.
255. Borg-Stein J, Simons DG. Myofascial pain. *Arch Phys Med Rehabil.* 2002;83(3):S40-S47.
256. Hong CZ. Lidocaine injection versus dry needling to myofascial trigger point—the importance of the local twitch response. *Am J Phys Med Rehabil.* 1994;73(4):256-263.
257. Zink W, Graf BM. Local anesthetic myotoxicity. *Reg Anesth Pain Med.* 2004;29(4):333-340.
258. Komorowski TE, Shepard B, Økland S, Carlson BM. An electron microscopic study of local anesthetic-induced skeletal muscle fiber degeneration and regeneration in the monkey. *J Orthop Res.* 1990;8(4):495-503.
259. Peloso PM, Gross AR, Haines TA, et al. Medicinal and injection therapies for mechanical neck disorders: a Cochrane systematic review. *J Rheumatol.* 2006;33(5):957-967.
260. Marcus NJ, Gracely EJ, Keefe KO. A comprehensive protocol to diagnose and treat pain of muscular origin may successfully and reliably decrease or eliminate pain in a chronic pain population. *Pain Med.* 2010;11(1):25-34.
261. Van Tulder MW, Koes B, Seitsalo S, Malmivaara A. Outcome of invasive treatment modalities on back pain and sciatica: an evidence-based review. *Eur Spine J.* 2006;15(Suppl 1):S82-S92.
262. Chen Q, Basford J, An K-N. Ability of magnetic resonance elastography to assess taut bands. *Clin Biomech (Bristol, Avon).* 2008;23(5):623-629.
263. Sikdar S, Shah JP, Gebreab T, et al. Novel applications of ultrasound technology to visualize and characterize myofascial trigger points and surrounding soft tissue. *Arch Phys Med Rehabil.* 2009;90(11):1829-1838.
264. Park G-YMDP, Kwon DRMDP. Application of real-time sonoelastography in musculoskeletal diseases related to physical medicine and rehabilitation. *Am J Phys Med Rehabil.* 2011;90(11):875-886.
265. Hunter C, Dubois M, Zou S, et al. A new muscle pain detection device to diagnose muscles as a source of back and/or neck pain. *Pain Med.* 2010;11(1):35-43.
266. Marcus N. *End Back Pain Forever.* New York: Atria Books; 2012.
267. Rachlin ES, Rachlin IS. *Myofascial Pain and Fibromyalgia: Trigger Point Management.* 2nd ed. St. Louis: Mosby; 2002:437.

Pain Associated with Arterial and Venous Vascular Disease

Robert I. Cohen

By late middle age 5% of men and women will have developed peripheral arterial disease and within 5 years 25% of these will develop pain at rest, ulceration, and gangrene (critical limb ischemia).[1] Physicians who practice in the specialty of pain medicine need to be familiar with the causes and treatment of pain due to peripheral vascular disease because it has a high prevalence. Appropriate therapy and management can significantly improve the quality of life for patients. Pain medicine physicians, by encouraging secondary or tertiary preventive therapy, have the opportunity to improve the life expectancy of their patients with symptomatic peripheral vascular disease of whom more than 50% have disease of the coronary and/or carotid arteries. This chapter will outline the disease conditions and treatments for pain associated with peripheral vascular disease.[2]

The ischemic pain of peripheral vascular disease can be approximated by sustained tourniquet inflation on an extremity. In experimental studies, as time passes, tissue oxygenation levels fall, metabolic byproducts accumulate, reactive cellular agents are released, nociceptive signals entering the central nervous system (CNS) increase, and patients report increasing intensity of pain. The affective descriptors for this pain differ and are more difficult to tolerate than pain produced by other experimental modalities. Patients with peripheral vascular disease experience this type of pain without the ability to restore blood flow by releasing the tourniquet. Effective management of this pain can restore quality of life for these patients.

PAIN OF ARTERIAL ORIGIN

Arterial insufficiency is most commonly the result of occlusive diseases with atheroma formation (arteriosclerosis obliterans), but less commonly occurs in thromboangiitis obliterans (Buerger disease), Raynaud syndrome, diabetic arteritis, and arteritis associated with collagen disease. Other diseases with vascular-related causes such as migraine and cluster headache are discussed elsewhere (see Chapter 3).

ATHEROMA AND ITS CONSEQUENCES: ARTERIOSCLEROSIS

The role of lipids was suggested with the early appearance of fatty streaks in young soldiers during emergency surgery and at autopsy in the 1970s. The role of lipids distinguishes arteriosclerosis from other arterial disease. Primary and secondary prevention strategies are available to reduce the incidence and/or aggressively treat the known risk factors of hypercholesterolemia, hypertension, cigarette smoking, and poor control of diabetes. As the disease progresses, plaque formation tends to occur at bifurcations in large and medium-sized arteries where turbulence, alteration of laminar flow, and shear stress may provoke an endothelial and/or vascular smooth muscle response. Arteriosclerosis is a dynamic process that involves vascular and inflammatory tissue responses with decreased release of nitric oxide (NO) and other protective secretions, increased release of cytokines by inflammatory cells responding to exposed matrix, and release of growth factors from the endothelium, as well as platelet activation. Arteries may respond initially to this process with an increase in size, but arterial remodeling may not be sustained in the face of ongoing plaque accumulation. Although a full discussion of arteriosclerosis is beyond the scope of this chapter, understanding of the causes at the gene and cellular level will suggest effective treatment options.

PROGRESSION OF ATHEROMATOUS PLAQUES

Although arteriosclerosis is most prominent at bifurcations, the straight femoropopliteal segment is involved in 60% of lower limb disease; the upper limbs are less often involved. Initially, as vessel diameter decreases, flow can be maintained if velocity increases. Vessel size also may increase, specifically at the arteriolar level, forming a collateral supply. As vessel diameter continues to decrease beyond 70%, the patient may develop symptoms, especially if the process is affecting collateral vessels as well. Initial symptoms usually occur during exercise when the circulation is stressed. Even in patients with severe claudication, blood flow may be near normal at rest. With progression, critical limb ischemia develops with an incidence of 0.5 to 1 per 1000.[3]

MECHANISM OF PAIN FROM ARTERIAL DISEASE

Oxygen is the most flow-limited nutrient for muscle and skin. Striated muscle is capable of working anaerobically, with delayed repayment of the oxygen debt. Lactate and pyruvate levels rise as oxygen debt continues. It is assumed that the accumulation of these products of metabolism trigger firing of C-fiber nociceptors, thus triggering the pain cascade.

As oxygen tissue levels fall, hypoxia triggers altered Ca^{2+} signaling in vascular smooth muscle,[4] gene transcription for expression of inflammatory cytokines such as tumor necrosis factor,[5] Interleukin-1 and 10 (IL-1, IL-10),[6] and cytokine factors promoting vessel growth,[7,8] particularly growth of small vessels less than 200 microns in diameter.[9] Endothelial dysfunction is associated with altered release of a mediator such as NO, eicosanoid, endothelium-derived hyperpolarizing factor, endothelin, and angiotensin II.[10] Inflammatory cytokines also affect the coagulation system; for example, hypoxia-triggered release of IL-1 can decrease tissue plasminogen activator and stimulate release of plasminogen activator inhibitor-1.[11] Decreased release of NO leads to increased endothelial adhesiveness to circulating white blood cells.[12] Inflammatory mediators may both directly and indirectly trigger C-fiber nociceptor barrage into the CNS.

CLINICAL PICTURE OF OCCLUSIVE ARTERIAL DISEASE

The patient may have complaint of claudication and/or rest pain. Claudication is defined as pain in a muscle group (commonly the calf, less often the thigh, instep or buttock) that occurs while walking and forces the patient to stop. Pain is rapidly relieved by rest after which walking can be resumed. Walking distance typically decreases as the disease progresses. The diagnosis can often be made with a careful history. Another disease such as arthritis may produce infirmity so the patient is unable to tolerate exercise. In these patients the diagnosis may be made by examination. In patients with severe coronary disease, the angina linked to very low-effort walking may occur before claudication, masking this presentation of the disease. Often the reverse is true, and the presence of claudication may limit the patient's exercise tolerance so that even significant coronary disease may remain quiescent. Because 50% of patients with symptomatic peripheral vascular disease have coronary artery disease, patients with claudication have a 50% 10-year survival rate with most deaths due to myocardial infarction.[13] Patients with claudication should receive preventive treatment to reduce the risk of myocardial infarction.

The differential diagnosis of claudication includes venous and neurogenic claudication. The latter is often associated with stenosis of the central spinal canal. In spinal stenosis during walking or standing, the cauda equina can become constricted within the narrowed canal, with decreased perfusion causing progressively intense lower extremity. In this case, pain may be worse with trunk extension and better with flexion. Watch for this clinical pearl when the patient reports that walking downhill (extending the spine) is more painful than walking uphill, especially in the setting where peripheral pulses are strong on examination. Lack of spina canal stenosis on computed tomography (CT) or magnetic resonance imaging (MRI) makes this diagnosis less likely. If the history is adequate, the site of claudication may also indicate the level of occlusion (**Table 61-1**). Intermittent claudication is more common in men than in women in whom it is rare before menopause.

Pedal ischemia rest pain occurs in the toes or forefoot with or without ulceration or gangrene. The history of ischemic pain is invariably that of pain occurring at night (after a variable recumbent period), which causes the patient to arise and is relieved by limb dependency. The patient may indicate that sleep is better in a chair. As the condition progresses, pain becomes continuous and the toes deteriorate. Ulceration or gangrene may occur. Spontaneous tissue necrosis may occur in the most peripheral distribution and is likely to affect the toes. It may also occur following trauma, overzealous chiropody, or orthopedic procedures including bunionectomy and treatment for ingrown toenails. Usually preceded by claudication, pedal ischemia may appear in patients who have little or no claudication pain.

TABLE 61-1 Relation of Site Claudication to Level of Major Arterial Occlusion

Site of Claudication	Level of Occlusion
Instep	Popliteal bifurcation or below
Calf	Femoropopliteal
Thigh	Common femoral
Buttock	Aortoiliac

OTHER RELEVANT HISTORY

Arteriosclerosis is a systemic disease and the history may be positive for myocardial ischemia (infarcts or angina), stroke, hypertension, arrhythmias, and transient ischemic attacks (in the form of focal neurologic deficits resolving within 24 h). A careful medication history may reveal the extent to which secondary prevention efforts have been successful. The extent of aspirin use and monitoring of cholesterol concentration in a follow-up of patients in the British regional heart study showed that most patients with intermittent claudication without history of myocardial infarction (MI), angina, cerebrovascular accident (CVA), were not receiving appropriate secondary prevention.[14] Behavioral interventions may be helpful if a history of tobacco use is elicited and psychosocial stressors are present.[15] An excellent review of the effect of smoking and cessation on mortality, morbidity, and quality of life was published in 2010.[16] In an 11-hospital study, 711 consecutive Dutch patients with surgical treatment of peripheral arterial disease were followed prospectively for 5 years. Interestingly, there was a negative result for the primary aim among 5-year survivors.

PHYSICAL EXAMINATION

The general examination includes blood pressure measurement, cardiac auscultation, and funduscopy. Local examination will reveal ischemic tissue loss and poor capillary circulation. Low input arterial pressure can be enhanced by elevating the legs above the heart for 2 minutes while the patient repeatedly dorsoplantar flexes the ankles; this will produce elevation pallor.

All accessible pulses should be palpated and large vessels (e.g., femoral) should be auscultated for presence of a bruit as indication of proximal stenosis. The data should be charted, as shown in **Table 61-2**.

INVESTIGATIONS

The general assessment of the patient is aided by chest radiography, cardiography, complete blood count (CBC), and blood chemistries that include a lipid profile. Echocardiography[17] testing of coagulation activity includes prothrombin time (PT), partial prothrombin time (PTT), and international normalized ratio (INR) for patients on coumarin. Testing fibrinogen and plasminogen activator inhibitor-1 levels has been suggested.[18] Noninvasive localization of disease by technology such as combined echo-Doppler (duplex) is preferred both for diagnosis and choosing between surgery and percutaneous transluminal angioplasty

TABLE 61-2 Example of a Pulse Chart

Site	Right	Left
Carotid	+	+
Subclavian	+	+
Radial	+	+
Aorta	[+]	
Femoral	(+)	+
Popliteal	−	+
Dorsalis pedis	−	+
Posterior tibial	−	+
Perforating peroneal	−	−

Note: [ ] indicates aneurysm, ( ) indicates bruit. This patient had an abdominal aortic aneurysm, right iliac stenosis, and right femoropopliteal occlusion.

TABLE 61-3 Relationship of Severity of Disease to Doppler Ankle-to-Arm Pressure Ratio

Ankle-to-Arm	Severity of Disease
0.85–1.10	Normal
0.60–0.85	Mild claudication
0.30–0.60	Severe claudication
<0.30	Critical ischemia

(PTA).[19] Magnetic resonance technologies are capable of providing high quality noninvasive studies with sensitivity and specificity comparing favorably to digital subtraction angiography.[20] The standard test remains the ankle-to-arm ratio (ankle-brachial-index [ABI]). Systolic pressure at the ankle is compared with systemic arterial pressure measured in the arm. This measure is far more sensitive than pulse oximetry.[21] Observed values are related to clinical state (**Table 61-3**). When distal vessels are calcified and poorly compressible, the ABI may prove unhelpful and values greater than 1.50 may be obtained. Angiography is generally performed prior to reconstructive surgery.

MANAGEMENT OF MAJOR ARTERIAL OCCLUSION

Management of a patient with an ischemic lower limb is summarized in the flow chart

TREATMENT OF CLAUDICATION

Conservative treatment includes observation and treatment of associated conditions such as diabetes, anemia, or polycythemia. Efforts to assist patients with smoking cessation and to engage in regular exercise have been shown to improve outcome and quality of life.[22] Over 3 months of supervised treadmill exercise (at claudication threshold for 30 to 40 minutes three times each week), marked improvement was demonstrated with increased time to claudication, increased peak walking and improved endothelial function.[23] Thought to mediate these positive changes, NO concentration increases with exercise but for patients with claudication, a reduction in NO stores may limit this effect. Might it be possible to boost the benefit of exercise in these patients by increasing NO stores, for example by increasing the concentration of its immediate precursor, plasma nitrite (NO_2–)? This may be the case when increased oral consumption of dietary nitrates (NO_3–), converted by a salivary enzyme to (NO_2–), results in increased time to claudication and exhaustion, 32 and 65 seconds, respectively (**Fig. 61-1**).[24]

The severity of claudication, response (or lack of response) to medical management, impact on lifestyle, and quality of life must be weighed against the risks before proceeding with a surgical treatment or percutaneous transluminal angioplasty (PTA.) The PTA procedure has high success rates for large vessels with short lesions such as the common iliac, and may be performed as a same-day procedure. Stenting may improve success rates when lesions are more complex or repeat therapy is required. In smaller vessels, PTA is less effective so that, for example, prominent pedal ischemia mandates consideration of vascular surgery if it is technically feasible. Arterial reconstruction may utilize endarterectomy, in situ or reverse venous or synthetic grafting material. The many variations and details are beyond the scope of this chapter; however, the efficacy of bypass surgery for treatment of lower limb ischemia is supported by evidence-based medicine review.[25]

PAIN RELIEF MEASURES

SYMPATHECTOMY

Interruption of the lumbar sympathetic chain has a time-honored place in the treatment of peripheral ischemia. Before the advent of arterial

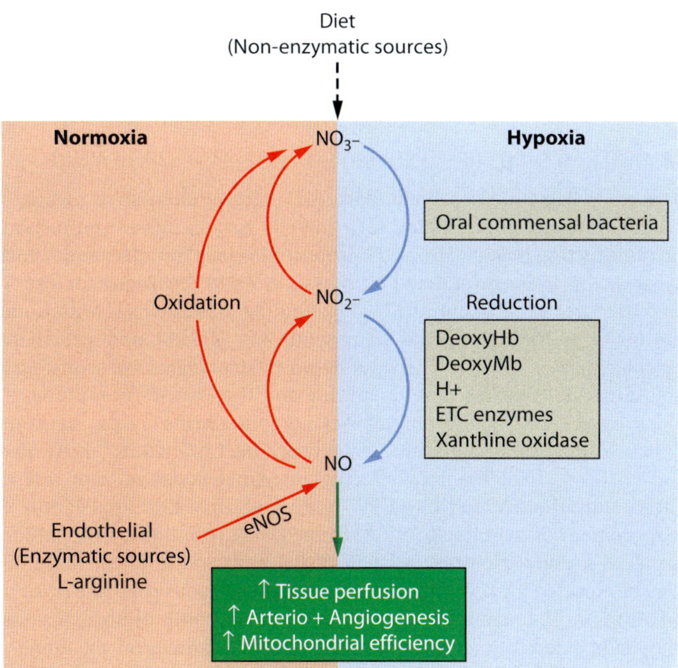

FIGURE 61-1. Nitrate-nitrite-nitric oxide formation/recycle pathways. In the presence of oxygen, endothelial nitric oxide synthase (eNOS) catalyzes the oxidation L-arginine to nitric oxide (NO). NO can exhibit biological effects and has been shown to increase tissue perfusion along with angio- and arteriogenesis in PAD models. NO may also be rapidly oxidized to nitrite (NO_{2}_) and nitrate (NO_{3}_). A secondary source of vascular NO is via diet. Consumption of foodstuffs high in inorganic nitrate (green leafy vegetables, beet root) has been shown to increase plasma nitrate which can be secreted in saliva and reduced to nitrite by commensal bacteria in the mouth. Nitrite can then be further reduced to NO (and other biologically active nitrogen oxides) via several mechanisms which are expedited under hypoxic conditions. Hence, although some of the circulating nitrate and nitrite are excreted in the kidneys, they are also able to be recycled back to NO. (Redrawn from Allen JD, Giordano T, Kevil CG. Nitrite and nitric oxide metabolism in peripheral artery disease. *Nitric Oxide.* 2012;26(4):217-22.)

reconstruction, it was the only surgical measure that produced pain relief. The indications for sympathectomy have diminished considerably over the last 50 years. Currently this treatment has a limited role.[26,27] Reports of the procedure performed successfully by laparoscopy and with chemical sympathectomy continue to appear in the literature.[28,29] Sympathectomy may improve blood flow to the foot and may improve rest pain, heal ulceration, and prevent skin necrosis.

If the affected foot is warmer than the unaffected foot, this suggests that autosympathectomy has occurred (especially in diabetic patients) and that the procedure will not be beneficial. However, there are patients who do not respond despite favorable characteristics. If the popliteal inflow index (Doppler inflow pressure in a popliteal artery vs. arm pressure) is 0.7 or greater, a good response can be predicted. It is unlikely that a favorable response will be obtained if the ankle to arm ratio is less than 0.35.[30]

Lumbar sympathectomy can be achieved by injection or surgery. The technique of lumbar sympathetic block is well described in the references.[31] An accurate block of the sympathetic chain at L3 may be adequate and it may not be necessary to use multiple needles; however, the use of radiographic control will make the procedure easier and safer. If repeated blocks with dilute local anesthetic solution produce appreciable circulatory improvement, a neurolytic block with 5 mL aqueous phenol 5% solution can be considered as an alternative to surgical sympathectomy.[32]

Operative sympathectomy may be completed by a relatively atraumatic extraperitoneal approach under general anesthesia in which lumbar ganglia 2, 3, and 4 are excised together with the chain connecting them. Post sympathectomy neuralgia, an aching pain in the femoral nerve distribution, is a complication that may resolve in 6 to 8 weeks. This is also a complication of chemical sympathectomy if the agent spreads through the prevertebral fascia to the level of the L-1 nerve root or through the psoas fascia to reach its major peripheral nerve.

OTHER METHODS OF IMPROVING THE PERIPHERAL CIRCULATION

Intravenous Regional Sympathetic Block An effective alternative means of producing sympathetic block in a limb is to administer intravenous agents affecting postganglionic neurons to produce noradrenergic block using an intravenous regional anesthesia (IVRA) technique. Before its manufacture was discontinued, guanethidine was used IV with some success in complex regional pain syndrome (CRPS) and peripheral vascular disease (PVD).[33,34] By acting on postganglionic neurons, guanethidine first releases norepinephrine and then causes noradrenergic block by preventing the reuptake of norepinephrine by the neurons. Other drugs such as clonidine,[35] phentolamine,[36] bretylium,[37] ketorolac, and corticosteroid, reported effective in management of pain due to CRPS and administered by IVRA technique, may find application in management of pain due to PVA. In the IVRA technique, a tourniquet is placed around the proximal part of the limb and inflated. The limb may be elevated for several minutes to enhance venous drainage prior to inflation of the tourniquet. The drug diluted in 50 mL of normal saline may be injected into an indwelling intravenous catheter in the affected leg or arm after tourniquet inflation. Lidocaine can be added to help the patient tolerate the tourniquet. The tourniquet is kept inflated for 15 minutes. The technique may be valuable for patients who are receiving anticoagulant therapy in whom paravertebral lumbar sympathetic block could cause significant hemorrhage. The technique can also be used for patients in whom the effects of operative lumbar sympathectomy are receding.

SPINAL CORD STIMULATION

Initial reports of the value of large fiber nerve stimulation suggested that patients with pain from peripheral arteriosclerotic disease who had not responded to arterial bypass surgery and/or sympathectomy might respond to stimulation of posterior spinal roots using implanted electrodes. Plethysmographic blood flow and skin temperature were also noted to increase. More recently it has been suggested that the primary effect may be occurring within the lamina of the dorsal horn of the spinal cord. Pain transmission in this layer is controlled by wide dynamic range neurons. Substance P was one of the first neuropeptides identified as modulating pain transmission, and may be particularly affected by descending traffic modulating pain transmission. It is likely there are multiple mechanisms involved. The stimulating electrodes may be introduced into the epidural space under direct surgical visualization or by means of a 15-gauge Tuohy needle with the electrodes placed between T 9 and T11.[38] This area of the spinal cord corresponds to lumbar segmental level output. Spinal cord stimulation at this level is associated with increased skin temperature, blood flow, decreased edema, and prolonged pain relief. The stimulating electrodes may be adjusted until stimulation of large fiber afferents produces a tingling paresthesia that overlies the painful region.[39] According to Augustinsson and coworkers, the vasodilating effects of spinal cord stimulation could be explained by (1) segmental inhibition of vasoconstrictor fibers, (2) antidromic activation of posterior root fibers, and (3) activation of ascending pathways to supraspinal autonomic centers. Interestingly, stimulation over lumbar spines or peripheral nerves was ineffective in these patients.[40,41] The long-term efficacy of spinal cord stimulation for pain from peripheral arteriosclerotic disease is reported to be excellent at 70% to 90% when compared to results of 50% to 70% for neuropathic pain.[42,43]

DRUG THERAPY

The search for a noninvasive treatment of peripheral ischemia has highlighted many drugs that, after a brief popularity, have vanished from our treatment armamentarium. The following discussion of drug therapy approaches include vasodilators, antithrombotic measures, fibrinolysis, phosphodiesterase inhibitors, antiplatelet drugs, metabolic agents, arachidonic acid derivatives, and gene therapy.[24]

VASODILATORS

Because the regulation of blood flow in the normal foot is affected by decreasing or increasing sympathetic tone, α-adrenergic blocking agents have been used, including thymoxamine, phentolamine, phenoxybenzamine, and clonidine. Other drugs have a local effect on vascular smooth muscle, which include papaverine and derivatives of nicotinic acid. Priscoline is an α-receptor blocker that has a direct effect.

Systemic use of vasodilators may reduce blood flow in the worst affected limb by shunting blood to healthier areas (the vasodilator paradox).[44] A local effect may be obtained by direct intra-arterial injection or by retrograde intravenous infusion (Bier technique). Ketanserin, a serotonin-2 receptor antagonist, and nifedipine, a calcium channel blocker, may play a role in therapy;[45] however, lowered systemic blood pressure and perfusion pressure to the ischemic tissue, and the maximal dilation of local vessels in the ischemic region suggest vasodilator treatment might not be effective.

ANTITHROMBOTIC MEASURES

Anticoagulant treatment has not been shown to be effective in peripheral vascular disease as thrombosis, when it occurs, is the final episode in the generation of the ischemic limb.

FIBRINOLYSIS

Fibrinogen is the substrate for thrombin that converts it to fibrin. Dissolution of fibrin can be achieved using streptokinase, urokinase, and tissue plasminogen activator. Although it would not affect the atheroma, and restenosis may follow cessation of therapy, it may delay progression and be a useful therapy in acute occlusion. Its use should be followed by arteriography to assess the need for reconstruction.

PHOSPHODIESTERASE INHIBITORS

Two drugs approved by the FDA for use in intermittent claudication are cilostazol and pentoxifylline. Both drugs exhibit phosphodiesterase inhibition that can increase the concentration of cyclic AMP leading to inhibition of platelet aggregation, thromboxane release, and increase in prostacyclin release. Unlike milrinone, which has similar effects on vessels and platelets, cilostazol does not display significant inotropic effect.[46] Pentoxifylline also affects blood rheology and specifically increases flexibility of red blood cells.

ANTIPLATELET DRUGS

Drugs such as aspirin, dipyridamole, ticlopidine, and prostacyclin inhibit release of thromboxane A and prevent platelet aggregation. Because the latter occurs in turbulent flow proximal or distal to atheromatous stenosis or occlusion, such treatment is of secondary importance in peripheral arterial disease. However, in conjunction with lipid-lowering drugs, antiplatelet drug therapy is the mainstay of secondary prevention to prevent myocardial infarction (MI) and stroke in patients with peripheral artery disease, even those who do not have signs or symptoms of coronary or carotid disease. Among drugs available in generic formulation, aspirin in low dose between 81 and 325 mg per day is efficacious and economical.

METABOLIC AGENTS

Naftidrofuryl was marketed first as a vasodilator, but it is purported to influence muscle metabolism beneficially through the Krebs cycle. Although a meta-analysis of seven randomized controlled trials involving 229 patients showed reduction in pain and analgesic consumption, the results were not statistically significant and in 1995 the drug was withdrawn in the United States for treatment of peripheral arterial disease.[47] Levocarnitine and propionyl levocarnitine are two drugs that may provide benefit by lessening the acylcarnitine metabolite build-up resulting from an impaired mitochondrial electron transport in ischemic muscle; however, propionyl levocarnitine is not FDA approved.[48]

ARACHIDONIC ACID DERIVATIVES

The term *prostaglandin* was first used by Von Euler[49] who discovered some of the pharmacologic effects of semen. Endoperoxides derived from cell membrane arachidonic acid are converted to thromboxane A_2 in platelets (vasoconstrictor and platelet aggregator) or to prostacyclin in blood vessel endothelium (vasodilator and inhibitor of platelet aggregation). The balance between these two classes of compounds maintains intravascular hemostasis.

The earliest report of the use of prostacyclin in ischemic feet used prostaglandin E_1 by intra-arterial infusion; the same team later administered the drug by the intravenous route. In both instances, they reported dramatic relief of rest pain in small groups of patients and healing of some ulcers.[50,51] Prostaglandin I_2 (PGI_2), also a platelet inhibitor and vasodilator, can be administered daily as an intravenous infusion (Iloprost), or given orally (Beraprost) with encouraging results.[52]

GENE THERAPY

Gene therapy may be helpful in restoring blood flow to ischemic extremities. A Boston group reported results in a small phase I study. Human DNA coded to make vascular endothelial growth factor (VEGF) was introduced into *Escherichia coli* plasmid which was grown in culture, purified, and administered by intramuscular injection into ischemic muscles of patients with critical limb ischemia. Ischemia is defined as rest pain with nonhealing ischemic ulcers in human volunteers identified as poor candidates for revascularization surgery. VEGF, secreted by endothelial cells, is the same protein as vascular permeability factor. It has binding sites limited to endothelial cells and therefore is site specific. Injection of plasmid VEGF DNA manufactured by *E. coli* produced significant transient edema in the limbs where it was injected. ELISA measured VEGF concentration also increased transiently and was associated in time with increased small blood vessel formation that persisted after VEGF levels returned to baseline, increased ankle-brachial index, healing of ulcers, increased exercise tolerance and resolution of rest pain. The authors cautiously interpreted their data as supportive for the strategy of IM gene therapy for therapeutic angiogenesis in patients with critical limb ischemia.[53]

PAIN DUE TO PERIPHERAL ARTERIAL DISEASE

RAYNAUD PHENOMENON

Raynaud phenomenon differs from other peripheral arteriopathies because it affects mainly the hands. It was described first by Maurice Raynaud[54] in 1862. Allen and Brown[55] advanced our understanding by separating affected patients into those with and without a known underlying cause.

Raynaud disease (also known as primary Raynaud phenomenon) includes the classic clinical picture of pallor in the distal two-thirds of the fingers (a result of arterial shutdown), cyanosis (from partial relaxation of arterial spasm and deoxygenation of blood), and rubor (reactive hyperemia); all occur in response to cold or emotion. As the condition progresses, the pain becomes more severe and continuous. The condition is more common in women than in men; usually it becomes apparent by the age of 40 years. It occurs much less often in the lower limbs. *Raynaud disease* describes patients in whom no underlying condition can be found.

Raynaud syndrome (also known as secondary Raynaud phenomenon) comprises those patients with Raynaud phenomenon secondary to underlying pathologic disorders (**Table 61-4**). Interestingly, 10% of patients with primary pulmonary hypertension may exhibit symptoms.[56]

Raynaud syndrome is particularly important because the associated condition may be treatable. However, the prognosis is worse, and patients may develop pathologic changes of ulceration, subungual infection, and pulp loss after digital arterial occlusion (**Fig. 61-2**). Porter and Rivers[57] reported 383 patients observed in a 10-year period. Of these, 162 had no associated disease and 137 had proven or suspected connective tissue disorder (57 of the latter had systemic sclerosis).

TABLE 61-4 Conditions Associated with Raynaud's Phenomenon
Immunologic and connective tissue disorders (such as systemic sclerosis, systemic lupus erythematosus, rheumatoid dermatomyositis, hepatitis-B associated vasculitis)
Arterial obstruction (e.g., thoracic outlet syndrome and Buerger disease)
Vibrating tool disease
Drug-induced (e.g., ergot, β-adrenergic blockers, cytotoxic drugs [vinblastine or bleomycin], oral contraceptives)
Miscellaneous (e.g., vinyl chloride disease, cold agglutinins, cryoglobulinemia)

RAYNAUD MANAGEMENT

General Measures Simple avoidance of cold, either of the body or of the hands, may be all that is required in mild cases. A change of occupation may be necessary if vibrating tools are used. Cessation of smoking has been advocated.

Sympathectomy Because nervous control of digital blood flow occurs simply as a result of increasing or decreasing sympathetic tone, pharmacologic or surgical sympathectomy has been used extensively. Drugs such as methyldopa, thymoxamine, reserpine, debrisoquine, and phentolamine have been administered orally and intra-arterially. Most of the studies are anecdotal, uncontrolled, or rely on subjective assessment. If no effect can be proved when a drug is given intra-arterially, it is unlikely that it will work systemically. The pain of Raynaud phenomenon has been controlled by IVRA sympathetic block with guanethidine (no longer manufactured). Agents used in IVRA to treat other pain syndromes may find application in Raynaud treatment as guanethidine alternatives are investigated (see section "Intravenous Regional Sympathetic Blocks").

Surgical sympathectomy can be done using an open procedure, but temporary and permanent Horner syndrome may occur. Transaxillary endoscopic coagulation to destroy thoracic ganglia 2 to 5 is another approach.[58] A thoracoscopic approach that is minimally invasive has also been described.[59,60] The immediate effect usually is good, although recurrence is common within 6 to 24 months and this treatment may be less effective than others.[61] Digital sympathectomy using microvascular techniques has also been reported.[62]

Sympathetic Blockade Where the condition is not severe and particularly if it is seasonal, a stellate ganglion block can be effective. A paratracheal approach at the C6 level reduces the risk of pneumothorax and

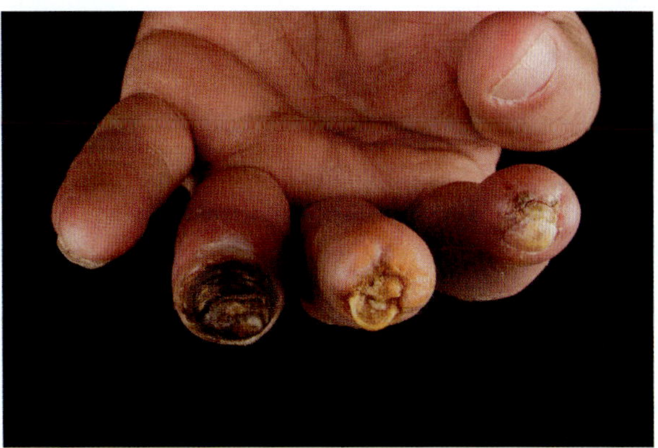

FIGURE 61-2. Digital ulceration in Raynaud disease. (Reproduced from Goldsmith LA, Katz SI, Gilchrest BA, Paller AS, Leffell DJ, Wolff K, eds. Fitzpatrick's Dermatology in General Medicine. 8th ed. New York, NY: McGraw-Hill;2012:1949. Copyright ©McGraw-Hill Education. All rights reserved.)

intravertebral artery injection. The accuracy may be increased by the use of radiographic control and a radiopaque dye that can identify the occurrence of dural cuff injection. A sympathetic block with local anesthetic does not tend to produce a sustained response.

Other Treatments Although Ketanserin was initially[63] considered to be a helpful therapy, recent reviews suggest no significant clinical effect.[64] Temperature biofeedback was recently shown to be inferior treatment in comparison with calcium antagonist.[65] Nifedipine or other calcium channel blockers are highly effective for patients who do not experience adverse effects. Interestingly, the dihydropyridine calcium channels are closely associated with the endothelin-1 receptor, suggesting endothelin-1, found in higher concentration in Raynaud patient serum, may be a neuron-independent vasoconstrictor.[66] Prostacyclin infusion and administration of a stable oral preparation may be effective and were described above. As noted above, spinal cord stimulation could be of value.

BUERGER DISEASE

Thromboangiitis obliterans was the name Leo Buerger[67] gave to a specific arterial disease which he believed was confined largely to Eastern Europeans. This disease subsequently was shown to be prevalent in Sri Lanka, Korea, and Japan where it was the most common form of arterial pathology. By the 1970s it was reported that 75% of 1641 cases of femoropopliteal occlusion were caused by this condition.[68] A gradual decrease in the incidence has been reported.[69]

Clinical Picture More than 90% of Buerger disease sufferers are men younger than 40 years of age who are smokers. They have instep claudication or painful ischemic changes in the feet. Less than 50% of patients have manifestations in their upper limbs, usually thrombophlebitis or minor ischemic changes. Upper extremity circulation may be assessed with an Allen test. The patient makes a fist while occluding radial and ulnar arteries at the wrist. The hand is relaxed and ulnar arterial pressure is released. Failure of the hand to regain color constitutes a positive test. The test is repeated for patency of radial artery. In these patients, foot pulses and later popliteal pulses are absent.

Buerger disease is an inflammatory process; the affected artery is surrounded by fibrosis whereas the normal structure of the vessel wall may be preserved, in contrast to the typical disruption of internal elastic lamina and media in arteriosclerosis and other systemic vasculitides.[70] The pathology is specific with thrombosis in crural arteries and veins. Giant cells are a histologic feature, even in early cases.

Management Universally, it is accepted that for smokers, treatment must begin with smoking cessation. If patients stop smoking, this alone may be sufficient to provide relief.

Local treatment is directed toward debridement and draining infections. Prostaglandin in the form of iloprost may provide benefit particularly during the period when patients first discontinue smoking.[71] Sympathectomy and spinal cord stimulators are used in management of difficult cases. As with arteriosclerosis, gene therapy may offer promise.[72]

VENOUS DISEASE

Venous disease may occur as acute (deep venous thrombosis [DVT]; thrombophlebitis) or chronic (DVT with recanalization or gravitational disease). Deep venous thrombosis occurs when normal venous flow is disturbed according to the Virchow triad: (1) diminished flow velocity after illness, operation, childbirth; (2) alteration in the characteristics of the contained blood producing increased viscosity, such as polycythemia, abnormal plasma protein fractions, leukemia, or thrombocythemia; and (3) local intimal damage. In most patients, more than one factor is responsible. The disease apparently arises spontaneously in healthy people; however, a search for underlying condition (such as malignancy or collagen-vascular disease) should be undertaken. Often without initial symptomatology, the disease may present with death due to pulmonary embolism. The focus should be on prevention rather than treatment, particularly for patients at increased risk due to immobility, including patients admitted to the hospital for surgery. For further information about venous thromboembolism, see the excellent discussion by Geerts et al.[73]

ACUTE VENOUS DISEASE

The clinical diagnosis of DVT is made by the triad of local tenderness, swelling, and color change. Clinical diagnosis alone does not detect the more subtle changes and may overdiagnose the condition. In the presence of atheroma, false-positive and false-negative results comprise 50% of tests.

When edema is present, it implies that the deep veins are occluded; embolization is less likely, but local sequelae are more likely. The clinical picture is either the white leg (milk leg), which is pale and shows infragenicular pitting edema, or the blue leg, which involves the entire leg as far proximally as the root of the limb. The former is a result of femoropopliteal obstruction; the latter indicates iliac-caval obstruction. The blue leg causes much discomfort, and if tissue pressure continues to rise, peripheral gangrene may supervene.

Acute thrombophlebitis is easily recognizable because there is visible swelling and tenderness along the course of a superficial vein. Apart from the underlying conditions already mentioned, the condition may be the harbinger of carcinoma of the pancreas or lung.

CHRONIC VENOUS DISEASE

Occlusion of the major veins is followed by recanalization with valve destruction. This allows transmission of the full force of the column of blood from the right atrium to the heel (+ 80 to 90 torr). The patient may have complaint of a resting pain in the calf, which, when associated with walking, is known as venous claudication.

Gravitational changes are more serious because of their reputation for intractability. These changes include pigmentation, distended intracutaneous veins (in the inframalleolar position, so-called venous flare), edema, liposclerosis, and ulceration (Fig. 61-2). The pain of a venous ulcer may be excruciating; it usually is worse at night and is unrelated to ulcer size. Investigation of venous disease is directed toward the following:

1. *Proving the diagnosis.* Isotope studies may be helpful in diagnosis of acute DVT. Duplex ultrasonography and impedance plethysmography are useful in establishing the diagnosis. The "gold standard" investigation is venography, which should be universally available. Testing for the D-dimer fibrin degradation product combined with clinical criteria has a high sensitivity and low false-negative results.[74,75]
2. *Demonstrating an underlying cause.* A complete blood count (CBC), erythrocyte sedimentation rate (ESR), chest x-ray (CXR), liver diagnostic tests, urinalysis, renal function tests, serum proteins, and immunoglobin level tests and tests for lupus erythematosus, rheumatoid, and other collagenoses may be required.

Management of Venous Disease

Acute Deep Venous Thrombosis The classical mainstay of treatment used to be a 5000 unit bolus of heparin followed by a continuous intravenous infusion in a dose of 40,000 units in 24 hours. This treatment was designed to prevent the spread of the thrombus and embolization until the clot became adherent and stabilized. In the absence of bleeding complications, therapy was maintained for 5 days, the last 3 of which overlap with the commencement of oral anticoagulation therapy with coumarin which was maintained for 3 months. Vitamin K antagonist treatment to maintain an INR of 2.5 is the most frequent secondary treatment for patients with venous thromboembolism. In four studies with 1500 patients, a meta-analysis revealed reduction for risk of recurrent events as long as treatment was maintained. As the risk of recurrent event may decrease over time, this benefit may eventually become outweighed by the risk of hemorrhagic complication that does not decrease over time.[76]

The availability of a low-cost outpatient management option has resulted in shortened hospital stays with many cases in the United States being treated with subcutaneous injections of low molecular weight heparin. A meta-analysis of 4754 patients in 14 randomized prospective controlled studies showed low molecular weight heparin was as effective as unfractionated intravenous heparin in preventing recurrent DVT. The risk of hemorrhage was lower during treatment and mortality at follow-up was also lower for the outpatient treatment protocol.[77]

ACUTE THROMBOPHLEBITIS

This usually is a self-limited condition that can be treated by local warm compresses and an anti-inflammatory drug (such as ibuprofen.) If the process involves the saphenous vein in the thigh, it may be necessary to ligate it at the groin to prevent the thrombosis from spreading into the femoral vein.

Chronic Venous Insufficiency The venous hypertension that follows extensive valvular obstruction after DVT includes various stigmata in the gaiter area of the leg, the most disabling of which is ulceration. There are a number of causes of leg ulceration, and it is important to exclude concomitant arterial disease, diabetes, and rheumatoid disease because these will render standard treatment ineffective. The linchpin of venous ulcer treatment is effective graded dynamic elastic compression to oppose the harmful effects of venous hypertension. Topical therapies include antibiotics, corticosteroids, and enzymes. However, they are all largely ineffective. They also may be expensive and can produce sensitization reactions that may be worse than the original condition.

Pain control with analgesic drugs during the healing phase is important; a decreasing need for analgesia is a good indication of progress toward healing.

SUMMARY

Interestingly, services for patients with pain due to peripheral vascular disease are delivered by a multitude of specialists including vascular surgeons, radiologists, anesthesiologists, rheumatologists, cardiologists, internists, dermatologists, primary care physicians, and podiatrists. The explosion of basic science and clinical research promises improved understanding and additional management options for these severely disabling diseases. Meanwhile, the author encourages the reader, irrespective of specialty, to take every opportunity to encourage smoking cessation, regular daily exercise, and other preventive measures that produce so much benefit to so many.

REFERENCES

1. Smith FB. Intravenous Naftidrofuryl for critical limb ischemia (Cochrane Review). *The Cochrane Library*. 2001;Issue 2.
2. Swerdlow M, Schraibman IG. Peripheral Vascular Disease. In: Warfield CA, ed. *Principles and Practice of Pain Management*. New York, NY: McGraw-Hill; 1993.
3. European Working Group on Critical Leg Ischemia. Second European consensus document on chronic critical leg ischemia. *Circulation*. 1991;84(suppl IV):IV-1-IV-26.
4. Sayeed MM. Signaling mechanisms of altered cellular responses in Trauma, Burn, and Sepsis: role of Ca2+. *Arch Surg*. December 2000;135(12):1432-1442.
5. Tani T, Fujino M, Hanasawa K, Shimizu T, Endo Y, Kodama M. Bacterial translocation and tumor necrosis factor-[alpha] gene expression in experimental hemorrhagic shock. *Crit Care Med*. November 2000;28(11):3705-3709.
6. Silvestre J-S, Mallat Z, Duriez M, Tamarat R, Bureau MF, Scherman D, et al. Antiangiogenic effect of interleukin-10 in ischemia-induced angiogenesis in mice hindlimb. *Circ Res*. September 15, 2000;87(6):448-452.
7. Forsythe JA, Jiang BH, Iyer NV, Agani F, Leung SW, Koos RD, et al. Activation of vascular endothelial growth factor gene transcription by hypoxia-inducible factor 1. *Mol Cell Biol*. 1996;16:4604-4613.
8. Akeno N, Czyzyk-Krzeska MF, Gross TS, et al. Hypoxia induces vascular endothelial growth factor gene transcription in human osteoblast-like cells through the hypoxia-inducible factor-2alpha. *Endocrinol (United States)*. Feb 2001;142(2):959-962.
9. Isner JM. Tissue responses to ischemia: local and remote responses for preserving perfusion of ischemic muscle. *J Clin Invest*. September 2000;106(5):615-619.
10. Cohen RA. The role of nitric oxide and other endothelium-derived vasoactive substances in vascular disease. *Prog Cardiovasc Dis*. 1995;38:105-128.
11. Opal S, Thijs L, Cavaillon J-M, Cohen J, Fourrier F. Roundtable I: relationships between coagulation and inflammatory processes. *Crit Care Med*. September 2000;28(9 Supplement):S81-S82.
12. Kullo IJ, Simari RD, Schwartz RS. Vascular gene transfer: from bench to bedside. *Arteriosclerosis, Thrombosis & Vascular Biology*. February 1999;19(2):196-207.
13. Creager MA, Dzau VJ. Vascular disease of the extremities. In: Braunwald E, Fauci AS, Kasper DL, et al., eds. *Harrisons Text Book of Medicine*. 15th ed. New York, NY: McGraw-Hill; 2001: 1036.
14. Vass A, Leng G, Papacosta O, Walker M, Lennon L, Whincup PH. Secondary prevention may help intermittent claudication. *BMJ*. 2001;322(7287):673.
15. DeBenetittis G, Panerai AA, Villamari MA. Effects of hypnotic analgesia and hypnotizability on experimental ischemic pain. *Int J Clin Exp Hypn*. January 1989;37(1):55-69.
16. Hoogwegt MT, et al. Smoking cessation has no influence on quality of life in patients with peripheral arterial disease 5 years post-vascular surgery. *Eur J Vasc Endovasc Surg*. 2010;40(3):355-362.
17. Kapral MK, Silver FL, with the Canadian Task Force on Preventive Health Care. Preventive health care, 1999 update: 2. Echocardiography for the detection of a cardiac source of embolus in patients with stroke. *CMAJ*. 1999;161(8):989-996.
18. Philipp CS, Cisar LA, Kim HC, Wilson AC, Saidi P, Kostis JB. Association of hemostatic factors with peripheral vascular disease. *Am Heart J*. 1997;134(5):978-984.
19. Kitslaar PJ, Wollersheim H, Zwiers I. Consensus noninvasive diagnosis of peripheral arterial vascular diseases. Central Guidance Organization for Peer Review. *Ned Tijdschr Geneeskd (Netherlands)*. 1995;139(22):1133-1136.
20. Huber A, Heuck A, Baur A, et al. Dynamic contrast-enhanced MR angiography from the distal aorta to the ankle joint with a step-by-step technique. *AJR Am J Roentgenol (United States)*. Nov 2000;175(5):1291-1298.
21. Jawahar D, Rachamalla HR, Rafalowski A, et al. Pulse oximetry in the evaluation of peripheral vascular disease. *Angiol (United States)*. August 1997;48(8):721-724.
22. Tan KH, de Cossart L, Edwards PR. Exercise training and peripheral vascular disease. *Br J Surg*. 2000;87(5):553.
23. Allen JD, et al. Plasma nitrite flux predicts exercise performance in peripheral arterial disease after 3 months of exercise training. *Free Radic Biol Med*. 2010;49(6):1138-1144.
24. Allen JD, Giordano T, Kevil CG. Nitrite and nitric oxide metabolism in peripheral artery disease. *Nitric Oxide*. 2012;26(4):217-222.
25. Leng GC, Davis M, Baker D. Bypass surgery for chronic lower limb ischaemia (Cochrane Review). In: *The Cochrane Library*. 2;2001.
26. Belkin M, et al. Peripheral arterial occlusive disease. In: Courtney D, et al., ed. *Sabiston Textbook of Surgery*. 16th ed. W. B. Saunders Company; 2001: 1375.

27. Wronski J. Lumbar sympathectomy performed by means of videoscopy. *Cardiovasc Surg.* October 1998;6(5):453-456.
28. Lee BY, Rangraj MS, Waisbren S. Laparoscopic retroperitoneal lumbar sympathectomy in the treatment of lower extremity reflex sympathetic dystrophy and ischemia. *Contemp Surg.* 1998;52:21-26.
29. Gleim M, Maier C, Melchert U. Lumbar neurolytic sympathetic blockades provide immediate and long-lasting improvement of painless walking distance and muscle metabolism in patients with severe peripheral vascular disease. *J Pain Symptom Manage (United States).* February 1995;10(2):98-104
30. Yao J, Bergan JJ. Predictability of vascular reactivity relative to sympathetic ablation. *Arch Surg.* 1973;107:676-679.
31. Breivik H, Cousins MJ, Lofstrom JB. Sympathetic neural blockade of the upper and lower extremity. In: Cousins MJ, Bridenbaugh PO, eds. *Neural Blockade in Clinical Anesthesia and Pain Management.* 3rd ed. Philadelphia, PA: Lippincott-Raven; 1998:411-447.
32. McCollum PT, Spence VA, Marcrae B, Walker WF. Quantitative assessment of the effectiveness of chemical lumbar sympathectomy. *Br J Anaesth.* 1985;57:1146-1149.
33. Hannington-Kiff JG. Antisympathetic drugs in limbs. In: Wall Pd, Melzack R, eds. *Textbook of Pain.* Edinburgh: Churchill Livingstone; 1984:566-577.
34. Stumpflen A, Ahmadi A, Atteneder M, Gschwandtner M, Hofmann S, Maca, et al. Effects of transvenous regional guanethidine block in the treatment of critical finger ischemia. *Angiol.* February 2000;51(2):115-122.
35. Sruben SS, Steinberg RB, Madabhushi L, Rosenthal E. Intravenous regional clonidine in the management of sympathetically maintained pain. *Anesthesiol.* 1998;89(2):527-530.
36. Malik VK, Inchiosa MA, Mustafa K, Sanapati MR, Pimentel MC, Frost EA. Intravenous regional phenoxybenzamine in the treatment of reflex sympathetic dystrophy. *Anesthesiol.* 1998;88(2):823-827.
37. Hogan QH, Abram SE. Neural blockade for diagnosis and prognosis: a review. *Anesthesiol.* January 1997;86(1):216-241.
38. Tesfaye S, Watt J, Benbow SJ, Pank KA, Miles J, MacFarlane IA. Electrical spinal-cord stimulation for painful diabetic peripheral neuropathy. *Lancet.* 1996;9043(348):1698-1701.
39. Stanton-Hicks M, Salamon J. Stimulation of the Central and Peripheral Nervous System for the Control of Pain. *Journal of Clinical Neurophysiology. Neurophysiology of Pain.* January 1997;14(1):46-62.
40. Augustinsson LE, Carlsson CA, Holm J, et al. Epidural electrical stimulation in severe limb ischemia: Pain relief, increased blood flow, and a possible limb-saving effect. *Ann Surg.* 1985 Jul;202:104-110.
41. Naver H, Augustinsson LE, Elam M. The vasodilating effect of spinal dorsal column stimulation is mediated by sympathetic nerves. *Clin Autonom Res.* 1992;2:41-45.
42. Augustinsson LE, Linderoth B, Mannheimer C, Eliasson T. Spinal cord stimulation in cardiovascular disease. *Neurosurg Clin North Am.* January 1995;6(1):157-165.
43. Jivegard LE, Augustinsson LE, Holm J, Risberg B, Ortenwall P. Effects of spinal cord stimulation (SCS) in patients with inoperable severe lower limb ischaemia: a prospective randomised controlled study. *Eur J Vasc Endovasc Surg.* May 1995;9(4):421-425.
44. Gillespie JA. The case against vasodilator drugs in occlusive vascular disease of the legs. *Lancet.* 1959;2:955.
45. Tjon JA. Treatment of intermittent claudication with pentoxifylline and cilostazol. *Am J Health Syst Pharm.* March 15, 2001;58(6):485-493; quiz 494-6.
46. Cone J, Wang S, Tandon N, et al. Comparison of the effects of cilostazol and milrinone on intracellular cAMP levels and cellular function in platelets and cardiac cells. *J Cardiovasc Pharmacol.* 1999;34:497-504.
47. Smith FB, Bradbury AW, Fowkes FGR. Intravenous naftidrofuryl for critical limb ischaemia (Cochrane Review). *The Cochrane Libary.* 2001;Issue 2.
48. Hiatt WR. Drug therapy: medical treatment of peripheral arterial disease and claudication. *N Engl J Med.* 2001;344(21):1608-1621.
49. Von Euler US. Uber der spezfishe blutdrucks enkende substanz des menshilichen Prostata-und samen blasensckretes. *Klin Wochenschr.* 1935;14:1182.
50. Carlson LA, Erickson I. Femoral artery infusion of prostaglandin E_1 in severe peripheral vascular disease. *Lancet.* 1973;1:155-156.
51. Carlson LA, Erickson I. Intravenous prostaglandin E_1 in severe peripheral vascular disease. *Lancet.* 1976;2:810.
52. Lievre M, Morand S, Besse B, Fiessinger JN, Boissel JP. Oral beraprost sodium, a prostaglandin I_2 analogue, for intermittent claudication: a double-blind, randomized, multicenter controlled trial. *Circulation.* 2000;102:426-431.
53. Baumbartner I. Constitutive expression of phVEGF165 after intramuscular gene transfer promotes collateral vessel development in patients with critical limb ischemia. *Circulation.* 1998;97:1114-1123.
54. Raynaud M. *De l'asphyxie locale et de la gangrene symmetrique des extremes.* Paris: Righoux; 1862.
55. Allen EV, Brown GE. Raynaud's disease—a critical review of the minimal requirements for diagnosis. *Ann J Jed Sci.* 1932;183-187.
56. Gaine S. Pulmonary hypertension. *JAMA.* December 27, 2000;284(24):3160-3168.
57. Porter JM, Rivers SP. Management of Raynaud's syndrome. In: Bergan JJ, Yao J, eds. *Evaluation and Treatment of Upper and Lower Extremity Circulatory Disorders.* Orlando, FL: Grune & Stratton; 1984:182.
58. Malone RS, Cameron AEP, Rennie JA. Endoscopic thoracic sympathectomy in the treatmnet of upper limb hyperhydrosis. *Ann R Coll Surg Engl.* 1986;68:93-94.
59. Colt HG. Thoracoscopy*: window to the pleural space. *Chest.* November 1999;116(5):1409-1415.
60. Krasna MJ, Jiao X, Sonett J, Gamliel Z, King K. Thoracoscopic sympathectomy. *Surg Laparosc, Endosc Percutan Tech.* October 2000;10(5):314-318.
61. Ho M, Belch JJ. Raynaud's phenomenon: state of the art 1998 [editorial]. [Review] [37 refs]. *Scand J Rheumatol.* 1998;27:319-322.
62. Yee AM, Hotchkiss RN, Paget SA. Adventitial stripping: a digit saving procedure in refractory Raynaud's phenomenon. *J Rheumatol (Canada).* February 1998;25(2):269-276.
63. Stranden R, Roald OK, Krohg K. Treatment of Raynaud's phenomenon with the 5-HT_2-receptor antagonist ketanserin. *BMJ.* 1982;285:1069-1071.
64. Pope J, et al. Ketanserin for Raynaud's phenomenon in progressive systemic sclerosis. *The Cochrane Library.* 1999;Issue 3.
65. Raynaud's Treatment Study Investigators. Comparison of sustained-release nifedipine and temperature biofeedback for treatment of primary Raynaud phenomenon: results from a randomized clinical trial with 1-year follow-up. *Arch Intern Med.* April 24, 2000;160(8):1101-1108.
66. Dowd P, Goldsmith P, Bull H, Burnstock G, Foreman J, Marshall I. Raynaud's phenomenon. *Lancet.* July 29, 1995;346(8970):283-290.
67. Buerger L. Thrombo-angiitis obliterans. A study of the vascular lesions leading to presenile gangrene. *Ann J Med Sci.* 1909;136:562.
68. Mishima Y. Curent status of femoropopliteal occlusion in Japan. *J Cardiovasc Surg.* Suppl 1970;11(3):97.
69. Matsushita M, Nishikimi N, Sakurai T, et al. Decrease in prevalence of Buerger's disease in Japan. *Surgery (United States).* Sep 1998;124(3):498-502.

70. Olin JW, Lie JT. Thromboangiitis obliterans (Buerger's disease). In: Loscalzo J, Creager MA, Dzau VJ, eds. *Vascular Medicine*. 2nd ed. Boston: Little, Brown; 1996:1033-1049.

71. Fiessinger JN, Schafer M. Trial of iloprost versus aspirin treatment for critical limb ischaemia of thromboangiitis obliterans: the TAO Study. *Lancet*. 1990;335:555-557.

72. Isner JM, Baumgartner I, Rauh G, et al. Treatment of thromboangiitis obliterans (Buerger's disease) by intramuscular gene transfer of vascular endothelial growth factor: preliminary clinical results. *J Vasc Surg*. 1998;28:964-973.

73. Geerts WH, Heit JA, Clagett GP, Pineo GF, Colwell CW, Anderson FA, et al. Prevention of venous thromboembolism. *Chest*. January 2001;119(1 Suppl):132S-175S.

74. Aschwanden M, Labs KH, Jeanneret C, et al. The value of rapid D-dimer testing combined with structured clinical evaluation for the diagnosis of deep vein thrombosis. *J Vasc Surg (United States)*. November 1999;30(5):929-935.

75. Wells PS, Anderson DR. Diagnosis of deep-vein thrombosis in the year 2000. *Curr Opin Pulm Med (United States)*. July 2000;6(4):309-313.

76. Hutten BA, Prins MH. Duration of treatment with vitamin K antagonists in symptomatic venous thromboembolism (Cochrane review). *Cochrane Database Syst Rev (England)*. 2000;(3):CD001367.

77. van Den Belt AG, Prins MH, Lensing AW, et al. Fixed dose subcutaneous low molecular weight heparins versus adjusted dose unfractionated heparin for venous thromboembolism. *Cochrane Database Syst Rev (England)*. 2000;(2):CD001100.

CHAPTER 62 Advances in the Management of Ischemic Pain

Janice E. Gellis
Gilbert J. Fanciullo

The heart asks pleasure first,
And then, excuse from pain.

—Emily Dickinson

Ischemic pain affects millions of people worldwide. It is a detriment to quality of life and carries with it significant morbidity and mortality. Ischemic pain occurs when there is obstruction of the circulation to an area of the body. The myocardium, lower extremities, and mesentery can be affected primarily from the development of atherosclerosis obliterans. Pain management centers are becoming more involved in the care of patients with ischemic diseases because the centers can offer interventional procedures applicable to these diseases. This chapter provides a review of the pathophysiology of ischemic disease, existing and emerging therapies available and their efficacy, and the role of the pain specialist in the management of patients with peripheral, coronary, and mesenteric ischemic disease.

PERIPHERAL ARTERY DISEASE

CHARACTERISTICS

Limb ischemia can be caused by atherosclerosis obliterans as well as atheroembolic or thromboembolic disease, vasculitis, trauma, and other disease processes. Limb ischemia affects macrovascular and microvascular circulation. Peripheral artery disease (PAD) is a marker for cardiovascular disease (CVD) and affects 8 million Americans.

TABLE 62-1 Differential Diagnosis for Intermittent Claudication

1. Atherosclerosis obliterans
2. Thromboangiitis obliterans
3. Acute arterial embolism
4. Entrapment syndrome
5. Acute deep venous occlusion
6. Lumbar spinal stenosis
7. Osteoarthritis of the hip and back

Ischemic pain in PAD is insidious and gradual in onset. The pain is described as an aching and cramping sensation that is worse at night and improves when the legs are in a dependent position, which improves blood flow. Most patients have atherosclerotic changes for 5 to 10 years before they have symptoms. Intermittent claudication is the earliest sign of vascular insufficiency, which is characterized by cramping, tightness, and heaviness that increase with exercise. The pain is relieved with rest and the claudication distance remains fairly constant until further progression of the disease. The differential diagnosis for intermittent claudication is listed in **Table 62-1**.

In the early stages of PAD, collateral circulation develops and may maintain adequate perfusion to the affected limb, but may not provide sufficient blood flow to prevent symptoms, especially during exercise. Approximately 25% of patients with intermittent claudication will progress to critical ischemia and pain at rest, secondary to the primary and collateral vessels becoming stenotic or occluded. When rest pain occurs, the degree of vascular insufficiency is severe. When ischemic pain at rest, tissue necrosis, and/or gangrene develop, patients fall into the category of critical limb ischemia (CLI) and will likely require surgery or endovascular procedures for pain control, limb salvage, and wound healing. Diagnosis and treatment is essential to minimize these sequelae (**Table 62-2**).

The most common sites of atherosclerosis obliterans are the femoropopliteal arterial segment and the aortoiliac vessels, causing pain in the calves and buttocks, respectively. With progression of the disease, gangrene, ischemic ulcers, and trophic changes can occur in the more distal locations, namely the distal foot and toes. Ischemic ulcers can occur spontaneously; however, trauma is usually the inciting event leading to ulcer formation. The injury is unable to heal due to poor perfusion. Trophic changes, specifically dry scaly skin, loss of hair, and thick nails, are signs of arterial insufficiency.

TREATMENT

Management of PAD includes risk factor modification, antiplatelet, and antithrombotic drugs. Critical limb ischemia necessitates the addition of interventional treatments such as bypass surgery or angioplasty. Patients with CLI, refractory to or not amenable to surgery, or those seeking an alternative treatment, may be candidates for spinal cord stimulation (SCS).

MEDICAL

Current guidelines recommend smoking cessation which may include pharmacotherapy and/or enrollment in a smoking cessation program. Patients with PAD who continue to smoke have a greater risk of amputation, death, myocardial infarction (MI), and lower patency rates with angioplasty or surgical revascularization.[1]

Diabetes contributes significantly to morbidity and mortality in patients with PAD. Additionally, diabetic patients are 20% to 30% more likely to develop PAD. Severity of diabetes and symptoms of PAD are directly correlated. Managing comorbidities such as hyperlipidemia, hypertension, and obesity are integral to the care of patients with PAD. Hypertension is associated with the development of atherosclerosis. Statins have been shown to diminish symptoms of claudication in patients with dyslipidemia and cardiac disease.[2] Protective and

TABLE 62-2 Diagnostic Methods for Peripheral Artery Disease

TEST	DESCRIPTION	INTERPRETATION	LIMITATIONS
Ankle-brachial index (ABI)	Expressed as a percentage, measures the systolic ankle pressure and divides it by the brachial artery systolic pressure; PAD symptomatology is inversely proportional to ABI	**NL**: 1.00-1.40 **BORDERLINE**: 0.91-0.99 **ABNORMAL**: < 0.90 **NONCOMPRESSIBLE ARTERY**: >1.40 (CLI is an ABI below 0.90)	Inability to detect PAD in presence of noncompressible vessels
Toe-brachial index	Systolic pressure is measured from the great toe (small cuff and Doppler)	**ABNORMAL:** 0.70	
Segmental pressure examination	Plethysmographic cuffs are placed over **brachial arteries** and **various points on lower limb** (upper and lower thigh, upper calf, and ankle)	**UNDERLYING STENOSIS:** 20 mmHg gradient between adjacent levels.	Inability to detect PAD in presence of noncompressible vessels
Pulse volume recordings	Cuff system incorporates a plethysmograph to detect volume changes in the limb throughout the cardiac cycle; can be helpful in assessment of status of small vessels	**NL WAVEFORM:** steep upstroke, sharp sys peak, narrow pulse width, dicrotic notch, downslope bowing to baseline **ABNL WAVEFORM:** flattened upstroke, rounded peak with wider pulse width, dicrotic notch disappears, downslope bows away from baseline	

prophylactic care of the feet including good hygiene, avoidance of trauma, pressure points, and poorly fitting shoes is imperative to prevent ischemic ulceration and gangrene. Keeping the feet clean, dry, and free from infection is also important.

Antiplatelet therapy is a component of treatment of PAD to reduce risk of MI, stroke, and vascular death. Aspirin is recommended in doses of 75 to 325 mg per day. Clopidogrel can be used as an alternative to aspirin. The combination of these medications can also be used to decrease the aforementioned risks. Unless a patient has another proven indication for warfarin, it is not recommended as an addition to antiplatelet therapy.

INTERVENTIONAL/SURGICAL

In spite of these measures to slow the progression of atherosclerotic occlusive disease, 25% to 50% of patients will require more aggressive treatment.

The bypass versus angioplasty in severe ischemia of the leg (BASIL) trial is considered the most comprehensive randomized controlled trial to date.[3] The study contrasted angioplasty to surgical vascular bypass examining overall survival and amputation-free survival. There was no significant difference after 2 years in amputation-free survival between the two arms of the study; however, bypass surgery, the first study, was associated with a significant increase in overall survival. Stenting and atherectomy are additional endovascular treatment options for patients with PAD.

For patients who are not candidates for surgical intervention, pain control, tissue salvage, and maintenance of an independent lifestyle are important issues. Unfortunately, limb amputation, which may have high perioperative mortality, may be the ultimate treatment option for some patients.

The success and efficacy of percutaneous transluminal angioplasty (PTA) has increased the number of patients treated for occlusive arterial disease who were not surgical candidates because of concomitant disease processes and substantial risk factors associated with surgery. PTA is a minimally invasive procedure that has fewer associated costs, shorter hospital stays, and fewer risks to the patient. The primary concern with PTA of the lower extremities is the long-term patency of the vessel.

Long-term success of iliac artery PTA is dependent on certain predictors as shown in Table 62-2. The early success rates of PTA for the iliac arteries range from 90% to 99% patency with 2-year patency rate of 80% to 95%. Angioplasty for femoropopliteal disease has a 2-year patency rate of 89% and a 4-year rate of 67%. Data indicate that PTA is a valuable and durable alternative to surgical revascularization (**Table 62-3**).

INTERVENTIONAL PAIN MANAGEMENT

Spinal Cord Stimulation A large body of evidence now exists supporting the use of epidural SCS in the treatment of limb-threatening peripheral vascular disease as well as for intractable angina pectoris. SCS is now considered in patients who do not have surgical or other interventional options. The patients may have significant relief of their ischemic symptoms by undergoing this minimally invasive procedure with few risks to the patient with multiple comorbidities. The technique involves placement of the electrode at high lumbar or low thoracic levels.

Spinal cord stimulation was first used by Shealy et al in 1967.[4] Early trials were plagued by equipment failures and malfunctions such as lead fracture and electrode movement. Patient selection was also poor because the specific mechanism of analgesia produced by SCS was and still is elusive. Regardless of the etiology of the pain, SCS was used in virtually any patient. The increase in the success rate of SCS over the ensuing years is a result of improved technology and better patient selection.

In the 1970s Cook et al used SCS to treat pain in patients with multiple sclerosis and noted that these patients had a significant improvement in lower extremity blood flow and a feeling of warmth in their lower extremities.[5] Further studies showed clinical improvement in pain, microcirculation, and healing of ischemic ulcers in patients with inoperable peripheral vascular disease. Claudication distance, temperature, limb salvage rates, and exercise tolerance were substantially improved. Relief of ischemic pain appears to correlate well with an increase in microcirculatory changes and success rates of 70% to 100% pain relief are common. Macrocirculatory changes do not correlate well with relief of symptoms.

The most common use for SCS in the United States is for back pain with a predominant radicular component. The indications that may have the highest success rates are inoperable angina pectoris, peripheral vascular disease, and complex regional pain syndrome.

There are multiple theories as to how SCS improves blood flow in CLI. One postulated reason for benefit is improvement in microcirculation or nutritional blood flow. There is also support for suppression of efferent sympathetic activity causing peripheral vasodilation and secondary relief of pain. There may also be antidromic mechanism, whereby dorsal root

TABLE 62-3 Predictors of Success of Percutaneous Transluminal Angioplasty

1. Site of PTA
2. Indication for PTA (claudication vs limb salvage)
3. Severity of the lesion (stenosis was better than occlusion)
4. Presence of runoff vessels

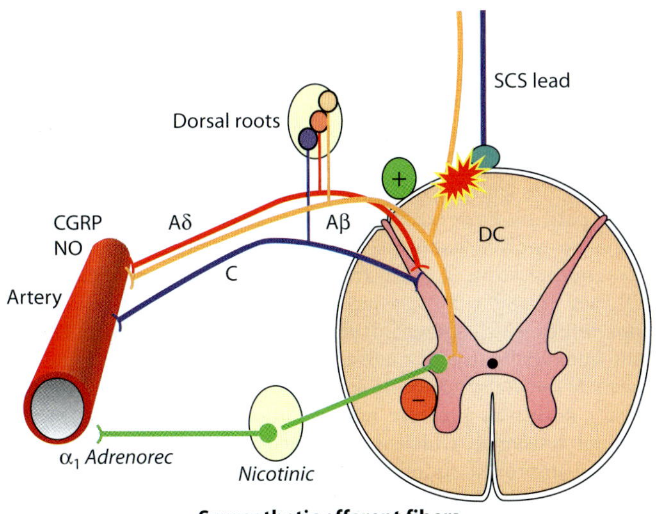

FIGURE 62-1. In alleviation of ischemic pain reduction of ischemia is the primary event. Also here multiple mechanisms seem to participate. Antidromic activation on hitherto unknown neuronal circuits reducing sympathetic outflow is one mechanism. The autonomic efference in question seems to be using nicotinic ganglionic receptors and mainly a1-adrenoreceptors at the neuro-effector junction. Another mechanism active at even low SCS intensities is the antidromic vasodilatation via activation of primary efferent fibers leading to peripheral release of CGRP with subsequent vasodilatation. The exact circuitry is not established but the presence of NO is required. Which mechanism that dominates seems to depend on the activity level of the sympathetic system. At low sympathetic tonus the antidromic activation dominates, but at higher levels, especially the later phase of vasodilatation seems to depend on sympathetic inhibition. (Redrawn after Linderoth and Foreman (1999).)

stimulation causes activation of primary efferent fibers leading to peripheral release of CGRP and subsequent vasodilation[6-8] (**Fig. 62-1**).

Ubbink and Vermeulen analyzed all randomized controlled trials evaluating the effectiveness of SCS patient with nonreconstructable chronic critical leg ischemia. They concluded that there is evidence that SCS is better than conservative treatment to decrease amputation risk. There was a finding of benefit on ulcer healing and pain relief. It was found that limb salvage with SCS was comparable to distal bypass surgery. They intimated that future studies may include SCS versus bypass surgery in reconstructable CLI. Additional studies show pain reduction in patients with CLI.[8]

EMERGING THERAPIES

Future treatment therapies may include gene therapy, growth factors, and cellular therapy to stimulate collateral blood vessel growth into ischemic tissues. These therapies are currently investigational. Current research is also directed to the use of autologous endothelial progenitor cell transplantation.[9]

ANGINA PECTORIS

CHARACTERISTICS

Angina pectoris results from an imbalance in myocardial oxygen consumption and myocardial oxygen supply. The disease process can produce severe incapacitating pain, pressure in the chest, arms, neck, and jaw. Atherosclerotic coronary artery disease (CAD) is a leading cause of morbidity and mortality in Western countries. The prevalence of angina pectoris in the United States is 3.9%, affecting about 9 million people.[10]

The arteries most commonly affected by atherosclerosis are the large epicardial arteries; however, small vessel disease may contribute to the overall clinical picture. Atherosclerosis may affect a single vessel and cause a discrete lesion, or it may affect multiple vessels diffusely. There appears to be no correlation between the severity of anginal pain and the severity of atherosclerosis. A single lesion in the left artery descending may produce extreme pain and disability, whereas multiple diffuse

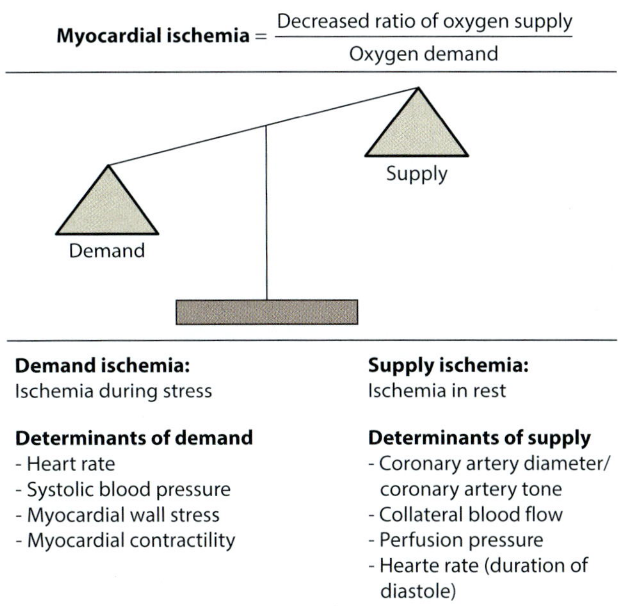

FIGURE 62-2. Schematic representation of myocardial ischemia and determinants of oxygen supply/demand ratio (see text for details). Redrawn from DeJongste MJ, Furman RD. Spinal cord stimulation for refractory angina. In: Krames ES, ed. *Neuromodulation*. 1st ed. 2009: 831-843, with permission, from Elsevier.

lesions affecting several vessels may produce mild to moderate anginal symptoms or no symptoms (**Fig. 62-2**).

TREATMENT

Medical Antianginal therapies have focused on decreasing myocardial oxygen consumption while increasing oxygen delivery to restore the natural balance between supply and demand. The long-term goals of antianginal therapy are to decrease the frequency of anginal attacks, reduce the severity of attacks, and prevent the ischemic event from progressing to myocardial damage. Control of anginal symptoms not only preserves the independence and lifestyle of patients, but can also improve their long-term prognosis.

Treatment for atherosclerotic CAD has focused on risk factor modifications, drug therapy, percutaneous coronary intervention, surgical revascularization, transmyocardial laser revascularization, and SCS. The mainstays of pharmacologic treatment are antiplatelet therapy, oral anticoagulant therapy, nitrates, β-adrenergic blockers and calcium channel blockers, renin-angiotensin-aldosterone therapy, and ranolazine. Beta blockers decrease myocardial oxygen demand and oxygen consumption by decreasing ventricular wall tension, heart rate, and myocardial ionotropic state. Calcium channel blockers inhibit the reuptake of calcium in slow calcium channels, thereby producing vasodilation. The vasodilatory effect works to increase coronary artery perfusion and oxygen supply. Vasodilation also decreases afterload and increases cardiac output and, in effect, reduces cardiac work. Nitroglycerin acts as a vasodilator, and it not only dilates coronary arteries, but also reduces afterload and preload secondary to its venous pooling effects. Nitrates and calcium channel blockers both relieve vasospasm, which may contribute to ischemic attacks. Ranolazine is used for treatment of chronic angina pectoris; it improves ventricular diastolic tension via an indirect effect on sodium-dependent calcium current during ischemic conditions. It also partially disrupts the consequences of cell hypoxia during transient myocardial ischemia via an effect on sodium influx. It decreases calcium overload in the ischemic monocyte. These drugs may also be used for patients who have anginal pain but no objective signs of ischemia and normal coronary arteriograms. This syndrome, known as syndrome X, may be the result of small vessel disease and/or coronary vasospasm.

Interventional/Surgical Patients who do not respond to medication and risk factor modification may need to consider percutaneous coronary intervention (PCI) or coronary artery bypass grafting (CABG). In 2009, Serrys et al performed the SYNTAX study (Synergy Between Percutaneous Coronary Intervention with TAXUS [stent] and Cardiac Surgery). The multicenter study randomly assigned 1800 patients with three-vessel or left main CAD to undergo CABG or PCI. It is recognized as one of the most comprehensive comparisons of PCI and CABG. Information gathered from this study, including the SYNTAX score (an angiographic tool to grade the complexity of CAD), has been incorporated into the recommendations for ischemic heart disease guidelines.[11] The SYNTAX score revealed that a percutaneous approach should be avoided in patients with high scores. Whether a patient undergoes CABG or PCI depends on many factors including degree of CAD, ventricular function, setting of acute ST segment elevation myocardial infarction (STEMI), and comorbidities. Percutaneous coronary intervention includes procedures such as catheter balloon dilation, coronary artery stent placement (metal and drug eluting), atherectomy, and laser angioplasty (**Table 62-4**).

Transmyocardial laser revascularization (TMLR) is a surgical treatment developed in the 1980s. The technique is based on the fact that myocardial perfusion comes from not only the epicardial arteries but also from ventriculocoronary anastomoses. Anginal symptoms are decreased by using CO_2, Ho:YAG, or XeCl excimer laser to create transmural channels in the myocardium. Thoracotomy or sternotomy is necessary and the laser is directed at the epicardial surface of the left ventricle in regions of viable myocardium. In 2009, the procedure was evaluated by Briones et al as a Cochrane review that studied results of seven randomized controlled trials (RCTs) published between 1999 and 2004.[12] They concluded that there was insufficient evidence to demonstrate that the clinical benefits of TMLR outweighed the potential risks secondary to a fourfold increase in early postoperative mortality. They also concluded that more robust studies were needed. Conclusions have been supported by other studies including Pratali et al, who found a high incidence of deaths (primarily from MI) and return of angina often within 3 years.[13] The conclusion regarding TMLR is found in other studies as well. The ACCF/AHA/ACP/AATS/PCNA/SCAI/STS Guidelines mention the use of TMLR combined with CABG in patients who had some myocardial segments perfused by arteries not considered amenable to grafting. In the studies mentioned, there was no increase in mortality compared with CABG alone. When used as a sole therapeutic approach, CABG is reserved for patients with angina refractory to medication who do not have other therapeutic options.

Percutaneous myocardial laser revascularization (PMLR) is an alternative to TMLR. It eliminates the need for sternotomy or thoracotomy. Ho:YAG laser is applied to the endocardial surface of the left ventricle via a flexible cather. Laser firing is synchronized during systole. Nontrasmural channels are created in regions of the left ventricle with reversible ischemia. Proposed mechanisms of decreasing anginal symptoms include direct perfusion, micorvascuaar angiogenesis, and cardiac afferent denervation. PMLR appears to have an improved safety profile compared with TMLR. McGillion, Cook et al[14] reviewed published and unpublished RCTs of PMLR from January 1999 to June 2009. Five trials, including patients with refractory angina, published in peer-reviewed journals btween 2001 and 2006 met inclusion criteria. They concluded that PMLR is a safe treatment with promise for improvement of anginal symptoms and quality of life.

TABLE 62-4 Indications for Percutaneous Transluminal Coronary Angioplasty

1. Unstable angina pectoris
2. Acute MI
3. Multivessel disease
4. Saphenous vein bypass graft stenosis
5. Acute complete coronary artery occlusion

An increased population of patients comprises the category of refractory angina (RFA), which is characterized by severe, unremitting cardiac pain resistant to all conventional treatments for CAD, including medical therapy, CABG, and PCI. The pain is chronic, peristing for more than 3 months. Patients experience severely impaired health-related quality of life including poor general health, psychologic stress, activity restriction, difficulties with activities of daily living, as well as severe pain.

These patients, however, do have treatments available to them, which continue to evolve. Noninvasive treatments include enhanced external counterpulsation (EECP) and intermittent thrombolytic therapy. EECP uses inflatable cuffs applied to the lower extremities to increase venous return and augment diastolic blood pressure (BP). The cuffs inflate sequentially from the calves to the thigh muscles during diastole and deflate during systole. The augmentation during diastole increases coronary perfusion pressure and deflation during systole decreases peripheral resistance, which is associated with improved LV diastolic filling and improved endothelial function. Mechanisms described for effectiveness of this treatment include recruitment of collateral circulation, release of substances that promote angiogenesis, and a peripheral training effect. This treatment is contraindicated in severe PAD, severe aortic regurgitation, and decompensated heart failure.

Intermittent thrombolytic therapy has primarily used urokinase. Urokinase activates circulating and bound plasminogen, which is converted to plasmin. Plasmin degrades fibrin, producing thrombolysis and improving blood rheology. Its use was first explored in the 1990s. Urokinase may also initiate regression of coronary plaques. It is no longer recommended as a treatment for stable ischemic heart disease (SIHD) in the ACCF/AHA/ACP/AATS/PCNA/SCAI/STS Guidelines. It is mentioned in the Canadian Guidelines for the Management of Patients with Refractory Angina as a promising treatment; however, additional randomized controlled studies are necessary to confirm safety and efficacy.[15]

Interventional Pain Management Interventional techniques, provided by interventional pain physicans, have emerged as treatment options for patients with refractory angina (RFA).

Spinal Cord Stimulation Spinal cord stimulation (SCS) has been found to have efficacy in treatment of intractable angina pectoris in patients refractory to medical therapy who are not candidates for further revascularization procedures. In 2002, Joint Study Group of the European Society of Cardiology recommended SCS as a first-line therapeutic alternative for patients with RFA based on positive effects on symptoms and ischemia and favorable side effect profile. It is a treatment option for patients with RFA per the ACCF/AHA/ACP/AATS/PCNA/SCAI/STS guidelines because of benefits of significant symptoms relief, greater exercise durationwith lower mortality, compared to surgical options for high-risk patients.

The mechanism by which SCS relieves anginal pain is a subject of much speculation and appears to be multifactorial. Interestingly, the mechanism of action varies when SCS is used for peripheral neuropathic pain, ischemic limb pain, and anginal pain.

Theories suggest that SCS works through a spinothalamic mechanism, which may inhibit neuronal transmission at a segmental level. It is possible that SCS inhibits sympathetic outflow and decreases circulating levels of epinephrine, which, in turn, reduces cardiac work load and myocardial oxygen consumption. Because the myocardium is innervated by sympathetic fibers, it is reasonable to extrapolate that stimulation of the thoracic spinal cord can induce changes in myocardial blood flow. It has been shown that SCS augments coronary or cardiac blood flow and redistributes flow to ischemic myocardium. The sympatholytic effect may also act directly or indirectly through stimulation of large dorsal column nerve fibers, which inhibit the smaller pain-transmitting fibers. It likely, therefore, also has a direct inhibitory effect on cardiac nociception. It may be that SCS induces protective changes in the myocardium making it more resistant to critical ischemia. SCS improves myocyte viability. Additionally, there appears to be an effect on arrhythmia control via stabilization of the intrinsic cardiac nervous system. Several studies have shown that SCS increases tolerance to

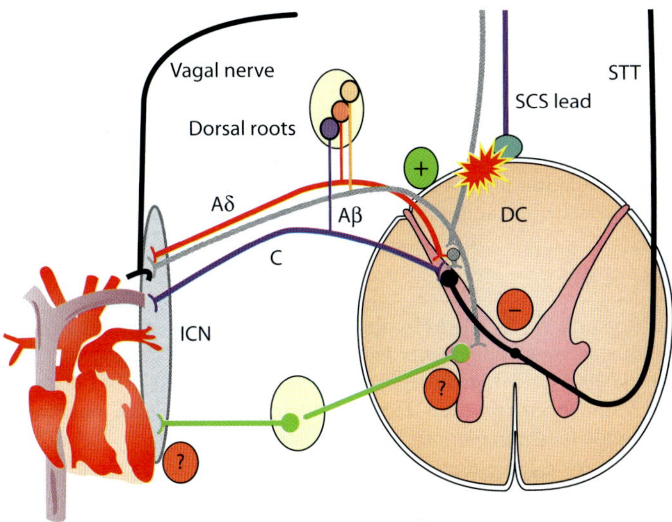

FIGURE 62-3. The circuitry active behind the beneficial effects of spinal cord stimulation in coronary ischemia. The exact mechanisms are still largely unknown (as outlined by the question marks) but as indicated in the text the intrinsic cardiac neurons form the "final common path" in the interaction between the CNS and the heart. Reprinted from Linderoth B. Spinal cord stimulation: a brief update on mechanisms of action. *Eur J Pain Suppl*. 2009; 3:89-93, with permission, from John Wiley and Sons.

pacing, myocardial lactate metabolism, and decreases the duration and magnitude of ST changes during maximal pacing with SCS (**Fig. 62-3**).

The stimulating electrode for angina is placed with the distal electrode of the lead at C7-T1, slightly left of midline. When paresthesia is elicited, the goal is to have perception in the usual anginal region of pain. In the protocol used by DeJongste and Foreman,[16] most patients are advised to stimulate for 1 hour, three times per day, and stimulate additionally when they are experiencing angina. They do also have patients, though who stimulate for 2 hours, four times per day, and others who use the stimulator continuously. Settings that are commonly used are listed in **Table 62-5**.

Thoracic Epidural Infusion High thoracic epidural infusion of local anesthetic has been used to treat unstable and refractory angina. Its antianginal effect is related to decreased myocardial ischemia secondary to blockade of afferent and efferent cardiac sympathetic fibers. This is associated with decreased myocardial oxygen demand and increased myocardial blood flow. Richter et al studied 152 patients for a period of 10 years who were treated with thoracic epidural infusions. These patients had epidural catheters placed at T 2, 3, 4, or 5. After initial hospitalization, these patients self-administered bupivicaine 0.25% twice per day, with allowance for some as needed boluses; 95% felt that they had benefited from the epidural treatment. There was a significant decrease in anginal episodes and significant improvement in anginal class. There was one serious complication (epidural hematoma in a patient with undiagnosed bleeding defect). There were no other serious complications or CNS infections; however, 53% had issues with catheter displacement.[17]

TABLE 62-5 Average Settings in Patients with Refractory Angina Treated with Unipolar Spinal Cord Stimulation

Stimulation Settings	Average (range)
Pulse width	210 (180–250) μs
Frequency	60 (30–110) Hz
Output amplitude	4.6 (2.2–10.5) V (comfortable paresthesia)
Stimulation protocol	3 × 1 h; 4 × 2 h; continuously at own discretion
Unipolar/bipolar	10%/90%

From DeJongste MJ, Furman RD. Spinal cord stimulation for refractory angina. In: Krames ES, ed. *Neuromodulation*. 1st ed. 2009: 831-843, with permission, from Elsevier.

Emerging Therapies Treatment options for refractory angina (RFA), which are currently investigational, include shock wave therapy, coronary sinus reducer, myocardial cryotherapy, and gene and stem cell therapy. Further randomized controlled studies are necessary to confirm safety and efficacy.[15]

CHRONIC MESENTERIC ISCHEMIA

Chronic mesenteric ischemia (CMI), also known as abdominal or intestinal angina, is caused by chronic arterial insufficiency and ischemia of the mesenteric circulation. It can be very difficult to diagnose, because patients often have vague complaints and unremarkable physical findings. It accounts for about 5% of all cases of intestinal ischemia, but has significant clinical consequences.

CHARACTERISTICS

The predominant cause of CMI is stenosis or occlusion of the mesenteric arterial circulation. This is most commonly caused by atherosclerotic disease, primarily as an extension of progression of atherosclerosis of the aorta. Commonly multiple vessels are involved. A number of conditions that can cause CMI are listed in **Table 62-6**.

The primary pathology of CMI is reduction of blood flow to the mesenteric circulation to meet demands of the intestinal tissue in the postprandial period. This can occur either from occlusion or adjacent arterial steal. Patients can have symptoms even before food reaches the small intestine secondary to arterial steal from the stomach.

Patients most commonly have pain in the postprandial period. Patients suffer from significant weight loss, nausea, and vomiting, and may develop a fear of eating. The pain often begins about 15 to 60 minutes after eating and may last from 1 to 6 hours. The pain is described as colicky and dull, often in the epigastrium with occasional radiation to the back. Pain can vary with different types of foods. Patients may report eating several small meals per day. The history may be difficult to differentiate from biliary disease. Although many patients eliminate foods from the diet and do experience food avoidance with subsequent weight loss, CMI can occur in the absence of weight loss. Patients with

TABLE 62-6 Causes of Chronic Mesenteric Ischemia

- Atherosclerosis
- Celiac artery compression syndrome
- Fibrovascular dysplasia
- Visceral vasculitis
  - Takayasu arteritis
  - Giant cells arteritis
  - Polyarteritis nodosa
  - Systemic lupus erythematosus
  - Thromboangiitis obliterans (Buerger disease)
- Radiation-induced vascular injury
- Ergotamine intoxication (commonly from use for headache)
- Colonic carcinoma
- Mesenteric venous thrombosis
  - Heritable disorders of coagulation
  - Hematologic disorders
  - Pancreatitis and peritonitis
  - Inflammatory bowel disease
  - Cirrhosis
  - Portal hypertension
  - Paraneoplastic disorders
  - Postoperative states
  - Trauma
  - Diverticulitis

TABLE 62-7 Diagnostic Testing for Chronic Mesenteric Ischemia

- Conventional interventional angiography
- Duplex ultrasonography
- CT angiography
- Magnetic resonance angiography
- Tonometry

this disorder often have a history of heavy tobacco use. On examination, there may be no specific findings. Pain may be present, but not localized. It is often out of proportion to findings on physical examination. A variety of diagnostic testing is outlined in **Table 62-7**.

TREATMENT

Management of CMI may involve medical and/or surgical options. Other gastrointestinal pathology should be ruled out. Upper endoscopy is usually recommended. Once a diagnosis is established, the decision tree includes whether the patient requires surgical intervention, open or percutaneous.

INTERVENTIONAL/SURGICAL

Transaortic endarterectomy has been used to obtain primary revascularization in acute and chronic mesenteric ischemia. Surgical bypass is an option. This is performed as anterograde or retrograde reconstruction. Autogenous or prosthetic grafts are used. Endovascular therapy has been used increasingly over the years. It is ideal with patients with short segments of stenosis (<10 cm) secondary to atherosclerosis near the ostia of the superior mesenteric artery or celiac artery.

MEDICAL

Medical management has a smaller role, given that definitive therapy is preferred to minimize potential serious consequences such as bowel infarction. Some patients may have disorders of coagulation and may be treated with warfarin and/or antiplatelet drugs. Antispasmodic agents may be used. Medical management should include smoking cessation. Eating small meals and the use of proton pump inhibitors have also been advocated. Proton pump inhibitors decrease the oxygen demands of the gastric mucosa.

INTERVENTIONAL PAIN MANAGEMENT

Spinal Cord Stimulation Spinal cord stimulation (SCS) may have a role in the management of patients with CMI, but to date, research has been limited. It is likely that pain control is achieved via dorsal midline and lateral spinal pathways transmitting visceral nociception. There is very little information regarding the mechanism of attenuation of visceral nociception with SCS.

Ceballos et al published a case report[18] of a 78-year-old man with a 9-year history of mesenteric ischemic pain, refractory to medical management. The patient was ineligible for surgery. Spinal cord stimulator was placed which provided the patient with complete pain control, without further need for analgesics. He remained symptom free in a 12-month follow-up. There have been other case reports and a limited number of studies utilizing SCS for refractory abdominal pain but further research is necessary to determine the efficacy.[19,20] Limitations exist in studying CMI because of the rarity of the diagnosis.

SUMMARY

Ischemic pain affecting the coronary, peripheral, and mesenteric circulation can be debilitating to patients and can significantly impact quality of life. These disease processes carry significant morbidity and mortality and often are interrelated secondary to the involvement of widespread atherosclerotic vascular disease. Initial management of CAD and PAD includes risk modification and institution of medical therapy. Interventions such as bypass surgery and endovascular procedures are utilized when management is not successful. Mesenteric ischemia involves procedural intervention as first-line treatment after which therapy may be centered on symptomatic and limited medical management.

The role of the pain physician in management of ischemic pain has emerged over the years, particularly for patients refractory to medical therapy, surgical and percutaneous endovascular treatment. Spinal cord stimulation plays a role with an ability to affect nociceptive pain, decrease ischemia, and improve outcomes for these patients.

REFERENCES

1. Rooke TW. ACCF/AHA focused update of the guideline for the management of patients with peripheral artery disease (updating the 2005 guideline): a report of the American College of Cardiology Foundation/American Heart Association Task Force on Practice Guidelines. *Circulation*. 2011;124:2020-2045.
2. Clair D, Shah S, Weber J. Current state of diagnosis and management of critical limb ischemia. *Curr Cardiol Rep*. 2012;14:160-170.
3. Bradbury AW, Adam DJ, Bell J, Forbes JF, Fowkes FGR, Gillespie I, et al. Bypass versus angioplasty in severe eschaemia of the leg (BASIL) trial: an intention-to-treat analysis of amputation-free and overall survival in patients randomized to a bypass surgery-first or a balloon angioplasty-first revascularization strategy. *J Vasc Surg*. 2010;51:5S-17S.
4. Shealy CN, Mortimer JT, Reswick JB. Electrical inhibition of pain by stimulation of the dorsal columns: preliminary clinical report. *Anesth Analg*. 1967;46:489-491.
5. Cook A, Oygar A. Baggenstos R, Pacheco S, Kleriga E. Vascular disease of extremities electrical stimulation of spinal cord and posterior roots NY State. *J Med*. 1976;76:366-368.
6. Wu M, Linderoth B, Foreman RD. Putative mechanisms behind effects of spinal cord stimulation on vascular diseases: a review of experimental studies. *Auton Neurosci*. 2008;138:9-23.
7. Pedrini L, Magnoni F. Spinal cord stimulation for lower limb ischemic pain treatment. *Interact Cardiovasc Thorac Surg*. 2007;6:495-500.
8. Ubbink DT, Vermeulen H. Spinal cord stimulation for non-reconstructable chronic critical leg ischaemia. *Cochrane Database Syst Rev*. 2013;1-22.
9. Lara-Hernandez R, Lozano-Vilardell P, Blanes P, Torreguitart-Mirada N, Galmes A, Besalduch J. Safety and efficacy of therapeutic angiogenesis as a novel treatment in patients with critical limb ischemia. *Ann Vasc Surg*. 2010;24:287-294.
10. Roger VL, Go AS. Heart disease and stroke statistics-2012 update: a report from the American Heart Association. *Circulation*. 2012:218.
11. Serruys PW, Morice MC, Kappetein AP, Colombo A, Holmes DR, Mack MJ, et al. Percutaneous coronary intervention versus coronary-artery bypass grafting for severe coronary artery disease. *N Engl J Med*. 2009;360:961-972.
12. Briones E, Lacalle JR, Marin I. Transmyocardial laser revascularization versus medical therapy for refractory angina. *Cochrane Database Syst Rev*. 2009:CD003712.
13. Pratali S, Chiaramonti F, Milano A, Bortolotti U. Transmyocardial laser revascularization 12 years later. *Interactive Cardiovascular and Thoracic Surgery*. 2010;11:480-481.
14. McGillion M, Cook A, Victor JC, Carroll S, Weston J, Teoh K, et al. Effectiveness of percutaneous laser revascularization therapy for refractory angina. *Vasc Health Risk Manage*. 2010;6:735-747.
15. McGillion M, Heather MA. Management of patients with refractory angina: Canadian Cardiovascular Society/Canadian Pain Society Joint Guidelines. *Can J Cardiol*. 2012;28:21.
16. DeJongste MJL, Foreman RD. Spinal cord ctimulation for refractory angina. In: Elliot SK, Peckham PH, Ali R, RezaiA2 - Elliot S. Krames

PHP, et al., eds. *Neuromodulation*. San Diego, CA: Academic Press; 2009:831-843.

17. Richter A, Cederholm I, Fredrikson M, Mucchiano C, Traff S, Janerot-Sjoberg B. Effect of long-term thoracic epidural analgesia on refractory angina pectoris: a 10-year experience. *J Cardiothorac Vasc Anesth*. 2012;26:822-828.
18. Ceballos A, Cabezudo L, Bovaira M, Fenollosa P, Moro B. Spinal cord stimulation: a possible therapeutic alternative for chronic mesenteric ischaemia. *Pain*. 2000;87:99-101.
19. Tiede JM, Ghazi SM, Lamer TJ, Obray JB. The use of spinal cord stimulation in refractory abdominal visceral pain: case reports and literature review. *Pain Pract*. 2006;6:197-202.
20. Kapural L, Nagem H, Tlucek H, Sessler DI. Spinal cord stimulation for chronic visceral abdominal pain. *Pain Med*. 2010;11:347-355.

ADDITIONAL READING

Begelman SM, Jaff MR. Noninvasive diagnostic strategies for peripheral arterial disease. *Cleve Clin J Med*. 2006;73(Suppl 4):S22-S29.

Jacobs MJ, Jorning PJ, Beckers RC, Ubbink DT, van Kleef M, Slaaf DW, et al. Foot salvage and improvement of microvascular blood flow as a result of epidural spinal cord electrical stimulation. *J Vasc Surg*. 1990;12:354-360.

Claeys LG, Berg W, Jonas S. Spinal cord stimulation in the treatment of chronic critical limb ischemia. *Acta Neurochir Suppl*. 2007;97:259-265.

Pepine CJ, Nichols WW. The pathophysiology of chronic ischemic heart disease. *Clin Cardiol*. 2007;30:I4-I9.

Chaitman BR, Sano J. Novel therapeutic approaches to treating chronic angina in the setting of chronic ischemic heart disease. *Clin Cardiol*. 2007;30:I25-I30.

Parker JD, Parker JO. Stable angina pectoris: the medical management of symptomatic myocardial ischemia. *Can J Cardiol*. 2012;28:S70-S80.

Fihn SD, Gardin JM, Abrams J, Berra K, Blankenship JC, Dallas AP, et al. ACCF/AHA/ACP/AATS/PCNA/SCAI/STS Guideline for the diagnosis and management of patients with stable ischemic heart disease: a report of the American College of Cardiology Foundation/American Heart Association Task Force on Practice Guidelines, and the American College of Physicians, American Association for Thoracic Surgery, Preventive Cardiovascular Nurses Association, Society for Cardiovascular Angiography and Interventions, and Society of Thoracic Surgeons. *J Am Coll Cardiol*. 2012;60:e44-e164.

Sianos G, Morel MA, Kappetein AP, Morice MC, Colombo A, Dawkins K, et al. The SYNTAX Score: an angiographic tool grading the complexity of coronary artery disease. *Euro Intervent*. 2005;1:219-227.

Tavris DR, Brennan JM, Sedrakyan A, Zhao Y, O'Brien SM, Peterson ED, et al. Long-term outcomes after transmyocardial revascularization. *Ann Thorac Surg*. 2012;94:1500-1508.

Mannheimer C, Camici P, Chester MR, Collins A, DeJongste M, Eliasson T, et al. The problem of chronic refractory angina: report from the ESC Joint Study Group on the treatment of refractory angina. *Eur Heart J*. 2002;23:355-370.

Falowski S, Celii A, Sharan A. Spinal cord stimulation: an update. *Neurotherapeutics*. 2008;5:86-99.

Linderoth B. Spinal cord stimulation: a brief update on mechanisms of action. *Eur J Pain Suppl*. 2009;3:89-93.

Cameron T. Safety and efficacy of spinal cord stimulation for the treatment of chronic pain: a 20-year literature review. *J Neurosurg*. 100:254-267.

Gramling-Babb P, Miller MJ, Reeves ST, Roy RC, Zile MR. Treatment of medically and surgically refractory angina pectoris with high thoracic epidural analgesia: initial clinical experience. *Am Heart J*. 1997;133:648-655.

Rosengart TK, Bishawi MM, Halbreiner MS, Fakhoury M, Finnin E, Hollmann C, et al. Long-term follow-up assessment of a phase 1 trial of angiogenic gene therapy using direct intramyocardial administration of an adenoviral vector expressing the VEGF121 cDNA for the treatment of diffuse coronary artery disease. *Hum Gene Ther*. 2013;24:203-208.

Biolato M, Miele L, Gasbarrini G, Grieco A. Abdominal angina. *Am J Med Sci*. 2009;338:389-395.

Sickle-Cell Disease

Natalie Moryl

INTRODUCTION

Sickle-cell disease (SCD) is the most prevalent single-gene disorder, affecting about 100,000 Americans. Sickle-cell disease is a debilitating condition associated with chronic anemia, stroke, splenic and renal dysfunction, susceptibility to bacterial infections in children, acute chest syndrome, and pain crises. Each year in the United States, an average of 75,000 hospitalizations are due to SCD, costing approximately $475 million. Despite a decrease in mortality in children with SCD over the last 25 years, median life expectancy for most SCD patients remains less than 50 years of age. Although tremendous resources have been invested in finding a cure, barriers to analgesia in SCD remain and stereotyping of patients persists. Major barriers to pain management are misconceptions regarding patients' report of pain, use of opioids and other pain medications, and perception of addiction. This chapter discusses the correlation between SCD pain and mortality; mistrust between patients and health care providers (HCPs) as one reason for undertreated pain; patients' perceptions of health care system response to their needs; and the need for clinical guidelines to provide appropriate comprehensive care to patients with SCD.

HISTORICAL PERSPECTIVES

Sickle-cell disease was identified in the United States in 1910, when sickle-shaped red blood cells were found in the blood of a medical student from Africa. Autosomal dominant inheritance was identified in 1923, and oxygen deprivation of tissues was shown to provoke sickling in 1927. Single amino acid substitution of glutamic acid for valine in the sixth amino acid position of the B chain of hemoglobin (Hb) was demonstrated to be responsible for physicochemical features of altered Hb. Further studies demonstrated that both altered erythrocytes and endothelial cells express surface molecules that mediate intracellular adhesions, leading to polymerization of deoxygenated sickle-cell hemoglobin (HbS) and vaso-occlusion. Advances in basic and clinical research did not significantly change the outcomes for patients until recently, when antibiotics, hydroxyurea, and bone marrow transplantation (BMT) were introduced. Bone marrow transplantation, first performed in 1998, is currently available as a cure for a selected group of patients only. Pain management and supportive care have been the cornerstones of the treatment of SCD since its discovery and remain the best intervention to reduce morbidity and improve the quality of life for most patients.

PREVALENCE

The Centers for Disease Control and Prevention (CDC) estimates that

- SCD affects 90,000 to 100,000 Americans.
- SCD occurs in about 1 in every 500 black or African-American births.
- SCD occurs in about 1 in 12 blacks or African Americans.[1]

MORTALITY

In 1973, the average life span for individuals with SCD was only 14 years.[2] Current life expectancy for SCD patients is 50 years and more.[3] Women with SCD live longer than men.

Vaso-occlusion resulting from Hb polymerization and erythrocyte rigidity, as well as chronic anemia, hemolysis, and vasculopathy, is central to the pathophysiology of this disease. Early death is associated with acute chest syndrome, renal failure, seizures, persistent leukocytosis, and depressed fetal hemoglobin (HbF) levels.[4] Recurrent episodes of vaso-occlusion and inflammation result in progressive damage to most organs, including the brain, with risk of cognitive impairment, increased prevalence of infections, and impairment in the functions of kidneys, lungs, bones, and the cardiovascular system, which become apparent with increasing age.

Sickle cell-related death among black or African American children younger than 4 years of age decreased by 42% from 1999 through 2002. The decrease coincided with the introduction in 2000 of a vaccine that protects against invasive pneumococcal disease.[1]

Relative to the rate for the period 1983 through 1986, the SCD mortality rate for the period 1999 through 2002 decreased by

68% at 0 through 3 years of age;

39% at 4 through 9 years of age; and

24% at 10 through 14 years of age.[1]

Pain episodes often signal life-threatening complications, such as sepsis, acute chest syndrome, stroke, blood and fat pulmonary embolism, autosplenectomy, gallstones, leg ulcers, priapism, and others. Among patients older than 20 years of age, the rate of pain episodes correlates with mortality. As many as 22% of deaths in patients with SCD follow acute pain episodes.[4–6]

ECONOMIC COSTS

During 2005, medical expenditures for children with SCD averaged $11,702 for children with Medicaid coverage and $14,772 for children with employer-sponsored insurance. Approximately 40% of both groups had at least one hospital stay.[1]

Sickle-cell disease is a major public health concern. From 1989 through 1993, an average of 75,000 hospitalizations caused by SCD occurred in the United States, costing approximately $475 million.[1]

PAIN

Pain is the most common symptom experienced by patients with SCD.[7,8] Pain profoundly impairs patients' functioning at home and work, their social interactions, their families, and their careers. Despite the high prevalence of pain episodes, correlating with morbidity and mortality, sickle-cell anemia (SCA) pain remains underestimated and undertreated.

Frequency of pain episodes was shown to be a risk factor for early death as long as 20 years ago.[5] The research to duplicate results continues. A recent study sought to determine the association between frequent vaso-occlusive crises (VOCs) and mortality.[9] A cohort of 264 adult SCA patients were monitored for 12 months and followed up for 5 years. The frequency of VOCs, ED visits, and hospitalization for acute pain correlated with laboratory data indicating disease severity (hematocrit, ferritin, and HDL cholesterol). Mortality was shown to be higher in patients who required frequent ED visits/hospitalizations for pain. Pain, a subjective experience, similar to the objective findings of higher tricuspid regurgitation, elevated ferritin, and lower glomerular filtration rate, was shown to be a marker predictive of early mortality. The authors concluded that in the contemporary setting, severe painful VOC is a marker for SCA disease severity and premature mortality. The authors suggested that frequency and severity of pain is a prognostic indicator that could identify high-risk patients for disease-modifying therapies.[9]

SICKLE-CELL DISEASE AND HEALTH CARE PROVIDERS

The complex cluster of symptoms and potential for life-threatening complications of SCD, as well as instability of the clinical manifestations, indicate the need for specialized centers to educate, prevent, diagnose, and treat life-threatening complications and pain. Historically, health care provided to patients with SCD was considered to be the responsibility of SCD centers; however, few patients have access to SCD specialists. Both children and adults have limited access to experts in SCD.[10] In a study of children enrolled in Medicaid programs in four states in 1989 through 1992, only 36% of those with SCD had equal to or more than one visit with a subspecialist in a given year.[11]

Limited access to specialized care brings SCD patients to EDs and general medicine clinics, which introduce them to HCPs who may have limited experience and expertise in SCD. Limited experience of nonspecialists and lack of updated guidelines permit wide variations in attitudes toward SCD patients that can result in delays in treatments and unnecessary suffering.

Distrust between SCA patients with pain and HCPs has been described extensively. Patients have reported that HCPs are at times insensitive and often do not understand or believe the patient's self-reports of pain.[12] Patients with SCD see the mistrust as a barrier and often avoid health care visits and end up in the ED only after their pain becomes unbearable and they are in crisis.[13,14]

In addition, some HCPs lack the skills, training, and preparation to accurately assess and manage SCD-related pain.[14,15] Limited knowledge of the principles and appropriateness of opioid therapy; a lack of evidence-based research on pain control; and misconceptions and prejudices about drug abuse and addiction contribute to this educational void. In a recent review, only 21% of medical textbooks presented treatment regimens that were consistent with available guidelines.[16] Treatment with hydroxyurea to decrease the frequency of VOCs is defined completely in 2 of 19 textbooks.[16] Not surprisingly, this lack of education about hydroxyurea translates into a staggering deficiency of its use: It is estimated that 30% or less of eligible patients are treated with hydroxyurea, a disease-modifying therapy for SCD.[3] Thus, most medical texts provided no adequate information for the treatment or prevention of pain caused by VOC in SCD.[16]

Upon examination of patients who report severe pain and seek pain medications including opioids, HCPs and hospital administrators may suspect "high utilizers of the ED" and stigmatize "high utilizers" as opioid seeking. To understand and address these suspicions, "low utilizers" were compared with "high utilizers" in a multicenter trial.[16] The authors compared demographics, pain characteristics, health data, psychosocial characteristics, and quality of life of patients who are "high utilizers of the ED" with other SCD patients. Eighty-two (35.5%) of 232 patients were found to be high ED utilizers. Clinically important and statistically significant differences between high ED utilizers and other SCD patients demonstrated that ED visits were legitimately associated with significant anemia, transfusions, pain days, frequency of pain crises, higher mean pain and distress, and worse quality of life on Medical Outcome Study 36 Item Short Form physical function summary scales. A striking outcome of the study was that after controlling for severity and frequency of pain, high ED utilizers did not use opioids more frequently than other SCD patients. The conclusion of the study was in favor of patients: Patients who presented to an ED more frequently were more severely ill, had more pain, and had a lower quality of life.[16]

Based on prior studies, we know that mortality correlates with frequency of pain crises: 50% of adult patients with more than three VOCs per year survive to 40 years of age, whereas patients with less than one VOC per year have a 50% chance of survival to 55 years of age.[4]

Data have been available for years but have not yet translated into change of behavior. Pervasive delays in administration of analgesics to SCD patients in EDs have been demonstrated recently in a prospective, multisite longitudinal cohort study performed in three midwestern EDs.[17] Three sites formed a multidisciplinary team charged with improving analgesic management for patients with SCD, and each site developed a nurse-initiated analgesic protocol for SCD patients. Despite clinicians' dedication and interest in the problem, the median time to initial analgesic for the cohort in the study was 74 minutes (IQR = 48–135 min). Even in this group of patients, delay in the initial analgesia was from three-fourths of an hour to more than 2 hours. Differences between choice of analgesic agent and route selected were evident between sites. For the cohort, 680 initial analgesic doses were given (morphine sulfate, 42%; hydromorphone, 46%; meperidine, 4%; morphine sulfate and ibuprofen or ketorolac, 7%) using the following routes: oral (2%), intravenous (IV) (67%), subcutaneous (SC) (3%), and intramuscular (IM) (28%). Patient satisfaction with pain was suboptimal. The patients in this study desired their level of pain to be at or below 4 points on 0 to10 pain scale; however, they were discharged with a pain level of 6.

Without widely accepted treatment protocols, pain management in an ED remains a function of attitudes and experiences of HCPs that have been shown to be handicapped with stereotyping and misperceptions.[18] National guidelines are necessary to empower the staff and hospital administration to provide sufficient resources, including trained staff, medications, and access to the SCD expert. National guidelines are needed to break the barriers and ensure comprehensive pain assessment and timely treatment of patients with SCD pain in EDs. Without such guidelines, despite knowledge obtained in research, pervasive delay in pain treatment remains a barrier.

MANAGEMENT OF SICKLE-CELL DISEASE, QUALITY OF LIFE, AND PALLIATIVE CARE

Components of the management of SCD include prevention and treatment of complications, as well as the potential cure for the disease. Most interventions do not lead to cure but are palliative, only aimed at harm reduction and improving quality of life in patients with significantly shortened life and high morbidity.

- **Prevention of complications**. Primary prevention of the acute complications of SCD includes routine health management with a hematologist or an HCP with expertise in SCD. Initial prevention of complications includes penicillin prophylaxis initiated in the newborn period, appropriate immunizations, and blood transfusions for those at risk for stroke.
- **Hydroxyurea** is a potent inducer of HbF with documented efficacy for both adults and children with SCA. In a randomized, double-blind, placebo-controlled study among 299 patients with three or more pain crises a year, hydroxyurea effected a significant decrease in pain crises and acute chest syndrome by increasing HbF to 20% and greater.[19] Taking hydroxyurea was associated with a 40% decrease in mortality. More recently, the results were confirmed in a phase III study of hydroxyurea administered to infants for 2 years (BABY HUG), which resulted in significant benefits for pain, acute chest syndrome, hospitalizations, and transfusions.[20] Current reports document the benefits of hydroxyurea on reducing mortality in adults and children: patients with HbS/β-thalassemia and hydroxyurea exposure had improved 10-year overall survival (OS) compared to patients without hydroxyurea exposure (87% vs 54%), and HbSS patients receiving hydroxyurea had a 10-year OS of 100% compared to 10% in those without hydroxyurea exposure.[21] The treatment is considered mostly safe. Concerns about long-term genotoxicity and specifically possible carcinogenicity with long-term exposure have been addressed by clinical investigators. Recent results from the HUSTLE protocol suggest minimal genotoxicity or carcinogenicity with long-term hydroxyurea exposure.[22]
- **Blood transfusions** are commonly used to treat worsening anemia and SCD complications. A sudden worsening of anemia due to an infection or enlarged spleen is a common reason for a blood transfusion. Blood transfusion remains the most common form of disease modification by suppression of HbS production.[23]
- In a recent Cochrane group review, prevalence of stroke in SCD patients receiving regular blood transfusions was significantly reduced. The review analyzed randomized and quasi-randomized controlled trials comparing blood transfusion as prophylaxis for stroke in persons with SCD to alternative or no treatment.[24] Regular blood transfusions not only reduced the risk of stroke, but stopping transfusions returned the patients to the baseline high-risk status for a stroke. The combination of hydroxyurea and phlebotomy is shown to be less effective than "standard" transfusion and chelation in preventing secondary stroke and iron overload.
- **Pain prevention**. The only US Food and Drug Administration (FDA)-approved agent to prevent pain episodes in SCD is hydroxyurea to reduce sickle hemoglobin polymerization process by increasing the production of HbF.
- **Treatment of complications**. A number of treatments are available for complications of SCD, such as hydration, administration of oxygen, pain medications for VOCs, and antibiotics for infection.
  1. General supportive measure. Because dehydration is a trigger of VOC, hydration is the most consistent intervention listed in each SCD guideline.[25] Supplemental oxygen should be administered if hypoxia is determined.
  2. Permanent organ damage resulting from VOC needs to be evaluated and treated by specialists.
     - Retinal injury
     - Strokes
     - Acute chest syndrome
     - Liver failure
     - Kidney injury/insufficiency
     - Multiple organ failure
     - Leg ulcers (may need skin grafts)
     - Gallstones
     - Priapism
- **Cure**. A cure for SCD is available only by means of hematopoietic stem cell transplantation (HSCT). However, HSCT is limited to individuals younger than 16 years of age because of the risk of severe toxicities and death among individuals older than 16 years of age with a human lymphocyte antigen (HLA)-matched sibling transplant. In a selected population, overall and disease-free survival following HSCT is 90% and 95%, respectively. Multicenter trials are now evaluating the safety and efficacy of unrelated HLA-matched transplantation in children and modified myeloablative programs for adults; however, the results are mixed.[26]

Early BMT may offer the obvious advantages. However, SCA poses a challenge with prognostication: It is impossible to select the individuals with potentially severe SCA early on. Accurate predictors of future severity of SCA on case-by-case basis are lacking. The role of early transplantation for the reversible complications of SCD needs to be defined.

In addition to prognostication, other barriers to early BMT exist. In a study of availability of potential donors and families' interest in BMT, a pediatric SCA cohort receiving chronic transfusions between July 2004 and January 2011 was analyzed.[27] Among 113 patients, 35% had an unaffected full sibling who could serve as a BMT donor. The families of 58% patients agreed to HLA-type sibling, 35% of whom were matched. Common reasons to decline HLA typing or transplantation included fear of the process, toxicities of the procedure, and comfort with current quality of life on transfusions. Ultimately, only 7% were eligible for matched BMT, and only 3% underwent HLA-matched transplantation. Two unmatched children received haploidentical transplantation. In this study, when a matched sibling was identified, most families declined to proceed with matched-sibling transplantation.

Other supportive medications. Corticosteroids remain a controversial modality because these agents were shown to shorten the duration of

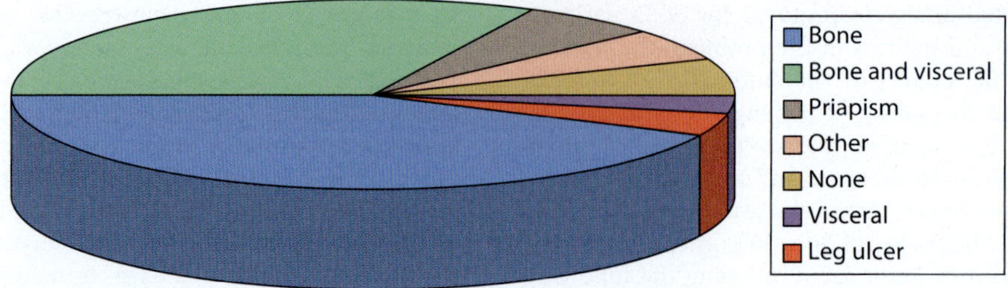

FIGURE 63-1. Distribution of pain symptoms among 117 adults with sickle cell anemia. (Adapted from Payne R. Pain Management in sickle cell anemia. *Anesthesiol Clin North Am.* 1997;15[20:305]).

analgesia requirement but after discontinuation led to more episodes of recurrent pain.[28] A recent study did not support the association between discontinuing steroids and recurrent VOCs.

PAIN ASSESSMENT IN SICKLE-CELL DISEASE

The International Association for the Study of Pain defines pain as "an unpleasant sensory and emotional experience associated with actual or potential tissue damage."[27]

Pain is the reason for up to 90% of hospital admissions in a patient with SCD.[30] Rate of pain is highest in patients between 19 and 39 years of age. Frequency of pain crises correlates with mortality of SCD. Pain was reported to be more severe than pain after major surgery. Typical crisis in adults lasts 10.3 days.[30]

PAIN ASSESSMENT RULES

- The patient, not the observer, should complete the scale.
- Measure pain with a numeric pain intensity scale of 0 to10, a verbal rating scale, or a visual analog scale that can be used for children or adults.
- Pain scale needs to be age- and development-appropriate.
- In younger children, the Face Pain Rating Scale should be used.[31,32]

Pain can be diffuse or localized. A number of sites can be involved that determine the complexity of clinical presentation. Pain syndromes encountered in SCA are listed in **Figure 63-1**.

Pain in SCD can be classified according to the time frame and continuity as chronic, acute, and recurrent pain and severity and frequency of pain episodes. An estimated 20% of patients have pain rarely, 60% have one or two episodes a year, and 20% have more than two episodes of pain per month and are considered severely affected.

Traditional classification of pain is based on extensive research of postsurgical and cancer pain (**Table 63-1**).

As with any chronic pain, repetitive injury accentuates pain transmission and perception with each repeated injury. This is commonly referred as a "wind-up phenomenon" that causes untreated pain to get worse. Both peripheral nerves and central nervous system are "trained" to transmit pain signals better. The experience of pain involves multiple mechanisms serving to locate and quantify pain (sensory response), change the affect of the patient (motivational change), and change the behavior (cognitive response). The reticular formation and limbic system in particular control the emotional and affective response to pain. Chronic pain is not a persistent acute pain condition but a disorder resulting from reorganization of central and peripheral nervous system. These changes have been confirmed by recent studies involving brain imaging demonstrating a cortical reorganization of white and gray matter in patients suffering from chronic pain.[34,35]

Patients with SCA often have both acute and chronic pain as well as increased sensitivity to new pain (decreased pain threshold). Chronic inflammation evident by increased inflammatory markers seen in SCD and recurrent acute pain episodes lead to pervasive activation of multiple pain mechanisms and ultimately central sensitization or cellular and gene up-regulation in the central nervous system of the patients with SCD.[36,37] These episodes result in increased pain sensitivity (hyperalgesia) and allodynia (pain from nonpainful stimulation, such as touch). Understanding of the mechanisms of hyperalgesia and allodynia is extremely important to clinical pain management of SCD pain. Without understanding of central sensitivity, hyperalgesia, and allodynia,

TABLE 63-1 Sickle-Cell Anemia Pain Syndromes

Pain Syndromes	Clinical Signs and Symptoms	Underlying Cause	Special Characteristics
Acute pain	• Sudden • Localized	• Vaso-occlusion • Endothelial damage • Inflammation	• Unpredictable • All ages
Acute hand-foot syndrome (dactylitis)	• Painful dorsal swelling of hands and feet	• Symmetrical • infarcts of metacarpal and metatarsal bones	• Children
Acute arthritis	• Painful swollen joints	• Vaso-occlusion • Inflammation • Infection • Gout	• May accompany dactylitis or aseptic arthritis
Acute chest syndrome	• Chest pain • Fever, tachypnea, hypoxia	• Pulmonary infiltrate • Infarction, infection or hemorrhage	• May require transfusion and can be fatal • May precede death
Splenic sequestration	• Left upper-quadrant pain • Splenomegaly • Anemia	• Splenic sequestration	• Can be acute in children • Insidious onset in adults
Hepatic sequestration	• Right upper-quadrant pain • Hepatomegaly • Anemia	• Hepatic sequestration	• More common in adults
Abdominal pain	• Jaundice • Diffuse pain • Splenomegaly	• Cholelithiasis • Gastritis • Constipation • Splenic infarction	• Can precede acute chest syndrome • May need surgery
Priapism	• Painful erection	• Sickling in sinusoids of penis	• Chronic or recurrent
Avascular necrosis of large joints	• Prolonged, constant bone pain • Large joint pain	• Bone infarction • Arthritis	
Chronic neuropathic pain	• Pain is diffuse • Spontaneous • Burning • Lancinating	• Degenerative disease of the spine • Iron overload neuropathy • Hyperalgesia and allodynia from recurrent pain	• Neuropathic pain agents • Chronic pain

TABLE 63-2 Correlation of the Location of Pain with Emergency Department Visits, Pain Crises, and Chronicity

Pain location	Sternum	Clavicle	Chest	Arm, shoulder	Upper back	Pelvis	Lower back	Knee	Hip
More likely to be the reason for ED visit	x	x	x						
More likely to cause pain crisis	x	x	x	x	x	x			
More likely to be chronic							x	x	x

(Data from McClish DK, Smith WR, Dahman BA, et al. Pain site frequency and location in sickle cell disease: the PiSCES project. *Pain. 2009*;145:246-251.)

misinterpreting reports of pain as "drug seeking" through exaggeration or fabrication of pain complaints is a real possibility.[38] The report of moderate to severe pain when only mild pain is expected (blood pressure cuff, blood drawing, repositioning in bed) or the report of severe pain when a nonpainful stimulation is applied (touching skin over the painful area) results not from exaggeration or faking but from a biological process of hypersensitization. This knowledge may allow HCPs more empathy and improve communications between patients and clinicians and ultimately improve pain control.

The location of pain varies considerably both within and between subjects and has some predictability for pain evolution: pain becoming chronic and even becoming a pain crisis that brings the patient to the ED.[39] In a study of 308 adults with SCD, patients kept diaries for 6 months, the results of which are summarized in **Table 63-2**.

1. Pain should become a routinely measurable vital sign, using a simple, preferably universal, scale.
2. Patient self-report should be the primary source of assessment, using age- and development-appropriate scales including behavioral cues in infants.
3. Pain should be reassessed frequently.
4. Pain control and medication side effects should be evaluated frequently (as often as every 20 minutes for severe pain and less frequently for mild to moderate pain) and pain medications adjusted as needed.
5. A comprehensive psychosocial assessment may need to be done by interdisciplinary team, with frequency determined by psychosocial conditions and support systems of the patient.
6. Disparity between the patient's report and clinician's observation should be evaluated professionally with the help of multidisciplinary team and in consultation with SCD specialist, and until proved otherwise, the patient's self-report should be considered objective.

TREATMENT OF PAIN

Comprehensive guidelines of SCA pain management are outlined in Sickle Cell Disease; Critical Elements of Care produced by The Center for Children with Special Needs, Seattle Children's Hospital, Seattle, Washington.[40] The guidelines give comprehensive recommendations for pain management, for the use of nonsteroid analgesics and opioids with doses, frequency of administrations, and recommendations for dose adjustment. These recommendations are congruent with guidelines of American Pain Society and guidelines for cancer pain management.[41,42]

Pain management in SCA follows WHO stepwise ladder approach (**Table 63-3**).[43]

TABLE 63-3 The World Health Organization (WHO) Analgesia Ladder

• Step 1. For mild pain, use acetaminophen, NSAIDs, or another adjuvant analgesic.
• Step 2. For mild to moderate pain, or persistent pain, add a lower potency opioid (codeine) or a low dose of a stronger opioid (morphine).
• Step 3. For moderate to severe pain, or worsening pain, use strong opioids (morphine, hydromorphone, or fentanyl).
Combinations of opioid and non-opioid agents are available; however, NSAIDs and acetaminophen limit the amount of the opioid that can be safely administered to the patient. Opioids on the other hand have no "ceiling effect" as their dose may be titrated up as needed.

(Data from World Health Organization. *Cancer Pain Relief with a Guide to Opioid Availability*, 2nd ed. Geneva, Switzerland: World Health Organization; 1996.)

OPIOIDS TREATMENT GUIDELINES

Acute Pain As in cancer pain, constant IV infusion appears to have better results than intermittent dosing, and the best results were obtained using patient-controlled analgesia (PCA) via IV route, which is preferable for most patients. One study showed that inpatient IV, rapidly changed to oral morphine given at home, reduced the number of admissions by 44%, the total number of inpatient days decreased by 57%, the length of hospital stay decreased by 23%, and the number of repeat ED visits decreased by 67%. The study used treatment with IM meperidine as a control.[42]

Step 1. Start opioids for moderate to severe pain with close supervision (**Table 63-4**):

- In opioid-naïve patients, start with IV morphine 2.5-5 mg as needed (or an equivalent) or equivalent dose given via IV PCA
- In opioid-tolerant patients, start with 20% of the daily dose IV every 20 min-2 h as needed
- In elderly patients, or those with severe liver or renal disease, start with one-half of the usual dose.

Opioid-naïve refers to a patient who has been taking opioids for less than 1 week and total dose of less than 60 mg oral morphine a day or its equivalent.

Step 2. After determining the effective daily dose (sum of doses given within the last 24 h), give the opioid around the clock AND 10-20% total daily dose every 3-4 h as needed.

Route. For acute pain, IV route is preferred.

Step 3. Adjust baseline upward daily based on total amount as needed.

Step 4. When dose escalation of an opioid is limited by side effects and pain remains uncontrolled, an opioid rotation should be considered.

- When converting from one opioid to another, reduce the equianalgesic dose by one-half (except for methadone in which dose reduction of approximately 90% should be considered).

Chronic Pain Step 1. Continue opioids for moderate to severe pain, with close supervision.

Step 2. Give the opioid around the clock AND 10-20% total daily dose every 3-4 h as needed.

- Route:

For chronic opioids therapy oral route is preferable, then transcutaneous, then SC, then IV.

Step 3. Adjust the dose upward to treat exacerbation of chronic pain (chronic opioids do not prevent new pain and do not "mask" new nociceptive injuries).

TABLE 63-4 Usual Opioid Starting Doses

Medication	Adults >50 kg; for opioid-naïve patients (*1/2 dose for elderly, or severe renal or liver disease) PARENTERAL	PO
Morphine	2.5-5 mg SC/IV q3-4h (*1.25-2.5 mg)	5-15 mg (IR or PO solution) q3-4h (*2.5-7.5 mg)
Oxycodone	Not available	5-10 mg q3-4h (*2.5 mg)
Hydromorphone	0.2-0.6 mg SC/IV q2-3h (* 0.2 mg)	2 mg q3-4h (*0.5-1 mg)
Fentanyl	25-50 μg IM/IV q1-3h (*12.5-25 μg)	Transdermal patches are contraindicated in opioid-naïve patients
Meperidine	75 mg SC/IM q2-3h (*25-50 mg) Generally not recommended	50 mg
Codeine	15-30 mg IM/SC q4h (*7.5-15 mg)	30-60 mg q3-4h (*15-30 mg)
Hydrocodone	Not available	5 mg/325 mg acetaminophen q4h (*2.5 mg)

Abbreviations: h, hour; q, every; IM, intramuscular; IV, intravenous; SC, subcutaneous.

Adapted from *Drug Facts and Comparisons 2008*, 62nd ed., by Facts & Comparisons, 2007, Philadelphia, PA: Lippincott Williams &Wilkins; and *Principles of Analgesic Use in the Treatment of Acute Pain and Cancer Pain*, 6th ed., by the American Pain Society, 2009, Glenview, IL: American Pain Society.

Step 4. When side effects of an opioid limit needed dose escalation and pain remains uncontrolled, an opioid rotation should be considered.[44–46]

- When converting from one opioid to another, reduce the equianalgesic dose by one-half (except for methadone in which dose reduction of approximately 90% should be considered).
- Use equianalgesic opioid tables to determine opioid rotation dose ratios (**Table 63-5**).

Pain Management in a Patient with Addiction

- Consider multidisciplinary team approach and a consultation with an addiction specialist.

Opioid Adverse Side Effects

- Constipation (no tolerance), nausea/vomiting (tolerance develops in 3-7 d), urinary retention, hypogonadism, sedation, respiratory depression (only after the onset of sedation), myoclonus, delirium, seizures, respiratory arrest, and death.

Opioid Overdose

- Manifestations: Respirations less than 6/min, myoclonic twitching, constricted pupils, skeletal muscle flaccidity, cold or clammy skin.
- Stop administering opioids, wait for the medication to wear off, stimulate patient.
- Naloxone 0.4 mg diluted in 10 mL NS, give 1 mL every 5 min until reversal of respiratory depression or severe sedation; infusion may be needed to counteract the effect of long-acting methadone or fentanyl patch.

TABLE 63-5 Variability in Dose Ratios When Switching Oral Morphine, Oral Hydromorphone, and Transdermal Fentanyl to Methadone

Morphine dose	Morphine→methadone ratio[44]
30-90 mg/24 h	4:1
91-300 mg/24 h	9:1
>300 mg/24 h	12:1
Hydromorphone dose	**Hydromorphone→methadone ratio[45]**
<330 mg hydromorphone/24 h	0.95:1
>330 mg hydromorphone/24 h	1.6:1
Fentanyl dose	**Fentanyl→methadone ratio[46]**
50 μg/h- 2500 μg/h	250 μg/h: 1 mg/h

Data From Ripamonti C, Groff L, Brunelli C, et al. Switching from morphine to oral methadone in treating cancer pain: what is the equianalgesic dose ratio? *J Clin Oncol*. 19980ct;16(10):3216-3221[44]; Bruera E, Pereira J, Wantanabe S, et al. Opioid rotation in patients with cancer pain: a retrospective comparison of dose ratios between methadone, hydromorphone, and morphine. *Cancer*. 1996;78(4):852-871[45]; Santiago-Palma J, Khojainova N, Kornick C, et al. Intravenous methadone in the management of chronic cancer pain: safe and effective starting doses when substituting methadone for fentanyl. *Cancer*. 2001;92(7):1919-1925.[46]

Adjuvant Analgesics

- Antidepressants (TCA, SSRI): for visceral and neuropathic pain, time to effect 3 to 7 days after reaching therapeutic level (e.g., for amitriptyline 75-125 mg/d).
- Anticonvulsants (gabapentin, pregabalin): for neuropathic pain, time to analgesia 3 to 7 days after reaching therapeutic levels (gabapentin 2400-3600 mg/d).
- NSAIDs: for bone pain; side effects: GI and renal toxicity, HTN, leg swelling.
- Steroids: for bone pain; side effects: GI toxicity, osteoporosis, insomnia, weight gain, infection.

BARRIERS TO PAIN MANAGEMENT IN SICKLE-CELL DISEASE

Common misconceptions about dependence and addiction deserve mentioning.

1. Concern about addiction is widespread among patients, families, and HCPs. Overestimated risk of adverse side effects and opioid addiction, combined with incomplete assessment of patients regarding physical, psychological, social, and spiritual dimensions of pain, and failure to review the effectiveness of the opioid regimen and make appropriate dose adjustment, can result in inadequate pain control.
2. Cross-racial and cross-cultural communication difficulties may reflect societal conflicts between the patient who is often disabled, has physical limitations, and is socially disadvantaged and the physician who is high-functioning and often white.
3. Often needed rehabilitation, social, spiritual, vocational, and other nonpharmacologic interventions may be unavailable or unaffordable, or not covered by the insurance.
4. Clinicians' limited training and understanding of SCA, pain syndrome, and its management, leading to disbelief of pain complaints and insufficient analgesics prescriptions, contributes to the challenge of sickle-cell management.
5. Lack of universally accepted guidelines setting standards for good pain management.
6. Lack of 24-hour-a-day availability of sickle-cell specialists and tertiary level consultations to patients and their families or to the primary care and ED physicians.

CONCLUSION

There are three major issues in the treatment of SCA with frequent pain crises:

1. Medical. Improved medical knowledge concerning SCD and the modalities of treatment, including disease-modifying modalities, their availability, as well as pain management, and supportive care, is needed.
2. Social. Concern about addiction, drug-seeking behavior, withdrawal, and tolerance should not overcome efforts to palliate the symptoms, provide support, and restore function in society, family, and work.
3. Financial. The reduction of pain-related disability that enables patients to return to work and to function in society would relieve a substantial financial burden on society, especially in view of the prevalence of the disease. Adequate pain control reduces hospital stay, doctors' visits, and so forth. Access to SCD specialists, proactive care, and innovative approaches such as day hospitals will reduce the financial burden on the society by reducing ED visits and hospital readmissions.

Wide distribution of the disease, marked reduction of life span, high morbidity, and adverse effects of chronic and recurrent pain on professional, social, and spiritual life to the extent of social isolation constitute the objective evidence of the need for large, controlled, prospective trials, and future research.

REFERENCES

1. http://www.cdc.gov/ncbddd/sicklecell/index.html
2. Diggs LM. Anatomic lesions in sickle cell disease. In: Abramson H, Bertles JF, Wethers DL, eds. *Sickle Cell Disease: Diagnosis, Management, Education and Research*. St Louis: C.V. Mosby; 1973:189-229.
3. http://www.cdc.gov/ncbddd/sicklecell/about.html
4. Platt OS, Brambilla DJ, Rosse WF, et al. Mortality in sickle cell disease. Life expectancy and risk factors for early death. *N Engl J Med*. 1994;330:1639.
5. Smith WR, Scherer M. Sickle-cell pain: advances in epidemiology and etiology. *Hematol Am Soc Hematol Educ Program*. 2010; 2010:409-415.
6. Vichinsky EP, Neumayr LD, Earles AN, et al. Causes and outcomes of the acute chest syndrome in sickle cell disease. National Acute Chest Syndrome Study Group. *N Engl J Med*. 2000;342: 1855-1865.
7. Field JJ, DeBaun MR. Acute pain management in adults with sickle cell disease. In: Landaw SA, ed. *UpToDate*. Waltham, MA: UpToDate; 2010.
8. http://www.cdc.gov/ncbddd/sicklecell/treatments.html
9. Darbari DS, Wand Z, Kwak M, et al. Severe painful vaso-occlusive crises and mortality in a contemporary adult sickle cell anemia cohort study. *PLoS One*. 2013;8(11):e79923.
10. Grosse SD, Schechter MS, Kulkarni R, et al. Models of comprehensive multidisciplinary care for individuals in the United States with genetic disorders. *Pediatrics*. 2009;123(1):407-412.
11. Kuhlthau K, Ferris TG, Beal AC, et al. Who cares for Medicaid-enrolled children with chronic conditions? *Pediatrics*. 2001;108(4):906-912.
12. Pack-Mabien A, Haynes J, Jr. A primary care provider's guide to preventive and acute care management of adults and children with sickle cell disease. *J Am Acad Nurse Pract*. 2009 May;21(5):250-257.
13. Aisiku IP, Smith WR, McClish DK, et al. Comparisons of high versus low emergency department utilizers in sickle cell disease. *Ann Emerg Med*. 2009 May;53(5):587-593.
14. Booker MJ, et al. Pain management in sickle cell disease. *Chron Illness*. 2006;2(1):39-50.
15. Pack-Mabien A, Labbe E, Herbert D, Haynes J, Jr. Nurses' attitudes and practices in sickle cell pain management. *Appl Nurs Res*. 2001;14(4):187-192.
16. Solomon LR. Treatment and prevention of pain due to vaso-occlusive crises in adults with sickle cell disease: an educational void. *Blood*. 2008;111(3):997.
17. Darbari DS, Wang Z, Kwak M, et al. Severe painful vaso-occlusive crises and mortality in a contemporary adult sickle cell anemia cohort study. *PLoS One*. 2013;8(11):e79923.
18. Payne R. Sickle cell anemia and pain: will data prevail over beliefs? *Ann Emerg Med*. 2009 May;53(5):596-597.
19. Charache S, Terrin ML, Moore RD, et al. Effect of hydroxyurea on the frequency of painful crises in sickle cell anemia. Investigators of the Multicenter Study of Hydroxyurea in Sickle Cell Anemia. *N Engl J Med*. 1995;332:1317.
20. McGann PT, Ware RE. Hydroxyurea for sickle cell anemia: what have we learned and what questions still remain? *Recent Findings: Curr Opin Hematol*. 2011 May;18(3):158-165.
21. Voskaridou E, Christoulas D, Bilalis A, et al. The effect of prolonged administration of hydroxyurea on morbidity and mortality in adult patients with sickle cell syndromes: results of a 17-year, single-center trial (LaSHS). *Blood*. 2010;115(12):2354-2363.
22. McGann PT, Flanagan JM, Howard TA, et al. Geoxicity Genotoxicity associated with hydroxyurea exposure in infants with sickle cell anemia: results from the BABY-HUG Phase III Clinical Trial. *Pediatr Blood Cancer*. 2012 Aug;59(2):254-257.
23. Davies SC, Roberts-Harewood M. Blood transfusion in sickle cell disease. *Blood Rev*. 1997;11:57.
24. Wang WC, Dwan K. Blood transfusion for preventing primary and secondary stroke in people with sickle cell disease. *Cochrane Database Syst Rev*. 2013;11:CD003146. doi:10.1002/14651858.CD003146.pub2.
25. Okomo U, Meremikwu MM. Fluid replacement therapy for acute episodes of pain in people with sickle cell disease. *Cochrane Database Syst Rev*. 2012 Jun13;6:CD005406. doi:10.1002/14651858.CD005406.pub3.
26. Kamani NR, Walters MC, Carter S, et al. Unrelated donor cord blood transplantation for children with severe sickle cell disease: results of one cohort from the phase II study from the Blood and Marrow Transplant Clinical Trials Network (BMT CTN). *Biol Blood Marrow Transplant*. 2012 Aug18(8):1265-1272. doi:10.1016/j.bbmt.2012.01.019.
27. Hansbury EN, Schultz WH, Ware RE, Aygun B. Bone marrow transplant options and preferences in a sickle cell anemia cohort on chronic transfusions. *Pediatr Blood Cancer*. 2012 Apr;58(4):611-615.
28. Griffin TC, McIntire D, Buchanan GR. High-dose intravenous methylprednisolone therapy for pain in children and adolescents with sickle cell disease. *N Engl J Med*. 1994;330:733.
29. Turk DC, Rudy TE. The robustness of an empirically derived taxonomy of chronic pain patients. *Pain*. 1990;43:27.
30. Brozovic M, Davies SC, Brownell AI. Acute admissions of patients with sickle cell disease who live in Britain. *Br Med J*. 1987;294:1206.
31. Hicks CL, von Baeyer CL, Spafford P, van Korlaar I, Goodenough B. The Faces Pain Scale–Revised: toward a common metric in pediatric pain measurement. *Pain*. 2001;93:173-183.
32. Bieri D, Reeve R, Champion GD, Addicoat L, Ziegler J. The Faces Pain Scale for the self-assessment of the severity of pain experienced

by children: development, initial validation and preliminary investigation for ratio scale properties. *Pain*. 1990;41:139-150.

33. Shapiro BS, Dinges DF, Orne EC, et al. Home management of sickle cell-related pain in children and adolescents: natural history and impact on school attendance. *Pain*. 1995;61:139.
34. Ivo R, Nicklas A, Dargel J, et al. Brain structural and psychometric alterations in chronic low back pain. *Eur Spine J*. 2013;22(9):1958-1964.
35. Kuchinad A, Schweinhardt P, Seminowicz DA, Wood PB, Chizh BA, Bushnell MC. Accelerated brain gray matter loss in fibromyalgia patients: premature aging of the brain? *J Neurosci*. 2007;27(15):4004-4007.
36. Holdcroft A, Power I. Recent developments: management of pain. *Br Med J*. 2003;326:635-639.
37. Reichling DB, Levine JD. Clinical role of nociceptor plasticity in chronic pain. *Trends Neurosci*. 2009;32:611-618.
38. Wright J, Ahmedzai SH. The management of painful crisis in sickle cell disease. *Cur Opinion Supportive and Palliative Care*. 2010;4(2):97-106.
39. McClish DK, Smith WR, Dahman BA, et al. Pain site frequency and location in sickle cell disease: The PiSCES project. *Pain*. 2009;145:246-251.
40. The Center for Children with Special Needs, Seattle Children's Hospital, Seattle, WA. Sickle Cell Disease; Critical Elements of Care, 5th ed. 2012. http://www.nwsicklecell.org.
41. http://www.americanpainsociety.org/library/content/guideline-for-the-management-of-acute-and-chronic-pain-in-sickle-cell-disease.html.
42. Brookoff D, Polomano R. Treating sickle cell pain like cancer pain. *Ann Intern Med*. 1992;116:364.
43. World Health Organization. *Cancer Pain Relief with a Guide to Opioid Availability*, 2nd ed. Geneva, Switzerland: World Health Organization; 1996.
44. Ripamonti C, Groff L, Brunelli C, Polastri D, Stavrakis A, De Conno F. Switching from morphine to oral methadone in treating cancer pain: what is the equianalgesic dose ratio? *J Clin Oncol*. 1998 Oct;16(10):3216-3221.
45. Bruera E, Pereira J, Wantanabe S, Belzile M, Kuehn N, Hanson J. Opioid rotation in patients with cancer pain: a retrospective comparison of dose ratios between methadone, hydromorphone, and morphine. *Cancer*. 1996;78(4):852-871.
46. Santiago-Palma J, Khojainova N, Kornick C, et al. Intravenous methadone in the management of chronic cancer pain: safe and effective starting doses when substituting methadone for fentanyl. *Cancer*. 2001;92(7):1919-1925.

SECTION E

Pediatric and Geriatric Pain

Acute Pain Management in Infants and Children

Christine D. Greco
Jean C. Solodiuk
Alyssa A. LeBel

Over the past two decades, there has been significant progress in the understanding of neuroanatomy, physiology, and the pharmacology of analgesics in children, which has led to considerable advancements in pediatric pain management. This chapter discusses developmental anatomy and neurochemistry, pain assessment, pharmacologic treatment of pain, and techniques for providing pain relief.

DEVELOPMENTAL ANATOMY AND NEUROCHEMISTRY

The Infants and fetuses in the last trimester are neurologically sophisticated in their ability to transmit pain signals and respond to stress.[1] Cutaneous sensory nerve terminals are present in the perioral region at 7 weeks' gestation and spread to all body areas by 20 weeks' gestation. Nerve growth factors regulate the extension of peripheral nociceptive fibers into the dorsal spinal cord, with the larger A fibers entering prior to the C fibers at 8 to 12 weeks' gestation. At birth, A and C fiber territories overlap in the developing substantia gelatinosa.[2] Therefore, the neonatal response to a nonspecific sensory stimulus is low-threshold, nonspecific, and poorly organized, as are the well-defined neonatal motor reflexes.[3,4] Noxious and non-noxious stimuli produce similar physiologic and behavioral infant responses, which complicate an accurate assessment of pain.[5]

In the central nervous system (CNS), the full complement of cortical neurons, approximately 1000 million, is present at 20 weeks' gestation. Pain transmission pathways complete myelination in the spine and brain stem between 22 and 30 weeks' gestation. Myelination extends to the thalamus by 30 weeks, and to the cortex by 37 weeks or term. Research using near-infrared spectroscopy (NIRS) shows activation of somatosensory cortex in preterm infants after noxious stimulation.[5,6] Cortical descending inhibition develops post-term. Excitatory and inhibitory neurotransmitters and neuromodulators are present in the fetus, with the balance favoring excitation. Calcitonin gene-related peptide (CGRP), substance P, and the glutamate-NMDA systems are present at 8 to 10 weeks' gestation. Enkephalins and vasoactive intestinal peptide (VIP) appear at 10 to 14 weeks' gestation. Catecholamines are present in late gestation, and serotonin at 6 weeks' postnatal. Of note, the receptors for excitatory neurotransmitters are numerous and widely distributed in the neonate, regressing toward an adult system in the postnatal months. As well, in the developing nervous system, inhibitory chemicals, such as γ-aminobutyric acid (GABA) and glycine, may act as excitatory transmitters. In an experimental murine model, the spinal cord concentration of *N*-methyl-D-aspartate (NMDA) receptors, and their ligand-affinity, is greater in neonates than in older animals. Neurokinin 1 (NK_1) receptor density is also maximal in late fetal and early postnatal life; however, substance P levels are lower at birth than adult levels.[7]

In relation to stress responses, the functional neuroendocrine pathways between hypothalamus and pituitary are present at 21 weeks' gestation. Corticotropin-releasing factor (CRF) may stimulate fetal adrenocorticotropic hormone (ACTH) and β-endorphin from that time period, and cortisol and β-endorphin increases have been assayed following intrauterine sampling for exchange transfusion. Norepinephrine is present in paravertebral ganglia and adrenal chromaffin cells at 10 weeks' gestation and is released with intrauterine stress (asphyxia). A smaller amount of epinephrine is present after 23 weeks' gestation.[7]

The long-term consequences of untreated pain in the developing organism are currently being defined, and a number of studies suggest that early pain responses influence later pain behaviors.[8] In one murine model, skin wounds on rat pups caused increased innervation and lowered pain thresholds in the area of injury for 3 months postinjury. In the rats that had recurrent painful stimuli from birth, the changes in the receptive fields of the dorsal horn neurons were persistent.[9] Another study exposed rat pups to repeated hindpaw injections over several days. When compared with control pups and at adult age, the rats that experienced repeated noxious stimuli showed increased responses to painful and nonpainful stimuli relative to their controls. Pathologically, the experimental group showed a loss of nociceptive primary afferents.[10] A third study found that the pain-conditioned behaviors of rats differed according to the timing of the stimulus. Rat pups exposed to early, repetitive noxious stimulation had a decrease in pain threshold compared with control rats. Adult rats that were given repetitive painful stimuli showed greater stress responses, such as freezing and digging, than controls.[11]

In humans, pain in infancy influences plasticity in a number of pain transmission pathways, including peripheral nerve sprouting, dorsal horn sensitization, decreased descending inhibitory control, and priming of the stress/hypothalamo-pituitary-adrenal (HPA) axis.[12] Many but predominantly empiric studies show late behavioral effects of painful stimuli, and the balance of potential pharmacologic toxicity versus adequate pain control is an important consideration.[13] One report describes that neonatal males who received a eutectic mixture of topical local anesthetic prior to circumcision had 12% to 25% less facial grimacing and tachycardia than randomized control infants without treatment.[14]

An earlier study reported that males circumcised by 2 days of age had longer periods of crying and higher pain ratings than uncircumcised males.[15]

Another report compared 18 preterm infants, subject to repeated painful procedures in the neonatal intensive care unit (NICU), with matched full-term infants regarding their somatic complaints at 18 months of age. Twenty-five percent of mothers of preterm infants with prolonged NICU stays noted a significantly increased number of somatic complaints in their toddlers compared with zero percent of mothers of full-term infants briefly managed in the normal nursery.[16] Alternatively, a recent study of 24 preterm infants compared with matched full-term infants had similar behavioral pain scores when exposed to a finger prick at 4 months of age.[17]

In summary, the neonatal pain transmission system is adequately developed, centrally hyperexcitable, with the necessary components of central sensitization, but generally nonspecific in its response to stimuli. Neonates and infants feel pain, but assessment of the phenomenon remains challenging.[18,19,20] Long-term effects of neonatal pain are being investigated; however data support prevention and management of pain in the newborn.[21]

PAIN ASSESSMENT IN INFANTS AND CHILDREN

Pain assessment is a fundamental and essential part of pain treatment. The ability to assess pain reliably facilitates the diagnosis of painful conditions and to evaluate efficacy of pain relief methods. The assessment of pain in infants and children, however, is one of the most difficult challenges faced by health care providers (HCPs) in part because of differences in verbal and cognitive developmental abilities, differences in pain expression and perception, and the subjective nature of pain.

For these reasons pain assessment in infants and children requires a comprehensive approach that utilizes self-report when available, observations, and physiologic measures. As discussed, there is evidence to suggest that inadequately treated pain can have both short-term and long-term consequences. For example, it is well established that full-term and preterm infants develop physiologic stress responses to pain and inadequate anesthesia that can result in greater postoperative complications.[1,13-17] Self-report methods are considered to be the most reliable guides to pain assessment for most patients. However, infants and preverbal children are unable to communicate their experience of pain and must rely on caregivers to interpret signs of pain and distress. Pain assessment methods that combine self-report with other measures, such as behavioral and physiologic responses, may provide more accurate measures of pain. There can be limitations in the use of behavioral and physiologic indices for pain assessment. The distinction between pain and distress may be difficult in young children. For example, a young child may cry and exhibit characteristic facial grimacing during an ear examination because of fear and anxiety rather than pain. Physiologic signs may also mislead measures of pain in certain situations. For example, patients who are septic, hypoxic, or receiving vasopressors may exhibit increase in heart rate or blood pressure that reflect other processes not related to pain. Most pain scales are designed for assessment of acute pain and tend to underestimate persistent or chronic pain in children.[22]

Most pain assessment scales used for infants and preverbal children rely on behavioral observation and physiologic parameters to guide assessment. Observational measures alone may not represent pain intensity accurately because HCPs tend to underestimate pain when compared with a patient or parent report.[23,24] Parent report also tends to underestimate children's pain but to a lesser extent than report by HCPs.[25] Behavioral parameters typically used are facial grimacing, cry, body movement, and sleep pattern. The typical pain facial expression of eyes tightly closed, furrowed brows, and square mouth is considered to be one of the most consistent signals of pain in infants.[26] Physiologic parameters such as heart rate, oxygen saturation, blood pressure, and palmar sweating provide objective evidence of pain.

The Premature Infant Pain Profile (PIPP) (**Fig. 64-1**) and CRIES (**Fig. 64-2**) are pain scales used for preterm and full-term infants, respectively, that combine behavioral observations and physiologic criteria to assess pain.[27,28]

The PIPP was specifically designed to assess acute pain in preterm infants with consideration to gestational age. The CRIES scale, an acronym for *C*rying, *R*equires O_2, *I*ncreased vital signs, *E*xpression, and *S*leepless, consists of five behavioral and physiologic parameters designed to rate postoperative pain in neonates.

The FLACC scale combines five types of pain behaviors, including facial expression, leg movement, activity, cry, and consolability which have been shown to have good interrater reliability and validity in children (**Fig. 64-3**). It is widely used because it is quick, versatile, and can be applied to infants and older children, including those with developmental disabilities.[29]

Children aged 3 to 7 years become increasingly able to communicate their experience of pain to parents and caregivers. Children in this age group may not understand the abstract concept of pain, but most are able to indicate pain intensity using either pictographic or faces scales[30,31,32] (**Figs. 64-4, 64-5**). Although self-report measures are most reliable, a number of factors may alter a child's report of pain.[33] For example, children with inadequately treated persistent pain from cancer or surgery may appear very quiet, still, and withdrawn, giving a false impression of adequate analgesia. Some children may underreport or deny pain for fear of receiving a painful analgesic "shot." Numeric scales are not useful in this age group because although many are proficient at counting, children younger than 7 years do not understand the quantitative significance of numbers. Several self-report methods have been developed that are validated and reliable in children as young as 4 years of age.[34,35,36] The Bieri faces scale is a series of facial expressions depicting degrees of pain and was found to be preferred by most children.[37,38]

Children aged 8 years and older generally can use standard "0 to 10" visual analog scales accurately, but many of the scales used in younger children such as the Bieri faces can also be used. Children in this age group may have concerns over loss of control, or may fear painful injections of analgesics that can distort their self-report. Older children and adolescents have the cognitive ability to understand the meaning of pain and tend to use behavioral coping strategies for pain.

Pain assessment in children with developmental disabilities is particularly challenging for parents and caregivers. Pain assessment in this

Indicators	0	1	2	3
GA in weeks	≥ 36 weeks	32 to 35 weeks and 6 days	28 to 31 weeks and 6 days	< 28 weeks
Observe the NB for 15 sec				
Alertness	Active Awake Opened eyes Facial movements present	Quiet Awake Opened eyes No facial movements	Active Sleep Closed eyes Facial movements present	Quiet Sleeping Closed eyes No facial movements
Record HR and SpO_2				
Maximal HR	↑ 0 to 4 bpm	↑ 5 to 14 bpm	↑ 15 to 24 bpm	↑ ≥ 25 bpm
Minimal saturation	↓ 0 to 2.4%	↓ 2.5 to 4.9%	↓ 5 to 7.4%	↓ ≥ 7.5%
Observe NB for 30 sec				
Frowned forehead	Absent	Minimal	Moderate	Maximal
Eyes squeezed	Absent	Minimal	Moderate	Maximal
Nasolabial furrow	Absent	Minimal	Moderate	Maximal

Absent is defined as 0 to 9% of the observation time; minimal, 10% to 39% of the time; moderate, 40% to 69% of the time; and maximal as 70% or more of the observation time. In this scale, scores vary from 0 to 21 points. Scores equal or lower than 6 indicate absence of pain or minimal pain; scores above 12 indicate the presence of moderate to severe pain. GA – Gestational Age. NB – Newborn.

FIGURE 64-1. Premature infant pain profile.

Crying Requires Oxygen Increased Vital Signs Expression Sleeplessness (CRIES)						
Date/Time						
Crying - Characteristic cry of pain is high pitched. 0 – No cry or cry that is not high-pitched 1 – Cry high pitched but baby is easily consolable 2 – Cry high pitched but baby is inconsolable						
Requires O_2 for SaO_2 <95% - babies experiencing pain manifest decreased oxygenation. Consider other causes of hypoxemia, e.g., oversedation, atelectasis, pneumothorax 0 – No oxygen required 1 – <30% oxygen required 2 – >30% oxygen required						
Increased vital signs (BP* and HR*) - Take BP last as this may awaken child making other assessments difficult 0 – Both HR and BP unchanged or less than baseline 1 – HR or BP increased but increase in <20% of baseline 2 – HR or BP is increased >20% over baseline						
Expression - The facial expression most often associated with pain is a grimace. A grimace may be characterized by brow lowering, eyes squeezed shut, deepening naso-labial furrow, or open lips and mouth. 0 – No grimace present 1 – Grimace alone is present 2 – Grimace and non-cry vocalization grunt is present						
Sleepless - Scored based upon the infant's state during the hour preceding this recorded score. 0 – Child has been continuously asleep 1 – Child has awakened at frequent intervals 2 – Child has been awake constantly						
Total Score						

FIGURE 64-2. CRIES pain scale.

population of children must be based on the child's individual abilities. Some children with developmental disabilities can self-report and should be given this opportunity. Others require behavioral or physiologic measures of pain. In the last decade, several pain assessment tools have been developed addressing the specific needs for this patient population.[39,40,41]

In general, pain assessment is best accomplished by correlation of self-report, behavioral, and physiologic measures with the child's overall clinical picture. The choice of pain assessment scale should be individualized and based on a child's age, clinical condition, environment, cognitive abilities, and coping style. Often, explanation and practice of the

	Scoring		
Categories	0	1	2
Face	No particular expression or smile	Occasional grimace or frown, withdrawn, disinterested	Frequent to constant quivering chin, clenched jaw
Legs	Normal position or relaxed	Uneasy, restless, tense	Kicking, or legs drawn up
Activity	Lying quietly, normal position, moves easily	Squirming, shifting back and forth, tense	Arched, rigid or jerking
Cry	No cry (awake or asleep)	Moans or whimpers; occasional complaint	Crying steadily, screams or sobs, frequent complaints
Consolability	Content, relaxed	Reassured by occasional touching, hugging or being talked to, distractable	Difficult to console or comfort

Each of the five categories (F) Face; (L) Legs; (A) Activity; (C) Cry; (C) Consolability is scored from 0-2, which results in a total score between 0 and 10.

FIGURE 64-3. FLACC scale.

Faces Pain Scale - Revised (FPS-R)

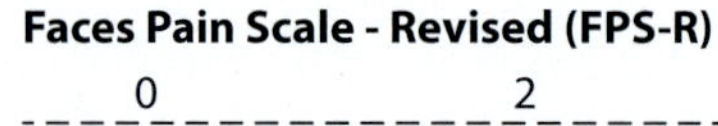

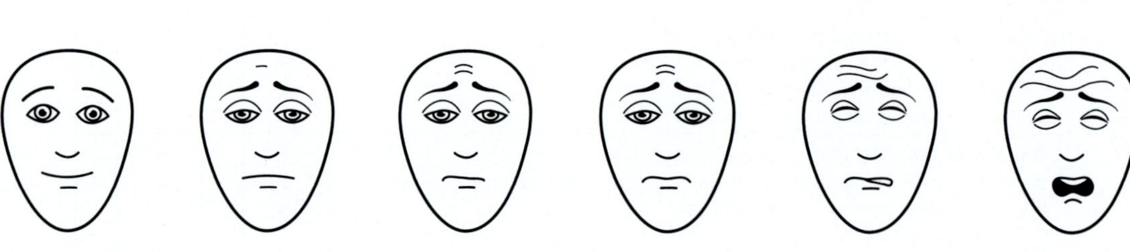

FIGURE 64-4. Bieri faces scale. (From Bieri D, et al. The Faces Pain Scale for the self-assessment of the severity of pain experienced by children: development, initial validation, and preliminary investigation for ratio scale properties. *Pain.* 1990;41:139)

Faces: Wong-Baker Pain Rating Scale
0
No hurt
2
Hurts
little bit
4
Hurts
little more
6
Hurts
even more
8
Hurts
whole lot
10
Hurts
worst

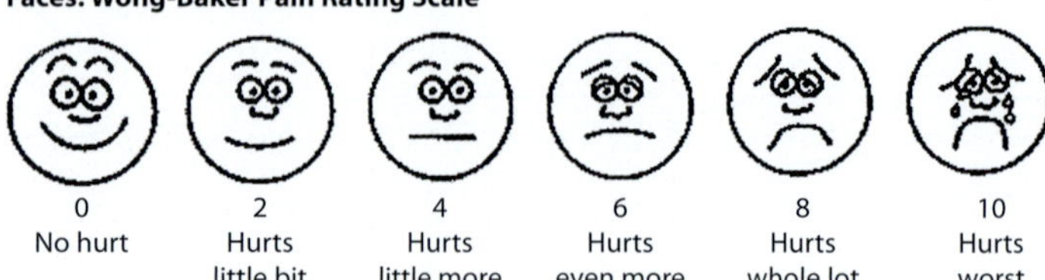

FIGURE 64-5. Wong-Baker pain rating scale. (Reprinted, with permission, from Hockenberry M, Wilson D, Winkelstein ML. *Wong's Essentials of Pediatric Nursing*, 8th ed. Copyright 2009, Mosby, St. Louis)

chosen pain assessment scale during the preoperative visit can facilitate the child's use after surgery.

PHARMACOLOGIC GUIDELINES IN THE NEWBORN AND INFANT

Infants and young children have age-related differences in the pharmacokinetics and pharmacodynamics of analgesics which are relevant to the safe and effective dosing of analgesics in this age group. Analgesics with high-water solubility have a larger volume of distribution, sometimes resulting in the need for larger initial dosing. However, neonates and young infants have immature hepatic enzyme systems involved in conjugation, glucuronidation, and sulfation of analgesics such as opioids and amide local anesthetics, which cause prolongation of elimination half-life and increase the risk of drug accumulation. Most infants and young children will have maturation of hepatic enzyme systems by 6 months of age; however, there is considerable variation in maturation rates. Neonates have decreased plasma-protein binding due to decreased levels of albumin and α_1 acid glycoprotein, resulting in increased free pharmacologically active drug and greater first-pass toxicity. Renal function, including glomerular filtration and renal tubular secretion, is decreased in the first few weeks of life compared with adults. Renal immaturity also results in the slower elimination of glucuronides of morphine, hydromorphone, and of monoethylglycinexylidide (MEGX), a principal metabolite of lidocaine. In addition, infants, particularly premature infants have immature ventilatory reflexes in response to hypoxia and hypercarbia and have increased risk of hypoventilation in response to opioids. Because of the developmental pharmacokinetic and pharmacodynamics differences in neonates and young children, dosing of opioids and local anesthetics require careful titration and increased vigilance for side effects.

PHARMACOLOGIC TREATMENT OPTIONS

NON-OPIOID ANALGESICS

Non-opioid analgesics include acetaminophen, nonsteroidal anti-inflammatory drugs (NSAIDs), and selective cyclooxygenase (COX-2) inhibitors. Analgesic effect occurs from peripheral and central actions involving inflammatory processes in the spinal cord and brain.[42,43] Because of their opioid-sparing effect, non-opioid analgesics are often first-line treatment for mild to moderate pain in children.

Acetaminophen is the most commonly and widely used analgesic in children and has a good safety record in children of all ages.[44] The analgesic and antipyretic effects of acetaminophen are largely via sites within the CNS through action at cyclooxygenase (COX-3 and COX-2) isoenzymes, cannabinoid receptors, and on tyrosine-related protein (TRPV1) receptors.[45,46] Although a weak analgesic, acetaminophen is a useful adjuvant for acute pain treatment and is often combined, synergistically, with opioids. The elimination of acetaminophen is primarily through glucuronidation and sulfation; elimination rates are similar among infants, children, and adults.[47] The recommended single dose is 15 to 20 mg/kg and 10 to 15 mg/kg with repeated dosing. Maximum daily dosing is 100 mg/kg/day in children, 75 mg/kg/day in term infants, and 40 mg/kg/day in preterm infants. Inadvertent overdosing can lead to fulminant hepatic failure.[48,49] Acetaminophen is available in several routes of administration—intravenous (IV), tablets, capsules, suspensions, and suppositories. Concentrated infant drops have been discontinued to reduce inadvertent overdosing.[50,51] The IV dosing in children 2 to 12 years is 15 mg/kg every 6 hours or 12.5 mg/kg every 4 hours with a maximum daily dose of 75 mg/kg/day. The rectal dose is 35 to 40 mg/kg initially followed by 20 mg/kg every 6 to 8 hours; absorption is low and variable. Rectal absorption peaks at 70 minutes.[52,53]

Nonsteroidal anti-inflammatory drugs (NSAIDs) are commonly used for mild-to-moderate pain and are often combined with opioids to improve analgesia and to help reduce opioid side effects. The use of NSAIDs has been shown to reduce postoperative opioid use by approximately 30% to 40%.[54] The anti-inflammatory effect of NSAIDs is through reversible inhibition of COX-1 and COX-2 isoenzymes and inhibition of the conversion of arachidonic acid to prostanoids.[55] The clearance of ibuprofen, ketorolac, and several other NSAIDs is more rapid in toddlers and preschool children compared with adults.[56] NSAIDs in general have a good safety margin in children 6 months of age and older, particularly with short-term use. A large-scale study in children administered short-term use of ibuprofen showed a very low overall risk of severe side effects.[57] There are limited safety data on the use of NSAIDs in neonates and young infants.[58,59] Much of the pharmacokinetic and safety data of NSAIDs in use in neonates come from the use of ibuprofen and indomethacin to facilitate closure of patent ductus arteriosus. Ibuprofen is associated with less risk of renal toxicity and hyponatremia compared with indomethacin in this age group. Significant bleeding caused by NSAIDs is relatively uncommon in healthy children. There are mixed data regarding the risk of NSAIDs use in children after tonsillectomy procedures.[60-62] Although analgesic trials show good analgesia, due to the potential risk of life-threatening bleeding after tonsillectomy procedures, the practice at this institution is to avoid NSAIDs in the perioperative period for children undergoing tonsillectomies. There is evidence in adult patients to suggest that NSAID use can impair bone healing after orthopedic surgeries that involve osteoclast activation and new bone formation. Children are less likely to have impairment of new bone formation; however, it is reasonable to avoid use of

TABLE 64-1 Dosing Guidelines for Non-Opioid Analgesics[a]

	Dose < 60 kg	Dose > 60 kg
Acetaminophen	10–12.5 mg/kg q4h PO or IV	650 mg q4h PO or IV
Ibuprofen	6–10 mg/kg q6–8h PO	400–600 mg q6h PO
Naproxen	5 mg/kg q12h PO	250–500 mg q12h PO
Celecoxib	2–4 mg/kg q12h PO	100–200 mg q12h PO
Ketorolac	0.5 mg/kg q6–8h IV, not for > 5 d	30 mg q6–8h IV, not for > 5 d

[a]Dosing guidelines listed refer to children > 2 years of age

Further modifications in dosing are required for use of these agents in term and preterm neonates and infants

Abbreviations: PO, orally; IV, intravenous; q, every

NSAIDs in children after orthopedic surgeries requiring significant active bone formation. **Table 64-1** lists dosing of commonly used non-opioid analgesics.

OPIOIDS

Opioids are widely used for the treatment of infants and children with moderate-to-severe pain. Safe and effective administrations of opioids require careful patient selection, an understanding of age-related differences in metabolism, dose titration, and aggressive treatment of opioid side effects.

As discussed, opioids are associated with an increased risk of respiratory depression and apnea and a prolonged duration of action in neonates and infants, particularly in premature infants, because of delayed hepatic enzyme maturation and immature renal excretion. Neonates and young infants also have reduced protein binding as a result of developmental changes in the expression of P-glycoproteins in the gastrointestinal tract and in the blood-brain barrier. Data from infant rat models show immature opioid receptor sites in the peri-aqueductal gray matter and descending pathways. Studies of use of opioids for procedural pain in neonates have shown mixed results; randomized trials assigning ventilated neonates to receive morphine infusions versus placebo infusions have not shown clear advantages in the morphine infusion groups.[63,64] In addition to neonates and young infants, others at risk for opioid-induced respiratory depression include children with obstructive sleep apnea, children with craniofacial abnormalities, and children with neurologic conditions. Dose reduction with careful dose titration, cardiorespiratory electronic monitoring, and close observation are necessary for safe and effective opioid treatment in neonates, infants, and children at risk for respiratory side effects.

Codeine Evidence indicates that codeine is ineffective as an analgesic and is associated with significant side effects.[65-68] Codeine is a pro-drug and is converted to morphine through the CYP2D6 enzyme pathway. There is significant polymorphism of CYP2D6 enzymes, leading to patients who are poor metabolizers, rapid metabolizers, and ultra-rapid metabolizers.[69,70] Pharmacogenic data show that 30% of children are poor metabolizers and unable to convert codeine to morphine, making codeine inactive in these patients.[71] Gene duplication in ultra-rapid metabolizers increases the amount of morphine metabolized from codeine. There have been fatalities and life-threatening events due to opioid overdose among children who were ultra-rapid metabolizers.[70,72] Breast-fed infants are at risk of overdose when their lactating mothers, having been prescribed codeine-containing products for postpartum analgesia, are ultrarapid metabolizers.[73] As a result of the safety and efficacy concerns for codeine, our institution has removed codeine from its formulary and from all medical record prescription software.[74,75]

Oxycodone Oxycodone is widely used in children with moderate pain, particularly in the postoperative setting when transitioning from IV opioids to oral opioids. It is metabolized via CYP3A4 to inactive metabolites, although a secondary pathway involving CYP2D6 generates potent oxymorphone, which is renally eliminated and has been associated with increased risks among ultrarapid metabolizers.[76,77] Pharmacokinetic data of oxycodone in children show significant variability in clearance and elimination half-life, particularly in neonates.[78] Our prevailing impression is that oxycodone is associated with fewer side effects in children compared with codeine. Typical starting doses are 0.05 to 0.1 mg/kg every 4 hours as needed for mild pain and 0.1 to 0.2 mg/kg every 4 hours as needed for moderate to severe pain. Oxycodone is available in an elixir form for children unable to swallow pills. Sustained-release preparation of oxycodone (OxyContin) is used for older children with chronic pain requiring opioids.

Morphine Morphine is often the first-line opioid considered for parenteral use in children. There is extensive pharmacokinetic data for morphine in children of all ages.[79-82] Metabolism occurs primarily in the liver via glucuronidation to morphine-3-glucuronide which has neuroexcitatory properties such as delirium, myoclonus, and agitation; and to morphine-6-glucuronide which has analgesic, sedative, and respiratory depressant actions. Glucuronides are renally eliminated and can accumulate in children with renal failure. Data suggest that morphine is metabolized preferentially to morphine-3-glucuronide in neonates, increasing the potential risk of seizures in this age group. Elimination half-life of morphine is prolonged in infants and neonates, particularly in premature infants whereas clearance of morphine is reduced, increasing the risk of opioid side effects.[82,83]

Hydromorphone Due to similar duration of action to morphine, hydromorphone is often used for patient-controlled analgesia (PCA) in children. It is metabolized primarily in the liver via glucuronidation and is five times more potent than morphine when given IV in steady-state dosing.[84] Hydromorphone is metabolized to glucuronides that can accumulate in patients with renal failure. There is little data about the metabolism of hydromorphone in neonates. Randomized blinded comparisons between morphine and hydromorphone have found few differences in the frequency of side effects.[85]

Methadone Methadone has a long elimination half-life with a prolonged duration of action; however, there is significant variability in elimination half-life, ranging from 6 to 30 hours. The bioavailability is approximately 70% to 90%.[86,87] Methadone can produce analgesia similar to that achieved by continuous infusion of other opioids when administered at prolonged dosing intervals. It can also be given orally in liquid form to young children in place of sustained-release preparations that are in pill form. The action of the d-isomer of methadone resulting in NMDA receptor antagonism is the basis for its use in the treatment of neuropathic pain.[88] Because of incomplete cross-tolerance, dose conversion between methadone and other mu opioids is often complex and different for opioid-naïve versus opioid-tolerant patients such that opioid-tolerant patients are likely to require much less methadone for equianalgesic dosing when switching from other mu (μ) opioids.[89,90] This is particularly relevant when converting morphine to methadone in children with advanced cancer and when weaning nonventilated children from prolonged opioid therapy.[91] For acute postoperative pain management in opioid-naïve children, our practice is to use an every 4 hour "sliding scale" of 0.025 mg/kg for mild pain, 0.05 mg/kg for moderate pain, and 0.075 mg/kg for severe pain. Patients are then converted to regular scheduled dosing after the first 24 hours. Because of its unique pharmacokinetic properties of prolonged but variable elimination half-life and incomplete cross-tolerance, methadone requires careful titration and vigilance to avoid overdosage.

Fentanyl Fentanyl is highly lipophilic and is 70 to 100 times more potent than morphine when given as a single dose. It is primarily metabolized in the liver to inactive metabolites, making it useful for patients with renal failure. The brief effect of a single dose of fentanyl is due largely to redistribution; however, with a continuous infusion or with repeated doses, the effect is much more prolonged and is more determined by elimination rather than redistribution.[92] The context-sensitive half-life of fentanyl is particularly prolonged in neonates receiving continuous infusions.[93]

Because single dosing of fentanyl has a rapid onset and brief duration, it is often used for procedural sedation in children undergoing lumbar punctures, bone marrow biopsies, dressing changes, and other brief painful procedures either alone or in combination with benzodiazepines or general anesthesia.[94,95] Doses of 0.5 to 1 µg/kg titrated every 3 to 5 minutes typically provide effective procedural sedation. Rapid administration may cause glottis and chest wall rigidity which can be particularly prominent in neonates; treatment may require assisted ventilation, and in some cases neuromuscular blockade and naloxone. Oral transmucosal fentanyl is also used for brief painful procedures in children and for children with cancer pain.[96] The bioavailability is approximately 50% since the oral transmucosal dose is partially absorbed through the buccal mucosa and partially swallowed.[97] Most children tolerate oral transmucosal dosing; however, almost 90% of children experience facial pruritus. Transdermal fentanyl is used in select opioid-tolerant children with cancer pain, chronic pain requiring opioids, and in select opioid-tolerant children with limited IV access.[98,99] After initial patch application or with dose changes, approximately 12 to 24 hours are needed to reach steady-state thus making transdermal fentanyl not effective for treating rapidly fluctuating pain. Adverse events including death have been reported with transdermal fentanyl use for opioid-naïve patients, particularly when used for acute postoperative pain.[100]

Intravenous Opioid Administration Intermittent IV bolus dosing is a common method of opioid administration; however, it is associated with wide swings in plasma opioid concentrations and fluctuations in analgesia and opioid side effects. Plasma opioid concentration is typically low prior to a bolus dose, resulting in suboptimal analgesia but with relatively few opioid side effects. After the bolus dose is administered, patients experience effective analgesia but often with significant side effects because plasma opioid concentrations are sometimes supratherapeutic. Continuous opioid infusions tend to provide stable levels of analgesia with steady-steady plasma opioid concentration; however, this method does not account for changes in pain intensity such as with chest physiotherapy or with coughing. Patient-controlled analgesia (PCA) takes into account individual variations in opioid pharmacokinetics and fluctuations in pain intensity. It is widely used for postoperative pain control in children as well as in the treatment of cancer pain and pain due to vaso-occlusive crises. Most children older than 6 years of age can use PCA effectively; there is a higher incidence of failure among younger children because of the inability to understand the causal relationship between pushing the PCA button and receiving medication for pain. Nurse-controlled analgesia (NCA) has been shown to be safe and effective and is commonly used for infants, young children not able to understand how to use PCA, children with cognitive limitations and those with physical limitations.[101] Morphine, hydromorphone, and fentanyl are most commonly used in PCA. There is evidence that basal infusions tend to improve sleep and pain scores although other data show an increased risk of hypoventilation, respiratory pauses, and nighttime oxygen desaturation.[102,103]

Our practice is to use demand dose only for children who received peripheral nerve catheters for postoperative pain and for those who are expected to have mild-to-moderate postoperative pain. Children expected to have severe postoperative pain such as those having spinal fusions and major hip surgery typically receive a basal infusion for the first 1 to 2 days postoperatively. Children with cancer pain and with painful vaso-occlusive crises generally receive approximately 40% of their total opioid dose through a basal infusion. Parent-controlled analgesia is primarily reserved for select cases of children in palliative care setting.

Safe opioid administration requires protocols to detect oversedation, signs of respiratory depression and impending respiratory failure. Protocols should include regular nursing assessments to document level of pain and sedation, vital signs, and the use of cardiorespiratory monitoring when indicated. In general, we recommend cardiorespiratory monitoring for children younger than 6 months, infants with history of apnea and bradycardia, opioid-naïve children receiving a continuous opioid infusion, and other children with neurologic or structural anomalies that increase the risk of respiratory depression. Typical starting doses for PCA are listed in **Table 64-2**.

TABLE 64-2 Typical Starting Doses for Patient-Controlled (Nurse-Controlled) Analgesia

Drug	Bolus dose (µg/kg)	Continuous rate (µg/kg)	4-hour limit (µg/kg)
Morphine	20	4–15	300
Hydromorphone	5	1–3	60
Fentanyl	0.25	0.15	4

Treatment of Opioid Side effects All opioids produce side effects that in some cases can be as distressing to children as pain. Infants and preverbal children experiencing intolerable pruritus or nausea from opioids can present with crying, irritability, and other behaviors that may be interpreted by caregivers as pain. Side effects occur by actions at both peripheral and central sites. For example, opioid-induced nausea and vomiting involve activation of receptors in the brainstem and the gastrointestinal tract.[104] Some opioids produce pruritus by peripheral release of histamine; however, small doses of intrathecal morphine are associated with profound pruritus, supporting a neurogenic central cause involving signaling and neurotransmission in the spinal dorsal horn and nucleus caudalis. Standardized protocols and ordersets for treatment of opioid side effects allow for prompt initiation of therapy. Data show that low-dose infusions of naloxone are effective in children for the treatment of opioid-induced nausea, vomiting, and pruritus without reversing analgesia.[105] A study measuring plasma levels of naloxone and morphine found comparable levels in children who had good relief of side effects compared with those who failed therapy suggesting that the effectiveness of naloxone in treating opioid side effects was unrelated to plasma levels.[106]

Methylnaltrexone is a peripherally constrained opioid antagonist that blocks opioid actions in the gastrointestinal tract and can be effective in treating opioid-induced constipation in children.[107,104] **Table 64-3** outlines the treatment of common opioid side effects in children.

TABLE 64-3 Management of Common Opioid Side Effects

Side effect	Comments	Drug dosage
Nausea	Consider switching to different opioid	Ondansetron 10–30 kg: 1–2 mg IV q 8 h >30 kg: 2–4 mg IV q 8 h Naloxone infusion 0.25–1 µg/kg/h Metoclopramide 0.1–0.2 mg/kg PO/IV q 6 h
Pruritus	Exclude other causes (e.g., drug allergy) Consider switching to different opioid	Nalbuphine 10–20 mg/kg/dose IV q 6 h Naloxone infusion 0.25–1 µg/kg/h
Sedation	Add nonsedating analgesic (e.g., ketorolac) and reduce opioid dose Consider switching to different opioid	Methylphenidate 0.05–0.2 mg/kg PO bid (morning and midday dosing) Dextroamphetamine 5–10 mg every day
Constipation	Regular use of stimulant and stool softener laxatives	Methylnaltrexone Docusate Child: 10–40 mg PO daily Adults: 50–200 mg PO daily Dulcolax Child: 5 mg PO/PR daily Adult: 10 mg PO/PR daily

Abbreviations: q, every; bid, twice a day; PO, orally; PR, rectally

REGIONAL ANESTHESIA AND LOCAL ANESTHETICS IN INFANTS AND CHILDREN

Over the past 30 years, pediatric applications of postoperative regional anesthesia and analgesia have expanded rapidly.[108] Regional anesthesia techniques are also used for the diagnosis and treatment of a variety of chronic pain conditions. In contrast to adults who are able to report paresthesias, severe pain with needle insertion and symptoms of local anesthetic toxicity, most regional anesthesia in children is performed under deep sedation or general anesthesia. A number of motivated, older children may require sedation only for certain blocks. There are prospective and retrospective safety studies that support the safe and widespread practice of performing regional anesthesia under general anesthesia in children.[109-111] A multi-center consortium of pediatric centers in the United States (Pediatric Regional Anesthesia Network) prospectively collected data on all regional blocks and showed overall very good safety of neuraxial and peripheral blocks in infants and children performed by clinicians in the participating hospitals.[111] Totals of nearly 15,000 blocks were performed in a 3-year period. Ninety percent of blocks were placed under general anesthesia. There were no deaths or complications with sequelae lasting greater than 3 months. Respiratory depression in several patients receiving neuraxial opioids was detected by respiratory monitoring, which stresses the importance of electronic respiratory monitoring and vigilance required in patients receiving neuraxial opioids. There were no cases of local anesthetic toxicity; however, there were several cases of positive test doses. Our provisional recommendations for epidural analgesia in anesthetized children:

1. Limit epinephrine dosing to the test dose (0.5 μg/kg in 0.1 mL/kg)
2. Prevent or promptly treat severe hypotension
3. Consider severe hypertension following a test dose to possibly indicate severe pain response to intraneural placement
4. Perform loss of resistance to saline, not air
5. Use dilute local anesthetic solutions for intraoperative epidural solutions; inject bolus doses slowly
6. In the postanesthetic care unit, document degree of sensory and motor blockade. If blockade appears dense, stop the infusion and assess for clear regression.

EPIDURAL ANALGESIA

Epidural analgesia is widely used for infants and children undergoing a number of surgical procedures, such as lower extremity and pelvic orthopedic surgery, major abdominal surgery, thoracic procedures and for certain chronic pain conditions such as Complex Regional Pain Syndrome.

Bupivacaine, ropivacaine and, in select cases, chloroprocaine are most frequently used local anesthetics for continuous epidural infusions in infants and children (**Table 64-4**). Pharmacokinetic studies of bupivacaine in children older than 6 months have reported good safety for infusion rates of bupivacaine of below 0.4 mg/kg/h with plasma bupivacaine levels in a safe range of less than 2 to 3 μg/mL.[112] Neonates have reduced clearance of bupivacaine and pharmacokinetic studies in neonates receiving continuous bupivacaine infusions have shown a continuous rise in plasma bupivacaine levels after the first 48 hours.

Our practice is to use a maximum dose of 0.4 mg/kg/h of bupivacaine for continuous epidural infusions in children over the age of 6 months. For children younger than 4 to 6 months of age, we restrict the dose of bupivacaine to 0.2 mg/kg/h. Pharmacokinetic studies in infants and children receiving single boluses of epidural ropivacaine show that as with bupivacaine, clearances for ropivacaine are reduced in infants. Overall, infusion rates of 0.4 mg/kg/h in older infants and children and 0.2–0.3 mg/kg/h in neonates and younger infants appear to be safe.[113-115]

Because of the limitations in dosing of amide local anesthetics in young infants, we typically use adjuvants such as opioids and clonidine to epidural infusions for synergistic effect. Studies of combinations of epidural clonidine with local anesthetics in children have shown a low side-effect profile.[116] Epidural infusions containing hydromorphone are rarely used in infants younger than 6 months due to increased risk of respiratory depression. Chloroprocaine is used as an alternative to amide local anesthetics for continuous epidural infusions in neonates and very young infants to avoid the toxicity of amide local anesthetics and to safely permit sufficient epidural infusion rates. Even in neonates, chloroprocaine is rapidly metabolized with an elimination half-life of less than 6 minutes, making it an attractive choice for continuous epidural infusions in neonates. Studies of continuous epidural chloroprocaine infusions in term and preterm infants have shown good sensory blockade with no signs of neurotoxicity.[117]

All patients with continuous epidural infusions require electronic monitoring, careful nursing observation and regular assessment of level of sedation, pain score and measurement of vital signs. Table 64-4 lists recommended doses for epidural infusions.

TABLE 64-4 Recommended Epidural Infusion Rates (mL/kg/h)[a]

Solution	< 1 month	1–4 months	> 4 months[b]
Bupivacaine 0.1%	rarely used	0.2	0.4
+/− Fentanyl 2 μg/mL			
+/− Clonidine 0.4 μg/mL			
Ropivacaine 0.1%	rarely used	0.3	0.4–0.5
+/− Fentanyl 2 μg/mL			
+/− Clonidine 0.4 μg/mL			
Bupivacaine 0.1% + hydromorphone 10 μg/mL	rarely used	rarely used	0.3–0.4
Ropivacaine 0.1% + hydromorphone 10 μg/mL	rarely used	rarely used	0.3–0.4
Chloroprocaine 1.5%	0.5 (mid-thoracic)	0.5 (mid-thoracic)	rarely used
+/− Fentanyl 0.2 μg/mL	0.6–.7 (lumbar and low thoracic)	0.6–0.7 (lumbar and low thoracic)	rarely used
+/− Clonidine 0.04 μg/mL			

[a]Infusion rates and solutions should be modified according to clinical circumstances. Little information is available on how best to adjust these rates based on degrees of prematurity. Rates shown reflect upper end of usual infusion rates, based largely on systemic accumulation of local anesthetics and on expected extent of sensory and/or motor blockade. Solutions containing hydrophilic opioids such as hydromorphone may pose a higher risk for delayed respiratory depression; therefore, appropriate frequency of observation and continuous electronic monitoring are recommended.

[b]Weight-scaled infusion rates should plateau at values recommended for patients weighing about 45 kg, i.e., maximum infusion rates for larger patients should rarely exceed 15 mL/h.

PERIPHERAL NERVE BLOCKS

Prospective and retrospective data have demonstrated the safety of peripheral nerve blocks in children with very good postoperative pain management. Advances in the use of ultrasound and an increased understanding of age-related pharmacology of local anesthetic have greatly increased the use of peripheral nerve blocks in children. A general trend of clinical trials of regional blocks is an observation of effective analgesia with low adverse events that compares favorably to systemic opioids or epidural infusions. In a randomized trial comparing popliteal block with epidural analgesia for foot and ankle surgery, popliteal block results in superior analgesia with reduced incidences of nausea, vomiting, and urinary retention.[118] Peripheral nerve catheters are used increasingly in infants and children for a number of upper and lower extremity and truncal surgical procedures, as well as in select patients with chronic neuropathic pain to facilitate physical therapy. Multicenter prospective registry will provide ongoing monitoring of adverse events, data on techniques and outcome data.

PAINFUL CONDITIONS IN PEDIATRIC HOSPITAL CARE

Cancer Pain Infants and children with cancer experience a number of types of pain related to cancer treatment and to their disease process. Pain from cancer treatment can result from painful mucositis, post-amputation pain, repeated painful needle procedures, and peripheral neuropathies. Tumor-related is often present as disease progresses to bone, spinal cord, and neural plexuses. Children with hematologic malignancies often experience bone pain from bone marrow infiltration and abdominal pain from capsular stretch of liver and spleen. Evidence suggests that as successful chemotherapeutic protocols, radiation therapy and surgical techniques have evolved for pediatric cancers, pain related to cancer treatment accounts for the more predominant source of pain and suffering in infants and children.[119]

Infants and children undergoing treatment for cancer frequently require diagnostic and sometimes painful procedures such as lumbar punctures, radiation therapy, bone marrow biopsies and central line insertions and removals. Topical analgesia should be used routinely for minor needle procedures such as IV line insertions and assessing implanted vascular access ports. Cognitive-behavioral interventions such as hypnosis and relaxation techniques have shown to be effective for procedural pain.[120] Conscious sedation or general anesthesia is used for more invasive needle procedures such as bone marrow biopsies and lumbar punctures and for radiation therapy requiring immobility.

Mucositis is painful inflammation of the mucosa and is a common side effect in children receiving chemotherapy or radiation. Mucositis is especially severe and prolonged with bone marrow transplantation. Topical agents are often used but with limited data regarding efficacy. Parenteral opioids through PCA or NCA are generally used for moderate to severe pain from mucositis. Data support the safety and efficacy of opioid infusions and PCA for the treatment of mucositis.[121,122]

Our practice is to administer approximately 60% of the total daily opioid dose through a basal infusion to provide sustained analgesia and without requiring the patient to use the PCA button repeatedly during the day and night. There are data showing efficacy of low-dose ketamine infusion for children with severe mucositis pain not relieved by standard PCA or NCA.[123-125]

Many children will have resolution of cancer pain after initial chemotherapy induction; however, some children will continue to experience pain due to tumor invasion of solid organs, bone, nerves and plexuses. Morphine, hydromorphone and other opioids are titrated to effect as pain escalates.[126] Oral opioids are generally used when possible. For children with persistent pain, it is useful to use a long-acting opioid such as methadone or sustained-release preparations of opioids. Short-acting morphine, hydromorphone, oxycodone, or other opioids are added for breakthrough pain. Oral methadone is a long-acting opioid available as an elixir formulation and is useful for children unable to swallow pills. Parenteral opioids are used for patients whose pain is rapidly escalating, are unable to tolerate oral opioids due to nausea, vomiting, painful mucositis, or are unable to swallow. Continuous infusions and PCA or NCA allow rapid titration for escalating pain. Opioid side effects should be aggressively treated. We frequently prescribe anticonvulsants and antidepressants for children who experience neuropathic pain although this practice is extrapolated from adult data.[127,128] Children with advanced cancer have a number of overlapping symptoms including fatigue, somnolence, sleep disturbance, and depressed mood.[129] Fatigue and sedation can be a result from the use of opioids and other sedating medications or from the underlying disease process.

Dose escalation of opioids effectively treats cancer pain for most children. However, some children will continue to experience unremitting pain despite massive doses of opioids. Refractory pain not well controlled by massive dose escalation of opioids is typically seen in children with exquisite neuropathic pain from tumor invasion to spinal cord and major nerves. Low-dose ketamine infusion can be used in this setting; rates below 0.2 mg/kg/h are generally well-tolerated with low rates of dysphoria and dissociation.[125] Our approach to persistent refractory neuropathic pain in this setting is to use regional anesthetic techniques such as implanted intrathecal ports with the catheter advanced to the dorsal horn level nearest the patient's location of pain. We prefer intrathecal route rather than epidural placement because epidural dosing of local anesthetics is limited by systemic toxicity.

CHILDREN WITH CYSTIC FIBROSIS

Patients with cystic fibrosis (CF) experience a range of pain including chronic back pain, abdominal pain, and limb pain. The incidence of chronic pain, particularly headache and chest pain increases sharply during the last 6 months of life.[130]

Chest pain is the most commonly reported pain among children with CF, regardless of the severity of lung disease and is usually multifactorial. Recurrent coughing and increased work of breathing result in chronic musculoskeletal chest pain. Severe coughing can produce rib fractures and severe pleuritic chest pain.

Greater than 50% of patients with CF report chronic headaches. Causes of headaches in this patient population include chronic hypoxia and hypercarbia, migraines, chronic musculoskeletal strain from coughing, and chronic sinusitis. Sinus disease is found in most patients with CF; surgery can help to treat underlying sinus disease and reduce pain for some patients. As disease progresses, headaches due to hypercarbia, hypoxia, and constant coughing are common.

The treatment of chronic pain in patients with CF depends on the nature of pain, the severity of lung disease and disease progression, as well as individual patient responses to NSAIDs and opioids. NSAIDs are often used in combination with opioids for opioid-sparing effect. There may be a role for COX-2 inhibitors in patients with pain and frequent hemoptysis. Because patients with CF experience a high incidence of constipation with opioids, aggressive use of stimulant laxatives and methylnaltrexone should be considered. We commonly use thoracic epidural analgesia or bilateral paravertebral catheter infusions for patients with CF undergoing lung transplantation. Many patients with CF who require lung transplantation have severe chronic chest pain and we typically use slightly more concentrated infusions of local anesthetics to achieve optimal analgesia. Patients with CF and severe pain from rib fractures may benefit from thoracic epidural catheter or from thoracic paravertebral catheter infusions.

PAIN ASSOCIATED WITH SICKLE CELL VASO-OCCLUSIVE EPISODES

Children with sickle hemoglobinopathies experience pain from acute vaso-occlusive episodes as well as pain from compression fractures, avascular necrosis, acute cholecystitis, splenic sequestration, priapism, and stroke. Painful vaso-occlusive episodes are the most common causes of pain in children with sickle cell disease and can occur in children as young as 6 months of age as the protective effect of fetal hemoglobin decreases. Painful vaso-occlusive crises are typically unpredictable in severity and location and can range from mild episodes managed at home with oral analgesics to frequent and severe exacerbations requiring numerous hospitalizations and IV opioid administration. Children with severe pain or escalating pain generally require hospitalization and treatment with PCA and NSAIDs.[131,132]

Surveys suggest that even with generous opioid dosing, pain scores remain high for a considerable percentage of patients.[133] Patients with severe chest pain high despite doses of opioids may experience excessive somnolence, inability to cough effectively leading to worsening hypoxia, and further pulmonary decline. For selected patients, continuous epidural analgesia or paravertebral catheter infusions can result in improved analgesia while decreasing systemic opioids and somnolence.

SUMMARY

Over the past 20 years, there have been significant clinical advances in the treatment of acute pain in children. Improved analgesics, better understanding of pediatric pharmacology and neurodevelopment, and increased experience in regional techniques in children have led to these clinical advances. Optimal management of acute pain requires reliable assessment of pain and aggressive management of pain and side effects with consideration to emotional and social factors contributing to pain. Multicenter clinical trials will be helpful for conducting adequately powered research for many forms of acute and chronic pain in pediatrics.

REFERENCES

1. Anand KJS, Hickey PR. Pain and its effects in the human neonate and fetus. *N Engl J Med*. 1987;317:1321.
2. Fitzgerald M, Anand KJ. Developmental neuroanatomy and neurophysiology of pain. In:Schecter N, Berde C (eds.) *Pain in Infants, Children and Adolescents*. Baltimore, MD: Williams & Wilkins, 1993:11-32.
3. Cornelissen L, Fabrizi L, Patten D, Worley A, Meek J, Boyd S, Slater R, Fitzgerald M. Postnatal temporal, spatial and modality tuning of nociceptive cutaneous flexion reflexes in human infants. *PLoS One*. 2013 Oct 4;8(10):e76470. doi:10.1371.
4. Koch SC, Fitzgerald M. The selectivity of rostroventral medulla descending control control of spinal sensory inputs shifts postnatally from A-fibre to C-fibre evoked activity. *J Physiol*. 2014 Apr 1;592(Pt7):1535-1544.
5. Slater R, Cantarella A, Gallella S, Worley A, Boyd S, Meek J, Fitzgerald M. Cortical pain responses in human infants. *J Neurosci*. 2006 Apr 5;26(14):3662-3666.
6. Bartocci M, Bergqvist LL, Lagercrantz H, Anand KJ. Pain activates cortical areas in the preterm newborn brain. *Pain*. 2006 May;122(1-2):109-117.
7. Morton NS. Development of pain perception. In:MortonNS (ed.) *Acute Pediatr Pain Manage*. Philadelphia, PA: WB Saunders, 1998:13-32.
8. Goubet N, Clifton RK, Shah B. Learning about pain in preterm newborns. *J Dev Behav Pediatr*. 2001;22:418.
9. Reynolds M, Fitzgerald M. Long-term sensory hyperinnervation following neonatal skin wounds. *J Comp Neurol*. 1995;358:487.
10. Reynolds M, et al. Neonatally wounded skin induces NGF-independent sensory neurite outgrowth in vitro. *Brain Res*. 1997;102:275.
11. Anand KJ, et al. Long-term behavioral effects of repetitive pain in neonatal rat pups. *Physiol Behav*. 1999;66:627.
12. Schwaller F, Fitzgerald M. The consequences of pain in early life: injury-induced plasticity in developing pain pathways. *Eur J Neurosci*. 2014 Feb;39(3):344-352.
13. Anand KJ. Effects of perinatal pain and stress Prog. *Brain Res*. 2000;122:117-129.
14. Taddio A, Ilersich AL, Koren G. Effect of neonatal circumcision on pain response during subsequent routine vaccination. *Lancet*. 1997;349:599.
15. Taddio A, Ipp M, et al. Effect of neonatal circumcision on pain responses during vaccination in boys. *Lancet*. 1995;345:291.
16. Grunau RV, Whitfield MF, Petrie JH. Pain sensitivity and temperament in extremely low-birth-weight premature toddlers and preterm and full-term controls. *Pain*. 1994;58:341.
17. Oberlander TF, Grunau RV, Whitfield MF. Biobehavioral pain responses in former extremely low-birth-weight infants at 4 months' corrected age. *Pediatrics*. 2000;105:6.
18. Anand KJ, International Evidence-Based Group for Neonatal. Consensus statement for the prevention and management of pain in the newborn. *Arch Pediatr Adoles Med*. 2001;155:173.
19. Johnston CC, Stevens BJ. Experience in a neonatal intensive care unit affects pain response. *Pediatrics*. 1996;98:925.
20. Fitzgerald M, deLima J. Hyperalgesia and allodynia in infants. In: Finley G, McGrath P, eds. *Acute and Procedural Pain in Infants and Children*. Seattle, Wash: IASP Press, 2000:1-12.
21. Anand KJ. Consensus statement for the prevention and management of pain in the newborn. *Arch Pediatr Adolesc Med*. 2001 Feb;155 (2):173-180.
22. Rohan AJ. The utility of pain scores obtained during 'regular reassessment process' in premature infants in the NICU. *J Perinatol*. 2014 Jul;34(7):532-537.
23. Romsing J, et al. Postoperative pain in children. A comparison between ratings of children and nurses[Danish]. *Ugeskrift Laeger*. 1997;159:422.
24. Romsing J. Assessment of nurses' judgement for analgesic requirements of postoperative children. *J Clin Pharm Ther*. 1996;21:159.
25. Jylli L, Olsson GL. Procedureal pain in a paediatric surgical emergency unit. *Acta Paediatr Scand*. 1995;84:1403.
26. Craig KD. The facial display of pain in infants and children. *Pain Res Manage*. 1998;10:103.
27. Krechel SW. CRIES: a new neonatal postoperative pain measurement score: initial testing of validity and reliability. *Pediatr Anaesth*. 1996;5:53.
28. Gibbins S, Stevens BJ, Yamada J, Dionne K, Campbell-Yeo M, Lee G, Caddell K, Johnston C, Taddio A. Validation of the Premature Infant Pain Profile-Revised (PIPP-R). *Early Hum Dev*. 2014 Apr;90(4):189-193.
29. Malviya S, Voepel-Lewis T, Burke C, Merkel S, Tait AR. The revised FLACC observational pain tool: improved reliability and validity for pain assessment in children with cognitive impairment. *Paediatr Anaesth*. 2006 Mar;16(3):258-265.
30. Tomlinson D, von Baeyer CL, Stinson JN, Sung L. A systematic review of faces scales for the self-report of pain intensity in children. *Pediatrics*. 2010 Nov;126(5):e1168-e1198.
31. Chang J, Versloot J, Fashler SR, McCrystal KN, Craig KD. Pain assessment in children: validity of facial expression items in observational pain scales. *Paediatr Anaesth*. 2013 Feb;23(2):156-161.
32. Cravero JP, Fanciullo GJ, McHugo GJ, Baird JC. The validity of the Computer Face Scale for measuring pediatric pain and mood. *Paediatr Anaesth*. 2013 Feb;23(2):156-161.
33. Beyer JE, McGrath PJ, Berde CB. Discordance between self-report and behavioral pain measures in children aged 3-7 years after surgery. *J Pain Symptom Manage*. 1990;5(6):350.
34. Beyer J, et al. The creation, validation, and continuing development of the Oucher: a measure of pain intensity in children. *J Pediatr Nurs*. 1992;7:335.
35. Bieri D, et al. The Faces Pain Scale for the self-assessment of the severity of pain experienced by children: development, initial validation, and preliminary investigation for ratio scale properties. *Pain*. 1990;41:139.
36. Garra G, Singer AJ, Domingo A, Thode HCJr. The Wong-Baker pain FACES scale measures pain, not fear. *Pediatr Emerg Care*. 2013 Jan;29(1):17-20.
37. Bieri D, et al. The Faces Pain Scale for the self-assessment of the severity of pain experienced by children: development, initial validation, and preliminary investigation for ratio scale properties. *Pain*. 1990;41:139.
38. Keck J, et al. Reliability and validity of the Faces and Word Descriptor Scales to measure procedural pain. *J Pediatr Nurs*. 1996;11(6):368.
39. de Bildt A, Kraijer D, Sytema S, Minderaa R. The psychometric properties of the Vineland Adaptive Behavior Scales in children and adolescents with mental retardation. *J Autism Dev Disord*. 2005;35:53-62.
40. Breau L. The science of pain measurement and the frustration of clinical pain assessment: does an individualized numerical rating

scale bridge the gap for children with intellectual disabilities? *Pain.* 2010;150:213-214.

41. Breau LM, Burkitt C. Assessing pain in children with intellectual disabilities. *Pain Res Manag.* 2009;14:116-120.
42. Dong L, Smith JR, Winkelstein BA. Ketorolac reduces spinal astrocytic activation and PAR1 expression associated with attenuation of pain after facet joint injury. *J Neurotrauma* 2013 May 15;30(10):818-825.
43. Telleria-Diaz A, Schmidt M, Kreusch S, Neubert AK, Schache F, Vazquez E, et al. Spinal antinociceptive effects of cyclooxygenase inhibition during inflammation: involvement of prostaglandins and endocannabinoids. *Pain.* 2010 Jan;148(1):26-35.
44. Lesko SM, Mitchell AA. The safety of acetaminophen and ibuprofen among children younger than two years old. *Pediatrics.* 1999 Oct;104(4):e39.
45. Jóźwiak-Bebenista M, Nowak JZ. Paracetamol: mechanism of action, applications and safety concern. *Acta Pol Pharm.* 2014 Jan-Feb;71(1):11-23.
46. Andersson DA, Gentry C, Alenmyr L, Killander D, Lewis SE, Andersson A, Bucher B, Galzi JL, Sterner O, Bevan S, Högestätt ED, Zygmunt PM. TRPA1 mediates spinal antinociception induced by acetaminophen and the cannabinoid Δ(9)-tetrahydrocannabiorcol. *Nat Commun.* 2011 Nov 22;2:551.
47. Strassburg CP, Strassburg A, Kneip S, Barut A, Tukey RH, Rodeck B, et al. Developmental aspects of human hepatic drug glucuronidation in young children and adults. *Gut.* 2002 Feb;50(2):259-265.
48. Heubi JE, Barbacci MB, Zimmerman HJ. Therapeutic misadventures with acetaminophen: hepatoxicity after multiple doses in children. *J Pediatr.* 1998 Jan;132(1):22-27.
49. Xie Y, McGill MR, Dorko K, Kumer SC, Schmitt TM, Forster J, et al. Mechanisms of acetaminophen-induced cell death in primary human hepatocytes. *Toxicol Appl Pharmacol.* 15 Sep 2014;279(3): 266-274.
50. Mitka M. FDA asks physicians to stop prescribing high-dose acetaminophen products. *JAMA.* 2014 Feb 12;311(6):563.
51. Dart RC, Rumack BH. Intravenous acetaminophen in the United States: iatrogenic dosing errors. *Pediatrics.* 2012;129(2):349-353.
52. Birmingham PK, Tobin MJ, Henthorn TK, Fisher DM, Berkelhamer MC, Smith FA, et al. Twenty-four-hour pharmacokinetics of rectal acetaminophen in children: an old drug with new recommendations. *Anesthesiology.* 1997 Aug;87(2):244-252.
53. Montgomery CJ, McCormack JP, Reichert CC, Marsland CP. Plasma concentrations after high-dose (45 mg.kg-L) rectal acetaminophen in children. *Can J Anaesth.* 1995 Nov;42(11):982-986.
54. Collins SL, Moore RA, McQuay HJ, Wiffen PJ, Edwards JE. Single dose oral ibuprofen and diclofenac for postoperative pain. *Cochrane Database Syst Rev.* 2000;(2):CD001548.
55. Boynton CS, Dick CF, Mayor GH. NSAIDs: an overview. *J Clin Pharmacol.* 1988 Jun;28(6):512-517.
56. Kauffman RE, Lieh-Lai MW, Uy HG, Aravind MK. Enantiomer-selective pharmacokinetics and metabolism of ketorolac in children. *Clin Pharmacol Ther.* 1999 Apr;65(4):382-388.
57. Kokki H, Hendolin H, Maunuksela EL, Vainio J, Nuutinen L. Ibuprofen in the treatment of postoperative pain in small children. A randomized double-blind-placebo controlled parallel group study. *Acta Anaesthesiol Scand.* 1994 Jul;38(5):467-472.
58. Cohen MN, Christians U, Henthorn T, Vu Tran Z, Moll V, Zuk J, Galinkin J. Pharmacokinetics of single-dose intravenous ketorolac in infants aged 2-11 months. *Anesth Analg.* 2011 Mar;112(3):655-660.
59. Lynn AM, Bradford H, Kantor ED, Andrew M, Vicini P, Anderson GD. Ketorolac tromethamine: stereo-specific pharmacokinetics and single dose use in postoperative infants aged 2–6 months. *Paediatr Anaesth.* 2011 March;21(3):325-334.
60. Moiniche S, Romsing J, Dahl JB, Tramer MR. Nonsteroidal anti-inflammatory drugs and the risk of operative site bleeding after tonsillectomy: a quantitative systematic review. *Anesth Analg.* 2003 Jan;96(1):68-77.
61. Marret E, Flahault A, Samama CM, Bonnet F. Effects of postoperative, nonsteroidal, antiinflammatory drugs on bleeding risk after tonsillectomy: meta-analysis of randomized, controlled trials. *Anesthesiol.* 2003 Jun;98(6):1497-1502.
62. Lewis SR, Nicholson A, Cardwell ME, Siviter G, Smith AF. Nonsteroidal anti-inflammatory drugs and perioperative bleeding in paediatric tonsillectomy. *Cochrane Database Syst Rev.* 2013 Jul 18;7:CD003591.
63. Anand KJ, Hall RW, Desai N, Shephard B, Bergqvist LL, Young TE, et al. Effects of morphine analgesia in ventilated preterm neonates: primary outcomes from the NEOPAIN randomised trial. *Lancet.* 2004;363(9422):1673-1682.
64. Carbajal R, Lenclen R, Jugie M, Paupe A, Barton BA, Anand KJ. Morphine does not provide adequate analgesia for acute procedural pain among preterm neonates. *Pediatrics.* 2005;115(6):1494-1500.
65. Whittaker MR. Opioid use and the risk of respiratory depression and death in the pediatric population. *J Pediatr Pharmacol Ther.* 2013 Oct;18(4):269-276. Review
66. Magos TA, Syed MI, Montague ML. More codeine fatalities after tonsillectomy in North American children: time to revise prescribing practice!*Clin Otolaryngol.* 2014 Feb;39(1):69.
67. Kaiser SV, Asteria-Penaloza R, Vittinghoff E, Rosenbluth G, Cabana MD, Bardach NS. National Patterns of Codeine Prescriptions for Children in the Emergency Department. *Pediatrics.* 2014 May; 133(5):e1139-e1147.
68. Friedrichsdorf SJ, Nugent AP, Strobl AQ. Codeine-associated pediatric deaths despite using recommended dosing guidelines: three case reports. *J Opioid Manag.* 2013;9(2):151-155.
69. Crews KR, Gaedigk A, Dunnenberger HM, Leeder JS, Klein TE, Caudle KE, et al. Clinical Pharmacogenetics Implementation Consortium. Clinical Pharmacogenetics Implementation Consortium guidelines for cytochrome P450 2D6 genotype and codeine therapy: 2014 update. *Clin Pharmacol Ther.* 2014 Apr;95(4):376-382.
70. Gasche Y, et al. Codeine intoxication associated with ultrarapid CYP2D6 metabolism. *N Engl J Med.* 2004;351, 2827-2831.
71. Williams DG, Patel A, Howard RF. Pharmacogenetics of codeine metabolism in an urban population of children and its implications for analgesic reliability. *Br J Anaesth.* 2002;89(6):839-845.
72. US Food and Drug Administration. FDA drug safety communication: safety review update of codeine use in children; new boxed warning and contraindication on use after tonsillectomy and/or adenoidectomy. Issued February 20, 2013.
73. Madadi P, Koren G, Cairns J, et al. Safety of codeine during breastfeeding: fatal morphine poisoning in the breastfed neonate of a mother prescribed codeine. *Can Fam Physician.* 2007;53(1):33-35.
74. Kaiser S, Asteria-Penaloza R, Vittinghoff E, Rosenbluth G, Cabana MD, Bardach NS. National patterns of codeine prescriptions for children in the emergency department. *Pediatrics.* 2014;133(5): e1139-e1147.
75. Woolf AD, Greco C. Why can't we retire codeine? *Pediatrics.* 2014 May;133(5):e1354-e1355.
76. Söderberg Löfdal KC, Andersson ML, Gustafsson LL. Cytochrome P450-mediated changes in oxycodone pharmacokinetics/ pharmacodynamics and their clinical implications. *Drugs.* 2013 May;73(6):533-543.

77. Samer CF, Daali Y, Wagner M, et al. Genetic polymorphisms and drug interactions modulating CYP2D6 and CYP3A activities have a major effect on oxycodone analgesic efficacy and safety. *Br J Pharmacol.* 2010;160(4):919-930.

78. Pokela ML, Anttila E, Seppala T, Olkkola KT. Marked variation in oxycodone pharmacokinetics in infants. *Paediatr Anaesth.* 2005 Jul;15(7):560-565.

79. Krekels EH, Tibboel D, Danhof M, Knibbe CA. Prediction of morphine clearance in the paediatric population: how accurate are the available pharmacokinetic models? *Clin Pharmacokinet.* 2012;51(11):695-709.

80. Bouwmeester NJ, Anderson BJ, Tibboel D, Holford NH. Developmental pharmacokinetics of morphine and its metabolites in neonates, infants and young children. *Br J Anaesth.* 2004;92(2):208-217.

81. Anand KJ, Anderson BJ, Holford NH, Hall RW, Young T, Shephard B, et al. Morphine pharmacokinetics and pharmacodynamics in preterm and term neonates: secondary results from the NEOPAIN trial. *Br J Anaesth.* 2008;101(5):680-689.

82. Knibbe CA, Krekels EH, van den Anker JN, DeJongh J, Santen GW, van Dijk M, et al. Morphine glucuronidation in preterm neonates, infants and children younger than 3 years. *Clin Pharmacokinet.* 2009;48(6):371-385.

83. Bouwmeester NJ, Hop WC, van Dijk M, Anand KJ, van den Anker JN, Tibboel D. Postoperative pain in the neonate: age-related differences in morphine requirements and metabolism. *Intensive Care Medicine.* 2009;29(11):2009-2015.

84. Collins JJ, Geake J, Grier HE, Houck CS, Thaler HT, Weinstein HJ, Twum-Danso NY, Berde CB. Patient-controlled analgesia for mucositis pain in children: a three-period crossover study comparing morphine and hydromorphone. *J Pediatr.* 1996 Nov;129(5):722-728.

85. Hong D, Flood P, Diaz G. The side effects of morphine and hydromorphone patient-controlled analgesia. *Anesth Analg.* 2008 Oct;107(4):1384-1389.

86. Berde CB, Beyer JE, Bournaki MC, Levin CR, Sethna NF. Comparison of morphine and methadone for prevention of postoperative pain in 3- to 7-year-old children. *J Pediatr.* 1991 Jul;119(1 (Pt 1)):136-141.

87. Fredheim OM, Moksnes K, Borchgrevink PC, Kaasa S, Dale O. Clinical pharmacology of methadone for pain. *Acta Anaesthesiol Scand.* 2008 Aug;52(7):879-889.

88. Davis AM, Inturrisi CE. d-Methadone blocks morphine tolerance and N-methyl-D-aspartate-induced hyperalgesia. *J Pharmacol Exp Ther.* 1999 May;289(2):1048-1053.

89. Mercadante S, Casuccio A, Fulfaro F, Groff L, Boffi R, Villari P, et al. Switching from morphine to methadone to improve analgesia and tolerability in cancer patients: a prospective study. *J Clin Oncol.* 2001 Jun 1;19(11):2898-2904.

90. Benitez-Rosario MA, Salinas-Martin A, Aguirre-Jaime A, Perez-Mendez L, Feria M. Morphine-methadone opioid rotation in cancer patients: analysis of dose ratio predicting factors. *J Pain Symptom Manage.* 2009 Jun;37(6):1061-1068.

91. Berens RJ, Meyer MT, Mikhailov TA, Colpaert KD, Czarnecki ML, Ghanayem NS, et al. A prospective evaluation of opioid weaning in opioid-dependent pediatric critical care patients. *Anesth Analg.* 2006 Apr;102(4):1045-1050.

92. Singleton M, Rosen J, Fisher D. Plasma concentrations of fentanyl in infants, children and adults. *Can J Anaesth.* 1987;34:152-155.

93. Santeiro ML, Christie J, Stromquist C, Torres BA, Markowsky SJ. Pharmacokinetics of continuous infusion fentanyl in newborns. *J Perinatol.* 1997;17(2):135-139.

94. Nagel K, Willan AR, Lappan J, Korz L, Buckley N, Barr RD. Pediatric oncology sedation trial (POST): a double-blind randomized study. *Pediatr Blood Cancer.* 2008 Nov;51(5):634-638.

95. Anghelescu DL, Burgoyne LL, Faughnan LG, Hankins GM, Smeltzer MP, Pui CH. Prospective randomized crossover evaluation of three anesthetic regimens for painful procedures in children with cancer. *J Pediatr.* 2013 Jan;162(1):137-141.

96. Schechter N, Weisman S, Rosenblum M, Bernstein B, Conard P. The use of oral transmucosal fentanyl citrate for painful procedures in children. *Pediatrics.* 1995;95(3):335-339.

97. Lötsch J, Walter C, Parnham MJ, Oertel BG, Geisslinger G. Pharmacokinetics of non-intravenous formulations of fentanyl. *Clin Pharmacokinet.* 2013 Jan;52(1):23-36.

98. Zernikow B, Michel E, Anderson B. Transdermal fentanyl in childhood and adolescence: a comprehensive literature review. *J Pain.* 2007 Mar;8(3):187-207.

99. Hadley G, Derry S, Moore RA, Wiffen PJ. Transdermal fentanyl for cancer pain. *Cochrane Database Syst Rev.* 2013 Oct 5;10.

100. Jumbelic MI. Deaths with transdermal fentanyl patches. *Am J Forensic Med Pathol.* 2010 Mar;31(1):18-21.

101. Monitto CL, Greenberg RS, Kost-Byerly S, Wetzel R, Billett C, Lebet RM, et al. The safety and efficacy of parent-/nurse-controlled analgesia in patients less than six years of age. *Anesth Analg.* 2000 Sep;91(3):573-579.

102. Anghelescu DL, Burgoyne LL, Oakes LL, Wallace DA. The safety of patient-controlled analgesia by proxy in pediatric oncology patients. *Anesth Analg.* 2005 Dec;101(6):1623-1627.

103. Voepel-Lewis T, Marinkovic A, Kostrzewa A, Tait AR, Malviya S. The prevalence of and risk factors for adverse events in children receiving patient-controlled analgesia by proxy or patient-controlled analgesia after surgery. *Anesth Analg.* 2008 Jul;107 (1):70-75.

104. Berde C, Nurko S. Opioid side effectsmechanism-based therapy. *N Engl J Med.* 2008 May 29;358(22):2400-2402.

105. Maxwell LG, Kaufmann SC, Bitzer S, Jackson EV, Jr., McGready J, Kost-Byerly S, et al. The effects of a small-dose naloxone infusion on opioid-induced side effects and analgesia in children and adolescents treated with intravenous patient-controlled analgesia: a double-blind, prospective, randomized, controlled study. *Anesth Analg.* 2005 Apr;100(4):953-958.

106. Koch J, Manworren R, Clark L, Quinn CT, Buchanan GR, Rogers ZR. Pilot study of continuous co-infusion of morphine and naloxone in children with sickle cell pain crisis. *Am J Hematol.* 2008 Sep;83(9):728-731.

107. Rodrigues A, Wong C, Mattiussi A, Alexander S, Lau E, Dupuis LL. Methylnaltrexone for opioid-induced constipation in pediatric oncology patients. *Pediatr Blood Cancer.* 2013 Oct;60(10):1667-1670.

108. Willschke H, Marhofer P, Machata AM, Lonnqvist PA. Current trends in paediatric regional anaesthesia. *Anaesthesia.* 2010;65(Suppl 1):97-104.

109. Bernards CM, Hadzic A, Suresh S, Neal JM. Regional anesthesia in anesthetized or heavily sedated patients. *Reg Anesth Pain Med.* 2008;33:449-460.

110. Ecoffey C, Lacroix F, Giaufré E, Orliaguet G, Courrèges P, Association des Anesthésistes Réanimateurs Pédiatriques d'Expression Française (ADARPEF). Epidemiology and morbidity of regional anesthesia in children: a follow-up one-year prospective survey of the French-Language Society of Paediatric Anaesthesiologists (ADARPEF). *Paediatr Anaesth.* 2010 Dec;20(12):1061-1069.

111. Polaner D, Taenzer A, Walker B, Bosenberg A, Krane E, Suresh S, Wolf C, Martin L. Pediatric Regional Anesthesia Network (PRAN): a multi-institutional study of the use and incidence of complications of pediatric regional anesthesia. *Anesthesia & Analgesia.* December 2012;115(6):1353-1364.

112. Luz G, Wieser C, Innerhofer P, Frischhut B, Ulmer H, Benzer A. Free and total bupivacaine plasma concentrations after continuous epidural anaesthesia in infants and children. *Paediatr Anaesth.* 1998;8(6):473-478.

113. Bosenberg AT, Thomas J, Cronje L, Lopez T, Crean PM, Gustafsson U, et al. Pharmacokinetics and efficacy of ropivacaine for continuous epidural infusion in neonates and infants. *Paediatr Anaesth.* 2005 Sep;15(9):739-749.

114. Hansen TG, Ilett KF, Lim SI, Reid C, Hackett LP, Bergesio R. Pharmacokinetics and clinical efficacy of long-term epidural ropivacaine infusion in children. *Br J Anaesth.* 2000 Sep;85(3):347-353.

115. McCann ME, Sethna NF, Mazoit JX, Sakamoto M, Rifai N, Hope T, et al. The pharmacokinetics of epidural ropivacaine in infants and young children. *Anesth Analg.* 2001 Oct;93(4):893-897.

116. De Negri P, Ivani G, Visconti C, De Vivo P, Lonnqvist PA. The dose-response relationship for clonidine added to a postoperative continuous epidural infusion of ropivacaine in children. *Anesth Analg.* 2001 Jul;93(1):71-76.

117. Henderson K, Sethna NF, Berde CB. Continuous caudal anesthesia for inguinal hernia repair in former preterm infants. *J Clin Anesth.* 1993 Mar-Apr;5(2):129-133.

118. Dadure C, Bringuier S, Nicolas F, Bromilow L, Raux O, Rochette A, et al. Continuous epidural block versus continuous popliteal nerve block for postoperative pain relief after major podiatric surgery in children: a prospective, comparative randomized study. *Anesth Analg.* 2006 Mar;102(3):744-749.

119. Collins JJ, Devine TD, Dick GS, Johnson EA, Kilham HA, Pinkerton CR, et al. The measurement of symptoms in young children with cancer: the validation of the Memorial Symptom Assessment Scale in children aged 7-12. *J Pain Symptom Manage.* 2002;23(1):10-16.

120. Birnie KA, Noel M, Parker JA, Chambers CT, Uman LS, Kisely SR, McGrath PJ. Systematic review and meta-analysis: distraction and hypnosis for needle-related pain and distress in children and adolescents. *J Pediatr Psychol.* 2014 Sep;39(8):783-808.

121. Anghelescu DL, Burgoyne LL, Oakes LL, Wallace DA. The safety of patient-controlled analge sia by proxy in pediatric oncology patients. *Anesth Analg.* 2005 Dec;101(6):1623-1627.

122. Ruggiero A, Barone G, Liotti L, Chiaretti A, Lazzareschi I, Riccardi R. Safety and efficacy of fentanyl administered by patient controlled analgesia in children with cancer pain. *Support Care Cancer.* 2007 May;15(5):569-573.

123. White MC, Hommers C, Parry S, Stoddart PA. Pain management in 100 episodes of severe mucositis in children. *Paediatr Anaesth.* 2011 Apr;21(4):411-416.

124. James PJ, Howard RF, Williams DG. The addition of ketamine to a morphine nurse- or patient-controlled analgesia infusion (PCA/NCA) increases analgesic efficacy in children with mucositis pain. *Paediatr Anaesth.* 2010 Sep;20(9):805-811.

125. Finkel JC, Pestieau SR, Quezado ZM. Ketamine as an adjuvant for treatment of cancer pain in children and adolescents. *J Pain.* 2007 Jun;8(6):515-521.

126. World Health Organization. *Principles of Acute Pain Management for Children.* Geneva: WHO; 2012.

127. Anghelescu DL, Faughnan LG, Jeha S, Relling MV, Hinds PS, Sandlund JT, et al. Neuropathic pain during treatment for childhood acute lymphoblastic leukemia. *Pediatr Blood Cancer.* 2011 Dec 15;57(7):1147-1153.

128. Friedrichsdorf S, Postier Nugent A. Management of neuropathic pain in children with cancer. *Curr Opin Support Palliat Care.* 2013;7:131-138.

129. Ullrich CK, Dussel V, Hilden JM, Sheaffer JW, Moore CL, Berde CB, et al. Fatigue in children with cancer at the end of life. *J Pain Symptom Manage.* 2010 Oct;40(4):483-494.

130. Ravilly S, Robinson W, Suresh S, Wohl ME, Berde CB. Chronic pain in cystic fibrosis. *Pediatrics.* 1996;98(4 Pt 1):741-747.

131. Kavanagh PL, Sprinz PG, Vinci SR, Bauchner H, Wang CJ. Management of children with sickle cell disease: a comprehensive review of the literature. *Pediatrics.* 2011 Dec;128(6):e1552-e1574.

132. Brandow AM, Weisman SJ, Panepinto JA. The impact of a multidisciplinary pain management model on sickle cell disease pain hospitalizations. *Pediatr Blood Cancer.* 2011 May;56(5):789-793.

133. Jacob E, Miaskowski C, Savedra M, Beyer JE, Treadwell M, Styles L. Quantification of analgesic use in children with sickle cell disease. *Clin J Pain.* 2007 Jan;23(1):8-14.

Chronic Pain in Infants and Children

Yuan-Chi Lin
Christine D. Greco

Children may experience a variety of recurrent chronic pain, such as headache or abdominal pain. Chronic pain is more common in children than persistent pain and is less likely to be associated with underlying organic disease. Some common conditions that may turn chronic pain into persistent pain include rheumatoid arthritis, malignancies, sickle-cell disease (SCD), and neuropathic pain syndromes.

The management of chronic pain is an important part of pediatric practice. It requires an understanding of pediatric illnesses as well as the psychosocial aspects of chronic pain conditions experienced by children. Most of the pediatric pain and related problems are undertreated. Because of the complex nature of chronic pain, treatment is often approached from a broad-based, comprehensive medical model that utilizes the expertise of psychologists, neurologists, anesthesiologists, nurses, and other health care providers (HCPs). This chapter evaluates some common types of recurrent and persistent pain in infants and children and summarizes treatment strategies, including pharmacologic and nonpharmacologic therapies.

HEADACHES

Recurrent headaches are an exceedingly common form of recurrent pain in pediatric patients. The most common types of headaches children experience include migraine, tension headache, and combined migraine-tension headache. Up to 10% of all children experience recurrent headaches.[1] The prevalence of nonmigrainous headache in childhood and adolescence is 10% to 25%.[2] Migraine headaches are more commonly experienced by boys than girls in early childhood but become more common in girls upon reaching puberty. There is usually a strong family history of migraine headaches. Children typically report an abrupt onset of unilateral or bilateral severe, throbbing headache pain, which is often associated with nausea and vomiting. Although some children experience classic visual or auditory auras of migraine, many experience more subtle premonitory signs such as pallor, irritability, and fatigue.[3] Patients typically experience relief after sleep. Tension headaches are most common among adolescents. Typically, there is no associated aura, nausea, or vomiting. These headaches are usually described as a squeezing pain located circumferentially around the head. It is not uncommon for patients with tension headaches to experience them daily. Children with combined headaches experience both chronic tension headache and episodic acute migraine headache and their associated abdominal pain, nausea, and vomiting. The diagnosis of chronic daily headache is made when headache has been present for more than 15 days per month, with a duration of 3 months or longer.

Chronic progressive headache is most likely the result of a secondary etiology, such as changes in intracranial pressure, infection, or neoplasm.[4]

Most headaches in children are not associated with serious underlying intracranial pathology or organic disease. A thorough history and physical examination are essential and should include a careful neurologic with funduscopic examination. A psychosocial history is also beneficial in helping to determine whether family stressors or maladaptive behaviors might play a causative role in reinforcing pain behaviors. A history of personality changes, visual disturbances, fever, and headaches associated with neurologic deficits are signs that neuroimaging is indicated. Chronic progressive headache or focal symptoms on neurologic examination warrant neuroimaging to investigate for structural abnormalities or malignancies. The routine use of diagnostic studies is not indicated when the clinical history reveals no associated risk factors and the child's examination is normal.[5]

Treatment for headaches in children includes the use of both pharmacologic and nonpharmacologic therapies. Patient and family education should be provided, along with reassurance that a most worrisome cause of headaches is unlikely and that reevaluation will be ongoing. Often, a diary will be kept by the patient, documenting the characteristics of the headaches, medications tried, diet, and stress level at the time of onset to identify aggravating factors. Modifications or any disruptions to the patient's lifestyle such as increasing physical activity as the patient can tolerate it, improving school attendance, and restoring sleep hygiene are important. In addition, cognitive-behavioral interventions can alleviate headache pain and promote functional and adaptive behavior.

Combinations of analgesics, antiemetics, and 5-HT serotonin agonists are commonly used abortive migraine therapies for children. Nonsteroidal anti-inflammatory drugs (NSAIDs) are often first-line agents for migraines, tension headaches, and combined headaches.[6] Patients should be instructed about proper dosing, as excessive use of NSAIDs, acetaminophen, and combination drugs such as Fioricet can cause rebound headaches.[7] Systematic reviews of NSAIDs among adult patients report little difference in their clinical effectiveness. However, parenteral NSAIDs such as ketorolac are often used in patients with persistent vomiting who cannot tolerate oral intake. In a randomized crossover study, ibuprofen was found to be more effective than acetaminophen for interruptive therapy.[7] Ibuprofen in suspension form is commonly used for abortive headache therapy in children who are unable to swallow pills. The recommended pediatric doses are between 6 and 10 mg/kg, taken orally. The 5-HT serotonin agonists, such as sumatriptan, zolmitriptan, and rizatriptan, have been shown to be effective abortive therapies in patients with severe migraines.[8-10] Chronic opioid use is generally not recommended for the treatment of recurrent or chronic headaches.[11]

Antidepressants, beta-blockers, and anticonvulsants are frequently used for prophylactic migraine therapy. Low-dose tricyclic antidepressants, such as amitriptyline and nortriptyline, may provide effective migraine prophylaxis. Typical starting dose in children is 0.2 mg/kg, administered at bedtime, to promote improved sleep. The doses are titrated, based on the clinical response and any side effects the patient may experience. Trazodone has been shown to be more effective than placebo in a crossover trial but should be avoided in teenaged boys because of the potential for priapism.[12] Propranolol is often used in doses of 1 to 2 mg/kg daily; however, controlled studies in pediatric headache management have shown equivocal results.[13,14] Gabapentin 5 to10 mg/kg/day, with a maximum dose of 2400 to 3600 mg, is commonly prescribed for patients with chronic headache. Several studies have shown positive clinical results from treatment with calcium channel blockers. Coenzyme Q10 supplement 25 to 300 mg/day can be effective in the prevention of migraine.[15] Occipital nerve blocks and botulinum toxin injection can control some intractable headaches.

Nonpharmacologic therapies and treatments for chronic headache in children include cognitive-behavioral therapy, biofeedback, relaxation, guided imagery, self-hypnosis, family therapy, and acupuncture. Evidence supports the effectiveness of biobehavioral headache management, when compared to pharmacologic agents, for certain types of headaches in children.[14,16] Through biofeedback, guided imagery, and progressive muscle relaxation, patients learn to shift their cognitive focus away from the pain, thereby decreasing their experience of pain. These skills reduce stress and anxiety, which are precipitating factors in many children with headaches. Cognitive-behavioral strategies help patients improve coping skills, return to school, recognize maladaptive behaviors, and reinforce more functional lifestyles. Acupuncture may be a valuable tool for patients with frequent, episodic, or chronic tension-type headaches.[17] Available studies suggest that acupuncture is at least as effective as, or possibly more effective than, prophylactic drug treatment and has fewer adverse effects.[18]

CHEST PAIN

Chest pain in children and adolescents is a common presenting symptom in emergency rooms, general pediatric practices, and pediatric pain clinics. Because chest pain is often an ominous symptom among adults, it causes much distress to children and their parents. It is, however, not commonly associated with heart disease in children. Of 67 patients referred to a pediatric cardiology clinic with chest pain, only 6% were found to have underlying cardiac disease.[19] The most common causes of chest pain in children include costochondritis, idiopathic causes, muscle pain from coughing, and other musculoskeletal causes.[20,21] Additional causes of chest pain in children include slipping rib syndrome and abdominal and gastroesophageal disease.[22]

A thorough medical history and physical examination help identify cardiac symptoms. Selbst and colleagues found that organic causes of chest pain in children were more common when associated with abnormal findings on physical examination or when symptoms were present in a younger child.[20] A history of syncope, presyncopal episodes, or a history of palpitations warrants further evaluation. Gastroesophageal reflux or esophageal spasm may cause referred pain in the chest.

In the absence of worrisome findings on history or physical examination, education and reassurance that heart disease is not a likely cause for the pain are helpful in resolving the symptoms in the long term.[19,23] A trial of NSAIDs may be helpful for patients with musculoskeletal causes such as costochondritis. Nonpharmacologic therapies such as physical therapy, transcutaneous electrical nerve stimulation (TENS), heat, and relaxation therapies are helpful for many pediatric patients experiencing chest pain.

FUNCTIONAL ABDOMINAL PAIN

Abdominal pain is a common painful condition in infants, children, and adolescents. Functional abdominal pain (FAP) is recurrent episodic pain with no evidence of structural or inflammatory origin.[24] It is a common condition among school-aged children. Several studies report that up to 25% of school-aged children experience recurrent abdominal pain, with the highest prevalence among girls.[25] Many children with FAP can maintain normal activities; the patients seen at pediatric pain clinics are typically those with more severe patterns of pain and disability. In most cases, there is no clear identifiable cause of FAP in school-aged children.[25,26]

A number of clinical characteristics distinguish benign FAP from other types of childhood abdominal pain. In general, children with FAP are between 4 and 16 years of age, experience episodic abdominal pain interspersed with pain-free periods, and are otherwise thriving and medically well. Children with FAP frequently describe diffuse periumbilical pain that is poorly localized. It rarely radiates to the back or chest. Pain is often worse at night but rarely awakens the child from sleep. Many children experience other chronic symptoms, such as headaches, nausea, and dizziness.

In the majority of cases, FAP is functional, which refers to the lack of an identifiable biochemical, structural, or other organic cause. However, the lack of a readily identifiable cause does not imply psychogenic origin. Most children with FAP are generally medically and psychologically well.[27] A subgroup of patients will have a recognizable underlying disease, such as lactose intolerance, constipation, ureteropelvic junction obstruction, inflammatory bowel disease, or endometriosis.[28-32] For many children, however, an underlying etiology is not diagnosed. Some studies suggest that FAP may be a precursor to irritable bowel syndrome (IBS) in adults, and that some children and adolescents may progress to meet the standardized criteria for IBS as adults.[33,34] In a study of 200 children with recurrent abdominal pain, somatic causes were found in 26%. Laxative therapy was successful in 46%, resulting in nearly all patients with functional abdominal pain becoming pain free. Eventually, 99% became pain free using a therapeutic intervention protocol.[35]

The diagnosis of FAP should be based on thorough history, physical examination, and review of symptoms. A psychosocial history is essential to learn how the child and family cope with pain and to identify issues, such as school avoidance and reinforcers of pain. A history of fever, weight loss, growth failure, rash, or other symptoms of systemic illness should prompt further investigation of organic causes.[36,37] Occurrence of persistent pain or recurrent abdominal pain in children younger than 4 years of age is also of concern. Physical examination should include a rectal examination with stool guaiac, evaluation for undescended testes, hernias, and abdominal masses. Findings on history and physical examination suggesting a possible underlying organic disorder should serve as a guide to laboratory and diagnostic testing. In general, extensive routine screening tests such as endoscopies, barium studies, and other radiographic studies are of low yield, particularly when there are no specific clinical suspicions from history or physical examination. In addition to careful history and physical examination, baseline complete blood count, sedimentation rate, and urinalysis are reasonable screening tests to help rule out occult organic disease. A family history of inflammatory bowel disease in a child with chronic abdominal pain warrants further laboratory and possibly diagnostic testing. In children who experience chronic persistent abdominal pain rather than the more characteristic episodic pain of FAP, laparoscopy identifies treatable conditions in a high percentage of cases.[38,39] In a study of 104 children with FAP, parents were randomly assigned and trained to interact with their children according to one of three conditions: attention, distraction, or no instruction. Parents of the pain patients rated distraction as having greater negative impact on their children than attention.[40]

A significant component of treatment is education and reassurance that no serious organic illness is likely. It should be emphasized that the child's pain is genuine and that clinical reassessments will be ongoing. Treatment is based on improving function and reducing maladaptive pain behaviors through emphasis on cognitive-behavioral therapies.[41-44] Underlying anxiety or depression should also be addressed. A return to school and participation in normal family and social activities is essential. Extensive diagnostic testing and referrals to multiple subspecialists may heighten patient and parental anxiety and reinforce a patient's "sick role." Although the study indicated no significant difference between amitriptyline and placebo after 4 weeks of treatment,[45] tricyclic antidepressants are commonly used. Antispasmodics are sometimes used; however, there are limited data on the efficacy of drug therapy. The routine use of pain medications should be avoided. Hypnotherapy can be used for children with FAP.[46]

Longitudinal studies show that only 30% of children with FAP have resolution of pain within 5 years and 25% to 50% continue to experience symptoms as adults. Walker and colleagues found that in a 5-year follow-up, only 1 in 31 children with FAP was eventually diagnosed with a definable "organic" disease.[47] A meta-analysis of 10 controlled studies regarding the effectiveness of psychological therapies for pain reduction in children with recurrent abdominal pain showed that psychological therapies are effective in treating children with chronic abdominal pain.[48]

PELVIC PAIN

Endometriosis is a common cause of pelvic pain among adolescents, affecting 45% to 70% of adolescents with chronic pelvic pain.[49,50] In general, endometriosis affects women of reproductive age, but adolescent girls can experience pain from endometriosis prior to the onset of menses. Laufer and colleagues studied adolescent patients with chronic pelvic pain which was unresponsive to conservative medical treatment using oral contraceptives and NSAIDs and determined that 70% of patients had endometriosis upon diagnostic laparoscopy.[49] A variety of other medical conditions such as painful musculoskeletal disorders, constipation, urologic conditions, and irritable bowel syndrome may present as chronic pelvic or abdominal pain.

Many adolescent patients with endometriosis report both cyclic and acyclic pelvic pain. Some patients experience more severe pain at midcycle and with menstruation, but many will experience pain throughout the month. There is evidence to suggest that the severity of endometriosis seen on laparoscopy does not necessarily correlate with the severity of pain.[51]

Treatment of chronic pelvic pain and endometriosis can include hormonal suppression of endometriosis, surgical treatment, effective pain control, and minimizing disability. Hormonal therapy with oral contraceptives and gonadotropin-releasing hormone (GnRH) agonists suppress the growth of endometriosis and inhibit progression of disease. Surgical resection of endometriosis has been shown to provide both immediate and long-term relief from chronic pelvic pain.

Chronic pelvic pain in female adolescents can lead to significant disability. Over 90% of adolescent women with chronic pelvic pain referred to the Pain Treatment Services at Boston Children's Hospital have been diagnosed with endometriosis. A comprehensive approach consisting of biobehavioral therapy, physical therapy, acupuncture, and selected medication trials has been helpful for many patients. As with the treatment of recurrent abdominal pain, emphasis is placed on school attendance, participation in social and family activities, and recognition of maladaptive behaviors. Patients should be evaluated for other conditions in addition to endometriosis that may contribute to pelvic pain, such as constipation, irritable bowel symptoms, and urolithiasis. Medication trials of tricyclic antidepressants may be helpful, particularly for patients with sleep disorders, although there are few data on efficacy. Opioids are rarely used for long-term treatment. There is evidence to suggest that an integrated approach to chronic pelvic pain with attention to organic causes as well as psychosocial factors early in the course of treatment may improve long-term outcome.[52]

NEUROPATHIC PAIN

Neuropathic pain conditions in children are most commonly a result of postsurgical nerve injury, extremity trauma, malignancies, complex regional pain syndromes, and congenital and traumatic amputation. Diabetic peripheral neuropathy and trigeminal neuralgia seen in adult patients are rarely seen in children. Clinical features of neuropathic pain in children include allodynia, hyperpathia, and hyperalgesia to noxious, mechanical, and thermal stimuli. Some children will also experience autonomic dysregulation and motor weakness. Children often have difficulty describing neuropathic pain, and report pain that is "strange" or "weird."

A thorough history and physical examination, including a careful neurologic examination, is essential when evaluating a child with neuropathic pain. A broad-based evaluation may provide clues to less common causes of neuropathic pain such as underlying cancer, neurodegenerative disorders, and metabolic diseases. Nerve conduction studies are insensitive to abnormalities of C and A-δ fibers, and therefore may be normal in patients with certain neuropathic pain conditions. Quantitative sensory testing (QST), which assesses thermal and vibratory thresholds, may be especially useful in evaluating pediatric patients because it is painless and does not require the use of sedation.[53]

The use of medications in the treatment of neuropathic pain in children is based on data extrapolated from adult studies. Randomized controlled studies of tricyclic antidepressants have shown effectiveness in treating neuropathic pain conditions in adults, including diabetic neuropathy and postherpetic neuralgia.[54-57] Nortriptyline and amitriptyline are antidepressants most commonly used in children, although desipramine is sometimes a useful alternative if excessive sedation is experienced with other tricyclic antidepressants. Because children metabolize tricyclic antidepressants more efficiently than adults, twice-daily dosing is sometimes necessary, with a larger portion of the dose administered in the evening to improve sleep disturbances and minimize daytime somnolence. As a result of rare case reports of sudden death attributed to cardiac dysrhythmia in children treated with tricyclics, a thorough cardiac history, physical examination, and baseline electrocardiogram are recommended prior to initiation of therapy.[58] Antidepressants such as selective serotonin reuptake inhibitors (SSRIs) are occasionally used in the treatment of neuropathic pain; however, additional studies are needed to determine efficacy. SSRIs can be useful for patients who have neuropathic pain associated with depressed mood or anxiety.

Adult clinical trials have shown effectiveness of anticonvulsants such as carbamazepine, phenytoin, valproic acid, and gabapentin for the treatment of various neuropathic pain conditions.[59-61] Gabapentin has a lower side effect profile and fewer severe adverse effects than other anticonvulsants, and monitoring of serum levels is not necessary. The most frequent side effects include dizziness and somnolence. Gabapentin may also be effective in the treatment of mood disorders.

The 5% lidocaine transdermal (Lidoderm) patch is safe for neuropathic pain. It penetrates the skin to act locally on dysfunctional nerve fibers. The patch measures 10 × 14 cm and contains 700 mg of lidocaine mixture with a nonwoven polyethylene backing. The patch can be cut to the desired size. A 12-hour-on and 12-hour-off schedule is recommended with a maximum of three patches at a time applied to intact skin at or beside the area of the neuropathic pain.[62] Most patients who are responsive to the Lidoderm patch experience relief within a few days of application. A trial of 2 weeks is recommended.

The use of opioids in the treatment of neuropathic pain remains controversial. Some evidence supports their ineffectiveness in treating neuropathic pain or their effectiveness only at doses that produce intolerable side effects.[63] Other studies suggest that opioids can provide effective pain relief in patients with neuropathic pain from cancer, limb amputation, and other causes without producing unremitting side effects.[64,65] In general, the use of opioids in selected patients with neuropathic pain not caused by cancer or other terminal illnesses should include a treatment plan emphasizing ongoing cognitive-behavioral therapy and maintenance of school and peer activities.

COMPLEX REGIONAL PAIN SYNDROMES

Complex regional pain syndrome type 1 (CRPS 1) is a condition characterized by persistent neuropathic limb pain with cyanosis, coldness, swelling, atrophy, or other signs of neurovascular abnormalities without an associated nerve injury. Complex regional pain syndrome type 2 (CRPS 2) refers to this clinical syndrome with a definable nerve injury.

The clinical presentation of CRPS in children differs from that in adults. Most children with CRPS are female with a lower limb affected. In the adult presentation, gender differences are not significant and upper and lower extremities are equally affected. CRPS in children occurs most frequently at 10 to 12 years of age and rarely before the age of 6 years. In a report by Wilder and colleagues of 70 children with CRPS, each of the subjects was able to identify a specific injury prior to developing symptoms, and some developed similar symptoms in a second extremity without additional injury.[66] Many patients experienced eating disorders and were involved in highly competitive sports, such as ballet and gymnastics.

Conservative treatment with aggressive physical therapy and cognitive-behavioral therapy results in marked improvement of symptoms in children with CRPS.[67,68] A noninvasive approach with physical therapy, TENS, and cognitive-behavioral therapy was effective in improving function and reducing pain scores in over 50% of patients.[66] Other studies have emphasized sympathetic blockade.[69] A prospective, randomized, controlled trial by Lee and colleagues[70] showed that most children had clinical improvement with a regimen that emphasized physical therapy and cognitive-behavioral therapy.

The approach at the Boston Children's Hospital includes an initial outpatient trial of active physical therapy and cognitive-behavioral therapy. Physical therapy is based on a rehabilitative approach involving desensitization techniques, weight-bearing exercises, and a gradual return to function. Cognitive-behavioral interventions typically include biofeedback training, relaxation techniques, and family and individual counseling. Education of both patients and parents is essential regarding the nonproductive nature of pain with CRPS and instructing that movement of the affected limb will ultimately diminish pain and dysfunction. Regular school attendance and participation in family and peer activities is emphasized. Often, a home diary that records pain scores and measures of function helps track response to therapy.

Commonly used medications in the treatment of CRPS in children include antidepressants, anticonvulsants, local anesthetic-like drugs, and opioids. There is significant individual variation in response to medication trials. Opioids are used in a selected group of patients. Sympathetic blockade is reserved for patients who do not improve with outpatient therapy and who continue to experience significant pain and limitations of limb mobility. Sympathetic blockade is also used for patients who have severe circulatory impairment with ischemic complications. Typically, sympathetic blockade is performed using continuous catheter techniques, combined with an intensive rehabilitative 5- to 7-day hospitalization.

Over the past 15 years, more than 650 children with CRPS have been treated at the Boston Children's Hospital. Over 85% of patients have experienced pain reduction and improvement in limb function. Less than 5% of patients have received spinal cord stimulation trials or implantations. Fewer than 1% over the past 15 years have received operative or chemical sympathectomies. In all cases, the patients who underwent sympathectomies did so to preserve limb circulation rather than for pain control.

AMPUTATION PAIN

Historically, it was assumed that children who have congenital absence of a limb or who experienced amputation early in life rarely experience phantom sensations. However, results of several case studies suggest that most children with limb amputations, as well as burn patients, do experience phantom sensations and pain.[71-74] In a retrospective study of children who had undergone amputation, Krane and Heller determined that 100% of patients reported phantom sensations and 75% experienced phantom pain.[71] A study by Melzack and colleagues[72] showed that approximately 20% of patients who had congenital limb absence and 50% of patients who had amputations at an early age experienced phantom limb sensations. There is some evidence to suggest that the children who receive chemotherapy prior to amputation are more likely to experience phantom limb pain than children with amputations who were not exposed to chemotherapy.[75]

Children describe a variety of phantom sensations such as persistent itching, burning, pain, or a perception of the presence of the missing limb. Some patients will experience allodynia and dysesthesia of the stump.

Studies of tricyclic antidepressants, anticonvulsants such as gabapentin and clonazepam, and opioids have shown effectiveness in treating amputation pain; however, there are limited data on the best treatment among adult and pediatric amputees.[76] Medication trials, biobehavioral techniques, physical rehabilitation, and the early use of prosthesis have been helpful for many patients.[76] Studies examining whether preoperative neurologic blockade reduces the severity or incidence of phantom pain have shown inconsistent results.[77-79]

CYSTIC FIBROSIS

Patients with cystic fibrosis (CF) suffer a variety of recurrent and chronic pains, particularly as lung disease becomes more advanced.[80] Recurrent chest pain is common and may occur from chest wall muscle strain, costochondritis, and spontaneous pneumothorax. Severe coughing may produce painful rib fractures that can significantly compromise respiratory function. Frequent headaches can be caused by sinus disease or by the intense contraction of muscles caused by coughing. As respiratory function declines with advanced disease, hypercarbia and hypoxia can contribute to headaches.[80] Other causes of pain in patients with CF include back pain from compression fractures, arthritis pain, and abdominal pain from pancreatitis.[81,82]

Treatment of recurrent and chronic pain of CF should provide optimal analgesia without further impairing respiratory function. Opioids may provide effective pain relief without inducing excessive sedation and respiratory depression in selected patients.[80] Because patients with CF frequently experience constipation with opioid use, laxatives should be used early in the course of treatment. Selective COX-2 inhibitors may provide analgesia without causing respiratory depression and constipation and cause less risk of hemoptysis than conventional NSAIDs. Continuous thoracic epidural infusions can provide effective analgesia for rib fractures or pneumothoraces and for postoperative pain control. Intercostal blockade is preferred less than epidural analgesia because of short duration of effect and a considerable risk of pneumothorax.

SICKLE CELL PAIN

Sickle cell pain ranges from acute vaso-occlusive episodes to chronic, daily pain. Acute painful episodes are characterized by an abrupt and usually unpredictable onset of severe ischemic pain. Vaso-occlusive episodes typically produce pain in extremities, chest, lower back, and abdomen and may be caused by a variety of factors such as infection, dehydration, hypoxia, and acidosis. Often, there is no obvious cause. Acute episodes of pain account for most hospitalizations and emergency room visits. In a prospective study, Platt and colleagues reported that 5% of patients with sickle cell hemoglobinopathy experienced over 30% of all painful episodes and that the patients with the highest rates of painful episodes tended to die earlier than the patients with lower rates of painful episodes.[83] Chronic pain may develop as episodic pain and become more frequent and severe, ultimately resulting in persistent daily pain. Bone infarction or necrosis may result in debilitating chronic pain conditions such as aseptic necrosis of the hip, vertebral compression fractures, and chronic low back pain.

Home management of vaso-occlusive episodes is encouraged through the use of NSAIDs and orally administered opioids. Day treatment programs may provide effective alternatives to hospitalizations or emergency room visits for some patients.[84] Hospitalization is necessary for patients who are unable to tolerate oral opioids because of vomiting or for patients with severe, escalating pain requiring rapid control with intravenous analgesics. Patient-controlled analgesia enables patients to rapidly titrate opioids according to the wide fluctuations in pain intensity common in vaso-occlusive episodes. A low-dose basal opioid infusion, in addition to on-demand doses, may provide effective analgesia, particularly during severe episodes of pain. However, there is some evidence that this regimen may increase the risk of hypoxemia at night.[85] Continuous epidural analgesia can provide effective analgesia and maintenance of respiratory drive in patients with acute chest syndrome.[86] It has not been established how frequently epidural analgesia should be chosen for patients with frequent, painful episodes. Self-report pain scales should be used as much as possible for pain assessment. Close nursing observation and monitoring is necessary, especially for patients at risk for opioid-induced respiratory depression and hypoxemia.

A multidisciplinary approach to sickle cell pain integrates pharmacologic therapy and cognitive-behavioral techniques to provide effective pain control, maintenance of normal functioning, and optimal quality of life. There is often excessive concern among HCPs and families about addiction to opioids, which has led to inadequate analgesia in some cases. Education is necessary regarding the use of opioids, home management strategies, and avoidance of precipitating factors of painful episodes. Cognitive-behavioral treatment such as biofeedback, hypnosis, guided imagery, and family therapy can improve coping mechanisms and prevent maladaptive behaviors.[87]

SUMMARY

A central component of the treatment of pain and distress in children is an in-depth understanding of pediatric diseases and the psychological and social dynamics involved in treatment of chronic pain conditions. Analgesics and specialized techniques should be combined with lifestyle changes and nonpharmacologic approaches to provide optimal care. Additional prospective clinical trials are necessary in the understanding and treatment of chronic pain conditions in children. The multidisciplinary pediatric pain service would allow pediatric patients and family to be seen in a single visit by a number of pain specialists, including pain physician, child psychologist, physical therapist, and complementary medical therapy providers. This comprehensive approach for pediatric pain management would allow pediatric pain patients to obtain optimal care with the least disruption for patients and their families.

REFERENCES

1. Bille B. Migraine and tension-type headache in children and adolescents. *Cephalalgia*. 1996;16(2):78.
2. Anttila P. Tension-type headache in childhood and adolescence. *Lancet Neurol*. 2006;5(3):268-274.
3. Barlow CF. Migraine in childhood. *Res Clin Stud Headache*. 1978;5:34-46.
4. Lipton RB, et al. Classification of primary headaches. *Neurol*. 2004;63(3):427-435.
5. Lewis DW, et al. Practice parameter: evaluation of children and adolescents with recurrent headaches: report of the Quality Standards Subcommittee of the American Academy of Neurology and the Practice Committee of the Child Neurology Society. *Neurol*. 2002;59(4):490-498.
6. Hamalainen ML, et al. Ibuprofen or acetaminophen for the acute treatment of migraine in children: a double-blind, randomized, placebo-controlled, crossover study. *Neurol*. 1997;1:103-107.
7. Symon DN. Twelve cases of analgesic headache. *Arch Dis Child*. 1998;78(6):555-556.
8. Linder SL. Subcutaneous sumatriptan in the clinical setting: the first 50 consecutive patients with acute migraine in a pediatric neurology office practice. *Headache*. 1996;36(7):419-422.
9. Ueberall MA, Wenzel D. Intranasal sumatriptan for the acute treatment of migraine in children. *Neurol*. 1999;52(7):1507-1510.
10. Hamalainen ML, Hoppu K, Santavuori P. Sumatriptan for migraine attacks in children: a randomized placebo-controlled study. Do children with migraine respond to oral sumatriptan differently from adults? *Neurol*. 1997;48(4):1100-1103.
11. Ziegler DK. Opioids in headache treatment. Is there a role? *Neurol Clin*. 1997;15(1):199-207.
12. Battistella PA, et al. A placebo-controlled crossover trial using trazodone in pediatric migraine. *Headache*. 1993;33(1):36-39.
13. Lutschg J, Vassella F. The treatment of juvenile migraine using flunarizine or propranolol. *Schweiz Med Wochenschr*. 1990;120(46):1731-1736.
14. Olness K, MacDonald JT, Uden DL. Comparison of self-hypnosis and propranolol in the treatment of juvenile classic migraine. *Pediatr*. 1987;79(4):593-597.
15. Hershey AD, et al. Coenzyme Q10 deficiency and response to supplementation in pediatric and adolescent migraine. *Headache*. 2007;47(1):73-80.
16. Sartory G, et al. A comparison of psychological and pharmacological treatment of pediatric migraine. *Behav Res Ther*. 1998;36(12):1155-1170.
17. Linde K, et al. Acupuncture for tension-type headache. *Cochrane Database Syst Rev*. 2009(1):CD007587.
18. Linde K, et al. Acupuncture for migraine prophylaxis. *Cochrane Database Syst Rev*. 2009;(1):CD001218.
19. Fyfe DA, Moodie DS. Chest pain in pediatric patients presenting to a cardiac clinic. *Clin Pediatr (Phila)*. 1984;23(6):321-324.

20. Selbst SM. Consultation with the specialist. Chest pain in children. *Pediatr Rev.* 1997;18(5):169-173.

21. Selbst SM, Ruddy R, Clark BJ. Chest pain in children. Follow-up of patients previously reported. *Clin Pediatr (Phila).* 1990; 29(7):374-377.

22. Mooney DP, Shorter NA. Slipping rib syndrome in childhood. *J Pediatr Surg.* 1997;32(7):1081-1082.

23. Lababidi Z, Wankum J. Pediatric idiopathic chest pain. *Mo Med.* 1983;80(6):306-308.

24. Baber KF, et al. Rome II versus Rome III classification of functional gastrointestinal disorders in pediatric chronic abdominal pain. *J Pediatr Gastroenterol Nutr.* 2008;47(3):299-302.

25. Apley J, Naish N. Recurrant abdominal pains: a field survey of 1,000 school children. *Arch Dis Child.* 1958;33:165.

26. Apley J. *The Child with Abdominal Pains.* London: Blackwell; 1975.

27. Astrada CA, et al. Recurrent abdominal pain in children and associated DSM-III diagnoses. *Am J Psychiatry.* 1981;138:687-688.

28. Feldman W, et al. The use of dietary fiber in the management of simple, childhood, idiopathic, recurrent, abdominal pain: results in a prospective, double-blind, randomized, controlled trial. *Am J Dis Child.* 1985;139(12):1216-1218.

29. Webster RB, DiPalma JA, Gremse DA. Lactose maldigestion and recurrent abdominal pain in children. *Dig Dis Sci.* 1995;40(7):1506-1510.

30. Wewer V, et al. The prevalence and related symptomology of Helicobacter pylori in children with recurrent absominal pain. *Acta Pediatr.* 1998;87(8):830-835.

31. Olafsdottir E, et al. Impaired accommodation of the proximal stomach in children with recurrent abdominal pain. *J Pediatr Gastroenterol Nutr.* 2000;30(2):157-163.

32. Khetan N, et al. Endometriosis: presentation to general surgeons. *Ann Royal Coll Surg Engl.* 1999;81(4):255-259.

33. Hyams JS, et al. Charachterization of symptoms in children with recurrent abdominal pain: resemblance to irritable bowel syndrome. *J Pediatr Gastroenterol Nutr.* 1995;20(2):209-214.

34. Walker LS, et al. Recurrent abdominal pain: a potential precursor of irritable bowel syndrome in adolescents and young adults. *JPediatr.* 1998;132(6):1010-1015.

35. Gijsbers CF, et al. Recurrent abdominal pain in 200 children: somatic causes and diagnostic criteria. *Acta Paediatr.* 2011;100(11):e208-e214.

36. Stein MT, et al. Challenging case: chronic disease-developmental and behavioral implications. *Pediatr.* 2001;107(4).

37. Boyle JT. Recurrent abdominal pain: an update. *Pediatr Rev.* 1997;18(9):310-320; quiz 321.

38. Stylianos S, et al. Laparoscopy for diagnosis and treatment of recurrent abdominal pain in children. *J Pediatr Surg.* 1996;31(8):1158-1160.

39. Stringel G, et al. Laparoscopy in the management of children with chronic recurrent abdominal pain. *JSLS: Soc Laparoendoscop Surg.* 1999;3(3):215-219.

40. Walker LS, et al. Parent attention versus distraction: impact on symptom complaints by children with and without chronic functional abdominal pain. *Pain.* 2006;122(1-2):43-52.

41. Gold N, et al. Well-adjusted children: an alternate view of childtren with inflammatory bowel disease and functional gastrointestinal complaints. *Inflamm Bowel Dise.* 2000;6(1):1-7.

42. Compas BE, Thomsen AH. Coping and responses to stress among children with recurrent abdominal pain. [Review]. *J Dev Behav Pediatr.* 1999;20(5):323-324.

43. Fritz GK, Fritsch S, Hagino O. Somatoform disorders in children and adolescents: a review of the past 10 years. [Review]. *J Am Acad Child Adolesc Psychiatry.* 1997;36(10):1329-1338.

44. Sanders M, et al. The treatment of recurrent abdominal pain in children: a controlled comparison of cognitive-behavioral family interventions and standard pediatric care. *J Consult Clin Psychol.* 1994;62:306-314.

45. Saps M, et al. Multicenter, randomized, placebo-controlled trial of amitriptyline in children with functional gastrointestinal disorders. *Gastroenterol.* 2009;137(4):1261-1269.

46. Vlieger AM, et al. Hypnotherapy for children with functional abdominal pain or irritable bowel syndrome: a randomized controlled trial. *Gastroenterol.* 2007;133(5):1430-1436.

47. Walker L, et al. Long term health outcomes in patients with recurrent abdominal pain. *JPediatr Psychol.* 1995;20:233-245.

48. Sprenger L, Gerhards F, Goldbeck L. Effects of psychological treatment on recurrent abdominal pain in children—a meta-analysis. *Clin Psychol Rev.* 2011;31(7):1192-1197.

49. Laufer MR, et al. Prevalence of endometriosis in adolescent girls with chronic pelvic pain not responding to conventional therapy. *J Pediatr Adolesc Gynecol.* 1997;10(4):199-202.

50. Laufer MR, Sanfilippo J, Rose G. Adolescent endometriosis: diagnosis and treatment approaches. *J Pediatr Adolesc Gynecol.* 2003; 16(3 Suppl):S3-S11.

51. Fedele L, et al. Stage and localization of pelvic endometriosis and pain. *Fertil Steril.* 1990;53(1):155-158.

52. Peters AA, et al. A randomized clinical trial to compare two different approaches in women with chronic pelvic pain. *Obstet Gynecol.* 1991;77(5):740-744.

53. Meier PM, et al. Quantitative assessment of cutaneous thermal and vibration sensation and thermal pain detection thresholds in healthy children and adolescents. *Muscle Nerve.* 2001;24(10):1339-1345.

54. Max MB, et al. Amitriptyline relieves diabetic neuropathy pain in patients with normal or depressed mood. *Neurol.* 1987;37(4):589-596.

55. Bowsher D. The effects of pre-emptive treatment of postherpetic neuralgia with amitriptyline: a randomized, double-blind, placebo-controlled trial. *J Pain Symptom Manage.* 1997;13(6):327-331.

56. McQuay HJ, et al. A systematic review of antidepressants in neuropathic pain. *Pain.* 1996;68(2-3):217-227.

57. Sindrup SH, Jensen TS. Efficacy of pharmacological treatments of neuropathic pain: an update and effect related to mechanism of drug action. *Pain.* 1999;83(3):389-400.

58. Varley CK. Sudden death related to selected tricyclic antidepressants in children: epidemiology, mechanisms and clinical implications. *Paediatr Drugs.* 2001;3(8):613-627.

59. Mellick GA, Mellick LB. Reflex sympathetic dystrophy treated with gabapentin. *Arch Phys Med Rehabil.* 1997;78(1):98-105.

60. Ross EL. The evolving role of antiepileptic drugs in treating neuropathic pain. *Neurol.* 2000;55(5 Suppl 1):S41-S46; discussion S54-S58.

61. Backonja MM. Anticonvulsants (antineuropathics) for neuropathic pain syndromes. *Clin J Pain.* 2000;16(2 Suppl):S67-S72.

62. Gammaitoni AR, Alvarez NA, Galer BS. Safety and tolerability of the lidocaine patch 5%, a targeted peripheral analgesic: a review of the literature. *J Clin Pharmacol.* 2003;43(2):111-117.

63. Arner S, Meyerson BA. Lack of analgesic effect of opioids on neuropathic and idiopathic forms of pain. *Pain.* 1988;33(1):11-23.

64. Portenoy RK, Foley KM, Inturrisi CE. The nature of opioid responsiveness and its implications for neuropathic pain: new hypotheses derived from studies of opioid infusions. *Pain.* 1990; 43(3):273-286.

65. Huse E, et al. The effect of opioids on phantom limb pain and cortical reorganization. *Pain*. 2001;90(1-2):47-55.

66. Wilder RT, et al. Reflex sympathetic dystrophy in children. Clinical characteristics and follow-up of seventy patients. *J Bone Joint Surg Am*. 1992;74(6):910-919.

67. Sherry DD, et al. Short- and long-term outcomes of children with complex regional pain syndrome type I treated with exercise therapy. *Clin J Pain*. 1999;15(3):218-23.

68. Stanton RP, et al. Reflex sympathetic dystrophy in children: an orthopedic perspective. *Orthoped*. 1993;16(7):773-779; discussion 779-780.

69. Kesler RW, et al. Reflex sympathetic dystrophy in children: treatment with transcutaneous electric nerve stimulation. *Pediatr*. 1988;82(5):728-732.

70. Lee BH, et al. Physical therapy and cognitive-behavioral treatment for complex regional pain syndromes. *J Pediatr*. 2002; 141(1):135-140.

71. Krane EJ, Heller LB. The prevalence of phantom sensation and pain in pediatric amputees. *J Pain Symptom Manage*. 1995; 10(1):21-29.

72. Melzack R, et al. Phantom limbs in people with congenital limb deficiency or amputation in early childhood. *Brain*. 1997;120 (Pt 9):1603-1620.

73. Wilkins KL, et al. Phantom limb sensations and phantom limb pain in child and adolescent amputees. *Pain*. 1998;78(1):7-12.

74. Thomas CR, et al. Phantom limb pain in pediatric burn survivors. *Burns*. 2003;29(2):139-142.

75. Smith J, Thompson JM. Phantom limb pain and chemotherapy in pediatric amputees. *Mayo Clin Proc*. 1995;70(4):357-364.

76. Lotze M, et al. Does use of a myoelectric prosthesis prevent cortical reorganization and phantom limb pain? *Nat Neurosci*. 1999;2(6):501-502.

77. Bach S, Noreng MF, Tjellden NU. Phantom limb pain in amputees during the first 12 months following limb amputation, after preoperative lumbar epidural blockade. *Pain*. 1988;33(3):297-301.

78. Nikolajsen L, et al. Randomised trial of epidural bupivacaine and morphine in prevention of stump and phantom pain in lower-limb amputation. *Lancet*. 1997;350(9088):1353-1357.

79. Nikolajsen L, Ilkjaer S, Jensen TS. Effect of preoperative extradural bupivacaine and morphine on stump sensation in lower limb amputees. *Br J Anaesth*. 1998;81(3):348-354.

80. Ravilly S, et al. Chronic pain in cystic fibrosis. *Pediatr*. 1996; 98(4 Pt 1):741-747.

81. Schidlow DV, et al. Arthritis in cystic fibrosis. *Arch Dis Child*. 1984;59(4):377-379.

82. Littlewood JM. Abdominal pain in cystic fibrosis. *J R Soc Med*. 1995;88(Suppl 25):9-17.

83. Platt OS, et al. Pain in sickle cell disease: rates and risk factors. *N Engl J Med*. 1991;325(1):11-16.

84. Benjamin LJ, Swinson GI, Nagel RL. Sickle cell anemia day hospital: an approach for the management of uncomplicated painful crises. *Blood*. 2000;95(4):1130-1136.

85. Shapiro BS, Cohen DE, Howe CJ. Patient-controlled analgesia for sickle-cell-related pain. *J Pain Symptom Manage*. 1993; 8(1):22-28.

86. Yaster M, et al. Epidural analgesia in the management of severe vaso-occlusive sickle cell crisis. *Pediatr*. 1994;93(2):310-315.

87. Gil KM, et al. Follow-up of coping skills training in adults with sickle cell disease: analysis of daily pain and coping practice diaries. *Health Psychol*. 2000;19(1):85-90.

CHAPTER 66

Cancer Pain and Palliative Care in Children

Alyssa A. LeBel
Christine D. Greco
Charles B. Berde

The prognosis of cancer in children has improved dramatically over the past 40 years. Unlike many adult cancers, pediatric malignancies are often responsive to initial aggressive chemotherapy, radiation, and surgery. Currently, the estimated survival rate for a child (age 0-19) with cancer is 80%. However, these therapies often produce acute and chronic pain problems, such as mucositis, graft versus host disease (GVHD), peripheral and central neuropathic pain, phantom limb pain, prolonged postdural puncture headache, radiation dermatitis, and visceral hyperalgesia. Although treatment-related pain generally exceeds tumor-associated pain in pediatric cancer patients, tumor-associated pain is prevalent and may involve bone, viscera, nerves, and other tissues. In the most common diagnostic category of pediatric cancer, leukemia, presenting in children 2 to 6 years of age, bone pain is secondary to rapid growth of precursor cells in the bone marrow. In adolescents, malignant bone tumors and lymphomas produce most tumor-related pain. The most common solid tumor diagnosed during childhood, central nervous system (CNS) tumor, may induce headache caused by increased intracranial pressure (ICP).

Following the often successful treatment protocols for children with cancer, there is increasing risk of delayed and chronic complications of treatment, such as secondary malignancies, skeletal disorders, cardiac and pulmonary insufficiency, neurocognitive disability, and pain. At present, the estimated number of childhood cancer survivors in the United States is greater than 300,000, and there is a 75% risk of a chronic health disorder 30 years postdiagnosis. Early recognition and treatment of medical and psychological issues in children treated for cancer are a public health care concern.

As the assessment of pain in children is guided by the child's cognitive and behavioral development and individualized coping skills,[1] the treatment of cancer pain in children should involve a multidimensional approach that uses medications for pain and symptom management and also cognitive-behavioral interventions and other nonpharmacologic therapies. This approach provides optimal pain control and addresses patients' complex emotional needs related to grief and sense of loss.

TREATMENT-RELATED PAIN

In contrast to adults, children with cancer experience pain more frequently related to aspects of cancer treatment. This is in part because of higher rates of remission in children after initial chemotherapy induction and improved long-term survival rates in childhood cancers.[1,2]

Procedures such as bone marrow biopsies and aspirates, lumbar punctures, and central venous line insertions are common sources of distress and pain in children with cancer. Pain related to the treatment of cancer includes painful mucositis, amputation pain, and painful neuropathies from surgery and chemotherapeutic agents.

Every attempt should be made to minimize distress, fear, and pain in children undergoing brief needle procedures and more invasive procedures because traumatic experiences with initial procedures make subsequent procedures more distressing. Treatment of procedure-related pain is combination of cognitive-behavioral interventions, local anesthesia, conscious sedation, and general anesthesia.

Evidence supports the use of cognitive-behavioral strategies in the management of procedure-related pain in children with cancer. Guided imagery, progressive muscle relaxation, and hypnosis can direct patients' focus away from pain and the procedure to reduce their experience of pain, fear, and discomfort. Young children or those with developmental deficiencies, however, may not have the cognitive abilities to use these strategies. Explaining the procedure in age-appropriate terms can gain the child's trust and confidence.

Local anesthetics and conscious sedation combined with cognitive-behavioral strategies can make procedures less terrifying for children. Traditional agents utilized as topical anesthetics for pediatric needlestick procedures include eutectic mixture of local anesthetics (EMLA), various lidocaine formulations, and vapocoolants. Newer agents and novel drug-delivery systems include lidocaine/tetracaine heating patches and pressurized lidocaine delivery systems (J-Tip, Zingo). Application of topical anesthetics to overlying intravenous (IV) catheter-insertion sites or lumbar puncture sites can decrease pain from needle insertion into the skin. This allows less painful infiltration of local anesthetics deep to the dermis. For more invasive procedures or for children who experience significant distress during brief needle procedures, conscious sedation or general anesthesia should be used. *Conscious sedation* is a level of sedation in which a child is comfortable but is able to maintain airway reflexes and spontaneous ventilation. Conscious sedation is often performed by pediatric subspecialists and is widely used for bone marrow aspirates or biopsies, lumbar punctures, and central venous line removals (**Table 66-1**). Consultation with a pediatric anesthesiologist is indicated for more invasive procedures or for children with certain risks of conscious sedation, such as airway anomalies, obstructive sleep apnea, and significant gastroesophageal reflux disease.

Centers that provide care for children with cancer often have a two-tiered approach in which specific procedures are performed under conscious sedation by pediatric subspecialists, such as oncologists and radiologists. Sedation protocols guide the choice of sedative, dosing, monitoring, and indications when a pediatric anesthesiologist is required. For young infants, or for patients with specific cardiac, neurologic, or airway diseases that increase risk, sedation or general anesthesia by pediatric anesthesiologist is indicated.

TABLE 66-1 Drugs Used for Conscious Sedation in Children

Drug	Dose	Comments
Midazolam	0.05 mg/kg IV q5-10 min titrated to clinical effect up to 3-5 doses 0.1-0.2 mg/kg IM (maximum dose 10 mg) 0.3-0.6 mg/kg PO (maximum dose 20 mg)	Good anxiolytic. Can be reversed with flumazenil. Use caution when combining with opioids.
Fentanyl	0.5 μg/kg IV titrated q5 min up to 3-5 doses	May cause chest wall rigidity. Increased risk of respiratory depression when combined with other sedatives.
Pentobarbital	1 mg/kg IV titrated q10 min up to 3 doses 2-4 mg/kg IM 4-6 mg/kg PO	Provides no analgesia. Often used for radiologic procedures.
Ketamine	0.2-0.5 mg/kg IV titrated q10 min up to 3 doses	Causes increased secretions, which may increase risk of laryngospasm.
Dexmedetomidine	1-2 μg/kg IM 1 μg/kg/dose IV over 10 min up to max of 160 μg	May cause hypotension. Should be administered by physicians with airway expertise.

Physicians with airway expertise and airway equipment should be readily available. Close observation and monitoring of patients is necessary.

Data from Greco C, Berde B. Pain management in children. In: Berhman R, Kliegman R, Jenson H, eds. *Nelson Textbook of Pediatrics*, 16th ed. W.B. Saunders Company, 2000.

Mucositis is painful mucosal inflammation and necrosis caused by chemotherapy or radiation therapy. Although mucositis is a self-limiting condition in most patients, it causes significant pain and distress in children. Mucositis associated with bone marrow transplantation can be especially prolonged and painful. Topical therapies such as diphenhydramine, viscous lidocaine, antacids, and sucralfate may be used to provide symptomatic relief; however, there is little evidence to support efficacy. Patient-controlled analgesia (PCA) is frequently used in addition to topical agents. Some children, however, continue to experience significant pain despite aggressive opioid dosing. PCA permits dose titration and treatment of acute exacerbations associated with mouth or perineal care. Several studies have shown lower pain scores, fewer side effects, and lower opioid use in treating mucositis with PCA compared with staff-controlled analgesia.[3]

Vincristine is an antineoplastic agent associated with peripheral neuropathies such as sensory deficits, gastrointestinal dysmotility, and paresthesias. Some children treated with vincristine experience burning neuropathic pain of the lower extremities. Additional studies are needed to determine the best treatment strategy; however, opioids, tricyclic antidepressants (TCAs), and anticonvulsants are often used. In most patients, symptoms improve gradually but may recur with repeated use of vincristine. Chemotherapeutic agents associated with potential neuropathic pain include cisplatin, etoposide, and paclitaxel.

TUMOR-RELATED PAIN

Most children experience tumor-related pain at initial diagnosis. A survey by Miser and colleagues showed that 62% of children reported pain prior to receiving an initial diagnosis of cancer.[4] Additional studies show that 25% of outpatient pediatric patients with cancer report experiencing daily pain.[5] Tumors can produce different types of pain through stretch or involvement of bone, viscera, nerves, and other tissues. Leukemia can produce constant, aching bone pain caused by proliferation of malignant cells in marrow causing compression of the marrow space. Bone pain can also result from metastasis of solid tumors to localized areas of bone. The involvement of lymphoma, leukemia, and neuroblastoma in solid viscera such as spleen and liver can cause abdominal pain by distension and capsular stretch. Tumors can spread to plexuses, peripheral nerves, or the epidural space, causing lancinating and sometimes refractory neuropathic pain. Children with brain tumors and increased ICP often present with headaches and, in some cases, focal neurologic signs or seizures. Spinal cord tumors or the extension of tumors into the intrathecal space typically cause back or neck pain.[6]

The assessment of pain in children with cancer can be challenging. Children with inadequately treated cancer pain may withdraw from their environment and may erroneously appear comfortable to health care providers (HCPs). Pain assessment scales developed to assess acute pain frequently underrate pain when used to assess persistent cancer pain. Physiologic signs such as blood pressure and heart rate may habituate with persistent pain. Gauvain-Piquard and colleagues designed an observational pain scale specifically for young children with cancer that includes depression and anxiety-like descriptors often reported by patients.[7]

Cancer pain is often best treated using a multidisciplinary approach that combines the aggressive use of pharmacologic agents, psychosocial support, cognitive and behavioral therapy, and nerve blocks. The World Health Organization (WHO) has developed an analgesia ladder to guide physicians in treating cancer pain. A study of children with terminal malignancies showed that over 90% of patients had effective pain relief when managed according to standard escalations based on WHO guidelines.[8] According to this treatment guide, non-opioid analgesics such as acetaminophen or nonsteroidal anti-inflammatory drugs (NSAIDs) are a "Step 1" therapy. Selective COX-2-inhibitors may be used for children with platelet dysfunction or for children who experience gastric side effects with NSAIDs. Weak opioids, such as low-dose oxycodone, often combined with acetaminophen are "Step 2" in managing mild pain. Recommended oral dosing of oxycodone is 0.5 to 1 mg/kg every 4 hours. Patients tend to experience more nausea and other side effects with higher doses of codeine compared with other opioids. In addition, some patients lack sufficient enzyme activity to *O*-demethylate codeine to morphine, causing a marked reduction in analgesic effect.[9] Dosing of acetaminophen and opioid combination preparations is usually limited by the maximum recommended acetaminophen dose. Weak opioids have a "ceiling effect" whereby escalation of dose typically causes increased side effects without improving analgesic effect. Strong opioids such as morphine, hydromorphone, and fentanyl used for moderate to severe pain, or worsening pain are "Step 3."

With progression of cancer pain, μ-opioid agonists are the cornerstone of treatment (**Table 66-2**). Oral dosing of opioids is preferable where possible. Regular scheduled dosing of opioids should be used for patients who have continued pain in order to avoid breakthrough pain. Morphine is the most widely used opioid for treating cancer pain in children. Younger infants have an increased risk of hypoventilation with opioids because of both pharmacokinetic factors, such as diminished hepatic conjugation, and pharmacodynamic factors, such as immature ventilatory reflex response to hypoxemia and hypercapnia. A typical starting dose for immediate-release morphine in opioid-naïve patients is 0.3 mg/kg orally every 4 hours. Sustained-release preparations of morphine and oxycodone are frequently used and are effective alternatives to frequent dosing of short-acting agents. A significant number of children are unable to swallow pills, which limits the use of sustained-release preparations in these patients.

Methadone has a prolonged duration of action because of slow hepatic metabolism. The elimination half-life of methadone is approximately 19 hours, and the oral bioavailability ranges from 60% to 90%. Elixir preparations are therefore useful for children with continued pain who are unable to swallow pills. Intermittent IV dosing can provide sustained analgesia without the need for a continuous infusion pump or PCA device.[10] Because of the prolonged effect and a slow but variable clearance, the dose-response to methadone can be variable.

Methadone dosing is also complicated because it is a combination drug: the l-isomer is a μ-opioid and the d-isomer of methadone is an antagonist at the *N*-methyl-D-aspartate (NMDA) subgroup of glutamate receptors.[11] NMDA receptor antagonists have been shown to prevent tolerance to opioids. The result is that methadone shows incomplete cross-tolerance, meaning that its relative potency for both analgesia and respiratory depression compared with other opioids is much greater in opioid-tolerant patients than in opioid-naïve patients.[12,13] Because of incomplete cross-tolerance and variable dose-response, frequent assessment and careful titration of methadone is necessary to avoid oversedation and hypoventilation. After adequate analgesia is achieved, the dose of methadone should be reduced or the dosing interval extended to avoid drug accumulation.

Hydromorphone is similar to morphine in onset of action and duration; it is used as an alternative when patients experience dose-limiting side effects with morphine. In a double-blind, randomized, crossover trial comparing morphine with hydromorphone in PCA for children with mucositis, hydromorphone was well tolerated and had an approximate potency ratio of 6:1 relative to morphine.

Meperidine is most commonly used for rigors following the administration of amphotericin or blood products. Normeperidine, the major active metabolite of meperidine, can cause dysphoria, CNS excitation, and seizures, thus limiting the use of meperidine in the management of pain in children.

Fentanyl is approximately 50 to 100 times as potent as morphine. It is frequently used for brief needle procedures because of its rapid onset and short duration of action caused by rapid redistribution. However, with continuous infusions or multiple dosing, the clinical duration of action becomes significantly more prolonged. Fentanyl is commonly used in PCA for children who have excessive side effects from morphine.

Mixed μ-agonists/antagonists and agonists with activity at κ (kappa) receptors, including buprenorphine, butorphanol, and nalbuphine, have limited use in the treatment of cancer pain compared with μ-agonists. Some of these agents may exhibit a ceiling effect with escalated doses, can cause dysphoria, and can precipitate withdrawal in opioid-tolerant patients. Buprenorphine provides prolonged analgesia and may be a useful agent in countries with limited access to μ-agonists.

TABLE 66-2 Recommended Initial Opioid Dosing Guidelines[a]

Drug	Starting IV or SC Dose <50 kg	Starting IV or SC Dose ≥50 kg	Ratio of Parenteral to Oral Dose	Starting PO Dose <50 kg	Starting PO Dose ≥50 kg
Morphine	Bolus: 0.1 mg/kg q2-4 h Infusion: 0.03 mg/kg/h	Bolus: 5-8 mg q2-4 h Infusion: 1.5 mg/h	1:3 chronic use 1:6 single dose	Immediate release: 0.3 mg/kg q3-4 h Sustained release: 10-15 mg q8-12 h	Immediate release: 15-20 mg q3-4 h Sustained release: 30-45 mg q8- h
Codeine	N/A	N/A	1:2	0.5-1 mg/kg q3-4 h	30-60 mg q3-4 h
Oxycodone	N/A	N/A	N/A	0.1-0.2 mg/kg q3-4 h	5-10 mg q3-4 h
Methadone[b]	0.1 mg/kg q4-8 h	5-8 mg q4-8 h	1:2	0.1–0.2 mg/kg q4-8 h	5-10 mg q4-8 h
Hydromorphone	Bolus: 0.02 mg/kg q2-4 h Infusion: 0.006 mg/kg/h	Bolus: 1 mg q2-4 h Infusion: 0.3 mg/h	1:4	0.04-0.08 mg/kg q3-4 h	2-4 mg q3-4 h
Fentanyl	Bolus: 0.5-1 μg/kg q1-2 h Infusion: 0.5-2 μg/kg/h	Bolus: 25-50 μg q1-2 h Infusion: 25-100 μg/h	N/A	N/A	N/A

[a]For infants younger than 6 months of age, initial dose should be reduced to approximately 25% of the above weight-scaled doses.

[b]Methadone requires careful vigilance because of potential for drug accumulation.

Adapted from Berde C, Sethna N. Analgesics for the treatment of pain in children. *N Engl J Med*. 2002;347:1094-1098.

ROUTES OF OPIOID ADMINISTRATION

The optimal route of analgesic administration varies in children with cancer. Oral administration of opioids is convenient and relatively easy; however, some children are either unwilling to swallow pills or unable to tolerate oral drugs because of painful swallowing from mucositis, vomiting, or lethargy associated with terminal disease. Oral analgesics are generally not effective for rapidly escalating pain. In these patients, other routes of administration such as IV, subcutaneous, or transdermal are indicated.

Intravenous administration allows for rapid titration in the setting of moderate to severe fluctuating pain. Many children with cancer have indwelling venous catheters, which can facilitate opioid administration. PCA is widely used in children to manage cancer pain and is useful for both inpatients and outpatients. Nurse-controlled analgesia (NCA) is used for infants or toddlers or those who are unable to press the PCA button. In a palliative care setting, parents often participate in PCA dosing. The use of parent-controlled analgesia in the nonpalliative care setting is more controversial.[14] If parent-controlled analgesia is to be considered in a nonpalliative care setting, we would advocate formal programs for parent education and standardized protocols for respiratory depression. Morphine is the most commonly used drug in PCA; however, hydromorphone and fentanyl are frequently used alternatives. The addition of a basal infusion appears to provide more consistent analgesia and can promote restful sleep when used at night.

Subcutaneous opioid infusions can be used for children who have limited IV access.[15,16] Typically, a 22- or 24-gauge catheter or butterfly needle is inserted in the subcutaneous tissue of the chest or abdomen, with the site changed every 3 to 7 days as needed. Concentrated solutions of morphine or hydromorphone are most commonly used. PCA, NCA, continuous infusions, and intermittent boluses can be administered through subcutaneous catheters.

Transdermal fentanyl patches can provide continuous opioid delivery without the need for IV access or PCA devices. Since steady state is reached in approximately 12 to 24 hours after initial patch application, titration by other routes is usually necessary during this time. Transdermal fentanyl patches are not useful for patients who have fluctuating pain intensity. The lowest dose available in the United States is 25 μg per hour, which may be excessive for some children, particularly for opioid-naïve patients.

MANAGEMENT OF OPIOID SIDE EFFECTS

The successful use of opioids in the treatment of cancer pain requires aggressive management of side effects (**Table 66-3**). Unremitting nausea, vomiting, and pruritus can be as distressing as pain to some children. Constipation should be anticipated and can be prevented and treated through the early use of stimulant laxatives. 5HT-3 antagonists, antihistamines, and phenothiazines can be effective for opioid-induced nausea in children. Pruritus can be treated with antihistamines or by switching to a different opioid. Sedation can be troublesome to patients as well as parents. The daytime use of dextroamphetamine or methylphenidate can provide additional analgesia and can allow patients to be more alert and interactive during the day. A trial of a different opioid should be considered in managing opioid-induced side effects because patients may experience fewer side effects with one opioid versus another. In general, tolerance to nausea, sedation, and pruritus develops within 1 to 2 weeks after initial opioid dosing. A recent retrospective study of parents' recollections following care of children with terminal malignancy suggested that nonpainful symptoms, including sedation, fatigue, dysphoria, and sleep disturbances, were as important sources of suffering as pain itself.[17] Attention should be directed toward improving methods for management of these symptoms.

TABLE 66-3 Management of Common Opioid Side Effects

Side Effect	Comments	Drug Dosage
Nausea	Exclude other processes (e.g., bowel obstruction) Consider switching to different opioid Antiemetics	Metoclopramide 0.1-0.2 mg/kg PO/IV q6h Ondansetron 10-30 kg: 1 mg IV q6h >30 kg: 2 mg IV q6h Prochlorperazine 10-40 mg: 2.5 mg PR 1-3 times/day Adult: 2.5-10 mg IV/IM q12h 25 mg PR q12h
Pruritus	Exclude other causes (e.g., drug allergy) Consider switching to different opioid Antipruritic	Diphenhydramine 0.5-1 mg/kg PO/IV q6h Nalbuphine 10-20 μg/kg/dose IV q6h Hydroxyzine Child: 0.5-1 mg/kg PO q6h Adult: 25-75 mg/dose PO/IM q6h
Sedation	Add nonsedating analgesic (e.g., ketorolac) and reduce opioid dose Consider switching to different opioid	Methylphenidate 0.05-0.2 mg/kg PO bid (morning and midday dosing) Dextroamphetamine
Constipation	Regular use of stimulant and stool softener laxatives	Ducosate Child: 10-40 mg PO daily Adults: 50-200 mg PO daily Dulcolax Child: 5 mg PO/PR daily Adult: 10 mg PO/PR daily

Topical anesthetics have advanced the treatment of pediatric procedural pain, with many dosage forms available, including gels, sprays, creams, ointments, and patches. Depending on the preparation, absorption through the skin for dermal afferent binding is enhanced by eutectic mixture, liposomal preparation, and iontophoresis (EMLA, LMX-4, Synera). Direct placement of a combination of lidocaine, epinephrine, and tetracaine (LET) into open lacerations/wounds may obviate the need for local injection (lidocaine 20%; Racemic epinephrine 2.25%; and tetracaine 2%).

EMLA: eutectic mixture of 2.5% of lidocaine and prilocaine

LMX-4: liposomal delivery system of 4% lidocaine

Synera: mixture of 7% tetracaine and lidocaine in a heated patch

	EMLA	LMX-4	Synera	LET (open wound)
Time to use (min)	60	20-30	20	20
Duration	4 h	1 h	3 h	21 min
Issues	Methemoglobin; use in pts less than 37 weeks gestation	Tegaderm occlusion; no methemoglobin	Heating agent; use in pts >3 yr	Need to mix solution; replaces TAC

ADJUVANT MEDICATIONS

Children with cancer can experience neuropathic pain from tumor invasion of nerves, chemotherapeutic agents, postsurgical trauma, and radiation. Neuropathic pain can range from mild symptoms to severe, lancinating pain that can be refractory to opioids and other medications (see Part 5, Section A: Neuropathic Pain). There is a subgroup of patients with neuropathic pain for whom opioids do provide effective analgesia. In other patients, however, doses of opioids that improve pain also cause intolerable side effects. Tricyclic antidepressants are used frequently in children to treat neuropathic pain; however, additional studies are needed to determine efficacy in children. Nortriptyline and amitriptyline are most commonly used. Typically, a bedtime dose is started and titrated according to clinical response and side effects. Plasma levels can help guide titration. A baseline electrocardiogram should be obtained to screen for rhythm disturbances prior to initiating TCAs. Intravenous administration of amitriptyline has been used for patients who cannot tolerate oral routes.[18] Selective serotonin reuptake inhibitors (SSRIs) are considered less effective for treating neuropathic pain; however, they are associated with fewer side effects than TCAs. Some children experience good analgesic effect with SSRIs, which may be especially helpful for patients with pain and depressed mood. SSRIs have shown some efficacy for patients with depression-related fatigue and those with fibromyalgia.

Anticonvulsants such as gabapentin, valproate, phenytoin, and carbamazepine are used for the treatment of neuropathic pain and are considered to be particularly effective for lancinating, paroxysmal pains. Gabapentin is usually well tolerated and, unlike other anticonvulsants, does not require monitoring of serum blood levels.

Corticosteroids are used as adjuvant analgesics for selected types of cancer pain such as headaches caused by increased ICP, spinal cord compression, and metastatic bone pain.[19] Dexamethasone effectively penetrates cerebral spinal fluid and is most frequently used for pain relief from brain tumors and spinal cord compression. Prolonged use of corticosteroids can result in immunosuppression, mood and behavior disturbances, and fractures.

REGIONAL TECHNIQUES FOR CANCER PAIN MANAGEMENT IN CHILDREN

Despite aggressive opioid dose escalation, some children with cancer experience intractable pain, particularly as the disease becomes widely metastatic. Regional blockade and neurodestructive procedures may be helpful for selected patients with refractory neuropathic pain, unremitting bone pain, severe chest or abdominal pain, and tumor involvement of the spine.[20-22] Pharmacologic, nonpharmacologic, and adjuvant therapies should be optimized when considering interventional approaches.

For pain that is below the umbilicus, we have found most success by placement of subarachnoid catheters. The subarachnoid route provides great flexibility in escalating local anesthetic dosing without producing toxic plasma levels. We prefer placement of thoracic epidural catheters for pain in upper abdominal and higher dermatomes. Epidural tumor involvement may result in technical difficulty in placing epidural catheters and may interfere with adequate spread of local anesthetics. Most children will require general anesthesia or deep sedation. Fluoroscopic guidance and use of contrast solution ensure proper catheter placement and determine spread of local anesthetics. Tunneling of the catheters facilitates skin care and prevents dislodgement. We generally tunnel catheters at initial placement rather than use the two-step process of a temporary catheter followed by an implanted catheter commonly used for adult patients.

The choice of neuraxial solution should be individualized and based on the nature and site of pain, location of catheter tip, and side effects with consideration of a child's additional symptoms, such as excessive sedation and air hunger. In our experience, local anesthetics applied to an appropriate dermatologic location provide improved analgesia; neuraxial opioids alone rarely provide sufficient improvement in therapeutic index relative to systemic opioids. If neuraxial opioids produce persistent pruritus, nausea, ileus, or urinary retention, clonidine may be useful because it provides synergistic analgesia with neuraxial local anesthetics and does not typically produce the side effects of neuraxial opioids. In home care of children with subarachnoid or epidural infusions, it is essential that families have the resources to manage issues related to the catheters, pumps, infusions, and side effects that may occur.

Neurolytic blockade is less commonly used in children with cancer pain; however, it can provide excellent analgesia for some children in terminal stage of the disease. Celiac plexus blockade can provide dramatic pain relief for children with upper abdominal pain caused by tumor involvement of viscera.[23,24]

NEURODEGENERATIVE DISEASES

A number of neurologic and neuromuscular diseases in children cause chronic pain, physical and cognitive impairments, and a shortened life span. Although there is a wide spectrum of clinical expression, children with these diseases require long-term symptom management, palliative care, and end-of-life care. For example, children with Duchenne muscular dystrophy and spinal muscle atrophy have intact cognition but have varying degrees of motor impairment. Some children will experience slowly progressive muscle weakness whereas others suffer from profound motor devastation, cardiomyopathy, and early death. Tay-Sachs disease causes severe cognitive and motor impairments and death early in life.

A number of factors make symptom management and palliative care challenging in these patients. A disease may have a variable prognosis and an unpredictable clinical course, which makes long-term care decisions difficult. Cognitive and motor impairments can make diagnosis of causes of pain, agitation, and distress difficult. Children may have persistent screaming and agitation without a clearly identifiable cause, which can be extremely distressing to parents and caregivers. Common causes of pain are usually excluded first, such as hip dislocations and gastrointestinal reflux. Therapeutic trials of opioids and sedatives are often used, but many patients have unremitting agitation. Baclofen and anticonvulsants trials are used with varying success.

Improved methods of assisted ventilation enable children with myopathies to have enhanced quality of life and improved life span. Some children require nasal or mask positive pressure devices only at night, without the need for a tracheostomy. However, as motor weakness progresses, many children will require more invasive mechanical ventilation. The decision to provide ventilatory support for patients with advanced neuromuscular disease is invariably difficult and must take into account individual variation. If the decision is made to forgo assisted ventilation, opioids and anxiolytics may have a role in the treatment of terminal air hunger.

CYSTIC FIBROSIS

Cystic fibrosis (CF) is a multisystem disease that affects the pancreas, lung, liver, sinuses, and sweat glands. The associated chronic obstructive lung disease, however, causes the most pain and suffering. There has been considerable increase in life-expectancy of patients with CF. Lung transplantation and heart-lung transplantation offer hope of improved quality of life; however, hope is limited by a shortage of organ donors and a significant early mortality caused by infection and acute rejection.

Patients with CF suffer from a variety of pain and distressing symptoms. A study by Ravilly and colleagues reported that many patients with advanced disease experience daily pains, including headaches and chest pain.[25,26] Chronic hypoxemia and hypercarbia and frequent strain of head and neck muscles from violent coughing contribute to chronic daily headaches. In addition, chronic sinusitis can exacerbate headaches.

Chest pain is a common symptom and can be caused by intercostal muscle strain from coughing and an increased work of breathing. Patients may experience severe chest pain from pneumothoraces or fracture ribs from violent coughing episodes.

Patients with CF die from progressive respiratory failure. In the final stages of life, patients experience a spectrum of distressing symptoms. Fatigue, air hunger, severe dyspnea, headache, and chest pain are predominant symptoms in children with advanced lung disease. Most patients experience daily headaches and chest pain in the final 6 months of life. Opioids can provide relief; however, they may exacerbate headaches by increasing hypercarbia. Benzodiazepines may help reduce anxiety associated with dyspnea in some patients. Sleep is often disturbed because of air hunger and anxiety and may be improved with use of TCAs at bedtime. Tetracyclics, such as trazodone, may be useful if anticholinergic effects of TCAs are bothersome.

Terminal care of patients with advanced disease varies. Prior to the possibility of lung transplantation, patients in our institution died in an in-patient adolescent unit. With the hope of transplantation, many patients in our institution now die in the intensive care unit awaiting a transplant.[26] Many of our patients fear suffocation and intractable pain and choose to be in a hospital setting for end-of-life care rather than home care. Other centers report higher patient preference for end-of-life care at home.[27]

TERMINAL CARE

Home care, hospices, or hospital-based programs are chosen by patients and families for end-of-life care. The choice is an individual one based on several factors, including the level of care required, the degree of support for families and caregivers, and the connection to pediatric subspecialists. Home care can provide a secure and comfortable environment for children, free from the anxiety associated with hospital care. Optimal care requires careful individual planning for availability of supplies and medications, with ongoing support from nurses, physicians, and pharmacists. Some children and families develop close connections with subspecialists and HCPs at tertiary care institutions throughout the course of the child's illness and prefer to remain in this environment in the terminal stage of disease.

Although free-standing hospices are commonly used in adult palliative care, they are used less often for children. More commonly, the choices are among home care, comfort-oriented care at their tertiary pediatric center, and comfort-oriented care at a local community hospital. Where pediatric hospices are available, they often combine care of children with advanced cancer, care of infants and children with advanced HIV disease who lack family support, and respite care or end-of-life care for children with neurodegenerative disorders.

Children with cancer, neurodegenerative conditions, and other life-threatening diseases require individualized treatment plans (ITPs) for symptom management through the use of pharmacologic agents, regional techniques, and psychological support. Consideration for quality of life is necessary in all stages of disease. For the terminal stage, optimal care should emphasize patient comfort in an emotionally and spiritually supportive environment, which may include home, hospital, or hospice care.

REFERENCES

1. Miser A, et al. The prevalence of pain in a pediatric and young adult cancer population. *Pain*. 1987;29:73.
2. Elliot S, et al. Epidemiologic features of pain in pediatric cancer patients: a co-operative community-based study. *Clin J Pain*. 1991; 7:263.
3. Zucker TP, et al. Patient-controlled versus staff-controlled analgesia with pethidine after allogeneic bone marrow transplantation. *Pain*. 1998;75:305.
4. Miser A, et al. Pain as a presenting symptom in children and young adults with newly diagnosed malignancy. *Pain*. 1987;29:85.
5. Elliott SC, et al. Epidemiologic features of pain in pediatric cancer patients. A cooperative community-based study. North Central Cancer Treatment and Mayo Clinic. *Clin J Pain*. 1991;7:263.
6. Hahn Y, McLone D. Pain in children with spinal chord tumors. *Child's Brain*. 1984;11:36.
7. Gauvain-Piquard A, et al. Pain in children aged 2–6 years: a new observational rating scale elaborated in a pediatric oncology unit—preliminary report. *Pain*. 1987;31:177.
8. Collins J, et al. Control of severe pain in children with terminal malignancy. *J Pediatr*. 1995;126:653.
9. Caraco Y, Sheller J, Wood AJ. Impact of ethnic origin and quinidine coadministration on codeine's disposition and pharmacodynamic effects. *J Pharmacol Exp Ther*. 1999;290:413.
10. Berde C, et al. A comparison of morphine and methadone for prevention of postoperative pain in 3 to 7 year old children. *J Pediatr*. 1991;119:136.
11. Davis AM, Inturrisi CE. d-Methadone blocks morphine tolerance and *N*-methyl-D-aspartate-induced hyperalgesia. *J Pharmacol Exp Ther*. 1999;289:1048.
12. Ripamonti C, et al. Equianalgesic dose/ratio between methadone and other opioid agonists in cancer pain: comparison of two clinical experiences. *Ann Oncol*. 1998;9:79.
13. Ripamonti C, et al. Switching from morphine to oral methadone in treating cancer pain: what is the equianalgesic dose ratio? [see comments]. *J Clin Oncol*. 1998;16:3216.
14. Monitto CL, et al. The safety and efficacy of parent-/nurse-controlled analgesia in patients less than six years of age. *Anesth Analg*. 2000;91:573.
15. Grimshaw D, et al. Subcutaneous midazolam, diamorphine and hyoscine infusion in palliative care of a child with neurodegenerative disease. *Child Care Health Dev*. 1995;21(6):377.
16. Miser AW, et al. Continuous subcutaneous infusion of morphine in children with cancer. *Am J Dis Child*. 1983;137:383.
17. Wolfe J, et al. Symptoms and suffering at the end of life in children with cancer. *N Engl J Med*. 2000;342:326.
18. Collins JJ, et al. Intravenous amitriptyline in pediatrics. *J Pain Symptom Manage*. 1995;10:471.
19. Watanabe H, Bruera E. Corticosteroids as adjuvant analgesics. *J Pain Symptom Manage*. 1994;9:442.
20. Collins JJ, et al. Regional anesthesia for pain associated with terminal pediatric malignancy. *Pain*. 1996;65:63.
21. Eisenach JC, et al. Epidural clonidine analgesia for intractable cancer pain. The Epidural Clonidine Study Group. *Pain*. 1995;61:391.
22. Plancarte R, et al. Superior hypogastric plexus block for pelvic cancer pain. *Anesthesiology*. 1990;73:236.
23. Berde CB, et al. Celiac plexus blockade for a 3-year-old boy with hepatoblastoma and refractory pain. *Pediatrics*. 1990;86:779.
24. Staats P, Kost-Byerly S. Celiac plexus blockade in a 7-year-old child with neuroblastoma. *J Pain Symptom Manage*. 1995;10:321.
25. Ravilly S, et al. Chronic pain in cystic fibrosis. *Pediatrics*. 1996; 98:741.
26. Robinson WM, et al. End-of-life care in cystic fibrosis. *Pediatrics*. 1997;100:205.
27. Westwood A. Terminal care in cystic fibrosis: hospital vs home? *Pediatrics*. 1998;102:436.

CHAPTER 67

Pain in the Elderly

William McCarberg

INTRODUCTION

It is well known that we are an aging society with 20% of the population reaching 65 years or older by the year 2030.[1] Older Americans have more chronic conditions such as osteoarthritis, atherosclerosis, cancer, and diabetes, contributing to increased health care costs, one-third of the total annual health budget today. In the older patient population, pain is the most common symptom noted when consulting a physician.[2] There are multiple sites and causes of these painful conditions, including lower back (40%), arthritis (24%), previous fractures (14%), and neuropathies (11%).[3]

Despite the well known association of aging and chronic painful conditions, pain remains underreported and undertreated. Reasons for undertreatment are related to fear, bias, and education from health care providers (HCPs) and from patients themselves. Patients often believe that pain is inevitable, a normal part of aging, and they fear adverse effects from treatment. They are apprehensive about underlying cancer and addiction to analgesics. Health professionals may mistakenly believe that older patients have a higher pain tolerance and fail to inquire about pain. Many of the chronic conditions manifesting pain in older patients are not curable; however, there must be a focus on the management of the pain associated with these chronic conditions.

The American Geriatrics Society and American Medical Directors Association have published guidelines for the assessment, treatment, and monitoring of chronic pain in older patients, advocating individualized pain management, which is vital to patients with multiple underlying chronic diseases.[4,5] A number of treatment modalities have been demonstrated to be effective for older persons. Pharmacologic and nonpharmacologic options should be considered in the context of the patient's beliefs, goals, and desires. Combining these options helps keep drug effects lower.[6] With advancement in research and newer treatment options, regimens can target chronic pain while addressing comorbid conditions specific to the older patient.

This chapter will explore pain in the older patient. We address the neurophysiology, assessment of pain in cognitively intact and nonintact patients, and psychosocial issues associated with pain in this clinical population. Traditional treatments including pharmacologic and nonpharmacologic treatments are discussed; complementary and alternative methods for pain treatment, as well as extended care facilities and pain at the end of life, are also reviewed.

PAIN AND AGING

Age-related functional, structural, and biochemical changes of the pain pathways have been reported.[7] The effects of age on the human brain are extensive, involving changes in structure, neurochemistry, and function.[8] Excitatory and inhibitory mechanisms in the nervous system exert differential effects that contribute to the experience of pain and depend on complex communications among neural systems. There is strong evidence of progressive, age-related loss of serotonergic and noradrenergic neurons in the dorsal horn, suggesting impairment of the pain inhibitory system.[9,10] Functional consequences of structural age-related changes are difficult to extrapolate because of the highly integrated nature of pain processing; however, several patterns have emerged from the literature. Unmyelinated and myelinated peripheral nerves decrease with age, and increasing age shows signs of related damage or degeneration of sensory fibers.[11,12] Neurotransmitters of primary sensory nerves, substance P, and calcitonin gene-related protein are found at lower levels with increasing age, reflecting a reduction in the density or functional integrity of nociceptive nerves.[13]

Decreased acuity for pain may place older people at greater risk of tissue damage.[14] Despite these changes, age does not produce a change in the pain stimulus-response curve.[15] Reports of increasing pain with age occur when stimuli are intense or persist for longer periods. The widely held belief that older persons do not experience pain with the same intensity as younger persons is not supported by the literature. Increased pain threshold to noxious thermal, mechanical, and electrical stimuli with age has been shown in more than 40 studies, yet there was no agreement among studies. An increased pain threshold could result in less time between the alerting pain and the onset of tissue injury, which puts the older patient at greater risk.

Nerves that have been injured by trauma or disease can become more sensitive. Older persons are more likely to have slow resolution of peripheral sensitization despite tissue healing that leads to prolonged pain states not seen in younger persons. In addition to their prolonged time to heal, older persons are more likely to demonstrate slower resolution of hyperalgesia.[16] Under circumstances where pain is likely to persist, older persons are especially vulnerable to the negative impacts of pain.

PAIN ASSESSMENT IN THE OLDER PATIENT

Assessment of pain in the older patient is difficult because patients commonly have physical limitations with loss of vision and hearing, and some patients present with cognitive impairments or dementia. Nevertheless, these patients have need of adequate pain assessment as they have many sources and reasons for pain related to aging. Taking the time to teach the older patient how to use the assessment scale and use of a pain assessment scale that meets the patient's needs can provide a fairly accurate rating for pain intensity.

Older patients who have pain may fear the pain they are experiencing because it means a disease is progressing or is a new disease. Many older patients want to be seen as good patients and feel that the pain they are having is just a part of the aging process and do not report pain concerns. Pain can also be a threat to independent living, leisure activities, and self-esteem, leaving patients feeling less worthwhile if they admit to having pain every day.[17]

Creation of a sense of trust is important to obtain the salient information needed for a good pain assessment. Reassuring the patient that he or she needs to report pain and that the reports of pain will be respected can go a long way in determining the best way to treat the patient's pain.

The basic elements of pain assessment can be used effectively with the older person. Asking the patient about the location and duration of the pain, intensity, description, aggravating or alleviating factors, functional impairment, and cognitive impairment can provide the base for the assessment.[17,18] In the older patient cognitive impairment and functional impairment may be key indicators for pain. Pain may be interfering with sleep, which may make it much more difficult for patients to concentrate and may cause the patient to appear disheveled in appearance or seem confused.[17]

Most cognitively intact older persons can use the numeric rating scale (NRS) based on ratings of 0-no pain to 10-worst pain possible. A systematic review found that single item pain ratings were a reliable and valid measure of pain intensity.[19] The NRS is best used to determine if pain interventions have been successful in reducing pain levels. If the patient reports a decreased pain rating of 2 points on the NRS or 30%, the decrease is considered to be clinically significant.[20] If using a written pain assessment scale, using off-white paper with larger, bolder print will make it easier for the older patient to see what is written.

When the older patient has chronic pain, a comprehensive pain assessment tool such as the brief pain inventory (BPI) or the McGill Pain Questionnaire (MPQ) not only can help determine the intensity of the pain but also provide information on activity and pain medications as well as determine descriptions. One helpful element of these tools is the use of a pain diagram where the patient can mark the location of the pain on a body diagram.[17]

There are pain assessment scales using pain behaviors that have been developed to assess pain in patients who cannot self-report pain. Before using a behavioral scale recommendations include asking the patient to self-report the pain intensity, attempting to identify any potential causes of pain, taking time to observe the patient especially with movement, asking the family or caregivers about behaviors that would indicate pain, and attempting an analgesic trial to see if the behaviors resolve.[18,21]

Behaviors identified as indicating pain include vocalizations, facial grimacing, bracing, rubbing, restlessness, vocal complaints such as moaning, changes in interpersonal behaviors such as resisting care and being disruptive, and changes in mental status such as confusion, irritability, and distress.[22,23,24]

Although the behavioral tools we are currently using to assess pain in the older patient are not as good as they will be with more research, they provide a method for assessment of pain in the nonverbal older patient. A behavioral tool currently used is the Modified FLACC scale, which uses facial expression, restlessness, and body tension that are rated using a 0 to 10 pain intensity composite rating. The Pain Assessment in Advanced Dementia Scale (PAINAD) is a behavioral tool designed for use with Alzheimer patients. The tool uses breathing, negative vocalizations, facial expression, body language, and consolability that is rated to derive a 0 to 10 pain intensity rating.[25] Additional pain assessment tools for older persons include Pain Assessment Checklist for Seniors with Limited Ability to Communicate (PACSLAC), Functional Pain Scale (FPS), and Dolophus-2.[18]

PSYCHOSOCIAL ISSUES ASSOCIATED WITH PAIN IN THE OLDER PERSON

Older patients with pain can feel depressed, isolated, and at risk for loss of independence. If pain is not adequately treated, older patients may find that they cannot function as well as they did prior to the onset of pain. Overall functionality can be impaired, resulting in deconditioning. Some older patients feel that pain is just a part of normal aging. Although patients may have a higher number of comorbidities that can produce painful conditions such as diabetic neuropathy, they should be afforded the opportunity for pain management to reduce pain and the unwanted effects of unrelieved pain.

Financial concerns also impact the way older patients report and treat pain. Patients who cannot afford clinic visits and medications will have untreated pain that can heavily impact functionality. This can lead to undertreated or untreated pain that results in depression, anxiety, decreased socialization, disturbed sleep, impaired ambulation, increased health care utilization and subsequent costs, impaired cognition, and altered nutrition.[24,26] Assessment of older patients for depression and other psychosocial effects at clinic visits can help pinpoint the effects of untreated pain and identify patients' needs.

TREATMENT OF OLDER PEOPLE WITH PAIN BASED UPON PATHOPHYSIOLOGY

Choosing treatment options for older patients requires considerations such as mental capacity to comprehend how to take medications, impaired kidney and liver functions where medication clearance may be affected, and age-related differences in muscle-to-fat ratios that may affect the binding ability of medications.[17] Absorption of medication may be slowed by increased gastric pH, decreased intestinal blood flow, and delayed gastric emptying.[26]

In studies comparing the efficacy and tolerability of opioids with both younger patients and those older than 65 years of age, findings indicate that older patients responded as well as, if not better than, younger patients when fentanyl, morphine, and buprenorphine were used.[27] For patients with cognitive impairment or difficulty with compliance, a sustained-release preparation is recommended although aging may cause higher concentrations of drug at the receptor sites, delayed elimination of the drug, and bizarre or atypical reactions to pain medications.[27]

Differences in medication utilization in older patients include

- A wide variety of comorbid diseases and potential for polypharmacy that can cause medication interactions resulting in increased adverse effects.
- Decrease in hepatic and renal function that can affect the rate of elimination, drug half-life, and onset of action related to decreased liver mass, decreased microsomal enzyme activity, and decreased hepatic blood flow.
- A 30% to 40% reduction in elimination of medications metabolized by the liver.
- Reduced glomerular filtration rates can increase the half-life of drugs eliminated through the kidneys.
- Age-related decrease in body water and increased body fat can cause a decrease in volume distribution of lipophilic drugs such as fentanyl and increase the volume of distribution of hydrophilic drugs such as morphine.[17,26,28]

The best base to use for medication choices is the World Health Organization (WHO) analgesia ladder. Although originally designed to treat cancer pain, the ladder has been used in many other settings successfully.[29] There are three steps of the ladder divided by the level of pain the patient is reporting (**Fig. 67-1**).

- Step 1 consists of medications for mild pain, intensity levels 1 to 3. Recommended medications include acetaminophen and nonsteroidal anti-inflammatory drugs (NSAIDs). For older patients the use of acetaminophen and NSAIDs can be contraindicated if comorbidities such as liver impairment or cardiovascular risk factors are present. Because older patients can have changes in liver function, decreasing the maximum recommended dose of acetaminophen that can be used daily to 2000 mg is an option. For older patients who are using aspirin as a cardiac prophylaxis, NSAIDs such as naproxen and diclofenac can interfere with the inhibitory effects of the aspirin.[30,31] Higher doses of NSAIDs in older persons are associated with increased risk of gastrointestinal bleeding.[32]
- Step 2 consists of medications for mild to moderate pain, intensity levels 4 to 6. Recommended combination medications include acetaminophen combined with hydrocodone, oxycodone, or codeine. Additionally, oxycodone alone, oxymorphone, tramadol, and tapentadol are listed on this step of the ladder.

Older patients can tolerate opioids but must have careful monitoring for adverse effects and toxicity; doses may have to be adjusted downward

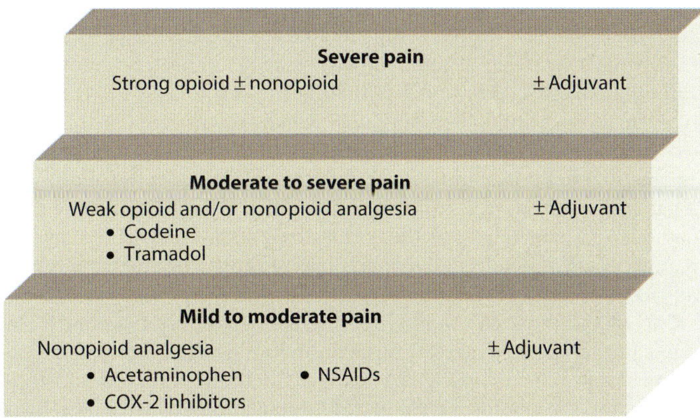

COX = cyclooxygenase; NSAIDs = nonsteroidal anti-inflammatory drugs.
Berry PH, et al, eds. *Pain: Current Understanding of Assessment, Management, and Treatments*. Reston, Va: National Pharmaceutical Council, Inc; 2001.

FIGURE 67-1. WHO step approach to cancer pain. (Reprinted, with permission, from Berry PH, et al, eds. *Pain: Current Understanding of Assessment, Management and Treatments*. Reston, VA: National Pharmaceutical Council, Inc. 2001.

to accommodate the patient's ability to tolerate adverse effects such as sedation, nausea, and dizziness. Tapentadol, a medication combining an opioid action with an antidepressant, can lower seizure threshold and has adverse effects such as sedation, nausea, and somnolence, making it more difficult to use in the older patient[17,33]

- Step 3 consists of pure opioids for moderate to severe pain, or pain intensity levels 7 to 10. Recommended medications include morphine, hydromorphone, fentanyl, and methadone. Older patients can tolerate these medications, but doses must be adjusted carefully for opioid-tolerant patients, and for opioid-tolerant individuals there should be careful monitoring for oversedation, nausea, and constipation.

In addition to the medications on the WHO analgesia ladder, there are medications specifically suited to older individuals. Targeted topical analgesics such as analgesic balms, creams, and patches can be used alone or as added pain relief options. Lidocaine patches with 5% lidocaine have been shown to be effective for postherpetic neuralgia and may help low back pain as well. Capsaicin cream can be used for neuropathic pain. Its main action is regression of C fibers in peripheral nerve endings. More recently, NSAIDs have been made into patches and gels that can be used on localized areas of pain such as sprains and strains for the patches and large joints such as knees for the gels. Older patients like this option as it gives them more control over pain relief.

Older patients may exhibit adverse effects of opioids, including respiratory depression, constipation, urinary retention, nausea and vomiting, dizziness, confused thinking, and sedation. Frequent and close monitoring of older patients using opioids is recommended as well as use of a laxative regimen for patients who are prescribed opioids.

Recommendations for use of pain medication for older patients:

- Use shorter-acting medications at the onset of therapy to determine if any adverse effects will occur.
- Reduce the beginning opioid dose by 25% to 50% to decrease the potential for oversedation.
- When patients have consistent and persistent pain, schedule medications to reduce the need for breakthrough or additional medication.
- Carefully monitor patients who are started on opioids at least daily if not more frequently.[34]

COMPLEMENTARY AND ALTERNATIVE MEDICINE

Older persons like using complementary and alternative medicine (CAM) for pain relief. A home remedy such as ice, heat, or an over the counter analgesic cream, can give them more control and be cost effective. The most common conditions for which patients use CAM include back pain, neck pain, joint pain, arthritis, and headache.[35] In primary care many practitioners do not ask about CAM therapies but about 40% of patients volunteer this information at office visits.[36] Complementary methods for pain relief are those that the patient uses with standard treatment, whereas alternative therapies are those that the patient uses in place of standard therapy.[37]

Two of the most common CAM therapies used are heat and cold. Using a heat pack can increase circulation to the affected area, decrease stiffness, and relieve muscle spasms.[17] A Cochrane review found little support for the use of heat and cold applications to treat low back pain.[38,39] Many older patients prefer heat to cold as they find the cold sensation uncomfortable.

Other types of CAM are attractive to the older patient. Massage may help muscle pain while providing relaxation. Older patients can benefit from physical therapy for reconditioning and improving balance.[24,26] Acupuncture can be used for pain related to fibromyalgia, osteoarthritis, and cancer.[40,41] The older patient can also benefit from movement therapy such as yoga or Tai Chi that improves functionality, balance, flexibility, and range of motion.

Some older patients can use cognitive behavioral strategies to relieve pain although others find them too difficult to master. Relaxation, imagery, meditation, and biofeedback can help reduce pain. Relaxation exercises can be provided using tapes, breathing exercises, or in class settings. The Arthritis Self Management Program (ASMP) provides techniques that older patients can use to reduce pain. Recommended techniques include education, cognitive restructuring, physical activity, problem solving, relaxation, and development of communication skills to interact with health care professionals.[42] For older patients the value of relaxation and cognitive behavioral techniques is an improved sense of well-being and higher scores on quality of life scales.[41]

EXTENDED CARE FACILITIES

There are about 20,000 nursing homes in the United States caring for almost 2 million older persons who are typically poor and very disabled. The average length of stay in a nursing home is about 2 years, 20% of individuals stay for longer than 5 years, and 20% of discharges are secondary to death. The goals of nursing home care vary widely from short-term rehabilitation, to short-term hospice care, to long-term custodial care. It has been estimated that for each resident in a nursing home, there are three more similarly disabled persons living at home relying on family caregivers and community resources for their health and dependency needs.[17]

Extended care facilities vary greatly in the amount of health care they may provide. Because of regional differences, categories of care in these facilities differ dramatically, which makes generalizations difficult. Most of what is known about health care in long-term care facilities has come from data generated in nursing homes where undertreatment of pain has been reported to be as high as 85%.[17] Similar to outpatient care, treatment may be withheld due to concerns about falling, diminished cognition, addiction, and constipation. Depression, anxiety, decreased socialization, sleep disturbance, impaired ambulation, and increased health care utilization are associated with the presence of pain in older people.[17] Deconditioning, gait disturbances, and falls result from poor pain management.

Pain is often overlooked, in part because identification of pain requires specific assessment skills not utilized by many long-term care facilities. Cognitively impaired older persons are even more at risk. In a study done by Won, 74% of a demented, older long-term care population suffered from inadequately treated pain.[22] Although cancer is a source of severe distress among patients and for staff, it is not nearly as common as arthritis and other musculoskeletal sources. Major causes of pain include low back pain, crystal-induced arthropathies, leg cramps, headaches, and claudication. Despite liberal treatment of cancer pain, an analysis of Medicare and Medicaid data showed that 25% of nursing home residents with severe cancer pain did not receive analgesic medication.[3]

Unique challenges are present in pain management for older residents in extended care facilities not seen in younger patients. The spectrum of complaints, manifestations of distress, and differential diagnosis is often difficult and challenging. Recovery from illness is less dramatic and slower to occur. Many of the medical problems are irreversible and expectations for cure or recovery lead to disappointments. Despite the progressive and incurable nature of many conditions in older residents, the discomfort or disability they produce can often be modified. Aggressive testing or complicated treatment is less important than comfort and effective symptom management, especially near the end of life.[17]

Assessment of acute and chronic pain is complicated by incomplete medical records and lack of access to laboratories, x-rays, and consultants. Transportation for medical workup results in missed meals, medications, and social interactions. For some patients, the alternative is referral to the emergency department, hospitalization, and repetition of tests that have substantial risk for these frail residents.[17]

Nursing homes are already highly burdened by local, state, and federal policies that regulate licensure and eligibility for reimbursement. Most of the care is delivered by nursing assistants with little or sometimes no formal medical education. Physicians see patients monthly and with an often unorganized staff where turnover can exceed 150% per year. Physicians often play a minor role in directing resources and quality improvement in many facilities. Despite Joint Commission for Accreditation of Health Care Organizations (JCAHO) adoption of pain indicators in its review process, only 5% of nursing homes submit themselves for JCAHO review. JCAHO is not required or substituted for yearly state licensure surveys or Medicaid and Medicare surveys.[17]

CONCLUSION

Pain in older patients is often underreported, underdiagnosed, and undertreated. Clinicians who care for patients receiving long-term care services must establish a treatment plan that is reasonable given the limited resources and skills available. Treatment must address the root cause of the pain as well as its severity, while taking into account comorbid conditions and concomitant medications. A pharmacologic regimen for older patients must combine sufficient analgesia, and be simplified as much as possible yet have safety precautions. Long-acting medications should be used whenever possible to provide longer durations of comfort and fewer doses for nurses or other caregivers to administer. The primary goal must be to control pain and prevent suffering. Extended care facilities must adopt contingency plans for pain management. These plans will prevent delays in pain care during medication changes or dosage adjustments. Nonpharmacologic strategies require further investigation for this highly disabled population. In an elderly population, that goal should be combined with safety considerations to avoid adverse effects that may not occur as often in younger patients. As the need for health systems for frail older persons continues to grow, it is our most important obligation to provide comfort and effective pain control appropriate for these new settings.

REFERENCES

1. Centers for Disease Control and Prevention. *Healthy Aging: Preventing Disease and Improving Quality of Life Among Older Americans.* Atlanta, GA: CDC; 2001. Available at: http://www.cdc.gov/mmwr/preview/mmwrhtml/mm5221a1.htm. Accessed October 25, 2011.
2. Otis JAD, McGeeney B. Managing pain in the elderly. *Clin Geriatr.* 2001;9:82-88.
3. Ferrel BA, Ferrel BR, Osterweil D. Pain in the nursing home. *J Am Geriatr Soc.* 1990;38:409-414.
4. American Geriatrics Society Panel on Chronic Pain in Older Persons. AGS clinical practice guidelines: the management of chronic pain in older persons. *J Am Geriatr Soc.* 1998;46:635-651.
5. American Medical Directors Association. *Chronic Pain Management in the Long-Term Care Setting: Clinical Practice Guideline.* Columbia, MD: AMDA; 1999.
6. Jacox A, Carr DB, Payne R, et al. Management of Cancer Pain. Clinical Practice Guideline Number 9. Rockville, MD: Agency for Health Care and Policy Research; US Department of Health and Human Services. 1994: AHCPR Publication No. 94-0592.
7. Verdu E, Ceballos D, Vilches JJ, Navarro X. Influence of aging on peripheral nerve function and regeneration. *J Peripher Nerv Syst.* 2000;5(4):191-208.
8. Hunskaar S, Fasmer OB, Hole K. Acetylsalicylic acid, paracetamol and morphine inhibit behavioral responses to intrathecally administered substance P or capsaicin. *Life Sci.* 1985;37:1835-1841.
9. Ko ML, King MA, Gordon TL, Crisp T. The effects of aging on spinal neurochemistry in the rat. *Brain Res Bull.* 1997;42(2):95-98.
10. Iwata K, Fukuoka T, Kondo E, et al. Plastic changes in nociceptive transmission of the rat spinal cord with advancing age. *J Neurophysiol.* 2002;87(2):1086-1093.
11. Knox CA, Kokmen E, Dyck PJ. Morphometric alteration of rat myelinated fibres with aging. *J Neuropathol Exp Neurol.* 1989;48(2):119-139.
12. Kakigi R. The effect of aging on somatosensory evoked potentials following stimulation of the posterior tibial nerve in man. *Electroencephalogr Clin Neurophysiol.* 1987;68:227-286.
13. Hukkanen M, Platts LA, Corbett SA, et al. Reciprocal age-related changes in GAP-43/B-50, substance P and calcitonin gene-related peptide (CGRP) expression in rat primary sensory neurones and their terminals in the dorsal horn of the spinal cord and subintima of the knee synovium. *Neurosci Res.* 2002;42(4):251-260.
14. Birren JE, Schroots JF. History, concepts, and theory in the psychology of aging. In: Birren JE, Schaie KW, eds. *Handbook of the Psychology of Aging.* 4th ed.. San Diego, CA: Academic Press; 1995.
15. Chakour M, Gibson SJ, Bradbeer M, Helme RD. The effect of age on A delta and C fibre thermal pain perception. *Pain.* 1996;64:143-152.
16. Gagliese L, Melzack R. Age differences in nociception and pain behaviours in the rat. *Neurosci Biobehav Rev.* 2000;24(8):843-854.
17. D'Arcy Y. *How to Manage Pain in the Elderly.* Indianapolis IN: Sigma Theta Tau International; 2010.
18. Hadjistavropoulos T, Herr K, Turk D, et al. An interdisciplinary expert consensus statement on assessment of pain in older persons. *Clin J Pain.* 2007;23(1):S1-S43.
19. Jensen MP. The validity and reliability of pain measures in adults with cancer. *J Pain.* 2003;4(1):2-21.
20. Gordon D, Pellino T, Miaskowski C, et al. A 10 year review of quality improvement monitoring in pain management: recommendations for standardized outcome measures. *Pain Manage Nurs.* 2002;3(4):116-130.
21. Herr K, Bjoro K, Decker S. Tools for assessment of pain in nonverbal older adults with dementia: a state of the science review. *J Pain Sympt Manage.* 2006;31(2):170-192.
22. Feldt KS. The checklist of non-verbal pain indicators (CNPI). *Pain Manage Nurs.* 2000;1(1):13-21.
23. Feldt KS, Ryden MB, Miles S. Treatment of pain in cognitively impaired compared with cognitively intact older patients with hip fractures. *J Am Geriatr Soc.* 1998;46:1079-1085.
24. American Geriatric Society (AGS). The management of persistent pain in older persons. *J Am Geriatr Soc.* 2002;50:S205-S224.
25. Lane P, Kumtupis M, MacDonald S, McCarthy P, Panke JA, Warden V, et al. A pain assessment tool for people with advanced Alzheimer's and other progressive dementias. *Home Health Nurse.* 2003;21(1):32-37.
26. Brukenthal P, D'Arcy Y. Assessment and management of pain in older adults: a review of the basics. *Top Adv Pract eJ.* 2007;7(1). Available at: http://www.medscape.com/viewarticle/556382. Accessed June 20, 2014.
27. Pergolizzi J, Borger R, Budd K, Dahan A, Erdine S, Hans G, et al. Opioids and the management of chronic severe pain in the elderly: consensus statement of an international expert panel with focus on the six clinically most often used World Health Organization step III opioids. *Pain Pract.* 2008;8(4):287-313.
28. Horgas A. Pain management in elderly adults. *J Infus Nurs.* 2003;26(3):161-165.
29. Dalton JA, Youngblood R. Clinical application of the World Health Organization analgesic ladder. *J Intraven Nurs.* 2001;23(2):118-124.
30. Capone ML, Sciulli MG, Tacconelli S, et al. Pharmacodynamic interaction of naproxen with low dose aspirin in healthy subjects. *J Coll Cardiol.* 2005;45:1295-1301.
31. Catella-Lawson F, Reilly M, Kapoor S, et al. Cycloxygenase inhibitors and antiparticle effect of aspirin. *N Engl J Med.* 2001;345:1809-1817.

32. Perez-Gutthann S, Rodriguez L, Raifoed D. Individual non-steroidal anti-inflammatory drugs and other risk factors for upper gastrointestinal bleeding and perforation. *Epidemiol.* 1997;8:18-24.

33. American Pain Society (APS). *Principles of Analgesic Use in the Treatment of Acute Pain and Cancer Pain.* Glenview Il: The Society; 2009.

34. McLennon S. Persistent pain management. National Guidelines Clearinghouse 2005. Available at: http://www.guideline.gov. Accessed June 20, 2014.

35. Pierce B. A nonpharmacologic adjunct for pain management. *NursePract.* 2009;34(2):10-13.

36. O'Hara DA. Pain Management in P Iyer (Ed) *Medical Legal Aspects of Suffering.* Tucson AZ: Lawyers & Judges Publishing; 2003.

37. National Center for Complementary and Alternative Medicine. *Expanding Horizons of Health Care Strategic Plan 2005–2009.* Bethesda, MD: U.S. Department of Health and Human Services. National Institutes of Health; 2004. Available at: http://www.nccam.nih.gov. Accessed June 20, 2014.

38. D'Arcy Y. *Pain Management: Evidence Based Tools and Techniques for Nursing Professionals.* Marblehead MA: HcPro, Inc.; 2007.

39. French SD, Cameron M, Walker BF, Reggars JW, Esterman AJ. Superficial heat or cold for low back pain. *Cochrane Database Syst Rev.* 2006;(2).

40. American Pain Society. *Guideline for the Management of Fibromyalgia Pain Syndrome in Adults and Children.* Glenview IL: American Pain Society; 2005.

41. Dillard J, Knapp S. Complementary and alternative pain therapy in the emergency department. *Emerg Med Clin North Am.* 2005;(23):529-549.

42. Khatta, M. A complementary approach to pain management. *TopAdv Pract Nurs eJ.* 2007;7(1). Available at: http://www.medscape.com/viewarticle/556408. Accessed June 20, 2014.

PART 6

Pain Therapies

SECTION A
Pharmacologic Treatments

CHAPTER 68 Opioid Pharmacotherapy

Arthur G. Lipman

"Among the remedies which it has pleased almighty God to give to man to relieve his sufferings, none is so universal and efficacious as opium."

—Sir Thomas Sydenham, 1680

Analgesics are drugs that relieve pain without significant loss of other sensations. The word *analgesic* is from the Greek *an*, without + *algesis*, sensation of pain. Opioid analgesics are the most effective and commonly used pharmacotherapy for moderate to severe pain.[1] Not all pain patients benefit from opioid therapy; however, more patients benefit from strong analgesics when the drugs are used as an element of multimodal therapy.

Opioids include all compounds that bind to opioid receptors; these include exogenous opioid receptor agonists and antagonists as well as the endogenous opioid peptides. The term *opiate* originally was used to describe a drug derived from opium but now includes the natural opium products (e.g., morphine), the semisynthetic derivatives (e.g., hydromorphone), and completely synthetic congeners (e.g., methadone).

The differences between exogenous opioids, such as morphine, and endogenous opioids, such as β-endorphin, do not justify differing terminology. Opioid accurately describes both types of compounds and is generally considered the preferred term in both clinical and scientific dialogue.

Narcotic, from the Greek *narkotikos*, benumbing, was originally used to describe opium derivatives. Today, narcotic has become a legal term that includes a broad range of sedating and potentially abused drugs, many of which are not related to opium. Because the word *narcotic* has negative connotations, physicians should *not* use it when talking with patients.

The last 30 years have seen a marked increase in our knowledge of the sites and mechanisms of action of opioids.[1] New analytical methods reveal pharmacokinetic (PK) data on the disposition and fate of opioids in humans. Recently elucidated opioid receptor-related genetic polymorphisms provide a greater understanding of how genetics can help predict responses to opioids.[2]

BRIEF HISTORY OF OPIOID ANALGESICS

The word *opium* is derived from the Greek *opion*, poppy juice. Opium is the milky exudation derived from the unripe capsules of the opium poppy, *Papaver somniferum*. Opium contains over 20 different alkaloids and has been used to control human discomfort for over five millennia. Opium was used clinically in the early days of European medicine, but it fell into disfavor because of toxic outcomes from nonstandardized forms that were not used with necessary care. Paracelsus repopularized the use of opium in the 16th century, and by the second half of that century, clinical use of opium was understood and adopted by physicians throughout the continent.

The French pharmacist Jean-François Derosne isolated a crystalline precipitate from opium in 1803, a mixture of morphine and narcotine. It was not until 3 years later that the German pharmacist Friedrich Wilhelm Sertürner isolated morphine, the pure alkaloid, and named it after Morpheus, the Greek god of dreams. Other opium alkaloids including papaverine and codeine were soon isolated, and within a few decades, the pure alkaloids replaced crude opium in clinical practice.

By the mid-19th century, many of the patent medicines sold as panaceas contained opioids. Steadily increasing federal and state control of opioids in the United States began with the passage of the Harrison Narcotic Act in 1914. The federal Bureau of Narcotics was created in the 20th century to address use of potentially abused drugs. In recent decades, political and law enforcement demands, rather than scientific or clinical findings, have defined the control system for opioid use in the United States. Creation of the Drug Enforcement Administration (DEA) by the Controlled Substances Act of 1970 assured that control of opioids and other controlled substances would be driven by law enforcement, not a patient care focus. Numerous initiatives, both within and outside of government, have worked to emphasize that opioids are important and frequently underused medications. These include the 1979 Report to the White House of the federal Interagency Committee on New Therapies for Pain and Discomfort, the 1985 report of the federal Interagency Committee on Pain and Analgesia,[3] and the 1986 National Institutes of Health Consensus Development Conference Report titled "The Integrated Approach to the Management of Pain."[4] It may be that serious opioid underuse in the latter decades of the 20th century has been replaced by overuse in the early 21st century.[5]

OPIOID PHARMACOLOGY

It is not logical that the human body should contain specific receptors for alkaloids derived from a plant. The presence of endogenous opioids was postulated to explain the presence of opioid receptors before the endogenous substances were isolated. Cloning studies have identified three groups of endogenous opioid peptides; the enkephalins, endorphins, and dynorphins appear to function as neurotransmitters, neuromodulators, and neurohormones. These peptides are found within the central nervous system (CNS), adrenal medulla, nerve plexi, gastric exocrine glands, and intestines.

PHARMACODYNAMICS – MECHANISM OF ACTION

Opioid drugs manifest analgesic effects primarily by binding to and activating (agonizing) opioid receptors. Opioid receptors are found in the CNS and gastrointestinal (GI) tract and, to a lesser degree, in peripheral tissues. The interaction of exogenous opioid medications and opioid receptors mimics the interaction when endogenous opioid peptides (dynorphins, endorphins, enkephalins) bind with these same receptors.[6] The three major classes of opioid receptors are the mu (μ), delta (δ), and kappa (κ) receptors.[7] Sigma (σ) and epsilon (ε) receptors were formerly classified as opioid receptors because opioids can bind to them. However, neither is currently considered an opioid receptor because activation does not necessarily result in analgesia and neither of these receptor types is opioid-specific.

Opioid receptors are composed of glycoproteins found in cellular membranes. These receptors are coupled to G proteins that modulate potassium and calcium ion conduction[8] (**Fig. 68-1**). At μ- and δ-opioid receptors, opioids open a potassium ion channel, increasing potassium conductance. Hyperpolarization inhibits neuronal activity. In contrast, κ-receptor activation inhibits calcium entry via a calcium ion channel. Activation of opioid receptors decreases transmission of signals from primary peripheral afferent sensory neurons to higher CNS centers, as well as the processing of the pain stimulus.

Administration of an opioid agonist activates opioid receptors, producing both analgesia and adverse effects. The three opioid receptor types have known subtypes (**Table 68-1**). Two μ subtypes have been elucidated. Activation of μ_1 leads to supraspinal analgesia, whereas μ_2 activation is associated with the adverse sequelae of opioid administration. Activation of κ and δ receptors produces spinal analgesia. However, κ_3 receptors are thought to mediate supraspinal analgesia.[9] Activation of δ receptors may potentiate μ-receptor-induced analgesia, but no δ agonists are available for clinical use. Clinical implications of the δ- and κ-receptor subtypes are not fully understood.

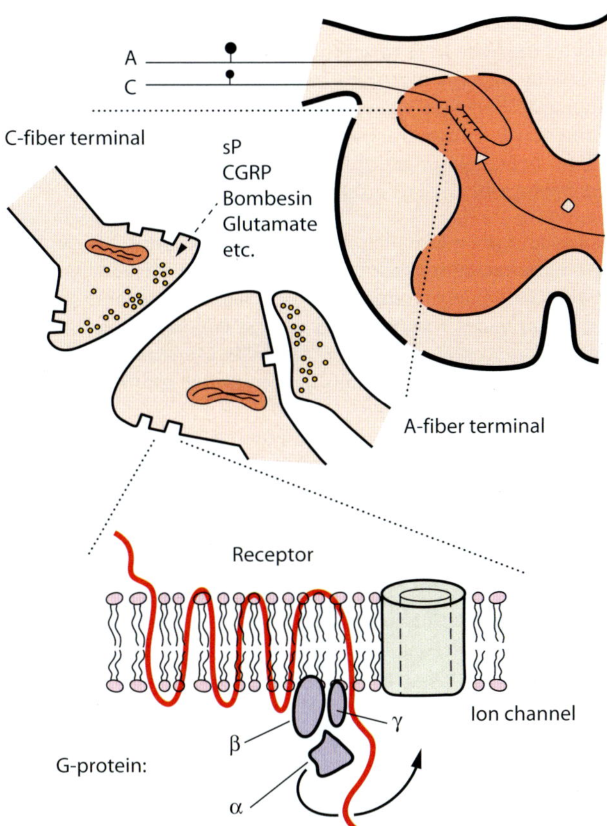

FIGURE 68-1. Illustration of synapse A δ and C fibers with second-order neurons in the dorsal horn of the spinal cord and proposed opioid receptor demonstrating the G protein subunits and close approximation to an ion channel. (Adapted with permission from Sabbe and Yaksh.[17])

Peripheral μ and κ opioid receptors in peripheral tissues can effect inflammation and exert antihyperalgesic activity.[10] Topical and intraarticular opioids have been used to treat pain in soft tissue and joints. The clinical significance of the peripheral effects of opioids is not yet well understood.

Most opioids used as analgesics are μ agonists which bind primarily at μ opioid receptors (MORs) and also may bind to a lesser degree at κ receptors. Kappa opioid receptor ligands provide a few drugs; however, their clinical pharmacology is complicated by concurrent μ opioid receptor antagonist activity. Delta opioid receptor ligands have been in clinical investigation for years, but none was available for clinical use at the time of this writing. Most analgesics which are predominantly μ agonists also have some ability to bind at κ receptors. Some recent literature has suggested that μ agonists with some preferential κ binding capacity may be advantageous in visceral pain. Oxycodone displays that characteristic.[11]

Opioid receptors generate nerve signals through a second messenger, cyclic adenosine monophosphate (cAMP), or an ion channel.[1] Alterations in the levels of cAMP and the transcription factor CREB (cAMP response element binding protein) during chronic morphine treatment are associated with numerous cellular changes, some of which can produce tolerance and physical dependence.[12] Molecular genetics approaches have used gene-targeting (knockout) technology to disrupt the gene that codes for each of the three types of opioid receptors. Mice given morphine that lack the μ opioid receptor (MOR-deficient mice) do not experience analgesia, respiratory depression, constipation, physical dependence, reward behaviors, or immunosuppression.[13] μ opioid receptors are evident in the periphery following inflammation, in presynaptic and postsynaptic spinal cord dorsal horn sites, and in the brainstem, thalamus, and cortex. These locations constitute the ascending pain transmission system. These receptors also reside in midbrain periaqueductal gray, the nucleus raphe magnus, and the rostral ventral medulla. Those sites constitute the descending inhibitory system that modulates spinal cord pain transmission.[14] μ agonists bind at MORs in the colon, causing opioid-induced constipation.[15] Opioids also decrease presynaptic neurotransmitter release through calcium channel inhibition and increase potassium ion efflux, causing hyperpolarization of postsynaptic neurons and decreasing synaptic transmission. An additional mechanism of action of opioids is inhibition of GABAergic transmission within the CNS. The net effect is descending inhibitory circuit excitation.

Animal studies suggest that the reinforcing and rewarding properties of opioids (e.g., euphoria) that are associated with opioid abuse involve the mesolimbic dopamine system, not the supraspinal systems most prominently involved in the production of analgesia and physical dependence.[16]

TABLE 68-1 Opioid Receptors, Subtypes, and Physiologic Effects

Receptor	Subtypes	Effects
μ	μ1 μ2	Supraspinal analgesia Physical dependence Euphoria Sedation Respiratory depression Constipation Orthostatic hypotension Arteriolar/venous vessel dilation
Delta	Delta 1, 2	Spinal analgesia Euphoria Potentiates μ receptor analgesia
κ	κ1, 2, 3	Spinal analgesia Sedation Miosis Supraspinal analgesia (K3)

CENTRAL NERVOUS SYSTEM OPIOID EFFECTS

Analgesia Pain relief from μ agonist opioids is relatively selective; other senses are not affected. After opioid administration, some patients still perceive pain, but they generally report it as being less uncomfortable than it was before receiving the drug. Pain includes both sensory-discriminative aspects (e.g., perception of the location, type, and intensity) and an emotional dimension sometimes described as unpleasantness. Sensory-discriminative aspects are processed in the somatosensory cortex (SSC), while the affective component is processed in the anterior cingulate cortex (ACC). μ opioid receptors (MORs) are found in both of these areas of the brain. Non-opioid analgesics have dose-dependent analgesic effect ceilings; morphine-like opioids do not. However, dose-related adverse events produce a functional ceiling. These include sedation, obtundation, nausea, vomiting, and respiratory depression. The clinical dose needed for analgesia varies with the type of pain and among patients. As result, the most important clinical principle is titration of the opioid dose to response. Some patients will prefer less analgesia to retain a more intact sensorium; others prefer mental clouding if it is accompanied by pain relief.

Mood Effects μ agonists can alter mood, including the relief of anxiety, euphoria, and—more commonly dysphoria. Chronic pain patients often report initial relief of depression, at least some of which may be due to decreased pain, which frequently proceeds to worsened depression in days to weeks. Reinforcing and rewarding properties of opioids in opioid abusers involve the mesolimbic dopamine system and differ from the systems which produce analgesia and physical dependence.

Nausea and Vomiting μ agonists produce nausea and vomiting by stimulating the chemoreceptor trigger zone (CTZ) in the medullary area postrema. These adverse effects occur more frequently in ambulatory patients due to motion exacerbating vestibular sensitivity. Opioid-induced nausea and vomiting varies among drugs and among patients. Patients who cannot tolerate GI adverse effects from one opioid may tolerate another and find tapentadol better tolerated than pure μ agonists. Central antiemetics such as phenothiazines (e.g., prochlorperazine), a gastrokinetic drug (e.g., metoclopramide), or a 5-HT receptor antagonist (e.g., ondansetron) can be helpful.

Sedation μ agonists are sedating and these effects are additive to those of other CNS depressants. Opioids are additive to respiratory depressants including alcohol, benzodiazepines, and other sedative-hypnotics. A central stimulant (e.g., methylphcnidate, modafinil) helps to counteract opioid sedative effects. Tolerance to opioid-induced sedation typically occurs to some degree within a few days.

Respiratory Depression Respiratory depression with initiation of opioid pharmacotherapy for acute pain is potentially the most serious adverse opioid effect. The μ agonists act at brainstem respiratory centers. The effect is dose-related and sensitivity varies among individuals. Therapeutic morphine doses can depress respiratory rate, minute volume, and tidal exchange. As CO_2 accumulates, it stimulates central chemoreceptors, causing a compensatory increase in respiratory rate that masks respiratory depression. Respiratory depression and CO_2 retention produce cerebral vasodilation and increased cerebrospinal fluid pressure unless the PCO_2 is normalized by artificial ventilation. Respiratory depression occurs most commonly in opioid-naive patients after acute opioid administration and is associated with other signs of CNS depression, including sedation and obtundation. Tolerance to these effects develops rapidly, and the risk of the effects is relatively low with chronic opioid use in chronic pain management. Obstructive sleep apnea is common in obese patients and presents risk for opioid-induced respiratory depression, especially when the patients are sleeping. Opioids, and perhaps more so methadone, may induce potentially life-threatening central sleep apnea Respiratory depression can be reversed by prompt administration of the opioid antagonist naloxone. In patients chronically receiving opioids who develop respiratory depression, naloxone diluted 1:10 should be titrated carefully to prevent the precipitation of severe withdrawal symptoms while reversing the respiratory depression.

Three mixed agonist-antagonists, pentazocine, nalbuphine, butorphanol, and the partial agonist buprenorphine have different dose-response characteristics for their respiratory depression curves from the morphine-like opioids. While therapeutic doses of pentazocine produce respiratory depression equivalent to that of morphine, increasing the dose does not ordinarily produce a proportional increase in respiratory depression. Whether this apparent ceiling to respiratory depression offers any significant clinical advantage has not been determined. Naloxone reversal of the respiratory depression produced by buprenorphine requires relatively large doses (5-10 mg) and is delayed in onset.

Constriction of the Pupil Opioids produce miosis through stimulation of the parasympathetic nucleus of the oculomotor nerve. Pinpoint pupils, respiratory depression, and loss of consciousness are the three signs of opioid overdose. All of these effects can be reversed with naloxone. Severe anoxia causes mydriasis.

Antitussive Effect Opioids depress the cough centers in the medulla, depressing the cough reflex. Different mechanisms depress cough than produce analgesia. As a result, the dextrorotatory isomers of opioids (e.g., dextromethorphan), which do not bind to opioid receptors, are antitussive.

Hypothalamic Effects Morphine alters hypothalamic heat regulation, lowering body temperature. Corticotrophin-releasing hormone (CRH) and gonadotropin-releasing hormone (GnRH) are inhibited, resulting in lowered luteinizing hormone (LH), follicle stimulating hormone (PSH), and adrenocorticotropic hormone (ACTH). Prolactin and antidiuretic hormone release are increased. Tolerance to these effects appears to occur.

Opioid-induced androgen deficiency (OPIAD) describes clinically meaningful decrease in testosterone levels that occurs in the majority of men receiving ongoing morphine or other potent μ agonist opioid pharmacotherapy. Worsening of pain, depressed mood, and refractoriness to treatment are common in such patients. Trials of androgen supplements have been helpful and this phenomenon also appears to occur in women, presumably due to progesterone suppression.

Central Nervous System Excitation In addition to being CNS depressants, opioids can be excitatory. Normeperidine, a major metabolite of meperidine produces anxiety, tremors, myoclonus, and generalized seizures when it accumulates with repeated dosing. Naloxone does not reverse, and may even exacerbate, this hyperexcitability. Other high-dose μ agonists can produce multifocal myoclonus in opioid-tolerant patients.[18]

CLINICAL USES

Opioids remain the most effective analgesics available; as such, they are essential in clinical medicine for the management of moderate to severe pain in many cases. However, the misuse of prescription opioids resulting in morbidity and mortality has produced controversy over opioid availability and control.[19] Opioids are clinically useful in treating diarrhea and GI hypermotility because activation of opioid receptors in the intestines slows peristalsis. Opioids decrease respiratory activity which can be useful in anesthetized patients and to help manage air hunger, especially in end-of-life care. Opioids also can lessen anxiety and excitation and induce a feeling of well-being.

Much opioid pharmacology learned by health care professional students is based on studies conducted in lower animals or isolated tissues. Those rarely address the profound cognitive effects of pain and analgesia that greatly influence outcomes of opioid therapy in humans. Serious misunderstanding among health care providers results from failure to recognize the great differences between acute opioid toxicity and that seen with long-term therapy. Incorrect assumptions and beliefs about opioid toxicity, addiction potential, and tolerance to analgesic effects have led to poor use of these effective drugs in many clinical settings. This has led to widespread *opiophobia,* the irrational and undocumented fear that appropriate use of opioids causes addiction.[20]

OPIOID AVAILABILITY AND USE

Balance in opioid availability and use is essential for good patient care outcomes and the public health. Well-designed guidelines have helped to define that balance.[21-23]

Opioid pharmacotherapy for chronic nonmalignant pain was considered controversial by many physicians well into the 1990s despite numerous published studies that documented the safety and efficacy of opioids in the management of a variety of chronic nonmalignant pain states, such as neuropathic, myofascial, arthritic, and osteoporosis pain.[24] In 2002, the Federation of State Medical Boards of the United States published "Model Policy for the Use of Controlled Substances in the Treatment of Pain."[25] This authoritative publication clearly documents that opioids have a place in the management of many patients' chronic nonmalignant pain.

Many physicians are more willing to use opioids in patients with cancer pain than noncancer pain. The fact that opioids are seriously underused was underscored by a study of opioid prescribing for cancer pain patients that was published in the *Journal of the American Medical Association* in 1998.[26] Researchers evaluated the records of 13,625 cancer patients discharged from hospitals to Medicare or Medicaid certified nursing homes during the 4-year period 1992 to 1995 in five states. A total of 4003 patients reported and had multiple factors independently associated with daily pain. Only 26% of patients received morphine or another opioid considered to be on level 3 of the World Health Organization (WHO) analgesic ladder[27] (**Fig. 68-2**). Only 32% of patients received a step 2 analgesic, and 26% received only acetaminophen or a nonsteroidal anti-inflammatory drug (NSAID) for analgesia.

The WHO analgesic ladder that was developed to guide analgesic therapy for cancer patients in developing countries has been shown

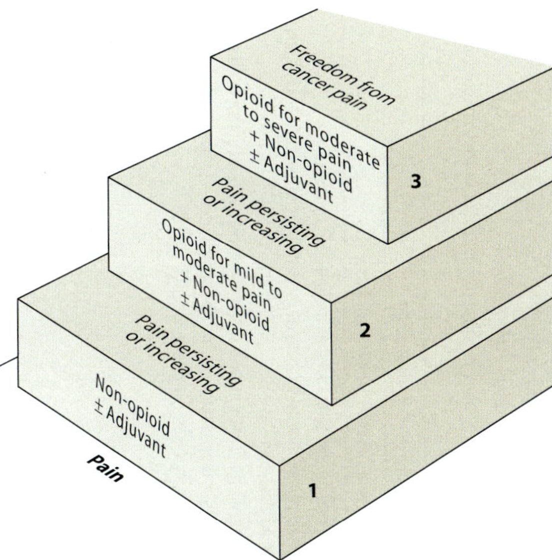

FIGURE 68-2. World Health Organization analgesic ladder: a progression of analgesics and doses to be used to manage pain of varying intensities.

to be applicable in most pain management in most societies. This approach describes three levels of analgesia. It suggests that pharmacologic management of mild to moderate pain should include a NSAID or acetaminophen unless there is a contraindication as a first step. When pain persists or increases, add an opioid as the second step. The third step consists of increasing the opioid dose to treat persistent moderate to severe pain. This is not a stepped approach in which prior steps must be tried before initiating more aggressive therapy. Analgesia should be started at the level appropriate for the patient's pain. For cancer pain, a fourth step including palliative radiation and chemotherapy, nerve blocks, and various other modalities exists in developed countries.

Equianalgesic dose tables often use parenteral morphine 10 mg every 4 hours as the standard for comparison. Equianalgesic doses are listed in **Table 68-2**. The dose tables will not apply to all patients because of interpatient variances in response to opioids. The tables do provide an approximation of equally effective doses, but patients must often be retitrated to response when the opioids they are taking are changed. It is important to differentiate among the pure μ-opioid receptor agonists, mixed agonist-antagonists (which are κ-opioid receptor agonists and either antagonistic or neutral at μ receptors), and partial agonists. There is no proven difference in analgesic activity among the pure μ agonists. Greater potency does not imply higher activity. Potency differences simply mean that different amounts of drug must be used to obtain the same activity. PK differences can be clinically important.

PHARMACOKINETICS

Pharmacokinetic parameters to consider include peak serum level (C_{max}), time to peak serum level (T_{max}), and elimination half-life ($T_{1/2}$). Oral-to-parenteral dose ratios also vary among opioids (**Table 68-3**). Also, differences in metabolism (biotransformation) may sometimes make one opioid preferable to another, especially in a patient with impaired metabolism or elimination. Opioids may be long acting due to inherent pharmacologic factors, for example, methadone, levorphanol, or a pharmaceutical formulation. Each type has advantages and disadvantages. The PKs of commonly used opioids have been well described at all phases of human life.[28-30]

CURRENTLY AVAILABLE OPIOIDS

Opioids can be administered by oral, intramuscular, intravenous, subcutaneous, rectal, sublingual, transdermal, transmucosal, epidural, and intrathecal routes. The intramuscular route is now discouraged because it is painful and the subcutaneous route provides similar PK. **Table 68-4** lists commercially available μ-agonist opioids. While several new dosage forms of previously available opioids were introduced in recent years, only one new opioid chemical entity per se has become available in the past quarter century. Tapentadol is a mixed μ agonist, norepinephrine reuptake inhibitor. Because these two mechanisms are synergistic, tapentadol can provide comparable analgesia to other potent opioids with less μ agonist activity, resulting in a fewer GI adverse effects. In some patients who experience GI intolerance to traditional opioids, this can be an advantage.[10]

The μ agonists can be divided into three categories based on their duration of action: short-acting, long-acting, and ultra–short-acting. Morphine and other opioids with short half-lives require frequent administration to maintain analgesia. Immediate-release morphine products provide about 4 hours of pain relief and need to be dosed every 4 to 6 hours to maintain analgesia. Pharmaceutical sustained-release formulations (e.g., MS Contin, Oramorph-SR, Kadian, Avinza, OxyContin, Opana ER, Nucynta ER orally; Duragesic transdermally),

TABLE 68-2 Dosing Comparison for Common Opioids

Drug	Approximate Equianalgesic Oral Dose (mg)	Approximate Equianalgesic IM Dose (mg)	Approximate Time to Onset PO-parenteral (minutes)		Dosing Interval (hours)
Morphine	30 Regular schedule 60 PRN dosing	10	20	15	4-6
Methadone	20	10	30	20	6-8
Levorphanol	4	2	30	20	6-8
Hydromorphone	4–6	1.5–2	20	15	4
Meperidine	150–250*	75–100	15	10	2.5-3.5
Codeine	130***	75	20	15	4-6
Buprenorphine	not available	0.3–0.4**	—	25	6-8
Butorphanol	not available	2**	—	20	3-4
Nalbuphine	not available	10**	—	20	3-6
Pentazocine	150**	60**	20	15	3-6
Oxycodone	10 mg is clinically equivalent to 10–20 mg of oral morphine. The maximum safe daily dose of oxycodone 5 mg/acetaminophen 325 mg is 12 tablets (~4 g of acetaminophen) due to potential for hepatotoxicity. Plain oxycodone can be titrated to higher doses much like morphine. OxyContin labeling recommends a dose ratio of oxycodone to morphine of 1:2. A ratio of 3:4 may be more accurate				
Fentanyl, transdermal	a 50 μg/hr patch provides similar analgesia to 10 mg of oral morphine on a regular q 4-hr schedule which is equal to 30 mg of sustained acting morphine administered q 12 hr. Patients with fever (e.g., tumor fever) may get only about 48 hr of analgesia from a patch; fever or exogenous heat, 9 (e.g., heat lamps, electric blankets) may accelerate drug release. The patch requires a mean of 17 hr to reach peak blood levels and effects remain for 12-24 hr after removing a patch. Therefore, patches cannot be used effectively to titrate doses.				

* Meperidine is not recommended for pain management >2 days due to adverse effects from metabolite.

* Agonist-antagonist analgesics are not recommended when pain may increase due to dose ceiling effect

** Codeine doses >65 mg are usually not appropriate due to diminishing incremental analgesia with increasing doses but continually increasing constipation side effect.

Published tables vary in suggested equianalgesic doses. Clinical response is the criterion that must be applied for each patient. There is not complete cross tolerance among these drugs; in patients whose pain is well controlled it is usually necessary to use 10%-20% less than equianalgesic doses when changing drugs and then retitrate to response. If pain is not well controlled, use equianalgesic or 10%-20% higher than equianalgesic doses of the new opioid drug and retitrate to response.

TABLE 68-3 Opioid Metabolites*

Parent Drug (% excreted unchanged)	Analgesic Duration (hours)	Metabolites (% if known)	Metabolite Half-lives (hours)	Metabolite Route Elimination	Comment
Morphine (~7.2% - IV) (~3.7% - PO)	4-6				Elimination of morphine is not affected by renal failure, however, volume of distribution may be smaller, resulting in increased plasma concentrations; enterohepatic circulation of morphine and glucuronides occurs
		Morphine-3-glucuronide (57-74)	2.8-4	Renal	Half-life is 41-141 hor in renal failure; 5-20 times more potent than morphine in causing hyperalgesia, EEG spiking, agitation, seizures in animals; possibly by a non-opioid receptor mechanism
		Morphine-6-glucuronide (4.7-12)	Duration of action 2 times longer than parent	Renal	Half-life is 89-136 hr in renal failure; may be responsible for narcosis in patients with renal failure; by IT administration is 100 times more potent than morphine; accumulates with chronic dosing
		Morphine-3-ethereal sulfate (5-10)			
		Normorphine (3.5)			May have toxic effects (myoclonus, allodynia)
		morphine-N-oxide			
Codeine 11.1%	4-6				
		Codeine-6-glucuronide			Primary elimination pathway; profound narcosis has occurred in chronic renal failure
		Norcodeine		Renal	Equipotent to codeine in analgesic activity
		Morphine (10)			May account for analgesic activity of codeine
Fentanyl (<10)	1-2				May be extensively liver metabolized
		Norfentanyl		Renal, hepatic	Metabolized to despropionyl fentanyl
					May cause neurotoxic adverse effects
					Structurally similar to normeperidine
		4-*N*-anilinopiperidine			
Hydromorphone (5.6%)					Clearance dependent on hepatic blood flow
		Hydromorphone-3-glucuronide			Shown to accumulate in renal failure in one patient
		Hydromorphone-6-glucuronide		Renal	Formed from intermediate metabolites, dihydroisomorphine and dihydromorphine
		Nor-metabolites			Significance not known
Levorphanol	6-8	Levorphanol glucuronide		Renal	Liver metabolized by glucuronide conjugation
Meperidine	2.5-3.5				Bioavailability increases from 50%- 80% in cirrhosis
5% (uncontrolled urine pH)					Half-life of meperidine and normeperidine prolonged in cirrhosis
					Urinary pH effects elimination of unchanged meperidine in urine 25% in acidic urine vs. 1%-2% in alkaline urine
		Normeperidine (5-30)	15-30	Renal, hepatic	Half-life prolonged significantly in renal failure (>30 hr); twice as potent in CNS stimulatory effects as meperidine; one-half the analgesic effect of meperidine; urinary excretion pH dependent: uncontrolled pH $f_e = 0.05$-0.06, acidic urine $f_e =$ 0.30, alkaline urine $f_e < 0.031$
		Meperidinic acid			Inactive metabolite

Methadone 21% (acidic urine increases the fraction of elimination [f_e])	4-6 initially;				In one anephric patient, 98% of methadone was found in feces as metabolite, suggesting a shift in metabolism from renal to fecal urinary excretion of methadone and metabolites is dose dependent and is the major route of elimination in doses >55 mg/d; 10%-45% of methadone is eliminated in feces as metabolites
	6-12 after steady state (1-2 d)				
		1,5-demethyl-2-ethyl-3,3-iphenyl-1-pyrroline		Renal, biliary	Unpredictable half-life with chronic dosing long-term analgesia is 10 times that of morphine; major metabolite $f_e = 0.30$
		2-ethyl-5-methyl-3,3-diphenyl-1-pyrroline		Renal, biliary	Minor metabolite
		Methadone-*N*-oxide			Minor metabolite
Oxycodone	3-6				Renally excreted, primarily as metabolites
		Noroxymorphone			
		Oxymorphone		Hepatic, renal	Active metabolite; renally excreted as oxymorphone-glucuronide
		Noroxycodone			
Propoxyphene 1.5%	4-6				May depress cardiac conduction secondary to anesthetic properties; half-life not altered in renal failure
		Norproproxyphene (25)	22.9-36.6	Renal	Local anesthetic properties; cardiac conduction abnormalities can result with accumulation (not reversed by naloxone); not hemodialyzable
Buprenorphine	6-8				One source says it is almost completely metabolized in the liver; another says the majority is excreted unchanged in feces Undergoes enterohepatic circulation with metabolites
		Glucuronidation products		Renal	
		Norbuprenorphine		Renal	May have weak analgesic properties. Primary route of elimination is renal; hepatic, biliary, and fecal routes also involved
Butorphanol 5%	3-4				Extensively liver metabolized; Cl_{Cr} <30 mL/min half-life increased from 5.75-10.5 hr in single-dose, intranasal administration
		Norbutorphanol		Biliary	No analgesic activity
		Hydroxybutorphanol		Renal	Analgesic activity; major metabolite; 60%-80% renally excreted
Nalbuphine	3-6				Hepatic metabolism; metabolites and parent compound excreted in urine and feces
7%					Major route of elimination is biliary secretion
Pentazocine 4.9%	3-6				(l) isomer responsible for analgesic activity; large interpatient variability in metabolism and oral bioavailability Bioavailability in cirrhotic patients increased to 60-70%
		Alcoholic and carboxylic acid metabolites		Renal	Inactive metabolites
		Pentazocine glucuronide		Renal	Inactive metabolite

*Developed in collaboration with the Drug Information Service, Department of Pharmacy Services, University Hospitals and Clinics, University of Utah Health Sciences Center.

Data from: References 76–79.

TABLE 68-4 Commercially Available Opioids

Generic (Proprietary) Name	Dosage Forms Available	Comments
μ Agonists		
Alfentanil (Alfenta)	Injectable: 500 μg/mL	
Codeine (others)	Injectable: 50 μg/mL	
Also available in combinations	Tablets: 15, 30, 60 mg	
Fentanyl (Sublimaze, Duragesic, Fentanyl Oralet, Actiq, others)	Injectable: 50 μg/mL Transdermal patch: 25, 50, 75, 100 μg/hr (Duragesic) Transmucosal: 100, 200, 300, 400 μg (Fentanyl Oralet) Transmucosal: 200, 400, 600, 800, 1200, 1600 μg (Actiq)	
Hydromorphone (Dilaudid, others)	Injectable: 1, 2, 3, 4, 10 mg/mL Tablets: 1, 2, 3, 4, 8 mg Oral liquid: 5 mg/5 mL Suppositories: 3 mg	
Levorphanol (Levo-Dromoran)	Injectable: 2 mg/mL Tablets: 2 mg	
Meperidine (Demerol, others)	Injectable: 10, 25, 50, 75, 100 mg/mL Tablets: 50, 100 mg Oral liquid: 50 mg/mL	Meperidine with Phenergan (Mepergan Fortis) Capsules: 50 mg with 25 mg promethazine
Methadone (Dolophine, others)	Injectable: 10 mg/mL Tablets: 5, 10 mg Dispersible tablets: 40 mg Oral liquid: 5 mg/5 mL, 10 mg/5 mL, 10 mg/10 mL Oral concentrate: 10 mg/mL	
Morphine (MSIR, MS Contin, Oramorph SR, Kadian, others)	Injectable: 0.5, 1, 2, 3, 4, 5, 8, 10, 15, 25, 50 mg/mL Tablets: 15, 30 mg Soluble tablets: 10, 15, 30 mg Controlled-release tablets: 15, 30, 60, 100, 200 mg (MS Contin) Oral liquid: 10 mg/5 mL, 10 mg/2.5 mL, 20 mg/5 mL, 20 mg/mL, 100 mg/5 mL Suppositories: 5, 10, 20, 30 mg	
Oxycodone (Roxicodone, OxyContin, others)	Tablets: 5 mg Controlled-release tablets: 10, 20, 40 mg (OxyContin) Oral liquid: 5 mg/5 mL Oral concentrate: 20 mg/mL	Available in combination with aspirin (Percodan) and acetaminophen (Percocet, Roxicet, others)
Oxymorphone (Numorphan)	Injectable: 1, 1.5 mg/mL Suppository: 5 mg	
Propoxyphene (Darvon, Darvon-N, others)	Tablets (as HCl): 32, 65 mg Tablets (as napsylate): 100 mg	Available in combination with acetaminophen (Darvocet N-100)
Sufentanil (Sufenta, others)	Injectable (as Citrate): 50 μg/mL	Solution contains no preservatives
Partial μ Agonist Buprenorphine (Buprenex)	Injectable: 0.3 mg/mL	
Mixed Agonist-Antagonists Butorphanol (Stadol, Stadol NS)	Injectable: 1, 2 mg/mL Nasal Spray: 10 mg/mL	
Dezocine (Dalgan)	Injectable: 5, 10, 15 mg/mL	
Nalbuphine (Nubain, various)	Injectable: 10, 20 mg/mL	
Pentazocine (Talwin NX, Talwin)	Injectable: 30 mg/mL Tablet: 50 mg (with 0.5 mg naloxone)	Also in combination with aspirin (Talwin Compound) and acetaminophen (Talacen)

require less frequent administration. Methadone is a pharmacologically long-acting opioid, allowing dosing every 8 hours for analgesia at a much lower cost than most pharmaceutically long-acting opioids. Because methadone has atypical PK, it should be used by physicians familiar with its pharmacology and in patients who are adherent to prescribed regimens. Deaths have resulted from overly rapid titration of methadone and possibly due to increased risk of central sleep apnea.

The fentanyl series is highly lipophilic, which allows these drugs to be used differently from the other μ agonists. Their rapid onset of action facilitates use as preoperative and intraoperative agents. High lipophilicity facilitates transdermal and subcutaneous administration. When administered through or under the skin, these medications deposit in subcutaneous fat. Medication is released from the fat slowly. Conversely, when these medications are administered transmucosally or sublingually, they are rapidly absorbed due to the lack of the buccal and sublingual fat. Rapid absorption following transmucosal and sublingual administration makes these drugs useful in managing breakthrough pain.

OPIOID DOSING

Although most μ-opioid agonists are similar pharmacodynamically, they differ in PK properties, which effects dosing. All except codeine normally provide the same level of analgesia when dosed appropriately on average. For several reasons, including genetic polymorphism, some patients respond better to some opioids than others. Clinical trial is the only way to determine a preferred alternative if a patient does not respond as expected to the initial choice. Pharmacokinetic properties and controlled-release formulations play major roles in the drugs' fate in the organism. As long as an opioid-responsive noxious nociceptive stimulus is present, these drugs should be used on a regular schedule or time-contingent basis. Undertreated acute pain predisposes to chronic pain syndromes.[31] Untreated or undertreated pain causes repeated stimulation of the CNS. Repeated stimulation of the afferent nociceptive neurons, producing the phenomenon known as physiologic windup, can sensitize these neurons and cells in the dorsal horn of the spinal cord, resulting in neuronal plasticity.[32] Such sensitization can induce neurologic changes that last long after the initial insult has healed. Neuronal plasticity, or changes in the CNS, may lead to hyperalgesia. Windup is the progressive increase in the frequency of elicited action potentials seen in neurons as a result of a slowly repeated stimulus of C fibers.[33] Long-term potentiation (LTP) is a high-frequency brief stimulus that increases the efficiency of synaptic transmission.[34] These processes lead to hyperalgesia as a consequence of central excitability. The use of around-the-clock opioids often breaks the cycle of pain and can decrease or eliminate the centrally mediated processes that complicate pain control. Thus, it may take less drug to prevent the recurrence of pain than would be required to treat recurring pain.

Morphine and other pure opioid agonists can provide analgesia in most acute and chronic malignant pain patients and many chronic nonmalignant pain patients. There is no *a priori* maximum dose for any pure μ agonists. Patients require individual titration of medication regimens. Morphine dose requirements for comfort following similar noxious stimuli may vary 50- to 100-fold among chronic malignant pain patients,[35] and 10- to 20-fold among acute pain patients.[36]

In addition to regularly scheduled opioid doses, supplemental doses should be available for management of breakthrough pain. Breakthrough pain can be defined as transitory increases in pain greater than moderate intensity, occurring in addition to baseline pain of moderate or less intensity.[37] Breakthrough pain regimens should be based on the background (time-contingent) dose, not on fixed doses. Sufficient rescue doses of the opioid should be available to the patient as immediate-release dosage forms to provide comfort when breakthrough pain occurs. Incidental pain often occurs predictably when a patient ambulates, gets tired, or undergoes medical procedures. In such cases, an additional dose of an oral, immediate-release dosage form should be administered to provide effective levels about one-half hour before the anticipated pain increase. For unpredictable breakthrough pain, a typical rescue dose is one-half of the every 4-hour scheduled dose (1/6 of the every 12-hour scheduled controlled-release dose) permitted every 2 hours as needed. When a patient with chronic pain requires more than two to three rescue doses for more than 2 to 3 days in succession, an increase in the time-contingent dose should be considered.

When increased doses are warranted, increase the dose as a percentage of the current regimen, not a set number of milligrams. Increases of 50% should be made as soon as steady-state serum levels are achieved (5 half-lives, which is equal to ~10 hr for morphine) after 5 days of scheduled opioid therapy. An increase from 30 mg every 4 hours to 45 mg every 4 hours would be appropriate. If the inadequate dose is 300 mg every 12 hours, the increase should be to 450 mg every 12 hours.

Physicians should carefully evaluate concerns of increased pain or diminished analgesic effect in patients whose analgesia was adequate before simply increasing the opioid dose. Clinical tolerance to opioid analgesia in itself is uncommon once comfort has been achieved and maintained for a few days. Ineffective analgesia often results from factors that increase pain or compromise analgesic efficacy. These include progressive disease, new disease, increased or excessive activity, poor adherence, changed medication formulation or brand, drug interactions, and opioid addiction or diversion.

Methadone affords analgesia for 8 hours once steady-state serum levels are achieved. Less frequent dosing protects against opioid withdrawal but does not provide ongoing analgesia. While low methadone serum levels can protect from withdrawal for 24 hours or more following a single dose, the levels are too low after 8 hours to provide analgesia. Because of the long and variable half-life of methadone, physicians should exercise caution. Patients may achieve adequate analgesia initially, but with continued use they may become toxic due to accumulation of methadone and its metabolites (**Fig. 68-3**). Methadone is not recommended in acute pain due to its extended half-life.

ROUTES OF ADMINISTRATION

Most currently available μ agonists can be given orally, rectally, parenterally, transdermally, and transmucosally. The mixed agonist-antagonists are available in parenteral dosage forms. Pentazocine also is available in an oral tablet, and butorphanol in a nasal spray. For most patients taking time-contingent opioids, oral dosage forms are preferred agents. The oral route is easy to use, is relatively inexpensive, does not signal increasing disease to the patient or family, and is effective. Incomplete bioavailability is easily overcome by increasing the dose. The only advantage of parenteral over oral administration for a patient able to take a drug orally is more rapid onset. The time difference to analgesic onset and peak levels between oral administration and intramuscular or subcutaneous injections is often negligible. With appropriate scheduling, each dose of opioid can be administered sufficiently in advance of the prior dose to prevent recurrence of pain.

Rectal administration is an option for patients unable to tolerate oral drugs, especially in short-term and terminal care. Hydromorphone, morphine, and oxymorphone are commercially available in rectal suppositories. Controlled-release oral morphine tablets have been used effectively via the rectal route[38] (**Table 68-5**). Mucosal irritation may occur in fewer patients with rectally administered oral controlled-release morphine tablets than with commercial morphine suppositories.[39] No local adverse effects were noted in a report of controlled-release oral morphine administered rectally.[40] Suppositories and tablets should be inserted just above the anal sphincter to minimize first-pass metabolism. The inferior and middle rectal veins do not drain into the portal circulation as do the superior rectal veins. Administration higher into the rectal vault could induce a partial first-pass effect, which would lessen the effectiveness of the dose. As with any rectal administration, patients receiving opioids by this route should lie quietly on their sides for about 15 minutes after administration to aid absorption and minimize risk of rectal expulsion of the dose. Rectal administration of oral liquids may be an option in some patients limited by acceptable rectal fluid volumes and esthetics.

An effective and noninvasive route for opioid administration is transdermal. Fentanyl and butorphanol are available for transdermal administration. Transdermal fentanyl patches are indicated for management of chronic pain in patients tolerant to the respiratory depressant effects of opioids. They provide 72 hours of clinically effective CNS opioid levels in most cases, but some patients obtain only about 48 hours of relief from a patch. Although the patches are more expensive than oral dosage forms, they are a convenient and cost-effective alternative to parenteral opioids. Transdermal fentanyl can be used by patients unable or unwilling to use oral or rectal opioids. The patch can also be useful for patients with noncompliant behaviors, for example, patients who cannot remember to take their opioid. As mentioned previously, this dosage form can be problematic in patients who require rapid-dose titration or have rapidly changing analgesic requirements.[41,42] Transdermal buprenorphine patches available in 5, 10, and 20 μg/hr strengths provide up to 7 days of continuous analgesia.[43]

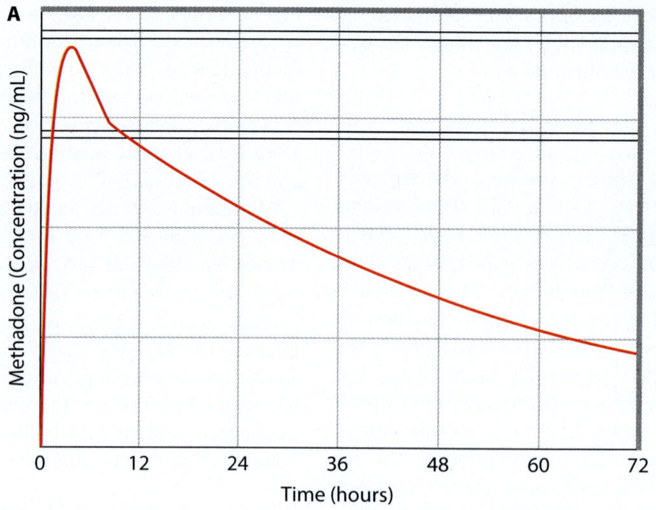

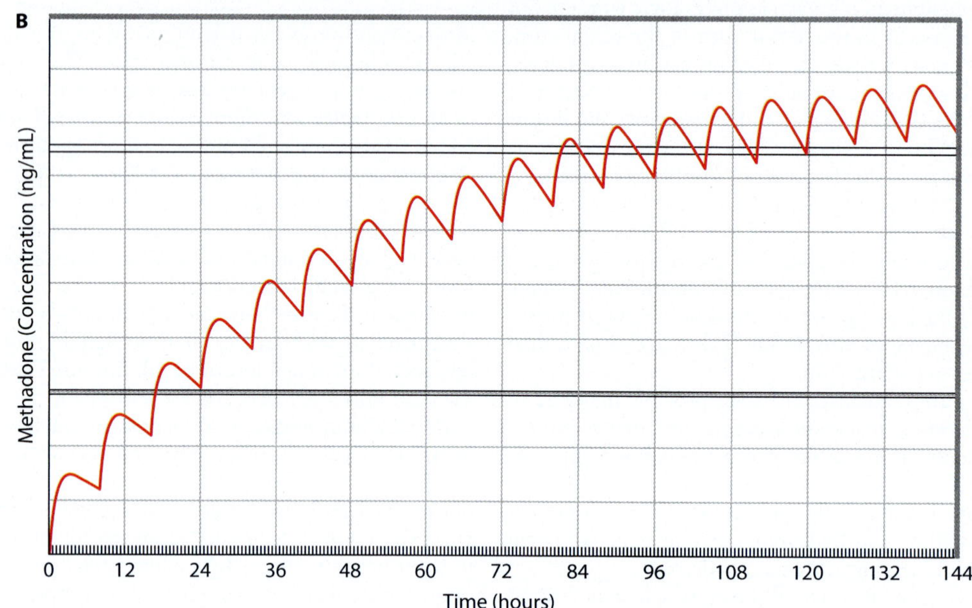

FIGURE 68-3. Methadone dose-response curve (**A**) and accumulation risk (**B**). Computer simulation of methadone dose response for a single dose at steady state and multiple doses administered at 12-hour intervals. The therapeutic window (effective analgesic concentration) is indicated by the double solid lines. (**A**) The dose response curve for a single dose of methadone after steady-state serum levels are achieved. Analgesic concentrations are seen in the alpha elimination phase. Long-lasting subanalgesic levels are seen in the beta elimination phase. (**B**) Accumulation of the beta elimination contribution to the total serum level may produce toxic serum levels after several days of therapy.

The subcutaneous route is an easy and inexpensive way to administer opioids. It is common in palliative care, where it provides a good alternative to the intravenous route. Intravenous opioid administration is especially useful following surgery and trauma. Intravenous patient-controlled analgesia (PCA) is routinely used in many acute settings, especially for postoperative analgesia. While intravenous opioids are warranted when GI function is limited (e.g., postoperative ileus), the intravenous route can negatively reinforce the sick role in patients with chronic pain and those requiring end-of-life care. The major advantage of intravenous PCA over regularly scheduled injections is the sense of control PCA provides to the patient. PCA offers no pharmacologic advantage over regularly scheduled oral opioids for patients able to tolerate oral medications.[44]

Spinal administration of opioids is warranted in a small number of patients. It avoids the toxicity associated with the systemic delivery of these medications. The epidural and intrathecal routes each have advantages and disadvantages. Epidural administration allows opioid placement at any dermatomal level and does not require puncturing of the dura. Larger doses, however, are required and systemic effects may occur with epidural administration, increasing the risk of adverse effects. For morphine, intrathecal doses are only one-tenth of those needed for an equianalgesic epidural dose. Intrathecal administration requires puncturing of the dura and placing the drug closer to the spinal cord receptors. Drawbacks to intrathecal use include increased potential for meningitis and risk of postdural puncture headaches. Dose-related problems associated with spinal analgesia include pruritus, urinary retention, and delayed respiratory depression. Spinal analgesia is discussed in depth in Chapter 81.

Sublingual opioid administration has been used extensively in palliative care. Advantages include ease of administration, low expense (with oral, not parenteral, solutions), avoidance of hepatic first pass, and rapid onset of action (~5-15 min). Disadvantages include relatively low bioavailability, potential for poor taste acceptance, and the need to avoid drinking anything for about 15 minutes following administration. Simple aqueous solutions are most appropriate for this route. The volume of a dose should not exceed 1 mL to minimize medication trickling down the throat. If a larger amount of medication is needed than will readily dissolve in 1 mL of water, a second dose can be given after 5 to 10 minutes. In a study of the percentage of sublingual opioid absorbed after 1 mL of

TABLE 68-5 Rectal Opioid Times to Peak and Duration of Action

Morphine immediate-release oral tablets	
Peak	1.1 hr
Duration	<6 hr
Morphine controlled-release oral tablets	
Peak	5.4 hr
Duration	8-12 hrs
Morphine oral solution	
Peak	0.5 hr
Duration	4-6 hr
Morphine rectal suppositories	
Peak	1.1 hr
Duration	<6 hr
Hydromorphone rectal suppositories	
Peak	1 hr
Duration	4-6 hr
Methadone oral tablets	
Peak	not known
Duration	6-8 hr
Oxycodone oral tablets and solution	
Peak	3.1 hr
Duration	8-12 hr

Adapted from Warren D. Practical use of rectal medications in palliative care. *J Pain Symptom Manage.* 1996;11:378.

an aqueous solution was held in the mouth for 10 minutes at pH 6.5, absorption was greater for lipophilic than hydrophilic opioids. Results from that study are listed in **Table 68-6**. As the mouth pH increased, absorption increased. Opioids often taste bitter, but many patients find overly sweet solutions even less palatable. Mild citrus or bland flavors are usually most acceptable. Changes in the oral mucosa, stomatitis, increased keratinization, decreased salivary flow, and changes in salivary pH due to disease, trauma, radiation or chemotherapy, as well as the overall condition of the mouth, influence absorption from sublingual, buccal, and oral transmucosal administration.

Nebulization into the lungs and intravaginal use of oral tablets and rectal suppositories have been reported. Nebulized morphine can be useful in dyspnea (air hunger), especially in terminally ill patients.[45] However, systemic opioids may be required to effectively treat cough.[46] Because of the unpredictable bioavailability resulting from vaginal delivery, this route is not recommended.[47] Intrastromal administrations have been used with reported success by some hospice programs. Drug level data from this route have not been reported.

DRUG INTERACTIONS

Opioids interact with a variety of medications (**Table 68-7**). Most opioid drug interactions are a consequence of additive effects, that is, pharmacodynamic interactions. Increased sedation can be seen when

TABLE 68-6 Sublingual Opioid Bioavailability

Drug	% Absorbed
Morphine	22
Methadone	34
Fentanyl	51
Buprenorphine	55

1 mL sublingual; held for 10 minutes at pH 6.5.

Adapted from Weinberg D, Inturrisi C, Reidenberg B, et al. Sublingual absorption of selected opioid analgesics. *Clin Pharmacol Ther.* 1988;44:335.

TABLE 68-7 Clinically Important Opioid Drug Interactions

Opioid(s)	Interacting drug(s)	Description
Codeine	Quinidine	Inhibition of conversion to morphine; decreased analgesia
Meperidine	Monoamine oxidase inhibitors (e.g., phenelzine, tranylcypromine)	Excitatory response (including seizures, arrhythmias, hyperpyrexia, and coma); potentially fatal interaction
Meperidine	Sibutramine	May induce serotonin syndrome
Meperidine	SSRIs	No evidence, but potential for serotonin syndrome should be considered
Meperidine, morphine	Cimetidine	Inhibition of opioid metabolism; Increased opioid effects
Methadone	Carbamazepine Erythromycin Phenytoin	Increased opioid metabolism; may induce withdrawal
Methadone, morphine	Desipramine	Inhibition of desipramine metabolism; toxicity possible
Opioids, (controlled-release) (e.g., MS Contin, Oramorph SR, OxyContin)	Metoclopramide	Earlier peak plasma concentration; increased sedation
Opioids (class)	Antihistamines (e.g., hydroxyzine, diphenhydramine)	Increased sedation
Opioids (class)	Butyrophenones (e.g., haloperidol)	Increased sedation
Opioids (class)	Tricyclic antidepressants (e.g., amitriptyline, desipramine doxepin, nortriptyline)	Increased sedation and potentiation of opioid Induced respiratory depression
Propoxyphene	Carbamazepine	Increased carbamazepine levels, potential for toxicity
Propoxyphene	Doxepin	Increased doxepin levels, potential for toxicity
Propoxyphene	Metoprolol, propranolol	Increased plasma levels of these β blockers

Data from: Maurer P, Bartkowski R. Drug interactions of clinical significance with opioid analgesics. *Drug Safety.* 1993;8:30; Quinn D, Day R. Drug interactions of clinical importance. An updated guide. *Drug Safety.* 1995;12:393; Hansten PD, Horn JR. *Drug Interactions Analysis and Management.* Vancouver, Wash: Applied Therapeutics, Inc.

opioids are administered with alcohol, benzodiazepines, butyrophenones, phenothiazines, sedative hypnotics, and tricyclic antidepressants. Midazolam may decrease the effect of fentanyl. Antinociceptive activity may be impaired by benzodiazepine administration from inhibition of the descending inhibitory control pathways.[48]

Methadone withdrawal has been precipitated by a number of agents known to induce hepatic microsomal enzymes.[49] This PK interaction increases methadone metabolism. Opioids can inhibit metabolism of other agents, leading to increases in serum levels of affected drugs. Desipramine plasma levels may be increased by coadministration with methadone or morphine.[49]

PRINCIPLES OF OPIOID USE

A World Health Organization (WHO) Expert Committee defined five principles of opioid use in 1986 to manage cancer pain in developing countries. Those principles have been validated numerous times in undeveloped, developing, and developed countries, including the United States.[50-58] Federal clinical practice guidelines published by the U.S. Department of Health and Human Services in the 1992[59] and for cancer pain by the government in 1994[60] and by the American Pain Society in 2005[61] validated these principles in both acute pain and chronic cancer pain. These principles may be summarized as:

1. Use oral or other noninvasive routes whenever possible.
2. Individualize doses by titrating to response.
3. Select analgesics according to needs as described on the analgesic ladder.
4. Maintain effective drug levels in the body as long as there is a noxious stimulus.
5. Use indicated adjuvants.

The usefulness of this approach has been studied in over 2100 cancer patients treated over a period of 10 years for a total of 140,478 treatment days. Drugs on step 1 of the WHO analgesic ladder provided adequate analgesia for only 11% of the days, step 2 for 31% of the days, and step 3 for 49% of the treatment days. Fifty-six percent of the patients received morphine. Co-analgesics, including antidepressants, anticonvulsants, and corticosteroids, were used on 37% of the treatment days and drugs for other symptoms, such as laxatives, were used on 79% of the treatment days. In their final days of life, 84% of the patients rated their pain as moderate or less.[57]

A 1998 study of over 4000 cancer patients with documented daily pain who were residents in over 1400 nursing homes in five Midwestern American states revealed serious underuse of opioids in managing pain. Sixteen percent received only acetaminophen or an NSAID, 32% received WHO analgesic ladder step 2 drug therapy, and only 26% received morphine. Fully 26% of these patients received no analgesia.[26] Although the WHO and AHCPR guidelines on use of opioids have been available for so long, it is difficult to understand how such inadequate use of these drugs continues.

MYTHS AND MISCONCEPTIONS

Many health care professionals subscribe to false beliefs about opioids. Unnecessary fears of addiction, dependence, tolerance, and toxicity often deter prescribing and taking of these important medications.

ADDICTION AND DEPENDENCE

Until recently, much of what was known about opioid addiction was based on the experience of drug abusers, not patients. Opioids more commonly cause dysphoria than euphoria among opioid-naive individuals. Patients in pain seek comfort, not a drug-induced high. Patients with a recent (not necessarily remote) history of substance abuse and certain psychiatric disorders, notably bipolar disease and personality disorders, may be at greater risk of drug misuse. Studies of the incidence of iatrogenic opioid addiction show that this phenomenon is uncommon. The Boston Collaborative Drug Surveillance Program study reported only four cases of iatrogenic addiction among 11,882 patients without prior history of substance abuse who received opioids for a broad range of indications and were followed for up to 2 years.[62] A national survey of over 10,000 burn patients without prior histories of drug abuse who received opioids for extended periods revealed no cases of addiction.[63] Only 3 of 2369 chronic headache patients, most of whom had access to opioids, abused the analgesics.[64] Although the studies were retrospective and may have underestimated the true prevalence of iatrogenic addiction, they certainly support the contention that this phenomenon is far less common than many physicians believe.

Addiction was defined by an international panel in 1988 as the compulsive use of a substance resulting in physical, psychological, or social harm and continued use despite that harm.[65] More recently, addiction was defined by a consensus committee of the American Pain Society, the American Academy of Pain Medicine, and the American Society of Addiction Medicine as a primary, chronic, neurobiologic disease with genetic, psychosocial, and environmental factors influencing its development and manifestations that is characterized by behaviors that include one or more of the following: impaired control over drug use, compulsive use, continued use despite harm, and craving.[66] Drug-seeking behavior does not in itself indicate addiction.

Pseudo-addiction has been defined as drug-seeking behavior due to inadequate analgesia, not substance abuse.[67] The American Society of Addiction Medicine said in its April 1997 Public Policy Statement that "Individuals who have severe, unrelieved pain may become intensely focused on finding relief for their pain. Sometimes, such patients may appear to observers to be preoccupied with obtaining opioids, but the preoccupation is with finding relief of pain, rather than using opioids, per se. This phenomenon has been termed pseudoaddiction."[68]

Dependence is defined as a physiologic phenomenon characterized by an abstinence syndrome upon abrupt discontinuation, substantial dose reduction, or administration of an antagonist.[65,66] Dependence occurs predictably among patients who take opioids on a regular basis for more than a few days. It also occurs predictably among patients taking steroids and many other common drugs. Opioid dependence can usually be ended by tapering the dose over 5 to 10 days when the drug is no longer needed. It should not be a barrier to use of the drugs when they are indicated. Neither dependence nor tolerance is indicative of or a predisposing factor to addiction.

TOLERANCE

Tolerance to opioids is widely misunderstood. Three distinct types of tolerance occur with opioids. Tolerance to the respiratory depressive effects and other manifestations of CNS depression normally occurs within 5 to 7 days of continuous, regularly scheduled opioid use. Such patients are referred to as *opioid-tolerant*. Tolerance to the constipating effects of opioids does not occur. Activated μ-opioid receptors in the colon inhibit peristalsis. Stimulating laxatives, (e.g., senna, bisacodyl) are needed to induce colonic emptying. Stool softeners alone are not effective. Because of the risk of severe constipation and fecal impaction, prophylaxis with stimulating laxatives may be indicated when opioid therapy is started.[69] However, about one-half of patients with severe opioid-induced constipation do not respond adequately to stimulating laxatives with increased water and fiber intake.[70] The peripherally acting μ opioid antagonist methylnaltrexone is now available to manage the potentially severe adverse effect of opioid pharmacotherapy.[71]

It often is necessary to increase the opioid dose over the first few days or week of therapy while finding the effective dose. Tolerance to analgesia does not occur in most patients once the effective dose of opioid is identified and administered regularly. Neither up nor down regulation of opioid receptors occurs with regularly scheduled dosing. Most patients remain comfortable on a consistent opioid dose unless another variable occurs. When an otherwise stable opioid dose ceases to be effective, pseudotolerance due to increasing or new pathology, excessive physical activity after the pain decreases, drug interactions, noncompliance, or other nonpharmacologic factors should be considered.[72]

MULTIPLE PAIN COMPLAINTS

Many physicians conclude that patients are opioid abusers when the patients have complaint of new pain after their initial pain is controlled. In a study of 955 advanced cancer patients, 34% experienced two or more different types of pain, and 80% reported pain resulting from two or more different causes.[73] Similar findings have been reported for AIDS patients.[69] More severe pain tends to mask less intense pain. When the former is effectively treated, masked pain that requires additional treatment often becomes evident.

SAVE OPIOIDS UNTIL THEY ARE REALLY NEEDED

A common belief of patients is that use of opioids relatively early in the course of a progressive disease will render them less useful later, when they may be needed more. That is not true. Pure μ opioids are effective over a broad clinical dosage range (**Fig. 68-4**). When pain increases, doses can be increased without loss of effectiveness.

OPIOIDS ARE EFFECTIVE FOR ALL TYPES OF PAIN

Opioids are effective analgesics for most nociceptive and much neuropathic pain. However, all pain is not opioid-responsive. Some pain that is opioid-responsive should not be managed with opioids, for example, constipation pain. The underlying cause of the pain should be treated before considering the sole use of opioids to control it. Examples of this

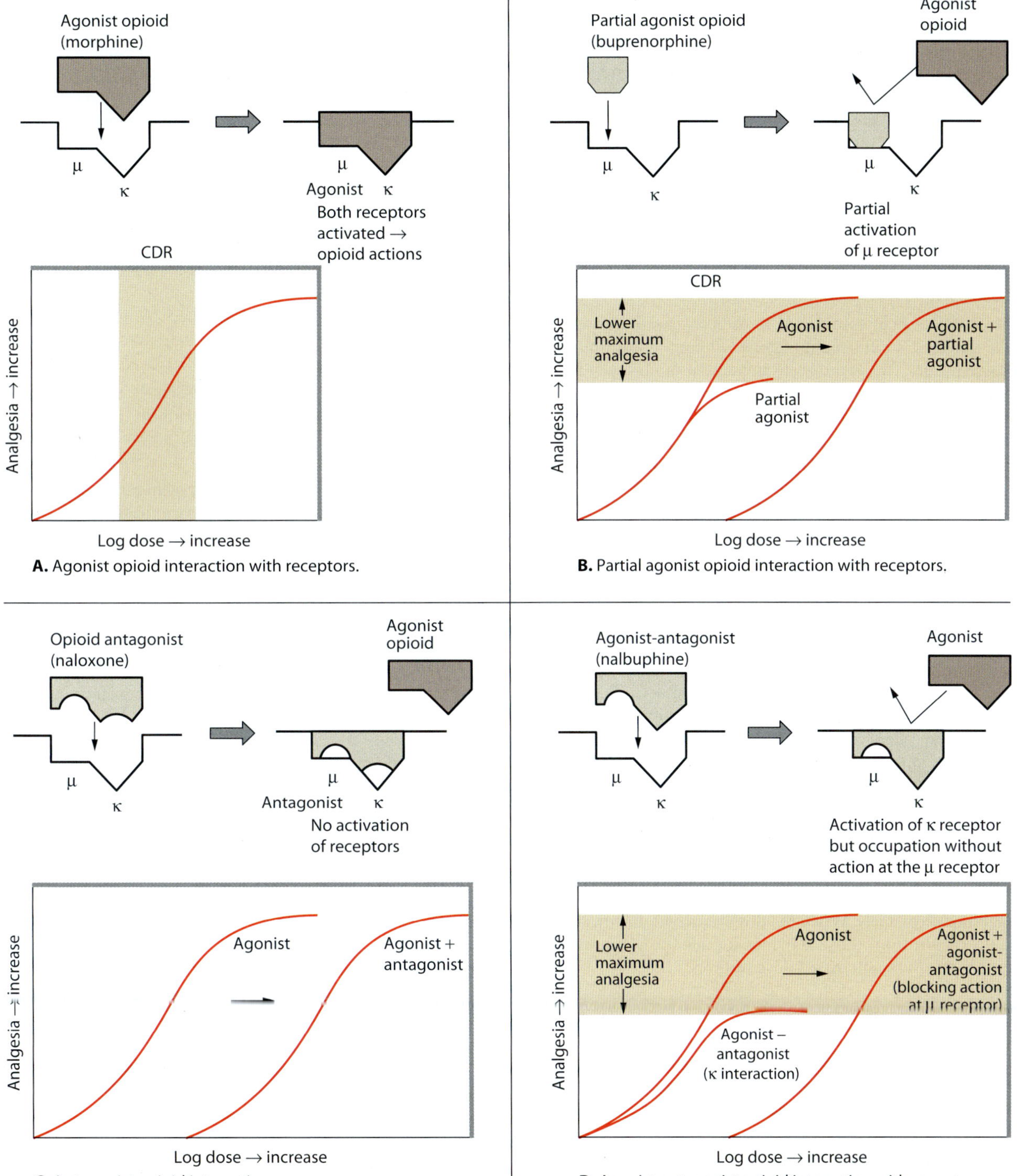

FIGURE 68-4. Receptor interactions of opioids. The various opioid-receptor interactions are illustrated, both in terms of a key-lock diagram with two receptor sites, mu (μ) and kappa (κ), and a representative dose-response (DR) curve of analgesic effects. (**A**) The agonist opioid such as morphine may stimulate both the μ and κ receptors. The steep portion of the DR curve is in the clinical dose range (CDR) = unlimited analgesia. (**B**) Partial agonists such as buprenorphine combine with the μ receptor, but they have only limited activity. The DR curve is flatter, with a lower maximum effect. The partial agonist will shift the DR curve for an agonist to the right. (**C**) The opioid antagonist naloxone can occupy both μ and κ receptors, but it has no intrinsic activity. The antagonist will shift the DR curve for an agonist to the right. (**D**) The agonist-antagonist opioids, e.g., nalbuphine, may have mixed effects at the μ and κ receptor. Analgesia occurs because of interaction with κ receptor while blockade with no activity occurs at the μ receptor. This naloxone-like effect would shift the DR curve for a μ-agonist to the right. (Adapted with permission.[20])

include neuropathic pain, for which tricyclic antidepressants, anticonvulsants, and nerve blocks may be indicated; painful infectious cysts, for which incision and drainage followed by anti-infectives may be indicated; and GI spasm, for which anticholinergic agents may be most effective.[74]

PARENTERAL OPIOIDS ARE MORE POTENT AND EFFECTIVE THAN ORAL DOSES

Many patients believe that parenteral opioids are more effective than analgesics administered by oral or other noninvasive routes. As discussed earlier, this is not true. Furthermore, use of parenteral routes signals advancing disease to many patients and may be psychologically disadvantageous. Potency is commonly misunderstood. Potency indicates only the amount of drug needed for effect. For example, 10 mg of oral morphine is approximately equal to 1.5 to 2 mg of oral hydromorphone. Hydromorphone is therefore about five times more potent, but no more effective, than morphine. When patients ask for more potent drugs, they usually mean more effective drugs.

DOSE INCREMENTS SHOULD BE CONSERVATIVE

Fear of opioids causes many physicians to use conservative dose increments. This can lead to treatment failure. Opioid doses should be increased to response. The appropriate increment is normally 50% of the dose, and this can be increased every five half-lives (twice a day for morphine). This percentage of increase applies no matter what the prior dose. When a patient knows that the opioid dose has been increased but adequate analgesia does not result, anxiety often increases. This increases the pain perception, which in turn increases the opioid dose requirement further. It is often better to err slightly in the direction of too much than too little opioid. Initial sedation may be advantageous when a patient is very anxious and experiencing a sleep deficit from the pain.

OPIOIDS PREVENT SAFE DRIVING DUE TO IMPAIRED JUDGMENT AND PSYCHOMOTOR FUNCTION

Opioids can markedly impair judgment and psychomotor function when therapy is initiated. Similar adverse effects can occur when doses are increased. But once a patient has been continuously receiving opioids on a regular schedule for about a week, these effects usually diminish markedly. There was no significant difference in the number of motor vehicle crashes that involved 24 drivers who were taking opioids on a regular schedule for long-term pain management than among the general population of Finland.[75] A systematic review of the world literature confirmed this finding.[76] If the patient is experiencing no observable opioid-induced impairment and the opioid dose has been consistent for a week or more, the patient can usually drive or carry out other normal functions safely. When the dose is increased, however, the patient should refrain from those activities for about a week and until any impairment due to the increased dose resolves.

CONCLUSION

Opioids are important and commonly underused analgesics. However, there is real concern about misuse and overuse of prescribed opioids as well. Health care professionals, patients, and care givers often harbor irrational fears about these drugs. Opiophobia has been defined as "irrational and undocumented fear that appropriate use of opioids causes addiction." As a result, opioids are often underprescribed, underdosed, taken irregularly in spite of instructions to the contrary, and stopped abruptly. Inappropriate beliefs about opioids have been documented among physicians,[77] nurses,[78] and pharmacists.[79] Societal barriers to the use of opioids are now being refuted by professional organizations and regulatory agencies. Concurrently, concerns about opioid misuse, overuse, and diversion are increasing. Physicians must use opioids with caution, but should not hesitate to use these important medications when they are clinically indicated. It is tragic that many physicians avoid opioids in their practices due to concerns about regulatory oversight; this works to the detriment of their patients. Unlike nonsteroidal anti-inflammatory drugs and even acetaminophen, long-term opioid use rarely causes end-organ toxicity.

Opioids delivery systems including oral controlled-release, iontophoretic, implanted, transdermal, and transmucosal dosage forms are currently under development. Combination dosage forms of opioids with other drugs also are being investigated. Some of these new forms may make opioid analgesia easier. However, excellent analgesia can be provided with the drugs and dosage forms currently available. Pain physicians can and should work to overcome opioid myths and misconceptions and should encourage appropriate use of opioids when they are indicated.

REFERENCES

1. Inturrisi CE. Clinical pharmacology of opioids for pain. *Clin J Pain*. 2000;12:S3-S13.
2. Diatchenko L, Robinson JE, Maixner W. Elucidation of mu-opioid gene structure: how genetics can help predict responses to opioids. *Eur J Pain Suppl*. Nov 11, 2011;5(2):433-438.
3. The Interagency Committee on New Therapies for Pain and Discomfort: Report to the White House. US Department of Health Education and Welfare, Public Health Service, National Institutes of Health, May 1979.
4. Pinkert T. Report from the Interagency Committee on Pain and Analgesia: a Public Health Service initiative. *J Pain Symptom Manage*. 1986;1:174.
5. Paulozzi LJ, Kilbourne EM, Shah NG, et al. A history of being prescribed controlled substances and risk of drug overdose death. *Pain Med*. Jan 2012;13(1):87-95.
6. Ferrante F. Principles of opioid pharmacotherapy: practical implications of basic mechanisms. *J Pain Symptom Manage*. 1996;11:265.
7. Yaksh T. Pharmacology and mechanisms of opioid analgesic activity. *Acta Anaesthesiol Scand*. 1997;41:94.
8. Pasternak GW. Pharmacological mechanisms of opioid analgesics. *Clin Neuropharmacol*. Feb 1993;16(1):1-18.
9. Farley P. Should topical opioid analgesics be regarded as effective and safe when applied to chronic cutaneous lesions? *J Pharm Pharmacol*. Jun 2011;63(6):747-756.
10. Arendt-Nielsen L, Olesen AE, Staahl C, et al. Analgesic efficacy of peripheral kappa-opioid receptor agonist CR665 compared to oxycodone in a multi-modal, multi-tissue experimental human pain model: selective effect on visceral pain. *Anesthesiology*. Sep 2009;111(3):616-624.
11. Lotsch J, Geisslinger G. Current evidence for a genetic modulation of the response to analgesics. *Pain*. 2006;121:1-5.
12. Angst MS, Clark JD. Opioid-induced hyperalgesia: a qualitative systematic review. *Anesthesiology*. 2006;104:570-587.
13. Nestler EJ. Molecular mechanisms of drug addiction. *Neuropharmacology*. 2004:47(suppl 1):24-32.
14. Terman GW, Bonica JJ. Spinal mechanisms and their modulation. In: Loeser JD. Butler SH, Chapman CR, Turk DC, eds. *Bonica's Management of Pain*. 3rd ed. Philadelphia: Lippincott Williams and Wilkins; 2001:73-152.
15. Kornetsky C, Porrino LJ. Brain mechanisms of drug-induced reinforcement. *Res Publ Assoc Res Nerv Ment Dis*. 1992;70:59-77.

16. Walker JM, Farney RJ, Rhondeau SM, et al. Chronic opioid use is a risk factor for the development of central sleep apnea and ataxic breathing. *J Clin Sleep Med.* 2007;3(5):455-461.

17. Webster LR, Choi Y, Desai II, et al. Sleep-disordered breathing and chronic opioid therapy. *Pain Med.* 2008;9(4):425-432.

18. McCann S, Yaksh TL, von Gunten CF. Correlation between myoclonus and the 3-glucuronide metabolites in patients treated with morphine or hydromorphone: a pilot study. *J Opioid Manag.* Mar-Apr 2010;6(2):87-94.

19. Lipman AG. Opioid overdose deaths: reactions and overreactions. *J Pain Palliat Care Pharmacother.* 2012;26(1).

20. Morgan J. American opiophobia: customary underutilization of opioid analgesics. *Adv Alcohol Subst Abuse.* 1985;5:163.

21. Chapman CR, Lipschitz DL, Angst MS, et al. Opioid pharmacotherapy for chronic non-cancer pain in the United States: a research guideline for developing an evidence-base. *J Pain.* Sep 2010;11(9):807-829.

22. Chou R, Fanciullo GJ, Fine PG, Miaskowski C, Passik SD, Portenoy RK. Opioids for chronic noncancer pain: prediction and identification of aberrant drug-related behaviors: a review of the evidence for an American Pain Society and American Academy of Pain Medicine clinical practice guideline. *J Pain.* Feb 2009;10(2):131-146.

23. Rolfs RT, Johnson E, Williams NJ, Sundwall DN. Utah clinical guidelines on prescribing opioids for treatment of pain. *J Pain Palliat Care Pharmacother.* Sep 2010;24(3):219-135.

24. Portenoy RK. Opioid therapy for chronic nonmalignant pain: a review of the critical issues. *J Pain Symptom Manage.* 1996;11:203.

25. The Federation of State Medical Boards of the United States. Model Policy for the Use of Controlled Substances for the Treatment of Pain, 2002.

26. Bernabei R, Gambassi G, Lapane K, et al. Management of pain in elderly patients with cancer. *JAMA.* 1998;279:1877.

27. World Health Organization. *Cancer Pain Relief and Palliative Care: Report of a WHO Expert Committee.* Technical Report Series 804. Geneva, Switzerland: World Health Organization, 1990.

28. Lugo RA, Satterfield KL, Kern SE. Pharmacokinetics of methadone. *J Pain Palliat Care Pharmacother.* 2005;19(4):13-24.

29. Lugo RA, Kern SE. The pharmacokinetics of oxycodone. *J Pain Palliat Care Pharmacother.* 2004;18(4):17-30.

30. Lugo RA, Kern SE. Clinical pharmacokinetics of morphine. *J Pain Palliat Care Pharmacother.* 2002;16(4):5-18.

31. Kehlet H, Jensen TS, Woolf CJ. Persistent postsurgical pain: risk factors and prevention. *Lancet.* May 13, 2006;367(9522):1618-1625.

32. Coderre T, Katz J, Vaccarino A, Melzack R. Contribution of central neuroplasticity to pathological pain: review of clinical and experimental evidence. *Pain.* 1993;52:259

33. Woolf C. Windup and central stimulation are not equivalent. *Pain.* 1996;66:105.

34. Pockett S. Spinal cord synaptic plasticity and chronic pain. *Anesth Analg.* 1994;80:173.

35. Twycross R. Morphine and diamorphine in the terminally ill patient. *Acta Anaesth Scand.* 1984;74:128.

36. Hill HF, Mather LE. Patient-controlled analgesia. Pharmacokinetic and therapeutic considerations. *Clin Pharmacokinet.* Feb 1993; 24(2):124-140.

37. Portenoy R, Hagen N. Breakthrough pain: definition, prevalence and characteristics. *Pain.* 1990;41:273.

38. Warren D. Practical use of rectal medications in palliative care. *J Pain Symptom Manage.* 1996;11:378.

39. Kaiko R, Fitzmartin R, Thomas G, Goldenheim P. The bioavailability of morphine in controlled-release 30-mg tablets per rectum compared with immediate-release 30-mg rectal suppositories and controlled-release 30-mg oral tablets. *Pharmacotherapy.* 1992; 12:107.

40. Maloney C, Kesner R, Klein G, et al. The rectal administration of MS Contin: clinical implications of use in end stage cancer. *Am J Hospice Care.* 1989;6:34.

41. Lipman AG, Ashburn MA. Titration with TTS fentanyl systems for previously uncontrolled cancer pain: in response. *Anesth Analg.* 1994;79:613.

42. Ashburn MA, Lipman AG. Management of pain in the cancer patient. *Anesth Analg.* 1993;76:402.

43. Plosker GL. Buprenorphine 5, 10 and 20 μg/h transdermal patch: a review of its use in the management of chronic non-malignant pain. *Drugs.* Dec 24, 2011;71(18):2491-509.

44. Kleiman R, Lipman AG, Hare B, MacDonald S. A comparison of morphine administered by patient-controlled analgesia and regularly scheduled intramuscular injection in severe postoperative pain. *J Pain Symptom Manage.* 1988;3:15.

45. Weinberg D, Inturrisi C, Reidenberg B, et al. Sublingual absorption of selected opioid analgesics. *Clin Pharmacol Ther.* 1988;44:335.

46. Stein W, Min Y. Nebulized morphine for paroxysmal cough and dyspnea in a nursing home resident with metastatic cancer. *Am J Hosp Palliat Care.* 1997;14:52.

47. Ostrop N, Lamb J, Reid G. Intravaginal morphine: an alternative route of administration. *Pharmacotherapy.* 1998;18:863.

48. Maurer P, Bartkowski R. Drug interactions of clinical significance with opioid analgesics. *Drug Saf.* 1993;8:30.

49. Quinn D, Day R. Drug interactions of clinical importance. An updated guide. *Drug Saf.* 1995;12:393.

50. Takeda F. Results of field-testing in Japan of the WHO draft interim guidelines on relief of cancer pain. *Pain Clin.* 1986;1:83.

51. Ventafridda V, Tamburini M, Caraceni A, et al. A validation study of the WHO method for cancer pain relief. *Cancer.* 1987;59:850.

52. Walker V, Hoskin P, Hanks G, et al. Evaluation of the WHO analgesic guidelines for cancer pain in a hospital based palliative care unit. *J Pain Symptom Manage.* 1988;3:145.

53. Vijayaram S, Bhargava K, Ramamani, et al. Experience with oral morphine for cancer pain relief. *J Pain Symptom Manage.* 1989; 4:130.

54. Giosis A, Giorini M, Ratti R, et al. Application of the WHO protocol on medical therapy for oncologic pain in an internal medicine hospital. *Tumori.* 1989;75:470.

55. Schug S, Zech D, Dorr U. Cancer pain management according to the WHO analgesic guidelines. *J Pain Symptom Manage.* 1990;5:27.

56. Grond S, Zech D, Schug S, et al. Validation of the World Health Organization guidelines for cancer pain relief during the last days and hours of life. *J Pain Symptom Manage.* 1991;6:411.

57. Zech D, Grond S, Lynch J, et al. Validation of the World Health Organization guidelines for cancer pain relief: a ten year prospective study. *Pain.* 1995;63:65.

58. Rappaz O, Tripiana J, Rapin C, et al. Soins palliatifs et traitement de la douleur cancereuse en geriatrie. Notre experience institutionnelle. *Ther Umsch.* 1985;42:843.

59. Acute Pain Management Guideline Panel. *Clinical Practice Guideline. Acute Pain Management: Operative or Medical Procedures and Trauma*. Rockville, Md: US Dept of Health and Human Services, Agency for Health Care Policy and Research; 1992. AHCPR publication 92-0032.

60. Jacox A, Carr DB, Payne R, et al. *Clinical Practice Guideline Number 9. Management of Cancer Pain*. Rockville, Md: US Dept of Health and Human Services, Agency for Health Care Policy and Research; 1994. AHCPR publication 94-0592.

61. Miaskowski C, Cleary J, Barney R, Coyne, P, Finley R, Foster R, et. al. *Guideline for the Management of Cancer Pain in Adults and Children*. Glenview IL: American Pain Society; 2005.

62. Porter J, Jick H. Addiction rare in patients treated with narcotics [letter]. *N Engl J Med*. 1980;302:123.

63. Perry S, Heidrich G. Management of pain during debridement: a survey of US pain units. *Pain*. 1982;13:267.

64. Medina J, Diamond S. Drug dependency in patients with chronic headache. *Headache*. 1977;17:12.

65. Rinaldi R, Steindler E, Wilford B, et al. Clarification and standardization of substance abuse terminology. *JAMA*. 1988;259:555.

66. Heit HA. Addiction, physical dependence, and tolerance: precise definitions to help clinicians evaluate and treat chronic pain patients. *J Pain Palliat Care Pharmacother*. 2003;17(1):15-29.

67. Weissman DE, Haddox JD. Opioid pseudoaddiction—an iatrogenic syndrome. *Pain*. 1989;36:363.

68. The American Society of Addiction Medicine. Public Policy Statement on Definitions Related to the Use of Opioids in Pain Treatment. Available at http://www.asam.org. Accessed April 1997.

69. Levy M. Pain management in advanced cancer. *Semin Oncol*. 1985;12:394.

70. Tuteja AK, Biskupiak J, Stoddard GJ, Lipman AG. Opioid-induced bowel disorders and narcotic bowel syndrome in patients with chronic non-cancer pain. *Neurogastroenterol Motil*. Apr 2010;22(4):424-430.

71. Zhukovsky D, Thomas J, Lipman AG, Slatkin N. Treatment of opioid-induced constipation with methylnaltrexone in patients with CNS metastases. *Supportive Care in Cancer*. 2007;15(6).

72. Pappagallo M. The concept of pseudotolerance to opioids. *J Pharm Care Pain Symptom Control*. 1998;6:95.

73. Twycross R, Fairfield S. Pain in far-advanced cancer. *Pain*. 1982;14:303.

74. Lipman AG. Comments on Fitzgibbon and Galer [letter]. *Pain*. 1995;63:135.

75. Vainio A, Ollila J, Matikainen E, et al. Driving ability in cancer patients receiving long-term morphine analgesia. *Lancet*. 1995; 346:667.

76. Fishbein DA, Cutler RB, Rosonoff HL, Rosonoff RS. Can patients taking opioids drive safely: a structured evidence-based review. *J Pain Palliat Care Pharmacotherap*. 2002;16:9–28.

77. Elliot T, Murray D, Elliot B, et al. Physician knowledge and attitudes about cancer pain management: a survey from the Minnesota Cancer Pain Project. *J Pain Symptom Manage*. 1995;10:495.

78. Rankin M, Snider B. Nurses' perceptions of cancer patients' pain. *Cancer Nurs*. 1984;7:149.

79. Doucette W, Mays-Holland T, Memmott H, et al. Cancer pain management: pharmacist knowledge and practices. *J Pharm Care Pain Symptom Control*. 1997;5:17.

Rising Standards for Risk Management in Opioid Use for Chronic Pain

Richard Scott Stayner
Scott M. Fishman

Similar to treatments that carry substantial risks and must be used with great care, the drug group collectively known as opioid analgesics can be therapeutically desirable for treating severe acute pain, pain at the end of life, and other pain conditions in which the benefits of use outweigh the potential risks. Despite the need for cautious use of opioids, prescribing has become pervasive and excessive. Although opioids are one of many legitimate and diverse options for treating pain, they represent a large share of risk.

Chronic pain is a common reason patients seek medical care. A significant challenge in treating patients with chronic pain is that no perfect method exists to assess the existence or intensity of pain that a patient experiences. It remains impossible to prove that a patient does or does not have pain or pain relief. Prescribers with limited background in pain management and scarce resources may feel pressured to lean too heavily on opioids as the first or only option for chronic pain management. For many prescribers, pain management and opioids have become synonymous, as if prescribing opioids is equivalent to adequate pain management or withholding them were equivalent to undertreatment.

Over the past decade, interrelated public health trends have developed as a result of the prevalence of and difficulty in treating patients with pain syndromes. First, increased clinical attention was directed across all medical specialties to the undertreatment of pain. This was followed by more frequent and escalating prescribing of opioids. The improved comfort and quality of life seen with aggressive opioid therapy for patients with terminal cancer was extrapolated to patients with chronic pain. Moreover, predictions of safety with chronic use of opioids were founded on low-quality data. The increased availability of opioid medications was followed by a shift in patterns of drug abuse from illicit to prescription drugs—most notably a dramatic increase in diversion and nonmedical use of opioid pain medications within the United States. A paradigm shift is under way that emphasizes safety and a more limited role for opioids in overall chronic pain care. Major policy changes have also emerged that every prescriber should be well aware of.

Addiction and abuse are pivotal concerns associated with using opioids. However, opioids have a wide range of adverse effects that can result in serious morbidity and mortality. Additionally, opioid medications are not universally effective for all types of chronic pain or all patients.[1] A major risk associated with opioids is respiratory depression resulting from unintended overdose. The risk for respiratory depression is heightened in older persons, those with mental illness, those with impaired renal or hepatic function, and individuals with cardiopulmonary disorders such as chronic obstructive pulmonary disease (COPD), congestive heart failure (CHF), and sleep apnea. Patients who combine opioids with other respiratory depressants such as alcohol, benzodiazepines, barbiturates, or sedative-hypnotics are also at increased risk for respiratory depression. Chronic opioid use also has a negative impact on endocrine function and possibly heightened fracture risk related to effects on bone metabolism,[2,3] potential birth defects in unborn children,[4] and potential facilitation of tumor growth in cancer.[5,6,7]

Prescriptions for opiates increased from 76 million in 1991 to 207 million in 2013; the United States was the largest consumer of opioid medications.[8] Hydrocodone is the most prescribed drug in the United States, which consumes 99% of the world's supply.[8] Factors that contribute to the increase in opioid prescribing include the introduction of long-acting formulations and novel delivery systems, as well as prescriber concerns about the dangers of non-opioid analgesics such as nonsteroidal anti-inflammatory drugs (NSAIDS) and acetaminophen. These factors are seen in a much different light as the United States confronts an epidemic of opioid prescription abuse:

- Between 1998 and 2008, the rate of opioid abuse increased 400%.[9]
- More than 6 million Americans abuse prescription drugs—more than the number estimated to abuse cocaine, heroin, hallucinogens, and inhalants combined.[10]
- Emergency-department visits related to pharmaceutical opioids doubled between 2004 and 2008.[11]
- Between 1998 and 2012, a tenfold increase was noted in drug treatment admissions for prescription opioids.[12]
- The number of deaths nationwide attributable to prescription opioid analgesics nearly quadrupled between 1999 and 2012.[13]
- From 1999 to 2005, the number of poisoning deaths mentioning methadone increased 468%.[14]
- Drug abuse is now a leading cause of accidental death in America, exceeded only by car crashes; in many states opioid overdose is the leading cause of accidental death.[15]

These alarming statistics have led some to propose extreme measures to curb opioid misuse. A number of physicians have chosen to stop treating chronic pain in patients altogether even though the problem of unrelieved pain is significant. In the United States, the incidence of chronic pain is estimated at 100 million people,[16] greater than that of diabetes, heart disease, and cancer combined.[17,18] The cost of treating patients with chronic pain is estimated to be up to $635 billion.[16]

Regardless of the need for comfort, prescribers must weigh the benefits versus the risks of pain management. Clinical guidelines, policy statements, and organizational goals generally accept the following principles of pain treatment:[19]

- Pain management is integral to good medical practice for all patients.
- Opioid therapy to relieve pain and improve function is a legitimate medical practice for acute and chronic pain of both cancer and noncancer origin.
- The use of opioids for other than legitimate medical purpose poses a threat to the individual and to society.
- Prescribers have a responsibility to minimize the potential for the abuse and diversion of controlled substances.

UPDATED POLICIES AND REGULATIONS REGARDING OPIOID PRESCRIBING

The Food and Drug Administration (FDA) announced in September 2013 that it would require more specific language regarding patient risks in the labeling of extended-release/long-acting opioid medications.[20] Manufacturers are now required to include language to emphasize potential for misuse and abuse, neonatal opioid withdrawal syndrome (NOWS), addiction, overdose, and death.[21] In addition to new labeling requirements, the FDA released strong recommendations advising prescribing physicians to carefully weigh the risks and benefits of opioid medications for the treatment of chronic pain, stopping short of recommending that opioid medications not be used for chronic pain.

THE NEW FDA LABELING FOR LONG-ACTING/EXTENDED-RELEASE (LA/ER) OPIOIDS WILL CHANGE IN THE FOLLOWING WAYS:

- "Indicated for the management of pain severe enough to require daily, around-the-clock, long-term opioid treatment and for which alternative treatment options are inadequate."
- LA/ER opioids are not intended for use as an "as-needed" pain reliever.
- Other, less potentially addictive, treatment options should be considered first ["Because of the risks of addiction, abuse and misuse with opioids, even at recommended doses, and because of the greater risks of overdose and death with extended-release opioid formulations, LA/ER opioids should be reserved for use in patients for whom alternative treatment options (e.g., non-opioid analgesics or immediate-release opioids) are ineffective, not tolerated, or would be otherwise inadequate"].
- Patients in pain should be assessed not only by rating on a pain intensity scale but also *based on a more thoughtful determination that their pain—however it may be defined—is severe enough to require daily, around-the-clock, long-term opioid treatment*, and for which alternative treatment options are inadequate.
- The new labeling will provide increased detail and elevate the risk of neonatal opioid withdrawal syndrome (NOWS) to the most prominent position in labeling—a boxed warning. It will emphasize the symptoms of NOWS, including poor feeding, rapid breathing, trembling, and excessive or high-pitched crying [FDA-approved labeling previously described the effects on newborns of exposure to these drugs while in the mother's womb and warned against use by women during pregnancy and labor and nursing.].
- Manufacturers of LA/ER opioids will be required to fund and conduct longer-term post-market studies and trials of LA/ER opioid pain relievers that evaluate long-term use and assess known serious risks, including misuse, abuse, addiction, overdose, death, and increasing sensitivity to pain.
- Patient/consumer education will be required that will target risk reduction. Educational materials for patients and health care professionals (HCPs) will be modified to reflect new labeling for ER/LA opioids and LA/ER opioid manufacturers will revise a paper handout that patients will receive with their prescription.
- The ER/LA Opioid Risk Evaluation and Mitigation Strategies program for LA/ER opioids, which offers voluntary education on risks and risk management associated with opioid use that is funded by manufacturers, will be updated to reflect the new labeling.

The FDA is not alone among regulatory agencies and medical organizations in publishing policy and regulation changes regarding the use of opioid medications. Other organizations such as the Centers for Disease Control (CDC), the Office of National Drug Control Policy (ONDCP), the Federation of State Medical Boards, the American Society for Interventional Pain Physicians (ASIPP), the American Pain Society (APS) and the American Academy of Pain Medicine have recently published new or updated previous versions of guidelines in response to reports of increases in opioid-related deaths with concomitant increases in the rate of opioid prescribing.[22,23,24]

FEDERATION OF STATE MEDICAL BOARDS:

REVISED MODEL POLICY FOR THE USE OF OPIOID ANALGESICS IN THE TREATMENT OF CHRONIC PAIN

The Model Policy for the Use of Opioid Analgesics in the Treatment of Chronic Pain, published by the Federation of State Medical Boards (FSMB), was revised in August 2013.[25] The policy assists state medical boards in advising and regulating physicians with regard to medically appropriate prescribing practices when using opioid medications for the treatment of chronic pain. It was updated to address dramatic increases in rates of abuse, misuse, and diversion of opioid medications with increased morbidity and mortality in the United States.[22] The updated policy emphasizes the need to assess and treat chronic pain as well as promote access to substance abuse and addiction treatment for high-risk patients. It recommends that physicians screen patients for history of abuse, misuse, or opioid addiction prior to and subsequent to prescribing opioid medications.

The 2013 FSMB revised model policy describes expectations for prescribing of opioids and stresses areas where opioid prescribing would be departures from accepted best clinical practices:

- Inadequate assessment to determine that opioids are clinically indicated.
- Inadequate determination of risks associated with opioid use.
- Inadequate monitoring of outcomes during the use of potentially abusable medications.
- Inadequate education of patients.
- Failure to obtain substantive informed consent.
- Escalation of dose without adequate attention to risks or alternative treatments.
- Excessive reliance on opioids, particularly high-dose opioids, for chronic pain management.
- Failure to make use of available tools for risk mitigation.

The revised FSMB model policy emphasizes that competent physicians must be capable of managing patients with chronic pain with appropriate assistance from specialists when necessary. Although opioid medications may be used to provide pain relief, the use of such medications for purposes other than prescribed puts the patient, physician, and society at risk for harm. The policy indicates that physicians are responsible for minimizing risks of abuse and diversion of prescription opioids by prescribing to carefully selected patients only for whom opioid therapies will provide benefit and by reevaluating periodically the benefits versus the risks of their continued use.

Although it is intended to support the work of state medical boards, the FSMB model policy can be a tool to educate physicians in appropriate use of opioid medications as part of a comprehensive chronic pain treatment plan for their patients. The model policy is not intended for use as a rigid algorithm from which deviation will be penalized by state medical boards. However, deviations from the general recommendations contained within the model policy should be supported with documentation of sound medical justification. Additionally, it is expected that assessment of the benefits versus risks of the treatment plan for a specific patient be recorded in the medical record.

The FSMB model policy is divided into the following categories:

- Patient evaluation and selection.
- Development and documentation of a treatment plan.
- Informed patient consent, agreement, and initiation of treatment.
- Periodic review of the treatment plan and monitoring.
- Consultation and referral.
- Discontinuation of opioid therapy.
- Maintenance of the medical record.

FSMB MODEL POLICY: PATIENT EVALUATION AND SELECTION

Accurate assessment, diagnosis of pain generators, and effective treatment of pain are essential for the patient with chronic pain. Evaluation is key to identification of patients with chronic pain who may need and benefit from opioid therapy for pain. An in-depth evaluation will explore the risks and benefits of a proposed therapy, including treatment with opioid medications. Such an evaluation should include a medical history and systems review, physical examination, review of pertinent imaging studies, and review of laboratory results as dictated by symptomatology and patient history.

The physician should assess the nature and intensity of pain and the effect that pain has on the patient's daily life (functional impact). Issues such as sleep, mood, relationships, and ability to participate in recreational activities should be reviewed and documented. Validated brief assessment tools such as the three-question "Pain, Enjoyment and General Activity Score" (PEG)[26] may be helpful in determining the global effect of chronic pain on a patient's life. Particular attention should be paid to evidence of untreated preexisting or onset of mental health illness, such as depression. This is important because patients with mental health comorbidities are at increased risk for abuse, misuse, and overdose of controlled medications.

As use of prescription opioid medications for illicit purposes such as recreation, diversion, or related to chemical dependency is higher than previously thought, the FSMB model policy emphasizes that opioid prescribers must protect the patient and the community at large from harm related to opioid misuse or abuse. Patients may not be forthright about their motivations for seeking opioid therapies for pain relief for various reasons. A detailed history of present and past alcohol, illicit and prescription drug abuse as well as history of physical, emotional, and sexual abuse should be obtained. Such information can be helpful, though not conclusive, to identify a particular patient's risk for misuse of opioid-based medications and chemical dependency. It may be helpful to corroborate a patient's health and behavior history with close friends or family members. Screening tools such as the Screener and Opioid Assessment for Patients with Pain (SOAPP-R)[27] and the Opioid Risk Tool (ORT)[28] can assist the physician in assessing a patient's potential risk for opioid misuse. The use of prescription drug monitoring programs (PDMPs) and confirmatory tests such as urine drug screening are also expected to be useful when available.

The treatment of a patient with both chronic pain and chemical dependency issues presents a unique challenge. It is now advised that patients who have an active substance abuse disorder, with the exception of tobacco, should be considered unsuitable candidates for opioid therapy until they have enrolled in, and preferably completed, a substance abuse treatment program.[29] Other non-opioid therapies, however, should be pursued as viable options.

FSMB MODEL POLICY: DEVELOPMENT AND DOCUMENTATION OF A TREATMENT PLAN

The FSMB model policy emphasizes early and ongoing treatment planning centered on reasonable and objectively demonstrable goals. Treatment goals include attainable function, improvement in symptoms such as sleep disturbance, and the avoidance of unnecessary medication use. Particular attention should be paid to mental health goals such as reduction in anxiety and depression as these are often associated with chronic pain. The patient should be counseled that opioid medications are not considered the primary treatment for any of the above-mentioned treatment goals. In some patients, judicious use of opioid medications may supplement pharmacologic and nonpharmacologic therapies as part of a comprehensive treatment plan. The efficacy of a treatment plan is enhanced by the incorporation of a multidisciplinary team approach; however, referrals and consultations to appropriate specialists should also be included. In order to evaluate progress, the treatment plan, as well as appropriate goals, should be documented and reviewed frequently. To accommodate changes in the patient's overall health and pain-generating conditions, prescribers are encouraged to review the full breadth of employed and available therapeutic modalities as well as the objectives of treatment.

FSMB MODEL POLICY: INFORMED PATIENT CONSENT, TREATMENT AGREEMENT, AND INITIATION OF TREATMENT

The FSMB model policy states that patients must be informed of the benefits and risks of treatment for a medical condition, which is most important for opioid-based therapies. When a trial of opioid medications for treatment of chronic pain is agreed upon, it is recommended that an agreement outlining the elements of informed consent and treatment conditions be written. The document is sometimes referred to as a "treatment contract." The agreement should be signed by the prescribing physician, the patient, or the patient's legal guardian and ideally the patient's primary care physician if another provider is prescribing opioid medications. The treatment contract formally documents the shared decision between the patient and treating physician(s) that, after careful consideration of the risks and benefits, a trial of opioids will be administered. The treatment contract also documents informed consent and specifics of the treatment agreement.

The informed consent portion of the treatment contract outlines the following patient education points:

- Risks and anticipated benefits of chronic opioid therapy.
- Potential short-term and long-term adverse events such as constipation and cognitive dysfunction.
- Likelihood of tolerance and physical dependence.
- Risks of drug interactions, oversedation, and potential respiratory arrest.
- Risk of impaired motor skills, including the ability to drive safely.
- Risk of opioid misuse, dependence, addiction, and overdose
- Limited evidence regarding the benefit of long-term opioid therapy.
- Prescribing policies and expectations, including the number and frequency of prescription refills, as well as the physician's policy on early refills and replacement of lost or stolen medications.
- Specific reasons for which drug therapy may be changed or discontinued (including violation of the policies and agreements written in the treatment contract).

The treatment contract documents the following joint responsibilities of the treating physician(s) and patient:

- Goals of treatment in terms of pain management, restoration of function, and patient safety.
- Patient's responsibility for safe medication use, such as not using more medication than prescribed or using opioid medications in combination with alcohol, storing medications in a secure location, and safe disposal of any unused medication.
- Patient's responsibility to obtain prescribed opioids from single physician or practice.
- Patient's agreement to periodic confirmatory drug testing.
- Physician's responsibility to be available to care for unforeseen problems and prescribe scheduled refills.

After a decision is made that benefits of treatment outweigh risks, and all appropriate screening, workup, and informed consent/treatment contract are completed, opioid medications should be tested for a trial period, usually no longer than 90 days. To minimize risk, the lowest dose of a short-acting medication should be used in the early phase, especially for opioid-naïve patients. Doses can be carefully titrated to effect and, if desirable, may be converted to long-acting preparations while incorporating nonpharmacologic modalities to minimize dose escalations. Regular evaluations should be performed throughout the trial period to assess the progress in achieving treatment goals and to determine the beneficial and harmful effects of opioids on the patient's pain experience, function, and quality of life. The decision to continue therapy beyond the trial period should be made after careful evaluation of the progress in achieving treatment goals and any risks or adverse events during the trial period.

FSMB MODEL POLICY: PERIODIC REVIEW OF THE TREATMENT PLAN AND MONITORING

It is important to regularly evaluate and adapt the treatment plan based on individual circumstances and any changes in risk or adverse events. Physician should regularly review the patient's health record, obtain collateral information from family members or close friends, and review the state PDMP. Gathering information from as many sources as possible will aid in determining the patient's response to the overall treatment plan, including opioid medications. Evaluations should be most frequent at the initiation of treatment as dose adjustments and modifications to the treatment plan may need to be made. However, ongoing vigilant follow-up is expected throughout the course of treatment and arrangements must be made for patients to obtain follow-up, review of outcomes, and a reasonable process for refills of medication.

The decision to continue, modify, or eliminate opioid medications from the treatment plan should be based on assessment of the patient's progress toward treatment goals and satisfactory responses to treatment, as well as evidence of adverse events, including diversion, overdose, or other misuse. Evidence of satisfactory response to treatment is indicated by reduced pain, increased function, and reports from the patient, caregivers, or other collateral sources regarding overall increased quality of life. One way to assess these variables is the "5As" of chronic pain management,[30] which should be assessed at each follow-up visit:

- Analgesia. Determination of whether the patient is experiencing a reduction in pain
- Activity. Demonstrated improvement in level of function
- Adverse effects. Negative side effects caused by medication
- Aberrant behaviors. Substance-related behavior and compliance with the treatment plan
- Affect. Mood of the individual

Patient or caregiver reports and observation of patient behavior in follow-up visits may be adequate to detect some problems with compliance but not others. Periodic pill counts and consultation with the state PDMP can be useful in monitoring adherence to the therapeutic plan. PDMPs can be invaluable for identifying patients who have multiple prescribing episodes ("doctor shopping") related to controlled substances.

Periodic drug testing is an important monitoring tool to detect the use of prescribed and nonprescribed or illicit drugs. Frequency of drug testing is determined by the clinical judgment of the treating physician. However, drug testing is imperative for patients if concerns for addiction, abuse, or diversion are heightened and should be performed as frequently as necessary to support risk management. Although there are many methods of drug testing available, urine drug screen testing is convenient and cost effective.[31] The testing performed for monitoring chronic pain patients does not usually follow forensic standards for collection, such as observed collection of the sample or following chain-of-custody protocols, but is still helpful in monitoring adherence to an agreed treatment plan. Point of care (POC) immunoassay testing often provides only identification of drug classes. Follow-up confirmatory testing, such as gas chromatography/mass spectroscopy (GC-MS), is often necessary for identification of specific drugs. When ordering confirmatory drug testing, it is useful to document the prescription medications that the patient should be taking as this will assist in a more accurate interpretation of the results by the laboratory.

Aberrant test results should be discussed with the patient in a positive and supportive manner. Regardless of the changes made regarding the continued use of opioid medications to treat chronic pain, the physician should reassure the patient that he or she will be treated with the best and safest care. A supportive physician-patient relationship can facilitate positive behavioral changes in the patient. Test results and details of subsequent discussion with the patient should be documented in the medical record.

Physicians who prescribe opioid therapies should be experienced in the identification of substance abuse and physical dependence and the diagnosis of substance abuse disorders. Patient behaviors such as recurring misuse, unauthorized dose increases, deteriorating function, evidence of forged prescriptions, and documented diversion are particularly worrisome and require immediate intervention by the physician. Failure to act can place the patient at risk for harm from accidental overdose, injury to self or others, arrest, incarceration, and even death.

FSMB MODEL POLICY: CONSULTATION AND REFERRAL

Treatment of patients with chronic pain can be complex with many challenges. Consultation with others who have greater knowledge and specialization related to the needs of a patient (i.e., psychiatry, neurology, PM&R, pain management, addiction medicine, physical therapy, psychology, social work) is an expected component of safe chronic pain management. Consultation with specialists may be needed for patients with comorbidities such as mental health disorders, addiction, and physical deconditioning.

FSMB MODEL POLICY: DISCONTINUATION OF OPIOID THERAPY

The FSMB model policy emphasizes that decrease or discontinuation of opioid therapy is a treatment option, which is especially true if continued use of opioid medications poses greater risk than benefit. Recent studies suggest that when opioids are significantly reduced or stopped, some chronic pain sufferers do no worse in terms of reported pain and function, whereas others may even improve.[1,32] Reasons for discontinuation of opioid therapy include resolution of pain, intolerable adverse effects, inadequate analgesia or hyperalgesia, deteriorating function, and evidence of medication abuse, misuse, or diversion.

Patients who have used opioids for more than a short time should be expected to have some degree of physical dependence. Tapering or discontinuing opioids in such patients may require slow downward titration and the assistance of an addiction specialist. It should be emphasized that the decision to discontinue opioid medications does not constitute a discontinuation of pain treatment. Use of opioid medications should be one component of a multimodal treatment plan. Other non-opioid modalities should continue to be viable options.

FSMB MODEL POLICY: MAINTENANCE OF MEDICAL RECORDS

Physicians should maintain medical records documenting treatment plans as they treat a medical condition. Documentation is most important when prescribing opioid medications to treat patients for chronic pain. The medical record should reflect the medical decisions that led to choosing opioids (risks vs benefits), the risk assessment, and the risk management plan. Documentation includes all orders for medications, especially opioid medications and other controlled substances. Documentation of instructions given to the patient regarding appropriate medication use (e.g. timing of doses, indications for taking medication for break through pain, avoidance of alcohol while using opioid medications, etc.) should also be written in the medical record. The name, address, and telephone number of the patient's pharmacy should also be recorded for easy reference in case questions arise.

The following elements are to be included in the medical record:

- Instructions to the patient and others caring for the patient, which include discussions of risks and benefits of opioid therapy.
  - A copy of signed treatment agreements or consents should be included.
- Documentation of patient progress (or lack of progress) in terms of pain management and functional improvement.
- Notes regarding evaluations and consultations with specialists.
- Information used to support the initiation, continuation, revision, or termination of opioid-based treatment and the steps taken in response to any aberrant medication use behaviors.
  - These may include medical records, notes from past hospitalizations, and treatments by other providers.
- Authorization for release of information to other treatment providers.

All records should be ready for immediate review if necessary. If a desired outcome is not achieved, complete documentation of the treatment plan and follow-up is needed to protect the physician and patient.

CENTERS FOR DISEASE CONTROL: GUIDANCE FOR OPIOID PRESCRIBING

Data released by the Centers for Disease Control and Prevention (CDC) show that the number of opioid-related poisonings doubled between 2001 and 2011[23] and opioid prescriptions quadrupled over the same time period.[23,24] The CDC had previously offered guidance for opioid prescribing to health care providers (HCPs) based on expert opinion:[33]

- Use opioid medications for acute or chronic pain only after determining that alternative therapies do not deliver adequate pain relief. The lowest effective dose of opioids should be used.
- In addition to behavioral screening and use of patient contracts, consider random, periodic, targeted urine testing for opioids and other drugs for any patient younger than 65 years old with noncancer pain who is being treated with opioids for more than 6 weeks.
- If a patient's dosage has increased to greater than 120 morphine milligram equivalents per day without substantial improvement in pain and function, request consultation with a pain specialist.
- Do not prescribe long-acting or controlled-release opioids (e.g., OxyContin, fentanyl patches, and methadone) for acute pain.
- Periodically request a report from your state prescription drug monitoring program

SUBSTANCE ABUSE AND MENTAL HEALTH SERVICES ADMINISTRATION: OPIOID SAFETY TOOLKITS

Data that clarify the substantial risks associated with prescription opioid use have prompted the Substance Abuse and Mental Health Services Administration (SAMHSA) to publish a collection of opioid safety toolkits.[34] Individual toolkits target prescribers, patients, first responders, general community members, and opioid overdose survivors and their families. Each SAMSHA toolkit addresses topics pertinent to a target audience such as signs and symptoms of acute opioid overdose, proper storage of medications, utilization of Prescription Drug Monitoring Programs (PDMPs), and other methods to reduce harm associated with the misuse of prescription opioid medications. The toolkits offer several strategies for minimizing the risk of unintended overdose death related to prescription opioids:

- STRATEGY 1. Encourage providers, persons at high risk, family members, and others to learn methods to prevent and manage opioid overdose (OD).
- STRATEGY 2. Ensure access to treatment for individuals misusing or addicted to opioids or with other substance use disorders.
- STRATEGY 3. Ensure ready access to naloxone.
- STRATEGY 4. Encourage the public to call 911.
- STRATEGY 5. Encourage prescribers to use state Prescription Drug Monitoring Programs (PDMPs).

The SAMHSA toolkits provide specific instructions for HCPs for administration of naloxone to treat acute opioid overdose. Specific instructions regarding naloxone coincide with increased support from certain states that are taking steps to allow HCPs to make naloxone available to a person at risk of an opioid-related overdose or a family member, friend, or other person in a position to assist a person at risk of an opioid-related overdose.[35]

Individuals with the greatest need for prescribing naloxone along with opioids include individuals who are:

- Taking high doses of opioids for long-term management of chronic malignant or nonmalignant pain.

- Receiving rotating opioid medication regimens and are thus at risk for incomplete cross-tolerance.
- Discharged from an emergency department following opioid intoxication or poisoning.
- At high risk for overdose because of a legitimate medical need for analgesia, coupled with a suspected or confirmed history of substance abuse, dependence, or nonmedical use of prescription or illicit opioids.
- Completing mandatory opioid detoxification or abstinence programs.
- Recently released from incarceration and a past user or abuser of opioids (and presumably with reduced opioid tolerance and high risk of relapse to opioid use).

The SAMHSA tool kits go further in recommending that at the time of prescribing, *clinicians should inform their patients that it is illegal to sell, give away, or otherwise share medication with others, including family members. The clinician's role as a patient educator is highlighted with emphasis placed on explaining patients' significant obligation to keep their medication in a safe place such as a locked cabinet. Patients must be instructed that access to controlled substances must be restricted and disposal of any unused supply must follow safety guidelines.*

For additional information on prescribing opioids for chronic pain, SAMHSA recommends the following websites:

- www.opioidprescribing.com
  - Sponsored by the Boston University School of Medicine, with support from SAMHSA
- www.pcss-o.org
  - Sponsored by the American Academy of Addiction Psychiatry in collaboration with other specialty societies and with support from SAMHSA
- http://www.medscape.org/viewarticle/770687 and http://www.medscape.org/viewarticle/770440
  - Course modules sponsored by NIDA &posted on MedScape.com

RESCHEDULING HYDROCODONE

Hydrocodone is regarded by some physicians as a "safer" opioid medication because of its classification as a schedule III drug rather than schedule II drug as are most other opioid medications. The fact that hydrocodone is combined in formulations containing acetaminophen or aspirin may have led some to believe it has less potential for abuse because of the widely recognized risk of hepatotoxicity and acetaminophen overdose. However, the Drug Enforcement Administration (DEA) has reported that hydrocodone is the second most abused prescription opioid in the US.[36]

The FDA has announced support for reclassification of hydrocodone-acetaminophen products from schedule III to schedule II.[37] Such a reclassification provides recognition that hydrocodone has equivalent or greater risk for misuse compared with other opioid medications. As this is the most prescribed drug in the United States, the reclassification sends a clear message that, regardless of its compounding, hydrocodone prescribing requires the same level of vigilance as any high-risk opioid. In August 2014, hydrocodone was reclassified as a controlled-substance schedule II drug. The FDA has also approved a new single entity, long-acting hydrocodone preparation.[38]

OTHER LEGAL AND REGULATORY ISSUES

Opioid medications are classified as controlled substances because of their high potential for abuse and are regulated by a complex set of federal and state policies, laws, and regulations. At the federal level, prescribers must have a firm grasp of the laws articulated in the Controlled Substances Act (CSA). Under this act, licensed professionals can prescribe, dispense, and administer controlled substances for legitimate medical purposes. Schedule I drugs such as heroin have no accepted medical use. Most opioid drugs used in medical practice are schedule II medications. Hydrocodone has been rescheduled from schedule III to schedule II.

In 2006, the Drug Enforcement Agency (DEA) released an updated Practitioner's Manual that summarizes and explains the basic requirements for prescribing, administering, and dispensing controlled substances under the CSA (www.deadiversion.usdoj.gov). In the fall of 2007, the DEA issued a final ruling that amends its regulations to allow practitioners to provide individual patients with multiple prescriptions to be filled sequentially for the same Schedule II medication. This ruling allows prescribers to write sequential prescriptions for up to a 90-day supply of a particular controlled substance. These prescriptions must be dated the day the prescriptions are written and would have sequential and nonoverlapping fill dates [one could be for immediate filling]. For example, a prescriber might state "do not fill until 30 days from prescription date" or "do not fill until 60 days from a prescription date" (www.deadiversion.usdoj.gov/fed_regs/rules/2007/fr1119.htm). In 2010, the DEA adopted new rules for allowing prescribers registered with the DEA to prescribe scheduled substances electronically and allow pharmacies to receive, dispense, and archive electronic prescriptions. (www.deadiversion.usdoj.gov/ecomm/e_rx/).

CONCLUSION

As the number of patients seeking medical care for chronic pain increases, demand for safe and effective pain management will increase. Prescribers must remain aware of new medication regulations, policies, and sanctioned recommendations by professional medical organizations in order to make informed decisions about best practices for opioid prescribing to protect their patients and the members of the communities they serve.

Pain is one of the most common reasons a patient will seek medical help. However, treating a patient with chronic pain can be a difficult challenge. The use of opioid medications in the treatment of chronic, noncancer pain is controversial because of the increase in prescription drug abuse. Initiating and continuing opioid therapy is a serious endeavor that requires complex medical decision making and substantial risk management. Prescribers who hold to the risk and benefit analysis will find that the evidence of benefit of chronic opioid prescribing for chronic pain is weak and the evidence for risk is clear, significant, and mounting.

Current professional guidelines for prescribing opioids are increasingly detailed and prescriptive as to their requirements for risk management and sound and shared medical decision-making. They provide a basic framework by which clinicians and regulatory boards can determine that a particular practice is within the current standard of care. The guidelines require an informed and engaged clinician and patient, with each able to initially and continually assess the risks and benefits of various treatment modalities. Clinicians must continually seek updated information regarding advances in research and drug development as well as changes in state or federal regulations while maintaining adequate vigilance for potential opioid misuse by patients. The guidance from regulatory groups such as the FDA, FSMB, and SAMHSA enables clinicians to formulate a treatment plan for patients with chronic pain that reduces reliance on opioids.

REFERENCES

1. Chen L, Vo T, Seefeld L, et al. Lack of correlation between opioid dose adjustment and pain score change in a group of chronic pain patients. *J Pain*. 2013;14:384-392.

2. Solomon DH, Rassen JA, Glynn RJ, Lee J, Levin R, Schneeweiss S. The comparative safety of analgesics in older adults with arthritis. *Arch Intern Med.* 2010;170:1968-1976.
3. Miller M, Sturmer T, Azrael D, Levin R, Solomon DH. Opioid analgesics and the risk of fractures in older adults with arthritis. *J Am Geriatr Soc.* 2011;59:430-438.
4. Broussard CS, Rasmussen SA, Reefhuis J, et al. Maternal treatment with opioid analgesics and risk for birth defects. *Am J Obstet Gynecol.* 2011;204:314.e1-e11.
5. Gach K, Wyrebska A, Fichna J, Janecka A. The role of morphine in regulation of cancer cell growth. *Naunyn Schmiedebergs Arch Pharmacol.* 2011;384:221-230.
6. Afsharimani B, Cabot P, Parat MO. Morphine and tumor growth and metastasis. *Cancer Metastasis Rev.* 2011;30:225-238.
7. Tavare AN, Perry NJ, Benzonana LL, Takata M, Ma D. Cancer recurrence after surgery: direct and indirect effects of anesthetic agents. *Int J Cancer.* 2012;130:1237-1250.
8. Volkow ND. America's Addiction to Opioids: Heroin and Prescription Drug Abuse | National Institute on Drug Abuse (NIDA) 2014. Available from: http://www.drugabuse.gov/about-nida/legislative-activities/testimony-to-congress/2014/americas-addiction-to-opioids-heroin-prescription-drug-abuse. Accessed 4/12/2015.
9. Substance Abuse and Mental Health Services Administration (SAMHSA). *Substance Abuse Treatment Admissions Involving Abuse of Pain Relievers: 1998 and 2008.* Available at: http://oas.samhsa.gov/2k10/230/230PainRelvr2k10Web.pdf. Accessed April 15, 2015.
10. United States Department of Justice, Drug Enforcement Administration (DEA), Office of Diversion Control. *DEA Diversion Control—Practitioner's Manual.* Available at: http://www.deadiversion.usdoj.gov/pubs/manuals/pract/pract_manual012508.pdf. Accessed April 15, 2015.
11. Substance Abuse and Mental Health Services Administration (SAMHSA). *Trends in Emergency Department Visits Involving Nonmedical Use of Narcotic Pain Relievers.* Available at: http://www.oas.samhsa.gov/2k10/DAWN016/OpioidED.htm. Accessed April 15, 2015.
12. Substance Abuse and Mental Health Services Administration (SAMHSA). Treatment Episode Data Set (TEDS) 1998 – 2008. National Admissions to Substance Abuse Treatment Services Available at: http://wwwdasis.samhsa.gov/teds08/TEDS2k8NatWeb.pdf. Accessed April, 15, 2015. Substance Abuse and Mental Health Services Administration, Center for Behavioral Health Statistics and Quality. Treatment Episode Data Set (TEDS): 2002-2012. National Admissions to Substance Abuse Treatment Services. Available at: http://www.samhsa.gov/data/sites/default/files/TEDS2012N_Web.pdf. Accessed April, 15, 2015.
13. Warner, Margaret. Hedegaard, Holly. Chen, Li-Hui. Trends in Drug-poisoning Deaths: United States, 1999 – 2012. Available at: http://www.cdc.gov/nchs/data/hestat/drug_poisoning/drug_poisoning.htm. Accessed April 15, 2015.
14. Fingerhut L. *Increases in Poisoning and Methadone-Related Deaths: United States, 1999-2005.* Available at: http://www.cdc.gov/nchs/data/hestat/poisoning/poisoning.pdf. Accessed April 15, 2015.
15. Centers for Disease Control and Prevention (CDC*). Unintentional Drug Poisoning in the United States.* Available at: http://www.cdc.gov/homeandrecreationalsafety/pdf/poison-issue-brief.pdf. Accessed April 15, 2015.
16. Institute of Medicine. Relieving Pain in America: A blueprint for transforming prevention, care, education, and research. Report Brief. Available at: http://www.iom.edu/~/media/Files/Report%20Files/2011/Relieving-Pain-in-America-A-Blueprint-for-Transforming-Prevention-Care-Education-Research/Pain%20Research%202011%20Report%20Brief.pdf. Accessed April 15, 2015.
17. American Cancer Society (ACS). *Cancer Facts & Figures-2012.* Available at: http://www.cancer.org/acs/groups/content/@epidemiologysurveilance/documents/document/acspc-031941.pdf. Accessed April 15, 2015.
18. Centers for Disease Control and Prevention-National Center for Health Statistics. *Health, United States, 2007 With Chartbook on Trends in the Health of Americans* (November 2007) - hus07.pdf Available at: http://www.cdc.gov/nchs/data/hus/hus07.pdf. Accessed April 15, 2015.
19. Veteran's Affairs/Department of Defense. *Clinical Practice Guidelines: Summary Management of Opioid Therapy for Chronic Pain 2010.* Available at: http://www.va.gov/painmanagement/docs/cpg_opioidtherapy_summary.pdf. Accessed April 15, 2015.
20. Liscinsky M. FDA announces safety labeling changes and post-market study requirements for extended-release and long-acting opioid analgesics: *New boxed warning to include neonatal opioid withdrawal syndrome.* Available at: http://www.fda.gov/NewsEvents/Newsroom/PressAnnouncements/ucm367726.htm. Accessed April 15, 2015.
21. US Food and Drug Administration. *Goal of Label Changes: Better Prescribing, Safer Use of Opioids.* Available at: http://www.fda.gov/ForConsumers/ConsumerUpdates/ucm367660.htm. Accessed April 15, 2015.
22. Office of National Drug Control Policy (ONDCP). *Epidemic: Responding to America's Prescription Drug Abuse Crisis.* Washington, DC: Executive Office of the President, The White House; 2011.
23. Centers for Disease Control and Prevention (CDC), National Center for Health Statistics. CDC WONDER Online Database. Available at: http://wonder.cdc.gov/mortsql.html. Accessed April 15, 2015.
24. Harvard Medical School. Painkillers fuel growth in drug addiction: Opioid overdoses now kill more people than cocaine or heroin. *Harvard Ment Hlth Let.* 2011;27:4-5.
25. Model Policy for the Use of Opioid Analgesics in the Treatment. Federation of State Medical Boards of the United States Inc.; 2013.
26. Krebs EE, Lorenz KA, Bair MJ, et al. Development and initial validation of the PEG, a three-item scale assessing pain intensity and interference. *J Gen Intern Med.* 2009;24:733-738.
27. Butler SF, Budman SH, Fernandez K, Jamison RN. Validation of a screener and opioid assessment measure for patients with chronic pain. *Pain.* 2004;112:65-75.
28. Webster LR, Webster RM. Predicting aberrant behaviors in opioid-treated patients: preliminary validation of the Opioid Risk Tool. *Pain Med.* 2005;6:432-442.
29. Center for Substance Abuse Treatment (CAST), Substance Abuse and Mental Health Services Administration (SAMHSA). *Treatment Improvement Protocol (TIP) 54: Managing Chronic Pain in Adults With or in Recovery From Substance Use Disorders* . Rockford, MD: CSAT, SAMHSA; 2012;(SMA) 12-4671.
30. Gourlay DL, Heit HA, Almahrezi A. Universal precautions in pain medicine: a rational approach to the treatment of chronic pain. *Pain Med.* 2005;6:107-112.
31. Christo PJ, Manchikanti L, Ruan X, et al. Urine drug testing in chronic pain. *Pain Physician.* 2011;14:123-143.
32. Chang G, Chen L, Mao J. Opioid tolerance and hyperalgesia. *Med Clin North Am.* 2007;91:199-211.
33. Institute of Clinical Systems Improvement (ICSI*). Health Care Guideline: Assessment and Management of Chronic Pain 2011.* Available at: https://www.icsi.org/_asset/bw798b/ChronicPain.pdf. Accessed April 15, 2015.

34. Substance Abuse and Mental Health Services Administration (SAMHSA). *Opioid Overdose Prevention Toolkit.* Available at: http://store.samhsa.gov/product/Opioid-Overdose-Prevention-Toolkit/SMA13-4742. Accessed April 15, 2015.
35. American Medical Association. *New State Laws Aim to Avert Opioid Overdose Deaths.* Available at: http://www.ama-assn.org/ama/pub/ama-wire/ama-wire/post/new-state-laws-aim-avert-opioid-overdose-deaths. Accessed April 15, 2015.
36. Drug Enforcement Administration, Office of Diversion Control. *Hydrocodone Fact Sheet.* Available at: http://www.deadiversion.usdoj.gov/drug_chem_info/hydrocodone.pdf. Accessed November 24, 2013.
37. Woodcock J. Statement on Proposed Hydrocodone Reclassification from Janet Woodcock, MD, Director, Center for Drug Evaluation and Research. Available at: http://www.fda.gov/drugs/drugsafety/ucm372089.htm. Accessed November 24, 2013.
38. Liscinsky M. FDA approves extended-release, single-entity hydrocodone product: first to have updated labeling now required for all ER/LA opioid analgesics. Available at: http://www.fda.gov/newsevents/newsroom/pressannouncements/ucm372287.htm. Accessed November 24, 2013.

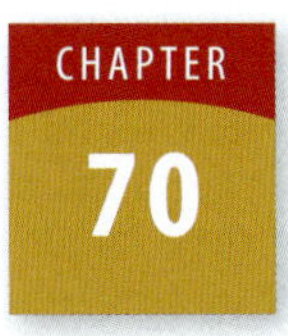

CHAPTER 70 The Interface of Pain Management and Chemical Dependency

Alan A. Wartenberg

INTRODUCTION

With the passage of the Harrison Narcotics Tax Act in 1914, the United States federal government put states, as well as physicians, nurses, and patients, on notice that treatment of those with "narcotic addiction" with drugs, specifically opiates and cocaine, was outside the purview of medical practice and was henceforth illegal.[1] Those who championed the Harrison Act saw a distinction between those with addiction and those with pain and saw the law as necessary to halt what many in the United States saw as a headlong slide into producing generations of opioid, cocaine, and marijuana addicts. Several years later, a political coalition of many of the same advocates saw the Volstead Act ratified as a Constitutional amendment banning the use of alcohol for recreational purposes. That "Great Experiment" lasted barely 13 years; drug prohibition, however, has continued.[2]

It was not until 60 years later with the adoption of the Narcotic Addict Treatment Act of 1974 that physicians could prescribe opioids to those with opioid addiction, but only in the context of federal and state licensed methadone treatment programs. In the interim 60 years, the use of prescribed opioids to treat pain was generally limited to acute pain of injury or surgery and in patients with chronic pain related to cancer and other terminal conditions. Even for these latter groups, great concern was expressed about the addictive nature of these medications, and such drugs were used sparingly.

In the last four decades, however, there has been a growing movement to extend pain treatment, particularly with opioids (as well as sedatives/benzodiazepines and other potentially dependency-producing medications) to those with nonterminal painful conditions.[3,4] In the last 10 years, the prescribing of opioids has increased fourfold, with a similar increase in overdose deaths, with grave concerns among the public, government officials, and the medical profession about these trends. A growth industry of pain clinics, many of which were no more than for-profit opioid and benzodiazepine dispensaries, has prompted some law enforcement and regulatory action, with calls for more.[5-7]

Original concerns expressed about the increasing availability of opioids for pain treatment were muted by assertions from experts that the prevalence of addiction in those who were treated for pain was astonishingly low.[4] Portenoy et al. asserted that undertreatment of pain and specifically "opiophobia" were greater concerns than overprescribing.[3,8] The Joint Commission on Accreditation of Health Care Organizations (JCAHO) declared pain as "the fifth vital sign" and judged hospitals by how well they addressed it.[9] However, in recent years, many experts have expressed concerns and admitted that overprescription and misuse, as well as outright abuse, have become significant problems, with associated mortality and morbidity[5-7] They advocate specially trained physicians to prescribe opioids in long-term nonmalignant pain,[10-11] and/or to develop risk evaluation and mitigation strategies for opioid prescribers.[12-14]

As a physician specializing in the treatment of patients with chemical dependency (CD), the author has developed some expertise in pain management and has treated a number of patients with both addiction and pain. A number of pain physicians may feel the need to recognize and assist in the management of CD in their patients, and some have become experts in this field as well. Many of our colleagues in CD treatment, including anesthesiologists, psychiatrists, internists, family physicians, and others, are now active in both treatment and research in this area.

A new interface in CD and addiction treatment came with the approval of buprenorphine alone (Subutex and generics) and with naloxone (Suboxone®, Zubsolv®, BunavailR and generics). Although buprenorphine is not approved for the treatment of pain except for the preparation for injection; however, for patients with the combination of pain and actual or potential opioid addiction, it has proved helpful in the management of both problems.[15,16]

This chapter will: 1) describe the diagnostic criteria for CD; 2) assist those who treat pain to set up practices which will discourage and perhaps eliminate those "drug-seekers" who attempt to obtain medications solely for diversion and profit; 3) educate pain physicians about appropriate screening measures to detect those who are chemically dependent or at high risk of developing CD; 4) discuss methods to detect the development of aberrant behaviors associated with addiction; 5) present the importance of appropriate referral for CD treatment, including the importance of determining that referral sources are expert in the appropriate management of these patients; and 6) describe potential tools available to pain physicians that will assist in the management of patients with CD.

IDENTIFICATION OF CHEMICAL DEPENDENCY

The Diagnostic and Statistical Manual of the American Psychiatric Association, 5th edition (DSM-5), is the American standard for the diagnosis of CD.[17] The DSM-5 shows particular concern regarding the differentiation of physical dependency, which occurs in virtually all patients who regularly take drugs that produce receptor dysregulation, from substance use disorders (SUDs), including abuse and dependency. The differentiation between abuse and dependency may be changed in the new edition, perhaps with the use, once more, of the term "addiction."[18]

It is important to emphasize that the amount of drug used and frequency of use are not the dominant issues in CD; it is rather the effects of the drug use on the individual and society, in a persistent and consistent manner, and the inability of these individuals to change their maladaptive behaviors. Of course, as drug use escalates and becomes more frequent, one commonly sees these behavioral issues, and ultimately pathological physical and mental changes. However, there are individuals who may use larger amounts of a particular drug without ill effects, while others who use smaller amounts, perhaps even less frequently, still develop serious problems with its use.

DSM-5 eliminates the sometimes confusing distinction between the "Dependency" and "Abuse" categories, replacing them with a unitary "Substance Use Disorder" category for each class of drugs, where the

TABLE 70-1 Aberrant Behaviors

YELLOW FLAGS – Behaviors less suggestive of addiction

1. Aggressive complaining about the need for more drug
2. Drug hoarding during periods of reduced symptoms
3. Requesting specific drugs
4. Openly acquiring similar drugs from other medical sources
5. Unsanctioned dose escalation or other non-adherence with therapy on one or two occasions
6. Unapproved use of the drug to treat another symptoms
7. Reporting psychic effects not intended by the clinician (e.g., increased energy, euphoria)
8. Mildly impaired cognition or subtle signs of impaired function

RED FLAGS – Behaviors probably more suggestive of addiction

1. Selling prescription drugs
2. Prescription forgery
3. Stealing or "borrowing" drugs from others
4. Injecting oral preparations
5. Obtaining prescription drugs from non-medical sources
6. Concurrent abuse of alcohol or illicit drugs
7. Multiple dose escalations or other non-adherence with therapy despite warnings
8. Multiple episodes of prescription "loss"
9. Repeatedly seeking prescriptions from other clinicians or from emergency rooms without informing prescriber or after warnings to desist
10. Evidence of deterioration in the ability to function at work, in the family, or in society that appear to be related to drug use
11. Repeated resistance to changes in therapy despite clear evidence of adverse physical or psychological effects from the drug

Adapted from Portnoy R. Acute and chronic pain. In: Ruiz P, Strain E, eds. *Substance Abuse: A Comprehensive Textbook,* 5th ed. Philadelphia, PA: Lippincott Williams and Wilkins; 2011:701.

criteria are put together into the 11 existing criteria, with the replacement of recurrent legal problems with the criterion of "drug craving." The specifiers are "absent" for 0 to 1 criterion, "mild" for a total of 2 to 3 criteria, "moderate" for 4 to 5 criteria, and "severe" for 6 or more criteria.[16] The moderate to severe category may become synonymous with "addiction." The presence of only tolerance and withdrawal in a patient taking appropriately prescribed medications in an adherent manner will not result in a SUD diagnosis.[18]

The use of screening instruments, such as the screener and opioid assessment for patients with pain (SOAPP), is discussed elsewhere (Chapter 19), and tables of "aberrant behaviors" often divided into "yellow flags" and "red flags" (**Table 70-1**) are based on criteria that are enunciated in the DSM criteria for CD. The diagnosis of CD, however, should not be based on screening tools but on application of the DSM-5 criteria. However, the pain physician must be aware that many of the behaviors associated with addiction can also be present in pain patients (so-called "pseudo-addiction"), particularly in those who have been previously undertreated with opioids, as well as those who have had adverse experience with opioid tapers.[19,20] These behaviors may include drug hoarding, doctor shopping, lack of adherence to dosing schedules, and others.

THE "DRUG-SEEKING" PATIENT

This term "drug-seeking" patient has become so widely and inappropriately used as to become meaningless. All pain patients are concerned with relief of their pain, and often that relief involves a number of drugs; some patients are inordinately fixated on obtaining those medications. However, the term "drug-seeking" refers here to individuals who are not patients, do not have pain problems, and who attempt to obtain opioids and other controlled substances solely for the purpose of abusing the drugs for euphoria and/or diverting them for profit. Individuals who are solely diverting and selling these drugs are criminals and can and should be referred to appropriate authorities.

Drug-seeking patients who attempt to obtain opioids from physicians solely with the intent of abusing them for euphoria, however, are very likely to be CD. In some cases, patients may be obtaining medications and selling them to obtain their drug of choice. Although these activities are illegal, efforts to direct these patients to CD treatment should be encouraged. Unlike the former group of diverting individuals, patients, if successfully treated, are far less likely to reoffend. Drug courts that specialize in drug-related nonviolent crime may be very useful in motivating patients into treatment, with a very high rate of successful completion.

It is recommended that the pain physician has a "no prescription" policy on a patient's first appointment. The referring physician and/or patient calling for appointment who is self-referred is informed that, if the patient is on controlled substances, those prescriptions *must* cover the patient through the evaluation process and that the pain physician will not write such prescriptions except under emergency circumstances, if at all. Unfortunately this is not always possible, but a clear statement of such a policy and its emphasis found in telephone directories and websites may discourage pure "drug-seekers" from seeking their drugs at your practice.

Physicians should be alert to the creative ways that patients create "emergencies," for example, stating that they are visiting from out of town, or calling late on Friday afternoons or weekends, calling only when on-call physicians are available, and many other techniques. Physicians and their staffs should not be persuaded by these urgent requests and insist on a proper intake process, including contact with prior prescribers. If such patients are referred to emergency facilities, a clinical member of the staff should contact the emergency department and speak to the triage nurse or physician regarding concerns.

An interesting study looked at the number of lifetime aberrant behaviors manifested by patients in pain treatment programs and found that the total of aberrant behaviors was a better predictor than the specifics of each aberrant behavior. Patients who manifested four or more aberrant lifetime behaviors were highly likely to have an underlying SUD and have current illicit drug use, whereas those with three or fewer lifetime aberrant behaviors were extremely unlikely to have SUD and current drug use (9.9% vs 1.1%). A positive urine cocaine toxicology test was associated with a fourteenfold increased rate of a SUD.[21]

Pain programs should also utilize state prescription monitoring programs (PMPs) in states where they exist, and physicians should work with colleagues to encourage other states to create them and have them available only to the medical profession (some have only been available to law enforcement and not to physicians, but most are now available to both). PMPs are web-based programs that allow appropriately credentialed individuals to review the prescription records for controlled substances of both new and current patients and can determine whether they are receiving additional prescriptions from other providers, including dates and numbers of pills. This can be enormously helpful in identifying doctor-shoppers and drug-seekers.

Drug testing is also appropriate at the first visit. Toxicology monitoring is dealt with elsewhere in this text (Chapter 19). However, urine or salivary screens, with confirmation of results by more advanced methods, are used to provide confirmation of patients' statements about what they are being prescribed to look for nonconcordance with toxicology results. In patients on certain drugs (e.g., methadone, fentanyl, oxycodone), assays for the measurement of serum concentrations of the drugs are commercially available and provide information as to whether patients are taking the approximate doses which they state are being prescribed. In some cases, proportions of metabolites may indicate the original drug used by the patient. However, many factors may impact the serum concentrations of these drugs.

PATIENTS WITH CHEMICAL DEPENDENCY AND THOSE "AT-RISK"

Many addiction medicine physicians hold to a "unitary model" of addiction, in which a patient who has developed addiction to any drug, including alcohol, is at high risk of development of addiction to other mood-altering or dependency-prone drugs, whereas others (including the author) believe that there is a spectrum of risk in these patients. At lowest risk of addiction are those with a distant history of CD other than opioids, followed by those who are using mood-altering substances or medications in appropriate and controlled ways. At intermediate risk of addiction are those who actively abuse mood-altering drugs, including tobacco, alcohol, and marijuana, as are those with past histories of opioid abuse. At highest risk of addiction are those who are actively abusing illicit opioids or illicitly obtaining licit opioids.

A. PATIENTS WITH PRIOR CHEMICAL DEPENDENCY HISTORY OF DRUGS OTHER THAN OPIOIDS

Patients with a history of CD, particularly those who have been involved in self-help treatment, particularly 12-step programs, may identify themselves initially as being "in recovery" and express their concerns regarding dependency or addiction on pain medications or anxiolytic agents. Other patients may not identify their addiction or dependency and may go to some lengths to deny a prior history. Denial may be in part because of their shame regarding the stigma of a CD diagnosis and in part because of their fear that pain physicians may not be accepting of their pain history and/or believe that they are drug seeking.

Patients with prior histories of CD may be at higher risk of abuse of opioids and benzodiazepines. Although it is important for all patients to explore maximizing nonpharmacologic treatment as well as non-opioid pharmacotherapy, it is most important for patients with prior history of alcohol, cocaine, and/or other stimulants, cannabis, or other CD. Again, many patients will urge doing so. Some patients will resist starting opioids or benzodiazepines even when clearly indicated.

The pain physician, when working with a patient in recovery, should review the patient's support system. If the patient is not involved in active counseling or a self-help group (including a sponsor and a "home" group), the physician should urge the patient to increase the level of support. If the patient's family system is intact, involving and educating the significant other(s) to the risks of opioid or benzodiazepine abuse may be of benefit. Although informed consent of all patients involves a frank discussion or risks/benefits, particularly those of physical dependency and addiction, this discussion is important in the patient with prior CD history.

In a patient with prior alcohol abuse, the pain physician should consider following the patient not only with usual toxicology studies but also with existing biomarkers for alcohol abuse, including a baseline CBC (with MCV), uric acid, triglycerides, ALT/AST, and γ-glutamyl transpeptidase (GGT). Newer biomarkers, commercially available, include carbohydrate-deficient transferrin (CDT), a reliable indicator of recent heavy alcohol consumption even if the individual has been abstinent for several days before the test. A test, which can be obtained together with a urine toxicology test, is the measurement of ethyl glucuronide (EtG), which can detect alcohol consumption for up to 48 hours prior to testing; ethyl sulfide (EtS) is complementary test and may be used instead of or in addition to EtG, with a slightly longer period of detection.[22]

It has been the author's practice to recommend that the patient who is actively involved in a 12-step program inform his or her sponsor or obtain a sponsor if one is needed and have the sponsor be actively involved in the patient's care. For patients in another support system (e.g., SMART Recovery, LifeRing, Women for Sobriety, and others), a more senior treatment "colleague" or the facilitator of their group may be similarly helpful.[23] For patients not so involved, discussion of the risks of relapse should include strong recommendation for developing a professional therapeutic relationship, either individual or group with a CD support group or with a pain support system. Some addiction programs have developed combination pain/addiction support groups.

Pain practices vary in their approaches to "social" drinking in patients receiving opioids. In patients with a prior history of alcohol abuse, any "social" use is significant and indicates relapse, with the likelihood of heavier drinking in the future. Many programs recommend total abstinence because of potential synergistic effects of alcohol with opioids and benzodiazepines, as well as drug-drug interactions secondary to alcohol effects on P-450 cytochrome enzymes. However, few programs routinely inquire about alcohol use at each visit; fewer still do any testing for alcohol metabolites or effects. Use of urinary EtG and/or EtS tests may indicate alcohol consumption within the 1 to 3 days prior to testing, which may be useful if the levels are high or if the patient has not given a history of alcohol use. Low levels of EtG and EtS may, however, occur with exposure to mouthwashes, alcohol in medications or foods, or even inhaling the vapors of alcohol-based skin sanitizers, which are over 60% ethyl alcohol.

Patients with prior histories of abuse of other drugs, particularly cocaine and amphetamines, as well as men younger than 35 years of age, are at higher risk of developing addiction to opioids. Treatment agreements clearly state that use of nonprescribed controlled substances or illicit substances will result in potential detoxification or immediate discharge; therefore, follow-up of those with prior histories should include ongoing toxicology studies, perhaps on a more frequent basis, including random call-backs (often with a 24-hour window) for toxicology studies, sometimes with pill counts.

A particularly difficult and controversial area involves patients who are using forms of cannabis, including marijuana and hashish. Many states have "medical marijuana" laws that permit patients to receive a "prescription" from medical professionals to allow them this use without state or local authorities charging them with criminal offenses. In some states, marijuana "dispensaries" are licensed where patients with medical marijuana cards can purchase it legally. However, others (particularly in states without dispensaries) obtain marijuana through the illegal sales systems.

Many pain physicians are concerned that patients who are using marijuana "medically" are still engaging in illegal activity by purchasing it, as well as having contact with other illicit drugs which may be sold by the same individuals. Others are concerned about the violation of federal laws by such patients. Still others have concerns about the potential for drug-drug interactions. Finally, many programs are concerned about DEA surveillance and prescribing controlled substances to those who are using cannabis or any illicit drug.[24,25] Some patients have prescriptions for medical dronabinol (Marinol), which makes determining the origin of positive THC urine drug screens problematic. Prescribing for opioids and other controlled substances for those using cannabis products remains a judgment call for each health professional.

B. PATIENTS ACTIVELY ENGAGED IN SUBSTANCE ABUSE

Patients who actively engage in substance abuse, whether with alcohol or with other substances, may present with serious painful conditions either from the underlying disorder (e.g., chronic pancreatitis, neuropathy from medications used to treat HIV) or from the causes of chronic pain. Some patients may be functional when abusing drugs and alcohol, and detection may be difficult. Standard screening instruments (e.g., AUDIT, MAST, DAST) may be helpful in some patients,[26] as well as screening tools developed to look for those at risk of abusing medications prescribed for pain, such as the SOAPP-R.[27] Pain physicians, specifically those in general medical practices who treat pain in their patients, may continue to treat patients who are known to be abusing other substances, depending on the severity of the abuse and drug(s) involved. However, these physicians do not use controlled substances in their treatment and focus on nonpharmacologic treatment and non-opioid pharmacologic treatment, as well as avoiding benzodiazepines and other sedatives.

In most cases, it is appropriate to refer such individuals to a treatment facility for CD. In those who are without physical dependency or withdrawal risks and who do not need a higher level of care, outpatient treatment may be appropriate. For those with more significant CD, referral to either free-standing or hospital-based detoxification facilities may be necessary. Upon discharge, there should be consideration for the use of anticraving drugs which are available for alcohol and for other drugs as well. Both detoxification and these agents are further discussed in the section on termination later in the chapter. One option for opioid treatment of pain in at-risk patients for chemical dependency, is the use of buprenorphine. While this can be done in the form of transdermal preparations approved for the treatment of pain, the use of buprenorphine or buprenorphine/naloxone sublingual preparations can also be considered off-label (Heit, H. DEA letter, personal communication, 2004). There may be insurance or pharmacy issues with such off-label prescribing.

C. PATIENTS WITH PRIOR HISTORY OF OPIOID ABUSE

The American Pain Society (APS), the American Academy of Pain Medicine, and the American Society of Addiction Medicine issued a joint policy statement in 2004, asserting that although physicians knowingly giving opioids to patients at high risk of diversion and/or abuse without medical necessity is inappropriate, it is equally problematic to deny appropriate treatment to patients with past or current histories of opioid abuse.[28] Of course, appropriate evaluation as well as careful monitoring is necessary in these patients.

As with patients with histories of other types of CD, every effort should again be made to maximize the use of nonpharmacologic therapies, as well as non-opioid drug therapy. The pain physician should inquire as to the patient's support system, and as with others with CD, every effort should be made to have the patient in appropriate treatment. For those already in a program, whether formal or informal (e.g., 12-step programs, SMART Recovery), recommendations to obtain and involve a sponsor and/or therapist, as well as appropriate family and friends, may be helpful in providing support during what will likely be an increased likelihood for craving and relapse. If the patient feels he or she is not in need of treatment, the physician may consider requiring the patient entering and remaining in treatment as part of the initial treatment agreement, or it may be presented initially as a contingency at the first sign of aberrant behaviors.

In patients with a prior opioid abuse history, it may be advisable to avoid use of the primary drug that the patient abused, particularly forms of oxycodone, as they have little hepatic first pass, can easily be used by nasal insufflations, and cross the blood-brain barrier rapidly, producing more euphoria. The patient's drug(s) of choice may also be triggers, further increasing the chance of abuse. The use of slow-acting agents such as continuous-release (CR) morphine or transdermal fentanyl should be considered when long-acting drugs are needed. Similarly, use of drugs with slower blood-brain barrier passage for acute or breakthrough pain, such as immediate release (IR) morphine, should be considered if such agents are required. Methadone can be legally prescribed for pain, and buprenorphine (an off-label use except for the injectable and transdermal forms) may be an option and is discussed in more detail later in the chapter.

D. PATIENTS WITH ACTIVE USE OF ILLICIT OPIOIDS

Chronic treatment of patients who are actively abusing opioids or other dependency-prone medications, is rarely, if ever appropriate. In the presence of moderate to severe acute pain, administering or dispensing an opioid for relief may be appropriate, but long-term prescribing is fraught with hazard. Such patients are likely to take excessive doses at shorter intervals or may divert licit opioids to obtain their drugs of choice. The clinical, ethical, and medical-legal implications make such prescribing dangerous for the patient and prescriber. In cases where patients are found to be actively abusing illicit opioids (or obtaining licit drugs illicitly), as is the case with other dependency-producing drugs, consideration of the level of use and the likelihood of a withdrawal syndrome should require referral to an appropriate detoxification program. Not all programs are equal, and further discussion of this matter can be found in the section on termination later in the chapter.

In cases involving patients who are taking opioids, pain physicians may want to assess them in an opioid-free state to determine the status of their pain. In those patients who are illicitly using "street" opioids (heroin) and those who are inappropriately using prescribed opioids (e.g., multiple prescribers, frequent early refills, obtaining licit drugs from nonmedical sources), referral to a detoxification facility should also be considered. Such determination may be made on the basis of the level of admitted use and/or the appearance of withdrawal signs and symptoms, as well as their severity. Conventional opinion holds that opioid withdrawal, although uncomfortable, rarely if ever has severe morbidity or mortality; however, the author has seen many cases of severe withdrawal resulting in vomiting, aspiration, pneumonia, myocardial infarction, Mallory-Weiss syndrome, and severe dehydration with renal failure. This is particularly true in older or more debilitated patients (HIV disease, hepatitis C). This is further discussed below.

E. PATIENTS ON OPIOID AGONIST THERAPY

A potentially more difficult decision involves the treatment of pain in opioid-dependent patients who are in treatment, particularly those in methadone agonist treatment. Many pain physicians are not aware of the strictures under which methadone maintenance treatment programs (MMTPs) operate. The basic requirement for admission to MMTPs is that the patient be Opioid Dependent by the old DSM-IV standards, which involves more than physical dependence and essentially labels the patient as a "narcotic addict." There are many other requirements as well, including being able to pay for the treatment, which may range from $4000 to $6000 per year, usually payable by the week. Most private insurance, despite the recent passage of federal mental health/substance abuse parity acts, will not pay for methadone treatment or will pay only for a brief detoxification. In addition, MMTPs are specifically enjoined from using methadone in the primary treatment of pain.

Methadone is given once daily in MMTPs, which is rarely, if ever, adequate for pain treatment. Patients must come daily for dosing until and unless they earn "take-home" privileges, in which they are initially given one take-home dose and then every 60-90 days may earn an additional take-home. Take-home doses require complete adherence to all clinic rules and regulations. Methadone programs may "split" the doses in patients who are hypermetabolizing the drug, such as pregnant women in their second or third trimester or patients on P-450 enzyme-inducing medications; however, there are legal restrictions on doing this, and it must be approved by both state and federal authorities on a case-by-case basis. Therefore, opioid-dependent patients dismissed from pain treatment who are admitted to MMTPs may continue to experience significant pain. In addition, being in a program with those using heroin and other street drugs may be entirely unacceptable to many patients.

The management of such patients represents a challenge to the pain physician, the MMTP, and the patients themselves. Many of these patients have significant real pain but cannot be depended upon to take medication safely and as directed without dose escalation and without the use of other drugs of abuse. Unfortunately, many of these patients, particularly those in treatment for HIV and hepatitis C complications, receive opioids from their other physicians with little or no consultation with the MMTP medical staff. In addition, opioids may be readily available from nonmedical sources or unscrupulous providers in so-called "pill mills."

The prescription of long-acting opioids in these patients can result in overlapping peak levels of both methadone and the other prescribed opioid, with risks of oversedation, overdose, and death. In addition, the program is often unable to use urine drug screens effectively, because most program budgets do not permit use of gas chromatography/mass spectroscopy (GC-MS) or other confirmatory tests, so that it becomes difficult or impossible to determine if the patient is taking only the prescribed drugs. Use of short-acting, rapidly absorbed opioids for breakthrough pain similarly makes monitoring the patient for illicit use problematic.

There is a certain irony in individuals who are in methadone treatment programs precisely because they have abused street drugs, whether heroin or illicitly obtained prescription drugs, and cannot be trusted to manage their medication who then receive as much as a month's worth of drugs similar or identical to their drugs of choice. In many cases, patients are selling the prescribed drugs in order to obtain their drugs of choice, particularly heroin, cocaine, or methamphetamine.

As stated above, all physicians treating pain in patients with addiction should exhaust all nonpharmacologic and non-opioid drug treatments in the management of chronic pain. If opioids are needed for acute pain, prescribers need to be aware of methadone-induced tolerance, which will likely require a higher dose of opioid. If the prescription is for fixed-dose acetaminophen combinations, the patient may escalate the dose and have potential problems with acetaminophen toxicity, as well as opioid-related issues. Every effort should be made to contact the MMTP and consult with its medical or nursing staff. Prescribers also need to be aware that prescribing mixed agonist-antagonists in these patients may result in both hyperalgesia and withdrawal. The author has seen several cases of this with tramadol and, more recently, tapentadol (Nucynta®).

Increasing the dose of methadone is rarely an effective means of treating acute pain both because methadone takes 2 to 4 hours to peak and because reaching a steady state of the increased dose will not take place for 4 to 7 days. Treating acute pain in an emergency department or medical office setting is not generally problematic; however, prescriptions of opioid medication for a week or longer is not without significant risk for these patients. The lowest effective dose should be given for the shortest possible time, with reevaluation every 2 to 3 days. The MMTP nurse and/or physician should be notified as soon as possible of such prescription; ideally, consultation with MMTP staff should be considered prior to prescribing.

For subacute and chronic pain, treatment of methadone-maintained patients should involve collaboration with the MMTP medical staff. In cases of socially rehabilitated MMTP patients who have been in treatment for several years and have extended take-home status and particularly in those with severe and potentially life-threatening medical problems, consideration should be given to turning over the opioid prescribing entirely to the pain physician. Intermediate steps, such as providing split doses, may be possible but are again associated with legal restrictions. Lower-risk opioids, such as methadone (in divided doses), CR morphine, and fentanyl transdermal patches (all of which have potential for abuse), may provide replacement for the methadone dose as well as satisfactory analgesia.

Patients who are on either methadone or buprenorphine preparations for treatment of their narcotic addiction present particular challenges in the treatment of significant pain.[25] In the case of methadone, tolerance may be very high, and patients may require doses of either other longer-acting opioids or short-acting rapidly absorbed opioids that are many times higher than the usual patients' doses. In some cases, it is both medically and logistically more logical to include the maintenance dose with the added needed doses for pain together, through the pain physician, either by using methadone as the maintenance pain drug or by converting the methadone dose into the dose of the other drug being used. Such conversions may be difficult, and equivalency tables are notoriously inaccurate, because individual absorption, tolerance, and metabolism play significant roles, often affected by pharmacogenomic differences among patients. "Starting low and going slow," always an appropriate paradigm, is appropriate for these titrations.

Buprenorphine presents difficulties in addition to tolerance. Unlike methadone, which does not block other opioids—it only increases tolerance to them—buprenorphine has such high receptor affinity and slow receptor dissociation that it keeps other opioids from acting at receptor sites. It will even displace prior opioids from those same sites, and because buprenorphine has lower receptor activity despite its high affinity, the end result can be the development of a withdrawal syndrome in patients on other opioid agonists who are given buprenorphine. This is mistakenly thought to be secondary to the naloxone component but is directly attributable to buprenorphine, particularly since no significant amount of naloxone is absorbed transmucosally or by ingestion.

Physicians prescribing either methadone or buprenorphine should have a preliminary discussion with their patients regarding contingencies for increased pain. If patients are facing elective procedures that will likely produce at least moderate pain, it is the author's preference to have a discussion with the proceduralist or the anesthesiologist regarding pain management in patients on methadone or buprenorphine. In patients on methadone, the task is relatively simple. The maintenance dose of methadone should be continued in a single morning dose when possible. If the patient is to have nothing by mouth, methadone can be given intramuscularly, but the total dose should be approximately half the oral dose, because of a 50% hepatic first-pass metabolism, and then given in divided doses (e.g., an individual on 120 mg of oral methadone who is NPO may receive a total of 60 mg, given as 15 mg every 6 h or 20 mg every 8 h).

The patient can then be given the acute pain drug the physician prefers, but required doses may be at least 50% higher than usual and are often two to three times the usual doses for opioid-naïve patients (and occasionally may be even higher). If the pain is likely to be of relatively short duration, the maintenance dose of methadone may not need to be changed; however, if the patient is on appreciable doses of short-acting drugs for several weeks, an adjustment in methadone dose may need to be ordered as the acute pain drug is tapered. Giving multiple long-acting opioids has the potential for overlapping peaks and producing oversedation and should be avoided when possible. If multiple long-acting drugs are used, patient education regarding the timing of the doses is important.

There are several strategies which may be successful in the treatment of short-term pain in the methadone or buprenorphine maintained patient.[29] The simplest of these is to maintain the buprenorphine dose prior to and through the period of postoperative or traumatic pain while adding a very high affinity, high potency opioid (fentanyl, sufentanil, hydromorphone), usually in significantly elevated doses, although it should be carefully titrated, starting at doses 50% to 100% higher than usual, and evaluating response and adjusting accordingly. This may particularly be appropriate in patients maintained on relatively low doses of buprenorphine, from 2 mg to 12 to16 mg per day.

In patients on higher doses of buprenorphine (i.e., >16 mg per d), it is thought best to discontinue buprenorphine, tapering it so that the last dose is given at least 48 hours (and the author's experience has shown that 72 hours or longer is desirable) prior to the planned procedure. The patient may then be maintained on a standard agonist, such as oxycodone IR, in doses ranging from 5 to 30 mg four times daily. Following the procedure, higher doses or a more potent drug (sufentanil, fentanyl, hydromorphone) can be used for analgesia. When the need for the acute pain treatment has passed, the medication may be tapered, and the patient referred back to the buprenorphine provider to resume treatment.

A third option is to use buprenorphine itself for pain treatment in these patients. However, this is rarely successful in patients already on higher doses of buprenorphine (24-32 mg/d) because of the ceiling effect of the drug and because buprenorphine is not as effective in moderate-severe to severe pain. However, in patients undergoing dental surgery or other moderately painful procedures or in those who are trauma victims, the use of additional buprenorphine 4 to 8 mg sublingually every 4 to 6 hours may be an effective pain management tool if the total dose does not exceed approximately 32 mg per day. One drawback to this strategy is that if buprenorphine is not effective in treating the pain, very high doses of fentanyl, sufentanil, or hydromorphone may be necessary to manage the pain. In some cases, patient monitoring with careful attention to respiratory rate and effort, as well as oxygenation, may become critical.

Patients on agonist treatment for addiction are at very high risk of relapse to "street" opiates or their other drugs of choice during these times of both severe pain and high stress. Involvement of supportive family and/or significant others, sponsors, and therapists may be important proactively, with the patient having a "safety plan" spelled out in advance.

Acute trauma may be more difficult to deal with because of the immediacy of the issue and the inability to plan in advance. It is wise to have the patient carry an emergency card or have a Medicalert® bracelet to provide treaters with necessary information, as well as an emergency number to contact the involved medical personnel. The use of injectable nonsteroidal anti-inflammatory drugs, such as ketorolac, as well as local anesthetic in regional or field blocks, may all be highly useful. The rapid titration of short-acting opioids such as fentanyl or hydromorphone can provide appropriate analgesia, starting near usual doses and escalating as needed, even in patients on high doses of methadone or buprenorphine. In severe cases, conscious sedation or achieving a light anesthetic state with benzodiazepines may be necessary, and rarely general anesthesia is required to achieve control of pain and pain-related behaviors. Again, careful monitoring of respiratory status, oxygenation, and mental status may be necessary. One particularly difficult group of patients is those who are on buprenorphine and present with major trauma or the need for emergency major surgery. Because tapering of buprenorphine is not an option, the buprenorphine may be stopped on admission and pain treated with high doses of potent opioids. However, these patients need close monitoring since they will be susceptible to respiratory depression when the buprenorphine wears off.

CONTRACT VIOLATION AND TREATMENT TERMINATION

The author has given a series of talks for many years titled "Don't put people on meds you don't know how to take them off of" but has settled on the shorter and perhaps more elegant title "Don't take off when you don't know how to land." Pain physicians and those dealing with patients with opioid addiction have had very different experiences in discontinuing opioids (and other dependency-producing drugs, especially benzodiazepines) in their patients. Review articles and textbooks frequently recommend relatively short tapering schedules for patients having opioids reduced and discontinued. This may be particularly effective in patients with opioid-induced hyperalgesia, where dose reduction may actually result in improved pain relief.

It has been the author's experience that patients with CD are far more sensitive to the dysphoria as well as to the physical manifestations of opioid withdrawal. The average patient undergoing therapeutic methadone detoxification may be withdrawn over a period of 6 to 12 months. However, shorter periods of detoxification may be well tolerated, but rarely at reductions of more than 10% of the dose per week, resulting in an approximately 3-month taper. This becomes an issue in those patients who are being dismissed because of problematic or aberrant behaviors, when continued prescribing is deemed unwise and/or dangerous.

Every pain physician or program should and must come up with treatment agreements that fit the needs of patient and the program. Sometimes, however, pain physicians do not differentiate between "yellow" flags, which should require refinement of the treatment agreement, and the use of predescribed contingencies (e.g., increased visits, more urine screens, involvement in counseling, or others), and "red" flags that may require dismissal from treatment. The period of dismissal may range from immediate and without detoxification for severe infractions to 30-day supplies of medication with instructions to find a different provider.

There is a widespread and incorrect assumption that opioid withdrawal is relatively minor and has few medical consequences. It is frequently compared with having a moderate viral syndrome, with diffuse pain, myalgias, arthralgias, shaking chills, nausea, vomiting, and diarrhea, and lasting a relatively short time. This may be true for younger, healthier patients taking only short-acting opioids. However, in older and more medically/psychiatrically complex patients, and in particular with the use of longer-acting SR opioids in higher doses, withdrawal may be severe and protracted, lasting weeks and even months.

Elevated pulse and blood pressure may be present and result in cardiac decompensation in those with underlying heart disease, including the development of angina and myocardial infarction. Vomiting may be severe and result in aspiration, esophageal tears with bleeding (Mallory Weiss syndrome), volume contraction, and severe electrolyte and acid-base balance issues, including acute tubular necrosis with renal failure. This may also occur with severe diarrhea. True informed consent should require that the prescribing pain physician discuss these possibilities with patients early in the treatment course and when treatment agreement violations are noted so that it may have a deterrent effect on further aberrant behaviors.

An issue that may result in treatment agreement violation is that of positive urine or salivary drug screens. Such positive screening tests should be subjected to appropriate confirmatory testing before taking action, as appropriate. Gas chromatography and mass spectroscopy (GC-MS) are the usual confirmatory tests, but other tests (such as double liquid chromatography followed by mass spectroscopy or in some cases thin layer chromatography, depending on the substance involved) may be appropriate. Chain of custody issues and false-positives from interfering substances should be considered as well. Drug testing is ideally an adjunctive test, and in cases where the clinical behaviors have not been aberrant and a positive drug test occurs with the patient denying its validity, consideration should be given to the potential for a false-positive.

Termination, particularly without detoxification, should be the final decision when no safe and effective treating of the patient remains. Adjunctive medications to ameliorate withdrawal, such as the use of α-2 agonists (clonidine, guanfacine, and guanabenz), as well as antidiarrheal and antiemetic agents, should be strongly considered and prescribed.[30-32] If a 30-day supply of opioid medication is given, it may be appropriate that it be written in a tapering dose schedule over that period of time. If benzodiazepines are prescribed, tapering doses of longer-acting, more slowly absorbed agents such as clonazepam or chlordiazepoxide may be indicated. Use of diazepam, alprazolam, and lorazepam, which are more rapidly absorbed and have high abuse potential, should be avoided. Anticonvulsants, such as carbamazepine, valproic acid, and gabapentin, in usual therapeutic doses for seizures, may also be used to aid patients in withdrawal from benzodiazepines.[33-35]

It is not uncommon for patients to be referred to a detoxification facility. If this occurs, it is worthwhile for the pain physician to have determined programs in advance that would meet the patients' needs. Many detoxification settings are managed by nursing staff, often licensed practical nurses with registered nurse supervision, having an off-site physician and prewritten protocols, with very little ability to individualize care. The author has seen hundreds of patients on appreciable doses of SR morphine, oxycodone, and other opioids given the same 5-day protocols using methadone, at doses no higher than 30 mg, then tapered over an additional few days. Such tapers are rarely, if ever, effective and leave patients with a moderate to severe and often protracted course of opioid withdrawal.

Many physicians are not aware of the nature of free-standing (so-called "public") detoxification facilities. Patients are evaluated and treated by nursing staff (often licensed practical nurses, with no registered nurses on site) on the basis of standing orders, and many, perhaps most (or even all) patients in these programs are not seen by a physician. The facility may have a very limited formulary, so that patients on medications they do not stock have to arrange to bring these medications, or have them brought by friends or family. Many facilities take a "one size fits all" approach and will take patients off all dependency-producing medications even if one or more of those medications has not been problematic (e.g., the physician may refer the patient because of benzodiazepine or alcohol abuse and the patient has been adherent to the opioid treatment; however, the program will taper them off of all their drugs, including the opioids).

There are generally hospital-based detoxification programs with on-site physicians and stronger nursing presence where a more individualized approach to these complex patients can be taken. Pain physicians and programs should take the time and effort to familiarize themselves with appropriate detoxification settings and trained physicians in their community, or within referral distance, where there is a greater likelihood of a safe and successful outcome. The American Society of Addiction Medicine (www.asam.org), the American Academy of Addiction Psychiatry (www.aaap.org), and the American Osteopathic Academy of Addiction Medicine (www.aoaam.org) have listings of members on their websites for referral.

In patients for whom opioids have been effective in management of pain but where the patient self-escalates doses or engages in other aberrant behaviors necessitating treatment termination, consideration should be given to referral to a buprenorphine prescriber. In some pain programs, the pain physicians have colleagues who have taken an approved buprenorphine training course and have a prescribing waiver. The sublingual forms of buprenorphine, Suboxone (available now only in the proprietary filmtab), and Subutex (available recently as a generic preparation), are not approved for pain treatment. However, in the patient with combined pain and addiction, they may prove useful in overall patient management, and as long as the patient has documentation of opioid dependency, buprenorphine can be legally prescribed. The combined buprenorphine/naloxone preparation is thought to be safer and less likely to be misused/abused, particularly by injection, and should be the first choice of most patients.

The author has treated many patients who were difficult or impossible to manage with usual SR opioids (particularly OxyContin and generic immediate-release and/or sustained-release oxycodone preparations), who became well managed without dose escalation and with tremendous improvement in compliance and quality of life with the use of usual doses of buprenorphine. In management of addiction, buprenorphine can usually be given once daily, but as with methadone, pain management is better accomplished with multiple divided doses. Again, combination buprenorphine/naloxone (Suboxone filmtabs) is considered safer, has less abuse potential, and is preferred.

Pain physicians may prescribe sublingual buprenorphine for pain, with or without a waiver, as an off-label use of the medication. However, it must be emphasized that there are few studies of its use for this indication, and full informed consent by the patient is important. In addition, both insurance companies and pharmacists may be unwilling to dispense the medication when the prescriber does not have a federal buprenorphine waiver or if it is for an off-label indication However, since these patients have both pain AND addiction, appropriate prescribing can generally be accomplished. Therefore, writing the words "for pain" on the prescription may be helpful. A letter from the Drug Enforcement Agency (DEA) to the chair of the ASAM pain committee indicated that physicians may legally use buprenorphine for pain treatment off label and without a special waiver.[36]

TOOLS FOR DEALING WITH PATIENTS WITH CHEMICAL DEPENDENCY

Unfortunately, it has been all too frequent in the author's experience that the identification of past or present CD is tantamount to dismissal of the patient as inappropriate for a pain management program. Such identification should ideally lead to the creation of an appropriate treatment agreement that applies the necessary contingencies so that these patients can be safely managed. As has been previously stated, the American Pain Society, the American Academy of Pain Management, and the American Society of Addiction Medicine in a common public policy statement, emphasized this point several years ago.[28] Fear of regulatory action, legal problems, and civil lawsuits are not adequate reasons to deprive patients in need of adequate pain management. Strategies for doing so have been discussed in the appropriate sections above.

There has been a dramatic increase in the number of medications available to treat chemically dependent patients for many different drugs of choice. While most of the approved drugs have been for combating alcohol use and craving (**Table 70-4**), there are several approved for opioids as well (buprenorphine and methadone have been discussed). Several medications have been studied for other forms of CD, such as cocaine and other stimulants, which have not yet been approved but are available off-label, and may be useful in specific patients. **Table 70-2** lists the approved medications for treatment of opioid dependency, as well as investigational agents for other indications. There are several excellent reviews of these medications.[37,38]

A. ALCOHOL

Disulfiram The oldest medication developed for the treatment of alcohol craving and abuse is disulfiram (Antabuse). This medication works by blocking acetaldehyde dehydrogenase, which is produced by alcohol dehydrogenase in the metabolism of alcohol to acetic acid

TABLE 70-2 Drugs Used in the Treatment of Other Chemical Dependencies

Opioids		
Methadone	FDA-approved 1974 for use in opioid dependency	Must be licensed program. Usual opioid SEs. Many drug interactions.
Naltrexone (ReVia, generics)	FDA-approved 1992 for opioids	Hepatic black box warning: nausea, vomiting, diarrhea. Monitor LFTs; patients must be fully detoxified from opioids.
Buprenorphine (Suboxone, Subutex)	FDA-approved 2003	Special training, DEA waiver. Usual opioid SEs, fewer drug interactions; may precipitate opioid withdrawal in patients dependent on pure agonists; ceiling dose 16-24 mg/d for addiction treatment, may be higher (>32 mg/d) in divided doses for pain.
Naltrexone ER (Vivitrol)	FDA-approved 2010 for opioids	Same as Naltrexone above; patients must be fully detoxified from opioids or severe/protracted withdrawal may occur.
Cocaine and Stimulants		
Topirimate (Topamax)	**OFF LABEL FOR THIS INDICATION.**	Multiple studies have shown significant reduction in craving and use of cocaine and other stimulants, including methamphetamine.
N-Acetylcysteine (Mucomyst)	**OFF LABEL FOR THIS INDICATION.**	Limited studies show modest reduction in craving and use of cocaine.
Baclofen (Lioresal)	**OFF LABEL FOR THIS INDICATION.**	Limited studies show modest reduction in craving and use of cocaine.
Cocaine vaccine		Investigational, early results promising.

and water. Acetaldehyde accumulates and causes nausea, vomiting, headache, flushing, and lightheadedness and may result in significant hypotension and syncope.[39,40]

Disulfiram does not have direct effects on craving but rather works as a deterrent to drinking. However, studies of self-administration have shown little effect, and in order to be effective, disulfiram should be monitored by a third party, which may be a motivated spouse, friend, supervisor, or coworker. Disulfiram should be prescribed only when there is no ethyl alcohol present; a blood alcohol concentration (BAC) should be checked, or a minimum of 24 hours should have passed since the last drink.

Although it is generally effective in a dose of 250 mg daily, patients may require doses of 500 mg per day. In monitored settings, disulfiram may be given in doses of 500 mg on Monday and Wednesday, with 750 mg on Friday. However, GI intolerance, with nausea, vomiting, and diarrhea, may increase at higher dose levels. It is critical to discuss with prospective patients disulfiram side effects and to warn against accidental alcohol exposure, which may be associated with foods (wine vinegar, alcohol used in cooking), liquid medications preserved with ethyl alcohol (cough and cold medications and others), and rarely exposure to alcohol in perfumes and colognes. In addition, breathing in the fumes of alcohol-based skin sanitizers (Purell and others) by washing hands close to the face, can result in absorption of alcohol.

Unsupervised disulfiram treatment has relatively poor results.[39] However, monitored treatment where a responsible individual in the home, workplace, or elsewhere directly observes the patient taking the medication daily (or three times weekly in higher doses) may have better results. This has been especially effective in impaired professional programs, in which physicians, nurses, and other health care professionals with alcohol addiction are mandated by their licensing boards to take disulfiram under supervision.

Disulfiram reactions are usually self-limited but in severe cases may require IV fluids, and there are anecdotal reports of the benefit of antiemetics, antihistamines, and ascorbic acid; the author has had good experience giving sublingual aspirin.[41] In individuals with underlying coronary heart disease, peripheral arterial disease, and cerebrovascular disease, however, hypotension associated with disulfiram reactions may be more problematic. Disulfiram also blocks dopamine β-hydroxylase, an enzyme involved in cocaine metabolism, and there are ongoing studies of its use for this indication.

Acamprosate Acamprosate is a homotauric acid derivative that modulates glutamatergic transmission by antagonizing the *N*-methyl-D-aspartate (NMDA) pathway in the CNS and appears to reduce the severity of postacute withdrawal syndromes in newly recovering alcoholics. This has an important effect on reducing alcohol craving. Several studies[42,43] have shown benefit of acamprosate. However, a large multisite study, Project Combine, failed to show statistically significant benefits of acamprosate.[44] The author believes that acamprosate resulted in a higher level of complete abstinence in a smaller group of individuals, while naltrexone (see below) resulted in more sustained reduction in drinking in a larger group of patients; however, there was a lower rate of total abstinence.

Acamprosate is remarkably free of side effects, with mild GI symptoms only, which generally abate. However, it has to be taken as 666 mg (two 333-mg tablets) three times daily for efficacy. It has no known drug interactions and may be combined with disulfiram or naltrexone to increase effects on alcohol craving. Although there are no published studies showing benefit of such drug combinations, the author has used them in many patients with good effect.

Naltrexone Naltrexone has been discussed above and obviously is contraindicated in patients who are receiving opioids or for whom opioid treatment is contemplated. However, in alcoholic patients at high risk for relapse in whom non-opioid pain treatment is contemplated, naltrexone may be very useful in preventing relapse.[44-46] Although the mechanism is not clear, it appears that alcohol works, in part, by the production of adduction products, tetrahydroisoquinolones (THIQs), which have opioid activity. Blocking this effect reduces the reinforcing activity of consuming alcohol, and individuals on naltrexone, if they have a brief drinking episode (a "slip" or "lapse"), are far less likely to develop a full relapse (a fall). Doses of 50 mg daily, or 100 mg on Monday and Wednesday with 150 mg on Friday in a monitored setting, are generally effective. Nausea and vomiting are the major side effects, and these decrease with continuing use in most patients.

While there is a "black box" liver warning in the prescribing information, there are no reported cases, of this drug causing hepatic toxicity in current doses; prior studies using 250 to 500 mg per day were associated with rare cases of very high transaminase levels, and it is recommended that ALT/AST be monitored prior to administration and that three times upper limits of normal (ULN) be considered a relative contraindication to prescribing or continuing naltrexone.

Naltrexone is also available as a SR injection (Vivitrol®), which is given every 4 weeks. It is a deep IM injection, generally given in the gluteus maximus muscle, and injection site pain, swelling, and rarely infection may occur.[47,48] The monthly injection has fewer gastrointestinal (GI) side effects and is generally well tolerated and eliminates the compliance issues with daily use of the medication. Pain in those on naltrexone can be treated similarly to that described for patients taking methadone and buprenorphine (see above and reference 29).

Additional Medications While disulfiram, naltrexone, and naltrexone ER (Vivitrol®) are approved for the treatment of alcoholism, there are several medications in clinical trials that have shown benefit but would be off-label if given for that indication. Topirimate has been extensively studied for alcohol[49] and cocaine and other stimulant abuse.[50,51] Dosing for topirimate is similar to that used in treatment for seizure disorders and migraine prophylaxis, and the side effects and precautions are similar. Ondansetron has had results comparable to naltrexone, but only in Cloninger type 2 (Babor type B) alcoholics (e.g., men with strong family histories of alcoholism, early onset disease, and high levels of psychopathology and criminality).[52]

A large number of medications and herbal preparations have shown some effects in small, open label studies (e.g., St. John's Wort, kudzu root), but the risk/benefit ratios for these are unknown, and they should all be considered investigational at this time. Combinations of antidepressants (particularly SSRI and SNRI agents) with anticraving drugs have been used successfully, particularly in patients with underlying mood disorders. Studies of combinations of gabapentin and naltrexone have also yielded positive results. However, many of these studies are smaller, open-label trials and have not been replicated in larger multicenter randomized controlled trials. Caution is indicated, and these agents should not be first-line considerations at this time.

COCAINE AND OTHER STIMULANTS

There are no approved medications for individuals who abuse cocaine and stimulants. Psychosocial treatment, with medication as needed supportively (e.g., brief use of anxiolytics), and treatment of underlying psychiatric disorders are the standards of care. In individuals whose triggers to abuse cocaine and stimulants are other drugs, such as alcohol or opioids, the use of agents to reduce craving may result in reduction of cocaine and stimulant use.

Topirimate has shown positive early results in trials for decreasing cocaine use and craving[50] as well as methamphetamine use.[51] In patients who may have alternative indications for topirimate, such as a seizure disorder or migraine prophylaxis, it may be more of a first-line drug in the presence of cocaine or other stimulant abuse. Disulfiram, described above for alcohol dependence treatment, may have utility in reducing cocaine craving, perhaps secondary to its effects on blocking dopamine-β-hydroxylase as well as acetaldehyde dehydrogenase.[53]

The use of amantadine, rimantadine, bromocriptine, and tricyclic antidepressants (particularly desipramine) has waned because of little evidence of sustained effects from any of these agents. There is ongoing investigation of *N*-acetylcysteine,[54] baclofen,[55] and other agents, but their use is considered investigational at this time. Early work on a cocaine vaccine has yielded positive results.[56] A large number of agents have been tried with initial success in small, open-label studies, but positive results have not been found in larger, randomized, controlled studies. The physician is encouraged to follow the current literature.

DRUGS USEFUL IN TREATING OPIOID-DEPENDENT PATIENTS

In opioid-dependent patients who are in treatment for pain where prior experience has shown that opioids cannot be used safely or for those patients in recovery from opioid dependency who would prefer not to receive opioids, consideration can be given to opioid-blocking agents (Table 70-4). Oral naltrexone has been approved for this indication since 1992. The depot IM form (Vivitrol) was approved for this indication in 2010. Although oral naltrexone has a significant number of studies indicating its long-term safety and efficacy in this population,[57,58] the depot form was approved on the basis of relatively limited studies[59,60] and its long-term effects have not been reported, with caution being urged.[61] It is critically important with both agents (oral and IM naltrexone) that patients are completely detoxified from opioids prior to administration, because each may precipitate a severe and potentially life-threatening withdrawal syndrome in the incompletely detoxified patient. Precipitated withdrawal is different from naturally occurring withdrawal, with delirium, seizures, severe agitation, vomiting, aspiration, and other complications, all of which have been witnessed by the author.

In patients who are leaving long-term residential treatment or those who have been incarcerated for long periods of time, the use of depot naltrexone may be useful in promoting abstinence from opioids, with no risk of precipitated withdrawal. However, in more recently detoxified individuals, the author has seen several cases of severe, intractable, and psychotic depression in patients receiving depot naltrexone; the cause, however, is not clear. In addition, the use of these agents may foreclose the option of using opioid treatment, particularly with the depot form, since the blockade may last 4 or more weeks. However, techniques as described above can be used to treat acute or subacute moderate to severe pain in these patients.[29]

Physicians who prescribe opioids to patients on long-term agonist therapy should be aware that there may be a receptor hypersensitization in these patients, with exaggerated responses to even small, therapeutic doses of opioids. If patients who have been on naltrexone or depot naltrexone are to be treated with opioids, caution should be used, with very low doses of medication prescribed, even lower than those given to opioid-naïve patients. A recent event in the Boston area involved a physician who had prescribed depot naltrexone to several hundred patients and had to leave his practice immediately. A number of the patients were unable to locate alternative prescribers and relapsed to opioid use. There were several anecdotal reports of serious overdoses in these patients, sometimes with extremely modest doses of opioid.

MISCELLANEOUS DRUGS OF ABUSE

Other drugs, including cannabinoids, hallucinogens, inhalants, and others, generally do not require detoxification, and no approved medications are shown to improve outcomes. Treatment of target symptoms, using neuroleptic agents, benzodiazepines, and supportive human contact in a calming environment, is generally sufficient. In most cases, intoxication is self-limited, and drug craving is treated supportively. Again, careful evaluation and treatment for underlying psychiatric disorders are essential. In addition, many drugs can produce neuropsychiatric abnormalities, and therefore, specialized evaluation and testing may be necessary.

CONCLUSION

The world of patients with pain and the world of patients with CDs are not two separate universes but rather a Venn diagram with significant overlap. Many patients develop CD as a response to unremitting chronic pain. A number of patients being treated for pain have underlying CD or its risk factors or develop CD during their pain treatment. The pain physician and the addiction medicine/psychiatry practitioner need to develop and use the tools to deal with the alternative problem in their patient population.

This requires both types of practitioners to develop a greater expertise in both areas than might be expected of the average generalist. It also should require a familiarity with the needed expertise that is available in the immediate vicinity of the practitioner in the form of individuals and programs that are well suited for the management of addiction in the pain patient and pain in the patient with addiction. Because neither pain programs nor addiction programs are created equal, it is well worth the time and effort to familiarize oneself with the available resources and refer to the most appropriate resource when needed.

There has been exciting progress in the development of personal medicine, with evidence that response to some anticraving medications may relate to genetic host factors. The efficacy of naltrexone, for example, differs among individuals with different single nucleotide polymorphisms (SNPs) of the dopamine gene.[62] Pain and addiction treatment clinicians should remain current with progress in this important area. All too often, the recognition of underlying or newly developed CD in a patient in a pain program is seen as an indication for dismissal rather than as a challenge and an opportunity to treat both issues. Pain physicians and addiction medicine physicians need to interact formally and informally to a far greater degree than is now the case in most programs. The prescription drug epidemic, which has increased since the late 1990s, will not allow for a fragmented approach to this population. It is hoped that this chapter will contribute in some way to that increased collaboration.

REFERENCES

1. Terry CE. The Harrison Anti-Narcotic Act. *Am J Public Health.* 1915;5:518.
2. Asbury H. *The Great Illusion: An informal History of Prohibition.* Garden City, NY: Doubleday; 1950.
3. Portenoy RK, Foley KM. Chronic use of opiate analgesics in non-malignant pain: report of 38 cases. *Pain.* 1986;25:171-186.
4. Porter J, Jick H. Addiction rare in patients treated with narcotics. *N Engl J Med.* 1980;302:123.
5. CDC Grand Rounds. Prescription drug overdoses: A U.S. epidemic. *MMWR.* 2012;61:10-13.
6. Manchikanti L, Fellow B, Ailinani H, et al. Therapeutic use, abuse, and nonmedical use of opioids: A ten-year perspective. *Pain Physician.* 2010;13:401-435.
7. Office of the President of the United States. *Epidemic: Responding to the Prescription Drug Abuse Crisis.* Available at http://www.whitehouse.gov/sites/default/files/ondcp/policy-and-research/rx_abuse_plan. Accessed October 22, 2012.
8. Portenoy RK, Dole V, Joseph H, et al. Pain management and chemical dependency: evolving perspective. *J Am Med Assn.* 1997;284:592-593.

9. JCAHO. *Pain Assessment and Management Standards [online]*. Available at http://www.jcaho.org/standard/pm 2002. Accessed October 22, 2012.
10. Fishman S, Gallagher RM, Carr D, et al. The case for pain medicine as a medical specialty. *Pain Med.* 2004;5:281-286.
11. Gourlay DH, Heit H. Universal precautions: a matter of mutual trust and responsibility. *Pain Med.* 2006;7:210-211.
12. United States Department of Health and Human Services, Food and Drug Administration. *Risk Evaluation and Mitigation Strategy (REMS) for Extended-Release and Long-Acting Opioids*. Available at http://www.fda.gov/Drugs/DrugSafety/InformationbyDrugClass/ucm163647.htm. Accessed October 2, 2012.
13. Okie S. A flood of opioids, a rising tide of deaths. *N Engl J Med.* 2010;363:1981-1985.
14. Perrone J, Nelson LS. Medication reconciliation for controlled substances — an "ideal" prescription-drug monitoring program. *N Engl J Med.* 2012;366:2341-2343.
15. Rosenblum A, Cruciani RA, Strain EC, Cleland CM, et al. Sublingual buprenorphine/naloxone for treatment of chronic pain in at-risk patients: investigation and pilot test of a clinical protocol. *J Opioid Manag.* 2012;8(6):369-382.
16. Roux P, Sullivan MA, Cohen J, Fugon L, Jones JD, et al. Buprenorphine/naloxone as a promising therapeutic option for opioid using patients with chronic pain: reduction of pain, opioid withdrawal symptoms, and abuse potential of oral oxycodone. *Pain.* 2013 Aug;154(8):1442-1448.
17. *Diagnostic and Statistical Manual, edition 4-TR (Text Revision)*. Arlington VA: American Psychiatric Association. 2000;192-199.
18. *Diagnostic and Statistical Manual, edition 5*. Arlington VA: American Psychiatric Association, 2014.
19. Weissman DE, Haddox JD. Opioid pseudoaddiction—an iatrogenic syndrome. *Pain.* 1989;36(3):363-366.
20. Weissman DE. Understanding pseudoaddiction. *J Pain Sympt Manage.* 1994;9(2):74
21. Fleming MF, Davis J, Passik SD. Reported lifetime aberrant drug-taking behaviors are predictive of current substance use and mental health problems in primary care patients. *Pain Med.* 2008;9:1098-1106.
22. Kissack JC, Bishop J, Roper AL. Ethylglucuronide as a biomarker for ethanol detection. *Pharmacotherapy.* 2008;28:769-81.
23. Volpicelli J, Szalavitz M. *Recovery Options: The Complete Guide*. New York, NY: John Wiley and Sons; 2004.
24. Heit HA. Healthcare professionals and the DEA: trying to get back in balance. *Pain Med.* 2006;7:75.
25. Covington E. The DEA and pain practitioners: Common goals, adversarial stance. *Pain Med.* 2006;7:75.
26. US Department of Health and Human Services, National Institutes of Health. Screening for alcohol use and alcohol-related problems. *Alcohol Alert.* 2005;65:1-7.
27. Butler SF, Fernandez K, Benoit C, et al. Validation of the revised Screener and Opioid Assessment for Patients with Pain (SOAPP-R). *J Pain.* 2008;9:360-372.
28. American Academy of Pain Medicine, American Pain Society, and the American Society of Addiction Medicine. Public Policy Statement on the rights and responsibilities of health care professionals in the use of opioids in the treatment of pain: A consensus document. *Pain Med.* 2004;5:301-302.
29. Alford DP, Compton P, RN, Samet JH. Acute pain management for patients receiving maintenance methadone or buprenorphine therapy. *Ann Intern Med.* 2006;144:127-134.
30. O'Connor PG, Fiellen DA. Pharmacologic treatment of heroin-dependent patients. *Ann Intern Med.* 2001;133:40-54.
31. Kleber HD, Topazian M, Gaspari J, et al. Clonidine and naltrexone in outpatient treatment of opioid withdrawal. *Am J Drug Alcohol Abuse.* 1987;13:1-18.
32. Wartenberg AA. Treatment considerations in the treatment of opioid dependent patients. *Health and Medicine/Rhode Island.* 1999; 82:91-94.
33. Zullino DF, Khazaal Y, Hattenschwiller J, et al. Anticonvulsant drugs in the treatment of substance withdrawal. *Drugs Today.* 2004;40:603-619.
34. Rickels K, Demartinis N, Rynn M, et al. Pharmacological strategies for discontinuing benzodiazepine treatment. *J Clin Psychopharmacol.* 1999;19(6 Suppl 2):125-165.
35. Oude Voshaar RC, Couvee JE, van Balkom AJ, et al. Strategies for discontinuing long-term benzodiazepine use. *Br J Psychiatry.* 2006;189:213-220.
36. Good, P. Letter to Dr. Howard Heit, published in ASAM News 2007. and accessed October 22, 2012 at https://www.naabt.org/links/DEA_Bup_for_pain_letter.pdf.
37. Petrakis H. A rational approach to the pharmacotherapy of alcohol dependence. *J Clin Psychopharmacol.* 2006;26(Suppl 1):3-12.
38. Swift RM. Drug therapy of alcohol dependence. *N Engl J Med.* 1999;340:1482-1490.
39. Fuller RK, Branchey L, Brightwell DR, et al. Disulfiram treatment of alcoholism: a Veterans Administration cooperative study. *JAMA.* 1986;256:1449-1455.
40. Brewer C, Meyers RJ, Johnsen J. Does disulfiram help to prevent relapse in alcohol abuse. *CNS Drugs.* 2000;14:329-341.
41. Liepman MR, Wartenberg AA, Nirenberg TD, et al. Treatment of the disulfiram-ethanol reaction with aspirin: report of a case. *Alcoholism: Clin Exp Res.* 1988;12:333.
42. Mann K, Lehert P, Morgan MY. The effects of acamprosate in the maintenance of abstinence in alcohol-dependent individuals: results of a meta-analysis. *Alcohol Clin Exp Res.* 2004;28:51-63.
43. Mason BJ, Goodman AM, Chabac S, et al. Effect of oral acamprosate on abstinence in patients with alcohol dependence in a double-blind, placebo-controlled trial: the role of patient motivation. *J Psychiatr Res.* 2006;40:383-393.
44. Anton RF, O'Malley SS, Ciraulo DA, et al. Combined pharmacotherapy and behavioral interventions for alcohol dependence: The COMBINE study: a randomized controlled trial. *JAMA.* 2006;295: 2003-2017.
45. Bouza C, Angeles M, Munoz A, et al. Efficacy and safety of naltrexone and acamprosate in the treatment of alcohol dependence: a systematic review. *Addiction.* 2004;99:811-828.
46. Streeton C, Whelan G. Naltrexone, a relapse prevention maintenance treatment of alcohol dependence: a meta-analysis of randomized controlled trials. *Alcohol Alcohol.* 2001;36:544-552.
47. Kranzler HR, Wesson DR, Billot L. Naltrexone depot for treatment of alcohol dependence: a multicenter, randomized, placebo-controlled clinical trial. *Alcohol Clin Exp Res.* 2004;28:1051-1059.
48. O'Malley SS, Garbutt JC, Gastfriend DR, et al. Efficacy of extended release naltrexone in alcohol-dependent patients who are abstinent before treatment. *J Clin Psychopharmacol.* 2007;27:501.
49. Johnson BA, Rosenthal N, Capece JA, et al. Topirimate for treating alcohol dependence: a randomized clinical trial. *JAMA.* 2007;298:1641-1651.
50. Kampman KM, Pettinati H. Lynch KG, et al. A pilot trial of topirimate for the treatment of cocaine dependence. *Drug Alcohol Dep.* 2004;75:233-240.

51. Elkashef A, Kahn R, Yu E, et al. Topiramate for the treatment of methamphetamine addiction: a multi-center placebo-controlled trial. *Addiction*. 2012 July;107(7):1297-30.

52. Johnson BA, Roache JD, Javors MA, et al. Ondansetron for reduction of drinking among biologically predisposed alcoholic patients: a randomized controlled trial. *JAMA*. 2000;284:963-71.

53. Malcolm R, Olive MF, Lechner W. the safety of disulfiram for the treatment of alcohol and cocaine dependence in randomized clinical trials: guidance for clinical practice. *Expert Opin Drug Safety*. 2008;7:459-472.

54. LaRowe SD, Mardikian P, Malcolm R, et al. Safety and tolerability of N-acetylcysteine in cocaine-dependent individuals. *Am J Addict*. 2006;15:105-110.

55. Shoptaw S, Yang X, Rotheram-Fuller EJ, et al. Randomized placebo-controlled trial of baclofen for cocaine dependence: preliminary effects for individuals with chronic patterns of cocaine use. *J Clin Psychiatry*. 2003;64:1440-1448.

56. Shen XY, Orson FM, Kosten TR. Vaccines against drug abuse. *Clin Pharmacol Ther*. 2012 Jan;91(1):60-70.

57. Church SH, Rothenberg JL, Sullivan MA, et al. Concurrent substance use and outcome in combined behavioral and naltrexone therapy for opiate dependence. *Am J Drug Alcohol Abuse*. 2001;27(3): 441-452.

58. Gonzales JP, Brogden RN. Naltrexone: a review of its pharmacologic and pharmacokinetic properties and therapeutic efficacy in the management of opioid dependence. *Drugs*. 1988;35(3):192-213.

59. Krupitsky E, Nunes EV, Ling W, Illeperuma A, Gastfriend DR, Silverman BL. Injectable extended-release naltrexone for opioid dependence: a double-blind, placebo-controlled, multicentre randomised trial. *Lancet*. 2011;377:1506-1513.

60. Wolfe D, Carrieri MP, Dasgupta N, et al. Injectable extended-release naltrexone for opioid dependence—Authors' reply. *Lancet*. 2011;378:666.

61. Mannelli P, Peindl KS, Wu LT. Pharmacological enhancement of naltrexone treatment for opioid dependence: a review. *Subst Abuse Rehabil*. June 2011;2: 113-123.

62. Ashenhurst JR, Bujarski S, Ray LA. Delta and kappa opioid receptor polymorphisms influence the effects of naltrexone on subjective responses to alcohol. *Pharmacol Biochem Behav*. 2012 Aug 27;103(2):253-259.

ADDITIONAL GENERAL READINGS IN ADDICTION MEDICINE/PAIN

The following are the three major American textbooks on substance abuse and addiction medicine. The most recent editions now have several chapters on pain management in the patient with addiction, the neurobiological connections of addiction and pain, and other topics of interest. I have also listed a very widely used handbook on the prescribing of opioids.

Ruiz P, Strain E, eds. *Substance Abuse: A Comprehensive Textbook*. 5th ed. Philadelphia, PA: Lippincott Williams & Wilkins; 2011.

Galanter M, Kleber HD, Brady KT, eds. *Textbook of Substance Abuse Treatment*. 5th ed. Washington, DC: American Psychiatric Publishing; 2015.

Ries RK, Fiellin DA, Miller SC, Saitz R, eds. *The ASAM Principles of Addiction Medicine*. 5th ed. Philadelphia, PA. Wolters Kluwers; 2014.

Fishman SM. *Responsible Opioid Prescribing*. Washington, DC: FSMB Foundation, Waterford Life Sciences; 2007.

Urine Drug Testing

Howard S. Smith
Zahid H. Bajwa

INTRODUCTION

Urine drug testing (UDT) is considered one of the mainstays of adherence monitoring in conjunction with prescription monitoring programs and other screening tools; however, UDT is associated with multiple limitations secondary to potential pitfalls related to drug metabolism, reliability of the tests, and the knowledge of the pain physician.[1] The practice of UDT is more common in a noncancer pain setting than in an oncology or primary care setting; however, it may be utilized in a punitive manner in efforts to "catch" the patient with an inappropriate positive or negative screen result. Unfortunately, this often results in dismissal of the patient from the practice. Drug testing is most commonly used for two reasons: to identify substances that should not be present in the urine (forensic testing) and to detect the presence of prescribed medications (compliance testing).

URINE DRUG TESTING IN CHRONIC PAIN PATIENTS ON CHRONIC OPIOID THERAPY

The use of UDT to monitor patients on chronic opioid therapy (COT) treated in a pain clinic is reasonable; however, this testing is not mandatory for all patients on COT in all settings. The use of UDT should be based on the clinical judgment of the prescribing clinician; however, some clinicians and/or clinics test all patients on COT sporadically based on policy. Katz and Fanciullo[2] propose that although further research is needed, it may be easier and more uniform to conduct routine urine toxicology testing in all patients with chronic pain treated with opioids. By adopting a uniform policy of testing, stigma is reduced while ensuring that those persons dually diagnosed with pain and substance use disorders receive optimal care. With careful explanation of the purpose of testing, patient concerns can be easily addressed.[3,4]

Abnormal UDT results of patients on COT in a chronic pain clinic generally include absence of the prescribed opioid, presence of nonprescribed drugs, presence of illegal drugs, and adulterated urine specimens.[5]

Fishbain and colleagues gathered urine toxicology results among 122 patients who were prescribed opioids for noncancer pain and found abnormal results in 43% of this sample.[6] Michna and colleagues published a report on 226 patients primarily with chronic back pain and found 46.5% of the sample to have abnormal urine toxicology.[5] In a retrospective study of 470 patients, 4 of 10 patients prescribed opioids also had abnormal urine toxicology.[2] In 2003, Katz and colleagues reported that approximately 20% of patients with persistent pain on COT who seem compliant will test positive for an illicit drug and/or another nonprescribed opioid.[7] Cone et al. analyzed a large number (n = 10,922) of urine samples from patients with persistent pain on COT and found that the overall prevalence of illicit drug use was 10.9%.[8] The illicit drugs found in the urine of these patients most often were marijuana, cocaine, and ecstasy-related drugs.[8] Couto and colleagues reported that over 30% of UDT results in chronic pain patients contained at least one other controlled substance in addition to the prescribed opioid.[9] These studies underscore the importance of urine toxicology testing along with behavioral observation and self-report measures to help identify aberrant drug-related behaviour.[10]

METHODS OF URINE DRUG TESTING

The health care professional (HCP) must know which drugs to test for and by what methods, as well as the expected use of the results. Manchikanti and colleagues[11] studied the diagnostic accuracy of POC testing with immunoassay compared to laboratory testing with chromatography in 1000 patients. Compared with laboratory testing for opioids and illicit drugs, immunoassay in-office testing has high specificity and agreement but variable sensitivity, which demonstrates the value of immunoassay drug testing; however, a cautious approach is advocated. Agreement for prescribed opioids was high with the index test (80.4%). The reference test of opioids improved the accuracy by 8.9% from 80.4% to 89.3%. Urine drug testing should not be confrontational, but rather both clinicians and patients should view UDT like any other laboratory test. Because UDT may support or trigger the clinician's suspicions about aberrant drug-taking, it is information that the clinician must view with other factors to see "the whole picture." The clinician must be aware of the limitations of these tests (e.g., low sensitivity of immunoassay for semisynthetic and synthetic opioids). Confirmatory tests should be specifically requested. If the purpose of testing is to find unprescribed or illicit drug use, combination techniques such as gas chromatography and mass spectrometry (GC/MS) or high-performance liquid chromatography (HPLC) are most specific for identifying individual drugs or their metabolites.[12]

Caveats to the use of UDT include the following:

1. Ensure the proper collection, handling, and documentation of the urine specimen.
2. Be knowledgeable regarding interpretation of UDT results.
3. Know specifically what your patient consumed and when it was consumed prior to the urine collection.
4. Know what you are looking for and what you will do when various results come back.

One of the most common urinary drug screens involves fluorescence polarization immunoassay, which detects the "federal five" of marijuana metabolite (delta-9-THC), cocaine metabolite (benzoylecgonine), opiates, phencyclidine (PCP), and amphetamines/methamphetamines. The test has a relatively low sensitivity for semisynthetic and synthetic opioids (e.g., hydrocodone, oxycodone, fentanyl). Therefore, if the test on the patient's urine is negative for the presence of one of these drugs, it does not exclude use. Furthermore, even if the test is positive for a specific drug, a confirmatory test should follow. The confirmatory UDT is based on principles of GC/MS or HPLC. The gold standard is considered to be the GC/MS. The expanded "federal ten" also tests for methadone, propoxyphene (no longer available), methaqualone, benzodiazepines, and barbiturates.

High-performance liquid chromatography (HPLC) uses a stationary phase (usually hydrophobic saturated carbon chains) contained in a stainless steel column in order to help separate, identify, and quantify compounds based on their particular polarities and interactions with the column's stationary phase. Other components may involve a pump providing high pressure to move the mobile phase (e.g. buffered organic solvent mixture) and a detector. The analyte retention times are variable and may be affected by the strength of interactions with the stationary phase as well as the ionic strength and flow rate of the mobile phase. When coupled with multiple mass spectrometers [MS] (e.g., HPLC/MS/MS), these techniques may be particularly effective to identify compounds in UDT.

Care must be taken in the collection of the urine specimen and in ensuring that the "handling chain"/"chain of custody process" to the lab is executed and documented properly. The collection facility should be a private area with no sink basin or access to water/liquids, and the toilet should have pigmented toilet water (e.g., blue). Measurements of urinary creatinine, pH, specific gravity, and temperature should also be ordered and recorded to assist with results interpretation and to increase specimen reliability. To confirm reliability and authenticity of the urine sample, values for each of the variables should be within the following limits:

- Temperature (within 4 minutes of voiding): 90°F to 100°F
- Urinary pH: 4.5 to 8.0
- Urinary creatinine: 20 mg/dL

Additionally, Specimen Validity Testing (SVT) to determine if adulterants/foreign substances were added to urine or if the specimen was substituted should occur (e.g., testing for nitrite, pyridine, glutaraldehyde, bleach, soap). Adulterated specimens may be suspected if nitrate is ≥500 mcg/mL, or pH is ≥11, or exogenous substances are present, or substances are present at significantly higher concentrations than normal physiologic concentration (e.g., chromium + 6 in significant supraphysiologic concentrations).

Appropriate interpretation of UDT is vitally important. Clinicians should appreciate the potential metabolites of the various opioids that their patients are taking (**Table 71-1**). Reisfield and colleagues concluded that family physicians who ordered UDT to monitor patients with persistent pain on COT were not proficient in their interpretation.[13] Nafziger and Bertino described the following factors that may affect the results of UDT: cutoff selection; pharmacogenetics [ultra-rapid metabolizers]; laboratory technology; and subversion/adulteration of the urine specimen[14] (**Table 71-2**).

URINE DRUG TESTING IN CLINICAL PRACTICE

Starrels and colleagues performed a systematic review of treatment agreements and UDT in efforts to reduce opioid misuse in patients with chronic pain and found that evidence was weak in supporting the effectiveness of opioid treatment agreements and UDT in reducing opioid misuse by patients with chronic pain.[15] Although there does not exist robust/rigorous evidence that UDT positively affects outcomes, a number of authors[5,6,8,16-19] demonstrate that UDT provides valuable

TABLE 71-1 Major Opioid Metabolites

Opioid	Major Metabolites	Bioactive Metabolite	Major Metabolic Enzymes
Morphine	Morphine-3-glucuronide	I	UGT2B7
Morphine	Morphine-6-glucuronide	A	UGT2B7
Hydromorphone	Hydromorphone-3-glucuronide	I	UGT2B7
	Hydromorphone-6-glucuronide	A	UGT1A3
Oxycodone	Noroxycodone	A	CYP3A4
Oxycodone	Oxymorphone	A	CYP2D6
Codeine	Codeine-6-glucuronide	A	UGT2B7
Codeine	Morphine	A	CYP2D6
	Norcodeine	A	CYP3A4
Hydrocodone	Norhydrocodone	A	CYP3A4
	Hydromorphone	A	CYP2D6
Oxymorphone	Oxymorphone-3-glucuronide	I	UGT2B7
Oxymorphone	6-hyroxy-oxymorphone	A	U.C.
Propoxyphene	Norpropoxyphene	A	CYP3A4
Meperidine	Normeperidine	A	CYP3A4, CYP2B6, CYP2C19
Fentanyl	Norfentanyl	I	CYP3A4
Buprenorphine	Norbuprenorphine	A	CYP3A4
Methadone	EDDP	I	CYP2B6
Tramadol	O-desmethyl tramadol (M1)	A	CYP2D6
Tapentadol	Tapentadol-O-glucuronide	I	UGT1A9 UGT2B7

I = inactive for analgesia; A = active for analgesia; U.C. = uncertain

TABLE 71-2 Urine drug testing: Typical screening and confirmation cut-off concentrations and detection times for drugs of abuse[1]

Drug	Screening Cut-off Concentrations ng/mL Urine	Confirmation Cut-off Concentrations ng/mL (Nonregulated)	Confirmation Cut-off Concentrations ng/mL (Federally regulated)	Urine Detection Time
Opioids				
Morphine	300	50	2000	3–4 days
Codeine	300	50	2000	1–3 days
Hydrocodone	300	50	2000	1–2 days
Oxycodone	100	50	2000	1–3 days
Methadone	300	100	2000	2–4 days
Benzodiazepines	200	20-50	NA	Up to 30 days
Cocaine	300	50	150	1–3 days
Marijuana	50	15	15	1–3 days for casual use; up to 30 days for chronic use
Amphetamine	1000	100	500	2–4 days
Methamphetamine	1000	100	500	2–4 days
Heroin*	10	10	NA	1–3 days
Phencyclidine	25	10	25	2–7 days for casual use; up to 30 days for chronic use

*6-MAM, the specific metabolite is detected only for 6 hours

information to make clinical decisions and care for patients with persistent pain on COT. Opioid misuse in patients with persistent pain on COT may have a variable and wide-ranging prevalence of 3% to 40%.[20-22] Manchikant et al. gave evidence that UDT has good diagnostic accuracy; is helpful in identifying noncompliance, opioid misuse, and/or use of illicit drugs; and may decrease prescription drug abuse or illicit drug use for patients with persistent pain on COT.[23]

Gupta and colleagues retrospectively reviewed physician opioids prescribing practices in patients with aberrant behaviors for patients at an academic center's chronic pain outpatient clinic and assessed what occurred after they interpreted the patient's UDT results.[24] The urines were categorized as having urine screens that were normal (expected findings based on their prescribed drugs) or abnormal. Abnormal findings were those with: 1) absence of a prescribed opioid; 2) presence of an additional nonprescribed controlled substance; 3) detection of an illicit substance; 4) adulterated urine sample.

When an aberrance occurred, it was most likely in the form of an abnormal UDT, followed by the presence of an illicit drug, and then self-escalating doses, with other types of aberrance comprising a small fraction of the total.[24] Health care provider (HCP) responses to this aberrance generally took the form of five basic types, with a smaller percentage of patients not returning to the clinic and therefore effectively discharging themselves. Of note, the preferred response to the discovery of aberrant behavior was to continue to prescribe opioids. This occurred approximately 55% of the time.[24] Discontinuation of opioid therapy was a distant second at roughly 20% of the responses (**Fig 71-1**) (even with instances in which the same patient had aberrant behavior on multiple occasions). Thus, it appeared that despite their interpreting UDT as abnormal with the presence of an illicit drug, most physicians continued COT without significant changes in treatment.

Barth and colleagues retrospectively reviewed medical records of patients on chronic opioids for longer than than 22 months in a primary care clinic and determined that patients on chronic opioids who have a UDT positive for an illicit opioid or unprescribed opioids are more likely to respond to monitored opioid pharmacotherapy.[25] Patients with a UDT positive for cocaine, alone or in combination, are less likely to resolve aberrant behavior within the structure of a monitored opioid pharmacotherapy program and are more likely to be discharged electively or administratively from the program without significant transition to addiction treatment.[25]

Physicians, specifically those in pain management settings, often believe that UDT may be helpful when utilized routinely to establish baseline information regardless of how much information is available from physicians, prescription monitoring programs, and other sources. In 2008, the Biomedical Research and Education Foundation (BREF) conducted a study based on a questionnaire distributed to 250 attendees of the American Congress of Pain Medicine in New York City.[26] Forty-nine attendees completed it ($n = 49$), most consisting of anesthesiologists, primary care physicians, and physiatrists. When selecting patients for urine testing, some respondents tested all patients who were being prescribed a controlled substance, while others tested a subset of that group. Seven respondents (14%) did not use UDT, 34 (69%) tested only patients who displayed aberrant behavior/drug-taking, and 25 (51%) tested patients that they were considering prescribing a controlled substance for.

The patient population subjected to urine drug testing varied from 0% to 25% of patients (testing practice of 38.8% of respondents) to testing 76% to 100% of patients (22.4% of respondents). The frequency of testing in the survey appears to be most frequently random ("other" as opposed to a calendar-oriented schedule—23 respondents [47%]), but some respondents reported testing monthly (16%)[27] or quarterly (10%).[27] Five respondents performed biannual testing and six (12%) said they tested annually. Testing was sometimes scheduled, but might also be driven by a specific patient action or change in treatment.[26]

Caution must be exercised in interpreting UDT results in a pain practice. True negative urine results for prescribed medication may indicate a pattern of bingeing rather than drug diversion. However, the clinician must not jump to the conclusion that because the laboratory reports a negative test result for the opioid for which the patient is being prescribed, the patient is not taking the opioid. Possible scenarios to explain this include the patient is an ultra-rapid metabolizer of this opioid, bacterial contamination lead to a lower opioid level in the specimen, and a random urine sample with a slightly lower specific gravity (e.g., if the concentration of the opioid is subthreshold, such as 199 ng/mL with a cutoff of 200 ng/mL, the test will be negative for that opioid). If the concentration of the opioid is roughly one-half that of the expected value, possible scenarios include the patient is a rapid metabolizer of the opioid, or the patient is taking a lower dose of opioid because of miscommunication, or the patient is doing well with less pain and decreased the dose but did not inform the pain specialist, or the patient is taking one-half his or her dose and selling the rest. Time of last use of

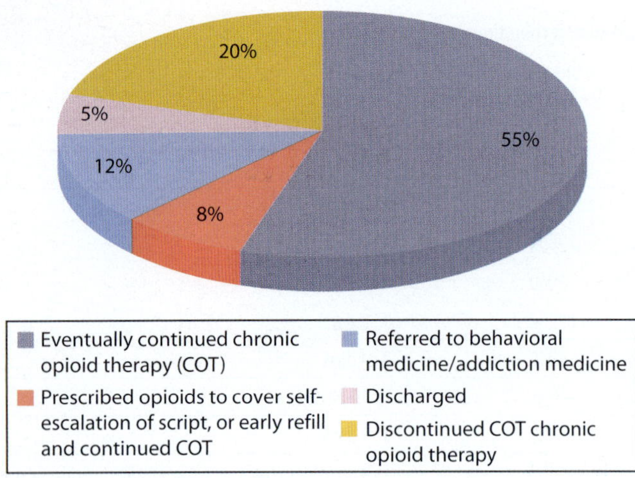

FIGURE 71-1. Estimates of health care provider action breakdown by percent.

the drug(s) and/or serum drug testing for the opioid prescribed can be helpful in interpretation of the results.

In specific patients, UDT may detect traces of unexplained opioids secondary to drug metabolism. For example, a patient taking codeine may show trace quantities of hydrocodone (≥11%) unrelated to hydrocodone use.[28] Detection of small amounts of hydrocodone in urine containing a high concentration of codeine should not be interpreted as evidence of hydrocodone misuse. In a patient who is prescribed hydrocodone, quantities of hydromorphone may also be detected due to hydrocodone metabolism.[3] Morphine may be metabolized to produce small amounts of hydromorphone (≥10%) through a minor metabolic pathway.[29] Quetiapine (Seroquel) may produce false methadone-positive urine drug screens.[30]

Normetabolites such as norcodeine, norhydrocodone, and noroxycodone are metabolites that are not available commercially. Consequently, detection of normetabolite in specimens not containing parent drug provides conclusive evidence that the parent drug was consumed.[31] Cone and colleagues analyzed 2654 urine specimens of pain patients in a chronic pain clinic treated with COT. For specimens containing normetabolite, the prevalence of norcodeine, norhydrocodone, and noroxycodone in the absence of parent drug was 8.6%, 7.8%, and 9.4%, respectively. From one-third to two-thirds of these specimens also did not contain other metabolites that could have originated from the parent drug. The authors concluded that norcodeine, norhydrocodone, and noroxycodone may be useful in interpretation of opiate drug source and may reduce false-negative results that would occur without tests for these unique metabolites.[31]

Urine drug testing may be useful to identify patients who are "poor metabolizers" or "ultra-fast metabolizers." Yee et al. evaluated the metabolism of oxycodone to oxymorphone in a pain patient population using a quantitative liquid chromatography-tandem mass spectrometry analysis of 32,656 urine specimens obtained from pain patients between March 2008 and February 2010.[32] Urine samples containing oxycodone without oxymorphone allowed an estimation of the proportion of poor metabolizers (2.4 ± 2.1%) in the population. A similar analysis of samples containing oxymorphone without oxycodone gave an estimate of the proportion of ultra-rapid metabolizers (1.8 ± 1.1%) in the population; and showed that it may be possible to identify fast or slow metabolizers who may be at risk for adverse events.[32]

SUMMARY

If UDT is utilized, it is crucial to avoid inappropriate interpretation of results, which may adversely affect clinical decision making. The HCP should not infer patient noncompliance or misuse of opioids based on positive or negative detection of opioid in the urine. Results of CDT in conjunction with other tools and clinical information are used when deciding whether to alter the treatment plan.

There is no uniform strategy to deal with specific abnormal results of UDT. Unexplained results should be verified and the discussed with the patient. Each practice should be comfortable dealing with abnormal results in a specific way, but it should be consistent for each practice. Patients found to have substance abuse problems should be referred immediately to an addiction medicine specialist for counseling and treatment. If COT is to be discontinued, it should be tapered gradually and replaced with non-opioid analgesic medications. Algorithms for UDT are available that may help certain clinicians/practices.[1,33] Furthermore, the options of what to do with abnormal results should be known in advance, and patients should be informed of these plans when they first become part of the practice (as long as the clinicians "stick to what they state").

REFERENCES

1. Christo PJ, Manchikanti L, Ruan X, et al. Urine drug testing in chronic pain. *Pain Physician.* 2011;14(2):123-143.
2. Katz N, Fanciullo G. Role of urine toxicology testing in the management of chronic opioid therapy. *Clin J Pain.* 2002;18 (4 Suppl):576-582.
3. Heit HA, Gourlay DL. Urine drug testing in pain medicine. *J Pain Symptom Manage.* 2004;27(3):260-267.
4. Heit HA. *Use of Urine Toxicology Tests in a Chronic Pain Practice.* 3rd ed. Chevy Chase, MD: American Society of Addiction Medicine; 2003.
5. Michna E, Jamison RN, Pham LD, et al. Urine toxicology screening among chronic pain patients on opioid therapy: frequency and predictability of abnormal findings. *Clin J Pain.* 2007;23(2): 173-179.
6. Fishbain DA, Curlter RB, Rosomoff HL, Rosomoff RS. Validity of self-reported drug use in chronic pain patients. *Clin J Pain.* 1999;15(3):184-191.
7. Katz N, Sherburne S, Beach M, et al. Behavioral monitoring and urine toxicology testing in patients receiving long-term opioid therapy. *Anesth Analg.* 2003;97(4):1097-1102.
8. Cone EJ, Caplan YH, Black DL, Robert T, Moser F. Urine drug testing of chronic pain patients: licit and illicit drug patterns. *J Anal Toxicol.* 2008;32(8):530-543.
9. Couto JE, Rommey MC, Leider HL, Sharma S, Goldfarb NI. High rates of inappropriate drug use in the chronic pain population. *Popul Health Manage.* 2009;12(4):185-190.
10. Jamison RN, Serraillier J, Michna E. Assessment and treatment of abuse risk in opioid prescribing for chronic pain. *Pain Res Treat.* 2011;2011:941808.
11. Manchikanti L, Malla Y, Wargo BW, Fellows B. Comparative evaluation of the accuracy of immunoassay with liquid chromatography tandem mass spectrometry (LC/MS/MS) of urine drug testing (UDT) opioids and illicit drugs in chronic pain patients. *Pain Physician.* 2011;14(2):175-188.
12. Vandevenne M, Vandenbussche H, Verstraete A. Detection time of drugs of abuse in urine. *Acta Clin Belg.* 2000;55(6):323-333.
13. Reisfield GM, Webb FJ, Bertholf RL, Sloan PA, Wilson GR. Family physicians' proficiency in urine drug test interpretation. *J Opioid Manag.* 2007;3(6):333-337.

14. Nafziger AN, Bertino JS. Utility and application of urine drug testing in chronic pain management with opioids. *Clin J Pain.* 2009;25(1):73-79.

15. Starrels JL, Becker WC, Alford DP, et al. Systematic review: treatment agreements and urine drug testing to reduce opioid misuse in patients with chronic pain. *Ann Intern Med.* 2010;152(11):712-720.

16. Kahan M, Srivastava A, Wilson L, Gourlay D, Midmer D. Misuse of and dependence on opioids. *Can Fam Physician.* 2006;52(9):1081-1087.

17. Heit HA, Gourlay DL. Urine drug testing in pain medicine. *J Pain Symptom Manage.* 2004;27(3): 260-267.

18. Passik SD, Kirsh KL. Opioid therapy in patients with a history of substance abuse. *CNS Drugs.* 2004;18(1):13-25.

19. Macario A, Pergolizzi JV Jr. Urine drug testing in chronic pain patients taking opioids: a clinical practice update. *Int J Pain Med Palliat Care.* 2005;4:133-139.

20. Fishbain DA, Cole B, Lewis J, Rosomoff HL, Rosomoff RS. What percentage of chronic nonmalignant pain patients exposed to chronic opioid analgesic therapy develop abuse/addiction and/or aberrant drug-related behaviors? A structured evidence-based review. *Pain Med.* 2008;9(4):444-459.

21. Hoffmann NG, Olofsson O, Salen B, Wickstrom L. Prevalence of abuse and dependency in chronic pain patients. *Int J Addict.* 1995;30(8):919-927.

22. Trescot AM, Boswell MV, Arluri SL, et al. Opioid guidelines in the management of chronic non-cancer pain. *Pain Physician.* 2006;9(1):1-39.

23. Manchikanti L, Abdi S, Arluri S, et al. American Society of Interventional Pain Physicians (ASIPP) Guidelines for Responsible Opioid Prescribing in Chronic Non-cancer Pain: Part I—Evidence Assessment. *Pain Physician.* 2012; In Press.

24. Gupta A, Patton C, Diskina D, Cheatle M. Retrospective review of physician opioid prescribing practices in patients with aberrant behaviors. *Pain Physician.* 2011;14(4):383-389.

25. Barth KS, Becker WC, Wiedemer NL, et al. Association between urine drug test results and treatment outcome in high-risk chronic pain patients on opioids. *J Addict Med.* 2010;4(3):167-173.

26. Pegolizzi J, Pappagallo M, Stauffer J, et al. The Integrated Drug Compliance Study Group. The role of urine drug testing for patients on opioid therapy. *Pain Pract.* 2010;10(6):497-507.

27. CMS Manual System. (2004)Pub 100-04 medicare claims processing, transmittal 1884. [WWW document]. URLhttp://www.cms.hhs.gov/transmittals/downloads/R1884CP.pdf. Accessed June 4, 2012.

28. Oyler JM, Cone EJ, Joseph RE Jr, et al. Identification of hydrocodone in human urine following controlled codeine administration. *J Anal Toxicol.* 2000;24(7):530-535.

29. Cone EJ, Heit HA, Caplan YH, et al. Evidence of morphine metabolism to hydromorphone in pain patients chronically treated with morphine. *J Anal Toxicol.* 2006;30(1):1-5.

30. Cherwinski K, Petti TA, Jekelis A. Falsemethadone-positive urine drug screens in patients treated with quetiapine. *J Am Acad Child Adolesc Psychiatry.* 2007;46(4):435-436.

31. Cone EJ, Zichterman A, Heltsley R, et al. Urine testing for norcodeine, norhydrocodone, and noroxycodone facilitates interpretation and reduces false negatives. *Forensic Sci Int.* 2010; 198(1-3):58-61.

32. Yee DA, Best BM, Atayee RS, Pesce AJ. Observations on the urine metabolic ratio of oxymorphone to oxycodone in pain patients. *J Anal Toxicol.* 2012;36(4):232-238.

33. Koyyalagunta D, Burton AW, Toro MP, Driver L, Novy DM. Opioid abuse in cancer pain: report of two cases and presentation of an algorithm of multidisciplinary care. *Pain Physician.* 2011;14(4): E361-E371.

CHAPTER 72 Novel Opioid Formulations

Lynn R. Webster

INTRODUCTION: WHY NOVEL FORMULATIONS?

The medical profession recognizes the clinical value of prescribed opioids in treating noncancer pain that is persistent and recalcitrant to other therapies.[1] However, the clinical benefit of conventional opioid formulations falls short of the need. Although analgesia from opioids is often limited to a subset of patients who achieve benefit, long-term analgesic efficacy is uncertain, and discontinuation of therapy due to adverse events or inadequate analgesia is common.[2]

Furthermore, opioids are dangerous when used inappropriately. Statistics reveal a trend toward unintended harm involving opioids:

- 5.1 million persons in the United States used opioids nonmedically in 2010, and 2 million persons tried nonmedical opioids for the first time.[3]
- Nonmedical prescription opioid use is responsible for more than 305,000 emergency department visits per year.[4]
- Prescribed and diverted opioids were involved in more than 14,800 fatal poisonings in 2008, a nearly fourfold increase from 1999.[5]

The accurate number of deaths caused by prescription drugs is difficult to confirm because data collected by medical examiners and eventually recorded by the Centers for Disease Control and Prevention (CDC) are inadequate to understand the cause of death in many patients.[6] Nevertheless, the rise in the number of unintentional overdose deaths is alarming.

Harm from opioids affects two dissimilar populations: patients who are prescribed opioids, sometimes for a long-term, to treat a pain problem, and nonpatients who use opioids without a prescription. Patients who are prescribed opioids may engage in *medical misuse* (e.g., overusing, mixing with unauthorized substances, and unlawful sharing with others). *Nonmedical use* by nonpatients can include experimentation, recreation, or use to self-medicate pain or psychiatric disorders. The spectrum of opioid misuse ranges from patients who use an extra pill in search of greater pain relief to patients and nonpatients who are suffering from the disease of addiction and who go to extreme, even illegal, lengths to obtain opioids (**Fig 72-1**).[7]

Motives for misuse, short of addiction, vary. Based on the self-reports of 80 nondependent, recreational users of opioids, the most common feelings obtained from opioids were to feel relaxed or mellow (80%),

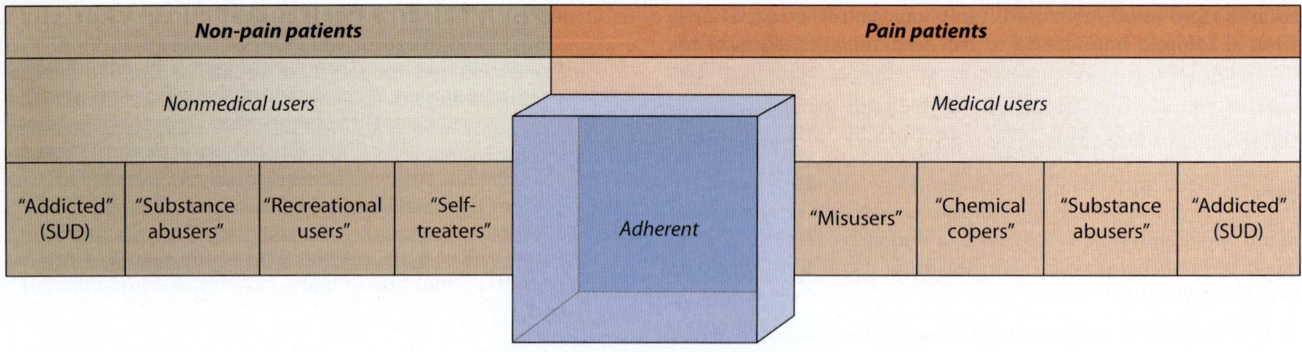

FIGURE 72-1. The Spectrum of Opioid Misuse: Patients and Non-Patients. The spectrum of misuse involves two different populations—patients and nonpatients—with behaviors that range from mild to severe. Motivations for nonpatients range from using non-prescribed opioids to self-treat pain, to recreation, to serious substance-use disorders. Although most patients are strictly adherent, some misuse opioids by taking them other than as directed, to self-treat uncontrolled pain, to chemically cope with a psychiatric disorder, or because of addiction.[7]

happy or pleasant (71%), and calm or less nervous (63%) (**Fig 72-2**). Most participants (55%) first took an opioid to treat pain; however, 38% first took an opioid for the purpose of getting high (**Fig 72-3**).[8]

The pharmaceutical industry has responded to the rise in opioid-related harm by developing several formulations that employ technologies to resist or deter misuse and to boost analgesic efficacy. Methods include modifying the route of delivery, combining opioid agonists with opioid antagonists or aversive agents that become active if altered, and targeting intracellular or molecular processes within the body. Most formulations are still in development, and none has yet been proved to deter substance abuse in real-world settings.

NEW DELIVERY SYSTEMS

BIOERODIBLE MUCOADHESIVE BUPRENORPHINE FORMULATION

First introduced via a buccal fentanyl product to treat breakthrough pain,[10] BEMA (BioErodible MucoAdhesive) technology is now being applied to other opioids. The technology is a small, bilayered, bioerodable, polymer film consisting of a backing layer and a muco-adhesive layer which contains the active drug.[11] Designed to cling to oral mucosa in less than 5 seconds and dissolve within 15 to 30 minutes; the developers claim the product optimizes delivery across the mucosa.

A formulation now in development combines BEMA technology with buprenorphine, a partial μ (mu) agonist and a κ (kappa) antagonist with a high affinity for μ opioid receptors.[12] Buprenorphine (monotherapy or in combination with naloxone) has a long history as an addiction treatment but is often used off-label for pain control and—as a Schedule III medication—is considered to have a lower propensity for misuse than other opioids. A randomized, placebo-controlled, Phase 3 clinical study of BEMA buprenorphine for the management of moderate to severe pain failed to meet the primary efficacy endpoint of pain-intensity difference compared with placebo.[13] Investigators cited a large placebo response in new opioid users compared with experienced users and planned a follow-up efficacy study.

BUPRENORPHINE FILM

A sublingual film formulation of combination buprenorphine/naloxone is currently available for the treatment of opiate dependence and is also expected to be used off-label as a treatment for pain with less presumed misuse and diversion potential. The film is placed under the tongue where it dissolves in approximately 5 minutes.[14] Clinical testing has established comparable safety and efficacy to the tablet form of buprenorphine/naloxone medication.[14]

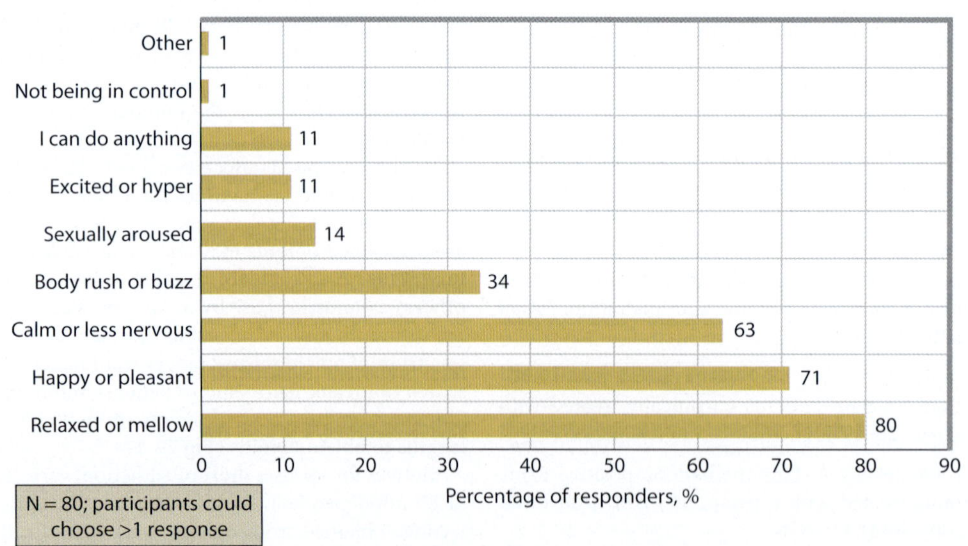

FIGURE 72-2. Motives for Misuse: How Would You Describe the Feeling of "High" From Prescription Opioids? Nondependent, recreational opioid users explain the effect(s) they seek in misusing opioids.[8]

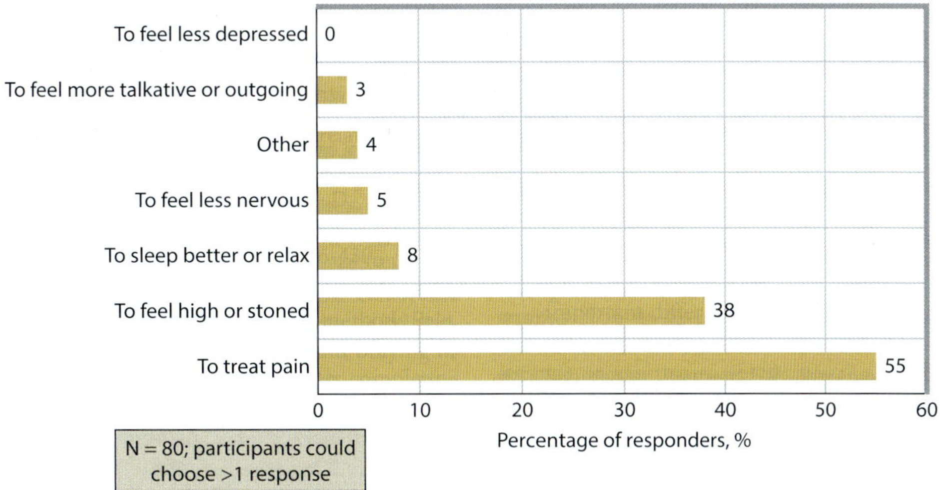

FIGURE 72-3. Initial Exposure: Why Did You Take an Opioid the First Time? Nondependent, recreational opioid users describe their initial reason(s) for taking an opioid.[8] Many opioid misusers chemically or physically alter the formulation (e.g., chewing, crushing, dissolving in alcohol or water) before ingesting in order to defeat controlled-release (CR) formulations and gain access to a full dose at once. Data from the Treatment Episode Data Set (TEDS) through the Substance Abuse and Mental Health Services Administration (SAMHSA) show that most persons admitted for substance-abuse treatment because of opioids took the medication orally (72%).[9] Other routes included inhaling (16%), injecting (10%), smoking (2%), and other (1%).

TRANSDERMAL BUPRENORPHINE

A transdermal buprenorphine that delivers a systemic dose through a patch that is changed every 7 days is approved for the treatment of moderate to severe pain. The formulation has not been studied for addiction treatment. Patient applies the patch to the upper outer arm, upper chest, upper back, or the side of the chest to receive a steady, continuous dose via an adhesive polymer matrix. Transdermal buprenorphine demonstrated equal analgesia with greater tolerability and fewer side effects compared with sublingual buprenorphine[15] and has an efficacy and tolerability profile comparable to twice-daily tramadol.[16]

TRANSMUCOSAL FENTANYL SPRAY

A sublingual fentanyl spray is in development for the treatment of breakthrough pain in opioid-tolerant cancer patients. A phase 3, randomized, double-blind, placebo-controlled multicenter study showed a statistically significant difference in the sum of pain intensity scores at 30 minutes, which was the primary endpoint, and at all other time points measured (5, 10, 15, 45, and 60 min).[17] Significant pain relief at 5 minutes postdose appears particularly well matched to treat the sudden flares of intense pain that characterize breakthrough pain.[18]

PRODRUGS

A completely different approach uses prodrugs or less soluble opioid salts that remain inert until a molecular process occurs in the body, thus releasing the active ingredient. In some formulations, the process occurs within the gastrointestinal (GI) tract, and in others, only when the ingredient enters a cell.

An example of prodrug technology uses a Bio-Activated Molecular Delivery system to release an active opioid at the molecular level only if the drug is ingested with no effects from inhaling, chewing, or injecting.[19] An additional feature of the formulation is meant to provide protection against oral overdose in that ingesting multiple pills would not equal a dose-proportional increase in active opioid exposure. A phase 1 human proof-of-concept study using hydromorphone confirmed the dose-proportional release of the opioid.[19] The study also demonstrated that the emergency department pharmacokinetic profile is intrinsic to the molecule, in contrast to other opioid products that reformulate opioids with physical matrices that may be circumvented. Further testing of these technologies is due with oxycodone and hydrocodone.

This category of formulations may prove useful for the most difficult-to-help category of medication misusers—those who do not tamper with or alter a pill but instead take an extra pill because of inadequate analgesia. Theoretically, prodrug formulations have potential to mitigate misuse but are expensive to develop.

FIRST-GENERATION FORMULATIONS WITH REDUCED MISUSE POTENTIAL

The first generation of novel opioid formulations was developed to resist or deter misuse when the formulation is altered. These formulations consist of the same opioid molecule contained in available prescription medications reformulated in combination with agents intended to act as physical or chemical barriers. Therefore, these formulations are principally aimed at deterring recreational or other nonmedical users who are attempting to convert a controlled-release (CR) formulation into an immediate-release (IR) formulation.

Based on the regulatory response thus far, the Food and Drug Administration (FDA) appears to view many first-generation formulations as offering little proven protection against opioid misuse. A large drawback is the lack of defense against oral overconsumption when swallowed whole. Thus, the relevance of many first-generation formulations to the needs of patients who are prescribed opioids is uncertain.

PHYSICAL BARRIERS

Strategies to limit opioid misuse are aimed at reducing the individual's ability to crush or dissolve the pill in order to snort or inject the full dose. One approach is to house the active pharmaceutical ingredient within a capsule that is tamper resistant. For example, a CR oxycodone formulation in a viscous base that is difficult to crush or chemically alter is currently in development (**Fig 72-4**).[20,21] The liquid matrix resists crushing, chewing, and extracting with liquid solvents and also resists injection because it cannot be drawn into or expressed from needles. At press time, the FDA had not approved the formulation for the market.[22]

A similar formulation combines IR oxycodone with a tamper-resistant gelling agent that resists extraction of the active ingredient. The formulation, which also contains sodium lauryl sulphate as a nasal irritant to prevent snorting, was approved by the FDA on June 17, 2011, for the treatment of acute and moderate to severe chronic pain.[23]

An available CR hydromorphone formulation uses patented OROS technology to deliver a steady once-daily dose through push-pull osmotic pressure.[24] The bilayer tablet appears to have tamper-resistant qualities, although no such claims are made on the product's label.

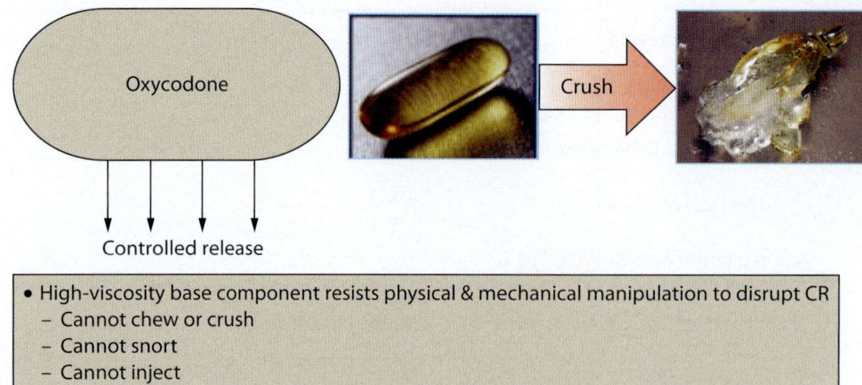

FIGURE 72-4. A Tamper-Resistant Opioid Formulation: Gelatin-Capsule, Controlled-Release Oxycodone. Viscous gel-cap base resists fracturing in order to preserve CR of oxycodone. *Source*: Pfizer Inc./Pain Therapeutics, Inc.

A reconstituted form of CR oxycodone containing polyethylene oxide as a tamper-resistant agent has been developed and approved by the FDA.[25] The polyethylene oxide forms a gel in the presence of moisture so that the pills resist crushing. No specific misuse-resistant claims are made, but postmarketing epidemiological data will be collected to determine whether the new formulation reduces the tampering and misuse observed with the company's conventional CR oxycodone formulation.

Yet another sustained-release (SR) oxycodone formulation (COL-003) consists of a capsule containing particles of the opioid in a waxy excipient base. This is known as DETER$_X$ technology, and the particles are designed to maintain SR properties even if crushed or chewed. Pharmacokinetic testing in 12 volunteers indicated that chewing the formulation did not compromise the SR mechanism but resulted in similar plasma levels to intact COL-003.[26]

CHEMICAL BARRIERS

Chemical barriers are formed when agents with deterrent properties are combined with an opioid. As with formulations that use physical barriers, the goal is to limit the attractiveness of opioids for nonmedical use.

One chemical strategy is to combine an opioid antagonist with an agonist. In one such formulation, an extended-release (ER) morphine pellet contains a sequestered core of naltrexone that remains inert unless the drug is altered, at which time the naltrexone blocks the opioid receptors, limiting euphoric effects (**Fig 72-5**). Safety testing indicated that failure to take the formulation as directed may precipitate withdrawal or lead to reduced efficacy.[27] The formulation was approved by the FDA but later voluntarily withdrawn due to a stability problem identified during routine testing.[28] The FDA confirmed that these issues were resolved and reapproved the medication in 2014.[29]

Another approach to agonist-antagonist formulations releases both agents together. A 2:1 ratio of oxycodone and naloxone, an antagonist with an extensive first-pass metabolism, is available in Europe.[30] This was intended to limit opioid-induced constipation by blocking opioid receptors in the GI tract, and pharmacokinetic testing found the formulation also could induce withdrawal symptoms if crushed and ingested intranasally.[31] Therefore, the mechanism is that of a combination drug when taken as directed and a chemical barrier if the drug is manipulated.

Yet another chemical barrier can be introduced by adding an aversive agent that releases during tampering and ingestion, causing discomfort to the user. One such formulation combines niacin with an IR oxycodone hydrochloride. The niacin is intended to cause heat and flushing during conditions of alteration and misuse, such as crushing and snorting. However, the FDA has found that the niacin effects could be mitigated by food and nonsteroidal anti-inflammatory drugs and deemed the evidence for abuse deterrence inadequate.[32]

PROBLEMS ADDRESSED IN A LIMITED POPULATION

Figure 72-6 illustrates two categories of individuals who use opioids in ways outside of medical direction: medical misusers and nonmedical misusers. The spectrum of medical misusers ranges from patients who infrequently swallow an extra pill or a pill prescribed for someone else to frequent misusers, including those who suffer from the disease of addiction. A high percentage of medical misusers occupy the center box, which

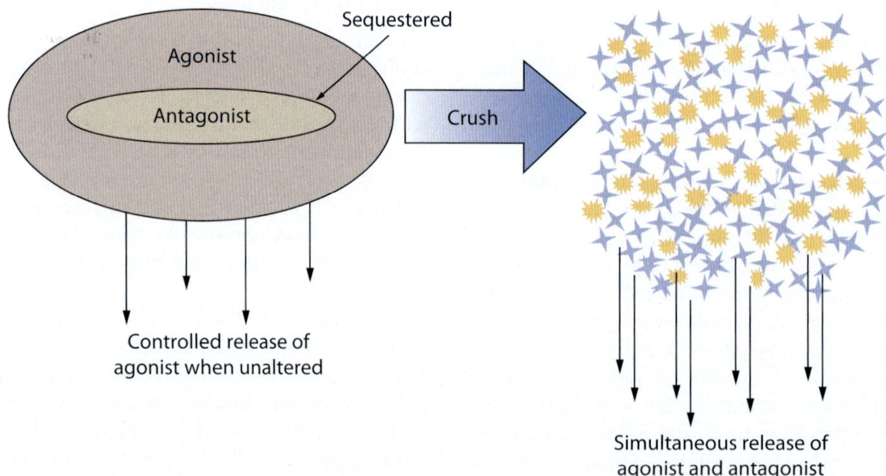

FIGURE 72-5. An Opioid Agonist-Antagonist Formulation: Extended-Release Morphine with Sequestered Naltrexone. A CR of morphine contains sequestered naltrexone that remains inert unless manipulated. Crushing releases naltrexone, reversing opioid effects. *Source*: Pfizer Inc./King Pharmaceuticals, Inc.

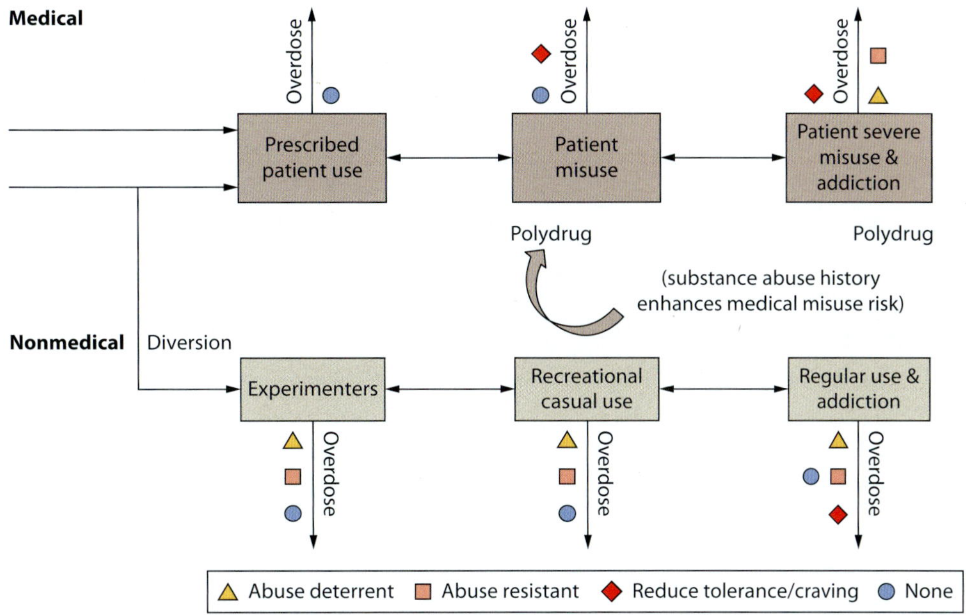

FIGURE 72-6. Populations Most Likely to Realize Benefit from Newer Opioid Formulations. First-generation formulations that incorporate physical and chemical properties to reduce misuse liability work only in users who perform deliberate extraction (i.e., nonmedical users and medical users who demonstrate the most severe misuse behaviors).

is less easily characterized. The lower half of Fig 72-6 illustrates that all nonmedical use follows from the criminal act of diversion. The spectrum of misuse for nonmedical users ranges from one end to the other in severity, with the main distinction being one of frequency of misuse.

Formulations that contain physical (abuse-resistant) and chemical (abuse-deterrent) barriers work only if the misuser has tampered to increase the potency of the formulation and the speed of effect onset. Therefore, chemical and physical barriers protect only those who seek to gain immediate access to the full strength of a CR dose. These include nonmedical users and patients who display the most extreme behaviors related to misuse and (possibly) addiction. For example, a formulation containing a sequestered antagonist may reverse respiratory depression but only if the formulation is crushed.

Limited evidence indicates that a low dose of a nonsequestered opioid antagonist, one that is released during adherent ingestion with the opioid agonist, may slow the pace of tolerance, leading to less craving and less need to escalate doses to overcome inadequate analgesia.[33] However, the research is inconclusive and the clinical significance of such a finding is unclear. Combination agonist-antagonist formulations have shown clinical utility in treating opioid-induced constipation.[31] Additionally, a low dose of a nonsequestered antagonist might help prevent overdose, but no evidence supports such an assertion.

THE LARGEST UNMET NEED

The principal shortcoming of the first generation of opioid formulations is the failure to block the primary method of overuse and overdose, which is ingesting the pill orally without crushing or tampering with it.[9] Currently, to gain protection from one of the newer formulations that incorporate physical and chemical barriers, a would-be misuser must perform an intentional act of extraction. This lack of protection has relevance along the entire spectrum of opioid misuse. A recreational user who decides to experiment can die from the one time he or she uses nonmedical opioids orally.

THE PROGRESS OF NOVEL FORMULATIONS

Table 72-1 shows the progress of a number of newer opioid formulations and delivery systems through the pharmaceutical development pipeline. The list is not meant to be comprehensive but represents a sample of the most interesting research in this area.

A sublingual buprenorphine/naloxone indicated for addiction treatment and a transdermal buprenorphine patch for moderate to severe pain have been approved by the FDA. Three formulations that incorporate physical barriers to misuse are also currently available. In some cases the FDA has challenged proof of misuse deterrence or asked for more data. No product using prodrug technology is yet on the market.

ISSUES THAT REMAIN

WHO WILL BENEFIT FROM NEWER OPIOID FORMULATIONS?

A question that remains is who should receive these medications. Webster (the current author) and Fine argued for considering newer opioid formulations a component of universal precautions to be applied to all long-term opioid patients.[34] The argument is that to do so would mitigate the greatest quantity of opioid-related harm in the event such formulations are approved, are introduced to market, and demonstrate true reduced misuse liability through postmarketing surveillance.

THE POTENTIAL BURDEN TO ADHERENT PATIENTS

Emerging formulations have the potential to ease the public health burden of opioid-related harm; however, to accomplish this goal would involve removal of conventional, alterable formulations from the market. The scientific support for such a far-reaching move is not yet adequate. Newer formulations frequently demonstrate less misuse liability compared with conventional formulations and analgesic efficacy over placebo in industry-supported clinical trials, but it is unknown whether clinical trial success would translate to real-world benefit. Dedicated substance abusers are highly adaptive when presented with novel technologies, and new extraction methods or simple overuses are still possible.

In light of these uncertainties, the question remains whether it is fair to ask adherent pain patients who achieve analgesia and improved quality of life using conventional opioids to shoulder potential burdens such as increased costs to cover drug development. Perhaps, instead, society could consider sharing costs more broadly given the widespread societal harm from opioid misuse and overdose. Such an approach would require robust scientific evidence that newer formulations bring true benefit in reversing trends of opioid misuse.

TABLE 72-1 Development Status of Novel Opioids

Formulation	Technology	Company	Development
New Delivery Systems:			
Sublingual buprenorphine/naloxone	Dissolvable film	Reckitt Benckiser Pharmaceuticals, Inc	FDA approved (for addiction treatment)
Transdermal buprenorphine	7-day adhesive patch	Purdue Pharma LP	FDA approved
Sublingual fentanyl	Sublingual spray	INSYS Therapeutics, Inc	NDA submitted
Buccal buprenorphine	Bilayer, dissolvable, polymer film	BioDelivery Sciences International, Inc.	Phase III
Prodrug at molecular level	Bioactivated molecular delivery + overdose protection	PharmacoFore, Inc.	Phase 1
Chemical Barriers:			
Oxycodone + naloxone (2:1)	Combination drug if taken intact/Induces withdrawal if crushed	Mundipharma International Limited	Available in Europe
SR morphine + naltrexone	Sequestered antagonist	Pfizer/King	Withdrawn by manufacturer/ reapproved 2014
IR oxycodone + niacin	Aversive agent (niacin)	Pfizer/Acura/King	Rejected by FDA panel
Physical Barriers:			
IR oxycodone	Gelling agent	Pfizer/Acura	FDA approved
CR hydromorphone	Osmotic push-pull technology	Covidien	FDA approved
CR oxycodone	Turns viscous with moisture	Purdue Pharma LP	FDA approved
CR oxycodone	Viscous gel	Pfizer/Pain Therapeutics	NDA submitted
SR oral oxycodone (COL-003)	Microparticle formulation	Collegium Pharma, Inc./Endo Pharma, Inc.	Phase III

SR, Sustained release; IR, Immediate release; CR, Controlled release; NDA, New drug application.

The impact of newer opioid formulations is still unknown. Follow-up research should focus on

- Patterns of appropriate or inappropriate use over time and in various populations.
- Treatment-emergent adverse events.
- Effects on analgesia, function, and quality of life in long-term medical users.
- Effects on nonmedical users.

Such effects can be measured only after a drug has been introduced to the market. It is the responsibility of drug developers to examine misuse liability and other effects for the entire life cycle of the product.

A PUBLIC SAFETY ANALOGY: THE SEAT BELT

The automobile seat belt provides an analogy to the current state of innovative opioid formulations. Seat belts were introduced to the American public nearly 80 years ago; however, their common usage was brought about only by legislation and a cultural shift. Seat belts save lives: 13,250 lives in 2008 and more than 75,000 lives during the 5-year period from 2004 to 2008.[35] However, arguments against their widespread use are similar to conversations today concerning opioids formulated to resist misuse (**Table 72-2**).

Critics of mandatory seat belt usage cited overregulation, additional costs, infringement of individual liberties, overestimation of lives saved, and the risk of greater danger because of a false sense of security. Proponents of *risk compensation* theory, who hold that individuals change to riskier behaviors as their perception of risk decreases, point to evidence that drivers increased speed and followed other cars more closely when they were belted.[36]

However, seat belts reduce costs to all of society. Accident victims who did not use seat belts had emergency department costs that were 25% higher than seat belt wearers and were more likely to be admitted to the hospital afterward, according to a University of Wisconsin study.[37] Furthermore, the conversation regarding infringement of individual rights cuts both ways as seat belt proponents argue that non-seat-belt wearers could be forced by an impact into seat belt wearers, injuring them.

To continue the analogy in the language of innovation, research into novel opioid formulations is now in the stage of the lap belt rather than the three-point harness (which provides far greater safety). Further innovations in novel opioid development will be needed to save the most lives from inadvertent overdoses, to improve analgesic effectiveness, and to realize the greatest dollar savings while fairly sharing the costs of implementing the changes.

THE FUTURE OF INNOVATION

The advances of opioid research are encouraging but fall short of the need. Major innovations in development must address motives of persons who over-ingest, including understanding the overuse and misuse patterns of medical compared with nonmedical users. For example, some persons misuse opioids for the psychoactive effect because they suffer from anxiety or depressive disorders.[38] Innovations that selectively target intracellular pathways so as to block specific opioid effects (e.g., respiratory depression, euphoria) while enabling the effect of analgesia should provide the basis of future research. Such a goal is well within the purview of science. To achieve this goal would revolutionize pain control and negate the necessity of pitting the interests of pain medicine against the need to control opioid-related harm.

TABLE 72-2 Comparison of Automobile Seat Belts to Novel Opioid Formulations

Issue	Automobile Seat Belts	Novel Opioid Formulations
Regulation of manufacturers	Federal standards	Risk evaluation and mitigation strategy
Cost	Beneficiary and nonbeneficiary	Beneficiary and nonbeneficiary
Compulsory use	By state	None
Potential risk behaviors	Increased speed, close following	Increased prescribing
Major risk group	Adolescents	Adolescents

SUMMARY

A number of novel opioid formulations aimed at reducing society's exposure to opioid-related harm are currently on the market or in development. Technologies include nonconventional delivery systems, tamper-resistant physical properties, chemical deterrents to achieving a quick release of the active pharmaceutical ingredient, prodrugs that require a biological process to activate the opioid, and—eventually—targeted therapies that provide analgesia while bypassing central psychoactive effects. Still unknown is whether real-world reduced liability and greater efficacy would follow clinical trial success, whether overuse or innovative extraction methods would still occur, and whether the costs of new drug development can be fairly shared by the larger society.

ACKNOWLEDGMENT

Dr. Webster wishes to acknowledge the contribution of medical writer, Beth Dove, Dove Medical Communications, Salt Lake City, Utah, in the preparation of this manuscript.

REFERENCES

1. Chou R, Fanciullo GJ, Fine PG, et al. Clinical guidelines for the use of chronic opioid therapy in chronic noncancer pain. *J Pain*. 2009;10(2):113-130.
2. Noble M, Treadwell JR, Tregear SJ, et al. Long-term opioid management for chronic noncancer pain. *Cochrane Database Syst Rev*. 2010;(1):CD006605.Review.
3. Substance Abuse and Mental Health Services Administration. Results from the 2010 National Survey on Drug Use and Health: Summary of National Findings, NSDUH Series H-41, HHS Publication No. SMA 11-4658. Rockville, MD: Substance Abuse and Mental Health Services Administration; 2011.
4. Substance Abuse and Mental Health Services Administration, Center for Behavioral Health Statistics and Quality. (2011). Drug Abuse Warning Network, 2008: National Estimates of Drug-Related Emergency Department Visits. HHS Publication No. SMA 11-4618. Rockville, MD.
5. Centers for Disease Control and Prevention (CDC). Vital signs: overdoses of prescription opioid pain relievers United States, 1999–2008. *MMWR Morb Mortal Wkly Rep*. 2011;60:1487-1492.
6. Webster LR, Dasgupta N. Obtaining adequate data to determine causes of opioid-related overdose deaths. *Pain Med*. 2011;12(S2):S86-S92.
7. Passik SD, Kirsh KL. The interface between pain and drug abuse and the evolution of strategies to optimize pain management while minimizing drug abuse. *Exp Clin Psychopharmacol*. 2008;16(5):400-404.
8. Setnik B, Roland CL, Cleveland JM, Goli V, Webster LR. Self reports of prescription opioid misuse, abuse and diversion in a sample of dependent, recreational opioid users. Presented at the 10th Annual American Society of Regional Anesthesia and Pain Medicine Annual Meeting; November 17-20, 2011; New Orleans, LA.
9. Substance Abuse and Mental Health Services Administration, Office of Applied Studies. Treatment Episode Data Set (TEDS): 1997-2007. National Admissions to Substance Abuse Treatment Services, DASIS Series: S-47, DHHS Publication No. (SMA) 09-4379, Rockville, MD, 2009.
10. Davies A, Finn A, Tagarro I. Intra- and interindividual variabilities in the pharmacokinetics of fentanyl buccal soluble film in healthy subjects: a cross-study analysis. *Clin Drug Investig*. 2011;31(5):317-324.
11. BioDelivery Sciences International, Inc. BEMA Technology. Available at: http://www.bdsi.com/BEMA_Technology.aspx. Accessed Nov. 29, 2011.
12. Lutfy K, Cowan A. Buprenorphine: a unique drug with complex pharmacology. *Curr Neuropharmacol*. 2004;2(4):395-402.
13. BioDelivery Sciences International, Inc. BioDelivery Sciences announces results from Phase 3 efficacy study for BEMA buprenorphine in chronic pain. Raleigh, NC: PRNewswire. Sept. 28, 2011.
14. SUBOXONE Sublingual Film [package insert]. Richmond, VA: Reckitt Benckiser Pharmaceuticals Inc; August 2010.
15. James IG, O'Brien CM, McDonald CJ. A randomized, double-blind, double-dummy comparison of the efficacy and tolerability of low-dose transdermal buprenorphine (BuTrans seven-day patches) with buprenorphine sublingual tablets (Temgesic) in patients with osteoarthritis pain. *J Pain Symptom Manage*. 2010;40(2):266-278.
16. Karlsson M, Berggren AC. Efficacy and safety of low-dose transdermal buprenorphine patches (5, 10, and 20 µg/h) versus prolonged-release tramadol tablets (75, 100, 150, and 200 mg) in patients with chronic osteoarthritis pain: a 12-week, randomized, open-label, controlled, parallel-group noninferiority study. *Clin Ther*. 2009;31(3):503-513.
17. Reynolds L, Geach J, Parikh N, et al. Safety and efficacy of fentanyl sublingual (SL) spray in the treatment of breakthrough cancer pain. [Abstract]. *J Pain*. 2011;12(suppl 4): S50.
18. Rauck R, Stearns L, Scherlis M, Parikh N, Dillaha L. Fentanyl sublingual (SL) spray: reduction of breakthrough cancer pain 5-minutes post dose. [Abstract]. *J Pain*. 2011;12(4 Suppl):S50.
19. PharmacoFore: Moderate-to-Severe Pain. PharmacoFore's Solution: Bio-Activated Molecular Delivery Technology. Available at: http://www.pharmacofore.com/view.cfm/39/Moderate-to-Severe-Pain. Accessed Nov. 29, 2011.
20. Setnik B, Roland CL, Cleveland JM, Webster L. The abuse potential of Remoxy, an extended-release formulation of oxycodone, compared with immediate- and extended-release oxycodone. *Pain Med*. 2011;12(4):618-631.
21. Friedmann N, Klutzaritz V, Webster L. Efficacy and safety of an extended-release oxycodone (Remoxy) formulation in patients with moderate to severe osteoarthritic pain. *J Opioid Manag*. 2011;7(3):193-202.
22. Pfizer Inc. and Pain Therapeutics, Inc. *FDA complete response letter received for Remoxy*. New York, NY, and Austin, TX: Business Wire; June 24, 2011.
23. Acura Pharmaceuticals, Inc.: Abuse Deterrent Products. Oxecta tablets. Available at: http://acurapharm.com/products/acurox-without-niacin-tablets. Accessed Nov. 29, 2011.
24. Coluzzi F, Mattia C. OROS® hydromorphone in chronic pain management: when drug delivery technology matches clinical needs. *Minerva Anestesiol*. 2010;76(12):1072-1084.
25. FDA Advisory Committee Briefing Document on NDA 22-272 (reformulated OxyContin tablets), Purdue Pharma L.P.;Sept. 24, 2009.
26. Fleming A, Noonan P, Wheeler A. (281) Abuse-deterrent properties and pharmacokinetics of a novel sustained release formulation of oxycodone for the treatment of moderate to severe pain. *J Pain*. 2008;9(4)(suppl2):S46.
27. Webster LR, Brewer R, Wang C, et al. Long-term safety and efficacy of morphine sulfate and naltrexone hydrochloride extended release capsules, a novel formulation containing morphine and sequestered naltrexone, in patients with chronic, moderate to severe pain. *J Pain Symptom Manage*. 2010;40(5):734-746.
28. Jeffrey S. Morphine/naltrexone combo temporarily withdrawn. *Medscape Today*. March 15, 2011.
29. FDA Approves Labeling with Abuse-Deterrent Features for Embeda (morphine/naltrexone). October 17, 2014. Available at: http://www.drugs.com/newdrugs/fda-approves-labeling-abuse-deterrent-features-embeda-morphine-naltrexone-4101.html.
30. Mundipharma International Limited. Targin (oral oxycodone/naloxone prolonged-release tablet) now launching across Europe to

control severe chronic pain with significantly reduced risk of opioid-induced constipation. Cambridge, UK: PRNewsire Jan. 26, 2009.

31. Decentralised Procedure. Public Assessment Report. Targin 5 mg/2.5 mg, 10 mg/5 mg, 20 mg/10 mg, 40 mg/20 mg prolonged release tablets. DE/H/1612/01-04/DC, BfarM.
32. Acurox (oxycodone HCl and niacin). Briefing information for a joint meeting of the anesthetic and life support drugs advisory committee and drug safety and risk management advisory committee. NDA 22-451. April 22, 2010.
33. Webster LR. Oxytrex: an oxycodone and ultra-low-dose naltrexone formulation. *Expert Opin Investig Drugs.* 2007;16(8):1-7.
34. Webster LR, Fine PG. Approaches to improve pain relief while minimizing opioid abuse liability. *J Pain.* 2010;11(7):602-611.
35. Traffic safety facts: Lives saved in 2008 by restraint use and minimum drinking age laws. Crash Stats. DOT HS 811 153. Washington, DC: National Highway Traffic Safety Administration; May 2010.
36. Janssen W. Seat-belt wearing and driving behavior: an instrumented-vehicle study. *Accid Anal Prev.* 1994;26(2):249-261.
37. Ceraso M, Frisch K, Hargarten S, Corden T. Primary enforcement of seatbelt laws: a means for decreasing injuries, deaths and crash-related costs in Wisconsin. *University of Wisconsin Population Health Institute Issue Brief.* 2006;7(1).
38. Wasan AD, Butler SF, Budman SH, Benoit C, Fernandez K, Jamison RN. Psychiatric history and psychologic adjustment as risk factors for aberrant drug-related behavior among patients with chronic pain. *Clin J Pain.* 2007;23(4):307-315.

CHAPTER 73 Opioid-Induced Hyperalgesia

Lucy Chen
Jianren Mao

Opioid analgesics are among the most powerful pain medications used to treat a variety of pain conditions. Activation of opioid receptors produces analgesia, euphoria, respiratory depression, decreased gastrointestinal motility, and cardiovascular effects. Exposure to opioids also can lead to opioid tolerance and opioid-induced hyperalgesia (OIH). The concept of OIH refers to a pronociceptive state induced by exposure to opioids with a paradoxical increase in nociceptive sensitization through changes at the cellular and system level. This chapter will review evidence of OIH from preclinical and clinical studies and discuss the issues relevant to clinical diagnosis and management of OIH.

EVIDENCE FOR OPIOD-INDUCED HYPERALGESIA: ANIMAL STUDIES

An original preclinical study by Mao et al. showed that baseline nociceptive threshold was progressively reduced, assessed by using a foot-withdrawal test, in rats receiving repeated intrathecal morphine administration (10-20 μg) over a 7-day period.[1] This finding was later supported by a series of animal studies. For example, **1)** the reduced baseline nociceptive threshold was observed in animals receiving subcutaneous fentanyl boluses using the Randall-Sellitto test in which a constantly increasing pressure was applied to a rat's hindpaw. The decreased baseline nociceptive threshold lasted 5 days after the cessation of four fentanyl bolus injections;[2] **2)** the reduced baseline nociceptive threshold was detected in animals with repeated heroin administration as well;[3] **3)** rats exposed to morphine also developed a latent sensitization of visceral hyperalgesia with a shift of the morphine dose-response curve to the right;[4] **4)** exposure to methadone induced hyperalgesia in rats, which was not prevented by a weak NMDA receptor antagonist (memantine);[5] and **5)** a partial μ-receptor agonist buprenophine produced a dose-related OIH.[6]

These findings indicate that repeated opioid administration can lead to a progressive and lasting reduction of baseline nociceptive threshold, referred as OIH.[7-9] This phenomenon differs from previous preclinical observations in which a large dose of intrathecal morphine resulted in hyperalgesic response[10,11] because OIH developed in response to a clinically relevant dose. It is of interest to note that OIH was observed in animals even when an opioid infusion continues via an implanted osmotic pump, suggesting the involvement of active cellular mechanisms in the process.[12] Therefore, a prolonged opioid treatment can result in not only a loss of the opioid antinociceptive effect, a negative sign of system adaptation (desensitization), but also activation of a pronociceptive system manifested as the reduced nociceptive threshold, a positive sign of system adaptation (sensitization).

CELLULAR MECHANISMS OF OPIOD-INDUCED HYPERALGESIA

A considerable number of recent studies have explored the neurobiological basis of OIH, revealing a divergent range of cellular elements contributory to OIH. For example, *N*-methyl-D-aspartate (NMDA) receptors have long been implicated in the cellular mechanism of OIH.[7-9,13] A recent study indicates that the periaqueductal gray may be a site of systemic morphine action on NMDA receptors and protein kinase C (PKC) in relation to the development of OIH.[14] In addition, calcium/calmodulin-dependent protein kinase IIα also has been involved in the initiation and maintenance of OIH.[15] Magnesium is an endogenous blocker at NMDA receptor-coupled calcium channels. In one study, intraperitoneal magnesium prevented or retarded the development of fentanyl-induced OIH in rats.[16] In an animal study of remifentanil-induced postoperative hyperalgesia, there was a marked increase in NR2B phosphorylation at Tyr1472 in the superficial spinal cord dorsal horn, which was attenuated by the pretreatment of the NMDA receptor antagonist ketamine.[17] Pretreatment with ketamine diminished morphine-induced OIH in a mouse model of orthopedic pain.[18] Systemic lidocaine also prevented remifentanil-induced OIH through the inhibition of PKCγ membrane translocation in the rat's spinal cord dorsal horn.[19] Coadministration of dextromethorphan (10 mg/kg), an NMDA receptor antagonist, with morphine produced antinociception and inhibited morphine-induced OIH.[20]

Inhibitory G-proteins played a role in OIH induced by a low opioid dose[21] and GPR3, an orphan G-protein-coupled receptor, contributed to the development of neuropathic pain and morphine-induced OIH.[22] Another study showed that G-inhibitory protein-mu receptor coupling might be necessary for morphine-induced acute OIH because, when a compound that inhibits Gβγ dimmer-dependent signaling was administered, low dose morphine-induced acute OIH was completely prevented.[23] Moreover, 5-HT receptors also have been involved in the cellular mechanism of OIH because the 5-HT_3 antagonist ondansetron given systemically or intrathecally prevented and reversed OIH.[24] NK-1 receptors have been shown to be critically involved in modulation of fentanyl-induced OIH through the ascending and descending pathways.[25] A possible mechanism of NK-1 involvement is that NK-1-expressing neurons may play a critical role in morphine-induced neuroplastic changes. Ablation of NK-1-expressing cells may eliminate the ascending limb of a spinal-bulbospinal loop that results in descending facilitation.[26]

Three potential cellular elements are neuropeptide FF (NPFF), Nitric oxide (NO), and TRPV1 receptors. (1) NPFF has been proposed to play a role in pain modulation. When the potent and selective NPFF receptor antagonist RF9 was co-administered with heroin, paradoxical heroin-induced OIH was completely prevented.[27] (2) Deletion of the inducible NO synthase gene attenuated remifentanil-induced OIH. Of interest is that in NO synthase mutant mice, remifentanil was still effective in enhancing incisional pain, but its pronociceptive effect was significantly attenuated as compared to wild-type mice,[28] suggesting a possible differential effect of opioid on antinociception and OIH. (3) A recent study suggests that TRPV1 is an essential peripheral mechanism in the expression of OIH.[29] This finding suggests that opioid-related long-term potentiation in the spinal cord may be induced by a pre-synaptic event in which TRV1-expressing primary afferents played a significant role.[30]

Intrathecal administration of nifedipine, an L-type calcium channel blocker, antagonized morphine-induced OIH. Furthermore, pretreatment with the selective PKC inhibitor chelerythrine resulted in prevention of OIH, whereas the PKA inhibitor KT 5720 had no effect.[31,32] Gabapentin, a proposed inhibitor of the $\alpha 2\delta$ subunit of voltage-gated calcium channels, prevented a delayed fentanyl-induced OIH in a dose-dependent manner.[33] When combined with ketamine, gabapentin produced the antihyperalgesic effect as well as an additive effect on the prevention of OIH.[34,35] It is of interest to note that 50% nitrous oxide (N_2O) was shown to prevent high dose fentanyl-induced OIH.[36] OIH was found to be associated with the increased expression of c-Fos or zif268 proteins in the amygdala receiving projections from the ascending spino-parabrachio-amygdaloid nociceptive pathway.[37] In another study, spinal NADPH oxidase, a source of endogenous superoxide, is also implicated in the development of OIH and morphine antinociceptive tolerance.[38] It has been reported that variants of the Abcb1b gene and the β_2-AR gene may be partially responsible for the inter-strain differences in OIH.[39,40] Gene expression studies also showed the involvement of opioid-induced SDF1/CXCR4 signaling in long-lasting OIH.[41]

Another interesting observation is that dynorphin A, a κ-opioid receptor, given into the centromedial amygdala resulted in the decreased tail-flick latency, which was blocked by the NMDA receptor antagonist MK-801 but not κ-opioid receptor antagonist nor-binaltorphimine.[42] In addition, OIH appears to be present in opioid receptor triple knockout (KO) mice that lack all three genes encoding μ-, δ-, and κ-opioid receptors, although the opioid antinociceptive effects were abolished in these mice.[43] Similar findings of OIH are reported in opioid receptor triple knock-out mice after fentanyl bolus or infusion and the NMDA receptor antagonist MK-801 reversed OIH under this condition.[44] It has also been reported that both low-dose and high-dose morphine induced OIH but the onset of OIH was earlier and OIH lasted longer in female rats. An NMDA receptor antagonist reversed the low-dose morphine-induced OIH in both male and female rats but reversed high-dose morphine-induced OIH only in male rats, suggesting that the neural substrate contributing to this phenomenon is morphine dose-dependent.[45] Ovariectomy without estrogen replacement treatment diminished this sex difference in OIH.[46]

The increasing number of preclinical studies in the area of OIH indicates that 1) there is an enormous and growing interest in the field with regard to the cellular mechanisms of OIH and, 2) the current evidence points to a progressive sensitization process within the central nervous system that involves a constellation of cellular elements such as NMDA receptors similar to those contributory to the mechanisms of pathologic pain.

EVIDENCE FOR OPIOD-INDUCED HYPERALGESIA: HUMAN STUDIES

Although preclinical studies can measure changes in baseline nociceptive threshold in a controlled setting, it is difficult to assess whether changes in pain threshold occur clinically following opioid administration.[9] It is indeed challenging to distinguish pharmacologic tolerance from OIH when the outcome of opioid therapy is primarily based on subjective pain scores. Despite the challenge, an increasing number of anecdotal case reports and clinical studies have suggested that OIH is likely to be a significant factor in clinical opioid therapy.[47-50,51-54]

In a large scale study of 1,620 patients, remifentanil was used for general anesthesia and the incidence of postoperative remifentanil-induced hyperalgesia was reported to be 16.1%. This study found that age (a higher rate in patients <16y old), sex (male >female), operation duration (higher in duration >2h), and remifentanil dose (higher in dose >30 μg/kg) are the factors that have had an impact on the incidence of OIH.[55] Alternately, heroin or opioid addicts not only demonstrated OIH, but also had prolonged symptoms of OIH after detoxification from opioids for at least 1 month.[56] In those chronic pain patients without opioid dependence, significantly lower pain threshold and lower pain tolerance were detected using pressure pain stimulation.[57] It appears that the sensitivity of detecting OIH in the clinical setting may be influenced by the modality of sensory stimulation.[58] A major caveat of these clinical observations is that OIH was not defined objectively, an issue that remains to be addressed.

In a prospective preliminary study of six patients with chronic low back pain, hyperalgesic response was detected after 1 month of oral morphine therapy in a cold pressor test but not in a heat pain test.[59] In a prospective, randomized, placebo-controlled, 2-way crossover study in healthy volunteers conducted by the same investigators, the development of OIH was quantified as changes in the average radius of the area of secondary hyperalgesia generated by electrical pain stimulation. A 23.6% increase in the area of secondary hyperalgesia over baseline was detected following the remifentanil infusion. The same study showed that endogenous opioids did not seem to have an effect on OIH because a single bolus of naloxone did not change the size of secondary hyperalgesic.[60]

To date, a number of clinical studies have examined clinical approaches to preventing OIH in human subjects, although the results remain inconclusive. (1) Treatment with morphine (150 μg/kg) prior to remifentanil infusion did not prevent the development of remifentanil-induced OIH.[61] (2) Infusion of propofol with remifentanil both delayed and attenuated remifentanil-induced OIH.[53] (3) Intraoperative administration of 70% N_2O appears to reduce postoperative OIH following an intraoperative remifentanil-propofol anesthesia regimen.[62] (4) Preventive administration of parecoxib significantly diminished OIH after withdrawal from remifentanil. In contrast, parecoxib given together with remifentanil did not prevent OIH, suggesting that pretreatment may be more meaningful in preventing OIH.[63] Other NSAIDs administered preemptively also appear to prevent remifentanil-induced OIH.[64] (5) Intraoperative magnesium administration reduced postoperative opioid consumption and OIH in subjects receiving intraoperative remifentanil-based anesthesia.[65,66] Intraoperative adenosine infusion also prevented acute opioid tolerance and remifentanil-induced OIH.[67] (6) Continuous intraoperative infusion of ketamine, an NMDA receptor antagonist, significantly lowered postoperative VAS and morphine use.[68] (7) In a randomized, double-blind, placebo-controlled study of 90 patients who underwent total abdominal hysterectomy, cumulative morphine consumption was significantly greater in subjects with fentanyl alone than those with saline alone, ketamine alone, ketamine with fentanyl, or fentanyl with lornoxicam at 3, 6, and 12 hours postoperatively.[69] (8) In a double-blind, randomized, placebo-controlled study of 40 patients undergoing elective shoulder surgery, clonidine was given intraoperatively with a remifentanil/propofol-based anesthesia. The results showed that clonidine did not reduce postoperative morphine consumption and pain score in these patients.[70] However, dexmedetomidine, another α_2 receptor agonist, substantially reduced baseline opioid doses in hospitalized patients with OIH.[71]

DETECTING OIH WITH QUANTITATIVE SENSORY TESTING

Despite the increasing effort, diagnostic tools for OIH are yet to be developed. However, many clinical studies have used quantitative sensory testing (QST) as a useful tool to assess OIH.[72,73] In a recent study, QST was used to compare pain threshold, pain tolerance, and the degree of temporal summation of second pain in response to thermal stimulation among three groups of subjects: Group 1 (no pain and no opioid), Group 2 (chronic pain but no opioid treatment), and Group 3 (both chronic pain and opioid therapy). Group 3 subjects displayed a decreased heat pain threshold and exacerbated temporal summation of second pain to thermal stimulation as compared with both group 1 and group 2 subjects. There were no differences in cold or warm sensation among all three groups. Among clinical factors, daily opioid dose consistently correlated with the decreased heat pain threshold and exacerbated temporal summation of second pain in group 3 subjects.[72] Another study investigated the sensitivity to cold pain and the magnitude of diffuse noxious inhibitory control (DNIC) using QST in subjects with or without opioid therapy. Pain threshold, intensity, and tolerance in response to cold pressor (1°C) were measured. It was found that oral opioid use did not result in abnormal sensitivity to cold pain but altered pain modulation as detected by DNIC.[74] Of importance is to recognize the limitation of QST such as the lack of a consensus baseline value for QST parameters in normal subjects. QST is likely to be most valuable when applied in within-subject longitudinal follow-ups and considered in the context of other clinical factors as discussed later in this chapter.

INFLUENCE OF OPIOID REGIMEN ON OPIOD-INDUCED ANALGESIA

Opioid regimen including the type of opioid analgesic and dose may influence the development of OIH. Anecdotal clinical observations have suggested that the degree of OIH may vary according to opioid analgesics.[75] Although the exact relationship between the dose regimen and the development of OIH remains to be determined, it is conceivable that OIH would be more likely to develop in patients receiving high opioid doses with a prolonged treatment course; however, OIH has been demonstrated in patients receiving a short course of highly potent opioid analgesics.[76] Moreover, patients with a pathologic pain condition (e.g., neuropathic pain) treated with opioid therapy may be more susceptible to developing OIH, because both pathologic pain and OIH may share a common cellular mechanism.[77]

If OIH develops following exposure to one opioid, can switching to a different opioid diminish OIH?[78] If cross-pain sensitivity does not develop between different opioids, switching to a different opioid would be justified, a similar rationale for opioid rotation to overcome opioid tolerance. This issue is yet to be investigated.

IMPLICATION OF OPIOD-INDUCED ANALGESIA ON PREEMPTIVE ANALGESIA

Despite the ongoing debate on the clinical effectiveness of preemptive analgesia in pain management, use of opioid analgesic as the sole agent for preemptive analgesia may not be desirable for three reasons. First, a large dose of intraoperative opioid could activate a pronociceptive mechanism leading to the development of postoperative OIH.[79] This may confound the assessment of postoperative pain and counteract the opioid analgesic effect. Second, preemptive analgesia calls for preemptive inhibition of neuroplastic changes mediated through multiple cellular mechanisms such as the central glutamatergic system. Paradoxically, opioid may activate the central glutamatergic system as discussed above. Third, the neural mechanism of opioid tolerance and OIH may interact with that of pathologic pain and pathologic pain could be exacerbated following opioid administration.[80,81] Nonetheless, this issue needs to be investigated in future studies.

IMPACT OF OIH ON OPIOID THERAPY

Until recently, a decreased opioid analgesic effect following opioid therapy (apparent opioid tolerance) is often considered to result from pharmacologic opioid tolerance (i.e., desensitization of the responsiveness of an opioid receptor and its cellular mechanism) and/or a worsening clinical pain condition (**Fig. 73-1**). If so, opioid dose escalation would be a logical approach to regaining the analgesic effectiveness of opioids. This concept needs to be re-considered in light of OIH (see Fig. 73-1). That is, apparent opioid tolerance in the clinical setting could result from pharmacologic tolerance, worsening pain condition due to disease progression, and/or OIH. Since the management for each of these elements of apparent opioid tolerance would be different, it is important to distinguish the elements of apparent opioid tolerance through differential diagnosis.[82]

DIFFERENTIAL DIAGNOSIS OF OIH

As listed in **Table 73-1**, a number of issues should be taken into consideration.

(1) The quality, location, and distribution pattern of pain due to OIH would be different from a pre-existing pain condition. Because opioid analgesics are often administered systemically, changes in pain quality would be diffuse as compared to the pre-existing pain condition. Since the mechanism of OIH has many in common with that of pathologic pain such as neuropathic pain, changes in pain threshold, tolerability, and distribution patterns seen in OIH would be similar to those seen in neuropathic pain patients. Moreover, QST may be a useful tool to detect such changes.

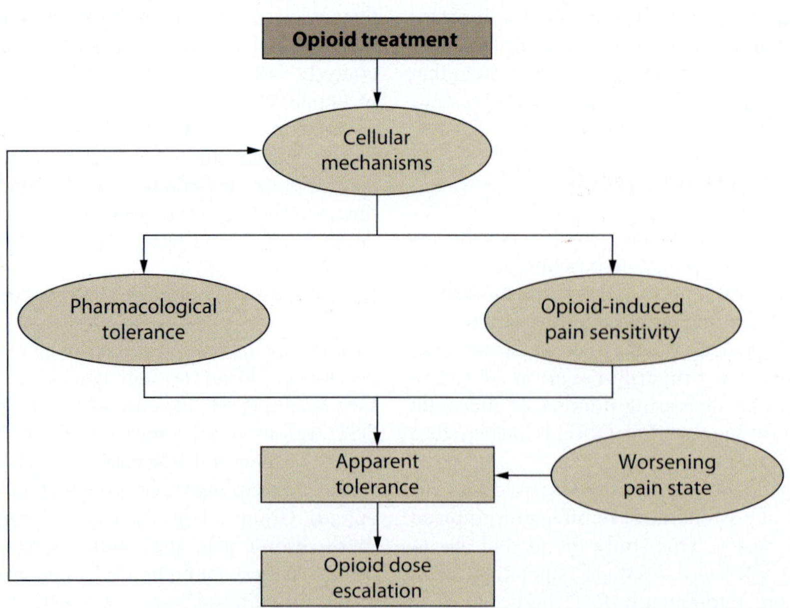

FIGURE 73-1. Flowchart illustrating possible causes of apparent opioid tolerance in the clinical setting and possible outcomes of opioid dose escalation.

TABLE 73-1 Differential Diagnosis of Opioid-Induced Hyperalgesia and Opioid Tolerance

	OIH	Opioid Tolerance
Opioid dose (the higher, the more likely)	Yes	Yes
Duration of opioid therapy (the longer, the more likely)	Yes	Yes
Dose escalation	Limited improvement in clinical pain and QST responses	Improvement in pain relief
Dose reduction	Improved opioid analgesia	Reduced opioid analgesia
Pain quality	Spontaneous, burning, diffuse pain similar to neuropathic pain	No change (from preexisting pain)
Pain location	Possibly beyond the dermatome distribution of the preexisting pain	No change (from preexisting pain)
Pain intensity	Similar or greater than the pre-existing pain	Similar to the pre-existing pain condition
QST Exacerbated temporal summation of second pain	Yes	No
Decreased pain threshold	Yes	No
Decreased pain tolerance	Yes	No

(2) OIH could exacerbate a preexisting pain condition. Therefore, overall pain intensity (VAS) would conceivably be increased above the level of pre-existing pain in the absence of disease progression. Opioid dose escalation could only transiently and minimally reduce pain intensity in such a setting, with a subsequent increase in pain intensity due to OIH.

(3) When a diagnosis is uncertain, a trial of opioid dose escalation or dose decrease may be used to differentiate tolerance from OIH. In an under-treated, worsening pain condition due to disease progress and/or pharmacologic opioid tolerance, improved pain control may well be an outcome after a trial of opioid dose escalation. On the other hand, opioid dose escalation may exacerbate pain condition due to OIH, whereas a supervised opioid tapering may reduce OIH and improve clinical pain. In this regard, if a patient is on a low opioid dose regimen and complains of unsatisfactory pain relief, a trial of opioid dose escalation may be appropriate. If a patient is already on a meg-dose of opioid analgesic, further dose escalation is rarely justified and may exacerbate OIH.

(4) It is important to remember that the clinical outcome of opioid therapy is a dynamic balance among the opioid analgesic effect, OIH, and worsening pain due to disease progression. While any opioid dose escalation may transiently increase the analgesic effect, albeit being small in many cases, the real issue is whether the dose escalation may also exacerbate OIH that could quickly overtake the transient improvement in opioid analgesia. Therefore, clinical judgment is fundamentally important and all clinical conditions related to opioid therapy need to be taken into consideration in this decision making process.

In summary, it is important to consider various aspects of a differential diagnosis when the decreased opioid analgesic effect is encountered during a course of opioid therapy. If the increased nociceptive input (e.g., disease progression) and/or psychological issues can be ruled out as the primary contributor to a state of increased pain, differentiating between pharmacologic tolerance and OIH should be considered. It seems reasonable to have a trial of opioid dose escalation at this point. If pain improves, the lack of opioid analgesic efficacy is more likely due to tolerance. However, if pain worsens or does not proportionally respond to the dose escalation, OIH could be the cause. This clinical diagnostic process could be aided by using QST and considering other clinical features of OIH as discussed above.

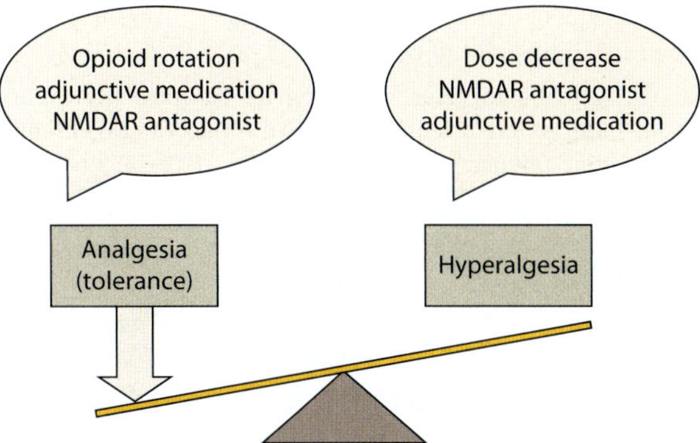

FIGURE 73-2. Possible measures for reducing opioid-induced hyperalgesia and increasing opioid analgesic effects.

CLINICAL MANAGEMENT OF OIH

If OIH is suspected, either dose decrease or taper-off would be a reasonable approach (**Fig, 73-2**). Alternatively, opioid rotation could be a feasible step if opioid therapy is considered to be necessary regardless of OIH. Patients may get better pain relief with a different opioid medication, often at a lower equal-analgesic dosage. Adjuvant non-opioid pain medications have been highly recommended in combination with opioid treatment to reduce the amount of opioid usage, minimize opioid side effects, and reduce the risk of opioid tolerance and OIH. Lastly, one should also consider the history of the patient's pain and its response to opioids. A patient who was previously on a stable opioid regimen and now complains of worsening pain is much different from the one whose pain never was improved with that opioid regimen. In the latter case, instead of having continued dose escalation, the patient would be better off if that opioid is weaned off, a non-opioid regimen is considered, and/or a different opioid is used for rotation.

SUMMARY

Opioids should be considered when the adjustment of opioid dose is contemplated if a) prior opioid dose escalation failed to provide the expected analgesic effect and b) there is unexplainable pain exacerbation following an initial period of effective opioid analgesia. Although in some cases increasing opioid doses lead to some improvement in pain management, in other cases less opioid may lead to more effective pain reduction. This goal may be accomplished by initiating a trial of opioid tapering, opioid rotation, adding adjunctive medications, or combining an opioid with a clinically available N-methyl-D-aspirate receptor antagonist. Continuing opioid therapy with endless dose escalations in the absence of clinical evidence of improved pain management is neither scientifically sound nor clinically justified.

REFERENCES

1. Mao J, Price DD, Mayer DJ. Thermal hyperalgesia in association with the development of morphine tolerance in rats: roles of excitatory amino acid receptors and protein kinase C. *J Neurosci.* 1994;14(4):2301-2312.
2. Celerier E, Rivat C, Jun Y, et al. Long-lasting hyperalgesia induced by fentanyl in rats: preventive effect of ketamine. *Anesthesiology.* 2000;92(2):465-472.
3. Laulin JP, Maurette P, Corcuff JB, Rivat C, Chauvin M, Simonnet G. The role of ketamine in preventing fentanyl-induced hyperalgesia

and subsequent acute morphine tolerance. *Anesth Analg.* 2002; 94(5):1263-1269, table of contents.

4. Lian B, Vera-Portocarrero L, King T, Ossipov MH, Porreca F. Opioid-induced latent sensitization in a model of non-inflammatory viscerosomatic hypersensitivity. *Brain Res.* 2010;1358:64-70.
5. Hay JL, Kaboutari J, White JM, Salem A, Irvine R. Model of methadone-induced hyperalgesia in rats and effect of memantine. *Eur J Pharmacol.* 2010;626(2-3):229-233.
6. Wala EP, Holtman JR Jr. Buprenorphine-induced hyperalgesia in the rat. *Eur J Pharmacol.* 2011;651(1-3):89-95.
7. Mao J, Sung B, Ji RR, Lim G. Chronic morphine induces downregulation of spinal glutamate transporters: implications in morphine tolerance and abnormal pain sensitivity. *J Neurosci.* 2002;22(18):8312-8323.
8. Mao J, Sung B, Ji RR, Lim G. Neuronal apoptosis associated with morphine tolerance: evidence for an opioid-induced neurotoxic mechanism. *J Neurosci.* 2002;22(17):7650-7661.
9. Mao J. Opioid-induced abnormal pain sensitivity. *Curr Pain Headache Rep.* 2006;10(1):67-70.
10. Woolf CJ. Intrathecal high dose morphine produces hyperalgesia in the rat. *Brain Res.* 1981;209(2):491-495.
11. Yaksh TL, Harty GJ, Onofrio BM. High dose of spinal morphine produce a nonopiate receptor-mediated hyperesthesia: clinical and theoretic implications. *Anesthesiology.* 1986;64(5):590-597.
12. Vanderah TW, Ossipov MH, Lai J, Malan TP Jr, Porreca F. Mechanisms of opioid-induced pain and antinociceptive tolerance: descending facilitation and spinal dynorphin. *Pain.* 2001;92(1-2):5-9.
13. Zhao M, Joo DT. Enhancement of spinal *N*-methyl-D-aspartate receptor function by remifentanil action at delta-opioid receptors as a mechanism for acute opioid-induced hyperalgesia or tolerance. *Anesthesiology.* 2008;109(2):308-317.
14. Ghelardini C, Galeotti N, Vivoli E, et al. Molecular interaction in the mouse PAG between NMDA and opioid receptors in morphine-induced acute thermal nociception. *J Neurochem.* 2008;105(1):91-100.
15. Chen Y, Yang C, Wang ZJ. Ca_2+/calmodulin-dependent protein kinase II alpha is required for the initiation and maintenance of opioid-induced hyperalgesia. *J Neurosci.* 2010;30(1):38-46.
16. Van Elstraete AC, Sitbon P, Mazoit JX, Conti M, Benhamou D. Protective effect of prior administration of magnesium on delayed hyperalgesia induced by fentanyl in rats. *Can J Anaesth.* 2006; 53(12):1180-1185.
17. Gu X, Wu X, Liu Y, Cui S, Ma Z. Tyrosine phosphorylation of the *N*-methyl-D-aspartate receptor 2B subunit in spinal cord contributes to remifentanil-induced postoperative hyperalgesia: the preventive effect of ketamine. *Mol Pain.* 2009;5:76.
18. Minville V, Fourcade O, Girolami JP, Tack I. Opioid-induced hyperalgesia in a mice model of orthopaedic pain: preventive effect of ketamine. *Br J Anaesth.* 2010;104(2):231-238.
19. Cui W, Li Y, Li S, et al. Systemic lidocaine inhibits remifentanil-induced hyperalgesia via the inhibition of cPKCgamma membrane translocation in spinal dorsal horn of rats. *J Neurosurg Anesthesiol.* 2009;21(4):318-325.
20. Gupta LK, Gupta R, Tripathi CD. *N*-methyl-D-aspartate receptor modulators block hyperalgesia induced by acute low-dose morphine. *Clin Exp Pharmacol Physiol.* 2011;38(9):592-597.
21. Bianchi E, Galeotti N, Menicacci C, Ghelardini C. Contribution of G inhibitory protein alpha subunits in paradoxical hyperalgesia elicited by exceedingly low doses of morphine in mice. *Life Sci.* 2011;89(25-26):918-925.
22. Ruiz-Medina J, Ledent C, Valverde O. GPR3 orphan receptor is involved in neuropathic pain after peripheral nerve injury and regulates morphine-induced antinociception. *Neuropharmacology.* 2011;61(1-2):43-50.
23. Bianchi E, Norcini M, Smrcka A, Ghelardini C. Supraspinal gbetagamma-dependent stimulation of PLCbeta originating from G inhibitory protein-mu opioid receptor-coupling is necessary for morphine induced acute hyperalgesia. *J Neurochem.* 2009;111(1):171-180.
24. Liang DY, Li X, Clark JD. 5-hydroxytryptamine type 3 receptor modulates opioid-induced hyperalgesia and tolerance in mice. *Anesthesiology.* 2011;114(5):1180-1189.
25. Rivat C, Vera-Portocarrero LP, Ibrahim MM, et al. Spinal NK-1 receptor-expressing neurons and descending pathways support fentanyl-induced pain hypersensitivity in a rat model of postoperative pain. *Eur J Neurosci.* 2009;29(4):727-737.
26. Vera-Portocarrero LP, Zhang ET, King T, et al. Spinal NK-1 receptor expressing neurons mediate opioid-induced hyperalgesia and antinociceptive tolerance via activation of descending pathways. *Pain.* 2007;129(1-2):35-45.
27. Simonin F, Schmitt M, Laulin JP, et al. RF9, a potent and selective neuropeptide FF receptor antagonist, prevents opioid-induced tolerance associated with hyperalgesia. *Proc Natl Acad Sci U S A.* 2006;103(2):466-471.
28. Celerier E, Gonzalez JR, Maldonado R, Cabanero D, Puig MM. Opioid-induced hyperalgesia in a murine model of postoperative pain: role of nitric oxide generated from the inducible nitric oxide synthase. *Anesthesiology.* 2006;104(3):546-555.
29. Vardanyan A, Wang R, Vanderah TW, et al. TRPV1 receptor in expression of opioid-induced hyperalgesia. *J Pain.* 2009;10(3):243-252.
30. Zhou HY, Chen SR, Chen H, Pan HL. Opioid-induced long-term potentiation in the spinal cord is a presynaptic event. *J Neurosci.* 2010;30(12):4460-4466.
31. Esmaeili-Mahani S, Shimokawa N, Javan M, et al. Low-dose morphine induces hyperalgesia through activation of G alphas, protein kinase C, and L-type ca 2+ channels in rats. *J Neurosci Res.* 2008;86(2):471-479.
32. Esmaeili-Mahani S, Fereidoni M, Javan M, Maghsoudi N, Motamedi F, Ahmadiani A. Nifedipine suppresses morphine-induced thermal hyperalgesia: evidence for the role of corticosterone. *Eur J Pharmacol.* 2007;567(1-2):95-101.
33. Van Elstraete AC, Sitbon P, Mazoit JX, Benhamou D. Gabapentin prevents delayed and long-lasting hyperalgesia induced by fentanyl in rats. *Anesthesiology.* 2008;108(3):484-494.
34. Van Elstraete AC, Sitbon P, Benhamou D, Mazoit JX. The median effective dose of ketamine and gabapentin in opioid-induced hyperalgesia in rats: an isobolographic analysis of their interaction. *Anesth Analg.* 2011;113(3):634-640.
35. Wei X, Wei W. Role of gabapentin in preventing fentanyl- and morphine-withdrawal-induced hyperalgesia in rats. *J Anesth.* 2011.
36. Bessiere B, Richebe P, Laboureyras E, Laulin JP, Contarino A, Simonnet G. Nitrous oxide (N_2O) prevents latent pain sensitization and long-term anxiety-like behavior in pain and opioid-experienced rats. *Neuropharmacology.* 2007;53(6):733-740.
37. Hamlin AS, McNally GP, Osborne PB. Induction of c-fos and zif268 in the nociceptive amygdala parallel abstinence hyperalgesia in rats briefly exposed to morphine. *Neuropharmacology.* 2007;53(2):330-343.
38. Doyle T, Bryant L, Muscoli C, et al. Spinal NADPH oxidase is a source of superoxide in the development of morphine-induced hyperalgesia and antinociceptive tolerance. *Neurosci Lett.* 2010;483(2):85-89.

39. Liang DY, Liao G, Wang J, et al. A genetic analysis of opioid-induced hyperalgesia in mice. *Anesthesiology*. 2006;104(5):1054-1062.

40. Liang DY, Liao G, Lighthall GK, Peltz G, Clark DJ. Genetic variants of the P-glycoprotein gene Abcb1b modulate opioid-induced hyperalgesia, tolerance and dependence. *Pharmacogenet Genomics*. 2006;16(11):825-835.

41. Wilson NM, Jung H, Ripsch MS, Miller RJ, White FA. CXCR4 signaling mediates morphine-induced tactile hyperalgesia. *Brain Behav Immun*. 2011;25(3):565-573.

42. Terashvili M, Wu HE, Schwasinger E, Tseng LF. Paradoxical hyperalgesia induced by mu-opioid receptor agonist endomorphin-2, but not endomorphin-1, microinjected into the centromedial amygdala of the rat. *Eur J Pharmacol*. 2007;554(2-3):137-144.

43. Juni A, Klein G, Pintar JE, Kest B. Nociception increases during opioid infusion in opioid receptor triple knock-out mice. *Neuroscience*. 2007;147(2):439-444.

44. Waxman AR, Arout C, Caldwell M, Dahan A, Kest B. Acute and chronic fentanyl administration causes hyperalgesia independently of opioid receptor activity in mice. *Neurosci Lett*. 2009;462(1):68-72.

45. Juni A, Cai M, Stankova M, et al. Sex-specific mediation of opioid-induced hyperalgesia by the melanocortin-1 receptor. *Anesthesiology*. 2010;112(1):181-188.

46. Juni A, Klein G, Kowalczyk B, Ragnauth A, Kest B. Sex differences in hyperalgesia during morphine infusion: Effect of gonadectomy and estrogen treatment. *Neuropharmacology*. 2008;54(8):1264-1270.

47. Forero M, Chan PS, Restrepo-Garces CE. Successful reversal of hyperalgesia/myoclonus complex with low-dose ketamine infusion. *Pain Pract*. 2011.

48. Vorobeychik Y, Chen L, Bush MC, Mao J. Improved opioid analgesic effect following opioid dose reduction. *Pain Med*. 2008;9(6):724-727.

49. Cortinas Saenz M, Geronimo Pardo M, Cortinas Saenz ML, Hernandez Vallecillo MT, Ibarra Marti ML, Mateo Cerdan CM. Acute opiate tolerance and postoperative hyperalgesia after a brief infusion of remifentanil managed with multimodal analgesia. *Rev Esp Anestesiol Reanim*. 2008;55(1):40-42.

50. Siniscalchi A, Piraccini E, Miklosova Z, Taddei S, Faenza S, Martinelli G. Opioid-induced hyperalgesia and rapid opioid detoxification after tacrolimus administration. *Anesth Analg*. 2008;106(2):645-6, table of contents.

51. Okon TR, George ML. Fentanyl-induced neurotoxicity and paradoxic pain. *J Pain Symptom Manage*. 2008;35(3):327-333.

52. Axelrod DJ, Reville B. Using methadone to treat opioid-induced hyperalgesia and refractory pain. *J Opioid Manag*. 2007;3(2):113-114.

53. Singler B, Troster A, Manering N, Schuttler J, Koppert W. Modulation of remifentanil-induced postinfusion hyperalgesia by propofol. *Anesth Analg*. 2007;104(6):1397-1403, table of contents.

54. Hallett BR, Chalkiadis GA. Suspected opioid-induced hyperalgesia in an infant. *Br J Anaesth*. 2012;108(1):116-118.

55. Ma JF, Huang ZL, Li J, Hu SJ, Lian QQ. Cohort study of remifentanil-induced hyperalgesia in postoperative patients. *Zhonghua Yi Xue Za Zhi*. 2011;91(14):977-979.

56. Pud D, Cohen D, Lawental E, Eisenberg E. Opioids and abnormal pain perception: new evidence from a study of chronic opioid addicts and healthy subjects. *Drug Alcohol Depend*. 2006;82(3):218-223.

57. Fishbain DA, Lewis JE, Gao J. Are psychoactive substance (opioid)-dependent chronic pain patients hyperalgesic? *Pain Pract*. 2011;11(4):337-343.

58. Hay JL, White JM, Bochner F, Somogyi AA, Semple TJ, Rounsefell B. Hyperalgesia in opioid-managed chronic pain and opioid-dependent patients. *J Pain*. 2009;10(3):316-322.

59. Chu LF, Clark DJ, Angst MS. Opioid tolerance and hyperalgesia in chronic pain patients after one month of oral morphine therapy: a preliminary prospective study. *J Pain*. 2006;7(1):43-48.

60. Chu LF, Dairmont J, Zamora AK, Young CA, Angst MS. The endogenous opioid system is not involved in modulation of opioid-induced hyperalgesia. *J Pain*. 2011;12(1):108-115.

61. McDonnell C, Zaarour C, Hull R, et al. Pre-treatment with morphine does not prevent the development of remifentanil-induced hyperalgesia. *Can J Anaesth*. 2008;55(12):813-818.

62. Echevarria G, Elgueta F, Fierro C, et al. Nitrous oxide (N_2O) reduces postoperative opioid-induced hyperalgesia after remifentanil-propofol anaesthesia in humans. *Br J Anaesth*. 2011;107(6):959-965.

63. Troster A, Sittl R, Singler B, Schmelz M, Schuttler J, Koppert W. Modulation of remifentanil-induced analgesia and postinfusion hyperalgesia by parecoxib in humans. *Anesthesiology*. 2006; 105(5):1016-1023.

64. Tuncer S, Yalcin N, Reisli R, Alper Y. The effects of lornoxicam in preventing remifentanil-induced postoperative hyperalgesia. *Agri*. 2009;21(4):161-167.

65. Lee C, Song YK, Jeong HM, Park SN. The effects of magnesium sulfate infiltration on perioperative opioid consumption and opioid-induced hyperalgesia in patients undergoing robot-assisted laparoscopic prostatectomy with remifentanil-based anesthesia. *Korean J Anesthesiol*. 2011;61(3):244-250.

66. Song JW, Lee YW, Yoon KB, Park SJ, Shim YH. Magnesium sulfate prevents remifentanil-induced postoperative hyperalgesia in patients undergoing thyroidectomy. *Anesth Analg*. 2011;113(2):390-397.

67. Lee C, Song YK, Lee JH, Ha SM. The effects of intraoperative adenosine infusion on acute opioid tolerance and opioid induced hyperalgesia induced by remifentanil in adult patients undergoing tonsillectomy. *Korean J Pain*. 2011;24(1):7-12.

68. Hong BH, Lee WY, Kim YH, Yoon SH, Lee WH. Effects of intraoperative low dose ketamine on remifentanil-induced hyperalgesia in gynecologic surgery with sevoflurane anesthesia. *Korean J Anesthesiol*. 2011;61(3):238-243.

69. Xuerong Y, Yuguang H, Xia J, Hailan W. Ketamine and lornoxicam for preventing a fentanyl-induced increase in postoperative morphine requirement. *Anesth Analg*. 2008;107(6):2032-2037.

70. Schlimp CJ, Pipam W, Wolrab C, Ohner C, Kager HI, Likar R. Clonidine for remifentanil-induced hyperalgesia: a double-blind randomized, placebo-controlled study of clonidine under intraoperative use of remifentanil in elective surgery of the shoulder. *Schmerz*. 2011;25(3):290-295.

71. Belgrade M, Hall S. Dexmedetomidine infusion for the management of opioid-induced hyperalgesia. *Pain Med*. 2010;11(12):1819-1826.

72. Chen L, Malarick C, Seefeld L, Wang S, Houghton M, Mao J. Altered quantitative sensory testing outcome in subjects with opioid therapy. *Pain*. 2009;143(1-2):65-70.

73. Bannister K, Dickenson AH. Opioid hyperalgesia. *Curr Opin Support Palliat Care*. 2010;4(1):1-5.

74. Ram KC, Eisenberg E, Haddad M, Pud D. Oral opioid use alters DNIC but not cold pain perception in patients with chronic pain—new perspective of opioid-induced hyperalgesia. *Pain*. 2008;139(2):431-438.

75. Compton P, Charuvastra VC, Ling W. Pain intolerance in opioid-maintained former opiate addicts: effect of long-acting maintenance agent. *Drug Alcohol Depend*. 2001;63(2):139-146.

76. Vinik HR, Kissin I. Rapid development of tolerance to analgesia during remifentanil infusion in humans. *Anesth Analg*. 1998;86(6):1307-1311.

77. Mao J, Price DD, Mayer DJ. Mechanisms of hyperalgesia and morphine tolerance: a current view of their possible interactions. *Pain*. 1995;62(3):259-274.

78. Sjogren P, Jensen NH, Jensen TS. Disappearance of morphine-induced hyperalgesia after discontinuing or substituting morphine with other opioid agonists. *Pain*. 1994;59(2):313-316.

79. Guignard B, Bossard AE, Coste C, et al. Acute opioid tolerance: intraoperative remifentanil increases postoperative pain and morphine requirement. *Anesthesiology*. 2000;93(2):409-417.

80. Angst MS, Clark JD. Opioid-induced hyperalgesia: a qualitative systematic review. *Anesthesiology*. 2006;104(3):570-587.

81. Baron MJ, McDonald PW. Significant pain reduction in chronic pain patients after detoxification from high-dose opioids. *J Opioid Manag*. 2006;2(5):277-282.

82. Mao J. Opioid-induced abnormal pain sensitivity: implications in clinical opioid therapy. *Pain*. 2002;100(3):213-217.

CHAPTER 74 Nonsteroidal Anti-inflammatory Drugs

Lee S. Simon

NONSTEROIDAL ANTI-INFLAMMATORY DRUGS

Nonsteroidal anti-inflammatory drugs (NSAIDs) are anti-inflammatory, analgesic, and antipyretic agents. They are used to reduce pain, decrease stiffness, and improve function in patients with osteoarthritis (OA), rheumatoid arthritis (RA), and other forms of arthritis. They are also used for the treatment of pain including headache, dysmenorrhea, and postoperative pain.[1-3] It is not known whether NSAID effectiveness results from the anti-inflammatory or analgesic effects or from other possible mechanisms.[4] There are at least 20 different NSAIDs currently available in the United States (**Table 74-1**). Cyclooxygenase-2 selective inhibitors (COX-2 inhibitors [celecoxib]), have similar efficacy but with significantly decreased gastrointestinal (GI) and platelet effects.[5-7] Several topical NSAIDs including diclofenac or salicylates for chronic pain have been approved in the United States; however, similar drugs have been available in Europe for a number of years. One study of a diclofenac liquid included an oral diclofenac comparator demonstrating no difference in efficacy from the topical agent in chronic dosing in treatment of the pain of osteoarthritis of the knee.[8]

NSAIDs are the most commonly used classes of drugs. It has been reported that more than 17 million Americans use these agents on a daily basis for the relief of pain and, at times, swelling related to inflammation.[9] With the aging of the US population, the Centers for Disease Control and Prevention (CDC) predict a significant increase in the prevalence of painful degenerative and inflammatory rheumatic conditions and thus an increased use of NSAIDs.[9,10] Approximately 60 million NSAID prescriptions are written each year in the United States; the number for elderly patients exceeds those for younger patients by approximately 3.6-fold.[10] Aspirin, ibuprofen, naproxen, and ketoprofen are also available over the counter (OTC). At equipotent doses, the clinical efficacy and tolerability of the various NSAIDs are similar; however, individual responses are highly variable.[1,11,12] It is believed that if a patient fails to respond to an NSAID from one class it is reasonable to put the patient on another NSAID from a different class; however, no one has studied this in a prospective controlled manner.[11,12] There are topical NSAIDs available including diclofenac and salicylate patches that have been demonstrated to work on single joints in osteoarthritis and soft tissue sprains and strains.

Sodium salicylic acid was discovered in 1763 but more impure forms of salicylates had been used as analgesics and antipyretics throughout the previous century. Once purified and synthesized, the acetyl derivative of salicylate, acetylsalicylic acid (ASA) was found to provide more anti-inflammatory activity than salicylate alone; however, it increased the incidence of toxicity, particularly related to the upper GI tract. Phenylbutazone, an indoleacetic acid derivative, was introduced in the early 1950s. This drug was a weak prostaglandin synthase inhibitor, which induced uricosuria, and was found useful in patients with ankylosing spondylitis and gout. However, because of concerns related to bone marrow toxicity, particularly in women older than 60 years of age, this compound now is rarely prescribed. Indomethacin, an indoleacetic acid derivative, was subsequently developed in the 1960s to substitute for phenylbutazone. It had the potential for significant toxicity as well, and the search for safer (particularly GI safer) and at least equally effective NSAIDs ensued. Other clinical issues have driven the development of newer agents, such as once or twice daily dosing to improve compliance.

MECHANISM OF ACTION

Some of the variability in clinical response of these drugs may be explained by the spectrum of inhibition of prostaglandin synthesis. Several NSAIDs appear to be potent inhibitors of prostaglandin synthesis, while others more prominently affect other nonprostaglandin-mediated biologic events.[1,2,13-16] Different responses have also been attributed to variations in the enantiomeric state of the drug or its pharmacokinetics and/or pharmacodynamics.[1,2,11,12] Although variability can be explained in part by absorption, distribution, and metabolism, potential differences in mechanism of action must be considered as possibly important to explain observed variable effects.[11,12]

The NSAIDs are primarily anti-inflammatory and analgesic by decreasing production of prostaglandins of the E series.[17] Many of these prostanoic acids are proinflammatory, and increase vascular permeability and sensitivity to the release of bradykinins. Decreasing the synthesis of these mediators leads to decreased pain, swelling, and edema in the peripheral tissues. In addition, there is accumulating evidence that central effects of pain modulation may be as important as the effects on the peripheral tissues. The hypothesis is that prostaglandin synthesis is upregulated in the brain with peripheral stimulation of pain particularly associated with inflammation, and those NSAIDs that are more lipophilic penetrate better into the central nervous system (CNS) and inhibit both synthesis of peripheral and central prostaglandins.[18]

NSAIDs have also been shown to inhibit the formation of prostacyclin and thromboxane, resulting in complex effects on vascular permeability and platelet aggregation in peripheral tissues, which undoubtedly contributes to the overall clinical effects of these compounds.

These prostaglandins are derived from polyunsaturated fatty acids that are constituents of all cell membranes. They exist in ester linkage in the glycerols of phospholipids and are converted through multiple enzymatic steps to prostaglandins or leukotrienes first through the action of phospholipase A_2 or phospholipase C.[17] Free arachidonic acid, which is released by the phospholipase from the fatty acids, acts as a substrate for the PGH synthase complex that includes cyclooxygenase (COX) and peroxidase. These enzymes catalyze the conversion of arachidonic acid to the unstable cyclic-endoperoxide intermediates, PGG_2 and PGH_2, which are then converted to the more stable PGE_2 and PGF_2 compounds by specific tissue prostaglandin synthases. NSAIDs specifically inhibit COX and thereby reduce the conversion of arachidonic acid to PGG_2.

At least two isoforms of the COX enzymes have now been identified. They are products of two different genes yet share 60% homology in the amino acid sequences considered important for catalysis of arachidonic acid. The differences are primarily in their regulation and expression.[19,20] COX-1, or prostaglandin synthase H_1 (PGHS-1), regulates normal cellular (physiologic) processes and is stimulated by hormones or growth

TABLE 74-1 Nonsteroidal Anti-Inflammatory Medications

Medication	Proprietary (trade) Name	Usual Daily Dose (adults)	Serum Half-Life (hours)	Approved Use*
Nonselective NSAIDS				
Carboxylic Acid Derivatives				
Aspirin (acetylsalicylic acid)	Multiple	2400–6000 mg/24h in 4-5 divided doses	4-15	RA, OA, AS, JCA, ST
Buffered aspirin	Multiple	Same	Same	Same
Enteric-coated salicylates	Multiple	Same	Same	Same
Salsalate	Disalcid	1500–3000 mg/24h bid	Same	Same
Diflunisal	Dolobid	0.500-1500 mg/24h bid	7–15	Same
Choline magnesium trisalicylate†	Trilisate	1.500-3000 mg/24h bid-tid		RA, OA, pain, JCA
Propionic Acid Derivatives				
Ibuprofen†	Motrin, Rufen, OTC	OTC: 200-400 mg qid Rx: 400, 600, 800, maximum: 3200 mg	2	RA, OA, JCA
Naproxen†	Naprelan, Anaprox, Naprosyn EC	250, 375, 500 mg bid	13	RA, OA, JCA, ST
Fenoprofen	Nalfon	300-600 mg qid	3	RA, OA
Ketoprofen	Orudis	75 mg tid	2	RA, OA
Flurbiprofen	Ansaid	100 mg bid-tid	3-9	RA, OA
Oxaprozin	Daypro	600-1800 mg/24h	40-50	RA, OA, pain
Tolmetin	Tolectin	400, 600, 800 mg; 800-2400 mg	1	RA, OA, JCA
Acetic Acid Derivatives				
Indomethacin†	Indocin, Indocin SR Indocin SR	25-50 mg tid or qid SR: 75 bid; rarely >150 mg/24h	3-11	RA, OA, G, AS
Tolmetin	See above		1	
Sulindac	Clinoril	150, 200 mg bid to tid	16	RA, OA, AS, ST, G
Diclofenac	Voltaren, Arthrotec	50 mg tid, 75 mg bid	1-2	RA, OA, AS
Etodolac	Lodine	200-300 mg bid-tid-qid maximum: 1200 mg	2-4	OA, pain
Ketorolac	Toradol	20-40 mg	2	Pain
Fenamates				
Meclofenamate	Meclomen	50-100 mg tid-qid	2-3	RA, OA
Mefenamic acid	Ponstel	250 mg qid	2	RA, OA
Enolic Acid Derivatives				
Piroxicam	Feldene	10, 20 mg qd	30-86	RA, OA
Phenylbutazone	Butazolidin	100 mg tid up to 600 mg/24h	40-80	G, AS
Meloxicam	Mobic	7.5-15 mg qd	20	OA
Naphthylkanones				
Nabumetone	Relafen	500 mg bid up to 1500 mg/24h	19-30	RA, OA
COX-2 Selective NSAIDS				
Celecoxib	Celebrex	100, 200 mg bid, 200 mg qd	11	RA, OA

*FDA approved.

†Available in liquid form.

RA, rheumatoid arthritis; OA, osteoarthritis; AS, ankylosing spondylitis; G, gout; JCA, juvenile chronic arthritis; ST, soft tissue injury.

factors. It is constitutively expressed in most tissues, and is inhibited by all NSAIDs to varying degrees depending on the applied experimental model system used to measure drug effects.[21-24] It has an important role in maintaining the integrity of the gastric and duodenal mucosa, and many of the toxic effects of the NSAIDs on the GI tract are attributed to its inhibition.[25-30] It has been described as a "housekeeping enzyme."

The other isoform, COX-2, or prostaglandin synthase H_2 (PGHS-2) is an inducible enzyme and is usually undetectable in most tissues. Its expression is increased during states of inflammation or experimentally in response to mitogenic stimuli. In monocyte/macrophage systems, endotoxin stimulates COX-2 expression; in fibroblast studies various growth factors, phorbol esters, and interleukin-1 do so.[19,31] This isoform is also constitutively expressed in the brain, specifically the cortex and hippocampus, in the female reproductive tract, the male vas deferens, in bone, and in some models, in human kidney.[19,20] In the brain it appears that COX-2 is upregulated with increased inflammation-induced pain impulses; thus, the inhibition of COX-2 in the brain is thought to be an important modulator of pain in states of inflammation.[18] The expression of COX-2 is inhibited by glucocorticoids.[19,20,31] COX-2 is also inhibited by all of the currently available NSAIDs to a greater or lesser degree, and its inhibition leads to a decrease in those prostanoid products associated with increased pain and swelling.[20-23] Therefore, we have observed the effects of prolonged inhibition of COX-2 for the last 25 years as we have used traditional nonselective NSAIDs.

The in vitro systems used to define the actions of the available NSAIDs are based on using cell-free systems, pure enzyme, or whole cells systems.[21] Each drug studied to date has demonstrated different measurable effects within each system. As an example, it appears that nonacetylated salicylates inhibit the activity of COX-1 and COX-2 in whole cell systems but are not active against either COX-1 or COX-2 in recombinant enzyme or cell membrane systems. This suggests that salicylates act early in the arachidonic acid cascade similar to glucocorticoids, perhaps by inhibiting enzyme expression rather than direct inhibition of cyclooxygenase.

Recent accumulated evidence has demonstrated that several NSAIDs are selective and inhibit the COX-2 enzyme more so than the COX-1 enzyme. For example, in vitro effects of etodolac and meloxicam demonstrate primary inhibition of COX-2 compared with COX-1, at low doses.[32,33] However, at higher approved therapeutic doses this effect appears to be mitigated, as both COX-1 and COX-2 are inhibited to variable degrees. Very potent, selective COX-2 inhibitors that have no measurable effect on COX-1 mediated events at therapeutic doses are now available such as celcoxib.[34] This COX-2 selective inhibitor (or COX-1 sparing drug) has been shown as effective at inhibiting osteoarthritis pain, dental pain, and the pain and inflammation associated with rheumatoid arthritis as naproxen at 500 mg twice daily, ibuprofen 800 mg three times daily, and diclofenac 75 mg twice daily, without endoscopic evidence of gastroduodenal damage and without affecting platelet aggregation.[5-8,34,35] Unfortunately, because of the design of the randomized controlled trials, many important questions regarding the renal effects of the selective COX-2 inhibitors remain unanswered.[19,20] Three other COX-2 selective drugs have been removed from the market throughout the world: rofecoxib due to concerns regarding increased incidence of hypertension and cardiovascular risk; valdecoxib due to increased risk of Stevens Johnson syndrome; and lumiracoxib due to increased risk of serious hepatotoxic adverse reactions. Etoricoxib and an IV form of valdecoxib, parecoxib, are still available elsewhere in the world but not in the United States.

Other possible mechanisms of action that may explain the clinical effects of the NSAIDs include several physicochemical properties of these drugs. The NSAIDs are variably lipophilic and become incorporated in the lipid bilayer of cell membranes and thereby may interrupt protein-protein interactions important for signal transduction.[13,14] For example, stimulus response coupling, which is critical for recruitment of phagocytic cells to sites of inflammation, has been demonstrated in vitro to be inhibited by some NSAIDs.[14] There are data suggesting that NSAIDs inhibit activation and chemotaxis of neutrophils as well as reduce toxic oxygen radical production in stimulated neutrophils.[36,37] There is also evidence that several NSAIDs scavenge superoxide radicals.[36]

Salicylates have been demonstrated to inhibit phospholipase C activity in macrophages. Several NSAIDs have been shown to affect T-lymphocyte function experimentally by inhibiting rheumatoid factor production in vitro. Another newly described action not directly related to prostaglandin synthesis inhibition includes interference with neutrophil-endothelial cell adherence, which is critical to migration of granulocytes to sites of inflammation. These data demonstrate that expressions of L-selectin are decreased.[16] NSAIDs have been demonstrated in vitro to inhibit NF-kB (nitric oxide transcription factor) dependent transcription, thereby inhibiting inducible nitric-oxide synthetase.[15] Anti-inflammatory levels of ASA have been shown to inhibit expression of inducible nitric-oxide synthetase and subsequent production of nitrite in vitro. At pharmacologic doses, sodium salicylate, indomethacin, and acetaminophen when studied had no effect, but at suprapharmacologic doses, sodium salicylate inhibited nitrite production.[15]

It has also been described that prostaglandins inhibit apoptosis (programmed cell death) and that NSAIDs, via inhibition of prostaglandin synthesis, may reestablish more normal cell cycle responses.[19,20] There is evidence suggesting that some NSAIDs may reduce PGH synthase gene expression, thereby supporting the clinical evidence of differences in activity in NSAIDs in sites of active inflammation.

The NSAIDs have been demonstrated to have variable effects on many biologic processes; however, how important some of these effects are clinically remains unknown. Although nonacetylated salicylates have been shown in vitro to inhibit neutrophil function and to have equal efficacy in patients with rheumatoid arthritis,[38] no clinical evidence exists to suggest that these biologic effects are more important than prostaglandin synthase inhibition.

PHARMACOLOGY

The NSAIDs are efficiently absorbed after oral administration, but absorption rates may vary in patients with altered GI blood flow or motility. Certain NSAIDs when taken with food have decreased absorption.[1,2] Enteric coating may reduce direct effects of NSAIDs on the gastric mucosa but may also reduce the rate of absorption.

Most NSAIDs are weak organic acids; once absorbed they are over 95% bound to serum albumin. This is a saturable process. Clinically significant decreases in serum albumin levels or institution of other highly protein-bound medications may lead to an increase in the free component of NSAID in serum. This may be important in patients who are elderly or are chronically ill, especially those with associated hypoalbuminemic states. Importantly, as a result of increased vascular permeability in localized sites of inflammation, this high degree of protein binding may result in delivery of higher levels of NSAIDs.

NSAIDs are metabolized predominantly in the liver by the cytochrome P-450 system and the CYP 2C9 isoform, and excreted in the urine. This must be taken into consideration when prescribing NSAIDs for patients with hepatic or renal dysfunction. Several NSAIDs (e.g., indomethacin, sulindac, piroxicam) have a prominent enterohepatic circulation, resulting in a prolonged half-life and should be used with caution in elderly patients. In patients with renal insufficiency, some inactive metabolites may be resynthesized in vivo to the active compound. Diclofenac, flurbiprofen, and celecoxib are metabolized in the liver. These agents should be used with care and at lowest possible doses, if used at all, in patients with clinically significant liver disease, including patients with cirrhosis with or without ascites, prolonged prothrombin times, falling serum albumin levels, and important elevations in liver transaminases in blood.

Salicylates are the least highly protein bound NSAID: approximately 68%. Zero order kinetics is dominant in salicylate metabolism. Thus, increase of the dose of a salicylate is effective over a narrow range, but once the metabolic systems are saturated, incremental dose increases may lead to very high serum salicylate levels. Thus, changes in salicylate doses need to be carefully considered at chronic steady-state levels, particularly in patients with altered renal or hepatic function.

Significant differences in plasma half-lives of the NSAIDs may be important in explaining their diverse clinical effects. Those with long half-lives typically do not attain maximum plasma concentrations quickly and important clinical responses may be delayed. In most chronic conditions that are appropriate for the use of these drugs, the acute effects are not as important as in the treatment of headache or acute pain. Plasma concentrations can vary widely because of differences in renal clearance and metabolism. Piroxicam has the longest serum half-life of currently marketed NSAIDs: 57 ± 22 hours. In comparison, diclofenac has one of the shortest: 1.1 ± 0.2 hours (see Table 74-1). Although drugs have been developed with very long half-lives to improve patient adherence with therapy, in the older patient it is sometimes preferable to use drugs of shorter half-life so that, when the drug is discontinued, any unwanted effects may more rapidly disappear.

Sulindac and nabumetone are "prodrugs" in which the active compound is produced after first-pass metabolism through the liver. In theory, prodrugs were intended to decrease the exposure of the GI mucosa to the local effects of the NSAIDs. Unfortunately, as noted, with adequate inhibition of COX-1 the patient is placed at substantial risk of an NSAID-induced upper GI event as long as COX-1 activity is inhibited. This is true for drugs such as ketorolac given as an injection or by these prodrugs when given at adequate therapeutic doses.[39]

Other pharmacologic properties may be important clinically. NSAIDs that are highly lipid soluble in serum will penetrate the CNS more effectively and occasionally may produce striking changes in mentation, perception, and mood.[40,41] Indomethacin has been associated with these side effects, even after a single dose, particularly in elderly persons.

ADVERSE EFFECTS

MECHANISM-BASED ADVERSE EFFECTS

Risk for Anaphylaxis and Pulmonary Effects Many adverse effects attributed to NSAIDs are due to inhibition of prostaglandin synthesis in local tissues (**Table 74-2**). For example, patients with allergic rhinitis, nasal polyposis, and/or a history of asthma, in whom all NSAIDs effectively inhibit prostaglandin synthase, are at increased risk for anaphylaxis. In high doses, even nonacetylated salicylates may sufficiently decrease enough prostaglandin synthesis to induce an anaphylactic reaction in sensitive patients.[42] Although the exact mechanism for this effect remains unclear, it is known that E prostaglandins serve as bronchodilators. When COX activity is inhibited in at risk-patients, decrease in synthesis of prostaglandins that contribute to bronchodilation result. Another explanation implicates enzymatic pathways that utilize the arachidonate pool after it is converted from phospholipase, whereby shunting of arachidonate into the leukotriene pathway occurs when cyclooxygenase is inhibited.[43] The leukotriene pathway converts arachidonate by 5-lipoxygenase, leading to products such as LTB4 as well as others clearly associated with anaphylaxis. This explanation implies that large stores of arachidonate released in certain inflammatory situations lead to excess substrate for leukotriene metabolism. This then results in release of products that are highly reactive, leading to increased bronchoconstriction and the risk for anaphylaxis in the right patient. Whether the main mechanism of effect is inhibition of prostaglandin synthesis or shunting of arachidonate into conversion by 5-lipoxygenase or a combination of the two, it is clear that patients who are sensitive are at great risk when NSAIDs are used. The nonacetylated salicylates as a group have been considered a safe choice for these patients because they are known to possess anti-inflammatory activity, but are relatively weak cyclooxygenase inhibitors.

Platelet Effects Platelet aggregation and thus the ability to clot are primarily induced through stimulating thromboxane production with activation of platelet COX-1. There is no COX-2 in the platelet. NSAIDs and aspirin inhibit the activity of COX-1 but the COX-2 selective inhibitors (or COX-1 sparing drugs) have no effect on COX-1 at clinically effective therapeutic doses.[19,20]

The effect of the nonsalicylate NSAIDs on platelet function is reversible and related to the half-life of the drug; whereas the effect of ASA is to acetylate the COX-1 enzyme, thereby permanently inactivating it. Since platelets cannot synthesize new cyclooxygenase enzyme after exposure to ASA, the platelet does not function appropriately for its lifespan. Therefore, the effect of ASA on the platelet does not wear off as the drug is metabolized as with the nonsalicylate NSAIDs. This then is why low-dose aspirin is used as a therapeutic to prevent recurrent cerebrovascular accidents and myocardial infarctions (MIs) in appropriate patients.[44] Patients awaiting surgery should therefore stop their NSAIDs at a time determined by 4 to 5 times their serum half-life; whereas ASA

TABLE 74-2 Adverse Reactions of Nonsteroidal Anti-Inflammatory Drugs

1. Nonspecific reactions
   - A. Rash: fixed drug eruptions, photosensitivity, exfoliative erythroderma, urticaria, Stevens-Johnson syndrome, and others.
   - B. Stomatitis
   - C. Nausea, vomiting; constipation, diarrhea
   - D. Central nervous system
     - (1) Headaches, dizziness, confusion, depression
     - (2) Depersonalization reactions, seizures, syncope
     - (3) Hallucinations, personality change, inability to concentrate, forgetfulness, sleeplessness, irritability, paranoid ideation (particularly in elderly persons)
     - (4) Tinnitus—almost always reversible, decrease in hearing may be the most prominent symptom; less likely evident at the extremes of age
     - (5) Aseptic meningitis—particularly with ibuprofen, including OTC ibuprofen
     - (6) Ocular
       - a. toxic amblyopia
       - b. asymptomatic crystals (of drug) in cornea
   - E. Interference with response to infections; Decrease in neutrophil chemotaxis and lysosomal enzyme release
   - F. Bone marrow suppression
   - G. Competition with other drugs for protein binding sites
2. Hypersensitivity reactions
   - A. Asthma/urticaria syndrome
     - (1) Triad of vasomotor rhinitis, nasal polyposis, asthma; may be seen only with history of asthma
       - a. Due to inhibition of bronchodilating prostaglandins
       - b. Due to shunting into lipoxygenase pathway
3. Platelet effects
   - A. Inhibits platelet cyclooxygenase
     - (1) ASA inhibits the enzyme irreversibly. Needs 7-14 days to repopulate platelet population
     - (2) All others reversible but dependent on half-life of drug: 4-5 × Short half-life: may need only 24 hours. Long half-life: may need days (e.g., piroxicam may need 8 d)
4. Reversal of effects of antihypertensive drugs. Greatest effect on ACE inhibitors than Beta Blockers; Least effect on diuretics
5. Increased cardiovascular risk of stroke, MI, sudden death
6. Renal effects
   - A. Interstitial disease and/or modify tubular function
     - (1) Occasionally observe typical hypersensitivity reaction fever, rash, eosinophilia
   - B. Glomerulopathy
     - (1) May be in association with interstitial disease
     - (2) Typically membranous in type
   - C. Rarely intratubular precipitation of either urate or drug metabolite
   - D. Modify intrinsic renal plasma flow leading to increased BUN, and serum creatinine
   - E. Modify water and electrolyte balance
7. Gastrointestinal (GI) effects
   - A. Nonspecific
     - (1) Dyspepsia, nausea/vomiting, diarrhea, constipation, anorexia
   - B. Specific
     - (1) Bleeding, gastritis, duodenitis, gastroduodenal ulcers with/without signs and symptoms
     - (2) Obstruction of small bowel
     - (3) Hepatotoxicity

needs to be discontinued 1 to 2 weeks before the planned procedure to allow for repopulation of platelets that have been unexposed to ASA.

Although there is little information about the use of the COX-2 selective inhibitors in patients at risk for thrombosis,[19] there is clear evidence that adequate inhibition of COX- 2 enzyme activity in the right patient, may lead to an increased risk of thrombogenic events. This is particularly well defined in mouse models.[45,46] The randomized clinical trials of the COX-2 selective inhibitors were not designed to address this question[47]

Furthermore, we have little information demonstrating that the traditional NSAIDs are safer or more useful than the COX-2 selective inhibitors in this regard. Only aspirin has been studied prospectively, and low-dose aspirin (<325 mg/d) should be given concomitantly with either NSAIDs or selective COX-2 inhibitors in patients at risk for thrombosis.[44] Secondary prophylaxes of cardiovascular events with aspirin has been shown to be important. There is approximately a 23% to 33% decrease in atherothrombotic events in patients with a history of ischemic heart disease when they are treated with more than 325-mg aspirin per day.[44] There are less data about the effectiveness of low-dose aspirin in primary prophylaxis.

There is little evidence that the nonaspirin NSAIDs have a role in primary or secondary prophylaxis of cardiovascular or cerebrovascular events. Because of the additive ulcerogenic potential associated with the use of multiple NSAIDs, it would be advisable to use selective COX-2 inhibitors with aspirin with or without gastroprotection, in the appropriate patient, when considering combination cardioprotective and anti-inflammatory therapies. In the two large bleeding trials describing the effects of celecoxib and rofecoxib, there was a statistically significant difference between the incidence of acute MIs with rofecoxib (0.4%) and naproxen (0.1%), whereas there was no difference in the incidence of acute MIs with celecoxib as compared with diclofenac or ibuprofen.[48,49] As noted above, in the study to decrease recurrent spontaneous GI polyps both drugs revealed an increased risk for acute MI. This was observed with rofecoxib at 25 mg per day and with celecoxib at 400 mg twice a day but not with 400 mgs as needed per day or 200 mgs as needed per day.[50-53]

In addition, the COX-2 selective drugs used for acute postoperative pain (parecoxib) or chronic pain (valdecoxib) have been associated in certain patients after endovascular cardiac surgery with an increased risk for thromboembolism[54-56]

Gastrointestinal Tract The most clinically significant NSAID-induced adverse effects occur in the GI tract, damage to the GI mucosa.[48,49,57-66] These events appear to be due to local or systemic inhibition of prostaglandin synthesis. NSAIDs cause a wide range of GI problems including symptoms of intolerance such as dyspepsia, nausea, vomiting, as well as esophagitis, esophageal stricture, gastritis, mucosal erosions, hemorrhage, peptic ulceration and/or perforation, obstruction, and death.[27,48,49,67-71] The unpleasant symptoms may be observed in about 40% to 60% of patients but are not related to COX-1 inhibition in the GI mucosa.[27,28] The exact cause of these symptoms remains unknown; however, use of H_2-receptor antagonists and proton pump inhibitors typically alleviates these unpleasant effects. Erosions and ulcers as well as ulcer complications are predominantly due to the effects of NSAID-induced systemic inhibition of COX-1, thus those prostaglandins that serve to protect the stomach mucosa from luminal toxins. This protection consists of a mucous layer serving as a barrier, a bicarbonate gradient serving to buffer the mucosa layer from the effects of the extremely acidic lumen, developing glutathione to serve as a scavenger of superoxides, prostaglandin-mediated inhibition of gastric acid, and prostaglandin-mediated increases in mucosal blood flow. All of these effects are inhibited by the NSAIDs by the inhibition of COX-1 activity. However, in an experiment with mice both COX-1 and COX-2 have to be inhibited in order for mice to have an ulcer. The exact effect of inhibiting COX-2 in this experiment is unknown, but some investigators have speculated that COX-2 plays an important role in healing of mucosal lesions.[72,73]

The mucosa of the large and small bowel may also be affected by NSAIDs. These agents in the small or large bowel may also induce stricture formation,[13,27,61-63,70-72] which may manifest as diaphragms leading to small or large bowel obstruction, and can be hard to detect on contrast radiographic studies.

Additionally, there is evidence to suggest that NSAIDs interfere with permeability of the GI mucosa. The weakly acidic NSAIDs rapidly penetrate the superficial lining cells of the GI mucosa leading to oxidative uncoupling of cellular metabolism, local tissue injury, and ultimately cell death. This can result in local erosions, hemorrhages, and formation of clinically significant ulcers in the right patients.[13]

Endoscopic studies have demonstrated that NSAID administration results in shallow erosions and/or submucosal hemorrhages that are observed in the stomach near the prepyloric area and the antrum, although they may occur at any site in the GI tract.[27,74] Typically, these lesions are asymptomatic, making prevalence data difficult to determine.[67] As a result, we do not know the number of lesions that spontaneously heal or which will progress to ulceration, frank perforation, gastric or duodenal obstruction, serious GI hemorrhage, or subsequent death. Risk factors for the development of GI toxicity in patients receiving NSAIDs include age older than 60 years, prior history of peptic ulcer disease, prior use of antiulcer therapies for any reason, concomitant use of glucocorticoids, particularly in patients with rheumatoid arthritis, comorbidities such as significant cardiovascular disease, or patients with severe rheumatoid arthritis (**Table 74-3**).[25,27,48,49,75,76] Other risk factors include increasing dose of specific and singular NSAIDs.

The magnitude of risk for GI adverse events is controversial. The US Food and Drug Administration (FDA) report an overall risk of 2% to 4% for NSAID-induced gastric ulcer development and its complications.[25,27,28] In general, based on multiple clinical trials, the relative risk is estimated to be 4.0 to 5.0 for gastric ulcer, 1.1 to 1.6 for duodenal ulcer, and 4.5 to 5.0 for clinically significant gastric ulcers with hemorrhage, perforation, obstruction, or death. The accurate absolute risk is harder to determine.

As noted, other sites in the GI tract, including the esophagus and small and large bowel, may also be affected. Exposure to NSAIDs is likely a major factor in the development of esophagitis and subsequent stricture formation.[58,59] Effects on small and large bowel have increasingly been reported.[27,53] An autopsy study on 713 patients showed that small bowel ulceration defined as ulcers greater than 3 mm in diameter were observed in 8.4% of patients exposed to NSAIDs compared with 0.6% of nonusers of NSAIDs.[61] Ulcerations of stomach and duodenum were observed in 22% of NSAID users compared with 12% of nonusers.

Before the COX-2 selective inhibitors became available, epidemiologic studies suggested that the nonacetylated salicylates are least likely to result in a NSAID-induced adverse GI event. Agents such as nebumatone are usually considered to be less likely to induce effects.[65,66] However, as higher doses of "safe" NSAIDs are used, then more GI damage is reported.[66] Thus at equally efficacious doses the non-selective NSAIDs all induce ulcers at variable rates, and any of these ulcers in the right patient could develop a complicated course. NSAIDs with prominent enterohepatic circulation and significantly longer half-lives such

TABLE 74-3 Risk Factors for NSAID-Induced Upper Gastrointestinal Toxicity

1. Older than 60 years of age
2. History of previous GI bleed, peptic ulcer disease, perforation, or obstruction
3. History of previous NSAID-induced GI toxicity
4. Concomitant illnesses such as cardiovascular disease leading to increased disability
5. Dose of the NSAID
6. Combinations of NSAIDs
7. Concomitant glucocorticoids
8. For bleeding: concomitant warfarin
9. Concomitant need for antacids of all types
10. Independent: infection with *Helicobacter pylori*, tobacco use, alcohol

as sulindac and piroxicam have been linked to increased potential for GI toxicity attributed to prolonged re-exposure of gastric and duodenal mucosa to bile reflux and the active moiety of the drug.[27]

Endoscopic data from large numbers of patients treated with COX-2 selective inhibitors strongly suggest that ulcers occur at the same rate as in patients who received placebo; whereas the traditional NSAID active comparators induced ulcers (as documented by endoscopy) in 15% (diclofenac 75 mg twice daily, ibuprofen 800 mg three times daily) to 19% (naproxen 500 mg twice daily) following 1 week of treatment in healthy volunteers and in 26% (naproxen 500 mg twice daily) of patients with OA and RA after 12 weeks of treatment.[5-8] Two large outcome trials with rofecoxib and celecoxib are published and demonstrate that rofecoxib and celecoxib both at suprapharmacologic doses (two to four times the treating doses) are associated with about two- to three-fold fewer GI complications than naproxen or ibuprofen, respectively, at standard therapeutic doses.[48,49] These data clearly show that compared with the effects of two widely used NSAIDs (ibuprofen 1.2%, naproxen 1.6%), that the COX-2 inhibitors induce bleeding complications at a lower rate (celecoxib 0.4%, rofecoxib 0.6%).[48,49] It is possible that patients with preexisting ulcer may experience delay in healing when treated with a COX-2 selective inhibitor, but only long-term outcome clinical trials will clarify if this is a risk.[72] There have been further publications confirming the benefit of the COX 2 selective drugs.[73,74]

Approach to the Patient at Risk for NSAID-induced GI Adverse Events The approach to the patient with pain and or inflammation who is about to embark on the use of a NSAID is partly related to dose, consistency, and planned length of therapy. For most patients who will take standard doses of nonselective NSAIDs for less than 10 days, there is little risk unless they have multiple significant risk factors noted previously. However, for the patient with OA or other chronic conditions at risk for an NSAID-induced GI event, the decision remains somewhat controversial. Many patients with dyspepsia or upper GI distress have superficial erosions evident on endoscopy that frequently heal spontaneously without change in therapy. It is more difficult to determine whether cytoprotective agents alter NSAID-associated symptoms, which may or may not predict significant GI events. Although one clinical study demonstrated that >80% of patients who developed significant NSAID-induced endoscopic abnormalities were asymptomatic,[67] several prospective observational trials indicated that patients were more symptomatic with NSAID-induced substantive mucosal damage than previously thought.[64]

The patient who develops a gastric or duodenal ulcer while taking NSAIDs should have treatment discontinued and therapy for ulcer disease, either H_2-antagonist or proton pump inhibitors, instituted.[27-29] If NSAIDs must be continued concomitantly, then the patient will be required to receive antiulcer therapy for longer periods.[28] Typically, most patients with uncomplicated gastric or duodenal ulcers will heal within 8 weeks of initiating H_2-antagonists. If NSAID treatment is continued, then perhaps 16 weeks of therapy may be necessary for adequate healing. Diagnostic tests to determine if the patient is *Helicobacter pylori* positive should be performed, and if the patient has positive studies, then specific antibiotic therapy to eradicate the infection should be administered.[79]

Prophylaxis to prevent NSAID-induced gastric and duodenal ulcers is more complicated. To date there has been no evidence that agents other than concomitant misoprostol therapy will prevent NSAID-induced gastric ulceration and its complications.[75-83] Although high-dose H_2-antagonists or proton pump inhibitors have been demonstrated to prevent NSAID-induced gastric and duodenal ulcers, prevention of ulceration complications has not been clearly shown[79-83]. Endoscopic trials have shown that famotidine at twice the approved dose (40 mg twice daily) significantly decreased the incidence of both gastric and duodenal ulcers.[81,82] Similarly, an endoscopy trial demonstrated that treatment with omeprazole (a proton pump inhibitor) decreased gastroduodenal ulcers.[83] Both H_2-antagonists and proton pump inhibitors decrease dyspeptic symptoms quite effectively. Combination drugs of either ibuprofen with high dose famotidine or enteric coated naproxen with a proton pump inhibitor have become available. Both drugs have been shown to decrease the incidence of gastroduodenal ulcers by endoscopy trials.[80,81]

Misoprostol is a prostaglandin analogue, believed to locally replace prostaglandins whose synthesis in the gastroduodenal mucosa is inhibited by the nonselective NSAIDs.[64-66] A large prospective trial evaluated 8,843 patients with rheumatoid arthritis to determine whether misoprostol would decrease the incidence of ulcers and their complications.[64,65] Patients received various NSAIDs and were followed for 6 months either on misoprostol co-therapy or placebo. The study was powered on the basis of endoscopic observations of an 80% decrease with concomitant misoprostol therapy in endoscopically proven ulcers larger than 0.3 to 0.5 cm in diameter in the gastric and duodenal mucosa.[66] Misoprostol successfully inhibited development of ulcer complications such as bleeding, perforation, and obstruction. There was a 40% reduction in patients treated with misoprostol in contrast to those receiving placebo.[64] Further analysis demonstrated that patients with health assessment questionnaire (HAQ) scores >1.5 (thus worse disease) had an 87% reduction in risk for a NSAID-induced toxic event if concomitantly treated with misoprostol.[65]

These data suggest that high-risk patients may benefit from concomitant misoprostol therapy if NSAID treatment is indicated. Gabriel et al have demonstrated the pharmacoeconomic utility of such therapy in the high-risk patient.[70] Unfortunately, the major adverse event causing withdrawal in approximately 10% of patients was diarrhea, and 30% of patients complained of diarrhea. Therefore medications such as stool softeners and cathartics should be stopped. There are data suggesting that concomitant treatment with misoprostol once an ulcer develops will allow the ulcer to heal.[68] As with famotidine and proton pump inhibitors, there is a combination product of diclofenac with misoprostol available around the world.[82,83]

Renal Adverse Effects The NSAIDs also have effects on the kidneys. The effects of the NSAIDs on renal function include changes in the excretion of sodium, changes in tubular function, the potential for interstitial nephritis, and reversible renal failure due to alterations in filtration rate and renal plasma flow.[84-86] Prostaglandins and prostacyclins are important for maintenance of intrarenal blood flow and tubular transport. All NSAIDs, except nonacetylated salicylates, have the potential to induce reversible impairment of glomerular filtration rate; this effect occurs more frequently in patients with congestive heart failure; established renal disease with altered intrarenal plasma flow including diabetes, hypertension, or atherosclerosis; and with induced hypovolemia, salt depletion or significant hypoalbuminemia.[19,84-86] Triamterene-containing diuretics, which increase plasma renin levels, may predispose patients prescribed NSAIDs to acute renal failure. NSAIDs have been implicated in the development of acute and chronic renal insufficiency, due to inhibition of vasodilating prostaglandins, thereby reducing renal blood flow.

NSAID-associated intersitial nephritis is typically manifested as nephrotic syndrome, characterized by edema or anasarca, proteinuria, hematuria, and pyuria. The usual stigmata of drug-induced allergic nephritis such as eosinophilia, eosinophiluria, and fever may not be present. Interstitial infiltrates of mononuclear cells are seen histologically with relative sparing of the glomeruli. Phenylproprionic acid derivatives, such as fenoprofen, naproxen, and tolmetin and the indoleacetic acid derivative indomethacin, are most commonly associated with the development of interstitial nephritis.

Inhibition of prostaglandin synthesis intrarenally by NSAIDs decreases renin release and thus produces a state of hyporeninemic hypoaldosteronism with resulting hyperkalemia.[84] This effect may be amplified in patients taking potassium-sparing diuretics. Salt retention precipitated by some NSAIDs leading to peripheral edema in some patients is likely due to both inhibition of intrarenal prostaglandin production, which decreases renal medullary blood flow and increases tubular reabsorption of sodium chloride, as well as other direct tubular effects. NSAIDs are also reported to increase antidiuretic hormone effects, thereby reducing excretion of free water, resulting in hyponatremia.[84] Thiazide diuretics may produce an added effect on the NSAID-induced hyponatremia. All NSAIDs have been demonstrated to interfere with medical management of hypertension and heart failure.

All NSAIDs, including the COX-2 inhibitors with the exception of the nonacetylated salicylates, are associated with increases in mean blood pressure in hypertensive patients but not in patients with normal blood pressure.[87] Patients receiving antihypertensive agents including β-blockers, ACE inhibitors, thiazide, and loop diuretics must be checked regularly when initiating therapy with a new NSAID to ensure that there are no significant continued and sustained rises in blood pressure.

The mechanism of acute renal failure induced in the at-risk patient treated with NSAIDs is believed to be prostaglandin mediated.[84-86] However, the role of COX-2 in maintenance of renal homeostasis in the human remains unclear. COX-2 activity is notably present in the macula densa and tubules in animals and humans, and is upregulated in salt-depleted animals.[88] In humans, COX-1 is an important enzyme for control of intrarenal blood flow. It is believed that COX-2 activity importantly modulates salt and water homeostasis, whereas COX-1 activity seems important in modulating renal plasma flow. In the patient who has decreased renal plasma flow, both COX-1 and COX-2 are upregulated and therefore there is not sufficient evidence to indicate that the COX-2 selective inhibitors will be safer than traditional NSAIDs in terms of renal function. Until the appropriate clinical trials are done, any patient at high risk for renal complications should be monitored very carefully. No patient with a creatinine clearance of less than 30 mL per minute should be treated with an NSAID or a COX-2 selective inhibitor.

NONMECHANISM-BASED ADVERSE EVENTS

Hepatotoxicity Elevations in hepatic transaminase levels induced by NSAIDs are not uncommon, although it occurs more often in patients with juvenile rheumatoid arthritis or systemic lupus erythematosus. Unless elevations exceed two to three times the upper limit of normal, or serum albumin falls, or prothrombin times are altered, these effects are usually not considered clinically significant.[89-91] Nonetheless, overt liver failure has been reported following use of many NSAIDs, including diclofenac, flurbiprofen, and sulindac.[90,91] Of all NSAIDs, sulindac has been associated with the highest incidence of cholestasis.[89] Therefore it is recommended that patients at risk for liver toxicity be followed very carefully. When initiating NSAID treatment, patients should be evaluated again within 8 to 12 weeks and serious consideration given to performing a blood analysis for serum transaminase changes.

Idiosyncratic Adverse Effects Many of the toxic effects of NSAIDs are related to their mechanism of action via prostaglandin inhibition, but there are also important potential idiosyncratic effects. A typical nonspecific reaction includes skin rash and photosensitivity, which is associated with all currently available NSAIDs, particularly the phenylproprionic acid derivatives.[92] This same class of NSAID derivative may also induce aseptic meningitis, especially in patients with systemic lupus erythematosus. The underlying mechanism of action remains unknown. Ibuprofen has also been associated with a reversible toxic amblyopia.[92]

Owing to the antiplatelet effects of all NSAIDs, except the nonacetylated salicylates, concomitant therapy with warfarin (Coumadin) puts patients at greater risk for bleeding. As concomitant NSAID therapy would displace warfarin from its albumin binding sites, the prothrombin time may be prolonged. In addition, given the increased relative risk for NSAID-induced gastroduodenal ulcers and bleeding, there is an increased risk for bleeding when the NSAIDs are used concomitantly with warfarin. In that the COX-2 selective inhibitors do not cause ulcers of the GI tract, nor do they alter platelet function, the patient on warfarin would have less risk for a significant GI bleed when treated with these drugs than traditional nonselective NSAIDs. Effects such as these may also be seen with dilantin or other highly protein-bound drugs such as antibiotics.

The NSAIDs inhibit the renal excretion of lithium and should be used with caution in patients taking this drug. Cholysteramine, an anion-exchange resin, reduces the rate of NSAID absorption and its bioavailability.

The CNS side effects of NSAIDs include aseptic meningitis, psychosis, and cognitive dysfunction.[1,41,42] These side effects are more commonly seen in elderly patients treated with indomethacin, whereas the phenylproprionic acid derivatives are more commonly associated with the development of aseptic meningitis and toxic amblyobia. Tinnitus is a common problem with higher doses of salicylates as well as the nonsalicylate NSAIDs. The mechanism is unknown. Interestingly, young patients and elderly patients may not complain of tinnitus but only of hearing loss. Other NSAIDs may also induce tinnitus in specific patients. Decreasing the dose often alleviates the effect.

It has been shown that COX-2 is important for ovulation through the PPRA l receptor.[19] In addition, COX-2 is upregulated with implantation of a fertilized ovum or in decidualization. Although there are a few case reports of reversible infertility associated with the use of NSAIDs, given the large numbers of patients who regularly use NSAIDs there does not appear to be a generalized epidemic of infertility.[93]

Use of NSAIDs does not lead to osteoporosis.[94,95] The role of COX-1 remains unclear. Although inflammation in the joint leads to juxtaarticular osteopenia, this is the result of increased prostaglandin synthesis in the inflamed joint, which is likely directly related to increased COX-2 activity.

Some of the early available NSAIDs have been associated with an increased risk for bone marrow failure. This is particularly true of phenylbutazone and indomethacin. Strom et al have described the incidence of neutropenia as a toxic effect of the NSAIDs.[96] In a case-controlled study performed using Medicaid claims data, investigators defined that the adjusted odds ratio for neutropenia in patients treated with NSAIDs is 4.2 (confidence interval (CI), 2.0-8.7). When patients treated with either phenylbutazone or indomethacin were excluded, the odds ratio for the development of neutropenia remained robust: 3.5 (CI 1.6-7.6). Because of the common use of NSAIDs, the risk of neutropenia is quite low.

There are little data documenting the effects of the NSAIDs on pregnancy or the fetus. In animal models, the NSAIDs have been shown to increase the incidence of dystocia, postimplantation loss, as well as delay of parturition and miscarriage.[93] The effect of prostaglandin inhibition may result in premature closure of the ductus arteriosus. ASA has been associated with smaller babies and neonatal bruising; however, it has been used for many years in the treatment of patients who require NSAIDs while pregnant. Typically, therapy with ASA is stopped about 8 weeks prior to delivery to decrease the risk for interfering with ductus closure. In animals, there is no evidence that ASA is a teratogen. The NSAIDs are excreted in breast milk. It is believed that salicylates in normally recommended doses are not considered dangerous to nursing infants.

SUMMARY

Although NSAIDs are known to decrease pain and inflammation and to be antipyretic, they have not been shown to decrease erosions in rheumatoid arthritis, to retard osteophyte formation in osteoarthritis, or to protect cartilage from mechanical or inflammatory injury. However, they continue to be important drugs for the palliation of acute and chronic pain and inflammation. Newer forms of COX-2 inhibitors are in development and are considered better analgesics because of rapid uptake in the CNS. Time will tell the ultimate role these drugs will play as more is learned about their complex physiologic effects.

REFERENCES

1. Brooks PM, Day RO. Nonsteroidal antiinflammatory drugs: differences and similarities. *N Engl J Med.* 1991;324:1716-1725.
2. Furst DE. Are there differences among nonsteroidal antiinflammatory drugs? Comparing acetylated salicylates, nonacetylated salicylates, and nonacetylated nonsteroidal antiinflammatory drugs. *Arthritis Rheum.* 1994;37:1-9.

3. Abramson SB, Weissman G. The mechanisms of action of nonsteroidal antiinflammatory drugs. *Arthritis Rheum*. 1989;32:1-9.
4. Simon LS. Actions and toxicities of the NSAIDs. *Curr Opin Rheum*. 1996.
5. Simon LS, Lanza FL, Lipsky PE, et al. Preliminary study of the safety and efficacy of SC-58635, a novel cyclooxygenase 2 inhibitor: efficacy and safety in two placebo-controlled trials in osteoarthritis and rheumatoid arthritis, and studies of gastrointestinal and platelet effects. *Arthritis Rheum*. 1998;41:1591-1602.
6. Simon LS, Weaver AL, Graham DY, et al. The anti-inflammatory and upper gastrointestinal effects of celecoxib in rheumatoid arthritis: a randomized, controlled trial. *JAMA*. 1999;282:1921-1928.
7. Hawkey CJ. COX-2 inhibitors. *Lancet*. 1999;353:307-314.
8. Simon LS, Grierson LM, Naseer Z, et al. Efficacy and safety of topical diclofenac containing dimethyl sulfoxide (DMSO) compared with those of topical placebo, DMSO vehicle and oral diclofenac for knee osteoarthritis. *Pain*. 2009;143(3):238-245.
9. Baum C, Kennedy DL, Forbes MB. Utilization of nonsteroidal antiinflammatory drugs. *Arthritis Rheum*. 1985;28:686-691.
10. Phillips AC, Polisson RP, Simon LS. NSAIDs and the elderly. Toxicity and economic implications. *Drugs Aging*. 1996 Feb;8(2):84-88.
11. Walker JS, Sheather-Reid RB, Carmody JJ, et al. Nonsteroidal antiinflammatory drugs in rheumatoid arthritis and osteoarthritis: support for the concept of "responders" and "nonresponders." *Arthritis Rheum*. 1997;40:1944-1954.
12. Simon LS, Strand V. Clinical response to nonsteroidal antiinflammatory drugs. *Arthritis Rheum*. 1997;40:1940-1943.
13. Mahmud T, Rafi SS, Scott DL, et al. Nonsteroidal antiinflammatory drugs and uncoupling of mitochondrial oxidative phosphorylation. *Arthritis Rheum*. 1996;39:1998-2003.
14. Abramson SB, Leszczynska-Piziak J, Clancy RM, et al. Inhibition of neutrophil function by aspirin-like drugs (NSAIDs): requirement for asembly of heterotrimeric G proteins in bilayer phosopholipid. *Biochem Pharmacol*. 1994;47:563-572.
15. Amin AR, Vyas P, Attur M, et al. The mode of action of aspirin-like drugs: effect on inducible nitric oxide synthase. *Proc Natl Acad Sci USA*. 1995;92:7926-7930.
16. Díaz-González F, González-Alvero I, Companero MR, et al. Prevention of in vitro neutrophil-endothelial attachment through shedding of L-selectin by nonsteroidal antiinflammatory drugs. *J Clin Invest*. 1995; 95:1756-1765.
17. Smith WL. Prostanoid biosynthesis and mechanisms of action. *Am J Physiol*. 1992;263:F181-F191.
18. Samad TA, Moore KA, Sapirstein A, et al. Interleukin-1beta-mediated induction of COX-2 in the CNS contributes to inflammatory pain hypersensivity. *Nature*. 2001;410:471-475.
19. Crofford LJ, Lipsky PE, Brooks P, et al. Basic biology and clinical application of cyclooxygenase-2. *Arthritis Rheum*. 2000;43:4-13.
20. Dubois RN, Abramson SB, Corfford L, et al. Cyclooxygenase in biology and disease. *FASEB J*. 1998;12:1063-1073.
21. Mitchell JA, Akarasereenont P, Thiemermann C, et al. Selectivity of nonsteroidal antiinflammatory drugs as inhibitors of constitutive and inducible cyclooxygenase. *Proc Natl Acad Sci USA*. 1994;90:11693-11697.
22. Patrignani P, Panara MR, Greco A, et al. Biochemical and pharmacological characterization of the cyclooxygenase activity of human blood prostaglandin endoperoxide synthases. *J Pharmacol Exp Ther*. 1994; 271:1705-1712.
23. Meade EA, Smith WL, Dewitt DL. Differential inhibition of prostaglandin endoperoxide synthase (cyclooxygenase) isoenzymes by aspirin and other non-steroidal anti-inflammatory drugs. *J Biol Chem*. 1993; 268(9):6610-6614.
24. Laneuville O, Breuer DK, DeWitt DL, et al. Differential inhibition of human prostaglandin endoperoxide H synthases-1 and -2 by nonsteroidal antiinflammatory drugs. *J Pharmacol Exp Ther*. 1994;271: 927-939.
25. Fries JP, Miller SR, Spitz PW. Toward an epidemiology of gastropathy associated with nonsteroidal antiinflammatory drug use. *Gastroenterology*. 1989;96:647-655.
26. Gabriel SE, Jaaklimainen L, Bombadier C. Risk for serious gastrointestinal complications related to use of nonsteroidal antiinflammatory drugs: a meta-analysis. *Ann Intern Med*. 1991;115:787-796.
27. Wolfe MM, Lichtenstein DR, Singh G. Gastrointestinal toxicity of the nonsteroidal antiinflammatory drugs. *N Engl J Med*. 1999;340:1888-1899.
28. Scheiman JM. NSAIDs, gastrointestinal injury, and cytoprotection. *Gastroenterol Clin North Am*. 1996;25:279-298.
29. Laine L. Nonsteroidal antiinflammatory drug gastropathy. *Gastrointest Endosc Clin North Am*. 1996;6:489-504.
30. Hollander D. Gastrointestinal complications of nonsteroidal antiinflammatory drugs: prophylactic and therapeutic strategies. *Am J Med*. 1994;96:274-281.
31. Charleson S, Cartwright M, Frank J, et al. Characterization of prostaglandin G/H synthase 1 and 2 in rat, dog, monkey, and human gastrointestinal tracts. *Gastroenterology*. 1996;111:445-454.
32. DeWitt DL, Meade EA, Smith WL. PGH synthase isoenzyme selectivity: the potential for safer nonsteroidal antiinflammatory drugs. *Am J Med*. 1993;95(suppl 2A):40S-44S.
33. Glaser K, Sung M-L, O'Neill K, et al. Etodolac selectively inhibits human prostaglandin G/H synthase 2 (PGHS-2) versus human PGHS-1. *Eur J Pharmacol*. 1995;281:107-111.
34. Lipsky PE, Abramson SB, Crofford L, et al. The classification of cyclooxygenase inhibitors [editorial]. *J Rheumatol*. 1998;25: 2298-3003.
35. Bensen WG, Fiechtner JJ, McMillen JI, et al. Treatment of osteoarthritis with celecoxib, a cyclooxygenase-2 inhbitor: a randomized controlled trial. *Mayo Clin Proc*. 1999;74:1095-1105.
36. Friman C, Johnston C, Chew C, Davis P. Effect of diclofenac sodium, tolfenamic acid and indomethacin on the production of superoxide induced by *N*-fromyl-methionyl-leucyl-phenylalanine in normal human polymorphonuclear leukocytes. *Scand J Rheumatol*. 1986;15:41-46.
37. Gay JC, Lukens JN, English DK. Differential inhibition of neutrophil superoxide generation by nonsteroidal antiinflammatory drugs. *Inflammation*. 1984;8:209-222.
38. Bombardier C, Peloso PM, Goldsmith CH. Salsalate, a nonacetylated salicylate, is as efficacious as diclofenac in patients with rheumatoid arthritis. Salsalate-diclofenac study group. *J Rheumatol*. 1995;22:617-624.
39. Litvak KM, McEvoy GK. Ketorolac, an injectable non-narcotic analgesic. *Clin Pharm*. 1990;9:921-935.
40. Saag KG, Rubenstein LM, Chrischilles EA, Wallace RB. Nonsteroidal antiinflammatory drugs and cognitive decline in the elderly. *J Rheumatol*. 1995;22:2142-2147.
41. Hoppmann RA, Peden JG, Ober SK. Central nervous system side effects of nonsteroidal antiinflammatory drugs. Aseptic meningitis, psychosis, and cognitive dysfunction. *Arch Intern Med*. 1991;151: 1309-1313.
42. Stevenson DD, Hougham AJ, Schrank PJ, et al. Salsalate cross-sensitivty in aspirin-sensitive patients with asthma. *J Allergy Clin Immunol*. 1990;86:749-758.

43. Robinson DR, Skosliewicz M, Bloch KJ, et al. Cyclooxygenase blockade elevates leukotriene E4 production during acute anaphylaxis in sheep. *J Exp Med.* 1986;163:1509-1517.
44. Antiplatelet Trialists Collaboration Collaborative. Overview of randomised trials of antiplatelet therapy, I: prevention of death, myocardial infarction, and stroke by prolonged antiplatelet therapy in various categories of patients. *BMJ.* 1994;308:81-106.
45. Yu Y, Ricciotti E, Scalia R, Tang Sy, Grant, G, Yu Z, et al. Vascular COX-2 modulates blood pressure and thrombosis in mice Sci Transl ed 4, 132ra54 (2012); DOI:10.1126/scitranslmed.3003787
46. Yu Z, Crichton I, Tang SY, Hu Y, Ricciotti E, Levin MD, et al. Disruption of the 5-lipoxygenase pathway attenuates the atherogenesis consequent to COX-2 deletion in mice. *PNAS.* 2012; 109:6727-6732.
47. Strand V Are COX-2 Inhibitors preferable to non-selective non-steroidal anti-inflammaotry drugs in patients with risk of cardiovascular events taking low-dose aspirin? *Lancet.* 2007 370: 2138-2151.
48. Silverstein FE, Faich G, Goldstein JL, et al. Gastrointestinal toxicity with celecoxib vs nonsteroidal anti-inflammatory drugs for osteoarthritis and rheumatoid arthritis: the CLASS study-a randomized controlled trial. *JAMA.* 2000;284:1247-1255.
49. Bombardier C, Laine L, Reicin A, et al. Comparison of upper gastrointestinal toxicity of rofecoxib and naproxen in patients with rheumatoid arthritis. *N Engl J Med.* 2000;343:1520-1528.
50. Bresalier RS, Sandler RS, Quan H, et al. Adenomatous polyp prevention on Vioxx (APPROVe) Trial Investigators. Cardiovascular events associated with rofecoxib in a colorectal adenoma chemoprevention trial. *N Engl J Med.* 2005;352:1092-1102.
51. Solomon SD, McMurray JJV, Pfeffer MA et al, on behalf of the Adenoma Prevention with Celecoxib (APC) Study Investigators Cardiovascular risk associated with celecoxib in a clinical trial for colorectal adnoma prevention *N Engl J Med.* 2005; 352: 1071-80
52. Solomon SD, Pfefer MA, McMurray JJV et al. for the APC and PreSAP Trial Investigators. Effect of celecoxib on cardiovascular events and blood pressure in two trials for the prevention of colorectal adenomas. *Circulation.* 2006;114:1028-1035.
53. ADAPT Research Group. Cardiovascular and cerebrovascular evetns in the randomized, controlled Alzheimer's Disease Anti-Inflammatory Prevention Trial (ADAPT). *PLoS Clin Trials.* 2006;1:E33. doi:10.371/journal.pctr.0010033.
54. Ott E, Nussmeier N, Duke P, and the Multicenter Study of Perioperative Ischemia (McSPI) Research Group. Ischemia Research and Education Foundation (IREF) Investigators: efficacy and safety of the cyclooxygenase 2 inhbitors parecoxib and valdecoxib in patients undergoing coronary bypass surgery. *J Thorac Cardiovasc Surg.* 2003;125:1481-1492.
55. Nussmeier NA, Whelton AA, Brown MT et al. Complications of the COX -2 inhibitors parecoxib and valdecoxib after cardiac surgery. *N Engl J Med.* 2005; 352: 1081-91.
56. US FDA Advisory Committee Briefing Document. Celecoxib and valdecoxib cardiovascular safety. FDA Arthritis and Drug Safety and Risk Management Advisory Committee Briefing Package, Feb 16-18, 2005-4090b1-01.htm.
57. Garcia Rodriguez LA, Walker AM, Perez Gutthann S. Nonsteroidal antiinflammatory drugs and gastrointestinal hospitalizations in Saskatchewan: a cohort study. *Epidemiology.* 1992;3:337-342.
58. Griffin MR, Piper JM, Daugherty JR, et al. Nonsteroidal anti-inflammatory drug use and increased risk for peptic ulcer disease in elderly persons. *Ann Intern Med.* 1991;114:257-263.
59. Garcia Rodriguez LA. Nonsteroidal antiinflammatory drugs, ulcers and risk: a collaborative meta-analysis. *Semin Arthritis Rheum.* 1997;26(suppl):16-20.
60. Bjarnason I, Thjodleifsson B. Gastrointestinal toxicity of nonsteroidal anti-inflammatory drugs: the effect of numesulide compared with naproxen on the human gastrointestinal tract. *Rheumatology.* 1999;38(suppl):24-32.
61. Holt S, Rigoglioso V, Sidhu M, et al. Nonsteroidal antiinflammatory drugs and lower gastrointestinal bleeding. *Dig Dis Sci.* 1993;38:1619-1623.
62. Wilcox CM, Alexander LN, Cotsonis GA, Clark WS. Nonsteroidal antiinflammatory drugs are associated with both upper and lower gastrointestinal bleeding. *Dig Dis Sci.* 1997;42:990-997.
63. Wallace JL, Bak A, McKnight W, et al. Cyclooxygenase I contributes to inflammatory reponses in rats and mice: implications for gastrointestinal toxicity. *Gastroenterology.* 1998;115:101-109.
64. Singh G, Ramey DR, Morfeld D, et al. Gastrointestinal tract complications of nonsteroidal antiinflammatory drug treatment in rheumatoid arthritis. A prospective observational study. *Arch Intern Med.* 1996;156:1530-1536.
65. Simon LS, Zhao SZ, Arguelles LM, et al. Economic and gastrointestinal safety comparisons of etodolac, nabumetone and oxaprozin from insurance claims data from patients with arthritis. *Clin Ther.* 1998;1218-1235; discussion, 1192-1193.
66. Agrawal NM, Caldwell J, Kivitz AJ, et al. Comparison of the upper gastrointestinal safety of Arthrtoec 75 and nabumetone in osteoarthritis patients at high risk for developing nonsteroidal anti-inflammatory drug-induced gastrointestinal ulcers. *Clin Ther.* 1999;21:659-674.
67. Larkai EN, Smith JL, Lidsky MD, Graham DY. Gastroduodenal mucosa and dyspeptic symptoms in arthritic patients during chronic nonsteroidal anti-inflammatory drug use. *Am J Gastroenterol.* 1987;82:1153.
68. Minocha A, Greenbaum DS. Pill-esophagitis caused by nonsteroidal antiinflammatory drugs. *Am J Gastroenterol.* 1991;86:1086-1089.
69. Eng J, Sabanathan S. Drug-induced esophagitis. *Am J Gastroenterol.* 1991;86:1127-1133.
70. Allison MC, Howatson AG, Torance CJ. Gastrointestinal damage associated with the use of nonsteroidal antiinflammatory drugs. *N Engl J Med.* 1992;327:749-754.
71. Reuter BK, Asfaha S, Buret A, et al. Exacerbation of inflammation-associated colonic injury in rat through inhibition of cyclooxygenase-2. *J Clin Invest.* 1996;98:2076-2085.
72. Mizuno H, Sakamoto C, Matsuda K, et al. Induction of cyclooxygenase 2 in gastric mucosal lesions and its inhibition by the specific antagonist delays healing in mice. *Gastroenterology.* 1997;12:387-397.
73. Chan FK et al. Celecoxib versus omeprazole and diclofenac in patients with osteoarthritis and rheumatoid arthritis (CONDOR): a randomised trial. *Lancet.* Jul 17, 2010;376(9736):173-179.
74. Cryer B, Li C, Simon LS, Singh G, Stillman MJ, Berger MF. GI-REASONS: A novel 6-month, prospective, randomized, open-label, blinded endpoint (PROBE) trial. *Am J Gastroenterol.* 2013;108:392-400; doi:10.1038/ajg.2012.467; published online 12 February 2013.
75. Silverstein, FE, Graham, DY, Senior, JR, et al. Misoprostol reduces serious gastrointestinal complications in patients with rheumatoid arthritis receiving nonsteroidal anti-inflammatory drugs. *Ann Intern Med.* 1995;123:214.
76. Simon LS, Hatoum HT, Bittman RM, et al. Risk factors for serious nonsteroidal-induced gastrointestinal complications: regression analysis of the MUCOSA trial. *Fam Med.* 1996;28:202-208.
77. Moore A, Bjarnson I, Cryer B, Garcia-Rodriguez L, Goldkind L, Lanas A, et al. Evidence for endoscopic ulcers as meaningful

surrogate endpoint for clinically significant upper gastrointestinal harm. *Clin Gastroentero Hepatol.* 2009;7:1156-1163.

78. Graham DY, White RH, Moreland LW, et al. Duodenal and gastric ulcer prevention with misoprostol in arthritis patients taking NSAIDs. *Ann Intern Med.* 1993;119:257-262.
79. Levine LR, Cloud ML, Enas NH. Nizatidine prevents peptic ulceration in high-risk patient taking nonsteroidal anti-inflammatory drugs. *Arch Intern Med.* 1993;153:2449-2454.
80. Hawkey CJ, Karrasch JA, Szczepanski L, et al. Omeprazole compared with misoprostol for ulcers associated with nonsteroidal antiinflammatory drugs. *N Engl J Med.* 1998;338:727-734.
81. Taha AS, Hudson N, Hawkey CJ, et al. Famotidine for the prevention of gastric and duodenal ulcers caused by nonsteroidal anti-inflammaotry drugs. *N Engl J Med.* 1996;334:1435-1439.
82. Schiff M, Peura D. HZT-501 (Duexis®; ibuprofen 800 mgs/famotidine 26.6 mgs) gastrointestinal protection in the treatment of the signs and symptoms of rheumatoid arthritis and osteoarthritis. *Expert Rev Gastroenterol Hepatol.* 2012;6:25-35.
83. Public Assessment Report of the Medicines Evaluation Board in the Netherlands; EU Procedure Number: NL/H/1848/001/DC Registration Number in the Netherlands: RVG 106235 17 January 2011.
84. Schlondorff D. Renal complications of nonsteroidal anti-inflammatory drugs. *Kidney Int.* 1993;44:643-653.
85. Whelton A. Renal and related cardiovascular effects of conventional and COX-2 specific NSAIDs and non-NSAID analgesics. *Am J Ther.* 2000;7:63-74.
86. Bennett WM, Henrich WL, Stoff JS. The renal effects of NSAIDs: summary and recommendation. *Am J Kidney Dis.* 1996; 28:56-62.
87. Pope JE, Anderson JJ, Felson DT. A meta-analysis of the effects of nonsteroidal anti-inflammatory drugs on blood pressure. *Arch Intern Med.* 1993;153:477-484.
88. Harris RC, McKanna JA, Aiai Y, et al. Cyclooxygenase-2 is associated with the macula densa of rat kidney and increases with salt restriction. *J Clin Invest.* 1994;94:2504-2510.
89. Garcia Rodriguez LA, Williams R, Derby LE, Dean AD, Jick H. Acute liver injury associated with nonsteroidal antiinflammatory drugs and the role of risk factors. *Arch Intern Med.* 1994;154:311-316.
90. Walker AM. Quantitative studies of the risk of serious hepatic injury in persons using nonsteroidal antiinflammatory drugs. *Arthritis Rheum.* 1997;40:201-208.
91. Helfgott SM, Sandberg-Cook J, Zakim D, Nestler J. Diclofenac-associated hepatotoxicity. *JAMA.* 1990;264:2660-2662.
92. Simon LS, Mills JA. Drug therapy: nonsteroidal antiinflammatory drugs. *N Engl J Med.* 1980;302:1179-1185, 1237-1243.
93. Nielsen GL, Sorensen HT, Larsen H, Pedersen L. Risk of adverse birth outcome and miscarriage in pregnant users of NSAIDs: population based observational study and case-control study. *BMJ.* 2001;322:266-270.
94. Kawaguchi H, Pilbeam CC, Harrison JR, Raisz LG. The role of prostaglandins in the regulation of bone metabolism. *Clin Orthop.* 1995; 313:36-46.
95. Pilbeam CC, Fall PM, Alander CB, Raisz LG. Differential effects of nonsteroidal anti-inflammatory drugs on constitutive and inducible prostaglandin G/H synthase in cultured bone cells. *J Bone Miner Res.* 1997;12:1198-1203.
96. Strom BL, Carson JL, Schinnar R, et al. Nonsteroidal anti-inflammatory drugs and neutropenia. *Arch Intern Med.* 1993;153: 2119-2124.

Cannabinoids in Pain Management

Christopher Noto
Mark S. Wallace

HISTORY AND CONTROVERSY OF MEDICAL MARIJUANA

Cannabis has been utilized as a medicine and in various cultural practices for millennia with accounts of its use dating back over 5000 years.[1] There is reference to the use of cannabis for the treatment of headache from the sixth and seventh centuries.[2] In the mid-1800s, reports of the therapeutic potential of cannabis entered the medical literature and its use became more widespread.[3] However, in the early twentieth century, cannabis was increasingly scrutinized for its psychoactive effects and recreational use, and it was removed from the US Pharmacopoeia in 1942.[4] Nonetheless, preclinical studies continued and many neurobehavioral tests confirmed its analgesic effects.[5-8] In addition to its use for analgesia, cannabis is under investigation for use in a number of neurological disorders, glaucoma, and as an antiemetic and appetite stimulant.

In the United States, the use of medical marijuana continues to be a politically charged issue. In November 1996, voters in the states of California and Arizona passed referenda designed to permit the use of marijuana as a medicine, though Arizona's referendum was invalidated 5 months later. Since then, several states have passed ballot initiatives in support of medical marijuana. In January 1997, the White House Office of National Drug Control asked the Institute of Medicine to conduct a review of scientific evidence to assess the health risks and benefits of marijuana. The 1999 Institute of Medicine report contained several recommendations regarding medical marijuana which stated: 1) research should continue into the physiologic effects of synthetic and plant-derived cannabinoids; 2) development of new delivery systems should be pursued;3) the psychological effects of cannabis should be evaluated; 4) studies to define health risks of smoked marijuana should be conducted, and; 5) clinical trials should involve short-term use, reasonable expectations of efficacy, and approval by an Institutional Review Board. The report stated that short-term use of smoked cannabis for patients with debilitating symptoms must meet the following conditions: (1) failure of approved medications, (2) reasonable expectation of efficacy, (3) administration under medical supervision, and (4) inclusion of an oversight strategy.[9]

1999 Institute of Medicine Recommendations for Research Focus of Medical Marijuana

1. Physiologic effects of synthetic and plant-derived cannabinoids
2. Development of new delivery systems
3. Psychological effects of cannabis
4. Health risks of smoked marijuana

CANNABINOID BACKGROUND

The two cannabinoid receptors are CB1 and CB2.[10,11] The term cannabinoid refers to a variety of compounds which are (1) derived from cannabis plants (phytocannabinoids), (2) endogenous cannabinoids (referred to as endocannabinoids), and (3) synthetic cannabinoids.[12]

Cannabis is a genus of flowering plants that contain three species: *Cannabis sativa* (the largest variety), *C indica*, and *C ruderalis*. The popular name, marijuana, refers to the dried leaves and flowers of *C sativa*, which are most commonly smoked.[4] Marijuana contains nearly 500 known compounds, of which more than 80 are classified as cannabinoids.[13] The main psychoactive compound in cannabis is Δ^9-tetrahydrocannabinol (THC).[14] Additional cannabinoids in the cannabis plant are cannabidiol (CBD) and cannabinol (CBN). CBD is the second most abundant compound in cannabis following THC.[15] It is less psychoactive than THC and has a low affinity for the CB1 and CB2 receptors.[16,17]

CBD appears to enhance the effects of THC but it is unclear if this is due to a pharmacokinetic or pharmacodynamic interaction.[18] CBN is found in trace amounts in cannabis and is a metabolite of THC.[19-22] It has weak CB receptor affinity but because of its higher affinity for the CB2 over CB1 receptor, it may have more anti-inflammatory effects.

A cannabis-based medicine extract (CBME) is derived by extraction of compounds from the marijuana plant. Two CBMEs have undergone clinical trials: Cannador and nabiximols (Sativex). Cannador is a CBME delivered in oral capsules with differing THC:CBD ratios.[23] Nabiximols is a sublingual spray that contains THC and CBD currently in phase III trials for cancer pain.[16-18,24]

The two major endocannabinoids are anandamide and 2-arachidonoyl-glycerol (2-AG) and are discussed in the endocannabinoid system.

Cannabinoid Sources

Phytocannabinoids

a. Cannabis-based plant extracts

- i. Nabiximols
- ii. Cannador

Endocannabinoids

b. Anandamide

c. 2-arachidonoylglycerol (2-AG)

Synthetic cannabinoids

d. Synthetic THC (dronabinol)

e. Synthetic analog of THC (ajulemic acid)

f. Semisynthetic analog of THC (nabilone)

Three synthetic cannabinoids have undergone clinical trials: dronabinol (Marinol), nabilone (Cesamet), and ajulemic acid (CT3). The synthetic Δ^9-THC analog dronabinol has been marketed in the United States since 1985 for treatment of nausea associated with chemotherapy and as an appetite stimulant in HIV/AIDS. It is currently available as generic, which eliminates some of the cost that precluded its use in the treatment of pain. Nabilone is a semisynthetic Δ^9-THC analog approximately 10 times more potent than dronabinol with a longer duration.[25] In the United States, nabilone is FDA-approved for treatment of chemotherapy-induced nausea. Ajulemic acid is a synthetic Δ^9-THC analog currently undergoing clinical trials for treatment of pain.

THE ENDOCANNABINOID SYSTEM

The endocannabinoid system refers to the ligands anandamide and 2-AG, enzymes involved in their synthesis and breakdown, and the CB1 and CB2 receptors[26] (**Fig. 75-1**). CB1 is located in the brain, spinal cord and on primary sensory nerve terminals. CB2 is found on microglia, monocytes, macrophages, B, and T lymphocytes. Both receptors belong to the G-protein coupled receptor superfamily. As such they contain seven transmembrane spanning domains. CB1 and CB2 receptors are coupled through $G_{i/o}$ proteins, negatively to adenylate cyclase (inhibiting the production of cyclic AMP; cAMP) and positively to mitogen-active protein kinase (MAPK).[27] Additionally, CB1 has been shown to be coupled positively to inwardly rectifying and A-type outward potassium channels, and negatively to N-type and P/Q type calcium channels. The endocannabinoid, 2-AG, is synthesized in postsynaptic neuron and acts as a retrograde signaling molecule. This synthesis results from the activation of the glutamate receptor which in turns activates the phospholipase C–diacylglycerol lipase pathway to generate 2-AG from membrane phospholipid precursors. Anandamide is an amide of ethanolamine and arachidonic acid. It is generated from its membrane precursor, N-arachidonoyl phosphatidylethanolamine (NAPE) through cleavage by phospholipase D. 2-AG is degraded in the presynaptic terminal by monoacylglycerol lipase (MAG). Anandamide is degraded in the postsynaptic terminal by fatty acid amino hydrolase (FAAH) and is a low-efficacy agonist similar to Δ^9-THC. 2-AG is far more abundant than anandamide and is considered a high-efficacy agonist.[28]

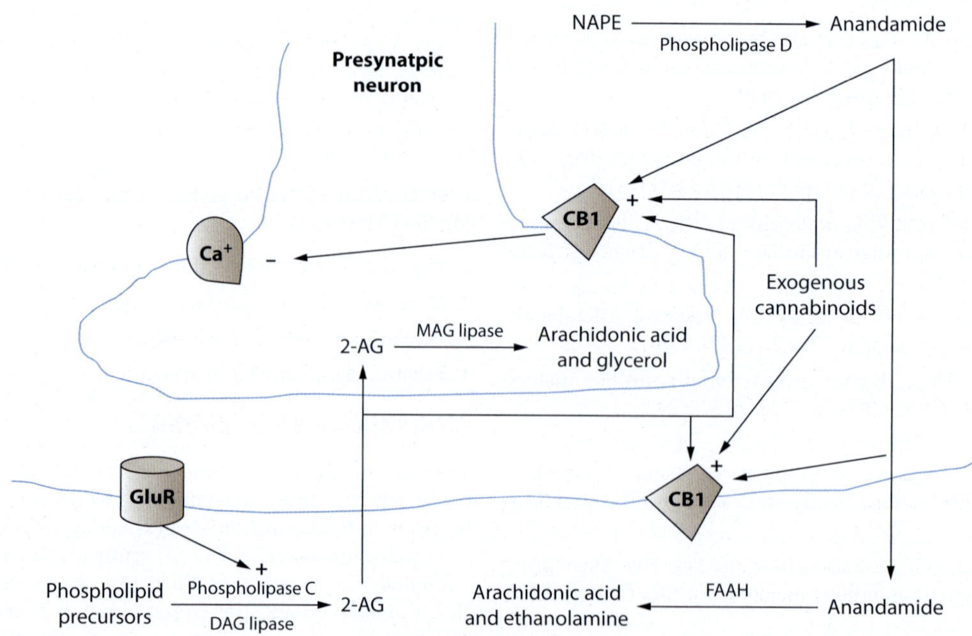

FIGURE 75-1. The endocannabinoid system.2-arachidonyl glycerol (2-AG) and anandamide are endocannabinoids that activate the presynaptic CB1 receptor. Activation of the glutamate receptor (GluR) stimulates phospholipase C. 2-AG is produced from the hydrolysis of phosphatidylinositol by phospholipase C and diacylglycerol lipase (DAG lipase) in the postsynaptic neuron. 2-AG is transported into the synaptic cleft where it activates the CB1 receptor. It is also transported into the presynaptic neuron where monoacylglycerol lipase (MAG lipase) degrades into arachidonic acid and glycerol. Anandamide is produced from the hydrolysis of N-arachidonoyl phosphatidylethanolamine (NAPE) by phospholipase D to stimulate the presynaptic CB1 receptor. It is then transported into the postsynaptic membrane and degraded by fatty acid amino hydrolase (FAAH) into arachidonic acid and ethanolamine. Activation of the CB1 receptor by exogenous cannabinoids, 2-AG, and anandamide reduce pain transmission in the dorsal horn through mechanisms summarized in Table 75-1.

2-AG and anandamide bind to presynaptic CB1 receptors with a resultant decrease in neurotransmitter (both excitatory and inhibitory) release. Activation of CB1 receptors on the peripheral terminal of primary sensory afferents has been shown to decrease terminal excitability and the release of proinflammatory mediators. Activation of CB2 on peripheral cells has been shown to decrease inflammatory cell mediator release, plasma extravasation, and the sensitization of afferent terminals. Additionally, activation of CB receptors by agonists leads to a reduction of elevated terminal excitability otherwise induced by local injury and inflammation.[28]

In the rat dorsal horn, the CB1 receptor has been demonstrated to be partially co-localized with TRPV1 on the presynaptic terminals of peptidergic and nonpeptidergic primary afferents.[28] Activation of CB1 by agonists leads to decreased influx of calcium through N/P/Q voltage-sensitive calcium channels that results in decrease in neurotransmitter release from the primary afferent. In the postsynaptic neuron, CB1 mRNA has been demonstrated in Laminae I-V and X. CB1 agonists that bind to postsynaptic CB1 receptors lead to increase conductance through potassium channels, with a resultant membrane hyperpolarization and decreased excitability.[28]

CB1 receptors in the brain are found in the periaqueductal gray, basolateral amygdala, and rostroventral medulla. Activation of CB receptors in these regions can have local effects on nociceptive processing and affect bulbospinal pathways which regulate dorsal horn excitability.

PHARAMCOLOGY AND CHARACTERISTICS OF MARIJUANA

Concentrations of THC and other cannabinoids in marijuana vary widely depending on growing conditions, plant genetics, and processing after harvest.[13] Naturally occurring marijuana has THC concentrations from 0.3% to 4% by weight; however, specially grown marijuana can contain 15% or more THC.[29,30]

Compared with other psychoactive drugs, THC is quite potent. Despite potent psychoactivity and pharmacologic actions on multiple organ systems, cannabinoids have remarkably low lethal toxicity and lethal doses in humans are not known.[31,32] There is a significant difference in the pharmacology of THC between smoking and oral administration.

INHALED VERSUS ORAL VERSUS SUBLINGUAL DELIVERY OF CANNABINOIDS

THC is extremely lipid soluble. The bioavailability and pharmacokinetics of THC from smoked marijuana are substantially different from those of the oral form. When marijuana is smoked, aerosolized THC in the inhaled smoke is absorbed within seconds and delivered to the brain. The absorption kinetics is typical of a very lipid-soluble drug with peak venous blood levels occurring soon after initiating smoking. A serum level absorption curve of THC when marijuana is smoked is similar to IV administration. The bioavailability averages about 30%[33-35]

By contrast, with oral administration, maximum THC and other cannabinoid blood levels are reached only 1 to 3 hours after an oral dose and the onset of psychoactive and other pharmacologic effects are much slower. Bioavailability is 5% to 20% due to erratic absorption from the stomach and small intestine and a large first pass metabolism by the liver.[29,30,36]

Nabiximols is a sublingual spray that contains the CBME combination of THC and CBD. It is approved in Canada to treat spasticity related to multiple sclerosis and is in phase III trials in the United States for treatment of cancer-related pain. Each spray delivers 2.7 mg of THC and 2.5 mg of CBD. As discussed, CBD appears to enhance the effects of THC; however, it is unclear if this is due to a pharmacokinetic or pharmacodynamics interaction.[37,38] Sublingual spray formulation has been developed to improve bioavailability above the oral delivery. However, the bioavailability and pharmacokinetics of both sublingual spray and oral delivery are similar.[36]

EFFECTS OF Δ^9-TETRAHYDROCANNABINOL: ACUTE AND CHRONIC

Cannabis induces an acute, psychoactive, mildly euphoric, relaxing intoxication or "high" that leads to slight changes in psychomotor and cognitive function. In limited cases, cannabis can also induce unpleasant effects including anxiety, panic, and paranoia. In rare cases, it may lead to acute psychosis involving delusions and hallucinations. Although CBD is not psychoactive, it has significant anticonvulsant, sedative, and other pharmacologic activities likely to interact with THC.[39,40,41]

The effect of chronic use of marijuana is the subject of much investigation. Forty studies reviewed on the use of cannabis could not detect consistent evidence for persisting neuropsychological deficits in cannabis users. Twenty of the 40 studies reported at least some subtle impairment. Another study reviewed 11 articles providing data for a total of 623 cannabis users and 409 nonusers or minimal users. It concluded that there might be decrements in the ability to learn and remember new information, whereas other cognitive abilities are unaffected. There is concern that the chronic use of cannabis in adolescents may affect brain development.[42-44]

There has been recent concern over the adverse effects of cannabis on adolescent brain development. Studies have suggested that long-term cannabis use is associated with harm to a person's intelligence if started younger than 18 years of age.[45,46] However this was challenged in a subsequent analysis of the data stating that when socioeconomic status was factored, the true effect was closer to zero.[47] In addition, a study at the University of California, San Diego, failed to show any adverse effects on the adolescent brains from cannabis use. The researchers compared brain scans for subjects 16 to 20 years old that used alcohol and those that used cannabis. They observed that alcohol but not cannabis resulted in a reduction in white matter in scanned brains.[48]

EFFICACY AND THE RESULTS OF PRECLINICAL AND CLINICAL STUDIES

PRECLINICAL STUDIES

Preclinical studies have confirmed the analgesic effect of cannabis. Cannabis has been shown to have antinociceptive properties in preclinical models of acute, inflammatory, neuropathic, and visceral pain. The largest antinociceptive effect of CB1 is mediated at the spinal level. CB2 effects are more prominent in states of inflammatory and visceral pain and are mediated more in the periphery than at the spinal level.[49-51]

CLINICAL STUDIES

Careful interpretation of human studies involving cannabinoids is necessary as there are a number of variables that can affect outcomes. Variables include the route of administration (oral or inhaled), the drugs studied (synthetic Δ^9-THC, other synthetic cannabinoids, or inhaled cannabis), and the dosages of studied drugs. Other factors include the study design and if it involves experimental pain or clinical pain.[31]

Studies in Healthy Volunteers Studies in healthy volunteers that involve experimentally induced pain have produced mixed results. Several studies demonstrated that cannabis increases the pain threshold suggesting an analgesic effect. Other studies have found either no effect on pain thresholds or even an increase in pain (a lowering of the pain threshold).[52-57] A randomized controlled trial (RCT) conducted by Wallace et al. demonstrated dose-dependent effects of smoked cannabis on capsaicin-induced pain and hyperalgesia in healthy volunteers. Compared with placebo, cannabis cigarettes with 2% THC produced no effect on pain, 4% THC significantly decreased pain, and 8% THC significantly increased pain.[58] Abrams et al. used the 4% THC dose to evaluate effects on capsaicin-induced pain in HIV patients. They showed a significant effect on both neuropathic pain and experimental pain.[59] These studies suggest that there is a therapeutic window for cannabis and emphasize that dosage and route of administration are likely to have a substantial effect on the results of a study. The therapeutic window observed in these studies is consistent with the phase II results of nabiximols in which the low dose but not the high dose met the primary endpoint.

Studies in Clinical Pain Clinical studies that are well designed are limited. A comprehensive literature review identified only 14 studies that used a randomized, double-blind, and placebo-controlled design. They vary in the cannabinoid studied, dosages used, and routes of administration. They are discussed and grouped following according to the type of pain that was studied.

CANCER PAIN

Clinical studies with cannabinoids were first conducted in patients with cancer pain and account for the largest number of human studies. One study involved 10 patients with various cancers who were administered oral THC at 5, 10, 15, and 20 mg dosages. The results showed pain relief significantly better than placebo at dosages of 15 and 20 mg, but also noted that these dosages produced substantial confusion and sedation.[60] Another study by the same authors examined 36 patients with various cancers and compared oral THC at 10 and 20 mg dosages to codeine.[61] THC at 10 and 20 mg was found to be equianalgesic to 60 and 120 mg codeine, respectively. Again, 20 mg THC produced unpleasant drowsiness and mental cloudiness, but 10 mg THC was relatively well tolerated.

Two studies investigated the effects of 4 mg of benzopyranoperidine, a synthetic analog of THC in patients with cancer pain. The first study found benzopyranoperidine superior to placebo and equivalent to 50 mg codeine; the second study found it superior to both placebo and secobarbital. Sedation was the largest adverse effect, but it occurred with similar instances for both the study drug and the comparison drugs.[62] In contrast, a study in which benzopyranoperidine was compared to codeine and placebo in patients with cancer pain, found that at dosages of 2 and 4 mg, benzopyranoperidine was less effective than 60 and 120 mg codeine and was no more effective than placebo.[63] The authors reported that pain was augmented by benzopyranoperidine and found an incidence of sedation similar to codeine. It is difficult to draw conclusions from these studies as the patient population was heterogenous (i.e., suffering from different forms of cancer).

A phase III RCT in opioid-tolerant cancer patients with intractable pain (N = 177) compared nabiximols, THC, and placebo. Nabiximols but not THC was superior to placebo suggesting the benefits of the THC:CBD combination.[64] A phase IIb study in opioid-treated cancer pain failures (N = 360) compared 3 doses of nabiximols to placebo. The study failed to meet the 30% responder rate primary endpoint; however, average daily pain to end of study for the low and medium dose but not the high dose were better than placebo.[65]

NEUROPATHIC PAIN

The synthetic cannabinoid ajulemic acid (CT-3) was studied on 21 patients with chronic neuropathic pain and was compared to placebo. Patients received 40 mg for 4 days and then 80 mg for 3 days. CT-3 use provided significant pain relief at 3 hours compared to placebo, with less of a response at 8 hours. Adverse effects included mild dry mouth and sedation.[66]

Nabiximols has been evaluated in several studies in patients with neuropathic pain. In an RCT, nabiximols, THC, and placebo were evaluated in 48 patients with neuropathic pain due to brachial plexus root avulsion.[67] Both drugs resulted in small but significant improvements in pain over placebo as well as in quality of sleep. Adverse effects were reported as mild to moderate and included sleepiness and dizziness. Despite a small reduction in pain, most patients said it was enough that they would like to continue to use the study drugs. Using a crossover design in 20 patients with neurogenic pain, nabiximols was superior to placebo.[68] A placebo-controlled study in 66 multiple sclerosis patients with central neuropathic pain showed that nabiximols was superior to placebo.[69] A study in 125 patients with peripheral neuropathic pain and allodynia showed that nabiximols was superior to placebo in reducing both spontaneous and evoked pain to stroking and punctate stimuli.[70]

A phase III RCT evaluated Cannador on spasticity in multiple sclerosis. Although there were no effects on spasticity, there was an improvement in spasticity-related pain.[71,72]

Several studies evaluated the efficacy of inhaled cannabis on neuropathic pain. Fifty patients with HIV-related peripheral neuropathy smoked either 3.56% THC cannabis cigarettes or placebo cigarettes three times a day for 5 days. Smoked cannabis significantly reduced pain by 34% compared to 17% with placebo. Adverse effects were mild and included sedation and anxiety.[59] A similar study in HIV neuropathy evaluated cannabis smoked four times a day over 5 days and titrated to effect (range of 1% to 8%). The primary endpoint, descriptor differential scale (DDS), significantly improved over placebo. Of the cannabis subjects 46% versus 18% of the placebo subjects achieved above 30% pain reduction.[73] Ware et al. studied varying doses of inhaled cannabis ranging from 0% to 9.4% in 23 patients with chronic neuropathic pain. The cannabis was smoked three times per day for 5-day cycles. Only the high dose separated from placebo.[74] Wilsey et al. studied two single doses of cannabis (7% and 3.5%) versus placebo in 38 patients with neuropathic pain of varying etiologies. The high dose only was superior to placebo.[75]

ACUTE PAIN

Several studies have evaluated the effects of cannabinoids on acute pain. Cannador was evaluated in a multicenter dose escalation study in 30 patients with postoperative pain and showed a dose-dependent reduction in pain.[76] Two studies with the synthetic cannabinoids, dronabinol (abdominal hysterectomy) and nabilone, failed to show any effect on postoperative pain.[77,78] Another synthetic cannabinoid, levonantradol, was compared to placebo in 56 patients with acute pain.[79] Four dosages (1.5, 2, 2.5, and 3 mg IM) provided significant analgesia, but the authors were unable to produce a significant dose-response curve. Adverse effects were mild with drowsiness the most frequent.

THC was administered intravenously (IV) in dosages of 0.22 and 0.44 mg/kg and compared with diazepam (Valium) and placebo for postoperative pain in 10 patients undergoing dental extraction.[80] Analgesia from the low dose of THC was superior to placebo but less than diazepam, whereas the high dose of THC provided less analgesia than both placebo and diazepam. This effect is consistent with healthy volunteer studies that show an increase in pain with higher doses of the cannabinoids (**Tables 75-1** and **75-2**).

TABLE 75-1 Cannabinoid Receptor Effects

Receptor	Peripheral Cells	Peripheral Terminal	Dorsal Horn	Supraspinal	Nonneuronal
CB1		↓ Terminal excitability	↓ Presynaptic Ca^+ conductance	Bulbospinal pathway activation	Unknown
		↓ Terminal proinflammatory peptide release	↓ Presynaptic neurotransmitter release	↓ Dorsal horn excitability	
			↑ Postsynaptic K^+ conductance		
			↑ Postsynaptic hyperpolarization		
			↓ Postsynaptic excitability		
CB2	↓ Inflammatory mediator release				Unknown
	↓ Plasma extravasation				
	↓ Sensitization of afferent terminals				

TABLE 75-2 Summary of Published Studies on Cannabinoid Analgesic Efficacy

Study Population	Agent	Delivery Method	Outcome	Adverse Effects	Reference
Healthy volunteers	Marijuana	Smoked	+	mild	Greenwald, 2000
Healthy volunteers	Marijuana	Smoked	+	mild	Milstein, 1975
Healthy volunteers	Marijuana	Smoked	0 low dose + moderate dose − high dose	mild	Wallace, 2007
Healthy volunteers	THC	Oral	0	mild	Naef, 2003
Healthy volunteers	THC	Oral	0	mild	Zeidenberg, 1973
Healthy volunteers	Marijuana	Smoked	−		Hill, 1974
Healthy volunteers	Marijuana	Smoked	−		Clark, 1981
Cancer pain	THC	Oral	+	Yes	Noyes, 1975
Cancer pain	THC	Oral	+	Yes (20 mg but not 10 mg)	Noyes, 1975
Cancer pain	benzopyranoperidine	Oral	+	Yes (similar to codeine)	Staquet, 1978
Cancer pain	benzopyranoperidine	Oral	−	Yes (similar to codeine)	Jochimsen, 1978
Cancer pain	Nabiximols	Sublingual spray	+ Sativex −THC	mild	Johnson, 2010
Cancer pain	Nabiximols	Sublingual spray	+ low and middle dose 0 high dose	mild	Portenoy, 2012
Neuropathic pain	CT-3	Oral	+	mild	Karst, 2003
Neuropathic pain	Nabiximols	Sublingual spray	+	mild	Berman, 2004
Neuropathic pain	Nabiximols	Sublingual spray	+	mild	Wade, 2003
Neuropathic pain	Nabiximols	Sublingual spray	+	mild	Rog, 2005
Neuropathic pain	Nabiximols	Sublingual spray	+	Mild	Nurmikko, 2007
Neuropathic pain	Cannador	Oral	+	Mild	Zajicek, 2003, 2005
Neuropathic pain	Marijuana	Smoked	+	Mild	Abrams, 2007
Neuropathic pain	Marijuana	Smoked	+ (high dose)	2 cases of toxic psychosis	Ellis, 2009
Neuropathic pain	Marijuana	Smoked	+ (high dose)	Mild	Ware, 2010
Neuropathic pain	Marijuana	Smoked	+ (high dose)	Mild	Wilsey, 2008
Acute pain	Cannador	Oral	+ (dose dependent)	Mild	Holdcroft, 2006
Acute pain	THC	Intravenous	+ low doses high doses	Moderate	Raft, 1977
Acute pain	Levonantradol	Intramuscular	+	Mild	Jain, 1981
Acute pain	THC (dronabinol)	Oral	0	Mild	Buggy, 2003
Acute pain	THC analog (nabilone)	Oral	−	Mild	Beaulieu, 2006
Arthritis	THC/CBD	Sublingual spray	+	Mild	Blake, 2005
Chronic pain	THC	Sublingual spray	+	Mild	Notcutt, 2004
Chronic pain	THC/CBD	Sublingual spray	+	Mild	Notcutt, 2004
Chronic pain	CBD	Sublingual spray	0	Mild	Notcutt, 2004
Chronic pain	Nabiximols	Sublingual spray	+	Mild	Narang, 2008

+, decrease pain; 0, no effect; −, increase pain

CHRONIC PAIN

A study using single daily doses of dronabinol, 10 and 20 mg, in 30 patients with chronic pain showed a dose-dependent increase in total pain relief.[81]

Effects of nabiximols were compared to placebo in 58 patients with chronic pain due to rheumatoid arthritis. Nabiximols produced significant pain relief with movement and at rest, improved quality of sleep, but did not decrease morning stiffness. Adverse effects were mild to moderate with dizziness the most common.[82] Another study evaluated the effects of a sublingual spray containing either 2.5 mg THC alone, 2.5 mg CBD alone, or a combination of the two, and compared them to placebo in 34 patients with chronic pain due to a number of different causes. The sprays containing THC alone, and THC with CBD were shown to be significantly better than placebo for relieving pain. The three sprays were significantly better than placebo for improving quality of sleep. The most frequent adverse effects were dry mouth, dysphoria, and sedation.[83]

REPORTS ON SMOKED CANNABIS

Several case series have been published discussing patients who self-medicate with cannabis. One study interviewed 15 patients who smoked cannabis for therapeutic reasons and noted that 12 reported improvements in pain and mood, and 11 reported improvement in sleep.[84] Another study performed a cross-sectional analysis of 209 chronic noncancer pain patients and found that 15% reported using cannabis to treat pain. The patients reported improvements in pain, mood, and sleep, and stated side effects were primarily dry mouth and euphoria.[85] A study in chronic pain patients on oral opioids evaluated 3.2% inhaled cannabis and showed a 27% reduction in pain.[86]

A study of 30 patients who used medical marijuana at a pain center in Canada found that 93% reported moderate or greater pain relief. Adverse effects were reported by 76% of patients which included increased appetite, weight gain, and slowed thoughts.[87] In the Netherlands, a questionnaire was sent to 300 patients who received medical marijuana for various reasons. Of the 107 patients who responded, 8.6% reported they used it primarily for pain.[88]

FUTURE DIRECTIONS

Because of the concerns with the psychoactive adverse effects of the cannabinoids, future research is likely to focus on peripherally acting CB1 agonists that do not cross the blood brain barrier. Preclinical studies with peripherally acting CB agonists show promise.[89] Other phytocannabinoids with less psychoactive properties such as CBD, are also attractive.[90]

Inhibition of endocannabinoid hydrolysis with inhibitors of the degradation enzymes fatty acid amide hydrolase (FAAH) and monoacylglycerol lipase (MGL) show promise. This would result in increased levels of anandamide and 2-AG and pain relief. Enzyme inhibitors restricted to the periphery would result in pain relief without the psychoactive effects.[91,92]

There is a pipeline of other phytocannabinoids and terpenoids that have noncannabinoid analgesic mechanisms such as TRPV, GABA, α-2, serotonin and opioid-receptor interactions, prostaglandin inhibition, and sodium channel blockade. However, the efficacy of these interactions on analgesia has yet to be determined.[93-100]

REFERENCES

1. Mechoulam R. The pharmacohistory of *Cannabis sativa*. In: Mechoulam, R. ed. *Cannabinoids as Therapeutic Agents*. Boca Raton, FL: CRC Press. 1986:1-19.
2. Russo E. Cannabis for migraine treatment: the once and future prescription? An historical and scientific review. *Pain*. 1998;76 (1-2):3-8.
3. Iversen L. Medical uses of marijuana. Fact or fantasy? In: L. Iversen, ed. *The Science of Marijuana*. Oxford: Oxford University Press; 2000:121-175.
4. Amar MB. Cannabinoids in medicine: a review of their therapeutic potential. *J Ethnopharmacol*. 2006;105:1-25.
5. Bicher HI, Mechoulam R. Pharmacological effects of two active constituents of marijuana. *Arch Int Pharmacodyn Ther*. 1968;172:24-31.
6. Sofia RD, et al. Antiedema and analgesic properties of D9 tetrahydrocannabinol. *J Pharmacol Exp Ther*. 1973;186:646-654.
7. Kosersky, DS, Dewey WL, Harris L. Antipyretic analgesic and antiinflammatory effects of delta-9-tetrahyodrocannabinol in the rat. *Eur J Pharmacol*. 1973;24:1-7.
8. Bloom AS, et al. 9-nor-9β-hydroxyhexahydrocannabinol a canabiniod with potent antinociceptive activity: comparisons with morphine. *J Phamacol Exp Therap*. 1977;200:263-270.
9. Joy JE, Watson SJ, Benson JA. *Marijuana and Medicine: Assessing the Science Base*. Institute of Medicine National Academy Press; 1999.
10. Di Marzo V, Melck D, Bisogno T, De Petrocellis L. Endocannabinoids: endogenous cannabinoid receptor ligands with neuromodulatory action. *Trends Neurosci*. 1998;21(12):521-528.
11. Howlett AC, et al. Classification of cannabinoid receptors. *Pharmacol Rev*. 2002:54:161-202.
12. Russo EB, Hohmann AG. Role of cannabinoids in pain management. In: *Comprehensive Treatment of Chronic Pain by Medical, Interventional, and Integrative Approaches: The American Academy of Pain Medicine Textbook on Patient Management*. New York, NY: Springer; 2013:181-197.
13. de Meijer E. The breeding of cannabis cultivars for pharmaceutical end uses. In: Guy GW, Whittle BA, Robson P, eds. *Medicinal uses of cannabis and cannabinoids*. London: Pharmaceutical Press; 2004:55-70.
14. Gaoni Y, Mechoulam R. Isolation, structure and partial synthesis of an active constituent of hashish. *J Am Chem Soc*. 1964;86(8):1646-1647.
15. Grlić Ljubiša. A comparative study on some chemical and biological characteristics of various samples of cannabis resin. *Bulletin on Narcotics (UNODC)*. 1962;(3):37-46.
16. Mechoulam R, Peters M, Murillo-Rodriguez E, Hanus, L. O. Cannabidiol – recent advances. *Chemistry & Biodiversity*. 2007; 4(8):1678-1692.
17. Pertwee RG. The diverse CB1 and CB2 receptor pharmacology of three plant cannabinoids: delta-9-tetrahydrocannabinol, cannabidiol and delta-9-tetrahydrocannabivarin. *Br J Pharmacol*. 2008;153(2):199-215.
18. Hayakawa K, Mishima K, Hazekawa M, Sano K, Irie K, Orito K, Egawa T, Kitamura Y, Uchida N, Nishimura R, Egashira N, Iwasaki K, Fujiwara M. 2008.
19. Karniol IG, Shirakawa I, Takahashi RN, Knobel E, Musty RE. Effects of delta9-tetrahydrocannabinol and cannabinol in man. *Pharmacology*. 1975;13(6):502-512.
20. McCallum ND, Yagen B, Levy S, Mechoulam R. Cannabinol: a rapidly formed metabolite of delta-1- and delta-6-tetrahydrocannabinol. *Experientia*. May 1975;31(5):520-521.
21. Mahadevan A, Siegel C, Martin BR, Abood ME, Beletskaya I, Razdan RK. Novel cannabinol probes for CB1 and CB2 cannabinoid receptors. *J Med Chem*. October 2000;43(20): 3778-3785.
22. Petitet F, Jeantaud B, Reibaud M, Imperato A, Dubroeucq MC. Complex pharmacology of natural cannabinoids: evidence for partial agonist activity of delta-9-tetrahydrocannabinol and antagonist activity of cannabidiol on rat brain cannabinoid receptors. *Life Sciences*. 1998;63(1):PL1-PL6.
23. Russo EB, Guy GW. A tale of two cabanninoids: the therapeutic rationale for combining tetrahydrocannibinol and cannabidiol. *Med Hypotheses*. 2006;66(2):234-246.
24. Ashton CH, Moore PB, Gallagher P, Young AH. Cannabinoids in bipolar affective disorder: a review and discussion of their therapeutic potential. *J of Psychopharmacol* (U.K.) 2005.
25. Lemberger L, Rubin A, Wolen R, et al. Pharmacokinetics, metabolism and drug-abuse potential of nabilone. *Cancer Treat Rev*. 1982;9(Suppl B):17-23.

26. Pacher P, Batkai S, Kunos G. The endocannabinoid system as an emerging target of pharmacotherapy. *Pharmacol Rev.* 2006;58(3):389-462.

27. Pagotto U, Marsicano G, Cota D, Lutz B, Pasquali R. (2006). The emerging role of the endocannabinoid system in endocrine regulation and energy balance. *Endocr Rev.* 27(1):73-100.

28. Demuth D, Molleman A. Cannabinoid signalling. *Life Sci.* 2006;78(6):549-563.

29. Adams IB, Martin BR. Cannabis: pharmacology and toxicology in animals and humans. *Addiction.* 1996;91:1585-1614.

30. Agurell S, et al. eds. *The Cannabinoids: Chemical Pharmacologic, and Therapeutic Aspects.* New York, NY: Academic Press; 1984.

31. Walker JM, Huang SM. Cannabinoid analgesia. *Pharmacol Ther.* 2002;95(2):127-135.

32. Jones RT. Drug of abuse profile: Cannabis. *Clin Chem.* 1987;33(11 Suppl):72B-81B.

33. Huestis, MA, et al. Absorption of THC and formation of 11-OH-THC and THC COOH during and after smoking marijuana. *J Anal Toxicol.* 1992a;16:276-282.

34. Huestis, MA, et al. Characterization of the absorption phase of marijuana smoking. *Clin Pharmacol Ther.* 1992b;52:31-41.

35. Goulle JP, Saussereau E, Lacroix C. Delta-9-Tetrahydrocannabinol Pharmacokinetics. *An Pharm Fr.* 2008;66(4):232-244.

36. Karschner EL, Darwin WD, Goodwin RS, Wright S, Huestis MA. Plasma cannabinoid pharmacokinetics following controlled oral delta-9-tetrahydrocannabinol and oromucosal cannabis extract administration. *Clin Chem.* Jan 2011;57(1):66-75. doi: 10.1373/clinchem.2010.152439. Epub 2010 Nov 15.

37. Guy GW, Robson P. A phase I, double-blind, three-way crossover study to assess the pharmacokinetic profile of cannabis based medicine extract (CBME) administered sublingually in variant cannabinoid ratios in normal healthy male volunteers (GWPK02125). *J Cannabis Ther.* 2003:3(4):121-125.

38. Karschner EL, Darwin WD, McMahon RP, et al. Subjective and physiological effects after controlled Sativex and oral THC administration. *Clin Pharmacol Ther.* 2011:89(3):400-407.

39. Kumar RN et al. Pharmacological actions and therapeutic uses of cannabis and cannabinoids. *Anaesthesia.* 2001;56:1059-1068.

40. Mechoulam, R, ed. *Marijuana: Chemistry, Pharmacology, Metabolism and Clinical Effects.* New York: Academic Press; 1973.

41. Agurell S, et al. Pharmacokinetics and metabolism of delta 1-THC and other cannabinoids with emphasis on man. *Pharmacol Rev.* 1986;38:21-43.

42. Gonzalez R, et al. Nonacute neuropsychological effects of cannabis use. *J Clin Pharm.* 2002, 42:48S-57S.

43. Grant I, et al. Non-acute neurocognitive effects of cannabis use: a meta-analytic study. *J Internat Neuropsych Soc.* 2003;9:679-689.

44. Hohmann AG, Briley EM, Herkenham M. Pre- and postsynaptic distribution of cannabinoid and mu opioid receptors in rat spinal cord. *Brain Res.* 1999:822:17-25.

45. Meier MH, et al. Persistent cannabis users show neuropsychological decline from childhood to midlife. *PNAS.* 2012;109(40):E2657.

46. Zalesky A, et al. Effect of long-term cannabis use on axonal fibre connectivity. *Brain.* 2012;135(7):2245-2255.

47. Rogeberg O. Correlations between cannabis use and IQ change in the Dunedin cohort are consistent with confounding from socioeconomic status. *PNAS.* 2013;110(11):4251-4254.

48. Bava S, Jacobus J, Thayer RE, Tapert SF. Longitudinal changes in white matter integrity among adolescent substance users. *Alcohol Clin Exp Res.* 2013.

49. Welch SP, Stevens DL. Antinociceptive activity of intrathecally administered cannabinoids alone and in combination with morphine in mice. *J Phamacol Exp Therap.* 1992;262:10-18.

50. Martin WJ, et al. An examination of the central sites of action of cannabinoid-induced antinociception in the rat. *Life Sci.* 1995;56: 2103-2109.

51. Richardson J, Kilo S, Hargreaves KM. Cannabinoids reduce hyperalgesia and inflammation via interaction with peripheral CB1 receptors. *Pain.* 1998;75:111-119.

52. Greenwald MK, Stitzer ML. Antinociceptive, subjective and behavioral effects of smoked marijuana in humans. *Drug Alcohol Depend.* 2000;59:261-275.

53. Milstein SL, et al. Marijuana-produced impairments in coordination. Experienced and nonexperienced subjects. *J Nerv Ment Dis.* 1975;161:26-31.

54. Naef M, et al. The analgesic effect of oral delta-9-tetrahydrocannabinol (THC), morphine, and a THC-morphine combination in healthy subjects under experimental pain conditions. *Pain.* 2003;105:79-88.

55. Zeidenberg P, et al. Effect of oral administration of delta-9-tetrahydrocannabinol on memory, speech, and perception of thermal stimulation: results with four normal human volunteer subjects. *Comp Psychiatry.* 1973;14:549-556.

56. Hill SY, et al. Marihuana and pain. *J Phamacol Exp Therap.* 1974;188:415-418.

57. Clark WC, et al. Effects of moderate and high doses of marihuana on thermal pain: a sensory decision theory analysis. *J Clin Pharmacol.* 1981;21:299S-310S.

58. Wallace M, Schulteis G, Atkinson JH, et al. Dose-dependent effects of smoked cannabis on capsaicin-induced pain and hyperalgesia in healthy volunteers. *Anesthesiology.* 2007;107(5):785-796.

59. Abrams DI, et al. Cannabis in painful HIV-associated sensory neuropathy. *Neurology.* 2007;68:515-521.

60. Noyes RJ, et al. The analgesic properties of delta-9-tetrahydrocannabinol and codeine. *Clin Pharmacol Ther.* 1975a;18:84-89.

61. Noyes RJ, et al. Analgesic effect of delta-9-tetrahydrocannabinol. *J Clin Pharmacol.* 1975b;15:139-143.

62. Staquet M, Gantt C, Machin D. Effect of a nitrogen analog of tetrahydrocannabinol on cancer pain. *Clin J Pharm Therap.* 1978;23:397-401.

63. Jochimsen PR, et al. Effect of benzopyranoperidine a delta-9-THC congener on pain. *Clin J Pharm Therap.* 1978;24:223-227.

64. Johnson JR, Burnell-Nugent M, Lossignol D, Ganae-Motan ED, Potts R, Fallon MT. Multicenter, Double-Blind, Randomized, Placebo-Controlled, Parallel-Group Study of the Efficacy, Safety, and Tolerability of THC:CBD Extract and THC Extract in Patients with Intractable Cancer-Related Pain. *J Pain Symptom Manage.* February 2010;39(2):167-179.

65. Portenoy RK, Ganae-Motan ED, Allende S, Yanagihara R, Shaiova L, Weinstein S, et al. Nabiximols for opioid-treated cancer patients with poorly-controlled chronic pain: a randomized, placebo-controlled, graded-dose trial. *J Pain.* 2012;13(5):438-449.

66. Karst M, et al. Analgesic effect of the synthetic cannabinoid CT-3 on chronic neuropathic pain. *JAMA.* 2003;290:1757-1762.

67. Berman JS, Symonds C, Birch R. Efficacy of two cannabis based medicinal extracts for relief of central neuropathic pain from brachial plexus avulsion: results of a randomized controlled trial. *Pain.* 2004;112(3):299-306.

68. Wade DT, Robson P, House H, Makela P, Aram J. A preliminary controlled study to determine whether whole-plant cannabis extracts can improve intractable neurogenic symptoms. *Clin Rehabil.* 2003;17:18-26

69. Rog DJ, Nurmiko T, Friede T, Young C. Randomized controlled trial of cannabis based medicine in central neuropathic pain due to multiple sclerosis. *Neurology*. 2005;65(6):812-819.
70. Nurmikko TJ, Serpell MG, Hoggart B, Toomey PJ, Morlion BJ, Haines D. Sativex successfully treats neuropathic pain characterized by allodynia: a randomized, double-blind, placebo-controlled clinical trial. *Pain*. 2007;133(1-3):210-220.
71. Zajicek J, Fox P, Sanders H, et al. Cannabinoids for treatment of spasticity and other symptoms related to multiple sclerosis (CAMS study): multicenter randomized placebo-controlled trial. *Lancet*. 2003;362:1517-1526.
72. Zajicek J, Sanders H, Wright DE, et al. Cannabinoids in multiple sclerosis (CAMS) study: safety and efficacy data for 12 months follow up. *J Neurol Neurosurg Psychiatry*. 2005;76(12):1664-1669.
73. Ellis RJ, Toperoff W, Vaida F, et al. Smoked medicinal cannabis for neuropathic pain in HIV: a randomized, crossover clinical trial. *Neuropsychopharmacology*. 2009;34(3):672-80.
74. Ware MA, Wang T, Shapiro S, et al. Smoked cannabis for chronic neuropathic pain: a randomized controlled trial. *CMAJ*. 2010;182(14):E694-E701.
75. Wilsey B, Marcotte T, Tsodikov A, et al. A randomized, placebo controlled, crossover trial of cannabis cigarettes in neuropathic pain. *J Pain*. 2008(6);506-521.
76. Holdcroft A, Maze M,Dore C, Tebbs S, Thompson S. A multicenter dose-escalation study of the analgesic and adverse effects of an oral cannabis extract (Cannador) for postoperative pain management. *Anesthesiology*. 2006;104(5):1040-1046.
77. Buggy DJ, Toogood L, Maric S, Sharpe P, Lambert DG, Rowbotham DJ. Lack of analgesic efficacy of oral delta-9-tetra hydrocannabinol in postoperative pain. *Pain*. 2003;106(1-2):169-172.
78. Beaulieu P. Effects of nabilone, a synthetic cannabinoid, on postoperative pain. *Can J Anaesth*. 2006;53(8):769-775.
79. Jain AK, et al. Evaluation of intramuscular levonantradol and placebo in acute postoperative pain. *J Clin Pharmacol*. 1981;21:320S-326S.
80. Raft D, et al. Effects of intravenous tetrahydrocannabinol on experimental and surgical pain. *Clin Pharmacol Ther*. 1977; 21:26-36.
81. Narang S, Gibson D, Wasan AD, et al. Efficacy of dronabinol as an adjuvant treatment for chronic pain patients on opioid therapy. *J Pain*. 2008;9(3):254-264.
82. Blake DR, et al. Preliminary assessment of the efficacy, tolerability and safety of a cannabis-based medicine (Sativex) in the treatment of pain caused by rheumatoid arthritis. *Rheumatology*, 2005.
83. Notcutt W, et al. Initial experiences with medicinal extracts of cannabis for chronic pain: results from 34 "N of 1" studies. *Anaesthesia*. 2004;59:440-452.
84. Ware MA, et al. Cannabis for chronic pain: case series and implications for clinicians. *Pain Res Manag*. 2002;7:95-99.
85. Ware MA, et al. Cannabis use for chronic non-cancer pain: results of a prospective survey. *Pain*. 2003;102:211-216.
86. Abrams DI, Couey P, Shade SB, Kelly ME, Benowitz NL. Cannabinoid-opioid interaction in chronic pain. *Clin Pharmacol Therap*. 2011;90(6):844-851.
87. Lynch ME, Young J, Clark AJ. A case series of patients using medicinal marihuana for management of chronic pain under the Canadian Marihuana Medical Access Regulations. *J Pain Sympt Manage*. 2006;32:497-501.
88. Gorter RW, et al. Medical use of cannabis in the Netherlands. *Neurology*. 2005;64:917-919.
89. Yu XH, Co CQ, Martino G, et al. A peripherally restricted cannabinoid receptor agonist produces robust anti-nociceptive effects in rodent models of inflammatory and neuropathic pain. *Pain*. 2010;151(2):337-344.
90. Izzo AA, Borrelli F, Capasso R, Di Marzo V, Mechoulam R. Nonpsychotropic plant cannabinoids: new therapeutic opportunities from an ancient herb. *Trends Pharmacol Sci*. 2009;30 (10):515-527.
91. Clapper JR, Moreno-Sanz G, Russo R, et al. Anandamide suppresses pain initiation through a peripheral endocannabinoid mechanism. *Nat Neurosci*. 2010;13:1265-1270.
92. Schlosburg JE, Blankman JL, Long JZ, et al. Chronic monoacylglycerol lipase blockade causes functional antagonism of the endocannabinoid system. *Nat Neurosci*. 2010;13(9):1113-1119.
93. De Petrocellis L, Starowicz K, Moriello AS, Vivese M, Orlando P, Di Marzo V. Regulation of transient receptor potential channels of melastatin type 8 (TRPM8): effect of cAMP, cannabinoid (CB1) receptors and endovanilloids. *Exp Cell Res*. 2007;313(9):1911-1920.
94. Cascio MG, Gauson LA, Stevenson LA, Ross RA, Pertwee RG. Evidence that the plant cannabinoid cannabigerol is a highly potent alpha2-adrenoreceptor agonist and moderately potent 5HT1A receptor antagonist. *Br J Pharmacol*. 2010;159(1):129-141.
95. Banerjee SP, Snyder SH, Mechoulam R. Cannabinoids: influence on neurotransmitter uptake in rat brain synaptosomes. *J Pharmacol Exp Ther*. 1975;194(1):74-81.
96. Evans AT, Formukong E, Evans FJ. Activation of phospholipase A2 by cannabinoids. Lack of correlation with CNS effects. *FEBS Lett*. 1987;211(2):119-122.
97. Bolognini D, Costa B, Maione S, et al. The plant cannabinoid delta9-tetrahydrocannabivarin can decrease signs of inflammation and inflammatory pain in mice. *Br J Pharmacol*. 2010;160(3):677-687.
98. Rao VS, Menezes AM, Viana GS. Effect of myrcene on nociception in mice. *J Pharm Pharmacol*. 1990;42(12):877-878.
99. Basile AC, Sertie JA, Freitas PC, Zanini AC. Anti-inflammatory activity of oleoresin from Brazilian Copaifera. *J Ethnopharmacol*. 1988;22(1):101-109.
100. Gertsch J, Leonti M, Raduner S, et al. Beta-caryophyllene is a dietary cannabinoid. *Proc Natl Acad Sci USA*. 2008;105(26):9099-9104.

CHAPTER 76

Psychotropic Medications

Robert M. McCarron
Shannon Suo

Chronic pain is frequently comorbid with both anxiety and mood disorders. Although many pain medicine practitioners may not manage psychiatric conditions, it is increasingly important to have at least a rudimentary familiarity with first-line psychiatric medications used to treat anxiety and mood disorders, a class of medications that is commonly encountered by pain specialists.

The mnemonic AMPS, or anxiety, mood, psychosis, and substance abuse, can be used to describe which psychiatric conditions are more commonly seen in the outpatient setting. In this chapter, we focus on the medication management of anxiety and mood (including major depressive disorder and bipolar spectrum disorders) because these disorders often influence the short- and long-term prognosis of those with chronic and unexplained pain. Antipsychotic medications are also discussed because there is much overlap with this class and the treatment of bipolar disorder. **Tables 76-1** and **76-2** provide a practical overview of these medications.

TABLE 76-1 Overview of the First-Line Antidepressants

Class	Initial Dose (mg/day)	Therapeutic Dose (mg/day)	Clinical Highlights
Selective Serotonin Reuptake Inhibitors			
Sertraline	50	50–200	Serotonin and dopamine reuptake inhibition Possible early and temporary diarrhea and dyspepsia Relatively low chance for drug interactions
Paroxetine	20	20–60	High anticholinergic and antihistamine side effect profile
Paroxetine CR	12.5–20	25–75	High risk for sedation, weight gain, and dry mouth Short half-life with more risk for discontinuation syndrome High chance for drug interactions Unsafe during pregnancy (Category D)
Fluoxetine	20	20–60	Long half-life and ideal for intermittently compliant patients Relatively inexpensive High chance for drug interactions
Citalopram	20	20–40	Structurally similar to escitalopram Decreased chance for drug interactions Warning for QTc prolongation above 40 mg/day
Escitalopram	10	10–20	Structurally similar to citalopram Decreased chance for drug interactions Warning for QTc prolongation
Vilazodone	10	40	Increase dose every week by 10 mg, as tolerated and to effect Must be taken with a meal in order to be fully bioavailable Moderate-to-high potential for CYP 3A4 drug interactions
Serotonin–Norepinephrine Reuptake Inhibitors			
Venlafaxine XR	37.5	75–225	Structurally similar to desvenlafaxine (do not use concurrently) Dual action on serotonin and norepinephrine receptors Not consistently "activating" but usually does not cause sedation Sometimes used as an adjunct for chronic pain Avoid in those with difficult-to-treat hypertension Short half-life with more risk for discontinuation syndrome Reduce dose with renal insufficiency
Desvenlafaxine	50	50–100	Structurally similar to venlafaxine (do not use concurrently) Dual action on serotonin and norepinephrine receptors Not consistently "activating" but usually does not cause sedation Avoid in those with difficult-to-treat hypertension Short half-life with more risk for discontinuation syndrome Sometimes used to treat neuropathic pain syndromes Reduce dose with renal insufficiency
Duloxetine	30	20–60	Dual action on serotonin and norepinephrine receptors Not consistently "activating" but usually does not cause sedation Approved for treatment of pain conditions Short half-life with more risk for discontinuation syndrome Increased risk for drug interactions
Atypical			
Bupropion XL	150	300–450	Given once daily with likely increased adherence to treatment Dual action on dopamine and norepinephrine receptors Contraindicated with seizure and eating disorders Increased risk for seizures in those with alcohol or benzodiazepine withdrawal Not used for anxiety disorders May worsen anxiety associated with depression No serotonin activity and no related sexual side effects
Mirtazapine	15	15–45	Dual action on serotonin and norepinephrine receptors Decreased frequency of sexual side effects Increased sedation and sleepiness at mainly *lower* doses May be associated with significant increase in appetite and weight gain Although not indicated for anxiety disorders, it may be helpful

TABLE 76-2 Overview of the Mood Stabilizers

	Starting Dose*	Target Serum Level	Titration Schedule	Side Effects	Monitoring
Lithium	300 mg BID/TID May be dosed QHS if tolerated	0.6–1.2 mEq/L (acute mania)	Steady-state level reached in 4–5 days Increase by increments of 300–600 mg/day, as tolerated	Nausea or vomiting, diarrhea, tremor, fatigue, polyuria, acne, worsened psoriasis, diabetes insipidus ECG changes (mainly benign T-wave changes) Hypothyroidism Toxicity (confusion, ataxia, dysarthria, coma) High caution in those with renal insufficiency Potentially lethal because of its narrow therapeutic window Pregnancy Category D	Check lithium level 5–7 days after each dose change Every 3 months: lithium level, TSH, metabolic panel Lithium toxicity risk increased by: 1. Drugs that decrease GFR will increase lithium levels (NSAIDs, ACE inhibitors, diuretics) 2. Conditions that cause volume depletion or "dehydration" (e.g., severe vomiting or diarrhea)
Valproate/ divalproex Indicated for prophylactic treatment of migraine headaches	500–1000 mg BID (25 mg/kg/ day for acute mania) ER dosed 500–2000 mg QHS	85–125 μg/mL	Steady-state level reached in 3–5 days Increase by 500–1000 mg/day, as tolerated	Sedation Tremor Weight gain Hypersensitivity Thrombocytopenia Transaminitis Hyperammonemia Encephalopathy Polycystic ovary syndrome Pancreatitis Pregnancy Category D	Baseline, 3-month, 6-month, and annually thereafter: VPA level, CBC, AST, and ALT
Carbamazepine Indicated for trigeminal neuralgia	ER 200 mg BID	6–10 μg/mL	Steady-state level reached in 3–4 days Increase by 200 mg/day (up to 1600 mg/day), as tolerated	Dizziness Somnolence Stevens Johnson syndrome Hyponatremia (SIADH) Leukopenia, pancytopenia, thrombocytopenia Hepatitis Drug interactions are common Pregnancy Category D	Baseline, 3-month, 6-month, and annually thereafter: carbamazepine level, CBC, serum chemistry, liver enzymes
Oxcarbazepine	300 mg BID	Not established for bipolar disorder	Increased by 300 mg/day, as tolerated	Fatigue Ataxia Hyponatremia Stevens Johnson syndrome Pregnancy Category C	Serum sodium during maintenance treatment (interval not established; consider every 3–4 months)
Lamotrigine[†]	25 mg/day	Not established for bipolar disorder	25 mg/day for 2 weeks, then 50 mg/day for 2 weeks, then 100 mg/day for 1 week, then 200 mg/ day (dose titration pack available), as tolerated[‡]	Rash, Stevens Johnson syndrome Hepatitis Anemia, leukopenia, thrombocytopenia Pregnancy Category C	Signs of rash

*Starting dose is for average adult patients. Elderly patients and patients with hepatic and renal disease should have lower starting doses. Frequent monitoring is required for those who have severe symptoms.

[†]For bipolar depression and maintenance; not for acute bipolar mania.

[‡]Even slower titration when used with valproate and hepatic enzyme–inducing drugs (alternate dose titration pack is available).

ACE, angiotensin-converting enzyme; ALT, alanine transaminase; AST, aspartate aminotransferase; BID, twice a day; CBC, complete blood count; ECG, electrocardiogram; ER, extended release; GFR, glomerular filtration rate; NSAID, nonsteroidal anti-inflammatory drug; QHS, every night; SIADH, syndrome of inappropriate antidiuretic hormone secretion; TID, three times a day; TSH, thyroid-stimulating hormone; VPA, valproic acid.

Adapted from *Physician's Desk Reference*; (65th ed., 2011). Montvale, NJ: PDR Network.

The following list illustrates the importance of including evidence-based psychiatric screening strategies and initiating timely and effective treatment for patients with depression and anxiety, within the context of providing care for those who have a severe or refractory pain condition(s).

- At least one-half of all those referred for outpatient mental health care do not connect with a mental health provider. There are many reasons for this, including poor access to care and mental health–related stigma.[1]
- Treatments of anxiety and mood disorders relieve "mental pain" and often have a therapeutic effect on "physical pain" disorders.
- Some psychotropic medications are used as to treat primary pain conditions (e.g., norepinephrine reuptake inhibitors). A complete understanding of the indications for use, mechanism of action, and possible side effects is critical for pain medicine practitioners.[2]
- The combination of severe and chronic pain, coupled with untreated depression and anxiety, can result in significant disability or possibly suicide. About one-half of all those who complete suicide have seen their non–mental health, medical provider 30 days before their death. About one-half of these cases result in litigation.[3]

ANTIDEPRESSANTS

SELECTIVE SEROTONIN REUPTAKE INHIBITORS/SEROTONIN ANTAGONIST AND REUPTAKE INHIBITORS

Indications The selective serotonin reuptake inhibitors (SSRIs) were developed in the 1980s and saw an explosion of use as safe, well tolerated, and effective treatments for depression. Now the SSRIs are indicated for a wide range of depressive and anxiety disorders, including major depression, obsessive-compulsive disorder (OCD), panic disorder, generalized anxiety disorder (GAD), posttraumatic stress disorder (PTSD), social phobia, premenstrual dysphoric disorder, and bulimia nervosa. Since the introduction of Prozac in 1987, antidepressant prescribing has quadrupled, and antidepressants have become the third most commonly prescribed class of medications among Americans and the most commonly prescribed class among Americans aged 18 to 44 years. Psychiatrists prescribe less than one-third of these medications. Depression occurs comorbid with chronic pain in up to 60% of patients and can complicate the treatment and worsen the prognosis of pain. On the other hand, the successful treatment of depression can reduce pain perception. The safety and tolerability of the SSRIs make them an important tool for the pain practitioner.

Regardless of the drug, medication therapy is effective in the majority of moderate to severe cases of depression. Within approximately 6 weeks, one-half of persons receiving antidepressants have at least a 50% reduction in symptoms.[4] In the Sequenced Treatment Alternatives to Relieve Depression (STAR*D) study, 30% of patients achieved full remission after 12 weeks of treatment with citalopram, and 10% to 15% more showed significant improvement. One-quarter of patients who failed citalopram responded when switched to sertraline, venlafaxine, or bupropion. A similar number responded when bupropion was added to citalopram.[5] Benefits of antidepressant therapy may take as little as 1 week or as long as 6 to 8 weeks to see. Unless intolerable, medications should not be changed or discontinued in the first 6 weeks of therapy for depression or anxiety (see Table 76-1).

Mechanism of Action As suggested by their name, the SSRIs inhibit the reuptake of serotonin (5HT) by presynaptic neurons. The targeted neurons are located in the midbrain raphe but can be found throughout the body, leading to side effects. Pre- and postsynaptic 5-HT receptors downregulate over time, however, reducing side effects. The monoamine hypothesis of depression assumes a deficit of serotonin at pre- and postsynaptic neurons, which SSRIs may restore. Given the dynamic nature of receptors and autoreceptors, though, this is likely an oversimplification of how SSRIs work. In addition to serotonin reuptake activity, vilazodone is a partial agonist of 5HT-1A; nefazodone and trazodone are 5HT-2 antagonists, making them serotonin antagonist and reuptake inhibitors (SARIs). SSRIs/SARIs also have individual effects on other neurotransmitters to lesser degrees.

Class Dosing Considerations The SSRIs have varying therapeutic ranges and strength. Sertraline, particularly, needs to be started very gradually at 25 mg/day and increased by 25- to 50-mg increments weekly to avoid significant gastrointestinal (GI) upset. Escitalopram, the S-enantiomer of citalopram, should generally be considered twice as potent. Therefore, a dose of 10 mg of escitalopram is roughly equivalent to 20 mg of citalopram. Citalopram has been associated with dose-dependent prolonged QTc, so doses above 40 mg are not recommended. Trazodone's antidepressant effects are seen around 400 mg in divided doses, 600 mg in divided doses in severe cases, but sleep initiation can be induced at much lower doses. Drugs with shorter half-lives, such as sertraline, paroxetine, or nefazodone, may need to be tapered to avoid symptoms of withdrawal or discontinuation syndrome.

Adverse Reactions The most significant advantages that SSRIs have over the tricyclic antidepressants (TCAs) are their enhanced tolerability and better safety. The SSRIs are considered relatively safe in overdose, with serotonin syndrome as their biggest risk. Nonetheless, patients may experience dry mouth, daytime sedation, insomnia, GI upset (particularly with sertraline), constipation, tremors, weight gain, and sexual dysfunction (decreased libido, decreased arousal, anorgasmia). Some of these side effects remit within a few weeks. Serzone was withdrawn from the U.S. market in 2004 after several fatalities associated with fulminant liver failure. Generic nefazodone remains available, however. Trazodone is a potent α_1 antagonist and is associated with orthostatic hypotension and (less commonly) priapism. The sedation associated with trazodone has relegated it to use primarily as a sleep agent. The Food and Drug Administration (FDA) has a "black box" warning to monitor children, adolescents, and young adults for development of suicidal ideation. All patients should also be screened for presence of mania before starting any antidepressant.

Interactions Paroxetine and fluoxetine show potent inhibition of cytochrome P450 enzyme 2D6, and fluoxetine, fluvoxamine, and nefazodone can potentially inhibit 3A4 as well. Citalopram is considered the least likely of the SSRIs to interact with P450 enzymes, but it does show some inhibitory effect at 2D6. If using concomitant TCAs, be aware that TCAs are metabolized by 2D6, and inhibition can lead to supratherapeutic or even toxic levels at low doses. Do not combine SSRIs with monoamine oxidase inhibitors (MAOIs) or St. John's Wort because serotonin syndrome is more likely to occur. The same risk exists for tramadol, triptans, or serotonin–norepinephrine reuptake inhibitors (SNRIs) combined with SSRIs but is less frequently encountered.

Serotonin syndrome is a clinical presentation of hyperserotonemia. Symptoms include agitation or altered mental status, diarrhea, hyperthermia, ataxia, myoclonus, hyperreflexia, and autonomic instability. There is considerable overlap of symptoms with neuroleptic malignant syndrome (NMS), but it is generally distinguishable by the recent introduction or increase of a serotonergic agent (vs. antipsychotic or antiemetic seen with NMS). Care is supportive, but cyproheptadine may be used to block further serotonin production.

Use in Pain Medicine The SSRIs may be useful as adjuncts for comorbid depression but have shown little effect on most types of pain.[6]

SEROTONIN–NOREPINEPHRINE REUPTAKE INHIBITORS

Indications The SNRIs have indications for major depression, social phobia, panic disorder, generalized and anxiety disorder and in the case of duloxetine, fibromyalgia, diabetic peripheral neuropathy, and chronic musculoskeletal pain.

Mechanism of Action As with the SSRIs, the SNRIs inhibit reuptake of serotonin but also norepinephrine from the synaptic cleft. The noradrenergic activity of venlafaxine increases with dose, acting primarily like an SSRI at lower doses. Desvenlafaxine, an active metabolite compound of venlafaxine, by contrast, shows greater in vitro inhibition of norepinephrine uptake.[7]

Class Dosing Considerations Venlafaxine has a very short half-life (5 hours), and even extended-release formulations only extend how slowly the medication is introduced into the bloodstream, not affecting half-life. It requires gradual titration from 37.5 mg, increasing the dose at weekly intervals. Similarly, venlafaxine must be gradually discontinued to avoid severe withdrawal, or discontinuation syndrome. Desvenlafaxine can be started at its therapeutic dose of 50 mg/day. Duloxetine may be started at 20 or 30 mg and then increased to 60 mg after 1 week.

Adverse Effects Not surprisingly, many of the side effects of the SNRIs are similar to those of the SSRIs. Some of the more prominent or unique effects of the SNRIs include nausea (particularly with duloxetine in the first week), hypertension (particularly with venlafaxine), and diaphoresis. As with the SSRIs, do not combine SNRIs with MAOIs or St. John's Wort and use caution with tramadol, triptans, or SSRIs.

Use in Pain Medicine The SNRIs remain a useful adjunct for treatment of depression, but given their effect on norepinephrine, it is not surprising they can also be helpful for chronic and neuropathic pain. These agents may be a safer and better tolerated alternative to TCA–SSRI combined therapy.

ATYPICAL ANTIDEPRESSANTS

So named for their unique pharmacologic profiles, the "atypical" antidepressants are a miscellaneous category of antidepressants that do not fit other molds described earlier, nor are they similar to TCAs or MAOIs. Note that serotonin antagonist and reuptake inhibitors (SARIs) are sometimes classified as atypical antidepressants.

Indications Indications include major depression, smoking cessation, and seasonal affective disorder (SAD).

Mechanism of Action Bupropion is a prodrug that is converted to an active metabolite that acts as a dopamine and norepinephrne reuptake inhibitor. Its effects are concentrated in the brain. Mirtazapine is an α_2 antagonist that leads to increased norepinephrine and serotonin release while blocking 5HT-2A, 5HT-2C, and histamine receptors (H1).

Class Dosing Considerations Immediate-release formulations of bupropion are all but abandoned because of the greater convenience, tolerability, and safety of sustained- or extended-release forms. Immediate-release bupropion requires twice- to thrice-daily dosing; sustained-release bupropion is only taken twice daily, and extended-release bupropion is only taken once. Patients taking bupropion should be advised to take the first dose in the morning, and if taking the sustained-release form, to take the second dose no later than mid-afternoon to avoid problems with insomnia. Because the risk of seizure is dose related, doses above 450 mg of bupropion are not recommended. Mirtazapine is best administered at night, but the sedating properties tend to diminish with increased dose.

Adverse Effects The most well known of all the side effects of bupropion is increased risk of seizure. The immediate-release formulations carry the highest risk, but at dosages at or below 450 mg/day, the risk of seizure is 0.4% or less. To minimize the risk of seizure, bupropion should not be used in patients with a history of seizures, head trauma, eating disorders, or abruptly discontinuing alcohol or benzodiazepines (BZDs). Other more common side effects include tachycardia, hypertension, headache, insomnia, dry mouth, and agitation. Sexual dysfunction and weight gain are uncommon with bupropion, and sometimes bupropion is used with another serotonergic agent to reverse sexual dysfunction. Mirtazapine, by contrast, commonly causes increased appetite and weight gain, as well as dry mouth and sedation. Bupropion has been known to cause false-positive urine drug screen results for amphetamines, but results should be negative with confirmatory gas chromatography. As with SSRIs, do not combine these drugs with MAOIs or St. John's Wort.

Use in Pain Medicine The atypical antidepressants are not indicated for pain conditions.

TRICYCLIC ANTIDEPRESSANTS

Indications Although originally discovered while developing treatments for schizophrenia, the TCAs have obtained a wide spectrum of indications for mood problems over the years, treating multiple forms of depression, including those secondary to other disorders, dysthymia, and anxiety. Individual TCAs are approved for use for nocturnal enuresis (imipramine), insomnia (doxepin), pruritus (doxepin), and OCD (clomipramine).

Mechanism of Action Generally speaking, the TCAs block serotonin and norepinephrine reuptake but at different ratios that range from more serotonergic (clomipramine) to more noradrenergic (desipramine, maprotiline, nortriptyline, protriptyline). Their blockade of α_1, H1, and muscarinic anticholinergic receptors account for most of their side effects.

Class Dosing Considerations The TCAs have a narrow therapeutic index, and doses that are therapeutic for depression can be toxic in overdose at even three times the daily dose. Fortunately, pain-relieving properties can be observed at much lower doses, even 1/10th to 1/30th of their FDA-approved maximum. TCA levels for either the parent compound or active metabolite may be helpful in guiding dosing for depression.

Adverse Effects The TCAs can cause multiple side effects, some of which can be beneficial such as sedation. Others, such as constipation, dry mouth, sexual dysfunction, and weight gain, may be treatment limiting. The TCAs are arrhythmogenic and may induce seizures in overdose. Check a baseline electrocardiogram and watch for widening of the QRS.

Use in Pain Medicine The TCAs have some of the best established evidence for chronic pain relief. Consider them incomplete analgesics whose benefits must be weighed against their significant side effects and risks. Analgesia may require moderate to high doses and weeks to see benefits. Consider that at high doses, they have some antidepressant effect as well.

MOOD STABILIZERS

The medications used as classic mood stabilizers were initially developed as anticonvulsants. Valproate, carbamazepine, and lamotrigine, as well as lithium, will be discussed. Nonapproved anticonvulsants are not discussed in this chapter because studies have found them not clearly effective for stabilization of bipolar disorder.

LITHIUM

Indications Lithium is an unusual drug compared with other mood stabilizers and even other psychotropic medications because it is only indicated for one purpose: treatment of bipolar disorder. It has been shown to lower the risk of suicide in bipolar disorder in some studies.

Mechanism of Action Lithium's mechanism of action is unknown. It is known to have effects on second messenger systems, including phosphatidyl inositol, adenyl cyclase, and G proteins. How these systems influence mood is unclear. Lithium inhibits thyroid hormone release and can both replace and increase uptake of iodine in the thyroid. Clinical hypothyroidism, or less frequently, hyperthyroidism is a possible result. Lithium has direct effects on the kidneys, including tubulointerstitial nephritis, renal tubular acidosis, minimal change disease, and focal segmental glomerulonephritis. As a metal salt, lithium commonly causes diabetes insipidus, replacing sodium intracellularly and concentrating there to have secondary effects on sodium and water transport.

Class Dosing Considerations Caution must be used with lithium, especially in elderly adults and medically compromised patients, because it has a very narrow therapeutic index. Therapeutic (trough) levels should be kept between 0.6 and 1.2 mEq/L. Usually a thrice-daily medication, extended-release formulations allow dosing to be decreased to only twice daily.

Adverse Effects Commonly seen side effects include tremor, polyuria, metallic taste, nausea, and diarrhea. Toxicity is accompanied by confusion, ataxia, and even coma. Avoid use of nonsteroidal anti-inflammatory drugs and use caution with diuretics (especially thiazide type) and angiotensin-converting enzyme inhibitors because these agents can dramatically increase lithium to toxic levels.

Lithium has been suggested as helpful in cluster headache and spinal cord injury.

ANTICONVULSANTS AND MOOD STABILIZERS

Indications The anticonvulsants have a number of different uses based on their individual actions. Obviously, they are all indicated for seizures of various types and are used for bipolar disorder (particularly manic and mixed states), but of interest for pain practitioners, they are also approved for migraines, glossopharyngeal neuralgia, and trigeminal neuralgia. A number of other anticonvulsants have been studied in bipolar disorder but have not been found to be consistently effective enough to obtain FDA indications for bipolar disorder. Among them is oxcarbazepine, a structural analog of carbamazepine. Despite its similarity to carbamazepine, it has failed to obtain FDA indication for use in bipolar disorder. However, because of its improved tolerability and decreased drug interaction profile compared with carbamazepine, it is frequently used off label (see Table 76-2).

Mechanism of Action Not much is known about the mechanism of action for anticonvulsants in the treatment of mood disorders. They are known to inhibit sodium channels, which may increase the effect of γ-aminobutyric acid (GABA) or decrease glutamate release.

Class Dosing Considerations Lamotrigine has strict dosing guidelines based on its risk of serious rash. Risk is minimized (1/1250) when lamotrigine is started at 25 mg/day for 2 weeks and then increased to 50 mg for another 2 weeks before increasing to 100 mg. These guidelines assume no interference by interacting medications. If coadministered with valproate, dosing must be cut in half because valproate inhibits the metabolism of lamotrigine and essentially doubles the serum concentration. By contrast, taking lamotrigine with oral contraceptives or carbamazepine can speed up its metabolism by twofold, requiring a doubling of the standard dosing regimen: 50 mg/day for the first 2 weeks, then 100 mg, and so on. Valproate can be "loaded" in acutely manic (usually hospitalized) patients at 20 to 30 mg/kg to achieve steady-state levels within 3 to 5 days. More stable outpatients do not tolerate rapid loading but can be started at 500 to 1000 mg/day and gradually increased over 7 to 10 days to achieve a target level of 85 to 125 μg/mL. Carbamazepine is not typically used as a first-line mood stabilizer because of poor tolerability and multiple drug interactions, but suggested effective levels are between 6 and 10 μg/mL. Oxcarbazepine can be started at 300 mg twice daily and increased in 300-mg increments. Levels are not routinely obtained for lamotrigine or oxcarbazepine.

Adverse Effects Valproate, carbamazepine, and lamotrigine all share a risk of serious rash, including Stevens Johnson syndrome and toxic epidermal necrolysis, but lamotrigine's risk appears to be the highest. Other common side effects of lamotrigine include benign rash (7%) and headache. However, unlike other mood stabilizers, lamotrigine is generally weight neutral and is pregnancy Category C. Carbamazepine is associated with somnolence, blood dyscrasias, liver enzyme elevations, and has multiple drug interactions because of induction of cytochrome P450 enzymes. Although structurally similar, oxcarbazepine does not have the same interactions. Side effects seen with valproate include weight gain, tremor, thrombocytopenia, and liver enzyme elevations. Rarer side effects include hyperammonemia and resultant encephalopathy.

Use in Pain Medicine Carbamazepine has indications for glossopharyngeal and trigeminal neuralgias, and valproate is indicated for migraine headaches. Additionally, valproate has shown benefit in postherpetic neuralgia.

ANTIPSYCHOTICS

INDICATIONS

Both first-generation (FGA) and second-generation antipsychotic (SGA) medications are indicated for the treatment of schizophrenia. These medications are not curative but are mainly used more to manage the symptoms associated with schizophrenia. Some of the SGA medications are used to treat bipolar disorder (depression, mania, and mixed episodes), hyperactive delirium, and other types of agitation and secondary forms of psychosis.

The FGA medications are dopamine receptor antagonists and are classified by their potency to block dopamine (D) receptors. This older group of medications will not be discussed in detail because they are infrequently used secondary to receptor non specificity and a heightened potential for extrapyramidal symptoms (EPS), sedation, weight gain, cardiac conduction abnormalities (mainly QTc prolongation), and increased prolactin levels.

The SGA medications or serotonin-dopamine antagonists are used mainly for the treatment of schizophrenia and bipolar disorder. They generally have a more targeted receptor specificity and are therefore less likely to cause EPS, increased prolactin levels, and cardiac conduction abnormalities. They do, however, carry the risk for serious metabolic derangements, including weight gain, glucose dysregulation, and dyslipidemia.

MECHANISM OF ACTION

The FGA medications work mainly on D1, D2, and D4 receptors to attenuate the positive symptoms of schizophrenia, which include hallucinations and delusions. They have little to no serotonergic receptor activity and, therefore, have a minimal effect on the negative symptoms associated with schizophrenia (e.g., cognitive slowing and depressed mood).

The SGA medications antagonize dopamine and serotonin receptors, which often improve both positive and negative symptoms. SGA medications also are less likely to block H1, cholinergic receptors, and D2 receptors, with a relative decrease in sedation, anticholinergic symptoms, and EPS, respectively.

CLASS DOSING CONSIDERATIONS

Most of the SGA medications have a similar dosing regimen when used to treat schizophrenia and bipolar disorder. In elderly adults, it is best to start at a relatively low dose and slowly increase the dose to effect and tolerability.

All SGAs have the potential to cause metabolic abnormalities. Patients should be screened for obesity, dyslipidemia, and glucose dysregulation before taking an antipsychotic medication for any reason. These same screening procedures should be used again at 3 and 12 months, with annual monitoring thereafter.

ADVERSE REACTIONS

Up to 60% of those taking antipsychotic medications stop within a 2-year period because of both a lack of efficacy and intolerability. Patients should be closely monitored for EPS, symptoms suggestive of an increased serum prolactin level, and metabolic abnormalities. Patients with dementia-related psychosis have increased all-cause morbidity associated with the use of SGA medications. This class of medications should be used with great caution in this patient population. Last, about 10% of those with schizophrenia commit suicide. It is important to monitor risk for suicide in those who have schizophrenia.

PAIN MEDICINE CONSIDERATIONS

There is currently no widely accepted indication for using antipsychotic agents in those who have chronic pain.

ANXIOLYTICS

SEROTONIN–NOREPINEPHRINE REUPTAKE INHIBITORS AND SELECTIVE SEROTONIN REUPTAKE INHIBITORS

Indications Up to 50% of those with chronic pain or unexplained physical pain experience a level of anxiety that impairs a significant level of functioning. SSRIs and SNRIs are often used to treat moderate to severe anxiety that has been present for 1 month or longer. Of the first-line antidepressants, bupropion and mirtazapine are the only medications not indicated for the treatment of anxiety disorders. The SSRIs and SNRIs may be helpful in the treatment of GAD, panic disorder social phobia (SP), PTSD, and OCD. Cognitive and supportive psychotherapy usually augment medication management for anxiety disorders.

Mechanism of Action Although the mechanism of action is unclear, it is believed that both serotonergic and norepinephrine receptors positively affect the emotional component of anxiety at the limbic area of the brain and the cognitive component of anxiety at the cortical level. Patients who have comorbid depression do better on these medications.

Class Dosing Considerations When using an SSRI or SNRI for the treatment of anxiety, it is best to start with the lowest dose possible, which is usually lower than the standard starting dose for the treatment of depression. Starting any higher or escalating the dose too quickly could paradoxically intensify anxious feelings. For those who have moderate to severe anxiety, it is recommended to start a low-dose SSRI or SNRI and increase slowly over 6 to 8 weeks. During this time, unless contraindicated, a low-dose, long-acting benzodiazepine (BZD) may be used during this titration period. For example, if a patient has GAD or panic disorder, one may consider the following titration schedule for sertraline, as tolerated: 25 mg for

2 weeks, 50 mg for 2 weeks, 100 mg for 2 weeks, 150 mg for 2 weeks, and 200 mg in the morning. Clonazepam, 0.25 to 0.5 mg twice per day, may be used during this titration upward and discontinued at week 8. There is no need to wean the patient off clonazepam because it has a long half-life and is used at a relatively low dose. Short-term psychotherapy may also be used, if indicated and available.

Adverse Reactions If used improperly, the SSRIs and SNRIs may worsen anxiety. Also, in those younger than 24 years of age or at high risk of suicide, it is important to monitor periodically for increased risk of suicide or harm to self. As a class, the SSRIs and SNRIs are relatively safe but may cause xerostomia, fatigue, sexual dysfunction, or weight gain.

Pain Medicine Considerations The SNRIs are often used to treat neuropathic pain and fibromyalgia. The SSRIs are generally not used to address chronic pain. See "Antidepressants" for more details about pain medicine considerations.

BENZODIAZEPINES

Indications The BZDs are indicated for the treatment of most anxiety disorders. Generally, they can be used for short-term and intermittent "as needed" treatment, daily short-term treatment, or long-term treatment for refractory and severe anxiety disorders. The latter situation should be referred for ongoing psychiatric care.

In most cases, the BZDs should not be used as monotherapy but should be augmented with an SSRI, SNRI, or psychotherapy. The BZDs can be quite effective when using a long-acting, low-dose medication for a short period of time.

Mechanism of Action The BZDs are GABA agonists, with resultant sedative, hypnotic, amnestic, anxiolytic action.

Class Dosing Considerations The BZDs should be used with much caution, if at all, in patients who abuse alcohol or take moderate to high doses of opioids. These combinations can result in respiratory depression, motor vehicle accidents, memory problems, and other adverse consequences. The lowest effective dose should be used, and it is relatively contraindicated in those who have cognitive disorders, including delirium, traumatic brain injury, and dementia.

Adverse Reactions About 30% of patients taking BZDs do not respond to treatment, and many who take moderate to high doses often develop tolerance. Retrograde amnesia is common and is not necessarily dose dependent. As noted earlier, caution must be used when combined with other medications or drugs that might suppress the respiratory drive. The BZDs have either pregnancy Category D or X, which means they are contraindicated for women who are pregnant or wish to become pregnant.

Pain Medicine Considerations The BZDs are not commonly used to treat chronic pain. They can be helpful in those who have pronounced anxiety, in the context of a well-defined pain condition. Although clonazepam is not FDA approved for the treatment of pain conditions, some case reports indicate that it may be helpful for some cases of neuropathic pain. Diazepam has some muscle relaxant properties and may be beneficial for those who have subacute or chronic muscle spasms and resultant pain.

BUSPIRONE

Indications Buspirone is indicated only for GAD. It has not been shown to be effective for any other anxiety disorder.

Mechanism of Action Buspirone is a serotonin 5-HT_{1A} receptor partial agonist and has minimal side effects. It has minimal H1 blockade and therefore is less likely to cause sedation.

Class Dosing Considerations The starting dosage is 5 mg three times per day. The usual effective daily dosage is 20 to 30 mg/day in divided doses. The maximum daily dose is 60 mg.

Adverse Reactions Buspirone has a wide therapeutic index, with minimal potential for the development of tolerance or withdrawal. Common side effects include headache, fatigue, and dizziness.

Pain Medicine Considerations Buspirone is not normally used to treat pain conditions.

SUMMARY

Pain medicine practitioners increasingly use psychotropic medications. The diagnosis and effective treatment of commonly encountered psychiatric conditions is critical to the treatment of those who have comorbid pain disorders. Assessment and treatment using the AMPS model is the easiest approach to use in the ambulatory pain clinical setting.

REFERENCES

1. Schulberg HC, Katon W, Simon GE, et al. Treating major depression in primary care practice: an update of the Agency for Health Care Policy and Research Practice Guidelines. *Arch Gen Psychiatry.* 1998;55:1121-1127.
2. Shah TH, Moradimehr A. Bupropion for the treatment of neuropathic pain. *Am J Hosp Palliat Care.* 2010;27(5):333-336.
3. National Center for Health Statistics. *Health, United States, 2010: With special feature on death and dying. Table 95: Selected prescription drug classes used in the past month, by sex and age: United States, selected years 1988–1994 through 2005–2008.* Hyattsville, MD: Author; 2011.
4. Trivedi MH, Fava M, Wisniewski SR, et al. Medication augmentation after the failure of SSRIs for depression. *N Engl J Med.* 2006;354:1243-1252.
5. Rush AJ, Trivedi MH, Wisniewski SR, et al. Bupropion-SR, sertraline, or venlafaxine-XR after failure of SSRIs for depression. *N Engl J Med.* 2006;354:1231-1242.
6. Max MB, Lynch SA, Muir J, et al. Effects of desipramine, amitriptyline, and fluoxetine on pain in diabetic neuropathy. *N Engl J Med* 1992;326:1250–1256.
7. Thase ME. Introduction. *Prim Psychiatry.* 2009;16:5(Suppl 4):4-7, 15.

Antiepileptics for Pain

Zahid H. Bajwa
Charles C. Ho

INTRODUCTION

- Antiepileptic drugs (AEDs) have been used in the treatment of chronic pain syndromes for more than 50 years.[1-4] Phenytoin, in particular, has been extensively used for the treatment of neuropathic pain during that time.[5-9] Carbamazepine was the first AED used and extensively studied specifically for the treatment of trigeminal neuralgia.[10-12] Since then a variety of neuropathic syndromes have been treated with AEDs, including:
  - Diabetic neuropathy
  - Postherpetic neuralgia
  - Glossopharyngeal neuralgia
  - Postsympathectomy neuralgia
  - Postthoracotomy pain syndromes[1-4]

The AEDs include the older drugs such as phenytoin, carbamazepine, and valproic acid and newer agents such as gabapentin, lamotrigine, felbamate, topiramate, vigabatrin, tiagabine, levetiracetam, zonisamide, and oxcarbazepine.

The individual AEDs are briefly reviewed here, and general guidelines for their use in pain control are provided.

PATHOGENESIS OF NEUROPATHIC PAIN AND ANTIEPILEPTIC DRUG USE

Neuropathic pain is defined as pain caused by dysfunction of the nervous system in the absence of ongoing tissue damage.[13]

- The pain typically is characterized as sharp, shooting, or burning and is usually felt in the area of sensory deficit.
- The pain is typically worsened by mild stimuli that normally would not produce pain, such as light touch or cool air.
- The pain tends to be chronic and causes considerable patient discomfort.

These symptoms have led to various hypotheses about the pathophysiologic mechanisms of neuropathic pain with relevance to AEDs.[14] When peripheral nerves become damaged, axons grow toward the formerly innervated area directed by an intact connective tissue sheath. If this sheath is also damaged, then axon extensions grow without any direction and become tangled into a structure called a neuroma.

Neuromas can generate ectopic electrical impulses at the regenerating tips in the damaged primary nociceptive afferents at various levels in the nervous system, from the dorsal root ganglia to demyelinated regions of a root or nerve.[15] Because nerves have been damaged, there is a potential disruption in the balance of the excitatory (e.g., glutamate) and inhibitory (e.g., γ-aminobutyric acid [GABA]) neurotransmitters. This disruption leads to hyperexcitability of the neuronal membrane sodium channels and voltage-dependent calcium channels, causing rapid ectopic firing. The AEDs have varying mechanisms of action, many of which are directed at sodium and calcium-dependent channels and GABA metabolism.

Although the AEDs provide at least partial pain relief in a large percentage of patients with a variety of neuropathic pain syndromes, their use is limited by side effects in a substantial percentage of patients. In addition, the older AEDs (phenytoin, carbamazepine, and valproic acid) also require monitoring of blood counts and liver function tests (LFTs) because of their hematologic and hepatic toxicity, leading to poor compliance. The newer AEDs (with the exception of felbamate) generally are not associated with life-threatening side effects and are easier to use.

ANTIEPILEPTIC DRUGS

PHENYTOIN

Phenytoin (5,5-diphenyl-2,4-imidazolidinedione) is an AED used to control generalized tonic-clonic and complex partial seizures. For years it was the most commonly used AED for the treatment of a wide variety of pain syndromes.

Phenytoin has been reported to be effective in the treatment of the following:

- Diabetic neuropathy
- Trigeminal neuralgia
- Neuropathic cancer pain
- Postherpetic neuralgia
- Complex regional pain syndrome (CRPS) types 1 and 2
- Postsympathectomy neuralgia[5-9]

The proposed mechanism of action is reduction of neuronal hyperexcitability by decreasing the activity of sodium channels, thereby stabilizing the neural membrane.[16]

Phenytoin is supplied as 30- and 100-mg capsules. The recommended dosage of phenytoin for epilepsy in most patients is 300 mg/day. An exact dosage needed to achieve adequate analgesia has not been defined. Use of phenytoin as a neuropathic analgesic should follow the guidelines for its use for epilepsy. Phenytoin has the advantage of once-a-day dosing and is relatively inexpensive. Absorption orally is slow and variable; peak concentrations may occur as early as 3 hours or as long as 12 hours. It is about 90% bound to plasma proteins and is metabolized primarily by the liver. Phenytoin has a half-life of 20 to 60 hours at therapeutic concentrations. However, a narrow therapeutic window and its short- and long-term side effects limit use.

Fosphenytoin (5,5-diphenyl-3-[(phosphonooxy)methyl]-2,4-imidazolidine-dione disodium salt) is a prodrug of phenytoin. It is indicated for short-term parenteral administration when other means of phenytoin administration are unavailable.[17]

Complete blood counts (CBCs), LFTs, and serum drug levels need to be closely monitored, particularly in the first 6 months. Long-term use can result in cosmetic side effects (e.g., gingival hyperplasia, hirsutism, coarsening of the facial features) and, rarely, cerebellar atrophy and peripheral neuropathy.

CARBAMAZEPINE

Carbamazepine (5H-dibenz(b,f)azepine-5-carboxamide) is considered to be a primary drug for partial and tonic-clonic seizures. It has structural similarities to the tricyclic antidepressants, making it a particularly desirable drug for treating chronic pain syndromes.

- It has been widely prescribed as the drug of choice for trigeminal neuralgia[10-12] and is considered the best neuropathic analgesic for lancinating or electric-like pain.[15]
- Carbamazepine is effective in other neuropathic pain syndromes such as glossopharyngeal neuralgia, diabetic neuropathy, and pain syndromes associated with multiple sclerosis.[18-21]
- It has also been used for the treatment of migraine headaches in pediatric populations.[22]

Carbamazepine enhances antidepressant effects and is an effective mood stabilizer. Its mechanism of action is similar to that of phenytoin in stabilizing neuronal membranes.

Carbamazepine is available as 100-mg chewable tablets; 100-, 200-, and 400-mg extended-release tablets; and 100 mg/5 mL suspension. The initial starting dosage of carbamazepine is between 100 and 200 mg/day; the dosage can be slowly increased over several weeks as needed to a maximum total dose of 1200 mg/day. It is absorbed slowly orally, and peak concentrations may be observed in 4 to 8 hours but may be delayed 24 hours. It is about 75% bound to plasma proteins. Carbamazepine is metabolized to 10,11-epoxycarbamazepine, which is an active metabolite. Its half-life is between 10 and 20 hours depending on induction of hepatic enzymes. Carbamazepine, similar to phenytoin, has a narrow therapeutic window. Before initiating therapy, a baseline CBC and LFTs should be obtained, with frequent monitoring thereafter, particularly in the first 6 months.

Agranulocytosis and aplastic anemia rarely occur; patients should be advised to report any episodes of fever while taking the drug so that a CBC can be checked. Other side effects of concern are hypersensitivity reactions manifesting as Stevens-Johnson syndrome with lymphadenopathy and rare cases of liver failure.

OXCARBAZEPINE

Oxcarbazepine (10,11-dihydro-10-oxo-5H-dibenz[b,f]azepine-5-carboxamide) is a new antiepileptic that is chemically similar to carbamazepine and may prove to be a neuropathic analgesic.[23] Oxcarbazepine is a prodrug, which means its metabolite is the active substance. It is indicated for monotherapy or adjunctive therapy in the treatment of partial seizures.[24]

Oxcarbazepine blocks voltage-sensitive sodium channels, resulting in stabilization of hyperexcited neural membranes, inhibition of repetitive neuronal firing, and diminution of synaptic impulse propagation.[25] It may modulate high-voltage activated calcium channels and increase potassium conductance.

- A small study demonstrated the efficacy of oxcarbazepine in trigeminal neuralgia.[26]
- Further controlled studies are under way to determine its efficacy and optimal dose in the treatment of neuropathic pain.

Oxcarbazepine is available as 150-, 300-, and 600-mg tablets. The starting dosage of oxcarbazepine is 150 to 600 mg/day divided into two doses, up to a maximum of 2400 mg/day. Monitoring of hepatic enzymes or hematologic parameters is not required with oxcarbazepine to the same degree as with carbamazepine. It does not extensively undergo oxidative metabolism and has low protein binding (40%). Oxcarbazepine is metabolized to 10,11-dihydro-10-hydroxy-5H-dibenz[b,f]azepine-5-carboxamide (MHD), which is responsible for the pharmacologic effects of oxcarbazepine. The peak serum levels of oxcarbazepine and MHD are reached in 4.5 hours after oral administration. The half-life of MHD is 9 hours.

Side effects associated with oxcarbazepine are primarily related to the nervous system and digestive system. The symptoms are somnolence, headache, dizziness, diplopia, ataxia, nystagmus, abdominal pain, anorexia, nausea, vomiting, and rash.

VALPROIC ACID

Valproic acid (n-dipropylacetic acid) is a broad-spectrum AED used to treat a number of epileptic syndromes; although it has been used in the management of chronic pain.[27]

- It has been mainly indicated in the preventive treatment of migraine, cluster, and tension-type headaches.[28,29]

Valproic acid has several proposed mechanisms of action, including increasing GABA brain concentrations by inhibition of GABA aminotransferase and succinic semialdehyde dehydrogenase (enzymes involved in the synthesis and degradation of GABA), selectively enhancing postsynaptic GABA responses, direct effects on neuronal membranes, and reduction of excitatory transmission by aspartate.[30] Valproic acid, similar to carbamazepine, is an effective mood stabilizer.

Valproic acid is available as 250-mg capsules and 250 mg/5 mL syrup. The starting dosage of valproic acid is usually 250 mg/day; it is titrated slowly upward to a maximum dosage of 1000 to 2000 mg/day, usually in divided doses. Valproic acid is absorbed rapidly orally, and peak concentrations are observed in 1 to 4 hours. It is about 90% bound to plasma proteins. It is metabolized hepatically with potent antiseizure metabolites. Valproic acid has an approximately 15-hour half-life.

Limitations for the use of this agent include drug interactions and drug-related side effects, such as central nervous system (CNS) depression, and hepatic and hematologic toxicity. Frequent monitoring of these parameters should continue during the first year of therapy and occasionally thereafter.

CLONAZEPAM

Clonazepam (5-(o-chlorophenyl)-1,3-dihidro-7-nitro-2H-1,4-benzodiazepin-2-one) is a benzodiazepine that has been used successfully in providing relief for both chronic malignant and nonmalignant pain syndromes:

- Headaches
- Temporomandibular joint dysfunction
- Phantom limb pain[31-33]

Clonazepam acts by enhancing GABA receptor–mediated chloride channels. It is particularly effective when used in combination with other neuropathic analgesics and in patients with prominent anxiety disorder and insomnia.

Clonazepam is available as 0.5-, 1-, and 2-mg tablets. The dose of clonazepam should initially be 0.5 mg at bedtime, with the dose being slowly increased to 0.5 to 1 mg three times per day. Dosages of up to 20 mg/day have been used in epilepsy; 1 to 6 mg/day is generally successful in treating headache and pain. It is absorbed rapidly orally with peak concentrations in 1 to 4 hours. Clonazepam is approximately 85% bound to plasma proteins. It is metabolized hepatically and has a half-life of about 24 hours.

The most common side effects are drowsiness, dizziness, fatigue, and sedation. As with other benzodiazepines, clonazepam may produce physical and psychological dependence; abrupt discontinuation is prohibited.

GABAPENTIN

Gabapentin (1-(aminomethyl)cyclohexanacetic acid) is one of the newer AEDs that has been approved for adjunctive treatment of partial seizures. In recently published anecdotal reports followed by multicenter, randomized, placebo-controlled studies, the drug was effective in the treatment of the following:

- Postherpetic neuralgia
- Diabetic neuropathy
- Refractory CRPS type 1
- Migraine headaches[34-41]

The efficacy and safety of gabapentin in treating a variety of chronic pain states have renewed interest and enthusiasm in trying new and old antiepileptics in the treatment of chronic pain.

The precise mechanism of action of gabapentin is unknown. It is structurally related to the inhibitory neurotransmitter GABA and is postulated to increase the level of GABA in the nervous system. However, gabapentin does not interact with any of the GABA receptors, nor is it converted to GABA, and it does not affect the metabolism of GABA in neurons. It does not act at or bind to most receptors tested, including *N*-methyl-D-aspartate (NMDA) and kainate receptors and does not directly act at the calcium or sodium channels.

Gabapentin is available as 100-, 300-, 400-, 600-, and 800-mg capsules and 250 mg/5 mL syrup. Patients have generally reported adequate relief with gabapentin dosages ranging from 900 to 2400 mg/day. It is generally well tolerated at even higher doses. Gabapentin is well absorbed orally and largely unbound to plasma proteins. It is not metabolized and is renally excreted. Gabapentin has a half-life of 5 to 9 hours.

The most common adverse effects include somnolence, diarrhea, mood swings, ataxia, fatigue, nausea, and dizziness.

LAMOTRIGINE

Lamotrigine (3,5-diamino-6-(2,3-dichlorophenyl)-1,2,4-triazine) is a novel antiepileptic, which is chemically different from other antiepileptics. It is an adjunctive treatment for partial seizures in adults but is approved for children only in the treatment of Lennox-Gastaut syndrome. No published placebo-controlled studies have evaluated the efficacy of lamotrigine in treating neuropathic pain; however, there have been anecdotal reports.

- A large series has been done of the successful use of lamotrigine in the treatment of refractory trigeminal neuralgia and facial pain[42,43] when used as adjunctive treatment with carbamazepine or phenytoin.

The precise mechanism of action of lamotrigine is unknown. It does not affect NMDA or GABA receptors directly. Lamotrigine, however, is thought to stabilize neuronal membranes through the inhibition of sodium channels[44] and reduces the release of excitatory neurotransmitters such as glutamate and aspartate.

Lamotrigine is available as 25-, 100-, 150-, and 200-mg tablets. There are also chewable dispersible tablets in 2-, 5-, and 25-mg strengths. Lamotrigine doses range from 200 to 500 mg/day in two divided doses for epilepsy therapy, but there are no defined doses for the treatment of neuropathic pain. The starting dosage of lamotrigine is 25 to 50 mg/day; it should be increased slowly to 100 mg twice per day. Caution is required when lamotrigine is used in a patient taking valproic acid because the latter significantly slows the clearance of lamotrigine. The dose should be cut by at least 50% in this circumstance and should not exceed 150 mg/day. It is well absorbed after oral administration, and peak serum levels are reached in 1 to 4 hours. It is metabolized by glucuronic acid conjugation and primarily excreted in the urine. Lamotrigine is 55% protein bound, and its half-life is 13 to 30 hours.

Rash is the most common side effect associated with lamotrigine and requires discontinuation of the drug. Patients should be instructed to inform their physicians about any rash or hypersensitivity reaction; these can result in life-threatening complications such as Stevens-Johnson syndrome and toxic epidermal necrolysis. Patients also should be warned of the possibility of dizziness, ataxia, nausea, and vomiting, which are dose-related side effects. Long-term use of lamotrigine can lead to its accumulation and binding to melanin-rich tissues in the body, including the eye, resulting in blurred vision.

FELBAMATE

Felbamate (2-phenyl-1,3-propanediol dicarbamate) has been successful in controlling partial seizures in adults and Lennox-Gastaut syndrome in children who are unresponsive to other medications.[45,46] In a neurobiologic study in rats, felbamate was found to reduce mechanoallodynia and hyperalgesia as well as heat hyperalgesia.[47]

- Because of the epileptiform nature of certain neuropathic pain states, felbamate has been reported effective for controlling pain in trigeminal neuralgia.[48]

Felbamate has multiple mechanisms of action, including inhibition of NMDA and AMPA (α-amino-3-hydroxy-5-methyl-4-isoxazolepropionic acid)/kainate receptors, potentiating GABA receptor–mediated chloride channels, and inhibiting spontaneous discharges from the voltage-dependent sodium channels.

Felbamate is available as 400- and 600-mg tablets and 600 mg/5 mL suspension. Felbamate provides effective seizure control at doses of 1200 to 2400 mg/day in three divided doses.

However, felbamate is rarely used except for patients who are refractory to all other AEDs because of its association with aplastic anemia and fulminant hepatic failure. Patients taking felbamate should have frequent monitoring with CBCs and LFTs.

TOPIRAMATE

Topiramate (2,3:4,5-bis-O-(1-methylethylidene)-β-D-fructopyranose sulfamate) is a novel AED approved as adjunctive therapy for partial seizures and generalized tonic-clonic seizures. No published placebo-controlled trials have examined the efficacy of topiramate in neuropathic pain syndromes.

- It has, however, been anecdotally reported to relieve pain in postthoracotomy pain syndrome, intercostal neuralgia, headaches, and other neuropathic pain states.[49-51]
- Further studies are needed to define its role in the treatment of neuropathic pain and such trials are currently underway.

Pharmacologic studies postulate at least three mechanisms of action for topiramate: blocking voltage-dependent sodium channels, potentiating the action of inhibitory GABA transmission, and blocking excitatory AMPA/glutamate receptors.[52]

Topiramate is available as 25-, 100-, and 200-mg tablets. The usual starting dosage of topiramate for the treatment of partial seizures is 25 to 50 mg/day; the dosage can be increased to 400 mg/day in two divided doses over 8 weeks. However, the optimal dosage for neuropathic pain is unknown.

Side effects of topiramate include anorexia and weight loss. Patients taking topiramate for prolonged periods may develop kidney stones because of the inhibition of carbonic anhydrase.

VIGABATRIN

Vigabatrin is a novel AED reported to be effective in the treatment of complex partial seizures; it is not currently marketed in the United States.[53]

It appears to act by increasing GABA levels through the inhibition of GABA metabolism in the nervous system. It causes an irreversible enzyme inhibition of GABA transaminase. Thus, like many of its predecessors that work through similar mechanisms in controlling neuropathic pain, vigabatrin can be postulated to be an effective alternative to other AEDs for patients who fail to achieve adequate analgesia.[54]

- The precise role of vigabatrin in pain management, however, has yet to be defined because there are currently no published randomized controlled trials reporting its efficacy in neuropathic pain.

Vigabatrin is well tolerated in patients treated for epilepsy with minimal CNS side effects. Unlike the older antiepileptics, vigabatrin is not metabolized through the liver and therefore has minimal drug interactions with other medications. It is available in 500-mg tablets. Vigabatrin has been shown to be effective in controlling epilepsy in dosages ranging between 1 and 4 g/day. It is rapidly absorbed orally with peak plasma concentrations in 2 hours. Vigabatrin is not extensively bound by plasma proteins, and its half-life is approximately 5 to 8 hours.

Common side effects include drowsiness, tiredness, headaches, stomach upset, weight gain, and vision problems.

TIAGABINE

Tiagabine ((−)-(R)-1-[4,4-Bis(3-methyl-2-thienyl)-3-butenyl]nipecotic acid hydrochloride), another new AED, is effective as adjunctive therapy for the treatment of complex partial seizures.[55]

Tiagabine increases the concentration of GABA by inhibiting the uptake catabolism pathways in presynaptic neurons and thereby prolonging the effect of this neurotransmitters.[56] This mechanism of action suggests the drug may be effective for the treatment of neuropathic pain.[57]

- Some anecdotal reports suggest tiagabine's effectiveness in the treatment of neuropathic pain, and controlled multicenter trials are currently underway.

Tiagabine is available as 2-, 4-, 12-, 16-, and 20-mg tablets. The adult maintenance dosage of tiagabine ranges from 32 to 56 mg/day in two to four divided doses for the treatment of epilepsy. It is rapidly absorbed with peak plasma concentrations occurring at approximately 45 minutes. Tiagabine is 96% bound to plasma proteins.

Side effects of tiagabine are generalized weakness, binding in the eye and other melanin-containing tissues, and rash.

ZONISAMIDE

Zonisamide (1,2-benzisoxazole 3-methanesulfonamide) is used for adjuvant therapy for partial seizures.[58] It is chemically classified as a sulfonamide and is unrelated to other antiepileptic agents.

Zonisamide blocks sodium channels and reduces voltage-dependent T-type calcium currents, stabilizing neuronal membranes and suppressing neuronal hypersynchronization.[59,60] It binds to the GABA-benzodiazepine receptor and facilitates both dopaminergic and serotonergic neurotransmission.

- There are no published reports of zonisamide's efficacy in treating headache and pain, but analgesic efficacy trials are currently underway.

Zonisamide is available in a 100-mg capsule. Its dosing is daily or twice a day. The starting dosage is 100 mg/day and can be increased up to 400 to 1200 mg/day. Drug interactions with carbamazepine and phenytoin have been noted. Peak serum levels are reached in 2 to 6 hours after oral administration. Zonisamide is metabolized by the liver but does not affect cytochrome P450 metabolism. It is excreted by the kidneys. Zonisamide is 40% protein bound but does not affect protein binding of other drugs such as phenytoin, phenobarbital, or carbamazepine. Zonisamide binds extensively to erythrocytes, resulting in higher concentrations in red blood cells (RBCs) than plasma. It has a half-life in plasma of 63 hours and half-life in RBCs of 105 hours.

Zonisamide is contraindicated in patients with hypersensitivity to sulfonamides. Side effects experienced with zonisamide are anorexia, nystagmus, ataxia, abdominal pain, confusion, and fatigue. There was concern that development of nephrolithiasis was related to zonisamide, but further investigation is required.

LEVETIRACETAM

Levetiracetam ([S]-α-ethyl-2-oxo-1-pyrrolidine acetamide) is indicated for adjunctive therapy for partial seizures and may be useful for photosensitive epilepsy.[61,62] It was initially developed as a cognition-enhancing agent for the treatment of Alzheimer's disease. It possesses antiepileptic, anxiolytic, and cognitive-enhancing properties.

It has no significant affinity for GABA or benzodiazepine receptors. Levetiracetam appears to act via an unknown binding site in the brain. It stimulates several neurochemical systems, including glutamatergic, dopaminergic, and cholinergic neurotransmission.

- There are no published reports of its efficacy in treating headache and pain at this time.

Levetiracetam is available in 250-, 500-, and 750-mg tablets. The recommended starting dosage is 1000 mg/day divided into two doses; the maximum recommended dosage is 3000 mg/day. Levetiracetam is rapidly absorbed after oral administration. Peak serum concentrations occur from 0.6 to 1.3 hours after administration. It is transformed by enzymatic hydrolysis of the acetamide group in the blood to inactive metabolite and renally excreted. Approximately 66% of levetiracetam is excreted unchanged. It is largely unbound to plasma protein, and its half-life is about 6 to 8 hours.

Adverse effects include drowsiness, memory impairment, depression, nausea, and ataxia.

PREGABALIN

Pregabalin, (S)-3-(aminomethyl)-5-methylhexanoic acid, is indicated to treat fibromyalgia, diabetic nerve pain, spinal cord injury nerve pain, and pain after shingles.[63]

Pregabalin binds with high affinity to the α2-δ site (an auxiliary subunit of voltage-gated calcium channels) in CNS tissues.[64] Although the mechanism of action of pregabalin has not been fully elucidated, results with genetically modified mice and with compounds structurally related to pregabalin (e.g., gabapentin) suggest that binding to the α2-δ subunit may be involved in pregabalin's antinociceptive and antiseizure effects in animals. In animal models of nerve damage, pregabalin has been shown to reduce calcium-dependent release of pronociceptive neurotransmitters in the spinal cord, possibly by disrupting α2-δ containing calcium channel trafficking or reducing calcium currents (or both). Evidence from other animal models of nerve damage and persistent pain suggest the antinociceptive activities of pregabalin may also be mediated through interactions with descending noradrenergic and serotonergic pathways originating from the brainstem that modulate pain transmission in the spinal cord.

Pregabalin has been approved by the U.S. Food and Drug Administration for the treatment of neuropathic pain in the following:

- Diabetic peripheral neuropathy[65]
- Postherpetic neuralgia[66]
- Fibromyalgia[67]

Pregabalin is available in 25-, 50-, 75-, 100-, 150-, 200-, 225-, and 300-mg capsules plus 20 mg/mL oral solution. The recommended dosage of LYRICA is 75 to 150 mg two times a day or 50 to 100 mg three times a day (150–300 mg/day) in patients with creatinine clearance of at least 60 mL/min. Begin dosing at 75 mg two times a day, or 50 mg three times a day (150 mg/day). The dose may be increased to 300 mg/day within 1 week based on efficacy and tolerability. Pregabalin is eliminated from the systemic circulation primarily by renal excretion as unchanged drug with a mean elimination half-life of 6.3 hours in subjects with normal renal function. Mean renal clearance was estimated to be 67.0 to 80.9 mL/min in young healthy subjects.

Adverse effects include angioedema, hypersensitivity, peripheral edema, dizziness, and somnolence.

RECOMMENDATIONS

Despite the increase in the number of AEDs available, the rule of "old is gold" continues to be applicable in developing a general strategy to treat neuropathic pain syndromes. Phenytoin, the "grandfather" of the modern day antiepileptics, should be tried first for four major reasons:

- Availability in both oral and injectable forms, which could be helpful in providing immediate pain relief
- Lower cost
- Established safety
- Relative ease of use

The major exception to this rule is in patients with trigeminal neuralgia, a disorder that generally has responded better to carbamazepine than to the other agents. For classic trigeminal neuralgia, carbamazepine followed by lamotrigine, topiramate, gabapentin, and oxcarbazepine should be tried either alone or in combination.

Among the newer AEDs, gabapentin appears to be the most effective and best tolerated. It probably should be considered first after phenytoin for most neuropathic pain states other than trigeminal neuralgia. Gabapentin has the added advantage of easy use in combination with other AEDs that have failed as single agents because it does not interact with these agents.

Other AEDs such as pregabalin, valproic acid, lamotrigine, tiagabine, clonazepam, and topiramate should be tried if the above either do not provide adequate pain relief or are not tolerated. In particular, preliminary data indicate that topiramate is a promising neuropathic analgesic, but results of randomized, placebo-controlled studies are not yet available. AEDs such as vigabatrin, levetiracetam, zonisamide, and oxcarbazepine have not yet demonstrated proven efficacy in controlled trials of the treatment of neuropathic pain. Felbamate should only be used as a last resort because of its association with aplastic anemia and fulminant hepatic failure.

An important point to keep in mind is that these medications are AEDs first rather than true analgesics and are limited by adverse effects, especially when used long term. Their use for neuropathic pain should generally follow the same dosing and monitoring guidelines used for seizure control, although in our experience, many patients benefit from low doses that are considered subtherapeutic in treating epilepsy; monitoring drug levels may not be necessary.

REFERENCES

1. Sindrup SH, Jensen TS. Efficacy of pharmacological treatments of neuropathic pain: an update and effect related to mechanism of drug action. *Pain*. 1999;83:389.
2. McQuay H, Carroll D, Jadad AR, et al. Anticonvulsant drugs for management of pain: a systematic review. *BMJ*. 1995;311:1047.
3. Ross EL. The evolving role of antiepileptic drugs in treating neuropathic pain. *Neurology*. 2000;55(Suppl 1):S41.
4. Backonja MM. Anticonvulsants (antineuropathics) for neuropathic pain syndromes. *Clin J Pain*. 2000;16(Suppl 2):S67.
5. Saudek CD, Werns S, Reidenberg M. Phenytoin in the treatment of diabetic symmetrical polyneuropathy. *Clin Pharmacol Ther*. 1977;22: 196.
6. Camtor FK. Phenytoin treatment of thalamic pain. *Br Med J*. 1972; 4: 590.

7. McCleane GJ. Intravenous infusion of phenytoin relieves neuropathic pain: a randomized, double-blinded, placebo-controlled, crossover study. *Anesth Analg*. 1999;89:985–988.
8. Chang VT. Intravenous phenytoin in the management of crescendo pelvic cancer-related pain. *J Pain Symptom Manage*. 1997;13:238.
9. Ellenberg M. Treatment of diabetic neuropathy with diphenylhydantion. *N Y State J Med*. 1968;68:2653.
10. Campbell FG, Graham JG, Zilkha KJ. Clinical trial of carbamazepine (Tegretol) in trigeminal neuralgia. *J Neurol Neurosurg Psychiatry*. 1966;29:265.
11. Amols W. Facial pain. Treatment with carbamazepine. *N Y State J Med*. 1970;70:2429.
12. Zakrzewska JM, Patsalos PN. Drugs used in the management of trigeminal neuralgia. *Oral Surg Oral Med Oral Pathol*. 1992;74:439.
13. Bennett GJ. Neuropathic pain. In: Wall PD, Melzack PD, Melzack R, eds. *Textbook of Pain*. 3rd ed. Edinburgh, Scotland: Churchill Livingstone; 1994:201.
14. Woolf CJ, Mannion RJ. Neuropathic pain: aetiology, symptoms, mechanisms, and management. *Lancet*. 1999;353:1959.
15. Burchiel KJ. Carbamazepine inhibits spontaneous activity in experimental neuromas. *Exp Neurol*. 1988;102:249.
16. Yaari Y, Devor M. Phenytoin suppresses spontaneous ectopic discharge in rat sciatic nerve neuromas. *Neurosci Lett*. 1985;58:117.
17. Fischer JH, Patel TV, Fischer PA. Fosphenytoin: clinical pharmacokinetics and comparative advantages in the acute treatment of seizures. *Clin Pharmacokinet*. 2003;42(1):33-58.
18. Rull JA, Quibrera R, Gonzalez-Millan M, Castaneda OL. Symptomatic treatment of peripheral diabetic neuropathy with carbamazepine (Tegretol): double blind crossover trial. *Diabetologia*. 1969;5:215.
19. Smith PF, Darlington CL. Recent developments in drug therapy for multiple sclerosis. *Multiple Sclerosis*. 1999;5:110.
20. Minagar A, Sheremata WA. Glossopharyngeal neuralgia and MS. *Neurology*. 2000;54:1368.
21. Ekbom KA, Westerberg CE. Carbamazepine in glossopharyngeal neuralgia. *Arch Neurol*. 1966;14:595.
22. Clancy RR. New anticonvulsants in pediatrics: carbamazepine and valproate. *Curr Probl Pediatr*. 1987;17:133.
23. Grant SM, Faulds D. Oxcarbazepine. A review of its pharmacology and therapeutic potential in epilepsy, trigeminal neuralgia and affective disorders. *Drugs*. 1992;43:873.
24. Schachter SC, Vazquez B, Fisher RS, et al. Oxcarbazepine: double-blind, randomized, placebo-control, monotherapy trial for partial seizures. *Neurology*. 1999;52:732.
25. McLean MJ, Schmutz M, Wamil AW, et al. Oxcarbazepine: mechanisms of action. *Epilepsia*. 1994;35(Suppl 3):S5.
26. Zakrzewska JM, Patsalos PN. Oxcarbazepine: a new drug in the management of intractable trigeminal neuralgia. *J Neurol Neurosurg Psychiatry*. 1989;52:472.
27. Guieu R, Mesdjian E, Rochat H, Roger J. Central analgesic effect of valproate in patients with epilepsy. *Seizure*. 1993;2:147.
28. Norton J. Use of intravenous valproate sodium in status migraine. *Headache*. 2000;40:755.
29. Rothrock JF. Clinical studies of valproate for migraine prophylaxis. *Cephalalgia*. 1997;17:81.
30. Johannessen CU. Mechanisms of action of valproate: a commentary. *Neurochem Int*. 2000;37:103.
31. Caccia MR. Clonazepam in facial neuralgia and cluster headache. *Eur Neurol*. 1975;13:560.
32. Bartusch SL, Sanders BJ, D'Alessio JG, Jernigan JR. Clonazepam for the treatment of lancinating phantom limb pain. *Clin J Pain*. 1996;12:59.
33. Harkins S, Linford J, Cohen J, et al. Administration of clonazepam in the treatment of TMD and associated myofascial pain: a double-blind pilot study. *J Craniomandib Disord*. 1991;5:179.
34. Mellick LB, Mellick GA. Successful treatment of reflex sympathetic dystrophy with gabapentin. *Am J Emerg Med*. 1995;13:96.
35. Mellick GA, Mellick LB. Gabapentin in the management of reflex sympathetic dystrophy. *J Pain Symptom Manage*. 1995;10:265.
36. Novel Applications of AEDS: Current Research. Express report from the American Academy of Neurology 48th Annual Meeting; 1996.
37. Magnus L. Nonepileptic uses of gabapentin. *Epilepsia*. 1999;40 (Suppl 6):S66.
38. Kanazi GE, Johnson RW, Dworkin RH. Treatment of postherpetic neuralgia: an update. *Drugs*. 2000;59:1113.
39. Perez HE, Sanchez GF. Gabapentin therapy for diabetic neuropathic pain. *Am J Med*. 2000;108:689.
40. Backonja MM. Gabapentin monotherapy for the symptomatic treatment of painful neuropathy: a multicenter, double-blind, placebo-controlled trial in patients with diabetes mellitus. *Epilepsia*. 1999;40 (Suppl 6):S57.
41. Di Trapani G, Mei D, Marra C, et al. Gabapentin in the prophylaxis of migraine: a double-blind randomized placebo-controlled study. *Clin Ter*. 2000;151:145.
42. Lunardi G, Leandri M, Albano C, et al. Clinical effectiveness of lamotrigine and plasma levels in essential and symptomatic trigeminal neuralgia. *Neurology*. 1997;48:1714.
43. Zakrzewska JM, Chaudhry Z, Nurmikko TJ, et al. Lamotrigine (Lamictal) in refractory trigeminal neuralgia: results from a double-blind placebo controlled cross-over trial. *Pain*. 1997;73:223.
44. Brodie MJ, Richens A, Yuen AW. Double-blind comparison of lamotrigine and carbamazepine in newly diagnosed epilepsy. *Lancet*. 1995;345:476.
45. Canger R, Vignol A, Bonardi R, Guidolin L. Felbamate in refractory partial epilepsy. *Epilepsy Res*. 1999;34:43.
46. Jensen PK. Felbamate in the treatment of Lennox-Gastaut syndrome. *Epilepsia*. 1994;35(Suppl 5):S4.
47. Imamura Y, Bennett GJ. Felbamate relieves several abnormal pain sensations in rats with an experimental peripheral neuropathy. *J Pharmacol Exp Ther*. 1995;275:177.
48. Chesire WP. Felbamate relieved trigeminal neuralgia. *Clin J Pain*. 1995;11:139.
49. Potter D, Edwards KR. Potential role of topiramate in relieving pain in patients with clinically refractory neuropathies. *Neurology*. 1998;50(Suppl):A-255.
50. Bajwa ZH, Sami N, Warfield CA, Wootton J. Topiramate relieves refractory intercostal neuralgia. *Neurology*. 1999;52:1917.
51. Zvartau-Hind M, Din MU, Gilani A, et al. Topiramate relieves refractory trigeminal neuralgia in MS patients. *Neurology*. 2000;55:1587.
52. Shank RP, Gardocki JF, Streeter AJ, Maryanoff BE. An overview of the preclinical aspects of topiramate: pharmacology, pharmacokinetics, and mechanism of action. *Epilepsia*. 2000;41(Suppl 1):S3.
53. Gidal BE, Privitera MD, Sheth RD, Gilman JT. Vigabatrin: a novel therapy for seizures disorders. *Ann Pharmacother*. 1999;33:1277.
54. Alves ND, de Castro-Costa CM, de Carvalho AM, et al. Possible analgesic effect of vigabatrin in animal experimental chronic neuropathic pain. *Arq Neuropsiquiatr*. 1999;57:916.
55. Tiagabine (Gabitril) [package insert] Abbott Laboratories, Abbott Park, IL, Aug 1999.

56. Meldrum BS, Chapman AG. Basic mechanisms of Gabitril (tiagabine) and future potential developments. *Epilepsia*. 1999;40(Suppl 9):S2.
57. Ipponi A, Lamberti C, Medica A, et al. Tiagabine antinociception in rodents depends on GABA(B) receptor activation: parallel antinociception testing and medial thalamus GABA microdialysis. *Eur J Pharmcol*. 1999;368:205.
58. Leppik IE. Zonisamide. *Epilepsia*. 1999;40(Suppl 5):S23.
59. Peters DH, Sorkin EM. Zonisamide. A review of its pharmacodynamic and pharmacokinetic properties, and therapeutic potential in epilepsy. *Drugs*. 1993;45:760.
60. Tomlinson DR, Malcangio M, Patel J, et al. Effects of zonisamide on mechanically-induced nociception in rats with streptozotocin-diabetes. Research supported by Elan Pharmaceuticals. In Worldwide Pain Conference Proceedings, Program and Abstract of the Worldwide Pain Conference, 2000, pp. 15-21.
61. Patsalos PN. Pharmacokinetic profile of levetiracetam: toward ideal characteristics. *Pharmacol Ther*. 2000;85:77.
62. Kasteleijn-Nolst Trenite DG, Marescaux C, Stodieck S, et al. Photosensitive epilepsy: a model to study the effects of antiepileptic drugs: evaluation of the piracetam analogue, levetiracetam. *Epilepsy Res*. 1996;25:225.
63. Tassone DM, Boyce E, Guyer J, et al. Pregabalin: a novel gamma-aminobutyric acid analogue in the treatment of neuropathic pain, partial-onset seizures, and anxiety disorders. *Clin Ther*. 2007; 29(1):26-48.
64. Taylor CP, Angelotti T, Fauman E. Pharmacology and mechanism of action of pregabalin: the calcium channel alpha2-delta subunit as a target for antiepileptic drug discovery. *Epilepsy Res*. 2007;73(2):137-150.
65. Rosenstock J, Tuchman M, LaMoreaux L, et al. Pregabalin for the treatment of painful diabetic peripheral neuropathy: a double-blind, placebo-controlled trial. *Pain*. 2004;110(3):628-638.
66. Cappuzzo KA. Treatment of postherpetic neuralgia: focus on pregabalin. *Clin Interv Aging*. 2009;4:17-23.
67. Mease PJ, Russell IJ, Arnold LM, et al. A randomized, double-blind, placebo-controlled, phase III trial of pregabalin in the treatment of patients with fibromyalgia. *J Rheumatol*. 2008;35(3):502-514.

CHAPTER 78

Muscle Relaxants and α_2 Agonists for Pain Management

Jennifer A. Elliott

INTRODUCTION

Skeletal muscle relaxants are frequently used in patients with both acute and chronic pain when a component of muscle spasm is thought to be contributing to pain symptomatology. They are also used in the management of disorders in which spasticity is a prominent feature, such as multiple sclerosis, cerebral palsy, and after spinal cord injury or stroke with paresis. A wide variety of muscle relaxants are available, and selection of an agent for use may be influenced by factors such as cost, perceived potency, side effect profile, chronicity of pain, and addictive potential (or lack thereof). Commonly used muscle relaxants in the United States include baclofen, carisoprodol, chlorzoxazone, cyclobenzaprine, dantrolene, diazepam, metaxalone, methocarbamol, orphenadrine, and tizanidine.

The α_2 agonists are well known historically for their use in the management of hypertension, but more recently, these agents have been found effective in a variety of pain management, anesthesia, and critical care applications. These applications include use in perioperative sedation and as adjuncts to regional and neuraxial anesthesia for pain management, including the treatment of refractory cancer pain. α_2 Agonists have also been used in the palliative care setting to reduce pain and the distress of the dying and to facilitate withdrawal of ventilatory support. Additionally, they may be useful in the management of opioid-induced hyperalgesia and opioid and nicotine withdrawal. α_2 Agonists currently in clinical use include clonidine, tizanidine, and dexmedetomidine.

MUSCLE RELAXANTS

Muscle relaxants are most often used in the management of acute musculoskeletal pain but are also commonly combined with other analgesic agents in some chronic pain management regimens. These agents should be distinguished from the nondepolarizing and depolarizing muscle relaxants that are used to provide paralysis of skeletal and respiratory muscles during general anesthesia and act by production of blockade of neuromuscular conduction. The mechanism of action of the "muscle relaxant" agents used for managing muscle spasm is not fully understood, but in general, most of these drugs act centrally by suppressing polysynaptic reflexes in the spinal cord and via depressant effects on the central nervous system (CNS). This section describes the pharmacologic profile of the currently available skeletal muscle relaxants.

BACLOFEN

Baclofen is marketed in the United States under the brand name Lioresal. It is labeled for use in the management of disorders in which spasticity is present, such as multiple sclerosis and spinal cord injury. Unlabeled indications for the use of baclofen include intractable hiccups and trigeminal neuralgia and for the relief of intractable pain.[1] Baclofen is available for oral and intrathecal use. Baclofen is thought to act by inhibition of monosynaptic and polysynaptic reflex transmission at the level of the spinal cord, possibly through hyperpolarization of primary afferent nerve terminals.[1] It is derived from γ-aminobutyric acid (GABA), an inhibitory neurotransmitter thought to play an important role in pain transmission.[2] This may explain why baclofen seems to have analgesic properties that make it useful in the treatment of conditions such as trigeminal neuralgia.[3] The usual dosing of baclofen is 5 to 10 mg orally three times daily, which may be titrated to 80 mg/day if needed for the management of spasticity. Caution should be used in prescribing baclofen to patients who are elderly, who have severe renal impairment, and who have a history of seizures.[1] The most frequently observed side effects of baclofen include drowsiness, ataxia, hypotonia, vertigo, insomnia, psychiatric disturbances, and weakness. Less commonly, patients may experience hypotension, confusion, fatigue, headache, rash, nausea, constipation, or polyuria with baclofen use. Withdrawal, which may be life threatening, can occur with abrupt discontinuation of baclofen, particularly if it is being administered intrathecally.[1] Baclofen is rapidly absorbed after oral administration has a half-life of 3.5 hours. It undergoes hepatic metabolism (15%) and renal and fecal excretion (85% as unchanged drug).[1]

CARISOPRODOL

Carisoprodol is marketed in the United States under the brand name Soma. It is indicated for short-term use (2–3 weeks) in the treatment of acute musculoskeletal pain.[4] The mechanism of action of carisoprodol is not completely understood, but it appears to have central depressant actions and anxiolytic and sedative effects related to its metabolism to meprobamate.[4] Metabolism to meprobamate may explain the abuse potential associated with carisoprodol.[5,6] In the past few years, increasing concerns about the abuse of carisoprodol and a growing number of reports of emergency department visits and deaths associated with carisoprodol use led to an effort for it to be classified as a controlled substance. After a review of data regarding carisoprodol abuse, the Drug Enforcement Administration ruled on December 12, 2011, that carisoprodol be placed into schedule IV of the Controlled Substances

Act, effective January 11, 2012.[7] Caution is warranted when carisoprodol is used in patients with a history of drug abuse.[8] Carisoprodol is dosed from 250 mg to 350 mg three times per day and at bedtime. As with other muscle relaxants, carisoprodol should be used with caution in elderly patients. Side effects seen in more than 1% of users of carisoprodol include drowsiness, dizziness, and headache.[4] After ingestion, carisoprodol takes effect within 30 minutes and has a duration of action of 4 to 6 hours. It is hepatically metabolized and has an active metabolite (meprobamate), which is renally excreted. Whereas the half-life of carisoprodol is 2 hours, that of meprobamate is 10 hours.[4]

CHLORZOXAZONE

Chlorzoxazone is marketed in the United States under the brand name Parafon Forte It is indicated for use in the management of muscle spasm and pain caused by acute musculoskeletal conditions.[9,10] It is thought to act by depressing polysynaptic reflexes in the spinal cord and subcortical areas of the brain. The dosing of chlorzoxazone is 250 to 750 mg three to four times daily. It should be used with caution among elderly patients, with lower dosing regimens suggested. Some adverse effects associated with the use of chlorzoxazone are drowsiness, dizziness, lightheadedness, malaise, nausea, rash, paradoxical stimulation, and liver toxicity (sometimes fatal).[9,10] Chlorzoxazone has an onset within 1 hour after ingestion and a duration of action of 6 to 12 hours. It is hepatically metabolized via glucuronidation, and the conjugates are renally excreted.[9]

CYCLOBENZAPRINE

Cyclobenzaprine is marketed in the United States under the trade names Flexeril, Fexmid, and Amrix (an extended-release version). Cyclobenzaprine is indicated for short-term use (2–3 weeks) in the relief of muscle spasm. It is thought to reduce tonic somatic motor activity in both α and γ motor neurons and is chemically related to the tricyclic antidepressants (TCAs).[11] It is dosed at 5 to 10 mg three times a day (immediate release) or 15 to 30 mg/day (extended release). Use of the extended-release version is not recommended in elderly adults or patients with any significant hepatic impairment.[11] Cyclobenzaprine is structurally related to TCAs and should not be used within 14 days of monoamine oxidase inhibitors. It is also contraindicated for use in individuals with hyperthyroidism, a recent history of myocardial infarction, congestive heart failure, cardiac arrhythmias, or conduction block.[11] Side effects observed in more than 1% of users are drowsiness, dizziness, dry mouth, fatigue, headache, confusion, irritability, decreased mental acuity, nervousness, dyspepsia, nausea, constipation, diarrhea, abdominal pain, unpleasant taste, weakness, blurred vision, pharyngitis, and acute respiratory infection.[11] Cyclobenzaprine is hepatically metabolized and renally and fecally excreted. Its elimination half-life is approximately 18 hours (immediate release) to 33 hours (extended release).[11]

DANTROLENE

Dantrolene is marketed in the United States under the trade names Dantrium and Revonto. It is well known for its use in the prevention and management of malignant hyperthermia. It is also used in the treatment of spasticity caused by upper motor neuron disorders such as spinal cord injury, stroke, cerebral palsy, and multiple sclerosis.[12] It is not indicated for the management of muscle spasm caused by rheumatic disorders.[13] Dantrolene works by preventing release of calcium from the sarcoplasmic reticulum in skeletal muscle, preventing excitation-contraction coupling. Dosing of oral dantrolene is initiated at 25 mg/day and may be titrated up to a maximum of 400 mg/day over several weeks if needed to treat spasticity. Dantrolene has a black box warning because of the potential for hepatotoxicity with its use.[14] It is recommended that dantrolene be discontinued after 45 days of therapy if no benefit is observed with its use because the onset of hepatitis is most common between 3 and 12 months of therapy.[12,13] Periodic monitoring of liver function tests is recommended when dantrolene is used in the management of spasticity, and its use is contraindicated in patients with preexisting liver disease.[13] Caution should be used when prescribing dantrolene to women older than 35 years of age because hepatotoxicity occurs most frequently among this population.[13] The most commonly observed side effects of dantrolene are dizziness, drowsiness, weakness, general malaise, fatigue, and diarrhea.[13] Photosensitivity has also been reported with the use of dantrolene.[12,13] Dantrolene is hepatically metabolized, has an elimination half-life of 4 to 8 hours, and is eliminated fecally (45%–50%) and renally (25 % unchanged drug and metabolites).[12]

DIAZEPAM (BENZODIAZEPINES)

Diazepam (Valium) is the prototypical benzodiazepine used in the management of muscle spasm and spasticity. Clonazepam (Klonopin) and Lorazepam (Ativan) have also been used in the treatment of these conditions. These agents are also known for their use in the management of seizures, anxiety and panic disorders, ethanol withdrawal, and sedation in critically ill or perioperative patients. Benzodiazepines are thought to act by enhancing GABA inhibition of neuronal excitability. This effect occurs as a result of increased neuronal membrane permeability to chloride ions, which causes hyperpolarization of the neuronal membrane and thereby reduces the likelihood of action potential propagation.[15] Benzodiazepines are schedule IV controlled substances. Diazepam is dosed at 2 to 10 mg orally three to four times daily when used as a skeletal muscle relaxant. Diazepam must be dose reduced (by 50%) in the setting of hepatic impairment because its half-life may be prolonged significantly in this setting. Significant renal impairment may also result in prolonged effects from diazepam and its metabolites. Long-acting benzodiazepines such as diazepam are not recommended for use in elderly adults because of an increased risk of falls.[15] The benzodiazepines are associated with teratogenic effects, and they are category D medications for use in pregnancy. Side effects that may be observed with the use of benzodiazepines include anterograde amnesia, somnolence, paradoxical psychiatric reactions (e.g., agitation, hallucinations, or psychosis), and hypotension and in large doses, respiratory depression.[15] With prolonged use, abrupt discontinuation may result in a withdrawal syndrome that, if severe, could involve seizures and be life threatening. Diazepam plasma concentrations peak 30 to 90 minutes after administration, and it has a terminal half-life of 1 to 2 days. It is hepatically metabolized to several active metabolites, which are renally excreted.[16]

METAXALONE

Metaxalone is marketed in the United States under the trade name Skelaxin. It is indicated for use in the relief of pain from acute musculoskeletal conditions.[17] It is thought to act through CNS depressant effects and does not have a direct effect on skeletal muscle.[17] Metaxalone is dosed at 800 mg three to four times daily. Its use is contraindicated in patients with significant hepatic or renal impairment. As with other muscle relaxants, it should be used with caution in elderly adults. Side effects associated with the use of metaxalone include dizziness, drowsiness, headache, irritability or nervousness, nausea, vomiting, and gastrointestinal (GI) upset.[17,18] Hemolytic anemia, leukopenia, and jaundice have also been reported with its use.[17] Metaxalone is hepatically metabolized and renally excreted. Metaxalone has an onset of action of approximately 1 hour and a duration of action of 4 to 6 hours. Its elimination half-life is 4 to 14 hours.[17]

METHOCARBAMOL

Methocarbamol is marketed in the United States under the trade name Robaxin. It is indicated for use in the treatment of muscle spasm related to acute musculoskeletal conditions and in the management of tetanus.[19] It is a derivative of guaifenesin that is thought to act through CNS depressant effects and has no action directly on skeletal muscle.[20] It is dosed at 1500 mg four times daily initially (the first 48–72 hours of treatment) with a maintenance dose of 1000 mg four times a day.[20] Because of its short half-life, it may be preferred over other muscle relaxants when used in elderly adults, although caution in this population is still warranted.[19] Side effects that may be associated with the use of methocarbamol include hypotension, bradycardia, flushing, syncope, amnesia, confusion, diplopia, dizziness, drowsiness, insomnia, nystagmus, vertigo, seizures, headache, rash, urticaria, fever, pruritus, angioneurotic edema, leukopenia, jaundice, metallic taste, dyspepsia, nausea, and vomiting.[19,20] The onset of action of methocarbamol is approximately 30 minutes after ingestion. It has an elimination half-life of 1 to 2 hours and is hepatically metabolized and renally excreted. Its half-life may be significantly extended in the presence of hepatic or renal impairment.[20]

ORPHENADRINE

Orphenadrine is marketed in the United States under the trade name Norflex. It is indicated for the treatment of muscle spasms caused by acute musculoskeletal conditions. It is thought to exert its effects centrally by atropine-like action on cerebral motor centers or on the medulla.[21,22] It has anticholinergic, antihistaminic, analgesic, and euphorigenic properties with associated potential for abuse.[21-23] Dosing of orphenadrine is 100 mg twice daily. Its use is contraindicated in patients with glaucoma, obstruction of the GI tract, stenosing peptic ulcers, myasthenia gravis, cardiospasm, prostatic hypertrophy, and bladder neck obstruction.[21,22] Caution is warranted when orphenadrine is used in elderly adults and in patients with significant cardiac disease. It is advised that patients receiving long-term orphenadrine therapy undergo periodic monitoring of blood cell counts and hepatic and renal functions.[22] Adverse effects associated with the use of orphenadrine include tachycardia, palpitations, dizziness, drowsiness, hallucinations, euphoria, agitation, headache, confusion, urticaria, pruritus, nausea, vomiting, dry mouth, constipation, stomach upset, urinary retention, blurry vision, increased intraocular pressure, papillary dilation, nystagmus, and (rarely) aplastic anemia.[21,22] Orphenadrine undergoes extensive hepatic metabolism, and its metabolites are renally excreted.[21,22] Its effects peak 2 to 4 hours after ingestion, its duration of action is 4 to 6 hours, and its elimination half-life is 14 to 16 hours.[21,22]

TIZANIDINE

Tizanidine is marketed in the United States under the trade name Zanaflex. It is an α_2-adrenergic agonist that is labeled for use in the management of spasticity. Unlabeled indications include management of tension headaches, low back pain (LBP), and trigeminal neuralgia.[24] It acts centrally with effects on the spinal cord to decrease excitatory input to α motor neurons.[24] Dosing is usually started at 4 mg at bedtime and gradually titrated to relief of symptoms in 2- to 4-mg increments to a maximum daily dose of 36 mg in divided doses. Use of tizanidine should be avoided in patients with hepatic impairment, and it should be dose reduced in patients with creatinine clearances less than 25 mL/min because its clearance is decreased by more than 50% in this setting.[24] Caution should be used when tizanidine is administered to elderly patients because of the potential for orthostatic hypotension and reduced renal clearance in this population.[24] Because use of tizanidine has been associated with visual hallucinations, its use in patients with a history of significant psychiatric disorders should be carefully considered. Adverse effects reported in more than 1% of patients taking tizanidine include hypotension, somnolence, dizziness, dry mouth, weakness, bradycardia (with large doses), nervousness, speech disorder, visual hallucinations, constipation, vomiting, urinary tract infection, increased urinary frequency, dyskinesia, blurred vision, pharyngitis, rhinitis, infection, flu-like syndrome, and elevated liver enzymes.[24] Liver enzyme elevations to greater than three times the upper limit of normal have been reported in approximately 5% of patients taking tizanidine.[25] Because of the rare risk of fulminant hepatic failure during tizanidine administration, it is recommended by the manufacturer that liver enzymes be measured at baseline and then 1, 3, and 6 months after it is initiated with further periodic monitoring as needed.[25] If discontinuation of tizanidine is desired in patients who have received prolonged therapy, it is recommended that gradual tapering be undertaken to minimize the potential risk of withdrawal symptoms, which could include rebound hypertension, tachycardia, and hypertonia.[24] Tizanidine is hepatically metabolized with extensive first-pass effect and undergoes fecal (60%) and renal (20%) excretion.[24] It has a duration of action of 3 to 6 hours and an elimination half-life of 2.5 hours. Tizanidine is available in both capsule and tablet forms, which are bioequivalent in the fasted state but differ in their pharmacokinetic profiles when ingested with food. Because of the variation in pharmacokinetics that occurs with being fasted or fed, it is recommended that patients using tizanidine always consume it consistently in either the fasting or fed state and that capsules and tablets not be interchanged.

EFFICACY OF MUSCLE RELAXANTS FOR PAINFUL MUSCULAR CONDITIONS: THE EVIDENCE

Muscle relaxants have been widely used in the treatment of both acute and chronic back pain and other painful conditions. It is estimated that in primary care settings, 35% of patients presenting with symptoms of acute LBP are prescribed muscle relaxants.[26] Despite their long-standing, widespread use, however, good-quality studies evaluating the efficacy of these agents are relatively sparse in the medical literature. One systematic review concluded that there was fair evidence for the efficacy of cyclobenzaprine, carisoprodol, orphenadrine, and tizanidine in the treatment of patients with musculoskeletal conditions such as back or neck pain.[27] The same review found there to be limited or inconsistent data to support the use of baclofen, chlorzoxazone, dantrolene, metaxalone, or methocarbamol for these conditions.[27] A meta-analysis of cyclobenzaprine in the treatment of back pain indicated that patients receiving cyclobenzaprine for a period of 14 days were five times as likely to report improvement than subjects receiving placebo for their back pain.[28] In this study, one subject reported modest improvement in local pain, muscle spasm, tenderness to palpation, range of motion, and activities of daily living per every three subjects exposed to cyclobenzaprine.[28] This degree of improvement, however, was accompanied by a significant occurrence of side effects, the most frequently reported being drowsiness (20% incidence).[28] A Cochrane review of muscle relaxants for nonspecific LBP found that there is strong evidence of efficacy of nonbenzodiazepines for acute LBP and that this treatment may reduce discomfort and accelerate recovery in this patient population. The evidence to support the use of benzodiazepines for acute LBP and nonbenzodiazepines for chronic LBP was less robust in this review.[26] This review also found that although muscle relaxants are effective for short-term relief of acute and chronic LBP, their use is associated with a high incidence of side effects such as dizziness and drowsiness.[26] The authors of the review suggested that muscle relaxants might best be used as adjunctive therapy along with nonsteroidal anti-inflammatory drugs (NSAIDs) and other analgesics in the management of back pain.[26] They also indicated a need for large, high-quality trials to further evaluate muscle relaxants in comparison with other analgesic agents such as NSAIDs for this purpose.[26] Unfortunately, another Cochrane review of cyclobenzaprine in the management of myofascial pain concluded that evidence to support its use for this indication was insufficient.[29] This was attributable to a paucity of clinical studies in this area. The authors indicated a need for additional large, high-quality studies to further evaluate the use of cyclobenzaprine in the management of myofascial pain before any solid inferences can be made regarding its efficacy and safety in this condition.[29]

α_2 AGONISTS

The α_2 agonists are known to create effects of sympatholysis, anxiolysis, analgesia, and sedation. These properties have made the α_2 agonists useful adjuncts in veterinary anesthesia for many years, especially because they lack respiratory depressant effects, which allows for anesthetization in spontaneously breathing animals. Additionally, these drugs have been found to have anesthetic and analgesic-sparing effects in numerous human clinical studies. The α_2 agonists are imidazoline compounds that exert their effects by binding to G protein–coupled receptors on cell membranes. Activation of these receptors on neuronal cell membranes causes membrane hyperpolarization, which results in decreased release of neurotransmitters and consequently reduces nerve impulse transmission. Hyperpolarization of neuronal cell membranes caused by

α_2 receptor activation occurs as a result of decreased 3′-5′-cyclic adenosine monophosphate (cAMP) formation, opening of potassium (K^+) channels to allow potassium efflux from cells, and reduced opening of voltage-gated N-type calcium (Ca^{2+}) channels.[30] Other mechanisms that may also be involved in α_2 agonist–mediated nociception include activation of phospholipase C second messenger systems and alkalinization of cells caused by accelerated sodium–hydrogen ion exchange across neuronal membranes.[30-32]

There are three α_2 receptor subtypes, α_{2A}, α_{2B}, and α_{2C}. α_2 Agonist–associated antinociception and α_2 agonist–opioid synergy appear to be mediated by the α_{2A} and α_{2C} receptor subtypes, with the α_{2A} subtype predominating.[33-36] The binding affinities of the α_2 agonists at spinal α_2 receptors correlates with their antinociceptive potency. In this regard, dexmedetomidine is the most potent of the available α_2 agonists; tizanidine is the least potent. Clonidine, which has been in use for decades for the treatment of hypertension, is perhaps the most well-known member of this drug class. Preclinical animal models and human study data of acute and chronic pain conditions using α_2 agonists have demonstrated their analgesic efficacy.[34,37-47] See **Table 78-1** for a summary of the pharmacologic properties of the clinically available α_2 agonists.[48]

As a class, the α_2 agonists share some potential adverse effects and drug interactions, and their use may warrant precautions in certain patient populations. These agents may cause side effects of hypotension, bradycardia, heart block, sedation, dizziness, dry mouth, asthenia, orthostasis, rash, and nausea. They should be used with caution in patients with known cardiac conduction defects and may compound sedation when used with other drugs that have sedative effects. Caution is advised when these drugs are combined with beta-blockers, calcium channel blockers, and digitalis because of the increased potential for heart block. **Table 78-2** provides further information about drug-specific drug interactions, precautions, and adverse effects of the α_2 agonists currently in clinical use.[48]

CLONIDINE

Clonidine is marketed in the United States under the brand names Catapres, Catapres-TTS, Kapvay, and Duraclon. It has an α_1:α_2 affinity ratio of 200:1.[49] Clonidine preparations are available for oral, transdermal, and neuraxial administration in the United States. Indications for which clonidine has Food and Drug Administration approval include the management of hypertension and pediatric attention deficit hyperactivity disorder and the treatment of severe cancer-associated pain unrelieved with opioids alone (when epidurally administered in conjunction with opioids). Other applications for which clonidine has been used include the management of opioid and alcohol withdrawal, smoking cessation, dysmenorrhea, diarrhea, glaucoma, vasomotor symptoms associated with menopause (hot flashes), as an adjunct for the management a variety of painful conditions, and in prophylaxis of migraine headaches.[50] After oral administration, clonidine levels peak within 3 to 5 hours, and it has an elimination half-life of 12 to 16 hours. When administered transdermally, it may take 2 days to achieve peak plasma levels of clonidine.[51] After epidural administration, peak plasma and cerebrospinal fluid levels of clonidine are achieved in 19 and 26 minutes, respectively.[52] Clonidine is hepatically metabolized with 40% to 60% being excreted unchanged in the urine and 20% being fecally excreted.[50] Its elimination may be delayed in patients with severely impaired renal function, and dose reduction may be necessary in this patient population. Typical dosing of clonidine is 0.1 mg orally twice daily, which may be titrated to a maximum daily dose of 2.4 mg. Transdermal clonidine is usually dosed at 0.1 mg (total daily delivered dose) and titrated to 0.6 mg as needed. Patches are changed on a weekly basis. Epidural clonidine infusions are usually initiated at a rate of 30 mcg/hr and titrated to 40 mcg/hr as needed. Single doses of as much as 700 mcg have been administered epidurally, but little literature exists regarding use of infusion rates exceeding 40 mcg/hr.[52,53] Sudden discontinuation or rapid dose reduction of clonidine can result in a withdrawal syndrome characterized by rebound hypertension, nervousness, agitation, headache, and tremor, with rare cases of associated hypertensive encephalopathy, cerebrovascular accidents, and death.[53] Clonidine doses should be gradually tapered before discontinuation, regardless of route of administration, because of this possible adverse outcome of abrupt dose reduction.

A substantial volume of literature exists that supports the use of clonidine in the management of a variety of painful conditions and as an adjuvant in general and regional anesthetic techniques. When used as an anesthetic adjuvant, clonidine may attenuate the stress response to surgery, including cortisol and norepinephrine release as well as the occurrence of perioperative hypertension.[54] It is also beneficial in the management of postoperative pain and has been shown to enhance the analgesic effects of neuraxially administered opioids.[55-57] When used in conjunction with patient-controlled analgesia, clonidine has been found to enhance

TABLE 78-1 Pharmacologic Properties of α_2 Agonists

Drug	Clonidine	Tizanidine	Dexmedetomidine
Formulations available	Oral immediate release: Catapres Oral extended release: Kapvay* Transdermal: Catapres TTS Epidural: Duraclon	Oral: tablet, capsule (Zanaflex)	Intravenous (Precedex)
Time to peak effect	Oral: 3–5 hours; extended release 7-8 hours Transdermal: 48 hours Epidural: 19 minutes	1 hour (fasted state) 1.5–3 hours (fed state)	60 minutes
Half-life	Elimination: 12–16 hours	2–2.5 hours	Distribution: 6 minutes Elimination: 2 hours
Route of metabolism or elimination	Hepatic: 50% Renal: 40%–60%	Hepatic: 95% with renal (60%) and fecal (20%) excretion of metabolites	Hepatic (nearly 100%)
Dosage	Oral immediate release: 0.2–2.4 mg/day Oral extended release: Kapvay* 0.1–0.4 mg/day Transdermal: 0.1–0.6 mg/day Epidural: 30–40 mcg/hr; maximum single dose, 700 mcg	4–36 mg total per day (limited information exists for long-term use of single doses >8–12 mg or total daily doses >24-36 mg)	Loading: 1 mcg/kg Maintenance: 0.2–0.7 mcg/kg/hr

*This formulation is relatively new, and little information is available regarding its use for pain management applications.

Reproduced with permission from Elliott JA. α_2-Agonists. In: Smith HS, ed. *Current Therapy in Pain*. Philadelphia: Saunders Elsevier; 2009:476-480.

TABLE 78-2 Drug Interactions, Precautions, and Adverse Effects of the α_2 Agonists

Drug interactions	General: sedatives (enhanced sedation); beta-blockers, calcium channel blockers, digitalis (increased risk of heart block)
	Clonidine: local anesthetics (prolonged sensory and motor block); cyclosporine (increased serum levels of cyclosporine or cyclosporine toxicity); TCAs (decreased antihypertensive action of clonidine)
	Tizanidine: oral contraceptives, fluvoxamine, ciprofloxacin, zileuton, amiodarone, mexiletine, propafenone, verapamil, cimetidine, famotidine, acyclovir, ticlopidine (increased serum tizanidine levels, decreased tizanidine clearance caused by CYP1A2 inhibition)
	Dexmedetomidine: no specific interactions (except as above in general drug interactions with α_2 agonists)
Precautions	General: pregnancy (category C), use in patients with known cardiac conduction defects
	Clonidine: potential for rebound hypertension with abrupt discontinuation regardless of route of administration; cautious use in obstetric patients because of the potential for hypotension; cautious use in patients with cerebrovascular disease, chronic renal failure, coronary artery disease, or recent myocardial infarction (because of potential for hypotension)*
	Tizanidine: dose reduction is advised in patients using oral contraceptives or with renal insufficiency (because of decreased clearance of tizanidine); avoid use in the presence of liver disease (because of risk of hepatotoxicity)
	Dexmedetomidine: use for periods exceeding 24 hours is not recommended (although several reports of use for longer periods have been described); because of its ability to blunt sympathetically mediated blood pressure and heart rate responses, there may be an increased risk of failure to detect signs of awareness under anesthesia if this drug is incorporated into an anesthetic regimen
Adverse effects	General: hypotension, bradycardia, heart block, sedation, dizziness, dry mouth, asthenia, orthostasis, rash, nausea
	Clonidine: depression, constipation, nervousness or agitation
	Tizanidine: elevation of LFTs (5%) with rare incidence of fulminant hepatic failure, hallucinations, muscle spasm, fever, abdominal pain, diarrhea, dyspepsia, depression
	Dexmedetomidine: sinus arrest, hypertension (with rapid infusion or loading dose administration); fever, tachycardia, anemia, hypoxia, atrial fibrillation

*May apply to α_2 agonists in general but is especially relevant to the use of clonidine.

CYP, cytochrome P-450; LFT , liver function test; TCA, tricyclic antidepressant.

Reproduced with permission from Elliott JA. α_2-Agonists. In: Smith HS, ed. *Current Therapy in Pain*. Philadelphia: Saunders Elsevier; 2009:476-480.

analgesia, reduce opioid requirements, decrease nausea and vomiting, and improve patient satisfaction.[58,59]

Neuraxial clonidine has been used in the management of both acute and chronic pain. Epidural clonidine has been shown to dose dependently control hemodynamic changes associated with surgical stimulation and also produce dose-dependent analgesia when used as the sole analgesic agent during and after abdominal surgery.[60] It also compared favorably with epidural bupivacaine when used as a sole analgesic during and after abdominal surgery.[61] Intrathecal clonidine has been shown to have analgesic effects that extend beyond the immediate postoperative period when used as part of an analgesic regimen for patients undergoing colonic surgery.[62] In addition to reducing postoperative opioid consumption, intrathecal clonidine appeared to effect a reduction in secondary hyperalgesia around the surgical wound that persisted when these patients were followed-up after 6 months. These patients reported less residual pain than subjects who had not received intrathecal clonidine as part of their perioperative analgesic regimen.[62] With regards to chronic pain management using neuraxial clonidine, epidurally administered clonidine is useful in the treatment of intractable, opioid-refractory cancer pain, especially that with neuropathic characteristics (a labeled indication).[63] Intrathecally administered clonidine is commonly used as an adjuvant in implanted drug delivery systems used to treat a variety of chronic, refractory pain disorders.[64]

In addition to the oral, transdermal, and neuraxial routes, clonidine has also been administered intraarticularly, in conjunction with local anesthetics for peripheral nerve blocks, as part of peribulbar blocks for eye surgery, and as part of intravenous regional anesthesia.[65-71]

TIZANIDINE

The pharmacology of tizanidine has been discussed in the previous section on muscle relaxants (within this chapter). In addition to its use in the treatment of spasticity and muscular and myofascial pain, tizanidine has been used in the management of a number of other pain diagnoses. Tizanidine has been used in the management of acute back pain caused by paravertebral muscle spasm, comparing favorably to diazepam in this setting.[72] When use of tizanidine in combination with ibuprofen for the treatment of LBP was studied, it was found that fewer patients experienced GI side effects compared with patients receiving ibuprofen with placebo.[73] Thus, it appears that in addition to potentiating the antinociceptive and anti-inflammatory effects of NSAIDS, tizanidine also improves the GI tolerability of these agents.[74] Tizanidine has been used in the treatment of headache disorders and facial pain with evident benefit. It has been shown to decrease the frequency, intensity, and duration of chronic daily headaches whether migrainous or tension type in nature.[75-78] Tizanidine has also been used in the management of cluster headaches and in detoxification from analgesic rebound headaches with some success.[79,80] When used for the treatment of neuropathic pain, tizanidine at a mean daily dose of 23 mg has demonstrated efficacy in nonresponders to other medications such as amitriptyline and gabapentin.[81] Tizanidine may also be useful as an anesthetic adjuvant because perioperative administration of tizanidine has been shown to reduce the minimum alveolar concentration of sevoflurane by nearly 20%.[82]

DEXMEDETOMIDINE

Dexmedetomidine is marketed in the United States under the trade name Precedex. Its current labeled indications are for use in the sedation of intubated patients in an intensive care unit (ICU) setting as well as nonintubated patients before and during surgical or other medical procedures.[83] Dexmedetomidine has minimal effects on respiratory function, making it a potentially useful adjunct for the management of pain in patients at risk of opioid-induced respiratory depression such as morbidly obese patients and in patients with possible airway management issues.[84-87] Dexmedetomidine decreases anesthetic and perioperative analgesic requirements.[88-95] It has also been used to reduce distress in dying patients and to facilitate ventilator withdrawal in the palliative care population.[96-98] Additionally, it may provide analgesia in palliative care patients refractory to treatment with other analgesic modalities.[99] It may also enhance the quality of anesthesia and reduce analgesic requirements when added to lidocaine for intravenous regional anesthesia.[100,101] The sedative effects of dexmedetomidine resemble those of normal physiologic sleep, likely a result of its actions on the locus ceruleus.[102] When used in an ICU setting, dexmedetomidine has been demonstrated to significantly reduce requirements for other sedatives such as midazolam and analgesics such as morphine.[103,104] It may also play a role in the management of the increasingly recognized phenomenon of opioid-induced hyperalgesia, a condition in which paradoxical pain hypersensitivity occurs in the setting of escalating opioid dosing.[105]

REFERENCES

1. Lexi-Comp Online: Baclofen. Lexi-Drugs Online, Hudson, Ohio: Lexi-Comp, Inc.; 2011. Accessed November 2, 2011.
2. Levy RA, Proudfit HK. The analgesic action of baclofen [β-(4-chlorophenyl)-γ-aminobutyric acid]. *J Pharmacol Exp Ther.* 1977;202(2):437-445.
3. Fromm GH, Terrence CF, Chattha AS. Baclofen in the treatment of trigeminal neuralgia: a double-blind study and long-term follow-up. *Ann Neurol.* 1984;15(3):240-244.
4. Lexi-Comp Online: Carisoprodol. Lexi-Drugs Online, Hudson, Ohio: Lexi-Comp, Inc.; 2011. Accessed November 2, 2011.
5. Reeves, RR, Burke RS. Carisoprodol: abuse potential and withdrawal syndrome. *Curr Drug Abuse Rev.* 2010;3(1):33-38.
6. Dougherty RJ. Carisoprodol should be a controlled substance (letter). *Arch Fam Med.* 1995;4:582.
7. Schedules of controlled substances: placement of carisoprodol into schedule IV, Final Rule. Federal Register 76 (December 12, 2011):77330-77360.
8. Drugs.com: Carisoprodol. Available at: http://www.drugs.com/monograph/carisoprodol.html. Accessed December 9, 2011.
9. Lexi-Comp Online: Chlorzoxazone. Lexi-Drugs Online, Hudson, Ohio: Lexi-Comp, Inc.; 2011. Accessed November 2, 2011.
10. Daily Med: Parafon DSC (chlorzoxazone) tablet. Available at: http://dailymed.nlm.nih.gov/dailymed/druginfo.cfm?id=15262. Accessed December 9, 2011.
11. Lexi-Comp Online: Cyclobenzaprine. Lexi-Drugs Online, Hudson, Ohio: Lexi-Comp, Inc.; 2011. Accessed November 2, 2011.
12. Lexi-Comp Online: Dantrolene. Lexi-Drugs Online, Hudson Ohio: Lexi-Comp, Inc.; 2011. Accessed November 2, 2011.
13. Drugs.com: Dantrolene. Available at: http://www.drugs.com/pro/dantrolene.html. Accessed December 14, 2011.
14. Schneider R, Mitchell D. Dantrolene hepatitis. *JAMA.* 1976; 235(15):1590-1591.
15. Lexi-Comp Online: Diazepam. Lexi-Drugs Online, Hudson, Ohio: Lexi-Comp, Inc.; 2011. Accessed November 2, 2011.
16. Medsafe: Diazepam. Available at: http://www.medsafe.govt.nz/profs/datasheet/d/dpamtab.htm. Accessed December 15, 2011.
17. Lexi-Comp Online: Metaxalone. Lexi-Drugs Online, Hudson, Ohio: Lexi-Comp, Inc.; 2011. Accessed November 2, 2011.
18. Drugs.com: Metaxalone. Available at: http://www.drugs.com/monograph/metaxalone.html. Accessed December 15, 2011.
19. Lexi-Comp Online: Methocarbamol. Lexi-Drugs Online, Hudson, Ohio: Lexi-Comp, Inc; 2011. Accessed November 2, 2011.
20. Drugs.com: Methocarbamol. Available at: http://www.drugs.com/pro/methocarbamol.html. Accessed December 9, 2011.
21. Lexi-Comp Online: Orphenadrine. Lexi-Drugs Online, Hudson, Ohio: Lexi-Comp, Inc.; 2011. Accessed November 2, 2011.
22. Drugs.com: Orphenadrine Citrate. Available at: http://www.drugs.com/monograph/orphenadrine-citrate.html. Accessed December 15, 2011.
23. Schifano F, Marra R, Magni G. Orphenadrine abuse (letter). *South Med J.* 1988;81(4):546-547.
24. Lexi-Comp Online: Tizanidine. Lexi-Drugs Online, Hudson, Ohio: Lexi-Comp, Inc.; 2011. Accessed November 2, 2011.
25. Product information: Zanaflex, tizanidine hydrochloride. South San Francisco, CA: Athena Neurosciences (Elan Pharmaceuticals), 2000.
26. Van Tulder MW, Touray T, Furlan AD, et al. Muscle relaxants for non-specific low-back pain (review). *Cochrane Database Syst Rev.* 2003;(4):CD004252.
27. Chou R, Peterson K, Helfand M. Comparative efficacy and safety of skeletal muscle relaxants for spasticity and musculoskeletal conditions: a systematic review. *J Pain Symptom Manage.* 2004;28:140-175.
28. Browning R, Jackson JL, O'Malley PG. Cyclobenzaprine and back pain: a meta-analysis. *Arch Intern Med.* 2001;161:1613-1620.
29. Leite FMG, Atallah AN, El Dib RP, et al. Cyclobenzaprine for the treatment of myofascial pain in adults (review). *Cochrane Database Syst Rev.* 2009;(3):CD006830.
30. Docherty JR. Subtypes of functional $alpha_1$ and $alpha_2$-adrenoceptors. *Eur J Pharmacol.* 1998;361:1-15.
31. Childers MK. How $alpha_2$ adrenergic agonists relieve pain. In: Childers, MK, ed. *Use of $Alpha_2$ Adrenergic Agonists in Pain Management.* Columbia: Academic Information Systems; 2001:13-27.
32. Khan ZP, Ferguson CN, Jones RM. $Alpha_2$ and imidazoline receptor agonists. *Anesthesia.* 1999;54:146-165.
33. Fairbanks CA, Stone LS, Kitto KF, et al. $Alpha_{2c}$-adrenergic receptors mediate spinal analgesia and adrenergic-opioid synergy. *J Pharmacol Exp Ther.* 2002;300:282-290.
34. Stone LS, MacMillan LB, Kitto KF, et al. The $alpha_{2A}$ adrenergic receptor subtype mediates spinal analgesia evoked by $alpha_2$ agonists and is necessary for spinal adrenergic-opioid synergy. *J Neurosci.* 1997;17(18):7157-7165.
35. Millan MJ. α2-adrenergic mechanisms of analgesia: strategies for improving their therapeutic window and identification of the novel, potent α2A-adrenergic receptor agonist, S 18616. *Adv Pharmacol.* 1998;42:575-579.
36. Giovannoni MP, Ghelardini C, Vergelli C, et al. α2-agonists as analgesic agents. *Med Res Rev.* 2008;29(2):339-368.
37. Yaksh TL, Pogrel JW, Lee YW, et al. Reversal of nerve ligation-induced allodynia by spinal alpha-2 adrenoceptor agonists. *J Pharmacol Exp Ther.* 1995;272:207-214.
38. Reddy SV, Maderhut JL, Yaksh TL. Spinal cord pharmacology of adrenergic agonist-mediated antinociception. *J Pharmacol Exp Ther.* 1980;213:525-533.
39. Takano Y, Yaksh TL. Characterization of the pharmacology of intrathecally administered alpha-2 agonists and antagonists in rats. *J Pharm Exp Ther.* 1992;261:764-772.
40. Hunter JC, Fontana DJ, Hedley LR, et al. Assessment of the role of α-2 adrenoceptor subtypes in the antinociceptive, sedative, and hypothermic action of dexmedetomidine in transgenic mice. *Br J Pharmacol.* 1997;122:1339-1344.
41. Puke MJ, Wisenfeld-Hallin Z. The differential effects of morphine and the alpha-2-adrenoceptor agonists clonidine and dexmedetomidine on the prevention and treatment of experimental neuropathic pain. *Anesth Analg.* 1993;77:104-109.
42. Pan HL, Chen SR, Eisenach JC. Intrathecal clonidine alleviates allodynia in neuropathic rats: interaction with spinal muscarinic and nicotinic receptors. *Anesthesiology.* 1999;90:509-514.
43. Kawamata T, Omote K, Yamamoto H, et al. Antihyperalgesic and side effects of intrathecal clonidine and tizanidine in a rat model of neuropathic pain. *Anesthesiology.* 2003;98:1480-1483.
44. Eisenach JC, Lysak SZ, Viscomi CM. Epidural clonidine analgesia following surgery: phase I. *Anesthesiology.* 1989;71:640-646.
45. Mendez R, Eisenach JC, Kashtan K. Epidural clonidine analgesia after cesarean section. *Anesthesiology.* 1990;73:848-852.

46. Glynn C, O'Sullivan K. A double-blind randomized comparison of the effects of epidural clonidine and lignocaine in patients with chronic pain. *Pain.* 1996;64:337-343.
47. Siddall PJ, Molloy AR, Walker S, et al. The efficacy of intrathecal morphine and clonidine in the treatment of pain after spinal cord injury. *Anesth Analg.* 2000;91:1493-1498.
48. Elliott JA. α2-Agonists. In: Smith HS, ed. *Current Therapy in Pain.* Philadelphia: Saunders Elsevier; 2009:476-480.
49. Kamibayashi T, Harasawa K, Maze M. Alpha-2 adrenergic agonists. *Can J Anaesth.* 1997;44(5):R13-R18.
50. Drugs.com: Clonidine. Available at: http://www.drugs.com/monograph/clonidine.html. Accessed December 21, 2011.
51. Lexi-Comp Online: Clonidine. Lexi-Drugs Online, Hudson, Ohio: Lexi-Comp, Inc; 2011. Accessed December 22, 2011.
52. Product information: Duraclon®, clonidine hydrochloride injection. Columbus, OH: Roxane Laboratories; 2000.
53. Product information: Catapres®, clonidine HCl. Ridgefield, CT: Boehringer Ingelheim; 1996.
54. Schneemilch CE, Bachmann H, Ulrich A, et al. Clonidine decreases stress response in patients undergoing carotid endarterectomy under regional anesthesia: a prospective, randomized, double-blinded, placebo-controlled study. *Anesth Analg.* 2006;103(2):297-302.
55. Goyagi T, Nishikawa T. Oral clonidine premedication enhances the quality of postoperative analgesia by epidural morphine. *Anesth Analg.* 1999;89:1487-1491.
56. Goyagi T, Nishikawa T. Oral clonidine premedication enhances the quality of postoperative analgesia by intrathecal morphine. *Anesth Analg.* 1996;82:1192-1196.
57. Motsch J, Graeber E, Ludwig K. Addition of clonidine enhances postoperative analgesia from epidural morphine: a double-blind study. *Anesthesiology.* 1990;73:1067-1073.
58. Park J, Forrest J, Kolesar R, et al. Oral clonidine reduces postoperative PCA morphine requirements. *Can J Anaesth.* 1996;43(9):900-906.
59. Jeffs SA, Hall JE, Morris S. Comparison of morphine alone with morphine plus clonidine for postoperative patient-controlled analgesia. *Br J Anaesth.* 2001;89(3):424-427.
60. De Kock M, Wiederker P, Laghmiche, et al. Epidural clonidine used as the sole analgesic agent during and after abdominal surgery. *Anesthesiology.* 1997;86:285-292.
61. De Kock M, Gautier P, Pavlopoulou A, et al. Epidural clonidine or bupivacaine as the sole analgesic agent during and after abdominal surgery. *Anesthesiology.* 1999;90:1354-1362.
62. De Kock M, Lavand'homme P, Waterloos H. The short-lasting analgesia and long-term antihyperalgesic effect of intrathecal clonidine in patients undergoing colonic surgery. *Anesth Analg.* 2005;101:566-572.
63. Eisenach JC, DuPen S, Dubois M, et al. Epidural clonidine analgesia for intractable cancer pain. *Pain.* 1995;61:391-399.
64. Dunbar SA. Alpha$_2$-adrenoceptor agonists in the management of chronic pain. *Bailiere's Clin Anaesthesiol.* 2000;14(2):471-481.
65. Eisenach JC, De Kock M, Klimscha W. Alpha$_2$-adrenergic agonists for regional anesthesia. *Anesthesiology.* 1996;85:655-674.
66. Buerkle H, Huge V, Wolfgart M, et al. Intra-articular clonidine analgesia after knee arthroscopy. *Eur J Anaesthesiol.* 2000;17(5):295-299.
67. Brill S, Plaza M. Non-narcotic adjuvants may improve the duration and quality of analgesia after knee arthroscopy: a brief review. *Can J Anaesth.* 2004;51(10):975-978.
68. El Saied AH, Steyn MP, Ansermino JM. Clonidine prolongs the effect of ropivacaine for axillary brachial plexus blockade. *Can J Anaesth.* 2000;47(10):962-967.
69. Gabriel JS, Gordin V. Alpha 2 agonists in regional anesthesia and analgesia. *Curr Opin Anaesthesiol.* 2001;14:751-753.
70. Sciard DA, Saint Raymond S, Matuszczak M. Clonidine combined peribulbar anaesthesia in vitreoretinal surgery. *Reg Anesth Pain Med.* 2001;26(2):S:S47.
71. Lauretti GR, Barioni MF, Lauretti-Fo A. Clonidine as coadjuvant in eye surgery: comparison of peribulbar versus oral administration. *Reg Anesth Pain Med.* 2001;26(2)S:S68.
72. Fryda-Kaurimsky Z, Mueller-Fassbender H. Tizanidine (DS 103-282) in the treatment of acute paravertebral muscle spasm: a controlled trial comparing tizanidine and diazepam. *J Int Med Res.* 1981;9:501-505.
73. Berry H, Hutchinson DR. Tizanidine and ibuprofen in acute low-back pain: results of a double-blind multicentre study in general practice. *J Int Med Res.* 1988;16:83-91.
74. Jain NK, Kulkarni SK, Singh A. Modulation of NSAID-induced antinociceptive and anti-inflammatory effects by alpha$_2$-adrenoceptor agonists with gastroprotective effects. *Life Sci.* 2002;2857-2869.
75. Saper JR, Lake AE, Cantrell DT, et al. Chronic daily headache prophylaxis with tizanidine: a double-blind, placebo-controlled, multicenter outcome study. *Headache.* 2002;42:470-482.
76. Lake AE, Saper JR. Chronic headache: new advances in treatment strategies. *Neurology.* 2002;59(Suppl 2):S8-S13.
77. Freitag FG. Preventative treatment for migraine and tension-type headaches. *CNS Drugs.* 2003;17(6):373-381.
78. Rapoport AM, Bigal ME. Preventive migraine therapy: what is new. *Neurol Sci.* 2004;25:S177-S185.
79. D'Alessandro R. Tizanidine for chronic cluster headache (letter). *Arch Neurol.* 1996;53:1093.
80. Smith TR. Low-dose tizanidine with nonsteroidal anti-inflammatory drugs for detoxification from analgesic rebound headache. *Headache.* 2002;42:175-177.
81. Semenchuk MR, Sherman S. Effectiveness of tizanidine in neuropathic pain: an open-label study. *J Pain.* 2000;4:285-292.
82. Wajima Z, Yoshikawa T, Ogura A, et al. Oral tizanidine, an alpha$_2$-adrenoceptor agonist, reduces the minimum alveolar concentration of sevoflurane in human adults. *Anesth Analg.* 2002;95:393-396.
83. Lexi-Comp Online: Dexmedetomidine. Lexi-Drugs Online, Hudson, Ohio: Lexi-Comp, Inc; 2011. Accessed December 22, 2011.
84. Hofer RE, Sprung J, Sarr MG, et al. Anesthesia for a patient with morbid obesity using dexmedetomidine without narcotics. *Can J Anaesth.* 2005;52(2):176-180.
85. Feld JM, Hoffman WE, Stechert MM, et al. Fentanyl or dexmedetomidine combined with desflurane for bariatric surgery. *J Clin Anesth.* 2006;18:24-28.
86. Ramsay MAE, Saha D, Heber RF. Tracheal resection in the morbidly obese patient: the role of dexmedetomidine. *J Clin Anesth.* 2006;18:452-454.
87. Ramsay MAE, Luterman DL. Dexmedetomidine as a total intravenous anesthetic agent. *Anesthesiology.* 2004;101:787-790.
88. Aantaa R, Kanto J, Scheinin M, et al. Dexmedetomidine, an alpha$_2$-adrenoceptor agonist, reduces anesthetic requirements for patients undergoing minor gynecologic surgery. *Anesthesiology.* 1990;73:230-235.
89. Peden CJ, Prys-Roberts C. Dexmedetomidine—a powerful new adjunct to anesthesia [editorial]?. *Br J Anaesth.* 1992;68:123-125.
90. Aho MS, Erkola OA, Scheinin H, et al. Effect of intravenously administered dexmedetomidine on pain after laparoscopic tubal ligation. *Anesth Analg.* 1991;73:112-118.
91. Gurbet A, Basagan-Mogol E, Turker G, et al. Intraoperative infusion of dexmedetomidine reduces perioperative analgesic requirements. *Can J Anaesth.* 2006;53(7):646-652.

92. Arain SR, Ruehlow RM, Uhrich TD, et al. The efficacy of dexmedetomidine versus morphine for postoperative analgesia after major inpatient surgery. *Anesth Analg*. 2004;98:153-158.
93. Weinbroum AA, Ben-Abraham R. Dextromethorphan and dexmedetomidine: new agents for the control of perioperative pain. *Eur J Surg*. 2001;167:563-569.
94. Unlugenc H, Gunduz M, Guler T, et al. The effect of pre-anesthetic administration of intravenous dexmedetomidine on postoperative pain in patients receiving patient-controlled morphine. *Eur J Anaesthesiol*. 2005;22:386-391.
95. Wahlander S, Frumento RJ, Wagener G, et al. A prospective, double-blind, randomized, placebo-controlled study of dexmedetomidine as an adjunct to epidural after thoracic surgery. *J Cardiothorac Vasc Anesth*. 2005;19(5):630-635.
96. Kent CD, Kaufman BS, Lowy J. Dexmedetomidine facilitates the withdrawal of ventilatory support in palliative care. *Anesthesiology*. 2005;103(2):439-441.
97. Soares LG, Naylor C, Martins MA, et al. Dexmedetomidine: a new option for intractable distress in the dying (letter). *J Pain Symptom Manage*. 2002;24(1):6-8.
98. Jackson KC, Wohlt P, Fine PG. Dexmedetomidine: a novel analgesic with palliative medicine potential. *J Pain Palliat Care Pharmacother*. 2006;20(2):23-27.
99. Roberts SB, Wozencraft CP, Coyne PJ, et al. Dexmedetomidine as an adjuvant analgesic for intractable cancer pain. *J Palliat Med*. 2010;14(3):371-373.
100. Memis D, Turan A, Karamanioglu B, et al. Adding dexmedetomidine to lidocaine for intravenous regional anesthesia. *Anesth Analg*. 2004;98:835-840.
101. Esmaoglu A, Mizrak A, Akin A, et al. Addition of dexmedetomidine to lidocaine for intravenous regional anesthesia. *Eur J Anaesthesiol*. 2005;22:447-451.
102. Nelson LE, Lu J, Guo T, et al. The alpha$_2$-adrenoceptor agonist dexmedetomidine converges on endogenous sleep-promoting pathway to exert its sedative effects. *Anesthesiology*. 2003;98:428-436.
103. Venn RM, Bradshaw CJ, Spencer R, et al. Preliminary UK experience of dexmedetomidine, a novel agent for postoperative sedation in the intensive care unit. *Anaesthesia*. 1999;54:1136-1142.
104. Arain SR, Ebert TJ. The efficacy, side effects, and recovery characteristics of dexmedetomidine versus propofol when used for intraoperative sedation. *Anesth Analg*. 2002;95:461-466.
105. Belgrade M, Hall S. Dexmedetomidine infusion for the management of opioid-induced hyperalgesia (case report). *Pain Med*. 2010;11:1819-1826.

CHAPTER 79

NMDA Receptor Antagonism in Pain Therapy

Alexander F. DeBonet

NMDA RECEPTOR STRUCTURE AND FUNCTION

The synapse between the primary afferent and secondary afferent neurons in the dorsal horn of the spinal cord is a critical site for the modulation of ascending pain pathways. Glutamate is the primary excitatory amino acid (EAA) involved in excitation of the secondary afferent neuron and is primarily stored in the presynaptic vesicles of the primary afferent neuron. Upon membrane depolarization, glutamate is released and targets postsynaptic receptors, which can be either metabotropic or ionotropic. Ionotropic glutamate receptors are ligand-gated channels that regulate ion conductance of calcium and sodium. There are three major subclasses of ionotropic receptors: a-amino-3-hydroxy-5-methyl-4-isoxazolepropionic acid (AMPA), kainate, and *N*-methyl-D-aspartate (NMDA). The discovery of several pharmacologic agents, beginning with compound (+) MK-801, that are highly selective antagonists for specific subtypes of glutamate receptors has helped clarify the characteristics and functions of the various glutamate receptors and in particular the role of the NMDA calcium channel in the central nervous system (CNS).[1]

Among various locations in the CNS, NMDA receptors are found on the postsynaptic terminal of second-order afferent neurons in the dorsal horn of the spinal cord that are involved in the transmission of pain signals. With the cloning of individual NMDA receptor subunit DNA sequences, it was ultimately discovered that NMDA receptors consist of glycine-binding GluN1 subunit and glutamate-binding GluN2 subunits. NMDA receptors are calcium ion channels composed of four individual subunits, including two GluN1 subunits and two GluN2 subunits, and the receptor requires coactivation by two ligands, glutamate and glycine. There is considerable diversity among receptor subtypes, which imparts distinct functional and pharmacologic properties to the NMDA receptor.[1] A unique property of the NMDA receptor is that in addition to being ligand activated, its activation is also voltage dependent, that is, dependent on the resting cell potential. At a normal resting membrane state, the NMDA calcium channel is blocked by magnesium and is in an inactive state. When the resting membrane potential of the afferent neuron is changed as a result of prolonged stimulus, the channel loses the magnesium ion block, and calcium moves into the cell, raising the membrane potential, resulting in neuronal hyperexcitability.[2]

Sound in vivo evidence indicates that peripheral tissue or nerve injury causes not only an increase in the sensitivity of primary afferent nociceptors at the site of tissue injury but also leads to NMDA receptor–mediated central changes in synaptic excitability and, consequently, on a clinical level, a reduction in opioid responsiveness, hyperalgesia, and allodynia.[3,4]

WINDUP AND CENTRAL SENSITIZATION

The NMDA receptor is a key component in the modulation of the strength of synaptic pathways, a property referred to as *synaptic plasticity*. This is demonstrated in its involvement in the states of windup and central sensitization. *Windup* refers to reversible synaptic changes that can result in neuronal hyperexcitability in response to a progressive or sustained noxious stimulus. In response to a sustained C-fiber or nociceptive stimulus, primary afferents express synaptic glutamate and other neurotransmitters, such as substance P, which then traverse the synapse to reach NMDA and other glutamatergic receptors on the secondary afferent neuron. The summation of these repeated synaptic discharges produces a crescendo depolarization of the secondary afferent neuron that leads to the loss of the magnesium ion blockade in voltage-gated NMDA receptors, allowing increased calcium conduction and more sustained depolarization of the secondary afferent neuron. When this process is sustained, it contributes to a cascade of phosphorylation and other intracellular transcription and translational events that potentiate the more established hyperexcitable state of central sensitization. Clinically, this sustained robust synaptic transmission leads to a reduction in pain threshold, an augmentation of pain responses, and an expansion of pain sensitivity to tissue regions that have not been injured.[5,6]

Clearly, the involvement of the NMDA receptor in the establishment and fortification of robust pain transmission pathways exposes a potential target for pain therapy. Several NMDA antagonist medications have been developed and extensively researched and are now becoming more broadly clinically applied, offering considerable benefit in the prevention of pain in both acute perioperative and chronic neuropathic clinical settings.

The NMDA receptor is found in many different levels of the CNS, including not only the afferent pain pathways in the dorsal horn of the spinal cord but also regions of the brain involved in motor and cognitive processes. As it is prominently involved in controlling synaptic plasticity, NMDA receptors have been determined to have a critical role in cognition and memory function.[6,7] NMDA receptor antagonists, therefore, expectedly, have multiple sites of action. Unfortunately, because NMDA receptor antagonists also impair normal synaptic transmission in nonpathologic processes, they can cause numerous side effects such as memory impairment, psychotomimetic effects, ataxia, and motor incoordination.

A major goal in pharmacologic development is the development of agents that have specificity for NMDA receptors that are involved in pathologic processes and do not interfere with normal physiologic roles in non–pain-related centers. NMDA channel blockers act in a noncompetitive manner that is use dependent, that is, they can only access their target subunit binding site and block the channel in its open conformation. These agents differ from each other in their binding affinities for their target subunits sites on the NMDA receptor, which result in different pharmacologic and physiologic characteristics. It has been clarified that NMDA antagonist agents with high affinity for the receptor subunits are more likely to disrupt normal physiologic processes and that noncompetitive agents with lower affinity for the receptor subunit target binding sites offer a better therapeutic benefit to side effect profile. Currently, available agents, such as memantine, ketamine, and dextromethorphan (DM), are clinically used agents that meet this lower affinity profile.[2-4]

KETAMINE

Ketamine is an NMDA receptor antagonist that has, arguably, the most clearly defined clinical utility. It has been available for research purposes for nearly 50 years and has been available in clinical practice for more than 30 years. It has various industrial names such as Ketalar and Ketajet as well as street names for illicit use such as Special K and Vitamin K. Ketamine has multiple target receptors, including NMDA, AMPA, and kainate. Ketamine is involved in the inhibition of voltage-gated sodium and potassium channels and serotonin and dopamine reuptake inhibition and has weak agonist properties at nicotinic receptors and antagonist properties at muscarinic receptors. Ketamine is available as a racemic mixture of the S and R isomers. The S isomer appears to cause greater unwanted psychic side effects than the R isomer.

Ketamine has several cardiovascular effects. It is a direct myocardial depressant; however, this effect is generally overridden by its sympathetic stimulation as well as the release of and reuptake inhibition of catecholamines. Ketamine generally causes an increase in systemic arterial pressure, heart rate, and cardiac output unless a patient is depleted of catecholamines in which case myocardial depression can be appreciated.

Ketamine has effects on the pulmonary system. Most important, it is a bronchial smooth muscle relaxant. The effect of ketamine on bronchial smooth muscle is as effective as inhalational agents in preventing bronchospasm; however, it must be acknowledged that ketamine causes an increase in pulmonary arterial pressure and in the acute care setting causes an increase in salivary and tracheobronchial secretions.

Ketamine has several important effects on the neurologic examination. Most prominently, nystagmus is noted frequently at doses of 0.25 to 0.5 mg/kg. Ketamine does not alter the seizure threshold, but it does increase the cerebral metabolic rate of oxygen ($CMRO_2$) as well as cerebral blood flow, and critically, it can cause an increase in intracranial pressure.

Ketamine has high (93%) bioavailability with intravenous (IV) administration yet because of high first-pass metabolism has a low oral bioavailability of 16%. However, because of a significantly higher accumulation of norketamine with the oral route, the effective oral dose is roughly one-third the effective IV dose. The metabolism of ketamine occurs via *N*-demethylation to norketamine primarily via the CYP384 system and less so via the CYP2B6 and CYP2C9 cytochrome systems. The metabolite norketamine has been shown to have 20% to 30% of the physiologic activity of ketamine. The metabolite norketamine is eventually hydroxylated to hydroxynorketamine and conjugated with glucuronate and finally is excreted into urine, where 80% is eliminated as the conjugated derivatives of ketamine.

Clinical research has revealed several major therapeutic advantages of ketamine use, including decreased opioid requirements in the postsurgical setting, attenuated opioid tolerance, the suppression of the onset of opioid-induced hyperalgesia.[8]

In a 2006 review, Bell et al. reviewed the role of perioperative ketamine usage in the management of acute postoperative pain. A total of 37 trials were reviewed, including 2240 participants and including randomized controlled trials (RCTs) of patients treated with perioperative ketamine versus placebo. The authors concluded that subanesthetic doses of ketamine indeed reduced the need for rescue analgesia doses, reduced overall pain intensity scores, reduced postoperative Patient-controlled morphine consumption, and reduced postoperative nausea and vomiting; adverse effects were found to be mild or even absent.[9]

In 2005, Joly et al. published a study involving 75 patients who underwent major upper abdominal surgery. Treatment groups were randomized to receive intraoperative remifentanil in two different groups of eightfold dosage difference plus a third group receiving a remifentanil plus ketamine infusion of 0.5 mg/kg/min initiated just after incision followed by an infusion for 48 hours of 2 μg/kg/min. Results demonstrated that hyperalgesia in the high-dose remifentanil group was substantially greater than hyperalgesia in the other two groups. Furthermore, it was shown that this hyperalgesia can be prevented by low-dose ketamine infusions.

In 2005, a study by Adam et al. involved 40 patients undergoing total knee arthroplasty under general anesthesia and continuous femoral nerve block. Treatment groups were randomized to involve a ketamine 0.5-mg/kg bolus before skin incision followed by infusion at 3 μg/kg/min until emergence from anesthesia followed by infusion at 1.5 μg/kg/min for 48 hours; a second group received only blinded placebo. Results demonstrated that the ketamine group required less overall morphine, reached 90-degree flexion more rapidly, and was able to achieve these goals without any additional side effects from ketamine therapy.[11]

A 2004 study by Kwok et al. involved 135 patients in three separate treatment groups investigating the role of ketamine as a preemptive analgesic. Group 1, the preincision group, received ketamine at 0.15 mg/kg immediately before induction of anesthesia; group 2, the postoperative group, received ketamine 0.15 mg/kg only after wound closure; and group 3 received placebo. Compared with groups 2 and 3, results demonstrated that group 1, the preincision and preemptive ketamine group, had lower pain scores, had a longer time to first request for rescue analgesia postoperatively, and required a lower overall total morphine consumption in the perioperative period. This was demonstrated with no difference in hemodynamic variables or other adverse effects during the study.[12]

In 2010, Goldberg et al. investigated the pharmacodynamic responses to racemic ketamine and norketamine in patients with complex regional pain syndrome (CRPS). Ketamine was titrated from 10 to 40 mg/hr in patients with CRPS and maintained at such levels for 5 days. Serum ketamine and norketamine concentrations were determined at several intervals during and after the conclusion of the 5-day infusion. Ketamine concentrations were found to peak at 4 to 5 hours. Norketamine concentrations were lower and peaked on day 2 of the infusion. Significant pain relief was achieved by day 2 of the infusion and correlated with the maximum plasma levels of ketamine and norketamine. Pain continued to improve over the 5-day infusion and was found to peak when serum ketamine concentrations of 200 to 225 ng/mL and norketamine levels of 9220 ng/mL were reached.[13]

When considering therapy of chronic pain using ketamine, one must take into consideration what little information is available about the clinical effects of long-term ketamine exposure. To investigate the clinical effects of long-term ketamine exposure, there are two major available cohorts. First, there are patients receiving ketamine for legitimate therapeutic reasons, generally in the perioperative setting. Second, there are abusers of ketamine in the community. Studying this second group provides a unique opportunity to gather data about long-term ketamine exposure on relatively larger cohorts. It must be acknowledged that this particular cohort is very heterogeneous, and there is frequently concomitant polysubstance abuse.[8] Ketamine is classified as a schedule 3 drug under the Controlled Substances Act; however, very few deaths have been associated with ketamine overdoses. Ketamine is frequently abused using routes of administration such as swallowing, snorting, smoking, or injecting into the muscles and veins.

Chronic ketamine use has been demonstrated to have deleterious effects on learning and memory as well as neuronal histology. A study in 2001 by Curran et al. compared 18 frequent users with an average of 13.5 days per month with 19 infrequent users with an average use of once per month in a single-dose trial. Compared with control participants, frequent users demonstrated marked memory impairments, some evidence of schizophrenia-like dissociative symptoms, and effects on memory that were shown to correlate progressively with increasing use. The authors theorize that ketamine causes disruption of long-term potentiation in the hippocampus, a process thought to be crucial for certain aspects of learning and memory.[14]

In 2001, Morgan et al. performed a study with 150 individuals who were divided into five groups stratified by the frequency of ketamine abuse. Participants underwent cognitive tasks involving spatial working memory, pattern recognition memory, and simple vigilance and verbal and category fluency. Results demonstrated that frequent ketamine users had impaired spatial working memory and pattern recognition memory. It was also demonstrated that frequent users showed increased dissociative and schizotypal symptoms. Delusional symptoms correlated positively with the amount of ketamine use. The authors concluded that the frequent use of ketamine is associated with impairments of working memory, episodic memory, and aspects of executive function as well as reduced psychological well-being.[15]

In a 2010 study, Liao et al. visited the question of whether chronic ketamine use has a lasting impact on brain structure and function. White matter integrity can be studied by examining a key index called fractional anisotropy on tensor magnetic resonance imaging (MRI). Reduced fractional anisotropy has been found to be characteristic of disrupted or damaged white matter. This study sampled 41 ketamine-dependent subjects and 44 aged matched healthy volunteers recruited from drug rehabilitation centers. Diffuse tensor imaging was performed on a 3-Tesla Siemens scanner. MRI findings revealed white matter abnormalities in ketamine-dependent patients in the bilateral frontal, corpus callosum, anterior cingulate cortex, and left temporal parietal white matter. It was also determined that greater cumulative ketamine use was positively correlated with a greater degree of white matter disruption.[16]

In a 2009 study by Zao et al., rats were administered 5, 10, or 20 mg/kg of ketamine at hourly intervals on postnatal day 7, and brain tissue samples were examined for neurotoxic effects using electron microscopy. Evidence for direct neuronal tissue injury was identified: apoptotic characteristics in frontal cortex tissue samples as well as increased cell death in other brain regions. Apoptosis continued to occur even after brain levels of ketamine returned to baseline levels. The authors concluded that ketamine administration results in a dose-related and exposure time–dependent increase in neuronal cell death during development that is apoptotic in nature.[17]

Chronic ketamine use has been implicated in the development of renal and biliary comorbidities. In 2007, Shahani et al. published an initial study of nine patients who presented with a 6-month history of painful hematuria, dysuria, urgency, and postmicturition pain. These symptoms began only after the onset of daily ketamine use. None of the nine patients used other illicit drugs. Urine cultures, urinalysis, and urine cytology results were negative. Cystoscopy and abdominal and pelvic computed tomography (CT) showed marked inflammatory changes as well as very small bladder capacities in these patients. Bladder biopsies demonstrated substantially denuded uroendothelial mucosa within a thin layer of reactive and regenerating epithelial cells. The superficial lamina propria was damaged with numerous dilated blood vessels and scattered inflammatory cells. Overall, biopsies showed the changes of chronic cystitis. Antibiotic and steroid therapy provided no benefit in controlling the symptoms. All patients benefited from the cessation of ketamine use. Thus, a new clinical phenomenon termed *ketamine-associated ulcerative cystitis* was identified. This syndrome is thought to be caused by the migration of eosinophils and release of damaging enzymes as well as potentially by the formation of active metabolites of ketamine. Long-term consequences include the potential development of fibrotic, small capacity, noncompliant bladders.[18]

In 2007, Wong et al. described several cases of ketamine abusers with epigastric pain after chronic ketamine use. Liver function tests (LFTs) demonstrated elevated alkaline phosphatase and alanine aminotransferase levels with normal bilirubin. Ultrasonography demonstrated dilated common bile ducts within normal gallbladders. CT scans demonstrated fusiform dilatation of the entire length of the common hepatic and common bile duct with no identifiable obstructions. The patients stopped taking ketamine, and symptoms gradually resolved with normalization of LFT and imaging results.[19]

DEXTROMETHORPHAN

Dextromethorphan is a low-affinity noncompetitive NMDA receptor antagonist that is widely used as an antitussive agent in syrup preparations generally at adult doses of 10 to 30 mg three to six times daily. DM, which was originally synthesized as a pharmacologic alternative to morphine nearly 50 years ago, is the D-isomer of levorphanol, a codeine analogue; however, in contrast to levorphanol, it has no action at opioid receptors. DM has no major opioid like respiratory or histamine release complications, nor does it have the hemodynamic side effects seen with ketamine administration. DM is rapidly absorbed in the gastrointestinal (GI) tract with peak serum levels reached at approximately 2 to 2.5 hours after oral administration. At therapeutic doses, its onset of action is 15 to 30 minutes, and its duration of action is 5 to 6 hours.[20-22] At doses substantially higher than recommended, DM has CNS depressant properties and has some abuse potential. DM is rapidly metabolized in the liver, where it is metabolized to dextrorphan, which has more potent NMDA antagonist properties than the parent compound.[21,23]

The clinical studies evaluating the role of DM as a therapeutic agent that reduces perioperative pain scores and opiate requirements are conflicting. An example of positive findings was in an initial study by Kawamata et al. that showed a single DM premedication dose of 30 or 45 mg administered 1 hour before tonsillectomy in adults was effective in reducing posttonsillectomy pain and reduced postprocedural analgesic requirements for 1 week after surgery.[24] However, in a contrasting study by McConaghy et al., 27 mg of oral DM was given twice preoperatively and three times on postoperative day 1 after total abdominal hysterectomy. Compared with placebo, results showed no benefit in patient pain complaints determined by visual analog scale (VAS) scores and morphine consumption over placebo at 24 or 48 hours after surgery or 1 month later.[25] Some researchers have argued that the negative results for DM in the acute setting are due to insufficient dosing caused by the relatively poor bioavailability of DM.[26] Other studies have demonstrated that GI effects such as nausea and neurologic side effects (e.g., euphoria, drowsiness, dizziness) become too prominent at higher dosages and limit its potential therapeutic value.[27]

As seen in the setting of acute perioperative pain, the clinical utility of DM in the setting of chronic neuropathic pain has been explored with disappointing findings. In 2000, Weinbroum et al. reviewed several trials of DM at various dosages and administration intervals in patients with chronic neuropathic pain of various etiologies, including postherpetic neuralgia and painful diabetic neuropathy, as well as experimentally induced pain with temporary induced limb ischemia and capsaicin.[23] Unfortunately, the overall conclusion is that there is limited clinical utility of the routine administration of DM at clinically tolerable doses for the management of chronic neuropathic pain.[23] A study of cancer-related pain by Mercadante et al. found no benefit from the addition of DM to an established regimen of multipharmacologic therapy.[22]

Further clinical trials are necessary to determine the role of DM in various pain pathologies and to clarify the optimal dosing regimens that are required for efficacy as well as minimizing adverse effects.

MEMANTINE

Memantine is a low-affinity, noncompetitive NMDA receptor antagonist that was discovered in the 1960s that has been available clinically for nearly 30 years in Germany, initially for the treatment of CNS diseases such as Parkinson's disease and Alzheimer's disease. In the United States, memantine received Food and Drug Administration approval in 2003 for the treatment of Alzheimer's disease but has been widely prescribed for treatment of dementia. Its off-label use in the treatment of chronic pain is relatively new. Compared with the earlier NMDA receptor antagonist ketamine, it demonstrates better patient tolerability with minimal psychogenic side effects. This more tolerable side effect profile is thought to relate to the elimination half-life of oral memantine of 60 to 80 hours compared with a half-life of 2.5 hours for oral or IV ketamine, which results in a slower onset of peak serum levels and less significant psychomimetic effects.[28]

There have been mixed results in studies using memantine to treat chronic pain. A 2007 preliminary series by Sinis et al. involved six patients with CRPS of one upper extremity treated with memantine for 8 weeks with at dosages of least 30 mg/day. Six months after treatment with memantine, all patients showed a significant decrease in their levels of pain, which coincided with an improvement in motor symptoms and autonomic changes.[29]

A 2004 study investigated the effect of memantine administered at 30 mg/day on the intensity of chronic phantom limb pain (PLP) in eight patients in a placebo-controlled, double-blinded, crossover trial of 4 weeks' duration per trial. The intensity of PLP was rated hourly by the patients on a VAS during baseline and both treatment periods. The data indicated that at the studied dosage, the NMDA receptor antagonist memantine is ineffective in the treatment of chronic PLP.[30]

In contrast, the prevention of acute PLP with memantine was also investigated in a randomized, double-blind, placebo-controlled trial of 19 patients with memantine 20 to 30 mg/day initiated immediately after upper limb amputation. Patients received postoperative analgesia by continuous brachial plexus ropivacaine infusion for 1 week. After cessation of ropivacaine infusion, patients were maintained on memantine 30 mg/day for 4 weeks postoperatively and demonstrated a nearly fourfold decrease in the incidence of PLP at 6 months from 38% to 10%.[31]

An additional dramatic case series supports the potential role of memantine in the prevention of PLP when administered in the early stages of the process. Hackworth et al. described two young soldiers who were treated successfully with memantine initiated within 2 months after the onset of severe PLP. Dramatically, in addition to multiple adjuvant analgesics, both patients were weaned from large requirements of IV hydromorphone of nearly 100 mg/day after commencing memantine at 20 to 45 mg/day.[32]

METHADONE

Methadone is a synthetic opioid analgesic first synthesized in the late 1930s in Germany and originally applied as a potential spasmolytic. It has been commercially available in the United States since the 1940s with the trade name Dolophine. The oral bioavailability of methadone is 85% with a IV potency that is twice that of the oral route. The analgesic half-life of methadone, 4 to 8 hours, differs critically from the plasma half-life, which ranges from 13 to 50 hours. This difference between the analgesic and plasma half-lives of methadone, upon repetitive doses for analgesia, potentiates a significant risk of toxicity and respiratory depression because substantial plasma drug accumulation can occur.[33] An additional critical adverse effect of methadone is its effect on the QT interval on the electrocardiogram (ECG). QTc prolongation is a risk factor for developing polymorphic ventricular tachycardia or torsades de pointes and has been associated with multiple medications, including methadone. QTc intervals of 0.500 seconds or greater are associated with an increased risk of torsades de pointes, and patients should be routinely screened for QT interval prolongation with ECG before initiation of methadone therapy and annually with continued therapy.[34]

Unique within the opiate class, methadone has an additional property as an NMDA receptor antagonist.[35] Methadone is commonly clinically available as a racemic mixture of two enantiomeric forms, the d and l isomers. The l isomer possesses analgesic activity; the d isomer is a weaker opioid agonist. Both the d and the l isomers bind to the noncompetitive site of the NMDA receptor with similar affinities.[36]

The NMDA activity of methadone may offer therapeutic benefits, including improved analgesia over other opiates in neuropathic and cancer pain states. Results of studies aiming to identify a clear advantage of methadone over conventional opiate therapy, however, have been inconsistent. A case series by Moulin et al. involved 50 consecutive noncancer pain patients with intractable neuropathic pain conditions, including CRPS, peripheral neuropathies, and central pain conditions. All patients had failed treatment with tricyclic antidepressants and conventional opioid analgesics with a mean maximal morphine equivalents of 384 mg/day and were then changed to oral methadone. A total of 22 of 50 (44%) had moderate or better relief with methadone with tolerable side effects and improved quality of life in 14 (28%) over a long follow-up period (mean, 21.3 months).[37] A contrasting study in 2004 by Bruera et al. sought to compare the effectiveness and side effects of methadone and morphine as first-line opioids for cancer pain in patients with and without a neuropathic pain syndrome. In the randomized, double-blind study that lasted for 4 weeks, 103 patients in palliative care programs with pain requiring opioid therapy were randomly assigned to receive methadone 7.5 mg orally every 12 hours and 5 mg every 4 hours as needed or morphine 15 mg sustained release every 12 hours and 5 mg every 4 hours as needed. The authors found that despite the additional NMDA activity of methadone, it did not produce superior analgesic efficiency or an improved side effect profile at 4 weeks compared with morphine.[38]

A recent Cochrane review in 2007 examined RCTs of methadone against active opiate agents such as morphine in patients with cancer pain as well as neuropathic and non-neuropathic pain. The review included 392 completing patients in nine RCTs, six of which were double blinded, as well as two crossover studies. All of the studies involved active opioids such as morphine in control groups with different dosing and titration schedules and various pain scoring scales. The author concluded that in addition to a higher rate of adverse effects, including the additional risk of dose accumulation, methadone does not offer superior analgesic efficacy to morphine in cancer pain nor in neuropathic pain.[39]

Theoretically, methadone has the potential to reduce tolerance to opioids as well as provide analgesia through its NMDA receptor blocking action. These potential benefits of methadone are attractive, but they have yet to be clinically supported in other than anecdotal reports.

CONCLUSION

The critical role of the NMDA receptor in the fortification and augmentation of acute pain processes as well as in the establishment of chronic pathological pain states clearly poses a tremendous target opportunity for therapeutic advancement. Because of the multiple nonspecific effects of the most effective available agent, ketamine, its use is largely limited to the tertiary pain center and hospital settings. Considering the somewhat limited clinical advantages of the other, better tolerated, available NMDA receptor antagonists, it is clear that the therapeutic route of NMDA antagonism is still broadly underexploited in current clinical practice. There is an extraordinary need for research and development of additional, more specific agents that can target individual NMDA receptor subunits with biophysical characteristics that minimize interference with normal physiologic processes such as cognition and memory while providing the considerable benefits of the attenuation of opiate-induced hyperalgesia, opiate tolerance, and establishment of central sensitization. Additionally, there is a tremendous need for well-designed studies to investigate the currently available agents to clearly define patient selection criteria for the therapy and optimal dosing regimens to maximize the potential benefit they may offer. The therapeutic mechanism of NMDA antagonism is indeed in its infancy and has the potential to offer extraordinary future benefits to patients with acute and chronic pain.

REFERENCES

1. Ogden KK, Traynelis SF. New advances in NMDA receptor pharmacology. *Trends Pharmacol Sci.* 2011;32(12):726-733.
2. Quibell R, Prommer E, Mihalyo M, et al. Therapeutic reviews: ketamine. *J Pain Symptom Manage.* 2011;41(3):640-640.
3. Dickenson AH. A cure for wind up: NMDA receptor antagonists as potential analgesics. *Trends Pharmacol Sci.* 1990;11:307-309.
4. Parsons Chris G. NMDA receptors as targets for drug action in neuropathic pain. *Eur J Pharmacol.* 2001;429:71-78.
5. Ji R, Kohno T, Moore K, Woolf CJ. Central sensitization and LTP: do pain and memory share similar mechanisms? *Trends Neurosci.* 2003;26(12).
6. Woolf CJ. Central sensitization uncovering the relation between pain and plasticity. *Anesthesiology.* 2007;106:864-867.
7. Zhuo M. A synaptic model for pain: long-term potentiation in the anterior cingulate cortex. *Moll Cells.* 2007;23(3): 259-271.
8. Hocking G, Cousins M. Ketamine in chronic pain management: an evidence-based review *Anesth Analg.* 2003;97:1730-1739.
9. Bell RF, Dahl JB, Moore RA, Kalso E. Perioperative ketamine for acute postoperative pain. *Cochrane Database Syst Rev.* 2006;3:1-61.
10. Joly V, Richebe P, Guignard B, et al. Remifentanil-induced postoperative hyperalgesia and its prevention with small-dose ketamine. *Anesthesiology.* 2005;103:147-155.
11. Adam F, Chauvin M, DaManoir B, et al. Small-dose ketamine infusion improves postoperative analgesia and rehabilitation after total knee arthroplasty. *Anesth Analg.* 2005;100:475-480.
12. Kwok RFK, Lim J, Chan MTV, et al. Preoperative ketamine improves postoperative analgesia after gynecologic laparoscopic surgery. *Anesth Analg.* 2004;98:1044-1049.
13. Goldberg ME, Torjman MC, Schwartzman RJ, et al. Pharmacodynamic profiles of ketamine (R)- and (S)- with 5-day inpatient infusion for the treatment of complex regional pain syndrome. *Pain Physician.* 2010;13(4):379-387.
14. Curran HV, Monaghan L. In and out of the K-hole: a comparison of the acute and residual effects of ketamine in frequent and infrequent ketamine users. *Addiction.* 2001;96:749-760.
15. Morgan CJA, Ricelli M, Maitland CH, Curran HV. Long-term effects of ketamine: evidence for a persisting impairment of source memory in recreational users. *Drug Alcohol Depend.* 2004;75:301-308.
16. Liao Y, Tang J, Ma M, Wu Z, et al. Frontal white matter abnormalities following chronic ketamine use: a diffusion tensor imaging study. *Brain.* 2010;133:2115–2122.
17. Zou X, Patterson TA, Sadovov N, et al. Potential neurotoxicity of ketamine in the developing rat brain. *Toxicol Sci.* 2009;108(1):149-158.
18. Shahani R, Streutker C, Dickson B, Stewart R. Ketamine-associated ulcerative cystitis: a new clinical entity. *Urology.* 2007;69(5).
19. Wong SW, Lee KF, Wong W, et al. Dilated common bile ducts mimicking choledochal cysts in ketamine abusers. *Hong Kong Med J.* 2009;15(1).
20. Pender ES, Parks BR. Toxicity with dextromethorphan-containing preparations: a literature review of two additional cases. *Pediatr Emerg Care.* 1991;7:163-165.
21. Siu A, Drachtman R. Dextromethorphan: a review of N-methyl-D-aspartate receptor antagonist in the management of pain. *CNS Drug Reviews.* 2007;13(1):96-106.
22. Mercadante S, Casuccio A, Genovese G. Ineffectiveness of dextromethorphan in cancer pain. *J Pain Symptom Manage.* 1998;16:317-322.
23. Weinbroum A, Rudick V, Paret G, Ben-Abraham R. The role of dextromethorphan in pain control. *Can J Anesth.* 2000;47(6):585-596.
24. Kawamata T, Omote K, Kawamata M, Namiki A. Premedication with oral dextromethorphan reduces postoperative pain after tonsillectomy. *Anesth Analg.* 1998;86:594-597.
25. McConaghy PM, McSorley P, McCaugey W, Campbell WI. Dextromethorphan and pain after total abdominal hysterectomy. *Br J Anaesth.* 1998;81:731-736.
26. Wong CS, Wu CT, Yu JC, et al. Preincisional dextromethorphan decreases postoperative pain and opioid requirement after modified radical mastectomy. *Can J Anesth.* 1999;46:1122-1126.
27. Nelson KA, Park KM, Robinovitz E, et al. High dose oral dextromethorphan versus placebo in painful diabetic neuropathy and post-herpetic neuralgia. *Neurology.* 1997;48:1212-1218.
28. Johnson JW, Kotermanski SE. Mechanism of action of memantine. *Curr Opin Pharmacol.* 2006;6:61-67.
29. Sinis N, Birbaumer N, Gustin S, et al. Memantine treatment of complex regional pain syndrome: a preliminary report of six cases. *Clin J Pain.* 2007;23(3):237-243.
30. Wiech K, Kiefer RT, Tapfner S, et al. A placebo-controlled randomized crossover trial of the N-methyl-D-aspartic acid receptor antagonist, memantine, in patients with chronic phantom limb pain. *Anesth Analg.* 2004;98(2):408-413, table of contents.
31. Schley M, Topfner S, Wiech K, et al. Continuous brachial plexus blockade in combination with the NMDA receptor antagonist memantine prevents phantom pain in acute traumatic upper limb amputees. *Eur J Pain.* 2007;11:299-308.
32. Hackworth RJ, Tokarz KA, Fowler IM, et al. Profound pain reduction after induction of memantine treatment in two patients with severe phantom limb pain. *Anesth Analg.* 2008;107(4):1377-1379.
33. Inturrisi CE. Clinical pharmacology of opioids for pain. *Clin J Pain.* 2002;18:S3-S13.
34. Nordt SP, Zilberstein J, Gold B. Methadone-induced torsade de pointes. *Am J Emerg Med.* 2011;29:476.e1-476.e2.
35. Ebert B, Andersen S, Krogsgaard-Larsen P. Ketobemidone, methadone and pethidine are non-competitive N-methyl-D-aspartate (NMDA) antagonists in the rat cortex and spinal cord. *Neurosci Lett.* 1995;187:165-168.
36. Gorman AL, Elliott KJ, Inturrisi CE. The d- and l-isomers of methadone bind to the non-competitive site on the N-methyl-D-aspartate (NMDA) receptor in rat forebrain and spinal cord. *Neurosci Lett.* 1997; 223:5-8.
37. Moulin DE, Palma D, Watling C, Schulz V. Methadone in the management of intractable neuropathic noncancer pain. *Can J Neurol Sci.* 2005;32:340-343.
38. Sandoval JA, Furlan AD, Mailis-Gagnon A. Oral methadone for chronic noncancer pain: a systematic literature review of reasons for administration, prescription patterns, effectiveness, and side effects [review]. *Clin J Pain.* 2005;21(6):503-512.
39. Bruera E, Palmer JL, Bosnjak S, et al. Methadone versus morphine as a first-line strong opioid for cancer pain: a randomized, double-blind study. *J Clin Oncol.* 2004;22(1):185-192.
40. Ilkjaer S, Dirks J, Brennum J, et al. Effect of systemic N-methyl-D-aspartate receptor antagonist dextromethorphan. on primary and secondary hyperalgesia in humans. *Br J Anaesth.* 1997;79:600-605.

41. Trujillo KA. Are NMDA receptors involved in opiate-induced neural and behavioral plasticity? A review of preclinical studies. *Psychopharmacology*. 2000;151, 121-141.

42. Mao JR, Price DD, Mayer DJ. Experimental mononeuropathy reduces the antinociceptive effects of morphine: implications for common intracellular mechanisms involved in morphine tolerance and neuropathic pain. *Pain*. 1995;61:353-364.

43. Carlton SM, Coggeshall RE. Inflammation-induced changes in peripheral glutamate receptor populations. *Brain Res*. 1999; 820:63-70.

44. Morgan CJA, Muetzelfeldt L, Valerie Curran H. *Ketamine Use, Cognition and Psychological Wellbeing: A Comparison of Frequent, Infrequent and Ex-Users with Polydrug and Non-Using Controls.* Clinical Psychopharmacology Unit, University College London, London, UK Addiction; 2001

45. Nicholson AB. Methadone for cancer pain. *Cochrane Database Syst Rev* [review]. 2007;(4):CD003971.

CHAPTER 80 Steroids

John C. Keel
Anna Serels
Jason C. Wu

INTRODUCTION

The main caveat of this chapter is that *all steroids are systemic.* Steroids, that is, corticosteroids, may be the first or second most commonly used class of medication in pain clinics, as well as orthopedic and other musculoskeletal clinics. The primary aim of this chapter is to detail the potential adverse events associated with corticosteroids themselves and to briefly review corticosteroid pharmacology and technical aspects. Clinical efficacy evidence is not reviewed here because it has been done extensively elsewhere; instead, a review of steroid-specific risks is presented to aid decision making on whether a steroid should even be used in the first place. If all steroids are systemic, then any adverse event related to steroids could potentially result from steroids administered in the pain clinic, whether or not such has been reported in the literature. Let not steroids be understood the least by those who use them the most.

Spinal injections containing steroids are generally safe. Recent events have focused attention on these procedures, such as the fungal meningitis outbreak caused by contaminated steroids and the recent Food and Drug Administration (FDA) Safety Alert, both of which are explained in detail in this chapter. However, a 7-year retrospective of 4265 epidural steroid injections (ESIs) in 1857 patients found no major complications and a minor complication rate of 2.4%, consisting mostly of increased pain or pain at the injection site or persistent numbness.[1] The ASA Closed Claims study reports 114 major complications, including nerve injury, infection, headache, worse pain, brain damage, and death.[2] However, in truth, we do not know the complication rate because there is no mandated reporting.[3]

MECHANISM AND METABOLISM

Cortisone was first isolated from the adrenal gland in 1935.[4] As initiates, we may cringe at the word "cortisone" when that is the limit of one's self-report of medical history. "Steroid" for purposes here refers to corticosteroid medications, which are now usually synthetic derivatives of the endogenous corticosteroids produced by the adrenal cortex in response to stimulation by adrenocorticotropic hormone (ACTH). All corticosteroids have mineralocorticoid and glucocorticoid potency in varying proportions and may have metabolic effects on every organ system. As part of the glucocorticoid effect, corticosteroids have powerful anti-inflammatory action.

ACTH is a 39–amino acid peptide cleaved from a larger precursor protein, pro-opiomelanocortin (POMC), and it exerts actions via the melanocortin receptor subtypes (MC2R in the adrenal cortex). ACTH from the pituitary stimulates adrenal cortex production and release of glucocorticoids, mineralocorticoids, and dehydroepiandrosterone. In clinical practice, a synthetic ACTH analog, cosyntropin, is given in a high dose to test the ability of the hypothalamic–pituitary–adrenal (HPA) axis response of increased cortisol production.

The HPA is a cooperation of these three organs in maintaining glucocorticoid levels. Three HPA mechanisms are: (1) diurnal rhythm or fluctuation in steroidogenesis, (2) negative feedback loop wherein excess glucocorticoid decreases ACTH, and (3) positive stress response wherein steroidogenesis is increased. Corticotropin-releasing hormone (CRH) from the hypothalamus is transported to the anterior pituitary, where it binds receptors on corticotrope cells, resulting in ACTH production. Arginine vasopressin (AVP), also from the hypothalamus, stimulates release of ACTH. In negative feedback, glucocorticoid binds glucocorticoid receptors on pituitary corticotropes and inhibits release of ACTH and production of its precursor, POMC. The stress response can trump negative feedback, and although the mechanisms are less known, the immune system is involved. Administered corticosteroids suppress ACTH release from the pituitary; as a result, the adrenal gland is less stimulated to produce cortisol.

Pharmacologic effects of corticosteroids include anti-inflammatory and neural blockade, and ultimately, pain relief. Corticosteroids decrease the inflammatory cascade by inhibiting phospholipase A2, resulting in decreased release of arachidonic acid. With less arachidonic acid to act as substrate for cyclooxygenase, production of leukotrienes and prostaglandins is reduced. Pharmaceutical corticosteroids are metabolized by the hepatic P450 cytochrome; topical, injected, and inhaled steroids bypass the liver initially.[5] Such corticosteroids include ESIs. Steroids may also prolong the effects of local anesthetics.[6,7]

Commonly cited steroid dose equivalencies are estimates based on systemic glucocorticoid effects (e.g., hydrocortisone 20 mg prednisone or prednisolone 5 mg ≈ dexamethasone 0.75 mg). The physiologic level of corticosteroid production is often cited as equivalent to 20 to 30 mg/day of hydrocortisone (**Tables 80-1** and **80-2**).

Adverse effects are common in patients treated chronically with corticosteroids even at low doses. Adverse events are seen after any route, including oral, intraarticular, epidural, inhaled, nasal, ocular, and topical.[5] More than 90% of such patients treated for 60 or more days reported adverse effects, and 55% reported serious events, including weight gain, cataracts, and fractures.[8] Certain populations well known to be at risk from chronic steroid treatment have been studied more, and there are even guidelines to suggest prevention and management of corticosteroid-induced side effects. For the spine and pain clinic population, it is possible that some guidelines are needed as well. For example, guidelines are available on the prevention and management of steroid-induced osteoporosis and diabetes.[9,10] Timing of steroid doses in the morning is suggested as a way to mimic the natural pattern and reduce adverse effects. For patients with diabetes, recommendations include more frequent monitoring and medication adjustment. For those with osteoporosis, guidelines include bone density assessment and treatment.

TABLE 80-1 Steroid Potency Relative to Cortisol

Steroid	Anti-inflammatory	Mineralocorticoid	Duration (hr)
Triamcinolone	5	0	12–36
Methylprednisolone	5	0	12–36
Dexamethasone	25+	0	36+

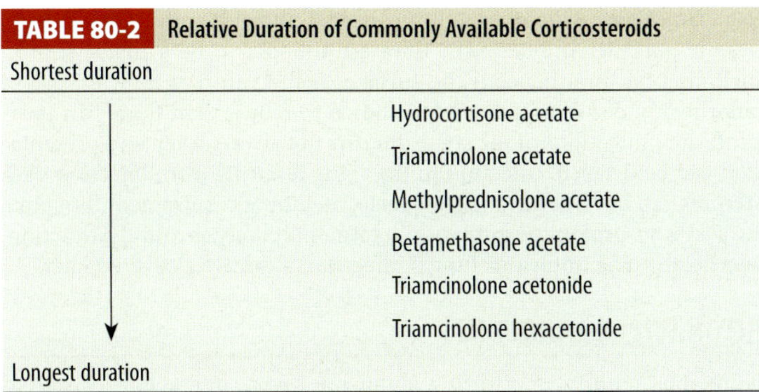

TABLE 80-2 Relative Duration of Commonly Available Corticosteroids

Shortest duration	
↓	Hydrocortisone acetate
	Triamcinolone acetate
	Methylprednisolone acetate
	Betamethasone acetate
	Triamcinolone acetonide
	Triamcinolone hexacetonide
Longest duration	

MUSCULOSKELETAL AND NEUROLOGIC EFFECTS

ADVERSE EFFECTS AND OSTEOPOROSIS

Glucocorticoids inhibit calcium absorption in the gastrointestinal tract, decrease renal tubule calcium reabsorption, and stimulate bone resorption. They decrease cellular activity and the viability of osteoblasts, including induction of apoptosis.[9] These actions contribute to steroid-induced osteoporosis. In a retrospective study of postmenopausal women treated with spinal injections for pain, exposure to less than 200 mg total dose of triamcinolone in 1 year may not increase the risk of osteoporosis.[11] Another retrospective study showed an increased risk of osteoporosis in postmenopausal women receiving more than 400 mg of triamcinolone, or about 14 injections, over a 3-year period.[12] A prospective observational study showed that a single ESI in postmenopausal women is followed by decreased bone mineral density of the hip.[13] Mitra advocates a 3-month interval between steroid injections because the relative risk of fracture decreases after cessation of steroid treatment, back toward the baseline risk, mostly within 3 months.[14]

Steroid-induced myopathy, characterized by proximal muscle weakness, has been reported after ESIs.[15]

CARDIAC AND RENAL EFFECTS

ADVERSE EFFECTS

Corticosteroids' mineralocorticoid activity causes sodium (and water) retention and potassium excretion.[5] These may lead to fluid retention, weight gain, hypertension, and congestive heart failure, which have been reported after ESIs.[15-18]

DIABETES

BLOOD SUGAR ELEVATION

Glucocorticoids cause insulin resistance, thereby causing blood glucose elevation.[10] Specifically, the liver secretes more glucose, and muscle and fat decrease glucose uptake because these tissues respond less to insulin. Steroid-induced diabetes is diagnosed and treated with the same American Diabetes Association guidelines. Spinal and other injections with steroids are likely to cause a temporary elevation in blood glucose, and patients should be cautioned. A prospective cohort of 12 patients with diabetes demonstrated blood glucose increase of about 106 mg/dL after ESI, but the elevation only lasted 3 days.[19] Another prospective cohort of 30 patients with diabetes demonstrated blood glucose increase from 160 to 286 mg/dL after ESI, but the elevation only lasted 2 days, and there was no rise in Hgb A1C.[20] A single observational study with only five subjects showed no change in glucose tolerance in patients with diabetes receiving an ESI.[21] These studies are limited because they have few subjects, and they screened for well-controlled diabetes. In the authors' experience, blood glucose elevation can persist for the duration of action of the steroid, perhaps a few weeks, and sometimes is significant enough to require medical attention.

TABLE 80-3 Cushing's syndrome

Rapid weight gain
Truncal obesity
Buffalo hump
Moon face
Hyperhidrosis
Thin skin, striae, acne
Alopecia or hirsutism
Insomnia
Impotence
Irregular menses
Mood or sleep disturbance
Hypertension
Diabetes
Lipidemia
Hypokalemia
Immune suppression

CUSHING'S DISEASE

Exogenous glucocorticoids in excess may result in Cushing's *syndrome* (**Table 80-3**). Recall that exogenous steroids suppress pituitary ACTH expression. In contrast, Cushing's disease is a primary pituitary cause of increased ACTH and then increased cortisol production. Secondary adrenal suppression and adrenal insufficiency may result from excess exogenous steroid. These have been reported after ESIs.[15-18]

WITHDRAWAL AND ADRENAL INSUFFICIENCY

Steroid used for acute flareups of pain is often supplied orally as a "taper" of several days' duration; there are many forms of a short course of oral glucocorticoids. If given for less than 1 week, no long-term tapering is typically required. Exogenous steroids administered longer than 1 week begin to inhibit hypothalamic CRH and pituitary ACTH release. The resulting atrophy of the adrenal glands can take weeks to months to recover. During the time while the adrenal glands are weakened, there is a risk of adrenal insufficiency. For this reason, long tapers of low-dose steroids are used while the adrenal glands recover, and higher "stress doses" may be used in times of need during recovery (**Table 80-4**).

FACIAL FLUSHING AND TACHON'S SYNDROME

Facial flushing is the abrupt development of erythema typically in the face but also in the trunk and limbs, and it may be accompanied by warm sensations. Facial flushing may occur in 1.4% to 9.3% of cases of steroid injections. It is a self-limited, benign condition that typically resolves within 3 days, is not a true allergy, and is not a contraindication to future injections, although the facial flushing may recur.[22]

It is possible that the facial flushing is related to Tachon's syndrome, which is acute intense malaise often associated with pain in the chest, thorax, and back. Tachon's syndrome begins immediately after steroid injection and is associated with facial flushing in 64% of cases. Tachon's syndrome is rare, but 39% of cases may occur after epidural injection. There may also be an association with soluble steroid such as dexamethasone, so we may be seeing more of this.[23]

TABLE 80-4 Addison's Disease or Adrenal Insufficiency Symptoms

Orthostasis
Weakness
Fatigue
Crisis (an emergency): profound weakness; severe pain in trunk, back, or legs; renal failure; shock; fever

HICCUPS

Numerous cases of persistent hiccups have been reported after spine injections with steroids. Mechanisms proposed for this include volume effects from injectate and effect on cerebrospinal fluid flow, unusual medication interaction, sympathetic block, and parasympathetic overactivity.[24-27]

MENSES AND BREASTFEEDING

Patients sometimes report dramatic abnormality in menses after epidural or other steroid injections, including heavy bleeding. Corticosteroids may alter the hypothalamic–ovarian axis and decrease luteinizing hormone and follicle-stimulating hormone, resulting in a blunted progesterone spike.[28,29] Temporary loss of breast milk production has been reported after steroid injection.[30]

EPIDURAL LIPOMATOSIS

Epidural lipomatosis is accumulation of fat in the epidural space. It is associated with diabetes, obesity, and other disorders. It may cause compression of nerve pathways, resulting in symptomatic stenosis. Cushing's syndrome, systemic steroids, and injected steroids (including ESI) can exacerbate epidural lipomatosis.[31-34]

HYPOPIGMENTATION

Hypopigmentation may occur at areas of corticosteroid injection, and discoloration may track in a linear fashion from the injection site, perhaps because of vascular or lymphatic spread of steroid. The hypopigmentation may be long lasting but may resolve spontaneously, usually by 9 months. It is more likely to be noticeable on darker skin. It can be distressing to patients but is not dangerous in itself unless accompanied by local tissue atrophy. Hypopigmentation is more likely when the steroid has been deposited superficially, as in musculoskeletal injections to relatively superficial targets such as de Quervain's tenosynovitis.[35] However, this author is aware of cases related to spine injections in which the steroid was tracked through the skin (this should be avoided). Biopsies suggest that decreased local melanocyte function is the mechanism of hypopigmentation.[36]

MELANOMA

Melanoma causes the majority of skin cancer deaths, and its incidence is on the rise. Immunosuppression has been associated with development of cancer, including immunosuppression with exogenous steroids. Lazarus and Kaufman describe a case of melanoma recurrence after localized injection of triamcinolone.[37] Corticosteroids affect cytokine production in T lymphocytes and thereby erode the body's defense against cutaneous melanoma. The immunologic effects of steroids should be considered carefully in the setting of melanoma history.

INFECTION

A potentially devastating effect of steroid injections around the spine is infection, such as epidural abscess, discitis, osteomyelitis, and meningitis. It is rational to avoid steroid injection to an area of the spine or through skin that has had recent infection because steroids suppress immune responses and could lead to reactivation of latent nidus. When does such a danger expire? It is not truly known; there is likely always a risk. What about in the case of spinal implants or at spinal locations previously infected? In this author's opinion, in such cases, once infected equals always infected (so I avoid injections of steroids there). It is rational to avoid steroid injection if there is a chance of systemic bacteremia, with potential for introduction into the spine with localized immune suppression. Such caveats may not be as applicable if injections are done without steroids; after all, is it not common to biopsy spinal areas thought to be infected, and is this not simply a spinal injection (because local anesthetic would usually be used)? Why do infections happen despite good technique? Skin flora are thought to be a major source, including bacteria beneath the surface, such as in hair follicles; use of chlorhexidine skin prep has been shown to reduce skin flora.[38] In postprocedure infections of the spine, there is not always fever, and presentation can be delayed. Infection in the spine resulting from injection with steroids can have devastating sequelae, including requirement for spinal surgery and prolonged antibiotic treatment, paralysis and dysfunction, and death.[3] The notorious fungal infection outbreak is covered later.

RITONAVIR: A LANDMINE

Numerous reports are swirling about the severe interaction of steroid injections in the setting of concurrent ritonavir. The interaction is especially noted with triamcinolone. Ritonavir comes alone as Norvir or is also a component of Kaletra, along with lopinavir. Ritonavir is a powerful protease inhibitor with extremely potent cytochrome P450 3A4 inhibition and is used as a boosting agent in the treatment of HIV. Ritonavir inhibits the metabolism of triamcinolone and greatly amplifies the effective exposure. Case reports describe severe Cushing's, emergency adrenal crisis, and hip avascular necrosis after as few as one or two triamcinolone injections while a patient is taking ritonavir.[39] Theoretically, it seems possible that other steroid injection preparations could also interact; there are reports of other steroids by other routes interacting. All HIV-positive patients need to be asked specifically about ritonavir.

OPHTHALMIC COMPLICATIONS

The most common ophthalmic complications include posterior subcapsular cataracts and glaucoma with the incidence ranging from 6% to 40% of patients developing one or the other after ESI. There are also reports of blindness and intraocular hemorrhage after steroid injection into the epidural space.[40] Glucocorticoids and Cushing's have been strongly implicated as pathogenic factors in central serous chorioretinopathy, including ESIs.[41] Hardwig et al. case series also reports a case of recurrence of ophthalmic ciliochoroidal melanoma associated with ESI.[41] Acute retinal necrosis has been reported after ESI.[42] It is hypothesized that the acute retinal necrosis could have been caused by reactivation of herpes virus infection in the retina as has been described in relation to local injection and systemic steroid effects (**Table 80-5**).

PARTICULATES AND PRESERVATIVES

Other causes of adverse effects of steroids include particulates, preservatives, and contaminants. The debate over particulate versus nonparticulate steroid formulations is ongoing. Particulate steroids are hypothesized to be a cause of a most feared but rare complication of spine injections: spinal cord injury. Especially in transforaminal epidural injections, particulate steroids are believed to enter the arterial supply to the cord and then embolize the spinal cord itself. It is hypothesized that nonparticulate steroids such as dexamethasone and betamethasone sodium phosphate do not embolize. Recent studies suggest the noninferiority of soluble steroids compared with particulate in terms of treatment effect.[43,44]

Spinal cord infarction has been reported at sacral, lumbar, thoracic, and cervical spine levels after transforaminal injections. In one of the earliest case series, Houten and Errico reported three cases of paraplegia after left and right L3 to L4 and left S1 transforaminal injections.[45] Kennedy et al. reported two cases of injury after right and left L3 to L4 transforaminal injections.[46] Glaser and Falco reported paraplegia after left T12 to L1 transforaminal injection.[47] Many cases of central nervous system infarction have now been reported after cervical transforaminal injections.[48,49] Embolism and infarction have not been described after caudal and interlaminar injections.[3]

It has been hypothesized that particulate size may play a role in embolic injuries after steroid injections. Derby et al. measured commonly used steroid particulates under light microscopy compared with red blood

TABLE 80-5 Ophthalmic complications

More serious or more common
- Posterior subcapsular cataracts
- Monocular vision loss
- Glaucoma
- Central serous chorioretinopathy
- Retinal hemorrhage
- Epiblepharon

Less serious or less common
- Ptosis
- Retinal embolic phenomenon
- Decreased resistance to infection
- Mydriasis
- Myopia
- Uveitis
- Exophthalmos
- Atrophy of eyelid skin
- Diplopia
- Ocular infections
- Papilledema
- Corneal ulceration
- Myasthenic neuromuscular blocking effect
- Ocular muscle palsy
- Delayed corneal wound healing
- Refractive changes
- Translucent blue sclera
- Scleral thinning and thickening
- Eyelid or conjunctival changes
- Pseudotumor cerebri
- Microcysts
- Hypertensive retinopathy
- Hordeolum
- Moon facies with ptosis
- Epiblepharon
- Chemosis and lid swelling
- Decreased tear lysozyme

cell (RBC) size and assessed particulate aggregation and solubility.[50] Dexamethasone particles measured smaller than 0.5 μm, far smaller than RBCs, and did not aggregate into larger particles. Betamethasone and triamcinolone had variable particle size, but extensive clumping was observed into aggregates larger than 100 μm, more than 12 times the size of erythrocytes. Betamethasone tended to have smaller particles and less aggregation than triamcinolone. Methylprednisolone had more consistent particle size and less aggregation, and the size of particles was generally smaller than the RBC size. Smaller particulate and aggregate size may be less likely to cause embolic injury (**Table 80-6**). MacMahon et al. found comparable particle and aggregate sizes, and dynamic imaging showed aggregates maintained integrity, allowing them to act as potential embolization agents.[51]

Preservatives in steroids may cause adverse reactions. Preservatives include benzoyl alcohol and polyethylene glycol. For example, methylprednisolone acetate, or Depo-Medrol, may contain polyethylene glycol 30 mg/mL. Injection of this in the region of the spine may cause severe disabling, and even sometimes fatal meningitis or arachnoiditis.[52] However, most of the reports of arachnoiditis related to steroid injection have been in patients with multiple sclerosis treated with repeated intrathecal methylprednisolone acetate injections.[3]

TABLE 80-6 Particle and Aggregate Sizes of Steroid Preparations

Smaller	<0.5 μm	Decadron (dexamethasone Na phosphate)
	<7.6 μm	Depo-Medrol (methylprednisolone)
RBC size	7.5–7.8 μm	
	A few >100 μm	Celestone Soluspan (betamethasone Na phosphate/betamethasone acetate)
Larger	>100 μm	Kenalog (triamcinolone acetonide)

CONTAMINANTS

FUNGI

Tragically, lack of preservatives has also been associated with devastating outcomes. In September 2012, a multistate outbreak of fungal infections took place, attributed to contaminated preservative-free steroids from the New England Compounding Center. The fungal infections included meningitis, paraspinal infections, epidural abscess, arachnoiditis, and peripheral joint infections. The contaminant was *Exserohilum rostratum*, except in the index case, who had *Aspergillus fumigatus*. A total of 751 cases of fungal infection occurred across 20 states, and 64 deaths resulted from this outbreak. (The Centers for Disease Control and Prevention's website notes that no changes to case counts were anticipated after October 23, 2013.) This outbreak caused tremendous suffering of patients and families. What followed were a massive recall of steroid medications, news media frenzy, and new regulation of compounding pharmacies. Many of us as pain physicians were involved in this catastrophe and had the misfortune to be supplied with the contaminated steroid or knew colleagues who had been. We all experienced the no shows, the erosion of trust in the medical profession, and the sinking confidence in the practice of pain and spine injections.[53]

FOOD AND DRUG ADMINISTRATION WARNING

In April 2014, the FDA distributed a Safety Alert consisting of vague warnings that ESIs did not have safety and efficacy, that steroid preparations were not FDA approved for epidural injections, and the FDA would now require a "warning" on the drug labels of injectable corticosteroids.[54] The FDA warning has been criticized for inaccuracies.[55] For example, the FDA has cited limited literature, consisting mostly of case reports, including a high proportion of cervical injection and transforaminal injection complications, which may be biased compared to current practice. The FDA focuses on rare adverse events and does not cite the numerous lessons learned and techniques refined that have contributed to safety. Most ominously, the FDA seems to be moving in the direction of regulating the practice of medicine. More will come on this, per the FDA, on April 23, 2014:

FDA's Safe Use Initiative convened a panel of experts, including pain management experts to help define the techniques for such injections which would reduce preventable harm. The expert panel's recommendations will be released when they are finalized. FDA will convene an Advisory Committee meeting of external experts in late 2014 to discuss the benefits and risks of epidural corticosteroid injections and to determine if further FDA actions are needed.

CONCLUSION

All steroids are systemic. Any complication from systemic steroids could theoretically arise from an injected steroid, including spine injections. This means that a patient who goes to the shoulder doctor to get an injection, then the knee doctor to get an injection, and then gets a trochanter injection in the spine surgeon's office before coming to you has likely had his or her yearly allotment of steroids already. There are many "landmines" out there that we have not covered in the limits of this chapter, and there are many we likely do not know yet. For example, is the steroid-related rebound effect in poison ivy a concern for us in pain clinics? Should we prescribe oral steroid tapers? We recommend that physicians read the entire physician package inserts for medications they use, including injected steroids. For now, it seems that soluble dexamethasone is in the lead as the steroid of choice for injection. However, Dr. Huntoon may be prescient when he writes in "Back to the Future: The End of the Steroid Century?" that we may "return to an earlier time ... in the 1930s, they were doing caudal epidurals with local anesthetic only ..."[56]

REFERENCES

1. McGrath J, Schaefer M, Malkamaki D. Incidence and characteristics of complications from epidural steroid injections. *Pain Med.* 2011;12:726-731.
2. Fitzgibbon D, Posner K, Caplan R, et al. Chronic pain management: American Society of Anesthesiologists Closed Claims Project. *Anesthesiology*. 2004;100:98-105.
3. Cohen SP, Bicket MC, Jamison D, et al. Epidural steroids: a comprehensive, evidence-based review. *Reg Anesth Pain Med.* 2013;38(3):175-200.
4. Kendall EC. *Nobel Lecture: The Development of Cortisone as a Therapeutic Agent.* http://www.nobelprize.org/nobel_prizes/medicine/laureates/1950/kendall-lecture.html. Accessed July 15, 2014.
5. Ericson-Neilsen W, Kaye AD. Steroids: pharmacology, complications, and practice delivery issues. *Ochsner J.* 2014;14(2):203-207.
6. Yilmaz-Rastoder E, Gold MS, Hough KA, et al. Effect of adjuvant drugs on the action of local anesthetics in isolated rat sciatic nerves. *Reg Anesth Pain Med.* 2012;37(4):403-409.
7. Parrington SJ, O'Donnell D, Chan VW, et al. Dexamethasone added to mepivacaine prolongs the duration of analgesia after supraclavicular brachial plexus blockade. *Reg Anesth Pain Med.* 2010;35(5):422-426.
8. Curtis JR, Westfall AO, Allison J, et al. Population-based assessment of adverse events associated with long-term glucocorticoid use. *Arthritis Rheum.* 2006;55(3):420-426.
9. Pereira RM, Carvalho JF, Canalis E. Glucocorticoid-induced osteoporosis in rheumatic diseases. *Clinics (Sao Paulo).* 2010; 65(11):1197-1205.
10. Lansang MC, Hustak LK. Review glucocorticoid-induced diabetes and adrenal suppression: how to detect and manage them. *Cleve Clin J Med.* 2011;78(11):748-756.
11. Kang SS, Hwang BM, Son H, et al. Changes in bone mineral density in postmenopausal women treated with epidural steroid injections for lower back pain. *Pain Physician.* 2012;15(3):229-236.
12. Kim S, Hwang B. Relationship between bone mineral density and the frequent administration of epidural steroid injections in postmenopausal women with low back pain. *Pain Res Manag.* 2014;19(1):30-34.
13. Al-Shoha A, Rao DS, Schilling J, et al. Effect of epidural steroid injection on bone mineral density and markers of bone turnover in postmenopausal women. *Spine (Phila Pa 1976).* 2012;37(25):E1567-E1571.
14. Mitra R. Adverse effects of corticosteroids on bone metabolism: a review. *PM & R.* 2011;3:466-471.
15. Boonen S, Van Distel G, Westhovens R, et al. Steroid myopathy induced by epidural triamcinolone injection. *Br J Rheumatol.* 1995;34(4):385-386.
16. Stambough J, Booth R, Rothman R. Transient hypercorticism after epidural steroid injection. *J Bone Joint Surg.* 1984;66A:1115-1116.
17. Tuel SM, Meythaler JM, Cross LL. Cushing's syndrome from epidural methylprednisolone. *Pain.* 1990;40(1):81-84.
18. Horani MH, Silverberg AB. Secondary Cushing's syndrome after a single epidural injection of a corticosteroid. *Endocr Pract.* 2005;11(6):408-410.
19. Gonzalez P, Laker SR, Sullivan W, et al. The effects of epidural betamethasone on blood glucose in patients with diabetes mellitus. *PM & R.* 2009;1(4):340-345.
20. Even JL, Crosby CG, Song Y, et al. Effects of epidural steroid injections on blood glucose levels in patients with diabetes mellitus. *Spine (Phila Pa 1976).* 2012;37(1):E46-E50.
21. Zufferey P, Bulliard C, Gremion G, et al. Systemic effects of epidural methylprednisolone injection on glucose tolerance in diabetic patients. *BMC Res Notes.* 2011;4:552.
22. DeSio JM, Kahn CH, Warfield CA. Facial flushing and/or generalized erythema after epidural steroid injection. *Anesth Analg.* 1995; 80(3):617-619.
23. Berthelot JM, Le Goff B, Maugars Y. Side effects of corticosteroid injections: what's new? *Joint Bone Spine.* 2013; 80(4):363-367.
24. Abbasi CM, Roque-Dang G, Malhotra G. Persistent hiccups after interventional pain procedures: a case series and review. *PM & R.* 2012;4:144-151.
25. Beyaz SG. Persistent hiccup after lumbar epidural steroid injection. *J Anaesthesiol Clin Pharmacol.* 2012;28(3):418-419.
26. McAllister RK, McDavid AJ, Meyer TA, et al. Recurrent persistent hiccups after epidural steroid injection and analgesia with bupivacaine. *Anesth Analg.* 2005;100(6):1834-1836.
27. Slipman CW, Shin CH, Patel RK, et al. Persistent hiccup associated with thoracic epidural injection. *Am J Phys Med Rehabil.* 2001;80(8):618-621.
28. Gitkind AI, Shah B, Thomas M. Epidural corticosteroid injections as a possible cause of menorrhagia: a case report. *Pain Med.* 2010;11(5):713-715.
29. Çok OY, Eker HE, Çok T, et al. Abnormal uterine bleeding: is it an under-reported side effect after epidural steroid injection for the management of low back pain? *Pain Med.* 2011;12(6):986.
30. McGuire E. Sudden loss of milk supply following high-dose triamcinolone (Kenacort) injection. *Breastfeed Rev.* 2012;20(1):32-34.
31. Tok CH, Kaur S, Gangi A. Symptomatic spinal epidural lipomatosis after a single local epidural steroid injection. *Cardiovasc Intervent Radiol.* 2011;34:S250-S255.
32. Fogel GR, Cunningham PY 3rd, Esses SI. Spinal epidural lipomatosis: case reports, literature review and meta-analysis. *Spine J.* 2005;5(2):202-211.
33. Sandberg DI, Lavyne MH. Symptomatic spinal epidural lipomatosis after local epidural corticosteroid injections: case report. *Neurosurgery.* 1999;45(1):162-165.
34. McCullen GM, Spurling GR, Webster JS. Epidural lipomatosis complicating lumbar steroid injections. *J Spinal Disord.* 1999; 12(6):526-529.
35. Saour S, Dhillon BS, Ho-Asjoe M, et al. Ascending hypopigmentation of the forearm following injection of triamcinolone. *J Plast Reconstr Aesthet Surg.* 2009;62(12):e597-e598.
36. Venkatesan P, Fangman WL. Linear hypopigmentation and cutaneous atrophy following intra-articular steroid injections for de Quervain's tendonitis. *J Drugs Dermatol.* 2009;8(5):492-493.
37. Lazarus M, Kaufman H. An association between corticosteroid use and melanoma recurrence: a case report and review of the literature. *Med Oncol.* 2012;29:2018-2020.
38. Simopoulos TT, Kraemer JJ, Glazer P, et al. Vertebral osteomyelitis: a potentially catastrophic outcome after lumbar epidural steroid injection. *Pain Physician.* 2008;11(5):693-697.
39. Fessler D, Beach J, Keel J. Iatrogenic hypercortisolism complicating triamcinolone acetonide injections in patients with HIV on ritonavir-boosted protease inhibitors. *Pain Physician.* 2012;15(6):489-493.

40. Serels A, Keel JC. Poster 451 Ophthalmic Complications of Steroid, Spine Injections: Case Series and Review, *PM&R*, 2014;9(6):S343-S344.

41. Hardwig PW, Silva AO, Pulido JS. Forgotten exogenous corticosteroid as a cause of central serous chorioretinopathy. *Clin Ophthalmol.* 2008;2(1):199-201.

42. Browning DJ. Acute retinal necrosis following epidural steroid injections. *Am J Ophthalmol.* 2003;136(1):192-194.

43. Ahadian FM, McGreevy K, Schulteis G. Lumbar transforaminal epidural dexamethasone: a prospective, randomized, double-blind, dose-response trial. *Reg Anesth Pain Med.* 2011;36(6):572-578.

44. Dreyfuss P, Baker R, Bogduk N. Comparative effectiveness of cervical transforaminal injections with particulate and nonparticulate corticosteroid preparations for cervical radicular pain. *Pain Med.* 2006;7(3):237-242.

45. Houten JK, Errico TJ. Paraplegia after lumbosacral nerve root block: report of three cases. *Spine J.* 2002;2(1):70-75.

46. Kennedy D, Dreyfuss P, Aprill C, Bogduk N. Paraplegia following image-guided transforaminal lumbar spine epidural steroid injection: two case reports. *Pain Med.* 2009;10:1389-1394.

47. Glaser S, Falco F. Paraplegia following a thoracolumbar transforaminal epidural steroid injection. *Pain Physician.* 2005;8:309-314.

48. Brouwers PJAM, Kottnik EJBL, Simon MAM, Prevo RL. A cervical anterior spinal artery syndrome after diagnostic blockade of the right C6-nerve root. *Pain.* 2001;91:397-399.

49. Tiso R, Cutler T, Catania J, et al. Adverse central nervous system sequelae after selective transforaminal block: the role of corticosteroids. *Spine J.* 2004;4:468-474.

50. Derby R, Lee SH, Date ES, et al. Size and aggregation of corticosteroids used for epidural injections. *Pain Med.* 2008;9(2): 227-234.

51. MacMahon PJ1, Shelly MJ, Scholz D, et al. Injectable corticosteroid preparations: an embolic risk assessment by static and dynamic microscopic analysis. *AJNR.* 2011;32(10):1830-1835.

52. Nelson DA. Dangers from methylprednisolone acetate therapy by intraspinal injection. *Arch Neurol.* 1988;45:804-806.

53. Centers for Disease Control and Prevention. *Multistate Outbreak of Fungal Meningitis and Other Infections.* October 23, 2013. http://www.cdc.gov/hai/outbreaks/meningitis.html. Accessed Sept. 2, 2014.

54. US FDA. *Epidural Corticosteroid Injection: Drug Safety Communication—Risk of Rare But Serious Neurologic Problems. U.S. Food and Drug Administration.* April 23, 2014. http://www.fda.gov/safety/medwatch/safetyinformation/safetyalertsforhumanmedicalproducts/ucm394530.htm. Accessed September 2, 2014.

55. Manchikanti L, Candido KD, Singh V, et al. Epidural steroid warning controversy still dogging FDA. *Pain Physician.* 2014;17(4): E451-E474.

56. Huntoon MA, Burgher AH. Back to the future: the end of the steroid century? *Pain Physician.* 2008;11:713-716.

SECTION B

Injections and Neurolytic Therapies for Pain

Spinal Injections (Including Epidural Steroids and Medial Branch Blocks)

Douglas Keene

OVERVIEW

Spinal injections have been performed for many years, most often for the management of axial, paraspinal, and radicular pain. They have evolved over the years with increasing popularity, with the number of epidural steroid injection procedures doubling from 2000 to 2008,[1] and have become essential therapies for the pain management clinician. Spinal injections can be used therapeutically, for treatment, or diagnostically, for the localization and identification of potential painful targets. As a result of their increasing use in pain management and their economic impact, they have been studied extensively, and their efficacies have been challenged. Despite controversy and contradicting results of numerous outcome studies, spinal interventional therapies will likely continue to play a significant role in interdisciplinary pain care.

The purpose of this chapter is to discuss commonly performed spinal interventions, especially epidural steroid injections and facet injections, with an emphasis on information that is clinically relevant to pain management specialists.

HISTORY OF SPINAL INJECTIONS

Spinal injections of substances for the treatment of low back and lower extremity pain[2,3] and for inoperable cancer of the rectum[4] were described in 1901,[5] with the use of medications, including cocaine and procaine, via multiple routes of administration, including epidurally, intrathecally, and via the sacral hiatus. In 1909, reports were published on the use of epidural anesthesia for the treatment of sciatica[6] followed in the 1920s and 1930s by emerging treatments for sciatica with varying degrees of benefit and duration.[7,8]

With the discovery of Compound E (cortisone) in 1936[9-11] and by 1950 its improvement of conditions, including rheumatoid arthritis,[12] and with the beneficial intraarticular effects of a longer acting steroid, Compound F (hydrocortisone),[13] including the histologically confirmed reduction of synovial membrane inflammation, the stage was set for numerous anti-inflammatory pain management procedures along with continuing investigations of its efficacy and mechanisms of actions.[14-20] By the 1950s, many pain management clinics were in operation,[21,22] and today, many interdisciplinary pain treatment facilities are in existence.

CLASSIFICATION OF SPINAL INJECTIONS

Spinal injections for pain management have been performed for many years, both for diagnostic and therapeutic purposes. They can be functionally categorized both by location (i.e., cervical, thoracic, lumbar, or sacral) and by purpose: (i.e., diagnostic or therapeutic). A significant proportion of procedures performed at modern pain clinics include epidural steroid injections and facet joint injections. Other common interventions include sympathetic blocks, provocative discography, and medial branch radiofrequency neurotomy. Epidural steroid injections can be subcategorized by the route of administration of medication, usually via transforaminal, interlaminar, or caudal approaches, with or without the use of a catheter.

Zygapophyseal or facet injections that are therapeutic in nature tend to be intraarticular, and although they can be therapeutic and diagnostic, medial branch blocks are usually performed to provide diagnostic information and to predict the potential benefit of facet denervation via radiofrequency neuroablation.

LOW BACK PAIN

EPIDURAL STEROID INJECTIONS

Epidural injections of glucocorticoids may be helpful in some patients for the treatment of axial lumbar, thoracic, and cervical pain, and radicular lower and upper extremity and thoracic radicular pain. Historically, injection of steroids into the epidural space followed the observation of the beneficial effects of intraarticular injection of steroids into osteoarthritic joints,[23] with the first use of hydrocortisone in 1952 periradicularly[24] and in 1953 caudally.[25]

The emergence of interventional pain management as a specialty has led to a significant increase in the use of interventional techniques, prompting continuous review and the establishment of evidence-based practice guidelines for the management of spinal pain.[26] With hospital-based and dedicated pain treatment facilities performing these and other types of injections[27] and with a 100% increase in the frequency of epidural injections between 1998 and 2003[28] and between 2000 and 2008, epidural steroid injections are the most commonly performed intervention used in the United States to manage chronic and subacute low back pain (LBP).[29]

Various causes of sciatic pain have been proposed, including pressure on the spinal nerve by disc fragment or bone spur;[30] however, nerve root compression does not always produce pain, and patients without a history of sciatic pain have had disc protrusion or herniation found on postmortem examination.[31] Additionally, myelographic and magnetic resonance imaging (MRI) abnormalities have been found in asymptomatic individuals,[32,33] and surgical decompression does not relieve symptoms in every case. Confusing the picture even more, many patients with sciatic pain have no imaging-based evidence of nerve root compression. This may suggest that radicular pain is multifactorial.

Although mechanical nerve root compression can cause sensory and motor dysfunction, inflammation may also be a source of neural pain.[34] Structures in the vicinity of the nerve root, including injured disc tissue,[35] injured vertebral endplates leading to disc degeneration,[36] degenerated lumbar intervertebral discs per se,[37] facet joints, and epidural tissues, may each modulate neural activity, leading to increased sensitivity and pain-generating discharges and heightened sensitivity to pressure.[38] Current imaging modalities may be unable to demonstrate anatomic abnormalities responsible for spinal or radicular pain, especially if the abnormalities are not macroscopic.

In 1950, inflammation and edema was noted in nerve root biopsy samples from patients undergoing laminectomy,[39] and it was observed that swollen nerve roots shrank as sciatic symptoms improved.[40] Similar observations were found in patients treated with intramuscular dexamethasone.[41] Increased concentrations of inflammatory and neurochemical mediators found in intervertebral discs, including phospholipase A_2,[42] and pain-related neuropeptides in nerve endings in the discs and epidural structures[43,44] may contribute to axial or radicular symptoms. Cells from degenerated disc fragments produce numerous inflammatory mediators, including tumor necrosis factor (TNF) and inflammatory cytokines,[45] and the released inflammatory mediators and TNF may penetrate within intraneural capillaries, causing axonal ischemia, which is responsible for nerve root pain.[46]

Glucocorticoids inhibit the synthesis or release of many inflammatory substances[47] and may prevent cell-mediated inflammation that can stimulate nociceptive nerve endings.[48] In radicular pain, glucocorticoids may mitigate early effects of inflammation, including edema, fibrin deposition, capillary dilation, leukocyte aggregation, and phagocytosis, and late effects such as capillary and fibroblast proliferation, collagen deposition, and scar formation.[27] LBP per se may respond to the effects of glucocorticoid through its reduction of inflammation specifically in the posterior longitudinal ligament and the outer annulus of the intervertebral disc.[27] Injecting glucocorticoid near the sites of inflammation achieves a higher concentration than that obtained by systematic administration.

Many studies have investigated the efficacy of epidural steroid injections in the cervical, thoracic, and lumbar regions, reporting conflicting results, likely because of the difficulty in studying pain treatment modalities. Significant variations exist with regard to the numerous mechanisms of pain generation and the natural course of acute and chronic back and upper and lower extremity pain. Factors that must be considered in these investigations include injection variability, the route of administration (transforaminal vs. interlaminar), the use of fluoroscopic guidance and contrast, operator experience, spinal anatomy, degenerative change, surgical hardware or granulation tissue affecting the spread of medication, timing and frequency of administration, and prior surgical procedures.

Results from one systematic review of lumbar interlaminar epidural steroid injections show a significant reduction of pain scores in patients with lumbar radiculitis compared with no therapy and compared with conservative management without injection therapy.[49] In the cervical region, a study regarding immediate pain score after a single image-guided cervical transforaminal epidural steroid injection does not predict the long-term effectiveness of the procedure.[50] The literature supporting or refuting the use of epidural steroid injections for the treatment of chronic mid and upper back pain caused by disc herniation, radiculitis, and other causes is scant.[51]

There will likely continue to be emerging and sometimes conflicting evidence on the cost effectiveness[52] and efficacy[53-58] of epidural steroid injections or the choice of medications, routes of administration, and the timing of injections.

ZYGAPOPHYSEAL JOINT INJECTIONS

Sources of axial spinal pain (cervical, thoracic, and lumbar) are numerous. These include intervertebral discs, nerve root dura, facet joints, ligaments, muscles, and fascia; in the lumbar region, the sacroiliac joints; and in the cervical region, the atlanto-axial and atlanto-occipital joints. The lumbar facet joint was suspected as a source of LBP, spinal instability, and leg pain in 1911,[59] and by 1933, the lumbar facet joint was recognized by Ghormley as part of a distinct LBP syndrome "facet syndrome."[60] Provocative intraarticular facet joint injections of hypertonic saline were used and described in 1976[61] to investigate lumbar facet–mediated pain patterns. Medical literature has identified the lumbar, thoracic, and cervical facet joints as independent pain generators.

Inflammation within the joint capsule can decrease thresholds of nerve endings in the facet capsules with resulting elevated baseline discharge rates, and stretch or excessive stretch may damage axons or the joint capsule, with activation of nociceptors leading to prolonged neural discharges.[62] In the lumbar region, facet-mediated pain may present with axial spinal, paraspinal, buttock, or leg distribution patterns;[63] similarly, cervical facet–mediated pain may present as axial and paraspinal pain with radiation to the upper extremities or as headache.[64] In the thoracic region, based on experience with cervical and lumbar facet joints, thoracic facet–mediated pain can be axial or paraspinal, with radiation to the upper back and chest wall.[65] Because facet-mediated pain may coexist with other sources of axial pain or radicular pain, in clinical practice, it may be helpful to consider each component individually.

The diagnostic and therapeutic utility of cervical, thoracic, and lumbar facet injections has been investigated in numerous studies. Medial branch blocks, named for targeting the sensory innervations of facet joints, are frequently performed for diagnostic purposes to determine the role of the facet joint as a mediator of pain in lumbar, thoracic, and cervical regions. Localizing the facet joints to target may be difficult with two facet joints at each vertebral level (left and right), and the potential variations in symptoms, historical, imaging and physical examination information may be helpful.

To establish a consensus among interventional pain management specialists in the diagnosis and management of spinal pain, particularly specifics of treatment techniques (treatment modality, medication, frequency of administration), an algorithmic approach for the clinical management of chronic spinal pain based on evidence-based guidelines has been suggested.[65]

In facetogenic pain, diagnostic blocks targeting suspected painful joints can identify sources of lumbar, thoracic, and cervical pain. Medial branch blocks can also aid in the selection of patients who might respond to facet radiofrequency denervation. For LBP, a systematic review[66] of 122 studies, leading to the inclusion of 11 randomized trials and observational studies concluded that the evidence is good for radiofrequency neurotomy and fair to good for lumbar facet joint nerve blocks for short- and long-term improvement. Evidence for intraarticular injections and pulsed radiofrequency neurotomy is limited.

In the cervical region, a systematic review[67] including four randomized trials and six observational studies concluded that evidence for cervical radiofrequency neurotomy and medial branch blocks is fair, and evidence for cervical intraarticular injections with local anesthetic and steroid is limited. However, the study noted a paucity of published literature for cervical facet joint injections. In the thoracic region, there is evidence that the facet joints are responsible pain generators for thoracic pain[68] and that the diagnostic accuracy of controlled facet joint blocks is strong for cervical and lumbar facet joints and moderate for thoracic facet joints.[69]

STEROID MEDICATIONS

OVERVIEW

Corticosteroids are steroid hormones produced in the adrenal cortex, and this class consists of glucocorticoids and mineralocorticoids. Mineralocorticoids, such as aldosterone, are responsible for regulation of electrolyte and fluid balance.[70] Glucocorticoids (named for their modulation of the metabolism of carbohydrates) exert their action via the glucocorticoid receptor (GR).[71]

With respect to their use in pain management, corticosteroids can be compared pharmacologically with focus on each medication's mineralocorticoid and glucocorticoid potency, duration of action, and particulate size.

Glucocorticoids have been useful in the treatment of inflammatory diseases for more than 50 years, but their usefulness has been limited by complications and side effects. These include, but are not limited to, suppression of the hypothalamic–pituitary–adrenal (HPA) axis and the immune system, exacerbation of diabetes, hypertension, and osteoporosis.[72-78] Pharmacologic research has focused on modifying the chemical structure of glucocorticoids in hopes of increasing their potency while decreasing the likelihood of side effects. The separation of anti-inflammatory activity from the systemic side effects of glucocorticoids has been difficult. The anti-inflammatory potency of steroids is related to the GR binding affinity.[79] While steroid preparations are typically injected in proximity to regions of inflammation, they cross into the systemic circulation and affect every major organ system in the body.[80]

STEROID MECHANISM OF ACTION

The mechanism of action of the glucocorticoids is complex but in part involves the inhibition of phospholipase A2 activity with a resulting reduction in the release of arachidonic acid from membrane phospholipids.[81] Arachidonic acid is the precursor for the synthesis of eicosanoids (including prostaglandins, thromboxanes, leukotrienes, and lipoxins), which mediate a wide range of inflammatory responses. Additionally, methylprednisolone has been shown in the rat to suppress transmission in thin unmyelinated C-fibers but not in myelinated A-β fibers, suggesting a direct membrane effect of the steroid per se.[82] Thus, inhibiting phospholipase A2 reduces the presence of inflammatory mediators, some of which cause hyperalgesia,[83] edema, and decreased blood flow.

STEROID PREPARATIONS USED FOR INJECTIONS

Although adverse events relating to neuraxially administered steroid medications are rare, their severity, especially with regard to brain and spinal cord infarction with regard to transforaminal administration, has prompted numerous reviews.[84] Studies have investigated particulate size, route of administration, and the use of sedation because embolic phenomena have resulted in spinal cord injuries, stroke, and deaths.[85-89] Etiologies for the sequelae have been postulated to include embolic infarction secondary to particulate injection into an arterial vessel; direct vascular injury causing spasm, trauma, or compression; or neurotoxicity from medications injected or the vehicle or additives to the preparation.[90]

Corticosteroids used for injection that are commercially available in the United States can be categorized as soluble, insoluble, or a combination of both. Insoluble corticosteroid preparations (methylprednisolone, triamcinolone) are typically corticosteroid esters and offer theoretical advantages in their longer duration of action because they require hydrolysis by cellular esterases for the active steroid moiety to be released.[91] Additionally, preparations of insoluble crystalline powder in aqueous suspensions are less likely to be absorbed soon after injection in comparison with soluble preparations.[92] Soluble steroid preparations (dexamethasone, betamethasone) are taken up rapidly by cells and have a quicker onset but reduced duration of action.[93] Betamethasone is unique in its availability as a water-soluble ester, betamethasone sodium phosphate, or as the practically water-insoluble salt, betamethasone phosphate. One formulation containing both betamethasone ester and salt (Celestone Soluspan; Schering, Kenilworth, NJ) may offer both a rapid onset and longer duration of action.

There are substantial variations in the size of the crystals found in insoluble corticosteroid preparations, and this has been demonstrated in numerous in vitro studies.[94-98] Ester corticosteroid preparations tend to contain larger particulate sizes, and because of variations in crystal concentrations and physical characteristics and with mixture with other injected medications or with plasma,[99] crystals may aggregate into larger particles. This phenomenon is of extreme importance given the potential for these particles, injected intravascularly, to cause distal embolization and tissue injury.

STEROID PARTICULATE SIZE AND MECHANISMS FOR SERIOUS ADVERSE EVENTS

Infarction of central nervous system (CNS) tissue has been postulated to be secondary to embolic occlusion by particulate steroid.[100-102] Particulate size may influence the degree of arterial occlusion and size and variability of particles in the injectate have been investigated,[103-106] as well as their dilution or mixture with other medications.[107] In comparison to the red blood cell, particles larger than the lumen of an arteriole may occlude arterioles, however collateral blood supply may decrease the likelihood of tissue damage.[108,109]

Particles smaller than an arteriole but greater than the size of a red blood cell may occlude terminal arterial vessels and cause infarction. The diameter of an arteriole ranges from 100 to 500 μm, and that of vertebral arteries ranges from 600 to 2600 μm. The size of corticosteroid ester particles can exceed 500 μm, and particles can aggregate or precipitate in the vascular space or in blood to form larger particles.

Use of nonparticulate steroid preparations (pure betamethasone, dexamethasone) may decrease the risk of embolic phenomena and may strengthen the postulate that embolic occlusion is the source of CNS damage. Ongoing investigations are looking at the incidence and clinical presentations of major complications associated with cervical transforaminal epidural steroid injections to make evidence-based recommendations.[110] Based on animal studies of the serious CNS sequelae after injection of insoluble methylprednisolone acetate versus no noticeable deficits after the injection of soluble dexamethasone phosphate,[111] MacMahon et al. suggest no longer performing transforaminal epidural steroid injections in the cervical, thoracic, or lumbar regions with insoluble corticosteroid preparations and believe that this reduces, if not removes, the risk of CNS embolization during the procedure.[112]

Additionally, two case reports describe significant CNS injury (bilateral lower extremity paralysis with neurogenic bowel and bladder) after a fluoroscopically guided (left L3–L4) lumbar transforaminal epidural steroid injection with betamethasone and a computed tomography–guided (right L3–L4) transforaminal injection of methylprednisolone, with MR images consistent with spinal cord infarction without evidence of intraspinal mass or hematoma.[113] In each of these cases, the use of particulate corticosteroid with embolization in a radicular artery is asserted as a likely mechanism of injury, and statements discuss reducing or eliminating this risk by the utilization of particulate-free steroids and testing for intraarterial injection with digital subtraction angiography and a preliminary injection of local anesthetic.

An alternative mechanism of injury suggests retrograde flow into a common arterial trunk with subsequent antegrade flow into vulnerable arteries and should be considered as a possible mechanism by which spinal cord or brain injury may occur.[114] Spinal cord infarction has also been reported after a (right L2–L3) transforaminal epidural steroid injection with spinal angiography demonstrating occlusion of the right L2 segmental artery with reconstitution of the radicular branch from collaterals. The artery of Adamkiewicz was presumably occluded by steroid injection.[115]

Numerous case reports and reviews describe and attempt to quantify both minor and devastating neurologic complications of epidural steroid injections and their mechanisms. Although embolic phenomena may be responsible for tissue infarction, direct injury to the vessel may also be problematic. Perineural hematoma after lumbar transforaminal steroid injection was described in a case report and demonstrated by MRI after the observation of progressive motor and sensory loss.[116] Although digital subtraction angiography (DSA) has been suggested as an adjunct to aid in the identification of vascular compromise during interventional neuraxial procedures, irreversible paraplegia was reported after a lumbar transforaminal epidural steroid injection despite the administration of a local anesthetic test dose and the use of DSA.[117]

Suggestions made from this case report include the use of blunt or larger bevel needles in place of sharp, cutting needles and the consideration of eliminating the use of particular steroids for transforaminal epidural steroid injections. In contrast, however, despite the use of an atraumatic pencil-point needle, simultaneous epidural and radicular artery spread were observed fluoroscopically during a cervical transforaminal corticosteroid injection using a 25-gauge Whitacre spinal needle,[118] although no complications were associated with the procedure.

An additional study comparing the use of sharp versus blunt tip needles in transforaminal epidural steroid injections[119] showed a statistically significantly higher incidence of vascular penetration with the sharp tip but no statistical difference with respect to the occurrence of paresthesias, dural puncture, and headache. The authors concluded that blunt needles seem to be more advantageous.

An additional case report describes the subdural spread of local anesthetic in a selective transforaminal cervical nerve root block, after which transient flaccid paralysis developed.[120] This underscores the risk of serious complication and the need for emergency airway management, ventilation, and cardiovascular support.

Although many serious reported adverse outcomes involve the transforaminal injections of local anesthetics and corticosteroids, a case report describes paraplegia after a low lumbar epidural steroid injection via the interlaminar route.[121] Although the mechanism was unclear, theories suggested ischemia caused by accidental interruption of the medullary blood supply by direct damage to a medullary artery, arterial spasm, or corticosteroid-induced occlusion caused by undetected intra-arterial injection.

A prospective evaluation[122] of more than 10,000 fluoroscopically guided epidural procedures of the cervical, thoracic, and lumbar spine via interlaminar, transforaminal, and caudal approaches and including percutaneous adhesiolysis procedures reported overall event rates of intravascular penetration of 4.3%; dural puncture of 0.5%, with post-dural puncture headache of 0.05%; and transient nerve root irritation and transient spinal cord irritation of 0.08%. The infection and abscess rates were both 0.0%, and there were no major complications.

ROUTE OF ADMINISTRATION

Because there are different routes to administer steroid medications, studies have attempted to evaluate and compare outcomes based on variables. These include the medications and their dosages; their timing in relation to the onset of symptoms; their frequencies; the routes and methods of administration (transforaminal, interlaminar, caudal) and condition treated (LBP, radicular pain), and cause (disc herniation, spinal stenosis). Evidence of the efficacy of lumbar epidural steroid injections is difficult to summarize.[123]

Of the available approaches to access the lumbar epidural space, the interlaminar approach is the most commonly used versus the transforaminal and caudal approach,[124-126] and blind or nonimage-guided interlaminar approaches do not represent contemporary interventional pain management practice.[127] The transforaminal approach offers an advantage of selectivity and can provide valuable diagnostic information in the treatment of radiculopathy to identify symptomatic nerve roots.[128] Numerous studies summarized in a recent, comprehensive evidence-based review of epidural steroid injections[129] support the general consensus by pain management practitioners that the transforaminal approach is superior to the interlaminar or caudal approaches. Previous surgical interventions, the presence of surgical hardware, or particular spinal anatomy may preclude one approach or favor another.

Caudal epidural steroid injections may offer alternative anatomic approaches to treating LBP and sciatica and may be less technically demanding to perform.[130]

INFECTION

Although generally considered safe and performed under strict aseptic conditions, the potential for infection after spinal injections exists and can lead to devastating consequences. Infections resulting from spinal injections have been considered rare. Overall infection rates have been reported to occur in 1% to 2% of spinal injections, and severe infections have been reported with an incidence of 0.01% to 0.1% of all spinal injections.[131] Causes may be bacterial, including the most common organism being *Staphylococcus aureus*, introduced via the skin through needle puncture, usually because of poor sterile technique.[132] Gram-negative infections may occur theoretically secondary to needle penetration into the intestine or the pelvic cavity,[133] which may occur most easily anatomically via S1 to S2 transforaminal injections.[134]

Pyogenic arthritis of the spinal facet joint, although rare, has been reported after intraarticular steroid injections[135] and can lead to epidural and paraspinal abscess formation.[136] Vertebral osteomyelitis has been reported in an immunocompromised diabetic male patient after lumbar epidural steroid injections.[137]

Fungal infections have also been reported and have been brought to light after recent outbreaks. In 2002, two occurrences of *Exophiala* meningitis, one leading to death, after epidural injections of methylprednisolone acetate prepared by a compounding pharmacy after the medication became difficult to obtain from the manufacturer; unopened vials from this pharmacy were analyzed by the Centers for Disease Control and Prevention.[138] Similarly, in 2012, an investigation of fungal infections associated with the injection of preservative-free methylprednisolone purchased from a compounding pharmacy in Massachusetts led to the discovery of fungal contamination from unopened vials. In April 2013, a Subcommittee on Oversight and Investigations reported a total of 733 cases of fungal meningitis and 53 deaths as a result of this contamination.

The potential effects of epidural glucocorticoid injections in modulating the immune system are not well described,[139] and data show that prolonged high-dose systemic glucocorticoid therapy for immunosuppression is a risk factor for invasive aspergillosis.[140]

STEROID-RELATED SIDE EFFECTS

Despite the therapeutic anti-inflammatory effects of corticosteroid therapy, their use can lead to obesity, diabetes, osteoporosis, insulin resistance, hyperglycemia, hyperlipidemia,[141] dermatologic conditions, peptic ulcer formation, and Cushing's syndrome.[142] The mechanisms underlying the side effects of short- or long-term use of steroid medications are complex; certain side effects are mediated via transactivation (e.g., diabetes, glaucoma), transrepression (e.g., suppression of the HPA axis), or both (e.g., osteoporosis).[143]

Side effects from intraarticular and epidural steroid injections may be underrecognized, and symptoms arising from the systemic absorption of steroids, such as a hormonal profile suggestive of hypopituitarism or Cushing's syndrome, may divert historical investigation of the iatrogenic cause, leading to expensive investigation, false diagnoses, and unnecessary treatment.[144]

Some side effects from chronic steroid therapy have direct implications in the differentiation of symptoms of LBP, radiculopathy, or paraparesis, as described in a case report of chronic steroid therapy–induced spinal epidural lipomatosis with MRI findings of accumulations of fatty deposits in the spinal canal not resolving with surgical intervention.[145] Neuropsychiatric effects of glucocorticoids range in scope, including the most severe psychotic symptoms designated as steroid psychosis,[146] can occur rapidly after exposure even to low doses from oral, epidural, or intraarticular administration.[147] Identifying patients at risk for steroid psychosis can be difficult because the neuropsychiatric effects of glucocorticoids are unpredictable.

Factors to consider in the evaluation of changes in mental status in the pain management setting include the current or recent use of steroids for pain or non–pain-related conditions, the dosage (including the timing and frequency and cumulative quantity of steroid), the presence of preexisting neuropsychiatric conditions, and a history of previous adverse reactions to steroid administrations.

Other studies have investigated the role of administrations of corticosteroid on glucose metabolism. Studies have shown that glucose metabolism can be disturbed in nondiabetic and diabetic patients after *intraarticular* injections of corticosteroids[148,149] secondary to the diffusion of medication into the systemic circulation. The degree of systemic absorption varies based on the degree of inflammation within the joint and the solubility and dosage of the injected steroid.[150]

Single-session intraarticular injections of methylprednisolone have been shown to cause impaired adrenocorticortical reserve, with most patients recovering after 1 to 2 weeks.[151] A recent study compared the effect of intraarticular versus epidural steroid injection in patients with diabetes and the diffusion of steroid in the two procedures.[152] The glycemic profile remained unchanged after epidural administration versus an increase in blood glucose in the 2 days after intraarticular injections of 80 mg of methylprednisolone. The study suggests that methylprednisolone injected epidurally remains mostly local.

In contrast, a prospective cohort study showed that epidural steroid injections caused a significant increase in blood glucose levels in patients with diabetes without correlation between preinjection blood glucose control represented by Hgb A1C levels.[153] Documentation of previous responses of blood glucose levels after epidural steroid injections may help to adjust changes in blood glucose monitoring regimen in the immediate postinjection period.

ANTICOAGULATION AND NEURAXIAL INJECTIONS

Performing diagnostic and therapeutic neuraxial injections carries the risk of iatrogenic hemorrhagic complications, although the actual incidence of neurologic dysfunction from these complications is unknown.[154] The incidence of these complications is rare, Horlocker and Wedel report it as less than one per 150,000 in epidurals and one per 220,000 for spinal anesthetics,[155] the incidence may be increasing and may be as high as one per 12,000 in epidurals for chronic pain relief.[156] Given the potential consequences of compressive hematomas, a great deal of effort has been made to understand the incidence, and much information has been gathered from the historical analysis of spinal and epidural injections, including catheter insertions, for the initiation and maintenance of regional anesthesia[157-160] and more recently through the investigation of complications occurring as a result of pain management–related neuraxial injections.[161,162] The potential for bleeding and hematoma formation can result from damage to vessels by the injection needle, either at the time of or after the injection. Although the use of contrast during fluoroscopy can help to identify intravascular needle placement, situations in which a vessel had been pierced before the injection of contrast would not be visualized.

The likelihood of bleeding and hematoma formation increases with primary coagulopathy and conditions associated with coagulopathy, such as liver disease, and in patients taking medications with anticoagulant properties. Factors predictive of difficulty in the performance of neuraxial blocks, such as anatomic variations, morbid obesity, prior spinal surgery, the presence of spinal hardware, severe degenerative change, or previous unsuccessful attempts, may influence the decision to perform neuraxial blocks. The risks associated with performing neuraxial procedures in patients receiving medications that affect components of the clotting system must be considered on an individual basis; factors to be considered include the consequences of temporary discontinuation of anticoagulants. As new medications with anticoagulant properties emerge, it is imperative that a careful review of these medications is performed before each neuraxial procedure. In contrast to the performance of neuraxial anesthesia for patients undergoing nonelective surgical procedures, the pain management clinic must facilitate all aspects of periprocedural care to optimize chances for success and minimize risk. Guidelines for performing spinal procedures in patients taking anticoagulants have been established by the American Society of Regional Anesthesia,[163] and specific recommendations regarding the time after discontinuing specific medications before neuraxial procedures are available.[164]

Just as important as optimizing coagulation status is recognizing signs of compressive hematoma. Neurologic changes that occur after neuraxial procedures must be investigated immediately. In the pain management setting, where neurologic deficits are common, documentation of baseline neurologic function is critical to compare postprocedure outcomes, and spinal imaging as soon as possible is vital in the differential diagnosis of neurologic changes. Neurosurgical consultation can help to assess the role of decompressive surgery as soon as possible.

Because neurologic outcome is linked to early diagnosis and intervention, it is critical to obtain radiographic imaging, preferably MRI, as soon as possible. Consultation with a neurosurgeon should also occur as soon as possible to determine the urgency of surgery.

REFERENCES

1. Manchikanti L, Pampati V, Falco FJ, Hirsch JA. Growth of spinal interventional pain management techniques: analysis of utilization trends and Medicare expenditures 2000 to 2008. *Spine*. 2013;38(2):157-168.
2. De Pasquier M, Leri M. Injections intra et extra-durales de cocaine a dose minime dans le traitement de la sciatique. Valeur comparee des deux methods: resultats immediats et tardifs. *Bull Gen Ther*. 1901;142:196-223.
3. Sicard MA. Les injections medicamenteuse extraduraqles per voie saracoccygiene. *Comptes Renues des Senances de la Societe de Biolgie et de ses Filliales*. 1901;53:396-398.
4. Cathelin MF. Mode d'action de la cocaine injectee dans l'espace epidural par le procede du canal sacre. *CR Soc Biol (Paris)*. 1901;53:478-479.
5. Manchikanti L. Role of neuraxial steroids in interventional pain management. *Pain Physician*. 2002;5(2):182-199.
6. Caussade G, Queste P. Traitement de al neuralgie sciatique par la mèthode de Sicard. Rèsultats favorables même dans les cas chroniues par la cocaïne à doses élevées et répétées à intervalles raproches. *Bull Soc Med Hosp Paris*. 1909; 28:865.
7. Viner N. Intractable sciatica: the sacral epidural injection: an effective method of giving relief. *Can Med Assoc J*. 1925;15: 630-634.
8. Evans W. Intrasacral epidural injection in the treatment of sciatica. *Lancet*. 1930;16:1225-1228.
9. Mason HL, Myers CS, Kendall EC. The chemistry of crystalline substances isolated from the suprarenal gland. *J Biol Chem*. 1936;114:613-631.
10. Mason HL, Myers CS, Kendall EC. Chemical studies of the suprarenal cortex II. The definition of a substance which possesses the qualitative action of Cortin; its conversion into a diketone closely related to androstenedione. *J Biol Chem*. 1936;116:267-276.
11. Hench PS, Kendall EC, Slocumb CH, et al. The effect of a hormone of the adrenal cortex (17-hydroxy-11-dehydrocorticosterone: compound E) and of pituitary adrenocorticotropic hormone on rheumatoid arthritis; preliminary report. *Proc Staff Meet Mayo Clin*. 1949;24:181-197.
12. Hench PS, Kendall EC, Slocumb CH, et al. Effects of cortisone acetate and pituitary ACTH on rheumatoid arthritis, rheumatic fever and certain other conditions. *Arch Intern Med*. 1950;85:545-566.
13. Hollander JL. The local effects of compound F (hydrocortisone) injected into joints. *Bull Rheum Dis*. 1951;2:3-4.
14. Gifford RH. Corticosteroid therapy for rheumatoid arthritis. *Med Clin North Am*. 1973;57:1179-1189.
15. Wilkens RF, Dahl SL. *Therapeutic Controversies in the Rheumatic Diseases*. Orlando: Grune and Stratton; 1987:72-78.
16. Maddison PJ, Isenberg DA, Woo P, et al. *Oxford Textbook of Rheumatology*. Oxford: Oxford University Press; 1993:334-336.
17. McCarty DJ, Koopman WJ. *Arthritis and Allied Conditions. A Textbook of Rheumatology*. Philadelphia: Lea and Febiger; 1993:715-718.
18. Schimmer BP, Parker KL. Adrenocorticotropic hormone; adrenocortical steroids and their synthetic analogs; inhibitory of the synthesis and actions of adrenocortical hormones. In: Hardman JG, Limbird LE, eds. *Goodman and Gilman's The Pharmacological Basis of Therapeutics*. 9th ed. New York: McGraw-Hill; 1996: 1459-1479.
19. Wilder RL. Corticosteroids. In: Kooperman WJ, ed. *Arthritis and Allied Conditions*. 13th ed. Baltimore: Williams and Wilkins; 1997:731-747.
20. Nelson DA, Landau WM. Intraspinal steroids: history, efficacy, accidentality, and controversy with review of United States Food and Drug Administration reports. *J Neurol Neurosurg Psychiatry*. 2001;70:433-443.
21. Jacobsen L, Mariano A, Chabal C, et al. Beyond the needle. Expanding the role of anesthesiologist in the management of chronic non-malignant pain. *Anesthesiology*. 1997;87:1210-1218.
22. Ruben JE. Experience with a pain clinic. *Anesthesiology*. 1951; 5:574-582.
23. Benoist M, Boulu P, Hayem G. Epidural steroid injections in the management of low-back pain with radiculopathy: an update of their efficacy and safety. *Eur Spine J*. 2012;21(2):204-213.

24. Robechhi A, Capra R, L'idrocortisone. Prime esperienze cliniche in campo reumatologico. *Minerva Med.* 1952; 98:1259-1263.
25. Lievre JA, Block-Michel H, Pean G, et al. L'hydrocortisone en injection locale. *Rev Rhumat Mal Osteoartic.* 1953; 20:310-311.
26. Boswell MV, Trescot AM, Datta S, et al. Interventional techniques: evidence-based practice guidelines in the management of chronic spinal pain. *Pain Physician.* 2007;10(1):7-111.
27. McLain RF, Kapural L, Mekhail NA. Epidural steroids for back and leg pain: mechanism of action and efficacy. *Cleve Clin J Med.* 2004;71(12):961-970.
28. Manchikanti L. The growth of interventional pain management in the new millennium: a critical analysis of utilization in the Medicare population. *Pain Physician.* 2004;7:465-482.
29. Gharibo C, Koo C, Chung J, et al. Epidural steroid injections: an update on mechanisms of injury and safety. *Tech Reg Anesth Pain Manag.* 2009;13:266-271.
30. Lindblom K, Rexed B. Spinal nerve injury in dorsolateral protrusions of lumbar disks. *J Neurosurg.* 1948;5:413-432.
31. McRae DL. Asymptomatic intervertebral disc protrusions. *Acta Radiol.* 1956; 46:9-27.
32. Hitselberger WE, Witten RM. Abnormal myelograms in asymptomatic patients. *J Neurosurg.* 1968; 28:204-206.
33. Boden SD, Davis DO, Dina TS, et al. Abnormal magnetic resonance scans of the lumbar spine in asymptomatic subjects. *J Bone Joint Surg.* 1990;72A:403-408.
34. Howe JF, Loeser JD, Calvin WH. Mechanosensitivity of dorsal root ganglia and chronically injured axons: a physiological basis for the radicular pain of nerve root compression. *Pain.* 1977;3: 25-41.
35. Byun WM, Ahn SH, Ahn MW. Significance of perianular enhancement associated with anular tears on magnetic resonance imaging in diagnosis of radiculopathy. *Spine.* 2008;33(22):2440-2443.
36. Dudli S, Haschtmann D, Ferguson SJ. Fracture of the vertebral endplates, but not equienergetic impact load, promotes disc degeneration in vitro. *J Orthop Res.* 2012;30:809-816.
37. Ozawa T, Ohtori S, Inoue G, et al. The degenerated lumbar intervertebral disc is innervated primarily by peptide-containing sensory nerve fibers in humans. *Spine.* 2006;31(21):2418-2422.
38. Murphy RW. Nerve roots and spinal nerves in degenerative disc disease. *Clin Orthop.* 1977;129:46-60.
39. Ozawa T, Ohtori S, Inoue G, et al. The degenerated lumbar intervertebral disc is innervated primarily by peptide-containing sensory nerve fibers in humans. *Spine.* 2006;31(21):2418-2422.
40. Berg A. Clinical and myelographic studies of conservatively treated cases of lumbar intervertebral disc protrusion. *Acta Chir Scand.* 1953;104:124-129.
41. Green LN. Dexamethasone in the management of symptoms due to herniated lumbar disc. *J Neurol Neurosurg Psychiatry.* 1975; 38: 1211-1217.
42. Saal JS, Franson RC, Dobrow R, et al. High levels of inflammatory phospholipase A2 activity in lumbar disc herniations. *Spine.* 1990;15:674-678.
43. Weinstein JN, Claverie W, Gibson S. The pain of discography. *Spine.* 1988;13:1344-1348.
44. Bogduk N. The innervation of the lumbar spine. *Spine.* 1983; 8:286-293.
45. Olmarker K, Rydevik B. Disc herniation and sciatica: the basic science platform. In: Gunzburg R, Szpalski M, eds. *Lumbar Disc Herniation.* Philadelphia: Lippincott Williams and Wilkins; 2002.
46. Benoist M, Boulu P, Hayem G. Epidural steroid injections in the management of low-back pain with radiculopathy: an update of their efficacy and safety. *Eur Spine J.* 2012;21(2):204-213.
47. DiRosa M, Calignano A, Carnuccio R, et al. Multiple control of inflammation by glucocorticoids. *Agents Action.* 1985; 17: 284-289.
48. Cronstein BN, Kimmel SC, Levin RI, et al. A mechanism for the anti-inflammatory effects of corticosteroids: the glucocorticoid receptor regulates leukocyte adhesion to endothelial cells and expression of endothelial-leukocyte adhesion molecule-1 and intercellular adhesion molecule-1. *Proc Natl Acad Sci USA.* 1992; 89:9991-9995.
49. Benyamin RM, Manchikanti L, Parr AT, et al. The effectiveness of lumbar interlaminar epidural injections in managing chronic low back and lower extremity pain. *Pain Physician.* 2012;15(4): E363-E404.
50. Wald JT, Maus TP, Geske JR, et al. Immediate pain response does not predict long-term outcome of ct-guided cervical transforaminal epidural steroid injections. *AJNR.* 2013;34(8):1665-1668.
51. Benyamin RM, Wang VC, Vallejo R, et al. A systematic evaluation of thoracic interlaminar epidural injections. *Pain Physician.* 2012;15(4):E497-E514.
52. Whynes DK, McCahon RA, Ravenscroft A, Hardman J. Cost effectiveness of epidural steroid injections to manage chronic lower back pain. *BMC Anesthesiol.* 2012;12(1):26.
53. Cohen SP, Bicket MC, Jamison D, et al. Epidural steroids: a comprehensive, evidence-based review. *Reg Anesth Pain Med.* 2013;38(3):175-200.
54. Benoist M, Boulu P, Hayem G. Epidural steroid injections in the management of low-back pain with radiculopathy: an update of their efficacy and safety. *Eur Spine J.* 2012;21(2):204-213.
55. Iversen T, Solberg TK, Romner B, et al. Effect of caudal epidural steroid or saline injection in chronic lumbar radiculopathy: multicentre, blinded, randomised controlled trial. *BMJ.* 2011;343:d5278.
56. Gelalis ID, Arnaoutoglou E, Pakos EE, et al. Effect of interlaminar epidural steroid injection in acute and subacute pain due to lumbar disk herniation: a randomized comparison of 2 different protocols. *Open Orthop J.* 2009;3:121-124.
57. Huston CW. Cervical epidural steroid injections in the management of cervical radiculitis: interlaminar versus transforaminal. A review. *Curr Rev Musculoskelet Med.* 2009;2(1):30-42.
58. Valat JP, Giraudeau B, Rozenberg S, et al. Epidural corticosteroid injections for sciatica: a randomised, double blind, controlled clinical trial. *Ann Rheum Dis.* 2003;62(7):639-643.
59. Goldthwaite GE. The lumbosacral articulation: An explanation of many cases of lumbago sciatica and paraplegia. *Boston Med Surg J.* 1911; 164:365-372.
60. Ghormley RK. Low back pain with special reference to the articular facets, with presentation of an operative procedure. *JAMA.* 1933; 101:1773-1777.
61. Mooney V, Robertson J. The facet syndrome. *Clin Orthop.* 1976; 115:149-156.
62. Cavanaugh JM, Lu Y, Chen C, Kallakuri S. Pain generation in lumbar and cervical facet joints. *J Bone Joint Surg Am.* 2006;88(Suppl 2): 63-67.
63. Falco FJ, Manchikanti L, Datta S, et al. An update of the effectiveness of therapeutic lumbar facet joint interventions. *Pain Physician.* 2012;15(6):E909-E953.
64. Falco FJ, Datta S, Manchikanti L, et al. An updated review of the diagnostic utility of cervical facet joint injections. *Pain Physician.* 2012;15(6):E807-E838.

65. Manchikanti L, Helm S, Singh V, et al. An algorithmic approach for clinical management of chronic spinal pain. *Pain Physician.* 2009;12(4):E225-E264.
66. Falco FJ, Manchikanti L, Datta S, et al. An update of the effectiveness of therapeutic lumbar facet joint interventions. *Pain Physician.* 2012;15(6):E909-E953.
67. Falco FJ, Manchikanti L, Datta S, et al. Systematic review of the therapeutic effectiveness of cervical facet joint interventions: an update. *Pain Physician.* 2012;15(6):E839-E868.
68. Manchikanti L, Singh V, Pampati V, et al. Evaluation of the prevalence of facet joint pain in chronic thoracic pain. *Pain Physician.* 2002;5(4):354-359.
69. Sehgal N, Shah RV, McKenzie-Brown AM, Everett CR. Diagnostic utility of facet (zygapophysial) joint injections in chronic spinal pain: a systematic review of evidence. *Pain Physician.* 2005; 8(2):211-224.
70. Pippal JB, Fuller PJ. Structure-function relationships in the mineralocorticoid receptor. *J Mol Endocrinol.* 2008;41(6):405-413.
71. Oakley RH, Cidlowski JA. Cellular processing of the glucocorticoid receptor gene and protein: new mechanisms for generating tissue-specific actions of glucocorticoids. *J Biol Chem.* 2011;286(5): 3177-3184.
72. Khalil MA, Kwon T, Lee HJ. *Curr Topic Med Chem.* 1993;1:173.
73. Avery MA, Woolfrey JR. *Medicinal Chemistry and Drug Discovery.* New York: John Wiley & Sons; 1997:281.
74. Timofeevski SL, Panarin EF, Vinogradov OL, Nezhentsev MV. Anti-inflammatory and antishock water-soluble polyesters of glucocorticoids with low level systemic toxicity. *Pharm Res.* 1996;13(3):476-480.
75. Rosen J, Miner JN. The search for safer glucocorticoid receptor ligands. *Endocr Rev.* 2005;26(3):452-464.
76. Martin-Du Pan RC, Vonlanthen MC, Dubuis JM. [Growth and collagen synthesis disorders in asthmatic children treated with inhaled steroids]. *Rev Med Suisse Romande.* 1999;119(6): 475-479.
77. Lipworth BJ. Systemic adverse effects of inhaled corticosteroid therapy: a systematic review and meta-analysis. *Arch Intern Med.* 1999;159(9):941-955.
78. Geddes DM. Inhaled corticosteroids: benefits and risks. *Thorax.* 1992;47(6):404-407.
79. Khan MO, Lee HJ. Synthesis and pharmacology of anti-inflammatory steroidal antedrugs. *Chem Rev.* 2008;108(12): 5131-5145.
80. Lansang MC, Farmer T, Kennedy L. Diagnosing the unrecognized systemic absorption of intra-articular and epidural steroid injections. *Endocr Pract.* 2009;15(3):225-228.
81. Di Rosa M, Calignano A, Carnuccio R, et al. Multiple control of inflammation by glucocorticoids. *Agents Actions.* 1986;17(3-4): 284-289.
82. Johansson A, Hao J, Sjölund B. Local corticosteroid application blocks transmission in normal nociceptive C-fibres. *Acta Anaesthesiol Scand.* 1990;34(5):335-338.
83. Gonzales R, Goldyne ME, Taiwo YO, Levine JD. Production of hyperalgesic prostaglandins by sympathetic postganglionic neurons. *J Neurochem.* 1989;53(5):1595-1598.
84. MacMahon PJ, Shelly MJ, Scholz D, et al. Injectable corticosteroid preparations: an embolic risk assessment by static and dynamic microscopic analysis. *AJNR.* 2011;32(10):1830-1835.
85. McMillan MR, Crumpton C. Cortical blindness and neurologic injury complicating cervical transforaminal injection for cervical radiculopathy. *Anesthesiology.* 2003;99:509-511.
86. Rozin L, Rozin R, Koehler SA, et al. Death during a transforaminal epidural steroid nerve root block(C7) due to perforation of the left vertebral artery. *Am J Forensic Med Path.* 2003;24:351-355.
87. Tiso RL, Cutler T, Catania JA, Whalen K. Adverse central nervous system sequelae after selective transforaminal block: the role of corticosteroids. *Spine J.* 2004;4:468-474.
88. Brouwers PJAM, Kottnik EJBL, Simon MAM, Prevo RL. A cervical anterior spinal artery syndrome after diagnostic blockade of the right C6-nerve root. *Pain.* 2001;91:397-399.
89. Baker R, Dreyfuss P, Mercer S, Bogduk N. Cervical transforaminal injection of corticosteroids into a radicular artery: a possible mechanism for spinal cord injury. *Pain.* 2003;103:211-215.
90. MacMahon PJ, Shelly MJ, Scholz D, et al. Injectable corticosteroid preparations: an embolic risk assessment by static and dynamic microscopic analysis. *AJNR.* 2011;32(10):1830-1835.
91. MacMahon PJ, Shelly MJ, Scholz D, et al. Injectable corticosteroid preparations: an embolic risk assessment by static and dynamic microscopic analysis. *AJNR.* 2011;32(10):1830-1835.
92. Cole BJ, Schumacher HR. Injectable corticosteroids in modern practice. *J Am Acad Orthop Surg.* 2005;13(1):37-46.
93. MacMahon PJ, Eustace SJ, Kavanagh EC. Injectable corticosteroid and local anesthetic preparations: a review for radiologists. *Radiology.* 2009;252(3):647-661.
94. Tiso RL, Cutler T, Catania JA, Whalen K. Adverse central nervous system sequelae after selective transforaminal block: the role of corticosteroids. *Spine J.* 2004;4(4):468-474.
95. Benzon HT, Chew TL, McCarthy RJ, et al. Comparison of the particle sizes of different steroids and the effect of dilution: a review of the relative neurotoxicities of the steroids. *Anesthesiology.* 2007;106(2):331-338.
96. Gazelka HM, Burgher AH, Huntoon MA, et al. Determination of the particulate size and aggregation of clonidine and corticosteroids for epidural steroid injection. *Pain Physician.* 2012;15(1): 87-93.
97. Derby R, Lee SH, Date ES, et al. Size and aggregation of corticosteroids used for epidural injections. *Pain Med.* 2008;9(2): 227-234.
98. Francis BA, Chang EL, Haik BG. Particle size and drug interactions of injectable corticosteroids used in ophthalmic practice. *Ophthalmology.* 1996;103(11):1884-1888.
99. MacMahon PJ, Shelly MJ, Scholz D, et al. Injectable corticosteroid preparations: an embolic risk assessment by static and dynamic microscopic analysis. *AJNR.* 2011;32(10):1830-1835.
100. Rathmell JP, Aprill C, Bogduk N. Cervical transforaminal injection of steroids. *Anesthesiology.* 2004;100:1595-1600.
101. Baker R, Dreyfuss P, Mercer S, Bogduk N. Cervical transforaminal injection of corticosteroids into a radicular artery: a possible mechanism for spinal cord injury. *Pain.* 2003;103:211-215.
102. McMillan MR, Crumpton C. Cortical blindness and neurologic injury complicating cervical transforaminal injection for cervical radiculopathy. *Anesthesiology.* 2003;99:509-511.
103. Lee JW, Park KW, Chung SK, et al. Cervical transforaminal epidural steroid injection for the management of cervical radiculopathy: a comparative study of particulate versus non-particulate steroids. *Skeletal Radiol.* 2009;38(11):1077-1082.
104. Bainbridge JS. Betamethasone: friend (soluble), foe (particulate), or either?. *Pain Med.* 2009;10(2):420.
105. Derby R, Lee SH, Date ES, et al. Size and aggregation of corticosteroids used for epidural injections. *Pain Med.* 2008; 9(2):227-234.

106. Benzon HT, Chew TL, McCarthy RJ, et al. Comparison of the particle sizes of different steroids and the effect of dilution: a review of the relative neurotoxicities of the steroids. *Anesthesiology.* 2007;106(2):331-338.

107. Gazelka HM, Burgher AH, Huntoon MA, et al. Determination of the particulate size and aggregation of clonidine and corticosteroids for epidural steroid injection. *Pain Physician.* 2012;15(1):87-93.

108. MacMahon PJ, Eustace SJ, Kavanagh EC. Injectable corticosteroid and local anesthetic preparations: a review for radiologists. *Radiology.* 2009;252(3):647-661.

109. Hurst RW, Rosenwasser RH. *Interventional Neuroradiology.* Boca Raton, FL: CRC; 2007.

110. Benny B, Azari P, Briones D. Complications of cervical transforaminal epidural steroid injections. *Am J Phys Med Rehabil.* 2010;89(7):601-607.

111. Okubadejo GO, Talcott MR, Schmidt RE, et al. Perils of intravascular methylprednisolone injection into the vertebral artery. An animal study. *J Bone Joint Surg Am.* 2008;90(9):1932-1938.

112. MacMahon PJ, Crosbie I, Kavanagh EC. Reducing the risk of spinal cord infarction during transforaminal steroid injections. *AJNR.* 2010;31(3):E32.

113. Kennedy DJ, Dreyfuss P, Aprill CN, Bogduk N. Paraplegia following image-guided transforaminal lumbar spine epidural steroid injection: two case reports. *Pain Med.* 2009;10(8):1389-1394.

114. Yin W, Bogduk N. Retrograde filling of a thoracic spinal artery during transforaminal injection. *Pain Med.* 2009;10(4):689-692.

115. Lyders EM, Morris PP. A case of spinal cord infarction following lumbar transforaminal epidural steroid injection: MR imaging and angiographic findings. *AJNR.* 2009;30(9):1691-1693.

116. Desai MJ, Dua S. Perineural hematoma following lumbar transforaminal steroid injection causing acute-on-chronic lumbar radiculopathy: a case report. *Pain Pract.* 2014;14(3):271-277.

117. Chang Chien GC, Candido KD, Knezevic NN. Digital subtraction angiography does not reliably prevent paraplegia associated with lumbar transforaminal epidural steroid injection. *Pain Physician.* 2012;15(6):515-523.

118. Smuck M, Leung D. Inadvertent injection of a cervical radicular artery using an atraumatic pencil-point needle. *Spine.* 2011;36(3):E220-E223.

119. Özcan U, Şahin Ş, Gurbet A, et al. Comparison of blunt and sharp needles for transforaminal epidural steroid injections. *Agri.* 2012;24(2):85-89.

120. Tofuku K, Koga H, Komiya S. Subdural spread of injected local anesthetic in a selective transforaminal cervical nerve root block: a case report. *J Med Case Rep.* 2012;6(1):142.

121. Thefenne L, Dubecq C, Zing E, et al. A rare case of paraplegia complicating a lumbar epidural infiltration. *Ann Phys Rehabil Med.* 2010;53(9):575-583.

122. Manchikanti L, Malla Y, Wargo BW, et al. A prospective evaluation of complications of 10,000 fluoroscopically directed epidural injections. *Pain Physician.* 2012;15(2):131-140.

123. Rho ME, Tang CT. The efficacy of lumbar epidural steroid injections: transforaminal, interlaminar, and caudal approaches. *Phys Med Rehabil Clin N Am.* 2011;22(1):139-148.

124. Boswell MV, Trescot AM, Datta S, et al. Interventional techniques: evidence-based practice guidelines in the management of chronic spinal pain. *Pain Physician.* 2007;10(1):7-111.

125. Abdi S, Datta S, Trescot AM, et al. Epidural steroids in the management of chronic spinal pain: a systematic review. *Pain Physician.* 2007;10(1):185-212.

126. Bogduk N, Christophidis N, Cherry D. Epidural use of steroids in the management of back pain. Report of working party on epidural use of steroids in the management of back pain. National Health and Medical Research Council. Canberra, Commonwealth of Australia, 1994:1-76.

127. Parr AT, Diwan S, Abdi S. Lumbar interlaminar epidural injections in managing chronic low back and lower extremity pain: a systematic review. *Pain Physician.* 2009;12(1):163-188.

128. Landa J, Kim Y. Outcomes of interlaminar and transforminal spinal injections. *Bull NYU Hosp Jt Dis.* 2012;70(1):6-10.

129. Cohen SP, Bicket MC, Jamison D, et al. Epidural steroids: a comprehensive, evidence-based review. *Reg Anesth Pain Med.* 2013;38(3):175-200.

130. Murakibhavi VG, Khemka AG. Caudal epidural steroid injection: a randomized controlled trial. *Evid Based Spine Care J.* 2011;2(4):19-26.

131. Windsor RE, Storm S, Sugar R. Prevention and management of complications resulting from common spinal injections. *Pain Physician.* 2003;6(4):473-483.

132. Goodman BS, Posecion LW, Mallempati S, Bayazitoglu M. Complications and pitfalls of lumbar interlaminar and transforaminal epidural injections. *Curr Rev Musculoskelet Med.* 2008;1(3-4):212-222.

133. Windsor RE, Storm S, Sugar R. Prevention and management of complications resulting from common spinal injections. *Pain Physician.* 2003;6(4):473-483.

134. Goodman BS, Posecion LW, Mallempati S, Bayazitoglu M. Complications and pitfalls of lumbar interlaminar and transforaminal epidural injections. *Curr Rev Musculoskelet Med.* 2008;1(3-4):212-222.

135. Lee JC, Doh HW, Cho YI, et al. Pyogenic arthritis and paraspinal abscess following facet joint steroid injection: a case report. *J Korean Soc Spine Surg.* 2003;10:196-201.

136. Rhyu KW, Park SE, Ji JH, et al. Pyogenic arthritis of the facet joint with concurrent epidural and paraspinal abscess: a case report. *Asian Spine J.* 2011;5(4):245-249.

137. Simopoulos TT, Kraemer JJ, Glazer P, Bajwa ZH. Vertebral osteomyelitis: a potentially catastrophic outcome after lumbar epidural steroid injection. *Pain Physician.* 2008;11(5):693-697.

138. *Exophiala* infection from contaminated injectable steroids prepared by a compounding pharmacy—United States, July-November 2002. *MMWR Morb Mortal Wkly Rep.* 2002;51(49):1109-1112.

139. Pettit AC, Pugh ME. Index case for the fungal meningitis outbreak, United States. *N Engl J Med.* 2013;368(10):970.

140. Walsh TJ, Anaissie EJ, Denning DW, et al. Treatment of aspergillosis: clinical practice guidelines of the Infectious Diseases Society of America. *Clin Infect Dis.* 2008;46(3):327-360.

141. Ferris HA, Kahn CR. New mechanisms of glucocorticoid-induced insulin resistance: make no bones about it. *J Clin Invest.* 2012;122(11):3854-3857.

142. Benyamin RM, Vallejo R, Kramer J, Rafeyan R. Corticosteroid induced psychosis in the pain management setting. *Pain Physician.* 2008;11(6):917-920.

143. Schäcke H, Döcke WD, Asadullah K. Mechanisms involved in the side effects of glucocorticoids. *Pharmacol Ther.* 2002;96(1):23-43.

144. Lansang MC, Farmer T, Kennedy L. Diagnosing the unrecognized systemic absorption of intra-articular and epidural steroid injections. *Endocr Pract.* 2009;15(3):225-228.

145. Gupta R, Shah M, Reese CM. Steroid induced spinal epidural lipomatosis—case report and review of the literature. *W V Med J.* 2011;107(4):20-22.

146. Dubovsky AN, Arvikar S, Stern TA, Axelrod L. The neuropsychiatric complications of glucocorticoid use: steroid psychosis revisited. *Psychosomatics*. 2012;53(2):103-115.

147. Ross DA, Cetas JS. Steroid psychosis: a review for neurosurgeons. *J Neurooncol*. 2012;109(3):439-447.

148. Uboldi F, Carlo-stella N, Belloli L, et al. Glucose blood levels after intra-articular steroid injection in diabetic and non-diabetic patients. *Clin Rheumatol*. 2009;28(4):491-492.

149. Habib G, Safia A. The effect of intra-articular injection of betamethasone acetate/betamethasone sodium phosphate on blood glucose levels in controlled diabetic patients with symptomatic osteoarthritis of the knee. *Clin Rheumatol*. 2009;28(1):85-87.

150. Habib GS, Bashir M, Jabbour A. Increased blood glucose levels following intra-articular injection of methylprednisolone acetate in patients with controlled diabetes and symptomatic osteoarthritis of the knee. *Ann Rheum Dis*. 2008;67(12):1790-1791.

151. Mader R, Lavi I, Luboshitzky R. Evaluation of the pituitary-adrenal axis function following single intraarticular injection of methylprednisolone. *Arthritis Rheum*. 2005;52(3):924-928.

152. Zufferey P, Bulliard C, Gremion G, et al. Systemic effects of epidural methylprednisolone injection on glucose tolerance in diabetic patients. *BMC Res Notes*. 2011;4:552.

153. Even JL, Crosby CG, Song Y, et al. Effects of epidural steroid injections on blood glucose levels in patients with diabetes mellitus. *Spine*. 2012;37(1):E46-E50.

154. Horlocker TT. Regional anaesthesia in the patient receiving antithrombotic and antiplatelet therapy. *Br J Anaesth*. 2011;107 (Suppl 1):i96-i106.

155. Horlocker TT, Wedel DJ. Anticoagulation and neuraxial block: historical perspective, anesthetic implications, and risk management. *Reg Anesth Pain Med*. 1998;23(6 Suppl 2):129-134.

156. Pitkänen MT, Aromaa U, Cozanitis DA, Förster JG. Serious complications associated with spinal and epidural anaesthesia in Finland from 2000 to 2009. *Acta Anaesthesiol Scand*. 2013;57(5): 553-564.

157. Tryba M. [Epidural regional anesthesia and low molecular heparin: Pro]. *Anasthesiol Intensivmed Notfallmed Schmerzther*. 1993;28(3):179-181.

158. Stafford-Smith M. Impaired haemostasis and regional anaesthesia. *Can J Anaesth*. 1996;43(5 Pt 2):R129-R141.

159. Vandermeulen EP, Van Aken H, Vermylen J. Anticoagulants and spinal-epidural anesthesia. *Anesth Analg*. 1994;79(6):1165-1177.

160. Horlocker TT, Wedel DJ, Benzon H, et al. Regional anesthesia in the anticoagulated patient: defining the risks (the second ASRA Consensus Conference on Neuraxial Anesthesia and Anticoagulation). *Reg Anesth Pain Med*. 2003;28(3):172-197.

161. Goodman BS, Posecion LW, Mallempati S, Bayazitoglu M. Complications and pitfalls of lumbar interlaminar and transforaminal epidural injections. *Curr Rev Musculoskelet Med*. 2008;1(3-4):212-222.

162. Pitkänen MT, Aromaa U, Cozanitis DA, Förster JG. Serious complications associated with spinal and epidural anaesthesia in Finland from 2000 to 2009. *Acta Anaesthesiol Scand*. 2013;57(5):553-564.

163. Horlocker TT, Wedel DJ, Rowlingson JC, et al. Regional anesthesia in the patient receiving antithrombotic or thrombolytic therapy: American Society of Regional Anesthesia and Pain Medicine Evidence-Based Guidelines (Third Edition). *Reg Anesth Pain Med*. 2010;35(1):64-101.

164. Horlocker TT. Regional anaesthesia in the patient receiving antithrombotic and antiplatelet therapy. *Br J Anaesth*. 2011;107(Suppl 1): i96-i106.

Intraarticular Injections

John C. Keel
Jennifer Earle

INTRODUCTION

Ideally, the comprehensive interdisciplinary pain center would combat the scourge of fragmented musculoskeletal care. Chronic musculoskeletal pain is prevalent in 50% of adults and is the leading cause of disability in the United States [1=Burden MSK dz].[1] Systemic corticosteroid treatment of musculoskeletal pain began soon after the discovery and synthesis of cortisone in the 1940s.[2] Intraarticular steroid injections followed shortly thereafter, and in 1951, Hollander published the results of a large series of patients treated with corticosteroid joint injections.[3] Corticosteroid injections continue to play an important role in the diagnosis and management of acute and chronic musculoskeletal pain. Pain physicians who recognize joint pain versus spine pain and who are proficient in multimodal management of both are well suited to coordinate reasonable utilization of intraarticular injections.

The spectrum of treatment options for painful joints includes tincture of time, education and counseling, activity and physical treatments, orthoses, medications, imaging, injections, and surgery. This chapter covers indications, techniques and anatomic details, sensitivity, specificity, outcomes, and associated adverse events of the most common intraarticular injections, as well as information on less frequently performed injections. Spine joint (facet and sacroiliac) intraarticular and certain nonarticular musculoskeletal injections are included. This chapter does not cover ultrasound-guided injections, a topic unto itself; please refer to the ultrasound chapter for more detail.

GENERAL PRINCIPLES

INDICATIONS AND CONTRAINDICATIONS

General principles favored by the authors are highlighted in the rules of **Table 82-1**. Indications for joint injections include (1) treatment of the painful joint, (2) for diagnosis to assess response to blockade of the joint, (3) for diagnosis to obtain joint fluid, or (4) for treatment to drain

TABLE 82-1 Rules for Joint Injections

1. Any joint *can* be injected (but *should* it be?).
   Search literature and texts for previously described techniques.
2. Indicated for diagnostic (clinical response and joint fluid sample) and therapeutic purpose
3. Contraindicated in my clinic:
   Active or very recent illness, infections
   Allergy, adverse drug reactions (ADRs) (but can use alternate medications)
   Pregnant or trying, breastfeeding
4. Use or adapt image guidance; surface landmark techniques can be adapted for imaging.
5. Avoid:
   Articular cartilage, labrum, implants
   Neurovascular bundles
   Viscera
6. "All steroid is systemic."
7. "Once infected, always infected" (e.g., surgical implants).
8. If there might be other treatments, get the consult.
   Surgical
   Rheumatologic
9. "Do not inject steroid near the Achilles tendon."
10. For peripheral joints, anticoagulation within therapeutic range is not a contraindication.

excess joint fluid causing pain. Corticosteroid injections are used for osteoarthritis (OA), rheumatoid arthritis (RA), psoriatic arthritis, lupus, crystalline arthritis (gout and pseudogout), reactive arthritis (Reiter's syndrome), and more. Other conditions include bursitis, tendonitis, and enthesopathy. Contraindications may include (1) infection, localized or systemic, or other immunity issues; (2) allergy or adverse reaction potential to substances involved; and (3) pregnancy or breastfeeding because of safety profiles of medications and radiation exposure. Infection in a joint may itself be a reason to access the joint with a needle to obtain fluid, but placing steroid there would not be done. Surgical implants give pause; truly consider the risk-to-benefit ratio. Pain in a joint that has been replaced is not likely to be cured with an injection. Anticoagulation is not a contraindication (see later discussion).

IMAGING AND LANDMARKS

As technology for image guidance has become more routinely available, it has been increasingly applied to interventional pain procedures previously performed with surface landmarks, and the trend of studies suggests increased accuracy in medication placement when using image guidance. The sterility and other rigorous protocols of the procedure suite may also benefit patients. For example, studies of major joint injections (knee, hip, and shoulder) have shown significant rates of failure to localize the joint when fluoroscopy was not used.[4] Blind injection of the osteoarthritic hip joint can be inaccurate even with careful technique, traditional methods are not reliable, and image guidance during the injection seems to be necessary.[5]

Preprocedure imaging (e.g., joint radiography or magnetic resonance imaging [MRI]) is not routinely required.

MEDICATIONS

The most commonly used injectable steroids include betamethasone sodium phosphate/acetate (Celestone Soluspan; Schering-Plough, Kenilworth, NJ), methylprednisolone (Depo-Medrol; Upjohn, Kalamazoo, MI), triamcinolone acetonide (Kenalog; Bristol-Meyers Squibb, Princeton, NJ), and triamcinolone hexacetonide (Aristospan; Sandoz, Princeton, NJ).[6] Triamcinolone hexacetonide has the longest duration of action, approximately 3 to 6 weeks, and pharmacokinetic studies have shown it to be absorbed from the joint over a period of 2 to 3 weeks.[7] The duration of clinical effect of corticosteroid is longer if it has lower aqueous solubility (**Table 82-2**).

Mechanisms for pain relief due to corticosteroids include anti-inflammatory action, analgesic effect, systemic effects after systemic uptake, and action on local neurons. Corticosteroids reduce synovial inflammation in patients with RA[8] and may reduce osteophyte formation in those with OA.[9] Injected corticosteroids suppress neural discharge in inflamed nerves and neuropathic pain states.[10] In synovial joints, corticosteroids promote secretion of phospholipid that may contribute to improved joint mobility.[11]

Local anesthetics frequently used for joint and soft tissue injections are bupivacaine (Hospira; Lake Forest, IL, and Sensorcaine; AstraZeneca, Wilmington, DE) and lidocaine (Xylocaine; AstraZeneca, Wilmington, DE). Methylparaben-free and preservative-free anesthetics reduce clumping or flocculation of particulates.

TABLE 82-2 Relative Durations of Commonly Available Corticosteroids

Shortest Duration	Hydrocortisone acetate
	Triamcinolone acetate
	Methylprednisolone acetate
	Betamethasone acetate
	Triamcinolone acetonide
Longest Duration	Triamcinolone hexacetonide

Viscosupplementation is the intraarticular injection of hyaluronic acid derivatives. The technique of injection is the same as with steroid injections. A decreased concentration of hyaluronic acid in the synovial fluid of osteoarthritic joints results in decreased viscosity, which reduces its protective function. Numerous varieties of viscosupplementation are now on the market, including hyaluronan (Sinovial, Yaral, Intragel), 1% sodium hyaluronate (Euflexxa), cross-linked hyaluronate (Gel-One), sodium hyaluronate (Hyalgan), high-molecular-weight hyaluronic acid (Orthovisc), sodium hyaluronate (Supartz), hylan G-F 20 (Synvisc), and hylan G-F 20 (Synvisc One). For example, Synvisc, extracted from chicken combs, is supplied in 2-mL prefilled syringes and is administered as a series of three intraarticular knee injections over 3 weeks. Utilization has drifted now to other joints, but the evidence basis for viscosupplementation is mixed, with enthusiastic results tempered by a meta-analysis of controlled trials suggesting that effect size may be clinically irrelevant and risks may be underappreciated.[12]

Other medications are sometimes used for intraarticular injections. Ketorolac 40-mg vials are often used for intraarticular injection. Intraarticular ketorolac and intraarticular opiates have been studied for perioperative analgesia in joint surgery.[13] Intraarticular botulinum toxin has had surprisingly positive results for shoulder and knee pain.[14,15] Literature search will reveal studies on numerous substances injected intraarticularly, including radiopharmaceuticals, precious metals, laser-absorbing agents, and more, not in common use.

Contrast agents are typically the same as for other interventional techniques. The authors prefer Isovue 300M or Magnevist in case of allergy.

ANTICOAGULATION

Anticoagulation is not routinely discontinued before peripheral joint and soft tissue injections. A prospective study of 32 injections and aspirations performed in patients taking therapeutic warfarin resulted in no cases of joint or soft tissue hemorrhage.[16] In a retrospective review of 640 injections in patients anticoagulated on warfarin, none had hemarthrosis, and only one had clinically significant bleeding postprocedure. A prospective cohort of 15 injections on anticoagulated patients resulted in one frank hemarthrosis, in a patient with an international normalized ratio of 5 and taking concurrent nonsteroidal anti-inflammatory drugs (NSAIDs). In a practice survey including more than 1000 rheumatologists, only 1% had observed bleeding events after shoulder injections in patients taking aspirin compared with 10% in patients taking vitamin K antagonists.[17]

COMPLICATIONS

Several large series have demonstrated the risk of infection to be one in 50,000 injections or less with joint injections.[18] The authors use strict aseptic technique and copious prep and drape.

Systemic absorption occurs following corticosteroid joint injection. Refer to the chapter on steroids for more detail. Possible systemic side effects after injection include any effect of systemic steroid administration. Using the lowest effective dose and limiting the number of injections minimizes the risk. Patients with diabetes may see a temporary (about 2-week) rise in blood glucose level. Corticosteroid injection may transiently suppress the hypothalamic–pituitary–adrenal (HPA) axis. Fluid retention, weight gain, and facial flushing have been reported following corticosteroid injection.[19] Common steroid injection side effects also include postinjection flare and skin and fat atrophy.[20] Tissue damage, such as tendon rupture, cartilage breakdown, skin depigmentation, and fat atrophy, is often attributed to steroid injections; however, as noted earlier, there is also some evidence of protective effect of steroid in OA. Achilles tendon rupture is strongly associated with steroid injection. See the chapter on steroids for more detail.

Chondrocyte toxicity is an emerging concern with intraarticular injections. An in vitro study on effects of single-dose local anesthetic showed decreased chondrocyte viability with 1% lidocaine but not 0.25% bupivacaine or 0.5% ropivacaine.[21] An in vitro study on effects of local anesthetic in combination with typical single injection doses of steroid showed decreased chondrocyte viability with 1% lidocaine or 0.25% bupivacaine combined with betamethasone sodium phosphate or betamethasone acetate or 1% lidocaine combined with methylprednisolone acetate or triamcinolone acetonide.[22] Bupivacaine and triamcinolone, alone or in combination, have demonstrated chondrotoxicity in vitro.[23] These studies may not reflect in vivo conditions.

JOINT REPLACEMENT INFECTION

Although it may not be true, the common belief persists that intraarticular steroid injections in the hip predispose to later infection in primary hip arthroplasty of that joint. A retrospective of 40 patients who had received such hip injections 2 to 23 months before hip replacement revealed no infections in the follow-up of 11 to 37 months.[24] A survey of 36 patients who had received hip injections 5 to 19 months before hip replacement revealed no infections in the follow-up of 7 to 10 years.[25] A retrospective of 175 patients who had received hip injections within 1 year before hip replacement compared with controls revealed no increased risk of infections associated with hip injection before hip replacement.[26] A retrospective of 90 patients who had received knee injections before knee replacement compared with control participants revealed no increased risk of infections associated with knee injection before knee replacement.[27] An analysis of 38 patients with and 352 patients without postoperative infection after knee arthroplasty revealed that steroid injection did not increase the incidence of infection.

JOINT FLUID ANALYSIS

Joint fluid may be sent to a laboratory for assessment. Note the macroscopic appearance of the fluid, including color, clarity, and viscosity. (1) Crystals, (2) cell count (white blood cell count and PMN), (3) Gram stain, (4) culture, and (5) glucose are typically requested. Monosodium urate crystals of gout have strong negative birefringence under polarized light. The crystals of calcium pyrophosphate disease have weak positive birefringence.[28] See **Table 82-3** for description of the types of synovial fluid.

SPECIFIC INJECTIONS

UPPER LIMB

Shoulder

Technique Approaches for the shoulder include the anterior and posterior glenohumeral and subacromial. The acromioclavicular joint is also sometimes injected. Shoulder injection with surface landmarks is performed with the patient sitting on the examination table at a height comfortable for the clinician. With fluoroscopy, the patient is recumbent on the procedure table, prone for a posterior approach and supine for an anterior approach.

For the posterior approach, the arm is slightly internally rotated, and the scapula spine is palpated to find indentation just lateral to its edge to mark the entry spot. Then the coracoid process is identified anterior, and the needle insertion is directed toward the tip of the coracoid process. For the subacromial approach, the needle is inserted in the space posterolateral to the acromion process, parallel to the examination table, at a depth of approximately 3 cm.[29] The techniques are similar when fluoroscopic guidance is used.

For the anterior approach, the shoulder is slightly externally rotated. The point of entry is marked just medial to the head of the humerus and just below (inferolateral) the coracoid process (**Figs. 82-1** and **82-2**). The technique is similar when fluoroscopic guidance is used.

Subacromial bursa injection can be performed using the above posterior approach or the lateral approach. Using the lateral approach, the needle entry site is marked on the lateral shoulder just inferior to the acromion. The needle is advanced toward the inferior border of the lateral acromion (see Fig. 82-1). After the needle contacts the acromion,

TABLE 82-3 Synovial Fluid

Fluid	Crystals	WBC Count	Gram Stain and Culture	Glucose
Noninflammatory (osteoarthritis)	NA	<2000	Negative	Normal
Inflammatory	May be present	>2000	Negative	Normal usually
Septic	NA	>100,000	Positive	Low
Hemorrhagic	NA	NA	Negative	Normal

NA, not applicable; WBC, white blood cell.

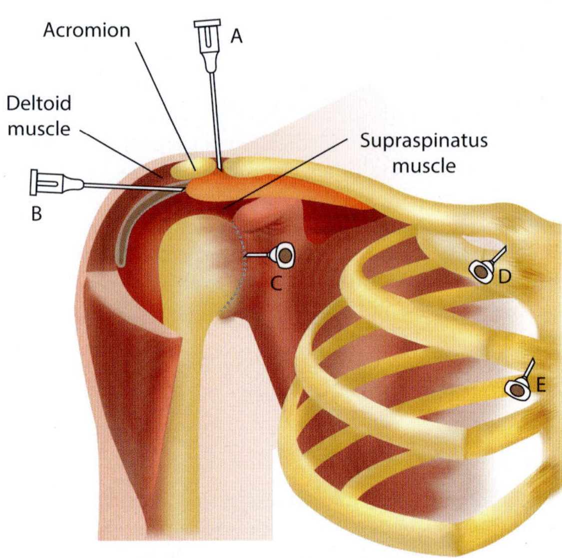

FIGURE 82-1. Shoulder and chest injections. Needle A demonstrates needle trajectory and placement for injections of the acromioclavicular joint. Needle B demonstrates needle placement for the lateral approach to the subacromial bursa injection. Needle C demonstrates needle placement for the anterior approach to the shoulder joint. Needle D demonstrates the needle approach to the sternoclavicular joint. Needle E demonstrates the needle approach to the costosternal joint.

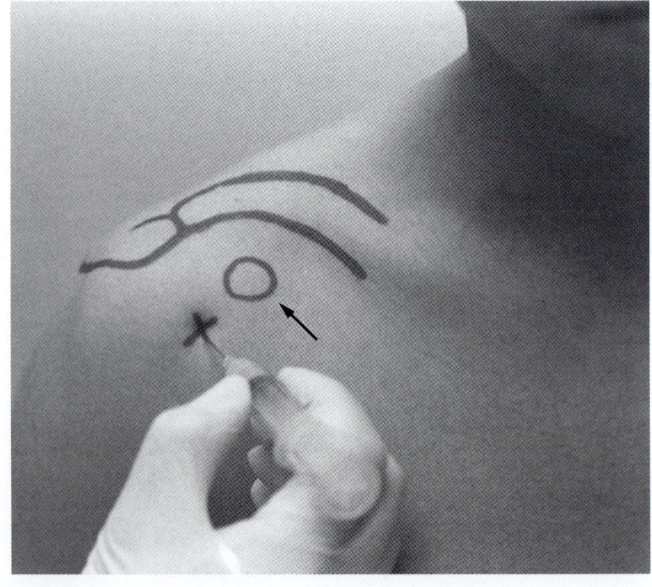

FIGURE 82-2. Anterior approach to intraarticular shoulder injection. Entry site is just inferior and lateral to the coracoid process (arrow).

it is "walked" inferiorly until it slips off the inferior edge of the acromion. Then it is advanced perhaps 0.5 to 1.0 cm to where medication is injected. The technique is similar when fluoroscopic guidance is used.

The acromioclavicular joint space entry site is identified as a groove or depression between the acromion and clavicle. This can be done with palpation or fluoroscopy.

Evidence Steroid injections are well tolerated and result in short-term relief of tendonitis.[30] Imaging-guided subacromial steroid injection may have short-term benefit in clinically and MRI-proven subacromial impingement; 83% of 69 patients reported symptom relief at 6-month follow-up evaluation. With a shorter duration of symptoms and minor-grade MRI findings, there is improved outcome.[31] A meta-analysis of steroid injection for painful shoulder found that subacromial injections are effective for rotator cuff tendonitis up to a 9-month period. A dose–response association has been reported for subacromial steroid injection for rotator cuff tendonitis.[32] In contrast, a randomized controlled trial (RCT) investigating corticosteroid dose in subacromial injection found no difference.[32] In an RCT of patients with rotator cuff tears, injection of triamcinolone improved night and activity pain compared with control participants. Two injections at a 21-day interval compared with a single dose offered no potentiating or prolonged effect.[33] Other studies have found that subacromial injection for rotator cuff pathology results in small benefit compared with placebo but no benefit compared with NSAIDs, but for adhesive capsulitis, there is possible benefit of injection over placebo but with less conclusive evidence.[34-38]

In an RCT, subacromial injection improved pain and disability and decreased range of motion (ROM) from poststroke hemiplegic shoulders.[37] In a prospective study, fluoroscopic-guided intraarticular steroid injection reduces pain and increases ROM in frozen shoulder syndrome.[38]

Other Adverse Events One study reported no significant effect of shoulder corticosteroid injection on blood glucose levels in patients with diabetes.[39] There is one reported case of steroid-induced psychosis from shoulder and interventional spine injections.[40a] There is one reported case of livedoid dermatitis after shoulder injection.[40b] There is also one reported case of fatal necrotizing fasciitis after steroid injection of the shoulder.[41]

Other Upper Limb

Elbow Injection The elbow joint is injected using a lateral approach. The radial humeral joint can easily be palpated laterally at the level of the skin crease of the elbow.

The lateral epicondyle of the humerus is the most identifiable landmark. Identify and palpate the groove between the epicondyle and the plateau of the radius. Mark this spot as the needle entry point (**Figs. 82-3** and **82-4**). The needle is advanced to contact the epicondyle. Then walk the needle distally until it slides off the epicondyle and into the joint space. Advance the needle about 0.5 cm and inject the medication. If an ulnar paresthesia is elicited during needle placement, the needle is too dorsal, and a more volar approach should be used.

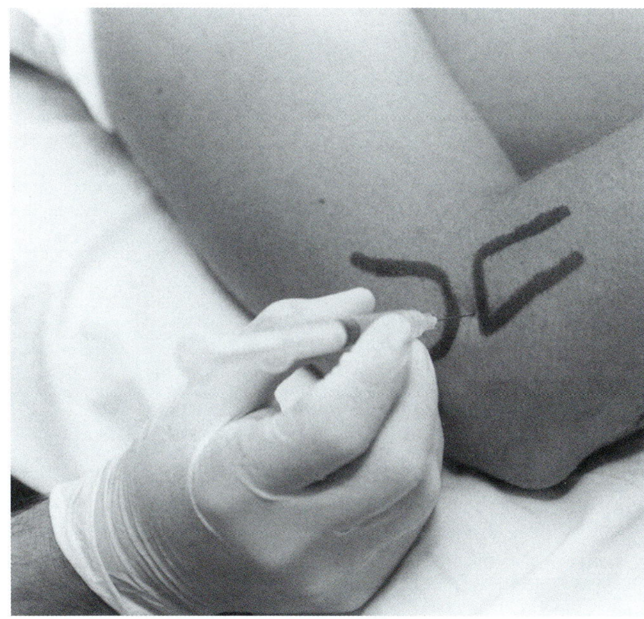

FIGURE 82-4. Lateral approach to the elbow joint injection

Olecranon Bursa Injection The olecranon bursa lies between the soft tissue and the olecranon process of the ulna. It is injected with the needle advanced in a direction perpendicular to the olecranon (see Fig. 82-3) until the olecranon surface is contacted. Then the needle is withdrawn approximately 1 to 2 mm to the site where medication is injected. To avoid a subcutaneous injection, do not withdraw the needle too far after contacting the olecranon.

Finger Joint Injections The carpometacarpal (CMC), metacarpophalangeal (MCP), and interphalangeal (IP) joints commonly are affected by RA and OA flare-ups and are amenable to injection therapy. The specific joint to be injected can easily be palpated. For the IP joints, a lateral or medial approach is used. For the MCP or CMC joints, a dorsal approach is used. It is best to avoid the more richly innervated volar (palmar) surface of the hand because these injections are more painful. The needle only needs to enter the superficial joint, just through the capsule (**Figs. 82-5** and **82-6**). Inject a small amount, perhaps 0.5 mL of anesthetic and corticosteroid solution.

Wrist Injections A dorsal approach to the radiocarpal and ulnocarpal joints is preferred. These joints can easily be palpated and the needle entry site marked (**Figs. 82-5** and **82-7**). Care should be taken to avoid the

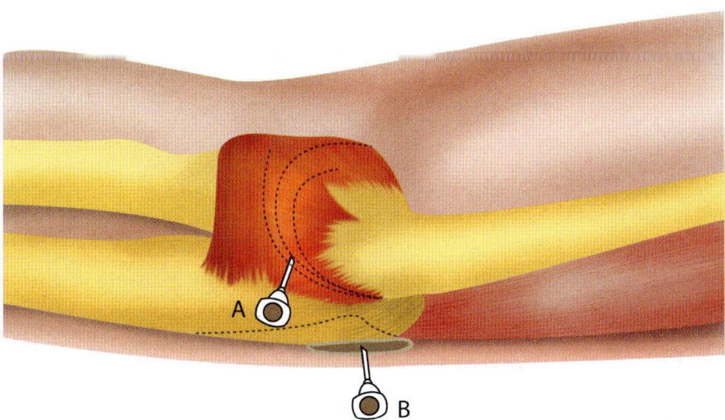

FIGURE 82-3. Elbow injections. Needle A demonstrates the lateral approach to the elbow joint. Needle B demonstrates olecranon bursa injection.

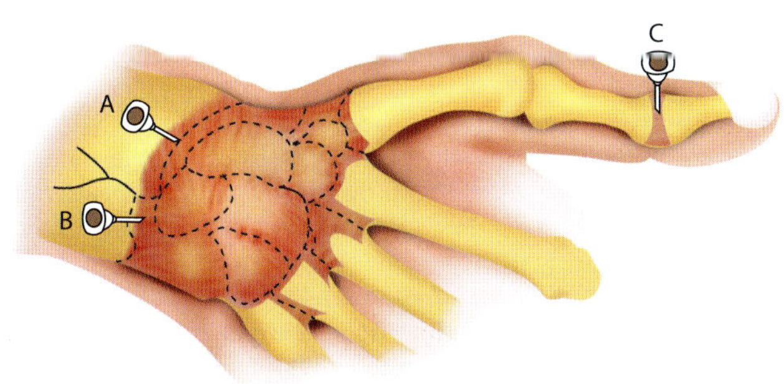

FIGURE 82-5. Hand and wrist injections. Needles A and B demonstrate the dorsal approach to the radiocarpal and ulnocarpal joints. Needle C demonstrates the needle approach to an interphalangeal joint.

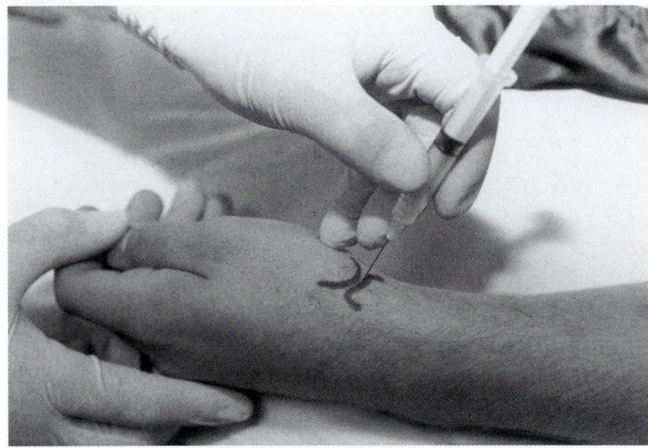

FIGURE 82-6. Needle approach to the carpometacarpal joint of the thumb.

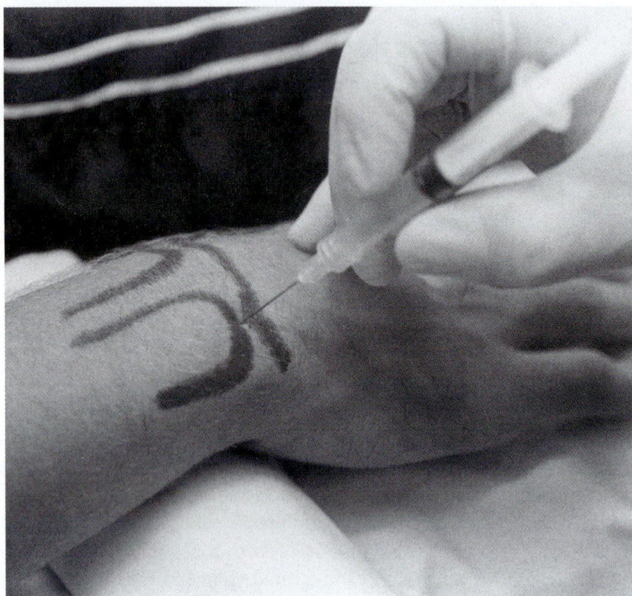

FIGURE 82-7. Dorsal approach to the wrist joint injection.

extensor tendons. The joint space can be "opened up" slightly by placing the wrist in 45 degrees of flexion. The needle is advanced into the joint superficially, and 1 to 2 mL of solution is injected.

LOWER LIMB

Hip (Femoroacetabular)

Technique Hip pain from the femoroacetabular joint can be confounded with spine, sacroiliac, or soft tissue processes in the same area. Intraarticular injection can be both diagnostic and therapeutic.[41] Blind injection with surface landmarks can be inaccurate and unreliable; image guidance during the injection is preferred.[5]

An anterior or anterolateral approach is the most frequently used method of intraarticular hip injection. The patient is supine on the fluoroscopy table with the hip internally rotated; the femoral pulse is palpated and marked. The suggested skin entry site is 8 to 10 cm under the inguinal ligament, with the needle angled toward the femur head. This minimizes risk of vessel or femoral nerve injury.[42] A more lateral approach has been demonstrated as safer in regards to potential neurovascular injury compared with the anterior approach.[43] The needle target is the lateral aspect of the femoral bone at the head–neck junction (**Figs. 82-8** and **82-9**).

The authors favor a posterior approach with the patient in the usual prone position, with the buttocks uncovered. This region is sterilely prepped with confidence. This approach easily avoids neurovascular bundles and allows down-the-beam advancement of the needle. It also may be more specific diagnostically because it does not directly target the psoas bursa. The needle target is the midpoint of the width of the femoral neck junction with the femoral head.

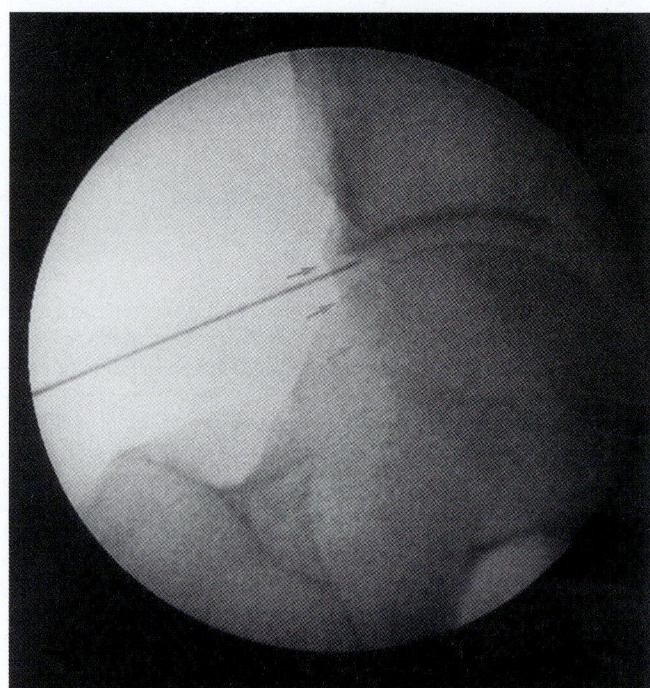

FIGURE 82-8. Hip joint injection. Needle placement for the lateral approach to the hip joint. The white arrows outline the margin of the acetabulum.

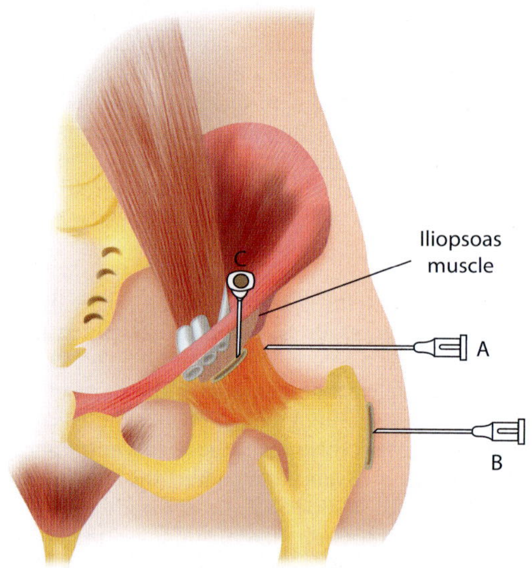

FIGURE 82-9. Hip injections. Needle A demonstrates needle orientation and trajectory for a lateral approach to the hip joint. Needle B demonstrates the lateral approach to the trochanteric bursa injection. Needle C demonstrates the approach to iliopsoas bursa injection.

Evidence The duration of pain relief after intraarticular corticosteroid hip injection typically is 1 to 3 months in patients with symptomatic OA.[44] Pain relief after intraarticular hip injection correlates with radiographic severity of OA.[45] Intraarticular hip injection after total hip arthroscopy has been shown to decrease opioid use and pain and increase rehabilitation activities.[46] In one study, injection volumes ranging from 3 to 9 mL did not result in different outcomes.[47]

Other Adverse Events There is one documented case of systemic septicemia after hip injection.[48]

OTHER HIP GIRDLE INJECTIONS

Greater Trochanter Trochanter injection may be performed with the patient lying on the asymptomatic side so the painful lateral hip area is superior and exposed. The area of greatest pain should be marked. Injection is targeted at this site.[28] Except when there is successful fluid aspiration, radiographic guidance is needed to ensure accuracy during trochanteric bursa injection.[48] However, the use of fluoroscopy may not improve outcomes in patients with greater trochanteric pain syndrome who receive corticosteroid injections. Comparable success rates were found for intra- and extrabursal injections.[49] A prosthetic joint is considered a relative contraindication by some authors[50] however, use of image guidance facilitates avoiding a surgical implant.

Evidence Patients show improvement in trochanteric pain at short-term follow-up after corticosteroid injection, although improvement does not persist for the long term.[51] Corticosteroid injection improves pain at 1 month of follow-up, but this effect does not persist, as noted in a study comparing injection, shockwave therapy, and home exercise.[52] Trochanteric pain improved with corticosteroid injection, with greater relief experienced with higher steroid doses.[53]

Other Adverse Events Necrotizing fasciitis has been reported as a complication of injection into the greater trochanteric bursa.[54]

Iliopsoas Bursa Injection The iliopsoas bursa is the largest bursa in the body and lies between the iliopsoas muscle and the anterior hip capsule (see **Fig. 82-8**). It is a common but often overlooked cause of groin pain.[55,56] There may be direct communication between the bursa and the joint.

The injection is performed with the patient supine. The needle entry site is just below the inguinal ligament and 1 to 2 cm lateral to the neurovascular bundle (femoral artery pulsation) to avoid needle trauma to the femoral nerve and vessels (see Fig. 82-8). The needle is advanced perpendicular to the skin and advanced until the anterior bone of the acetabulum is contacted. The needle is then withdrawn 3 to 5 mm, and after careful aspiration, medication is injected. If blood is aspirated, or a femoral nerve paresthesia occurs during needle placement, the needle is redirected laterally. Be sure to check the patient for femoral nerve anesthesia before allowing ambulation.

Knee

Technique Knee injection can be performed by having the patient lie supine, with a rolled towel under the lower thigh to angle the knee. Medial and lateral approaches may be done. Knee bursae are also sometimes injected. For a medial approach, palpate along the medial aspect of the patella from superior to inferior. Identify an indentation at around the 3 o'clock position and mark it for needle entry. The needle is inserted here parallel to the undersurface of the patella. Backpressure should be provided to determine if joint fluid is present and to ensure a blood vessel is not contacted.[29]

The lateral approach is quite similar, with skin entry at the analogous position laterally. Lateral midpatellar injection (an injection into the patellofemoral joint) was intraarticular 93% of the time and was more accurate than other methods in one study.[58] A benefit of lateral approach includes avoiding the medial neurovascular bundle.

The anterior approach, easily used with fluoroscopy, uses a needle entry medial and inferior to the patella, and the target is the medial femoral condyle of medial joint compartment.

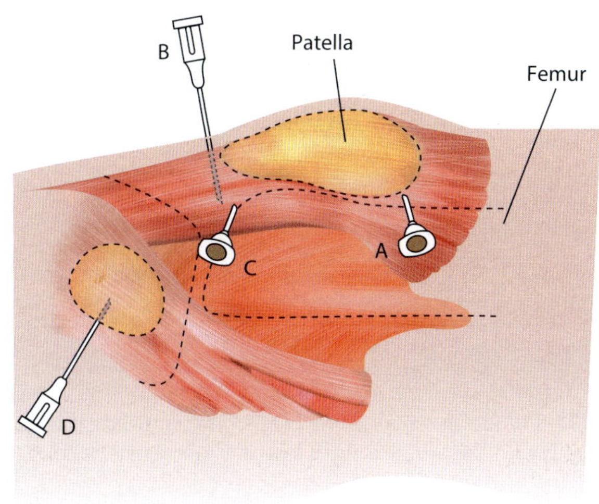

FIGURE 82-10. Knee injections. Needle A demonstrates the approach to the patellar bursa. Needle B demonstrates the anterior approach to intraarticular knee joint injection. Needle C demonstrates the medial approach to intraarticular knee joint injection. Needle D demonstrates the approach to the anserine bursa injection.

The prepatellar bursa lies between the patella and the overlying soft tissue. The anserine bursa lies between the medial knee joint and the pes anserinus (tendons of the semitendinous, gracilis, and sartorius muscles) and is found by palpating the area of maximal tenderness over the medial tibial plateau. Prepatellar bursitis and anserine bursitis are common causes of knee pain and respond well to injection. Local injection is rather superficial in each case: the needle is advanced until it contacts bone (**Fig. 82-10**) and is then withdrawn slightly, and the medication is injected.

Evidence Common indications for knee injection include OA, Baker's cyst, and pes anserine bursitis. Literature review supports the use of intraarticular corticosteroid injections for RA, OA, and juvenile idiopathic arthritis.[59] RCTs support the long-term safety of intraarticular steroid injections for patients with symptomatic knee arthritis. No deleterious effects of the long-term administration of steroids on the anatomic structure of the knee were noted in one trial.[60] Moreover, long-term treatment of knee arthritis with repeated steroid injections appears to be clinically effective for the relief of symptoms of the disease. Studies have demonstrated short-term pain relief and improved periarticular muscle strength in patients after intraarticular corticosteroid injection of a symptomatic rheumatoid joint.[61] Injection can provide short-term relief (2–4 weeks) in patients with symptomatic OA, allowing time for participation in an appropriate rehabilitation program.[62]

Other Adverse Events The risk of septic arthritis from intraarticular injections is less than 0.03%.[63] Case reports have identified rare but severe adverse events include septic arthritis and osteonecrosis.[64,65]

Other Lower Limb

Ankle Injection The ankle joint may be entered from an anterior approach to the joint between the tibia and the talus. The patient is positioned supine with the leg–foot angle placed at 90 degrees. The point of entry is just medial to the anterior tibial and extensor hallucis longus tendons on a line drawn between the medial and lateral malleoli (**Figs. 82-11** and **82-12**). These tendons can be easily identified by having the patient dorsiflex the foot and great toe. The needle is advanced directly posteriorly until contacting bone. The needle is then walked inferiorly until it slips between the tibia and talus. A total of 1 to 2 mL of solution is injected. Joints between the tarsal bones are best injected by using fluoroscopic guided injection.[66]

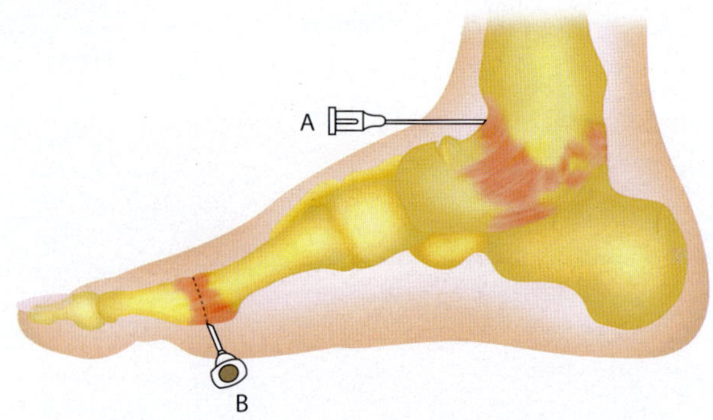

FIGURE 82-11. Foot and ankle injections. Needle A demonstrates the anterior approach to ankle joint injection. Needle B demonstrates metatarsophalangeal joint injection.

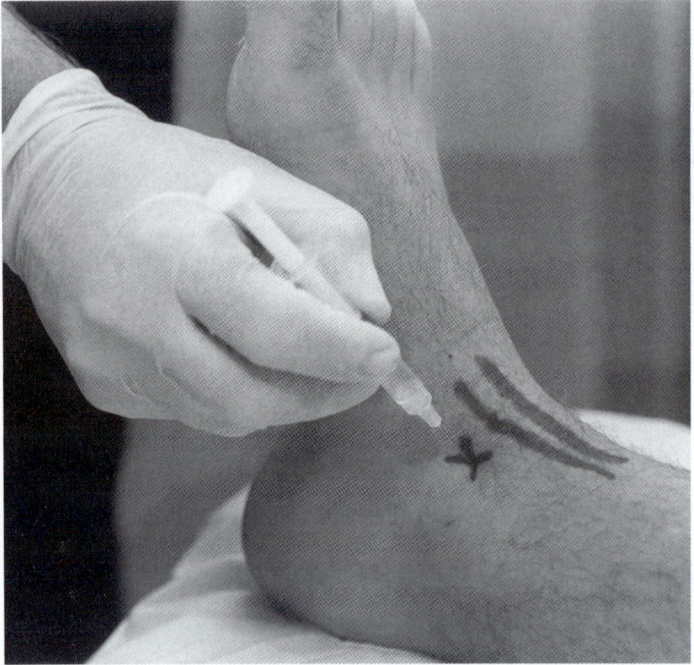

FIGURE 82-12. Anterior approach to ankle joint injection. The two parallel lines represent the anterior tibialis and extensor hallucis longus tendons.

Forefoot Injections The injection technique for metatarsal, phalangeal, and IP joints is exactly the same as the techniques described for the IP and MCP joints on the hand (see Fig. 82-11). Again, a lateral or dorsal approach is usually favored over the more painful plantar approach.

Spine Joint The paravertebral spine joints include zygapophyseal or facet joints, sacroiliac joints, and costovertebral joints. The costosternal and sternoclavicular joints are included here for convenience, although they are not spine joints.

Atlantoaxial Joint Injection The first cervical facet joint, the atlantoaxial or C1 to C2 joint is markedly different from the remaining five cervical facet joints and the cervical–thoracic facet joint. This joint is responsible for at least 50% of axial rotation in the normal cervical spine. Suboccipital pain with rotation of the head to the left or right often is indicative of C1 to C2 joint pathology.

The C1 to C2 joint may be injected using a lateral or posterior approach.[67-70] Because the vertebral artery courses along the lateral edge of the joint, the posterior approach is preferred. The patient is positioned prone on the fluoroscopy table, and the fluoroscopy beam is positioned in a posteroanterior (PA) projection (**Fig. 82-13**). Because the teeth and jaw frequently project over the upper cervical spine, it is usually necessary to have the patient open the mouth. Once a clear view of the joint is obtained by adjusting the fluoroscopy column, the entry point is marked, sterilized, and anesthetized. Then a 3½-in, 22- or 25-gauge needle is advanced directly toward the joint with the target being the junction of the lateral one third and the medial two thirds of the joint. The needle is advanced to contact the bony edge of the joint at C2. The needle is then walked off the bone into the joint and advanced no more than 1 to 2 mm. Intraarticular placement is confirmed by the injection of 0.25 to 0.5 mL of radiopaque contrast. An appropriate arthrogram should be identifiable (**Fig. 82-14**), and there should not be any intravascular uptake or neuraxial spread. This is followed by the injection of a mixture of 0.25 mL of anesthetic (1% lidocaine is recommended) and 0.25 mL of corticosteroid. The C2 nerve root runs across the posterior surface of the joint (**Fig. 82-15**). If a paresthesia is obtained during needle placement, it is advisable to choose a slightly different trajectory. It is usually best to make the initial needle puncture sight slightly more caudad. Potential complications include intravascular injection, spinal axis injection, needle trauma to the nerve root or spinal cord, and vascular injury. Since most injectable corticosteroids are particulate, cerebral embolism is a risk.

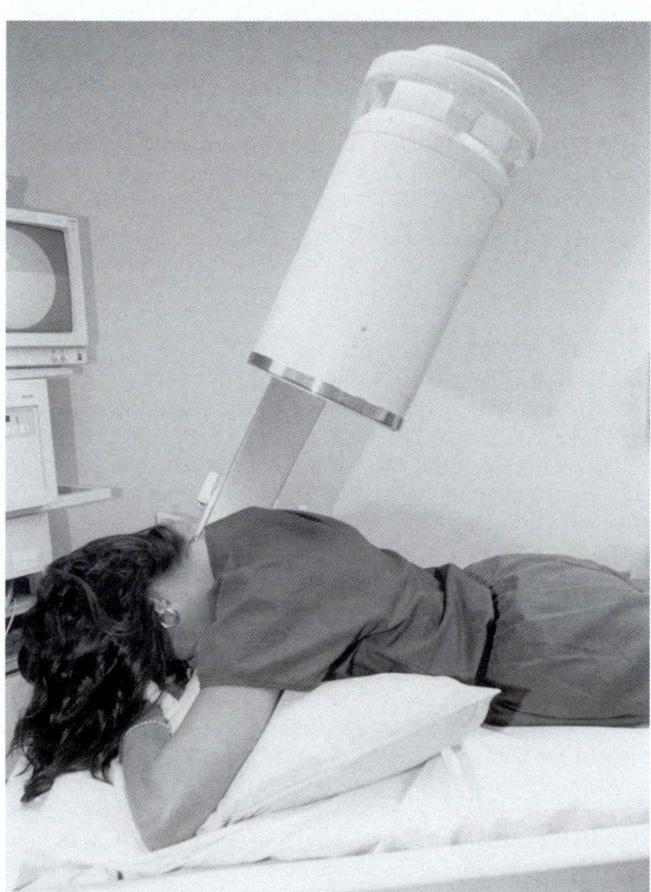

FIGURE 82-13. Patient positioning for posterior cervical facet joint injection.

Cervical Facet Joint Injection The C2 to C3 through C6 to C7 joints can be injected using a posterior approach or a lateral approach.[71,72] The posterior approach is safer but technically more difficult because of the marked cephalocaudal angulation of the joints. The lateral approach is technically easier but more risky because the advancing needle can pass through the joint and into the spinal canal. This can be prevented by frequent PA and lateral fluoroscopic views.

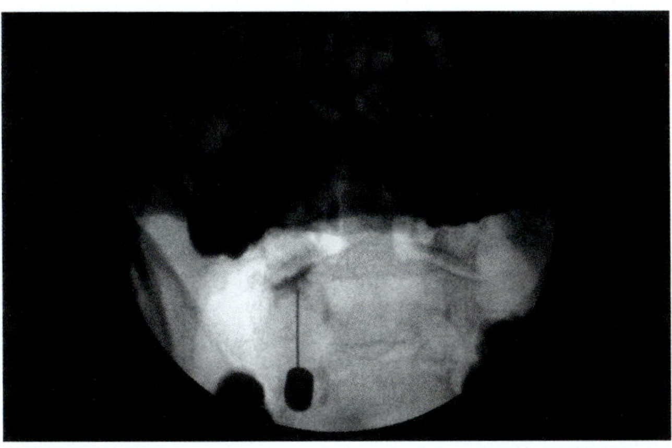

FIGURE 82-14. C1 to C2 facet joint injection. Fluoroscopic view was obtained with the mouth wide open. The right C1 to C2 joint is clearly visualized and contrast outlines the left C1 to C2 joint.

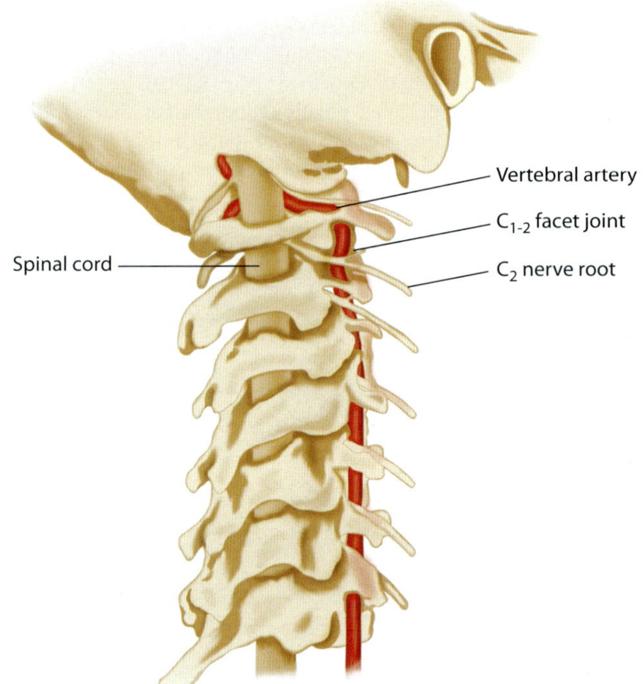

FIGURE 82-15. The relationship of the vertebral artery and C2 nerve root to the C1 to C2 joint are illustrated in this oblique view of the cervical spine.

For the posterior approach, the patient is prone, and the neck is slightly flexed (see Fig. 82-13). The fluoroscopy column is adjusted to identify the target joint(s). The needle entry site should be marked one level below the target joint. This allows angulation of the needle at an angle that will facilitate entry into the cephalocaudal oriented cervical facet joints. A 3½-in, 22- or 25-gauge needle is advanced into the joint under fluoroscopic guidance. Intraarticular placement is confirmed with PA and lateral fluoroscopy by injecting 0.25 to 0.5 mL of contrast. After proper needle placement is confirmed and following negative aspiration, a mixture of 0.25 mL of anesthetic plus 0.25 to 0.50 mL of corticosteroid is injected.

For the lateral approach, the patient may be positioned prone, lateral, or even supine. Lateral positioning usually is preferred by the patient and is convenient for the physician (**Fig. 82-16**). The target joint is identified and marked using fluoroscopy. After sterile preparation and local anesthesia, a 1½- to 2½-in, 25-gauge needle is advanced to contact bone at the inferior edge of the joint. The needle is walked off the bone and advanced 2 to 3 mm into the joint (**Fig. 82-17**). Posteroanterior fluoroscopy is used to confirm that the needle is in the lateral one third of the joint. The needle is withdrawn slightly if the tip is beyond the lateral one third of the joint. Injection is performed as described for the posterior approach.

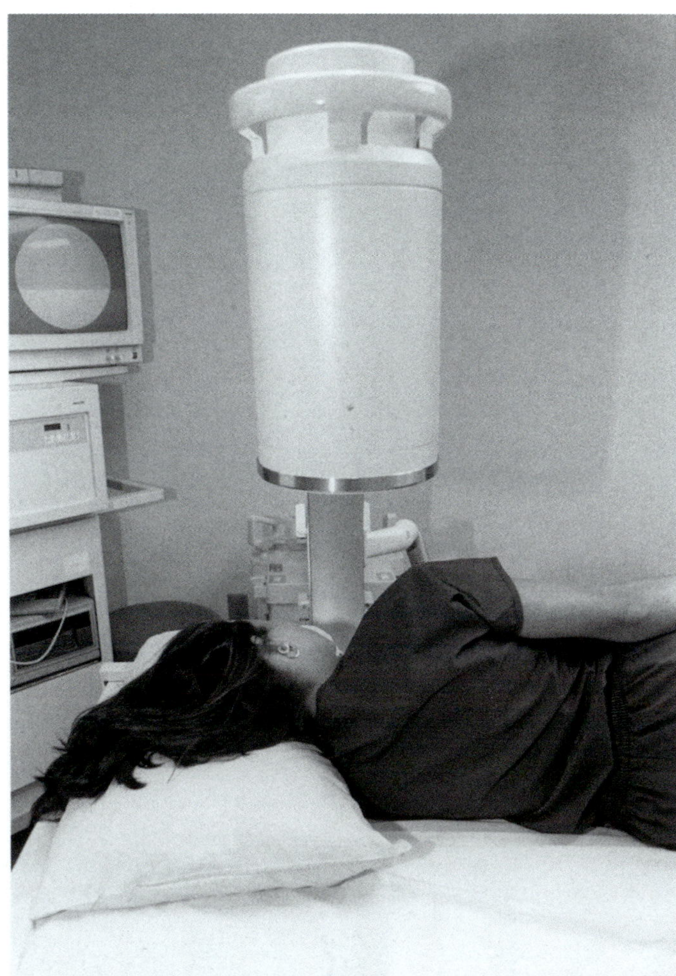

FIGURE 82-16. Patient positioning for lateral cervical facet joint injection.

Complications and side effects from cervical facet blocks include intravascular injection, spinal axis injection, joint trauma, nerve root and spinal cord trauma, infection, and side effects from the injected corticosteroid.

Thoracic Facet Joint Injection Thoracic facet joint pain is not a common clinical problem. The thoracic facet joints are not as prone to arthritic involvement as are the cervical and lumbar facet joints. The most common cause of thoracic facet pain is trauma. For example, thoracic facets may be a source of pain around a previous compression fracture.

Similar to the lower cervical facets, the thoracic facets have a marked cephalocaudal angulation. The average angle of incline from the horizontal plane is 60 degrees in the midthoracic region. Accordingly, the technique for thoracic facet injection is very similar to the posterior approach to the cervical facet joint.[73] The patient is placed prone, and the fluoroscopy tube is angled in order to get the best view of the target joint. The needle entry site is one to two segments below the target joint to allow angulation of the needle to facilitate joint entry (**Fig. 82-18A** and **82-18B**). The remainder of the technique is as described for posterior cervical facet injection.

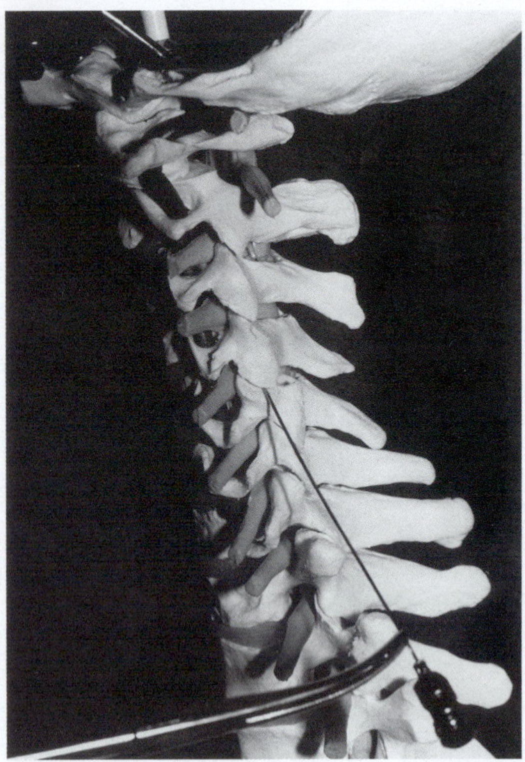

FIGURE 82-17. Lateral approach to the C4 to C5 facet joint.

Costovertebral Joint Injections The pain related to costovertebral and costotransverse joints usually is unilateral, beginning in a paravertebral location, and often radiates in a bandlike fashion around the thorax.[74,75] The pain is described as aching and burning and is usually worse in the morning. It is also worsened by deep inspiration, coughing, and twisting or rotation of the torso.

The injection is performed with fluoroscopy guidance to minimize the risk of pneumothorax. The patient is placed in the prone position, and the lateral tip of the transverse process of the level in question is identified. The skin is entered just cephalad and lateral to this point, with the needle directed medially. The needle is advanced until contact is made with the vertebral body, which indicates that the needle tip is in the intertransverse space. The needle tip placement is then adjusted cephalad or caudad until it lies within the joint or pierces the articular capsule. At this point, 0.5 to 1 mL of medication is injected.

Pneumothorax is the most feared complication of this block, although the incidence should be low with proper technique and fluoroscopic guidance.

Lumbar Facet Joint Injection Because of the prevalence of low back pain, lumbar facet injection is one of the most commonly performed pain management procedures. Intraarticular facet injections can be performed for diagnostic or therapeutic purposes.[76-78] Because of the oblique orientation of the lumbar facet joints, especially the lower two levels, it often is helpful to position the patient in a slightly oblique position with the side to be injected rotated up 30 to 45 degrees (**Fig. 82-19**).

With the patient appropriately positioned, the target joint is identified with fluoroscopic guidance, and the skin is marked. It is best to identify the level by starting at the lumbosacral junction and then working up

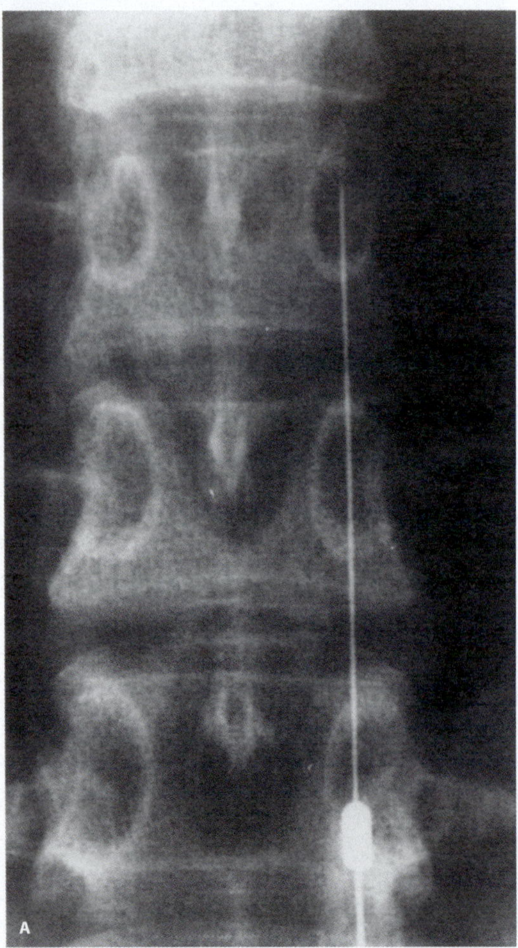

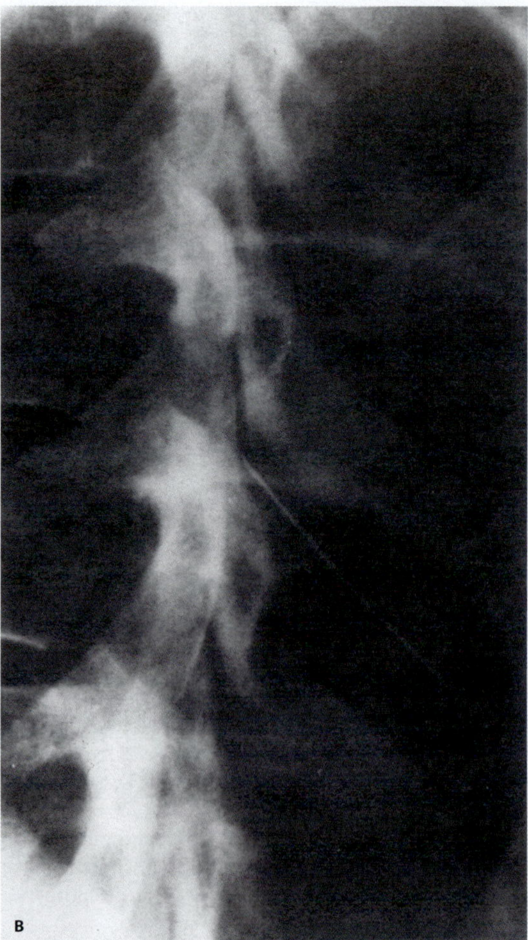

FIGURE 82-18. (**A**) Posteroanterior fluoroscopic view of thoracic facet joint injection. (**B**) Lateral fluoroscopic view of thoracic facet joint injection. (Reproduced, with permission, from Dreyfuss P, Tibiletti C, Dreyer S. Thoracic zygapophyseal joint pain patterns: a study in normal volunteers. *Spine* 1994;9:807-811.)

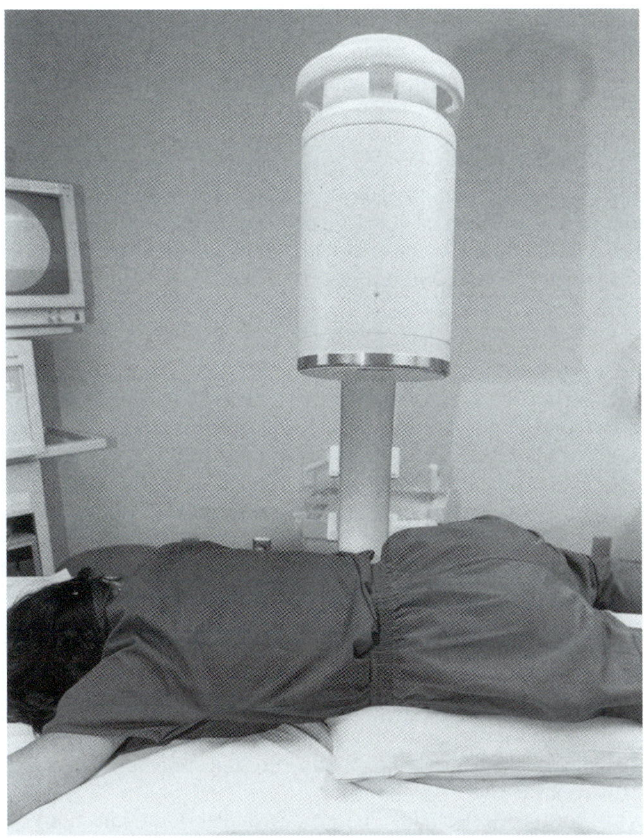

FIGURE 82-19. Patient positioning for a lateral approach to lumbar facet injection.

to the thoracolumbar junction. Lumbosacral anomalies and transitional levels are common. To make communication among practitioners clear, it is important to specify the presence of any abnormalities and how it influences the counting and reporting of the level or levels injected.

The needle is advanced under fluoroscopic guidance toward the target joint until it contacts the bony edge and is then walked off the bone to slip into the facet joint.

In patients with severe OA, the joint space may be narrowed to the point that needle entry is not possible. A periarticular injection can be performed in this situation for therapeutic purposes, but a periarticular injection may be of less diagnostic value. Intraarticular position is confirmed by injecting a tiny amount of contrast. A typical lumbar facet arthrogram is shown in **Figure 82-20**.

It is not unusual for the facet capsule to have small fenestrations. The injectate may spread to contiguous structures, including the epidural space or intervertebral foramen. It is important to identify such spread during the contrast injection. **Figure 82-21** is an example of contrast spreading from the L5 to S1 facet joint to the adjacent S1 nerve root. Arthrography is followed by the diagnostic or therapeutic injection. Typically, 0.25 to 0.50 mL of anesthetic is mixed with 0.25 to 0.50 mL of corticosteroid for each joint.

Complications after facet joint injection are uncommon and include intravascular injection, spinal injection, infection, and needle trauma to the joint or adjacent nerve root.

Sacroiliac Joint Injection Diagnostic sacroiliac injections are considered an important part of the diagnostic workup for mechanical low back pain because history and physical examination are notoriously unreliable.[79] Sacroiliac joint injection can be performed with or without the use of fluoroscopy; however, when fluoroscopy is not used, there is a significant rate of failure to enter the joint. Therefore, if the block is being performed for diagnostic reasons, fluoroscopy or computed tomography guidance should be used.

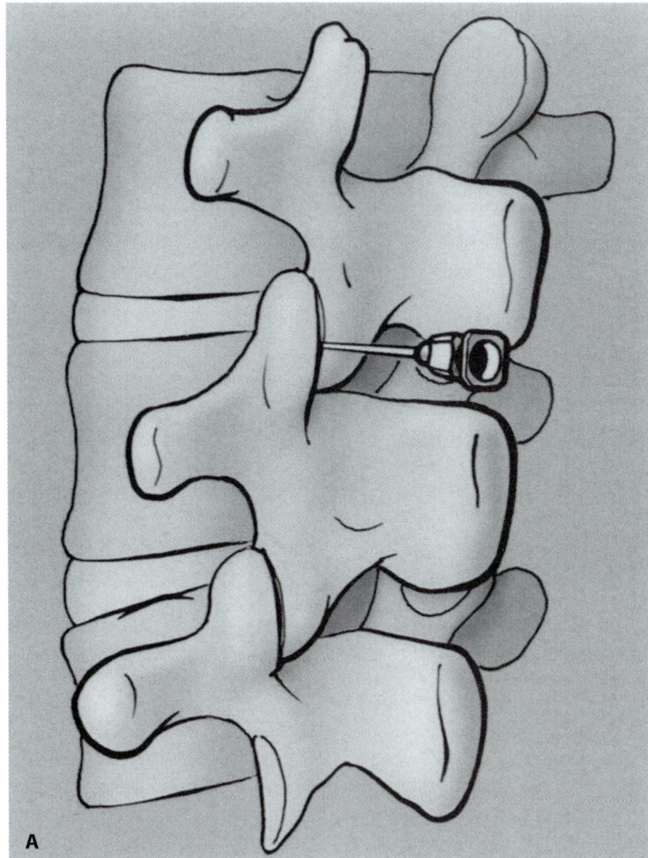

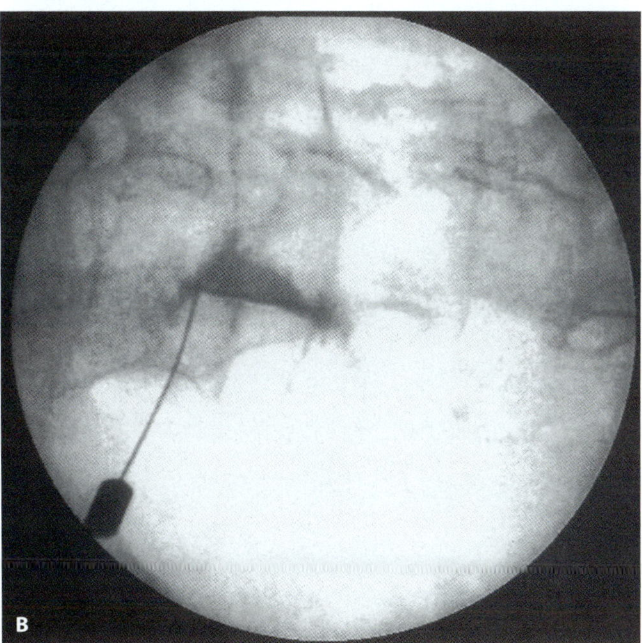

FIGURE 82-20. (**A**) Posterolateral approach to the lumbar facet joint. (**B**) Posterolateral fluoroscopic view of lumbar facet joint injection with contrast.

For this injection, the patient is placed in the prone position. The sacroiliac joint is most accessible to injection at the most caudal or inferior portion of the joint.[80,81] Attempts to enter the synovial cavity of the joint at the middle and cranial or superior portions of the joint have a higher failure rate. Using fluoroscopy, or by palpation, the posterior superior iliac spine (PSIS) is identified. The needle entry site

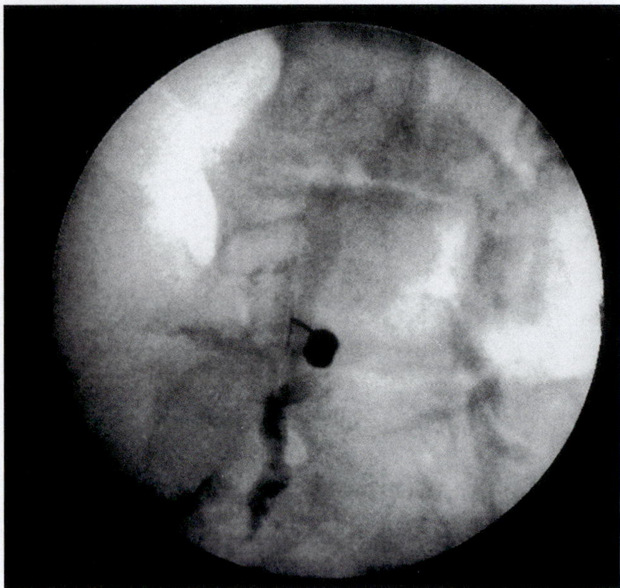

FIGURE 82-21. L5 to S1 facet injection with contrast. The injectant has spread beyond the ventral aspect of the joint to surround the first sacral nerve root in this patient with previous lumbar spine surgery.

is approximately 1 cm below the PSIS (**Fig. 82-22A** and **82-22B**). The needle is simply advanced toward the joint, with needle angle typically 20 to 30 degrees lateral from the sagittal plane (if using AP view). Upon initial entry, the needle will traverse through the thick and tough posterior sacroiliac ligament (**Fig. 82-23**). The needle must be advanced through this ligament to reach the synovial joint cavity. This joint cavity may be obliterated or replaced by fibrous tissue in some patients. If fluoroscopy is used, 1 to 2 mL of radiopaque contrast can be injected to confirm an intraarticular dye pattern (**Fig. 82-24**). This is followed by an injection of medication.

Costosternal Joint Injection Costosternal joint pain can be posttraumatic or inflammatory in nature. The costosternal joints are synovial joints; however, the joint space can be obliterated or replaced by fibrous tissue.

The patient is placed supine, and the affected joint (or joints) is identified by palpation. The joint space is usually identifiable by palpating a groove between the costal cartilage and the sternum. After it is identified, the affected joint is injected with 0.5 to 1.0 mL of local anesthetic or corticosteroid (or both) using a 25-gauge short (e.g., 1-in) needle (see Fig. 82-2).

Sternoclavicular Joint Injection The patient is placed in the supine position, and the gap between the medial end of the clavicle and the sternum is palpated. The joint is entered with a 25-gauge, 1-in needle, and 1 mL of local anesthetic and/or depot steroid is injected (see Fig. 82-2). There should be little resistance to injection. If resistance is encountered, the needle tip is most likely in the meniscal cartilage and should be withdrawn slightly or repositioned until the injectate flows freely.

If posterior sternoclavicular pain is suspected, the posterior ligament of the sternoclavicular joint may be injected. There are two ways to approach this ligament. With the patient in the supine position, a slightly longer 25-gauge needle may be passed completely through the joint, until ligamentous resistance is felt, and then 1 mL of local anesthetic and/or depot steroid is injected around the ligament. The alternate approach is to enter the skin above the superior aspect of the clavicle and walk the needle off the posterior aspect of the clavicle in a slightly medial direction. Again, the injection is carried out as described earlier.

With both costosternal and sternoclavicular joint injections, care must be taken to have the needle enter the skin perpendicularly in order to diminish the possibility of pneumothorax. With sternoclavicular joint injections, there is also the possibility of puncture of the subclavian artery or vein with a misplaced needle. Careful attention to technique and use of short needles should minimize these complications.

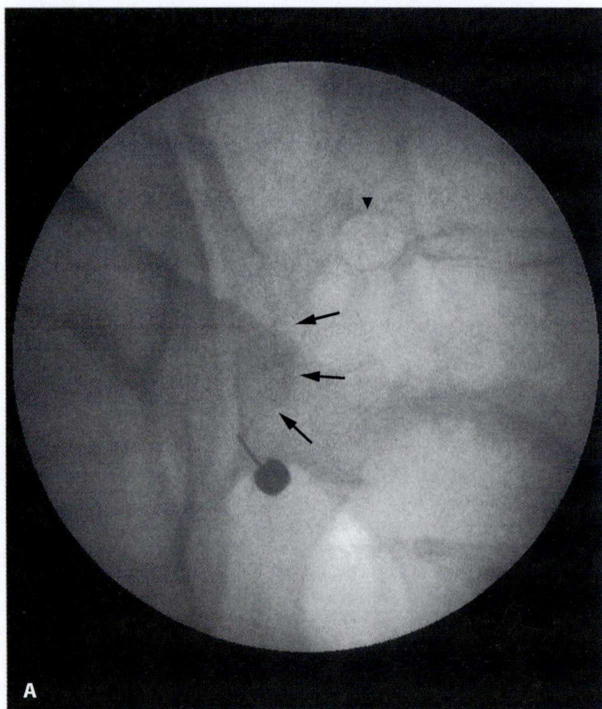

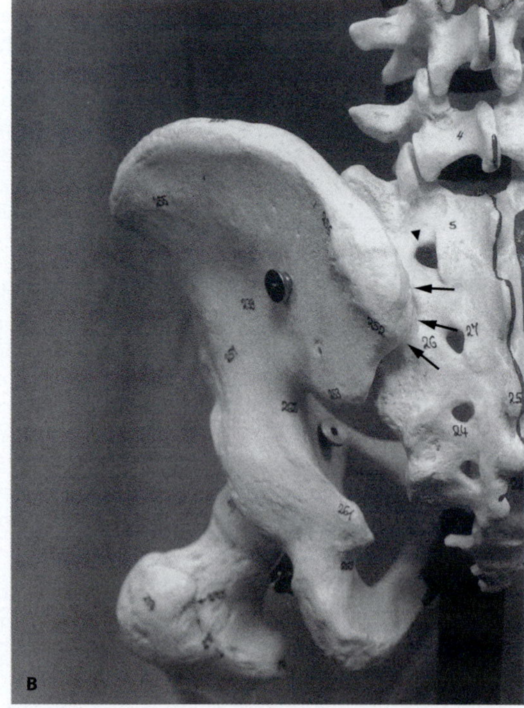

FIGURE 82-22. (**A**) Needle placement for sacroiliac joint injection. Small arrows outline the posterior superior iliac spine (PSIS). The large arrow is at the first sacral foramen. (**B**) Skeletal model showing corresponding landmarks. Small arrows again outline the PSIS. The large arrow is at the first sacral foramen.

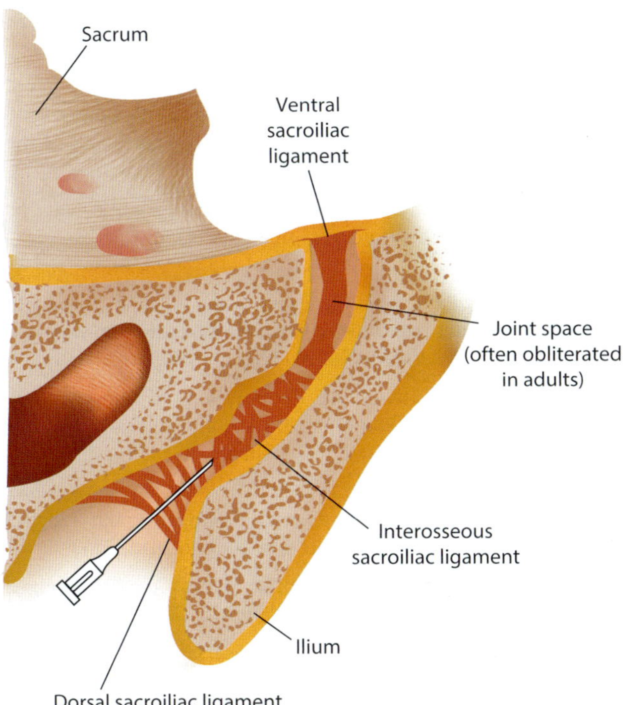

FIGURE 82-23. Diagram of sacroiliac injection.

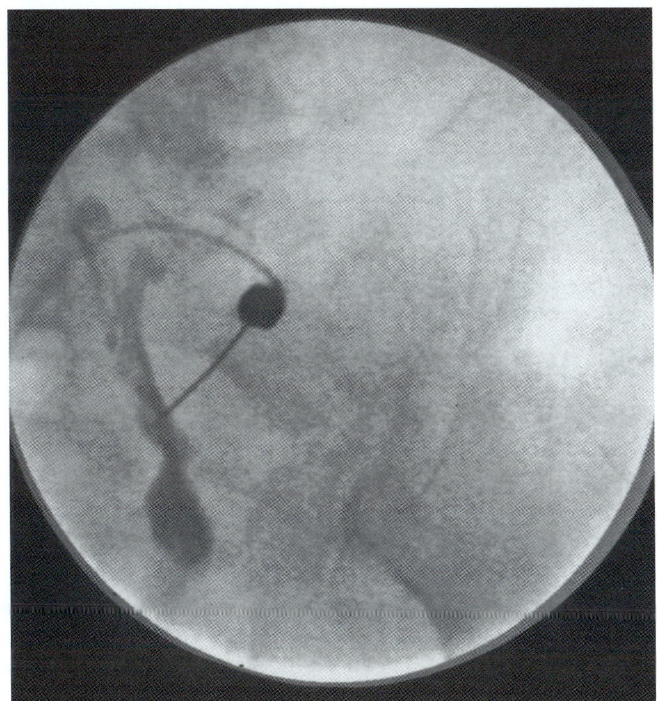

FIGURE 82-24. Contrast spread after sacroiliac injection.

REFERENCES

1. Woolf AD, Pfleger B. Burden of major musculoskeletal conditions. *Bull World Health Organ*. 2003;81(9):646-656.
2. Hench PS, Kendall EC, Slocumb CH, Polley HF. The effect of a hormone of the adrenal cortex (17-hydroxy-11-dehydrocorticosterone) and of pituitary adrenocorticotrophic hormone on rheumatoid arthritis. *Proc Staff Meet Mayo Clin*. 1949;24:181.
3. Hollander JL. The local effects of compound F (hydrocortisone) injected into joints. *Bull Rheum Dis*. 1951;2:3.
4. Partington PF, Broome GH. Diagnostic injection around the shoulder: hit and miss? A cadaveric study of injection accuracy. *J Shoulder Elbow Surg*. 1998;7:147.
5. Diraçoğlu D, Alptekin K, Dikici F, et al. Evaluation of needle positioning during blind intra-articular hip injections for osteoarthritis: fluoroscopy versus arthrography. *Arch Phys Med Rehabil*. 2009;90(12):2112-2115.
6. Centeno LM, Moore ME. Preferred intraarticular corticosteroids and associated practice: a survey of members of the American College of Rheumatology. 1994;7(3):151-155.
7. Derendorf H, Mollmann H, Grüner A, et al. Pharmacokinetics and pharmacodynamics of glucocorticoid suspensions after intra-articular administration. *Clin Pharmacol Ther*. 1986;39:313.
8. Firestein FS, Paine MM, Littman BH. Gene expression in rheumatoid arthritis and osteoarthritis synovium: quantitative analysis and effect of intra-articular corticosteroids. *Arthritis Rheum*. 1991; 34:1094.
9. Williams JM, Brandt KD. Triamcinolone hexacetonide protects against fibrillation and osteophyte formation following chemically induced articular cartilage damage. *Arthritis Rheum*. 1985; 28:1267.
10. Johansson A, Bennet G. Effect of local methylprednisolone on pain in nerve injury model. *Reg Anesth*. 1997;22:59.
11. Hills BA, Ethell MT, Hodgson DR. Release of lubricating synovial surfactant by Intraarticular steroid. *Br J Rheum*. 1998;37:649.
12. Rutjes AW, Jüni P, da Costa BR, et al. Viscosupplementation for osteoarthritis of the knee: a systematic review and meta-analysis. *Ann Intern Med*. 2012;157(3):180-191.
13. Axelsson K, Gupta A, Johanzon E, et al. Intraarticular administration of ketorolac, morphine, and ropivacaine combined with intraarticular patient-controlled regional analgesia for pain relief after shoulder surgery: a randomized, double-blind study. *Anesth Analg*. 2008;106(1):328-333.
14. Singh JA, Fitzgerald PM. Botulinum toxin for shoulder pain: a Cochrane systematic review. *J Rheumatol*. 2011;38;409-418.
15. Singh JA, Mahowald ML, Noorbaloochi S. Intraarticular botulinum toxin A for refractory painful total knee arthroplasty: a randomized controlled trial. *J Rheumatol*. 2010;37:2377-2386.
16. Thumboo J, O'Duffy JD. A prospective study of the safety of joint and soft tissue aspirations and injections in patients taking warfarin sodium. *Arthritis Rheum*. 1998;41:736.
17. Goupille P, Thomas T, Noël E. A practice survey of shoulder glucocorticoid injections in patients on antiplatelet drugs or vitamin K antagonists. *Joint Bone Spine*. 2008;75(3):311-314.
18. Gray RG, Tenenbaum J, Gottlieb NK. Local corticosteroid injection treatment in rheumatic disorders. *Semin Arthritis*. 1981;10:231.
19. Koehler BE, Urowitz MB, Killinger DW. Systemic effects of intra-articular corticosteroid. *J Rheumatol*. 1974;1:117.
20. Cole BJ, Schumacher HR Jr. Injectable corticosteroids in modern practice. *J Am Acad Orthop Surg*. 2005;13(1):37-46.
21. Dragoo JL, Braun HJ, Kim HJ, et al. The In vitro chondrotoxicity of single-dose local anesthetics. *Am J Sports Med*. 2012;40:794.
22. Braun HJ, Wilcox-Fogel N, Kim HJ, et al. The effect of local anesthetic and corticosteroid combinations on chondrocyte viability. *Knee Surg Sports Traumatol Arthrosc*. 2012;20:1689-1695.

23. Syed HM, Green L, Bianski B, et al. Bupivacaine and triamcinolone may be toxic to human chondrocytes. A pilot study. *Clin Orthop Relat Res.* 2011;469:2941-2947.
24. Sankar B, Seneviratne S, Radha S, et al. Safety of total hip replacement following an intra-articular steroid hip injection–an audit. *Acta Orthop Belg.* 2012;78(2):183-186.
25. McMahon SE, Lovell ME. Total hip arthroplasty after ipsilateral intra-articular steroid injection: 8 years follow up. *Acta Orthop Belg.* 2012;78(3):333-336.
26. Meermans G, Corten K, Simon JP. Is the infection rate in primary THA increased after steroid injection? *Clin Orthop Relat Res.* 2012;470:3213-3219.
27. Desai A, Ramankutty S, Board T, et al. Does intraarticular steroid infiltration increase the rate of infection in subsequent total knee replacements? *The Knee.* 2009;16:262-264.
28. Courtney P, Doherty M. Joint aspiration and injection and synovial fluid analysis. *Best Pract Res Clin Rheumatol.* 2009;23(2):161-192.
29. Wittich CM, Ficalora RD, Mason TG, et al. Musculoskeletal injection. *Mayo Clin Proc.* 2009;84(9):831-836; quiz 837.
30. Gaujoux-Viala C, Dougados M, Gossec L. Efficacy and safety of steroid injections for shoulder and elbow tendonitis: a meta-analysis of randomised controlled trials. *Ann Rheum Dis.* 2009;68(12):1843-1849.
31. Hambly N, Fitzpatrick P, MacMahon P, et al. Rotator cuff impingement: correlation between findings on MRI and outcome after fluoroscopically guided subacromial bursography and steroid injection. *AJR Am J Roentgenol.* 2007;189(5):1179-1184.
32. Hong JY, Yoon SH, Moon do J, et al. Comparison of high- and low-dose corticosteroid in subacromial injection for periarticular shoulder disorder: a randomized, triple-blind, placebo-controlled trial. *Arch Phys Med Rehabil.* 2011;92(12):1951-1960.
33. Arroll B, Goodyear-Smith F. Corticosteroid injections for painful shoulder: a meta-analysis. *Br J Gen Pract.* 2005;55(512):224-228.
34. Gialanella B, Prometti P. Effects of corticosteroids injection in rotator cuff tears. *Pain Med.* 2011;12(10):1559-1565.
35. Buchbinder R, Green S, Youd JM. Corticosteroid injections for shoulder pain. *Cochrane Database Syst Rev.* 2003;(1):CD004016.
36. Dogu B, Yucel SD, Sag SY, et al. Blind or ultrasound-guided corticosteroid injections and short-term response in subacromial impingement syndrome: a randomized, double-blind, prospective study. *Am J Phys Med Rehabil.* 2012;91(8):658-665.
37. Rah UW, Yoon SH, Moon do J, et al. Subacromial corticosteroid injection on poststroke hemiplegic shoulder pain: a randomized, triple-blind, placebo-controlled trial. *Arch Phys Med Rehabil.* 2012;93(6):949-956.
38. Lorbach O, Kieb M, Scherf C, et al. Good results after fluoroscopic-guided intra-articular injections in the treatment of adhesive capsulitis of the shoulder. *Knee Surg Sports Traumatol Arthrosc.* 2010;18(10):1435-1441.
39. Habib GS. Systemic effects of intra-articular corticosteroids. *Clin Rheumatol.* 2009;28(7):749-756.
40a. Benyamin RM, Vallejo R, Kramer J, et al. Corticosteroid induced psychosis in the pain management setting. *Pain Physician.* 2008;11(6):917-920.
40b. Van Linthoudt D, Kurmann PT. Livedoid dermatitis of the shoulder after a repeated subacromial corticosteroid injection. *Praxis (Bern 1994).* 2006;95(39):1499-1503.
41. Unglaub F, Guehring T, Fuchs PC, et al. Necrotizing fasciitis following therapeutic injection in a shoulder joint. *Orthopade.* 2005;34(3):250-252.
42. Masala S, Fiori R, Bartolucci DA, et al. Diagnostic and therapeutic joint injections. *Semin Intervent Radiol.* 2010;27(2):160-171.
43. Leopold SS, Battista V, Oliverio JA. Safety and efficacy of intraarticular hip injection using anatomic landmarks. *Clin Orthop Relat Res.* 2001;(391):192-197.
44. Crawford RW, Gic GA, Ling RSM, Murray DW. Diagnostic value of intra-articular anaesthetic in primary osteoarthritis of the hip. *J Bone Joint Surg.* 1998;80B:279.
45. Plant MJ, Borg AA, Dziedzic K, et al. Radiographic patterns and response to corticosteroid hip injection. *Ann Rheum Dis.* 1997; 56:476.
46. Deshmukh AJ, Panagopoulos G, Alizadeh A, et al. Intra-articular hip injection: does pain relief correlate with radiographic severity of osteoarthritis? *Skeletal Radiol.* 2011;40(11):1449-1454.
47. Liu W, Cong R, Li X, et al. Reduced opioid consumption and improved early rehabilitation with local and intraarticular cocktail analgesic injection in total hip arthroplasty: a randomized controlled clinical trial. *Pain Med.* 2011;12(3):387-393.
48. Young R, Harding J, Kingsly A, et al. Therapeutic hip injections: is the injection volume important? *Clin Radiol.* 2012;67(1):55-60.
49. Apyan P, Rudd J. Methicillin-sensitive Staphylococcus aureus infection after steroid hip injection. *Orthopedics.* 2012;35(1):e94-e96.
50. Cohen SP, Narvaez JC, Lebovits AH, et al. Corticosteroid injections for trochanteric bursitis: is fluoroscopy necessary? A pilot study. *Br J Anaesth.* 2005;94(1):100-106.
51. Cohen SP, Strassels SA, Foster L, et al. Comparison of fluoroscopically guided and blind corticosteroid injections for greater trochanteric pain syndrome: multicentre randomised controlled trial. *BMJ.* 2009;338:b1088.
52. Stephens MB, Beutler AI, O'Connor FG. Musculoskeletal injections: a review of the evidence. *Am Fam Physician.* 2008;78(8):971-976.
53. Brinks A, van Rijn RM, Willemsen SP, et al. Corticosteroid injections for greater trochanteric pain syndrome: a randomized controlled trial in primary care. *Ann Fam Med.* 2011;9(3):226-234.
54. Rompe JD, Segal NA, Cacchio A, et al. Home training, local corticosteroid injection, or radial shock wave therapy for greater trochanter pain syndrome. *Am J Sports Med.* 2009;37(10):1981-1990.
55. Hofmeister E, Engelhardt S. Necrotizing fasciitis as complication of injection into greater trochanteric bursa. *Am J Orthop (Belle Mead NJ).* 2001;30(5):426-427.
56. Johnston CAM, Wiley JP, Lindsay DM, Wiseman DA. Iliopsoas bursitis and tendonitis. *Sports Med.* 1998;25:271.
57. Toohey AK, LaSalle TL, Martinez S, Polisson RP. Iliopsoas bursitis: clinical features, radiographic findings, and disease associations. *Semin Arthritis Rheum.* 1990;20:41.
58. Jackson DW, Evans NA, Thomas BM. Accuracy of needle placement into the intra-articular space of the knee. *J Bone Joint Surg Am.* 2002;84-A(9):1522-1527.
59. Cheng OT, Souzdalnitski D, Vrooman B, et al. Evidence-based knee injections for the management of arthritis. *Pain Med.* 2012;13(6):740-753.
60. Raynauld JP, Buckland-Wright C, Ward R, et al. Safety and efficacy of long-term intraarticular steroid injections in osteoarthritis of the knee: a randomized, double-blind, placebo-controlled trial. *Arthritis Rheum.* 2003;48(2):370-377.
61. Geborek P, Monsson B, Wollheim FA, Montz U. Intra-articular corticosteroid injection into rheumatoid arthritis knees improves extensor muscle strength. *Rheumatol Int.* 1990;9:265.
62. Jones A, Doherty M. Intra-articular corticosteroids are effective in osteoarthritis but there are no clinical predictors of response. *Ann Rheum Dis.* 1996;55:829.

63. Charalambous CP, Tryfonidis M, Sadiq S, et al. Septic arthritis following intra-articular steroid injection of the knee–a survey of current practice regarding antiseptic technique used during intra-articular steroid injection of the knee. *Clin Rheumatol.* 2003;22(6):386-390.

64. Shemesh S, Heller S, Salai M, et al. Septic arthritis of the knee following intraarticular injections in elderly patients: report of six patients. *Isr Med Assoc J.* 2011;13(12):757-760.

65. Kontovazenitis PI, Starantzis KA, Soucacos PN. Major complication following minor outpatient procedure: osteonecrosis of the knee after intraarticular injection of cortisone for treatment of knee arthritis. *J Surg Orthop Adv.* 2009;18(1):42-44.

66. Lucas PE, Hurwitz SR, Kaplan PA, et al. Fluoroscopically guided injections into the foot and ankle: localization of the source of pain as a guide to treatment. *Radiology.* 1997;204:411.

67. Dreyfuss P, Michaelsen M, Fletcher D. Atlanto-occipital (AO) and lateral atlanto-axial (AA) joint pain patterns. *Spine.* 1990;19:1125.

68. Lamer TJ. Ear pain due to cervical spine arthritis: treatment with cervical facet injection. *Headache.* 1991;31:682.

69. Racz GB, Sanel H, Diede JH. Atlanto-occipital and atlantoaxial injections in the treatment of headache and neck pain. In: Waldman SD, Winnie AP, eds. *Interventional Pain Management.* Philadelphia: WB Saunders, 1996:220-222.

70. Busch E, Wilson P. Atlanto-occipital and atlanto-axial joint injections in the treatment of headache and neck pain. *Reg Anesth.* 1989;14:45.

71. Dory MA. Arthrography of the cervical facet joints. *Radiology.* 1983;148:379.

72. Wedel DJ, Wilson PR. Cervical facet arthrography. *Reg Anesth.* 1985;10:7.

73. Dreyfuss P, Tibilette C, Dreyer SJ. Thoracic zygapophysial joint pain patterns: a study in normal volunteers. *Spine.* 1994;19:807.

74. Benjamou C, Roux C, Tourliere D, et al. Pseudovisceral pain referred from costovertebral arthropathies. *Spine.* 1993;18;790.

75. Raney F. Costovertebral-costotransverse joint complex as the source of local or referred pain. *J Bone Joint Surg.* 1996;48A;1451.

76. Marks R. Distribution of pain provoked from lumbar facet joints and related structures during diagnostic spinal infiltration. *Pain.* 1989;39:37.

77. Schwarzer AC, Aprill CN, Derby R, et al. The relative contributions of the disc and zygapophysial joint in patients with chronic low back pain. *Spine.* 1995;20:907.

78. Schwarzer AC, Aprill CN, Derby R, et al. Clinical features of patients with pain stemming from the lumbar zygapophysial joints: is the lumbar facet syndrome a clinical entity? *Spine.* 1994;19:1132.

79. Dreyfuss P, Michaelson DC, Pauza K. The value of medical history and physical examination in diagnosing sacroiliac joint pain. *Spine.* 1996;21:2594.

80. Ebraheim N, Rongming X, Nadaud M, et al. Sacroiliac joint injection: a cadaveric study. *Am J Orthop.* 1997;26:338.

81. Maldjian C, Mesgarzadeh M, Tehranzedeh J. Diagnostic and therapeutic features of facet and sacroiliac joint injection. *Radiol Clin North Am.* 1998;36:497.

SUGGESTED READINGS

Ahmed I, Elie Gertner E. Safety of arthrocentesis and joint injection in patients receiving anticoagulation at therapeutic levels. *Am J Med.* 2012;125:265-269.

Devor M, Govrin-Lippman R, Raber P. Corticosteroids suppress neural discharge originating in experimental neuromas. *Pain.* 1985;22:127

Habib GS, Abu-Ahmad R. Lack of effect of corticosteroid injection at the shoulder joint on blood glucose levels in diabetic patients. *Clin Rheumatol.* 2007;26(4):566-568.

Salvati G, Punzi L, Pianon M. Frequency of the bleeding risk in patients receiving warfarin submitted to arthrocentesis of the knee. *Reumatismo.* 2003;55(3):159-163.

Shbeeb MI, O'Duffy JD, Michet CJ Jr, et al. Evaluation of glucocorticosteroid injection for the treatment of trochanteric bursitis. *J Rheumatol.* 1996;23(12):2104-2106.

CHAPTER 83 Sympathetic Blocks

Jatinder S. Gill

INTRODUCTION

The autonomic nervous system (ANS) is a powerful system that has important homeostatic functions. Disorders of this system can lead to many disease states and may contribute to some pain disorders such as complex regional pain syndrome (CRPS). Having a good working knowledge of the anatomy and physiology of the ANS is of paramount importance when considering sympathetic blocks. The higher neural centers in the brainstem, the hypothalamus, and the prefrontal cortex have nerve cells that tightly control the function and the output of the ANS. The ANS is composed of the sympathetic and parasympathetic nervous systems. The parasympathetic outflow has cranial (several cranial nerves), vagal (mainly via the vagus nerve, which innervates many intrathoracic and intraabdominal structures), and sacral outflow that controls the urinary and reproductive organs. The sympathetic nervous system is formed by neurons in the intermediolateral cell column of the thoracolumbar spinal cord. These are in turn modulated by descending autonomic projections from the hypothalamus, the suprachiasmatic nucleus, and the supraparaventricular nucleus.[1] Axons from these neuron cells exit the spinal cord by the anterior spinal roots and white rami communicantes to the sympathetic chain ganglia located along the left and right anterolateral margins of the spinal column. Upon reaching these paravertebral ganglia, the preganglionic sympathetic axons may synapse, pass cephalad or caudad for variable distances within the sympathetic chain before synapsing, or continue uninterrupted to a more distant ganglion or plexus, such as the celiac or hypogastric plexus.

Nerves from the cervical and thoracic ganglia innervate the head and neck and control the blood supply to these structures. The nerves from the thoracic ganglia control the function of the heart and lungs. The nerves that bypass paravertebral sympathetic chain ganglia to more distant ganglia (celiac, hypogastric) are called splanchnic nerves. Splanchnic nerves are the primary sympathetic fibers that innervate visceral organs. Nerves from the lumbar ganglia innervate the legs and control the blood supply to the legs.

The A-δ and C fibers transmit pain and discomfort sensations from the visceral organs to the spinal cord dorsal horn lamina. These fibers develop from the dorsal root ganglion cells and travel along the blood vessels, ganglia, and mesenteric nerves. Hence, blockade of the sympathetic nerves not only causes sympatholysis but also sensory denervation of the abdominal organs.

Kappis originally used paravertebral sympathetic blocks[2] as treatment for severe pain and visceral pain syndromes. Mandl[3] first introduced

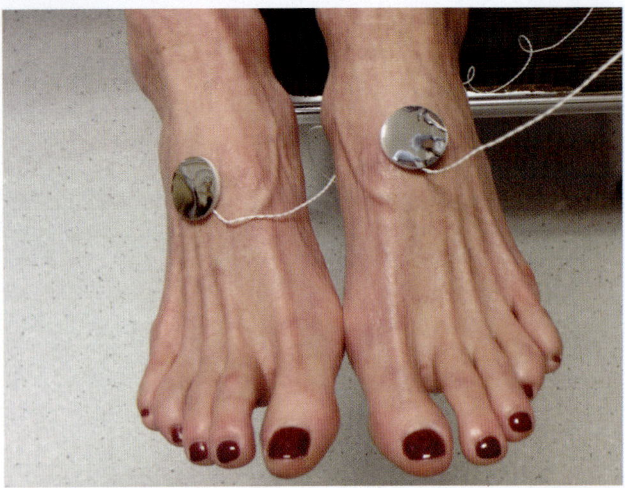

FIGURE 83-1. Temperature probe placed on bilateral feet before a lumbar sympathetic nerve block.

percutaneous interruption of the sympathetic chain in the early 20th century, and for many years thereafter it was a mainstay therapy for vascular insufficiency of the lower extremities. Sympathetic nervous system blocks may be performed to diagnose sympathetically mediated pain (SMP), to diagnose visceral abdominal pain (by blocking splanchnic afferents), and for short-term benefit in conditions of pathologic vasoconstriction (e.g., Raynaud's disease)[4] or when sympathectomy can provide therapeutic benefit (e.g., digit reimplantation, limb ischemia). Stellate ganglion block has also been successfully used to treat recurrent ventricular tachycardia.[5]

PATIENT PREPARATION

The patient should not be overly sedated during the procedure because verbal contact with the patient is extremely valuable and is needed to assess the response to the block, especially when the diagnostic phase is to be followed by neurolysis such as celiac neurolysis. Monitoring and intravenous (IV) access should be used. For sympathetic blocks involving the limbs, skin temperature probes are placed bilaterally on the extremities undergoing sympathetic block (**Fig. 83-1**). The block is considered adequate if cutaneous temperature of the treated limb approaches core temperature.[6] A careful evaluation of placebo effects, systemic uptake of drug, and blockade of somatic nerves must be performed in patients who have obtained relief after a sympathetic block. As with any invasive procedure, resuscitation equipment and drugs should be readily available. Major contraindications to sympathetic blocks include coagulopathy and patient refusal.

STELLATE GANGLION BLOCKS

ANATOMY

The cervical chain is composed of a superior, middle, and inferior cervical ganglion; the inferior ganglion is fused with the first thoracic ganglion, resulting in a "starlike" (stellate) appearance. It receives preganglionic sympathetic fibers via white rami communicantes from the intermediolateral cell column of T1 to T6 in the spinal cord. It is an oval-shaped structure approximately 2 cm long, 1 cm wide, and about 0.5 cm thick. The ganglion lies anterior to the transverse process of C7 and extends along the C7 to T1 interspace. It is bound inferiorly by the dome of the pleura, posteromedially by the longus colli muscle and laterally by the scalene muscles. It is also bound anteriorly in part by the subclavian artery and posteriorly by the transverse processes of C7

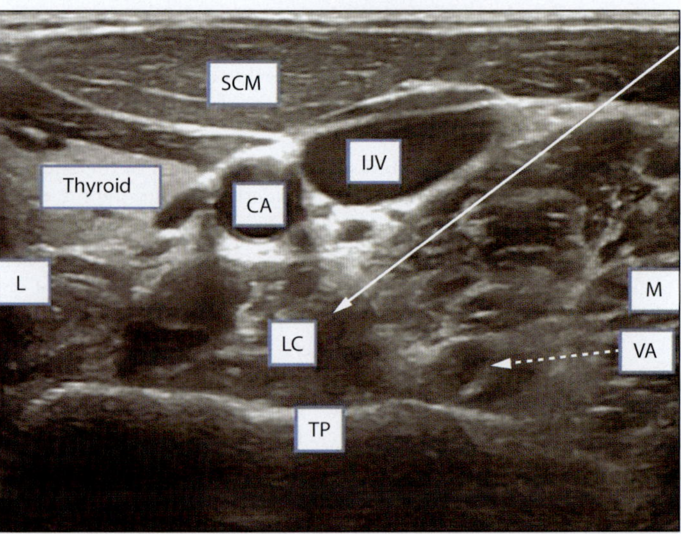

FIGURE 83-2. Ultrasound image at C7. The transverse process (TP) is not prominent. The vertebral artery (VA) lies posterolateral to the stellate ganglion. The arrow shows the trajectory of the needle insertion as well as the target. CA, carotid artery; IJV, internal jugular vein; L, lateral; LC, longus colli; M, medial; SCM, sternocleidomastoid.

and T1 (**Figs. 83-2** and **83-3**). The prevertebral fascia, which originates posterior to the sympathetic chain in the cervical region, is pierced by the chain around C7 and becomes anterior to the stellate ganglion as the fascia forms a transition from the neck to the chest. Superior to the stellate ganglion is the transverse process of the sixth cervical vertebrae, or Chassaignac's tubercle, a prominence that is easily palpable along the paratracheal region of the neck (**Figs. 83-4** and **83-5**).

One must remember that although Chassaignac's tubercle is the major landmark for performing the anterior paratracheal block of the stellate

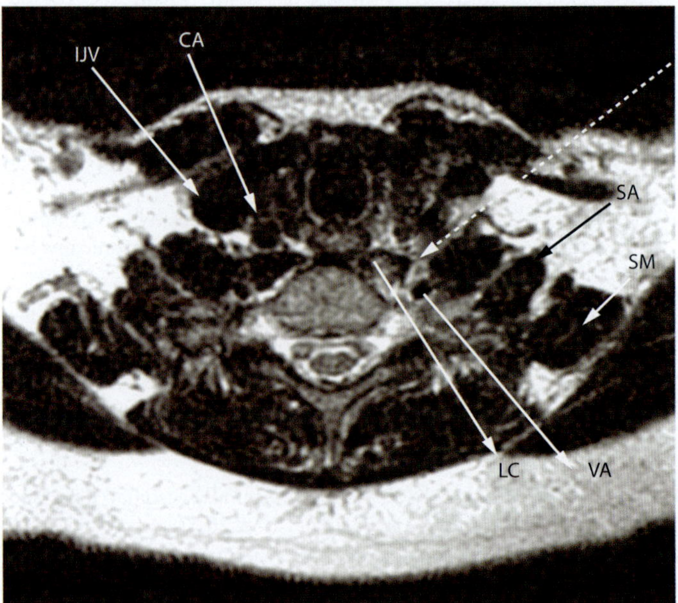

FIGURE 83-3. Magnetic resonance imaging, axial cut at the C7 level. The vertebral artery (VA) lies posterior and lateral to the longus colli (LC) muscle. The stellate ganglion lies anterior to the LC muscle and is posterior to and bounded by the prevertebral fascia. The anterior tubercle is not prominent. The needle is placed in-plane lateral to medial, and local anesthetic injected posterior to the prevertebral fascia and anterior to the LC muscle. CA, carotid artery; IJV, internal jugular vein; SA, scalenus anterior; SM, scalenus medius.

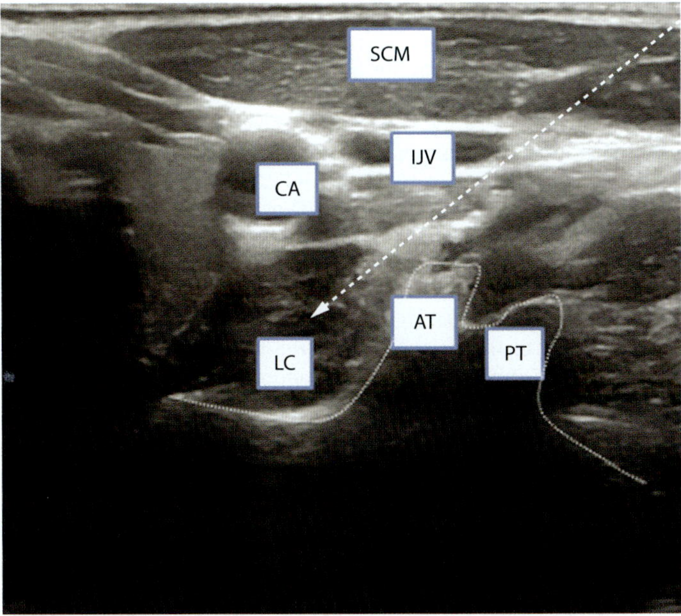

FIGURE 83-4. Ultrasound image at C6. Same structures as ultrasound at C7. The transverse process is prominent (Chassaignac's tubercle), and the carotid artery (CA) has entered the foramen transversarium. The dotted arrow shows the trajectory of needle insertion and the target. AT, anterior tubercle, IJV; internal jugular vein; LC, longus colli; PT, posterior tubercle; SCM, sternocleidomastoid muscle.

ganglion, the location of the ganglion itself is inferior to the tubercle. Interestingly enough, ultrasonography and magnetic resonance imaging studies suggest that local anesthetic spread to the ganglion does not occur; rather, the spread occurs anterior to the ganglion.[7,8] Other radiographic and injection studies have supported this finding as well.[9-12] This anterior spread likely relates to prevertebral fascia being in the same plane as Chassaignac's tubercle at the C6 vertebra but then becomes more anterior at the stellate ganglion, thus preventing the spread of injectate onto the ganglion. The presence of this fascia also promotes mediastinal and even contralateral spread of injectate.[8] Therefore, sympathetic neural blockade during stellate ganglion block may take place at sites other than the stellate ganglion.

INDICATIONS

The stellate ganglion block is used to diagnose facial and upper extremity SMP. It may be repeated as a therapeutic measure when prolonged pain relief response lasting several weeks is seen. This period may then be helpful to facilitate physiotherapy and desensitization. A positive response with pain relief in CRPS may also predict a favorable response to spinal cord stimulation.[13] Other indications include circulatory insufficiency such as Raynaud's disease (short-term improvement), thromboembolic or vasospastic event, or conditions in which sympatholysis is highly desirable (e.g., digit reimplantation surgery).

TECHNIQUE

The block may be performed under fluoroscopic control or with ultrasound guidance with all sterile precautions.

With fluoroscopic assistance, the junction of the transverse process with the vertebral body (C6 or C7) is visualized. The patient is placed in supine position, and an IV line is started. Standard monitors are placed. A 3.5-in, 25-gauge needle is advanced to the junction of the transverse process with the vertebral body and then slightly withdrawn (**Fig. 83-6**). Under real-time fluoroscopy 1 to 5 mL of contrast agent is injected, and linear spread of the agent along the gutter confirms adequate placement. A total of 5 mL of local anesthetic without epinephrine is deposited there, and the needle is withdrawn. Because of the risk of particulate steroid embolization causing infarction, no adjuvant particulate steroid should be used. The amount of contrast agent and local anesthetic injected is determined by the spread.

Gofeld et al. describe ultrasound-guided stellate ganglion block based on cadaver studies.[14] When using ultrasound guidance, Chassaignac's tubercle is identified by its characteristic shadow, and the transverse process at this level is clearly identified (Fig. 83-4). The transducer is translated inferiorly to assess if the C7 transverse process can be identified (Fig. 83-2). Injection at lower level will be in closer proximity to the stellate ganglion. When the transverse process is clearly identified, the longus colli muscle is seen overlying this and underlying the carotid artery. A 3.5-in, 25-gauge needle is advanced to this point in an in-plane approach. Thereafter, 5 to 6 mL of local anesthetic without additional epinephrine is injected, making sure it is underlying the prevertebral fascia. As with fluoroscopic guidance, because of the risk of particulate

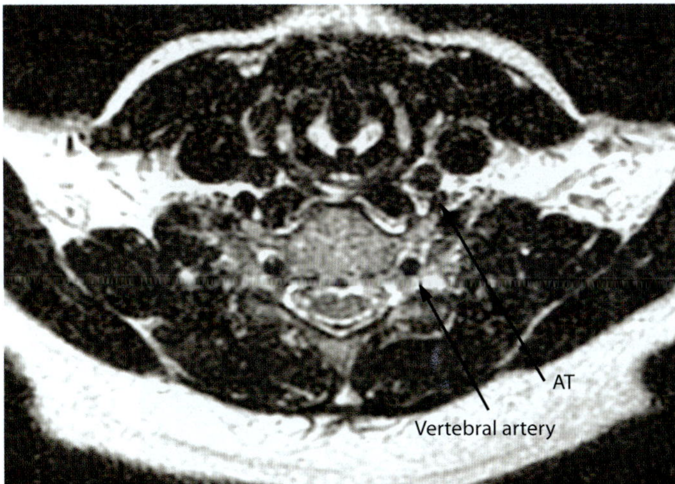

FIGURE 83-5. Magnetic resonance imaging, axial cut at the C6 level. Same structures as at the C7 level, but the vertebral artery is in the foramen transversarium and well protected from the needle tip. The anterior tubercle (AT) of C6 (Chassaignac's tubercle) is prominent. If block is performed at this level, the needle is placed in-plane lateral to medial and local anesthetic injected anterior to longus colli muscle and posterior to the carotid artery.

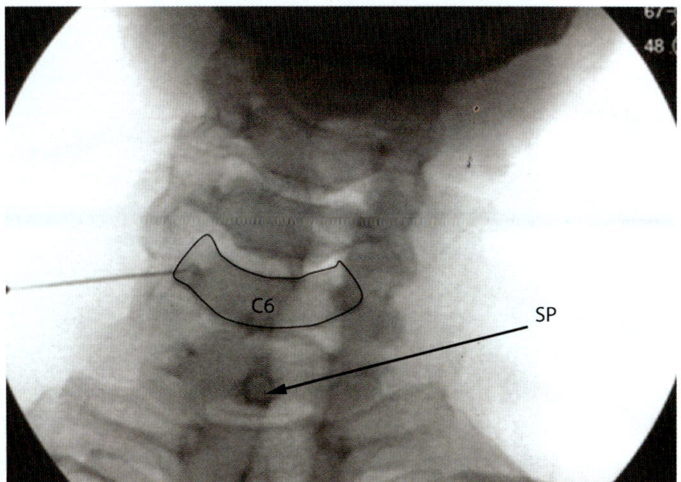

FIGURE 83-6. The needle is placed at the junction of the C6 transverse process with the vertebral body. This needle was placed under ultrasound guidance, and fluoroscopy is used to confirm the location. SP, spinous process.

steroid embolization causing infarction, no adjuvant particulate steroid should be used.

Evaluation for the presence of sympathectomy must be performed. Although a Horner's sign (ipsilateral ptosis, miosis, anhydrosis, and conjunctival engorgement) is indicative of a sympathectomy of the head and face, it in no way suggests a sympathectomy of the arm and hand. Skin surface temperature probes placed bilaterally at the palmar thenar regions are simple yet effective. A 1.0° to 1.5°C increase in the blocked side or, perhaps more specifically, an increase in temperature toward core temperature that exceeds that of the contralateral side[15,16] is strongly suggestive of a successful sympathetic block of the arm. Somatic block of the arm must also be ruled out.

COMPLICATIONS

Minor complications are common. Because of the proximity of laryngeal nerves to the stellate ganglion, dysphagia and hoarseness are common with the anterior approach. Transient central nervous system events such as seizures, aphasia, blindness, loss of consciousness, and hemiparesis can occur after injected doses as low as 15 mg of lidocaine or 2.5 mg of bupivacaine.[17-21] Other complications include pneumothorax and seizure (vertebral artery injection). The incidence of complications can be reduced by using lower volumes, meticulous technique, aspiration before injection, and slow injection. Appropriate resuscitation equipment should be readily available and used as the clinical scenario dictates. Use of ultrasound guidance might further help reduce the complications because the needle and the target are well visualized.

CELIAC PLEXUS AND SPLANCHNIC NERVE BLOCKS

ANATOMY

The celiac plexus is a dense matrix of diffuse nerve fibers and ganglia located around the abdominal aorta and periaortic space at the level of the T12 and L1 vertebrae. The most distinct feature of the celiac plexus are the paired semilunar ("celiac") ganglia that lie immediately superior to the pancreas in the midline and are flanked in close approximation by the adrenals. These "paired" ganglia can actually vary in number and size.[22] The aorta is surrounded by the plexus, which makes this large vascular structure an important landmark in performing the block. In fact, transgression of the aorta has been used in identifying needle placement.[23] In addition to the celiac ganglia, the components of the celiac plexus include the greater, lesser, and least (also called lowest) splanchnic nerves; there are also contributions from the aorticorenal ganglia and aortic and superior hypogastric plexus. It is important to realize that the celiac plexus is not a distinct entity but a diffuse network that varies in size, network, and position. The most consistent landmark is the celiac artery because these elements intertwine around the base of this artery (**Fig. 83-7**).

There are sympathetic, parasympathetic, and visceral afferent contributions to the celiac plexus. The sympathetic fibers originate from the thoracic sympathetic chain via the greater and lesser splanchnic nerves, and the visceral afferents have cell bodies that originate from the dorsal root ganglion of the spinal cord and travel with the sympathetic nerves. The parasympathetics originate from the vagus nerve. The nerves of the celiac plexus innervate most of the abdominal viscera to include the pancreas, liver, kidneys, biliary tract, spleen, adrenals, intestines, and omentum.

INDICATIONS

The celiac plexus block is indicated for patients in pain from upper abdominal tumors such as pancreatic cancer. Pain relief rates vary from 70% to 100%, with an average of 85% of patients that experience at least temporary pain relief.[24,25] Pain from these tumors can be severe, and opioid therapy is often limited by the sedation and constipation that accompany the high doses required to manage the patient's discomfort. Neurolytic celiac plexus blocks in these patients can provide superior pain relief for up to 3 to 4 months. In most patients, relief will be immediate and effective. Furthermore, they can lessen the severity of opioid-induced side effects by decreasing requirements of these drugs. Gastrointestinal (GI) motility is also improved by the sympathectomy caused by the block. The predictive value of a neurolytic celiac plexus block can be determined by the degree of tumor invasion. Akhan et al.[26] found that the grade of tumor as measured by invasion of periaortic and paracaval fat planes was a good predictor for successful neurolytic celiac plexus block. More than 50% invasion of the fat planes correlated with little pain relief. Age and history of laparotomy, chemotherapy, or radiation therapy have not been shown to decrease the efficacy of neurolytic celiac plexus blocks.

Benign conditions such as acute and chronic pancreatitis may also respond to celiac plexus blocks. As with pancreatic cancer patients, acute pancreatitis is often resistant to opioid therapy; furthermore, the disease process may be improved by decreasing the ductal and sphincter spasm

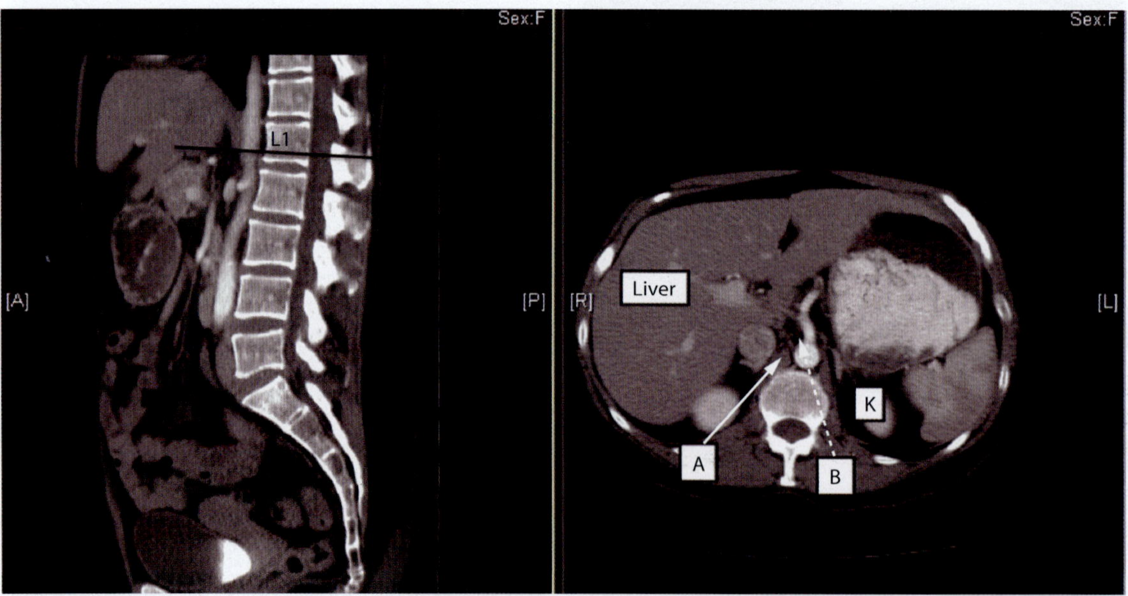

FIGURE 83-7. Computerised tomograph with contrast at L1 level. The kidney (K) is appearing. Arrow A shows the trajectory and target retrocrural and transcrural location; arrow B shows the trajectory and target for transaortic celiac plexus block just anterior to the aorta on the left.

thought to be associated with acute pancreatitis. Addition of steroids to the local anesthetic injectate has been shown to decrease the severity of the attack,[27] but use of particulate steroids is no longer advisable given the embolic risk if intraarterial uptake occurs in this sensitive location. Continuous catheter techniques can be effective in chronic alcoholic patients diagnosed with acute pancreatitis who were previously unresponsive to epidural analgesia. Rykowski et al.[28] used 0.5% bupivacaine, 20 mL every 6 to 12 hours as intermittent injection, or 0.5% bupivacaine at 6 mL/hr with good results. Overall, celiac plexus blocks have shown to be an effective adjunct in managing chronic pancreatitis pain.[29] Using celiac plexus blocks, especially neurolytic celiac plexus blocks in chronic pancreatitis, is however controversial. Although 4 to 6 months of relief can be obtained from neurolytic celiac plexus blocks, a subset of alcoholic patients may view their pain-free state as an opportunity to resume the consumption of alcoholic beverages. Furthermore, because this block also interrupts the visceral afferents from abdominal organs, it may mask pain related to intraabdominal emergencies. Given the chronic recurrent nature of chronic pancreatitis and associated morbidities, including the psychological effects of pain, central sensitization, and the availability of other modalities (medications, epidural), celiac plexus block is now rarely used for acute pain control in chronic pancreatitis. Given the short-lasting benefit from neurolysis, this also is not an effective strategy for the management of pain in these patients.

TECHNIQUE

A variety of techniques can be used to approach the splanchnic nerves or celiac plexus. In general, they can be summarized as posterior or anterior approaches. The posterolateral approach has become the most practiced and proven technique by anesthesiologists, whereas the anterior techniques using computed tomography (CT) or ultrasound guidance are preferred by invasive radiologists. In recent years, endoscopic ultrasound guided celiac plexus neurolysis has become increasingly prevalent.[30] In all cases, noninvasive monitoring should be used, and an IV line should be established. IV vasoactive agents, volume expanders (crystalloid or colloids), and sedative and analgesics should be made available for use as needed. Procedure is performed with sterile precautions and resuscitation equipment available. The fragile condition of some of these patients should be taken into account.

Posterolateral Approaches Posterolateral techniques allow access to both the splanchnic nerves and the celiac plexus. The posterolateral approach is one originally defined by Kappis and refined by Moore.[31] Frequently used variations of the posterolateral approach include the transcrural approach, the transaortic approach, and the retrocrural or deep splanchnic approach.

The patient is placed in a prone position with a pillow placed at the midsection of the abdomen. This minimizes the lumbar lordosis and aids in patient comfort. Occasionally, the abdominal pain can be so severe that the prone position is not tolerated, and analgesics must be used or the patient must be positioned in the lateral decubitus position. The arms are underneath behind the head or allowed to hang off the table. An IV line is placed to provide light sedation if necessary, and a 200- to 500-mL crystalloid bolus may be administered depending on patient condition, to offset the sympathectomy-induced hypotension caused by the block. Anatomic landmarks are identified and marked in ink. Agents typically used for the celiac plexus block include 0.25% to 0.5% bupivacaine, 6% to 10% phenol, and 50% to 100% alcohol. Volumes are described for each technique (see the following sections).

The classic posterior approach is a two-needle technique; needle placement is similar for both sides. The needle is placed under radiologic control. The oblique fluoroscopic projection is used so that the tip of the L1 transverse overlies the vertebral body. The insertion points lie 6 to 9 cm from the midline and usually correspond to the junction of the paraspinal muscles and the 12th rib. After administering local anesthetic to create a skin wheal at this point, a 12- to 20-cm, 20- to 22-gauge subarachnoid needle is inserted percutaneously The needle is inserted in a coaxial approach . The needle may be "walked off" the lumbar body or

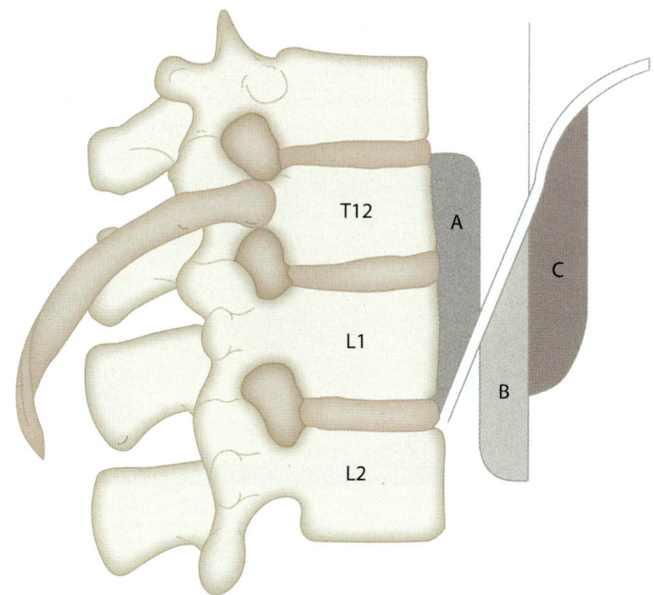

FIGURE 83-8. (**A**) Retrocrural (spreads within and slightly outside the margin of the vertebral body on anteroposterior (AP) view. (**B**) Transcrural (confined to the margins of the vertebral body on AP view. (**C**) Transaortic (midline spread).

placed directly sliding adjacent to the vertebral body. The final placement of the needle tip is 1.0 to 1.5 cm anterior to the vertebral margin. The needle pulsation occurs on the left side because the final position of the needle tip is often close to the aorta. The second needle is placed on the right side using the same technique as the first; depth is guided by the final needle depth used on the left side. Contrast agent is seen on fluoroscopy will indicate retrocrural, transcrural, transaortic, or intradiaphragmatic injection of agent (**Figs. 83-8** and **83-9**). If CT imaging is used, needle paths are traced from the skin to the celiac plexus to avoid injury to renal or vascular structures.

For the transcrural approach, advancing the needle tips an additional 1 to 2 cm will pierce the diaphragmatic crus and place the needle tip anterior to the diaphragm. A loss of resistance is usually felt as the crus is pierced. The anteroposterior (AP) and lateral radiographs with contrast will show a linear spread in the left lateral preaortic area. If contrast spread is predominately cephalad and appears to collect around the L1 vertebral body, the needle tip is likely to be retrocrural. Lateral radiographs can confirm that the contrast is posterior and superior to the diaphragm, also suggesting retrocrural spread. The procedure can then be performed as a deep splanchnic nerve block (see later section), or the needle is advanced to pierce the diaphragmatic crus (thus transcrural). If muscle striations are seen following contrast injection, the needle tip is likely contained within diaphragmatic muscle and should be advanced about 1 cm. On lateral fluoroscopy, contrast agent is typically seen to spread in a craniocaudal direction anterior to the vertebral body, but agent spread is limited to below the diaphragm (**Fig. 83-8B**). After negative aspiration of each needle, 10 mL of local anesthetic is injected through each needle. The patient is watched for more than 10 minutes for pain relief and to rule out somatic nerve block. If neurolysis is planned, then 10 to 25 mL of local anesthetic or neurolytic agent is injected through each needle in divided doses.

The transaortic approach is a single needle, left-sided technique that is also transcrural.[23] The intent of this approach is to pierce the aorta with the needle to ensure that the needle tip is anterior to the aorta. Placement of the injectate anterior to the aorta can minimize the risk of neurologic complications caused by unintended spread of neurolytic agents to the lumbar plexus. Needle placement is the same as for the transcrural approach, but the needle is advanced until aortic wall penetration occurs and free-flowing blood is aspirated. The needle is then

A

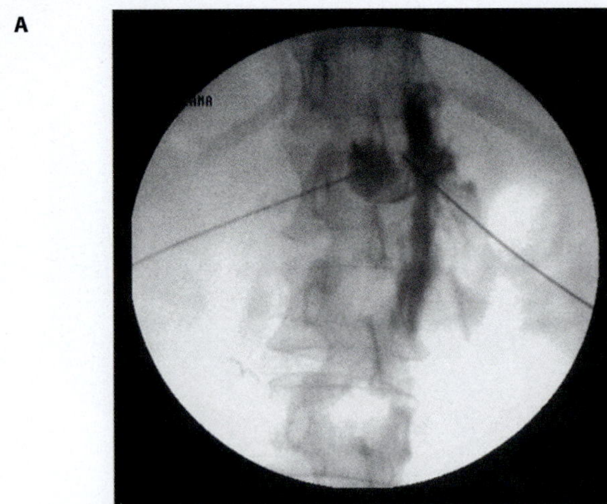

B

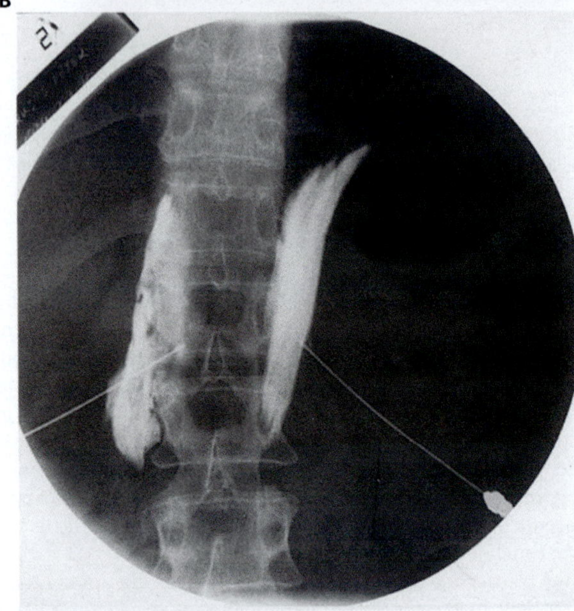

FIGURE 83-9. (**A**) The needle on the left transaortic demonstrates midline contrast. The needle on the right is transcrural with no significant paraspinal spread of contrast. (**B**) The needle on the left shows retorcrural spread (some paraspinal spread), and the needle on the right demonstrates injection into the diaphragm.

advanced further through the anterior wall of the aorta until no blood is aspirated.

A 5-mL loss of resistance syringe filled with saline can be used to identify anterior aortic wall penetration. Once blood is aspirated through the block needle, the loss of resistance syringe is attached to the needle, and constant pressure is applied to the syringe plunger. A resistance to injection will be felt when the anterior aortic wall has been contacted followed by loss of resistance once the needle tip has entered the anterior periaortic space. After negative aspiration, contrast agent is injected and will appear anterior to the vertebral bodies (Figs. 83-8C and 83-9A). Local anesthetic, steroid, or neurolytic agent is then injected. A smaller total volume of agent (12–15 mL) is used for this technique.

Anterior Approach With the anterior approach, a 12- to 15-cm, 22-gauge needle is passed through the midline epigastrium until the body of L1 is contacted. The needle is then withdrawn 1.0 to 1.5 cm, and placement is confirmed using fluoroscopy or CT imaging.[32,33] Patient comfort is a major advantage to this approach, especially when the patient is unable to lie prone. Only one needle is used with this technique, so there is less pain from posterior two-needle approaches. Furthermore, the risk of needle-related injury to motor nerves is significantly reduced compared with posterior approaches.

Splanchnic Nerve Blocks An alternative technique to achieve abdominal sympathectomy and visceral nerve block is the splanchnic nerve block. The splanchnic nerve block specifically interrupts the sympathetic input to the celiac plexus without blocking the abdominal parasympathetics. The final position of the needle tip is superior to the diaphragm; the intention is to block the greater, lesser, and least splanchnic nerves before they traverse the diaphragm into the abdomen. The advantages of performing sympathectomy and visceral nerve block are multifold. GI motility is improved compared with the celiac plexus block because the parasympathetics (which join the splanchnics at the level of the celiac ganglia) are left unopposed. Also, because the lumbar sympathetics are not blocked by this technique, hypotension is decreased. Last, with the classic splanchnic nerve block, a smaller volume of local anesthetic or neurolytic agent can be used.

For the deep splanchnic approach[34,35] (also known as the retrocrural celiac plexus block), landmarks and needle approach are similar to the transcrural celiac plexus block. The needle is walked off the vertebral body and advanced until the needle pulsates (because of the proximity of the needle tip to the aorta) on visual inspection and tactile analysis. When the block is performed correctly, 3- to 5-mL injection of contrast will remain within the retrocrural space and migrate primarily cephalad (Figs. 83-8A and 83-9B). On fluoroscopic AP view, the contrast will be confined along the lateral border to the L1 vertebral body . On lateral view, layering of the contrast in a narrow line along the anterior vertebral column should be seen. The procedure is then repeated on the right side. Fifteen milliliters of local anesthetic or neurolytic agent is injected through each needle. Parasympathetics and the lumbar sympathetic chain are not blocked with this technique.

The classic splanchnic nerve block is performed in a manner similar to the deep splanchnic approach, but the needle is directed toward the anterolateral margin of T12 vertebral body. Radiographic contrast patterns are similar to the deep splanchnic nerve block. The disadvantages of this block relate to final position of the needle tips; compared with the transcrural and transaortic blocks, the needle tips lie posterior and cephalad to the diaphragm, which increases the risk of chylothorax and pneumothorax (**Fig. 83-10**).

COMPLICATIONS

The incidence of major complications with neurolytic celiac plexus blocks is 0.15% to 1.0%.[36,37] These complications typically occur from transgression of structures during needle placement or unintentional spread of neurolytic or local anesthetic solutions. Inadvertent injury to structures can result in pneumothorax, chylothorax (secondary to thoracic duct injury), genitourinary injury, somatic nerve injury, and retroperitoneal hematoma; complications secondary to inadvertent spread of agent include sexual dysfunction, groin neuralgia, paraplegia, retroperitoneal fibrosis after repeated neurolytic blocks,[38] and pleural effusion.[39] Complications are often self-limited. In a study of 136 cases after celiac plexus block, Brown et al. describe two cases of pneumothorax, neither requiring thoracostomy as therapy.[25] Renal perforation can occur, albeit typically without sequelae, especially if the block needles are placed more than 7.5 cm from the midline. When inserted lateral to this point, renal impalement can occur in 10% of cases.[40] Paraplegia has been described secondary to injury to the artery of Adamkiewicz during block placement[41] and from arterial vasospasm causing anterior spinal artery syndrome.[42] Paraplegia can also occur from incorrect needle placement and subsequent injection in the subarachnoid or epidural space or from intrapsoas muscle injection with blockade or neurolysis of the lumbar plexus. Radiographic imaging (biplanar fluoroscopy or CT) can minimize these risks.

Minor sequelae inherent to the celiac plexus block are relatively common. The most common side effects of the block include local pain (96%), hypotension (38%), and diarrhea (44%).[36] Systolic blood

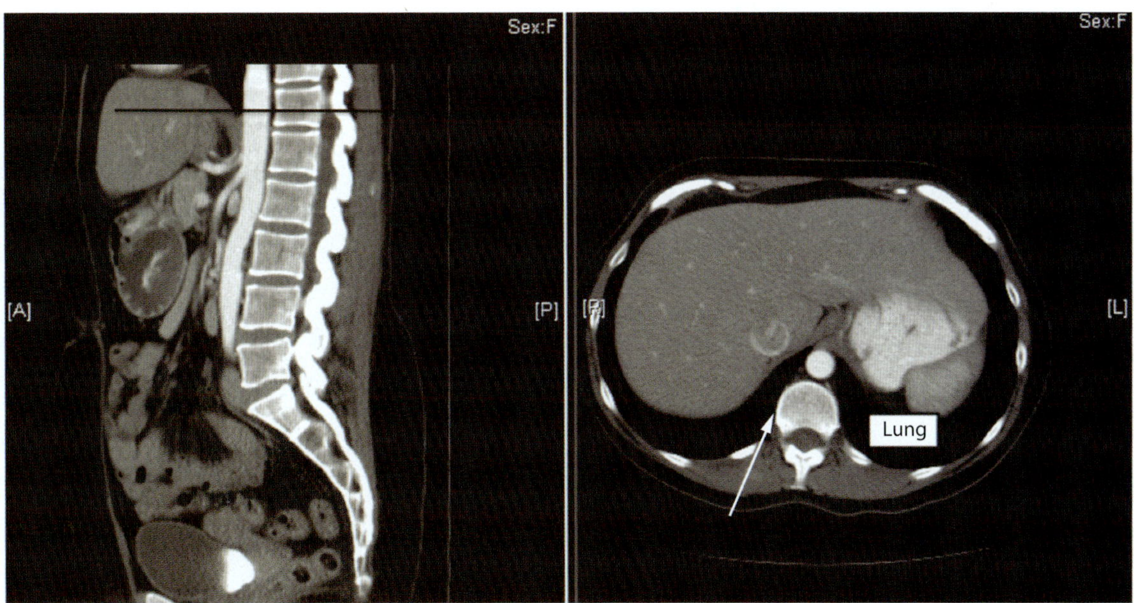

FIGURE 83-10. Computerised tomograph at T12. Very low volumes are used for splanchnic neurolysis, and the needle stays posterior. This is more amenable to radiofrequency ablation. There is risk of pneumothorax. The needle stays medial to the 12th rib, hugging the vertebral body.

pressure decreases of 30 to 40 mm Hg are not uncommon and are usually seen when the patient assumes an upright or sitting position after celiac plexus block. The hypotension is caused by blood pooling in the splanchnic vessels after sympathectomy; this can be minimized by an IV fluid bolus at the time of block placement. Compensatory reflexes usually appear by 48 hours. Diarrhea is thought to be caused by unopposed parasympathetic activity; impairment of α-adrenergic stimulation to enterocytes that increase intestinal secretory activity as well as decrease absorptive processes may also play a role. Intractable diarrhea may respond to clonidine patches or to octreotide 0.1 mg subcutaneously twice a day.[43,44] The increase in GI activity can be used in a therapeutic manner. Weinstabl et al. used bupivacaine celiac plexus blocks to reduce the intestinal dysfunction (as measured by decreased gastric volumes) in several patients in a neurosurgical intensive care unit.[45] Nausea and vomiting can occur from the hypotension caused by the block or from alcohol intoxication when excessive amounts of neurolytic alcohol are absorbed at the block site. Chest pain can also occur after celiac alcohol block. It usually resolves within 1 hour.[46]

SUPERIOR HYPOGASTRIC PLEXUS BLOCKS

ANATOMY

The superior hypogastric plexus is a retroperitoneal structure located bilaterally between the level of the lower third of the fifth lumbar vertebral body and the upper third of the sacral promontory; it is inferior to the bifurcation of the abdominal aorta and in proximity to the bifurcation of the common iliac vessels (**Fig. 83-11**). The superior hypogastric

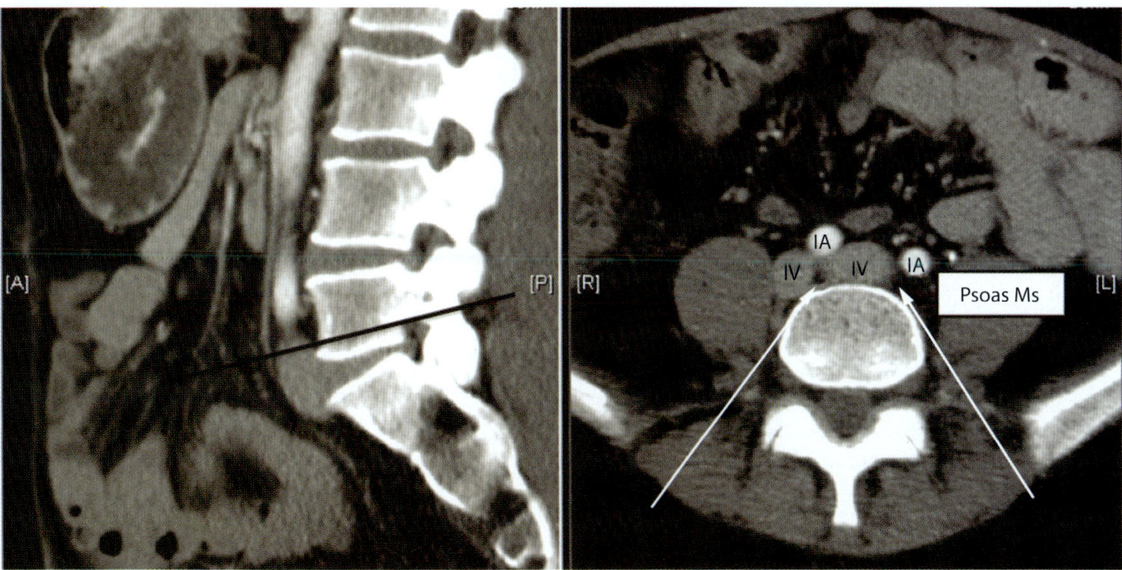

FIGURE 83-11. Computerized tomograph at L5. The arrows show the trajectory and the target for superior hypogastric block. The anesthetic is deposited just anterior to the vertebral body after passing through the psoas muscle. IA, iliac artery; IV, iliac vein.

plexus along with the left and right inferior hypogastric plexus and the pelvic plexus comprise the hypogastric plexus; this network provides innervation to the pelvic viscera. The superior hypogastric plexus receives postganglionic sympathetic contributions from the inferior mesenteric ganglion and from the hypogastric nerves (lumbar splanchnics) that course along with the abdominal aorta.[47] Parasympathetic innervation arises from the second, third, and fourth sacral segments and contributes to the plexus via the pelvic nerve. Finally, visceral afferents from the pelvic organs course through the hypogastric plexus and enter the spinal cord via the L1 or L2 spinal nerve roots or via the sacral segments S2, S3, or S4. Pelvic organs innervated by the hypogastric plexus include the rectum, bladder, perineum, prostate, and uterus. Pain associated with these ganglia will often cause patients to complain of pain in the lower abdominal wall around the pubic region.

INDICATIONS

Pelvic pain secondary to neoplasm can be successfully managed by superior hypogastric plexus blocks. Lee et al. reported that surgical interruption of the hypogastric plexus (presacral neurectomy) can provide pain relief in various malignant and nonmalignant painful conditions.[48,49] Plancarte et al. then devised a reliable means to percutaneously block nerves in this region.[50] They showed that in patients with advanced pelvic neoplasms (to include cervical, prostate, and testicular cancers), pain scores are reduced up to 90% using superior hypogastric plexus blocks and nonopioid analgesics. As with other block techniques, the superior hypogastric plexus block is performed using local anesthetic to determine efficacy and then repeated as needed using a neurolytic agent.

TECHNIQUE

The patient is placed in the prone position with a pillow beneath the lower abdomen and hip to reduce the lumbosacral lordosis. This region is then prepared and draped in sterile fashion, and fluoroscopy is used to identify the L4 to L5 interspace. Oblique fluoroscopy with cranial tilt is used to visualize the anterolateral margin of vertebral body and this entry point is marked on the skin and a skin wheal raised. A 15- to 20-cm, 22-gauge needle is inserted through one of these skin wheals, and the needle advances in a caudad fashion medial to the iliac crest and inferior to the L5 transverse process and walked off the L5 vertebral body. Advancing the tip 1 cm past the vertebral body may result in a loss of resistance or "pop," suggesting that the needle tip has traversed the anterior fascia of the psoas muscle. This typically occurs at a depth of 8 to 12 cm. A second block needle is inserted on the opposite side to the first, and the angles of entry and the depth of the first needle are then used as a guide. Needle tip placement is confirmed by using 3 to 5 mL of water-soluble contrast dye and fluoroscopy. On the lateral view, the dye is seen to spread in a smooth contour anterior to the L5 vertebral body and sacral promontory; on the AP view, the contrast medium should be confined to the midline (**Fig. 83-12**). Eight to ten milliliters of 0.25% bupivacaine or 1% lidocaine is injected through each needle. Six to eight milliliters of aqueous 10% phenol should be injected through each needle if neurolysis is desired.

Variations to the above technique include a single-needle approach, a transdiscal approach, and a transarterial approach. A single-needle approach follows the same technique as that described earlier; however, only one needle is placed, and a larger volume (20–30 mL) of local anesthetic is used. A transdiscal approach is another single-needle approach.[51] Occasionally, the needle trajectory results in needle passage through part of the L5 to S1 disc; when this occurs, the final position of the needle tip is very close to the anterior border of the disc. Confirmation of needle placement with contrast agent is performed. A discogram is seen if the needle tip remains in the intervertebral disc. When the appropriate contrast pattern is achieved, a smaller volume of local anesthetic or neurolytic solution (10–15 mL) is then used. The transarterial approach is used when arterial blood is aspirated from the block needle. Aspirated blood suggests that the needle has inadvertently entered the iliac artery. The needle is then advanced until blood can no longer be aspirated. Because the iliac arteries are retroperitoneal and are in the same tissue plane as the superior hypogastric plexus, a loss of resistance technique (similar to the transaortic celiac plexus block) can then be used to confirm that the needle tip has traversed the anterior wall of the artery. Contrast dye followed by local anesthetic or neurolytic agent is then injected.

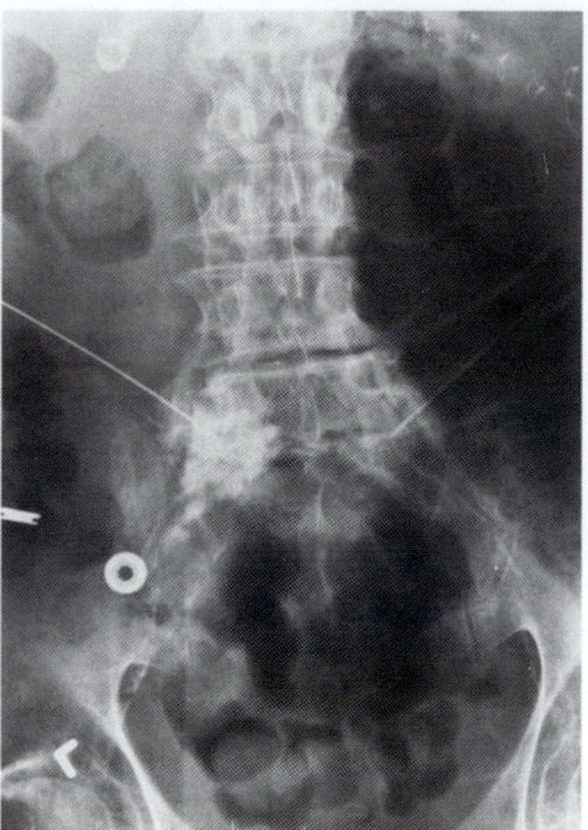

FIGURE 83-12. Superior hypogastric block: The contrast is confined to the midline and lies in front of the L5 vertebral body.

COMPLICATIONS

Complications are rarely serious and include hematoma from puncture of the iliac vessels, back pain and spasm from needle trauma, and intramuscular or intraperitoneal injection of local anesthetic or neurolytic solution. Other complications include inadvertent somatic block from subarachnoid or epidural injection, somatic nerve injury, and ureteral or renal puncture. According to Racz, if neurolytics are used, phenol at concentrations less than 6% should be used to minimize ureteral injury. He also notes that his experience in men is limited to unilateral blocks and recommends that bilateral neurolytic blocks in men should not be performed because of the possibility of sexual dysfunction.[52] Proper technique with the use of fluoroscopy should negate these risks.

LUMBAR SYMPATHETIC BLOCKS

ANATOMY

The lumbar sympathetic chain is easily blocked with few complications compared with other levels of the sympathetic chain. This is primarily because of the consistent position of the chain next to the lumbar vertebrae as well as its relative separation from somatic nerves. When the sympathetic trunk extends into the abdomen, it assumes a prevertebral position compared with the paravertebral position occupied in the thorax. On the right side, it lies posterior to the inferior vena cava, and on the left side, it lies lateral and slightly behind the abdominal aorta. The lumbar sympathetic chain consists of several ganglia (average three per side) between the L1 and L5 vertebral bodies.[53] The ganglia are most frequently found at the level of the lower third of the second lumbar vertebra to the middle third of the third vertebra on both the right and left sides.[53,54] Most importantly, the psoas muscle always lies posterior to the sympathetic chain, thus separating the chain from the lumbar somatic roots. This separation of the sympathetic chain from the somatic lumbar plexus minimizes the spread of local anesthetic or neurolytic agent to these nerves during percutaneous lumbar sympathetic blocks. As a result, the untoward side effects are minimal and infrequent.

INDICATIONS

The common indications for lumbar sympathetic blocks are to diagnose SMP (CRPS) and vascular insufficiency. If the pain is relieved in a prolonged fashion, then this block may be repeated with the recurrence of pain. Pain relief with sympathectomy may also bode well for spinal cord stimulation therapy.[13] In the past, means to achieve prolonged sympathetic blockade included the use of neurolytic agents[55] and radiofrequency lesioning,[56] but these practices have now fallen out of favor. It is important to ensure that sympathectomy therapy of the lower (and upper) extremity is complemented by aggressive physical therapy to optimize treatment success.

TECHNIQUE

The classic lumbar sympathetic block is performed by placing a needle at the anterolateral border of the L2, L3, and L4 vertebral bodies or higher volume deposited at one location, L2 or L3 (in case of foot) (**Fig. 83-13**). Patient positioning is similar to that used in the posterolateral approach to the celiac plexus block. The patient is placed prone with a pillow beneath the lower abdomen and hip. Oblique fluoroscopy is used to determine the entry point. The L2 or L3 transverse process tip is made to overlie the edge of the vertebral body. A local anesthetic skin wheal is raised at the entry point. A 15-cm, 22-gauge needle is advanced directly toward the anterolateral aspect of the vertebral body. Once the needle tip is positioned along the anterolateral aspect of the selected vertebral body, the needle is aspirated for cerebrospinal fluid or blood. Contrast agent (1–5 mL) is then injected and a characteristic longitudinal spread of contrast dye can be seen. Injected contrast will appear striated and spread in a diagonal pattern if the needle tip is in the psoas muscle; a "psoas stripe" can be seen. This is easily corrected by advancing the needle tip an additional 0.5 to 1.0 cm; injection of contrast is then repeated. The appropriate spread is in a craniocaudal direction and appears rather thin when seen in a lateral view with fluoroscopy. A 2-mL test dose of 1% lidocaine or 0.25% bupivacaine is injected, and the patient is evaluated for untoward side effects. About 5 mL of local anesthetic is then injected through the needle; the procedure is then repeated at the other two (L3 and L4) lumbar sites.

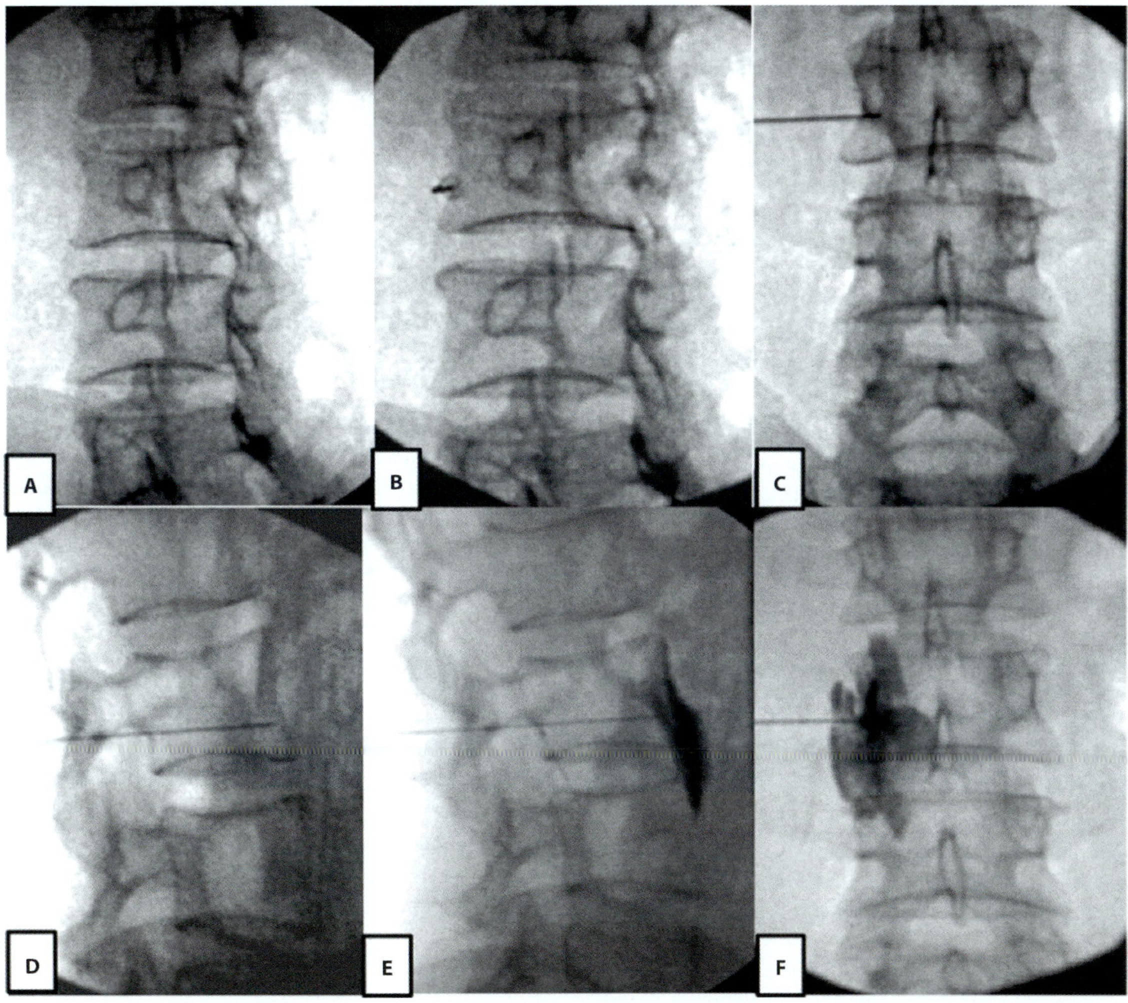

FIGURE 83-13. Lumbar sympathetic block for foot pain. (**A**) The ipsilateral oblique view of L3 is obtained such that the tip of the transverse process overlaps the vertebral body margin. (**B**) The needle is advanced coaxially to just before the anterior margin of the vertebral body. (**C**) The anteroposterior (AP) view shows that needle is just medial to the lateral margin of the vertebral body. (**D**) The lateral view shows the needle just behind the anterior margin of the vertebral body. (**E**) Contrast spread anterior and in a craniocaudad orientation. There is no evidence for posterior extravasation into the psoas muscle. (**F**) The AP view shows the contrast medial to the lateral margin of the vertebral body and 10 mL of local anesthetic injected here. There is some extravasation laterally as well. This patient had a 7°C increase in temperature after sympathetic block with no new sensory or motor deficits.

Alternatively, a single-injection technique can be performed using the same approach except that when the appropriate depth is obtained, a larger volume (10–20 mL) of local anesthetic is injected.[57] Because the ganglia are most often found at the lower portion of the second lumbar vertebral body to the middle of the third vertebral body, this area becomes the most favorable when using a single-needle technique. The advantage of a single-needle technique is decreased postprocedure pain and muscle spasm as a result of less needle trauma through the paraspinal and psoas muscles[53,54] A paradiscal, extraforaminal approach based on cadaveric study has also been described.[58]

COMPLICATIONS

Serious complications are rare and are minimized with the use of radiographic imaging. The most common sequela is backache, typically related to needle trauma that usually responds to conservative therapy such as short-term oral opioids, nonsteroidal anti-inflammatory drugs, or ice and heat therapy. Somatic nerve block can occur from inadvertent injection of local anesthetic into the psoas muscle (psoas compartment block); it can also occur after posterior spread of local anesthetic along tendinous arches that bridge the concave sides of the lumbar vertebrae, thus blocking somatic nerves roots.[59] Hematuria occasionally occurs from needle puncture of the kidney or ureter. Although this finding usually resolves spontaneously after 2 to 3 days, the hematuria can be very distressing to the patient. Kidney puncture is avoided by limiting injections to below the L2 vertebral body.[60]

Genitofemoral neuralgia occurs with an incidence of approximately 20% after fluoroscopically guided neurolytic lumbar sympathetic block.[50] This incidence is decreased by using smaller volumes of neurolytic agent (thus minimizing the spread of agent to the genitofemoral nerve) and injecting cranial to the L4 vertebral body.[61] The symptoms consist of a burning dysesthesia in the anteromedial area of the upper thigh; the pain is frequently severe and can last 6 to 8 weeks but is usually controlled with neuropathic pain medications.[62]

Because incidental genitofemoral nerve block is common, it is important to consider whether the pain syndrome in question unsuspectingly involves the genitofemoral nerve or the L1 nerve root. A "diagnostic" lumbar sympathetic block that unintentionally blocks the genitofemoral nerve may yield the false diagnosis that the pain syndrome was sympathetically maintained. Such a situation may exist when a somatic pain syndrome is present in the genitofemoral or anterior thigh area and the following sequence occurs: a lumbar sympathetic block is performed to diagnose SMP, an unintentional genitofemoral nerve block occurs that then alleviates the somatic pain, and the syndrome is incorrectly identified as involving sympathetic elements. Performing a sympathetic block at L2 may avoid this scenario by preferentially sparing the genitofemoral nerve.[61]

Other complications occur from inadvertent needle placement. Needle entry into the dural cuff of a somatic nerve can result in an epidural or subarachnoid block.[63] A case report of retroperitoneal hemorrhage has also been described with paravertebral blocks.[64]

ALTERNATIVES FOR REGIONAL SYMPATHETIC BLOCKS

Certain conditions preclude pain specialists from using regional sympathetic blocks. These include coagulopathy, infection, and postsurgical changes in the region of interest (e.g., radical neck surgery or aortic graft placement). Alternatives to regional sympathetic blocks include peripheral nerve or plexus blocks and epidural administration of local anesthetic. Other options to nerve blocks include regional or systemic IV techniques, oral therapy, and surgical sympathectomy.

Even in the absence of contraindications, epidural block and peripheral nerve blocks (e.g., brachial plexus blocks) may be better options when prolonged sympathectomy is desired (e.g., digit reimplantation), and there is a lot more experience in using infusions in these locations.[65]

Intravenous regional sympathetic blocks have been performed using guanethidine, bretylium, and reserpine. Complications of IV regional sympathectomy include transient syncopal episodes with apnea,[66] orthostatic hypotension, pain with administration, nausea, and vomiting.

Varying success rates have been reported with these agents; as a result, the use of IV regional sympathectomy is somewhat controversial.[67–72] In 1983, Bonelli et al. reported that in patients with reflex sympathetic dystrophy, IV regional guanethidine blocks provided comparable pain relief with a longer duration to stellate ganglion block therapy.[70] In a 10-year follow-up study of neuralgia in the hand, Wahren and colleagues noted that guanethidine therapy can provide 2 weeks to 6 months of prolonged pain relief.[71]

Hord et al. showed in a double-blind, randomized trial that IV regional bretylium also provided effective analgesia of reflex sympathetic dystrophy; however, a review of their data reveal that only a 30% improvement of pain relief was considered significant.[73] In contrast, randomized, double-blind studies evaluating the use of guanethidine[72,74] and reserpine[74] did not show any improvement in pain scores compared with IV regional therapy with placebo. A mechanism of tourniquet-induced analgesia may play a role.[74]

Phentolamine infusion has gained some popularity as an alternative to diagnosing sympathetically maintained CRPS.[75,76] Incremental dosing of IV phentolamine to supine patients under a monitored setting can be safely performed[77]; the total dose given over 30 to 60 minutes is 0.5 to 1.0 mg/kg. IV phentolamine can help determine responsiveness to the oral α-adrenergic blocking agents such as phenoxybenzamine. Pain relief of at least 50% or untoward effects such as hypotension, dizziness, or headache are the usual end points to this diagnostic test. Complications are rare and typically self-limited and include sinus tachycardia, premature ventricular beats, or wheezing.

Infusions to diagnose and treat SMP are now infrequently used and are more of historical significance.

NEUROLYTIC AGENTS

Neurolytic agents are used to provide long-term pain relief. Before injecting a neurolytic agent, a local anesthetic test block is useful to assess the feasibility of a "permanent" block. It should be noted, however, that a successful test block does not always predict the outcome of a neurolytic celiac plexus block.

Alcohol and phenol are the two neurolytic agents most commonly used. Alcohol is used in concentrations from 50% to 100%. The mechanism of neurolysis is via extraction of cholesterol and phospholipid from neural membranes. There is also precipitation of lipoproteins and mucoproteins. Alcohol probably provides more intense nerve destruction than phenol. Alcohol diffuses more rapidly through biological tissue, thereby increasing the degree of somatic nerve damage. Of note, although no controlled studies comparing the two agents exist, there may be an increased incidence of L1 neuralgia during lumbar sympathetic block when alcohol is used versus phenol.[55] Sedation, dysphoria, and nausea and vomiting can occur from excessive systemic absorption of injected alcohol. The plasma alcohol level can be measured, but levels are highly variable and depend on concentration, volume, and the metabolic rate of the patient. Phenol is usually used in concentrations of 6% to 10%. Phenol causes protein coagulation and necrosis of nerves. The higher concentrations of phenol must be made soluble in a glycerin base; as a result, the heavier viscosity makes it difficult to inject. The primary advantage of phenol is its inherent local anesthetic effect, which precludes pain on injection; in contrast, alcohol typically causes a severe, transient pain on injection. Phenol has a slower onset of action, is less efficacious, and is of shorter duration than alcohol.

REFERENCES

1. Ruud M Buijs. autonomic nervous system. *Handb Clin Neurol.* 2013;117:1-11.
2. Kappis M. Weitere Erfahrungen mit der Sympthektomic. *Klin Wehr.* 1923;2:1441.

3. Mandl F. Die parvertibrale Injection. J. Springer, Vienna, 1926. In: Stanton-Hicks M. Treatment of sympathetically maintained pain. *Reg Anesth*. 1995;20:1.
4. Lowell RC1, Gloviczki P, Cherry KJ Jr, et al. Cervicothoracic sympathectomy for Raynaud's syndrome. *Int Angiol*. 1993;12(2):168-172.
5. Patel RA1, Priore DL, Szeto WY, Slevin KA. Left stellate ganglion blockade for the management of drug-resistant electrical storm. *Pain Med*. 2011;12(8):1196-8.
6. Treede R-D, Davis KD, Campbell JN, et al. Plasticity of cutaneous hyperalgesia during sympathetic ganglion blockade in patients with neuropathic pain. *Brain*. 1992;115:607.
7. Kapral S, Krafft P, Gosch M, et al. Ultrasound imaging for stellate ganglion block: direct visualization of puncture site and local anesthetic spread. A pilot study. *Reg Anesth*. 1995;20:323–328.
8. Hogan QH, Erickson SJ, Haddox JD, et al. The spread of solutions during stellate ganglion block. *Reg Anesth*. 1992;17:78.
9. Lofstrom JB. Stellate ganglion block. In Ericksson E, ed. *Illustrated Handbook in Local Anaesthesia*. Philadelphia: WB Saunders; 1980:141.
10. Hardy P, Wells J. Extent of sympathetic blockade after stellate ganglion block with bupivacaine. *Pain*. 1989;36:193.
11. Grodinsky M, Holyyoke EA. The fasciae and fascial spaces of the head, neck, and adjacent regions. *Am J Anat*. 1938;63:367.
12. Guntamukkala M, Hardy PAJ. Spread of injectate after stellate ganglion block in man: an anatomical study. *Br J Anaesth*. 1991;66:643.
13. Hord ED, Cohen SP, Cosgrove GR, et al. The predictive value of sympathetic block for the success of spinal cord stimulation. *Neurosurgery*. 2003;53(3):626-32; discussion 632-3.
14. Gofeld M, Bhatia A, Abbas S, et al. Development and validation of a new technique for ultrasound-guided stellate ganglion block. *Reg Anesth Pain Med*. 2009;34(5):475-9.
15. Hogan QH, Taylor ML, Goldstein M, et al. Success rates in producing sympathetic blockade by paratracheal injection. *Clin J Pain*. 1994;10:139.
16. Stevens RA, Stoltz A, Kao T-C, et al. The relative increase in skin temperature after stellate ganglion block is predictive of a complete sympathectomy of the hand. *Reg Anesth Pain Manage*. 1998;23:266.
17. Wulf H, Maier CH. Complications of stellate ganglion blockade: results of a questionnaire. *Anaesthesist*. 1992;41:146–151.
18. Korevaar WC, Burney RG, Moore PA. Convulsions during stellate ganglion block: a case report. *Anesth Analg*. 1979;58:329.
19. Szeinfeld M, Laurencio M, Pallares VS. Total reversible blindness following attempted stellate ganglion block. *Anesth Analg*. 1981;60:689.
20. Schot DL, Ghia JN, Teeple E. Aphasia and hemiparesis following stellate ganglion block. *Anesth Analg*. 1983;62:1038.
21. Kozody R, Ready L, Basra JM, et al. Dose requirement of local anesthetic to produce grand mal seizure during stellate ganglion blockade. *Can J Anaesth*. 1982;29:489.
22. Ward EM, Rorie DK, Nauss LE, et al. The celiac ganglion in man: normal anatomic variations. *Anesth Analg*. 1979;58:461.
23. Ischia S, Luzzani A, Ischia A, et al. A new approach to the neurolytic block of the coeliac plexus. The transaortic technique. *Pain*. 1983;16:333.
24. Lebovits AH, Lefkowitz M. Pain management of pancreatic carcinoma: a review. *Pain*. 1989;36:1.
25. Brown DL, Bulley CK, Quiel EL. Neurolytic celiac plexus block for pancreatic cancer pain. *Anesth Analg*. 1987;66:869.
26. Akhan O, Altinok D, Ozman MN, et al. Correlation between the grade of tumoral invasion and pain relief in patients with celiac plexus block. *AJR Am J Roentgenol*. 1997;168:1565.
27. Kune GA, Cole R, Bell S. Observations on the relief of pancreatic pain. *Med J Aust*. 1975;2:789.
28. Rykowski JJ, Hilgier M. Continuous celiac plexus block in acute pancreatitis. *Reg Anesth*. 1995;20:528.
29. Bell SN, Cole R, Roberts-Thompson IC. Coeliac plexus block for control of pain in chronic pancreatitis. *Br Med J*. 1980;281:1604.
30. Seicean A1, Cainap C, Gulei I, et al. Pain palliation by endoscopic ultrasound-guided celiac plexus neurolysis in patients with unresectable pancreatic cancer. *J Gastrointestin Liver Dis*. 2013;22(1):59-64.
31. Moore DC. Regional block. *A Handbook for Use in the Clinical Practice of Medicine and Surgery*. 4th ed. Springfield, IL: Charles C. Thomas; 1965:145.
32. Lieberman RP, Nance PN, Cuka DJ. Anterior approach to celiac plexus block during interventional biliary procedures. *Radiology*. 1988;167:562.
33. Montero MA, Vidal LF, Aguilar SJ, et al. Percutaneous anterior approach to the celiac plexus, using ultrasound. *Br J Anaesth*. 1989; 62:637.
34. Singler R. An improved technique for alcohol celiac plexus nerve block. *Anesthesiology*. 1982;56:137.
35. Weber JG, Brown DL, Stephens DH, et al. Celiac plexus block: retrocrural CT anatomy in patients with and without pancreatic cancer. *Reg Anesth*. 1996;21:407.
36. Davies DD. Incidence of major complications of neurolytic celiac plexus block. *J R Soc Med*. 1993;86:264.
37. Thompson G, Moore DC, Bridenbaugh LD, et al. Abdominal pain and alcohol celiac plexus nerve block. *Anesth Analg Curr Res*. 1977;56:1.
38. Pateman J, Williams MP, Filshie J. Retroperitoneal fibrosis after multiple celiac plexus blocks. *Anaesthesia*. 1990;45:309.
39. Fujita Y, Takaori M. Pleural effusion after CT-guided alcohol celiac plexus block. *Anesth Analg*. 1987;66:911.
40. Moore DC, Bush WH, Burnett LL. Celiac plexus block: a roentgenographic, anatomic study of technique and spread of solution in patients and corpses. *Anesth Analg*. 1981;60:369.
41. Woodham MJ, Hanna MH. Paraplegia after coeliac plexus block. *Anaesthesia*. 1989;44:487.
42. Wong GY, Brown DL. Transient paraplegia following alcohol celiac plexus block. *Reg Anesth*. 1995;20:352.
43. Mercadante S. Clinical note—octreotide in the treatment of diarrhoea included by coeliac plexus block. *Pain*. 1995;61:345.
44. Chan VWS. Chronic diarrhea: an uncommon side effect of celiac plexus block. *Anesth Analg*. 1996;82:205.
45. Weinstabl C, Porges P, Plainer B, et al. Coeliac plexus block with bupivacaine reduces intestinal dysfunction in neurosurgical ICU patients. *Anaesthesia*. 1993;48:162.
46. Abram SE, Hogan Q. Complications of nerve block. In: Benumof JL, Saidman LJ, eds. *Anesthesia and Perioperative Complications*. St Louis: Mosby-Year Book; 1992:52.
47. Crafts RC. *A Textbook of Human Anatomy*. 3rd ed. New York: John Wiley and Sons; 1985.
48. Lee RB, Stone K, Magelssen D, et al. Presacral neurectomy for chronic pelvic pain. *Obstet Gynecol*. 1986;68:517.
49. Frier A. Pelvic neurectomy in gynecology. *Obstet Gynecol*. 1965; 25:48.
50. Plancarte R, Amescua C, Patt RB, et al. Superior hypogastric plexus block for pelvic cancer pain. *Anesthesiology*. 1990;73:236.
51. Ina H, Kitoh T, Kobayashi M, et al. New technique for the neurolytic celiac plexus block: the transintervertebral disc approach. *Anesthesiology*. 1996;85(1):212-7.

52. Raj PP, Rauck RL, Racz GB. Autonomic nerve blocks. In: Raj PP, ed. *Pain Medicine—A Comprehensive Review*. St Louis: Mosby-Year Book; 1996:227.
53. Rocco AG, Palombi D, Racke D. Anatomy of the lumbar sympathetic chain. *Reg Anesth*. 1995;20:13.
54. Umeda S, Arai T, Hatano Y, et al. Cadaver anatomic analysis of the best site for chemical lumbar sympathectomy. *Anesth Analg*. 1987;66:643.
55. Cousins MJ, Reeve TS, Glynn CJ, et al. Neurolytic lumbar sympathetic blockade: duration of denervation and relief of rest pain. *Anaesth Intens Care*. 1979;7:121.
56. Rocco AG. Radiofrequency lumbar sympatholysis: the evolution of a technique for managing sympathetically maintained pain. *Reg Anesth*. 1995;20:3.
57. Hatangdi WS, Boas RA. Lumbar sympathectomy: a single needle technique. *Br J Anaesth*. 1985;57:285.
58. Sukdeb Datta MD, Umeshraya Pai MD. Paradiscal extraforaminal technique for lumbarsympathetic block: report of a proposed new technique utilizing a cadaver study. *Pain Physician*. 2004;7:53-57.
59. Bryce-Smith R. Injection of the lumbar sympathetic chain. *Anaesthesia*. 1991;6:150.
60. Brown VM, Kunjappan V. Single-needle approach for lumbar sympathetic block. *Anesth Analg*. 1975;54:725.
61. Sayson SC, Ramamurthy S, Hoffman J. Incidence of genitofemoral nerve block during lumbar sympathetic block: comparison of two lumbar injection sites. *Reg Anesth*. 1997;22:569.
62. Raskin ND, Levinson SA, Hoffman PM, et al. Postsympathetectomy neuralgia: amelioration with diphenylhydantoin and carbamazepine. *Am J Surg*. 1974;28:75.
63. Gay GR, Evans JA. Total spinal anesthesia following lumbar paravertebral block. A potentially lethal complication. *Anesth Analg*. 1971;50:344.
64. Learned LO, Calhoun R. Retroperitoneal hemorrhage as a complication of lumbar paravertebral injection. Report of three cases. *Anesthesiology*. 1951;12:391.
65. Ilfeld BM. Continuous peripheral nerve blocks: a review of the published evidence. *Anesth Analg*. 2011;113(4):904-925.
66. Woo R, McQueen J. Apnea and syncope following intravenous guanethidine bier block in the same patient on two different occasions. *Anesthesiology*. 1987;67:281.
67. Ford SR, Forrest WH, Eltherington L. The treatment of reflex sympathetic dystrophy with intravenous regional bretylium. *Anesthesiology*. 1988;68:137.
68. Hannington-Kiff JE. Intravenous regional sympathetic block with guanethidine. *Lancet*. 1974;1:1019-1020.
69. Hanowell LH, Kanefield JK, Soriano SG. A recommendation for reduced lidocaine dosage during intravenous regional bretylium treatment for reflex sympathetic dystrophy. *Anesthesiology*. 1989;71:811.
70. Bonelli S, Conoscente F, Movilia PG, et al. Regional intravenous guanethidine vs. stellate ganglion block in reflex sympathetic dystrophies: a randomized trial. *Pain*. 1983;16:297.
71. Wahren LK, Gordh T, Torebjork E. Effects of regional intravenous guanethidine in patients with neuralgia in the hand; a follow-up study over a decade. *Pain*. 1995;62:379.
72. Ramamurthy S, Hoffman J, the Guanethidine Study Group. Intravenous regional guanethidine in the treatment of reflex sympathetic dystrophy/causalgia: a randomized, double-blind study. *Anesth Analg*. 1995;81:718.
73. Hord AH, Rooks MD, Stephens BO, et al. Intravenous regional bretylium and lidocaine for treatment of reflex sympathetic dystrophy: a randomized, double-blind study. *Anesth Analg*. 1992;74:818.
74. Blanchard J, Ramamurthy S, Walsh N, et al. Intravenous regional sympatholysis: a double-blind comparison of guanethidine, reserpine, and normal saline. *J Pain Symptom Manage*. 1990;5:357.
75. Arner S. Intravenous phentolamine test: diagnostic and prognostic use in reflex sympathetic dystrophy. *Pain*. 1991;46:17.
76. Raja SN, Treede RD, Davis KD, et al. Systemic alpha-adrenergic blockade with phentolamine: a diagnostic test for sympathetically maintained pain. *Anesthesiology*. 1991;74:691.
77. Shir T, Cameron LB, Raja SN, et al. The safety of intravenous phentolamine administration in patients with neuropathic pain. *Anesth Analg*. 1993;76:1008.

Peripheral Nerve Blocks

Jatinder S. Gill

INTRODUCTION

The peripheral nervous system consists of numerous individual nerves, nerve trunks, nerve plexuses, and ganglia. This chapter discusses the blockade of somatic peripheral nerves. The sympathetic and visceral nerve blocks are discussed separately. The blockade of peripheral somatic nerves is the hallmark of regional anesthesia. This may be done for the facilitation of surgery as a sole technique or in combination with general anesthesia. Peripheral nerve blocks can be continued into the postoperative period via infusion through catheters for the purpose of continued postoperative pain relief. Excellent perioperative analgesia may help reduce the possibility of development of chronic pain.[1,2] Additionally, some evidence indicates that regional anesthesia may have a role in reducing the recurrence of disease in patients undergoing oncologic surgery.[3]

In the field of chronic pain management, peripheral nerve blocks are useful in the diagnosis of pain conditions. At times these may provide pain relief beyond the duration of the local anesthetic itself and hence serve a therapeutic purpose.[4] Various adjuvants such as clonidine, steroids, and vasoconstrictors may be added to the local anesthetic to prolong the duration of the nerve block. In some select circumstances, once the pain generating nerve is identified, neurolysis of the nerve via chemical or thermal techniques can be done. Chemical neurolysis is often done with alcohol or phenol, and in general, use of these agents is reserved for patients with terminal illness because of the risk of recurrent pain that may be worse, as well as the risk of permanent neurologic sequelae. Thermal techniques such as medial branch thermal neurotomy and cryoablation of neuromas are useful in the management of chronic pain.[5]

Historically, peripheral nerve blocks were often performed as a blind technique using surface anatomy landmarks, as well as feel. The introduction of nerve stimulation techniques was instrumental in improving the success of peripheral nerve blockade. With this technology, the proximity of the needle tip to the neural tissue can be objectively verified. Recently, with the introduction of ultrasound, the nerve can be visually identified and a needle placed next to it in real time. The spread of the medication around the nerve can also be visualized in real time. The availability of portable ultrasound machines has led to exponential use of this modality in the performance of peripheral nerve blocks. There has been increased use of ultrasound guidance in the field of chronic pain management as well. Interventional pain management, however, has a strong reliance on fluoroscopy in the performance of peripheral nerve blocks near the spine because bony landmarks serve well to predict the location of the nerve, and ultrasound has limited utility.

The success of a nerve block depends on several factors. First, it is key that the purpose of performing the nerve block is clearly understood both by the patient and the physician. Second, in the case of diagnostic blocks, knowledge of the factors contributing to a false-positive result or a false-negative result is essential, along with attempts to minimize their influence. Third, the physician should have an excellent knowledge of the anatomy of the nerve and the anticipated effects of the block. Fourth, appropriate preparation is done to deal with any untoward effects of the block. Fifth, appropriate technology such as ultrasound, fluoroscopy, etc. is used when needed to improve the technical success of the procedure. Last, the results of the nerve block and inferences thereof should be clearly documented.

INDICATIONS FOR THE USE OF NERVE BLOCKS

Nerve blocks can be broadly divided into three categories, anesthetic blocks to facilitate surgery, diagnostic blocks for identifying the pain generator, and therapeutic blocks for prolonged benefit.

Diagnostic blocks are performed when the cause of a pain condition is suspected but not confirmed. Some examples of these include medial branch blocks to identify facet pain, lateral branch blocks to identify sacroiliac joint pain, ilioinguinal nerve blocks to differentiate ilioinguinal neuralgia from genitofemoral neuralgia, and transversus abdominis plane (TAP) blocks to differentiate abdominal wall somatic pain from visceral abdominal pain.

Blocks are considered therapeutic when prolonged meaningful relief of pain occurs beyond the duration of the nerve block itself or when permanent denervation is the intended outcome such as radiofrequency ablation of the medial branches.[4,5]

NEUROPHYSIOLOGY AND PHARMACOLOGY

Neuronal membranes are characterized as semipermeable, double-thickness walls composed of lipid molecules with interspaced globular proteins. Small channels allow ions such as sodium and potassium to pass between the internal and external compartments of nerve membranes. Sensory stimulation causes a sudden influx of sodium ions, which results in depolarization of the nerve membrane. Local anesthetics such as lidocaine or bupivacaine produce temporary impairment of conduction of neural impulses by blocking sodium nerve channel conductance and maintaining the nerve in a polarized state.[6] This effect on nerve membranes is temporary and reversible. The size of the nerve fiber affects its sensitivity to local anesthetics, with smaller, thinner, unmyelinated fibers being most susceptible. Peripheral nerves are composed of three types of nerve fibers:

- A fibers are the largest myelinated somatic nerve fibers. These are further subdivided into motor and sensory. The motor fibers are α, β, and γ fibers and innervate the muscle spindle. The sensory fibers are α (muscle sense, high conduction velocity), β (touch), and γ (pain and cold temperature) fibers.
- B fibers are myelinated preganglionic autonomic nerves. B fibers innervate vascular smooth muscle and are the most readily blocked nerve fiber. Successful blockade results in a sympathectomy, with increased warmth caused by increased blood flow and decreased sweating.
- C fibers, the thinnest nonmyelinated fibers, are the slowest conducting nerve fibers. They transmit postganglionic pain and temperature sensation.
- The two types of pain fibers, Aδ myelinated and nonmyelinated C fibers, have slightly different functions. Aδ fibers transmit sharp pain, while C fibers are responsible for the dull pain and burning sensations that accompany many chronic pain syndromes.

The choice of local anesthetic used will affect the density of the nerve block as well as the duration. Small nerve fibers (Aδ) and unmyelinated fibers (C fibers) can be interrupted with low concentrations of local anesthetic, with minimal effect on the larger myelinated efferent fibers. The subsequent nerve block would produce analgesia without any limb weakness. In contrast, a higher concentration of local anesthetic would produce a motor block, resulting in temporary limb weakness.

The duration of the analgesic effect depends on the choice of local anesthetic used. Lidocaine has a relatively short duration of action compared with bupivacaine, which typically lasts much longer. The addition of a vasoconstrictor such as epinephrine would prolong the duration of the nerve block by decreasing the absorption of the drug into the vascular system.

PRINCIPLES AND GUIDELINES FOR REGIONAL ANESTHESIA AND NERVE BLOCKS

PATIENT ASSESSMENT

Patients with chronic pain should always undergo a thorough evaluation before any interventional procedure. Patients may have numerous other medical problems that need to be addressed before deciding if a procedure is warranted. Examples of common medical problems include poorly controlled diabetes, asthma, and hypertension, to name a few. Elements of the patient workup and assessment should include:

- A history from the patient and any other records or diagnostic studies
- Psychological factors if any
- Details of type of pain, location, and duration, as well as exacerbating and relieving factors
- Medication and allergy review, including details of anticoagulant use with doses and indications (The performing physician should have a good knowledge of the anticoagulants used and the indications for the use. A risk-to-benefit ratio should be done on a case-by-case basis before stopping the anticoagulants and in concert with the primary care physician or the specialist).
- Measurement of pain
- Physical examination with clear documentation of neurologic findings

COMMUNICATION AND INFORMED CONSENT

Communication with the patient is equally important. The description of the procedure should be discussed, including why it is being performed, alternatives to it, expected outcome, and possible side effects. Sedation may be offered to minimize any discomfort, which should also be discussed. Oversedation and general anesthesia is not recommended as it is useful to maintain communication with the patient. Finally, the postprocedure recovery period should be discussed (e.g., return to work, physical activity).

LIMITATIONS AND CONTRAINDICATIONS OF NERVE BLOCKS

Nerve blocks can play an integral part in a comprehensive approach to pain management, but it is important that limitations are well understood. The placebo response can dramatically affect the positive predictive value.[7] The spillover of the local anesthetic from the target structure, thus anesthetizing other structures, can also create false–positive results.[8] Failure to appropriately anesthetize the nerve can give rise to false-negative results. Other causes of false-negative results include vascular uptake of the local anesthetic, improper technique, and inadequate amount of active agent to create nerve blockade. The results of the block need to be carefully interpreted. The mere absence of pain relief after successful blockade of the painful area does not necessarily imply psychogenic pain but may point toward a more central pain generator.[9] Improper patient selection, psychological factors, compensation, and litigation issues can also create complexities in the interpretation of the results of a nerve blockade.

CONTRAINDICATIONS TO PERFORMING NERVE BLOCKS

Absolute contraindications are as follows:

- Infection at the proposed site of injection
- Local anesthetic allergy (Allergies to ester local anesthetics (procaine, tetracaine, and chloroprocaine) are known; however, these

solutions are rarely used for regional nerve blocks. Amide local anesthetic allergy (lidocaine, bupivacaine, and ropivacaine) is rare. Some patients may report an allergic reaction after a dental procedure. Further investigation may be warranted to see if it was a true local anesthetic allergy or simply a reaction to epinephrine).

Relative contraindications are as follows:

- Blood clotting abnormalities secondary to intrinsic disease or extrinsic use; management is decided case by case
- Patients with systemic infection or hemodynamic instability
- Situations in which a single or continuous nerve block may mask other pathology, such as limb ischemia from a compartment syndrome that may develop after fractures or crush injuries

PERFORMANCE AND ASSESSMENT OF NERVE BLOCKS

The physician performing the procedure should possess the technical knowledge, experience, and expertise pertinent to the specific procedure. Knowledge of relevant anatomy, potential side effects, and complications of the procedure are essential in preventing adverse outcomes. The expertise to handle immediate serious complications related to the nerve block is also critical. Appropriate technology such as nerve stimulator, fluoroscopy, and ultrasonography should be available as needed to improve the technical success of the procedure.

Discomfort during the procedure may be minimized by using short-acting opioids such as fentanyl. Anxiolytics or short-acting agents such as midazolam are also useful intravenous (IV) medications for minimizing anxiety or discomfort during needle placement. Excess sedation may make accurate assessment of diagnostic or therapeutic blocks difficult.

Appropriate monitoring and resuscitation equipment should be available to manage the effects of the block or any untoward complications. Thus, an IV line should be in place when a large amount of local anesthetic is to be used. Additional intralipid and resuscitation equipment should be available.[10] These preparations may not be needed when a low-volume block such as an occipital nerve block is being performed.

Before and after regional anesthesia, baseline pain measurements should be obtained. Various indicators or scales such as the visual analog scale can be used to help document baseline pain level and response to treatment.[11] For more specific nerve blocks, additional information may be helpful. For somatic nerve blocks, sensory and motor deficits should be consistent with the anticipated region or dermatome blocked.

The duration and onset of the physiologic effect of the block and its correlation with the duration of pain relief are important for several reasons. If the duration of pain relief is shorter than expected, it may indicate inaccurate needle placement, an incomplete or partial nerve block, or possibly an alternate pain source. If the duration is longer than expected or the onset much quicker than expected, a potential placebo effect should be considered.

SIDE EFFECTS AND COMPLICATIONS OF REGIONAL ANESTHESIA

Effects of the block may include physiological sequelae or side effects such as hypotension after sympathectomy or dizziness after occipital nerve block. Vagal stimulation can cause syncope; this is often seen in young patients. Other effects may relate to complications of the nerve block such as direct needle injury (pneumothorax after intercostal nerve block) or intravascular injection (seizure during a stellate ganglion block), and these remain specific to each block.

Large volume of local anesthetic can cause cardiac arrest, and intralipids should be available to manage this catastrophic complication when large volumes of local anesthetic are to be used.[10] To safeguard against this, intermittent aspiration should be done to rule out intravascular placement. When using fluoroscopy, real-time contrast injection is useful in detecting this. When using ultrasound, the local anesthetic spread around the needle tip should be visualized in real time.

NEEDLE PLACEMENT AND POSITIONING

Utmost care should be taken when positioning the patients, and all pressure points should be checked. This is especially important in older individuals.

Needle advancement should be done slowly and incrementally in a goal-directed fashion. This is to reduce patient discomfort and to help minimize multiple redirections. This can take some practice. When approaching important structures, only small changes should be made. If the patient reports pain, determination as to local pain versus paresthesia is important. One necessitates more local anesthetic, whereas the other may require needle withdrawal or redirection. One important point is to refrain from injecting anything if the patient reports pain when the needle is in the vicinity of an important neural structure and to rather gently withdraw it. When using ultrasound the more perpendicular the needle is to the beam, the better it is visualized.[12,13]

SPECIFIC NERVE BLOCKS

HEAD AND NECK

The skin of the face is supplied by the three divisions of the trigeminal nerve. The scalp is supplied by various divisions of the occipital nerve posteriorly and the auriculotemporal nerve in the temporal region. The branches from the dorsal rami of the cervical nerves supply the neck posteriorly, and the branches of the superficial cervical plexus supply the neck anteriorly. Various neuralgia can affect these nerves. In addition, different branches can be peripherally blocked for the provision of surgery such as dental surgery. Blockade of superficial pericranial nerves may also provide relief to patients with intractable headache.[4]

Trigeminal Nerve

Anatomy The trigeminal nerve consists of three divisions: the ophthalmic nerve (V1), maxillary nerve (V2), and mandibular nerve (V3). These three branches supply sensation to most of the face. Trigeminal nerve blocks are used mainly to treat severe pain from trigeminal neuralgia and various malignancies affecting the face.

Gasserian Ganglion Block (Fig. 84-1)

Anatomy The gasserian or trigeminal ganglion lies within the medial cranial fossa across the superior border of the petrous temporal bone. The posterior two-thirds is fully covered by dura mater. This posterior portion lies within a small recess called *Meckel's cave*. This invagination of the dura surrounding the posterior two-thirds of the ganglion allows direct continuity with the cerebrospinal fluid.

Indications This block is used for intractable pain from trigeminal neuralgia and involves neurolysis of one or two divisions of the trigeminal nerve via thermal radiofrequency lesioning or glycerol rhizotomy. Neurodestructive procedures are usually reserved for older individuals who are poor surgical risks and have intractable pain unresponsive to multiple neuropathic medications. The V1 branch is not a candidate for neurolysis because of the risks of corneal insensitivity.

Technique The foramen ovale is visualized on an anteroposterior view of the skull. The entry point for the needle is lateral to the lateral margin of the mouth medial to the masseter muscle.[14] A 22-gauge, 10-cm needle is advanced to the foramen ovale in the plane of the pupil and directed cephalad toward the auditory meatus. As the foramen is entered, a mandibular paresthesia is perceived.

Complications Subarachnoid injection can cause unconsciousness or seizures. The internal carotid artery lies medially at this location. Radiofrequency ablation of V1 will lead to corneal anesthesia, leading to loss of corneal sensation and corneal ulcers.

Mandibular and Maxillary Nerve Block at the Coronoid Notch

Anatomy The trigeminal nerve divides into three branches that can be individually blocked at the coronoid notch. The V3 division is posterior

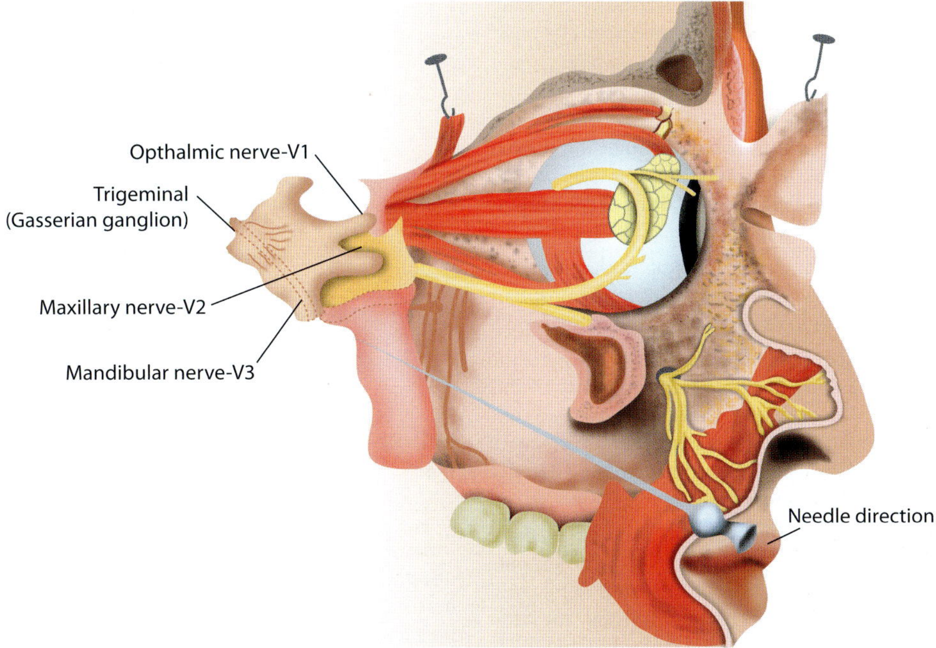

FIGURE 84-1. Trigeminal nerve block. (Adapted with permission from MediClip, Williams & Wilkins.)

at the pterygoid plate, whereas the V1 and V2 divisions are anterior. The mandibular nerve splits to form two divisions. The anterior division supplies the muscles of mastication, and the posterior division is sensory to the jaw, tongue, and the teeth, forming the alveolar, auriculotemporal, and lingual nerves. The maxillary nerve is mainly a sensory nerve to the nasal cavity, upper teeth, and middle of the face.

Indications This block is used for diagnosis and treatment of neuralgia of these nerves or in trigeminal neuralgia. It provides the ability to block individual nerves. Anesthesia to the areas of nerve innervation can also be provided.

Technique The coronoid notch is identified by having the patient open and close the mouth. A 25-gauge, 3.5-in needle is advanced through the midpoint of the coronoid notch inferior to the zygomatic arch to contact the pterygoid plate. If both the nerves are to be blocked, an injection with 7 to 10 mL of local anesthetic may be performed here. For the mandibular nerve, the needle is then slightly withdrawn and directed posteriorly and inferiorly and about 1 cm deeper to block the V3 branch; 3 to 5 mL of local anesthetic is injected here. To block the V2 nerve, the needle is redirected in a similar fashion but anteriorly and superiorly. Higher volumes injected at this anterior location can also block the V1 nerve.

Particulate steroids should not be used.

Complications Possible complications include spread to additional nerves, intravascular injection, hematoma, and bleeding.

Supraorbital and Supratrochlear Nerve Block

Anatomy This is a peripheral branch of the V1 division with sensory innervation to the forehead.

Indications This block is used for diagnosis and treatment of neuralgia of the nerve and in management of patients with chronic intractable migraine often requiring multiple blocks in the management.[15]

Technique The skin is cleaned with alcohol. The supraorbital notch is identified by palpation, and a 30-gauge, 1-in needle is advanced to this location. A total of 1 to 2 mL of local anesthetic is injected in a fan-shaped manner. To block the supratrochlear nerve, the needle is then advanced medially to the apex of the nose, and local anesthetic is injected here as well. Do not mix with steroids, as steroids can leave a mark on the face resulting from lipoatrophy.[16]

Complications Possible complications include local bruising and neuritis.

Infraorbital Nerve Block

Anatomy This is a peripheral branch of the V2 division with sensory innervation to the region below the eye.

Indications This block is used for the diagnosis and treatment of neuralgia of the nerve and management of intractable headaches.[15]

Technique The infraorbital ridge of the maxillary bone is identified, and the foramen is palpated. A 30-gauge, 1-in needle is advanced to this location. A total of 1 to 2 mL of local anesthetic is injected in a fan-shaped manner. Do not mix with steroids, as steroids can leave a mark on the face resulting from lipoatrophy.[16]

Complications Possible complications include local bruising and neuritis.

Auriculotemporal Nerve Block

Anatomy This is a peripheral branch of the V3 division with sensory innervation to the area of the temple, external auditory canal, tympanic membrane, and a few articular branches to the temporomandibular joint.

Indications This block is used for the diagnosis and treatment of auriculotemporal neuralgia and in the management of chronic intractable migraine often requiring multiple blocks in the management.[15]

Technique Field block in the region of the auriculotemporal nerve as it emerges above the zygomatic arch. A total of 1 to 2 mL of local anesthetic is injected. Do not mix with steroids, as steroids can leave a mark on the face resulting from lipoatrophy.[16]

Complications Possible complications include local bruising and neuritis.

Mental Nerve Block

Anatomy This is a peripheral branch of the V3 division emerging from the mental foramen with sensory innervation to the anterior mandible.

Indications This block is used for the diagnosis and treatment of neuralgia of the mental nerve.

Technique The foramen lies about 2 cm from the midline and can often be palpated. A 30-gauge, 1-in needle advanced to this location with care taken not to enter the foramen. A total of 1 to 2 mL of local anesthetic is injected in a fan-shaped manner. Do not mix with steroids, as steroids can leave a mark on the face resulting from subcutaneous tissue atrophy.[16]

Complications Possible complications include local bruising and neuritis.

Glossopharyngeal Nerve Block

Anatomy The glossopharyngeal nerve exits the skull through the jugular foramen located posterior to the tip of the mastoid process. The glossopharyngeal nerve supplies sensation to the posterior third of the tongue, the palatine tonsils, and the pharyngeal wall.

Indications This block is used for glossopharyngeal neuralgia characterized by clusters of severe lancinating, electric shock–like pain in the oropharynx and tonsils with possible radiation to the ear. It is usually unilateral.[17]

Technique An imaginary line is drawn from the mastoid process to the angle of the jaw. The styloid process lies just below the midpoint of this line. A 25-gauge, 1.5-in needle is inserted and the styloid process contacted within 3 cm. The needle is withdrawn and inserted posteriorly to lie just past the styloid process and local anesthetic injected here. Do not use particulate steroid because of the embolic risk.

Complications Possible complications include dysphagia from paralysis of the pharyngeal muscles and weakness or partial paresis of the tongue. The block should only be performed unilaterally because a bilateral block will produce complete paralysis of the pharyngeal muscles. Weakness in the trapezius muscle can also be seen caused by blockade of the spinal accessory nerve.

Occipital Nerve Block (Figs. 84-2 and 84-3)

Anatomy The greater occipital nerve is formed from the dorsal primary ramus of the second and third cervical nerves. It supplies sensation to the medial-posterior portion of the scalp. This nerve is usually located 2 to 3 cm lateral to the external occipital protuberance and just medial to the occipital artery, which serves as a reliable landmark. A 25-gauge, 1.5-in needle is identified, and 2 to 5 mL of local anesthetic is deposited in this location. The lesser occipital nerve arises from the ventral primary ramus of the second and third cervical nerves passing along the posterior border of the sternocleidomastoid muscle. It is located approximately 2.5 cm lateral to the occipital artery.

Indications This block is used for the diagnosis and treatment of neuralgia of the nerve and in the management of chronic intractable migraine often requiring multiple blocks.[15]

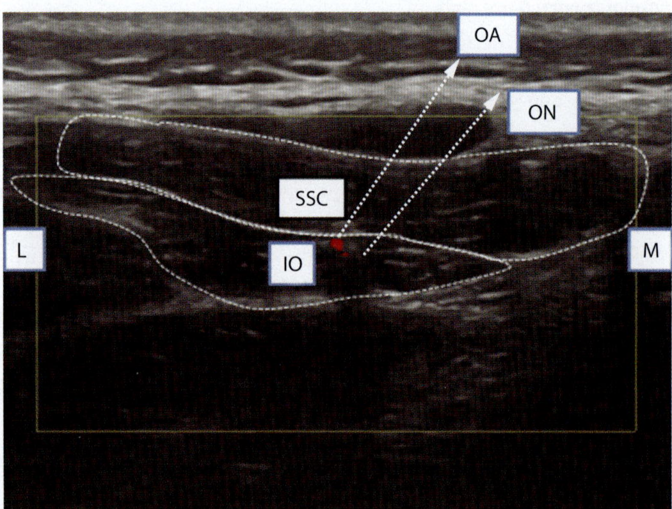

FIGURE 84-2. Ultrasound image of the occipital region. The occipital artery (OA) is visualized in the center with the help of color Doppler. The nerve usually lies medial to it. The needle is inserted in an in-plane approach, and real-time injection of local anesthetic is used to block the nerve. The probe is placed horizontally to obtain a cross-section view of the artery. IO, internal oblique; L, lateral; M, medial; ON, occipital nerve; SSC, semispinalis capitis.

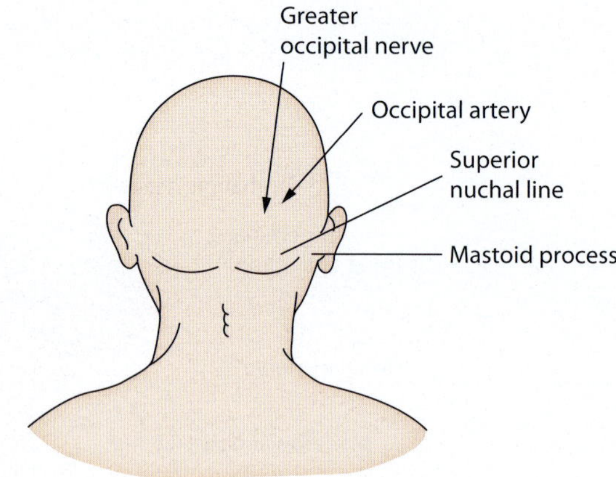

FIGURE 84-3. Occipital nerve block. (Adapted with permission from MediClip, Williams & Wilkins.)

Technique The occipital nerve is blocked at the superior nuchal line about one-third of the distance from the external occipital protuberance to the mastoid process. The lesser occipital nerve is blocked as a field block posterior to the mastoid process. An ultrasound-guided occipital nerve block has been described.[18]

Complication A possible complication is local bruising.

Deep Cervical Plexus Block (Fig. 84-4)

Anatomy The plexus is formed by the ventral rami of C1 to C4. These divide into ascending and descending branches, forming series of three loops called the cervical plexus. Each loop gives a superficial and deep branch. The superficial branches form the superficial cervical plexus. Blockade of the deep cervical plexus blocks both the deep and superficial branches.

Indications This block is used to provide surgical anesthesia over the anterior neck for procedures such as neck dissection, thyroidectomy, and carotid endarterectomy.

Technique Traditionally, the block is done by multiple injections at C2, C3, C4 or by single injection technique at C4. A line is drawn from the mastoid process to the C6 anterior tubercle. The C2, C3, and C4 transverse processes are marked at 1.5, 3, and 4.5 cm caudad to the mastoid process, respectively. A needle is inserted medially and caudally at these points to contact the transverse process at 1.5 to 2 cm, and 3 to 5 mL of local anesthetic is injected at each point.[19] Recently an ultrasound-guided technique has also been described.[20,21]

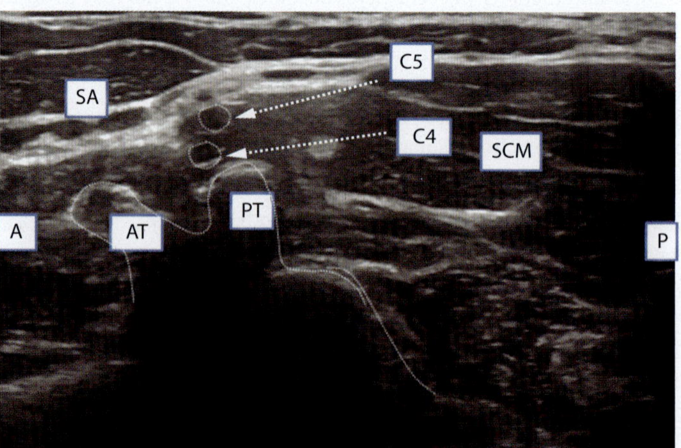

FIGURE 84-4. Deep cervical plexus block. The needle is inserted in plane posterior to anterior. The probe is placed transversely between the mastoid and the C6 tubercle to obtain a cross-sectional view of the nerves. A, anterior; AT, anterior tubercle; P, posterior; PT, posterior tubercle; C4 and C5, nerve roots; SA, scalene anterior; SCM, sternocleidomastoid.

Complications Possible complications include epidural or spinal spread and consequent effects, phrenic nerve paralysis, and intravascular injection. Do not use particulate steroid because of the embolic risk.

Superficial Cervical Plexus Block

Anatomy The superficial branches of the cervical plexus emerge approximately in the middle of the posterior margin of the sternocleidomastoid muscle and provide cutaneous innervation via supraclavicular, transverse cutaneous (anterior), greater auricular, and lesser occipital nerves.

Indications This block is used to provide surgical anesthesia over the anterior neck for procedures such as neck dissection and carotid endarterectomy.

Technique Field block is done in the midsternocleidomastoid region posteriorly. A total of 5 mL of local anesthetic is injected subcutaneously, and then 2 to 3 mL of local anesthetic is injected in a fan-shaped manner superiorly and inferiorly. An ultrasound-guided technique is also described.[22]

Complications Possible complications include hematoma and bruising if the external jugular vein is injured.

SHOULDER AND UPPER EXTREMITY

Brachial Plexus Block

Anatomy The brachial plexus is formed from the ventral primary rami of the fifth (C5), sixth (C6), seventh (C7), and eighth (C8) cervical nerves along with the first thoracic nerve (T1). The C4 and T2 spinal nerves may also contribute to the plexus. These roots pass between the anterior and middle scalene muscles in the neck before passing into the arm. The roots combine to form upper, middle, and lower trunks that subdivide into anterior and posterior divisions. These divisions then form the cords. Within the axilla, near the lateral border of the axilla, the cords divide into the peripheral nerves of the upper extremity.

- The long thoracic nerve contains fibers from C5, C6, and C7.
- The suprascapular nerve contains fibers from C4, C5, and C6.
- Peripheral branches of the lateral cord form the musculocutaneous nerve and lateral root of the median nerve formed from C5, C6, and C7.
- Peripheral branches of the medial cord (C8 and T1) form the medial root of the median nerve, the ulnar nerve, and the medial cutaneous branches of the arm and forearm.
- Peripheral branches of the posterior cord form the axillary, radial, and subscapular nerves.

Indications

- Anesthesia for upper extremity surgery
- Postoperative pain relief and rehabilitation
- Manipulation of frozen shoulder
- Continuous sympathetic nerve blockade to improve blood flow to the affected extremity (i.e., Raynaud's disease)

TYPES OF BRACHIAL PLEXUS BLOCKS

Interscalene Block (Fig. 84-5)

Anatomy The roots combine to form upper, middle, and lower trunks that lie in the interscalene groove.

Indications This block is used as anesthesia for surgery on the shoulder, catheters for postoperative pain relief, and for shoulder manipulation in case of frozen shoulder. It is not ideal for forearm surgery because ulnar sparing is seen.

Technique The block is usually done with ultrasound guidance or with the help of a nerve stimulator. A combined technique is often used. With the stimulator technique, a 22-gauge, 1.5-in stimulating needle is inserted into the interscalene groove after rolling of the anterior scalene muscle. The needle is inserted perpendicular to the skin, and stimulation of the brachial plexus is sought. After obtaining stimulation, 10 to 15 mL of local anesthetic is injected here. When using ultrasonography, the probe is placed in transverse plane, and the needle is advanced using an in-plane approach from posterior to anterior; the local anesthetic is deposited between the middle and the lower trunk. With ultrasound guidance, low volumes of local anesthetic can provide adequate coverage and in one study has been shown to allow for shorter procedure times and fewer skin and vascular punctures.[23] Lower volumes might decrease the incidence of phrenic nerve blockade.

Complications Possible complications include neuritis, intravascular injection, and phrenic nerve block. Major neurologic complications are rare.

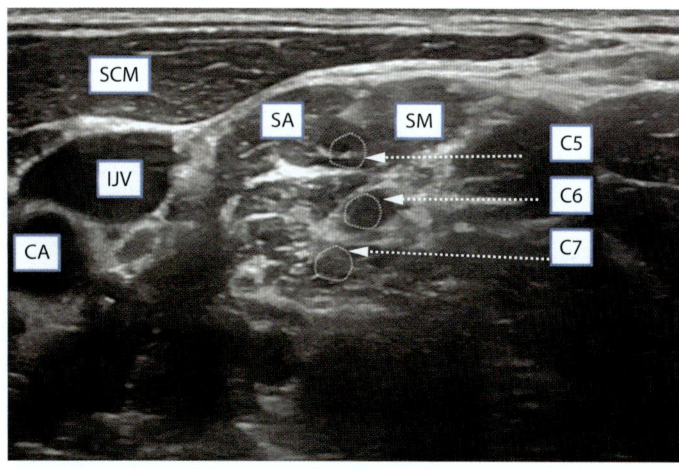

FIGURE 84-5. Interscalene block. The probe is placed transversely at about the C6 to C7 level to get a cross-sectional view of the nerve roots, and the needle is inserted in plane posterior to anterior. CA, carotid artery; C5 to C7, nerve roots; IJV, internal jugular vein; SA-scalenus anterior; SCM, sternocleidomastoid muscle; SM, scalenus medius.

Supraclavicular Block (Fig. 84-6)

Anatomy The divisions of the trunks lie in the supraclavicular fossa. A block at this location anesthetizes the entire arm from shoulder to the hand.

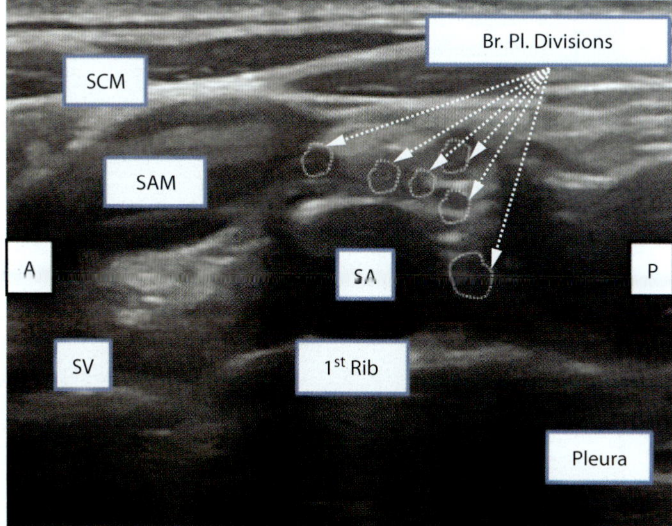

FIGURE 84-6. Supraclavicular block. The probe is placed transversely posterior (P) to anterior (A) to get a cross-sectional view of the nerve roots, and the needle is inserted in plane posterior to anterior. Infiltration is started in the sheath between the subclavian artery (SA) and the first rib. Br. Pl. Divisions, brachial plexus divisions; SAM, scalenus anterior muscle; SCM, sternocleidomastoid; SV, subclavian vein.

Indications This block is used for anesthesia for surgery on the shoulder and arm. The advantage of this block may be less likelihood of phrenic nerve block; however, the interscalene block is still preferred for shoulder surgery.

Technique The block is usually done with ultrasound guidance or with the help of a nerve stimulator. A combined technique is often used. With the stimulator technique, a 22-gauge, 5-cm stimulating needle is inserted perpendicular to the skin and lateral to the subclavian artery in a direction aimed at the first rib. After obtaining stimulation, 10 to 15 mL of local anesthetic is injected here. When using ultrasound the probe is placed in transverse plane, and the needle is advanced using an in-plane approach from posterior to anterior, the local anesthetic is deposited around the brachial plexus divisions. With ultrasound guidance, low volumes of local anesthetic can provide adequate coverage.

Complications Possible complications include neuritis, intravascular injection, and phrenic nerve block, pneumothorax. Major neurologic complications are rare.

Infraclavicular Block (Fig. 84-7)

Anatomy The cords of the brachial plexus are formed at and below the clavicle. With this block, the axillary nerve may be spared.

Indications This block is used for anesthesia for surgery on the elbow and forearm. Shoulder and upper arm is spared.

Technique The block is usually done with ultrasound guidance or with the help of a nerve stimulator. Often combined technique is used. With the stimulator technique 22-gauge, 10 cm stimulating needle is inserted perpendicular to the skin 2 cm medial and 2 cm inferior to the coracoid process. Stimulation of the posterior cord is sought. After obtaining stimulation 15-30 mL of local anesthetic is injected here. When using ultrasound the probe is placed in a vertical plane to visualize the cross section of the subclavian artery and the surrounding brachial plexus cords and the needle advanced using an in-plane approach from superior to inferior. The local anesthetic is deposited around the posterior cord from where it spreads to the other cords or these may also be blocked individually. With ultrasound guidance low volumes of local anesthetic can provide adequate coverage.

Complications Possible complications include neuritis, intravascular injection, hematoma, and pneumothorax. Major neurological complications are rare.

Axillary Block (Fig. 84-8)

Anatomy The branches of the brachial plexus lie beyond the axillary fold. At this location musculocutaneous sparing may occur, and a separate injection to cover may be needed.

Indications This block is used for anesthesia for surgery on the forearm and hand. Shoulder and upper arm sparing occurs. Musculocutaneous sparing occurs and is blocked separately.

Technique The block is usually done with ultrasound guidance or with the help of a nerve stimulator. A combined technique is often used. When using ultrasound, the probe is placed in a transverse plane to visualize the cross-section of the subclavian artery and the surrounding brachial plexus branches, and the needle is advanced using an in-plane approach from lateral to medial. The musculocutaneous nerve is blocked separately. With ultrasound guidance, low volumes of local anesthetic can provide adequate coverage.

Complications Possible complications include neuritis, intravascular injection, and hematoma. Major neurological complications are rare.

Suprascapular Nerve Block (Fig. 84-9)

Anatomy The suprascapular nerve arises from C4, C5, and C6 contributions from the upper trunk of the brachial plexus. It passes beneath the trapezius muscle to the superior border of the scapula, where it passes through the suprascapular notch. The suprascapular nerve is the major sensory supply to the shoulder joint and motor supply to the supraspinatus and infraspinatus muscles.

Indications This block is used to treat arthritis or bursitis of the shoulder joint in addition to intra- and periarticular injections. It is also used diagnostically to confirm suprascapular nerve irritation or entrapment.

The technique is done with fluoroscopic[24] or ultrasound guidance.[25] With fluoroscopic guidance, the patient lies in a prone position, and the C-arm image intensifier is tilted cranially and with medial obliquity to visualize the notch. The needle is then directed inferior to the notch and then slid in. With ultrasound guidance, it may be more reliable to block the nerve in a supraclavicular position.[25]

Complications Possible complications include pneumothorax with improper technique and neuritis.

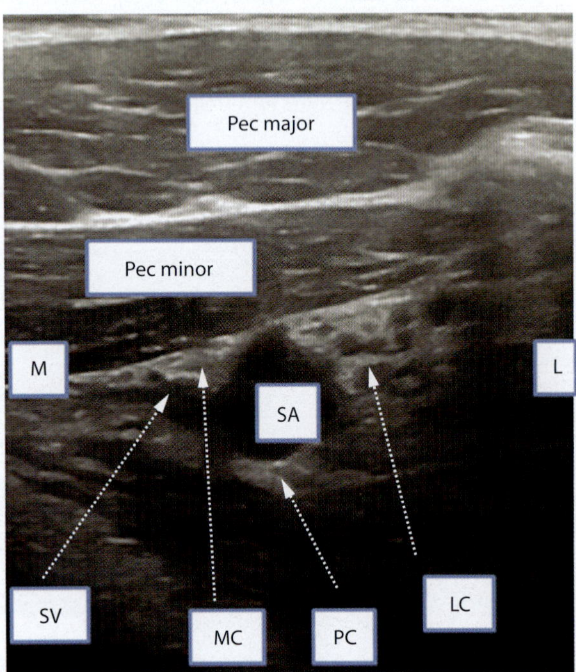

FIGURE 84-7. Infraclavicular block. The probe is placed vertically medial to the coracoid process to get a cross-sectional view of the nerve roots and the subclavian vessels. Medial (M) scanning is done to outline the extent of the pleura medially. The needle is inserted in plane superior to inferior, and infiltration around the posterior cord (PC) is done. Medial cord infiltration may be needed if the medication does not spread there from the PC. L, lateral; LC, lateral cord; MC, medial cord; SA, subclavian/axillary artery; SV, subclavian vein.

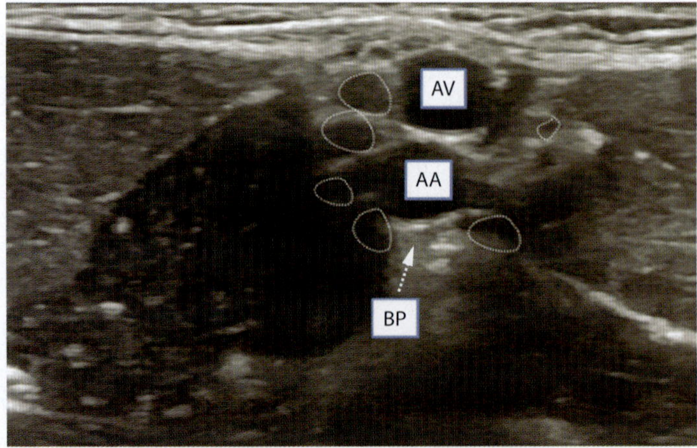

FIGURE 84-8. Axillary nerve block. The circles drawn outline the nerves. The probe is placed horizontally to get a cross-sectional view of the nerve roots, and the needle is inserted in plane. AA, axillary artery; AV, axillary vein; BP, brachial plexus.

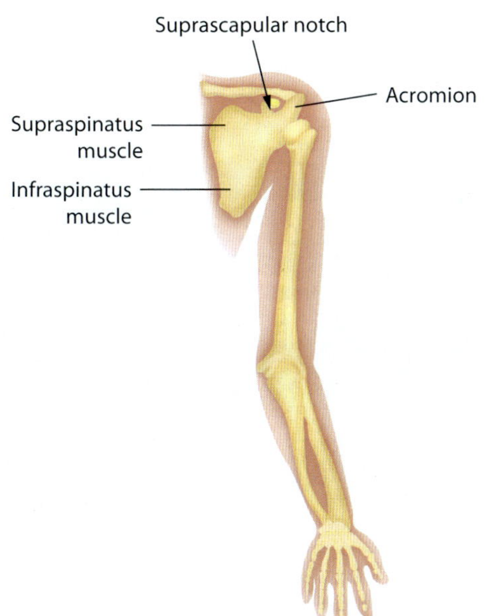

FIGURE 84-9. Suprascapular nerve block. (Adapted with permission from MediClip, Williams & Wilkins.)

UPPER EXTREMITY: ELBOW AND WRIST

Median Nerve Block (Fig. 84-10)

Anatomy The median nerve, formed from the lateral and median roots of the brachial plexus, contains fiber from C5 through T1. There are no branches in the upper arm, and it descends with the brachial artery, being slightly medial to it at the elbow. It crosses the elbow anteriorly and passes between the two heads of the pronator teres. It courses through the wrist deep to the palmaris longus tendon.

Indications This block is used to supplement a brachial plexus block or as a diagnostic and therapeutic block for carpal tunnel syndrome.[26]

Technique The nerve can be easily visualized in the forearm and the wrist, and the block is accomplished with ultrasound guidance. A total of 2 to 3 mL of local anesthetic is enough to block the nerve when using ultrasound.

Complications Major neurological complications are rare.

Ulnar Nerve Block

Anatomy The ulnar nerve is formed from the C7, C8, and T1 roots. At the elbow, it lies behind the medial epicondyle in the ulnar groove.

Indications This block is used to supplement brachial plexus anesthesia[27] or as a diagnostic and therapeutic block for ulnar nerve injury such as compression or entrapment neuropathies.

Technique The nerve can be easily visualized in the forearm and the wrist and the block accomplished with ultrasound guidance. A total of 2 to 3 mL of local anesthetic is enough to block the nerve when using ultrasound.

Complications Major neurological complications are rare.

Radial Nerve Block

Anatomy The posterior cord (C5–T1) gives rise to the radial nerve.

Indications This block is used to supplement a brachial plexus block.[27] It is also used to diagnose and treat neuralgia.

Technique The nerve can be easily visualized and the block accomplished with ultrasound guidance. A total of 2 to 3 mL of local anesthetic is enough to block the nerve when using ultrasound.

Complications Major neurological complications are rare.

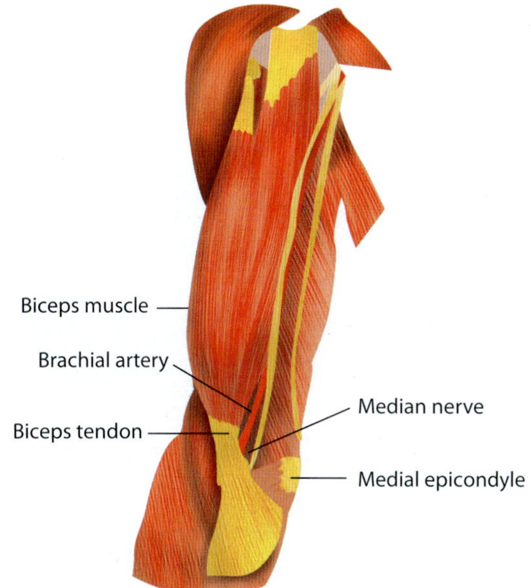

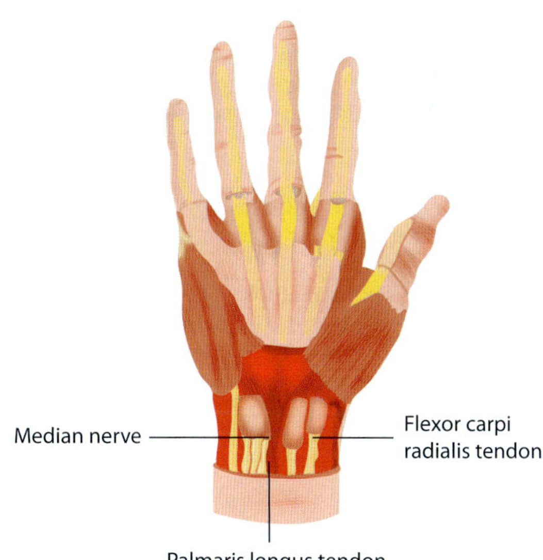

FIGURE 84-10. Median nerve block. (Adapted with permission from MediClip, Williams & Wilkins)

TRUNK

Paravertebral Nerve Block (Fig. 84-11)

Anatomy In the thoracic area, the paravertebral space is a potential space that surrounds the somatic nerves as they course from the spine to the thoracic wall to form the intercostal nerves. It is bounded laterally by the pleura and medially by the intervertebral foramen. Injection of local anesthetics into this space is efficacious in blocking multiple somatic nerves. In the lumbar area, the anatomy is different, and a block here is essentially a block of the lumbar plexus.

Indications This block is used for intraoperative and postoperative analgesia for breast, thoracic, and upper abdominal surgery. It has been shown that paravertebral block can provide superior analgesia compared with an epidural infusion.[28] It can also serve a diagnostic role in distinguishing somatic from visceral pain.

The lumbar paravertebral block is used for intraoperative and postoperative analgesia for hip and leg surgery where epidural or spinal analgesia is either not feasible or not desirable. Postoperative catheter infusions are often used.

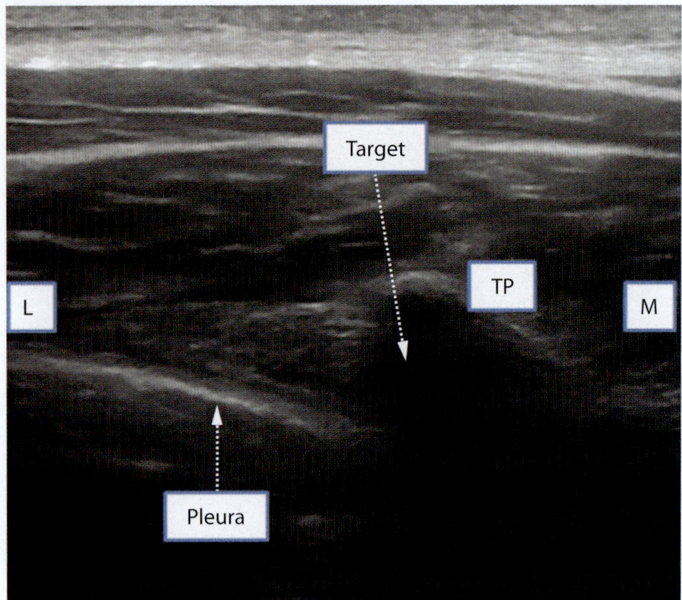

FIGURE 84-11. Paravertebral block. The probe is placed transversely between the ribs and parallel to the ribs, and the view of the pleura diving under the transverse process is obtained. The needle is inserted in plane lateral (L) to medial (M). When the injectate is in the correct plane, the pleura is seen to push down. TP, transverse process.

Technique This block may be accomplished by landmarks, often with the help of a stimulator to identify the nerve or with ultrasound guidance.

A single injection of 10 to 20 mL of local anesthetic may be done in the midpoint of the incision or multiple injections (2 to 5 mL per site) to cover all the dermatomes. The superior margin of the thoracic spinous process is marked. A needle is inserted perpendicular to all planes and 2.5 cm lateral to the spinous process to contact the transverse process. It is then slightly withdrawn and advanced caudad to lie at the lower edge of the transverse process and then advanced 1 cm past the caudad edge of the transverse process.[29,30]

Ultrasound guidance can also be used to accomplish this block. The needle is advanced in an in-plane approach to lie ventral to the transverse process and dorsal to the pleura, which is clearly identifiable with the use of ultrasound.[31]

A lumbar plexus or lumbar paravertebral block is usually accomplished at the L3 or L4 level.[32,33] The patient is placed on the side with the side to be blocked being nondependent. A 22-gauge, 10-cm needle is inserted 3 to 4 cm off the midline (4–5 cm at the L4 level) at about the superior margin of the corresponding spinous process, advanced to contact the transverse process, and then walked off cephalad 1.5 cm beyond the transverse process. A total of 20 to 30 mL of local anesthetic solution is injected here. If a twitch monitor is used, a twitching of the thigh muscles can be visualized. The sciatic nerve and the sacral plexus are usually spared, requiring a separate sciatic nerve block.[34]

In a recent study, sonoanatomy of the lumbar paravertebral block was described as a prelude to developing an ultrasound-guided technique.[35]

Complications Possible complications include intravascular injection, neuritis, pneumothorax, and spinal or epidural spread and consequent effects.

Transversus Abdominis Plane Block (Fig. 84-12)

Anatomy The somatic nerves in the abdominal wall run in a plane between the internal oblique and transverse abdominis muscle. Injection into this plane between the internal oblique and the transverse abdominis muscle leads to blockade of these nerves.[36]

Indications This block is used for surgical anesthesia for abdominal wall procedures and to differentiate abdominal wall pain from visceral pain.

Technique The technique can be performed with feel or with ultrasound guidance. The block is performed above the iliac crest anterior to the latissimus dorsi muscle. A blunt needle is advanced and a pop is perceived as the needle pierces the fascia of the external oblique muscle. A second pop is perceived as the needle pierces the fascia of the internal oblique muscle and lies in the transverse abdominis muscle. A total of 20 mL of local anesthetic is deposited here.[36] This block is commonly accomplished with ultrasound guidance. A 22-gauge, 10-cm needle is carefully advanced with ultrasound guidance in an in-plane approach to the plane that lies between the internal oblique and the transverse abdominis muscle.[37] A total of 15 mL of local anesthetic is deposited here.[38]

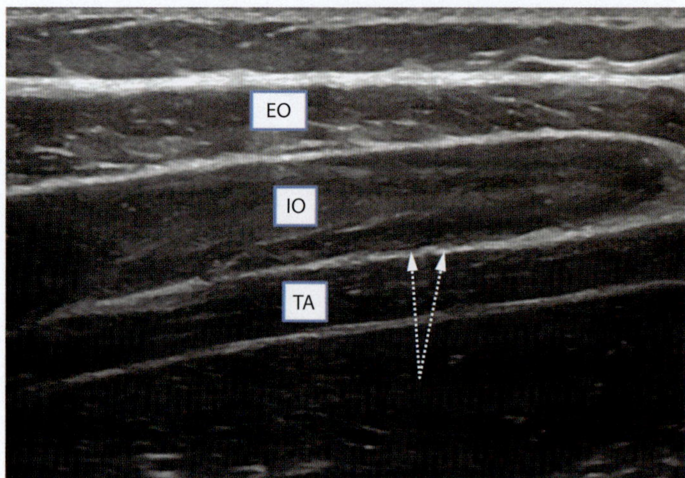

FIGURE 84-12. Transversus abdominis (TA) plane block. The probe is placed transversely and scanned medial to lateral beyond the rectus abdominis and as far lateral as possible. The target is the fascial band (arrows) between the internal oblique and the transverse abdominis. The needle is inserted in plane. EO, external oblique; IO, internal oblique.

Complications Possible complications include intravascular injection and intraperitoneal injection.

Anterior Cutaneous Nerve Block (Fig. 84-13)

Anatomy The somatic abdominal nerves run between the internal oblique and the transverse abdominis muscle to the junction with the rectus abdominis. Slightly medial to the linea semilunaris, these nerves pierce through the rectus muscle and provide cutaneous innervation.

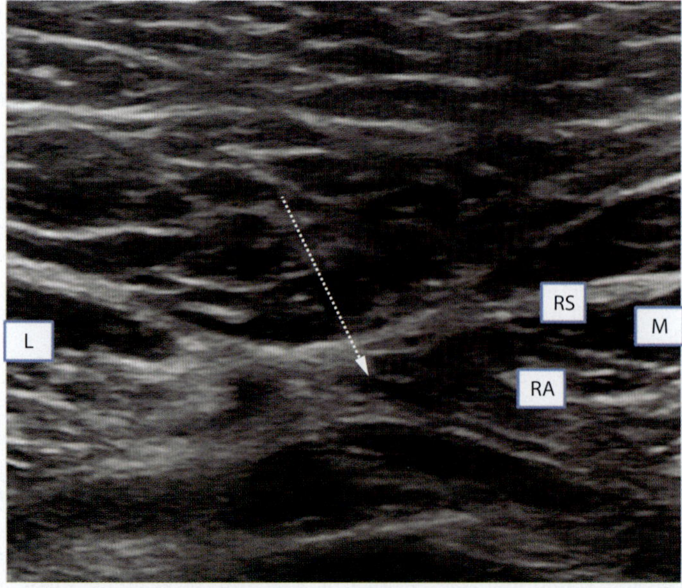

FIGURE 84-13. Anterior cutaneous nerve block. The arrow points to the target for the block as the nerves ascend medial (M) to the area semilunaris. The needle is inserted in plane. L, lateral; RA, rectus abdominis; RS, rectus sheath.

Indications This block is used for the diagnosis and treatment of anterior cutaneous nerve entrapment syndrome.[39]

Technique Infiltration of the rectus muscle may be done by feel. Ultrasound is commonly used. The point of maximal tenderness is determined, and usually there is positive Carnett sign at this location. The hyperechoic nerve within the rectus muscle is identified just medial to the linea semilunaris.[40] A 22-gauge, 1.5-in needle is inserted in an in-plane approach, and 2 to 3 mL of local anesthetic is injected here.

Complications Possible complications include neuritis and intravascular or intraperitoneal injection.

Intercostal Nerve Block (Fig. 84-14)

Anatomy The intercostal nerves lie in a groove under the rib in close association with the vein and the artery. In addition to supplying the intercostal muscles, three cutaneous branches supply the posterior, lateral, and anterior skin.[41]

Indications This block is used for temporary relief of rib fracture pain, to diagnose and treat neuralgia, and to augment surgical analgesia.

Technique In the classic approach, the nerve is blocked posteriorly about 7 to 10 cm from the midline. The lower edge of the rib is identified by feel while the patient lies in a prone position with the arms hanging down. A 22-gauge, 1.5-in needle is advanced 3 to 5 mm beyond the margin of the rib. Thereafter, 3 to 5 mL of local anesthetic is injected at each level.[41] The technique may need to be modified if the patient is unable to stay in this position. Alternately, ultrasound may be used and the needle advanced under the rib but above the pleura.[42]

Complications Possible complications include intravascular injection, neuritis, and pneumothorax.

PELVIS

Ilioinguinal and Iliohypogastric (Fig. 84-15)

Anatomy The ilioinguinal and iliohypogastric nerves originate from the L1 nerve root. A small contribution from T12 can also exist. The iliohypogastric nerve courses between the transverse and internal or internal and external oblique abdominis. It divides into lateral and anterior cutaneous branches at the level of the iliac crest. The lateral branch provides sensation to the posterolateral gluteal area. The anterior branch sends sensory fibers to the skin of the abdomen around the pubis.

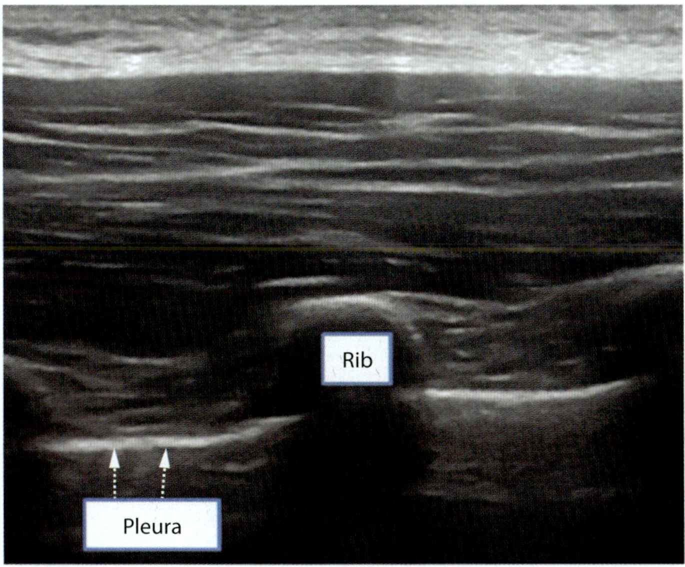

FIGURE 84-14. Intercostal nerve block: The needle is inserted in an in-plane approach under the rib just above the pleura. The in-plane approach helps with needle tip visualization, which is critical to avoid entering the lung.

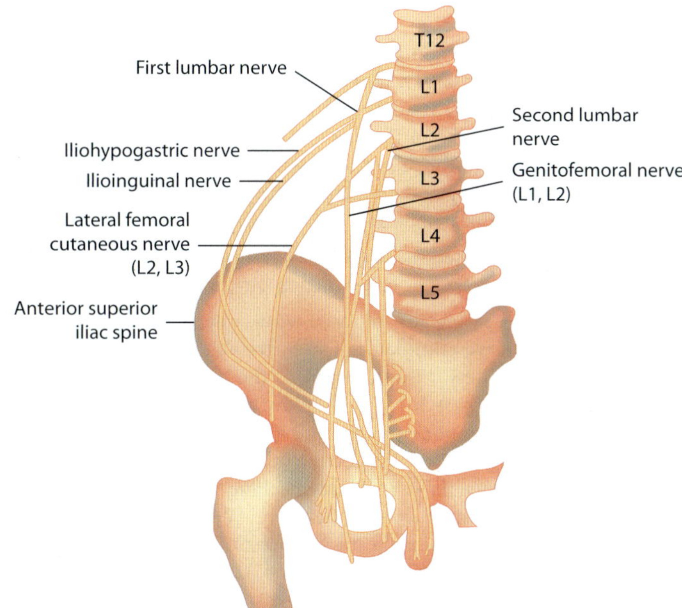

FIGURE 84-15. Lateral femoral cutaneous nerve, ilioinguinal and iliohypogastric nerve block. (Adapted with permission from MediClip, Williams & Wilkins.)

The ilioinguinal nerve is typically smaller. It lies slightly lateral to the iliohypogastric nerve, traversing the internal oblique muscle following the spermatic cord into the inguinal canal. Sensation is provided to the inner thigh, upper part of the scrotum in men, and mons pubis and lateral labia in women.

Indications This block is used for inguinal hernia operations and to diagnose and treat postherniorrhaphy nerve entrapment as well as diagnosis of groin pain.

Technique A blunt 22-gauge, 1.5-in needle is inserted 2 cm medial and 2 cm superior to the anterior superior iliac spine. A total of 2 to 4 mL of local anesthetic is injected as the first pop is felt, representing the needle passing through external oblique fascia. A second pop is felt as the needle pierces through the second fascial layer and lies between the internal oblique and the transversus abdominis. Another 2 to 4 mL of local anesthetic is injected here. The same maneuver is repeated by fanning the needle medially and laterally from this point. Alternately, ultrasound guidance may be used, and the nerve is visualized as a hypoechoic structure splitting the fascial layer and in close vicinity to the ascending branch of the deep circumflex artery.[43]

Complications Possible complications include neuritis and intraperitoneal injection. Major complications are rare.

Lateral Femoral Cutaneous (see Fig. 84-15)

Anatomy The lateral femoral cutaneous nerve is formed from the posterior divisions of L2 and L3 within the psoas muscle. It passes into the thigh slightly medial to the anterior superior iliac spine and beneath the inguinal ligament. It provides sensation to the anterolateral thigh and buttock.

Indications This block is used for the diagnosis and treatment of meralgia paresthetica.

Technique A 22-gauge, 1½-in needle is inserted approximately 2.5 cm medial and distal to the anterior iliac spine and just inferior to the inguinal ligament. The needle is inserted perpendicular to the skin and advanced slowly until a paresthesia is obtained. Then 5 to 10 mL of local anesthetic solution can be injected deep to the fascia lata. Sensory response using a nerve stimulator might improve the accuracy of the block.

Alternately, ultrasound may be used to better identify the nerve, and 2 to 3 mL of local anesthetic is injected around the nerve.[44]

Complications Possible complications include neuritis. Major complications are rare.

Sciatic Nerve Block (Fig. 84-16)

Anatomy The sciatic nerve contains most of the sensory and sympathetic fibers of the leg. It is the largest nerve in the body, originating from anterior divisions of L4, L5, S1, S2, and S3. This nerve leaves the pelvis through the sciatic notch below the piriformis muscle and then courses between the greater trochanter of the femur and ischial tuberosity. In the thigh, it branches to the hamstring and adductor magnus muscles before dividing into the common peroneal and tibial nerves behind the head of the fibula.

Indications This block is used for surgery or manipulation of the leg below the knee. It may be blocked at times during piriformis injection.

Technique The nerve is usually blocked with ultrasound guidance or with the use of a nerve stimulator. The nerve can be visualized in the subgluteal region, posterior thigh as well as the popliteal fossa and may be blocked in any of these locations. Below the division, the common peroneal and tibial components can be blocked separately. The probe is placed transversely, and a cross-section view of the nerve is obtained. A 22-gauge, 10-cm needle is inserted in-plane lateral to medial, and local anesthetic is deposited around the nerve. When using a stimulator, the patient is placed on the side for the subgluteal approach, and the needle is inserted parallel to the skin at the subgluteal crease between the greater trochanter and the ischial tuberosity, and stimulation of the foot is obtained. At the popliteal fossa, the block is usually performed in a prone position. The needle is inserted perpendicular to the skin and slightly laterally at the apex of the popliteal fossa until stimulation of the nerve can be obtained. A total of 15 to 30 mL of local anesthetic is injected. Much lower volumes will suffice when using ultrasonography.

Complications Possible complications include neuritis and intravascular injection. Major neurological complications are rare.

Femoral Nerve Block

Anatomy The femoral nerve is formed by the dorsal divisions of the anterior rami of the second (L2), third (L3), and fourth (L4) lumbar segments. It emerges from the psoas muscle and is primarily responsible for extension of the thigh. It passes into the thigh underneath the inguinal ligament and just lateral to the femoral artery. The femoral nerve sends branches to the sartorius, quadriceps femoris, and pectineus muscles along with sensory branches to the skin overlying anteromedial thigh. It terminates in the lower leg as the saphenous nerve, which supplies sensation to the skin on the medial aspect of the leg.

Indications This block can be combined with a sciatic nerve block for surgical manipulation of the leg. It is also used to diagnose and treat neuralgia.

Technique This block is performed with a nerve stimulator below the inguinal ligament. The patient is in a supine position, and the needle is inserted below the inguinal ligament and lateral to the femoral artery pulsation until contraction of the quadriceps is visualized. A total of 10 to 15 mL of local anesthetic is deposited. Ultrasound is commonly used. The probe is placed transversely below the inguinal ligament, and the femoral nerve is identified lateral to the femoral artery. The needle is inserted in an in-plane approach from lateral to medial. Lower volumes can be used when ultrasound is used.

Complications Possible complications include intravascular injection and hematoma. Nerve injury is rare.

LOWER EXTREMITY: KNEE

Common Peroneal and Tibial Nerve Block (see Fig. 84-16)

Anatomy The common peroneal and the tibial nerve are the two major peripheral branches of the sciatic nerve. This nerve enters the lower leg behind the head of the fibula, where it then courses laterally around the neck of the fibula before dividing into the deep peroneal and superficial peroneal nerves.

Indications This block is generally used in combination with tibial and saphenous nerve blocks for analgesia of the lower leg. It is also used to diagnose and treat neuralgia.

Technique The nerves can be identified with ultrasound and confirmed with stimulation. A total of 5 to 10 mL local anesthetic is sufficient to block the nerve using ultrasound.

Complications Possible complications include injury to the nerve adjacent to the neck of the fibula.

LOWER EXTREMITY: ANKLE

Deep Peroneal Nerve Block (Fig. 84-17)

Anatomy The common peroneal nerve branches into the deep and superficial peroneal nerves. This nerve enters the foot lateral to the tendon of the hallucis longus muscle and in close relationship to the dorsalis pedis artery. It supplies fibers to the tarsal and metatarsal joints and the skin adjacent to the first and second toes.

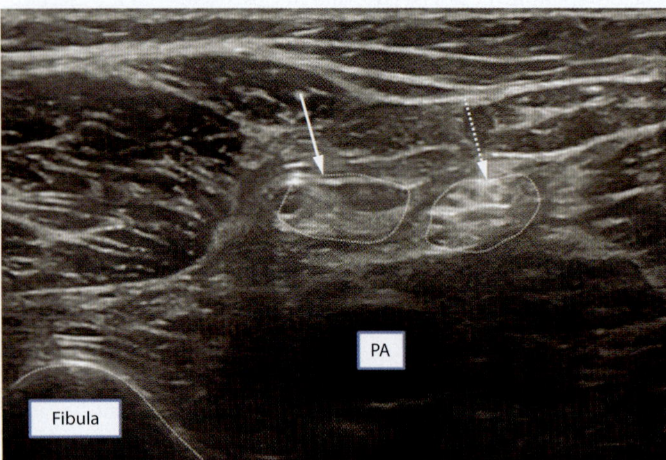

FIGURE 84-16. Sciatic nerve block. The bold arrow points to the common peroneal nerve, and the dashed arrow points to the tibial nerve. The nerves can be blocked individually in the popliteal fossa or together as sciatic nerve at the apex of the fossa or higher in the thigh or the subgluteal region. The probe is placed transversely to bisect the vessels and nerves, and the needle is inserted in-plane lateral to medial. PA, popliteal artery.

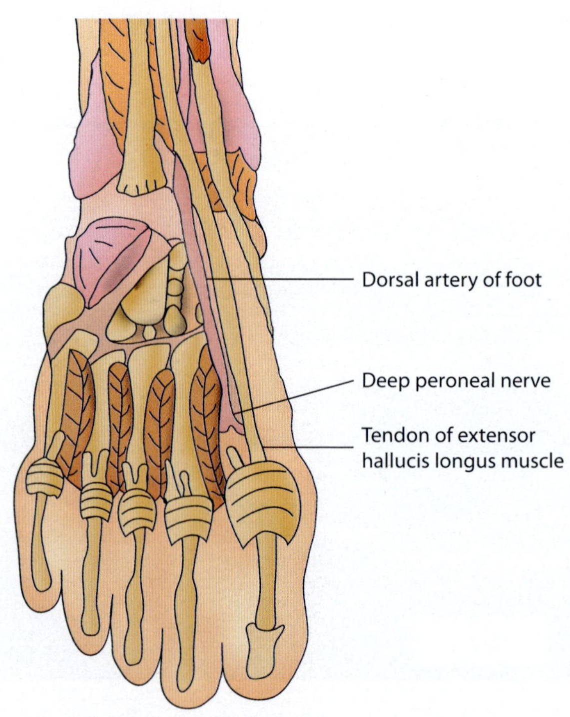

FIGURE 84-17. Deep peroneal nerve block. (Adapted with permission from MediClip, Williams & Wilkins.)

Indications When combined with a tibial nerve block, almost complete analgesia and sympathetic blockade of the foot is possible. It is also used to diagnose and treat neuralgia.

Technique A 25-gauge, 1.5-in needle is inserted slightly lateral to the groove of extensor hallucis longus and the dorsalis pedis artery. The needle is advanced until the bone is contacted and then slightly withdrawn. A total of 3 to 5 mL of local anesthetic is then deposited.

Complications Possible complications include injury to the nerve.

Superficial Peroneal and Saphenous Nerve Block (see Fig. 84-17)

Anatomy After branching from the common peroneal, the superficial peroneal nerve travels adjacent to the extensor digitorum longus muscle before dividing into terminal branches just above the ankle. It supplies sensation to the dorsum of the foot and first through fifth toes. The saphenous nerve supplies the skin over medial malleolus anteriorly and may extend to the foot. At this level, it exists as superficial branches in the subcutaneous area.

Indications This block is usually combined with other nerve blocks around the ankle for surgical anesthesia. It is used for therapeutic interventions on the feet or toes. It is also used to diagnose and treat neuralgia.

Technique The superficial peroneal nerve can be blocked by subcutaneous infiltration of 5 mL of local anesthetic from the lateral malleolus to the tibial ridge. Another 5 mL of local anesthetic is injected subcutaneously, extending medially to the medial malleolus and toward the Achilles tendon to block the saphenous nerve.

Complications Possible complications include neuritis.

Tibial Nerve Block (Fig. 84-18)

Anatomy After branching off from the sciatic nerve, this nerve courses through the popliteal fossa into the lower leg deep between the heads of the gastrocnemius muscle, which it supplies. This nerve becomes superficial at the ankle, passing between the medial malleolus and Achilles tendon before dividing into the lateral and medial plantar nerves. It supplies sensation to the skin of the heel and medial sole of the foot.

Indications This block is used to supplement inadequate sciatic block for lower extremity interventions. It is also used to diagnose and treat neuralgia.

Technique The nerve can be blocked with a landmark approach. The nerve lies deep to the fascia midway between the posterior margin of the malleolus and the Achilles tendon. A 25-gauge, 1.5-in needle is placed at this location until bone is contacted. The needle is then slightly withdrawn, and 2 to 5 mL of local anesthetic is injected. The nerve lies posterior to the tibial artery, and this is an important landmark when ultrasound is used. A paresthesia can sometimes be elicited.

Complications Possible complications include neuritis.

Sural Nerve Block (Fig. 84-18)

Anatomy The sural nerve branches from the posterior tibial nerve entering the foot between the lateral malleolus and the Achilles tendon. It provides sensation to the posterior lateral aspect of the lower calf, lateral side of the foot, and small toe.

Indications This block is used for operative and therapeutic interventions on the foot and toes. It is also used to diagnose and treat neuralgia.

Technique A total of 5 mL of local anesthetic is subcutaneously infiltrated from the lateral malleolus to the Achilles tendon.

Complications Neuritis is rare.

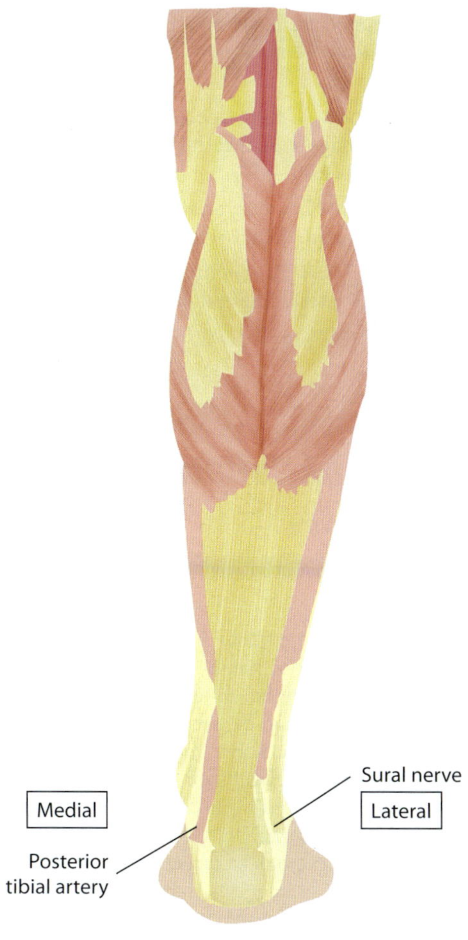

FIGURE 84-18. Common peroneal and sural nerve block. (Adapted with permission from MediClip, Williams & Wilkins.)

REFERENCES

1. Kehlet H, Jensen TS, Woolf CJ. Persistent postsurgical pain: risk factors and prevention. *Lancet*. 2006;367(9522):1618-16125.
2. Andreae MH, Andreae DA. Regional anaesthesia to prevent chronic pain after surgery: a Cochrane systematic review and meta-analysis. *Br J Anaesth*. 2013;111(5):711-720.
3. Snyder GL, Greenberg S. Effect of anaesthetic technique and other perioperative factors on cancer recurrence. *Br J Anaesth*. 2010;105(2):106-115.
4. Lambru G, Abu Bakar N, Stahlhut L, et al. Greater occipital nerve blocks in chronic cluster headache: a prospective open-label study. *MS Eur J Neurol*. 2014;21(2):338-343.
5. Lord SM, Barnsley L, Wallis BJ, et al. Percutaneous radio-frequency neurotomy for chronic cervical zygapophyseal-joint pain. *N Engl J Med*. 1996;335(23):1721-1726.
6. Butterworth JF, Strichartz GR. Molecular mechanisms of local anesthesia: a review. *Anesthesiology*. 1990;72:711-734.
7. Pollo A, Benedetti F. The placebo response: neurobiological and clinical issues of neurological relevance. *Prog Brain Res*. 2009;175: 283-294.
8. Cohen SP, Strassels SA, Kurihara C, et al. Randomized study assessing the accuracy of cervical facet joint nerve (medial branch) blocks using different injectate volumes. *Anesthesiology*. 2010;112(1): 144-152.
9. Bowsher D. Central pain: clinical and physiological characteristics. *J Neurol Neurosurg Psychiatry*. 1996;61(1):62-69.
10. Picard J, Ward SC, Zumpe R, et al. Guidelines and the adoption of 'lipid rescue' therapy for local anaesthetic toxicity. *Anaesthesia*. 2009;64(2):122-125.
11. Miller MD, Ferris DG. Measurement of subjective phenomena in primary care research: the Visual Analog Scale. *Fam Pract Res J*. 1993;13:15-24.
12. Sites BD, Brull R, Chan VW, et al. Artifacts and pitfall errors associated with ultrasound-guided regional anesthesia. Part I:

understanding the basic principles of ultrasound physics and machine operations. *Reg Anesth Pain Med.* 2007;32(5):412-418.

13. Sites BD, Brull R, Chan VW, et al. Artifacts and pitfall errors associated with ultrasound-guided regional anesthesia. Part II: a pictorial approach to understanding and avoidance. *Reg Anesth Pain Med.* 2010;35(2 Suppl):S81-S92.
14. Brown DL. Trigeminal ganglion block. In: Brown DL, ed. *Atlas of Regional Anesthesia,* 4th ed. Philadelphia: Saunders, 2010, pp. 151-156.
15. Levin M. Nerve blocks in the treatment of headache. *Neurotherapeutics.* 2010;7(2):197-203.
16. Ahmed I. Post-injection involutional lipoatrophy: ultrastructural evidence for an activated macrophage phenotype and macrophage related involution of adipocytes. *Am J Dermatopathol.* 2006;28(4):334-337.
17. Blumenfeld A, Nikolskaya G. Glossopharyngeal neuralgia. *Curr Pain Headache Rep.* 2013;17(7):343.
18. Vanderhoek MD, Hoang HT, Goff B. Ultrasound-guided greater occipital nerve blocks and pulsed radiofrequency ablation for diagnosis and treatment of occipital neuralgia. *Anesth Pain Med.* 2013;3(2):256-259.
19. Pappas JL, Kahn CH, Warfield CA. Cervical plexus blockade In. Waldman SD, Winnie AP, eds. *Interventional Pain Management.* 1996:247-265.
20. Usui Y, Kobayashi T, Kakinuma H, et al. An anatomical basis for blocking of the deep cervical plexus and cervical sympathetic tract using an ultrasound-guided technique. *Anesth Analg.* 2010;110(3):964-968.
21. Saranteas T, Kostopanagiotou GG, Anagnostopoulou S, et al. A simple method for blocking the deep cervical nerve plexus using an ultrasound-guided technique. *Anaesth Intensive Care.* 2011; 39(5):971-972.
22. Herring AA, Stone MB, Frenkel O, et al. The ultrasound-guided superficial cervical plexus block for anesthesia and analgesia in emergency care settings. *Am J Emerg Med.* 2012;30(7):1263-1267.
23. Danelli G, Bonarelli S, Tognú A, et al. Prospective randomized comparison of ultrasound-guided and neurostimulation techniques for continuous interscalene brachial plexus block in patients undergoing coracoacromial ligament repair. *Br J Anaesth.* 2012;108(6): 1006-1010.
24. Bennett DL, Cronin AM, Palmer WE, et al. Optimization and standardization of technique for fluoroscopically guided suprascapular nerve blocks. *AJR Am J Roentgenol.* 2014;202(3):576-584.
25. Siegenthaler A, Moriggl B, Mlekusch S, et al. Ultrasound-guided suprascapular nerve block, description of a novel supraclavicular approach. *Reg Anesth Pain Med.* 2012;37(3):325-328.
26. Ustün N, Tok F, Yagz AE, et al. Ultrasound-guided vs. blind steroid injections in carpal tunnel syndrome: a single-blind randomized prospective study. *Am J Phys Med Rehabil.* 2013;92(11):999-1004.
27. Dufeu N, Marchand-Maillet F, Atchabahian A, et al. Efficacy and safety of ultrasound-guided distal blocks for analgesia without motor blockade after ambulatory hand surgery. *J Hand Surg Am.* 2014;39(4):737-743.
28. Raveglia F, Rizzi A, Leporati A, et al. Analgesia in patients undergoing thoracotomy: epidural versus paravertebral technique. A randomized, double-blind, prospective study. *J Thorac Cardiovasc Surg.* 2014;147(1):469-473.
29. Moore D. *A Handbook for Use in Clinical Practice of Medicine and Surgery.* 4th ed. Springfield, IL: Charles C. Thomas; 1965.
30. Klein SM, Bergh A, Steele SM, et al. Thoracic paravertebral block for breast surgery. *Anesth Analg.* 2000;90(6):1402-1405.
31. Cowie B, McGlade D, Ivanusic J, Barrington MJ. Ultrasound-guided thoracic paravertebral blockade: a cadaveric study. *Anesth Analg.* 2010;110(6):1735-1739.
32. Winnie AP, Ramamurthy S, Durrani Z. The inguinal paravascular technique of lumbar plexus anesthesia: the "3-in-1" block. *Anesth Analg.* 1973;52:989-996.
33. Chayen D, Nathan H, Chayen M. The psoas compartment block. *Anesthesiology.* 1976;45:95-99.
34. Parkinson SK, Mueller JB, Little WL, Bailey SL. Extent of blockade with various approaches to the lumbar plexus. *Anesth Analg.* 1989;68(3):243-248.
35. Karmakar MK, Li JW, Kwok WH, et al. Sonoanatomy relevant for lumbar plexus block in volunteers correlated with cross-sectional anatomic and magnetic resonance images. *Reg Anesth Pain Med.* 2013;38(5):391-397.
36. McDonnell JG, O'Donnell BD, Farrell T, et al. Transversus abdominis plane block: a cadaveric and radiological evaluation. *Reg Anesth Pain Med.* 2007;32(5):399-404.
37. Hebbard P, Fujiwara Y, Shibata Y, Royse C. Ultrasound-guided transversus abdominis plane (TAP) block. *Anaesth Intensive Care.* 2007;35(4):616-617.
38. Moeschler SM, Murthy NS, Hoelzer BC, et al. Ultrasound-guided transversus abdominis plane injection with computed tomography correlation: a cadaveric study. *J Pain Res.* 2013;6:493-496.
39. Applegate WV. Abdominal cutaneous nerve entrapment syndrome. *Am Fam Physician.* 1973;8(3):132-133.
40. Kanakarajan S, High K, Nagaraja R. Chronic abdominal wall pain and ultrasound-guided abdominal cutaneous nerve infiltration: a case series. *Pain Med.* 2011;12(3):382-386.
41. Waldman SD. Intercostal nerve block. In: Waldman SD, ed. *Atlas of Interventional Pain Management*, 4th ed. Philadelphia: Elsevier, 2015, pp. 336-343.
42. Shankar H, Eastwood D. Retrospective comparison of ultrasound and fluoroscopic image guidance for intercostal steroid injections. *Pain Pract.* 2010;10(4):312-317.
43. Gofeld M, Christakis M. Sonographically guided ilioinguinal nerve block. *J Ultrasound Med.* 2006;25(12):1571-1575.
44. Ng I, Vaghadia H, Choi PT, Helmy N. Ultrasound imaging accurately identifies the lateral femoral cutaneous nerve. *Anesth Analg.* 2008;107(3):1070-1074.

CHAPTER 85 Cranial Peripheral Nerve Blocks

Paul G. Mathew

The practice of headache medicine has evolved over time, and the use of peripheral nerve blocks has been gradually increasing among practitioners. Peripheral nerve blocks are generally safe, well-tolerated office-based procedures that can be performed for the acute treatment of numerous headache disorders. For reasons that are less clear, nerve blocks can have prolonged effects beyond the duration of the injected anesthetic, at times lasting weeks to months.[1] As such, nerve blocks can also be used for preventive treatment.

Although peripheral nerve blocks target peripheral nerves, the duration of benefit in some cases suggests that these procedures likely also have effects on central pain–modulating structures. One study that supports the theory of peripheral nerve blocks causing central pain modulation demonstrated that after performing occipital nerve blocks in the setting of an acute migraine, migraine pain, brush allodynia in the trigeminal nerve distribution, and photophobia improved.[2]

In a survey study conducted by the American Headache Society, occipital neuralgia and chronic migraine were the most common indications for performing peripheral nerve blocks. Clinicians were more likely to perform nerve blocks if the patient had local tenderness in the region where the nerve block was performed.[3]

The greater occipital nerve is the most commonly targeted nerve for peripheral nerve blockade. Some other common peripheral nerve block targets are the lesser occipital nerve, supratrochlear nerve, supraorbital nerve, and auriculotemporal nerve. Nerve blocks can be performed using various techniques, volumes, and drugs. Lidocaine and bupivacaine are the most commonly used anesthetics for these procedures.[3] These anesthetics can be injected with or without steroids. The use of steroids in peripheral nerve blocks is controversial for different headache disorders, but some of the most compelling evidence for steroid use is for the treatment of both episodic and chronic cluster headaches.[4] In addition to the use of anesthetic combined with steroid, one study demonstrated that betamethasone injections without anesthetic were more effective than placebo for the treatment of cluster headache.[5] The use of anesthetic combined with steroids is usually preferred because this combination tends to generate a more rapid analgesic effect than steroids alone.

Steroids should be used with caution given the potential for Cushing's syndrome, glaucoma, cutaneous atrophy, and alopecia.[6, 7] Because of these possible complications, steroid use should be avoided in nerve blocks around face, especially given the risk of significant cosmetic disfigurement. These local cutaneous changes can have an additive effect when serial nerve blocks with steroids are performed within a relatively short time period. If repeat injections with steroids are indicated based a beneficial patient response, examination of the injection site should be performed before the procedure is repeated to look for signs of cutaneous atrophy and alopecia. If present, steroid use should be avoided. In clinical practice, steroids are typically used in nerve blocks no more frequently than once every three months.

A basic principle for any medical procedure is that both the patient and the practitioner should be in a comfortable position. Following this principle often leads to improved patient tolerance of the procedure and a reduction of practitioner fatigue. Although practitioner fatigue may seem trivial, it can be a significant issue in the setting of a prolonged procedure or when multiple patient procedures are scheduled for a single clinic session. Even the simplest procedures can be complicated by patient anxiety, low pain tolerance, and excessive bleeding.

Although some practitioners perform nerve blocks with patients in a seated position, supine and prone positions certainly have some advantages. In the supine and prone positions, the patient's head tends to be more fixed compared with the head movement that can more easily occur with the seated position. Movement of the patient's head can lead to injecting in the wrong area, injury to the patient, and accidental needle sticks to the provider. In addition, nerve blocks have been associated with syncope and less frequently seizures, which could potentially lead to more significant injury while in the seated position compared with lying flat.

OCCIPITAL NERVE BLOCKS

The patient is placed in the prone position with a pillow under the chest. Using palpation, the inion and the mastoid process are identified on the skin, and a line is drawn using a surgical marker connecting these points while remaining superior to the occipital ridge. The skin is prepped with alcohol in the midpoint of this line. Next, using a 2-in, 21-gauge needle, a solution consisting of 6 cc of 0.75% bupivacaine and 20 mg of triamcinolone is injected from the midpoint of this line connecting the inion to the mastoid process, with the practitioner being careful to stay above bone and superficial throughout the entire process (**Fig. 85-1**).

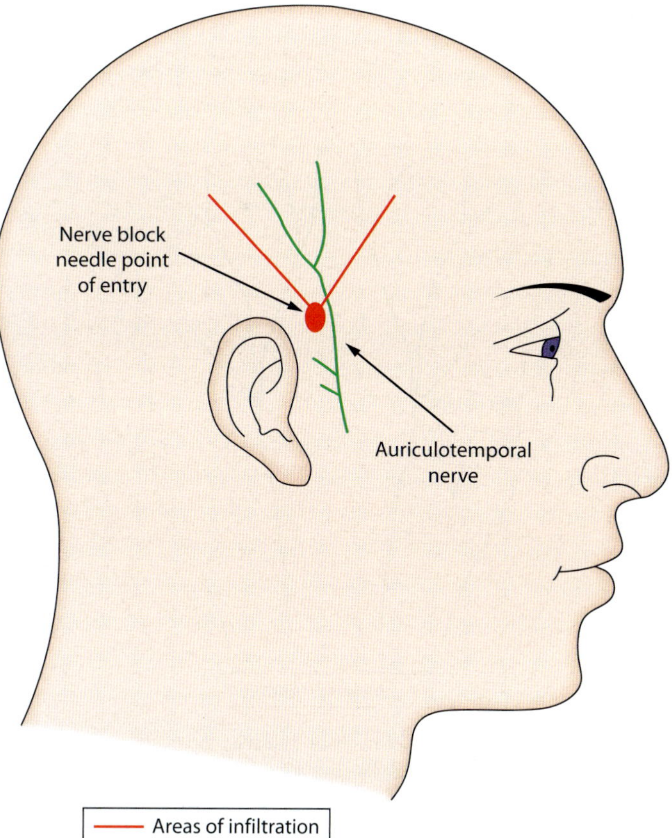

FIGURE 85-1. Lateral view of the head illustrating the course of the auriculotemporal nerve, as well as needle entry point and areas of infiltration for an auriculotemporal nerve block. (Artwork by Paul G. Mathew, MD, FAHS.)

AURICULOTEMPORAL NERVE BLOCKS

The patient is placed in the supine position. Using direct palpation, the temporal artery pulse is located, and the skin is prepped with alcohol. Using a 1-in, 30-gauge needle, 0.2 cc of 0.75% bupivacaine is injected anterior to the temporal artery above the posterior portion of the zygoma, with the practitioner being careful to remain superficial throughout the entire process. The needle is then advanced at a 45-degree angle anterior and superior to the point of entry, and 0.4 cc of 0.75% bupivacaine is injected. The needle is then retracted without exiting the skin. The needle is then advanced at a 45-degree angle posterior and superior to the point of entry, and another 0.4 cc of 0.75% bupivacaine is injected for a total volume of 1 cc (**Fig. 85-2**).

SUPRAORBITAL NERVE BLOCKS

The patient is placed in the supine position. Using direct palpation, the supraorbital foramen is identified, and the skin is prepped with alcohol. Next, using a 1 inch 30-gauge needle, 0.2 cc of 0.75% bupivacaine is injected just superior to the foramen. The needle is then advanced superiorly about 0.5-1 cm, and 0.3 cc of 0.75% bupivacaine is injected for a total volume of 0.5 cc.

SUPRATROCHLEAR NERVE BLOCKS

The patient is placed in the supine position. Using direct palpation, the supratrochlear foramen is identified, and the skin is prepped with alcohol. Next, using a 1-in, 30-gauge needle, 0.2 cc of 0.75% bupivacaine was injected just superior to the foramen. The needle is then advanced

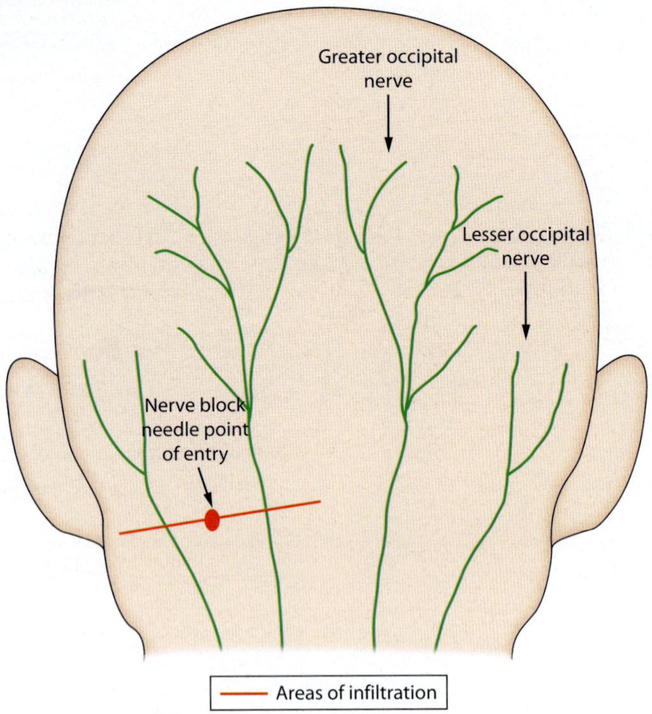

FIGURE 85-2. Posterior view of the head illustrating the course of the greater and lesser occipital nerves, as well as needle entry point and areas of infiltration for occipital nerve blocks. (Artwork by Paul G. Mathew, MD, FAHS.

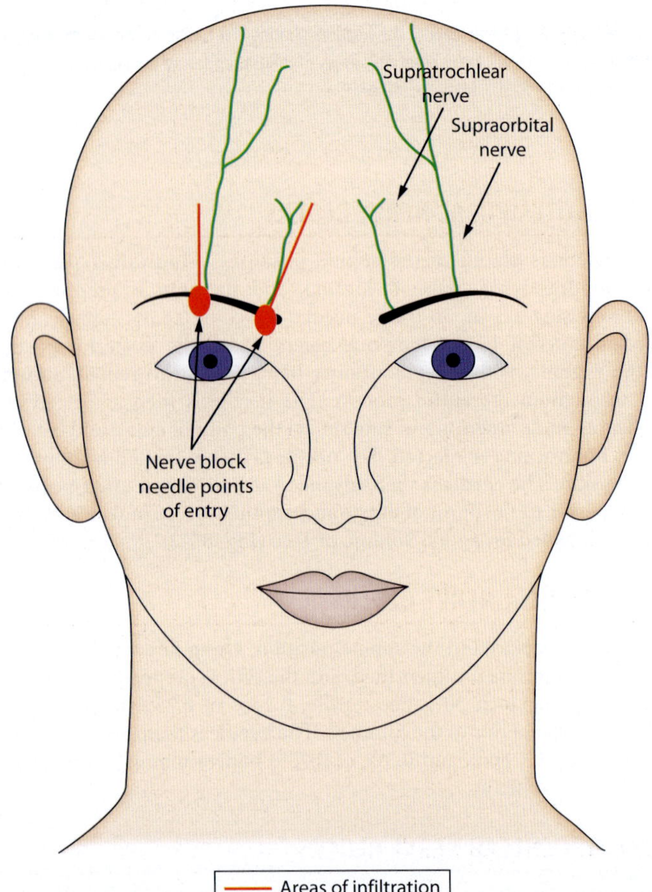

FIGURE 85-3. Anterior view of the head illustrating the course of the supraorbital and supratrochlear nerves, as well as needle entry points and areas of infiltration for supraorbital and supratrochlear nerve blocks. (Artwork by Paul G. Mathew, MD, FAHS.)

superiorly about 0.5 to 1 cm, and 0.3 cc of 0.75% bupivacaine is injected for a total volume of 0.5 cc (**Figure 85-3**).

REFERENCES

1. Afridi SK, Shields KG, Bhola R, Goadsby PJ. Greater occipital nerve injection in primary headache syndromes—prolonged effects from a single injection. *Pain*. 2006;122(1-2):126-129.
2. Young W, Cook B, Malik S, et al. The first 5 minutes after greater occipital nerve block. *Headache*. 2008;48:1126-1128.
3. Blumenfeld A, Ashkenazi A, Grosberg B, et al. Patterns of use of peripheral nerve blocks and trigger point injections among headache practitioners in the USA: Results of the American Headache Society Interventional Procedure Survey (AHS-IPS). *Headache*. 2010;50(6):937-942.
4. Lambru G, Abu Bakar N, Stahlhut L, et al. Greater occipital nerve blocks in chronic cluster headache: a prospective open-label study. *Eur J Neurol*. 2014;21(2):338-343.
5. Ambrosini A, Vandenheede M, Rossi P, et al. Suboccipital injection with a mixture of rapid- and long-acting steroids in cluster headache: a double-blind placebo-controlled study. *Pain*. 2005;118(1-2):92-96.
6. Lambru G, Lagrata S, Matharu MS. Cutaneous atrophy and alopecia after greater occipital nerve injection using triamcinolone. *Headache*. 2012;52(10):1596-1599.
7. Tripathi RC, Parapuram SK, Tripathi BJ, et al. Corticosteroids and glaucoma risk. *Drugs Aging*. 1999;15(6):439-450.

CHAPTER 86 Local Anesthetics

Lance J. Lehmann

ORIGINS AND HISTORY

Cocaine is a naturally occurring compound. It was the first anesthetic to be discovered and is the only naturally occurring local anesthetic; all others are synthetically derived. Cocaine was introduced in Europe in 1860 after its isolation from coca leaves by German chemist Albert Niemann (1834–1861). Sigmund Freud (1856–1939), the noted Austrian psychoanalyst, was an early proponent of its medicinal uses. He encouraged a physician colleague, Dr. Carl Koller (1857–1944) to experiment with its analgesic properties.

The origins of local anesthesia date back to 1884 when Koller introduced cocaine to the field of ophthalmology in Vienna. He discovered that cocaine instilled into his conjunctival fornix produced localized insensitivity to touch and pain.[1] The news quickly spread around the world and to the United States after publication of Koller's paper on September 18, 1887. William Stewart Halsted (1852–1922) and his colleague Richard John Hall (1856–1897) were the first to report the use of cocaine for nerve blocks in the United States in 1884.[2] Halsted injected cocaine into the lower jaw of a patient and extracted a tooth with no pain or sensation reported by the patient. Halsted and Hall developed various nerve and regional blocking techniques.

On August 16 1898, August Bier performed the first surgery under spinal anesthesia at the Royal Surgical Hospital by injection of 15 mg of cocaine intrathecally. In 1908, Bier pioneered the technique for intravenous regional anesthesia (IVRA)[3] commonly known as "Bier block" (**Fig. 86-1**).

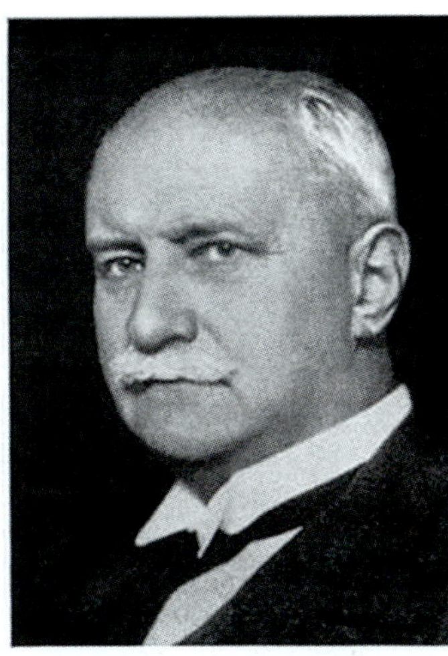

August Bier.

FIGURE 86-1. August Bier (1861-1949).

After the adverse effects of cocaine (toxicity, addiction, and others) became more widely known, new anesthetic drugs were sought to replace it (**Fig. 86-2**).

The first successful attempt came on November 27, 1904, when German chemist Alfred Einhorn (1856–1917) patented 18 para-aminobenzoic derivatives that were developed in Hesse, Germany.[4] One of the compounds was given the name *novocaine*, from the Latin *nov*,-new + *caine*, a common ending for alkaloids used as anesthetics. In 1905, in an article by Heinrich Braun, novocaine was compared with other local anesthetics being developed.[5] Novocaine was found to be safe and quickly became the standard for local anesthesia; it then was renamed procaine in the United States during World War I. The drug needed to be combined with high concentrations of adrenaline for optimal affect. In addition, some patients were highly allergic to it. These drawbacks prompted searches for stronger anesthetic agents with fewer allergic side effects.

Lidocaine, the first amino amide-type local anesthetic was synthesized under the name *xylocaine* by Swedish chemist Nils Lofgren in 1943. His colleague Bengt Lundquist self-administered the first local anesthetic injection experiments.[6] Lidocaine has a different chemical composition from novocaine yet proved to be safe, with a stronger effect and much less allergic activity. It became the most widely used local anesthetic during World War II and was widely marketed in 1948.

Additional amide-type local anesthetics were quickly developed and reported: mepivacaine[7] in 1956 followed by prilocaine, which was synthesized in 1960.[8] Bupivacaine was developed in 1963,[7] etidocaine in 1972,[9] and articaine, which was first developed and described in an article published in 1972.[10]

CHEMICAL STRUCTURE

Local anesthetic agents conform to a similar molecular configuration consisting of a lipophilic aromatic ring connected to a hydrophilic amine group. The linking chain may be used to classify an agent as an ester or amide.

Two types of local anesthetics exist: the amino amides and the amino esters. Amino amides (lidocaine) have an amide link between the intermediate chain and the aromatic end, whereas amino esters (procaine) have an ester link between the intermediate chain and the aromatic end (**Fig. 86-3**).

Amino esters differ from amino amides in several respects. Amino esters are metabolized in the plasma via pseudocholinesterase, whereas amino amides are metabolized in the liver. Amino esters are unstable in solution, but amino amides are very stable in solution. Amino esters are much more likely than amino amides to cause allergic hypersensitivity reactions.

Commonly used amino amides include lidocaine, mepivacaine, prilocaine, bupivacaine, etidocaine, ropivacaine, articaine, and levobupivacaine. Commonly used amino esters include cocaine, procaine, tetracaine, 2-chloroprocaine, and benzocaine. An easy way to remember which drug belongs in which category is that all the amino amides generally contain the letter "I" twice, as does the term "amino amides."

The newest additions to clinically available local anesthetics, ropivacaine and levobupivacaine, represent exploitation of the S enantiomer of these chemicals to create anesthetics which are less toxic, more potent, and longer acting.

ESTER LOCAL ANESTHETICS

Cocaine

CH_3 CO_2CH_3 N O O

Cocaine

Cocaine (2-B-carbomethoxy-3-B-benzoxytropane) is an ester of benzoic acid and is found naturally in the leaves of *Erythroxylum coca* or *Erythroxylum truxillensis*, which are indigenous to Bolivia and Peru.[11]

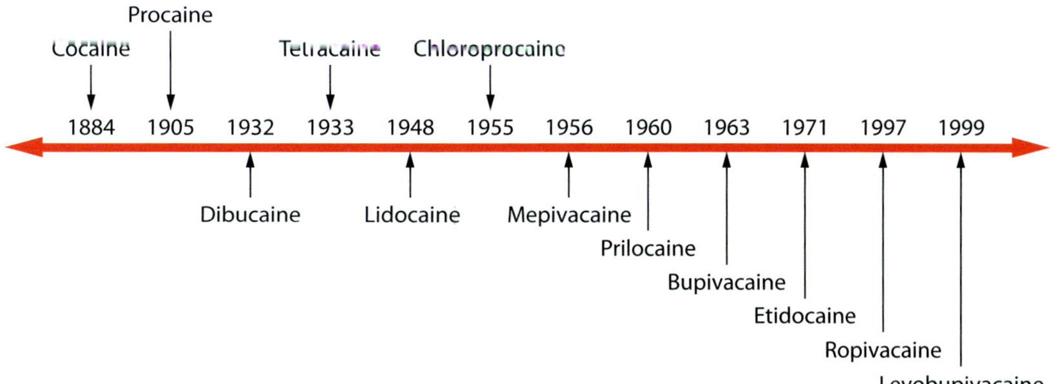

FIGURE 86-2. Timeline for local anesthetic discovery and introduction.

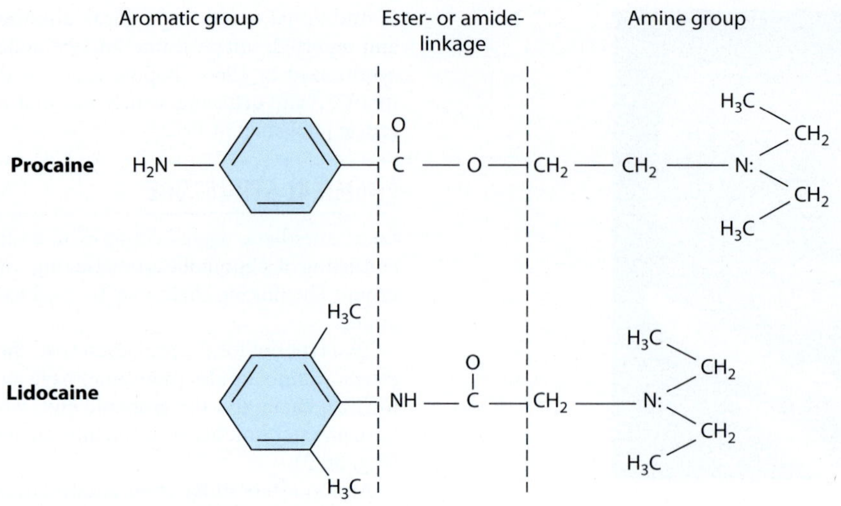

FIGURE 86-3. Chemical structure of the two classes of local anesthetics: amino esters and amino amides.

It is a colorless crystalline compound only slightly water soluble but soluble in most organic solvents. In addition to local anesthetic action on nerve membranes, it is also able to block the reuptake of norepinephrine at sympathetic neurons, thus potentiating the effects of catecholamines and causing intense vasoconstriction. When used as a topical anesthetic it is absorbed well from mucous membranes. Concentrations of 1% to 10% are currently used for procedures involving the nasal mucosa. Overdoses can produce hypertension, tachyarrhythmia, and tachypnea, as well as central nervous system (CNS) effects. Toxicity is partly related to the fact that it is metabolized more slowly than other ester local anesthetics.

Procaine (Novocain®)

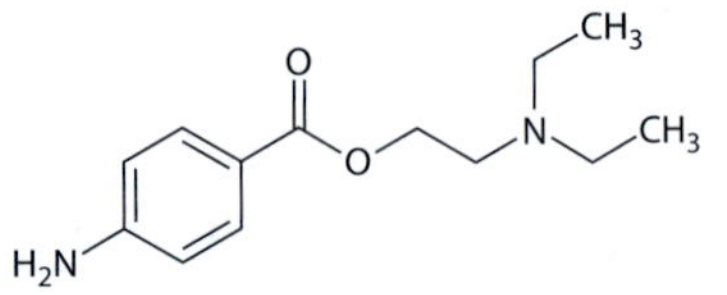

Procaine (2-diethyl-4-aminoethyl-p-aminobenzoate) was the first synthetic local anesthetic, developed by Alfred Einhorn in 1905. This ester local anesthetic was less toxic than cocaine, but it was a weaker agent with slow onset and short duration of action. Concentrations of 0.25% were used for infiltration, increasing to 5% for epidural anesthesia. It is metabolized by hydrolysis to diethyl-aminoethanol and *p*-aminobenzoic acid.

2-Chloroprocaine (Nesacaine®)

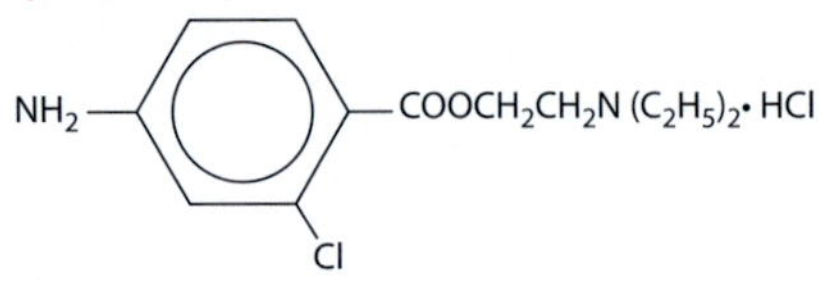

NH_2—(ring, Cl)—$COOCH_2CH_2N\ (C_2H_5)_2 \cdot HCl$

The low potency of procaine led to the development of 2-chloroprocaine (2-diethlyaminoethyl-4-amino-2-chlorobenzoate) in 1952. Clinically it had a rapid onset and short duration of action. This agent was more lipid soluble, more potent and required lower concentrations 2% to 3%.

Tetracaine (Pontocaine)

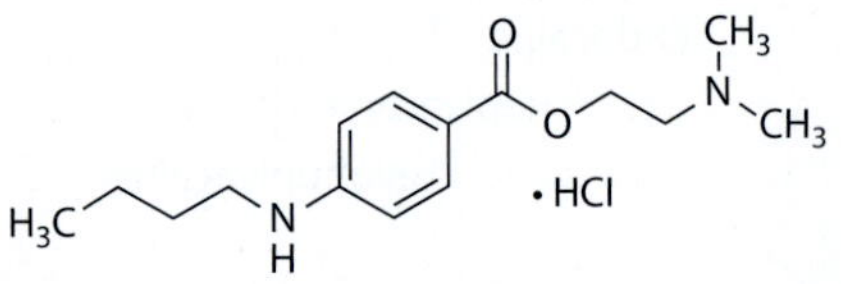

Synthesized by Eisleb in 1928, tetracaine was first used clinically in 1931. It has a moderate onset of action and prolonged duration. It has been used for spinal anesthesia, but its use today is mainly restricted to ophthalmic procedures.

Benzocaine (Americaine®)

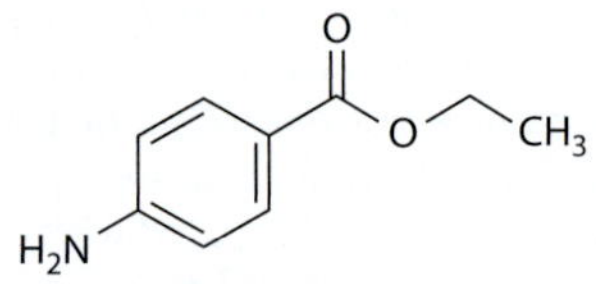

Benzocaine (ethyl p-aminobenzoate) is a derivative of procaine with no amino terminus. It is not very water soluble, so its primary use is topically due to its slow absorption. Formulations include gel or lozenges for dentistry or mucosal irritation.

AMIDE LOCAL ANESTHETICS

Lidocaine (Xylocaine®)

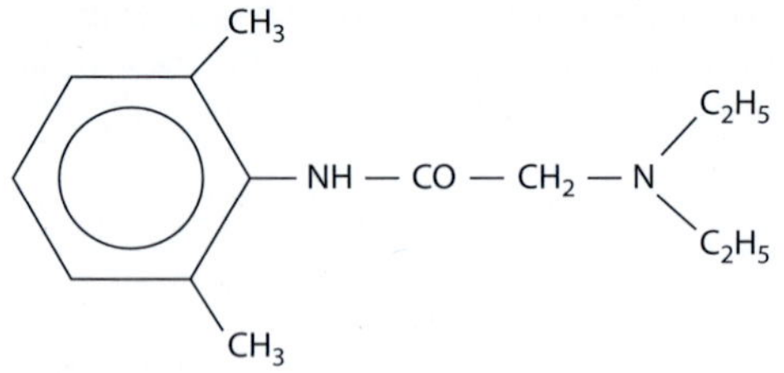

Synthesized by Lofgren and Lundquist in Sweden in 1943 and introduced clinically in 1947, lidocaine (diehtylaminoacetyl-2-6-xylidine) is the tertiary amine derivative of diethyl amino-acetic acid. It is one of the most widely used local anesthetics in the world at concentrations of 0.5% to 2%. Rapid onset of sensory and motor block contributes to the popularity of lidocaine for use in regional anesthesia. Higher concentrations (5%) were used for spinal anesthesia until reports suggested this concentration caused transient radicular irritation.[12] Some laboratory data indicate that even lower concentrations may result in neurotoxicity, although there are no data supporting this in humans.[13] Protein binding is low, lending to intermediate duration of action, and tachyphylaxis occurs with repeated injection. Lidocaine is also use intravenously as a class 1b anti-arrhythmic drug.

In addition to its local anesthetic and antiarrhythmic effects, lidocaine has also been studied as a tinnitus-suppressing drug. Following the accidental discovery of the tinnitus-suppressing effect of procaine described by Barany in 1935, extensive research was conducted on the intravenous administration of lidocaine as a treatment for tinnitus.

In 1992, Murai et al. reported that 40% to 80% of patients with tinnitus had a reduction in their tinnitus with the intravenous administration of lidocaine.[14] Unfortunately, problems with systemic toxicity limit the practicality of lidocaine as an effective treatment for tinnitus.

Research suggests that lidocaine suppresses some forms of tinnitus in either the cochlea or the central auditory system, or potentially in both locations, depending on the kind of tinnitus and the mode of application. The inferior colliculus may be a central target of lidocaine. Evidence indicates that various molecular channels and receptors in this area that are linked to tinnitus are affected by lidocaine. As the specific mechanism of tinnitus inhibition by lidocaine is elucidated, new pharmacological targets for the treatment of tinnitus may be devised.

Mepivacaine (Carbocaine®, Polocaine®)

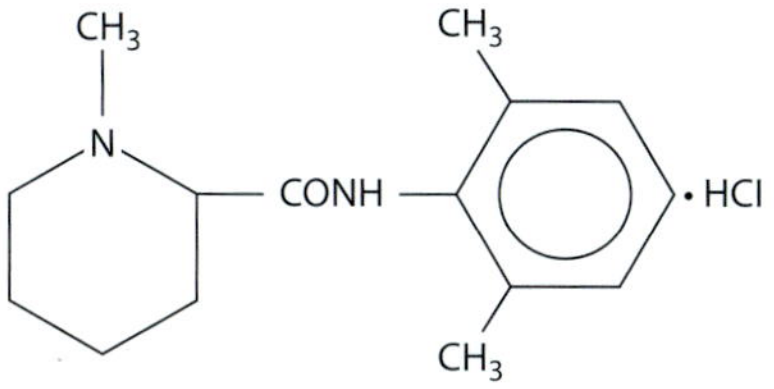

CH_3 CH_3 N CONH • HCl CH_3

Mepivacaine (1-methyl-2-[2, 6-xylylcarbamoyl]-piperidine) is structurally related to bupivacaine and ropivacaine. It was synthesized in 1956 by Ekenstam and Egner and was the second amide local anesthetic to be introduced clinically. It has a fast onset that is similar to that of lidocaine; however, it has a longer duration of action due to its lack of vasodilator activity. Used in concentrations of 0.5% to 2% it has a reliable safety record and is used for a wide range of regional anesthetic techniques as well as IVRA.

Bupivacaine (Marcaine®, Sensorcaine®)

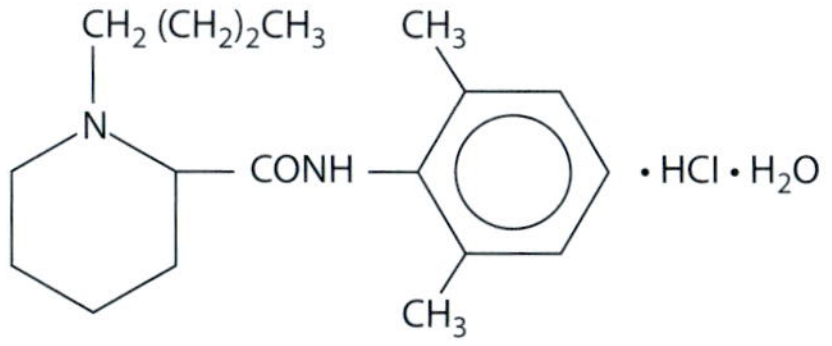

$CH_2(CH_2)_2CH_3$ CH_3 N CONH • HCl • H_2O CH_3

Bupivacaine (1-butyl-2-[2, 6-xylycarbamoyl]-piperidine]) was introduced in 1963. It is structurally related to mepivacaine and ropivacaine and available in concentrations of 0.1% to 0.75% with a slow onset of action. As a result of its prolonged duration of action bupivacaine is a popular choice for peripheral nerve blocks. Concerns about toxicity and difficult resuscitation led to the removal of higher concentrations of bupivacaine (0.75%) from obstetrical anesthesia.[15]

Ropivacaine (Naropin®)

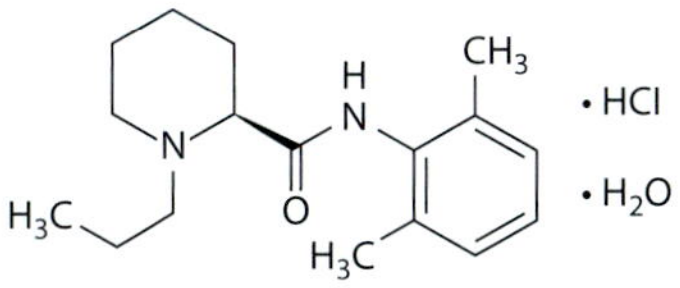

N H N CH_3 • HCl • H_2O H_3C O H_3C

First synthesized in the 1950s, it was introduced into clinical use in 1996. Ropivacaine (N-*n*-propyl-2, 6-pipecoloxylidide) is the propylderivative of N-alkylpipecoloxylidine, the third in the mepivacaine, bupivacaine series.[16] Its onset and duration of action are similar to bupivacaine but less potent, requiring concentrations up to 1%. Lower concentrations of ropivacaine can provide a differential sensory and motor block which disappears at higher concentrations. The preservation of motor function is appealing in cases in which ambulation is desired. This duel effect may be due to decreased lipid solubility, thus preventing ropivacaine from penetrating the larger AB fibers. The commercially available form of ropivacaine is the *S*(-) isomer. This isomer has reduced cardiovascular and CNS toxicity when compared to the racemic bupivacaine preparation, and adverse events following accidental intravascular injection may be easier to treat.[17] Relative to other agents the toxicity of ropivacaine is intermediate between bupivacaine and lidocaine; however, the toxicity advantages over bupivacaine may be offset by its reduced potency.

Etidocaine (Duranest®)

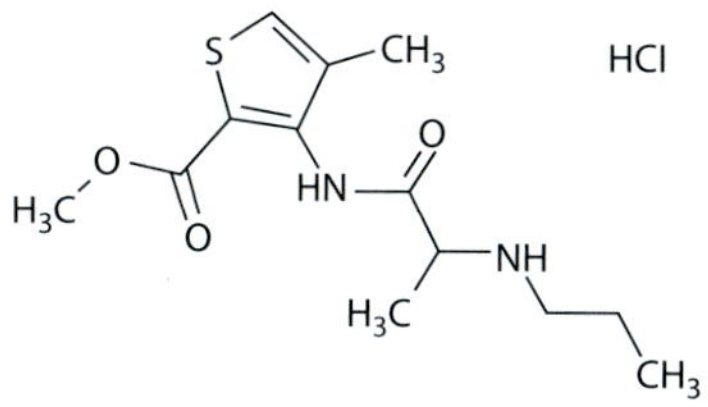

S CH_3 HCl O H_3C O O HN O NH H_3C CH_3

Etidocaine (2-[N-ethylpropylamino]-butyro2, 6-xylidine) has a structure similar to lidocaine and was first described by Adams in 1972. Clinically, its rapid onset of action is similar to lidocaine, but with a more prolonged duration. It is highly lipid soluble, resulting in a very intense motor block. Concentrations of 0.25% to 1.5% are typically used, and its profound motor block does not make it suitable for certain types of regional anesthesia in which ambulation may be required.

Prilocaine (Citanest®)

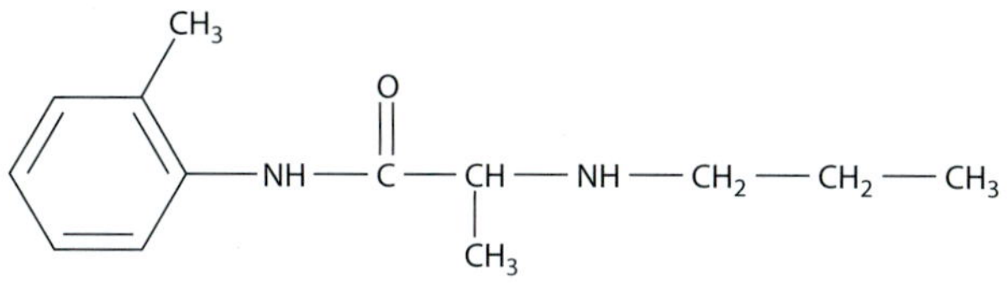

CH_3 O NH — C — CH — NH — CH_2 — CH_2 — CH_3 CH_3

Originally described by Lofgren and Tegner in 1960, prilocaine (N-[2-propylaminopropionyl]-O-toluidine) is a secondary amide analog of lidocaine with similar onset of action but longer duration. The O-toluidine structure lacks an aromatic methyl group, which is present in most other amides. Properties include rapid tissue uptake and metabolism, so plasma levels will quickly fall. These characteristics make it a popular choice for IVRA. Ortho-toluidine, a breakdown product of prilocaine metabolism converts ferrous iron to ferric iron in hemoglobin, causing methemoglobinemia. Treatment of this condition requires high-concentration oxygen and intravenous methylene blue (1 mg/kg).

Prilocaine is contained in a eutectic mixture of local anesthetic (EMLA) cream. This oil/water emulsion contains 2.5% procaine and 2.5% lidocaine. Room temperature is cool enough to allow the EMLA to exist as a cream which then liquefies when it comes in contact with skin. EMLA easily penetrates the skin making it useful for pain reduction in pediatric patients. Application to broken or inflamed skin use should be avoided because of potentially greater absorption; large amounts of EMLA are reported to cause meth-hemaglobulinemeia.[18]

Articaine (Carticaine®)

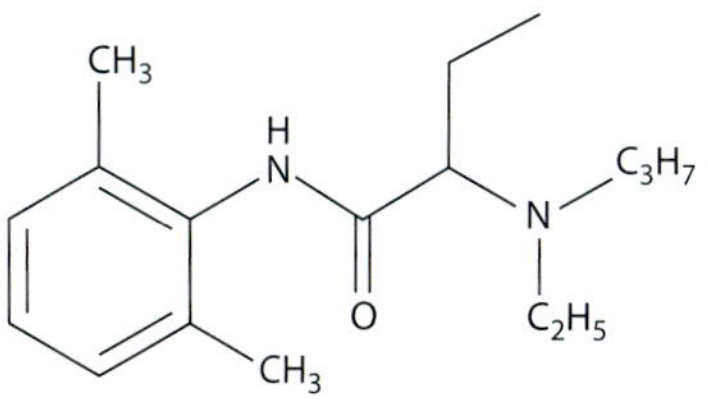

CH_3 H N C_3H_7 N O C_2H_5 CH_3

Articaine (4-methyl-3-[2-{propylamino} propionamidol]-2-thiophene-2-carboxylate), was synthesized by Rusching in 1969 and began clinical use in the early to mid-1970s. Unlike the other amide local anesthetics articaine has a thiophene ring which increases its lipid solubility to a value close to prilocaine. The primary use of articaine is in ophthalmology, and its quick metabolism allows for rapid return of ocular movement after surgery. Unlike other amide local anesthetics articaine contains an additional ester group so that metabolism occurs by nonspecific plasma cholinesterases as well as in the liver.

MECHANISM OF ACTION

Local anesthetics produce anesthesia by inhibiting excitation of nerve endings or by blocking conduction in peripheral nerves. Neuronal conduction is interrupted by inhibiting the influx of sodium ions through channels or ionophores within neuronal membranes. This is achieved by anesthetics reversibly binding to the D4-S6 part of the α-subunit of the voltage-gated sodium channel in the nerve membrane. The site of action is intracellular, requiring the local anesthetic to diffuse across the lipophilic lipoprotein membrane (**Fig. 86-4**).

Local anesthetic is administered in an acidic solution that maintains most of the drug in the ionized soluble form. Once injected, it must be converted into the neutral unionized form in order to enter the nerve cell. The proportion of drug that is converted will depend upon the local anesthetic pK_a and the pH of the tissue. Once inside the cell, the lower intracellular pH regenerates the ionized form, which blocks the sodium channel receptor. Sodium influx is reduced, resulting in decreased depolarization and an increased excitability threshold that prevents action potentials from forming, and impulse conduction stops.[19] Local anesthetic action can be augmented by blockade of potassium channels, calcium channels, and G-protein coupled receptors.[20] Local anesthetics have greater affinity when the sodium channel is open (activated or inactive) and lesser affinity when the channel is closed (deactivated and resting). Therefore, neural fibers with more rapid firing rates are more susceptible to local anesthetic action. In addition, smaller fibers are generally most susceptible because a given volume of local anesthetic can more readily block the requisite number of sodium channels to interrupt impulse transmission. Because of this the tiny rapid-firing autonomic fibers are most sensitive, followed by sensory fibers and finally somatic motor fibers. As the block proceeds, different sensory modalities are lost in the order of pain, temperature, touch, deep pressure, and motor function. During recovery from neuronal blockade the opposite is true, with the patient being able to void (autonomic control) returning last.

PHYSIOLOGIC ACTIVITY

Physiologic activity of local anesthetics is a function of their lipid solubility, affinity for protein binding, percent ionization at physiologic pH, and vasoactive properties.

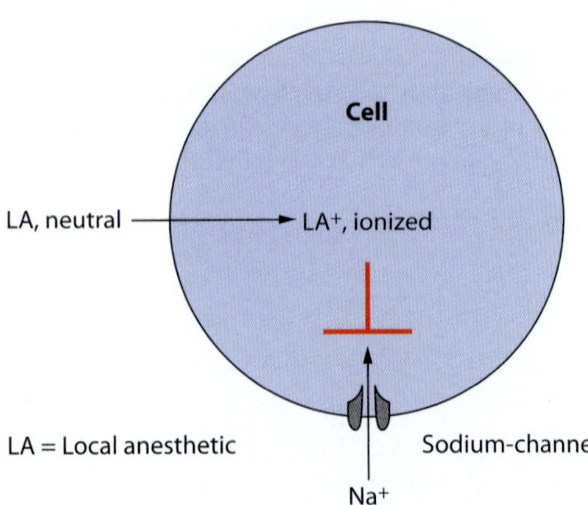

FIGURE 86-4. Intracellular action of local anesthetic after ionization.

LIPID SOLUBILITY

Lipid solubility is an important characteristic. Potency is directly related to lipid solubility, because 90% of the nerve cell membrane is composed of lipid. Lipid solubility is measured by a partition coefficient. The higher the partition coefficient is, the higher the lipid solubility, and the greater the local anesthetic potency will be. Local anesthetics vary in their potency, allowing for concentrations that typically range from 0.5% to 4%. Increased lipid solubility leads to faster nerve penetration and blockade of sodium channels. This property is determined by the aromatic ring and its substitutions, along with those added to the tertiary amine. For example, bupivacaine is more lipid-soluble and potent than articaine, allowing it to be formulated as a 0.5% concentration (5mg/mL) rather than a 4% concentration (40 mg/mL).

PROTEIN BINDING

Protein binding has been shown to correlate with the duration of action. Like most drugs, local anesthetics reversibly bind to plasma proteins circulating in the bloodstream. This property is expressed as the percentage of circulating drug that is protein bound and has been found to correlate with the anesthetic's affinity within sodium channels as well. The more firmly the local anesthetic binds to the protein of the sodium channel, the longer the duration of action. For example, bupivacaine exhibits 95% protein binding compared with 55% for mepivacaine. Local anesthetics bind to plasma (albumin, α1-acid glycoprotein) and tissue proteins. Albumin is considered high volume, low affinity, whereas α1-acid glycoprotein is high affinity but low volume. Factors that have an effect on duration of action include potency, dose administered, addition of vasoconstrictors, tissue vascularity, and rate of metabolism. Protein binding may vary, increasing in cases of trauma, major surgery, chronic inflammation, cancer and uremia.[21] Conversely, protein binding decreases during pregnancy, in newborns, and with the use of oral contraceptives.

IONIZATION

Local anesthetics exist in ionized and nonionized forms, the percentage of which varies with the pH of the environment. The pK_a is the pH at which ionized and unionized fractions of a substance are present in equal amounts. The ratio of ionized to neutral base varies and is calculated according to the Henderson-Hasselbalch equation:

$$\log \frac{\text{Cationic form}}{\text{Uncharged form}} = pK_a - = pH$$

- Mode of entrance of local anesthetic into cells
- The pK_a of most local anesthetics is 8.0–9.0, so in the body they exist as cations
- The cationic form is the most active form at the receptor site because it cannot exit from the closed channel
- Local anesthetics are less effective when injected into infected (acidic) tissue

The nonionized portion is the form that is capable of diffusing across nerve membranes and blocking sodium channels. Anesthetics with presence of greater nonionized portions have a faster onset of action. Local anesthetics differ in respect to the pH at which the ionized and nonionized forms are present at equilibrium, but this pH is generally in the range of 7.6–8.9. The more closely the equilibrium pH for a given anesthetic approximates the physiologic pH of tissues (7.35–7.45), the more rapid the onset of action.

A decrease in pH shifts equilibrium toward the ionized form, delaying onset of action. This explains why local anesthetics are slower in onset of action and less effective in the presence of inflammation, which creates a more acidic environment with lower pH. The addition of sodium bicarbonate is used clinically to increase the pH of local anesthetic solutions, thereby enhancing onset of action. Overzealous alkalinization, however, can cause local anesthetic molecules to precipitate from solution.

VASOACTIVITY

Local anesthetics, with the exception of cocaine, are vasodilators. In addition ropivacaine has a pronounced vasoconstrictor effect at low concentrations, which may reduce the requirement for adding vasoconstrictors.[22] Vasodilatation occurs via direct relaxation of peripheral arteriolar smooth muscle fibers. The greater the vasodilator activity of a local anesthetic is, the faster the absorption, and thus there is a shorter duration of action. To counteract this vasodilatation, epinephrine is often included in local anesthetic solutions. Isometric differences have also been noted, with L-bupivacaine having greater vasoconstrictor activity than R-bupivacaine.

ABSORPTION AND DISTRIBUTION

After intravenous administration, local anesthetics are distributed first to highly perfused organs, including brain, kidneys, and heart. Distribution then occurs in less perfused areas, including skin, skeletal muscle, and fat. Local anesthetic absorption into various organs is affected by lipid solubility, pK_a, protein binding, tissue-binding affinity, and clearance. Patient factors such as cardiac output, metabolic status, and site of local injection anesthetic need to be considered. The highest peak level can be seen following intercostal or caudal injection routes, followed by lumbar epidural, brachial plexus, sciatic, and femoral injections.[23] During this first pass through the lungs a significant amount of local anesthetic is temporarily extracted from the circulation. The lower pH of lung tissue relative to plasma may result in a degree of ion trapping. Consequently, the lungs may be able to attenuate toxic sequelae after accidental intravenous injection of local anesthetics.[24] The local anesthetic is then slowly released back into the circulation after lung absorption.

Local anesthetics may also diffuse across the placenta; however, ester local anesthetics are quickly hydrolyzed in the blood, so significant placental transfer does not occur. Amide local anesthetics vary considerably in their speed of placental transfer and the degree of protein binding. Increased protein binding in the mother decreases the amount of local anesthetic available to diffuse across the placenta. Conversely, the fetus has low levels of α_1-acid glycoprotein, allowing a reduced concentration of local anesthetic binding sites. Fetal pH is lower than maternal pH, resulting in ion trapping of local anesthetics with higher pK_a values. Local anesthetic distribution across the placenta can be measured by the ratio of local anesthetic in the umbilical vein versus maternal arterial blood. The transfer of local anesthetic into breast milk has been reported with lidocaine being detected in patients.[25]

CLEARANCE

Ester local anesthetics undergo rapid hydrolysis in the plasma by nonspecific esterase. The metabolites are inactive as local anesthetics, but a derivative such as para-aminobenzoic acid (PABA) is an allergen; therefore, the amino esters are more likely to cause a true allergic reaction.[26] The quick degradation affects the safety of these agents as plasma levels will fall quickly after injection. Patients who have atypical cholinesterase may be at higher risk for developing toxicity as a result of slow or absent plasma hydrolysis. Cocaine is the exception to plasma hydrolysis and is more slowly metabolized in the liver.

Amide local anesthetics are more stable in the blood compared with esters (lidocaine half-life = approximately 90 minutes vs. prilocaine = 6 minutes). Clearance occurs by both hepatic and renal metabolism. Biotransformation occurs in the liver via cytochrome p450 enzymes followed by renal excretion. Phase I involves hydroxylation, N-dealkylation, and methylation, followed by phase II, in which metabolites are conjugated with amino acids into inactive metabolites. The rate of metabolism is highly dependent on liver blood flow and differs among agents. The most rapidly metabolized are prilocaine and etidocaine, lidocaine and mepivacaine are intermediate, and ropivacaine and bupivacaine are the slowest. Prilocaine clearance is thought to occur via the liver as well as the lungs.

ADMINISTRATION OF LOCAL ANESTHETICS

For proper administration of local anesthetics, consider the individual characteristics of the patient, dose of local anesthetic to be administered, presence or absence of epinephrine, speed of administration, local tissue vascularity, and technique of administration.

In each case, physicians should strive to find the smallest dose possible administered over the longest period of time in order to achieve adequate anesthesia. Dosages are presented in **Table 86-1**.

To calculate the maximum dose, consideration should include the local anesthetic being used, patient weight, and history of heart disease. Dilution of the concentration of local anesthetic may aid in decreasing the total dose required to establish adequate anesthesia. Commercial preparations of local anesthetics are typically provided in bottles of 1% or 2% concentrations. These concentrations are higher than those required to produce the desired effect in most individuals.

Addition of epinephrine to the local anesthetic solution may improve safety and allow administration of lower doses of local anesthetic. Since local anesthetics are vasodilators, they tend to be absorbed into the bloodstream from the operative field because of vasodilatation of peripheral arterioles. Epinephrine induces vasoconstriction, delaying absorption of the local anesthetic for a longer duration of action at the site of injection. By delaying absorption, epinephrine also increases the safe dose of local anesthetic that may be administered.

Epinephrine has its own toxicities and should be used with caution in certain patients. Cardiac arrhythmias may be produced in patients with heart disease. Hypertension may develop in patients with a preexisting history of hypertension or with hyperthyroidism. In some cases, hypertension may be severe and actually trigger a hypertensive crisis. Epinephrine has been demonstrated to be detrimental to the survival of delayed or expanded flaps, since the new vessels present in these flaps appear to be exquisitely sensitive to the effects of epinephrine.

Bicarbonate is another drug that is commonly added to local anesthetic solutions, particularly when the patient is awake. Because the pH of local anesthetic solutions is generally 4–5, patients often experience burning on injection. Addition of 1 cc of a 1 mEq/mL solution of bicarbonate for every 9 cc of local anesthetic can alleviate burning and improve patient comfort.

Speed of administration is also important because toxicity develops as a result of peak serum concentration. When multiple areas are to be anesthetized with local anesthetic, inject each site sequentially rather than all at once at the beginning of the procedure

Tissue vascularity is another important consideration. Nasal mucosa, oral mucosa, the scalp, and the skin of the head and neck have a tremendous blood supply. This leads to rapid absorption of local anesthetics into the serum, which may precipitate an adverse reaction. When

TABLE 86-1 Clinical Characteristics of Local Anesthetics

Agent	Onset	Duration	Maximum Dose	Maximum Dose With Epinephrine
Bupivacaine	5-10 min	200 min + (>540 min with epinephrine)	2.5 mg/kg	3 mg/kg
Lidocaine	<2 min	30-60 min (longer with epinephrine)	3 mg/kg	5mg/kg
Articaine	2-3 min	180-360 min	7 mg/kg	7 mg/kg
Mepivacaine	3-5 min	45-90 min	5-6 mg/kg	5 mg/kg
Prilocaine	5 min	30-90 min	5 mg/kg	7 mg/kg
Ropivacaine	5-15 min	200 min +	3 mg/kg	3 mg/kg
Procaine	10-20 min	40 min	7 mg/kg	Not applicable

working in these areas, inject the area more slowly and wait longer between injections.

Technique of injection is important for safety reasons and for patient comfort. Always aspirate before injecting. This prevents inadvertent direct intravascular injection of the local anesthetic, which leads to an abrupt rise in serum levels and may precipitate an adverse reaction. Using the smallest needle possible decreases the pain of injection. Warming the local anesthetic solution and injecting slowly may decrease patient discomfort, since much of the discomfort is produced by rapid distention of tissues by the volume of the local anesthetic solution.

ADVERSE REACTIONS AND THEIR MANAGEMENT

Systemic toxicity attributed to local anesthetics is dose-dependent; however, an understanding of these doses is not always a simple matter. Circulating levels are determined by the rates of absorption, distribution, and metabolism, all of which vary considerably from agent to agent. The question of what systemic serum concentration follows the administration of a particular dose of local anesthetic was addressed by Scott in 1972.[27] The fact that serum concentrations were found to vary according to the relative vascularity of the tissues in which the local anesthetic was injected was not surprising. Additional variables addressed by Scott and his colleagues were that the dosage and speed of injection were directly related to serum concentration. A solution's concentration (2% vs. 4%) was not relevant; serum concentrations were related to the total dosage. For example, administering 20 mL of 2% or 10 mL of 4% (400 mg) produced the same serum concentration.

Contrary to popular thought, the age or weight of a patient does not predict systemic serum concentration following doses calculated as milligrams per age (years) or milligrams per kilogram. However, in managing pediatric patients, maximum dosages are expressed in mg/kg, and should be followed as a precaution. For adults this is less relevant, and one should follow guidelines showing the maximum allowable dose in milligrams, regardless of age or weight.

The distribution of local anesthetic after absorption into the bloodstream occurs in three phases. Initially, uptake occurs by highly vascular tissues such as the lungs and kidneys. Subsequently, the local anesthetic appears in less vascularized tissues such as muscle and fat. Finally, the drug is metabolized.

Metabolism of local anesthetics depends on the chemical structure. Amino esterases are degraded primarily by plasma pseudocholinesterases. Amino amides are cleared primarily by hepatic metabolism with renal excretion.

Adverse reactions may occur after administration of local anesthetics and usually result from administration of too much drug. As local anesthetics are absorbed from the injection site, their concentration in the bloodstream rises and the peripheral nervous system and CNS are depressed in a dose-dependent manner. Adverse reactions may also occur after injection of very vascular sites or from accidental direct intravascular injection of the drug. Deaths after local anesthetic administration are always a result of overdosage. Treatment with intravenous lipid emulsions (Intralipid) has been shown to reverse or attenuate the effects of local anesthetic toxicity.[28]

Tissue toxicity can be achieved by all local anesthetics if "high" concentrations are used. Adverse reactions occur primarily in the CNS (neurotoxicity) and cardiovascular system (myotoxicity) because these tissues are also composed of excitable membranes, the target of local anesthetic action.

In the CNS, a progression of signs and symptoms may be observed in the patient. The patient may report light-headedness, tinnitus, circumoral numbness, a metallic taste, or double vision. Upon examination, the patient may become drowsy and slur speech, and nystagmus may develop. At higher levels of anesthetics, the patient may become anxious and develop fine tremors of the muscles of the hands and/or face. Tremors may worsen and precipitate a grand mal seizure. Convulsive seizures are the initial life-threatening consequence of local anesthetic

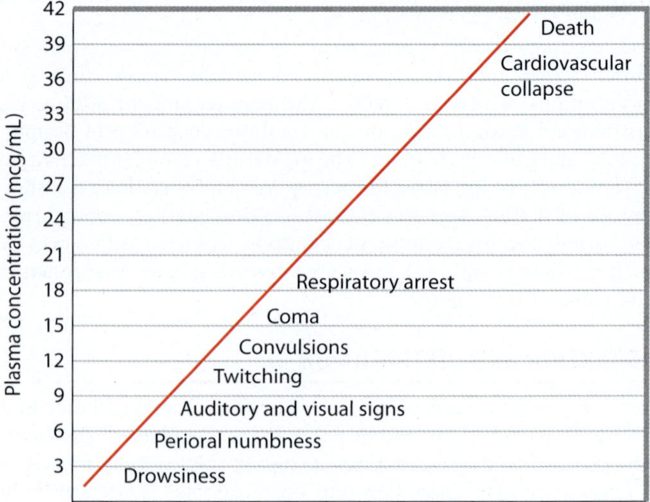

FIGURE 86-5. Serum concentrations and systemic effect of lidocaine.

overdose. This is presumed to be due to selective depression of central inhibitory tracts, which allow the excitatory tracts to remain uninhibited. As serum concentrations continue to rise further, all pathways are inhibited, resulting in CNS depression and coma, respiratory arrest, and finally cardiovascular collapse (**Fig. 86-5**).

It is essential that local anesthetics be respected as CNS depressants and that they can potentiate any respiratory depression associated with sedatives and opioids. In addition, serum concentrations required to produce seizures are lower if hypercarbia is present.

Although all local anesthetics carry comparable risk for CNS toxicity, it should be noted that bupivacaine exhibits greater potential for direct cardiac toxicity than other agents. This is thought to be related to the fact that bupivacaine has greater selectivity for the inactive and resting sodium channels and dissociates more slowly from these channels. This delays recovery from action potentials, rendering cardiac tissues susceptible to arrhythmias. Local anesthetics decrease the rate of depolarization of cardiac tissue, which is the rationale behind the use of lidocaine for the treatment of ventricular arrhythmias. At higher concentrations, amplitude of the cardiac action potential is decreased, and the velocity of conduction is reduced. At toxic doses, the negative inotropic effects of local anesthetics may lead to bradycardia, ventricular fibrillation, or asystole. Imminent toxicity may be seen on EKG with a prolonged PR interval and widened QRS complexes. Other cardiovascular effects include hypotension, which occurs via the direct vasodilating effects of local anesthetics on peripheral arteriolar smooth muscle.

Recognizing signs and symptoms of an adverse reaction to local anesthetics and administering emergency care in relation to the severity of the reaction are essential. With severe life-threatening reactions, immediately discontinue the procedure. Activate advanced cardiac life support (ACLS) protocols immediately, including intubation and defibrillation if indicated. Hypotension may require intravenous fluids and vasoconstrictor drugs for circulatory support. Control seizure activity with diazepam 5–10 mg IV. Succinylcholine may be required to stop ongoing tremors, but its use requires intubation and mechanical ventilation. Atropine or epinephrine may be indicated to treat bradycardia and hypotension.

Above all, seek help immediately. In a hospital setting, assistance is usually close by. In the office surgery setting, call 911 immediately. The physician must direct resuscitation until assistance arrives. This requires that any physician using local anesthetics in the office be familiar with ACLS protocols and have proper equipment on hand should an emergency situation arise. The American Society of Regional Anesthesia and Pain Medicine (ASRA), has a checklist for the treatment of local anesthetic systemic toxicity titled "The pharmacologic treatment of local anesthetic systemic toxicity (LAST)."

HYPERSENSITIVITY REACTIONS

Although very rare, hypersensitivity reactions may occur with use of local anesthetics. This is usually a reaction to the preservative used in the solution such as methylparaben or antioxidants (sulfites).[29] Allergic reactions are uncommon in the amino ester group and extremely rare in the amino amide group. Most reactions to local anesthetics are actually caused by anxiety, panic attacks, vasovagal responses, accidental intravascular injection, or the addition of epinephrine. True allergic reactions occur in less than 1% of all reactions to local anesthetics.

The cause of hypersensitivity reactions is believed to be a breakdown product created by the action of serum pseudocholinesterases on the amino ester PABA. PABA is very antigenic and is capable of sensitizing lymphocytes and eliciting formation of antibodies for a humoral immune response.

Hypersensitivity reactions were first categorized by Gell and Coombs as types I through IV, based on distinct immunologic mechanisms.[30] Type I reactions occur within minutes and are mediated by antibodies or immunoglobulin E (IgE) produced by B lymphocytes. This type of reaction is most common, manifested by a range of symptoms from local or systemic urticaria to anaphylactic shock. Type IV reactions are delayed for several days after provocation and are mediated by sensitized T lymphocytes. This type of reaction to local anesthetic rarely occurs.

Severe allergic manifestations include: hypotension, tachycardia, hives, angioedema, dyspnea, and bronchospasm with wheezing. These symptoms should be evaluated and treated immediately. Ceasing the surgery or procedure immediately at the onset of any signs or symptoms of a severe allergic reaction is important. Antihistamines and corticosteroids are first-line treatments, to be administered concomitantly with activation of ACLS protocols and the Emergency Medical Services (EMS) system.

If a patient has a reaction to a local anesthetic, assuming that he or she is also sensitive to other agents in the same class is the safest route. Most patients with a hypersensitivity reaction to an amino ester can probably be treated safely with an amino amide. However, many commercial amino amide preparations contain methylparaben as a preservative. Methylparaben is chemically similar to PABA and is capable of eliciting a hypersensitivity reaction. The extremely rare cases of hypersensitivity reactions to amino amides may be related to the methylparaben preservative rather than to the amino amide itself. Mepivacaine commercial preparations do not contain methylparaben and can usually be substituted safely in this situation.

If any question exists regarding a prior hypersensitivity reaction to local anesthetics, initially administer a test dose prior to proceeding with the intended therapeutic amount. Alternatively, referral to an allergist can help elucidate a suspected allergy to a local anesthetic.

REFERENCES

1. Koller C. Historical notes on the beginning of local anesthesia. *JAMA*. 1928;90:1742-1743.
2. Hall RJ. Hydrochlorate of cocaine. *N Y Med J*. 1884;40:643-644.
3. Wulf HFW. The centennial of spinal anesthesia. *Anesthesiology*. 1998;89(2):500-506.
4. Link WJ. Alfred Einhorn, SC D: Inventor of novocaine. *Dent Radiog Photog*. 1959;32:1-20.
5. Braun H. Ueber einige neue ortliche anaesthetica (Stovain, Alypin, Novocain). *Dtsch Med Wochenschr*. 1905;31:1667-1671.
6. Lofgren N, Lundquist B. Studies on local anesthetics: II. *Svenks Kem Tidskr*. 1946;58:206-217.
7. Ekenstam B, Egner B, Petterson G. Local anaesthetics: I. N-alkyl pyrrolidine and N-alkyl piperidine carboxylic acid amides. *Acta Chem Scand*. 1957;11:1183-1190.
8. Lofgren N, Tegner C. Studies on local anesthetics: XX. Synthesis of some alpha-monoalklyamino-2-methylpropionanilides: a new useful local anesthetic. *Acta Chem Scand*. 1960;14:486-490.
9. Adams HJ, Kronberg GH, Takman BH. Local anesthetic activity and acute toxicity of (+) 2-(N-Ethylpropylamino)-2',6'-butyroxylidide, a new long-acting agent. *J Pharm Sci*. 1972;61:1829-1831.
10. Winther JE, Nathalang B. Effectivity of a new local analgesic Hoe 40 045. *Scand J Dent Res*. 1972;80:272-278.
11. Loza-Balsa G. Monografia sobre la coca. La Paz, Bolivia, Edita Sociedad Geografica de la Paz, 1992:ix:x, xiv, xv, 3.
12. Hiller A, Karjalainen K, Rosenberg P. Transient neurological symptoms after spinal anesthesia with hyperbaric 5% lidocaine or general anesthesia. *Br J Anaesth*. 1999;82:575-579.
13. Kanai Y, Katsuki H, Takaski M. Lidocaine disrupts axonal membrane of rat sciatic nerve in vitro. *Anesth Analg*. 2000;91:944-948.
14. Murai K, Tyler RS, Harker LA, et al. Review of pharmacologic treatment of tinnitus. *Am J Otol*. Sep 1992;13(5):454-464.
15. Albright G. Cardiac arrest following regional anesthesia with etidocaine or bupivicaine. *Anesthesiology*. 1979;51:285-287.
16. McClure J. Ropivicaine. *Br J Anaesth*. 1996;76:300-307.
17. Feldman HS, Arthur GR, Pitkanen M, et al. Treatment of acute systemic toxicity after rapid intravenous injection of ropivicaine and bupivicaine in the conscious dog. *Anesth Analg*. 1991;73: 373-384.
18. Hahn I, Hoffman R, Nelson L. EMLA-induced methemaglobinanemia and systemic topical anesthesia toxicity. *J Emerg Med*. 2004;26:85-88.
19. Heavner JE. Local anesthetics. *Curr Opin Anaesthesiol*. Aug 2007;20(4):336-342.
20. Olschewski A, Hemplemann G, Vogel W. Blockade of Na+ currents by local anesthetic in the dorsal horn neurons of the spinal cord. *Anesthesiology*. 1998;88:172-179.
21. Tucker G. Local anestheticdrugs: mode of action and pharmacokinetics. In: Nimmo W, Rowbotham D, Smith G, eds. *Anaesthesia*. Oxford, England:Blackwell Scientific;1994:1371.
22. Dahl JB, Sinonsen L, Mogensen T, et al. The effect of 0.5% ropivacaine on epidural blood flow. *Acta Anaesthesiol Scand*. 1990;34:308-310.
23. Tucker GT, Moore DC, Brindenbaugh PO, Brindenbaugh LD, Thompson GE. Systemic absorption of mepivacaine in commonly used regional block procedures. *Anesthesiology*. 1972;37:277-287.
24. Kietzmann D, Foth H, Geng WP, Rathgeber J, et al. Transpulmonary disposition of prilocaine, mepivacaine, and bupivacaine in humans in the course of epidural anesthesia. *Acta Anaethesiol Scand*. 1995;39:885-890.
25. Zeisler J, Gaarder T, De Mesquita S. Lidocaine excretion in breast milk. *Drug Intell Clin Pharm*. 1986;20:691-693.
26. Tezlaff JE. The pharmacology of local anesthetics. *Anesthesiol Clin North Am*. Jun 2000;18(2):217-233.
27. Scott DB, Jebson PJR, Braid DP, et al. Factors affecting plasma levels of lignocaine and prilocaine. *Brit J Anaesth*. 1972;44:1040-1049.
28. Picard J, Ward SC, Zumpe R, Meek T, et al. Guidelines and the adoption of "lipid rescue" therapy for local anesthetic toxicity. *Anaesthesia*. Feb 2009;64(2):122-125.
29. Schatz M. Adverse reactions to local anesthetics. *Immunol Allergy Clin North Am*. 1992;12:585-609.
30. Gell PGH, Coombs RRA. Classification of allergic reactions responsible for clinical hypersensitivity and disease. In: Gell PGH, Coombs RRA, Hachmann PJ, eds. *Clinical Aspects of Immunology*. 3rd ed. Oxford, England: Blackwell Scientific; 1975.

CHAPTER 87

Use of Botulinum Toxins in Pain Syndromes

Atif B. Malik
Soorena Khojasteh
Zahid H. Bajwa

Botulinum toxins (BTX) are potent neurotoxins produced by the bacterial spores of *Clostridium botulinum.* The major effect of BTX is at the neuromuscular junction, where they block the release of acetylcholine, preventing muscle contraction and causing dose-dependent weakness (rather than titanic weakness caused by tetanus toxin, a related clostridial protein). This blockade results in a temporary loss or reduction in activity in the target organ (muscle, sweat gland, and sphincter) with minimal risk of systemic adverse effects. However, BTX work not only work at the neuromuscular junction but also alter the sensory input, producing secondary changes at the central level. Clinical use of BTX depends on the multiple direct and indirect effects that the toxin exerts in the peripheral nervous system and the central nervous system (CNS).

HISTORICAL BACKGROUND AND EARLY CLINICAL DEVELOPMENT

C. botulinum was identified as a causative agent in food poisoning by Van Ermengem after a fatal outbreak in 1895.[1] In the 1920s, additional outbreaks led to the isolation of a relatively crude form of BTX,[2] the neurotoxin responsible for botulism.

Development of BTX began during World War II in the study of the nature of certain toxins, including BTX, and ways of protecting against them.[3] Although much of the early work focused on BTX-A, also studied were BTX types B, C, D, and E. The purpose was to develop a polyvalent toxoid for immunization purposes. After the war, a crystallized form of BTX-A became available and stimulated considerable scientific interest. Alan B. Scott, of the Smith-Kettlewell Eye Research Foundation, initiated efforts to study BTX in a monkey model of strabismus in the late 1960s.[4] Sufficient data were collected by 1978 to file an investigational new drug (IND) application for human clinical studies.[5] The passage of the Orphan Drug Act of 1983 and FDA approval aided clinical development of BTX-A as an orphan drug in December 1989.

In 1989, the U.S. Food and Drug Administration (FDA) approved BTX-A (Botox) for the treatment of strabismus, blepharospasm, and hemifacial spasm. In 2000-2001, both BTX-A and BTX-B (Myobloc) were FDA-approved for treatment of cervical dystonia, and in 2002, Botox was approved by the FDA for treatment of glabellar frown lines. In addition to the FDA-approved indications in the United States, BTX-A has been used for treatment of a number of painful conditions, including achalasia, anismus, benign prostatic hypertrophy, dysphonia, other dystonias, tremor, hyperhidrosis, kyphoscoliosis, low back pain, migraine and tension-type headache, myofascial pain syndrome (MPS), pancreatitis, pelvic floor pain, anal fissures, sialorrhea, spasticity, temporomandibular joint disorder, sphincter dysfunction, wrinkles, and other movement disorders.

PHARMACOLOGY OF BTX

There are several BTX preparations available in the US: Botox (BTX-A, Allergan, Inc.) and Myobloc. Botox is currently FDA-approved for the treatment of overactive bladder, detrusor overactivity associated with a neurologic condition (e.g., spinal cord injury [SCI], multiple sclerosis [MS]), chronic migraine, upper limb spasticity, blepharospasm, strabismus, hemifacial spasm, cervical dystonia, primary axillary hyperhidrosis, and glabellar frown lines in patients older than 12 years of age. BTX-B was FDA-approved in December 2000 for the treatment of cervical dystonia and is presently in clinical trials for other conditions. Dysport (Botulinum toxin type A, Ipsen Ltd, Berkshire, UK) is available only in Europe.

MECHANISM OF ACTION, AND PHARMACOLOGY OF BTX

Although there are many reviews of BTX in the recent literature,[6,7] optimal clinical use of BTX as a therapeutic agent depends on a clear understanding of its mechanism of action, as well as dosing, chemistry, techniques of administration, and side effects.

As the clinical uses of BTX expand, it is important to understand the basic properties of the various serotypes (A, B, C_1, D, E, F, and G) of BTX with sequence homology amounting to approximately 50% across the serotypes. The subtypes are most similar in regard to their larger structural features and certain functional sites and more diverse regarding the finer details of function as well as antigenic cross-reactivity.[8] Lyophilized BTX-A supplied as a pharmaceutical agent is a bipartite protein that is synthesized in bacterial culture as a single long-chain protein and subsequently nicked by bacterial proteases to form the free toxin. The free toxin consists of one heavy chain (H-chain; 100 kDA) and one light chain (L-chain; 50 kDA) bound together by at least one disulfide bond and additional noncovalent forces (**Fig. 87-1**). When secreted into culture medium by *C. botulinum,* BTX is complexed with two other proteins, a nontoxin nonhemagglutinin protein (150 kDA) and a hemagglutinating protein (600 kDA); the additional proteins enhance the stability of BTX complex.[9] Most relevant to clinical use is BTX-A, which appears to be the most potent of the subtypes and, when injected clinically, has the longest duration of action.[10–14] Although BTX-B and BTX-F have seen limited clinical use, and others are the subject of further study, many differences observed thus far suggest that the subtypes are not interchangeable.[15–18] For this reason and because much of the preclinical and clinical literature employs BTX, this chapter presents results obtained primarily from BTX-A.

MECHANISMS OF ACTION

Pharmacologic effect of BTX-A occurs in three stages, with control of each stage assigned to one of three functional units existing on either the H-chain or the L-chain of the toxin. Each chain performs the functions associated with it in applicable model systems even when separated from the other; however, the component chains do not block neurotransmission when applied separately.[19]

The binding of BTX-A to the motor end plate presynaptic membrane is a two-stage process, with concentration of the toxin occurring through a relatively nonspecific affinity for ganglioside-containing, lipid-rich presynaptic membrane, followed by specific binding to a protein-containing receptor.[20–22] Binding is irreversible but not itself toxic to the neuron[23] (**Fig. 87-2**).

Internalization of the bound toxin occurs by receptor-mediated endocytosis.[24] Once formed, the contents of the endosome become increasingly acidic, most likely by normal cellular mechanisms. The decrease in pH within the endosome prompts a configurational change in the toxin, which then forms a channel through the membrane. The channel allows all or part of the toxin to enter the cytosol.[25–27]

Once in the cytosol, the L-chain of BTX effects a long-lasting inhibition of acetylcholine (ACh) release, which current evidence suggests is

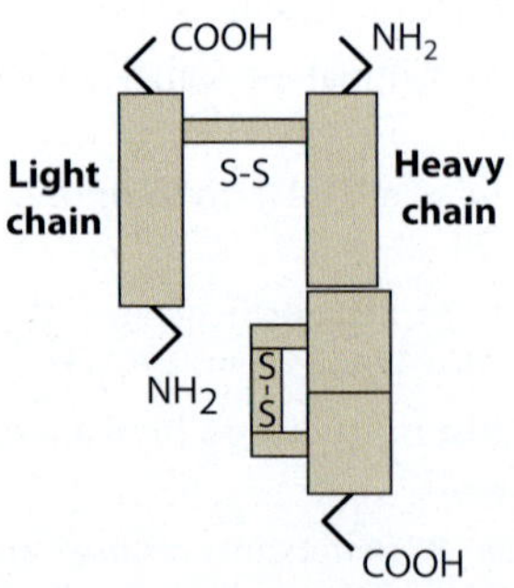

FIGURE 87-1. Diagram of botulinum toxin A free toxin. (© Allergan Inc. with permission.)

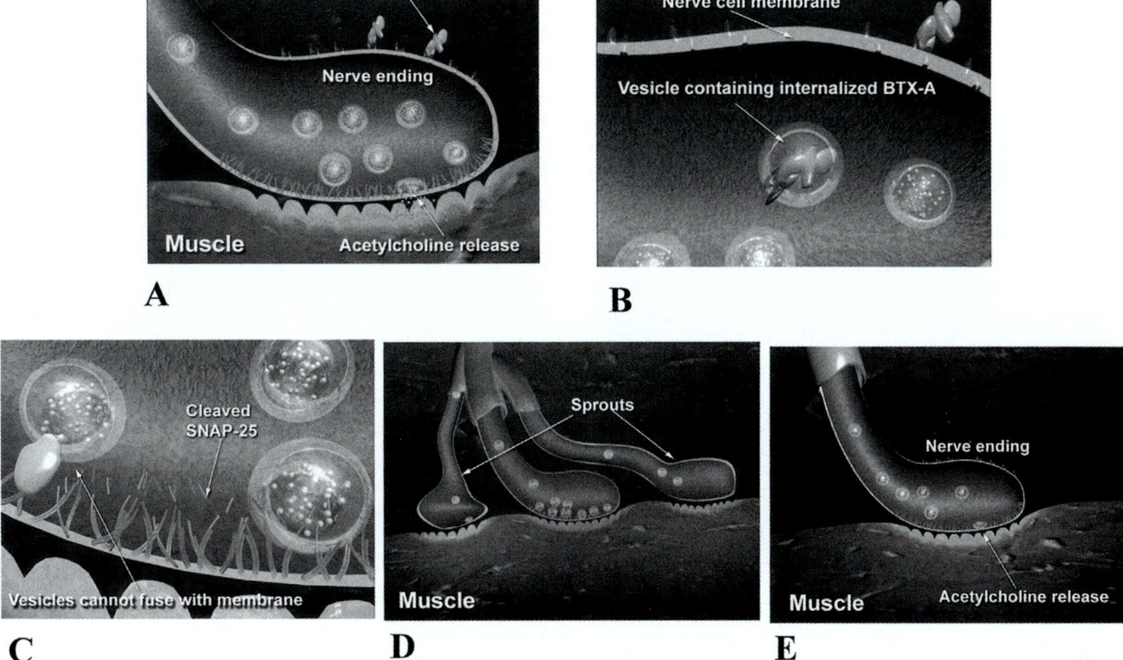

FIGURE 87-2. Representation of the sequential events that lead to the blockade of the neurotransmitter release of the neurotoxin. (**A**) The neurotoxin binds to the receptor (*arrow* on the presynaptic membrane) via the heavy chain. (**B**) Internalization of the neurotoxin, which is now in the endosome. Acidification occurs at this stage, which allows the formation of channels that allows the light chain to egress from the vesicle. (**C**) The light chain cleavages SNAP-25 (synaptosomal-associated protein, 25 kDA) by enzymatic action and does not allow the vesicle to fuse with the membrane; thus, the acetylcholine is prevented from release. (**D**) New sprouts of the nerve endings create new neuromuscular junction in response to the botulinum toxin action. (**E**) After return of function at the neuromuscular junction the sprouts recede and the new nerve ending is created. (© Allergan Inc. with permission.)

accomplished by the cleavage of the SNAP-25 (synaptosomal-associated protein, 25 kDA) proteins necessary for the release of ACh by synaptosomes.[8] Although all toxin subtypes evidence a high degree of sequence homology associated with a functioning zinc-endopeptidase on the L-chain, and proteolytic activity can be found in all BTX subtypes except C_2, each toxin subtype has a characteristic specificity for cleaving a certain spectrum of proteins involved in synaptosomal function.[8]

PHARMACOLOGY

When injected intramuscularly at therapeutic doses, BTX-A induces a localized chemical denervation. With appropriate dose and proper localization of the target muscle, the injected muscle is only partially denervated, and therefore involuntary contracture diminishes without complete paralysis. Depending upon the underlying condition, dose, and site of injection, onset of effect of BTX varies from a few days to 2 weeks. This corresponds roughly to the time it takes for the toxin to reach the cytosol of the targeted synapses and begin its enzymatically mediated cholinergic blockade. Functional denervation is observable from 6 weeks to 6 months after injection but typically lasts 3 to 4 months. During peak effect, muscle histology shows evidence of atrophy and increased variation of fiber size after BTX administration. Recovery of functional innervation is associated with histologic evidence of neuronal sprouting, reinnervation, and enlargement of some end plates, as well as the formation of new smaller end plates.[10,28,29] There is an increase in the number of muscle fibers innervated per axon, with some fibers being innervated by more than one axon.[10] Recovery is complete after allowing sufficient time for regrowth.[30,31] Fiber size and presumably neuromuscular function return to normal even after multiple cycles of injection and recovery.[32] Botulinum toxin therapy is reported to alleviate pain associated with various conditions with or without accompanying muscle contractions. An extensive review of the literature also indicates that BTX-A is effective in reducing pain caused by trigger points, myofascial pain, back pain, and headaches. The degree of response to BTX-A therapy in chronic pain has been variable and warrants further controlled investigations. The potential mechanism of action of BTX in pain relief is discussed in the following paragraph.

Botulinum toxin (types A, B, C_1, and F) have an inhibitory effect on the in vitro neuropeptide release from rat embryonic dorsal root ganglia neurons and from isolated rabbit iris sphincter and dilatory muscles.[33–35] In addition, BTX-A was reported to inhibit in vitro release of acetylcholine and substance P (but not norepinephrine) in rabbit ocular tissue.[35] Based on these in vitro and limited in vivo observations, it is hypothesized that BTX treatment reduces the local release of nociceptive peptides either from cholinergic neurons or from C- or Ad fibers in vivo. This reduction in neuropeptide release would prevent local sensitization of nociceptors and reduce the local perception of pain. A reduction of nociceptive signals from the periphery could result in reduced central sensitization associated with chronic pain. Preclinical investigation on the local antinociceptive effects of BTX-A was reported by Cui at the Society of Neuroscience annual meeting in 2000, and a follow-up report was submitted more recently by Aoki at the American Academy of Neurology annual meeting in 2003.[36] To investigate the mechanism of the antinociceptive effect of subcutaneous BTX-A (Allergan, Inc.), its effect on formalin-induced local glutamate release, electrophysiological activities of dorsal horn neurons, and the spinal expression of c-fos, an indicator of activation of neurons, were assessed in the rat model for inflammatory pain (formalin model). Formalin (5%, 50 μL subcutaneous) OK produces prolonged distinct biphasic excitations (spikes) of dorsal horn neurons, which correspond to early (acute nociceptive) and late (tonic nociceptive) phases of the behavioral formalin pain response. Pretreatment of rats with BTX-A (1 day, sc) significantly inhibited the formalin-induced electrophysiological activities in the late phase but not in the early phase. BTX-A, also dose-dependent, inhibited formalin-induced glutamate release in the paw and the expression of c-fos in the dorsal horn of the spinal cord. These results demonstrate that the inhibition of neurotransmitter release from primary sensory neurons by subcutaneous BTX-A mediates at least some of its antinociceptive effect. Local administration of BTX-A directly inhibits the peripheral sensitization produced by local neurotransmitter release, which then results in an indirect reduction in central sensitization. Inhibition of nociceptive processing at the peripheral site and at the spinal cord level may underlie the mechanism of BTX-A effect in alleviation of certain chronic pain conditions. In conclusion, the preclinical (in vitro and in vivo) data, coupled with clinical observations, strongly support the theory that botulinum toxin (especially BTX-A) may have antinociceptive properties distinct from its well-documented effects on the neuromuscular junction and other cholinergic nerves.

BTX-B (Myobloc) is produced by fermentation of *C. botulinum* type B (Bean strain) as a noncovalently associated neurotoxin complex with hemagglutinin and nonhemagglutinin proteins. After the fermentation process, the neurotoxin complex is purified through a series of precipitation and chromatography steps. Myobloc is marketed as a clear to light yellow solution in 3.5-mL glass vials with 5000 units BTX-B per mL in 0.05% human serum albumin, 0.01 M sodium succinate, and 0.1 M sodium chloride at a pH of about 5.6. Although biological activity is maintained at room temperature for 6 months, recommended storage guidelines are for refrigeration at temperatures of 2°C to 8°C, with stability maintained for 2 years. For Myobloc, one unit corresponds to the calculated median lethal intraperitoneal dose for female Swiss Webster mice weighing 18 to 20 g. The specific activity of Myobloc ranges between 70 and 130 U/ng. However, units of biological activity of BTX-B cannot be compared to or converted into units of another BTX. Extrapolation from animal data should not be done because of differences in species sensitivity to BTX neurotoxin serotypes. Until adequate studies are done, extrapolation from human cervical dystonia dosing data to other conditions in which BTX might be used in an off-label manner is not prudent.

The most commonly reported adverse events associated with BTX-B in clinical trials were dry mouth, dysphagia, dyspepsia, and injection site pain, with dry mouth and dysphagia the most common reasons for discontinuation. Doses up to 25,000 units were studied, but most patients received 12,500 units or less. Dysphagia increased with increasing doses injected into the sternocleidomastoid muscle. Dry mouth showed some dose-related increases with injections into the splenius capitis, trapezius, and sternocleidomastoid muscles. Additionally, dry mouth appeared to be much less of a problem with repeat dosing, even when higher doses were used.

ANTIBODY FORMATION

Tsui reported on the incidence of antibody formation in 32 patients with spasmodic torticollis who received repeated injections of BTX-A.[46] Four patients (12.5%) produced antibodies after 2 to 9 months of treatment. Because the dose range used in blepharospasm is much less than that used in cervical dystonia/spasmodic torticollis, the incidence of antibody formation is far less. Based on data from a number of studies, the incidence of antibody formation with BTX-A for the treatment of cervical dystonia is probably less than 5%.[37] The current BTX-A (Botox) formulation is "cleaner" (5 ng vs. 25 ng protein) than the older formulation used in much of the published data discussing antibody formation. As a result of its lower neurotoxin complex load, current BTX-A exposes cervical dystonia patients to approximately 12 ng of protein per treatment (or 48 ng of protein per year based on treatment every 3 months) based on a mean effective dose of 236 units. Hatheway and Dang reported that an annual exposure 125 ng or less of BTX-A would result in higher than 5% of patient population with neutralizing antibodies.[38] Based on current data, general guidelines of keeping the dose as low as is necessary (300-600 U for BTX-A) and injecting no more frequently than every 3 months remain. The BTX-B product from Elan Pharmaceuticals contains 50 ng of neurotoxin complex per 5000 units. As a result, BTX-B exposes cervical dystonia patients to approximately 100 ng of protein per treatment cycle based on the most effective dose of 10,000 units published in two double-blind studies.[39,40] According to the BTX-B product insert (Myobloc, US Product Insert, Elan), at 10,000 units, 18% of patients treated for 18 months developed neutralizing antibodies. There were no data regarding efficacy of this neutralizing activity. The reasons for such rapid development of neutralizing antibodies remain unclear and may be a result of previous exposure of the patients to BTX-A or the high content of protein in this product. Factors that may influence the risk of BTX antibody formation include the overall exposure to neurotoxin complex protein, protein load per effective dose of the toxin, and, most important, the frequency of exposure.

Because BTX-A and BTX-B display quite different chemical compositions, it has long been felt that the antibody cross-reactivity between the two is extremely small.[41] Nonetheless, concern has been expressed over the potential problem of neutralizing antibody formation with lower potency and shorter-acting BTX serotypes.[42] Preliminary data based on the amino acid sequences of botulinum neurotoxin serotypes and tetanus toxin, which provide the molecular basis for cross-reactivity, indicate that there is a molecular basis for cross-reactivity between the proteins. However, the exact clinical significance of these findings has yet to be determined.[43] Although BTX-A and BTX-F have similar potency, increasing doses of BTX-F to increase duration of response to that seen with BTX-A may increase antibody formation to BTX-F. This was demonstrated in a study by Chen et al, who reported that 4 of 18 (22%) cervical dystonia patients treated with BTX-F became nonresponsive to BTX-F after 12 to 66 months of treatment.[44]

PAIN ABATEMENT IN CLINICAL STUDIES WITH BOTULINUM TOXIN TYPE A

Botulinum toxin therapy is reported to alleviate pain associated with various conditions with or without accompanying muscle contractions. Early reports in cervical dystonia patients treated with BTX-A suggested that the pain relief was much greater than the benefits gained by decreasing excess muscle contraction.[28,39,45,46] Pain associated with myoclonus of spinal cord origin was also treated successfully with BTX-A.[47] Furthermore, pain from tension-type headaches was reported to improve after BTX-A therapy.[48-52] Intramuscular BTX-A administered prior to adductor release surgery in children with cerebral palsy resulted in significant antinociceptive effects. The children treated with BTX-A reported a reduced need for narcotics, were discharged earlier, and had better outcomes than the placebo group. The results of this trial were so dramatic that the trial was terminated earlier than scheduled.[53] An extensive review of the literature also indicates that BTX-A is effective in reduction of pain caused by trigger points, myofascial pain, back pain, and headaches. The degree of response to BTX-A therapy in chronic pain has been variable and therefore warrants further controlled investigations.

This section organizes the burgeoning number of clinical studies of BTX into a few medically useful categories into which the same or similarly classified patients have been grouped for treatment. It is thereby hoped to make evident the essential features of BTX use in a particular subcategory and also to identify principles of practice that may guide the use of BTX for neuromuscular pain. The first general principle for the rational use of BTX in pain management is a precondition: The patient must be experiencing chronic pain of a known or highly probable etiology for which there is no curative treatment and for which other conservative and noninvasive pain relief strategies have been considered and exhausted.

Pain related to involuntary or excessive muscle contraction can be produced by a wide range of clinical conditions, some of which are associated with movement disorders, and others in which pain, spasm, and cramping are the only symptoms present. Case studies describing the use of BTX-A in musculoskeletal pain can be placed into two categories based on 1) the predominance of a movement disorder, primarily the focal dystonias, and 2) the predominance of spasticity, primarily of CNS origin. Myofascial pain syndrome (MPS) is considered in a distinct category.

FOCAL DYSTONIAS WITH PAIN

Dystonia, generalized or focal, is a condition of increased muscular tone that leads to abnormal fixed postures or shifting postures resulting from irregular, forceful twisting movements of the trunk and extremities.

The mobile spasms of generalized dystonia are similar to those of athetosis but are usually slower and involve the larger muscle groups of the trunk, extremities, and neck. Dystonic movements increase during volitional motor activity, nervousness, and emotional stress and diminish during relaxation and sleep.[53]

Focal dystonias are more common than generalized dystonias and include disorders such as cervical dystonia, writer's cramp (occupational dystonia), blepharospasm, and spastic dysphonia. In the focal dystonias, a single area of the body is affected. Focal dystonias occur more frequently in adults than in children, remain stable over time, and rarely spread to involve other body parts.[54]

Both generalized and focal dystonias may be associated with pain resulting from the extremes of posture, excessive tendon and joint tension, or muscle contraction. The focal dystonias are more readily treated with BTX than are the generalized dystonias because of the greater number of muscles involved and consequent larger doses required in the treatment of the latter; larger doses may cause systemic toxicity and possibly lead to development of resistance. Nevertheless, if pain can be localized to one or two muscle groups, BTX may prove beneficial even in the generalized dystonias. The focal dystonias for which there is an extensive literature detailing treatment with BTX and for which pain represents an important element of response include cervical dystonia (spasmodic torticollis) and occupational dystonia (writer's cramp).

Cervical Dystonia Cervical dystonia is the most common focal dystonia. There are intermittent or continuous spasms of the sternocleidomastoid, trapezius, and other cervical muscles, usually more prominent on one side than on the other. Approximately 70% of patients with cervical dystonia report pain as the main complaint. Controlled clinical trials in cervical dystonia suggest a dramatic effect of BTX injections in controlling the pain component of this syndrome; not surprisingly, objective improvements in movement were similarly improved. Supporting these findings is a survey of 19 studies in which BTX was used for the treatment of cervical dystonia.[55] The mean weighted percent of patients reporting an improvement in pain was 76% (range: 50% to 100% for the 16 studies reporting pain results; N = 938 patients). Per-muscle doses of BTX ranged from 40 to 120 mU (Botox), and per-treatment doses ranged between 100 and 374 mU (Botox).

Writer's cramp, now considered a focal dystonia, is the most common form of occupational dystonia.[56] Similar disorders have been described in musicians and others whose daily work involves frequent repetitive movements of the hands.[57,58] In one large survey, the incidence of writer's cramp accounted for 25% of all focal dystonias, with an incidence of 2.7 per million population.

Writer's cramp typically begins with a feeling of clumsiness during writing or other fine motor activity, and there is a loss of speed and fluency of movement. The grip may be too tight, causing the hand to become quickly fatigued. Tightness and aching can extend to the forearm or shoulder, and abnormal muscle contraction may lead to a distortion of normal posture. In some cases, the wrist flexes or extends and the fingers curl into the palm or pull away, so that there cannot be a proper grasp, as in cervical dystonia, but it is significant in some patients. Spontaneous remission is rare and probably occurs in fewer than 5% of patients. Writer's cramp responds poorly to conventional drug, physical, and behavioral therapy.[59] Of the many pharmacotherapies tried in this focal dystonia, the most effective appear to be systemic anticholinergics. Unfortunately, these medications rarely work and must frequently be used at such high doses that the side effects become intolerable. In contrast, numerous studies of BTX in the occupational dystonias have shown that it proved effective in relieving hyperactive muscle contracture and provided pain relief when pain was associated with this condition.

In an early study of dystonia of diverse forms, one patient with writer's cramp showed modest motor improvement along with significant pain relief after injection with BTX.[60] A subsequent larger study showed improvement in 16 of 19 patients (84%).[61] The results of three open-label trials indicate that 83% to 92% of patients with focal hand dystonia derive at least subjective benefit of BTX therapy; the third trial showed pain abatement in all 12 subjects who reported pain as a feature of their condition.[61–65] When patients have been observed long enough, some have continued to respond to BTX for as long as 6 years.[66]

Three published double-blind trials in writer's cramp have shown some degree of response as well; however, pain was not assessed in these studies. In one such study of 17 patients, subjective improvement was noted after 53% of the BTX injections, compared to only one patient (7%) after placebo injection.[66] Subjective improvement lasted for 1 to 4 months in 82% of the patients after a single dose of toxin; however, objective assessments based on videotapes of patient performance failed to demonstrate a significant difference between toxin and placebo. A second double-blind study with a crossover design treated 20 patients with writer's cramp with either BTX or placebo, administered in random order. Patients were assessed subjectively and by three objective tests of pen control and writing. Of these 20 patients, 6 had subjective improvement in writing, 7 had improved writing speed, 4 had improved writing by "blinded" rating, and 12 had better pen control on quantitative testing.[67] A third study in 10 patients employed a similar double-blind, crossover design, and 80% of patients showed both a subjective and objective response.[68]

Considering that pain is relatively infrequently mentioned in studies of writer's cramp, it is interesting to note that most attempts at the efficacy of BTX in this form of dystonia showed better response with subjective responses than with objective ones, even in the double-blind studies. Nevertheless, BTX-A appears to be the best treatment available at present for writer's cramp and especially for patients who also experience pain.

SPASTIC DISEASE STATES WITH PAIN

Two subgroups of pain patients are those in whom there is a known cause of spasticity tracing its origin to the peripheral nervous system or to the CNS. Peripheral nervous system lesions may cause MPS. CNS dysfunction may cause the sometimes painful spasticity in patients with cerebral palsy, multiple sclerosis, stroke, and traumatic brain injury.

Upper Motor Neuron Disease Syndromes and Pain Patients experiencing acute or long-standing insults and degenerative processes of the CNS display a wide variety of signs that constitute the upper motor neuron syndrome. Spasticity, a velocity-dependent increase in muscle tone characterized by hyperactive stretch reflexes, is one sign. Additional positive and negative signs characterize the syndrome. Positive signs include hyperactive tendon reflexes, increased resistance to passive movement, flexed posture in the arm and extension in the leg, excessive contraction of antagonistic muscles, and stereotypic movement synergies; negative signs include weakness, lack of dexterity, and paresis.[68]

Until recently, spasticity was viewed as a consequence of overactive muscle spindles or fusimotor fibers, resulting from disruption of descending inhibitory tracts, the corticospinal and corticobulbar tracts, and sensory afferents.[69] Dimitrijevic et al suggest that this view is no longer entirely accurate.[70] Spastic paresis or spastic dystonia is better understood as an imbalance of inhibition and excitation occurring at the motor neuron level of the spinal cord, not unlike focal hypertonia with dystonic features.[71,72] The fundamental component of this sequence is the abnormal intraspinal response to sensory input. Modulation of local spinal cord activity occurs via the descending pathways, such as the rubrospinal tract.[73,74] Positive signs such as hyperreflexia are generally caused by the disinhibition of local cord excitatory circuits. Negative signs, such as paresis and loss of dexterity, reflect dysfunction of corticospinal pathways. The positive signs of spasticity interfere with the activities of daily living, can cause fractures or contractures, can increase the frequency of pressure sores, and are often associated with pain.[75] Although they can interfere with rehabilitation, positive signs are more amenable to clinical intervention than negative signs.

Spasticity as described above is a prominent clinical feature of several important afflictions of the CNS, including stroke, cerebral palsy, multiple sclerosis, Parkinson disease, and traumatic brain injury. For chronic or degenerative states, the management of spasticity is an ongoing task which is best begun with conservative measures and accelerated as needed.[76–79] Initially, physical therapeutic modalities should be tried, such as avoidance of noxious stimuli, passive movement exercises, thermal agents, vibratory treatment, and serial inhibitive casting.[79] Oral medications can be tried in conjunction with physical measures or alone; however, neither neural depressants (e.g., oral or intrathecal baclofen, benzodiazepines, clonidine, tizanidine) nor muscle relaxants (e.g., dantrolene) have proved satisfactory because of limited efficacy and intolerable side effects.[80–82] For the more seriously affected or unresponsive patient, invasive procedures such as phenol and alcohol nerve blocks cord stimulation, rhizotomies, and intrathecal baclofen administration have been tried.[75,83–88]

The cost of prolonged care and lack of benefit from conservative management have resulted in the recommendation that BTX be attempted in the management of spasticity. BTX can be used therapeutically to produce a reversible, partial chemical denervation when injected directly into a contracted muscle. Because of its potentially pronounced paralytic action, BTX can be as effective as surgeries used currently for the management of spasticity; moreover, it has the advantage of being reversible and generally repeatable as needed in accord with the fluctuating state of the patient.

A number of preliminary studies with BTX have been reported in spasticities of varying etiology. Although the focus of this chapter is on pain management, it is worthwhile to note that all of these studies have shown a clinical benefit in the control of muscle tone in patients with severe spasticity. Three studies followed a randomized, double-blind, placebo-controlled design, and in these studies, the results were statistically significant.

Pain is a variable feature of spasticity, dependent on the degree of impairment and the specific regions of the anatomy affected. Although there are at least 12 studies reporting the benefits of BTX in the improvement of muscle tone in spastic conditions, fewer than 6 include formal measures of pain relief. Even in the studies that include formal measures of pain relief, the number of patients experiencing pain at the start of study was frequently lower than the number of patients studied. There were a total of 130 patients treated in six studies. Of these, 106 (82%; range: 25% to 100%) had clinically significant pain at the start of study. Within the group experiencing significant pain at the start of treatment, 77% (range: 63% to 90%) obtained relief. The study of Parkinson disease patients was notable in that it contained a relatively large sample of patients similarly affected by a particularly painful lower leg cramp. In this sample, 70% of patients reported complete pain relief and the balance appeared to have obtained significant reduction in pain. Taken together, results support the use of BTX for pain relief in spastic conditions in which it has been tested. Approximately 75% of patients may expect to obtain pain relief.

Myofascial Pain Syndrome Many therapies are available to patients with MPS. The condition is associated with regional pain and is most typically revealed by deep palpation of highly localized hyperirritable spots known as trigger points. Trigger points appear as nodular masses within taut bands of skeletal muscle and cause referred pain upon palpation.

The etiology of MPS associated with trigger points is incompletely understood and may result from an acute episode of muscle overload or from chronic repetitive muscle overload. Active myofascial trigger points which cause pain can exhibit marked localized tenderness and often refer pain to distant sites and disturb motor function. Additionally, myofascial trigger points may produce autonomic changes. Chronic MPS is one of the most common finding in patients presenting at pain clinics, varying between 30% and 85% of people presenting to pain clinics, and is more prevalent in women than in men.[89] The locations of tender nodules in MPS are remarkably constant; they are found most frequently at the base of the head and in the neck, shoulders, extremities, and lower back. Nodules in similar locations may be present in normal persons but are not tender (latent trigger points).

The differential diagnosis of MPS is critical because MPS can mimic the signs of diseases, such as chronic headache, shoulder bursitis, or, more seriously, lumbar herniated disc with radiculopathy, angina pectoris, and appendicitis.[90]

The trigger points found in MPS should also be distinguished from the tender sites found in fibromyalgia because treatment strategies are different. The most important distinction is that the tender sites of fibromyalgia represent a widespread, nonspecific, soft-tissue pain and, when palpated, cause only local pain.[91] The nodular trigger points of MPS are thought to develop after trauma or after overuse or prolonged spasm of muscles and cause local and referred pain when palpated. Fibromyalgia is a systemic disease process, possibly caused by dysfunction of the limbic system and/or neuroendocrine axis and responding to a multidisciplinary treatment approach, including psychotherapy, low-dose antidepressant medication, and a moderate exercise program. The trigger points of MPS often respond to structured medical management. If there is doubt, injection of local anesthetic into a suspected trigger point will relieve the pain of MPS, and confirm the diagnosis. Curiously, injection into trigger points with analgesics, saline, and even distilled water can produce temporary relief.[92,93]

In a small but carefully designed double-blind, crossover study of six patients with MPS, injections of BTX-A or placebo showed a clear benefit of BTX-A.[94] Patients were selected on the basis of focal pain involving the cervical paraspinal or shoulder girdle muscles, and had discrete trigger points which when palpated reproduced a typical pattern of radiating pain for that patient. Patients with diffuse pain or neurological deficits were excluded. Patients were randomly injected with either BTX-A (50 mU in 4 mL normal saline) or normal saline alone on two occasions separated by at least 8 weeks. Trigger points were injected identically in the two or three sites affected on both occasions. Subjects were not told when to expect relief and were followed up at weekly intervals for 4 weeks and at 8 weeks after treatment. During the study, additional medications for pain relief were not permitted. In addition to investigator palpation and grading of trigger points, pain was assessed both subjectively (visual analog scale [VAS]) and by the application of a pressure algometer to determine pain threshold in kilograms. A positive response was defined as a reduction from baseline of more than 30% on at least two occasions. Four of six patients responded in this manner. Onset of response occurred within the first week after BTX-A injection but not at the 30-minute observation time. Mean duration of response was 5 to 6 weeks. One subject responded to both BTX-A and saline, and one subject's pain threshold after BTX-A had not returned to baseline by the time of the placebo injection. Results between the two treatment regimens were statistically significant in favor of BTX, suggesting that additional clinical testing for this indication is warranted.

The goal of treatment in MPS is restoration of function. Circumspect measures consisting of massage and physical therapy, preferably without using narcotic or nonnarcotic analgesics, are preferred, with the addition of lifestyle change to reduce psychosocial stressors in the home and at work where needed. If these measures fail, local anesthetics with steroids should be injected up to a maximum of three times in 6 weeks. If the pain is relieved but returns quickly, a trial of BTX injection therapy may provide longer-lasting benefit. Besides providing a longer period of pain relief, this strategy may facilitate physical therapy and promote long-term improvement in quality of life.

Thoracic Outlet Syndrome Thoracic outlet syndrome (TOS) is a symptom complex characterized by pain, paresthesia, and functional impairment caused by compression of the neurovascular supply to the upper limb. Impingement may occur at the interscalene triangle, and both anesthetic blockade and chemodenervation of the scalene muscles have shown improvement of symptoms of TOS in nonrandomized controlled trials. Nonsurgical techniques to decrease compression in the interscalene triangle including injections of anesthetic agents and steroids[95-100] indicate that anesthetic block of the anterior scalene muscle could be used to help determine which patients may potentially benefit from decompressive surgery for TOS. They used electrophysiological (EMG) guidance to successfully demonstrate the location of the anterior scalene muscle in all 122 subjects. Using this technique they proceeded with injection of anesthetic agent and found that 90% of those with a clinical diagnosis of TOS had a positive outcome. Of 38 patients who went on to have surgical decompression, 30 of 32 (94%) with a positive block had a positive outcome compared with 3 of 6 (50%) who underwent surgery in spite of a negative block. The authors suggest that blocking the anterior scalene muscle under EMG guidance may predict the patients who will benefit from surgical decompression of the thoracic outlet. BTX-A has shown promise to provide more sustained symptom relief for patients with neurogenic TOS (NTOS) and has a significant advantage over temporary anesthetic blockade.[101] This comparison may not be an accurate one as anesthetic blockade has been used primarily to enhance the assessment as opposed to treatment of NTOS. The rationale for BTX-A injections is that weakening the muscles that specifically impinge upon the brachial plexus trunks and cords may lead to symptom reduction.[102] Jordan et al. injected 100 units of Botox distributed throughout the anterior and middle scalene muscles and trapezius. This study used electrophysiologically and fluoroscopically guided selective injection of the scalene muscles with BTX-A. Sixty-four percent of the 22 patients had greater than 50% reduction of symptoms. The results had a mean duration of symptom relief of 88 days. Two patients in the study experienced symptoms of mild subjective dysphagia. No other complications were found. BTX-A may help in the prediction of individuals who may benefit from scalenectomy as a surgical option.[103] The role of BTX-A as a predictor of a good surgical outcome is supported by a previous study that demonstrated a 94% surgical success rate in those patients who had previously shown temporary improvement with anesthetic and steroid injection into the scalene muscles.[104,105] A study by Torrianni et al of 41 individuals diagnosed with NTOS who underwent ultrasound guided BTX-A injections into anterior scalene, pectoralis minor, and subclavius muscles showed encouraging results. Twelve units of BTX-A was injected to the scalene muscle and subclavius muscle and 15 units was injected to the pectoralis minor muscle. Symptom improvement as measured on a visual analogue scale (VAS) for pain indicated that 69% had significant improvement, with a mean reduction in the VAS after the procedure of 4 cm. The mean duration of symptom improvement was 31 days. There were no complications in this study.

In summary, there is a growing body of evidence that BTX has a role in the management of pain and in the treatment of TOS. The decision to treat a patient with BTX should be undertaken carefully as there are potential complications resulting from this injection, such as muscle weakness, dysphagia, and dysphonia. Additionally, many patients would require repeat injections as the effect of the BTX wears off, and this may put them at an increased risk for development of antibodies to the BTX and make subsequent treatment less effective. However, in the appropriate patient population this treatment may help those patients avoid or postpone surgery or act as an outcome predictor for surgical intervention in the future.

Refractory Chronic Low Back Pain As discussed in Chapter 38 of this book, chronic low back pain is a multifactorial condition that affects many patients. Refractory chronic low back pain includes patient who have failed other interventions both medical and procedural, including spinal surgery. A number of studies have examined the role of botulinum neural toxin A in treatment of the myofascial component of lumbar back pain. One study by Jabbari et al looked at both the short-term and long-term effects of Botox injections to the lumbar paraspinal muscles. Although there was significant variation in the dosing of Botox, 53% of patients who received Botox injections to the lumbar paraspinal muscles achieved significant pain relief at 2 months. Moreover, of those patients, 91% continued to have significant pain relief with subsequent injections out to 14 months.[106]

Cervicothoracic Muscle Pain Secondary to migraines, cervical degenerative disc disease, cervical spine injury, or shoulder pathology, cervicothoracic muscle pain is commonly encountered in both the primary care and pain clinic settings. Because of the beneficial role of Botox for treatment of migraine headaches, it is hypothesized that the administration of Botox to the cervicothoracic paraspinal muscles may provide pain relief more than traditional techniques such as trigger points with local anesthetic and trigger points with a mixture of local anesthetic and corticosteroid. Diffuse studies have examined this hypothesis. In a randomized double-blind crossover study, Graboski et al looked at Botox versus bupivacaine trigger point injections for the treatment of MPS. With a study size of only 18 patients the authors failed to find any difference between Botox in 0.5% bupivacaine regarding duration or magnitude of pain relief. Kamanli et al showed similar findings when comparing Botox to lidocaine trigger point injections. A study of Botox versus methylprednisolone for the treatment of MPS and muscle spasm, found slightly improved results in patients who received BTX-A. Lastly, Freund and Schwartz found increased range of motion and decreased pain score in patients suffering from whiplash associated neck pain after receiving BTX-A.[107-109]

PIRIFORMIS MUSCLE SYNDROME

Piriformis muscle syndrome is a controversial myofascial pain condition that presents with seemingly unusual symptoms. The condition is more common among women with history of history of trauma to the buttocks or pelvis (usually from a fall) and complaint of deep pain in the buttocks and hip, radiating into the thigh or even into the leg and foot. Characteristic signs and symptoms may be from sciatic nerve compression by a contracted piriformis muscle as the nerve passes through the pelvis. On clinical examination, pressure over the buttocks at a point midway between the sacrum and greater trochanter of the hip elicits the pain. Since the piriformis muscle is deep, a number of physicians recommend palpation of the trigger point by rectal or vaginal examination. Palpation of the trigger point on the posterolateral portion of the rectal (or vaginal) vault elicits pain at the site of compression and refers pain either into the thigh or down the leg.

If conservative treatment of piriformis syndrome fails, local injections of anesthetics and/or steroids should be considered. Surgical resection of the piriformis muscle is an additional option; however, some patients may gain short-term benefits from local tryptophan (TrP) injections into the muscle without responding to treatment for long-term pain control. This subset of patients may benefit from treatment with Botox. A small number of studies assessed the efficacy of BTX in the treatment of piriformis syndrome.[110]

In one study, Childers reported findings from a double-blind placebo-controlled crossover pilot study of BTX-A injection for refractory piriformis syndrome in nine subjects. All patients in this study reported pain intensity greater than 3/10 on VAS for pain after at least 3 months of failed conservative treatment prior to enrollment. Symptomatic muscle in each patient was injected with 100 units BTX-A or placebo (saline), using fluoroscopic and electromyographic guidance. Ten weeks postoperatively, saline or BTX-A injections were repeated. The main outcome measures were VAS of pain intensity, distress, spasm, and interference with daily activities.

At baseline, no differences were detected between groups, yet significant ($P < .05$) differences were observed between the average of 2 minimum VAS at baseline and the average of 2 minimum VAS (in all categories) under the 10-week treatment (BTX-A) arm but not the 10-week placebo arm. In addition, Botox-A treatment average was improved significantly ($P = .0273$), from baseline/washout average in VAS of daily activities. Data also suggested that a significant ($P = .0547$) improvement in VAS in muscle spasm ($P = .0547$) occurred in the BTX-A group but not in the placebo group. Taken together, the findings demonstrated that compared to intramuscular saline, BTX-A injections reduced some, but not all, reports of pain attributed to chronic piriformis syndrome.[111]

Neuropathic Pain Neuropathic pain includes the discomfort associated with conditions such as diabetic peripheral neuropathy and postherpetic neuralgia, as well as phantom limb pain. Recently studies have looked at using Botox to treat refractory cases of these conditions. In a randomized double-blind and placebo-controlled study, Xiao et al looked at 60 patients with postherpetic neuropathy and distributed them into one of three groups: Botox, lidocaine, and placebo. When comparing VAS pain scores at day 7 and 3 months posttreatment, the Botox group decreased most significantly compared to the lidocaine and placebo groups at the same time points. Sleep quality improved in all three groups, most significantly in the Botox group. Lastly, opioid use posttreatment was significantly less in the Botox group compared to the lidocaine and placebo groups. Similarly, Yuan et al. used a double-blind crossover trial to examine the effect of Botox in diabetic neuropathic pain. Again, the Botox group was shown to have increased pain relief at 4 weeks, 8 weeks, and 12 weeks postinjection compared with the placebo group. In addition, at the 4-week postinjection stage, sleep quality was improved in the Botox group. Regarding phantom limb pain, one randomized double-blind pilot study was done looking at 14 amputees with intractable phantom limb pain who failed conventional treatment. The study amputees were randomized to either a Botox injection group or a combination of local anesthetic and corticosteroid injection group. Not only did both groups exhibit immediate pain relief, the treatment effect was sustained for 6 months in both groups, with no significant statistical difference between the groups.[112-114]

DOSING CONSIDERATIONS

Once the decision is made to consider BTX for the treatment of MPS or headache, the key questions are which patient will best benefit from this therapy, what dose to administer (in what concentration and in what diluent), and how to do it. Unfortunately, the answers to these questions are still uncertain. Until more studies are performed, only general guidelines are available in the currently available literature.

Whom to Inject? As with any new therapy, especially one that is expensive, it makes sense to use BTX-A only in more refractory cases until the treatment becomes established and pharmacoeconomics data are supportive. In the case of headache management, avoidance of a single emergency department visit or multiple office visits or significant reduction in expensive triptan use could easily sway the economic balance to use BTX if preliminary study results are confirmed in subsequent trials. In MPS, the potential for significant reduction in medication use and complete resolution of symptoms in the majority of refractory cases is a strong argument in support of BTX use. In both conditions, quality of life and functional improvement can be measurably improved.

Where to Inject? With MPS, most investigators have injected active trigger points directly or used a grid pattern (Lang method) around them to get more diffuse spread through the involved muscle.[42] Scalene or psoas compartment injections under fluoroscopic guidance can be used with success to target adjacent muscles. In the lower back, trigger points in deeper paraspinals are not as easily felt and the limited studies that have been published have *chased tenderness* or *spasm* as their guide for which muscles to inject. In tension-type headache management, most investigators have *chased the tenderness* and injected posterior neck muscles (upper trapezius, levator scapulae, and suboccipitals), and, if tender, temporalis, frontalis, suboccipitals have been injected.

How Much to Inject? Cervical and VII nerve dystonia data have been used as a starting point for BTX-A dose calculations with adjustments depending upon the size of the muscle and degree of spasm. Extensive clinical experience with BTX-A supports this extrapolation to MPS/headache, but with BTX-B, it will be important to be cautious and start at a maximum of 2500 to 5000 units and move upward, depending upon clinical response until data from current studies provide dose-response information.

The total maximum dose per visit for BTX (Botox) typically should not exceed 300 to 400 units (although many have gone as high as 600-700 U safely for numerous involved muscles as in diffuse spasticity/dystonia) and intervals between doses should be no less than 3 months. Following these general guidelines will reduce adverse events (primarily weakness) and antibody formation. Few data are available to help one decide on BTX-B dosing outside of cervical dystonia. It appears to be about 40 to 50 times less potent than BTX-A, with very few patients having received doses at or above 20,000 U, although these doses appear to be well tolerated. In the cervical dystonia data, BTX-B produced duration of effect between 12 and 16 weeks.

Larger volumes of injectant and doses of neurotoxin may influence the tendency for excess BTX to diffuse to nontargeted sites (adjacent muscles or remote sites). This becomes a concern especially with anterior neck injections where electromyogram guidance and low volumes of injectant (BTX-A 100 U/cc or BTX-B 5,000 U/cc) should be used. The technique of using multiple injection sites within the muscle appears to reduce unwanted side effects as does using electromyogram guidance to target motor end plates, thus allowing one to use fewer toxins.

What to Use as Diluent? Allergan recommends that only preservative-free saline (PFNS) is used as the diluent and that once it is added to reconstitute Botox, it should be used within 4 hours because of concerns of compromised sterility and infection risk. Elan Pharmaceuticals also recommends that PFNS be used if one desires a more dilute concentration of Myobloc than 5,000 U/cc, and although the unopened toxin is stable for months at room temperature, once opened, the toxin should be used within 4 hours because of infection concern.

The use of preservative-free local anesthetic as a diluent, although outside of labeling from the manufacturers, does not denature the protein (as long as bicarbonate is not added to neutralize the acidic pH of the local anesthetic) and certainly helps to decrease local injection pain.[95,115] In MPS, a number of studies document that local anesthetics seem not to interfere with toxin efficacy, although studies comparing local anesthetics versus PFNS have not been done. Additionally, whether volume of diluent makes a difference in efficacy is not known, although studies are in progress to answer this question.[1,96]

Is Targeting of Injections Needed? The use of fluoroscopic or electromyogram guidance to identify the muscle or localize the motor end plate prior to injections appears to be a benefit in some situations (particularly in the anterior neck and the deep paraspinal muscles, and possibly to reduce unwanted remote spread by targeting motor end plates with lower toxin doses), but other clinicians have not shown that this technique is necessary when the muscles and trigger points are easily palpable.

CONCLUSION

BTX appears to be a useful treatment in refractory MPS and headache. Presumably BTX works by breaking the spasm–pain cycle, giving the patient a "window of opportunity" for traditional conservative measures to have a greater beneficial impact, but several studies suggest that a direct antinociceptive effect distinct from any reduction in muscle spasm may be at play. The major benefit of BTX compared with standard therapies is duration of response.

We do not advocate that BTX be used as a first-line treatment for MPS or headache. However, in refractory cases where nothing else has worked, it may offer a chance for improvement or cure not otherwise available. Data from studies currently being conducted will help us decide where to place BTX in our pain treatment continuum. For now, it remains an off-label, but increasingly accepted, approach in patients with refractory myofascial pain and headache who despite multidisciplinary approaches continue to suffer.

ACKNOWLEDGMENT

We are grateful to Mike A. Royal, MD, OK for allowing us to take excerpts from his article "The use of botulinum toxins in the management of pain and headache" (*Pain Practice* 2001;1(3):215–235).

Dr. Prithvi Raj and Dr. Sara Sangha contributed to this chapter in the previous edition.

REFERENCES

1. Van Ermengem E. A new anaerobic bacillus and its relation to botulism. *Rev Infect Dis.* 1979;1:701-719.
2. Snipe PT, Sommer H. Studied on botulinus toxin. 3. Acid precipitation of botulinus toxin. *J Infect Dis.* 1928;43:152-160.
3. Shantz EJ. Historical perspective. In: Jankovic J, Hallett M, eds. *Therapy with Botulinum Toxin.* New York, NY: Marcel Dekker; 1994:23-36.
4. Scott AB, Rosenbaum AL, Collins CC. Pharmacologic weakening of extra-ocular muscles. *Invest Ophthalmol.* 1973;12:924-927.
5. Scott AB. Botulinum toxin injection into extra-ocular muscles as an alternative to strabismus surgery. *Ophthalmology.* 1980;87: 1044-1049.
6. Tsui JKC. Botulinum toxin as a therapeutic agent. *Pharmacol Ther.* 1996;72:13-24.
7. Jankovic J, Hallett M, eds. *Therapy with Botulinum Toxin.* New York, NY: Marcel Dekker; 1994.
8. DasGupta BR. Structures of botulinum neurotoxin, its functional domains, and perspectives on the crystalline type A toxin. In: Jankovic J, Hallett M, eds. *Therapy with Botulinum Toxin.* New York, NY: Marcel Dekker; 1994:15-39.
9. Hesse S, Lucke D, Malezic M, et al. Botulinum toxin treatment for lower limb extensor spasticity in chronic hemiparetic patients. *J Neurol Neurosurg Psychol.* 1994;57:1321-1324.
10. Sellin LC, Thesless S, Dasgupta BR. Different effects of types A and B botulinum toxin on transmitter release at the rat neuromuscular junction. *Acta Physiol Scand.* 1983;119(2):127-133.
11. Sellin LC, Kauffman JA, Dasgupta BR. Comparison of the effects of botulinum neurotoxin types A and E at the rat neuromuscular junction. *Med Biol.* 1983;61(2):120-125.
12. Kauffman JA, Way JF, Siegel LS, Sellin LC. Comparison of the action of types A and F botulinum toxin at the rat neuromuscular junction. *Toxicol Appl Pharmacol.* 1985;79(2):211-217.
13. Schantz EJ, Johnson EA. Preparation and characterization of botulinum toxin type A for human treatment. In: Jankovic J, Hallett M, eds. *Therapy with Botulinum Toxin.* New York, NY: Marcel Dekker; 1994:41-49.
14. Sugiyama H. Clostridium botulinum neurotoxin. *Microbiol Rev.* 1980;44:419-448.
15. Moyor E, Settler PE. Botulinum toxin type B: experimental and clinical experience In: Jankovic J, Hallett M, eds. *Therapy with Botulinum Toxin.* New York, NY: Marcel Dekker; 1994:71-86.
16. Borodic GE, Pearce LB, Smith KL, et al. Botulinum B toxin as an alternative to botulinum A toxin: a histology study. *Ophthal Plast Reconstr Surg.* 1993;9:182-190.
17. Greene P, Fahn S. Use of botulinum toxin type F injections to treat torticollis in patients with immunity to botulinum toxin type A. *Mov Disord.* 1993;8:479-483.
18. Ludlow CL, Hallett M, Rhew K, et al. Therapeutic use of type F botulinum toxin. *N Engl J Med.* 1992;326:349-350.
19. DasGupta BR. Structure and biological activity of botulinum neurotoxin. *J Physiol (Paris).* 1990:84:220-228.
20. Montccucco C. How do tetanus and botulinum toxins bind to neuronal membranes? *Trends Biochem Sci.* 1986:11:314-317.
21. Evans DM, Williams RS, Shone CC, Hambleton P, Melling J, Dolly JO. Botulinum neurotoxin type B: its purification, radioiodination and interaction with rat-brain synaptosomal membranes. *Eur J Biochem.* 1986:154:409-416.
22. Black JD, Dolly JO. Interaction of 125I-labeled botulinum neurotoxins with nerve terminals. I. Ultrastructural autoradiographic localization and quantitation of distinct membrane acceptors for types A and B on motor nerves. *J Cell Biol.* 1986:103: 521-534.
23. Burgen AS, Dickens VF, Zatman LJ. The action of botulinum toxin on the neuromuscular junction. *J Physiol (London)* 1949;109:10-24.
24. Simpson LL. The study of clostridial and related toxins: the search for unique mechanisms and common denominators. *J Physiol (Paris).* 1990;84:143-151.
25. Poulain B, Tauc L, Maisery EA, et al. Neurotransmitter release is blocked intracellularly by botulinum neurotoxin, and this requires uptake of both toxin polypeptides by a process mediated by the larger chain. *Proc Natl Acad Sci USA.* 1988;85:4090-4094.
26. Finkelstein A. Channels formed in phospholipid bilayer membranes by diphtheria, tetanus, botulinum and anthrax toxin. *J Physiol (Paris).* 1990;84:188-190.
27. Schiavo G, Boquet P, DasGupta BR, Montecucco C. Membrane interactions of tetanus and botulinum neurotoxins: a photolabelling study with photoactivatable phospholipid. *J Physiol (Paris).* 1990;84:180-187.
28. Duchen LW, Strich SJ. The effects of botulinum toxin on the pattern of innervation of skeletal muscle in the mouse. *Q J Exp Physiol.* 1968;53:84-89.
29. Elston JS. Botulinum toxin treatment of blepharospasm. In: Fahn S, Marsden CD, eds. *Dystonia 2.* New York, NY: Raven Press; 1988: 579-581.
30. Borodic GE, Ferrante R. Histologic effects of repeated botulinum toxin over many years in human orbicularis oculi muscle. *J Clin Neuroophthalmol.* 1992;12:121-127.
31. Harris CP, Alderson K, Nebeker J, et al. Histology of human orbicularis muscle treated with botulinum toxin. *Arch Ophthalmol.* 1991;109:393-395.
32. Borodic GE, Ferrante RJ, Pearce LB, Alderson K. Pharmacology and histology of the therapeutic application of botulinum toxin. In: Jankovic J, Hallett M, eds. *Therapy with Botulinum Toxin.* New York, NY: Marcel Dekker; 1994:119-157.
33. Purkiss J, Welch M, Doward D, Foster K. Capsaicin-stimulated release of substance P from cultured dorsal root ganglion neurons: involvement of two distinct mechanisms. *Biochem Pharmacol.* 2000;59:1403-1406.
34. Welch MJ, Purkiss JR, Foster KA. Sensitivity of embryonic rat dorsal root ganglia neurons to Clostridium botulinum neurotoxins. *Toxicon.* 2000;38:245-258.
35. Ishikawa H, Mitsui Y, Yoshitomi T, et al. Presynaptic effects of botulinum toxin type A on neuronally evoked response of albino and pigmented rabbit iris sphincter and dilator muscles. *Jpn J Ophthalmol.* 2000;44:106-109.
36. Cui ML, Khanijou S, Rubino J, Aoki KR. Botulinum toxin A inhibits the inflammatory pain in the rat formalin model. Poster 246.2. Presented at the Society for Neuroscience Annual Meeting; New Orleans, LA; 2000.
37. Porta M, Perretti A, Gamba M, Luccarelli G, Fornari M. The rationale and results of treating muscle spasm and myofascial syndromes with botulinum toxin type A. *Pain Digest.* 1998;8:346-352.
38. Hatheway CL, Dang C. Immunogenicity of neurotoxins of Clostridium botulinum. In: Jankovic J, Hallett M, eds. *Therapy with Botulinum Toxin.* New York, NY: Marcel Dekker; 1994:93-107.
39. Brin MF, Fahn S, Moskowitz C, et al. Localized injections of botulinum toxin for the treatment of focal dystonia and hemifacial spasm. *Mov Disord.* 1987;2:237-254.

40. Lew MF, Adornato BT, Duane DD, et al. Botulinum toxin type B: a double-blind placebo-controlled, safety and efficacy study in cervical dystonia. *Neurology*. 1997;49:701-707.
41. Abrams BM. Tutorial 36: myofascial pain syndrome and fibromyalgia. *Pain Digest*. 1998;8:264-272.
42. Lang AM. Botulinum toxin for myofascial pain. In: *Advancements in the Treatment of Neuromuscular Pain*. Ch 5. Baltimore, MD: Johns Hopkins University Office of Continuing Medical Education Syllabus; 1999:23-28.
43. Atassi MZ, Oshima M. Structure, activity and immune (T and B cell) recognition of botulinum neurotoxins. *Crit Rev Immunol*. 1999;19:219-260.
44. Chen R, Karp BI, Hallett M. Botulinum toxin type F for treatment of dystonia: long-term experience. *Neurology*. 1998;51:1494-1496.
45. Jankovic J, Schwartz K, Donovan DT. Botulinum toxin treatment of cranial-cervical dystonia, spasmodic dysphonia, other focal dystonias and hemifacial spasm. *J Neurol Neurosurg Psychiatry*. 1990;53:633-639.
46. Tsui JKC, Eisen A, Stoessl HA, et al. Double-blind study of botulinum toxin in spasmodic torticollis. *Lancet*. 1986;2:245-247.
47. Polo KB, Jabbari B. Botulinum toxin A improved the rigidity of progressive supranuclear palsy. *Ann Neurol*. 1994;35:237-239.
48. Porta M. A comparative trial of botulinum toxin type A and methylprednisolone for the treatment of myofascial pain syndrome and pain from chronic muscle spasm.
49. Relja M. Botulinum toxin type A in the treatment of tension-type headache. Presented at the 9th World Congress on Pain; Vienna, Austria; August 22–27, 1999, and at the International Conference 1999: Basic and Therapeutic Aspects of Botulinum and Tetanus Toxins; Orlando, FL; November 16–18, 1999.
50. Schulte-Mattler WJ, Wieser T, Zierz S. Treatment of tension-type headache with botulinum toxin: a pilot study. *Eur J Med Res*. 1999;4:183-186. These data were also presented at the International Conference 1999: Basic and Therapeutic Aspects of Botulinum and Tetanus Toxins; Orlando, FL; November 16–18, 1999.
51. Smuts JA, Baker MK, et al. Botulinum toxin type A as prophylactic treatment in chronic tension-type headache. Presented at the International Conference 1999: Basic and Therapeutic Aspects of Botulinum and Tetanus Toxins; Orlando, FL; November 16–18, 1999. See also: Smuts JA, Baker MK, Smuts HM, et al. Prophylactic treatment of chronic tension-type headache using botulinum toxin type A. *Eur J Neurol*. 1999;6(suppl 4):S99-S102.
52. Wheeler AH. Botulinum toxin A, adjunctive therapy for refractory headaches associated with pericranial muscle tension. *Headache*. 1998;38:468-471.
53. Barwood S, Baillieu C, Boyd R, et al. Analgesic effects of botulinum toxin A: a randomised, placebo trial. *Dev Med Child Neurol*. 2000;42:116-121.
54. Fish DR, Sawyers D, Allen PJ, et al. The effect of sleep on the dyskinetic movements of Parkinson's disease, Gilles de la Tourette syndrome, Huntington's disease, and torsion dystonia. *Arch Neurol*. 1991;48:210-214.
55. Poewe W, Wissel J. Experience with botulinum toxin in cervical dystonia. In: Jankovic J, Hallett M, eds. *Therapy with Botulinum Toxin*. New York, NY: Marcel Dekker; 1994:267-278.
56. Sheehy MP, Marsden CD. Writer's cramp—focal dystonia. *Brain*. 1982;105:461-480.
57. Hunter D. *The Diseases of Occupations*. 6th ed. London, UK: Hodder & Stoughton; 1978.
58. Gowers WR. *A Manual of Diseases of the Nervous System*. Philadelphia, PA: P. Blakiston; 1888.
59. Albanese A, Bentivoglio AR, Cassetta E, et al. Review article: the use of botulinum toxin in the alimentary tract. *Aliment Pharmacol Ther*. 1995;9(6):599-604.
60. Cohen LG, Hallett M, Celler BD, Hochberg F. Treatment of focal dystonia of the hand with botulinum toxin injections. *J Neurol Neurosurg Psychaiatry*. 1989:52:355-363.
61. Cole RA, Cohen LG, Hallett M. Treatment of musician's cramp with botulinum toxin. *Med Probl Performing Artists*. 1991;6:137-143.
62. Poungvarin N. Writer's cramp: the experience with botulinum toxin injections in 25 patients. *J Med Assoc Thai*. 1991;74:239-247.
63. Rivest J, Lees AJ, Marsden CD. Writer's cramp: treatment with botulinum toxin injections. *Mov Discord*. 1991:6:55-59.
64. Jankovic J, Schwartz KS. Use of botulinum toxin in the treatment of hand dystonia. *J Hand Surg*. 1993;18A:883-887.
65. Karp BI, Cole RA, Cohen LG, et al. Long-term botulinum toxin treatment of focal hand dystonia. *Neurology*. 1994;44:70-76.
66. Tsui JKC, Bhatt M, Calne S, Clane DB. Botulinum toxin in the treatment of writer's cramp: a double-blind study. *Neurology*. 1993;43:183-185.
67. Cole R, Hallett M, Cohen LG. Double-blind trial of botulinum toxin for treatment of focal hand dystonia. *Move Discord*. 1995;10:466-471.
68. Young RR. Treatment of spastic paresis. *N Engl J Med*. 1989:320:1553-1555.
69. Burke D. Critical examination of the case for or against fusimotor involvement in disorder of muscle tone. In: Desmedt JE, ed. *Motor Control Mechanisms in Health and Disease*. New York, NY: Raven Press; 1983:133-150.
70. Dimitrijevic MR. Spasticity and rigidity. In: Jankovic J, Tolosa E, eds. *Parkinson's Disease and Movement Disorders*. 2nd ed. Baltimore, MD: Williams and Wilkins; 1993:443-453.
71. Simpson DM, Alexander DN, O'Brien CF, et al. Botulinum toxin type A in the treatment of upper extremity spasticity: a randomized, double-blind, placebo-controlled trial. *Neurology*. 1996;46(5):1306-1310.
72. Gordon J. Spinal mechanisms of motor coordination. In: Kandel ER, Schwartz JH, Jessell TM, eds. *Principles of Neural Science*. 3rd ed. Norwalk, CT: Appleton & Lange; 1991:581-595.
73. Delwaide PJ, Yoiung (Young) RR, Eds. *Clinical Neurophysiology in Spasticity*. Amsterdam, The Netherlands: Elsevier; 1985.
74. Young RR. Physiologic and pharmacologic approaches to spasticity. *Neurol Clin*. 1987;5:529-539.
75. Katz RT. Management of spasticity. *Am J Phys Med Rehabil*. 1988:67:108-116.
76. Gans BM, Glenn MB. Introduction. In: Glenn MB, Whyte J, eds. *The Practical Management of Spasticity in Children and Adults*. Philadelphia, PA: Lea & Febiger; 1990:1-7.
77. Mayer NH. Functional management of spasticity after head injury. *J Neurol Rehab*. 1991;5:S1-S4.
78. Lehmkuhl LD, Thoi LL, Baize C, Kelley CJ, Krawcryk L, Bontke CF. Multimodality treatment of joint contractures in patients with severe brain injury: cost, effectiveness, and integration of therapies in the application of seria Vinhibitive casta. *J Head Trauma Rehabil*. 1990;5:23-42.

79. Carthidge NE, Hudgson P, Weightman D. A comparison of baclofen and diazepam in the treatment of spasticity. *J Neurol Sci.* 1974:23:17-24.

80. Whyte J, Robinson KM. Pharmacologic management. In: Glenn MB, Whyte J, eds. *The Practical Management of Spasticity in Children and Adults.* Philadelphia, PA: Lea & Febiger; 1990:201-226.

81. Chan CH. Dantrolene sodium and hepatic injury. *Neurology.* 1999;40:1427-1432.

82. Reeves KD, Baker A. Mixed somatic peripheral nerve block for painful or intractable spasticity: a review of 30 years of use. *AJPM Am J Phys Med Rehabil.* 1992;2:205-210.

83. Glenn MB. Nerve blocks. In: Glenn MB, Whyte J, eds. *The Practical Management of Spasticity in Children and Adults.* Philadelphia, PA: Lea & Febiger; 1990:227-258.

84. Kasdon KL, Abromovitz JN. Neurosurgical approaches. In: Glenn MB, Whyte J, eds. *The Practical Management of Spasticity in Children and Adults.* Philadelphia, PA: Lea & Febiger; 1990:259-267.

85. Albright AL, Barron WB, Fasick MP, Polinko P, Janosky J. Continuous intrathecal baclofen infusion for spasticity of cerebral origin. *JAMA.* 1993;270:2476-2477.

86. Bowers DN, Averill A. Intrathecal baclofen for Intractable spasticity due to severe traumatic brain injury (abstract). *Arch Phys Med Rehabil.* 1991;72:816.

87. Meythaler JM. Use of intrathecal baclofen in brain injury patients (abstract). *Arch Phys Med Rehabil.* 1994;75:1036.

88. Shaari CM, Sanders I. Assessment of the biological activity of botulinum toxin. In: Jankovic J, Hallett M, eds. *Therapy with Botulinum Toxin.* New York, NY: Marcel Dekker; 1994:159-170.

89. Han SC, Harrison P. Myofascial pain syndrome and trigger-point management. *Reg Anesth.* 1995;65:167-170.

90. Flax HJ. Myofascial pain syndromes—the great mimicker. *Bol Asoc Med P R.* 1995;65:167-170.

91. Schneider MJ. Tender points/fibromyalgia vs. trigger points/myofascial pain syndrome: a need for clarity in terminology and differential diagnosis. *J Manipulative Physiol Ther.* 1995;65:398-406.

92. Tschopp KP, Gysin C. Local injection therapy in 107 patients with myofascial pain syndrome of the head and neck. *ORL J Otorhinolaryngol Relat Spec.* 1996;58:306-310.

93. Wreje U, Brorsson B. A multicenter randomized controlled trial of injections of sterile water and saline for chronic myofascial pain syndromes. *Pain.* 1995;65:441-444.

94. Cheshire WP, Abashian SW, Mann JD. Botulinum toxin in the treatment of myofascial pain syndrome. *Pain.* 1994;59:65-69.

95. Jordan SE, Machleder HI. Diagnosis of thoracic outlet syndrome using electrophysiologically guided anterior scalene blocks. *Ann Vasc Surg.* 1998;12:260-264. and BTX-A.

96. Torriani M, Gupta R., Donahue, D. Botulinum toxin injection in neurogenic thoracic outlet syndrome: results and experience using an ultrasound-guided approach. *Skeletal Radiol.* 2010; 39:973-380.

97. Christo PJ, Christo DK, Carinci AJ, Freischlag JA. Single CT-guided chemodenervation of the anterior scalene muscle with botulinum toxin for neurogenic thoracic outlet syndrome. *Pain Med.* 2010;11:504-511.

98. Danielson K, Odderson IR. Botulinum toxin type A improves blood flow in vascular thoracic outlet syndrome. *Am J Phys Med Rehabil.* 2008;87:956-959. Toxins 2012.

99. Jordan SE, Ahn SS, Freischlag JA, Gelabert HA, Machleder HI. Selective botulinum toxin chemodenervation of the scalene muscles for treatment of neurogenic thoracic outlet syndrome. *Ann Vasc Surg.* 2000;14:365-369.

100. Jordan SE, Machleder HI. Diagnosis of thoracic outlet syndrome using electrophysiologically guided anterior scalene blocks. *Ann Vasc Surg.* 1998;12:260-264.

101. Le EN, Freischlag JA, Christo PF, Chhabra S, Wigley FM. Thoracic outlet syndrome secondary to scleroderma treated with botulinum toxin injection. *Arthritis Care Res.* 2010;62:430-433.

102. Jordan SE, Machleder HI. Diagnosis of thoracic outlet syndrome using electrophysiologically guided anterior scalene blocks. *Ann Vasc Surg.* 1998;12:260-264.

103. Danielson K, Odderson IR. Botulinum toxin type A improves blood flow in vascular thoracic outlet syndrome. *Am J Phys Med Rehabil.* 2008;87:956-959.

104. Jordan SE, Ahn SS, Gelabert HA. Combining ultrasonography and electromyography for botulinum chemodenervation treatment of thoracic outlet syndrome: Comparison with fluoroscopy and electromyography guidance. *Pain Physician.* 2007;10:541-546.

105. Torriani M, Gupta R, Donahue D. Botulinum toxin injection in neurogenic thoracic outlet syndrome: Results and experience using an ultrasound-guided approach. *Skeletal Radiol.* 2010;39: 973-380.

106. Jabbari B, Ney J, Sichani A, Monacci W, Foster L, Difazio M. Treatment of refractory, chronic low back pain with botulinum neurotoxin A: an open-label, pilot study. *Pain Med.* 2006 May-Jun;7(3): 260-264.

107. Graboski CL, Gray DS, Burnham RS. Botulinum toxin A versus bupivacaine trigger point injections for the treatment of myofascial pain syndrome: a randomised double blind crossover study. *Pain.* 2005 Nov;118(1-2):170-175. Epub 2005 Oct 3.

108. Kamanli A, Kaya A, Ardicoglu O, Ozgocmen S, Zengin FO, Bayik Y. Comparison of lidocaine injection, botulinum toxin injection, and dry needling to trigger points in myofascial pain syndrome. *Rheumatol Int.* 2005 Oct;25(8):604-611. Epub 2004 Sep 15.

109. Freund BJ, Schwartz M. Treatment of whiplash associated neck pain [corrected] with botulinum toxin-A: a pilot study. *J Rheumatol.* 2000 Feb;27(2):481-484.

110. Jeynes LC, Gauci CA. Evidence for the use of botulinum toxin in the chronic pain setting—a review of the literature. *Pain Pract.* Jul-Aug 2008;8(4):269-276.

111. Childers MK, Wilson DJ, Gnatz SM, et al. Botulinum toxin type A use in piriformis muscle syndrome: a pilot study. *Am J Phys Med Rehabil.* Oct 2002;81(10):751-759.

112. Yuan RY, Sheu JJ, Yu JM, et al. Botulinum toxin for diabetic neuropathic pain: a randomized double-blind crossover trial. *Neurology.* 2009 Apr28;72(17):1473-1478. doi:10.1212/01.wnl.0000345968.05959.cf. Epub 2009 Feb 25.

113. Xiao L, Mackey S, Hui H, Xong D, Zhang Q, Zhang D. Subcutaneous injection of botulinum toxin A is beneficial in postherpetic neuralgia. *Pain Med.* 2010 Dec;11(12):1827-1833. doi:10.1111/j.1526-4637.2010.01003.x.

114. Wu H, Sultana R, Taylor KB, Szabo A. A prospective randomized double-blinded pilot study to examine the effect of botulinum toxin type A injection versus Lidocaine/Depomedrol injection on residual and phantom limb pain: initial report. See comment in PubMed Commons below. *Clin J Pain.* 2012 Feb;28(2):108-112. doi:10.1097/AJP.0b013e3182264fe9.

115. Holz RW, Fisher SK. Synaptic transmission and cellular signaling; an overview. In: Siegal GJ, Siegel, GJ et al., eds. *Basic Neurochemistry: Molecular, Cellular and Medical Aspects.* 6th ed. Ch 10. Lippincott-Raven OK Publishers; 1999:191-212.

CHAPTER 88

Ultrasound in the Diagnosis and Treatment of Pain

Einar Ottestad
Abhishek Gowda

OVERVIEW

Ultrasound imaging technology has become prevalent and easily accessible to the pain physician. In the past 20 years, there has been a significant increase in the use of ultrasound-guided pain procedures to the point that even procedures once relegated to fluoroscopic approaches are now able to be done sufficiently with ultrasound techniques. The advancement of ultrasound technology and clarity of imaging currently available give an additional advantage to the ultrasound-based pain physician in terms of soft-tissue visualization for diagnostic and therapeutic purposes. Ultrasound-based procedures are cost-efficient and when performed appropriately are safe because the medium allows visualization of muscles, tendons, ligaments, soft tissues, and neurovascular structures in a real-time, dynamic manner. Furthermore, because of the lower cost, lack of radiation, and smaller physical footprint, ultrasound imaging can be provided within the outpatient clinical setting, thus reducing the need for specialized surgical centers and fluoroscopic imaging.

The goal of this chapter is to provide a framework for the pain physician to gain basic knowledge and understanding of ultrasound-based procedures. We will begin with a comparison of ultrasound imaging and traditional imaging and the advantages and disadvantages of each. Thereafter, we will provide a short discussion on specific types of available ultrasound equipment and specific technical factors necessary for appropriate ultrasound use. We will also review basic techniques of scanning and needle localization using ultrasound and optimization of imaging. Finally, we will provide overviews on specific ultrasound-based procedures for neuronal structures pertinent to the pain medicine physician followed by a review of ultrasound-guided major joint injections.

COMPARISON OF ULTRASOUND, FLUOROSCOPY, AND OTHER IMAGING MODALITIES

Traditionally, the pain physician has used fluoroscopy as the primary imaging modality for various procedures throughout the body. Although fluoroscopy is an invaluable tool, the equipment is expensive and cumbersome, exposes the physician and patient to radiation, and requires a specialized procedure suite. Additionally, fluoroscopy is able to visualize osseous structures only. In order to see the soft-tissue targets, more cumbersome and expensive technology is required such as computed tomography (CT) or magnetic resonance imaging (MRI) guidance. With the advent of ultrasound imaging, many procedures can be done more efficiently with better visualization of regional structures without the unnecessary exposure to radiation and the technical precautions that must be instituted with their use. However, there are limitations of ultrasound use compared to traditional imaging approaches. **Table 88-1** provides an outline as to advantages and disadvantages of three imaging modalities used for pain procedures: ultrasound, fluoroscopy and CT (Table 88-1).

BASICS OF ULTRASOUND

A full review of ultrasound technology and knobology is beyond the scope of this chapter. That stated, some technical knowledge and understanding of the specific vocabulary of ultrasound is necessary. Ultrasound transducers contain piezoelectric crystals which have the capability to generate sound waves from electricity. The sound waves travel through body tissues and depending on the physical properties of the tissues, a certain proportion of this energy is absorbed, refracted, or reflected. The ultrasound transducer is then able to capture the reflected ultrasound wave energy and in turn generate electricity, which, after computer processing, is displayed on the screen.

The wavelength and frequency of ultrasound are inversely related. Higher-frequency, linear-array probes (5–12 MHz) provide greater resolution and better visualization of superficial structures. Lower-frequency, curved-array probes (2–5 MHz) have less resolution but much better penetration for visualization of deeper structures. As such, the first step is to choose the correct probe for the depth of the procedure.

The second step is to optimize the image. First, choose the correct depth to visualize the target. Next, adjust the gain on the machine. Gain is essentially the brightness of the image and simply amplifies the electrical signal from the transducer. The third step is to move the focus of the ultrasound beam to the depth of the target. Moving the focus to the target optimizes the lateral resolution at that depth making the target more visible. Most ultrasound instruments will also have a color Doppler function that allows visualization of blood vessels (**Table 88-2**).

TABLE 88-1 Advantages and Disadvantages of Three Imaging Modalities

	Anatomy Visualized	Radiation Exposure	Cost	Efficiency	Neuraxial Blocks	Patient Body Habitus
Ultrasound (US)	Soft tissue	None	Affordable	Procedures can be done quickly	Difficult to visualize bony anatomy and landmarks in spine	Difficult visualization with obese patients
	Ligament		Can be done by single physician			
	Tendon, neurovascular structures					
Fluoroscopy	Bony anatomy only		Moderate	Moderate	Can use contrast to visualize concerns for intravascular flow of medication	Good visualization but operating table may have weight limit in excess of 300 lb
	No visualization of soft-tissue structures	Moderate exposure	Requires technical expertise with fluoroscopy technician		Digital subtraction angiography is added advantage	
Computed tomography (CT) guidance	Soft-tissue and bony anatomy visualization	Significant	Expensive equipment and requires radiology input, need separate facility to house CT scanner	Time-consuming procedures with having to step out of the room for each scan and difficult access	Good visualization for soft-tissue and bony anatomy for neuraxial blockade	Difficult to place in scanner if patient is larger than 400 lb

TABLE 88-2 Color Doppler Function and Definitions of Axis and Plane Functions for Ultrasound

Term	US Reflection	Screen Color	Example Tissue
Anechoic	Minimal	Black	Fluid, blood vessels, local anesthetic
Hypoechoic	Some	Gray	Muscle, nerve, tendon
Hyperechoic	Extensive	White	Bone, calcifications, particulate steroids

Short-axis	US probe perpendicular to target	Probe sees small slice of target
Long-axis	US probe parallel to target along its length	Probe sees 2-3 contiguous cm of target
In-plane	Needle is parallel to the long axis of US probe	Entire needle is visualized in the US beam
Out-of-plane	Needle is perpendicular to the long axis of US probe	Only a cross-section of needle is visualized as a dot

Abbreviation: US, ultrasound.

PERIPHERAL NERVE BLOCKS OF HEAD AND NECK

Table 88-3 is a list of the structures used for identifying the peripheral nerve blocks and joint injections discussed below.

GREATER OCCIPITAL NERVE BLOCK

Anatomy The greater occipital nerve (GON) has its origin from the second and third cervical spinal nerves. It emerges below the posterior arch of the atlas and wraps around the obliquus capitis inferior muscle and runs lateral to medial at the level of C1. The obliquus capitis inferior muscle originates at the C2 spinous process and inserts at the C1 transverse process. The GON then penetrates through the semispinalis capitis, the splenius capitis, and the trapezius muscles. Its sensory distribution is the medial aspect of the posterior scalp to the base of the scalp.

Ultrasound The patient is placed in a prone position with the head flexed forward. A linear transducer is placed over the superior nuchal ridge with a transverse view to identify the hyperechoic line of the occiput. The ultrasonographer then scans caudad from the skull to identify a deep, rounded, and irregular arch of C1 followed by the superficial, bifid spine of the C2 spinous process (**Fig. 88-1**). Next the transducer is translated laterally so only a single spine of the C2 spinous process is visible, and then the lateral aspect of the probe is obliqued cephalad (**Fig. 88-2**). In this view, the obliquus capitis inferior muscle should be visualized extending from the C2 spinous process, over C2 lamina, and inserting at the C1 transverse process. Superficial to the obliquus capitis inferior one will see the semispinalis capitis and then the trapezius muscle. The suboccipital artery often travels in the plane between the

TABLE 88-3 Structures Used to Identify Peripheral Nerve Blocks and Joint Injections (Legend for Figures 88-1 to 88-31)

Structures to identify for greater occipital nerve (GON) block
C1 transverse process
C2 spinous process
Superior nuchal ridge
Occipital artery
Obliquus capitis inferior Muscle (OCI)
Structures to identify for stellate ganglion block
Thyroid gland (Th)
Trachea (Tr)
Vertebral artery
Esophagus (E)
Lung pleura
Longus colli muscle (LC)
Anterior tubercle of C6 (AT)
Monitoring for successful stellate ganglion block
Unilateral Horner syndrome
Guttman sign
Facial warmth
Increase of temperature in upper extremity by at least 1°C
Structures to identify for suprascapular nerve block
Posterior triangle of the neck
Suprascapular artery and vein
Scapular spine
Acromion
Coracoid process
Transverse scapular ligament
Supraspinatus muscle
Infraspinatus muscle
Cubital tunnel block
Humerus, radius, ulna, olecranon
Fat pad
Radial nerve
Ulnar nerve
Brachioradialis muscle
Supinator muscle
Carpal tunnel block
Flexor digitorum superficialis: 4 tendons (FDS)
Flexor digitorum profundus: 4 tendons (FDP)
Flexor carpi radialis
Flexor pollicis longus
Flexor carpi ulnaris
Flexor retinaculum
Median nerve
Ulnar nerve
Intercostal nerve block
Angle and costal groove of the target thoracic rib
External intercostal muscle
Internal intercostal muscle
Lung pleura
Lateral femoral cutaneous nerve (LFCN) of the thigh
Psoas muscle
Anterior superior iliac spine (ASIS)
Tensor fascia lata
Iliaca (I)

(*continued*)

TABLE 88-3 Structures Used to Identify Peripheral Nerve Blocks and Joint Injections (Legend for Figures 88-1 to 88-31) (*continued*)

Sartorius
Ilioinguinal and iliohypogastric nerves
Transversus abdominus (TA)
Internal oblique (IO)
External oblique (EO)
Inguinal ligament
Peritoneum (P)
Deep circumflex iliac artery
Saphenous nerve block
Sartorius (S)
Femoral artery (FA)
Popliteal artery
Vastus medialis (VM)
Superficial peroneal nerve block
Peroneus longus and peroneus brevis (PB)
Extensor digitorum longus (EDL)
Fibular head
Sural nerve block
Gastrocnemius
Lateral malleolus
Achilles tendon
Kagel fat pad
Posterior tibial nerve
Medial malleolus
Achilles tendon
Tibial artery (TA)
Tibialis posterior (TP)
Flexor hallucis longus (FHL)
Glenohumeral joint injection
Glenoid labrum (GL)
Humeral head (HH)
Glenohumeral ligaments
Subscapular bursa
Spine of the scapula
Intraarticular hip injection
Greater trochanter
Femoral head (FH)
Fibrocartilage labrum
Intraarticular knee injection
Patella (P)
Femur (F)
Quadriceps (Q)
Prefemoral fat pad (PFF)
Quadriceps fat pad (QFF)

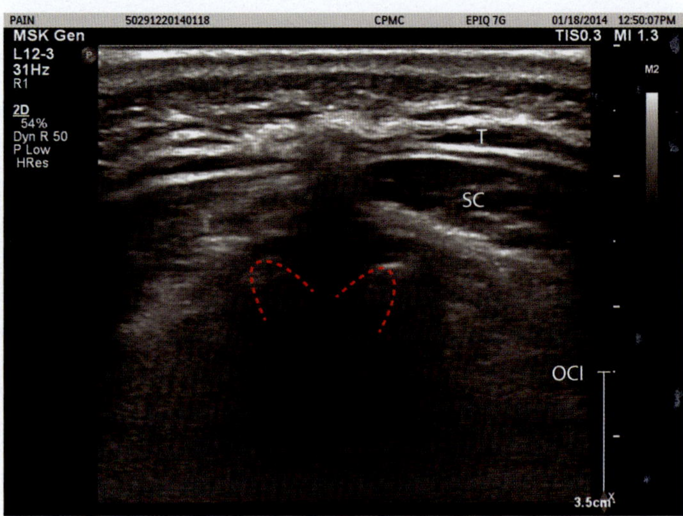

FIGURE 88-1. Greater occipital nerve (C2 spinous process in midline).

semispinalis capitis and the obliquus capitis inferior and is visible using color Doppler imaging. Deep to the obliquus capitis inferior one can sometimes see the vertebral artery as it courses toward the C1 transverse foramen. The needle technique should be an in-plane approach from a lateral to medial with an end point in the plane between the semispinalis capitis and the obliquus capitis inferior approximately 1.5 to 2 cm from the midline. Nerve stimulation can also be instituted in order to determine typical pain emanating from the greater or lesser occipital nerve, and the injectate can be adjusted accordingly secondary to patient input.

STELLATE GANGLION BLOCK

Anatomy The cervical sympathetic chain is made up of the superior, middle, and inferior cervical ganglia. The stellate ganglion is formed by a fusion of the inferior cervical and first thoracic ganglion and arises on the anterior and the lateral surface of the longus colli muscle between the inferior margin of the seventh cervical transverse process and the first rib. As it ascends in the neck, the cervical sympathetic chain travels from lateral to medial over the longus colli, deep to the prevertebral fascia. The trachea, esophagus, recurrent laryngeal nerve, carotid artery, jugular vein, vertebral artery, inferior thyroid artery, and spinal nerves

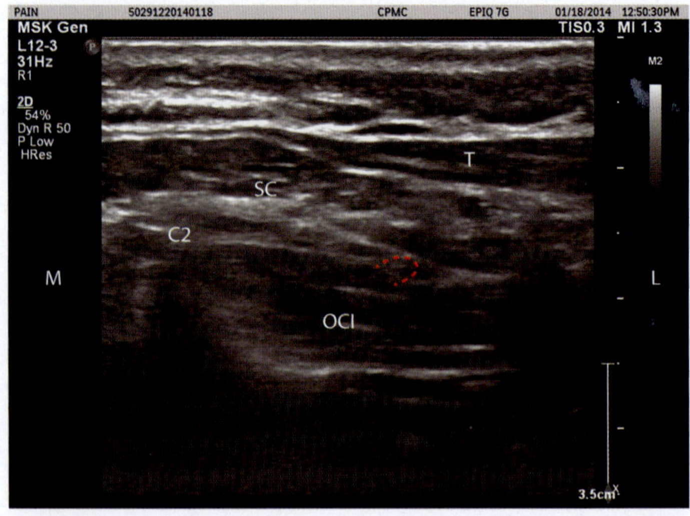

FIGURE 88-2. Greater occipital nerve.

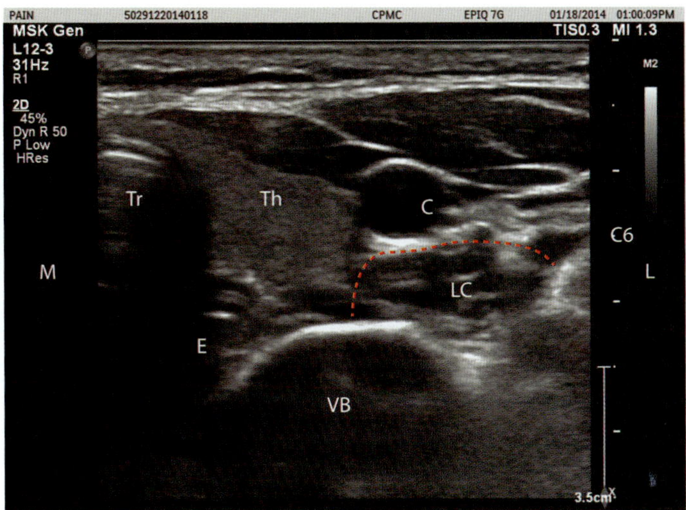

FIGURE 88-3. Stellate ganglion at C6 and its relation to the trachea, thyroid, and vertebral artery.

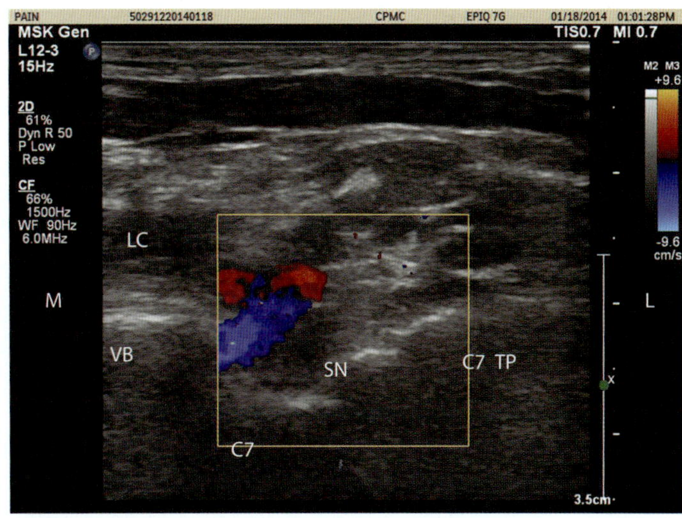

FIGURE 88-5. Stellate ganglion at C7 level with Doppler rendering of vertebral artery. Note its posterior location.

are important anatomic structures in the area that can be visualized and avoided by using ultrasound. The block is performed at the level of C6 since the vertebral artery is protected by the C6 transverse foramen. At C7 the vertebral artery will be close to the target location. In order to identify these landmarks using ultrasound it is important to note that the C7 transverse process has a single posterior tubercle with a visible vertebral artery and the C6 transverse process has both anterior and posterior tubercles with no vertebral artery visible.

Ultrasound Approach The patient is positioned in a supine manner with the head and neck tilted to the contralateral side of the injection. Transverse ultrasound is then used to identify trachea, thyroid, esophagus, carotid sheath, and the anterior cervical spine (**Fig. 88-3**). Scanning laterally identifies the cervical transverse processes. At this point, scanning cephalad and caudad over the transverse processes will allow the identification of the single tubercle of C7 (**Figs. 88-4** and **88-5**) versus the anterior and posterior tubercles of C6 (**Fig. 88-6**). Once C6 is identified, the longus colli muscle is identified adjacent and medial to the anterior tubercle. Color Doppler is mandatory as this is a very vascular area. The needle is placed lateral to medial, superficial to the anterior tubercle of C6, with an end point over the muscle and deep to the prevertebral fascia. Once this location is confirmed by live injection of local anesthetic, 5 mL of solution will block the cervical sympathetic chain. Using this posterior and lateral approach to the stellate ganglion allows the physician to avoid trauma to the thyroid, esophagus, and other midline structures (**Fig. 88-7**).

The stellate ganglion block is an advanced ultrasound approach, and there are associated risks with the procedure in general (see Fig. 88-5). Complications include bleeding, pneumothorax, intravascular injection into the carotid and/or the vertebral artery, soft-tissue injury to the esophagus and trachea, and nerve injury to the phrenic nerve, the brachial plexus, and the recurrent laryngeal nerve.

PERIPHERAL NERVE BLOCKS OF UPPER EXTREMITIES

SUPRASCAPULAR NERVE BLOCK

Anatomy The suprascapular nerve is a peripheral nerve that is derived from the fifth and sixth cervical nerve roots. It has both motor and sensory fibers and courses through the lateral aspect of the upper trunk of the brachial plexus. It pierces through the posterior triangle of the neck,

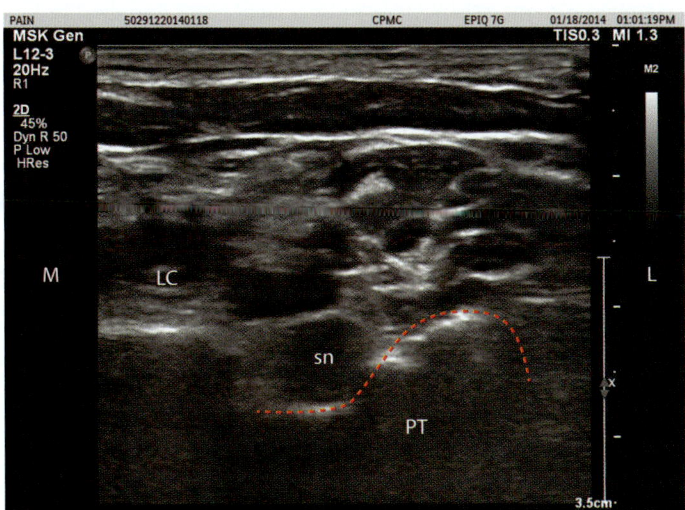

FIGURE 88-4. Stellate ganglion at C7.

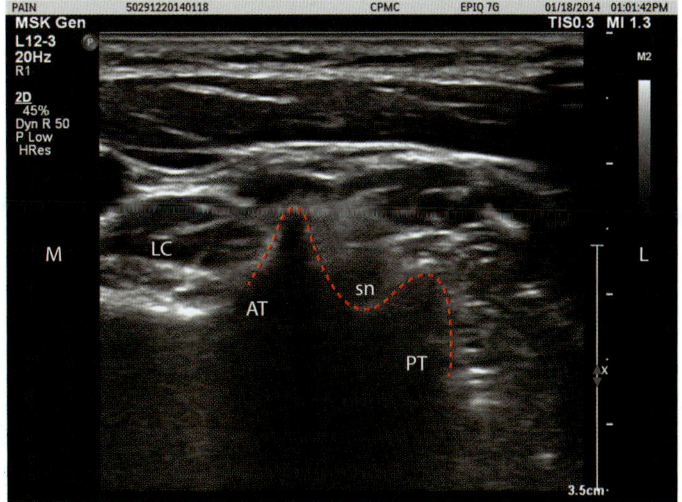

FIGURE 88-6. Stellate ganglion approach at C6.

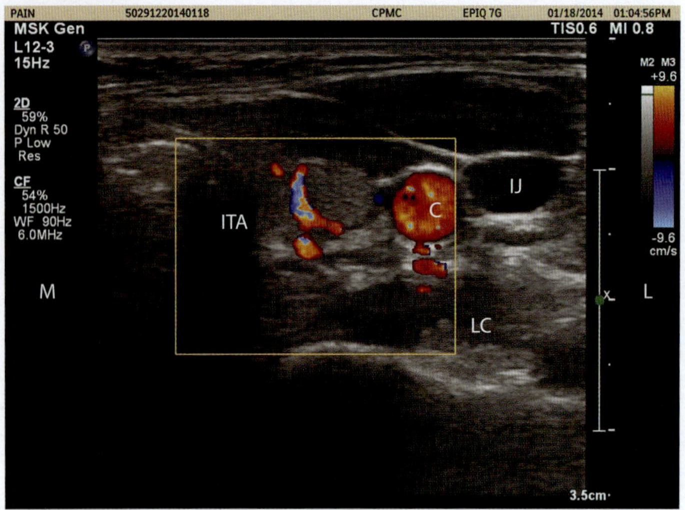

FIGURE 88-7. Stellate ganglion with Doppler flow rendering of inferior thyroidal artery.

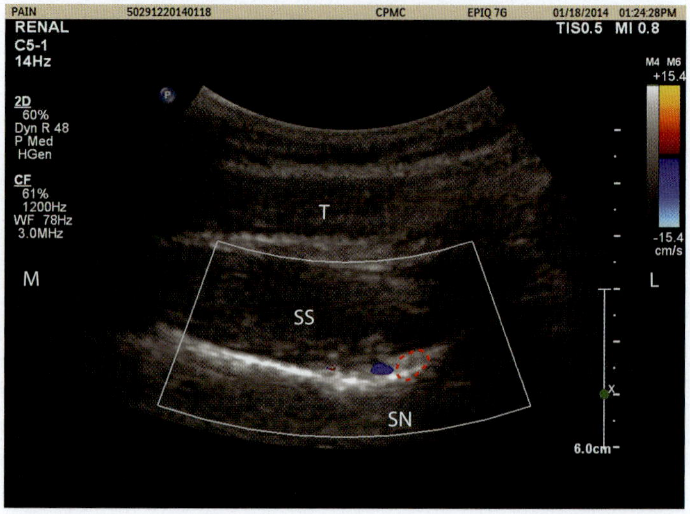

FIGURE 88-9. Suprascapular nerve in relation to suprascapular artery with Doppler flow.

deep to the trapezius and omohyoid, and enters the supraspinous fossa through the suprascapular notch underneath the superior transverse scapular ligament. The suprascapular artery and vein pass above the ligament. In the supraspinous fossa, the nerve is in direct contact with bone and exits the suprascapular fossa to infrascapular fossa lateral to the spinoglenoid notch.

Through the suprascapular notch, the suprascapular nerve has two branches. One is the motor nerve for the supraspinatus muscle, and the other is the sensory superior articular branch. The latter branch supplies the coracoclavicular and coracohumeral ligaments, the AC joint, the glenohumeral joint, and the subacromial bursa.

Ultrasound The patient is placed in a prone or sitting position and the scapular spine, acromion, and coracoid process are palpated and determined. A curved transducer is placed over the spine of the scapula and then moved cephalad into the supraspinatus fossa, revealing the scapula with supraspinatus and trapezius muscles overlying. Scanning medial to lateral will reveal the suprascapular notch (**Fig. 88-8**). Using Doppler enhancement, the suprascapular artery and vein should also be visualized (**Fig. 88-9**). The needle is generally placed in-plane with the ultrasound probe medial to lateral with an end point in the suprascapular notch.

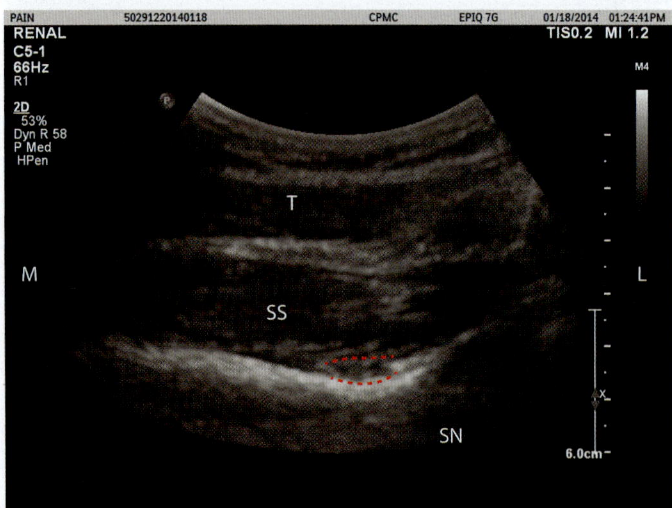

FIGURE 88-8. Suprascapular nerve.

CUBITAL TUNNEL BLOCK

Anatomy The elbow joint comprises of the association of the humerus, radius, and ulna. The ulnar-humeral joint is a hinge whereas the radioulnar and radiohumeral joints allow for rotation. Three fat pads are common sites of compression.

At the elbow, the ulnar nerve runs between the olecranon process and the medial epicondyle. The radial nerve is located laterally under the brachioradialis, where it gives off its deep and superficial branches. The median nerve lies anteriorly, superficial to the brachialis muscle and medial to the brachial artery.

Ultrasound The patient is placed facing away from the physician with elbow in neutral support, with either foaming or a pillow. A linear transducer is then placed over the cubital tunnel, visualizing the medial epicondyle, olecranon, and ulnar nerve between. Often the ulnar nerve is easier to visualize immediately proximal to the cubital tunnel (**Fig. 88-10**), and it can then be traced into the cubital tunnel proper (**Fig. 88-11**). Either a medial to lateral or lateral to medial needle technique is appropriate depending on patient and physician positioning. Individual nerve blocks of the ulnar and radial nerve can also be done and performed most effectively using nerve stimulation proximal to the elbow. The spiral groove of the humerus is an excellent target for the radial nerve, and the 2 to 3 cm proximal to the ulnar groove is ideal for the ulnar nerve.

CARPAL TUNNEL BLOCK

Anatomy The carpal tunnel is located at the wrist and is composed of the median nerve, four tendons of the flexor digitorum superficialis, four tendons of the flexor digitorum profundus, and one tendon of the flexor pollicis longus. The median nerve is located below the common flexor retinaculum above the flexor pollicis longus, medial to the flexor carpi radialis, and lateral to the flexor digitorum superficialis. Carpal tunnel syndrome is the most common entrapment syndrome of a peripheral nerve.

Ultrasound Approach The patient is positioned seated up with the wrist and hand in a supine position underneath an elbow rest. A linear transducer is used for this superficial structure. The median nerve can be difficult to distinguish from the flexor tendons on a static ultrasound image. As such, it is easier to identify the median nerve in the distal forearm when it is traveling between the deep and superficial flexor muscles than to trace it distally into the carpal tunnel median nerve in forearm (**Fig. 88-12**). Once identified, a lateral to medial in-plane technique can be used to place the needle tip deep to the retinaculum and close to but not inside the nerve. It is often helpful to inject a small amount

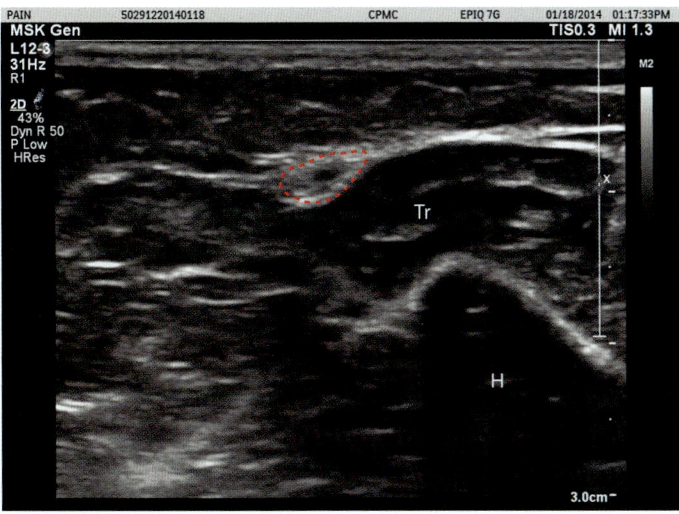

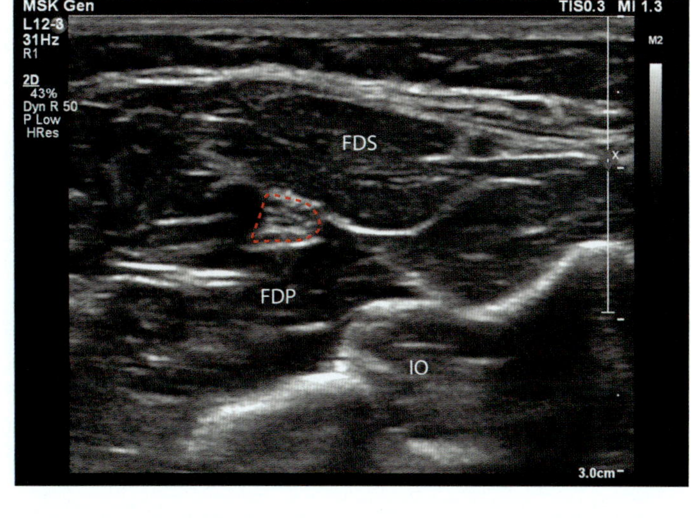

FIGURE 88-10. Proximal cubital tunnel.

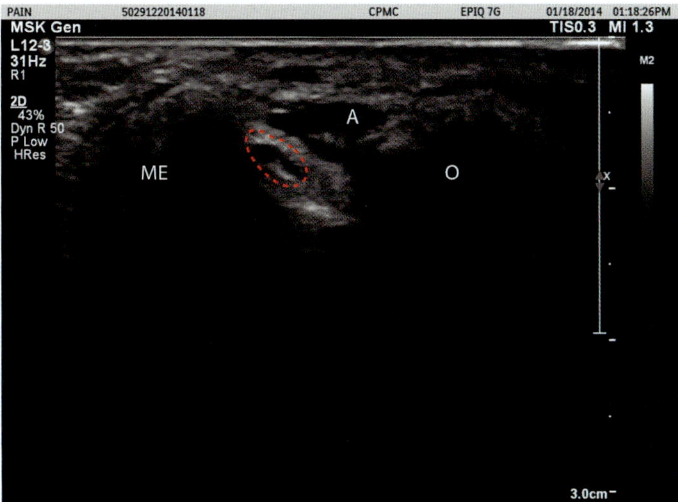

FIGURE 88-11. Cubital tunnel.

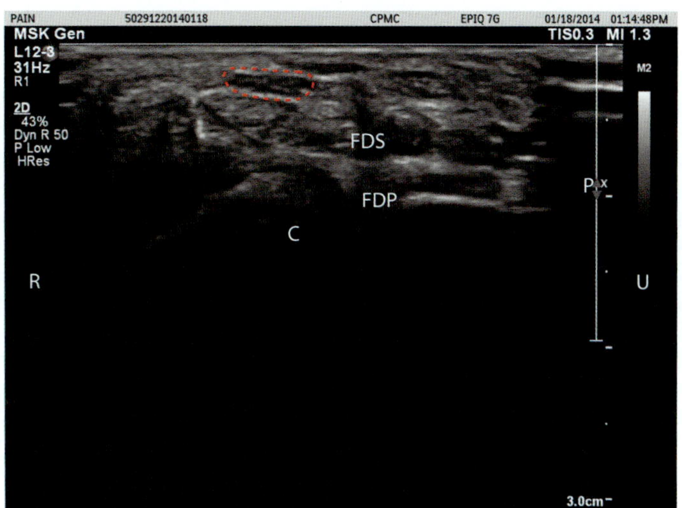

FIGURE 88-12. Carpal tunnel.

of nonparticulate fluid to hydrodissect and create space for particulate steroids. After the procedure, the patient is asked to extend the fingers to draw up the injectate fully into the carpal tunnel.

PERIPHERAL NERVE BLOCKS OF THORAX AND PELVIS

INTERCOSTAL NERVE

Anatomy The intercostal nerves are a continuation of the anterior division of the thoracic paravertebral nerve and have four major branches. The first includes the unmyelinated postganglionic fibers of the gray rami communicantes, which influence the sympathetic chain. The second is the posterior cutaneous branch, which innervates the paraspinal muscular region. The third is the lateral cutaneous division, which arises in the axilla. The fourth is the anterior cutaneous branch, which supplies sensation to the midline of the chest and abdominal wall. The 12th nerve is the subcostal nerve and is unique in that it gives a branch to the first lumbar nerve and gives a branch to the lumbar plexus. The intercostal nerve is a mixed sensory-motor nerve.

The intercostal nerve travels with the intercostal artery and vein caudad to each rib. Between each pair of ribs there are three layers of intercostal muscles: external, internal, and innermost. The neurovascular bundle is located between the internal and innermost intercostal muscles (**Fig. 88-13**).

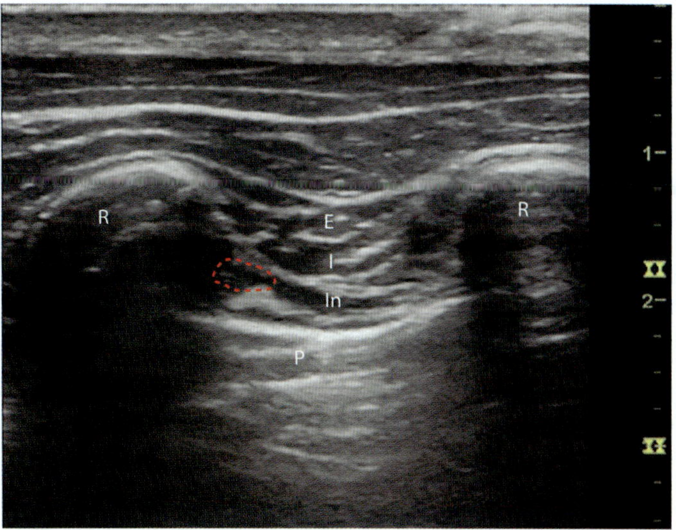

FIGURE 88-13. Intercostal nerve in transverse plane.

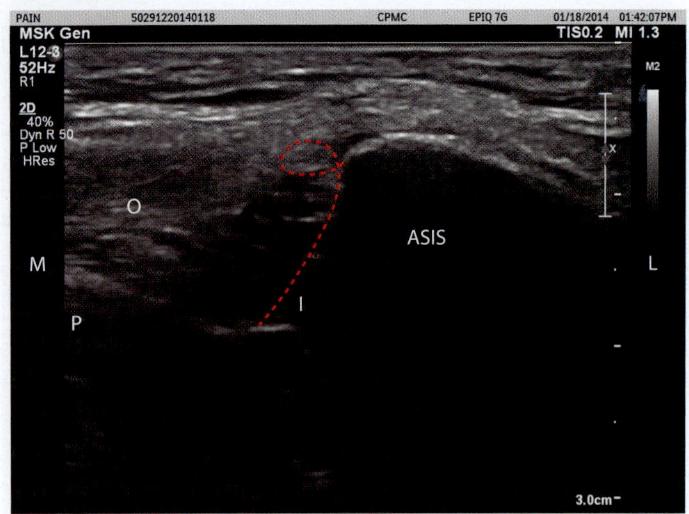

FIGURE 88-14. Lateral femoral cutaneous nerve of the thigh at the anterior superior iliac spine.

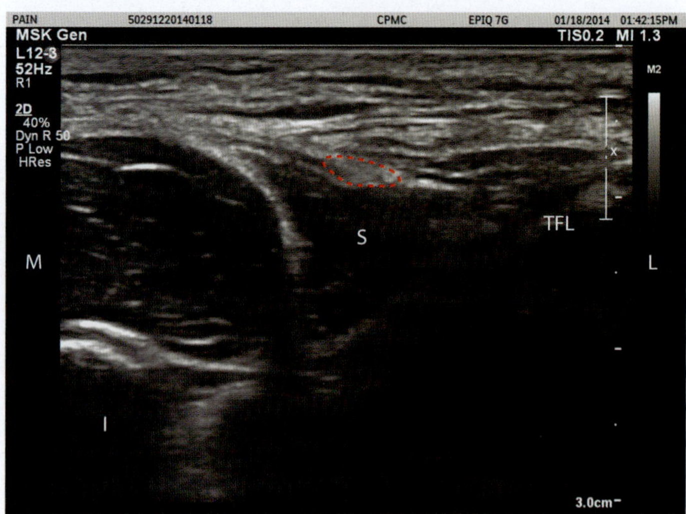

FIGURE 88-15. Lateral femoral cutaneous nerve of the thigh at the level of the sartorius muscle.

Ultrasound Approach The patient is placed in the prone position. A linear transducer is placed in a sagittal fashion approximately 5 centimeters from the midline over the posterior thorax (**Fig. 88-13**). Scanning medial to lateral will help identify the angle of the rib in that this should be the point at which the rib is most superficial, allowing for a safer injection. Identifying the intercostal muscles is of utmost importance in addition to monitoring the pleura, which appears as a bright, hyperechoic line with each respiration. The needle is placed in-plane with the transducer oriented from caudad to cephalad, with an end point between the internal and innermost intercostal muscle. As a safety measure, it is frequently helpful to intermittently inject a small amount of solution to ascertain the location of the needle tip and avoid pleura.

After the block is completed, the probe can be used to check for pneumothorax by placing the wand in a nondependent area. The pleura should appear to glide with respiratory movement. When a pneumothorax is present, the pleura will not glide with respiration.

LATERAL FEMORAL CUTANEOUS NERVE OF THE THIGH

Anatomy The lateral femoral cutaneous nerve (LFCN) of the thigh branches from the lumbar plexus and receives its proximal innervation from the L2 and L3 nerve roots. There is anatomic variability with contributions in some individuals from combinations of nerve roots extending from L1 to L3.

The LFCN emerges lateral to the psoas major muscle above the crest of the ilium and travels in that course inferiorly across the iliacus muscle. The LFCN then descends on the superficial aspect of the iliacus toward the medial anterior superior iliac spine (ASIS) where it penetrates the inguinal ligament and then courses laterally over sartorius. The sartorius is generally identified as an inverted triangle caudad to the ASIS. After the nerve passes laterally over the superficial aspect of the sartorius, it is often easily visible in the fat pad between sartorius and tensor fascia lata.

The LFCN provides sensory innervation to the lateral thigh most notably.

Ultrasound Approach The patient is positioned supine, and the ASIS is noted. A linear ultrasound probe is placed over the ASIS and the inguinal ligament is identified (**Fig. 88-14**). If the nerve is visible here, a simple in-plane needle technique can be used for the block. However, if the nerve is not readily identified at the level of the inguinal ligament, it needs to be found as it traverses the sartorius toward the tensor fascia lata more distally (see **Fig. 88-15**). When the ASIS has been identified, slowly scanning caudad will reveal the triangular sartorius muscle coming off the ASIS medially and the tensor fascia lata coming off laterally. Dynamic scanning cephalad and caudad over the sartorius and tensor fascia lata will reveal the small nerve as it moves medial to lateral in this plane. In most patients the nerve is very difficult to visualize in the actual inguinal ligament.

ILIOINGUINAL AND ILIOHYPOGASTRIC NERVES

Anatomy The ilioinguinal and iliohypogastric nerves supply the intersection between the abdomen and the thigh and are often subject to injury from surgical interventions such as laparoscopy. Originating from the T12 and L1 ventral rami, the ilioinguinal and iliohypogastric nerves course across the lateral border of the psoas major, behind the medial arcuate ligament and anteriorly and laterally to the quadratus lumborum. Above the level of the ASIS, they penetrate the transversus abdominis.

The iliohypogastric nerve courses between the transversus abdominis and internal oblique and has branches in the lateral and anterior cutaneous distribution. The lateral cutaneous branch runs between the internal and external oblique above the iliac crest and gives sensation to the posterolateral gluteal skin. The anterior cutaneous branch runs medial to the ASIS, extending through the external oblique aponeurosis above the superficial inguinal ring and innervating the skin in the suprapubic region.

The ilioinguinal nerve pierces through the internal oblique, traversing the inguinal canal below the spermatic cord. It terminates through the superficial inguinal ring to innervate the medial skin of the thigh. It innervates the superficial skin of the genitalia of males and females.

Normal anatomic variations exist wherein the iliohypogastric and ilioinguinal may coalesce which gives variation in dermatomal patterns.

Ultrasound Approach The patient is positioned supine, and a high-frequency linear probe is obtained to provide optimal field scope. Initially, the ASIS is scanned posteriorly and superiorly. When the probe is placed perpendicular to the direction of the ilioinguinal and iliohypogastric nerves (ASIS laterally and pointing toward umbilicus medially), the iliac crest appear hyperechoic and three abdominal muscle layers may be observed including the external oblique, internal oblique, and transversus abdominus (**Fig. 88-16**). If the muscle layer anatomy is not clear at the ASIS, one should identify the transversus abdominis plane more laterally over the iliac crest and then translate the fascial plane between

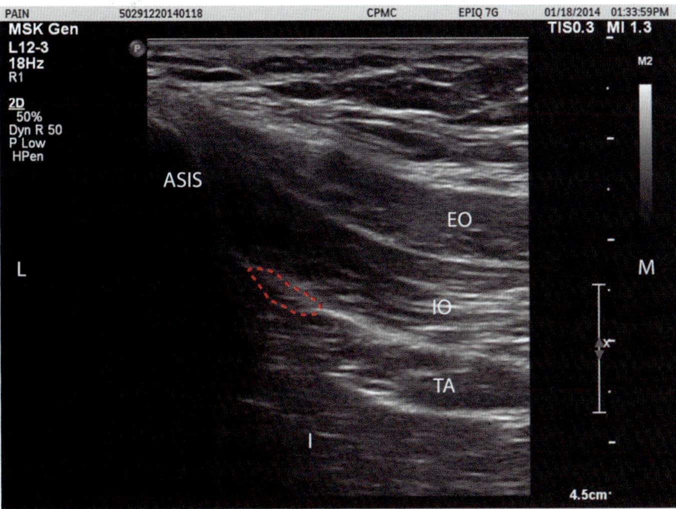

FIGURE 88-16. Ilioinguinal and iliohypogastric nerve in transverse abdominis plane.

internal oblique and transversus abdominis to the medial aspect of the ASIS. Adjusting the probe caudally or cephalad may optimize the view. The peritoneum can be clearly visualized underneath the transversus abdominis medially, and the iliacus muscle is noted deep to the transversus abdominis laterally near the iliac crest. As the muscles are visualized, the ilioinguinal and iliohypogastric nerves can be noted to run between the fascia of the internal oblique and transversus abdominis layer and are usually within 1.5 cm of the iliac crest at this site with the ilioinguinal nerve closer to the iliac crest. Identifying the deep circumflex iliac artery can be helpful in identifying the target nerves as they generally lie on either side of the artery (**Fig. 88-17**). Doppler flow visualization can be especially helpful.

Using an in-plane medial to lateral technique for injection is optimal as this decreases the risk for bowel injury if the needle is advanced too far.

PERIPHERAL NERVE BLOCKS OF LOWER EXTREMITIES

SAPHENOUS NERVE BLOCK

Anatomy The saphenous nerve is a purely sensory, terminal branch of the femoral nerve which itself originates from the L3 and L4 spinal nerves. During its anatomic course, the saphenous nerve is a branch of the posterior division of the femoral nerve and descends through the femoral triangle, lateral to the femoral sheath, and lateral to the femoral artery, behind the adductor canal (also known as Hunter's canal). It remains in the adductor canal on the superolateral surface of the femoral artery throughout most of the thigh until the adductor hiatus approximately 10 cm cephalad of the patella. At this point the femoral artery dives deeper and becomes the popliteal artery. The saphenous nerve then follows the descending genicular artery of the knee as it becomes superficial through the sartorius, between the sartorius and gracilis, or between the sartorius and vastus medialis. At the medial aspect of the knee, the saphenous nerve descends posterior to the sartorius and becomes subcutaneous. At this location the saphenous nerve gives off its infrapatellar branches, which innervate and cross the knee. The saphenous nerve then travels along the medial aspect of the tibia and divides into two branches at the distal third of the leg. One branch innervates the medial aspect of the tibia and stops at the ankle and the other branch passes anteriorly to the ankle and innervates the medial aspect of the foot and great toe.

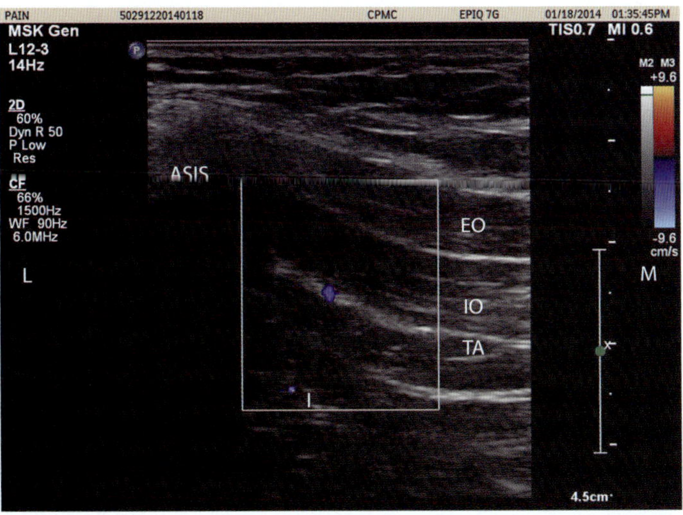

FIGURE 88-17. Ilioinguinal and iliohypogastric nerves with Doppler rendering demonstrating deep circumflex iliac artery.

Ultrasound Approach Optimum positioning for the patient is in the supine position with a slight abduction of the leg with external rotation. Exposure of the medial thigh to the knee is of utmost importance. The nerve is optimally localized in the middle third of the thigh on the medial aspect of the knee. This ensures capture of the saphenous nerve in the adductor canal before it gives off infrapatellar branches to the knee. This nerve is optimally blocked using an in-plane approach with a high-frequency linear ultrasound (7–12 MHz). The probe is placed transverse for initial scanning to identify the femur. Anterior to the femur the vastus intermedius and rectus femoris muscles are seen. The probe is then slowly moved medially, and one can see the rectus femoris transitioning into sartorius and the vastus intermedius transitioning into the vastus medialis (**Fig. 88-18**). The femoral artery is clearly seen deep to the sartorius muscle, with the saphenous nerve lying on its superolateral surface (**Fig. 88-19**). The femoral motor branch to the vastus medialis is also located in the adductor canal and can be visualized and blocked here. It is generally deep to the saphenous nerve.

The saphenous nerve can also be localized at the level of the ankle. The main landmarks in this area are the medial malleolus and the greater saphenous vein. Sometimes a tourniquet can be applied to the leg to improve visualization of the vein and the nerve can be identified near it.

SUPERFICIAL PERONEAL NERVE BLOCK

Anatomy The superficial peroneal nerve is a terminal branch of the sciatic nerve that innervates the peroneus longus and peroneus brevis muscles in the leg. It then emerges from the anterolateral compartment

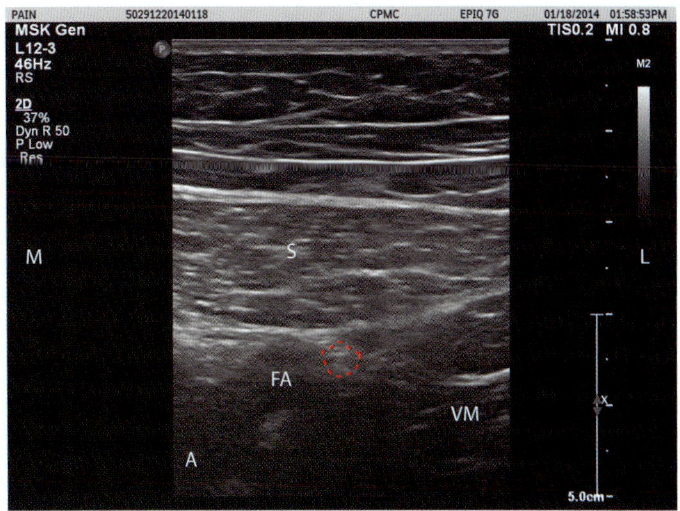

FIGURE 88-18. Saphenous nerve in transverse plane.

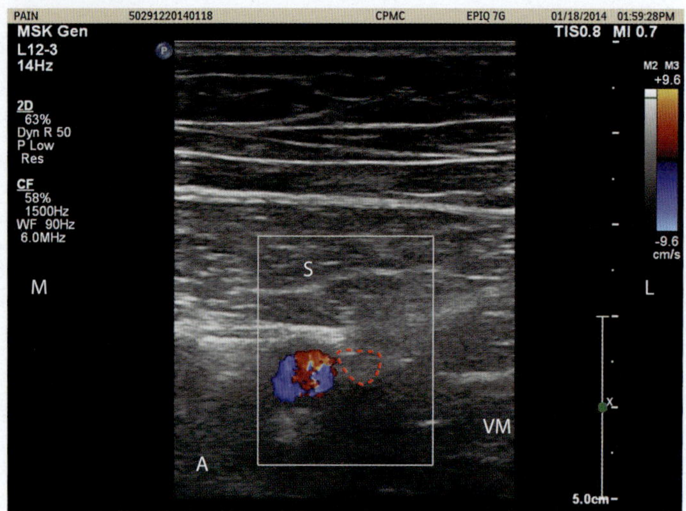

FIGURE 88-19. Saphenous nerve with Doppler flow rendering.

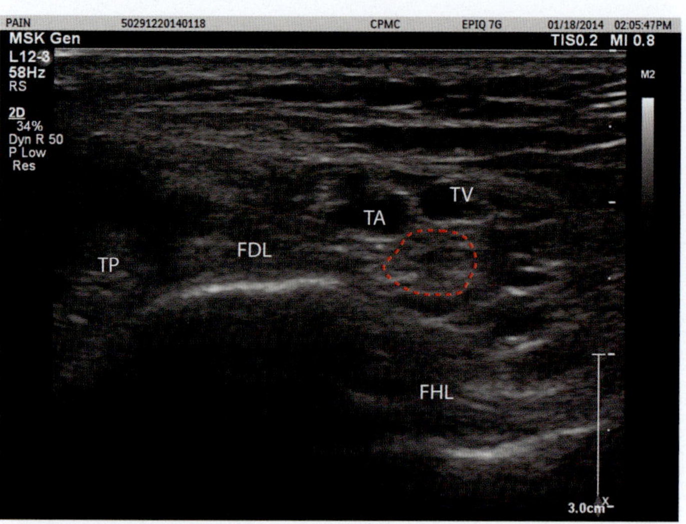

FIGURE 88-21. Tarsal tunnel in transverse plane.

of the lower part of the leg and penetrates the crural fascia above the lateral malleolus and divides into the medial and intermediate dorsal cutaneous nerves. These nerves provide pure sensory innervation to the dorsum of the foot and communicate with the saphenous nerve medially and the deep peroneal nerve in the first webspace as well as the sural nerve on the lateral aspect of the foot.

Ultrasound Approach The patient is placed in a supine position. A linear ultrasound probe is used with a transverse plane to identify the fibula, peroneus brevis, and extensor digitorum longus muscles deep to the crural fascia 10 to 12 cm cephalad to the lateral malleolus (**Fig. 88-20**). Careful scanning cephalad and caudad can identify the point at which the nerve traverses the crural fascia and divides into its terminal branches. One can ask the patient to wiggle the toes and evert the foot to delineate the extensor digitorum longus and peroneus brevis, respectively. The injection is easily performed using an in-plane approach to the nerve.

SURAL NERVE BLOCK

Anatomy The sural nerve is a pure sensory nerve formed by the conglomeration of the lateral sural nerve (a branch of the common peroneal nerve) and the medial sural nerve (a branch of the tibial nerve). Both of these nerves emerge in the popliteal area then decend in the leg and join at a variable location in the leg prior to reaching the ankle. The sural nerve travels between the heads of the gastrocnemius posteriorly and emerges about 10 cm above the lateral malleolus at the level of the lateral Achilles tendon. Here it provides lateral calcaneal branches to the heel, descends behind the lateral malleolus and provides sensation to the Achilles tendon and ankle joint, and terminates on the lateral aspect of the foot, innervating the skin, subcutaneous tissue, fourth digit webspace, and fifth toe.

Ultrasound The patient is placed in a prone position and the linear transducer is placed in short axis across the Achilles tendon laterally, approximately 4 to 5 cm above the posterior heel. A tourniquet is applied to the patient's leg to enhance identification of the lesser saphenous vein. In this position the achilles tendon is located superficial and medial with the lateral malleolus deep and lateral. Between these two structures one will also see the peroneus tendons inside their sheath. The sural nerve is best identified by dynamic scanning near the lesser saphenous vein in this location. An in-plane lateral to medial approach should be undertaken as well as nerve stimulation localization because this nerve is small and often difficult to find.

TIBIAL NERVE

Anatomy The tibial nerve runs behind the medial malleolus and is located laterally and posteriorly to the tibial artery (**Fig. 88-21**). Distal to the medial malleolus, the nerve terminates into the calcaneal nerve and medial/lateral plantar nerves (**Fig. 88-22**). This nerve provides sensation

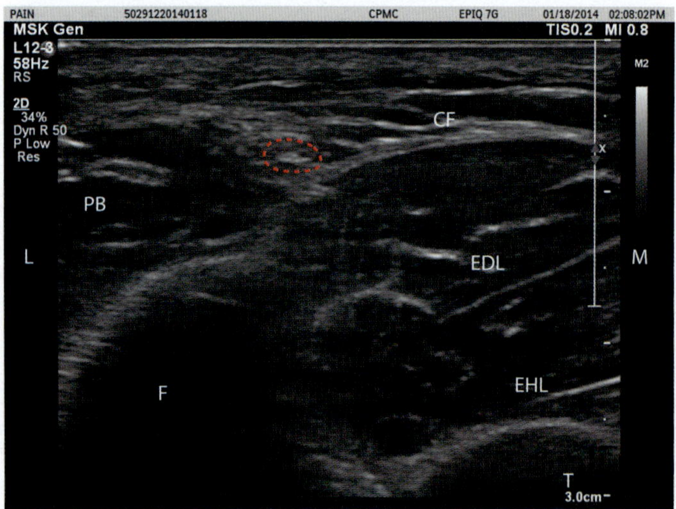

FIGURE 88-20. Superficial peroneal nerve in transverse plane.

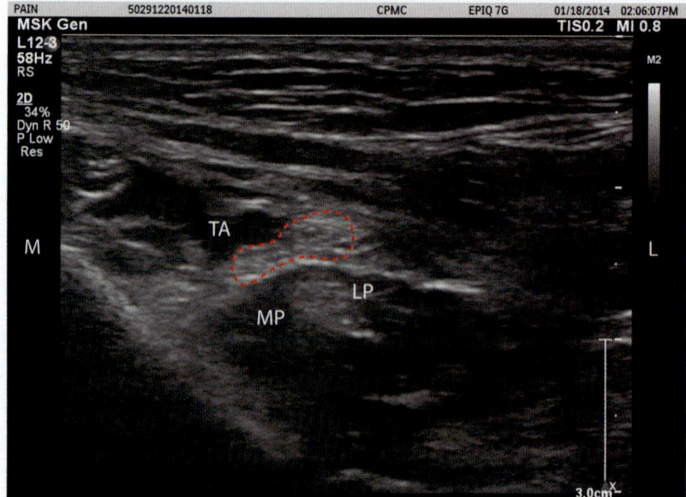

FIGURE 88-22. Tarsal tunnel.

to the Achilles tendon, the inner aspect of the heel, the posterior third of the sole, and the skin in its distribution.

Ultrasound Approach The patient is placed in a supine position and a 10 to 15 MHz linear transducer is placed at the medial ankle between the Achilles tendon and the medial malleolus. The medial malleolus is identified and Doppler may be used to help identify the posterior tibial artery. The tibialis posterior tendon is seen closest to the medial malleolus, followed by the flexor digitorum longus and then the neurovascular bundle. The flexor hallucis longus tendon is generally deep to the neurovascular complex. The posterior tibial nerve is generally medial and posterior to the posterior tibial artery. An in-plane approach is used with nerve stimulation as needed in a lateral to medial approach.

MAJOR JOINT INJECTIONS

GLENOHUMERAL JOINT INJECTION

Anatomy The glenohumeral joint is the conglomeration point of the glenoid cavity and the proximal humeral head. The glenoid labrum, which is cartilaginous, allows the surface area of the joint to expand. The overall articular capsule is weak, although it is strengthened by three glenohumeral ligaments. The joint synovium extends to the bicipital sheath into the intertubercular groove. There is a subacromial bursa which also communicates with the joint capsule.

Ultrasound Approach The patient is positioned facing away from the ultrasonographer and the shoulder is approached posteriorly. A linear transducer is placed along the posterior shoulder with a goal of identifying the humerus in a short-axis view. Once the humerus is identified, the probe is translated cephalad until one sees the humerus broaden and expand into the humeral head, which then inserts into the glenoid cavity (**Fig. 88-23**). The labrum is visualized as a triangular hyperechogenicity coming off the glenoid. The infraspinatus muscle is seen inserting on the greater tubercle of the humerus as well.

Injection of the joint is accomplished by using a posteromedial approach with the humerus adducted across the thorax. A lateral to medial approach is ideal and the target zone is between the humeral head and the glenoid labrum. If the labrum is not well observed, targeting the needle to the humeral head is optimal to avoid damaging labrum. Injectate should be observed coursing through the joint space, not extending into different muscle planes.

Other easily identified targets include the biceps tendon anteriorly (**Fig. 88-24**), the acromioclavicular joint superiorly (**Fig. 88-25**), the subdeltoid subacromial bursa laterally (**Fig. 88-26**), and the axillary nerve posteriorly (**Fig. 88-27**).

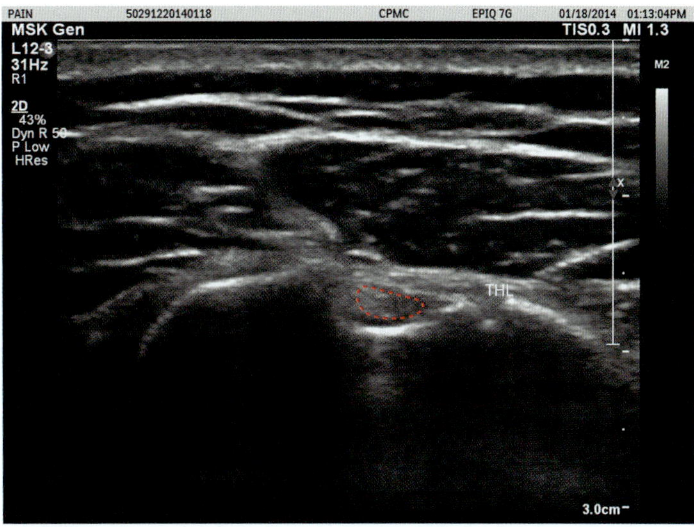

FIGURE 88-24. Biceps tendon.

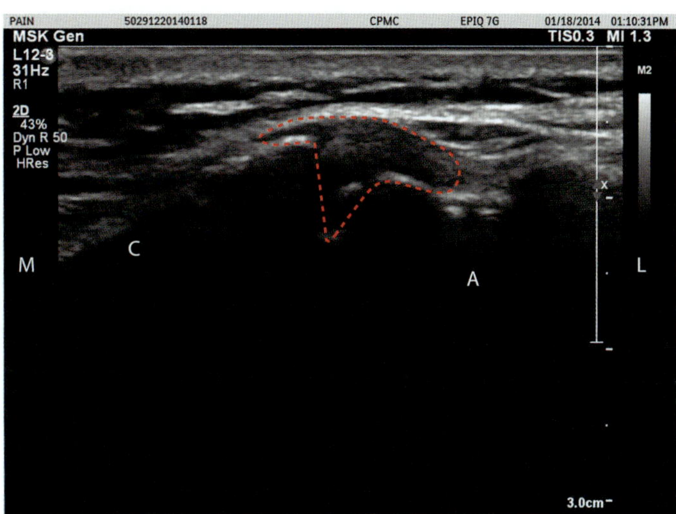

FIGURE 88-25. Acromioclavicular joint.

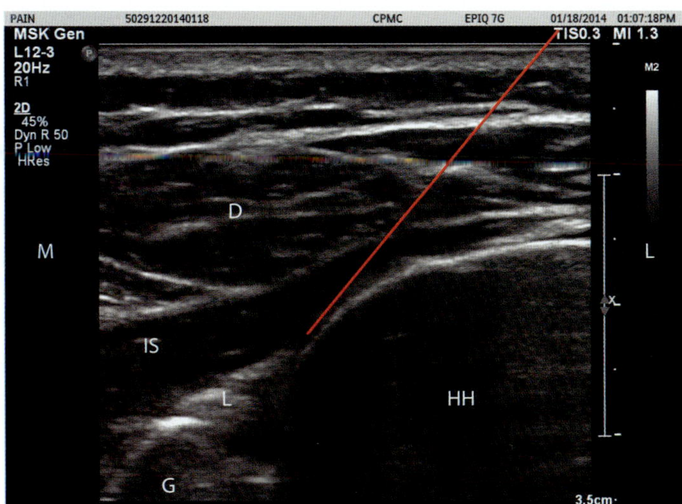

FIGURE 88-23. Glenohumeral joint.

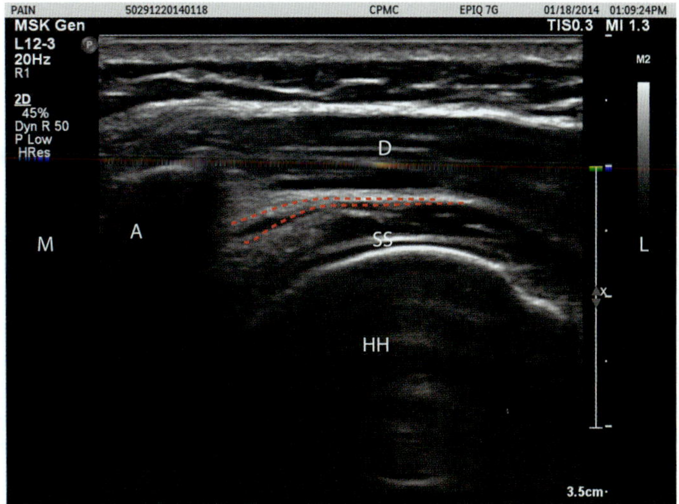

FIGURE 88-26. Subdeltoid and subacromial bursa.

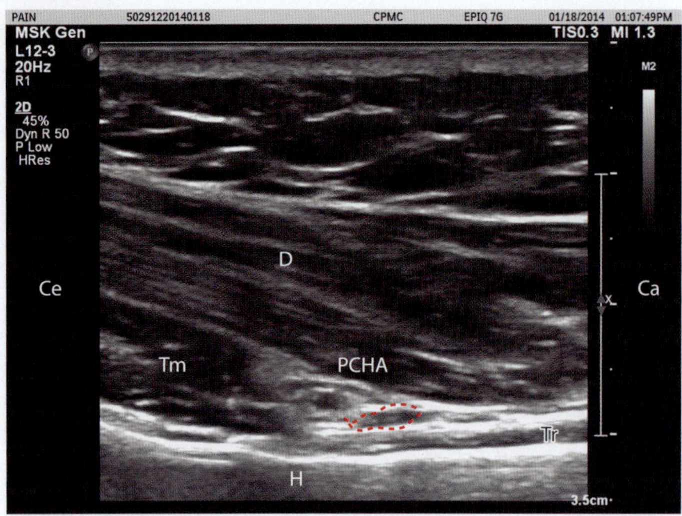

FIGURE 88-27. Axillary nerve.

INTRAARTICULAR HIP INJECTION

Anatomy The hip is a synovial joint that permits a wide range of motion due to its ball and socket conformation between the acetabulum and the femoral head. The labrum deepens the cavity of the acetabulum and permits extensive movement. Multiple ligaments traverse the joint as well, including the iliofemoral, ischiofemoral, and pubofemoral. The head of the femur attaches to the acetabulum by the ligamentum teres femoris.

Ultrasound Approach The patient is placed in a supine position with the hip in a neutral position. A curvilinear probe is utilized with the injection target at the anterior synovial recess at the junction between the femoral head and the femoral neck. Initially a short-axis view of the femur is obtained. The probe is moved cephalad, and the femur is monitored as it broadens and expands into the greater trochanter. At this point, the medial aspect of the transducer is pointed cephalad toward the acetabulum, and minor movements should bring the junction of the femoral neck and femoral head into view (**Fig. 88-28**). Superiorly, the labrum can be observed as a triangular structure. Use of Doppler flow should be utilized to avoid the anterior circumflex femoral artery on the trajectory of the needle (**Fig. 88-29**). The needle approach is in-plane inferolateral to superomedial with an end point at the juncture of the femoral neck and head.

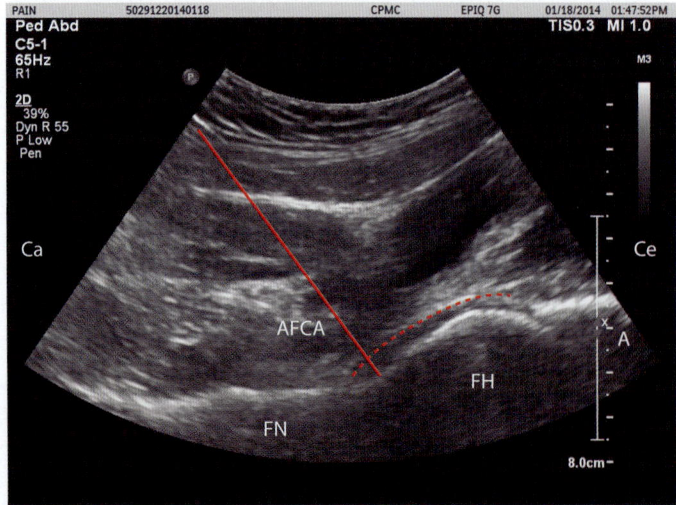

FIGURE 88-28. Intra-articular hip approach.

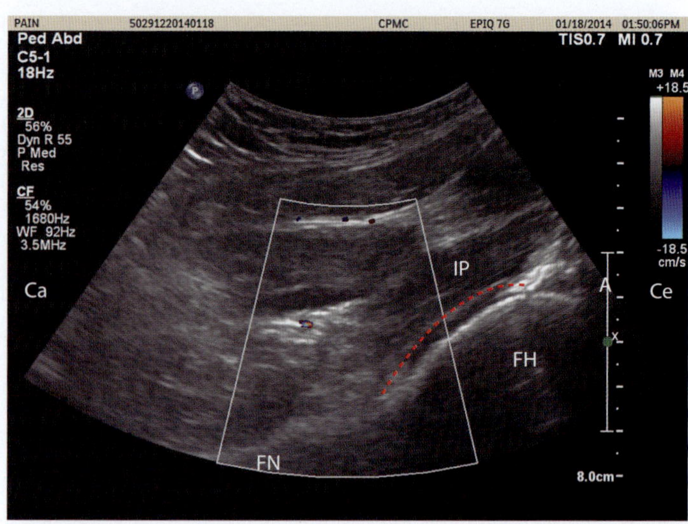

FIGURE 88-29. Doppler approach to intra-articular hip injections.

INTRAARTICULAR KNEE INJECTION –SUPRAPATELLAR APPROACH

Anatomy The knee joint is made up of the culmination of the femur and the tibia and the association of the femur and patella. It is a hinge joint, allowing flexion and extension with a modicum of movement with internal and external rotation. Of greatest importance to the ultrasonographer is the fact that the suprapatellar recess is contiguous with the synovial cavity of the knee joint. This allows access to the joint without traversing bony structures (patella). Important structures to visualize include the vastus tendons inserting on the patella, the patella, the prepatellar fat pad, the prefemoral fat pad, the femur, and the suprapatellar recess.

Ultrasound Approach The patient is placed supine with the knee flexed 30 to 40 degrees, with a foam padding or pillow placed underneath the knee. A high-frequency linear probe is utilized in order to observe these superficial structures. The quadriceps tendon is visualized by first placing the probe in a long-axis fashion over the suprapatellar area (**Fig. 88-30**). The prepatellar fat pad is visualized deep to the tendon, over the suprapatellar recess, and cephalad of the patella. Deep to the suprapatellar recess is the prefemoral fat pad and femur. The suprapatellar recess is generally sigmoid-shaped from patella to quadriceps tendon.

In order to minimize the risk of quadriceps tendon damage, the intra-articular injection is best done after changing from a long-axis

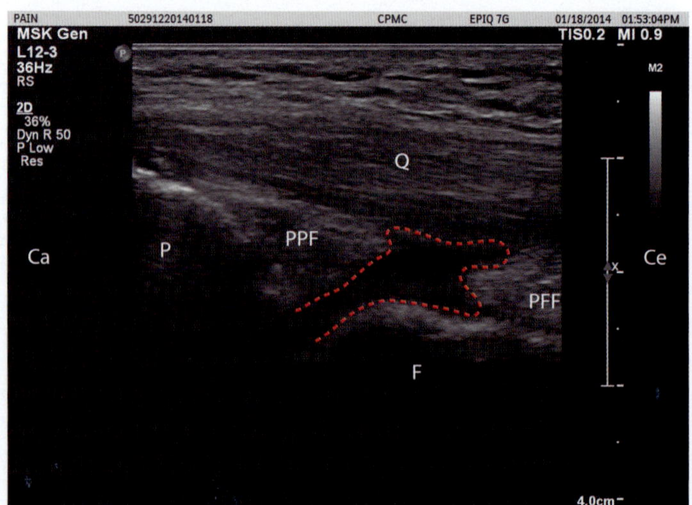

FIGURE 88-30. Intra-articular knee approach sagittal approach.

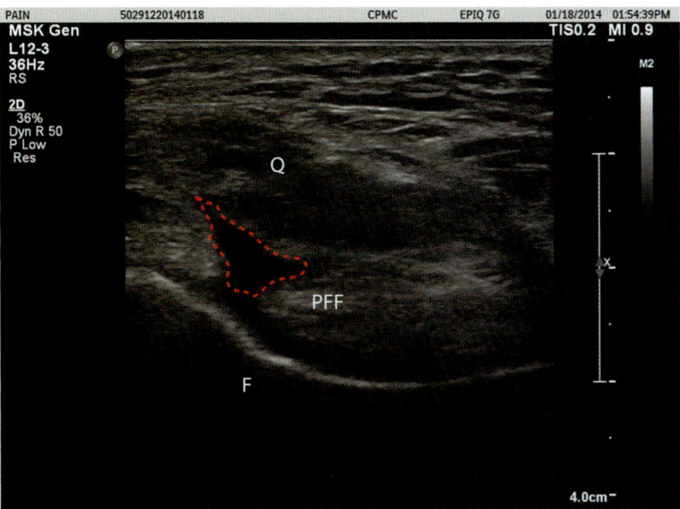

FIGURE 88-31. Intra-articular knee approach in transverse plane.

view (see Fig. 88-30) to a short-axis view over the suprapatellar recess (**Fig. 88-31**). Then a lateral to medial in-plane approach can easily be taken to enter the suprapatellar recess.

CONCLUSION

Although fluoroscopy may be the gold standard for the pain physician, ultrasound imaging has many advantages, especially in soft-tissue diagnostics and therapeutics. Rather than reliance on bony landmarks using fluoroscopy or direct nerve stimulation using a nerve stimulator, ultrasound allows direct visualization of most soft tissues to allow more specific delivery of medication.

Benefits of ultrasound include low cost of the technology, low footprint in clinic, portability, ability for dynamic scanning, enhanced soft-tissue visualization, lack of ionizing radiation to patient and physician, and real-time needle guidance. The inability of ultrasound to see through bone or recognize intravascular injection with injection of intravenous contrast means that fluoroscopy will remain the preferred imaging modality for most pain physician procedures.

CHAPTER 89

Intrathecal Drug Delivery: An Overview of Modern Concepts in Advanced Pain Care

Jason E. Pope
Timothy R. Deer

HISTORY OF THE THERAPY

The concept of placement of drugs into the cerebral spinal fluid (CSF) to impact a patient's perception or sensation is not a novel concept. In the early 19th century scientists and physicians sought this route to impact health care. Early pioneers of this therapy can be traced back to the origins of spinal anesthesia, and many people are responsible for the current state of the art.[1] In 1885, Corning performed the first "spinal block." This was followed by August Bier in Germany, who was a self-volunteer for a spinal injection. In 1898, the first spinal anesthetic was documented using cocaine as the drug, followed in 1901 with the first epidural used for pain treatment. The use of corticosteroids for treatment of pain occurred in 1952. Development of newer agents slowed at this point, with no major advances until the 1980s when intrathecal morphine and intrathecal baclofen were approved for the treatment of chronic pain and spasticity, respectively.[2] Ziconotide received US Food and Drug Administration (FDA) approval in 2004 as a non-opioid intrathecal alternative for treatment of pain. Current studies have been conducted on hydromorphone, gabapentin, octreotide, and new calcium channel blocking drugs, but no new positive reports have been noted. The history of intrathecal therapy has been shaped by a series of consensus conferences that have given guidance based on information provided by experts in the field. The history to be written in the next decade will most likely focus on new drugs and improved safety.

INTRODUCTION

Intrathecal drug delivery (IDD) has undergone a renaissance in the last few years, positioning the therapy as less of a salvage therapy in the pain care algorithm and earlier in patients who fail more conservative therapies. Advances in the platform technology, including patient-controlled bolusing, as well as new medications positioned as monotherapy, including ziconotide, suggest that intrathecal therapy will continue to be an important strategy in the pain care armamentarium. This chapter focuses on methods to improve outcomes and to position drugs properly in the pain treatment algorithm. The abuse of opioids given by the oral route has made this a particularly timely issue, since proper use of intrathecal administration of opioids may deter the escalating use of opioids and thus may reduce morbidity and mortality from currently used strategies.

As with any therapy, outcomes depend largely on patient selection. This chapter will discuss pharmacokinetics and pharmacodynamics of the intrathecal space, patient indications, candidacy, methodology for trialing and therapy initiation, maintenance strategies, efficacy, and comorbidities associated with intrathecal therapy and then comment on future directions.

OVERVIEW

Simply stated, IDD is a platform to deliver medication into the intrathecal space. It does not define a specific therapy. The theoretical advantages of intrathecal therapy, in contrast to systemic therapy, include delivery of medications largely to the site of action, i.e., the dorsal horn of the spinal cord, thus avoiding systemic exposure, increasing potency, and reducing the required dose. A reduction in dose and systemic exposure reduce side effects[3] (**Table 89-1**).

In order to use chronic intrathecal therapy strategies the physician implants a device in the subcutaneous tissues to act as a drug reservoir. This reservoir houses the medication and is depleted through infusion into the intrathecal space. This drug delivery mechanism and subsequently the volume delivered are controlled by programmable reservoir or, in the case of nonprogrammable pumps, occur via constant pressure on the reservoir. As medication is depleted from the reservoir, it requires replacement, necessitating a refill procedure. Most of the morbidity and mortality associated with intrathecal therapy centers on iatrogenic causes, specifically around the refill and reprogramming of the device.[4] The refill procedure is commonly done blindly, without image guidance. When accessing the reservoir fill port is difficult, image guidance is suggested and can be accomplished by ultrasound or fluoroscopy.[5]

TABLE 89-1 Comparison of Intrathecal and Systemic Drug Delivery

Intrathecal Drug Delivery	Systemic Drug Delivery
Medication delivered near site of action pharmacodynamically	Systemic delivery via blood to spinal cord
Low systemic exposure	High serum blood concentration
Drug potency increased	Dose needed commonly has side effects

(From Yaksh TL, De Kater A, Dean R, Best BM, Miljanich GP. Pharmacokinetic analysis of ziconotide (SNX-111), an intrathecal N-type calcium channel blocking analgesic, delivered by bolus and infusion in dog. *Neuromodulation.* 2012;15:508-519.)

The duration of the battery within the reservoir is typically 7 to 10 years, and although the mechanics behind the deployment of volume from the reservoir differ based on the manufacturer, the refill procedure is largely the same. Battery life can vary dependent upon the flow rates of the device, and the complexity of the programming. External variables include pressure on the catheter within the spine, development of granuloma, and impact of drugs on the internal pump catheter and rotor.

DEVICES

The Synchromed II by Medtronic is an implantable, programmable device.[6] It has a geared, rotor mechanism. The programming allows for simple continuous rate, flex dosing (dosing with variable increases in volume of delivery), and has a patient-activated bolusing strategy, termed the patient therapy manager, which functions like patient-controlled analgesia (PCA) in the inpatient setting. It is magnetic resonance imaging (MRI)-compatible, with the advisory to read the pump before and after the scan, without the need to remove medication from the internal tubing or reservoir. If the pump were to malfunction during MRI scan, a motor stall could occur, without restarting, causing an abrupt withdrawal of the therapy potentially creating loss therapy and/or withdrawal symptoms. The failure to restart the pump could be a critical event in a patient, but should be enthusiastically pursued in those with ongoing baclofen infusion since withdrawal of this drug can lead to significant morbidity and potential death. The abrupt withdrawal of clonidine can lead to hypertension and other issues, so vigilance for patients with this drug infusing is critical.

Medtronic has improved Synchromed II by making sutureless connectors, a new catheter, and an anchor that can be injected around the catheter. The impact of these features on the outcome of the device has not been evaluated (**Fig. 89-1**).

The Prometra pump by Flowonix is an implantable, programmable pump.[7] The accuracy, efficacy, and safety of the Prometra pump were assessed in clinical trials, demonstrating an accuracy of 97.1%, with a 90% confidence interval of 96.2% to 98.0%.[8,9] The Prometra pump employs a valve-gated dose regulation system, in contrast to the peristaltic pump roller system. Evidence suggests improved volume delivery accuracy of Prometra compared with the Medtronic Synchromed II.[8] The pump is MRI-compatible only after removal of the medication completely from the reservoir and could result in inadvertent overdose. There currently is no PCA dosing strategy available. In the informed consent process the patient should be made aware of the MRI precautions. Noncompliance of patients with the instructions can lead to overdose and morbidity and mortality. Flowonix is actively pursuing a new generation of pumps that have similar MRI properties to Medtronic and have PCA properties. These features are not currently approved by the FDA (**Fig. 89-2**).

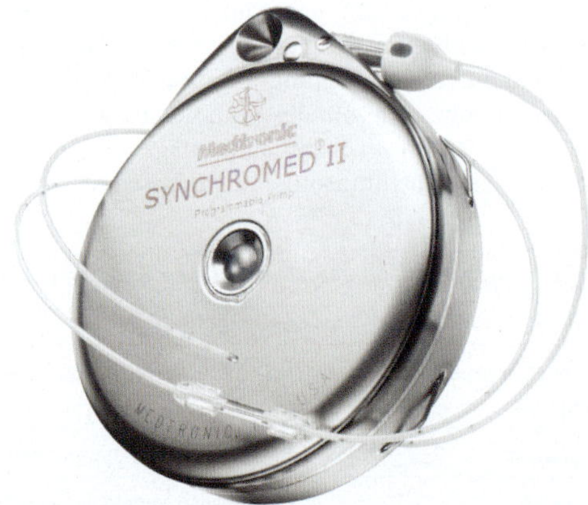

FIGURE 89-1. Medtronic Synchromed II Intrathecal Pump, the health care provider programmer and the patient therapy manager. (Courtesy of Medtronic)

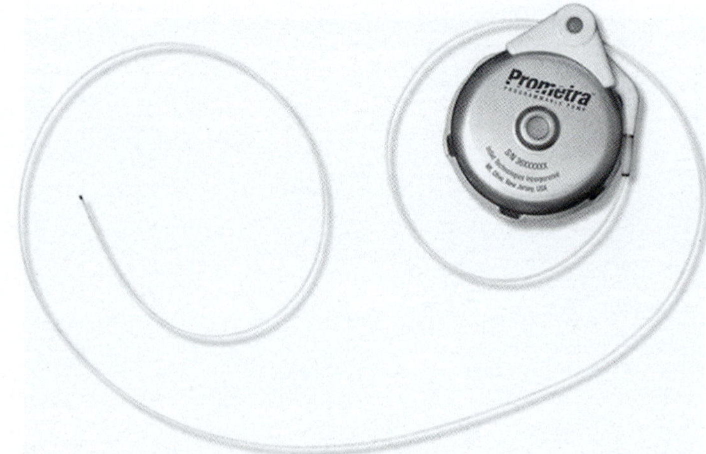

FIGURE 89-2. Flowonix Prometra Pump with Programmer. (From Rauck R, Deer T, Rosen S, Padda G, Barsa J, Dunbar E, et al. Accuracy and efficacy of intrathecal administration of morphine sulfate for treatment of intractable pain using the prometra programmable pump. *Neuromodulation*.)[8]

The Codman 3000 pump is a constant flow device that does not require a battery and in theory does not require replacement because it works on a pressurized constant flow platform.[10] The use of this device has been limited in the United States because of the limitation in adjusting dose, and to making changes without changing the drug in the reservoir. In some countries with limited health care resources, nonprogrammable pumps are still in favor, but the cost analysis may be adverse since the cost of changing the drug at more frequent intervals can be inefficient and costly (**Fig. 89-3**).

Codman has developed a programmable pump for use in the United States and in International markets, termed the Medstream programmable infusion system. The advances targeted by this device include a mechanism that does not involve a rotor, a "fuel" gauge that will give actual pump volumes rather than set volumes, and certification for use in 3-Tesla MRI systems. Clinical experience with this device is currently limited, so conclusions regarding accuracy and efficacy would be premature. There was a recall regarding the fill level sensor, with errors occurring casing the low reservoir alarm to sound too early or too late[11] (**Fig. 89-4**).

PHARMACODYNAMICS AND PHARMACOKINETCS

A great deal of debate has occurred over the years regarding the way that drugs disperse after intrathecal catheter delivery. In many circumstances, "experts" lectured on drug dispersion with actual poor modeling of the events that occurred in the human or even in the animal model. With this background it is reassuring that the understanding of pharmacokinetic modeling with intrathecal drug administration has gained considerable traction in recent years. It is well characterized that there is very little bulk CSF flow, and rather oscillatory movement with

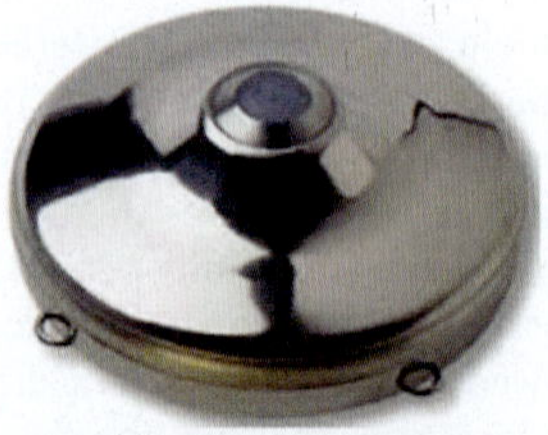

FIGURE 89-3. Codman 3000 image. (From http://www.accessdata.fda.gov/scripts/cdrh/cfdocs/cfpma/pma.cfm?start_search=1&sortcolumn=do_desc&PAGENUM=500&pmanumber=P890055)[10]

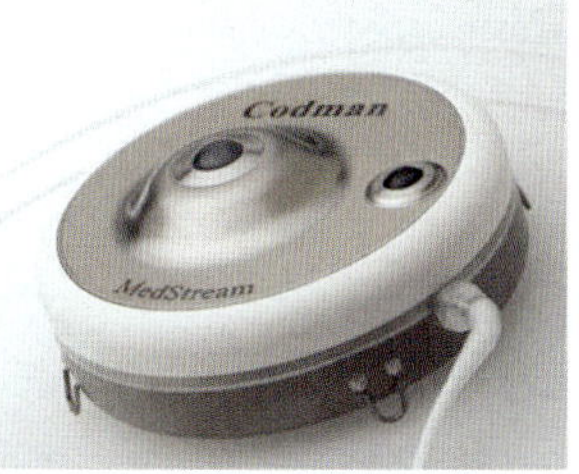

FIGURE 89-4. Codman Medstream.

locomotives of cardiac and pulmonary origin.[11-14] Further, the intrathecal space is nonhomogenous, allowing for complex mixing in different anatomic regions of the spine, as demonstrated by radiographic, biochemical, and mathematical modeling,[11,12,15] suggesting an interregional poorly mixed system.[16]

It is important to understand intrathecal pharmacokinetics in the large animal model in order to make extrapolations to the human. In recent upright and horizontal pig models, with volumes delivered commonly by IDD per day, suggests that the spread from the catheter tip is limited.[17] In addition, the physiochemical properties of the drug delivered play a large role in the dispersion from the catheter tip[17-19] (**Fig. 89-5**).

As demonstrated, drug spread is dependent on the rate and volume delivered. Once placed, the injectate is dispersed because of the oscillatory mixing, as well as a second elimination phase out of the intrathecal compartment. The second phase is contingent on the physiochemical properties of the medication, as well as ongoing local dilution, and redistribution out of the CSF. Larger molecules within the CSF are cleared by rostral bulk-flow and absorbed in the arachnoid granules and onto venous drainage.[20,21]

Ziconotide is very large, hydrophilic, and hypobaric at clinically useful concentrations.[22] Currently there is a great deal of debate over the impact of pulsed delivery on dispersion in opposition to constant delivery of drug. The debate involves both efficacy and the development of high concentrations that may contribute to the formation of inflammatory masses (granuloma) at or near the catheter tip.

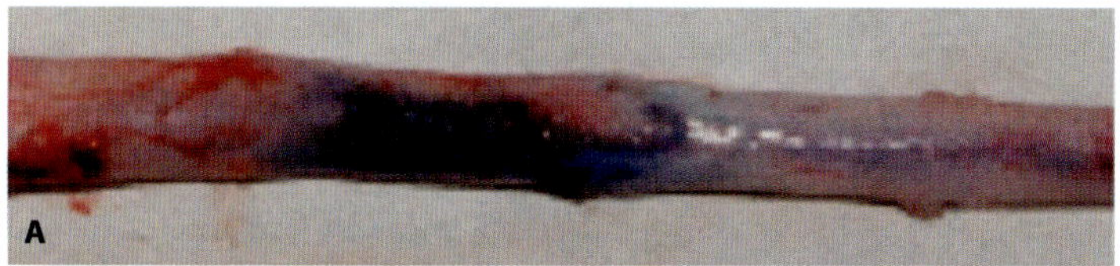

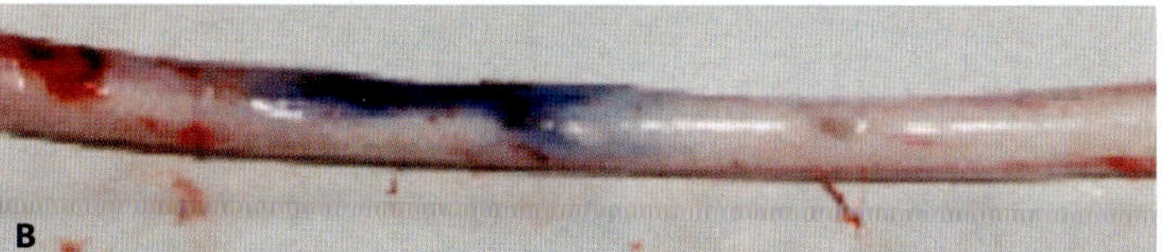

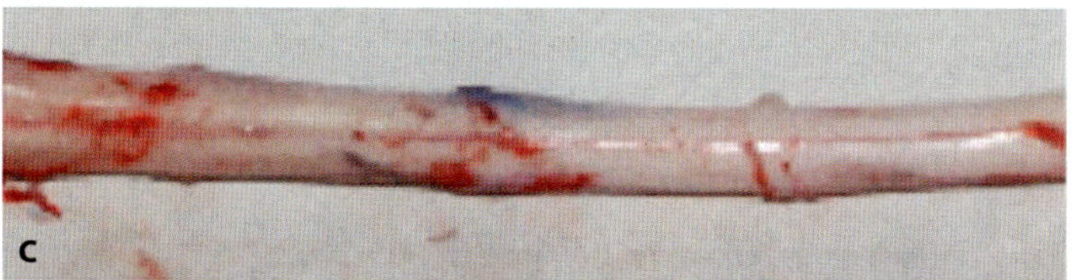

FIGURE 89-5. Dispersion of methylene blue delivered at rate of 20 μL/h for 8 h. This shows most dispersion on posterior portion (A), then lateral (B), with very little anteriorly (C). (From Bernards, CM. Cerebrospinal fluid and spinal cord distribution of baclofen and bupivacaine during slow intrathecal infusion in pigs. *Anesthesiology*. 2006;105:169-78.).[17]

MEDICATIONS

Initially, the choice of medication appears to be a simple decision. For physicians practicing in the United States, the FDA has approved only preservative-free morphine and ziconotide for treatment of chronic pain and baclofen for treatment of spasticity and movement disorders. This simplification does not represent best clinical practice nor does it lead to good outcomes in many patients.[23] Two surveys have been published involving the use of intrathecal therapies.[24,25] The surveys showed that in over 60% of patient case histories, morphine as an initial intrathecal therapy failed to produce pain relief or included unacceptable side effects. Failure of initial therapy led to the use of other agents and polyanalgesia.[24] Initially this was done in a disorganized, unsafe, and often illogical manner. A panel of experts, led by Samuel Hassenbusch and Russell Portenoy, provided guidance to the field. The panel was termed the Polyanalgesic Consensus Conference (PACC), and first met in 1999. The recommendations of this panel have led to improved safety, uniformity with algorithmic care, and have set standards for best practices in care. Recent panels have been chaired by one of the authors of this chapter (Deer), and have addressed recent issues to decrease incidence of morbidity and mortality, improve efficacy, and ensure proper trialing methods. Notwithstanding, the main goals of group are to encourage safe and proper use of drug algorithms.[26-29]

In order to address the current state of the art we should consider the most recent version of this expert work group.[29] Recommendations concerning drug choice, concentration limits, and starting doses, were outlined by the PACC in 2012.[29] A panel of experts on behalf of the International Neuromodulation Society (INS) convened on intrathecal therapy to promote safety and efficacy. For the first time in the history of the PACC, the medications tiers were designed based on nociceptive or neuropathic pain. The panel created an algorithmic table for the use of proper drug selections **Tables 89-2** and **89-3**. In order to improve patient safety and to decrease incidence of morbidity and mortality, the PACC recommended conservative starting doses. This was based on

TABLE 89-2 PACC Recommendations or Medication Algorithm for Neuropathic Pain Management[21]

Line 1	Morphine	Ziconotide		Morphine + bupivacaine
Line 2	Hydromorphone	Hydromorphone + bupivacaine or Hydromorphone + clonidine		Morphine + clonidine
Line 3	Clonidine	Ziconotide + opioid	Fentanyl	Fentanyl + bupivacaine or Fentanyl + clonidine
Line 4	Opioid + clonidine + bupivacaine		Bupivacaine + clonidine	
Line 5	Baclofen			

Line 1: Morphine and ziconotide are approved by the US Food and Drug Administration for intrathecal therapy and are recommended as first-line therapy for neuropathic pain. The combination of morphine and bupivacaine is recommended for neuropathic pain on the basis of clinical use and apparent safety.

Line 2: Hydromorphone, alone or in combination with bupivacaine or clonidine, is recommended. Alternatively, the combination of morphine and clonidine may be used.

Line 3: Third-line recommendations for neuropathic pain include clonidine, ziconotide plus an opioid, and fentanyl alone or in combination with bupivacaine or clonidine.

Line 4: The combination of bupivacaine and clonidine (with or without an opioid drug) is recommended.

Line 5: Baclofen is recommended on the basis of safety, although reports of efficacy are limited.

TABLE 89-3 PACC Recommendations or Medication Algorithm for Nociceptive Pain Management[21]

Line 1	Morphine	Hydromorphone	Ziconotide	Fentanyl
Line 2	Morphine + bupivacaine	Ziconotide + opioid	Hydromorphone + bupivacaine	Fentanyl + bupivacaine
Line 3	Opioid (morphine, hydromorphone, or fentanyl) + clonidine			Sufentanil
Line 4	Opioid + clonidine + bupivacaine		Sufentanil + bupivacaine or clonidine	
Line 5	Sufentanil + bupivacaine + clonidine			

Line 1: Morphine and ziconotide are approved by the US Food and Drug Administration for Intrathecal therapy and are recommended as first-line therapy for nociceptive pain. Hydromorphone is recommended on the basis of widespread clinical use and apparent safety. Fentanyl has been upgraded to first-line use by the consensus conference.

Line 2: Bupivacaine in combination with morphine, hydromorphone, or fentanyl is recommended. Alternatively, the combination of ziconotide and an opioid drug can be employed.

Line 3: Recommendations include clonidine plus an opioid (i.e., morphine, hydromorphone, or fentanyl) or sufentanil monotherapy.

Line 4: The triple combination of an opioid, clonidine, and bupivacaine is recommended. An alternate recommendation is sufentanil in combination with either bupivacaine or clonidine.

Line 5: The triple combination of sufentanil, bupivacaine, and clonidine is suggested.

the need to eliminate postimplant respiratory depression. Adherence to these starting doses can lead to improved patient safety. **Table 89-4**.

In the same spirit, the PACC recommended limiting the high limits of drug concentrations. The theory behind this recommendation is that by limiting concentration we can improve safety. First, intrathecal granuloma is directly linked to high drug concentrations, particularly of morphine and hydromorphone. Second, excessive increases in concentration can lead to difficulty with compounding, specifically the drug can precipitate and lead to catheter and pump issues. The daily dose has also been limited in these recommendations as a further attempt to improve safety **Tables 89-5** and **89-6**.

In addition to specific drug recommendations the PACC recommended a vigilance to detail when using compounding pharmacies. This

TABLE 89-4 PACC Recommended Starting Doses of Intrathecal Therapy

Morphine	0.1–0.5 mg/d
Hydromorphone	0.02–0.5 mg/d
Fentanyl	25–75 µg/d
Bupivacaine	1–4 mg/d
Clonidine	40–100 µg/d
Ziconotide	0.5–2.4 µg/d

TABLE 89-5 PACC Recommended Maximum Concentrations of Intrathecal Agents

Morphine	20 mg/mL
Hydromorphine	15 mg/mL
Fentanyl	10000 µg/mL
Bupivacaine	30 mg/mL
Clonidine	1000 µg/mL
Ziconotide	100 µg/mL

TABLE 89-6 PACC Recommended Maximum Dose Per Day of Intrathecal Agents

Morphine	15 mg/d
Hydromorphine	10 mg/d
Fentanyl	None
Bupivacaine	10 mg/d
Clonidine	600 µg/d
Ziconotide	19.2 µg/d

includes using pharmacies that are accredited by the proper certifying agencies, employing proper quality and quantitative analysis.

As noted earlier, when discussing IDD in the United States, two medications are approved by the FDA to treat chronic pain: Infumorph (morphine) and Prilat (ziconotide). Morphine delivered within the intrathecal space works pharmacodynamically at the opioid receptors within the dorsal horn, whereas ziconotide, a non-opioid based medication, antagonizes the N-type calcium channels within the dorsal horn.[30,31] Medtronic recently released a statement regarding nonlabeled drugs use within the Synchromed II pump, describing a statistically significant higher incidence of motor rotor malfunction when nonlabeled medications were employed as monotherapy or in combination.[32] If combination therapy is chosen, as suggested as early as line 2 of the PACC, innately some points deserve mention. Literature suggests the stability of medications within the reservoir in mono or combination therapy, should be replaced every 3 to 4 months.[33-38] Further, combination therapy has been demonstrated to slow dose escalation when initiated at onset of intrathecal therapy.[39] Clinical data supports the use of bupivacaine as an adjuvant to opioid to reduce the total required dose of opioid.[40] The combination may lead to a reduction in pump function from 97 months on average to 91 or 92 months based on the Medtronic communication. These risks must be weighed against the risks of therapy failure, granuloma, and dose escalation.[41] The mechanism of early pump failure appears related to internal tubing and rotor stalling. These problems may be resolved going forward with new pump mechanisms.

INDICATIONS

Intrathecal therapy may be used to treat chronic moderate to severe cancer and noncancer pain uncontrolled by more conservative measures. The indications for intrathecal therapy include chronic intractable pain with failure of conservative medical care. The failure may result from lack of efficacy, unacceptable dose escalation or side effects at any dose including very low doses. Conservative care strategies include physical therapy, pharmacotherapy, and lesser interventional care. With the advances in neurostimulation therapies, intrathecal therapy has been positioned commonly following these stimulation strategies;[42] however, it should be positioned as an alternative therapy because it serves a different patient population. In nonmalignant pain, intrathecal therapy is less often positioned as a salvage therapy to treat patients with escalated opioid medications. Elderly patients who suffer from axial back pain and are unresponsive to more conservative therapy or have analgesic benefit from systemic opioids but with intolerable side effects should be considered. In cancer patients, intrathecal therapy is demonstrated to reduce side effects and improve treatment outcomes, with improvement using the Karnofsky Performance Index.[3,44] Common disease processes that lead to pump implantation are listed in **Table 89-7**.

TRIALING AND IMPLANT PROCEDURES

PSYCHOLOGICAL CLEARANCE

Prior to proceeding with a trial for the potential placement of IDD system, an evaluation by psychiatry or psychology is recommended. This evaluation should determine if the patient is stable enough to

TABLE 89-7 Indications for Intrathecal Therapy

Axial back pain
Multiple compression fractures • Discogenic pain • Spinal stenosis • Facet arthropathy
Abdominal pain
Complex regional pain syndrome (CRPS)
Trunk pain • Postherpetic neuralgia
Cancer pain
Analgesic efficacy with systemic opioid delivery with intolerable side effects

undergo the procedure, has a concept of their situation, and has coping skills and support structures to participate in the health care process.[44]

TRIAL PROCEDURE

IDD systems allow a trial period to evaluate potential success of the therapy. The trial procedure is typically performed in one of two ways. Both trialing methods require a 23-hour inpatient observation to determine efficacy and monitor for untoward events, specifically respiratory depression. Awareness of predictable side effects can mitigate complications. Side effects are dose-related, but not linearly. Success is gauged by at least 50% reduction of pain with no intolerable side effects. The physician can measure functional progress during the trial and include this in the decision process. Variables to measure include walking distance, sleep quantity, range of motion, and global perceived impact.

SINGLE-SHOT TRIAL PROCEDURE

Patients are positioned prone or in the lateral decubitus in an operating room or injection suite and strict sterile precautions and drape are followed. Using fluoroscopy, after appropriate topicalization, a 3.5-inch 22-gauge or 25-gauge needle is advanced using anteroposterior (AP) and lateral guidance to enter into the intrathecal space at the L1-2 interspace. After free flow CSF is obtained, 1–2 cc of Isovue is injected to demonstrate myelogram and to survey the intrathecal space for filling defects. Medication is then injected with barbotage. The needle is removed, a small adhesive bandage is placed over the puncture site, and patient is monitored for 23 hours with an opioid injection. In cases where a single-injection of ziconotide or baclofen is given, the physician may determine it is safe and within the standard of care to discharge the patient at 8 hours postinjection if stable. Postinjection spasticity assessment up to 6 to 8 hours is recommended with baclofen trialing.

$$\text{Dose calculation opioids} = \frac{\left(\dfrac{\text{Oral route converted to morphine equivalents}}{300}\right)}{2^{*}}$$

Typical intrathecal morphine dose trials range from 0.1 to 0.5 mg. Conversion from morphine to other opioids is provided. Conversions are not exact and require clinical judgment.

Morphine (mg)	Dialudid (mg)	Fentanyl (μg)
0.1 mg	0.02 mg	10 μg

*the denominator of the equation will increase with escalating doses of medications.

TABLE 89-8 Intrathecal Medication Side Effects

Opioids	Pruritis, urinary retention, pedal edema, sedation, respiratory depression
Ziconotide	Nausea, headache, urinary retention, confusion, dizziness, sedation, psychosis (rare), hallucinations (rare)

Ziconotide dosing typically is initiated as a 2 μg bolus and increased in intervals to a maximum dose of 8 μg with each subsequent trial. Some physicians prefer a single shot of 3 μg, but initial doses should be limited with this as the maximum in most cases. Most common side effects in the immediate injection period with ziconotide include hypotension, urinary retention, and headache (**Table 89-8**). Intravenous hydration is recommended in the periprocedural period with this drug.

CATHETER TRIAL PROCEDURE

Patient preparation positioning is the same as for single shot-procedure. Under AP and lateral fluoroscopic guidance, a 17-gauge Touhy needle is advanced into the epidural space with the standard "loss of resistance" technique, localizing the epidural space. Careful attention to paresthesias is needed during needle placement in patients who have conditions that allow positioning without the need for deep sedation. Some physicians prefer to do the neuro-axial trial in the epidural space. In these patients the procedure is completed at this point once confirmed with preservative-free contrast. Other physicians prefer to trial intrathecally. In these patients, the needle is advanced until CSF is obtained. When CSF flow is adequate, a flexible catheter is threaded, avoiding paresthesias, and the needle is removed. It is important not to withdraw the catheter back into the needle since catheter shearing has been reported. After the needle is removed, the catheter is secured with anchors, suture, and adhesives. Sterile dressings are placed and the patient is covered again. A slow infusion of medication is initiated and titrated to clinical effect up to a reasonable clinical dose. The trial period may be very brief or may require drug and dose manipulation lasting several days. The trial ends when the physician and patient determine the goals have been achieved or, in some patients, goals are not obtainable. If a trial is successful, a permanent implant is considered.

IMPLANT PROCEDURE

After a successful trial, the patient should be reevaluated to determine the willingness, desire and appropriateness to move forward with a permanent implant. The patient returns to the office setting to discuss the trial results with the physician or member of the pain medicine care team. At this visit all questions are answered, the procedure is explained and other patient education is completed. Prior to the procedure, the patient is give chlorhexidine to bathe in the morning of surgery. The patient also undergoes preadmission testing and evaluation by the anesthesia care team. On the day of surgery, the patient is examined and body marking is made to determine placement of the catheter and device. All available films are evaluated before surgery and details of the trial are reviewed. At this point the patient is brought to the operating room and positioned in the lateral decubitus position, with the back flush to the end of the table. The patient is marked and draped and widely prepped with proper sterilizing solution. The procedure is performed with assistance employing fluoroscopic guidance. The steps of the procedure are shown in (**Figs. 89-6** and **89-7**).

After appropriate topicalization, a 3.5-inch incision overlying the paraspinal site and carried down to the lumbodorsal fascia using blunt dissection and electrocautery. It is identified by the glossy fascia appearance. A Weitlaner is commonly used to aid in visualization. After this is accomplished, a small pocket is formed by horizontal dissection along the fascia to accommodate the anchor and stress relief loop.

Using AP and lateral fluoroscopic guidance, an introducer needle is placed contacting the lamina of the vertebral body ipsilateral to the reservoir site. It is then walked off cephalad and medial into the intrathecal

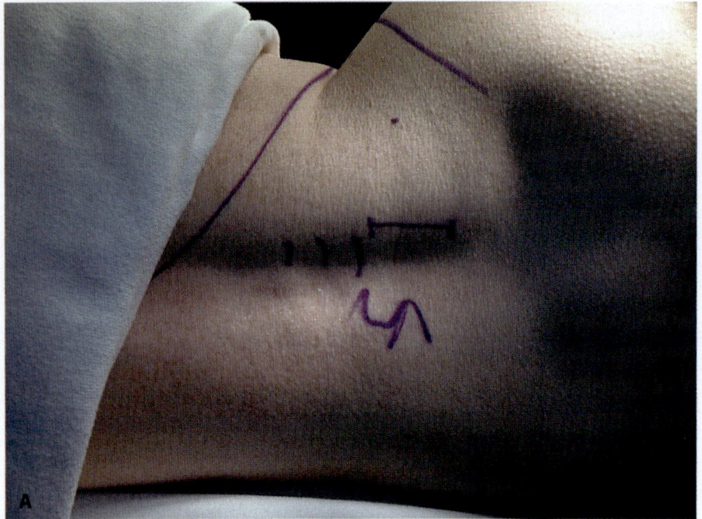

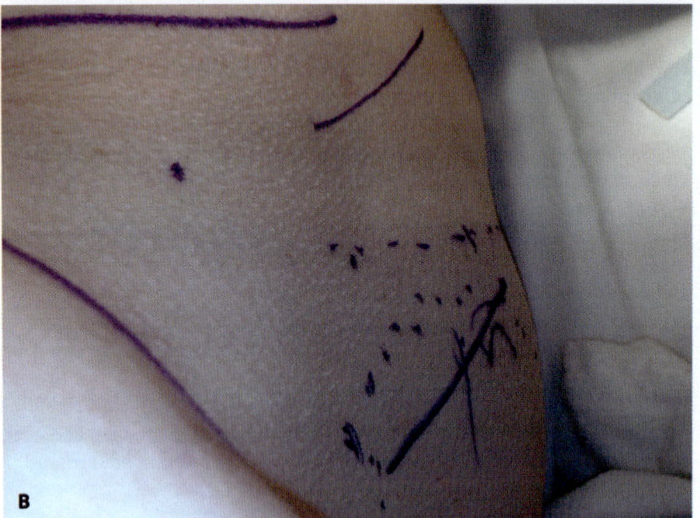

FIGURE 89-6. Preoperative marking of the catheter insertion (A), and reservoir site (B).

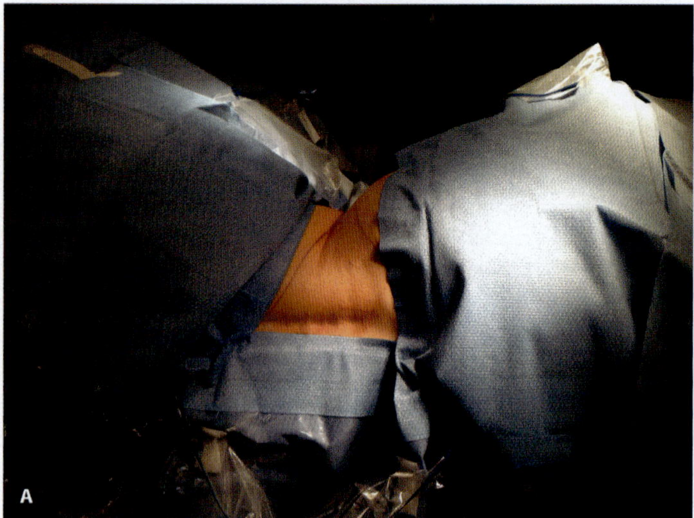

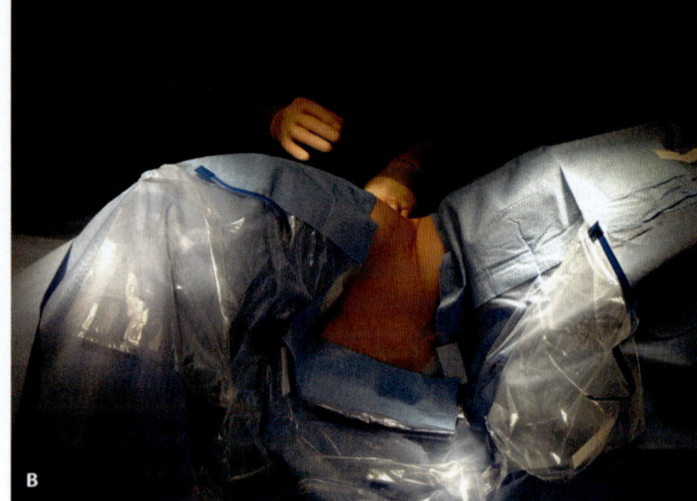

FIGURE 89-7. Sterile prep (A), and drape (B).

space with serial checks in the lateral projection to determine depth while the patient is conversant. Once free flow CSF has been obtained, the catheter is advanced into the CSF again, in the ideal setting, while the patient is conversant (**Fig. 89-8**).

If paresthesias are felt, the catheter is withdrawn and repassed after a fresh needle stick. If resistance is met while threading the catheter, the catheter is withdrawn. After the catheter is in place, the needle and stylet are removed, leaving the catheter within the CSF. It is then secured to the lumbodorsal fascia using an anchor and a nonabsorbable suture. The catheter distal end is then clipped to the drape, and a sterile wet laparotomy pad is placed within the incision (**Fig. 89-9**).

Attention is then directed to the reservoir site. A 5- to 6-cm incision is created to accommodate the diameter of the intrathecal pump. Small rake retractors are used on the caudal side of the incision and pulled outward to create a dissection plane to Scarpas fascia, then replaced by army-navy retractors on either side of the formed pocket. After the pocket is created to accommodate the pump, hemostasis is confirmed, and a saturated lap is placed inside the incision. The tunneling tool is utilized to pass the catheter from the reservoir site to the paraspinal incision. The catheter segments are clipped, measured by the device representative, and the segments are anastomosed (**Fig. 89-10**).

Attention is then directed to the pump for preparation. Commonly, the pump is shipped with sterile water within the reservoir. The water should be removed entirely and discarded. The pump is refilled with the designed therapeutic medication, prior to implant. The catheter is connected to the pump. The incisions are copiously irrigated, the pump internalized, and a layered incision is recommended. Wound closure is an important part of the procedure and attention to proper skin alignment is a priority. A sterile dressing is applied and an abdominal

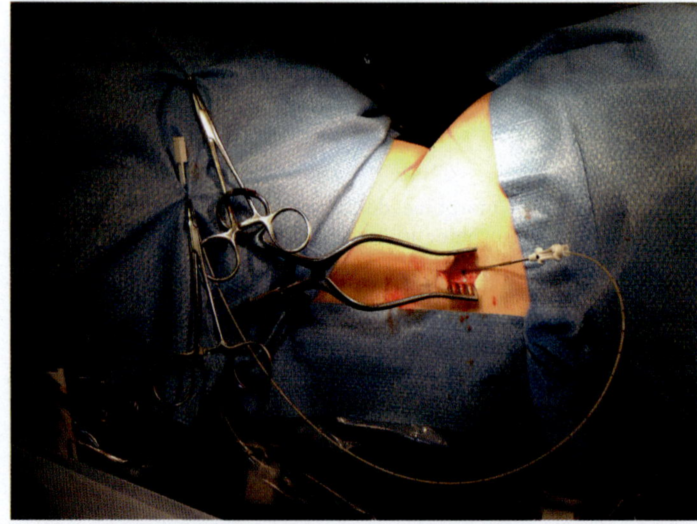

FIGURE 89-8. Catheter placement.

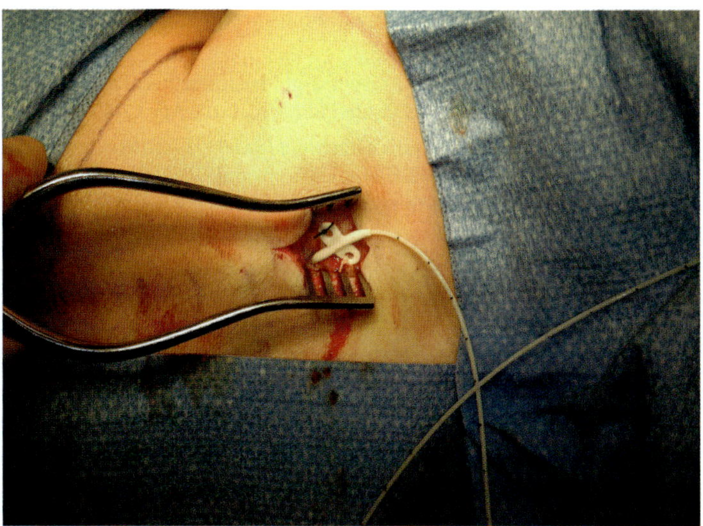

FIGURE 89-9. Securing the catheter with the anchor sutured to the lumbodorsal fascia.

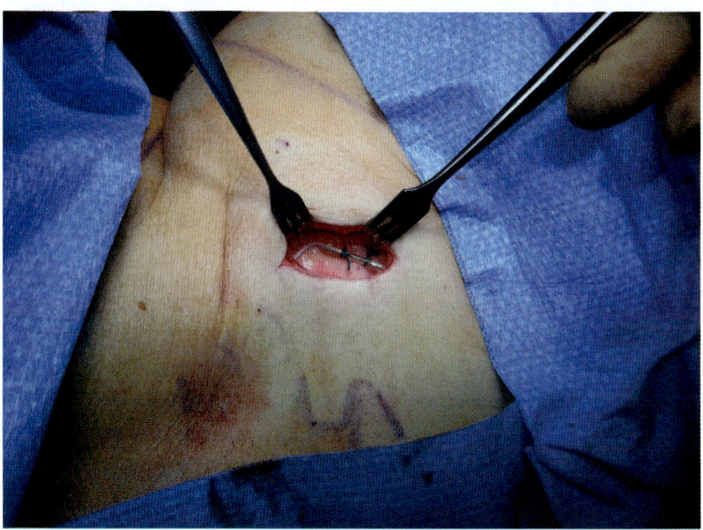

FIGURE 89-10. Anastomosed spinal and pump segments.

binder is placed. Postoperative antibiotics and 23-hour hospitalization are warranted.

MAINTENANCE

Chronic pain requiring IDD should be viewed much like diabetes or hypertension. It is a disease requiring long-term therapy. Care of these patients requires evaluation, assessment, and constant monitoring of the situation. The pump device requires careful titration and attention to determine system integrity. The reservoir requires refill with strict sterile technique and meticulous programming. Much of the morbidity and mortality of intrathecal therapy centers around predictable, although unanticipated, iatrogenic events.[4] The refill procedure requires confirmation of needle placement within the reservoir, either by tactile feel and serial aspiration, visual confirmation under fluoroscopy or ultrasound, or ideally, a combination. In some patients the body habitus leads to pump "flipping" or slipping. In these patients refill may become impossible even with imaging assistance,[5] which is an indication for surgical pump revision.

Catheter evaluations or rotor examinations are performed to confirm the integrity of the drug delivery platform. Under fluoroscopy, the side port is accessed and aspiration attempts are made, to a volume of 2 mL. It is important to note that an unaspiratable side port does not indicate a faulty system, but rather suggests a system integrity issue. In some patients, a catheter that cannot be aspirated is due to scarring near the tip that makes it impossible to aspirate, but the system may still be patent. If the catheter is unaspiratable, it is recommended to avoid injection of Isovue and to inspect for catheter breaks secondary to a potential inadvertent bolus of the medication within the external catheter thus causing an overdose scenario. If the catheter can be aspirated, a myelogram is performed to evaluate flow. If the catheter cannot be aspirated, surgical inspection and revision or ongoing monitoring of volumes and effect may be indicated.

EFFICACY

Intrathecal therapy is well documented to improve pain control and improve function in both cancer and noncancer pain.[45] Intrathecal therapy has level II-2 evidence and level II-3 evidence for cancer and noncancer pain, respectively, as described by the United States Preventative Services Task Force (USPSTF) criteria for evidence-based medicine.[46,47] Landmark work has been done in cancer patients showing superiority of IDD over Comprehensive Medical Management (CMM) in regard to fatigue, and side effects, while achieving relatively better pain relief. The study also showed a trend towards improved survival in the IDD group.[3] This type of landmark study in noncancer patients has not yet been performed. The authors have proposed an IDD versus CMM study in failed back surgery patients, but to date this has not been funded.

RISKS AND COMPLICATONS

In many patients, oral and transdermal opioids lead to side effects such as somnolence, fatigue, anorexia, and malaise that can be reduced or eliminated with much smaller doses given in equianalgesic doses in the intrathecal space. All consequences of long-term systemic opioid therapy are not remedied by intrathecal therapy. Endocrinopathic and immunologic sequelae occur, as well as tolerance and physical dependence.[48] Common opioid related side effects intrathecally include endocrinopathy, urinary retention, pruritus, and fluid retention.[48] Because the device is an implanted therapy, typical perioperative risks are present and should be addressed prior to proceeding. The importance of a communicative patient during needle placement within the intrathecal space and catheter deployment and positioning is paramount. Optimization of the clinical context for placement of the intrathecal device is important. If the patient is unable to tolerate positioning secondary to pain, deeper sedation or analgesia may be required.

Common device-related side effects include infection, bleeding, wound-healing issues, and catheter malfunction. Catheter malfunction is the most common problem; and rarely pump, rotation or flipping, preventing reservoir refill. Biologic-related side effects include infection, bleeding, and seroma.[28] As mentioned, much of the reported morbidity and mortality associated with intrathecal therapy is related to iatrogenic error regarding device maintenance.[4] Further, depositing the medication inadvertently outside of the reservoir (pocket fill) can cause overdose that require hospital admission and vigilant care.

Granuloma is the development of a noninfectious inflammatory mass in the area of the catheter tip that can contribute to cord compression and neurological sequelae. Most commonly these issues occur at concentrations of medications that are elevated outside of the PACC recommendations, although exceptions arise. A granuloma is a noninfectious collection of cells near the catheter tip that can become compressive in nature. Granulomagenic medications include most of the commonly employed intrathecal medications, and are often associated with opioids. There have been no reports of granuloma formation with monotherapy employing ziconotide or fentanyl. If granuloma is suspected secondary to loss of therapy efficacy or new neurologic findings, a plain radiograph should document catheter tip and then a MRI should be performed at that level.[49] Further, a catheter evaluation could be performed prior to revision. Treatment includes cessation of the granulomagenic medication and replacement of catheter, and extremely rarely, a formal neurosurgical decompression is required.

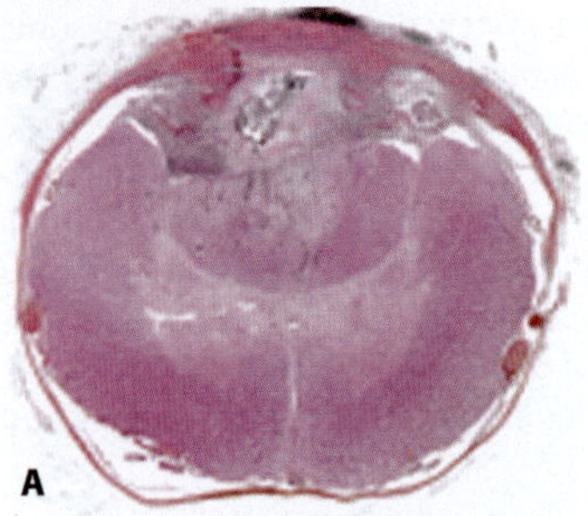

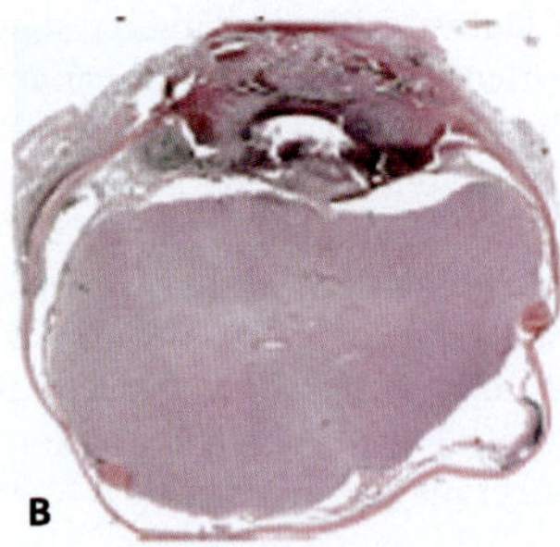

FIGURE 89-11. Granuloma formation with infusion of morphine (A), and hydromorphone (B).[51] (From Allen JW, Horais KA, Tozier NA, Yaksh TL. Opiate pharmacology of intrathecal granulomas. *Anesthesiology*. 2006;105(3):590-598.)

The histological characterizations of these lesions have been well described by Yaksh and colleagues.[50] The figure below shows the histological make up of these lesions (**Fig. 89-11**).

FUTURE DIRECTIONS

The future of IDDS is reassuring, although uncertain. The evaluation of this therapy going forward can be segmented into innovations in the device, the delivery strategy, medications, and expansion of indications.

The device can be seemingly miniaturized, mechanism of propulsion improved, as well as improvement in anchoring and catheter durability. Medtronic has developed a new catheter and anchoring system, and prospective date to gauge improved outcomes is needed. Further, software improvements with greater flexibility in dosing strategies are needed. The opportunity to advance drugs in this field is promising, as evidenced by the failures and sequela associated with opioids and admixtures. Work is currently being done on new drugs that may provide hope to many that suffer. Some of the working drug groups include growth factors, glial activating factors, nitric oxide, gene transfer mechanisms, gastrodin, growth hormone analogs, specific trophic factors, and antiRNA.[52-61] The opportunity to treat chronic pain is well described. Additional positive extensive work has been done for movement disorders. In the area of disease advancement recent interest has been shown in treating seizure disorder, depression, amyotrophic lateral sclerosis, and other degenerative diseases of the neurological system. The advancement in these areas will be based on new drug development, a commitment to clinical research and collaboration between industry, physicians, and scientists.

CONCLUSION

The use of IDDS has become a part of the mainstream algorithm for the treatment of chronic pain of both cancer and noncancerous origin. The proper selection of patients, attention to detail in trialing, excellence in implant techniques, and vigilance in follow up and maintenance can lead to good long-term outcomes. Future research on refining the devices, developing new drugs, and improving best practices for safety may lead to repositioning the therapy away from salvage therapy and placed appropriately earlier in the pain care algorithm.

REFERENCES

1. Deer TR. History of intrathecal drug delivery. Atlas of implantable therapies for pain management. 2011; New York, NY: Springer; 139-141.
2. Krames ES. A history of intraspinal analgesia, a small and personal journey. *Neuromodulation: Technology at the Neural Interspace*. 2012;15(3):172-193.
3. Smith TJ, Staats PS, Deer T, et al. Randomized clinical trial of an implantable drug delivery system compared with comprehensive medical management for refractory cancer pain: impact on pain, drug-related toxicity, and survival. *J Clin Oncol*. 2002;20(19):4040-4049.
4. Coffey RJ, Owens ML, Broste SK, et al. Mortality associated with implantation and management of intrathecal opioid drug infusion systems to treat noncancer pain. *Anesthesiology*. 2009;111:881-891.
5. Gofeld M, McQueen CK. Ultrasound-guided intrarthecal pump access and prevention of the pocket fill. *Pain Med*. 2011 Apr;12(4):607-611.
6. http://www.fda.gov/MedicalDevices/Safety/ListofRecalls/ucm271492.htm (Website of the FDA, US Food and Drug Administration, US Department of Health and Human Services, www.fda.gov)
7. http://www.fda.gov/MedicalDevices/ProductsandMedicalProcedures/DeviceApprovalsandClearances/Recently-Approved Devices/ucm293502.htm (Website of the FDA, US Food and Drug Administration, US Department of Health and Human Services, www.fda.gov)
8. Rauck R, Deer T, Rosen S, et al. Accuracy and efficacy of intrathecal administration of morphine sulfate for treatment of intractable pain using the Prometra Programmable Pump. *Neuromodulation*. 2010 Apr; 13:102-108.
9. Allen JW, Horais KA, Tozier NA et al. Opiate pharmacology of intrathecal granulomas. *Anesthesiology*. 2006;105:590-598.
10. http://www.accessdata.fda.gov/scripts/cdrh/cfdocs/cfpma/pma.cfm?start_search=1&sortcolumn=do_desc&PAGENUM=500&pmanumber=P890055; http://www.fda.gov/MedicalDevices/Safety/ListofRecalls/ucm362016.htm (Website of the FDA, US Food and Drug Administration, US Department of Health and Human Services, www.fda.gov)
11. Battal B, Kocaoglu M, Bulanski N et al. Cerebrospinal fluid flow imaging by using phase-contrast MR technique. *Brit JfRadiol*. 2011;(84):758-765.
12. Bulat M, Klarica M. Recent insights into the hydrodymanics of the cerebrospinal fluid. *Brain Rese Rev*. 2011;65:99-112.
13. Henry-Feugeas MC, Idy-Peretti I, Baledent O, et al. Origin of subarachnoid cerebrospinal fluid pulsations: a phase-contrast MR analysis. *Magn Reson Imaging*. 2000;(18):387-395.
14. Friese S, Hamhaber U, Erb M, et al. The influence of pulse and respiration on spinal cerebrospinal fluid pulsation. *Invest Radiol*. 2004;39:120-130.
15. Stockman HW. Effect of anatomic fine structure on the flow of cerebrospinal fluid in the spinal subarachnoid space. *JBiochem Eng*. 2006;128:106-114.
16. Degrell I, Nagy E. Concentration gradients for HVA, 5-HIAA, ascorbic acid, and uric acid in cerebrospinal fluid. *Biol Psychiatry*. 1990;t 27:891-896.
17. Bernards, CM. Cerebrospinal fluid and spinal cord distribution of baclofen and bupivacaine during slow intrathecal infusion in pigs. *Anesthesiology*. 2006;105:169-178.
18. Flack SH, Bernards CM. Cerebrospinal fluid and spinal cord distribution of hyperbaric bupivacaine and baclofen during slow intrathecal infusion in pigs. *Anesthesiology*. 2010;112:165-175.
19. Flack SH, Anderson CM, Bernards CM. Morphine distribution in the spinal cord after chronic infusion in pigs. *Anesth Analg*. 2011;112(2):460-464.
20. Hejtmanek MR, Harvey TD, Bernards, CM. Measured density and calculated baricity of custom-compounded drugs for chronic intrathecal infusion. *Reg Anesth Pain Med*. January-February 2011;36(1):7-11.
21. Yaksh TL, De Kater A, Dean R, Best BM, Miljanich GP. Pharmacokinetic analysis of ziconotide (SNX-111), an intrathecal N-type calcium channel blocking analgesic, delivered by bolus and infusion in dog. *Neuromodulation*. 2012;15:508-519.
22. Pope JE, Deer TR. Ziconotide: a clinical update and pharmacologic review. *Expert Opinion Pharmacother*. 2013 May;14(7):957-966.
23. Portenoy RK, Savage SR. Clinical realities and economic considerations: special therapetic issues in intrathecal therapy-tolerance and addiction. *J Pain Symptom Manage*. 1997;14(3, Supplement 1):S27-S35.

24. Hassenbusch SJ, Portenoy RK. Current practicies in transpinal therapy—a survey of clinical trends and decision making. *J Pain Symptom Manage.* Aug 2000;20(2):S4-S11.

25. Deer TR, Krames E, Levy RM, Hassenbusch SJ 3rd, Prager JP. Practice choices and challenges in the current intrathecal therapy environment: an online survey. *Pain Med.* 2009 Mar;10(2):304-309.

26. Bennett G, Burchiel K, Buchser E, et al. Polyanalgesic Consensus Conference 2000: clinical guidelines for intraspinal infusion: report of an expert panel. *J Pain Symptom Manage.* 2000;20:S37-S43.

27. Hassenbusch SJ, Portenoy RK, Cousins M, et al. Polyanalgesic Consensus Conference 2003: an update on the management of pain by intraspinal drug delivery:report of an expert panel. *J Pain Symptom Manage.* 2004;27:540-563.

28. Deer T, Krames ES, Hassenbusch SJ, et al. Polyanalgesic Consensus Conference 2007: recommendations for the management of pain by intrathecal (intraspinal) drug delivery: report of an interdisciplinary expert panel. *Neuromodulation.* 2007;10:300–328.

29. Deer TR, Prager J, Levy R, Rathmell J, Buchser E, Burton A, et al. Polyanalgesic Consensus Conference 2012: Recommendations for the management of pain by intrathecal (intraspinal) drug delivery: report of an interdisciplinary expert panel. *Neuromodulation.* 2012.

30. Westenbroek RE, Hoslins L, Cattarall WA. Localization of Ca 2+ channel subtypes on rat spinal motor neurons, interneurons, and nerve terminals. *J Neurosci.* 1998;18(16):6319-6330.

31. Kerr LM, Filloux F, Olivera BM, et al. Autoradiographic localization of calcium channels with [125I] omega-conotoxin in rat brain. *Eur J Pharmacol.* 1988;146:181-183.

32. Medtronic Update: Increased risk of motor stall and loss of or change in therapy with unapproved drug formulations. November 2012.

33. Shields DE, Aclan J, Szatkowski A. Chemical stability of admixtures containing 25 mcg/mL ziconotide and 10 mg/mL or 20 mg/mL morphine sulfate during simulated intrathecal administration. *Int J Pharm Compd.* 2008;12:552-557.

34. Shields D, Montenegro R, Ragusa M. Chemical stability of admixtures combining ziconotide with morphine or hydromorphone during simulated intrathecal administration. *Neuromodulation.* 2005;8:257-263.

35. Shields D, Montenegro R, Aclan J. Chemical stability of admixtures combining ziconotide with baclofen during simulated intrathecal administration. *Neuromodulation.* 2007;10(suppl 1):12-17.

36. Shields D, Montenegro R. Chemical stability of ziconotide-clonidine hydrochloride admixtures with and without morphine sulfate during simulated intrathecal administration. *Neuromodulation.* 2007; 10(suppl 1):6-11.

37. Shields D, Montenegro R, Aclan J. Chemical stability of an admixture combining ziconotide and bupivacaine during simulated intrathecal administration. *Neuromodulation.* 2007;10(suppl 1):1-5.

38. Shields DE, Aclan J, Szatkowski A. Chemical stability of admixtures combining ziconotide with fentanyl or sufentanil during simulated intrathecal administration. *Int J Pharm Compd.* 2008 Sept-Oct;12(5):463-466.

39. Veixi IE, Hayek SM, Narouze S, Pope JE, Mekhail N. Combination of intrathecal opioids with bupivacaine attenuates opioid dose escalation in Cchronic noncancer pain patients. *Pain Med.* 2011;12(10):1481-1489.

40. Deer TR, Caraway DL, Kim CK, Dempsey CD, Stewart CD, McNeil KF. Clinical experience with intrathecal bupivacaine in combination with opioid for the treatment of chronic pain related to failed back surgery syndrome and metastatic pain of the spine. *Spine J.* 2002 Jul-Aug;2(4):274-278.

41. Deer, Kloth editorial PP this month.

42. Deer TR. A critical time for practice change in the pain treatment continuum: we need to reconsider the role of pumps in the patient algorithm. *Pain Med.* 2010;11:987-989.

43. Hollen PJ, Gralla RJ, Kris MG, et al. Measurement of quality of life in patients with lung cancer in multicenter trials of new therapies. *Cancer.* 1994;73(8):2087-2098.

44. Deer TR, Smith HS, Cousins M, Doleys DM, Levy RM, Rathmell JP, Staats PS, et al. Consensus guidelines for the selection and Iimplantation of Ppatients with noncancer pain for intrathecal drug delivery. *Pain Pysician.* 2010;13:E175-E213.

45. Hayek SM, Deer TR, Pope JE, Panchal SJ, Patel VB. Intrathecal therapy for cancer and noncancer pain. *Pain Physician.* 2011;14(3):219-248.

46. Harris RP, Helfand M, Woolf SH, et al. Current methods of the US Preventive Services Task Force: a review of the process. *Am J Prev Med.* 2001;20(suppl 3):21-35.

47. Guayatt GH, Sackett DL, Sinclair JC, Hayward R, Cook DJ, Cook RJ. Users' guides to the medical literature: IX. A method for grading health care recommendations. *JAMA.* 1995;274(22):1800-1804.

48. Benyamin R, Trescot AM, Datta S, et al. Opioid complications and side effects. *Pain Physician.* 2008;11(suppl 2):S105-S120.

49. Phillips JA, Escott EJ, Moosy JJ, Kellemier HC. Imaging appearance of intrathecal catheter tip granulomas: three case and review of literature. *Am J Roentgenol.* December 2007;189(6):W375-W381.

50. Yaksh TL, Allen JW, Veesart SL, Horais KA, Malkmus SA, Scadeng M, et al. Role of meningeal mast cells in intrathecal morphine-evoked granuloma formation. *Anesthesiology.* 2013 Mar;118(3):664-678.

51. Allen JW, Horais KA, Tozier NA, Yaksh TL. Opiate pharmacology of intrathecal granulomas. *Anesthesiology.* 2006;105(3):590-598.

52. Wang R, Guo W, Ossipov MH, Vanderah TW, Porreca F, Lai J. Glial cell Line derived neurotrophic factor normalizes neurochemical changes in injured dorsal root ganglion neurons and prevents the expression of experimental neuropathic pain. *Neuroscience.* 2003;(121):815-824.

53. Aveill S, Michael GJ, Shortland PJ, Leavesley RC, King VR, Bradbury EJ, et al. NGF and GDNF ameliorate the increase in ATF3 expression which occurs in dorsal root ganglion cells in response to peripheral injury. *Eur J Neurosci.* 2004;19:1437-1445.

54. Lin CR, Chen KH, Yang CH, Cheng JT, Sheen-Chen SM, Wu CH, et al. Sonoporation-mediated gene transfer into adult rat dorsal root ganglion cells. *J Biomed Science.* 2010;17:44.

55. Yu H, Fischer G, Jia G, Reiser J, Park F, Hogan QH. Lentivirial gene transfer into the dorsal root ganglion of adults rats. *Mol Pain.* 2011 Aug 23;7:63.

56. Milligan E. Inflammatory mediators for pain. Paper presented at North American Neuromodulation Society Meeting. December 3, 2011; Las Vegas, NV.

57. Jin Y, Kim J, Kwak J. Activation of the cGMP/Protein Kinase G Pathway by nitric oxide can decrease TRPVI activity in cultured rat dorsal root ganglion neurons. *Korean J Physiol Pharmacol.* 2012 Jun;(16):211-217.

58. Kwak J. Capsaicin blocks the hyperpolarization-activated inward currents via TRPV1 in the rat dorsal root ganglion neurons. *Exp Neurobiol.* 2012 Jun;21(2):75-82.

59. Sun W, Miao B, Wang XC, Duan JH, Ye X, Han WJ, et al. Gastrodin inhibits allodynia and hyperalgesia in painful diabetic neuropathic rats by decreasing excitability of nociceptive primary sensory neurons. *PLoS ONE.* 2012 Jun (7)6: e39647.

60. Samad OA, Tan AM, Cheng X, Foster E, Dib-Hajj SD, Waxman SG. Virus-mediated shRNA knockdown of Nav1. 3 in rat dorsal root ganglion attenuates nerve injury-induced neuropathic pain. *Molecular Therapy.* 2013;21(1):49-56.

61. Xu Q, Chou B, Fitzsimmons B, Miyanchara A, Shubayev V, Santucci C, et al. In vivo gene knockdown in rat dorsal root ganglio mediated by self-complementary adeno-associated virus serotype 5 following intrathecal delivery. March 2012;3(3):e32581.

CHAPTER 90

Neuromodulation for Pain

Jennifer A. Elliott
Thomas T. Simopoulos

INTRODUCTION

Neurostimulation techniques have been used in the management of pain for close to 50 years. Transcutaneous electrical nerve stimulation (TENS) represents one of the most widely utilized external neuromodulation devices. Over the past several decades, more complex forms of neurostimulation devices and techniques have been developed and implemented in pain management practice for permanent human implantation. These include peripheral nerve stimulation (PNS), peripheral nerve field stimulation (PNFS), spinal cord stimulation (SCS), and intracranial stimulation (ICS). More patients suffering from intractable pain elect to undergo neurostimulation device implantation after failure of conservative management techniques for pain control. The advantages from a patient's perspective include an essentially side-effect free device under direct patient control that can be dynamically self-adjusted to his or her level of pain and activity.

For physicians, electrical implantable therapies have gained popularity because of safety, long-term efficacy, and cost savings.

The inspiration for development of these technologies came from the landmark "gate control theory" introduced by Melzack and Wall in 1965.[1] Although this model fails to explain certain phenomena seen in painful conditions and cannot account for all of the observed effects of neurostimulation, the gate control theory remains the primary paradigm used to describe how neurostimulation acts to modify pain transmission. The gate control theory is based on the presence of interneurons in the dorsal horn of the spinal cord that receive afferent signals from peripheral C fibers (which convey painful stimuli) as well as nonnociceptive sensory fibers. When pain signals reach these dorsal horn interneurons, a "gate" is activated, allowing painful impulses to propagate along ascending fibers to the brain and resulting in conscious awareness of pain. Wall and Melzack proposed that the "gate" could be closed to transmission of painful impulses by means of selective activation of nonnociceptive sensory fibers. With this hypothesis, the notion of using neurostimulatory devices to preferentially activate nonnociceptive sensory fibers as a means of diminishing pain was born.

The application of neurostimulation has expanded dramatically since C. Norman Shealy implanted the first spinal cord stimulator in 1967. Current indications for the use of these devices (worldwide) include failed back surgery syndrome (FBSS), complex regional pain syndrome (CRPS), peripheral vascular disease (PVD) with critical limb ischemia, refractory angina pectoris, deafferentation syndromes, isolated peripheral nerve injuries, spinal cord injury related pain, interstitial cystitis, and trigeminal neuralgia. The range of painful conditions amenable to treatment with these techniques continues to broaden with more recent studies suggesting the potential for these devices to provide relief of chronic visceral pain, headaches, and poststroke pain. In addition to treatment of pain, neurostimulation may also be useful as a means to monitor evoked potentials during thoracoabdominal aneurysm repair[2] and in the treatment of movement disorders (dystonia, Parkinson disease, and essential tremor), Tourette syndrome, major depression, and obsessive-compulsive disorder.

PERIPHERAL NEUROSTIMULATION

TAXONOMY, ANATOMIC TARGETS, APPLICATIONS AND MECHANISMS OF ACTION

The use of electrical stimulation of peripheral nerves for pain relief was first reported more than 40 years ago by Wall and Sweet based on the aforementioned gate control theory.[3] The basic goal is to place a lead (an assembly of stimulating contacts, wires and insulators) that can depolarize the axons of a peripheral nerve in order to render comfortable paresthesias within the sensory distribution of that nerve and override pain and dysesthesias. The lead may be placed on the nerve or in the subcutaneous tissues along the course of the target nerve.

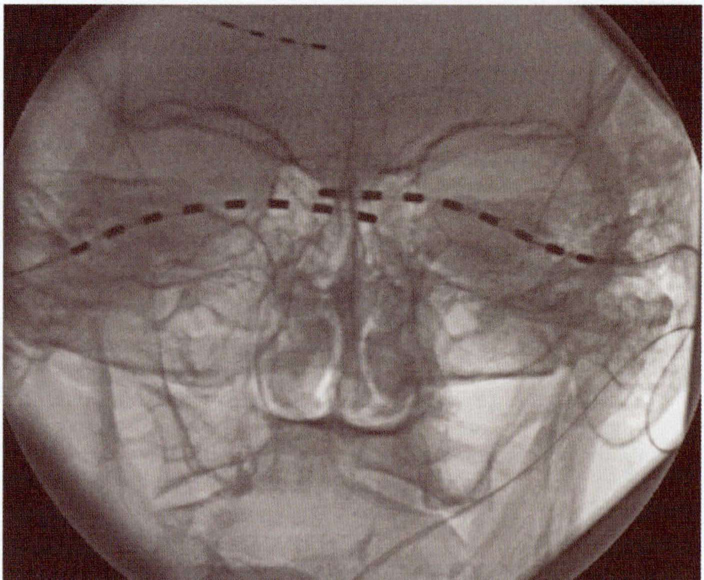

FIGURE 90-1. Combined epicranial nerve stimulation of the left supraorbital/supratrochlear nerve (4 contact lead) with bilateral greater and lesser occipital nerves (8 contact leads) for the treatment of refractory chronic migraine.

The popularity of PNS began in the 1990s with the introduction of occipital nerve stimulation for headache secondary to occipital neuralgia by Reed and Wiener.[4] Since then, epicranial PNS of the various sensory scalp nerves has been explored by a number of authors as treatments for chronic migraine, chronic cluster headache, and neuralgias of the supraorbital and occipital nerves (**Fig. 90-1**).[5-8] Similarly, PNS for the extremities and trunk has been reported primarily in anecdotal form for the treatment of a variety of neuralgias[9-11] (**Fig. 90-2**). **Tables 90-1** and **90-2** summarize the reports of PNS for the management of multiple

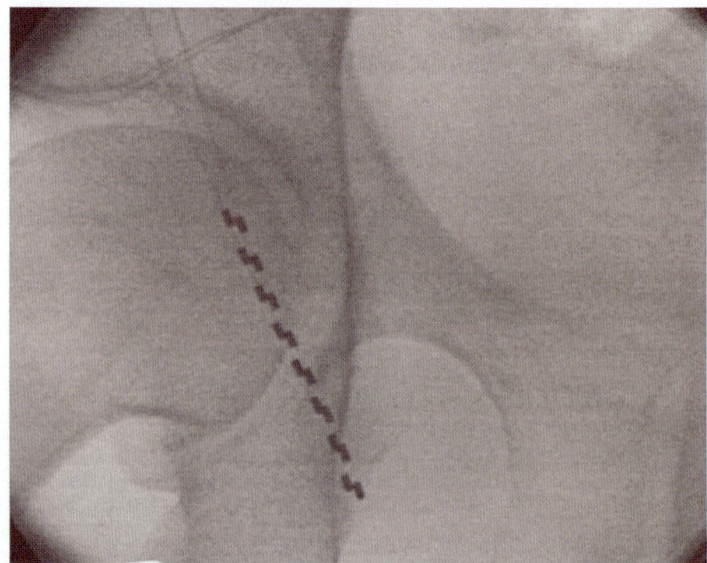

FIGURE 90-2. Genitofemoral nerve stimulation with dual 8 contact electrodes for the treatment of postherniorrhaphy pain.

TABLE 90-1 Selected Cases of Epicranial Peripheral Nerve Stimulation

Headache Condition	Number of Patients	Outcome
Chronic migraine	7	100% of patients with marked reduction in headache frequency and severity with normal function using SONS and ONS.[13]
	25	ONS resulted in 90% average improvement in migraine disability scores at 18-month follow-up.[14]
	8	All patients reported more than 50%-75% reduction in headache frequency and intensity with ONS or SONS.[15]
Chronic cluster	14	ONS patients with a mean follow-up of 17 months resulted in cluster reduction for 3 (90%), 3 (50%), 4 (30%), and 4 patients with no change.[16]
	8	ONS with median follow-up 20 months for attack frequency, 2 patients with 90%, 3 with average of 50%, and the rest with little to no response.[17]
	8	Therapeutic ONS rendered two patients pain free, 2 with a 90% attack frequency reduction, 2 with 40% reduction in attack frequency, and 2 no response over mean 15- month follow-up.[18]
	1	SONS rendered remission of symptoms after 2 months and lasted over 14 months at last follow-up.[19]
Hemicrania continua	1	Left ONS resulted in the patient being pain free at 3 months follow-up.[20]

ONS, occipital nerve stimulation; SONS, supraorbital nerve stimulation

refractory chronic pain conditions. The Food and Drug Administration (FDA) has approved PNS only for neuropathic pain of the extremities and trunk.[12]

In contrast to PNS, PNFS is applied to the region of the body where pain is perceived and not a specific nerve or its sensory distribution. PNFS targets a very specific pain distribution and usually cannot be relied upon to spread much beyond the active portions of the length and width of the lead.[30] Some authors have reported that PNFS can be expanded with the addition of a second lead in order to create interlead stimulation (cross talk) to cover a pain topographical area up to 377 square centimeters, while others have not found such cross talk influential.[31,32] However, PNS produces paresthesias beyond the active electrode dimensions and often follows in the sensory distribution of the stimulated peripheral nerve.[33] Because paresthesias must be felt in the area of pain in order to render relief, PNFS is believed to stimulate distal branches of peripheral nerves that are too small to be specifically distinguished. As with PNS, PNFS involves placing the leads in the subcutaneous space in order to create deep and soothing paresthesia sensations. PNFS is most frequently applied to painful regions of the axial spine that are difficult to treat with SCS, in particular the low back (**Fig. 90-3**).[30]

The mechanism(s) for PNS and PNFS are complex and incompletely understood. PNS is thought to activate low threshold A-β (beta) fibers that inhibit nociceptive A-Δ (delta) and C-fibers at the level of the dorsal horn.[34] A-β fibers may also propagate signals via medial lemniscal tracts to the level of the thalamus in the ventroposteromedial nucleus.[35] At this location, PNS may modulate the activity of ascending spinothalamic tracts at the third order neuron level. Another potential mechanism may include impulse interruptions by collision that may be important for inhibiting excessive peripheral nerve activity, for example in a case of neuroma.[36] PNFS has been thought to have similar mechanisms to PNS but also include altering local blood flow, local

TABLE 90-2 Selected Cases of Peripheral Nerve Stimulation and Peripheral Nerve Field Stimulation for the Trunk

Medical Condition	Number of Patients	Clinical Outcome
Low back pain	13	PNFS resulted in a 50% pain intensity reduction at 7-month follow-up.[21]
	6	PNFS with a 50% reduction in pain level.[22]
Neck pain	1	PNFS provided 100% pain alleviation at 9-month follow-up for midaxial symptoms.[23]
Thoracic pain	1	PNFS for postthoracotomy related pain, 90% improvement.[24]
	2	PNFS in postherpetic neuralgia of the chest wall gave reduction in medication and marked improvement.[16]
Inguinal pain	3	PNS in all patients gave greater than 75% relief at follow-up out to 12 months.[26]
Abdominal pain	2	PNFS applied in one patient with chronic pancreatitis and one with abdominal wall pain following liver transplantation, follow-up at 9 months with marked pain score reduction.[27]
Shoulder pain	1	PNFS allowed for 95% pain reduction from traumatic scapular fracture, engaged in physical therapy, and discontinued all oral medications.[29]

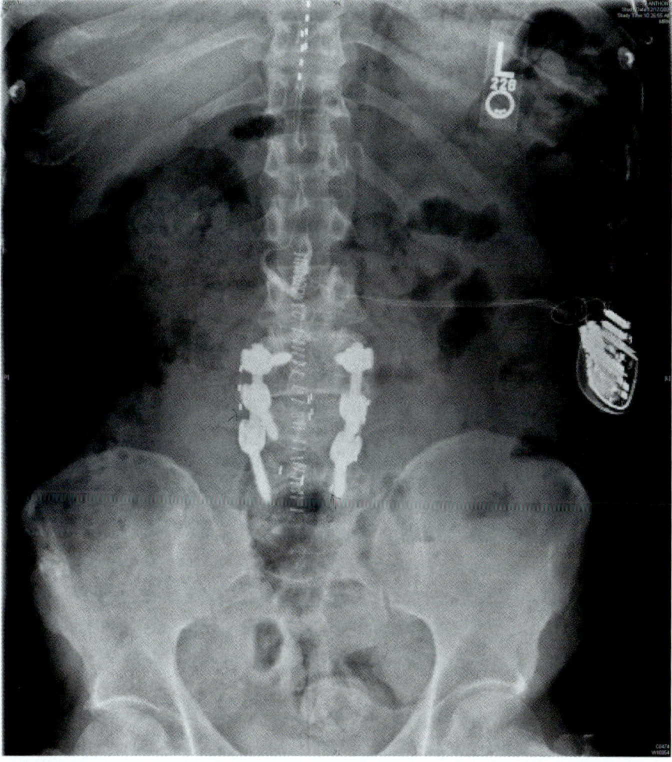

FIGURE 90-3. Axial back pain related to hardware treated successfully with peripheral nerve field stimulation (PNFS) with overlapping dual 4 contact leads. N.B. Anterograde spinal cord stimulator leads (T10 level) alleviated bilateral radiating leg pain but failed to deliver adequate paresthesia coverage at the L3-5 level.

endorphins, as well as blockade of cell membrane depolarization.[30] Interruption of nociceptive traffic by PNS along afferents that traverse the calvaria at suture lines may be an underlying mechanism of how epicranial stimulation alleviates primary headache syndromes.[37] Thus, there is little preclinical work to guide a quickly growing clinical interest in these techniques.

OUTCOMES, COMPLICATIONS AND FUTURE DIRECTIONS

As would be expected, most studies are anecdotal series reporting 60-70% of patients having analgesic and/or functional improvement with PNS.[38] A recent prospective observational trial following 100 patients over 1 year consisted of: 40-craniofacial pain, 8-thoracic, 44-lumbosacral, 3-abdominal, and 5 groin/pelvis.[39] The average pain reduction was just over 40% in pain intensity, with secondary outcomes including 72% of patients reducing analgesic consumption, and chronic low back pain patients having significant improvement in the Oswestry Disability Index (ODI). In patients with chronic migraines, occipital nerve stimulation (ONS) reduced the headache days per month by 50% or headache intensity by 3 points or more at 3-month follow-up in 39% of drug-resistant patients.[40] The study was prospective, multicenter, randomized, blinded, placebo-controlled, and contained optimal inclusion/exclusion criteria. It concluded that response to occipital nerve block failed to predict the outcome from PNS. Ultimately, 61% of chronic migraine patients did not achieve a positive response in this study, suggesting the need for better selection criteria given the costs of this technology.

PNS and PNFS are frequently applied to patients with favorable psychological profiles who have conditions that are difficult to stimulate using conventional SCS techniques. Unanswered questions about these techniques remain and should be resolved prior to undertaking prospective randomized control trials. These include:

- Defining the optimal surgical technique, including lead depth (avoiding painful dermal or muscle stimulation) and anchoring.
- Determining optimal lead and pulse generator–lead configuration, durability, and generator energy output with specific stimulation modes and parameters for the PNS.
- Defining the patients who would most likely benefit from these techniques. Presently, patients who have failed all other measures with a favorable psychological profile are selected.
- Selecting the optimal trial interval that balances infectious risks while ruling out a placebo effect.

Presently, the equipment used for stimulating nerves in the periphery is for an "off label" use of spinal cord stimulator devices. Thus, there is little by way of modeling studies and preclinical work to determine the optimal device design. Most complications for PNS/PNFS are minor and easily treated. Two frequent problems are lead migration and skin erosion. Although the blame can be laid on surgical technique, it is important not to lose sight of the fact that insertion techniques, lead size, and anchors were not designed with stimulation of the periphery in mind.

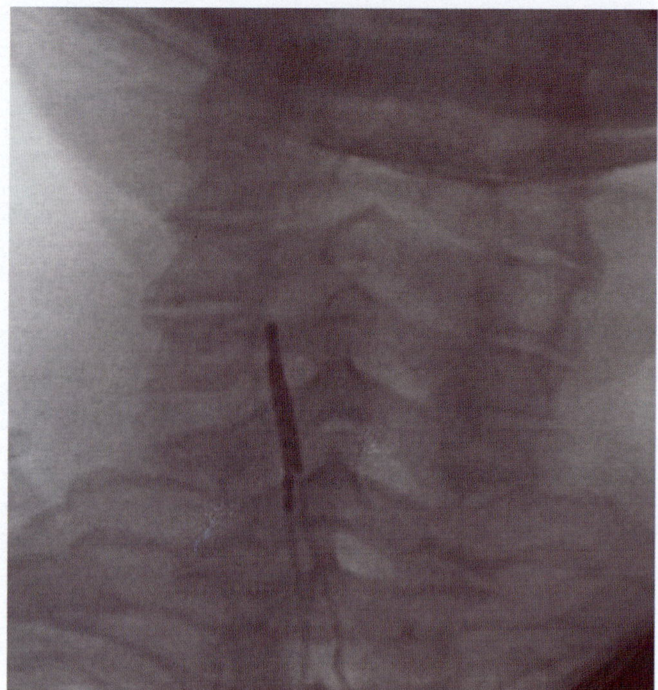

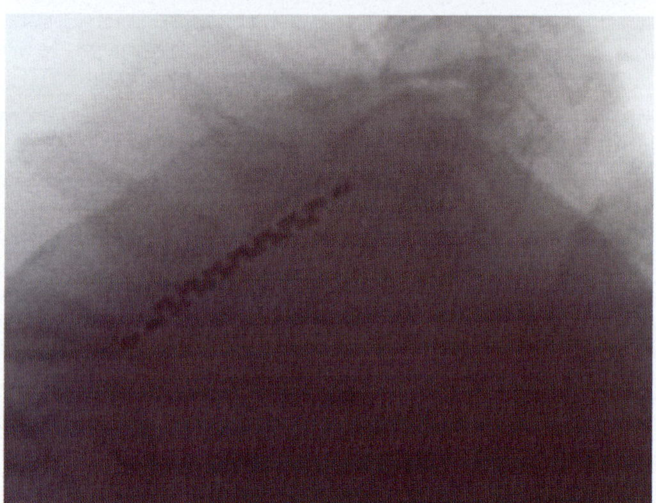

FIGURE 90-4. Dual stimulating 8 contact electrodes placed in the cervical periforaminal region with stimulating targets of the dorsal root entry zones and the corresponding exiting nerve roots in anteroposterior view. N.B. The lateral image reveals the stimulating lead on the mid-point of the facet pillars (compare/contrast to Figure 90-7 lateral view).

SPINAL NEUROSTIMULATON

ANATOMIC TARGETS

Over the past two decades, electrical stimulation of structures in the epidural space has gone beyond the dorsal columns. These structures include the dorsal horn, dorsal root entry zone (**Fig. 90-4**), dorsal root ganglia (**Fig. 90-5**), and posterior nerve roots (**Fig. 90-6**).[29] Classic anterograde epidural SCS targets the dorsal columns (**Fig. 90-7**), resulting in large myelinated A-β fiber axons undergoing depolarization. Antidromic activation of large myelinated tracts inhibits overactive wide dynamic range neurons of the dorsal horn via activation of interneurons in neuropathic pain states.[41] Similar mechanisms are thought to occur with A-β fiber activation in the nerve root/dorsal root ganglion. Additional potential anatomic targets include dorsolateral funiculus and the activation of a supraspinal negative feedback loop. Although direct activation of the dorsolateral funiculus is debated, the orthodromic activation of the dorsal columns can result in excitation of the anterior pretectal nucleus from which the dorsal horn is inhibited by the descending dorsolateral funiculus, which releases serotonin and norepinephrine.[42] The neuromodulation of these targets is thought to result in suppression of allodynia, hyperesthesia, and constant pain. Lastly, alteration in sympathetic activity is noted in patients who have an SCS device that results in inhibition and increased blood flow to the periphery.[43] Preclinical studies support the modulatory effects of SCS on the sympathetic nervous system as determined by pharmacological inhibitors of sympathetic outflow.[44,45]

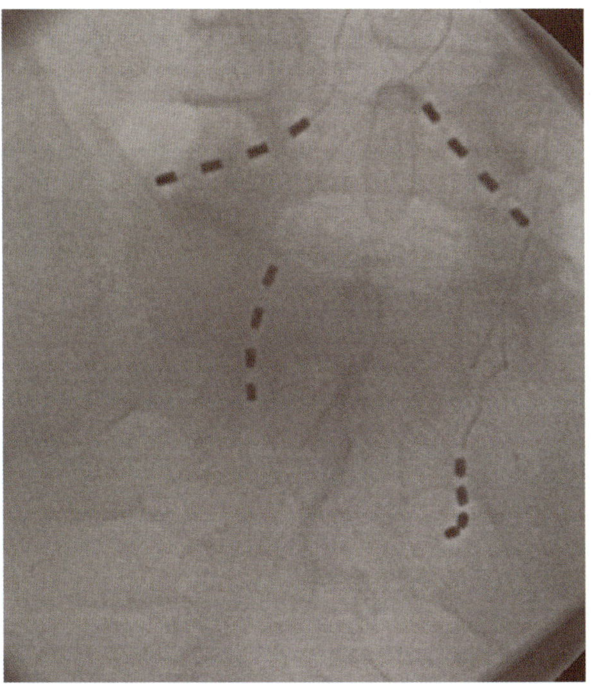

FIGURE 90-5. Anteroposterior fluoroscopic view depicting 4-contact leads in proximity of the L5 and S1 dorsal root ganglia. The right 4-contact lead that is in the most inferior location is placed transforaminally and is stimulating the S1 ventral ramus.

BEYOND GATE CONTROL: NEUROHUMORAL BASIS OF SPINAL CORD STIMULATION

Although the gate control theory may explain the primary mechanism by which SCS works, it cannot account for some of the clinically observed effects of SCS. Some researchers have proposed that SCS inhibits transmission of painful impulses partly by inducing a differential conduction block of afferent nociceptive fibers via antidromic stimulation. That the effects of stimulation can outlast the duration of the stimulation would seem, however, to indicate that this is not the only mechanism by which neurostimulation influences pain transmission.

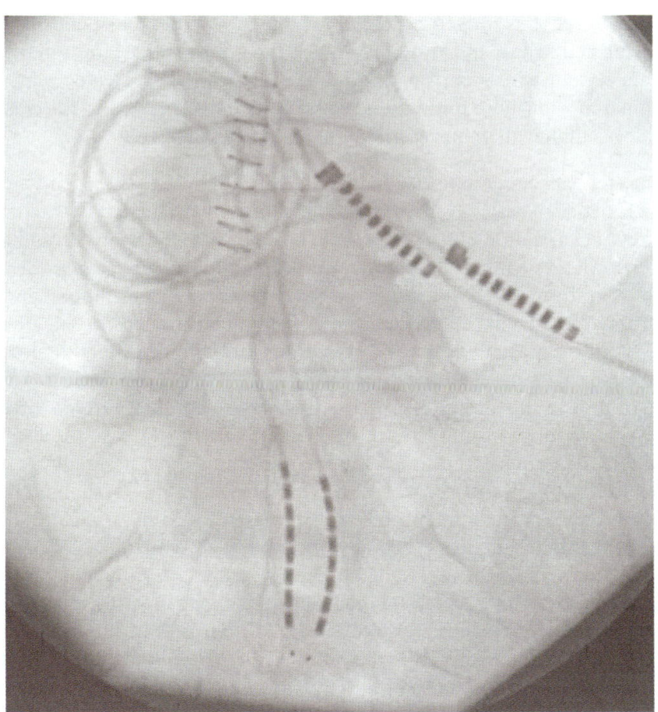

FIGURE 90-6. Dual 8 contact leads placed in a retrograde fashion, dorsally over the sacral nerves mid-line and preferentially to the right for pelvic pain related to interstitial cystitis.

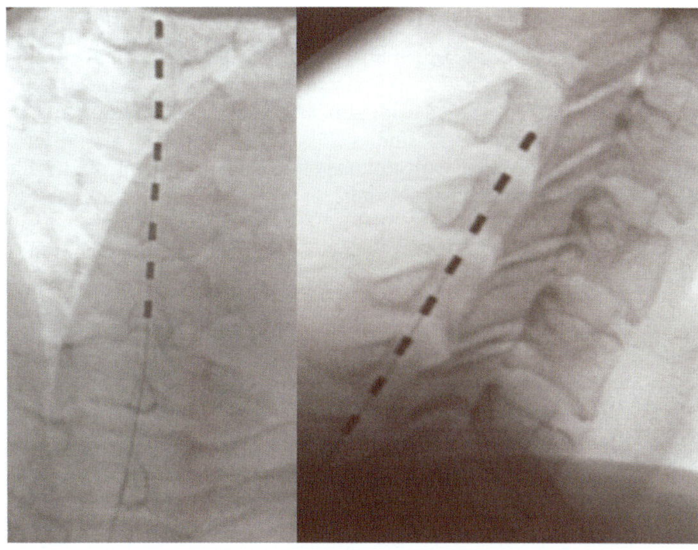

FIGURE 90-7. Fluoroscopic images anteroposterior and lateral of a right-sided cervical 8-contact lead targeting the dorsal columns. Notice the lateral view depicts the lead up to C3 with the lead posterior to the cervical facet pillars.

Investigators have speculated that neurohumoral mechanisms are also involved. Studies have been conducted to elucidate which mediators may contribute. Substances that have been purported to be involved in the neuromodulatory effects of SCS include endogenous opioids, (γ)-[gamma] aminobutyric acid (GABA), adenosine, substance P, serotonin, calcitonin gene-related peptide (CGRP), acetylcholine, and nitric oxide. Several mediators may also play a role in the sympathetic inhibitory effects of SCS. **Table 90-3** summarizes the role of putative neurotransmitters in the neurochemistry of SCS mechanisms.

TABLE 90-3 Neurotransmitters in Putative Neurochemical Mechanisms of Spinal Cord Stimulation as Determined in Preclinical Studies

Neurotransmitter	Proposed Modulatory Effect
Opioid receptors (μ, κ)	No reversal of SCS analgesia but of low frequency transcutaneous electrical stimulation (TENS).[46]
γ-aminobutyric acid (GABA)	Suppression of allodynia and hyperalgesia correlate with release in dorsal horn by electrical stimulation.[47,48] Baclofen, a GABA agonist enhances SCS analgesic effects.[49] GABA release suppresses the release of excitatory amino acids.[50]
Adenosine	Experiments that parallel those used to evaluate the role of GABA in the allodynia-suppressing effect of SCS have been done using adenosine agonists and antagonists.[51-53]
Serotonin	Elevation in dorsal horn results in diminution of tactile and cold hyperalgesia.[54]
Substance P	Marked increase in the dorsal horn with SCS in the cat functioning as an inhibitor of pain signaling.[55]
Calcitonin-gene related peptide	Antidromic stimulation of the dorsal roots results in peripheral release and subsequent vasodilation.[56]
Nitric oxide	Blockade of nitric oxide synthase diminishes peripheral vasodilation independent of SNS.[57]

APPLICATIONS AND OUTCOMES OF SPINAL CORD STIMULATION

Systematic reviews of the use of SCS for FBSS, CRPS, PVD, and chronic angina have demonstrated its efficacy in pain relief and, in most cases, cost-effectiveness compared with standard conservative treatments. A 20-year literature review (49 studies, 2520 subjects) assessing long-term (>6 months) pain relief with the use of SCS for treatment of chronic pain revealed a pooled success rate of 67%.[58] As data continues to accrue demonstrating the potential benefits of SCS in the management of refractory pain, case reports of new applications of this technology appear in the medical literature regularly.

Failed Back Surgery Syndrome Patients who have undergone surgical procedures such as laminectomies to treat back pain and radiculopathy may continue to experience pain postoperatively or redevelop pain at a later date. Patients who appear to have successful correction of spinal anatomical derangements and experience recurrent pain are said to be suffering from FBSS. A number of patients may demonstrate residual or recurrent disc herniations or epidural scarring/fibrosis although others may have no visibly demonstrable lesions causing pain. In the United States FBSS may afflict up to 40% of patients treated with back surgery and is costly to treat.[59,60] When surgically remediable lesions have been excluded or reoperation for identified lesions is not desired, SCS may be considered for ongoing pain management. In addition to relief of pain, outcome measures such as reduced analgesic consumption, increased physical activity levels, loss of neurologic function, and return of the previously physically disabled to work have been examined in a number of studies.[61-63] These studies have demonstrated that patients who derived pain relief from SCS often decreased their use of analgesics or discontinued them completely. In addition, most patients in these studies were able to perform more routine daily activities, and some who had been unfit to work were able to regain employment.

When SCS is considered in the management of FBSS, the presence of a number of indicators may predict a greater likelihood of success with SCS. These indicators include early treatment (initiated 0-3 yr after failed back surgery), the predominant presence of neuropathic leg pain, and the absence of major psychological disturbances such as depression.[45]

North et al, have conducted studies comparing SCS to reoperation in refractory FBSS patients with surgically remediable nerve root compression and radicular pain.[59,64] They found that aside from being reversible, less invasive, and having a lower associated morbidity, SCS was also more effective and less expensive than reoperation among selected patients with FBSS.[59] Most patients randomized to reoperation (62%) crossed over to SCS by follow-up at a mean of 3.1 years; however, fewer subjects (26%) randomized to SCS crossed over to reoperation by the time of follow-up. None of the patients who crossed over to reoperation after spinal cord stimulator implant achieved successful pain relief. After reviewing the outcomes and associated treatment costs, North, et al, concluded that SCS is most-cost effective when patients forego reoperation and therefore recommended that SCS be considered as the therapy of choice in this population.[59]

In the Prospective Randomized Controlled Multicenter Trial of the Effectiveness of Spinal Cord Stimulation (PROCESS), Kumar, et al, evaluated patients undergoing SCS for FBSS primarily for reduction in leg pain by 50% or more. They found that SCS offered superior pain relief and improved health-related quality of life and functional capacity compared with conventional medical management at 6 months.[60] When these patients were followed-up at 24 months, improved pain control, health-related quality of life, and functional capacity were sustained, with 93% of patients reporting satisfaction with therapy and indicating that, based upon their experience thus far, they would again elect to undergo SCS.[60]

In a systematic review by Taylor, et al, pooled data from 72 case series studies of 3427 patients implanted with SCS for FBSS demonstrated that 62% of patients achieved a reduction in pain of at least 50%.[65] Frey, et al, concluded that the level of evidence for SCS in the long-term management of FBSS is II-1 or II-2 with a 1B or 1C/strong recommendation (using criteria developed by the American College of Chest Physicians Task Force criteria) for use based upon systematic analysis that included 2 randomized trials and 10 observational studies.[66]

Complex Regional Pain Syndromes Chronic complex regional pain syndromes type I and II (CRPS I, II), are characterized by the presence of severe pain that persists long after an inciting noxious event respectively resolves. Spinal cord stimulation has long been used as a treatment for this condition, especially when conservative management including sympathetic blocks and medications has failed. Early treatment may provide the best chance of functional restoration in the affected limb(s). Therefore, some authors have recommended consideration of SCS in the treatment of CRPS I if 12 to 16 weeks of conservative medical management is unsuccessful in controlling symptoms.[45] A number of studies have demonstrated a high degree of CRPS I patient satisfaction with SCS.[58,67-70]

Systematic reviews of SCS for the treatment of CRPS I have shown that the number needed to treat (NNT) with a trial of SCS is 3 to have one CRPS I patient subjectively report being greatly improved after 6 months, or to achieve a rating of 6 on the global perceived effect scale.[70,71] A summary of the findings of one systematic review, which included one randomized controlled trial (level 1b evidence) and 14 observational studies (level 4 evidence), indicated that SCS for the treatment of CRPS I unresponsive to conservative medical management is effective (grade B/C recommendation).[70] In another systematic review assessing clinical outcomes and cost-effectiveness of SCS for CRPS, the authors concluded that SCS, used in conjunction with physical therapy, is both clinically and cost effective in patients with CRPS I (grade A recommendation).[69]

Peripheral Vascular Disease Peripheral vascular disease is among the common indications for the use of SCS worldwide. Patients with advanced PVD that is not amenable to revascularization procedures may be candidates for SCS.[72,73] One systematic review of the use of SCS for PVD included 9 trials with 444 patients. Pooled data indicated that limb salvage among the SCS group was significantly greater than in patients undergoing only conventional medical management at 12 months.[74] It was determined that the NNT with SCS in PVD to avoid one major amputation was 8.[74] Additionally, in patients with chronic critical limb ischemia, 3 patients had to be treated with SCS for one to improve to a Fontaine stage 2 classification of ischemia (mild to severe claudication), and pain relief as judged by visual analog pain scores was better in the SCS treated group at 3 months. Pooled data, however, did not demonstrate benefit with regard to wound healing in the SCS treated patients compared with those undergoing conservative treatment, and the cost of SCS was higher than conventional medical management.[74]

Intractable Angina Pectoris As with patients suffering from end-stage PVD, patients with severe coronary syndromes that are not amenable to revascularization may find relief through SCS. These patients have often undergone multiple prior coronary angioplasties or coronary artery bypass grafting (CABG) and are receiving maximal medical therapy with continued recurrent angina despite aggressive treatment. Most patients are fairly incapacitated by their symptoms and fall into functional classifications III and IV of the New York Heart Association (NYHA). The use of SCS in this group of patients with severe coronary artery disease serves not only to diminish their pain, but also to decrease the overall number of ischemic episodes they experience. This is thought to be due, in large part, to a reduction in sympathetic nervous system activity induced by SCS. A number of studies have evaluated the impact of SCS on myocardial ischemia. Generally, the studies revealed that use of SCS in patients with intractable angina pectoris may lead to a reduction in angina episodes and decreased requirements for short-acting nitrates.[75,76]

It also appears that exercise tolerance is increased in these patients, likely due to alterations in myocardial oxygen supply-to-demand ratio and possibly through redistribution of coronary blood flow to ischemic areas. Several studies have used techniques of atrial pacing to determine how anginal thresholds are affected by SCS.[77-79] Patients were paced to angina before and after turning on their spinal cord stimulators.

After initiating stimulation, patients were able to tolerate pacing to higher heart rates than prior to stimulation. It was noted that these patients would still experience angina when being paced maximally. The findings are of considerable importance in this arena, as some critics have expressed concern that SCS may only mask the symptoms of ischemia, thereby eliminating a key warning signal for these patients. It would seem, therefore, that instead of masking ischemia, SCS actually enhances coronary perfusion and ionotropic performance.[80]

In one study, patients receiving SCS for refractory angina experienced improvement in the Canadian Cardiovascular Society (CCS) angina class (similar to the NYHA) by 1 or more classes (80% of patients) or 2 or more classes (42% of patients).[81] Patients demonstrated improved exercise tolerance (increased exercise duration and time to angina), decreased nitrate consumption, reductions in ischemic episodes at rest and with exercise, and decreased rates of hospitalization and lengths of stay.[81]

Similar findings were noted in a study in which patients who had previously undergone CABG and were not candidates for additional revascularization procedures were offered SCS therapy for refractory disabling angina.[82] Patients responding to SCS (88.2% of the study subjects) experienced a reduction greater than 50% in weekly anginal episodes and also had significant improvements in quality of life and CCS angina classification.[82] When use of SCS was compared with percutaneous myocardial laser revascularization (PMR), both procedures had similar efficacy in the management of refractory angina.[83]

Further, patients who are not candidates for treatments such as PMR because of thin myocardium or poor left ventricular function, SCS may be considered as an effective alternative.[83] In a study of the long-term effects of SCS and CABG on quality of life and survival in patients with refractory angina deemed unlikely to have prognostic benefit from CABG, improvements in quality of life and survival rates were comparable between the two groups at 3-year and 5-year follow-ups.[84] A recent systematic review of the subject of SCS versus CABG or PMR in the management of refractory angina involved 7 randomized controlled trials with 210 patients.[85] When SCS was compared to "no stimulation" controls, significant improvements were seen in exercise capacity and health-related quality of life, which was similar to the outcomes seen in subjects undergoing CABG or PMR.[85] At 2-year follow-up, it appeared that SCS was associated with lower health care costs than CABG, and the findings of the review overall provided support for the American College of Cardiology/American Heart Association level B recommendation for the use of SCS in refractory angina.[85]

New and Emerging Indications Case reports and case series have appeared in the literature regarding the use of SCS in the management of chronic abdominal pain from various etiologies. Diagnoses for which SCS has been used successfully in the treatment of refractory abdominal pain include mesenteric ischemia, chronic nonalcoholic pancreatitis, familial Mediterranean fever, irritable bowel syndrome, and chronic visceral abdominal pain due to adhesions after various abdominal surgical procedures.[86-91] Many patients experienced temporary relief with celiac plexus block or differential epidural blocks prior to placement of SCS. In addition, many were able to substantially reduce or discontinue opioid therapy after initiation of SCS.

Contraindications to Spinal Cord Stimulation As with other pain management techniques targeting the neuraxis, placement of a SCS system is contraindicated in the presence of active coagulopathy, systemic or localized infection, and patient refusal. Formerly, the presence of an implanted pacemaker or automatic implantable cardioverter defibrillator (AICD) was considered a contraindication for SCS. Concerns about the combination of SCS and these cardiac devices center on the potential for interference, which could theoretically cause a failure to pace in pacemaker-dependent patients or delivery of an inappropriate shock if SCS triggers the discharge of an AICD. Because many more patients with serious cardiac conditions are considered for treatment with both devices for management of coronary disease related angina syndromes and arrhythmias, case reports involving their combined use have become more frequent over the past decade.[92-96] Collectively, case reports indicate that SCS and pacemakers/AICDs can be used together safely if both devices are bipolar, but it is important that they be tested together to ensure noninterference. Reprogramming of either device should always include retesting for continued device compatibility.

COST EFFECTIVENESS OF SPINAL CORD STIMULATION

Several systematic reviews of SCS have been performed looking at cost effectiveness of this treatment in addition to evaluating clinical effectiveness. In the treatment of FBSS, North, et al, in 2007 reported that the cost per successful outcome was $48,357 for SCS, $105,928 for reoperation, $117,901 for SCS after unsatisfactory results with reoperation, and $260,584 in patients reoperated after unsuccessful SCS.[59] Notably, none of the patients who underwent reoperation after failed SCS in this review experienced improvement with reoperation, indicating that despite the use of considerable financial resources, benefit is unlikely if patients proceed to reoperation after failure of SCS in FBSS.[59] A separate systematic review of the cost-effectiveness of SCS found that SCS is more effective and less costly than usual care long-term despite the initial high cost of device implantation and maintenance.[97] Another systematic review determined that in comparison with other common treatments, SCS is economically favorable in the medium- to long-term (1-3 yr) in patients with FBSS, CRPS and refractory angina pectoris.[98] The authors of this review concluded that over time, reductions in health care expenditures for drug therapies, physician visits, and hospitalizations offset the initial acquisition costs of SCS.[98] In a comparative study of SCS and CABG in patients with severe angina pectoris likely to have no prognostic benefit from CABG, SCS was found to be less expensive than CABG with no significant difference in survival rates between the groups at 2-year follow-up.[99]

SCREENING OF PROSPECTIVE CANDIDATES FOR SPINAL CORD STIMULATION

General criteria should be considered for selection of patients for SCS implantation. Criteria include the presence of nonmalignant pain that has responded poorly to at least 6 months of conservative treatment; no corrective surgery is possible or advisable; no major psychological disorders, including somatization, are present; no ongoing litigation or secondary gain is involved; no inappropriate drug use at the time of planned implantation; and the patient is capable of providing informed consent.[45]

Spinal cord stimulators and related neurostimulation devices are used increasingly in the management of refractory pain. To ensure maximal efficacy of these technologies, appropriate patient selection is crucial. The selection process should involve a review not only of the condition to be treated, but also individual patient factors that may impact the likely success of these techniques. Psychological screening of potential candidates for SCS is considered standard practice prior to proceeding with the trial and implant in many centers and is required by many third party payers during authorization process for SCS implantation.

It has been noted that 25% to 50% of patients who have had a successful trial of SCS report decreased efficacy of SCS within 12 to 24 months of implantation despite evidence that their devices are functioning appropriately.[100,101] Psychological factors may underlie the loss of device efficacy over time in many of these patients. The psychological profiles most predictive of long-term failure of SCS therapy remain debated. Some have suggested that the presence of the so-called "conversion V" pattern on Minnesota Multiphasic Personality Inventory (MMPI) testing, consisting of elevated hypochondriasis and hysteria scores relative to depression scores, may indicate a significant psychogenic component to pain and portends a negative outcome with SCS.[100] Conversely, others have noted that lower hypochondriasis and hysteria scores in conjunction with elevated depression scores are more commonly seen among patients refractory to treatment than in patients successfully managed with SCS for chronic pain.[100] Several studies have implicated depression as a negative predictive factor for the efficacy of SCS.[101] The impact of depression on the effectiveness of SCS for chronic pain may depend on whether depression is a preexisting disorder or results from the pain for which SCS is being prescribed.[101] If depression is caused by ongoing pain and associated disability, effective control of pain via SCS may result in an improvement in depressive symptoms.[101]

Most experts agree that the presence of certain psychological conditions such as active psychosis, suicidality or homicidality, severe mood disturbances, somatization, and uncontrolled drug or alcohol abuse contraindicate the use of SCS.[100] Additional factors that may make one hesitant to employ SCS include a history of noncompliance, poor social support, ongoing litigation or unresolved worker's compensation issues, the presence of significant cognitive deficits, and overly optimistic expectations regarding the outcome of treatment with SCS.[100]

TRIAL OF SPINAL CORD STIMULATION

The standard SCS trial duration remains variable. In the United States, a temporary trial of SCS typically lasts 2 to 7 days. In Europe, trials are more commonly performed for a 3-week duration whereby the trial lead is contained within the incision and a temporary trial extension is externalized via stab skin incision. A successful trial is measured by an average pain intensity reduction of 50% and paresthesia overlap with 80% of the somatotopic pain distribution.

COMPLICATIONS OF SPINAL CORD STIMULATION

Complications of SCS may relate to the surgical procedure for device placement or technical failures of equipment. Surgical complications include infection, pain, postdural puncture headache, cerebrospinal fluid leak, and seroma formation at the pulse generator pocket site. Technical failures may involve lead migration or fracture, loss of stimulation, and battery failure, which may require the patient to undergo additional surgery for correction.

INTRACRANIAL STIMULATION

TAXONOMY, ANATOMIC TARGETS, APPLICATIONS AND MECHANISMS OF ACTION

Stimulation within the cranium consists of two main modalities, deep brain stimulation (DBS) and motor cortex stimulation (MCS). Stimulation of the thalamus for pain relief dates back to 1960.[102] The targets of DBS are the ventroposteromedial (VPM) nucleus, ventroposterolateral (VPL) nucleus, internal capsule, and central medial nucleus to cause depolarization and induce paresthesias in order to relieve deafferentation (central) neuropathic pain.[103] In chronic pain states, these nuclei maintain an abnormal firing pattern, and electrical stimulation may restore the appropriate level of inhibitory surround.[104,105] These thalamic nuclei project via the dorsolateral funiculus to inhibit the lamina I neurons. Stimulation of the periaqueductal gray (PAG) matter and the periventricular gray (PVG) matter has been shown to have efficacy in nociceptive pain.[106,107] The PVG sends projections to the amygdala and the cingulate cortex, and therefore influences limbic system pain responses. The analgesic effects are in part mediated by endogenous opioid release and have been shown to be significantly antagonized by the opioid antagonist, naloxone.[108] Combining stimulation of the PVG/PAG with the thalamic nuclei/internal capsule offers the best chance of relief in chronic neuropathic pain states.

More recently, DBS of the posterior hypothalamus has been reported to effectively treat refractory chronic cluster headaches.[109] Patients with cluster headaches have increased amounts of tissue in this region with high levels of spontaneous activity, and therefore this region was chosen to be the target for neuromodulation. As would be expected, the mode of analgesic action is largely unknown. Hypothalamic stimulation does not affect the neurohypophyseal hormones or the circadian rhythm of melatonin secretion. There is no change or reduction of pain perception in the trigeminal system. Interestingly, chronic cluster patients treated with active DBS systems become resistant to the well-known attack-triggering agent, nitroglycerin.

MCS has been shown to be beneficial in poststroke pain, traumatically induced neuropathic pain, atypical facial pain, and trigeminal deafferentation neuralgia.[110,111] The motor cortex projects extensively to the thalamus and therefore is a neuromodulatory target for influencing thalamic neuronal activity. Indeed, MCS can improve glucose metabolism in the ipsilateral thalamus in poststroke pain patients.[112] MCS can increase blood flow to the ventrolateral thalamus, medial thalamus, insula, orbitofrontal, cingulated gyrus, and upper brain stem.[113] Epidural MCS is therefore a convenient modality to reach and modulate deep brain structures in an inhibitory fashion.

OUTCOMES, COMPLICATIONS AND FUTURE DIRECTIONS

In a meta-analysis, DBS was found to be more successful in the long-term management of nociceptive pain (63%) than deafferentation pain (47%).[114] Reviews and cases series as well as meta-analyses indicate that the low back in FBSS responds very favorably with up to 80% of patients reporting significant improvement. Poststroke pain has responded in about 50% of patients with marked reduction in the burning pain component.[115] An additional small study suggested that cortical stroke may respond better than a subcortical stroke, with an average 50% reduction in 70% of patients, which was highly variable at 2-year follow-up.[116] Stimulation of the PAG in combination with the PVG or PVG/PAG and the VPM/VPL tended to result in more durable pain relief in the long run. In another long-term follow-up study of DBS patients, failed back surgery patients and CRPS II patients showed a high percentage of satisfaction, while patients with spinal cord injury and anesthesia dolorosa pain did not.[117] Finally, 11 of 16 chronic intractable cluster headache patients were rendered pain free at a mean follow-up of 23 months.[118] In conclusion, DBS seems to consistently benefit peripheral mixed neuropathic/nociceptive pain such as FBSS and CRPS II. Although most patients with cluster headaches appear to obtain relief, patients with poststroke pain, phantom limb pain, and deafferentation pain show variable responses over the long run.

The surgical techniques of DBS have improved significantly so that complications are relatively rare. A review found that intracranial hemorrhage or paralysis is far less common than hardware malfunction analogous to SCS.[119] One case series of DBS for cluster headache also suggests that placement of electrodes in the posterior hypothalamus raises concern for intracerebral hemorrhage.[120] A further consideration for DBS patients is the safety of magnetic resonance imaging (MRI) because of a recent report of intracranial radiofrequency lesions produced by heating of the DBS electrode with catastrophic results.[121] Currently, MRI can be performed only on DBS patients with strict adherence to the manufacturers' recommendations (Medtronic, Inc, Minneapolis, MN).[122]

Over the past 20 years, MCS has shown promise in central poststroke pain, trigeminal neuropathic pain, phantom limb pain, brachial plexus lesions, and spinal cord injury. The invasive form of MCS is the most common approach, which uses an "off label" application of SCS paddle-style electrodes that is over-laid epidurally on the motor cortex using anatomical and electrophysiologic guidance. The initial average response rate (pain reduction by 50%) as determined by a meta-analysis of reported cases series is at a mean of 64% and long-term fell modestly to 54.6% suggesting durable responses.[123] Noninvasively, transcranial magnetic stimulation (TMS) can render appreciable responses in 40% of patients. A recent randomized crossover trial for refractory neuropathic pain confirmed these response rates.[124] The complications of TMS are uncommon because of the epidural placement of the electrodes; however, these may include epidural hematoma, subdural effusion, infection, and seizures. Development of electrodes designed specifically to stimulate the motor cortex may improve efficacy, safety, and long-term outcomes.

REFERENCES

1. Melzack R, Wall P. Pain mechanisms: a new theory. *Science*. 1965;150:971-978.
2. North RB, Drenger B, Beattie C, et al. Monitoring of spinal cord stimulation evoked potentials during thoracoabdominal aneurysm surgery. *Neurosurgery*. 1991;28:325-330.

3. Wall PD, Sweet WH. Temporary abolition of pain in man. *Science.* 1967;155:108-109.
4. Weiner RL, Reed KL. Peripheral neurostimulation for control of intractable occipital neuralgia. *Neuromodulation.* 1999;2:217-222.
5. Popeney CA, Alo KM. Peripheral neurostimulation for the treatment of chronic, disabling transformed migraine. *Headache.* 2003;43(4):369-375.
6. Burns B, Watkins L, Goadsby PJ. Treatment of medically intractable cluster headache by occipital nerve stimulation: long-term follow-up of eight patients. *Lancet.* 2007;369(9567):1099-1106.
7. Amin S, Buvanendan A, Park KS, Kroin JS., Moric M. Peripheral nerve stimulator for the treatment of supraorbital neuralgia: a retrospective case series. *Cephalalgia.* 2008;28(4):355-359.
8. Johnstone CSH, Sundaraj R. Occipital nerve stimulation for the treatment of occipital neuralgia-eight case studies. *Neuromodulation.* 2006;9(1):41-47.
9. Kourouki I, Neofytos D, Panaretou V, Zompolas D, Papstergiou V, et al. Peripheral subcutaneous stimulation for the treatment of intractable postherpetic neuralgia: two case reports and literature review. *Pain Prac.* 2009;9(3):225-229.
10. Rauchwerger JJ, Giordano J, Rozen D, Kent JL, Greenspan J, Closson CWF. On the therapeutic viability of peripheral nerve stimulation for ilioinguinal neuralgia: putative mechanisms and possible utility. *Pain Prac.* 2008;8(2):138-143.
11. Mobbs RJ, Nair S, Blum P. Peripheral nerve stimulation for the treatment of chronic pain. *J Clin Neuro Sci.* 2007;14:216-221.
12. U.S. Food and Drug Administration Code of Federal Regulations. Title 21, Volume 8, 21CFR882.5870.
13. Reed Kl, Black SB, Banta CJ, Will KR. Combined occipital and supraorbital neurostimulation for the treatment of chronic migraine headaches: initial experience. *Cephalalgia.* 2011;30(3);260-271.
14. Popeney CA, Alo KM. Peripheral neurostimulation for the treatment of chronic, disabling transformed migraine. *Headache.* 2003;43(4):369-375.
15. Matharu MS, Bartsch T, Ward N, et al. Central neuromodulation in chronic migraine patients with suboccipital stimulators: a PET Study. *Brain.* 2003;127:220-230.
16. Burns B, Watkins L, Goadsby PJ. Treatment of intractable chronic cluster headache by occipital nerve stimulation in 14 patients. *Neurology.* 2009;72:341-345.
17. Burns B, Watkins L, Goadsby PJ. Treatment of medically intractable cluster headache by occipital nerve stimulation: long-term follow-up of eight patients. *Lancet.* 2007;369:1099-1106.
18. Magis D, Allena M, Bolla M, De Pasqua V, Remacle JM, Schoenen J. Occipital nerve stimulation for drug-resistant chronic cluster headache: a prospective pilot study. *Lancet Neurol.* 2007;6:314-321.
19. Narouze SN, Kapural L. Supraorbital nerve electrical stimulation for the treatment of intractable chronic cluster headache: a case report. *Headache.* 2007;Jul/Aug:1100-1102.
20. Shwedt TJ, Dodick DW, Trentman TL, Zimmerman RS. Occipital nerve stimulation for chronic cluster headache and hemicrania continua: pain relief and persistence of autonomic features. *Cephalagia.* 2006;26:1025-1027.
21. Verrills P, Mitchell B, Vivian D, Sinclair C. Peripheral nerve stimulation: a novel treatment in chronic low back pain and failed back surgery syndrome? *Neuromodulation.* 2009;12(1):68-75.
22. Paicius RM, Bernstein CA, Lempert-Cohen C. Peripheral nerve stimulation for the treatment of chronic low back pain: Preliminary results of long-term follow-up: a case series. *Neuromodulation.* 2007;10(3):279-290.
23. Lipov EG, Joshi JR, Snaders S, Slavin KV. Use of peripheral subcutaneous field stimulation for the treatment of axial neck pain: a case report. *Neuromodulation.* 2009;12(4):292-295.
24. Desai M, Jacob L, Leiphart J. Successful peripheral nerve stimulation for thoracic radiculitis following Brown-Sequard syndrome. *Neuromodulation.* 2011;14:249-252.
25. Kouroukli I, Neofytos D, Panretou V, Zompolas V, Papastergiou D, et al. Peripheral subcutaneous stimulation for the treatment of intractable postherpetic neuralgia: two case reports and literature review. *Neuromodulation.* 2009;9(3):1-5.
26. Stinson LW, Roderer GT, Cross NE, Davis BE. Peripheral subcutaneous electrostimulation for control of intractable post-operative inguinal pain: a case series. *Neuromodulation.* 2001;4(3):99-104.
27. Paicus RM, Bernstein CA, Lempert-Cohen C. Peripheral nerve field stimulation in chronic abdominal pain. *Pain Phys.* 2006;9:261-266.
28. Theodosiadis P, Salmoladas E, Grosomanidis V, Goroszeniuk T, Kothari S. A case of successful treatment of neuropathic pain after a scapular fracture using subcutaneous targeted neuromodulation. *Neuromodulation.* 2008;11(1):62-65.
29. Holsheimer J. Which neuronal elements are activated directly by spinal cord stimulation. *Neuromodulation.* 2002;5:25-31.
30. Abejon D, Deer T, Verrills P. Subcutaneous stimulation: how to assess optimal implantation depth. *Neuromodulation.* 2011;14:343-348.
31. Falco FJE, Berger J, Vrable A, Onyewu O, Zhu J. Cross talk: a new method for peripheral nerve stimulation. An observational report with cadaveric verification. *Pain Phys.* 2009;12:965-983.
32. Burgher AH, Huntoon MA, Turley TW, Doust MW, Stearns LJ. Subcutaneous peripheral nerve stimulation with inter-lead stimulation for axial neck and low back pain: case series with review of the literature. *Neuromodulation.* 2012;15(2):100-107.
33. Trentman TL, Zimmerman RS, Seth N, Hentz JG, Dodick DW. Stimulation ranges, usage ranges, and paresthesia mapping during occipital nerve stimulation. *Neuromodulation.* 2011;(1):56-61.
34. Rauchwerger JJ, Giordano J, Rozen D, Kent JL, Greenspan J, Closson CWF. On the therapeutic viability of peripheral nerve stimulation for ilioinguinal neuralgia: putative mechanisms and possible utility. *Pain Prac.* 2008;8(2):138-143.
35. Giordano J. The neuroscience of pain and analgesia. In: Boswell M, ole BE, eds. *Weiner's Pain Management: A Guide for Clinicians.* 7th ed. Boca Raton, FL: CRC Press; 2005:15-34.
36. Huntoon MA, Burgher AH. Review of ultra-sound guided peripheral nerve stimulation. *Tech Reg Anesth Pain Manag.* 2009;13:121-127.
37. Simopoulos TT, Bajwa ZH, Lantz G, Lee S, Burstein R. Implanted auriculotemporal nerve stimulation for the treatment of refractory chronic migraine. *Headache.* 2010;50(60):1064-1069.
38. Hassenbusch SJ, Stanton-Hicks M, Schoppa D, Walsh JG, Covington EC. Long-term results of peripheral nerve stimulation for reflex sympathetic dystrophy. *J Neurosurg.* 1996;84:415-423.
39. Verrills P, Vivian D, Mitchell B, Barnard A. Peripheral nerve field stimulation for chronic pain: 100 cases and review of the literature. *Pain Med.* 2011;12:1395-1405.
40. Saper JR, Dodick DW, Silberstein SD, McCarville S, Sun M, Goadsby PJ. Occipital nerve stimulation for the treatment of intractable chronic migraine headache: ONSTIM feasibility study. *Cephalagia.* 2011;31(3):271-285.
41. Guan Y, Wacnik PW, Yang F, Carteret AF, Chung CY, Meyer RA, et al. Spinal cord stimulation-induced analgesia: electrical stimulation of dorsal column and dorsal roots attenuates dorsal horn neuronal excitability in neuropathic rats. *Anesthesiology.* 2010;113:1392-1405.
42. Roberts MHT, Rees H. Physiological basis of spinal cord stimulation. *Pain Rev.* 1994;1:184-198.

43. Oakley JC, Prager JP. Spinal cord stimulation: mechanism of action. *Spine*. 2002;27(22):2574-2583.
44. Linderoth B, Herregodts P, Meyerson BA. Sympathetic mediation of peripheral vasodilation induced by spinal cord stimulation: animal studies of the role of cholinergic and adrenergic receptor subtypes. *Neurosurgery*. 1994;35:711-719.
45. Lee AW, Pilitsis JG. Spinal cord stimulation: indications and outcomes. *Neurosurg Focus*. 2006;21(6):1-6.
46. Han JS, Chen XH, Sun SL, et al. Effect of low- and high-frequency TENS on metenkephalin-Arg-Phe and dynorphin A immunoreactivity in human lumbar CSF. *Pain*. 1991; 47:295-298.
47. Linderoth B, Foreman RD. Physiology of spinal cord stimulation: a review and update. *Neuromodulation*. 1999; 2:150-164.
48. Stiller CO, Cui JG, O'Connor WT, et al. Release of gamma aminobutyric acid in the dorsal horn and suppression of tactile allodynia by spinal cord stimulation in mononeuropathic rats. *Neurosurgery*. 1996; 39:367-375.
49. Cui JG, Linderoth B, Meyerson BA. Effects of spinal cord stimulation on touch evoked allodynia involve GABAergic mechanisms. an experimental study in the mononeuropathic rat. *Pain*. 1996; 66:287-295.
50. Cui JG, O'Connor WT, Ungerstedt U, et al. Spinal cord stimulation attenuates augmented dorsal horn release of excitatory amino acids in mononeuropathy via a GABAergic mechanism. *Pain*. 1997; 73:87-95.
51. Cui JG, Sollevi A, Linderoth B, Meyerson BA. Adenosine receptor activation suppresses tactile hypersensitivity and potentiates spinal cord stimulation in mononeuropathic rats. *Neurosci Lett*. 1997; 173-176.
52. Cui JG, Meyerson BA, Sollevi A, Linderoth B. Effect of spinal cord stimulation on tactile hypersensitivity in mononeuropathic rats is potentiated by simultaneous GABAB and adenosine receptor activation. *Neurosci Lett*. 1998; 247:183-186.
53. Meyerson BA, Cui JG, Yakhnista V, et al. Modulation of spinal pain mechanisms by spinal cord stimulation and the potential role of adjuvant pharmacotherapy. *Stereotactic Funct Neurosurg*. 1997; 68:129-140.
54. Song Z, Ultenius C, Meyerson BA, Linderoth B. Pain relief by spinal cord stimulation involves serotonergic mechanisms: an experimental study in a rat model of mononeuropathy. *Pain*. 2009;147:241-248.
55. Linderoth B, Gazelius B, Franck J, Brodin E. Dorsal column stimulation induces release of serotonin and substance P in the cat dorsal horn. *Neurosurgery*. 1992;31:289-297.
56. Croom JE, Foreman RD, Chandler MJ, Barron KW. Cutaneous vasodilation during dorsal column stimulation is mediated by dorsal roots and CGRP. *Am J Physiol*. 1997;272:H950-H957.
57. Croom JE, Foreman RD, Chandler MJ, et al. Role of nitric oxide in cutaneous blood flow increases in the rat hind paw during dorsal column stimulation. *Neurosurgery*. 1997;40:565-571.
58. Cameron T. Safety and efficacy of spinal cord stimulation for the treatment of chronic pain: a 20-year literature review. *J Neurosurg (Spine 3)*. 2004;100:254-267.
59. North RB, Kidd D, Shipley J, et al. Spinal cord stimulation versus reoperation for failed back surgery syndrome: a cost effectiveness and cost utility analysis based on a randomized, controlled trial. *Neurosurgery*. 2007;61(2):361-369.
60. Kumar K, Taylor RS, Jacques L, et al. The effects of spinal cord stimulation in neuropathic pain are sustained: a 24-month follow-up of the prospective randomized controlled multicenter trial of the effectiveness of spinal cord stimulation. *Neurosurgery*. 2008;63:762-770.
61. North RB, Ewend MG, Lawton MT, et al. Failed back surgery syndrome: 5 year follow-up after spinal cord stimulator implantation. *Neurosurgery*. 1991;28:692-699.
62. Turner JA, Loeser JD, Bell KG. Spinal cord stimulation for chronic low back pain: a systematic literature synthesis. *Neurosurgery*. 1995. 37:1088-1096.
63. Wetzel FT, Hassenbusch S, Oakley JC, et al. Treatment of chronic pain in failed back surgery patients with spinal cord stimulation: a review of current literature and proposal for future investigation. *Neuromodulation*. 2000;3:59-74.
64. North RB, Kidd DH, Lee MS, Paintodosi S. A prospective, randomized study of spinal cord stimulation versus reoperation for failed back surgery syndrome: initial results. *Stereotactic Funct Neurosurg*. 1994;62:267-272.
65. Taylor RS, Van Buyten J-P, Buchser E. Spinal cord stimulation for chronic back and leg pain and failed back surgery syndrome: a systematic review and analysis of prognostic factors. *Spine*. 2005;30:152-160.
66. Frey ME, Manchikanti L, Benyamin RM, et al. Spinal cord stimulation for patients with failed back surgery syndrome: a systematic review. *Pain Physician*. 2009;12:379-397.
67. Oakley JC, Weiner RL. Spinal cord stimulation for complex regional pain syndrome: a prospective study of 19 patients at two centers. *Neuromodulation*. 1999;2:47-50.
68. Bennett DS, Alo KM, Oakley J, et al. Spinal cord stimulation for complex regional pain syndrome I [RSD]: a retrospective multicenter experience from 1995 to 1998 of 101 patients. *Neuromodulation*. 1999;2:202-210.
69. Taylor RS, Van Buyten J-P, Buchser E. Spinal cord stimulation for complex regional pain syndrome: a systematic review of the clinical and cost-effectiveness literature and assessment of prognostic factors. *European Journal of Pain*. 2006;10:91-101.
70. Grabow TS, Tella PK, Raja SN. Spinal cord stimulation for complex regional pain syndrome: an evidence-based medicine review of the literature. *The Clinical Journal of Pain*. 2003;19(6):371-383.
71. Turner JA, Loeser JD, Deyo RA, et al. Spinal cord stimulation for patients with failed back surgery syndrome or complex regional pain syndrome: a systematic review of effectiveness and complications. *Pain*. 2004;108:137-147.
72. Huber SJ, Vaglienti RM, Huber JS. Spinal cord stimulation in severe, inoperable peripheral vascular disease. *Neuromodulation*. 2000;3:131-143.
73. Claeys LG. Spinal cord stimulation in the treatment of chronic critical limb ischemia: a review of clinical experience. *Neuromodulation*. 2000;3:89-96.
74. Ubbink DT, Vermeulen H, Spincemaille GHJJ, et al. Systematic review and meta-analysis of controlled trials assessing spinal cord stimulation for inoperable critical leg ischemia. *Br JSurg*. 2004;91:948-955.
75. Jessurun GAJ, DeJongste MJL, Blanksma PK. Current views on neurostimulation in the treatment of cardiac ischemic syndromes [review]. *Pain*. 1996;66:109-116.
76. Eliasson T, Augustinsson LE, Mannheimer C. Spinal cord stimulation in severe angina pectoris—presentation of current studies, indications and clinical experience [review]. *Pain*. 1996;65:169-179.
77. DeJongste MJL. Efficacy, safety and mechanisms of spinal cord stimulation used as an additional therapy for patients suffering from chronic refractory angina pectoris. *Neuromodulation*. 1999;2:188-192.
78. DeJongste MJL. Spinal cord stimulation for ischemic heart disease. *Neurol Res*. 2000;22:293-298.
79. Sanderson JE, Brooksby P, Waterhouse D, et al. Epidural spinal electrical stimulation for severe angina: a study of its effects on symptoms, exercise tolerance and degree of ischaemia. *Eur Heart J*. 1992;13:628-633.

80. Sagher O, Huang D-H. Mechanisms of spinal cord stimulation in ischemia. *Neurosurg Focus.* 2006;21(6):1-5.

81. Di Pede F, Lanza GA, Zuin G, et al. Immediate and long-term clinical outcome after spinal cord stimulation for refractory stable angina pectoris. *Am J Cardiol.* 2003;91:951-955.

82. Lapenna E, Rapati D, Cardano P, et al. Spinal cord stimulation for patients with refractory angina and previous coronary surgery. *Ann Thorac Surg.* 2006; 82:1704-1708.

83. McNab D, Khan SN, Sharples LD. An open-label, single-centre, randomized trial of spinal cord stimulation vs. percutaneous myocardial laser revascularization in patients with refractory angina pectoris: the SPiRiT trial. *Eur Heart J.* 2006;27:1048-1053.

84. Ekre O, Eliasson T, Norrsell H, et al. Long-term effects of spinal cord stimulation and coronary artery bypass grafting on quality of life and survival in the ESBY study. *Eur Heart J.* 2002;23:1938-1945.

85. Taylor RS, De Vries J, Buchser E, et al. Spinal cord stimulation in the treatment of refractory angina: systematic review and meta-analysis of randomised controlled trials. *BMC Cardiovasc Disord.* 2009;9:13.

86. Ceballos A, Cabezudo L, Bovaira M, et al. Spinal cord stimulation: a possible therapeutic alternative for chronic mesenteric ischaemia. *Pain.* 2000;87:99-101.

87. Kapural L, Rakic M. Spinal cord stimulation for chronic visceral pain secondary to chronic non-alcoholic pancreatitis. *J Clin Gastroenterol.* 2008;42(6):750-751.

88. Krames E, Mousad DG. Spinal cord stimulation reverses pain and diarrheal episodes of irritable bowel syndrome: a case report. *Neuromodulation.* 2005;8:82-88.

89. Kapur S, Mutagi H, Raphael J. Spinal cord stimulation for relief of abdominal pain in two patients with familial Mediterranean fever. *Br J Anaesth.* 97(6):866-868.

90. Kapural L, Nagem H, Tlucek H, et al. Spinal cord stimulation for chronic visceral abdominal pain. *Pain Med.* 2010;11:347-355.

91. Tiede JM, Ghazi SM, Lamer TJ, et al. The use of spinal cord stimulation in refractory abdominal visceral pain: case reports and literature review. *Pain Pract.* 2006;6(3):197-202.

92. Monahan K, Casavant D, Rasmussen C, et al. Combined use of a true-bipolar sensing implantable cardioverter defibrillator in a patient having a prior implantable spinal cord stimulator for intractable pain. *Pace.* 1998;21:2669-2672.

93. Hoelzer BC, Burgher AH, Huntoon MA. Thoracic spinal cord stimulation for post-ablation cardiac pain in a patient with permanent pacemaker. *Pain Practice.* 2008;8(2):110-113.

94. Kosharskyy B, Rozen D. Feasibility of spinal cord stimulation in a patient with a cardiac pacemaker. *Pain Physician.* 2006;9:249-252.

95. Ferrero P, Grimaldi R, Massa R, et al. Spinal cord stimulation for refractory angina in a patient implanted with a cardioverter defibrillator. *Pace.* 2007;30;143-146.

96. Ekre O, Borjesson M, Edvardsson N, et al. Feasibility of spinal cord stimulation in angina pectoris in patients with chronic pacemaker treatment for cardiac arrhythmias. *Pace.* 2003;26:2134-2141.

97. Bala MM, Riemsma RP, Nixon J, et al. Systematic review of the (cost-)effectiveness of spinal cord stimulation for people with failed back surgery syndrome. *Clin J Pain.* 2008;24(9):741-756.

98. Taylor RS, Taylor Rj, Van Buyten J-P, et al. The cost effectiveness of spinal cord stimulation in the treatment of pain: a systematic review of the literature. *J Pain Symptom Manage.* 2004;27:370-378.

99. Andrell P, Ekre O, Eliasson T, et al. Cost-effectiveness of spinal cord stimulation versus coronary artery bypass grafting in patients with severe angina pectoris—long-term results from the ESBY study. *Cardiology.* 2003;99:20-24.

100. Doleys DM. Psychological factors in spinal cord stimulation therapy: brief review and discussion. *Neurosurg Focus.* 2006;21(6):1-5.

101. Sparkes E, Raphael JH, Duarte RV, et al. A systematic literature review of psychological characteristics as determinants of outcome for spinal cord stimulation therapy. *Pain.* 2010;150:284-289.

102. Mazars G Roge R, Mazars Y. Stimulation of the spinothalamic fasciculus and their bearing on the pathophysiology of pain. *Rev Neurol.* 1960;103:136-138.

103. Hosobuchi Y, Asams J, Rutkin B. Chronic thalamic stimulation for the control of facial anesthesia dolorosa. *Arch Neurol.* 1973;29:158-161.

104. Hirayama T, Dostrovsky J, Gorecki J. et al. Recordings of abnormal activity in patients with deafferentation and central pain: proceedings of the microelectrode meeting. *Stereotactic Funct Neurosurg.* 1989;52:120-126.

105. Lenz F, Tasker R, Dostrovsky J, et al. Abnormal single-unit activity recorded in the somatosensory thalamus of a quadriplegic patient with central pain. *Pain.* 1987;31:225-236.

106. Richardson DE, Akil H. Pain reduction by electrical brain stimulation in man, Part I. Acute administration in periaqueductal and periventricular sites. *J Neurosurg.* 1977;47:178-183.

107. Richardson DE, Akil H. Pain reduction by electrical brain stimulation in man, Part II. Chronic self-administration in the periventricular gray matter. *J Neurosurg.* 1977;47:184-194.

108. Hosobuchi Y, Adams JE, Linchitz R. Pain relief by electrical stimulation of the central gray matter in humans and its reversal by naloxone. *Science.* 1977;81:76-85.

109. Schoenen J, Di clenete L, Vandenheede M, Fumal A, De Pasqua V, et al. Hypothalamic stimulation in chronic cluster headache: a pilot study of efficacy and mode of action. *Brain.* 2005;128:940-947.

110. Brown JA, Pilitsis JG. Motor cortex stimulation for central and neuropathic facial pain: a prospective study of 10 patients and observation of enhanced sensory and motor function during stimulation. *Neurosurgery.* 2005;56:290-297.

111. Rasche D, Ruppolt M, Stirppich C, Unterberg A, Tronnier VM. Motor corterx stimulation for long-term relief of neuropathic pain: A 10-year experience. *Pain.* 2006;121:32-52.

112. Ito M, Kuroda S, Shiga T, Tamaki N, Iwasaki Y. Motor cortex stimulation improves local cerebral glucose metabolism in the ipsilateral thalamus in patients with poststroke pain: case report. *Neurosurg.* 69(2):E462-E469.

113. Garcia-Larrea L, Peryron R. Motor cortex stimulation for neuropathic pain: from phenomenology to mechanisms. *Neuroimage.* 2007;37(suppl 1):S71-S79.

114. Bittar RG, Kar-Purkayastha I, Owen SL, Bear RL, Green A, et al. Deep stimulation for pain: A meta-analysis. *J Clin Neurosci.* 2004;12(5):515-519.

115. Owen SL, Green L, Nandi D, Bittar RG, Wang SY, Aziz TZ. Deep brain stimulation for neuropathic pain. *Neuromod.* 2006;9(2): 100-106.

116. Owen SL, Green AL, Stein JF, Aziz TZ. Deep brain stimulation for the alleviation of post-stroke neuropathic pain. *Pain.* 2005;120 (1-2):202-206.

117. Rasche D, Rinaldi PC, Young RF, Tronnier VM. Deep brain stimulation for the treatment of various chronic pain syndromes. *Neurosurg Focus.* 2006;21(6):1-8.

118. Leone M, Franzini A, Broggi G, Bussonce G. Hypothalamic stimulation for intractable cluster headache: long-term experience. *Neurology.* 2006;67(1):151-153.

119. Hariz MI. Complications of deep brain stimulation surgery. *Movement Dis.* 2002;17(3):S162-S166.

120. Schoenen J, Di Clemente L, Vandenheede M, Fumal A. et al. Hypothalamic stimulation chronic cluster headache: a pilot study of efficacy and mode of action. *Brain*. 2005;128:940-947.

121. Henderson JM, Tkach J, Philips M, Baker K, Shellock FG, Rezai AR, Permanent Neurological deficit related to magnetic resonance imaging in a patient with implanted deep brain stimulation electrodes for Parkinson's disease: a case report. *Neurosurg*. 2005;57(5):E1063-E1066.

122. Rezai AR, Baker K, Tkach JA, Philips M, Hrdlicka G, Sharan AD, et al. Is magnetic resonance imaging safe for patients with neurostimulation systems used for deep brain stimulation? *Neurosurg*. 2005;57(5):1056-1062.

123. Lima MC, Frengi F. Motor cortex stimulation for chronic pain: systematic review and meta-analysis of the literature. *Neurology*. 2008;70:2329-2337.

124. Lefaucheur JP, Drouot X, Cunin P, Bruckert R, Lepetit H, et al. Motor cortex stimulation for the treatment of refractory peripheral neuropathic pain. *Brain*. 2009;132:1463-1471.

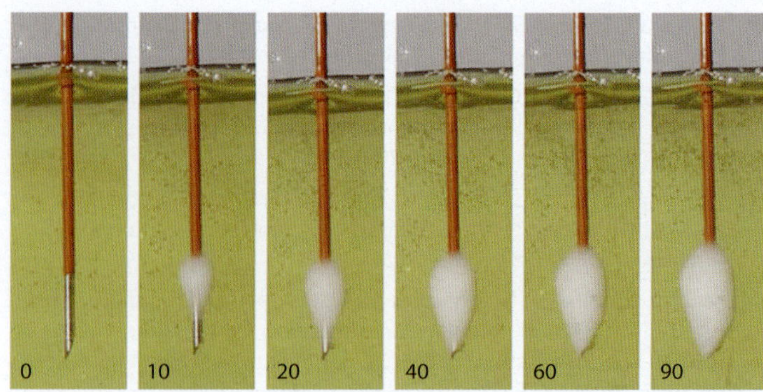

FIGURE 91-1. A 22-gauge, 10-cm SMK radiofrequency cannula with a 5-mm active tip is immersed in egg white, and conventional radiofrequency ablation is applied at 80°C for 90 seconds. The radial size of the lesion is maximal near the midportion of the active tip. Thus, for optimal application of conventional radiofrequency ablation treatment, the shaft of the needle's active tip is optimally placed adjacent to the target. The size of the lesion is near maximal by 60 seconds of treatment.[118] Notably, however, egg white immersion setups, although useful for illustrative purposes, can also underestimate heating at the distal end of the electrode because fluid convection causes heated egg white to flow upward. (Used with permission from and image courtesy of Dr. James Rathmell from *Atlas of Image-Guided Intervention in Regional Anesthesia and Pain Medicine*.[5])

Cryoanalgesia and Radiofrequency Ablation

Josemaria Paterno
James P. Rathmell
Chris Gilligan

BACKGROUND AND EVOLUTION OF RADIOFREQUENCY TREATMENT

Radiofrequency ablation (RFA) has an established and expanding role in the treatment of a myriad of pain conditions. As early as the 1930s, the application of electric current for neural ablation was reported in the medical literature. Clinicians initially used large (12–14 gauge) electrodes emitting *direct* current, which risked mechanical injury and produced unpredictable lesions.[1] However, investigators soon discovered that alternating current in the radiofrequency (RF) range between 300 and 500 KHz created more predictable lesions.[2,3] In the early 1950s, the first commercial RF lesion generator became available through the collaboration between electrical engineer Bernard Cosman and neurosurgeon Thomas Sweet at the Massachusetts General Hospital. In 1975, RFA was first described in the literature for the treatment of back pain.[1,4] Over the subsequent decades, RFA has become a widespread and effective treatment to create significant and sustained pain relief. Current and expanding clinical applications of RFA include facial; cervical, thoracic, and lumbar facet; spinal radicular; sacroiliac joint (SIJ); lumbar discogenic; peripheral nerve; intraarticular joint; and sympathetically mediated pain. The bulk of clinical data involves conventional RFA; however, over the past decade, modified forms of RF treatments have emerged. Today four forms of RFA predominate in clinical use: conventional (i.e. continuous) RFA (CRF), pulsed RFA (PRF), water-cooled RFA (WCRF), and bipolar RFA (BRF) (**Fig. 91-1**):

Conventional RFA (CRF): RF current is administered continuously for 60 to 150 seconds at a specific temperature, usually 80°C.

Pulsed RFA (PRF): Intermittent brief pulse (20 ms/pulse) of RF current is administered every half second. Lesion temperatures are often maintained at 42°C, which is below the thermocoagulation threshold.

Water-cooled RFA (WCRF): Continuous RF current that involves a specialized cannula needle that has cool water circulating within the electrode to prevent surrounding tissue from reaching excessive temperatures. It permits larger lesions to be created, which can also extend distal to the electrode tip.

Bipolar RFA (BRF): Involves two electrode tips placed side by side so that current density and electric fields are focused between the two. When spaced properly, the result is a single lesion larger than that created by two monopolar electrodes alone.

CONVENTIONAL RADIOFREQUENCY TREATMENT

The essence of CRF treatment involves the precise placement of an RF electrode probe on a specific target nerve followed by the application of RF alternating current in order to interrupt a nociceptive pathway. With only 90 to 150 seconds of treatment, the RF current alters the adjacent neural environment via thermal and electromagnetic-induced cellular changes.

Creating effective RF lesions requires understanding determinants of lesion consistency and predictability. RF lesions are prolate ellipsoidal in shape, the dimensions of which depend on static and dynamic factors.[6] Static factors include the length and gauge of the electrode active tip, the surrounding vasculature, and the characteristics of adjacent tissue. Dynamic factors include the amount of RF energy delivered, which is influenced by the electric field strength (proportional to voltage), heat accumulation, and total lesion time. Two recently published studies have also implicated fluid preinjection before RF treatment with 0.5 to 1 cc of normal saline, glucose solution, or hydroxyethyl starch as increasing lesion size compared with control or water preinjection.[7,8] Although still preliminary and not incorporated into routine practice, preinjection may enhance electrical and thermal conductivity to the surrounding tissues.

Earlier studies demonstrated that a 45° to 50°C threshold temperature is needed to create neuronal damage.[2,9] As the temperature increases, thermocoagulation of target nerve fibers commences. The volume of coagulated tissue further expands as temperature increases to 80°C. Studies indicate that after 60 to 90 seconds at 80°C, a lesion approaches maximum size.[10] Monitoring the electrode temperature enables consistent lesion size and avoids unnecessary tissue injury. The electrode itself is heated only passively as it induces heat generated in the surrounding tissue. As the electrode tip absorbs heat, the electrode thermocouple sensor represents the temperature of the hottest tissue adjacent to it.

Because larger 14- to 16-gauge electrodes led to a higher risk of mechanical injury and side effects such as deafferentation pain and bleeding, smaller diameter electrodes (e.g., 18–22 gauge) have emerged as the leading probe of choice in the majority of clinical applications. Larger gauge electrodes may be applied for specific targets such as the SIJ.

Notably in CRF, the elliptoid RF lesion extends only 1 to 2 mm both distal and proximal to the electrode's active end. The bulk of a lesion's volume is spread circumferentially around the long axis of the uninsulated active tip, usually approximately 4 to 5 mm as demonstrated in RF heating of egg whites (see **Fig. 91-1**). This lesion pattern has significant implications for electrode tip placement: Satisfactory lesion creation necessitates an electrode positioned parallel to the targeted nerve tissue, as opposed to perpendicular. This requirement highlights the anatomic technical accuracy required for electrode placement to lesion a target nerve adequately.

Factors Affecting the Size of a Radiofrequency Lesion

- Electrode active tip length
- Electrode active tip diameter
- Lesion time
- Tip temperature
- Local tissue characteristics (impedance of surrounding tissue).

NEUROBIOLOGY OF RADIOFREQUENCY LESIONS

The exact mechanism behind RFA has been debated but generally attributed to two key factors: the effects of thermal destruction and electrical field exposure. Because continuous RF current generates electric fields immediately adjacent to the probe, charged particles in the tissue such as free ions and proteins succumb to ionic agitation and friction from the high-frequency alternating current. Over the 60 to 150 seconds of treatment, the oscillation of charged molecules generates heat and ultimately results in protein denaturation, cellular membrane disruption, and increased membrane permeability, a neurodestructive process resulting in thermocoagulation.[11-13]

Because of thermocoagulation, CRF is *indiscriminately* neurodestructive. Early in the history of RFA, initial studies in cats hinted at the possibility of selective destruction of smaller nerve fibers, but subsequent animal data in cats, goats, and dogs showed an indiscriminate and nonselective destruction of both small and large myelinated fibers.[3,9] Even CRF lesions created at temperatures of 55°C, 65°C, and 75°C showed no specific selectivity for particular nerve fibers.[2] A minimum threshold of 45° to 50°C can produce some irreversible neuronal injury.[2,14] However, to maximize clinical efficacy, most practitioners today have adopted target temperatures at about 80°C, well above the neurodestructive threshold but below 95° to 100°C, which produces unwanted sequelae such as charring, tissue adherence to the probe, hematoma, gas formation, and extended damage to adjacent structures.

The mode of action of RF was initially attributed solely to the thermocoagulation of nerve fibers, but recent data point to mechanisms other than temperature-mediated destruction. Indeed, the electric field itself, *independent of heat*, can cause neuromodulatory changes that may affect pain transmission pathways. Data over the past decade have highlighted the influence of the electric field on neurobiology and have led to an interest in PRF technology.

PULSED RADIOFREQUENCY TREATMENT

Pulsed RF was first introduced in the mid 1990s. In PRF, the same high-frequency alternating current as in CRF (~300–500 KHz) is delivered but only in brief intermittent pulses. A typical application consists of two 20-ms bursts of RF current delivered per second, which represents a *pulsed* delivery cycle of 2 Hz. During one cycle, the delivery phase of 20 ms is followed by a rest period of 480 ms. Pulsed cycling prevents thermal buildup by allowing adequate time for heat washout. Thus, the total time of current delivery in PRF is only 4% (40 ms out of 1000 ms) that of CRF. Because the total time of current delivery is much shorter, PRF can deliver higher voltages than CRF (~45 volts in PRF compared with ~20 volts in CRF), all without raising the average temperature of adjacent tissue past the denaturation threshold of 45°C. With these higher voltages, PRF produces stronger electrical fields than CRF (**Fig. 91-2**). Thus, PRF maximizes electrical energy delivery through higher voltages while minimizing the risk of thermal destruction.

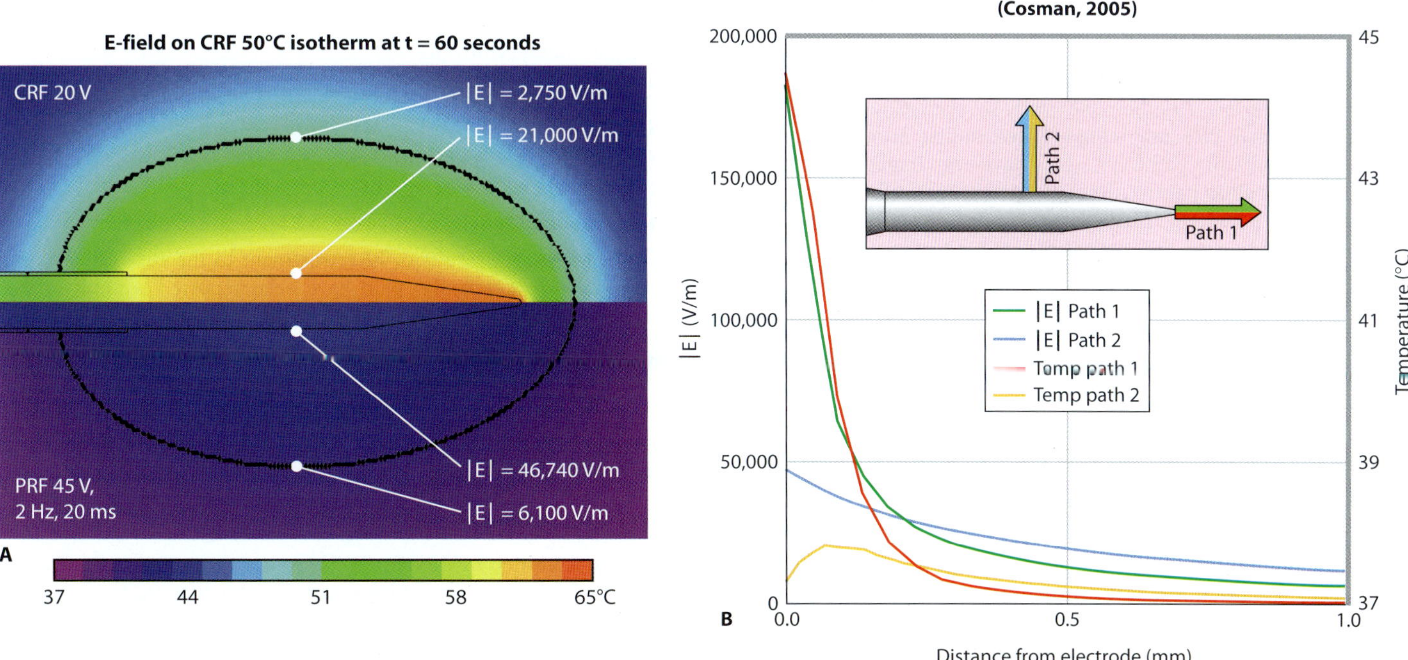

FIGURE 91-2. **A,** In conventional radiofrequency ablation, higher temperature gradients dominate, but in pulsed radiofrequency ablation (PRF), the higher voltage results in much stronger electric fields. **B,** During PRF, although the electric field is maximal within approximately 0.2 mm of the electrode point, it declines quickly ahead of the tip, so that beyond about 0.2 mm, its magnitude is smaller ahead of the tip than it is lateral to the shaft. (Used with permission from and image courtesy of Dr. Eric Cosman from *Manual of Radiofrequency Techniques*.[5])

The evolving evidence of minimal neurodestructive effects is a key appeal of PRF. With CRF, a neurodestructive thermal lesion increases the risk of weakness from damage to nearby motor nerves and deafferentation pain from complete loss of sensory input. Deafferentation syndrome results in dysesthesias and can evolve into a neuropathic syndrome.[15] Thus, PRF represents an alternative to CRF, especially in higher-risk anatomic locations such as the cervical dorsal root ganglion (DRG), where CRF studies have reported significant postprocedural pain or weakness.[16]

ELECTRIC FIELD NEUROMODULATION

A key unanswered question is the exact mechanism behind clinical pain relief in PRF. Without significant heat-induced tissue destruction, pain relief is posited to result from electromagnetic field– (EMF-) induced changes within the nerve cells.[17] Neurobiology studies have demonstrated the effect of electric fields on cellular activity at the transcription factor level. For example, C-Fos, an early transcription factor gene product that indicates neuronal activation and is possibly important in neuronal plasticity, has been demonstrated to be present 7 days after stimulation from *both* PRF and CRF. The implication is sustained neuronal activation of a pain-inhibiting process.[18] Interestingly, when comparing CRF with PRF at maximum electrode temperatures of only 38°C (well below thermocoagulation threshold of 45°–50°C), *only PRF* results in upregulation of c-FOS in DRG cells.[19] The inferred causative factor could be the stronger electric fields of PRF because of the higher applied voltage.

In PRF, the electric field is at its maximum within 0.2 mm distal to the electrode active tip point. Within this very short distance, it is speculated some minimal amount of neurodestruction is possible. However, overall, PRF produces *transient* histologic and structural changes not on the same destructive scale as CRF. Animal studies have demonstrated that when comparing PRF at 42°C with CRF (either at 67°C or 80°C), PRF-treated DRG cells exhibit signs of transient cellular stress, such as endoneurial edema, collagen deposition, fibroblast activation, increased cytoplasmic vacuolization, and enlarged endoplasmic reticulum. But these cells do *not* demonstrate signs observed in CRF such as Wallerian degeneration or mitochondrial and nuclear membrane damage.[12,20]

Additionally, a recent study suggests PRF may have selective effects on small-diameter unmyelinated C fibers and small myelinated A-δ-fibers.[21] When PRF was applied close to the DRG, staining of ATF3 (activating transcription factor 3), a neuronal activation marker, was significantly and selectively upregulated in the small- and medium-caliber DRG neurons. Another 2009 study by Hagiwara and colleagues demonstrated that PRF may enhance descending noradrenergic and serotonergic inhibitory pathways, which have been implicated in modulation of neuropathic pain.[22] Although speculation still dominates our understanding of how electric fields affect pain perception, a reasonable hypothesis may be that PRF activates an inhibitory state of excitatory pain fibers (e.g., C fibers) with resulting long-term depression. This inhibition could temporarily raise the nociceptive threshold and delay long-term potentiation of pain pathways.

PULSED RADIOFREQUENCY: PARALLEL (SIDE ON) VERSUS PERPENDICULAR (POINT ON) APPROACH

The optimal positioning of the PRF probe relative to its target nerve still remains a topic of controversy. With CRF, most clinicians prefer the electrode positioned adjacent and parallel to the target nerve to achieve the largest volume of thermal neurodestruction. PRF, however, permits some flexibility in placing the probe tip perpendicular to the target nerve because the goal is neuromodulation via the electric field, not neurodestruction. However, beyond 0.2 mm distal to the electrode active tip point, the electric field intensities drop dramatically,[23] which may create uncertainty in clinical efficacy with little margin for error if the target nerve is too distal and beyond an optimal zone of electric field influence. The advantage of the parallel approach with CRF also applies to PRF—electric field intensity declines less abruptly lateral to the electrode shaft; thus, side-by-side targeting exposes a bigger nerve volume to stronger electric fields (see **Fig. 91-2**).[23] Further studies and clinical trials are needed to determine PRF's optimal probe positioning.

EFFICACY OF PULSED VERSUS CONVENTIONAL RADIOFREQUENCY

Lacking a clear mechanistic understanding of PRF also raises the question of efficacy and sustainability of pain control compared with established CRF applications. It is possible that thermal neurodestruction would logically have longer-lasting results than electric field neuromodulation in targeting a nociceptive source. Although the evidence supporting the clinical efficacy of PRF continues to evolve, some studies indicate that PRF may be less effective or no better than CRF in specific applications, such as in patients with lumbar facet pain and trigeminal neuralgia (TGN).

In 2007, Tekin et al. compared PRF with CRF in a randomized controlled trial (RCT) for lumbar facet pain.[24] In 40 patients with lumbar facet pain, the PRF group did *not* show a decrease in visual analog scale (VAS) and Oswestry Disability Index (ODI) score, but the CRF group did at 6- and 12-month follow-ups. In a 2008 randomized, double-blinded, prospective study on lumbar facet pain, Kroll et al. demonstrated significantly improved pain scores with *both* CRF and PRF. However, there was no difference in outcome between the two groups, and the magnitude of improvement appeared greater in the CRF group.[25] Finally, for idiopathic TGN, Erdine et al. demonstrated that nearly all patients in the CRF group experienced significant sustained pain relief, but only 2 out of 20 patients in the PRF group had similar results.[26]

Nevertheless, PRF may be the RF modality of choice for targets such as the cervical DRG, where the risk of motor nerve destruction is high and potentially devastating. In 2007, Van Zundzert demonstrated PRF's efficacy for cervical radicular pain. Although PRF was not compared directly with CRF, PRF was compared with a sham control procedure, and the PRF group showed significantly better global perceived effect (GPE) and VAS scores.

If PRF does exhibit selectivity for smaller diameter fibers,[21] this may also explain some of PRF's temporal limitations. CRF-mediated neurodestruction necessitates neural regeneration and axonal regrowth, whereas recovery from the transient cellular stresses of PRF neuromodulation likely occurs over a shorter period. Further studies involving PRF are ongoing and encompass diverse applications in which CRF is contraindicated, such as the suprascapular nerve for rotator cuff pain and carpal tunnel syndrome.

- PRF clinical effects are temperature *independent* and largely through electrical field–induced cellular changes.
- PRF produces transient histologic stress changes in neural cells but not the destruction seen in CRF.
- PRF exhibits selectivity for C- and A-δ nociceptive fibers.
- Significant lasting results of PRF treatment to the cervical DRG for chronic cervical radicular pain have been reported without neurologic complications.
- In head-to-head comparison trials, evidence exists that PRF is not as effective as CRF for lumbar facet pain and TGN.
- Although the mechanism of PRF is yet to be fully elucidated, PRF may represent a minimally neurodestructive alternative to CRF heat lesions.

WATER-COOLED RADIOFREQUENCY

Lesion size is limited in CRF by the risk of tissue immediately adjacent to the cannula tip reaching temperatures greater than 90°C, which can cause charring, gas formation, and irregular unpredictable lesions. Invented in the 1990s for tumor ablation,[27] the third modality of RF technology involves internally cooling the shaft of the treatment cannula with a continuous flow of water. The cooled cannula acts as a heat sink to absorb thermal energy from the immediately adjacent tissue. This removes the constraint of proximal tissue reaching excessive

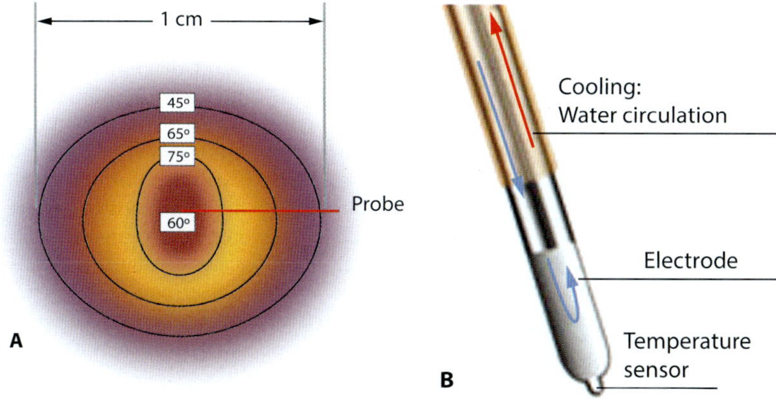

FIGURE 91-3. A water-cooled radiofrequency electrode enables creation of larger volume lesions without excessive heating adjacent to the electrode. The spherical lesion shape allows for perpendicular or oblique probe placement at the target site. (Used with permission from and image courtesy of Bayliss Medical.)

temperatures but allows distal tissue to accumulate thermal energy and reach target temperatures. With effective thermocoagulation extended a greater distance than in CRF, the size and sphere of an effective lesion are modestly increased (**Fig. 91-3**).

Water-cooled probes can lead to a substantial increase in lesion size for WCRF systems used in tumor ablation, where the peak temperature is allowed to exceed 100°C. For WCRF systems used in the spine, where the peak tissue temperature is limited to 75°C, the heat lesion size has a more modest but still clinically appreciable increase compared with CRF probes. For example, a WCRF electrode with a 17-gauge spinal introducer produces a heat lesion that is 10 mm in diameter, and a larger 16-gauge CRF electrode also produces a heat lesion 10 mm in diameter.[28,29]

Importantly, the ability to delivery greater energy to surrounding tissue also results in lesions that *extend distal* to the active tip. Therefore, using cooled RF, the cannula can be placed perpendicular to the course of the nerve to be treated and, in this position, can be expected to incorporate the nerve within the resulting lesion. In this system, the tissue immediately adjacent to the tip is kept at 60°C, and tissue beyond experiences a gradient from 75°C to 45°C. The most significant published application to date is for SIJ pain.[30] Clinical studies are under way for thoracic facet applications. Though promising as a relatively new RF delivery system, WCRF clinical data are still limited, and further studies are needed.

BIPOLAR RADIOFREQUENCY

CRF, PRF, and WCRF fall under the category of monopolar RF in which a circuit is completed by electrical current passing from the active electrode through surrounding tissues to a large reference ground pad placed on the patient's skin. The large area of the grounding pad helps to disperse the electric current density to safe and tolerable levels.

Bipolar RF involves two electrode tips precisely placed side by side so that current density and electric fields are focused between the two. When optimally spaced, the result is a lesion larger than that created by two monopolar electrodes alone (**Fig. 91-4**). Ex vivo lesion studies have estimated the optimal space between two electrodes to be 6 to 10 mm depending on the cannula gauge, tissue tested, and experimental conditions.[31,32] The size of one bipolar lesion can approximate three monopolar CRF lesions created side by side. Modern RF generators are required to adjust and coordinate the energy output level so that neither electrode's tip exceeds a target temperature. Bipolar lesions have been used to create elongated "strip" lesions for difficult targets such as the SIJ.

RADIOFREQUENCY DEVICE FEATURES

To perform RF treatment safely and effectively, an RF generator should also be capable of nerve stimulation and monitoring of electrode temperature, impedance, voltage, and lesion time.

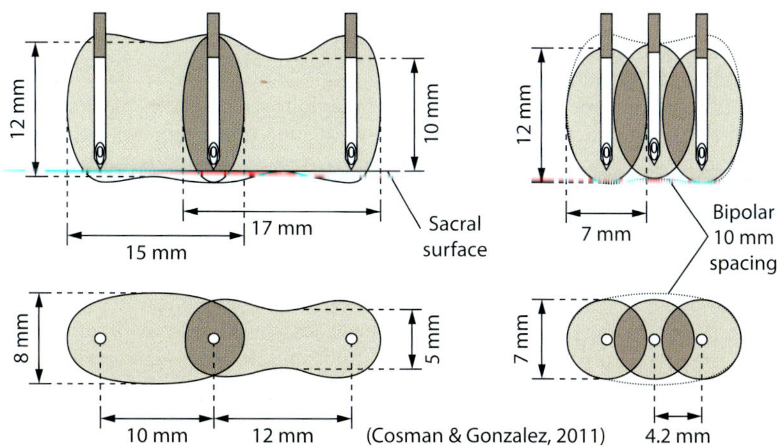

FIGURE 91-4. Bipolar lesion geometry with 10-mm active tips for 10- and 12-mm intertip spacings, 0-mm tip-to-sacrum distance, 90°C set temperature, and 3-minute lesion time. Three monopolar lesions, created using 90°C set temperature and 3-minute lesion time, are required to approximate a single bipolar lesion for 10-mm tip spacing and the same radiofrequency parameters (shown by the dotted outline). Lesions are in both lateral (top) and tunnel (bottom) views. (Used with permission from and image courtesy of Dr. Eric Cosman from *Manual of Radiofrequency Techniques*.[23])

TABLE 91-1 Summary of Impedance Changes and Differential During Radiofrequency Treatment

Impedance Changes	Differential
Very high impedance (resembles open circuit)	• Disconnected cables • Grounding pad not properly connected to patient
Rising impedance	• Broken temperature probe and tissue boiling • If thoracic procedure, concern for entry into pleural cavity and pneumothorax
Decreasing impedance to 150–250 ohms	• Dural sleeve perforation with CSF contact or intravascular penetration
Very low impedance (resembles short circuit)	• Contact of electrode with metallic implant • Contact with grounding pad

CSF, cerebrospinal fluid.

Temperature monitoring is accomplished by a thermocouple sensor at the tip of the electrode. For CRF, most practitioners raise the temperature 1°C/sec. Raising the temperature too quickly risks cavitation and unpredictably shaped lesions. Highly vascular areas can result in the dissipation of heat away from the contacted tissue, a phenomenon termed *heat washout*. Tissues that are better insulated (e.g., bone) can maintain the higher temperatures and experience less heat washout.

Nerve stimulation helps determine electrode to nerve distance. Sensory testing confirms that one is *close enough* to the target nerve, and motor testing ensures one is *far enough away* from any important motor innervation. To test sensory stimulation, 50 Hz of electrical current should produce pain or tingling with less than 0.5 to 0.6 V. For motor stimulation, electrical current is set at 2 Hz, and muscle contractions are observed with voltages greater than two to three times the sensory voltage threshold. Especially in spinal applications, the interventionalist is not concerned with localized motor contractions that represent direct muscle stimulation but rather with true motor nerve stimulation observed as distal twitches in the upper or lower extremities.

Impedance is an overall measure of tissue resistance to electrical current and helps characterize the adjacent tissue environment. During any RF treatment procedure, impedance should remain relatively constant. For facet and DRG treatments, impedance is typically between 250 and 700 ohms. A changing or abnormal impedance can provide a differential for the culprit clinical situation (**Table 91-1**). For example, a very high impedance resembles an open circuit, meaning that cable connections could be loose or disconnected or the patient grounding pad not properly applied. A very low impedance indicates low resistance to flow and could denote electrode contact with a metallic implant if applicable to the patient (e.g., nearby spinal instrumentation or spinal cord stimulator) or any kind of direct contact between an electrode component and the grounding pad, indicating a short circuit. Additionally, any impedance drop to approximately 200 ohms or less could indicate an intravascular probe, electrode probe or the occurrence of dural puncture and cerebrospinal fluid (CSF) contact. Conversely, if the impedance has been stable but then steadily rises, this could be a failsafe warning sign of boiling tissue combined with a broken temperature sensor because electrical current cannot easily be conducted through air and boiling gas bubbles.[23]

PATIENT SELECTION, DIAGNOSTIC BLOCKS, AND CONTRAINDICATIONS FOR RADIOFREQUENCY INTERVENTION

Before one embarks on RF treatment, the appropriate history, physical examination, and ancillary studies must have been completed. Computed tomography (CT) and magnetic resonance imaging (MRI) rarely give a clear indication for RF treatment but help rule out other conditions and the need for surgery. RFA is an elective procedure that is not an alternative to a clear surgical indication. The reported pain should be of a chronic nature, and conservative treatment should have already been fully explored.

The successful diagnostic block of a target nerve is the currently accepted standard indication for RF treatment. This typically entails pain relief of greater than 50% to 70% after a targeted nerve block. For some interventions such as lumbar facets, many guidelines and position papers from leading pain societies[33,34] have advocated for double blocks because of the high number of false positives after a single diagnostic block. However, recent analyses have argued against the double block paradigm because of the significant false-negative rate and speculated lack of cost effectiveness.[35] Clearly, double blocks have a role in clinical trials in need of strict selection criteria and do result in the highest success rate for RF denervation. However, many practices and even recently published trials have used single blocks before RF treatment.[36,37] The topic of single versus double diagnostic blocks remains a point of controversy among practitioners.

A range of contraindications for RF procedures exist, some of which require clinical judgment. Clear contraindications include coagulopathies, therapeutic anticoagulation, ongoing sepsis, or the presence of nearby invasive lesion such as tumor or infection. Relative contraindications include inadequately treated psychiatric conditions, psychopathology, previous failed RFA to the same target nerve, unrealistic expectations, and associated neuropathic or deafferentation pain syndromes. Anatomic abnormalities may also present a contraindication, especially with the presence of prior surgical instrumentation.

Additionally, patients with a pacemaker or spinal cord stimulator must be carefully monitored because of the risk of interaction with the RF equipment. As a consequence of RF lesioning, sensing pacemakers may mistakenly interpret RF signal as intrinsic atrial activity and fail to pace, which would result in asystole for pacemaker-dependent patients. Knowledge of the pacemaker features, an available magnet for override mode, and continuous electrocardiographic monitoring are prudent preventive measures. Patients with spinal cord stimulators should have the devices turned off for the remote chance RF current travels through the stimulator and directly involves the spinal cord. Also, the grounding pad should be placed so as to draw current away from the device.

Emergency resuscitation equipment such as a defibrillator and bag valve mask with oxygen source should be readily available in any interventional suite. Anaphylactic reactions are a rare but possible reaction to either local anesthetic or contrast agent. In some procedures, direct trauma to the spinal cord or unintended intrathecal administration of local anesthetic could result in respiratory compromise and hypotension. Finally, current leakage and serious burns are extremely rare with RF procedures, but one must be aware of the small chance of generator malfunction, electrical fault, or insulation cracks in the RF electrodes.

ZYGAPOPHYSEAL (FACET) JOINT RADIOFREQUENCY TREATMENT

Zygapophyseal or facet joints are paired structures that arise from the articulation of the superior articular process (SAP) of one vertebra with the corresponding inferior articular process (IAP) of the above vertebra. Each facet joint is a true joint encased by a fibrous capsule and lined by a synovial membrane with opposing articular cartilage surfaces. The facet joint structures are densely innervated and highly sensitive to mechanical forces.

Facet joints are innervated by the medial branch nerve (MBN), which provides sensation to the joint and also innervates the paraspinal multifidus muscle. Each vertebral level possesses a spinal nerve that departs from the intervertebral foramen and divides into a posterior (dorsal) and anterior (ventral) ramus. The MBN originates from its respective posterior ramus with the subsequent course depending on the anatomic vertebral level. Facet joints may be a source of chronic pain in 15% to 30% of patients with chronic low back pain (LBP) and 30% to 50% of patients with chronic neck pain.[38,39] Facet pain may present with a pseudoradicular pattern, making the underlying diagnosis difficult to confirm without the use of diagnostic blocks. Presently, facet interventions are the second most common type of interventional procedure performed in pain management clinics in the United States.[40]

CERVICAL FACET RADIOFREQUENCY TREATMENT

Between 30 - 50% of chronic axial neck pain originates from the facet joint.[38] It manifests with any combination of neck, arm, shoulder girdle, and upper back pain as well as possible paravertebral tenderness to palpation. Headache caused by the involvement of C1 to C3 nerve roots is known as cervicogenic headache, which projects unilaterally from the neck and occiput. The differential diagnosis of chronic axial neck pain also includes cervical muscle strain, spinal stenosis, and discogenic pain.

The two most common etiologies of cervical facet pain are degenerative disease and traumatic injury. In hyperextension whiplash injury, cervical facet pain is the single most common cause of chronic neck pain with a prevalence as high as 80% in motor vehicle accident injuries.[41] The traumatic mechanism relates to ligamentous sprain and ultimately periosteal tearing within the densely innervated facet joint. The cervical facet joints are innervated by articular nerves originating from the medial branches of the cervical dorsal rami.[42] At the cervical levels, the MBN curves through a groove at the lateral margin of the articular pillar. However, the C1 to C2 facet (atlanto-occipital/axial joint) is *not* innervated by cervical dorsal rami but by branches of the C1 and C2 ventral rami. Additionally, the C3 dorsal ramus has *two* medial branches: the C3 superficial medial branch is actually the third occipital nerve, innervating the C2 to C3 facet joint, and the second or deep medial branch innervates the C3 to C4 facet articular surface (**Fig. 91-5**).

Imaging studies often do not correlate with symptoms. About 20% to 30% of asymptomatic subjects have abnormal MRIs of the cervical spine depending on age.[43] Although neck pain is a challenging clinical entity, estimating a central focus of pain by examination and history helps target segmental levels for diagnostic blocks and subsequent RF treatment. Common manifestations are bilateral pain at the same segmental level and pain from consecutive segments. The false-positive rates from single diagnostic injection range from 27% to 66%, again adding to the controversy over single versus double blocks before the RF treatment decision.[44,45]

Cervical Facet Radiofrequency Posterior Approach (Fig. 91-6) The cervical facets may be targeted by both a posterior and a posterolateral approach; the latter is a useful approach for PRF. The posterior technique is described first. Minimal sedation is used to maintain constant communication with the patient because of the risk of inadvertent injury to the spinal cord or nerve root. With the patient prone, the level to be lesioned is identified in the anteroposterior (AP) view. The C-arm is rotated 25 to 35 degrees caudally to align the fluoroscope with the axis of the facet joints. The target area is the lateral margin of the articular pillar, midway between the IAP and SAP. This is seen as an invagination or "waist" of the articular pillar. Local anesthetic is applied, and an angiocatheter is placed in "gun-barrel" fashion (i.e., the needle is coaxial with the x-ray path). A 10-cm SMK cannula with a 5-mm curved active tip is advanced just medial to the lateral margin of the articular pillar until

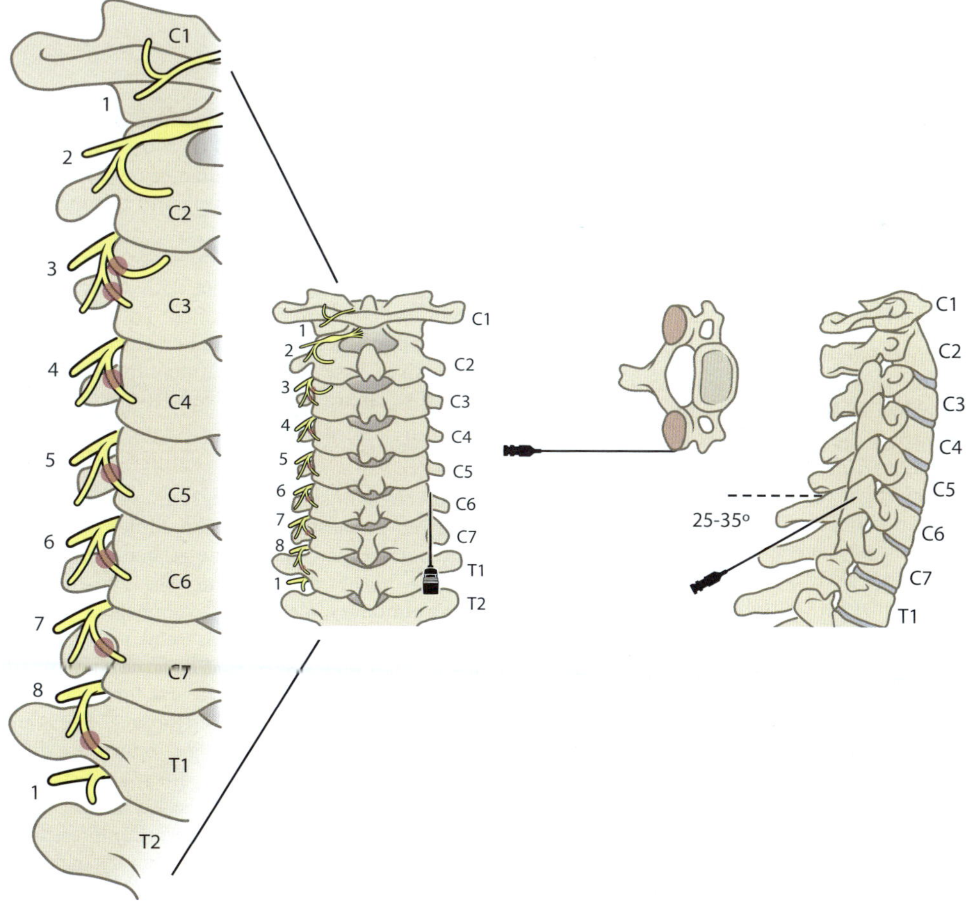

FIGURE 91-5. Cervical medial branch (MB) nerve anatomy. Cannula entry for cervical MB blocks and radiofrequency (RF) treatment (posterior approach). A 22-gauge, 10-cm SMK RF cannula with a 5-mm active tip is advanced in a plane 25 to 35 degrees caudal to the axial plane toward the midpoint between the superior articular process and inferior articular process of the target facet. This point appears as an invagination or "waist," where the lateral margin of the facet column dips medially between articular surfaces. Note that treatment of the C3 third occipital nerve requires an additional cannula placed toward the superior aspect of the C3 articular pillar overlying the C2 to C3 facet joint. (Used with permission from and image courtesy of Dr. James Rathmell from *Atlas of Image-Guided Intervention in Regional Anesthesia and Pain Medicine.*[5])

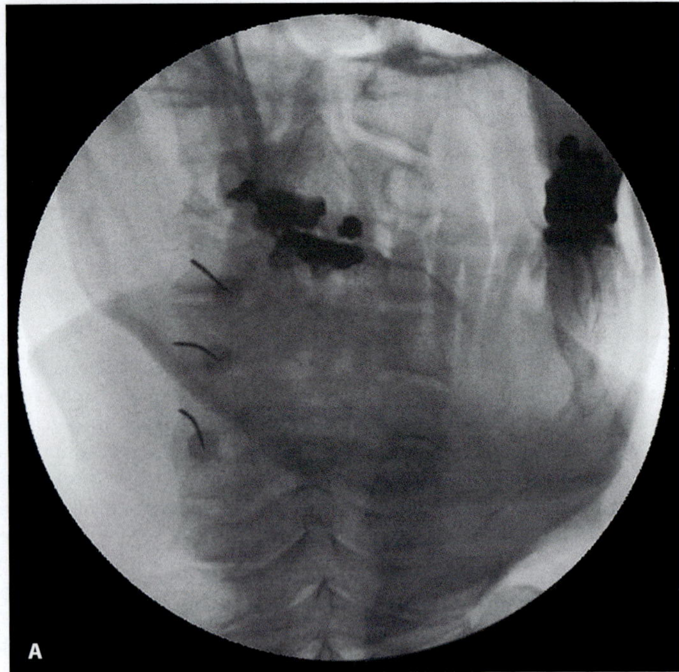

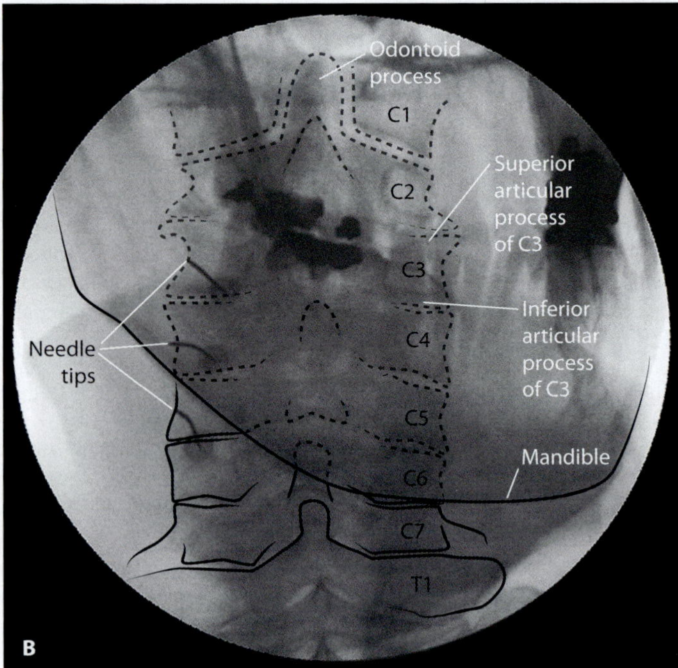

FIGURE 91-6. Cervical facet radiofrequency (RF) posterior approach. Three RF cannulae placed in the middle of the facet pillar at C3, C4, and C5 on the left, midway between the superior articular process and inferior articular process at each level. The caudad angulation of 25 to 35 degrees brings the facet joints into clear view and allows placement of the cannulae along the course of the medial branch nerves. Image with anatomic labels superimposed. (Used with permission from and image courtesy of Dr. James Rathmell from *Atlas of Image-Guided Intervention in Regional Anesthesia and Pain Medicine.*[5])

bony resistance of the back of the pillar is encountered. It is imperative that bony contact be made to prevent overinsertion. After the back of the pillar is contacted, the needle is walked off laterally in small increments until a loss of bony resistance allows the needle to gently slip forward 2 to 3 mm, as tangential to the pillar as possible. Here the cannula is adjacent and parallel to the MBN. Sensory and motor testing is performed as described. 0.5 cc of 2% lidocaine is administered and impedance is monitored while CRF is applied for 60 to 90 seconds at 80°C.

Cervical Facet Radiofrequency Posterolateral Approach If pulsed RF is desired, one can approach the MBNs laterally. The patient lies in the lateral decubitus position with a pillow to keep the neck in neutral position. The C-arm is placed directly over the patient's neck without rotation or angulation. The left and right articular pillars must be perfectly superimposed over each other. Any slight rotation of the neck can place the left and right facets in different radiographic positions. If the cannula is advanced anteriorly toward the contralateral facet by mistake, the spinal cord may be injured. This is more likely if the patient is slightly rotated toward the treatment side such that the contralateral facet appears more anterior. The tip of a PRF probe (5-cm cannula with a 5-cm active tip) is placed in the center of the trapezoid of the target facet under gun-barrel technique until bony contact is made, midway between articular surfaces and midway between the anterior and posterior extent of the facet column. After sensory and motor testing and application of 0.5 cc of 2% lidocaine, impedance is monitored, and PRF is applied at 45 V and 42°C for 90 seconds.

EVIDENCE FOR CERVICAL FACET RF TREATMENT

Reports have shown that between 50% and 90% of chronic neck pain patients treated by cervical RF ablation experienced at least 40% pain relief.[46-48] In 1996, Lord et al. established the efficacy of cervical facet RF treatment.[49] In this randomized, double-blind, controlled study, 24 patients with whiplash injury were enrolled. The experimental group ($n = 12$) received CRF at 80°C for 60 to 90 seconds, and the control group ($n = 12$) underwent the same procedure using CRF at only 37°C. Patients treated with CRF at 80°C experienced at least 50% pain relief for a median of 263 days. In the control group, 50% pain relief was experienced for a median of only 8 days. Some studies report that with proper selection criteria and technique, a 70% response rate can be expected.[48,50]

The Lord et al. trial and three other observational studies have yielded positive results for patients with chronic cervical facet pain.[46,51,52] A significant proportion of these patients had pain caused by cervical facet whiplash injury. To date, controlled prospective studies have not exclusively assessed RF treatment for cervical neck pain from degenerative disc disease, but positive retrospective data have been published.[51,52]

THORACIC FACET RADIOFREQUENCY TREATMENT

Thoracic pain symptoms account for roughly 5% to 6% of the patients referred to an outpatient pain clinic.[53,54] With thoracic pain, important etiologies other than spine-related pain must be ruled out such as angina, herpes zoster, aneurysms, and neoplastic disease (encompassing pulmonary, mediastinal, esophageal, and pleural tumors). Although thoracic disc herniations account for only 1% of all disc herniations, many are underappreciated because they manifest as anterolateral disc protrusions caused by the reverse lordosis or kyphotic curve of the thoracic spine (thus, force on the thoracic disc is anterior rather than posterior). Because many radiologic reports are directed posteriorly to areas encompassing nerve roots, pain specialists should be cognizant of any thoracic degenerative disc disease or disc protrusion because any disc space narrowing may lead to facet compression, inflammation, and pain.

Among those with localized thoracic pain, the prevalence of thoracic facet pain was estimated between 42% and 48%.[45] The symptoms of thoracic facet pain are often described as paravertebral pain that worsens with prolonged facet loading such as standing, hyperextension, or rotation of the thoracic spine. The thoracic spine is relatively immobile compared with its cervical and lumbar counterparts. The thoracic facet joints are also more vertically positioned than the lumbar facet joints. Lateral bending is extremely limited, and flexion/extension is only 10 degrees.

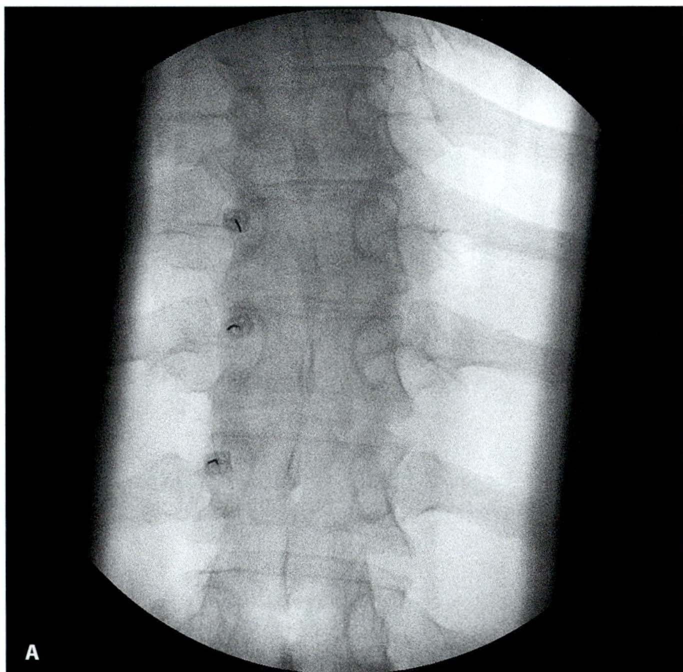

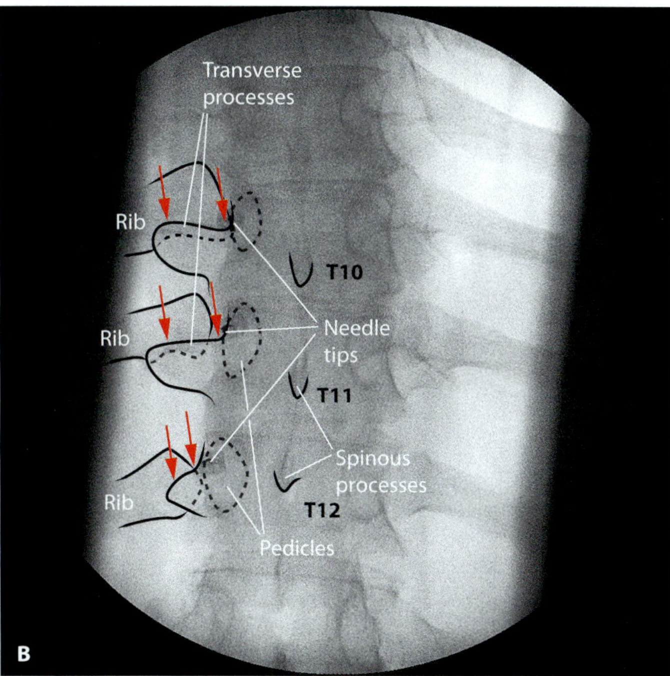

FIGURE 91-7. Anteroposterior radiograph of the thoracic spine with cannula placed along the superolateral margin of the left T10, T11, and T12 transverse processes. **B,** Labeled image. The *arrows* indicate the range, from medial to lateral extremes, where the medial branch nerves may pass over the superior margin of the transverse process. Unlike the predictable location of the nerve near the junction of the TP and superior articular process at lumbar spinal levels, the position of the nerve is less predictable at thoracic levels. (Used with permission from and image courtesy of Dr. James Rathmell from *Atlas of Image-Guided Intervention in Regional Anesthesia and Pain Medicine.*[5])

Although expert opinion varies on the precise course, the thoracic MBN is unique compared with its lumbar counterpart. Whereas the predictable lumbar MBN courses immediately over the junction of the transverse process and SAP, extensive anatomic dissections have demonstrated a more lateral path of the thoracic MBN (**Fig. 91-7**). In fact, the thoracic MBN often extends as far as the superolateral corner of the transverse process before travelling medially and inferiorly across the posterior surfaces of the transverse processes before innervating the multifidus muscles.[55] And notably, at midthoracic levels T5-T8, the curved inflection of the nerve occurs slightly *above* the superolateral corner of the transverse process. In 84 cadaveric thoracic medial branches studied under the dissecting microscope, these nerves did not cross the junction between the SAP and transverse process,[55] the classic targets of lumbar facet pain.

Thoracic Facet Radiofrequency Technique The patient is prone, and the C-arm is positioned directly over the thoracic spine. A 10-cm SMK cannula with a 5-mm active tip is advanced toward the superolateral margin of the TP in a coaxial fashion (gun-barrel approach). When the cannula rests on the superior margin of the TP, it is walked superolaterally off the TP and advanced 2 to 3 mm (see **Fig. 91-7**). Depth is confirmed on lateral view. The probe is parallel and adjacent to the MBN. Sensory and motor testing is performed, and 0.5 cc of 2% lidocaine is administered. Impedance is monitored, and RF lesioning is performed. Of note, important anatomic structures such as the pleural space and artery of Adamkiewicz are in proximity to this region. With the probe properly positioned, the pleural membrane still lies approximately 15+ mm anterior to the tip depending on body habitus. Usually between T9 and T12, the artery of Adamkiewicz originates from the aortic trunk and curves around the vertebral bodies to the anterior spinal cord. The practitioner should be aware of this artery's course and the theoretical danger of not just pneumothorax but also serious neurologic injury with a malpositioned cannula.

In a 1993 retrospective study, Stolker et al. evaluated 40 patients who underwent thoracic facet CRF treatment. A total of 82% of these patients had greater than 50% reduction in pain symptoms 2 months after the procedure.[56] A 2000 retrospective study by Tzaan and Tasker of 119 all-level facet procedures reported a 40% success rate in the 15 patients who were treated with one level thoracic facet-CRF at 6-month follow-up.[57] Further investigation is needed in how to best effectively target the thoracic MBN because of its unique course, particularly between T5 and T8. Thus, RF modalities that enable larger lesion size such as WCRF are currently in clinical trials.

LUMBAR FACET RADIOFREQUENCY TREATMENT

Lumbar facet pain conservatively affects 15% to 40% of patients with mechanical LBP.[54,58] The L1-L4 MBNs descend from their respective L1-L4 posterior rami. Each facet joint receives dual innervation from the MB nerve at the same level and the MB nerve one level *above* the facet joint. For example, the L3-L4 facet is innervated by the L3 MB (the same level nerve) and the L2 MB (the above level nerve) (**Fig. 91-8**). The L1-L4 MBNs curve around the base of the SAP and then subsequently under the mamillo-accessory ligament. It then courses medially and innervates the multifidus muscle, which lies adjacent to the spinous processes and deep to the spinal erectors. Of note, for L5, it is the posterior ramus itself that is targeted, as it courses along the junction between the sacral ala and articular process of the sacrum.

Direct palpation over the facet joint may induce localized tenderness. Patients may also have occasional diffuse radiation to the posterior thigh and buttock but without other spinal root radicular signs or associated weakness. Facet-loading maneuvers often exacerbate or recreate the pain. For lumbar facets, single diagnostic blocks have been shown to be associated with a false-positive rate as high as 35%.[59]

Lumbar Facet Radiofrequency Technique (Fig. 91-9) The patient is placed in the prone position and the lumbar level identified in the AP view. The x-ray beam is aligned with the L4-L5 disc to eliminate parallax of the disc end plates. Then the C-arm is rotated 15 to 25 degrees ipsilaterally in the oblique view to visualize the facet joint and the junction between the TP and SAP (the "Scottie dog"). Local anesthetic is subcutaneously

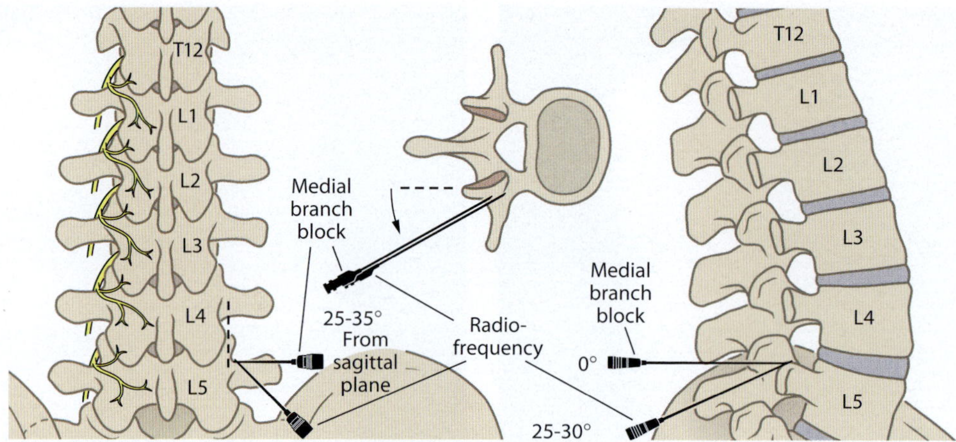

FIGURE 91-8. Angle and position of needle entry for lumbar medial branch (MB) block and radiofrequency (RF) treatment. A 22-gauge, 10-cm SMK RF cannula with a 5-mm active tip is advanced toward the base of the TP, where it joins with the superior articular process (SAP). Cannula placement for conventional RF treatment should be carried out with 25 to 30 degrees of caudal angulation of the C-arm to bring the axis of the active tip parallel to the course of the MB in the groove between the TP and the SAP. The MB target nerve points for RF treatment are illustrated on the left. (Used with permission and image courtesy of Dr. James Rathmell from *Atlas of Image-Guided Intervention in Regional Anesthesia and Pain Medicine.*[5])

injected over the "eye" of the Scottie dog. The C-arm is then rotated 25 to 35 degrees caudally to align the RF active tip with the course of the MB nerve. A 10-cm RF cannula with a 5-mm active tip is advanced in "gun-barrel" fashion at the junction between the superior margin of the TP and the inferior aspect of the SAP (the "ear" of the "Scottie dog"). The needle is advanced to periosteum and then "walked off" in the lateral superior direction immediately above the superior margin of the TP. The catheter is advanced 2 to 3 mm so that it is immediately adjacent and parallel to the MB nerve. In the lateral view, this should be noted to be at the level of the facet column line, posterior to the foraminal line and below the level of the disk. Sensory and motor testing is performed. Lesioning is preceded by injection of 0.5 cc of 2% lidocaine. The CRF lesion is made at 80°C for 60 to 90 seconds.

EVIDENCE FOR LUMBAR FACET RADIOFREQUENCY TREATMENT

Lumbar facet RF is an accepted standard treatment for facetogenic pain, and previous reviews have affirmed the evidence for the efficacy of lumbar facet RFA.[60-62] Crucial elements of high-quality lumbar facet RF studies include patient selection, correct anatomic targeting, and correct electrode placement. Earlier randomized trials that showed limited clinical effectiveness[63] have been criticized for flaws in incorrect needle positioning or poor diagnostic selection criteria.[64]

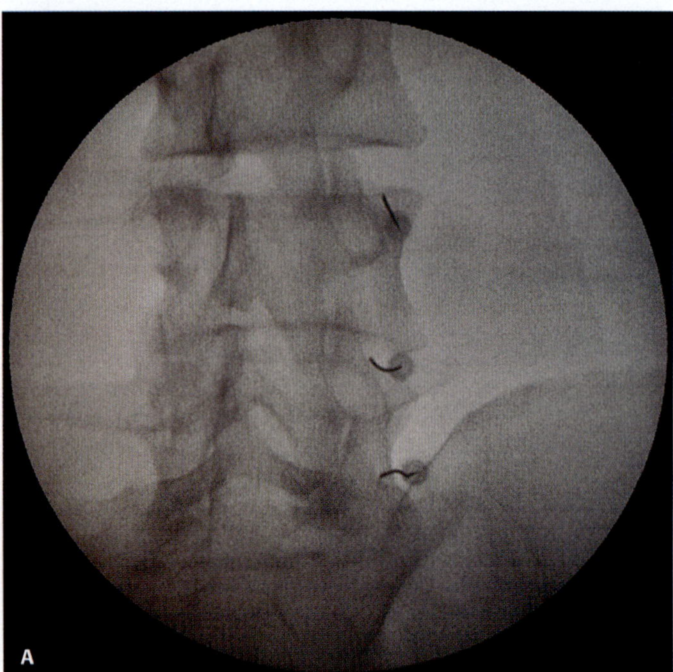

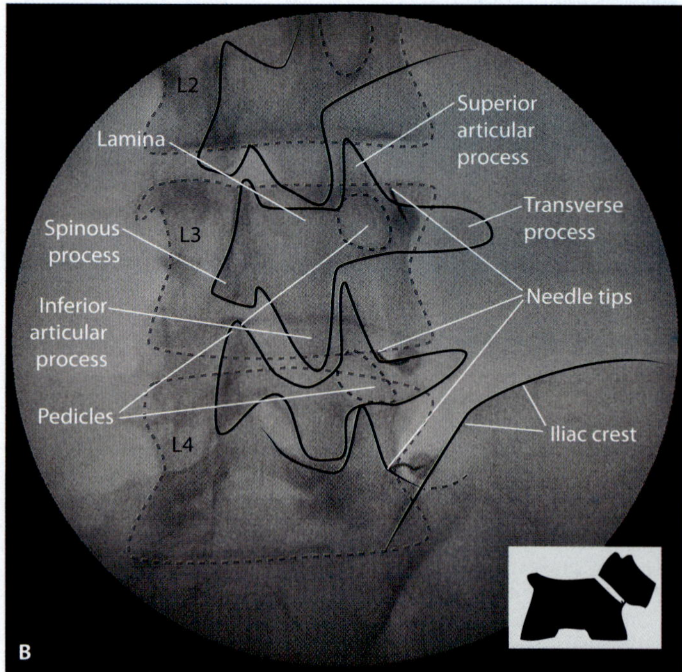

FIGURE 91-9. Left, Oblique radiograph during lumbar facet radiofrequency (RF) treatment. Three RF cannulae are in place at the base of the TP and superior articular process at the L3, L4, and L5 levels on the right. Right, Image with anatomic labels superimposed. The contours of the posterior bony elements on the oblique projection resemble the silhouette of a Scottish terrier or "Scotty dog." Compare the outlined areas of the radiograph with the contour of an actual Scottish terrier shown in the inset lower right corner. (Used with permission and image courtesy of Dr. James Rathmell from *Atlas of Image-Guided Intervention in Regional Anesthesia and Pain Medicine.*[5])

Multiple descriptive, prospective, and retrospective studies have indicated successful short- and long-term pain relief.[47,60,65] In 1999, Van Kleef et al. performed a double-blind RCT of 31 patients with a 1-year history of chronic LBP with positive diagnostic blocks.[37] The patients were divided into an 80°C CRF group ($n = 15$) and a sham procedure control group ($n = 16$). At 8 weeks, 10 of 16 patients in the CRF group had significant improvement compared with 6 of 16 in the sham control group by GPE and VAS scores. This statistical significance was maintained at the 6- and 12-month follow-up periods.

In 2008, Nath et al. also performed a double-blind RCT in 40 patients with chronic lower back pain.[66] Inclusion criteria were notable for three separate controlled positive diagnostic facet blocks. Twenty control patients received a sham procedure, and 20 patients received CRF treatment. The authors noted that for each MBN targeted, four separate lesions were performed to account for any anatomic variation in MBN course. Outcomes were assessed at 6 months and demonstrated significant improvement in pain VAS scores and functional ability.

Another prospective audit showed that with accurate technique and controlled diagnostic blocks, 60% of patients receive 90% relief from their pain, and nearly 90% reach at least 60% relief after lumbar facet CRF treatment at 12 months.[67] Lumbar facet RF has been one of the most studied RF applications and is currently considered the "gold standard" for treating lumbar facetogenic pain.[62]

DORSAL ROOT GANGLION RADIOFREQUENCY TREATMENT

Radiofrequency lesions adjacent to the DRG have been performed since the late 1970s.[68] Located in proximity to the respective intervertebral foramen, the DRG contains cell bodies of afferent spinal nerves and appears as an enlargement of the dorsal spinal root. Radicular pain is attributed to compression of the spinal nerve root, most often by a herniated disk that causes nerve root irritation and release of inflammatory cytokines. Such cytokines affect ion channels, causing repetitive and prolonged firing of the relevant sensory axons.[69] These sustained discharges have been linked to heightened mechanical sensitization of the spinal dorsal horn cells and a resulting hyperalgesic and potentially neuropathic state.

Radiofrequency treatment of the DRG was applied in the 1980s as an alternative to surgical rhizotomy for chronic refractory pain. Initially, surgical rhizotomy was shown to lead to great short-term pain relief in various pain syndromes. However, the long-term effects of surgery diminished and severe adverse effects, such as neuroma formation, were noted with substantial denervation.

The sine qua non for performing RF-DRG is based on a diagnostic nerve root block that suggests a monoradicular pain syndrome. As with facet pain, physical examination findings and imaging can be variable. The procedure is not without risk because of the potential for deafferentation syndrome, neuritis, and accidental lesioning of motor nerve fibers.[68,70] Because of these risks as well as alternative conservative treatments and surgical options, RF-DRG is less commonly performed in pain clinics, especially compared with RF-facet treatments. Additionally, to avoid unintended sequelae, most studies using CRF set a target lesion temperature of 67°C rather than 80°C. DRG fibers are anatomically distinct from motor fibers, and electrode placement may be tested by motor and sensory stimulation. Compared with CRF, some advocate for the exclusive use of PRF for the DRG because of the greater procedural comfort, lower risk of neurodestruction and motor nerve damage, and prevention of neuropathic pain exacerbation.

CERVICAL DORSAL ROOT GANGLION

Cervical radicular pain is a common pain syndrome that 10% to 12% of people experience at some time in their lives and has an annual incidence of 1 in 1000.[71,72] Cervical radicular pain can be classically described by the level affected—whereas C5 radicular pain extends into the upper arm, that from C6 and C7 extends from the neck and shoulder into the forearm and hand. In both instances, the pain occurs in the lateral upper limb, but C7 pain extends more onto the posterior aspect. Trials have demonstrated the efficacy of DRG RF treatment for patients with intractable cervical radicular pain adequately selected by diagnostic blocks and for whom surgery has failed or is contraindicated.

For the cervical DRG PRF technique (for cervical roots C3 and below), the patient is supine. After the appropriate level in the AP view is identified, the C-arm is rotated 30 degrees oblique to view the foramina. The approach is analogous to a cervical facet lateral approach in the supine position; however, the 10-cm cannula with a 5-mm active tip is advanced to the 6 o'clock position into the posteriormost aspect of the vertebral canal. This dorsal position is used to avoid the anterior vertebral artery. Frequent AP views are obtained to assure the needle does not pass medial to the midfacet line. Sensory and motor stimulation must be done meticulously. Confirmation may be done with the injection of 0.5 mL of water-soluble, nonionic contrast dye. As with any DRG RF lesion, sensations elicited at less than 0.4 V may indicate intraganglionic position and warrant needle repositioning to avoid any adverse sensory deafferentation from intraganglionic lesioning. Impedance is monitored as previously described, and PRF is then performed at 42°C for 90 to 120 seconds.

EVIDENCE FOR CERVICAL RADIOFREQUENCY DORSAL ROOT GANGLION

Retrospective and observational clinical studies have reported efficacy of cervical RF-DRG treatment.[61,73,74] According to two RCTs and two systematic reviews, cervical CRF DRG is more effective than placebo for chronic cervical radicular pain.[61,70,75,76] In 1996, Van Kleef performed the first RCT in 20 patients with at least 1 year of chronic intractable cervical radicular pain. Selection criteria included at least three diagnostic segmental nerve blocks in each patient. CRF was used at 67°C, and outcomes were assessed by various pain scales at 8 weeks. The investigators reported significant ($P = 0.0027$) 8-week efficacy in the 67°C CRF-DRG group compared with the sham control group.

The second trial, by Slappendel et al. in 1997, sought to determine the relevance of lesion temperature in CRF-DRG. CRF-DRG was performed at both 67°C and 40°C. Efficacy between the two groups was equal. Reduction in VAS greater than 2 occurred in 47% of the 67°C group and 51% of the 40°C group. Even though there was no sham control group, the 51% response rate in the 40°C CRF "control" group is significantly higher than the response rate of sham control procedures in other trials and historical control participants. Thus, this early study actually highlighted the importance of the electric field, rather than temperature, in RF neuromodulation.

In 2007, a high-quality RCT was published using PRF-DRG for the treatment of cervical radicular pain. This trial by Van Zundert et al.[77] had a positive result for short-term clinical efficacy of PRF-DRG. The PRF group showed a significantly better outcome by global perceived effect (GPE >50% improvement) and VAS (> 2) score compared with the sham group.

For cervicogenic headache, the only RCT of CRF-DRG was performed by Haspeslagh et al.[78] This trial concluded that CRF treatment of the facet joints and the DRG were only as effective as but not better than local nerve blocks in the treatment of cervicogenic headaches.

THORACIC DORSAL ROOT GANGLION

Thoracic radicular pain is characterized by unilateral radiating segmental pain originating from intercostal innervation. Because different levels overlap, it can be difficult to relate the pain pattern to a specific level involved. The etiology of thoracic radicular pain is often postsurgical and known as chronic postsurgical thoracic pain (CPTP). Culprit surgical procedures include thoracotomy, mastectomy, and sternotomy. Because CPTP presents a major therapeutic challenge in patients with chronic pain, the DRG has been targeted for refractory cases.

The exact technique depends on the thoracic level.[79] In low thoracic regions below T7, a posterolateral approach is used. The intervertebral foramen is identified by adjusting the C-arm to the 10- to 20-degree oblique position. Under AP view, the cannula is inserted caudal to the lateral half of the pedicle, roughly 1 cm medial to the angle of the ribs. On lateral view, the final position of the probe tip is in the craniodorsal part of the intervertebral foramen. Above T7, the technique is more specialized and is described in detail by Van Kleef et al.[79] A dorsal approach is chosen mainly because of anatomic interference from the angle of the ribs. A special drill hole is made using Kirschner wire through the lamina through which the RF cannula can pass to reach the DRG. Careful sensory and motor testing is performed. Contrast should exclude epidural spread or vascular penetration. CRF or PRF is performed.

Evidence for Thoracic Radiofrequency Dorsal Root Ganglion Three retrospective studies have examined the use of RF for thoracic radicular pain by targeting the DRG. Stolker et al.'s 1994 retrospective study of 45 patients with thoracic radicular pain reported 70% of patients with significantly reduced pain 1 to 3 years after the procedure.[80] Van Kleef et al. reported, out of 43 patients with a 6-month history of unilateral segmental thoracic pain selected by two or more diagnostic blocks, 52% of patients had long-term relief at 9 months after CRF at 67°C for 60 seconds.[53] Finally, in 2006, Cohen et al. reported retrospective data on 49 patients comparing PRF-DRG versus PRF of the intercostal nerve for thoracic radicular pain.[81] A total of 54% of patients in the PRF-DRG group had greater than 50% pain relief at 3 months after the procedure compared with only 7% in the PRF intercostal nerve only group.

LUMBAR DORSAL ROOT GANGLION

Lumbar radicular pain is classically described as a sharp, shooting pain that radiates down the length of the leg. The most frequent causes of lumbar radicular pain are herniated discs with nerve compression, foraminal stenosis (from bone spurs or osteoarthritis), nerve root injuries, and scar tissue from previous spine injuries compressing the nerve root. In general, the procedure has been reserved for patients with intractable pain who are not surgical candidates.

Many saw promise in RF lumbar DRG because the efficacy of RF cervical DRG had been reported in randomized trials. Even initial prospective and retrospective RF lumbar DRG studies showed promising results with success rates up to 60%.[73,82] However, evidence of efficacy from RCTs failed to show any benefit. A well-regarded 2003 RCT by Guerts et al. using CRF of the lumbar DRG showed no difference compared with the control group.[83] Only 16% of patients in the CRF lumbar DRG group but 25% in the sham treatment group had successful results. Although once performed with greater frequency in United States and Europe, routine RF lumbar DRG for lumbosacral radicular pain is no longer advocated.

SACROILIAC RADIOFREQUENCY TREATMENT

The SIJ is the largest axial joint in the human body and is formed by the articulation of the lateral sacrum with the medial surface of the ilium. SIJ pain is increasingly recognized as the cause of chronic LBP in 15% to 25% of patients but remains challenging to diagnose.[84,85] SIJ mechanical pain often presents with referred generic complaints such as low back (72%), buttock (94%), and lower extremity pain (50%).[86] Anatomic abnormalities may be absent on imaging.[87]

> **Box Summary**
>
> Evidence for Dorsal Root Ganglia Radiofrequency Treatment[69]
>
> - Cervical radicular pain ⟶ limited evidence in favor of CRF and PRF treatment
> - Cervicogenic headaches ⟶ unclear benefit of CRF treatment.
> - Lumbar radicular pain ⟶ limited evidence *against* use of CRF treatment.

Injury occurs with chronic or traumatic axial or rotational overloading. The extraneous compression and shearing forces result in *extraarticular* ligamentous damage and inflammation as well as *intraarticular* pathology. With certain chronic conditions such as osteoarthritis, pain may primarily originate from an intraarticular origin. In a study of 54 patients with SIJ syndrome (diagnosed by intraarticular local anesthetic injection), 44% were related to trauma, 21% attributed to repeated joint stress, and 35% idiopathic.[88] Variable patient populations are at risk. Repeated joint stress encompasses the wear and tear of aging, manual labor, or repeated athletic endeavors. Special at risk populations include peri- or postpartum patients and those with HLA B27 seronegative spondyloarthropathies such as psoriatic arthritis.

There is variance of practice in diagnosis of SIJ pain. Commonly, the diagnosis is made by intraarticular local anesthetic block. Although lumbar facet blocks have a false-positive rate greater than 35%,[59] one study concluded a smaller 17% false-positive rate for SIJ blocks.[89] Notably, the SIJ innervation is complex and variable. The lumbosacral plexus, specifically the posterior rami of L1–S2, and the superior gluteal and obturator nerve contribute to sensory innervation of the *anterior* SIJ. The *posterior* SIJ is innervated by the posterior rami of L4–S3 (L4-L5 medial branches and S1-S3 lateral branches). The S1–S3 lateral branches exit from the sacral foramina and traverse the sacrum in sometimes unpredictable fashion. Additionally, because of anatomic constraints, the SIJ is difficult to target with CRF treatment. Owing to the flat plane of the posterior sacrum, the interventionalist is unable to place the probe truly parallel and adjacent to the sacral foramina lateral branches. Rather, the tip of the cannula reaches these target nerves at a more perpendicular angle. Because CRF lesions are unable to be fully realized distal to the active tip, failure to ablate the target nerve adequately is common.

One notable caveat to SIJ-RFA procedures is that pain originating from the *anterior/ventral* SIJ may not be adequately addressed despite a perfect approach and technique, especially if, as some suspect, the obturator and superior gluteal nerve contribute to anterior SIJ sensory innervation. Although imaging is not a perfect correlate to pain, one study showed that anterior/ventral capsular pathology accounted for 69% of CT pathology in 13 patients with block confirmed SIJ pain.

Innovation with Radiofrequency Sacroiliac Joint Treatment Over the past decade, innovative RF techniques such as WCRF and bipolar strip lesioning have been explored for SIJ pain with promising results. With WCRF because tissue immediately adjacent to the probe is cooled, the thermal buildup in more distal tissue can "catch up" to approach effective lesioning thresholds. Consequently, lesions extend further distally, relative to the active tip, which helps compensate for the perpendicular orientation of the probe. With BRF, an elongated strip lesion can be created by a *leapfrog* or *palisade* arrangement of electrodes as demonstrated by Cosman and Gonzalez,[32] Burnham and Yasui,[90] and Ferrante et al.[91] Bipolar lesions strip lesions can be created either along the posterior aspect of the joint capsule or lateral to the sacral foramina to target the sacral lateral branch nerves.

Bipolar Radiofrequency Technique of the Sacroiliac Joint The patient is prone, and the C-arm is rotated 25 to 35 degrees caudally from the axial plane to place the posterior-superior iliac spine and iliac crest along the line of the SIJ. The C-arm is rotated obliquely 0 to 30 degrees toward the contralateral side until the posterior inferior aspect of the SIJ is clearly visible. Using 10-cm SMK cannulae with 5-mm active tips, the first cannula is placed at the inferiormost aspect of the joint, and then a second cannula is placed 6 to 7 mm above the first cannula (**Fig. 91-10**). To ensure optimal lesions, the active tips are placed in parallel, so care must be taken to ensure the cannulae are at the same depth. Important functional nerves are not in this area, so sensory and motor testing is not performed. 0.5 cc of 2% lidocaine is administered through the cannula. Bipolar lesions are created with a target temperature of 90°C for 3 minutes. Sequential bipolar lesions are performed cephalad maintaining the 6- to 7-mm intertip spacing. Modern RF generators have multiple outputs, so two or three bipolar lesions can be created at once. Depending

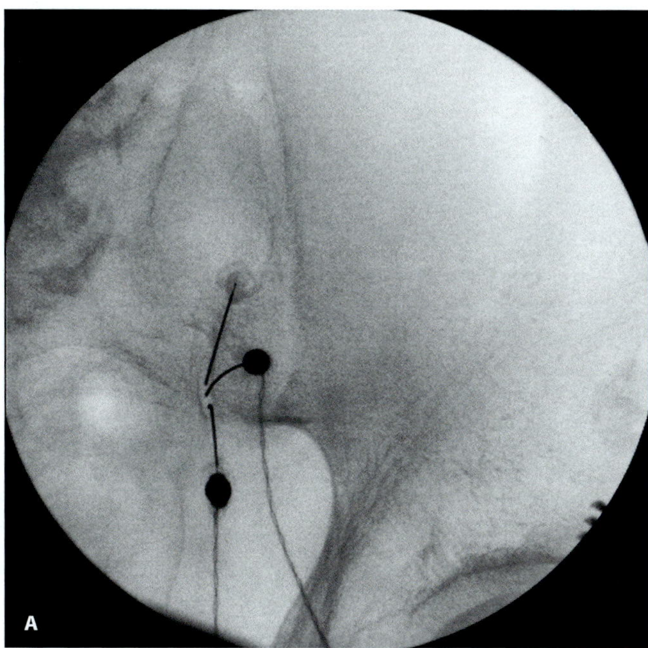

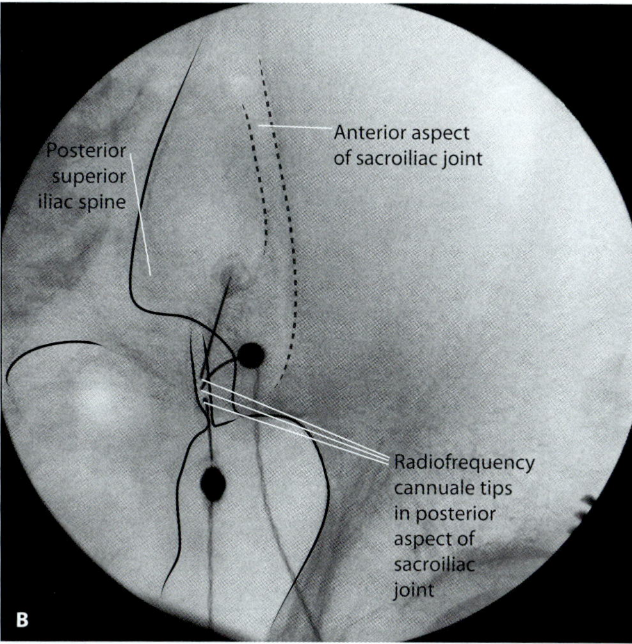

FIGURE 91-10. **A,** Anteroposterior radiograph of the sacroiliac joint (SIJ) during bipolar radiofrequency (RF) treatment. Three separate 22-gauge, 10-cm SMK cannulae with 5-mm active tips are in position over the posterior-inferior aspect of the right SIJ. One cannula is attached to the active output from the RF generator and the other to the ground port. A third cannula is in position 6 mm cephalad to the second cannula. The superior limit of the treatment is limited by access to the SIJ, which is blocked by the posterior superior iliac spine. **B,** Labeled image. (Used with permission and courtesy of Dr. James Rathmell from *Atlas of Image-Guided Intervention in Regional Anesthesia and Pain Medicine.*[5])

on body habitus, six to eight lesions may be created in total until the posterior superior iliac spine is encountered. Of note, some practitioners use 10-mm active tips for bipolar SIJ lesions, which, as Cosman et al. have demonstrated, can extend intertip spacing to 10 mm.[32]

Water-Cooled Radiofrequency Technique The L4 MBN and L5 primary dorsal rami are treated by CRF as described previously. To target the S1–S3 foramina lateral branches by WCRF, 17-gauge electrodes with 4-mm active tips are inserted between 2 and 4 mm from the lateral border of the foramina in a *contiguous periforaminal* fashion. For the S1 and S2 foramen, this corresponds to a superolateral, lateral, and inferolateral lesion for each foramen or is also described as the 2:30, 4:00, and 5:30 positions based on a clock face superimposed over each foramen (**Fig. 91-11**). Depending on anatomic spacing and patient size, the S3 and S4 foramen may be treated with two or three similar lesions. WCRF lesions are set for a 60°C electrode tip temperature for 2.5 minutes at each level. In some patients, the S4 foramen is well below the SIJ, and its corresponding sacral lateral branches would not need treatment.

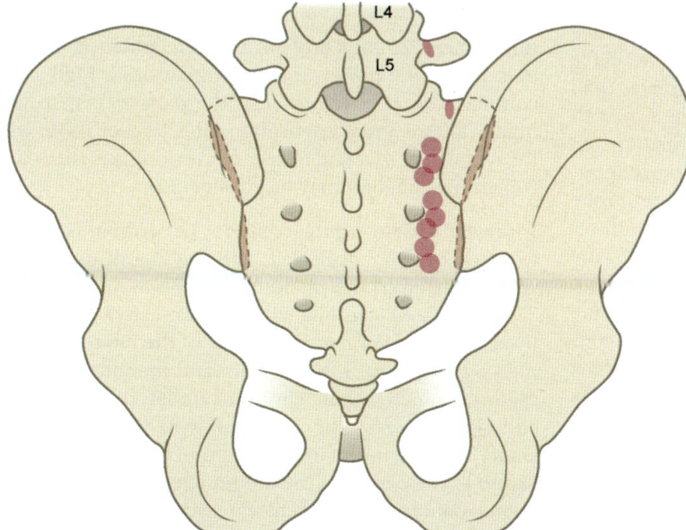

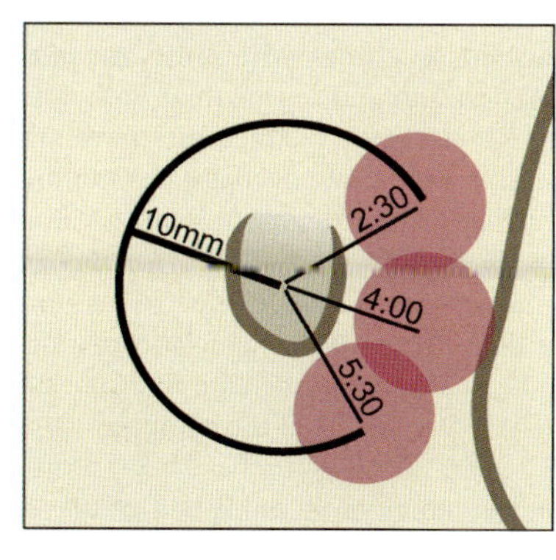

FIGURE 91-11. Target points and the anticipated lesions for right-sided conventional (L4 and L5) and cooled (S1-S3) radiofrequency denervation at the junction of the L5 superior articular and transverse processes (L4 primary dorsal ramus), the sacral ala (L5 primary dorsal ramus), and S1-S3 foramina (lateral branches). Inset: Lesions should be placed at the 2:30, 4:00, and 5:30 positions relative to the face of a clock approximately 10 mm lateral to the center of each foramen. (Used with permission and courtesy of Dr. James Rathmell from *Atlas of Image-Guided Intervention in Regional Anesthesia and Pain Medicine.*[5])

TABLE 91-2 Summary of Sacroiliac Joint Radiofrequency Trials with Radiofrequency Mode and Technique Approaches

Authors	Study Design	Patients (*n*)	RF Mode	Technique	% Patients with >50% Relief at ≥3 Months
Buijs et al. (2004)[6]	Prospective observational	38	CRF	L4-L5 dorsal ramus and "three-puncture technique" lateral upper quadrant of S1-S3 dorsal foraminaLesion time, 60 seconds at 80°C	63
Yin (2003)[120]	Retrospective	14	CRF	Sensory-stimulation guided CRF S1-S3 lateral branches; 20-gauge electrodes with 10-mm active tipsLesion time, 90 seconds at 80°C	64
Gevargez et al. (2002)[93]	Prospective observational	38	CRF	CT-guided CRF to L5 dorsal ramus and posterior interosseous SI ligaments; 23-gauge electrodes with 5-mm active tipsLesion time, 90 seconds at 90°C	66
Cohen et al. (2008)[95]	Randomized placebo controlled	14	CRF + WCRF	CRF to L4-L5 dorsal ramus and WCRF to S1-S3 lateral branches; 18-gauge electrodes with 4-mm active tips (17-gauge cannula)Lesion time, 2.5 minutes at 60°C probe temperature	64
Cohen and Abdi (2003)[94]	Retrospective	9	CRF	CRF to L4-L5 dorsal ramus and S1-S3 lateral branches; 22-gauge electrodes with 5-mm active tipsLesion time, 90 seconds at 80°C	89
Ferrante et al. (2001)[91]	Retrospective	33	BRF	Leapfrog technique along posterior SIJ; 20- or 22-gauge cannula spaced <10 mmLesion time, 90 seconds at 90°C	36
Kapural (2008)[121]	Retrospective	26	WCRF	Lateral edges of S1-S3 sacral foramina; 18-gauge electrodes with 4-mm active tips (17-gauge cannula) spaced ~10 mm apart	50
Burnham and Yasui (2007)[90]	Prospective observational	9	BRF	L4-L5 dorsal ramus + BRF strip lesions to S1–S3; for BRF, 20-gauge electrodes with 10-mm active tips spaced 4–6 mm apartLesion time, 90 seconds at 80°C	67
Cohen et al. (2009)[85]	Retrospective	77	CRF + WCRF	CRF to L4-L5 dorsal ramus and WCRF to S1-S3 lateral branches; 18-gauge electrodes with 4-mm active tips (17-gauge cannula) spaced ~10 mm apart	52
Vallejo (2004)[122]	Prospective observational	22	PRF	PRF to MB of L4, dorsal ramus of L5, lateral branches of S1 and S2; 22-gauge electrodes with 10-mm active tipsPRF 42°C at 45 V for 120 seconds	73

BRF, bipolar radiofrequency ablation; CRF, conventional radiofrequency ablation; CT, computed tomography; MB, medial branch; PRF, pulsed radiofrequency ablation; RF, radiofrequency; SI, sacroiliac; SIJ, sacroiliac joint; WCRF, water-cooled radiofrequency ablation.

RADIOFREQUENCY SACROILIAC JOINT EVIDENCE

Despite some heterogeneity in anatomic approach and technique, multiple trials have demonstrated positive results with sacroiliac joint CRF, WCRF, and BRF treatments (**Table 91-2**).[87,92-95] The recent randomized trial by Cohen et al. in 28 patients demonstrated clinical efficacy with WCRF targeting L4–L5 primary dorsal rami and S1–S3 lateral branches.[95] A total of 79% of patients experienced greater than 50% pain relief at 1 month, which decreased to 57% at 6 months. A 2010 meta-analysis also concluded that at 3 and 6 months, RFA was an effective treatment for SIJ pain.[96] Using weighted pooled averages from available trials, approximately 60% of patients at 3 months showed a greater than 50% improvement in pain, and 50% of patients reached the 6-month mark. The diminished outcomes with time are likely related to the expected nerve regeneration and regrowth as with any RFA procedure.

Other emerging RF electrode technologies have innovated on probe and electrode design to save time, decrease the number of probe placements, and facilitate targeting the variable innervation of the SIJ. The flexible Simplicity III probe replicates the natural anatomic curve of the SIJ and has three separate active RF electrodes along the shaft of the curved probe. The probe permits navigation from a single percutaneous entry site and can be customized to create multiple strip lesions for the sacral lateral branches. The results of the company sponsored pilot study of 30 patients and 3 years of follow-up have been positive, but these data are preliminary and independently published studies are needed before widespread clinical adoption.

TRIGEMINAL GANGLION RADIOFREQUENCY TREATMENT

The trigeminal (gasserian) ganglion may be targeted for clinical conditions such as TGN, atypical facial pain, and even intractable cluster headaches. TGN typically affects patients older than 50 years of age and has a 2:1 female predominance. Demyelinating diseases, such as multiple sclerosis, also greatly increase the risk of TGN. Triggers are unpredictable but often related to a small sensitive area of touch. Paroxysmal pain episodes most commonly occur in the second (maxillary) and third (mandibular) trigeminal divisions. Many cases are idiopathic. Vascular compression injury of the trigeminal root may trigger trigeminal neuron hypersensitivity and ultimately lead to this neuropathic state. TGN also may be caused by a compressive primary nerve tumor.

Carbamazepine and oxcarbazepine have demonstrated success as first-line pharmacologic therapy. But for those refractory to medications, the first choice of invasive treatment is microvascular decompression in the posterior fossa, which has a high success rate and low complication rate. However, if the pain recurs, reoperation has much higher failure and complication rates.[97,98] For those who are too frail or for whom microvascular decompression has failed, RF lesioning of the trigeminal ganglion may be considered.

Trigeminal Radiofrequency Technique The patient is placed supine, and the foramen ovale is visualized with the C-arm until it appears as an oval shape, medial to the mandibular process and lateral to the maxilla. A SMK 10-cm RF cannula with a 2-mm active tip is used. The cannula is inserted 2 cm lateral to the corner of the mouth aimed toward the foramen ovale to treat the maxillary and mandibular branch. For the ophthalmic branch, needle entry is 3 cm lateral to the corner of the mouth and aimed toward the medial part of the foramen ovale. If one only wants to treat the mandibular branch, the needle entry point is 1 cm lateral to the corner of the mouth and on the lateral foramen ovale. The appropriate motor and sensory testing is performed. After appropriate paresthesia, a 60°C CRF treatment is performed for 60 to 90 seconds. After this, the corneal reflex is tested, and the patient is evaluated for hypoesthesia. If well tolerated, some advocate a second lesion at 70°C.[99]

Although rare, RF of the TGN has the potential for serious complications. In Kanpolat et al.'s retrospective study of 1600 patients, serious events included two patients with permanent cranial nerve VI palsy, two patients with CSF leakage, one patient with carotid-cavernous fistula, and one case of aseptic meningitis.[100] Loss of facial sensation or paresthesias account for 80% of the side effects of CRF-TGN. Other complications involve masseter weakness and paralysis (4.1%), dysesthesias (1%), and transient paralysis of cranial nerves III and IV (0.8%).[100] Additionally, the trigeminocardiac reflex can produce hypotension and bradycardia upon stimulation of the trigeminal nerve, necessitating careful monitoring of vital signs during the procedure.

EVIDENCE

Despite the lack of a sham-controlled randomized trials, there is extensive clinical experience with RF treatment for TGN. The 25-year retrospective review from Kanpolat et al. of 1600 patients who received RF neurotomy of the gasserian ganglion for idiopathic TGN reported eventual pain relief in 97%.[100] A total of 76% patients achieved pain relief after a single procedure. Even at 5 years of follow-up, 58% had ongoing successful results. Furthermore, Erdine et al. published an RCT with 40 patients indicating clear superiority of CRF over PRF for the management of idiopathic TGN (only 2 of 20 patients in the PRF group experienced any benefit).[26]

CRYOANALGESIA

Since the time of Hippocrates and the ancient Egyptians, cryoanalgesia has been described as an effective method of pain control. Most of these early historical applications used topical cold therapy to create a neural conduction block, analogous to a temporary local anesthetic. However, in a manner similar to RF treatment, modern cryolesioning achieves analgesia by the focal application of subfreezing temperatures, resulting in cryoneurodestruction of a target nerve. Modern cryoneurolysis was developed in 1961 by Cooper, who designed the first cryoprobe needle with liquid nitrogen to create temperatures as low as −190°C. Instead of liquid nitrogen, today's cryoprobes rely on the Joules-Thompson gas expansion principle through the use of carbon dioxide or nitrous oxide gas. Cryoneurolysis has been trialed in a variety of nerve targets often for postoperative analgesia such as postthoracotomy and herniorrhaphy pain.

PHYSICS AND NEUROBIOLOGY OF CRYONEUROLYSIS

Studies have demonstrated that a threshold temperature below −20°C is needed to create an effective cryolesion.[101,102] The mechanism of cryoneurolysis likely includes the instantaneous formation of large ice crystals within the neural vasculature. Ice crystals disrupt the sensitive microvasculature, compromise the blood supply, and increase endoneural pressure. Subsequently, protein denaturation, membrane rupture, and ischemic necrosis result in neurolysis. Axons and myelin disintegrate at the cryolesion site and then undergo wallerian degeneration distal to the cryoinjury. Notably, the endoneurium, perineurium, and epineurium stay intact, which permits nerve regeneration.[103]

In thermodynamic physics, the Joule-Thompson principle states that as a gas rapidly expands, it cools its surroundings and creates lower temperatures. To accomplish this, a modern cryoprobe is composed of a tube within a tube. Highly pressurized gas at 600 to 800 psi is driven through the smaller inner tube and then allowed to escape from a very small distal slit into the low-pressure (10–15 psi) larger outer tube. The escaping gas expands into the outer lumen following the large pressure gradient. This expanding gas absorbs heat from its immediate environment and produces subfreezing temperatures radially in the surrounding tissue. The expansion of a compressed gas through a small orifice can generate temperatures of −50°C to −70°C. The size of the freeze zone for a gas expansion cryoprobe is two to three times the probe's diameter. A 2.0-mm diameter probe (~14 gauge) forms a 5.5-mm-diameter ice ball; a 1.4-mm probe forms a 3.5-mm ice ball. The typical size of a cryoprobe ranges from 12 to 16 gauge.

Studies in rat sciatic nerves showed that a minimum temperature of −20°C was necessary for prolonged sensory loss and that further decreases in temperature did not greatly influence the duration of sensory loss.[104] The size of the cryolesion is also important because saltatory conduction is still possible in myelinated fibers when only short interruptions in axonal continuity exist. In cats, a cryogenic injury of 3 to 6 mm in length can prevent saltatory conduction.[105]

CRYOLESIONING TECHNIQUE

As with RF ablation, localization of the target nerve must be precise and fluoroscopy may be used when needed. Sensory and motor stimulation is performed after the probe is properly positioned. Gas flows between 10 and 12 L/min are set for the larger 2-mm probe and 8 and 10 L/min for the 1.4-mm probe. Previous studies showed that repeat freeze-and-thaw cycles help maximize the size of the final cryolesion.[102,106] Practitioners often use two or three freeze cycles consisting of 2 to 3 min/freeze cycles with 30 to 45 seconds of defrosting between cycles. More than one freeze cycle is needed because with each subsequent freeze, the size of the freeze zone increases slightly. However, ice can act as its own insulation; hence, freeze cycles longer than 3 minutes or more than three total cycles will not increase the size of the final lesion. When lesioning is complete, the physician must ensure that the ice ball has completely thawed before removing the probe to avoid tissue trauma.

Similar to RF, cryoneurolysis is best suited for conditions in which the nerve to be lesioned is small and well localized. Contraindications include presence of adjacent motor nerve, coagulopathies, and failed diagnostic nerve block. Cryoneurolysis has been trialed in a variety of surgical procedures to provide postoperative analgesia. For postherniorrhaphy pain, the ilioinguinal nerve can be easily identified and cryolesioned with good efficacy.[107,108] Small trials of cryoneurolysis have been published for target nerves in TGN, other facial pains, and facet joints.[109-113]

POSTTHORACOTOMY CRYOLESIONING

Of all published applications, cryolesioning of the intercostal nerve after thoracotomy has been the most extensively evaluated. Optimal pain control after thoracotomy facilitates extubation and adequate pulmonary toilet to prevent respiratory complications. Narcotics alone can blunt the cough reflex, lower respiratory rate, and cause further respiratory complications. Intercostal nerve blocks with local anesthetic are temporary and insufficient to provide adequate postoperative analgesia. Thus, cryoablation of the relevant intercostal nerves before closure of the thoracotomy incision has been trialed. The intercostal nerves at two levels above and below the incision are dissected away from the intercostal vessels and cryoablated, a process that can add 15 to 20 minutes of operative time.

In the 1980s, three studies of intraoperative intercostal cryoneurolysis were shown to be effective in decreasing postoperative pain and the amount of total analgesics consumed postprocedure.[114-116] However, those studies compared cryolesioning only with temporary local anesthetic block or narcotic usage. Of 11 randomized trials evaluating intercostal cryoanalgesia for thoracotomy pain, only the three initial studies, which did not use thoracic epidural analgesia, showed greater benefit with cryoanalgesia. Today, thoracic epidural analgesia is the current preferred practice for thoracotomy pain control.

Recent trials have demonstrated lack of clear efficacy and adverse events associated with intercostal nerve cryolesioning. An RCT in 2004 showed that cryoneurolysis was not more effective than intravenous analgesia in improving pulmonary function tests, lessening postthoracotomy pain, or reducing analgesia consumption.[117] Furthermore, a 2008 RCT by Ju et al. demonstrated that cryolesioning of intercostal nerves was not more effective than thoracic epidural analgesia.[118] Intercostal cryolesioning actually resulted in a higher incidence of allodynia and neuropathic postthoracotomy pain that was statistically significant at 6 and 12 months of follow-up.

TABLE 91-3 Summary of Evidence of Radiofrequency Procedures.

Clinical Indication	Level of Evidence	RF Mode	Implication
Lumbar facetogenic pain	1B+	CRF	Positive recommendation: more than one RCT with demonstrable effectiveness
• SIJ pain: sacral lateral branches (S1-S3) • CRPS: lumbar sympathetic ganglion • Whiplash-associated cervical facet pain • Discogenic pain: lumbar ramus communicans • Trigeminal neuralgia: gasserian ganglion	2B+	WCRF CRF CRF CRF CRF	Positive recommendation: one or more RCTs with some weaknesses
• Lumbosacral radicular pain: lumbar PRF-DRG • Degenerative cervical facet joint pain • SIJ pain: L5 dorsal ramus and lateral branches of S1-S3 • SIJ pain: L5 dorsal ramus and lateral branches of S1-S3 • Thoracic radicular pain: thoracic DRG • Thoracic facet pain • Idiopathic facial pain: sphenopalatine • Cluster headache: pterygopalatine ganglion	2C+	PRF CRF PRF CRF/BRF PRF/CRF CRF PRF CRF	Recommended with careful consideration: effectiveness only demonstrated in observational studies
• Cervicogenic headache: RF cervical dorsal rami	2B+/-	CRF	Recommended with careful consideration: RCTs with contradictory results
• Discogenic pain: RF thermocoagulation • Trigeminal neuralgia: gasserian ganglion	2B-	CRF PRF	Negative recommendation: one or more RCTs with some weaknesses in which treatment was not superior to control
• Lumbosacral radicular pain: lumbar CRF-DRG	2A-	CRF	Negative recommendation: RCT of good quality in which treatment did not exhibit any clinical effect

BRF, bipolar radiofrequency ablation; CRF, conventional radiofrequency ablation; CRPS, complex regional pain syndrome; DRG, dorsal root ganglion; PRF, pulsed radiofrequency ablation; RCT, randomized controlled trial; RF, radiofrequency; SI, sacroiliac; SIJ, sacroiliac joint; WCRF, water-cooled radiofrequency ablation.

Based on evidence guidelines developed by Guyatt et al. and adapted by Van Kleef for EBM Series 2009-2010 Pain Practice.

Although cryoneurolysis is a relatively safe and often effective method of pain control, clinical trial data are poor, and other modalities of neuroablation such as RF treatment appear to have gained more mainstream adoption. The growing use of RF with its advantages of shorter procedure time and smaller gauge probes has made it somewhat more attractive in targeting peripheral sensory nerves.

CONCLUSION

Cryoanalgesia and RF represent an evolution in pain practice, providing practitioners a proven method of targeting specific nerves safely and reliably. The major advantage of these techniques compared with other forms of neurolysis are controlled and reproducible lesion dimensions produced in a minimally invasive manner. The current state of evidence supporting RF treatment for the multitude of clinical conditions and anatomic sites is summarized in **Table 91-3**.

REFERENCES

1. Shealy CN. Percutaneous radiofrequency denervation of spinal facets. Treatment for chronic back pain and sciatica. *J Neurosurg.* 1975;43(4):448-451.
2. Smith HP, McWhorter JM, Challa VR. Radiofrequency neurolysis in a clinical model: neuropathological correlation. *J Neurosurg.* 1981;55(2):246-253.
3. Uematsu S, Udvarhelyi GB, Benson DW, Siebens AA. Percutaneous radiofrequency rhizotomy. *Surg Neurol.* 1974;2(5):319-325.
4. Shealy CN. Facet denervation in the management of back and sciatic pain. *Clin Orthop Relat Res.* 1976; (115):157-164.
5. Rathmell J. *Atlas of Image-Guided Intervention in Regional Anesthesia and Pain Medicine*: Philadelphia: Lippincott Williams & Wilkins; 2006.
6. Buijs EJ, van Wijk RM, Geurts JW, et al. Radiofrequency lumbar facet denervation: a comparative study of the reproducibility of lesion size after 2 current radiofrequency techniques. *Reg Anesth Pain Med.* 2004;29(5):400-407.
7. Provenzano DA, Lassila HC, Somers D. The effect of fluid injection on lesion size during radiofrequency treatment. *Reg Anesth Pain Med.* 2010;35(4):338-342.
8. Bruners P, Muller H, Gunther RW, et al. Fluid-modulated bipolar radiofrequency ablation: an ex-vivo evaluation study. *Acta Radiol.* 2008;49(3):258-266.
9. Letcher FS, Goldring S. The effect of radiofrequency current and heat on peripheral nerve action potential in the cat. *J Neurosurg.* 1968;29(1):42-47.
10. Bogduk N, Macintosh J, Marsland A. Technical limitations to the efficacy of radiofrequency neurotomy for spinal pain. *Neurosurgery.* 1987;20(4):529-535.
11. Van Zundert J, Raj P, Erdine S, van Kleef M. Application of radiofrequency treatment in practical pain management: state of the art. *Pain Pract.* 2002;2(3):269-278.
12. Erdine S, Yucel A, Cimen A, et al. Effects of pulsed versus conventional radiofrequency current on rabbit dorsal root ganglion morphology. *Eur J Pain.* 2005;9(3):251-256.
13. Sluijtel ME, Teixeira A, van Duijn B. Comment on: Erdine S et al.; Ultrastructural changes in axons following exposure to pulsed radiofrequency fields. *Pain Pract.* 2010;10(3):262; author reply 262-263.
14. Cosman ER Jr., Cosman ER Sr. Electric and thermal field effects in tissue around radiofrequency electrodes. *Pain Med.* 2005;6(6):405-424.
15. Kornick C, Kramarich SS, Lamer TJ, Todd Sitzman B. Complications of lumbar facet radiofrequency denervation. *Spine (Phila Pa 1976).* 15 2004;29(12):1352-1354.
16. van Boxem K, van Eerd M, Brinkhuizen T, et al. Radiofrequency and pulsed radiofrequency treatment of chronic pain syndromes: the available evidence. *Pain Pract.* 2008;8(5):385-393.
17. Sluijter ME. Pulsed radiofrequency. *Anesthesiology.* 2005;103(6):1313; author reply 1313-1314.
18. Van Zundert J, de Louw AJ, Joosten EA, et al. Pulsed and continuous radiofrequency current adjacent to the cervical dorsal root

ganglion of the rat induces late cellular activity in the dorsal horn. *Anesthesiology*. 2005;102(1):125-131.

19. Higuchi Y, Nashold BS Jr, Sluijter M, et al. Exposure of the dorsal root ganglion in rats to pulsed radiofrequency currents activates dorsal horn lamina I and II neurons. *Neurosurgery*. 2002;50(4):850-855; discussion 856.
20. Podhajsky RJ, Sekiguchi Y, Kikuchi S, Myers RR. The histologic effects of pulsed and continuous radiofrequency lesions at 42 degrees C to rat dorsal root ganglion and sciatic nerve. *Spine (Phila Pa 1976)*. 2005;30(9):1008-1013.
21. Hamann W, Abou-Sherif S, Thompson S, Hall S. Pulsed radiofrequency applied to dorsal root ganglia causes a selective increase in ATF3 in small neurons. *Eur J Pain*. 2006;10(2):171-176.
22. Hagiwara S IH, Takeshima N, Noguchi T. Mechanisms of analgesic action of pulsed radiofrequency on adjuvant-induced pain in the rat: roles of descending adrenergic and serotonergic systems. *Eur J Pain*. 2008;3(13):249-252.
23. Cosman ER Sr CEJ. *The Physics of Pulsed Radiofrequency (Manual of RF Techniques*. 3rd Edition; 2011.
24. Tekin I, Mirzai H, Ok G, et al. A comparison of conventional and pulsed radiofrequency denervation in the treatment of chronic facet joint pain. *Clin J Pain*. 2007;23(6):524-529.
25. Kroll HR, Kim D, Danic MJ, et al. A randomized, double-blind, prospective study comparing the efficacy of continuous versus pulsed radiofrequency in the treatment of lumbar facet syndrome. *J Clin Anesth*. 2008;20(7):534-537.
26. Erdine S, Ozyalcin NS, Cimen A, et al. Comparison of pulsed radiofrequency with conventional radiofrequency in the treatment of idiopathic trigeminal neuralgia. *Eur J Pain*. 2007;11(3):309-313.
27. Goldberg SN, Gazelle GS, Solbiati L, et al. Radio-frequency tissue ablation: increased lesion diameter with a perfusion electrode. *Acad Radiol*. 1996;3:636-644.
28. Cosman ER, Nashold BS, Bedenbaugh P. Stereotactic radiofrequency lesion making. *Appl Neurophysiol*. 1983;46(1-4):160-166.
29. Cosman ER, Nashold BS, Ovelman-Levitt J. Theoretical aspects of radiofrequency lesions in the dorsal root entry zone. *Neurosurgery*. 1984;15(6):945-950.
30. Rupert MP, Lee M, Manchikanti L, et al. Evaluation of sacroiliac joint interventions: a systematic appraisal of the literature. *Pain Physician*. 2009;12(2):399-418.
31. Pino CA, Hoeft MA, Hofsess C, Rathmell JP. Morphologic analysis of bipolar radiofrequency lesions: implications for treatment of the sacroiliac joint. *Reg Anesth Pain Med*. 2005;30(4):335-338.
32. Cosman ER Jr., Gonzalez CD. Bipolar radiofrequency lesion geometry: implications for palisade treatment of sacroiliac joint pain. *Pain Pract*. 2011;11(1):3-22.
33. Bogduk N. International Spinal Injection Society guidelines for the performance of spinal injection procedures. Part 1: Zygapophysial joint blocks. *Clin J Pain*. 1997;13(4):285-302.
34. Bogduk N. Evidence-informed management of chronic low back pain with facet injections and radiofrequency neurotomy. *Spine J*. 2008;8(1):56-64.
35. Cohen SP, Williams KA, Kurihara C, et al. Multicenter, randomized, comparative cost-effectiveness study comparing 0, 1, and 2 diagnostic medial branch (facet joint nerve) block treatment paradigms before lumbar facet radiofrequency denervation. *Anesthesiology*. 2010;113(2):395-405.
36. van Wijk RM, Geurts JW, Wynne HJ, et al. Radiofrequency denervation of lumbar facet joints in the treatment of chronic low back pain: a randomized, double-blind, sham lesion-controlled trial. *Clin J Pain*. 2005;21(4):335-344.
37. van Kleef M, Barendse GA, Kessels A, et al. Randomized trial of radiofrequency lumbar facet denervation for chronic low back pain. *Spine (Phila Pa 1976)*. 1999;24(18):1937-1942.
38. Aprill C, Bogduk N. The prevalence of cervical zygapophyseal joint pain: a first approximation. *Spine (Phila Pa 1976)*. 1992;17(7):744-747.
39. Barnsley L, Lord S, Bogduk N. Comparative local anaesthetic blocks in the diagnosis of cervical zygapophysial joint pain. *Pain*. 1993;55(1):99-106.
40. Manchikanti L. The growth of interventional pain management in the new millennium: a critical analysis of utilization in the Medicare population. *Pain Physician*. 2004;7(4):465-482.
41. Barnsley L, Lord S, Bogduk N. Whiplash injury. *Pain*. 1994;58(3):283-307.
42. Bogduk N. The clinical anatomy of the cervical dorsal rami. *Spine (Phila Pa 1976)*. 1982;7(4):319-330.
43. Teresi LM, Lufkin RB, Reicher MA, et al. Asymptomatic degenerative disk disease and spondylosis of the cervical spine: MR imaging. *Radiology*. 1987;164(1):83-88.
44. Barnsley L, Lord S, Wallis B, Bogduk N. False-positive rates of cervical zygapophysial joint blocks. *Clin J Pain*. 1993;9(2):124-130.
45. Manchikanti L, Boswell MV, Singh V, et al. Prevalence of facet joint pain in chronic spinal pain of cervical, thoracic, and lumbar regions. *BMC Musculoskelet Disord*. 2004;5:15.
46. Sapir DA, Gorup JM. Radiofrequency medial branch neurotomy in litigant and nonlitigant patients with cervical whiplash: a prospective study. *Spine (Phila Pa 1976)*. 2001;26(12):E268-E273.
47. Manchikanti L, Singh V, Vilims BD, et al. Medial branch neurotomy in management of chronic spinal pain: systematic review of the evidence. *Pain Physician*. 2002;5(4):405-418.
48. Manchikanti L, Manchikanti KN, Damron KS, Pampati V. Effectiveness of cervical medial branch blocks in chronic neck pain: a prospective outcome study. *Pain Physician*. 2004;7(2):195-201.
49. Lord SM, Barnsley L, Wallis BJ, et al. Percutaneous radio-frequency neurotomy for chronic cervical zygapophyseal-joint pain. *N Engl J Med*. 1996;335(23):1721-1726.
50. Boswell MV, Colson JD, Spillane WF. Therapeutic facet joint interventions in chronic spinal pain: a systematic review of effectiveness and complications. *Pain Physician*. 2005;8(1):101-114.
51. Barnsley L. Percutaneous radiofrequency neurotomy for chronic neck pain: outcomes in a series of consecutive patients. *Pain Med*. 2005;6(4):282-286.
52. McDonald GJ, Lord SM, Bogduk N. Long-term follow-up of patients treated with cervical radiofrequency neurotomy for chronic neck pain. *Neurosurgery*. 1999;45(1):61-67; discussion 67-68.
53. van Kleef M, Barendse GA, Dingemans WA, et al. Effects of producing a radiofrequency lesion adjacent to the dorsal root ganglion in patients with thoracic segmental pain. *Clin J Pain*. 1995;11(4):325-332.
54. Manchikanti L. Facet joint pain and the role of neural blockade in its management. *Curr Rev Pain*. 1999;3(5):348-358.
55. Chua WH, Bogduk N. The surgical anatomy of thoracic facet denervation. *Acta Neurochir (Wien)*. 1995;136(3-4):140-144.
56. Stolker RJ, Vervest AC, Groen GJ. Percutaneous facet denervation in chronic thoracic spinal pain. *Acta Neurochir (Wien)*. 1993;122(1-2):82-90.
57. Tzaan WC, Tasker RR. Percutaneous radiofrequency facet rhizotomy--experience with 118 procedures and reappraisal of its value. *Can J Neurol Sci*. 2000;27(2):125-130.

58. Bogduk N, Schwarzer A. Facet joint pain. *Aust Fam Physician.* 1995;24(5):924.

59. Schwarzer AC, Aprill CN, Derby R, et al. The false-positive rate of uncontrolled diagnostic blocks of the lumbar zygapophysial joints. *Pain.* 1994;58(2):195-200.

60. Boswell MV, Colson JD, Sehgal N, et al. A systematic review of therapeutic facet joint interventions in chronic spinal pain. *Pain Physician.* 2007;10(1):229-253.

61. Geurts JW, van Wijk RM, Stolker RJ, Groen GJ. Efficacy of radiofrequency procedures for the treatment of spinal pain: a systematic review of randomized clinical trials. *Reg Anesth Pain Med.* 2001;26(5):394-400.

62. van Kleef M, Vanelderen P, Cohen SP, et al. 12. Pain originating from the lumbar facet joints. *Pain Pract.* 2010;10(5):459-469.

63. Leclaire R, Fortin L, Lambert R, et al. Radiofrequency facet joint denervation in the treatment of low back pain: a placebo-controlled clinical trial to assess efficacy. *Spine (Phila Pa 1976).* 2001;26(13):1411-1416; discussion 1417.

64. Lau P, Mercer S, Govind J, Bogduk N. The surgical anatomy of lumbar medial branch neurotomy (facet denervation). *Pain Med.* 2004;5(3):289-298.

65. Royal MA, Bhakta B, Gunyea I, et al. Radiofrequency neurolysis for facet arthropathy: a retrospective case series and review of the literature. *Pain Pract.* 2002;2(1):47-52.

66. Nath S, Nath CA, Pettersson K. Percutaneous lumbar zygapophysial (Facet) joint neurotomy using radiofrequency current, in the management of chronic low back pain: a randomized double-blind trial. *Spine (Phila Pa 1976).* 2008;33(12):1291-1297; discussion 1298.

67. Dreyfuss P, Halbrook B, Pauza K, et al. Efficacy and validity of radiofrequency neurotomy for chronic lumbar zygapophysial joint pain. *Spine (Phila Pa 1976).* 2000;25(10):1270-1277.

68. Sluijter M, Racz G. Technical aspects of radiofrequency. *Pain Pract.* 2002;2(3):195-200.

69. Malik K, Benzon HT. Radiofrequency applications to dorsal root ganglia: a literature review. *Anesthesiology.* 2008;109(3):527-542.

70. van Kleef M, Liem L, Lousberg R, et al. Radiofrequency lesion adjacent to the dorsal root ganglion for cervicobrachial pain: a prospective double blind randomized study. *Neurosurgery.* 1996;38(6):1127-1131; discussion 1131-1122.

71. Bland JH. Pain in the head and neck; where does it come from? *Cranio.* 1989;7(3):167-169.

72. Radhakrishnan K, Litchy WJ, O'Fallon WM, Kurland LT. Epidemiology of cervical radiculopathy: a population-based study from Rochester, Minnesota, 1976 through 1990. *Brain.* 1994;117 (Pt 2):325-335.

73. Pevzner E, David R, Leitner Y, et al. [Pulsed radiofrequency treatment of severe radicular pain]. *Harefuah.* 2005;144(3): 178-180, 231.

74. van Kleef M, Spaans F, Dingemans W, et al. Effects and side effects of a percutaneous thermal lesion of the dorsal root ganglion in patients with cervical pain syndrome. *Pain.* 1993;52(1):49-53.

75. Slappendel R, Crul BJ, Braak GJ, et al. The efficacy of radiofrequency lesioning of the cervical spinal dorsal root ganglion in a double blinded randomized study: no difference between 40 degrees C and 67 degrees C treatments. *Pain.* 1997;73(2): 159-163.

76. Niemisto L, Kalso E, Malmivaara A, et al. Radiofrequency denervation for neck and back pain: a systematic review of randomized controlled trials. *Cochrane Database Syst Rev.* 2003;(1):CD004058.

77. Van Zundert J, Patijn J, Kessels A, et al. Pulsed radiofrequency adjacent to the cervical dorsal root ganglion in chronic cervical radicular pain: a double blind sham controlled randomized clinical trial. *Pain.* 2007;127(1-2):173-182.

78. Haspeslagh SR, Van Suijlekom HA, Lame IE, et al. Randomised controlled trial of cervical radiofrequency lesions as a treatment for cervicogenic headache [ISRCTN07444684]. *BMC Anesthesiol.* 2006;6:1.

79. van Kleef M, Stolker RJ, Lataster A, et al. 10. Thoracic pain. *Pain Pract.* 2010;10(4):327-338.

80. Stolker RJ, Vervest AC, Ramos LM, Groen GJ. Electrode positioning in thoracic percutaneous partial rhizotomy: an anatomical study. *Pain.* 1994;57(2):241-251.

81. Cohen SP, Sireci A, Wu CL, et al. Pulsed radiofrequency of the dorsal root ganglia is superior to pharmacotherapy or pulsed radiofrequency of the intercostal nerves in the treatment of chronic postsurgical thoracic pain. *Pain Physician.* 2006;9(3):227-235.

82. van Wijk RM, Geurts JW, Wynne HJ. Long-lasting analgesic effect of radiofrequency treatment of the lumbosacral dorsal root ganglion. *J Neurosurg.* 2001;94(2 Suppl):227-231.

83. Geurts JW, van Wijk RM, Wynne HJ, et al. Radiofrequency lesioning of dorsal root ganglia for chronic lumbosacral radicular pain: a randomised, double-blind, controlled trial. *Lancet.* 2003;361(9351):21-26.

84. Cohen SP. Epidemics, evolution, and sacroiliac joint pain. *Reg Anesth Pain Med.* 2007;32(1):3-6.

85. Cohen SP, Strassels SA, Kurihara C, et al. Outcome predictors for sacroiliac joint (lateral branch) radiofrequency denervation. *Reg Anesth Pain Med.* 2009;34(3):206-214.

86. Schwarzer AC, Aprill CN, Bogduk N. The sacroiliac joint in chronic low back pain. *Spine (Phila Pa 1976).* 1995;20(1):31-37.

87. Hansen HC, McKenzie-Brown AM, Cohen SP, et al. Sacroiliac joint interventions: a systematic review. *Pain Physician.* 2007;10(1):165-184.

88. Chou LH, Slipman CW, Bhagia SM, et al. Inciting events initiating injection-proven sacroiliac joint syndrome. *Pain Med.* 2004;5(1):26-32.

89. Maigne JY, Planchon CA. Sacroiliac joint pain after lumbar fusion: a study with anesthetic blocks. *Eur Spine J.* 2005;14(7):654-658.

90. Burnham RS, Yasui Y. An alternate method of radiofrequency neurotomy of the sacroiliac joint: a pilot study of the effect on pain, function, and satisfaction. *Reg Anesth Pain Med.* 2007;32(1): 12-19.

91. Ferrante FM, King LF, Roche EA, et al. Radiofrequency sacroiliac joint denervation for sacroiliac syndrome. *Reg Anesth Pain Med.* 2001;26(2):137-142.

92. Slipman CW, Whyte WS 2nd, Chow DW, et al. Sacroiliac joint syndrome. *Pain Physician.* 2001;4(2):143-152.

93. Gevargez A, Groenemeyer D, Schirp S, Braun M. CT-guided percutaneous radiofrequency denervation of the sacroiliac joint. *Eur Radiol.* 2002;12(6):1360-1365.

94. Cohen SP, Abdi S. Lateral branch blocks as a treatment for sacroiliac joint pain: a pilot study. *Reg Anesth Pain Med.* 2003;28(2): 113-119.

95. Cohen SP, Hurley RW, Buckenmaier CC 3rd, et al. Randomized placebo-controlled study evaluating lateral branch radiofrequency denervation for sacroiliac joint pain. *Anesthesiology.* 2008;109(2):279-288.

96. Aydin SM, Gharibo CG, Mehnert M, Stitik TP. The role of radiofrequency ablation for sacroiliac joint pain: a meta-analysis. *PM R.* 2010;2(9):842-851.

97. Sekula RF Jr., Frederickson AM, Jannetta PJ, et al. Microvascular decompression for elderly patients with trigeminal neuralgia: a prospective study and systematic review with meta-analysis. *J Neurosurg*. 2011;114(1):172-179.

98. Zakrzewska JM, McMillan R. Trigeminal neuralgia: the diagnosis and management of this excruciating and poorly understood facial pain. *Postgrad Med J*. 2011;87(1028):410-416.

99. van Kleef M, van Genderen WE, Narouze S, et al. 1. Trigeminal neuralgia. *Pain Pract*. 2009;9(4):252-259.

100. Kanpolat Y, Savas A, Bekar A, Berk C. Percutaneous controlled radiofrequency trigeminal rhizotomy for the treatment of idiopathic trigeminal neuralgia: 25-year experience with 1,600 patients. *Neurosurgery*. 2001;48(3):524-532; discussion 532-524.

101. Evans PJ, Lloyd JW, Green CJ. Cryoanalgesia: the response to alterations in freeze cycle and temperature. *Br J Anaesth*. 1981;53(11):1121-1127.

102. Evans PJ. Cryoanalgesia. The application of low temperatures to nerves to produce anaesthesia or analgesia. *Anaesthesia*. 1981;36(11):1003-1013.

103. Sunderland SS. *Nerves and Nerve Injuries*. 2nd ed. London: Churchill Livingstone; 1978.

104. Saberski LR. *Cryoneurolysis in Clinical Practice*. Philadelphia: WB Saunders; 1996.

105. Douglas WW, Malcolm JL. The effect of localized cooling on conduction in cat nerves. *J Physiology*. 1955(130):63-71.

106. Gill W, Fraser J, Carter D. Repeated freeze-thaw cycles in cryosurgery. *Nature*. 1968;219:410-413.

107. Wood GJ, Lloyd JW, Bullingham RE, et al. Postoperative analgesia for day-case herniorrhaphy patients: a comparison of cryoanalgesia, paravertebral blockade and oral analgesia. *Anaesthesia*. 1981;36(6):603-610.

108. Wood GJ, Lloyd JW, Evans PJ, et al. Cryoanalgesia and day-case herniorrhaphy. *Lancet*. 1979;2(8140):479.

109. Goss AN. Peripheral cryoneurotomy in the treatment of trigeminal neuralgia. *Aust Dent J*. 1984;29(4):222-224.

110. Goss AN. Cryoneurotomy for intractable temporomandibular joint pain. *Br J Oral Maxillofac Surg*. 1988;26(1):26-31.

111. Barnard D, Lloyd J, Evans J. Cryoanalgesia in the management of chronic facial pain. *J Maxillofac Surg*. 1981;9(2):101-102.

112. Zakrzewska JM, Nally FF. The role of cryotherapy (cryoanalgesia) in the management of paroxysmal trigeminal neuralgia: a six year experience. *Br J Oral Maxillofac Surg*. 1988;26(1):18-25.

113. Schuster GD. The use of cryoanalgesia in the painful facet syndrome. *Neural Orthop Surg*. 1982;3:271-274.

114. Katz J, Nelson W, Forest R, Bruce DL. Cryoanalgesia for post-thoracotomy pain. *Lancet*. 1980;1(8167):512-513.

115. Nelson KM, Vincent RG, Bourke RS, et al. Intraoperative intercostal nerve freezing to prevent postthoracotomy pain. *Ann Thorac Surg*. 1974;18(3):280-285.

116. Brynitz S, Schroder M. Intraoperative cryolysis of intercostal nerves in thoracic surgery. *Scand J Thorac Cardiovasc Surg*. 1986;20(1):85-87.

117. Gwak MS, Yang M, Hahm TS, et al. Effect of cryoanalgesia combined with intravenous continuous analgesia in thoracotomy patients. *J Korean Med Sci*. 2004;19(1):74-78.

118. Ju H, Feng Y, Yang BX, Wang J. Comparison of epidural analgesia and intercostal nerve cryoanalgesia for post-thoracotomy pain control. *Eur J Pain*. 2008;12(3):378-384.

CHAPTER 92

Vertebral Augmentation

Ronil V. Chandra
Vinil Shah
Thabele M. Leslie-Mazwi
James D. Rabinov
Albert J. Yoo
Joshua A. Hirsch

KEY POINTS

1. Vertebral compression fractures are a common cause of pain and loss of independence in middle-aged and elderly adults.
2. Vertebroplasty and kyphoplasty are minimally invasive, image-guided vertebral augmentation procedures that involve the injection of cement into a fractured vertebral body. The primary goal of augmentation is pain relief and enhanced functional status with the secondary goals of vertebral body stabilization in cases of fracture.
3. Although two recent high-profile trials in the *New England Journal of Medicine (NEJM)* found no benefit to vertebroplasty, more recent randomized controlled trials of vertebral augmentation versus conservative therapy for both osteoporotic and malignant fractures have demonstrated significant improvements in back pain, reduction in disability, and improvement in quality of life in favor of vertebral augmentation.
4. Complications are rare and generally result from unrecognized extraosseous leakage of the injected cement. These include radiculopathy, paralysis, and pulmonary embolism. These risks can be minimized and vertebral augmentation safely performed by experienced operators using high-quality imaging, preferably with biplane fluoroscopy.

CLINICAL RELEVANCE

Osteoporosis is a prevalent disease that affects 200 million women worldwide.[1] Approximately one in two women and one in four men older than the age of 45 years will experience an osteoporotic fracture. Most of these are asymptomatic or have tolerable symptoms, with only one-third of new fractures resulting in medical attention.[2] In the vast majority, acute back pain symptoms subside over a period of 6 to 8 weeks as the fracture heals.[3] Vertebroplasty and kyphoplasty are minimally invasive, image-guided procedures that involve the injection of cement into a vertebral body. The majority of these vertebral augmentation procedures are performed for a small subset of these patients with symptomatic osteoporotic compression fractures that are refractory to conventional medical therapy. The primary goals of augmentation are pain relief and enhanced functional status with the secondary goal of vertebral body stabilization.

Augmentation for neoplastic fractures, in particular from multiple myeloma or osteolytic metastasis or symptomatic neoplasm or vascular tumor, is also common. The spine is affected by osteopenic or osteolytic bone disease in 70% of those with multiple myeloma.[4] Sixty-five percent of patients experience a fracture during the course of the disease,[5] with 30% of patients sustaining a vertebral compression fracture.[6] The vertebral column is the most common site for bone metastasis.[7] Osteolytic metastases weaken bony integrity and are at higher risk of compression fracture compared with osteoblastic lesions. Although up to 70% of the patients who die of cancer have spinal metastases at autopsy, only 14% have symptomatic lesions during their illness.[8] Vertebral augmentation is used in a small cohort with symptomatic vertebral involvement or pathological fractures that are refractory to conventional medical therapy.

MEDICAL MANAGEMENT

The goals of conservative therapy are pain reduction (with analgesics, bed rest, or both), improvement in functional status (with orthotic devices and physical therapy), and prevention of future fractures (with vitamin D, calcium supplementation, and bisphosphonate therapy).

Although conservative management for those with mild pain or limitation of function is appropriate, conservative treatment for those with more severe pain or limitation of function is not benign. In this cohort, conservative therapy often involves a period of bed rest, which may lead to undesirable side effects such as bone mass and muscle strength loss, decubitus ulceration, and venous thromboembolic (VTE) disease, all of which can prolong the recovery period and result in loss of independence. Bone loss occurs at approximately 2% per week, most rapidly in the first 12 weeks of immobilization, with these patients unlikely to regain lost bone mass.[9] Muscle strength reduces by 10% to 15% each week, with almost one-half of normal strength lost within 3 to 5 weeks of immobilization.[10] Prolonged bed rest can lead to decubitus ulcers; infectious complications can lead to septicemia and osteomyelitis. The presence of fracture or malignancy combined with bed rest also elevates the risk of VTE. Overall, the complications of prolonged bed rest, combined with opioid narcotic use and associated side effects, can result in a vicious cycle of physical deconditioning, poor nutrition, and subsequent increased risk of vertebral insufficiency in an elderly cohort with inherent poor physiological reserve.

Indications

- Treatment of symptomatic osteoporotic vertebral body fractures refractory to medical therapy
- Treatment of symptomatic vertebral bodies weakened or fractured caused by neoplasia, refractory to medical therapy
- Failure of medical therapy is variably defined but can be considered if pain persists at a level that severely compromises mobility or activities of daily living despite analgesic therapy or if unacceptable side effects such as confusion, sedation, or constipation occur as a result of medication doses required to reduce pain to tolerable levels.

Contraindications

Absolute Contraindications

1. Active systemic infection, particularly, spinal infection
2. Uncorrectable bleeding diathesis
3. Insufficient cardiopulmonary health to safely tolerate sedation or general anesthesia
4. Myelopathy resulting from fracture retropulsion or epidural tumoral extension
5. Known allergy to bone cement

Relative Contraindications

These substantially increase the risk and technical difficulty of the procedure and should only be treated by experienced practitioners.

- *Marked loss of vertebral body height* (>75% height loss) makes the procedure more difficult because there may be little space for cannula placement.
- *Vertebroplasty above T5* is challenging because of the small size of the vertebral bodies and pedicles. The shoulders often limit fluoroscopic imaging at these levels. Computed tomographic (CT) guidance is best to ensure accurate needle trajectories.
- *Severe osteopenia resulting in poor visualization of osseous structures on fluoroscopy* increases the risk of improper needle placement and cement leakage. This can be overcome with the use of CT.
- *Disruption of the posterior cortex* increases the risk of posterior cement leakage and therefore the risk of spinal cord or nerve root compression. Although rare in osteoporotic compression fractures, this feature is frequently seen in burst fractures and neoplasm. The integrity of the posterior cortex is best evaluated with CT scanning.
- *Substantial canal narrowing* (without neurologic dysfunction) increases the risk that even a small amount of cement leakage will produce neurologic compromise. However, even in the setting of spinal cord deformity on preprocedural magnetic resonance imaging (MRI), the procedure can be performed with a high rate of pain relief and without adverse neurologic sequelae.[11]
- *Retropulsion of fracture fragments* are at risk of further canal compromise with vertebral augmentation, particularly if the posterior vertebral body wall is unstable. Most practitioners limit treatment to those in which retropulsion is less than 20% of canal diameter.[12] Hiwatashi et al. have demonstrated that vertebroplasty can be safely performed in fractures with retropulsion, without new neurologic dysfunction.[13]
- *Epidural extension of tumor* in the setting of pathologic fractures results in significantly higher rates of spinal canal leakage compared with osteoporotic fractures. Saliou et al. have demonstrated that vertebroplasty can be safely performed in this setting, even when epidural tumor results in neurologic dysfunction.[14]

Preprocedural Workup This should identify patients who will likely benefit from vertebral augmentation and screen for the above-mentioned contraindications.

History

- These fractures may occur with little or no trauma.
- Classic symptoms:
  - Deep pain with sudden onset
  - Midline location
  - Exacerbation by axial mechanical loading (worsening with standing or weight bearing and often at least partially relieved by recumbency)
  - Exacerbation by motion (especially flexion)
  - Referred lateral radiation in a dermatomal pattern may be present.
- It is important to document failure of conventional medical therapy, which includes pain that is not adequately controlled by bed rest and analgesics, and intolerance to analgesics (e.g., adverse reaction, constipation). The trial of conservative therapy should not extend beyond 4 to 6 weeks because pain from compression fracture usually resolves within this time.[15] There has been a growing trend to earlier treatment with vertebral augmentation (within days), especially for patients that require hospitalization and parenteral narcotics.[15,16]
- Also determine whether the patient is taking anticoagulants, which may need to be ceased.
- Physical examination:
  - The classic physical finding is point tenderness at the spinous process of the fractured vertebra. However, up to 30% of patients may have subjective off midline pain or tenderness over nontarget vertebrae and still gain significant benefit.[17] Localization to a specific level, if possible, is important in targeting treatment in patients who have multiple compression fractures, some of which may be healed and do not require treatment.
  - If there is a clear disparity between the examination findings and imaging or a clear alternate source of back pain, augmentation should not be performed.
  - Assessment of lower extremity neurologic function is especially important in patients with symptoms suggestive of myelopathy, radiculopathy, or spinal stenosis.
- Laboratory evaluation:
  - Preprocedural laboratory studies screen for infection, coagulopathy, and metabolic abnormality.
  - Additional tests such as the performance of a urinalysis, electrocardiogram (ECG), or chest radiography are left to the discretion of the practitioner and local practice patterns.

- Imaging:
  - Imaging of the spine is undertaken in all cases to confirm the clinical diagnosis, aid in the identification and assessment of acuity of the acute painful fracture, identify potential technical difficulties, and plan the procedure.
  - Radiographs can serve as the initial imaging evaluation. When recent prior radiographs are available for comparison, new compression fractures can be identified. In addition, there may be a fracture cleft or evidence of intraosseous vacuum phenomena.
  - MRI is the test of choice for further evaluation and should be obtained on all patients if not contraindicated. The single most useful sequence is a short tau inversion recovery (STIR) or T2-weighted sequence with fat saturation, on which unhealed fractures show hyperintense signal consistent with edema within the bone marrow. The role of the MRI is to identify the unhealed fracture level as well to identify other levels that may be fractured and not evident on less sensitive modalities such as plain radiography or CT (**Fig. 92-1**). MRI also distinguishes between benign osteoporotic and pathologic fractures and assesses the degree of fracture retropulsion, epidural tumor extension, spinal canal compromise, and compression of the spinal cord or nerve roots. Fracture clefts appear as a linear band of T1 hypointensity and T2 hypo- or hyperintensity within the vertebral body.
  - In patients who cannot undergo MRI (e.g., those with a pacemaker), nuclear scintigraphic bone scan is the test of choice. It allows for the differentiation of healed and unhealed fractures; the unhealed fractures will take up the injected ^{99m}Tc-MDP tracer in much higher concentrations. Bone scan highly predicts a positive clinical response to vertebral augmentation.[18] The major disadvantage is the poor spatial resolution, which can result in imprecise localization. Single-photon emission computed tomography (SPECT) imaging can be helpful in this regard and is highly predictive of good clinical response to augmentation.[19]
  - CT can be particularly useful for preprocedural evaluation of the integrity of the posterior vertebral body cortex. This may be important in the setting of burst fracture or metastasis, in which a fracture through the posterior cortex increases the risk of posterior leakage of cement or posterior displacement of bone or tumor during the procedure.[20] In patients with metastatic fractures, CT also helps to define the extent of sclerosis, which in turn increases the technical challenges associated with the procedure.[21]

TECHNIQUE

Sedation Analgesia is necessary for vertebroplasty and kyphoplasty. In the majority of cases, this is achieved with a combination of local analgesics (e.g., bupivacaine or lidocaine with bicarbonate) and moderate sedation (intravenous [IV] midazolam and fentanyl). In some cases, general anesthesia is needed to provide adequate comfort and safety, particularly in patients who are at high risk of airway or respiratory complications with prone positioning or those with significant preprocedural narcotic analgesic requirements. However, having the patient awake is desirable because it allows feedback (e.g., increasing pain, neurologic dysfunction) that can alert the operator to potential complications. In all cases, continuous monitoring is performed with a minimum of ECG, blood pressure measurements, and pulse oximetry.

Patient Positioning Prone is the ideal patient position for thoracic and lumbar procedures. In practical terms, we allow patients an amount of freedom to place themselves in the prone oblique position if it promotes greater comfort throughout the procedure. This can introduce 10 to 15 degrees of obliquity depending on the patient's position. This position with proper cushion support under the upper chest and lower abdomen maximizes extension of the fractured segments, promoting kyphosis reduction[22] (**Fig. 92-2**). The patient's arms should be placed sufficiently toward the head to keep them out of the path of the fluoroscope. Analgesia should be considered before placement on the table because this part of the procedure may be quite painful. Particular care must be

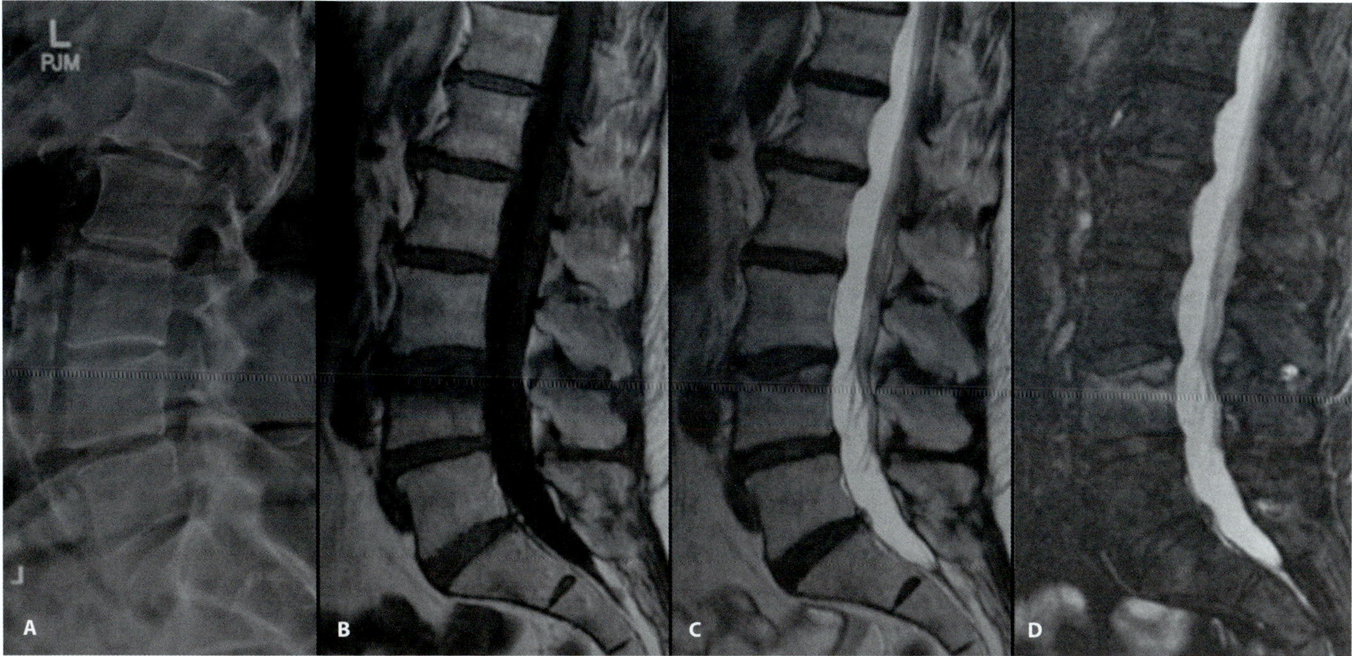

FIGURE 92-1. Magnetic resonance imaging (MRI) reveals an acute L4 compression fracture. (**A**) Lateral radiographic image. No definitive vertebral fracture is evident to explain lower back pain. (**B**) Sagittal T1-weighted MRI image. Reduced signal intensity in the L4 vertebral body from marrow edema. (**C**) Sagittal T2-weighted MRI image. Focal linear low-intensity signal adjacent to the superior endplate of the L4 vertebral body represents the acute fracture line. (**D**) STIR (short-tau inversion recovery) MRI image. Increased signal intensity in the L4 vertebral body adjacent to the fracture line, confirming the acute nature of the fracture.

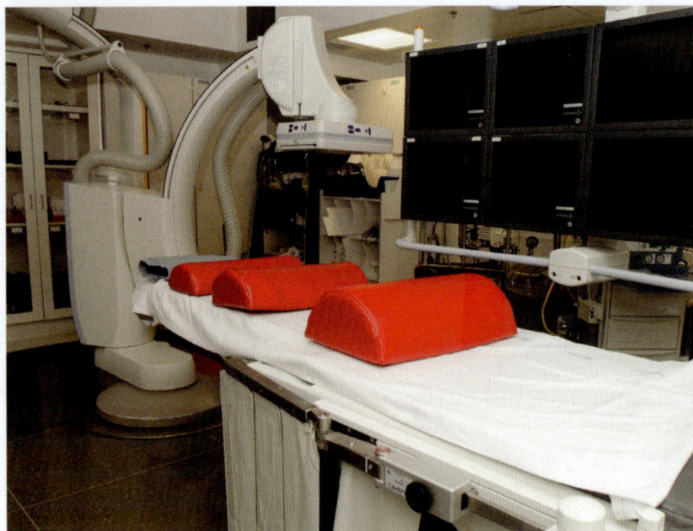

FIGURE 92-2. Cushioning support for prone positioning. Proper cushion support under the upper chest and lower abdomen maximizes fracture extension, which may widen fracture clefts and allow cement penetration.

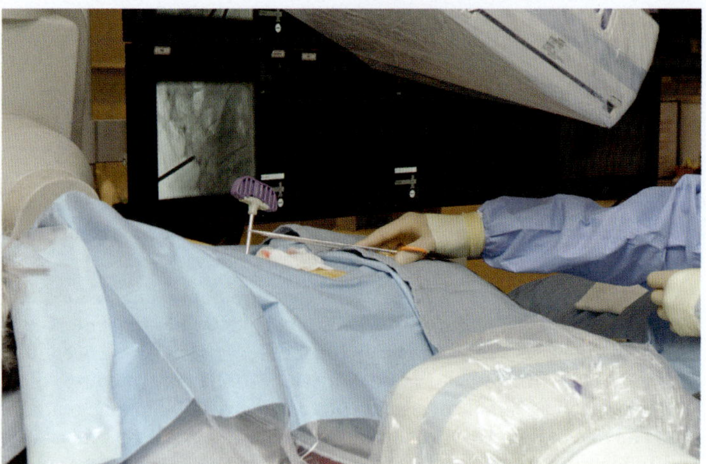

FIGURE 92-3. The diamond-tip needle is placed and the trajectory assessed under fluoroscopy. Note the use of sterile long forceps to hold the cannula in place to minimize radiation dose to the operator's hands.

taken when transferring patients who are older, have osteoporosis, or have myelomatous infiltration because patient transfer may result in new rib or vertebral fractures.

Antibiotic Prophylaxis and Skin Preparation The risk of infection is minimized with the use of standard operating room guidelines for sterile preparation of the skin; draping; operator scrub; and sterile gowns, masks, and gloves. Antibiotic prophylaxis for these procedures comes in one of two forms. An intravenous antibiotic such as cefazolin (1 g) or clindamycin (600 mg if there is a penicillin allergy) may be administered before skin incision. Alternatively, the polymethylmethacrylate (PMMA) may be mixed with an antibiotic, such as tobramycin (1.2 g). There is little data to support or oppose antibiotic administration, but there are reports of spine infections after these procedures,[15,23] and the presence of the PMMA makes these infections difficult to treat successfully.

Needle Placement The most important aspect of needle placement is to keep the needle trajectory lateral to the medial cortex and superior to the inferior cortex of the pedicle. This prevents entry of the needle into the spinal canal or the neural foramen. The needle may be placed via a transpedicular or parapedicular approach. The transpedicular approach takes the needle from the posterior surface of the pedicle, through the length of the pedicle, and into the vertebral body. The long intraosseous path protects the postganglionic nerve roots and other soft tissues. However, the pedicle configuration can limit one's ability to achieve a final needle tip position near the midline. The parapedicular approach takes the needle along the lateral surface of the pedicle, penetrating the pedicle along its path or the vertebral body at its junction with the pedicle. This approach may permit a more medial tip placement.

For either of these approaches, there are multiple potential image guidance strategies, typically an anteroposterior (AP) view, or an end-on ("down-the-barrel") view. The "down-the-barrel view" uses ipsilateral oblique positioning to place the fluoroscopy beam and needle tract perfectly parallel to each other.

- The image intensifier is first rotated to a true AP position, aligning the spinous process midway between the pedicles.
- The craniocaudad angulation is changed to bring the pedicles to the midportion of the vertebral body. Use of lateral fluoroscopy can aid in the determination of the correct craniocaudad adjustment required.
- For the end-on view, the image intensifier is rotated approximately 20 degrees ipsilateral to the target pedicle so that the medial cortex of the pedicle is at the middle third of the vertebral body. The vertebra adopts the "Scotty dog" configuration. The needle will be placed so that it is "end on" to the image intensifier and appears as a dot.
- The trocar trajectory should be planned. The trocar entry position should be at the 3 o'clock position of the right pedicle or 9 o'clock position of the left pedicle for the transpedicular approach. For the parapedicular approaches, an entry position just lateral to the 3 or 9 o'clock positions of the pedicular cortex is best.
- The skin and periosteum are anesthetized with subcutaneous lidocaine or bupivacaine.
- A small vertical skin incision is made (allows easier craniocaudal needle angulation), and an 11- or 13-gauge diamond-tip needle stylet (sheathed in a cannula) is placed (**Fig. 92-3**).
- When the needle has been advanced to the bone surface, small corrections in the craniocaudad angulation can be made using a true lateral view. For the parapedicular approach, the position at which bone is encountered (i.e., at the junction of the pedicle and vertebral body) is more anterior on the lateral view (**Fig. 92-4**).
- In the bone, the needle is advanced by carefully tapping the needle handle with an orthopedic hammer.
- If the end-on view was used initially, the needle is kept as a dot through the initial placement through the pedicle. The needle must remain lateral to the medial cortex of the pedicle until it has traversed the entire pedicle on the lateral view.
- After the needle has traversed the pedicle, the diamond-tip needle may be replaced with a straight bevel-tip needle or a curved needle for better maneuverability. The needle is advanced farther using the lateral view to the anterior one-third to one-quarter of the vertebral body.

Additional Steps for Kyphoplasty For vertebroplasty, the PMMA is delivered through the cannula after the above-described needle placement. Kyphoplasty involves the additional steps of balloon tamp insertion and inflation to create a cavity within the bone. For kyphoplasty, the cannula is pulled back to the posterior aspect of the vertebral body to allow for the insertion of the balloon tamp. After the needle stylet is removed, the balloon tamp is inserted through the cannula and is slowly inflated with iodinated contrast. The balloon is attached to a locking syringe with digital manometer. The inflation is monitored both with the pressure transducer and intermittent fluoroscopy. Inflation continues until one of two conditions is met: the system reaches significant pressure or maximum balloon volume or the further inflation results in patient

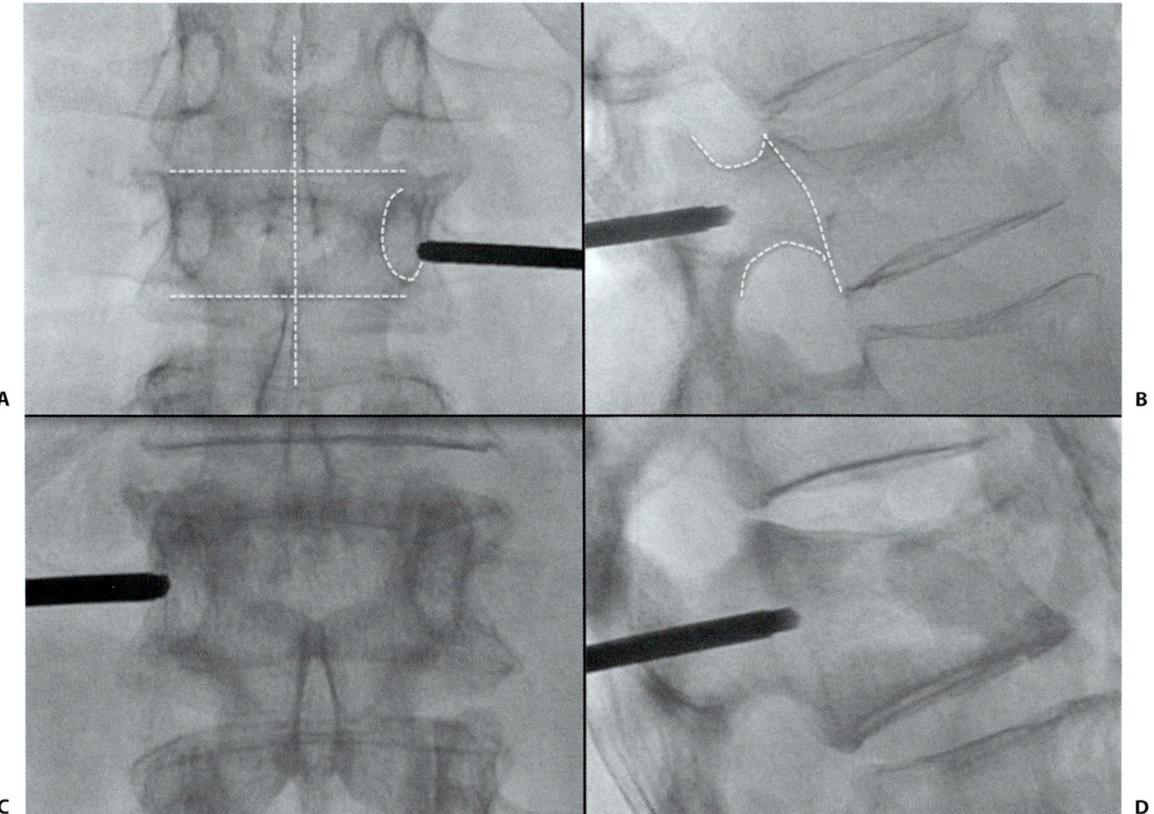

FIGURE 92-4. Initial positioning for needle trajectory for transpedicular (**A** and **B**) and parapedicular (**C** and **D**) approaches. (**A**) Anteroposterior (AP) fluoroscopic image. The image intensifier is first rotated to a true AP position, aligning the spinous process midway between the pedicles (vertical dotted line). The craniocaudad angulation is changed to bring the pedicles to the midportion of the vertebral body (horizontal dotted lines). The needle tip lies at 3 o'clock of the target right pedicle. (**B**) Lateral fluoroscopic image. The image intensifier is rotated to a true lateral position by overlapping the cortices of both pedicles and ensuring that the posterior margin of the vertebral body is aligned (dotted lines). The needle tip lies at the junction of the pedicle and the posterior vertebral arch. (**C**) AP fluoroscopic image. A true AP position with appropriate craniocaudad angulation achieved. The needle tip lies at 9 o'clock of the target left pedicle. (**D**) Lateral fluoroscopic image. With the parapedicular approach, the needle tip enters bone more anteriorly, at the junction of the pedicle and vertebral body.

discomfort. This can be done in a unipedicular or bipedicular fashion. The balloon tamp is then deflated and removed.

Cement Placement The consistency of the cement, when ready for injection, is similar to toothpaste. Wong et al. recommend a drip test, in which the cement should ball up at the end of the needle and not drip downward, resulting in a cement that is slightly more viscous than toothpaste.[24] Working time varies from 10 to 20 minutes, depending on temperature and the specific PMMA formulation being used. A variety of delivery systems are available for the cement. These systems vary from a few 1-cc syringes with a spatula and a mixing bowl to self-contained delivery devices. A screw-syringe injector with long, flexible delivery tubing has the advantage of minimizing radiation exposure to the operator.[25]

Vertebroplasty

- After the needle stylet is removed, the cannula is filled with saline to prevent pressurized injection of air and air embolus. The delivery system is connected to the cannula, and the cement is slowly injected.
- Careful fluoroscopic monitoring is performed to ensure that the cement remains within the vertebra. Posterior or posterolateral leakage could result in irritation of or damage to the spinal cord or nerve roots and should be avoided. New pain with a different character should prompt additional views.
- The end points for cement injection include passage of cement beyond the marrow space or cement reaching the posterior quarter of the vertebral body on the lateral projection. In the case of cement leakage, one may wait 1 to 2 minutes to allow the cement to harden and then reinject it to see if the cement is redirected within the vertebral body.[26] Ideally, the cement will extend across the midline and to the opposite pedicle by the end of the injection. The optimal volume of cement remains a matter of controversy.
- The final portion of cement may be delivered by inserting the needle stylet. Alternatively, the cement may be allowed to harden and the needle removed with a gentle rocking motion to ensure that the cement within the cannula separates at the cannula tip.

Kyphoplasty

- The cavity created by the balloon tamp allows for injection of a cement that is more viscous than that typically used for vertebroplasty. The cavity and more viscous cement theoretically minimize the risk of cement extravasation. Sufficient time is allowed for the cement to reach a doughy consistency, with loss of the "sheen" of the initially mixed cement.
- Many practitioners use manual bone filler devices to inject cement, although one can also use injector systems. The delivery system is connected to the cannula, and the cement is slowly injected under fluoroscopic guidance. The cement fills the cavity from anterior to posterior, matching or slightly exceeding the volume of the inflated balloon tamp (**Fig. 92-5**).

CONTROVERSIES AND SPECIAL TOPICS

Bipedicular Versus Unipedicular Approach Vertebroplasty and kyphoplasty can be performed with the placement of bilateral needles or a single needle.[27] In either case, the goal is to place cement across the midline within the vertebral body; we use placement of PMMA to the opposite pedicle as our general landmark. Therefore, the use of a single needle

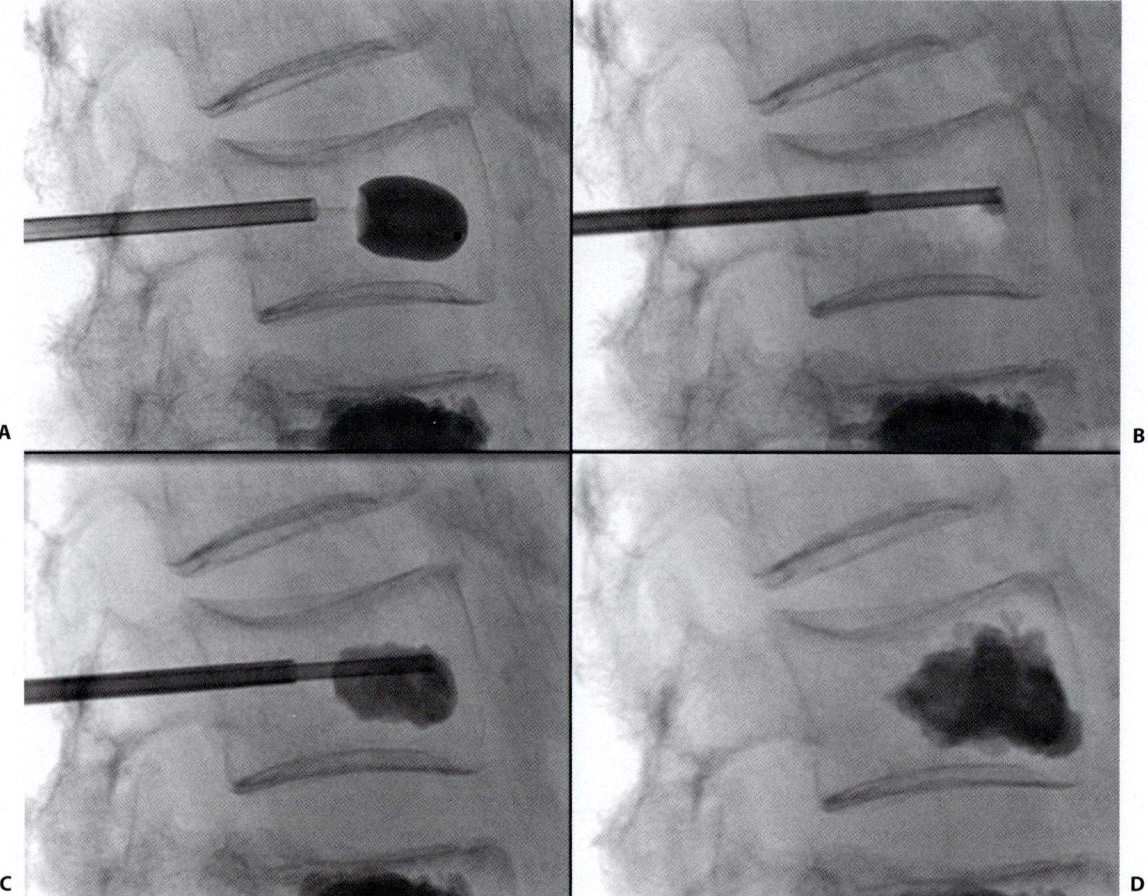

FIGURE 92-5. Cavity creation with balloon kyphoplasty. (**A**) Lateral fluoroscopic image. The kyphoplasty balloon is inflated to create a cavity within the vertebral body. (**B**) Central bony lucency (dotted line) at the site of balloon inflation confirming successful cavity creation. Note that the cavity appears slightly smaller than maximal balloon inflation achieved, a common finding. (**C**) Cement injection initially opacifies the bony cavity. (**D**) Further polymethylmethacrylate (PMMA) injection extends beyond the initial cavity created.

with a relatively medial needle tip position is sufficient in many cases (**Fig. 92-6**). If a unilateral approach is attempted during kyphoplasty and balloon expansion does not cross the midline, a second system may then be placed on the other side, depending on the distribution of cement fill. In many cases, cement fill will continue across the midline. Moreover, hemivertebral fill (cement traverses <10% of the contralateral unfilled vertebra) has been shown to be as efficacious in reducing pain and improving function without an increased risk of fracture.[28]

Importantly, there is no statistically significant difference in pain relief achieved between the unipedicular and bipedicular vertebroplasty[29] or kyphoplasty.[30] There are advantages to each approach. The advantages of a unipedicular approach include decrease in procedure time and elimination of the risk associated with a second needle placement. A unipedicular approach is also associated with lower rates of cement leakage.[31] The major advantage of a bipedicular approach is that access is typically transpedicular with a less aggressive lateral–medial approach that may result in less paravertebral vessel and nerve injury.

Volume of Cement Injection The optimal volume of cement is a matter of controversy, with some practitioners advocating injection of maximal amounts of cement to completely fill the vertebral body and others advocating lower cement volumes with an emphasis on safety. The theoretical goal of more complete filling is to achieve restoration of biomechanical strength within the vertebral body to prevent refracture without creating excess stiffness that may be transmitted to the adjacent levels. Based on an in vitro biomechanical study, Mathis and Wong recommend cement filling of 50% to 70% of the residual volume of the vertebral body.[32] However, much smaller amounts of cement (as little as 0.5 cc) appear to result in similar clinical outcomes in terms of pain relief compared with larger volume injections, with no association between the volume of cement injected and the clinical outcomes of pain and medication use.[31] The decreased risk of cement extravasation with smaller volume injections and meticulous attention to the end of injection criteria outlined recommend a smaller cement volume approach.

Vertebra Plana When the vertebral body loses 70% of its original height, needle placement becomes a challenge. According to Stallmeyer et al., at least 8 mm of residual height is required for cannula placement.[16] The vertebra plana often adopts a bow tie configuration, in which the center is compressed the most. This usually requires a lateral needle position with the placement of bilateral needles.[33] Only a small amount of cement is needed to achieve pain relief.[34] If there is a cystic cleft within the fracture (Kummel disease), the needle may be placed near the midline within the cleft with the hopes of height expansion during needle placement and cement injection.

Fractures with Intraosseous Vacuum Phenomenon (Kummel Disease) The intraosseous vacuum phenomenon is thought to be related to osteonecrosis. A fluid-filled cleft seen on MRI is an equivalent finding. Pain in this setting is believed to arise from motion between the unhealed fracture fragments. In some cases, this motion can even be seen under fluoroscopy as the height of the vertebral body changes with respiration. Prone positioning during the procedure promotes height restoration because of the traction placed across the vertebral body. The needle should be placed into or as close to the cleft as possible so that the cement will fill the cleft. Vertebral augmentation yields significant rates of pain relief in the setting of intraosseous vacuum phenomenon[35,36] and, in our experience, can provide considerable height restoration. It

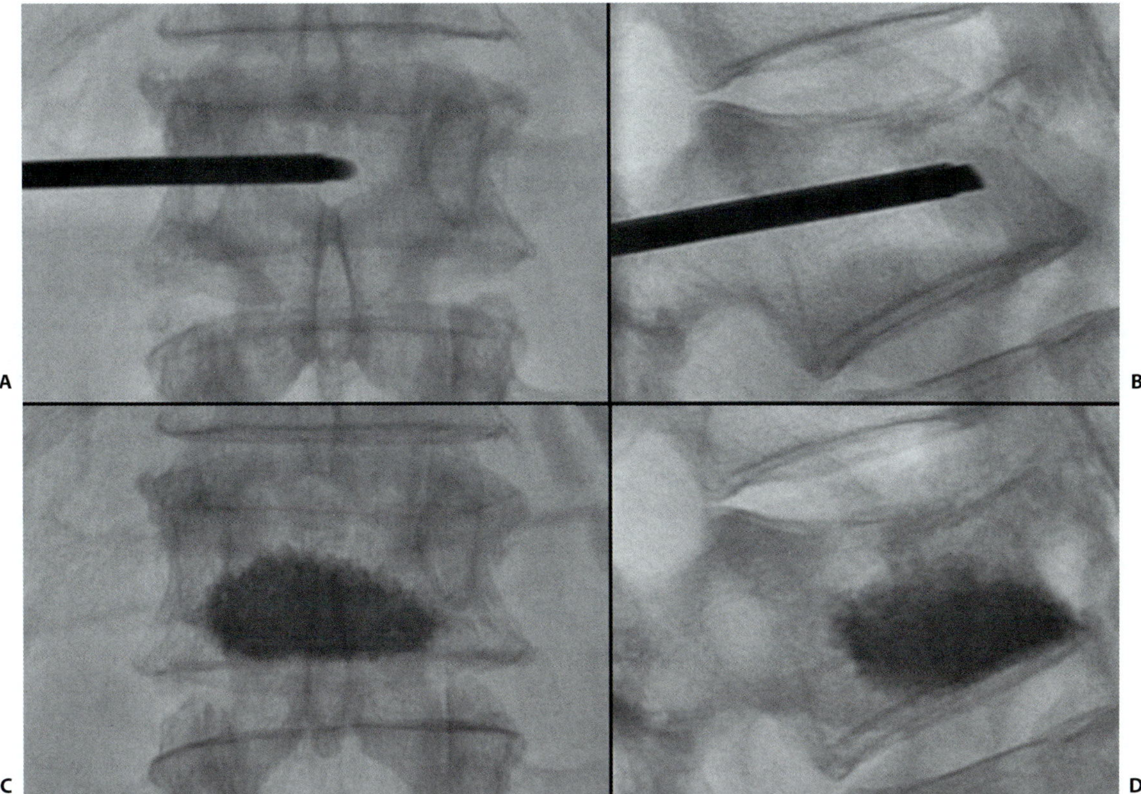

FIGURE 92-6. Unipedicular approach. Anteroposterior (AP) (**A**) and lateral (**B**) fluoroscopic images demonstrating a unipedicular approach with the needle tip achieving midline position in the anterior third of the L1 vertebral body. AP (**C**) and lateral (**D**) fluoroscopic images demonstrating a midline column of cement within the anterior two-thirds of the L1 vertebra.

is important to keep the patient prone for 15 to 20 minutes after the cement injection to allow the cement to harden within the cleft before moving the patient off the fluoroscopy table.

Malignant Fractures with Posterior Wall Osteolysis or Epidural Tumor Extension Although vertebral augmentation may be performed in the setting of posterior wall osteolysis or epidural tumor extension, there should be heightened awareness of the potential neurologic complications related to epidural extension of cement or posterior displacement of tumor. In a study of 51 patients with epidural extension treated with vertebroplasty, 30% had preprocedural symptoms of partial or complete cord compression or cauda equina syndrome.[14] Although no further clinical deterioration was observed in this subgroup after vertebroplasty, one of the 36 patients without neurologic symptoms developed a cauda equina syndrome 2 days after vertebroplasty and required surgical decompression.[14] This was the only symptomatic cement leak. Analgesic efficacy was impressive—94% (48 of 51 patients) at day 1, 86% (31 patients) at 1 month, 83% (19 patients) at 6 months, and 92% (11 patients) after 1 year (data are from surviving patients).[14] Safeguards to prevent complications in this cohort include performing the procedure with the patient awake because new pain may be the first sign of dangerous cement leakage and more modest cement injection compared with routine cases. Limiting the cement to the anterior two-thirds of the vertebral body may be a good rule of thumb as well as injection of thicker cement, which may in turn reduce the risk of epidural cement leakage.[37]

Safety of Multilevel Treatment The patient presenting for vertebral augmentation may have multiple fractures that require treatment. Ideally, all of the levels would be treated at one time. However, treating an excessive number of levels in a single session raises many concerns, including PMMA toxicity, difficulty for elderly patients to lie prone and cooperate for the extended amounts of time this would require, and fat emboli being extruded from the marrow during the cement injections. There have been two reported deaths in patients who received vertebral augmentation at eight or more levels.[38] Although there is no established guideline, a good rule of thumb is to treat a maximum of three levels per session.[39,40]

OUTCOMES

The mechanism by which vertebroplasty and kyphoplasty relieve pain is uncertain.[41] Hypotheses include mechanical stabilization of mobile fracture fragments, thermal or chemical neurolysis, or inherent tumoricidal or cytotoxic effects on malignant fractures. A cadaveric study has also demonstrated new bone formation after PMMA injection.[42]

There have been two highly publicized placebo-controlled randomized clinical trials on vertebroplasty published in the *NEJM*. Both trials used a sham procedure in the placebo arm, which involved local anesthetic injection down to the periosteum of the pedicle[43] or local anesthetic injection combined with passage of a 13-gauge needle to rest on the lamina.[44] Both studies found that there was no significant reduction in pain or pain-related disability in patients undergoing vertebroplasty compared with the sham procedure.

The Investigational Vertebroplasty Safety and Efficacy Trial (INVEST) trial included 131 patients, with 68 patients randomized to vertebroplasty and 63 to the sham procedure.[43] Although at 1 month, there was a trend toward a higher rate of clinically meaningful improvement in pain (30% decrease from baseline), there was no statistical difference in regard to pain scores, back pain–related disability, or quality of life.[43] Buchbinder et al. studied 78 patients, with 38 patients randomized to vertebroplasty and 40 to the sham procedure.[44] After the procedure, both groups had similar improvements in pain, physical functioning, and quality of life. There were no significant differences between groups at 1 week, 1 month, 3 months, and 6 months of follow-up.[44]

These reports were in contrast to previous retrospective case series that had documented impressive rates of pain relief from these procedures.[45] The *NEJM* trials were criticized for potential inclusion of patients with chronic fractures of up to 12 months in duration. The average back pain duration was 18 weeks in INVEST, with one-third of all patients randomized having pain for longer than 6 months. Although the Buchbinder et al. trial had only four patients randomized after 6 months, only 25 patients (one-third of the study group) were randomized less than 6 weeks from symptom onset. Moreover, there was little use of advanced imaging for selection. In the INVEST trial, marrow edema on MRI or increased uptake on bone scanning was only required for fractures of an uncertain age (rate of usage was not reported); in the Buchbinder et al. trial, MRI-demonstrated marrow edema or a fracture line was required; however, the determination of bone marrow edema was not described. Further criticisms include inconsistent use of physical examination, difficulties in recruitment, and absence of a control group without intervention.

Since then, the VERTOS II investigators[46] performed a nonblinded randomized trial in 202 patients with severe back pain for 6 weeks or less, focal tenderness at the fracture level, and MRI-demonstrated bone edema, equally into vertebroplasty or conservative arms. All patients were prescribed analgesics that were individually titrated, bisphosphonates, calcium, and vitamin D supplements. Vertebroplasty was performed at a mean of 5.6 weeks after symptom onset. There were statistically significant reductions in mean visual analog scale (VAS) scores in favor of vertebroplasty at 1 month ($P < 0.0001$), with the benefit persistent at 1 year ($P < 0.0001$).[46] There were significant reductions in use of drugs compared at conservative treatment at 1 day ($P < 0.0001$), 1 week ($P = 0.001$), and 1 month ($P = 0.033$).[46] Moreover, significant pain relief (VAS reduction of ≥3 points) was achieved earlier and in more patients after vertebroplasty (29.7 days; 95% confidence interval [CI] 11.45–47.97) than with conservative treatment (115.6 days, 95% CI 85.87–145.40).[46] Notably, the same investigators have already planned VERTOS IV, a prospective, multicenter, randomized controlled trial (RCT) designed to compare pain relief after vertebroplasty with a sham intervention in patients with an acute osteoporotic vertebral compression fracture using the same strict inclusion criteria as in VERTOS II.[47]

The Fracture Reduction Evaluation (FREE) trial was another large trial supporting the efficacy of vertebral augmentation. A total of 300 patients were randomized to receive kyphoplasty ($n = 149$) or conservative therapy ($n = 151$).[48] Fractures were to have a minimum of 15% height loss and have MRI evidence of edema. Although both osteoporotic and malignant fractures were included, 96% of fractures were related to primary osteoporosis. At randomization, fractures were a mean of 6 weeks old, kyphoplasty was performed at a mean of 7 days after randomization, and patients with fracture ages older than 3 months were excluded. The primary outcome measure was the mean short-form (SF)-36 physical component summary (PCS) scale, a validated global quality-of-life measure weighted on physical abilities.[48] There were statistically significant improvements in the SF-36 PCS scores in favor of kyphoplasty at 1 month ($P <0.0001$) and 12 months ($P = 0.0004$). There were greater reductions in the Roland-Morris disability questionnaire (RDQ) scores in favor of kyphoplasty at 1 month ($P <0.0001$) and 12 months ($P = 0.0012$).[48] Patients in the kyphoplasty group also had greater reductions in back pain scores, lower rates of narcotic analgesic use, and fewer days of restricted activity than those managed with conservative therapy.[48] By 12 months, these differences between the conservative therapy arm and kyphoplasty group were diminished, most likely as a result of fracture healing.[48]

Further RCT evidence comes from the Cancer Patient Fracture Evaluation (CAFE) study, which reported benefit of kyphoplasty over conservative therapy for malignant painful vertebral compression fractures.[49] CAFE recruited 134 patients with malignant fractures at 22 sites in Europe, the United States, Canada, and Australia. Approximately 50% of patients had breast, lung, or prostate cancer metastases, and 40% had multiple myeloma–related fractures. Patients with osteoblastic tumors or primary bone tumors such as osteosarcoma or a plasmacytoma at the index compression fracture were excluded. Patients were randomly assigned to kyphoplasty ($n = 70$) or conservative therapy ($n = 64$). The median estimated symptomatic fracture age was 3·5 months [Inter-quartile range (IQR) 1.2–6.8]; 87 of 129 patients had edema on MRI. The primary end point was back-specific functional status as measured by the RDQ at 1 month. There was a statistically significant reduction in the RDQ scores in favor of kyphoplasty at 1 month ($P <0.0001$).[49] The mean RDQ score in the kyphoplasty group reduced from 17.6 at baseline to 9.1 at 1 month; the mean score in the control group changed from 18.2 to 18.0; the kyphoplasty treatment effect on RDQ was −8.4 points at 1 month (95% CI −7.6 to −9.2; $P <0.0001$). Patients in the kyphoplasty group also had greater reductions in back pain—both groups had baseline mean back pain scores of 7.3; the mean score at 7 days was 3.5 compared with 7.0 in the conservative arm ($P <0.0001$). This remained significant at 1 month ($P <0.0001$). In addition, there were significant reductions in analgesic use, days of bed rest, improvement in quality of life (measured by SF-36 PCS), and Karnofsky performance status in the kyphoplasty group compared with the conservative arm. These improvements in pain, overall functional status, and quality of life continued for the 12 months of the study period.[49]

With regard to longer term outcomes, there is little data. Two-year outcome data from the FREE trial revealed that although there were no longer statistically significant differences in the SF-36 PCS or RDQ scores at 24 months, there remained a statistically significant reduction in back pain scores for patients in the kyphoplasty arm compared with conservative therapy at 24 months ($P = 0.009$).[50] A similar benefit was also reported at 36 months after kyphoplasty from a smaller prospective nonrandomized study of 60 patients.[51]

For height restoration, the results are less dramatic. Studies have shown that magnitude of partial height restoration after vertebroplasty ranges from 2.5 to 8.4 mm and is overall similar to that reported after kyphoplasty.[52] However, many of these studies did not report the incidence of fracture clefts. Overall, height restoration appears to relate to dynamic mobility of fracture fragments from the presence of a fracture cleft.[53] Dynamic mobility refers to a change in vertebral body height during changes in position, typically an increase in vertebral body height with supine or prone positioning compared with the erect position; this typically occurs in fractures at the thoracolumbar junction (T11–L1), where the relatively fixed thoracic spine joins the more mobile lumbar spine. A study of 65 vertebral compression fractures referred for vertebroplasty revealed dynamic mobility in one-third of treated levels.[54] All fractures that were mobile had a fracture cleft; all fractures that were fixed did not have a fracture cleft. Fractures that were mobile had an average absolute increase of anterior vertebral height of 8.4 mm (range, 2.0–17.4 mm) and a decreased kyphosis angle of 7.2 degrees (40%) after vertebroplasty. There was no height restoration or kyphosis correction in fixed fractures.[54] In general, restoration of vertebral body height and kyphosis correction may be desirable to improve postural endurance, reduce abdominal crowding, and improve overall pulmonary capacity; however, it remains unclear whether these results have any clinical significance.[52]

COMPLICATIONS

With adherence to careful technique and optimal visualization, the risk of morbidity or mortality from vertebral augmentation is small. The potential complications that should be explained to the patient before consent include cement leakage, nerve or spinal cord damage resulting in paralysis or bowel or bladder dysfunction[38,55,56], pulmonary embolus (secondary to cement or fat emboli),[38,57,58]) infection (osteomyelitis, epidural abscess[23]), paraspinal hematoma, fracture (of rib, pedicle, or vertebral body[15,57]), hypotension or depressed myocardial function (secondary to free PMMA monomer or fat emboli[38,57]), pneumothorax (for thoracic levels), and worsened pain or failure to treat. Death from cardiovascular collapse or anaphylaxis to the cement has also been reported.[59]

For benign osteoporotic fractures, complication rates are approximately 1%.[40] Not surprisingly they are higher for inexperienced practitioners or those attempting the procedure without adequate image guidance or cement opacification.[40] In the VERTOS II trial, the only complications referable to vertebroplasty occurring in the 101 patients treated were a urinary tract infection (UTI) in one patient and asymptomatic cement deposition in a segmental pulmonary artery in another.[46] Similarly, in the FREE trial, complications referable to kyphoplasty in the 149 patients treated were one soft tissue hematoma and one UTI.[48] Of note, almost all kyphoplasties performed in the FREE trial were performed under general anesthesia, and in neither cohort were the rates of urinary catheterization reported. In our experience, both vertebroplasty and kyphoplasty can be performed with local anesthesia and conscious sedation in most cases, and urinary catheterization is not required.

The risks are greater for malignancy-related fractures, with an overall complication rate of 5% to 10% reported.[58] In the CAFE trial, of the 70 patients treated with kyphoplasty for malignancy-related fractures, the only complications referable to kyphoplasty were one superficial wound infection and one patient with a cement leakage to the adjacent disc who had an adjacent fracture the day after the procedure.[49] There were no serious adverse events that were deemed device related. Importantly, kyphoplasty was not performed on those who had vertebral fracture morphology deemed unsuitable as determined by the treating physician. Thus, patients with vertebra plana, comminuted fractures, fractures that had posterior wall involvement, or those with epidural involvement, which would incur higher risk, were excluded.

Extraosseous passage of cement is an important source of complications during vertebral augmentation (**Fig. 92-7**). For vertebroplasty for osteoporotic fractures, small amounts of cement leakage are very common—in VERTOS II, 72% of treated vertebral bodies demonstrated cement leaks on postprocedural CT, with the majority discal or into segmental veins; none were into the spinal canal.[46] All patients remained asymptomatic. There was one patient (1%) with an asymptomatic cement segmental pulmonary embolus.[46]

For kyphoplasty, a large low resistance cavity is created and will fill first, theoretically resulting in a lower rate of cement leakage.[60-63] In FREE, cement extravasation occurred in 27% of treated vertebrae, but this was assessed with intraoperative fluoroscopy and postoperative radiographs.[48] Most were endplate or discal leakages; there was one foraminal leakage, none were into the spinal canal, and there were no cement embolisms. All patients remained asymptomatic.[48] In a small retrospective series with postprocedural CT, the rate of local leakage of bone cement was 87.5% (21 of 24) for percutaneous vertebroplasty and 49.2% (29 of 59) for kyphoplasty.[64]

Cement leaks are also common in pathologic fractures.[57,58,65] A recent retrospective study of CT-guided vertebroplasty for 331 malignant vertebral lesions revealed a local cement leak in 59% (194 of 331 vertebrae).[66] Although osteolysis of the posterior wall was evident in 49% (162 of 331 vertebrae), only 6% (15 of 331) of leaks were into the spinal canal through the posterior cortex. Pulmonary cement emboli were detected in 1 of 53 (2%) chest radiographs and 10 of 88 (11%) chest CT scans.[66] A large single-center study of 106 patients with multiple myeloma treated with vertebroplasty revealed CT-detected cement extravasation in 23% of treated vertebrae, mainly into perivertebral veins (85%) and epidural veins (9%). In 5 patients (5%) cement emboli were detected in the lungs. All leaks were asymptomatic.[67]

Although most extraosseous cement produces no symptoms or long-term morbidity, even small amounts of PMMA adjacent to a nerve root, including cement within the foraminal veins, can produce radicular pain.[58] When radiculopathy is produced by cement leakage, the pain can be treated with nerve root block or systemic steroids. The need for surgical decompression is rare[39] but may be necessary when there is sufficient foraminal cement to cause frank root compression or when sufficient cement has been placed in the spinal canal to cause cord compression or cauda equina syndrome.[14]

POSTPROCEDURE AND FOLLOW-UP CARE

Immediately after the procedure, manual compression is applied over the needle access sites for 5 minutes to promote clotting and prevent paraspinal soft tissue bleeding complications. Transfer to a stretcher may be performed immediately after the procedure except in the setting of a vertebral cleft, in which we keep the patient prone on the fluoroscopy table for 15 to 20 minutes. The patient is positioned supine and flat in bed for 2 hours followed by another hour in a 30-degree head-up position after the procedure. To alleviate immediate postprocedural pain, the patient may be given 15 to 30 mg of IV ketorolac unless the patient has renal insufficiency. The majority of patients can be discharged later the same day or can be observed overnight in the hospital. Assessment of the patient shortly after the procedure commonly reveals improvement of the back pain. Often, the patient will discriminate a new procedure-related pain, which is typically treated with nonsteroidal anti-inflammatory drugs and should resolve over 24 to 72 hours. In the setting of clinical deterioration suspicious for cement leakage, cross-sectional imaging should be performed.

Postprocedure follow-up of the patient is important. The patient should be seen in follow-up in the near term after the procedure (e.g., 3 weeks). At that time, the patient is assessed with regard to pain and mobility levels and need for pain medication. It is important to counsel the patient to report any sudden increase in back pain or new back pain because it may indicate a new fracture. Imaging should be performed in this case to help elucidate the cause of the patient's new pain. Importantly, up to one-third of patients will sustain a repeat fracture within 1 to 3 years, with the greatest risk in steroid-induced osteoporosis.[68,69] Thus, prevention of future fractures (with vitamin D and calcium supplementation and bisphosphonate therapy) is particularly important. Although the vast majority of recurrent fractures occur at new levels, a small percentage of patients that sustain recurrent fracture at a previously treated level and may gain pain relief from repeat vertebral augmentation.[70] This being said, caution should be taken when interpreting marrow edema at a previously treated level because according to one study, normal MRI findings after vertebroplasty include persistent or progressive marrow edema at the treated level in up to one-third of patients and up to 6 months after the procedure.[71]

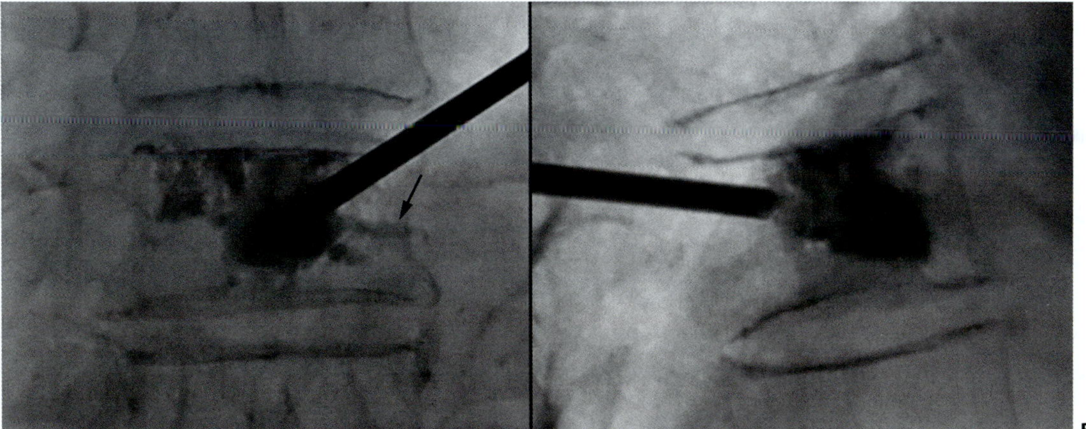

FIGURE 92-7. Importance of biplane fluoroscopy during cement injection. (**A**) Anteroposterior (AP) fluoroscopic images demonstrating paraspinal venous extravasation clearly evident on the AP projection. (**B**) This cannot be identified on the lateral projection, highlighting the importance of good biplane fluoroscopy. Cement injection was ceased, and no further venous penetration occurred. The patient remained asymptomatic.

REFERENCES

1. Iqbal MM. Osteoporosis: epidemiology, diagnosis, and treatment. *South Med J*. 2000;93:2-18.
2. Cooper C, O'Neill T, Silman A. The epidemiology of vertebral fractures. European vertebral osteoporosis study group. *Bone*. 1993;14(Suppl 1):S89-S97.
3. Kawaguchi S, Horigome K, Yajima H, et al. Symptomatic relevance of intravertebral cleft in patients with osteoporotic vertebral fracture. *J Neurosurg Spine*. 2010;13:267-275.
4. Durie BG, Kyle RA, Belch A, et al. Myeloma management guidelines: a consensus report from the scientific advisors of the international myeloma foundation. *Hematol J* 2003;4:379-398.
5. Vogel MN, Weisel K, Maksimovic O, et al. Pathologic fractures in patients with multiple myeloma undergoing bisphosphonate therapy: incidence and correlation with course of disease. *AJR Am J Roentgenol*. 2009;193:656-661.
6. Hussein MA, Vrionis FD, Allison R, et al. The role of vertebral augmentation in multiple myeloma: International Myeloma Working Group consensus statement. . 2008;22:1479-1484.
7. Aaron AD. The management of cancer metastatic to bone. *JAMA*. 1994;272:1206-1209.
8. Perrin RG. Metastatic tumors of the axial spine. *Curr Opin Oncol*. 1992;4:525-532.
9. Babayev M, Lachmann E, Nagler W. The controversy surrounding sacral insufficiency fractures: to ambulate or not to ambulate? *Am J Phys Med Rehabil*. 2000;79:404-409.
10. Dittmer DK, Teasell R. Complications of immobilization and bed rest. Part 1: Musculoskeletal and cardiovascular complications. *Can Fam Physician*. 1993;39:1428-1432.
11. Appel NB, Gilula LA. Percutaneous vertebroplasty in patients with spinal canal compromise. *AJR Am J Roentgenol*. 2004;182:947-951.
12. Jensen ME, Dion JE. Percutaneous vertebroplasty in the treatment of osteoporotic compression fractures. *Neuroimaging Clin N Am*. 2000;10:547-568.
13. Hiwatashi A, Westesson PL. Vertebroplasty for osteoporotic fractures with spinal canal compromise. *AJNR Am J Neuroradiol*. 2007;28:690-692.
14. Saliou G, Kocheida el M, Lehmann P, et al. Percutaneous vertebroplasty for pain management in malignant fractures of the spine with epidural involvement. *Radiology*. 2010;254:882-890.
15. Kallmes DF, Jensen ME. Percutaneous vertebroplasty. *Radiology*. 2003;229:27-36.
16. Stallmeyer MJB, Zoarski GH, Obuchowski AM. Optimizing patient selection in percutaneous vertebroplasty. *J Vasc Interv Radiol*. 2003;14:683-696.
17. Rad AE, Kallmes DF. Pain relief following vertebroplasty in patients with and without localizing tenderness on palpation. *AJNR Am J Neuroradiol*. 2008;29:1622-1626.
18. Maynard AS, Jensen ME, Schweickert PA, et al. Value of bone scan imaging in predicting pain relief from percutaneous vertebroplasty in osteoporotic vertebral fractures. *AJNR Am J Neuroradiol*. 2000;21:1807-1812.
19. Sola M, Perez R, Cuadras P, et al. Value of bone SPECT-CT to predict chronic pain relief after percutaneous vertebroplasty in vertebral fractures. *Spine J*. 2011;11:1102-1107.
20. Weill A, Chiras J, Simon JM, et al. Spinal metastases: indications for and results of percutaneous injection of acrylic surgical cement. *Radiology*. 1996;199:241-247.
21. Calmels V, Vallee JN, Rose M, et al. Osteoblastic and mixed spinal metastases: evaluation of the analgesic efficacy of percutaneous vertebroplasty. *AJNR Am J Neuroradiol*. 2007;28:570-574.
22. Teng MM, Wei CJ, Wei LC, et al. Kyphosis correction and height restoration effects of percutaneous vertebroplasty. *AJNR Am J Neuroradiol*. 2003;24:1893-1900.
23. Yu SW, Chen WJ, Lin WC, et al. Serious pyogenic spondylitis following vertebroplasty—a case report. *Spine*. 2004;29:E209-E211.
24. Wong W, Mathis J. Is intraosseous venography a significant safety measure in performance of vertebroplasty? *J Vasc Interv Radiol*. 2002;13:137-138.
25. Komemushi A, Tanigawa N, Kariya S, et al. Radiation exposure to operators during vertebroplasty. *J Vasc Interv Radiol*. 2005;16:1327-1332.
26. Mathis JM, Ortiz AO, Zoarski GH. Vertebroplasty versus kyphoplasty: a comparison and contrast. *AJNR Am J Neuroradiol*. 2004;25:840-845.
27. Ortiz AO, Zoarski GH, Beckerman M. Kyphoplasty. *Tech Vasc Interv Radiol*. 2002;5:239-249.
28. Knavel EM, Rad AE, Thielen KR, et al. Clinical outcomes with hemivertebral filling during percutaneous vertebroplasty. *AJNR Am J Neuroradiol*. 2009;30:496-499.
29. Kim AK, Jensen ME, Dion JE, et al. Unilateral transpedicular percutaneous vertebroplasty: initial experience. *Radiology*. 2002;222:737-741.
30. Song BK, Eun JP, Oh YM. Clinical and radiological comparison of unipedicular versus bipedicular balloon kyphoplasty for the treatment of vertebral compression fractures. *Osteoporos Int*. 2009;20:1717-1723.
31. Kaufmann TJ, Trout AT, Kallmes DF. The effects of cement volume on clinical outcomes of percutaneous vertebroplasty. *AJNR Am J Neuroradiol*. 2006;27:1933-1937.
32. Mathis JM, Wong W. Percutaneous vertebroplasty: technical considerations. *J Vasc Interv Radiol*. 2003;14:953-960.
33. O'Brien JP, Sims JT, Evans AJ. Vertebroplasty in patients with severe vertebral compression fractures: a technical report. *AJNR Am J Neuroradiol*. 2000;21:1555-1558.
34. Guglielmi G, Andreula C, Muto M, et al. Percutaneous vertebroplasty: indications, contraindications, technique, and complications. *Acta Radiol*. 2005;46:256-268.
35. Lane JI, Maus TP, Wald JT, et al. Intravertebral clefts opacified during vertebroplasty: pathogenesis, technical implications, and prognostic significance. *AJNR Am J Neuroradiol*. 2002;23:1642-1646.
36. Peh WC, Gelbart MS, Gilula LA, et al. Percutaneous vertebroplasty: treatment of painful vertebral compression fractures with intraosseous vacuum phenomena. *AJR Am J Roentgenol*. 2003;180:1411-1417.
37. Basile A, Cavalli M, Fiumara P, et al. Vertebroplasty in multiple myeloma with osteolysis or fracture of the posterior vertebral wall. Usefulness of a delayed cement injection. *Skeletal Radiol*. 2011;40:913-919.
38. Nussbaum DA, Gailloud P, Murphy K. A review of complications associated with vertebroplasty and kyphoplasty as reported to the Food and Drug Administration medical device related web site. *J Vasc Interv Radiol*. 2004;15:1185-1192.
39. Zoarski GH, Snow P, Olan WJ, et al. Percutaneous vertebroplasty for osteoporotic compression fractures: quantitative prospective evaluation of long-term outcomes. *J Vasc Interv Radiol*. 2002;13:139-148.
40. Mathis JM, Barr JD, Belkoff SM, et al. Percutaneous vertebroplasty: a developing standard of care for vertebral compression fractures. *AJNR Am J Neuroradiol*. 2001;22:373-381.
41. Deramond H, Wright NT, Belkoff SM. Temperature elevation caused by bone cement polymerization during vertebroplasty. *Bone*. 1999;25:17S-21S.

42. Braunstein V, Sprecher CM, Gisep A, et al. Long-term reaction to bone cement in osteoporotic bone: new bone formation in vertebral bodies after vertebroplasty. *J Anat.* 2008;212:697-701.
43. Kallmes DF, Comstock BA, Heagerty PJ, et al. A randomized trial of vertebroplasty for osteoporotic spinal fractures. *N Engl J Med.* 2009;361:569-579.
44. Buchbinder R, Osborne RH, Ebeling PR, et al. A randomized trial of vertebroplasty for painful osteoporotic vertebral fractures. *N Engl J Med.* 2009;361:557-568.
45. Eck JC, Nachtigall D, Humphreys SC, et al. Comparison of vertebroplasty and balloon kyphoplasty for treatment of vertebral compression fractures: a meta-analysis of the literature. *Spine J.* 2008;8:488-497.
46. Klazen CA, Lohle PN, de Vries J, et al. Vertebroplasty versus conservative treatment in acute osteoporotic vertebral compression fractures (VERTOS II): an open-label randomised trial. *Lancet.* 2010;376:1085-1092.
47. Firanescu C, Lohle PN, de Vries J, et al. A randomised sham controlled trial of vertebroplasty for painful acute osteoporotic vertebral fractures (VERTOS IV). *Trials.* 2011;12:93.
48. Wardlaw D, Cummings SR, Van Meirhaeghe J, et al. Efficacy and safety of balloon kyphoplasty compared with non-surgical care for vertebral compression fracture (free): a randomised controlled trial. *Lancet.* 2009;373:1016-1024.
49. Berenson J, Pflugmacher R, Jarzem P, et al. Balloon kyphoplasty versus non-surgical fracture management for treatment of painful vertebral body compression fractures in patients with cancer: a multicentre, randomised controlled trial. *Lancet Oncol.* 2011;12:225-235.
50. Boonen S, Van Meirhaeghe J, Bastian L, et al. Balloon kyphoplasty for the treatment of acute vertebral compression fractures: 2-year results from a randomized trial. *J Bone Miner Res.* 2011;26:1627-1637.
51. Kasperk C, Grafe IA, Schmitt S, et al. Three-year outcomes after kyphoplasty in patients with osteoporosis with painful vertebral fractures. *J Vasc Interv Radiol.* 2010;21:701-709.
52. McKiernan F, Faciszewski T, Jensen R. Does vertebral height restoration achieved at vertebroplasty matter? *J Vasc Interv Radiol.* 2005;16:973-979.
53. Sun G, Jin P, Li M, et al. Height restoration and wedge angle correction effects of percutaneous vertebroplasty: association with intraosseous clefts. *Eur Radiol.* 2011;21:2597-2603.
54. McKiernan F, Jensen R, Faciszewski T. The dynamic mobility of vertebral compression fractures. *J Bone Miner Res.* 2003;18:24-29.
55. Yazbeck PG, Al Rouhban RB, Slaba SG, et al. Anterior spinal artery syndrome after percutaneous vertebroplasty. *Spine J.* 2011;11:e5-e8.
56. Ratliff J, Nguyen T, Heiss J. Root and spinal cord compression from methyl methacrylate vertebroplasty. *Spine.* 2001;26:E300-E302.
57. Laredo JD, Hamze B. Complications of percutaneous vertebroplasty and their prevention. *Skeletal Radiol.* 2004;33:493-505.
58. Barragan-Campos HM, Vallee JN, Lo D, et al. Percutaneous vertebroplasty for spinal metastases: complications. *Radiology.* 2006;238:354-362.
59. Childers JC, Jr. Cardiovascular collapse and death during vertebroplasty. *Radiology.* 2003;228:902-903.
60. Coumans JV, Reinhardt MK, Lieberman IH. Kyphoplasty for vertebral compression fractures: 1-year clinical outcomes from a prospective study. *J Neurosurg.* 2003;99:44-50.
61. Ledlie JT, Renfro M. Balloon kyphoplasty: one-year outcomes in vertebral body height restoration, chronic pain, and activity levels. *J Neurosurg.* 2003;98:36-42.
62. Lieberman IH, Dudeney S, Reinhardt MK, et al. Initial outcome and efficacy of "kyphoplasty" in the treatment of painful osteoporotic vertebral compression fractures. *Spine.* 2001;26:1631-1638.
63. Theodorou DJ, Theodorou SJ, Duncan TD, et al. Percutaneous balloon kyphoplasty for the correction of spinal deformity in painful vertebral body compression fractures. *Clin Imaging.* 2002;26:1-5.
64. Lee IJ, Choi AL, Yie MY, et al. CT evaluation of local leakage of bone cement after percutaneous kyphoplasty and vertebroplasty. *Acta Radiol.* 2010;51:649-654.
65. Hodler J, Peck D, Gilula LA. Midterm outcome after vertebroplasty: predictive value of technical and patient-related factors. *Radiology.* 2003;227:662-668.
66. Trumm CG, Pahl A, Helmberger TK, et al. CT fluoroscopy-guided percutaneous vertebroplasty in spinal malignancy: technical results, PMMA leakages, and complications in 202 patients. *Skeletal Radiol.* 2012.
67. Anselmetti GC, Manca A, Montemurro F, et al. Percutaneous vertebroplasty in multiple myeloma: prospective long-term follow-up in 106 consecutive patients. *Cardiovasc Intervent Radiol.* 2012;35(1): 139-145.
68. Harrop JS, Prpa B, Reinhardt MK, et al. Primary and secondary osteoporosis incidence of subsequent vertebral compression fractures after kyphoplasty. *Spine.* 2004;29:2120-2125.
69. Tanigawa N, Kariya S, Komemushi A, et al. Percutaneous vertebroplasty for osteoporotic compression fractures: long-term evaluation of the technical and clinical outcomes. *AJR Am J Roentgenol.* 2011;196:1415-1418.
70. Gaughen JR, Jr., Jensen ME, Schweickert PA, et al. The therapeutic benefit of repeat percutaneous vertebroplasty at previously treated vertebral levels. *AJNR Am J Neuroradiol.* 2002;23:1657-1661.
71. Dansie DM, Luetmer PH, Lane JI, et al. MRI findings after successful vertebroplasty. *AJNR Am J Neuroradiol.* 2005;26:1595-1600.

Percutaneous and Endoscopic Disc Procedures

Atif B. Malik
Sandeep Sherlekar
Said Osman
Sania Mahmood

INTRODUCTION

Minimally invasive treatments have undertaken all areas of the spine over the past 50 years. The majority of these minimally invasive techniques use a small passage to access the appropriate anatomical area thereby minimizing the resultant injury to the neural, muscular, and ligamentous soft tissues. Spinal disc disease has been treated with chemonucleolysis, percutaneous discectomy, laser discectomy, intradiscal thermoablation, and other minimally invasive microdiscectomy techniques. The goals of minimally invasive spinal procedures embody achieving clinical outcomes comparable to conventional open surgery while reducing the risk of iatrogenic complications. With the advent of modern surgical technologies such as digital fluoroscopy image guidance, high-resolution endoscopy, and minimally invasive surgical tools, less invasive approaches have become popular over the past decade among interventional pain physicians, neurosurgeons, and orthopedic spine specialists.

Percutaneous and endoscopic techniques, such as those used for cholecystectomy by general surgeons, have evolved into procedures performed by spinal surgeons for discectomy and fusion. Fluoroscopy image systems have been adapted to facilitate pedicle screw placement with great accuracy and to treat compression fractures with vertebroplasty and kyphoplasty. The progression of endoscopy and video image guidance systems, microscopy, radiofrequency, and laser technology along with percutaneous technique provide the foundation on which minimally invasive spinal surgery is based. Further improvement in optics and imaging resources, development of biologic agents, and introduction of instrumentation systems designed for endoscopic procedures will inevitably lead to further applications in minimally invasive spine surgery that will continue to challenge interventional pain management and spine surgeons.

HISTORICAL PERSPECTIVES

In the 1930s, Mixter and Bar recognized the relationship between disc herniation and sciatica.[1] In 1964, Smith was able to dissolve the nucleus pulposus via chemonucleolysis in a rabbit model via percutaneous enzymatic applications; this technique was later successfully applied in humans and later abandoned because of complications.[2,3] In 1973, Kambin and Gellman initiated a percutaneous indirect spinal canal posterolateral extracanal nonvisualized approach through an anatomically safe triangle appropriately named Kambin's triangle (see **Fig. 93-1**).[4] Then Hijikata et al. in 1975 reported the first percutaneous nucleotomy for posterolateral lumbar disc herniations using arthroscopic techniques.[5-7] Kambin and Gellman reported a 72% success rate for 136 patients treated with a percutaneous lateral technique similar to method adopted by Hijikata.[8] This success was due to a reduction of intradiscal pressure by forming fenestrations in the outer annulus. In 1983, Frost and Hausmann first introduced a modified arthroscope into the intervertebral disc space.[9] In 1985, Onik et al. described the automated percutaneous lumbar discectomy using a 2-mm blunt-tipped suction cutting probe.[10] Additionally, percutaneous laser discectomy was introduced by Choy et al. in the late 1980s.[11] Kambin published the first intraoperative discoscopic views of herniated nucleus pulposus in 1988.[12]

The first percutaneous vertebroplasty technique was developed in 1984 by Galibert and Deramond in which polymethylmethacrylate (PMMA) was injected into the vertebral body through the pedicles.[13] In 2001, kyphoplasty was developed to restore the height of collapsed vertebrae using an inflatable bone tamp before injecting PMMA.[14] In the late 1990s, Saal and Saal reported intradiscal electrothermal therapy to treat discogenic axial back pain.[15] In 2001, Knight et al. described the technique of endoscopic foraminoplasty using a side-firing holmium:yttrium-aluminum-garnet (Ho:YAG) laser.[16] Yeung and Tsou[17], in 2002, retrospectively evaluated the efficacy of endoscopic discectomy in 307 patients and reported it to be comparable to conventional open surgery. Nowadays, with the addition of video imaging to standard endoscopy, fluoroscopy and percutaneous minimally invasive instruments have gained rapid use and diversification in clinical application.

CERVICAL SPINE

The first anterior cervical cord decompression was described by Key in 1838.[18] With significant advancement Over the past decade, percutaneous endoscopic cervical discectomy (PECD) has been keenly used to treat soft disc herniation among spinal endoscopists. Establishing a safe

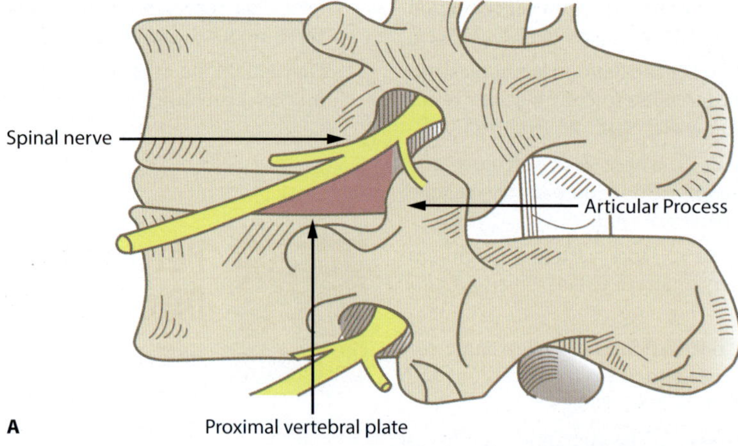

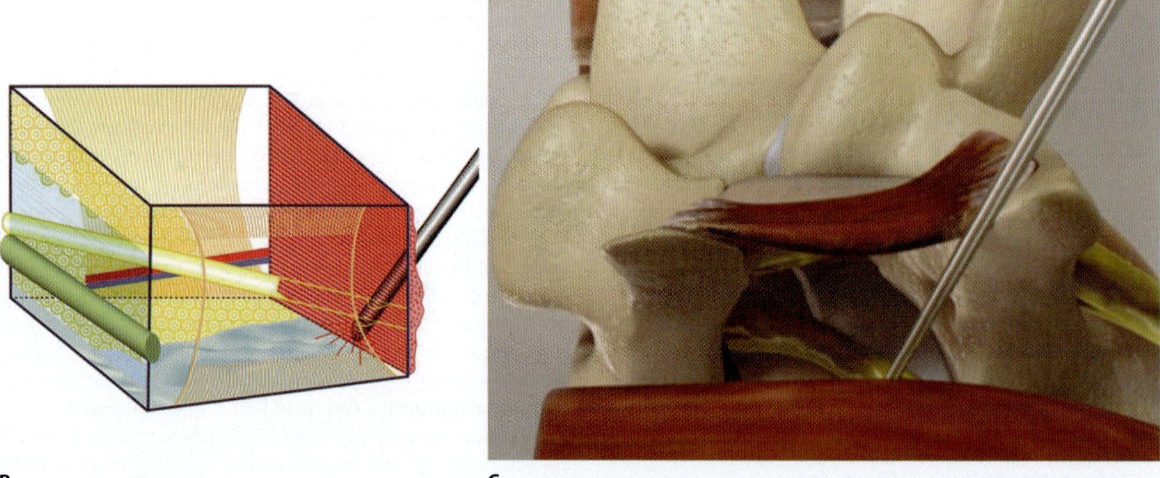

FIGURE 93-1. A. Instrumentation approximating the sagittal plane, in the Kambin's triangle risks injury to the traversing nerve. The boundries of Kambin's triangle are the spinal nerve, articular process, and proximal vertebral plate. **B** and **C**. The conceptual and corresponding spinal anatomical space respectively, to portray the angles for instrumentation through Kambin's triangle in 3D and proximity to surrounding nerves and structures.

corridor percutaneously to the anterior cervical spine can be difficult and can carry the risk of potential injury to the carotid artery, jugular vein, esophagus, trachea, thyroid, and laryngeal nerves. The standard anterior cervical discectomy and fusion, artificial disc replacement, and posterior microdiscectomy have considerable comorbidity. Thus, using sequential dilating tubular approaches to access the anterior cervical spine are often less traumatic to surrounding tissue, vessels and integument than conventional open methods.

The first descriptions of cervical percutaneous discectomies by Tajima et al. were mainly performed at the center of the disc, and the clinical application was limited.[19] Since then, the use of chemonucleolysis with chymopapain, automated percutaneous cervical discectomy, and laser percutaneous cervical decompression have been explored and introduced.[20-25] However, it is the recent advancements in percutaneous endoscopic cervical discectomy (PECD) which have been most beneficial by allowing decompression of the cervical nerve root through a direct and small endoscopic visualization, with subsequent visual removal of the herniated mass and shrinkage of the nucleolus pulposus with the use of microforceps with or without Ho:YAG laser.[25]

Recent studies by Ruetten et al. have been carried out comparing the endoscopic anterior cervical decompression with the open anterior decompression and fusion in 120 patients. The study concluded that there was no significant statistical difference in the clinical outcomes between the two groups. Postoperatively, 85.9% of the patients who received endoscopic anterior cervical decompression did not report axial pain or radiculopathy, and 10.1% had occasional axial pain. There was no significant statistical difference concerning adjacent disc degeneration or kyphosis angle in the operated segment between the two groups. Furthermore, the authors did not find a relation between kyphosis, the height of the intervertebral space, and the clinical outcome.[26] The percutaneous technique has been used not only to treat soft disc pathology but also calcified fixed bony pathology through the anterior cervical foraminotomy approach in an effort to avoid adjacent segment disease which is common after fusion procedures.[27] The use of percutaneous endoscopic approach for cervical spine procedures preserves healthy tissues, decreases intra- and post-operative complication rates, and leads to a faster recovery while preserving the range of motion of the cervical spine.

THORACIC SPINE

Thoracic disc herniation is a challenging entity clinically. The clinical presentation is often vague and may mimic other syndromes.[28-30] The literature also illustrates a 20- to 24-month delay in treatment due mostly to the vague presentation, difficulty in clinical diagnosis, and concern about morbidity associated with current surgical treatment options.[30] A literature review shows that the incidence of thoracic disc herniation ranges from 0.15% to 4% of all symptomatic disc protrusions. Thoracic discectomies account for 0.2% to 1.8% of all discectomies of symptomatic herniations.[31-33] The standard treatment has been transthoracic discectomy.[28,34] This approach to the thoracic disc requires a thoracotomy. The alternative method with comparable results is costotransversectomy.[30,35,36] Both of these transthoracic procedures involve deflating the lung for access to the spine, and postoperative thoracic drainage is necessary; postoperative morbidity can be significant.

In light of catastrophic complications that have occurred in patients who underwent thoracic laminectomies for thoracic disc herniations, as well as complications associated with transthoracic approaches to the spine, there was justifiable hesitance to operate on the thoracic disc in the past unless there was imminent danger of paralysis.[44,45] Other less destabilizing and extrathoracic approaches include costotransversectomy and the retropleural approach. Bohlman and Zdeblick reviewed 22 patients who underwent transthoracic decompression and costotransversectomy and showed that 16 patients had excellent or good results.[34] Currier et al. reviewed 19 patients who underwent transthoracic decompression and fusion. Twelve had excellent or good results.[46]

In an effort to minimize complications related to surgical trauma, in the past 20 years, there has been a shift toward less invasive procedures. Thoracoscopic discectomy has reduced some of the complications associated with thoracotomy, notably chronic chest pain and shoulder stiffness.[37-39] However, the procedure, although reducing the size of the incision and related pain, still relies on the deflation of the lungs and rib excision to access the discs; the risk of intrathoracic complications is not eliminated. Furthermore, there is a need for intrathoracic drainage tubes postoperatively until the lung reinflates, and monitoring in the intensive care unit (ICU) is often necessary until the patient is deemed out of danger. McAfee et al. reviewed 100 patients who had video-assisted thoracoscopic surgery of the spine and reported that, on average, patients had chest tubes in place for 1.44 days, 32% of the patients needed ICU monitoring, and the length of hospital stay was 5 days.[40] Simpson et al. noted that the mean length of hospital stay was 6.8 days.[30]

Over the past couple of decades, a less invasive approach, video-assisted thoracoscopic discectomy, has gained increasing application.[37-39] Although the surgical trauma is not as severe as with the open approach, the potential for intrathoracic complications is similar to the thoracotomy approach.[40] More recently, an extracavitary, posterolateral technique has been reported with encouraging results.[41] In 1994, Osman and Marsolais demonstrated the posterolateral endoscopic approach to the thoracic disc in a cadaveric experiment.[42] In this approach, access channels were posterior to the rib neck and head, with the two acting as barriers against penetration into the retropleural space and the thoracic cavity, thus minimizing trauma to the lungs and the major vessels. Osman and Marsolais went on to demonstrate this procedure successfully in patients with thoracic disc herniations in 1994.[43]

Khoo et al. described a posterolateral approach using a 20-mm-diameter tubular access channel docked at the junction of the transverse process and the facet joint.[41] Decompression of the disc and fusion were carried out without violation of the pleural cavity. Thirteen patients who had myelopathy caused by 15 noncalcified thoracic disc herniations underwent the procedures. The short operating time and minimal blood loss are impressive. The mean length of hospital stay was 3.1 days. One dural leak, four transient paresthesias, and one case of abdominal wall weakness occurred.

The procedure consists of posterolateral arthroscopic decompression, and the evolution of this technique mirrors the evolution of knee arthroscopy from a uniportal operating arthroscope to current independent arthroscope and instrument portals. Maintaining the intraforaminal location of the arthroscope cannula permits safely monitoring the spinal cord and nerve roots during the decompression procedure.

In most cases, The patients are able to go home at less than 24 hours postoperatively. Blood loss is consistently minimal, as well as surgical trauma. The access to the disc is often through the soft tissue, but—as described by Osman and Marsolais in their cadaveric study—at T5 to T6, T6 to T7, and T7 to T8, the rib heads tend to articulate with the discs, obstructing access to the posterolateral corner of the disc.[43] In this situation, instead of walking or tilting the instruments more medially and risking injury to the cord, the dorsal part of the rib head and neck is reamed out with a trephine to gain access to the disc. This leaves the angle of the rib and rib neck as a protection against penetration into the pleural cavity or retropleural space. Another important anatomic finding from the cadaveric study is the posterolateral and rostral course the nerve root takes as it approaches the costal groove of the rib. This is in contradistinction to the lumbar nerve root, which courses ventrolaterally and caudally. These courses of the nerves make the former less likely to undergo injury by a small-diameter cannula and the latter more vulnerable to compression by the instrumentation.

Although retropleural procedures are in their infancy, the published results are promising. Posterolateral arthroscopic thoracic decompression is extrapleural, is less disruptive to normal anatomy, and is a cost-effective way of treating thoracic disc pathology on an outpatient basis.

LUMBAR SPINE

Almost everyone will experience acute low back pain at least once during their lifetime. The lumbar disc may herniate secondary to acute injury to an otherwise normal disc in an adolescent spine or in a degenerated disc, without an obvious injury in an aged spine. In the majority of cases, symptoms subside over a period of several weeks to months with nonoperative measures. A small percentage of patients require surgical intervention either electively, or in case of severe neurologic deficit urgently, as in the case of cauda equina syndrome. The standard surgical treatment is removal of the offending herniated nuclear material impinging on the nerve root. The method of removal has varied over the past several decades, but at the disc level, essentially treatment has remained the same—removal of the offending herniated nuclear material. Whatever the approach, the result is usually immediately gratifying for the patient and the surgeon. The disc, despite symptomatic relief after surgery, continues to deteriorate and may sustain recurrent herniation in the future or degenerate much faster, producing symptoms of spondylosis and stenosis. The challenge for the medical profession today is to prevent further deterioration and even possibly restoration of normal anatomy and function of the vertebrae.

A number of surgical options currently exist,[47-51] most of the newer options being less invasive than the conventional open discectomy. With the emergence of the new technologies and increasing cost of treatment, there is increasing demand for evidence-based treatment for spine patients. Superiority of one method over another should be based on published reports of the various options. Prospective randomized controlled trials (RCTs; level I evidence) are generally best relied on, but as recent controversy on bone morphogenetic protein (BMP) studies show,[52] all RCTs are not the equal, and even the evidence provided by thoroughly well-conducted studies[53-55] often is not good enough to convince third-party payers about the superiority of one surgical approach over another. As will be discussed later, disc herniation is not a monolithic entity; rather, there are variations in the pathoanatomy of the herniation, and there may be abnormalities of the other structures of the spinal motion segment, namely the facet, the ligamentum flavum, and the spinal alignment. Each of these structures may contribute to the symptoms, and certain patient attributes may bias the surgical result one way or another. It is imperative that the technique for evidence gathering is comprehensively refined to take all these variables into account, to determine the superiority or otherwise of the approaches as accurately as the science and the technology will permit.

PATHOANATOMY

DISC DISEASE

The intervertebral disc is the largest avascular structure in the body, mainly nourished by diffusion across the vertebral end plates and annular periphery.[56] Postmortem studies show that disc degenerations start early in adulthood.[57] Quite early in the degeneration cascade,[58] histologic and biochemical changes demonstrate reduced cellularity and decrease in nuclear water content.[59] These intranuclear changes are generally thought, although not universally agreed upon, to lead to intranuclear fragmentation which leads to annular fissuring and eventual rupture and herniation through the annulus.[60,61] The most common area for disc herniation is paracentral. The most plausible explanation for this feature appears to be the anatomy of the posterior longitudinal ligament. The posterior longitudinal ligament has tough fibers that run longitudinally and centrally. At the disc level, fibers run transversely from the deeper layer of the ligament and attach firmly to the annulus of the disc in the foraminal space but not centrally or paracentrally to the disc annulus. This is the weakest area of the disc, where herniation is most common. The fibers of the posterior longitudinal ligament are not attached to the vertebral body; hence, extraannular (free fragment) herniation can track cephalad or caudad between the two. The annulus has multiple lamellae of fibers, The fibers provide the strongest disc attachment to the outer cortical ring of the vertebral end plate and the annulus resists tension from the disc nucleus within. The lumbar disc nucleus is placed slightly posteriorly in a kidney-shaped disc configuration. The annulus is rather thin posteriorly and posterolaterally—causing these areas to also be prone to rupture. The peridural membrane extends laterally and dorsally from underneath the posterior longitudinal ligament.[62] This structure is most likely what is encountered wrapped around the nuclear free fragment in the spinal canal.

FACET DISEASE

The facet joint is a diarthrodial joint formed by the anterolaterally facing convex inferior articular process, posteromedially facing concave superior articular process and a ligamentous capsule that encloses the joint space. The opposing articular cartilage surfaces of the facet joint provide a low-friction environment. When the herniation occurs in a disc of normal height and configuration, chances are that the facet anatomy is normal. On the other hand, when the disc is collapsed secondary to degeneration and the facet joint is normal, the loss of disc height would lead to a degree of retrolisthesis because of the combined effects of facet joint inclination posterocaudally and the normal articular cartilage thickness. Conversely, if the disc is of relatively normal height and the facet joint is degenerate with loss of articular cartilage space, a low-grade spondylolisthesis will result as the rostral vertebral disc slides anteriorly secondary to loss of cartilage space in the facet joint. A degenerated, collapsed disc may rupture and aggravate an already narrowed lateral recess and foraminal canal by virtue of direct effect of the herniation or by further collapse of the disc height and increased bulging of the disc. The combined effect of the hypertrophied superior articular process and collapsed disc causes impingement on the exiting nerve root, foraminal stenosis, and lateral recess narrowing. The combined effect of bulging or herniated disc and hypertrophy of the inferior articular process is stenosis of the central canal.

LIGAMENTUM FLAVUM

The thickness of normal ligamentum flavum is variable, and its absolute thickness may not be an indication of abnormality as long as there is no encroachment on the spinal canal. Haig et al.[63] concluded that although the ligamentum flavum appears to get thicker with age, other factors, including clinical diagnosis, pain, and function, do not appear to relate to the ligamentum flavum width. On the other hand, a collapsed motion segment usually associated with hypertrophied inferior articular process may lead to pathologic thickening and infolding of the ligamentum flavum. This will cause trefoil deformity of the lateral walls of the spinal canal on axial magnetic resonance imaging (MRI) view. The symptomatic aspect of this finding definitely needs to be defined as one contemplates treatment options.

SPINAL CANAL

In cross section, the spinal canal may appear as circular, ovoid, or triangular. The average lumbar central canal has a midsagittal diameter (anteroposterior [AP]) greater than 13 mm, with an area of 1.45 cm^2. Relative stenosis is said to exist when the AP canal diameter measures between 10 and 13 mm. Absolute stenosis of the lumbar canal exists anatomically when the AP measurement is 10 mm or less.[64] The spinal canal is divided into the central canal and lateral recesses. The lateral recess has an average AP width of 5 mm. A width of less than 3 to 4 mm is considered stenotic. The impingement on the nerve root in this area is usually by posterolateral disc herniation or facet hypertrophy.[65] The encroachment on the spinal canal space by the structures in its walls leads to neurologic signs and symptoms. Disc herniation, depending on its magnitude and location, may cause compression on a specific nerve route or the cauda equina itself. The hypertrophied and subluxed facet joint, hypertrophied ligamentum flavum, and malalignment of the spinal motion segment may contribute, individually or in combination, to the narrowing of the spinal canal and entrapment of the nerves. These anatomic abnormalities have to be addressed in addition to removal of herniated disc to ensure a satisfactory surgical outcome.

INTERVERTEBRAL FORAMEN

The foraminal canal is divided into three regions: the entrance (medially), foraminal canal, and extraforaminal area (laterally). The foraminal boundaries (see **Fig. 93-2**) are: anteriorly, the rostral vertebral body, intervertebral disc (IVD), and caudal vertebral body; posteriorly, the pars interarticularis, superior articular processes, joint capsule and

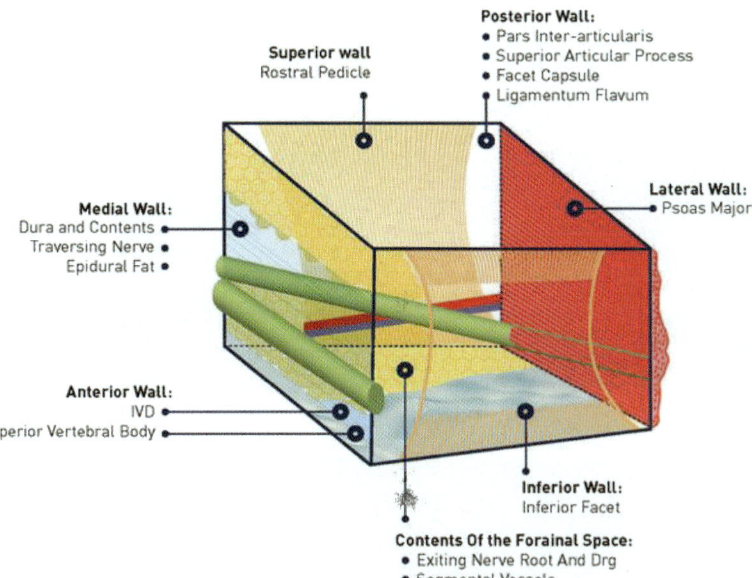

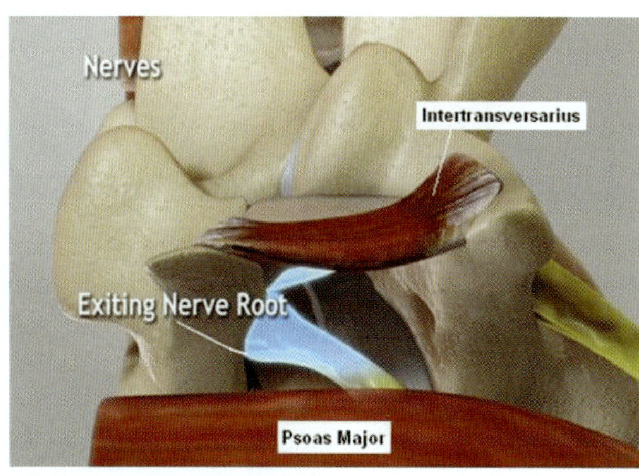

FIGURE 93-2. Boundaries of the lumbar foraminal space.

ligamentum flavum, and intertransverse ligaments and muscles; superiorly, the rostral pedicle; inferiorly, the caudal pedicle; medially, the dura and traversing nerve; and laterally, the psoas major muscle. In the lumbar spine, the intervertebral foramen (IVF) is in the shape of an inverted tear drop, being widest superiorly and narrowest inferiorly. The heights of the normal lumbar IVF range 17.73 to 24.43 mm, and the AP diameters in the mid- and superior portions of the IVF may vary from 1.64 to 11.6 mm.[66] The AP narrowing is the least tolerated by the exiting nerve whose dimensions may approximate the AP diameter of the foramen.

NEURAL STRUCTURES

In an adult lumbar spine, the spinal cord terminates at the conus medullaris, usually at the level at the level of L1 vertebra. The cauda equina, made up of the lumbar and sacral nerve roots, emerges from the spinal cord giving off a pair of nerve roots at each spinal level. The nerve roots emerge from the dural sac about one level cephalad to their exit levels. The outpocketing of the pia, arachnoid, and dura matter that encase the nerve root as it emerges from the cauda equine form the nerve root canal. This sheath blends with the epineurium of the nerve as it exits from the foraminal canal. The traversing nerve travels caudally and laterally, crossing over the dorsum of the disc and anterior to the superior articular process in the lateral recess. In this location, the nerve is at risk of impingement by the herniated disc or hypertrophied superior articular process and the attached capsule and ligaments. The dorsal and ventral nerve roots of the exiting nerve enter the foraminal canal 1.5 mm caudal to the superior pedicle and 5.3 mm cephalad to the inferior pedicle. The dura is, on average, 1.5 mm medial to the pedicle.[67] The roots fuse within the foramen or in the subarticular space and exit the foramen as a spinal nerve. The dorsal root ganglion (DRG) may be in the lateral recess, within the foramen, or within the extraforaminal space.[68] In the foraminal canal or extraforaminal location, there is an increased risk of pressure on the DRG during transforaminal endoscopic surgery, especially when the foraminal space is collapsed, leading to distressing postoperative dysesthesia. In a cadaver study, Osman and Marsolais[69] determined that the distance from the superior margin of annulotomy site to the inferior edge of the exiting nerve was 2 to 3 mm.

PATHOPHYSIOLOGY OF SPINAL AND RADICULAR PAIN

The roles played by mechanical compression[70,71] and biochemical irritation[72,73] in pain generation must be appreciated by the treating surgeon to intervene effectively. Chemical irritation by tumor necrosis factor released by disc chondrocytes and upregulated by the local Schwann cells and endoneurial cells[74] along with other cytokines such as interleukin-6 play a major role in the generation of sciatic pain even without physical compression by the herniated disc nucleus. In a human and animal study, Smyth and Wright[75] showed that pure compression of nonirritated nerve produced motor and sensory deficit but no radicular pain. These findings support the fact that other factors aside from mechanical compression contribute to pain.

ENDOSCOPIC SURGICAL ANATOMY

MORPHOLOGY AND TOPOGRAPHY OF THE DISC LESION

The most frequently practiced endoscopic discectomy techniques are transforaminal and interlaminar approaches. Recently, Osman et al. have introduced the transiliac approach.[76,77] Because of variation in patient characteristics, level of disc herniation, foraminal anatomy, herniation topography and morphology, choosing the appropriate approach and location for portal entry is critical to optimally address the pathology. For this reason the authors have, as part of a new treatment-based classification, modified the current classification of the disc morphology and topography as follows: Morphologically, the disc may be classified as an intraannular or extraannular tear of an otherwise normal looking disc (T1 and T2, respectively) or an intraannular or extraannular tear of a degenerated disc (T4 and T5) and globally bulging degenerated disc (T3) as seen on the MRI images (**Fig. 93-3**). The herniated free fragment is further classified as retroannular (directly posterior to the torn annulus), rostral displacement, caudal displacement, retrodural displacement (displaced posterior to the dural sac), or foraminal displacement.

Topographically, the disc lesion is classified as central (L1 = midline herniation), paracentral-predural (L2 = extending from midline to one side or the other), paracentral-axillary (L3 = between dura and traversing nerve), preradicular (L4 = ventral to the traversing nerve), or intra- or extraforaminal (L5 = in or outside the foramen). In the axillary location, the surgeon may find it prudent to approach translaminarly or transforaminally and transdiscally, but a transforaminal, transepidural approach can adequately expose the herniation, although manipulation of the laterally placed traversing nerve may be necessary. A preradicular disc herniation lies directly ventral to the traversing nerve often stretching it and causing the nerve to be draped over the herniation. A transforaminal approach tends to be the most appropriate for this type of abnormality as well as intra- and extradural herniations (**Fig. 93-4**).

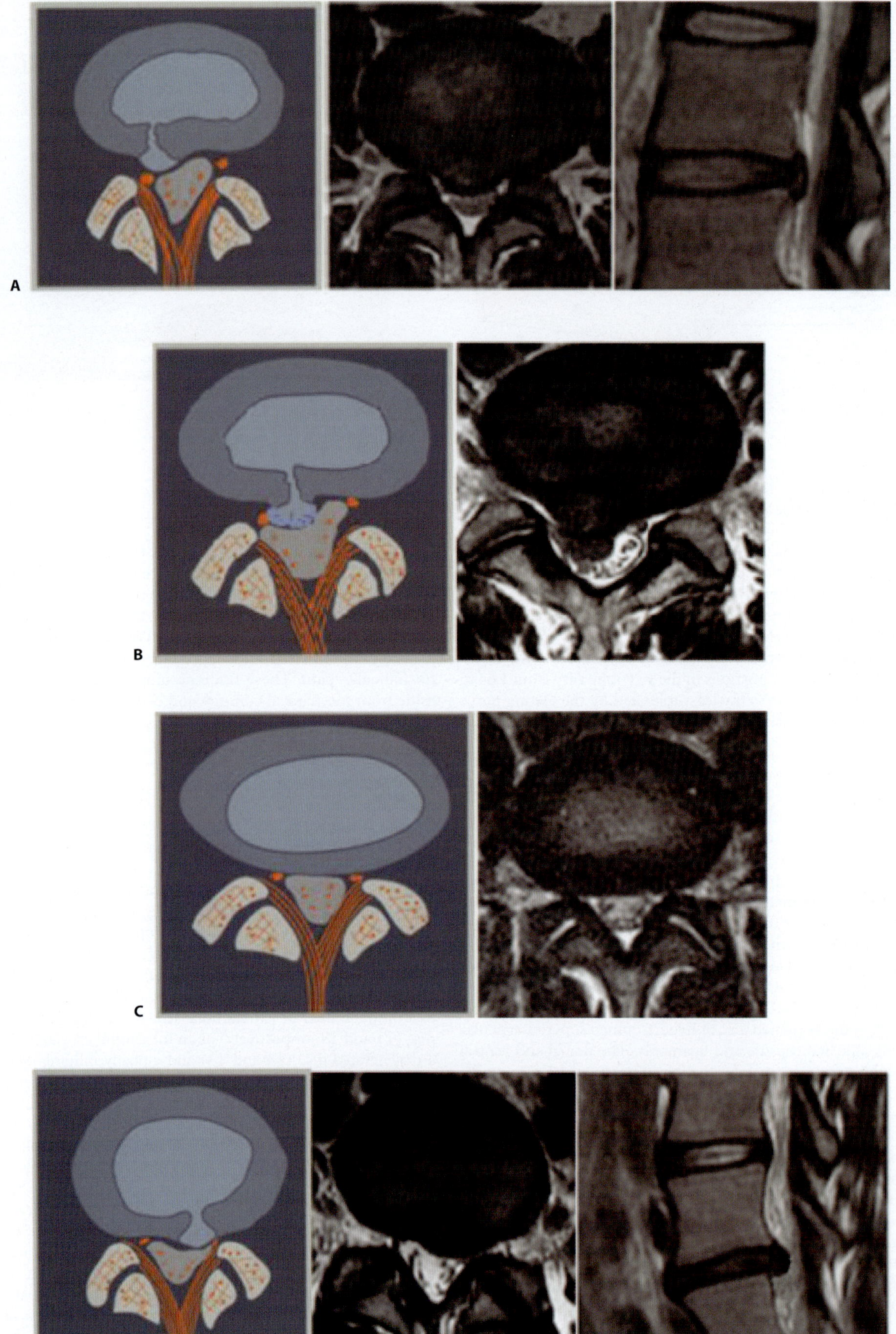

FIGURE 93-3. (**A**) Acute intraannular tear (T1). (**B**) Acute extraannular tear (T2). (**C**) Global disc bulge (T3). (**D**) Intraannular herniation, degenerated disc (T4) (*continues*).

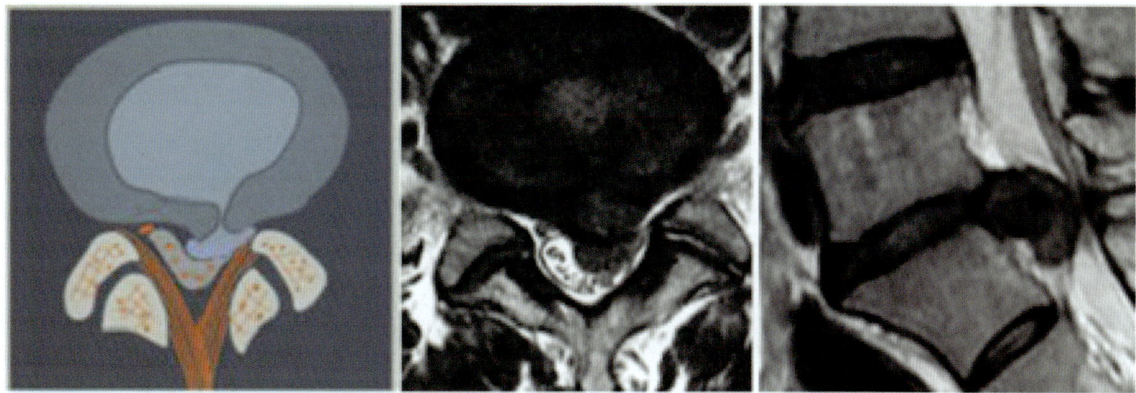

FIGURE 93-3. *Continued.* (**E**) Extraannular herniation, degenerated disc (T5).

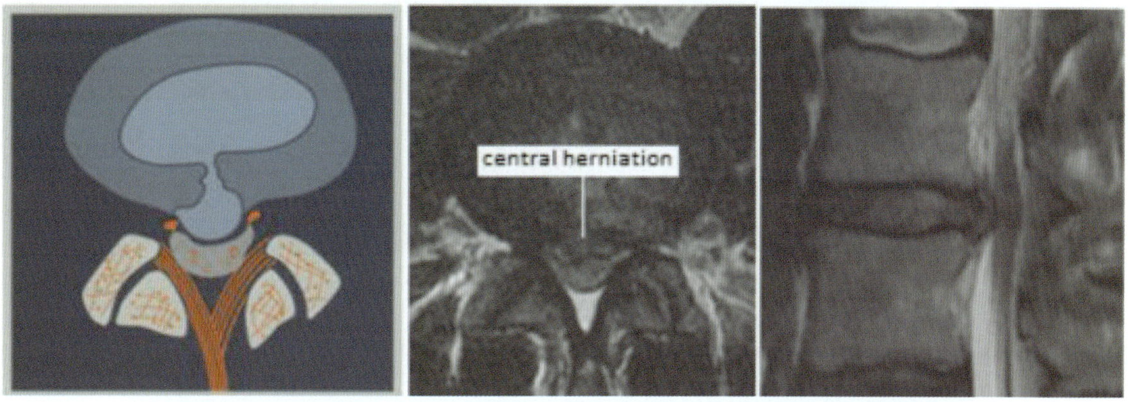

A

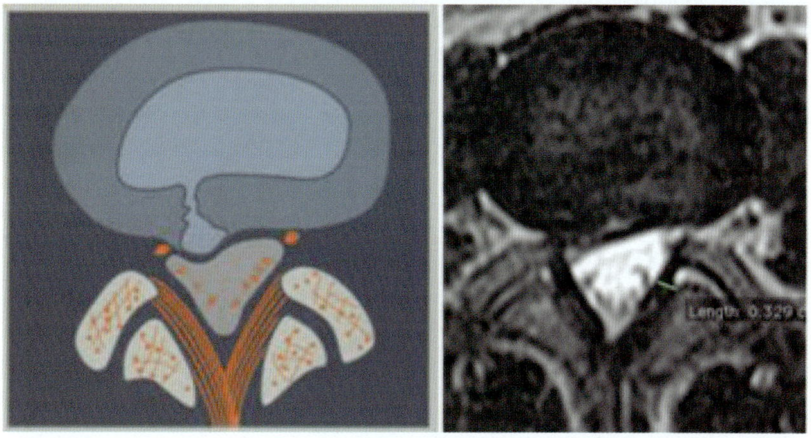

central herniation

B

Traversing nerve

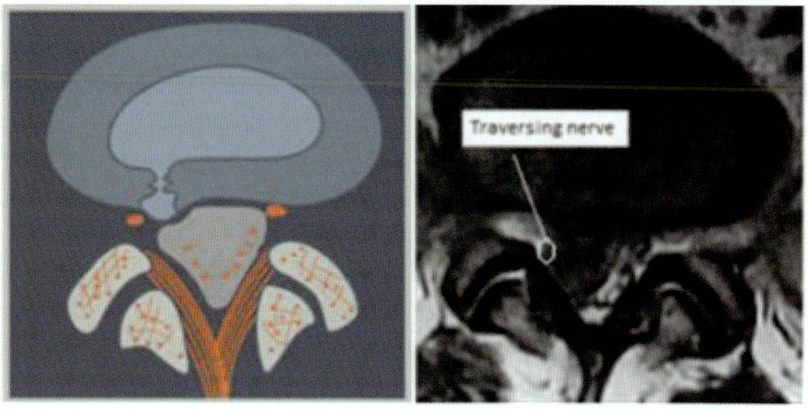

C

FIGURE 93-4. (**A**) Central herniation (L1). (**B**) Paracentral, predural herniation (L2). (**C**) Paracentral, axillary herniation (L3) (*continues*).

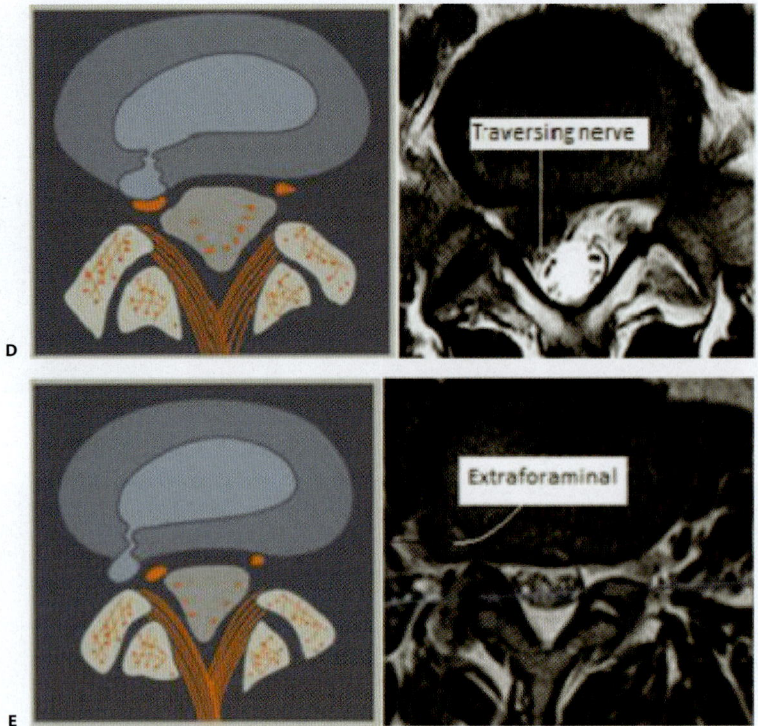

FIGURE 93-4. *Continued.* **(D)** Paracentral, preradicular herniation (L4). **(E)** Intra- or extraforaminal herniation (L5).

The percutaneous transforaminal access channel traverses several tissue layers before it reaches the intervertebral disc. Because the surgeon does not see the traversed structures, it is imperative for the beginner to have sound anatomic knowledge of the area to avoid injuries to the paraspinal as well as intraspinal structures. **Figure 93-5** illustrates structures traversed:

1. Skin and subcutaneous tissue: There are venous channels that may cause troublesome bleeding if perforated.
2. Thoracolumbar fascia: This is fibrous and invests the paraspinal muscles. After passage of instruments through the skin, resistance is encountered as this fascia is penetrated.

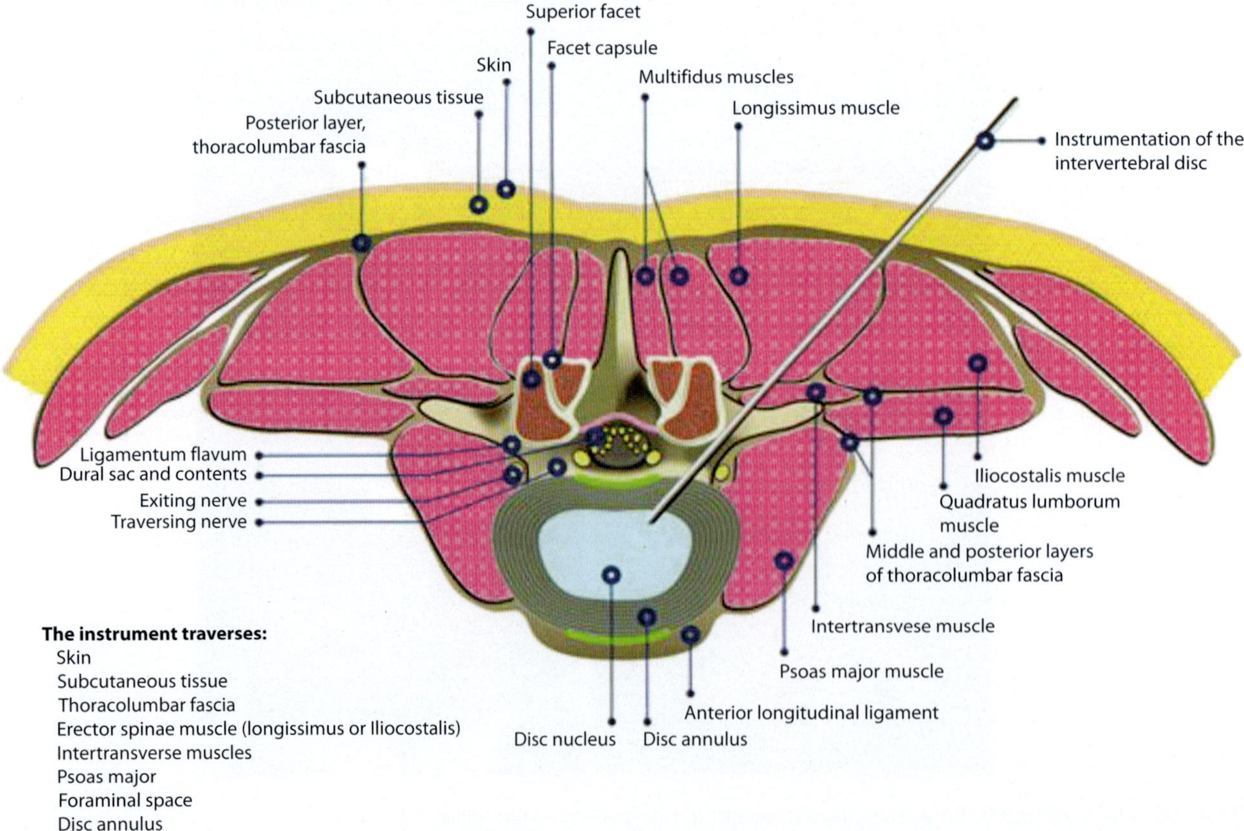

FIGURE 93-5. Anatomic relationship of the percutaneous transforaminal portal.

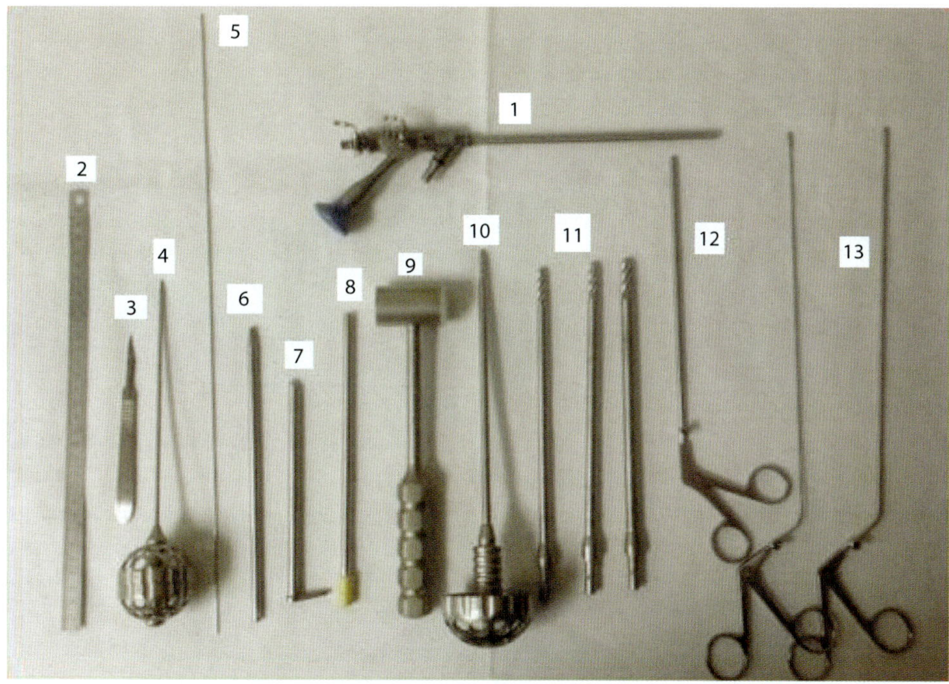

FIGURE 93-6. 1, Endoscope; 2, ruler; 3, #11 scalpel; 4, TOMsShidi® needle; 5, guidewire; 6, obturator (dilator); 7, cannula; 8, trephine; 9, mallet; 10, reamer on a handle; 11, reamers; 12, pituitary rongeurs; and 13, endoscopic pituitary rongeurs.

3. Latissimus dorsi in the lower lumbar region (L4 to the sacrum): The instruments are likely to pass through the aponeurosis of the latissimus dorsi. But from L3 cephalad, the instruments would most likely traverse muscle fibers running obliquely cephalad and laterally.
4. Serratus posterior inferior (SPI): Between L3 and T11 deep to the latissimus dorsi, the SPI runs obliquely cephalad and lateral to insert into the lower four ribs.
5. Erector spinae: Deep to the SPI and the latissimus dorsi lie the erector spinae muscles consisting of the spinalis, longissimus, and iliocostalis lumborum. Most posterolateral approaches would traverse either the longissimus or the iliocostalis
6. Intertransverse muscles: The instrument would then pass through the deep layer of the thoracolumbar fascia and the intertransverse muscles and intertransverse ligament as it enters the foraminal space.
7. Foraminal canal: When done properly the disc annulus is contacted between the exiting nerve laterally, traversing nerve medially, and the margin of the caudal vertebral body.

TRANSFORAMINAL INSTRUMENTATION

There are many manufacturers of endoscopic instruments. Although most of the instruments are very similar, they do offer different cutting options, including reamers and drills. Reamers and drills are used to shave down osteophyte complex and remove hypertrophic superior articular process to decompress the lateral recess as well as work within the disc. **Figure 93-6** is a sample set of instruments for transforaminal endoscopy.

TRANSFORAMINAL INSTRUMENTATION TRAJECTORY

The foraminal space is bordered by the rostral and caudal pedicles superiorly and inferiorly; medially by the traversing nerve, dura, and epidural fat; laterally by the psoas major; dorsally by the pars interarticularis, superior articular process, facet capsule, and ligamentum flavum; and ventrally, the foramen is bordered by the rostral vertebral body, intervertebral disc, and superior aspect of the caudal vertebral body (see Fig. 93-2).

The distance of the portal site from midline and the angle of instrument insertion into the foraminal space are determined based on the patient's body habitus, the location of the disc herniation, and the pathoanatomy of the facet joint. The objective is to instrument Kambin's triangle without injuring the traversing nerve, the exiting nerve, and the posterosuperior margin of the caudal vertebral body. Osman et al.'s publication on a cadaver study gives some guideline for the instrumentation.[76]

Instrumentation at 40 to 65 degrees from the vertical (sagittal plane) at the appropriate portal site would bring the instruments to the posterolateral annulus safely within the Kambin's triangular working space within the lower lumbar region for the majority of patients (**Fig. 93-7**).

Approximating the coronal plane (**Fig. 93-8**): Insertion of the instruments at an angle (to the sagittal plane) larger than 65 degrees risks penetration medially into the epidural space and possibly injuring the dura or the traversing nerve (or both). This trajectory is necessary for excision of the more central disc herniation, but the surgeon needs to exercise extreme care.

Approximating the sagittal plane (see Fig. 93-1): The safe angle of insertion into the disc varies with the motion segment. A cadaver study revealed that at an angle less than 45-degree to the sagittal plane of the spine, there is an increased likelihood that the instrument will miss the triangular zone and hit the disc lateral to or through the exiting nerve.

KAMBIN'S TRIANGLE

DISTANCES OF NEURAL ELEMENTS FROM THE TRANSFORAMINAL ANNULOTOMY

In a cadaver study conducted by Osman et al,[76] the distance of the traversing nerve to the medial edge of the midinterpedicular annulotomy ranged from 9 to 14 mm. The superior edge of annulotomy to the exiting nerve ranged from 2 to 3 mm (**Fig. 93-9**).

CLINICAL PICTURE

Surgery for lumbar disc disease may involve discectomy alone, discectomy with some degree of facetectomy, decompression and fusion, or decompression and dynamic stabilization. The choice of surgical

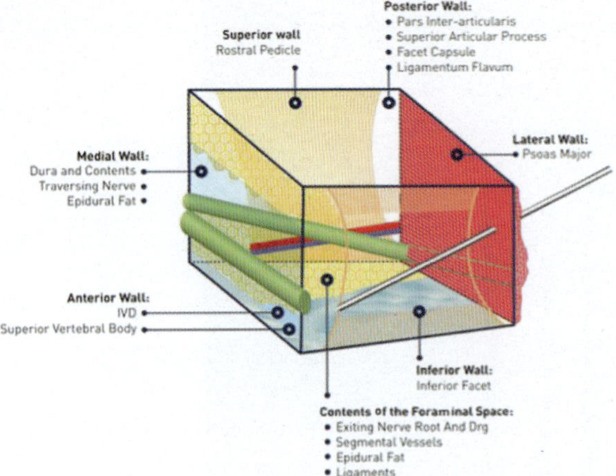

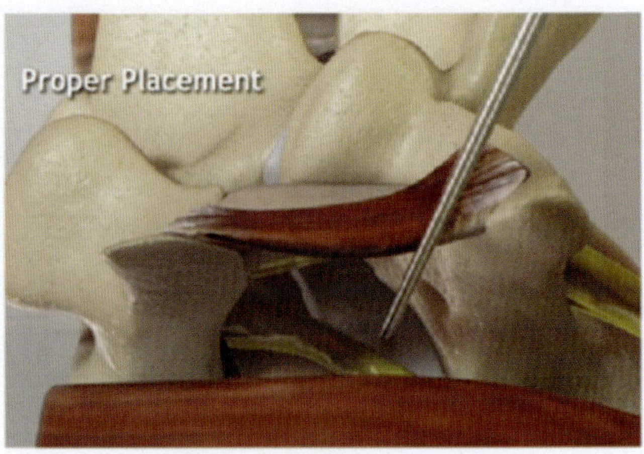

FIGURE 93-7. Transforaminal instrumentation at a 40- to 65-degree angle to the sagittal plane, in the disc plane, will likely safely enter the Kambin working space without risk on neural injury.

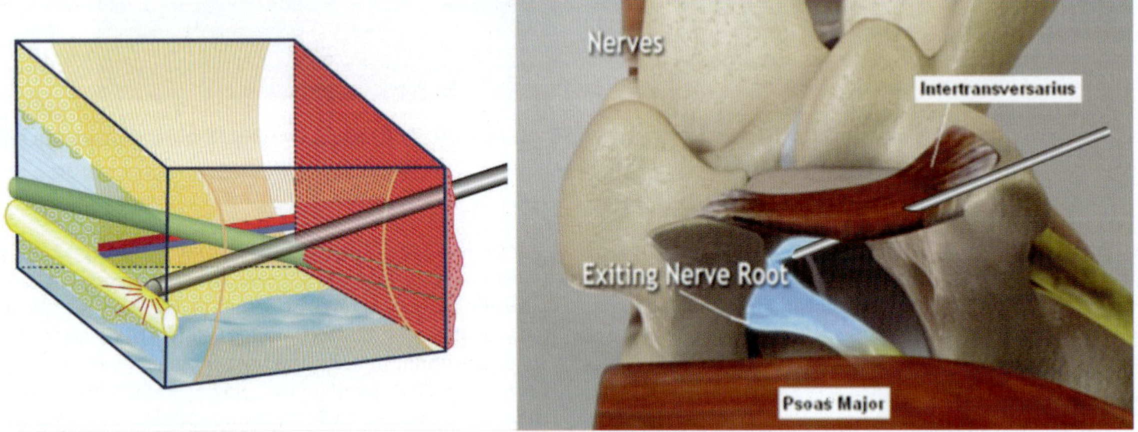

FIGURE 93-8. More than 65-degree angle to the sagittal plane may risk injury to the traversing nerve.

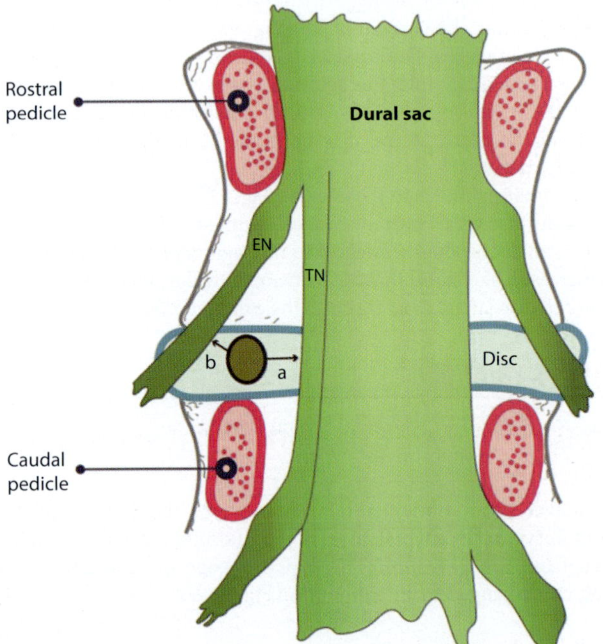

FIGURE 93-9. The distance from the annulotomy to the lateral edge of the traversing nerve (a) ranged 9 to 14 mm. Annulotomy to the traversing caudal edge of the exiting nerve (b) ranged between to 2 to 3 mm. EN = exiting nerve; TN = traversing nerve.

intervention depends on the symptoms and signs relating to the spine, imaging studies, and other attributes of the patient. In the simplest form, a young, healthy individual with no previous history of spinal problem presents with acute onset of back pain with radiation into a lower extremity after bending and lifting. The radicular symptoms include sharp and shooting pain; numbness and paresthesia in a specific dermatome; and some degree of weakness in appropriate myotomes, with or without associated deep tendon reflex deficit. When the disc is the only pain generator, sitting aggravates both the back and radicular pain. In this situation, the imaging studies such as MRI often show an otherwise normal spine, with well-defined rupture of an intervertebral disc. The clinical picture becomes more complicated in an older individual with long-standing history of back and leg pain, weakness, and lack of relief in any given position. Objective findings are indicative of complex motion segment disease, and the images may show disc rupture in the setting of degeneration, hypertrophic facet degeneration, alignment abnormality, and hypertrophy of the ligamentum flavum, compromising the spinal canal. Such complex spinal pathology may be in the setting of a patient who has other comorbidities that preclude certain or all surgical interventions. Therefore, it is imperative that the surgeon evaluates all of these factors with appropriate tools, including neurophysiologic studies, diagnostic and therapeutic injections, and laboratory studies, to exclude other pathologic entities.

TREATMENT OPTIONS

After the diagnosis of disc rupture has been made, the first approach should be conservative measures since a large number of these cases resolve without surgical intervention.[77,78] Activity modifications, oral pain medications, oral steroids, therapeutic injections, and physical therapy must be given adequate time to work. However, in a rare case of severe motor deficit or cauda equina syndrome, an early surgical intervention is mandated.

SURGICAL OPTIONS

In the majority of cases, discectomy is the appropriate surgery for a herniated disc when nonoperative measures have failed. More importantly, when comorbid conditions exist, debilitating disc herniations must be addressed to avoid further aggravation of concurrent conditions that may be destabilizing the patient but without compromising other spine motion segments.[79]

STRATEGIC PLANNING FOR ENDOSCOPIC APPROACHES

Based on the clinical findings and the classification described earlier, the endoscopic approach to the herniation is planned as laid out in **Table 93-1**. Most types of disc herniations can be accessed and removed through an endoscopic transforaminal approach. The location and angle of instrumentation depend on the topography and morphology of the herniation. If the disc is the only diseased structure, the portal location tends to be closer to the midline of the spine and the angle of instrumentation closer to the sagittal plane for herniations in the lateral recess and foraminal space. A central herniation and those associated with facet hypertrophy require portal placement farther away from the midline and at an angle approaching the coronal plane for transepidural approach to the disc lesion and foraminoplasty, respectively.

In axillary disc herniation, retrodurally migrated free fragment, and some cases of caudally or rostrally migrated herniations, an endoscopic interlaminar approach may be the best approach to address the pathology while avoiding neural injury. At the L5 to S1 level, most lateral recess and intra- or extraforaminal herniations are accessible through an endoscopic transforaminal approach; however, for patients with deep-seated L5 to S1 disc herniations, the standard transmuscular (suprailiac) approach may not be able to access the lesion. In this situation, a properly placed portal and the appropriate angular trajectory will place the

TABLE 93-1 Surgical Strategies for Lumbar Disc Herniation

Type of Herniation	Grade	Surgical Strategy
Intraannular Herniation	T1, T4	Strategy is to remove the protruding nucleus and preserve the remaining disc with as little additional damage as possible, preferably using an endoscopic approach.
1. Central	L1	1. Endoscopic transforaminal approach, far posterolateral portal in the disc equator, shallow insertion angle (approaching coronal plane) 2. Disc instrumentation at medial interpedicular line 3. Intradiscal approach for contained herniation; transepidural approach, if preferred 4. May need foraminoplasty to facilitate central instrumentation 5. Endoscopic transiliac approach for L5–S1 segment
2. Paracentral		
a. Predural	L2	1. Endoscopic transforaminal: far/medium posterolateral, in the disc equator, instrument disc at mid-interpedicular line 2. Disc instrumentation at medial interpedicular line 3. Intradiscal approach for contained herniation; transepidural approach if preferred 4. May need foraminoplasty to facilitate central instrumentation 5. Endoscopic transiliac approach for L5–S1 segment
b. Axillary	L3	1. Endoscopic interlaminar versus endoscopic posterolateral: medium posterolateral 2. Midinterpedicular disc instrumentation 3. Intradiscal or transepidural approach 4. Endoscopic transiliac: at L5–S1 level with tall iliac wing
c. Preradicular	L4	1. Endoscopic transforaminal: medium posterolateral portal 2. Midinterpedicular disc instrumentation 3. Intradiscal approach 4. Identify and protect the traversing nerve 5. Endoscopic transiliac: at L5–S1 level with tall iliac wing
3. Intra- or extraforaminal	L5	1. Endoscopic interlaminar approach: uniportal vs. ipsilateral biportal 2. Medium to near posterolateral portal 3. Midinterpedicular discoscopy through hernial summit. *Watch out for the exiting nerve for extraforaminal. Best handled with double-portal, unilateral approach.* 4. Endoscopic transiliac: at L5–S1 level with tall iliac wing
Extraannular Herniation	T2, T5	The strategy is to remove the free fragment through endoscopic transforaminal epiduroscopy or endoscopic interlaminar and to avoid additional trauma to the disc.
1. Retroannular	RA	1. Endoscopic transforaminal: far posterolateral portal in disc equator 2. Medial interpedicular disc instrumentation if needed; transepidural approach preferred 3. Will need foraminoplasty with superior articular process (SAP) shaving 4. Transiliac for L5–S1
2. Caudal displacement	CD	1. Endoscopic interlaminar vs endoscopic transforaminal: far-, medium-posterolateral portal 2. Caudad trajectory; may need to shave off the SAP and the upper edge of the caudal pedicle 3. Transepidural, transdiscal approach 4. Rigid vs. flexible endoscope for transforaminal 5. Endoscopic transiliac approach at L5–S1 may be necessary
3. Rostral displacement	RD	1. Endoscopic interlaminar approach: ipsilateral biportal 2. Endoscopic transforaminal (rigid endoscope): far lateral portal, cephalad trajectory, transepidural or transdiscal, retract nerve root 3. Endoscopic transforaminal approach (flexible endoscope): medium posterolateral portal; transepidural technique 4. Will need foraminoplasty (lateral partial facetectomy) 5. Flexible endoscopy
4. Dorsal (retrodural) displacement	DRD	1. Endoscopic interlaminar approach: ipsilateral biportal 2. Endoscopic transforaminal: far posterolateral portal in disc equator; most likely will need foraminoplasty with superior articular process (SAP) shaving, transepidural approach 3. Endoscopic transiliac approach at L5–S1 may be necessary
5. Extra- or intraforaminal displacement	FD	1. Endoscopic transforaminal: medium/near lateral portal. Lateral interpedicular line; watch out for the exiting nerve. 2. Uni-, biportal, unilateral approach 3. Endoscopic transiliac approach at L5–S1 may be necessary

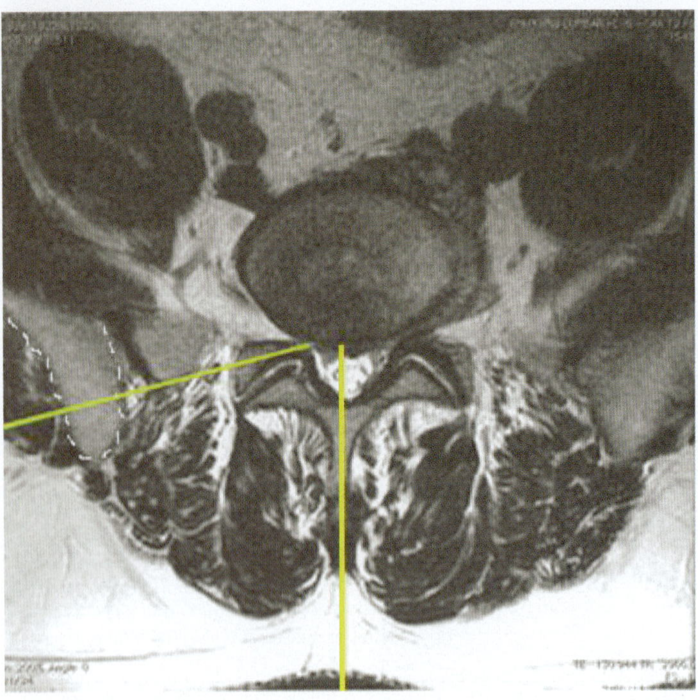

FIGURE 93-10. Preoperative determination of the posterolateral portal site and angle of instrumentation of the disc.

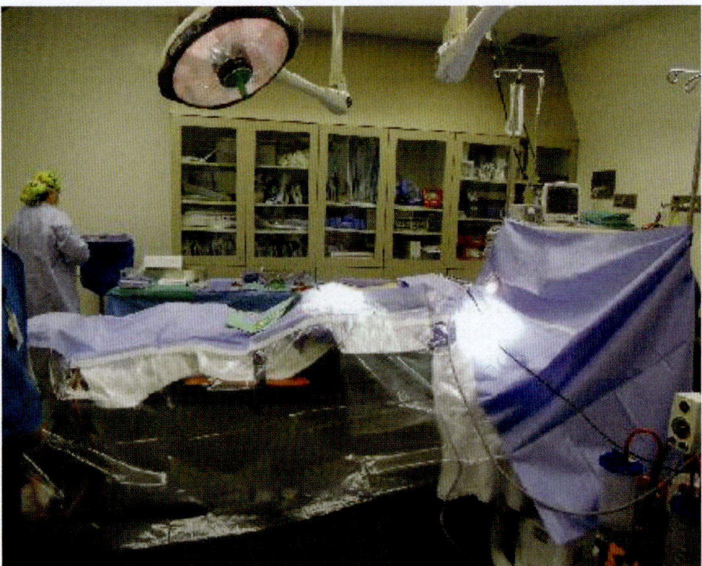

FIGURE 93-11. The patient in prone position on a Kambin Frame. The transparent sides of the surgical drape permit visualization of the foot pedals on the floor in lateral position of the fluoroscope.

iliac wing in the path of the disc instrumentation. Furthermore, even in cases of normal iliac anatomy, a more central disc herniation and facet hypertrophy or foraminal stenosis may prevent instrumentation and impede access to the disc pathology. To access the disc herniations in this situation, a transiliac approach is appropriate.[76,77]

Preoperative planning of the transforaminal approach includes the determination of the portal location and the angle of instrumentation to reach the disc herniation. Using the preoperative axial MRI slice through the disc equator, a line is drawn from the herniation, through the foramen, to exit through the skin. Another line is drawn from the midline of the disc to exit the skin posteriorly. The distance between the two lines at the skin and the angle subtended between them will be the distance of the portal from midline and the angle of instrumentation, respectively. At the L5 to S1 level, the line may traverse the iliac wing, in which case a transiliac window may be necessary (**Fig. 93-10**).

ENDOSCOPIC TRANSFORAMINAL LUMBAR DISCECTOMY

SURGICAL TECHNIQUE

The procedure is performed with the patient in a prone position on a Wilson or Kambin Frame on a radiolucent table under sedation and local anesthesia or, rarely, general anesthesia. Neuromonitoring is recommended and fluoroscopic guidance is essential. Disc instrumentation is performed through the Kambin's triangular working space. Surgery is aimed at relieving the neural compression.

After skin preparation, a transparent drape with wide aperture exposing the operative field is applied. The minimally invasive surgery transparent drape is used to enable the surgeon to visualize the fluoroscope as it is placed in lateral position and to be able to see foot pedals on the floor with the fluoroscope in a lateral position (**Fig. 93-11**).

A radiopaque marker is used to determine the midline of the spine with the fluoroscope in anteroposterior or Ferguson position. With the end plates bordering the disc parallel to each other and the anterior and posterior margins of each end plate superimposed on one another, the disc line is drawn at the equator of the disc. The portal site is marked at the preoperatively determined site, and after infiltrating the skin with 0.5% bupivacaine with epinephrine, a stab incision is made with a # 11 blade (**Fig. 93-12A**).

The presumed access track is infiltrated with 0.5% bupivacaine with epinephrine. If there is need for foraminoplasty, the periosteum of the superior articular process is infiltrated with a small amount of local anesthetic. An 18-gauge spinal needle is then inserted through the 8-mm stab incision made at portal site. Depending on the location of the disc lesion, the needle is aimed to contact the posterolateral annulus at mid- (for a lateral disc lesion) or medial-interpedicular line (for a more central disc lesion). The needle placement is controlled with biplanar fluoroscopy. When satisfactory intradiscal placement of the needle is confirmed, the stylet is removed, and the mixture of radiopaque dye mixed with Indigo Carmine is injected under fluoroscopic control. This is done to determine the distribution of the injectate in the disc as well as to stain the disc nucleus for excision at the endoscopy stage. Instrumentation with a guidewire, obturator, and cannula is then performed in sequential fashion (**Figs. 93-12B** and **93-13**).

Needle placement is a crucial step in the instrumentation of the disc through Kambin's triangle. For most intraannular disc herniations, the instrumentation should be at the mid- or medial interpedicular line (**Fig. 93-14**).

Needle placement medial to the medial interpedicular line may cause injury to the traversing nerve root (**Fig. 93-15**).

A more vertical instrumentation will risk injury to the exiting nerve laterally (**Fig. 93-16**).

If there is hypertrophy of the superior articular process (SAP) obstructing the path of instrumentation, partial lateral facetectomy (foraminoplasty) becomes necessary. The guidewire is docked into the SAP, and cannulated hand reamers are used to remove the hypertrophied bone under fluoroscopic control. Care is taken that the reamer does not advance beyond the medial interpedicular line on the AP view, and it should engage the superior articular process, as visualized on lateral view (**Fig. 93-17**). The reamer should be on the caudal half of the SAP at the disc level, and may be directed cephalad or caudad, depending on the migration of a free fragment herniation.

An automated bur may be used endoscopically with an operating endoscope or using a unilateral biportal endoscopic approach (**Fig. 93-18**).

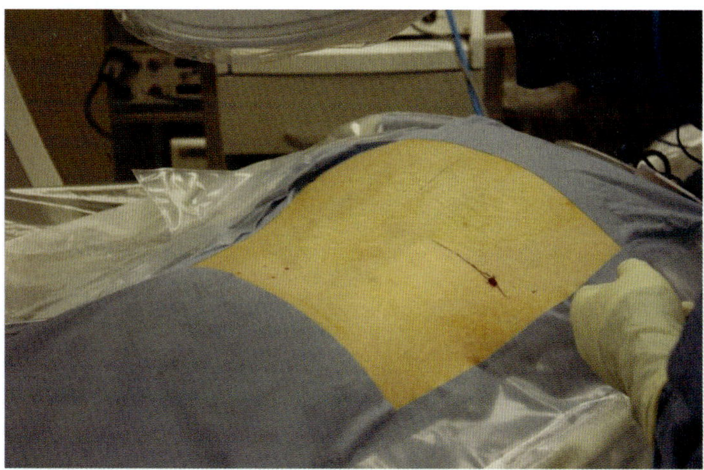

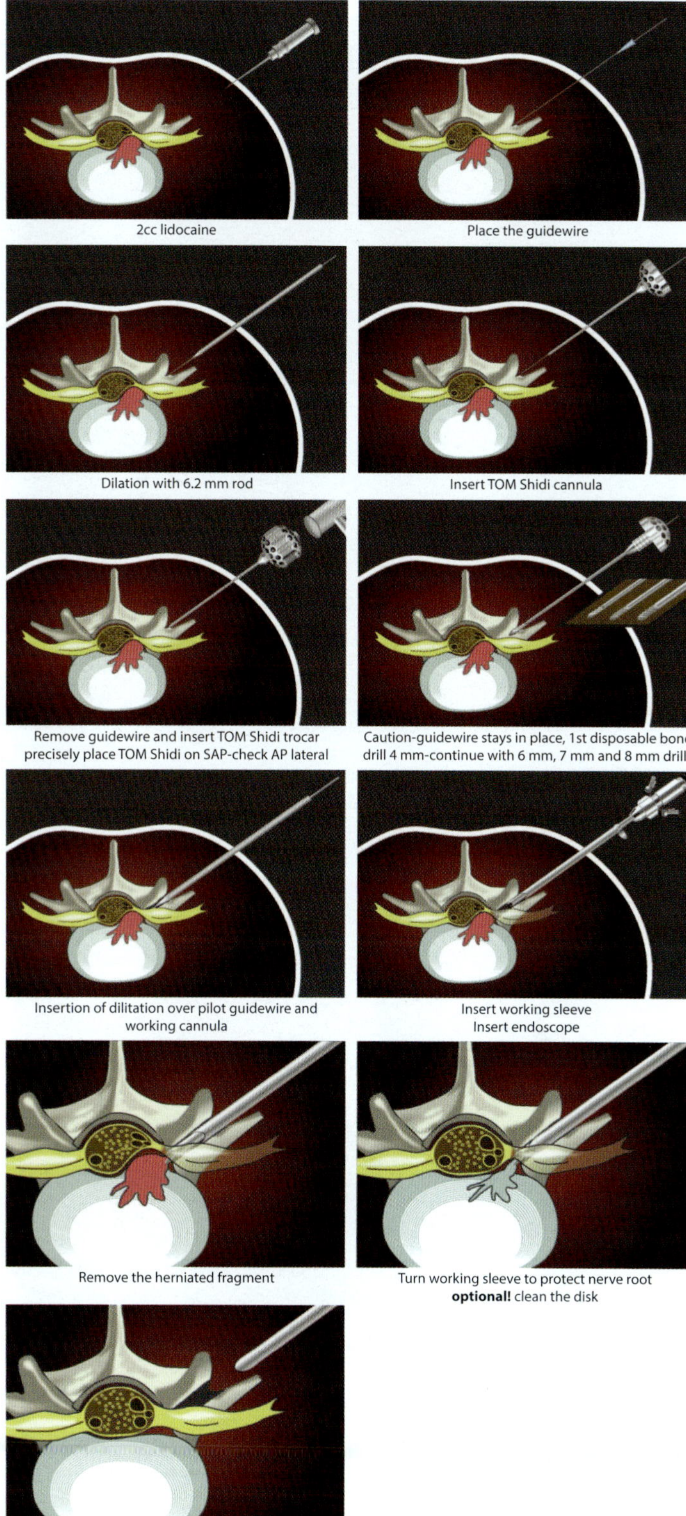

FIGURE 93-12A. Stab incision on the disc line on the left side of the spine.
FIGURE 93-12B (Right). Animation of the lumbar endoscopic discectomy procedure.

Osman et al.,[78] revealed that an increase in the foraminal area is significantly larger, and the spinal stability is not as affected after transforaminal decompression compared with conventional laminectomy, in which increased extension and axial rotation were produced.

For intraannular herniation requiring an intradiscal approach, the cannula is docked into the disc through or close to the herniation. A beveled cannula, with the bevel facing the epidural space, is preferred to ensure that the extruded nucleus, as shown by the blue staining, is completely removed. A trephine may be necessary if the annulus is calcified or hard to penetrate with the #4 Penfield probe. A plug of calcified annulus is then removed with a pituitary rongeur. The endoscope is then inserted and further discectomy is performed under the endoscopic visualization with pituitary forceps. Other tools, including a laser and radiofrequency probe, may be used to ablate annular fragments or calcified disc protrusion. At the conclusion of the discectomy, annuloplasty is performed with a radiofrequency probe to stabilize the annulotomy. The exiting and traversing nerve roots are visualized to ensure the adequacy of the decompression before the endoscope and cannula are withdrawn. The surgeon injects platelet-rich plasma into the disc and foraminal space for hemostasis and postoperative pain control.

For extraannular herniations with or without migration, a transepidural approach may be adequate. A far posterolateral portal is necessary, as is lateral partial facetectomy. The beveled cannula is inserted as described earlier, but for this approach, the cannula may not need docking into the disc. Epidural fat and vascular network may be encountered before the herniation is visualized. The fat and the vascular channels may be cauterized to expose the herniated disc. A flexible bipolar diathermy probe is ideal for this work. Pituitary rongeurs are used to remove the herniated material. Further loose nuclear material is removed from the disc interior as necessary. Care is taken to protect the neural structures and the dura during the excision of the disc. The long side of the cannula bevel may be rotated to shield the nerve root while the disc fragments are removed. Other tools, such as the Penfield #4 probe, may be used to manipulate the loose disc material while protecting the nerve root.

POSTOPERATIVE CARE

This is an outpatient procedure. Lumbar support is prescribed for the first couple of weeks, at which time comprehensive physical therapy is instituted.

ENDOSCOPIC TRANSILIAC APPROACH TO L5 TO S1 DISC AND FORAMEN

Surgical anatomy of the transiliac access channel (Fig. 93-19): The access portal traverses the skin, subcutaneous tissue, and gluteus maximus plus or minus the gluteus medius before contacting the iliac wing. The iliac window is 4.8 cm cephalad to the superior gluteal neurovascular bundle. The transiliac window is about 1.6 cm caudal to the iliac crest and 4.16-cm ventrolateral to the posterosuperior iliac spine. An appropriately placed track passes posterior to the sacral ala and sacroiliac joint. The track passes ventral to the iliolumbar ligament and cephalad to the superior articular process of S1.

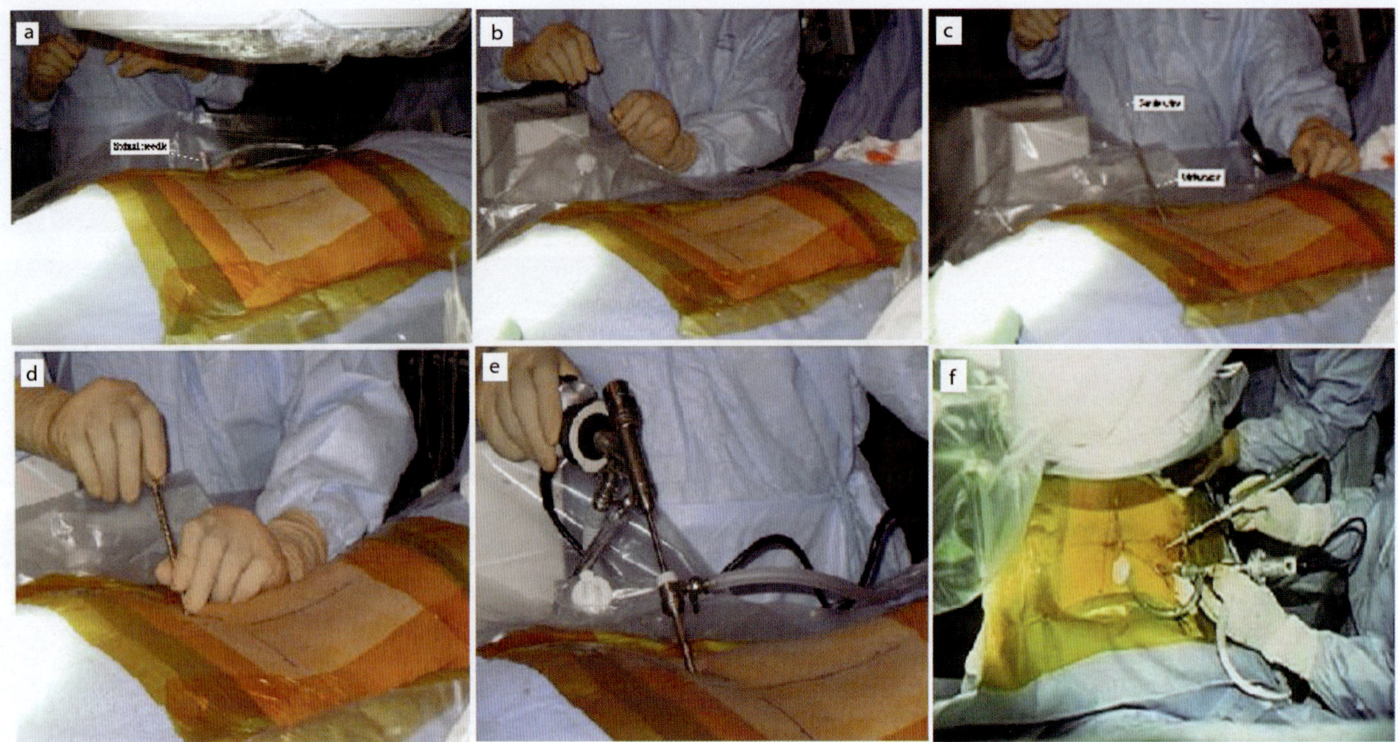

FIGURE 93-13. a, Placement of the spinal needle; b, guidewire insertion through the needle; c, insertion of the obturator over the guidewire after removal of the needle; d, insertion of the cannula over the obturator and the guidewire; e, insertion of the endoscope through the cannula after removal of the obturator and the guidewire; f, biportal, unilateral foraminal instrumentation.

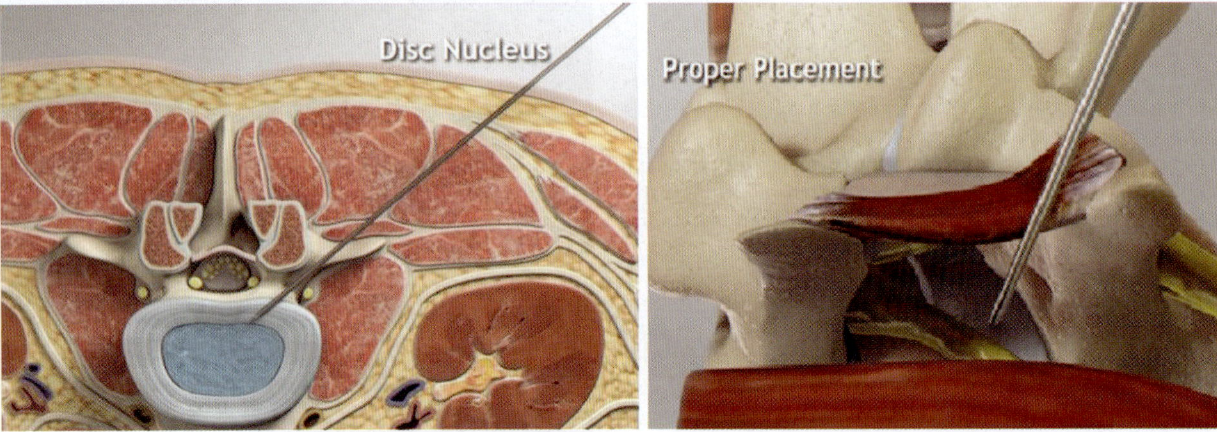

FIGURE 93-14. Proper disc instrumentation in Kambin's triangle.

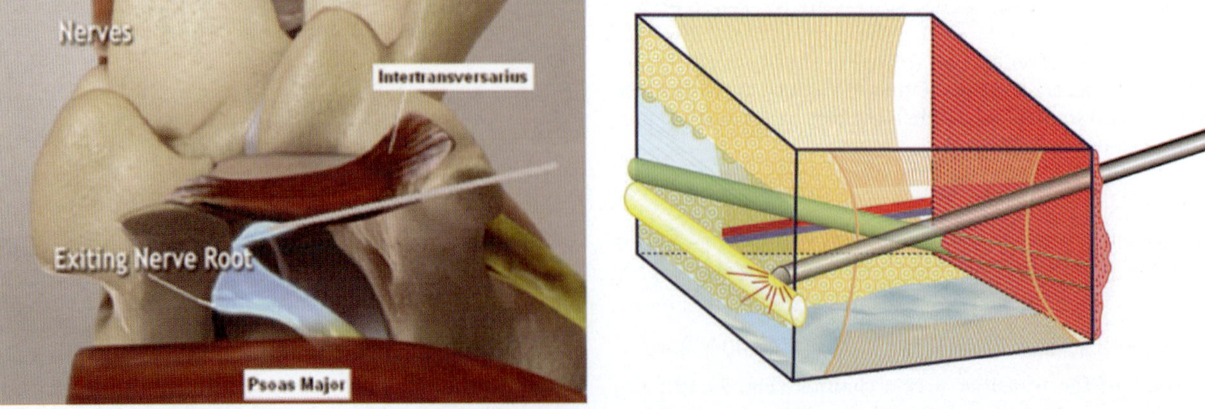

FIGURE 93-15. Medially placed instrumentation causing impingement on the traversing nerve root.

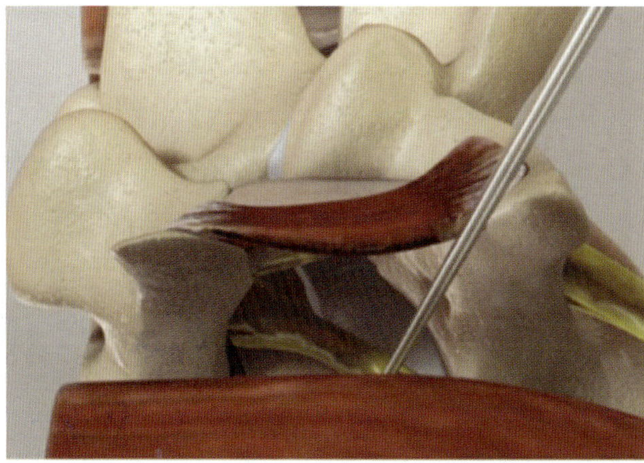

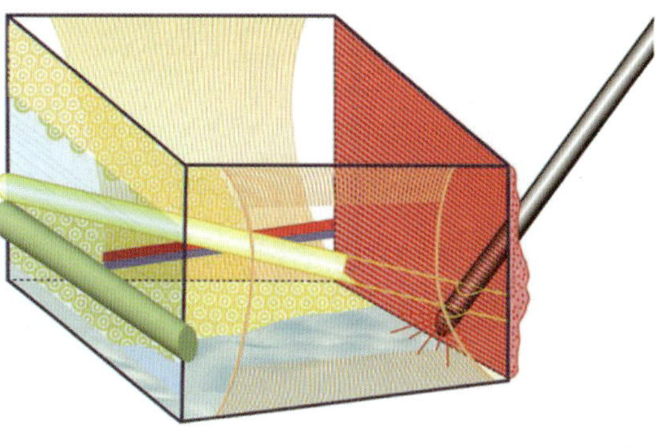

FIGURE 93-16. Laterally placed instrumentation causing impingement on the exiting nerve root.

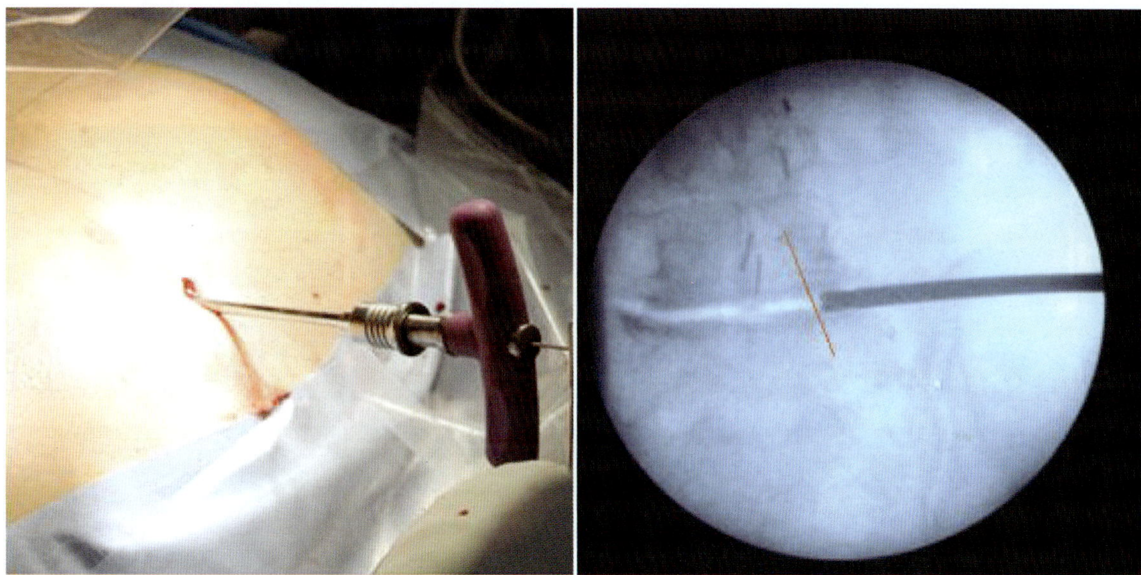

FIGURE 93-17. Foraminoplasty being performed with a manual reamer. The reamer should contact the disc annulus (on the lateral fluoroscopic view) laterally or at the medial interpedicular line as illustrated.

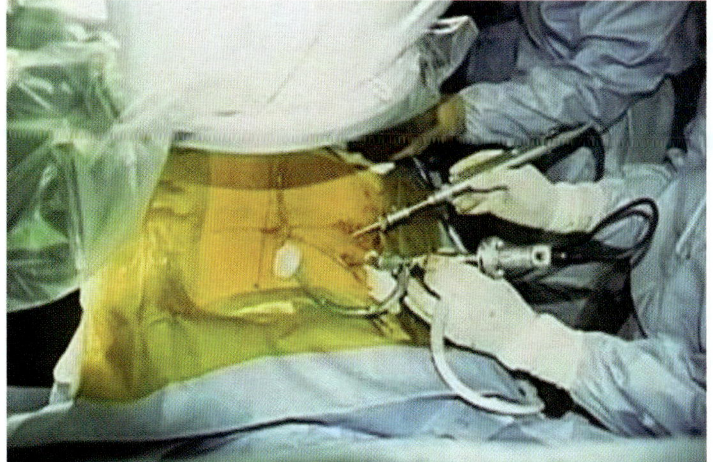

FIGURE 93-18. Unilateral biportal endoscopic foraminoscopy showing the endoscope in the left hand and the foraminoplasty bur in the right hand.

INDICATIONS FOR THE TRANSILIAC APPROACH

Indications for this approach include a high iliac wing, facet hypertrophy with foraminal stenosis, central or paracentral disc pathology, and the indications for endoscopic transforaminal approach described earlier.

PREOPERATIVE PLANNING

1. Determine the morphology and topography of the herniated disc—intra- or extraannular; central, paracentral, axillary, preradicular, or intra- or extraforaminal.
2. Determine the portal location and angle of instrumentation on the preoperative axial MRI slice of the target disc.
3. Based on the portal site and angle of instrumentation, determine if the track will be transiliac.

SURGICAL TECHNIQUE

1. Anesthesia: The procedure is usually done under monitored sedation and local anesthesia or, occasionally, under general endotracheal anesthesia.

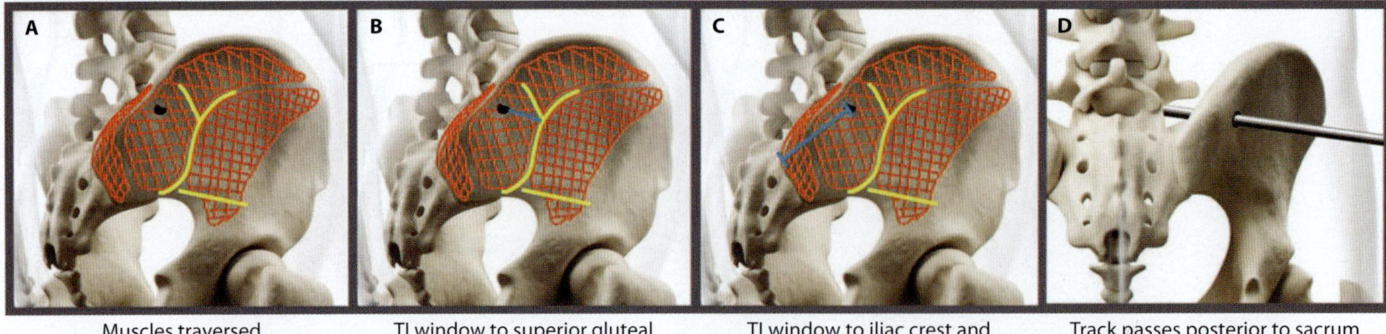

Muscles traversed | TI window to superior gluteal neurovascular bundle | TI window to iliac crest and PSIS | Track passes posterior to sacrum and rostral to SAP of S1

FIGURE 93-19. (**A**) Muscles traversed. (**B**) TI window to superior gluteal neurovascular bundle. (**C**) TI window to the iliac crest and posterior superior iliac spine. (**D**) The track passes posterior to the sacrum and rostral to the SAP of S1.

2. Neuromonitoring: This is used to monitor the integrity of the nerve roots in the vicinity of instrumentation.
3. A sequential compression device is attached for intraoperative prophylaxis of deep venous thrombosis.
4. Position on the operating table and draping are as described earlier for endoscopic transforaminal discectomy.
5. Under fluoroscopic control in Ferguson projection, the level of the disc is marked on the skin with the aid of radiopaque object. The L5 and S1 end plates must be parallel. The predetermined portal entrance is marked on the disc line (**Fig. 93-20A**).
6. The access track is infiltrated with local anesthetic (0.5% bupivacaine with epinephrine). A stab incision is made to create the portal (see **Fig. 93-20A**).

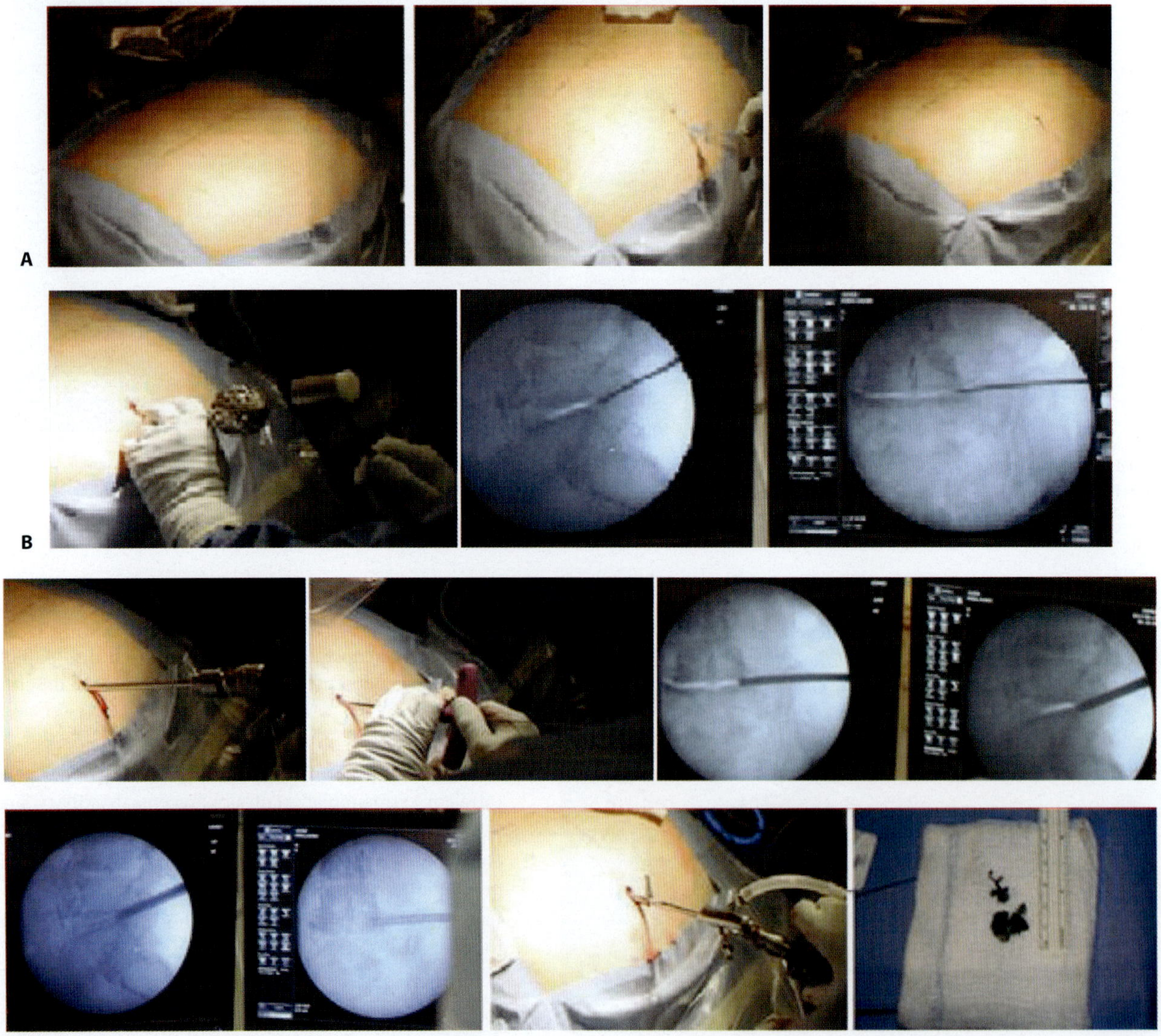

FIGURE 93-20. (**A**) Predetermined portal entrance marked on patients skin prior to incision. (**B**) Guidewire is powerdrilled through ileum, visualized in two different fluoroscopic views. (**C**) Bone core is removed with a cannulated trephine or cannulated power drill. (**D**) Instrumentation through the passage created in the ileum, and towards L5 or S1 intervertebral space. Last frame shows Indigo blue labeled fragments from the discectomy.

7. A TOM Shidi needle or guidewire on a power drill is driven through the ilium in the predetermined angle aiming for the target site in the L5 to S1 foramen on the disc or superior articular process (**Fig. 93-20B**). Biplanar fluoroscopy is used to introduce the guidewire to ensure the appropriate trajectory is maintained.
8. A cannulated power drill or cannulated trephine is used to remove a core of bone around the trans iliac guidewire (**Fig. 93-20C**). The core of bone so obtained with the trephine may be used as a graft.
9. After the transiliac window has been established, instrumentation proceeds as described earlier for lumbar endoscopic discectomy (**Fig. 93-20D**). A suprailiac portal may be established simultaneously for biportal endoscopy of the L5 to S1 endoscopy.

ENDOSCOPIC INTERLAMINAR APPROACH

a. Indications: These are similar to those mentioned earlier, including central canal stenosis, caudal, rostral, and retrodural displacement of herniated disc material.
b. Anatomy of interlaminar approach: The access portal traverses the skin, subcutaneous tissue, the thoracolumbar fascia and the multifidus muscles before it contacts the laminae and intervening ligamentum flavum. Laterally is the inferior process of the rostral vertebra and the facet capsule. Depending on the pathologic state, the laminae may overlap, and the ligamentum flavum may be hypertrophied. There may be hypertrophy of the inferior articular process with osteophytes as well. Deep to the ligamentum flavum, there may be a variable amount of epidural fat. The dura and underlying disc may be visualized by retracting the epidural fat and the dura respectively. Discectomy is performed under endoscopic visualization.
c. Treatment-based classification and preoperative strategy are as discussed earlier.
d. Surgical technique:
    1. Anesthesia: The procedure is usually done under monitored sedation and local anesthesia or occasionally, under general endotracheal anesthesia.
    2. Neuromonitoring: This is used to monitor the integrity of the nerve roots in the vicinity of instrumentation.
    3. A sequential compression device is attached for intraoperative prophylaxis of deep venous thrombosis.
    4. The patient is placed in a prone position on a Wilson or Kambin frame on a radiolucent table. Care is taken to minimize lordosis at the site of the herniation. Pressure points are checked and rendered safe.
    5. The skin is prepared, and draping is performed using a transparent drape with a pouch to house the fluoroscope in a lateral position. The transparent drape also allows the surgeon to see foot pedals, including diathermy and automated tools on the floor, especially when the fluoroscope is in the lateral position.
    6. The level of the disc is marked on the skin with the aid of a radiopaque marker. Two portal sites are marked on the skin. The instrumentation site is made at the disc line slightly to the side of the midline and cephalad to the arthroscope portal.
    7. After infiltrating the portal sites with local anesthetic, stab incisions are made and blunt ended dilators are inserted under fluoroscopic control triangulating on the interlaminar space over the ligamentum flavum. The cannulas are inserted over the dilators until the laminae and the ligamentum flavum are contacted. If beveled cannulas are used, the bevels are oriented such that the visualization of the instruments is maximized.
    8. The soft tissue over the interlaminar space is excised with shavers and or radiofrequency ablation to expose the ligamentum flavum.
    9. The spherical bur is used to perform medial facetectomy and remove the inferior edge of the rostral lamina to expose the lateral margin of the ligamentum flavum. Care is taken to avoid injury to underlying dura.
    10. The lateral ligamentum is excised with shavers and small Kerrison rongeurs (**Fig. 93-21A**). The cannulas are docked into the epidural space. The nerve root overlying the herniation may be mobilized with a modified nerve hook (**Fig. 93-21B**). After the nerve has been rendered safe, serial dilation of the annular fibers (in the case of intraannular herniation) with cone-tipped probes may be performed before pituitary rongeurs are inserted to remove the herniated material (**Fig. 93-21C**).
    11. When the ligamentum flavum is not hypertrophied and the motion segment is not collapsed, a single portal may be used for the operating arthroscope. In this situation, the portal is made at the level of the disc, and after the cannula is docked in to the interlaminar space as described, the soft tissue over the ligamentum is removed and laminotomy may be necessary. Blunt-tipped conical probes are used to separate the fibers of the ligamentum flavum until the obturator and the cannula are docked. From this point discectomy proceeds as described next.
    12. With the aid of the nerve root retractor, the traversing nerve is retracted medially to expose the disc.
    13. The disc annulus is incised with a series of conical probes if the herniation is intraannular, and the pituitary rongeurs are used to perform discectomy. A unipolar diathermy probe is used to control epidural hemostasis.

OUTCOMES

In an RCT, Ruetten et al.[53] compared full-endoscopic interlaminar and transforaminal lumbar discectomy versus conventional microsurgical technique and demonstrated that surgical trauma, postoperative back pain, duration of rehabilitation, and complication rates were significantly less in patients who had endoscopic procedures. In further RCTs, Ruetten et al. demonstrated the superiority of endoscopic interlaminar and transforaminal discectomies compared with conventional

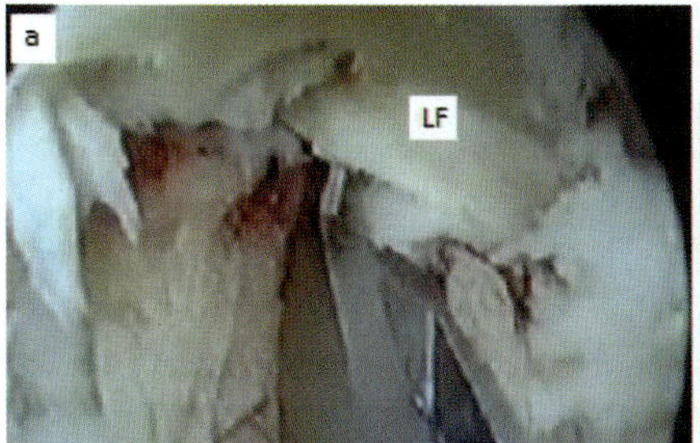

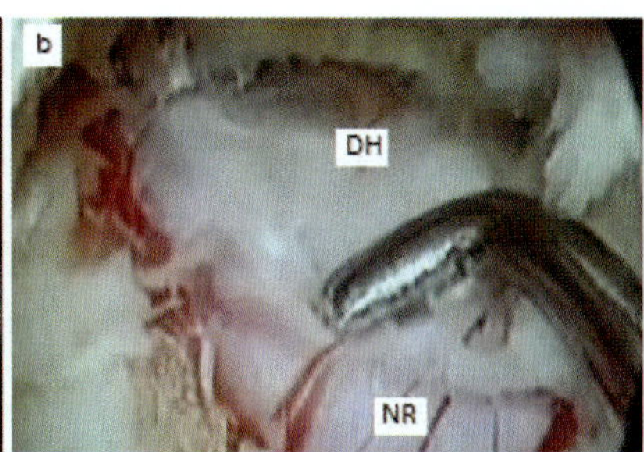

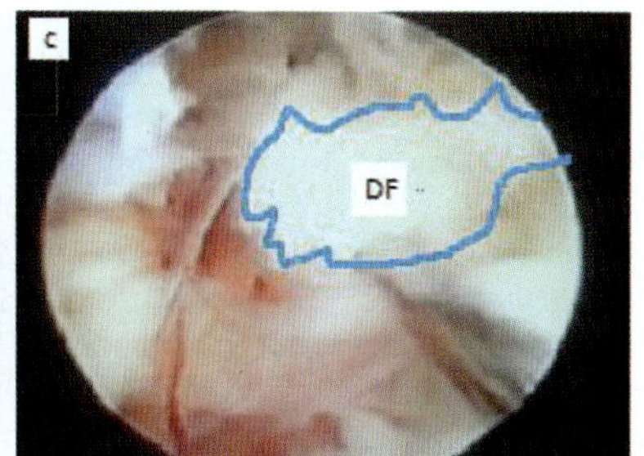

FIGURE 93-21. (**A**) Kerrison rongeur being used to remove ligamentum flavum and trim the inferior articular process. (**B**) Mobilization of the nerve root to expose the preradicular herniation. (**C**) The herniated nuclear material being removed. DH, disc herniation; LF, ligamentum flavum.

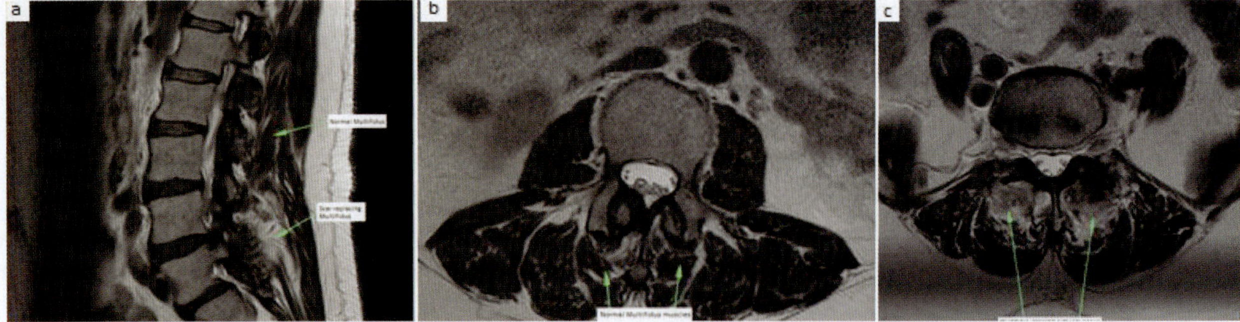

FIGURE 93-22. **(A)** Sagittal magnetic resonance imaging (MRI) view of the lumbar spine. The upper arrow shows the normal multifidus muscle, and the lower arrow shows scar tissue, which has replaced the multifidus muscle. **(B)** Axial MRI view of normal multifidus muscle corresponding to the upper arrow in A. **(C)** Axial MRI view corresponding to the lower arrow in A.

open discectomies for recurrent disc herniations.[79] In another RCT by Hermantin et al. comparing open discectomy and arthroscopic (transforaminal) microdiscectomy, it was also concluded that although the rate of satisfactory outcomes was approximately the same in both groups, the patients who underwent arthroscopic microdiscectomy had a shorter duration of postoperative disability and used narcotics for a shorter period of time. In a recent unpublished prospective case study of transiliac L5 to S1 endoscopic discectomies followed up for 10.9 months, the authors[35,81] revealed that the mean total operating time (access to skin closure) was 41.7 minutes, access time (AT; exposure and closure time) was 19.8 minutes, and cure time (CT; time spent on removal of the disc and associated procedures) was 21.4 minutes. The AT-to-CT ratio was 0.9. The visual analog scale for back and leg pain reported significant improvement in pain for all patients. The Oswestry Disability Index (ODI) dropped by an average of 46.4% postoperatively (55.3% to 8.9%). Blood loss was minimal (<10 mL). Apart from mild postoperative dysesthesia, which resolved within 2 weeks in four patients, there were no other complications in this short series.

DISCUSSION

There is decisive movement, albeit rather slow, toward endoscopic spine surgery. The slow pace of transition toward endoscopy, especially in North America, is in part due to the steep learning curve, and partly because of the litigious practice environment. Medical insurance companies generally consider endoscopic spine procedures experimental, although the techniques have been in practice for more than 2 decades. Today there are anatomic, surgical, biochemical, biomechanical, and socioeconomic evidence of the superiority of the endoscopic lumbar disc surgery to conventional open discectomy. The subperiosteal dissection of the multifidus, laminotomy, and often partial facetectomy required by the open discectomy are anatomically required in open discectomies and distinguish the open from endoscopic discectomies. Most of the other distinguishing features flow from differences in tissue disruption. Rahman et al.[54] and Harrington and French[55] compared operating times and blood loss in conventional laminotomy and microdiscectomy; the conventional open procedures took significantly longer operating times and resulted in larger amounts of blood loss. Ruetten et al., in very well-structured RCTs,[53,82] demonstrated that the endoscopic techniques had advantages in operating time, complication rates, surgical trauma, and brief rehabilitation. Damage to the multifidus, as evidenced by postoperative serum elevation of cytokine, was shown to be higher in patients who underwent conventional posterior decompression as compared with muscle-sparing procedures.[83] In a literature review, Kim[84] revealed the structurally damaging effect of surgical trauma on the multifidus muscle and subsequent clinical and physiologic impact. Dramatic postoperative changes in the multifidus muscles after open laminotomy are seen in MRI films of the spine. Comparisons of the operated and nonoperated levels are shown in **Fig. 93-22**.

As stated earlier, Osman et al.[78] demonstrated in a cadaver study, that transforaminal decompression achieves a larger area of foraminal decompression without any significant effect on the range of motion of the functional spinal unit unlike the laminectomy and partial facetectomy, which produced significant increases in axial rotation and extension while offering a smaller area of foraminal decompression. Although firm data is still in the works at this time, personal experience and the literature are bearing testament to the fact that overall, the cost of endoscopic disc surgery is cheaper than conventional open discectomy.[85]

CONCLUSION

Endoscopic spine surgery, in the hands of a properly trained interventionalist is safe, anatomically less disruptive, and effective in appropriately selected cases; is associated with brief rehabilitation; and is socioeconomically less disruptive. What is sorely missing is the comprehensive curriculum for education in spine endoscopy. Furthermore, even in the RCTs, often the selection criteria do not take into account all factors that significantly influence the outcome of surgical intervention. A simple example is when one case may have evidence, albeit mild, of abnormalities of the facet joint, malalignment and disc degeneration in addition to disc herniation. Thus, stratification based on the pathology, in addition to other patient attributes, including age, body mass index, and other comorbid status, is necessary to make a meaningful comparison of the outcomes.

REFERENCES

1. Mixter WJ, Barr JS. Rupture of intervertebral disc with involvement of the spinal canal. *N Engl J Med*. 1934;211:210-215.
2. Smith L. Enxyme dissolution of the nucleus pulposus in humans. *JAMA*. 1964;197:137-140.
3. Smith L. Chemonucleolysis: personal history, trials and tribulations. *Clin Orthop*. 1993;287:117-124.
4. Kambin P, Gellman H. Percutaneous lateral discectomy of the lumbar spine. A preliminary report. *Clin Orthop*. 1983;174:127-132.
5. Hijikata S, Yamagishi M, Nakayma T. Percutaneous discectomy: a new treatment method for lumbar disc herniation. *J Tokyo Den-ryoku Hosp*. 1975;5:39-44.
6. Hijikata S. Percutaneous nucleotomy. A new concept technique and 12 years' experience. *Clin Orthop*. 1989;238:9-23.
7. Hijikata S, Yamagishi M, Nakayama T, et al. Percutaneous nucleotomy: a new treatment method for lumbar disc herniation. *J Toden Hosp*. 1975;5:5-13.
8. Kambin P, Gellman H. Percutaneous lateral discectomy of the lumbar spine. A preliminary report. *Clin Orthop*. 1983;174:127-132.
9. Forst R, Hausmann G. Nucleoscopy: a new examination technique. *Arch Orthop Trauma Surg*. 1983;101:219-221.

10. Onik G, Helms CA, Ginsburg L, et al. Percutaneous lumbar discectomy using a new aspiration probe. *AJR Am J Roentgenol.* 1985;6: 290.
11. Choy DS, Case RB, Fielding W, et al. Percutaneous laser nucleolysis of lumbar disks. *N Engl J Med.* 1987;317:771-772.
12. Kambin P. Percutaneous lumbar microdiscectomy (Triangular working zone): Current Practice. *Surgical Rounds in Orthopaedics.* 1988:31-35.
13. Galibet P, Deramond H, Rosat P, et al. Preliminary note on the treatment of vertebral angioma by percutaneous acrylic vertebroplasty. *Neurochirurgie.* 1987;33:166-168.
14. Belkoff SM, Mathis JM, Jasper LE, et al. An ex vivo biomechanical evaluation of an inflatable bone tamp used in the treatment of compression fracture. *Spine.* 2001;26:151-156.
15. Saal JA, Saal JS. Intradiscal electrothermal treatment for chronic discogenic low back pain. *Spine.* 2000;25:2622-2627.
16. Knight MTN, Goswami AKD. Endoscopic laser foraminoplasty. In: Savitz MH, Chiu JC, Yeung AT, eds. *The Practice of Minimally Invasive Spinal Technique.* Vol. 42, 1st ed. Richmond, VA: AAMISMS Education, LLC; 2000:337-40.
17. Yeung AT, Tsou PM. Posterolateral endoscopic excision for lumbar disc herniation: Surgical technique, outcome, and complications in 307 consecutive cases. *Spine* (Phila Pa 1976), 2002;27(7):722-731.
18. Key C. Mr. Aston Key on paraplegia. *Guy's Hospital Reports.* 1838;3:17-34.
19. Bonaldi G, Minonzio G, Belloni G, et al. Percutaneous cervical diskectomy: preliminary experience. *Neuroradiology.* 1994;36(6): 483-6.
20. Tajima T, Sakamoto H, Yamakawa H. Diskectomy cervicale percutanee. *Rev Med Orthop.* 1989;17:7-10.
21. Hoogland T, Scheckenbach C. Low-dose chemonucleolysis combined with percutaneous nucleotomy in herniated cervical disks. *J Spinal Disord.* 1995;8(3):228-232.
22. Richaud J, Lazorthes Y, Verdie JC, Bonafe A. Chemonucleolysis for herniated cervical disc. *Acta Neurochir (Wien).* 1988;91(3-4):116-119.
23. Courtheoux F, Theron J. Automated percutaneous nucleotomy in the treatment of cervicobrachial neuralgia due to disc herniation. *J Neuroradiol.* 1992;19(3):211-216.
24. Ahn Y, Lee SH, Chung SE, et al. Percutaneous endoscopic cervical discectomy for discogenic cervical headache due to soft disc herniation. *Neuroradiology.* 2005;47(12):924-930.
25. Ahn Y, Lee SH, Shin SW. Percutaneous endoscopic cervical discectomy: clinical outcome and radiographic changes. *Photomed Laser Surg.* 2005;23(4):362-368.
26. Ruetten S, Komp M, Merk H, Godolias G. Full-endoscopic anterior decompression versus conventional anterior decompression and fusion in cervical disc herniations. *Int Orthop.* 2009;33(6):1677-1682.
27. Snyder GM, Bernhardt M. Anterior cervical fractional interspace decompression for treatment of cervical radiculopathy. A review of the first 66 cases. *Clin Orthop.* 1989;246:92-99.
28. Epstein JA. The syndrome of herniation of the lower thoracic intervertebral discs with nerve root and spinal cord compression: a presentation of four cases with a review of the literature, methods of diagnosis, and treatment. *J Neurosurg.* 1954;11:525-538.
29. Tahmouresie A. Herniated thoracic intervertebral disc—an unusual presentation (case report). *Neurosurgery.* 1980;7:623-625.
30. Simpson JM, Silveri CP, Simone FA. Thoracic disc herniation (re-evaluation of the posterior approach using a modified costotransversectomy). *Spine.* 1993;13:1872-1877.
31. Abbott KH, Retter RH. Protrusions of thoracic intervertebral disks. *Neurology.* 1956;6:1-10.
32. Alvarez O, Roque CT, Pampati M. Multilevel thoracic disc herniations: CT and MRI studies. *J Comput Assist Tomogr.* 1988;12:649-652.
33. Arce CA, Dohrmann GJ. Herniated thoracic discs (improved diagnosis with computed tomographic studies and review of the literature). *Surg Neurol.* 1985;23:356-361.
34. Bohlman HH, Zdeblick TA. Anterior excision of herniated thoracic discs. *J Bone Joint Surg Am.* 1988;70:1038-1047.
35. Arce CA, Dohrmann GJ. Herniated thoracic disks. *Neurol Clin.* 1985; 3:383-392.
36. Benson MKD, Byrnes DP. The clinical syndromes and surgical treatment of thoracic disc prolapse. *J Bone Joint Surg Br.* 1975; 57:471-477.
37. Regan JJ, Mack MJ. Endoscopic anterior thoracic discectomy: a prospective evaluation of the first thirty-six cases. Presented at the 10th North American Spine Society Annual Meeting, Seattle, WA, October 18-21, 1995.
38. Regan JJ, Mack MJ, Picetti GD. A technical report on video-assisted thoracoscopy in thoracic spinal surgery (preliminary description). *Spine.* 1995;20:831-837.
39. Rosenthal D, Rosenthal R, de Simone. Removal of a protruded thoracic disc using microsurgical endoscopy (a new technique). *Spine.* 1994;19:1087-1091.
40. McAfee PC, Regan JR, Zdeblick T, et al. The incidence of complications in endoscopic anterior thoracolumbar spinal reconstructive surgery (a prospective multicenter study comprising the first 100 consecutive cases). *Spine.* 1995;20:1624-1632.
41. Khoo LT, Smith ZA, Asgarzadie F, et al. Minimally invasive extracavitary approach for thoracic discectomy and interbody fusion: 1-year clinical and radiographic outcomes in 13 patients compared with a cohort of traditional anterior transthoracic approaches. *J Neurosurg Spine.* 2011;14:250-260.
42. Osman GO, Marsolais EB. Posterolateral arthroscopic discectomies of the thoracic and lumbar spine. *Clin Orthop Relat Res.* 1994;304:122-129.
43. Osman GO, Marsolais EB. Posterolateral endoscopic discectomies and fusion of the thoracic spine. Presented at the 12th North American Spine Society Annual Meeting, New York, October 22-25, 1997.
44. Fisher RG. Protrusions of thoracic disc (the factor of herniation through the dura mater). *J Neurosurg.* 1965;22:591-593.
45. Logue V. Thoracic intervertebral disc prolapsed with spinal cord compression. *J Neurol Neurosurg Psychiatry.* 1952;15:227-242.
46. Currier BL, Eismont JF, Green BA. Transthoracic disc excision and fusion for herniated thoracic discs. *Spine.* 1994;19:323-328.
47. White AH, von Rogov P, Zucherman J, et al. Lumbar laminectomy for herniated disc: a prospective controlled comparison with internal fixation fusion. *Spine.* 1987;12:305-307.
48. Soldner F, Hoelper BM, Wallenfang T, Behr R. The translaminar approach to canalicular and -dorsolateral lumbar disc herniations. *Acta Neurochir.* 2002;144(4):315-320.
49. Tullberg T, Isacson J, Weidenhielm L. Does microscopic removal of lumbar disc herniation lead to better results than the standard procedure? Results of a one-year randomized study. *Spine.* 1993; 18(1):24-27.
50. Yeung AT, Tsou PM. Posterolateral endoscopic excision for lumbar disc herniation: surgical technique, outcome, and complications in 307 consecutive cases. *Spine.* 2002;27(7):722-731.
51. Choi G, Prada N, Modi HN, et al. Percutaneous endoscopic lumbar herniectomy for high-grade down-migrated L4-L5 disc through an L5-S1 interlaminar approach: a technical note. *Minim Invasive Neurosurg.* 2010;53(3):147-152.

52. Carragee EJ, Hurwitz EL, Weiner BK. A critical review of recombinant human bone morphogenetic protein-2 trials in spinal surgery: emerging safety concerns and lessons learned. *Spine J.* 2011;11(6):471-491.
53. Ruetten S, Komp M, Merk H, Godolias G. Full-endoscopic interlaminar and transforaminal lumbar discectomy versus conventional microsurgical technique: a prospective, randomized, controlled study. *Spine.* 2008;33(9):931-939.
54. Rahman M, Summers LE, Richter B, et al. Comparison of techniques for decompressive lumbar laminectomy: the minimally invasive versus the "classic" open approach. *Minim Invasive Neurosurg.* 2008;51(2):100-105.
55. Harrington JF, French P. Open versus minimally invasive lumbar microdiscectomy: comparison of operative times, length of hospital stay, narcotic use and complications. *Minim Invasive Neurosurg.* 2008;51(1):30-35.
56. Urban JP, Holm S, Maroudas A, Nachemson A. Nutrition of the intervertebral disc: effect of fluid flow on solute transport. *Clin Orthop Relat Res.* 1982;(170):296-302.
57. Miller JAA, Schmatz C, Schultz AB. Lumbar disc degeneration: correlation with age, sex, and spine level in 600 autopsy specimens. *Spine.* 1988;13:173.
58. Kirkaldy-Willis WH. The epidemiology and natural history of low back pain and spinal degeneration. In: *Managing Low Back Pain.* 2nd ed. Churchill Livingston; 1988:3-13.
59. Adams P, Eyre DR, Muir H. Biochemical aspects of development and ageing of human lumbar intervertebral discs. *Rheumatol Rehabil.* 1977;16:22.
60. Adam MA, Hulton WC. Gradual disc prolapse. *Spine.* 1985;10:524.
61. Brinkmann P, Porter RW. A laboratory model of lumbar disc protrusion: fissure and fragment. *Spine.* 1994;19228.
62. Dommissee G. Morphological aspects of the lumbar spine and lumbosacral regions. *Orthop Clin North Am.* 1975;6:163-175.
63. Haig AJ, Adewole A, Yamakawa KS, et al. The ligamentum flavum at L4-5: relationship with anthropomorphic factors and clinical findings in older persons with and without spinal disorders. *PM R.* 2012;4(1):23-29.
64. Herbiest H. The significance and principles of computed axial tomography in the idiopathic developmental stenosis of the bony lumbar vertebral canal. *Spine.* 1979;4:369-378.
65. Lee CK, Rauschning W, Glenn W. Lateral lumbar spinal stenosis: classification, pathologic anatomy and surgical decompression. *Spine.* 1980;13:313-320.
66. Hasegawa T, An HS, Haughton VM, Nowicki BH. Critical heights of the intervertebral discs and foramina. A cryomicrotome study in cadavera. *J Bone Joint Surg Am.* 1995;77A:32-38.
67. Ebraheim NA, Xu R, Darwich M, Yeasting RA. Anatomic relation between the lumbar pedicle and the adjacent neural structures. *Spine.* 1997;15:2338-2341.
68. Hasue M, Kunogi J, Konno S, Kikuchi S. Classification by position of dorsal root ganglia in the lumbosacral region. *Spine.* 1989;14:1261-1264.
69. Osman SG, Marsolais EB. Posterolateral arthroscopic discectomies of the thoracic and lumbar spine. *Clin Orthop Rel Res.* 1994;304:122-129.
70. Olmarker K, Rydevik B, Nordborg C. Nutrition and function of the porcine cauda equina compressed in vivo. *Acta Orthop Scand Suppl.* 1991;242:1-27.
71. Olmarker K, Holm S, Rosenqvist AL, Rydevik B. Experimental nerve root compression: experimental nerve root compression: a model of acute, graded compression of the porcine cauda equina and an analysis of neural and vascular anatomy. *Spine.* 1991;16:61-69.
72. Olmarker K, Rydevik B, Nordborg C. Autologous nucleus pulposus induces neurophysiologic and histologic changes in porcine cauda equina nerve roots. *Spine.* 1993;18:1425-1432.
73. Olmarker K, Nordborg C, Larsson K, Rydevik B. Ultra-structural changes in spinal nerve roots induced by autologous nucleus pulposus. *Spine.* 1996;21:411-414.
74. Olmarker K, Larsson K. Tumor necrosis factor alpha and nucleus-pulposus-induced nerve root injury. *Spine.* 1998;23:2538-2544.
75. Smyth MJ, Wright VJ. Sciatica and the intervertebral disc: an experimental study. *J Bone Joint Surg (A).* 1958;40:1401.
76. Osman SG, et al. Endoscopic transiliac approach to L5-S1 disc and foramen—a cadaver study. *Spine.* 1997;22(11):1259.
77. Osman SG, et al. *Endoscopic Transiliac Approach to L5-S1 Disc and Foramen A Report of Clinical Experience.* ISASS13 , Vancouver, April 2013.
78. Osman SG, Nibu K, Panjabi MM, et al. Transforaminal and posterior decompressions of the lumbar spine. A comparative study of stability and intervertebral foramen area. *Spine.* 1997;22(15):1690-1695.
79. Ruetten S, Komp M, Merk H, Godolias G. Recurrent lumbar disc herniation after conventional discectomy: a prospective, randomized study comparing full-endoscopic interlaminar and transforaminal versus microsurgical revision. *J Spinal Disord Tech.* 2009;22(2):122-129.
80. Hermantin FU, Peters T, Quartararo L, Kambin P. A prospective, randomized study comparing the results of open discectomy with those of video-assisted arthroscopic microdiscectomy. *J Bone Joint Surg Am.* 1999;81(7):958-965.
81. Osman SG, *Endoscopic Trans-iliac Approach to L5-S1 Disc and Foramen—A Report on Clinical Experience.* ISASS14, Miami, 2014.
82. Ruetten S, Komp M, Merk H, Godolias G. Surgical treatment for lumbar lateral recess stenosis with the full-endoscopic interlaminar approach versus conventional microsurgical technique: a prospective, randomized, controlled study. *J Neurosurg Spine.* 2009;10(5):476-85.
83. Huang TJ, Hsu RW, Li YY, Cheng CC. Less systemic cytokine response in patients following microendoscopic versus open lumbar discectomy. *J Orthop Res.* 2005;23(2):406-411.
84. Kim CW. Scientific basis of minimally invasive spine surgery: prevention of multifidus muscle injury during posterior lumbar surgery. *Spine.* 2010;35(26 Suppl):S281-S286.
85. Gibson JN, Cowrie JG, Orenburg M. Transforaminal endoscopic spinal surgery: the future 'gold standard' for discectomy? A review. *Surgeon.* 2012;10(5):290-296.

Destructive Neurosurgical Procedures for Treatment of Chronic Pain

Joshua M. Rosenow
Konstantin V. Slavin

Destructive interventions on the nervous system are a valuable method to obtain control of otherwise intractable pain. Before the relatively recent development of augmentative techniques, such as intrathecal drug delivery and electrical neurostimulation (both peripheral and central), these were the mainstay of neurosurgical pain treatment. Options exist for lesioning the nervous system at multiple levels, including the brain and brainstem, cranial nerves, spinal cord, and peripheral nerves. Although the rise of these newer therapies has pushed aside many ablative procedures, these are still valuable components of the neurosurgical armamentarium.

GENERAL COMMENTS

The interruption of peripheral or central nervous system (CNS) pathways carrying pain has always seemed the most direct and logical manner to solve the problem of medically intractable pain, whether benign or malignant in origin. The targets for these interventions include the peripheral nerves and ganglia, the ascending spinothalamic tract and central aspects of the spinal cord, and the trigeminothalamic tract. Supratentorial structures such as the thalamus and cingulate gyrus have also been destroyed in the quest for pain control. Unfortunately, the results of these interventions have not been as straightforward as the theories behind them use, again demonstrating that the physiology underlying the development and maintenance of chronic pain is more complex than we understand.

Several methods have been used to lesion the nervous system. The easiest is a simple mechanical interruption via avulsion, transaction, or resection of a peripheral nerve, a cranial nerve branch, a ganglion, or a segment of the spinal cord. Thermocoagulation or radiofrequency (RF) lesioning has been most often used in the CNS, including the creation of ganglionic, spinal cord, and intracerebral lesions. Cryoablation found some favor in the mid 20th century but is rarely used today. Other alternatives include laser, radiation, and focused ultrasound.

Patients selected for these procedures should have chronic pain that has failed to adequately respond to multiple other conservative nonsurgical treatments. These prior treatments should include rehabilitation, oral medications (anti-inflammatories, opioids, anticonvulsants, antidepressants), and injections. Given the advances in neurostimulation and intrathecal drug delivery, it is also reasonable to conduct a trial of these therapies before considering ablative procedures. This is true both for patients with pain from late stage malignancies (because of their higher medical risk in undergoing surgery) and those with pain from nonmalignant causes (because of the risk of permanent neurologic morbidity from the procedures).

It is just as important to carefully select the correct ablative procedure for the patient, considering both the etiology of the pain and its location within the nervous system, so as to maximize the chance of achieving pain relief. For instance, central neuropathic pain is not expected to respond well to a peripheral neurectomy or dorsal root ganglion lesion.

This chapter reviews the published experience with several neuroablative procedures, beginning with those that are still most commonly in use. Certain destructive procedures (e.g., trigeminal ganglionic lesions and spinal facet denervation) are not included in this chapter.

DORSAL ROOT ENTRY ZONE LESIONS AND NUCLEUS CAUDALIS DORSAL ROOT ENTRY ZONE

The dorsal horn of the spinal cord serves as both a relay center and an integration site for sensory signaling. Sindou and Jeanmonod[1] (via coagulation in 1972) and Nashold and Ostdahl[2] (via RF energy in 1974) pioneered lesioning of the dorsal root entry zone (DREZ) of the spinal cord as a method of removing the portions of the CNS that had already undergone central sensitization in response to a peripheral lesion, such as malignancy or nerve injury. The lesions are intended to destroy Lissauer's tract and preserve fibers subserving proprioception and certain aspects of touch that travel in the dorsal rootlets to the dorsal columns. It continues to have clinical application primarily for the treatment of pain caused by traumatic brachial plexus root avulsions.

In this procedure, the intended anatomic levels are exposed first via complete laminectomy or hemilaminectomy and dural opening. Microsurgical dissection of the dorsal rootlets (if they are present) is performed to separate and isolate them from each other. If the rootlets are absent, a line is drawn between existent rootlets above and below the avulsion level. After the correct anatomic levels are identified, either by electrical stimulation or the absence of avulsed rootlets, lesions are created on the inferolateral aspect of the rootlet entry zone. The small, lightly myelinated or unmyelinated fibers that carry pain signals to the dorsal horn enter from the lateral aspect of the DREZ while the medial side contains primarily fibers destined for the dorsal columns. Lesions are created either by coagulating and opening the pia on the lateral aspect of the dorsal rootlets followed by microbipolar coagulation of the DREZ (Sindou's method) or by using a DREZ RF needle (0.25 mm diameter) to make 1-mm-spaced lesions at 75°C for 15 seconds. Laser[3] and ultrasonically[4] created lesions have also been described.

For the treatment of facial pain, the lesions may be made in the trigeminal nucleus caudalis (so-called nucleus caudalis DREZ lesions). This is essentially a cranial continuation of the dorsal horn, extending from the brainstem down into the upper cervical spinal cord, and receives much of the nociceptive signaling from the trigeminal system. As pioneered by Bernard et al.[5] based on the initial work of Sjoqvist,[6] these lesions are made from the upper rootlets of C2 to a point just above the obex. In the nucleus caudalis, cells receiving input from the first division are located in a more ventrolateral position, and cells receiving input from the third division are located in a more dorsomedial position. Moreover, following so-called "onion-skin" distribution, perioral sensation is only represented in the more cranial aspect of the nucleus while representation of the more lateral aspects of the face is located below the level of the obex down to C2.[7]

Great care must be exercised in targeting DREZ lesions because of the presence of the corticospinal tract just lateral to the dorsal horn. Moreover, the size and angulation of the DREZ and dorsal horn vary depending on the spinal level, being much thinner in the thoracic region. Moreover, the inherently tenuous vascular supply to the spinal cord must not be disrupted. Motor complications range from 0% to 69%.[8]

Percutaneous trigeminal tractotomy may be done with the help of computed tomography (CT) guidance;[9] it represents a less invasive alternative for open caudalis DREZ procedure. Here the trigeminal tract and nucleus caudalis are approached via percutaneously inserted needle that is placed at occipital–C1 interspace, entering skin 1 to 2 cm off the midline with the patient in a prone position. The RF electrode is inserted into the uppermost aspect of the spinal cord, and the RF thermal lesion is performed after testing somatotopy of the nucleus by electrical stimulation.[9]

RESULTS

Larger series show reasonable rates of pain control. Dreval published results of 124 patients with brachial plexus avulsion pain followed a mean of 47.5 months after DREZ and reported an 87% rate of good pain control.[4] This has traditionally been the main indication for DREZ lesioning, and most series for this indication note good pain relief in a majority of patients (usually between 50% and 80% of the cohort). The limited series of results of DREZ lesioning for phantom limb pain show less favorable outcomes (14%–67% good pain relief). Outcomes to these are similar for DREZ lesioning when used for pain caused by spinal cord injury and truncal postherpetic pain.[8] It is worth noting that in spinal cord injury patients, DREZ myelotomy works only for "end-zone" pain and does not help with pain below the injury level.

Caudalis DREZ procedure was initially associated with a high incidence of postoperative ataxia (up to 90%) because of the location of the nucleus caudalis deep to the spinocerebellar tract. Nashold et al. developed new angled, insulated RF needles specifically for this procedure that protected this pathway from damage during lesioning of the nucleus caudalis, reducing the ataxia complication rate down to 39%.[10] As opposed to spinal DREZ, the best indication for caudalis DREZ is postherpetic facial pain (71% excellent to good relief in the Duke series[11]). However, this procedure is rarely performed at this point. The main indication for nucleus caudalis DREZ, in the authors' experience, is the trigeminal anesthesia dolorosa that develops following previous surgical interventions for treatment of trigeminal neuralgia.[7]

PERIPHERAL NEURECTOMY

Resection of a peripheral nerve found its most significant use in the treatment of trigeminal neuralgia[12-15] and painful peripheral neuromas.[16,17] Although it is not often used for the former indication, it remains a mainstay of treatment for the latter.

Avulsion of the peripheral branches of the ophthalmic nerve (supraorbital and supratrochlear nerves) was often used in the treatment of trigeminal neuralgia in this region so as to selectively cause cutaneous anesthesia while avoiding the corneal anesthesia that often results from RF trigeminal gangliolysis aimed at the fibers of the first trigeminal nerve branch. This has also been applied to the branches of the maxillary and mandibular nerves in patients deemed inappropriate candidates for other procedures for relief of trigeminal pain.

Supraorbital neurectomy is most commonly performed via an incision through the eyebrow, while infraorbital neurectomy uses a transcutaneous approach with a small horizontal incision or transorally via the gingivolabial margin. After the nerve is located, it is wound around a small instrument and avulsed.

RESULTS

Grantham and Segerberg[18] reported an average duration of pain relief from these procedures of 33.6 months. Oturai et al.[19] compared RF coagulation and neurectomy and found that only 51% of patients undergoing neurectomy were pain free postoperatively and 78% had pain recurrence compared with a pain-free rate of 83% of the RF cohort, with only 49% pain recurrence.

Neurectomy has also been used for orbital pain,[20] thoracic pain,[21] shoulder pain,[22] and pelvic pain.[23-25] It is sometimes applied as a treatment of postherniorrhaphy pain seen in 5% to 8% of people undergoing hernia repair.[26] Among the 26 patients with postherniorrhaphy pain reported by Zacest et al.,[27] 19 had significant initial pain improvement after ilioinguinal neurectomy, but 13 experienced recurrence of pain. Pappalardo et al.[28] demonstrated that the long-term results for this procedure are not durable. The best results from the procedure seem to be reported either in only small series of patients[29] or series with only limited follow-up time.[30]

GANGLIONECTOMY

Ganglionectomy is intended to avoid the issue of peripheral nerve regeneration, which may follow peripheral RF ablation or avulsion. Although selecting patients who will benefit most from the procedure remains a challenge, most investigators agree that diagnostic anesthetic nerve blocks of the prospective target root should produce significant temporary pain relief.

The dorsal root ganglion contains the cell bodies of the sensory neurons whose central projections enter the dorsal horn of the spinal cord. The ganglion itself lies in the lateral aspect of the neural foramen, distal to the termination of the subarachnoid space in the nerve root sleeve. It may be exposed by resection of the lateral portion of the facet joint and inferior aspect of the lamina of the superior vertebral segment overlying the target root. Opening the root sleeve exposes the ganglion, which can be separated from the underlying ventral root and resected.

The C2 ganglion (alone or with C3 ganglion) has been resected as a therapy for intractable occipital neuralgia. In this procedure, the C2 ganglion is located ventral to the prominent venous plexus in between the laminae of C1 and C2. The inferior aspect of the C1 lamina must sometimes be removed to gain access to the ganglion.

RESULTS

Results from ganglionectomy have been highly variable. In Taub et al.'s[31] large series of 61 patients who underwent ganglionectomy for persistent radicular pain following lumbar surgery, 59% of patients achieved good pain relief. Strait and Hunter[32] reported that 66% of their patients who had both the L5 and S1 ganglia resected for this same indication were pain free. However, of the 37 patients in Wetzel et al.'s[33] series followed at least 2 years after ganglionectomy, only 19% of patients had durable pain relief from the procedure. North et al[34] published even more disappointing results, with only 1 of the 13 patients reporting greater than 50% pain relief at 5.5 years postoperatively. There was little effect on medication intake and minimal functional improvement in the cohort.

Despite these issues, ganglionectomy may yet have a role to play. Young[35] and Arbit et al.[36] both published series of patients treated with ganglionectomy for cancer pain. In the latter series, 13 of 14 patients had excellent or good results following thoracic ganglion resection for malignant chest wall pain. However, the median follow-up period was only 22 weeks (longest, 45 weeks), which may provide one explanation for the greater utility of the procedure in cancer pain.

Acar et al.[37] found that the procedure may also be useful for treatment of intractable occipital neuralgia in patients who received good temporary relief from selective C2 and C3 blocks. At final follow-up (mean, 42.5 months), 60% of patients reported either excellent or moderate pain relief. In Lozano et al.'s[38] series, 80% of patients with neuropathic or posttraumatic occipital pain reported an excellent or good response to the procedure. Not surprisingly, individuals who had undergone peripheral neurectomy or RF ablation procedure before ganglionectomy did not obtain additional pain relief from the ganglionectomy.

SYMPATHECTOMY

Palmar hyperhidrosis is the most common contemporary indication for sympathectomy. However, interruption of the sympathetic chain has long been performed for treatment of a variety of pain syndromes, such as complex regional pain syndrome (CRPS, types I and II) and angina pectoris, as well as painful vasospastic disorders such as syndrome X and Raynaud's syndrome.

The mechanisms by which the sympathetic nervous system either generates or maintains neuropathic pain syndromes are still not well understood despite significant research in this area.[39,40] Conditions thought to have sympathetically mediated pain often have a pain distribution that does not conform to traditional peripheral nerve or dermatomal innervation patterns and whose intensity is out of proportion to the inciting event or imaging findings. Vascular and dystrophic changes often accompany the pain.

In determining a patient's candidacy for sympathectomy, a determination must be made as to the relative contributions of sympathetically mediated pain and sympathetically independent pain the overall level of pain. Most commonly this is determined by observing the clinical response to local anesthetic sympathetic blocks. Intravenous phentolamine (α_2-adrenergic blockade) and guanethidine Bier block (adrenergic depletion) may also be used to this end. Sympathectomy is offered to those patients with appropriate pain syndromes who have failed other therapies and have demonstrated substantial temporary relief from these injections.

Surgical sympathectomy may be performed via several routes, depending on the region of the chain to be disrupted. Thoracic sympathectomy is most commonly performed by resecting the T2 and T3 ganglia for the treatment of upper extremity pain. This region is approached either anteriorly via a small thoracotomy or, most typically, via thoracoscopic approaches. The sympathetic chain runs on the paramedian posterior thoracic wall. The chain is coagulated and sectioned above and below the intended ganglia, and the specimen is removed. Costotransversectomies at T2 and T3 may be performed to access the chain from a posterior approach. The chain is located over the pleura near the lateral vertebral body and may be clipped/coagulated and resected. The ganglia from T9 to T12 may be resected, along with the splanchnic nerves, for relief of neuropathic visceral pain (such as in chronic pancreatitis) that has responded temporarily to splanchnic blockade. This most frequently is performed as a bilateral procedure.

The ganglia at L2 and L3 may be resected for relief of pain in the lower extremities. These may be approached via an open, muscle-splitting retroperitoneal approach through a flank incision, sweeping the peritoneal sac away from the vena cava or aorta (depending on the side of symptoms). The chain is found at the junction of vertebral body and psoas muscle.

Wilkinson[41] has pioneered RF thoracic sympathectomy. This involves fluoroscopically placing RF needlelike electrodes at the levels of the T2 and T3 sympathetic ganglia. The ganglion is located near the dorsal half of the vertebral body near the craniocaudal midpoint of the vertebral body. Multiple lesions are created in the craniocaudal direction to ensure appropriate lesioning. Intraprocedural monitoring of limb temperature may be used to determine the procedural endpoint. A 2°C rise in temperature in the ipsilateral limb is considered significant. Complications from thoracic procedures include pneumothorax, Horner's syndrome, vascular injury, and intercostal neuralgia. Lumbar sympathectomy carries the risk of ejaculation problems in men. Rarely, patients may experience "postsympathectomy neuralgia," a constant, aching pain in the proximal portion of the targeted limb. This is almost always self-limited to several months.

RESULTS

Series of patients undergoing thoracic sympathectomy for pain[42-45] have reported rates of 65% to 100% at achieving significant pain relief, at least initially. Success rates for lumbar sympathectomy are similar.[46,47]

Wilkinson[48] performed 37 RF sympathectomies for pain in 27 patients (3 bilateral). Eight were diagnosed with reflex sympathetic dystrophy (CRPS type 1) and 14 with causalgia (CRPS type 2). Useful pain relief was initially noted in 93% of targeted regions, but this declined to 69% at 1-year follow-up. In his entire series of 110 patients undergoing RF sympathectomy for a variety of indications, there were 6 symptomatic pneumothoraces. Two patients developed persistent Horner's syndrome, and 7 patients had transient intercostal neuralgia.

CORDOTOMY

The none-too-subtle premise of cordotomy is the interruption of the spinothalamic and spinoreticular pathways in the anterolateral quadrant of the cord carrying pain inputs to the brain from the periphery. These lesions are intended to preserve fine touch and proprioceptive tracts. Within the spinothalamic tract, the sacral fibers are located more dorsolaterally and the cervical fibers more ventromedially. Moreover, at any spinal level, axons comprising the spinothalamic tract are primarily projections from cells located in the contralateral cord beginning two or three spinal segments below the specific level. Therefore, a lesion should produce pain relief beginning two or three dermatomes below the level of the lesion on the contralateral side. Caution must be taken in lesioning the upper cervical cord, however, because of respiratory fibers of the reticulospinal tract lying medial to the spinothalamic tract. For this reason, bilateral upper cervical cordotomy is often not performed, and patients with tenuous respiratory function are often considered unsuitable candidates. This procedure has found most utility in the treatment of refractory malignant pain. Although open cordotomy was first performed by Spiller in 1912, Mullan[49-51] pioneered the percutaneous approach, which enabled even medically fragile patients with advanced malignancies to undergo the procedure.

In performing an open cordotomy, intradural exposure is first accomplished after laminectomy followed by sectioning of the dentate ligament at the appropriate level. Grasping the free end of the dentate ligament allows the surgeon to gently rotate the cord away from the operative side and expose the ventral cord. A cordotomy hook with a 45-degree angle or a dedicated surgical instrument (the cordotome) is inserted into the anterolateral quadrant just under the anterior pia before sweeping ventrally. Care is taken to not violate the ventral pia and risk injury to the anterior spinal vessels. Keeping the lesion ventral to the dentate ligament assists in reducing the chance of inadvertent lesioning of the corticospinal tract.

Percutaneous cordotomy is often performed in the upper cervical (C1–C2) region to treat hemibody malignant pain. This may be done using either CT or fluoroscopic guidance combined with contrast myelography. Following dural puncture from a lateral approach, contrast is instilled into the cerebrospinal fluid, allowing identification of the dentate ligament and definition of the ventral hemicord. We usually start with injecting myelographic dye through a standard lumbar puncture in prone or lateral decubitus position and then proceed with C1 to C2 lateral puncture in a supine position. A stimulating or lesioning electrode is advanced through the needle, and impedance mapping is used to signal entry into the cord. Pial penetration is heralded by an increase in the impedance from around 300 ohms to more than 500 ohms. Patients may also report minor neck pain with this maneuver. Low-frequency electrical stimulation is used to obtain a motor threshold for approximation of the distance to the corticospinal tract. High-frequency stimulation should produce contralateral sensations covering the painful region. Serial RF lesions are then created until the area of pinprick analgesia encompasses the patient's area of pain.

Computed tomography–guided cordotomy, described by Kanpolat et al.,[52] features direct radiographic visualization of the electrode tip inside the spinal cord, allowing the surgeon to determine the depth of electrode insertion. A recently introduced endoscopic guidance for cordotomy[53] provides additional means of orientation within subarachnoid space, allowing for precise placement of the electrode anterior (ventral) to the dentate ligament.

RESULTS

The majority of the outcomes literature regarding cordotomy deals with percutaneous procedures. Sindou et al.[54] culled 2022 patients from the literature and personal experience who underwent cordotomy for malignant pain and reported a 75% success rate at 6 months and 40% at 1 year. Tasker[55] noted that he could complete the procedure with a single lesion 95.5% of the time, with 94.4% of patients achieving an adequate result and dropping to 84% at last follow-up. The most common complications are ataxia or paresis caused by collateral lesioning of the nearby spinocerebellar and corticospinal tracts, respectively. This is transient in a significant percentage of patients (2.9–100%) but permanent in a minority (1%–20%). Severe respiratory failure was noted in 0.5% to 27% of patients, and some[56] have advocated an anterior transdiscal approach in the lower cervical region as a method of avoiding this complication. This approach, however, is more technically challenging and has not gained wide acceptance. Unfortunately, one particularly devastating complication is the late onset of new pain following cordotomy. Of Nagaro et al.[57] series of 45 patients who underwent cordotomy, 33 experienced this problem. In 28 patients, the new pain was in the mirror-image location of the original pain and could often be abolished by blockade of the nerves subserving the original pain. This type of pain has been reported as affecting 1% to 16% of patients in various series. Bowsher[58] suggested that this was due to destruction of pathways providing unilateral inhibition of nociceptive cells with naturally bilateral receptive fields.

Regarding open cordotomy, Cowie and Hitchcock[59] report of 56 patients listed a 95% immediate pain-free result, which diminished to 55% at 1-year follow-up. For patients with nonmalignant pain, the success rate was 85% initially but only 35% at 1 year and 20% at 3 years. Two patients died from respiratory failure.

COMMISSURAL MYELOTOMY

Commissural myelotomy involves severing the fibers of the spinothalamic tract where they cross the spinal cord in the anterior commissure. It is expected that interrupting the flow of nociceptive information in this fashion will produce analgesia at the spinal level of the myelotomy and just below. However, the extent of pain relief is often larger than would be predicted by the simple neurophysiology. This phenomenon is believed to be due to the presence of extralemniscal nociceptive pathways. Given that myelotomy does produce some damage to the dorsal columns, even in the most talented of hands, and that the dorsal columns already carry multimodality sensory information, this is a leading contender for the location of this collateral pathway.[60-62] Myelotomy is considered primarily for patients with intractable pain in the lower body and pelvis.

The spinal cord is exposed over the spinal neural level (rather than the bony spinal segment) corresponding to the pain. A small probe is inserted just lateral to the fibrous septum in the dorsal midline between the posterior columns. Traditionally, this is then used to carefully section the midline-crossing fibers until the anterior cleft of the cord is noted, taking care not to injure the ventrally located anterior spinal artery and other epidural veins. For lower body and pelvic pain, the cord is often exposed via a T9 laminectomy.

Nauta et al.[63] and others have reduced the exposure and depth of dissection required for this procedure. In their technique, which may be performed either openly or stereotactically,[64] a single punctate lesion is made in the dorsal midline of the cord. Given the theory that pain relief from this procedure is due to the lesioning of a dorsal column nociceptive pathway, some surgeons[65] perform bilateral lesions of the paramedian dorsal columns without sectioning of the deeper midline-crossing fibers.

Similar to CT-guided cordotomy, CT-guided midline myelotomy has also been described by Kanpolat's group.[66]

RESULTS

Given that the patient population considered eligible for this procedure is rather small (and smaller still in the era of neurostimulation), extant series are all rather small. Most patients are suffering from intractable malignant pain and have a limited life expectancy following the procedure. In Hirshberg et al.'s[62] series of eight patients, survival ranged from 3 to 11 months following myelotomy, and all had significant pain relief up until death. One patient experienced new leg weakness following the procedure. Nauta et al.'s[63] group of six patients who underwent punctate midline myelotomy had similar results. However, in Kim and Kwon's[67] cohort of eight patients undergoing high thoracic myelotomy for visceral pain from gastric cancer, three developed new pain at other sites (with relief of the preoperative pain), and one developed proprioceptive deficits and paresthesias. Across the published series, the outcomes from punctate and traditional techniques do not differ much.

INTRACEREBRAL LESIONS

Moving the site of lesioning cranially is often intended to accomplish one of several well-defined goals: capture pain involving the face, head, and neck that cannot be treated with spinal ablative lesions; treat a wider area of the body; treat the affective nature of pain; or reduce hormonal drivers of malignancy.

MIDBRAIN TRACTOTOMY

First performed in 1938 by Dogliotti and then reported in 1942 by Walker, section of the spinothalamic tract in the midbrain is intended to produce hemibody analgesia in patients with intractable pain that involves the head and neck.[68] Unfortunately, its utility has been severely hampered by disturbing postoperative dysesthesias and other complications, such as auditory disturbances caused by the approach through the colliculus. Moreover, the technical difficulty of the exposure was also a hindrance. Wycis and Spiegel described a stereotactic, rather than open, technique for the procedure.[69] This and other series[70,71] reported more than 150 patients undergoing the procedure. Pain relief was highly variable and complications plentiful. The most common complications were dysesthesias (15%–40%), gaze palsy, and hemiparesis. Attempts to minimize complications and improve pain relief included moving the lesion more cranially to avoid the auditory and visual problems inherent in lesioning the brainstem near the colliculi. Colombo[72] noted that the disturbing dysesthesias are often associated with abolition of the somatosensory evoked potential signals, indicating unintended lesioning of the medial lemniscal fibers in addition to the spinothalamic fibers. Intraoperative stimulation may help identify the spinothalamic fibers from the lemniscal fibers by the painful sensations evoked by stimulating the former and the more vibratory or pleasant sensations from stimulating the latter tract. Lesioning includes not only the spinothalamic tract proper but often also a second lesion just medial to the first that includes the periaqueductal gray matter.

THALAMOTOMY

The thalamus serves as the main deep relay nucleus for most motor and sensory functions. Several thalamic nuclei have been targeted, either singly or in isolation, to achieve pain control, including the medial/intralaminar thalamus, ventrocaudal nucleus (Vc), and pulvinar. Cells in the Vc nucleus subserving anesthetic body regions have a higher likelihood of exhibiting an abnormal bursting firing pattern as compared with Vc cells subserving areas of normal sensation.[73] In the medial thalamus, the central lateral (CL) and centromedian/parafascicular complex (CM/Pf) are most commonly lesioned because of their large input from the spinothalamic tract and diffuse cortical projections.[40] These nuclei are more difficult to identify because of the lack of specific somatotopic physiologic responses evoked with intraoperative stimulation, unlike what is observed when targeting the Vc nucleus. Of 913 patients undergoing medial thalamotomy for pain reported in the literature, 73% had some initial pain relief with a recurrence rate of approximately 25%. Lesioning other nuclei in addition to the medial thalamus did not appear to increase the chance of clinical success.[74] Stimulation of the Vc thalamus produces a paresthetic sensation akin to that of spinal cord stimulation. This is frequently evoked as part of the medial-lateral targeting process during surgery to implant thalamic stimulating electrodes in the ventral intermediate (Vim) nucleus for tremor control. Several groups have reported that stimulation of the CM and Pf nuclei may be associated with unpleasant and even painful sensations.[75]

Lesioning the medial thalamic complex (CL or CM/Pf) does not produce sensory deficits. The largest series have been published by Jeanmonod et al. Their initial paper[76] described 69 patients who underwent CL thalamotomy. Two-thirds of these patients achieved at least 50% pain relief. This group later expanded the series to 85 patients, 52% of whom experienced greater than 50% pain relief with a mean follow-up period of 3 years.[74] One-third of patients had no pain relief. Interestingly, patients with only constant pain (without superimposed paroxysms) were more likely to fail the procedure. Young et al.[77] performed radiosurgical medial thalamotomy for intractable pain in 19 patients (24 lesions). After a mean of 12 months, 4 patients were pain free, and 5 others had greater than 50% pain relief. However, in both the series of Urabe and Tsubokawa[78] as well as that of Sugita et al.,[79] approximately 15% of patients had significant postoperative confusion.

Mark and Ervin[80] and Mark et al.[81] reported results of Vc thalamotomy in 28 patients; 18 obtained good pain relief. They defined several patterns of postoperative neurologic changes. Patients with "VPL sensory syndrome" exhibited significant hypesthesia but little pain relief. Those with intralaminar or Pf nucleus syndrome had good pain relief without significant sensory changes. Tasker[82] reviewed the literature on Vc thalamotomy for pain and noted significant complications in 32% of patients and only a similar percentage with good pain relief. Postoperative dysesthesias were common. He stated that lesioning this target is not very useful for eliminating burning pain and recommended a trial of neurostimulation in this region rather than lesioning.

Lesions in the pulvinar, located posterior to the CM/Pf complex, have also been created for the treatment of intractable pain. These lesions produce pain relief in a minority of patients and appear to be better for relief of oncologic pain and less so for those with neuropathic pain of nonmalignant origin. As has been noted with other ablative procedures for pain, the clinical benefit tends to substantially fade with time.[83]

HYPOPHYSECTOMY

This procedure was a logical extension of the work by Huggins[84] and others that demonstrated that hormonal deprivation slowed the growth of prostate and breast cancers. Olivecrona and Luft's series[85] of 12 patients was the first demonstration of the utility of pituitary ablation for control of prostate and breast cancer with relief of severe pain in one patient. Thompson et al.[86] reported results of 47 patients undergoing the procedure for prostate cancer. Interestingly, 60% had significant initial pain relief, but only 14% had oncologic control. However, only 16% maintained this pain relief at 1 year postoperatively. Among the 203 breast cancer patients undergoing hypophysectomy in Fracchia et al.'s[87] series, 90% had initial pain relief, and 101 were still alive and pain free 1 year later. Other series[88] showed similar dramatic initial results that often were lost as the cancer progresses. No significant series of the use of this technique for pain have been published in more than 20 years except for radiosurgical hypophysectomy using Gamma Knife.[89]

The pituitary gland may be ablated via either a standard craniotomy or a less invasive transsphenoidal approach. The gland is destroyed via direct resection, instillation of alcohol into the sella, RF, cryotherapy, or interstitial brachytherapy. Stereotactic radiosurgery may also be considered, but the variable time to onset of clinical effect with this technique may limit its utility in patients with a limited life expectancy and urgent problems. The complications of the panhypopituitarism produced by this technique are not surprising.

CINGULOTOMY

Lesions of the anterior cingulate gyrus target the affective components of pain rather than the pain transmission itself. Freeman and Watts[90] anecdotally noted that some patients undergoing prefrontal lobotomy for psychiatric indications also experienced significant pain relief. Autopsy studies revealed involvement of the cingulate gyrus. The procedure typically involves bilateral stereotactically placed RF or radiosurgical lesions in the bilateral anterior cingulate gyrus. Foltz and White[91] published the first series of 12 patients undergoing stereotactic (as opposed to open) cingulotomy for pain. Of the 16 patients reported, 4 of 11 with bilateral lesions had an excellent result, and 5 of 11 had a fair result. Most reported series are retrospective analyses of small cohorts.[92-98] The largest series is that of Ballantine et al.,[99] who reported results on 133 patients undergoing cingulotomy for pain relief. Pain relief was initially obtained by 20 of the 35 patients with malignant pain, but this waned significantly over several months. However, 62% of patients with failed back surgery syndrome obtained significant and durable pain relief. Grouping together multiple series, the procedure shows a modest benefit, with slight majorities of patients with malignant (52%) and benign (53%) etiologies obtaining useful pain relief.[100]

CONCLUSION

Although not commonly used, certain ablative neurosurgical techniques continue to have a role in the management of medically intractable pain. Moreover, they all have a role to play in our understanding of the pathophysiology behind the generation and maintenance of chronic pain states. With the rise in neurostimulation as a treatment of many types of neuropathic pain, there is significant concern that some of these valuable treatments will be lost forever. Physicians who treat patients with chronic pain must continue to be educated in these procedures to ensure that they continue to be available for carefully selected patient populations. It is even more important for the neurosurgical community not to lose the experience in performing these procedures in an era of device implants for neurostimulation and intrathecal drug delivery. Moreover, introduction of new technologies, such as magnetic resonance imaging–guided focused ultrasound,[101] may resurrect some interest in ablative procedures, making them perceived as less invasive by the suffering patients.

REFERENCES

1. Sindou M, Jeanmonod D. Microsurgical DREZ-otomy for the treatment of spasticity and pain in the lower limbs. *Neurosurgery*. 1989;24:655-670.
2. Nashold BS Jr, Ostdahl RH. Dorsal root entry zone lesions for pain relief. *J Neurosurg*. 1979;51:59-69.
3. Sindou M. Laser-induced DREZ lesions. *J Neurosurg*. 1984; 60:870-871.
4. Dreval ON. Ultrasonic DREZ-operations for treatment of pain due to brachial plexus avulsion. *Acta Neurochir (Wien)*. 1993;122:76-81.
5. Bernard EJ Jr, Nashold BS Jr, Caputi F, Moossy JJ. Nucleus caudalis DREZ lesions for facial pain. *Br J Neurosurg*. 1987;1:81-91.
6. Sjoqvist O. Studies on pain conduction in the trigeminal nerve: a contribution of the surgical treatment of facial pain. *Acta Psychiat Scand [Suppl]*. 1938;17:1-139.
7. Grigoryan YuA, Slavin KV, Ogleznev Kya. Ultrasonic lesion of the trigeminal nucleus caudalis for deafferentation facial pain. *Acta Neurochir (Wien)*. 1994;131:229-235.
8. Iskandar BJ, Nashold BS. Spinal and trigeminal DREZ lesions. In: Gildenberg P, Tasker R, eds. *Textbook of Stereotactic and Functional Neurosurgery*. New York: McGraw-Hill; 1998:1573-1583.
9. Kanpolat Y, Deda H, Akyar S, et al. CT-guided trigeminal tractotomy. *Acta Neurochir (Wien)*. 1989;100:112-114.
10. Nashold BS Jr, el-Naggar AO, Ovelmen-Levitt J, Abdul-Hak M. A new design of radiofrequency lesion electrodes for use in the caudalis nucleus DREZ operation. Technical note. *J Neurosurg*. 1994;80:1116-1120.
11. Gorecki JP, Nashold BS Jr, Rubin L, Ovelmen-Levitt J. The Duke experience with nucleus caudalis DREZ coagulation. *Stereotact Funct Neurosurg*. 1995;65:111-116.
12. Cerovic R, Juretic M, Gobic MB. Neurectomy of the trigeminal nerve branches: clinical evaluation of an "obsolete" treatment. *J Craniomaxillofac Surg*. 2009;37:388-391.
13. Mason DA. Peripheral neurectomy in the treatment of trigeminal neuralgia of the second and third divisions. *J Oral Surg*. 1972;30:113-120.
14. Quinn JH, Weil T. Trigeminal neuralgia: treatment by repetitive peripheral neurectomy. Supplemental report. *J Oral Surg*. 1975;33:591-595.
15. Sung RR. Peripheral neurectomy as treatment for incipient trigeminal neuralgia. *Oral Surg Oral Med Oral Pathol*. 1951;4:296-302.
16. Koch H, Haas F, Hubmer M, et al. Treatment of painful neuroma by resection and nerve stump transplantation into a vein. *Ann Plast Surg*. 2003;51:45-50
17. Williams HB. The painful stump neuroma and its treatment. *Clin Plast Surg*. 1984;11:79-84.
18. Grantham EG, Segerberg LH. An evaluation of palliative surgical procedures in trigeminal neuralgia. *J Neurosurg*. 1952;9:390-394.
19. Oturai AB, Jensen K, Eriksen J, Madsen F. Neurosurgery for trigeminal neuralgia: comparison of alcohol block, neurectomy, and radiofrequency coagulation. *Clin J Pain*. Dec 1996;12(4):311-315.
20. Trowbridge WV, French JD, Bayless AE. Greater superficial petrosal neurectomy for orbitofacial pain; preliminary report *Neurology*. 1953;3:707-713.
21. Lai YY, Chen SC, Chien NC. Video-assisted thoracoscopic neurectomy of intercostal nerves in a patient with intractable cancer pain. *Am J Hosp Palliat Care*. 2006-2007;23:475-478.
22. Nizlan NM, Skirving AP, Campbell PT. Arthroscopic suprascapular neurectomy for the management of severe shoulder pain. *J Shoulder Elbow Surg*. 2009;18:245-250.
23. Chen FP, Soong YK. The efficacy and complications of laparoscopic presacral neurectomy in pelvic pain. *Obstet Gynecol*. 1997;90:974-977.
24. Griffiths M, Reginald PW. A simplified method of laparoscopic presacralneurectomy for the treatment of central pelvic pain due to endometriosis. *Br J Obstet Gynaecol*. 1993;100:499-500.

25. Jedrzejczak P, Sokalska A, Spaczyński RZ, et al. Effects of presacral neurectomy on pelvic pain in women with and without endometriosis. *Ginekol Pol.* 2009;80:172-178.
26. Aasvang EK, Kehlet H. The effect of mesh removal and selective neurectomy on persistent postherniotomy pain. *Ann Surg.* 2009;249:327-334.
27. Zacest AC, Magill ST, Anderson VC, Burchiel KJ. Long-term outcome following ilioinguinal neurectomy for chronic pain. *J Neurosurg.* 2010;112:784-789.
28. Pappalardo G, Frattaroli FM, Mongardini M, et al. Neurectomy to prevent persistent pain after inguinal herniorrhaphy prospective study using objective criteria to assess pain. *World J Surg.* 2007;31:1081-1086.
29. Whiteside JL, Barber MD. Ilioinguinal/iliohypogastric neurectomy for management of intractable right lower quadrant pain after cesarean section: a case report. *J Reprod Med.* 2005;50:857-859.
30. Giger U, Wente MN, Büchler MW, et al. Endoscopic retroperitoneal neurectomy for chronic pain after groin surgery. *Br J Surg.* 2009;96:1076-1081.
31. Taub A, Robinson F, Taub E. Dorsal root ganglionectomy for intractable monoradicular sciatica. A series of 61 patients. *Stereotact Funct Neurosurg.* 1995;65:106-110.
32. Strait TA, Hunter SE. Intraspinal extradural sensory rhizotomy in patients with failure of lumbar disc surgery. *J Neurosurg.* 1981;54:193-196.
33. Wetzel FT, Phillips FM, Aprill CN, et al. Extradural sensory rhizotomy in the management of chronic lumbar radiculopathy: a minimum 2-year follow-up study. *Spine (Phila Pa 1976).* 1997;22:2283-2291; discussion 2291-2292.
34. North RB, Kidd DH, Campbell JN, Long DM. Dorsal root ganglionectomy for failed back surgery syndrome: a 5-year follow-up study. *J Neurosurg.* 1991;74:236-242.
35. Young RF. Dorsal rhizotomy and dorsal root ganglionectomy In: Youmans JR, ed. *Neurological Surgery* 4th ed. Philadelphia: WB Saunders; 1996:3442-3451.
36. Arbit E, Galicich JH, Burt M, Mallya K. Modified open thoracic rhizotomy for treatment of intractable chest wall pain of malignant etiology. *Ann Thorac Surg.* 1989;48:820-823.
37. Acar F, Miller J, Golshani KJ, et al. Pain relief after cervical ganglionectomy (C2 and C3) for the treatment of medically intractable occipital neuralgia. *Stereotact Funct Neurosurg.* 2008;86:106-112.
38. Lozano AM, Vanderlinden G, Bachoo R, Rothbart P. Microsurgical C-2 ganglionectomy for chronic intractable occipital pain. *J Neurosurg.* 1998;89:359-365.
39. Roberts WJ. A hypothesis on the physiological basis for causalgia and related pains. *Pain.* 1986;24:297-311.
40. Rosenow JM, Henderson JM. Anatomy and physiology of chronic pain. *Neurosurg Clin North Am.* 2003;14:445-62.
41. Wilkinson HA. Percutaneous radiofrequency upper thoracic sympathectomy: a new technique. *Neurosurgery.* 1984;15:811-814.
42. Olcott C 4th, Eltherington LG, Wilcosky BR, et al. Reflex sympathetic dystrophy—the surgeon's role in management. *J Vasc Surg.* 1991;14:488-495.
43. Herz DA, Looman JE, Ford RD, et al. Second thoracic sympathetic ganglionectomy in sympathetically maintained pain. *J Pain Symptom Manage.* 1993;8:483-491.
44. AbuRahma AF, Robinson PA, Powell M, et al. Sympathectomy for reflex sympathetic dystrophy: factors affecting outcome. *Ann Vasc Surg.* 1994;8:372-379.
45. Robertson DP, Simpson RK, Rose JE, Garza JS. Video-assisted endoscopic thoracic ganglionectomy. *J Neurosurg.* 1993;79:238-240.
46. AbuRahma AF, Thaxton L, Robinson PA. Lumbar sympathectomy for causalgia secondary to lumbar laminectomy. *Am J Surg.* 1996;171:423-426.
47. Schwartzman RJ, Liu JE, Smullens SN, et al. Long-term outcome following sympathectomy for complex regional pain syndrome type 1 (RSD). *J Neurol Sci.* 1997;150:149-152.
48. Wilkinson HA. Percutaneous radiofrequency upper thoracic sympathectomy. *Neurosurgery.* 1996;38:715-725.
49. Mullan S. Percutaneous cordotomy for pain. *Postgrad Med.* 1969;45:114-118.
50. Mullan S. Percutaneous cordotomy for pain. *Surg Clin North Am.* 1966;46:3-12.
51. Mullan SF. Cordotomy and rhizotomy for pain. *Clin Neurosurg.* 1983;31:344-350.
52. Kanpolat Y, Akyar S, Cağlar S, et al. CT-guided percutaneous selective cordotomy. *Acta Neurochir (Wien).* 1993;123:92-96.
53. Fonoff ET, de Oliveira YS, Lopez WO, et al. Endoscopic-guided percutaneous radiofrequency cordotomy. *J Neurosurg.* 2010;113:524-527.
54. Sindou M, Jeanmonod D, Mertens P. Ablative neurosurgical procedures for the treatment of chronic pain. *Neurophysiol Clin.* 1990;20:399-423.
55. Tasker RR. Percutaneous cordotomy for persistent pain. In: Gildenberg P, Tasker R, eds. *Textbook of Stereotactic and Functional Neurosurgery.* New York: McGraw-Hill; 1998:1491-1505.
56. Raslan AM. Percutaneous computed tomography-guided transdiscal low cervical cordotomy for cancer pain as a method to avoid sleep apnea. *Stereotact Funct Neurosurg.* 2005;83:159-164.
57. Nagaro T, Adachi N, Tabo E, et al. New pain following cordotomy: clinical features, mechanisms, and clinical importance. *J Neurosurg.* 2001;95:425-431.
58. Bowsher D. Contralateral mirror-image pain following anterolateral cordotomy. *Pain.* 1988;33:63-65.
59. Cowie RA, Hitchcock ER. The late results of antero-lateral cordotomy for pain relief. *Acta Neurochir (Wien).* 1982;64:39-50.
60. Foreman RD, Beall JE, Coulter JD, Willis WD. Effects of dorsal column stimulation on primate spinothalamic tract neurons. *J Neurophysiol.* 1976;39:534-546.
61. Vierck CJ Jr, Hamilton DM, Thornby JI. Pain reactivity of monkeys after lesions to the dorsal and lateral columns of the spinal cord. *Exp Brain Res.* 1971;13:140-158.
62. Hirshberg RM, Al-Chaer ED, Lawand NB, et al. Is there a pathway in the posterior funiculus that signals visceral pain? *Pain.* 1996;67(2-3):291-305.
63. Nauta HJ, Soukup VM, Fabian RH, et al. Punctate midline myelotomy for the relief of visceral cancer pain. *J Neurosurg.* 2000;92(2 Suppl):125-130.
64. Vilela Filho O, Araujo MR, Florencio RS, et al. CT-guided percutaneous punctate midline myelotomy for the treatment of intractable visceral pain: a technical note. *Stereotact Funct Neurosurg.* 2001;77:177-182.
65. Gildenberg PL, Hirshberg RM. Limited myelotomy for the treatment of intractable cancer pain. *J Neurol Neurosurg Psychiatry.* 1984;47:94-96.
66. Kanpolat Y, Atalağ M, Deda H, Siva A. CT guided extralemniscal myelotomy. *Acta Neurochir (Wien).* 1988;91:151-152.
67. Kim YS, Kwon SJ. High thoracic midline dorsal column myelotomy for severe visceral pain due to advanced stomach cancer. *Neurosurgery.* 2000;46:85-92.
68. Gorecki J. Stereotactic midbrain tractotomy. In: Gildenberg PL, Tasker RR, eds. *Textbook of Stereotactic and Functional Neurosurgery.* New York: McGraw-Hill; 1998:1651-1660.

69. Wycis HT, Spiegel EA. Long-range results in the treatment of intractable pain by stereotaxic midbrain surgery. *J Neurosurg.* 1962;19:101-107.
70. Voris HC, Whisler WW. Results of stereotaxic surgery for intractable pain. *Confin Neurol.* 1975;37:86-96.
71. Zapletal B. Open mesencephalotomy and thalamotomy for intractable pain. *Acta Neurochir (Suppl).* 1969, 18:11-119.
72. Colombo F. Somatosensory-evoked potentials after mesencephalic tractotomy for pain syndromes. Neuroradiologic and clinical correlations. *Surg Neurol.* 1984;21:453-458.
73. Lenz FA, Kwan HC, Dostrovsky JO, Tasker RR. Characteristics of the bursting pattern of action potentials that occurs in the thalamus of patients with central pain. *Brain Res.* 1989;496:357-360.
74. Dougherty PM, Lee JI, Dimitrou T, Lenz FA: Medial thalamotomy. In: Burchiel KJ, ed. *Surgical Management of Pain.* New York: Thieme; 2002:795-805.
75. Sano K. Intralaminar thalamotomy (thalamolaminotomy) and postero-medial hypothalamotomy in the treatment of intractable pain. *Prog Neurol Surg.* 1977;8:50-103.
76. Jeanmonod D, Magnin M, Morel A. Chronic neurogenic pain and the medial thalamotomy. *Schweiz Rundsch Med Prax.* 1994;83:702-707.
77. Young RF, Jacques DS, Rand RW, et al. Technique of stereotactic medial thalamotomy with the Leksell Gamma Knife for treatment of chronic pain. *Neurol Res.* 1995;17:59-65.
78. Urabe M, Tsubokawa T. Stereotaxic thalamotomy for the relief of intractable pain—CEM-thalamotomy. *Tohoku J Exp Med.* 1965;85:286-298.
79. Sugita K, Mutsuga N, Takaoka Y, Doi T. Results of stereotaxic thalamotomy for pain. *Confin Neurol.* 1972;34:265-274.
80. Mark VH, Ervin FR. Role of thalamotomy in treatment of chronic severe pain. *Postgrad Med.* 1965;37:563-571.
81. Mark VH, Ervin FR, Yakovlev PI. Correlation of pain relief, sensory loss, and anatomical lesion sites in pain patients treated with stereotactic thalamotomy. *Trans Am Neurol Assoc.* 1961;86:86-90.
82. Tasker RR. Thalamotomy. *Neurosurg Clin North Am.* 1990;1:841-864.
83. Gorecki JP. Thalamotomy for cancer pain. In: Gildenberg PL, Tasker RR eds. *Textbook of Stereotactic and Functional Neurosurgery.* New York: McGraw-Hill; 1998:1431-1441.
84. Huggins C. Endocrine control of prostatic cancer. *Science.* 1943;97:541-544.
85. Olivecrona H, Luft R. Experiences with hypophysectomy in cancer of the breast. *Ann R Coll Surg Engl.* 1957;20:267-279.
86. Thompson JB, Greenberg E, Pazianos A, Pearson OH. Hypophysectomy in metastatic prostate cancer. *N Y State J Med.* 1974;74:1006-1008.
87. Fracchia AA, Farrow JH, Miller TR, et al. Hypophysectomy as compared with adrenalectomy in the treatment of advanced carcinoma of the breast. *Surg Gynecol Obstet.* 1971;133:241-246.
88. Polin RS, Laws ER Jr , Shaffrey ME.. Hypophysectomy for intractable pain from metastatic carcinoma: a historical perspective. In: Burchiel KJ, ed. *Surgical Management of Pain.* New York: Thieme; 2002:821-827.
89. Hayashi M, Taira T, Ochiai T, et al. Gamma knife surgery of the pituitary: new treatment for thalamic pain syndrome. *J Neurosurg.* 2005;102(Suppl):38-41.
90. Freeman W, Watts JW. Psychosurgery for pain. *South Med J.* 1948;41:1045-1049.
91. Foltz EL, White LE Jr. Pain "relief" by frontal cingulumotomy. *J Neurosurg.* 1962;19:89-100.
92. Foltz EL, White LE. The role of rostral cingulotomy in "pain" relief. *Int J Neurol.* 1968;6:353-373.
93. Hassenbusch SJ, Pillay PK, Barnett GH. Radiofrequency cingulotomy for intractable cancer pain using stereotaxis guided by magnetic resonance imaging. *Neurosurgery.* 1990;27:220-223.
94. Pillay PK, Hassenbusch SJ. Bilateral MRI-guided stereotactic cingulotomy for intractable pain. *Stereotact Funct Neurosurg.* 1992;59:33-38.
95. Wong ET, Gunes S, Gaughan E, et al. Palliation of intractable cancer pain by MRI-guided cingulotomy. *Clin J Pain.* 1997;13:260-263.
96. Wilkinson HA, Davidson KM, Davidson RI. Bilateral anterior cingulotomy for chronic noncancer pain. *Neurosurgery.* 1999;45:1129-1136.
97. Yen CP, Kung SS, Su YF, et al. Stereotactic bilateral anterior cingulotomy for intractable pain. *J Clin Neurosci.* 2005;12:886-890.
98. Brotis AG, Kapsalaki EZ, Paterakis K, et al. Historic evolution of open cingulectomy and stereotactic cingulotomy in the management of medically intractable psychiatric disorders, pain and drug addiction. *Stereotact Funct Neurosurg.* 2009;87:271-291.
99. Ballantine HT, Cosgrove GR, Giriunas IE. Surgical treatment of intractable psychiatric illness and chronic pain by stereotactic cingulotomy. In: Schmidek HH, Sweet WH eds. *Operative Neurosurgical Techniques.* Philadelphia: WB Saunders; 1995:1423-1430.
100. Abdelaziz OS, Cosgrove GR. Stereotactic cingulotomy for the treatment of chronic pain. In: Burchiel KJ, ed. *Surgical Management of Pain.* New York: Thieme; 2002:812-820.
101. Jeanmonod D, Werner B, Morel A, et al. Transcranial magnetic resonance imaging-guided focused ultrasound: noninvasive central lateral thalamotomy for chronic neuropathic pain. *Neurosurg Focus.* 2012;32(1):E1.

Radiation and Imaging Radiation Safety for the Pain Specialist*

Howard S. Smith
Samir J. Sheth
David J. Copenhaver
Scott M. Fishman

INTRODUCTION

A fundamental knowledge of radiation effects and safety is essential for any pain management specialist who performs fluoroscopically guided procedures. It is sobering to note that practitioners of fluoroscopy and radiography in the first half of the twentieth century had the highest incidence of cancer-related death among all physicians. Although a complete review of this topic is beyond the scope of this chapter, the following outlines some of the most important details of working in an x-ray environment. These include basic principles of radioactivity, potential adverse effects to patients and physicians, and preventive measures for maintaining effective radiation safety.

*This chapter is dedicated to the memory of our dear colleague Howard Smith who was a trusted friend, a renaissance clinician trained in multiple fields and disciplines, a scholar with boundless energy, and a compassionate professional who strived to reduce pain in all of his many endeavors.

RADIATION FUNDAMENTALS

Radiation is the process by which energy in the form of waves or particles is emitted from a source. Electromagnetic radiation (EMR) has no mass and no charge. Common types of EMR include gamma rays, x-rays, ultraviolet visible light, infrared, radar, microwaves, and radio waves. This list is in order of increasing wavelength.

X-rays are one of the most common potential radiation hazards in health care. The hazard is mainly due to potential harmful biological effects resulting from x-rays passing through matter with enough energy to remove electrons (ionizing radiation) from atoms, which can result in ionized atoms and free radicals (atoms with an unpaired electron in the outer shell). This risk of biological damage from radiation exposure can exist even with low doses. Biological effects of radiation exposure depend on two major factors: dose and duration. Greater exposure is associated with greater risk.

Radiation is both naturally occurring and man-made. It occurs all around us and cannot be completely avoided ("background" radiation.) We are also exposed to radiation through medically necessary testing (e.g., dental x-rays, nuclear medicine, and radiology procedures). Typically, the average individual is exposed to roughly 3.6 mSv per year or 360 mrem per year (see terminology in following section), of which 15% is due to medically necessary procedures.

A BRIEF REVIEW OF RADIATION PROTECTION TERMINOLOGY

Exposure (E) is the ability of energy to ionize air (source-related). The unit is the roentgen (R), which is the amount of radiation that produces ionization of one electrostatic unit (ESU) of either positive or negative charge per cc of air at 0°C and 760 mm Hg (STP). In SI units, it is coulombs (C)/kg (1R = 2.58 × 10).

Absorbed Dose (D) is a measure of the energy absorbed in a unit mass of material from radiation. It depends on the characteristics of the absorbing medium. The unit is the radiation absorbed dose or the rad (1 rad = 100 erg/g absorber). In SI units, gray (Gy) is the unit of radiation absorbed dose and is given by 1 Gy = 100 rad = 1 J/kg absorber. D = f × E (is the f-factor or roentgen-to-rad conversion factor). At diagnostic x-ray energies, the f-factor for air and soft tissues is close to 1.

Dose Equivalent (DE) is a measure of the biological damage that is likely to result from the absorbed energy. The unit is roentgen equivalents man, or rem. In SI units, the Sievert (Sv) is the unit of dose equivalent and is given by 1 Sv = 100 rem.

$$\mathbf{DE} = \mathrm{D} \times \mathrm{QF} \times \mathrm{N}$$

QF is the quality factor and related to linear energy transfer (LET) of the radiation in a given medium. It represents the effectiveness of the radiation to cause biologic or chemical damage. For pain specialists, it is important to note that the QF of x-ray is roughly equivalent to 1.0 such that rad × QF = rem. Moreover, 1R ≅ 1rad ≅ 1rem.

N is the modifying factor of the radiation and related to absorption coefficient of the absorbing material (assumed to be unity).

LET is defined as the amount of energy deposited per unit length of the path by the radiation and is measured in kiloelectron volts per micrometer. LET is proportional to the square of the particle charge and is universally related to particle kinetic energy. LET is the measure of the effectiveness of a particular radiation to cause biological damage. X-rays are considered low LET radiation.

Time is the amount of time a worker is exposed to radiation. (This should be as short as possible.)

Distance is the distance from the source (should be as far as practicable.)

Inverse Square Law is radiation exposure that varies inversely as the square of the distance. Therefore, if the distance from the source is doubled, the exposure rate is reduced by one-fourth.

Shielding is the use of appropriate materials to diminish exposure from a given source. Designing shielding for radiation protection must take into account the *half-value layer* (HVL), which is defined as the amount of shielding that reduces exposure from a radiation source by half. HVL is dependent on both the energy of the radiation and the atomic number of the absorbing material.

As a rough guideline using x-rays or fluoroscopy for the clinician, the units rad and rem are approximately equivalent (e.g., interchangeable). *Rad* refers to the radiation dose of the incident beam delivered to the air (i.e., what is coming) out of the fluoroscopy machine. *Rem* refers to the radiation dose (energy) deposited inside the patient and more closely reflects potential biological damage.

Scatter radiation is essentially any radiation other than the direct incident beam that comes out of the fluoroscopy machine.

INTERACTION OF X-RAYS AND MATTER

The absorption of energy from radiation in living matter may lead to molecular excitation, releasing significant amounts of energy that is capable of breaking strong chemical bonds. Ionizing radiation is generally classified as either particulate (e.g., protons, alpha particles) or electromagnetic (e.g., x-rays, gamma rays). X-rays are generally produced in an electrical device that accelerates electrons from a cathode to high energy and then stops them abruptly in a target (e.g., tungsten-anode). Part of the kinetic energy of the electrons is converted into x-rays.

The process by which x-ray photons are absorbed depends on the energy of the particular photons and the chemical composition of the absorbing material. Two major processes occur for photon energies commonly used in diagnostic radiology: the Compton process and the photoelectric process. Each of these causes a transfer of energy from photon to electron. In this way, a mark is made that can ultimately serve as an image. It is also important to note that *scattered* radiation from the Compton process and the photoelectric effect are responsible for inducing untoward side effects and therefore require the practitioner to wear special equipment for protection.

BIOLOGICAL EFFECTS OF RADIATION

X-rays are scattered by the atoms of patients, leading to scattered radiation. No amount of radiation can be considered safe for living matter. The maximum permissible dose (MPD) is the upper limit of radiation dose that one should be "allowed" to receive. Radiation exposure below this level probably only carries remote chances of clinically significant adverse effects.

The radiation dose from an average chest x-ray is approximately 10 to 20 mrad compared with 300 mrad for an average 2-second fluoroscopy scan. Whole-body total radiation dose exceeding 1 Sv (100 rem) can lead to problems that often first affect the most rapidly multiplying cells such as mucosa, bone marrow, and skin. Common radiation-related illnesses include radiation sickness, nausea, fatigue, hematopoietic disturbances, intestinal problems, alopecia, cataracts, and radiation dermatitis. The International Commission on Radiological Protection has determined that the risk of death from radiation-induced cancers or hereditary disorders of radiation is roughly 1/100 per sievert (100 rems) absorbed.

Since actively dividing cells are particularly affected by radiation, fetuses are at special risk. It is suggested that, except in emergencies, women of reproductive capacity should be x-rayed only in the first 10 days of their menstrual cycles (i.e., before ovulation has occurred—the 10-day rule). It may be most prudent to display warnings about risk to pregnancy for female patients and clinicians.

Two major long-term risks of radiation exposure are an increased incidence of cancer and chromosomal abnormalities. Early effects may present as a skin reaction. Patients should be informed that there have been patients who have developed skin erythema and even second-degree burns from fluoroscopy ("lead foot" practitioner). **Table 95-1**

TABLE 95-1 Radiation Dosages That May Produce Biological Effects after Acute Exposure

Target Organ	Radiation Dose rad (Gy)	Results	Rough No. of Equivalent
Eye lens	200 (2)	Cataract formation	10,000
Skin	500 (5)	Erythema	25,000
Skin	700 (7)	Permanent alopecia	35,000
Whole body	200–700 (2–7)	Death from infection caused by hematopoietic failure (4–6 weeks)	10,000–35,000
Whole body	700–5000 (7–50)	Death from gastrointestinal failure (3–4 days)	35,000–250,000
Whole body	5000–10,000 (50–100)	Death from cerebral edema (1–2 days)	250,000–500,000

lists radiation dosages that may produce biological effects after acute exposure. **Table 95-2** lists recommended occupational dose limits per year from the National Council on Radiation Protection for comparison; 1 minute of fluoroscopy with typical exposure of 2 R/min is roughly 130 chest x-rays. Although fluoroscopic guidance for a lumbar epidural steroid injection may involve exposures as low as 0.03, academic settings have been shown to have increased exposure times, and it is therefore imperative to stress the dangers of radiation throughout clinical training.

A major concern for those being exposed to radiation is cataract formation. A cataract is an opacification of the normally transparent lens. Dividing cells are limited to the pre equatorial region of the epithelium, and progeny of these mitotic cells differentiate into lens fibers and accumulate at the equator. If dividing cells are injured by radiation, the resulting abnormal fibers are not removed from the lens but migrate toward the posterior poles. Since they are not translucent, they may evolve into a cataract. The minimum dose required to produce a progressive cataract is over 200 rad in a single exposure, with larger doses necessary in a fractionated regimen. Exposure in excess of 800 rem have been linked to inducing cataracts. The latent period between irradiation and the appearance of lens opacities is dose related but is roughly 8 years. The use of "leaded" glasses worn correctly should reduce eye exposure from minimal to nondetectable.

FLUOROSCOPY

Radiation exposure from fluoroscopy is a significant risk. Entrance skin exposure rates generally range from 1 to 10 rad/min but can escalate as high as 40 rad/min with continuous cine operating modes, which are commonly used in cardiology and angiography. Collimators limit the area where the beam exits. Skin dose estimates can be calculated for patients (and are required in many institutions) based predominantly on total fluoroscopy time.

The maximum National Council on Radiation Protection limit for entrance skin exposure is 10 rad/min and should be less than 5 rad/min. Fluoroscopic systems with "high-dose" options usually have a 5-rad/min manual mode dose maximum but no limit for high-dose options. These options need special activation mechanisms that include visual or audible signals to indicate that the high-dose options are being used.

The skin is often a primary sign of radiation toxicity because organ doses are usually much less than skin doses secondary to soft tissue attenuation. **Table 95-3** lists common radiation-induced skin injuries. Irresponsible use of high-dose fluoroscopy may produce very high doses that lead to disorders such as skin erythema or epilation. Reducing fluoroscopy time and radiation field area can minimize exposure. Additionally, whenever possible, the use of "last image hold" should be used. This "freezes" the image on the monitor after the radiation exposure has been turned off.

The maximum dose rate with conventional fluoroscopy is 10 rad/min. However, individual fluoroscopy imaging typically uses much less than this. Image quality significantly improves when increasing from 0.75 to 3 rad/min, but beyond this, further increases do not dramatically improve image quality.

There are usually no limits placed on doses delivered in high-dose mode. High-dose mode should be used extremely sparingly and only for a few minutes at a time. All fluoroscopy machines are not equal. Newer machines have improved safety measures. Generally, older machines yield more radiation than newer machines, which have improved changes such as tube design and image intensifier, but each system may differ markedly. Most modern fluoroscopy machines have an image intensifier that brightens the image enough so that it can be displayed on a TV screen. Non intensified fluoroscopy produces inferior image quality while yielding higher radiation exposures than fluoroscopy with an intensifier. Each state differs in terms of how frequently fluoroscopy machine testing (kerma rates) are required, but generally, annual inspections are recommended.

Conventional fluoroscopy has often been compared with computed tomography (CT) fluoroscopic-guided techniques. By example, epidural steroid injections under conventional fluoroscopy versus CT fluoroscopic guidance have been reported to have considerable differences in the effective dose of radiation. The effective dose of CT-guided fluoroscopic epidural steroid injections has been demonstrated to be 50% less than conventional fluoroscopy. This reduction in effective dose is highly variable but primarily predicated on reduced fluoroscopy times. However, the overall radiation dose for CT-fluoroscopic guided epidural steroid injections can be up to four times greater when performed as part of a full diagnostic lumbar CT. The planning portion of the lumbar CT can also add considerable amounts of radiation to the procedure when compared with conventional fluoroscopy. It may be advisable for practitioners who perform CT-fluoroscopic guided lumbar spine procedures to take measures to reduce the radiation dose of the preliminary lumbar spine CT scan.

TABLE 95-2 Recommended Occupational Dose Limits per Year

Area or Organ	Annual Maximum Permissible Dose
Thyroid	50 rem
Extremities	50 rem
Lens of the eye	15 rem
Gonads	50 rem
Whole body	5 rem
Pregnant women	0.5 rem* To fetus*

*Data from the National Council on Radiation Protection.

TABLE 95-3 Radiation-Induced Skin Injuries

Skin Effects	Rads	Normal Mode (10 R/min)
Early transient erythema	200	20
Temporary epilation	300	30
Basal cell erythema	600	60
Permanent epilation	700	70
Dry desquamation	1000	100

PRACTICAL RADIATION PROTECTION

Table 95-4 lists practical tips for protecting oneself from radiation. The Nuclear Regulatory Commission (NRC) and most other agencies endorse the concept of implementing the ALARA (as low as reasonably achievable) program, which states that all exposures that can be prevented should be prevented. The International Committee on Radiation Protection (2006) has recommended the maximal permissible annual dose (MPD) to be 2 rem per year. This is not usually a clinically significant problem for interventional pain physicians who are careful and follow appropriate ALARA principles. Ideally, most radiation workers should not receive more than 10% of the MPD.

A minimum amount of filtration is used to remove low-energy x-rays. Each system has inherent filtration to "harden" the incident beam in order to produce an incident beam of consistent energy level. This helps to diminish the amount of scatter. Generally, the scatter dose level at 1 m from patients is roughly 0.1% of the entrance skin dose (e.g., if the patient entrance skin exposure rate is 3 rad/min, the operator exposure at 1 m would be about 3 mrad/min). Low-energy x-rays only enter and do not exit the patient. Basic protection includes minimizing time of exposure, maximizing the distance away from the source, proper shielding, using freeze frames instead of real time whenever possible, and using collimation whenever possible.

Optimizing protective safety equipment and avoiding placing hands in the beam can reduce operator radiation exposure. Lead aprons absorb between 90% and 95% of the scattered radiation reaching exposed fluoroscopy clinicians. As noted earlier, shielding is defined as HVL because it is gauged by the amount of protection that reduces exposure from a radiation source by half. HVL ratings of thyroid shields and aprons can be found on labels sewn inside of the protective shielding. Although the use of thyroid collar shields and leaded safety glasses is not required unless exposure to the thyroid or eye could exceed 5 rem per year, all physicians using fluoroscopy should wear these at all times. Additionally, when performing numerous interventional procedures with fluoroscopy, shielded surgical gloves with radiation attenuation offer further protection. Annual physical examinations should include careful thyroid examination. If exposed physicians are asymptomatic, there is no need for routine complete blood counts or thyroid function testing.

TABLE 95-4 Radiation Protection Tips
• Personnel in the fluoroscopy suite should wear lead aprons of at least 0.5 mm lead equivalent.
• During fluoroscopy, only essential workers should be in the room.
• Radiation workers should never hold a patient for a study.
• Everyone in the room should have protection before beginning fluoroscopy.
• Prior to any radiation exposure, the primary clinician should signal (e.g., "is everyone shielded, fluoro starting").
• Maintain scatter dose level at 1 m from patients at less than 0.1% of the entrance skin dose.
• Leakage radiation from tube housing should be less than 0.1 R/h at a distance of 1 m.
• For C-arm fluoroscopy units, it is preferable to locate the x-ray tube underneath the patient. (Radiation transmitted through the patient is usually about 5%–10% of the entrance dose.)
• Total fluoroscopy time exceeding 30 minutes may lead to radiation-induced skin injury, and patients should be counseled regarding this if they are exposed for more than ½ hour.
• The lowest radiation dose and the sharpest image result from keeping the image intensifier as close to the patient as possible.
• Keep the collimators (which cover the x-rays after they are produced) "closed" to as small an exposed field size as possible (just the region of interest).

RADIATION EXPOSURE MONITORS

The NRC is an independent federal regulatory agency responsible for ensuring that workers and the public are protected from unnecessary or excessive exposure to radiation. If you work near radiation sources, the amount of radiation exposure that you are permitted to receive may be limited by the NRC. Additionally, employers are required to advise employees of their annual exposure. Thus, regulations must stipulate that practitioners using fluoroscopy wear radiation detection devices (RDDs).

The Code of Federal Regulations (10 CFR19) requires workers to receive radiation safety training and states that workers have a right to ask questions, are required to wear RDDs if they are likely to receive more than 50 mrem/year, and must receive an annual report with their exposure levels. RDDs should preferably be worn at collar level on the outside of clothes. They should not be stored in warm or humid areas where x-ray equipment is used and should generally be changed monthly.

Although protective garments are common, it is not uncommon to find some clinicians without RDDs or radiation monitors (e.g., film badges) while performing fluoroscopic procedures. Film badges may become obsolete by the next decade, replaced by thermoluminescent dosimeters and/or detectors of aluminum oxides. The newer RDDs are more sensitive and reliable and can be read any time but probably only once reliably. Without diligently wearing these monitors and proper documentation, there is no precise way to determine how much exposure an individual has had. Some practitioners with significant exposure in cardiac catheterization laboratories wear them inside the lead apron monitors, external monitors, and ring monitors (on their fingers). If a practitioner uses fluoroscopy only rarely, a pocket dosimeter may be a convenient monitoring option. The question of when to be concerned (e.g., how many fluoroscopic procedures should practitioners do?) cannot be answered without the use of radiation monitors. Total fluoroscopy time per week should be kept as low as reasonably possible. Because exposure is cumulative, an effective strategy can be to limit the fluoroscopy time for each individual patient and holding all cases to less than 5 minutes.

Some clinicians attach a monitor (radiation detector device) to their personal thyroid collar shield and keep the thyroid shield in a shielded locker or any radiation-protected location near the fluoroscopy suites. Of course, if a RDD is on the practitioner's thyroid shield, he or she has to remember to wear the shield whenever he or she is involved with fluoroscopy or other diagnostic imaging sources of x-rays.

PATIENT INFORMED CONSENT FOR RADIATION EXPOSURE

Any procedure with known radiation exposure requires obtaining informed consent from the patient. Thus, performing fluoroscopy must include a discussion with the patient concerning the risks and benefits, as well as the alternatives, to radiation exposure from fluoroscopy. Documenting informed consent is another critical variable. Patients should be informed that radiation exposure will be kept to ALARA to properly perform the procedure. If contrast is going to be injected, the risks and benefits must be explained and documented (e.g., hypersensitivity, allergic-type reactions). Depending on the procedure and anticipated scope and duration of radiation exposure, the patient might be advised that although it is impossible to know the exact amount of radiation exposure, it is usually somewhere between chest x-ray and a CT scan. There is less risk when a focal area is exposed versus a whole-body exposure. Because skin reaction may reflect early radiation toxicity; patients should be informed that skin erythema and even second-degree burns are possible from fluoroscopy. A separate standardized consent form for patients undergoing fluoroscopy may be useful.

SUMMARY

Maintaining safe radiation practice is a critical component of interventional pain practices that use fluoroscopy (see Table 95-4). Safe measures include practicing the basic principles of ALARA, time, distance, and shielding. A healthy respect for EMR, continued radiation safety education, radiation monitoring, and safe "commonsense" practices will minimize the risks to patients and clinicians. Each institution should have a radiation safety officer (RSO)[1] who can offer in-depth information regarding personal protection, the safety of a particular fluoroscopic suite or machine, and how to obtain additional training or radiation safety.

SUGGESTED READINGS

Broadman LM, Navalgund YA, Hawkinberry DW. Radiation risk management during fluoroscopy for interventional pain medicine physicians. *Curr Pain Head Rep*. 2004;8:49-55.

Fishman SM, Smith H, Meleger A, Seibart JA. Radiation safety in pain medicine. *Reg Anesth Pain Med*. 2002;27:296-305.

Hall EJ. *Radiobiology for the Radiologist*. 4th ed. Philadelphia: JB Lippincott; 1993.

Hoang JK, Yoshizumi TT, Toncheva G, et al. Radiation dose exposure for lumbar spine epidural steroid injections: a comparison of conventional fluoroscopy data and CT fluoroscopy techniques. *Am J Roentgenol*. 2011;197(4):778-782.

National Council on Radiation Protection and Measurements (NCRP) Report No. 100: Exposure of the US Population from Diagnostic Medical Radiation. Washington, DC: National Council on Radiation Protection and Measurements; 1989.

Pizarello DJ, Witcofski RL. *Medical Radiation Biology*. 2nd ed. Philadelphia: Lea & Febiger; 1982.

Sprawls P Jr. *Physical Principles of Medical Imaging*. 2nd ed. Gaithersburg, MD: Aspen; 1993.

Wolbarst AB. *Physics of Radiology*. Norwalk, CT: Appleton & Lange; 1993.

Zhou Y, Singh N, Abdi S, et al. Fluoroscopy radiation safety for spine interventional pain procedures in university teaching hospitals. *Pain Physician*. 2005;8:49-53.

[1]Note: Further information about radiation safety for your particular environment can usually be obtained by contacting the RSO at your institution.

SECTION C

Physical Treatments for Pain

CHAPTER 96

Physical Medicine and Rehabilitation

Donna Bloodworth
Martin Grabois

The objectives of this chapter are to review the literature for articles about skilled therapy services applied to treat painful conditions; report primary outcomes of therapy participation (improved flexibility, strength, and endurance); and report secondary outcomes of therapy participation, including improved pain, disability, and quality of life. When the literature is informative, patient and provider attributes that guide patient selection for therapy are discussed. The terms "physical therapy for chronic pain" and "human," were used to search the literature from January 1999 to January 2013. The search yielded 4940 articles, of which 200 were selected because they describe the application of licensed physical therapy[1] or the use of multidisciplinary programs[2] or functional restoration[3,4] as treatment for a painful disorder. That Cochrane reviews, systematic reviews, meta-analyses, randomized controlled trials (RCTs), and small series are included. Licensed physical therapy, as defined by the Centers for Medicare and Medicaid Services (CMS), is under the scope of PM&R and is a therapeutic activity funded by CMS and other payers in the United States. For articles not written in the United States, articles were selected that implied that a medical professional with an equivalent educational and licensing level of "licensed physical therapist" provided therapy services. Excluded were articles pertaining to exercise done at home or in a commercial gym, club, or spa, biofeedback, complementary and alternative medicine ([CAM]: homeopathy, acupuncture, hydrotherapy, massage), chiropractic manipulation, Tai Chi, Qi Gong, yoga, Pilates exercises, spas, balneotherapy (warm springs), mindfulness therapy, and cognitive-behavioral therapy (CBT) independent of a multidisciplinary program. Also excluded were articles that described exercise administered in nonmedical settings (commercial gyms or spas or home) and by trainers, instructors, certified trainers, "qualified lab personnel," and kinesiologists. These exclusions were made because these activities, settings, or personnel do not fall under the scope of PM&R (e.g., CBT alone) or are activities that neither require medical prescription nor are reimbursed by medical insurance.[5] (**Fig. 96-1**).

Discussions of rehabilitation applications for pain in the low back, knee, neck and pain caused by fibromyalgia and chronic regional pain syndrome, which were covered in the second edition chapter, are updated here. The current literature review permits a discussion of PM&R treatments for pain in the head and pelvic regions and for pain due to Achilles tendinopathy. The constructs of "back schools," multidisciplinary programs, and functional restoration are also discussed.

BACKGROUND

The PM&R chapter in the second edition[6] described the scope and philosophy of PM&R, explained the components of a detailed therapy script, and outlined basic prescriptions for various painful diagnoses. Simply put, PM&R focuses on function and performance and on restoring or compensating ability despite disease and impairment. The practice of PM&R spans the settings of home health, inpatient, outpatient, and community reentry. Our literature search confirms that most PM&R services that are accessed to treat pain are delivered in the outpatient setting.

The practice of PM&R has a long multidisciplinary tradition in which the physician works in concert with physical therapists (PTs), occupational therapists (OTs), and speech therapists, as well as social workers, nurses, pharmacists, psychologists, and recreational and vocational (or child life) specialists. Physical therapists help patients with gait or alternative mobility and trunk and lower limb strengthening, and OTs help patients with upper limb dexterity and strength, self-care, and activities of daily living. The literature search confirms that treatment of simple pain disorders may require only the physician and PT or OT; however, complex chronic pain disorders that cause severe disability and handicap may require treatment in a multidisciplinary program or a

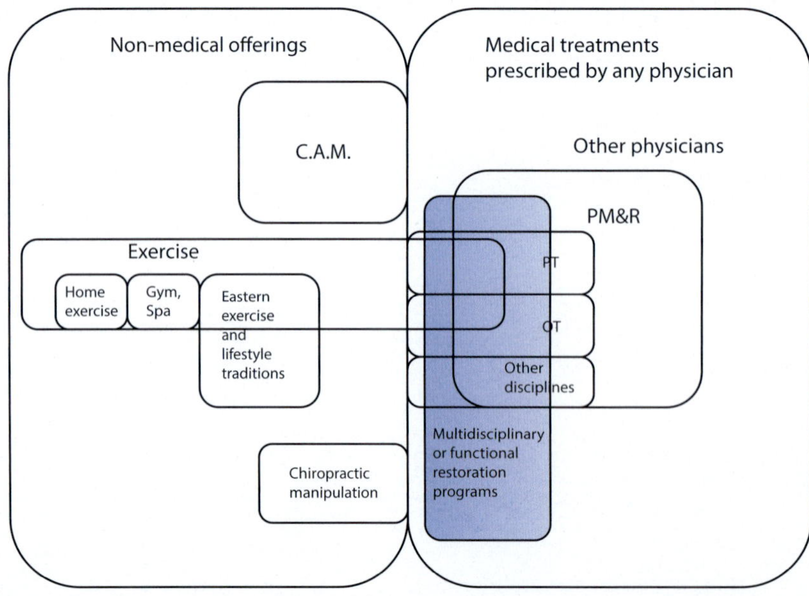

FIGURE 96-1. Exercises and modalities identified in the literature to treat pain: Not all exercises or modalities fall within the scope of PM&R; this chapter considers skilled therapy services and multidisciplinary programs shaded in blue.

functional restoration program in which the services of a psychologist, nurse, or social worker are enlisted.

A physician writes a prescription to communicate the specifics of treatment to another allied health care provider, the medical record, and also the patient. There is no gold standard for what a therapy prescription should include, but Currie and Marberger[7] suggest patient name and diagnosis, goals of treatment, discipline of the treating therapist (T, OT, speech therapist), precautions, and date of reevaluation. A physician familiar with options provided by a PT, OT, or speech therapist may elect specific types of exercise or treatments (**Table 96-1**). However, precautions, contraindications, or limitations to exercise are most important and should be discussed first.

A prudent physician pauses before prescribing a therapeutic moiety and, in the case of PM&R, considers any attribute of the patient that contraindicates participation in exercise or use of a thermal or electrical modality. It is second nature for a physician to ask about allergies prior to prescribing a medication. Exercise allergy is possible even when the antigen is unknown.[8] Exercise mobilizes leukocytes and induces an initial inflammatory response; albeit rare, derangements of this inflammatory response, up to and including anaphylaxis, as well as exercise-induced asthma, and exercise-induced urticaria are possible.[8] Medical and surgical conditions may limit, delay, or preclude exercising a patient. Writing about resistance exercises, Wai states that unstable medical or surgical conditions preclude participation.[9] Wai cites the American Heart Association (AHA) article that recommends that persons with unstable ischemic, valvular, hypertensive, or arrhythmic conditions should not participate in resistance (strengthening) exercises[10] (**Table 96-2**). Persons with these untreated or unstable diagnoses should not participate in aerobic,[11,12] aquatic, or flexibility exercises. Resources from the American College of Sports Medicine (ACSM) note other unstable medical conditions, including metabolic disorders (e.g., uncontrolled diabetes), hematologic disorders (e.g., acute deep venous thrombosis, severe anemia, coagulopathies, disorders of hemostasis), open wounds and certain skin eruptions, and unstable or untreated spinal or extremity fractures[11,12] (see Table 96-2). May notes that the exclusion criteria of studies may inform decisions about patients "felt to be unfit for physical therapy treatment," for example, individuals with fracture, grade III or IV spondylolisthesis, malignancy, inflammatory arthropathies, pregnancy, significant neurologic loss, and prior spine surgery.[13] In order to avoid burns, hot or cold modalities should never be used on insensate or vascularly compromised skin.[6] In the United States, millions of people access PM&R services annually, but a complete history and physical examination are requisite to confirm diagnoses and conditions that limit, delay, or proscribe exercise participation. If there is a question regarding the patient's ability to participate in an exercise program or how to adjust an exercise program so that a patient may participate, consultation with a PM&R physician may be in order.

A physician familiar with the spectrum of treatments provided by a PT, OT, or speech therapist may elect to specify certain types of exercise or treatments (see Table 96-1). The goal of the second edition chapter was to familiarize physicians with exercise options. The ACSM guidelines are excellent resources for information about the medical prescription and monitoring of exercise and applied exercise physiology.[11,12]

Stretch and flexibility are initial steps in an exercise program and prevent injury to soft tissue.[6] Slow sustained stretch held for 60 seconds is optimal.[6] The activity of stretching may not distend the myotendonous unit as much as increase tolerance of the activity. Discussing hamstring stretch, Halbertsma demonstrates no change in the length or elasticity

TABLE 96-1 Physical Therapeutics Useful in the Treatment of Pain

Stretch
Exercise Strengthening methods: McKenzie; Graded; Core Strengthening; Extension bias Strengthening physiologic styles: Isometric (stiffening a muscle at a fixed length) Isotonic ("weight lifting") Concentric (lifting the weight) Eccentric (putting down the weight in a controlled fashion) Isokinetic (weight machines with a fixed axis and fixed torque) Endurance (also known as aerobic): brisk walking, jogging, running, swimming, jumping rope, biking)
Aquatic therapy: may combine flexibility, endurance, and strengthening
Modalities Thermal Superficial heat: hot packs, paraffin, heat lamps Deep heat: ultrasound Superficial cold: ice massage, ice packs, vapo-coolant spray and stretch Electrical: TENS
Bracing: Resting or functional
Assistive devices: mobility (cane, walker, crutches, wheelchair) Activities of daily living (bedside commode, reacher)
Patient education: anatomic instruction, simplification and conservation techniques

TABLE 96-2 Unstable Medical and Surgical Conditions That Contraindicate or Limit Participation in Exercise

Baseline or new onset fever, tachycardia or bradycardia,[12] hypo- or moderate hypertension, hypoxia, tachypnea; dizziness, dyspnea, palpitations, claudication, unusual fatigue, edema[12]
NO THERMAL MODALITIES ON INSENSATE SKIN
History of anaphylaxis with vigorous physical activity
Unstable angina[10,12] Acute myocarditis, pericarditis[12]
Uncontrolled hypertension (SBP >160 mmHg and/or DBP >100 mmHg)[10,12]
Uncontrolled dysrhythmias[10,12]
Untreated congestive heart failure[10,12] Poor left ventricular function[10]
Severe stenotic or regurgitant valvular disease[10,12]
Hypertrophic cardiomyopathy[10]
Aortic dissection[12]
Angina or ischemia at low workloads[10] (5-6 METs, e.g., climbing one flight of stairs)
Acute fracture,[9,13] joint dislocation[9] Unstabilized spinal or appendicular fracture[11]
Grade III or IV spondylolisthesis[13] Spinal disorders with significant neurological loss[13] Prior spine surgery[12]
Acute infection[9,12] (e.g., osteomyelitis, pneumonia, cellulitis)
Diagnosis of tumor or cancer/bony metastases[9]/malignancy[13]
Unstable metabolic disorders (e.g., uncontrolled diabetes, diabetic ketoacidosis, untreated new onset hypothyroidism, Addison disease)[11]
Unstable hematologic disorders (e.g., acute deep venous thrombosis or pulmonary embolus[12], severe anemia, coagulopathies, disorders of hemostasis, severe thrombocytopenia)[11]
Open wounds[11] and skin contagious eruptions (impetigo,[11] scabies,[11]shingles)
Exercise-induced asthma[11]
Inflammatory arthropathies[13]
Pregnancy[13]

of hamstrings with applied stretch; rather increased tolerance of stretching activity occurs.[14] The presence of tubes, wires (new spinal stimulator implantation), and lines may limit participation. Stretching has been shown to relieve pain at least briefly. Lewitt studied patients with myalgic pain and found that stretch applied immediately after an isometric contraction gave immediate pain relief in 94% of patients.[15]

Strength refers to the ability of a muscle group to apply force.[16] There are three types of muscle contractions and three types of strength training: isometric, isotonic, and isokinetic. The first type, isometric ("same length") contraction occurs when the muscle is hardened, or "set," and the length of the muscle does not change.[6] The body builder posing with his elbows flexed and biceps contracted is an example of isometric contraction. In contrast to static isometric contraction, isotonic contraction has motion and contracts a muscle through all or part of its normal range of motion (ROM) while lifting a constant amount of weight. Lifting a dumbbell as the elbow moves from full extension to full flexion is an example of an isotonic contraction of the biceps. There are two types of isotonic contractions: shortening, that is, concentric contraction, and lengthening that is, eccentric contraction. Concentric strengthening creates power, but eccentric strengthening increases tendon tensile strength or lengthens tendon or the myotendonous junction.[17] The third type, isokinetic contraction, occurs when the muscle contracts against a fixed torque. Club machines with cams and fixed axes or a heavy door on a hydraulic governor provide examples if one pulls against them. Strength training improves the force production of a group of muscles by any of the following mechanisms: an increase in the number of motor units activated, an increase in the rate of activation, an increase in the synchronization of motor units firing, or the hypertrophy of muscle fibers.[16]

Strengthening occurs as long as exercise continues to the point of fatigue. The various formulas for strength training involve lifting some percentage of the "one-repetition-maximum" that a muscle group can move and doing repetitions to the point of fatigue. For example, if the heaviest dumbbell an individual can lift (safely) with the biceps is 20 pounds, the one repetition maximum, then a strengthening strategy might be lifting 10 pounds for 10 repetitions and then 15 pounds for 10 repetitions or less if fatigue occurs. When weights are handled through a set of repetitions, additional weights can be added. For strengthening to be accomplished, strengthening regimens of each target muscle group must be performed to fatigue about three to five times per week.[6]

Contraindications and precautions for strength training exist.[6] Strengthening exercise is contraindicated in the presence of fracture; the orthopedic surgeon should prescribe permitted activity and denote prohibited activity for a fractured limb and the contiguous joints.[6] If this is not specified, the primary physician or health care provider should ask the orthopedist to determine allowed ROM, weight-bearing, and exercises permitted. Strengthening exercise acutely increases blood pressure, and this vital sign needs to be monitored in patients with hypertension.[6] Persons should have a "spotter" or partner when performing strengthening exercises, especially with free weights.[6] Strengthening exercises are contraindicated in the presence of acute or unstable cardiopulmonary disease.[6]

The last exercise type is endurance, also known as aerobics, which involves the rapid repeated motion of large muscle groups under low load, often to accomplish locomotion (jogging, swimming, biking) for a prolonged period. Endurance is the time that a person can maintain either a static force or a power level involving a combination of concentric and eccentric muscle actions.[18] Endurance is "the ability to continue a prescribed task in the desired manner."[19] Although strengthening exercise increases muscle force, endurance exercise increases aerobic capacity, or maximal oxygen uptake (VO_2). As a result of endurance training, the number and size of mitochondria in muscle increase, the activity of mitochondrial enzymes increases, and blood flow to muscles increases because of increased numbers of capillaries and improved efficiency of blood flow shunting.[18] Adaptations in the heart and vasculature include increased stroke volume, expanded blood volume, decreased resting heart rate, and decreased resting systolic and diastolic blood pressure.[18]

To achieve an endurance effect, the patient needs to participate in 15 to 60 minutes of continuous aerobic activity three to five times per week at sufficient intensity to raise heart rate to 60 to 90% of maximum.[6] A maximal exertion exercise treadmill test can determine maximal heart rate; however, an easy approximation of maximal heart rate for a given age is arrived at by subtracting the patient's age from 220.

Howley writes about the classification of leisure and occupational activity in terms of aerobic and metabolic physiologic expenditures.[20] Patients often report that they get "plenty of exercise" in this manner. However the randomness of both the vector and intensity of work and leisure activity although it may expend calories, may not achieve strength, flexibility or cardiac endurance above the demand requirements the individual encounters and may expose the individual to risk and injury not inherent in isolated measured exercise.

To reiterate, this chapter is a review of the recent literature for articles pertaining to PM&R applications, that is, supervised exercise by a licensed therapist or multidisciplinary and functional restoration programs for the treatment of painful disorders, and to assess and report the effectiveness of these treatments. There are limitations for the review, and Mayer elegantly comments "that studies on therapeutic exercises often fail to provide details on the specific exercise techniques used and the exact exercise protocol that was prescribed or followed (e.g., dose, timing, intensity) and guidelines and systematic reviews frequently combine various forms of therapeutic exercise and ignore important differences among the types of exercise."[21] Exercise to relieve pain and applied at home or a commercial gym or the effectiveness of Eastern exercise and lifestyle traditions for the relief of pain is a different topic and not answered in this chapter.

NECK PAIN

In the second edition, a physical therapy prescription for neck pain that included corner stretches, cervical-thoracic stabilization exercises, and postural correction of head thrust position was described.[6] The literature review for this edition supports that stretching for chronic neck pain is effective[22] (**Table 96-3**). The literature finds that low-intensity postural neck exercise is not supported.[23,24] Deep cervical flexor (DCF) strengthening, which is believed to affect head and neck posture, does show correlations between improved electromyographic readings (a proxy for strength) decreased neck pain, and disability[25-29] (see Table 96-3). The review article by Ylinen reports that the effectiveness of long-term isotonic and isometric strengthening exercises of the neck and shoulders for chronic and recurring neck disorders was supported.[23] Pain and disability due to chronic neck pain are significantly improved not only by strengthening but also by endurance and coordination regimens[30] (see Table 96-3). The treatment of acute and chronic whiplash with exercise modalities continues to be problematic.[31-33] Only one study was found that evaluated the predictors of poor short-term and long-term outcomes for patients undergoing a rehabilitation program for chronic neck pain: Cecchi et al. concluded that poor outcome was predicted by pain-related medication intake in the short term and long term and by catastrophizing in the long-term.[34]

A Cochrane review on applied exercise for mechanical neck disorders concludes that combinations of cervical and scapulothoracic stretching and strengthening for chronic neck pain improved function in the short and intermediate term.[35] However, chronic neck pain does not respond to upper extremity stretching and strengthening or a general exercise program.[35] Neck strengthening exercise in acute cervical radiculopathy relieves pain in the short term.[35] Many, but not all, studies analyzed in the Cochrane review describe the administration of an exercise program by a PT; however, some exercise regimens were self-administered or administered by a nonrehabilitation practitioner such as a chiropractor, which are applications outside the scope of PM&R.[35] The studies subsequently discussed are performed by a PT within a PM&R setting.

Cunha et al. found that stretching significantly reduces neck pain immediately and at 6 weeks.[22]

TABLE 96-3 Effects of Various Exercise Regimens on Chronic Neck Pain

	Exercise	Physiologic Change	Change Pain	Change Disability
Cunha[22]	Stretching	Improve flexion, 10.5 degrees $P < .000$	7.2 decreased to 1.6 (VAS) $P < .000$	
Jull[26]	Cervicocranial flexion strengthening	Increased EMG amplitude $P < .0001$	4.5 +/− 1.6 decreased by 1.7 +/− 2.0 $P < .001$	11.0 +/− 2.7 decreased by 5.0 +/− 4.2 $P < .05$
	versus neck strengthening		4.2 +/− 2.1 decreased by 1.0 +/− 3.3 $P < .001$	9.6 +/− 3.1 decreased by 3.5 +/− 2.3 $P < .001$
Falla[28]	Cervicocranial flexion strengthening	Increased EMG amplitude $P < .0001$	4.1 +/− 1.7 decreased to 2.3 +/− 2.3 $P < .01$	10.2 +/− 2.7 decreased to 5.5 +/− 4.4 $P < .001$
Falla[27]	Endurance-strength neck flexion	Increased MVC AS and SCM 10.1 +/− 17.3 N P .05	Decreased VAS 1.1 +/− 2.8	Decreased NDI 2.8 +/− 4.0
	versus cervicocranial flexion strengthening	Change 1.8 +/− 10.6 N	Decreased VAS 0.9 +/− 2.3	Decreased NDI 3.5 +/− 4.8
O'Leary[30]	Endurance	Improved endurance $P < .02$	29.9 +/− 14.5 decreased to 20.9 +/− 18 (10 wk) and 21.7 +/− 13.0 (26 wk)	11.0 +/− 2.2 decreased to 6.1 +/− 4.3 (10 wk) and 3.5 +/− 4/.1 (26 wk)
	Mobility		30.6 +/− 14.5 decreased to 20.5 +/− 11.1 (10 wk) and 16.9 +/− 11. (26 wk)	10.5 +/− 2.52 decreased to 7.6 +/− 3.3 (10 wk) and 7.3 +/− 3.7 (26 wk)
	Coordination	Improved coordination $P < .01$	33.2 +/− 13.0 decreased to 14.0 +/− 10.2 (10 wk) and 22.6 +/− 16.5 (26 wk)	9.80 +/− 2.1 decreased to 5.4 +/− 3.0 (10 wk) and 7.3 +/− 3.1 (26 wk)
Nikander[36]	Strength		VAS 57 decreased to 18	NDI 35 decreased to 12
	Endurance		VAS 57 decreased to 23	NDI 38 decreased to 16
	Control		VAS 58 decreased to 42	NDI 38 decreased to 26
Ylinen[37]	Strength		69% decrease VAS (average baseline 58)	
	Endurance		61% decrease VAS (average baseline 58)	
	Control		28% decrease VAS (average baseline 58)	

Cunha et al. compared prolonged stretch (15 min) with manual therapy (pommage) versus conventional stretch after pommage, performed twice weekly for 6 weeks.[22] Both were equally and significantly effective in reducing pain and improving the ROM and quality of life of women patients with chronic neck pain immediately after treatment (VAS 6.6 to 2, combination and 7.2 to 1.6 conventional stretch only , $P > .000$) and at a 6-week follow-up (VAS 3.2 combination, and 2.7 conventional stretch only)[22] (see Table 96-3). The authors concluded that stretching exercises should be prescribed to chronic neck pain patients.[22]

The literature review identified one active comparator trial[24] and one review article[23] regarding postural correction. The active comparator trial by Griffiths suggests that although posture exercises alone or combined with neck stabilization exercises (four sessions over 6 wk) may show a trend toward improving disability.[24] A significant finding in Griffiths's study is that neck stabilization groups were less likely to be taking pain medication at 6-week follow-up ($P < .02$).[24] Ylinen concludes that the effectiveness of postural and proprioceptive low-intensity exercise regimens for chronic neck pain is not supported.[23]

Jull et al.[26] discuss imbalance or impaired function of the deep cervical flexors (DCF) associated with chronic neck pain. Impaired function of the DCF may allow extension in the upper cervical segments and flexion in the lower segments and a head-forward posture. Rudolfsson et al. studied sagittal movement of persons with chronic neck pain and reported reduced extension in the upper cervical levels and reduced flexion for the lower levels.[29] Additional altered ratios between ROM for the upper and lower levels was observed with less contribution of motion of lower cervical levels to the total sagittal ROM compared with pain-free controls, but the findings were not explained by greater forward head posture.[29] These sagittal changes may relate to DCF weakness. Strengthening the DCF results in improved pain rating[25] and neck disability scores[25,26] and in improved muscle strength as indicated by electromyographic proxy.[25-28]

In an RCT of low-load exercises of the DCF, C-CF versus higher load neck flexion exercises, Jull et al.[26] report improved electromyographic (EMG) amplitude DCF after C-CF training as well as decreased EMG amplitude of the superficial flexors (scalenes and sternocleidomastoid). The relative latency between the activation of the deltoid and the DCF during rapid arm movement in the C-CF group shortened compared to the strength group ($P < .05$).[26] Average pain intensity (C-CF decreased 1.7+/−2.0 and strength group decreased 1.0 +/− 3.3, both $P < .001$)) and neck disability index score significantly decreased in both exercise groups (C-CF −5.0 +/− 4.2 ($P < .05$) and strengthening group −3.5 +/− 2.3, $P < .001$) (see Table 96-3). Baseline pain on a scale of 10 was 4.5 +/− 1.0 in the C-CF and 4.2 +/− 1.0 in the strength group while baseline disability on a 50 point scale was 11.0 +/− 2.7 and 9.6 +/− 3.1, respectively.[26] O'Leary evaluated change in pain (visual analog scale [VAS]) and change in pain pressure threshold (PPT) after a single performance of C-CF versus neck flexion exercises.[25] He found an immediate small but significant improvement in pain and in PPT (change on 10 cm VAS 0.42 cm vs. 0.11 cm, $P < .04$) (PPT increase of 21% ($P < .001$)) in the C-CF group.[25] Falla et al. undertook a prospective strengthening program for the DCF 14 subjects with supervision from a PT once a week for 6 weeks with home repetition twice a day.[28] The activation of the DCF increased ($P < .0001$) most in patients with the lowest amplitude of DCF EMG at baseline.[28] A significant ($P < .05$) relationship existed between initial pain intensity, change in pain level with training, and change in EMG amplitude for the DCF during C-CF.[28] Pain decreased with the exercise regimen from 4.1 +/− 1.7 to 2.3 +/− 2.3 ($P < .01$) VAS 0-10) and neck disability index (possible 50) decreased from 10.2 +/− 2.7 to 5.5 +/− 4.4, $P < .001$) (see Table 96-3). The baseline characteristics of some test subjects demonstrated only moderate pain and disability related to chronic neck pain, but for persons with similar symptomatology C-CF exercises demonstrated efficacy for reducing pain and disability.

Another controlled trial by Falla et al.[27] used C-CF low load exercises as a comparator versus a neck flexion endurance-strength regimen for the cervical flexors to evaluate if superficial cervical flexor muscle fatigue could be improved in patients with chronic nonsevere neck pain. Maximal voluntary contraction of the anterior scalenes and sternocleidomastoid was significantly improved in the endurance-strength group (10.1 +/− 17.3 N, baseline 75.5 +/− 17.9 N) versus the C-CF group (1.8 +/− 10.6 N, baseline 78.2 +/− 19.1 N) ($P < .05$)[27] Average intensity of pain about 1 point on a 10 point scale in each group (baseline ~4) and neck disability index score decreased about 3 points in both intervention groups (baseline ~10).[27] Falla et al. note that these changes although small are significant. This study underscores the specificity of exercise for both targeted muscle (in this study, the superficial flexors) and type of exercise; that is, strength-endurance regimens improved strength-endurance.[27] Pain improves regardless of the exercise regimen, and the authors draw no conclusions about the interaction or directionality of improved pain and improved strength endurance.[27]

O'Leary et al. compare mobility, endurance, and coordination exercises showed training specific benefits with between-group comparisons revealed significantly greater gains in endurance ($P < .02$) by the endurance group, and significantly greater gains in coordination ($P < .01$) by the coordination training group. However, all three groups had improvement in pain ($P < .01$) and disability ($P < .01$) (see Table 96-3).[30] The authors comment that subjects with mild to moderate symptoms are recruited so that the study regimens can be completed but they hypothesize that patients with more severe symptoms might benefit.

A RCT to determine the dose or intensity of exercise required to decrease chronic neck pain was accomplished by Nikander.[36] Patients in the control group received baseline strength measurements and several days of instruction in stretching with a recommendation to complete aerobics activities three times a week. Patients in the two active groups were trained by a PT for 12 days in strength or endurance exercises and continued the exercise program at home for 1 year.[36] Strength and endurance training (compared to the control group) decreased perceived neck pain and disability.[36] Declines in neck pain and disability correlated positively with the amount of specific training, and specifically neck, shoulder, and upper-extremity training for more than 8.75 metabolic equivalent of task (MET)-hours per week was an effective training dose for decrease of neck pain.[36] One MET-hour of training per week accounted for a 0.8-mm decrease of neck pain on a VAS (100 range VAS) and a 0.5-mm decrease on a disability index.[36] Improvements in pain and disability occurred in both the strength and endurance-training groups. The pain and disability baselines in this study indicate a more symptomatic group.

Ylinen et al. studied isometric strengthening versus dynamic endurance training trained over four sessions with a PT and then carried over at home for 12 months. In the strength training and aerobic training groups the greatest gains in neck strength, as well as decrease in neck pain and disability, were achieved during the first 2 months, and improvements continued up to 12 months.[37] The isometric strengthening group achieved the greatest strength gains at all follow-ups, and change in neck pain and disability indices correlated with the isometric neck strength.[37] The baseline VAS of the subjects was 58 (VAS range 100) and at 12 months, the strength group improved 69%, the endurance group improved 61%, and the control group improved only 28% ($P < .001$)[37] (see Table 96-3). Ylinen et al. crossed the control group who had only minor changes in pain and functional measures in this study over high-intensity strength training.[38] Significant decreases in neck pain and disability indices occurred, and maximal isometric neck strength increased in flexion and rotation and extension at the 2-year follow-up.[38]

Other PM&R strategies applied to treat neck pain include grade exercise, a multidisciplinary rehabilitation program, and a multidisciplinary or functional restoration type program with exercise and fear avoidance training. Pool et al.[39] studied behaviorally graded progressive exercises (BGA) versus manual therapy each applied by PT for the treatment of subacute (4-12-wk duration) neck pain. Pain and function were improved about 90% of the time.[39] The statistically significant overall effect was found on the NDI in favor of the BGA treatment.[39] An active comparator trial of multimodal group rehabilitation practicing stability, strengthening, and proprioceptive exercises with an educational program, 1 hour a week for 6 weeks, was compared to control group treated as deemed appropriate by their physiotherapist.[40] Both groups significantly improved in both function and pain scores (4.6 +/− 2.3 and 4.5 +/− 2.2, $P < 0.01$). There was no significant difference in improvements in disability or pain between groups.[40] No comparison based on program cost or patient time expenditure or convenience was made. Taimela et al.[41] compared a functional restoration type program to an active comparator of home exercise with two educational sessions to an inactive control group of education alone for the treatment of chronic neck pain. The exercise regimen for chronic neck pain, administered by a physiotherapist, which included 24 sessions of cervicothoracic stabilization, relaxation training to reduce unnecessary muscle tension, behavioral support to reduce anxiety and fear, and seated wobble-board training to improve postural control, yielded a significant reduction in neck symptoms and improvement in general health and self-reported working ability at 3 and 12 months.[41] A trend of improved psychological well-being was observed at 3 and 12 months but was not significant.[41]

Little regarding modalities and neck pain was identified in our literature search. A study group in Hong Kong found that TENS (150 us square pulses at 80 Hz) applied over acupressure points for 30 minutes was as effective as strengthening exercise (twice a week for 6 weeks) compared to infrared radiation (heat lamp for 20 min) to improve disability, isometric neck muscle strength, and pain at 6 weeks and at the 6-month follow-up.[42]

Lastly, the literature suggests that the neck disorder whiplash, both in acute and chronic states, has limited PM&R treatment options. Regardless of active or inactive treatment of acute whiplash Kongsted et al. showed 50% of subjects with pain at 1 year.[31] The randomized parallel group trial for acute whiplash showed no differences among three treatment groups lasting 6 weeks. The treatment arms included immobilization with a neck collar for 2 weeks and then mobilization, "act-as-usual," or mobilization, with weekly evaluation and instruction by a PT in ROM and exercise completed at home.[31] The progressive mobilization was based on principles of mechanical diagnosis and therapy (MDT), which are based on repetitive movements directed by pain response. At 1 year, about one-half of subjects reported considerable neck pain and disability and one-seventh had not returned to work.[31] A RCT for chronic whiplash demonstrated that exercise and advice was significantly more effective than advice alone to reduce pain intensity and pain annoyance and improve function at 6 weeks; however, the effect did not persist at 12 months.[32] In the exercise group, activities included aerobic exercise (e.g., a walking or cycling program), stretches, functional activities, activities to build speed, endurance and coordination, and trunk and limb strengthening exercises, all performed with the PT two to three sessions per week for 6 weeks.[32] Greater treatment effect was observed with patients with higher levels of initial pain or disability.[32] A review of RCT and non-RCT analyzing the effect of defined physical therapy protocols or multidisciplinary programs on whiplash associated disorder (WAD) support the use of interdisciplinary interventions and chiropractic manipulation but not strongly.[33] Regarding exercise the review concluded that more effective regimens were supervised, and started earlier but aggressive subacute programs like work hardening could be counterproductive.[33]

In considering PM&R treatments for neck pain, whiplash may be a distinct entity because of its less favorable outcome after these interventions. However for patients with moderate chronic neck pain and related disability, stretch, strengthening, endurance training, and deep neck flexor strengthening supervised in a PM&R setting have demonstrated significant improvement.

KNEE ARTHRITIS AND OTHER KNEE PAIN SYNDROMES

In the second edition, a physical therapy prescription was outlined including instruction in cane use and joint protection, hamstring stretch and progressive strengthening of the quadriceps, and low-impact or pool aerobics, as well as the use of TENS or ice for pain.[6] The interim literature for the third edition chapter yielded five review articles (two on exercise,[42,43] two on TENS,[44,45] and one on bracing[46]) and four controlled trials (two on exercise,[47,48] one on exercise with bracing,[49] and one on diathermy[50]) for the treatment of knee pain, generally due to osteoarthritis but also anterior knee pain.[49] Strengthening and aerobic types of exercise improve pain and function,[42] walking pain and locomotor function,[43] and pain and strength[47] in osteoarthritis. The Jessep study compared cost of individual supervised therapy to cost of activity and education administered at a community center with simple equipment and found no differences at 12 months in clinical outcomes (WOMAC pain and function, HADS anxiety and depression, and aggregated physical performance); however, there was significant (50%) cost savings with the community center approach[48] (**Table 96-4**). Regarding patient selection, only the Brakke review article noted that patient traits that predict a response to physical therapy include "milder disease (i.e., unilateral OA, symptoms for less than 1 year, and a 40-m self-paced walking test faster than 25.9 seconds)" and those who rate their pain 6 or greater on the numerical pain rating scale.[42] Fatalism and fear that activity can worsen arthritis may bode work against a positive physical therapy outcome.[42] Overall the interim literature does not support the use of TENS in knee arthritis.[42,45] Bracing may be helpful, but compliance after 6 months declines.[46]

Exercise continues to be a primary PM&R treatment for knee arthritis, and Brakke et al.[42] conclude that "strength training, aquatic therapy, and balance and perturbation therapy were the most beneficial with respect to reducing pain and improving function." Bennell and Hinman[43] reviewed application of exercise for primarily knee osteoarthritis across the spectrum of self-administered to therapist-supervised scenarios and reported that strengthening improves strength, pain, and physical function while aerobic exercise benefits pain, joint tenderness, functional status, and respiratory capacity. Bennell and Hinman also caution that the literature does not clarify the optimal exercise modality and dosage for osteoarthritis of the knee and the existing literature has not compared exercise regimens on the basis of exercise modality, intensity, duration, and/or frequency.[43] Specific to therapist administered exercise, Bennell and Hinman cite an 8-week program that led to significantly greater improvements in locomotor function and walking pain long-term at 12 months. Bennell and Hinman also report a smaller treatment effect with regimens fewer than 12 sessions but 12 or more supervised sessions having a moderate effect.[43] One study comparing types of exercise showed isokinetic exercise to improve strength and pain better than isometric exercise of the knee.[47] Hernandez-Rosa et al. compared 8 weeks of isometric to isokinetic strengthening applied every third day.[47] Isokinetic exercises had greater effectiveness for strength gains and pain relief (see Table 96-4), but ROM was similar.[47]

TABLE 96-4 Effects on Pain and Function of Various Exercise Regimens for Knee Arthritis

	WOMAC Pain index	Womac Functional Index
Jessep[48]		
Supervised individualized physical therapy, mean 4 sessions	5.7 +/− 3.2 decreased to 4.2 +/− 4	15.9 +/− 10.4 decreased to 12.2 +/− 13.9
ESCAPE community center, approximately 8 visits	5.6 +/− 3.4 decreased to 3.2 +/− 3.3, no group difference, $P < .27$	16.1 +/− 11.8 decreased to 11.5 +/− 12.1, no group difference, $P < .06$
Hernandez-Rosa[47]	WOMAC pain index, maximal score 20	
Isokinetic exercise	11.53 +/− 3.42 decreased to 5.5 +/−2.17 at 8 wk	
Isometric exercise	10.5 +/− 4.19 decreased to 7.48 +/− 3.77 at 8 wk	

The Jessep article highlights cost-efficiency in the delivery of skilled therapy services.[48] The community-based ESCAPE program starts with patient education and group discussions and instruction and supervision in the performance of an exercise set with the PT.[48] Over time the ESCAPE patients become independent with the carryover of the regimen. Patients in the ESCAPE paradigm were compared with patients receiving individualized therapy.[48] Although the authors use inconsistent terms to describe the number of visits, the authors suggest that the ESCAPE patients had about twice as many (8, presumed median) visits for strengthening exercise as the individualized therapy group (median 4) at about one-half the cost, £583 (currency expressed as pounds) per subject for the individualized group versus £320 for an ESCAPE subject.[48] Outcomes on the Western Ontario and McMaster Universities Osteoarthritis (WOMAC) pain and function indices, the Hospital Anxiety and Depression Scale (HADS), and the aggregated functional performance time (AFPT) for four tasks were similar between groups.[48] In sum, aerobic and strengthening (preferably isotonic or isokinetic) exercises improve pain and function related to symptomatic knee arthritis. Twelve or more visits may have a more substantial dose effect than fewer than 12 visits for this diagnosis. The setting in which supervised therapy is delivered did not affect outcome, and paradigms for economical therapy service delivery exist.

In addition to osteoarthritis other painful conditions of this joint exist. For refractory anterior knee pain, Schneider[49] described a study comparing 8 weeks of proprioceptive neuromuscular facilitation with 16 exercises to a training program using a special resistance-controlled knee splint for 15 minutes three times daily. Increased electromyographic activity in the vastus medialis muscle increased in both groups but a significant improvement in pain was observed only in those treated by knee splint.[49]

A Cochrane review in 2000 reported that TENS and acupuncture-like TENS were more effective than placebo for the relief of pain and stiffness due to knee osteoarthritis.[44] However the updated review in 2009 of interim smaller studies of questionable quality did not confirm that TENS is effective for pain relief.[45] Brakke also concludes that electrical stimulation likely has little impact for knee osteoarthritis and also that evidence regarding manual therapy is equivocal.[42]

A modality for knee osteoarthritis includes diathermy (433.92 MHz microwave), and Giombini et al. showed that the modality reduces pain and improves physical function in patients with moderate knee arthritis symptoms when applied 30 minutes three times a week for 4 weeks and compared to sham treatment.[50] The last review article of physical therapy interventions for knee pain due to unicompartmental arthritis reported that patellar taping reduces pain and knee unloader braces improve symptoms; however, about one-half of patients discontinue brace use within 6 months.[46]

ACHILLES TENDINOPATHY

Achilles tendinopathy is one of the most common foot and ankle complaints related to sports and overuse injuries. A discussion of the exercise treatment of Achilles tendinopathy is included because the clinical complaint is common and the regimen is simple. In contrast to other painful diagnoses discussed in this chapter, Achilles tendinopathy and its treatment fall in the realm of sports medicine, in which a primary goal of intervention is the expedient return of the athlete to his or her sport, whether at the level of a professional athlete or as a tenacious weekend warrior. Unlike patients with chronic pain who may need supervision and education to overcome fear avoidance and kinesiophobia, athletes may require supervision and education to allow adequate healing and to improve techniques to prevent reinjury and safe return to play.

Eccentric training for chronic Achilles tendinopathy is described in the literature. After initial supervised instruction with a PT, the exercises can be performed independently. Petersen et al. demonstrate the technique that compared eccentric stretching to an ankle bracing device to both treatments.[51] Eccentric training can be done with the patient standing on tiptoe, that is, the foot plantar flexed, on a step edge and slowly lowering the heel to achieve maximal dorsiflexion at the ankle.[51] Petersen et al. reported that Air Heel brace was as effective as eccentric exercise for pain relief, but no synergistic effect with a combination of bracing and exercise was observed.[51]

Eccentric stretching has not been found to be harmful, and one study demonstrated improved microcirculatory tendon levels without any evidence of adverse effects in both midportion and insertional Achilles tendinopathy.[52] A review of the literature on eccentric stretch for Achilles tendinopathy by Kingma et al. concluded that because of the methodologic limitations of the trials, the effects of eccentric overload training are inconclusive but promising.[53]

Verrall et al. studied athletes with chronic Achilles tendinopathy and reported that after 6 weeks of stretching, pain significantly decreased (VNS 7.2 to 2.9, $P < .01$).[54] Patient satisfaction was rated as excellent for 80% of athletes, and average time to return to premorbid activity was 10 weeks.[54] However, long-term results may be limited. In a 5-year follow-up of Alfredson heel drop exercises, about 40% of patients were pain-free; however, about 50% of patients had elected other therapies.[55] Subjects were average age 50 years, and about 70% engaged in sports or recreational activities. Additional PM&R treatments for Achilles tendinopathy include supportive night splints, but no recent literature was located on this topic.

CHRONIC REGIONAL PAIN SYNDROME

In the second edition, a physical therapy prescription for chronic regional pain syndrome (CRPS) included instruction in pacing activity and admonitions to withhold therapy if vasomotor sudomotor instability worsened.[6] Passive and active ROM and stretch were recommended.[6] Four review articles or treatment guidelines[56,59] summarize older PMR as well as medical strategies to treat CRPS and introduce newer therapy strategies.[58,59] A Canadian review summarized medications and injection therapies as well as physical therapeutics for CRPS.[56] Contrast baths and stress loading are older techniques and are discussed in a review by Li et al.[57] Stress loading has patients do "scrubbing" and "carrying."[57] A recent review of therapy techniques used in the treatment of CRPS include graded exposure to activity, movements, and light touch; pain-adapted exercises and desensitization activities, exercise with stretching and active ROM, water therapy, stress loading, and mirror visual feedback.[58] British guidelines for the treatment of CRPS recommend referral to PT and integrated interdisciplinary treatment and the use of newer therapy paradigms such as graded motor imagery and mirror therapy.[59] Articles are reviewed for current treatment strategies with motor imagery programs or graded motor imaging, mirror therapies, pain exposure physical therapy (PEPT), and interdisciplinary programs for adults and children.

Motor imagery program (MIP) described by Moseley[60] is an exacting technique and uses 2 weeks each of recognition of hand laterality with pictures and then imagined and then mirrored movements.[60] This specific order of the component treatments needs to be maintained in order to improve pain and disability as was shown in later research with sequence changes that were unsuccessful.[61] Moseley compared the MIP technique to a control group who received twice to three times weekly active and passive mobilization of the limb, systematic desensitization, and hydrotherapy in a department of physical therapy.[60] Compared to conventionally treated subjects, the MIP group reported significantly less pain and the neuropathic pain scale (NPS) (**Table 96-5**), finger circumference and response time to recognize the affected hand significantly improved ($P < .01$), and the beneficial effects of treatment were replicated when the conventionally treated controls were crossed over to the MIP group.[60] No improvement was noted in the control group while they were receiving conventional therapy. Twelve weeks after the study four patients in the initial MIP group and two patients in the crossover MIP group no longer fulfilled the criteria for CRPS.[60] Moseley concludes that response to MIP supports the hypothesis that cortical abnormalities are involved in the development of this disorder.[60] Because a specific sequence of activity is required, Moseley postulated that a sequential activation of cortical motor networks may occur.[61] However, motor graded imagery (GMI) did not show improvement in pain outcomes in a prospective clinical audit of "real world" patients with CRPS treated in physical therapy clinics.[62] Average pain intensities did not change from pre- to posttreatment, and 3 of 32 patients reported that pain had decreased by at least one-half.[62] However, a secondary outcome of pain interference with activities of daily life was significantly improved at one center.[62]

Moseley et al. studied mirror therapies to evaluate if tactile training resulted in improvement in tactile acuity (as determined by two-point discrimination[TPD]); when patients watched the reflected image of their unaffected limb in a mirror during training, they looked toward the stimulated (CRPS) body part and could see the skin of the opposite body part in the mirror.[63] TPD was 8 mm less 2 days after training compared with before training ([95% CI = 1.5-14.3 mm], $P < .001$).[63] Reduction in pain and change in TPD over the session were strongly related ($R = .83$, $P < .001$). However the effect is short-lived and there was no residual effect on pain at 2-day follow-up.[63]

Van de Meent et al. explain pain exposure physical therapy (PEPT) as "treatment for patients with chronic regional pain syndrome type 1 (CRPS-1) that consists of a progressive-loading exercise program and management of pain-avoidance behavior without the use of specific CRPS-1 medication or analgesics."[64] Ek et al.[65] studied an application of physical therapy of the affected CRPS limb that ignored or neglected pain and was directed at functional improvement only and normal use of the limb despite pain.[65] The authors emphasize that

TABLE 96-5 Effects on Pain and Function of Various Exercise Regimens for Chronic Regional Pain Syndrome

	NPS baseline, pain intensity and total score	6 weeks	12 weeks
Moseley[63]			
MIP group	6.6 +/− .5 and 46 +/− 4.2	3 (2.6–5.4) and 20 +/− 9.9	3 (2.8–5.6) and 22 +/− 8.6
Conventional treatment group	6.0 +/− 1.1 and 44 +/− 4.3	Not given	Not given
Ek[65]			
Pain exposure PT (PEPT)	VAS decreased from 4.9 (SEM .24) to 2.7 (SEM 0.27) $P < .0001$	76 patients VAS decreased, 14 increased and 12 unchanged	
Van de Meent[64]			
PEPT	VAS 58.2 +/− 3.2 decreased to 25.1 +/− 3.2 at 12 mo, $P < .001$	DASH 71.7 +/− 16.2–45.7 +/− 18.2 at 12 mo, $P < .001$	Grip strength difference 100% between sides decreased to 48% of the original difference $P < .001$
Lee[67]			
PT one or three times weekly (children)	VAS both groups improved 6.4 to .6	Allodynia after treatment was/approximated zero, both groups	Recurrence 50%; progression to sympathetic blockade 33%

extensive explanation and disclosure is required with this methodology. Additionally, the subjects included were considered "end stage" and had failed multiple prior treatments and had symptoms of CRPS longer than 9 months. Activities included traction and translation of the stiff joints, assisted or active movement of the joint combined with passive stretching of contiguous muscles, and manual friction of tender points if needed. The patients underwent about four treatments over 3 months with encouragement to use the limb normally between sessions. It should be noted that the authors did not obtain institutional review board review prior to performing this study, rationalizing that the patients had already failed all available treatments. The function of the affected arm or leg improved in 95 patients and full functional recovery (defined outcome) was experienced in 49 (18 upper limb and 31 lower limb) (46%).[65] However, functional improvement did not imply a reduction in pain, and in 23 patients functional recovery but pain also increased.[65] Seventy-six patients had a significant reduction in pain.[65] At completion pain increased in 14 patients and did not change in 12. Four patients dropped out of the study related to pain increase.[65] No harm or injury from this therapy regimen is reported. Van de Meent et al.[64] studied the safety of PEPT in 20 patients and found that the physical signs of CRPS did not worsen (edema, color change, temperature, and joint mobility). The mean and mode for the number of sessions was five, and the maximum number allowed was six. Pain, upper and lower limb disability and function, and quality of life improved significantly at 12 months. Visual analog scale (57% decrease at 12 months from baseline, $P < .001$), pain intensity (48%), muscle strength (Newton) (improved 52% (upper limb) and 59% (lower limb) of the difference at baseline between affected and normal limb), arm/shoulder/hand disability (improved 36%, 71.7 +/− 16.2 at baseline 5.7 +/− 18.2, $P < .001$) (disability of arm, shoulder, and hand [DASH] measure), 10-meter walking speed (improved 29%), pain disability index (improved 60% 37.8 +/− 9.4 improved to 15.3 +/− 13.7 at 12 months ($P < .001$), kinesiophobia (18%) (Tampa Scale of Kinesiophobia), and the domains of perceived health change in the SF-36 survey (26.9% [corrected]) improved. Three patients initially showed increased vegetative signs but improved. Two patients had increased edema that resolved.[64] No injuries were reported.

The frequently cited Oerleman article is a RCT of PT versus OT versus a control group (social service interview) on 135 subjects with upper limb CRPS of less than 1 year's duration.[66] Therapy regimens and frequencies were individualized for the patient, but the goals of PT were increasing pain control and optimizing coping and extinguishing the source of the ongoing pain and improving skills while the goals for OT were reducing symptoms of inflammation and/or protecting and supporting the hand in the most functional and comfortable position and normalizing sensibility and improving functional abilities of the hand and improving independence in activities of daily living.[66] Outcome measures were ROM and pain evaluation with VAS and the McGill pain questionnaire (MPQ). Results indicated that PT improved VAS pain scores somewhat faster than OT and significantly faster than the control group.[66] PT significantly improved scores on the McGill pain questionnaire (MPQ) compared with OT and the control group at 1 year.[66] Raw scores are not provided. Physical therapy or pursuit of the treatment goals assigned to that discipline in this study's methodology (increasing pain control, optimizing coping, extinguishing the source of the ongoing pain, and improving skills) improved the symptomatology of upper limb CRPS more than OT or pursuit of its assigned treatment goals.

The Lee[67] pediatric CRPS article is often cited to indicate the frequency of therapies for CRPS.[8] Twenty children with lower limb CRPS received physical therapy once a week for 6 weeks or three times a week for 6 weeks and both groups received six sessions of CBT.[8] All patients were treated with transcutaneous electrical nerve stimulation (TENS), progressive weight-bearing, tactile desensitization, massage, and contrast baths.[67] All measures of pain and function improved significantly in both groups after treatment: VAS pain improved from 6.4 to 0.6; VAS effect improved from 5.4 to 0.6; allodynia (7-point Likert scale) improved from 5 to 7 (7 is anchored to no allodynia, 1 is anchored to extreme allodynia); stair climbing impairment score and gait impairment score also improved.[67] Sustained benefit was observed in most patients at long-term follow-up (average 66 weeks), but was not permanent as the authors note that recurrent episodes of CRPS were reported in one-half of subjects and about one-third eventually received sympathetic blockade.[67] The possibility of recurrence is noted in a review article by Bialocerkowski and Daly.[68] The review of the treatment of CRPS in children with PT or OT concluded that "low volume and poor to fair quality evidence which suggests that physiotherapy prescribed with other interventions may lead to short-term improvement in the signs and symptoms of CRPS-1 or functional ability in children with CRPS and relapse rate may be moderately high."[68]

Additional treatment strategies for children with CRPS include an interdisciplinary day hospital program.[69] The day hospital program described by Logan et al. demonstrated clinically and statistically significant improvements from admission to discharge in pain intensity ($P < .001$), functional disability ($P < .001$), subjective report of limb function ($P < .001$), timed running ($P < .001$), occupational performance ($P < .001$), medication use ($P < .01$), use of assistive devices ($P < .001$), and emotional functioning (anxiety, $P < .001$; depression, $P < .01$), and functional gains were maintained or further improved at follow-up (range 2-24 mo).[69] Treatment consisted of intensive daily physical, occupational, and psychological therapies 8 hours a day, 5 days a week for an average of 3 weeks.[69]

Singh et al.[70] reported on a prospective study of 4 weeks of interdisciplinary management for adult patients with CRPS. The treatment consisted of 20 sessions of PT, 20 sessions of OT, 12 sessions of water therapy, 20 sessions of group psychotherapy, stellate ganglion blocks, and drug therapy that resulted in significantly improved upper limb function for weight tolerance and fine and gross motor skills and physical activity evaluated as maximum isometric force and endurance.[70] The MPQ was administered but does not appear to have been an outcome measure.[70] Results seem to be largely observational. After 2 years, 11 of 12 subjects could be contacted and 9 were employed, 8 had the same or less pain, 4 reported the spread of pain, and 5 reported using opioids.[5]

CRPS remains a difficult pain disorder to treat. Old treatment strategies like desensitization, contrast baths, and stress loading are still referred to in the literature. Newer treatment paradigms such as motor imagery program (MIP) which requires exact sequencing of therapy stages have had significant results in the laboratory but have not translated into real world practice. Mirror therapy alters sensory discrimination but has only short-lived effects on pain. It appears that PEPT significantly improves pain and function in patients with upper and lower limb CRPS and have not been shown to cause harm; however, it is indicated only for end stage patients who have failed available treatments. Children with CRPS show significant response to physical therapy given one or three times per week, but improvement may not be lasting and recurrence of CRPS happens one-half the time and one-third of patients opt for interventional treatment.

PRIMARY FIBROMYALGIA SYNDROME

In the second edition, a physical therapy prescription for primary fibromyalgia syndrome (PFS) included generalized upper and lower limb flexibility and aerobic activity to a heart rate of over 70% predicted maximum.[6] A review of exercise for fibromyalgia by Busch et al.[71] catalogs the self-administered, community-based, and skilled-therapy exercise for fibromyalgia. Exercise regimens applied to treat PFS include stretch, stretching in a warm pool, Pilates, lifestyle exercise, Tai Chi, yoga, aquatic breathing, Nordic walking, vibration boards, aerobics, strengthening combinations of flexibility, aerobics, strengthening, aquatics, and multidisciplinary programs.[71] Nijs recommends "primary care physical therapy" for patients with FMS that includes education, aerobic exercise, and strengthening exercise.[72] Nijs recommends against passive treatments, activity management, and relaxation, citing less evidence supporting use as primary treatment.[72] The search strategy used for this chapter yielded few examples[73-75] of physician-prescribed and physical therapy-supervised exercise for the treatment of fibromyalgia; a secondary literature search of references from the Busch article[71] and others was also undertaken, but few additional examples of PT-supervised exercise for PFS were identified.

Although the descriptions of exercise to treat fibromyalgia in the literature are frequent, the specific trials of skilled PT within the prescriptive authority of a physician are not. It is not clear why skilled therapy does not seem to be used as often, or at least reported in the literature as often, with PFS patients compared to patients with other pain disorders. It is possible that the patients do not select skilled therapy services. The Valencia group commenting on their dropout rate during a stretching trial (25%) postulate that "sometimes, an fibromyalgia patient's idea of how a rehabilitation program should be, or how it is going to affect their pathology, is often a wishful thinking; and their expectations are poorly satisfied."[76] It is possible that the straightforward regimens described, for example walking 45 minutes three times a week or cycling for 60 minutes, do not require the skilled and more expensive attention of a PT. Busch et al.[71] have observed that for patients with PFS, exercises with self-selected intensity appear well tolerated; by contrast, Busch et al. also note that PFS symptoms, like stiffness, may increase or new symptoms, like plantar pain, may emerge if the patient adheres to vigorous and even moderate-intensity exercise.[71] They recommend "supervised programs encouraging PFS participants to perform short bouts of self-selected physical activity" as an initial exercise endeavor, but they then encourage progression to "self-efficacy," "mastery," and "modeling" of exercise for the ongoing management of PFS symptoms through instruction and practiced behavioral techniques.[71] The recent review[71] and Cochrane review[77] by Busch et al are recommended for the physician seeking a detailed discussion of exercise applications for PFS, and caveats for the exercise of PFS patients are provided. If the physician prescribes physical therapy for the treatment of fibromyalgia, aerobic, strengthening, and flexibility exercises may be specified; however, it is best to proceed slowly, to rest and repeat, and to advance weight, duration, or speed of exercise in a slower manner than might be expected for the patient's age. Education about pacing and about carrying over exercise, and discrimination of old symptoms (tender points) from new ones (e.g., plantar fasciitis) or from postexertional myalgia, and about self-treatment with ice or heat should be reviewed. Patients who wish to pursue alternatives like Tai Chi, Nordic walking, yoga, and aquatic- or gym-based offerings do not require prescription and may not be reimbursed by medical insurance, but advice about pacing, proper athletic and foot wear, and exertional myalgia can be offered as counsel.

Valencia et al. evaluated stretching regimens to treat fibromyalgia.[76] Patients were randomized to a program of kinesiotherapy and active muscular stretching (self-administered) or to techniques of Meziere's Global Myofascial Physiotherapy[76] (global stretching postures and manual myofascial and articular mobilization in relation to the patient's respiratory dynamics).[78] Both treatment arms were twice weekly for 150 minutes per week for 12 weeks; with 20 total participants whose average duration of symptoms was 7 years, one-fourth dropped out (3 from control and 2 from Meziere). Both groups achieved a statistically significant reduction in the severity of the disease as measured by fibromyalgia impact questionnaire (FIQ) (**Table 96-6**) during treatment but then significantly worsened in the follow-up period.[76] Regarding tender points, while both groups showed improved counts, only the control group's change was significant; both groups returned to baseline at follow-up (see Table 96-6).[76] Significant improvement in flexibility was demonstrated in both groups during treatment, and significant improvements remained in the Meziere group at follow-up (see Table 96-6).[76] Stretching in either form yielded short-term improvement for number of tender points and disease impact with a notable return to baseline in the intermediate term while short- and intermediate-term effects were noted for flexibility.

Aerobic exercise improves cardiovascular fitness, pain, tender points, function, depression, and quality of life in patients with PFS. Articles about aerobic exercise to treat fibromyalgia largely describe exercise programs administered by trainers or fitness instructors; these personnel are outside the scope of skilled therapy and PM&R. The Hauser meta-analysis of aerobic exercise for fibromyalgia describes 35 studies and notes that aerobic exercise was supervised by a "trainer" in 32 studies.[79] McCain[80] describes cycling three times per week for 60 minutes for 20 weeks to an intensity to sustain elevated heart rate, supervised by "medical fitness instructors," improved pain thresholds of tender points, and improved cardiovascular fitness. Busch et al. conclude that aerobic exercise interventions reduce pain and improve physical fitness, as in the McCain article, and also reduce fatigue and depression and improve health-related quality of life.[71] Thomas similarly concludes that there is moderate evidence that aerobic exercise for the treatment of fibromyalgia improves physical function and possibly improves tender points and pain and benefits the management of PFS.[81] Busch cautions that the dropout rate for subjects in the aerobic exercise arm of studies is double

TABLE 96-6 Effects on Pain and Function of Various Exercise Regimens for Fibromyalgia

	Tender points	FIQ (severe >70)	Sit and reach	Sit, reach 24-wk follow-up
Valencia[7]				
Control	13.3 +/− 2.5 decreased to 10.7 +/− 2.2, $P < .005$	48.9 +/− 10.9 decreased to 28.0 +/− 15.8, $P < .01$	−2.6 +/− 8.2 increased to 5.7 +/− 4.8 at 12 wk, $P < .007$	5.7 +/− 4.8 decreased to 2.8 +/− 5.9
Mezieres stretch	14.8 +/−2.9 decreased to 12.5 +/− 2.7, p <.15	49.4 +/0 11.6 decreased to 38.6 +/− 8.1, $P < .04$	−8.8 +/− 6.7 increased to 1.1 +/− 7.5at 12 wk, $P < .0007$	1.1 +/− 7.5 decreased to −2.2 +/− 7.4, $P < .03$, start to 24 wk $P < .02$
Kingsley[84]	Tender points	FIQ	Myalgic score	
Strengthening BIW	13 +/− 3 decreased to 8 +/− 4	52 +/− 17.5 decreased to 41.6 +/− 15.5	13.3 decreased to 8 +/− 4	
Hakkinen[85] Strengthening	Pain	Neck pain	Depression	
Fibro Exercise	48 +/− 25 decreased to 24 +/− 19 (no P value)	45 +/−19 decreased to 22 +/− 29 , $P < .05$	6.4 =/− 5.1 decreased to 3.6 +/− 3.1, $P < .05$	
Fibro controls	35 +/− 19 increased to 60 +/− 27	56 +/−33 decreased to 51 +/− 35	6.6 +/− 4.9 increased to 7.5 +/− 4.9	
Sanudo[87]	BDI (Beck depression inventory)	FIQ	SF 36	
Aerobic	Improved 8.5 +/− 8, $P < .001$	Improved 8.8+/− 14, $P < .02$	Improved 8.9 +/− 10	
Combination	Improved 6.4 +/−4, $P < .001$	Improved 8.8+/− 12, $P < .02$	Improved 8.4 +/− 11	

(22% vs. 10%) the drop-out rate of control subjects.[71] However, Lemos et al. report that PFS patients who complete an aerobic program can tolerate and be trained within the anaerobic threshold at 75% to 85% of predicted maximum heart rate and predicted using either (208 – [0.7 × age]) or (220 – age).[82] In this study, PFS patients were enrolled in a walking program 45 minutes three times weekly for 20 weeks. No patient drop-out was described.[82] The same work group led by Valim[83] compared the aerobic walking program to a stretching control. Valim et al.[83] reported a drop-out rate of 16 of 76 subjects (20%). Attributes of subjects who dropped out of the study included a higher pain score (29.86 +/− 15.71 drop-out versus 23.5 _+/− 8.57 completing study, $P < .03$) and significantly higher vitality and mental health (MH) on the SF-36 in the dropout group (vitality 48.46 +/− 24.36 dropout vs. 31.18 =/− 18.95 completing study, $P < .007$; MH 56 +/− 23.26 dropout vs. 42.83 +/− 19.19).[83] The aerobic group was superior to stretching for improvement of aerobic capacity, function, depression, pain, and emotional and mental health domains of the SF-36.[83] Aerobic exercise is superior to stretching to improve pain and function in persons with PFS. Patients who do not drop out of an aerobic excise program can be exercised to a target heart rate of 75% of (220 − age). The supervision of a PT is not warranted for the participation in a basic regimen such as timed walking or cycling.

The effect of resistance exercises on fibromyalgia was evaluated by Kingsley in a prospective controlled trial administered in a rheumatology department research.[84] Thirty-minute training sessions twice weekly involved resistance, that is, weight training, of the upper and lower body at an initial intensity set at 50% to 60% of 1RM (one repetition maximum) in weeks 1 to 8 and progressing to 75% to 85% of the 1RM in weeks 8 to 12.[84] Both the control and fibromyalgia women had significant increases in maximal strength ($P < .05$) after strength training. In the fibromyalgia subjects, the number of active tender points, myalgic score, and FIQ score were significantly decreased ($P < .05$)[84] (Table 96-6). Hakkinen studied strength training in premenopausal women with fibromyalgia at an initial intensity of 40% to 60% of 1RM (one repetition maximum) and progressing to 70% to 80% of the 1RM over 21 weeks.[85] Subjects with PFS increased maximal and explosive strength and EMG activity as much as healthy controls, and there were significant immediate benefits on subjectively perceived fatigue, depression, and neck pain of training patients with FM.[85] The study does not indicate that the strengthening program was administered in a therapy setting. A study of similar design of elderly subjects (average 59 yr) showed that older women with fibromyalgia also benefited from strength training.[86] Significant increases in maximal isometric and concentric forces, muscle cross-sectional area, and EMG activity were observed.[86] The strengthening group also reported a significant decrease (16–14) in the number of tender points after strength training but pain, sleep quality, fatigue, and general wellbeing only showed a tendency toward but not a significant decrease.[86] The study does not indicate that the strengthening program was administered in a therapy setting although exercise was "supervised." Strengthening exercise improves pain, tender points, depression, and function in persons with PFS, and the patients can be exercised intensively enough to gain strength. The supervision of a physical examination may not be warranted for the participation in weight-training program.

Sanudo compared and "supervised" a combined aerobic, flexibility and strengthening program (15 min aerobic exercise to HR 70% maximum plus strengthening of 8 muscle groups, 10 repetitions of 1- 3 kg weights) to aerobic exercise (45 min at HR of 60 to 80% maximum) to no exercise.[87] Dropout was 4, 4, and 1 respectively, in groups of 22, 21, and 21 subjects. Improvements in more individual SF-36 domains were observed after the combined intervention with significant improvements in SF-36 Physical Functioning ($P < .003$) and Bodily Pain ($P < .003$) domains and Vitality ($P < .002$) and Mental Health ($P < .04$) domains.[87] Compared to inactive controls, combined exercise and aerobic-only exercise significantly improved total FIQ score from baseline (about 15 5%; $P < .02$) and Beck depression inventory (BDI) scores decreased significantly ($P < .001$, aerobic 8.5 decrease and combined 6.5).[87]

Suman reported on a 3-week intensive residential multidisciplinary treatment program for fibromyalgia patients whose symptoms before treatment were constant.[74] At 1 year subjects still demonstrated improved pain area and intensity and aerobic fitness.[74] The authors' perception is that physical exercise was adopted as a coping strategy for chronic pain acceptance.[74] An outpatient multidisciplinary program by Carbonell-Baeza et al.[75] studied 75 women with fibromyalgia who participated in a 3-month (3 times/week) multidisciplinary (pool, land-based, and psychological session) (n = 41) or to a usual care group (n = 34). Post hoc analysis revealed significant improvements in total score of FIQ ($P < .001$), fatigue ($P < .001$), stiffness ($P < .001$), anxiety ($P < .011$), depression ($P < .008$), physical role ($P < .002$), bodily pain ($P < .001$), vitality ($P < .001$), and social functioning ($P < .001$) in the multidisciplinary group.[75] The control group showed significant worsening in the subscale depression ($P < .006$) and social functioning ($P < .019$).[75] Compared to no treatment, patients in a multidisciplinary treatment show decrease in pain and other symptoms, anxiety and depression, and functioning whereas the control group worsens for mood and function.

Lastly, Mannerkorpi et al. studied of the effects of pool therapy on PFS.[73] One hundred and thirty-four women with fibromyalgia and 32 with chronic widespread pain were randomized to a 20-session pool exercise program supervised by a PT and a six-session education program or to a control group undertaking the same education program.[73] Patients who had participated in at least 60% of the exercise sessions showed significantly improvement ($P < .05$) for the FIQ total and FIQ pain and the 6-minute walk test. Analyses within the subgroups showed that patients with milder stress, pain, or depression improved most by treatment on the FIQ total (effect size >.50, $P < .05$) compared with controls.[73]

In sum, stretching yields short-term improvement for number of tender points and disease impact and intermediate-term improvements to flexibility. Aerobic exercise is superior to stretching to improve pain and function in persons with PFS. Patients who do not drop out of an aerobic excise program can be exercised to a target heart rate of 75% of (220 – age). The supervision of a PT is not warranted for the participation in simple aerobic programs. Strengthening exercise improves pain, tender points, depression and function in persons with PFS, and the patients can be exercised intensively enough to gain strength. The supervision of a physical examination may not be warranted for the participation in weight training program. Variations on the basic exercise types, including combination programs, aquatic version, and multidisciplinary programs, improve pain, function, and mental health.

PELVIC PAIN

Myofascial physical therapy (MPT) for pelvic pain targets internal (pelvic) and external trigger point work, focusing on the muscles and connective tissues of the pelvic floor, hip girdle, and abdomen.[88] Sacroiliac dysfunction (hypermobility) and transverse abdominal muscle weakness may contribute to pelvic floor dysfunction and may be targets of physical therapy interventions.[89] Doggweiler and Stewart[90] review the evaluation and available treatments for chronic pelvic pain. Kavvadias et al.[91] review neurostimulation, physical therapy, oral agents and hydrodistension, and intravesical instillations for the treatment of females with pelvic pain. Cox and Neville[92] detail the physical therapy strategies for vulvodynia:

"Myofascial release and connective tissue massage performed on the inner thighs, labia majora, perineum, superficial genital muscles, and associated trunk, abdominal, and hip muscles;

Trigger point release performed on the levator ani, superficial genital muscles, and obturator internus muscles intravaginally or intrarectally and on associated trunk, abdominal, and hip muscles;

Visceral mobilization Improve mobility and motility of bladder and urethra and neural mobilization to improve mobility of the pudendal nerve at Alcock canal."

PTs who do pelvic myofascial work may seek a certificate of achievement as well as postgraduate offerings in this specific therapy application.

Patients who seek physical therapy treatment for pelvic floor dysfunction are primarily were female (92%), younger than 65 years of age, and with symptoms present longer than 90 days.[93] Urinary problems were reported two-thirds of the time, 25% had bowel problems, and 39% had pelvic pain.[93] Bladder and bowel problems included leakage and constipation.[93] About one-third had the constellation of all three problems (bowel, bladder, and pain).[93]

FitzGerald et al. studied 47 patients (23 men, 24 women) with chronic prostatitis/chronic pelvic pain syndrome (CP/CPPS) or interstitial cystitis/painful bladder syndrome (IC/PBS) who were randomized to global therapeutic massage (GTM) or myofascial physical therapy (MPT). Forty-four patients (94%) completed the study.[88] MPT treatment targets internal (pelvic) and external trigger point work, focusing on the muscles and connective tissues of the pelvic floor, hip girdle, and abdomen whereas GTM is a nonspecific somatic treatment with full-body Western massage and was included as a comparison treatment arm.[88] Patients were scheduled for 10 weekly treatments of 1 hour each; 87% of patients received at least 7 treatments. For home practice, the patients were instructed in a double voiding maneuver to improve pelvic proprioceptive awareness and drop the pelvic floor. The main outcome measure, global response assessment (markedly or moderately improved), was significantly higher (57%, 13 subjects) in the myofascial physical therapy group than the rate of 21% (5 subjects) in the global therapeutic massage treatment group ($P < .03$).[88] Five (21%) patients in the GTM group and 12 (52%) patients in the MPT group reported adverse events, primarily increased pain by 14 (30%) subject.[86] Three adverse events for pain were rated as severe (1 in GTM group and 2 in MPT group).[88] Other adverse events were arrhythmia, infection, and constitutional symptom.[86] Of note a significant difference of response to GTM was noted between the IC/PBS group and CP/CPPS group since many patients with CP/CPPS responded to GTM with improved domains of pain, quality of life, and ICSI (O'Leary-Sant IC Symptom Index) ($P < .05$).[88] One IC/PBS patient responded to GTM. In the IC/PBS group, pain, urinary urgency and frequency MPT significantly decreased (all 11 point scales) on average from about 7 +/−2.0 to 4 +/− 2.5. The IC symptom index, IC problem index, and female sexual health index also significantly improved.[88] Different pain and urinary symptom scales were used in the CP/CPPS group (21-point pain scale and 10-point urinary scale from NIH-CPSI), but pain decreased from 14 +/− 2.5 to 8 +/− 5.7 and the urinary scale decreased from 8.9 +/−1.4 to 5 +/− 2.8.[88] (**Table 96-7**) Tenderness of the anterior and posterior levator, and obturator internus but not the urogenital diaphragm was significantly decreased by MPT but not by GTM in both IC and CP patients.[88] The appendix of exclusion criteria for this study is extensive and includes pregnancy, active infection including prostatitis or urinary, calculi, painful lower abdominal scars, unilateral orchialgia, pelvic mass or suspicious prostate, etc.

Anderson et al. used a different study design to evaluate the effectiveness of MPT for pelvic pain in 200 men who had had pain for an average of 4.8 years, average age 47 years.[94] Male urologic pain syndromes include interstitial cystitis, isolated testicular pain, pudendal neuralgia, and levator ani syndrome.[94] Male subjects who had failed traditional therapies for chronic pelvic pain were recruited for a 6-day intensive (immersion) treatment protocol including training of participants in self-treatment of intrapelvic and extrapelvic myofascial trigger point release therapy, and training in paradoxical relaxation including some cognitive behavioral methods.[94] The therapy method was detailed:

"For 5 consecutive days the same PT performed myofascial trigger point release and trained patients in the self-administration of the method. This consisted of placing the patient in a semilateral, prone position with pillows under the abdomen after external abdominal and pelvic muscles had been examined. Using a gloved finger the sphincter ani, internal posterior and anterior pelvic muscles were examined, turning the patient as necessary. A traditional palpation force of approximately 4 kg/cm2 for tender points (recommended for examination of fibromyalgia) was used for the assessment of pain. The therapist treated individual muscle groups and released TrPs with applied pressure (details have been previously described). Therapy was delivered in 30 to 60-minute sessions each day, and patients were also instructed how to stretch and enhance relief of muscle tension."[94]

Outcome measures were National Institutes of Health Chronic Prostatitis Symptom Index (NIH-CPSI), global response assessment, and a psychological query.[94] At 6 months 116 patients (about 60% of 200 self-referrals) were included in the data assessment. Global response assessment (the same primary outcome as the Fitzgerald trial[88]) showed that 60% reported marked to moderate improvement.[94] Symptom index scores decreased by 30% (average score 26 +/− 4 decreased to 19 +/− 6, maximal possible score 43) ($P < .001$) at follow-up. (see Table 96-7) For comparison in the FitzGerald trial[88] NIH-CPSI decreased on average from 33.5 +/− 4.3 to 19 +/− 11.1 ($P < .003$). Domains of pain (decreased from 12 to 9), urinary dysfunction (decreased from 4 to 2), and quality of life showed significant improvement ($P < .001$).[94]

Patients with urologic chronic pelvic pain syndrome (UCPPS) who referred themselves for an intensive 6-day PT and relaxation therapy

TABLE 96-7 Effects on Pain and Function of Myofascial Physical Therapy for IC/PBS and CP/CPPS

	Pain IC/PBS	Urinary Urgency IC/PBS	Urinary frequency/ IC/PBS	Anterior levator tenderness	Posterior levator tenderness	Obturator internus tenderness
FitzGerald[8]						
MTP	6.8 +/− 1.4 decreased to 4.2 +/− 2.9, $P < .005$	6.8 +/− 1.4 decreased to 4.0 +/− 2.7, $P < .01$	7.2 +/− 1.4 decreased to 3.5 +/− 2.5, $P < .003$	3.62 decreased to 2.0, $P < .003$	3.83 decreased to 2.0, $P < .09$	3.17 decreased to 1.73, $P < .001$
GTM	6.7 +/− 1.6 decreased to 5.9 +/− 2.0, $P < .09$	6.7 +/− 2.0 decreased to 6.3 +/− 2.5, $P < .26$	7.6 +/− 1.7 decreased to 6.8 +/− 1.8 $P < .09$	3.21 decreased to 2.75, $P < .64$	3.29 decreased to 2.42, $P < .12$	3.07 decreased to 2.3, $P < .10$
	Pain CP/CPPS	Urinary CP/CPPS				
MTP	14.2 +/− 2.5 decreased to 8.0 +/−5.7, $P < .0007$	8.9 +/− 1.4 decreased to 5.0 +/− 2.8, $P < .002$		3.72 decreased to 1.64, $P < .003$	2.45 decreased to 1.27, $P < .09$	2.36 decreased to 0.55, $P < .001$
GTM	12.7 +/− 2.8 decreased to 8.2 +/− 5.6, $P < .39$	4.6 +/− 2.7 decreased to 3.9 +/− 2.4, $P < .007$		3.1 decreased to 2.0, $P < .02$	2.9 decreased to 0.78, $P < .001$	2.6 decreased to 1.11, $P < .13$
Anderson[94]	Pain CP/CPPS	Urinary CP/CPPS				
	12 decreased to 9, $P < .001$	4 decreased to 2, $P < .001$				
Goldfinger[96]	Pain	Pain threshhold				
	5.23 +/− 2.05 decreased to 2.06 +/− 1.67, $P < .01$	49.46 +/− 78.32 improved to 134.61 +/− 153.19, $P < .05$				

program were invited to participate in a study to evaluate the safety of a personal wand that enables a patient's self-treatment of internal myofascial trigger points in the pelvic floor.[95] The Anderson group is from the same facility; the patients may overlap from the preceding study: Enrollment in the preceding study was from 2004 to 2009[94] and, in this study, 2008 to 2009.[95] The average age of patients was 41 years, and 93% were men.[95] Baseline median sensitivity VAS score (1 to 10, 10 = most sensitive) was 7.5 and decreased significantly at 6 months to 4 ($P < .001$).[95] Most patients (95.5%) reported the wand as very or moderately effective in alleviating pain.[95] No serious adverse events occurred; 44 of 157 patients withdrew from the study but not because of adverse events.[95]

Pelvic floor physical therapy has also been shown in provoked vestibulodynia (PVD), the most common form of chronic vulvar pain, to significantly increase vestibular pain thresholds and significantly lower pain ratings during the gynecologic examination and during intercourse.[96] Goldfinger[96] studied 13 patients with PVD. The treatment protocol describes eight treatment sessions of 60 to 75 minutes each. The sessions began with a discussion of interim pain and exercise adherence, followed by a series of intravaginal manual techniques (e.g., trigger point release, massage) carried out by the PT that progressed over the course of the treatment program (e.g., progressed from one to two fingers, more pressure applied), and then biofeedback with practiced exercises, and progressive dilation occurred.[96] The subjects' mental health did not improve significantly; however, pain catastrophizing and pain-related anxiety significantly decreased.[96] Vestibular pain significantly decreased from 5.23 +/− 2.05 to 2.06 +/− 1.67, ($P < .01$) and point tenderness significantly decreased[96] (see Table 96-7).

The use of devices at home or during therapy in the treatment of pelvic pain is described above. Additionally, a trial of TENS on 24 patients with chronic prostatitis revealed a significant effect of TENS on chronic prostatitis pain ($P < .05$).[97]

Male and female patients with chronic pelvic pain respond moderately to markedly to MPT over half the time, and pain, tenderness, and urinary symptoms significantly decreased; a thorough review of systems should occur prior to prescribing this therapy to determine there are no contraindications. Devices and techniques to use at home are available.

TEMPOROMANDIBULAR JOINT DYSFUNCTION AND HEADACHE PAIN

PM&R strategies have been described to treat temporomandibular joint pain, tension headache, and myofascial facial pain. Treatment regimens utilize oral appliances, stretching and relaxing exercises, and thermal modalities.

Cuccia et al.[98] compared osteopathic manipulation to conventional physical therapy for the treatment of temporo-mandibular joint dysfunction (TMJD). One group was treated with specific manipulative procedures performed by an osteopath, and a second group with conventional treatment by a physiotherapist with an oral appliance, physical therapy (gentle muscle stretching and relaxing exercises), thermal therapies such as hot or cold packs (or both), and TENS.[98] Patients were treated every 2 weeks for 24 weeks. After treatment the use of medication was greater in the conventional therapy group (14 using medication) than in the osteopathic group (6 using medication); however, both treatments led to significantly decreased pain. The osteopathic treatment significantly increased mouth opening range.[98] The authors concluded that both osteopathic manipulation and conventional physical therapy stretching, relaxation, and modalities improved TMJD symptoms during the 6-month trial.[98]

Soderberg et al. compared strength training for neck flexion, shoulder elevation, arm row, arm extension, and latissimus pull down to acupuncture with specified insertions to relaxation training to improve central nervous system symptoms (e.g., tranquility, self-confidence, mental fatigue, concentration, and quality of sleep) in chronic tension headache in 90 patients.[99] Sessions were conducted weekly for 8 to 10 weeks.[99] The outcome measure was the minor symptom evaluation profile (MSEP), which was significantly improved in the physical training group compared with the acupuncture group at 2 months ($P < .036$).[99] No significant difference was found among the three treatment groups at baseline or immediately after treatment. At 3-month follow-up the physical training group had significantly better MSEP score that the acupuncture and relaxation group, and improvement continued to 6-month follow-up.[99] On specific subscales of vitality and sleep both were significantly better at 6 months in the relaxation group compared to the acupuncture and exercise groups ($P < .04$). The authors conclude that moderate physical training has a long-lasting positive effect on collective central nervous system symptoms of chronic tension headache; however, relaxation training specifically affords long-term improvement in vitality and sleep in patients with chronic tension headache.

Doepel et al. concluded that effectiveness of the prefabricated appliance is similar to that of the stabilization appliance in the long term in treating patients with myofascial pain.[100]

The use of prefabricated or stabilization oral appliances is effective in the treatment of myofascial facial pain. Eighty-one percent of patients with a prefabricated appliance improved to "better" to "symptom-free" and 64% in the group with stabilization appliances.[100] At the 12-month follow-up, graded chronic pain, functional limitation of the jaw, nonspecific physical symptoms, and depression showed statistically significant reduction at 12-month follow-up in both groups.[100]

BACK PAIN

In the second edition,[6] sample physical therapy prescriptions were suggested for:

- Axial low back pain (LBP) (back education, flexibility, flexion bias, e.g., "crunch" strengthening)
- Spondylolisthesis (similar)
- Radicular LBP (back education, flexion or extension bias exercise to centralize pain)
- Exercise after laminotomy (exercise regimens discussed began 1 year after surgery)
- Discectomy (variable, from no restrictions, to walking and passive ROM, to leg strengthening)
- Osteoporotic compression fracture (education, bracing as needed, thoracic extension, and scapular stabilization).

The search strategy for this chapter identified 100 articles concerning PM&R and physical therapy applications for LBP. There is no therapy regimen, temporal phase, or specific diagnosis in the catchment of LBP that is the agreed upon gold standard comparator in clinical trials.[101] Comprehensive reviews, PM&R applications, and LBP include Cochrane reviews of exercise for LBP,[102] back schools,[103] multidisciplinary programs for LBP,[104] exercise after lumbar surgery,[105] and TENS for LBP;[106] review articles of lumbar stabilization exercises,[107] general physical activity and other life style modifications,[9] lumbar extension,[21] McKenzie exercises,[13] and TENS and other modalities;[108] and reviews of the treatment of LBP[109] by the Philadelphia panel.[110]

A number of exercise techniques have been proffered and trialed in the literature for the treatment of LBP.[21]

- Activity as usual (sometimes a control group)
- Community-based commercial offerings (e.g., Pilates, Tai Chi)
- Aerobic (repetitive movement of large muscle groups to achieve locomotion usually to a target heart rate)
- Aquatic (pool activities to achieve unweighting of painful limbs, resistance with "buoyant weights" or difficult end-of-range motion aided by buoyancy)
- Directional preference (e.g., McKenzie)
- Flexibility (e.g., yoga)
- Proprioceptive/coordination (e.g., wobble board, stability ball)

Stabilization (e.g., low-load isometric or restricted ROM exercise targeting abdominal and spinal trunk muscles)

Strengthening (e.g., lifting weights or progressive resistive exercises)

Lumbar extensor strengthening (e.g., "Roman chairs" targeting the lumbar erector spinae and multifidus)

Back school and multidisciplinary programs.

The European guidelines for the management of nonspecific CLBP note that the "active ingredient" of exercise programs is unknown;[111] however, the guidelines recommend supervised exercise and back schools as well as brief educational interventions and multidisciplinary (biopsychosocial) treatment for the condition of nonspecific chronic low back pain (CLBP).[111] Van Middelkoop et al. commented that no type of exercise has been shown to be more effective than others and subtypes of LBP or patients with specific attributes may respond differently to various exercise therapies, but the correct match of patient with exercise is not known.[112] Van Middelkoop et al. observe that adherence to exercise prescription is usually poor, so supervision by a therapist is recommended."[112] This said, therapy cannot and should not continue indefinitely. The goal of a therapy program should be transition to a home exercise program.

Therapy benefits should not be squandered; in 2012 in the Unites States, CMS capped outpatient therapy services at $1880 per annum; this equates to probably 10 to 14 visits to achieve specified therapeutic goals for your patient.[113] Useful information regarding costs and coverage as well as benefits and harms of physical activity for LBP were found.[3,9,13,21,107,108,114] Uniquely, this series of articles in *The Spine Journal* discusses coding and reimbursement for the skilled-therapy exercise programs and this information may be useful when discussing options with patients.

Quality reviews about nonspecific exercise programs for LBP and their outcomes were found. A Cochrane review concludes that exercise chronic LBP is slightly effective for reducing pain and increasing function and that in subacute back pain there is some evidence of effectiveness of graded-activity exercises.[102] In acute LBP, exercise was not better than no treatment or other conservative measures.[102] More positively, the Wai review[9] reported moderate benefit for aerobic, strengthening, or water exercise versus no activity to reduce disability, and improve pain in low back conditions.[9] Wai et al. reported limited evidence supporting home aerobics to improve worst pain, medication use, work status, and mood.[9] No harm of exercise was found.[9]

The Spine Journal series of articles on lumbar extension exercise,[21] McKenzie method,[13] and lumbar stabilization[107] provide an opportunity to compare the features, outcomes, and risks of these different exercise methods and are highly recommended for perusal. Specific studies of **lumbar extension exercises** with both active and wait listed controls demonstrated significant benefits in the short term (3–6 mo) for endpoints including lumbar extensor strength and cross sectional area, pain, disability, physical impairment, and psychosocial function.[21] The cited literature demonstrates no clear benefit of lumbar extensor strengthening exercises compared with other exercise programs.[21] Potential harms of extension exercises include delayed onset muscle soreness, and rare complications such as fracture or disc herniation.[21] May's article in *The Spine Journal* reviews the McKenzie method is an approach to CLBP that includes an assessment and an intervention component.[13] The assessment component of the McKenzie method, also called mechanical diagnosis and therapy (MDT), attempts the assessment of a pattern of pain response called "centralization," which refers to the decrease or eradication of radiating symptoms of a back pain complaint in response to a single direction—"directional preference"—of repeated movements or sustained postures.[13] Side effects or adverse events to the McKenzie method have not been documented, but May et al. note that, as a clinical assessment method, failure to alter symptom distribution (non-centralization) predicts negative outcomes and poor behavioral responses to back pain.[13] The Standaert article[107] on **lumbar stabilization exercises**, also called core stabilization, motor control exercises, or segmental stabilization, has a therapeutic goal of improving the neuromuscular control, strength, and endurance of muscles central to maintaining dynamic spinal and trunk stability, including the transversus abdominis (TrA), lumbar multifidi, and regional musculature from the diaphragm to pelvis and paraspinals to abdominals. Andrusaitis[115] explains that the term "stabilization," based on co-contraction of the abdominal and multifidus muscles, is a generalization describing any type of exercise that challenges the stability of the spine while training muscle activity patterns in a variety of positions and postures that ensure sufficient stability without unnecessarily overloading tissue. Standaert et al. note trials comparing general exercise to lumbar stabilization; both yield significant improvements in function, pain, and quality of life over baseline, and there were no significant differences between groups and no additional benefit of lumbar stabilization.[107] No serious harms result from lumbar stabilization exercise, but the authors are careful to note that exclusion criteria in studies listed patients "felt to be unfit for physical therapy treatment" including subjects with fracture, Grade III or IV spondylolisthesis, malignancy, inflammatory arthropathies, pregnancy, significant neurological loss," and other unstable medical conditions and prior spine surgery.[107] A review of exercise to evaluate the duration of benefit found that trials which reported on pain scales at 6-month follow-up found significant differences in favor of exercise.[116]

The Cochrane reviews and *The Spine Journal* articles on back schools,[103,114] functional restoration,[3] and multidisciplinary programs[104] provide an opportunity to compare the features, outcomes, and risks and are highly recommended for perusal. Back school is a Swedish concept from 1969 that initially instructed participants how to protect spinal structures in daily activities but later added exercises for the back.[103,114] Back school involves **group** education about fear-avoidance and kinesiophobia and exercise, delivered in an occupational setting or as part of a multidisciplinary rehabilitation program.[114] The Cochrane review on back school[103] concluded that moderate evidence suggests that back schools, in an occupational setting and when compared with exercises, passive therapies, or wait list, improve function and return to work for patients with chronic and recurrent LBP status in the short and intermediate term. Brox et al. concluded evidence for back school was too conflicted to recommend it as an intervention.[114] While back school started as an educational strategy that evolved to add an exercise component, multidisciplinary programs consist of a physician consultation as well as at least one additional psychosocial or vocational evaluation and intervention. A Cochrane review of multidisciplinary programs[104] concluded that moderate evidence of positive effectiveness of multidisciplinary rehabilitation for subacute LBP exists and that a workplace visit increases the effectiveness. The same Cochrane review characterized multidisciplinary programs as an inpatient or outpatient rehabilitation program that consisted of a physician's consultation plus either a psychological, social, or vocational intervention or a combination of these.[104] Functional restoration is a more complex treatment that addresses the biopsychosocial complexity of chronic LBP that is disabling. Functional restoration that is metric and outcome focused distinguishes itself from back school, which is on the surface task-defined, and multidisciplinary programs which on the surface are personnel defined. Developed and described by Gatchel and Mayer in the 1990s, components of functional restoration include:

1. "formal, repeated quantification of physical deficits to guide, individualize, and monitor physical training progress;
2. psychosocial and socioeconomic assessment to guide, individualize, and monitor pain, disability, behavior and outcomes;
3. multimodal disability management programs using cognitive-behavioral therapy approaches;
4. psychopharmacological interventions for any required detoxification and psychosocial management;
5. ongoing outcome assessment using standardized outcome criteria and objective data collection through structured interviews; and
6. interdisciplinary, medically directed team approach with formal staff meetings and frequent conferences."[3]

Differing from other treatment approaches, functional restoration has been shown to prevent chronic disability for persons with LBP compared to usual treatment and also to have a long-term effect that other interventions lack. Bendix et al.[117] note "functional restoration" programs for the treatment of LBP may have a full-day schedule lasting 3 to 6 weeks. Bendix et al.[117] explain that personnel are multidisciplinary and patients are treated in groups with "intensive physical and ergonomic training, psychological pain management, back school, and instruction in social- and work-related issues," including "acceptance of the pain, activity, and self-responsibility," and quantitative functional evaluation "to make participants aware of physical improvement." Gatchel et al.[3] report patients with acute LBP at risk for chronicity were enrolled in a functional restoration program (FRP) and, compared to "usual treatment," (UT) at one year were significantly more likely to return to work (91% vs. 69%, P 0.027), utilized about half as much health care (12 visits vs. 25, $P < .004$) and medication (27% vs. 43%, $P < .02$) , and had less self-reported pain (VAS 26 vs. 43, $P < .001$)."[118] If lost wages related to sick days ($7K FRP vs. $18.9 K UT) are included in costs, FRP treatment (program $3.8K plus health care and medication and lost wages = $12.7K) is about 60% of the cost of no treatment ($21.8K).

Systematic reviews of therapeutic modalities for the treatment of pain were reviewed. For treatment of CLBP a recent Cochrane review concluded the evidence was conflicting about whether TENS was beneficial in reducing back pain intensity.[106] TENS was not shown to improve back-specific functional status, work status, or the use of medical or the Sickness Impact Profile.[106] The Poitras article in *The Spine Journal* also concluded there is little evidence to support the use of TENS in LBP.[108] He concluded TENS does not appear to have an impact on perceived disability or long-term pain.[108] Skin irritation and even burns are possible with TENS with inappropriate electrode placement.[108]

STRETCH

Stretch and flexibility are the first steps in an exercise program and prevent injury to soft tissue.[6] Slow sustained stretch held 60 seconds is optimal.[6] The new implantation of subcutaneous portions of stimulators or implanted pumps may be a contraindication for a time specified by the implanting physician. No peer reviewed literature was found regarding activity restriction after the implantation of spinal cord stimulators. Recommendations to avoid lifting, bending, and twisting for 6 to 8 weeks after implantation to allow the tract site to scar down was found searching the internet for "patient information" or "restrictions" after the procedure.[119]

The conservative treatment includes flexibility exercises, especially of the hamstrings. The rationale is that hamstring tightness during tasks of lumbar flexion restricts motion and introduces shear among the vertebral segments and risk for injury.[120] Johnson et al. evaluated hamstring flexibility and hip and lumbar joint excursions during forward-bending tasks in persons with LBP compared to persons recovered from LBP, but no significant correlation was found.[120] The authors conclude that hamstring flexibility is not strongly related to the amount of lumbar flexion used to perform forward-reaching tasks in participants who have chronic LBP or who have recovered from LBP.[120] Halbertsma's work demonstrates no change in the length or elasticity of hamstrings occurs with applied stretch but stretching increases tolerance of the activity.[14] Stretching has been shown to reduce pain at least briefly.[15] However, how stretching helps pain is not clear and seems to be more complex than the presumed rationale of tissue distension or improved lumbar mechanics.

WALKING AND AEROBIC EXERCISE

Walking is a basic human ability requiring no equipment other than appropriate clothing and comfortable footwear. It does not require the supervision of a physiotherapist. Unless performed briskly enough to elevate heart rate to 70% of maximal predicted heart rate, it does not constitute aerobic exercise. However, even at a slow pace, if continued for 30 minutes five times per week aerobic exercise has shown benefits to bone density.[121] Walking is simple and in the spectrum of treatments for the individual suffering with LBP, walking (similar to stretch) has been shown to lessen pain following the activity and in combination with other treatments.[122] Hendrick et al.[122] systematically reviewed the literature comparing walking to exercise or physiotherapy for the relief of back pain and cited four articles comparing preferred speed walking to fast walking, vertical traction (VT) alone to VT plus walking, exercise versus thermal modalities, and traction versus walking and core stabilization versus supported walking. Hendrick et al. report that preferred walking speed significantly relieved pain ($P < .02$) and fast walking did not; VT plus walking and VT alone relieved pain but the combined program was significantly better, but in the other three-arm study with an exercise arm and a traction and modalities arm, both relieve pain significantly better compared to walking. Lastly stabilization exercise with supported walking had a notable dropout rate at 45% but pain decreased in 50% of patients completing the study and function improved in 80%. No study found walking to be detrimental, but it is probably complementary at best.[122] Compared to interventions with higher costs or burdens of travel, expense, or personnel, walking may not be as effective at relieving pain; however, for its simplicity, walking as a start in the spectrum of treatments for LBP has an initial economical and uncomplicated place.

One study, Chan et al.,[123] found aerobic exercise to be administered under the supervision of a PT, that is, within the context of PM&R. Other studies were found in which subjects performed aerobic exercise in a fitness center or individually, but these settings are outside this chapter's inclusion criteria. Compared to conventional physiotherapy (modalities, mobilization, stabilization exercise, and education for 8 weeks), the addition of aerobic exercise (starting at 40% of predicted heart rate and progressing to 85% over 8 weeks) to conventional treatment shows a significant decrease in pain and disability at 2 and 12 months in both groups, with no significant difference between groups.[123] Conventional therapy alone and aerobic plus conventional therapy both significantly improve pain reports.[123] For clinical applications, if the individual patient has specific aerobic conditioning goals, an aerobic prescription might be added to the usual prescription for strengthening and education but will not further improve pain.

CORE STABILIZATION, MOTOR CONTROL EXERCISES, SEGMENTAL STABILIZATION, AND LUMBAR STABILIZATION

Core stabilization, as a strengthening strategy, is known by a variety of terms and targets the transversus abdominis, and multifidi as well as abdominal muscles, paraspinals and pelvic girdle muscles. The deepest abdominal muscle, transversus abdominis, interacting with the lumbar fascia is believed to contribute to lumbar stability and vertebral constraint.[124] Altered timing and changes in muscle contraction thickness and slide in the deep abdominal muscles has been found in LBP patients.[124] The significance and contribution of the excursion and timing of the transversus abdominis in dynamic tasks in patients with LBP is debated.[125,126]

Some studies have found that improvement in these measurements after core stabilization exercise parallels improved pain reports in patients with LBP. Unsgaard-Tondel et al.[124] report that transversus abdominis lateral slide (excursion of the muscle border between rest and contraction as determined on ultrasonography) that was low at baseline improves after an 8-week exercise program and is associated with a VAS improvement of 2 or greater ("clinically important pain reduction") through 1 year follow-up compared to participants with small baseline slide and no improvement in slide. They did not find a correlation with muscle thickness, which was also measured, but Ferriera et al did.[126]

Ferreira et al. compared three supervised therapy regimens, motor control (core stabilization exercise versus general exercise versus manipulative therapy, found that subjects with chronic LBP who received motor control exercise had a greater improvement in recruitment (as measured by increased thickness on ultrasonography) of transversus abdominis (7.8%) than participants receiving general exercise

(4.9% reduction) or spinal manipulative therapy (3.7% reduction).[126] Similar to Unsgaard-Tondel in which poor performers who improved had better pain relief, Ferreira et al. observed that the effect on pain reduction was greater in motor-control participants who had a poor ability to recruit transversus abdominis at baseline.[126] There was a significant, moderate correlation between improved recruitment of transversus abdominis and a reduction in disability.[126] A third study showed no correlation with deep abdominal muscle function (as measured by thickness on ultrasound) and exercise although subjects improved clinically.[127] Mannion et al. observe that although significant improvements in pain and disability occurred after a 9-week physiotherapy program of stabilization exercises (once a week with therapist and daily home exercise), neither baseline transversus abdominis (TrA) muscle function nor its improvement after the exercise intervention was a statistical predictor of a good clinical outcome.[127]

Improved outcome measures include a decreased disability (Roland Morris, RM) score from 8.9 ± 4.7 to 6.7 ± 4.3 (P <.01), and decreased pain from 4.7 ± 1.7 to 3.5 ± 2.3 (P <.01), increased voluntary activation of the TrA by 4.5% (P <.045).[127] The authors report, but not available in tablature, that changes only, presumably improvements, in catastrophizing (P <.003) and in fingertip-to-floor distance (P <.006) explain the variance in the improved RM scores.[127]

While excursion and thickness of the deep abdominal muscles may show a relation to pain, the onset of firing of the muscle group during standardized dynamic tasks does not. Additionally, although exercise shows an ability to improve "muscle slide" and thickness, exercise does not affect the onset of firing relative to other muscles during a standardized task. Vasselgen et al.[128] used arm swing as a proxy for testing lumbar stability dynamically. Comparing low-load core strengthening to high-load sling exercise and to general exercise, the group reports that abdominal muscle onset in coordination with an arm swing task was largely unaffected by any 8-week strengthening program, and there was no association between change in faster or slower onset of firing of the transversus abdominis and arm movement and LBP.[128]

The multifidi are believed to be strengthened both by core strengthening and by lumbar extension strengthening strategies. Chan et al.[129] have observed that the multifidus, as measured by ultrasonography methods, is stiffer, smaller, and possesses higher fat content in chronic LBP patients compared to asymptomatic controls. Different multifidus cross-sectional area were identified in relation to upright compared to lumbar flexed postures in both normals and subjects with LBP having smaller cross-sectional areas in all positions.[129] Beneck et al. report that even active persons with LBP when compared to active pain-free controls showed considerable localized, bilateral multifidus atrophy.[130] The authors hypothesize that impaired size of the multifidus reduces its capacity to control intersegmental motion and increases susceptibility to further injury.[130] A poor ability to contract multifidus was related to poor transversus abdominis contraction.[131] Changes in the firing pattern of other muscles in persons with LBP has been noted. Higher activation of global and lower activation of local abdominal muscles in patients with CLBP has been noted, and the authors interpret this as a pain-related change to neuromuscular control, with the increased activity of extensor muscles during trunk flexion contributing to stability and controlling flexion.[132]

Andrusaitis et al.[117] studied the effect of stabilization exercises versus general strengthening of the abdominals and pelvic and back muscles or versus normal volunteers assessed at baseline for 40-minute sessions three times weekly for 5 weeks. The stabilization group demonstrated significant reductions in both pain intensity (VAS decreased from 5.08 to 0.23, P <.043) and pain frequency (VAS decreased from 6.19 to 2.09, P <.043) and disability (measured by the Oswestry Disability Questionnaire [ODQ], decreased from 11.8 to 3.4) (P <.05) after the treatment while the strengthening group did not show any significant changes (pain intensity 4.83 decreased to 3.59, intensity from 8.74 to 5.31, and Oswestry 19.8 decreased to 18.2, P >.05).[117] Kumar et al.[133] compared stabilization exercises versus general strengthening and had similar results showing certain functional activities and pain were significantly (P <.01) improved with stabilization more than with strength training, and rate of improvement was significantly (P <.01) higher in the stabilization group. Franca et al. evaluated 30-minute sessions twice weekly for 6 weeks, showing similar results.[134] Franca et al.[134] compared segmental stabilization, with exercises targeting the transversus abdominis and lumbar multifidus muscles, versus superficial strengthening, with exercises targeting the rectus abdominis, abdominus obliquus internus, abdominus obliquus externus, and erector spinae. Outcome measures included pain (VAS and MPQ), functional disability, ODQ, and transversus abdominis muscle activation capacity (pressure biofeedback unit [PBU]). Both treatments were effective in relieving pain and improving disability (P <.001), but the segmental stabilization group had significant gains for all variables when compared to the standard exercise group (P <.001).[134] From a perspective of not only efficacy but also cost, Critchley et al.[135] compared stabilization exercises versus general strengthening versus PT-led pain management education were found to significantly reduce disability [Roland Disability Questionnaire score improved from 11.1 (9.6–12.6) to 6.9 (5.3–8.4) with usual outpatient physiotherapy, 12.8 (11.4–14.2) to 6.8 (4.9–8.6) with spinal stabilization, and 11.5 (9.8–13.1) and to 6.5 (4.5–8.6) following pain management classes]; and also reduce pain and time off work, improve quality of life.[135] In this cost analysis study, PT-led pain management was the most cost effective intervention (£165 [British pounds]); the stabilization was just over twice as expensive (£379), and the individual strengthening physiotherapy almost three times as expensive (£474).[135]

Compared to graded exercise, motor control (stabilization) exercises showed no significant difference at 2, 6, and 12 months for pain over the previous week (numeric rating scale) and function (Patient-Specific Functional Scale) or disability (24-item Roland-Morris Disability Questionnaire), global impression of change (Global Perceived Effect Scale), and quality of life (36-Item Short-Form Health Survey questionnaire [SF-36] in a study by Macedo.[136] The outcome measures improved in both treatment groups: Pain Numeric rating decreased from 6.1 to 3.7 in both groups at 12 months; function (Patient-Specific Functional Scale) improved from about 3.6 to about 6.0 in both groups; and disability (Roland Morris Disability Questionnaire (RMDQ) decreased from about 11.3 to 8.0 in the Graded exercise group and 7.4 in the motor control group.[136] Additionally the authors provide a useful comparison of the two exercise approaches.[136] The authors explain **graded activity** as time contingent, paced progressive exercises that aim to reduce pain and disability by addressing pain-related fear, kinesiophobia, and unhelpful beliefs and behaviors about back pain while correcting physical impairments such as reduced endurance, muscle strength, or balance, whereas **motor control exercises** are general and focal strengthening exercises focused on correcting the activation of muscles and motor patterns and on the correction of posture and coordination.[136] Adverse effects included temporary exacerbation of pain (27 of 176), increased pain of preexisting musculoskeletal condition such as knee arthritis (n = 7), development of shin splints (n = 1), and hip bursitis.[136]

Compared with an educational booklet or manual therapy, stabilization exercises have been shown to be significantly better at improving pain and dysfunction at 6 months and, at 1 year, reduction in medication usage, dysfunction, and disability (Oswestry).[137] Another study comparing sham modalities to motor control exercises demonstrated improved activity and patient's global impression of recovery in the motor control group, but this did not clearly reduce pain at 2 months.[138]

Motor control or core stabilization exercises are believed to strengthen, and increase excursion and hypertrophy deep abdominal flexors including the transversus abdominis and multifidus through low load, limited excursion strengthening exercises of the trunk. Pain and disability have variably been shown to correlate with improvements in these physiologic outcomes. Studies have not clearly shown a relationship with pain or dynamic coordination with other muscle groups in studies of arm swing. Motor control core stabilization exercises have been shown in several studies to be superior to general exercise regimens for pain and disability outcomes and on a par in one study. Motor control exercises were as effective as graded exercise to improve function, pain, and disability and superior to written educational materials or manual therapy alone. Adverse effects are not reported for the most part but when reported seem to be minor.

GENERAL EXERCISE AND STRENGTHENING REGIMENS

Nassif et al.[139] evaluated assembly line workers with chronic LBP doing 60-minute sessions of muscle strengthening, flexibility, and endurance training with a physiotherapist in an occupational environment performed three times per week during 2 months. A significant beneficial effect (*P* <.025) for the experimental group at 2 months (program end) was observed in pain parameters (numerical rating scale (NRS) decreased from 4.54 to 2.76, *P* <.001), specific flexibility tests, and back function and disability (Tampa Scale of Kinesiology decreased from 46.71 to 41.59, *P* <.001; RMDQ decreased from 13.91 to 9.75, *P* <.001; Quebec Back Pain Disability Questionnaire decreased from 40.85 to 26.5, *P* <.001) subscales of the Dallas Pain Questionnaire significantly improved); the effect persisted at 6-month follow up.[139] No changes were noted in the control group at 2 months except a change in persons engaged in physical activity.[139] Significant improvement at 6 months in the control group (education or seek aid on own) was observed for NRS (4.92 decreased to 3.53, *P* <.01), anterior flexion, flexibility of quadriceps, and Dallas Pain Questionnaire's work recreational score.[139] The authors concluded that multiple health benefits of physical activity and physical therapy modalities in the workplace exist for employees with chronic LBP.[139]

Smeets compared general aerobic and strengthening exercise versus cognitive behavioral training or a combination versus "wait list" and observed significantly reduced functional limitations, reduced "patient's main complaints" and decreased pain intensity for all three active treatments.[140] Self-rated treatment effectiveness and satisfaction was higher in the three active treatments.[140] The two active treatments with an exercise intervention, but not CBT, significantly improved physical performance tasks of walking and stair climbing.[140] The authors conclude that either active program is effective, arguing against a more expensive combination program.[140]

Isokinetic strengthening compared to usual strengthening, flexibility, and endurance training by a physiotherapist was found to improve significantly the VAS fingertip-to-floor test, disability (Modified ODQ), and BDI scores compared to the baseline, which persisted through the end of the study (7 weeks) (*P* <.05).[141] Exercises were done 10 times a day for 1 month.[141]

The most beneficial dose, frequency, and duration of exercise have not been elucidated in the literature. Kell et al.[142] attempted to discern the optimal frequency of a strengthening program. Patients were randomly assigned to groups receiving exercise 4 days per week, 3 days per week, 2 days per week, or no training with an exercise program that progressively overloaded muscle groups for 16 weeks.[142] The 4 days per week training volume significantly (*P* <.05) outperformed all other training volumes by weeks 9 and 13 on the relief of pain, Oswestry Disability Index, and SF-36, although all groups improved.[142] All training volumes made significant (*P* <.05) improvements in strength, but the 4-day training pattern consistently demonstrated the largest effect size.[142] Limke et al.[143] assessed the benefit of one versus two sets of progressive resistive exercises (PRE). Exercises on various equipment were performed twice weekly for 6 weeks for about 1 hour, one or two sets of PRE.[143] At discharge there was no statistical difference between the group completing one set and the group completing two sets of PRE for pain, disability, or strength measures, which suggests that there is no additional benefit to completing a second set of PRE in patients with LBP.[143] A review article on strengthening exercise for LBP arrived at similar conclusions to this section.[144] Trunk strengthening appears effective compared with no exercise, but compared with aerobics or McKenzie exercises is not shown to be better.[144] Increasing exercise intensity, which differs from increasing the number of sets or times per week, and adding motivation increase treatment effects.[144]

MCKENZIE METHOD

McKenzie is a methodology to "centralize" peripheral pain and exercise the patient in the "direction" that accomplishes that goal. Al-Obaidi evaluated patients in a physical therapy setting using the McKenzie method, and outcomes measures for pain-related disability and fear beliefs, as well as time to complete various mobility tasks were obtained.[145] Patients were then treated with McKenzie intervention for 12 visits at a minimum frequency of three per week.[145] Patients showed significant (*P* <.001) improvement in pain and related fear and disability beliefs and functional task completion at the end of the treatment and throughout the 10-week follow up period.[145] McKenzie exercises perform similarly to a back school paradigm for improvement of pain and disability. Garcia compared four sessions of back school versus four sessions of McKenzie directional preference exercises that showed improvements in pain intensity and disability.[146] The results of the two groups do not seem to have been considered separately, but patients regardless of the treatment arm improved; pain intensity (0–10) decreased from 6.4 to 4 (*P* <.005) and RMDQ decreased from 13 to 7.8 (*P* <.001).[146] Paatelma compared six sessions of McKenzie exercise to six sessions of manual therapy to one advice-education session.[147] At 3 months there was no significant difference in any group for leg or back pain, but at 6 months back pain (*P* <.009), leg pain (*P* <.03) and disability (*P* <.003) were significantly improved in the McKenzie group compared with the advice group, and disability continued to be significantly improved in the McKenzie group compared with the advice group at 12 months (*P* <.028).[147] The manual therapy group trended toward improved leg pain over the advice group at 6 months (*P* <.075) and disability trended toward improved at 12 months in the manual therapy group compared to advice (*P* <.068).[147] The authors note there was no significant difference between the McKenzie and manual therapy groups.[147] The authors concluded that the McKenzie method is only marginally better than advice[147] but the McKenzie regimen appeared to perform significantly better in the long term (6–12 months). A meta-analysis of outcomes subsequent to the McKenzie method and intervention by Machado et al.[148] echoed Paatelma's conclusions. Machado et al.[148] conclude that "some evidence that the McKenzie method is more effective than passive therapy for acute LBP exist; however, the magnitude of the difference suggests the absence of clinically worthwhile effects. There is limited evidence for the use of McKenzie method in chronic LBP."[148]

LUMBAR EXTENSION

Progressive resistive exercise in extension demonstrated significant reductions in pain and improved muscle strength, endurance, and joint mobility in patients with LBP.[149] The optimal frequency and duration of the various exercise regimens to treat LBP has not been determined. One study of lumbar extension exercise evaluated the difference in outcomes between one and two sessions per week supervised by a therapist.[150] The results (pre vs. post) showed significant increases in maximal strength and ROM and reductions in pain for both training groups, and Bruce-Low et al. concluded that one lumbar extension training session per week is sufficient for strength gains and reductions in pain in LBP in CLBP patients.[150] Investigators have also tried to discern whether high load or low load extension exercises are more therapeutic. Harts et al.[151] evaluated whether 8 weeks of high-intensity strengthening (10 sessions, 10 to 15 repetitions, start 50% maximal extensor strength and add 2.5 kg if able to complete 20 repetitions) of the isolated lumbar extensors was more effective than low-intensity strengthening (fixed 20% maximal extensor strength) or no strengthening. Of interest, while the SF-36 was 7% better and the self-assessed decrease of back symptoms was on average 39% in the high intensity group, no other differences were found at the 8-week conclusion or 24-week follow-up, and the authors concluded that the results of this study of high-intensity strengthening program of the isolated lumbar extensor muscles do not clearly support the generally claimed beneficial influence of lumbar extension exercise for chronic nonspecific LBP at any intensity.[151] Review of the tabulated data show a RMDQ baseline in the high intensity of 6.2 (similar in the low-intensity group and wait list controls) with improvement at 8 weeks to 3.4. The range on the RMDQ is 24; other studies have enrolled patients with "more" disability. The exercise program may show weak effect due to patients with low disability being enrolled in the first place. Harts comments on this as a limitation of "voluntary" recruitment and bias.[151]

GRADED EXERCISE

Graded activity exercises were developed based on studies suggesting that counterproductive belief systems delayed recovery from back pain and increased levels of disability in patients with chronic pain. Therefore, graded activity exercises address pain-related fear, kinesiophobia, and unhelpful beliefs and behaviors about back pain while increasing strength and endurance.[136] Graded activity programs target activities the patient does not feel he or she can do, having the patient perform submaximal exercises while the supervisor ignores illness behaviors and reinforces wellness behaviors.[136] In a systematic review Bunzli et al. reviewed 15 trials that included over 3700 subjects and found moderate evidence supporting the application of graded (physiotherapist-provided operant conditioning) for the treatment of LBP.[152] Graded exercise was not inferior to any comparators in reducing disability, and there was moderate evidence that graded exercise is more effective than other behavioral interventions in reducing long-term disability in chronic LBP.[152] In subacute LBP the authors found moderate evidence that operant exercise may be more effective than other treatments in reducing posttreatment fear avoidance beliefs and more effective than a placebo intervention in reducing short-term pain.[152]

Macedo et al. compared graded exercise and motor control (core stabilization) exercise for the treatment of LBP and found no significant difference between treatments for outcomes of average pain over the previous week and function or disability, global impression of change and quality of life.[136] Rasmussen-Barr et al.[153] compared weekly supervised graded core stabilization exercise with an education component to daily 30-minute walks and education about the benefits of walking. The primary outcome was perceived disability and pain at 12-month follow-up, but secondary outcomes included physical health, fear-avoidance, and self-efficacy beliefs.[153] Perceived disability ($P < .01$), pain ($P < .001$), and physical health improved significantly in both groups ($P < .001$), but fear-avoidance and self-efficacy beliefs improved significantly only in the exercise group ($P < .001$).[153] Significant differences in favor of the exercise group for perceived disability at 6-, 12-, and 36-month follow-up were found.[153] Pain showed greater reduction for the exercise group after the intervention.[153]

Smeets et al.[154] compared graded exercise plus problem solving training to active physical training (lumbar extension strengthening) or a combination of graded exercise and physical training for 10 weeks. Their objective was to determine any long-term benefits at 1 year follow-up. None of the treatments showed a clinically relevant reduction of pain and depression or improvement of performance tasks at 1 year.[154] They found that there were no significant differences between each single treatment and the combination treatment on disability and pain, depression, and task performance at 1 year.[154] Graded exercise and active physical training, compared with the combination, showed a higher, but both statistically and clinically insignificant, reduction of disability.[154] Smeets et al. did not endorse a combination treatment.[154]

Graded exercise compared to graded exposure was included the 3- to 5-week, seven-hour-a-day interdisciplinary treatment of patients with chronic LBP in a study by George et al.[155] In the graded exercise process the PT first determined tolerance to a particular exercise and determined the baseline target intensity and increased the exercise based on a quota system with positive reinforcement if the quota was met or additional education if the quota was not met.[155] The graded exposure process was described as determining the exercise and activity that were fearful to the patient and was determined using the Fear of Daily Activities Questionnaire.[155] Two feared activities were then incorporated into the patient's exercise regime, initially at a nonthreatening level and progressed with positive reinforcement and increase of intensity or education and maintenance of intensity, depending on the patient's ability to complete the task.[155] Statistically significant ($P < .01$) improvements were observed for pain intensity and disability at discharge in both goups.[155] Interestingly, Tampa Scale of Kinesiophobia scores did not change significantly in either group. Change in depressive symptoms was associated with change in pain intensity, while change in pain catastrophizing was associated with change in disability.[155]

Graded exercise is as effective to reduce pain and disability as lumbar stabilization exercise. However, in a comparison to general exercise, either treatment was found to be clinically significant. Effects on fear avoidance and kinesiophobia, which this treatment theoretically targets, are mixed.

BACK SCHOOL

Back school started as an education intervention in the late 1960s and then an exercise component was added. A systematic review by van Middelkoop et al.[156] concluded that there are insufficient data to draw firm conclusions on the clinical effect of back schools. Brox et al.[114] reviewed the literature on back school, brief education, and fear avoidance training and concluded that evidence supporting back school as treatment for LBP was conflicting and back school as a treatment was not recommended.

The literature cited in this section reviews back school compared to general physical therapy, and suggests patient attributes that may improve patient selection for this therapy.

Van der Roer et al.[157] compared exercise with operant conditioning (graded exercise) combined with back school education (10 individual and 20 group sessions) to guideline-driven therapy treatment (session frequency and number determined by therapist) for the treatment of patient with LBP that had lasted over 12 weeks. Multilevel analysis did not show significant differences between the treatment groups on any outcome measures in the intermediate (26-weeks) or long term (52 weeks) except that the operant conditioning back school group showed more reduction in pain intensity (NRS decreased from 6.2 to 4.1 vs. 5.9 to 4.8 in the comparator group) at 26 weeks.[157] Other outcome measures show trends in improvement, but some return to or toward baseline occurs at 1 year.[157] Functional status as measured by Roland Morris Disability Questionnaire (RMDQ) decreases from 11.6 to 6.7 in the operant conditioning back school group while the guideline group decreases for 12.1 to 7.1; however fear avoidance as measured by Tampa Scale of Kinesiophobia at baseline was 37.9 with a nadir of 35.6 at 13 weeks and return to 37.9 at 52 weeks in the operant conditioning back school group; the control group values have a similar shape.[157] The authors note that the differences in groups are small and insignificant at 1 year but the operant back school group "tended to be more effective in reducing pain, coping and self-efficacy" and perceived improvement (45%) than the guideline-driven group in which 32% perceived improvement.[157] They note that at the level of the individual patient 48% of the operant back school group (vs. 375 in control group) achieved a clinically significant decrease in pain (change of 2 points on NRS) and 57% achieved a clinically significant improvement in RMDQ (30% change) compared to 48% in the control group.[157] In the balance the program was noted to be more expensive than the guideline-driven comparator and the authors' overall conclusion is that this specific program is not recommended to be implemented in primary care physical therapy.[157]

Sahin et al.[158] compared physical therapy alone (TENS, hot packs, flexion and extension exercise, and stretching, twice weekly for 5 weeks) to back school (twice weekly education for 2 weeks) combined with therapy and found that VAS and ODQ were significantly reduced at the conclusion of therapy ($P < .01$) in both groups.[158] However, between groups, there was significantly greater improvement in VAS ($P <.01$ post-treatment, and $P <.002$ at 3 months) and ODQ in the back school group (VAS baseline 5.69 +/− 2.14 decreased to 4.9 +/− 0.11 decreased to 3.6 +/− 0.15; ODQ baseline 54.50 +/− 14.13 decreased to 41.01 +/− .59 decreased to 36.13 +/− 0.69) compared with the control group (VAS baseline 6.52 +/− 1.12 decreased to 5.35 +/− 0.11 decreased to 4.31 +/− 0.15; ODQ baseline 55.65+/− 11.80 decreased to 44.76 +/− .59 decreased to 39.93 +/− 0.69)at the end of therapy and 3 months post-treatment ($P <.001$ for both time frames).[158] Sahin et al.[158] concluded that the addition of back school was more effective than physical therapy and exercises alone for patients with chronic LBP.

Yang et al.[159] reported on a 4-week back school program with typical educational topics and core strengthening exercise and concluded that less use of relaxation (odds ratio _ 2.11. 95%, P _.001) and more use of exercise and stretching (odds ratio _ 2.39, P _.001) as coping strategies were significantly predictive of the success of back school programs. Based on the scores of the Oswestry Disability Index patients were subclassified as very improved, somewhat improved, or not improved (change <6 points) and compared.[159] As a group, participants improved, pretreatment to posttreatment, significantly in terms of back-specific disability ($P <.005$), worst pain ($P <.001$), and mean pain ($P <.005$), SF36 subscales bodily pain ($P <.001$), mental health ($P <.005$), vitality ($P <.001$), and social functioning ($P <.001$).[159] In long-term follow-up, the much-improved group showed significant improvement in chronic pain coping inventory (CPCI 9) scores for relaxation, task persistence, and exercise; however, the coping strategies of those in the somewhat improved and not improved groups did not change significantly over the course of treatment.[159] At the baseline, patients who had used relaxation less as an initial coping strategy were more likely to succeed in the back school program (CPCI relaxing subscale most improved 1.6+/− 1.0 increased to 2.6 +/−1.1; somewhat improved baseline 2.4+/− 1.7 with no change 2.6 +/− 1.4; unimproved 2.8 +/− 1.2 decreased to 2.0 +/−1.8). The exercise/stretching coping score after back school increased significantly in the much-improved group compared with the slightly improved or unimproved group; of interest the most improved group, as with relaxing, was least likely to use this strategy before the treatment (CPCI exercise subscale most improved 3.11.1 increased to 5.2 +/−1.9; somewhat improved baseline 3.7+/− 1.2 with no change 3.6 +/− 1.6; unimproved 3.8 +/− 1.7 decreased to 3.0 +/−2.0) ($P <.035$).[159] The patients who benefit most from the program are the ones who need to learn the coping strategies. The authors comment that "these findings suggest that a low level of wellness-focused coping skills at baseline could be predictive of better outcome."[159]

The effectiveness of back school for improvement of pain, disability, and return to work conflicts in the literature but a subgroup of patients who could benefit from instruction on coping with pain by relaxing or exercise may be most helped by this format.

MULTIDISCIPLINARY PROGRAMS

Stanos provides an excellent review and explanation of multidisciplinary pain programs within the context of the biopsychosocial model for the treatment of chronic pain.[2] He notes that in the collaborative spectrum of patient treatment there exists "parallel, collaborative, coordinated, multidisciplinary, interdisciplinary, and integrative approaches."[2] Multidisciplinary treatments often involve one or two physician specialists or practitioners directing the services of a number of team members, who often have independent goals.[2] Stanos notes that interdisciplinary programs use cognitive and behavioral approaches to provide outcome-focused, coordinated, goal-oriented services to team members who work together for a common goal and make collective therapeutic decisions in team meetings.[2,160] Stanos reports that participation in a well-established interdisciplinary pain treatment programs decreases pain disability scores by about half.[160] Multidisciplinary pain treatment centers may seek accreditation by the Commission on Accreditation of Rehabilitation Facilities (CARF).

Several studies have investigated patient traits that may affect outcome in these programs. Pieh et al.[161] studied gender differences and response to treatment of chronic pain in multidisciplinary settings and found that women improved more in pain-related disabilities in daily life than men. These distinctions are not due to differences in pain duration, received medication, psychiatric comorbidities, pain chronicity stage, or application for a disability pension.[161] MacLaren et al.[162] studied the effect of opioids on patient outcome and noted that significant improvements from pretreatment to posttreatment were shown on all psychological and physical measures for both opioid users and nonusers. Additionally opioid use did not affect or return-to-work outcomes.[162] However, Howard et al.[163] found that opioid use as well as other factors predicted drop out from multidisciplinary treatment for chronic pain. Persons who dropped out had a longer duration of total disability between injury and admission to treatment (completers, 20 mo vs. noncompleters, 13 mo; $P <.001$).[163] Also patients, who were opioid-dependent were 1.5 times more likely to drop out of rehabilitation, and patients diagnosed with a socially problematic Cluster B Personality Disorder were 1.6 times more likely to drop out.[163] The multivariate logistic regression analysis was found to be significant with the addition of each block. In sum, women may fare better in this therapeutic environment than men. The effect of opioid use on participation is debatable. Longer duration of disability (20 months) and Cluster B personality disorder (Narcissistic, Borderline, Anti-social with dramatic, erratic, or emotional attributes) may suggest patients less suited for this treatment.

A systematic review by van Middlekoop et al.[156] found that multidisciplinary treatment reduced pain intensity in patients with CLBP at short-term but not long-term follow-up compared to both no treatment/waiting list controls and active treatments; evidence was moderate. A systematic review by Scascighini et al.[164] implied that multidisciplinary treatment is a more effective treatment model than other treatments for LBP and they systematically reviewed the literature about multidisciplinary treatment in order to develop the minimum standards for an effective program that should serve as an international model. Scascighini et al.[164] recommend:

> *"a minimum standard of multidisciplinary therapy can be currently established from these data, namely ideally: specific individual exercising, regular training in relaxation techniques, group therapy led by a clinical psychologist (1.5 hr) per week, patient education sessions once a week, two physiotherapy treatments per week (CBT) for pacing strategies, medical training therapy, and neurophysiology information given by trained physician."*

Scascighini et al.[164] found moderate evidence of greater effectiveness for multidisciplinary interventions compared to active treatment. Compared to no treatment, strong evidence supporting the effectiveness of multidisciplinary treatments was found.[164] Moderate evidence supported that inpatient programs were more beneficial than outpatient programs.[164] Multidisciplinary programs were more effective for patients with more specific diagnoses like fibromyalgia and chronic back pain, compared to patients with nonspecific diagnoses like chronic pain.[164]

Demoulin studied the effects of a semi-intensive (>30 hr but <100 hr) multidisciplinary program in which patients participated in thirty-six 2-hour sessions at a rate of about twice to three times weekly in a program with PTs and OTs, a physiatrist, and a psychologist.[165] Study outcomes significantly improved, including "pain intensity was decreased by 44%, functional impairment by 40%, and kinesiophobia by 11% whereas knowledge was improved by 59%, back-sparing technique by 95%, trunk muscle strength by 40% on average, trunk extensor muscle endurance by 90%, mobility by 8%, and aerobic capacity by 18%."[1] Compared to an inpatient or all-day outpatient program, this program allows the patient to continue work.[165]

Dufour et al.[166] describe a 12-week 73-hour multidisciplinary program of physical therapy and occupational therapy and education, in comparison to 12 weeks of twice weekly supervised exercise for 1 hour.[166] With regard to pain there were significant improvements in both groups with no difference between groups for the degree of pain improvement (20-30%) and there was no difference in medication usage to relieve pain.[166] Improvements were maintained throughout the 24-month follow-up period.[166] Based on the SF36, both groups improved significantly (P <.05) in all dimensions except for the "General Health" and "Role Limitation Emotional."[166] Between groups, the improvement in "Physical functioning" and "Physical component summary" was significantly greater in the multidisciplinary group throughout the 24-month follow-up.[166] Scores on the RMDQ significantly improved (P <.05) in both groups, but between groups the multidisciplinary group had a more significant change of 24% versus a 12% change in the exercise-only group.[166] Adverse events included a fall and concussion, herniated disc and surgery, and delayed onset muscle soreness.[166] Based on the study, Dufour et al.[166] conclude that both approaches are effective, with the multidisciplinary group approach being less costly but more time consuming and the individual exercise being more expensive but efficient.

A similar study by Kaapa et al.[167] compared 120 female working subjects in a 70-hour multidisciplinary program consisting of physical therapy and occupational therapy and education to a 10-hour supervised exercise program, with follow-up after the program and at 6, 12, and 24 months. Outcomes measures included: back pain and sciatic pain intensity, disability, sick leaves, health care consumption, symptoms of depression, and beliefs of working ability. In both groups all measures improved; however, P-values do not appear in the text or tables of the article and it is not clear that the improvements have statistical weight.[167] For, example the pain rating changes from 4.6 to 3.5 in the multidisciplinary group and from 5.0 to 4.0 at 24-month follow-up in the control group. There are no differences between groups. The Oswestry score in both groups is approximately 24 at baseline (on a scale to 100) and improves in both groups to about 19 at 24-month follow-up. The authors note that the mild to moderate symptoms of the patients may limit the study design, finding significant differences between the treatments. As in the previous study the authors did not find a significant preference to either treatment but note the low cost of the multidisciplinary program and the time flexibility of the individual therapy program.[167]

Monticone et al.[168] compared patients with LBP randomly assigned to a multidisciplinary program consisting of CBT and exercise training versus exercise training alone administered over the course of 1 year. Monticone et al.[168] found that the multidisciplinary program reduced disability, fear-avoidance beliefs, and pain and enhanced the quality of life of patients significantly better than exercise alone for group and time (P <.001) and group-time interaction (P <.001, except SF-36-Physical function, P .002; SF-36-Physical role, P .007; and SF-36-Emotional role, P .01) for up to 1 year. Roche-Leboucher[169] compared a multidisciplinary program versus exercise only to see if the number of sick days differed as a result of treatment. The multidisciplinary group was treated in groups of 6 to 8, and met 6 hours a day, 5 days a week, for 5 weeks.[169] The patients were evaluated and treated by OTs, a physiatrist, psychologist, and dietician, and work site consultation for ergonomic advice from an occupational physician was available.[169] A private-practice physiotherapist treated individual subjects in the exercise group 1 hour 3 times a week, during 5 weeks.[169] There was no difference between groups regarding the number of sick-leave days during the 2 years preceding treatment. In both groups, the number of sick-leave days in the 12 months after treatment decreased significantly but the reduction was significantly greater in the multidisciplinary group (-101.2 ± 126.5 d vs. -79 ± 143.9 d; P <.001). Other functional and physical outcomes included fingertip-to-floor distance, Sorensen test, ito test, intensity of pain on VAS, Dallas daily activities score, Dallas work and leisure score, Dallas anxiety and depression score, and the Dallas sociability score.[169] All physical and functional criteria were significantly improved in both groups except for the Dallas anxiety and depression score and sociability score in the exercise group.[169] The multidisciplinary program had a more robust effect on the outcome of sick days.

Moradi et al.[170] assessed the effect size of multidisciplinary treatment, which was found to be moderate for the treatment of chronic LBP. The program was an inpatient treatment lasting 3 weeks, 8 hours per day, 5 days per week for a total of 120 hours of treatment, consisting of physical exercises, ergonomic training, psychotherapy, patient education, behavioral therapy, and workplace-based interventions on an individual basis and in group sessions.[170] There was no placebo or active comparator group. Medium effect sizes ($d = 0.6$ to 0.7) were shown for VAS after treatment and at 6 months, indicating clinically relevant pain relief.[170] Pain-related disability ($d = 0.8$) and quality-of-life subscales on SF-36 for physical function, vitality, and mental health ($d = 0.5$ to 0.8) showed a strong treatment effect immediately after treatment.[170] Low to medium effect sizes were shown for functional capacity ($d = 0.4$-0.5). Depression improved significantly with strong effect sizes of $d = 0.7$.[170] Demographically, females, the age group 30 to 39 years, and patients with low physical job exposure showed the most effect size for VAS, based on comparison of effect size.[170] An increase in number of pain locations and severity of accompanying pain in other body areas significantly impaired therapy outcome.[170] Compared to effect sizes reported in the literature, the authors concluded that effect sizes are higher than for monodisciplinary treatments and had the highest effect size for pain-related disability, mental health-related quality of life, and depression.[170]

Aftercare following multidisciplinary rehabilitation programs (MRP) has been evaluated. Henchoz et al. compared a 3-month exercise program following MRP versus "usual care" after MRP.[171] They found that just after MRP (start of the 3-month exercise program or care-as-usual) there was no difference between groups, and, at 1 year, there was no difference between groups for the outcome measures of physical functioning, physical role, bodily pain, general health perception, vitality, emotional role, mental health, and physical component score and mental component score.[171] In both groups quality of life significantly improved at 1-year follow-up.[171] No additional benefit to quality of life parameters was found by adding an aftercare exercise program.[171] The same group evaluated effects on physical function and found that at the 3-month and 1-year follow-up, both groups maintained improvements in all outcome measures except cardiovascular endurance.[172] No differences between groups were found except the aftercare-exercise group showed significant improvement in disability score and trunk muscle endurance.[172] The authors concluded that after completing a functional multidisciplinary rehabilitation, patients simply need advice to stay active in order to reach long-term improvements. Henchoz et al.[172] recommend that although disability score and trunk muscle endurance improve as a result of additional prescribed exercise, identification of patients receive this limited benefit requires further research.

Multidisciplinary pain treatment programs are an effective treatment model to reduce disability and pain and other outcomes like sick days, kinesiophobia, and physical functioning. Multidisciplinary programs have greater effect sizes than monotherapies, and the highest effect size for pain-related disability, mental health-related quality of life, and depression. A program schedule which is flexible enough to allow the patient to continue to work is probably optimal since more time consuming formats have not been found to be superior. Women may do particularly well in this type of program. Patients with Cluster B personality disorders may not do as well.

FUNCTIONAL RESTORATION

Huge et al. comment that functional restoration programs for CLBP have been shown to be more effective in improving function than in reducing pain.[173] They compared the outcomes of a 4-week, 6 to 8 hours per day outpatient functional restoration program (education, physical therapy, psychological counseling and relaxation training and ergonomics) to "treatment as usual" with a PT, psychologist, and relaxation.[173] The authors found that compared with the "treatment as usual" group, pain and disability were significantly improved in patients completing the functional restoration program, and a significant reduction in depression and improvement in quality of life was also observed.[173] No changes were detected in the "treatment as usual" group.[173] The authors conclude that a functional restoration program for CLBP significantly improves health-related quality of life and decreases the perception of pain and pain-related disability even in patients with a long history of CLBP.[173]

Beaudreuil studied patients with LBP who had been on sick leave for over 3 months.[174] Patients participated in a 5-week, 5 days per week day hospital program and then the patients were followed for one year.[174] After 1 year, two-thirds of the patients had returned to work and sick leave was decreased by 50% compared to the previous year.[174] Patients who remained on sick leave after 1 year were older and had higher scores on the Dallas Pain Questionnaire's anxiety and depression subscale.[174] The authors conclude that functional restoration returns most patients to work.[174] The argument could be made that if more of the patients were older or more anxious or depressed the return to work rate would not have been as robust. However within the group that did return to work, the program did seem to effect a lower rate of absenteeism.[174]

Bendix et al.[117] compared a 3-week, 8-hour-a-day functional restoration program (aerobic and strength training, occupational work hardening, psychology, education, stretching, and recreational activity) to an 8-week, three times weekly 1.5-hour aerobic and strengthening program. Review of the statistics confirms the authors' comment the expensive functional treatment had relatively poor results compared with the results from the less expensive physical therapy treatment.[117] Work capability increased in both groups; the functional restoration group increased from 28 to 36 of 48 patients ($P < .08$) and the outpatient therapy group increased from 21 to 35 of 51 patients ($P < .005$).[117] The authors posited that the control program may have been too substantial or the patient sample may have been "acute" enough that they would have improved regardless of treatment.[117]

Functional restoration programs significantly improve pain and disability and, like multidisciplinary programs, return to work rates. Older patients or persons with attributes of depression or anxiety may be less likely to return to work.

AQUATIC THERAPY

Aquatic therapy adapts any of the main exercise types, stretching, aerobics, and strengthening, in a buoyant environment. Buoyancy can help a patients achieve an end-ROM that they are unable to achieve on land in gravity. Aqua-running with a weight belt is a common sports medicine technique. Air-filled bladders that offer resistance in the water can be used for strengthening. Persons with arthritis just seeking to walk may do so more comfortably in waist to chest deep water.

A systematic review of aqua-therapy concluded that there was sufficient evidence to suggest that therapeutic aquatic exercise is potentially beneficial to patients suffering from CLBP and pregnancy-related LBP.[175] Review of the seven included trials does not clarify whether the study participants were in a pool setting supervised by a licensed therapist or not.[175] One case report described the use of pool therapy progressing to land based walking over a 26-week period in a patient 10 status after a multilevel spinal fusion for spinal stenosis and reporting high levels of persistent postoperative pain with minimal activity.[176] The progression of the pool program started as pool exercise only, five times per week for 6 weeks, and then brief land based walking followed by pool exercise, five times per week for 8 weeks and the last phase for 11 weeks was land-based walking only, 5 days per week, completely phasing out the pool once the patient could walk about one mile.[176] At 10 months the patient's surgical wound would be healed. However, it is important to note that pool therapy could not commence before complete healing of any open wounds or surgical was complete.

Dundar et al.[177] compared physical therapy supervised water therapy with flexibility, aerobic, and strengthening components that convened five times a week for 4 weeks to a land-based home exercise program.[177] At 12-week follow-up statistically significant improvements were detected in both groups, compared with baseline, for lumbar flexion, extension and rotation tests, pain at rest, with movement and at night, for disability (Modified ODQ and the SF36).[177] However, improvement in disability questionnaire and physical function and role limitations subscales of the Short-Form 36 Health Survey were better in aquatic exercise group ($P < .05$).[177] The authors concluded that a water-based exercise program produced improvement in disability and better quality of life.[177]

Cuesta-Vargas et al.[178] compared PT-supervised deep water running three times per week for 4 months to an educational booklet only as treatments for nonspecific CLBP.[178] At 1 year findings included significantly more improved VAS ($P < .05$), disability ($P < .05$), physical health ($P < .05$), and mental summary component of the SF-12 ($P < .05$) in favor of the deep water running group.[178] The authors found this treatment to be significantly better for the relief of pain and disability and improvement of quality of life. Cuesta-Vargas et al.[179] in a different study added 20 minutes of deep-water running to and education and physical therapy program but found no added benefit of the deep water running. Both interventions (PT + education vs. PT + education + deep water running) resulted in significant improvements in pain, disability, and physical health.[179]

Baena-Beato evaluated the dose response of water aerobic activity and found that groups participating in water exercise twice or three times a week for 8 weeks had a significant decrease in levels of back pain and disability, increased quality of life, and improved health-related fitness in adults with CLBP without effects in body composition.[180] Dose-response effects were observed in some parameters, with greater benefits when exercising 3 days per week compared with 2 days per week.[180]

Compared to a booklet, aquatic therapy improves pain, disability, and quality of life significantly more. Aquatic therapy is better than home exercise but par with supervised physical therapy for improvements in pain disability and quality of life for persons with chronic back pain. A dose response is noted between twice and three times weekly therapies.

NOVEL APPROACHES TO PHYSICAL THERAPY

A case series (n = 3) on Sensorimotor Retraining which involves graphesthesia training and a variety of exercise maneuvers, some with a applied sensory feedback component, was reported by Wand et al.[181]

Significant improvement in pain level, disability, and pain interference was reported.[181]

Gatti et al. reported on the effectiveness of trunk balance exercises versus trunk strengthening to improve pain intensity, disability, and quality of life.[182] The authors note that the patients with CLBP have difficulty maintaining balance, especially under challenging conditions such as single-limb support.[182]

The experimental group performed trunk balance exercises in addition to standard trunk flexibility exercises, and the control group performed strengthening exercises in addition to the same standard trunk flexibility exercises.[182] A significant difference in scores on the Roland-Morris Questionnaire ($P < .011$) and the physical component of the 12-Item Short-Form Health Survey ($P < .048$) was noted in the time-by-group analysis, and between groups for pain reduction ($P < .03$). The number of participants reaching the minimal clinically important difference for the RMDQ and reduction of painful positions ($P < .03$) was in favor of the experimental treatment.[182] Medication use decreased in both groups but was not significant.

Pozo-Cruz evaluated the effectiveness of the vibration therapy, done twice weekly for 12 weeks, and compared to activity as normal, for the treatment of LBP. Vibration therapy entails the use of oscillatory muscle stimulation.[183] The authors explain that a foot is placed on a platform that vibrates at a predetermined frequency and amplitude, which are then transmitted throughout the body, eliciting reflexive muscle stimulation, with the short and fast changes in muscle length detected by different proprioceptive organs.[183] Significant improvements in the vibration group included anterior posterior stability ($P < .031$), ODQ ($P < .013$), RMDQ ($P < .001$), quality of life ($P < .042$), and 24.13% improvement in VAS in back pain ($P = 0.006$).[183] Proprietary devices to provide the therapy as well as perform follow-up measurements may be limitations to this therapeutic strategy.

Telephone coaching of patients with low to moderate expected responses from physical therapy intervention by therapists trained in health coaching yielded significant improvement in the Patient Specific Functional Scale and recovery expectation at 12 weeks.[184] The billing code for this service would need clarification to make this service economically viable in a busy rehabilitation outpatient service.

PREDICTING OUTCOME

Very little is known about factors that predict treatment outcome.[185] A systematic review by Wessels et al. to discern the predictors of nonoperative treatments of CLBP showed that functional coping mechanisms and pain reduction, but not physical performance factors, were associated with a decrease in disability and increase in return to work.[186] Decreases in disability and functional coping mechanisms as well as physical performance factors were associated with pain reduction.[186] In obese patients with LBP referred for physical therapy, pain-related fear of movement predicted self-reported disability with walking and overall Oswestry scores despite similar pain ratings to normal weight patients.[187] Participants with recurrent LBP currently working participated in an 8-week exercise program; ratings of poor self-efficacy for physical activity, greater disability, and higher pain ratings were the most consistent independent predictors of long-term poor outcome of disability and pain.[188]

Both the components of the treatment program as well as patient characteristics can affect outcome. The characteristic that best predicted improved pain in patients who participated in an adaptive community based exercise program for one year was adherence to the exercise program (participation >75% of session) In the same group, presence of depressive symptoms and poor self-rated health best predicted no improvement in pain at one year.[189] Among the patients with improved pain and adherence to the program, factors that correlated with adherence were proximity of exercise facilities, positive perception of exercise trainer, and positive perceived health and functional status.[189]

SUMMARY

In the end, skilled physical therapy alone or in combination with other allied health professionals in a multidisciplinary program is in the spectrum of possible treatments for a person experiencing pain. Exercise does not "cure" pain, and like the other moieties we prescribe there are responders and nonresponders and, among responders, the effect is, most often, only partial. For example, if the pain numerical rating scale is reported at six, a successful therapy intervention may decrease the NRS to three or four. The tabulated data of many of the papers reviewed was included in the tables and texts of this chapter not to provoke ennui but to allow the physician or provider reading this chapter to gauge whether the "significant outcome" described in the specific paper is applicable to the physician or provider's own patients, and, if so, how much improvement as a result of skilled therapy the patient can expect.

REFERENCES

1. § 484.4 Personnel qualifications. Centers for Medicare & Medicaid Services, HHS In Authenticated Government Information, Government Printing Office at http://www.gpo.gov/fdsys/pkg/CFR-2011-title42-vol5/pdf/CFR-2011-title42-vol5-sec484-4.pdf. Accessed February 28, 2013.
2. Stanos S, Houle T. Multidisciplinary and Interdisciplinary Management of Chronic Pain. *Phys Med Rehabil Clin N Am.* 2006;17:435-450.
3. Gatchel RJ, Mayer TG. Evidence informed management of chronic low back pain with functional restoration. *Spine J.* 2008;8:65-69.
4. Bendix T, Bendix A, Labriola M, et al. Functional restoration *versus* outpatient physical training in chronic low back pain—a randomized comparative study. *Spine.* 2000;25(19):2494-2500.
5. Paying for CAM Treatment. National Center for Complementary and Alternative Medicine. National Institutes of Health. U.S. Department of Health and Human Services at http://nccam.nih.gov/health/financial. Accessed February 28, 2013.
6. Schramm-Bloodworth DM, Grabois M. Physical medicine and rehabilitation. In: Warfield C, Bajwa ZH, eds. *Principles and Practice of Pain Medicine.* 2nd ed. New York, NY: McGraw-Hill; 2004:792-810.
7. Currie DM, Marburger RA. Writing therapy referrals and treatment plans and the interdisciplinary team. In: DeLisa JA, et al., eds. *Rehabilitation Medicine: Principles and Practice.* 2nd ed. Philadelphia, PA: JB Lippincott; 1993:145-157.
8. Cooper DM, Radom-Aizik S, Schwindt C, et al. Dangerous exercise: lessons learned from dysregulated inflammatory responses to physical activity. *J Appl Physiol.* 2007;103:700-709.
9. Wai EK, Rodriguez S, Dagenais S, et al. Evidence-informed management of chronic low back pain with physical activity, smoking cessation, and weight loss. *Spine J.* 2008;8:195-202.
10. Pollock M, Franklin B, Balady G, et al. AHA Science Advisory. Resistance exercise in individuals with and without cardiovascular disease: benefits, rationale, safety, and prescription: an advisory from the Committee on Exercise, Rehabilitation, and Prevention, Council on Clinical Cardiology, American Heart Association; Position paper endorsed by the American College of Sports Medicine. *Circulation.* 2000;101:828-833.
11. American College of Sports Medicine. *ACSM's Handbook for the Team Physician.* Baltimore, MD; Philadelphia, PA: Williams & Wilkins; 1996.
12. American College of Sports Medicine. *ACSM's Guidelines for Exercise Testing and Prescription.* Philadelphia, PA: Lippincott Williams & Wilkins; 2013.
13. May S, Ronald Donelson R. Evidence-informed management of chronic low back pain with the McKenzie method. *Spine J.* 2008; 8:134-141.
14. Halbertsma JPK, Goeken LNH. Stretching exercises: effect on passive extensibility and stiffness in short hamstrings of healthy subjects. *Arch Phys Med Rehabil.* 1994;75:976-981.
15. Lewit K, Simons DG. Myofascial pain: relief by post-isometric relaxation. *Arch Phys Med Rehabil.* 1984;65:452-456.
16. Musculoskeletal function. In: Pollock ML, Wilmore JH. eds. *Exercise in Health and Disease: Evaluation and Prescription for Prevention and Rehabilitation.* 2nd ed. Philadelphia, PA: W.B. Saunders; 1990;202-237.
17. Standish W, Curwin S, Mandell S. Eccentric exercise in chronic tendinopathy. *Clin Orthop Related Res.* 1986;208:65-68.
18. Frontera WR. Exercise in physical medicine and rehabilitation. In: Grabois M, Garrison SJ, Hart T, et al. eds. *Physical Medicine and Rehabilitation: The Complete Approach.* Malden, MA: Blackwell Science; 2000:487-503.
19. DeLateur BJ. Therapeutic exercise. In: Braddom RL, ed. *Physical Medicine and Rehabilitation.* 2nd ed. Philadelphia: W. B. Saunders Co; 2000:392-412.
20. Howley ET. Type of activity: resistance, aerobic and leisure versus occupational physical activity. *Med Sci Sports Exerc.* 2001;33:S364-S369.
21. Mayer J, Mooney V, Dagenais S. Evidence-informed management of chronic low back pain with lumbar extensor strengthening exercises. *Spine J.* 2008;8:96-113.
22. Cunha ACV, Burke TN, França FJR, Marques AP. Effect of global posture reeducation and of static stretching onto pain, range of motion, and quality of life in women with chronic neck pain: a random clinical trial. *Clinics.* 2008;63:763-770.
23. Ylinen J. Physical exercises and functional rehabilitation for the management of chronic neck pain. *Eura Medicophys.* 2007;43:119-132.

24. Griffiths SC, Dziedzic K, Waterfield J, et al. Effectiveness of specific neck stabilization exercises or a general neck exercise program for chronic neck disorders: a randomized controlled trial. *J Rheumatol.* 2009;36:390-397.

25. O'Leary S, Falla D, Hodges PW, et al. Specific therapeutic exercise of the neck induces immediate local hypoalgesia. *J Pain.* 2007;8(11):832-839.

26. Jull GA, Falla D, Vicenzino B, et al. The effect of therapeutic exercise on activation of the deep cervical flexor muscles in people with chronic neck pain. *Manual Ther.* 2009;14:696-701.

27. Falla D, Jull GA, Hodges P, et al. An endurance-strength training regime is effective in reducing myoelectric manifestations of cervical flexor muscle fatigue in females with chronic neck pain. *Clin Neurophysiol.* 2006;117:828-837.

28. Falla D, O'Leary S, Farina D, et al. The change in deep cervical flexor activity after training is associated with the degree of pain reduction in patients with chronic neck pain. *Clin J Pain.* 2012;28:628-634.

29. Rudolfsson T, Björklund M, Djupsjöbacka M. Range of motion in the upper and lower cervical spine in people with chronic neck pain. *Manual Ther.* 2012;17:53-59.

30. O'Leary S, Jull G, Kim M, et al. Training mode-dependent changes in motor performance in neck pain. *Arch Phys Med Rehabil.* 2012;93:1225-33.

31. Kongsted A Qerama E, Kasch H, et al. Neck collar, "act-as-usual" or active mobilization for whiplash injury? A randomized parallel-group trial. *Spine.* 2007;32:618-626.

32. Stewart MJ, Maher CG, Refshauge KM, et al. Randomized controlled trial of exercise for chronic whiplash-associated disorders. *Pain.* 2007;128:59-68.

33. Teasell RW, McClure JA, Walton D, et al. A research synthesis of therapeutic interventions for whiplash-associated disorder (WAD): Part 3–interventions for sub-acute WAD. *Pain Res Manage.* 2010; 15(5):305-312.

34. Cecchi F, Molino-Lova R, Paperini A, et al. Predictors of short- and long-term outcome in patients with chronic non-specific neck pain undergoing an exercise-based rehabilitation program: a prospective cohort study with 1-year follow-up. *Intern Emerg Med.* 2011;6:413-421.

35. Kay TM, et al. Exercises for mechanical neck disorders. *Cochrane Database System Rev.* 2012;8. Art. No.: CD004250. doi:10.1002/14651858.CD004250.pub4.

36. Nikander R, Malkia E, Parkkari J, et al. Dose-response relationship of specific training to reduce chronic neck pain and disability. *Med Sci Sports Exerc.* 2006;38(12):2068-2074.

37. Ylinen J, Hakkinen AH, Takala E, et al. Effects of neck muscle training in women with chronic neck pain: one-year follow-up study. *J Strength Cond Res.* 2006;20(1):6-13

38. Ylinen J, Takala E, Nykanen MJ. Effects of twelve-month strength training subsequent to twelve-month stretching exercise in treatment of chronic neck pain. *J Strength Cond Res.* 2006;20(2):304-308.

39. Pool JJM, Ostelo RWJG, Knol DL, et al. Is a behavioral graded activity program more effective than manual therapy in patients with subacute neck pain? Results of a randomized clinical trial. *Spine.* 2010;35:1017-1024.

40. Hudson JS, Ryan CG. Multimodal group rehabilitation compared to usual care for patients with chronic neck pain: a pilot study. *Manual Ther.* 2012;15:552-556.

41. Taimela S, Takala E, Asklo T, et al. Active treatment of chronic neck pain: a prospective randomized intervention. *Spine.* 2000; 25(8):1021-1027.

42. Brakke R, Singh J, Sullivan W. Physical therapy in persons with osteoarthritis. *PMR.* 2012;4:S53-S58.

43. Bennell KL, Hinman RS. A review of the clinical evidence for exercise in osteoarthritis of the hip and knee. *J Sci Med Sport.* 2011; 14:4-9.

44. Osiri M, Welch V, Brosseau L, Shea B, et al. Transcutaneous electrical nerve stimulation for knee osteoarthritis. *Cochrane Database System Rev.* 2000;4. Art. No.: CD002823. Doi:10.1002/14651858. CD002823.

45. Rutjes AWS, Nüesch E, Sterchi R, et al. Transcutaneous electrostimulation for osteoarthritis of the knee. *Cochrane Database System Rev.* 2009; 4. Art. No.: CD002823. DOI:10.1002/14651858. CD002823.pub2.

46. Page CJ, Hinman RS, Bennell KL. Physiotherapy management of knee osteoarthritis. *Int J Rheum Dis.* 2011;14:145-151.

47. Hernández-Rosa U, Velásquez-Tlapanco J, Lara-Maya C, et al. Comparison of the effectiveness of isokinetic vs. isometric therapeutic exercise in patients with osteoarthritis of knee. *Reumatol Clin.* 2012;8(1):10-14.

48. Jessep SA, Walsh NE, Ratcliffe J, et al. Long-term clinical benefits and costs of an integrated rehabilitation programme compared with outpatient physiotherapy for chronic knee pain. *Physiotherapy.* 2009;95:94-102.

49. Schneider F, Labs K, Wagner S. Chronic patellofemoral pain syndrome: alternatives for cases of therapy resistance. *Knee Surg, Sports Traumatol, Arthrosc.* 2001;9:290-295. doi:10.1007/s001670100219.

50. Giombini A, Di Cesare A, Di Cesare M, et al. Localized hyperthermia induced by microwave diathermy in osteoarthritis of the knee: a randomized placebo-controlled double-blind clinical trial. *Knee Surg Sports Traumatol Arthrosc.* 2011;19:980-987. doi:10.1007/s00167-010-1350-7.

51. Petersen W, Welp R, Rosenbaum D. Chronic achilles tendinopathy: a prospective randomized trial comparing the therapeutic effect of eccentric training, and air heel brace and the combination of both. *Am J Sports Med.* 2007;35(10):1659-1667.

52. Knobloch K. Eccentric training in Achilles tendinopathy: is it harmful to tendon microcirculation? *Br J Sports Med.* 2007;41:e2-e7.

53. Kingma JJ, de Knikker R, Wittink HM, et al. Eccentric overload training in patients with chronic Achilles tendinopathy: a systematic review. *Br J Sports Med.* 2007;41:e3-e8. Retrieved from http://www.bjsportmed.com/cgi/content/full/41/6/e3. doi:10.1136/bjsm.2006.030916.

54. Verrall G, Schofield S, Brustad T. Chronic Achilles tendinopathy treated with eccentric stretching program. *Foot Ankle Int.* 2011;32(9):843-849.

55. van der Plas A, de Jonge S, de Vos RJ, et al. A 5-year follow-up study of Alfredson's heel-drop exercise programme in chronic midportion Achilles tendinopathy. *Br J Sports Med.* 2012;46:214-218. doi:10.1136/214bjsports-2011-090035.

56. Tran DQH, Duong S, Bertini P, et al. Treatment of complex regional pain syndrome: a review of the evidence. *Can J Anesth/J Can Anesth.* 2010;57:149-166. doi:10.1007/s12630-009-9237-0.

57. Li Z, Smith BP, Smith TL, et al. Diagnosis and management of complex regional pain syndrome complicating upper extremity recovery. *J Hand Ther.* 2005;18:270-276.

58. Veizi E, Chelimsky TC, Janata JW. Chronic regional pain syndrome: what specialized rehabilitation services do patients require? *Curr Pain Headache Rep.* 2012;16:139-146. doi:10.1007/s11916-012-0253-3

59. Turner-Stokes L, Goebel A. Complex regional pain syndrome in adults: concise guidance. *Clin Med.* 2011;11(6):596-600.

60. Moseley G. Graded motor imagery is effective for long standing complex regional pain syndrome: a randomized controlled trial. *Pain*. 2004;108:192-8.
61. Moseley GL. Is successful rehabilitation of complex regional pain syndrome due to sustained attention to the affected limb? A randomised clinical trial. *Pain*. 2005;114(1-2):54-61.
62. Johnson S, Hall J, Barnett S, et al. Using graded motor imagery for complex regional pain syndrome in clinical practice: failure to improve pain. *Eur J Pain*. 2012;16:550-561.
63. Moseley GL, Wiech K. The effect of tactile discrimination training is enhanced when patients watch the reflected image of their unaffected limb during training. *Pain*. 2009;144:314-319.
64. van de Meent H, Oerlemans M, Bruggeman A, et al. Safety of "pain exposure" physical therapy in patients with complex regional pain syndrome type 1. *Pain*. 2009;152(6):1431-1438.
65. Ek JW, van Gijn JC, Samwel H, et al. Pain exposure physical therapy may be a safe and effective treatment for longstanding complex regional pain syndrome type 1: a case series. *Clin Rehabil*. 2009;23(12):1059-1066.
66. Oerlemans HM, Oostendorp RA, de Boo T, Goris RJ. Pain and reduced mobility in complex regional pain syndrome. I: Outcome of a prospective randomised controlled clinical trial of adjuvant physical therapy versus occupational therapy. *Pain*. 1999;83:77-83.
67. Lee BH, Scharff L, Sethna NF, et al. Physical therapy and cognitive-behavioral treatment for complex regional pain syndromes. *J Pediatr*. 2002;141:135-140.
68. Bialocerkowski AE, Daly A. Is physiotherapy effective for children with complex regional pain syndrome type 1? *Clin J Pain*. 2002;28:81-91.
69. Logan DE, Carpino EA, Chiang G, et al. A day-hospital approach to treatment of pediatric complex regional pain syndrome: initial functional outcomes. *Clin J Pain*. 2012;28:766-774.
70. Singh G, Willen SN, Boswell MV, et al. The value of interdisciplinary pain management in complex regional pain syndrome type I: a prospective outcome study. *Pain Physician*. 2004;7:203-209.
71. Busch AJ, Webber SC, Brachaniec M, et al. Exercise therapy for fibromyalgia. *Curr Pain Headache Rep*. 2011;15:358-367. doi:10.1007/s11916-011-0214-2.
72. Nijs J, Mannerkorpi K, Descheemaeker F, Van Houdenhove B. Primary care physical therapy in people with fibromyalgia: opportunities and boundaries within a monodisciplinary setting. *Phys Ther*. 2010;90:1815-1822.
73. Mannerkorpi K, Nordeman L, Anna Ericsson A, et al. Pool exercise for patients with fibromyalgia or chronic widespread pain: a randomized controlled trial and subgroup analyses. *J Rehabil Med*. 2009;41:751-760.
74. Suman AL, Biagi B, Biasi G, et al. One-year efficacy of a 3-week intensive multidisciplinary non-pharmacological treatment program for fibromyalgia patients. *Clin Exp Rheumatol*. 2009;27(1):7-14.
75. Carbonell-Baeza A, Aparicio VA, Chillón P, et al. Effectiveness of multidisciplinary therapy on symptomatology and quality of life in women with fibromyalgia. *Clin Exp Rheumatol*. 2011;29(6 Suppl 69):S97-S103. Epub 2012 Jan 3.
76. Valencia M, Alonso B, Alvarez MJ, et al. Effects of 2 physiotherapy programs on pain perception, muscular flexibility, and illness impact in women with fibromyalgia: a pilot study. *J Manipulative Physiol Ther*. 2009;32:84-92.
77. Busch AJ, Barber KA, Overend TJ, et al. Exercise for treating fibromyalgia syndrome. *Cochrane Database Syst Rev*. 2007;CD003786. doi:10.1002/14651858.CD003786.pub2.
78. Postgraduate Mézières Method. Global Physiotherapy Myofascial Presentation. Universitat Internacional Catalunya. Retrieved from http://www.uic.es/en/physiotherapy-miofascial. Accessed March 3, 2013.
79. Hauser W, Klose P, Langhorst J, et al. Efficacy of different types of aerobic exercise in fibromyalgia syndrome: a systematic review and meta-analysis of randomised controlled trials. *Arthritis Res Ther*. 2010;12:R79. Retrieved from http://arthritis-research.com/content/12/3/R79.
80. McCain GA, Bell DA, Mai FM, Halliday PD. A controlled study of the effects of a supervised cardiovascular fitness training program on the manifestations of primary fibromyalgia. *Arthritis Rheum*. 1988;31:1135-1141.
81. Thomas EN, Blotman F. Aerobic exercise in fibromyalgia: a practical review. *Rheumatol Int*. 2010;30:1143-50.
82. Lemos MC, Valim V, Zandonade E, et al. Intensity level for exercise training in fibromyalgia by using mathematical models. *BMC Musculoskelet Disord*. 2010;11:54. Retrieved from http://www.biomedcentral.com/1471-2474/11/54.
83. Valim V, Oliveira L, Suda A, et al. Aerobic fitness effects in fibromyalgia. *J Rheumatol*. 2003;30:1060-1069.
84. Kingsley JD, McMillan V, Figueroa A. The effects of 12 weeks of resistance exercise training on disease severity and autonomic modulation at rest and after acute leg resistance exercise in women with fibromyalgia. *Arch Phys Med Rehabil*. 2010;91:1551-1557.
85. Hakkinen A, Hakkinen K, Hannonen P, Alen M. Strength training induced adaptations in neuromuscular function of premenopausal women with fibromyalgia: comparison with healthy women. *Ann Rheum Dis*. 2001;60:21-26.
86. Valkeinen H, Hakkinen K, Pakarinen A, et al. Muscle hypertrophy, strength development, and serum hormones during strength training in elderly women with fibromyalgia. *Scan J Rheumatol*. 2005;34:309-114.
87. Sanudo B, Galiano D, Carrasco L, et al. Aerobic exercise versus combined exercise therapy in women with fibromyalgia syndrome: a randomized controlled trial. *Arch Phys Med Rehabil*. 2010;91:1838-1843.
88. FitzGerald MP, Anderson RU, Potts J, et al. Randomized multicenter feasibility trial of myofascial physical therapy for the treatment of urological chronic pelvic pain syndromes. 2009;182:570-580.
89. Clinton SC, George SE. Pelvic floor pain: physical therapy versus injections. *PMR*. 2011;3:762-770.
90. Doggweiler R, Stewart AF. Pelvic floor therapies in chronic pelvic pain syndrome. *Curr Urol Rep*. 2011;12:304-311. doi:10.1007/s11934-011-0197-x
91. Kavvadias T, Baessler K, Schuessler B. Pelvic pain in urogynecology. Part II: treatment options in patients with lower urinary tract symptoms. *Int Urogynecol J*. 2012;23:553-561. doi:10.1007/s00192-011-1649-z
92. Cox KJ, Neville CE. Assessment and management options for women with vulvodynia. *J Midwifery Womens Health*. 2012;57:231-240.
93. Wang Y-C, Hart DL, Mioduski JE. Characteristics of patients seeking outpatient rehabilitation for pelvic-floor dysfunction. *Phys Ther*. 2012;92:1160-1174.
94. Anderson RU, Wise D, Sawyer T, et al. 6-day intensive treatment protocol for refractory chronic prostatitis/chronic pelvic pain syndrome using myofascial release and paradoxical relaxation training. 2011;185:1294-1299.
95. Anderson R, Wise D, Sawyer T, et al. Safety and effectiveness of an internal pelvic myofascial trigger point wand for urologic chronic pelvic pain syndrome. *Clin J Pain*. 2011;27:764-768.

96. Goldfinger C, Pukall CF, Gentilcore-Saulnier E, etal. A prospective study of pelvic floor physical therapy: pain and psychosexual outcomes in provoked vestibulodynia. *J Sex Med.* 2009;6:1955-1968.

97. Sikiru L, Shmaila H, Muhammed SA. Transcutaneous electrical nerve stimulation (TENS) in the symptomatic management of chronic prostatitis/chronic pelvic pain syndrome: a placebo-control randomized trial. *Braz J Urol.* 2008;34(6):708-713; discussion 714.

98. Cuccia AM, Caradonna C, Annunziata V, et al. Osteopathic manual therapy versus conventional conservative therapy in the treatment of temporomandibular disorders: a randomized controlled trial. *J Bodywork Movement Ther.* 2010;14:179-184.

99. Soderberg EI, Carlsson JY, Stener-Victorin E, et al. Subjective well-being in patients with chronic tension-type headache: effect of acupuncture, physical training, and relaxation training. *Clin J Pain.* 2011;27:448-456.

100. Doepel M, Nilner M, Ekberg E, et al. Long-term effectiveness of a prefabricated oral appliance for myofascial pain. *J Oral Rehabil.* 2012;39:252-260.

101. Lehtola V, Luomajoki H, Leinonen V, et al. Efficacy of movement control exercises versus general exercises on recurrent sub-acute nonspecific low back pain in a sub-group of patients with movement control dysfunction: protocol of a randomized controlled trial. *BMC Musculoskel Disord.* 2012;13:55. Retrieved from http://www.biomedcentral.com/1471-2474/13/55.

102. Hayden J, van Tulder MW, Malmivaara A, Koes BW. Exercise therapy for treatment of non-specific low back pain. *Cochrane Database Syst Rev.* 2005;3. Art. No.: CD000335. Doi:10.1002/14651858.CD000335.pub2.

103. Heymans MW, van Tulder MW, Esmail R, et al. Back schools for non-specific low-back pain. *Cochrane Database Syst Rev.* 2004;4. Art. No.: CD000261. DOI: 10.1002/14651858.CD000261.pub2.

104. Karjalainen KA, Malmivaara A, van Tulder MW, et al. Multidisciplinary biopsychosocial rehabilitation for subacute low-back pain among working age adults. *Cochrane Database Syst Rev.* 2003;2. Art. No.: CD002193. DOI: 10.1002/14651858.CD002193.

105. Ostelo RWJG, Costa LOP, Maher CG, et al. Rehabilitation after lumbar disc surgery. *Cochrane Database Syst Rev.* 2008;4. Art. No.: CD003007. doi:10.1002/14651858.CD003007.pub2.

106. Khadilkar A, Odebiyi DO, Brosseau L, Wells GA. Transcutaneous electrical nerve stimulation (TENS) versus placebo for chronic low-back pain. *Cochrane Database Syst Rev.* 2008]4. Art. No.: CD003008. DOI: 10.1002/14651858.CD003008.pub3.

107. Standaert CJ, Weinstein SM, John Rumpeltes J, et al. Evidence-informed management of chronic low back pain with lumbar stabilization exercises. *Spine J.* 2008;8:114-120.

108. Poitras S, Brosseau L. Evidence-informed management of chronic low back pain with transcutaneous electrical nerve stimulation, interferential current, electrical muscle stimulation, ultrasound, and thermotherapy. *Spine J.* 2008;8:226-233.

109. Albright J, Allman R, Bonfiglio RP, et al. Philadelphia panel evidence-based clinical practice for low back pain guidelines on selected rehabilitation interventions. *Phys Ther.* 2001;81:1641-1674.

110. Albright J, Allman R, Bonfiglio RP, et al. Philadelphia panel evidence-based clinical practice guidelines on selected rehabilitation interventions for shoulder pain. *Phys Ther.* 2001;81(10):1719-1730.

111. Airaksinen O, Brox JI, Cedraschi C, et al. European guidelines for the management of chronic nonspecific low back pain. *Eur Spine J.* 2006;15(Suppl 2):S192-S300. doi:10.1007/s00586-006-1072-1.

112. van Middelkoop M, Rubinstein SM,Verhagen AP, et al. Exercise therapy for chronic nonspecific low-back pain. *Best Pract Res Clin Rheumatol.* 2010;24:193-204.

113. Centers for Medicare and Medicaid Services. Limits on therapy services. Retrieved from http://www.medicare.gov/Pus/pdf/10988.pdf. Accessed March 28, 2013.

114. Brox JI, Storheim K, Grotle M, et al. Evidence-informed management of chronic low back pain with back schools, brief education, and fear-avoidance training. *Spine J.* 2008;8:28-39.

115. Andrusaitis SF, Brech GC, Vitale GF, et al. Trunk stabilization among women with chronic lower back pain: a randomized, controlled, and blinded pilot study. *CLINICS.* 2011;66(9):1645-1650. doi:10.1590/S1807-59322011000900024.

116. Smith C, Grimmer-Somers K. The treatment effect of exercise programmes for chronic low back pain. *J Eval in Clin Pract.* 2010;16:484-491.

117. Bendix T, Bendix A, Labriola M, et al. Functional restoration versus outpatient physical training in chronic low back pain: a randomized comparative study. *SPINE.* 2000;25(19):2494-2500.

118. Gatchel RJ, Polatin PB Noe C, et al. Treatment and cost-effectiveness of early intervention for acute low back pain patients: one year prospective study. *J Occup Rehabil.* 2003;13(1):1-9.

119. Medtronic@ (Minneapolis, Minnesota) Chronic pain. After surgery-neurostimulators. Retrieved from http://www.medtronic.com/patients/chronic-pain/living-with/neurostimulators/after-surgery/index.htm. Accessed March 30, 2013.

120. Johnson EN, Thomas JS. Effect of hamstring flexibility on hip and lumbar spine joint excursions during forward-reaching tasks in participants with and without low back pain. *Arch Phys Med Rehabil.* 2010;91:1140-1142.

121. Coupland C. Cliffe SJ, Bassey EJ, et al. Habitual activity and bone mineral density in postmenopausal women in England. *Int J Epidem.* 1999;28:241-246.

122. Hendrick P, Te Wake AM, Tikkisetty AS, et al. The effectiveness of walking as an intervention for low back pain: a systematic review. *Eur Spine J.* 2010;19:1613-1620. doi:10.1007/s00586-010-1412-z.

123. Chan CW, Mok NW, Yeung EW. Aerobic exercise training in addition to conventional physiotherapy for chronic low back pain: a randomized controlled trial. *Arch Phys Med Rehabil.* 2011;92:1681-1685.

124. Unsgaard-Tøndel M, Lund Nilsen TI, Magnussen J, et al. Is activation of transversus abdominis and obliquus internus abdominis associated with long-term changes in chronic low back pain? A prospective study with 1-year follow-up. *Br J Sports Med.* 2012;46:729-734. doi:10.1136/2of6bjsm.2011.085506.

125. Allison GT, Morris SL. Transversus abdominis and core stability: has the pendulum swung? *Br J Sports Med.* 2008;42:930-931. doi:10.1136/bjsm.2008.048637.

126. Ferreira PH, Ferreira ML, Maher CG, et al. Changes in recruitment of transversus abdominis correlate with disability in people with chronic low back pain. *Br J Sports Med.* 2010;44:1166-1172. doi:10.1136/1166bjsm.2009.061515.

127. Mannion AF, Caporaso F, Pulkovski N. Spine stabilisation exercises in the treatment of chronic low back pain: a good clinical outcome is not associated with improved abdominal muscle function. *Eur Spine J.* 2012;21:1301-1310. doi:10.1007/s00586-012-2155-9.

128. Vasseljen O, Unsgaard-Tøndel M, Westad C, et al. Effect of core stability exercises on feed-forward activation of deep abdominal muscles in chronic low back pain. *Spine.* 2012;37:1101-1108.

129. Chan ST, Fung PK, Ng NY, et al. Dynamic changes of elasticity, cross-sectional area, and fat infiltration of multifidus at different postures in men with chronic low back pain. *Spine J.* 2012;12:381-388.

130. Beneck GJ, Kulig K. Multifidus atrophy is localized and bilateral in active persons with chronic unilateral low back pain. *Arch Phys Med Rehabil.* 2012;(93):300-306.

131. Hides J, Stanton W, Mendis MD, et al. The relationship of transversus abdominis and lumbar multifidus clinical muscle tests in patients with chronic low back pain. *Manual Ther.* 2011;16:573-577.

132. Ershad N, Kahrizi S, Abadi MF. Evaluation of trunk muscle activity in chronic low back pain patients and healthy individuals during holding loads. *J Back Musculoskel Rehabil.* 22:165-172. doi:10.3233/BMR-2009-0230.

133. Kumar S, Sharma VP, Negi MPS. Efficacy of dynamic muscular stabilization techniques (DMST) over conventional techniques in rehabilitation of chronic low back pain. *J Strength Cond Res.* 2009;23(9):2651-2659.

134. França FR, Burke TN, Hanada ES, Marques AP. Segmental stabilization and muscular strengthening in chronic low back pain: a comparative study. *Clinics.* 2010;65(10):1013-1017.

135. Critchley DJ, Ratcliffe J, Noonan S, et al. Effectiveness and cost-effectiveness of three types of physiotherapy used to reduce chronic low back pain disability: a pragmatic randomized trial with economic evaluation. *SPINE.* 2007;32(14):1474-1481.

136. Macedo LG , Latimer J, Maher CG, et al. Effect of motor control exercises versus graded activity in patients with chronic non-specific low back pain: a randomized controlled trial. *Phys Ther.* 2012;92(3):363-379.

137. Goldby LJ, Moore AP, Doust J, et al. A randomized controlled trial investigating the efficiency of musculoskeletal physiotherapy on chronic low back disorder. *SPINE.* 2006;31(10):1083-1093.

138. Costa LOP, Maher CG, Latimer J, et al. Motor control exercise for chronic low back pain: a randomized placebo-controlled trial. *Phys Ther.* 2013;89(12):1275-1286.

139. Nassif H, Brosset N, Guillaume M, et al. Evaluation of a randomized controlled trial in the management of chronic lower back pain in a French automotive industry: an observational study. *Arch Phys Med Rehabil.* 2011;92:1927-36.

140. Smeets RJEM, Vlaeyen JWS, Hidding A, et al. Active rehabilitation for chronic low back pain: cognitive-behavioral, physical, or both? First direct post-treatment results from a randomized controlled trial [ISRCTN22714229]. *BMC Musculoskel Disord.* 2006;7:5. doi:10.1186/1471-2474-7-5.

141. Sertpoyraz F, Eyigor S, Karapolat H, et al. Comparison of isokinetic exercise versus standard exercise training in patients with chronic low back pain: a randomized controlled study. *Clin Rehabil.* 2009;23:238-247.

142. Kell RT, Risi AD, Barden JM. The response of persons with chronic nonspecific low back pain to three different volumes of periodized musculoskeletal rehabilitation. *J Strength Cond Res.* 2011;25(4):1052-1064.

143. Limke JC, Pena E, Rainville J, et al. Randomized trial comparing one set vs. two sets of resistance exercises for outpatients with chronic low back pain and leg pain. *J Eur Phys Rehabil Med.* 2008;(44):399-405.

144. Slade SC, Keating JL. Trunk-strengthening exercises for chronic low back pain: a systematic review. *J Manipulative Physiol Ther.* 2006;29:163-173.

145. Al-Obaidi SM, Al-Sayegh NA, Ben Nakhi H, et al. Evaluation of the McKenzie intervention for chronic low back pain by using selected physical and bio-behavioral outcome measures. *PM R.* 2011;3:637-646.

146. Garcia AN, Gondo FLB, Costa RA, et al. Effects of two physical therapy interventions in patients with chronic non-specific low back pain: feasibility of a randomized controlled trial. *Rev Bras Fisioter, São Carlos.* 2011;5(15):420-427.

147. Paatelma M, Kilpikoski S, Simonen R, et al. Orthopaedic manual therapy, Mckenzie method or advice only for low back pain in working adults: a randomized controlled trial with one year follow-up. *J Rehabil Med.* 2008;40:858-863.

148. Machado LA, von Sperling de Souza M, Ferreira PH, et al. The McKenzie method for low back pain a systematic review of the literature with a meta-analysis approach. *Spine.* 2006;31:E254-E262.

149. Carpenter DM, Nelson BW. Low back strengthening for the prevention and treatment of low back pain. *Med Sci Sports Exerc.* 1999;31(1):18-24.

150. Bruce-Low S, Smith D, Burnet S, et al. One lumbar extension training session per week is sufficient for strength gains and reductions in pain in patients with chronic low back pain ergonomics. *Ergonomics.* 2012;55:4, 500-507.

151. Harts CC, Helmhout PH, de Bie RA, et al. A high-intensity lumbar extensor strengthening program is little better than a low-intensity program or a waiting list control group for chronic low back pain: a randomised clinical trial. *Aust J Physiother.* 2008;54:23-31.

152. Bunzli S, Gillham D, Esterman A. Physiotherapy-provided operant conditioning in the management of low back pain disability: a systematic review. *Physiother Res Int.* 2011;16:4-19.

153. Rasmussen-Barr E, Ang B, Arvidsson I, et al. Graded exercise for recurrent low-back pain—a randomized, controlled trial with 6-, 12-, and 36-month follow-ups. *SPINE.* 2009;34(3):221-228.

154. Smeets RJEM, Vlaeyen JWS, Hidding A, et al. Chronic low back pain: physical training, graded activity with problem solving training, or both? The one-year post-treatment results of a randomized controlled trial. *Pain.* 2008;134:263-276.

155. George SZ, Wittmer VT, Fillingim RB, et al. Comparison of graded exercise and graded exposure clinical outcomes for patients with chronic low back pain. *J Orthop Sports Phys Ther.* 2010;40(11):694-670. doi:10.2519/jospt.2010.3396.

156. van Middelkoop M, Rubinstein SM, Kuijpers T, et al. A systematic review on the effectiveness of physical and rehabilitation interventions for chronic non-specific low back pain. *Eur Spine J.* 2011;20:19-39. doi:10.1007/s00586-010-1518-3.

157. van der Roer N, van Tulder M, Barendse J, et al. Intensive group training protocol versus guideline physiotherapy for patients with chronic low back pain: a randomised controlled trial. *Eur Spine J.* 2008;17:1193-1200. doi:10.1007/s00586-008-0718-6.

158. Sahin N, Ilknur Albayrak I, Durmus B, et al. Effectiveness of back school for treatment of pain and functional disability in patients with chronic low back pain: a randomized controlled trial. *J Rehabil Med.* 2011;43:224-229.

159. Yang EJ, Park W-B, Shin H-I, Lim J-Y. The effect of back school integrated with core strengthening in patients with chronic low-back pain. *Am J Phys Med Rehabil.* 2010;89:744-754.

160. Stanos S. Focused review of interdisciplinary pain rehabilitation programs for chronic pain management. *Curr Pain Headache Rep.* 2012;16:147-152. doi:10.1007/s11916-012-0252-4.

161. Pieh C, Altmeppen J, Neumeier S, et al. Gender differences in outcomes of a multimodal pain management program. *PAIN.* 2012;153:197-202.

162. MacLaren JE, Gross RT, Sperry JA, et al. Impact of opioid use on outcomes of functional restoration. *Clin J Pain.* 2006;22:392-398.

163. Howard KJ, Mayer TG, Theodore BR, et al. Patients with chronic disabling occupational musculoskeletal disorder failing to complete functional restoration: analysis of treatment-resistant personality characteristics. *Arch Phys Med Rehabil.* 2009;90:778-785.

164. Scascighini L, Toma V, Dober-Spielmann S, et al. Multidisciplinary treatment for chronic pain: a systematic review of interventions and outcomes. *Rheumatology.* 2008;47:670-678.

165. Demoulin C, Stéphanie Grosdent S, Lucile Capron L, et al. Effectiveness of a semi-intensive multidisciplinary outpatient rehabilitation program in chronic low back pain. *Joint Bone Spine.* 2010;77:58-63.
166. Dufour N, Thamsborg G, Oefeldt A, et al. Treatment of chronic low back pain: a randomized, clinical trial comparing group-based multidisciplinary biopsychosocial rehabilitation and intensive individual therapist-assisted back muscle strengthening exercises. *Spine.* 2010;35(5):469-476.
167. Kaapa EH, Frantsi K, Sarna S, et al. Multidisciplinary group rehabilitation *versus* individual physiotherapy for chronic nonspecific low back pain a randomized trial. *SPINE.* 2006;31(4):371-376.
168. Monticone M, Ferrante S, Rocca B, et al. Effect of a long-lasting multidisciplinary program on disability and fear-avoidance behaviors in patients with chronic low back pain: results of a randomized. *Clin J Pain.* 2013 Jan 25. [Epub ahead of print].
169. Roche-Leboucher G, Petit-Lemanac'h A, Bontoux L, et al. Multidisciplinary intensive functional restoration *versus* outpatient active physiotherapy in chronic low back pain a randomized controlled trial. *SPINE.* 2011;36(26):2235-2242.
170. Moradi B, Hagmann S, Zahlten-Hinguranage A, et al. Efficacy of multidisciplinary treatment for patients with chronic low back pain: a prospective clinical study in 395 patients. *J Clin Rheumatol.* 2012;18:76-82.
171. Henchoz Y, Pinget C, Wasserfallen JB, et al. Cost-utility analysis of a three-month exercise programme vs usual care following multidisciplinary rehabilitation for chronic low back pain. *J Rehabil Med.* 2010;42: 846-852.
172. Henchoz Y, de Goumoens P, Norberg M, et al. Role of physical exercise in low back pain rehabilitation a randomized controlled trial of a three-month exercise program in patients who have completed multidisciplinary rehabilitation. *SPINE.* 2010;35(12): 1192-1199.
173. Huge V, Schloderer U, Steinberger M, et al. Impact of a functional restoration program on pain and health-related quality of life in patients with chronic low back pain. *Pain Med.* 2006;7(6):501-508.
174. Beaudreuil J, Kone H, Lasbleiz S, et al. Efficacy of a functional restoration program for chronic low back pain: prospective 1-year study. *Joint Bone Spine.* 2010;77:435-439.
175. Waller B, Lambeck J, Daly D. Therapeutic aquatic exercise in the treatment of low back pain: a systematic review. *Clin Rehabil.* 2009;23:3. doi:10.1177/0269215508097856.
176. Pons T, Shipton EA. Multilevel lumbar fusion and postoperative physiotherapy rehabilitation in a patient with persistent pain. *Physiother Theory Pract.* 2011;27(3):238-245.
177. Dundar U, Solak O, Yigit I, et al. Clinical effectiveness of aquatic exercise to treat chronic low back pain a randomized controlled trial. *SPINE.* 2009;34(14):1436-1440.
178. Cuesta-Vargas AI, Adams N, Salazar JA, et al. Deep water running and general practice in primary care for non-specific low back pain versus general practice alone: randomized controlled trial. *Clin Rheumatol.* 2012;31:1073-1078.
179. Cuesta-Vargas AI, García-Romero JC, Arroyo-Morales M et al. Exercise, manual therapy, and education with or without high-intensity deep-water running for nonspecific chronic low back pain: a pragmatic randomized controlled trial. *Am J Phys Med Rehabil.* 2011;90:526-538.
180. Baena-Beato PA, Arroyo-Morales M, Delgado-Fernández M, et al. Effects of different frequencies (2–3 days/week) of aquatic therapy program in adults with chronic low back pain: a non-randomized comparison trial. *Pain Med.* 2013;14:145-158.
181. Wand BM, O'Connell NE, Di Pietro F, et al. Managing chronic nonspecific low back pain with a sensorimotor retraining approach: exploratory multiple baseline study of 3 participants. *Phys Ther.* 2011;91:535-546.
182. Gatti R, Faccendini S, Tettamanti A, et al. Efficacy of trunk balance exercises for individuals with chronic low back pain: a randomized clinical trial. *J Orthop Sports Phys Ther.* 2011;41(8):542-552. Epub 7 June 2011. doi:10.2519/jospt.2011.3413
183. del Pozo-Cruz B, Hernández-Mocholí MA, Adsuar HC, et al. Effects of whole body vibration therapy on main outcome measures for chronic non-specific low back pain: a single-blind randomized controlled trial. *J Rehabil Med.* 2011;43: 689-694.
184. Iles R, Taylor NF, Davidson M, et al. Telephone coaching can increase activity levels for people with non-chronic low back pain—a randomized trail. *J Physiother.* 2011;57(4):231-238. doi:10.1016/S1836-9553(11)70053-4.
185. Badke MB, Boissonnault WG. Changes in disability following physical therapy intervention for patients with low back pain: dependence on symptom duration. *Arch Phys Med Rehabil.* 2006;87:749-756.
186. Wessels T, van Tulder M, Sigl T, et al. What predicts outcome in non-operative treatments of chronic low back pain? A systematic review. *Eur Spine J.* 2006;15:1633-1644. doi:10.1007/s00586-006-0073-4.
187. Vincent HK, tOmli MR, Tim Day T, et al. Fear of movement, quality of life, and self-reported disability in obese patients with chronic lumbar pain. *Pain Med.* 2011;12: 154-164.
188. Rasmussen-Barr E, Campello M, Arvidsson I, et al. Factors predicting clinical outcome 12 and 36 months after an exercise intervention for recurrent low back pain. *Disabil Rehabil.* 2012;34(2):136-144. doi:10.3109/09638288.2011.591886. Epub 2011 Sep 29.
189. Hicks GE, Benvenuti F, Fiaschi V, et al. Adherence to a community-based exercise program is a strong predictor of improved back pain status in older adults: an observational study. *Clin J Pain.* 2012;28:195-203.
190. Chiu TTW, Hui-Chan CHY, Cheing G. A randomized clinical trial of TENS and exercise for patients with chronic neck pain. *Clin Rehabil.* 2005;19:850. doi:10.1191/0269215505cr920oa.

Physical Modalities, Orthoses, and Assistive Devices

Aaron J. Yang
Steven Stanos

PHYSICAL MODALITIES

Modalities are commonly used to produce a response in tissues and include heat, water, cold, sound, and electricity. These modalities should not be used as the primary mode of treatment but rather used in adjunct with the main intervention such as physical or occupational therapy. This chapter will discuss the more common modalities used as well as briefly discussing electrical stimulation. **Box 97-1** describes factors to consider prior to selection of a specific therapeutic modality.

HEAT

Therapeutic uses for heat are based on analgesia, increase in collagen elasticity, and hyperemia to decrease pain, reduce contractures and joint stiffness, and decrease muscle spasms.[1] Therapeutic range for heat is 40°

BOX 97-1

Considerations in Modality Selection

- Intended tissue location
- Depth and intensity of heating or cooling
- Comorbidities such as neuropathy, inflammatory conditions, cancer
- Age of the patient
- Pregnancy
- Body habitus
- Cognition

to 45°C and is commonly maintained for about 5 to 30 minutes. It is important to note that the temperature for pain threshold in humans is 45°C.[2] Heat can be divided by superficial and deep heat and is dependent on depth of heat and form of transfer of heat which include convection, conversion, conduction, and radiation. *Convection* is the contact between two surfaces at different temperatures with resultant flow through this medium to transport thermal energy. Examples include contrast baths and hydrotherapy. *Conduction* is the transfer of thermal energy between two bodies by contact at different temperatures with examples such as hot water and hot packs. *Conversion* is the transformation of energy to heat such as ultrasound and microwave diathermy. Lastly, *radiation* involves thermal radiation from any surface or body with temperature above absolute zero. General precautions for the use of heat are listed in **Box 97-2** but can include acute inflammation, ischemic locations, bleeding disorders, impaired sensation, malignancy, scar tissue, and those with inability to communicate or respond to pain.[3]

Superficial heat is considered to be 1 to 2 cm and deep heat generally involves increasing tissue temperature to a depth of 3 to 5 cm or more. Examples of superficial heat include heating pads, hydrocollator packs, whirlpool baths, and paraffin baths which achieve maximal tissue temperature in the skin and subcutaneous fat. Hot packs such as hydrocollator packs are commonly stored in heated water tanks and need to be wrapped in layers of insulation prior to being applied to the skin. Caution should be used as this type of modality is one of the most common reasons for burns in therapy sessions. Radiant heat in the form of heat lamps can also be used therapeutically and is usually placed 30- to 60 cm from the patient's body and is useful when the patient cannot tolerate the weight of the heating pads. Paraffin baths is another type of modality that is used with wax and mineral oil. Immersion technique has been shown to provide the greatest duration of temperature increase and is commonly applied in scleroderma patients.[4] Superficial heat is commonly used to treat low back pain, arthritic conditions, neck pain, and various chronic musculoskeletal injuries.[5]Examples of deep heat include ultrasound, shortwave, and microwave diathermy. These modalities transfer heat through conversion and the differences are outlined in **Table 97-1**. Ultrasound diathermy should not be confused with diagnostic ultrasound. Ultrasound heats the greatest at the bone-tissue interface while short wave diathermy heats fat more so than muscle. Ultrasound that is

BOX 97-2

Precautions for Use of Therapeutic Heat

- Acute inflammation
- Bleeding disorder or hemorrhage
- Malignancy
- Impaired sensation
- Vascular disease
- Scars or atrophic skin
- Inability to respond to pain

TABLE 97-1 Deep Heat Modalities

Ultrasound	Shortwave	Microwave
• Frequency: 0.8-1.1 MHz • Sound waves • Depth: 8 cm	• Frequency: 27.12 MHz • Radio waves • Depth: 4-5 cm	• Frequency: 915-2456 MHz • Microwaves • Depth: 1-4 cm

therapeutic in nature uses high frequency energy to produce a deeper tissue response and the most commonly used frequency is a range from 0.8 to 1.1 MHz. Thermal response in tissues involves energy absorption causing heat production in tissues whereas nonthermal responses cause distortion and movement of tissues.[6] Techniques for ultrasound application can vary with the most common technique involving stroking the probe over the affected site as opposed to static application. Contraindications for therapeutic ultrasound include areas over fluid-filled cavities, laminectomy sites due to concern for heating the spinal cord, open epiphysis in the growing adolescent, pacemakers, and prosthetic cements.[7]

Shortwave diathermy is used to treat deep muscles and joints and commonly uses a frequency of 27.12 MHz. This type of modality can involve two condenser plates placed on either side of the body part or induction coils that can be molded to the body part. Through conversion, electromagnetic energy converted to thermal energy travels between the coils or condensers to cause deeper heating of tissues. Contraindications for this type of treatment include pacemakers, metal objects, and heating over the eyes. General contraindications for the three modalities for deep heat are listed in **Table 97-2**

CRYOTHERAPY

Therapeutic uses for cold are based on immediate local vasoconstriction to reduce swelling and acute inflammatory response, decreased pain and muscle spasm, decreased spasticity, slowing of the nerve conduction velocity, and decrease in local metabolism. Cryotherapy is often used in acute musculoskeletal conditions as well as for spasticity management.[8] Mechanisms for cold transfer include conduction, convection, and evaporation. Examples of conduction include cold packs and ice massage; convection includes cold baths; and evaporation includes vapocoolant sprays. Cold packs can generally be applied for 20 to 30 minutes with external compression providing increased effectiveness of cooling.[9] Vapocoolant sprays are commonly combined with stretching of a contracted muscle to treat various musculoskeletal related conditions.[10]

General precautions and contraindications for cryotherapy are listed in **Box 97-3** and include cold intolerance or hypersensitivity, impaired sensation, communication or cognitive deficits, arterial insufficiency, and cryopathies such as paroxysmal cold hemoglobinuria or cryoglobulinemia. In general, cold application should be avoided over superficial nerves due to increased risk of affecting nerve conduction.

HYDROTHERAPY

The main forms of hydrotherapy are contrast baths, shower carts, and whirlpool baths with therapeutic use in arthritic conditions and also for burn injuries with gentle debridement. Whirlpool baths are commonly used for partial body immersion while Hubbard tanks are larger and used

TABLE 97-2 General Contraindications for Deep Heat

Ultrasound	Shortwave	Microwave
• Malignancy • Open epiphysis • Pacemaker • Near to heart; reproductive organs • Laminectomy site • Total hip prosthesis	• Metal • Contact lenses • Immature skeleton	• Immature skeleton • Fluid-filled cavities

BOX 97-3

Precautions for Use of Cryotherapy

- Impaired sensation
- Cold intolerance
- Ischemia
- Raynaud syndrome or phenomenon
- Cryopathies or cryoglobulinemia
- Poor cognition

for total body immersion. With increased body immersion and extremes in temperature change, there is increased potential for change in core body temperature. As mentioned previously, burns or infected areas of the skin can be therapeutically treated with antiseptic conditions with sodium hypochlorite most commonly used as an antibacterial solution. General contraindications for hydrotherapy include bowel and bladder incontinence, unstable blood pressure, and uncontrolled epilepsy.

Briefly, other modalities that may be encountered include iontophoresis and phonophoresis. Iontophoresis involves the use of an electrical field to move charged particles across a biologic membrane. For therapeutic purposes it is used to deliver medicines directly to soft tissues with a small electric current which limits systemic absorption.[11] The therapeutic medication is placed on the electrode of the same polarity with the opposite electrodes placed on the skin. A current is applied to drive the medication away from the electrode into the directed tissue target. Common diagnoses that are treated with this modality include various bursitis and plantar fasciitis. Phonophoresis involves the use of ultrasound on topically applied medicines to facilitate migration of the medication into the skin. Corticosteroids are the most common medications used and are indicated to treat bursitis, osteoarthritis, and contractures.

ELECTRICAL STIMULATION

One of the most common forms of electrical stimulation used for treatment of pain is transcutaneous electrical nerve stimulation (TENS). Based on the Gate Control theory proposed by Melzack and Wall in 1965, TENS stimulates the large Ia myelinated afferent nerve fibers "gating" or blocking afferent pain transmission at the dorsal horn, thus modulating ascending pain signals to the brain.[12] TENS units are often used as adjuvant therapy to a more active rehabilitation program including exercise, stretching, and strengthening. The most common and effective type of stimulation is a high-frequency, low-intensity stimulation which results in increased tolerance and shorter onset pain relief. On the other hand, low-frequency, high-intensity stimulation causes more immediate discomfort but more commonly leads to longer lasting analgesia. Contraindications include circulatory impairment, pregnancy, active hemorrhage, malignancy, and decreased skin sensation.

ORTHOSES

An orthosis is an external device applied to the body that can provide multiple different functions including support and stability, prevention or correction of a deformity, assistance in weak muscles, controlling spasticity, and limit range of motion or unload damaged joints. Orthotics assist for the spine as well as the upper and lower extremities. This section will focus on the more commonly encountered orthoses including spinal orthotics, ankle foot orthoses (AFO), knee orthosis, and static wrist-hand orthosis.

SPINAL ORTHOTICS

These orthoses can be subdivided into the more common cervical and thoracic and lumbar orthosis. The Philadelphia collar is a common cervical orthosis used for stable bony or ligamentous injuries with more control of flexion and extension. The Philadelphia collar is commonly used during emergency transport, after cervical fusion, or halo removal. The Philadelphia collar limits flexion and extension by 70% and less with rotation. This orthosis is used to wean off more rigid orthosis such as the sternal occipital mandibular immobilizer (SOMI) brace which is used for bedridden patients due to lack of posterior uprights, stabilizing the cervical and thoracic regions and limiting flexion by 75%. This brace is easier to don and doff in contrast to the halo vest which has a rigid headpiece secured by pins and posters that connect to a vest or plaster body cast. The halo device provides the best control of motion in all planes and is commonly used to treat unstable cervical fractures and dislocations. The halo is used for approximately 3 months and the pins should be checked for tightness every 1 to 2 days. **Table 97-3** shows normal cervical motion from the occiput to the first thoracic vertebra and the effect of different cervical orthoses on limiting motion.[13]

TABLE 97-3 Normal Cervical Motion

	Mean of Normal Motion (%)		
Cervical Orthosis	Flexion/Extension	Lateral Bending	Rotation
Normal	100	100	100
Soft collar	74.2	92.3	82.6
Philadelphia collar	28.9	66.4	43.7
SOMI brace	27.7	65.6	33.6
Halo device	4.0	4.0	1.0

Rigid truncal orthoses include the Jewett brace which uses a three-point pressure system to allow extension but limit flexion, leaving the abdomen free and applying pressure on bone prominences (i.e., sternum, pubis anterior, and the thoracolumbar junction posteriorly). It is typically used to treat lower thoracic or upper lumbar compression fractures or is used after surgical stabilization. The thoracolumbosacral orthosis (TLSO) extends from the sacrum to the inferior angle of the scapula and is commonly used to prevent progression of scoliosis and to stabilize the trunk from the middle thoracic segments to the lower lumbar spinal segments. It is most commonly used during postoperative stabilization from spine surgery. The TLSO is also used to decrease load on the spine by increasing intraabdominal pressure which decreases load on the spine. Lastly, the Taylor brace provides flexion and extension control similar to a TLSO and is primarily used to treat kyphosis from osteoporotic fractures.

ANKLE FOOT ORTHOSES

The ankle foot orthosis (AFO) is commonly used to assist the ankle joint that may be affected due to weakness or pain. The composition of the AFO may be plastic or metal with a plastic design being more advantageous because of its light weight, cosmetic appearance, and intimate fit whereas the metal AFO can accommodate fluctuating edema. The three most common types of plastic AFOs include the posterior leaf spring, semirigid plastic, and solid AFO. The posterior leaf spring AFO is composed of a thin plastic piece placed behind the ankle that allows the patient to push off or plantar flex at the ankle thus overpowering the brace when needed. This is typically used in patients with flaccid foot drop. The semirigid AFO provides much less motion than posterior leaf spring AFO and increases mediolateral stability at the ankle. The semirigid AFO is used when increased stability of the ankle is needed or there is foot drop with associated extensor tone. Lastly, the rigid plastic AFO is used when the patient exhibits high levels of spasticity or complete immobilization of the ankle is required. It is important that the calf band be at least 1 inch below the fibular neck in order to avoid compression of the common peroneal nerve.

KNEE ORTHOSES

Knee orthoses may be used to provide support of the knee and typically are used to either provide mediolateral stability or prevent hyperextension of the knee. They may be used during increased physical activity, unstable knees, or in the rehabilitation period. Knee orthoses are classified as *prophylactic*, *rehabilitative*, and *functional*. Prophylactic knee bracing helps to prevent or reduce severity of injuries although evidence for this is lacking.[14] Common types of prophylactic orthoses include flexible orthoses typically made from rubber to enhance proprioceptive feedback at the knee and provide minimal stability. More rigid and durable rehabilitative orthoses include the Swedish knee cage and Lenox-Hill derotation orthoses that not only provide structural protection but also limit knee hyperextension. Functional braces provide stability for unstable joints. They may be useful in stabilizing a laterally displacing patella or a weakened or torn anterior cruciate ligament (ACL).[15,16] Patients with advanced osteoarthritis may be fitted with a knee orthosis to unload increased pressures across the knee with a focus along the medial compartment of the knee. To date, bracing has shown a small beneficial effect with a recent Cochrane review demonstrating that the use of a knee brace may increase walking distance but does not lead to improvement in pain or function.[17]

STATIC WRIST-HAND ORTHOSIS

There are multiple types of upper limb orthoses used to immobilize, stabilize, support the joints, prevent contractures, and facilitate healing of different types of injuries. The static wrist-hand orthosis, also known as the resting hand splint, may be the most commonly encountered type of orthosis of the upper limb. This is commonly used to treat and rest an injured hand or prevent or stretch a contracture. It is usually applied to the volar surface of the arm and the wrist is usually placed in neutral with the thumb abducted and the metacarpal phalanges in flexion to 70°.

ASSISTIVE DEVICES

Assistive devices are tools that make a particular function or task easier to perform. They can aid persons with disabilities to perform their activities of daily living. This section will discuss mobility aids with a special focus on canes, walkers, and crutches. **Table 97-4** outlines general fitting guidelines for selected mobility aids. It should be noted that supervision or training with a therapist as well as strengthening of the upper extremities can enhance the benefits and safety of these devices.[18]

CANES

Canes are usually prescribed to improve balance, reduce weight-bearing forces of injured joints or structures, compensate for weakened muscles, and decrease pain. The cane can vary in the components from an inexpensive adjustable metal cane to a small or a wide-based quad cane provides a wider base of support. The function of the cane should be to increase the base of support, provide additional sensory feedback, and decrease loading on the lower limbs. In general, the cane should be held in the hand opposite of the affected lower limb and is advanced with the affected limb. This reduces the load on the affected limb 20% to 25%. The cane length should be from the bottom of the shoe heel to the height of the greater trochanters with the elbow flexed from 20° to 30°.[19] When climbing up and down stairs, patients should be counseled to ascend stairs with the strong and unaffected limb and to descend stairs with the affected limb.

TABLE 97-4 Fitting Guidelines for Selected Mobility Aids

Cane	Elbow should be flexed to 20°-30° with the tip of the cane at the level of the greater trochanter with the patient in an upright position
Walker	Walker should be placed 12 inches in front of the patient and the elbows should be flexed to 20° with the patient in an upright position
Axillary crutches	Length: Distance from anterior axillary fold to point 6 inches lateral to the foot with the patient in an upright position Handpiece: Elbow should be flexed to 30° with wrist in extension and fingers forming a fist

WALKERS

Compared to canes, walkers provide wider and more stable bases of support. The walker can allow up to 100% of weight-bearing relief of the affected lower limb and common indications can vary from bilateral lower extremity weakness or incoordination to general support to aid in mobility. One disadvantage of the walker is the slow and awkward gait pattern that may not only promote poor posture, but also cause difficulty maneuvering stairs and small spaces. A properly fitted walker is set with the elbows flexed to 20° with the patient standing straight and shoulders relaxed. The three most common types of walkers include the rolling walker, hemiwalker, and platform walker. The rolling walker is used for patients who cannot lift the upper limbs to advance the walker and also when a smoother reciprocal gait is desired. The hemiwalker is used by hemiplegics who need a wide base of support. The platform walker is used to allow weight bearing at the elbow without putting pressure on the distal upper extremities.

CRUTCHES

Crutches are more stable than canes because of the two points of contact with the body. Increased energy expenditure is needed to maneuver with crutches rather than canes and preparation with strengthening of the shoulder depressors such as the latissimus dorsi and other muscles such as the triceps, biceps, and hip extensor and abductors are crucial to avoid muscle fatigue. The most common crutches prescribed are the axillary, forearm (Lofstrand), and platform crutches. The axillary crutches are inexpensive and easier to use at the expense of requiring good strength and increased cardiac demand on the patient. Crutch length should be the distance from the anterior axillary fold to about 6 inches lateral to the foot with the patient standing. The hand piece should allow the elbow to be flexed to 30° with the wrist in extension and fingers forming a fist. The axillary nerve can be compressed with improper use; however, when used properly, the affected lower limb can be fully nonweight-bearing. Contrary to common belief, the axillary part of the crutch should not be padded as it is not designed to take on body weight as this can cause nerve injury. The patient should be able to raise the body 1 to 2 inches by extending the elbow. Forearm crutches are indicated when pressure on the axilla is contraindicated and also for freedom for hand activities. Unilateral forearm crutches may decrease body weight transmission by 40% to 50% to the opposite limb. However, they provide less trunk support than axillary crutches and may require more strength and skill to maneuver. Use of the bilateral forearm crutch may offload 80% of body weight on the affected limb.[20] Platform crutches are useful when the distal upper extremities are affected such as fractures of the wrist or hand because they avoid weight-bearing through the wrist and hand. However, they are heavy and may be difficult to maneuver. The patient's elbow should be flexed to 90° with the patient standing straight with shoulders relaxed.

REFERENCES

1. Falconer J, Hayes KW, Chang RW. Therapeutic ultrasound in the treatment of musculoskeletal conditions. *Arthritis Care Res*. Jun 1990;3(2):85-91.
2. Guy AW, Webb MD, Sorensen CC. Determination of power absorption in man exposed to high frequency electromagnetic fields by thermographic measurements on scale models. *IEEE Trans Biomed Eng*. Sep 1976;23(5):361-370.
3. Schmidt KL, Ott VR, Rocher G, Schaller H. Heat, cold and inflammation. *J Rheumatol*. Nov-Dec 1979;38(11-12):391-404.
4. Abramson DI, Tuck S, Jr., Chu LS, Agustin C. Effect of paraffin bath and hot fomentations on local tissue temperatures. *Archives of Phys Med Rehabil*. Feb 1964;45:87-94.

5. Lehmann JF, Warren CG, Scham SM. Therapeutic heat and cold. *Clin Orthop Relat Res.* Mar-Apr 1974(99):207-245.
6. Coakley WT. Biophysical effects of ultrasound at therapeutic intensities. *Physiotherapy.* Jun 1978;64(6):166-169.
7. Miller DL, Smith NB, Bailey MR, et al. Overview of therapeutic ultrasound applications and safety considerations. *J. Ultrasound Med.* Apr 2012;31(4):623-634.
8. Grant AE. Massage with ice (cryokinetics) in the treatment of painful conditions of the musculoskeletal system. *Arch Phys Med Rehabil.* May 1964;45:233-238.
9. Barlas D, Homan CS, Thode HC, Jr. In vivo tissue temperature comparison of cryotherapy with and without external compression. *Ann Emerg Med.* Oct 1996;28(4):436-439.
10. Kostopoulos D, Rizopoulos K. Effect of topical aerosol skin refrigerant (spray and stretch technique) on passive and active stretching. *J Bodyw Mov Ther.* Apr 2008;12(2):96-104.
11. Chien YW, Banga AK. Iontophoretic (transdermal) delivery of drugs: overview of historical development. *J Pharm Sci.* May 1989;78(5):353-354.
12. Melzack R, Wall PD. Pain mechanisms: a new theory. *Science.* Nov 19 1965;150(3699):971-979.
13. Johnson RM, Hart DL, Simmons EF, Ramsby GR, Southwick WO. Cervical orthoses. a study comparing their effectiveness in restricting cervical motion in normal subjects. *J Bone Joint Surg Am.* Apr 1977;59(3):332-339.
14. Rovere GD, Haupt HA, Yates CS. Prophylactic knee bracing in college football. *Am J Sports Med.* Mar-Apr 1987;15(2):111-116.
15. Draper CE, Besier TF, Santos JM, et al. Using real-time MRI to quantify altered joint kinematics in subjects with patellofemoral pain and to evaluate the effects of a patellar brace or sleeve on joint motion. *J Orthop Res.* May 2009;27(5):571-577.
16. Chew KT, Lew HL, Date E, Fredericson M. Current evidence and clinical applications of therapeutic knee braces. *Am J Phys Med Rehabil.* Aug 2007;86(8):678-686.
17. Brouwer RW, Jakma TS, Verhagen AP, Verhaar JA, Bierma-Zeinstra SM. Braces and orthoses for treating osteoarthritis of the knee. *Cochrane Database Syst Rev.* 2005(1):CD004020.
18. Hennessey WJ. Lower limb orthotic devices. In: Braddom RL, ed. *Physical Medicine and Rehabilitation.* 4th ed. Philadelphia, PA: Elsevier Saunders; 2011.
19. Joyce BM, Kirby RL. Canes, crutches and walkers. *Am Fam Physician.* Feb 1991;43(2):535-542.
20. Deathe AB HK, Winter DA. The biomechanics of canes, crutches, and walkers. *Crit Rev Phys Rehabil Med.* 1993;5:15-29.

SECTION D

Complementary and Alternative Therapies

CHAPTER 98 Acupuncture

Joseph F. Audette

INTRODUCTION

There has been growing interest in the West about the application of acupuncture to control pain since President Nixon's well-publicized trip to China in 1971. The fascination with this ancient medical modality was heightened when a member of the press corps, James Reston, received acupuncture during an appendectomy. The subsequent publication in 1998 of the National Institutes of Health (NIH) consensus statement on the clinical applications of acupuncture based on over 2000 scientific articles brought a degree of optimism that acupuncture would become a mainstay in the war against pain.[1]

There has been some dampening of the initial enthusiasm, however, with continued skepticism regarding the efficacy of acupuncture. This skepticism arose from the lack of high-quality randomized controlled clinical trials (RCTs); but the results of a number of recent large RCTs using sham acupuncture controls have nevertheless left many believing that acupuncture is just an elaborate placebo ritual.[2] As we shall discuss in more detail, the introduction of sham acupuncture has serious flaws but was based on the desire of researchers to filter the clinical practice of acupuncture through the mesh of standard placebo controlled methodology used in pharmacological research. Although clearly not a universal panacea for all pain syndromes, a more careful reading of the literature in fact does support that acupuncture is a cost-effective method for the treatment of pain.

The goal of this chapter is to lay the basic theoretical and physiological groundwork for understanding the clinical applications of acupuncture for pain. Then the current clinical data regarding the efficacy of acupuncture in various pain syndromes will be discussed. Attention will be given to understanding the pitfalls in devising a true placebo control for acupuncture trials, and our discussion of the literature will focus on the effect this has had on the outcomes of a number of large clinical trials for common pain conditions. Finally, a brief representation of some of the different treatment styles for common pain syndromes is outlined, and the chapter concludes by identifying further educational resources in this field.

BRIEF HISTORY OF ACUPUNCTURE

The term *acupuncture* is from the Greek *acus*, "needle," and *punctura*, "puncture"; it is the English translation of *chan* in Mandarin and *hari* in Japanese.

The clinical practice of inserting needles into the body (initially stone or flint needles) occurred in China by the 5th centuries BC and was followed some time later, between the 2nd and 3rd centuries BC, by the first written medical text on Chinese medicine, the *Huang Di Nei Jing*, or the *Yellow Emperor's Classic of Internal Medicine*. In this text, acupuncture was the most cited treatment method, with Chinese herbal therapies endorsed more cautiously because they were considered dangerous and potentially lethal if used incorrectly. In China, there was a slow evolution of practice, and by the 19th century, acupuncture had lost most of its support in the Imperial Court and herbal therapies were preferred. In the early 20th century, acupuncture had been eliminated from medical training colleges and was practiced mainly by itinerant healers with education provided through family traditions. In the 1930s Cheng Dan'an, a Western-trained Chinese physician, undertook to bring acupuncture out of its superstitious and metaphysical past and ground it on a more secure foundation based on Western concepts of anatomy and thereby bring it into the mainstream. His decision to pursue this effort was based on a personal experience that he had when his father had treated him with acupuncture for back pain. Cheng developed the seminal acupuncture text that is still used in China and is the basis for the acupuncture approach called Traditional Chinese Medicine (TCM) now practiced in the West.[3] With this modernized form of acupuncture, point combinations were often written for specific clinical presentations, in direct parallel to how herbal combinations were taught. This led to a proliferation of books giving point combinations that were thought of as canonical in the West but are actually the result of Western scientific and political influences on the evolution of acupuncture in China. In Japan, acupuncture has been practiced for over 500 years and has developed with an emphasis on using classical Chinese texts to guide practice, with less influence by the historical factors that led to the development of TCM in China. The use of TCM formulas has been readily adopted by Western researchers both because of the mistaken viewpoint that these formulas had an uninterrupted and ancient pedigree in China and because of the ease of maintaining scientific reproducibility. As discussed later in the chapter, this has had a significant adverse impact on study design and has led to some of the difficulties interpreting the results of recent large clinical trials in pain.

BASIC ACUPUNCTURE THEORIES

Chinese Taoist theories of yin and yang, or the balance of opposing influences in nature, underlie the theoretical framework used in acupuncture to understand human health. Human beings are seen as an integral part of a larger macrocosm that includes all the elements of the surrounding world. These elements are seen to have varying degrees of influence on the human organism, and factors such as weather, diet, and social environment are all taken to have significant effects on an individual's health. The dynamic balance of these external factors, together with the internal physical and emotional state of the organism, interacts in a complex way to influence health and disease. As a correlate to this holistic view of human health, Chinese medicine makes no distinction between mental and physical illness and largely bypasses the mind-body dualism that plagues Western medical traditions.

In this integrated framework, the workings and function of the internal organs are believed to have specific, observable effects on the external appearance of the individual. Subtle changes seen on the surface of the body are all seen to reflect accurately on the homeostasis of the internal organ system. For example, alterations in the skin color and skin texture, variations in the suppleness and compliance of underlying muscles, the quality of arterial pulses, and the appearance of the tongue and eyes are important factors that go into making a diagnosis and treatment plan.[2]

As an outgrowth of Taoist theories of health, forces were postulated to explain how the internal and external systems interrelated. This metaphysical construct led to the concept of *qi*, or *vital energy*. As a means of developing organized treatment strategies that could explain empirical observations of human health and disease, *qi* was postulated to flow in various channels or meridians in the body. There are 12 principal meridians, 8 extra meridians, and a total of 361 classic acupuncture points that are located on these proposed energy channels. Although an anatomical correlation to the meridians has not been located, the concept is useful to understand and treat symptoms seen in various disease and pain states and may provide clues about the deep organization of the nervous system (**Fig. 98-1**).

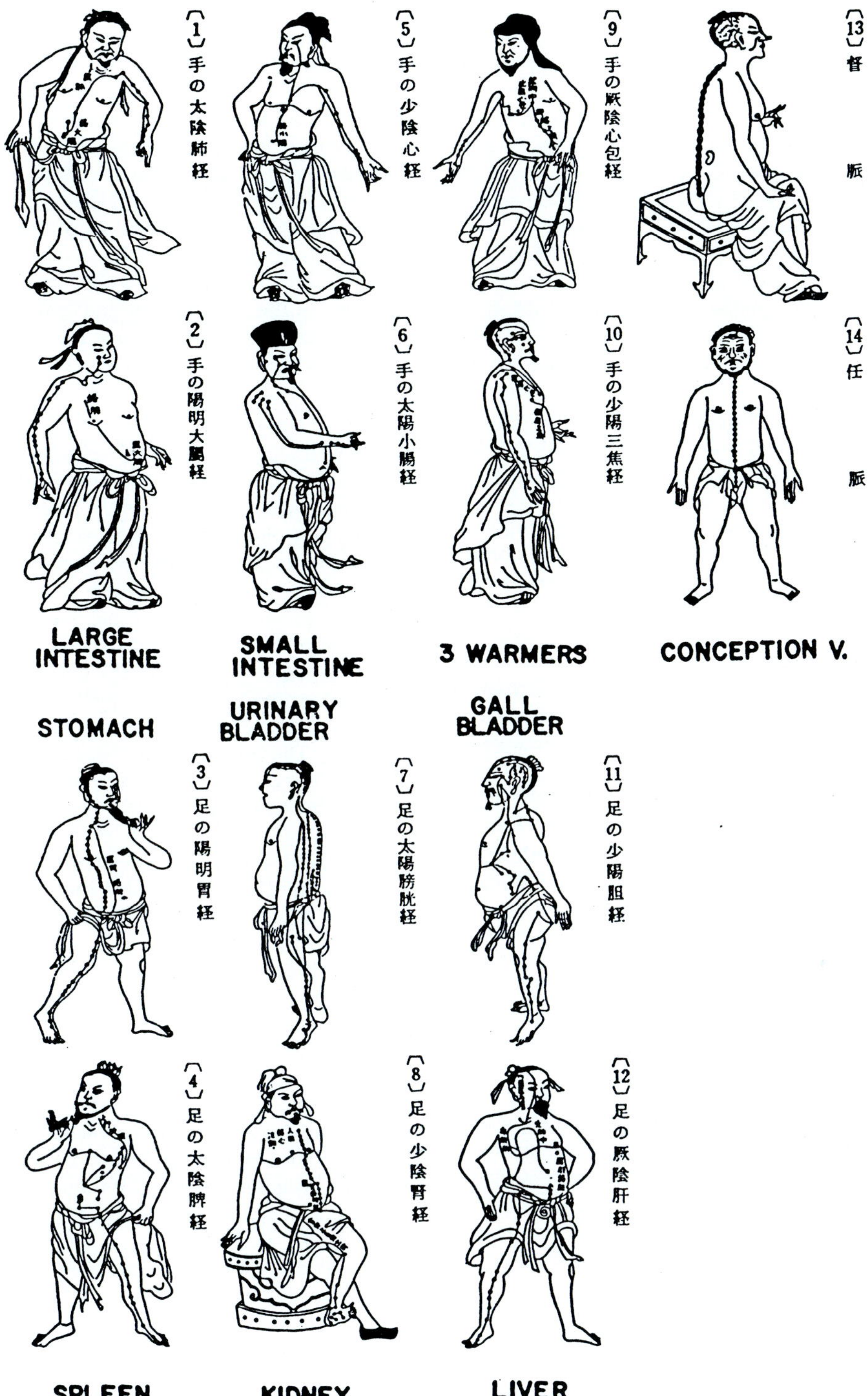

FIGURE 98-1. Diagrams of the 12 regular meridians and their organ correlates and two of the governing extraordinary meridians. (From Omura, Y. *Acupuncture Medicine: Its Historical and Clinical Background*. Tokyo, Japan: Japan Publications Inc; 1982. Used with permission by Dover Publications.)

The sine qua non of acupuncture treatment is for the practitioner to elicit the *de qi* response when inserting and manipulating the needle with a twisting and thrusting motion. This needle technique has been misinterpreted as a sensation that is as felt by the patient, indicating that the *qi* has been moved. This misinterpretation has been tacitly accepted in Western clinical research as a key component of ensuring the authenticity of the acupuncture treatment. Current clinical evidence strongly suggests that this phenomenon is not an adequate method of validating the treatment protocol.

SCIENTIFIC EVIDENCE

NEUROHUMORAL DATA

Over the last 30 years, a great deal of scientific evidence has accumulated to verify that both acupuncture point (AP) stimulation and electroacupuncture (EA) stimulation have reproducible physiologic effects. Three main lines of evidence are presented in the following discussion. All go to the heart of the neurologic mechanisms that are currently understood to modulate and influence pain.

The evidence for the release of endogenous opioids with AP and EA derives from the seminal work done by Pomeranz and Chiu[4] in animals and Mayer et al.[5] in humans in the 1970s. Since that time, a large body of evidence has developed to show that both AP and EA lead to the release of endorphins and enkephalins into the cerebrospinal fluid (CSF). Furthermore, the release of these neuropeptides has been demonstrated to play a role in the analgesic effect of acupuncture as evidenced by opioid-receptor antagonists that can abolish the analgesia obtained with acupuncture in both human and animal models of acute pain.

Since the initial studies, both the met-enkephalin-responding neurons in the dorsal column of the spinal cord and the endorphin and enkephalin active sites in the periaquaductal gray zone of the brain have been shown to be involved in acupuncture analgesia. Both the parameters of stimulation and the site of stimulation have significant effects on the type of chemical releases. In particular, antiserum to met-enkephalin abolished acupuncture analgesia but antiserum to dynorphin did not when a true acupuncture point was stimulated, whereas the reverse was true when a nonacupuncture or sham point was stimulated.[5] Manual acupuncture (MA) involves the insertion of an acupuncture needle into an acupuncture point followed by application of a stimulation technique, the most classic of which is a Chinese method of twisting the needle while thrusting up and down to elicit the *de qi* response. This method has been found to activate a broad range of afferent fibers, including Aβ, Aδ, and C.[6] In EA, a stimulating, alternating current via the inserted needle is delivered and has been found to activate Aβ and Aδ-fibers.[7] Centrally, the sensory information from acupuncture stimulation ascends through the spinal ventrolateral pathway to the brain with multiple effects that involve a network of brain regions, including the nucleus raphe magnus (NRM), periaqueductal gray (PAG), locus coeruleus, arcuate nucleus (Arc) of the hypothalamus, and the accumbens, caudate nuclei, and amygdale. There is a growing list of chemical releases that are felt to mediate acupuncture analgesia, including the opioid peptides (μ-, δ- and κ-receptors), glutamate (NMDA and AMPA/KA receptors), 5-hydroxytryptamine, and cholecystokinin octapeptide (CCK-8). Among these, the opioid peptides and their receptors in the descending pain modulatory pathway play an important role in mediating acupuncture analgesia.

One factor that may influence the response of a particular individual to acupuncture appears to involve CCK-8 receptor density.[8] Interestingly the blockade of CCK receptors also potentiates the placebo analgesic response.[9] Recently published evidence suggests that a patient's analgesic response to acupuncture may be related to the patient's genetic profile. In a Korean study using cDNA microarrays, investigators found that "high responders" had 375 genes that showed significant up- or downregulation compared to "low responders." Many of the genes that showed upregulation were related to signal related biomolecules and stress and immune function, suggesting that genetics may play a role in the patient's response to acupuncture.[10]

Electro-acupuncture stimulation has also been found to elevate levels of 5-hydroxytryptamine (5-HT) in the raphe nucleus, which enhances acupuncture analgesia presumably through descending inhibitory control mechanisms. Destruction of these neurons in the raphe nucleus of the midbrain or injection of paracholorophenylalanine, which lowers cerebral levels of 5-HT, will attenuate acupuncture analgesia, and injection of pargyline, which slows enzymatic degradation of 5-HT, enhances acupuncture analgesia.[11] There has been further elucidation of the specific subtypes of 5-HT receptors influenced by EA. In particular, intrathecal injection of antagonists of 5-HT1A and 5-HT3 receptors, but not 5-HT2A antagonists, significantly blocked EA-induced depression of cold allodynia in the neuropathic rat and reduced spontaneous pain behaviors.[12]

The hypothalamic-pituitary-axis and catecholamines are also influenced by EA and AP and may further influence the analgesic response to pain through both immune modulation and modulation of the sympathetic responses. It has showed that spinal α_2-adrenoceptors play a crucial role in inhibitory descending pain control by noradrenergic projections from supraspinal nuclei to the dorsal horn, particularly in modulating neuropathic pain.[13,14] Intrathecal injection of α_2 receptor antagonist yohimbine, but not α_1 receptor antagonist prazosin, significantly blocked EA analgesia in neuropathic rats.[12]

There is evidence to suggest that acupuncture analgesia may also work through blockade of NMDA and AMPA/KA receptors. In the rat spinal nerve ligation model, EA decreased nerve injury-induced mechanical allodynia.[15] Immunochemical studies revealed that nerve ligation increased the expression of NMDA receptor subtype NR1 immunoreactivity, which could be reduced by low-frequency EA.[16]

Spinal cord glia (microglia and astrocytes) make important contributions to the development and maintenance of inflammatory and neuropathic pain.[17] It appears that EA can also act to inhibit microglial activation in mice and rat models of chronic pain.[18,19]

NEUROIMAGING DATA

Recent technological advances in mapping brain activity using functional magnetic resonance scanning (fMRI) have begun to be applied to acupuncture. Comparison has been made between tactile sensation (tapping the skin with a wire at 2 Hz) and AP using a manual stimulation technique. The acupuncture stimulation used in this study involved twisting the needle at 2 Hz in L I4 (a point in the first dorsal interosseous muscle of the hand). Stimulation of an acupuncture point in this manner produces a *deqi* sensation, which is a full, aching feeling at the point of the needle and is believed to be important in obtaining the clinical effect with AP. The results of unilateral AP showed bilateral neural modulation of cortical and subcortical structures. The primary action was to decrease signal intensity in the limbic region and other subcortical areas. Tactile stimulation did not produce these changes in fMRI. In addition, if the needle was placed in the point and left at rest or placed subcutaneously and not in the muscle, fMRI signal decrease in these deep subcortical structures was not seen. This suggests that the response of the organism to AP depends on activation of the muscle sensory afferents and not the superficial afferents in the skin.[20]

Although most of the focus on the physiology of acupuncture has been on the release of endogenous opioids, the use of positron emission tomography (PET) has allowed the study of acupuncture effects on the opioid receptors themselves. In a study using 11C-carfentanil (an analog of the μ-opioid receptor) as the tracer, both short- and long-term increases in μ-opioid receptor binding potential in the cingulate, caudate, and amygdala were observed in patients receiving acupuncture therapy. In the comparison group that received sham acupuncture, the effects on μ-opioid receptor binding potential were not present, suggesting that acupuncture and sham acupuncture function by different mechanisms.[21]

PET has also allowed us to study the effects of acupuncture on brain metabolism. In a recent study by Park et al. using fluorodeoxyglucose (an analog of glucose) as the tracer, acupuncture stimulation was shown to increase glucose brain metabolism in the left insula, bilateral thalami, the superior frontal region of the right frontal lobe, and the inferior frontal region of left frontal lobe. At the same time, glucose metabolism was decreased in the cingulate and parahippocampal regions of the left limbic lobe. This study suggests that acupuncture changes regional brain glucose metabolism patterns in a very specific and specialized way based on the acupoints stimulated.[22]

These studies suggest that the grid of acupuncture points may be focused regions in the peripheral nervous system that represent a network of nodes that have profound and specific effects on modulating and regulating the activity of the central nervous system.

NEUROMODULATION DATA

It is still an open question whether acupuncture has an influence on pain and other disease states that goes beyond the direct effect of the chemical releases previously mentioned. The early data using fMRI suggest that the sensory stimulation provided by acupuncture may have direct and selective effects on CNS function. Although the demonstration that endogenous opioids can be consistently released in both animal and human experimental models has been an important step in verifying that acupuncture analgesia has a physiologic basis, there continues to be debate about whether this effect is sufficient to explain the observed clinical benefits. Humoral effects are nonspecific and short-lived and cannot explain why a certain treatment method for a particular condition would have a sustained or permanent disease-modifying result. The chemical releases observed with EA and AP may just be an epiphenomenon, indicating that there is an influence on the CNS without yet comprehending what the actual changes are. **Table 98-1** lists the problems with our current understanding of acupuncture analgesia.

An example of how the neurohumoral model fails to comprehend the clinical effect of AP is a recently published study using heat stimulation (moxabustion) of an acupuncture point on the fifth toe (B67) to turn breech babies after the 33rd week of pregnancy. The results of the study were profound, showing a significantly improved turning of the infants to the cephalic position at delivery compared with the control group. Of 130 fetuses in the intervention group, 98 (75.4%) were cephalic, compared with 62 (47.7%) of 130 fetuses in the control group ($P < .001$; relative risk = 1.58; 95% CI, 1.29–1.94).[23]

One theory that may help better explain the long-term effect of EA and AP is that by stimulating peripheral sensory afferents of the skin and muscle, sustained changes occur in the CNS through central neuromodulation. We are now just beginning to understand the basic mechanisms of pathologic neuromodulation that can lead to chronic pain. A fundamental concept that has emerged is that sustained nociceptive input can have profound effects on the CNS that cause adverse neuroplastic changes.[24] Interestingly, continuing along this line of argument, unlike transcutaneous electrical nerve stimulation (TENS), AP and EA do rely on a more "painful stimulation" of the peripheral nervous system.[25] In effect, through controlled stimulation of peripheral nociceptors, acupuncture may be causing a *reverse neuroplasticity* in the CNS.

A clue to the neuroplastic changes that may be occurring in the CNS with EP and AP is found in the literature looking at *c-fos* expression. The production of the *fos* protein in spinal cord and cerebral neurons is known to occur with painful peripheral nerve stimulation and is a guide to the location of neurons that have been activated by this noxious input. It is believed that the observed *c-fos* release in the CNS couples transient intracellular signals to long-term changes in the central processing of peripheral sensory input and heralds the initiation of adverse neuroplastic changes in response to nociceptive input.[26]

We now know that EP causes the expression of *c-fos* in certain cells of the CNS, but in cells that are different from those which express *c-fos* with noxious input.[27] In addition, EA has been shown to suppress *fos* expression in the spinal cord dorsal horn in response to mechanical noxious stimulation.[28] There is also evidence to suggest that point specificity is important. In a study of inflammatory pain in the hind foot of a rat, Gallbladder 30 produced significant anti-hyperalgesia, although Triple Warmer 5 (Waiguan) and sham points, an abdominal point and a point off meridian near GB30, did not.[29] These early data with animal models suggest that some form of reverse neuroplasticity is taking place with acupuncture stimulation.

There is a growing literature on maladaptive cortical changes in chronic pain leading both to regions of brain atrophy and to cortical sensitization.[30,31] In studies that used carpal tunnel syndrome as a model of peripheral nerve dysfunction, structural remodeling and neuroplasticity in cortical and subcortical regions of the brain were found. Acupuncture was found to have a conditioning effect on cortical sensitization.[32]

CORRESPONDENCE TO MYOFASCIAL TRIGGER POINTS

The previous section shows how basic research in acupuncture intersects with the current thrust of the work being done in understanding the physiology of pain. In addition, there is some evidence to suggest that EA and AP depend on stimulation of muscle sensory afferents. On the clinical side, the techniques developed for trigger-point injections and our understanding of their mechanisms of action are relevant to acupuncture techniques. Early on, Melzack demonstrated the high degree of point correlation between myofascial trigger points and acupuncture points.[33] The connection between myofascial pain and acupuncture is explained in terms more relevant to practitioners of acupuncture (**Table 98-2** and **Fig. 98-2**).[34]

Andersson has proposed that the key element underlying the physiologic effect of AP and EA is the sensory stimulation of the low- and high-threshold mechanoreceptors in muscle tissue, which occurs with trigger-point injection methods as well.[35] One can theorize that needle stimulation of the skin afferents tends to elicit a protective pain reflex that has as its main evolutionary goal to withdraw from danger. In contrast, needle stimulation of deeper afferents in muscle and tendons,

TABLE 98-1 Humoral Theories and Problems Associated with Acupuncture Analgesia

Humoral Theory of Acupuncture Analgesia	Problems
Endogenous opioid effect	Humoral effect short-lived.
Midbrain monoamines	Fails to explain importance of point selection and meridians.
Pituitary–hypothalamic-axis	Fails to explain disease modification and sustained analgesia obtained with acupuncture. Difficult to implement theory to explain effects of nonpain-related conditions such as stroke. Fails to capture neuromodulating effects of acupuncture.

TABLE 98-2 Acupuncture and Myofascial Trigger Point Correlations

Acupuncture Zone	Region of Body	Acupupoints	Muscles
Tai Yang	Dorsal zone: Frontal region of forehead to occiput. Down back to lateral ankles.	B 10 SI 9–14 B 11–25, 41–45 B 53, 54 B 31, 34	Suboccipital Scapular Thoracic and lumbar Paraspinals Gluteus medius Piriformis
Shao Yang	Lateral zone: Temporalis region of head to lateral arm to wrist extensors. Down flank to lateral aspect of leg.	GB 3–6, 8 GB 16 GB 20, 21 TH 9 GB 24–28 GB 29 GB 31	Temporalis Sternocleidomastoid and scalenes Upper trapezius Finger extensors Abdominal obliques Tensor fasciae latae Iliotibial band
Yang Ming	Ventral Zone: Mouth to anterior neck, anterior chest wall. Down abdomen to medial aspect of leg and foot.	ST 5–7 St 9,10 ST 14–18 ST 19–30 ST 31,32	Masseter Sternocleidomastoid Pectoral muscles Rectus abdominis Quadraceps muscles

Abbreviations: bladder, B; gallbladder, GB; small intestine, SI; triple heater, TH; stomach, ST.

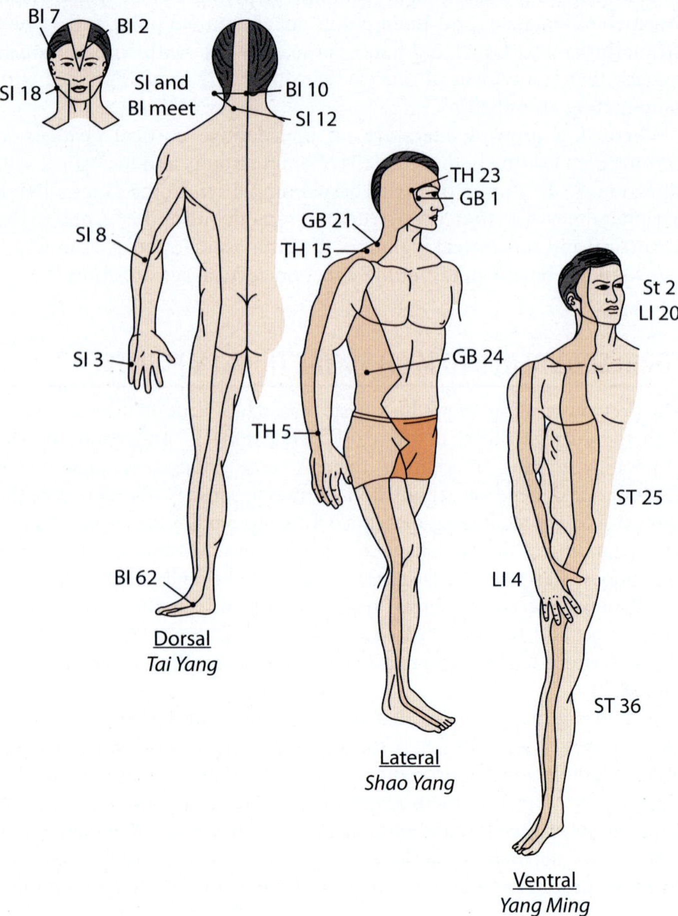

FIGURE 98-2. The Yang cutaneous zones are composed of the tendinomuscular, divergent, luo, and regular meridians of the regions diagramed. The zones act much like myofascial maps of muscular dysfunction and help organize both diagnosis and treatment of pain syndromes. (From Seem M. *A New American Acupuncture: Acupuncture Osteopathy, the Myofascial Release of the Bodymind Holding Patterns.* Boulder, CO: Blue Poppy Press; 1993. Used with permission.)

which are not normally involved in these protective reflexes, elicits a pain inhibitory rather than a pain-withdrawal reflex. Andersson makes the point that sustained, physical activity such as running also stimulates these muscle afferents, and many of the physiologic benefits of exercise might be related to the activation of the same mechanoreceptors that are stimulated with EA and AP.

Stimulation of the muscle mechanoreceptors also has distant effects on muscle tone that is not seen with cutaneous sensory stimulation. To illustrate this, EA of Large Intestine 4 and 11 (points in the first dorsal interosseous and extensor digitorum communis [EDC] muscles, respectively) has been shown to suppress the contralateral stretch reflex in the EDC, whereas painful subcutaneous stimulation in the same location had no effect.[36]

In a recent review, there have been a number of clinical trials showing that trigger-point injections and dry needling have similar efficacy and that the type of solution injected into the trigger point is irrelevant to clinical outcome. This suggests that the most important factor in relieving the pain associated with a trigger point is the needle stimulation of the muscle sensory afferents.[37] This is supported by many of the physiologic studies of EA and AP, in which the effect was achieved only when the needle stimulation occurred in the muscle underlying the acupuncture point, again showing the convergence of clinical experience with the work on myofascial trigger-point needling.

Recently, a group from the National Institute of Health has developed an acupuncture dialysis needle that allows in vivo sampling of the chemical milieu of an acupuncture point. A point in the neck, gall bladder 21 which corresponds to a common trigger point in the upper trapezius muscle was studied. In comparison of three groups, those with pain at rest in the region of gall bladder 21 with findings consistent with an active myofascial trigger point, those with no pain at rest but with evidence of a latent trigger point issue in the upper trapezius characterized by a taught band sensitivity to deep palpation, and healthy normal controls, the group with pain at rest had markedly elevated levels of substance P (SP), calcitonin gene-related peptide (CGRP), a lower pH, as well as other chemicals known to be involved with neurogenic inflammation and peripheral sensitization, including bradykinin, and tumor necrosis factor alpha (TNF-α).[38] This suggests that the physiology of an acupuncture point is not static and can change in response to various pathological states. When active, the effect of this process of peripheral sensitization can then make an acupuncture point more responsive to minimal needling techniques. The converse is suggested as well, in that in a healthy normal state, the acupuncture point gallbladder-21 may be minimally responsive to needling and requires more aggressive stimulation to produce any central physiological effect.

CLINICAL RESEARCH

An exhaustive review of the acupuncture literature was performed by a panel of experts convened by NIH, and their findings were published in the November 1998 edition of *JAMA*.[1] The conclusions of the review reveal that for many of the common pain conditions such as back pain, tendinitis, arthritis, headaches, and neuropathic pain, better-designed studies are needed to determine scientific efficacy. A series of meta-analyses have been published by Ernst on the effect of acupuncture for the treatment of back pain, osteoarthritis, and neck pain. Conclusions were similar in all cases: that in the studies that were deemed to be well-designed randomized controlled trials, acupuncture was often better than control treatments but inconsistently better than sham acupuncture treatments.[39-41] All of the studies reviewed suffered in general from small patient numbers, inconsistent use of outcome measures, and widely variable treatment strategies. Each of these methodologic problems makes it difficult to draw strong generalizations from these meta-analyses.

Sham needling is a means of introducing a placebo control into acupuncture research. Types of sham needling protocols used include inserting the needle a standard needling depth off meridian or on what are considered ineffective points without needling to obtain the *de qi* sensation. Other methods to make the technique more inert include minimal acupuncture where the needle is inserted into the subcutaneous fascia again without adding any additional needle stimulation. Streitberger and Kleinhenz and later Park developed placebo needle techniques in which the needle touches the patient's skin over a verum acupuncture point or a point off meridian but does not penetrate. In both of these research devices, the needle telescopes into the needle handle as it comes into contact with the skin, making it look to the patient as though the needle has penetrated through the skin.[42,43]

To correct these methodological deficits, a series of strongly powered RCTs have been published over the last 10 years, many from Germany, where acupuncture has been a covered service in the national health care system. This has led to a better understanding of the efficacy of acupuncture for common pain conditions as well as the effectiveness when this modality is delivered broadly by physician practitioners. However, important methodological issues continue to present difficulties. For example, a study by Leibina et al. in 2005 enrolled 150 subjects with chronic low back pain and randomized them to usual care versus usual care with verum acupuncture or usual care with sham acupuncture.

The verum acupuncture formula was developed by an expert, and treatment in both the verum and sham group was performed by the expert 5 times per week for 2 weeks, then once a week for 10 weeks, Although both the sham and verum acupuncture groups did significantly better than usual care, there was no statistical difference between the expert formula and sham groups. Patients in the verum group were needled at the same points and the practitioner used a needle technique to elicit the *de qi* response, yet the results were no better than putting the needles superficially into the subcutaneous fascia in locations 10 to 20 mm away from the official acupuncture points used in the study.[44] Contrast the result of this study with one performed by Molsberger's group in 2002 where he randomized 186 subjects with chronic low back pain into conventional orthopedic care (COT: physical therapy, diclofenac) versus COT with verum and COT with sham acupuncture. Subjects received three sessions per week for 12 weeks, and at the conclusion of treatment and at 3-month follow-up, the verum acupuncture group was significantly better than both COT and the sham with COT. A key difference in the acupuncture protocol used in the Molsberger study was that in addition to eliciting the *de qi* response at the points fixed by the protocol or formula, the acupuncturist was allowed the addition of 3 extra points that were individualized to the patient presentation.[45]

As a result of these trials, subsequent large trials sponsored by the German National Health Care system (GERAC initiative) devised a set of protocols to study patients with chronic low back pain, osteoarthritis of the knee, and headache.[46-48] The acupuncture protocol for each condition was designed by expert consensus and involved fixed points with the addition of a set of possible variable points that a practitioner could select based on the individual presentation. The trial design was multicenter with hundreds of physician acupuncturists enrolling patients in their practices across Germany. After patients were enrolled, they had the option to either be part of a randomized study comparing verum acupuncture to superficial sham points or be part of a large observational study comparing verum acupuncture to usual care. As in the Leibing study, the outcomes could not statistically distinguish between verum and sham, although both groups did significantly better than usual care. In a comprehensive meta-analysis that includes the above pain trials and groups the data from a number of large, well-designed trials from the United Kingdom, United States, Spain, and Sweden, a total of 14,597 patients were analyzed who were involved in trials with nonacupuncture controls and 5230 patients who were involved in studies in which the control was sham acupuncture.

Acupuncture was statistically superior to control for all analyses ($P < .001$), but the effect sizes were larger when the control group did not involve a sham acupuncture technique. The effect sizes in the analysis of nonacupuncture controlled studies were 0.55, 0.57, and 0.42 for spine-related pain, osteoarthritis, and chronic headache, respectively. The effect size when the control was sham acupuncture was by comparison 0.37, 0.26, and 0.15.[49] After review of data from controlled studies in which sham acupuncture was the control (superficially inserted needles into nonclassic locations), Lewith has argued that these sham locations for needle insertions are clearly not inert. It is likely that sham points that are not traditionally considered true acupuncture points have some efficacy, and he estimated that there is an analgesic effect from sham point stimulation in 40% to 50% of patients in comparison to an effectiveness in 60% of patients for true acupuncture point stimulation.[50]

Lundeberg argues that both sham needling and even use of a nonpenetrating placebo needle have physiological effects via such mechanisms as diffuse noxious inhibitory control (DNIC) that occurs any time tissue is traumatized (needle insertion) or if even the threat of trauma has occurred (needle in contact with skin).[51] There are styles of acupuncture, specifically Japanese techniques that utilize minimally invasive methods and even skin scratching techniques to effect a successful treatment.[52,53]

Part of the confusion about the consideration of minimal acupuncture methods as an inert placebo in acupuncture studies may come from the myriad of basic science studies on acupuncture analgesia using normal healthy animals and humans in contrast to clinical trials that are conducted on subjects with various chronic pain conditions. It is well known that in pathological pain states, the skin and deeper somatic tissues become sensitized as a result of both peripheral and central mechanisms.[54] Central sensitization leads to expanded receptive fields, resulting in a larger topographic distribution of responsiveness to small sensory inputs from the periphery. Even in visceral disease, there is evidence that by means of a process called dorsal root reflexes, a strong afferent drive to the dorsal horn can lead to retrograde release of neuropeptides such as substance P (SP) and calcitonin gene-related peptide (CGRP) into peripheral somatic and cutaneous tissue, leading to neurogenic inflammation. With tissue level peptide release, discrete areas of skin and muscle will become sensitized, leading to lower sensory thresholds and a greater responsiveness to minimal input.[55] In the early 1800s, Sir Henry Head characterized this phenomenon in humans in his seminal papers, in which he discusses patients who develop cutaneous allodynia and hyperalgesia in distinct multisegmental patterns in response to visceral disease.[56]

This leads to the concept of state dependent effects of acupuncture points, which has been clearly demonstrated with recent fMRI studies comparing healthy normal controls to individuals with pathological states. For example, in patients with carpal tunnel syndrome (CTS), the cortical brain response to needle stimulation at acupoint LI-4 in CTS patients compared with healthy controls (HC) was markedly different. CTS patients responded to verum acupuncture with greater activation in the hypothalamus and deactivation in the amygdala compared to HC. A similar difference was found between CTS patients at baseline and after 5 weeks of acupuncture therapy, suggesting that the brain response after a series of acupuncture treatments to needle stimulation at LI-4 became similar to that seen in HC.[57] In the same group of CTS patients, a nonnoxious stimulation to the affected hand led to a hyperactive response of the somatosensory cortex when compared to HC. Again after 5 weeks of acupuncture, this hyperactive response diminished and became similar to that seen in the HC. This supports the concept that in a pathological state like CTS, the system becomes sensitized and minimal peripheral input leads to an exaggerated cortical response that could be reversed with a course of acupuncture.[32] This supports Lundeberg's argument that in individuals with various pain conditions minimal or nonnoxious input with a sham acupuncture protocol can still have strong central effects on the central nervous system and is not an inert intervention.

A study at NIH strongly suggests that degree of responsiveness to needle stimulation may change dramatically based on the pathological state of an individual and that points not commonly thought to be classical acupuncture points may become active in response to disease by a process of neurogenic inflammation.[58]

TREATMENT PRINCIPLES

A number of treatment styles of acupuncture have influenced the practice of acupuncture in the United States. Many of these styles date back to prerevolution medical traditions prevalent in China prior to Mao and were exported to other Far East countries. One method commonly practiced in US is called *acupuncture energetics*. This technique evolved in Europe based on interpretations of the classic Chinese texts and was influenced by the Vietnamese in France. With this approach, point selection for pain is governed by the pattern of pain and symptoms presented by the patient and involves palpation of the areas of pain, much as one would do for assessing the location of trigger points. Japanese techniques rely heavily on palpation of soft tissue as well, with the exception of the needling technique, which is not as deep, and often there is no attempt to elicit the *de qi* response.

Postrevolutions styles of traditional Chinese medicine are strongly influenced by herbal treatment strategies. During the Communist revolution in China, an attempt was made to make acupuncture more systematic and uniform in technique and point location. This led to the use of diagnostic techniques developed by herbalists because it was felt by Mao to be more scientific.[3] An attempt is made to diagnose the state of balance of the internal organs by asking general questions and using pulse and tongue diagnosis. Palpation of the soft tissues is less common, and point selection is often directed at bringing the general state of health back to homeostasis rather than focusing on the specific local complaints of pain.

Other treatment techniques include Korean four-needle technique, where only four needles are placed regardless of the presenting condition, and Korean hand acupuncture that represents the whole body with extra points found in the hand. Auricular acupuncture is a more widely spread treatment technique that also takes a small part of the body—the ear—and represents the whole body in that region. A special aspect of this treatment method involves the use of a point localizer that is essentially an impedance meter.[59]

Unfortunately, there is no clinical research currently to guide treatment type or style for specific clinical conditions. From personal clinical experience, however, failure of one technique for a particular condition does not always imply total acupuncture failure, and there is some value in trying a few treatment techniques before labeling the acupuncture ineffective for the condition. In addition, although compared to many medical interventions, acupuncture is relatively safe; however, serious adverse effects have been reported, including serious infections, vascular injury, and pneumothorax, that require proper precautions.[60]

TRAINING OPTIONS

The accreditation of acupuncture educational programs is directed by the Accreditation Commission of Acupuncture and Oriental Medicine (ACAOM), formerly called the National Accreditation Commission for Schools and Colleges of Acupuncture and Oriental Medicine. The organization that credentials nonphysicians to practice acupuncture in the United States is the National Certification Commission of Acupuncture and Oriental Medicine (NCCAOM). The NCCAOM requires candidates to complete 1725 hours of formal didactics and 500 hours of clinical training in acupuncture. Candidates who meet these requirements are then eligible to sit for a national written and practical examination administered biannually. Despite these national standards, the practice of acupuncture is still further regulated by each state. Currently, 43 states and the District of Columbia license acupuncturists, and most follow the NCCAOM guidelines for nonphysicians.

The regulation of the practice of acupuncture by physicians and dentists also varies from state to state. As of 1999, 35 states permit physicians to practice acupuncture within the current scope of their license without requiring additional training. There are eight states that do require some additional training and certification (from 100 to 300 hours, depending on the state). Four states (Hawaii, Montana, Rhode Island, and Vermont) do not permit physicians to practice acupuncture within the scope of their license without the full training that nonphysicians are required to take.[61]

For full membership in the American Academy of Medical Acupuncturists (AAMA), individuals must have an active MD or DO license (or equivalent) to practice medicine under U.S. or Canadian jurisdiction, have completed a minimum of 220 hours of formal training in medical acupuncture (120 hours didactic, 100 hours clinical), and have 2 years of experience practicing medical acupuncture. Currently, most physicians are able to satisfy the educational and clinical requirements demanded by any state except the four previously mentioned by completing the training offered by the Helms Institute and through the Department of Medicine at the Brigham and Women's Hospital, both of which offer a 300-hour course in medical acupuncture that would satisfy both the AAMA requirements and most state requirements to practice acupuncture.

The federal Health Care Financing Administration (HCFA), which is responsible with administering the Medicare program, currently denies coverage for acupuncture pending establishment of the scientific efficacy of this modality. With a showing of such efficacy, HCFA may consider acupuncture as a "reasonable and necessary" service, at which time coverage would be authorized under the Federal Social Security Act 37.

CONCLUSIONS

As we move into the 21st century, the future of acupuncture for the treatment of pain is secure but still in need of better scientific validation. Acupuncture in many ways is out in front in the race to gain general scientific approval in comparison with other complementary and alternative treatment modalities. This is demonstrated by literature reviews and acceptance in many traditional Western medical hospital settings. But as the older sister in a family of holistic treatments, great responsibility still lies on those who are involved in this field and on those who will become involved in the future to help tear away the shroud of mystery that still clouds our view of this 2000-year-old treatment modality.

REFERENCES

1. NIH Consensus Conference. Acupuncture. *JAMA*. 1998;280:1518-1524.
2. Kerr CE, Shaw JR, Kaptchuk TJ, et al. Placebo acupuncture as a form of ritual touch healing: a neurophenomenological model. *Conscious Cogn*. 2011;20(3):787-791.
3. Andrews BJ. Acupuncture and the reinvention of chinese medicine. *APS Bulletin*. 1999;9(3).
4. Pomeranz B, Chiu D. Naloxone blockade of acupuncture analgesia: endorphins implicated. *Life Sci*. 1976;19:1757.
5. Mayer DJ, Price DD, Raffii A. Antagonism of acupuncture analgesia in man by narcotic antagonist naloxone. *Brain Res*. 1977;121:368.
6. Kim, JH, Min, BI, Park, DS, et al. The difference between electroacupuncture and acupuncture with manipulation on analgesia in rats. *Neurosci Lett*. 2000;279:149-152.
7. Leung A, Khadivi B, Yaksh T, et al. The effect of Ting point (tendinomuscular meridians) electroacupuncture on thermal pain: a model for studying the neuronal mechanism of acupuncture analgesia. *J Altern Complement Med*. 2005;11:653-661.
8. Chae Y, Park HJ, Lee H, et al. Individual differences of acupuncture analgesia in humans using cDNA microarray. *J Physiol Sci*. 2006;56:425-431.
9. Benedetti F. The opposite effects of the opiate antagonist naloxone and the cholevyctokinin antagonist proglumide on placebo analgesia. *Pain*. 1996;64:535-543.
10. Chae Y, Park HJ, Hahm DH, Yi SH, Lee HJ. Individual differences of acupuncture analgesia in humans using cDNA microarray. *Physiol Sci*. 2006;56(6):425-431.
11. Debreceni L. Chemical releases associated with acupuncture and electric stimulation. *Crit Rev Phys Rehab Med*. 1993;5: 247-275.
12. Kim SK, Park JH, Na HS, et al. Effects of electroacupuncture on cold allodynia in a rat model of neuropathic pain: mediation by spinal adrenergic and serotonergic receptors. *Exp Neurol*. 2005;195:430-436.
13. Millan MJ. Descending control of pain. *Prog Neurobiol*. 2002; 66:355-474.
14. Wiesenfeld-Hallin, Z. Long-term alleviation of allodynia-like behaviors by intrathecal implantation of bovine chromaffin cells in rats with spinal cord injury. *Pain*. 1998;74:115-122.

15. Huang C, Li HT, Han, JS, et al. Ketamine potentiates the effect of electroacupuncture on mechanical allodynia in a rat model of neuropathic pain. *Neurosci Lett.* 2004;368:327-331.

16. Sun, RQ, Wang HC, Wang Y, et al. Suppression of neuropathic pain by peripheral electrical stimulation in rats: A-opioid receptor and NMDA receptor implicated. *Exp Neurol.* 2004;187:23-29.

17. Watkins LR, Hutchinson MR, Johnston, IN, Maier SF. Glia: novel counterregulators of opioid analgesia. *Trends Neurosci.* 2005;28:661-669.

18. Kang JM, Park HJ, Lim S, et al. Acupuncture inhibits microglial activation and inflammatory events in the MPTP-induced mouse model. *Brain Res.* 2007;1131:211-219.

19. Sun S, Chen WL, Zhang YQ, et al. Disruption of glial function enhances electroacupuncture analgesia in arthritic rats. *Exp Neurol.* 2006;198:294-302.

20. Hui KK, Liu J, Makris N, et al. Acupuncture modulates the limbic system and subcortical gray structures of the human brain: evidence from fMRI studies in normal subjects. *Hum Brain Mapp.* 2000;9:13-25.

21. Harris RE, Zubieta JK, Napadow V, et al. Traditional Chinese acupuncture and placebo (sham) acupuncture are differentiated by their effects on mu-opioid receptors (MORs). *Neuroimage.* 2009; 47(3):1077-1085.

22. Park MS, Sunwoo YY, Chung YA, et al. Changes in brain FDG metabolism induced by acupuncture in healthy volunteers. *Acta Radiol.* 2010;51(8):947-952.

23. Cardini F, Weixin H. Moxibustion for correction of breech presentation: a randomized controlled trial. *JAMA.* 1998;280:1580-1584.

24. Woolf CJ, Salter MW. Neuronal plasticity: increasing the gain in pain. *Science.* 2000;9:1765-1769.

25. Woolf CJ, Thompson JW. Stimulation induced analgesic: transcutaneous electrical nerve stimulation (TENS) and vibration. In: Wall PD, Melzack R, eds. *Textbook of Pain.* 3rd ed. London, England: Churchill Livingstone, 1994.

26. Morgan JI, Curran T. Stimulus-transcription coupling in the nervous system: involvement of the inducible proto-oncogenes *fos* and *jun*. *Ann Rev Neurosci.* 1991;14:421-451.

27. Pan B, Castro-Lopes JM, Coimbra A. C-fos expression in the hypothalamo-pituitary system induced by electroacupuncture or noxious stimulation. *Neuroreport.* 1994;5:1649-1652.

28. Lee JH, Beitz AJ. The distribution of brain-stem and spinal cord nuclei associated with different frequencies of electroacupuncture analgesia. *Pain.* 1993;52:11-28.

29. Lao L, Berman BM, Ren K, et al. A parametric study of electroacupuncture on persistent hyperalgesia and Fos protein expression in rats. *Brain Res.* 2004;1020(1-2):18-29.

30. Apkarian AV, Hashmi JA, et al. Pain and the brain: specificity and plasticity of the brain in clinical chronic pain. *Pain.* 2011;152(3 Suppl):S49-S64.

31. Apkarian, AV, Sosa Y, Sonty S, et al. Chronic back pain is associated with decreased prefrontal and thalamic gray matter density. *J Neurosci.* 2004;24(46):10410-10415.

32. Napadow V, Hui KKS, Audette JF, et al. Somatosensory cortical plasticity in carpal tunnel syndrome treated by acupuncture. *Hum Brain Map.* 2007;28:159-171.

33. Melzack R, Stillwell DM, Fox EJ. Trigger points and acupuncture points for pain: correlations and implications. *Pain.* 1977;3(1):3-23.

34. Seem M. *A New American Acupuncture: Acupuncture Osteopathy, the Myofascial Release of the Bodymind Holding Patterns.* Boulder, Colo: Blue Poppy Press; 1993.

35. Andersson S. The functional background in acupuncture effects. *Scand J Rehab Med.* 1993;29(Suppl):31-60.

36. Milne RJ, Dawson NJ, Butler MJ, Lippold OC. Intramuscular acupuncture-like electrical stimulation inhibits stretch reflexes in contralateral finger extensor muscles. *Exp Neurol.* 1985;90:96-107.

37. Han S. Myofascial pain syndrome and trigger-point management. *Reg Anesth.* 1997;22:89.

38. Shah JP, Phillips TM, Danoff JV, Gerber LH. An in vivo microanalytical technique for measuring the local biochemical milieu of human skeletal muscle. *J Appl Physiol.* 2005;99(5):1977-1984.

39. Ernst E, White AR. Acupuncture for back pain. *Arch Intern Med.* 1998;158:2235-2241.

40. Ernst E. Acupuncture as a symptomatic treatment of osteoarthritis. *Scand J Rheumatol.* 1997;26:444-447.

41. White AR, Ernst E. A systematic review of randomized controlled trials of acupuncture for neck pain. *Rheumatology.* 1999;38:143-147.

42. Streitberger, K, Kleinhenz, J. Introducing a placebo needle into acupuncture research. *Lancet.* 1998;352(9125):364-365.

43. Park J, White A, Lee HJ, Ernst E. Development of a new sham needle. *Acupuncture in Medicine.* 1999;17(2):110-112.

44. Leibing E, Leonhardt U, Ramadori G, et al. Acupuncture treatment of chronic low-back pain—a randomized, blinded, placebo-controlled trial with 9-month follow-up. *Pain.* 2002;96(1-2):189-196.

45. Molsberger AF, Mau J, Pawelec DB, Winkler J. Does acupuncture improve the orthopedic management of chronic low back pain—a randomized, blinded, controlled trial with 3 months follow up. *Pain.* 2002;99(3):579-587.

46. Scharf HP, Mansmann U, Streitberger K, et al. Acupuncture and knee osteoarthritis: a three-armed randomized trial. *Ann Intern Med.* 2006;145(1):12-20.

47. Haake M, Muller HH, Schade-Brittinger C, et al. German acupuncture trials (GERAC) for chronic low back pain: randomized, multicenter, blinded, parallel-group trial with 3 groups. *Arch Intern Med.* 2007;167(17):1892-1898.

48. Diener HC, Kronfeld K, Boewing G, et al. Efficacy of acupuncture for the prophylaxis of migraine: a multicentre randomised controlled clinical trial. *Lancet Neurol.* 2006;5(4):310-316.

49. Vickers AJ, Cronin AM, Witt CM, et al. Acupuncture for chronic pain: individual patient data metaanalysis. *Arch Intern Med.* 2012;172(19):1444-1453.

50. Lewith G, Vincent C. Evaluation of the clinical effects of acupuncture: a problem reassessed and a framework for future research. *Pain Forum.* 1995;4:29-39.

51. Lundeberg T, Lund I, Naslund J, Thomas M. The emperor's sham—wrong assumption that sham needling is sham. *Acupunct Med.* 2008;26(4):239-242.

52. Ahn AC, Bennani T, Freeman R, Hamdy O, Kaptchuk TJ. Two styles of acupuncture for treating painful diabetic neuropathy—a pilot randomised control trial. *Acupunct Med.* 2007;25(l-2):ll-7.

53. Kawakita K, Shinbara H, Imai K, Fukuda F, Yano T, Kuriyama K. How do acupuncture and moxibustion act? Focusing on the progress in Japanese acupuncture research. *J Pharmacol Sci.* 2006; l00(5):443-459.

54. Lund I, Naslund J, Lundeberg T. Minimal acupuncture is not a valid placebo control in randomized controlled trials of acupuncture: a physiologist's perspective. *Chin Med.* 2009;4:1-9.

55. Peng HY, Chen GD, Lin TB, et al. Colon mustard oil instillation induced cross-organ reflex sensitization on the pelvic-urethra reflex activity in rats. *Pain.* 2009;142(1-2):75-88.

56. Beissner F, Henke C, Unschuld PU. Forgotten features of head zones and their relation to diagnostically relevant acupuncture points. *Evidence-Based Compl Altern Med Vol.* 2011:240653.

57. Napadow V, Audette J, Hui KKS, et al. Hypothalamus and amygdala response to acupuncture stimuli in carpal tunnel syndrome. *Pain.* 2007;130:254-266.

58. Shah JP, Danoff JV, Gerber LH, et al. Biochemicals associated with pain and inflammation are elevated in sites near to and remote from active myofascial trigger points. *Arch Phys Med Rehabil.* 2008;89(1):16-23.

59. Saku K, Mukaino Y, Ying H, Arakawa K. Characteristics of reactive electropermeable points on the auricles of coronary heart disease patients. *Clin Cardiol.* 1993;16:415-419.

60. Ernst E, White AR. Acupuncture may be associated with serious adverse events. *BMJ.* 2000;320:513.

61. Leake R, Broderick JE. Current licensure for acupuncture in the United States. *Altern Ther.* 1999;5(4):94-96.

SECTION E

Pain and Wellness

CHAPTER 99

Cognitive-Behavioral Treatment of Sleep Disorders in the Pain Patient

Lisa R. Strauss

INTRODUCTION

The physician treating either pain or sleep disorders is familiar with the comorbidity of complaints in the two domains. Inasmuch as sleep disturbances and pain each occur in a sizable proportion of the population,[1,2] it is to be expected that they would co-occur with some frequency even in the absence of mutual influence or common cause. However, estimates of their comorbidity[3,4] far exceed such expectations, and it is clear from both controlled experimentation and observational data that difficulty in one domain predisposes to difficulty in the other.

Whether the relationship between pain and disordered sleep is causative or coincidental for any given patient, it is beneficial for the pain physician to be acquainted with ameliorative strategies for impaired sleep and to know when to refer the patient to a sleep specialist. In the context of pain treatment, improved sleep may decrease pain per se, enhance the patient's ability to cope with pain, and confer long-term benefit on physical and mental health.[5-9] In some cases it may prevent development of chronic pain in acute-pain patients,[10] and may prevent regional pain from becoming more widespread.[11] Preventing, mitigating, or interrupting the influence of disturbed sleep on pain, or a vicious cycle in which pain and sleeplessness exacerbate each other, may not only benefit the individual, but also reduce lost-productivity costs to society.

Cognitive-behavioral interventions have long played an important role in the treatment of sleep disorders, and a developing body of research supports their efficacy in improving sleep in a pain population. Although studies of cognitive behavior therapy (CBT) for disordered sleep in patients with pain have focused on insomnia, there are a number of other sleep disturbances for which CBT is deployed in the general sleep-disordered population. The application of CBT to conditions other than insomnia, even if as yet unstudied specifically in the context of pain, bears some explication. Specific conditions (e.g., apnea) are known to exacerbate pain,[12] so their treatment might diminish the intensity and duration of pain. In addition, there is no a priori reason to surmise the failure of such techniques in patients with pain, especially considering that time-intensive and sometimes complex regimens for insomnia have been successfully applied in that population.[5,13-16]

CONFLUENCE OF PAIN AND SLEEP DISTURBANCE

The epidemiology of sleep disorders is complicated by a history of discrepant definitions of the most common disturbance, insomnia, estimates of whose prevalence range from 4% to 48% depending upon the stringency of defining criteria.[17,18] Sleep-disordered breathing and restless legs syndrome are the next most prevalent conditions.[1] At least one-third of the population is generally reported to suffer from some degree of sleep compromise and/or daytime sleepiness, and one out of ten to experience a clinically significant sleep disorder.[1] Estimates of the prevalence of chronic pain similarly vary widely depending upon definitions, populations, and methodologies, but 11% is a frequently cited figure for the adult population.[18]

More than 50% of patients seeking help for chronic pain report difficulties with sleep, with some estimates considerably higher.[3,19-22] Sleep-disordered breathing, periodic limb movements, and insomnia are among the sleep disturbances more prevalent in the presence of chronic pain,[23,24] and insomnia is especially common. In one study, 44% of respondents with chronic pain (versus 19% of pain-free controls) reported insomnia;[25] other studies offer higher estimates.[22,26] Patients with chronic pain also experience insomnia of greater chronicity and endorse more severe daytime consequences than nonpain controls,[27] as well as sleeping less than pain-free insomniacs.[24] In turn, a higher percentage of chronic insomniacs endorse chronic pain (50.4% vs. 18.2% of noninsomniacs) more than any other medical problem from a list of nine major categories of concern, including respiratory, neurological, and gastrointestinal difficulties.[26]

A wide gamut of chronic-pain conditions is associated with complaints of poor sleep, including arthritis, fibromyalgia, cephalgia, neck pain, back pain, temporomandibular pain, neuropathic pain, chronic widespread pain, and cancer pain.[5,18,19,22,24,28-30] Medical conditions that are not pain syndromes per se but that are associated with chronic pain, such as irritable bowel syndrome, are also associated with compromised sleep,[25,31] and far more prevalently than is the case for medical conditions more generally.[32,33] Sleep in patients with chronic pain may be noteworthy for its diminished quantity (as indexed by total sleep time, sleep latency, and duration of wakeful periods after sleep initiation) and/or diminished quality (i.e., sleep marked by fragmentation, insufficient slow-wave sleep, or other architectural abnormalities rendering it not fully restorative). For example, up to 75% of rheumatoid arthritis patients endorse sleep difficulties, significantly more than in a general medical population.[34] Fragmented sleep in rheumatoid arthritis patients is well documented, and may explain self-reports of nonrestorative sleep and daytime sleepiness in that population.[34] Rheumatoid arthritis patients also complain of difficulty initiating and maintaining sleep.[34]

Acute pain, too, is associated with compromised sleep, though the effects are usually short-term and reversible with alleviation of pain. For example, acute surgical pain is strongly associated with reduced sleep time and disturbances of sleep architecture.[35,36]

Among the risk factors for the development of sleep disturbance in a pain population are physiological and cognitive presleep arousal, depression or other mood disturbance, general anxiety, health anxiety, dysfunctional beliefs about sleep, greater pain and pain-related disability, inactivity, fatigue, age (with different age groups inclined to different sleep disorders), and the use of certain analgesics.[18,37] A number of pain medications suppress slow-wave and rapid eye movement (REM) sleep, much as pain itself does.[38] Tang et al.[22] found that affective pain ratings and health anxiety were the best predictors of insomnia severity in a chronic-pain population, accounting for 30% of the variance even after controlling for the effects of pain intensity, depression, and general anxiety. A later study of adults with pain and concomitant insomnia indicated that presleep cognitive arousal, but not presleep pain intensity, predicted a particular night's sleep quality,[37] a counterintuitive finding affirmed in an adolescent pain population by Lewandowski et al.[39] As reviewed in Smith and Haythornthwaite,[40] although pain patients experience disproportionate anxiety, depression, and other psychological and behavioral risk factors for the development of impaired sleep, a relationship between pain and sleep exists even in the absence of such factors.[3,41,42]

Insufficient sleep conversely serves as a risk factor for pain. Primary insomniacs report more spontaneous pain and evidence lower pain thresholds than matched controls.[43] Pain inhibition is also attenuated in insomnia subjects, though pain facilitation is not enhanced, seemingly because of a ceiling effect.[43] In a study of 424 patients with various pain disorders, disturbed sleep was one of three variables associated with reduced pain thresholds.[44] (The other two variables were depression and psychological distress.) Additional support for sleep disturbance as a risk factor for pain comes from studies showing that insufficient sleep interferes with analgesic treatment,[45] that pain patients who report concurrent insomnia endorse greater pain intensity than those who report normal sleep,[22] that severity of chronic pain is correlated with severity of sleep disturbance[4] (which equally supports pain as a risk factor for poor sleep), that sleep quality predicts next-day pain,[37] and that subjective sleepiness correlates with pain sensitivity.[46]

In the aftermath of acute injury, insomnia serves as an independent risk factor for the development of chronic pain[10,47] and for the evolution of widespread pain from regional pain.[11,48] One study examined the development of chronic pain after burn injury and found that insomnia at the time of discharge predicted more severe and less improved pain at long-term follow-up.[10] Sleep disturbance is also an independent predictor of physical and psychosocial disability in chronic-pain patients, above and beyond the effects of the pain itself or depression,[49] though there are data to the contrary for rheumatoid arthritis.[30] Still, depression itself is also a risk factor for pain. Patients with both major depression and insomnia experience chronic musculoskeletal pain more than do those with insomnia alone.[41]

Caveats in interpreting associations between sleep and pain include reliance on self-report measures in both domains, small sample sizes and insufficient controls in many studies, and the correlational nature of the data.

RECIPROCAL INFLUENCE OF SLEEP AND PAIN

A growing corpus of controlled studies supports the proposition that pain and sleep disturbances are causally related and mutually influential. Experimental manipulations argue that even short-term and not necessarily total sleep deprivation heightens propensity to acute pain in both humans and animals. For example, healthy volunteers develop spontaneous pain under conditions of partial or total sleep deprivation for 1 or more days,[50,51] and healthy women exhibit reduced capacity for pain inhibition after 3 nights of experimentally induced sleep fragmentation.[52] Several studies have restricted selected stages of sleep and demonstrated lower pain thresholds. Selective REM deprivation increases sensitivity to thermal pain,[53,54] although one study found such effects only with total sleep deprivation.[55] Selective slow-wave sleep deprivation decreases tolerance of pressure pain.[56] In general, hyperalgesia ensues under conditions of sleep restriction or disruption,[45]although there are data to the contrary.[57] Conversely, experimentally induced pain during sleep in healthy subjects effects disruptive changes to sleep architecture.[58,59]

There are three main pathophysiological hypotheses to explain the interrelationship between sleep and pain:[45] that pain enhances arousal, in turn disrupting sleep;[60] that a common neurobiologic system modulates both pain and sleep-wake patterns;[61] and, most recently and garnering significant support, that poor sleep affects pain processing.[52,62] These explanations are not necessarily mutually exclusive.

Sleep and pain are generally thought to exert mutual influence, whether unidirectionally or reciprocally.[18] One hypothesis as to why acute pain sometimes evolves into chronic pain is that a vicious cycle is established between sleep deprivation and pain.[18] A prospective study of women with fibromyalgia found, using self-report measures, that nighttime pain intensity predicted sleep quality, which in turn predicted pain intensity the next day.[63] Because insomnia after burn injury is a risk factor for chronic pain, greater pain in patients prior to hospital discharge is associated with a higher likelihood of chronic insomnia.[10] One study showed that sleep duration was highly predictive of next-day pain, which in turn predicted that night's sleep duration,[64] but again, there are data to the contrary regarding effects of presleep pain on sleep.[37,39] Other studies also corroborate the mutual influence of pain and sleep,[47,65] sometimes termed "bidirectional."[60,64]

Although pain and sleeplessness may be reciprocally influential, relief of pain may not be sufficient to relieve any insomnia precipitated by the pain, as insomnia can be maintained by a variety of factors once triggered.[66,67] It is therefore beneficial to offer relief from insomnia symptoms concurrent with the treatment of pain. In parallel, successful resolution of a sleep complaint in patients suffering from both pain and sleep difficulties may not provide sufficient relief of pain.[68]

COGNITIVE BEHAVIOR THERAPY AND ITS ROLE IN TREATING SLEEP DISORDERS

Cognitive behavior therapy[69,70] encompasses a family of techniques targeting distorted cognitions, maladaptive thought processes, and self-defeating behaviors symptomatic of and contributory to the genesis, maintenance, or exacerbation of susceptible conditions. Resolution of the problematic thoughts and behaviors can provide symptomatic relief and resiliency to future episodes.[71] CBT is grounded in the proposition that thought influences emotion, and in behavioral principles derived from the field of learning theory, including the precepts of classical and operant conditioning.[72]

The efficacy of CBT has been firmly established for both depression and anxiety,[73-76] both of which can serve as causes or emerge as sequelae of disturbed sleep.[77-83] Studies support its parity with antidepressant medication in the short run, and its superiority over the long term, perhaps because it imparts coping skills.[75,76,84] CBT is more effective than medication for anxiety disorders, and is considered the standard of care for such diagnoses.[85] Furthermore, CBT tends to be well accepted and well tolerated,[86-88] is usually without side effects, and can often be at least partially undertaken on a self-help basis.[89]

CBT has been adapted for use in the treatment of sleep disorders, having been especially well studied and validated for insomnia.[90-94] Among the other sleep-related concerns to which it is suited as at least an adjunct to medical care are intolerance of positive airway pressure in sleep-disordered breathing,[95-97] disorders of circadian rhythms,[98] parasomnias such as nightmares,[99] and even incontrovertibly biologically based syndromes such as narcolepsy, where coping with the diagnosis may be at issue, as may the need for structuring sleep opportunity.

The rationale for CBT targeting sleep symptoms in the pain patient extends beyond the general rationale for treating the sleep of those experiencing pain. There are multiple parallels and points of overlap in the cognitive distortions and maladaptive behaviors of those with pain and sleep difficulties such that CBT for one condition may have some carryover effect for alleviating or coping with the other. For example, Linton and MacDonald[100] point out parallels in the feelings, thinking, and behavior associated with both chronic pain and insomnia, including depressed mood and anxiety, hypervigilance, catastrophic thinking, ruminating about pain or sleep, and avoidance. Other shared pitfalls that may emerge as patients attempt to cope with or compensate for sleep or pain problems are spending excessive time in bed; lengthy naps; irregular sleep times; light exposure in the middle of the night; and habitual use of ethanol, caffeine, and prescription medications. These cognitive-behavioral factors can perpetuate sleep difficulties such that impaired sleep persists even after resolution of pain, making it imperative to offer independent treatment of sleep symptoms.

COGNITIVE BEHAVIOR THERAPY FOR INSOMNIA IN THE PAIN PATIENT

The term "insomnia" may refer to a symptom, a diagnosis, or both.[101] As a symptom, it is generally understood in contradistinction to hypersomnia to entail difficulty initiating or maintaining sleep, or achieving only nonrestorative sleep.[102] Informally, patients may think of it as difficulty initiating or reinitiating sleep. In an effort to systematize communication and redress often widely disparate criteria for insomnia in clinical and research contexts, the American Academy of Sleep Medicine has offered consensus guidelines for the definition of insomnia to include at least one sleep symptom (e.g., difficulty initiating sleep) and one waking symptom (e.g., fatigue), and has established that insomnia must entail a complaint of insufficient sleep in the context of sufficient opportunity and circumstances for sleep.[103] Insomnia is thereby differentiated from sleep deprivation, in which there exists insufficient opportunity or circumstances.

Insomnia as a nosological category subsumes several disorders, which differ depending upon the classification system in use. The most detailed taxonomic scheme is that found in the *International Classification of Sleep Disorders*, 3rd Edition (ICSD-3).[102] The new ICSD-3 no longer bases diagnoses on etiology. Other classifications are found in the *Diagnostic and Statistical Manual of Mental Disorders*, 5th Edition (DSM-5)[104] and the International Classification of Diseases, 10th Revision (ICD-10).[105]

Cognitive behavior therapy for insomnia (CBT-I) is a collection of techniques selectively applied in varying combinations depending upon symptomatology and suspected etiology. As its title suggests, CBT-I targets both thinking and behavior. It is essential to address both domains because insomnia is generally characterized by both maladaptive thinking and maladaptive behavior. The interventions detailed here and summarized in **Table 99-1** are usually offered in some combination rather than as monotherapies.[106,107]

STIMULUS CONTROL THERAPY

Stimulus control therapy, developed by Richard Bootzin in the 1970s,[108] requires the patient to use the bedroom only for sleep and sex, to come to bed only once drowsy, and to limit wakeful time in bed thereafter. If unable to sleep, the patient must get out of bed within 10 to 20 minutes and return upon becoming sleepy again, repeating this action as many times as necessary until sleep ensues. Additional instructions are to rise at an identical, reasonably early hour each morning regardless of how little one has slept, and to prohibit daytime napping. These last two recommendations enhance the homeostatic drive for sleep and address inconsistent timing of sleep that may undermine a stable and desirably timed circadian propensity for sleep and wakefulness, while the initial recommendations target maladaptive conditioned associations.

TABLE 99-1 Summary of Cognitive-Behavioral Interventions for Insomnia

Intervention	Description
Stimulus control therapy	• Use the bedroom only for sleep and sex. • Come to bed only once drowsy. • Limit wakeful time in bed. • Rise at the same time each morning. • Avoid napping.
Sleep restriction	• Establish a fixed rising time compatible with patient's current circadian rhythm. • Delay initial sleep time so that total sleep opportunity equals average time asleep plus about 30 minutes. • Gradually expand sleep window to optimize quantity and quality.
Cognitive restructuring	• Reappraise faulty cognitions using strategies such as examining evidence for and against propositions, identifying common errors in thinking, conducting cost-benefit analyses of holding to certain assumptions, and examining worst-case scenarios. • Alter maladaptive thought processes such as worry using techniques such as labeling anxious or negative thinking, scheduling "worry time," using imaginal worry exposure, and cultivating distraction.
Sleep hygiene	• Establish environmental conditions conducive to sleep, such as a cool, dark bedroom and a comfortable mattress and pillows. • Establish personal habits conducive to sleep, such as careful timing of caffeine, nicotine, or ethanol consumption; supportive timing of exercise; a warm bath 2 hours before bedtime; regular sleep hours; limited napping; and a substantial wind-down period each night.
Deep relaxation	• Meditation • Diaphragmatic breathing • Progressive muscle relaxation • Visualization • Hypnosis
Other approaches	• Psychotherapy as needed • Psychopharmacology as needed

Stimulus control therapy derives from an operant-conditioning paradigm in which a neutral stimulus serves as a signal that a behavioral contingency is in effect: in the presence of the stimulus, performing the behavior will elicit a reward (or punishment, depending upon the experiment). In the absence of the stimulus, no such reward for the behavior is forthcoming. The classic paradigm is one in which a pigeon is given a food reward for pecking a key only when a small light in its cage is illuminated; when the light is off, pecking the key brings no reward. The light serves as a so-called "discriminative stimulus."

In the treatment of insomnia, stimulus control therapy putatively helps patients establish bedtime and the bedroom environment as discriminative stimuli signaling that a rewarding, sleep-inducing contingency is in effect, thus occasioning a stronger association between response (e.g., lying in bed) and reinforcer (i.e., falling asleep). It is hypothesized that using the bedroom for myriad activities other than sleep both during the day (e.g., for paying bills or reading) and at night (e.g., for reading or watching television, or for lying awake while worrying about sleeplessness) prevents bedtime and the bedroom from signaling strongly that engaging in presleep behaviors then and there will be rewarded with sleep.

Classical conditioning may also or alternatively play a role in sleeplessness[109] in that the bedroom environment and activities occurring around bedtime become associated with states inconducive to sleep, such as anxious wakefulness. Such associations are a reasonable consequence of lying awake for long periods in bed while struggling with the frustration and toll of insomnia or while attempting to cope with pain, fatigue, and/or depression. Stimulus control therapy may work in part by extinguishing these associations and establishing competing ones between the bedroom and deep relaxation and drowsiness such that the bedroom comes to elicit relaxation and sleep.

A number of studies strongly support the efficacy of stimulus control therapy for insomnia,[110-112] and the therapy has been identified by the American Academy of Sleep Medicine as one of a small number of treatments for insomnia that outcome studies convincingly support as a standard of care.[107,113] Implementation can be challenging for patients[114] because the regimen must be adhered to strictly; because there is a delay in treatment response; because sleep may worsen at first; because the instruction to get out of bed whenever one can't sleep and the instruction to rise at the same time each day, though comforting to some, can stimulate anticipatory anxiety about sleep and a sense of pressure to sleep "or else" for others; and because being deprived of external means of relaxing and drowning out one's thoughts in bed (e.g., reading) may leave the patient feeling defenseless. Considerable support from the therapist and reassurance as to likely results are important during the few weeks it takes to overcome the problem, and capacity for adherence should inform treatment recommendations. It should be noted that the technique may need to be adapted if used in conjunction with sleep restriction therapy (see Sleep Restriction below), which may require staying awake beyond when one first feels sleepy to prevent sleep prior to a designated hour.

Stimulus control therapy may be of obvious benefit to the pain patient who attempts to mitigate and cope with discomfort by spending long hours in bed during the day or while awake at night, thereby establishing sleep-incompatible associations. Pigeon[115] points out that pain patients may thwart the instructions by noting their doctors' recommendations for bed rest or by feeling satisfied that "at least I am resting," or by invoking the reality that it can be physically challenging, painful, and antithetical to rest to get out of bed, perhaps repeatedly, and not to lie recumbent. Pigeon suggests coaching patients that "You may rest; you just need to do it somewhere other than the bedroom."

If pain is so severe or mobility so impaired that getting out of bed repeatedly would be intolerable or impractical, the patient should not attempt stimulus control therapy, but should instead come to bed only once drowsy and then remain there with the goals of relaxing body and mind, engaging in gentle distraction (e.g., by listening to audiobooks or reading under low lighting conditions), and relinquishing any tendency to "try" to sleep.

SLEEP RESTRICTION

Insomniacs often try to compensate for lost sleep by affording themselves lengthier than usual windows of opportunity for sleep.[67] For example, they may initiate sleep earlier or rise later than they did prior to the development of insomnia in order to make up for sleep lost in the middle of the night. Based on the principle that sleep-promoting, homeostatic mechanisms are best engaged by constraining total permissible hours for sleep, sleep restriction entails limiting the window of sleep opportunity.[116] Constraint is usually accomplished by establishing a fixed rising time compatible with the patient's current circadian rhythm, and delaying initial sleep time such that the window of time permitted for sleep equals the number of hours of sleep the patient actually tends to obtain on average plus about 30 minutes, though physicians may recommend less restrictive regimens to enhance acceptance and minimize anxiety. Sleep may alternatively or additionally be truncated at the morning end after comparison of current and premorbid sleep schedules. The sleep window is gradually expanded (usually in 15-minute increments every week) until sleep length and subjective depth are optimized and wakefulness and fragmentation are minimized. Some titration is usually required.

Sleep restriction, like stimulus control therapy, is highly effective for insomnia and meets stringent criteria set forth by the American Academy of Sleep Medicine as a recommended treatment.[113] As with stimulus control therapy, applicability to the pain patient obtains because of often excessive wakeful time spent in bed, though pronounced restriction should be prescribed cautiously due to a theoretical risk of increased pain. Sleep restriction may be poorly tolerated in any population for both physical and emotional reasons, but does tend to be well accepted when flexibly implemented as less restrictive "sleep compression."[117] Either method should be used judiciously in bipolar patients who are vulnerable to manic or hypomanic episodes with insufficient sleep and in patients with seizure disorders or other conditions, such as confusional states, that may dangerously flare with insufficient sleep.[40,118,119]

COGNITIVE RESTRUCTURING

It is not uncommon for insomnia patients to struggle with anxious and pessimistic thinking in anticipation of and during the night. Dysfunctional beliefs about sleep are more common in insomniacs than in normal controls.[120-122] Such thoughts emerge in response to failed efforts to sleep, and are almost certainly exacerbated by the challenge to coping posed by insufficient sleep itself. Although depression and anxiety are predisposing and sometimes precipitating factors in the development of insomnia, even patients without such predisposition can be vulnerable to negative and anxious thinking when confronted with insomnia. Such thinking in insomniacs is not usually symptomatic of a mood or anxiety disorder, although insomnia is a risk factor in the development of these disorders.[79,123,124]

Insofar as negative and anxious cognitions represent irrational or exaggerated appraisals of circumstances (e.g., "I could lose my job if I don't get some sleep" or "I cannot function at all if I have a bad night") and/or are undue objects of focus, they may maintain insomnia. Cognitions can function as perpetuating factors with respect to insomnia because sleep lends itself to performance anxiety,[106] and heightened concerns about sleep in turn heighten performance anxiety, thereby undermining performance. Anxiety about sleep also contributes to physiological and mental arousal, making it harder to relax enough for sleep. Pessimistic thinking (e.g., "I'll never get to sleep"), while perhaps protecting the patient from a continuing cycle of hope and disappointment, can itself fuel anxiety and can forestall adaptive efforts to improve sleep, as well as promote depression.

Although each insomniac is unique, there are certain anxieties commonly encountered in clinical practice, including but not limited to:

- Performance anxiety: insomniacs may believe it is their job to sleep, experience urgency to discharge that responsibility, pressure themselves to do so, and feel responsible for the consequences of failure.
- Anticipatory anxiety about the implications of insomnia for the next day or for the long term: insomniacs may anticipate feeling ill the next day; having difficulty functioning at work, school, or in caring for children; job loss; inability to cope; dependency on sleeping pills; being identifiably sleep-deprived and judged on that basis; lifelong difficulties with sleep; early death; and more.
- Anxiety about what the insomnia signifies about the sufferer: insomniacs may anxiously interpret sleep difficulties as a sign of potentially irremediable brain changes.

All of these anxieties may be exacerbated by common assumptions that bear reappraisal, such as "I need 8 hours of sleep to function"[125] or "My mistakes at work are due to my insomnia." The attendant anxieties may engender ill-advised strategies such as checking the clock or trying to sleep.[126] They may also foster hypervigilance about bedtime rituals and internal cues, as well as anticipatory anxiety hours before bedtime. Morin et al.[125] have developed the *Dysfunctional Beliefs and Attitudes about Sleep* scale (DBAS-16) to aid physicians in assessing which cognitions to target for a particular patient.

Patients must learn to relax excessive vigilance about sleep, relinquish intention to induce sleep, take sleeplessness and anxiety about it in stride, and appraise accurately the consequences and causes of sleep loss. The full complement of cognitive-behavioral strategies may be brought to bear on these aims.

Reappraisal of potentially faulty cognitions is achieved through methods such as examining evidence for and against propositions (which may entail gathering evidence from observation, published materials, interviewing others, or personal experimentation); identifying common errors in thinking (e.g., overgeneralization, "catastrophizing"); conducting cost-benefit analyses of holding to certain assumptions; and examining worst-case scenarios to recalibrate assessments of their severity and likelihood.[127] The patient who fears being fired from a job might be asked whether coworkers generally notice when he or she has not slept well, what the worst outcome might be if they did notice, what their most likely response would be, and whether he or she has come close to being fired due to the effects of sleep loss.

Maladaptive thought processes such as excessive worry can similarly be altered using a variety of approaches,[127] including labeling anxious or negative thinking as such; scheduling "worry time" to corral and organize a constructive approach to concerns; using imaginal worry exposure to defuse the impact of unsettling thoughts; cultivating distraction to provide relief and demonstrate that thoughts can be set aside; and practicing the deep relaxation techniques discussed below.

Psychoeducation is useful for introducing information patients do not already possess. For example, they may be taught that one can function on less than the optimal amount of sleep for long periods and that the suffering of insomnia need not equate with danger. Other distortions are best suited to formal cognitive-behavioral methods so that patients arrive at insights over which they feel ownership and so that they learn methods to employ if and as related anxieties arise. For example, pain patients might be invited to evaluate empirically the proposition that "bed rest is important after a night of insomnia."[106]

Pigeon[115] has identified certain other dysfunctional, sleep-related cognitions particular to pain patients, including doubt about their ability to achieve comfort, the belief that sound sleep will eventuate additional stiffness and soreness, the belief that pain will cause wakings and subsequent insomnia, and hopelessness about sleep related to lack of hope about the pain that precipitates the poor sleep. Additions to this list might include the belief that going to bed or to sleep is the best solution for pain, that changes to sleep habits will impede coping with pain, that pain will make it impossible to adhere to a treatment regimen, and that analgesics and sedative-hypnotics are more helpful to sleep than they actually are. Pigeon offers suggestions for how pain patients can be helped to reframe these cognitions by, for example, providing encouragement to optimize mattress and pillow comfort; inviting them to consider that morning stiffness would signify a restful night's sleep; advising them that it is normal to awaken from time to time even on good nights and that one can take that opportunity to change position; recommending stretching in the morning or during wakeful periods; and educating them regarding the severity or suddenness of pain required to occasion full wakefulness. They can also be educated that lying in bed or napping excessively to cope with pain can exacerbate insomnia. They can additionally be taught to identify maladaptive hypervigilance about pain and sleep, and to redirect their focus.

Patients are advised not to attempt detailed cognitive reappraisal or other complex cognitive interventions during the night when experiencing insomnia, but rather to deploy simple, reassuring, conclusory statements such as, "I'm feeling anxious right now, and that's okay. My job is just to get as peaceful as possible, whether or not I sleep well tonight." Soothing distraction may help during these wakeful periods, with many patients preferring judiciously selected audiobooks, which require little effort to consume, can be enjoyed in darkness, and afford ready redirection from anxious thoughts. If sound of even low volume is experienced as noxious, other forms of gentle, nonstimulating distraction should be considered.

SLEEP HYGIENE

Cultivating good sleep hygiene entails establishing environmental conditions and personal habits conducive to sleep.[128] Sleep-hygiene instructions vary but may include advice regarding timing of any caffeine, nicotine, or ethanol consumption (i.e., no caffeine after noon and no alcohol or nicotine in the hours before bedtime) and timing of exercise (late afternoon or early evening is best for many insomniacs); a warm bath 2 hours before bedtime; regular sleep hours; limited napping; a substantial wind-down period each night; and a cool, quiet, dark (until morning), and comfortable bedroom. Sleep-hygiene instructions, though helpful, tend not to be sufficient for treating insomnia.[107,110,129] It is generally considered best to offer them as part of an omnibus of interventions.[107] Selecting the particular behaviors that the patient needs to target and explaining their rationale may be more helpful and promote better compliance than just handing him or her a list.[115] Lengthy lists can also perpetuate a misconception that a complex and large number of behaviors must be mastered before sleep can ensue, fueling overeffort or resignation.

For the pain patient, sleep-hygiene advice might highlight the importance of a comfortable bed and pillows, extra pillows to prop limbs as needed, stretching at night, avoidance of bed during the day when in pain,[115] and encouragement to engage in relaxing and pleasurable nighttime activities outside the bedroom.

DEEP RELAXATION

Relaxation techniques are an effective component of therapy for insomnia,[113] an unsurprising finding given the autonomic hyperarousal and anxious thinking that characterize the syndrome. It is best to match the technique to the type of arousal: autonomic and/or cognitive.[106] Techniques include but are not limited to meditation,[130] which is helpful not only for relaxation but also for cultivating perspective on tendencies of mind such as worry or hypervigilance; diaphragmatic breathing; progressive muscle relaxation;[131] visualization;[132] and hypnosis. It is also best to match the technique to the patient's preferences and abilities.[106] For example, meditation may prove challenging for patients with limited commitment to regular practice, racing thoughts, or anxious attunement to their breathing, whereas persons who have been traumatized may feel threatened by techniques such as hypnosis that entail a sense of surrendering control.

Most techniques can be learned with self-help books, in special classes, through audio or video instruction, or in the office of a behaviorally oriented mental-health practitioner. With sufficient mastery and practice, the techniques are roughly equally effective in treating insomnia,[106] although they may need to be supplemented by other forms of stress management, self-care, mental-health care, or basic education in establishing relaxing regimens such as reading to wind down in the evenings.

Relaxation techniques are generally incorporated as part of a multicomponent treatment for insomnia, although evidence has accrued for their effectiveness on their own.[90,133,134] They are best applied with the aim of relaxation rather than sleep lest patients hijack them in the service of maladaptive goal orientation.[106] In fact, paradoxical intention not to sleep can sometimes usefully overcome the undermining effects of overeffort to sleep.[135] Time of day to implement the techniques varies, but most patients choose to practice at night. A key exception may be meditation, which can have an energizing effect.[136] Obviously, care must be taken in applying muscle-based techniques with the pain patient. Techniques may independently benefit both pain and sleep.[137]

OTHER APPROACHES

It is important to note that improvement in sleep habits and sleep-related cognitions is not always sufficient to cure insomnia, especially in patients with comorbid psychiatric conditions[8] or intense stress. The cognitive-behavioral therapist will assess the context in which symptoms are occurring so that insufficiencies and imbalances can be redressed in areas such as exercise, diet, social support, work/free-time balance, mental health, and use of substances to regulate mood, pain, and alertness. Self-defeating behaviors (e.g., lying in bed all day to cope with sleep loss, pain, and/or depression) are treated not only by challenging the thinking that reinforces them and through explicitly behavioral regimens targeting poor sleep habits and maladaptive conditioning, but also by addressing avoidance, low motivation, anhedonia, inadequate structure, and difficulty prioritizing self-care.[138] Key supplemental techniques include reinforcing positive behaviors through positive outcomes and self-reward; scheduling activities for pleasure and mastery; goal setting; and graded exposure to counter avoidance.[127,138]

Addressing mental-health concerns can be an essential part of successful treatment of insomnia. Among the psychiatric conditions associated with insomnia are unipolar and bipolar depression, posttraumatic stress disorder, generalized anxiety disorder, and obsessive-compulsive disorder.[77,78] Referral to a psychotherapist with expertise in the patient's condition may be indicated, as may referral to a psychopharmacologist.

Habitual use of sleeping pills may mask insomnia without treating its underlying cause, and may thereby hinder application of conventional cognitive-behavioral interventions. In such instances patients can be helped gradually to taper from their medications while concurrently implementing substitutive cognitive and behavioral strategies to rebuild their confidence and competence in achieving sleep without pharmacological aids. For many individuals, knowing that a pill is available can be sufficiently reassuring to permit use of nonpharmacological strategies.

OUTCOME STUDIES

CBT-I has been shown to be highly efficacious in treating insomnia in otherwise healthy patients, with improvements sustained and even enhanced at long-term follow-up and associated with reduced reliance on sleeping pills.[92,94,139,140] Some studies have extended CBT-I to patients with comorbid medical or psychiatric conditions and again demonstrated significant positive effects on sleep, but in these studies subjects have not been selected from an explicit pain population.[93,141] Case studies with chronic-pain patients argued that this population could benefit from CBT-I,[142,143] and four controlled studies with chronic-pain patients have evaluated this proposition.[5,13-16] All four support the efficacy of CBT-I in chronic-pain patients with results at least comparable to those seen in otherwise healthy insomniacs. All four studies employed stimulus control therapy and sleep restriction, with other components differing across studies. All are limited by use of self-report measures, which do not always conform to objective data, but such indices are standard and considered defensible in the study of insomnia.[144] Only one of the studies[15] demonstrated improvements in pain as a result of treating the sleep, and only once the data were reanalyzed.[5] Smith and Haythornthwaite[40] have speculated that greater increases in consolidated sleep over time, as seen at longer-term follow-up, might be required for pain reduction.

In the first study, Currie et al.[13] demonstrated reduced sleep latency and time awake after sleep onset (assessed with actigraphy as well as self-report measures) in subjects offered CBT-I in a group format relative to self-monitoring/wait-list controls. In the second study, Edinger et al.[14] compared fibromyalgia patients in three groups: those receiving individually administered CBT-I, those receiving sleep-hygiene instructions, and those receiving treatment as usual for fibromyalgia. They found reductions in the CBT-I group in self-reported sleep latency, total time awake, and sleep efficiency, which is defined as (time asleep/time in bed)*100. In the third study, Rybarczyk et al.[15] compared elderly patients with insomnia in three groups: those with chronic pain secondary to osteoarthritis, those with chronic obstructive pulmonary disease, and those with coronary artery disease. Patients were assigned either to a group CBT-I intervention or to a stress-management control group. All three medical groups demonstrated comparable improvements in self-reports of sleep latency, wake time after sleep onset, and sleep efficiency, and collectively, the medical groups reported significantly better sleep than the control group. In the fourth study, Jungquist et al.[16] recruited insomniacs with nonmalignant neck and/or back pain in whom the insomnia emerged after pain began, and assigned them either to individually administered and manualized CBT-I or to a contact/measurement control condition. Relative to controls, the CBT-I group evidenced significant improvement in sleep latency, wake time after sleep onset, number of awakenings, sleep efficiency, and sleep continuity as assessed by self-report measures.

COGNITIVE-BEHAVIORAL TECHNIQUES FOR INTOLERANCE OF CONTINUOUS POSITIVE AIRWAY PRESSURE IN THE PAIN PATIENT WITH OBSTRUCTIVE SLEEP APNEA

The ICSD-3[102] contains a category of diagnoses called "Sleep Related Breathing Disorders," the most common of which (occurring with 2% to 5% prevalence) is obstructive sleep apnea (OSA).[145] The respiratory events of OSA result in fragmentation of sleep. In severe cases, arousals occur as often as every other minute or more.[6] Daytime sequelae may include sleepiness and fatigue, cognitive impairment, depression, myalgia, and cephalgia.[12] Types of cephalgia associated with OSA include cluster, migraine, hypnic, and morning headaches.[12] The relationship between severity of OSA and severity of pain is equivocal.[146,147] OSA is more common in a pain population, probably in part because pain can occasion a sedentary lifestyle that promotes weight gain and because medications used in the context of pain (analgesic, muscle-relaxant, or hypnotic) may affect muscle tone in the airway during sleep.[115]

Continuous positive airway pressure (CPAP) is generally the first-line treatment for moderate to severe cases of OSA, reducing or eliminating obstructive events and consequent arousals, and preventing hypoxemia during sleep.[148] An additional advantage of CPAP in the OSA patient with comorbid pain is that CPAP has been shown to reduce sensitivity to pain in patients with severe OSA in a thermal nociception paradigm[6] and reportedly to reverse the pain response to stimulation of muscles associated with fibromyalgia.[12] Other treatments may include dental appliances that reposition the mandible, surgery, weight loss, and medications such as nasal steroids.[149]

Unfortunately, CPAP can be problematic for patients for a number of reasons,[149] including imperfect management of underlying symptoms, mechanical and ergonomic issues such as ill-fitting or leaky masks, attitudinal barriers such as perceiving the treatment as onerous or unnecessary, claustrophobia, cost, and insufficient family or clinical support. It is estimated that 18% of patients refuse to initiate treatment,[150] and that 25% discontinue treatment within 3 years[150] despite advances in mask and machine design. Only one-half use CPAP for longer than 4 hours per night.[151] Interestingly, level of adherence appears largely to be determined during the first week of treatment,[151] with 20 to 30% of the variance accounted for by patient perception of such factors as pros versus cons of use and self-efficacy.[152,153] Perceptions of symptomatic relief are also strongly linked to adherence,[150] but may take more than a week to coalesce. Other predictors of adherence include race and socioeconomic status.[154]

Psychological and educational interventions should theoretically be able to improve adherence by addressing such variables as pros (including outcome expectancy) versus cons, self-efficacy, social support, and claustrophobia. A review of 17 randomized trials examining educational, supportive, and behavioral interventions to enhance PAP adherence found that CBT fostered the greatest increase in usage, in part because more patients were willing to try PAP after intervention.[155] For example, one randomized, controlled study applied group cognitive therapy prior to CPAP initiation and yielded significantly greater usage as indicated by hours of use per night and total nights of use relative to a treatment-as-usual group.[95] The therapy addressed social support, self-efficacy, and outcome expectations, though this last variable proved not to increase with the intervention. Another randomized, controlled study increased usage through intensive support and CPAP supervision.[96] In contrast, a study providing regular telephonic support from a nurse did not yield positive results.[156] Therapy designed explicitly to enhance motivation has achieved promising results.[157] In vivo desensitization to CPAP in a claustrophobic patient was successfully applied in one published case study.[97]

Although no study has been published on the intervention, in clinical practice some CBT practitioners use desensitization to help nonclaustrophobic patients adapt to CPAP and the physical intrusion it entails using staged exposure to CPAP in situations gradually approximating the usual sleep environment, time, and circumstances. Accompanying psychological interventions include support; education; challenging maladaptive beliefs (e.g., "I could never sleep with CPAP"); identifying coping resources; troubleshooting; empathy; and other measures. For example, patients may be helped with emotional aversion to the machine eventuated by their being unconvinced they need it, despairing of its impact on their relationships, associating it with illness, or resenting its intrusion into sleep time.

Although the pain patient probably will not require much customization of these techniques, CPAP may be poorly tolerated in cases of orofacial pain, and much care should be taken to find a comfortable mask, to explore treatment alternatives as needed, and to help the patient participate collaboratively in treatment decisions. Knowing that treating apnea could diminish pain may serve as encouragement. Another challenge may be positional constraints imposed by CPAP, though these can often be overcome with appropriate hose length, a well-fitting mask, and arrangement of pillows. Empathy, support, and a collaborative approach may also and especially well serve the patient whose pain has taken such a toll that the added stress of an additional, difficult-to-assimilate treatment is overwhelming.

Because untreated sleep-disordered breathing may result in sleeping later than usual in compensation for a poor night's sleep, insomnia and circadian disruptions can ensue. In addition, startled wakings during the night may result in significant difficulty reinitiating sleep. Once sleep-disordered breathing is treated, there may therefore be residual insomnia or circadian symptoms resulting from a prolonged sleep window, conditioned anxiety, or other factors, and in these cases additional cognitive-behavioral interventions can help.

COGNITIVE BEHAVIOR THERAPY FOR DELAYED CIRCADIAN PHASE IN THE PAIN PATIENT

In the ICSD-3, Circadian Rhythm Sleep-Wake Disorders comprise a broad category of diagnoses describing a misalignment between endogenous sleep-wake rhythm and the 24-hour physical and social environment or an alteration in the circadian timekeeping system.[102] There may be phase delays, as in the so-called "night owl" who initiates sleep late at night and has difficulty awakening in the morning, phase advances (in "early birds" or "larks"), and other syndromes such as jet leg or a "free-running" type in which sleep rhythms shift clockwise day by day. Delayed sleep phase syndrome is the most commonly encountered in a sleep clinic[158]—though it is less prevalent than shift-work and jet-lag syndromes in the general population—and is probably the most likely to be encountered in the clinical pain setting because of characteristic, maladaptive coping strategies.

Of particular relevance to the pain patient is the influence of light on biological rhythms.[159,160] Insofar as patients lie awake at night due to pain and attendant poor sleep, they may have lights on, whether from the television, book lights, computers, smart phones, or room lights. Nonphotic influences on the circadian timing system are less well established in humans,[161] but if patients are engaging in exercise or social activity, or ingesting food during the desired sleep interval, circadian misalignment may be reinforced. Any of these activities may falsely signal to the biological clock that it is daytime, thus precipitating or perpetuating circadian shifts. In addition, certain types of pain are more likely to occur at night[162]—though not necessarily due to fundamental circadian variation in pain perception—and conceivably could alter the timing of sleep even in the absence of light exposure or activity.

Conventional therapy for delayed circadian phase,[163,164] summarized in **Table 99-2**, may include phototherapy, often with the use of a light box; strategically timed darkness and/or use of special glasses, filters for electronic screens, or computer or phone applications that selectively prevent exposure to short-wavelength light; chronotherapy, which involves successive delays in initial sleep time to effect clockwise arrival at the desired sleep time; successively earlier rising times followed by regularization of the sleep schedule; a shift in the timing of food intake; relaxation and distraction strategies not dependent on light exposure for use as needed late at night or in the middle of the night; customary insomnia interventions if warranted; and supportive lifestyle measures (e.g., restricting caffeine intake after noon despite late rising and bedtime, and limiting late-night social activities despite energy and interest). Some physicians adjunctively recommend melatonin or a melatonin agonist, which can act synergistically with light therapy.[165] There is evidence that strategically timed exercise can also assist in shifting or maintaining sleep schedules.[166] The treatment of most other circadian rhythm sleep-wake disorders employs the same basic toolkit, but with differences in the timing of interventions.

It is important to consult phase-response curves for light and[167] melatonin[168] before selecting their optimal timing, as it is common to prescribe melatonin too late to capture its maximal phase-shifting effects (which occur about 6 hours prior to sleep initiation) and to prescribe lights too early in the morning (i.e., prior to a core body temperature minimum) such that the patient's sleep phase shifts in the wrong direction. The phase-response curves guide the timing of lights and melatonin to achieve the desired magnitude and direction of phase shift. To assist in determining the patient's endogenous rhythm, physicians may employ sleep diaries, wrist actigraphs, salivary melatonin assays, core body temperature measurements, questionnaires assessing "morningness" versus "eveningness,"[169] or other phase markers.

TABLE 99-2 Summary of Methods for Shifting Sleep Phase

Phototherapy, often with a light box
Strategically timed darkness or use of short-wavelength-blocking glasses, filters, or applications
Chronotherapy to rotate schedule clockwise by means of successive delays in bedtime
Successively earlier rising times followed by regularization of sleep schedule
Relaxation and distraction strategies not dependent on light exposure
Customary insomnia interventions if warranted
Supportive lifestyle measures (e.g., restricting caffeine intake after noon, restricting late-night socializing)
Strategically timed exercise and meals
Chronobiotics such as melatonin or a melatonin agonist

Most of the standard recommendations for circadian rhythm sleep-wake disorders are behavioral, but they are not strictly speaking CBT in that they are not rooted in the principles of conditioning or in methodologies for correcting cognitive distortions. But as applied de facto in populations seeking help for these disorders, CBT can be adjunctively useful. For example, persons with delayed sleep phase often develop a component of conditioned insomnia as they endure sleep loss in an effort to adapt to work or school schedules, and may be awake for long periods with anxiety and despondency about chronic sleep loss, as well as overeffort to sleep. Furthermore, circadian misalignment may develop in the first place as a result of insomnia.[170] Other targets of CBT in the phase-delayed patient are the many lifestyle factors that can sustain the condition, for which motivation can figure heavily. For example, patients may be advised to adopt a constant rising time 7 days per week but resist this prescription and stay up late on weekends and during vacations. These challenges can be particularly marked in adolescents, who may seek treatment at the behest of adults. CBT was recently studied as an adjunct to conventional therapy for delayed sleep phase syndrome in adolescents, and was found to be helpful.[171]

COGNITIVE BEHAVIOR THERAPY FOR OTHER SLEEP DISORDERS IN THE PAIN PATIENT

Behavioral and psychological interventions are occasionally deployed in the treatment of other sleep disorders, typically by targeting accompanying stress, anxiety, or poor sleep habits in specially adapted ways. For example, a variety of parasomnias benefit from hypnosis incorporating suggestions for deep sleep.[99] Imagery rehearsal therapy, sometimes combined with exposure therapy or other interventions, can help with nightmares.[172] Stress management, improved sleep habits, and deep relaxation may help with bruxism, which can leave patients with morning cephalgia and jaw pain, though the role of stress is uncertain and bruxism does not necessarily interfere with daytime functioning.[12] Strategic napping and psychological support can help with narcolepsy symptoms[173] and coping with the diagnosis, respectively. Whether or not pain precipitates or exacerbates any of these conditions for any given patient, the psychological stress pain imposes may impede coping, and psychological or behavioral assistance may be indicated.

There are other sleep disorders that may exacerbate pain but that do not lend themselves to cognitive-behavioral intervention except insofar as patients develop secondary insomnia as a result of startled wakings and/or anxiety about sleep. These include restless legs syndrome and periodic limb movements.[12,174]

WHEN TO REFER TO A SLEEP SPECIALIST

Because chronic pain in a primary-care setting is associated with a broad range of sleep disorders,[26] it is important to screen pain patients for sleep disturbances. Any time there is suspicion of sleep-disordered breathing (e.g., apnea), periodic limb movements, restless legs syndrome, narcolepsy, or other biologically based sleep disorders, referral should be made to a physician specializing in sleep disorders.

The CBT techniques for sleep explicated in the foregoing sections are typically the purview of behavioral sleep specialists, though other practitioners can learn to use them. Behavioral sleep specialists are usually psychologists with expertise in applying behavioral and other psychological techniques to the treatment of sleep disorders. They collaborate with physician specialists (most often neurologists or pulmonologists), who may make referral once the patient has been assessed (through history-taking, examination, and often laboratory testing, including polysomnography), and once biologic and/or mechanical therapies have been introduced. When the behavioral sleep specialist is the patient's first contact, the patient will generally also be directed to evaluation by a sleep physician to prevent misdiagnosis. For example, sometimes a complaint of insomnia is caused by sleep-disordered breathing.

Some patients alternatively learn CBT techniques through bibliotherapy or other self-help resources, and may successfully treat their own symptoms. Others are well guided by health professionals who do not specialize in treating sleep disorders. The advantages of specialized professional intervention include the experienced behavioral sleep specialist's comfort with complex clinical presentations and strategies, his or her ability to customize techniques to the patient, accurate diagnosis, and troubleshooting. When the cognitive-behavioral regimen required for a patient is either complex or unclear, or when psychiatric disorder hinders improvement, it is especially important that treatment by a behavioral sleep specialist and/or other mental-health professional be initiated.

CONCLUSION

In summary, sleep and pain exert mutual influence, and treating sleep complaints in the pain patient may ameliorate both pain and sleep symptoms, enhance coping, and confer long-term health benefits. Cognitive, behavioral, and other psychological tools are effective adjuncts to the usual strategies available to the physician. Future directions include disseminating treatment to underserved populations using online tools,[175,176] and employing subtler findings from studies of learning and behavior to design even more effective interventions, as has been achieved for a number of other conditions.[177] For example, one promising new treatment called "intensive sleep retraining" uses principles of conditioning to remediate insomnia in a single night,[114] though its current reliance on access to expensive laboratory resources renders it impractical at present.

REFERENCES

1. Partinen M, Hublin C. Epidemiology of sleep disorders. In: Kryger MH, Roth T, Dement WC, eds. *Principles and Practice of Sleep Medicine*. 5th ed. St. Louis, MO: Elsevier; 2011:694-715.
2. Ruiz-Lopez R. The epidemiology of chronic pain. *Pain Digest*. 1995;5:67-68.
3. Morin CM, Gibson D, Wade J. Self-reported sleep and mood disturbance in chronic pain patients. *Clin J Pain*. 1998;14(4):311-314.
4. Smith MT, Perlis ML, Smith MS, Giles DE, Carmody TP. Sleep quality and presleep arousal in chronic pain. *J Behav Med*. 2000;23(1):1-13.
5. Vitiello MV, Rybarczyk B, Von Korff M, Stepanski EJ. Cognitive behavioral therapy for insomnia improves sleep and decreases pain in older adults with co-morbid insomnia and osteoarthritis. *J Clin Sleep Med*. 2009;5(4):355-362.
6. Khalid I, Roehrs TA, Hudgel DW, Roth T. Continuous positive airway pressure in severe obstructive sleep apnea reduces pain sensitivity. *Sleep*. 2011;34(12):1687-1691.
7. Theadom A, Cropley M, Humphrey KL. Exploring the role of sleep and coping in quality of life in fibromyalgia. *J Psychosom Res*. 2007;62(2):145-151.
8. Manber R, Edinger JD, Gress JL, et al. Cognitive behavioral therapy for insomnia enhances depression outcome in patients with comorbid major depressive disorder and insomnia. *Sleep*. 2008;31(4):489-495.
9. Walsh JK, Dement WC, Dinges DF. Sleep medicine, public policy, and public health. In: Kryger MH, Roth T, Dement WC, eds. *Principles and Practice of Sleep Medicine*. 5th ed. St. Louis, MO: Elsevier; 2011:716-724.
10. Smith MT, Klick B, Kozachik S, et al. Sleep onset insomnia symptoms during hospitalization for major burn injury predict chronic pain. *Pain*. 2008;138(3):497-506.
11. Gupta A, Silman AJ, Ray D, et al. The role of psychosocial factors in predicting the onset of chronic widespread pain: Results from a prospective population-based study. *Rheumatology (Oxford)*. 2007;46(4):666-671.
12. Chen G, Guilleminault C. Sleep disorders that can exacerbate pain. In: Lavigne G, Sessle BJ, Choinière M, Soja PJ, eds. *Sleep and Pain*. Seattle, WA: IASP Press; 2007, reprinted 2010:311-340.
13. Currie SR, Wilson KG, Pontefract AJ, deLaplante L. Cognitive-behavioral treatment of insomnia secondary to chronic pain. *J Consult Clin Psychol*. 2000;68(3):407-416.
14. Edinger JD, Wohlgemuth WK, Krystal AD, Rice JR. Behavioral insomnia therapy for fibromyalgia patients: A randomized clinical trial. *Arch Intern Med*. 2005;165(21):2527-2535.
15. Rybarczyk B, Stepanski E, Fogg L, et al. A placebo-controlled test of cognitive-behavioral therapy for comorbid insomnia in older adults. *J Consult Clin Psychol*. 2005;73(6):1164-1174.
16. Jungquist CR, O'Brien C, Matteson-Rusby S, et al. The efficacy of cognitive-behavioral therapy for insomnia in patients with chronic pain. *Sleep Med*. 2010;11(3):302-309.
17. Ohayon MM. Epidemiology of insomnia: What we know and what we still need to learn. *Sleep Med Rev*. 2002;6(2):97-111.
18. Lavigne G, Smith MT, Denis R, Zucconi M. Pain and sleep. In: Kryger MH, Roth T, Dement WC, eds. *Principles and Practice of Sleep Medicine*. 5th ed. St. Louis: Elsevier; 2011:1442-1451.
19. Foley D, Ancoli-Israel S, Britz P, Walsh J. Sleep disturbances and chronic disease in older adults: Results of the 2003 National Sleep Foundation Sleep in America Survey. *J Psychosom Res*. 2004;56(5):497-502.
20. Atkinson JH, Ancoli-Israel S, Slater MA, et al. Subjective sleep disturbance in chronic back pain. *Clin J Pain*. 1988;4:225-232.
21. Pilowsky I, Crettenden I, Townley M. Sleep disturbance in pain clinic patients. *Pain*. 1985;23(1):27-33.
22. Tang NK, Wright KJ, Salkovskis PM. Prevalence and correlates of clinical insomnia co-occurring with chronic back pain. *J Sleep Res*. 2007;16(1):85-95.
23. Alattar M, Harrington JJ, Mitchell CM, Sloane P. Sleep problems in primary care: a North Carolina Family Practice Research Network (NC-FP-RN) study. *J Am Board Fam Med*. 2007;20(4):365-374.
24. Okura K, Lavigne GJ, Huynh N, et al. Comparison of sleep variables between chronic widespread musculoskeletal pain, insomnia, periodic leg movements syndrome and control subjects in a clinical sleep medicine practice. *Sleep Med*. 2008;9(4):352-361.
25. Moldofsky H. Sleep and pain. *Sleep Med Rev*. 2001;5(5):385-396.
26. Taylor DJ, Mallory LJ, Lichstein KL, et al. Comorbidity of chronic insomnia with medical problems. *Sleep*. 2007;30(2):213-218.
27. Ohayon MM. Relationship between chronic painful physical condition and insomnia. *J Psychiatr Res*. 2005;39(2):151-159.
28. Moffitt PF, Kalucy EC, Kalucy RS, Baum FE, Cooke RD. Sleep difficulties, pain and other correlates. *J Intern Med*. 1991;230(3):245-249.
29. Smith MT, Wickwire EM, Grace EG, et al. Sleep disorders and their association with laboratory pain sensitivity in temporomandibular joint disorder. *Sleep*. 2009;32(6):779-790.
30. Luyster FS, Chasens ER, Wasko MC, Dunbar-Jacob J. Sleep quality and functional disability in patients with rheumatoid arthritis. *J Clin Sleep Med*. 2011;7(1):49-55.
31. Menefee LA, Cohen MJ, Anderson WR, et al. Sleep disturbance and nonmalignant chronic pain: A comprehensive review of the literature. *Pain Med*. 2000;1(2):156-172.
32. Sivertsen B, Krokstad S, Øverland S, Mykletun A. The epidemiology of insomnia: Associations with physical and mental health. The HUNT-2 study. *J Psychosom Res*. 2009;67(2):109-116.

33. Sutton DA, Moldofsky H, Badley EM. Insomnia and health problems in Canadians. *Sleep*. 2001;24(6):665-670.
34. Abad VC, Sarinas PS, Guilleminault C. Sleep and rheumatologic disorders. *Sleep Med Rev*. 2008;12(3):211-228.
35. Onen SH, Onen F, Courpron P, Dubray C. How pain and analgesics disturb sleep. *Clin J Pain*. 2005;21(5):422-431.
36. Roehrs T, Roth T. Sleep and pain: interaction of two vital functions. *Semin Neurol*. 2005;25(1):106-116.
37. Tang NK, Goodchild CE, Sanborn AN, et al. Deciphering the temporal link between pain and sleep in a heterogeneous chronic pain patient sample: a multilevel daily process study. *Sleep*. 2012;35(5):675-87A.
38. Cairns BE. Alteration of sleep quality by pain medication: an overview. In: Lavigne G, Sessle BJ, Choinière M, Soja PJ, eds. *Sleep and Pain*. Seattle, WA: IASP Press; 2007, reprinted 2010:371-390.
39. Lewandowski AS, Palermo TM, De la Motte S, et al. Temporal daily associations between pain and sleep in adolescents with chronic pain versus healthy adolescents. *Pain*. 2010;151(1):220-225.
40. Smith MT, Haythornthwaite JA. Cognitive-behavioral treatment for insomnia and pain. In: Lavigne G, Sessle BJ, Choinière M, Soja PJ, eds. *Sleep and Pain*. Seattle, WA: IASP Press; 2007, reprinted 2010:439-457.
41. Wilson KG, Eriksson MY, D'Eon JL, Mikail SF, Emery PC. Major depression and insomnia in chronic pain. *Clin J Pain*. 2002;18(2):77-83.
42. Smith MT, Perlis ML, Carmody TP, Smith MS, Giles DE. Presleep cognitions in patients with insomnia secondary to chronic pain. *J Behav Med*. 2001;24(1):93-114.
43. Haack M, Scott-Sutherland J, Santangelo G, et al. Pain sensitivity and modulation in primary insomnia. *Eur J Pain*. 2011 epub; *Eur J Pain*. 2012;16(4):522-533.
44. Chiu YH, Silman AJ, Macfarlane GJ, et al. Poor sleep and depression are independently associated with a reduced pain threshold. Results of a population based study. *Pain*. 2005;115(3):316-321.
45. Lautenbacher S, Kundermann B, Krieg JC. Sleep deprivation and pain perception. *Sleep Med Rev*. 2006;10(5):357-369.
46. Chhangani BS, Roehrs TA, Harris EJ, et al. Pain sensitivity in sleepy pain-free normals. *Sleep*. 2009;32(8):1011-1017.
47. Drewes AM, Nielsen KD, Hansen B, et al. A longitudinal study of clinical symptoms and sleep parameters in rheumatoid arthritis. *Rheumatology (Oxford)*. 2000;39(11):1287-1289.
48. Mikkelsson M, Sourander A, Salminen JJ, Kautiainen H, Piha J. Widespread pain and neck pain in schoolchildren: A prospective one-year follow-up study. *Acta Paediatr*. 1999;88(10):1119-1124.
49. McCracken LM, Iverson GL. Disrupted sleep patterns and daily functioning in patients with chronic pain. *Pain Res Manag*. 2002;7(2):75-79.
50. Haack M, Mullington JM. Sustained sleep restriction reduces emotional and physical well-being. *Pain*. 2005;119(1-3):56-64.
51. Haack M, Sanchez E, Mullington JM. Elevated inflammatory markers in response to prolonged sleep restriction are associated with increased pain experience in healthy volunteers. *Sleep*. 2007;30(9):1145-1152.
52. Smith MT, Edwards RR, McCann UD, Haythornthwaite JA. The effects of sleep deprivation on pain inhibition and spontaneous pain in women. *Sleep*. 2007;30(4):494-505.
53. Andersen ML, Silva A, Kawakami R, Tufik S. The effects of sleep deprivation and sleep recovery on pain thresholds of rats with chronic pain. *Sleep Sci*. 2009;2:82-87.
54. Roehrs T, Hyde M, Blaisdell B, Greenwald M, Roth T. Sleep loss and REM sleep loss are hyperalgesic. *Sleep*. 2006;29(2):145-151.
55. Azevedo E, Manzano GM, Silva A, et al. The effects of total and REM sleep deprivation on laser-evoked potential threshold and pain perception. *Pain*. 2011;152(9):2052-2058.
56. Onen SH, Alloui A, Gross A, Eschallier A, Dubray C. The effects of total sleep deprivation, selective sleep interruption and sleep recovery on pain tolerance thresholds in healthy subjects. *J Sleep Res*. 2001;10(1):35-42.
57. Drewes AM, Rössel P, Arendt-Nielsen L, et al. Sleepiness does not modulate experimental joint pain in healthy volunteers. *Scand J Rheumatol*. 1997;26(5):399-400.
58. Lavigne G, Zucconi M, Castronovo C, et al. Sleep arousal response to experimental thermal stimulation during sleep in human subjects free of pain and sleep problems. *Pain*. 2000;84(2-3):283-290.
59. Drewes AM, Nielsen KD, Arendt-Nielsen L, Birket-Smith L, Hansen LM. The effect of cutaneous and deep pain on the electroencephalogram during sleep: An experimental study. *Sleep*. 1997;20(8):632-640.
60. Smith MT, Haythornthwaite JA. How do sleep disturbance and chronic pain inter-relate? Insights from the longitudinal and cognitive-behavioral clinical trials literature. *Sleep Med Rev*. 2004;8(2):119-132.
61. Foo H, Mason P. Brainstem modulation of pain during sleep and waking. *Sleep Med Rev*. 2003;7(2):145-154.
62. Haack M, Scott-Sutheralns J, Sethna N, Mullington JM. Mechanisms of sleep loss-pain interactions. In: Lavigne G, Cistulli PA, Smith MT, eds. *Sleep Medicine for Dentists: A Practical Overview*. Hanover Park, IL: Quintessence Publishing; 2009: 155-160.
63. Affleck G, Urrows S, Tennen H, Higgins P, Abeles M. Sequential daily relations of sleep, pain intensity, and attention to pain among women with fibromyalgia. *Pain*. 1996;68(2-3):363-368.
64. Edwards RR, Almeida DM, Klick B, Haythornthwaite JA, Smith MT. Duration of sleep contributes to next-day pain report in the general population. *Pain*. 2008;137(1):202-207.
65. Lee YC, Chibnik LB, Lu B, et al. The relationship between disease activity, sleep, psychiatric distress and pain sensitivity in rheumatoid arthritis: a cross-sectional study. *Arthritis Res Ther*. 2009;11(5):R160.
66. Spielman A. Assessment of insomnia. *Clin Psychol Rev*. 1986;6: 11-25.
67. Spielman AJ, Caruso LS, Glovinsky PB. A behavioral perspective on insomnia treatment. *Psychiatr Clin North Am*. 1987;10(4):541-553.
68. Haynes PL. Is CBT-I effective for pain? *J Clin Sleep Med*. 2009;5(4): 363-364.
69. Beck AT. *Cognitive Therapy and the Emotional Disorders*. Madison, CT: Intl. Universities Press; 1975.
70. Beck, JS. *Cognitive Therapy: Basics and Beyond*. 2nd ed. New York, NY: Guilford; 2011.
71. Hollon SD, Stewart MO, Strunk D. Enduring effects for cognitive behavior therapy in the treatment of depression and anxiety. *Annu Rev Psychol*. 2006;57:285-315.
72. Shawe-Taylor M, Rigby J. Cognitive behaviour therapy: its evolution and basic principles. *J R Soc Promot Health*. 1999;119(4):244-246.
73. Butler AC, Chapman JE, Forman EM, Beck AT. The empirical status of cognitive-behavioral therapy: a review of meta-analyses. *Clin Psychol Rev*. 2006;26(1):17-31.
74. Hofmann SG, Smits JA. Cognitive-behavioral therapy for adult anxiety disorders: a meta-analysis of randomized placebo-controlled trials. *J Clin Psychiatry*. 2008;69(4):621-632.
75. DeRubeis RJ, Hollon SD, Amsterdam JD, et al. Cognitive therapy vs medications in the treatment of moderate to severe depression. *Arch Gen Psychiatry*. 2005;62(4):409-416.

76. Hollon SD, DeRubeis RJ, Shelton RC, et al. Prevention of relapse following cognitive therapy vs medications in moderate to severe depression. *Arch Gen Psychiatry*. 2005;62(4):417-422.
77. Peterson MJ, Benca RM. Mood disorders. In: Kryger MH, Roth T, Dement WC, eds. *Principles and Practice of Sleep Medicine*. 5th ed. St. Louis, MO: Elsevier; 2011:1488-1500.
78. Ramsawh H, Stein MB, Mellman TA. Anxiety disorders. In: Kryger MH, Roth T, Dement WC, eds. *Principles and Practice of Sleep Medicine*. 5th ed. St. Louis, MO: Elsevier; 2011: 1473-1487.
79. Johnson EO, Roth T, Breslau N. The association of insomnia with anxiety disorders and depression: exploration of the direction of risk. *J Psychiatr Res*. 2006;40(8):700-708.
80. Ohayon MM, Roth T. Place of chronic insomnia in the course of depressive and anxiety disorders. *J Psychiatr Res*. 2003;37(1):9-15.
81. Taylor DJ, Lichstein KL, Durrence HH, Reidel BW, Bush AJ. Epidemiology of insomnia, depression, and anxiety. *Sleep*. 2005;28(11):1457-1464.
82. Yates WR, Mitchell J, John Rush A, et al. Clinical features of depression in outpatients with and without co-occurring general medical conditions in STAR*D: Confirmatory analysis. *J Clin Psychiatry*. 2007;9(1):7-15.
83. Taylor DJ. Insomnia and depression. *Sleep*. 2008;31(4):447-448.
84. DeRubeis RJ, Gelfand LA, Tang TZ, Simons AD. Medications versus cognitive behavior therapy for severely depressed outpatients: mega-analysis of four randomized comparisons. Am *J Psychiatry*. 1999;156(7):1007-1013.
85. Westra HA, Stewart SH. Cognitive behavioural therapy and pharmacotherapy: Complementary or contradictory approaches to the treatment of anxiety? *Clin Psychol Rev*. 1998;18(3):307-340.
86. Ehlers A, Clark DM, Hackmann A, et al. Intensive cognitive therapy for PTSD: A feasibility study. *Behav Cogn Psychother*. 2010;38(4):383-398.
87. Morin CM, Gaulier B, Barry T, Kowatch RA. Patients' acceptance of psychological and pharmacological therapies for insomnia. *Sleep*. 1992;15(4):302-305.
88. Vincent N, Lionberg C. Treatment preference and patient satisfaction in chronic insomnia. *Sleep*. 2001;24(4):411-417.
89. Boudreau R, Moulton K, Cunningham J. *Self-Directed Cognitive Behavioural Therapy for Adults with Diagnosis of Depression: Systematic Review of Clinical Effectiveness, Cost-Effectiveness, and Guidelines*. Ottawa, Canada: Canadian Agency for Drugs and Technologies in Health; 2010.
90. Edinger JD, Wohlgemuth WK, Radtke RA, Marsh GR, Quillian RE. Cognitive behavioral therapy for treatment of chronic primary insomnia: A randomized controlled trial. *JAMA*. 2001;285(14): 1856-1864.
91. Espie CA, Lindsay WR, Brooks DN, Hood EM, Turvey T. A controlled comparative investigation of psychological treatments for chronic sleep-onset insomnia. *Behav Res Ther*. 1989;27(1):79-88.
92. Jacobs GD, Pace-Schott EF, Stickgold R, Otto MW. Cognitive behavior therapy and pharmacotherapy for insomnia: A randomized controlled trial and direct comparison. *Arch Intern Med*. 2004;164(17):1888-1896.
93. Lichstein KL, Wilson NM, Johnson CT. Psychological treatment of secondary insomnia. *Psychol Aging*. 2000;15(2):232-240.
94. Morin CM, Colecchi C, Stone J, Sood R, Brink D. Behavioral and pharmacological therapies for late-life insomnia: A randomized controlled trial. *JAMA*. 1999;281(11):991-999.
95. Richards D, Bartlett DJ, Wong K, Malouff J, Grunstein RR. Increased adherence to CPAP with a group cognitive behavioral treatment intervention: A randomized trial. *Sleep*. 2007;30(5):635-640.
96. Hoy CJ, Vennelle M, Kingshott RN, Engleman HM, Douglas NJ. Can intensive support improve continuous positive airway pressure use in patients with the sleep apnea/hypopnea syndrome? *Am J Respir Crit Care Med*. 1999;159(4 Part 1):1096-1100.
97. Edinger JD, Radtke RA. Use of in vivo desensitization to treat a patient's claustrophobic response to nasal CPAP. *Sleep*. 1993;16(7):678-680.
98. Lancee J, Spoormaker VI, Krakow B, van den Bout J. A systematic review of cognitive-behavioral treatment for nightmares: Toward a well-established treatment. *J Clin Sleep Med*. 2008;4(5):475-480.
99. Hauri PJ, Silber MH, Boeve BF. The treatment of parasomnias with hypnosis: A 5-year follow-up study. *J Clin Sleep Med*. 2007;3(4):369-373.
100. Linton SJ, MacDonald, S. Pain and sleep disorders: Clinical consequences and maintaining factors. In: Lavigne G, Sessle BJ, Choinière M, Soja PJ, eds. *Sleep and Pain*. Seattle, WA: IASP Press; 2007, reprinted 2010: 417-437.
101. Lichstein KL, Taylor DJ, McRae CS, Ruiter ME. Insomnia: Epidemiology and risk factors. In: Kryger MH, Roth T, Dement WC, eds. *Principles and Practice of Sleep Medicine*. 5th ed. St. Louis, MO: Elsevier; 2011: 827-837.
102. American Academy of Sleep Medicine. *International Classification of Sleep Disorders*. 3rd ed. Darien, IL: American Academy of Sleep Medicine; 2014.
103. Edinger JD, Bonnet MH, Bootzin RR, et al. Derivation of research diagnostic criteria for insomnia: Report of an American Academy of Sleep Medicine Work Group. *Sleep*. 2004;27(8):1567-1596.
104. American Psychiatric Association. *Diagnostic and Statistical Manual of Mental Disorders*, 5th ed. (DSM-5). Washington, DC: American Psychiatric Association; 2013.
105. World Health Organization. *International Statistical Classification of Diseases and Related Health Problems, Vol. 1, 10th rev. 2nd ed.* Geneva: Author; 2004.
106. Morin CM. Psychological and behavioral treatments for insomnia I: Approaches and efficacy. In: Kryger MH, Roth T, Dement WC, eds. *Principles and Practice of Sleep Medicine*. 5th ed. St. Louis, MO: Elsevier; 2011: 866-883.
107. Morin CM, Bootzin RR, Buysse DJ, et al. Psychological and behavioral treatment of insomnia: Update of the recent evidence (1998-2004). *Sleep*. 2006;29(11):1398-1414.
108. Bootzin RR. Stimulus control treatment for insomnia. *Proc Am Psychol Assoc*. 1972;7:395-396.
109. Perlis M, Shaw PJ, Cano G, Espie CA. Models of insomnia. In: Kryger MH, Roth T, Dement WC, eds. *Principles and Practice of Sleep Medicine*. 5th ed. St. Louis, MO: Elsevier; 2011: 850-865.
110. Morin CM, Culbert JP, Schwartz SM. Nonpharmacological interventions for insomnia: A meta-analysis of treatment efficacy. *Am J Psychiatry*. 1994;151(8):1172-1180.
111. Murtagh DR, Greenwood KM. Identifying effective psychological treatments for insomnia: A meta-analysis. *J Consult Clin Psychol*. 1995;63(1):79-89.
112. Riedel B, Lichstein K, Peterson BA, et al. A comparison of the efficacy of stimulus control for medicated and nonmedicated insomniacs. *Behav Modif*. 1998;22(1):3-28.
113. Morgenthaler T, Kramer M, Alessi C, et al. Practice parameters for the psychological and behavioral treatment of insomnia: An update. An American Academy of Sleep Medicine report. *Sleep*. 2006;29(11):1415-1419.
114. Harris J, Lack L, Kemp K, Wright H, Bootzin R. A randomized controlled trial of intensive sleep retraining (ISR): A brief conditioning treatment for chronic insomnia. *Sleep*. 2012;35(1):49-60.

115. Pigeon WR. Treatment of adult insomnia with cognitive-behavioral therapy. *J Clin Psychol.* 2010;66(11):1148-1160.

116. Spielman AJ, Saskin P, Thorpy MJ. Treatment of chronic insomnia by restriction of time in bed. *Sleep.* 1987;10(1):45-56.

117. Lichstein KL, Thomas SJ, McCurry SM. Sleep compression. In: Perlis M, Aloia M, Kuhn B, eds. *Behavioral Treatments for Sleep Disorders: A Comprehensive Primer of Behavioral Sleep Medicine Interventions.* London: Academic Press; 2011:55-59.

118. Fountain NB, Kim JS, Lee SI. Sleep deprivation activates epileptiform discharges independent of the activating effects of sleep. *J Clin Neurophysiol.* 1998;15(1):69-75.

119. Colombo C, Benedetti F, Barbini B, Campori E, Smeraldi E. Rate of switch from depression into mania after therapeutic sleep deprivation in bipolar depression. *Psychiatry Res.* 1999;86(3):267-270.

120. Carney CE, Edinger JD, Manber R, Garson C, Segal ZV. Beliefs about sleep in disorders characterized by sleep and mood disturbance. *J Psychosom Res.* 2007;62(2):179-188.

121. Edinger JD, Wohlgemuth WK. Psychometric comparisons of the standard and abbreviated DBAS-10 versions of the Dysfunctional Beliefs and Attitudes about Sleep questionnaire. *Sleep Med.* 2001;2(6):493-500.

122. Morin CM, Stone J, Trinkle D, Mercer J, Remsberg S. Dysfunctional beliefs and attitudes about sleep among older adults with and without insomnia complaints. *Psychol Aging.* 1993;8(3):463-467.

123. Neckelmann D, Mykletun A, Dahl AA. Chronic insomnia as a risk factor for developing anxiety and depression. *Sleep.* 2007;30(7):873-880.

124. Perlis ML, Smith LJ, Lyness JM, et al. Insomnia as a risk factor for onset of depression in the elderly. *Behav Sleep Med.* 2006;4(2):104-113.

125. Morin CM, Vallières A, Ivers H. Dysfunctional beliefs and attitudes about sleep (DBAS): Validation of a brief version (DBAS-16). *Sleep.* 2007;30(11):1547-1554.

126. Harvey AG. A cognitive model of insomnia. *Behav Res Ther.* 2002;40(8):869-893.

127. Burns DD. *When Panic Attacks: The New, Drug-free Anxiety Therapy That Can Change Your Life.* New York, NY: Three Rivers Press; 2007.

128. Hauri PJ. Can we mix behavioral therapy with hypnotics when treating insomniacs? *Sleep.* 1997;20(12):1111-1118.

129. Lacks P, Morin CM. Recent advances in the assessment and treatment of insomnia. *J Consult Clin Psychol.* 1992;60(4):586-594.

130. Ong JC, Shapiro SL, Manber R. Combining mindfulness meditation with cognitive-behavior therapy for insomnia: A treatment-development study. *Behav Ther.* 2008;39(2):171-182.

131. Jacobson E. *Progressive Relaxation.* Chicago, IL: University of Chicago Press; 1938.

132. Harvey AG, Payne S. The management of unwanted pre-sleep thoughts in insomnia: Distraction with imagery versus general distraction. *Behav Res Ther.* 2002;40(3):267-277.

133. Lichstein KL, Riedel BW, Wilson NM, Lester KW, Aguillard RN. Relaxation and sleep compression for late-life insomnia: A placebo-controlled trial. *J Consult Clin Psychol.* 2001;69(2):227-239.

134. Means MK, Lichstein KL, Epperson MT, Johnson CT. Relaxation therapy for insomnia: Nighttime and day time effects. *Behav Res Ther.* 2000;38(7):665-678.

134. Ascher LM, Turner RM. A comparison of two methods for the administration of paradoxical intention. *Behav Res Ther.* 1980;18(2):121-126.

136. Britton WB, Haynes PL, Fridel KW, Bootzin RR. Polysomnographic and subjective profiles of sleep continuity before and after mindfulness-based cognitive therapy in partially remitted depression. *Psychosom Med.* 2010;72(6):539-548.

137. Brown CA, Jones AK. Meditation experience predicts less negative appraisal of pain: Electrophysiological evidence for the involvement of anticipatory neural responses. *Pain.* 2010;150(3):428-438.

138. Beck AT, Rush J, Shaw BF, Emery G. *Cognitive Therapy of Depression.* New York, NY: Guilford; 1987.

139. Morin CM, Kowatch RA, Barry T, Walton E. Cognitive-behavior therapy for late-life insomnia. *J Consult Clin Psychol.* 1993;61(1):137-146.

140. Morgan K, Dixon S, Mathers N, Thompson J, Tomeny M. Psychological treatment for insomnia in the management of long-term hypnotic drug use: A pragmatic randomised controlled trial. *Br J Gen Pract.* 2003;53(497):923-928.

141. Rybarczyk B, Lopez M, Benson R, Alsten C, Stepanski E. Efficacy of two behavioral treatment programs for comorbid geriatric insomnia. *Psychol Aging.* 2002;17(2):288-298.

142. Morin CM, Kowatch RA, Wade JB. Behavioral management of sleep disturbances secondary to chronic pain. *J Behav Ther Exp Psychiatry.* 1989;20(4):295-302.

143. Morin CM, Kowatch RA, O'Shanick G. Sleep restriction for the inpatient treatment of insomnia. *Sleep.* 1990;13(2):183-186.

144. Riemann D. Insomnia research is coming of age. *Sleep.* 2012;35(2):175.

145. Young T, Peppard PE, Gottlieb DJ. Epidemiology of obstructive sleep apnea: A population health perspective. *Am J Respir Crit Care Med.* 2002;165(9):1217-1239.

146. Donald F, Esdaile JM, Kimoff JR, Fitzcharles MA. Musculoskeletal complaints and fibromyalgia in patients attending a respiratory sleep disorders clinic. *J Rheumatol.* 1996;23(9):1612-1616.

147. Sergi M, Rizzi M, Braghiroli A, et al. Periodic breathing during sleep in patients affected by fibromyalgia syndrome. *Eur Respir J.* 1999;14(1):203-208.

148. Gay P, Weaver T, Loube D, Iber C. Evaluation of positive airway pressure treatment for sleep related breathing disorders in adults: A review by the Positive Airway Pressure Task Force of the Standards of Practice Committee of the American Academy of Sleep Medicine. *Sleep.* 2006;29(3):381-401.

149. Buchanan P, Grunstein R. Positive airway pressure treatment for obstructive sleep apnea-hypopnea syndrome. In: Kryger MH, Roth T, Dement WC, eds. *Principles and Practice of Sleep Medicine.* 5th ed. St. Louis, MO: Elsevier; 2011: 1233-1249.

150. Engleman HM, Wild MR. Improving CPAP use by patients with the sleep apnoea/hypopnoea syndrome (SAHS). *Sleep Med Rev.* 2003;7(1):81-99.

151. Weaver TE, Kribbs NB, Pack AI, et al. Night-to-night variability in CPAP use over the first three months of treatment. *Sleep.* 1997;20(4):278-283.

152. Stepnowsky CJ Jr, Marler MR, Ancoli-Israel S. Determinants of nasal CPAP compliance. *Sleep Med.* 2002;3(3):239-247.

153. Aloia MS, Arnedt JT, Stepnowsky C, Hecht J, Borrelli B. Predicting treatment adherence in obstructive sleep apnea using principles of behavior change. *J Clin Sleep Med.* 2005;1(4):346-353.

154. Billings ME, Auckley D, Benca R, et al. Race and residential socioeconomics as predictors of CPAP adherence. *Sleep.* 2011;34(12):1653-1658.

155. Smith I, Nadig V, Lasserson TJ. Educational, supportive and behavioural interventions to improve usage of continuous positive airway pressure machines for adults with obstructive sleep apnoea. *Cochrane Dbse Syst Rev.* 2009;(2):CD007736.

156. Fletcher EC, Luckett RA. The effect of positive reinforcement on hourly compliance in nasal continuous positive airway pressure

users with obstructive sleep apnea. *Am Rev Respir Dis.* 1991;143(5 Part 1):936-941.

157. Aloia MS, Smith K, Arnedt JT, et al. Brief behavioral therapies reduce early PAP discontinuation rates in SAS: Preliminary findings. *Behavioral Sleep Med.* 2007;5(2):89-104.
158. Dagan Y, Eisenstein M. Circadian rhythm sleep disorders: Toward a more precise definition and diagnosis. *Chronobiol Int.* 1999;16(2):213-222.
159. Czeisler CA, Allan JS, Strogatz SH, et al. Bright light resets the human circadian pacemaker independent of the timing of the sleep-wake cycle. *Science.* 1986;233(4764):667-671.
160. Czeisler CA, Kronauer RE, Allan JS, et al. Bright light induction of strong (type 0) resetting of the human circadian pacemaker. *Science.* 1989;244(4910):1328-1333.
161. Czeisler CA, Buxton OM. The human circadian timing system and sleep-wake regulation. In: Kryger MH, Roth T, Dement WC, eds. *Principles and Practice of Sleep Medicine.* 5th ed. St. Louis, MO: Elsevier; 2011: 402-419.
162. Bentley, AJ. Pain perception during sleep and circadian influences: The experimental evidence. In: Lavigne G, Sessle BJ, Choinière M, Soja PJ, eds. *Sleep and Pain.* Seattle, WA: IASP Press; 2007, reprinted 2010: 123-136.
163. Reid KJ, Zee PC. Circadian disorders of the sleep-wake cycle. In: Kryger MH, Roth T, Dement WC, eds. *Principles and Practice of Sleep Medicine.* 5th ed. St. Louis, MO: Elsevier; 2011: 470-482.
164. Terman M, Terman JS. Light therapy. In: Kryger MH, Roth T, Dement WC, eds. *Principles and Practice of Sleep Medicine.* 5th ed. St. Louis, MO: Elsevier; 2011: 1682-1695.
165. Revell VL, Burgess HJ, Gazda CJ, et al. Advancing human circadian rhythms with afternoon melatonin and morning intermittent bright light. *J Clin Endocrinol Metab.* 2006;91(1):54-59.
166. Buxton OM, Lee CW, L'Hermite-Baleriaux M, Turek FW, Van Cauter E. Exercise elicits phase shifts and acute alterations of melatonin that vary with circadian phase. *Am J Physiol Regul Integr Comp Physiol.* 2003;284(3):R714-R724.
167. Khalsa SB, Jewett ME, Cajochen C, Czeisler CA. A phase response curve to single bright light pulses in human subjects. *J Physiol.* 2003;549(Part 3):945-952.
168. Burgess HJ, Revell VL, Molina TA, Eastman CI. Human phase response curves to three days of daily melatonin: 0.5 mg versus 3.0 mg. *J Clin Endocrinol Metab.* 2010;95(7):3325-3331.
169. Horne JA, Ostberg O. A self-assessment questionnaire to determine morningness-eveningness in human circadian rhythms. *Int J Chronobiol.* 1976;4(2):97-110.
170. Vaughn BV, O'Neill DF. Cardinal manifestations of sleep disorders. In: Kryger MH, Roth T, Dement WC, eds. *Principles and Practice of Sleep Medicine.* 5th ed. St. Louis, MO: Elsevier; 2011: 647-657.
171. Gradisar M, Dohnt H, Gardner G, et al. A randomized controlled trial of cognitive-behavior therapy plus bright light therapy for adolescent delayed sleep phase disorder. *Sleep.* 2011;34(12):1671-1680.
172. Lancee J, Spoormaker VI, Krakow B, van den Bout J. A systematic review of cognitive-behavioral treatment for nightmares: Toward a well-established treatment. *J Clin Sleep Med.* 2008;4(5):475-480.
173. Goswami M, Pandi-Perumal SR, Thorpy MJ, eds. *Narcolepsy: A Clinical Guide.* New York, NY: Springer; 2009.
174. Edinger JD, Fins AI, Sullivan RJ, et al. Comparison of cognitive-behavioral therapy and clonazepam for treating periodic limb movement disorder. *Sleep.* 1996;19(5):442-444.
175. Espie CA, Kyle SD, Williams C, et al. A randomized, placebo-controlled trial of online cognitive behavioral therapy for chronic insomnia disorder delivered via an automated media-rich Web application. *Sleep.* 2012;35(6):769-781.
176. Ritterband LM, Thorndike FP, Gonder-Frederick GA, et al. Efficacy of an Internet-based behavioral intervention for adults with insomnia. *Arch Gen Psychiatry.* 2009;66(7):692-698.
177. Schachtman TR, Reilly SS, eds. *Associative Learning and Conditioning Theory: Human and Non-Human Implications.* New York, NY: Oxford Univ. Press; 2011.

FURTHER READING

Burns DD. *When Panic Attacks: The New, Drug-free Anxiety Therapy That Can Change Your Life.* New York, NY: Three Rivers Press; 2007.

Jacobs GD. *Say Good Night to Insomnia.* New York, NY: Henry Holt and Co.; 1998.

Kryger MH, Roth T, Dement WC, eds. *Principles and Practice of Sleep Medicine.* 5th ed. St. Louis, MO: Elsevier; 2011.

Lavigne G, Sessle BJ, Choinière M, et al., eds. *Sleep and Pain.* Seattle: IASP Press; 2007, reprinted 2010.

Perlis ML, Jungquist C, Smith MT, Posner D. *Cognitive Behavioral Treatment of Insomnia: A Session-by-Session Guide.* New York, NY: Springer-Verlag; 2005.

Pigeon WR. Treatment of adult insomnia with cognitive-behavioral therapy. *J. Clin. Psychol.* 2010;66(11):1148-1160.

Lifestyle Choices in the Management of Chronic Pain

Katharine M. Larsson
Amaro J. Laria

In this chapter we will discuss the role of various factors associated with particular lifestyle choices in the management of chronic pain. Lifestyle choices will be grouped into the following four general categories: (1) weight, exercise, and nutrition; (2) common substances of daily living, specifically caffeine, tobacco, and alcohol; (3) sleep, and; (4) other lifestyle factors with variable degrees of choice, including social isolation/social support, employment-related factors, and religiosity/spirituality.

WEIGHT, EXERCISE, AND NUTRITION

WEIGHT

There is a solid body of research evidence that confirms a positive correlation between weight and chronic pain. Several studies have found that individuals with high body mass index (BMI) levels report higher levels of pain associated with various chronic pain conditions, including chronic widespread pain,[1] chronic low back pain (CLBP),[1-4] arthritic pain,[5,6] abdominal pain, headaches—both tension and migraines—and fibromyalgia (FMS),[1] among others. Moreover, the relationship appears to be incremental; that is, increasingly higher levels of weight lead to incrementally higher levels of pain. Using four target overweight categories, a large-scale study that gathered survey data through telephone interviews with over 1 million subjects found that "overweight" subjects (BMI >25) reported 20% higher rates of pain than subjects in the "low-normal weight group" (BMI = 18.5-24.9); 68% higher for subjects in the "Obese I" group (BMI = 30-34.9), 136% higher for the "Obese II" group (BMI = 35-39.9), and 254% higher for the "Obese III" group (BMI >40)[7]. Other studies have confirmed the incremental nature of this relationship.

In addition to higher levels of pain intensity, higher levels of BMI are also correlated with a higher prevalence of a number of chronic pain conditions. Moreover, there is evidence that the relationship between excess weight and chronic pain can be bidirectional. Although a chronic pain condition may lead to higher levels of inactivity that may result in weight gain, there is also evidence that excessive weight may lead to the onset and maintenance of chronic pain conditions. A prospective study by Heuch and colleagues[4] found that high levels of BMI were associated with subsequent prevalence of low back pain in individuals with no previous history of low back pain at baseline. Moreover, in this study the presence of a history of low back pain at baseline did not predict subsequent higher levels of BMI.

High BMI levels among chronic pain sufferers have also been associated with a negative quality of life, poor physical functioning, greater disability, and greater accident liability.[8,9] Psychological factors, mainly anxiety and depression, can also play a significant role in modulating the relationship between weight and pain. This relationship can also be bidirectional; whereas anxiety and depression may lead to significant weight gain, being overweight may reinforce feelings of anxiety and depression. However, regardless of the particular direction of causality, it in turn may exacerbate pain intensity.

Traditional theories to explain the relationship between excess weight and higher levels of pain intensity typically implicated the effect associated with extra strain placed on the body, primarily on the joints, by the extra weight. Recent research has explored other possible explanatory mechanisms, such as the role of inflammation. There is evidence that carrying extra weight in the body, a state often referred to as *adiposopathy* or "sick fat syndrome" is associated with a chronic systemic inflammatory state, which in turn can enhance pain intensity.[10] Other proposed mechanisms have looked at the role of associated factors like exercise and nutrition. Clearly, the relationship between excess weight and chronic pain is a complex and multifactorial one, and further research is needed to elucidate the specific nature.

There is some evidence that weight loss interventions may be effective in the management of chronic pain conditions. One study with knee osteoarthritis (OA) patients found that a weight reduction of at least 2 kg (4.4 lbs) in the previous 10 years was associated with a greater than 50% reduced likelihood of symptomatic OA.[11] The authors estimated that if overweight and obese OA sufferers lost an average of 5 kg (11 lbs) or reached a normal BMI, approximately 24% of surgery for knee OA might be avoided. Several other studies have confirmed these findings, showing that weight reduction, in particular through the combination of diet and exercise, may lead to a significant decrease in pain severity.[12] Another study showed that after having attained even modest weight loss during an 18-month period, knee OA sufferers undergoing a combination of diet plus exercise reported a significant improvement in pain and physical function.[13] The diet plus exercise group had a significantly better outcome than diet only, exercise only, and healthy lifestyle groups.

Similar positive outcomes of weight loss have been reported with CLBP and other chronic pain conditions. A study with FMS sufferers found that after completing a 20-week behavioral weight loss treatment and losing an average 9.2 lbs (4.4% weight reduction), participants reported a significant reduction of FMS symptoms, pain interference, higher quality of life, and greater body satisfaction.[14]

Clearly, being overweight plays a significant precipitating and maintaining role in the onset and course of chronic pain conditions. The ideal target goal for overweight and obese individuals should be to engage in a weight loss program to reach a BMI within the normal range (18.5–24.9). However, because most overweight and obese individuals struggle with a number of unsuccessful attempts to lose weight, it is important to highlight that even more realistic modest reductions in weight, short of reaching the ideal BMI, can have a significant positive impact on their chronic pain conditions. It is also clear that weight loss approaches that rely on a combination of diet and exercise yield far better outcomes for chronic pain sufferers than those that rely on diet alone. Moreover, because of the involvement of psychological and social factors in both weight and chronic pain problems, integrative behavioral weight management programs that address the interplay of biological, psychological, and social factors will probably yield the best results. For example, rather than focusing on a specific diet and exercise regimen only, it is essential to highlight the role of social contextual factors (e.g., socioeconomic and sociocultural factors, such as accessibility and affordability of healthy foods) and psychological factors (e.g., emotional eating, distorted cognitions about food) that reinforce maladaptive eating patterns. **Table 100-1** summarizes the basic recommendations for chronic pain patients with regard to weight.

TABLE 100-1 Practical Recommendations: *Weight*

- If you are overweight, loss of some weight will yield positive results in the management of your chronic pain.
- Avoid fad diets that make unrealistic promises of significant weight loss in a short amount of time. Follow a program that emphasizes slow, gradual, and consistent weight loss.
- Look for a behavioral weight management program that not only emphasizes diet and exercise but also examines social and situational factors that reinforce weight problems.
- Set realistic goals; any weight loss (even short of your ideal) is likely to yield positive results.

EXERCISE

There's a substantial body of research that confirms the inversely proportional relationship between levels of physical activity, or exercise, and chronic pain conditions. That is, higher levels of physical activity are associated with lower levels of pain and related dysfunction. One can reasonably argue that this relationship is to be naturally expected as individuals with greater pain intensity will tend to restrict physical activity to prevent reinjury and pain exacerbation. However, much of the research has focused on the subsequent effect of physical activity on disease course and severity among individuals suffering from preexisting chronic pain conditions. Thus, chronic pain sufferers who engage in higher levels of physical activity endorse subsequent lower levels of pain ratings and related disability. Although the estimated effect size of this relationship appears to be small to moderate based on various systematic reviews of the literature,[15] the observed positive effect of exercise is remarkably consistent.

Not surprisingly, most of the research that has explored the effects of exercise on chronic pain conditions has targeted musculoskeletal pain conditions. Among these, CLBP has received the most attention, followed by OA, most commonly knee and hip. Some studies have also looked at the effect of exercise on other pain conditions, such as FMS. In general, findings with musculoskeletal conditions have yielded pretty consistent results. Several studies, including various meta-analyses and systematic reviews of the literature, have confirmed the significant beneficial effect of exercise, primarily general aerobic and strengthening exercises.[15-17] Both aerobic and strengthening exercises have been associated with significant reductions in pain intensity ratings and associated disability. Although land-based programs have been studied substantially more than water-based ones, both types of exercise programs are found to be effective.

With regard to comparing the relative effectiveness of different exercise modalities, while some studies have found aerobic exercises to be more effective than localized conditioning exercises,[18] others have found them to be equally effective.[19,20] Studies with exercise combinations, typically general aerobic and strengthening exercises with more localized exercises that target the sufferers' particular pain conditions (e.g., trunk muscle conditioning and joint range of motion exercises, eye fixation and other balance exercises, etc.), have found these combinations to be effective.[15,17,21] In addition, the importance of including stretching/flexibility exercises in an exercise program has been noted, primarily to reduce the risk of reinjury. While more research is needed to solidly establish the relative contributions of various types of exercise, it seems reasonable to assume that a combination of stretching/flexibility, aerobic, and strengthening exercises (both general and localized as relevant) will probably yield optimal results. In addition to more conventional aerobic and strengthening exercises, there is evidence that supports the effectiveness of other less conventional physical activities, such as yoga and Tai Chi, in the treatment of musculoskeletal disorders.[17,22]

Both provider-supervised and nonsupervised ("home-based") exercise programs are found to be effective. However, it appears that provider supervision, at least during the initial stages of establishing an exercise routine, may lead to a greater adherence.[20] One particular recommendation is to include provider supervision for the first 12 workout sessions, with scheduled follow-up "booster" sessions to review progress and readjust goals.[22] It is also important to keep in mind the individual factors that are specific to each chronic pain sufferer's particular condition. Therefore, individual tailoring of an exercise program to the particular type of injury or condition is essential to minimize risk of new injury or reinjury from exercise. Overactivity (i.e., engagement in excessive amounts of activity or exercise) can also significantly exacerbate pain conditions and related disability.[23] And comparisons of individual versus group exercise programs have shown both modalities to be effective, with some evidence that group settings may reinforce adherence.[21,22] Moreover, groups have the added benefit of providing social support, which can have a significant impact on promoting mental health and social functioning, thus reducing functional disability.

Despite findings about the relative contributions of various exercise modalities, it is essential to keep in mind that the effectiveness of any exercise program will depend primarily on adherence to that program. The proven effectiveness of a wide range of exercise modalities allows the practitioner to tailor an exercise program to an individual's particular circumstances and preferences. This will significantly increase the likelihood that an individual will adhere to any exercise routine. There is also evidence that the positive effects of exercise on chronic pain are quickly lost once an exercise routine is discontinued, which further supports the need to promote ongoing adherence and maintenance.

As mentioned earlier, most of the research that has explored the relationship between levels of physical activity or exercise and chronic pain has focused on pain severity and related functional disability as the two most relevant outcome measures. However, positive outcomes of exercise have been observed in other variables that are relevant to pain, such as psychological status (i.e., depression, anxiety, stress, anger), cardiovascular health (heart rate, cholesterol), and work status, among others. The notions of fear avoidance and pacing have also been studied with regard to their role in the pain-exercise relationship. Fear avoidance, in the pain literature, refers to the commonly observed reduction in physical and other daily activities as a means to minimize pain escalation. It has been highlighted as a key variable moderating the observed relationship between significant reductions in physical activity and higher levels of pain severity and disability. Pacing is defined as a strategy to divide one's daily activities into smaller, more manageable portions, with planned and calculated increases in activity.[23] Pacing is regarded as an important strategy in striking an optimal compromise between minimizing the risk of injury with gradual progressions of increased physical activity while preventing fear avoidance and the resulting detrimental reduction in physical activity. There appears to be inconsistency in the literature regarding the effectiveness of pacing in the management of chronic pain. These discrepancies may stem from methodological issues that limit comparisons among various studies. Despite the inconsistent findings, most providers emphasize pacing as an important strategy in the management of chronic pain conditions.

Various theories have been proposed to explain the beneficial effects of exercise on chronic pain conditions. Clearly, improved muscle conditioning through exercise can have a significant impact on pain reduction and improved functioning. Exercise also encourages the release of endorphins, which are well known to have an analgesic effect. In addition, given the relationship between excess weight and chronic pain reviewed in the previous section, the potential role of exercise on weight loss can be of significant benefit in pain management. In addition to improved physical conditioning, enhancing physical fitness may promote a sense of confidence to engage in daily activities, thus reducing fear avoidance. This may also lead to improved social functioning, which in turn may help increase social support and reduce anxiety and depression. As discussed in previous chapters, anxiety, depression, and in particular anger and hostility have been implicated in reinforcing chronic pain conditions.

Based on findings from the literature reviewed, **Table 100-2** lists recommendations to develop an exercise program to assist in the management of chronic pain conditions.

TABLE 100-2 Practical Recommendations: *Exercise*

- Design an exercise program that combines stretching/flexibility (warm-up), general aerobic, and strengthening; include other specific exercises as relevant to particular pain condition (e.g., trunk muscle conditioning exercises, balance, etc.).
- Exercise at least 30 minutes per session; 4-5 times per week (include at least 1 rest day x wk).
- Exercise intensity should be tailored to individual's particular pain condition. The goal is to promote physical strength and endurance while minimizing risk of reinjury.
- Pace your activity level according to your capabilities and limitations, ensuring periodic reviews, and reset your goals according to the progress made.
- As can be tolerated, engage in moderate intensity physical activities (e.g., walking briskly, biking, dancing, recreational swimming) or more vigorous activities (e.g., lap swimming, cycling uphill, high-impact aerobic dancing).
- Individualize exercise program according to particular pain condition and professionally confirmed limitations and individual interests and preference.
- Be creative and enjoy your workout (yoga and Tai Chi have shown to be effective).
- Set realistic individual goals (initially under supervision); then periodically review and readjust goals (to maximize exercise potential and stay challenged and interested).
- Exercise program should be professionally supervised (at least initially); schedule periodic consultation sessions (to ensure appropriateness, prevent reinjury).
- If possible, include a social component (fitness club, friends, community program, etc.).
- If overweight, combine with weight loss program (based on healthy eating plus exercise).

NUTRITION

The role of nutrition in chronic pain conditions has received significant attention in recent years. However, given the myriad of popularly held misconceptions associated with nutrition as our society tends to look to foods and supplements as the magic cure for all health problems, this is an area where one needs to be very cautious to discern fad from science. This section reviews some of the nutrients, some ingested as foods or supplements or both, that have been studied scientifically and that show some evidence to support their potential influence, either detrimental or beneficial, on chronic pain conditions. After some general considerations of the potential role of certain nutrients with various chronic pain conditions, we will discuss some specific considerations relevant to migraine headaches.

Vitamin D One nutrient that has received significant attention in the pain literature is vitamin D. Although we can obtain vitamin D from some foods (e.g., oily fish such as salmon, mackerel, sardines, cod liver oil), our primary source comes from the sun's ultraviolet rays (UVB). It is estimated that a very large number of individuals worldwide suffer from vitamin D deficiency, which has been referred to as a largely unrecognized world epidemic. Obviously, individuals with least amount of sun exposure are at higher risk of vitamin D deficiency, but other risk groups include individuals with darker skin (high skin melanin levels interfere with absorption of UVB), obese individuals, and the elderly among others.

Vitamin D deficiency has been linked to a variety of diseases. Most specifically with relevance to chronic pain conditions, low level of vitamin D (typically <20 ng/mL) have been shown to be associated with the development of osteoporosis and rheumatoid arthritis (RA),[24] muscle weakness and other muscular-skeletal problems,[24-27] fractures resulting from falls among the elderly,[26] and chronic widespread pain,[28] among others.

Although randomized clinical trials of the effects of vitamin D therapy are more limited than studies documenting the adverse effects of its deficiency, results from some studies appear promising. A study with FMS patients with mild to moderate vitamin D deficiency (10–25 ng/mL) who underwent vitamin D_3 supplementation (50,000U/wk) for 8 weeks showed a significant improvement in FMS symptoms, especially symptoms of fatigue.[26,29] Improvements in pain intensity and analgesic use were also found in studies with RA patients taking large doses of vitamin D for 1 year[26] and in postmenopausal women with osteoporotic fractures who took vitamin D in conjunction with calcium and fluoride.[30]

The effects of vitamin D deficiency with particular relevance to pain appear to be related to its central role in the absorption of calcium. Vitamin D deficiency is associated with the marked suppression in intestinal calcium and the resulting disruption of calcium balance, which leads to low bone mineral and density. This in turn results in poor bone health and an increased risk of fractures, especially among the elderly. Given the close interplay with calcium, vitamin D supplementation based on results from blood serum levels needs to be determined in coordination with calcium levels. The IOM recommendations[31] for vitamin D supplementation are 600 IU daily for children and adults up to 70 years old and 800 IU for adults 71 years or older. However, it has been suggested that, without adequate sun exposure, children and adults may require higher doses between 800 and 1,000 IU per day.[24]

Polyunsaturated Fatty Acids Polyunsaturated fatty acids (PUFAs) have received a great deal of attention in recent years with regard to their role in a variety of health conditions, including pain. An important distinction is the contrast between the omega-3 (n-3 series) and omega-6 (n-6 series) PUFAs, given the observed anti-inflammatory effect of the former and the proinflammatory effect of the latter. A comprehensive review of the literature identified 17 randomized controlled studies (RCTs) that looked at omega-3 supplementation with individuals suffering from RA and joint pain secondary to inflammatory bowel disease (IBD).[32] The general picture from the findings is consistent, showing that omega-3 supplementation is associated with reduction in lower pain intensity, minutes of morning stiffness, number of painful joints, and use of nonsteroidal anti-inflammatory drugs (NSAIDs). In addition to RA and IBD, positive findings have also been reported with pain associated with dysmenorrhea and neuropathy.[33] The consistent results from these studies suggest that omega-3 PUFAs seem to play a central role in the modulation of pain, in particular conditions associated with inflammation. In addition to their anti-inflammatory action, they are antioxidants and are believed to promote intestinal calcium absorption.

In contrast to the clear picture that has emerged with omega-3 PUFAs, findings are less consistent with the omega-6 PUFAs. Some omega-6 PUFAs have a proinflammatory effect that can exacerbate pain, in particular when taken at a high ratio to omega-3 PUFAs. But, it appears some omega-6 PUFAs may also have an anti-inflammatory effect via the conversion of linoleic acid (LA) to gamma-linoleic acid (GLA). GLA can be found in rare oils such as black currant, borage, and hemp oil. Thus, the particular effect of omega-6 PUFAs on pain depends on the specific types and ratios of PUFAs consumed. Given the potential detrimental effect on pain by promoting inflammation and affecting bone health, one must exercise caution consuming omega 6-PUFAs with chronic pain conditions. The estimated current ratio of omega-6 to omega-3 PUFAs in most Western diets is 10 to 15:1, while the recommended ideal ratio is 1:1.[25] The daily recommended intake of omega-3 is 500 mg, which is much higher than the intake level in the typical diet of most industrialized countries. Given that most Western diets provide a much higher ratio of omega-6 to omega-3 PUFAs than the recommended daily intake, it seems reasonable to supplement omega-3 and limit omega-6 consumption. Foods that are rich sources of omega-3 PUFAs include walnuts, flaxseed, fish (especially high-fat fish like salmon, sardines, and tuna), vegetable oils (olive, canola), and beans, among others. Omega-6 PUFAs are commonly obtained from vegetable oils derived from corn, sunflower, safflower, soy, and cottonseed, among others.

Glucosamine and Chondroitin Sulfate Glucosamine is the most commonly used supplement by individuals suffering from OA. It is frequently taken alone and often in combination with chondroitin. However, studies with both supplements have yielded inconsistent results. Some comprehensive reviews concluded that glucosamine was effective in significantly reducing pain and improving joint space narrowing in OA sufferers.[34] However, other reviews have failed to confirm these findings. It has been suggested that some of the inconsistent findings can be explained by the lack of consistency with the type of glucosamine tested, as well as the particular assessment tools used in different research methodologies. There is suggestion that results may be more positive with glucosamine sulfate than with glucosamine hydrochloride.[35] Similarly, findings with chondroitin are mixed, and many studies have investigated its effect in combination with glucosamine, which makes it difficult to compare the effectiveness of chondroitin alone. Both glucosamine and chondroitin have been found to be relatively safe, with reported concerns appearing to be anecdotal at this time, and no significant negative side effects have been confirmed in well-designed research studies. Despite their apparent safety, it is important for a person deciding to take these supplements to consult with a physician in case of possible contraindications or reactions with medications. Greater consistency in future research methodologies may clarify the question of the effectiveness of these popular supplements.

Probiotics There has been a great deal of attention on the potential beneficial role of probiotics in the treatment of irritable bowel syndrome (IBS) and IBD. There is evidence that alterations of natural gastrointestinal microbiota may be involved in the pathophysiology of both IBS and IBD. Probiotics are live microbiologic organisms that live in foods with live active culture, such as yogurt and some fermented foods. There is some evidence that probiotics can reregulate microbiotic alterations that may be involved in IBS and IBD, in particular decreasing some of the elevations in proinflammatory bacteria. Some studies with IBS patients taking probiotics supplements have shown significant reductions in pain associated with IBS.[36-38] Results with IBD have been mixed, with suggestion that the effects of probiotics may be more effective in ulcerative colitis and pouchitis than in Crohn's disease.[37] An important caution with probiotics is that it appears that some types of probiotics may have specific effects on particular subtypes of IBS and IBD. For example, probiotics with the greatest efficacy data currently for treating IBS are *Bifidobacterium infantis* 35624 and *Escherichia coli* DSM 17252.[36] Moreover, *B. infantis* has been shown to be most effective in reducing pain in patients with diarrhea-predominant IBS. Although further research will help determine with greater specificity what types of probiotics may be most beneficial for what subtypes of gastrointestinal conditions given their apparent safety, there seems to be little risk in taking these supplements.

Other Supplements with Potential Value in the Treatment of Chronic Pain Conditions A variety of herbal products, spices, and other supplements have received attention given claims of their apparent effectiveness reducing pain and inflammation. Among these is "devil's claw" (*Harpagophytum procumbens*), an African plant that appears to have anti-inflammatory property. Some studies have reported positive findings decreasing pain in OA[35] and CLBP.[39] Although more research is needed before its effectiveness can be established, this supplement appears to hold potential value in the treatment of a number of chronic pain conditions.

Another supplement that has received attention for its anti-inflammatory property is turmeric, a spice derived from the plant *Curcuma longa*. Turmeric is commonly used in Indian cooking as a spice and coloring agent in curry powders and other foods. Curcumin is the substance that gives it its yellow color, and it is believed by some to be the major active therapeutic ingredient in turmeric. Both turmeric and curcumin have been used for years in Ayurvedic medicine to treat various health conditions. Research reveals that both appear to have antioxidant and anti-inflammatory properties. Preliminary clinical research has shown potential value in the treatment of RA.[27,40] However, more research is needed to determine its effectiveness in the treatment of OA and other chronic pain conditions.

A variety of other herbs and supplements have received attention given their potential value in the treatment of a variety of chronic pain conditions. What most of the supplements seem to have in common for the treatment of pain are their anti-inflammatory properties. A partial list of these includes flavonoids, magnesium, capsaicin, vitamin B_{12}, folate, SAMe, methylsulfonylmethane (MSM), ginger, red clover, carotenoids, white willow bark, cayenne, alpha-lipoic acid, acetyl-L-carnitine, and selenium, among others. Again, more research is needed in order to establish whether any of these can be indeed effective in the treatment of chronic pain.

Nutrition and Migraines Perhaps one of the chronic pain conditions most commonly associated with food triggers (besides IBS and IBD given their obvious gut involvement) is migraines. Popular lore has promoted a long list of foods that have been reported to act as significant triggers for migraine episodes, including sweeteners containing aspartame, aged cheese, chocolate, monosodium glutamate (MSG), tyramine-containing foods (e.g., processed meats, soy sauce), and others. Bernstein,[41] a migraine scientist and specialist, warned that the sensitivity of migraines to particular foods has likely been overemphasized, highlighting the marked individual differences in responses to particular food triggers. Moreover, the author proposed that abrupt episodes of hypoglycemia (typically following intake of foods with a high glycemic index) may account for many of the claimed food sensitivities by migraine sufferers. The following dietary recommendations followed this proposition to ensure effective management of migraines: (1) eating breakfast regularly, including protein-based foods, (2) having a meal that includes proteins every 4–6 hours, (3) ensuring an adequate amount of complex carbohydrates in the diet, (4) having healthy snacks with protein, (5) staying adequately hydrated, (6) keeping a food diary to carefully monitor and record particular individual sensitivities (not necessarily allergies) to foods, and (7) avoiding foods with a high glycemic index.

Conclusion Although there seems to be strong evidence that several foods and supplements have potential value in the treatment of chronic pain conditions, we are far from having attained a clear picture of what particular supplements are most effective for what conditions. The evidence appears strong to support the value of vitamin D and omega-3 PUFAs, in particular for treating neuromuscular conditions that can be significantly exacerbated by inflammatory mechanisms, and skeletal problems, such as those involved in RA and OA. There is also strong evidence to support the consumption of probiotics in the treatment of IBS, and possibly IBD. In addition, avoiding foods with a high glycemic index to prevent hypoglycemic episodes appears to be a sound preventive measure in the management of migraine headache. With regard to some of the other supplements discussed, although promising, further research is needed before their therapeutic value can be firmly established. In the meantime, personal decisions to include any of these supplements in a dietary regimen should be done after consultation with a physician to rule out any possible counter indications associated with existent medical conditions or interactions with medications. Perhaps the nutrition-related lifestyle change that bears greatest potential value in the management of chronic pain, as well as in many other health conditions, is to adopt a balanced diet following the recommendations made by the USDA (www.ChooseMyPlate.gov).[42] In other words, a low-fat, high-fiber, high-protein diet with adequate servings of fruits and vegetables, which are generally lacking in the typical diet of many highly industrialized and Western countries, will yield invaluable health benefits. Nutritional recommendations are summarized in **Table 100-3**.

COMMON SUBSTANCES OF DAILY LIVING

This section discusses the relationship between chronic pain and various substances commonly used by millions of individuals worldwide and intrinsically associated with their social lifestyles: caffeine, tobacco smoking, and alcohol.

TABLE 100-3 Practical Recommendations: *Nutrition*

- Eat a balanced diet, prioritizing fruits and vegetables over meats, oils, and fats.
- Monitor effects of particular foods on pain. Make relevant changes with foods that appear to intensify your pain.
- If vitamin D deficient, consider supplementing your diet with vitamin D.
- An adequate intake of omega 3 PUFAs may be beneficial for pain management.
- If you are taking or considering supplements for pain, consult your physician to identify possible contraindications.

CAFFEINE

Caffeine is a powerful psychoactive substance derived primarily from coffee beans and tea leaves. It is one of the most widely used psychoactive substances throughout the world and is commonly found in many drinks, including tea, carbonated beverages, energy drinks, and others. But by far the most common method of consuming caffeine is as a coffee drink. The use of coffee as a social drink, primarily for its stimulant effect, is believed to have originated in Ethiopia. From there, it was introduced to the Arab world via Egypt and Yemen, and subsequently to Italy, the rest of Europe, and the world. Today, coffee is one of the most common drinks consumed worldwide.

The relationship between caffeine consumption and pain is a complex one and has been a source of much controversy. The controversies stem primarily from evidence of caffeine's apparent positive and negative health effects. Similarly, with regard to its effect on pain, there appears to be evidence that caffeine may be both beneficial and detrimental to pain conditions. These apparently contradictory findings with regard to the effect of caffeine on pain and other health conditions have to do with the complex biochemical mechanisms involved, lack of consistency in research methodologies used (type of caffeine consumption, amounts consumed, etc.), and a general lack of well-designed randomized controlled trials on the effect of caffeine on human health. With regard to pain, it appears that, in general, the beneficial effects of caffeine are most evident with acute pain conditions, although the potentially detrimental effects may be more likely associated with both chronic pain and chronic caffeine use in very large amounts.

Most of the research documenting the positive health effects of caffeine on pain has been with headaches (both tension-type and migraine). A meta-analysis conducted by Sawynok[43] concluded that caffeine may be useful for headache relief. In a double-blind controlled prospective study, caffeine (100 mg) was found to significantly augment the analgesic effect of diclophenac (100 mg, oral) in patients with acute onset of migraines without auras.[44] In a clinical trial with patients suffering from tension headaches, a combination of ibuprofen (400 mg) plus caffeine (200 mg) yielded a more significant improvement of headaches than either ibuprofen or caffeine alone.[45] Caffeine alone showed similar improvement as ibuprofen alone, although patients on the caffeine group reported faster relief. In addition, both caffeine and ibuprofen brought about significantly more relief than a placebo condition. By contrast, there is some evidence that regular caffeine use may be associated with the development of migraines and daily chronic headaches, primarily in children and adolescents.[43,46]

In addition to headaches, there is some evidence that caffeine may potentiate the analgesic effect of morphine in oncology patients.[47] It has also been found to increase and prolong the analgesic effect of paracetamol or acetaminophen in postoperative pain.[48] There is less clarity regarding the effect of caffeine with other pain conditions. Besides its positive effect on pain, research evidence indicates that caffeine may be beneficial for the treatment of a variety of medical conditions, including congestive heart failure (treats associated edema given its diuretic effect), apnea in premature newborns, asthma (improves pulmonary function), depression, and type II diabetes, among others.[49] There is also evidence that caffeine may have a potential role in the prevention of hepatic cirrhosis, Alzheimer's, Parkinson's, and some types of cancer.

On the other side of the controversy, there is evidence that caffeine, especially when consumed in large amounts and for an increased period of time, may be detrimental to some gastrointestinal conditions (primarily gastroesophageal reflux, peptic ulcers, and gastritis), renal or hepatic function, some cardiovascular conditions (primarily arrhythmias, angina, and palpitations), anxiety, and irritability, among others. In pregnancy, caffeine consumption has been associated with increased risk of miscarriages, skeletal alterations, delayed intrauterine growth, congenital malformations, and low birth weight. Chronic exposure to large amounts of caffeine also appears to potentiate the action of glucocorticoids, which among other effects, may lead to decreased bone density.

With regard to its interaction with other drugs, as mentioned earlier, caffeine appears to increase the analgesic effect of ibuprofen and acetaminophen. It also appears to increase the analgesic effect of NSAIDs. However, caffeine potentiates the effect of nicotine and alcohol, increases the risk of serotonin syndrome with paroxetine, and increases the teratogenic effects of vasoconstrictors. It may also inhibit some of the analgesic effect of acupuncture and transcutaneous electrical nerve stimulation (TENS).[49]

Most of the effects, both positive and negative, of caffeine on humans have been linked to its pharmacokinetic property blocking the action of adenosine receptors. Its antinociceptive action has been associated more specifically with blockade of adenosine A2a and A2b receptors. Blocking the effect of adenosine leads to vasoconstriction, which may help explain, at least in part, the positive effect of caffeine in alleviating headaches. In addition to the biochemical mechanisms involved, it appears that the particular dose of caffeine intake may also help in part explain its potential positive or negative effects. For reference, an 8-ounce cup of brewed coffee (drip method) contains between 95 and 200 mg of caffeine, whereas a 1-ounce cup of espresso contains between 40 and 75 mg of caffeine; an 8-ounce cup of black tea 14-61 mg, and a 12 oz Coke ("Classic") between 30 and 35 mg. "Moderate consumers" are described as individuals who consume 128 to 595 mg daily (approx. 3 to 5 cups dripped coffee daily), while "major consumers" intake 1,020 to 1,035 mg daily (approx. 6 or more cups of dripped coffee daily).[49] Despite the marked inconsistency of caffeine dosing in research studies, in general, studies that document the beneficial health effects of caffeine tend to be based on moderate caffeine consumption, whereas evidence of risk is typically associated with major caffeine intake for a prolonged period of time.

In summary, it is clear that caffeine can have both significant beneficial and detrimental health effects on humans. Similarly, it may be of potential value in the treatment of some pain conditions, in particular acute headaches in adults. But, it can also exacerbate certain pain conditions, including headaches in children and adolescents. Future research will help clarify the specific conditions that can help us maximize the health-promoting effects of caffeine while minimizing its potential health risks. Until more specific data are available, it seems reasonable to assume that moderate amounts of caffeine consumption, while taking into consideration the counter indications mentioned earlier, may be a relatively safe practice and in some specific cases, potentially helpful in the management of some pain and other health conditions. At high levels of consumption (approximately more than 6 cups of coffee or daily equivalent), the potentially detrimental effects of caffeine will pose a greater health risk (**Table 100-4**).

TABLE 100-4 Practical Recommendations: *Caffeine*

- Consider abstinence or minimal use if you have any conditions that can be exacerbated by caffeine intake (e.g., gastritis, GERD, arrhythmias, palpitations, etc.).
- If your caffeine consumption is moderate (no more than 3 to 4 cups of coffee or equivalent daily), and you do not have a particular contraindication (as noted above), it is probably safe to maintain your regular caffeine intake, and there may be potential health benefits resulting from it.

SMOKING

Similar to the case of caffeine, there has been some controversy with regard to the relationship between tobacco smoking and pain. As with caffeine, there is an apparent paradox that stems from evidence of both detrimental and analgesic effects of tobacco smoking on pain. However, unlike the case of caffeine, the significant health risks associated with tobacco smoking, as well as its strong positive correlation with chronic pain conditions, substantially overshadow any potential beneficial effects. According to the CDC,[50] smoking is the leading preventable cause of morbidity and mortality in the U.S.A., accounting for approximately 443,000 deaths each year.[51] Moreover, it is estimated that smoking is associated with approximately $190 billion in annual medical expenses and lost productivity. It is well established that tobacco smoking represents a significant risk factor in the development of cardiovascular disease, some cancers (in particular lung cancer), and chronic respiratory disorders, among others.

Several comprehensive reviews of the literature have documented a solid body of evidence confirming the positive correlation between smoking and chronic pain disorders. Findings consistently show that smokers have a significantly higher incidence and prevalence of chronic pain disorders, higher ratings of pain intensity, and higher levels of associated functional impairment.[51-53] There is also evidence that former smokers have a higher prevalence of chronic pain disorders,[54] which suggests the possibility of long-lasting negative consequences of smoking. However there is also evidence that the positive association between smoking and chronic pain is reduced significantly among former smokers compared to current smokers.[55] One of the most alarming findings is that even nonsmokers who are passively exposed to environmental tobacco smoke report higher pain ratings than nonsmokers who are almost never exposed to environmental smoke.[56]

The particular types of chronic pain conditions that have been positively correlated with tobacco smoking include CLBP, RA, OA, headaches (tension, migraines and clusters), FMS, temporomandibular joint (TMJ) disorders, dyspepsia, menstrual pain, pregnancy-related pelvic pain, and others.[51] The observed relationship between tobacco smoking and chronic pain appears to be a complex one. One of the typical questions that surfaces with most correlational studies is whether any causal associations exist, and if so, what particular direction and temporality characterize these relationships. In other words, does smoking lead to an increased prevalence of chronic pain conditions and pain intensity, or are chronic pain sufferers more likely to smoke? Evidence suggests that smoking leads to a higher incidence and prevalence of chronic pain conditions, as well as higher pain intensity ratings and related dysfunction. However, there is also evidence that chronic pain sufferers may seek smoking as a coping mechanism and that smokers may engage in other unhealthy behaviors that either lead to or reinforce chronic pain conditions.

Several European prospective studies found evidence that smoking during adolescence or early adulthood predicted the incidence and severity of chronic pain conditions years later.[52] There is also evidence that chronic pain sufferers are more likely to smoke. One study reported a greater than twofold likelihood of smoking among chronic pain sufferers (54%) compared to the general population (25.7%).[9] Therefore, it appears that smoking and pain are involved in a bidirectional causal relationship.

As mentioned earlier, despite clear evidence of the detrimental effects of smoking on pain, there is also evidence that tobacco smoking may have an analgesic effect. Animal studies have consistently confirmed the pain-inhibitory effect of nicotine and tobacco smoke on pain. Although the analgesic effect of pain has been confirmed in some human studies, the evidence here is more mixed as some studies have failed to confirm this relationship. It appears as if the pain-inhibitory effect of nicotine and tobacco smoke on pain is explained, at least partly, by the activation of nicotinic acetylcholine receptors, primarily in the brainstem, which in turn activate spinal cord pain-inhibitory pathways.[41] Other mechanisms that have been proposed to explain the analgesic effect of smoking include the release of β-endorphins, increased cardiovascular reactivity leading to decreased pain sensitivity, and attentional narrowing that results in decreased awareness of pain sensation.

A variety of mechanisms have been proposed to explain the detrimental effects of smoking on chronic pain. These mechanisms involve complex interactions among biological, psychological, and social factors, suggesting that this relationship may be best understood from a biopsychosocial perspective. At the biological level, there is evidence that smoking is a risk factor for the development of osteoporosis, lumbar disc disease, and impaired bone healing.[53] This may be the result of decreased carboxyhemoglobin levels, which may impair oxygen delivery to tissues. In addition, the physiologic stress that results from pain activates the sympathetic nervous system and hypothalamic-pituitary-adrenal (HPA) axis, which in turn helps blunt pain perception. However, there is evidence that the HPA system is downregulated in long-term smokers, which may lead to an increased pain perception.

At the psychological level, both chronic pain and smoking have a positive correlation with affective disorders, primarily depression and anxiety, as well as substance abuse disorders. The significant associations among these variables suggest the existence of complex multidirectional feedback loops at play that may reinforce the detrimental effects of smoking on pain. Individuals who are anxious and/or depressed are more likely to smoke and use other psychoactive substances and experience higher rates and intensity of pain and related dysfunction. Chronic pain sufferers are more likely to be depressed and anxious and to be active smokers and substance abusers. Smokers are more likely to be depressed and anxious, abuse other substances, and experience significant pain. A variety of sociodemographic factors are also positively associated with both smoking and chronic pain. These include low socioeconomic status (SES), low educational level, unemployment, social isolation, and lack of social support. In other words, smokers, as well as chronic pain sufferers, are more likely to be poor, undereducated, unemployed (or underemployed), and divorced. Most likely, these associations are primarily mediated by the significant psychosocial stress that is associated with these sociodemographic factors and the lack of resources that could otherwise help buffer the resulting psychosocial stress.

Ditre and colleagues[51] proposed an "integrative reciprocal model of pain and smoking" that describes the complex smoking-pain interactions, highlighting the reciprocal feedback loops that maintain them. Once these complex multidirectional self-reinforcing feedback loops have been established among biological, psychological, and social factors, attempts to identify the original direction of causality and temporality of these relationships may be of relatively little clinical significance. It seems reasonable to assume that integrative interventions that target both biological and psychological factors may yield the best outcomes. In summary, given the established role that smoking plays in reinforcing pain conditions, as well as the clear health risks associated with smoking, it is quite clear that total abstinence, or smoking cessation, should be the ultimate goal of clinical interventions with chronic pain sufferers who smoke. Given the wide range of treatment options available for pain management, potential analgesic benefits of smoking are largely overshadowed by the significant health risks associated with such a highly toxic substance (**Table 100-5**).

ALCOHOL

There has been relatively little attention focused on the association between alcohol and pain, as compared to other substances of daily living such as caffeine and smoking. This is surprising given that alcohol is such a common coping strategy used by pain sufferers to manage their pain. As with the case of caffeine and smoking, there is controversy with regard to apparent findings of both positive and negative effects of alcohol on pain. But unlike the case of these other substances, there is much less clarity about what specific recommendations to follow based on the existent findings.

TABLE 100-5 Practical Recommendations: *Smoking*

- If you smoke tobacco, consider a smoking cessation program. There are no advantages from smoking, and there are significant health risks from this highly toxic substance.
- Behavioral smoking cessation programs that target behavioral modification techniques (e.g., CBT, hypnosis) can be of value to help you quit.

A review of the literature shows that a modest but positive correlation has been reported between alcohol and chronic pain conditions such as CLBP.[57] This relationship seems to be primarily evident with alcohol abuse and dependence, as opposed to regular alcohol consumption or use. However, several studies have failed to confirm a positive correlation between alcohol consumption and chronic pain. In fact, some studies, many of which were conducted in Europe, have reported a negative correlation, that is, lower alcohol consumption among chronic pain sufferers.[57-60] It is unclear whether cultural differences associated with alcohol usage and lifestyle among the diverse populations studied have had any influence on these disparate findings.

As with caffeine and smoking, there is evidence that alcohol may either have an analgesic effect or increase pain sensitivity. The analgesic effect of alcohol on pain appears to be most evident in acute pain conditions, whereas increased pain sensitivity is generally observed with prolonged pain and alcohol consumption. Moreover, long-term alcohol use is clearly associated with other detrimental health consequences, which, indirectly, may have a negative impact on chronic pain conditions.

Despite the controversies with regard to the role of alcohol in pain, it is well known that alcohol is used as a common coping strategy by chronic pain sufferers. There is also evidence that prolonged alcohol consumption increases pain sensitivity, thus lowering the pain threshold, in particular with alcohol abuse or dependence.[61] As seen with caffeine and smoking, alcohol abuse and dependence show a high correlation with disorders that involve affective dysregulation, in particular depression and anxiety. Rather than playing a confounding role, it appears that alcohol may play an important moderating role in the complex interactions that link these behavioral and psychological states in chronic pain sufferers. Egli and colleagues[62] proposed an interesting theoretical model that highlights the role of complex neurochemical interactions associated with sensory dysregulation in chronic pain sufferers, affective dysregulation in depression and anxiety, and prolonged alcohol consumption. Their model emphasizes a resulting self-reinforcing cycle among chronic stress, alcohol abuse, and pain.

Excessive alcohol consumption is commonly associated with a variety of sociodemographic factors that represent significant risk factors for chronic pain conditions, including low socioeconomic status, low educational level, and unemployment, among others. Future research will help elucidate the precise nature of the apparent complex interactions among these social, psychological, and biological factors. Much of the lack of clarity in our understanding of the alcohol-pain relationship also seems to stem from a lack of consistency in the variables studied, such as inconsistent criteria used to define "normal" versus "excessive" alcohol consumption, abuse and dependence, as well as long-term use. A study by Lawton and Simpson[63] found that among chronic pain patients, being male, having a high intensity affective pain experience, and lacking reliance on relaxation as a coping mechanism were all strong predictors of significant alcohol consumption. These findings suggest that we need to pay closer attention to the particular characteristics and circumstances that mediate the positive relationship between excessive alcohol consumption and chronic pain.

In conclusion, our knowledge of the role of alcohol on chronic pain based on the existent research seems quite inconsistent. Nonetheless, it seems reasonable to conclude that excessive alcohol consumption (i.e., meeting diagnostic criteria for alcohol "abuse" or "dependence" according to the DSM-5 or ICD-10) for a prolonged period of time has the potential to exacerbate the course of chronic pain. Moreover, the

TABLE 100-6 Practical Recommendations: *Alcohol*

- If you drink alcohol casually, it is probably safe to continue doing so (confirm with your physician that there are no interactions with your medications).
- If you drink in excess (i.e., meet criteria for abuse or dependency according to the DSM-5 or ICD-10), it is urgent that you completely abstain from or significantly reduce your alcohol intake.
- Substance abuse programs that integrate biological, psychological, and social aspects of your substance abuse are most likely to be effective.

significant detrimental health consequences that are associated with excessive and prolonged alcohol consumption, some of which may interact directly or indirectly with chronic pain conditions, further supports the significant health benefits that are associated with either complete abstinence or consuming alcohol with moderation (**Table 100-6**).

SLEEP

A substantial body of research confirms a very strong relationship between sleep and pain. The general picture shows that significant sleep disturbances are associated with high intensity and frequency of pain conditions, both acute and chronic, and other related functional impairment. There is also clear evidence that the relationship between sleep and pain is bidirectional, where pain can disrupt sleep and disrupted sleep can exacerbate pain. This relationship seems to be often mediated by other factors, such as psychiatric symptoms like depression and anxiety, fatigue, obesity, and psychosocial stress. These findings suggest that the best way to fully appreciate the pain-sleep relationship is from a multifactorial biopsychosocial perspective.

Studies with chronic pain sufferers have shown strong correlations with sleep disruptions. A comprehensive critical review of the literature of headaches and sleep found a very strong relationship between chronic headaches, both migraines and tension-type headaches, and significant sleep complaints, sleep disruptions, and short nocturnal sleep duration.[64] A similar relationship was reported with cluster headaches, although stronger correlations were found with episodic, in contrast to chronic cluster headaches.[65] Besides nighttime disturbances, chronic headaches have also been found to correlate significantly with daytime sleepiness.

Several studies have confirmed a significantly high level of sleep disruptions (i.e., sleep deprivation, clinical insomnia, poor quality of sleep, sleep-related functional impairment) among CLBP sufferers.[66] Similarly high correlations of sleep problems were found with other chronic pain conditions, including chronic neck pain, RA, OA, chronic neuropathic pain, FMS, and postoperative pain, among others.[66-68] Even studies with nonclinical populations have found that sleep deprivation can significantly increase pain sensitivity and cause generalized hyperalgesia in healthy subjects with no prior history of clinical pain conditions.[69]

With regard to the question of whether a causal relationship exists and, if so, which direction it takes, there is evidence to support bidirectional causality. Robust evidence comes from a longitudinal prospective cohort study conducted in Norway based on survey data from the Nord-Trøndelag Health Surveys HUNT-2 and HUNT-3.[70] The presence of insomnia at baseline in headache-free subjects predicted the prevalence and frequency of headaches, both migraine and tension-type, at follow-up 11 years later. Subjects who reported insomnia at baseline had a 40% increased risk for headaches 11 years later at follow-up, and the presence of insomnia-related work disability at baseline increased that risk to 60%. Moreover, the presence of headaches plus neuromuscular complaints at baseline significantly increased the risk of insomnia at follow-up. These data offer support for a bidirectional causal relationship between sleep and chronic headaches.

Conditions involving affective dysregulation, such as stress, depression, and anxiety, have been found to modulate the sleep-pain relationship. Although some studies have confirmed that the sleep-pain relationship holds strong, independent of the role of these psychological factors, their comorbid presence typically strengthens that relationship. Other factors that appear to modulate the sleep-pain relationship include fatigue,[71] obesity,[72] and functional impairment or disability.[70] Again, these findings suggest that a biopsychosocial model is best suited to fully understand the complex multifactorial relationship between sleep disturbances and chronic pain.

With regard to the mechanisms involved in the sleep-pain relationship, several models have been hypothesized. Some authors have highlighted the role of inflammatory processes that appear to underlie both sleep disturbances and some chronic pain conditions.[73] The potential role of melatonin has been explored, especially given its influence in regulating circadian rhythms and as an anti-inflammatory agent. Some studies have focused on the apparent dysregulation in short sleep waves and REM sleep that have been observed in migraine sufferers. Ong and colleagues[64] proposed an interesting biobehavioral model of chronic headaches and sleep that proposes three main interacting mechanisms: (1) common coping behaviors for headaches (e.g., sleep, naps, caffeine, sleep medication, lying down in a dark room) can precipitate and perpetuate sleep disturbance; (2) disruption in sleep physiology increases the propensity for headaches (mainly by decreasing short-wave sleep, which leads to increased pain sensitivity); and; (3) over time, coperpetuating interacting cycles transform episodic headaches into chronic headaches. It has also been proposed that alterations in pain modulation in the central nervous system may lead to pain amplification in patients suffering from RA. Although there seems to be some support for all of these theories, but further research is needed to clarify the specific nature of this relationship.

Some important observations have been made about the sleep-pain relationship with relevance to clinical implications for pharmacotherapy. Sleep deprivation appears to attenuate the analgesic effects of some medications. The importance of considering the diverse effects on sleep of opioid analgesics, in particular long-acting ones, has also been highlighted, as these may interfere with sleep and in turn exacerbate pain. Hajak[74] noted that since pain perception shows a strong circadian pattern exhibiting significant variation over the 24-hour sleep-wake period, this variation needs to be considered in prescribing pain medication. Ideally, intake of pain medication should follow circadian variations to assure sufficient pain reduction at early morning hours. In addition, ideal pain medication at night should have hypnotic properties that facilitate deep sleep, while daytime medications should be activating in order to promote good sleep the following night.

In contrast to the substantial body of research documenting the strong relationship between sleep disturbances and chronic pain, studies that have looked at the effect of interventions to improve sleep on pain are more limited. However, available findings seem to support the reasonable assumption that improving sleep quality can have a significant positive impact on the management of chronic pain. Pharmacological and behavioral approaches that target improving sleep quality can be invaluable in treating chronic pain conditions with comorbid sleep disturbances. In addition, given the significant comorbidities of sleep problems and chronic pain with stress, depression, and anxiety, effective treatment of these affective comorbidities needs to be central in pain management interventions. Behavioral medicine interventions that target stress management, such as relaxation training, meditation, cognitive-behavioral therapy (CBT), hypnosis, and others, can be of potential value to improve sleep quality and associated chronic pain. A comprehensive chronic pain assessment includes a thorough evaluation of sleep-related variables, such as total sleep duration, quality of sleep, nocturnal awakenings, energy level upon awakening, daytime sleepiness, and other sleep-related disturbances. Because a multifactorial biopsychosocial model can best help us understand the sleep-pain relationship, an integrative treatment approach that targets as many of these factors as possible will probably yield optimal treatment outcomes. Recommendations are summarized in **Table 100-7**.

TABLE 100-7 Practical Recommendations: *Sleep*
• Make sure that you get sufficient sleep quantity (~7-8 hr x night) and quality (feeling rested, refreshed, and energetic upon awakening). • If you have a specific sleep disturbance (e.g., insomnia, interrupted sleep, daytime sleepiness or drowsiness), seek treatment for this problem. • Ensure you undergo a comprehensive sleep evaluation to uncover the nature of the problem. • If there are significant affective problems present (e.g., depression, anxiety, severe stress), seek help for these from a specialist. • Regardless of the nature of psychological factors, a treatment that integrates pharmacological and behavioral approaches (e.g., sleep hygiene, relaxation) will likely yield the best results.

OTHER LIFESTYLE FACTORS WITH VARIABLE DEGREES OF "CHOICE"

There are a variety of lifestyle factors that play a significant role in the experience and course of chronic pain but which have variable degrees of personal choice. Among these are social isolation/social support, employment, and religiosity/spirituality. We will briefly discuss the role of these lifestyle factors.

SOCIAL SUPPORT/SOCIAL ISOLATION

A common thread that has clearly emerged throughout all of the previous sections is that a biopsychosocial model is best suited to conceptualize chronic pain conditions given the close interplay of biological, psychological, and social factors that influence the experience and course of chronic pain. Therefore, it should not be surprising that social support has been found to be a significant factor in chronic pain. Many studies have documented a positive effect of social support, the general picture being that chronic pain sufferers who report high levels of social support, particularly from significant others, tend to report lower pain intensity and related disability. Such positive effects have been documented with populations suffering from general chronic pain,[75] CLBP,[76,77] OA,[78] RA,[79] persons with disabilities,[80] and in particular with older adults.[81]

However, there has been controversy given some contradictory findings that show that high levels of social support may be associated with higher levels of pain intensity and disability.[82] These apparently conflictual findings have led to attempts among researchers to attain a greater level of specificity with regard to the construct of social support in order to better understand what type of support, and under what circumstances, may lead to positive or negative effects. It appears as if perceived social support that is experienced by the pain sufferer as validating, empowering, and emotionally empathic, while promoting independence and reliance on active coping strategies, leads to decreased pain intensity and higher levels of functioning. By contrast, social support that tends to be expressed primarily as direct solicitousness and providing compensation, often unsolicited, for pain-related limitations tends to be associated with higher levels of pain intensity and disability, also fostering dependency and passive coping strategies and reinforcing pain behaviors.

The other side of the coin of social support is social isolation. Several studies have looked at whether, for adults, being in a long-term relationship (i.e., married or "partnered") versus being alone has any influence on the experience of chronic pain sufferers.[78,79] The picture here seems to be much clearer; that is, being in a relationship, either marriage or partnering, that is described as satisfying, happy, or nondistressing, leads to significantly lower reports of pain intensity and related dysfunction than either being alone or in a relationship described as distressing, unhappy, or providing low satisfaction.

Another aspect of social support/isolation that has received much less attention in the literature has to do with the experience of social disadvantage. Studies show a very consistent strong relationship between being a member of socially disadvantaged groups (e.g., low socicoeconomic status, low educational level, ethnic/racial minority, etc.) and pain intensity and related disability.[76] Moreover, these effects are observed independent of participation in unhealthy behaviors (e.g., smoking, alcohol abuse, unhealthy diets), which has often being suggested as a possible explanation for these findings. Two explanations that have been proposed and are supported by research findings include: (1) the experience of severe chronic stress that is known to characterize living in a context of social disadvantage, and the well-established positive correlation between chronic stress and chronic pain, and (2) social limitations associated with the lack of availability, accessibility, and utilization of resources and adequate treatments for chronic pain management.

The fact that this area is generally underemphasized is probably explained at least in part, by the helplessness providers may feel about any likelihood of making significant changes in social ills that go beyond the power and scope of clinical interventions. Nonetheless, an awareness of these relationships may result in some concrete practical implications for clinical practice. First, assessing the need for interventions that address the severe psychosocial stress often experienced by members of socially disadvantaged groups needs to be set as a high priority in chronic pain treatments with this population. Second, it is important to ensure that interventions with members of socially disadvantaged groups take into consideration some of the barriers that may interfere with treatment adherence. For example, poor attendance in physical therapy programs, which are often several times a week, may result from the financial strain associated with missing work to attend therapy appointments. There is also some evidence that CBT, which has been promoted as the gold standard behavioral treatment for chronic pain, may have limited effectiveness with members of socially disadvantaged groups. Some of the reasons for resistance to treatment may have to do with sociocultural values underlying CBT, which assume that fatalistic cognitions represent distortions of reality that need to be corrected rather than accurate appraisals of a disheartening social situation. Members of socially disadvantaged groups also tend to feel little control over external events, which may interfere with therapeutic goals based on notions of self-control and self empowerment. Given the general absence of empirical evidence of interventions that are effective specifically with members of socially disadvantaged groups, a patient-centered approach that takes into consideration a particular patient's individual and social situation may yield the best results. **Table 100-8** summarizes recommendations with regard to social support and pain.

EMPLOYMENT-RELATED FACTORS

There is an extensive literature on the relationship between pain and a variety of factors associated with work or employment. Much of this literature is motivated by health economic and policy factors, thus prioritizing the understanding of the effects of pain, primarily acute pain, and related disability on the ability to work (i.e., productivity), and absenteeism or time elapsed before returning to work. Less attention has been given to understanding the effects of characteristics associated with the type of employment on the pain itself, in particular chronic pain. Nonetheless, some studies have looked at the role of work-related variables, such as job satisfaction and type of work on the experience and course of chronic pain.

TABLE 100-8 Practical Recommendations: *Social Support*
• Social relationships that are perceived as supportive, emotionally empathic, and validating of one's experience, while promoting independence and reliance on active coping strategies can facilitate pain management. • Being in an intimate/romantic relationship that is satisfying and nondistressing appears to have a buffering effect on the experience of chronic pain. • Patient-centered treatment approaches that take into account individual and social factors associated with a patient's pain experience should be prioritized with patients from socially disadvantaged groups because of the lack of empirical evidence of effective interventions with these populations.

Job Satisfaction There is some evidence that the degree of *job satisfaction* an individual feels is associated with chronic pain related disability. Low job satisfaction, in general, refers to perceptions held by an individual about how difficult job conditions and demands are. A landmark prospective study was conducted in this area with workers at the Boeing Company who were followed for 9 years.[83] Findings revealed that workers who reported they "hardly ever" enjoyed their jobs had a 2.5 times greater likelihood to report pain associated with acute back injuries than workers who "almost always" enjoyed their work. However, there have been mixed results with the research on job satisfaction; several studies, primarily with acute pain, failed to confirm this association.[84] It is possible that these discrepant results may be explained, at least in part, by a lack of consistency in defining the construct of job satisfaction and by the different measurement tools used.

Type of work There is evidence that *type of work* may be associated with the pain experience. Work with greater physical demands (i.e., "heavy work") is typically associated with greater disability in chronic pain patients.[77,84]

Availability for Modified Work/Work Autonomy Two other related factors that show a significant association with chronic pain intensity and related disability are the *availability for modified work* and *work autonomy*. The concept of modified work refers to the level of flexibility a job may have to make modifications in work demands in order to accommodate to limitations of the injured worker. The concept of work autonomy refers to how much control injured workers may have to set their own pace with work activities once they return to work after an injury. The presence of modified work and high levels of work autonomy have been shown to be associated with lower levels of chronic pain disability.[85]

In summary, although individuals may have little control or "choice" with regard to the particular conditions associated with the type of work that they perform, it is important to understand the role of these lifestyle factors in the experience and course of their pain. An important implication from these findings is that interventions with injured workers that focus primarily on finding the right kind of treatment to manage pain, in combination with actions to prevent fraud while minimizing the disincentive effects of benefits may be limited if they fail to also address the characteristics of the work itself that may influence the course of the pain. A supportive response from the workplace soon after an injury, coupled with flexibility to accommodate to the limitations of the worker once she or he can return to work, can have a significant positive effect toward helping minimize the pain experience and related disability (**Table 100-9**).

RELIGIOSITY/SPIRITUALITY

It has been estimated that more than 60% of chronic pain patients use prayer to help them cope with pain, and 40% of pain patients report becoming more religious or spiritual after the onset of a painful condition.[86] Moreover, some studies report that prayer is either the most common or the second most common coping strategy used by chronic pain sufferers.[87,88] Therefore, it is clear that religiosity/spirituality (R/S) is a relevant area in the study of pain. There is an extensive body of research that has explored the relationship between various aspects associated with R/S and pain. In general, various beliefs and practices associated with R/S used as a way of coping with pain appear to have a positive effect on pain severity, tolerance to pain, ability to control pain, and associated functioning.[86] However, there are some mixed findings in the literature given that several studies have found some aspects of R/S coping to be associated with negative outcomes.[87]

These apparently contradictory findings are probably explained by the general lack of definitional clarity and operational specificity of the R/S constructs. First, despite evidence of marked differences in the way individuals define religiosity and spirituality, these two constructs are typically lumped together in much of the literature. Second, assessment tools are quite limited in their ability to capture much of the complexity and multidimensionality of both religiosity and spirituality. These general constructs likely act as distal variables with regard to their association with pain; thus, there is a need to explore the more specific proximal variables and mechanisms that mediate this relationship.

One attempt to capture this complexity has led to the differentiation between "positive R/S coping" and "negative R/S coping."[89] Positive R/S coping is described as collaborative problem-solving with God, helping others, and/or seeking support from the R/S community or a higher power. Negative R/S coping refers to an attitude characterized by deferring responsibility to God, feeling abandoned by God, or blaming God for difficulties. Making this distinction, the relationship between R/S and pain becomes somewhat clearer, as positive R/S coping is generally associated with positive pain outcomes, and negative R/S coping with negative ones. Positive versus negative R/S coping strategies can be compared with active and passive pain coping strategies. Active coping strategies reinforce a sense of self-efficacy, whereas passive ones reinforce overdependency and helplessness. Research has confirmed that active coping is associated with more positive outcomes, and passive coping with more negative ones. These findings suggest that R/S coping can be associated with either adaptive or maladaptive pain coping strategies. Thus, assessment of high levels of R/S by itself does not provide us with much information about whether individuals may be using R/S coping in a way that is beneficial or detrimental to their pain experience. It is important to go beyond simple quantitative assessment tools of R/S in order to attain a deeper qualitative-contextual understanding of R/S coping strategies used by a chronic pain sufferer.

Pain physicians, like most practitioners, are generally quite reluctant to address topics associated with R/S in clinical sessions. This is probably explained by various factors. First, there is a general sense that R/S represents personal/private matters with little relevance to a clinical assessment or treatment of a pain condition. Physicians may also be hesitant to elicit topics in a clinical session that tend to be associated with strong personal feelings and potential divergent beliefs and values between the patient and physician. This could, in the physician's mind, undermine the development of a positive therapeutic relationship. Moreover, physicians may feel the need to be cautious to prevent imposing their own personal values onto a patient. In the quest to maintain objectivity and remain "scientific" physicians may worry about potentially losing some objectivity in their clinical work. In addition, physicians may also have personal biases and prejudices regarding R/S coping representing a more primitive (i.e., less "scientific") and therefore less effective way of coping with pain. Any of these reasons will lead to a failure to adequately assess invaluable information about one of the most common coping strategies that chronic pain sufferers rely on.

Prioritizing the assessment of R/S beliefs and practices in coping with pain can provide physicians with invaluable information in the treatment of chronic pain conditions. These beliefs and practices can be regarded as cognitions and behavioral patterns associated with the pain that can be quite useful in CBT interventions. Discerning the adaptive or maladaptive use of R/S coping can also help physicians encourage or discourage any of these practices, when they do so supported by empirically based scientific rationale rather than personal values. Another important therapeutic aspect of R/S coping may be associated with the social/spiritual support provided by a religious community and/or higher power. There is also evidence that particular ritualized R/S practices, such as prayer and meditation, may have a positive therapeutic effect on pain management.[87,88] Possible explanations

TABLE 100-9 Practical Recommendations: *Employment*

- In general, work that is perceived as satisfying and without posing heavy physical demands is associated with a better prognosis for workers who have suffered a work-related injury.
- Jobs in which employers display a supportive attitude toward an injured worker, offering flexibility for modified work upon returning to work, and with high levels of worker autonomy will facilitate the process of recovering from an injury and returning to work as soon as possible.

TABLE 100-10 Practical Recommendations: *Religiosity/Spirituality*

- Religious/spiritual coping strategies can be beneficial in the management of chronic pain conditions, especially if they promote active coping.
- Physicians should assess the role of a patient's R/S beliefs and practices on his or her pain; adaptive R/S coping strategies should be encouraged, whereas maladaptive R/S coping should be discouraged, while displaying sensitivity to the patient's values.

for this positive effect may include a relaxation/stress-management effect, a distraction technique, promoting greater psychosomatic awareness, enhancing a sense of self-efficacy, and the direct analgesic effect of particular psycho-physiological mechanisms associated with these practices, among others. Further research that better captures the complexity and multidimensionality of R/S coping and explores the effects of variables that mediate its relationship with pain will help elucidate more specific ways in which R/S coping may be used and prescribed to enhance the treatment of chronic pain. In the meanwhile, assessing patients' R/S beliefs and practices in relation to coping with chronic pain and a careful examination of the particular effects, positive or negative, resulting from these coping strategies will allow physicians to either encourage or discourage such practices in the service of effective chronic pain management (**Table 100-10**).

REFERENCES

1. Wright LJ, Schur E, Noonan C, Ahumada S, Buchwald D, Afari N. Chronic pain, overweight, and obesity: findings from a community-based twin registry. *J Pain*. 2010;11(7):628-635.
2. Shiri R, Karppinen J, Leino-Arjas P, Solovieva S, Viikari-Juntura E. The association between obesity and low back pain: a meta-analysis. *Am J Epidemiol*. 2010;171(2):135-154.
3. Heuch I, Hagen K, Heuch I, Nygaard O, Zwart JA. The impact of body mass index on the prevalence of low back pain: the HUNT study. *Spine (Phila Pa 1976)*. 2010;35(7):764-768.
4. Heuch I, Heuch I, Hagen K, Zwart JA. Body mass index as a risk factor for developing chronic low back pain: a follow-up in the nord-trondelag health study. *Spine (Phila Pa 1976)*. 2013;38(2):133-139.
5. Butterworth PA, Landorf KB, Smith SE, Menz HB. The association between body mass index and musculoskeletal foot disorders: A systematic review. *Obes Rev*. 2012;13(7):630-642.
6. Andersen RE, Crespo CJ, Bartlett SJ, Bathon JM, Fontaine KR. Relationship between body weight gain and significant knee, hip, and back pain in older americans. *Obes Res*. 2003;11(10):1159-1162.
7. Stone AA, Broderick JE. Obesity and pain are associated in the United States. *Obesity (Silver Spring)*. 2012;20(7):1491-1495.
8. Caldwell J, Hart-Johnson T, Green CR. Body mass index and quality of life: examining blacks and whites with chronic pain. *J Pain*. 2009;10(1):60-67.
9. Jamison RN, Stetson B, Sbrocco T, Parris WC. Effects of significant weight gain on chronic pain patients. *Clin J Pain*. 1990;6(1):47-50.
10. Seaman DR. Body mass index and musculoskeletal pain: is there a connection? *Chiropr Man Therap*. 2013;21(1):15-709X-21-15.
11. Coggon D, Reading I, Croft P, McLaren M, Barrett D, Cooper C. Knee osteoarthritis and obesity. *Int J Obes Relat Metab Disord*. 2001;25(5):622-627.
12. Anandacoomarasamy A, Caterson I, Sambrook P, Fransen M, March L. The impact of obesity on the musculoskeletal system. *Int J Obes (Lond)*. 2008;32(2):211-222.
13. Rejeski WJ, Focht BC, Messier SP, Morgan T, Pahor M, Penninx B. Obese, older adults with knee osteoarthritis: weight loss, exercise, and quality of life. *Health Psychol*. 2002;21(5):419-426.
14. Shapiro JR, Anderson DA, Danoff-Burg S. A pilot study of the effects of behavioral weight loss treatment on fibromyalgia symptoms. *J Psychosom Res*. 2005;59(5):275-282.
15. Wai EK, Rodriguez S, Dagenais S, Hall H. Evidence-informed management of chronic low back pain with physical activity, smoking cessation, and weight loss. *Spine J*. 2008;8(1):195-202.
16. Hendrick P, Te Wake AM, Tikkisetty AS, Wulff L, Yap C, Milosavljevic S. The effectiveness of walking as an intervention for low back pain: a systematic review. *Eur Spine J*. 2010;19(10):1613-1620.
17. May S. Self-management of chronic low back pain and osteoarthritis. *Nat Rev Rheumatol*. 2010;6(4):199-209.
18. Tritilanunt T, Wajanavisit W. The efficacy of an aerobic exercise and health education program for treatment of chronic low back pain. *J Med Assoc Thai*. 2001;84 (Suppl 2):S528-S533.
19. Mannion AF, Muntener M, Taimela S, Dvorak J. Comparison of three active therapies for chronic low back pain: results of a randomized clinical trial with one-year follow-up. *Rheumatology (Oxford)*. 2001;40(7):772-778.
20. Jordan JL, Holden MA, Mason EE, Foster NE. Interventions to improve adherence to exercise for chronic musculoskeletal pain in adults. *Cochrane Database Syst Rev*. 2010;(1):CD005956. doi(1):CD005956.
21. Crandall S, Howlett S, Keysor JJ. Exercise adherence interventions for adults with chronic musculoskeletal pain. *Phys Ther*. 2013;93(1):17-21.
22. Bennell KL, Hinman RS. A review of the clinical evidence for exercise in osteoarthritis of the hip and knee. *J Sci Med Sport*. 2011;14(1):4-9.
23. Andrews NE, Strong J, Meredith PJ. Activity pacing, avoidance, endurance, and associations with patient functioning in chronic pain: a systematic review and meta-analysis. *Arch Phys Med Rehabil*. 2012;93(11):2109-2121.e7.
24. Zhang R, Naughton DP. Vitamin D in health and disease: current perspectives. *Nutr J*. 2010;9:65-2891-9-65.
25. Bell RF, Borzan J, Kalso E, Simonnet G. Food, pain, and drugs: does it matter what pain patients eat? *Pain*. 2012;153(10):1993-1996.
26. Rosen CJ, Adams JS, Bikle DD, et al. The nonskeletal effects of vitamin D: an endocrine society scientific statement. *Endocr Rev*. 2012;33(3):456-492.
27. Nieves JW. Skeletal effects of nutrients and nutraceuticals, beyond calcium and vitamin D. *Osteoporos Int*. 2013;24(3):771-786.
28. Vandenkerkhof EG, Macdonald HM, Jones GT, Power C, Macfarlane GJ. Diet, lifestyle and chronic widespread pain: results from the 1958 British birth cohort study. *Pain Res Manag*. 2011;16(2):87-92.
29. Arvold DS, Odean MJ, Dornfeld MP, et al. Correlation of symptoms with vitamin D deficiency and symptom response to cholecalciferol treatment: a randomized controlled trial. *Endocr Pract*. 2009;15(3):203-212.
30. Grove O, Halver B. Relief of osteoporotic backache with fluoride, calcium, and calciferol. *Acta Med Scand*. 1981;209(6):469-471.
31. Institute of Medicine of the National Academies. Available at: http://www.iom.edu/Reports/2010/Dietary-Reference-Intakes-for-calcium-and-vitamin-D.aspx. Accessed August 19, 2013.
32. Goldberg RJ, Katz J. A meta-analysis of the analgesic effects of omega-3 polyunsaturated fatty acid supplementation for inflammatory joint pain. *Pain*. 2007;129(1-2):210-223.
33. Tokuyama S, Nakamoto K. Unsaturated fatty acids and pain. *Biol Pharm Bull*. 2011;34(8):1174-1178.
34. Goldenberg DL, Clauw DJ, Fitzcharles MA. New concepts in pain research and pain management of the rheumatic diseases. *Semin Arthritis Rheum*. 2011;41(3):319-334.

35. Gregory PJ, Sperry M, Wilson AF. Dietary supplements for osteoarthritis. *Am Fam Physician*. 2008;77(2):177-184.
36. Parkes GC, Sanderson JD, Whelan K. Treating irriBox bowel syndrome with probiotics: The evidence. *Proc Nutr Soc*. 2010;69(2):187-194.
37. Whelan K, Quigley EM. Probiotics in the management of irriBox bowel syndrome and inflammatory bowel disease. *Curr Opin Gastroenterol*. 2013;29(2):184-189.
38. Anastasi JK, Capili B, Chang M. Managing irriBox bowel syndrome. *Am J Nurs*. 2013;113(7):42-52.
39. Gagnier JJ, van Tulder MW, Berman B, Bombardier C. Herbal medicine for low back pain: a Cochrane review. *Spine (Phila Pa 1976)*. 2007;32(1):82-92.
40. Aggarwal BB, Sundaram C, Malani N, Ichikawa H. Curcumin: the indian solid gold. *Adv Exp Med Biol*. 2007;595:1-75.
41. Bernstein C, McArdle E. *The Migraine Brain: Your Breakthrough Guide to Fewer Headaches, Better Health*. Free Press, NY, New York; 2008.
42. www.cnpp.usda.gov/MyPlate. Accessed May, 2015.
43. Sawynok J. Caffeine and pain. *Pain*. 2011;152(4):726-729.
44. Peroutka SJ, Lyon JA, Swarbrick J, Lipton RB, Kolodner K, Goldstein J. Efficacy of diclofenac sodium softgel 100 mg with or without caffeine 100 mg in migraine without aura: a randomized, double-blind, crossover study. *Headache*. 2004;44(2):136-141.
45. Diamond S, Balm TK, Freitag FG. Ibuprofen plus caffeine in the treatment of tension-type headache. *Clin Pharmacol Ther*. 2000;68(3):312-319.
46. Zhang WY. A benefit-risk assessment of caffeine as an analgesic adjuvant. *Drug Saf*. 2001;24(15):1127-1142.
47. Mercadante S, Serretta R, Casuccio A. Effects of caffeine as an adjuvant to morphine in advanced cancer patients. a randomized, double-blind, placebo-controlled, crossover study. *J Pain Symptom Manage*. 2001;21(5):369-372.
48. Renner B, Clarke G, Grattan T, et al. Caffeine accelerates absorption and enhances the analgesic effect of acetaminophen. *J Clin Pharmacol*. 2007;47(6):715-726.
49. Tavares C, Sakata RK. Caffeine in the treatment of pain. *Rev Bras Anestesiol*. 2012;62(3):387-401.
50. Centers for Disease Control: Smoking and Tobacco Use. Available at: http://www.cdc.gov/tobacco/data_statistics/fact_sheets/fast_facts/. Accessed August 19, 2013.
51. Ditre JW, Brandon TH, Zale EL, Meagher MM. Pain, nicotine, and smoking: research findings and mechanistic considerations. *Psychol Bull*. 2011;137(6):1065-1093.
52. Shi Y, Hooten WM, Warner DO. Effects of smoking cessation on pain in older adults. *Nicotine Tob Res*. 2011;13(10):919-925.
53. Weingarten TN, Shi Y, Mantilla CB, Hooten WM, Warner DO. Smoking and chronic pain: a real-but-puzzling relationship. *Minn Med*. 2011;94(3):35-37.
54. Palmer KT, Syddall H, Cooper C, Coggon D. Smoking and musculoskeletal disorders: findings from a British national survey. *Ann Rheum Dis*. 2003;62(1):33-36.
55. Mitchell MD, Mannino DM, Steinke DT, Kryscio RJ, Bush HM, Crofford LJ. Association of smoking and chronic pain syndromes in Kentucky women. *J Pain*. 2011;12(8):892-899.
56. Pisinger C, Aadahl M, Toft U, Birke H, Zytphen-Adeler J, Jorgensen T. The association between active and passive smoking and frequent pain in a general population. *Eur J Pain*. 2011;15(1):77-83.
57. Ferreira PH, Beckenkamp P, Maher CG, Hopper JL, Ferreira ML. Nature or nurture in low back pain? Results of a systematic review of studies based on twin samples. *Eur J Pain*. 2013;17(7):957-971.
58. Thelin Bronner KB, Wennberg P, Kallmen H, Schult ML. Alcohol habits in patients with long-term musculoskeletal pain: comparison with a matched control group from the general population. *Int J Rehabil Res*. 2012;35(2):130-137.
59. Ekholm O, Gronbaek M, Peuckmann V, Sjogren P. Alcohol and smoking behavior in chronic pain patients: the role of opioids. *Eur J Pain*. 2009;13(6):606-612.
60. Rashiq S, Dick BD. Factors associated with chronic noncancer pain in the Canadian population. *Pain Res Manag*. 2009;14(6):454-460.
61. Stewart SH, Finn PR, Pihl RO. A dose-response study of the effects of alcohol on the perceptions of pain and discomfort due to electric shock in men at high familial-genetic risk for alcoholism. *Psychopharmacology (Berl)*. 1995;119(3):261-267.
62. Egli M, Koob GF, Edwards S. Alcohol dependence as a chronic pain disorder. *Neurosci Biobehav Rev*. 2012;36(10):2179-2192.
63. Lawton J, Simpson J. Predictors of alcohol use among people experiencing chronic pain. *Psychol Health Med*. 2009;14(4):487-501.
64. Ong JC, Park M. Chronic headaches and insomnia: working toward a biobehavioral model. *Cephalalgia*. 2012;32(14):1059-1070.
65. Barloese M, Jennum P, Knudsen S, Jensen R. Cluster headache and sleep, is there a connection? A review. *Cephalalgia*. 2012;32(6):481-491.
66. Artner J, Cakir B, Spiekermann JA, et al. Prevalence of sleep deprivation in patients with chronic neck and back pain: a retrospective evaluation of 1016 patients. *J Pain Res*. 2013;6:1-6.
67. Lee YC, Lu B, Edwards RR, et al. The role of sleep problems in central pain processing in rheumatoid arthritis. *Arthritis Rheum*. 2013;65(1):59-68.
68. Prados G, Miro E. Fibromyalgia and sleep: A review. *Rev Neurol*. 2012;54(4):227-240.
69. Schuh-Hofer S, Wodarski R, Pfau DB, et al. One night of total sleep deprivation promotes a state of generalized hyperalgesia: a surrogate pain model to study the relationship of insomnia and pain. *Pain*. 2013;154(9):1613-1621.
70. Odegard SS, Sand T, Engstrom M, Stovner LJ, Zwart JA, Hagen K. The long-term effect of insomnia on primary headaches: a prospective population-based cohort study (HUNT-2 and HUNT-3). *Headache*. 2011;51(4):570-580.
71. Bahouq H, Allali F, Rkain H, Hmamouchi I, Hajjaj-Hassouni N. Prevalence and severity of insomnia in chronic low back pain patients. *Rheumatol Int*. 2013;33(5):1277-1281.
72. Okifuji A, Donaldson GW, Barck L, Fine PG. Relationship between fibromyalgia and obesity in pain, function, mood, and sleep. *J Pain*. 2010;11(12):1329-1337.
73. Ranjbaran Z, Keefer L, Stepanski E, Farhadi A, Keshavarzian A. The relevance of sleep abnormalities to chronic inflammatory conditions. *Inflamm Res*. 2007;56(2):51-57.
74. Hajak G. CS03-02 - Sleep and chronic pain. *Eur Psychiatry*. 2011;26, Suppl 1(0):1775.
75. Lopez-Martinez AE, Esteve-Zarazaga R, Ramirez-Maestre C. Perceived social support and coping responses are independent variables explaining pain adjustment among chronic pain patients. *J Pain*. 2008;9(4):373-379.
76. Carr JL, Moffett JA. The impact of social deprivation on chronic back pain outcomes. *Chronic Illn*. 2005;1(2):121-129.
77. Steenstra IA, Verbeek JH, Heymans MW, Bongers PM. Prognostic factors for duration of sick leave in patients sick listed with acute low back pain: a systematic review of the literature. *Occup Environ Med*. 2005;62(12):851-860.
78. Taylor SS, Davis MC, Zautra AJ. Relationship status and quality moderate daily pain-related changes in physical disability, affect, and cognitions in women with chronic pain. *Pain*. 2013;154(1):147-153.

79. Reese JB, Somers TJ, Keefe FJ, Mosley-Williams A, Lumley MA. Pain and functioning of rheumatoid arthritis patients based on marital status: is a distressed marriage preferable to no marriage? *J Pain.* 2010;11(10):958-964.

80. Jensen MP, Moore MR, Bockow TB, Ehde DM, Engel JM. Psychosocial factors and adjustment to chronic pain in persons with physical disabilities: a systematic review. *Arch Phys Med Rehabil.* 2011;92(1):146-160.

81. Keefe FJ, Porter L, Somers T, Shelby R, Wren AV. Psychosocial interventions for managing pain in older adults: outcomes and clinical implications. *Br J Anaesth.* 2013;111(1):89-94.

82. Cano A, Barterian JA, Heller JB. Empathic and nonempathic interaction in chronic pain couples. *Clin J Pain.* 2008;24(8):678-684.

83. Bigos SJ, Battie MC, Spengler DM, et al. A prospective study of work perceptions and psychosocial factors affecting the report of back injury. *Spine (Phila Pa 1976).* 1991;16(1):1-6.

84. Teasell RW, Bombardier C. Employment-related factors in chronic pain and chronic pain disability. *Clin J Pain.* 2001;17(4 Suppl):S39-45.

85. Crook J, Moldofsky H, Shannon H. Determinants of disability after a work related musculoskeletal injury. *J Rheumatol.* 1998;25(8): 1570-1577.

86. Wachholtz AB, Pearce MJ. Does spirituality as a coping mechanism help or hinder coping with chronic pain? *Curr Pain Headache Rep.* 2009;13(2):127-132.

87. Rippentrop AE. A review of the role of religion and spirituality in chronic pain populations. *Rehabili Psychol.* 2005;50(3):278-284.

88. Koenig HG. Religion and medicine IV: Religion, physical health, and clinical implications. *Int J Psychiatry Med.* 2001;31(3):321-336.

89. Wachholtz AB, Pearce MJ, Koenig H. Exploring the relationship between spirituality, coping, and pain. *J Behav Med.* 2007;30(4):311-318.

PART 7

Pain, Administration, and the Law

SECTION A

Pain Practice

Setting Up a Pain Treatment Facility

Steven D. Waldman

INTRODUCTION

Over the past several years, there has been considerable interest in expanding the role of the pain management specialist as an integral member of the health care team. This interest has been stimulated in part by the increased availability of health care professionals with a special interest and advanced training in pain medicine, in part by the increasing societal awareness that undertreated and untreated pain have reached epidemic proportions, and in part by the unprecedented economic pressures of our rapidly evolving health care system. These economic pressures have forced many pain management specialists and hospitals to explore new avenues of revenue generation and to examine new strategies to help improve the efficiency and cost-effectiveness of the care they provide.

The purpose of this chapter is to serve as a guide for pain management specialists who may be considering setting up a pain treatment center or expanding the scope of services currently offered. Although many of the concepts presented are basic, failure to take them into consideration may lead to high levels of professional frustration and dissatisfaction, damage to the professional image of the pain management specialist, economic loss, and increased exposure to malpractice liability.

BASIC CONSIDERATIONS

SHOULD PAIN MANAGEMENT SERVICES BE OFFERED?

There is no question that there is a huge demand for quality pain management services. The 2011 Institute of Medicine report titled *Relieving Pain in America—A Blueprint for Transforming Prevention, Care, Education and Research* found that approximately 100 million American adults are affected by chronic pain.[1] This is more than the total number of American adults affected by cancer, heart disease, and diabetes combined.[2] The report estimated that the cost of the pain to the United States is more than $635 billion each year and is rising as Baby Boomers age. A recent study of pain patients in America by the National Center for Health Statistics revealed the four most common types of pain complaints are low back pain, headache, neck pain, and facial pain[3] (**Fig. 101-1**).

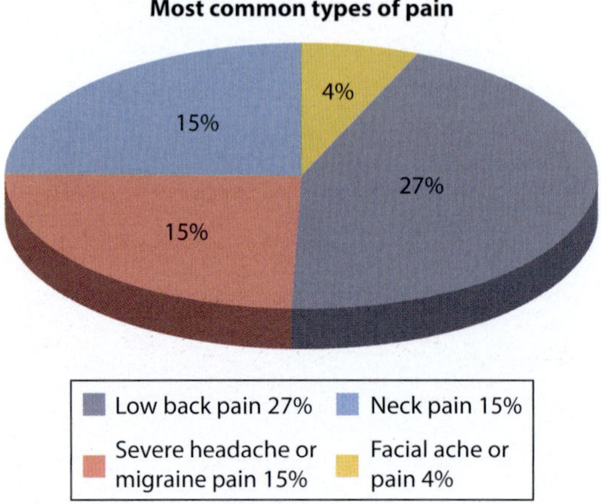

FIGURE 101-1. Most common types of pain.

In recognition of the pain epidemic the 2010 Patient Protection and Affordable Care Act requires that the Department of health and Human Services in partnership with the Institute of Medicine provide a comprehensive assessment of the science surrounding pain, care, research, and education and provide specific recommendations to improve performance in each of these areas.

From these data, it is obvious that there are a huge number of patients who could potentially benefit from quality pain management services.

INTERFACING PAIN MANAGEMENT SERVICES WITH EXISTING SERVICES

The first question that must be asked when considering the implementation or addition of new pain management services is how the addition of those new services will interface with existing professional activities. One must take into account the impact of such new services on existing care. The addition or expansion of pain management services requires a high level of commitment from *all* members of the health care team. Even if additional professional staff is added to provide pain management services, consideration must be given to such issues as call responsibilities, vacation coverage, and so forth.

As with all health care endeavors, there must be sufficient expertise to provide an ongoing level of quality care. One would not implement an open heart surgery program or start a burn unit without adequate expertise or additional training. Pain management requires the same level of training, expertise, and commitment. In addition to the clinical expertise required to provide quality pain management services, there must be administrative expertise if the endeavor is to be economically viable. This is especially important when setting up a pain treatment facility under the managed care paradigm and the new Affordable Care Act.[4,5]

ARE THERE ADEQUATE PERSONNEL TO PROVIDE QUALITY CARE?

When setting up a pain treatment facility, it is important that the pain management specialist recognize the high level of commitment in terms of the time and energy essential to providing quality pain management services. For this reason, the pain management specialist must ensure that there are adequate personnel to provide high-quality coverage for any new services that are contemplated or to cover the expansion of existing services.

There is a common misconception that pain management can be done at the convenience of the pain management specialist. This is simply not the case. This approach can only lead to high levels of dissatisfaction from both patients and referring physicians. Today's patient, or what has become affectionately known as today's "health care consumer," is unwilling to wait for extended periods in order to receive care. During the implementation of a new pain management facility or an expansion of an existing one, a realistic appraisal of the time required to provide the proposed care must be undertaken to assure the provision of care in a timely manner. Just as there must be an adequate number of health care professionals to provide high-quality pain management services, there must also be a high level of motivation in order for the pain facility to ultimately succeed.[6] All members of the health care team must be committed to quality and compassionate provision of pain management services. A lone pain management specialist, no matter how motivated and caring, can do little to make up for the disinterest and lack of support of the remainder of the pain management team. This statement applies not only to the clinical personnel but to the administrative personnel as well. A failure to adequately supervise midlevel providers can also lead to medical misadventures and high levels of patient dissatisfaction.[7]

IS THE SUPPORT STAFF ADEQUATE?

In setting up a pain treatment facility, care must be taken to be sure that the practice infrastructure is adequate to support a busy and growing pain management service. If the pain management specialist's existing billing office is unable to keep up with the volume of work generated from existing activities, the addition of billings from new or expanded pain management service may throw the entire office into disarray and adversely affect cash flow. Obviously, additional help can be added to alleviate this situation, but this should be done in a prophylactic manner.[8]

SERVICES OFFERED

Before setting up a new pain treatment facility, the first decision that needs to be made is which specific services (e.g., evaluation, neural blockade, drug management and detoxification) should be offered. To adequately delineate these services, the pain management specialist must take into account his or her existing expertise, experience, and preferences as well as those of other health care professionals providing pain management services within the group practice. The availability of support services such as physical therapy, occupational therapy, psychiatry, and radiology support services (e.g., computed tomography scanning, magnetic resonance imaging, ultrasound, and biplanar fluoroscopy) must also be considered.[9] Under the managed care paradigm, some services may not be reimbursed at levels adequate to justify their use from a purely economic viewpoint.

It is important to clearly define to patients as well as referring physicians what a new pain treatment facility can and cannot offer. Too often a pain management specialist with limited experience and training tries to hold him- or herself out as a specialist in all areas of pain management. This not only is academically dishonest but often leads to high levels of patient and referring physician dissatisfaction.[5] It may also place the pain management specialist, and those with whom he or she practices, in a potentially serious medicolegal situation. Services should not be advertised that are not available or cannot be provided with sufficient expertise to keep complications to a minimum.

TYPES OF PATIENTS SEEN

The second decision that needs to be made is delineating the types of patients that the pain management specialist believes are appropriate for the scope of pain management services he or she has chosen to offer at the new facility. The pain management specialist should determine if he or she is comfortable treating cancer pain, headache and facial pain, chemical-dependent problems, acute and postoperative pain, and so forth. As the enthusiasm for the prescribing of opioids for chronic nonmalignant pain wanes, a clear plan as to whether opioids will be prescribed in this clinical setting needs to be clearly defined.[10] The pain management specialist must also determine whether he or she will accept patients who are involved in workers' compensation claims and patients who are involved in litigation. Third, the pain management specialist must decide whether he or she will accept self-referred patients or if he or she will require patients to be evaluated and then referred by another physician (see section on physician referral). Finally, the pain management specialist will also have to decide whether he or she will accept primary responsibility for patients who are admitted to the hospital. This decision has specific implications that must be carefully thought out from a quality-of-care viewpoint because some pain management specialists may be incapable or unwilling to deal with the various medical problems that may occur while a patient is hospitalized under their care. Political issues as to the appropriateness of a pain management specialist providing primary care may also have to be addressed.[11,12]

FINANCIAL CONSIDERATIONS

The following issues must be handled according to each pain management specialist's existing financial situation, current policies, and prior contractual agreements with the hospital or third-party carriers, as well as his or her own philosophical and ethical viewpoints on providing indigent care.[13,14] To ignore these variables when starting a pain treatment facility is to ensure economic disaster.

For the pain management service to remain on a strong economic footing in this period of ever-decreasing revenues, financial considerations must be carefully considered.[8] Some pain management specialists have chosen to provide pain management services on a cash-only basis. Although this may work in some affluent communities, by and large, in view of the high cost of many of the modalities offered, this represents an impractical approach for most pain management specialists.

A decision must be made as to the desirability of accepting Medicare assignment as well as other third-party assignments of insurance benefits. Participation in managed care plans should also be carefully weighed.[4] It should be remembered that midlevel providers may be paid at lower levels than physicians, yet these midlevel providers are held to the same standards insofar as fraud and abuse issues are concerned.[15] Obviously, local factors have to dictate the variables to be taken into account in making this decision. The pain management specialist must also decide what provisions will be made for the indigent patient who has Medicaid or who is solely responsible for the payment of his or her health care costs. The pain management specialist is likely to be approached by attorneys who want care to be rendered on a contingency basis. The economic impact of these decisions cannot be overstated.

AVAILABILITY

It has been said that there are three "As" of a successful practice of pain management: ability, amiability, and availability. Obviously, from a patient-care viewpoint, ability is the most important issue. From a practice management viewpoint, however, there is no question that availability is the most important. When starting a pain treatment center, it is imperative that the clinical and administrative staff all agree on the appropriate levels of availability if the facility is to succeed. Most patients expect to see the same physician at each visit, and this fact has a specific impact on call schedule issues (e.g., days off after call, vacation scheduling, afternoons off). If *all* members of the pain management care team are not motivated to facilitate the provision of quality pain management services, it is impossible for a single member of the team to make the pain management service successful. This statement also applies to the midlevel providers and administrative staff. If the administrative staff refuses to work in additional patients or limits the hours of operation of the pain treatment facility, adverse economic consequences will often result.

Additional issues that need to be determined when setting up a pain treatment facility include the hours of operation for the pain management center. The availability of evening hours has become increasingly important and is increasingly expected by health care consumers in today's competitive market. Weekend coverage and holiday coverage must be also clearly defined for both patients and referring physicians. Expectations of the pain management specialist who is covering these periods should also be delineated to avoid friction between members of a group pain management practice and to assure appropriate availability from all members of the pain management care team. A clear protocol for how emergency referrals will be handled is mandatory in order to assure quality, compassionate care with a high level of satisfaction for both the patient and the referring physician.

How patient phone calls are handled will also have an impact on the ultimate success of the pain management specialist. Calls from referring physicians, the pharmacy, and patients, as well as support services, including laboratory, radiology, physical therapy, and occupational therapy, are the rule rather than the exception. Again, it must be clearly defined how these calls will be handled by all members of the pain management care team in order to provide consistent, quality care and avoid lost revenues through missed consults or unavailability. The use of answering machines and voice mail as a way to avoid dealing with patients and referring physicians is to be avoided and may require careful monitoring by the pain treatment facility management team.

Coupled with the need for the prompt returning of phone calls is the timeliness with which outpatient appointments and inpatient consultations are handled.[16,17] Although specific times may vary from community to community, seeing inpatient consults (other than emergencies) within 24 hours of being called works well in most situations. Any consult requested on an emergency basis should be seen as soon as possible. Seeing all routine consults that are received before 4:00 PM on the same day (this includes Saturdays, Sundays, and holidays) projects a strong message that the pain patient will not suffer needlessly while waiting for pain management service to be implemented. The same reasoning applies to the availability of outpatient consultation. When setting up a pain treatment facility, immediate appointments should be available on a same-day basis for patients with acute pain problems and pain emergencies.[18] Such appointments should allow appropriate screening and triage for such patients without disrupting the flow of previously scheduled patients.

This approach also makes good sense from a time management viewpoint. As the pain treatment facility grows busier, if inpatient and outpatient consultations are put off, a large backlog of patients waiting to be seen may result. Given the competitive nature of pain management services in most geographic areas, such delays will result in significant lost revenues and high levels of patient and referring physician dissatisfaction.

SUPPORT STAFF AVAILABILITY

Closely related to the issue of physician availability is the issue of support staff availability. How consultations and phone messages for the pain management service are to be handled is of paramount importance to the ultimate success of the pain practitioner. In many hospital-based pain treatment facilities, all scheduling activities have been made the responsibility of the hospital secretarial staff. Often this simply does not work, both in terms of efficiency as well as motivation, when applied to the pain management service. The hospital employee may not be willing or able to provide prompt and courteous handling of phone calls from referring physicians as well as patients. Messages may get misplaced or lost. Generally, the 7:00 AM to 3:30 PM staffing patterns of the hospital do not meet the needs of the referring physician, who is often in his or her office until 5:00 or 5:30 at night. For this reason, it is desirable as well as cost-effective to hire a high-quality secretary whose prime responsibilities are the administrative aspects of the pain management service. The use of 12-hour shifts may have some advantages.[19] This will ensure that the phone is answered courteously and promptly, phone messages are handled appropriately, patient records are readily available, and there is an appropriate level of motivation to work in add-on and emergency patients.

The pain management support staff must be available during regular clinic hours. The overuse of an answering machine and voice mail is strongly discouraged because most busy referring physicians are unwilling to make several calls trying to reach the pain management physician to discuss or schedule a patient. Provisions for phone coverage during lunch and break periods by the pain management support staff is mandatory.

PHYSICIAN-REFERRED VERSUS SELF-REFERRED PATIENTS

Pain management specialists have traditionally thought that physician-referred patients are desirable. In fact, many practitioners will not accept self-referred patients. There are distinct advantages and disadvantages to this philosophical viewpoint, as outlined in **Tables 101-1** and **101-2**.

The physician-referred patient *may* be appropriately worked up and carry a correct diagnosis. Conversely, the pain specialist has limited control over the appropriateness and quality of the evaluation and treatment of the physician-referred patient. The patient may be inadequately or inappropriately evaluated, which puts tremendous medicolegal responsibilities on the pain management physician to complete the evaluation. These problems can be magnified under the managed care paradigm because the managed care plan may want to save money by limiting diagnostic testing. Furthermore, the patient referral may not be appropriate for the services and expertise available at the pain treatment facility chosen by the referring physician or managed care plan.

Advantages of the self-referred patient include pain management specialist control over the evaluation and treatment and the choice of consultants needed to help him or her make the diagnosis; these consultants may be of a higher quality than those used by some referring physicians. The pain management specialist has control over treatment and the use of prescription medication (especially controlled substances) when providing care for self-referred patients. Furthermore, the pain management specialist may exercise a choice in diagnostic imaging facilities or for hospitals if admission for further evaluation is necessary. As an increasing number of patients under managed care have out-of-network or point-of-service benefits as part of their managed care contracts, such patients can choose the pain management

TABLE 101-1 Physician-Referred Patients

Advantages
1. The patient *may* be appropriately worked up.
2. The patient's condition *may* be appropriately diagnosed.
3. The patient *may* be familiar with pain management services and the reason he or she has been sent to the pain center.
4. The referral *may* be appropriate for the services and expertise of the pain center.
5. Patient acquisition is low cost relative to advertising for self-referred patients.
Disadvantages
1. The pain specialist has limited control over the appropriateness of the evaluation and treatment.
2. The patient may be inadequately worked up, which puts tremendous medicolegal responsibilities on the pain management physician to complete the evaluation.
3. The patient may be sent to the pain management specialist carrying the wrong diagnosis.
4. The patient may be an inappropriate referral to the pain clinic relative to the services being offered.
5. The pain management physician may inherit a patient who has been inappropriately treated by a referring physician and assume significant medical liability if he or she continues this treatment.

TABLE 101-2 Self-Referred Patients

Advantages
1. The pain management specialist may control the evaluation and treatment.
2. The pain management specialist may choose consultants needed to help him or her make the diagnosis who are of a higher quality than those chosen by the referring physician.
3. The pain management specialist has control over treatment and the use of prescription medication (especially controlled substances).
4. The pain management physician may exercise a choice in diagnostic imaging facilities or for hospitals if admission for further evaluation is necessary.
Disadvantages
1. The pain management specialist has sole responsibility for the evaluation and treatment.
2. The pain management specialist assumes the role of primary care physician.
3. When the patient is under the care of pain management specialist, transfer of the patient to a more appropriate specialist may be difficult if a problem arises.
4. Cost of patient acquisition is high relative to physician-referred patients if advertising is used.

physician or pain treatment facility despite the dictates of the managed care plan.[20,21] Such patients can represent a significant source of revenue for a pain treatment facility, and care should be taken to identify patients with such benefits before assuming they cannot be seen at a pain treatment facility.

Disadvantages of self-referred patients include the fact that the pain management specialist and pain treatment facility have sole responsibility for the evaluation and treatment, essentially assuming the role of primary care physician. After the patient is under the care of the pain management specialist and facility, transfer of the patient to a more appropriate specialist or facility may be difficult if a problem arises.

The pain management specialist and the pain treatment facility must weigh these variables to determine the best course to follow. If a pain management specialist decides to accept self-referred patients, he or she must recognize that in essence, he or she is assuming the role of primary care physician. Inherent in this role is an increase in responsibility with its attendant nighttime phone calls, emergencies, talking with family members, and so forth. Regardless of the pain management specialist's ultimate decision, it is the author's strong belief that a physician-referred patient requires the same level of vigilance and quality of evaluation that a self-referred patient does, especially under the managed care paradigm.

HOSPITAL-BASED VERSUS FREE-STANDING FACILITIES

As hospital administrators, government, managed care plans, and third-party payers seek to exert greater control over hospital-based physicians, pain management specialists have sought to limit their vulnerability to this situation (e.g., the opening of surgical centers, affiliating with rehabilitation centers).[22] An additional option is the development of a free-standing pain treatment facility. By developing such a facility, the pain management specialist may avoid the "label" associated with a given hospital. This can be good or bad depending on the public perception of a specific hospital. It should be remembered that these perceptions can change over time, and what may be a desirable hospital to practice in at one point may represent a negative practice location at another.

An additional advantage of starting a free-standing pain treatment facility is that the pain management specialist may choose its geographic location. This is advantageous if the pain management specialist's primary hospital practice is located at a less desirable geographic area of the city.[23] A free-standing pain treatment facility can use advertising to great advantage when seeking to increase market penetration at a new geographic location.[24]

In some localities, it is possible for the pain management specialist to bill not only for his or her professional fees but also for the drugs, trays, radiology services, laboratory services, and block room and recovery room charges. Some third-party carriers in specific geographic locations in the United States (e.g., the East Coast) allow a pain management specialist to charge 150% of his or her professional fee to cover the cost of drugs, trays, and room charges. In other areas, local or state law as well as policies of the third-party carriers may require that the facility be licensed and accredited as an ambulatory surgery center in order for a facility fee to be paid. At the time of this writing, Medicare is considering paying pain management physicians a higher professional fee if they provide care in an office setting rather than an ambulatory surgical center or hospital-based pain treatment facility. This may lead to a shift in where pain management services are provided in the future.

In the free-standing pain treatment facility, the pain management specialist will have greater control of the space, staffing, hours of operation, capital expenditures, and utilization review–quality assurance activities. Obviously, with this added control and flexibility, there comes an added measure of responsibility and risk.[25]

The major disadvantage of a free-standing pain treatment facility is cost. The pain management specialist can anticipate a large capital expenditure to provide adequate space, equipment, and personnel to implement pain management services at a free-standing location. In addition, the pain management specialist assumes the added liability and cost of malpractice insurance of the facility as well as the liability for professional services offered. The pain management specialist also inherits the liability for the actions of his or her staff. The advantages and disadvantages of a hospital-based pain management practice versus a free-standing pain center are summarized in **Tables 101-3** and **101-4**.

TABLE 101-3 Hospital-Based Pain Center

Advantages
1. The rent is free.
2. The personnel are free.
3. The equipment is free.
4. There is high visibility to referring physicians.
5. There is a high level of convenience for inpatients.
6. There is excellent emergency support if problems arise.
7. There is high-technology equipment readily available.
8. Support services (e.g., physical therapy, occupational therapy) are available.
Disadvantages
1. There may be a lack of adequate designated space.
2. The pain management specialist does not have control of staffing.
3. The hospital administration may be very unwilling to provide the capital expenditure necessary to provide appropriate diagnostic and therapeutic equipment.
4. If the hospital develops a negative perception in the community, this will be carried over to the pain management services.
5. The pain management specialist will be subject to hospital utilization review and quality assurance activities.
6. The pain management specialist is subject to medical staff rules that may limit his or her ability to use operating room facilities, admit patients, and so on.
7. The pain management specialist receives no portion of the revenues from the facility, laboratory, radiology, and support service fees generated.

TABLE 101-4 Free-Standing Pain Centers

Advantages
1. The pain management specialist can avoid the "label" of a specific hospital.
2. The pain management specialist can choose the location of the free-standing pain center.
3. The pain management specialist may bill for drugs, trays, radiology services, laboratory services, and block room and recovery charges.
4. The pain management specialist can control the space, staffing, hours of operation, capital expenditures, and utilization review–quality assurance activities.
Disadvantages
1. Cost
2. The pain management specialist assumes the added liability of the facility.
3. The pain management specialist assumes the added liability of the staff.
4. There is not a built-in referral source of patients.
5. There is no backup for emergencies.
6. There may not be high-technology equipment available to perform some procedures.

SUMMARY

Starting a pain treatment facility is a significant undertaking in terms of time as well as tangible expense. Although the risks are great, so can be the rewards if it is done properly. By addressing the previously mentioned issues as an integral part of the planning process, the pain management specialist will be better able to determine if setting up a pain treatment facility is the right decision.

REFERENCES

1. Institute of Medicine Report from the Committee on Advancing Pain Research, Care, and Education: *Relieving Pain in America, A Blueprint for Transforming Prevention, Care, Education and Research*. The National Academies Press; 2011.
2. Heart Disease and Stroke Statistics—2011 Update: A report from the American Heart Association. *Circulation*. 2011;123:e18-e209:20.
3. National Center for Health Statistics. Health, United States, 2014: With Special Feature on Adults Aged 55–64. Hyattsville, Maryland. 2015.
4. Waldman SD. Joining a managed care plan: a guide to the pain management specialist. *Am J Pain Manage*. 1992;2:215-218.
5. Smith MJ. Accountable disease management of spine pain. *Spine J*. 2011;11(9):807-815.
6. Waldman SD. Motivating the pain center employee. *Am J Pain Manage*. 1993;3:114-117.
7. Benedict DG. Walking the tightrope: chronic pain and substance abuse. *J Nurse Practitioners*. 2008;4(8):604-609.
8. Waldman SD. Hiring employees for the pain center. *Am J Pain Manage*. 1992;2:164-166.
9. Curatolo M, Eichenberger U. Ultrasound in interventional pain management. *Eur J Pain Suppl*. 2008;2(1):78-83.
10. Watson CPN. Chronic non-cancer pain and the long-term efficacy and safety of opioids: Some blind men and an elephant? *Scand J Pain*. 2012;3(1):5-13.
11. Waldman SD. The antitrust implications of medical staff credentialing—part I. *Am J Pain Manage*. 1997;7:22-27.
12. Waldman SD. The antitrust implications of medical staff credentialing—part II. *Am J Pain Manage*. 1997;7:66-69.
13. Crawley J. Chronic pain experiences described by African-American indigent adults. *Pain Management Nursing*. June 2011;12(2):e11.
14. Head B. Just give me hope: Lived experiences of Medicaid patients with advanced cancer (725). *J Pain Symptom Manage*. 2011;41(1):287.
15. DiSantostefano J. Medicare fraud and abuse issues. *J Nurse Practitioners*. January 2013;9(1):61-63.
16. Concato J, Feinstein AR. Asking patients what they like: overlooked attributes of patient satisfaction with primary care. *Am J Med*. April 1997;102(4):399-406.
17. Vermeulen IB, Bohte SM, Elkhuizen SG, et al. Adaptive resource allocation for efficient patient scheduling. *Artif Intell Med*. 2009;46(1):67-80.
18. Qu X, Shi J. Modeling the effect of patient choice on the performance of open access scheduling. *Int J Prod Econom*. 2011;129(2):314-327.
19. Ferguson SA, Dawson D. 12-h or 8-h shifts? It depends. *Sleep Med Rev*. 2012;16(6):519-528.
20. Waldman SD. Any willing provider laws—paradox or panacea. Part I. *Am J Pain Manage*. 1996;6:54-61.
21. Waldman SD. Any willing provider laws—paradox or panacea. Part II. *Am J Pain Manage*. 1996;6:93-96.
22. Waldman SD, Ford NA. Selling your medical practice–Part I. *Am J Pain Manage*. 1998;8:23-28.
23. Waldman SD, Ford NA. Selling your medical practice–Part II. *Am J Pain Manage*. 1998;8:53-60.
24. Waldman SD. Advertising pain management services. *Am J Pain Manage*. 1993;196-200.
25. Waldman SD. Total quality management for the pain center—an idea whose time has come. *Am J Pain Manage*. 1993;3:38-41.

CHAPTER 102 How to Manage a Pain Practice

Edgar L. Ross

INTRODUCTION

A well-managed pain management center is more than an economically successful pain clinic; it also provides high-quality multidisciplinary care that meets the changing needs of today's health care environment. Health care is in the initial stages of what is likely to be unprecedented change induced by unsustainable health care inflation and the growing realization that this level of expenditure has not led to uniformly world-leading outcomes.[1] The targeting of health care waste such as duplication of services; patient noncompliance; emphasis on doing, not preventing; and incentives that drive reactive care and utilization of services in an episodic manner are all mentioned as cost drivers. Just 1% of the U.S. population consumes 22% of health care expenditures. The magnitude for 5% and 10% of the U.S. population is also as striking.[2] There is also a widespread notion that chronic diseases such as heart disease, diabetes, and cancer are examples of cost drivers. Yet as recognized by Gaskin and Richard, chronic pain's cost exceeds the cost of heart disease, diabetes, and cancer combined.[3] Yet chronic pain is rarely recognized by health care policy debates for the impact it has on expenditures overall. According to the Institute of Medicine report, there are 100 million Americans with chronic pain at a cost of $635 billion per year for treatment and lost productivity. Yet there is only one pain specialist per 33,000 patients.[4] A forward-thinking pain management center that is prepared to deliver services in a timely, efficient manner and can provide high-quality services within the framework of rapidly changing delivery systems will have significant opportunities in this new era.

Earlier attempts at controlling the cost of health care using coordinated care models such as disease management programs did not work because of the cost needed to established and maintain these programs and the lack of coordination of care among specialties.[5,6]

For these changes to occur, a movement away from fee-for-service reimbursement schemes to a value-based reimbursement model needs to occur.[7] The insurance industry has initially been slow to adopt these changes. This inertia is beginning to break.[8] This transition period will be difficult for all practices but particularly for specialty practices such as pain management centers. More than ever, keeping track of outcomes and what value interventions bring to value-based care will be required for pain management programs.

Medical practices of all types will need to understand the implications of new types of organizations and payment models. The complexities of transitioning a practice from fee-for-service to these new care models will require in-depth planning and establishing new partnerships while closely tracking local trends and understanding the implications of regulatory implementation at a national level. Some of these new types of organizations and payment models include the following:

- **The patient-centered medical home (PCMH)** is a care delivery system that seeks to enhance the communication between high-cost patients and their primary care providers. PCMH has been suggested for primary care practices as a vehicle to take advantage of value-based reimbursement. The potential value of a PCMH is to control costs by keeping patients out of the hospital by improvement in care coordination and improvement in the management of their chronic diseases. Some commercial insurers have been willing to pay an enhanced per-member, per-month, or care management fee per patient in these PCMH practices. Practices interested in this new care delivery system often become certified by the National Council for Quality Assurance (NCQA) to achieve this designation. The following checklist for primary care doctors considering a change of practice focus to patient-centered care model has been suggested and reviewed.[9,10]

1. Access to care
   - Same-day appointments
   - Extended hours
   - Access to patient records 24/7
   - Freedom of patients to select their own physicians
   - Secure e-mail for communication with patients
   - Web portal for patients to request prescription refills, laboratory results, schedule appointments, and so on
   - Policies and procedures to overcome patient's barriers to care, such as transportation and cognitive barriers
   - Linguistically and culturally appropriate services
2. Engaging patients in decision making
   - Treatment options
   - Understanding patients' health goals and priorities
   - Providing and reviewing with patients condition-specific decision aids
   - Understanding patient treatment preferences and ensuring follow-up of these
3. Practice supports patient self-management
   - Document patient and caregiver self-management abilities
   - Motivational coaching for patients
   - Engage family and caregivers in care plans
   - Offer health coach support
4. Assess and improve patient's experience of care
   - Regular patient satisfaction surveys
   - Patient advisory panels to guide practice and quality improvement
   - Patient focus groups

- **Bundled payments** is a concept that seeks to reimburse different providers with a single payment that traditionally has not been paid together or is usually paid through different payment methodologies. Examples include hospital services paid by diagnosis-related groups and physician-paid fee-for-service. Bundled payment programs may make one payment to a hospital, which is then responsible for distributing a portion of that to the physicians taking care of the patient in a single admission. This bundled payment approach provides full reimbursement for a single episode of care and all the services that are required for this hospital admission, including even postdischarge care related to the admission. Some programs retroactively include any charges for diagnostic testing that occurred even before the admission.
- **Accountable care organizations (ACOs)** is a term used to describe an organizational structure that allows health insurers to share some cost savings with primary care practices. Physicians are still paid for charges in the usual manner, bundled payment, and percent of global capitation, episode of care payments, or some form of payment plus bonus if cost saving targets are met. If a cost savings threshold is achieved, the practice will share a portion of this savings with an insurance company or Medicare. Virtually all ACOs have entered in some form of bundled payment program and have integrated into their practice measurement of outcomes such as quality performance, practice efficiencies, or patient satisfaction. ACOs usually have a PCMH approach as part of the practice. ACOs have rapidly increased in number.[11] The primary reason for this has been demonstration of the bending the cost curve of care in dual eligible patients who are usually considered the most difficult patient populations for cost containment. These populations have a high incidence of emergent visits, controlled substance misuse, and problems with compliance and following through with treatment recommendations for their chronic diseases.

All of these new approaches have one thing in common: varying degrees of risk for outcomes are being shifted to providers. Yet patients with chronic diseases spend most of their time away from their doctor and health care systems, and most of our patients' decisions affecting their health are made outside the doctor's office away from physician's watchful eyes.[12]

Improving patient satisfaction is another area of increasing importance for all health care providers. High-quality pain management is a very important component of patient satisfaction.[13] Patients' satisfaction with their health care has been identified as an important outcome measure by Centers for Medicare and Medicaid Services. Both the Hospital Consumer Assessment of Healthcare Providers and Systems Survey (HCAHPS) and Consumer Assessment of Healthcare Providers and Systems (CAHPS) contain rules implementing health care consumer feedback. Results from this feedback will soon impact reimbursement for both inpatient and later outpatient visits.[1,14,15]

Pain management centers have had long-standing credibility issues with payers. Costs of care, narrowly focused specialty specific care, seemingly endless treatment without end points, and unsubstantiated subjective outcomes have resulted in chronic pain management programs being placed under increasing scrutiny.[16,17] Meanwhile, numerous studies have documented that multidisciplinary pain management centers have better outcomes. These studies have shown that multidisciplinary pain management centers provide improved care, are cost-effective, and have improved long-term outcomes.[18-20] Anesthesiology as a specialty is expanding beyond its traditional role in the operating room to provide leadership in the treatment of chronic pain.[21] Anesthesiologists have an opportunity to participate in the development of and provide leadership in the development of multidisciplinary pain management centers of excellence. To succeed in this role, anesthesiologists must recognize the complexity of chronic pain.[16,22,23]

The successful treatment of chronic pain requires the understanding that chronic pain is a multifaceted problem. Chronic pain is not only a sensory complaint; it also has profound impacts on a patient's affect, social circle, vocational pursuits, and cognitive abilities. Pain management centers of excellence understand the unique needs of each of their patients and provide cost-effective care based on those needs. A pain management center that seeks to develop its referral base to include ACOs and practices that support patient-centered care must have in place the resources and systems that will have the ability to provide expertise to treatment pain on site in the ACOs and efficiently accept patients that will underpin the goals of the practices.

The characteristics of a well-managed pain management center that is set up for success in this rapidly changing environment are:

- The recognition that chronic pain is a multifactorial problem that requires specialized care delivered by a team of specialized providers with a full-time commitment to the treatment of chronic pain
- The organization of the pain management center administration is set up to recognize that different patient groups are affected by chronic pain and understand new practice structures and their requirements for success
- Specific emphasis on accessibility and customer-focused initiatives that enhance treatment outcomes improve customer service and facilitate referrals
- Recognition and planning for outcome measures that understand and trace the specific outcome important to specific payer classes while also supporting local ACOs in their mission
- Creation of a network of mutually beneficial relationships that sustain the center's growth with the center's various customers, including hospital administration and payers
- Innovative products and services to help patients recover all aspects of their lives as part of a continuum of care
- The commitment to increase the visibility and viability of pain management as a specialty, working within care teams supporting global payments and supporting an institution's initiatives

Single-modality pain management centers that emphasize procedures and short-term relief that these blocks produce do not meet the previously mentioned objectives. An overemphasis on procedures for short-term relief serves only to enhance the perception of disability and does little for the long-term pain management problems that need to be solved for enhanced patient function. In addition, the economic viability of a single-modality approach is increasingly unlikely. Well-managed pain management centers are organizations that are equipped to manage all aspects of chronic patient disability. A broad focus such as this requires long-term commitments toward multidisciplinary team and program development.

Formulating a strategy is key for successful program development. Separating a multidisciplinary pain management center into smaller elements or key components can facilitate the developmental process. These elements are:

- Organizational structure and administration
- Physical facilities
- The medical treatment continuum
- Service lines
- Practice infrastructure
- Trained interdisciplinary team
- Key patient groups
- Information and outcomes management
- Fiscal management and business planning

KEY COMPONENTS OF A PAIN MANAGEMENT CENTER OF EXCELLENCE

In the following sections, each of these elements is examined; strategies are suggested that will lead an organization through the different stages of growth toward a pain management center of excellence.

ORGANIZATIONAL STRUCTURE AND ADMINISTRATION

More than ever, chronic pain management centers are under constant pressure to improve performance and integrate their unique specialized knowledge into developing multidisciplinary episodes of care, overcoming the image of procedural-based service that is viewed by many skeptical payer organizations as a large financial burden without appropriate returns. Chronic pain remains one of this country's primary public health problems. Centers of excellence provide the leadership and advocacy necessary to influence the attitudes of the local community about pain management services.

This component recognizes that the organizational foundation of a pain management practice is important to achieve these objectives. These objectives are achieved through the following:

1. Mission statement developed by the interdisciplinary team
2. Showing a complete commitment to the discipline of pain management with full-time staff and board certification such as the added qualifications in pain offered by the American Board of Anesthesiology and the American Academy of Pain Medicine
3. Developing key relationships with affiliated institutions and working toward complete integration of pain management services in all aspects of health care
4. Development of a governing body that includes members from various interest groups that are representative of patient groups treated by the pain center
5. Formation of a dedicated organization providing the foundation from which a pain management center can build

The pain management center must initially make the needed alliances to ensure that the appropriate resources are available. This can be in the form of informal professional contacts forming actual contractual links with pertinent organizations such as drug addiction treatment centers or vocational rehabilitation organizations. Developing an appropriate continuum of care requires not only considerable effort to identify appropriate personnel who have an interest in treating chronic pain; it also requires ongoing interactions with referral sources and payers to determine the necessary resources required to fund a treatment continuum. Determining the type of treatment to be included in the treatment continuum requires an understanding of the needs of the referral sources as well as the patients. Understanding this requires the tracking of referral sources, treatment outcomes, and patient satisfaction along with the demographics of all patients seen.

Intensive training in advances in pain management and allied interests, such as enhancing return-to-work rates, keeping patients out of emergency rooms (ER), strategies to identify patients early at risk for developing chronic pain, and research on adaptive appliances for disability, must be ongoing. This training also lends itself to team building, which is a vital component of a multidisciplinary center. The synergism that occurs during team building will improve outcomes and enhance customer satisfaction. Developing a pain management center of excellence requires a substantial investment in time and personnel to develop the needed resources as previously described to treat chronic pain.

THE PHYSICAL FACILITY

Processes of care for chronic pain require team interactions. The physical facility should be developed to enhance interdisciplinary team interaction. In addition, as the practice grows, the facility must have enough space that can be allocated to facilitate the integration of medical management services, various psychotherapies, and individual and group as well as rehabilitative therapies in one contiguous building. This integration of services or interdisciplinary treatment approach will have a positive impact on patient outcomes. Tight coordination will exist among the disciplines for patient conferences and team interaction. The facility should be designed to enhance patient comfort and confidentiality as well as convenient access for patients with disabilities. The physical facility should have enough space for family conferences so that family members can also participate in the rehabilitation process. Although a pain management program must have a home base, provision for outreach programs is increasingly important. Having only one central location can become a barrier to PCMH initiatives. Advanced planning is required to ensure that outreach programs are economically viable.

THE MEDICAL TREATMENT CONTINUUM

As the pain management center grows, clinical problems tend to increase in complexity. There becomes a need to customize a treatment plan for each patient. Rational customizing of treatment plans requires a framework to classify patients into similar groups and develop an understanding of their unique needs. The emphasis on treatment being both cost-effective and efficient must lead to an understanding of how to optimize the treatment to these groups of patients.[24] Treatment of chronic pain requires a triad of therapies: medical management, behavioral intervention, and physical rehabilitation. The assessment of a chronic pain patient must lead to an understanding of the patient's needs in each of these areas. This assessment could then lead to the classification of the pain syndrome using a combination of various tools available today. The International Association for the Study of Pain (IASP) taxonomy of pain provides both an axis tool and a list of chronic pain diagnoses that can provide a framework for the optimization of treatment plans. Because psychological factors often figure prominently in chronic pain diagnosis, additional understanding of patient subgroups requires a means of stratifying the IASP diagnostic groups. Many different evaluation tools exist that can quantify the impact of disease on the patient's physical and psychological functioning. Using this multidimensional approach allows further subclassification of patients.[25] The data collected allow efficient customization of an individual patient plan, as well as the accumulation of data along with outcome data that facilitates quality-improvement activities.

SERVICE LINES

A service line is a list of needed services required in the order of occurrence necessary to perform clinical evaluations and treatment. This list becomes a blueprint upon which these clinical processes can be developed. Service lines are useful concepts that can be used to evaluate outcomes and facilitate internal quality-improvement initiatives. Multidisciplinary teams enhance chronic pain management outcomes. But these multidisciplinary teams add greatly to the complexity of determining cost-effectiveness or treatment outcomes as well as determining best practices. Effective treatment requires that the patient be evaluated and treated systematically. This process can become complex to analyze when the many different individualized encounters are considered for the unique needs of each chronic pain patient. Yet, in order to achieve the efficiency and outcomes demanded by today's health care environment, these processes must be thoroughly understood, measured, and evaluated. Service lines facilitate the identification of the processes and systems that are used to treat patients. This identification process must involve the entire staff. Service lines lend the pain management center a valuable tool to understand the complex processes that must occur for a chronic pain patient to be successfully treated. A service line with a list of processes breaks the treatment continuum into manageable parts and allows analysis to occur that will optimize treatment outcomes. Service lines are used to track all of the clinical activities of the pain management center. The processes involved that support the clinical activities, as well as the clinical activities themselves, are listed in flow diagrams that allow the staff to understand the necessary activities to treat a patient. These flow charts are then used to form a framework to measure key outcomes that reflect the needs of referral sources and the values of the organization as articulated in the mission statement.

For example, a service line such as Evaluation and Assessment could be used to measure the speed at which a new referral patient is seen. Managed care places a premium on customer service and the importance of rapid response to patient concerns. Pain management centers working with managed care organizations could use the service line Evaluation and Assessment to understand the barriers to timely intervention and improve performance. Other service line examples are:

1. Limited Service Line is used to describe patients who need treatment plans with a smaller focus.
2. Comprehensive Pain Management Program is used to describe treatment plans that require comprehensive treatment such as returning a long-standing disabled worker to work or a high-cost patient who has repeated visits to the ER for his or her uncontrolled pain.
3. Research Service Line can be used to track the research activities of a pain management center. Integration of a clinical trial's center can be a useful tool to enhance expertise in the clinical staff, improve the image of expertise of the pain management center, and develop important referral sources.
4. Follow-up and Referral service line is used to track long-term outcomes of patients after they have left the active treatment program.

Service lines can be used to formulate outcomes as well as treatment costs that will allow the pain center to engage in creative managed care contracting, which gives the pain center a potentially competitive edge. Data using performance measures of these processes are used for quality-improvement activities directed toward meeting the specific needs of the pain management center's patients, referral sources, and payers. The data that are collected allow the pain center to become a strong advocate for its patients and their unique needs.[26]

PRACTICE INFRASTRUCTURE

The multidisciplinary nature of chronic pain management treatment requires extensive interaction and team building on an ongoing basis to achieve optimal outcomes. At times, this can make team building difficult, but it must occur nonetheless. In addition, the rapidly changing health care market demands that an organization be versatile, communicate effectively, and be able to innovate quickly and effectively. Regular meetings for pain management center personnel to identify issues as they occur and create solutions are a vital component of the success or failure of any pain management center. Meetings such as those devoted to performance improvement or customer service are examples of important skills that pain management centers must have. Other subcommittees may be formed within a pain management center to keep the organization vital; these can include a managed care committee, quality assurance, and various ad hoc committees to address new program development as the opportunities become apparent. When these meetings are held on a regular basis, all personnel within the pain management center begin to understand the intricacies and nuances of the varied professional backgrounds of the multidisciplinary team. This helps to strengthen the team and helps the team to understand the broad range of services that the pain management center can offer. The need to move away from modality based services such as repeated epidural steroid injections or facet joint injections to a more comprehensive outcome functionally orientated treatment plans should be apparent. Functionally oriented treatment plans are increasingly being demanded by managed care.

TRAINED INTERDISCIPLINARY TEAM

An interdisciplinary team forms the foundation of treatment of any chronic pain management center. The primary goal of any treatment plan is to provide for the unique needs of each individual. Patient satisfaction has been used to provide insight into treatment effectiveness.[27] With careful attention to patient experience, high rates of satisfaction can be reached even in a chronic pain population that has a high incidence of dissatisfaction with health care in general. Patients who report high satisfaction with their treatment are less likely to miss appointments, show better treatment compliance, and adopt a more active role in the treatment plan. These are all important success criteria for chronic pain management treatment plans. In addition, high patient satisfaction correlates with successful treatment outcomes. Payers are also increasingly looking for providers with consistently high patient satisfaction results with which to form relationships.

The foundation of successful outcomes begins when a patient makes an appointment. The professional interaction of the interdisciplinary team conveys trust and facilitates the transference that will lead to patient trust to change behavior. Ingrained behaviors such as long-term disability are difficult to change. Chronic pain management treatment plans often require multiple visits and intensive treatment regimens. Patient satisfaction and the resulting transference can provide the needed motivation for patients to radically depart from the norms they have come to rely on. High customer satisfaction means performing pain management center services in a manner that patients view as highly valid and appropriate. At times, pain can be overwhelming for a patient; accessibility and convenience are important elements of a customer-service-driven organization. In today's health care market, price for service seems to be the only criterion upon which one is evaluated. Customer satisfaction can be a key positioning point in negotiating for new referral sources. To achieve uniform high customer satisfaction ratings, the entire organization must be dedicated to that goal with a passion that is equaled only by the passion for high-quality care. It is important to understand that what a health care professional may determine is important for customer satisfaction is not necessarily the same for varied groups of patients that receive their treatment in a pain management center. Customer satisfaction means much more than timeliness of office appointments. Customer satisfaction may mean having services in a convenient location where a person may not need to miss work and varied services that will support patient needs such as letter writing to employers, disability evaluations, and general efficacy for a patient who has chronic pain.

KEY PATIENT GROUPS

A pain management center's influence should extend beyond the walls of the clinic. The roots of relationships that link the pain management center to the community are critical for survival. Focused efforts to enhance these relationships will result in an ongoing positive image in these areas. External relationships are necessary to track patients and to cultivate local, regional, and national referral sources. In addition, these interactions can help to improve reimbursement and generate community support and goodwill. Identification of key patient groups is very important in determining needs, patient treatment satisfaction, and successful outcomes.[28,29]

High-quality pain management services are recognized as a right in today's health care environment. However, providing these services effectively demands appropriate referrals and reimbursement. Relationships to address these concerns are vital. Positive internal relationships are imperative to keep the team, administration, and referral sources abreast of all new program development in the pain management center. External key customer relationships in a pain management center should include payers, referral sources, vendors of medical equipment, pain management center users (e.g., patients and case managers), and other health care institutions within the community with which the pain management center must interact. These entities can support the patient referrals, medical education, latest technology, reimbursement, and their external consultations that a pain management center needs in order to survive. Strong relationships with these entities are essential to the development and success of a pain management center.

Marketing is also another activity that is placed in this key component. Marketing not only involves activities to increase the visibility of the pain management center but also is used to identify specific patient needs, which may lead to restructuring of the pain management center described in earlier key components. For example, marketing for workers' compensation programs requires an understanding of what services are highly valued and will enhance the care for patients from these referral sources. For example, this may involve developing a seamless continuum of care that brings a patient through a pain management center that engages in specific rehabilitative needs and is able to refer immediately to a vocational training program so that back-to-work rates are optimized. Regular round table discussions with referral sources will be helpful to focus the pain management center's efforts and provide the necessary understanding to customize programs.

INFORMATION AND OUTCOMES MANAGEMENT

Ensuring the delivery of consistent high-quality medical care along with patient satisfaction has to become part of the culture of the pain management center. Activities have to be focused on achieving these goals. Concurrent program evaluation and identification of areas needing improvement leading to the design of new systems and processes is the key to reaching and maintaining consistent high-quality care. This evaluation, leading to innovation followed by implementation, is a constant cycle in any organization that is focused on becoming a center of excellence. All activities included in the pain center have to be understood by the team in the minutest detail, and evaluation systems must be put into place by the people who are responsible for these tasks. Appointing an "overseer" to run these activities can quickly destroy effective teamwork and lead to deterioration in morale, decreased staff effectiveness, and decreased customer satisfaction. Performance goals that are set by the team are much more meaningful and lead to more rapid improvement in quality of care. Continuous quality improvement is part of everyone's job. Appropriate outcomes for chronic pain management are often discussed. Examples such as back-to-work rates, perceived helpfulness, and physical activity scores are all used to define the value of chronic pain management programs. Increasingly, pain management programs are being called upon to justify expenditures and to control costs.[23] Determining program costs, cost-effectiveness, and cost–benefits of a program requires a thorough and complete understanding of the pain management center processes used to deliver care. Payers will require appropriate financial analysis of pain management center treatment.[11] Examples of this might include reduction of health care costs in patients frequenting EDs, reduction of length of stay for postoperative patients, or earlier ambulation of joint replacement patients. Evidence-based algorithms are the foundation for determining cost of care and calculating cost-effectiveness of treatment.[26] Algorithms should be diagnosis specific, evidenced-based, and inclusive enough to achieve pain center physician consensus. Algorithms are then used to standardize treatment for each specific diagnosis, thus permitting financial analysis and disease-specific outcome analysis. Using this structure, a center of excellence will be able to accumulate data to permit informed analysis of the entire treatment continuum for chronic pain management.

FISCAL MANAGEMENT AND BUSINESS PLANNING

In general, all managers must have the appropriate information to manage, and pain management centers should have access to theirs as well. Knowing the monetary impact a pain center can have on an institution's bottom line is vital. This is extremely important for success in negotiations with the institution. These financial reports should provide the pain management center with the necessary information to develop reimbursement strategies and search for new business opportunities that are ever developing in this rapidly changing health care environment. Meetings with payers to discuss their needs and develop new services along with them can provide valuable new insights and ensure successful program development. Appropriately structured pain management centers can provide services in a fiscally responsible manner and still achieve excellent patient outcomes. This perspective comes not only from the hospital itself and from payers and referral sources but from health care delivery systems at risk for cost control.

Any successful enterprise requires the development of a clearly written business plan. Although this will not guarantee that a practice will be a success, most successful businesses are based on well-developed business plans that are revised as required for changing conditions. The purpose of a business plan is to document in writing a brief description of the business and the market niche served by that business, as well as the infrastructure that is required to become a successful practice. Financial resources required to start, sustain, and staff the clinic as well as an outline of a marketing plan are also vital components of a business planning process. Developing a comprehensive outline and understanding of the reimbursement climates under which the pain center exists, including governmental managed care insurance companies and patients, is vital. This can occur in an accurate fashion only when a pain management center develops the solid internal and external relationships as described in an earlier key component.

CHANGING HEALTH CARE ENVIRONMENT

Managed care has become the most important force driving the health care market in the United States. Different areas of the country are in various stages of managed care penetration. For ease of description, managed care penetration has been placed in four stages. Each stage of change requires adaptations in the delivery of health care services to meet this challenge. These are known as the evolving stages of value.[28,29] Pain management centers are part of this evolving health care market and therefore must identify the stage of the local area in which they are operating. The evolving stages of value in the health care market occur at four levels:

- Stage 1, or the unstructured stage, describes a market with independent hospitals and physicians, few unsophisticated purchasers, and less than 10% penetration of managed care. The organizational source of value comes from its hard assets, quality is defined internally, and reimbursement is fee-for-service. Examples of chronic pain management care in this environment would be the intensive 6- to 8-week inpatient programs, with very little program customization for individual patient needs.

TABLE 102-1 Matrix of the Characteristics Key Components Through the Five Stages of Change

Key Components	Stage 1: Product-Focused Practice	Stage 2: Customer-Focused Practice	Stage 3: Market-Segment-Focused Practice	Stage 4: Opportunity-Focused Practice	Stage 5: Pain Management Center of Excellence
Organizational Structure/ Administration	• Create mission statement • Make commitment to become a pain center • Educate key relationships about pain management	• Build relationships with key advisors • Educate advisors on chronic pain and total quality management as it applies to pain	• Set up systems to expand and new service lines • Revisit mission statement • Establish and educate board	• Add administrative capability to support larger patient base • Expand relations with board	• Maintain strong active board • Build structure to allow rapid growth • Revisit mission statement
Physical Facilities	• Facility shared with other services	• Space dedicated to chronic pain services	• Offer inpatient and outpatient facilities • Offer transportation to pain center from other system locations • Design work areas that encourage interaction	• Maintain central treatment facility • Establish basic services in satellite locations	• Expand services in satellite locations • Facility reflects regional reputation
Medical Treatment Continuum	• Limited pain treatment offered • Broaden knowledge of chronic pain management • Build physician network to ensure full diagnosis • Begin collection of outcomes data • Offer patient education	• Commit to full treatment continuum • Establish basic treatment protocols • Execute contracts with external providers • Expand patient education	• Offer full range of medical treatments • Expand and refine treatment protocols • Analyze processes for better outcomes • Test patient education	• Able to treat all types of pain problems • Develop critical pathways • Develop protocols for different venues of care • Improve treatment processes • Institute follow-up care	• Offer full treatment continuum • Refine critical pathways • Continuous refinement of treatments for enhanced outcomes • Integrated patient education
Service Lines	• Basic chronic pain treatment offered • Broaden professional expertise • Essential feedback loops in place	• Identify basic service lines • Support service lines with documentation systems	• Design multidisciplinary service lines • Offer 24-hour service • Strengthen infrastructure • Ensure consistency of care	• Discover opportunities for new service lines • Customize service lines for payers and patients	• Create service line and extensions for niche markets • Create seamless delivery of health care for chronic pain • Essential customer feedback loops in place
Practice Infrastructure	• Establish regular team communication • Keep team focused and motivated	• Regular team meetings • Team building • Activities begin	• Team focused on patient assessment • Regularly scheduled team-building activities • Cross training is begun	• Activities to promote cohesive team • Continuous training for cohesive team	• Conduct ongoing team building
Trained Interdisciplinary Team	• Identify members of the core team	• Add to core team as required	• Team dedicated solely to pain management	• Full team in place	• Maintain strong team communication
Key Patient Groups	• Identify patient customer groups • Measure patient satisfaction	• Expand efforts to attract customers • Expand patient satisfaction surveys • Begin patient-oriented market research • Begin community education efforts	• Expand marketing efforts • Communicate with patients regularly • Establish clinicwide customer service policies • Begin community education	• Attract patients from wider service radius • Work toward exceeding customer expectations • Continue community education efforts	• Develop the ability to customize all aspects of patient care • Gather continuous customer feedback • Increase COE visibility • Broaden reputation
Information/ Outcomes Management	• Establish basic record-keeping systems • Develop basic patient treatment outcome parameters	• Expand patient treatment outcome parameters • Measure and report patient satisfaction • Educate team on continuous quality improvement	• Develop and track outcome studies • Create database • Implement continuous improvement cycles • Establish nonthreatening management systems	• Team proactively improves processes • Streamline information exchange • Work across department boundaries	• Team committed to strive for perfection • Management removes barriers for team improvement • Quality, not quantity, is measure of success
Fiscal Management/ Business Planning	• Create business plan • Conduct informal market research • Establish financial reporting systems	• Develop individual and team goals and action plans • Conduct market research for business planning • Develop a budget	• Conduct feasibility studies for new ventures • Create dedicated financial reports • Negotiate managed care contracts	• Create tactical plans • Conduct SWOT analysis • Maintain managed care links and contracts	• Team empowered to change workplace • Apply CQI to management systems • Management serves as advisors and facilitators

COE, Center of excellence; CQI, continuous quality improvement; SWOT, strengths, weaknesses, opportunities, and threats.

Data from Ross G, Kay M. *Toppling the Pyramids; Redefining the Way American Companies Are Run*. New York: Times Books; 1994.

- Stage 2, or the loose framework stage, is characterized by a growing presence of managed care, decreasing profit margins, and eroding hospital bottom lines. With the emphasis on outpatient care, hospitals have excess inpatient capacity. Joint ventures are beginning to form between the medical staff and health care facilities. Quality increasingly is defined by the near-term cost of care. Chronic pain management treatment plans in this environment require customization of treatment plans specific to each patient's needs, with an increasing emphasis on outpatient care and day programs.
- Stage 3, or the consolidation stage, is defined by the development of large health care systems and increasing emphasis on developing a complete integrated health system. Quality is defined by customer satisfaction, along with cost of care. Managed care is an important part of the market, with penetration now up to 50%. This stage is found in most major population centers in the United States. Pain management centers existing in this environment must also reengineer themselves to reflect these changes. Internally, the pain center must focus on outcomes, understand the needs of their referral sources, and design programs that address these needs. Pain management centers that work toward becoming part of an integrated delivery system will find many opportunities in this environment.
- Stage 4, or managed competition, is characterized by employer coalitions, which drive the market toward the formation of strategic alliances and the shifting of risk to the health care provider. The focus of these organizations on health status and quality is now defined by the health status of populations or covered lives. Health care systems are driven to provide the highest customer value, and the most important source of value comes from capability of the organization and its image. Risk sharing is an important consideration in this stage. Specific disease-specific episodes of care are developed for high-cost or high-volume diagnoses. Appearance of PCMH and ACOs with their specific needs also become part of the health care environment. Chronic pain in this stage has become a real cost that must be effectively and appropriately treated throughout all patient care sites, both inpatient and ambulatory.

Using the components and health care stages described in the preceding sections, five stages can be described that allow pain management centers to set goals and respond to the changes of the health care market. **Table 102-1** presents a matrix of the key components as well as characteristics of each of these five stages.

Health care is changing from a product-focused practice (fee-for-service reimbursement) in which reimbursement encourages utilization to much more sophisticated reimbursement schemes that emphasize outcomes and shift the risk of outcomes to providers.

It is important to note that as a pain management center begins to work itself through the stages of change, as outlined earlier, all nine key components must be coordinated to achieve progress. Planning time frames of years can be needed to achieve desired results. Only with total and complete commitment of the pain management staff can the pain center evolve into a center of excellence. The stages described are fluid, and changes in personnel and health care reimbursement strategies may cause the pain center at times to regress. A commitment to ongoing process improvement as described earlier will allow a pain management center to achieve and maintain leadership in the community. The key to achieving a center of excellence reputation is the full-time commitment of the medical staff. Pain management should not be viewed as an opportunity to earn supplementary income by providing procedure-oriented services. Reviewing Table 102-1, along with the previously described stages, will give a comprehensive understanding of the planning process that must take place for success to occur. Understanding these stages of change and using them as a framework for a methodical planning process and breaking the planning process into the key components described earlier will lead to a strong and dedicated organization with a passion to succeed and an ability to achieve the goal of becoming a well-managed pain management center known as a *pain management center of excellence*.

REFERENCES

1. Yong PL, Saunders RS, Olsen LA, eds. *The Healthcare Imperative: Lowering Costs and Improving Outcomes: Workshop Series Summary*. Washington, DC: 2010.
2. Blumenthal D. Performance improvement in health care–seizing the moment. *N Engl J Med*. 2012;366(21):1953-1955.
3. Gaskin DJ, Richard P. The economic costs of pain in the United States. *J Pain*. 2012;13(8)715-724.
4. Institute of Medicine. IOM calls for transformation of attitudes toward pain and its prevention and management. *J Pain Palliat Care Pharmacother*. 2012;26(1):40-43.
5. Burns LR, Pauly MV. Accountable care organizations may have difficulty avoiding the failures of integrated delivery networks of the 1990s. *Health Aff (Millwood)*. 2012;31(11):2407-2416.
6. Noble DJ, Casalino LP. Can accountable care organizations improve population health? Should they try? *JAMA*. 2013;309(11): 1119-1120.
7. Song Z, Lee TH. The era of delivery system reform begins. *JAMA*. 2013;309(1):35-36.
8. Song Z, Safran DG, Landon BE, et al. Health care spending and quality in year 1 of the alternative quality contract. *N Engl J Med*. 2011;365(10):909-918.
9. Miller WL, Crabtree BF, Nutting PA, et al. Primary care practice development: a relationship-centered approach. *Ann Fam Med*. 2010;8(Suppl 1):S68-S79, S92.
10. Nutting PA, Miller WL, Crabtree BF, et al. Initial lessons from the first national demonstration project on practice transformation to a patient-centered medical home. *Ann Fam Med*. 2009;7(3):254-260.
11. Luft HS. From small area variations to accountable care organizations: how health services research can inform policy. *Annu Rev Public Health*. 2012;33:377-392.
12. Asch DA, Muller RW, Volpp KG. Automated hovering in health care—watching over the 5000 hours. *N Engl J Med*. 2012;367(1):1-3.
13. Gupta A, Daigle S, Mojica J, Hurley RW. Patient perception of pain care in hospitals in the United States. *J Pain Res*. 2009;2:157-64.
14. New CMS guidelines for managing complaints. *Hosp Peer Rev*. 2006;31(1):5-6.
15. Hospital value-based purchasing: biggest bonuses and penalties. CMS percentage change in reimbursement based on process performance and patient satisfaction. *Mod Healthc*. 2013;43(1):34.
16. Loeser JD. The future. Will pain be abolished or just pain specialists? *Minn Med*. 2001;84(7):20-21.
17. Kulich R, Loeser JD. The business of pain medicine: the present mirrors antiquity. *Pain Med*. 2011;12(7):1063-1075.
18. Manchikanti L, Pampati V, Boswell MV, et al. Analysis of the growth of epidural injections and costs in the Medicare population: a comparative evaluation of 1997, 2002, and 2006 data. *Pain Physician*. 2010;13(3):199-212.
19. Manchikanti L, Singh V, Boswell MV. Interventional pain management at crossroads: the perfect storm brewing for a new decade of challenges. *Pain Physician*. 2010;13(2):E111-E140.
20. Lang E, Liebig K, Kastner S, et al. Multidisciplinary rehabilitation versus usual care for chronic low back pain in the community: effects on quality of life. *Spine J*. 2003;3(4):270-276.
21. Greene NM. The 31st Rovenstine Lecture. The changing horizons in anesthesiology. *Anesthesiology*. 1993;79(1):164-170.
22. Loeser JD. Pain: disease or dis-ease? The John Bonica Lecture: presented at the third World Congress of World Institute of Pain, Barcelona 2004. *Pain Pract*. 2005;5(2):77-84.

23. Loeser JD. Comprehensive pain programs versus other treatments for chronic pain. *J Pain*. 2006;7(11):800-801; discussion 804-806.

24. Turk DC, Swanson KS, Tunks ER. Psychological approaches in the treatment of chronic pain patients—when pills, scalpels, and needles are not enough. *Can J Psychiatry*. 2008;53(4):213-23.

25. Classification of chronic pain. Descriptions of chronic pain syndromes and definitions of pain terms. Prepared by the International Association for the Study of Pain, Subcommittee on Taxonomy. *Pain Suppl*. 1986;3:S1-S226.

26. Smith MJ. Accountable disease management of spine pain. *Spine J*. 2011;11(9):807-815.

27. Shirley ED, Sanders JO. Patient satisfaction: implications and predictors of success. *J Bone Joint Surg Am*. 2013;95(10):e69.

28. Kauer RT, Berkowitz E. Strategic positioning. Part 2: positioning challenges in an evolving health care marketplace. *Physician Exec*. 1997;23(8):46-51.

29. Kauer RT, Berkowitz E. Strategic positioning. Part 1: the sources of value under managed care. *Physician Exec*. 1997;23(6):6-12.

CHAPTER 103 The Evolution of Training and Certification in the Field of Pain Medicine

James P. Rathmell

Dr. John Bonica was a pioneer in establishing pain medicine as a medical discipline; he died on August 15, 1994, at the age of 77. His obituary in *The New York Times*,[1] in which he is described as a leader in the effort to understand and cope with pain, reads:

> He committed himself to the alleviation of pain while tending to the wounded of World War II. When his own wife almost died in childbirth, he took up a pioneering effort against the pain of childbirth, and was instrumental in developing epidural anesthesia. . . . Working at Tacoma General Hospital from 1947 to 1963, he established the first residency training program in anesthesiology in Washington State. He founded the University of Washington's Department of Anesthesiology in 1960 and headed it for 18 years. He retired as its chairman in 1978 to promote advanced treatments of acute and chronic pain worldwide. The recipient of many honors at home and abroad, he was a founder and past president of the International Association for the Study of Pain, which now has 6,000 members in 80 countries.[1]

Before his death, his wife, Emma, noted that one of the first things Dr. Bonica did at the University of Washington, in collaboration with a nurse, Dorothy Crowley, and a neurosurgeon, Lowell E. White, Jr., was to establish a multidisciplinary pain clinic. Dr. Bonica brought in research scientists; young anesthesiologists interested in pain management also were drawn to the clinic, which provided the first formalized training program in pain management. "This group of academic health care providers and researchers met regularly to discuss problem patients with chronic pain and to devise effective treatment strategies. . . . The University established the Multidisciplinary Pain Center in 1978, recognizing John's accomplishments and wishing to provide a broad base for its support beyond a single department. Health care providers of all types collaborated in this Pain Center."[2] Dr. Bonica clearly recognized the need for a group of physicians who dedicated their professional lives to the treatment of pain, and we must thank him for moving us so far toward that goal. This chapter looks back over how pain medicine came to be where it is today and sets out the next steps in further maturing this new young medical discipline, with a focus on training and certification of physicians.

ON MEDICAL SPECIALIZATION

It has become impossible for any physician to become an expert in every field. As knowledge expands and the need for detailed skills arises, the natural progression is for specialization to ensue. Yet there has long been a discomfort with specialization. The urge to both specialize and remain unspecialized dates back to the earliest recorded history of medicine. The first specializations were between the barber-surgeons and the internists, and a rivalry of sorts remains to this day. Writing about Ambroise Paré, the 16th-century physician who elevated the role of the barber-surgeons to that of other physicians, the present-day surgeon and historian Sherwin Nuland reflects on the ongoing distinction between internist and surgeon:

> Surgery is an exercise in the use of the intellect. Heckling internists, with tongues barely in check, would prefer that surgical specialists be viewed merely as dexterous craftsman who carry out the routing errands assigned to them by their more cerebrally endowed medical overseers. I attribute this teasing raillery to a kind of good-natured fraternal envy, not so much of our celebrity status, but rather of the visibility of the cures we surgeons achieve and the particular personal gratification we have while doing it.[3]

In the United States, anesthesiology has progressed toward further specialization, first with the establishment of critical care; then pain management (now pain medicine); and more recently, pediatric anesthesiology and cardiothoracic anesthesiology. With specialization comes a conscious effort to focus the practice and become intricately familiar with a more limited realm. The obvious result is a loss of the skills and knowledge needed to practice in the broader parent specialty. In pain medicine, many view theirs as a full-time vocation. The scientific meetings and journals that keep pain medicine specialists up to date have little overlap with those designed for anesthesiologists practicing in operating rooms. The only common thread in their technical skills is expertise with neural blockade, one of several important skill sets in pain medicine. The rapid expansion of knowledge in the causes and complications of acute and chronic pain, particularly in the neurobehavioral sciences, has led to a growing recognition that pain medicine practitioners must acquire a vastly different skill set than practicing anesthesiologists, including expanding their diagnostic skills.

THE EMERGENCE OF ANESTHESIA CLINICS FOR THERAPY OF PAIN

Much has been written about the origins of pain medicine as a distinct discipline, and anesthesiologists have played a primary role,[4-6] as have specialists in neurology, psychiatry, neurosurgery, and physical medicine and rehabilitation (PM&R).[7] Anesthesiology really started with the introduction of ether as an effective general anesthetic in the mid 19th century, when surgical pain could first be separated from operation. Toward the end of his tenure as chair of the Department of Anesthesiology at Columbia University, which extended from 1952 to 1969, Dr. Emmanuel "Manny" Papper wrote, "Events in the changing medical world have made it imperative that our functions be broadened and that we accept the challenge of pain occurring outside the surgical amphitheater. Such a concept fully justifies an anesthesia clinic on the therapy of pain."[8] This sentiment was echoed by a number of other leading anesthesiology chairs, including Leroy Vandam at Harvard, and the first dedicated pain treatment centers were born, largely in academic anesthesiology departments in major medical centers. Nearly 100 years after the introduction of ether came Dr. Bonica, an anesthesiologist. Although he began his practice with a focus on developing regional anesthesia techniques, he soon came to realize these were inadequate to meet the needs of his patients. These techniques alone could not incorporate the growing epidemiologic, basic, and clinical scientific evidence of the salience of neurobehavioral factors. Dr. Bonica himself came to believe that developing the field of pain as a separate clinical discipline and treating chronic pain competently required the intellectual input and clinical skills of several other specialties. To that end, he published the first edition of the seminal textbook *The Management of Pain* in 1953.[9] The International Association for the Study of Pain (IASP), which founded its U.S. chapter in 1974, the American Pain Society, and the journal *Pain* are legacies left by Dr. Bonica for our patients. From his life's work, we now have extensive ongoing efforts to recognize and treat pain effectively, to train subspecialists, and to conduct basic and clinical research to further our understanding of pain and its treatment. It is noteworthy that IASP presidents have backgrounds in anesthesiology, dentistry, neurology, neurophysiology, neurosurgery, psychiatry, and psychology. All share a common intellectual passion and achievement as well as clinical dedication to developing pain research, teaching, and clinical care in pain medicine.

THE ESTABLISHMENT OF FORMAL PAIN TRAINING PROGRAMS

Accredited fellowship training in pain medicine is a relatively recent development. Before 1992, training was frequently obtained in academic anesthesiology departments, including those led by Drs. Bonica, Philip Bridenbaugh, Harold Carron, Daniel Moore, Prithvi Raj, Alon Winnie, and others, and subsequently in programs run by their trainees. These unaccredited programs advanced the specialty, widened interest in pain medicine as a career, and propagated anesthesiology-based pain care in smaller and smaller communities across the country. Other specialists also contributed to the development of the practice model of pain care; they trained fellows in unaccredited programs as well. Multispecialty entrance into pain medicine training became a tradition in several cities, including Boston, under Daniel Carr (Harvard, Massachusetts General) and Carol Warfield (Harvard, Beth Israel); New York, under Kathy Foley, Russell Portenoy, and Bob Breitbart (Sloan-Kettering); and in Seattle, under John Loeser, Bonica's successor (University of Washington), among many others. Outside the United States, this type of informal training remains the rule for those seeking expertise in pain medicine. In the United States, the American Board of Anesthesiology (ABA) developed interest in certifying pain medicine training. The failure of the boards of Anesthesiology, Psychiatry and Neurology, Physical Medicine and Rehabilitation and Neurosurgery in 1990 to form a conjoint American Board of Medical Specialties (ABMS) board prompted the ABA, under the leadership of Bill Owens in his roles on both the ABA and the Accreditation Council for Graduate Medical Education (ACGME) Residency Review Committee (RRC), and through his representations of the subspecialty to the ABMS, to begin accrediting formal training programs in 1992 through the ACGME. Steve Abram and John Rowlingson were key members of the group who helped Dr. Owens move the new subspecialty forward.

The number of ACGME-accredited programs (**Fig. 103-1**) and the number of trainees in accredited programs have grown steadily over the past decade. In 1999, just under 100 training programs were turning out more than 300 new pain specialists each year (**Fig. 103-2**). The ABA, working in parallel with the ACGME, developed a subspecialty certification examination in pain medicine that was first named the "Certificate of Added Qualifications in Pain Management" and is now titled "Subspecialty Certification in Pain Medicine." The first examination was given in 1993. The number of physicians sitting for the examination has steadily grown (see Fig. 103-2).

THE EVOLUTION OF TRAINING AND CERTIFICATION IN PAIN MEDICINE

Dr. Bonica's original push to develop multidisciplinary pain care recently evolved into collaboration among four specialties for a single and unified set of program requirements for all ACGME-accredited pain fellowships regardless of sponsoring specialty. Consequently,

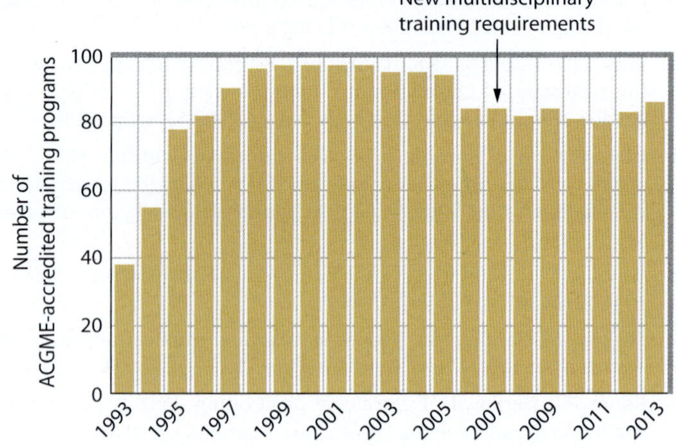

FIGURE 103-1. Trends in the number of pain medicine fellowship training programs accredited by the Accreditation Council for Graduate Medical Education since they were first established in 1992. (Data courtesy of the American Board of Anesthesiology, October 2013.)

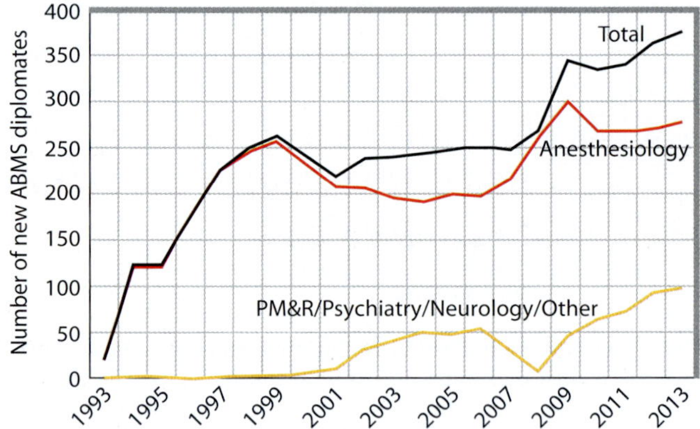

FIGURE 103-2. Trends in the number of newly subspecialty board-certified diplomats in pain medicine recognized by the American Board of Medical Specialties (ABMS) and their primary discipline of ABMS board certification. (Data courtesy of the American Board of Anesthesiology, October 2013.)

in 1999, the ABA invited representatives of the American Board of Psychiatry and Neurology (ABPN) and the American Board of Physical Medicine & Rehabilitation (ABPMR) to join the ABA's Pain Management Examination Committee in broadening the examination beyond regional anesthesia, and in 2000, the ABPN and ABPMR began issuing certificates of subspecialty certification in pain management to diplomats who passed the expanded ABA examination. Between 2002 and 2006, the ACGME, working in collaboration with the ABA, ABPN, and ABPMR, developed new program requirements for pain fellowship training programs aimed at improving the quality of education and promoting a multidisciplinary approach to care. The new program requirements were adopted in 2006, and the number of programs achieving ongoing accreditation under these broader and more rigorous requirements has declined by nearly 20% (see Fig. 103-1). Equally important in the evolution of the discipline is the creation of academic physicians who undertake research programs in the fellowships to add new knowledge to this needed field of medical practice.

Pain and its consequences draw on resources from all medical disciplines. Dr. Bonica's experiences treating soldiers during World War II suggested that each medical specialist had unique expertise to bring to patients suffering in pain. Thanks largely to Dr. Bonica, anesthesiology has led the development of formal training programs. Indeed, the majority of currently accredited training programs reside within academic anesthesiology departments, and most program directors are anesthesiologists. Specialists from other disciplines have also focused their clinical and research efforts on pain. The most obvious example is neurology, in which the majority of clinical treatment and research about headache and peripheral neuropathy has arisen. PM&R has also long had a focus and expertise in functional restoration, and physiatrists lead many chronic pain rehabilitation programs. And, of course, psychiatrists have been closely involved where pain, illness behavior, stress, depression, anxiety and substance abuse overlap. During the past decade, specialists from these other disciplines have been seeking subspecialty training in pain medicine with increasing regularity (Figs. 103-2 and **103-3**).

The range of practitioners declaring themselves as pain medicine specialists is extraordinary. From clinics that provide largely or solely cognitive-behavioral approaches to chronic pain through functional restoration programs, to the type of clinic that offers nothing more than a variety of injections, "interventional pain medicine" is a term that has been coined for techniques that involve minimally invasive treatments and minor surgery, including neural blockade and implantable analgesic devices. Despite the paucity of scientific evidence to guide pain practitioners, particularly evidence to support the use of interventional modalities, many techniques appear to have efficacy based on limited observational data, and many have been adopted into widespread use. As practitioners, we are left to choose among available treatment modalities, often with only anecdote and personal experience to guide us, in treating a group of desperate patients with intractable pain who are willing to accept almost any treatment, even those which remain unproven. There is no single practice pattern that a pain specialist can point to as the correct way to treat patients with chronic pain. Training programs vary widely in the scope of what they train practitioners to do. The best pain medicine practitioners strike a reasonable balance between interventional and noninterventional management. This practice pattern is sustainable, and those adopting a balanced style of practice will be able to adapt to evolving scientific evidence that supports pain treatment regardless of the type of treatment. A balance between or among treatment modalities also allows practitioners to switch from one mode to another or incorporate multiple treatment approaches simultaneously. Use of these interventional modalities is just a small part of the armamentarium of skilled pain medicine practitioners.

Primary specialty of pain medicine diplomates*

Family practice
Psychiatry & neurology
Neurological surgery
Surgery
Plastic surgery
Pediatrics
Radiology
(<1%)
Internal medicine (1%)
Psychiatry (1%)
Neurology (6%)
Physical medicine & rehabilitation (36%)
Anesthesiology (55%)

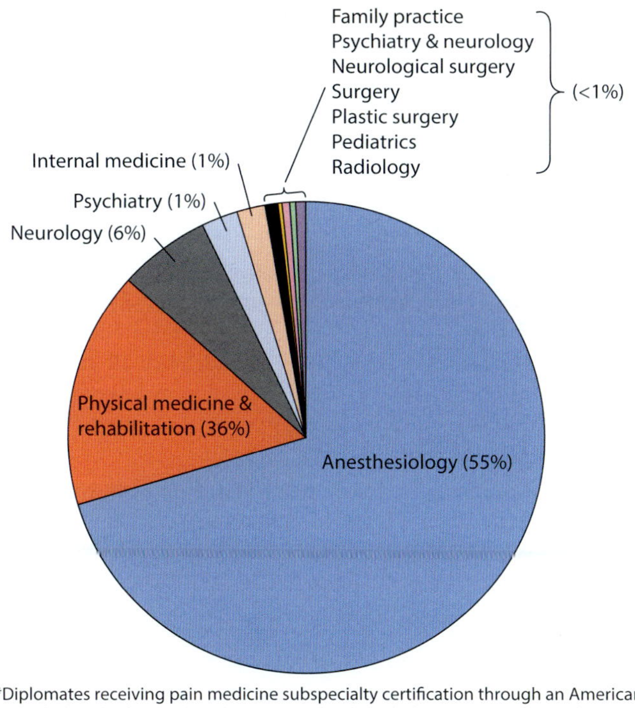

*Diplomates receiving pain medicine subspecialty certification through an American Board of Medical Specialties (ABMS) member board (the American Board of Anesthesiology, American Board of Physical Medicine and Rehabilitation, or the American Board of Psychiatry and Neurology).

FIGURE 103-3. Primary specialty of board certification of diplomats receiving subspecialty certification in pain medicine through a member board of the American Board of Medical Specialties (ABMS). Member boards offering pain medicine subspecialty certification include the American Board of Anesthesiology [ABA], the American Board of Physical Medicine and Rehabilitation [ABPMR], and the American Board of Psychiatry and Neurology [ABPN]). (All data provided by ABA, ABPMR, and ABPN, July 2010.)

THE FUTURE OF TRAINING AND CERTIFICATION IN PAIN MEDICINE

Two prominent forces have increased the urgency to reform our training programs in pain medicine. The first is the expanding breadth of this multidisciplinary subspecialty that now requires in-depth education in many medical disciplines beyond anesthesiology. The second is the emergence of evidence-based medicine as a new paradigm to guide practicing physicians.

As previously noted, the number of fellowship training programs achieving ongoing accreditation under these rigorous requirements has declined since 2006 (see Fig. 103-1). Nonetheless, many of the remaining programs have expanded fellowship training positions, helping to offset the decrease in programs. Under the ACGME's new Multidisciplinary Pain Medicine Program Requirements, trainees from disciplines other than anesthesiology are now assured access to subspecialty training. This ensures that the specialty of pain medicine does not fragment into numerous subspecialties with disparate views and practices. The same subspecialty certification offered for anesthesiologists through the ABA has been available to other physicians with primary certification by member boards of the ABMS through the ABPMR and ABPN since 2001. Board certification of Pain Medicine subspecialists is mostly in anesthesiology (55%) followed by PM&R (36%) and neurology (6%) (see Fig. 103-3).

The urgent need for expanded clinical research, coupled with the need for multidisciplinary education, makes it clear that the current 1-year fellowships cannot adequately offer the training and research needed in the field of pain medicine. So, what is the next and best step in improving education for pain medicine specialists? The ABA and the ACGME RRC for Anesthesiology are actively grappling with this question. In a recent position statement, the leadership of the American Board of Pain Medicine, an independent organization outside of the ABMS, argued that pain medicine should become a primary, 4-year residency in which training begins immediately after medical school.[10] This would sever the link to any primary medical specialty and create an entirely new discipline. However, we have no existing group of academic physicians in place to lead the training in these hypothetical new residency programs and little evidence that medical students are ready to commit to training in such a new field. We do have an extensive infrastructure in place that has already trained nearly 20 years of physician specialists in pain medicine, including the most prominent leaders in the discipline. Aside from creating new residency programs in pain medicine, perhaps there are different routes that can bridge the divide between the training available now and something more optimal.

One route to ensuring improved training for pain medicine specialists is simply to increase the duration of fellowship training to 2 years. This would provide the additional time needed to ensure exposure to all aspects of multidisciplinary pain care and leave time for research. Indeed, this is the route that pediatrics chose more than a decade ago for subspecialty training in neonatology and pediatric cardiology, among other areas: 3 years of general pediatrics followed by 3 additional years of subspecialty training that includes a mandatory research component. Extending pain medicine fellowships to 2 years would result in a total training period after medical school of 6 years (the clinical base year, 3 years of clinical anesthesiology, and 2 years of pain medicine fellowship). Many current fellowship program directors and other advocates of 2-year fellowships argue that this is a needed change. Opponents contend this would lead to a precipitous decline in the number of physicians entering pain medicine fellowships because graduating residents would weigh the benefits versus the additional year of training required compared with all other anesthesiology subspecialties.

Perhaps there exists a middle ground between creating primary residency programs in pain medicine and extending fellowships to 2 years. Several anesthesiology programs have developed a novel approach that combines anesthesiology residency with a critical care fellowship during the same 5-year period but also allows for more extensive critical care experiences throughout the entire 5 years of training. These programs have been approved through the ACGME's Innovative Programs pathway and have been in existence for several years at Oregon Health Sciences University; the University of Washington; the University of California, San Francisco; and Washington University. Trainees completing these Innovative Programs are eligible for primary board certification in anesthesiology as well as subspecialty certification in critical care medicine. Using such a combined approach seems well suited to pain medicine. Trainees could spend many core and elective months during the clinical base (postgraduate year 1) and clinical anesthesia (postgraduate years 2 to 4) years focusing on pain medicine, and this would add greatly to overall subspecialty pain training for medical students without detracting from their core training in anesthesiology. With interest and involvement of other core disciplines, including psychiatry, neurology, and PM&R, similar programs could be developed within these parent disciplines. Indeed, this may be the first logical step in the evolution toward an independent discipline, serving as a bridge between the existing infrastructure of pain medicine fellowships and some future infrastructure. Indeed, Dr. John Loeser, a neurosurgeon by training and the physician who succeeded John Bonica in leading the University of Washington's pain center, recently argued that pain medicine should remain as 1-year subspecialty training programs following completion of primary residency in a related discipline.[11] Loeser argued that complete core training is essential for physicians to gain competence in the broad skill sets required of physicians, including the technical skills required in disciplines such as anesthesiology and neurosurgery. However, he argued strongly for an independent and multidisciplinary group to oversee the review of training programs and the certification of subspecialists in pain medicine. This intermediate step between the current state and primary residency training programs in pain medicine may well be the most logical next step in the evolution of the discipline. The next step is to ensure that all key stakeholders with interest and expertise in this specialty work together to design a rational short- and long-term strategy for pain medicine to evolve as a cohesive and evidence-based discipline.

THE FUTURE OF PAIN MEDICINE AS A MEDICAL SPECIALTY

The urgent need for expanded clinical research in pain medicine (coupled with the recent efforts to improve multidisciplinary training) is straining the ability of training programs to adequately provide the needed education and research experiences for pain medicine fellows in the course of a 1-year fellowship. The ACGME and ABA are currently restructuring the pain medicine fellowship in order to accomplish these goals. The aim is to create a more homogeneous group of pain medicine specialists that emerges with similar knowledge and skills, regardless of the parent discipline in which they trained. This will move us toward improving the consistency and quality of care for patients with acute, chronic, and cancer-related pain.

ACKNOWLEDGEMENTS

Much of the material first appeared in the following article and is reproduced here with permission from the publisher and the American Society of Regional Anesthesia and Pain Medicine: Rathmell JP. American Society of Regional Anesthesia and Pain Medicine 2011 John J. Bonica Award Lecture: the evolution of the field of pain medicine. *Reg Anesth Pain Med.* 2012;37:652-656.

REFERENCES

1. *The New York Times*. August 20, 1994. Available at http://www.nytimes.com/1994/08/20/obituaries/john-j-bonica-pioneer-in-anesthesia-dies-at-77.html?pagewanted=2&src=pm. last accessed September 3, 2012.
2. Loeser JD. John J. Bonica 1917-1994. Emma B. Bonica 1915-1994. *Pain*. 1994;59:1-3.
3. Nuland SB. The gentle surgeon: Ambrose Paré. In: Nuland SB. ed. *Doctors: The Biography of Medicine*. New York: Knopf; 1988:94.
4. Rathmell JP, Brown DL. The evolution of training in pain medicine in the United States. American Society of Anesthesiologists Newsletter, November 2002.
5. Huntoon MC, Rathmell JP, Hidalgo NA. Update on Interdisciplinary Education in Pain Medicine, American Society of Anesthesiologists Newsletter, November 2009.
6. Rathmell JP. Next Steps in Improving Subspecialty Education in Pain Medicine, American Society of Anesthesiologists Newsletter, November 2010.
7. Gallagher RM. Pain education and training: progress or paralysis? *Pain Med.* 2002;3(3):196-197.
8. Papper EM. Regional anesthesia: A critical assessment of its place in therapeutics. E. A. Rovenstine Memorial Lecture. *Anesthesiology.* 1967;28:1074-1084.
9. Bonica JJ. *The Management of Pain*. Philadelphia: JB Lippincott; 1953.
10. Dubois MY, Gallagher RM, Lippe PM. Pain medicine position paper. *Pain Med.* 2009;10:972-1000.
11. Loeser JD. The education of pain physicians. *Pain Med.* 2014 Jan 8. doi:10.1111/pme.12335. [Epub ahead of print].

SECTION B

Legal and Ethical Issues

Disability Assessment of Pain-Impaired Patients

James Celestin
Joseph Rigby
Joseph F. Audette

CHAPTER OBJECTIVES

- Review key terminology (impairment, disability, and handicapped)
- Review American Medical Association and Social Security Administration guidelines for impairment and disability
- Contradictions of disability determination in chronic pain
- Functional assessment methods in pain patients
- Measuring pain intensity
- Determining functional impairment
- The role of diagnostic studies in disability assessment
- The role of psychological assessment tools in disability assessment
- Basics of disability evaluation

OVERVIEW

Approximately one-third of all Americans have a chronically painful condition; 50% to 60% of these individuals are partially or totally disabled. Cost estimates in the United States run as high as $79 billion a year in direct and indirect expenses, with 40 million physician visits annually because of chronically painful conditions.[1] Many of these costs are related to the disability process, including workers' compensation, litigation, personal indemnity, lost productivity, and Social Security Administration (SSA) payments. In the period from 1980 to 1994, there was a 73% increase in workers' compensation costs as a percentage of payrolls in the period from 1980 to 1994, and in the same period, the medical costs in compensation cases rose 1.5 times faster than did general health care costs in the United States.[2] Although from 1988 to 1996 the length of disability on workers' compensation decreased by 60.9% and the average cost per claim decreased by 41.4%, this probably reflects state policy changes with more aggressive case management.[3] Given that during this same period, applications for Supplemental Security Income (SSI) and Social Security Disability Insurance (SSDI) rose by more than 40% in 1992, one can assume that there may have been a shift from workers' compensation to federal compensation. Interestingly, pain was a factor in 40% to 60% of these SSA claims.[4] The reasons for this dramatic increase are multifactorial; increased social and vocational demands and change in work ethics may have contributed. Health care professionals themselves may be a significant cause of this change. In one study using the Health Care Providers' Pain and Impairment Relationship Scale (HC-PAIRS), community health care providers had much lower expectations regarding the functional performance of patients with chronic low back pain (LBP) than health care professionals who treated these patients with a functional restoration approach.[5] Perhaps we demand too little from our patients with chronic pain, therefore contributing to increased disability.

One question that is often raised is what distinguishes individuals with chronically painful conditions who are disabled from those who are not. Ideally, one would expect that there would be major differences in disease severity that could be assessed with the use of standard clinical methods. What is frustrating for many physicians dealing with the question of impairment and disability in chronic pain is that there are no generally accepted standards to assess these differences. The pain field lacks the tests and examination techniques that rise to the level of a gold standard to which all other clinical methods can be compared for validation. To illustrate the difficulty, it is all too common for a patient with severe congenital scoliosis who has undergone spinal fusion with instrumentation at multiple levels to have no pain and little in the way of functional limitations. Contrast this with another typical patient with a remote history of low back injury and minimal findings on examination and imaging studies who has, by self-report, severe disabling pain. Many of the instruments used to predict outcome that use the self-report of the patient in various domains of pain, function, and psychological distress have to be used with caution in a disability assessment, recognizing that "prediction of failure to return to work would be used as a predictor of certification of inability to work."[6]

We begin by analyzing the current definitions of impairment and disability and point out where these definitions break down when it comes to occult conditions such as chronic pain. We then present the advances that have been made in this field and propose a pragmatic, systematic approach to the functional evaluation of pain-impaired patients.

DEFINITIONS OF IMPAIRMENT, DISABILITY, AND HANDICAP

The terms *impairment*, *disability*, and *handicap* are commonly used in daily medical practice. Significant confusion, however, exists about the appropriate use of these terms. In addition to the well-known International Classification of Diseases (ICD), the World Health Organization (WHO) published the International Classification of Impairments, Disabilities, and Handicaps (ICIDH) in 1980.[7] Since that time, the WHO subsequently proposed a new International Classification of Function (ICF) model in 2001 to incorporate personal and environmental factors in the assessment and evaluation of disability (**Fig. 104-1**).

Because of dramatic demographic changes and technological advances, medical care in industrialized countries has had to address the increasing prevalence of chronic diseases, and this has led to a change from a disease- to an illness-consequence focus. This shift required an internationally accepted common language outside the traditional medical model to serve the needs of people with disabilities. It is no longer sufficient to record the occurrence of a disease and its consequences

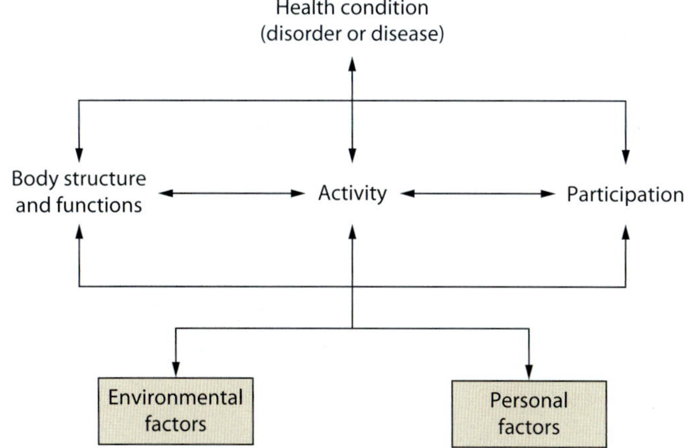

FIGURE 104-1. International Classification of Function model proposed by the World Health Organization in 2001 to incorporate personal and environmental factors in the assessment and evaluation of disability.

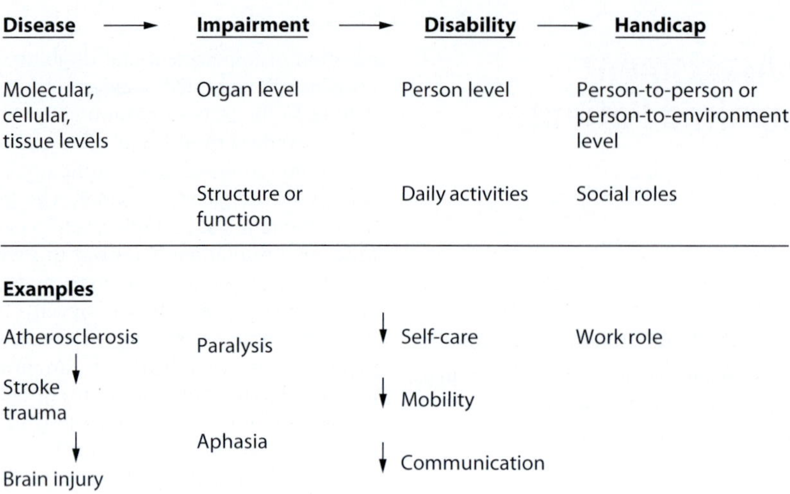

FIGURE 104-2. Schematic of the progression from a disease process to a disability and handicap.

solely in terms of complete recovery or death.[8] Many conditions, such as chronic pain, result in long-term functional limitations that are nonfatal and that call for a different theoretical framework. Since its introduction, the ICIDH has been a widely accepted framework for understanding the consequences of a disease for a person at the structural, individual, and societal level (**Fig. 104-2**).

Impairment is defined as "any loss or abnormality of psychological, physiological or anatomical structure or function." Examples of impairments are decreased range of motion (ROM) and loss of strength. Disability that results from an impairment is "any restriction or lack of ability to perform an activity in the manner or within the range considered normal for a human being" and is represented by activity limitations such as difficulties with community ambulation, inability to perform activities of daily living (ADLs), and disturbances in appropriate social behaviors. A handicap is caused by an impairment or disability that "limits or prevents the fulfillment of a role that is normal (depending on age, sex, and social and cultural factors) for that individual." For example, the inability to meet social obligations or fulfill occupational requirements may be a result of an impairment or disability.[9]

In summary, impairment is the result of an injury or disease at the level of the organ (e.g., decreased ROM or poor endurance), variables that can often be measured and compared for differences (**Fig. 104-3**).

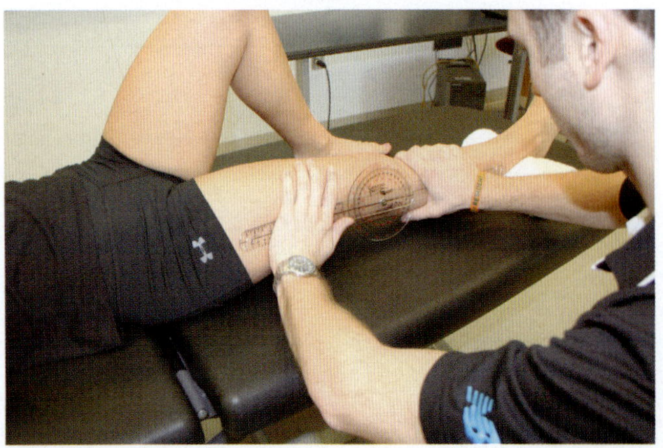

FIGURE 104-3. An example of impairment testing (range of motion of the knee).

Disability describes the possible effects of an impairment at the level of the individual such as the inability to walk or lift. A handicap characterizes the consequences of impairment and disability at the level of the environment and society, that is, the work role.

The new ICICH puts a greater emphasis on presenting a handicap as a description of the circumstances that people encounter because of the interaction between their impairment or disability and their physical and social environment. Disability is defined as an activity limitation rather than inability, and handicap as a participation restriction. One of the goals of the revised ICIDH is to provide a framework for functional diagnoses for persons with chronic limitations, similar to the medical diagnoses that constitute the ICD.[8] This is a concept that may be particularly helpful in addressing the problems of patients with chronic pain with occult impairments by focusing on the functional effects rather than the disease.

AMERICAN MEDICAL ASSOCIATION AND SOCIAL SECURITY ADMINISTRATION GUIDELINES

Although the goal of the ICIDH is the maximization of societal participation and improvement in the quality of life of people with disabilities and changes in social practices at the international level, the American Medical Association (AMA) uses impairment evaluations as a medicolegal tool to guide physicians to assess, report on, and communicate information about the impairments of human organ systems.[10] The purpose of the AMA evaluations is to estimate the severity of a person's impairment, for example, to assist in the settlement of workers' compensation cases, and therefore has entirely different implications than the ICIDH. Although the AMA definition of impairment closely parallels the WHO definition, one of the major criticisms of the AMA guidelines is that the rating of impairment is done in isolation without reference to the greater social context of potential disability and handicap. Physicians using the AMA guidelines determine impairment, but the matter of interest in medicolegal cases is disability or the patient's work capacity. Although the AMA guidelines recognize that an impaired individual is not necessarily disabled (i.e., a surgeon who loses his leg is impaired but not disabled from performing his or her job as a surgeon if fitted with an appropriate prosthesis), the impairment rating system breaks down when there is a paucity of impairments with severe disability such as is often seen in chronic pain states.

The SSA regulations define disability as an "inability to engage in any substantial gainful activity by reason of any medically determinable physical or mental impairment which can be expected to result in death or which has lasted or can be expected to last for a continuous period of not less than 12 months."[11] For the purposes of SSA, pain is a symptom, not an impairment, so it must be corroborated by medical signs or laboratory or imaging findings. In addition, chronic pain has been deemed not sufficient to demonstrate a mental impairment. As a result, what is assumed with the AMA guidelines is more overtly stated by the SSA, that disability is causally linked to impairment, and the greater the impairment found, the greater the disability.

An illustration of how the inference from impairment to disability can break down is well illustrated in the spinal cord injury (SCI) population. Up to 75% of SCI patients have chronic pain, with the intensity of pain being positively associated with greater disability, greater perceived stress, and lower measures of well-being. This is true despite the fact that greater pain intensity and disability in SCI have been shown to be negatively correlated with the degree of physical impairment as measured by accepted standards.[12]

We must keep in mind that disability determination is not in any straightforward way based solely on medical factors. Even from state to state, the environment in which disability is determined will vary markedly. For example, the court-determined percent disability for a man with LBP will vary on average from 9.4% in New Hampshire to 27% in Tennessee.[2] Ultimately, disability is inevitably tied to the incentives, values, and goals of both the patient and the society in which he or she lives.

CONTRADICTIONS OF DISABILITY DETERMINATION IN CHRONIC PAIN

As can be seen from the previous discussion, the current medical paradigm is not ideally suited for the assessment and determination of disability in patients with chronic pain. The problem is further complicated by the medicolegal construct, in which the identification of disability is meant to be static. Defining a certain level of disability may convey the message to the patient that the rehabilitation effort has ended and will be of no further benefit despite functional limitations that are quite effort-dependent in chronic pain conditions.[13] Identification of impairments with a level of disability may erroneously give the patient the idea that the disability is considered fixed and therefore will weaken the patient's motivation for recovery. Even in other catastrophic medical illnesses (e.g., stroke, myocardial infarction, and others), functional recovery, disability, and impairment are based both on the fixed lesions and on factors that are alterable, such as patient motivation, family support, cultural and environmental background, and the medical and social commitment of resources to rehabilitation. Hence, a disability determination may be countertherapeutic in a chronic pain patient if it negatively affects these alterable factors.

However, a disability rating that results in the settlement of a workers' compensation or a personal liability case may be necessary from a psychological point of view before a chronic pain patient gives his or her full effort to reach maximal functional improvement in a rehabilitation program. In this setting, secondary gain issues, whether conscious or unconscious, may be impeding the positive outcome of rehabilitation.[14]

In many cases, physicians end up sanctioning or reinforcing disability inappropriately, especially in cases in which the patient complains of pain and functional limitations and there has been a history of major pain-related surgery such as with *failed back syndrome*. This group of patients with chronic pain is at high risk for becoming disabled. The data are abysmal with high reoperation rates (17%–20% in an industrial setting) and low-return-to work rates (only 23%–43% return to work after disc surgery, and up to 51% of patients will still be on disability 3 years after spinal fusion). In this setting, physicians tend to "overmedicalize" the patient (repeat surgeries, overmedication, repeated invasive injection procedures) in an attempt to relieve pain because the pain report is generally believed, given the history of structural damage. This tends to lead the treating physician to sanction the reported disability of the patient because at least there is "objectively" something wrong with the patient's spine and none of the applied treatments have diminished the pain.[5] However, this inevitable path to permanent disability can be significantly reversed if the patient is given an aggressive functional restoration program that includes behavioral as well as physical treatment. The return-to-work rates for this group of *failed back* patients can be as high as 87% despite no change in the structural impairments.[15]

FUNCTIONAL ASSESSMENT METHODS IN PAIN PATIENTS

Disability assessment should be viewed as an attempt to determine the behavior or performance of an individual in a specific context.[16] Loss of a specific function such as the *inability* to bend to pick up a 15-lb box at work may coexist with the *ability* to bend and pick up a 30-lb, 3-year-old child. This functional dissonance can exist without conscious malingering because of the powerful differences between the absolute inability to perform a task and the inability to perform a certain task comfortably in a specific environmental context. This makes the differentiation of those who cannot work from those who do not want to work quite difficult. Pain is subjective and is influenced by environmental factors. Impairments and disabilities may fluctuate depending on the situation in which a chronic pain patient finds him- or herself.

A wide range of functional assessment methods are available, which vary from simple ROM measurements that can be easily performed in the office setting to sophisticated 2-day functional capacity evaluations (FCEs) that require expensive equipment and trained personnel. The most commonly used methods are pain measurement tools, functional assessments (by patient report or examination), psychological measurements, and information about the general health status. The use and combination of these different methods depends largely on the goal of the assessment. These goals may be a medicolegal disability rating in a workers' compensation case, identification of limitations to direct the patient to an appropriate therapy program, or for research purposes. **Table 104-1** gives an overview of the different categories and frequently used assessment methods in pain patients. The most widely used measurements are discussed in the following paragraphs. **Table 104-2** further shows some of the most frequently used pain questionnaires in the rehabilitative setting.

Moreover, in the physical therapy and rehabilitative setting, patients can be further classified by using the Childs Classification.

PAIN INTENSITY

Because pain is a multidimensional experience and is private and subjective in nature, it may be the most difficult measurement to perform in health assessment. Its results often do not follow the basic requirements of psychometric measurement, that is, reliability and validity. Pain measurement can capture two dimensions of the pain experience, namely, the sensory aspects of the pain and the person's emotional reaction to the pain. Although most clinical applications use fairly simple intensity scales, newer measurement methods are starting to evolve. Based on sensory decision theory, these methods attempt to distinguish the stimulus strength from the subjective response. It has been demonstrated, for example, that a placebo works as an analgesic primarily by reducing the respondent's tendency to label an experimental stimulus as "painful" rather than by altering the person's ability to feel it. Thus, the placebo seems to alter the affective response, not the perception of the stimulus.[17]

Most pain measurement methods can be divided into the following categories: pain questionnaires that record verbal or written responses to pain; behavioral measurements of pain that depend on observed pain behaviors of the subject; and analog methods, commonly used in laboratory studies, in which the respondent compares his or her pain with an experimentally induced pain stimulus of known intensity.[18] However, these different approaches measure different aspects of pain, and there appears to be little correlation among them.

TABLE 104-1 Categories and Examples of Commonly Used Assessment Methods in Pain Patients

Impairment Level
Pain Intensity
Visual analog scale
Verbal rating scale
Numerical rating scale
Pain drawing
Functional Tools
Standardized Assessment of Flexibility, Strength, Lifting, and Endurance
Psychological Measures
Minnesota Multiphasic Personality Inventory (MMPI)
Beck Depression Index (BDI)
Symptom Checklist 90 (SCL-90)
Illness Behavior Questionnaire (IBQ)
Pain Management Inventory (PMI)
Disability Level
Oswestry Low Back Pain Disability Questionnaire
Functional capacity evaluations
Medical Rehabilitation Follow Along
Pain Disability Index (PDI)
Waddell Disability Instrument
Multidimensional, General Health Status, and Quality-of-Life Measures
Short-Form Health Survey (SF-36)
Sickness Impact Profile (SIP)

The most commonly known and widely accepted questionnaires are the different subtypes of the visual analog pain rating scales. They provide a simple way to record a subjective estimation of pain intensity. Several types have been used, but the original scale, popularized by Huskisson, consisted of a straight line, 10 cm long, that represented the range of pain to be rated.[19] The visual analog scale (VAS) has been studied extensively, showing excellent reliability and adequate validity. In the comparison of different types of pain rating scales, it has been demonstrated that the numerical ratings are preferable to the verbal rating scales. For children and illiterate patients, a version showing faces is available. Overall, the VAS provides a robust, sensitive, and reproducible method of expressing pain severity that is applicable to a wide age range (children age 5 years and older to adults who are cognitively intact) and is easily applied in a clinical setting.

Melzack's McGill Pain Questionnaire (MPQ) is the most commonly used measurement to describe the diverse dimensions of pain. The MPQ was initially presented in 1975 as a preliminary method. However, the questionnaire continues to be used in its original form and is considered the gold standard against which other, newer instruments are compared.[18] An attempt to address three major dimensions of pain—sensory-discriminative, motivational-affective, and cognitive-evaluative—are represented on the MPQ. The complete MPQ includes the patient's history and diagnosis, drug regimen, and symptoms and the effects of pain on the patient. The most commonly used section, however, is the 102-word questionnaire in which the patient has to mark pain attributes (i.e., sharp, burning, lancinating, punishing), pain intensity, accompanying symptoms (i.e., headache, dizziness), sleep, food intake, activity, and time course. It also includes a dermatomal pain drawing.

Four different scoring methods have been described by Melzack. The reliability of the MPQ is only weak, and the validity is adequate. There have been considerable discussions about whether the selection and grouping of words reflects the dimensions he proposed.[20] Nevertheless, the importance of the MPQ is demonstrated by the incorporation of certain of its sections into several other scales and its use in many study protocols. The questionnaire takes about 15 to 20 minutes to administer and is therefore probably too long for a routine office visit, but it may be helpful for an initial evaluation.

FUNCTIONAL IMPAIRMENT

Limitations at the impairment level can be easily measured with the addition of a small number of functionally oriented examination techniques. Determining physical parameters such as ROM, strength, lifting, and endurance can be incorporated in routine office visits or evaluation protocols and enables numeric documentation of structural impairment. Waddell et al. studied the correlation between physical examination findings and self-reported disability in LBP patients, demonstrating that total lumbosacral flexion measured at the T12 to L1 interspace explained the greatest proportion of variance in disability scores compared with any other physical examination test performed to assess chronic LBP.[21] After impairments are identified, treatment can focus on improvement

TABLE 104-2 Self-reported Measures of Pain and Disability

Questionnaires	Reliability and Validity	Test Administration	Utility
Visual analog scale (VAS)		Patient makes a mark on a line to indicate pain level. Left is no pain, and right is worst pain ever experienced.	Measures pain intensity. According to Collins, on a 100-mm line, lines at 30 mm or more is moderate pain, and above 54 is severe pain.
Pain diagram	Highly reliable for locating patient's symptoms	Patient is given a body diagram on which to mark the area and type of pain.	Records location and type of pain.
Northwick Park Neck Pain Questionnaire (NPQ)	Shown to be valid for correlation with pain intensity	36 items on the test each scored on a 0 to 4 scale	Measures both perception of pain and disability from neck pain.
Patient Specific Functional Scale (PSFS)	Very high reliability; high specificity and sensitivity to change	Patient picks the most difficult activities and then rates their perceived level of dysfunction.	Great for clinical use because it allows clinician to evaluate individual patients over time.
Neck Disability Index (NDI)	High degree of validity and reliability and sensitive to change in population with neck pain	10 functional activities scored on a 0 to 5 scale	Good disability scale for patients with neck pain.
Tampa Scale for Kinesiophobia (TSK)	Has predictive and construct validity and high test–retest reliability	Questionnaire with 17 items, each scored on a 4-point scale	Assesses reinjury risk as well as fear of movement.
Fear Avoidance Beliefs Questionnaire (FABQ)	High test–retest reliability	Total of 16 items, 5 analyzing physical activities and 11 analyzing work activities	Quantifies fear with work and physical activities; often used in the low back pain population.

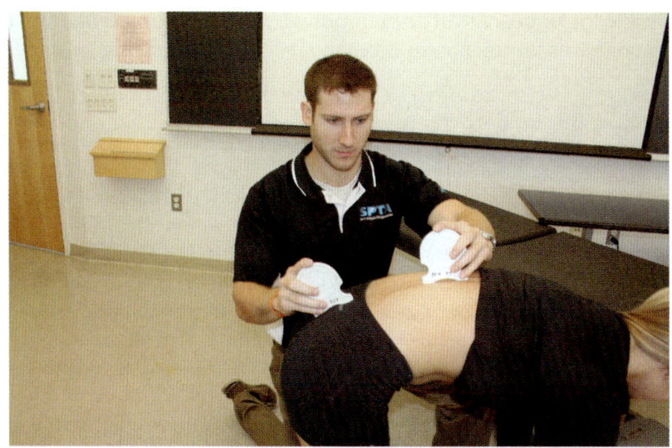

FIGURE 104-4. Demonstration of lumbosacral flexion using the inclinometer technique.

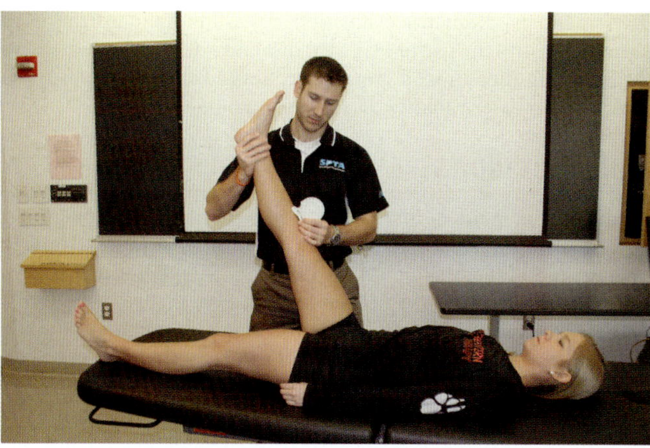

FIGURE 104-5. Demonstration of the straight-leg raise test using the inclinometer technique.

of these functions rather than pain reduction. This becomes increasingly important in patients with chronic pain, in whom a pain elimination treatment approach is rarely successful.

Inclinometer techniques have become increasingly popular (**Fig. 104-4**), especially in the physical assessment of patients with back pain, because these techniques are easy to apply.[22] They have become standard measurements in functional restoration programs for chronic back pain. Total lumbosacral flexion and extension can be assessed by placing a single inclinometer over the T12 to L1 spinous processes. Some also recommend using two-inclinometer technique over T12 and on the sacrum to get "true" lumbar flexion. Straight-leg raising can be tested by using the inclinometer placed on the tibial tuberosity (**Fig. 104-5**). Suggested normal ROM values for lumbosacral mobility are a minimum of 100 degrees of flexion and 25 degrees of extension, and for straight-leg raising, a minimum of 75 degrees. Recorded measurements can be documented on graphs for quick reference (**Fig. 104-6**). Initial measurements in pain patients are likely to be influenced by psychological issues as well as physical tolerances because patients may be inhibited by emotional distress, fear of injury, and pain. Therefore, although measurements may not represent true physiologic abilities, they still provide a numeric measure of the patient's psychophysical status and a meaningful starting point for treatment decisions.

The testing of strength, lifting, and endurance can be performed in a number of ways. None of the strength measure methods (isometric, isotonic, or isokinetic) is superior in this setting because all provide quantification of strength impairments. One relatively inexpensive method of lower back extension strength testing was developed using a standard back extension unit found in many fitness facilities.[23] The testing protocol determines the maximum amount of weight that a subject can lift for four repetitions. Testing weight is begun at 9 kg. The end points for the test are psychophysical (subjective maximum), form (poor performance), and safety (>120% of the body weight). Based on normative data, the trunk extensor strength for a nonimpaired person should be around 100% to 110% of ideal body weight.[23] Chronic back pain patients typically have an isometric extension strength that shows an approximate 50% reduction compared with nonimpaired persons. Although other measurements of impairments have been described in the literature, this method illustrates the basic concept that the effects of pain on physical performance rather than solely the pain intensity itself should be measured. Similar strategies should be adopted for other pain syndromes not related to the spine.

The role of FCEs has considerably increased over the past several years. They are used for work injury prevention and in rehabilitation to define an individual's functional abilities or limitations. When the patient is asked to perform a set of certain test activities, the individual's ability to meet the required work demands can be assessed. FCEs are increasingly used to determine a patient's ability to return to his or her workplace, for preemployment screening, for disability determinations, and to assist in determining case closure in medicolegal cases.[24] Although all systems share the common goal of attempting to measure work-related functional performance objectively, considerable differences in length

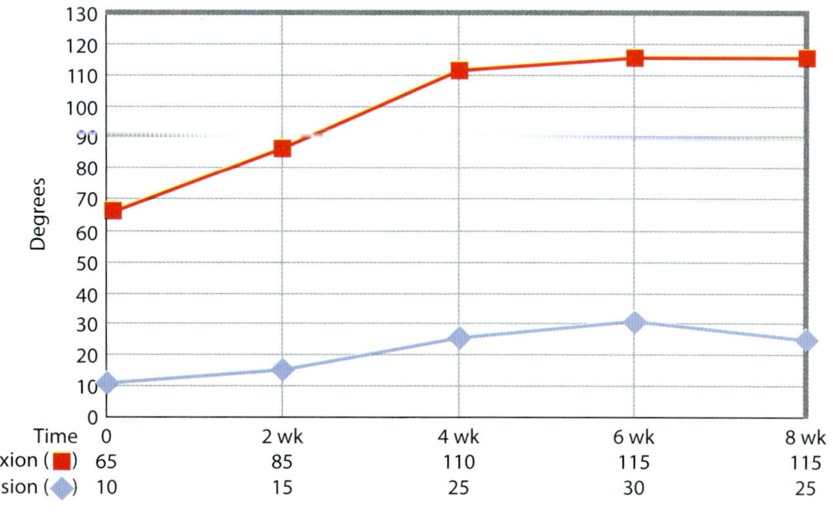

FIGURE 104-6. Graph for lumbosacral flexion and extension measured with the single-inclinometer technique.

of assessment, psychometric evaluation, costs, and standardization exist. Research to justify the use of FCEs for disability determination is sparse, and the testing measures of consistency should not be inappropriately used to make a determination of possible malingering.

DIAGNOSTIC STUDIES

There has been a marked increase in the use of diagnostic imaging over the past 10 years. Recent analysis of the data from the National Low Back Pain Study found that men receiving disability compensation were much more likely to have both computed tomography (CT)-myelogram and magnetic resonance imaging (MRI) performed compared with those with a comparable diagnosis who were not receiving compensation.[25] One possible explanation is that this overuse of imaging techniques in compensation patients is driven by the goal of finding a structural abnormality to justify the degree of reported disability because either imaging test alone would normally be sufficient to rule out serious injury or the need for surgery.

The perception that references to structural abnormalities necessarily increase objectivity in disability assessment is not supported by the literature. There is very poor correlation between objective structural deficits seen with various diagnostic studies and pain and functional loss. In a recent study of MRI findings of the lumbar spine in pain-free individuals, only 36% of asymptomatic individuals had a normal study.[26] Up to 70% of asymptomatic individuals have degenerative disc disease demonstrable on plain films.[27] The objective function of the spine, as measured by isokinetic trunk muscle strength for patients with chronic LBP, has been shown to be independent of the degree of degenerative changes seen on CT scans.[28] Conversely, the absence of findings on diagnostic testing of a patient with pain does not prove in any way that the pain syndrome lacks a physical cause. Numerous conditions have a paucity of objective findings on the diagnostic tests commonly available but nevertheless have accepted diagnostic criteria based on clinical examination techniques. Examples include myofascial pain, fibromyalgia, and complex regional pain syndromes. Should we then call all of these conditions *behavioral disorders* as has been recommended for nonspecific LBP by the International Association for the Study of Pain Task Force on Back Pain in the Workplace?[29]

Attempts to overcompensate for the lack of clear structural deviations in patients with chronic pain by excessive diagnostic testing to find something "objective" only reinforces illness behavior. Even when a test result is positive for some abnormality, the anatomic finding may have nothing to do with the functional losses observed, given the low specificity of most tests. Less common testing procedures such as thermograms and quantitative sensory testing are even less sensitive and specific and offer no help. In a survey of 80 pain specialist asked to rank the utility of various tests and procedures used to evaluate pain patients in order to develop a weighted ranking, the top seven ranked methods of evaluation were clinical examination procedures: examination of the nervous system, gait, spinal mobility, muscular function, soft tissue, and joint mobility were all ranked higher than any imaging or laboratory test.[30] The same authors have developed a total index of pathology (Medical Examination and Diagnostic Information Coding System, MEDICS) using 17 biomedical procedures commonly used to evaluate chronic pain conditions.

ILLNESS BEHAVIOR AND SECONDARY GAIN

The progression from acute to chronic pain can be viewed to occur in three stages[31]:

> Stage 1: Onset of pain produces an individual emotional reaction to pain.
>
> Stage 2: After pain persists more than 2 to 4 months, there is an increase in the emotional, behavioral, and physical maladaptation to the pain.

Preexisting psychosocial and socioeconomic factors may weigh heavily at this stage. Increased somatization and symptom magnification are probable for someone who is premorbidly hypochondriacal or who may have conscious or unconscious secondary gains from being disabled.

> Stage 3: Patient adopts a sick role and becomes accustomed to being relieved from normal responsibilities, social obligations, and financial responsibilities.

Attempts to develop a systematic approach to quantifying illness behavior in spine patients have been well established by Waddell (**Table 104-3**). This is further illustrated in **Table 104-4**.

A high Waddell score is defined as three of five positive signs, has been associated with poor performance on FCEs and poor outcomes in surgery, and is often used as an indication that a mental health consult is necessary. There is a less clear picture with regard to its prognostic relevance in determining degree of disability. A number of well-designed studies have shown that there was no predictive value in using the Waddell signs when looking at return to work, work retention, or posttreatment health care utilization after an intensive functional restoration program.[32] Others have found some utility in using the Waddell scores in screening of those who will do well in an intensive work-hardening rehabilitation program that did not have a behavioral treatment component.[33]

Does compensation status influence disability in pain patients? **Table 104-5** illustrates some of the socioeconomic factors that are predictive of disability. The majority of well-designed studies have demonstrated that patients receiving or seeking financial compensation exhibit greater levels of psychological distress and depression, higher levels of pain severity, and perceived disability.[14,34,35] In these studies, pain severity and perceived loss of function were independent of physical impairments. Is this all due then to problems of conscious secondary gain? Arguing against this is that these factors do not tend to be predictive of subsequent employment or health care utilization in prospective studies in which an appropriate rehabilitation intervention has been applied.[36] After the rehabilitation process, measures such as improved strength and ROM were correlated with reduced levels of pain and depression in both the compensation and noncompensation groups. In general, a traumatic onset of pain and lack of employment have been associated with higher levels of emotional distress and perceived disability and probably play an independent role in compensation cases.

TABLE 104-3 Waddell's Assessment Tools for Illness Behavior and Exaggerated Symptoms

Assessment Methods	Normal Illness Behavior	Abnormal Illness Behavior
Pain Drawing	Localized with appropriate neuroanatomic features	Magnified, covering diffuse regions of body
Pain Adjectives	Sensory	Affective, evaluative
Symptoms		
Pain	Localized	Whole-leg pain
Numbness	Dermatomal	Whole leg
Weakness	Myotomal	Whole leg giving away
Time pattern	Varies with time	Never free of pain
Response to treatment	Variable benefit	Intolerance of treatments, frequent emergency department visits
Signs		
Tenderness	Localized	Superficial, nonanatomic
Axial loading	No lumbar pain	Lumbar pain
Straight-leg raise	Limited on distraction	Improves with distraction
Sensory	Dermatomal	Regional
Motor	Myotomal	Jerky, give away weakness
Tenderness	Appropriate pain	Overreaction

TABLE 104-4 Waddell's Signs

Type of Nonorganic Signs	Nonorganic Sign	Description
Tenderness		Tenderness not related to a particular skeletal or neuromuscular structure; may be either superficial or nonanatomic.
	Superficial	The skin in the lumbar region is tender to light pinch over a wide area not associated with the distribution of a posterior primary ramus.
	Nonanatomic	Deep tenderness, which is not localized to one structure, is felt over a wide area and often extends to the thoracic spine, sacrum, or pelvis.
Stimulation tests		These tests give the patient the impression that a particular examination is being carried out when in fact it is not.
	Axial loading	Low back pain is reported when the examiner presses down on the top of the patient's head; neck pain is common and should not be indicative of nonorganic sign.
	Rotation	Back pain is reported when the shoulders and pelvis are passively rotated in the same plane as the patient stands relaxed with the feet together; in the presence of root irritation, leg pain may be produced and should not be considered indicative of a nonorganic sign.
Distraction tests		A positive physical finding is demonstrated in the routine manner, and this finding is then checked while the patient's attention is distracted; a nonorganic component may be present if the finding disappears when the patient is distracted.
	Straight-leg raising	The examiner lifts the patient's foot as when testing the plantar reflex in the sitting position; a nonorganic component may be present if the leg is lifted higher than when tested in the supine position.
Regional disturbances		Dysfunction (e.g., sensory, motor) involving a widespread region of body parts in a manner that cannot be explained based on anatomy; care must be taken to distinguish from multiple nerve root involvement.
	Weakness	Demonstrated on testing by a partial cogwheel "giving way" of many muscle groups that cannot be explained on a localized neurologic basis.
	Sensory	Include diminished sensation to light touch pinprick or other neurologic tests fitting a "stocking" rather than a dermatomal pattern.
Overreaction		May take the form of disproportionate verbalization, facial expression, muscle tension and tremor, collapsing, or sweating; judgments should be made with caution, minimizing the examiner's own emotional reaction.

Waddell G, McCulloch JA, Kummel E, Venner RM. Nonorganic physical signs in low-back pain. *Spine.* 1980; 5:117-125.

Unfortunately, both Waddell signs and questions of increased emotional distress with exaggerated ratings of pain severity and disability have been attributed to malingering or conscious secondary gain. This is not, however, a medical determination and is better left to a court of law. Ultimately, short of a surveillance videotape, we must rely on patient reports of pain and dysfunction and cannot make determinations of conscious falsification of the data based on observed pain behaviors or seemingly exaggerated complaints. Fishbain et al. point out that the concept of secondary gain is confused in any case and does not help distinguish true physical pathology from purely psychological pathology because both can have secondary gain issues.[37] The reality is that many of the secondary gains, conscious or not, are more than compensated for by the secondary losses related to chronic pain and thus the lack of utility in using this concept for predicting disability outcome. This is demonstrated by ample case experiences of patients whose cases are finally settled and who will still exhibit continued heightened pain behaviors and signs of emotional distress if not treated for their pain issues. Multiple signs on Waddell testing by Waddell's own analysis are not a test of credibility or malingering but rather indicate the need for further psychological assessment.[38]

TABLE 104-5 Data from National Health and Nutrition Epidemiologic Survey of 5202 Disabled Persons Age 24 to 70 Years[52]

Factors Associated with Disability	Comments
Demographic	
Age 55–65 years	Sharp rise in prevalence in age group from 45–55 years
Low income	Disability four times higher in <$7000/y group than in >$25,000 income group
Limited education	Highest rates with maximum 8 years of education, five times that of college educated
Widowed or divorced	Married individuals with lowest rates of disability
Socioeconomic	
Adverse work environment	Employees exposed to unpleasant conditions are two times as likely to be disabled

Data from Cats-Baril WL, Frymoyer JW. Demographic factors associated with the prevalence of disability in the general population: analysis of the NHANES I database. *Spine,* 1991;16:671-674.

PSYCHOLOGICAL ASSESSMENT

It is well accepted that a number of psychosocial factors contribute to poor functional outcomes in pain. These include attitudes, beliefs, cultural norms, mood, focus of attention, motivation, and personality traits. Although most patients with chronic pain are depressed and anxious, they seldom have a history of long-standing psychiatric problems. Rather, most of their symptoms reflect their current condition. Although patients with chronic pain may exhibit certain personality traits that potentially contribute to their inability to cope with a chronic condition, rarely are these traits suggestive of significant psychopathology.[39] Certain psychosocial risk factors have been identified that are more likely to result in poor treatment outcomes and the development of disabling pain if left untreated (**Table 104-6**). In New Zealand, comprehensive guidelines for the treatment of LBP were designed to assist health care professionals in recognizing these patients early and to ensure timely mental health referrals (**Table 104-7**).[47]

Nevertheless, the role of psychological assessment is still poorly understood by many pain specialists. The traditional notion that the lack of an easily identifiable physical or "organic" cause of pain implies that the pain must be psychogenic or "nonorganic" and deserves a mental health referral is erroneous logic. This type of faulty reasoning does the patient and society a disservice at many levels. Embracing such a dualistic view of the body in which there is an attempt to compartmentalize the painful sensations reported by a patient into either the body or the mind is wrong both philosophically as well as physiologically and therapeutically. The perception and interpretation of pain is just as important as the nociceptive input. The notion that we can come to a firm conclusion about the objective origins of a pain experience based on diagnostic testing, examination, and various diagnostic and therapeutic invasive treatments is not founded on science.[26,48] That a patient does not respond

TABLE 104-6 Factors Shown to Influence Poor Disability Outcome in Low Back Pain and Rheumatoid Arthritis

Domain (Study Reference)	External Factors	Internal Factors
Socioeconomic		
LBP (Cats-Baril[40])	Physical demands of job (heavy labor vs. sedentary)	Perception of compensable nature of injury
	Occupation	Job satisfaction or unpleasantness
	Benefits policy	Perception of fault
	Educational level	
	Past hospitalizations	
LBP (Lehmann[41])	Litigation status	
	Workers' compensation case status	
LBP (Gatchel[42])	Female	
	Workers' compensation or personal injury case status	
RA (Wolfe[43])	Education level	
Psychosocial		
LBP (Gatchel[42])		Pain severity
		Perceived disability
LBP (Dionne[44])		Somatization
		Depression
LBP (Sanders[45])	Low activity	Elevated hysteria
	Elevated pain behavior	Negative beliefs about pain and activity
		Depression
Upper extremity pain (Burton[46])	Previous history of psychopathology	Depressed mood
	Previous history of substance abuse	Pain severity
	Anxiety or borderline disorder	Perceived disability
	History of child abuse	
RA (Wolfe[43])		Perceived disability
		Pain severity

to treatment as expected often means we have not taken into sufficient account the myriad of psychosocial, socioeconomic, and physical factors that are influencing the patient's pain experience. The presence of emotional distress, anxiety, depression, and anger is often present in the chronic pain state, even in the absence of work disability, and does not signify the absence of nociceptive input. Functionally oriented treatment of patients with chronic pain even with elevated scores of hypochondriasis, depression, and hysteria as measured by the Minnesota Multiphasic Personality Inventory has been shown to be successful, and typically the posttreatment scores on these three scales drop significantly.[49] This indicates that it is not a fixed personality trait that predisposes patients to chronic pain but the pain itself that may underlie the emotional distress.

The value of a systematic psychological assessment is to try to determine the factors that, if left untreated, will ultimately lead to prolonged loss of function and disability. In a study of pain severity by Von Korff,[50] four grades of disability scores were developed from a population survey of a large health maintenance organization in Washington State:

Grade I: low disability score, low pain intensity score

Grade II: low disability score, high pain intensity score

Grade III: moderately limiting, high disability score

Grade IV: severely limiting, high disability score

The disability score was based on days missed from work over a 6-month period, and degree of limitation and pain severity were determined by self-report. Pain severity was not included in the grading of grades III and IV because these individuals uniformly reported elevated pain intensity. What is of interest is knowing what the differences were among individuals in the transition from grade II to III. These groups by definition had significant differences in degree of disability (3 days off work vs. on average 23 days off work in past 6 months) but no discernible differences in pain scores, persistence of pain, or recency of onset of pain. The largest differences turned on behavioral variables such as reported functional limitations, unemployment status, and health care utilization rather than differences in psychological variables such as depression and health status. Grade IV patients did show significantly higher levels of depression.[50] This suggests a gradient of dysfunction in chronic pain, in which many individuals may be disabled because of nonadaptive reinforcing patterns of behavior rather than overt emotional distress or psychological impairment. Psychological referral is appropriate both in cases of overt psychopathology and when the problem is more due to dysfunctional patterns of illness behavior.

TABLE 104-7 Psychosocial Risk Factors for Chronic Back Pain

- Maladaptive attitudes and beliefs concerning back pain
- Frequent display of pain behaviors
- Reinforcement of pain behavior by family members
- Heightened emotional reactivity
- Lack of social support
- Job dissatisfaction
- Compensation issues

Data from National Advisory Committee on Health and Disability. *Guide to Assessing Yellow Flags in Acute Low Back Pain*. Wellington, NZ: Ministry of Health; 1997.

BASIC SET OF INFORMATION FOR DISABILITY EVALUATION

In clinical practice, a screening method to quantify the three important areas of physical functioning, pain, and psychoaffective well-being is needed. A quick overview of these three areas could help the clinician in prescribing therapies for problems that most significantly affect the patient based on the degree of disability found. One approach, based on Internet technology, is the Medical Rehabilitation Follow Along (MRFA). This interactive tool has been designed to assist in patient screening, resource allocation, and outcome assessment for pain patients in the outpatient setting. The MRFA was developed by using major concepts from the Functional Assessment Screening Questionnaire, the Oswestry Scale, the short form of the McGill Pain Questionnaire, and the Brief Symptom Inventory.[51]

The administration of the self-report questionnaire takes approximately 15 minutes, and it can be filled out before every office visit. The scores of eight subcategories are summarized in the areas of physical functioning, pain experience, driving, and affective well-being. With the use of computer technology, the results are available to the treating physician within minutes. This allows the physician to tailor the treatment plan according to the results. The patient's profile can be compared with that of other patients from the database, especially during follow-up visits when the effectiveness of a therapy plan is assessed. Differences from a "normal" recovery process are recognized immediately, allowing immediate changes in the treatment strategies. This may permit identification of problematic patients early on in the recovery process, allowing intervention before disability develops from chronic pain.

Another strategy was developed as part of the recognition by the SSA of the growing problem with pain-related disability. The Commission on the Evaluation of Pain was formed, and together with the Institute of Medicine, a predictive tool was developed called the Multiperspective Multidimensional Pain Assessment Protocol (MMPAP). Similar to the MRFA, the MMPAP combines a number of recognized instruments (the McGill Pain Questionnaire, the Multidimensional Pain Inventory, and the Oswestry Pain Inventory) together with a structured functional assessment by the examining physician to rate patient's pain behavior, medical status, and rehabilitation potential. The MMPAP has been tested and validated with good interrater reliability when rehabilitation medicine specialists were given training in the use of the tool. Findings support that the individual's ability to adapt or cope with pain is a significant determinant of disability. The analysis also indicates that functionally oriented physician assessments can be predictive of future disability risk if the physicians are properly trained (**Table 104-8**).[4]

TABLE 104-8 From Analysis of Social Security Administration Applicants' Subsequent Employment and Pain Status Using Data from the Multiperspective Multidimensional Pain Assessment Protocol

	Assessed by Physician	Patient Report
Predictive Factors		
Subsequent employment status		
Frequency of pain	+	+
Degree to which patient verbalizes about pain	+	+
Length of pain-free periods		+
Unpleasantness of pain when severe		+
Hopelessness, depression		+
States: "Will never work again"		+
Difficulty with relationship with significant other		+
Gait abnormalities	+	
Joint deformities	+	
Functional limitations with ADLs	+	
Perception that FCE would require extreme effort	+	
Estimation of level of treatment needed	+	
Subsequent pain intensity		
Functional limitations with ADLs	+	+
Estimation of level of treatment needed	+	
Perception that pain complaints were exaggerated	+	
Nonpredictive Factors		
Subsequent employment status		
Functional limitations with ADLs		+
Social support network		+
Subsequent pain intensity		
Pain intensity		+
Unpleasantness of pain		+
Depression, hopelessness		+
Social support network		+

FCE, functional capacity evaluation; MMAP, Multiperspective Multidimensional Pain Assessment Protocol.

From Rucker KS, Metzler HM. Predicting subsequent employment status of SSA disability applicants with chronic pain. *Clin J Pain*. 1995;11:22-35.

CONCLUSION

Recent estimates reported in *Business Week* (March 1, 1999) of the costs for the treatment of pain are now rising to $100 billion a year in the United States with 515 million work days lost each year. In 2014, Congress voted to allocate $102 million to the National Institutes of Health for pain research, a 15% jump from the prior year. Despite this, chronic pain continues to grow, and as physicians, we must shift our attention from trying to *cure* these patients to finding ways of limiting loss of function and disability. To do this, the complex multidimensional nature of pain must be accepted as part of the territory. Physical, psychosocial, and socioeconomic factors must be included in the assessment to avoid being more a part of the problem than a part of the solution. We end by offering a minimal guide to the four domains of assessment that should be included in any pain evaluation (**Table 104-9**).

TABLE 104-9 Basic Contents of a Pain Evaluation

1. Pain-Related Medical History
   - Description of pain localization, quality, intensity, time course
   - Medications (past and current)
   - Diagnostic procedures
   - Therapies
   - Procedures
   - Surgeries
   - History of similar pain problems
   - Ever pain free?
   - Pain improved by
   - Pain worsened by
   - Pain drawing
   - Visual analog scale
2. Functional and Occupational History
   - Occupation
   - Education
   - Level of physical activity before onset of pain
   - Current level of activity: difficulties with:
     - Personal care (washing, dressing)
     - Lifting real life objects (groceries, small children)
     - Walking distance
     - Sitting time
     - Standing time
     - Traveling
   - Work-related or traumatic accident?
   - Job satisfaction?
   - Could you do your last job today?
   - If not, what type of jobs could you do now?
3. Psychosocial History
   - Marital status
   - Who lives with you?
   - Current social activity level (or desired level)
   - Primary social role (i.e., work, education, homemaking)
   - Current social role activity level (or desired level)
   - History of childhood abuse, family dysfunction
   - Depressive, anxious symptoms
   - History of psychological or psychiatric problems
   - Pain-related fears
   - Financial problems
   - General life satisfaction?
4. Physical Examination
   - General medical examination
   - Neurologic examination
   - Musculoskeletal examination, including assessment of muscular function (tone, mass, strength), joint motion, and soft tissue
   - Gait
   - Spinal mobility using inclinometer technique (or similar)
   - Dynamic strength examination (e.g., lifting of several predetermined weights)
   - Waddell signs (axial loading, straight-leg raise, sensory, motor, tenderness)

REFERENCES

1. Bonica JJ. General considerations of chronic pain. In: Bonica JJ, ed. *The Management of Pain*. Vol 1. Philadelphia: Lea & Febiger; 1990.
2. Durbin D. Workplace injuries and the role of insurance: claims costs, outcomes, and incentive. *Clin Orthop Rel Res*. 1997;336:18-32.
3. Hashemi L, Webster BS, Clancy EA. Trends in disability duration and cost of workers' compensation low back pain claims (1988–1996). *J Occup Environ Med*. 1998;40:1110-1119.
4. Rucker KS, Metzler HM. Predicting subsequent employment status of SSA disability applicants with chronic pain. *Clin J Pain*. 1995;11:22-35.
5. Rainville J, Bagnall D, Phalen L. Health care providers' attitudes and beliefs about functional impairments and chronic back pain. *Clin J Pain*. 1995;11:287-295.
6. Carey TS. Disability: how successful are we in determining disability? *Neurol Clin North Am*. 1999;17(1):167-178.
7. World Health Organization. *International Classification of Impairments, Disabilities, and Handicaps*. Geneva, Switzerland: WHO; 1980, 1993.
8. Thuriaux MC. The ICIDH: evolution, status and prospects. *Disabil Rehabil*. 1995;17:112-118.
9. deKleijn-deVrankrijker MW. The International Classification of Impairments, Disabilities, and Handicaps (ICIDH): perspectives and developments (Part 1). *Disabil Rehabil*. 1995;17:109-111.
10. *Guides to the Evaluation of Permanent Impairment*. 4th ed. Chicago: American Medical Association; 1995.
11. Social Security Act 42 USC, Section 423 as amended by Social Security Disability Reform Act of 1984, PL 98-460.
12. Rintala DH, Loubser PG, Castro J, et al. Chronic pain in a community-based sample of men with spinal cord injury: prevalence, severity, and relationship with impairment, disability, handicap, and subjective well-being. *Arch Phys Med Rehabil*. 1998;79:604-614.
13. Sullivan MD, Loeser J. The diagnosis of disability: treating and rating disability in a pain clinic. *Arch Intern Med*. 1992;152:1829-1835.
14. Rainville J, Sobel JB, Hartigan C, et al. The effect of compensation involvement on the reporting of pain and disability by patients referred for rehabilitation of chronic low back pain. *Spine*. 1997;22:2016-2024.
15. Mayer TG, McMahon MJ, Gatchel RJ, et al. Socioeconomic outcomes of combined spine surgery and functional restoration in workers' compensation spinal disorders with matched controls. *Spine*. 1998;23:598-605.
16. Fordyce WE. On the nature of illness and disability: an editorial. *Clin Orthrop Rel Res*. 1997;336:47-51.
17. Clark WC, Yang JC. Application of sensory decision theory to problems in laboratory and clinical pain. In: Melzack R, ed. *Pain Measurement and Assessment*. New York: Raven Press; 1983:15-25.
18. McDowell I, Newell C. *Measuring Health: A Guide to Rating Scales and Questionnaires*. 2nd ed. New York: Oxford University Press; 1996.
19. Huskisson EC. Measurement of pain. *J Rheumatol*. 1982;9:768-769.
20. Turk DC, Rudy TE, Salovey P. The McGill Pain Questionnaire reconsidered: confirming the factor structure and examining appropriate uses. *Pain*. 1985;21:385-397.
21. Waddell G, Somerville D, Henderson I, Newton M. Objective clinical evaluation of physical impairment in chronic low back pain. *Spine*. 1992;17:617-628.
22. Rainville J, Sobel JB, Hartigan C. Comparison of total lumbosacral flexion and true lumbar flexion measured by a dual inclinometer technique. *Spine*. 1994;19:2698-2701.
23. Rainville J, Sobel JB, Hartigan C, et al. Decreasing disability in chronic back pain through aggressive spine rehabilitation. *J Rehabil Res Dev*. 1997;34:383-393.
24. King PM, Tuckwell N, Barrett TE. A critical review of functional capacity evaluations. *Phys Ther*. 1998;78:852-866.
25. Ackerman SJ, Steinberg EP, et al. Patient characteristics associated with diagnostic imaging evaluation of persistent low back problems. *Spine*. 1997;22:1634-1641.
26. Jenson MC, Brandt-Zawadzki MN, et al. Magnetic resonance imaging of the lumbar spine in people without back pain. *N Engl J Med*. 1994;331:69-73.
27. Hadler NM. Regional musculoskeletal diseases of the low back. *Clin Orthop*. 1987;221:33-41.
28. Keller A, Johansen JG, Hellesnes J, Brox JI. Predictors of isokinetic back muscle strength in patients with low back pain. *Spine*. 1999;24:275-280.
29. Teasell RW, Merskey H. Chronic pain disability in the workplace. *Pain Forum*. 1997;6(4):228-238.
30. Rudy TE, Turk DC, Brena SF, et al. Quantification of biomedical findings of chronic patients: development of and index of pathology. *Pain*. 1990;42:167-182.
31. Gatchel RJ, Gardea MA. Psychosocial issues: their importance in predicting disability, response to treatment, and search for compensation. *Neurol Clin North Am*. 1999;17(1):149-166.
32. Polatin PB, Cox B, Gatchel RJ, Mayer TG. A prospective study of Waddell signs in patients with chronic low back pain: when they may not be predictive. *Spine*. 1997;22:1618-1621.
33. Werneke M, Harris D, Lichter R. Clinical effectiveness of behavioral signs for screening chronic low-back pain patients in a work-oriented physical rehabilitation program. *Spine*. 1993;18:2412-2418.
34. Cassisi, JE, Sypert GW, Laganá L, et al. Pain, disability, and psychological functioning in chronic low back pain subgroups: myofascial versus herniated disc syndrome. *Neurosurgery*. 1993;33:379-385.
35. Turk DC, Okifuji A. Perception of traumatic onset, compensation status and physical findings: impact on pain severity, emotional distress, and disability in chronic pain patients. *J Behav Med*. 1996;19:435-453.
36. Wright A, Mayer TG, Gatchel RJ. Outcomes of disabling cervical spine disorders in compensation injuries: A prospective comparison to tertiary rehabilitation response for chronic lumbar spine disorders. *Spine*. 1999;15:178-183.
37. Fishbain DA, Rosomoff HL, Cutler RB, et al. Secondary gain concept: a review of the scientific evidence. *Clin J Pain*. 1995;11:6-21.
38. Main CJ, Waddell G. Behavioral responses to examination: A reappraisal of the interpretation of "nonorganic signs." *Spine*. 1998;23:2367-2371.
39. Jamison RN. Psychological factors in chronic pain: assessment and treatment issues. *J Back Musculoskel Rehabil*. 1996;7:79-95.
40. Cats-Baril WL, Frymoyer JW. Identifying patients at risk of becoming disabled because of low-back pain: The Vermont Rehabilitation Engineering Center predictive model. *Spine*. 1991;16:671-674.
41. Lehmann TR, Spratt KF, Lehmann KK. Predicting long-term disability in low back injured workers presenting to a spine consultant. *Spine*. 1993;18:1103-1112.
42. Gatchel RJ, Polatin PB, Mayer TG. The dominant role of psychosocial risk factors in the development of chronic low back disability. *Spine*. 1995;20:2702-2709.
43. Wolfe F, Hawley DJ. The longterm outcomes of rheumatoid arthritis: work disability: a prospective 18 year study of 823 patients. *J Rheumatol*. 1998;25:2108-2117.
44. Dionne CE, Koepsell TD, Von Korff M, et al. Predicting long-term functional limitations among back pain patients in primary care settings. *J Clin Epidemiol*. 1997;50:31-43.

45. Sanders SH. Risk factors for the occurrence of low back pain and chronic disability. *Am Pain Soc Bull.* 1995;5:1-5.

46. Burton K, Polatin PB, Gatchel RJ. Psychosocial factors and the rehabilitation of patients with chronic work-related upper extremity disorders. *J Occup Rehabil.* 1997;7;139-153.

47. National Advisory Committee on Health and Disability. *Guide to Assessing Yellow Flags in Acute Low Back Pain.* Wellington, New Zealand: Ministry of Health; 1997.

48. North RB, Kidd DH, Zahurak M, Piantadosi S. Specificity of diagnostic nerve blocks: a prospective, randomized study of sciatica due to lumbosacral spine disease. *Pain.* 1996;65:77-85.

49. Barnes D, Gatchel RJ, Mayer TG, et al. Changes in MMPI profiles of chronic low back pain patients following successful treatment. *J Spinal Disord.* 1990;3:353-355.

50. Von Korff M, Ormel J, Keefe FJ, Dworkin SF. Grading the severity of chronic pain. *Pain.* 1992;50:133-149.

51. Baker JG, Granger CV, Ottenbacher KJ. Validity of a brief outpatient functional assessment measure. *Am J Phys Med Rehabil.* 1996;75:356-363.

52. Cats-Baril WL, Frymoyer JW. Demographic factors associated with the prevalence of disability in the general population: analysis of the NHANES I database. *Spine.* 1991;16:671-674.

Ethical Issues and Problems of Physician Trust in the Chronic Pain Patient

Steven H. Richeimer
Faye M. Weinstein
Lisa Victor

INTRODUCTION

The focus of the ethics literature regarding pain management has shifted from issues related to the treatment of patients experiencing terminal pain to the concept of pain management as a human right[1] for patients with nonmalignant pain. International, federal, and state initiatives; new guidelines and standards; and numerous studies that document the high costs of chronic pain have fueled this attention to untreated or undertreated pain in nonterminal patients. Thus, the new ethical pressure to provide pain medication to patients with nonmalignant pain may be experienced by physicians as putting them in legal jeopardy. This is complicated further by Hall and Boswell's[1] assertion that there is no clear legal or ethical basis for pain management as a right; others conclude that failure to treat pain is a breach of human rights.[2] Hellman[3] examines whether trusting patients even constitutes a legitimate and accepted medical practice, although she provides a compelling argument that doctors can be morally justified in trusting patients' reports of pain.

Crucial to the physician's ability to practice ethically in the current environment[2] is for the physician to be able to trust the patient. The two areas of trust that are needed are in the patient's self-report of pain level and in the patient's reporting of judicious use of pain medication.

In this chapter, we describe some of these ethical dilemmas and examine the underlying problems with physician trust in the patient with chronic pain. We then propose how a reconceptualization of pain clinic treatment systems might serve to diminish some of the ethical dilemmas in relation to the emerging standard of the human right for pain management.

Legal and ethical considerations relate not only to the concept of pain management as a right but also to the interactions between the patient and the doctor. Although the literature and research dealing with rights versus ethics is both thoughtful and influential, there is a remarkable void of attention on the common ethical and relationship issues that arise on a daily basis with the care of patients with chronic nonmalignant pain. An exception to this is literature about the patient–provider relationship that has largely focused on provider issues and the trust that patients have in their doctors. Patient trust in a physician has been identified as the expectation that the physician will behave in a way that allows the patient to take the risk of sharing personal information, and it can be a predictor of adherence, satisfaction with care, and health improvement.[4,5] Educational modules and standards are available for doctors to help promote trust, and several trust scales have been developed to assess the trust that patients have in their physicians.[6]

In contrast, consideration of the doctor's trust in the patient tends not to receive much of our attention;[7] however, the problems are real and common. Researchers have identified that physicians' trust in a patient stems from factors external to the patient, such as media events, racial bias, the practices of colleagues, and their own experiences.[8] This chapter focuses on the physician trust of the patient with chronic pain for the purpose of starting to identify the nature of underlying problems and to institute systems to minimize their frequency.

The following cases do not represent single individuals but composites of several. After reviewing a case history, we examine the ethical issues and later develop a methodology for building trust. We then apply this methodology to additional cases.

We have used a case-study format for discussion because it is common practice in both medical and ethics education and best affords the reader concrete examples of potential clinical and ethical dilemmas.

BACKGROUND

Ethical deliberation usually consists of the application of basic ethical *theories* that support and guide ethical decision making. Such philosophical theories, or models of deliberation, provide different approaches for analyzing basic ethical *principles* and how such principles are to be judged in relation to others. English[9] states that "an ethical theory attempts to achieve a general applicability to considerations of moral behavior, with as few exceptions as possible. Important characteristics of a theory include universalizability, comprehensiveness, and consistency." Because this is a chapter devoted to ethical issues in chronic pain management, readers should be aware of the relevant and predominant ethical theories that exist to guide them in ethical analysis. Of the three theories subsequently listed[10] (there are many more), we have adopted a more casuist approach for this chapter.

UTILITARIANISM

Utilitarianism, identified most closely with Jeremy Bentham (1748–1832) and John Stuart Mill (1806–1873), is the theory whereby the rightness of an act is judged by its ability to bring about the greatest good or benefit. Therefore, utilitarians judge actions by their consequences. In medicine, a physician is to maximize the benefits to his or her patients while minimizing the burdens of treatment.

DEONTOLOGY

Deontology is the study of duties that persons have toward one another. The most prominent of the classic deontologic theories is that developed by Immanuel Kant (1724–1804). Considered duty-based as opposed to action-based utilitarians, deontologists judge actions by the intent behind them instead of their consequences (however, consequences can be taken into account in decision making).

CASUISTRY

Casuistry was an influential ethical theory in medieval and early modern philosophy. "Rather than concentrate on rules and general principles that may be applied to specific cases, casuists insist that moral judgment must emerge from particular cases, or better still, from experience with a number of cases that can be compared to one another in various ways." Casuists regard ethics as a set of practices that arise from human moral experience.[8]

As mentioned earlier, there are many methodologies for analyzing clinical ethical dilemmas. Fins[11] and Loewy[12] have argued persuasively that a problem-solving approach—similar to developing a medical diagnosis and treatment plan—is more useful than the application of predetermined ethical principles. Their arguments apply primarily to the approach to each individual clinical-ethical problem. However, when examining a group of problems in an effort to search for common themes and possible solutions, it may still be useful to apply the template or framework of primary ethical principles. Most clinical ethical dilemmas involve a conflict between or among two or more of the following basic or primary ethical principles:

1. Respect for persons, which includes respect for the autonomy, or self-determination, of the patient and the need to protect patients with diminished autonomy
2. Beneficence, which includes the obligation to maximize possible benefits while minimizing the risks and the requirement to do no harm (nonmaleficence)
3. Justice, which includes the need to provide fair access to medical care and fair allocation of scarce resources[11]

Solutions to such dilemmas begin with a basic understanding of these concepts and the clinician's ability to incorporate these principles into his or her everyday clinical practice.

CASE EXAMPLES

CASE 1

A 41-year-old man is seen for a 3-month history of complex regional pain syndrome (CRPS, also known as reflex sympathetic dystrophy) of his left foot. He reports debilitating pain. Examination reveals classic features of CRPS, including severe allodynia. The patient's past medical history is significant for heroin abuse. He has not abused any drugs for the past year. For the past 2 months, his primary care physician has prescribed acetaminophen with codeine (30 mg), one tablet three times per day. The patient reports that this does not touch his pain. The physician refuses to provide more or stronger opioids. The pain clinic consultant develops a treatment plan. Many of the treatments yield slow and uncertain results. Meanwhile, in spite of concerns regarding potential drug abuse, the consultant establishes a pain medication agreement with the patient for the use of long-acting oral morphine: 15 mg two times per day. Five days later, the patient calls the clinic and reports that the new opioid prescription is better but still inadequate. The consultant believes that she has increased the opioid dose by a large amount and is not willing to increase it further at this time. She tells this to the patient.

Discussions with the consultant reveal that she is uncomfortable with a number of aspects of this case. She recognizes that her opinion regarding an appropriate drug dose is influenced by the patient's prior history of drug abuse. This history suggests that the patient may be at higher risk of developing an addiction. Furthermore, she finds herself uncertain about whether the patient is accurately reporting his pain levels even though his pain symptoms match those of classic CRPS. Finally, upon introspection, the consultant realizes that if this patient were suffering with pain from a malignancy, she would be more aggressive with her prescribing of analgesics, yet she knows that the pain of CRPS can be more intense than the pain associated with malignancy.

ANALYSIS

Within the framework of the basic bioethical principles described earlier, we can see that the scenario in Case 1 describes an infringement of the obligation to respect the patient, or more specifically to respect the autonomy of the patient. The consultant is assuming a paternalistic attitude—which typically is considered to be contrary to the principle of autonomy—and determines for the patient what is the appropriate amount of medication. However, according to English,[9] there are circumstances in which the initial status of respect for autonomy (of the patient) is overruled by, among other factors, the concept of *professional autonomy* (a professional is not obliged to act against personal or professional ethical convictions). Given the complicating factor of prior drug use in this case, it is possible that the consultant, concerned that this patient is at higher risk for developing another addiction that would be harmful, *could* use the concept of professional autonomy to justify at least a prudent delay in prescribing more or increasing the dose of opioids. Such concerns and reasoning should also be shared with the patient so that he or she may understand that the physician's concern is for his or her best interest, especially with regard to the patient's risk of developing another addiction. However, had this patient no prior history of drug abuse, the principle of professional autonomy would not be as applicable. The physician probably believes that her drug limits are required by the principle of nonmaleficence because she believes that higher doses of opioid medication significantly increase the risk of addiction. In her efforts to do no harm, however, the physician may not be following the other half of the principle of beneficence, that is, the requirement to maximize the potential benefits while minimizing the risks. Finally, this case may also demonstrate a violation of the principle of justice. By virtue of a previous medical problem (heroin addiction), the patient is now not receiving medication for the relief of pain equal to what would be prescribed for a patient without such a history. If this is the result of prejudice, as opposed to a considered assessment of the involved risks to the patient, then this would represent unfair limits on the access to medical resources (i.e., medications). Similarly, if the patient would receive more analgesic medication if the underlying cause of his pain was cancer and if the reason for more medication was simply a reflection of societal attitudes regarding cancer pain versus nonmalignant pain, then this too may reflect an ethically unjustifiable limit on the provision of medical care.

Without exploring the causes that underlie these dilemmas, resolution will be difficult. The physician is stuck trying to balance the potential benefits and risks of prescribing higher doses of opioids. Although evidence of past experience is commonly considered in placing trust, this often interferes with building trust in the person, a future-oriented endeavor.

Trust is, in fact, the critical element that underlies all of these problems. O'Neill[13] describes trust as a dynamic activity rather than a one-time judgment. She offers that trust is "given, built, conferred, refused and withdrawn in ways that fall short of the evidence." What O'Neill is describing as a trust is a partnership. As noted by Sass,[14] "medicine necessarily will have to shift attention from physician ethics toward patient ethics and a partnership in health care. From the perspective of trust-based communication and trust-based cooperation, it is only logical to strengthen the other side of the partnership and make difficult cases of clinical decision making an issue for trust-based decision making in partnership." Sass is not suggesting that we increase our blind trust in our patients but rather that we enable our patients to earn our trust and that such earned trust "safeguards all expert-lay interactions."[14]

On reexamination of the ethical problems in Case 1, we see that each of these problems is triggered by the physician's suspicion that she is being manipulated and that increasing the dosage implies that she is deliberately ignoring obvious implications that the patient is abusing drugs again. Because of this lack of trust, the consultant believes that she cannot rely on the patient's autonomy, in this case, the patient's ability to accurately determine his or her own need for medication or give a reliable report of pain level. At that point, the physician acts in a paternalistic fashion and determines her own limits for the medications because she has no gauge for judging when she has provided maximal benefit. For this doctor, without the ability to judge the degree of benefit, it was natural to rely more heavily on the nonmaleficence component of beneficence to minimize risk and harm.

Finally, lack of trust may often underlie the tendency to treat nonmalignant pain less aggressively than cancer-related pain. Vrancken[15] gives a telling description of the attitude of many pain physicians regarding cancer pain patients. "They really have something, it is also recognized by everybody that they really have something. Their problems are also very real which makes it easier for doctors as well as patients to face psychosocial factors too." Vrancken is telling us that cancer pain patients

TABLE 105-1 Recommendations to Avoid Relapse[17]

Education	The distinction between physical dependence, which is to be expected, and addiction, which should be avoided, should be clarified for the patient.
Social support	Encourage the patient to join or increase involvement in a recovery program or in individual psychological care in order to garner support and develop and bolster relapse prevention strategies.
Behavioral agreements	A behavioral agreement should be made to provide the patient with a clear definition of problematic use, misuse, and abuse behaviors, giving the patient the parameters to demonstrate reliability and responsibility.
Supervision	Physician provides close supervision, including frequent follow-up appointments, the use of only one prescribing physician and dispensing pharmacy, and toxicology screenings. Supervision at follow-up includes inquiry about referred care and review of the treatment plan.
Protective and preemptive prescribing	Long-acting opioids, or around-the-clock dosing, may be helpful in reducing the reinforcing, and therefore addictive, properties of these medications.

are trusted more than patients with nonmalignant pain. There is nothing inherent about nonmalignant pain that makes its sufferers less trustworthy; therefore, problems with trusting patients with nonmalignant pain may lead to violations of the ethical principle of justice. Other factors may also be involved for patients who "really have something." In a study of patient's with HIV-related chronic pain, Moskowitz et al.[16] highlighted how lack of trust undermines the principle of justice, leading to disparities in receiving care and treatment for pain despite a "real" diagnosis and similar psychosocial features. In a study of 169 patients with HIV, these researchers found that physician attitudes, trust, and prescribing decisions were different for patients of nonwhite race or ethnicity. In their study sample, trust was guided more by perceptions of the racial or ethnic group of the patient despite individual patients' medical diagnoses or history of opioid analgesic misuse.

Pappagallo and Heinberg[17] raise another point in regard to patients with chronic pain with a history of addiction, which is that they may not want opioids to manage their pain for the fear of relapse. Considering both potential responses from such patients, Pappagallo and Heinberg give further treatment suggestions for reducing the risk of relapse in dealing with patients with chronic pain with a past history of addiction. Their recommendations are outlined in **Table 105-1**.

In order to further employ the concept of justice, these recommendations would apply and be provided to all patients receiving opioid analgesics, not just those for whom addiction is a concern. By incorporating these recommendations as part of usual care, the physician can develop an ethical and clinically sound standard of practice for all patients and thereby help each patient increase autonomy through the support of his or her doctor.

Two additional cases are presented to illustrate how the method of analyzing trust may underlie potential infringements of basic bioethical principles as the lack of trust creates an unethical barrier to appropriate, unbiased treatment.

CASE 2

A 24-year-old woman is referred to the chronic pain clinic. The patient reports constant, severe midpelvic pain. She is unable to concentrate on her graduate school work. She has seen numerous specialists and has had extensive evaluations, including laparoscopy, all without result. After the laparoscopy, a new, burning pain developed in her left labia and inguinal area. The patient's gynecologist reported generalized vulvar and pelvic tenderness, with more exquisite pain responses with light touch of the left labium. The pain consultants thought that this newer pain was suggestive of ilioinguinal neuralgia. There is no apparent cause for the original pelvic pain. Even opioids have not helped. During the clinic evaluation, the patient reveals a childhood history of sexual abuse. Her affect is depressed and angry. She is very frustrated by all the previous failed diagnostic and therapeutic efforts and their apparent complications. The patient asks the pain clinic physicians to please do nerve blocks. The physicians are concerned about the patient's psychological health. They explain the potential for interaction between physical and emotional distress. They tell the patient that they will consider nerve block techniques for the left inguinal and labial pain, but the patient should first undergo psychological evaluation and treatment. The patient states that she is unwilling to do this. Efforts to address her concerns about the treatment plan fail. The patient continues to insist that nerve blocks be performed. The clinic physicians explain that they provide a comprehensive treatment plan and that they cannot proceed with only one element (the blocks) without the other elements (the psychotherapy). The patient is upset and leaves the clinic.

CASE 3

A 33-year-old man is being seen in the pain clinic for a 1-year history of incapacitating low back pain. The primary care doctor, orthopedic surgeon, and pain consultant are all unable to establish a cause for the patient's pain. Magnetic resonance imaging of the lumbar region reveals mild disk bulges, which would not be expected to cause the degree of discomfort that the patient reports. A psychological evaluation reveals mild depression and somatic preoccupation, findings common to most patients with chronic pain. Results of nerve conduction studies are normal. The patient reports that the pain interferes with his ability to concentrate, his relationships with colleagues, and his ability to maintain prolonged sitting or standing positions. Because of this, he has been unable to return to work. The workers' compensation insurance company now insists on a report on whether the pain clinic agrees with the patient's claim that he is totally disabled.

ANALYSIS

In Case 2, the primary ethical concern is regarding autonomy. The physicians were concerned that acceding to the patient's requests for nerve blocks without prior psychotherapy carried an unacceptably high risk of harm. Respect for autonomy requires that patients' decisions regarding care be made without coercion; however, the consultants verged on coercion by telling the patient that they would consider providing the treatment she desired (nerve blocks) only if she accepted a treatment that she did not want (psychotherapy). As noted by Whedon and Ferrell,[18] pain patients may be exceptionally susceptible to subtle coercion because they are so vulnerable to any offered possibility of relief. However, the more vulnerable the patient, the greater the obligations of the physicians to respect the patient's vulnerability by meeting it with trust.[3] The patient became especially vulnerable after she revealed a history of sexual abuse. Unfortunately, this revelation on top of the patient's new pain after laparoscopy, plus the patient's distressed affect, may have triggered the physicians to distrust the patient's judgment and insight. This lack of trust may have stopped the physicians from conveying their concerns that a block, given her experience with the laparoscopy, could worsen her condition. This patient became further upset because her request was refused and no other offers of pain relief were forthcoming. The perception that her pain needs were ignored was a further emotional trigger for her.[19] Although the doctors explained their perceptions of her psychopathology and how this might interact with experience of pain, they did not attempt to identify her beliefs, knowledge, or expectations about the connection between her abuse history and her current pain. Without this information, they could not identify what was needed to preserve her autonomy, which was a precondition to trust.

In Case 3, the clinician faces a dilemma. The patient may be malingering; however, this cannot be determined simply on the basis of lack of objective data. A report of disability may reinforce unconscious pain behaviors and diminish healthy, productive behaviors. Therefore, such a report may not be in the patient's best interests, yet a failure to report disability may cause the loss of the patient's only potential income. The bases and rationale for determining disability are complex and beyond the scope of this chapter; however, here, too, the core of the problem is a lack of trust. The clinicians recognize that the possibility of monetary gain may be consciously or unconsciously influencing the patient. Because they cannot enter the patient's reality, they look for objective evidence that might explain the patient's pain. When they cannot find such evidence, the concerns regarding the trustworthiness of the patient are heightened.

BUILDING TRUST

Problems with trust underlie many of the ethical problems that arise in the treatment of chronic nonmalignant pain. Trust is the overriding principle and virtue that establishes and safeguards all expert–layperson interactions, particularly in pain clinics.[14] With this understanding, we can reexamine our interactions with our patients. We can enable more of our patients to earn our trust and thereby prevent ourselves from acting with willful blindness.

Techniques with the potential for trust building are already widely used; however, the full potential of these techniques is not realized because they are not explicitly thought of in terms of trust building but rather in terms of contracts or patient compliance. Often, the patients are presented with paperwork they must sign before receiving medication, the physician's signature is absent, and the paperwork is brought out again only when the patient is suspected of misusing medications. Reframing the ideas of patient treatment agreements, monitoring of adherence and progress, and patient education are three approaches that may enable us to trust our patients and enable clinicians to more clearly recognize our obligation to those patients who have not earned our trust.

Patient treatment plan agreements are commonly used tools for educating our patients about the treatments that will be provided, the expectations regarding their participation, and the operating rules of the pain clinic. Patient treatment plans establish:

1. Which treatments are likely to be provided
2. Goals for increased function
3. Requirements
   a. For clinic attendance
   b. For use of medications
   c. For drug testing
   d. For adherence with all treatment modalities
   e. For having a primary physician to assume care when the treatment is completed

Such treatment plan agreements are a valuable first step to increase patient trust, and when properly used, they may help to address the dilemma between beneficence and autonomy. The agreement should *not* be presented with the underlying assumption that patients are untrustworthy.[20] A discussion should accompany the agreement and might start with an explanation that pain treatment programs rely heavily on both the patient and the physician being informed about the treatment process and progress and to have shared beliefs about goals and a similar investment in the treatment plan. The physician can then explain his or her goal of beneficence, especially in using potentially dangerous drugs and procedures and decisions regarding impairment and disability. This interaction is one way we meet our obligation to all of our patients for the opportunity to earn our trust while at the same time working to earn theirs. The discussion would continue with explanations showing how the treatment plan agreement will be reviewed at follow-up visits to demonstrate that patients can adhere to the plan, that barriers are addressed, and that the patient has an opportunity to demonstrate his or her effort and motivation to pursue multiple treatment modalities (e.g., physical therapy, psychotherapy, and medication use). Physicians consider effort and dependability signs of trustworthiness. Failure to identify these signs may indicate that we are unlikely to be able to help the patient.

Pain logbooks or diaries may also help to establish that the patient is a trustworthy reporter of his or her pain. However, patients who report maximal pain levels without variation are often perceived to be unlikely to be accurate and trustworthy reporters. This is where physician involvement and discussion can help. Including functional goals and the progress reports from other treatment modalities can give weight and context to the patient's pain reports. For example, a patient who reports more pain despite an increase in opioid dosage will be evaluated differently if he or she is also reporting an increase in time ambulating. Physicians are encouraged to include behavioral components in the pain scale. For instance, instead of identifying pain as "the worst pain imagined," a 10 would be interpreted for the patient as needing hospitalization, and a score of 8 or 9 means the patient is staying in bed.[21]

Upon reanalysis of Case 2, we can see the potential value in empowering the patient with education about the benefits and burdens of invasive procedures, for instance, the problems with injecting an already-inflamed area. Other treatment options to address immediate pain could have been offered to avoid collusion with the concept that only blocks are helpful. In addition, withholding treatment until the patient has a psychological evaluation is likely to sabotage any help the psychologist could offer because patients tend not to participate in treatment when forced. At this point, the patient has learned that revealing personal information leads to negative consequences and would be unlikely to trust the psychologist and therefore less likely to benefit from therapy. In addition, it would behoove physicians to have explanations on hand on what pain psychology can offer in terms of treatment of symptoms, thereby bypassing the judgment of the patient's pain as "all in her head." Such a discussion might have minimized any coercive aspects in the interaction.

In Case 3, it is critical to provide the patient the opportunity to demonstrate his efforts to get better if the physician sees there is this potential. It would be valuable to discuss that it is impossible to clearly establish disability on the basis of subjective complaints. However, the patient can earn our trust over a 4- to 6-month period by demonstrating his effort and adherence with a carefully tailored but demanding physical therapy and psychotherapy program (including homework assignments). This is an important opportunity to provide because often we forget that patients in pain exist in a system in which nontrustworthy behavior is created or reinforced. For instance, patients may always report high pain levels because their pain levels are ignored or they believe they will be denied medication or treatment if improvement is reported. Some patients believe that although they would like to go out and walk, they fear that if this is documented by workers' compensation investigators, they will be perceived as malingerers. A patient who appears depressed yet denies any mood problems may be perceived as lacking insight and thus might also be seen as an unreliable reporter of pain. Sometimes patients underreport depression because they have found that when they do report their depression, their physical concerns are dismissed.

A potential pitfall must be noted. It is reasonable to expect patients to be adherent and to demonstrate effort, but it is not reasonable to demand that patients get better. Treatment failure does not establish that the patient is not trustworthy; rather, it may imply misdiagnosis or the need for alternative treatments.

TRUST MUST BE MUTUAL

Patients are much more likely to accept our suggestions and treatment plans if they trust the physician. Failure to comply with treatment does not necessarily mean that the patient is not trustworthy, but it may indicate that the patient did not find the physician to be trustworthy. Chronic pain patients may be particularly prone to mistrust their providers because they have typically been through extensive, failed therapeutic efforts. When treatment efforts fail, the patient is then often treated in a dismissive or punishing manner. *Business & Health*[22] reported on what patients endure before referral to a comprehensive pain management center: litigation, insurance-related delays or denials, and loss of employment, and more than half have had at least one surgery or mood symptoms that reach the criteria for depression.

Physicians can and must earn the trust of the patient by (1) being there (within boundaries), (2) attempting to understand the problem, (3) being respectful, (4) pursuing the best interests of the patient (ignoring self-interest), (5) avoiding harm, (6) providing nonprejudicial care, and (7) maintaining knowledge and expertise.

Pursuing the best interests of the patient rather than professional self-interests means that physicians must carefully analyze their own motives to ensure that they are not affected by potential "secondary gains" such as financial reward, research benefits, the acquisition of experience, or the avoidance of anxiety regarding liability or legal regulations.

SUMMARY

Problems with trust underlie many of the daily ethical dilemmas that are seen in pain clinics. Reconceptualizing and refocusing the processes of patient education and treatment plan agreements may provide more patients with the opportunity to earn our trust. Trust building puts the patient and the provider in a working and supportive relationship and perhaps can avoid the need to argue the position of whether treatment of pain is a human right. In addition to monitoring levels of pain and function, now the clinician can also monitor the parameter of earned trust. We like to think that patients are our partners in the treatment process, but in fact, this is not always true. Attention to the parameter of earned trust may provide the clinician with a firmer basis for difficult treatment decisions.

REFERENCES

1. Hall JK, Boswell, MV. Ethics, law, and pain management as a patient right. *Pain Physician*. 2009;12:499-506.
2. Brennan F, Carr DB, Cousins M. Pain management: A fundamental human right. *Anesth Analg*. 2007;105:205-221.
3. Hellman D. Prosecuting doctors for trusting patients. *16 Geo Mason L Rev*. 701:2008-2009.
4. Thom DH, Wong ST, Guzman D, et al. Physician trust in the patient: development and validation of a new measure. *Ann Family Med*. 2011;9:148-154.
5. Jacobs EA, Rolle I, Ferrans C, et al. Understanding African Americans' views of the trustworthiness of physicians. *J Gen Intern Med*. 2006;21:642-647.
6. Pearson SD, Raeke LH. Patients' trust in physicians: many theories, few measures, and little data. *J Gen Intern Med*. 2000;15:509-513.
7. Rogers WA. Is there a moral duty for doctors to trust patients? *J Med Ethics*. 2002;28:77-80.
8. Gooberman-Hill R, Heathcote C, Reid CM, et al. Professional experience guides opioid prescribing for non-cancer pain in primary care. *Fam Pract*. 2010;0:1-8.
9. English DC. *Bioethics: A Clinical Guide for Medical Students*. New York: WW Norton & Company; 1994.
10. Ahronheim JC, Moreno J, Zuckerman C. *Ethics in Clinical Practice*. New York: Little, Brown and Company; 1994.
11. Fins JJ, Bacchetta MD, Miller FG. Clinical pragmatism: a method of moral problem solving. *Kennedy Inst Ethics J*. 1997;7:129-143.
12. Loewy EH. Suffering as a consideration in ethical decision making. *Cambridge Q Healthcare Ethics*. 1992;1(2):135-142.
13. O'Neill O. *Autonomy and Trust in Bioethics*. Cambridge, England: Cambridge University Press; 2002.
14. Sass HM. The clinic as testing ground for moral theory: a European view. *Kennedy Inst Ethics J*. 1996;6:351-355.
15. Vrancken MAE. Schools of thought on pain. *Soc Sci Med*. 1989;29:435-444.
16. Moskowitz D, Thom DH, Guzman D, et al. Is primary care providers' trust in socially marginalized patients affected by race? *J Gen Intern Med*. 2012;(8):846-851.
17. Pappagallo M, Heinberg L. Ethical issues in the management of chronic nonmalignant pain. *Semin Neurol*. 1997;17:203-211.
18. Whedon M, Ferrell BR. Professional and ethical considerations in the use of high-tech pain management. *Oncol Nurs Forum*. 1991;18:1135-1143.
19. Charlton JE, ed. *Core Curriculum for Professional Education in Pain*. 3rd ed. Seattle: IASP Press; 2005.
20. Victor L, Richeimer SH. Trustworthiness as a clinical variable: the problem of trust in the management of chronic, nonmalignant pain. *Pain Med*. 2005;6:285-391.
21. Whitten, CE, Evans, CM, Cristobal K. Pain management doesn't have to be a pain: working and communicating effectively with patients who have chronic pain. *Perm J*. 2005;9(2):41-48.
22. Special Report. *Business & Health*, Fall 1996.

SUGGESTED READINGS

Cain JM, Hammes BJ. Ethics and pain management: respecting patients' wishes. *J Pain Symptom Manage*. 1994;9:160-165.

The National Commission for the Protection of Human Subjects of Biomedical and Behavioral Research. *The Belmont Report: Ethical Principles and Guidelines for the Protection of Human Subjects of Research*. Washington, DC: US Government Printing Office; 1979.

Outcome Measurements in Pain Medicine

Harriët Wittink
Leonidas C. Goudas
Scott Strassels
Daniel B. Carr

The measurement of health is central to the evaluation of health care. Until the first part of the 20th century, *health* was defined as the absence of disease and was measured in terms of morbidity and mortality. This simple approach to health status was rejected in 1948 with the expansion of the concept of health by the World Health Organization (WHO), which defined health as "A state of complete *physical*, *mental* and *social* wellbeing and not merely the absence of disease or infirmity."[1] This definition reflected the multidimensionality of health and considered not only biologic markers but also the ability to perform physically, psychologically, and socially in the everyday environment.

This change in the definition of health gave rise to the current outcomes movement. Other factors, such as the reversal of the proportion of care rendered for acute illnesses versus chronic diseases, technological advancements in health care, rising health care costs, the emerging concept of quality of care, and increased recognition of the importance of patients' views about their care and health, have further fostered the growth of this movement. Conscientious health care providers use both individual clinical expertise and the best available objective, external evidence for treatment. The best available external evidence for treatment is defined as clinically relevant research, often from the basic sciences of medicine but especially from patient-based clinical research into the accuracy and precision of diagnostic tests (including the clinical examination); the power of prognostic markers; and the efficacy and safety of therapeutic, rehabilitative, and preventive regimens.[2] The integration of clinical expertise and best available external evidence for treatment is the practice of evidence-based medicine. With the plethora of current and relevant literature, it is impossible for most clinical care providers to keep abreast of the latest developments in their field. Because of this problem, structured approaches to literature synthesis, such as that organized by the Cochrane Collaboration, have arisen to summarize, with the least possible bias, the best available research on a specific topic (see later discussion). The goal is to make relevant information widely available and evidence-based practice unencumbered for all health care providers.

This chapter focuses on common terminology used in outcomes assessment and on outcomes measurement tools used in research on and treatment of patients with chronic noncancer pain because they are part of the foundation of what will become evidence-based practice and perhaps eventually guidelines for treatment. Although the comprehensiveness and validity of outcome measures for the treatment of all types of pain lag behind those of equally high-impact conditions that affect the public's health, this lag is even more pronounced for cancer pain than for noncancer pain.[3] Much more research has addressed functional assessment, and how pain management influences function, in patients with acute or chronic noncancer pain than in those whose pain results from malignancy.[4]

OUTCOMES RESEARCH

As health care providers, we treat patients to make them "better." How is "better" defined, and by whom? "Better" from the point of view of the practitioner, the patient, or society? Does "better" equate to less pain, increased physical functioning, decreased disability (as judged by a physical therapist), improved quality of life (as judged by the patient), or decreased cost of worker's compensation charges and fewer health care visits (as judged by payers)? Does the same intervention that benefits one patient benefit a group of patients with similar conditions? How do we know whether it does? These are questions that the outcomes assessment movement is trying to address.

Outcomes research studies the results of medical care.[5] It involves "the rigorous determination of what works in medical care and what does not" and states that "outcomes research, by informing the content of policy positions, payment rules, and practice guidelines, presumably solves both the problems of quality and cost that beset health care and does so by scientific rather than political means" (p. 1268).[6] Outcomes research is the foundation of evaluation of the quality and costs of health care delivery. Adoption of an evidence-based approach to health care, exemplified by the Cochrane Collaboration,[2,7,8] has been accompanied by a shift toward an emphasis on patient-centered health outcomes.[9] This broadened perspective has heightened the need for tools to monitor and adjust treatment and to approach clinical decision making from a viewpoint that is evidence based and patient centered.[10] The pressing need to know which treatments reduce chronic pain; which improve functional status (including return to work and social activities); whether they change pain intensity; and, in particular, which treatments are worth paying for has fueled the development of a number of instruments. These instruments are intended to capture in a simple, speedy, and robust fashion the health status of patients.[11]

HEALTH STATUS ASSESSMENT: DEFINITIONS AND TERMS

This section discusses common terminology used in outcomes assessment and provides several examples of assessment tools used in measuring outcomes during the treatment of patients with chronic noncancer pain. Health assessments focus on three broad categories of measures: traditional biologic, general (or generic), and disease specific.[12] Traditional biologic measures may be primary, such as morbidity and mortality, or surrogate, such as a decrease in blood pressure in patients given an antihypertensive drug. Measures used for patient-centered outcomes generally estimate persons' health-related quality of life (HRQOL) and their ability to function and to do the things they want to do. These measures may be generic, evaluating overall health status, or disease specific, focusing on the effect of a given condition on a person's life.

HRQOL assessment is the measurement or evaluation of the health of an individual or a patient. HRQOL may include biologic markers, but it emphasizes indicators of physical functioning; mental health; social functioning; and other health-related concepts, such as pain, fatigue, and perceived well-being.[13] Concepts included in some commonly applied HRQOL instruments are presented in **Table 106-1**.

Quality of life includes HRQOL but is a broader term that includes nonmedical aspects of life that reflect the aggregate impact of food, shelter, safety, living standards, and social and physical environmental factors.[13]

Patient-based outcome measures are indicators of patients' evaluations of both changes in patient health status, including HRQOL and mortality, and the quality of health care. The importance of patients' views has been increasingly recognized in health care.[14] One might even argue that the increased interest in palliative care and pain control in recent years is the direct result of a power shift in which patients and their families—the consumers of health care—have much greater autonomy and power than under the previous disease-centered model of care.[15] Clinicians' taking patients' views into account is associated with greater patient satisfaction with care,[16] better compliance with treatment programs,[17] and an increased likelihood of maintaining a continuous relationship during health care.[18]

The distinction between disease-based clinical investigation and patient-centered outcomes research is analogous to that between measures of efficacy and measures of effectiveness. In an ideal setting, such as a randomized, controlled clinical trial, the *efficacy* of a treatment may

TABLE 106-1 Domains Used in Health-Related Quality of Life Measurements

Domains	QWB	SIP	NHP	QLI	COOP	EQ-5D	DUKE	MOS SF-36
Physical functioning	X	X	X	X	X	X	X	X
Social functioning	X	X	X	X	X	X	X	X
Role functioning	X	X	X	X	X	X	X	X
Psychological distress		X	X	X	X	X	X	X
Health perceptions (general)			X	X	X	X	X	X
Pain (bodily)		X	X		X	X	X	X
Energy/fatigue	X		X				X	X
Psychological well-being							X	X
Sleep		X	X				X	
Cognitive functioning		X				X		
Quality of life					X			
Reported health transition					X			

COOP, Dartmouth Function Charts; DUKE, Duke Health Profile; EQ-5D, European Quality of Life; MOS SF-36, Medical Outcomes Study 36-item Short-Form Health Survey; NHP, Nottingham Health Profile; QLI, Quality of Life Index; QWB, Quality of Well-Being Scale; SIP, Sickness Impact Profile Index.

Modified from Ware J. The status of health assessment 1994. *Ann Rev Public Health.* 1995;16:327-354.

TABLE 106-2 Terms and Definitions Commonly Used in Outcomes Assessment

Term	Definition
Item	A single question (e.g., "In general, how would you say your health is?")
Scale	A range of available responses to an item Can be categorical (e.g., excellent, very good, good, fair, poor), be numerical, or consist of a visual analog scale
Domain	Identifies a particular focus of attention (e.g., physical functioning, mental or general health, patient satisfaction with care) and may consist of the response to a single item or responses to several related items May consist of one scale (a collection of related items) or multiple scales
Instrument	A group of items used for the collection of desired data May contain a single item or multiple items that may or may not be divided into domains
Domain- or dimension-specific instrument	A one-scale instrument (e.g., the McGill Pain Questionnaire)
Ceiling or floor effect	Indicates the lack of sensitivity of an instrument to discriminate differences at the higher or lower end of a scale used to measure this effect (e.g., a ceiling effect may be a 10/10 pain intensity that is now reported as a 12/10 by a patient)
Disease- or condition-specific tools	Instruments used exclusively for assessment of the health status of populations with a specific disease or condition (e.g., back pain, postherpetic neuralgia)
Generic HRQOL tools	Instruments that estimate an individual's overall health status that can be used to compare HRQOL among groups of patients with different diseases

HRQOL, health-related quality of life.

be derived from the dose-response relationship for a given physiologic effect assessed under well-controlled conditions. In controlled trials, the end points of interest are usually biologic measures, such as changes in blood glucose levels or blood pressure. However, equally important to practitioners and patients is the *effectiveness* of a treatment, which refers to the outcomes of this treatment when applied in typical practice settings, measured over the course of disease, and including measures that matter most to patients (i.e., patient-centered outcomes).[19] Outcomes research is more likely to be generalizable to typical medical practice than are controlled clinical trials. Terminology commonly used in outcomes research is presented in **Table 106-2**.

CHOICE OF INSTRUMENTS

Because the purpose of this overview is to present a few widely applied outcomes measurement tools and the context in which they are used, we next describe the criteria used to select one from among available instruments rather than how to create a new questionnaire.

Selection of a specific outcomes tool will depend on the population of interest and the ability of the measurement tool to detect changes within the domain of interest. The selection of an instrument consists of two phases. The first has to do with the condition(s) for which this instrument will be used; the second has to do with the psychometric properties of the instrument.

Choosing a domain-specific, condition-specific, or generic instrument depends on the aim of the study. If one specific domain is of interest, such as pain intensity or depression, a domain-specific instrument can be used (e.g., the McGill Pain Questionnaire [MPQ] or the Beck Depression Inventory). In general, a condition- (or disease-) specific instrument will have a narrow focus but will provide considerable detail in the area of interest. If the interest is in general HRQOL, comparison with different conditions, or comparison with healthy people, a generic instrument can be used. Generic and condition-specific HRQOL instruments can be used together to supplement the information collected.[20] Using a condition-specific survey or module together with a generic scale may provide more insight into aspects of health that are not well measured by either type of instrument.[21-23] Comparison of the impact of pain on health status with the impact of other chronic illnesses on general health status, for example, allows researchers to conduct trials of various treatments so as to make clinical decisions in medical practice and inform health care policy.[12]

Important psychometric properties to consider include the following:[24-26]

- *Test–retest reliability*: the extent to which the measure generates consistent results. How closely do the results of repeated applications agree with each other?
- *Internal reliability*: (quantitated by Cronbach α) the sensitivity of the number of items that make up the measure and the degree of intercorrelation between the items. A Cronbach α of 0.9 or higher is generally preferred for measurement in a single person, whereas a Cronbach α of 0.7 or higher is preferred for group measurement.[27]
- *Validity:* the extent to which the instrument actually measures what it claims (i.e., the correspondence between what the instrument reports and reality)
- *Responsiveness:* the ability of an instrument to detect changes, particularly clinically important changes, over time in individuals or in groups of subjects
- *Applicability:* the appropriateness of the instrument's use in the specific study population
- *Practicality:* the likelihood that an instrument can be applied readily, without excessive burden to patient or investigator and produce data that can be easily analyzed and applied

Cronbach α = a coefficient of reliability (or consistency) used to measure how well a set of items (or variables) measures a single unidimensional latent construct. It ranges from 0 to 1. (For details, see http://www.ats.ucla.edu/stat/spss/fqq/alpha.html.)

DESCRIPTIONS OF SELECTED GENERIC HEALTH-RELATED QUALITY OF LIFE INSTRUMENTS

Of the many generic instruments available to assess HRQOL, four validated, widely used questionnaires stand out. Brief descriptions of these instruments are given in **Table 106-3**.

PAIN-SPECIFIC OUTCOMES MEASUREMENT

Pain, in general, and chronic and persistent pain, specifically, is a unique challenge to outcomes research because of the importance of subjective information. Unlike the majority of other medical conditions, chronic pain may not involve a distinct organ system, pathophysiologic process, or specific discipline. Although pain is characterized as a symptom, it is, in fact, a subjective experience, a perception.[41] This perception not only depends on nociceptive transmission and modulation within the central nervous system but also is integrated with psychological, social, and other environmental factors.[42] Physical functioning, work, family, and social relationships are usually impaired by chronic pain. Comorbid conditions, such as depression and anxiety, often accompany chronic pain.[43] For these reasons, it is argued that the assessment of patients with chronic pain should be accomplished within a multidimensional framework.[44] Assessment of chronic pain should provide clinicians with relevant information to formulate a treatment plan and allow for measurement of the outcome of treatment interventions. The generic HRQOL instruments discussed earlier are mostly epidemiologic tools and as such are able to measure change in large samples of patients. By design, they are not intended, nor are they sufficiently sensitive, to measure changes in a single subject. Furthermore, these instruments do not

TABLE 106-3 Generic Outcomes Assessment Tools

Name of Instrument	Internal Reliability (Cronbach α)	Cross-Validation Instruments	Number of Items	Number of Domains	Time to Complete (min)	References
Nottingham Health Profile (NHP)	Cronbach α was reported as 0.77–0.85 for the first section and 0.44–0.86 for the second section in a sample of patients with OA	SIP SF-36 COOP WONCA EQ-5D	37	Six plus physical abilities, pain, sleep, social isolation, emotional reactions, and energy level A second section includes optional questions about work, social and sex life, interests and hobbies, and holidays	10–15	Hunt and McEwen,[28] Hunt et al.,[29] Essink-Bot et al.[30,31]
Medical Outcomes Study 36-item Short-Form Health Survey (SF-36)	Cronbach α in both general and chronic disease populations ranges from 0.78–0.93	Oswestry Disability Index SIP NHP EQ-5D Social Maladjustment Schedule WOMAC OA Index Chronic Pain grade Questionnaire	36	Eight scales of general health and functioning: physical functioning, role—physical (limitations in physical roles caused by health problems), bodily pain, general health, vitality, social functioning, role—emotional (limitations in emotional roles caused by health problems), and mental health	10–15	Tarlov et al.,[32] Stewart,[33] Ware,[34] McHorney et al.,[35] Stansfeld et al.,[36] Grevitt et al.[37] See also http://www.rand.org/health/totalsnav.html
Sickness Impact Profile (SIP)	Cronbach α = 0.94 Test–retest reliability r = 0.92	NHP SF-36 EQ-5D MMPI	136	12	20–30	Bergner et al.[38-40]
European Quality of Life (EQ-5D, Euro-QoL)	Test–retest reliability in stroke patients: κ 0.63–0.80	SF-36 NHP COOP WONCA	15	Five dimensions: mobility, self care, usual activities, pain/discomfort, and depression/anxiety The sixth item is a global evaluation of one's own health using a VAS of 0–100 (worst imaginable health to best imaginable health)	Few	Essink-Bot et al.[30,31] See also http://www.euroqol.org

COOP, Dartmouth Function Tests; ED-5D, European Quality of Life; MMPI, Minnesota Multiphasic Personality Inventory; NHP, Nottingham Health Profile; SF-36, Short-Form Health Survey; SIP, Sickness Impact Profile; OA, osteoarthritis; VAS, visual analog scale; WOMAC, Western Ontario and McMaster Universities Arthritis; WONCA, World Organization of Family Doctors.

provide information on items frequently assessed in pain management, such as solicitous responses,[45,46] coping ability,[47,48] fear avoidance,[49-51] and the extent of disablement from pain.

Many instruments are used to assess the impact of pain on patients' lives. Ideally, the instrument should provide relevant information to all clinicians within an inter- or multidisciplinary team, have a low respondent burden, and be sensitive enough to detect changes at both group and individual levels. Widely used methods to assess pain and its influence range from domain to condition specific. Some of the most frequently used tools are presented next.

DOMAIN-SPECIFIC MEASUREMENTS

Pain Intensity (or Pain Relief) The three most commonly used methods to assess pain intensity are the verbal rating scales, visual analog scales, and numerical rating scales (**Table 106-4**). Von Korff et al.[52] cautions that multiple factors influence patients' pain reports, including time of day. Aggregated pain measures have, therefore, been shown to be more reliable and more sensitive to treatment effects than single items.[53] Aggregated pain measures are scores that are created from multiple measures. For instance, the average of three concurrent responses to a 100-mm visual analog scale of pain intensity ratings of current, average, and best pain can be taken.[54] A composite measure shown in cancer pain patients to have high internal consistency (Cronbach α >0.8) consists of an average of ratings on a 0-to-10 scale of current, least, and average pain.[55] Jensen and colleagues[56] report that individual 0-to-10 pain intensity ratings have sufficient psychometric strength to be used in chronic pain research, especially in studies with large sample sizes, but composites of 0-to-10 ratings may be more useful when maximal reliability is necessary (i.e., in studies with small sample sizes or in the monitoring of an individual patient).

Verbal Rating Scales Verbal rating scales (VRSs) are positively and significantly related to other measures of pain intensity.[26] Jensen and colleagues[57] reported on the potential clinical utility of classifying pain as mild, moderate, or severe based on the impact of pain on quality of life. There is a nonlinear relationship between pain intensity and pain interference. Pain intensity begins to have a serious impact on functioning when it reaches a specific threshold: about 5 on a 0-to-10 scale in patients with cancer pain.[55] To explore in greater detail the relationship between pain severity and interference in patients with cancer pain, Serlin and

TABLE 106-4 Pain Intensity Scales

Scale	Description
Verbal rating scale (VRSs)	A list of adjectives describing different levels of pain intensity (e.g., 0 = no pain, 1 = slight pain, 2 = moderate pain, 3 = severe pain)
Visual analog scales (VASs)	Lines that are usually 100 mm long and represent the continuum of the symptom being rated, with labels at either end to represent the extremes of the symptom (e.g., 0 = "no pain," 100 = "pain as bad as it could be")
Numerical rating scales (NRSs)	Ascending sequences of numbers, each representing increasing levels of pain intensity (e.g., 11-point scale in which 0 = no pain, 10 = worst possible pain)

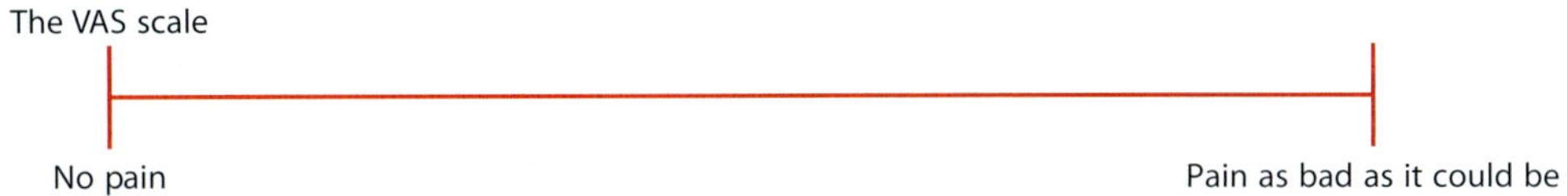

FIGURE 106-1. The visual analog scale.

colleagues[55] administered the Brief Pain Inventory (BPI) to a total of 1897 patients from numerous sites in the United States, France, China, and the Philippines. In this classic study, they gathered self-reported data on pain severity as well as interference by pain with enjoyment of life, activity, walking, mood, sleep, work, and relations with others. These four diverse populations had "fairly consistent patterns relating pain severity to pain interference." Statistical analyses showed that pain severity on a 0-to-10 verbal numerical rating scale could be stratified according to the degree of interference it produced as mild (1–4), moderate (5–6), and severe (7–10).

Visual Analog Scales These are simple tools to assess intensity and other dimensions of pain, such as anxiety, efficacy of treatment, and emotional responses[26,58,59] (**Fig. 106-1**). Patients mark the scale at a point that represents the severity of their pain at a specified time point or within a well-defined interval (e.g., the past 24 hours). Variations of these techniques request that patients circle a number from 0 to 10 or place a mark through one of these numbers. VASs are more sensitive and precise than descriptive scales. They are also easy to use and interpret; however, they are limited to expressing only one dimension of the complex experience of pain. It may be difficult for patients to imagine the worst pain imaginable, or they might report their pain as being outside the 0-to-10 limits, saying that it is a 20, for example.

The validity of VASs is supported by their positive relations to other measures of pain intensity.[24,60] They are sensitive to treatment effect and are distinct from measures of other subjective components of pain.[52]

Numerical Rating Scales Numerical rating scales (NRSs) were demonstrated to provide sufficient levels of discrimination for patients with chronic pain to describe their pain intensity.[61] Similar to VRSs and VASs, NRSs demonstrate positive and significant correlations with other measures of pain intensity.[26,60]

PAIN AFFECT

The McGill Pain Questionnaire The questionnaire provides estimates of the sensory, affective, and evaluative dimensions of pain.[62] It is one of the most frequently used instruments for pain measurement and is considered useful for evaluating pain treatments and as a diagnostic aid.[26,63-66] In addition to collecting information about diagnosis, drug therapy, pain and medical history, and other symptoms and modifying features, the MPQ contains a list of words that describe pain, divided into groups pertaining to the sensory, affective, and evaluative dimensions of the pain experience.

The MPQ is available in several languages, as well as extended (Dartmouth Pain Questionnaire, McGill Comprehensive Pain Questionnaire) and shortened versions. Components of the MPQ have been incorporated into other instruments.[26] Although the MPQ is one of the leading pain assessment tools and is considered the gold standard of pain assessment tools, it has some limitations.[67] For the purposes of this discussion, clinicians should keep in mind that it may be difficult to discriminate among types of pain syndromes in persons who are very anxious or who have other psychological morbidity.

Pain Distress Scales The Acute Pain Management Guideline Panel[68] recommends, among other tools, the use of the scales shown in **Figure 106-2**.

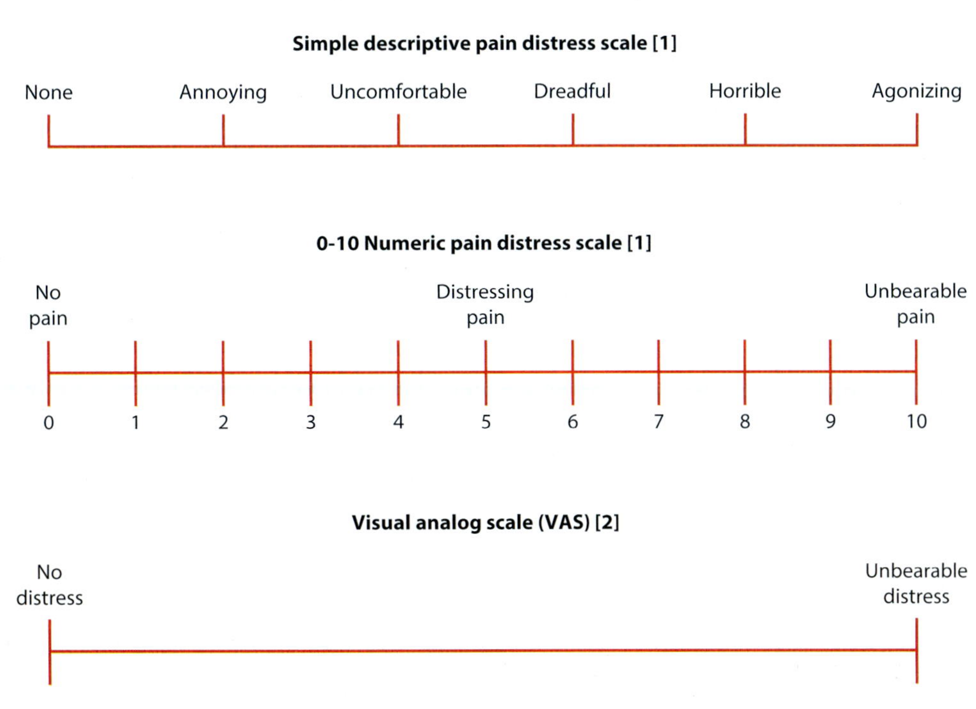

FIGURE 106-2. Examples of pain distress tools. From: AHCPR. Acute pain management guideline panel, (Carr et al., 1992).

MULTIDIMENSIONAL MEASUREMENTS

BRIEF PAIN INVENTORY

The BPI was originally developed for use in persons with cancer, although it is also used to assess pain in people with other diseases.[26] The purpose of the BPI is to assess the severity of pain and the impact of pain on daily functions. Assessment areas include severity of pain, impact of pain on daily function, location of pain, pain medications, and the amount of pain relief in the past 24 hours or the past week.[69] The internal consistency ranges from Cronbach α 0.77 to 0.91. The form takes about 10 minutes to complete. It is valid for use in Chinese (Mandarin),[70] Filipino, French, Hindi,[71] Italian,[72] Japanese, and Vietnamese, among other languages. It is also available in a shortened form, the BPI-SF,[73,74] that takes 5 minutes to complete. When applying the BPI to persons with chronic noncancer pain, the clinician should keep in mind that interpretation may be difficult if the questions asked do not reflect the patient's experience. Furthermore, questions about functioning are subject to both floor and ceiling effects. The BPI is copyrighted, but permission to use it is routinely granted at no cost after providing a short description of intended use. (Samples of the form, both the short and the long version, can be found at http://prg.mdanderson.org/bpicopy.htm.)

MULTIDIMENSIONAL PAIN INVENTORY

The MPI (formerly the West Haven-Yale Multidimensional Pain Inventory, or WHYMPI) was developed by Kerns and colleagues.[45] It is a 64-item self-report questionnaire consisting of three parts and 12 subscales. The first two parts are related to patients' appraisals of pain and its impact on different domains of their lives and patients' perceptions of the responses of significant others to their distress and suffering. The third part assesses how frequently patients perform 18 common daily activities. Internal consistency ranges from Cronbach α 0.70 for outdoor activities to 0.90 for interference.

Using cluster-analytic and multivariate classification methods, three homogeneous subgroups of patients with chronic pain have been identified and replicated across a wide range of medical diagnoses (i.e., back pain, temporomandibular disorders, headache). The three groups' distinct profiles were labeled "dysfunctional," "interpersonally distressed," and "adaptive coper."

Burton and colleagues[75] suggested that a psychometric battery consisting of the MPI and the BPI[76] was useful for both identifying problem areas that might impede treatment of patients with chronic pain and assessing treatment outcome. Moreover, the MPI has been shown to be predictive of chronicity of pain after acute symptom onset.[77,78] The MPI has demonstrated reliability and validity in patients with chronic low back pain (LBP).[79]

A recent study compared the redundancy, reliability, validity, and sensitivity to change among the Short-Form Health Survey (SF-36), Oswestry Disability Index (ODI; see later in the chapter), and MPI on a cross-sectional sample of 424 patients, with a follow-up sample of 87 patients with chronic pain, seen in an interdisciplinary pain clinic.[80] Cronbach α ranged from 0.69 to 0.92 for the MPI, ranged from 0.79 to 0.91 for the SF-36, and was 0.86 for the ODI. Three concepts overlapped between the SF-36 and the MPI: pain, interference or social functioning, and mental health. Both the SF-36 and the MPI contributed unique scales (e.g., the MPI "significant other" scales; R^2 range 0.03–0.16). Significant changes after treatment were observed for the MPI pain severity, interference, and outdoor work activities; the SF-36 physical and social functioning, bodily pain; and the ODI. The MPI is used widely and has been translated into Spanish, Portuguese, French, Swedish, Dutch, and Italian.[44,81,82]

TREATMENT OUTCOMES OF PAIN SYSTEM

Because, when applied to individual patients, the SF-36 lacked measurement reliability for assessment of treatment outcomes, lacked sensitivity to upper extremity or facial pathology, and failed to separate limitations of work versus everyday activity, two of us (Wittink and Carr) and colleagues conducted a two-part study to develop an outcomes instrument suitable for measurement of change in individual patients with chronic pain. A novel group of scales derived from responses to 61 questions (which include the SF-36) proved sufficiently reliable for routine follow-up of individual patients during treatment for chronic pain. This new instrument, the Treatment Outcomes of Pain System (TOPS), allows assessment of individual patient outcomes and aggregate or individual clinician performance during interdisciplinary treatment of chronic pain.[22,23]

In addition to the SF-36, this instrument contains demographic data and 14 scales of which 7 fit into the Nagi framework.[83] The remaining 7 scales are considered to be mediating factors among the domains of pain, functional limitation, and disability. The seven main scales include pain symptom, perceived and objective family disability, work limitations, objective work disability, and upper and lower body limitations. Cronbach α of these scales ranges from 0.70 for objective work disability to 0.92 for lower body functioning and 0.93 for perceived family/social disability. The mediating scales include fear avoidance, passive coping, life control, and solicitous responses. In addition, two scales measure patient satisfaction with care and outcomes. The final scale is the total pain experience scale, which is a composite of pain intensity, pain interference, physical functioning, and disability.

For evaluating a single patient, the TOPS pain symptom, perceived family/social disability, and total pain experience scales are considerably more sensitive to individual change than the SF-36 bodily pain (BP) scale. Their increased sensitivity can be attributed to their greater measurement reliability. For example, Cronbach α equals 0.93 for total pain experience compared with 0.84 for the SF-36 BP scale. The TOPS scales also provide a clearer and more clinically relevant set of concepts for a pain clinician who may have objectives apart from a simple reduction in pain intensity, such as the reduction of suffering or the reduction of disability in spite of pain. This high internal consistency allows for the measurement of change during treatment of an individual patient.[22]

Pain clinic normative values were established based on a sample of 1230 administrations of the tool in interdisciplinary pain clinics in Boston and Salt Lake City. The instrument was translated and validated in French Canadian and eight European languages.[84] The TOPS takes 10 to 15 minutes to complete.

INSTRUMENTS MEASURING MENTAL HEALTH AND COGNITIONS

Many patients with chronic pain learn to function normally despite their pain, continue to work productively, and rarely seek medical care. Factors such as coping ability,[85-87] fear avoidance,[49,88] self efficacy,[89,90] and catastrophizing[90-92] have been associated with adjustment differences in patients with chronic pain. The beliefs or cognitions that patients have regarding their pain problem are hypothesized to have a direct impact on mood. For instance, negative thoughts about pain are strongly related to depressive symptomatology.[93] Depression has been associated with high health care utilization and costs[94] and is prevalent in patients with chronic pain. Patients with chronic pain may develop a variety of psychological problems, including depression, anxiety, sleep disorders, and disruptions in family life. Because of the importance of psychological factors in the experience of chronic pain, adding an assessment of mental health and cognitive factors to generic and condition-specific HRQOL may help patients and health care providers work together more effectively toward their common goals of pain relief and improved functioning. Some commonly used mental health assessment tools are listed in **Table 106-5**.

Moderate to strong associations have been identified among coping responses, pain severity, psychological well-being, and physical functioning.[95,96] Fear avoidance beliefs correlated significantly with self-reported disability in activities of daily living (ADLs) and work loss[49] and were shown to be a significant predictor of chronic pain[40,97] in patients with musculoskeletal disorders. Catastrophizing was shown to predict depression,[86,90,91] perception of pain,[87,98] lower self-efficacy for

TABLE 106-5 Selected Mental Health Assessment Tools
Beck Depression Inventory (BDI)
Carroll Rating Scale for Depression
Center for Epidemiologic Studies Depression Scale (CES-D)
Depression Adjective Checklists
Geriatric Depression Scale
Hamilton Rating Scale for Depression
Millon Behavioral Health Inventory
Minnesota Multiphasic Personality Inventory (MMPI)
Montgomerysberg Depression Rating Scale
Multidimensional Health Locus of Control Scale
Self-Rating Depression Scale (Zung)
Symptom Checklist-90 (SL-90)

pain, lower spousal ratings of self-efficacy for control of fatigue or mood symptoms,[99] and disability.[100] Patients' beliefs and self-appraisals thus play a large part in shaping the outcome of treatment. Many instruments exist that measure patient beliefs; here we limit ourselves to discussing a few widely used tools.

COPING STRATEGIES QUESTIONNAIRE

Questionnaires that address cognitive factors include the widely used Coping Strategies Questionnaire (CSQ) and the Pain Beliefs and Perceptions Inventory (PBPI). The CSQ was designed to help identify methods of coping used by persons with chronic LBP.[101] It contains six types of cognitive strategies, two types of behavioral mechanisms, and two effectiveness ratings. The CSQ was found to be internally reliable when used to assess pain coping strategies. The authors also found that praying, hoping, and coping self-statements were used frequently, but others, such as reinterpretation of pain sensations, were not. Overall, cognitive coping and suppression, helplessness, and diverting attention or praying explained much of the variance in coping strategies. The CSQ has been studied widely to better describe its factor structure, its utility in persons with LBP or cancer pain, and its utility for prediction of patient and spouse ratings of patients' self-efficacy.[87,99,102-106]

PAIN BELIEFS AND PERCEPTIONS INVENTORY

The PBPI assesses three aspects of pain beliefs: self-blame, perception of pain as mysterious in origin, and beliefs about pain duration.[107] These authors found that the belief that pain will last is associated with greater pain intensity and decreased compliance with psychological and physical therapies. The PBPI contains only 16 items; thus, respondent burden is very low. Similar to the CSQ, the PBPI has been used widely and has been translated for use in the United Kingdom.[108-110]

FEAR AVOIDANCE BELIEFS QUESTIONNAIRE

The Fear Avoidance Beliefs Questionnaire (FABQ) is a 16-item instrument developed by Waddell and colleagues.[49] Within the 16 items are two fear-avoidance scales. The first scale (seven items) concerns fear-avoidance beliefs about work, and the second scale (four items) concerns fear-avoidance beliefs about physical activity. The internal consistencies (Cronbach α values) for these two scales were 0.88 and 0.77, respectively. Test–retest reliability had a κ equal to 0.74.

PAIN CATASTROPHIZING SCALE

The Pain Catastrophizing Scale (PCS) is a 13-item instrument developed in 1995 at the Dalhousie University Pain Research Centre to facilitate research on the mechanisms by which catastrophizing has an impact on the pain experience.[111] The items on the PCS were drawn from previous experimental and clinical research on catastrophic thinking in relation to pain experience.[101,112,113]

The PCS yields a total score and three subscale scores assessing rumination ("I can't stop thinking about how much it hurts"), magnification ("I worry that something serious might happen"), and helplessness ("There is nothing I can do to reduce the intensity of the pain").[114] A total PCS score of 38 represents a clinically relevant level of catastrophizing.[114]

Cronbach α for the total PCS is 0.87; for rumination, 0.87; for magnification, 0.66; and for helplessness, 0.78. Test–retest reliability across a 6-week period was $r = 0.75$.[111] The PCS takes about 5 minutes to complete. Support for good internal consistency and validity of the PCS was provided by others.[115,116]

DISEASE-SPECIFIC OUTCOMES MEASURES

Disease-specific instruments reflect particular limitations or restrictions associated with specific disease states. These instruments are designed to be sensitive in determining the effects of treatment on or the spontaneous longitudinal course of a single disease or condition. Disease-specific measures have been developed for almost every imaginable condition. For an overview of pain-specific tools, see **Table 106-6**.

TABLE 106-6 Selected Pain-Specific Health-Related Quality of Life Instruments
Arthritis Impact Measurement Scales (AIMS-2)
Back Pain Classification Scale (BPCS)
Brief Pain Inventory (BPI, BPI-SF; formerly Wisconsin Brief Pain Inventory)
Biobehavioral Pain Profile
Catastrophizing Scale
Family Pain Questionnaire
Fear Avoidance Beliefs Questionnaire (FABQ)
Fibromyalgia Impact Questionnaire (FIQ)
Graded Chronic Pain Scale (GCPS)
Illness Behavior Questionnaire
Low Back Pain Rating Scale
McGill Pain Questionnaire (MPQ, MPQ-SF)
Medical Outcomes Study Pain Measures
Multidimensional Pain Inventory (MPI; formerly West Haven-Yale Multidimensional Pain Inventory)
Neck Disability Index (NDI)
Neuropathic Pain Scale (NPS)
Oswestry Low Back Pain Disability Questionnaire
Pain and Distress Scale (PAD)
Pain Disability Index (PDI)
Pain Distress Scales
Pain and Impairment Relationship Scale (PAIRS)
Pain Perception Profile (PPP)
Patient Pain Questionnaire
Roland-Morris Disability Questionnaire (RDQ)
Somatic Input, Anxiety, and Depression (SAD) Index for the Clinical
Assessment of Pain
Treatment Outcomes of Pain System (TOPS)
Visual Analog Pain Rating Scales
Work Limitations Questionnaire (WLQ)

A few further examples of disease-specific instruments are instruments that measure the impact of migraine,[117] shoulder pain,[118-120] knee pain[121] (KOOS, a knee injury and osteoarthritis outcome tool, and Lysholm scales),[122] neck pain,[123] and back pain. Two of the most commonly used disease-specific tools for back pain are the ODI[124] and the Roland-Morris Disability Questionnaire (RDQ).[125] The ODI and RDQ scores are highly correlated, with similar test–retest reliability and internal consistency. Floor and ceiling effects determine the choice of instruments. A greater proportion of patients score in the top half of the distribution of RDQ sores than in the top half of the ODI scores. The ODI is, therefore, recommended in patients who are likely to have persistent severe disability, and the RDQ in patients who are likely to have relatively little disability.[126]

OSWESTRY DISABILITY INDEX

The ODI[124] is one of the most frequently used tools in back pain research. It consists of 10 sections that include pain intensity, personal care, lifting, walking, sitting, standing, sleeping, sex, social life, and traveling. Each section is scored on a 6-point scale (0–5), with 0 representing no limitation and 5 representing maximal limitation. The subscales combined add up to a maximum score of 50. The score is then doubled and interpreted as a percentage of patient perceived disability (the higher the score, the greater the disability).

The ODI has excellent test–retest reliability ($r = 0.99$,[124] ICC = 0.83,[127]) and clinical face validity. The internal reliability, Cronbach α, was found to be 0.71 for version 1.0.[128] Two studies that determined a Cronbach α of version 2.0 found it to be 0.76[14] and 0.87.[129]

ROLAND-MORRIS DISABILITY QUESTIONNAIRE

The RDQ[125] was derived from the Sickness Impact Profile (SIP). The generic SIP was modified to become disease specific by adding "because of my back pain" to each item. Twenty-four items were selected from the SIP by the original authors because they related specifically to physical functions that were likely to be affected by LBP. These items include walking, bending over, sitting, lying down, dressing, sleeping, self-care, and ADLs. Cronbach α for the scale has been estimated to be between 0.84 and 0.93.[126] The RDQ correlates well with the SF-36 physical subscales, the SIP,[130] and pain ratings.[131] It is available in 12 languages, and translations are available from the author (mroland@man.ac.uk).

WORK LIMITATIONS QUESTIONNAIRE

The WLQ was developed by Lerner and Amick with support from GlaxoWellcome, Inc. The WLQ is a 25-item self-administered questionnaire that evaluates the degree to which health problems interfere with ability to perform job roles. It was designed to assess groups of individuals who are currently employed. The WLQ indicates the degree to which health problems interfere with specific aspects of job performance (on-the-job disability) and the impact of these limitations on workers' productivity.

The WLQ items ask respondents to rate their level of difficulty (or, on one scale, their level of ability) to perform 25 specific job demands. These demands have four defining features: (1) a wide range of jobs in the United States include these demands, (2) a wide variety of physical and emotional health problems can make it difficult to perform these demands effectively, (3) the demands are considered important to their jobs by workers who hold these jobs, and (4) losses in individual work productivity are frequently related to the degree to which these job-related demands are not met.

Responses to the 25 items are combined into four work limitation scales: the Time Management scale (question 1), the Physical Demands scale (question 2), the Mental/Interpersonal Demands scale (questions 3 and 4), and the Output Demands scale (question 5). Cronbach α ranged from 0.88 for Output Demands to 0.91 for Mental/Interpersonal Demands. The WQL was shown to have high reliability and validity.[132] The instrument takes 5 to 10 minutes to complete. (For more information, contact wlq@lifespan.org.)

EVIDENCE-BASED RESEARCH AND GUIDELINES

The gold standard of current evidence-based literature synthesis is the Cochrane Collaboration. The Cochrane Collaboration was developed in response to a call by Archie Cochrane, a British epidemiologist, for systematic, up-to-date reviews of all randomized controlled trials (RCTs) on health care. Several centers have been established throughout the world, and collaborative review groups prepare and maintain systematic reviews. At the beginning of 1997, the existing and planned review groups (>40) covered most of the important areas of health care. Relevant to this chapter, Cochrane collaborative review groups have been formed to assess spine problems, musculoskeletal pathology, and pain (palliative and supportive care).[8] The Cochrane group's aims are "preparing, maintaining and disseminating systematic reviews of the effects of health care" to provide reliable, unbiased, up-to-date information to health care providers worldwide to permit informed decisions about the specific effects of health care interventions.[8] As stated earlier, in making decisions about the care of individual patients, the results of these reviews must be integrated with the clinician's expertise, which has been acquired through experience and practice. The results of the reviews must also be integrated with patients' understanding and preferences, which derive from their knowledge of their condition (particularly if it is a chronic or recurrent health problem), the treatments offered, and the responsiveness or otherwise of the former to the latter (http://www.cochrane.org/cochrane/cc-broch.htm#GDAHC). The integration of the results of the reviews, clinician expertise, and patient feedback and participation is considered evidence-based practice.

Methods for scoring the quality of research reviewed have been established.[133] If studies are combinable, a meta-analysis can be performed. A meta-analysis is a synthesis, usually understood to be quantitative, of the results of several studies.[2] The precision of such a meta-analysis is greater than that of any one of its component studies because of the aggregation of patient numbers. Cumulative meta-analysis recalculates aggregate treatment effects and confidence intervals as each new relevant study is published. This technique of ongoing recalculation permits early decisions as to whether a treatment is efficacious or not, thereby averting the need for subsequent unneeded, costly, time-consuming (and some would say unethical) clinical trials. Cumulative meta-analysis has documented that it may take years for statistically significant conclusions from RCTs to diffuse into textbooks and narrative review articles.[134]

One meta-analysis published outside of the Cochrane Library identified published studies of treatment in multidisciplinary pain clinics (MPCs) between 1960 and 1990.[135] These authors identified 65 studies that met inclusion criteria. They concluded that multidisciplinary pain treatment resulted in large effect sizes that were maintained for more than 6 months, that MPCs were efficacious, and that the effects were not limited to patients' perceptions but also extended to objective behavior, such as return to work or decreased use of health care resources. One analysis evaluated whether return to work could be predicted after MPC treatment.[136] These authors concluded that although prediction of return to work is an increasingly important topic, few of the studies they evaluated met appropriate design and statistical criteria. They were unable to clearly identify which variables were useful predictors of return to work.

One of the challenges unique to evaluating treatment at MPCs is that the criteria used to define success are often not uniform.[137] Despite this problem, Turk and colleagues[137] found that reported pain reduction ranged from 14% to 60% and that reductions appeared to be well maintained at follow-up, although some studies reported no improvement during treatment. Treatment was reported to result in decreased opioid use in nearly three-fourths of persons, whereas untreated people generally reported no change. Treatment was also noted to improve activity levels and return to work, lower use of the health care system (including hospitalization and surgery), and increase the percentage of disability claims that were settled. This last point suggests that many persons with chronic noncancer pain can return to work even after an extended period of being disabled.

Finally, one group of researchers performed a meta-analysis of meta-analyses.[138] These researchers concluded that MPC treatment is consistently effective for most outcomes, including return to work, although many different outcome variables were assessed in individual meta-analyses, and ultimately, it was "unclear what combination of treatments is necessary for an effective [treatment] package." Meta-analytic results depend, however, on the studies included within the analysis. Thus, owing to a variety of methodologic problems that affect pain treatment studies, the results of this literature synthesis should be interpreted cautiously. Indeed, some experts have argued that a single meta-analysis of heterogeneous trials of a single intervention applied to diverse groups of patients with a complex clinical condition may be frankly misleading.[139]

The College of Physicians and Surgeons of Ontario, Canada, was the first to publish guidelines on the treatment of chronic, noncancer pain based on the best available evidence in November 2000. (A PDF file of the entire guide is available at http://www.cpsbc.bc.ca/physician/documents/pain.htm.) Clinical practice guidelines have been defined as "systematically developed statements to assist practitioner and patient decisions about appropriate health care for specific clinical circumstances." In the establishment of guidelines, levels of evidence generally are stratified as follows:

Level I	Strong evidence from at least one systematic review of multiple well-designed randomized controlled trials
Level II	Strong evidence from at least one properly designed randomized controlled trial of appropriate size
Level III	Evidence from well-designed trials without randomization, single group pre–post, cohort, time series, or matched case-controlled studies
Level IV	Evidence from well-designed nonexperimental studies from more than one center or research group
Level V	Opinions from respected authorities based on clinical evidence, descriptive studies, or reports of expert committees

Often, guideline committees will add a second dimension that documents not only the nature of the evidence that forms the basis of the recommendations but also the strength and consistency of the evidence. Guidelines thus incorporate Cochrane or other systematic reviews when available but go one step further by making specific recommendations with the definite intent to influence what clinicians do. (Evidence reports and clinical practice guidelines can be found at http://www.ahrq.gov.)

PATIENT-CENTERED OUTCOMES RESEARCH AT THE POPULATION LEVEL

The Patient-Centered Outcomes Research Institute (PCORI) and PROMIS® (Patient-Reported Outcomes Measurement Information System) represent two developments in health outcomes research over the past several years. The PCORI's mission and vision emphasize information that can be used by patients and families, caregivers, payers, and policymakers to make decisions about health-related goals.[140] In comparison, the primary goal of PROMIS® is to provide valid measures to assess health and well-being from the patient's perspective, across all ages.[141]

THE PATIENT-CENTERED OUTCOMES RESEARCH INSTITUTE

The PCORI funds comparative effectiveness research related to three strategic goals and five national priorities.[142,143] These goals are to increase the amount and quality of timely comparative research, to move this research to application sooner, and to encourage other funders to make research more patient focused. The research priorities that PCORI emphasizes are:

- Assessment of prevention, diagnosis, and treatment options
- Improving health care systems
- Communication and dissemination of research
- Addressing disparities
- Accelerating patient-centered outcomes research and methodologic research

These research priorities are applicable to efforts to improve care for people with pain specifically, given the importance of the patient's perspective in this effort. Additionally, pain-related research fits well within other specific aims. For example, one study that PCORI has committed to support examines patient outcomes during the transition from hospital to home and the role of patient-centered medical homes and accountable care organizations.[142] Although this study is not necessarily specific to pain, there is evidence that pain is severe for a substantial proportion of people after surgery,[144] that postoperative pain can adversely affect functioning well after discharge to home,[145] and that analgesic gaps during this transition can result.[146] Furthermore, given that pain is a risk factor for readmission to the hospital[147] and is associated with decreased satisfaction with care (even in persons considered at low risk for having pain),[148] pain is an increasingly important outcome for patients, clinicians, payers, and policymakers.

THE PATIENT-REPORTED OUTCOMES MEASUREMENT INFORMATION SYSTEM

Begun in 2004 with funding from the National Institutes of Health, PROMIS consists of methods to develop patient-reported outcomes measures, a set of measures that meet these standards, and software to help clinicians and researchers use these instruments with patients.[149] The domains included in PROMIS questionnaires and surveys (broadly called "instruments") are related to self-reported health for children and adults, as well as for child care providers. The patient-reported outcomes structure for adults includes global, physical, mental, and social health,[150] whereas that for child self-reported proxy-reported health consists of physical, mental, and social health.[151] Pain-specific domains assessed in each of these groups include pain intensity, pain interference, pain behavior, and pain quality, and other domains that may be reasonably expected to be affected by pain (or vice versa) are also included. In adults, these areas include physical function, fatigue, sleep disturbance, sexual function, depression, anxiety, self-efficacy, and ability to participate in social roles and activities. In children and caregivers, the related counterparts include mobility, upper extremity function, fatigue, physical activity, sedentary behavior, depressive symptoms, anxiety, and peer relationships.

A search of the English-language biomedical literature conducted in July 2014 using the search strategy "PROMIS AND pain" resulted in 88 reports and articles. More than half of these articles were published since 2013, suggesting that use of the PROMIS framework to study pain and painful conditions is growing. The major categories of these papers included validation of item banks used to construct PROMIS instruments, evaluation of PROMIS in individuals with specific diseases or conditions (e.g., chronic noncancer pain, fibromyalgia, inflammatory bowel disease, chronic obstructive pulmonary disease, and multiple sclerosis), estimates of the epidemiology and effects of pain, and a report on research standards for chronic LBP.

One such study compared the prevalence of pain and pain interference in adults with physical disabilities with normative data from adults using PROMIS.[152] Individuals with neuromuscular disease, postpolio syndrome, or multiple sclerosis reported higher pain intensity and interference because of pain relative to individuals in the normative sample. Furthermore, impairment caused by pain did not decline with age.

Similar findings have been reported in cancer survivors and in children with cancer.[153,154] The purpose of the study of adults ($n = 170$) with head and neck, esophageal, gastric, or colorectal cancer was to assess pain and depression 6, 12, and 18 months after diagnosis. Younger adults reported higher pain intensity and greater interference with work and daily activities because of pain. In one study of children with cancer, investigators assessed the ability of 8- to 17-year-old patients in treatment for cancer or who were survivors to complete eight PROMIS measures. These investigators found that patients in this age group were able to complete the instruments and that participants in treatment reported worse functioning than survivors in seven measures, including pain interference. Fatigue, anger, and pain interference were worse for female study participants than for males.

Last, research has also been done to estimate the association between estimates derived from PROMIS instruments and other patient-reported tools. One such study was designed to assess pain interference as measured by the BPI compared with that assessed using the PROMIS pain interference short form in individuals with multiple sclerosis.[155] These researchers found that pain interference scores from these two instruments were similar and that previously collected data can serve as a starting point to compare data from newer studies using the PROMIS instruments.

CONCLUSION

This chapter has presented an overview of the terminology used in HRQOL outcomes assessment, examples of instruments that can be applied in clinical practice, and descriptions of PCORI and the PROMIS system and examples of how they apply to studying health care for people with pain. Systematic measurement and documentation of HRQOL is a useful, clinically relevant approach to incorporate patient preferences into front-line medical decision making. Doing so is expected to improve overall patient satisfaction with care.[10] No tool will be used if it is too burdensome (too long or too difficult to understand). Instruments must be easily understood, administered, and interpreted by both clinicians and patients. No instrument is ideal for all intended uses; questionnaires are available in a variety of forms, and many of them can be readily incorporated into clinical care and research. Outcomes assessment is a dynamic area, particularly as it stands at the interface between routine practice and new standards for pain assessment and treatment applied by The Joint Commission (formerly the Joint Commission for the Assessment of Healthcare Organizations). The dissemination of ever-simpler and more powerful means to capture data electronically in everyday health care opens new opportunities for understanding which treatments are effective and for whom and may provide irrefutable evidence that we who treat pain add patient-centered value to the health care enterprise.

WEBSITES TO VISIT FOR MEASUREMENT TOOLS

http://www.stat.washington.edu/TALARIA/talaria0/LS2.2.html: measurement of pain in children and patients with cancer pain

http://www.outcomes-trust.org/instruments/

http://www.york.ac.uk/inst/crd/welcome.htm

http://eircae.net/testcol.htm: test locator site

WEBSITES TO VISIT FOR EVIDENCE-BASED RESEARCH

http://www.cochrane.org: main site for the Cochrane Collaboration

www.med.unr.edu/medlib/netting.html: website containing evidence-based websites

http://www.herts.ac.uk/lis/subjects/health/ebm.htm: websites and databases

http://www.medicine.ox.ac.uk/bandolier/: Bandolier Evidence Based Medicine (EBM)

http://www.jr2.ox.ac.uk/bandolier/painres/painres.html: pain research at Bandolier EBM

http://www.iwh.on.ca/home.htm: Institute for Work and Health, Canada

http://www.ahcpr.gov/: Agency for Healthcare Research and Quality

WEBSITES TO VISIT FOR GUIDELINES ON MANAGING PAIN

http://www.ampainsoc.org/pub/bulletin/nov00/clin1.htm

http://www.guideline.govhttp://www.nlm.nih.gov/nichsr/hsrsites html: research on health care in general

REFERENCES

1. World Health Organization. *Constitution of the WHO, Basic Documents*. Geneva: WHO; 1948.
2. Sackett DL, Haynes RB, Rosenberg W, Richardson WS. *Evidence-Based Medicine: How to Practice and Teach EBM*. Orlando, FL: WB Saunders; 1997.
3. Goudas L, Carr DB, Bloch R, et al. Management of cancer pain. In: *Evidence Report/Technology Assessment No. 35*. Rockville, Md: Agency for Healthcare Research and Quality; 2001. AHRQ Publication No. 02-E002.
4. McQuay H, Moore A. *An Evidence-Based Resource for Pain Relief*. Oxford, England: Oxford University Press; 1998.
5. Foundation for Health Services Research. Health outcomes research: A primer [Association for Health Services Research]. 1994. Available at: http://www.ahsr.org. Accessed April 17, 2002.
6. Tanenbaum SJ. What physicians know. *N Engl J Med*. 1993;329: 1268-1271.
7. Mulrow CD, Oxman A, eds. Cochrane Collaboration Handbook [updated September 1997]. In: The Cochrane Library [database on disk and CDROM]. The Cochrane Collaboration. Oxford, England: Update software, issue 4; 1997.
8. Carr DB, Wiffen P, Fairman F, LeMaitre M. The Cochrane Collaboration and its Pain, Palliative, and Supportive care review group. In: Max M, ed. *Pain 1999—An Updated Review*. Refresher course syllabus. Seattle: IASP; 1999:399-410.
9. Gerteis M, Edgman-Levitan S, Daley J, Delbanco TL, eds. *Through the Patient's Eyes: Understanding and Promoting Patient-Centered Care*. San Francisco: Jossey-Bass; 1993.
10. Marvel MK, Epstein RM, Flowers K, Beckman HB. Soliciting the patient's agenda: have we improved? *JAMA*. 1999;281:283-287.
11. Rucker KS, Metzler HM, Kregel J. Standardization of chronic pain assessment: a multiperspective approach. *Clin J Pain*. 1996;12:94-110.
12. Ware J. The status of health assessment 1994. *Ann Rev Public Health*. 1995;16:327-354.
13. Greenfield S, Nelson EC. Recent developments and future issues in the use of health status assessment measures in clinical settings. *Med Care*. 1992;30:MS23-MS41.
14. Fisher K, Johnson M. Validation of the Oswestry low back pain disability questionnaire, its sensitivity as a measure of change following treatment and its relationship with other aspects of the chronic pain experience. *Physiother Theory Pract*. 1992;13:67-80.
15. Carr DB. The development of national guidelines for pain control: synopsis and commentary. *Eur J Pain*. 2001;5(Suppl A):91-98.
16. Hall JA, Roter DL, Katz NR. Meta-analysis of correlates of provider behavior in medical encounters. *Med Care*. 1988;26:657-675.
17. Becker MH. Patient adherence to prescribed therapies. *Med Care*. 1985;23:539-555.
18. Kaplan SH, Greenfield S, Ware JE. Assessing the effects of physician-patient interactions on the outcomes of chronic disease. *Med Care*. 1989;7(Suppl):S110-S127.
19. Pransky G, Himmelstein J. Outcomes research; implications for occupational health. *Am J Ind Med*. 1996;29:573-583.
20. Ware JE Jr. Conceptualizing and measuring generic health outcomes. *Cancer*. 1991;67(Suppl):774-779.
21. Wagner AK, Rogers WH, Sukiennik A, et al. Outcomes assessment in chronic pain treatment: The need to supplement the SF-36. American Pain Society, 1995 Annual Meeting Program; A-66.
22. Rogers W, Wittink HM, Wagner A, et al. Assessing individual outcomes during outpatient, multidisciplinary chronic pain treatment by means of an augmented SF-36. *Pain Med*. 2000;1:44-54.

23. Rogers WH, Wittink HM, Ashburn MA, et al. Using the "TOPS": an outcomes instrument for multidisciplinary outpatient pain treatment. *Pain Med.* 2000;1:55-67.
24. Jensen MP, Karoly P, Braver S. The measurement of clinical pain intensity: a comparison of six methods. *Pain.* 1986;27: 117-126.
25. Wood-Dauphinee S, Troidl H. Endpoints for clinical studies: Conventional and innovative variables. In: Troidl H, Spitzer WO, McPeek B, et al., eds. *Principles and Practice of Research: Strategies for Surgical Investigators.* 2nd ed. New York: Springer-Verlag; 1991:151-168.
26. McDowell I, Newell C. *Measuring Health: A Guide to Rating Scales and Questionnaires.* New York: Oxford University Press; 1996.
27. Nunnally J. *Psychometric Theory.* New York: McGraw-Hill; 1978.
28. Hunt SM, McEwen J. The development of a submissive health indicator. *Social Health Illness.* 1980;2:231-246.
29. Hunt SM, McKenna SP, Williams J. Reliability of a population survey tool for measuring perceived health problems: a study of patients with osteoarthrosis. *J Epidemiol Community Health.* 1981;35:297-300.
30. Essink-Bot ML, Krabbe PF, van Agt HM, Bonsel GJ. NHP or SIP—a comparative study in renal insufficiency associated anemia. *Qual Life Res.* 1996;5:91-100.
31. Essink-Bot ML, Krabbe PF, Bonsel GJ, Aaronson NK. An empirical comparison of four generic health status measures: The Nottingham Health Profile, the Medical Outcomes Study 36-item Short-Form Health Survey, the COOP/WONCA charts, and the EuroQol instrument. *Med Care.* 1997;35:522-537.
32. Tarlov AR, Ware JE Jr, Greenfield S, et al. The Medical Outcomes Study. An application of methods for monitoring the results of medical care. *JAMA.* 1989;262:925-930.
33. Stewart AL, Hays RD, Ware JE Jr. The MOS short-form general health survey: Reliability and validity in a patient population. *Med Care.* 1988;26:724-735.
34. Ware JE Jr, Sherbourne CD. The MOS 36-item Short-Form Health Survey (SF-36). I. Conceptual framework and item selection. *Med Care.* 1992;30:473-483.
35. McHorney CA, Ware JE, Raczek AE. The MOS 36-Item Short-Form Health Survey (SF-36): II. Psychometric and clinical tests of validity in measuring physical and mental health constructs. *Med Care.* 1994;31:247-263.
36. Stansfeld SA, Roberts R, Foot SP. Assessing the validity of the SF-36 General Health Survey. *Qual Life Res.* 1997;6:217-224.
37. Grevitt M, Khazim R, Webb J, et al. The Short Form-36 health survey questionnaire in spine surgery. *J Bone Joint Surg Br.* 1997;79:48-52.
38. Bergner M, Bobbitt RA, Carter WB, Gilson BS. The Sickness Impact Profile: development and final revision of a health status measure. *Med Care.* 1981;19:787-805.
39. Bergner M, Bobbitt RA, Kressel S, et al. The sickness impact profile: conceptual formulation and methodology for the development of a health status measure. *Int J Health Serv.* 1976;6:393-415.
40. Bergner M, Bobbitt RA, Pollard WE, et al. The Sickness Impact Profile: validation of a health status measure. *Med Care.* 1976; 14:57-67.
41. Chapman CR, Gavrin J. Suffering: the contributions of persistent pain. *Lancet.* 1999;353:2233-2237.
42. Brown J, Klapow J, Doleys D, et al. Disease-specific and generic health outcomes: a model for the evaluation of long-term intrathecal opioid therapy in noncancer low back pain patients. *Clin J Pain.* 1999;15:122-131.
43. Rudy TE, Kerns RD, Turk DC. Chronic pain and depression: towards a cognitive-behavioral mediation model. *Pain.* 1988; 35:129-140.
44. Lousberg R, Van B, Groenman NH, et al. Psychometric properties of the Multidimensional Pain Inventory, Dutch language version (MPI-DLV). *Behav Res Ther.* 1999;37:167-182.
45. Kerns RD, Turk DC, Rudy TE. The West Haven-Yale Multidimensional Pain Inventory (WHYMPI). *Pain.* 1985;23:345-356.
46. Romano JM, Turner JA, Jensen MP, et al. Chronic pain patient-spouse behavioral interactions predict patient disability. *Pain.* 1995;63:353-360.
47. Tan G, Jensen MP, Robinson-Whelen S, et al. Coping with chronic pain: a comparison of two measures. *Pain.* 2001;90:127-133.
48. Nielson WR, Jensen MP, Hill ML. An activity pacing scale for the chronic pain coping inventory: development in a sample of patients with fibromyalgia syndrome. *Pain.* 2001;89:111-115.
49. Waddell G, Newton M, Henderson I, et al. A Fear-Avoidance Beliefs Questionnaire (FABQ) and the role of fear-avoidance beliefs in chronic low back pain and disability. *Pain.* 1993;52:157-168.
50. Vlaeyen JW, Linton SJ. Fear-avoidance and its consequences in chronic musculoskeletal pain: a state of the art [review]. *Pain.* 2000;85:317-332.
51. Al Obaidi SM, Nelson RM, Al Awadhi S, Al Shuwaie N. The role of anticipation and fear of pain in the persistence of avoidance behavior in patients with chronic low back pain. *Spine.* 2000;25:1126-1131.
52. Von Korff M, Jensen MP, Karoly P. Assessing global pain severity by self-report in clinical and health services research. *Spine.* 2000;25:3140-3151.
53. Jensen MP, McFarland CA. Increasing the reliability and validity of pain intensity measurement in chronic pain patients. *Pain.* 1993;55:195-203.
54. Dworkin SF, Von Korff M, Whitney CW, et al. Measurement of characteristic pain intensity in field pain research. *Pain.* 1990;(Suppl 5):S290.
55. Serlin RC, Mendoza TR, Nakamura Y, et al. When is cancer pain mild, moderate or severe? Grading pain severity by its interference with function. *Pain.* 1995;61:277-284.
56. Jensen MP, Turner JA, Romano JM, Fisher LD. Comparative reliability and validity of chronic pain intensity measures. *Pain.* 1999;83:157-162.
57. Jensen MP, Smith DG, Ehde DM, Robinsin LR. Pain site and the effects of amputation pain: Further clarification of the meaning of mild, moderate, and severe pain. *Pain.* 2001;91:317-322.
58. Scott J, Huskisson EC. Graphic representation of pain. *Pain.* 1976;2:175-184.
59. Huskisson EC. Measurement of pain. *Lancet.* 1974;2:1127-1131.
60. Kremer E, Atkinson JH, Ignelzi RJ. Measurement of pain: patient preference does not confound pain measurement. *Pain.* 1981;10:241-248.
61. Jensen MP, Turner JA, Romano JM. What is the maximum number of levels needed in pain intensity measurement? *Pain.* 1994;58:387-392.
62. Melzack R. The McGill pain questionnaire: major properties and scoring methods. *Pain.* 1975;1:275-299.
63. Graham C, Bond SS, Gerkousch MM, Cook MR. Use of the McGill Pain Questionnaire in the assessment of cancer pain: replicability and consistency. *Pain.* 1980;8:377-387.
64. Keefe FJ, Wilkins RH, Cook WA, et al. Depression, pain, and pain behavior. *J Consult Clin Psychol.* 1986;54:665-669.

65. Melzack R. The McGill Pain Questionnaire. In: Melzack R, ed. *Pain Measurement and Assessment*. New York, NY: Raven Press; 1983:41-47.

66. Sternbach RA, Murphy RW, Timmermans G, et al. Measuring the severity of clinical pain. In: Bonica JJ, ed. *Advances in Neurology*. (Vol. 4). New York: Raven Press; 1974:281-288.

67. Turk DC, Melzack R, eds. *Handbook of Pain Assessment*. New York: Guilford Press; 1992.

68. Carr DB, Jacox AK, Chapman CR, et al. *Acute Pain Management: Operative or Medical Procedures and Trauma. Clinical Practice Guideline No. 1*. Rockville, MD: Agency for Health Care Policy and Research, Public Health Service, US Department of Health and Human Services; February 1992. AHCPR Pub. NO 92-0032.

69. Cleeland CS. Pain assessment in cancer. In: Osoba D, ed. *Effect of Cancer on Quality of Life*. Boca Raton, FL: CRC Press; 1991:293-305.

70. Uki J, Mendoza TR, Gao SZ, Cleeland CS. The Chinese version of the Brief Pain Inventory (BPI-C): its development and use in a study of cancer pain. *Pain*. 1996;67:407-416.

71. Saxena A, Mendoza T, Cleeland CS. The assessment of cancer pain in north India: the validation of the Hindi Brief Pain Inventory—BPI-H. *J Pain Symptom Manage*. 1999;17:27-41.

72. Caraceni A, Mendoza TR, Mencaglia E, et al. A validation study of an Italian version of the Brief Pain Inventory (Breve Questionario per la Valutazione del Dolore). *Pain*. 1996;65:87-92.

73. Cleeland CS, Ryan KM. Pain assessment: Global use of the Brief Pain Inventory. *Ann Acad Med Singapore*. 1994;23:129-138.

74. Cleeland CS, Syrjala KL. How to assess cancer pain. In: Turk D, Melzack R, eds. *Pain Assessment*. New York: Guilford Press; 1992: 360-387.

75. Burton HJ, Sline SA, Hargadon R, et al. Assessing patients with chronic pain using the basic personality inventory as a complement to the multidimensional pain inventory. *Pain Res Manage*. 1999;4:131-129.

76. Jackson DN. *The Basic Personality Inventory: The BPI Manual*. Port Huron, MI: Research Psychologists Press; 1989.

77. Epker J, Gatchel RJ. Prediction of treatment-seeking behavior in acute TMD patients: practical application in clinical settings. *J Orofacial Pain*. 2000;14:303-309.

78. Olsson I, Bunketorp O, Carlsson SG, Styf J. Prediction of outcome in whiplash-associated disorders using West Haven-Yale Multidimensional Pain Inventory. *Clin J Pain*. 2002;18(4):238-244.

79. Turk DC, Rudy TE. The robustness of an empirically derived taxonomy of chronic pain patients. *Pain*. 1990;43:27-35.

80. Wittink H, Turk DC, Carr DB, et al. Assessing chronic pain treatment outcomes: comparison of the SF-36, ODI, and MPI. *Clin J Pain*. 2004;20(3):133-142.

81. Walter L, Brannon L. A cluster analysis of the Multidimensional Pain Inventory. *Headache*. 1991;31:476-479.

82. Bergström G, Jensen IB, Bodin L, et al. Reliability and factor structure of the Multidimensional Pain Inventory–Swedish language version (MPI-S). *Pain*. 1998;75:101-110.

83. Nagi S. Disability concepts revisited: Implications for prevention. In: Pope AM, Tarlov A, eds. *Disability in America: Toward a National Agenda for Prevention*. Committee on a National Agenda for the Prevention of Disabilities, Division of Health Promotion and Disease Prevention, Institute of Medicine. Washington, DC: National Academies Press; 1991:309-327.

84. Nadjar A. *Personal communication*. Lyon, France: MAPI Research Institute; 2002.

85. Nicassio PM, Schoenfeld-Smith K, Radojevic V, Schuman C. Pain coping mechanisms in fibromyalgia: relationship to pain and functional outcomes. *J Rheumatol*. 1995;22:1552-1558.

86. Turner JA, Jensen MP, Romano JM. Do beliefs, coping, and catastrophizing independently predict functioning in patients with chronic pain? *Pain*. 2000;85:115-125.

87. Geisser ME, Robinson ME, Henson CD. The Coping Strategies Questionnaire and chronic pain adjustment: a conceptual and empirical reanalysis. *Clin J Pain*. 1994;10:98-106.

88. Lethem J, Slade PD, Troup JDG, Bentley G. Outline of a fear-avoidance model of exaggerated pain perceptions. *Behav Res Ther*. 1983;21:401-408.

89. Geisser ME, Robinson ME, Keefe FJ, Weiner ML. Catastrophizing, depression and the sensory, affective and evaluative aspects of chronic pain. *Pain*. 1994;59:79-83.

90. Keefe FJ, Lefebvre JC, Egert JR, et al. The relationship of gender to pain, pain behavior, and disability in osteoarthritis patients: the role of catastrophizing. *Pain*. 2000;87:325-334.

91. Keefe FJ, Brown GK, Wallston KA, Caldwell DS. Coping with rheumatoid arthritis pain: Catastrophizing as a maladaptive strategy. *Pain*. 1989;37:51-56.

92. Buckelew SP, Parker JC, Keefe FJ, et al. Self-efficacy and pain behavior among subjects with fibromyalgia. *Pain*. 1994;59:377-384.

93. Geisser ME, Roth RS, Theisen ME, et al. Negative affect, self-report of depressive symptoms, and clinical depression: Relation to the experience of chronic pain. *Clin J Pain*. 2000;16:110-120.

94. Engel CC, Von K, Katon WJ. Back pain in primary care: predictors of high health-care costs. *Pain*. 1996;65:197-204.

95. Jensen MP, Karoly P. Control beliefs, coping efforts, and adjustment to chronic pain. *J Consult Clin Psychol*. 1991;59:431-438.

96. Jensen MP, Turner JA, Romano JM, Karoly P. Coping with chronic pain: a critical review of the literature. *Pain*. 1991;47:249-283.

97. Klenerman L, Slade PD, Stanley IM, et al. The prediction of chronicity in patients with an acute attack of low back pain in a general practice setting. *Spine*. 1995;20:478-484.

98. Hassett AL, Cone JD, Patella SJ, Sigal LH. The role of catastrophizing in the pain and depression of women with fibromyalgia syndrome. *Arthritis Rheum*. 2000;43:2493-2500.

99. Keefe FJ, Kashikar-Zuck S, Robinson E, et al. Pain coping strategies that predict patients' and spouses' ratings of patients' self-efficacy. *Pain*. 1997;73:191-199.

100. Martin MY, Bradley LA, Alexander RW, et al. Coping strategies predict disability in patients with primary fibromyalgia. *Pain*. 1996;68:45-53.

101. Rosenstiel AK, Keefe FJ. The use of coping strategies in chronic low back pain patients: relationship to patient characteristics and current adjustment. *Pain*. 1983;17:33-44.

102. Riley JL, Robinson ME. CSQ: five factors or fiction? *Clin J Pain*. 1997;13:156-162.

103. Robinson ME, Riley JL, Myers CD, et al. The Coping Strategies Questionnaire: a large sample, item level factor analysis. *Clin J Pain*. 1997;13:43-49.

104. Swartzman LC, Gwadry FG, Shapiro AP, Teasell RW. The factor structure of the Coping Strategies Questionnaire. *Pain*. 1994;57:311-316.

105. Dozois DJA, Dobson KS, Wong M, et al. Predictive utility of the CSQ in low back pain: Individual vs. composite measures. *Pain*. 1996;66:171-180.

106. Lin CC. Comparison of the effects of perceived self-efficacy on coping with chronic cancer pain and coping with chronic low back pain. *Clin J Pain*. 1998;14:303-310.

107. Williams DA, Thorn BE. An empirical assessment of pain beliefs. *Pain*. 1989;36:351-358.

108. Williams AC, Richardson PH. What does the BDI measure on chronic pain? *Pain*. 1993;55:259-266.

109. Herda CA, Siegeris K, Basler H-D. The Pain Beliefs and Perceptions Inventory: further evidence for a 4-factor structure. *Pain.* 1994;57:85-90.

110. Morley S, Wilkinson L. The pain beliefs and perceptions inventory: a British replication. *Pain.* 1995;61:427-433.

111. Sullivan MJL, Bishop SR, Pivik J. The Pain Catastrophizing scale: development and validation. *Psychol Assess.* 1995;7:524-532.

112. Chaves JF, Brown JM. Spontaneous cognitive strategies for the control of clinical pain and stress. *J Behav Med.* 1987;10:263-276.

113. Spanos NP, Perlini AH, Robertson LA. Hypnosis, suggestion, and placebo in the reduction of experimental pain. *J Abnorm Psychol.* 1989;98:285-293.

114. Sullivan MJL. *The Pain Catastrophizing Scale Manual.* Halifax, Nova Scotia: Dalhousie University, Pain Research Centre; 2000.

115. Osman A, Barrios FX, Gutierrez PM, et al. The Pain Catastrophizing Scale: Further psychometric evaluation with adult samples. *J Behav Med.* 2000;23:351-365.

116. Osman A, Barrios FX, Kopper BA, et al. Factor structure, reliability, and validity of the Pain Catastrophizing Scale. *J Behav Med.* 1997;20:589-605.

117. Patrick DL, Hurst BC, Hughes J. Further development and testing of the migraine-specific quality of life (MSQOL) measure. *Headache.* 2000;40:550-560.

118. Beaton DE, Richards RR. Measuring function of the shoulder. A cross-sectional comparison of five questionnaires. *J Bone Joint Surg Am.* 1996;78:882-890.

119. Roddey TS, Olson SL, Cook KF, et al. Comparison of the University of California-Los Angeles Shoulder Scale and the Simple Shoulder Test with the shoulder pain and disability index: single-administration reliability and validity. *Phys Ther.* 2000;80:759-768.

120. van der Heijden GJ, van der Windt DA, de Winter AF, et al. The responsiveness of the Shoulder Disability Questionnaire. *Ann Rheum Dis.* 1998;57:82-87.

121. Roos EM, Roos HP, Lohmander LS, et al. Knee Injury and Osteoarthritis Outcome Score (KOOS)—development of a self-administered outcome measure. *J Orthop Sports Phys Ther.* 1998;28:88-96.

122. Lysholm J, Gillquist J. Evaluation of knee ligament surgery results with special emphasis on use of a scoring scale. *Am J Sports Med.* 1982;10:150-154.

123. Vernon H, Mior S. The Neck Disability Index: A study of reliability and validity. [erratum appears in *J Manipulative Physiol Ther* 1992;15]. *J Manipulative Physiol Ther.* 1991;14:409-415.

124. Fairbank J, Couper J, Davies J, O'Brien J. The Oswestry Low Back Pain Disability Questionnaire. *Physiotherapy.* 1980;66:271-273.

125. Roland M, Morris R. A study of the natural history of back pain. Part I: development of a reliable and sensitive measure of disability in low-back pain. *Spine.* 1983;8:141-144.

126. Roland M, Fairbank J. The Roland-Morris Disability Questionnaire and the Oswestry Disability Questionnaire. *Spine.* 2000;25:3115-3124.

127. Gronblad M, Hupli M, Wennerstrand P, et al. Intercorrelation and test-retest reliability of the Pain Disability Index (PDI) and the Oswestry Disability Questionnaire (ODQ) and their correlation with pain intensity in low back pain patients. *Clin J Pain.* 1993;9:189-195.

128. Strong J, Ashton R, Large RG. Function and the patient with chronic low back pain. *Clin J Pain.* 1994;10:191-196.

129. Kopec JA, Esdaile JM, Abrahamowitz ED, et al. The Quebec back pain disability scale: Conceptualization and development. *J Clin Epidemiol.* 1996;49:151-161.

130. Jensen MP, Strom SE, Turner JA, Romano JM. Validity of the Sickness Impact Profile Roland scale as a measure of dysfunction in chronic pain patients. *Pain.* 1992;50:157-162.

131. Beurskens AJ, de Vet HC, Koke AJ. Responsiveness of functional status in low back pain: a comparison of different instruments. *Pain.* 1996;65:71-76.

132. Lerner D, Amick BC, Rogers WH, et al. The Work Limitations Questionnaire. *Med Care.* 2001;39:72-85.

133. Jadad AR, McQuay HJ. Meta-analyses to evaluate analgesic interventions: a systematic qualitative review of their methodology. *J Clin Epidemiol.* 1996;49:235-243.

134. Lau J, Antman EM, Jimenez-Silva J, et al. Cumulative meta-analysis of therapeutic trials for myocardial infarction. *N Engl J Med.* 1992;327:248-254.

135. Flor H, Fydrich T, Turk DC. Efficacy of multidisciplinary pain treatment centers: A meta-analytic review. *Pain.* 1992;49:221-230.

136. Fishbain DA, Rosomoff HL, Goldberg M, et al. The prediction of return to the workplace after multidisciplinary pain center treatment. *Clin J Pain.* 1993;9:3-15.

137. Turk DC. Efficacy of multidisciplinary pain centers in the treatment of chronic pain. In: Cohen MJM, Campbell JN, eds. *Pain Treatment Centers at a Crossroads: A Practical and Conceptual Reappraisal.* (Vol. 7). Seattle: IASP Press; 1996:257-272.

138. Fishbain DA, Cutler RB, Rosomoff HL, Rosomoff RS. Status of chronic pain treatment outcomes research. In: Aronoff GM, ed. *Evaluation and Treatment of Chronic Pain.* 3rd ed. Baltimore: Williams & Wilkins; 1999:655-670.

139. Lau J, Ioannides JPA, Schmid CH. Summing up evidence: one answer is not always enough. *Lancet.* 1998;351:123-127.

140. Patient-Centered Outcomes Research Institute. Mission and Vision. Available at: http://www.pcori.org/about-us/mission-and-vision/. Accessed 7/26/14.

141. PROMIS Mission, Vision, and Goals. Available at: http://www.nihpromis.org/about/missionvisiongoals. Accessed 7/26/14.

142. Selby JV, Lipstein SH. PCORI at 3 years—progress, lessons, and plans. *N Engl J Med.* 2014;370:592-595.

143. PCORI National Priorities and Research Agenda. Available at: http://www.pcori.org/research-we-support/priorities-agenda/. Accessed 7/26/14.

144. Gan TJ, Habib AS, Miller TE, et al. Incidence, patient satisfaction, and perceptions of post-surgical pain: results from a US national survey. *Curr Med Res Opin.* 2014;30(1):149-60.

145. Strassels SA, McNicol E, Wagner AK, et al. Persistent postoperative pain, health-related quality of life, and functioning one month after hospital discharge. *Acute Pain.* 2004;6:95-104.

146. Ng A, Hall F, Atkinson A, et al. Bridging the analgesic gap. *Acute Pain.* 2000;3:194-9.

147. Coley KC, Williams BA, DaPos SV, et al. Retrospective evaluation of unanticipated admissions and readmissions after same day surgery and associated costs. *J Clin Anesth.* 2002;14:349-353.

148. Whelan CT, Jin L, Meltzer D. Pain and satisfaction with pain control in hospitalized medical patients: No such thing as low risk. *Arch Intern Med.* 2004;164:175-180.

149. PROMIS History. Available at: http://www.nihpromis.org/about/history. Accessed: 7/27/14., PROMIS®. Frequently Asked Questions. Available at: http://www.nihpromis.org/faqs. Accessed 7/27/14).

150. Domain Frameworks. PROMIS Adult Self-Reported Health. Available at: http://www.nihpromis.org/measures/domainframework1. Accessed: 7/27/14.

151. Domain Frameworks. PROMIS Pediatric Self- and Proxy-Reported Health. Available at: http://www.nihpromis.org/measures/domainframework2. Accessed: 7/27/14.

152. Molton I, Cook KF, Smith AE, et al. Prevalence and impact of pain in adults aging with a physical disability: comparison to a US general population sample. *Clinical Journal of Pain.* 2014;30(4): 307-15.

153. Moye J, June A, Martin LA, et al. Pain is prevalent and persisting in cancer survivors: differential factors across age groups. *Journal of Geriatric Oncology*. 2014;5(2):190-196.

154. Hinds PS, Nuss SL, Ruccione KS, et al. PROMIS pediatric measures in pediatric oncology: valid and clinically feasible indicators of patient-reported outcomes. *Pediatric Blood & Cancer*. 2013; 60(3):402-408.

155. Askew RL, Kim J, Chung H, et al. Development of a crosswalk for pain interference measured by the BPI and PROMIS pain interference short form. *Qual Life Res*. 2013;22(10):2769-2776.

SUGGESTED READINGS

Fischer D, Stewart AL, Bloch DA, et al. Capturing the patient's view of change as a clinical outcome measure. *JAMA*. 1999;282:1157-1162.

Galer BS, Jensen MP. Development and preliminary validation of a pain measure specific to neuropathic pain: The Neuropathic Pain Scale. *Neurology*. 1997;48:332-338.

Gill TM, Feinstein AR. A critical appraisal of the quality of quality-of-life measurements. *JAMA*. 1994;272:619-626.

Hunt SM, McKenna SP, McEwen J, et al. A quantitative approach to perceived health status: a validation study. *J Epidemiol Community Health*. 1980;34:281-286.

Meenan RF, Mason J, Anderson JJ, et al. The content and properties of a revised and expanded Arthritis Impact Measurement Scales Health Status Questionnaire. *Arthritis Rheum*. 1992;35:1-10.

Stewart AL, Greenfield S, Hays RD, et al. Functional status and well-being of patients with chronic conditions: Results from the Medical Outcomes Study [published erratum appears in *JAMA* 1989;262:2542]. *JAMA*. 1989;262:907-913.

Turk DC, Rudy TE. Toward an empirically derived taxonomy of chronic pain patients: integration of psychological assessment data. *J Consult Clin Psychol*. 1988;56:233-238.

World Health Organization. *International Classification of Impairments, Disabilities and Handicaps (ICIDH)*. Geneva, Switzerland: WHO; 1980.

Questions from Selected Chapters

CHAPTER 4 INFLAMMATION IN PAIN DISORDERS

1. Which of the following support the contrarian theory that inflammation has no role in painful disorders of the intervertebral disc?
   (a) The intervertebral disc is a relatively avascular structure.
   (b) The intervertebral disc is relatively free of sensory innervation, including nociceptors.
   (c) Discogenic pain does not respond to treatments targeting inflammation.
   (d) Disc herniations do not involve actual "swelling," per se.
2. The following are true about Celsus' cardinal signs of inflammation, except:
   (a) Dolor is pain, with biochemical substrates including substance P, bradykinin, TNF-α, and its receptor.
   (b) Rubor is redness, with biochemical substrates, including calcitonin gene–related peptide (CGRP).
   (c) Calor is heat, with biochemical substrates, including calcitonin gene–related peptide (CGRP).
   (d) Tumor is swelling, with biochemical substrates, including substance P.
   (e) Pallor is leukocytosis, with biochemical substrates, including the chemokines.
3. The following statements about complex regional pain syndrome (CRPS) and classic and neurogenic inflammation are true, except:
   (a) In CRPS, there may be increased local, systemic, and cerebrospinal fluid levels of proinflammatory cytokines such as TNF-α and IL-1, as well as decreased systemic levels of antiinflammatory cytokines such as IL-10.
   (b) CRPS is associated with alterations in circulating catecholamines and sympathetic nerve function.
   (c) Animal postfracture model of CRPS-I implicate substance P and TNF-α.
   (d) Genetic associations with CRPS include human leukocyte antigen alleles and a TNF-α promoter gene polymorphism.
   (e) Neurogenic inflammation involves increased systemic levels of proinflammatory neuropeptides such as CGRP, bradykinin, and substance P.
4. Which of the following statements are correct regarding tumor necrosis factor alpha (TNF-α) in relation to inflammation and pain?
   i. In animal models, injection of TNF-α into sciatic nerve causes neuropathic pain, and histologic changes in nerve are consistent with inflammation.
   ii. Animal and clinical studies demonstrate elevations of TNF-α as well as TNF-α receptors in neuropathic pain states.
   iii. TNF-α mediates pain due to herniated discs, and controlled clinical trials consistently demonstrate effect of epidural injection of TNF-α inhibitor to treat radicular pain due to herniated discs.
   iv. TNF-α and its receptor are specifically linked to the clinical phenomena of hyperalgesia and allodynia, as seen in neuropathic pain.
   (a) i, ii, iii
   (b) i, ii, iv
   (c) i and iv only
   (d) i and iii only

CHAPTER 8 EVALUATING THE PATIENT WITH CHRONIC PAIN

1. Detailed history on the first visit of a complex pain patient should include
   (a) Effect of stress on pain
   (b) Effect of pain on quality of life
   (c) Effect of pain on functioning at work
   (d) Associated sleep and mood disturbances
   (e) All of the above
2. A 63-year-old male presents with recent exacerbation of his chronic neck pain, with occasional radiation into the right shoulder and right arm. On examination, he has sensory deficits over the right medial forearm; decreased motor strength in finger flexors, finger extensors, and flexor carpi ulnaris. Strength is normal in the intrinsic muscles of the hand. Deep tendon reflexes are 2+ throughout the right arm. The most likely diagnosis is
   (a) Median nerve entrapment
   (b) Ulnar nerve compression
   (c) Radial nerve injury
   (d) C 8 radiculopathy
   (e) C 6 radiculopathy
3. A 41-year-old male presents with right hand pain and intermittent numbness/tingling for 6 months duration. On examination, he has sensory deficits to pin prick in the palm of the right hand (more prominent in the thumb and first finger), decreased motor strength in abductor pollicis brevis, finger flexors in fingers 1, 2 and 3 (with sparing of finger flexors 4, 5). Strength in abductor digiti minimi, finger extensors, and flexor carpi ulnaris is 5/5. Deep tendon reflexes are 2+ throughout the right arm. The most likely diagnosis is
   (a) C 8 radiculopathy
   (b) T 1 radiculopathy
   (c) Median neuropathy
   (d) Ulnar neuropathy
   (e) Radial neuropathy

4. A 27-year-old female presents with pain in the left shoulder and proximal left arm, which started acutely after a skiing injury three months ago, when she fell on an abducted left arm. On physical exam, she has motor weakness in the intrinsic hand muscles, finger flexors, wrist flexors, finger extensors, and flexor carpi ulnaris. Which of the following is the best initial diagnostic test for this patient?
   (a) MRI cervical spine without contrast
   (b) MRI cervical spine with and without contrast
   (c) MRI left shoulder
   (d) Nerve conduction study and Electromyography
   (e) Plain XR of the left shoulder and wrist
5. Multidimensional pain instruments are often used for in-depth evaluation of complex pain patients at multidisciplinary pain management centers. The following is an example of a multidimensional pain instrument
   (a) Minnesota Multiphasic Personality Inventory
   (b) Visual Analog Scale
   (c) Faces Pain Rating Scale
   (d) Verbal Descriptor Scale
   (e) Verbal Rating Scale

CHAPTER 10 RADIOLOGIC EVALUATION OF SPINAL DISEASE

1. Plain radiographs are helpful in the evaluation of all of the following except
   (a) spondylosis.
   (b) screening for nonspecific back pain.
   (c) scoliosis.
   (d) acute osteomyelitis.
2. Imaging of spine with CT/MRI is indicated in all of the following except
   (a) nonspecific symptoms.
   (b) when metastatic disease is suspected.
   (c) progression of neurologic symptoms.
   (d) evaluation of trauma.
3. Which is true regarding gadolinium-based contrast agents?
   (a) There is a risk of NSF.
   (b) Caution should be taken with pregnant patients.
   (c) Help differentiate disk herniation from scar tissue.
   (d) All of the above
4. Regarding spinal stenosis, all of the following are true except
   (a) it can be congenital or acquired.
   (b) the thecal sac AP dimension is less than 10 mm or the area is less than 100 mm^2.
   (c) it can be stenosis of central canal, lateral recess, or foramen.
   (d) patients with moderate-severe canal stenosis are always symptomatic.
5. In postoperative patients, MRI is useful in the assessment of
   (a) recurrent disc herniation.
   (b) arachnoiditis.
   (c) scar tissue.
   (d) All of the above

CHAPTER 11 ROLE OF ELECTRODIAGNOSTICS IN PAIN ASSESSMENT

1. A 30-year-old woman who just delivered a healthy baby last week presents with 5 to 6 weeks of neck pain and burning pain in the medial right arm and forearm. Neurological exam is nonfocal. Cervical x-ray reveals a cervical rib. Electrodiagnostic studies will likely reveal:
   (a) abnormal response of the lateral antebrachial cutaneous nerve.
   (b) reduced amplitude of compound muscle action potentials in the thenar muscles.
   (c) abnormal median sensory responses.
   (d) abnormal spontaneous activity on needle exam in the pronator teres muscle.
2. A 40-year-old man presents with severe back pain radiating to the top of the right foot. He reports total numbness in the leg and foot. This began 3 weeks ago, abruptly, after an unwitnessed fall at work. On exam, he is 6'0" tall, and motor exam demonstrates giveaway weakness in all right leg groups. Electrodiagnostic testing will show:
   (a) normal needle EMG without fibrillations or positive sharp waves in the gastrocnemius muscle, because there has not been time for Wallerian degeneration of axons.
   (b) normal sensory nerve conductions because he is malingering.
   (c) abnormal sensory nerve conductions because he has a pure sensory radiculopathy, as demonstrated by lack of proprioception and motor control.
   (d) normal sensory nerve conductions because there is definite nerve damage proximal to the dorsal root ganglion.
3. You are evaluating a 60-year-old man who has had two lumbar laminectomies in the past year for a right L5 radiculopathy. You suspect a recurrent right L5 radiculopathy, and needle EMG reveals 3+ positive sharp waves and fibrillations with decreased recruitment in the right tibialis anterior. The patient is having a difficult time tolerating the needle exam due to pain and will allow you to test only one more muscle. You would choose the:
   (a) extensor hallucis longus.
   (b) L5 paraspinals.
   (c) adductor longus
   (d) flexor digitorum longus.
4. Blink reflex studies can be useful in diagnosing which condition?
   (a) Myasthenia gravis
   (b) Fibromyalgia
   (c) Midpontine lesion
   (d) Motor neuron disease
5. A 50-year-old woman with diabetes mellitus type 1 is having an electrodiagnostic exam. She has had a prior laminectomy at L5 about 5 years ago. She has no other health problems. Her symptoms include chronic numbness and mild burning in the feet. She has more recent severe back pain and radiating right leg pain to the top of the foot, which started abruptly 3 weeks ago. She has a right Trendelenberg sign. Lumbar MRI shows diffuse multilevel degeneration that is not severe. All of the following are true in this case except:
   (a) electrodiagnostics are not necessary to make the diagnosis of peripheral neuropathy.
   (b) needle EMG of the paraspinal muscles would not be helpful.
   (c) needle EMG of the gluteus medius with fibrillations suggests chronic radiculopathy.
   (d) slight variations in room temperature will cool the limbs and wildly distort results.

CHAPTER 12 IMAGING PAIN

1. Functional brain imaging is currently a diagnostic modality for pain disorders.
   (a) True
   (b) False
2. Which functional imaging modality appears best suited for studying pain disorders and headache?
   (a) MEG
   (b) fMRI
   (c) PET
3. Which imaging technique examines white matter tract integrity by measuring microstructural changes in directional water diffusion in the brain?
   (a) fMRI
   (b) VBM
   (c) DTI
   (d) MEG
4. Which imaging techniques examines the blood oxygen level dependency (BOLD), measures changes in the local concentration of deoxyhemoglobin, and provides an indirect index of neuronal activity?
   (a) fMRI
   (b) PET
   (c) MEG
5. Functional imaging is capable of examining drug receptor interactions in real time.
   (a) True
   (b) false

CHAPTER 17 PSYCHOLOGICAL EVALUATION OF PATIENTS FOR SPINAL CORD STIMULATOR IMPLANTATION

1. Spinal cord stimulators are typically indicated for all of the conditions below except
   (a) failed back surgery syndrome.
   (b) postherpetic neuralgia (PHN).
   (c) interstitial cystitis.
   (d) complex regional pain syndrome (CRPS).
2. The following are typically regarded as exclusion criteria for SCS implantation except
   (a) somatization disorder.
   (b) extreme poverty.
   (c) untreated major mood disturbance.
   (d) alcohol or drug dependency.
3. The following are typically regarded as favorable inclusion criteria for SCS implantation except
   (a) type A personality.
   (b) appropriate expectations for outcome.
   (c) general psychological stability.
   (d) ability to comprehend instructions.
4. During the clinical interview, it is especially important to assess the patient's
   (a) readiness for change.
   (b) level of psychological adjustment.
   (c) history of trauma.
   (d) all of the above.
5. Psychological tests typically used in the assessment of candidates for neuromodulation include all except
   (a) Rorschach.
   (b) MMPI-2.
   (c) McGill Pain Questionnaire.
   (d) Beck Depression Inventory.

CHAPTER 20 WHEN PSYCHOTHERAPY IS INDICATED IN THE MANAGEMENT OF PAIN

1. Multidisciplinary treatment approaches to the management of chronic pain may be characterized by the following:
   (a) increased treatment effects or efficacy.
   (b) improved cost-effectiveness.
   (c) greater patient and provider satisfaction.
   (d) improved utilization of resources.
   (e) all of the above.
2. The new DSM-5 diagnostic category of somatic symptom and related disorders
   (a) does not replace the category of somatoform disorders in DSM-IV.
   (b) cannot be diagnosed concurrently with a medical disorder.
   (c) was conceived as an alternative to the medically unexplained nature of the somatoform disorders in DSM-IV.
   (d) cannot be diagnosed concurrently with mood disorders.
   (e) none of the above.
3. Criteria for prescribing individual psychodynamic psychotherapy for patients with chronic pain might reasonably include
   (a) a background of socioeconomic privilege.
   (b) a history of posttraumatic stress.
   (c) a concurrent diagnosis of depression.
   (d) a history of unresolved emotional conflicts.
   (e) both b and d.
4. The form of psychotherapy with the greatest demonstrated efficacy for patients with chronic pain is
   (a) psychodynamic psychotherapy.
   (b) supportive psychotherapy.
   (c) existential psychotherapy.
   (d) cognitive-behavioral psychotherapy.
   (e) drug counseling.
5. Group psychotherapy for patients with chronic pain
   (a) can incorporate cognitive-behavioral techniques.
   (b) is often more cost-effective than individual psychotherapy.
   (c) has demonstrated consistently positive treatment effects.
   (d) can include an educational component.
   (e) all of the above.

CHAPTER 21 MIND/BODY INTERVENTIONS IN THE MANAGEMENT OF CHRONIC PAIN

1. Analgesia occurs in mind–body therapies through
   (a) dissociation.
   (b) pain gate.
   (c) medications.
   (d) A and B
   (e) B and C
2. Psychosomatic conditions are difficult to diagnose because
   (a) DSM-IV-TR terms are vague.
   (b) pain experience is not really "real."
   (c) patients hide symptoms.
   (d) pain generator does not register in imaging studies.
   (e) all of the above.
3. Which of the following qualify as mind–body healing?
   (a) Behavioral changes
   (b) Physiological changes such as peripheral vasodilation
   (c) Negative emotions upregulating proinflammatory cytokines
   (d) All of the above
   (e) a and b
4. Hypnosis is helpful as a mind–body therapy because it
   (a) provides a way of communicating with the unconscious.
   (b) provides an "x-ray" of mental issues.
   (c) can allow for rapid pain relief
   (d) A and C
   (e) B and C
5. Biofeedback
   (a) is a tool.
   (b) is a treatment.
   (c) measures physiological reactivity.
   (d) A and B
   (e) A and C

CHAPTER 23 NEW PROSPECTS FOR ALLEVIATION OF ANGER IN THE CONTEXT OF CHRONIC PAIN

1. Which of the following is the best definition of anger?
   (a) A feeling related to appraised wrongdoing and motivation to resist or retaliate against that wrongdoing
   (b) A pattern of recurrent outbursts of annoyance or rage
   (c) Deliberately inflicting harm to a person or property
   (d) The mere intention to hurt a person physically or verbally
2. Anger in chronic pain patients is best explained as
   (a) neurophysiologically hardwired.
   (b) the product of classical conditioning.
   (c) occurring in a psychosocial context.
   (d) usually preceding the onset of pain.
3. Meta-analysis of cognitive-behavior therapy (CBT) for anger has shown
   (a) that recipients of CBT turn out the same as those receiving no treatment.
   (b) an effect size of about +0.70.
   (c) a worsening of anger.
   (d) an effect size of +2.0.
4. In contrast to CBT, CBAT for anger
   (a) supplements treatment with many more cognitive and behavioral techniques.
   (b) draws techniques from affective and experiential psychotherapy.
   (c) sequences techniques for use in a contingent fashion.
   (d) all of the above.
5. The conflict resolution model of anger is
   (a) Intrapsychic.
   (b) Relational.
   (c) theologically grounded.
   (d) none of the above.

CHAPTER 24 WORK DISABILITY AND CHRONIC PAIN

1. Which predictors control most of the variance in predicting work-related disability?
   (a) Permanent impairment ratings and medical diagnosis
   (b) Number of pain sites and fear avoidance of work tasks
   (c) Job satisfaction and results of a functional capacity assessment
   (d) Mild depression and a successful trial with spinal column stimulation
   (e) All of the above
2. The social and medical models of disability
   (a) take into account physical impairment and various barriers that may hinder the person's full and effective participation in society.
   (b) are recognized by the United Nations Convention on the Rights of People with Disabilities.
   (c) are commonly misunderstood by clinicians who work with chronic pain patients.
   (d) are plagued by methodological difficulties when trying to apply the models with cross-cultural assessment.
   (e) all of the above.
3. If return to work is a goal, a patient with chronic pain is best treated with
   (a) passive, supportive therapies that target pain relief.
   (b) active treatments in which the treatments are conducted at the work site.
   (c) pharmacotherapy treatments that target the underlying cause of the patient's complaint.
   (d) multidisciplinary approaches that include all possible treatments and provide support for the patient's physical concerns.
   (e) any approach that targets pain relief and returns the patient to the worksite after a resolution of the symptoms.
4. Psychiatric diagnoses that may predict work disability include
   (a) posttraumatic stress disorder.
   (b) substance use disorder.
   (c) chronic depression.
   (d) somatization disorder.
   (e) all of the above.

5. Self-report screening and outcome measures for work-related disability
   (a) are most effective when they address general measures of cognitive functioning such as self-efficacy.
   (b) can be used adjunctively to assist the clinician with an overall assessment.
   (c) can reliably assess whether a patient is malingering with respect to their report of pain.
   (d) can determine a patient's percent impairment for purposes of calculating a financial compensation award.
   (e) all of the above

CHAPTER 27 EPIDEMIOLOGY OF HEADACHES

1. Research indicates that approximately________ of individuals with migraine remain undiagnosed.
   (a) 10%
   (b) 25%
   (c) 50%
   (d) 80%
2. The World Health Organization ranks headache disorders in the top _________ most disabling conditions.
   (a) 10
   (b) 20
   (c) 50
   (d) 100
3. Which of the following are true of chronic migraine?
   (a) Prevalence peaks in middle age.
   (b) Prevalence is higher among women than men.
   (c) Headache-related disability is higher among women than men.
   (d) All of the above
4. Which of the following are true of tension-type headache?
   (a) Prevalence rates widely vary.
   (b) It is more common among men than women.
   (c) All of the above
   (d) None of the above
5. Research indicates what proportion of individuals with migraine are candidates for preventive medications?
   (a) 1 in 20
   (b) 1 in 10
   (c) 1 in 5
   (d) 1 in 4

CHAPTER 28 HISTORICAL FEATURES IN PRIMARY HEADACHE SYNDROMES

1. You see a 23-year-old woman with a 5-year history of unilateral throbbing headaches that are worse at the onset of her menses. She presents now with 2 weeks of severe headaches occurring two or three times per week that prevent her from working. The headaches are throbbing and unilateral. Is this a new headache or an old headache?
   (a) New
   (b) Old
2. What if her headache is bifrontal, nonthrobbing, mild, and does not disrupt her daily activities? Is this an old headache or a new headache?
   (a) New
   (b) Old
3. Which of the following features most accurately distinguishes migraine from tension-type headache?
   (a) Nausea
   (b) Throbbing pain
   (c) Photophobia
   (d) Unilateral pain
4. Which of the following types of migraine aura is least common?
   (a) Scintillating scotoma
   (b) Hemiparesis
   (c) Paresthesias
   (d) Aphasia
5. Which of the following statements regarding cluster headache is true?
   (a) The typical headache duration is 6 hours.
   (b) Women are affected more often than men.
   (c) There is often a circadian rhythm to the timing of headaches.
   (d) When lacrimation occurs, it can be either unilateral or bilateral.

CHAPTER 29 PATHOPHYSIOLOGY OF HEADACHES

1. The primary neurotransmitter for the transmission of head pain to the trigeminal nucleus caudalis is
   (a) calcitonin gene–related peptide.
   (b) glutamate.
   (c) substance P.
   (d) neurokinin A.
   (e) GABA
2. Pain transmission in the trigeminal nucleus caudalis can be modulated by projections from which of the following structures?
   (a) Rostral trigeminal nuclei
   (b) Periaqueductal gray matter
   (c) Nucleus raphe magnus
   (d) Descending cortical inhibitory systems
   (e) All of the above
3. Which statement regarding cortical spreading depression is true?
   (a) It is wave of neuronal depression followed by hyperexcitation that is observed to move across areas of contiguous cortex.
   (b) It cannot be triggered by chemical or mechanical perturbation.
   (c) It is accompanied by a transient increase in blood flow followed by blood flow reductions.
   (d) It is the cornerstone of the vasogenic theory of migraine.
4. Which of the following is not true regarding aura?
   (a) 25% of individuals with migraine experience aura.
   (b) Both positron emission computed tomography (PET) and functional magnetic resonance imaging (fMRI) studies have demonstrated that moderate blood flow reductions that spread across vascular territories likely play a role in aura.
   (c) These transient symptoms are typically characterized by a slow expansion of the area affected by the dysfunction followed by rapid resolution.
   (d) Typical auras last 1 hour or less

5. Which of the following is true regarding cluster headache?
   (a) There is a manifestation of pain primarily in the ophthalmic and mandibular divisions of the trigeminal nerve.
   (b) The lack of circadian rhythmicity of cluster headache is suggestive of hypothalamic involvement in headache generation.
   (c) Sweating of the forehead or face, ptosis, miosis, lacrimation, and nasal congestion are cluster headache features indicating sympathetic, but not parasympathetic, dysfunction.
   (d) Cavernous sinus anomalies have been associated with cluster headache.

CHAPTER 30 COMMON HEADACHE SYNDROMES

1. Which of the following are red flags in the diagnosis of migraine headaches?
   (a) Headache onset after the age of 30 years
   (b) New onset of headache during pregnancy or postpartum
   (c) Headache that is precipitated by exertion, bending over, coughing, or sneezing
   (d) Headache attacks that alternate sides from one attack to another
   (e) B and C
2. Which of the following triptans contains a sulfonamide group and are therefore contraindicated in patients with sulfa allergies?
   (a) Almotriptan and sumatriptan
   (b) Sumatriptan alone
   (c) Eletriptan
   (d) Frovatriptan
   (e) Rizatriptan
3. According to the 2000 US Headache Consortium Guidelines, when is it recommended to initiate migraine prophylaxis?
   (a) More than 2 headache days monthly regardless of impairment
   (b) 2 headache days monthly with severe impairment
   (c) 3 or more headache days monthly with severe impairment
   (d) 4 or more headache days monthly with at least some impairment
   (e) C and D
4. All of the following are diagnostic criteria of tension-type headache EXCEPT:
   (a) Nonpulsating quality
   (b) Mild or moderate intensity
   (c) Neither photophobia or phonophobia may be present
   (d) Bilateral location
   (e) No aggravation by routine physical activity
5. What is the range for duration of a cluster headache attack?
   (a) 4 to 72 hours
   (b) 30 minutes to 7 days
   (c) 5 to 240 seconds
   (d) 15 to 180 minutes
   (e) 2 to 30 minutes

CHAPTER 32 CHRONIC DAILY HEADACHE

1. What is the prevalence of daily headache in the general adult population?
   (a) 1%
   (b) 2%
   (c) 4%
   (d) 6%
2. What is the most common circumstance associated with the abrupt onset of chronic daily headache?
   (a) Head, neck, or back injury
   (b) Flulike illness or sinusitis
   (c) Medical illness
   (d) Surgical procedure
3. What is the average duration of the transition of headaches from intermittent to daily?
   (a) 1 year
   (b) 10 years
   (c) 11 years
   (d) 20 years
4. For how long may headaches improve following withdrawal from analgesics and vasoconstrictors?
   (a) 1 month
   (b) 3 months
   (c) 6 months
   (d) 12 months
5. In how many hours is full relief of headache accomplished in effective abortive treatment?
   (a) 1 hour
   (b) 2 hours
   (c) 3 hours
   (d) 4 hours

CHAPTER 33 HEADACHE THERAPEUTICS

1. A 24-year-old woman with a history of depression and gastritis is seen in your office for headaches. She has had rare headaches associated with nausea, photophobia, and phonophobia for the past 8 years. Recently, she has noticed that her headaches have become more frequent, but primarily occur during her menstrual cycle. When present, her headaches often prevent her from meeting her deadlines at work. What is the next best step in the management of this patient's care?
   (a) Start sumatriptan twice daily for 5 days during her cycle.
   (b) Start zolmitriptan twice daily for 5 days during her cycle.
   (c) Start rizatriptan twice daily for 5 days during her cycle.
   (d) Start frovatriptan twice daily for 5 days during her cycle.
   (e) Start naproxen twice daily for 5 days during her cycle.
2. Which of the following medications is *not* approved by the Federal Drug Administration (FDA) for the treatment of migraine?
   (a) Propranolol
   (b) Amitriptyline
   (c) Divalproex sodium
   (d) Topiramate
   (e) All of the above are FDA approved for the treatment of chronic migraine.

3. A 55-year-old man returns to your office for management of cluster headaches. He complained of worsening headache at his last office visit and met criteria for chronic cluster headache at that time. He was given an occipital nerve block, which terminated his cluster period for a few months. Today, his blood pressure is 96/64 and his heart rate is 56 beats per minute. Electrocardiogram showed first-degree atrioventricular block. What is the best choice for maintenance prevention of cluster headaches in this patient?
   (a) Amitriptyline
   (b) Indomethacin
   (c) Verapamil
   (d) Occipital nerve stimulator
   (e) Divalproex sodium
4. A 32-year-old woman presents to your office for evaluation of worsening headaches. She typically notices the headaches just before dinner. She describes the headaches as a bifrontal pressure pain without photophobia, phonophobia, or nausea. In the last 3 months, her headaches have increased in frequency so that she now gets them 3 to 4 days per week. They are mild to moderate in intensity. Although acetaminophen was initially helpful, she no longer gets benefit from this medication. What medication(s) would you suggest initiating at today's visit?
   (a) Cyclobenzaprine
   (b) Topiramate
   (c) Amitriptyline
   (d) Aaproxen sodium
   (e) Sumatriptan and naproxen sodium, taken together
5. Which of the following is not true about neuroleptics?
   (a) Promethazine is an antihistamine.
   (b) Metoclopramide is used to treat gastroparesis.
   (c) Metoclopramide is not available in a rectal formulation.
   (d) Hypertension is a known side effect of prochlorperazine.
   (e) Phenothiazines may precipitate acute dystonic reactions.

CHAPTER 35 FACIAL PAIN

1. Which two drugs have the best evidence for efficacy in treating trigeminal neuralgia?
   (a) Baclofen and carbamazepine
   (b) Carbamazepine and oxcarbazepine
   (c) Clonazepam and carbamazepine
   (d) Phenytoin and baclofen
2. Diagnostic confusion can easily occur between trigeminal neuralgia and
   (a) cluster headache.
   (b) hemicrania continua.
   (c) SUNCT/SUNA.
   (d) paroxysmal hemicrania.
3. The most effective medication for "jabs and jolts" (primary stabbing headache) is:
   (a) celecoxib.
   (b) carbamazepine.
   (c) oxcarbazepine.
   (d) indomethacin.
4. Raeder's paratrigeminal syndrome may be caused by:
   (a) carotid artery dissection.
   (b) ophthalmodynia periodica.
   (c) venous sinus thrombosis.
   (d) All of the above
5. Persistent idiopathic facial pain may be caused by:
   (a) occult dental pathology.
   (b) nasopharyngeal carcinoma.
   (c) lung cancer.
   (d) All of the above

CHAPTER 37 NECK PAIN

1. Choose the correct statement regarding thoracic outlet syndrome (TOS).
   (a) It is most frequently diagnosed in middle-aged women and involves neurologic symptoms of the C8, T1 nerve roots (ulnar distributions).
   (b) Pancoast tumors are a common cause of neurogenic TOS.
   (c) Because the diagnosis and treatment of TOS is controversial, spinal cord stimulation is a usual therapeutic modality for this syndrome.
   (d) The clavicle/first rib and the pectoralis minor/rib cage are the most common sites implicated in TOS.
2. Regarding establishing the diagnosis of cervical facet pain, which diagnostic modality has proven to have clinical validity?
   (a) Bone scan
   (b) Magnetic resonance imaging
   (c) Computed tomography
   (d) Cervical x-rays
   (e) Controlled diagnostic blocks of the medial branches supplying the cervical facets
3. Select the incorrect statement regarding chronic cervical discogenic pain.
   (a) Diagnosis is established by disc morphology on magnetic resonance imaging and by careful history and physical examination.
   (b) Cervical discography/disc stimulation is used to establish the diagnosis.
   (c) Cervical facet pain is ruled out by medial branch blocks prior to performing disc stimulation studies.
   (d) Symptoms related to cervical discogenic pain can mimic cervical radicular pain and refer pain to the occiput.
4. Common treatment options for chronic occipital neuralgia that have demonstrated to be safe and effective include each of the following except:
   (a) occipital nerve stimulation.
   (b) serial occipital nerve blocks.
   (c) tricyclic antidepressants.
   (d) botulinum toxin injections.
   (e) serial phenol injections.

5. True statements concerning whiplash associated disorders (WAD) include all of the following except:
   (a) WAD III and IV are commonly treated in pain management centers.
   (b) Cervical facet joint damage is implicated as a cause.
   (c) Psychological distress often resolves with successful treatment of pain—in particular, cervical facetogenic pain.
   (d) Chronic neck pain as a result of WAD not uncommonly persists even after litigation settlements.

CHAPTER 40 FAILED BACK SURGERY

1. A 35-year-old man failed to improve after a microdiscectomy for low back pain without significant leg pain. His MRI before surgery showed a desiccated disc with midline herniation at L5–S1 with no neural compression. The most likely cause of his low back pain is:
   (a) facet joint pain.
   (b) discogenic pain.
   (c) epidural fibrosis.
   (d) recurrent disc herniation.
2. A 74-year-old woman underwent bilateral wide decompression at L4–5 for leg pain, but almost no low back pain. Preoperative MRI showed central stenosis, disc narrowing and dessication, and fluid in the facet joints, all at L4–5. Her leg pain is better after surgery, but she now has significant low back pain, especially with walking. Her most likely diagnosis is:
   (a) neuropathic pain.
   (b) recurrent spinal stenosis.
   (c) epidural fibrosis.
   (d) instability due to spondylolisthesis.
3. Which of the following diagnoses are best viewed on plain x-rays with flexion and extension views:
   (a) Recurrent disc herniation
   (b) Spinal stenosis
   (c) Spondylolisthesis
   (d) Sacroiliac joint pain
4. A 71-year-old man presents with a 2-year history of progressive right gluteal and groin pain, minimal low back pain, and no pain distal to the proximal thigh. An MRI before surgery showed foraminal stenosis, and he underwent L4–5 decompression. His pain never improved. Which test is NOT likely to be helpful in making the correct diagnosis?
   (a) Facet joint injection
   (b) Sacroiliac joint injection
   (c) X-ray of the pelvis and hips while standing
   (d) MRI scan
5. A 39-year-old woman presents with right gluteal pain and groin pain that began after a motor vehicle accident 4 years ago. Preoperative MRI showed a bulging disc at L5–S1. She underwent L5–S1 discectomy, but there was no relief. Repeat MRI after surgery is unchanged except for surgical changes. Her most likely diagnosis is:
   (a) discogenic pain.
   (b) sacroiliac joint pain.
   (c) spinal stenosis.
   (d) neuropathic pain.

CHAPTER 41 PAIN MANAGEMENT IN RHEUMATOLOGIC DISEASES

1. Which of the following is not a risk factor for cardiovascular risks associated with NSAIDs?
   (a) Age > 80
   (b) History of cardiovascular disease
   (c) Rheumatoid arthritis
   (d) Renal disease
   (e) Female gender
2. What is the mechanism of effect on pain of tanezumab?
   (a) Activates and sensitizes peripheral c-nocireceptors
   (b) Anti-inflammatory effect
   (c) Serotonin and norepinephrine reuptake inhibitor
   (d) Binds to and inhibits nerve growth factor
3. Which one of these nonselective NSAIDs is least associated with gastrointestinal side effects?
   (a) Aspirin
   (b) Indomethacin
   (c) Diclofenac
   (d) Nonacetylated salicylate
   (e) Ibuprofen
4. What is the approximate half-life of hyalorunic acid in the synovial fluid postinjection?
   (a) Few hours to few days
   (b) 3 weeks
   (c) 4 weeks
   (d) 3 months
   (e) 6 months
5. What is the mechanism of increased cardiovascular risk with ibuprofen?
   (a) Cyclooxygenase-2 inhibitor selectivity
   (b) Increased cholesterol
   (c) Interfering with the protective role of aspirin
   (d) Increasing calcium deposits in coronary arteries plaques

CHAPTER 42 OSTEOARTHRITIS OF THE MAJOR JOINTS

1. Which of the following is not a risk factor for primary osteoarthritis of the elbow?
   (a) Manual labor
   (b) Female gender
   (c) Repetitive trauma
   (d) Genetic predisposition
2. Which of the following is not a recommended treatment modality for osteoarthritic pain of the hip?
   (a) Cane
   (b) NSAID
   (c) Synvisc® injection
   (d) Corticosteroid injection

3. What is the gold standard surgical treatment for tricompartmental osteoarthritis of the knee?
   (a) Chondroplasty
   (b) Arthroscopic lavage and débridement
   (c) Total knee replacement
   (d) Cartilage transplant
4. What is the recommended surgical treatment for severe primary elbow osteoarthritis in a high-demand patient?
   (a) Elbow arthrodesis
   (b) Total elbow arthroplasty
   (c) Ulnohumeral arthroplasty
   (d) Interposition arthroplasty
5. Which of the following treatments is an effective treatment modality for osteoarthritic pain of the knee?
   (a) Glucosamine
   (b) Chondroitin sulfate
   (c) Lateral shoe wedge
   (d) Arthroscopic debridement and lavage

CHAPTER 43 FOOT AND ANKLE PAIN

1. Which of the following are clinical characteristics of a plantar wart?
   (a) Spongy center
   (b) Pain with side-to-side compression
   (c) Black dots in center
   (d) Absence of skin lines across lesion
   (e) All of the above
2. What is the best imaging modality when evaluating a soft-tissue injury such as a neuroma or a tendon or ligament rupture?
   (a) X-ray
   (b) CT scan
   (c) MRI
   (d) Bone scan
3. Tendinosis is easier to treat than tendinitis and typically resolves with NSAIDs, rest, and immobilization.
   (a) True
   (b) False
4. Which of the following is not part of PRICE (five general principles a clinician can employ to minimize pain and swelling in an acute foot trauma)?
   (a) Protection
   (b) Resume regular activity
   (c) Ice
   (d) Compression
   (e) Elevate extremity
5. What is a good treatment plan for a patient with complex regional pain syndrome?
   (a) Nerve block injections
   (b) Psychology consult
   (c) Antiseizure medications
   (d) Physical therapy
   (e) Nerve transmission interference
   (f) All of the above

CHAPTER 44 PELVIC AND ABDOMINAL PAIN

1. Visceral nociceptors are:
   (a) polymodal.
   (b) sensitized after tissue insult.
   (c) often silent.
   (d) all of the above.
2. The most common cause of abdominal wall pain is:
   (a) xiphoidalgia.
   (b) abdominal wall hernia.
   (c) abdominal cutaneous entrapment syndrome.
   (d) abdominal scars.
3. The common areas of pudendal entrapment occur:
   (a) in the Alcock's canal.
   (b) at the junction of sacrotuberous and sacrospinaous ligaments.
   (c) near scar tissue from previous surgery or trauma.
   (d) All of the above.
4. Treatment of irritable bowel syndrome includes:
   (a) dietary modification.
   (b) antidepressants.
   (c) serotonin agonists and antagonists.
   (d) all of the above.
5. Treatment of osetits pubis includes:
   (a) nonsteroidal antinflammatory agents.
   (b) physical therapy.
   (c) local injections of steroid.
   (d) all of the above.

CHAPTER 45 PERINEAL PAIN

1. The perineum is innervated by which of the following (Mark all choices that apply.):
   (a) Sympathetic nervous system
   (b) Parasympathetic nervous system
   (c) Somatic nervous system
2. Mark all choices that apply to vulvodynia (vulvar pain syndrome).
   (a) Primary vulvar vestibulitis is defined as dyspareunia from the first attempt of sexual intercourse.
   (b) Subtypes of localized vulvodynia include vestibulodynia and clitorodynia.
   (c) Vulvodynia affects primarily women of Caucasian origin.
   (d) Vulvodynia has an infectious origin.
3. Mark all choices that apply to rectal pain and coccygodynia.
   (a) Chronic proctalgia can be caused by local disease of the anus or rectum, or it can be referred from the urogenital tract or lumbosacral spine.
   (b) Proctalgia fugax refers to paroxysms of pain in the rectal-anal area.
   (c) Surgery is the treatment of choice for coccygodynia.

4. Mark all correct choices.
   (a) Chronic pelvic pain syndrome is a generic term that covers all causes of pain perceived in the pelvis including cancer and infection.
   (b) Chronic pelvic pain syndrome is a condition of the female gender alone.
   (c) Chronic pelvic pain syndrome describes pain perceived in the pelvis without functional disorder of the pelvic organs.
   (d) The term chronic pelvic pain syndrome encourages an interdisciplinary and multispecialty approach to management.
5. Mark all choices that apply to urethral pain syndrome.
   (a) It is usually due to urethral stricture.
   (b) It is never due to infection.
   (c) It may occur in men and women.
   (d) It can cause significant emotional distress.

CHAPTER 50 PREEMPTIVE ANALGESIA

1. Which of the following best describes the concept of peripheral sensitization
   (a) Wind-up
   (b) Gate control theory
   (c) Tactile allodynia
   (d) Sunburn pain
   (e) Opioid-induced hyperalgesia
2. A 75-year-old man with a history of peripheral vascular disease is scheduled for a right side below-knee amputation. Which of the following preemptive analgesic techniques is most likely to provide postoperative pain relief?
   (a) Local anesthetic injected into the incision preoperatively
   (b) Cingulotomy
   (c) Epidural bupivacaine
   (d) Preoperative topiramate
   (e) Preoperative amitriptyline
3. Which of the following are risk factors for the development of chronic postsurgical pain?
   (a) Increasing age
   (b) Severe postoperative pain
   (c) Laparoscopic surgery
   (d) Operations of short duration
   (e) Primary surgical repair
4. Which of the following may reduce the incidence of chronic postsurgical pain
   (a) Preemptive analgesia
   (b) Preventative analgesia
   (c) Aminoglycoside antibiotics
   (d) Steroids
   (e) Gabapentin
5. Which of The following are associated with the development of chronic pain?
   (a) Reduced sodium channel expression
   (b) Microglial inactivation
   (c) Reduced glutamate release
   (d) Central sensitization
   (e) Reduced spontaneous neuronal discharge.

CHAPTER 55 MEDICAL MANAGEMENT OF CANCER PAIN

1. What dosage of daily morphine (for at least 1 week) defines "opioid tolerant?"
   (a) 15 mg/day
   (b) 30 mg/day
   (c) 45 mg/day
   (d) 60 mg/day
   (e) None of the above
2. The verbal rating scale (VRS)
   (a) is a visual analog scale.
   (b) is a scale that uses a 100-mm line for patients to mark pain intensity.
   (c) uses verbal descriptors for pain intensity
   (d) uses a numerical rating scale from 0 to 10 for pain intensity.
   (e) none of the above.
3. The tricyclic antidepressant (TCA) considered to be the *least* sedating is
   (a) trazodone.
   (b) desipramine.
   (c) nortriptyline.
   (d) amitriptyline.
   (e) imipramine.
4. Known side effects of corticosteroids for use in pain management include the following except
   (a) hyperglycemia.
   (b) Suppression of the hypothalamic–pituitary–adrenal axis.
   (c) hyperalgesia.
   (d) hypertension.
   (e) proximal myopathy.
5. What is the primary metabolite of morphine after hepatic biotransformation?
   (a) Morphine-3-glucuronide (M3G)
   (b) 6-Monoacetylmorphine (6-MAM)
   (c) Morphine-6-glucuronide (M6G)
   (d) Diacetylmorphine (DAM)
   (e) Morphine

CHAPTER 60 MUSCLE PAIN: PATHOPHYSIOLOGY, EVALUATION, AND TREATMENT

1. The following tissue does not refer pain to muscles:
   (a) skin.
   (b) nerve.
   (c) joint.
   (d) viscera.
   (e) muscle.

2. The following statement is false. Muscle pain afferents
   (a) are composed of group III and group IV fibers.
   (b) exclusively supply nerve endings responding to mechanical stimuli.
   (c) supplying free nerve endings are predominantly found in the adventitia of arterioles and venules.
   (d) supplying free nerve endings may be found more densely in peritendineum than in muscle tissue.
   (e) terminating in the dorsal horn appear to release both substance P and CGRP.
3. The following statement concerning central sensitization is true.
   (a) It does not produce muscle allodynia.
   (b) When present for long periods, it is easily reversible.
   (c) It results in expansion of muscle-induced excitation in the spinal cord.
   (d) It is easily differentiated from peripheral sensitization.
   (e) All of the above are true.
4. The following is true concerning muscle spasm.
   (a) Painful muscles generally produce spasm-like contractions.
   (b) During activities, the pain–spasm–pain vicious cycle predicts increased electromyographic activity in the muscle agonist.
   (c) Muscle spasm is a result of pain in a muscle.
   (d) The Lund hypothesis predicts increased activity in the antagonistic muscle during painful contractions.
   (e) All of the above are true.
5. Which of the following is true?
   (a) Concentric muscle contractions are less demanding than eccentric contractions.
   (b) Prolonged eccentric contractions may produce delayed-onset muscle soreness.
   (c) Muscle pain inhibits the activity of synergistic muscles.
   (d) Vastus medialis pain may impair knee joint control during walking.
   (e) All of the above are true.

CHAPTER 64 ACUTE PAIN MANAGEMENT IN INFANTS AND CHILDREN

1. You are asked to evaluate a 1-day-old male infant who had a duodenal atresia repair 6 hours ago. He remains on ventilatory support and appears agitated. You are called to determine if his epidural catheter is providing effective analgesia. How do you test his epidural catheter?
   (a) Give a lidocaine test dose and observe for response
   (b) Give chloroprocaine test dose and observe for a response
   (c) Inject contrast and obtain an x-ray
2. A 6-year-old with cerebral palsy has an epidural catheter for postoperative analgesia after having bilateral femoral osteotomies. He has developmental delay and seizures. His weight is 17 kg. He is receiving 0.1% bupivacaine with fentanyl 2 μg/mL at the maximum recommended rate of 6.8 mL/h (0.4 mg/kg/h bupivacaine). He has received no additional analgesics. He appears comfortable at rest but grimaces and cries with positioning. What are your options to optimize his analgesia?
   (a) IV morphine at 0.1 mg/kg q2h
   (b) PO oxycodone
   (c) Change the epidural solution to a hydromorphone containing solution
3. You are assessing a 2-year-old who had abdominal surgery 1 day ago. What is the best assessment tool to evaluate her degree of postoperative pain?
   (a) Ask her if she has a little or a lot of pain
   (b) Use the Faces scale
   (c) Use the FLACC scale
4. You are asked by the attending pediatric hematologist for your advice regarding pain management of a 9-year-old boy with sickle cell disease. He is having a pain crisis involving his chest as he has had previously and has just been admitted from the emergency department. Due to his underlying disease, he has mild renal insufficiency. When not in crisis, he takes only occasional PO acetaminophen or ibuprofen. What is the best option for management of his pain in this situation?
   (a) PO OxyContin
   (b) MSIR
   (c) IV PCA morphine with a low basal rate + demand dosing
   (d) Epidural local anesthetic
   (e) E IV ketorolac at 0.5 mg/kg q6h for up to 3 days
5. You are asked to provide analgesia for an 18-year-old female with cystic fibrosis. She has been an inpatient receiving treatment for a pulmonary exacerbation, possibly caused by a bacterial pneumonia. She is thin and malnourished appearing. She is afebrile. She has just had a chest tube placed to drain a pleural effusion and now has complaint of significant pain with each breath and is obviously splinting. She is unable to tolerate chest physiotherapy due to severe pain. Her pediatric pulmonologist requests help with her analgesia; he fears further splinting and subsequent respiratory decline might result in the need for ventilatory support. What is the best option to provide analgesia for this patient?
   (a) Paravertebral infusion of 0.2% ropivacaine
   (b) Thoracic epidural infusion of 0.2% ropivacaine
   (c) IV morphine at 0.1 mg/kg q2h
   (d) IV ketorolac 1.0 mg/kg q6h
   (e) Lidoderm patches over the chest tube site

CHAPTER 69 RISING STANDARDS FOR RISK MANAGEMENT IN OPIOID USE FOR CHRONIC PAIN

1. The single most prescribed opioid in the United States is:
   (a) Oxycodone
   (b) Methadone
   (c) Hydrocodone
   (d) Morphine
2. All of the following are true statements documenting the epidemic of prescription opioid abuse EXCEPT:
   (a) Between 1998 and 2008, a fivefold increase was noted in drug treatment admissions for prescription opioids.
   (b) More than 6 million Americans abuse prescription drugs — more than the number estimated to abuse cocaine, heroin, hallucinogens, and inhalants, combined.
   (c) From 1999 to 2005, the number of poisoning deaths mentioning methadone increased 200%
   (d) The number of deaths nationwide attributable to prescription opioid analgesics quadrupled between 1999 and 2007.

3. The Federation of State Medical Boards in its revised Model Policy for the Use of Opioid Analgesics in the Treatment of Chronic Pain (2013) states all of the following are deviations from best practices when prescribing opioid medications EXCEPT:
   (a) Excessive reliance on opioids, particularly high dose opioids, for chronic pain management
   (b) Escalating the dose of opioids to the extent patients become physically dependent on their medication
   (c) Inadequately assessing whether opioids are clinically indicated
   (d) Inadequately educating patients and failing to obtain substantive informed consent
4. The following statements are part of the five "As" mnemonic to assess efficacy of pain treatment at follow-up visits EXCEPT:
   (a) Activity
   (b) Aberrant behaviors
   (c) Analgesia
   (d) Allodynia
5. In setting functional goals to track the efficacy of opioid use for pain treatment, which of the following is MOST likely true?
   (a) Functional goals should be established using a standard applicable to all patients.
   (b) Doses of opioid medications should routinely be increased if patients do not meet their stated functional goals because of excessive pain.
   (c) Functional goals should be reassessed at regular intervals and modified on an individual basis.
   (d) Some patients simply cannot be expected to set and achieve functional goals because they have excessive pain.

CHAPTER 71 URINE DRUG TESTING

1. The opioid that if being orally administered and found in urine least likely to be confused with other opioids in metabolites is
   (a) Oxycodone
   (b) Oxymorphone
   (c) Hydrocodone
   (d) Tapentadol
   (e) Hydromorphone
2. The opioid that may be found in the urine of patients taking hydrocodone is
   (a) Morphine
   (b) Codeine
   (c) Hydromorphone
   (d) Oxymorphone
3. Confirmation testing of opioids in the urine should include
   (a) Point of care testing
   (b) Enzyme immunoassay
   (c) Enzyme-linked immunosorbent assay (ELISA)
   (d) Western blot
   (e) Gas chromatography/mass spectrometry (GC/MS) or high-performance liquid chromatography (HPLC)
4. The detection of normetabolites in UDT may
   (a) Help identify adulterated specimens
   (b) Help catch patients who are not compliant
   (c) Help identify potential false negative specimens
   (d) Help identify patients taking illicit drugs
   (e) Help identify patients selling their prescription opioids
5. Utilizing UDT for pain patients on COT:
   (a) Is mandated in many states
   (b) Should be interpreted cautiously in conjunction with other patient information, tools and history/physical examination
   (c) Is the best way to catch to catch patients who are addicted to opioids
   (d) Is the best way to check on whether or not the patient is compliant
   (e) Should be done on most visits

CHAPTER 72 NOVEL OPIOID FORMULATIONS

1. What is the most common reason nondependent, recreational opioid users first use an opioid?
   (a) To feel high
   (b) To feel less anxious
   (c) To fit in socially
   (d) To treat pain
2. New opioid delivery systems include
   (a) A biodegradable adhesive film
   (b) A buprenorphine transdermal patch
   (c) An oral buprenorphine prodrug
   (d) A molecular bio-erodible tablet
3. Transmucosal fentanyl spray
   (a) Is approved for noncancer breakthrough pain
   (b) Showed statistical difference in onset from other transmucosal fentanyl products
   (c) Can be used in opioid-naive patients
   (d) Provided pain relieve in 5 minutes
4. First-generation misuse-deterrent opioid formulations
   (a) Have been shown to protect against opioid misuse
   (b) Work best in patients who manipulate the formulation
   (c) Are considered major advances in addressing a public health crisis
   (d) Are safe and not associated with adverse effects
5. The largest unmet need with newer opioid formulations is
   (a) Failure to block the primary method of overuse
   (b) Failure to make the products available to everyone experiencing pain
   (c) Failure to prevent opioid-induced constipation with chronic use
   (d) Failure to provide adequate pain relief

CHAPTER 73 OPIOID-INDUCED HYPERALGESIA

1. What would be clinical indications of opioid-induced hyperalgesia?
   (a) Increasing pain despite opioid dose escalation
   (b) Diffuse pain beyond the distribution of preexisting pain condition
   (d) Evidence of hyperalgesia and allodynia that was not present before opioid therapy
   (e) All of the above
2. Potential mechanisms of opioid-induced hyperalgesia include
   (a) Increased spinal dynorphin release
   (b) Increased descending facilitation
   (c) Increased central glutamatergic activation
   (d) All of the above

3. Possible signs of opioid-induced hyperalgesia detected by quantitative sensory testing include
   (a) Decreased heat pain threshold
   (b) Decreased latency in cold pressor test
   (c) Increased temporal pain summation
   (d) All of the above
4. Apparent clinical opioid tolerance (lack of opioid effectiveness despite opioid dose escalation) may result from
   (a) Pharmacologic opioid tolerance
   (b) Opioid-induced hyperalgesia
   (c) Increased preexisting pain due to disease progression
   (d) All of the above
5. Possible tools to manage opioid-induced hyperalgesia include
   (a) Opioid dose reduction or opioid tapering
   (b) Adjunctive pain medications
   (c) Agents serving as NMDA receptor antagonists
   (d) All of the above

CHAPTER 75 CANNABINOIDS IN PAIN MANAGEMENT

1. Which of the following compounds in the marijuana leaf is the most psychoactive?
   (a) Δ^9-tetrahydrocannabinol (THC)
   (b) Cannabidiol (CBD)
   (c) Cannabinol (CBN)
   (d) Anandamide
2. Which of the following results from activation of the CB2 receptor?
   (a) Increased potassium conductance in the postsynaptic membrane
   (b) Reduced calcium influx into the presynaptic terminal
   (c) Reduced inflammatory mediator release from white blood cells
   (d) Reduced presynaptic terminal neurotransmitter release
3. A 45-year-old woman with severe rheumatoid arthritis is seen for evaluation in your office. She has failed a number of conservative therapies including DMARDs and opioids. She is interested in trying cannabis and asks your opinion on safety and efficacy. Which of the following is true?
   (a) There is an increase risk of multiple types of cancer
   (b) It is likely to result in major reductions in her pain
   (c) Bioavailability is better with ingestion than inhalation
   (d) It is likely to result in mild reductions in her pain
4. Which of the following is a CBME?
   (a) Nabiximols
   (b) Dronabinol
   (c) Ajulemic acid (CT-3)
   (d) Nabilone
5. Which of the following is true about clinical studies with cannabinoids to treat pain?
   (a) Results show a robust reduction in pain
   (b) There may be a therapeutic window with high doses increasing pain
   (c) Major adverse effects and poor tolerability limit use
   (d) Studies have only been effective in the treatment of acute pain

CHAPTER 80 STEROIDS

A 31-year-old man comes in, complaining about his acute L5 disc herniation. Should you treat him with an oral steroid taper? He usually just calls in to get it and does not understand why you, newly graduated from fellowship and just moved to town, insisted that he come for a clinic visit in person. He also has an extensive rash from poison ivy, he explains.

1. Should you prescribe the oral steroid taper?
   (a) Yes, for 7 days as it will treat both pain and poison ivy
   (b) Yes, for 5 days as it will treat both pain and poison ivy
   (c) No brief taper because there is risk of systemic reaction recurrence
   (d) No brief taper because there is no evidence for use in spine pain conditions
2. Arachnoiditis most likely caused by
   (a) inadvertent intrathecal injection of Kenalog during a LESI.
   (b) facet injections repeated every two months for five years with 80 mg DepoMedrol per joint each time.
   (c) disc herniation.
   (d) laminectomy and fusion.
3. Spinal cord injury from steroid injection can be avoided by
   (a) injections should be performed using image guidance and a test dose of contrast medium.
   (b) cervical interlaminar injections should preferably be performed at C7 to T1.
   (c) reviewing imaging studies that show there is adequate epidural space for needle placement at the target level.
   (d) injecting contrast medium under real-time fluoroscopy or DSA in a frontal plane before injecting any substance that may be hazardous to the patient.
   (e) all of the above.
4. A 31-year-old man comes in complaining about his acute L4 to L5 disc herniation. He has been sent to you directly from the spine surgeon, who is has just started a "spine center" in collaboration with the big hospital in town. You are newly graduated from fellowship and just moved here. The patient is leaving for vacation this afternoon and is eager to get his injection. Also, has a medical history of blindness in one eye from herpes retinitis. The other eye recovered, and he was warned not to get intravenous steroids ever again. The surgeon assured him that injection of steroid would be okay. What should you do?
   (a) Perform epidural steroid injection because there is no concern with a localized injection.
   (b) Perform epidural steroid injection with local anesthetic, as evidence demonstrates no benefit of addition of steroid.
   (c) Perform a thorough evaluation of the patient and provide coun seling; defer the invasive procedure because the patient will not be around for appropriate follow-up because of to his pending travels.
   (d) Prescribe gabapentin.

CHAPTER 86 LOCAL ANESTHETICS

1. All of the following influence duration of local anesthetic action EXCEPT:
   (a) Addition of vasopressor to the formulation
   (b) Dissociation constant (pK_a) of the local anesthetic
   (c) Relative protein binding affinity of the local anesthetic
   (d) Relative vasodilating property of the local anesthetic

2. The risk for direct neurotoxicity from local anesthetics is most closely associated with which of the following characteristics?
   (a) Greater concentration
   (b) Greater lipid solubility
   (c) Higher pH
   (d) Lower pK_a
3. Early signs of local anesthetic toxicity after intravenous administration include all of the following EXCEPT
   (a) tinnitus
   (b) hypotension
   (c) agitation
   (d) metallic taste
   (e) lightheadedness
4. Which of the following drugs is an amino ester local anesthetic?
   (a) Etidocaine
   (b) Ropivacaine
   (c) Mepivacaine
   (d) Tetracaine
5. Which local anesthetic is most likely to be associated with an allergic reaction?
   (a) Mepivacaine
   (b) Bupivacaine
   (c) Lidocaine
   (d) Tetracaine
   (e) Ropivacaine

CHAPTER 88 ULTRASOUND IN THE DIAGNOSIS AND TREATMENT OF PAIN

1. What advantage does use of ultrasound have over other common imaging modalities such as CT and fluoroscopy?
   (a) Ultrasound can visualize bony anatomy and define joint articulations completely.
   (b) With ultrasound, one can use contrast agents to define joint spaces and potential flow of medication in the neuraxis.
   (c) Ultrasound is the primary means of performing neuraxial blockades.
   (d) With ultrasound, there is no radiation exposure and it is highly user-dependent based on experience.
2. In the ultrasound guided stellate ganglion block, which cervical anterior tubercle is a necessary anatomical landmark to visualize for a safe approach?
   (a) C7
   (b) C4
   (c) C6
   (d) C5
3. Through which muscle layers does the iliohypogastric nerve travel?
   (a) Between external oblique and internal oblique
   (b) Between rectus abdominus and transversus abdominus
   (c) Between transversus abdominus and internal oblique
   (d) Between rectus abdominus and internal oblique
4. How does hyaline cartilage appear under ultrasound observation?
   (a) Fibrillar
   (b) Hypoechoic
   (c) Fascicular
   (d) Hyperechoic
5. What is the ideal transducer frequency necessary to visualize the hip joint?
   (a) linear 7-12 MHz
   (b) linear 10-15 MHz
   (c) curvilinear 7-12 MHz
   (d) curvilinear 1-6 MHz

CHAPTER 90 NEUROMODULATION FOR PAIN

1. The nerve fiber type purported to "close the gate" when activated by neurostimulation devices is
   (a) A-α (alpha) fibers
   (b) A-β (beta) fibers
   (c) A-Δ (delta) fibers
   (d) B fibers
   (e) C fibers
   (f) Γ (gamma) fibers
2. The most common indication for the use of spinal cord stimulation (SCS) in the United States is
   (a) Failed back surgery syndrome (FBSS)
   (b) Complex regional pain syndrome (CRPS)
   (c) Peripheral vascular disease (PVD) with critical limb ischemia
   (d) Intractable angina pectoris
3. When neurostimulation devices are used in conjunction with indwelling pacemakers or AICDs, theoptimal configuration to minimize device interference is
   (a) Unipolar neurostimulator and unipolar pacemaker/AICD
   (b) Unipolar neurostimulator and bipolar pacemaker/AICD
   (c) Bipolar neurostimulator and unipolar pacemaker/AICD
   (d) Bipolar neurostimulator and bipolar pacemaker/AICD
4. Motor cortex stimulation has been shown to be effective in the management of all of the following EXCEPT
   (a) Atypical facial pain
   (b) Cluster headache
   (c) Poststroke pain
   (d) Trigeminal deafferentation neuralgia
   (e) Traumatically induced neuropathic pain
5. Neurohumoral substances thought to be involved in mediating the effects of neurostimulators include all of the following EXCEPT
   (a) GABA
   (b) Endogenous opioids
   (c) Bradykinin
   (d) Serotonin
   (e) Nitric oxide

CHAPTER 91 CRYOANALGESIA AND RADIOFREQUENCY ABLATION

1. Select the True statement regarding Pulsed RF vs Conventional RF:
   (a) Compared to CRF, PRF clinical effects depend on *both* temperature *and* electrical field induced cellular changes
   (b) In Pulsed RF, the strength of the electric field tapers more abruptly lateral to the tip rather than distal to the tip.
   (c) Some studies have demonstrated that PRF exhibits selectivity for C and A delta nociceptive fibers
   (d) In typical clinical applications, CRF produces stronger electric fields than PRF
2. Which of the following represents standard settings for a pulsed RF treatment approach:
   (a) 100 ms RF pulses, 2 pulses/second, max temperature 50C
   (b) 20 ms RF pulses, 10 pulses/second, max temperature 50C
   (c) 20 ms RF pulses, 10 pulses/second, max temperature 42C
   (d) 20 ms RF pulses, 2 pulses/second, max temperature 42C
   (e) 100 ms RF pulses, 5 pulses/second, max temperature 42C
3 Select the True statement regarding evidence of radiofrequency treatment
   (a) Randomized clinical trials utilizing PRF have demonstrated efficacy for trigeminal neuralgia compared to CRF.
   (b) Evidence does not currently support the routine use of RF treatment of the lumbar DRG for chronic radicular pain
   (c) The 1996 randomized trial by Lord et al. assessed cervical facet RF treatment for patients with cervical neck pain due to degenerative disc disease.
4. Select the False statement regarding the anatomical relationships of the medial branch nerve (MBN):
   (a) The thoracic MBN courses immediately over the junction of the transverse process (TP) and superior articulating process (SAP) whereas the lumbar MBN courses over the superolateral corner of the transverse process.
   (b) At mid-thoracic levels (T5–T8), the course of the MBN curves *slightly above* the superolateral TP.
   (c) The L2 and L3 MBN innervate the L3-4 facet joint.
   (d) To target the C5 medial branch, the target is the lateral margin of the articular pillar, midway between the inferior articulating process (IAP) and superior articulating process (SAP).
5. Select the True statement regarding cryoanalgesia:
   (a) Modern crylolesioning is governed by the Joules-Thompson gas expansion principle and utilizes liquid nitrogen.
   (b) One freeze cycle is adequate to result in the final maximal size of a cryolesion.
   (c) Ice can act as its own insulation, hence freeze cycles greater than 3 minutes will not generally increase the size of a cryolesion
   (d) Animal studies demonstrated that a minimum temperature of negative 5-10°C was necessary to create an effective cryolesion and prolonged sensory loss.

CHAPTER 92 VERTEBRAL AUGMENTATION

1. The primary goal of vertebral augmentation is
   (a) vertebral body stabilization.
   (b) vertebral body height restoration.
   (c) pain relief and improved functional status.
   (d) tumoricidal effect in malignant fractures.
2. Which of the following is an absolute contraindication to vertebral augmentation?
   (a) Vertebraplana
   (b) Symptomatic urinary tract infection
   (c) Cervical spine vertebral augmentation
   (d) Vertebral body metastasis with posterior wall destruction
   (e) Tumor with epidural extension causing spinal canal narrowing
3. What is the single most useful imaging test in assessing osteoporotic patients for vertebral augmentation?
   (a) Plain radiographs
   (b) CT of the spine
   (c) Bone scan
   (d) MRI with T2 fat saturated imaging or STIR imaging
   (e) SPECT scans
4. When performing vertebral augmentation, which part of the pedicle must be clearly visualized at all times on anteroposterior fluoroscopy during needle placement?
   (a) The lateral and superior cortices of the target pedicle
   (b) The lateral and inferior cortices of the target pedicle
   (c) The medial and superior cortices of the target pedicle
   (d) The medial and inferior cortices of the target pedicle
   (e) The superior and inferior cortices of the target pedicle
5. With regard to vertebral augmentation for neoplastic fractures, which of the following statements is false?
   (a) Vertebral augmentation can be performed for both pathological fractures as well as nonfractured vertebrae involved by a painful vertebral metastasis.
   (b) Needle access into an osteolytic metastasis will be less challenging than an osteosclerotic metastasis.
   (c) Posterior wall integrity from a pathological vertebral fracture is best assessed with CT.
   (d) Complication rates are lower than augmentation for osteoporotic compression fractures.

CHAPTER 95 RADIATION AND IMAGING RADIATION SAFETY FOR THE PAIN SPECIALIST

1. What is the maximum permissible dose per year?
   (a) 2 rem
   (b) 20 rem
   (c) 200 rem
   (d) 0.2 rem
2. What radiation dose is safe with regards to increasing chances of developing cancer?
   (a) 3.6 mSv
   (b) 5 mSv
   (c) 400 mrem
   (d) Any amount of radiation is unsafe.
3. Which piece of equipment on the fluoroscopy machine helps to limit low-energy x-rays?
   (a) Thermoluminescent dosimeter
   (b) Image intensifier
   (c) Filters
   (d) None of the above.

4. In providing informed consent, it is reasonable to explain to the patient that the radiation exposure throughout the case is
   (a) between a chest radiograph and an abdominal radiograph.
   (b) between an abdominal radiograph and a lumbar spine radiograph.
   (c) between a lumbar spine radiograph and a computed tomographys.
   (d) between a chest radiograph and a computed tomography scan.
5. The effective dose of computed tomography–guided fluoroscopic epidural steroid injections has been demonstrated to be
   (a) 25% less than conventional fluoroscopy.
   (b) 50% less than conventional fluoroscopy.
   (c) 25% more than conventional fluoroscopy.
   (d) 50% more than conventional fluoroscopy.

CHAPTER 96 PHYSICAL MEDICINE AND REHABILITATION

1. Isometric, isotonic, and isokinetic resistance exercises are what type of exercise?
   (a) Strengthening
   (b) Aerobic
   (c) Flexibility
   (d) Balance
2. Regarding contraindications to exercise, the following is true:
   (a) There are no contraindications to exercise as it is beneficial to everyone
   (b) Anaphyaxis and urticaria are not possible immunologic responses to vigorous exercise
   (c) Unstable medical conditions, like angina, hypoxia, and severe hypertension, preclude exercise participation
   (d) After a fracture is stabilized, the patient can weight bear as tolerated
3. Pain exposure physical therapy (PEPT) consist of progressive loading exercises and the management of pain avoidance behaviors and is indicated for the treatment of what subset of patients with CRPS (complex regional pain syndrome):
   (a) Those who have failed multiple treatments
   (b) Those with new onset CRPS
   (c) Those in the pediatric age group
   (d) Those with multiple limb involvement
4. Physical therapy for the pelvic pain targets internal and external trigger points and focuses on muscles and connective tissues of the pelvic floor, hip girdle, and abdomen. Patients with the following diagnoses may be helped by this type of treatment:
   (a) Women with interstitial cystitis
   (b) Men with chronic prostatitis
   (c) Men with chronic pelvic pain syndrome
   (d) All of the above
5. The optimal frequency of strengthening exercise to improve signs and symptoms of CLBP is not known; however a study comparing four times weekly, three times weekly and two times weekly strengthening regimens concluded that:
   (a) Pain, disability, and strength did not improve in the two-times-a-week group
   (b) Pain, disability, and strength improved the most in the four-times-a-week group
   (c) Strength improved in the two-times-a-week group but not pain and disability
   (d) Pain and disability was not affected regardless of the frequency of exercise

CHAPTER 97 PHYSICAL MODALITIES, ORTHOSES, AND ASSISTIVE DEVICES

1. Which of the following is not a contraindication to application of cryotherapy?
   (a) Impaired sensation
   (b) Spasticity
   (c) Paroxysmal cold hemoglobinuria
   (d) Raynaud syndrome
2. You are evaluating a 28-year-old runner with plantar fasciitis. In addition to physical therapy, which modality would utilize an electrical field to deliver medication to limit systemic absorption?
   (a) Transcutaneous electrical nerve stimulation (TENS)
   (b) Phonophoresis
   (c) Short wave diathermy
   (d) Iontophoresis
3. You are evaluating a patient in your office with low back pain for the last 2 weeks. Which of the following modalities has been shown to improve pain and would be recommended to this patient?
   (a) Microwave diathermy
   (b) Transcutaneous electrical nerve stimulation
   (c) Superficial heat
   (d) Therapeutic ultrasound
4. Which of the following cervical orthoses is the most restrictive in terms of motion?
   (a) Halo device
   (b) Jewett brace
   (c) Philadelphia collar
   (d) SOMI brace
5. You are evaluating an 85-year-old man with history of gait imbalance who recently sustained a fall resulting in a right scaphoid fracture and cannot bear weight through the wrist. Which type of mobility aid would you recommend?
   (a) Rolling walker
   (b) Axillary crutches
   (c) Platform walker
   (d) Lofstrand crutches

CHAPTER 99 COGNITIVE-BEHAVIORAL TREATMENT OF SLEEP DISORDERS IN THE PAIN PATIENT

1. Which of the following best describes the relationship between pain and sleep?
   (a) Unidirectional: poor sleep occasions hyperalgesia and diminishes pain inhibition
   (b) Unidirectional: pain diminishes sleep quantity and quality
   (c) Mutually influential: pain and poor sleep are risk factors for one another
   (d) Independent: sleep and pain do not affect one another, but difficulty with one makes it more difficult to cope with the other
   (e) Contingently unidirectional: poor sleep causes hyperalgesia in chronic-pain patients, but not in normal controls
2. Stimulus control therapy
   (a) Entails condensing the allowable sleep window to the number of hours actually slept, and then gradually expanding it.
   (b) Encourages patients to rest peacefully in bed when unable to sleep.
   (c) Encourages patients to engage in enjoyable activities in the bedroom to re-associate that environment with ease and pleasure.
   (d) Requires patients to come to bed only when drowsy, to limit wakeful time in bed, and to adopt a constant rising time.
   (e) Combines analgesics with deep relaxation to promote a positive association between the bedroom and pain relief.
3. When treating pain patients for insomnia
   (a) Certain dysfunctional beliefs about sleep and pain may have to be addressed above and beyond those encountered in pain-free insomniacs.
   (b) They should be encouraged to remain awake for one full night to learn that nothing catastrophic happens and that their pain is no worse.
   (c) They should be discouraged from stretching at night.
   (d) They should be advised to read or watch television in the middle of the night if unable to sleep at that hour.
   (e) Bed rest should be encouraged during the day so that patients are not anxious about sleep at night.
4. Continuous positive airway pressure (CPAP) for obstructive sleep apnea
   (a) Is generally well tolerated due to advances in mask and machine design.
   (b) Is associated with low rates of adherence, although cognitive behavior therapy (CBT) can help.
   (c) Is slightly less efficacious than mandibular repositioning.
   (d) Lowers pain thresholds at first due to sleep-architecture changes.
   (e) Cannot generally be made tolerable to claustrophobic patients.
5. Delayed sleep phase syndrome
   (a) Is marked by successively later bedtimes each night.
   (b) Is most rapidly treated with bright light exposure in the middle of the night.
   (c) Is primarily treated by reducing anxious cognitions about sleep.
   (d) Is associated with a paradoxical reduction in pain despite reduced sleep quality.
   (e) Is sensitive to the timing of light, melatonin, and exercise.

CHAPTER 104 DISABILITY ASSESSMENT OF PAIN-IMPAIRED PATIENTS

1. If three of five Waddell signs are present, patient is malingering and should be treated accordingly.
   (a) True
   (b) False
2. True/False: Patients with low back pain should always be imaged to rule out potential neurologic complications.
   (a) True
   (b) False
3. The new International Classification of Impairments, Disabilities and Handicaps was adjusted to include which of the following factors?
   (a) Genetic tendencies
   (b) Personal and environmental contexts
   (c) Activity and participation restrictions
   (d) Waddell Signs
4. Which of the following is NOT considered one of the stages of progression from acute to chronic pain?
   (a) Onset of pain produces individual emotional reaction to pain.
   (b) After pain persists more than 2 to 4 months, there is an increase in the emotional, behavioral, and physical maladaptation to the pain.
   (c) The patient presents as positive to multiple pain questionnaires, including VAS and FABQ.
   (d) The patient adopts a sick role and becomes accustomed to being relieved from normal responsibilities, social obligations, and financial responsibilities
5. Which of the following is NOT an accepted measure of pain in patients?
   (a) Visual analog scale
   (b) Fear Avoidance Beliefs Questionnaire
   (c) Neck Disability Index
   (d) Florida Scale for Kinesophobia

Answers

CHAPTER 4 INFLAMMATION IN PAIN DISORDERS

1. a
2. e
3. b
4. b

CHAPTER 8 EVALUATING THE PATIENT WITH CHRONIC PAIN

1. e
2. d
3. c
4. d
5. a

CHAPTER 10 RADIOLOGIC EVALUATION OF SPINAL DISEASE

1. (**d**) Acute osteomyelitis.

   Plain radiographs are not sensitive in the detection of marrow changes that occur with acute osteomyelitis before bone destruction, although they show changes after a few weeks and can also demonstrate sequela of chronic osteomyelitis such as vertebral body collapse, sclerosis, etc.
2. (**a**) Nonspecific symptoms

   Imaging of the spine with CT/MRI is not indicated for nonspecific symptoms because it may not always improve the outcome or be cost-effective, can have deleterious effects such as exposure to radiation, and may result in unnecessary invasive treatment.
3. (**d**) All of the above.

   Gadolinium-based contrast agents should be used with caution in pregnant patients and those with risk of NSF; they help in differentiating recurrent disk herniation from scar tissue as scar tissue has some enhancement.
4. (**d**) 7% to 21% of patients with moderate to severe central canal stenosis can be asymptomatic.
5. (**d**) All of the above. MRI is useful in the assessment of postoperative complications including recurrent disk herniation, arachnoiditis, and scar tissue.

CHAPTER 11 ROLE OF ELECTRODIAGNOSTICS IN PAIN ASSESSMENT

1. (**b**) Commentary: Neurogenic thoracic outlet syndrome involves the lower trunk of the brachial plexus, therefore symptoms develop in the C8–T1 distribution including all ulnar innervated muscles, median C8-T1 innervated muscles, radial C8 innervated muscles, and sensory symptoms in the medial hand and arm (C8-T1 distribution which includes the medial antebrachial cutaneous nerve).
2. (**d**) This patient has L5 radiculopathy. The gastrocnemius innervation is most commonly attributed to S1. The only EMG finding that will immediately be seen in an acute radiculopathy is reduced recruitment, due to loss of some motor units. Changes on EMG occur in a proximal to distal pattern. Fibrillation potentials and positive waves may be seen in the paraspinals as early as 1 week (average 10 to 14 days) and in the extremities by 3–5 weeks. Reinnervation is a slow process that occurs by axon sprouting and takes a least 6 weeks to see increased amplitude and duration of muscle activity. Disc herniations most commonly injure the spinal nerve proximal to the DRG, so the peripheral sensory NCS are normal.
3. (**d**) To get the diagnosis of radiculopathy, there needs to be evidence of involvement in two muscles innervated by the same root but different peripheral nerves. The flexor digitorum has L5 root innervation and is innervated by the tibial nerve, so the presence of spontaneous activity in the flexor digitorum along with the spontaneous activity found in the tibialis anterior (peroneal nerve) would point toward a L5 radiculopathy. The extensor hallucis longus is also innervated by the peroneal nerve, and the adductor longus is innervated by the obturator nerve but not supplied by L5. Needling of the paraspinals is not useful in the postsurgical back due to the persistent presence of spontaneous activity in the paraspinals.
4. (**c**) Blink reflex studies, which are the electrodiagnostic equivalent to the clinical corneal reflex, can help assess facial and trigeminal nerve lesions as well as central lesions in the brain stem. Repetitive nerve stimulation is a better test to assess the neuromuscular junction disorders. Fibromyalgia should have an intact blink reflex. Motor neuron disorders such as amyotrophic lateral sclerosis do not typically affect the blink reflex.
5. (**c**) Electrodiagnostics may not be needed in cases of polyneuropathy of known cause, such as in diabetes. Needle EMG of the paraspinals is not useful in the postsurgical back due to the persistent presence of spontaneous activity in the paraspinals. Fibrillations are abnormal spontaneous activity that would indicate Wallerian degeneration and subacute or more recent radiculopathy in this case. Even slightly cool limbs will vastly distort nerve conduction values.

CHAPTER 12 IMAGING PAIN

1. b
2. b
3. c
4. a
5. a

CHAPTER 17 PSYCHOLOGICAL EVALUATION OF PATIENTS FOR SPINAL CORD STIMULATOR IMPLANTATION

1. **(c)** Although neuromodulation devices have been developed for the treatment of interstitial cystitis, these are not spinal cord stimulators.
2. **(b)** There are few data to suggest that socioeconomic status bears much influence on outcome in neuromodulation.
3. **(a)** Type A personality has not been found to be a desirable characteristic among SCS candidates.
4. **(d)** All three factors may influence the outcome.
5. **(a)** There are no studies to suggest that projective testing may prove helpful in the screening process for SCS candidates.

CHAPTER 20 WHEN PSYCHOTHERAPY IS INDICATED IN THE MANAGEMENT OF PAIN

1. **(e)** These are all well-established characteristics of the multidisciplinary approach to pain management.
2. **(c)** The category of somatic symptom and related disorders was conceived, in part, as a corrective measure to the somatoform disorders of DSM-IV, which specified a medically unexplained nature to the described symptoms and often heralded the closing of the door to further medical investigation and treatment.
3. **(e)** Psychodynamic psychotherapy may prove critical to uncovering and assisting the patient toward insight and adjustment, where a history of unresolved emotional conflicts is concerned—conflicts that may sometimes be expressed through posttraumatic stress. No studies have linked socioeconomic privilege to the success of psychodynamic psychotherapy, and depression usually can be addressed more expediently and effectively with cognitive-behavioral therapy.
4. **(d)** By far, the form of psychotherapy applied to chronic pain that has been most scrutinized, with consistently positive results, is cognitive-behavioral therapy.
5. **(e)** All are characteristics of group psychotherapy in the setting of chronic pain.

CHAPTER 21 MIND/BODY INTERVENTIONS IN THE MANAGEMENT OF CHRONIC PAIN

1. **(d)** Analgesia can occur through both dissociation and pain gate. Dissociation is a means through which hypnosis disconnects the conscious aspect of self from the sensory aspect. Medications are not included, because this is not a mind/body approach.
2. **(d)** In psychosomatic conditions, the patient's experience includes pain that does not result from tissue damage, neuropathology, or inflammation and does not register in imaging studies.
3. **(e)** Behavioral and certain physiological changes, such as peripheral vasodilation recorded via biofeedback, reflect aspects of mind/body healing.
4. **(d)** Hypnosis may be seen as a means of communicating with the unconscious and can allow for rapid pain relief when pain is an unconscious expression of intrapsychic conflict.
5. **(e)** The term biofeedback typically refers to the instrument: a tool used to assess or measure physiological changes or reactivity, such as skin temperature or EMG muscle tension.

CHAPTER 23 NEW PROSPECTS FOR ALLEVIATION OF ANGER IN THE CONTEXT OF CHRONIC PAIN

1. a
2. c
3. b
4. d
5. b

CHAPTER 24 WORK DISABILITY AND CHRONIC PAIN

1. **(b)** Both factors have been shown to predict to disability. Although the importance of physical diagnosis and objective diagnostic findings may be important for patient care, they are poor predictors of work disability. Similarly, measures such as impairment ratings serve other purposes and are relatively poor predictors for work disability. Job satisfaction is a predictor; however, the role of functional capacity assessment in predicting work disability is limited. Treatments such as spinal column stimulation may assist with pain, but success with SCS generally does not predict to a successful return to work.
2. **(e)** Although there are conflicts between those who espouse each model, a compromise continues to be supported across national and international agencies charged with assessment of disability. The assessment of disability remains a problem, especially in the cross-cultural context.
3. **(b)** Active approaches are preferred over passive treatments, with investigations supporting the efficacy of treatments closely tied to the worksite. Multidisciplinary treatments may be beneficial for return to work, although not all programs emphasize work as a primary goal. The other treatments listed may benefit the patient, although they are less likely to result in a successful return to work.
4. **(e)** Chronic psychiatric conditions are predictive of work disability, but this may vary across patients. Other psychosocial and environmental factors may be more predictive.
5. **(b)** Although self-report measures may be used adjunctively to conduct a comprehensive assessment of the patient, interview questions should focus on patient-specific barriers that may prevent returning to work. Work-specific measures may be better than general psychological questionnaires. Impairment assessments are conducted with assistance of a physical examination.

CHAPTER 27 EPIDEMIOLOGY OF HEADACHES

1. c
2. a
3. d
4. a
5. d

CHAPTER 28 HISTORICAL FEATURES IN PRIMARY HEADACHE SYNDROMES

1. **(a)** A new headache is either a headache of recent onset or the change in the character of a long-standing headache. In this case, although the headaches are more severe and frequent, the character of the headaches is the same. They are old headaches. Thus, the goal is to determine why the old headaches are more frequent (lifestyle factors and triggers) rather than to explore alternative diagnoses.
2. **(a)** In this instance, her headaches are less severe and nondisabling. However, the character is now different: the headaches are bifrontal and nonthrobbing. Therefore, even though the headaches are less severe, they are new headaches. The clinician must now consider a differential diagnosis that includes alternative diagnoses from

her long-standing headaches. One must not be misled by the mild headache into assuming that these are old headaches.

3. (**a**) Among clinical features, nausea most accurately distinguishes between migraine and tension-type headache. The positive LR and negative LR are 23 and 0.19, respectively. The features of the head pain itself, surprisingly, prove less helpful when faced with these two possible diagnoses. For example, unilateral pain and throbbing pain, although common in migraine, also occasionally are present in patients with tension-type headache. Thus, they are less valuable in distinguishing between the two diagnoses.
4. (**d**) Visual auras are the most common types of migrainous aura; they occur in 84% of patients who have migraine with aura. Among visual auras, stars or flashes are most common followed by scintillating scotoma (fortification spectra).Among features of migraine with typical aura, sensory aura are most common. These are commonly paresthesias in the hand and face. Aphasia is next most common, and motor features, including hemiparesis, are the least common type of aura, occurring in only 4% of patients who have aura.
5. (**c**) Cluster headache is the only primary headache syndrome that is more common among men than among women. The duration is shorter than that of migraine and commonly lasts less than 1 hour. The most common time of onset for cluster headaches is 2:00 in the morning. In individual patients, the time of onset is commonly the same with each occurrence. All of the associated autonomic symptoms, including lacrimation, are strictly unilateral and occur on the same side as the head pain.

CHAPTER 29 PATHOPHYSIOLOGY OF HEADACHES

1. (**b**) Although all of these neurotransmitters are involved in the transmission of nociceptive information from perivascular terminals through the trigeminal ganglia to project to second-order neurons within the trigeminal nucleus caudalis, glutamate is the primary neurotransmitter.
2. (**e**) Activity in the trigeminal nucleus caudalis can be modulated by projections from rostral trigeminal nuclei, the periaqueductal gray matter, and the nucleus raphe magnus, as well as by descending cortical inhibitory systems.
3. (**c**) Some studies have reported a transient increase in blood flow before the blood flow reductions as well as an apparent anterior spread of the blood flow decrements, which move across neurovascular boundaries. Spreading depression is a wave of neuronal hyperexcitation followed by suppression that is observed to move across areas of contiguous cortex in experimental animals after chemical or mechanical perturbation. The neurogenic theory of migraine holds that migraine is a brain disorder, and cortical spreading depression is the main event that triggers the vascular changes that occur during a migraine. This is in contrast to the vasogenic theory, which proposes that vascular changes are the main cause of the attack.
4. (**c**) Aura symptoms are typically characterized by a slow expansion of the area affected by the dysfunction followed by gradual resolution rather than rapid resolution. A total of 25% of individuals with migraine experience aura, which typically lasts 1 hour or less. Both PET and fMRI studies have demonstrated that aura is associated with moderate blood flow reductions, which cross vascular territories.
5. (**d**) Although a subject of some controversy, changes in the drainage pattern of the cavernous sinus have been reported in patients with cluster headaches. Fibers from the ophthalmic and maxillary trigeminal divisions converge with projections from the superior cervical and the sphenopalatine ganglia within the cavernous sinus. The mandibular division of the trigeminal nerve is not typically involved in cluster headache. The circadian rhythmicity of cluster headache is suggestive of hypothalamic involvement. Lacrimation and congestion are manifestations of parasympathetic dysfunction.

CHAPTER 30 COMMON HEADACHE SYNDROMES

1. e
2. b
3. e
4. c
5. d

CHAPTER 32 CHRONIC DAILY HEADACHE

1. c
2. b
3. c
4. b
5. b

CHAPTER 33 HEADACHE THERAPEUTICS

1. (**d**) The half-life of frovatriptan is about 26 hours, while zolmitriptan, rizatriptan, and sumatriptan all have half-lives between 2 to 3 hours. Menstrual dosing of naproxen sodium would also be a reasonable approach but should be avoided given her history of gastritis.
2. (**b**) Although amitriptyline is often prescribed for migraine prevention, particularly in patients with poor sleep, it is not approved by the FDA for treatment of chronic migraine.
3. (**e**) The first line maintenance prevention for chronic cluster headaches is verapamil. However, caution should be used in patients with atrioventricular block. Indomethacin is most effective for the hemicranias but is not typically used to treat chronic cluster headaches. Occipital nerve stimulators should only be considered when all other, more conservative therapies have failed. Divalproex sodium, lithium, and topiramate are second-line maintenance prevention agents.
4. (**c**) This patient is likely suffering from tension-type headaches (TTH). She now may benefit from preventive therapy because her headaches are now daily. The mainstays of TTH prevention are the tricyclic antidepressants. Cyclobenzaprine or muscle relaxants may have some role in some patients with predominant neck pain and spasm, but this is generally not a first-line treatment. Her headaches are not clearly migrainous in description, and therefore, a triptan may not be effective. Naproxen is an excellent therapy for episodic TTH, but chronic administration may put the patient at risk for gastritis.
5. (**d**) Prochlorperazine is a D2 dopamine antagonist. Orthostatic hypotension is a known side effect, along with extrapyramidal symptoms, akathisia, sedation, and, with long-term use, tardive dyskinesia. Phenothiazine drugs are a class of neuroleptics that include promethazine and prochlorperazine and can be associated with extrapyramidal side effects.

CHAPTER 35 FACIAL PAIN

1. b
2. c
3. d
4. a
5. d

CHAPTER 37 NECK PAIN

1. a
2. c
3. a
4. e
5. a

CHAPTER 40 FAILED BACK SURGERY

1. b
2. d
3. d
4. a
5. b

CHAPTER 41 PAIN MANAGEMENT IN RHEUMATOLOGIC DISEASES

1. e
2. d
3. d
4. a
5. c

CHAPTER 42 OSTEOARTHRITIS OF THE MAJOR JOINTS

1. b
2. c
3. c
4. c
5. c

CHAPTER 43 FOOT AND ANKLE PAIN

1. (**e**) – all of the above

   Plantar warts can be confused with calluses. Warts are found on any area and are not limited to weight-bearing surfaces. Also, calluses typically have a hard center with skin lines running through it. It is normal to pare down to bleeding tissue when sharply excising a wart because there are capillary ingrowths seen as dark spots in the spongy center. Also, warts have pain when squeezed, where a callus has pain on direct compression.

2. (**c**) – MRI

   Magnetic resonance imaging (MRI) is a useful modality to determine soft-tissue injuries in the foot and ankle. It shows great contrast between structures, and easily depicts an increase in fluid or inflammation as well as when soft-tissue structures are abnormal or ruptured. Another advantage is that it does not use ionizing radiation, though the cost of the exam is a deterrent.

3. (**b**) – False

   Tendinosis is likely more common than tendinitis, especially if chronic and caused from repetitive trauma to the tendon. It is more difficult to treat, and there may not be inflammation within the tendon. It can take months to heal, and treatment is guided toward stretching and strengthening to help reorganize collagen alignment and stimulate repair.

4. (**b**) – resume regular activity

   PRICE stands for protection, rest, ice, compression and elevation. By employing these principles, the clinician can help reduce pain and swelling following an acute trauma. Rest does not necessitate complete bed rest but includes modifying the regular activity that resulted in the injury. For athletes, this is important because complete bed rest can lead to an even longer recuperation.

5. (**f**) – all of the above

   Complex regional pain syndrome (CRPS) is very challenging to treat. The exact cause is unknown, and there may not be a predilection to who it affects—though there is some correlation with depression and anxiety. Upon reaching the diagnosis, the clinician should act quickly and use multiple treatments to help minimize symptoms and prevent extension proximally up the extremity and future loss of function.

CHAPTER 44 PELVIC AND ABDOMINAL PAIN

1. d
2. c
3. d
4. d
5. d

CHAPTER 45 PERINEAL PAIN

1. a, b, c
2. a & b
3. a & b
4. d
5. b, c, d

CHAPTER 50 PREEMPTIVE ANALGESIA

1. d
2. c
3. a
4. a
5. d

CHAPTER 55 MEDICAL MANAGEMENT OF CANCER PAIN

1. d
2. c
3. b
4. c
5. a

CHAPTER 60 MUSCLE PAIN: PATHOPHYSIOLOGY, EVALUATION, AND TREATMENT

1. a
2. b
3. c
4. d
5. e

CHAPTER 64 ACUTE PAIN MANAGEMENT IN INFANTS AND CHILDREN

1. **(b, c)** Because of the increased risks of amide local anesthetic local anesthetic toxicity on neonates, a chloroprocaine test dose can be used to test whether the catheter is effective. Both objective and subjective signs should be used to observe for a response. Physiologic parameters such as a return of heart rate and blood pressure to baseline levels help to provide objective evidence of pain control. Relaxed posture and calm facial appearance can provide subjective evidence. Alternatively, injecting contrast into the epidural catheter and observing for epidural spread can also help to confirm proper placement. It is important to recognize other, nonsurgical causes of pain that include endotracheal suctioning, nasogastric tubes, and IV and arterial lines.
2. **(c)** The best option to provide more effective analgesia is to change the epidural solution to bupivacaine-hydromorphone infusion to allow for more cephalad spread of hydromorphone. Alternatively, clonidine can be added to the bupivacaine-fentanyl solution. Giving additional IV or PO opioids will increase the risk of respiratory depression. All patient receiving neuraxial opioids should be cardiorespiratory monitoring and close observation for respiratory depression.
3. **(c)** It is most appropriate to assess pain in a 2-year-old by using the FLACC scale. Most 2-year-old children cannot reliably use self-report scales. The Face, Legs, Activity, Cry, and Consolability (FLACC) pain scale is validated for postoperative use among in children aged 2 to 7 years.
4. **(c, d)** Prior to institution of an analgesic regimen it is important to learn from the patient and his family what has been used previously and how successful those intervention have been. In general, oral analgesics are not the best choice for management of an acute vaso-occlusive crisis. PCA offers the advantages of rapid treatment of severe, escalating pain. Epidural analgesia may be effective for this patient, particularly if he experiences opioid-induced sedation, hypoventilation, and oxygen desaturation in the setting of inadequate analgesia. Given renal insufficiency, NSAIDs are best avoided.
5. **(a, b, c)** It is reasonable to give IV morphine and ketorolac. If patient continues to have severe pain resulting in a declining pulmonary status, a regional technique might be indicated. Due to her malnutrition secondary to malabsorption, she will have lowered serum albumin which may affect analgesic pharmacokinetics. The possibility of pneumonia and bacteremia may affect the choice of regional techniques, possibly favoring paravertebral catheter over epidural.

CHAPTER 69 RISING STANDARDS FOR RISK MANAGEMENT IN OPIOID USE FOR CHRONIC PAIN

1. c
2. c
3. b
4. d
5. c

CHAPTER 71 URINE DRUG TESTING

1. d
2. c
3. e
4. c
5. b

CHAPTER 72 NOVEL OPIOID FORMULATIONS

1. d
2. b
3. a
4. a
5. a

CHAPTER 73 OPIOID-INDUCED HYPERALGESIA

1. d
2. d
3. d
4. d
5. d

CHAPTER 75 CANNABINOIDS IN PAIN MANAGEMENT

1. a
2. c
3. d
4. a
5. b

CHAPTER 80 STEROIDS

1. c
2. d
3. e
4. a
5. c

CHAPTER 86 LOCAL ANESTHETICS

1. b
2. a
3. b
4. d
5. d

CHAPTER 88 ULTRASOUND IN THE DIAGNOSIS AND TREATMENT OF PAIN

1. d
2. a
3. c
4. b
5. b

CHAPTER 90 NEUROMODULATION FOR PAIN

1. a
2. a
3. d
4. b
5. c

CHAPTER 91 CRYOANALGESIA AND RADIOFREQUENCY ABLATION

1. c
2. d
3. b
4. a
5. c

CHAPTER 92 VERTEBRAL AUGMENTATION

1. c
2. b
3. d
4. d
5. d

CHAPTER 95 RADIATION AND IMAGING RADIATION SAFETY FOR THE PAIN SPECIALIST

1. a
2. d
3. c
4. d
5. b

CHAPTER 96 PHYSICAL MEDICINE AND REHABILITATION

1. a
2. c
3. a
4. d
5. b

CHAPTER 97 PHYSICAL MODALITIES, ORTHOSES, AND ASSISTIVE DEVICES

1. b
2. d
3. c
4. a
5. c

CHAPTER 99 COGNITIVE-BEHAVIORAL TREATMENT OF SLEEP DISORDERS IN THE PAIN PATIENT

1. c
2. d
3. a
4. b
5. e

CHAPTER 104 DISABILITY ASSESSMENT OF PAIN-IMPAIRED PATIENTS

1. (**b**) Three of five positive Waddell signs are indicative of a need for further psychological assessment, not necessarily malingering. The patient may still be experiencing pain, but the approach to pain treatment may need to be adjusted.
2. (**b**) Patients with low back pain and certain accompanying symptoms should be receive imaging to rule out more serious diagnoses, but up to 70% of asymptomatic individuals will show some form of degeneration in the spine. Imaging is currently being overused as a diagnostic technique.
3. b
4. c
5. d

Index

Note: Page numbers followed by b indicate boxed material; those followed by f indicate figures; those followed by t indicate tables.

P